ROSDAHL'S TEXTBOOK OF Basic Nursing

TWELFTH EDITION

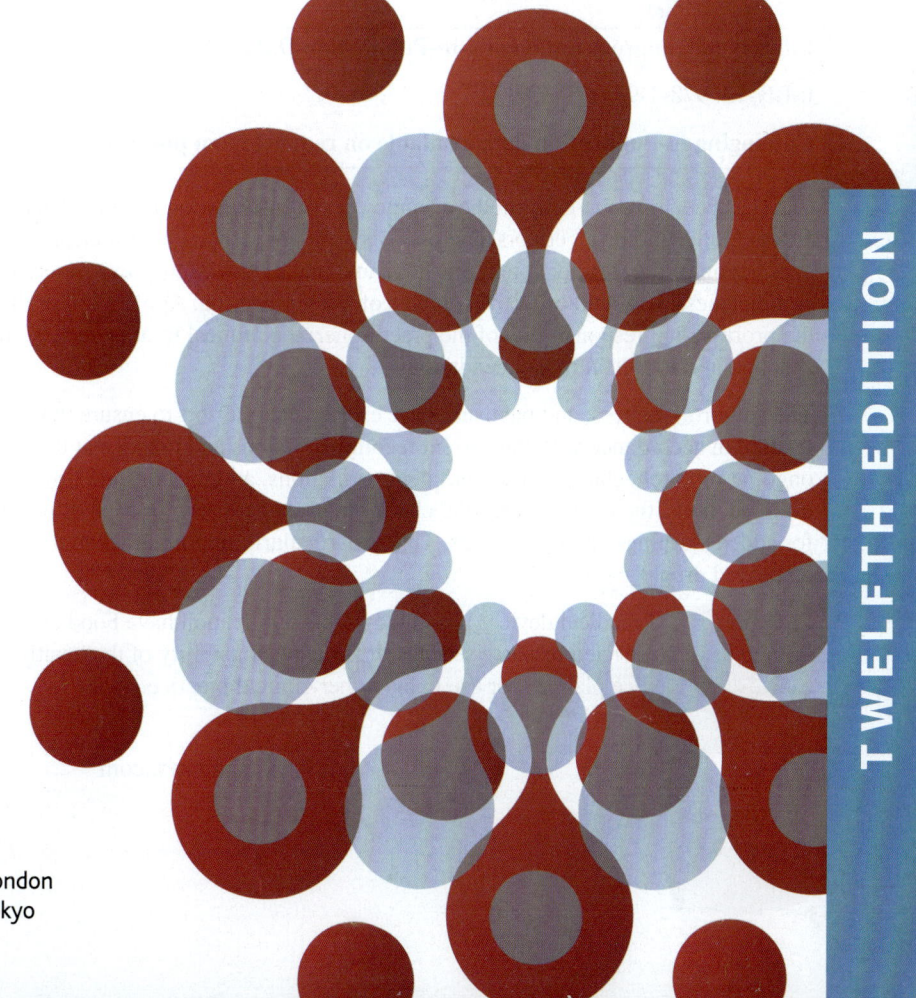

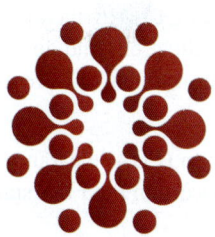

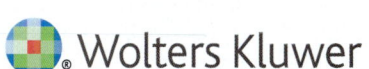

**Philadelphia • Baltimore • New York • London
Buenos Aires • Hong Kong • Sydney • Tokyo**

Vice President and Publisher: Julie K. Stegman
Manager, Nursing Education and Practice Content: Jamie Blum
Senior Acquisitions Editor: Jonathan Joyce
Associate Development Editor: Rebecca J. Rist
Editorial Coordinator: Michael Jeffery Cohen
Marketing Manager: Brittany K. Riney
Editorial Assistant: Molly Kennedy
Design Coordinator: Stephen Druding
Art Director, Illustration: Jennifer Clements
Senior Production Project Manager: Sadie Buckallew
Manufacturing Coordinator: Karin Duffield
Prepress Vendor: TNQ Technologies

12th edition

Copyright © 2022 Wolters Kluwer.

Copyright © 2017 by Wolters Kluwer. ©2012, 2008 Wolters Kluwer Health | Lippincott Williams & Wilkins. Copyright © 2003, 1999 by Lippincott Williams & Wilkins. Copyright © 1995, 1991, 1985, 1981, 1973, 1966 by J. B. Lippincott Company. All rights reserved. This book is protected by copyright. No part of this book may be reproduced or transmitted in any form or by any means, including as photocopies or scanned-in or other electronic copies, or utilized by any information storage and retrieval system without written permission from the copyright owner, except for brief quotations embodied in critical articles and reviews. Materials appearing in this book prepared by individuals as part of their official duties as U.S. government employees are not covered by the above-mentioned copyright. To request permission, please contact Wolters Kluwer at Two Commerce Square, 2001 Market Street, Philadelphia, PA 19103, via email at permissions@lww.com, or via our website at shop.lww.com (products and services). 7/2021

9 8 7 6 5 4 3 2 1

Printed in China

Library of Congress Cataloging-in-Publication Data

ISBN-13: 978-1-975171-33-9

Cataloging in Publication data available on request from publisher

---

Care has been taken to confirm the accuracy of the information presented and to describe generally accepted practices. However, the author(s), editors, and publisher are not responsible for errors or omissions or for any consequences from application of the information in this book and make no warranty, expressed or implied, with respect to the currency, completeness, or accuracy of the contents of the publication. Application of this information in a particular situation remains the professional responsibility of the practitioner; the clinical treatments described and recommended may not be considered absolute and universal recommendations.

The author(s), editors, and publisher have exerted every effort to ensure that drug selection and dosage set forth in this text are in accordance with the current recommendations and practice at the time of publication. However, in view of ongoing research, changes in government regulations, and the constant flow of information relating to drug therapy and drug reactions, the reader is urged to check the package insert for each drug for any change in indications and dosage and for added warnings and precautions. This is particularly important when the recommended agent is a new or infrequently employed drug.

Some drugs and medical devices presented in this publication have Food and Drug Administration (FDA) clearance for limited use in restricted research settings. It is the responsibility of the health care provider to ascertain the FDA status of each drug or device planned for use in his or her clinical practice.

shop.lww.com

Consultants and Contributors, 12th Edition

Renée L. Davis, DNP, APRN, CPNP-PC
Associate Professor
　Traditional BSN Program Coordinator
　Saint Louis University
　Trudy Busch Valentine School of Nursing
　Dr. Norman's Pediatrics
　St. Louis, Missouri

Judy R. Hyland, PhD, RN
Assistant Professor
　Houston Baptist University
　Houston, Texas

Naomi Lee, MSN, BSN, RN
Assistant Professor (retired)
　St. Louis, Missouri

Kelly Moseley, DHSc, MSN, RN
Assistant Professor
　Texas Tech University Health Sciences Center
　Odessa, Texas

Preface

Welcome to *Rosdahl's Textbook of Basic Nursing,* 12th Edition. This textbook has been an integral part of the education of thousands of practical/vocational nurses. In fact, it was the first nursing textbook that included behavioral objectives that later became the present-day Learning Objectives. In this textbook, the active, involved participant of nursing care is identified as the *client*, emphasizing that healthcare is a service that involves a knowledgeable consumer who makes personal choices and shares responsibilities relating to personal health. This textbook takes into consideration that both clients and nurses need to work in tandem to achieve well-being. Teaching the client strengthens the overall concepts of nursing and healthcare.

Rosdahl's Textbook of Basic Nursing is a student-friendly, cost-effective, all-in-one text that is responsive to the NCLEX-PN Test Plan and state-mandated curricular requirements. All program directors and instructors are encouraged to view the valuable resources to support this text located with the Instructor Resources found on thePoint at thepoint.lww.com/Rosdahl12e.

The reading level of *Rosdahl's Textbook of Basic Nursing* is designed to be understandable to the maximum number of students, including those for whom English is a second language. Key English-to-Spanish phrases are included in Appendix A and an audio glossary is also available on thePoint.

NEW TO THIS EDITION

Every effort has been made to keep up with the constantly changing world of nursing and its external regulation by various agencies. All of the descriptive material and nursing procedures have been updated, as needed.

Nutrition, discussed in Unit 5, was updated to match objectives in *Healthy People 2030*. It covers the latest government guidelines and incorporates illustrations of *MyPlate* and the *Nutrition Facts Label*, which help integrate nutritional concepts for students and consumers. Nutrition considerations are also integrated in specific chapters throughout the text. Additionally, significant content on *diet therapy* and *cultural considerations* are included.

In keeping with the NCLEX-PN test plan, the NCLEX-style Review Questions that appear at the end of each chapter include questions that are written at the application or higher levels of cognitive ability. Answers to the questions, with rationales that fully explain the correct answer as well as explanations of why answers are incorrect, are available to instructors in the Instructor Resources found on thePoint at thepoint.lww.com/Rosdahl12e. Instructors may use these questions as in-class instruction to help students develop the skills needed to fully apply content and to think through a problem.

Nursing Procedures appear in a special section at the end of selected chapters. The mnemonic "LPN WELCOME" phrase highlights important first steps that must occur before performing each procedure, and the mnemonic "ENDDD" phrase serves as an important memory aid for final steps that must always be performed with each procedure. Checklists for these procedures are offered in the Student Resources on thePoint to aid in student understanding.

The Appendices summarize useful and important aspects of medicine and nursing. They are available on thePoint to allow students to print and use them when needed.

TEXT ORGANIZATION

Instructors and students will appreciate the logical design and simple format of this book. *Rosdahl's Textbook of Basic Nursing* is divided into four main parts. Students will learn about the foundations of nursing, nursing care skills, and nursing throughout the life cycle. The book then examines the various settings and job opportunities available for the LVN/LPN nurse.

The parts are organized on a continuum from *general or simple to integrated or complex*. General healthcare issues and basic sciences introduced early in the book lead to the more complex and specific healthcare topics in later units. Normal anatomy and physiology provide the basis of comparison for abnormal etiologies in diseases and disorders.

Some critical topics as well as those that may be on the NCLEX-PN examination (e.g., *Maslow's Hierarchy of Needs, Erikson's Life Span Stages,* and *Kübler-Ross Stages of Death and Dying*) are discussed individually and also integrated within specific subject areas. Crucial contemporary points such as *privacy legislation, requirements of regulatory agencies, Standard Precautions, disposal of hazardous wastes, prevention of disease, electronic and traditional documentation,* and *nutrition* are thoroughly discussed as well.

As the role of the LVN/LPN is expanding in many settings, Unit 9 presents chapters relating to **Pharmacology and Administration of Medications**.

Nursing throughout the life cycle is covered in Units 10 through 13, in which topics such as the etiologies and disorders of anatomy and physiology are combined with pediatric and adult medical-surgical nursing. These units provide information relating to the onset of diseases and disorders, diagnostic testing and procedures, treatment, pertinent medications, and nursing considerations. *Changes relating to aging* for each faction of the body systems are presented in Unit 4 and Unit 13, **Gerontologic Nursing**, which visits the complexities of defining a*ging* and the issues of *geriatrics*.

Specific chapters with comprehensive information are also dedicated to the topics of *mental health* nursing and *substance use disorders*.

Many community settings are providing employment for growing numbers of practical/vocational nurses. The chapters in Unit 15 address and compare the situations and nursing needs for areas such as **Extended Care, Rehabilitation Nursing, Home Care Nursing, Ambulatory Healthcare,** and **Hospice Nursing**.

The *graduating nurse* obtains valuable information in the final unit of the book relating to employment opportunities in many of these areas and in acute care settings. A separate chapter on **Career Opportunities and Job-Seeking Skills** is included. Components of *teamwork, leadership,* and *supervision* are emphasized in specific chapters, as well as integrated throughout the text. The units in the book combine to provide a comprehensive education for the practical/vocational nurse.

SPECIAL FEATURES

The 12th edition of *Rosdahl's Textbook of Basic Nursing* contains numerous pedagogical features to help focus and enhance student learning. The section, *Using Rosdahl's Textbook of Basic Nursing*, 12th edition, highlights the important "In Practice" features found in the text.

Each chapter opens with **Learning Objectives**, **Important Terminology**, and **Acronyms** that provide a general overview of important content. The Student Synthesis section, which appears at the end of each chapter, contains **Key Points**, **Critical Thinking Exercises**, and **NCLEX-Style Review Questions** to help students integrate and summarize the content of each chapter. The Critical Thinking Exercises are designed for in-class discussions or individual student essays. Instructors may also use the NCLEX-Style Review Questions as in-class instruction to help students develop the skills needed to fully apply content and to think through a problem.

Additional features include the following:

- **NCLEX Alerts** that appear throughout the chapters providing practical ideas designed to help the student consider how chapter content might be used in a variety of NCLEX situations.
- **Nursing Alerts** that clarify important nursing actions used in daily nursing practice.
- **Special Considerations** that highlight key culture, lifespan, homecare, or nutrition information.
- **Key Concepts** that draw attention to important information for students regarding topics as they read the chapter.

STUDENT AND INSTRUCTOR RESOURCES

Rosdahl's Textbook of Basic Nursing includes a wide variety of resources for students and instructors to enhance the teaching/learning experience. All resources are available on thePoint at thepoint.lww.com/Rosdahl12e.

Student Resources

The student resources are free to students who purchase a new copy of *Rosdahl's Textbook of Basic Nursing*, 12th Edition. Simply use the one-time activation code in the front of the book to discover a wealth of information and activities.

- **Concepts in Action Animations** bring concepts to life and enhance student learning.
- **Watch and Learn videos** demonstrate specific skills to enhance student understanding of key nursing techniques.
- **Procedure Checklists** offer students step-by-step instruction for procedures in the text.
- Plus **Appendices, Heart and Breath sounds**, and more!

Instructor Resources

The following resources are available on thePoint at thepoint.lww.com/Rosdahl12e for instructors who adopt *Rosdahl's Textbook of Basic Nursing*, 12th Edition.

- **PowerPoint Presentations** provide an easy way for you to integrate the textbook with your students' classroom experience, either via slide shows or through handouts. Multiple-choice and true/false questions are integrated into the presentations to promote class participation and allow you to use i-clicker technology.
- **Case Studies** with related questions (and suggested answers) give students an opportunity to apply their knowledge to a client case similar to one they might encounter in practice.
- **Prelecture Quizzes** (and answers) are quick, knowledge-based assessments that allow you to check students' reading.
- **Guided Lecture Notes** walk you through the chapters, objective by objective, and provide you with corresponding PowerPoint slide numbers.
- **Discussion Topics** (and suggested answers) can be used as conversation starters or in online discussion boards.
- **Assignments** (and suggested answers) include group, written, clinical, and web assignments.
- An **Image Bank** lets you use the photographs and illustrations from this textbook in your PowerPoint slides or as you see fit in your course.
- **Answers to Questions in the Book** (Stop, Think, and Respond Exercises; Critical Thinking Exercises; and NCLEX-Style Review Questions) are provided for each chapter. Instructors are free to share these with their students to enhance student self-learning.
- A **sample Syllabus** provides guidance for structuring your medical-surgical nursing course.
- **Answer Key for the Workbook** supplies answers to the questions appearing in *Workbook for Rosdahl's Textbook of Nursing*, 12th Edition, the accompanying for-sale workbook.

Using Rosdahl's Textbook of Basic Nursing, 12th Edition

In order to help prepare nurses to practice safely, important *In Practice* features are provided. **Nursing Procedures** present step-by-step instructions.

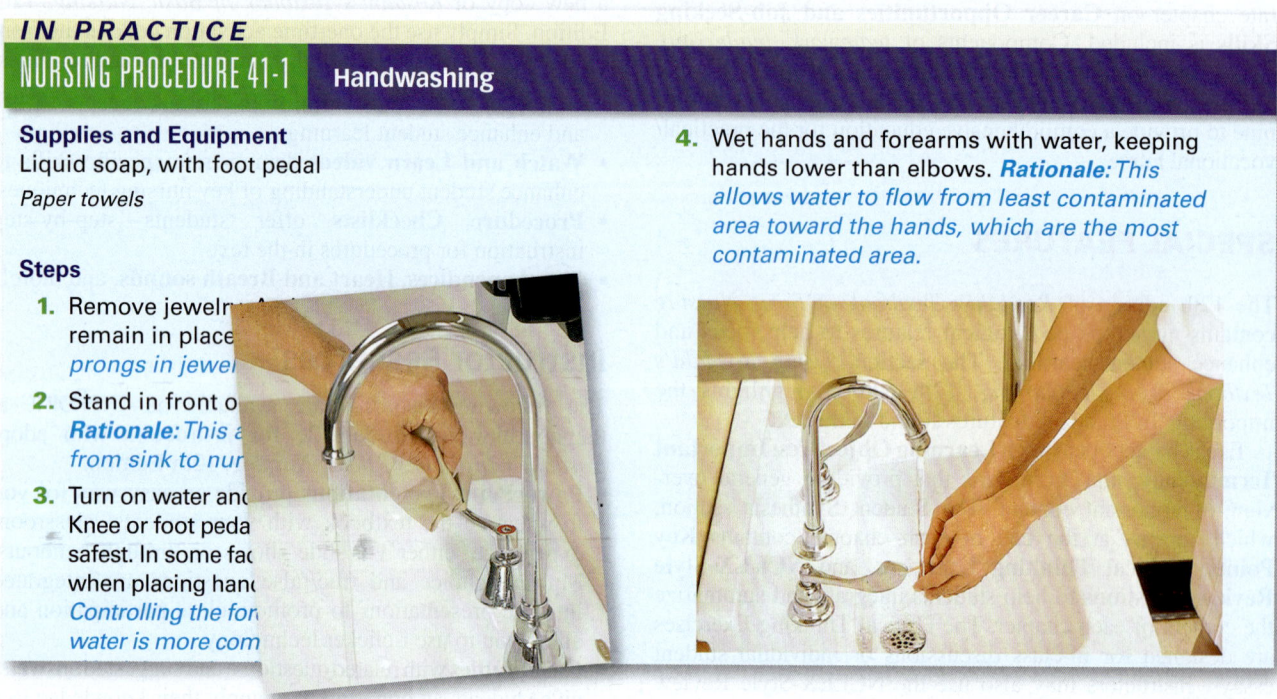

IN PRACTICE
NURSING PROCEDURE 41-1 — Handwashing

Supplies and Equipment
Liquid soap, with foot pedal
Paper towels

Steps
1. Remove jewelry. A ... remain in place ... *prongs in jewel...*
2. Stand in front o... *Rationale:* This a... from sink to nur...
3. Turn on water and... Knee or foot peda... safest. In some fa... when placing hand... *Controlling the for... water is more com...*
4. Wet hands and forearms with water, keeping hands lower than elbows. *Rationale:* This allows water to flow from least contaminated area toward the hands, which are the most contaminated area.

Educating the Client includes essential information for teaching clients.

Nursing Care Guidelines summarize important nursing considerations.

IN PRACTICE
EDUCATING THE CLIENT 57-2 — After Catheter Removal

Client education encourages cooperation and lessens anxiety. Teach the client to
- Drink plenty of fluids (to facilitate voiding).
- Report the urge to void for the first time after catheter removal.
- Understand that some discomfort may be felt with the first voiding.
- Report any severe pain or blood in the urine.

IN PRACTICE
NURSING CARE GUIDELINES 57-1 — Sterile Technique

- After sterile gloves (and/or gown) have been put on, the nurse cannot touch anything that is not sterile. Keep hands between nipple and waist level, whether or not a gown is worn.
- Reaching over a sterile field contaminates the sterile area, unless sterile clothing and gloves are being worn.
- If a sterile wrapper becomes wet, the wrapper *and its contents* are no longer sterile.
- If a mask becomes wet, it no longer screens out microorganisms; the mask must be changed for a new mask.
- When wearing sterile gloves to perform a sterile procedure, keep them in front, between the nipple

Important Medications inform about key medications for a specific disorder.

IN PRACTICE
IMPORTANT MEDICATIONS 56-1 — Examples of Importan[t]

Sedatives Used as Premedication Before Anesthesia
- Promethazine HCl (Phenergan)—used pre- or postoperatively, and in obstetrics
- Midazolam HCl—benzodiazepine, central nervous system (CNS) depressant, anxiolytic; causes some amnesia, can be used alone for IV moderate sedation (conscious sedation)

Sedatives Used to Assist Clients to Sleep
- Chlorpromazine (used in Canada)—especially to relieve preoperative apprehension, also antiemetic
- Secobarbital Na⁺ (Seconal Na⁺)—also can be premedication
- Temazepam (Restoril)—used pre- or postoperatively

Nursing Care Plan presents a sample care plan and its application.

IN PRACTICE
NURSING CARE PLAN 81-1 — The Person With an Acute

Medical History: C.F., a 37-year-old single white male a[dmitted with] crushing chest pain. Cardiac enzyme levels and an ECG [indicated] infarction of the left ventricle. He was admitted to the C[CU]. cannula and intravenous morphine were ordered. Card[iac monitoring] initiated.

Medical Diagnosis: Acute MI of anterior wall of the left [ventricle]

DATA COLLECTION/NURSING OBSERVATION

Client appears pale and diaphoretic. Skin is cool and clammy. States that chest pain is 5 on a 1–10 scale. Vital signs as follows: Temperature, 97.2 °F (37.2 °C); pulse, 120 bpm, irregular and thready; respirations, 26 breaths/min; blood pressure, 90/58 mm Hg

Data Gathering in Nursing offers important points in data collection.

IN PRACTICE
DATA GATHERING IN NURSING 47-1 — Gross Functioning of Cranial Nerves

The gross functioning of most of the cranial nerves can be observed by simple actions. For example, the examiner asks the client:

Action	Cranial Nerve Evaluated
To follow a moving finger with the eyes (with or without moving the head)	III Oculomotor IV Trochlear VI Abducens
To move or clench the jaw	V Mandibular branch of the trigeminal
To smile or make a funny face	VII Facial
To stand with the eyes closed	VIII Vestibular division of the vestibulocochlear

In addition, **Nursing Alerts**, **Key Concepts**, and **NCLEX Alerts** ensure that students obtain critical information to help them safely practice nursing as an LVN/LPN.

> **Nursing Alert** Before performing any catheterization, make sure the client is not allergic to latex (rubber). Although catheters today usually are not latex, the client with a latex allergy could also have a severe reaction to another type of catheter, even though a special nonallergenic catheter (e.g., polyurethane, Teflon, silicone) is used. If the client's allergy is severe, specific allergy testing must precede catheterization.

Nursing Process uses the steps of the nursing process to guide the nurse in data collection.

NURSING PROCESS

DATA COLLECTION

Carefully observe the individual with a cardiac or blood vessel disorder. Establish a baseline for future comparison to determine the presence of suspected cardiovascular complications. Report any changes in baseline observations.

A complete cardiovascular assessment begins on admission. The nursing assessment includes a complete nursing history, as well as observations. When taking the health history, ask about any potential risk factors, such as family history of cardiovascular disease, smoking, lack of exercise, or poor nutrition. Also include any issues, such as shortness of breath or fatigue, which might interfere with the client's ability to perform activities of daily living (ADL).

Key Concept

Healthcare professionals use medical terminology to communicate assessment findings, diagnostic test results, and other pertinent information.

NCLEX Alert

Understanding medical terminology is important when answering NCLEX questions. Appropriate and effective communication, as well as coordination of client care, is demonstrated by correct knowledge of the language of medicine.

Contents

PART A FOUNDATIONS OF NURSING

UNIT 1

The Nature of Nursing 1

1 The Origins of Nursing 1

Nursing's Heritage 1
Nursing in the United States 4
Nursing Insignia 6

2 Beginning Your Nursing Career 9

Healthcare: A Multidisciplinary Approach 9
Types of Nursing Programs 9
Approval and Accreditation of Nursing Programs 12
Licensure of Nurses 13
Theories of Nursing 13
Roles and Responsibilities of the Nurse 14
Nursing Organizations 15

3 The Healthcare Delivery System 19

Healthcare Trends in the 21st Century 19
Healthcare Settings and Services 21
Quality Assurance 23
Organization and Ownership of Healthcare Facilities 24
Financing Healthcare 25
Complementary Healthcare 28
Consumer Fraud 30

4 Legal and Ethical Aspects of Nursing 32

Legal Issues of Nursing Practice 32
Regulations of Nursing Practice 37
Advance Directives 40
Vulnerable Persons 41
Definitions of Death 41
Ethical Standards of Healthcare 42
Clients' Rights and Responsibilities 44

UNIT 2

Personal and Environmental Health 47

5 Basic Human Needs 47

Maslow's Hierarchy of Human Needs 47
Nursing's Relationship to Basic Needs 48
Overview of Individual Needs 49
Family and Community Needs 53

6 Health and Wellness 55

Health and Wellness 56
Inconsistencies in Healthcare 56
Morbidity and Mortality 56
Finances and Healthcare 58
Prevention and Healthcare 59
The Wellness–Illness Continuum 59
Lifestyle and Risk Factors 62
Education and Health Promotion 65
Age-Related Health Concerns 65
Categories of Disease and Disorders 69

7 Community Health 72

Healthcare Worldwide 72
Healthcare on the National Level 73
Healthcare at the State Level 78
Healthcare at the Local Level 79
The Environment 79

8 Transcultural Healthcare 83

Culture, Ethnicity, and Race 83
Cultural Sensitivity 86
Culturally Influenced Components 86
Religious/Spiritual Customs and Traditions 91
Implementing Culturally Competent Care 92

UNIT 3

Development Throughout the Life Cycle 97

9 The Family 97

Characteristics of the Family 97
Family Structure 99
Influence of Culture, Ethnicity, and Religion 100
Family Stages 100
Stress and Family Coping 103

10 Infancy and Childhood 106

Concepts of Growth and Development 106
Developmental Milestones and Developmental Delays 107
Growth and Development 107
The Newborn 110
Infancy: 1–12 Months 110
Toddlerhood: 1–3 Years 113
Preschool: 3–6 Years 116
School Age: 6–10 Years 118

11 Adolescence 122

Growth and Development Theories 122
Adolescent Growth and Development 123
In Practice 127

12 Early and Middle Adulthood 129

Erikson's Adult Growth and Development Theory 129
Early Adulthood 130
Middle Adulthood 132
Transition From Middle Adult to Older Adult 134

13 Older Adulthood and Aging 136

Words Related to Aging 136
Erikson's Adult Growth and Development Theory 137
Development in Older Adulthood 138

14 The End of Life: Death, Dying, Grief, and Loss 146

The Dying Process 146
Kübler-Ross Stages of Grief and Loss 149

UNIT 4

Structure and Function 155

15 Organization of the Human Body 155

Chemistry and Life 155
Medical Terminology 157
Anatomy and Physiology 157
Body Directions, Areas, and Regions 158
Structural Levels in the Body 161
Cells 161
Tissues 165
Organs and Systems 167

16 The Integumentary System 169

Structure and Function 169
Skin 169
Accessory Structures 172
System Physiology 174
Protection 174
Thermoregulation 174
Vitamin D Production 175
Maintenance of Healthy Skin 176

17 Fluid and Electrolyte Balance 179

Homeostasis 179
Body Fluids 180
Fluid and Electrolyte Transport 186
Fluid and Electrolyte Balance 190
Acid–Base Balance 190

18 The Musculoskeletal System 195

The Skeleton 195
Vertebral Column 204
Thoracic (Rib) Cage 204
The Muscles 207
Formation Of Bone Tissue 211
Muscle Contractions 212
Exercise 213
Mobility 213

19 The Nervous System 216

Structure and Function 216
Cells of the Nervous System 216
Divisions of the Nervous System 219
Transmission of Nerve Impulses 227
Reflexes 229

20 The Endocrine System 232

Structure and Function 233
System Physiology 243

21 The Sensory System 246

Structure and Function 246
The Eye 247
The Ear 249
Vision 252
Hearing 253
Balance and Equilibrium 253
Taste 254
Smell 254
Touch/Tactile Sense 255
Other Sensations 255

22 The Cardiovascular System 259

Structure and Function 259
Heart 259
Systemic Blood Vessels 263
Cardiac Conduction 266
Cardiac Cycle 267
Cardiac Output 268
Blood Pressure 268

23 The Hematologic and Lymphatic Systems 272

Blood 272
Lymph 279
Blood Circulation 282
Lymphatic Circulation 283

24 The Immune System 286
  Structure and Function 286
  Bone Marrow and Lymphocyte Production 286
  Lymphoid Organs 290
  The Mononuclear Phagocyte System 290
  Nonspecific Defense Mechanisms 290
  Specific Defense Mechanisms 290
  Antigen–Antibody Reaction 292

25 The Respiratory System 295
  Structure and Function 295
  Upper Respiratory Tract 295
  Lower Respiratory Tract 298
  Ventilation 299
  External (Pulmonary) and Internal (Tissue) Respiration 301
  Regulation of Acid–Base Balance 302
  Respiratory Reflexes 302
  Vocalization 302

26 The Digestive System 305
  Structure and Function 305
  Mouth 306
  Pharynx 308
  Esophagus 308
  Stomach 309
  Small Intestine 309
  Duodenum 310
  Jejunum and Ileum 310
  Large Intestine 310
  Cecum and Appendix 312
  Colon 312
  Rectum and Anus 313
  Accessory Organs 313
  System Physiology 315
  Metabolism 316
  Elimination 317

27 The Urinary System 320
  Kidneys 320
  Organs of Urine Storage and Elimination 325
  Blood Pressure Regulation 326
  Urine Formation 326
  Characteristics and Composition of Urine 327
  Micturition 328

28 The Male Reproductive System 331
  Testes 331
  The Ductal System 332
  Scrotum 333
  Penis 333
  Accessory Glands 334
  Hormonal Influences 334
  Sperm Cells and Spermatogenesis 334
  Copulation 335

29 The Female Reproductive System 337
  Reproductive Organs 337
  Breasts 339
  Hormonal Influences 340
  Egg Cells and Oogenesis 340
  Menstrual Cycle 341
  Female Sexual Response 342

UNIT 5

Nutrition and Diet Therapy 345

30 Basic Nutrition 345
  Nutrients 346
  Creating the Healthy Diet 368
  Nutrition Across the Lifespan 371

31 Transcultural and Social Aspects of Nutrition 377
  Regional Preferences 377
  Ethnic Heritage 377
  Cultural Groups 381
  Religious Beliefs and Practices 384
  Vegetarian Diets 384
  Sociocultural Factors 386

32 Diet Therapy and Special Diets 389
  Helping the Client Meet Nutritional Needs 389
  Serving Food 389
  The Client Who Needs Assistance With Eating 392
  House Diets 393
  Modified Diets 393
  Nutritional Support 400
  Food and Medication Interactions 404

PART B   NURSING CARE SKILLS

UNIT 6

The Nursing Process 411

33 Introduction to the Nursing Process 411
  Problem-Solving 411
  Critical Thinking 412
  The Nursing Process 412

34 Nursing Assessment 420
  Nursing Assessment 420
  Data Analysis 423

35 Nursing Diagnosis and Planning 428

Nursing Diagnosis 428
Planning Care 431

36 Implementing and Evaluating Care 435

Implementing Nursing Care 435
Evaluating Nursing Care 437

37 Documenting and Reporting 441

Documentation 441
Reporting 453

UNIT 7

Safety In the Healthcare Facility 455

38 The Healthcare Facility Environment 455

The Client Unit 455
Provision of Nursing Care 458
Healthcare Personnel and Services 461

39 Emergency Preparedness 466

Safety and Preparedness 466
The Disaster Plan 473
The Fire Plan 476

40 Introduction to Microbiology 479

Microorganisms 479
Metabolism and Growth 480
Infectious Disease 488
Response to Infection 491

41 Medical Asepsis 493

Standard Precautions 493
Medical Asepsis 494
Client and Family Teaching 503

42 Infection Control 508

Infection Control 508
Isolation 512
Antibiotic-Resistant Organisms and Special Infections 514

43 Emergency Care and First Aid 517

Principles of Emergency Care 517
Assessing the Person in an Emergency 522
Sudden Death and Life Support 525
First-Aid Measures 527

UNIT 8

Client Care 549

44 Therapeutic Communication Skills 549

Communication 549
Therapeutic Communication Techniques 557
Facilitating Communication in Healthcare 562

45 Admission, Transfer, and Discharge 564

Admission 564
Transfer to Another Unit 573
Discharge 574
Leaving the Healthcare Facility Against Medical Advice 576
Communications Among Healthcare Team Members 577

46 Vital Signs 581

The Graphic Record 581
Assessing Body Temperature 582
Determining Pulse 586
Assessing Respiration 589
Assessing Blood Pressure 591
Pulse Oximetry 595

47 Data Collection in Client Care 607

Medical and Nursing Diagnosis 607
Factors That Influence Data Collection 608
The Physical Examination 617

48 Moving and Positioning Clients 643

Body Mechanics 643
Positioning the Client 645
Joint Mobility and Range of Motion 651
Using Mobility Devices 658
Moving an Immobile Client 665
Using Client Safety Devices 666

49 Beds and Bed Making 687

Bed Making 687
Attachments and Accessories 689
Special Beds and Mattresses 691

50 Personal Hygiene 701

Mouth Care 701
Routine Eye Care 703
Ear Care 703
Care of Hands and Feet 704
Shaving 706
Hair Care 707
Skin Care 709
Skin Infestations 714

51 Elimination 733

Urinary Elimination 733
Bowel Elimination 737
Assisting With Toileting 738
Assisting With Urinary Elimination 740
Assisting With Bowel Elimination 747
Nausea and Vomiting 752

52 Specimen Collection 762

The Stool Specimen 768
The Sputum Specimen 769
Collecting Other Specimens 769

53 Bandages and Binders 777

Bandages 777
Binders 781

54 Heat and Cold Applications 788

Normothermia 788
Heat Therapy 788
Cold Therapy 792

55 Pain Management 801

Pain 801
Collection of Client Data About Pain 804
Pain Management 807

56 Preoperative and Postoperative Care 812

Perioperative Care 812
Preoperative Nursing Care 818
Intraoperative Nursing Care 824
Postoperative Nursing Care 827

57 Surgical Asepsis 841

Asepsis 841
Disinfection and Sterilization 841
Medical and Surgical Asepsis 842
Sterile Technique (Surgical Asepsis) 842
Procedures Requiring Sterile Technique 845

58 Special Skin and Wound Care 857

Wounds 857
Special Considerations 860
Wound Healing 867

59 End-of-Life Care 880

Stages of Dying 880
The Client's Wishes 880
Basic Needs, as Related to the Death Experience 883
Nursing Care of the Dying Client's Family 887
Signs of Approaching Death 888
Care Following the Death of a Client 888
Feelings of the Nurse 890

UNIT 9

Pharmacology and Administration of Medications 895

60 Review of Mathematics 895

Systems of Measurement 895
The Metric System 896
Dosage Calculation 897

61 Introduction to Pharmacology 903

Legal Aspects 903
Medication Preparations and Actions 906
Prescribed Medications 909

62 Classification of Medications 913

Interactions Between Food and Medications 913
Interactions Between Drugs (Drug–Drug Interactions) 914
Introduction to Drug Classifications 914
Antibiotics and Other Anti-Infective Agents 914
Medications That Affect the Integumentary System 921
Medications That Affect the Nervous System 921
Medications That Affect the Endocrine System 931
Medications That Affect the Sensory System 932
Medications That Affect the Cardiovascular System 932
Medications That Affect the Blood 937
Antineoplastic Medications 939
Medications That Affect the Immune System 939
Medications That Affect the Respiratory System 940
Medications That Affect the Gastrointestinal System 943
Medications That Affect the Urinary Tract 947
Medications That Affect the Reproductive Systems 948

63 Administration of Noninjectable Medications 951

Preparation for Administration 951
Safety 954
General Principles of Medication Administration 960
Enteral Administration Methods 962
Parenteral Administration Methods 964

64 Administration of Injectable Medications 978

Syringes and Needles 979
Preparations 981
Intradermal Injections 982
Subcutaneous (SubQ) Injections 982
Intravenous Administration 985
Administration of Intravenous Medications 992
Venipuncture 996

PART C NURSING THROUGHOUT THE LIFE CYCLE

UNIT 10

Maternal and Newborn Nursing 1023

65 Normal Pregnancy 1023

Defining Pregnancy as a Normal Process 1024
Healthcare During Pregnancy 1035
Preparing to Be a Parent 1045

66 Normal Labor, Delivery, and Postpartum Care 1052

Labor and Birth as Normal Processes 1052
Nursing Care During Labor 1061

67 Care of the Normal Newborn 1076

Important Concepts in Newborn Care 1077
Care of the Newborn Immediately After Birth 1077
Characteristics of the Normal Newborn 1081
Care of the Newborn After Delivery 1085
Daily Newborn Care 1089
Nutrition 1091
Discharge 1096

68 High-Risk Pregnancy and Childbirth 1104

Tests to Assess Fetal Status 1105
Interrupted Pregnancy 1106
Maternal Complications During Pregnancy 1108
Existing Disorders Complicating Pregnancy 1114
Disorders Affecting the Fetus 1115
Placental and Amniotic Disorders 1116
Other High-Risk Pregnancies 1118
Complications of Labor and Delivery 1118
Umbilical Cord Complications 1120
Considerations Related to Delivery 1121
Complications of the Postpartum Period 1123
When a Newborn Dies 1125

69 The High-Risk Newborn 1128

Categories of High-Risk Newborns 1129
Nursing Considerations for the High-Risk Newborn 1131
Potential Complications in the High-Risk Newborn 1136
Hemolytic Disease of the Newborn 1139
Intrauterine Disorders: Congenital and Acquired Infections 1140
Congenital Musculoskeletal Disorders 1141
Neural Tube Defects 1142
Congenital Cardiovascular Disorders 1142
Congenital Gastrointestinal Disorders 1143
Congenital Genitourinary Disorders 1143
Substance Misuse and the Newborn 1143

70 Sexuality, Fertility, and Sexually Transmitted Infections 1146

Human Sexuality 1147
Infertility 1150
Contraception 1153
Sexually Transmitted Infections 1162

UNIT 11

Pediatric Nursing 1175

71 Fundamentals of Pediatric Nursing 1175

Health Maintenance 1176
The Hospital Experience 1178
Basic Pediatric Care and Procedures 1181
Intermediate Pediatric Care and Procedures 1184
Advanced Pediatric Care and Procedures 1191
The Child Having Surgery 1194

72 Care of the Infant, Toddler, or Preschooler 1200

Communicable Diseases 1201
Parasitic Infestations 1208
Trauma 1209
Child Abuse 1213
Skin Disorders 1219
Musculoskeletal and Orthopedic Disorders 1219
Neurologic Disorders 1221
Metabolic and Nutritional Disorders 1224
Disorders of the Eyes 1225
Disorders of the Ears, Nose, Throat, and Mouth 1225
Cardiovascular Disorders 1229
Blood and Lymph Disorders 1233
Respiratory Tract Disorders 1237
Gastrointestinal Disorders 1239
Urinary System Disorders 1241
Reproductive System Disorders 1243
Nutritional Considerations in Young Children 1244

73 Care of the School-Age Child or Adolescent 1246

Communicable Diseases 1246
Skin Disorders 1250
Musculoskeletal Disorders 1253
Endocrine Disorders 1257
Vision Disorders 1257
Gastrointestinal Disorders 1259
Reproductive System Disorders 1260

Sleep Deprivation and Disorders 1261
Eating Disorders 1262
Nutritional Considerations 1263

74 The Child or Adolescent With Special Needs 1265

Disabilities and Disorders 1266
Special Learning Disabilities 1267
Etiology of Disabilities and Disorders 1269
Common Disorders 1270

UNIT 12

Adult Care Nursing 1289

75 Skin Disorders 1289

Diagnostic Tests 1290
Common Medical Treatments 1290
Common Surgical Treatments 1293
Acute and Chronic Skin Conditions 1295
Infections 1297
Parasitic Infestations 1298
Sebaceous Gland Disorders 1298
Burns 1299
Neoplasms 1306

76 Disorders in Fluid and Electrolyte Balance 1310

Diagnostic Tests 1310
Common Medical Treatments 1311
Maintenance of Fluid Balance 1312
Maintenance of Electrolyte Balance 1314
Maintenance of Acid–Base Balance 1318

77 Musculoskeletal Disorders 1321

Diagnostic Tests 1321
Common Medical Treatments 1323
Common Surgical Treatments 1323
Common Musculoskeletal Disorders 1325
Systemic Disorders With Musculoskeletal Manifestations 1332
Traumatic Injuries 1334
Trauma Care and Management 1335
Complications of Fractures or Bone Surgery 1344
Neoplasms 1349

78 Nervous System Disorders 1351

Diagnostic Tests 1351
Craniocerebral Disorders 1353
Nerve Disorders 1359
Spinal Cord Disorders 1362
Degenerative Disorders 1364

Inflammatory Disorders 1370
Head Trauma 1373
Neoplasms 1377

79 Endocrine Disorders 1382

Diagnostic Tests 1382
Common Medical and Surgical Treatments 1386
Pituitary Gland Disorders 1387
Thyroid Gland Disorders 1388
Parathyroid Gland Disorders 1391
Adrenal Gland Disorders 1391
Pancreatic Endocrine Disorders 1393

80 Sensory System Disorders 1413

Diagnostic Tests 1413
Common Medical Treatments 1415
Common Surgical Treatments 1415
The Eye and Vision Disorders 1422
Trauma to the Eye 1426
The Ear and Hearing Disorders 1427
Disorders of Other Special Senses 1431

81 Cardiovascular Disorders 1435

Diagnostic Tests 1436
Common Medical Treatments 1438
Common Surgical Treatments 1438
Abnormal Conditions That May Cause Cardiovascular Disease 1444
Heart Disorders 1445
Blood Vessel Disorders 1455

82 Blood and Lymph Disorders 1466

Diagnostic Tests 1466
Common Treatments 1470
Hematopoietic Stem Cell Transplantation 1472
Hematologic System Disorders 1473

83 Cancer 1486

Cancer Development 1486
Diagnostic Tests 1489
Treatment Modalities for Cancer 1492
Nursing Considerations for Clients With Cancer 1496

84 Allergic, Immune, and Autoimmune Disorders 1506

Diagnostic Tests 1506
Allergies 1508
Immune Disorders 1514
Autoimmune Disorders 1514

85 HIV and AIDS 1520

History of HIV/AIDS 1520
Transmission 1521
Signs and Symptoms of HIV Infection 1523

Acquired Immunodeficiency Syndrome 1525
HIV Exposure Guidelines 1531

86 Respiratory Disorders 1533

Diagnostic Tests 1533
Common Medical Treatments 1536
Common Surgical Treatments 1536
Infectious Respiratory Disorders 1544
Chronic Respiratory Disorders 1552
Trauma 1558
Neoplasms 1559
Disorders of the Nose 1559
Disorders of the Throat 1561

87 Oxygen Therapy and Respiratory Care 1566

Oxygen Provision 1566
The Client Who Is Having Difficulty Breathing 1569
The Client Who Is Unable to Breathe 1571

88 Digestive Disorders 1583

Diagnostic Tests 1583
Common Medical and Surgical Treatments 1588
Disorders of the Mouth 1599
Disorders of the Esophagus 1601
Disorders of the Stomach 1604
Disorders of the Small or Large Bowel 1609
Peritonitis 1615
Disorders of the Sigmoid Colon and Rectum 1616
Disorders of the Liver 1617
Disorders of the Gallbladder 1621
Disorders of the Pancreas 1623
Conditions of Overnutrition and Undernutrition 1623

89 Urinary Disorders 1629

Diagnostic Tests 1630
Urinary Incontinence 1635
Urinary Tract Infections 1637
Inflammatory Disorders 1639
Obstructive Disorders 1641
Urinary Tract Tumors 1646
Urinary Tract Trauma 1649
Renal Failure 1649

90 Male Reproductive Disorders 1656

Diagnostic Tests 1656
Common Medical Treatments 1657
Erectile Disorders 1657
Structural Disorders 1659
Inflammatory Disorders 1661
Neoplasms 1662

91 Female Reproductive Disorders 1670

Diagnostic Tests 1670
Common Surgical Treatments 1674
Disorders Related to the Menstrual Cycle 1676

Structural Disorders 1680
Inflammatory Disorders 1681
Cervicitis 1683
Neoplasms 1686

UNIT 13

Gerontologic Nursing 1697

92 Gerontology: The Aging Adult 1697

Geriatric Care Settings 1698
Helping the Older Adult Meet Basic Needs 1703
Helping the Older Adult Meet Emotional Needs 1707
Special Concerns of the Adult Related to Increasing Age 1710
Elder Abuse 1713

93 Cognitive Impairment in the Aging Adult 1715

Cognitive Impairment 1715
Aspects of Dementia 1718

UNIT 14

Mental Health Nursing 1735

94 Psychiatric Nursing 1735

Mental Health 1736
Mental Illness 1736
The Mental Healthcare Team 1742
Methods of Psychiatric Therapy 1746
The Client in an Inpatient Setting 1759
Mental Health Nursing Skills 1764

95 Substance Use Disorders 1778

Substance Use Disorders 1778
Nursing Care Measures 1781
Detoxification and Recovery 1783
Alcohol Use Disorder 1790
Other Substance Use Disorders 1794
Special Populations 1801

UNIT 15

Nursing In A Variety of Settings 1805

96 Extended Care 1805

Extended-Care Options 1806
The Concept of Transitional Care 1810

97 Rehabilitation Nursing 1813

Definitions of Rehabilitation 1813
Rehabilitation and Maslow Hierarchy of Needs 1813
Stages of Adjustment to a Disability 1814
The Rehabilitation Team 1814
Nursing Considerations in Rehabilitation 1815
Activities of Daily Living 1815
The Scope of Rehabilitative Services 1824
Community Resources 1826
Barriers to Rehabilitation 1827

98 Home Care Nursing 1830

Reasons for Home Care 1830
Types of Agencies and Services 1831
Telehealth 1832
Self-Management of Chronic Conditions 1832
Payment for Home Care 1832
Members of the Home Care Team 1833
Nursing Duties in Home Care 1834
Safety for the Home Care Team 1836
Suggestions for Primary Caregivers 1836

99 Ambulatory Nursing 1839

The Role of the Nurse 1839
Types of Ambulatory Facilities 1840
Use of the Electronic Health Record 1849

100 Hospice Nursing 1851

Evolution of the Hospice Movement 1851
The Hospice Concept 1852
Assisting the Hospice Client to Meet Basic Needs 1856
Pain Management 1860
Children in Hospice Programs 1865
When the Client Dies 1865

PART D   YOUR CAREER

UNIT 16

The Transition to Practicing Nurse 1869

101 From Student to Graduate Nurse 1869

Nursing Licensure 1869
Role Transition 1873
Personal Life 1880

102 Career Opportunities and Job-Seeking Skills 1883

Employment Opportunities 1883
Obtaining Employment Information 1889
Job-Seeking Skills 1890

103 Advancement and Leadership in Nursing 1898

Advancement in Nursing 1898
Leadership 1900

Bibliography 1907

Glossary 1927

Index 1983

The following Appendices can be found on **the**Point

Appendix A: Key English-to-Spanish Healthcare Phrases

Appendix B: Key Abbreviations and Acronyms Used in Healthcare

Appendix C: Medical Terminology: Prefixes, Roots, and Suffixes Commonly Used in Medical Terms

Summary of Special Displays

NURSING PROCEDURES

- 32-1 Inserting a Nasogastric (NG) Tube (Nasogastric Intubation) 405
- 32-2 Administering a Tube Feeding 409
- 41-1 Handwashing 505
- 41-2 Using Clean (Nonsterile) Gloves 506
- 41-3 Using a Mask 507
- 43-1 Applying a Sling 546
- 43-2 Assisting the Client Who Has a Nosebleed 547
- 43-3 Applying a Tourniquet 547
- 45-1 Undressing the Immobile Client 580
- 46-1 Measuring Body Temperatures 597
- 46-2 Measuring Radial Pulse Manually 601
- 46-3 Measuring Apical Pulse 601
- 46-4 Counting Respirations 602
- 46-5 Measuring Blood Pressure (Aneroid Manometer and Manual Cuff) 603
- 46-6 Using a Pulse Oximeter 605
- 48-1 Turning the Client to a Side-Lying Position 671
- 48-2 Logroll Turn 673
- 48-3 Performing Passive ROM Exercises 674
- 48-4 Using a Transfer Belt, With Metal-Toothed Buckle 675
- 48-5 Dangling 676
- 48-6 Helping the Client From Bed and/or Into a Chair 677
- 48-7 Pushing a Nonmotorized Wheelchair or Wheeled Stretcher/Gurney (Litter) 679
- 48-8 Walking With a Cane 680
- 48-9 Using a Walker 681
- 48-10 Moving the Client From Bed to Wheeled Stretcher/Gurney 682
- 48-11 Adjusting Pillows and Moving the Client Up in Bed 683
- 48-12 Using Client Safety/Protective Devices 684
- 49-1 Making an Unoccupied Bed 694
- 49-2 Making an Occupied Bed 696
- 49-3 Making a Postoperative Bed 698
- 49-4 Using a Bed Cradle 699
- 50-1 Routine Daily Mouth Care 717
- 50-2 Flossing the Teeth 718
- 50-3 Caring for Dentures 719
- 50-4 Special Mouth Care: The Dependent Client 720
- 50-5 Caring for Fingernails and Toenails 721
- 50-6 Giving a Foot Soak 722
- 50-7 Shaving a Client 723
- 50-8 Using the Shampoo Cap 724
- 50-9 The Bed Shampoo 725
- 50-10 Giving a Backrub 726
- 50-11 Assisting With a Tub Bath 727
- 50-12 Giving a Bed Bath 729
- 50-13 Assisting With Perineal Care 732
- 51-1 Giving and Removing the Bedpan and Urinal 755
- 51-2 Emptying the Urinary Drainage Bag 757
- 51-3 Bladder Retraining With Closed Urinary Drainage 757
- 51-4 Giving an Enema 758
- 51-5 Performing Manual Disimpaction 760
- 51-6 Assisting With Bowel Retraining 761
- 51-7 Helping to Relieve Flatus 761
- 52-1 Measuring Urinary Output 772
- 52-2 Measuring Urine Specific Gravity 773
- 52-3 Collecting a Single-Voided Specimen 773
- 52-4 Collecting a 24-hr Urine Specimen 774
- 52-5 Collecting a Urine Specimen From an Indwelling Catheter 774
- 52-6 Collecting a Stool Specimen 776
- 52-7 Collecting a Sputum Specimen 776
- 53-1 Applying Antiembolism Stockings (TED sox) 785
- 53-2 Applying Montgomery Straps 786
- 54-1 Using an Aquathermia (Aqua-K) Pad 796
- 54-2 Applying Warm, Moist Compresses and Packs 797
- 54-3 Administering a Therapeutic Soak to an Arm or Leg 798
- 54-4 Using a Sitz Bath 799
- 54-5 Applying an Icecap or Ice Collar 800
- 56-1 Receiving the Client From the Postanesthesia Care Unit (PACU) 839
- 57-1 Opening a Sterile Package 848
- 57-2 Putting on Sterile Gloves (Open Gloving) 850
- 57-3 Catheterizing the Female Client 851
- 57-4 Catheterizing the Male Client 854
- 57-5 Removing the Retention Catheter 856
- 58-1 Changing a Dry, Sterile Dressing 875
- 58-2 Performing a Sterile Wound Irrigation 878
- 59-1 Postmortem Care of the Body 892
- 63-1 Administering Oral Medications 969
- 63-2 Administering Medications Through a Gastrointestinal Tube 970
- 63-3 Administering a Rectal Suppository 972
- 63-4 Administering a Vaginal Suppository 972
- 63-5 Administering Eye Medications 973
- 63-6 Administering Ear Medications 975
- 63-7 Administering a Transdermal Patch 977
- 64-1 Drawing Medication From an Ampule or Vial 999
- 64-2 Administering Intradermal Injections 1001
- 64-3 Administering Subcutaneous or Intramuscular Injections 1002
- 64-4 Giving a Subcutaneous (SubQ) Injection 1003
- 64-5 Giving an Intramuscular (IM) Injection 1004
- 64-6 Changing the Intravenous (IV) Bag, Dressing, and/or Tubing 1005
- 64-7 Converting a Continuous Intravenous (IV) Infusion to an Intermittent Line (Saline Lock) 1008
- 64-8 Flushing the Saline Lock; Administration of Medications Via Saline Lock 1009
- 64-9 Discontinuing an Intravenous (IV) Infusion or Saline Lock 1010
- 64-10 Administration of IV Medications Via Piggyback Setup (Small Volume Delivery System) 1011

64-11	Administration of Medications Via Volume-Controlled Infusion 1013		43-5	Assisting the Client Who Feels Faint 537
64-12	Administration of Medications Into a Continuous Infusion (IV Push) 1014		43-6	Giving First Aid in Suspected Heart Attack (MI) 538
64-13	Venipuncture (Phlebotomy)/Obtaining a Blood Specimen 1015		43-7	Giving First Aid in Poisoning or Overdose 542
64-14	Initiating Intravenous Infusions 1018		44-1	Using Therapeutic Communication 550
65-1	Listening to Fetal Heart Tones (FHTs) 1051		47-1	Measuring Reflexes 620
66-1	Application of External Monitor 1074		48-1	Positioning the Client for Comfort 647
66-2	Fundal Massage 1075		48-2	Assisting the Client to Walk 658
67-1	Assisting a Newborn With Breathing 1099		48-3	Using Client Reminder or Protective (Safety) Devices 666
67-2	Prophylaxis for the Eyes of the Neonate 1100		50-1	Caring for a Client Who Wears Dentures or Other Mouth Appliances 702
67-3	Weighing a Neonate 1100		50-2	Caring for the Eyes 703
67-4	Measuring Head Circumference 1101		50-3	Caring for a Hearing Aid 705
67-5	Bathing a Neonate 1101		50-4	Performing Hand Massage 706
67-6	Performing a Heel Stick Procedure on a Newborn 1102		50-5	Caring for Hair 708
71-1	Collecting a Pediatric Urine Specimen 1198		50-6	Backrub 711
78-1	Assisting With a Lumbar Puncture 1380		50-7	Washing the Client's Face and Hands 712
79-1	Testing for Blood Glucose Level 1411		51-1	Straining Urine for Calculi 736
80-1	Using a Cotton-Tipped Applicator 1433		51-2	Listening for Bowel Sounds 738
80-2	Irrigating the Ear 1433		51-3	Performing Catheter Care 743
86-1	Suctioning to Remove Secretions 1564		51-4	Using External Catheter Systems 744
87-1	Supplying Oxygen With the Nasal Cannula 1578		51-5	Using the Ultrasound Bladder Scanner 747
87-2	Using the Simple Mask 1579		51-6	Administering the Harris Flush 749
87-3	Applying the Partial-Rebreathing Mask 1579		51-7	Administering an Enema 751
87-4	Applying the Venturi Mask 1580		51-8	Assisting the Client Who Is Nauseated or Vomiting 753
87-5	Assisting at a Tracheostomy 1580		52-1	Collecting Specimens and Samples 763
87-6	Suctioning and Providing Tracheostomy Care 1581		52-2	Collecting Urine Specimens 765
88-1	Irrigating the NG Tube 1627		52-3	Collecting Clean-Catch Midstream Urine Specimens 767
88-2	Changing the Ostomy Appliance 1628		53-1	Applying a Roller Bandage (Arm or Leg) 780
91-1	Performing a Vaginal Irrigation (Douche) 1695		53-2	Applying a Stretch-Net Dressing to a Finger 781
			53-3	Applying a T-Binder 782
			53-4	General Nursing Care of the Client With a Bandage or Binder 783

NURSING CARE GUIDELINES

32-1	Helping at Hospital Mealtimes 390		54-1	Applying Heat Therapy 789
32-2	Feeding Clients 391		54-2	Applying Cold Therapy 792
37-1	Change-of-Shift Reporting 453		54-3	Applying Cold Moist Compresses 793
38-1	General Guidelines for Performing Nursing Procedures 459		54-4	Giving a Tepid Sponge to Reduce Body Temperature 794
38-2	Guidelines for Performing Grouped Procedures 460		56-1	Caring for the Client Who Is Receiving Anesthesia 817
39-1	Preventing Accidents in the Healthcare Facility or Client's Home 467		56-2	Organizing Preoperative Nursing Care 819
41-1	Implementing Standard Precautions 493		56-3	Assisting the Client With Postoperative Exercises 833
41-2	Preventing Infection for Nursing Staff and Clients 497		57-1	Sterile Technique 843
42-1	Caring for the Body of a Deceased Person Who Was in Isolation 514		63-1	Setting Up Medications 953
			63-2	Administering Medications Safely 956
43-1	Treating Shock in an Emergency 522		63-3	Crushing or Splitting Tablets 963
43-2	Providing Emergency First Aid for Burns 533		63-4	Administering Orally Disintegrating Tablets 963
43-3	First Aid for Avulsed Teeth 535		63-5	Administering Aerosolized and Powdered Respiratory Medications 966
43-4	Giving First Aid for Eye Injuries 536		63-6	Administering Nasal Sprays or Drops 967
			64-1	Caring for the Client Receiving Intravenous (IV) Therapy 986

64-2	Managing Parenteral Nutrition 993	86-1	Assisting With Postural Drainage 1537
64-3	Administering Intravenous (IV) Medications 994	86-2	Caring for the Person Who Has Had Chest Surgery 1538
66-1	Postpartum Period 1070	86-3	Caring for the Person With Chest Suction 1540
67-1	Care of the Normal Newborn 1090	86-4	Caring for the Person With Pneumonia 1548
68-1	Assisting in an Emergency Delivery 1122	86-5	Caring for the Person Who Has Had Nasal Surgery 1561
71-1	Reducing Anxiety and Calming Children for Procedures 1180	87-1	Providing Oxygen 1567
71-2	Providing Pediatric Safety 1184	87-2	Nursing Care Priorities for the Client Receiving Mechanical Ventilation 1576
71-3	Using Pediatric Restraints 1185	88-1	Providing Care Before and After Barium Studies 1585
71-4	The Child and IV Therapy 1188	88-2	Giving Care for a Gastrostomy, Colostomy, or Ileostomy 1598
71-5	Giving an Infant a Bath 1189	88-3	Caring for the Client With a Liver Disorder 1618
71-6	General Considerations for Oxygen (O_2) Administration 1190	88-4	Caring for the Hospitalized Client Who is Obese 1624
71-7	Diagnostic Procedures 1192	89-1	Caring for the Client Receiving Dialysis 1654
71-8	Managing a Fever 1193	90-1	Managing Continuous TURP or Bladder Irrigation 1667
71-9	Administering Medications to Children 1193	93-1	Monitoring a Client's Hydration Status 1732
71-10	Preoperative Care for Children 1195	93-2	Communicating With the Person Who Has Dementia 1733
71-11	Postoperative Care for Children 1196	94-1	Caring for the Client Who Is to Have ECT 1749
74-1	Working With an Individual With Special Needs 1266	94-2	Administering Medication Therapy in the Mental Health Unit 1756
74-2	Feeding the Intellectually Impaired Child 1268	94-3	Maintaining the Client's Dignity in Mental Health Units 1760
75-1	Giving a Therapeutic Bath 1291	94-4	Supervised Visits 1760
75-2	Application of Moist Dressings 1292	94-5	Using Safety Devices for the Client With Mental Illness 1762
77-1	Preparing for Casting 1336	94-6	Suicide Prevention 1770
77-2	Performing Cast Care 1337	94-7	Care of the Client Who Is Manic/Hypomanic 1772
77-3	Caring for Clients in Traction 1342	94-8	Care of the Combative or Assaultive Client 1772
77-4	Caring for Clients With New Hip Replacements 1347	94-9	Assisting the Client Who Has Delusions or Hallucinations 1773
78-1	Maintaining the Client's Safety During a Seizure 1358	94-10	Assisting the Client Who Is Confused or Demented 1773
78-2	Caring for the Client With Paralysis 1365	94-11	Assisting the Client Who Is Withdrawn or Depressed 1774
78-3	Determining Cerebrospinal Fluid (CSF) in Drainage 1375	94-12	Assisting the Client Who Is Regressed 1774
81-1	Administering the Cardiotonic Drug Digoxin (Lanoxin) 1451	95-1	Caring for the Alcohol- or Drug-Using Person in the Emergency Department 1782
81-2	Caring for Clients With Peripheral Vascular Disease 1459	95-2	Nursing Care in Alcohol Withdrawal 1789
81-3	Communicating With the Client With Aphasia 1463	95-3	Nursing Considerations in Antabuse Therapy 1794
82-1	Precautions During Blood Transfusions 1471	100-1	Providing Care in Hospice Nursing 1857
82-2	Managing a Transfusion Reaction 1472		
82-3	Administering Iron Supplements 1475		
83-1	Providing Care for the Person Receiving Chemotherapy 1494		
83-2	Providing Care for Clients Receiving External-Beam Radiation Therapy 1497		
83-3	Providing Care for Clients With Implanted Radioactive Isotopes 1499		

The Nature of Nursing | UNIT 1

1 The Origins of Nursing

Learning Objectives

1. Explain how certain events in ancient and medieval times influenced the development of contemporary nursing.
2. Discuss Florence Nightingale's influence on modern nursing practice.
3. List at least 10 of Florence Nightingale's nursing principles that are still practiced today.
4. Identify important individuals who contributed to the development of nursing in the United States.
5. Name some pioneer nursing schools in the United States.
6. List important milestones in the history of practical nursing education.
7. Explain war-related developments in nursing.
8. Discuss current trends that are expected to influence the nursing profession in the 21st century.
9. Describe the importance of nursing insignia, uniforms, and the nursing school pin.

Important Terminology

Caduceus   Hippocratic oath   holistic healthcare   insignia   Nightingale lamp

You have chosen to become a nurse. The word *nurse* derives from the Latin word meaning *to nourish*. You are embarking on a career that combines scientific principles, technical skills, and personal compassion. Although people have been performing many nursing skills for centuries, nursing in its present form began to emerge only in the 19th century. Contemporary nursing continues to evolve as society and its healthcare needs and expectations change. Nursing must continue to adapt to meet society's goals and to provide needed services in the changing world.

Nursing is a practical and noble profession. It provides a stable career in the ever-changing world of healthcare, with plenty of career options.

Individual attributes required to be a nurse include a strong sense of responsibility and the highest standards of integrity. Personal conviction and flexibility are necessary foundations of a nurse. A nurse must be well educated and integrate the art and the science of working with people.

Nurses interact with a vast assortment of individuals, including numerous and varied healthcare personnel who have their own fields of expertise. Many of these healthcare fields were originally included in the broader roles and responsibilities of nursing. For example, the nurse was originally responsible for nutrition and diets. Nurses were also responsible for rehabilitative needs of the persons under their care. The role of the nurse became so important to the healthcare system that the functions of the nurse had to become diverse and specialized to meet fast-growing needs. Many of these duties were broken into specialties that are seen today, such as nutritionist, dietitian, physical therapist, or occupational therapist.

As the role of the nurse has evolved, so has the role of the person receiving care. When the physician was the primary manager or leader of health issues, the individual receiving care was typically called a *client*. During the 20th century, the client became more aware of his or her own health issues. Instead of being a passive participant, the client became a more knowledgeable consumer of healthcare and, as in other service industries, the consumer became a client of the primary care provider, nurse, and healthcare system. In the 21st century, all of these terms are currently used to describe the individual who receives healthcare. This textbook uses the term *client* because the term client reflects the roles of the nurse who actively interacts with individuals, families, and the healthcare system. In everyday conversations, the terms *patient*, *client*, and/or *consumer* may be heard.

NURSING'S HERITAGE

A detailed history of nursing is beyond the scope of this book. All nurses should become familiar with some important people and developments in the history of nursing. Several internet sites record nursing's heritage. As your nursing career develops, you will be part of nursing's ongoing history.

Early Influences

In ancient times, people often attributed illness to punishment for sins or to possession by evil spirits. Most primitive

1

tribes had a medicine man, or shaman, who performed rituals using various plants, herbs, and other materials, to heal the sick. Tribal rituals included dances, chants, and special costumes and masks. Some groups used human or animal sacrifices. Women had various folk roles in ancient health practices, depending on the culture and social customs. Women were often involved with assisting in childbirth.

Religious images of the nurse developed as care of the sick became associated with concepts that are discussed in the Bible, the Talmud, and other ancient texts. Centers in India and Babylonia provided care for the sick before the time of Christ. By 500 BC, the advanced Greek civilization had begun to acknowledge causes of disease other than punishment by God or demonic possession. Based on mythical figures, the caduceus and the staff of Aesculapius are the modern symbols of medicine (Fig. 1-1). The Greeks began to establish centers, sometimes called hostels or hospitals, for care of the sick and injured. They used warm and mineral baths, massage, and other forms of therapy that priestesses sometimes administered. Pregnant women or people with an incurable illness were not admitted to these hostels.

The Influence of Hippocrates

One of the early outstanding figures in medicine was Hippocrates, born in 460 BC on the Greek island of Kos. Hippocrates is the acknowledged "Father of Medicine." Hippocrates denounced the idea of mystical influence on disease. He was also the first person to propose concepts such as physical assessment, medical ethics, client-centered care, and systematic observation and reporting. By emphasizing the importance of caring for the whole person (holistic healthcare), he helped to lay the groundwork for nursing and medicine. Contemporary healthcare practitioners preserve the principles of Hippocrates. Typically, a physician will repeat the Hippocratic oath when graduating from a school of medicine. The Florence Nightingale pledge and Practical Nurses' pledge are based on this oath.

Early medical educators helped to solidify the need for practitioners to be well-educated individuals. Physicians were eventually required to obtain a university degree as a doctor of medicine (MD). Specialized healthcare education and training became standard as scientific knowledge increased. Modern medicine has multiple medical and surgical specializations; for instance, the client can be described as having heart and lung diseases, or injury and trauma. Nursing has developed a role of assistant to the physician, serving their needs and following orders regarding care of individuals.

Relatively unchanged from the beginning is the concept that the nurse must be aware of the whole client. The holistic approach translates into the nurse's attentiveness to a client's personal needs from various perspectives. The nurse is aware of the client's emotions, lifestyles, physical changes, spiritual needs, and individual challenges. Nursing is unique in this approach to healthcare.

The Roman Matrons

The first recorded history of nursing begins with Biblical women who cared for the sick and injured. Many were in the religious life. For instance, Phoebe, mentioned in the Epistle to the Romans (about 58 AD), is known as the first deaconess and visiting nurse.

Fabiola, a Roman woman, is credited with influencing and paying for the construction of the first free hospital in Rome in 390 AD. Another Roman woman, Saint Marcella, converted her beautiful home into a monastery, where she taught nursing skills. She is considered the first nursing educator. Saint Paula is credited with establishing inns and hospitals to care for pilgrims traveling to Jerusalem. She is said to be the first person to teach the philosophy that nursing is an art rather than a service. Saint Helena, the mother of the Roman Emperor Constantine, is credited with establishing the first gerontologic facility, or home for the aged.

Monastic and Military Nursing Orders

Beginning in the first century, several monastic orders were established to care for the sick. Sometimes, the monastery itself became the refuge for the sick; in other cases, members of a religious order founded a hospital. Both men and women of religious orders performed nursing care.

During the Crusades (1096–1291), female religious orders in northern Europe were nearly eliminated. Male military personnel, such as the Knights Hospitallers of St. John in Jerusalem, conducted most nursing care. Because these military men were required to defend the hospital as well as care for the sick, they wore suits of armor under their religious habits. The symbol for this order was the Maltese cross, which later became the symbol of the Nightingale School. This symbol was the forerunner of nursing school pins worn today.

The Reformation

In the 1500s, during the European religious movement called the Reformation, many monasteries closed and the work of

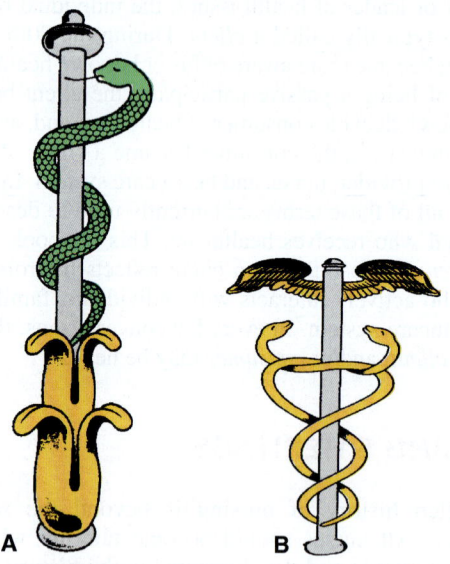

Figure 1-1 Symbols of medicine. **A.** Aesculapius, a mythical Greek god of healing and son of Apollo, had many followers who used massage and exercise to treat clients. This god is also believed to have used the magical powers of a yellow, nonpoisonous serpent to lick the wounds of surgical clients. Aesculapius was often pictured holding the serpent wrapped around his staff or wand; this staff is a symbol of medicine. **B.** Another medical symbol is the caduceus, the staff of the Roman god Mercury, shown as a winged staff with two serpents wrapped around it.

women in religious orders nearly ended. Until the 1800s, the few women who cared for the sick were prisoners or prostitutes. Nursing was considered the most menial of all tasks, and the least desirable. This period is called the *dark ages of nursing*.

Fliedner in Kaiserswerth

In 1836, Pastor Theodor Fliedner established the Kaiserswerth School for Nursing in his parish in Kaiserswerth, Germany. It was one of the first formally established schools of nursing in the world. Out of it grew the Lutheran Order of Deaconesses, which Fliedner directed. Its most famous student was Florence Nightingale.

By the late 1800s, many schools for trained nurses existed throughout Europe. The status of nursing began to improve, and many women, including members of religious orders, once again became involved in nursing care.

Florence Nightingale

Even during the days when nursing was considered menial and undesirable, some women continued to care for the sick. Probably the most famous was Florence Nightingale (Fig. 1-2). Most nurses before her time received almost no training. Not until she graduated from Kaiserswerth and began to teach her concepts did nursing become a respected profession.

Nightingale was born in Italy in 1820 to wealthy English parents. When she was still very young, her parents returned to England.

In 1851, Nightingale entered the Deaconess School in Kaiserswerth. She was 31 years old, and her family and friends were strongly opposed to her becoming a nurse. After her graduation in 1853, she became superintendent of a charity hospital for governesses. She trained her attendants on the job and greatly improved the quality of care. In 1854, the Crimean War began. Nightingale gained fame during

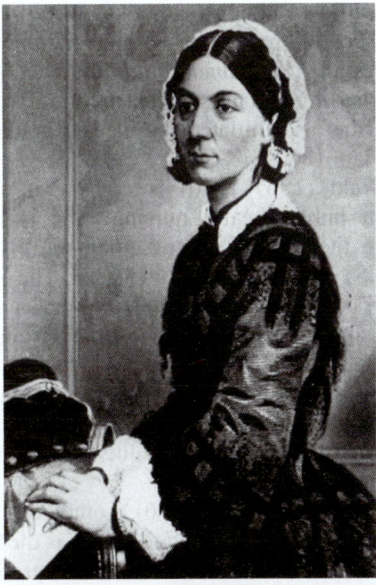

Figure 1-2 Florence Nightingale. (Photo courtesy of the Center for the Study of the History of Nursing.)

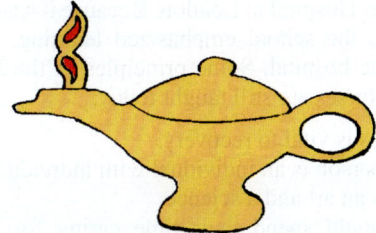

Figure 1-3 The "Nightingale lamp" (also known as the "Lamp of Nursing" or the "Lamp of Learning") is an insignia of nursing and nursing education. The lamp represents the warmth of caring. The light of the lamp symbolizes the striving for excellence. The oil represents the energy and commitment of the nurse to heal others.

this conflict. She entered the battlefield near Scutari, Turkey, with 38 other nurses and cared for the sick and injured. The nurses had few supplies and little outside support. Nonetheless, Nightingale insisted on establishing sanitary conditions and providing quality nursing care, which immediately reduced the mortality rate. Her persistence made her famous, and she and her nurses were greatly admired. Her dedicated service both during the day and at night, when she and her nurses made their rounds carrying oil lamps, created a public image of the lady with the lamp. In time, the Nightingale lamp or the "Lamp of Learning" (Fig. 1-3) became a symbol of nursing and nursing education. Today, many schools of nursing display a model of the lamp or a picture of Florence Nightingale carrying a lamp.

Nightingale's Definition of Nursing

Nightingale had definite and progressive ideas about nursing, as discussed in her book, titled *Notes on Nursing: What It is, and What It is Not* (published in 1859). These ideas remain foundations of contemporary nursing. Nightingale states:

> The very elements of what constitutes good nursing are little understood for the well as for the sick. The same laws of health or of nursing, for they are in reality the same, obtain among the well as among the sick.…If a patient is cold, if a patient is feverish, if a patient is faint, if he is sick after taking food, if he has a bed-sore, it is generally the fault not of the disease, but of the nursing.…I use the word nursing for want of a better. It (nursing) has been limited to signify little more than the administration of medicines and the application of poultices. It ought to signify the proper use of fresh air, light, warmth, cleanliness, quiet, and the proper selection and administration of diet—all at the least expense of vital power to the patient.

Nightingale specified five essential points that are necessary for the maintenance of health and the support of recuperation. These include clean air, clean water, efficient drainage, cleanliness, and light.

The Nightingale School

Building on the respect she had established in the Crimean War, Nightingale opened the first nursing school outside a hospital in 1860. The nursing course was 1 year in length and included both classroom and clinical experience, a major innovation at that time. Students gained clinical experience at St. Thomas Hospital in London. Because it was financially independent, the school emphasized learning, rather than service to the hospital. Some principles of the Nightingale School for Nurses are still taught today:

- Cleanliness is vital to recovery.
- The sick person is an individual with individual needs.
- Nursing is an art and a science.
- Nurses should spend their time caring for others, not cleaning.
- Prevention is better than cure.
- The nurse must work as a member of a team.
- The nurse must use discretion but must follow the physician's orders.
- Self-discipline and self-evaluation are important.
- A good nursing program encourages a nurse's individual development.
- The nurse should be healthy in mind and body.
- Teaching is part of nursing.
- Nursing is a specialty.
- A nurse does not graduate but continues to learn throughout his or her career.
- Nursing curricula should include both theoretical knowledge and practical experience.

The Nightingale School included other innovations:

- Establishment of a nurses' residence
- Entrance examinations and academic and personal requirements, including a character reference
- Records of each student's progress—later known as the "Nightingale plan," a model for current nursing programs
- Records of employment of students after graduation, or a formal register—the beginnings of nursing practice standards

> **NCLEX Alert**
>
> NCLEX questions are based on the contents of the official NCLEX-PN Test Plan. Students need to be aware of these general categories because specific questions, better referred to as *clinical scenarios*, can involve one or more components of the Plan. The answers provided by NCLEX are referred to as *options*. When taking the NCLEX, read the clinical scenario carefully and read all of the options. Keep in mind that more than one option may be correct. You must choose the BEST correct option.

NURSING IN THE UNITED STATES

Nursing in the colonial United States was primarily a family matter, with mothers caring for their own families or neighbors helping each other. Throughout the 19th and 20th centuries, historical and nursing developments interacted to build the foundation of modern nursing practice. The establishment and growth of a system of nursing education is the most important development that has shaped today's nursing.

The First Nursing Schools

The influence of Florence Nightingale and the Kaiserswerth School extended to the United States when Pastor Fliedner came to Pittsburgh, Pennsylvania, with four nurse-deaconesses. In 1849, he became involved with the Pittsburgh Infirmary, the first Protestant hospital in the United States. Today it is called Passavant Hospital. The four deaconesses trained other nurses and started the movement to educate American nurses. The Pittsburgh Infirmary was the first real school of nursing in the United States, although limited training existed in other hospitals in New York and Pennsylvania before 1849.

In 1873, three nursing programs based on the Nightingale plan were formally established: Bellevue Hospital School of Nursing in New York; Connecticut Training School in New Haven; and Boston Training School at Massachusetts General Hospital.

Notable American Nurses

With the onset of the Civil War (1861–1865), the public need for nurses became more evident. In 1861, the Union Army appointed Dorothea Lynde Dix (1802–1887) Superintendent of Female Nurses. Her job was to recruit volunteer nurses to treat men injured in the war. Dix is especially remembered for her campaign against the inhumane treatment of the mentally ill. One of Dix's volunteers was Louisa May Alcott (author of *Little Women*). Another was Clara Barton (1821–1912), who in 1881 founded the organization now known as the American Red Cross.

Melinda Ann (Linda) Richards (1841–1930) was the first trained nurse in the United States. She graduated in the early 1870s and organized the school of nursing at Massachusetts General Hospital, then called the Boston Training School.

Isabel Hampton Robb (1860–1910) was the founder of the school of nursing at Johns Hopkins University. She is credited with founding two national nursing organizations, one in 1911, which eventually emerged as the American Nurses Association (originally called the Alumnae Association). She and Lavinia Lloyd Dock (1858–1956) founded the American Society of Superintendents of Training Schools of Nursing in 1894, which in 1903 evolved into the Education Committee of the National League for Nursing. Robb wrote one of the earliest nursing textbooks, *Materia Medica for Nurses*, and coauthored a four-volume *History of Nursing*. Robb also founded the *American Journal of Nursing*. She introduced charting and nurse licensure to improve continuity of care. She also initiated the idea of graduate nursing study in the late 1800s.

Lillian Wald (1867–1940) is considered the founder of American public health nursing. She is best known for founding the Henry Street Settlement Visiting Nurse Society (VNS) in New York City in 1893. The Henry Street Settlement was a neighborhood nursing service that became a model for similar programs in the United States and other countries. Wald also convinced New York City schools to have a nurse on duty during school hours. She persuaded President Theodore Roosevelt to create a Federal Children's Bureau and insisted that nursing education occur in institutions of higher learning.

Mary E. Mahoney (1845–1926) promoted fair treatment of African Americans in healthcare. She was the first African American graduate nurse and promoted integration and better working conditions for minority healthcare workers in Boston.

Mary Breckinridge (1881–1965) was a pioneer as a visiting nurse-midwife to the mountain people of Kentucky in the early 1900s, often making her rounds on horseback. She also started one of the first midwifery schools in the United States.

Collegiate Nursing Education

In 1907, Mary Adelaide Nutting (1858–1947) and Isabel Robb were instrumental in establishing the first college-based nursing program at Teachers College of Columbia University. Nutting thus became the first nurse to be on a university staff. She was also instrumental in founding the International Council of Nurses.

In 1909, the University of Minnesota established the first continuous program to educate nurses at the university level, with an enrollment of four students. Isabel Robb strongly influenced the organization of this program, which is considered the beginning of nursing as a profession. This program, however, did not lead to a bachelor's degree until 1919, when several other schools had also initiated college- and university-based nursing programs.

The History of Practical Nursing Education

Practical nursing, also called vocational nursing, has existed for many years. Women often cared for others and called themselves practical nurses. Not until the 1890s, however, was formal education in practical nursing available.

Pioneer Schools

Curricula in all of the early practical nursing schools included child care, cooking, and light housekeeping, in addition to care of the sick at home. Hospital care was not necessarily included.

Ballard School
In 1892, the Young Women's Christian Association (YWCA) opened the first practical nursing school in the United States in Brooklyn, New York. Later, it was named the Ballard School because Lucinda Ballard provided the funding. Practical nursing (attendant nursing) was one of several courses offered to women. This program was a 3-month course to train women in simple nursing care, emphasizing care of infants and children, older adults, and the disabled in their own homes. The Ballard School closed in 1949 because of YWCA reorganization.

Thompson Practical Nursing School
Thomas Thompson, a wealthy man who lived in Vermont during the Civil War, learned that women were making shirts for the army at only a dollar a dozen. In his will, he left money to help them. Richard Bradley, his executor, was a public-spirited man and determined that the local citizens needed nursing service. In 1907, he used some of Thompson's money to establish the Thompson Practical Nursing School in Brattleboro, Vermont. This school still exists today.

Household Nursing School
In Boston, a group of women wanted to provide nursing care in the home for people who were sick. They called on Bradley for advice, and he encouraged them to follow Brattleboro's example. In 1918, the Household Nursing Association School of Attendant Nursing opened. The school was later renamed the Shepard-Gill School of Practical Nursing in honor of Katherine Shepard Dodge, the first director, and Helen Z. Gill, her associate and successor. This school operated until 1984.

In all, 36 practical nursing schools opened during the first half of the 20th century in the United States. Between 1948 and 1954, 260 additional programs had opened. Today, more than 1,500 practical nursing programs exist in the United States. There is a growing need for licensed vocational/licensed practical nurses (LVN/LPNs) in multiple healthcare settings. Many LVN/LPNs choose to continue their nursing education and become registered nurses (RNs) via utilization of resources, such as career ladder programs, which accept LVN/LPN curricula for RN programs. Chapter 2 discusses the education requirements for nurses in greater detail.

American Red Cross Training

In 1908, the American Red Cross began offering home nursing education to teach lay women appropriate nursing care for illnesses within their own families. Jane Delano (1862–1919) was an Army nurse who was instrumental in this movement. Chapter 7 discusses the Red Cross in more detail.

Practical Nursing in Vocational and Community Colleges

In the early part of the 20th century, nursing schools—training both practical nurses and registered nurses—were traditionally located in or affiliated with hospitals. In 1917, the U.S. Congress passed the Smith-Hughes Act, the funds from which gave impetus to vocational-technical and public education. In 1919, the first vocational school-based nursing program opened in Minneapolis at Minneapolis Vocational High School. Today, the majority of practical nursing and associate's-degree nursing programs are located in vocational education settings or in community colleges.

Other Milestones in Practical Nursing Education

The Association of Practical Nurse Schools was founded in 1941. It was later renamed the National Association of Practical Nurse Education and Service.

In 1914, Mississippi became the first state to designate LPNs. By 1955, all states had laws that regulated the licensure of practical nurses. The first state to have mandatory licensure for LPNs to practice was New York. Chapter 2 discusses permissive and mandatory licensure more fully.

During World War II, people realized that nurses needed a consistent curriculum. In 1942, the U.S. Office of Education planned and advocated the first practical nursing curriculum for the entire country.

In 1966, the Chicago Public School system's program was the first practical nursing program to be accredited by the National League for Nursing (NLN).

Nursing During Wartime

Nursing during wartime has long been important. From Florence Nightingale in the Crimean War to the American Civil War, Spanish–American War, Korea, Vietnam, and continuing to the wars of the 21st century, nurses have always played a vital role.

World War I marked the first emergency training of nurses. The Army School of Nursing was established; Annie W. Goodrich (1876–1955) wrote the curriculum. Hundreds of women were trained in this abbreviated program; however, nearly all of them left nursing and returned to homemaking after the war's end in 1918.

The U.S. Cadet Nurse Corps was established during World War II, with Lucile Petry Leone (1902–1999) as Director. More than 14,000 volunteer nurses graduated in about 2 years. Originally, the plan was to draft nurses into the Army. A major opponent to this idea was Katherine J. Densford (1890–1978), Director of the School of Nursing at the University of Minnesota. She promised to train expanded numbers of nurses in a short time, if the government abandoned the nurse draft. Because of Densford's efforts, the student population at the University of Minnesota multiplied by five in a matter of weeks; more than 1,200 cadets graduated from that school alone.

World War II also marked the first time that men as well as women were actively recruited into nursing. Male nurses were not given equal rank to female nurses in the Armed Forces, however, until 1954. By the war's end in 1945, the world had changed. Many cadet nurses remained in the field, especially in the military. This employment gave many women a measure of independence that they had not previously known. After this time, emphasis was placed on improved graduate education for nurses. Nurses also began to assume a broader, more responsible role—a trend that continues today.

Current Nursing Trends

Nursing evolved rapidly in the 20th century, which promoted the needs and status of nurses. Technology, economics, and healthcare access continue the evolution of nursing in the 21st century. Many factors influenced trends that are expected to continue in the 21st century. The responsibilities of the nurse have increased as a direct result of these trends. This book has been written with these trends in mind:

Higher Client Acuity in Hospital and Long-Term Settings

Because of limitations on payment for healthcare, hospital stays are markedly shorter than they were in the 20th century. Clients in all healthcare facilities are more acutely ill than in years past. Long-term care facilities also have seen an increase in clients with highly acute conditions because of the growth of home care for those with more manageable conditions. Such developments require nurses working in all care areas to have higher levels of skill, additional education, and more specialization.

Shift to Community-Based Care

Most clients now receive healthcare outside acute care settings. For example, much surgery is now done on an outpatient basis; many clients receive care for chronic or long-term conditions at home; and community clinics provide primary healthcare for many clients. Thus, today's nursing care is delivered in a much wider range of settings than in the past.

Technology

Nurses, clients, and family members often must learn to operate highly sophisticated equipment to manage conditions in the home. This equipment makes accuracy in diagnosis and treatment possible. The teaching role of nursing is emphasized to a greater extent.

Social Factors

Many clients experience homelessness, are unemployed, or are underemployed. Devastating diseases, such as the coronavirus disease 2019 (COVID-19) pandemic, acquired immunodeficiency syndrome (AIDS), tuberculosis, measles, or pertussis, are more prevalent. These factors create a need for more healthcare services in the public sector. National and state healthcare legislation are promoting the concepts of preventative treatment and universal availability of healthcare.

Lifestyle Factors and Greater Life Expectancy

Today's society and the healthcare industry emphasize prevention of disease, healthy lifestyles, and wellness programs. Many people are living much longer and are more active and healthy into their later years than in past generations. Greater life expectancy is causing huge growth in the areas of extended, long-term, and home care. This growth will require many more nurses to work in such fields.

Changes in Nursing Education

Today's nursing programs emphasize education over service to clinical sites; they identify specific objectives (outcomes) for students. An earlier edition of this textbook was the first to identify learning objectives in practical nursing. Many LVN/LPNs are returning to school to become RNs, and many "career ladder" programs are available.

Autonomy

The social concept that all people, regardless of gender, should have equal access to opportunities has influenced nurses, most of whom are women, to be more assertive and independent. Today's nursing role is to collaborate with others in the healthcare field. Primary care, previously delivered only by physicians, can be delivered by nurses who succeed in advanced educational opportunities and specialized clinical experiences.

NURSING INSIGNIA

An insignia is a distinguishing badge of authority or honor. The symbolism dates back to the 16th century in Europe, when only a nobleman could wear a coat of arms. Later this privilege was expanded to include members of guilds (craftsmen). Certain types of training schools, including religious nursing

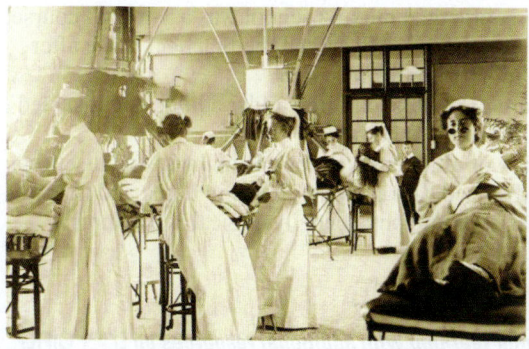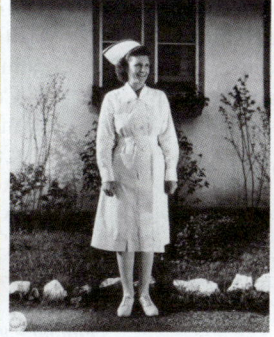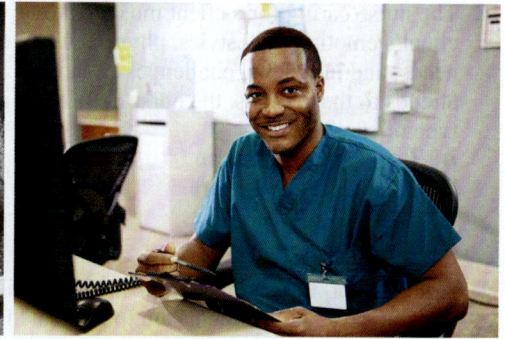

Figure 1-4 Nursing uniforms have changed throughout the years. (Courtesy of the National Institutes of Health/Department of Health and Human Services.)

orders, were also given the privilege. In the past, female nurses wore nursing caps and all nurses were awarded a school pin at graduation. Some schools also had distinguishing capes. The "Nightingale lamp," "Lamp of Nursing," or "Lamp of Learning" remain a standard of nursing insignia (see Fig. 1-3).

Nursing Uniforms

Although the style of uniform has changed throughout the years, nurses have always dressed professionally (Fig. 1-4). Clients usually feel more comfortable when nurses are easily identifiable and distinguishable from other staff. Today, a nametag, which includes your name, a current photo ID, and your job title, is required whenever you provide nursing care, no matter where you are employed.

The Nursing School Pin

You may receive a nursing pin at graduation that symbolizes your school of nursing. Early nursing symbols were usually religious in nature. Today, many nursing school pins bear some religious symbol, such as a cross (based on the Maltese cross) or a Star of David, even though the school may not be directly affiliated with a religious organization. The Nightingale lamp is also a common component of the nursing pin.

Key Concept

Remember that as you embark on your nursing career, you continue nursing's history and heritage.

STUDENT SYNTHESIS

KEY POINTS

- Medicine men and women and religious orders cared for the sick in early times.
- Florence Nightingale contributed a great deal to the development of contemporary nursing.
- Establishment of nursing schools in the United States began in the late 19th century.
- The first practical nursing school in the United States opened in 1892 in New York.
- Nursing during the World Wars I and II contributed to the profession's and to women's evolving roles in society.
- Many current societal and healthcare trends are influencing the nursing profession, including higher levels of client acuity in hospital settings, more community-based care, technological advances, changing lifestyles, greater life expectancy, changing nursing education, and more nursing autonomy.
- Nursing insignia, such as those found on nursing school pins, often symbolize nursing's history and heritage.

CRITICAL THINKING EXERCISES

1. Explain how the changing role of women in society helped contribute to the changing role of nursing.
2. Determine why established standards of nursing practice and education are so important to the development of nursing as a respected profession.
3. A friend interested in nursing asks you about the profession's history and its place in today's society. How would you answer your friend? What developments and milestones would you highlight?

NCLEX-STYLE REVIEW QUESTIONS

1. Which trends in nursing are expected to influence nursing in the 21st century? Select all that apply.
   a. Higher client acuity in hospital and long-term settings
   b. Traditional nursing education programs
   c. Shift to community-based care
   d. Advancements in technology
   e. Greater life expectancy

2. A client has been involved in a motor vehicle crash and has multiple injuries. Which guiding principles of Florence Nightingale would assist this client's recuperation and health maintenance? Select all that apply.
   a. Clean air and water
   b. Cleanliness
   c. Blood administration
   d. Light
   e. Efficient drainage

3. The nurse caring for a client must be attentive to the client's emotions, lifestyles, physical changes, spiritual needs, and individual challenges. When the nurse attends to these needs, the nurse is providing which type of care?
   a. Behavioral healthcare
   b. Specialized healthcare
   c. Caring healthcare
   d. Holistic healthcare

4. A nurse working in a mental healthcare facility understands that the clients are to be treated respectfully and their rights maintained. Which nurse was an advocate for the humane treatment of the mentally ill?
   a. Florence Nightingale
   b. Melinda Richards
   c. Isabel Robb
   d. Dorothea Dix

5. The first practical nursing school was a 3-month course. What was the primary role of the practical nurse after graduation from this program?
   a. Care of infants, children, older adults, and disabled in the client's home
   b. Care of all client populations in the hospital setting
   c. Advanced care of adult clients in home and hospital
   d. Assisting the physician in surgical procedures

CHAPTER RESOURCES

Enhance your learning with additional resources on thePoint*!*

Student Resources related to this chapter can be found at thePoint.lww.com/Rosdahl12e.

2 Beginning Your Nursing Career

Learning Objectives

1. Compare the education and level of practice between registered and practical nurses.
2. Explain the various types of educational programs that lead to licensure.
3. Identify the standards of the National Federation of Licensed Practical Nurses in relationship to each of the following: education, legal status, and practice.
4. Discuss the reasons for a nurse to seek licensure.
5. Identify the importance of the nurse's pledge.
6. Explain the importance of nursing theory and how a theoretical framework helps nurses in their learning, understanding, and practice.
7. List the roles of today's nurse, briefly explaining each one.
8. Discuss the importance of nurses projecting a professional image.
9. Discuss the goals of at least three nursing organizations and state at least two reasons why a student or a licensed nurse should join a professional organization.

Important Terminology

accreditation
advanced practice registered nurse
approval
career ladder
endorsement
licensure
mandatory licensure
nurse practice act
practical nurse
reciprocity
theoretical framework
vocational nurse

Acronyms

ANA
ANCC
CNS
HOSA
ICN
LPN
LVN
NALPN
NCLEX
NLN
NP
RN

Nursing provides service to help people meet the daily needs of life when they have difficulty satisfying these needs on their own. Students bring certain knowledge, skills, attitudes, and abilities to their nursing program. They will develop skills and knowledge in school. Their ability to act independently will depend on their professional background, motivation, and work environment. Defining all the specific roles of a nurse is difficult because these roles constantly change. Factors that influence nursing activity include new discoveries in the biomedical field, development of new healthcare knowledge, changes in patterns of health services and payment, and the relationships among healthcare team members.

This chapter discusses various programs for nursing education, approval and accreditation, licensure, the role and image of the nurse, and nursing organizations. Chapter 3 examines information about the healthcare system, and Chapter 6 discusses the concepts of health and wellness.

HEALTHCARE: A MULTIDISCIPLINARY APPROACH

The sophisticated healthcare system of the 21st century requires many trained individuals working together in a complex healthcare system (Box 2-1). Many contemporary healthcare positions originated as functions of either the physician or the nurse. For example, the duties of a hospital dietitian and the physical therapist started as functions of nursing. As knowledge of nursing and medicine grew, several segments of healthcare became their own professions. Healthcare has a tremendous variety of specialties and subspecialties. All healthcare positions have unique educational requirements.

To achieve licensure as a physician, an individual starts with a minimum of 4 years of undergraduate study and continues with 4 years of medical school, after which the graduate doctor must take a licensure examination before practicing. As a new doctor of medicine, the physician who wishes to specialize must continue their education as a resident, which requires another 2–6 years of study. These years can be followed by additional years of advanced study. The physician is responsible for diagnosing and treating clients. In this role, the physician often acts as a team leader (Fig. 2-1).

TYPES OF NURSING PROGRAMS

Nurses are an important part of the healthcare team. Four basic types of educational programs lead to a credential in nursing (Table 2-1). Three programs allow the graduate to take the licensure examination and to become a registered nurse (**RN**). The fourth, a practical or vocational nursing program, allows the graduate to take the licensure examination and to become a **licensed practical nurse** (**LPN**) or a **licensed vocational nurse** (**LVN**). California and Texas use the term

Box 2-1 Allied Health Professionals

Chiropractor—Manipulates the musculoskeletal system and spine to relieve symptoms
Dental hygienist—Trained and licensed to work with a dentist by providing preventive care
Dietitian—Trained nutritionist who addresses dietary needs associated with illness
Electrocardiograph technician—Assists with the performance of diagnostic procedures for cardiac electrical activity
Electroencephalograph technician—Assists with the diagnostic procedures for brain wave activity
Emergency medical technician—Trained in techniques of administering emergency care in route to trauma centers
Histologist—Studies cells and tissues for diagnosis
Infection control officer—Identifies situations at risk for transmission of infection and implements preventive measures
Laboratory technician—Trained in performance of laboratory diagnostic procedures
Medical assistant (administrative and/or clinical)—Assists the primary care provider in the front and/or back medical office, clinic, or other medical settings
Medical secretary—Trained in secretarial sciences with an emphasis on medical applications
Medical transcriptionist—Trained in secretarial sciences to make typed records of dictated medical information
Nuclear medical technician—Specializes in diagnostic procedures using nuclear devices
Occupational therapist—Evaluates and plans programs to relieve disorders that interfere with activities
Paramedic—Trained in advanced rescue and emergency procedures
Pharmacist—Prepares and dispenses medications by the primary care provider's order
Phlebotomist—Trained to perform venipunctures
Physical therapist—Plans and conducts rehabilitation procedures to relieve musculoskeletal disorders
Physician's assistant (PA)—Trained academically and clinically to practice medicine under the supervision of a doctor of medicine or osteopathy
Psychologist—Trained in methods of psychological assessment and treatment
Radiographer—Works with a radiologist or primary care provider to operate radiologic equipment for diagnosis and treatment
Respiratory therapist—Trained to preserve or improve respiratory function
Risk manager—Identifies and corrects potential high-risk situations within the healthcare field
Social worker—Trained to evaluate and improve social, emotional, and environmental problems associated with the medical profession
Speech therapist—Treats to prevent and correct speech and language disorders
Surgical technician or technologist—Assists primary care providers and nurses in the operating room
Unit clerk—Performs the administrative duties on a hospital client care unit

"vocational nurse" instead of "practical nurse". This text utilizes three different but interchangeable abbreviations: LPN, LVN, and LVN/LPN.

Registered Nurses

RNs spend from 2 to 4 years learning their profession. In addition, RNs may have special training that allows them to practice public health nursing or specialize in fields such as surgery. RNs are responsible for care of the acutely ill; teaching professional and practical nursing students; managing personnel; and taking charge in various healthcare settings. RNs also perform many duties that only physicians performed in the 20th century. For example, the RN may be the first assistant in surgery. RNs may continue their education to become nurse anesthetists, nurse-midwives, or advanced practice nurses.

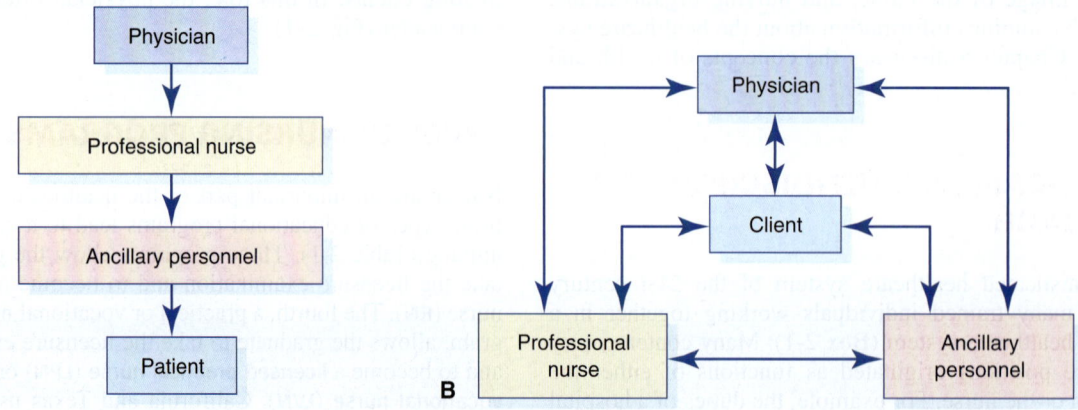

Figure 2-1 Traditional (A) and contemporary (B) views of healthcare practice.

TABLE 2-1 Nursing Practice and Educational Levels

CLASSIFICATION	FUNCTIONS AND ROLE	EDUCATIONAL REQUIREMENTS
Certified nursing assistant (CNA), state tested nursing assistant (STNA), unlicensed assistive personnel (UAP)	Provides basic nursing care for clients in a long-term care facility. Works under the supervision of an LVN, RN, or MD	2–6 months Educational requirements may differ between CNA, STNA, and the UAP
Licensed vocational/practical nurse (LVN/LPN)	Provides nursing care in long-term and acute care facilities. May also work in primary care providers' offices and clinic settings. Works under the supervision of an RN or MD	1–2 years
Registered nurse (RN)	Provides direct and indirect nursing care, supervision, and leadership in a wide variety of healthcare settings	2–4 years Associate's degree (AD) or bachelor's degree (BS or BA) or master's degree (MS or MA)
Advanced practice registered nurse (APRN), certified nurse specialist (CNS), or nurse practitioner (NP)	An RN who receives additional training in a specialized field, such as pediatrics, maternity, geriatrics, family practice, or mental health	RN with a master's degree plus additional and specific education and internship in the field of specialty

Basic Education
Three basic types of education lead to the RN license:

1. A student attends a 2-year program at a community or junior college and receives an associate's degree (AD) in nursing. This AD-RN is educated primarily as a bedside nurse and is sometimes called a *technical nurse*. In some states, some nursing groups are advocating different licensure for RNs who graduate from AD programs, as opposed to graduates of 4-year programs.
2. The 3-year program, or diploma program, was formerly sponsored by and based in a hospital. Most of today's 3-year programs, however, are affiliated with community and state colleges that grant college credits. Some states no longer have 3-year programs.
3. The 4-year program in a college or university leads to a baccalaureate or bachelor's degree in nursing. The graduate of this program may enter graduate school to study for an advanced master's degree or doctorate. Most of these programs aim to prepare professional nurses who will be teachers or administrators or who will assume other leadership positions. Many bachelor's degree graduates become certified as public health nurses and work in community health.

Some community colleges have programs that admit only LPNs, which, via a **career ladder** program, lead to an RN. The LPN is usually required to take general education courses before admission. Then, with approximately 1 additional year of education, an LPN becomes eligible to take the licensure examination and become an RN. This program leads to an AD.

Advanced Nursing Credentials
Several types of advanced certification are available to RNs. An **advanced practice** registered **nurse**, formerly called a nurse practitioner (NP), is an RN, usually with a bachelor's and/or master's degree, who has specialized in a particular field. A specific combination of classroom and clinical learning beyond that of a standard RN program plus the successful completion of an examination provided by a credentialing center is necessary for these credentials. The RN functions in a different role than does a nurse who does not have this type of specialization. The state issues a license to practice as an RN as provided by the state's Nurse Practice Act. Individual states define and grant authority to practice healthcare beyond that of the traditional RN. Advanced practice nurses assess clients, assist in the diagnosis and treatment of illness, and, in many states, are authorized to prescribe medications. The roles of nurses with other additional educational preparation, such as midwives and anesthetists, are described later in this book.

The American Nurses Credentialing Center (**ANCC**) of the American Nurses Association (**ANA**) grants several types of **NP** certifications and Clinical Nurse Specialist certifications as well as many specialty certifications. Examples of the NP certifications include Family NP, Adult-Gerontology, Acute Care NP, and Psychiatric Mental Health NP.

Practical Nurses/Vocational Nurses
Practical or vocational nurses are licensed under specific state laws (**Nurse Practice Act**) to care for clients in various settings in the same manner as does the RN. Generally, the LVN/LPN works under the direct or indirect supervision of an RN or physician. The functions and responsibilities of the LVN/LPN and the RN often coincide. Many LVN/LPNs supervise nursing assistants or aides.

Do not confuse the position of the individual who is called a nurse's aide, nursing assistant, certified nursing assistant, or unlicensed assistive personnel (UAP) with the LVN/LPN or RN. Although the aide may receive a certification by the state when completing a nurse aide training course, this individual is not licensed, and therefore not regulated by a state nurse practice act. A nursing assistant, aide, or UAP is a person who is taught via on-the-job training or in short-term programs to help clients and residents meet the needs of daily living, such as hygiene and dressing.

Current functions of the LVN/LPN include providing bedside care, doing wound care, administering prescribed medications, monitoring client status, and reporting reactions to medications or treatments to the RN or physician. Individual states or healthcare agencies may limit the LVN/LPN's care of intravenous lines, complex treatment and medication regimens, and functions related to primary or complex healthcare assessment of clients.

Standards of nursing practice of LVN/LPNs are promoted by the National Association for Practical Nurse Education and Service, an association for the representation of LVN/LPN's education and training. Another association, the National Association of Licensed Practical Nurses, Inc. (formerly known as National Federation of Licensed Practical Nurses [NFLPN]), also promotes standards of practice for the practical/vocational nurse. These two major nursing organizations are discussed later in this chapter.

According to the Bureau of Labor Statistics *Occupational Outlook Handbook* (2020), most practical/vocational nurses work full-time in long-term care facilities, acute care hospitals, physician offices/clinics, home healthcare services, outpatient care centers, and government agencies (e.g., correctional facilities or military reserve). Growth in employment opportunities for the LVN/LPN is projected for 2018–2028 to be 11% faster than the average for all occupations.

Practical/Vocational Nursing Education

Most practical/vocational nursing programs exist under the auspices of a high school, a vocational institute, a proprietary college, or a community college. Such diverse institutions as hospitals and universities administer some programs. The number of state-approved practical/vocational nursing programs has grown consistently in the 21st century. The growth of LVN/LPN programs is an indicator of the need for nurses, both LVN/LPNs and RNs. Because they depend on the availability of clinical sites, LVN/LPN and RN programs accept a limited number of students for each graduating class. In the late 20th century, some RN programs closed, as they were not cost-effective for the college or university. Some of these have reopened due to an ongoing nursing shortage and the federal and state availability of funds for nursing students and nursing programs. In addition to the nursing shortage, there is also a great shortage of nursing instructors in both LVN/LPN and RN programs. This has led to an alternate route to the RN licensure, via a career ladder, also known as an LVN/LPN to RN program. This approach has the dual benefit of allowing graduate LVN/LPNs to work as licensed practical/vocational nurses while attending RN programs.

Curricula are designed to include classroom theory in the various aspects of nursing. The student then has an opportunity to practice clinical skills in a hospital, nursing home, community health agency, or other health-related facility. Classroom theory and clinical practice are correlated as closely as possible to ensure maximum retention of skills. Most practical nursing programs are the equivalent of 12–18 months of full-time study. Many LVN/LPN to RN career ladder programs generally accept the LVN/LPN curricula in place of the first year of RN curricula, which often means that the LVN/LPN may not need to take the fundamental and/or beginning level RN courses of an RN program. Both LVN/LPN and RN programs require additional general education or specific science-related classes that enhance the content of nursing courses. Each school will have educational counselors or advisors who will be able to provide unique advice to each student in their choice of general educational or nursing-related courses.

APPROVAL AND ACCREDITATION OF NURSING PROGRAMS

Approved Nursing Programs

Nursing programs are very different from general college courses, such as history, mathematics, or English. Nursing schools must maintain specific educational standards that are defined by legislating bodies. As such, nursing programs must have **approval** from a specific state agency or nursing authority, which is usually a state, provincial, or territorial Board of Nursing. The approval agency visits the school and determines whether the students are receiving an appropriate education. Reapproval, or updating the original approval process, of the nursing program may be required on a regular schedule as determined by the agency.

The purpose of approval of a school's educational criteria is to protect the consumers of healthcare against unqualified nurses. A minimal standard of education is required. Approval is mandatory (required), meaning that a school must be approved or its graduates cannot be licensed.

The word *approved* tells you the following about a school:

- It teaches specific things a nurse must know.
- It has stated objectives and teaches to those objectives.
- It provides experience with the types of individuals the nurse will care for when practicing nursing.
- It employs qualified instructors to teach and to supervise the students' practice in the classroom, laboratory, and healthcare facility.
- It prepares graduates eligible for examination and licensure as LPNs, LVNs, or RNs.
- It has courses of the required minimum length.

Accredited Nursing Programs

Accreditation is voluntary and does not specifically concern licensure of graduates. A program can be approved without being accredited, but it cannot be accredited without first being approved by the state's Board of Nursing.

Accreditation is not a matter of law. The **accreditation** of a school means that an agency other than the state has reviewed the nursing program in detail. If a nursing program has been accredited, the program has met criteria established by that agency. Application for accreditation is voluntary on the part of the program; accreditation is not given to all programs. That a school is accredited gives further evidence of its excellence because the program must undergo a detailed evaluation to become accredited. A program need not be accredited for its graduates to become licensed. The National League for Nursing (**NLN**) has established standards of accreditation for nursing education for both RNs and LPNs.

As a nursing student, you must understand that a difference exists between *approval* and *accreditation* of a nursing program. Each state has a legislated Nurse Practice Act that defines the approval process. Nurse Practice Acts delineate or spell out the educational requirements, roles and functions, and disciplinary actions of a nurse.

Many nursing programs have entrance requirements. Most programs require entrants to be high school graduates. Nursing programs may also require their entrants to have taken certain courses, such as anatomy, physiology, nutrition, or pharmacology. Nursing students may also be required to be immunized against several diseases, such as hepatitis B. Drug testing, alcohol testing, and criminal background checks also can be mandated. Requirements are established to maintain client safety and may be required by the educational program or the clinical facilities in which the training occurs. Programs must consider applicants for admission without regard to gender, age, marital status, sexual preference, race, or religion. To graduate from a nursing program, a student nurse must meet the minimal standards of the approved nursing program.

LICENSURE OF NURSES

Licensing laws, often referred to as Nurse Practice Acts, protect the public from unqualified workers and establish standards for the profession or occupation. Licensing laws establish a minimal level of requirements for competence and practice. The Nurse Practice Act differs from one state to another. Obtaining licensure helps the public determine the difference between a qualified and an unqualified worker.

> **NCLEX Alert**
>
> NCLEX clinical scenarios include situations that will need you to select the appropriate healthcare individual (MD, RN, LVN/LPN, or assistive personnel). For example, who is responsible for the care of the client during the time of the clinical scenario? You must know the major legal differences and responsibilities for the levels of healthcare personnel.

The first licensure laws for nursing were passed in 1903 in North Carolina, New York, Virginia, and New Jersey. The first LPN law was passed in Mississippi in 1914. In 1940, fewer than 10 states had LPN laws, but by 1955 all states had LPN laws. Every state and the District of Columbia, Puerto Rico, Guam, American Samoa, the Virgin Islands, the Canadian provinces, and the North Mariana Islands now have licensing laws for both RNs and LPNs.

Any student who has graduated from an approved nursing program is eligible to take an examination provided by the National Council of State Boards of Nursing. The examination is called the National Council Licensure Examination (NCLEX). The NCLEX-RN is the licensing examination for registered nurses. The NCLEX-PN is for licensed practical/vocational nurses. Following the student's successful completion of the approved program, the school must submit documentation of completion to the state Board of Nursing. Graduates may be required by the state Board of Nursing to pay licensing fees and submit fingerprints before being allowed to schedule to take the NCLEX.

State licensing laws have individual variations, but all nurse practice laws state that it is illegal for any nurse to practice nursing for pay without a license. Practice acts differentiate between LVN/LPN and RN licenses. This regulation is called mandatory licensure. The mandatory law designates the functions, duties, and responsibilities of the nurse and use of the title "nurse." *Mandatory licensure* requires that a nurse cannot perform the functions designated as exclusive to nursing without proper licensure in that state. Healthcare consumers are protected because minimal competence levels are established and enforced by regulatory state agencies (i.e., the State Board[s] of Nursing). Chapter 4 discusses additional aspects of licensure and the legal issues surrounding it.

Often nurses move from one state to another. Regulations provide for the licensed nurse to continue their nursing practice in a new state without retaking the licensing examination. Endorsement is a form of agreement between states, particularly state licensing agencies. One state recognizes or endorses the qualifications of another state. However, each state Board of Nursing has its fees the individual pays for a license in that state. For example, an LVN in California can practice nursing in Minnesota as an LPN without retaking the NCLEX-PN, but the individual will have to apply and pay for the new Minnesota license. Reciprocity occurs when a mutual agreement is set in place by the Nurse Licensure Compact (NLC) between states who have agreed to grant a license to practice medicine to any person licensed by the state in which they have their permanent residency. The NLC makes it easier for nurses while maintaining standards of practice and protection for the public.

> **Key Concept**
>
> Licensure establishes a minimal level of competence for nursing. It ensures that a licensed nurse meets a basic level of excellence in practice and knowledge.

The Nurse's Pledge

All nurses are expected to practice ethically and conduct themselves appropriately as members of a specific group. As a nurse, you also accept responsibilities within the role delineated by licensure. Chapter 4 is devoted to a discussion of the legal and ethical aspects of nursing.

Many ethical principles are reflected in the Nurse's Pledge, which many students recite at graduation. Even if the pledge is not part of your graduation ceremony, it should serve as a guide for nursing practice. RNs recite the Florence Nightingale Pledge, and LPNs recite the Practical Nurse's Pledge (Box 2-2). The basic philosophy of nursing care espoused in both pledges is the same. Notice the similarity between them.

THEORIES OF NURSING

As a science, nursing is based on the theory of what nursing is, what nurses do, and why. Nursing is a unique discipline and is separate from medicine. It has its own body of knowledge on which delivery of care is based.

Box 2-2 Nursing Pledges

FLORENCE NIGHTINGALE PLEDGE

I solemnly pledge myself before God and in the presence of this assembly: To pass my life in purity and to practice my profession faithfully.

I will abstain from whatever is deleterious and mischievous, and will not take or knowingly administer any harmful drug.

I will do all in my power to maintain and elevate the standards of my profession, and will hold in confidence all personal matters committed to my keeping, and all family affairs coming to my knowledge in the practice of my profession.

With loyalty will I endeavor to aid the physician in his work, and devote myself to the welfare of those committed to my care.

THE PRACTICAL NURSE'S PLEDGE

Before God and those assembled here, I solemnly pledge:

To adhere to the code of ethics of the nursing profession.

To cooperate faithfully with the other members of the nursing team and to carry out faithfully and to the best of my ability the instructions of the physician or the nurse who may be assigned to supervise my work.

I will not do anything evil or malicious and I will not knowingly give any harmful drug or assist in malpractice.

I will not reveal any confidential information that may come to my knowledge in the course of my work.

And I pledge myself to do all in my power to raise the standards and the prestige of practical nursing.

May my life be devoted to service, and to the high ideals of the nursing profession.

Nursing programs usually base their curricula on one or more nursing theories. Such theories provide a skeleton on which to hang knowledge. This theoretical framework gives you and other students a basis for forming a personal philosophy of nursing. It also helps you to develop problem-solving skills systematically. A **theoretical framework** provides a reason and a purpose for nursing actions. Other factors also involved in nursing actions include ethics, safety, confidentiality, and culture. The theoretical framework on which this book is based is that of meeting basic human needs.

Throughout this book, you will learn ways to perform nursing procedures. You will also be presented with *rationales*, or reasons for these actions. These rationales are based on nursing's knowledge base. After you graduate and become more experienced, you will realize that more than one correct way exists to perform particular procedures. You must always follow the nursing protocols of the healthcare facility in which you are employed.

Nursing theories are often expressed in relationship to factors such as mind, body, spirit, and emotions. Most theories also include a definition of health. Be sure to consider all these factors when delivering nursing care so that you provide holistic care—care of the whole person. Among the many nursing theories are those of Florence Nightingale, Virginia Henderson, Dorothea Orem, Sister Callista Roy, and Betty Neuman. Table 2-2 outlines the general concepts related to these theories.

TABLE 2-2 Theories of Nursing

THEORIST	MODEL	CONCEPTS
Florence Nightingale (1859)	Natural-Healing	Nature alone cures. Nursing assists the person to an improved condition for nature to take its course. Health is "freedom from disease."
Virginia Henderson (1955)	Independent-Functioning	Mind and body are one. Nursing's role is to assist clients to perform functions they would perform unaided if they had the necessary strength, will, or knowledge. Functions vital to health are the ability to breathe normally, eat/drink adequately, eliminate wastes, move/position oneself, sleep, dress, maintain body temperature, maintain hygiene, and keep the skin intact. Safety, communication, worship, work, recreation, and learning are individualized. Health is the ability to function independently.
Dorothea Orem (1958)	Self-Care	Building on Maslow's "Hierarchy of Human Needs" (see Chapter 5), nursing assists clients to meet self-care needs necessary to maintain life, health, and well-being. Health is the ability to meet self-care needs, which are physiological, psychological, and sociological.
Sister Callista Roy (1964)	Adaptation	An individual's state of health/illness moves back and forth on a continuum (see Chapter 6). Nursing focuses on the body, mind, spirit, and emotions; and emphasis is on holistic healing, rather than curing. Each person's health status fluctuates because humans are constantly interacting in a dynamic (changing) environment.
Betty Neuman (1972)	Systems	Humans deal with forces in both internal and external environments. The goal of the whole person is stability and harmony. Health is "relative" in terms of psychological, sociocultural, developmental, and physiological factors.

ROLES AND RESPONSIBILITIES OF THE NURSE

Today's nurse functions in a number of roles. As a nurse, you have a responsibility to maintain your own health. You also will need to project a professional image to your clients, their families, and the general public. Doing so will help others have confidence in your nursing abilities.

Contemporary Nursing Roles

Nurses are respected as a healthcare resource in the community. Examine the following roles of the nurse (Fig. 2-2). As you progress through your nursing program, you may be able to think of other roles that nurses assume in their practice. For example:

The nurse is a care provider. Nurses help each person achieve the maximum level of wellness possible. In some cases, clients will achieve total wellness; in others, compromises must be made.

The nurse is an advocate. Nurses serve this important role by ensuring that clients receive necessary care, and by intervening when necessary. Nurses help clients understand their rights and responsibilities. Nurses listen to and support clients' concerns; and accurately report to the appropriate team members.

The nurse is a communicator. The nurse documents client care and the client's response. Professional nurses write care plans with input from other healthcare staff members—much of the staff uses this important plan. Nurses record information in daily flow sheets or nursing notes, record medications and treatments, and communicate with other healthcare team members in daily reports and team meetings to maintain continuity of care.

The nurse is a team member. Nurses work cooperatively with other healthcare professionals to provide the best care possible.

The nurse is a teacher. Professional nurses write teaching plans and assist people in preventing illness and injury before they occur. Other members of the healthcare team assist with teaching as well. Together, the healthcare team teaches clients and families about illness, surgical procedures, performed tests, and home care. Clients learn about medications, when and how to take them, expected side effects, and possible adverse reactions. Many nurses teach prenatal classes and assist with labor and delivery, providing encouragement and support during childbirth. Later, they often teach new mothers important self-care as well as care measures for the baby.

The nurse is a leader. Nurses must work with clients to motivate them to achieve important goals. Leadership inspires and empowers others, and nurses can use their skills to direct that empowerment for improvement, not only in their clients' health, but also in the facilities in which they work, the community, and for the entire healthcare system.

> **Key Concept**
> Always practice nursing ethically. When you recite your pledge at graduation, you are promising to abide by this code.

The Nurse's Image

Today's society is filled with information about leading a healthier lifestyle. Many people are working to change their behaviors to restore or maintain good health.

As a nursing student and as a nurse, you need to project a professional image. Remember that you represent not only yourself to the public, but also your school, the healthcare facility for which you work, and the entire healthcare system.

Your nursing program will give you specific guidelines to follow regarding style of dress and grooming when you conduct clinical nursing practice. Box 2-3 identifies some general considerations to help you project the image of the nurse. Remember that many of the measures listed in Box 2-3 are important not only to project a professional image, but also to maintain maximal levels of safety, hygiene, and protection for you and your clients.

Today's Nursing Student

Many of today's nursing students are returning to school after several years outside education. You may be one of these adult learners who has entered a nursing program with the additional responsibilities of a home, family, and outside job. Adult learners may need to master new skills in addition to learning their nursing skills. For example, some adult learners have not worked much with computers, email, or the Internet. All students, and especially those with multiple responsibilities, must plan a schedule that provides ample time for classes, household duties, studying, work, family, and personal time. Managing all of these responsibilities will be a challenge, but the rewards can be great.

NURSING ORGANIZATIONS

Nursing organizations provide professional forums for students, licensed nurses, and nursing faculty. Most organizations offer continuing education opportunities, publications, certifications in such areas as pharmacology or long-term care nursing, and monitoring of national and state legislation relating to healthcare. State and national conferences that

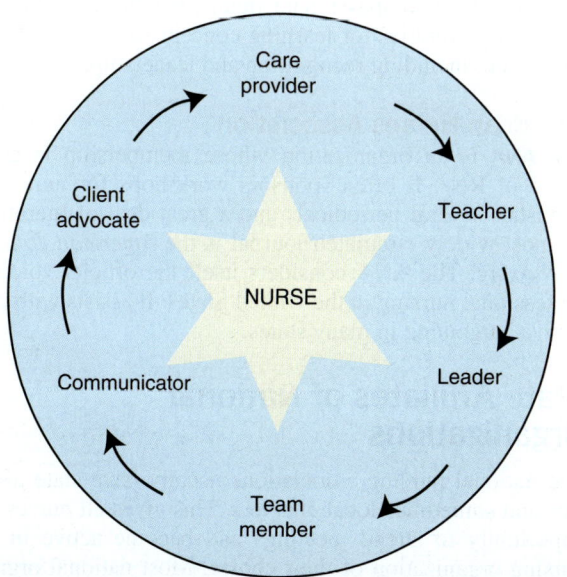

Figure 2-2 The roles of the nurse include, but are not limited to, care provider, communicator, teacher, advocate, leader, and team member.

Box 2-3 Projecting the Image of a Nurse

- Show respect for others, including your clients, your instructors, and the staff at your clinical sites.
- Follow general practices of good grooming and hygiene: bathe/shower daily, use deodorant, brush teeth, avoid bad breath (especially if you smoke).
- Keep hair clean, pulled away from the face, and off the neck.
- Wear a minimum of jewelry—it can harbor microorganisms and could injure a client.
- Clients may act out—protect yourself by keeping your hair short or pinned up, and avoiding large earrings, neckties, and necklaces.
- Keep moustaches and beards neatly trimmed.
- Avoid aftershave, cologne, and perfume. Clients may be allergic to them.
- Use a minimum of makeup. Artificial nails may not be permitted (Centers for Disease Control and Prevention [CDC] recommendation).
- Wash hands often. Make sure fingernails are short and clean. Clip hangnails. Nail polish is not recommended.
- Cover cuts or open wounds for your protection.
- Wear washable clothes/uniforms and sweaters.
- Wear pants long enough to reach your shoe tops.
- Keep skirts long and loose enough so you can bend and lift without embarrassment.
- Wear safe and comfortable shoes. Most facilities do not allow sandals or clogs.
- Always wear your ID Badge—it is part of your uniform.
- Follow guidelines in Chapter 6 for maintaining optimal health.
- Follow any additional guidelines specified by your school or clinical facility.

are presented or supported by nursing organizations are productive ways to network with peers, discuss concerns, and advocate for changes in all aspects of nursing. Continuing education seminars generally are part of the organizations' conferences. Nursing organizations can have major impacts on healthcare, nursing, and public policy legislation. Most professional organizations offer student members discounted membership fees, opportunities for scholarships, and discussion opportunities with peers on state and national levels. By being a member of nursing organizations, you can keep informed of healthcare trends; learn of legislation that will affect you as a nurse and receiver of healthcare; and provide opportunities for growth, development, and change in your field.

National Organizations

National Association for Practical Nurse Education and Service

Organized in 1941, the National Association for Practical Nurse Education and Service was the first national nursing organization to delineate goals for the development and improvement of practical nursing education. The organization's focus is on the professional practice, licensure, and education of LVN/LPNs.

National Association of Licensed Practical Nurses, Inc.

Started in 1949 in New York State, the **NFLPN** has become and is now known as the National Association of Licensed Practical Nurses, Inc. It is a professional organization providing structure nationally for practical nursing standards of care, promote continued education/certification, and interpret the role and function of LVN/LPNs. It is the only organization which is governed entirely *by* LVN/LPNs and *for* LVN/LPNs. The National Association of Licensed Practical Nurses, Inc. is recognized by other nursing organizations as the official voice of LVN/LPNs.

National League for Nursing

The designated purpose of the **NLN** is "to advance excellence in nursing education that prepares the nursing workforce to meet the needs of diverse populations in an ever-changing healthcare environment." The NLN has been a leader in the profession of nursing education since 1893. A major focus is providing accreditation to RN and LVN/LPN schools. The organization assesses, establishes goals, implements plans, and sets standards for:

- Nursing education
- Faculty development
- Research in nursing education
- Nursing needs in the work arena and education setting
- Services to the nursing community
- Public policy related to lifelong education

HOSA

Organized in 1976, **HOSA**-Future Health Professionals, formerly known as Health Occupations Students of America, is a vocational organization specifically designed for students in secondary and postsecondary/collegiate health occupational programs, including nursing. HOSA's mission is "to provide career opportunities in the healthcare industry and to enhance the delivery of quality healthcare to all people." Students in the field of health science technology are motivated to deliver compassionate, quality healthcare while providing opportunities for learning concepts of the healthcare profession, including recognition and leadership.

American Nurses Association

The **ANA** is an organization whose membership is composed of RNs. It often sponsors workshops for nurses. It publishes several periodicals and a great deal of literature. Its most widely circulated journal is the *American Journal of Nursing*. The ANA considers itself the official voice of professional nursing in the United States. It assists with collective bargaining in many states.

State Affiliates of National Organizations

The national nursing associations usually have state affiliates and sometimes local chapters. This gives all nurses the opportunity to attend meetings and become active in the nursing organization of their choice. Most national organizations also have student affiliates, so you can begin your professional membership as a student.

State organizations often publish newsletters of local interest. Sometimes scholarships, continuing education, and other services are available to members.

> **Key Concept**
>
> All nursing students and graduates should belong to an organization, so they will have a voice in the future of the profession.

International Council of Nursing

Started in 1899, the International Council of Nursing (**ICN**), based in Geneva, Switzerland, is the major international organization of nurses. The ICN has three key program areas listed as crucial to nursing:

1. Professional nursing practice with a focus on an International Classification for Nursing Practice (ICNP), advanced nursing practice, and specific health issues, such as human immunodeficiency virus/acquired immunodeficiency syndrome (HIV/AIDS), tuberculosis, malaria, women's health, family health, and safe water.
2. Regulation of the standards of nursing, including aspects related to credentialing, standards of competencies, and a code of ethics.
3. Socioeconomic welfare for nurses, which includes areas such as occupational health and safety, human resource planning and policies, remuneration, and career development.

This agency often works in concert with other organizations, such as the ANA or the Canadian Nurses Association (Association des Infirmières et Infirmiers du Canada).

STUDENT SYNTHESIS

KEY POINTS

- Differences exist in the education and level of nursing practice between RNs and LVN/LPNs.
- Several types of nursing education lead to licensure as an RN or as a practical/vocational nurse.
- Only graduates of state-, commonwealth-, territory-, or province-approved schools of nursing are eligible to take the licensure examination.
- All states have mandatory licensure laws for nurses. Nurse licensure is available in all states, territories, and Canadian provinces.
- Nurses promise to practice ethically when they recite pledges at graduation and when they receive their license to practice nursing.
- Many nursing programs base their curricula on nursing theories. These theoretical frameworks provide reasons and purposes for nursing actions.
- The nurse assumes many roles. Many responsibilities accompany the title of "nurse."
- Projecting a professional image is important. Such an image helps nurses properly represent their school, place of employment, and the healthcare industry. Moreover, it serves to protect and maintain safety for clients and for nurses themselves.
- Nursing organizations set standards of practice for RNs and LPNs. A primary nursing responsibility is to be familiar with these standards.
- Nursing organizations assist in continuing education and collective bargaining. Additionally, they offer a forum for discussion of nursing issues with peers.

CRITICAL THINKING EXERCISES

1. Discuss the difference in the roles, practices, and functions of the physician, the LPN, and the RN. If you started your nursing career as a nurse's aide, describe your experiences working with nurses.
2. Interview class members and have them relate an experience in healthcare. What events are significant in the individual's medical history and how did the members of the healthcare team affect the individual's perspective of the experience?
3. A nursing student in your group tells you that she cheated on an examination yesterday. What would you do and why? How does your response relate to nursing practice?
4. Ask your instructor for a copy of your program's "Philosophy and Objectives." Compare and contrast them with your own personal standards and philosophy of nursing. Do you find similarities? Differences?

NCLEX-STYLE REVIEW QUESTIONS

1. A high school student interested in becoming a nurse asks the nursing instructor what the role of the LVN/LPN is. Which are the **best** responses by the instructor? Select all that apply.
   a. The LVN/LPN provides bedside care.
   b. The LVN/LPN develops the plan of care for clients.
   c. The LVN/LPN performs wound care.
   d. The LVN/LPN supervises RNs.
   e. The LVN/LPN administers prescribed medications to clients.

2. The LVN/LPN is supervising a nursing assistant working in a long-term care facility. What task may be assigned to the nursing assistant by the LVN/LPN?
   a. Administer prescribed medication to a client.
   b. Change a sterile dressing.
   c. Assist with feeding a client.
   d. Insert a nasogastric tube in a client.

3. The student nurse in a practical nursing program asks the instructor what an RN does. Which are the **best** responses by the instructor? Select all that apply.
   a. The RN performs surgical procedures.
   b. The RN cares for acutely ill clients.
   c. The RN teaches professional and practical nursing students.
   d. The RN takes charge in various healthcare settings.
   e. The RN manages personnel.

4. The new RN graduate from a 4-year baccalaureate program would like to obtain an advanced practice degree as a family NP. What would this mean to the nurse after completing the program? Select all that apply.
   a. The NP would be responsible for performing advanced assessment techniques.
   b. The NP would be able to perform surgical procedures without assistance from the surgeon.
   c. The NP would assist in diagnosis and treatment of illness.
   d. The NP would be able to prescribe medication in many states.
   e. The NP would be able to practice independently without a physician in all states.

5. An LVN/LPN is moving to another state to practice nursing. After receiving a license to practice there, what is most important that the LPN do?
   a. Determine what the standards of practice are in that state.
   b. Take another NCLEX exam for that state.
   c. Sign up at the local community college to take review classes.
   d. Call the state Board of Nursing to let them know they are going to practice in that state.

CHAPTER RESOURCES

Enhance your learning with additional resources on thePoint!

Student Resources related to this chapter can be found at thePoint.lww.com/Rosdahl12e.

3 The Healthcare Delivery System

Learning Objectives

1. Discuss trends and challenges of healthcare in the 21st century. Relate these changes to the Affordable Care Act, the needs of nurses and healthcare practitioners, and the consumers of healthcare (clients).
2. Define and discuss differences between acute care and extended care facilities and identify the types of healthcare services provided in each type of healthcare facility.
3. Identify at least three services available to meet the healthcare needs of the community.
4. State at least two functions of a school nurse and an industrial nurse.
5. State at least two functions of The Joint Commission. Relate these functions to nursing standards of care.
6. Define the term *quality assurance* and state its function in healthcare facilities.
7. Explain the role of the client representative, advocate, or ombudsperson.
8. Describe at least six methods of payment for healthcare services.
9. Determine the role of complementary or holistic care in the delivery of healthcare.
10. Identify at least three negative impacts of consumer fraud on public wellness.

Important Terminology

acuity
Affordable Care Act
capitation fee
case management
chain of command
client
complementary healthcare
co-pay
holistic healthcare
home healthcare
hospice
incentive programs
managed care
managed care payment
Medicaid
Medicare
outcome-based care
patient
prospective payment
quality assurance
respite care
telehealth
The Joint Commission

Acronyms

CQI
DRG
ECF
HMO
ICF
ICU
OSHA
POS
PPO
QA
RUG
SNF
SSDI
UAP

> **Key Concept**
> Remember: The principles of excellent nursing care are universal.

This textbook primarily addresses nursing in the context of a healthcare facility that cares for the very ill or a facility that has services that provide long-term or extended care. Throughout the book you will note references to specific nursing situations, such as geriatrics, pediatrics, or home health.

Your school of nursing may provide clinical experiences in acute care and long-term care, as well as supplemental clinical experiences in ambulatory care settings such as clinics or home care. Field trips to specialty areas may be available (e.g., dialysis units, burn units, or rehabilitation centers).

This chapter discusses concepts related to basic healthcare service in the United States. The student and the consumer need to be aware of different types of healthcare facilities and payment plans, as well as the common types of healthcare services. Healthcare providers must be aware of the general concepts of the various aspects of healthcare service because the consumer (i.e., client) often relies on providers as preliminary reference sources. In other words, we are often asked where to go for further information, what to do next when a situation occurs, or how to obtain assistance.

Your student nursing experiences are individual and unique. It is the responsibility of the student to achieve the maximal benefits from each experience.

HEALTHCARE TRENDS IN THE 21ST CENTURY

Healthcare continues to change dramatically. Changes include an emphasis on wellness and individuals assuming more responsibility for their own health. Technology will continue to influence healthcare in direct and indirect ways. The cost of healthcare technology also remains a major consideration. The use of technology in healthcare will provide new avenues of diagnosis, treatment, and nursing care. Chapters 6 and 7 provide additional information in the areas of wellness and community health.

Before the 1980s, healthcare was primarily the concern of physicians who treated clients during times of illness. The less educated client was expected to be dependent on the advanced knowledge of a physician. Typically, clients were made aware of neither their vital sign readings nor the rationale for many aspects of treatment. The object of care was to treat existing health problems, such as diabetes, obesity, cardiac problems, and cancer. Enormous amounts of money were needed to care for clients with such existing health problems. Over time, views and concepts of preventive care evolved and the individual needed to learn the requirements for the avoidance of disease and disorder. As technology developed, it became possible to prevent problems or to find and treat disorders before extensive damage occurred. Preventive healthcare also revealed that health issues are often interrelated. Obesity, for example, was found in clients with diabetes, cardiac complications, visual problems, and acute and chronic infections. Prevention and early treatment literally affect a variety of immediate and long-term consequences, such as the quality of life, financial obligations, and family dynamics.

Research into the rising costs of healthcare determined that costs could be better managed by preventive care. Clients became consumers of healthcare; thus, the term "client" became more appropriate to the changing focus of responsibility. Starting in the 1980s, the concept of the client, in lieu of the word "patient," was implemented. Clients needed better health education with ongoing screening and monitoring of illness. Additionally, the focus of many aspects of health and healthcare could and should be the responsibility of the client rather than the domain of a healthcare provider.

Preventive care can keep health problems from developing. The benefits of preventive care for infants, children, and adolescents should be strongly encouraged by the healthcare professional. Preventive intervention includes a variety of methods, such as using well-baby clinics, encouraging clients to wear safety gear, or monitoring nutrition and weight. The benefits of remaining healthy are also extremely cost effective. The trend continues to evolve to prevent illness and accidents, as often as possible, before they occur.

> **Key Concept**
>
> Because healthcare recipients are involved in the management of their own health, they are often referred to as *clients*, rather than patients. *Client* implies active participation in the choice of the (healthcare) service. The client makes decisions regarding health in the same manner as any consumer who makes choices or decisions based on their existing level of knowledge, the type of resources available, the comments or referrals from others, and their personal, past experiences. The overall goal of this textbook is to focus on the aspects of the independent, health-educated, and consumer-aware aspects of the client.

Clients are now expected to participate in **managed care** or case management. Managed care is a plan for continual monitoring and maintenance of an individual's health that involves participation of both the healthcare provider and the individual receiving care. Managed care promotes wellness-focused care and preventive medicine. The consumer or client, who may still be referred to as a patient, remains an individual. A healthcare, that is, a managed care, organization standardizes goals for clients with similar disorders in order to manage costs of particular conditions. The client can still be treated on an individual case-by-case basis. A group of individuals can have similar goals or plans. For example, preventative services include immunization programs for infants and children, diabetic support groups, and cardiac rehabilitation.

Managed care plans are called many names, including *critical pathways, care maps, clinical pathways,* or *standard nursing care plans*. **Managed care payment** involves financial reimbursement for healthcare services by a third party, that is to say, all or part of the healthcare costs are billed to a designated agency or service, not the beneficiary (individual/client). The client accepts this type of payment for service when they join a group that offers the healthcare plan such as an employer or union.

Health maintenance organizations (**HMOs**) are examples of managed care systems. HMOs emphasize disease prevention and health promotion. Their goal is to avoid health problems by preventing conditions that could become more serious (and more costly). Clients are often treated on an outpatient basis, and hospitalizations are minimized. HMOs will be discussed in more detail later in this chapter.

Trends that differentiate HMOs from "traditional" healthcare have evolved. In the 21st century, healthcare involves discussion among a variety of healthcare practitioners, insurance providers who agree to pay for the treatment or therapy, and the client.

The role of the nurse is being redefined to meet the challenges of managed care and reimbursement regulations. In some cases, unlicensed assistive personnel (**UAPs**) are being hired to administer nursing care. This practice is becoming more common across the country and is often a subject of controversy. The standards of education for UAPs are generally much less stringent than the educational requirements for a licensed nurse.

As a result of financial constraints and the influence of managed care plans, clients may have treatment outside a hospital, such as in a wound care treatment center or a rehabilitation center. Clients can be admitted to the hospital, have a surgical procedure performed, and be discharged the same day.

To be admitted to an acute care facility, the client must meet a minimal level or need for healthcare services known as **acuity**. Clients admitted to acute care facilities have high levels of acuity. Thus, the person receiving care in the hospital is often more critically ill than such clients have been in the past. Hospitalizations are of shorter duration and—as a result—the client is often discharged while still in need of healthcare services.

As a result of specific changes in the delivery of healthcare services, extended care facilities (**ECFs**) and **home healthcare** services have restructured to meet the intermediate acuity needs of clients. In the recent past, ECFs were exclusively the "nursing home" or long-term care facility for the aging adult. Twenty-first century clients may be transitioned or transferred from one level of care (acuity) to another level of care. For example, a client may be discharged from an acute care hospital to be admitted into an ECF. At the ECF, the client may receive physical therapy (PT) and rehabilitation before being discharged to home. A client may be monitored at home by a home health nurse. Employment for nurses in all of these areas is projected to increase in the future.

The Affordable Care Act

The **Affordable Care Act** is a major effort in healthcare reform. Legislation, which may also be informally referred to as "Obamacare," was passed in 2010 and institutes significant changes in the availability and access to healthcare for Americans. Detailed information is available on the federal government's website, www.healthcare.gov. Included in the Act are rights and protections that apply to the available insurance policies found within a Health Insurance Marketplace. Individual coverage as well as options for job-based group insurance plans is available. Individual states may offer similar Health Insurance Marketplace insurance options. By 2014, overall goals of these expansive regulations included the following:

- The 2010 Patient's Bill of Rights (Chapter 4)
- Free preventive services for Medicare-eligible individuals and a 50% discount on brand-name drugs
- Access to health insurance options for all Americans
- Prohibition of denial of coverage of healthcare due to preexisting conditions
- Improving healthcare quality and lowering healthcare costs by reforming aspects of the insurance industry's previously existing policies
- Increasing access to individuals eligible for Medicaid
- Promoting an individual's responsibility to obtain health insurance or pay a fee to help offset the costs for caring for uninsured Americans (exemptions may apply)

The Nurse's Role

The myriad of changes in healthcare will continue to alter the role of nurses in the 21st century, whether they practice in acute/subacute, extended, community-based, or home care settings (which are discussed later in this chapter). As the healthcare system and methods of payment develop and change in this century, so will nurses' responsibilities and the facilities in which they work. Nurses must continue to be involved in planning for future healthcare service. Teamwork will remain important, but the methods of collaboration will change. Economic needs for healthcare facilities may require staffing changes and a subsequent change of the care for clients due to the limitations of duties of some healthcare personnel. For example, the increasing use of UAPs as care partners can affect and increase responsibilities for licensed practical nurses. Healthcare reform may result in profound effects on the delivery of healthcare.

Nursing plays a significant role in the attainment of client care outcomes. As a nurse, you will need to understand and articulate the value of a well-educated staff for the delivery of healthcare in the 21st century.

HEALTHCARE SETTINGS AND SERVICES

Acute Care Facilities

Acute Care Hospitals
Acute care hospitals are the most commonly known healthcare facility. Acute care implies that a client in the hospital has a serious condition that needs to be closely monitored by healthcare professionals, particularly nurses. Acute care facilities admit clients for short periods of time, usually only a matter of a few days. Clients are often very sick and need a great deal of nursing care. Box 3-1 summarizes services that are commonly found in acute care facilities.

Intensive Care Units
Intensive care units (**ICUs**) that care for the critically ill are found in acute care facilities. ICUs may specialize in medical,

---

Box 3-1 Services Commonly Found in an Acute Care Facility

- Administration
- Admitting and discharge
- Ambulatory care/outpatient surgery
- Dietary
- Emergency care
- Home health
- Intensive care unit
- Laboratory
- Medical unit
- Neonatal
- Obstetrics/gynecology
- Pediatrics
- Physical therapy
- Radiology
- Respiratory therapy
- Surgical unit
- Telemetry unit
- Transitional care/step-down units

---

surgical, respiratory, coronary, burn, neonatal, and pediatric care areas. ICUs provide care for clients by specially trained nurses, generally registered nurses (RNs). Many ICUs use high-tech equipment and health status monitors.

Subacute Care Facilities
Many hospitals have areas that are classified as *subacute care* or *step-down* units. A person may move to a subacute unit when the level of acuity of care has decreased. However, the client is not considered ready for discharge. A client may be transferred from an ICU to a step-down unit before being discharged from the hospital.

Outpatient Care Centers
Most general hospitals provide "same-day" surgery, also known as *outpatient* or *ambulatory care centers*. In the past, nearly all surgical procedures required hospital admission. Economic issues forced the increase of surgeries performed on an outpatient basis. The client can return home the same day to recuperate. Outpatient treatment centers have become very popular because they save the client time and money. Day surgery centers built by physician groups often compete with an acute care facility's outpatient department.

NCLEX Alert

Clinical scenarios describe care in different types of healthcare environments such as acute care, long-term care, rehabilitative care, or home-based hospice. To select the correct option on an NCLEX question, you may need to know what type of care is needed and select the agency that will best serve the client.

Specialized Hospitals
Specialized hospitals are facilities that admit only one type of client. Examples include government veteran hospitals, psychiatric, or pediatric hospitals. Specialized hospitals may

also have units for medical, surgical, or intensive care. Other types of specialized hospitals include facilities for the developmentally or mentally disabled. Some facilities care for specific conditions, such as head and spinal cord injuries or substance abuse.

Although its primary function is to provide healthcare, the hospital performs other functions. For example, your clinical facility has the added role of education, and many large hospitals, particularly those affiliated with a university, also play an important role in research.

With acute care facilities sending individuals home earlier to recover from surgery or illness, the need for home healthcare has increased. In some cases, nursing care is available 24 hours a day in the home. However, in most cases, the family and other lay caregivers need to take responsibility for some care. Nurses are vital in teaching individuals how to perform care in the home.

Home Healthcare

Home healthcare may be a service provided by an acute care facility or it may be a service provided by an agency that specializes in home healthcare (Fig. 3-1). Home healthcare focuses on the return of health using a recuperative environment that is familiar to the client. Services in the home often include intravenous medications, respiratory care, and wound care. Visits by the nurse may be one or more times per day, weekly, or monthly, as prescribed by the healthcare provider. The family or a significant other is often the main caregiver, with the nurse assisting using assessment/data-gathering skills, specialized training (e.g., in diabetes), or follow-up care (e.g., wound care). Nurses provide the specialized knowledge to treat diseases and disorders or postoperative therapies.

> **Key Concept**
> Many individuals prefer to be cared for at home. Home care is also less expensive than hospitalization. Individuals often have family or friends who can assist in their care. Home health nursing and hospice care have greatly enhanced the quality of healthcare available in the home.

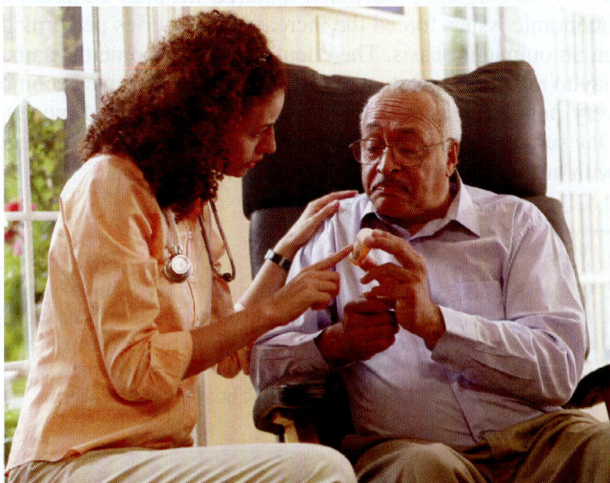

Figure 3-1 Taking time to teach clients about their medication and treatment program promotes interest and cooperation. Older adults who are actively involved in learning about their medication and treatment program and the expected effects may be more likely to adhere to the therapeutic regimen.

 SPECIAL CONSIDERATIONS **Lifespan**

The older adult clients who have dementia may have difficulty managing at home without assistance. Nurses, discharge planners, and primary care providers work as a team to provide safe and adequate care to those individuals living at home. Home health agencies and social services can assist in discharge planning and make arrangements for home care or public health nursing visits.

Hospice

Hospice care specializes in the care of the terminally ill. This service also may be part of the services available from an acute care facility or a separate private agency. Hospice care and home care share a similar nursing objective: taking care of a client in a home environment versus a traditional hospital setting. However, they are two different specialty areas of care. Hospice care focuses on the transition from life to death and works with the client, family, and significant others.

Respite Care

Healthcare services have recognized the need for **respite care**. Respite care provides part-time supervision of clients who have chronic conditions. Family or friends who are the primary caregivers for children and adults with serious, chronic medical conditions or mental illness need respite care. The client may be taken to a facility for part of the day. The client receives supervised care and has an opportunity for socialization outside the home. The caregiver has a chance to be relieved of the exhausting and constant responsibility and stress of caring for someone 24 hours a day.

Telehealth

Telehealth is a service that has developed a specific setting in healthcare due to the ongoing growth of the Internet, webcams, economic needs, and isolated locations of clients. The term "telehealth" refers to the ability to access a healthcare provider via telephone or computer audio/video link. Nurses can communicate and assist clients in numerous ways using distance communication modes. Frequent contact with clients helps to increase medication compliance and helps healthcare providers recognize potential problems before they become acute problems. Thus, unscheduled visits to the physician, the emergency room, and rehospitalization are decreased. Physicians use telehealth to contact other physicians or specialty facilities. Rural communities find the immediate contact with physician specialists a great asset in client care. This concept is discussed in more detail later in Chapters 98 and 102.

Extended Care Facilities

Some facilities admit clients for longer periods of time than is common in acute care hospitals. These ECFs include nursing homes, inpatient rehabilitation centers, inpatient treatment centers for chemical dependency, and facilities for chronic mental healthcare. Some facilities are attached to a general hospital; others are free-standing. More emphasis is being placed on returning people to their homes or other community-based living facilities as quickly as possible. Thus, the population in long-term care facilities is changing.

The federal government divides nursing homes into two categories: a skilled nursing facility (SNF) or an intermediate care facility (**ICF**). The **SNF** provides 24-hour nursing care under the supervision of an RN. The ICF provides 24-hour service from nursing assistants under the supervision of an LVN/LPN, with an RN as a consultant. Many rules and regulations apply to nursing homes. The employment opportunities for nurses continue to grow in this area.

Community Health Services

Community health services provide care for individuals and families within a specific area, such as a neighborhood, a small town, or a rural county. The costs of in-hospital medical care, along with governmental limits and regulations, have forced many people to be cared for in the community, rather than in a hospital.

One type of community health service is the public health service. Public health departments offer immunizations, well-baby checks, and treatment for specific diseases, such as tuberculosis or sexually transmitted diseases (STDs). Community health clinics offer low-cost healthcare services to the public. Prenatal and pediatric care, diabetic care, and general medical-surgical ambulatory care services may be offered by community health clinics. Chapter 7 discusses community health and community-based health services in more detail.

Independent living facilities may provide care for a small number of individuals in a house located in a community neighborhood. These facilities provide a stable, homelike environment for mentally challenged individuals, while still providing some degree of supervision.

Healthcare in School and Industry

Most school systems provide some healthcare services for students, particularly those with disabilities. A nurse may be on duty full time or divide time among several schools. In addition to assisting ill children or children in emergencies, the nurse provides preventive care by performing regular assessments, teaching, screening for common disorders, supervising the administration of immunizations and medications, and providing health counseling.

Children with special physical challenges receive more intensive nursing care, sometimes on a one-to-one basis. To provide total healthcare to students with challenges, some school systems provide comprehensive clinics as part of the educational facilities.

Industries in which machinery is operated usually employ a nurse for health promotion and interventions. Teaching is part of the nurse's responsibility, and prevention of accidents is a major goal. The industrial nurse often serves as liaison between the industry and the Occupational Safety and Health Administration (**OSHA**). OSHA is discussed in Chapter 7.

QUALITY ASSURANCE

Quality of care has become a major issue for both consumers and providers of healthcare. **Quality assurance** (**QA**) is defined as a pledge to the public that healthcare services will provide optimal achievable goals and maintain standard excellence in the services rendered.

Hospital Accreditation

Just as your nursing program can be accredited, a hospital or other healthcare facility also can be accredited. Accreditation implies that the facility has met rigid, minimal standards of service to the client and the community. The agency that assigns this recognition to hospitals is called **The Joint Commission** (formerly known as the Joint Commission for Accreditation of Healthcare Organizations or JCAHO). Other facilities have similar accreditation processes.

The Joint Commission has established rigid standards for an ongoing QA program in hospitals, as well as for community health centers, home care agencies, and various levels of ECFs. The Joint Commission requires objective and systematic monitoring and evaluation of the quality and appropriateness of client care. The QA procedure requires healthcare facilities to identify what they mean by "quality" and to define their evaluation methods.

> **NCLEX Alert**
>
> When reading an NCLEX question, look for the option that suggests the best possible action. Do not confuse the best NCLEX response with an action or shortcut that you might have witnessed while working in a similar situation. Correct nursing options should consider the safety of a situation, the quality of care, and the priorities of nursing care.

Components of Quality Care

Quality management requires that healthcare services be well planned and delivered in a manner that ensures good care. Adequate staff and support services, such as nursing care, must be available.

Quality control and QA focus on delivery of care. The process of care is important, as is the outcome. *Process* relates to how care is given. *Outcome* relates to the result, which is also known as **outcome-based care**.

Nurse accountability, which involves the delivery and accurate documentation of quality care, is vital. Healthcare facilities and agencies have contiguous (or continuous) quality improvement (**CQI**) committees that monitor the quality of ongoing care.

Standards for Quality Assurance

Each healthcare facility establishes individual standards of quality to guide the nursing staff in providing care. In general, these standards include the following:

- *Standards of nursing practice:* Procedures used in the delivery of care, the hospital policy book, textbooks, and other references. Sometimes the term *nursing protocol* is used.

Standards of nursing practice focus on the caregiver, the nurse, and on the nursing process (Unit 6).
- *Standards of client/patient care:* Activities determined by client expectations or by personal standards of care. What did the client expect? How well did nursing care meet the client's expectations? Standards of client care focus on the recipient of care, the client. The client participates in developing the nursing care plan. (The "case manager" is responsible for making sure the client's care is planned and carried out appropriately.)
- *Standards of performance:* How well the nurse performs, as compared with a job description. How well you meet standards of performance as a nursing student will change as you progress through the program. As you become more experienced, you will be expected to provide more complex nursing care.

The *nursing audit* committee or CQI committee evaluates care given to clients. *Peer review* allows nurses to constructively critique each other.

Client Representatives or Advocates

Many hospitals have initiated the position of client (patient) representative, advocate, liaison, or *ombudsperson*. This person's role is to act as consumer advocate. As an advocate, the ombudsperson assists the client and family by resolving concerns or problems. The goal is to focus on client care, needs, and concerns, not the problems that may be encountered during the hospital admission.

Client representatives often help clients and their families find needed services. They listen and answer questions. Representatives can help families find housing, restaurants, parking, child care, or chaplain services. During hospitalization, clients have the right to contact their representatives if they have a problem or concern. Each individual is informed about and receives a copy of the Patient's Bill of Rights. In preparation for discharge, the advocate can make sure the family knows where to purchase needed supplies and medications. The nursing *case manager* has overall responsibility for the client's care. The *advocate* assists as needed.

ORGANIZATION AND OWNERSHIP OF HEALTHCARE FACILITIES

Hospital Organization

Hospitals are almost always governed by a board of directors or trustees or, in the case of a university hospital, by a board of regents. This board appoints the administrators of the hospital. The hospital administrator in turn develops an organizational structure. Box 3-2 lists some of the numerous administrative individuals who are necessary in a modern healthcare facility.

It is important that the student and future employee learn the administrative structure of each healthcare facility. All facilities follow a **chain of command** or organizational reporting system. It is critical that the nurse use the appropriate system for communication (i.e., chain of command) with peers and supervisors.

Box 3-2 Administrative Individuals in a Healthcare Facility

Each healthcare facility requires numerous trained individuals working together. The *chain of command* binds the hospital team members into organized units:
- Chief executive officer
- Medical staff and services
- Nursing staff and services
- Financial officer
- Quality assurance
- Engineering and maintenance
- Environmental services
- Safety officer
- Medical records
- Purchasing
- Dietitian
- Human resources
- Billing and accounts
- Infection control
- Education

Key Concept

While you are in your nursing program, your chain of command begins with your instructor. Problems, concerns, or issues should first be directed to your immediate supervisor (instructor). Each program will have a designated chain of command for students to follow.

Teamwork is a critical component of healthcare. To provide care, members of the healthcare team collaborate in their assessments, planning, and delivery of care. Team members communicate with one another and with clients so that services are neither duplicated nor omitted. Their goal is to help clients maintain wellness. When they find problems, team members focus their energies on restoring clients to health. As a nurse or a nursing student, you are part of the team providing healthcare.

Hospital Ownership and Funding

In addition to types of clients served, healthcare facilities are classified in relation to ownership and funding structure. These lines are becoming blurred, as mergers occur between various types of hospitals.

Governmental Ownership

Governmental, public, or official hospitals are nonprofit organizations that are owned and operated by local, state, or federal units of government. These governmental agencies are also called *official* hospitals. Box 3-3 provides some examples.

Private Ownership

Private or voluntary hospitals are owned and operated by individuals or by groups, such as churches, labor unions, and fraternal organizations. These hospitals may be established as for-profit or not-for-profit organizations.

> **Box 3-3 Types of Ownership of Healthcare Facilities**
>
> **PROFIT-ORIENTED—PROPRIETARY**
> - Individual
> - Partnership
> - Corporation
>
> **NONPROFIT—VOLUNTARY**
> - Church associated (e.g., Loma Linda University Medical Center)
> - Private school associated
> - Foundation associated (e.g., Shriners Hospitals)
>
> **NONPROFIT—GOVERNMENT**
> - Federal (e.g., Veterans Administration, active duty military hospitals)
> - State (e.g., university hospital)
> - County (e.g., city or county hospital)
> - City (e.g., city or county hospital)
> - City-county (e.g., city or county hospital)

For-profit versus not-for-profit: A further classification of hospitals relates to distribution of their profits:

- *Proprietary, investor-owned,* or *for-profit* hospitals are those in which profits are returned to shareholders. Very few such hospitals exist today. Many nursing homes, however, fall into this category.
- *Not-for-profit* hospitals constitute the majority of all hospitals. In the not-for-profit hospital, profits are returned to the funding agency and are used for improvements to the facility, added equipment, and other related costs.

FINANCING HEALTHCARE

The costs of healthcare continue to be a concern. Various programs and legislation, such as the Affordable Care Act, have evolved to address this issue. Societal, legal, and ethical issues influence the costs of healthcare (Chapter 4). Healthcare expenses include not only the salaries of healthcare office and clinical personnel but also the ability to sustain the economics of supplies for the institution plus the need to pay for diagnostic and treatment resource technologies. Personal health choices, such as diet, tobacco use, or high-risk lifestyles, affect individual, family, and societal use of healthcare funds. Therefore, the nurse should consider the concept that healthcare for the 21st century must include the following priorities:

- Primary care services for medically underserved populations, especially those in rural or economically depressed areas
- Mobile services available in low-population areas, such as visits from mobile mammography, magnetic resonance imaging, or computed tomography scan units
- Multi-institutional systems for the coordination or consolidation of expensive or specialized health services (e.g., obstetrics, pediatrics, intensive care, radiation therapy)
- Development of institutions on a geographically integrated basis to prevent excessive duplication of services
- Multi-institutional arrangements for sharing support services (e.g., purchasing)
- Uniform cost accounting, simplified reimbursement, and utilization reporting systems
- Improved financial management procedures
- Cooperation and/or mergers of hospitals and other healthcare facilities
- Case management to oversee the administration and cost of healthcare services
- Improvements in the quality and ongoing quality assessment of healthcare
- Promotion of the nursing profession as a career
- Use of advanced practice nurses as independent providers, in collaboration with physicians
- Training and increased use of assistants to physicians
- Use of complementary care methods, such as acupuncture and herbal medicine
- Additional and early services for pregnant women and at-risk children
- Group medical practices, HMOs, and other organized systems of healthcare delivery
- Special healthcare screenings, immunizations, walk-in clinics, feeding programs, and other services—for clients experiencing homelessness, clients who have recently immigrated, and other high-risk populations
- Improved identification, screening, treatment, and management of the chronically chemically dependent population
- Disease prevention, including studies of nutritional and environmental factors and provision of preventive healthcare services
- Community-based care and services, rather than institutionalization, for clients with chronic and persistent mental health concerns and clients with profound intellectual disabilities
- Mainstreaming school-aged children with physical, emotional, and mental challenges; provision of healthcare to these children as needed
- Consideration of cultural differences in the planning and delivery of healthcare
- Effective methods of educating the public concerning proper healthcare and the effective use of available services
- Additional research and development of medications and treatments for devastating diseases, such as AIDS

Insurance and Healthcare

Healthcare coverage can be purchased by an individual or specific groups. Within the Health Insurance Marketplace, the Affordable Care Insurance Act provides a variety of insurance plans. Policies can be purchased according to a person's unique needs (e.g., young family, older adult, single individual, or a group of employees). Plans typically include various premiums, deductibles, co-payments, and out-of-pocket expenses. Table 3-1 compares general features of the main types of healthcare available in the United States.

Individual Private Insurance
An individual or a family can purchase private health insurance. The cost of private insurance tends to be higher than

TABLE 3-1 Comparison of Three Types of Healthcare Plans[a]

	TRADITIONAL INSURANCE OR FEE FOR SERVICE	HMO MANAGED CARE	PPO MANAGED CARE
Choice of primary healthcare providers (e.g., physicians, hospitals)	Personal selection of any healthcare provider (e.g., physician, nurse practitioner, hospital)	Selection of healthcare provider within HMO network. Use of healthcare provider outside of network is at member's own expense	Selection of healthcare provider within PPO network. Use of healthcare provider outside of network is partially paid, but at a higher expense
Choice of specialists	Personal selection of specialist. Some insurance policies may require preapproval for physician or procedure	HMO primary physician approves specialist. Use of specialist or procedures outside of network is at member's own expense	Selection of specialist within PPO network. Use of specialist or procedure outside of network may be partially paid, but at a higher expense
Additional costs (out-of-pocket costs)	Possible annual deductible. Co-pay ranges widely. Possible co-pay responsibility of 20% of costs; limit on co-pay costs may apply. Routine visits may not be covered	Co-pay for each visit and for prescription drugs. Co-pay ranges widely. Sometimes co-pay for hospital and emergency room visits (may be higher than office visit co-pay)	Co-pay for each visit and for prescription drugs. Co-pay ranges widely. For use of provider outside of PPO network, member pays a deductible and then the plan may pay a percentage of the costs

HMO, health maintenance organization; PPO, preferred provider organization.
[a]Healthcare plans are available for individuals or for specific groups. This table provides generalizations concerning some basic types of services.

---

group insurance. Individual policies can be obtained via the Health Insurance Marketplace or through a variety of health insurance companies or health insurance agencies. A person's policy can be designed around the individual's needs. For example, a younger, healthy person may elect to purchase a policy with a higher deductible than an older individual with chronic conditions.

Group Insurance
Group insurance offers coverage for people who belong to a certain group. Many companies, institutions, and fraternal organizations offer members group insurance benefits. The Affordable Care Act provides employers with criteria and provisions for an employee's group healthcare insurance. Group policies generally have standardized premiums and deductibles.

Fee-for-Service Plans
In a *fee-for-service* plan for either individual or group insurance, coverage is available for medical bills, hospitalization, and other related services, such as surgery or laboratory tests. Fee-for-service plans are the most traditional type of coverage. People may purchase coverage only for themselves, or they may purchase family coverage for members of the immediate family.

Many plans also offer insurance that pays a set amount if a person becomes unable to work due to illness or injury, known as long-term disability insurance.

Health Maintenance Organizations
HMOs offer health services for a fixed monthly charge called a *premium*. Members prepay for healthcare services generally through payroll deductions, governmental agencies (e.g., Medicare, Medicaid), or individual monthly fees. The fee or premium paid in advance to the HMO is called the **capitation** fee (also referred to as *capitated payment*). Members must use a healthcare provider within the HMO network. The healthcare provider uses medical services and specialty referrals that are provided by the HMO. Some HMOs have contracted healthcare facilities for their members.

Each plan will also have some type of additional financial obligation or predetermined **co-pay** that is charged to the client at the time of each visit. Typical services provided to the client by the HMO are listed in Box 3-4.

Box 3-4 Typical Services of a Managed Care System

Services provided vary from plan to plan, and not all services may be available. Some services may be available at additional costs:

- Dental examinations and routine care
- Diabetic care
- Family planning and birth control
- Health education (e.g., antismoking, substance abuse)
- Home healthcare
- Hospice care
- Immunizations
- Inpatient medical and surgical care
- Laboratory and x-ray services
- Long-term care
- Prenatal, labor and delivery, and childbirth care
- Prescription drugs
- Routine checkup
- Speech, hearing, and vision examinations
- Urgent care
- Well-child care

Some HMOs provide dental and optical services as well as medical and surgical services. The provider is responsible for managing the client in the most appropriate and cost-effective manner, to achieve desired outcomes.

Just as with any individual plan, HMO members can elect to go to any physician or seek any medical service that is not part of the HMO network. However, the HMO will generally not pay for this service unless it is preapproved by the administrators of the plan. Emergency room visits may be approved at the time of the client's need.

Features and Services Most HMOs Include

Most HMOs include the following services and features:

- *Group practice:* Several physicians and specialists practice together.
- *Prepayment:* A person or company pays a certain amount in advance (capitation fee) and then is entitled to whatever care is needed. Sometimes, the client pays a small added cost (co-pay) as well.
- *Prevention:* The emphasis is on preventing disease, rather than treating it after it develops.
- *Treatment:* When diseases or disorders occur, they are treated, but the HMO makes decisions as to the type of treatment.

Some states require that employees in large organizations be given a choice between group insurance and HMO membership.

Some employers have initiated **incentive programs** to encourage employees to practice healthy habits. Employers reward employees for smoking cessation, weight loss, and regular physical examinations. Employees are encouraged to be seen in an urgent care center for routine illnesses rather than the emergency room. Usually the co-pay is much higher in the emergency room if urgent care was available at the same time.

Preferred Provider Organizations

Similar to HMOs, preferred provider organizations (**PPOs**) are used to deliver healthcare within a "managed" system. PPOs are made up of groups of healthcare practitioners who contract with the PPO to provide services. PPOs refer clients among their groups, and they usually require that their clients receive healthcare services from a member of that group, unless a special exception is made.

PPO members may use any of the services of the PPO, or they can elect to go outside of the PPO network for service. However, the cost of the service outside of the PPO network is generally higher. For example, a PPO may pay 90% of the cost of a visit to a PPO physician, but only 70% of the cost to a physician who is not a PPO-contracted physician.

Point-of-service Plans

A point-of-service (**POS**) plan is similar to HMO and PPO plans, in that they are all types of managed care. The POS plan also contracts with physicians and other healthcare providers. The client is "managed" by a primary care doctor within the network of POS providers. In this plan, a client may seek care outside of the POS network but will pay a larger share of the healthcare costs. The percentage of cost outside of the POS varies. Often, the lines that define an HMO, PPO, and POS are indistinguishable.

Medicare

Medicare is a federal health insurance program that is available to most people aged 65 years and older, some people with disabilities younger than 65 years, and people with end-stage renal disease. Criteria for eligibility exist. Medicare consists of two parts: Part A, which is used for care in hospitals, SNFs, hospice care, and some home healthcare, and Part B, which helps pay for physicians' services, outpatient hospital care, and some medical services not covered by Part A. Various prescription benefits are available, which may be called Part D. Older adults, their spouses, and their families are encouraged to obtain a thorough understanding of the types of Medicare insurance and prescription coverage. Medicare is also available to younger people receiving Social Security Disability Insurance (**SSDI**) payments. SSDI is a type of insurance program for employees who have become unable to work. SSDI is administered by the Social Security Administration (SSA). Both employees and employers pay into the SSDI fund, and it is reflected in the FICA tax on payroll deduction forms.

SSDI is not the same program as workers' compensation. To be qualified to receive SSDI, employees must be totally incapacitated from gainful employment for at least a year. Workers' compensation benefits may pay for partial disabilities, and the benefits may be for a shorter period of time (Society for Human Resource Management, 2020).

Medicaid

Medicaid is a joint effort of federal and state governments. The federal government has set up guidelines for Medicaid, but individual states design their own programs. Regulations, eligibility requirements, and benefits vary among the 50 states. The Affordable Care Act contains provisions that can assist individuals who qualify. Generally, qualifications for Medicaid are based on income level. In addition to those who meet the criteria of low income, certain other groups may also receive Medicaid. For example, people older than 65 years, families and children, people who are pregnant, and people with disabilities can receive Medicaid. States are ensured access to preventive healthcare (prenatal care, immunizations, and health and developmental screening) for women, infants, and children through their Medicaid programs. The program is tax supported; thus, people who receive Medicaid benefits do not pay monthly premiums.

Medicaid pays for inpatient and outpatient services, including physician or advanced practice nurse services; laboratory and x-ray services; and screening, diagnosis, and treatment for children. It also pays for home care services and family planning. Some states support services, such as dental care and eye care, immunization clinics, well-child clinics, and various preventive medicine and rehabilitation programs.

Medicaid-waiver programs, including those for those with chronic disabilities, older adults, and people with AIDS, facilitate the ability of these participants to remain at home and within the community. Medicaid often waives some of the qualification criteria and regulations for these clients.

People who are eligible for Medicare and Medicaid can supplement one program with the other. Medicaid may pay expenses not covered by Medicare if a person is eligible for both programs.

> **Key Concept**
> Both Medicare and Medicaid are undergoing constant changes. These changes tend to be more visible to the public when they occur along with changes in the presidency or legislature. Be aware of the impact of these changes on clients, their families, and healthcare institutions.

Prospective Payment

In 1983, an amendment to the federal Social Security legislation changed the delivery of healthcare. This amendment created a **prospective payment system**, originally only affecting Medicare payments, but later adopted by other third-party payers. Prospective payment is a reimbursement system in which a predetermined amount is allocated for treating individuals with specific diagnoses.

The type of payment and reimbursement that existed in years past was called *retrospective payment*. This system reimbursed all actual costs of providing care. Many people felt that these costs were excessive, which contributed to the development of the system of prospective payment.

Diagnosis-Related Groups

Prospective payment is based on categories called diagnosis-related groups (**DRGs**) for hospitals and for home care. The term used in nursing homes and ECFs is resource utilization groups (**RUGs**).

The DRG system of prospective payment is based on medical diagnoses. Under this system, a federal agency has predetermined how much it "should" cost to treat a certain condition in a particular area of the United States. In this system, each client is classified according to the particular diagnosis (e.g., hip surgery, pneumonia, or heart attack). The costs for the client's care are based on federally determined standards for that diagnosis.

The amount paid to the healthcare facility is predetermined and is *without consideration of the actual costs of providing care to the client*. Thus, a hospital treating an individual with a serious illness or surgery will receive the same reimbursement whether the person is hospitalized for 5 days or for 25 days.

Because a preset or *prospective* amount of money is paid for each diagnosis, the healthcare facility loses money if an individual client's care costs more than average. The facility gains money, however, if a client's care costs less than the average.

At the beginning of the 1990s, healthcare in the United States was a big business and one of the top three industries in the country. Healthcare continues to be a big business, but the emphasis is shifting from inpatient to community-based care. With the implementation of DRGs, facilities must be run cost effectively or they will not survive. Not all states, however, continue to use DRGs. For example, in 1993, New Jersey deregulated, allowing the state to make more decisions itself.

Impact of Changes in Third-Party Payment

The evolving system of healthcare financing in the United States has greatly affected the delivery of healthcare. Changes include the following:

- Emphasis on wellness, disease prevention, and health promotion
- Greatly decreased length of hospital stays
- Use of hospitals for only the critically ill
- Higher levels of client acuity in nursing homes
- Fewer admissions for in client care
- Sicker people discharged from hospitals, needing more care at home
- Greater responsibility required of caregivers in the home
- Greater need for outpatient care because procedures formerly done in the hospital are done on an outpatient basis
- More community-based care and home care nursing
- More specialized care
- More diversified hospitals that rent medical equipment, provide home care, and have day surgery centers and ECFs—in addition to providing in client care
- Decentralized administration
- Greater need for cooperation among departments to maximize resources
- Mergers of several hospitals or nursing homes to form a large corporation
- Extensive use of computers for data collection and information processing
- Competition by hospitals for the use of their services involving advertising and marketing
- Competition for client satisfaction
- Loss of some healthcare facilities due to financial competition of healthcare services

COMPLEMENTARY HEALTHCARE

Many people believe that means other than traditional Western medicine can cure diseases and help them to achieve optimum health. These methods and beliefs are known as alternative healthcare or **complementary healthcare**. Several such modalities are discussed in the following sections. They may be used alone or in conjunction with other therapies; however, clients should only use qualified practitioners. Some practitioners must be licensed to practice legally.

Chiropractic, Physical, and Occupational Therapy

Chiropractic therapy uses manipulation of the spinal column and joints to treat pain and certain disorders. This therapy is based on the structure and function of the body. Chiropractors believe that the relationships between the spinal column and nervous system are important. Chiropractic adjustments seek to achieve a balance between these systems.

PT and occupational therapy (OT) are forms of rehabilitation after disease or injury. They use exercise, heat, cold, electrical muscle stimulation, splinting, ultraviolet radiation, and massage to improve circulation and to strengthen and retrain muscles. PT is also important in the management of chronic disorders such as arthritis. OT is important in teaching skills that will enable people to return to work, manage their homes, or care for themselves again.

Holistic Healthcare

Holistic healthcare was at the center of many beliefs and practices of ancient civilizations. Holism became accepted in North American healthcare within the last half of the 20th century. Holism is a philosophy that considers the "whole person," or the multidimensional aspects of the human being, to be in need of healthcare.

Holistic healthcare refers to comprehensive and total care of a person by meeting his or her needs in all areas: physical, emotional, social, spiritual, and economic. Rather than defining health in terms of disease, holistic healthcare emphasizes wellness.

Holistic healthcare teaches that individuals can be in control of their own life and health and that people can largely *determine* the quality of their life. Chapter 5 relates the concepts of holistic healthcare and wellness to Maslow's hierarchy of human needs.

> **NCLEX Alert**
>
> The concepts of Maslow's Hierarchy are fundamental components of clinical nursing. They can determine the importance of a nursing care situation. Therefore, it is critical to know these concepts. Often these concepts may answer which action should be taken first (prioritization).

Clients have the right to be actively involved in their own care. Rather than passively following the physician's orders, clients should consider the physician's advice and make informed decisions about care they wish to receive. Clients also have the right to refuse care. Part of your nursing responsibility is to teach clients and to answer their questions. You will also teach clients ways to prevent disease and to improve their health.

Nurses and other healthcare professionals should provide holistic care in a supportive and positive fashion to help clients maintain a self-image as a worthy human being. By sincerely caring about your clients and respecting their ways of life, you can strengthen their feelings of self-respect and dignity.

Herbalists and Vibrational Remedies

Herbalists promote health through the use of herbs and other plants (botanicals). In many cases, the use of herbs is combined with a healthful diet, exercise, and other healthy practices. "Vibrational remedies" include flower essences and homeopathy.

Acupuncture and Acupressure

Acupuncture, a healing method originating from Chinese medicine, is based on *Chi*, which is believed to be the energy of life. Acupuncture views health and its functions as energy balance—and disease as imbalance—in the body. Acupuncture therapy includes the use of very fine needles inserted into specific energy points underneath the skin to balance the body's flow of energy.

The use of this procedure is increasing in Western culture and is becoming more accepted by traditional allopathic medicine. It allows the body to heal naturally and does not involve the use of drugs, although herbal extracts and vitamins may be used. Acupuncture is often combined with meditation and exercise. It can be used for health promotion, such as weight control or smoking cessation, as well as for healing.

Clients can learn acupressure (external pressure applied to the energy points) for pain and symptom control between acupuncture treatments. PT and chiropractic therapy use many of the same energy and pressure points.

Relaxation and Imagery

Relaxation and imagery are becoming more common in many areas of healthcare. Therapeutic relaxation begins with the client sitting or lying in a comfortable position, with eyes gently closed and the body relaxed. The client breathes deeply and concentrates on systematically and progressively relaxing all the muscles in the body. The client may also visualize relaxing images, such as clouds or colors. Hypnosis and self-hypnosis make use of relaxation techniques.

Imagery involves calling up mental pictures or events, usually after the client completely relaxes. Although the client can use any of the senses, the most common is visual imagery. Imagery is often used in cancer therapy. For example, clients visualize their cells as being big and strong and the cancer as being small and weak, or clients picture the cancer cells being destroyed by their own white blood cells or visualize themselves as being well and whole. Other practitioners teach clients to "love the cancer out of existence." Imagery is also used in pain and spasm control, weight reduction, and smoking cessation.

Meditation

Many religious groups practice meditation, which consists of deep personal thought and breath control. The meditating person can keep his or her eyes open or closed. A word or phrase (mantra) may be repeated to aid concentration. Meditation strives to "clear or still the mind" through the art of "quiet thinking." Those who meditate change their concentration from the external world to the internal world, bringing mindfulness to oneself. Meditation helps decrease anxiety and enables people to better cope with stress. People can meditate while doing any relaxing activity: sitting, gardening, knitting, or walking.

Therapeutic Touch

Therapeutic touch is a specific noninvasive modality that does not require entering the body or puncturing the skin. Therapeutic touch grew out of the holistic healthcare movement. It is based on the ancient practice of "laying on of hands," although the skilled practitioner never actually touches the client. Therapeutic touch teaches that each person is surrounded by an energy field. This electromagnetic field can be detected by magnetic resonance imaging.

The practitioner first assesses the client's energy with the goal of *restoring harmony*. If the client's energy flow is obstructed, depleted, or disordered, the practitioner tries to unblock and balance the areas of disturbed flow. Therapeutic touch aids relaxation, lowers muscle tension, and may decrease the client's need for medication.

UNIT 1 The Nature of Nursing

CONSUMER FRAUD

Unlike complementary healthcare methods, which are acceptable modalities used in place of or along with conventional Western methods, many fraudulent healthcare practices and treatments are on the market.

The public spends an estimated $25 billion per year on "sure cures" for every imaginable ailment. The result is that ill people run the risk of delaying vital treatment until it is too late. Cancer, obesity, and arthritis "cures" are the most common subjects of frauds. If fraud is suspected, it should be reported to a reputable agency. The Internet is the most rapidly growing source of fraud. To protect yourself and your clients, be sure that healthcare claims are supported by valid research and consistently trustworthy organizations (Educating the Client 3-1).

Misleading the public (consumer fraud) is illegal. A great deal of money is at stake, so new schemes continue to develop. Why are so many people taken in by claims for a drug or other magic cure? People who are experiencing pain may be willing to try anything at any cost. Also, the general public often cannot tell the difference between true and false claims. As a nurse, you may be asked for your opinion about a questionable medical practice. Although people must make their own decisions, encourage them to find out all the facts before starting any untested healthcare measure.

IN PRACTICE
EDUCATING THE CLIENT 3-1 — Detecting Frauds

When teaching clients and families about consumer fraud, be sure to address the following concepts:

- Encourage people to develop their consumer awareness. Support groups are available for those who have been victims of fraud and for advocates of consumer rights. Help direct clients and families to such avenues, if appropriate.
- Warn clients and families to suspect products, treatments, or methods with the following advertising claims:
  - "Special formula"
  - Support by unrecognized "healthcare experts" or celebrities
  - Testimonials by those who have used the product ("It really works!!")
  - Attractive refund policy if not "completely satisfied"
- Discuss with clients their option to consult other qualified healthcare practitioners about their current treatment and prognosis (second opinion).
- Explain to clients that they have rights to information about their health and about any product or treatment measure that they use or are interested in pursuing.

STUDENT SYNTHESIS

KEY POINTS

- Many changes in the healthcare system in the 21st century will bring new and unknown challenges for nurses.
- The Affordable Care Act has brought about many changes within the healthcare insurance industry.
- Types of healthcare facilities include hospitals, which now primarily treat people with acute conditions; extended care facilities, where care is given for a longer time; and community services, which include outpatient care, walk-in care, home healthcare, and care in schools and industries. Employment opportunities for nurses exist in all these areas.
- The Joint Commission establishes quality and appropriate care standards.
- Many hospitals have established the position of client advocate (representative, ombudsperson) to help the client and family adapt to hospitalization.
- Third-party payment has been the method of payment for healthcare in the United States for a number of years. A variety of organizations provide this service.
- Complementary healthcare will play an increasing role in the healthcare delivery system in the United States in the future. Holism is a philosophy that views the "whole person."

CRITICAL THINKING EXERCISES

1. Relate Florence Nightingale's theory of nursing (Chapter 2) to modalities, such as therapeutic touch, meditation, and imagery.
2. Obtain a copy of a "critical pathway" or detailed nursing care plan from your healthcare facility. Analyze this document and its relationship to holistic healthcare.
3. Evaluate today's healthcare system and project forward about 25 years. How do you envision healthcare delivery? Relate your predictions to at least one theory of nursing, as presented in Chapter 2. Also relate your beliefs to the concept of holistic healthcare.

NCLEX-STYLE REVIEW QUESTIONS

1. A client no longer requires care in the coronary intensive care unit after coronary artery bypass graft surgery. Where should the nurse prepare to transfer the client?
   a. Subacute or step-down unit
   b. Skilled care unit
   c. Medical floor
   d. Long-term care facility

2. The nurse is caring for a terminally ill client that is to be discharged. Which referral should the nurse make with the client's and family's approval?
   a. Extended care
   b. Telehealth
   c. Respite care
   d. Hospice

3. A client that is homebound requires long-term intravenous antibiotic therapy. The insurance company refuses to keep the client in the hospital during this treatment regimen. Which services would best meet the needs of the client?
   a. Hospice
   b. Respite care
   c. Home healthcare
   d. Telehealth

4. The RN is developing the plan of care for a client with pneumonia. Who should the nurse include in the development of the care plan?
   a. Unit secretary
   b. Dietary
   c. The client
   d. Administration

5. The nurse is concerned about a newly developed policy regarding scheduling on the unit. Who is the appropriate person for the nurse to discuss the concerns with?
   a. The nurse manager
   b. The nurse's peers
   c. The chief nursing officer
   d. The board of directors

CHAPTER RESOURCES

Enhance your learning with additional resources on thePoint!

Student Resources related to this chapter can be found at **thePoint.lww.com/Rosdahl12e**.

4 Legal and Ethical Aspects of Nursing

Learning Objectives

1. Define and describe the legal and ethical standards of healthcare and how they relate to nursing.
2. Explain the implications for nurses for the concepts of false imprisonment, abandonment of care, invasion of privacy, and confidentiality.
3. Define and discuss the purpose of a Nurse Practice Act. Name the components of a Nurse Practice Act.
4. State at least three functions of a State Board of Nursing.
5. Name some commonsense precautions that nurses can take against lawsuits.
6. State the benefits and limitations of the Good Samaritan Act.
7. Discuss the concept of professional boundaries.
8. Define and discuss the three major types of advance directives.
9. Define the types of people who are vulnerable to deficient or harmful care.
10. Differentiate between biological death and brain death.
11. State the rights and responsibilities of healthcare clients.
12. List the major provisions of the HIPAA legislation and state the overall goal of this legislation. Describe how this impacts nursing care.

Important Terminology

advance directive
alias
assault
assisted suicide
battery
biological death
brain death
clinical death
crime
endorsement
ethics
euthanasia
felony
Good Samaritan Act
informed consent
law
legal death
liability
libel
malpractice
misdemeanor
negligence
Nurse Practice Act
slander
tort

Acronyms

AHA
AKA
AMA
CAT
CEH
CEU
CPR
EEG
EPHI
HIPAA
LVN/LPN
NCLEX-PN
NCLEX-RN
NCSBN
PHI
PSDA
RN
ROI
UNOS

Chapter 2 discussed standards of practice, the Nightingale Pledge, and the Practical Nurse's Pledge. Legal and ethical issues of nursing practice were introduced. This chapter further explores legal and ethical issues and relates them to the concepts of nursing and healthcare.

Laws are formal, written rules of behavior that govern conduct and are enforced by an authority. **Ethics** refers to philosophic studies that examine the actions, values, and moral principles of human behaviors and that provide the fundamental ideas of societal and cultural values of right versus wrong. Ethics and ethical standards evolve as changes in society occur. The issue of right and wrong affects actions, language, and spiritual beliefs. The healthcare system combines the practice of medicine and nursing within this complex system of laws, societal beliefs, and cultural values. Laws and ethics commonly overlap, and the relationship between them is complex.

The ethical standards of the healthcare profession and the laws of the United States and Canada are carefully designed to protect both you and those you serve. You are responsible for becoming familiar with these legal and ethical standards before caring for clients.

LEGAL ISSUES OF NURSING PRACTICE

In the course of your activities as a student and later as a licensed nurse, you are held responsible for maintaining established standards of nursing care. You will encounter many situations involving legal responsibilities. In addition to avoiding those acts that all citizens know are illegal, you must not violate other important laws that are specific to healthcare. Table 4-1 summarizes common sources of law and gives examples related to nursing and healthcare.

Legal issues encompass a variety of concerns. Listed below are some of the major concerns related to the legal and ethical aspects of the healthcare professions:

- Nurse practice acts, nursing standards, and nursing licensure
- Nursing practice and medical practice laws: similarities and differences
- Patient/client rights and nursing obligations regarding informed consent, protecting the individual's rights, and upholding privacy standards
- Malpractice, negligence, and nursing liability
- Nursing responsibilities in your professional versus your personal (off duty) life

TABLE 4-1	Common Sources of Law	
TYPE OF LAW	GENERAL PURPOSE	EXAMPLE OF LAW
Constitutional	Law written as part of a local, state, or federal constitution	Protection of right to free speech
Statutory	Any law enacted by a legislative body	Creation of Nurse Practice Act
Administrative	Empowers agencies to create and enforce rules and regulations	Development of State Boards of Nursing
Criminal	Laws that define offenses that violate the public welfare	Prosecution of violation of provisions of Nurse Practice Act
Civil	Protects civil rights such as freedom from invasion of privacy and freedom from threats of injury	Healthcare client charges nurse with invasion of privacy and violation of confidentiality laws

- Documentation: written or computer, errors and avoidance of errors
- Ethical issues, the law, societal needs, and healthcare practices

Legal Terminology

A *crime* is a wrong committed against a person or property or public good. A crime occurs when a law is violated. In a crime, intention to do wrong is also present. Crimes may be misdemeanors or felonies.

A **felony** is a serious crime. Healthcare workers can be convicted of felonies for such offenses as falsification of medical records, insurance fraud, theft of narcotics, or practicing without a license.

A **misdemeanor** is a crime that is considered not as serious as a felony. A misdemeanor is still a serious charge and may be the cause for revocation of a nursing license. Possession of controlled substances may be either a misdemeanor or a felony as defined by the local, state, or federal laws. Federal law requires that healthcare facilities keep records about the dispensing of narcotics. This law specifies that narcotics are to be given under the direction and supervision of a physician, osteopath, dentist, or veterinarian. In a hospital, all narcotics are kept double locked, and every dose or tablet must be accounted for. Violation of the Controlled Substances Act is a serious crime.

Liability is the legal responsibility for one's actions or failure to act appropriately. A crime may be the deliberate *commission* of a forbidden act or *omission* of an act required by law.

A nurse may be liable if a client receives the wrong medication and is harmed (an "act of commission"). Examples of other nursing *crimes of commission* would be participation in an illegal abortion, participation in **euthanasia** ("mercy killing"), and practicing nursing without a license or beyond the legal limits of your nursing practice.

A nurse also may be liable if a client did not receive a prescribed medication and was harmed (an "act of omission"). *Crimes of omission* include failure to perform a prescribed treatment, failure to report child or elder abuse, and failure to report a specified communicable disease or an animal bite.

A tort is an injury that occurred because of another person's intentional or unintentional actions or failure to act. The injury can be physical, emotional, or financial. A tort involves a breach of duty that one person owes another, such as the duty of a nurse to care for a client. Examples of intentional torts include assault, battery, false imprisonment, invasion of privacy, and defamation. The example of an unintentional tort is negligence. **Malpractice** is defined as professional negligence.

Negligence is defined as harm done to a client as a result of neglecting duties, procedures, or ordinary precautions. Negligence is one of the most common causes of lawsuits by healthcare clients. Negligence describes the failure to act as a reasonable person would have acted in a similar situation. Negligence takes into account your educational level and experience. Thus, negligence is balanced against what another nurse with similar education and experience would have done in a similar situation. A nurse can be found negligent and be sued for damages for any of the following reasons:

- Performing nursing procedures that have not been taught
- Failing to follow standard protocols as defined by the facility's policy and procedure manuals
- Failing to report defective or malfunctioning equipment
- Failing to meet established standards of safe care for clients
- Failing to prevent injury to clients, other employees, and visitors
- Failing to question a physician's order that seems incorrect

Malpractice is the improper, injurious, or faulty treatment of a client that results in illness or injury. Harm that results from a licensed person's actions or lack of actions can be called malpractice. A nurse commits malpractice when their conduct deviates from the normal or expected standard of behavior that would be performed by someone of similar education and experience in similar circumstances.

Healthcare professionals are held to higher standards than untrained individuals. Standards of practice are defined by a state's Nurse Practice Act, written agency policies and procedures, documented standards of care, such as a nursing care plan, and the testimony of expert witnesses. The nurse's personal life and actions may also be scrutinized according to the higher standards of nonnursing individuals. Additional information regarding Nurse Practice Acts is found in the next section of this chapter.

Assault is a threat or an attempt to do bodily harm. Assault includes physical or verbal intimidation. A gesture that the client may perceive as a threat is an assault if the client believes that force or injury may follow. For example, telling the client that you are going to restrain them in bed if they try to get out of bed without assistance is an assault.

Battery is physical contact with another person without that person's consent. Physical striking or beating is battery. Also considered to be battery may be the touching of a person's body, clothing, chair, or bed. A charge of battery can be made even if the contact did not cause physical harm.

Giving an injection that the client refuses is battery. Forcing the client to get out of bed can be considered both assault and battery. To protect nurses and other healthcare individuals from the charge of battery, clients sign a general permission for care and treatment. Before any special test, procedure, or surgery, clients sign another consent form. Informed consent is discussed below.

Consent for care is provided by the individual, parent, or guardian if the client is a minor, with intellectual disability, or mentally incompetent. In an emergency, the law assumes inferred consent. *Inferred consent* means that in life-threatening circumstances, the client would provide consent for care.

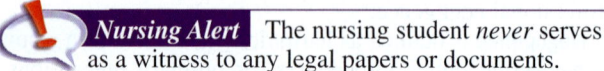

Nursing Alert The nursing student *never* serves as a witness to any legal papers or documents.

Informed consent means that tests, treatments, and medications have been explained to the person, as well as outcomes, possible complications, and alternative procedures. Before any client receives routine treatment, a specialized diagnostic procedure, an invasive procedure, special medical or surgical treatment, or experimental therapy, they must give informed consent. Usually, the physician explains the situation and obtains consent. The physician and all healthcare workers must be reasonably satisfied that the client understands what will be done and what the expected or adverse results are likely to be. All teaching must be documented.

Key Concept
All teaching must be documented.

The client or a legal guardian must understand and sign the consent form before the performance of any procedure. In certain extreme emergencies, no one may be available to give consent. In such cases, procedures may be performed without specific written or verbal consent; however, each facility will have specific protocols that will need to be followed. For example, if an unconscious client is admitted to an emergency room and needs immediate surgical intervention before family can be located, some facilities allow for two physicians to sign an emergency consent. In some cases, a court order to administer treatment is obtained.

The person who will perform any procedure is ultimately responsible for obtaining consent. As a nurse, you must confirm that the signed consent is in a client's health record before performing any procedure. In cases of serious surgery or life-threatening procedures, physicians usually obtain consent. *Students do not obtain consent or witness consent forms.*

Nonconsensual physical contact may be required if the client is mentally ill, intoxicated, or endangering the safety of self or others (Chapter 94 discusses care in the mental health unit.). Legal protection in this type of circumstance relies heavily on thorough documentation. It is critical for the healthcare provider to describe the behavior of the client that resulted in the use of force. The documentation should specify that the situation required the type of restraint that was used. Excessive force is never appropriate.

False imprisonment or restraint of movement may be charged in certain situations, such as the use of unnecessary restraints or solitary confinement. By law, a person cannot be restrained against their will unless the person has been convicted of a crime or a court order exists permitting restraint. False imprisonment may be a result of either physical or chemical limitations.

Libel and slander relate to personal integrity. **Libel** refers to a written statement or photograph that is false or damaging. Special precautions must be taken to avoid libel when using email communications. The Internet and electronic communications have the potential of carrying personal conversations into the public domain.

Slander is the term given to malicious verbal statements that are false or injurious. Clearly, nurses must avoid untrue and unwise statements at all times. Slander can take the form of gossip and exaggerations, such as "That nurse is lazy," "The supervisor doesn't know what they are doing," or "Doctor X's clients always have complications." *Defamation* is an act that harms a person's reputation and good name.

Abandonment of care is a legal term that implies that a healthcare professional has prematurely stopped caring for a client. For example, if a client cannot safely be left alone, you may be found liable if the client under your care is injured while unsupervised. If a home care client has an infection or stops taking medications, you may be found liable if you fail to report this information in a timely manner. To avoid the charge of abandonment, you NEVER leave your employment or clinical assignment, even in an emergency, without proper notification being given to your supervisors.

Invasion of privacy and confidentiality are of critical legal and medical concern. The *right to privacy* means that a client has the right to expect that their property will be left alone. Healthcare individuals may be charged with trespassing, illegal search and seizure, or releasing private information (even if the information is true). Remember, you are violating the law if you give out any information about a client without their written consent. Also, prevent clients and visitors from seeing other clients' health records and private information. For example, be careful not to pull client information onto the computer screen where other clients can see it (Fig. 4-1).

Student nurses are often assigned research projects that contain a client's medical history and personal information. Rather than using client names or initials, it is more prudent to use code numbers. If lost or misplaced, even your scratch notes can be the basis for a breach of confidentiality lawsuit. ALWAYS protect the client's confidentiality.

NCLEX Alert

Clinical situations on the NCLEX can include references to legal and ethical situations. To choose the correct option, you must understand the terms presented in this chapter, for example, negligence, liability, legal death, HIPAA, advance directive, etc. Your professional responsibility in these situations can be a component of the correct answer.

HIPAA and Client Privacy

In 1996, the Health Insurance Portability and Accountability Act (**HIPAA**), Title II, was passed and serves as federal privacy regulation. HIPAA protects clients' information and

CHAPTER 4 Legal and Ethical Aspects of Nursing

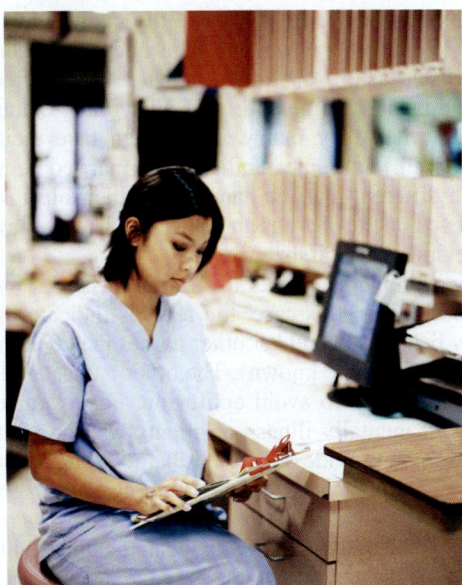

Figure 4-1 Computers are excellent tools for nurses, but they can be a source of loss of confidentiality for clients.

All clients or their caregivers are asked to sign an HIPAA statement on admission to a healthcare facility, whether an inpatient or an outpatient. This statement acknowledges that the client has seen the HIPAA regulations. The facility promises to abide by these regulations.

> **Key Concept**
>
> As a nursing student or staff nurse, you will most likely be asked to sign a HIPAA confidentiality statement each year. This certifies that you are familiar with HIPAA regulations and will follow their guidelines. Be aware that violation of HIPAA privacy practices is cause for termination of employment or of student status in most facilities.

Failure to Comply with These Standards May Result in Civil or Criminal Penalties

Detailed official information regarding this important legislation can be found on the Health and Human Services website. Because confidentiality is so important, as is legislated by HIPAA, state, and individual healthcare agencies, all providers of healthcare must take precautions in their verbal and written communications, such as avoiding gossip, restricting conversations regarding clients to private, professional settings, and preserving the privacy of your clients *at all times*.

Violation of confidentiality or misuse of the health record is a violation of privacy laws (Fig. 4-2). If a client requests anonymity, just acknowledging the person's hospitalization can be a violation of the law.

Effective January 2009, the Patient Safety and Quality Improvement Act of 2005, also known as the *Patient Safety Act*, establishes a voluntary reporting system that improves and enhances increased safety of clients. The goal of this act is to encourage the reporting and the subsequent analysis of medical errors and safety issues in a confidential manner without the fear of increased liability risk. As data are reported and analyzed, the information will yield a better understanding of what changes need to be made to promote client safety.

makes sure this information remains private. This legislation, although it protects clients, limits the ability to do medical research in some cases. It also adds to the facility's cost of providing care.

The "Security Rule" of this legislation deals specifically with (Electronic) Protected Health Information (**PHI/EPHI**). This information is defined as "any information concerning a client's health status" or "any part of an individual's medical record or payment history." The rule states that each facility must have written privacy procedures; supervision of these procedures must be documented. Each facility must name a privacy officer. Only employees who "need to know" can legally access any client's record. All employees must undergo documented ongoing confidentiality training and sign a confidentiality agreement annually. The facility must also have a contingency plan for emergency data backup, should a disaster occur. Internal audits must occur on a regular basis and disciplinary action taken against any staff member who violates privacy rules. In addition, severe financial penalties are levied against the facility if it does not follow these rules.

> **Nursing Alert** A healthcare facility can legally release PHI under certain circumstances, such as suspected child abuse or abuse of a client by a healthcare worker.

The HIPAA, Title II act

- Regulates who can have access to client information
- Sets standards for storage and transmission of client information
- Requires that healthcare facilities write policies allowing clients access to their own personal health information. (The client has the right to request correction of any errors.)

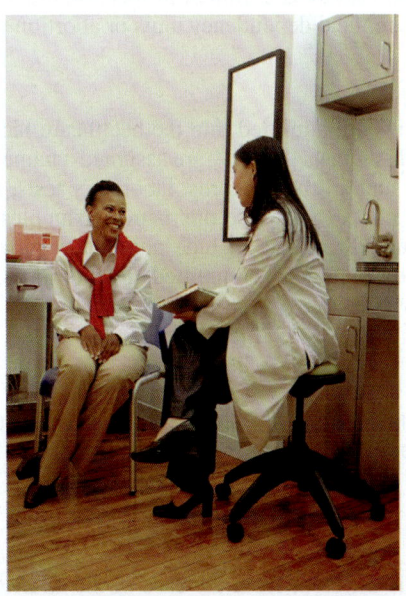

Figure 4-2 When interviewing clients, make sure to maintain privacy by waiting until visitors leave and closing doors.

Release of Client Information

No one can legally give out personal information about a client without a signed Release of Information (**ROI**) by the client. If a nurse is unsure about what information is acceptable to release, they should consult the team leader or charge nurse. For example, if someone calls to ask the client's condition, facility protocol may allow the nurse to state the condition listed in the record. If the caller wants more information, the client's written permission is required. The nurse must avoid revealing any information that destroys the confidentiality of the nurse–client or agency–client relationship.

Nursing Alert

- Before discussing a client with anyone other than the healthcare team, be sure to have a signed "Release of Information" form from the client.
- Make sure the person who is receiving information is authorized to receive it.
- In some cases, the client does not want anyone to know they are in the facility.
- Make sure you are within legal limits before giving out any information.
- When giving any information regarding a client, whether in person or by telephone, be sure you cannot be overheard by other clients or visitors.
- Protect the computer screen so no one can see the information.
- Always log off when leaving the computer.
- Protect the client's confidentiality at all times.

"No Information" Status

Any client can request "no information" status if they do not want anyone to know that they are in the healthcare facility. In this case, you cannot acknowledge that the client is there, and they do not receive mail, flowers, or visitors. The "no information" status is common in locations such as mental health or chemical dependency units or abortion clinics.

The Alias

Some clients are admitted into the healthcare facility under an **alias**. This means that they are assigned a name other than their own, and all their records, laboratory tests, room tags, diet slips, and so forth use this name. Examples of clients admitted under an alias include politicians, movie or rock stars, persons who have committed violent crimes, and other well-known people.

Key Concept

If a person is registered under an alias, it is important to use the alias when addressing them, even if you know their given name.

The AKA

The alias is different from the case of the AKA. The AKA occurs when a client's record is changed to reflect their new name. One example is a woman who marries and takes her husband's last name. In this case, the client's records are changed to reflect her new name. This client's previous name is often listed as an **AKA** (also known as) in the record, to avoid confusion. (Remember, not all women change their last name when they marry. Some men take their wife's name as well.) In some facilities, all married female clients with different married names have their birth (maiden) names listed on the chart as an AKA, even if they have never been previously hospitalized.

In addition, some clients use different names on different admissions. In this case, the records indicate the name currently being used and list other names the client has used in the past (if any are known). The other names are listed as AKA in the chart, to avoid confusion. For example, some clients with mentally illness or clients who are wanted by the police may provide a different name. Some clients give a false name on admission to the hospital. If their true name is later learned, it is added to the client's record as an AKA. Sometimes, the client's family is located and asked to make a positive identification.

In some cases, clients from other countries give their name on admission in a format that is different from Western names. For example, sometimes it is difficult to determine which is the client's first name and which is the client's last name, or both first and last names may be the same. It can be difficult to determine the English spelling of a non-English name. Therefore, a client's name may be spelled several different ways before it is determined which way is most accurate.

Key Concept

Sometimes, it is possible to help identify a person on the basis of his or her birth date. However, in some cultures, all people are considered to have been born on January 1. Therefore, it is impossible to differentiate certain clients by using birth date. In this case, it is also not known exactly how old the person is because their age could vary by nearly a year. Some people simply do not know their birth date and do not know how old they are.

John Doe Admissions

Sometimes an unidentified person is admitted to the healthcare facility, most often as an emergency admission. One practice in this case is to admit the person as "John Doe" or "Jane Doe." Some facilities admit as "unidentified," including race and sex (e.g., "unidentified Asian female"). When the identity of this person is established, the records are changed to indicate the person's name. In some cases, a family member or friend is located who can accurately establish the identity of the person.

Special Healthcare Concerns

The laws relating to healthcare are many and varied. A basic understanding of laws that apply to nursing is essential so that you can make informed decisions about your practice. The following are common healthcare issues that have particular legal and sometimes ethical implications:

- *Duty to provide treatment.* The person's ability to pay should not determine whether they receive care. Laws regulate the rights of the person and of the healthcare facility.

- *Abortion and sterilization.* State laws differ as to what types of consents are required, who must be notified, and who must sign the consent. The length of gestation for a legal abortion also differs among states.
- *Experimentation.* Stringent regulations govern research studies using human beings. All participants in such studies must give informed consent.
- *Release from liability.* A person may leave the healthcare facility against medical advice (**AMA**) or may refuse treatment. Laws specify the extent of the responsibility of the facility and of physicians and nurses.
- *Death in the hospice facility or during the hospice program at home.* When a person is expected to die (as in hospice), the laws relating to pronouncement of death are different from those in other situations.

> **Key Concept**
>
> Keep up to date on current legislation by reading nursing journals and attending continuing education classes. Ignorance of the law does not protect you from prosecution.

REGULATIONS OF NURSING PRACTICE

Legislation for the Practice of Nursing: the Nurse Practice Act

Nursing is a specific profession that has legal definitions as to scope or boundaries of practice. The laws for the practice of nursing are written by the legislature of each state or province. The law that defines and regulates the practice of nursing in the United States is called the **Nurse Practice Act**. In Canada, it is called the *Nurses (Registered) Act*. These laws define the title of "nursing" and regulate the many aspects of the field of nursing.

In some areas a single Nurse Practice Act is written to include both registered and practical nurses. In other areas, licensed practical nursing and registered nursing have completely separate Nurse Practice Acts.

Only individuals who are regulated by Nurse Practice Acts can legally be called nurses. Certified Nursing Assistants are not licensed personnel because they do not function under nurse practice legislation. However, many states require that they complete basic, minimal training by qualified instructors. When the training is complete, the individual may apply to the state for "certification." Currently, unlicensed assistive personnel (UAP) and medical assistants are not licensed personnel and may or may not have any formal healthcare training.

> **NCLEX Alert**
>
> When preparing for the NCLEX, utilize available NCLEX Review resources. These resources provide you with valuable practice clinical situations and options. The questions at the end of the chapter will help prepare you to think and to analyze the NCLEX's view of nursing concerns.

State Boards of Nursing

The legislative power to initiate, regulate, and enforce the provisions of the Nurse Practice Act is delegated to a specific state agency often known as the State Board of Nursing. The state governor may appoint Board members, but the criteria and credentials for Board members generally are written within the Nurse Practice Act. For example, in states with a single Board, the law usually requires that a specified number of licensed vocational/licensed practical nurses (**LVN/LPNs**) be Board members so that LVN/LPNs have a representative voice in affairs concerning them. The state nursing associations also make recommendations for Board appointments.

Boards are subject to legal parameters, but usually they have some leeway in interpreting aspects of the Nurse Practice Act. For example, the Board may define LVN/LPN limitations regarding working with intravenous lines and administering intravenous medications. The Boards work cooperatively with other regulating Boards, such as the Board of Medical Examiners and the Pharmacy Board. All state "Boards" may be part of one or more larger state agencies, such as the Department of Consumer Affairs or the Department of Health Services.

Sometimes, State Nursing Boards are known by other titles, such as the Board of Nurse Examiners. In the recent past, the State Boards of Nursing were responsible for the creation of the licensing examination (thus the name "Nurse Examiners"). However, the licensing examinations today are written by the National Council of State Boards of Nursing (NCSBN), which is discussed in this chapter.

Licensing laws vary from state to state in many respects. The goal of nurse planners is to establish uniform requirements so that a license issued in one state will be recognized in all states. A national nursing license has also been proposed.

The law or Nurse Practice Act in each state, province, or territory defines regulations for practical and registered nursing. Licensing and renewal fees generally provide revenue for the Boards.

The major concepts of the legislation of Nurse Practice Acts include the following:

- Definition of practical and registered nursing
- Nursing functions protected by the law
- Requirements for an approved school of nursing (e.g., length of program, curricula, admission requirements)
- Establishment of requirements for licensure (e.g., age, graduation from an approved course, criminal background screening checks)
- Process and procedures for becoming licensed in each state, territory, or province
- Procedures for maintaining licensure, including required continuing education
- Issuing and renewing nursing licenses
- Conditions under which a license may be suspended or revoked and conditions for reinstatement
- Procedures for transferring licenses from one state to another (interstate endorsement)

The facility in which you are employed has the right to limit the functions of a nurse. For example, a facility may state that only specially trained nurses may perform certain procedures—even if the Nurse Practice Act states that the nurse may legally do that procedure. However, a facility cannot allow a nurse to practice without a license or beyond the legal definitions of practice of that state.

Your employer may also require that you have additional education in specialized fields in order to work in that facility. Generally, training in cardiopulmonary resuscitation (**CPR**) is required by all clinical facilities. To work in specialty care units, such as geriatrics, wound care, intensive care, or pediatric care, your employer may require that you complete additional nursing courses. These advanced courses are generally not part of your nursing program and are not listed as educational requirements by the Nurse Practice Act. Education in nursing is a lifelong, continual process; a nurse never stops learning.

> **Key Concept**
> - Always practice within the limits of practical or registered nursing as you were taught.
> - Use good common sense and judgment.
> - Ask questions if you are unsure.
> - Report any errors immediately.
> - Report any defective equipment immediately.

Cause for Revoking or Suspending a License

The Nurse Practice Act defines conditions under which a license can be revoked. Such conditions include drug or alcohol abuse, fraud, deceptive practices, criminal acts, previous disciplinary action, and gross or ordinary negligence. For example, telling an employer that you are a registered nurse (**RN**) if you are actually an LVN/LPN is a deceptive practice and is cause for revoking the LVN/LPN license.

The Licensing Examination: the NCLEX

After successful completion of your nursing program, and before being able to practice as an LVN/LPN or RN, your first responsibility is to pass either the National Council Licensing Examination for Practical Nurses (**NCLEX-PN**) or the National Council Licensing Examination for Registered Nurses (**NCLEX-RN**).

The **NCSBN** is responsible for the NCLEX examinations. It is the National Council's responsibility to provide the State Boards of Nursing with a valid and reliable examination that can demonstrate that a licensure candidate has passed the examination with minimal competence to perform safe and effective entry-level nursing care. The purpose of the NCLEX-PN is to separate candidates into two groups: those who can pass with minimal entry-level knowledge and those who cannot.

The NCLEX-PN and NCLEX-RN are used by all 50 states, the District of Columbia, and the US territories of Guam, the Virgin Islands, American Samoa, Puerto Rico, and the Northern Mariana Islands. The NCLEX was first implemented in 1994 in a computerized form called computerized adaptive testing (**CAT**). Test questions are written by practicing clinical nurses and educators. Revisions to the CAT are made on a regular basis. Extensive surveys are conducted every 3 years to ensure that the test questions accurately reflect job tasks normally performed by the novice nurse. The NCLEX-PN has its most significant content areas in nursing process and client needs. Each of these two areas is further subdivided into specific subject areas. A further discussion of the NCLEX-PN plan is beyond the scope of this chapter.

Because of the nationwide utilization of the NCLEX, when a nurse moves from one state to another state, the nurse is not required to take another licensing examination. The nurse applies for licensure in the new state and may receive a license by the process of **endorsement**. Licensing fees and other fees may be required by the individual state, and the nurse may need to file specific documentation in the new state. The situation is similar in Canada, except in Ontario.

After you become licensed, you will be required to renew that license at specified intervals. Many states require both LVN/LPNs and RNs to take courses that document that you are maintaining currency in nursing. Continuing education classes must meet specified criteria. The classes are allotted continuing education units (**CEUs**) or continuing education hours (**CEHs**). The numbers of required units or hours are dictated by your State Board of Nursing and are commonly mandated for license renewal. Some states specify what courses must be taken. For example, Texas requires a course in jurisprudence and ethics; in New York, course content in child abuse is required for RN relicensure. On satisfactory completion of these courses, you will receive a certificate. You will be required to maintain your own records of continuing education courses. Your records may be audited by your State Board of Nursing.

Legal Responsibilities in Nursing

Safeguards for the Nurse and Student

Although as a practical or vocational nurse you are likely to work under the direction of other nurses and physicians, you are personally liable for any harm a client suffers as a result of your own acts. Healthcare facilities may also be legally liable for their employees' acts of negligence. Legal actions involving negligent acts by a person engaged in a profession may become malpractice lawsuits.

Commonsense Precautions
Follow Accepted Procedures
Protect yourself from possible lawsuits by always performing procedures as taught and as outlined in the procedure manual of your healthcare facility. If these policies are incorrect or inadequate, work to improve them through the proper channels.

Be Competent in Your Practice
You are always responsible for your own behavior. Refuse to perform procedures for which you have not been prepared. Ignorance is not a legal defense. Neither will lack of sleep nor overwork be accepted as a legal reason for carelessness about safety measures or mistakes.

Ask for Assistance
Always ask for help when you are unsure about how to perform a procedure. Do not assume responsibilities beyond those of your level. Admitting that you do not know how to

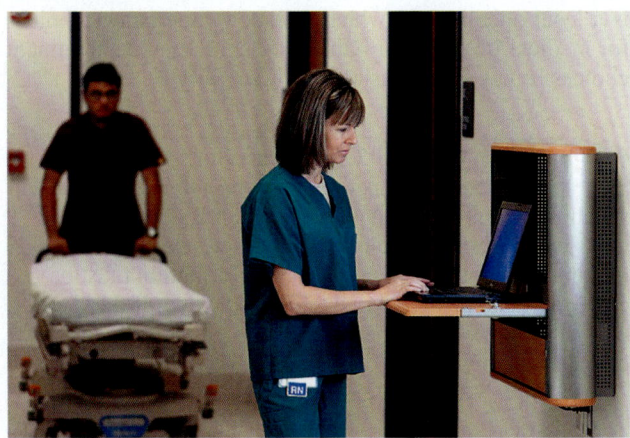

Figure 4-3 Careful documentation and reporting are nursing responsibilities and also help to maintain legal records (Weber, 2014).

perform a procedure is always better than attempting to do it and injuring someone. Also question any physician's order that you do not understand, cannot read, or in which you believe an error exists.

Document Well
The importance of keeping exact records of all treatments and medications, as well as a record of a client's reactions and behavior, cannot be overemphasized. The health record is the written and legal evidence of treatment. The record is to reflect facts only, not personal judgments. *Careful* and *accurate* documentation is vital for each client's welfare and your own (Fig. 4-3). Chapter 37 discusses documentation in detail.

> **Key Concept**
>
> Careful documentation is perhaps the most important thing you can do to protect yourself against an unjustified lawsuit. If you do not document a treatment or medication, legally the measure is considered not to have been done. You can be held accountable. Of course, you will be held accountable for performing an illegal or negligent act, whether or not you document it.

Do Not Give Legal Advice to Clients
The laws governing personal and property rights of an individual are many and complex. Never attempt to advise a client on legal rights or financial matters. Encourage clients to confer with their families and to consult an attorney.

Do Not Accept Gifts
Accepting gifts from clients is unwise for several reasons. Some clients are considered *vulnerable adults* (e.g., clients who are mentally ill or who have dementia). Exchange of gifts could compromise your professional position, and you could be accused of coercing the client. Some clients may feel that by accepting a gift, you now "owe" them special care or services. Because determining appropriate gift acceptance is difficult, the safest measure is to accept no gifts. An exception to this rule would be in the event that a client wishes to give candy or flowers to all staff on a hospital unit to share.

Do Not Help a Client Prepare a Will
Never attempt to help a client prepare a will or any other legal document. The law has formal requirements a will must meet to make it valid. As a graduate, you may be asked to witness the signing of a will. After the death of a client, you and other witnesses may be asked to testify as to the mental competence of the testator or to other conditions prevailing at the time of execution of the will.

Consider a Malpractice Insurance Policy
Malpractice insurance is available through private insurance companies and sometimes through the healthcare facility or a professional organization. The wise nurse carries malpractice insurance. Even if you are found innocent of charges in a case, preparing a defense still costs money. Malpractice insurance will cover these charges if you have practiced within the limits of your job description and level of training. Healthcare facilities usually carry umbrella liability insurance that covers the facility if an employee is named in a legal action. This insurance does not always protect the individual nurse; thus, having your own insurance is also important. Many professional and technical personnel protect themselves from paying court-imposed settlements by carrying private malpractice insurance.

Obtain the services of a lawyer specializing in medical/nursing malpractice at the first sign that you are involved in an illegal or negligent act or that you may be named in a lawsuit. Notify your malpractice carrier immediately because it may appoint an attorney for you. Insist on your legal rights. If you remember your limitations and practice within the scope of your education, you should have no difficulty with lawsuits and your clients will be safe. Box 4-1 gives examples of situations in which you may be held liable.

> **Key Concept**
>
> Malpractice insurance covers nurses only when they act "as any prudent nurse would." In other words, if you deliberately commit an illegal act or are negligent beyond accidental errors, your malpractice insurance and that of your employer will probably not be valid.

> **Box 4-1 Examples of Situations in Which Nurses Can Be Held Liable**
>
> - Burns, falls, or incorrect medications
> - Lack of common nursing judgment (e.g., using an oral thermometer for a confused or out-of-control client)
> - Failure to follow the policies of the healthcare facility to protect the client and their belongings
> - Allowing an unsafe condition to continue
> - Damages that arise from violation of the client's rights
> - Treatment without informed consent (can be considered assault and battery)
> - Stories, information, or photographs given without consent
> - Revelation of confidential information (HIPAA)[a]
> - Assault of one client by another client
>
> [a]Health Insurance Portability and Accountability Act of 1996.

Legal Concerns of Emergencies

In some states, the law requires any person who witnesses an automobile or other accident to give aid to persons injured in that accident. In most states, a person who has medical or nursing education is *required to assist*, if needed. In areas other than those to which this law applies, no person is legally obligated to render aid during an emergency. Each person who gives assistance should act as a reasonably prudent person would, within the limits of education and experience. Thus, as a nurse, you will be expected to render a higher level of emergency care than an untrained person. A law called the **Good Samaritan Act** is in effect in most states. This law protects you from liability if you give emergency care *within the limits of first aid* and if you act in a "reasonable and prudent manner."

Stay informed regarding legal issues surrounding all types of documentation.

Professional Boundaries

All healthcare personnel must maintain appropriate professional boundaries. Abstain from benefiting personally at the client's expense. Be sure to refrain from inappropriate involvement in the client's personal relationships. By doing so, you help to promote the client's independence. Remember the following important considerations:

- *Power versus vulnerability:* You, as a nurse, have power in your position and access to private client information. Do not exploit this power.
- *Boundary crossings:* Any questionable behavior should be brief, unintentional, and not repeated. Evaluate any such incidents immediately if they occur.
- *Boundary violations:* Excessive personal disclosures or asking clients to keep secrets are examples. Such actions can cause clients distress and are inappropriate.
- *Professional sexual misconduct:* Seductive, sexually demeaning, or harassing behavior is illegal and is a breach of the trust placed in you. Such misconduct constitutes just cause for dismissal from a job.

Remain helpful to clients without taking advantage of them. Your duty is to practice in the area of *therapeutic involvement*. Overinvolvement includes boundary crossings and violations, and sexual misconduct. Underinvolvement causes disinterest and client neglect.

Danger signals of overinvolvement include excessive self-disclosure, defensiveness about the relationship, believing that only you can meet a particular client's needs, spending excessive time with one client, flirting, or overt sexual acts. Evaluating each interaction you have with clients is vital to ensure that the relationship is helpful and that you are not over- or underinvolved. If you have questions, your nursing instructor or the facility's nursing supervisor can assist you.

ADVANCE DIRECTIVES

To preserve client's rights, all healthcare workers need to be aware of the client's wishes regarding continuing, withholding, or withdrawing treatment in the event the client cannot make these decisions for themselves. An **advance directive** is a legal document in which a person either states choices for medical treatment or names someone to make treatment choices if they lose decision-making ability.

> **Nursing Alert** Competent adults must speak for themselves. Another person cannot decide to withhold treatment, as long as the client is able to make decisions. If the client cannot talk, other means of communication may be used. Such information must be carefully documented, witnessed, and signed. If the person is legally incompetent, the court may make decisions about care.

The federal government passed the Patient Self-Determination Act (**PSDA**) in 1991. This law requires all healthcare institutions to comply with the provisions of this act or to forfeit reimbursement from Medicare and other types of funding. This legislation mandates an individual's right to some sort of advance directive. The law *requires* that all adults admitted to any healthcare facility must be asked if they have an advance directive and given assistance if they desire more information. Box 4-2 describes the nurse's role in carrying out mandates of this legislation.

Three major types of advance directives exist:

- Living will
- Directives to physicians
- Durable power of attorney for healthcare

Living Will

A *living will* is a written and legally witnessed document (but can be executed without an attorney) that requests no extraordinary measures to be taken to save a person's life in the event of terminal illness. The living will goes into effect only if the

---

Box 4-2 Advanced Directives and the Nurse's Responsibility

NURSING RESPONSIBILITIES INCLUDE
- Determining a client's understanding of the concepts of advance directives and the Patient Self-Determination Act *upon admission*.
- Providing pertinent literature/brochures that explain the functions and types of advance directives.
- Providing appropriate (nonnursing) assistance if client wishes to initiate or change an advance directive.
- Knowing that specific advance directives may apply to certain areas (e.g., in mental health units).
- Informing clients that they have the right to refuse treatment or can refuse life-prolonging measures but can still receive palliative care and pain control.
- Notifying healthcare providers of the existence of an advance directive.
- Placing the information in the designated records for the healthcare facility or agency.
- Maintaining copies according to protocols of the healthcare facility or agency.
- Documenting actions appropriately in the nursing records.

person becomes unable to make their own decisions regarding care. The living will may indicate life-sustaining treatments that the person does or does not want used and may specify comfort measures to be used or not used. Some form of living will legislation is in place throughout the United States. A great deal of controversy surrounds this issue. For example, in some states, living will legislation notes that artificial nutrition and hydration must be maintained, even if the person has previously requested that no artificial means be used to sustain life. In addition, various states have slightly different formats for living wills and do not necessarily recognize documents written in another state. A living will does not automatically expire in a certain length of time. It is in effect until the individual changes or revokes it. If a person has a living will, a copy is kept on file in the healthcare facility. Physicians and nurses are bound by the person's wishes.

> **Key Concept**
>
> If no documented evidence exists to the contrary, the healthcare team uses all means available to keep a person alive. Without a living will or other advance directive, a full "code" is called on all those who suffer a cardiac arrest, and full resuscitation efforts are made.

Directive to Physicians

A *directive to physicians* is another type of written document that can be useful for terminally ill adults who have no other person to name as their agent for making healthcare decisions. In this case, the person directs the healthcare provider to be their decision-maker. The physician must also agree, in writing, to accept this responsibility.

Durable Power of Attorney for Healthcare

In this written document, a client names another person to make healthcare decisions for them should the client become unable to do so. This designated person does not need to be a relative. Individuals should discuss *durable power of attorney* in advance with those they wish to designate as their decision-makers.

Mental Health Advance Declaration

In addition to the general advance declaration available to all persons, the *mental health advance declaration* establishes specific guidelines for psychiatric care. In this case, the mental health declaration specifies an individual's wishes concerning intrusive mental health treatment (e.g., electroconvulsive therapy and special types of medications called neuroleptics). Even if the person who refuses these treatments is committed as mentally ill or mentally ill and dangerous, these treatments may not be given without a specific court order.

VULNERABLE PERSONS

Children and some adults are considered vulnerable to deficient or harmful care. Reporting suspected child abuse or vulnerable adult abuse is mandatory in the United States and Canada. In addition, most states have laws protecting persons considered to be vulnerable, which includes almost any hospitalized individual. Laws protecting the vulnerable are particularly important for those who work with clients who have mental illness or have intellectual disabilities. Older people are often considered vulnerable adults. The law protects vulnerable persons from injury, abuse, or neglect while receiving care in a healthcare facility, nursing home, school, or their own home. Often, a person's isolation in their own home can increase the person's vulnerability. Families can also be charged with abuse under the vulnerable adult laws (Chapter 98 discusses home care issues.).

DEFINITIONS OF DEATH

Prior to the mid-20th century, the legal definition of death was universally accepted to be the loss of vital functions, that is, no pulse, no blood pressure, and no respirations. When technology was developed that could sustain an individual's heartbeat and respirations, confusion occurred. It now became possible for a machine to pump blood and to provide oxygenation (breathe) for the client. However, without this artificial intervention, it was possible that this same client would not have a blood pressure or oxygenation. Therefore, medical practice, the legal profession, and society needed alternate ways of defining death that would take into account the rapid advances in technological healthcare.

The traditional definition of **legal death** is the same as that for **clinical death** or **biological death**—that is, death due to the absence of respirations and the absence of a heartbeat.

With today's advanced life support systems, however, new criteria were needed other than the absence of breathing and heartbeat because in some cases the physical body may be kept functioning for long periods of time by artificial means.

The Uniform Determination of Death Act of 1980 is the accepted standard of brain death. In a unique collaboration, the American Medical Association, the American Bar Association, and the President's Commission for the Study of Ethical Problems in Medicine and Behavioral Research worked to differentiate death caused by the loss of vital functions or by the loss of neurological functions. The two major definitions of death are as follows:

1. Legal death—The legal definition of death states that an individual who is dead is one who has sustained loss of circulation and respiratory functions.
2. Brain death—Brain death considers the irreversible cessation of all neurological functions of the entire brain, including the brain stem, to signify death.

In brain death, the brain has a lack of response to stimuli, lack of cephalic reflexes (see below), and absent stimulation to breathe. Criteria for the diagnosis of brain death include the following:

- *Cessation of breathing* after artificial ventilation is discontinued (usually requires cessation for at least 3 minutes).
- *Cessation of heartbeat* without external stimuli.
- *Unresponsiveness* to external stimuli.

- *Complete absence of cephalic reflexes* (the lowest form of brain stem reflexes). Some states accept the absence of some cephalic reflexes.
- *Pupils fixed and dilated.* Some states accept pupils unresponsive to light, but not necessarily dilated.
- *Irreversible cessation of all functions of the brain.* In some states, this includes all functions of the brain stem as well. This brain and brain stem function can be assessed by evaluation of reflexes. In some cases, one or more electroencephalograms (EEG) are done to confirm the diagnosis of clinical death.

Brain death is also termed an *irreversible coma*. Many individuals have a condition called a *vegetative state* or a *permanent vegetative state*, and these individuals may also be considered to be brain dead even though some types of brain wave functions are seen on an EEG. When a client is in a vegetative state, they can seem to be awake because their eyes might be open. They can have spontaneous movement owing to muscle reflexes; however, these movements are not related to cognitive function or senescence. The person can be pronounced legally dead and be designated the "right to die" if nutrition or artificial physical methods are not used to sustain the organ systems.

> **Key Concept**
> Owing to technological interventions, death is defined more as a process of irreversible brain functioning than a specific condition of clinical demise. When defined by a qualified professional, a client, who has no brain activity, but who has functioning respiratory and circulatory systems, can be declared legally dead. Determination of clinical death is complex and controversial. Check the laws in your state.

A client with the diagnosis of brain death may be considered a donor candidate for organ transplantation. The diagnosis of death is a legal and ethical concern to healthcare providers. Before removal of organs or tissues for donation, especially when a person's vital processes are being maintained artificially, the wishes of the client and the family need to be in harmony with legal regulations.

Exceptions

In all cases that may involve the determination of death, the following *exceptions* are identified:

- Marked hypothermia (core body temperature below 90 °F [32.2 °C], such as might follow a near-drowning episode)
- Severe depression of the central nervous system (CNS) after drug overdose with a CNS depressant, such as a barbiturate

ETHICAL STANDARDS OF HEALTHCARE

Ethics is defined as conduct appropriate for all members of a group. Chapter 2 gives standards of nursing practice. A code of ethics builds on these standards. Today, healthcare workers confront many ethical issues that have arisen as a result of increased knowledge and technology, changing demographic patterns, and consumer demands.

Prejudice, Personal Values, and Nursing

Each individual brings personal values to the healthcare system. These values include beliefs about such concepts as life and death, a higher power, who should receive healthcare and what kind of care, and complex issues, such as abortion and euthanasia. Values are the culmination of heritage, culture, and one's family of origin, combined with life experiences. Values evolve as life situations change. A person's values may change when faced with illness, injury, and possible death. To be of optimal support to each client, you must undergo your own personal values clarification process.

Consciously examining your own values, beliefs, and feelings about life and healthcare issues is helpful because it provides you with a frame of reference. Your beliefs may be different from those of your peers and clients. Prejudice in nursing is imposing your beliefs and value system onto others. When practicing nursing, your personal beliefs and those of your clients may be radically different. Remember, however, that you must also allow clients the freedom to formulate and to express their own values. *Do not impose your values on clients.*

> **Key Concept**
> Be aware of your feelings and behavior. Always act in the client's best interests.

Quality of Life

Quality of life is a complicated ethical issue. At what point does the healthcare team decide that a person should receive treatment or not? For example, not enough donated organs or specialized facilities are available to serve everyone who needs them. How then is the decision made as to who receives lifesaving treatment and who does not? Healthcare ethics comes into play in such decisions.

Part of the discussion as to who receives treatment centers around the quality of life expected following treatment. Can treatment measurably improve the quality of a person's life or life expectancy? Would others benefit more? Who decides on the quality of another person's life? Who makes the decision as to who lives and who dies? What determines quality of life? Some suggested criteria include ability to work, ability to function physically, chronological age, contributions to society, happiness or satisfaction with life, ability to care for oneself, and the person and family's opinions.

> **Key Concept**
> The client's right to confidentiality is always important (Box 4-3).

Nurses' Role Regarding Ethics

You are expected to practice ethically. Because of the intimate nature of nursing, you are often the first person to recognize that an ethical problem exists. You are responsible for bringing forth these issues and for participating in decision making. Whether nursing practice occurs in the United States, Canada, or the international community, basic ideas remain the same.

> **Box 4-3 Right to Confidentiality**
>
> As delegated by the Health Insurance Portability and Accountability Act (HIPAA) of 1996, the client has the right to expect that their privacy will be protected. *Privacy* means that information is available to the client but not to the public. Information collected may be used to provide effective care, develop treatment guidelines, determine ability to pay for care, bill third-party payers, and anonymously conduct research studies. The client may refuse to give information, but in this case, the quality of care may be limited by lack of information.
>
> For detailed information regarding confidentiality rules, regulations, and issues, go to the Health and Human Services website (see Web Resources on thePoint).

Ethical Issues in Treatment

Examples of some major issues in healthcare ethics are presented below. Some issues that were mentioned in the legal section of this chapter are also issues for ethical debate.

Organ Transplantation

Many organs are successfully transplanted from person to person. In some cases, as in heart transplant, the donor must be pronounced legally dead before the organ can be removed. To keep the organ at its healthiest, however, it must be recovered at the moment the donor is pronounced clinically dead. In most cases, circulation and ventilation are artificially maintained until the organ is removed.

These situations involve such issues as defining clinical death and informed consent. Organ donation is a difficult decision for a family to make at such a traumatic time. A person can simplify matters in advance by designating that they wish to be an organ donor on an organ donor card or a driver's license.

The United Network of Organ Sharing (**UNOS**) was established to ensure fairness in the receipt of donated organs. This computerized network links all procurement organizations and maintains a list of potential organ recipients. UNOS has established specific criteria to determine which recipient will be eligible to receive a donated organ.

> *Key Concept*
>
> Even if a person designates themselves as a "donor" on a driver's license, the next of kin usually must give permission after death. If you wish to be an organ donor, discuss your feelings with your family now.

Criteria and Questions

Criteria of UNOS attempt to answer questions such as the follows: Who should receive treatment (i.e., donated organs)? Why should this client receive an organ and not another client? Who will pay for the treatment? Many questions and factors influence decisions to give or to withhold treatment; legal and ethical considerations may be part of the criteria. Organ donations can cost hundreds of thousands of dollars and who should have the responsibility of paying for the surgery as well as the long-term care of the client.

Refusal of Treatment

Additional concerns may involve the refusal of treatment. Can a client legally refuse treatment? Under what circumstances does the client lose the right to refuse treatment? Another consideration is should treatment be given, even against the person's will.

If the healthcare team makes the decision to provide treatment, it is called *beneficence*. If the client makes the decision, it is termed *autonomy*. Usually a person gives permission for treatment; thus, refusal is seen as reversal of that permission. States debate the individual's right to refuse lifesaving treatment. If any argument among family members or doubt on the part of the healthcare team exists, *treatment must be given* until the case is resolved in court.

Withholding Treatment

Withholding treatment means denial of treatment or care because treatment has been deemed inappropriate, not enough of a particular treatment is available, which may occur with donor kidneys or dialysis, or the client or family has refused it. In some circumstances, a court order must be obtained before treatment may be withheld or removed. If a person refuses treatment and it is illegally given, the healthcare team can be charged with battery.

The only time a person does not have the right to make the decision to refuse treatment is when the greater public interest would be in danger. For example, if a person has a communicable disease or is in immediate danger of harming self or others and refuses treatment, legal action may be taken.

Termination of Treatment

Termination of treatment, or withdrawal of treatment, involves the conscious decision to stop treatment once it has been started. The treatment may be withdrawn at the client's request or when the healthcare team determines brain death has occurred. Stopping treatment once it has begun is often more difficult legally than is withholding treatment altogether.

Euthanasia

In the past, euthanasia was called "mercy killing." It meant the deliberate taking of a person's life to put the individual out of misery. This definition has been amended to include the withdrawal or withholding of treatment. A great deal of discussion and controversy has occurred in recent years about **assisted suicide**. The laws surrounding this ethical problem differ among states.

The Ethics Committee

Healthcare facilities have ethics committees made up of healthcare professionals, chaplains, social workers, and others (Fig. 4-4). The chief functions of the ethics

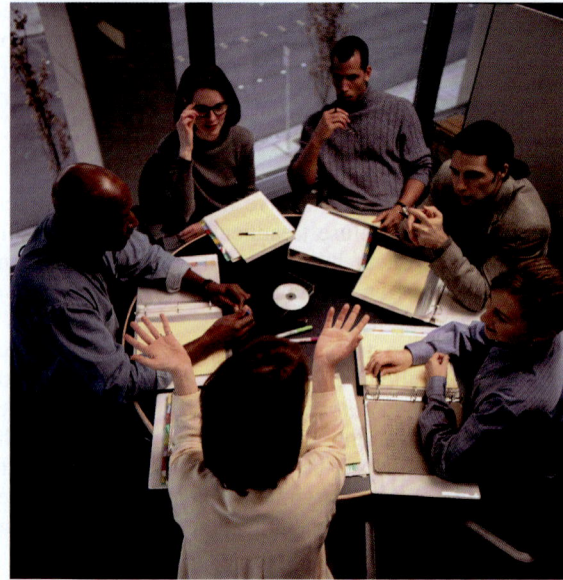

Figure 4-4 The ethics committee may be composed of nurses, physicians, social workers, religious leaders, and community members.

committee are education, policy-making, case review, and consultation. These committees are important because they bring together a variety of healthcare workers from various disciplines. They are able to share ideas and concerns related to their field. Many nurses bring a unique voice to the committee because they act as an advocate for their clients.

CLIENTS' RIGHTS AND RESPONSIBILITIES

Clients also have rights and responsibilities. The concept of clients' rights stems from the rise of the consumer movement. The public demands the right to quality care.

Clients' Rights

The rights of the individual, client, or patient were first formally addressed in 1972 by the American Hospital Association (**AHA**). The AHA adopted *A Patient's Bill of Rights*, which stated the rights of hospitalized individuals. Since then, other healthcare agencies and services have provided a variety of bills of rights specifically designed to address the needs of their clients. For example, bills of rights are available for Home Care or Hospice Care. Older bills of rights may still apply to the situations or environments for which they were written. The AHA, medical and nursing organizations, and other consumer/client agencies provide guidelines that serve as a basis for decision making in hospital care. The applicable bill of rights is generally posted per accrediting regulations in public viewing areas of the healthcare center.

The Affordable Care Act of 2010 initiated and updated a Patient's Bill of Rights with the focus on protecting clients from specific actions of the healthcare insurance industry.

The guidelines of the various versions of the assorted bills of rights help to ensure the concept of basic human rights and are widely accepted among healthcare providers. Consumer support and information may be found listed at www.cms.gov (the Center for Consumer Information and Insurance Oversight).

> **Key Concept**
>
> Clients are active participants in their own healthcare and need to be provided with information regarding their own health.

Clients' Responsibilities

In addition to the rights of a client, the *responsibilities* of the client have become a significant part of their self-care and welfare. Recognized as a priority, the client is an active participant in formulating their care plan and making healthcare decisions. The client also has a responsibility to participate in and cooperate with care given. Certain cooperative actions can be expected from clients. Your duties as a nurse are to help your clients understand their responsibilities, teach them how to enhance their recovery process, and assist them to attain their greatest level of health and wellness.

> **Key Concept**
>
> *In some cases*, the healthcare provider also has the right to bring charges against a client for an unlawful act, such as a physical attack.

To summarize various organizations' sets of identified responsibilities of the client, see the following bulleted list.

The client has the responsibility to

- Recognize that healthcare is a partnership among the client, the client's family/significant others, and all healthcare providers.
- Provide an accurate and up-to-date medical history including (but not limited to): current health status, past medical illnesses and surgeries, hospitalizations, medications and nonprescription drugs, allergies/sensitivities, results of previous therapies, and family histories.
- Request additional information and clarification about health status or treatment if the current information or instructions are not completely clear.
- Recognize the impact of personal lifestyle choices on health and to make positive lifestyle changes to improve their own health.
- Ensure that the healthcare institution has a copy of their written advance directive, if one is completed.
- Inform physicians and other caregivers if they anticipate problems in following prescribed treatment.
- Respect the facility's rules and regulations and responsibilities to other clients and the community.
- Provide necessary information and to assist in the process of payment for services.

STUDENT SYNTHESIS

KEY POINTS

- You are legally and ethically bound to practice nursing within the rules and regulations of your Nurse Practice Act and within the laws of your state, territory, or province.
- You must be knowledgeable about the concepts and terminology of the legal aspects of healthcare as well as the basic concepts of law.
- Several types of advance directives allow individuals to plan ahead and to make decisions in advance about healthcare to be received if they become incapacitated.
- Individuals have the right to accept or to refuse treatment in most situations.
- You will encounter many ethical decisions in healthcare. Some of these require the assistance of an ethics committee.
- The client has the responsibility to inform healthcare providers of pertinent information and to assist in their own care by accurately following treatment plans.

CRITICAL THINKING EXERCISES

1. Discuss how your personal values relate to your choice of nursing as a profession. Discuss how you think this will relate to your nursing practice in the future.
2. As you come on duty, you check your client's chart and notice that he received an injection of Demerol 100 mg at 2:00 PM and again at 3:30 PM today. Two different nurses administered these injections. Administration of the medication is ordered for every 4 hours.
   a. Which actions would you take and why?
   b. Which legal implications apply to this situation?
   c. Discuss this situation in relationship to the importance of documentation.
   d. Has a crime been committed? Why or why not?
3. You see a licensed nurse at the facility where you work take some money out of a coworker's backpack. Which actions would you take and why? How does this scenario affect your coworker's nursing license? How could it affect your nursing license (if you were licensed at this time)?
4. You are working part-time in a hospital while you attend school. A client there is being discharged tomorrow and asks you on a date next Saturday. (Assume that you are single and find the client attractive.)
   a. What is your response? Why?
   b. What are the legal implications of dating a client?

NCLEX-STYLE REVIEW QUESTIONS

1. A student nurse approaches the instructor and states, "the staff nurse told me to witness this surgical consent after the surgeon signs it." Which is the best response by the instructor?
   a. "Students are not to serve as a witness to legal papers. Let's explain this to the staff nurse so they may have it witnessed."
   b. "You will need another student to go with you to cosign the consent."
   c. "That is fine. Do you want me to come with you?"
   d. "This type of consent doesn't need to be witnessed."

2. The nurse is caring for a client that has been confused and climbing out of the bed. Which action should the nurse take if the nurse must leave the room to take care of another client?
   a. Place all four side rails up and come back and check on the client when finished with the other task.
   b. Place the client in soft wrist restraints so the client will not get out of the bed.
   c. Inform the client not to get out of the bed.
   d. Don't leave the client alone and request that another nurse sit one-on-one with the client.

3. A nurse discovers that a neighbor is a client on the unit in which the nurse works although the nurse is not assigned to care for that client. The nurse accesses the electronic medical record (EMR) to find out what the client's diagnosis is. Which action may clients take if they are aware of this type of incident?
   a. Report the incident as a HIPAA violation.
   b. Sue the nurse for libel.
   c. Sue the nurse for negligence.
   d. Report the nurse for defamation.

4. A staff nurse comes to work and accepts the assignment of clients. After a verbal altercation with the nurse manager about the assignment, the nurse states "I quit" and leaves the facility. Which action may the nurse manager take?
   a. Call to ask the nurse to come back.
   b. Report the nurse for abandonment of care.
   c. Have the police arrest the nurse.
   d. Let the nurse cool off and come back when ready.

5. A client is to be transferred from the acute care facility to a rehabilitation facility after suffering a stroke. The nurse is gathering papers to send to the accepting facility but is unsure what to send. Which action should the nurse take?
   a. Send the entire chart.
   b. Consult the charge nurse.
   c. Call the transferring physician and ask what to send.
   d. Only send the demographic information.

CHAPTER RESOURCES

Enhance your learning with additional resources on thePoint!

Student Resources related to this chapter can be found at **thePoint.lww.com/Rosdahl12e**.

Personal and Environmental Health | UNIT 2

5 Basic Human Needs

Learning Objectives

1. Describe and discuss the hierarchy of needs, from the simple to the complex, as developed by Maslow.
2. Define the term *regression* and explain at least two examples of regression.
3. List at least five physiologic needs of all people and animals.
4. Compare Maslow's hierarchy of needs with the more specific hierarchy of needs related to healthcare clients and nursing care.
5. List two examples of nursing activities that help an individual meet basic physiologic human needs.
6. List two examples of nursing activities that help an individual meet the needs of security and safety.
7. List two examples of nursing activities that help an individual obtain the goal of self-esteem.
8. List two examples of nursing activities that help an individual obtain the goal of self-actualization.
9. Address the deficiency or basic needs with the growth or aesthetic needs of individuals who are homeless, who have a terminal illness, or who have lost their jobs and source of income.
10. Relate at least three community or societal needs to the hierarchy of needs of an individual.

Important Terminology

deficiency needs	physiologic needs	psychological needs	secondary needs	social needs
growth needs	primary needs		self-actualized	survival needs
hierarchy of needs	priority needs	regression	self-esteem	

In 1943, psychologist Abraham H. Maslow described a theory of human needs that identified simple basic needs in relation to the more complex, higher level needs. These needs are common to all people regardless of age, sex, race, social class, and state of health (well or ill). Maslow asserted that people respond to needs and need satisfaction as whole and integrated beings.

Nursing has been defined as a helping relationship. As a nurse, you will help people to satisfy their basic needs and to reduce threats to this need fulfillment. Dorothea Orem's theory of nursing (see Chapter 2) and many nursing programs and textbooks are based on Maslow's theory of needs. This textbook incorporates Maslow's hierarchy of needs. Most types of nursing care are prioritized using the same hierarchy. This chapter summarizes Maslow's hierarchy of human needs and explains their relationship to health and nursing care.

MASLOW'S HIERARCHY OF HUMAN NEEDS

Maslow defined the basic needs of all people as a progression from simple survival—or physical—needs, called **deficiency** needs, to more complex needs related to personal fulfillment, called **growth needs**. We can refer to the deficiency or basic needs as priority needs. *Prioritization of needs is an extremely important concept of nursing.* A client must meet the needs within the foundation of the hierarchy (i.e., priorities), before working toward the higher level growth needs. For example, individuals must first meet needs related to deficiency, such as oxygen, food, safety, and belonging before being able to progress to the more abstract growth needs. Maslow called this progression a **hierarchy of needs**. On this hierarchy, typically illustrated by a pyramid (Fig. 5-1), needs are ranked from the lowest to the highest levels of importance to the individual's survival.

In the 1970s, the five stages of needs were expanded to eight steps. The additional steps are cognitive (#6), aesthetic (#7), and transcendence needs (#8). These addendum needs are generally used in advanced discussions of the original five steps. In the eight-step variation of the pyramid, the individual understands and explores life; appreciates symmetry, order, and beauty; and connects with the ability to help others to realize their potential. However, basic life-supportive measures remain the first, fundamental step of the hierarchy.

Meeting needs is a process; it is never static. In addition, needs are interrelated and some needs depend on others.

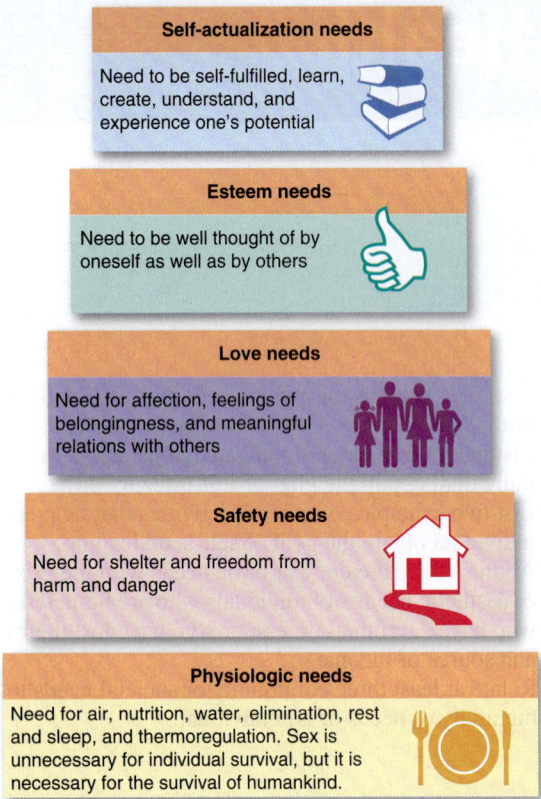

Figure 5-1 Hierarchy of needs. According to Maslow, basic physiologic needs, such as for food and water, must be met before a person can move on to higher level needs, such as security and safety. Nursing is based on helping people to meet the needs they cannot meet by themselves because of age, illness, or injury. (From Craven, R. F., & Hirnle, C. J. [2012]. *Fundamentals of nursing: Human health and function* [7th ed.]. Wolters Kluwer Health/Lippincott Williams & Wilkins.)

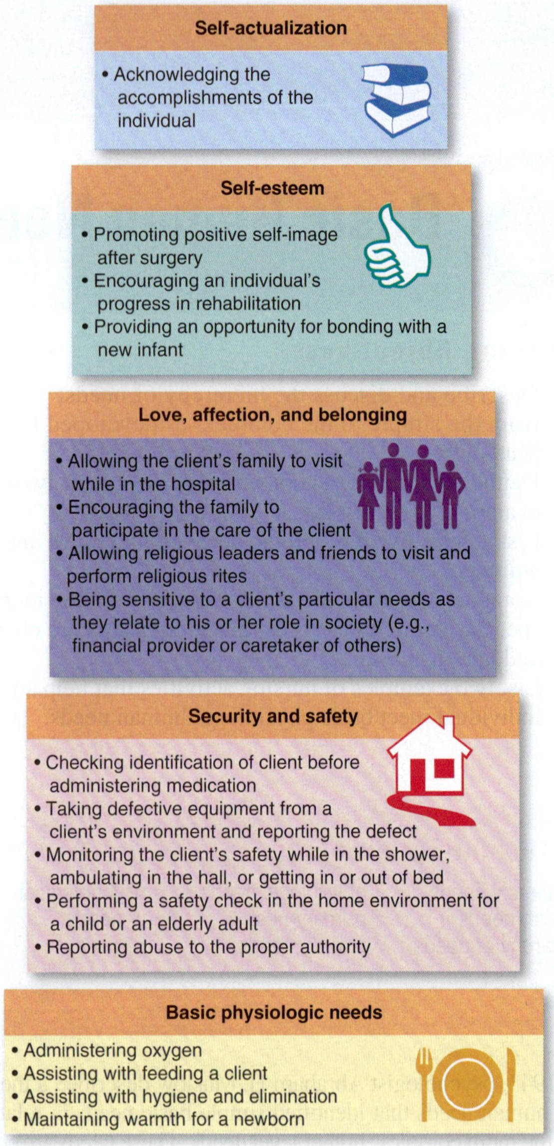

> **NCLEX Alert**
>
> The concepts within Maslow's hierarchy of needs are fundamental components of correct NCLEX options because they address priority needs. You may be given more than one correct response, but you must choose the best, most appropriate response. Maslow's hierarchy of priorities often presents clues to the correct answer.

Figure 5-2 Hierarchy of needs and nursing interventions. Nursing actions and Maslow's hierarchy can take many forms. This figure gives examples of nursing interventions that can assist a client to meet basic and aesthetic human needs. The hierarchy begins at the bottom and works upward.

NURSING'S RELATIONSHIP TO BASIC NEEDS

The nurse must remain aware that basic **survival needs** are the primary nursing priorities. When the survival needs are met, people can progress to more complex needs, such as safety, love, and self-esteem (Fig. 5-2). For example, people who are hungry will not be concerned about cleanliness (e.g., cleaning a wound) or learning (e.g., discharge planning) until they have a constant, reliable source of food. Individuals in pain will not be concerned about personal appearance or relationships with others until pain is relieved. Those facing surgery will not be able to learn about the operation unless they feel safe and secure. **Regression**, or focusing on a lower level need that has already been fulfilled, is common in illness or injury. For example, a client recovering from an illness will focus their physical and emotional energies on recovery (physical needs) before returning to employment (security).

Many situations will arise in which you will assist clients to meet their needs. You may feed an infant, provide full range of motion for a person who has had a stroke, administer a tube feeding to a person who cannot swallow, bathe a person who is in a full body cast, or play with a child. You may encourage the recovering person to attend to personal care, visit with someone who is lonely or frightened, or arrange for a social worker or a member of the clergy to visit. This text discusses issues common to all people, noting that individual needs may be unique. Illness may modify a person's perception of their needs. As a result, the client's "need priority" may differ from what you, the nurse, would expect. Illness or injury may present a block or obstacle to the meeting of needs. Nursing tries to help remove those obstacles.

In many cases, nursing priorities can be determined by observation. You may be able to determine the client's survival, safety, or belonging needs by looking at them. For example,

- Survival needs—is the client lacking oxygen? The nurse looks for cyanosis (blueness of skin) and difficulty breathing.
- Safety needs—is the client likely to fall? The nurse looks for an unsteady gait, bruising on the limbs, or a history of paralysis.
- Belonging needs—is the client crying, depressed, or angry? The nurse looks for isolation from others or an inability to control frustrations.

Listening to the client is also helpful. The client may tell the nurse that they are hungry, thirsty, or in pain.

> **Key Concept**
> Nursing is concerned with helping clients meet their physical, spiritual, and psychological needs. Much of nursing deals with assisting clients to meet basic physiologic needs that they cannot meet independently.

OVERVIEW OF INDIVIDUAL NEEDS

Basic Physiologic Needs

First-level needs are called **physiologic needs**, survival needs, or **primary or priority needs**. Without them, a person will die. *They take precedence over higher level needs.* Priority needs must be met to sustain life; **secondary needs** are met to give quality to life.

> **Key Concept**
> *Deficiency* or *physiologic needs* are priority needs and must be met first in order to maintain life. Growth needs are *secondary needs*, which must be met to maintain quality of life. Deficiency needs are the nurses' priority, but growth needs remain important concepts for the client and the nurse.

Oxygen

Oxygen is the most essential of all basic survival needs. Without oxygen circulating in the bloodstream, a person will die in a matter of minutes. Oxygen is provided to the cells by maintaining an open airway and adequate circulation.

As a nurse, you will constantly evaluate the oxygenation status of your clients. Various situations can threaten the body's oxygen supply. For example, emphysema, asthma, paralysis, or secretions may make breathing difficult; circulation may be impaired, thus preventing oxygen from reaching the cells. Some breathing difficulties also have an emotional component.

Water and Fluids

Water is necessary to sustain life. The body can survive only a few days without water, although certain conditions may alter this length of time. For example, the person in a very hot climate needs more water and fluids to sustain life than the person in a cold climate. The fluids in the body must also be in balance, or homeostasis, to maintain health.

Examples of conditions in which individuals may require assistance to meet their fluid needs include unconsciousness, inability to swallow, and severe mental illness. If the kidneys do not function, the body may retain water in the tissues (edema) or the body may not have enough water (dehydration). The nurse can assist in these conditions by measuring intake and output, weighing the client daily, and observing intravenous infusion of fluids.

Food and Nutrients

Nutrients are necessary to maintain life, although the body can survive for several days or weeks without food. Poor nutritional habits, inability to chew or swallow, nausea and vomiting, food allergies, refusal to eat, and overeating pose threats to a client's nutritional status. The nurse helps by feeding the client, monitoring calorie counts, or maintaining alternative methods of nutrition such as tube feedings or assisting with intravenous infusions.

Elimination of Waste Products

Elimination of the body's waste products is essential for life and comfort. The body eliminates wastes in several ways. The lungs eliminate carbon dioxide and water; the skin eliminates water and sodium; the kidneys eliminate fluids and electrolytes; the intestines discharge solid wastes and fluids. If the body should inappropriately allow wastes to accumulate, many serious conditions can result.

A bowel obstruction, bladder cancer, kidney disease, and gallbladder disease disrupt normal elimination. Difficulty in breathing, poor circulation, acid–base imbalance, allergies, cuts, wounds, diabetes, and infection also hinder adequate elimination.

The nurse may help the client eliminate wastes by giving an enema, catheterizing the client, or assisting with dialysis. You may assist with surgery to eliminate a bowel obstruction and administer medications to relieve diarrhea or constipation. You may give oxygen to assist with breathing. You may inject insulin for the diabetic client to aid in proper carbohydrate metabolism.

Sleep and Rest

Sleep and rest are important in maintaining health. The amount of sleep a client needs is influenced by factors such as pregnancy, age, and general health. The absence of sleep is not immediately life threatening, but it can cause various disorders if allowed to continue. For example, sleep deprivation aggravates some forms of mental illness.

The nurse can assist clients to get enough sleep and rest by providing safe, comfortable, and quiet surroundings. Various treatments such as a soothing back rub, warm tub bath, warm milk, and certain medications can also promote sleep.

Activity and Exercise

Activity stimulates both the mind and body. Exercise helps maintain the body's structural integrity and health by enhancing circulation and respiration. Mobility is not necessary for survival, but some form of exercise is needed to maintain optimum health.

The nurse can assist the client to obtain needed exercise in many ways. Examples include encouraging a person to walk after surgery, teaching a client to walk with crutches, providing passive range of motion, and teaching the person in a cast to do exercises. Clients in nursing homes are encouraged to exercise, even if they are confined to wheelchairs. Physical therapists and nurses work together to assist clients with rehabilitation of injured bones and muscles. The person who is paralyzed from the waist down can do push-ups in bed and many other upper body exercises. Turning the immobilized person often helps to prevent lung problems, skin breakdown, circulatory problems, bowel obstruction, and pressure wounds (bedsores).

Sexual Gratification

Sexual gratification is important; however, unlike other basic physiologic needs, sexual gratification may be sublimated. The need for sex is not vital to the survival of the individual, but it is vital to the survival of the species.

The nurse will need to be aware of sexuality issues when care is given. Perhaps an older male client is not comfortable with a younger male or female nurse. A client may also wish to discuss sexual problems with you. As part of the assessment, the nurse may learn that the client has concerns relating to sexual issues. For example, the client recovering from surgery may be concerned about the physical effects of sexual intercourse on a healing incision. Remember that age or physical disability usually does not eliminate a person's desire for sexual activity.

Temperature Regulation

Several factors can threaten the body's need for temperature regulation, including excessive external heat or cold or a high internal fever in response to an infection. The human body functions within a relatively narrow survival range of temperatures. Core temperature survival ranges for the human body (under usual circumstances) are given below using equivalent values from the Celsius and Fahrenheit scales:

- Celsius physiologic compatible range = 35 °C–41 °C;
    - "Average" oral temperature = 37 °C
- Fahrenheit physiologic compatible range = 95 °F to 106 °F;
    - "Average" oral temperature = 98.6 °F

The body has mechanisms to assist in temporary regulation of body temperature. These mechanisms include shivering, goose flesh, and perspiration. The nurse will assist

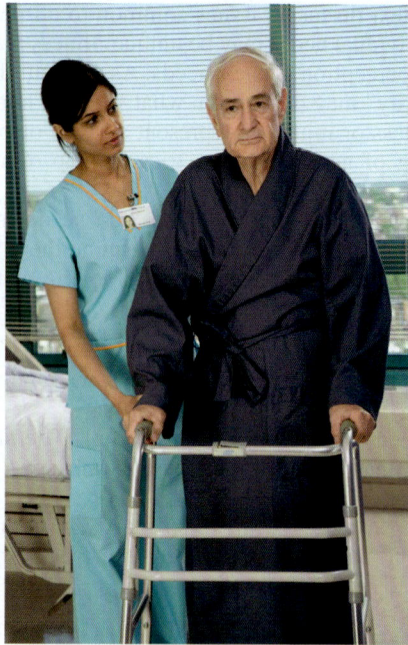

Figure 5-3 Security and safety needs can be met by helping the client ambulate using a walker. Notice how the nurse uses her body position and her arms to anticipate helping the client in case of loss of balance. (From Craven, R. F., & Hirnle, C. J. [2012]. *Fundamentals of nursing: Human health and function* [7th ed.]. Wolters Kluwer Health/Lippincott Williams & Wilkins.)

clients to meet the need for temperature regulation in cases such as a severe burn, a high fever, or exposure to extreme heat (heat stroke) or cold (hypothermia, frostbite) by monitoring the client's temperature and providing treatment for the effects of thermal damage.

Security and Safety Needs

The second level of Maslow's hierarchy of needs relates to safety. At this level, there are both physical and **psychological needs** (Fig. 5-3).

Freedom from Harm

People must feel safe and secure, both physically and emotionally, before being comfortable enough to move on to meet other needs. They must feel free from harm, danger, and fear. Characteristics of safety include predictability, stability, and familiarity, as well as feeling safe and comfortable and trusting other people. Financial security is also a component of this need.

Safety adaptations are made for age, whether the person is an older adult or an infant. The person who is physically challenged often needs special adaptations. The nurse may assist in removing threats to safety from the client's environment. Examples include using proper handwashing techniques, preventing wound infections by using sterile dressings, using a night light, disabling the gas stove in the home of a person with Alzheimer's disease, and locking up poisons in the home to safeguard small children. The nurse can explain to clients their surgical procedure before surgery, as well as any other treatments or medications. Such discussion can help clients feel safer and can aid in postoperative recovery.

> **Key Concept**
> Any type of abuse is a threat to the basic need for safety and security. If a person feels unsafe, they cannot pursue higher level needs.

Abuse

Abuse inside or outside a home has always existed. Society is becoming less tolerant of all types of abuse. Legal penalties for abuse are becoming more severe. Abuse may take the form of spousal or partner battering, child abuse, or rape by family members or others. Psychological abuse may have longer lasting scars than physical abuse. Often, people find it difficult to escape from abusive situations for many reasons. Resources within the community can assist victims. The nurse is legally bound to report any instances where it is suspected clients are experiencing abuse. Remember that abuse also can occur in the healthcare facility. Abuse must be reported immediately.

> **Nursing Alert** If you, as a nurse, do not report suspected abuse, you could be subject to arrest and civil penalties.

Healthcare

Consider higher level coping skills in relationship with planned versus unplanned healthcare. People whose incomes are below the federal poverty threshold, who experience food insecurity, or homelessness, or those who feel unsafe are unable to plan ahead for healthcare. In most cases, people in these situations become ill first and then seek healthcare. Such behaviors are concrete methods of dealing with illness, or emergency responses to the stimulus of illness (episodic healthcare). People in developing countries often have no access at all to healthcare. Their healthcare needs are unmet, thus shortening their life expectancy.

People in more comfortable situations are able to strive for wellness and prevention of illness (see Chapter 6). They experience a more abstract means of coping and of seeking healthcare. Abstract thinking and action require higher level skills, including planning and being able to understand the consequences of being unprepared.

Shelter

A lack of adequate shelter may not always be life threatening, but it will thwart the ability of a person to progress toward a higher level of needs. A person's shelter should provide the warmth necessary to maintain an adequate body temperature, in addition to helping the person feel safe.

A large number of Americans experience homelessness, including significant numbers of children. Often, healthcare providers are unaware that a client is experiencing homelessness. Be alert when interviewing clients; a comprehensive evaluation is often needed to uncover this situation because the person may be embarrassed or ashamed.

The person caring for children who experiences homelessness faces great challenges. Such individuals not only must find food and shelter for themselves, but for their children as well. Safety is an issue, because it is more difficult to protect themselves and their children at the same time. The children lack a sense of security because they do not know where they belong and often do not understand what is happening.

Those who experience homelessness spend most of their energy trying to cope with daily life. They may travel great distances by foot to locate food and other necessities. They face the constant dangers of disease, frostbite, or physical harm from others. They often must move from place to place, sometimes to avoid the law or to fulfill time limits in shelters. Many people who are homeless carry all their belongings with them to avoid theft. With all of these contributing factors, these individuals have little emotional energy left to worry about meaningful relationships, belonging to a group, maintaining cleanliness, or going to school. No time exists to be creative. Finding a permanent job without an address or telephone is almost impossible, adding to despair and hopelessness. These people are often mired at the lower levels of the basic needs hierarchy.

Healthcare for people who are homeless is a problem that many communities are addressing. Some community health and public agencies have nursing services that provide outreach, health assessment, and health monitoring programs for individuals and families. For example, screening these individuals for tuberculosis and other communicable diseases and giving immunizations to the children are important to the individual as well as to the health of the public.

Love, Affection, and Belonging

Societal Needs

Social needs are addressed in the third level of Maslow's hierarchy. The needs for love, affection, and belonging are fundamental human needs; however, people must meet survival and security needs before they can address social needs. Love and affection begin with bonding between the infant and mother at birth and must continue throughout life for a person to meet needs at this level. All people need to feel that they have meaningful relationships with others and that they belong to a group. People need the acceptance of their families and friends. Gang affiliation is one method of meeting the need to belong. The older adult and the young person in society often have much in common in that they may not feel a part of a group. They may feel that they are not useful or appreciated. Encouragement and assurance from loved ones can help to alleviate such anxieties.

When an ill or injured person is in a healthcare facility, they are often separated from friends and family. The person who is confined to home may also lack social contacts. Many people are very frightened and do not feel safe, especially when they are ill. The nurse can assist these people by encouraging visitors, cards, and telephone calls and by visiting with the client whenever possible. Explain to the client's family that the person needs more reassurance and acceptance if they are experiencing changes in physical appearance or ability. Clients being cared for at home need social support, stimulation, and encouragement from nurses and their loved ones. Do not forget the universal need for diversion, recreation, and social interactions.

> **Key Concept**
>
> A need at any given level of the hierarchy is more urgent to the person if the needs below it are satisfied. Thus, a person who is not preoccupied with obtaining oxygen and finding food will be able to be concerned with love and belonging.

Spiritual Needs

Many people believe in a higher power. This power takes many different forms, depending on one's religious background, ethnicity, and life experiences. The person who is ill or injured may find comfort in spirituality. The nurse can help clients meet their spiritual needs by assisting them to worship services, by providing reading or video materials, or by contacting the client's clergy person or the chaplain of the healthcare facility.

> **Key Concept**
>
> Basic needs are common to all people; thus, basic needs are universal. Individuals of all cultures have basic needs; in other words, basic needs are transcultural—across all cultures. Needs can be satisfied or they can be blocked during times of illness.

Self-Esteem Needs

The term **self-esteem** (self-image, self-respect) is related to the person's perception of self. Positive self-esteem is an appreciation of one's own personal worth. A person who feels that their contributions are appreciated by family, friends, and employers, for example, is more likely to have self-confidence. People meet their esteem needs when they think well of themselves by considering individual achievements, perception of self-adequacy, or self-competence. Self-esteem is related to how an individual is thought of by others through recognition, status, awards, or prestige.

Those who are ill or injured or who undergo surgery may have altered levels of self-esteem. This scenario is often true in situations that change a client's appearance and lifestyle, such as amputation of a limb or the presence of scars or acne. Many clients experience difficulty with their self-image after a hysterectomy or breast removal. As a nurse, you will be able to assist such individuals to regain positive self-esteem within their "new normal" by encouraging independence, by helping them with necessary lifestyle changes, and rewarding progress. Observe these clients for symptoms of regression, depression, overdependency, or a refusal to cooperate. Low self-esteem also directly relates to disorders such as chemical dependency. See Figure 5-2 for examples of nursing interventions throughout the hierarchy of needs.

Self-Actualization Needs

The **self-actualized** person has "reached their full potential." Thus, needs at this level are the highest order needs. The self-actualized person is comfortable enough to plan ahead and to be creative. It is common to think that great artists and musicians are functioning in the self-actualized sphere. However, any individual is able to advance to this level.

An individual incorporates all levels of the hierarchy to function as a self-actualized person. As with each level of Maslow's hierarchy, lower level needs must first be satisfied before a person can evolve to the self-actualization level. Some people function partially on this level, even though all other needs have not been completely met. Those who are comfortable with themselves and their place in the world have the emotional energy to plan, to learn, and to create.

The term *self-actualized* implies a fully functioning person. Maslow described this state as a comfortable relationship with the real world. The self-actualized individual is able to cope with life's situations, to deal with failure, and to be able to be free of anxiety. This person has a sense of humor, is self-controlled, and is able to deal with stress in productive ways. Self-actualization can take the form of being a better person, obtaining an education, being a good parent, or learning to grow roses.

It is probable that people reach this level many times throughout life, yet very few people believe they have reached the peak of self-actualization permanently. An individual who has met their highest goal is most likely to continue to create new personal or professional goals. Thus, the process of becoming self-actualized continually flows as new goals are born, develop, and are achieved. As a nursing student, you are striving toward self-actualization as well, and you will continue to strive toward new achievements as your career develops (Fig. 5-4).

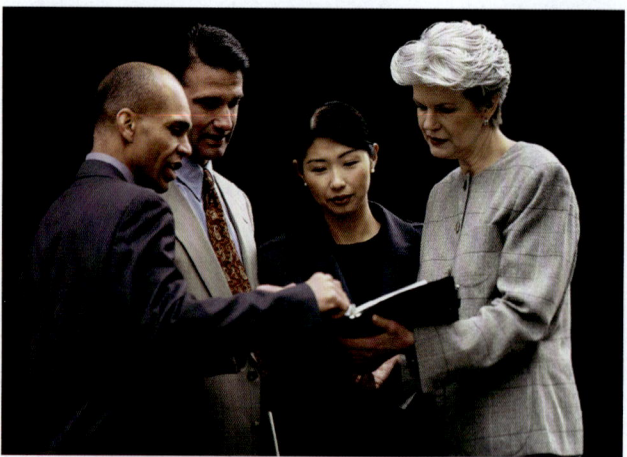

Figure 5-4 One way of achieving self-esteem is by having good working relationships with your peers. Self-actualization needs can be met by being successful in personal endeavors. Self-actualization can be reflected by presenting a professional appearance and working comfortably in team environments. Notice here the professional dress of these team members and their body language suggesting mutual cooperation.

While in your nursing program, you would be wise to think about Maslow's hierarchy of needs. For example, you will do much better in your nursing program if you do not have to worry about where you will live, whether or not you and your children are safe, or if you have enough money for food. Basic needs must be met first. When these primary needs are met, then the individual will have physical and psychological energy to reach the higher levels of the pyramid.

> **Key Concept**
>
> Homelessness is a threat to the person's basic need for warmth, shelter, and safety. If a person is responsible for others, such as children, the threats multiply. The higher needs of self-esteem or aesthetics cannot be addressed at all.

FAMILY AND COMMUNITY NEEDS

The family unit has needs that must be met for life to run smoothly. The special needs of the family include developmental tasks and functions to meet the needs of its members. The highly functioning family also works toward common goals as a group. Chapter 9 describes family development in more detail. Needs are met in a variety of family structures.

The community has basic needs concerning the welfare of all its residents. Among these needs are public health measures (immunization programs), access to healthcare (Affordable Care Act), maintenance services (water, electricity, waste disposal), environmental concerns (energy sources, pollution), safety (safety belts, police, highways), and emergency services (911 service, ambulances, disaster preparedness drills). Chapter 7 discusses issues involving community health.

STUDENT SYNTHESIS

KEY POINTS

- Physiologic needs drive all human beings and animals.
- Human needs are thought of in progressive levels, known as a *hierarchy*.
- Psychological needs are at a higher level than physiologic needs.
- A person must satisfy lower level needs before they can address higher level needs.
- Illness or injury can interfere with a person's ability to meet basic needs.
- Illness or injury can also cause a person to regress to a lower level of functioning.
- Nursing can assist a person in meeting needs or in eliminating potential threats to need satisfaction.
- Many factors, such as loss of income, illness, homelessness, and personal crises, threaten basic human needs.
- Health is a continually fluctuating and fluid state of physiological and psychological well-being.
- Relationships with others, including family and the community, are higher level needs that can be addressed only after basic physiologic needs are met.

CRITICAL THINKING EXERCISES

1. Describe how you are meeting your higher level needs while you are a nursing student.

2. Reflect on a time when you were unable to pursue higher level needs because one or more of your basic needs were not being satisfied. Examine ways you altered this situation to meet your needs.

3. Consider the care of a client who does not speak the same language as you. Discuss possible client needs that may be unmet. Determine any considerations for you to take to improve the quality of care.

4. Using Maslow's hierarchy of needs, discuss possible unmet needs for the following: a person who has been evicted, a client in a nursing home with no immediate family, a mother of triplets, a person who has difficulty breathing, and a nursing student during examination week.

NCLEX-STYLE REVIEW QUESTIONS

1. The nurse is caring for a client who is recovering from a recent stroke and is unable to move the left side of the body. Based on Maslow's hierarchy of needs, which nursing action will take priority in the care of this client?
   a. Ensuring the client is eating and drinking
   b. Instituting fall precautions
   c. Assisting with education regarding sexual activity
   d. Providing care with hygiene

2. The nurse is obtaining data from a 5-year-old child admitted with fractured ribs from an alleged fall. The child states to the nurse, "I was bad and my dad punished me by pushing me down the steps." Which action by the nurse is priority?
   a. Nothing. It will just create problems for the child.
   b. Report the statement to child protective services.
   c. Confront the parent with what the child stated.
   d. Talk to another coworker about the situation.

3. The nurse is observing a client to determine belonging needs. Which question will the nurse ask?
   a. "Which type of medications are you taking?"
   b. "Are you having difficulty breathing?"
   c. "Do you have a history of falling?"
   d. "Are you feeling isolated or upset?"

4. The nurse is assisting a client who is recovering from a hip replacement in the home setting. The nurse offers suggestions for safety adaptations. Which suggestions by the nurse would be most helpful in addressing the client's safety needs? Select all that apply.
   a. Encourage ambulation and exercise.
   b. Adjust the temperature in the home for comfort.
   c. Remove scatter rugs.
   d. Use a night light.
   e. Have a shower chair when bathing.

5. A client is having a surgical procedure. Which intervention provided by the nurse can help the client feel safe and aid in postoperative recovery?
   a. Explain the procedure before surgery.
   b. Inform the client that they will be alright.
   c. Call a family member prior to the client entering the surgical suite.
   d. Make sure all insurance information has been obtained.

CHAPTER RESOURCES

Enhance your learning with additional resources on thePoint!

Student Resources related to this chapter can be found at **thePoint.lww.com/Rosdahl12e**.

6 Health and Wellness

Learning Objectives

1. State the World Health Organization's definition of health.
2. List five components of health and describe how each is attained.
3. Define and differentiate the terms *morbidity* and *mortality*.
4. Discuss nursing and personal implications related to the costs of financing healthcare.
5. State preventive healthcare measures that have benefited American society.
6. Explain the wellness–illness continuum. Discuss the implications of acute and chronic illnesses as part of the continuum.
7. Relate the concept of wellness to Maslow's hierarchy of human needs.
8. Define and differentiate the terms *lifestyle factor* and *risk factor*. Describe lifestyle and risk factors that can directly affect health and the nursing considerations for these factors.
9. List sources of healthcare education and information.
10. Identify health concerns of each of the following age groups: infants, children, adolescents and young adults, mature adults, and older adults. State at least four nursing implications related to each.
11. Identify categories of diseases or disorders that are deviations from wellness.

Important Terminology

acute illness
atherosclerosis
benign
carcinogenic
chronic illness
congenital disorders
contagious
coronary artery disease
defense mechanisms
disease
domestic violence
dysfunctional
elder abuse
etiology
functional disease
health
hereditary
homeostasis
hypertension
illness
infection
lifestyle factor
local
malignant
metastasis
morbidity
mortality
neoplastic
organic disease
osteoporosis
prediabetes
preterm birth
risk factor
secondhand smoke
stress
systemic
wellness

Acronyms

BAC
CDC
CAD
CHD
COPD
CVA
DM
IPV
MI (AMI)
MVA
NCHS
PCP
SDG
SIDS
STD (also known as STI)
STI (also known as STD)
WHO

Chapters 6 and 7 discuss many concepts that will be important to you as both a provider and a consumer of healthcare. You will be a component of a complex healthcare system that involves local, state, national, and international health issues and trends. Nurses are affected directly and indirectly by these concerns.

Global health concerns are closely related to local health concerns because of ever-growing physical, environmental, and societal changes on a worldwide scale. The world's macrocosm is reflected in a community's microcosm. As an example of the intermingling of global issues, look to your own classroom and community. You probably have classmates with backgrounds originating from several countries. A country's physical boundaries do not isolate that country's governmental and societal issues, such as economy and the health of its citizens, from other nations. Global issues, such as health, illness, and healthcare services, are quite relevant to your local community concerns.

This chapter presents some general concepts that are pertinent to healthcare providers and show that these general concepts are linked to specific healthcare concerns.

All these concepts affect a nation's ability to provide healthcare to its citizens and the ability of individuals to provide healthcare for themselves. As a student and later in your career, you must be aware of the broadest issues affecting health, wellness, and healthcare. You should understand the issues that contribute to a healthy lifestyle and have good healthcare practices because you also serve as a model to your clients, family, and friends. Risk factors of health need to be recognized. You will need to understand your client's changing healthcare concerns throughout their lifetime. Nurses need to be able to answer a client's questions on multiple social and economic topics or be able to refer clients to appropriate resources when necessary. Your ability to facilitate solutions will be part of your nursing functions.

NCLEX Alert

NCLEX clinical situations commonly include the important concepts of acute or chronic needs of healthcare issues. You will need to choose the option that will reflect the appropriate action for the situation described.

HEALTH AND WELLNESS

The World Health Organization (**WHO**) was established by the United Nations in 1948 to improve worldwide health. Since then, the WHO has promoted a global social conscience of healthcare and flexible health reforms in an increasingly complex 21st century. This major influential agency believes that health is a shared global responsibility. Health issues include equitable access to essential personal healthcare as well as defense against transnational healthcare threats. Changes that need to be made to enhance health involve societal, physical, environmental, and economic issues. Direct linkages occur between a country's economics and the healthcare of its citizens. That is to say, health and healthcare services for individual citizens cannot be separated from a nation's economic health. An individual country's resources affect neighboring and distant nations. For example, mass migrations of individuals, as well as entire cultures, occur because the infrastructure of some countries cannot provide basic needs such as water, food, shelter, or personal safety. As a result, strain is placed on the healthcare services and financial resources of higher developed, technologically based countries. These issues are global trends that require massive internal change in many countries. Box 6-1 summarizes some of the global issues and potential resolutions—that is, *Sustainable Development Goals* (**SDGs**)—to these concerns. Your own healthcare community will be affected by these worldwide trends.

> **Key Concept**
>
> **Health**, according to the WHO, is a state of complete physical, mental, and social well-being, and not merely the absence of disease or infirmity.

Health is much more than physical well-being. Health includes the concepts of mind–body–spirit homeostasis. **Homeostasis** is the balance of all of the components of the human organism. Homeostasis implies continual adaptation to maintain a balance of sameness, that is to say, we must continuously adjust to our psychological, physical, and spiritual environment to maintain a balance. Another way of referring to homeostasis is to refer to an overall feeling of well-being or wellness. Wellness infers that the individual has a healthy balance of issues that affect the mind, body, and spirit.

> **Key Concept**
>
> The body adapts to change to maintain homeostasis.

Health influences everything in our lives. Our work, play, social, professional, and interpersonal relationships are influenced by our psychological, physical, and spiritual health. Health must be considered in its broadest, holistic sense, which includes the following components:

- *Physical health:* Physical fitness, the body functioning at its best
- *Emotional health:* Feelings and attitudes that make one comfortable with oneself
- *Psychological* or *mental health:* A mind that grows and adjusts, is in control, and is free of serious stress
- *Social health:* A sense of responsibility and caring for the health and welfare of others
- *Spiritual health:* Inner peace and security, comfort with one's higher power, as one perceives it

Disease is a change in the structure or function of body tissues, biologic systems, or the human mind. **Illness** is the response to disease that involves a change in function. **Infection** is a change in the structure and function of body tissues caused by invasion from harmful microorganisms.

> **Key Concept**
>
> A person responds to threats to one's well-being or wellness whether the threat is perceived, potential, or actual. A person seeks professional healthcare when they are unable to meet needs without assistance.

INCONSISTENCIES IN HEALTHCARE

Ideally, everyone receives the best healthcare services available. However, disparities or gaps in healthcare benefits exist. Many reasons account for the quality and quantity of these differences. Historically, disparities are related to existing social, political, economic, and geographic factors. Your physical environment and the location in which you live can make a big difference. Typically, rural areas have fewer healthcare resources, but urban areas have higher rates of violence, unintended pregnancies, and substance abuse. Many rural citizens must be able travel a long way for basic care and, often, even greater distances for specialized care. Individual responsibility is another factor; not everyone who has access to services and resources uses these services. Disease, injury, violence, and lack of healthcare opportunities could be minimized through changes in educational, social, and/or environmental conditions.

Educating the public influences healthcare. For example, in the 20th century, the public was made aware of the availability and advantages of preventive immunizations, food safety, nutrition, and accident prevention. However, inequities in education and the distribution of resources can result from discrepancies in income, race, ethnicity, gender, and disabilities. Students who leave high school before graduation are documented to have an increased dysfunction in their personal lives, which affects health issues in adulthood. Health risks, such as obesity, substance abuse, and violence, are more likely to develop. Higher levels of education are associated with a better quality of life (Centers for Disease Control, 2018).

MORBIDITY AND MORTALITY

Morbidity refers to the number of people with an illness or disorder relative to a specific population. For example, influenza morbidity rates (percentage of persons with the disease) are released every year. Thus, the morbidity rates for influenza may be 25% of the older population in any particular year, but only 2% of the younger population for that same year.

Box 6-1 WHO Health in the Millennium: Trends, Reforms, and Goals

The World Health Organization has documented specific trends, goals, and expected dates for reform. Reforms will affect healthcare for individual, national, and international relationships. These evolving changes include societal, cultural, physical, environmental, and economic issues. Global interactions demonstrate the direct linkages between a country's economics and the healthcare of its citizens. The WHO recognizes that mass migrations of individuals and entire cultures continue when the infrastructure of many nations cannot provide basic needs such as water, food, or shelter. The WHO also identifies that these survival needs must be met before the complex issues of healthcare can be addressed. Global trends show that issues that affect the health of one population can, and often do, evolve into stresses upon the societal and economic resources of other nations. The WHO attempts to address the complexity of healthcare, resources, and economic issues using an impressive variety of approaches. The identified trends listed below summarize the issues, goals, and reforms related to massive dynamic changes worldwide.

TRENDS IDENTIFIED BY THE WHO

The countries of the United Nations monitor disease indicators, risk factors to the individual, and factors that affect the citizens of its countries. The list below summarizes some of the UN/WHO's conclusions:

1. By the year 2050, there will be a 300% increase in the world's population.
2. Most adults younger than 25 years live in developing countries.
3. Preventable traffic injuries will increase by 65%.
4. Low- and middle-income countries will sustain hundreds of thousands of individuals who are victims of homicide, war, or commit suicide.
5. The leading cause of mortality in the age group 15–59 years will be HIV/AIDS, representing 15% of global deaths.
6. Maternal, newborn, and child deaths will be in the millions. Many of these deaths are related to vaccine-preventable diseases.
7. Tuberculosis and malaria kill millions of people annually. Of these deaths, 98% occur in developing countries.
8. Environmental contaminations, such as unsafe food and water, will continue to be the cause of death of hundreds of thousands of people.

UNITED NATIONS SUSTAINABLE DEVELOPMENT GOALS (SDGS)

The United Nations member states adopted the 2030 agenda for Sustainable Development, which consists of 17 goals to commit world leaders to combat poverty, hunger, disease, illiteracy, environmental degradation, and discrimination against women. The SDGs were built off of the Millennium Development Goals (MDGs), whose "deadline" was 2015 but still had progress to make. All SDGs have specific targets and indicators with the target date for these goals being 2030. The purpose of these goals is to

1. End poverty in all forms everywhere.
2. End hunger, achieve food security and improved nutrition and promote sustainable agriculture.
3. Ensure healthy lives and promote well-being for all at all ages.
4. Ensure inclusive and equitable quality education and promote lifelong learning opportunities for all.
5. Achieve gender equality and empower all women and girls.
6. Ensure availability and sustainable management of water and sanitation for all.
7. Ensure access to affordable, reliable, sustainable, and modern energy for all.
8. Promote sustained, inclusive, and sustainable economic growth, full and productive employment and decent work for all.
9. Build resilient infrastructure, promote inclusive and sustainable industrialization, and foster innovation.
10. Reduce inequality within and among countries.
11. Make cities and human settlements inclusive, safe, resilient, and sustainable.
12. Ensure sustainable consumption and production patterns.
13. Take urgent action to combat climate change and its impacts.
14. Conserve and sustainably use the oceans, seas, and marine resources for sustainable development.
15. Protect, restore, and promote sustainable use of terrestrial ecosystems, sustainably manage forests, combat desertification, and halt and reverse land degradation and halt biodiversity loss.
16. Promote peaceful and inclusive societies for sustainable development, provide access to justice for all and build effective, accountable, and inclusive institutions at all levels.
17. Strengthen the means of implementation and revitalize the global partnership for sustainable development.

From United Nations. (2015). *Sustainable Development Goals.* Copyright © 2015 United Nations. Reprinted with the permission of the United Nations. https://www.un.org/sustainabledevelopment/sustainable-development-goals/

Mortality refers to the chances of death associated with a particular illness or disorder. The Centers for Disease Control and Prevention (**CDC**) and the National Center for Health Statistics (NCHS), a branch of the CDC, monitor morbidity and mortality rates of many disorders in order that interventions and prevention may be instituted. For example, according to the NCHS, data showed that the mortality rate of women dying of lung cancer increased 400% from 1960 to 1990. This increase in mortality was investigated and found to be directly related to the increase in the number of women who started smoking during these years. Educational programs about the hazards of smoking were instituted as a result of these and other findings. The CDC is discussed further in Chapter 7.

The **NCHS** tracks the 15 leading causes of morbidity and mortality in the United States, as listed below. Mortality rates for these causes remain relatively stable:

1. Diseases of the heart such as coronary artery disease (**CAD**) and acute myocardial infarction (**MI or AMI**), also known as a heart attack
2. Malignant neoplasms (e.g., cancer)
3. Chronic lower respiratory disease, for example, chronic obstructive pulmonary disease (COPD)
4. Cerebrovascular disease, for example, a stroke, formerly known as a cerebrovascular accident or CVA.
5. Accidents or unintentional injuries, for example, motor vehicle accidents (**MVAs**)
6. Alzheimer's disease
7. Diabetes mellitus (**DM**)
8. Influenza and pneumonia
9. Nephritis, nephrotic syndrome, and nephrosis (e.g., chronic kidney diseases)
10. Intentional self-harm (suicide)
11. Septicemia (severe, body-wide, blood-borne infections)
12. Chronic liver disease and cirrhosis
13. Essential hypertension and hypertensive renal disease
14. Parkinson disease
15. Pneumonitis due to solids and liquids

The incidences of morbidity and mortality are influenced by one or more of the following: age, race, socioeconomic status, access to healthcare, education level, lifestyle, and risk factors. The varied types of cancer and their associated risk factors, morbidity, and mortality rates are discussed in Chapter 83. Alzheimer's disease and Parkinson disease incidences have increased due to age-related demographics. *Baby boomers* is the term for the large number of people born after World War II, in the years 1946 through 1964. As shown in Figure 6-1, baby boomers in the 21st century have become mature adults and represent a strategic spike in the number of older Americans who have age-related risk factors.

> **NCLEX Alert**
>
> When reading the NCLEX clinical scenario, it is important to consider all of the provided information such as past and present health issues, age of client, and stated lifestyle factors. Do not "read into" the scenario—use only the provided data when choosing the best option.

The CDC and the NCHS maintain extensive and comprehensive Websites of information. The CDC can provide information about specific diseases or disorders, statistics, educational supplements, and links to other Websites; this information is useful for the layperson and healthcare professionals, including students. Substantial medical information is available on the Internet, but the reader needs to maintain a cautious approach and use quality resources. The use of three or more Internet resources is highly recommended when searching for valid and reliable information.

FINANCES AND HEALTHCARE

Funding issues in healthcare are major concerns to clients and healthcare professionals. One factor is the willingness of the government to allocate funds to healthcare. The allocation of funds is often influenced by the political atmosphere and social priorities at a given moment. The Affordable Care Act (discussed in Chapter 3) is a major legislative step toward providing healthcare to all Americans.

Without finances, the technical advances that have occurred in industrialized countries in the late 20th century, such as the CT scanner shown in Figure 6-2, will not be able to continue. Premiums for healthcare, including private and public insurance sources, are affected. Actual costs of treatment to clients and healthcare providers are influenced by the practicality of financial support.

Countries that do not have financial resources have higher incidences of problems that could be cured or treated, for example, Ebola, malaria, tuberculosis (TB), or human

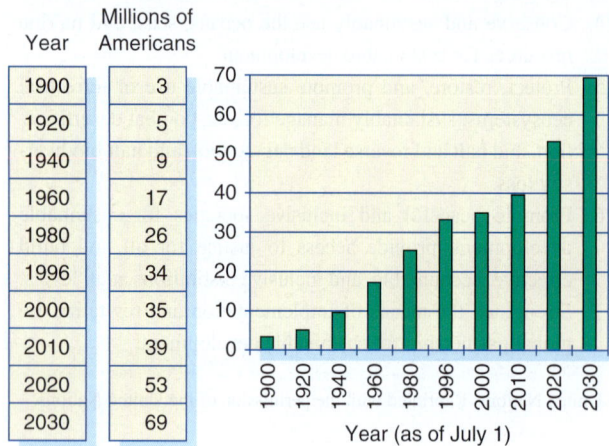

Figure 6-1 Demographics of the "baby boomer" generation. This table shows the estimated numbers of individuals in the United States who are 65 years and older from 1900 to 2030. Notice that nearly 70 million U.S. citizens will be aged 65 years or older during your nursing career. According to the WHO, during your time frame, the majority of adults younger than 25 years live in developing countries. Consider how the numbers of these two generations will affect issues such as employment, retirement, medical care, and birth rates. (Based on information adapted from the U.S. Bureau of the Census and the WHO. Percentages rounded to whole numbers.)

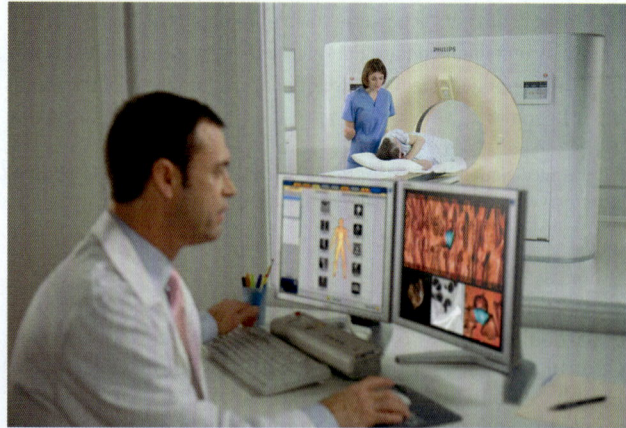

Figure 6-2 Computed tomography (CT) scanner. Healthcare technology has had many beneficial developments; however, they are often costly. (Photo courtesy of Philips Medical Systems.)

immunodeficiency virus/acquired immunodeficiency syndrome (HIV/AIDS). In our highly mobile global community, the health problems of other countries can and do become local health concerns.

Many individuals have lifelong, recurring problems that tend to worsen in severity over time. The costs of care for long-term or chronic illnesses, such as diabetes and obstructive lung diseases, are huge.

Another lifelong, chronic illness is HIV/AIDS (Chapter 85). About 40,000 individuals *every year* are infected with HIV in the United States. The United States spends billions of dollars every year on this one infection. Much of this financial cost provides for the medical care of the HIV/AIDS client. Some of the funds go to research and preventive educational programs, which have been effective in decreasing the morbidity rates of HIV/AIDS in the United States. More than a million people in the United States currently have HIV or AIDS. Unfortunately, 15%–20% of the people in this group do not know they have this infectious virus and, therefore, put others at risk. Expensive and powerful drugs have decreased the mortality rates of AIDS in the United States and other developed countries.

Healthcare trends are influenced by the continuously increasing wealth of scientific knowledge of health. Examples include the knowledge of the negative effects of tobacco products, the positive effects of good nutrition, and the negative lifetime effects of childhood obesity. Health research has resulted in many changes in healthcare knowledge and delivery. Cures for chronic illnesses could result in more money being available for illness prevention in the future.

Childhood immunizations represent a cost-effective and very efficient use of healthcare monies. The positive effects of childhood immunizations cannot be overstated. These advances were a result of combined financial and scientific resources, plus the relentless persistence of nurses, *primary care providers* (**PCPs**), and other healthcare professionals.

PREVENTION AND HEALTHCARE

Today's healthcare systems emphasize prevention rather than treatment of disease. Healthcare systems vary in different countries. The benefits of preventive education cannot be underestimated.

Changing lifestyle behaviors have resulted in improved maternal, neonate, and child healthcare statistics. Education of youth has resulted in fewer adult smoking-related problems. Healthcare providers, health insurance companies, life insurance companies, and numerous health-focused agencies, such as the American Diabetes Association and the American Dietetic Association, have become heavily involved in the campaign for improved health. These groups encourage healthier lifestyles through information campaigns designed to educate the public.

Primary healthcare services, or prevention services, have had significant positive effects on healthcare issues, such as prenatal care for mothers and infants, anti-smoking campaigns, and mammography for women. *Secondary healthcare services* provide individuals with specific medical or surgical therapies, generally in acute care settings. Rehabilitation or *tertiary services* have greatly enhanced the level of the health of clients with chronic illness or disability.

Statistics from the CDC and NCHS indicate that the United States has a higher percentage of immigrants and underrepresented groups than do many similar high-tech countries. Disparities are most evident in African American, Asian, Pan-Asian, and Latino communities. Certain segments of the population, including low-income families, individuals with chronic illnesses, the unemployed or underemployed, and those who live in rural areas encounter more difficulties getting to sites of healthcare. Individuals with physical and intellectual disabilities may have attainable resources but may not be physically or intellectually capable of using them.

Healthy People 2030 is a comprehensive set of 10-year national goals and objectives for improving the health of all Americans, developed by the U.S. Department of Health and Human Services and available on www.healthypeople.gov. These high-priority health issues, called Leading Health Indicators, reflect major health concerns and public health issues. The individual, the community, and healthcare professionals are challenged to take specific steps to ensure good health and long life by making improvements in the following areas:

- Access to healthcare
- Clinical preventative services
- Environmental quality
- Injury and violence
- Maternal, infant, and child health
- Mental health
- Nutrition, physical activity, and obesity
- Oral health
- Reproduction and sexual health
- Social determinants
- Substance abuse
- Tobacco use

The detailed Leading Health Indicators can be viewed on the Healthy People 2030 website (https://health.gov/healthypeople/objectives-and-data/leading-health-indicators). Box 6-2 summarizes areas of health promotion for several specific topics. Age, sex, genetics, and environment can minimize or enhance these preventive measures. The nurse, along with client input, will need to customize these suggestions to reflect individual healthcare needs.

> **Key Concept**
>
> A key to good health is for clients to assume personal responsibility for their health.

THE WELLNESS–ILLNESS CONTINUUM

Most people are not totally healthy or totally ill at any given time. An individual's daily state of health falls somewhere on a continuum from high-level wellness or *optimum health* to death. Figure 6-3 illustrates the basic concept of the wellness–illness continuum. The state of wellness or illness fluctuates depending on the individual.

The following components contribute to a state of wellness:

- Good physical self-care
- Prevention of illness/injury
- Using one's full intellectual potential
- Expressing emotions and managing stress appropriately
- Comfortable and congenial interpersonal relationships
- Concern about one's environment and conditions throughout the world

Box 6-2 — Health Promotion and Disease Prevention Measures

HEALTHY PREGNANCY
- Start your pregnancy with early prenatal care.
- Avoid tobacco, alcohol, and secondary smoke during and after pregnancy.
- Take dietary supplements, such as iron and folic acid.
- Avoid contact with individuals who have been exposed to measles or chickenpox.
- Use protective measures during sex to protect from sexually transmitted infections (STIs).
- Use caution with household chemicals.
- Avoid cleaning cat litter box.

CHILDHOOD INJURIES AND ILLNESSES
- Know the U.S. National Poison Control Number—1-800-222-1222. Visit the U.S. National Poison Control Website.
- Canada: Dial 911 or contact the Drug and Poison Information Control Center for the specific geographic area. A list of Canadian Poison Control Centers can be found at https://safemedicationuse.ca/tools_resources/poison_centres.html
- Baby/child-proof house, garage, yard, and vehicles.
- Encourage parenting classes for first-time and/or high-risk parents.
- Follow immunization programs.
- Provide instruction in first aid and CPR to caregivers (including babysitters).
- Use appropriate-sized car seats.
- Use helmets, elbow pads, and knee pads with appropriate toys.
- Detect and treat parasites early.
- For comprehensive child safety information, go to the Website of MedlinePlus, a service of the U.S. National Library of Medicine.

DENTAL HEALTH
- Schedule regular preventive dental care.
- Teach good dental hygiene at home (e.g., flossing, tooth brushing, use of fluoride toothpaste) as needed in your community.

VISION CARE
- Encourage preventive measures, such as regular checkups for early detection of visual problems, such as glaucoma and cataracts.
- Use fastidious handwashing and hygienic care for corrective lenses and contact lenses.
- Provide adequate lighting.
- Know the location of eyewash stations at employment or school laboratories.

HEART HEALTH
- Use preventive measures against cardiovascular disease, such as a low-fat diet and regular exercise.
- Maintain appropriate body weight.
- Avoid all tobacco products.
- Protect yourself and your children from the hazards of secondhand smoke.
- Monitor stress levels and use productive methods to protect self from unnecessary physical or mental stress.
- Consult with your healthcare providers regarding the need for laboratory studies, such as cholesterol levels.
- Be aware of your normal blood pressure and consult healthcare providers when blood pressure is not within your own averages.

SMOKING
- Encourage attendance at smoking cessation programs for those who use tobacco products.
- Encourage utilization of smoke-free environments.

DIABETES
- Encourage early detection of diabetes.
- Monitor the three critical elements: diet, exercise, and appropriate use of prescription medications.
- Encourage compliance to diabetic regimen, which can minimize diabetic complications.

HYPERTENSION
- Consult your physician about increased physical activity and be as active as is possible for your situation.
- Limit alcohol intake.
- Monitor sodium (salt) intake.
- Read food labels to determine sodium, sugar, and fat content.
- Monitor laboratory levels of potassium and eat sufficient natural sources, such as bananas, oranges, potatoes, or watermelon.
- Take prescribed blood pressure medications as indicated by healthcare providers.
- Notify healthcare providers of all changes or reactions to medications.
- Do NOT abruptly stop taking prescribed medications without professional guidance.
- Have regular healthcare, dental, and vision checkups.
- Learn to talk to your physician about any physical, emotional, financial, or lifestyle changes.

CHOLESTEROL
- Eat low-fat foods.
- Read food labels.
- Increase activity.
- Include the Website of MyPlate in your favorites list for comprehensive information on healthy dietary habits for men, women, children, and families.

CANCER
- Follow a low-fat diet.
- Have adequate fiber daily.
- Adhere to screening recommendations for prostate, colon, and breast cancers.
- Prevent sunburns in children.
- Protect the skin by wearing hats, scarves, or specifically made sun-protective clothing.

CHAPTER 6 Health and Wellness

Box 6-2 Health Promotion and Disease Prevention Measures (Continued)

- Use sun screens and reapply according to product directions.
- Avoid getting sunburns.
- Refrain from smoking.

REPRODUCTIVE HEALTH
- Discuss STI protective measures with your partner.
- Protect yourself from unplanned pregnancies.
- Use safer sex practices that are appropriate for your personal needs.
- Be aware that many safer sex practices do not protect from STIs.
- Get reproductive health checkups, including testing for HIV and STIs.

OSTEOPOROSIS
- Eat foods high in calcium and vitamin D.
- Exercise or include some physical activity.

ALCOHOL AND DRUGS
- Educate children and adults on how to detect and treat abuse.
- Avoid excessive alcohol use.

EATING DISORDERS
- Be aware of the possibilities of eating disorders for yourself, friends, and family.
- Research health maintenance programs related to obesity, anorexia nervosa, and bulimia.

MENTAL HEALTH
- Be aware of the stressors in your life.
- Include stress reduction activities in your daily life, such as exercise, reading, and listening to music.
- Recognize the symptoms of depression, anxiety, panic disorder, and seasonal affective disorder.
- Access suicide prevention and abuse hotlines and programs, if necessary.

REGULAR PHYSICAL EXAMINATIONS AND SELF-EXAMINATIONS
- Adhere to screening recommendations for mammograms, breast, intestinal, and testicular cancer, as well as for tuberculosis.
- Update and maintain immunizations throughout life.

Acute illnesses are illnesses that interfere with the wellness–illness continuum for a short period of time. Acute illnesses generally develop suddenly and resolve within a specified period of time. The common cold is an acute illness. You may be ill for a few days and then return to your normal state of health.

Chronic illnesses such as arthritis, asthma, or HIV/AIDS result in a long-term health disturbance. Individuals with chronic illnesses function within the wellness–illness continuum, but often are limited by their disorder.

A person may have an acute illness, a chronic illness, or both. It is very common for an individual with a chronic illness to become acutely ill. For example, a person might become acutely ill from a seasonal virus, or someone with a chronic illness may become unstable from an acute asthma attack. Older adults commonly have both acute and chronic illnesses. Figure 6-4 illustrates the possible fluctuations of acute and chronic illnesses.

Healthcare facilities are also known by the terms *acute care* or *long-term care*. Acute care hospitals provide short-term care for clients with serious illnesses. Long-term care facilities, such as rehabilitation centers or skilled nursing facilities, are responsible for the care of residents with chronic illness. Occasionally, a resident may become seriously ill and need to be transferred to an acute care facility.

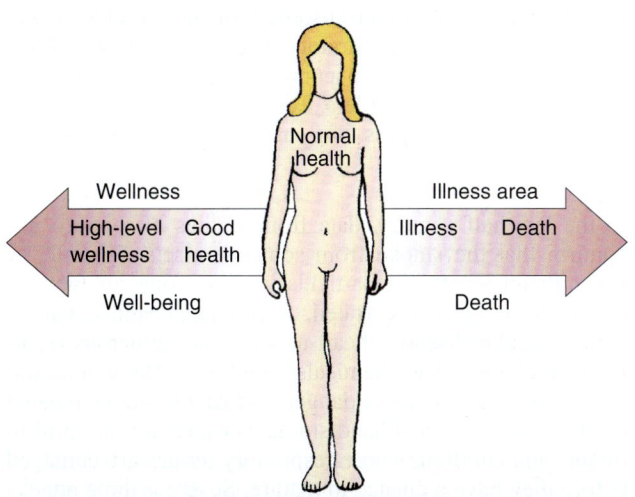

Figure 6-3 The wellness–illness continuum. Individuals function on a fluctuating continuum of health and illness.

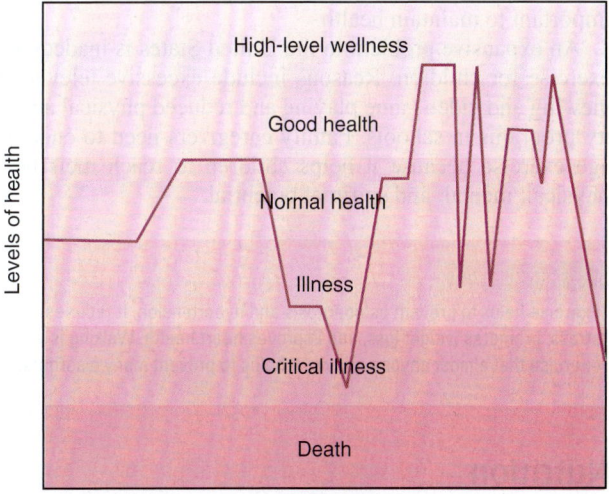

Figure 6-4 The wellness–illness continuum shows the different levels of health a person experiences over a lifetime.

> **NCLEX Alert**
>
> The concepts of Maslow's hierarchy (discussed in Chapter 5) and their relationship to nursing priorities and nursing care may be components of NCLEX-PN scenarios. The correct option, that is, response on the NCLEX, may be related to which level of wellness (acute, chronic, survival, self-esteem, etc.) pertains to the client's condition in the scenario.

LIFESTYLE AND RISK FACTORS

Lifestyle factors are patterns of living that we choose to follow, such as the amount and type of exercise performed by an individual. Nutrition, smoking, substance abuse, stress, and violence are also lifestyle factors an individual can control. These factors may also include risk factors. **Risk factors** may or may not be preventable. Smoking is a risk factor that is preventable. Our genetic makeup contains risk factors that we cannot control. Certain risk factors are related to our occupation, environment, or age.

> **NCLEX Alert**
>
> Lifestyles, inherited risk factors, preventive measures, and educational topics are frequently components of NCLEX clinical scenarios and options. These issues identify specific, individual healthcare priorities for a client.

Physical Activity

Physical activity is recommended for all people. Moderate physical activity enhances energy, reduces stress, and provides relaxation. Physical activity is essential in the management of chronic conditions such as diabetes and arthritis. It helps in weight control and decreases the percentage of body fat. Exercise increases the activity and health of the cardiovascular system. It improves flexibility, muscle tone, strength, and stamina. It helps to increase the levels of good cholesterol in the blood. In many individuals, exercise can minimize life-threatening conditions such as coronary heart disease (**CHD**), obesity, and cancer. Sleep and rest are also important to maintain health.

An expansive problem in the United States is inadequate exercise for children. Reasons include excessive television viewing and video game playing and reduced physical activity programs in schools. Family caregivers need to encourage exercise because it helps children to reach their best physical, mental, and spiritual potential.

> **Key Concept**
>
> Exercise helps to prevent osteoporosis and hypertension. It reduces stress, promotes weight loss, and improves heart health. Walking is an exercise that almost anyone can do. It helps to prevent many disorders.

Nutrition

In recent years, a great deal of attention has been given to nutrition. The U.S. Surgeon General has stated that 70% of illnesses are related to nutrition. Poor nutrition contributes to heart failure, cancer, obesity, and growth retardation in children. High sugar intake, pesticide use, fertilizer overuse, and food additives also contribute to disease. The major components of a healthy diet include reduced fat and sodium intake, adequate calcium intake, and increased intake of fiber and natural carbohydrates. Unit 5 covers nutrition and diet therapy.

Some programs to improve the American diet include nutrition education in schools, improved quality and choices in school lunches, worksite nutritional programs, and home-delivered meals for older adults. PCPs who educate and counsel clients on healthcare topics can provide additional help on nutritional issues, if needed. Laws now require basic informational labeling of food products, so consumers can be better informed. More reduced-fat foods are now available.

> **Key Concept**
>
> Some situations in combination dramatically increase risks. For example, the combination of high cholesterol and hypertension increases the risk of CHD up to six times. Add smoking to that combination and the risk increases up to 20 times.

Facts About Tobacco Use

More than 50 years of data collection and health studies have proven that *the use of tobacco is the single leading cause of preventable death and disease in the United States*. For every one of the nearly half a million U.S. citizens who die from tobacco-related illnesses *annually*, 20 additional people are affected and suffer from tobacco-related illnesses. Financially, tobacco costs the U.S. government, that is, your tax money, about $300 billion annually in direct medical expenses and lost productivity (Centers for Disease Control, n.d.).

More than 7,000 substances, including highly addictive nicotine, are found in tobacco smoke. At least 14 forms of cancer are caused by smoking alone. Chemicals that cause cancer are called **carcinogenic**. Smoking causes heart attacks, strokes, diabetes, and **COPD**. Smokeless tobacco is proven to cause oral cancer, for example, cancers of the lips, throat, and mucosa of the cheeks, as well as heart disease and pancreatic cancer. *All forms of tobacco are addictive*.

Other medical conditions that result from smoking include acute and chronic disorders of the circulatory and respiratory systems. Respiratory disorders include asthma, emphysema, bronchitis, pneumonia, and other acute and chronic respiratory disorders. Tobacco-related heart attacks and stroke deaths surpass lung cancer deaths each year.

Secondhand Smoke

In the last half century, data from studies of tobacco use confirm that the smoke from someone else's cigarette, or **secondhand smoke**, is particularly dangerous; in fact, its effects have been underrated. Secondhand smoke causes cardiovascular diseases, heart attacks, and numerous respiratory problems. The chemicals found in smoke that a non-smoker breathes are more dangerous than the smoke inhaled by the smoker. Secondhand smoke is especially harmful to infants and children, whose respiratory tissues are damaged before they have a chance to mature. Severe asthma attacks and ongoing respiratory infections are common side effects in children, as are ear infections and sudden infant death syndrome (SIDS). Acute and chronic pulmonary problems occur early in the lives of children of smokers and remain lifelong problems. *There is no risk-free level of exposure to secondhand smoke.* This and much more information can be found on www.smokefree.gov.

Other Hazards of Smoking

The highly addictive substance nicotine found in cigarettes makes platelets more sticky, which can injure heart arteries or form clots and cause a heart attack. Smoking contributes to heart disease because nicotine increases plaque buildup in arteries; it causes the insides of arteries to form rough, chapped places. Sticky cholesterol can attach there more easily and build up plaque, which can increase the chances of a heart attack.

Low-tar, filtered, and menthol cigarettes are just as dangerous as plain ones. Smokeless tobacco is also dangerous. Studies show it causes cancers of the lips, mouth, larynx, and mucosal linings of the oral cavity. Smokeless tobacco is strongly associated with heart disease and pancreatic cancer.

Electronic cigarettes, or e-cigarettes, are battery-powered devices that provide doses of nicotine and numerous other additives and flavorings (e.g., chocolate, mint) in a smokeless aerosol system. It is important for consumers to know that e-cigarettes are just as dangerous as standard tobacco products because they contain nicotine, which has harmful effects on the developing adolescent brain and on pregnant women.

Benefits of Smoking Cessation

Smoking cessation has an immediate effect on the improvement of health and reduces one's risk for disease and premature death. Quitting smoking has its greatest benefits on younger individuals (who have had less smoke-related damage); however, nonsmoking is beneficial to all ages. The health benefits of quitting smoking are much greater than the risks of weight gain that may occur. The health of families and friends of nonsmokers also improves because they are not exposed to the extensive hazards of secondhand smoke.

> **Key Concept**
> Smoking not only increases an individual's risk of having a heart attack but also increases that individual's risk of having a fatal heart attack.

Tobacco Use and Pregnancy

Concerns abound for the child of the pregnant woman who smokes. As listed on www.cdc.gov/reproductivehealth, smoking during pregnancy increases the risk of the following: **preterm births** (infants born before the expected due date); problems with the placenta (e.g., early separation, hemorrhage); low birth weight (a factor in infant sickness and death); stillborn babies and **SIDS**; birth defects (e.g., cleft lip or cleft palate); and miscarriage. Smoking also interferes with a woman's ability to get pregnant.

Substance Abuse

Three of every five Americans drink alcoholic beverages. Everyone who drinks alcohol is influenced to some extent. Therefore, each person has the potential for abusing alcohol.

The abuse of alcohol and other drugs contributes in many ways to decreased public health. Accidents and homicides are major causes of death. Alcohol and drugs often contribute to these events. Alcohol abuse also contributes to such disorders as cirrhosis of the liver and diverticulitis and mental health conditions such as depression and suicide.

Substance abuse contributes to family strife, domestic violence, work absenteeism, and unemployment. The crime rate statistically increases when "street" drugs invade communities. Substance abuse directly affects the physical and mental health of individuals, families, and societies.

Laws regulating substance use have become more stringent, but the appeal and habit-forming nature of many illegal drugs offset the effects of the laws in many cases. In addition, the huge amount of money to be made on drugs has rendered laws difficult to enforce. Chapter 95 describes chemical dependency treatment programs and the nurse's role in detoxification.

Stress

Stress is normal. It is the physical and mental wear and tear of life. **Stress** is a mental or physical tension exerted on an individual's homeostasis. It is often associated with change. Some stress is beneficial because it offers people a challenge that keeps them moving toward goals. Stress can also alert people to danger, helping them deal with emergencies. Sometimes stress is harmful and can interfere with homeostasis.

Often the stress is not the actual physical or emotional event, but rather our *reaction* to the event. For example, getting married is a highly emotional event. The preparations for marriage cause stress. This type of stress can be energizing or damaging to the individual.

Common physical responses to stress include the following:

- Tense muscles, causing headache, backache, or neck ache
- Jaw pain, caused by grinding of teeth or clenched jaw (*Note:* Jaw pain can also be associated with a myocardial infarction [MI or heart attack], *especially in women.*)
- Stomach distress (gas, bloating, nausea, mild pain)

Common psychological responses to stress include the following:

- Mood swings or irritability
- Impatience with others or oneself
- Forgetfulness
- Fatigue not due to any documented physical finding
- Difficulty sleeping
- Anxiety
- Anger
- Depression
- Helplessness
- Feelings of being out of control with oneself or life's situations
- Generalized tension

Cumulative stress leads to health problems. The individual may be able to adapt to a major change, such as moving to a new state or starting a nursing program. However, stress can progress from relatively annoying symptoms to much greater problems. Accumulated stress can lead to disruption in our daily personal, family, and social lives. Stress can be the precursor to major physical and emotional dysfunctions. As stress becomes more intolerable, often initiated by additional change, major, life-threatening problems develop. Individuals need to recognize that stress is insidious (sneaky) and often we do not recognize the symptoms until a crisis emerges.

Responses to cumulative stress are often the cause of maladaptive or negative **defense mechanisms**. **Defense mechanisms** are behaviors that provide protection from internal conflicts (things we do not want to think about), thoughts, or feelings that we are unable to resolve. Defense mechanisms develop subconsciously in both children and adults. Negative feelings can promote anxiety and lower self-esteem. Box 6-3 summarizes some common maladaptive behaviors. In the short-term, defense mechanisms can be beneficial; however, issues that linger often cause more than just emotional anxieties. Stress and its responses result in many disorders that lead to acute and chronic physical and emotional conditions. Unmanaged stress causes or aggravates disorders. Physical disorders are intermingled with emotional factors, for example:

- Overeating ←→ weight gain ←→ depression ←→ loss of self-esteem
- Anxiety ←→ tobacco use ←→ respiratory and cardiac disorders ←→ poor health
- Substance abuse ←→ mood swings ←→ loss of control ←→ failures of friendship and family

In summary, defense mechanisms are internal stress reducers, even though they may not be truthful or effective ways of adapting to a stressful situation. Defense mechanisms are also discussed in Chapter 94. Additional examples of defense mechanisms include the following:

- Denial—The unconscious refusal to accept facts or reality. Denial is one of the most common defense mechanisms used. For example, a student refuses to accept a failing grade thinking that the given score must be a mistake.
- Projection—Displacing unwanted feelings onto another individual, as if it is the other person who has the problem. For example, a student believes that the instructor made the examination too difficult.
- Repression—Moving the awareness of an unwanted idea or act by pushing it into the subconscious. For example, a student forgets that he/she did not study for an examination.

Box 6-3 Stress and Personal Responses

The following behaviors are common maladaptive (not helpful) reactions to chronic or acute stress:

- Drinking alcohol to relax
- Smoking or use of tobacco products
- Speaking or eating very fast
- Starting multiple projects but finishing none
- Working all the time
- Procrastinating (delaying) things that you need to do
- Sleeping too little, too much, or both
- Slowing down to the point of not doing anything
- Refusing to acknowledge that you have problems (denial)

- Regression—Reverting to an earlier stage of emotional development; becoming less mature. For example, a student stays in bed and refuses to come into class after failing an examination.

Violence and Abuse

Domestic violence is violence that occurs in the home, inflicted by a person (perpetrator) upon another, who is known to the victim. Also known as *intimate partner violence* (**IPV**), domestic violence is intentional physical, sexual, or psychological harm or threats of harm by words, gestures, or weapons by a current or former partner or spouse. The severity of abuse ranges from threats to blows to chronic and severe battering. The hostility can occur between same sex couples as well as heterosexual partners. Violence does not always include sexual intimacy. Domestic abuse occurs within all racial and ethnic groups and at all socioeconomic levels. Some cultures permit violence to women as a prerogative of the men.

Risk factors can be the same for both the victim and the perpetrator. For example, a person who has had childhood physical or sexual trauma is also at risk for becoming the future perpetrator of similar acts. Not all persons who have been victims or have significant risk factors become perpetrators of violence. Risk factors involved include individual experiences and relationship factors as listed below:

Individual Risk Factors

- Low self-esteem, low income, low academic achievement
- Age—young and older persons are at risk of experiencing violence
- Alcohol and drug use
- Anger and hostility, isolation, unemployment
- Aggressive, delinquent, or antisocial behaviors
- Depression, feelings of insecurity, and friendlessness
- Prior history of being physically or emotionally abused
- Desire for power and control in relationships
- Belief in strict gender roles (male dominance/female passivity)
- Dysfunctional family history or poor parenting skills
- History of having physical discipline and/or violence as a child

Relationship Risk Factors

- Economic stress, unemployment, or underemployment
- Dysfunctional family relationships and interactions
- Dominance and control of relationship by one partner over the other conflicts in relationships: arguments, tension, fights
- Instability of partnership: separations, divorce

Community violence is a concern for both the individual and the nation. Violence in the workplace reflects problems of society. Violence in schools can start at elementary levels and continue through the educational system. Increasing numbers of gang members and the use of drugs (e.g., crack cocaine) contribute greatly to rising violence—especially in young adults. Risk factors for committing violence in public settings can include combinations of the factors listed above for individuals and relationships, in addition to the following:

Community Risk Factors

- Income below the poverty threshold, overcrowding

- Acceptance of existing standards of maladaptive behaviors (limited or no sanctions)
- Unwillingness to initiate change or to interfere
- Acceptance of traditional or cultural gender-related norms
- Fear of retaliation

Elder abuse and neglect are problems that promise to increase in the 21st century. This form of abuse occurs to older adults. Many times, an older adult who is abused or neglected is dependent on the care of one or more family members. Physical abuse, poor nutrition, lack of medical care, and emotional abuse, such as threats, are examples of elder abuse.

People are living longer and many do not have the resources to care for the side effects of aging. These seniors will be using the healthcare system in the early 21st century in large numbers, perhaps more than can be adequately cared for with current resources (Fig. 6-1).

Abuse commonly occurs in families in which personal and financial resources have been exhausted. In many cases, older adults may not be receiving the care they need. This is a form of neglect. The isolation of living alone or with relatives sometimes allows abuse to continue without detection or reporting. Chapter 92 discusses the needs of older adults and the potential of elder abuse and neglect in more detail.

Conflict resolution and anger management programs attempt to reduce rates of violence. Your legal nursing responsibility is to report any cases of suspected abuse or violence. Victims of domestic violence can receive assistance at shelters, by using a telephone hotline or through individual counseling. Local law enforcement and social service agencies are other available resources.

> **Key Concept**
> Physical activity; having a well-balanced diet; maintaining a healthy body weight; and not smoking can reduce the incidence of many disorders.

EDUCATION AND HEALTH PROMOTION

One way to combat society's health problems is through extensive education. Education can be the leading source of prevention of disease and disabilities. Among the numerous sources of information available are, for example, formal courses in school (e.g., mine safety); informal courses (e.g., prenatal and birth courses); public service announcements and advertisements; informational flyers, brochures, and books; nonprofit organizations (e.g., American Cancer Society); healthcare providers; and Internet Websites.

> **Nursing Alert** Use caution when gathering information from Websites. Not all sites use information based on truth and documented fact. Double check your resources and use sites that have reliable, professional, and current information.

Individuals need to be aware of their risk and lifestyle factors. A person whose parents had high blood pressure (**hypertension**) may be at risk for this condition and its complications. Therefore, that person's lifestyle should include changes in diet, exercise, or use of medications in order to manage the inherited risk factor.

Many schools and healthcare facilities offer classes that emphasize child development and effective parenting. All levels of schooling offer age-appropriate health education courses. Special programs are often set up in worksites to educate employees on topics from the safe operation of equipment to the hazards of lifting heavy objects. Many of these educational resources are free. These courses are effective ways of educating individuals and preventing illness and injury, and thus the employer or facility may require that all employees attend. Acute and long-term healthcare facilities have voluntary and mandatory educational in-service programs for hospital staff.

Many insurance and pharmaceutical companies publish materials aimed at assisting people to live more healthy lives. Information is provided with all prescribed drugs. These companies also publish materials regarding selected disorders and their management, laboratory and other diagnostic tests, and surgical procedures. Such materials are often published in other languages in addition to English to better serve target populations. They are also available on audiotape and videotape for persons who cannot read. Students should use caution with some materials because they may be promotional, that is to say, used to advertise the product.

Social issues are affected by television programs, social media sites, and the advertising industry, which exist to try to forge social change and affect your habits. You, as a nurse and a consumer, need to be aware that advertisements are often exaggerations and commonly do not represent all of the facts. A good example of this is cigarette and alcohol advertising. Many programs are targeted at selected populations, such as teenagers, mothers with young children, and older adults. The media can also bring about positive cultural changes, for example, awareness of another's point of view, and promote acceptance of other ways of life.

> **Key Concept**
> If you understand the concepts of healthy living, you will be better able to teach your clients. Education of your clients and their care providers is an essential daily component of nursing care.

AGE-RELATED HEALTH CONCERNS

Health is a family concern. You are aware that if one person in the family has the common cold, then the rest of the family is more apt to get it as well. Healthy habits are also contagious. Simple examples, such as frequent handwashing and responsible eating habits, educate others in the ways to enhance health and to help prevent illness.

Avoidance of risk behaviors can be part of a family's healthy lifestyle. Children who see smoking in their home are more likely to develop the habit. Good eating habits become generational.

Specific concerns are related to each age group. Some of these concerns relate to avoidable risk and lifestyle factors. The CDC has summarized much information on age-related concerns that you will find helpful during your nursing program and after graduation, when you need educational information and resources for your clients. As you progress through the subjects of your curriculum, refer to Box 6-4.

> **Box 6-4 The Centers for Disease Control and Prevention**
>
> The Centers for Disease Control and Prevention or CDC has extensive resource information on its vast Website, www.cdc.com. Information is convenient, suitable, and practical. These valuable pages provide free data for the nursing student, clients, and the general population. It may be wise to keep this Website in mind when instructing clients, families, travelers, specific populations, or during current outbreaks of infectious diseases. Subject materials include fact sheets, disease and disorder discussions, or statistics. Examples of topics found within this Website are listed below.
>
> **LIFE STAGES**
> - Infants and Toddlers: Birth defects, healthy youth, immunizations, SIDS
> - Children: ADHD, autism, child development, growth charts, healthy youth, injury
> - Adolescents and Teens: Adolescent health, alcohol and drug use, nutrition, risk behavior, school health
> - Young Adults: College health and safety, folic acid healthy living, HIV and AIDS: Are You at Risk
> - Pregnancy: Folic acid, nutrition, pregnancy tips, vaccination, violence
> - Women: Bone health, breast cancer, heart disease, mammograms, reproductive health
> - Men: Alcohol use, HIV/AIDS, oral health, prostate cancer, reproductive health
> - Older Adults: Arthritis, cancer, falls, heart disease, stroke, older adult drivers
>
> **SPECIFIC POPULATIONS**
> - On the Job: Workplace hazards and illnesses, stress, injuries and health disorders, safety and prevention
> - Correctional Health: Criminal justice and public health, HIV/AIDS, MRSA, TB, viral hepatitis, STDs
> - Lesbian, Gay, Bisexual, and Transgender: Health resources for gay, lesbian, bisexual, and transgender individuals
> - Disabilities: Accessibility, autism, disability and health, hearing loss, intellectual disability
> - Minority Health: African American, health disparities, Hispanic, racial, and ethnic populations
> - Outbreaks: Pandemics, multistate foodborne outbreaks, public health alerts/advisories, emergency incidents/outbreaks, morbidity, and mortality data
> - Traveler's Information: Vaccines, medicines, traveler's health notices for specific health and age-related populations, country-specific health concerns (e.g., polio, measles)
>
> Adapted from material obtained at www.cdc.gov.

Infants

According to the CDC and NCHS, the United States has an average infant mortality rate of 0.6% (fewer than 6 of 1,000 newborns or infants die before 1 year of age). Asian and Pacific Islander newborn populations have the lowest mortality rate of less than 0.4%. The rate for Hispanic or Latino populations is less than 0.6%. The Black or African American mortality rate is about double that of the non-Hispanic White population.

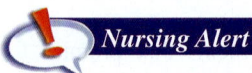

> ***Nursing Alert***
>
> - U.S. National Poison Control Number—1-800-222-1222
> - Canada: Dial 911 or specific poison control center for geographic area
> - General rule: Dial 911 if an individual is unconscious, having a seizure, difficulty breathing, or chest pain

The leading causes of infant mortality are congenital malformation, deformations, and chromosomal abnormalities. Other causes include short gestation and low birth weight, SIDS, maternal complications affecting pregnancy, and accidents. Newborn birth-related complications, sepsis, respiratory distress, diseases of the circulatory system, and hemorrhage summarize the top 10 causes. Chapter 72 discusses healthcare issues of the infant and toddler.

Two major factors, the education level and the financial resources of the mother, influence mortality rates. Many women do not obtain prenatal care. The reasons include lack of available finances (even though prenatal care can be free or income adjusted), lack of transportation to the facility, and lack of interest in obtaining prenatal care. Infants and mothers who have prenatal care have a significantly decreased morbidity and mortality rate. If prenatal care is neglected, the infant often has an unhealthy beginning. A healthy infant has a much better chance of growing and developing into a fulfilled adult.

Children

The number one cause of death in young children in America is accidental injury. Asthma is the leading cause of illness in children and can be life threatening. Asthma is most likely to occur in homes where tobacco and secondhand smoke are present. Asthma also is influenced by environmental conditions such as air pollution.

Lack of exercise and physical play activities is a major concern for the young. Obesity commonly begins in childhood. The CDC reports that there are significant racial and age disparities in obesity among children and adolescents. There are higher rates of obesity among Hispanic and non-Hispanic Black youths than non-Hispanic White youths. Children who are overweight are much more likely to develop health risk factors (e.g., CAD) in their youth, which will stay with them throughout their lifetime.

The great news is that major childhood infectious diseases are preventable. Six of the childhood scourges of the past have highly effective immunizations. Immunizations are available against measles, mumps, rubella, diphtheria, pertussis, and tetanus. Newer vaccines against hepatitis A and B, chickenpox, and other viruses are also eliminating illness in children. Because of the effectiveness of modern immunization programs, infectious diseases are no longer the problem they were in the past in countries with well-developed healthcare systems. The public must remain alert to these potential killers because these diseases have not been eliminated. They can only be prevented with proper and complete immunizations. Populations in transition across world borders are at high risk for acquiring and transmitting communicable childhood diseases. Measles and tetanus, which are vaccine-preventable diseases, are still responsible for hundreds of thousands of childhood deaths worldwide.

Adolescents and Young Adults

Risk behaviors are more prevalent in adolescents and young adults. For example, an individual is more likely to start smoking during adolescence than during adulthood. Substance abuse is another risk behavior common in adolescents and young adults.

Specific lifestyle factors influence this age group. Peer pressure is stronger in this age group than in others. In addition, this population has the lowest rate of utilization of healthcare, possibly because of the costs of healthcare, a high unemployment rate, and lack of healthcare insurance.

Motor Vehicle Accidents

Motor vehicle accidents (MVAs) are the leading cause of morbidity and mortality for children, adolescents, and young adults aged 5–34 years. MVAs are associated with alcohol and/or other abused drugs, the use of electronic devices (such as smartphones), and fatigue. Accidents are very often related to distractions, of which there are three types: (1) visual distraction—you take your eyes off the road; (2) manual distraction—you remove your hands from the wheel; and (3) cognitive distraction—your attention is diverted from driving.

Fortunately, public education, car safety features, child booster seats, and legislation have reduced unnecessary deaths due to MVAs. The health-related benefits of the mandated use of seat belts cannot be overstated. Motor vehicle safety has advanced due to aggressive educational national, state, and local campaigns. Prevention of MVAs could result in a significant decrease of injuries, pain, and work-related nonproductivity.

Firearms

The use and misuse of firearms has become a societal problem. Adolescents and young adults have shown an increase in mortality and morbidity often due to peer pressure and weapons. If a weapon is kept in the home, statistics show that a child is five times more likely to be injured or killed by a firearm. Firearms are the second leading cause of death for young adults aged 15–24 years. Homicide is the second leading cause of death in adolescents and young adults. It is the number one cause of death among African American youth.

Binge Drinking

Binge drinking is defined as a pattern of drinking that brings a person's blood alcohol concentration (**BAC**) to 0.08% or above. This BAC can happen when men consume five or more alcoholic drinks in about 2 hr. Women's BAC can reach 0.08% in 2 hour with four drinks. Weekend binge drinking is not uncommon in high school students and is very common in college students. Binge drinkers are not typically alcohol dependent. Alcohol is not metabolized in young adults as efficiently as in older adults. The effects of alcohol consumption are often tragic. Binge drinking is associated with the following:

- MVAs
- Violent acts
- Suicide
- Alcohol poisoning
- Sexually transmitted infections (Chapter 70)
- Unintended pregnancy
- Sexual dysfunction
- Fetal alcohol syndrome (Chapter 74)
- Hypertension and CVAs
- Cardiovascular disorders
- Liver disorders
- Neurologic damage
- Lack of control of diabetes

Prevention of binge drinking and its harmful consequences includes mounting aggressive educational campaigns that reach all ages, enforcing existing legislation, and holding individuals responsible who provide alcohol or ignore abuse of alcohol intake.

Suicide

Suicide is among the top 10 leading causes of death for U.S. citizens. The third leading cause of death among persons aged 15–25 years, or about 20% of that group, is suicide. Not included in these mortality rates is the prevalence of suicidal thoughts, suicide planning, and suicide attempts. Statistically, for every one suicide, 25 attempts are documented. Males commit suicide four times more often than do females. Females are more likely to have suicidal ideation (thoughts). The causes of suicide differ. Females tend to use some type of poisoning while males are most likely to use firearms. Some religions and cultures discourage suicide and support the instincts for self-preservation, while other groups view suicide as a noble act of sacrifice. Causes of self-intended harm are complex and include multiple factors. Box 74-1 summarizes Risk Factors for Suicide. Chapter 74 discusses suicide during youth; Chapter 94 examines suicide in adult clients. Suicide prevention includes a mixture of the following:

- Acknowledgment of risk factors, for example, anxiety, depression, mood swings, suicide attempt(s)
- Reduction of risk factors
- Easy access to clinical interventions
- Nonjudgmental family and community support
- Appropriate mental health drug therapies
- Educational awareness of mental health issues

Eating Disorders

Young women who begin dysfunctional eating habits often develop eating disorders between the ages of 12 and 25 years. Eating disorders include self-starvation, bingeing, purging, excessive exercise, and overuse of diuretics, laxatives, and diet pills.

Sexual Health and Safe Sex

Sexual health and safe sex concerns are a result of the peer pressure that exists for early sexual activity. Sexual activity involves consequences such as sexually transmitted infections (STIs). STIs may also be known as sexually transmitted diseases (**STDs**). Chapter 70 discusses sexuality and STIs in more detail.

The use of condoms is recommended for sexually active individuals, whether or not they use other fertility control measures. Condom use does not prevent all disease transmission. Therefore, the use of condoms is considered "safer" but not totally "safe" sex. The use of a dental dam is recommended for those who engage in oral sexual contact.

Abstinence is the only 100% effective way of preventing pregnancy, exposure to herpes, gonorrhea, syphilis, and other STIs.

Pregnancy

Pregnancy occurs most often to women in their 20s and 30s. The maternal and infant morbidity risks are significantly higher in teenage mothers and mothers over the age of 35 years. Prenatal care is imperative, especially with the higher-risk pregnancies. Unit 10 discusses pregnancy in detail.

Pregnant women who smoke or use cocaine, crack, heroin, marijuana, alcohol, or a number of other drugs also put their babies at high risk. Use of crack or cocaine, even one time, can cause learning disabilities, preterm birth, low birth weight, fetal stroke, miscarriage, and stillbirth. Cocaine use increases the chance of preterm birth by 25%.

Pregnant women should maintain a healthy weight, eat a balanced diet (with special modifications), continue physical activity, and avoid smoking and alcohol. Pregnant women should discuss all medications (including over-the-counter drugs) with their PCP.

Mature Adults

Heart Disease and Hypertension

Heart disease is the leading cause of death for both men and women in the United States. One in every four people dies of some form of heart disease, or about 600,000 people annually. Heart disease is a general term for several disorders that affect the heart, coronary arterial vessels, or systemic arterial blood vessels. Cholesterol deposits accumulate in the heart (**coronary artery disease** or **CAD**) and systemic arterial vessels, leading to strictures or narrowing of the arteries. The process of narrowing of the arteries over time by cholesterol is called **atherosclerosis**. Heart disorders due to CAD include myocardial infarctions (heart attacks), angina, heart failure, and strokes (formerly CVAs). Additional problems such as heart failure and arrhythmias can also occur. Heart disease is the leading cause of death for most racial and ethnic groups in the United States.

Hypertension or elevated blood pressure is common in the mature adult, which can be a risk factor in CVAs and MIs. Kidney damage often results. The incidence of hypertension is equal in men and women, although it is more common among African American individuals, especially men.

Many lifestyle factors increase the risk for heart disease and hypertension. For example, women who take birth control pills and smoke significantly increase their risk. Other contributing factors include a mixture of lifestyle choices, for example, smoking, alcohol intake, a lack of physical activity, excess body weight, and high salt (sodium) intake. Diabetes is a major contributing risk factor to CAD. Chapter 81 discusses cardiovascular diseases in more detail.

Diabetes Mellitus

DM is a disease that causes blood glucose levels to rise and remain above normal levels. Normally, the digestive tract breaks down food into glucose, which is sent to the bloodstream. The body needs the hormone insulin, which is formed in the pancreas, to usher circulating glucose into the body's cells. DM develops when your pancreas cannot make enough insulin or cannot use its body's insulin. If the circulating glucose remains in the blood vessels, the cells do not receive insulin and cannot use it to help metabolize sugars within the cells. Your body must have metabolized sugar in order to provide itself with energy. Without insulin or the ability to use insulin, serious complications result. Any part of the body can be affected by diabetes. In individuals with diabetes, many conditions that are typically associated with aging, for example, MI, CAD, and CVA, happen at a younger age; therefore, people with diabetes tend to die earlier than their nondiabetic counterparts.

Diabetes remains among the top 10 causes of death in the United States. The complications of diabetes are among the leading causes of death—heart disease, cancer, and kidney diseases. In fact, diabetes is the largest cause of kidney failure, blindness, and limb amputation in the United States. Signs and symptoms, risk factors, and complications of diabetes are discussed in more detail in Chapter 79, as well within broader discussions throughout the textbook.

Diabetes can be organized into different three main groups:

- Type 1—The client must take insulin to survive.
- Type 2—The client must adjust food intake, lose weight, and may be required to take blood glucose–lowering drugs but not insulin.
- Gestational—The client temporarily develops diabetes during pregnancy. The diabetes may disappear after birth, but the client is at a high risk for developing diabetes later in life.

Prediabetes is a condition of impaired fasting glucose or impaired glucose tolerance. Blood glucose levels are higher than normal but are not yet within the diagnostic range for diabetes. Individuals with prediabetes are at a high risk for developing type 2 diabetes and also have an increased risk of developing heart disease. Weight loss and increased physical activity are known to prevent or delay the onset of diagnosed diabetes. Individuals aged 45 years or older should consider getting tested for diabetes because approximately 30% of cases are undiagnosed. Left untreated, diabetes is fatal.

Diabetes is sometimes preventable and generally manageable, but not curable. The incidence of diabetes is prevalent in all ethnic groups but higher in African Americans, Hispanic Americans, Native Americans, and Asian Americans. Lifestyle changes, nutritional awareness, weight control, and exercise can offset many of these risks. Preventive education is important for every age group.

Men's Health

Men's health issues include the number 1 and 2 killers, which are heart disease and cancer. African American men are at highest risk of heart disease and hypertension. Men need to consider prevention of accidents, a leading cause of injuries and death in all male age groups. Prostate and lung cancer are the most common cancers in men.

Men should self-examine for testicular cancer. Careful observation for symptoms and regular examinations are the best preventive measures against prostate and testicular cancer. Specific issues related to men's health are discussed in Chapters 89 and 90.

Women's Health

Women's health issues include concerns related to reproduction and menopause. Maternal health is discussed in Unit 10. Menopause brings additional health challenges to women. **Osteoporosis** (loss of bone density) is the most prevalent bone disease in the world and causes more than one million fractures of the hip, spine, and wrist yearly in the United States. After menopause, the loss of the estrogenic hormones speeds bone density loss. Women lose bone density and have twice as many fractures as men, especially if they are slender or underweight. The incidence of osteoporosis is higher in White and Asian American women than in other races. Low calcium levels increase a woman's risk factor of developing osteoporosis.

Cardiovascular disorders in women often present with different symptoms than in men. Lack of exercise is a contributing factor, as are smoking, family history of osteoporosis in mother or sister, and removal of ovaries before age 50 years.

Cancer is a concern for women. Because of increases in smoking, lung cancer is a major contributor to increased mortality rates of cancer in women. Breast and ovarian cancers are among the leading causes of cancer deaths in women.

Women need to protect themselves through regular checkups, including mammography (for breast cancer) and Pap tests (for cervical cancer). Regular mammograms are considered an excellent preventive measure.

Older Adults

The major causes of death in the older population are heart disease, cancer, stroke, COPD, pneumonia, and influenza. Many chronic problems are also of concern because of their impact on a person's everyday life. These problems include arthritis, osteoporosis, incontinence, vision and hearing impairment, and dementia. Chapters 92 and 93 discuss aging in more detail.

CATEGORIES OF DISEASE AND DISORDERS

Disease

Diseases are categorized in several ways. Usually, they are classified according to their **etiology** (cause), the body system that they affect, the extent of their involvement in the organ or body, or the way they are acquired. Classifying diseases according to cause is not always satisfactory because more than one body system or dysfunction may be involved. The biologic etiology of some diseases is unknown. Even if one cause is the etiology (e.g., a bacteria, virus, or heredity), the consequences or symptoms of most disorders are not typically limited to a single outcome. Similar symptoms (e.g., pain, fever, loss of function) are associated with each etiology.

Organic and Functional Diseases

A disease is classified as organic or functional. **Organic disease** means that detectable structural change has occurred in one or more organs that also alters usual function. **Functional disease** is a disorder in which a structural cause cannot be identified. The person, however, experiences changes that affect his or her ability to conduct the usual activities of daily living. The person is said to be **dysfunctional** if he or she cannot perform usual activities.

Hereditary Disorders

One or both biologic parents may transmit a **hereditary** (genetic) disorder to an embryo, resulting in the child's physical impairment. For example, hemophilia (prolonged blood clotting time) is a hereditary disorder transmitted from mother to child. It appears mostly in male children because it is almost always carried on the X chromosome. The mother is the carrier and is generally free of symptoms.

Congenital Disorders

Congenital disorders are also present at birth. Unlike hereditary disorders, however, they are not necessarily transmitted through genes. Congenital disorders may be genetic or may be caused by another unfavorable condition that affects normal fetal development. For example, herpes virus in the mother can be transmitted through the placenta or during the birth process and can cause congenital defects. If a woman contracts rubella (German measles) during pregnancy, the disease may cause body abnormalities or defects in the infant. Consumption of alcohol or smoking by a pregnant woman can profoundly affect the fetus. Congenital heart disease and clubbed feet (deformities of bones in the feet) are examples of abnormal fetal development.

Infectious Diseases

A common cause of disease is invasion of the body by microorganisms, such as bacteria or viruses, or by animal parasites. This microscopic invasion is called an *infection*. Some infections are **local**, which means the area of invasion is limited to one area or organ. **Systemic** infections involve the whole body. Microorganisms that cause infections may or may not be **contagious**, which means the infection can be transferred from one person to another. Chapter 40 discusses microorganisms in more detail.

Deficiency Diseases

Deficiency diseases are disorders of nutrition that result from a lack of one or more dietary nutrients. For example, lack of vitamin C causes scurvy. A deficiency of several vitamins, or general malnutrition, is more common in the United States than is a single vitamin deficiency. If the body does not use nutrients properly (malabsorption syndrome), various disorders result. Deficiency diseases also may be seen in the immune system. An immunodeficiency syndrome caused by HIV/AIDS is often manifested in the body by infections, malignancies, and neurologic disease.

Metabolic Disorders

A disturbance of one or more of the endocrine glands causes metabolic disorders. Endocrine glands secrete hormones that regulate body processes (Chapter 20). For example, the thyroid hormone affects the rate of metabolism for the entire body, and insulin deficiency results in DM. Dysfunction occurs from hypersecretion (too much) or hyposecretion (too little) of a hormone.

Neoplastic Diseases

The growth of abnormal tissue or tumors is called **neoplastic**. These growths can be benign or malignant. A **benign** tumor results from the growth of cells similar to the tissue in which it appears. A benign tumor is often surrounded by a capsule. Once removed, the tumor usually does not recur. It may be disfiguring, but it is not dangerous unless it crowds other structures or robs surrounding tissues of their blood supply. A **malignant** tumor (e.g., cancer) is a wild and disorderly growth of cells that is unlike the tissue from which it arises. This cell growth robs normal tissues of nutrients. Malignant cells also tend to spread to other parts of the body, a process called **metastasis**.

Traumatic Injuries

Traumatic injuries are those injuries caused by external forces. Injuries incurred in automobile accidents and falls are examples. Mental trauma (e.g., emotional distress) also falls under this category.

Occupational Disorders

Certain occupational groups are subject to hazardous conditions particular to their jobs. Construction, firefighting, agriculture, and mining are examples of occupations with high rates of morbidity and mortality. High stress environments can exist in any occupation. Stress is a major factor of maladaptive behaviors such as overeating and smoking. Violence in any workplace is, unfortunately, not uncommon. Healthcare personnel may be required to receive self-protection training for possible or probable exposure to pathogens and violence in the workplace. Myocardial infarctions, injuries from falls, or injuries from equipment are examples of some of the numerous perilous aspects of occupational disorders.

Morbidity can also be related to occupational exposures to substances or environment. Employees who work around chemicals, radiation, smoke from fires, and other hazardous materials are more likely to be susceptible to acute and chronic conditions. People working in noisy areas for prolonged periods must wear protective devices to prevent permanent hearing loss. Prevention of occupational disorders begins with awareness and education of the hazards of the job. Equipment needs to be designed for safety. Enforcement of safety regulations is a priority.

STUDENT SYNTHESIS

KEY POINTS

- Although many definitions of health exist, optimum health includes physical, emotional, mental, social, and spiritual well-being.
- The state of one's health is on a continuum and is dynamic, changing from day to day.
- The concept of high-level wellness relates to the higher-level needs in Maslow's hierarchy.
- Lifestyle changes can have a major impact on health and wellness.
- The four most important wellness lifestyle factors are physical activity, healthy diet, maintenance of appropriate body weight, and not smoking.
- Some stress is beneficial, whereas too much stress can lead to physical and emotional disorders.
- Keys to changing behavior include health promotion, education, and community health awareness.
- Infant mortality remains a health concern in the United States.
- The major cause of death and disability in young children involves accidents.
- Accidents continue to be a major health concern for adolescents and young adults, along with homicide and suicide.
- Heart disease and cancer are the top causes of death in adults.
- Diabetes mellitus is a major healthcare concern to all ages; early diagnosis and treatment are suggested.
- The etiology of diseases and disorders may be organic, functional, hereditary, congenital, infectious, related to a deficiency, metabolic, neoplastic, traumatic, or related to an occupation.

CRITICAL THINKING EXERCISES

1. Based on the information provided in this chapter, relate how the health of citizens of other nations can affect your and your neighbors' health.
2. Describe "high-level wellness" in terms of your own lifestyle. What measures can you take to improve your own health?
3. Relate wellness and a healthy lifestyle to Maslow's hierarchy of needs.
4. In Africa, a child dies every 30 s of malaria, or about 3,000 children per day. Discuss what your community and your country would be expected to do if this statistic were true of any infection affecting you.

NCLEX-STYLE REVIEW QUESTIONS

1. The nurse is planning a community program with other healthcare providers in order to address prevention of the leading cause of death for men and women. Which program would take priority to address this issue?
   a. Early recognition and intervention of coronary artery disease
   b. Development of a support group for families of those affected by Alzheimer's disease
   c. Recognition of the early signs of Parkinson disease
   d. Recognition and intervention to prevent suicide

2. A client with diabetes asks the nurse, "If I can't do heavy exercise, what's the point in exercising?" Which response by the nurse regarding the benefits of exercise can encourage the client to perform moderate exercise? Select all that apply.
   a. Prevents the use of insulin.
   b. Prevents cancer.
   c. Enhances energy levels.
   d. Reduces stress.
   e. Provides relaxation.

3. A parent brings a toddler into the clinic with a strong odor of cigarette smoke on the toddler's clothing. Which information should the nurse discuss with the parent?
   a. Secondhand smoke may cause numerous health-related problems.
   b. If the parent continues to smoke around the child, the parent will be reported for child abuse.
   c. Continuing to smoke around the child can create childhood nicotine addiction.
   d. Seeing a parent smoke will lead to the child smoking.

4. A parent states that since the birth of a sibling, the older child is wetting the bed. How should the nurse respond to the parent?
   a. "This is referred to as regression and is a common defense mechanism."
   b. "The child is in denial and can't accept the fact that another child is part of the family."
   c. "The child is repressing feelings of anger."
   d. "The child is punishing the parent by soiling."

5. The nurse is gathering data from a client in the home setting for care of a pressure wound. The nurse observes multiple areas of ecchymosis in various stages of healing. The client states, "They do their best to care for me but get frustrated when I wet the bed." What priority action should the nurse take?
   a. Ask the family why they are abusing the client.
   b. Place the client in the car and take the client to the nearest emergency department.
   c. Ensure the client's safety and notify adult protective services.
   d. Call the police department and file a complaint.

CHAPTER RESOURCES

Enhance your learning with additional resources on thePoint!

Student Resources related to this chapter can be found at **thePoint.lww.com/Rosdahl12e**.

7 Community Health

Learning Objectives

1. Define the term *community*. State the relationship of a community to the health of that community. Identify types of communities.
2. Identify the health-related functions of the WHO and UNICEF.
3. State the achievements attributed to improvements in public health that resulted in an increase of lifespan in the 20th century.
4. Define and differentiate between the USPHS and the HHS.
5. Identify and discuss functions of the HHS, the CDC, and the FDA.
6. Discuss the purpose of the NIH and state the role of the NINR.
7. Identify the functions of OSHA and of the Social Security Agency.
8. Identify the role and functions of the National Safety Council, the Red Cross, and the VNA.
9. Differentiate between organizations that are related to specific disorders and organizations promoting specific health goals.
10. Identify at least seven programs that are common to state healthcare services.
11. Discuss primary care and functions of the community health center.
12. Identify the causes and discuss the significance of the various types of pollution.

Important Terminology

biohazardous
bionomics
community
community health
demography
ecology
plumbism
pollution
primary healthcare
radiation
radon
Standard Precautions
target population
Transmission-Based Precautions
worker's compensation

Acronyms

(*Note:* Each government agency has its own acronym and not all acronyms in this chapter are listed below.)

CDC	IFRC	UNICEF
DOA	MUA	USDA
DOL	NHIC	USPHS
EMS	NIH	VNA
EPA	NINR	WHO
FDA	NSC	WIC
FQHC	OSHA	
HHS	SSA	
ICRC	UN	

A group of individuals who interact with each other for the mutual benefit of their common interests to support a sense of unity or belonging is a **community**. You are a member of many communities: your family, school, place of employment, town or city, state or province, nation, and the world. Community can also refer to a smaller organization, such as a retirement home or a health maintenance organization.

Communities are studied as a part of **demography**, which is the study of populations. Demography examines the dynamic balances among population size, racial and ethnic distribution, economic opportunities, growth potential, and other indicators. Health concerns are based on a community's demographics as well as a nation's overall health and economy. World and national events influence state and local communities. The welfare and priorities of the individual are balanced against the needs and resources of a community.

Chapter 6 initiated discussions on health issues in general and how health issues relate to communities. **Community health** is the aggregate health of a population: a town, state, nation, or planet. A community's health is continuously monitored by numerous federal and state agencies using the Leading Health Indicators listed in Chapter 6 plus other factors, such as rates of birth, morbidity (illness), mortality (death), teen pregnancy, immunizations, sexually transmitted infections (STIs), prevalence of infectious diseases, and prevalence of cancer.

Other factors influencing societal health include crime and high school graduation rates, and juvenile justice statistics. The number of people living below the federal poverty threshold, population density, incidences of domestic violence, and adequate housing (rental and ownership) contribute to community health.

HEALTHCARE WORLDWIDE

Health promotion is a worldwide concern. The guidelines established by the World Health Organization (WHO) have become international standards for sanitation, chemical safety, water purification, immunizations, and infectious diseases. Box 6-1 in Chapter 6 reviews the trends and goals of this organization. As a part of the United Nations (UN) in New York City, WHO's objectives are to emphasize growth and development of significant internal, governmental changes in countries that currently have difficulty providing basic healthcare services to their citizens. Review the section in Chapter 6 on the United Nations and their Sustainable Development Goals.

The WHO sends healthcare professionals to nations to combat diseases and disorders at both the community and the individual level. Ebola, malaria, tuberculosis, HIV, and other diseases are major international health concerns. Women of childbearing age are of special concern. More than 228 million cases of malaria occurred worldwide in 2018, with 405,000 documented deaths (Centers for Disease Control, 2020). Although malaria was eliminated in the United States in the early 1950s, about 2,000 cases each year are reported. The CDC reports that these cases are almost always linked to recent travelers to countries with uncontrolled malaria.

> *Nursing Alert* Even if a disease such as Ebola or malaria is uncommon, it cannot be ruled out. You must be aware that a client's travel history is part of your nursing data collection.

The WHO also addresses other issues. Globally, public health officials are increasing their nations' efforts to decrease smoking. The diseases associated with the high-fat, high-salt, and high-calorie intake of Western industrialized countries—such as cardiac disease and hypertension—are noted. Mental health issues are also addressed.

Hundreds of international healthcare and nonhealthcare agencies are linked to the WHO. After events such as earthquakes, floods, or volcanic eruptions, a country may need extensive assistance to prevent starvation and widespread disease. The UN tailors specific programs to meet the needs that arise from natural disasters.

Another UN program, the United Nations Children's Fund (UNICEF) helps children, especially those in developing countries. Some of its goals include nutrition instruction, development of low-cost food supplements, support of general education, childhood immunization programs, procedures for supplying safe water, and infant rehydration programs.

> **NCLEX Alert**
>
> NCLEX scenarios may relate to changing, eliminating, or treating the effects of risk factors. Read the scenario carefully and select the best option available, which may be different from what you might want to do in a similar situation.

HEALTHCARE ON THE NATIONAL LEVEL

United States Public Health Service

The United States Public Health Service (USPHS) is about 220 years old. Since 1798, it has had many responsibilities, including investigation and control of communicable diseases, protection from disease carried by immigrants, control of sanitation, prevention of disease spread through interstate commerce, and control of the manufacture and sale of biologic products.

The achievements of the USPHS are truly impressive. Life expectancy in the early 1900s was about 45 years. Due to regulations and implementation of health safety and healthcare measures, the lifespan of Americans has increased to about 78 years in the 21st century. Advances in public health have contributed to at least 30 of those additional years. Eight of the most notable contributions to the increase in lifespan include:

- Vaccinations
- Motor-vehicle safety
- Safer workplaces
- Control of infectious diseases
- Declines in deaths from coronary artery disease and stroke
- Safer and healthier foods
- Healthier mothers and babies
- Recognition of tobacco use as a health hazard

Despite these improvements, however, in the United States, life expectancy for some ethnic or racial minorities, especially non-Hispanic black males, remains below that of others (Fig. 7-1).

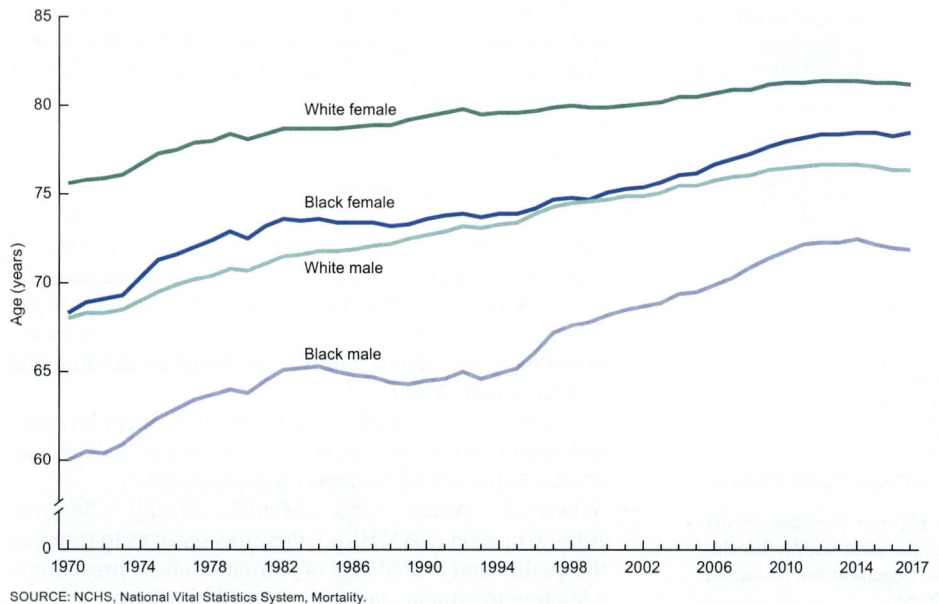

Figure 7-1 Comparative life expectancies at birth, 1970–2017. (Centers for Disease Control, 2019.)

SOURCE: NCHS, National Vital Statistics System, Mortality.

The USPHS was the forerunner of the U.S. Department of Health and Human Services (HHS). HHS was created by Congress and is one of the executive agencies of the U.S. president.

Department of Health and Human Services

The Department of HHS is a highly versatile agency that has a myriad of responsibilities. The agencies that constitute the branches of HHS are listed in Figure 7-2 and described below. Each of these programs provides a multitude of services. You may be familiar with some of these agencies, as they are often mentioned publicly and many individuals benefit from these resources. Three of the branches of HHS that will be discussed in further detail are the Centers for Disease Control and Preventions (CDC), the Food and Drug Administration (FDA), and the National Institutes of Health (NIH). The day-to-day effects of all of the HHS agencies on U.S., citizens, as well as on individuals in a global population, cannot be overstated. Box 7-1 summarizes the priorities of the HHS. You are encouraged to check the Websites of each component of the agencies of HHS.

> **Box 7-1 Priorities of the Department of Health and Human Services**
>
> The Department of Health and Human Services (HHS) is one of the larger U.S. institutions and includes the CDC, FDA, and NIH. Its aims are to identify healthcare challenges and to find solutions to these problems.
> - Health insurance marketplace
> - Affordable Care Act
> - Mental health
> - Stop bullying
> - Be tobacco free
> - Food safety
> - Getting vaccinated
> - Flu prevention
> - Raise healthier kids
> - Open government at HHS
> - Stop Medicare fraud
> - HHS digital strategy
> - Supporting military families
> - Fighting HIV/AIDS
>
> http://www.hhs.gov.

- Administration for Children and Families (ACF): Provides services and assistance to needy children and families
- Administration for Community Living: Provides assistance and support for aging persons and individuals with intellectual and developmental disabilities
- Agency for Healthcare Research and Quality (AHRQ): Provides research designed to improve quality of healthcare, including information on costs and client safety
- Agency for Toxic Substances and Disease Registry (ATSDR): Provides information, assessments, and educational training related to the U.S. Environmental Protection Agency's (EPA) national priorities list of hazardous substances and waste sites
- Centers for Medicare & Medicaid Services (CMS): Administers the Medicare and Medicaid programs and the Children's Health Insurance Program
- Health Resources and Services Administration (HRSA): Provides health resources for medically underserved populations, such as migrant workers, the homeless, and residents of public housing; oversees the national organ transplantation system; provides services to decrease infant mortality and to improve the health of children and of people with AIDS
- Indian Health Service (IHS): Provides a network of hospitals and health centers and stations for American Indians and Alaska Natives of 557 federally recognized tribes
- Substance Abuse and Mental Health Services Administration (SAMHSA): Provides services to improve the quality and availability of substance abuse prevention, addiction treatment, and mental health services

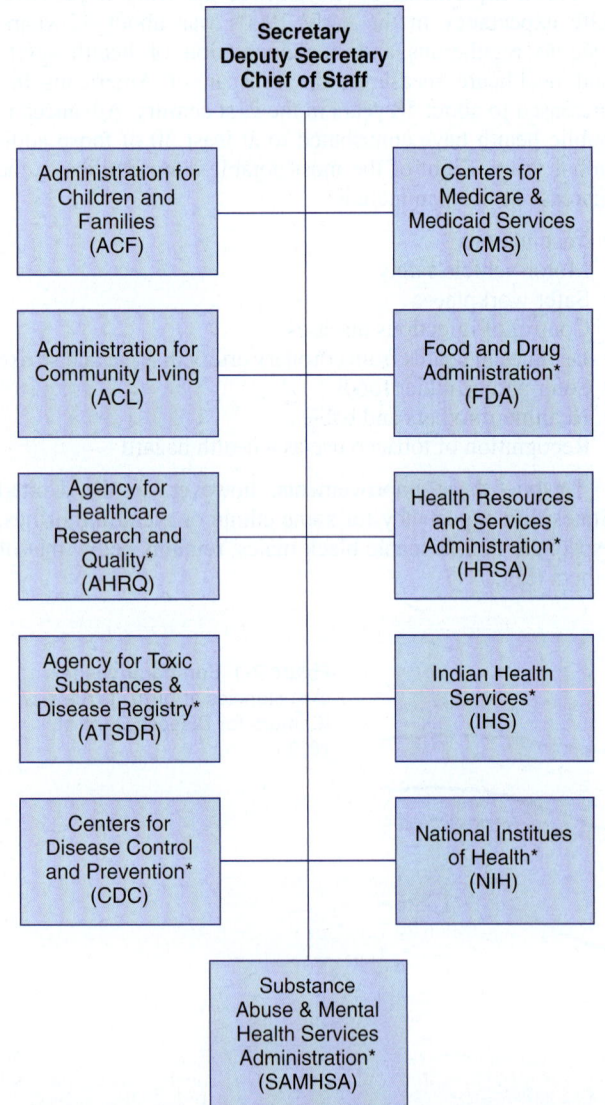

*Designates a component of the U.S. Public Health Service

Figure 7-2 Department of Health and Human Services (HHS) is an important government agency. Its agencies supply fundamental healthcare services to multiple populations. (Adapted from http://www.hhs.gov/about/orgchart/.)

- CDC: Provides health surveillance to monitor and prevent outbreaks of disease; guards against international disease transmission; maintains national health statistics; provides for immunization services; and supports research into disease and injury prevention
- FDA: Provides for the safety of foods and cosmetics, and the safety and effectiveness of pharmaceuticals, biologic products, and medical devices
- NIH: Provides for research projects in 27 separate institutes for thousands of health-related subjects

> **Key Concept**
>
> Health information is available from many sources. A referral service called the National Health Information Center (NHIC) provides health professionals and consumers with resource organizations. Visit the Center's Website (www.health.gov/nhic).

Centers for Disease Control and Prevention

The mission of the CDC is to promote health and quality of life by preventing and controlling disease, injury, and disability. This globally recognized agency is a major force in the protection of the health and safety of citizens of the United States. It also functions as an advocate for environmental health, health promotion, and education worldwide. Review Box 6-4 for more information.

CDC national headquarters is located in Atlanta, Georgia, but it also has health departments in most states and employees in many countries. It works with nearly 200 public health disciplines throughout the world to:

- Monitor health trends
- Detect local, national, or international outbreaks (e.g., avian flu), or occurrences of bioterrorism (e.g., anthrax, Ebola, influenzas)
- Investigate disease outbreaks
- Conduct research
- Enhance prevention
- Promote healthy behaviors
- Foster safe and healthy environments
- Provide current and accurate health-related information to the public
- Protect the public via direct actions (e.g., immunizations) and indirect actions (e.g., education)
- Foster cooperative relationships with global, national, state, and local organizations to combat dangerous environmental exposures, such as might occur in the air, the water, and the workplace

Due to the increases in transnational healthcare safety concerns, Global Disease Detection Centers have been developed throughout the world. The CDC has the scientific ability and resources to respond to infectious outbreaks, to identify infectious diseases, and to assist with the treatment of these problems. Examples of potential health threats that were prevented or controlled include anthrax in Scotland, cholera in Haiti and Africa, and legionella in Mexico. The CDC recognizes that a weakness in the health monitoring system in any one country can become a threat to all countries (CDC, 2020).

Food and Drug Administration

As an agency within the HHS, the FDA's mission is to promote and protect public health by helping safe and effective products reach the market in a timely way and by monitoring products for continued safety after they are in use. The FDA blends science and law to protect consumers. In some instances, its goal is to advance public health and safety by helping speed product innovations. Some of the specific duties of the FDA include *monitoring* the *safety, effectiveness,* and *quality* of the following: human drugs; veterinary drugs; tobacco products; vaccines and biologic products; medical devices; electronic products that give off radiation; cosmetics; dietary supplements; and food supply (with the exception of meat from livestock, poultry, and some egg products, which are regulated by the U.S. Department of Agriculture).

The headquarters for the FDA is in Washington, D.C., but it also has nearly 200 field offices. FDA's responsibilities extend to the 50 U.S. states, the District of Columbia, Puerto Rico, Guam, the Virgin Islands, American Samoa, and other U.S. territories and possessions.

Employees perform inspections, surveillance, laboratory studies, and education in industrial and public sectors. The FDA does not develop or test products itself. Scientists and medical personnel at the FDA carefully review marketing applications submitted by the laboratories and/or clinical trials of other agencies, for example, a pharmaceutical company. FDA accomplishments include:

- Requiring that new drugs and complex medical devices (e.g., cardiac pacemakers) be proved safe before they are put into a consumer market
- Reviewing or revising performance standards for products, such as x-ray machines, mammography equipment, and microwave ovens
- Requiring safety practices in blood banking
- Requiring accurate, truthful, and useful labeling for prescription drugs, over-the-counter medications, foods, and dietary supplements
- Conducting scientific research and providing standards and guidelines to make regulatory decisions
- Requesting or requiring that manufacturers recall unsafe products

National Institutes of Health

Another well-known component of the HHS is the NIH. The NIH is unique in that it is the nation's medical research agency. Its goals are to make medical and scientific discoveries that improve health and save lives. New knowledge will lead to better health for everyone. In Box 7-2, you will see the 27 separate institutes or centers that make up the NIH, each dedicated to a particular area of medical or nursing research. These individual institutes are located in 75 buildings on more than 300 acres in Bethesda, Maryland. Every center has a specific research agenda which focuses on specific diseases or body systems. The NIH also has

> **Box 7-2** **National Institutes of Health**
>
> The National Institutes of Health (NIH) is composed of 27 separate research institutes and centers. Throughout your nursing education and your nursing career, you will find these sites helpful. The NIH Website has detailed information on the functions of each institute.
>
> - Office of the Director (OD)
> - National Cancer Institute (NCI)
> - National Eye Institute (NEI)
> - National Heart, Lung, and Blood Institute (NHLBI)
> - National Human Genome Research Institute (NHGRI)
> - National Institute on Aging (NIA)
> - National Institute on Alcohol Abuse and Alcoholism (NIAAA)
> - National Institute of Allergy and Infectious Diseases (NIAID)
> - National Institute of Arthritis and Musculoskeletal and Skin Diseases (NIAMS)
> - National Institute of Child Health and Human Development (NICHD)
> - National Institute on Deafness and Other Communication Disorders (NIDCD)
> - National Institute of Dental and Craniofacial Research (NIDCR)
> - National Institute of Diabetes and Digestive and Kidney Diseases (NIDDK)
> - National Institute on Drug Abuse (NIDA)
> - National Institute of Environmental Health Sciences (NIEHS)
> - National Institute of General Medical Sciences (NIGMS)
> - National Institute of Mental Health (NIMH)
> - National Institute of Neurological Disorders and Stroke (NINDS)
> - National Institute of Nursing Research (NINR)
> - National Library of Medicine (NLM)
> - National Institute for Biomedical Imaging and Bioengineering (NIBIB)
> - National Institutes of Health Clinical Center (CC)
> - Center for Information Technology (CIT)
> - National Center for Complementary and Alternative Medicine (NCCAM)
> - National Center for Research Resources (NCRR)
> - National Center on Minority Health and Health Disparities (NCMHD)
> - John E. Fogarty International Center (FIC)
> - Center for Scientific Review (CSR)

National Institutes of Health, www.nih.gov.

its own and unique Clinical Center, which is the largest hospital in the world totally dedicated to clinical research. Each institute works in its specific field to accomplish the following goals:

- Conducting research on site or through universities, medical schools, hospitals, or other research institutions
- Training research investigators
- Promoting improved sharing of medical information

It is of special significance to nursing professionals that the NIH formally recognized nursing as a unique and important component of the healthcare system in 1993, when the National Institute for Nursing Research (NINR) was established. The NINR separates the funding for nursing research from other institute research funding, such as medicine.

The NINR supports research and establishes a scientific basis for the care of individuals across the lifespan. The focus of nursing research is to discover ways to benefit clients. These areas include:

- Managing clients during illness and recovery
- Reducing risks for disease and disability
- Promoting needs for underserved, high-risk clients, such as those with chronic illness and healthcare disparities
- Caring for individuals at the end of life
- Promoting the care of families within a community

Other Federal Agencies

Occupational Safety and Health Administration

Along with the HHS, the U.S. Department of Labor (DOL) is an Executive Agency of the federal government. Several subdivisions of the DOL gather information related to working conditions, occupational hazards, international child labor, and numerous other work-related issues.

The Occupational Safety and Health Administration (OSHA) is the subdivision of the DOL that works to prevent occupational injury and illness. OSHA regulations cover most of the private sector businesses as well as many public sector workers in all 50 states, plus certain territories and other jurisdictions under U.S. federal authority. OSHA has affiliations with individual state agencies that focus on occupational health and safety. OSHA accomplishments include:

- Standards for safety and health protection in the workplace
- Standards for occupational exposure to blood-borne pathogens
- Standards published to protect construction workers
- Ergonomic standards to prevent musculoskeletal disorders

Healthcare workers encounter a vast number of safety concerns. According to OSHA, the healthcare industry has one of the highest rates of work-related injuries and illnesses (OSHA, 2020). Healthcare has a very wide assortment of sources of possible injuries:

- Blood-borne pathogens
- Biologic hazards
- Chemical and drug exposures
- Waste anesthetic gas exposures
- Respiratory hazards, infectious respiratory pathogens
- Ergonomic hazards and repetitive tasks
- Musculoskeletal injuries from falls and other hazards
- Laser hazards
- Workplace violence, assaults
- Laboratory hazards and accidents
- Radioactivity material and x-ray exposure

OSHA has developed criteria for the education and protection of all levels of healthcare workers, in all settings, regarding blood-borne pathogens, particularly hepatitis B and HIV. These criteria are found in **Standard Precautions** and its supplement,

Transmission-Based Precautions (airborne, droplet, and contact). OSHA's standards mandate that all healthcare agencies and facilities develop policies, procedures, education, and training for staff, and encourage immunization of healthcare workers against hepatitis B. Ultimately, these standards serve to protect consumers as well. Chapter 42 and Table 42-1 provide detailed information regarding Standard Precautions and Transmission-Based Precautions.

> *Nursing Alert* Standard Precautions and Transmission-Based Precautions are fundamental procedures of healthcare. Everyone who works with client needs to understand and to use these guidelines for their own safety as well as prevention of cross-contamination of pathogens to the public sector.

Another subdivision of the DOL is the Bureau of Labor Statistics, which assists with worker's compensation. **Worker's compensation** provides financial compensation to a person who has been injured at work or who has contracted a disease that can be directly related to his or her job. The federal government supervises the program, and employers are required to contribute funds, based on the hazards of the particular occupation and the place of employment.

Social Security Administration
In 1995, the Social Security Administration (SSA) splits from the HHS to become an independent agency. The SSA provides retirement income for many people and financial assistance for healthcare to special populations.

Persons older than 62 or 65 years, and those of any age with special disabilities or handicaps, may receive financial support from this agency, as well as from Medicare and Medicaid (see Chapter 3), which the SSA oversees. Regular Social Security benefits are also available to persons younger than 62 years as a result of the death, disability, or retirement of a parent or spouse.

USDA: Women, Infants, and Children
The USDA is responsible for the control of insect- and animal-borne diseases, meat and other food inspections, and school lunch programs. The USDA also administers the Special Supplemental Nutrition Program for Women, Infants, and Children (WIC). The goal of this program is to improve the health of pregnant women, new mothers, and their infants. Most states also have a Department of Agriculture (DOA).

Other National and International Organizations

National Safety Council
Founded in 1913, the National Safety Council (NSC) is a nonprofit organization whose mission is to save lives by preventing injuries and deaths at work, in homes and communities, and on the road. The mission of the NSC is fostered by partnerships with businesses, government agencies, elected officials, and the public. The NSC relies on research to educate and influence society to adopt safety, health, and environmental policies, practices, and procedures that prevent and mitigate human suffering and economic losses arising from preventable causes.

The NSC analyzes causes of accidents, develops preventative measures, and disseminates information to industry, to the public, and for public highway usage. A recent focus of NSC advocacy has been distracted driving and teen driving. For example, highway and traffic laws protect everyone by requiring inspection of motor vehicles, licensing of drivers, establishing speed regulations, and providing highway markings. All states require seat belts and child safety seats.

Influenced by the NSC, building and electrical codes require mandatory sprinkler systems, automatic alarm systems, emergency lighting, and regular inspections, which reduce fires, accidents, and health hazards. Educational programs and training help to convert the information gained by the NSC into direct actions that affect community well-being.

The Red Cross and the Red Crescent
The *Red Cross* was originally formed in 1863 by a young Swiss man, Henry Dunant, whose efforts organized the local citizens in time of need to help fallen and injured soldiers. Later, this national organization grew into the *International Committee of the Red Cross* (ICRC). In many countries, the organization is known as the *Red Crescent*. Humanitarian needs during times of conflict and disaster have continued the need of the National Red Cross and Red Crescent Societies. Each unique local society works in its home country as an asset to their respective healthcare systems by providing emergency medical services (EMS). The American Red Cross is discussed below. Both of these national and international societies provide assistance to protect the life and dignity of the victims of national and global conflicts and community disasters.

The *International Federation Red Cross and Red Crescent Societies* (IFRC) is a humanitarian partnership between several global agencies. In the early 20th century, an international medical conference proposed the formation of international medical groups, such as the American Red Cross, International Red Cross, and the International Red Crescent societies. Millions of volunteers worked to assist with humanitarian activities on behalf of prisoners of war and combatants. Today, these societies are interlinked as the IFRC and are found in nearly every country in the world.

The American Red Cross
The *American Red Cross* was founded by nurse Clara Barton in 1881. Although not a federal agency, the American Red Cross provides national and international services. For example, local Red Cross chapters work with community health associations and public health departments to coordinate services during disasters. Globally, the American Red Cross has several strategically located facilities and supplies that are available for use when a disaster occurs. Services provided by the American Red Cross include:

- *Armed forces emergency services:* Communications, counseling, financial assistance
- *Biomedical services:* Blood, tissue, and plasma services in national testing laboratories
- *Community services:* Food and nutrition, homeless issues, and transportation

- *Health and safety services:* Swimming, youth programs, health and safety programs
- *International services:* Emergency disaster response, tracing individuals, and providing messages

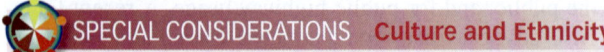

SPECIAL CONSIDERATIONS — Culture and Ethnicity

The symbol of a red cross was adopted by the International Red Cross Movement as a symbol of neutrality. However, some societies view the Red Cross emblem as a religious symbol. In Islamic countries, the symbol of a Red Crescent is used. In Israel, a symbol of the Red Shield of David designates the function of the Movement.

Visiting Nurse Association

The Visiting Nurse Association of America (VNA) is a nationwide, not-for-profit, community-based home health and hospice care agency. The VNA provides care to any person regardless of his or her ability to pay. VNAs collaborate with other health and social service agencies throughout the community, setting up health linkages and networks.

Health services may be provided in a person's home or in a senior residence, board-and-care home, or homeless shelter. Services may be therapeutic or preventive in nature. For example, a VNA may conduct tuberculin screening, immunizations for communicable diseases, or education programs about STIs. Refer to Chapters 98 and 100 for more information on these services. Direct care services provided by the VNA include:

- Skilled nursing
- Physical therapy
- Maternal and child care
- Medical social work
- Pain management
- Hospice
- Private duty nursing
- Enterostomal therapies
- IV and enteral therapies

Organizations Related to Specific Diseases

The American Cancer Society, the National Society for the Prevention of Blindness, the American Heart Association, the American Diabetes Association, the Cystic Fibrosis Foundation, the National Easter Seal Society, the March of Dimes, and numerous other organizations fulfill the need for funding and education devoted to specific diseases. These national voluntary agencies often have state or regional affiliates.

In many cases, volunteer organizations sponsor activities or conduct fund drives to raise money for treatment or research relating to their particular area of interest. They may also receive some funding from campaigns, such as those conducted by the United Way. Many organizations publish pamphlets, books, and audiovisual materials to educate the public. Clinics, waiting and reception areas, and physician's offices are often sources of free brochures, as depicted in Figure 7-3. One of your employment duties might be to ensure that waiting areas have educational materials available for the public.

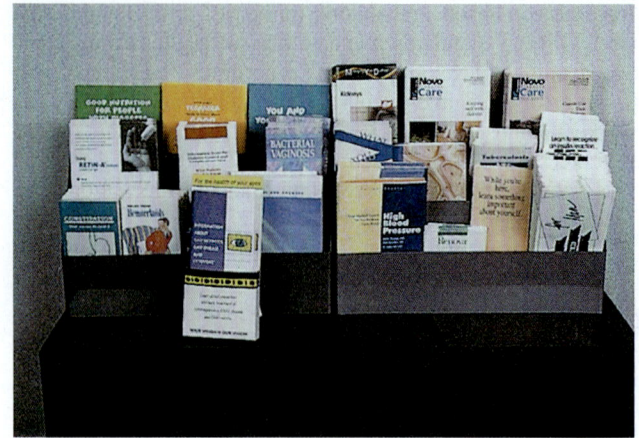

Figure 7-3 Clinics and physicians' offices are often sources of free brochures. Nurses have access to or receive quite a lot of free, educational materials. Be responsible and use these materials in your waiting or reception areas and give them to clients, friends, and families.

Voluntary health agencies include those that provide direct service and those that provide education and conduct fund-raising. Voluntary organizations can have a great impact. They may be able to provide a specific or unique service, or fill a healthcare gap.

Organizations That Promote Specific Health Goals

Some voluntary health agencies are concerned not with disease, but with the promotion of one aspect of health. For example, Planned Parenthood of America focuses on family planning and prevention of STIs. Their counselors, physicians, and nurses assist people by providing genetic counseling, abortion counseling, infertility examination, and birth control. They may also provide prenatal care. Another such organization, the La Leche League, advances maternal and newborn health by encouraging breastfeeding.

HEALTHCARE AT THE STATE LEVEL

State health laws must conform to federal laws, but states also have the right to make their own health laws, if necessary. Many state agencies are also affiliated with federal agencies such as OSHA. Sometimes funding for programs is derived from money received from both federal and state agencies, as is the case with Medicaid.

Typically, state healthcare services may be grouped into separate programs under a State Department of Health, or under broader umbrellas, such as a Department of Consumer Affairs or a Department of HHS. Regardless of the titles, the services that the states provide remain basically standard. However, the comprehensiveness of services in each state may differ widely. Programs or agencies on state levels address many specific healthcare concerns including:

- Aging
- Children's health
- Families in need
- Mental health

- Special populations, such as underrepresented ethnic groups and persons with disabilities (hearing and vision impaired, physical disabilities)
- Alcohol and substance abuse
- Environmental health
- Communicable diseases
- Safety and disability issues

In addition to services that are directly related to the healthcare of a community, state agencies provide certification and licensing requirements for healthcare professionals (nurse aides, nurses, and physicians). Additional regulatory agencies may be available for ancillary healthcare providers such as chiropractors, optometrists, midwives, pharmacists, or physical therapists.

State health departments serve as consultants to local health departments and exercise regulatory powers over them. State health departments often serve as surveyors to enforce federal health requirements, along with planning health requirements for their own jurisdictions.

HEALTHCARE AT THE LOCAL LEVEL

City, town, or county health departments focus on the health protection of persons within their jurisdiction. Usually the Department of Health operates under a Board of Health or Public Health Service. These departments carry out policies and regulations under the direction of a health officer. State regulations mandate requirements for health officer licensure; public health education is a prerequisite.

Health departments provide services dealing with conditions that affect all residents. Their personnel inspect places where food is sold and the people who handle food. They check water and milk supplies, housing, and sewage and other waste disposal facilities. They monitor and control air quality. They may provide school health services and health education, community clinics, or hospital/nursing home care.

The Community Health Center

Regional community health centers or family health centers may be formed using funds from the HHS. The regional centers, for example, state or local health departments, often sponsor community-based healthcare sometimes referred to as **primary healthcare**. The concepts of primary healthcare are to provide integrated, accessible healthcare services by clinicians who are responsible for addressing important healthcare needs of individual persons, families, and communities. Advanced practice nurses (nurse practitioners), working with physicians, often provide primary healthcare in community health centers. Available services include physical screenings, maternal and prenatal care, and specialized examinations for both men and women (Health Resources and Services Administration, n.d.).

Target populations are subgroups in a community with unique or special healthcare needs, such as those experiencing homelessness, older adults, younger individuals, migrant workers, or immigrants. Community health centers may provide healthcare services in locations where target populations are found. When health centers are located near the target population, individuals have easier access to healthcare. Compared with traditional medical clinics, community-based healthcare is generally designed to have resources for low-income households.

The community health center may provide testing for various disorders, including tuberculosis, STIs (including HIV), and lead poisoning. It provides immunizations and prenatal services.

> **NCLEX Alert**
>
> Use the ABC acronym as a guide for prioritization on the NCLEX. ABC = Airway, Breathing/Bleeding, and Circulation. Acute, life-sustaining needs always take precedence before chronic concerns (e.g., hygiene) or preventive needs (e.g., immunizations).

Infants and older adults are served in wellness programs or through nursing care and preventive services provided in the home. Other services of the community health center include programs for special clients, such as those with AIDS, the homeless, migrant workers, and teen parents. The centers refer clients as necessary to other providers for further care.

Centers with similar functions may be referred to as *public health centers* and function under the state's Public Health Department. The U.S. Public Health Service designates and monitors certain community health centers, called Federally Qualified Healthcare (FQHC). FQHCs provide healthcare in parts of the United States identified as medically underserved areas (MUA). Bilingual staff members are present in many centers, to better serve the varied populations in the local service area. The Public Health services and the CDC work collaboratively to address local, national, and international health issues.

THE ENVIRONMENT

Humanity is only one part of a complex system that depends on the balance of life, growth, and death of all living organisms on the planet. This growing recognition has awakened many concerned citizens to the need to preserve this balance. The study of mutual relationships between living beings and their environment is called **ecology** or **bionomics**. The federal EPA was established in an attempt to control problems relating to the environment and its ecology.

Pollution

The task of maintaining ecologic balances to preserve safe air to breathe, water to drink, and food to eat is complicated. **Pollution** (contamination and impurity) severely compromises the ecologic balance.

Air Pollution

Air pollution can be in the form of a solid, liquid droplets, or gases. They can be of natural or man-made origins. A pollutant can be of natural origin or man-made. Air pollution is greatest in industrial areas (e.g., factories), exhaust from motor vehicles, and smog. Smog results from vehicular and industrial emissions that interact with ultraviolet light from the sun. Every community has some air pollution, even though it may have comparatively few industries. The sources of air contaminants include:

- Natural gases, such as sulfur, nitrogen oxides, carbon monoxide
- Volatile organic compounds, such as methane or nonmethane gases
- Toxic metals, such as lead, mercury
- Chlorofluorocarbons, from air conditioners, aerosol sprays, refrigerators
- Ammonia, from fertilizers, agricultural processes
- Particulate matter (fine particles of solid or liquid suspended in a gas), from volcanoes, dust storms, forest fires, burning of fossil fuels

Air pollution is responsible for increases in respiratory infections, such as chronic bronchitis and emphysema. The incidence of asthma is increasing, especially in the young. Poor air quality, tobacco smoke, and numerous other pollutants are directly connected to asthma. Heavy pollution irritates the eyes, nose, and throat and may have other serious health effects as yet unknown. Polluted air damages plant life, including farm crops. Pollution is also destructive to building materials.

Pollution inside buildings is a concern. Persons who work in certain industrial environments must wear protective gear to prevent lung disorders. In addition, office buildings, hotels, and other public buildings are now tightly sealed, with air cooling, heating, and ventilation controlled mechanically. Such regulation may contribute to respiratory disorders, such as asthma and sinusitis, particularly if the air is not exchanged often enough. Smoking is not allowed in many public buildings. Furnaces or tuck-under garages may release carbon monoxide and other dangerous gases into a home's atmosphere. Homes should not be too tightly sealed, to avoid buildup of these gases. A carbon monoxide detector should be present in every home, along with a smoke detector.

Secondhand Smoke

Studies of the effects of random tobacco smoke in the environment, also known as secondhand smoke, have shown that any amount of smoke is potentially unhealthy to anyone breathing the polluted air. Even small amounts of secondhand smoke can be hazardous to one's health. This concern is of importance to all people, particularly families with small children, because secondhand smoke is likely to influence the development of disorders such as asthma and ear infections. Teenagers who were exposed to secondhand smoke in their younger years are highly likely to develop acute respiratory problems that will become lifelong chronic conditions. Older adults who inhale secondhand smoke are particularly susceptible to pneumonia—a leading cause of death among senior citizens.

Many companies, healthcare facilities, schools, and other public buildings are now smoke-free. Smoking is not allowed on commercial airline flights within the United States and on many international flights. Schools and healthcare facilities usually declare their buildings and grounds as totally nonsmoking premises; in many cases, this designation is mandated by law or by accrediting agencies. Most restaurants have nonsmoking areas, hotels have nonsmoking rooms, and smoke-free rental cars are available. Many facilities have policies banning the use of ecigarettes and vaping. See Chapter 6 for a discussion of the hazards of tobacco use and secondhand smoke.

Water Pollution

Water pollution is a serious and increasing health hazard. Contaminated water transmits a number of diseases, including typhoid fever, dysentery, and infectious hepatitis. Water pollution is a life-threatening hazard to all sources of water, such as individual wells, groundwater, aquifers, rivers, lakes, and oceans. All forms of life are disturbed and/or destroyed by water contamination, including all marine organisms and advancing through the food chain to humans. Nitrogen pollutes oceans and causes algal blooms, which deplete the dissolved oxygen killing marine life. The mercury level in water and seafood is particularly dangerous for pregnant women. Guidelines from public health officials establish amounts of seafood and fish from designated areas that can be eaten safely in a specified time.

Land Pollution

As the population grows, it produces more garbage and trash. Large cities have had to institute creative solutions to the lack of places for trash disposal. People often do not want landfills or incinerators in their neighborhoods. As a result, most communities have developed recycling programs, well-managed landfills, and pollution-free incinerators.

A new danger exists regarding landfills. As land near cities becomes increasingly scarce, homes and other buildings are being built on old landfill sites. This practice has been proven to contribute to diseases (including cancer), particularly in children.

Radon is a chemical element that occurs in nature as a by-product of the disintegration of radium. It contributes to diseases, including lung cancer. Radon can collect in spaces that are poorly ventilated, such as caves. It can also seep into homes through cracks in the foundation or the basement floor. The more tightly sealed a home is, the greater the danger of radon exposure. Each home should be tested periodically for radon and appropriate measures taken to eliminate it.

Noise Pollution

Damage to the delicate structures of the ear is caused by loud noise or music. Chronic exposure to loud noise, such as loud music, poses the greatest hazard to hearing. Noise pollution also causes stress. Laws are in place to regulate noise. OSHA requires workers in occupations that are extremely noisy to wear ear protection. Recreational activities such as target shooting require ear protection.

Other Types of Pollution

Other situations contribute to pollution and endanger the environment. An oil spill can kill countless fish and animals, and thus destroy environments and food sources for many lifetimes. Insecticides and agricultural chemicals pose a threat to water and clean air. Workers may bring hazardous substances home on their clothing, thereby endangering the health of their family members. For example, in addition to causing cancer that may affect the workers themselves, asbestos particles on clothing contribute to chronic obstructive pulmonary disease in the families of workers.

Lead Poisoning (Plumbism)

Lead poisoning (**plumbism**) continues to be a significant public health problem. It causes serious mental and physical disabilities, particularly in young children. Many cities have programs to test children for lead poisoning and to remove leaded paint and lead pipes from older buildings. Lead can also be present in the soil, partially as a result of exhaust from cars that used leaded gasoline. Lead can also be found in newspaper print and old toys with chipped paint. Plumbism is discussed further in Chapter 74.

Radiation

Citizens are concerned about **radiation** (ionizing waves of energy that penetrate objects). Many disputes between the public and power companies using nuclear fuel remain unresolved. One problem concerns the disposal of radioactive wastes. Repercussions from events such as Three Mile Island in 1979 in Pennsylvania, USA; Chernobyl in the Ukraine in 1986; and at the Fukushima nuclear power plant in northern Japan in 2011 continue to raise questions about the environmental, economic, and personal effects of dangerous radiation.

Biohazardous Waste Disposal

Proper and safe disposal of **biohazardous** medical wastes, which are infectious and harmful to humans or animals, is the responsibility of every institutional and individual healthcare provider. Policies and procedures dictate the processes by which the disposal of medical wastes should occur. These processes must meet the multiple-standard regulations of OSHA, the Department of Environmental Protection, and local and state health departments.

Nurses performing home care must be especially careful to dispose of medical waste properly and to teach clients and families correct disposal methods. Medical equipment companies can provide containers and bags for proper disposal of sharps and biohazardous materials.

Key Concept

You are part of the world community. Participate in protecting the world you live in. Teach others to protect the environment as well.

STUDENT SYNTHESIS

KEY POINTS

- You are a member of many communities and should serve as an advocate and educator to protect those communities.
- Healthcare services are provided on international, national, state, and local levels.
- Federal agencies include the United States Public Health Service and the Department of Health and Human Services. These agencies have many branches and numerous programs.
- The blood-borne pathogen standard established by OSHA has significantly affected nursing procedures and delivery of services in healthcare facilities.
- The Social Security Administration supervises the Medicare and Medicaid programs.
- Voluntary health agencies may be set up to provide direct service, education, or fund-raising to combat a particular disease or for specific health concerns.
- Public and private agencies often work together to provide healthcare services.
- Many primary healthcare services are provided at community health centers. These services include examinations, health screening, immunizations, education, support groups, and illness care.
- Community health is concerned with environmental issues, including air, water, land, and noise pollution; plumbism; radiation; and biohazardous waste disposal.

CRITICAL THINKING EXERCISES

1. Evaluate healthcare services provided in your community.
2. What types of pollution are a problem in your community? Discuss various ways that you can contribute to reducing the problem.
3. As a member of the healthcare industry, what special responsibilities do you feel you have toward the community? Are you responsible in special ways for the environment?

NCLEX-STYLE REVIEW QUESTIONS

1. A client is admitted to the acute care facility with a suspected case of malaria. Which question is a priority for the nurse to ask related to this diagnosis?
   a. "Have you had unprotected sex?"
   b. "Have you recently traveled out of the country?"
   c. "What medication are you taking?"
   d. "Do you take any street drugs?"
2. The nurse is caring for a group of clients. Which fundamental procedure of healthcare should the nurse include in the care?
   a. Sterile technique
   b. Having assistance from another healthcare worker
   c. Determining financial status
   d. The use of Standard Precautions

3. The nurse is visiting an older adult client in the home for a dressing change. When the nurse arrives, they find the client on the floor, unresponsive. Which is the priority action by the nurse?
   a. Notify the client's family members.
   b. Obtain the client's glucose level.
   c. Establish a patent airway.
   d. Take the client's blood pressure.

4. The nurse is assigned to care for a group of four clients. A client with which condition should be seen first?
   a. Shortness of breath with chest pain
   b. Incontinence of stool
   c. Requiring a flu vaccine
   d. Requesting a bath

5. Parents inform the nurse that they have chosen not to vaccinate their child. Which response by the nurse is best?
   a. "I can't believe you would knowingly expose your child to these illnesses."
   b. "Vaccinations increase life span. Can you tell me what your fears are?"
   c. "I am going to have to report this to child protective services."
   d. "I understand. If you are going to home school, it doesn't matter anyway."

CHAPTER RESOURCES

Enhance your learning with additional resources on thePoint!

Student Resources related to this chapter can be found at thePoint.lww.com/Rosdahl12e.

8 Transcultural Healthcare

Learning Objectives

1. Define and state the components of culture, subculture, race, ethnicity, and racial and ethnic underrepresented groups.
2. Define and give examples of prejudice, ethnocentrism, and stereotyping.
3. Identify facilitators and barriers to providing culturally competent nursing care.
4. List nursing considerations that need to be included as part of a cultural assessment.
5. Discuss ways in which each of the following influences nursing care: values and beliefs, taboos and rituals, concepts of health and illness, language and communication, diet and nutrition, elimination, and death and dying.
6. Assess the importance of religious and spiritual beliefs and practices for clients experiencing illness.
7. Compare and contrast the following belief systems: magico-religious, scientific/biomedical, holistic medicine (e.g., yin/yang theory, hot–cold).
8. Identify important qualifications for a professional interpreter.
9. Discuss cultural aspects of each of the following: personal space and touching, eye contact, diet and nutrition, elimination, and concepts of death and dying. Relate these aspects to the concepts of nursing care.

Important Terminology

beliefs	ethnicity	nirvana	racial and ethnic underrepresented group	subculture
cultural competence	ethnocentrism	norms		taboos
cultural diversity	imam	prejudice		transcultural nursing
cultural sensitivity	karma	priest	rituals	values
culture	minister	rabbi	shaman	yin/yang theory
curandero	mullah	race	stereotype	

In the late 20th century, nurse and anthropologist Madeleine Leininger helped develop the concept that a client has physical, spiritual, psychological, and socioeconomic needs that arise in response to our complex, diverse world.

As a nurse, you are responsible for becoming acquainted with the predominant cultures in your community. Remember to view each person within a group as an individual and to provide care in a nonjudgmental way. Individuals identify with their cultural, ethnic, racial, and religious backgrounds to various degrees. Nurses must be aware of their own beliefs and be sensitive to the beliefs of others.

CULTURE, ETHNICITY, AND RACE

Definitions of Culture

Culture is the accumulated learning for generational groups of individuals that includes the combination of knowledge, belief systems, and behaviors (National Institutes of Health, 2017). Individuals experience a cultural heritage with others. Heritage is learned through formal and informal experiences throughout the life cycle. Culture consists of the combined heritage of language and communication style, health beliefs and health practices, customs and rituals, and religious beliefs and practices. Culture is influenced by environment, expectations of society, and national origin. An individual's culture may be a mixture of many longstanding belief systems.

> **Key Concept**
> Remember that people are unique. Not everyone in a particular group follows all the practices or shares the same beliefs and characteristics.

The way an individual behaves in social groups and as an individual within that group is also part of one's culture. An individual learns, evaluates, and behaves according to specified values within a culture. Cultural concepts and beliefs provide the blueprints or guides for determining one's personal and societal values, individual beliefs, and lifelong practices. A pattern of values, attitudes, and social, political, economic, educational, and other behaviors emerges from the learned culture, and these values are shared in a defined group over time as an identifiable heritage. Box 8-1 presents some characteristics of culture.

Subcultures are groups within dominant cultures. Subcultures form because individuals share characteristics that belong to an identifiable group, such as occupations (nurse, teacher, politician), religions (Islam, Methodist, Baptist), geographic origins (New Englander, Midwesterner, Californian), or age (infant, adolescent, older adult). Of particular importance to healthcare is the aging population. Over the course of your nursing career, the nation's 65-and-older

Box 8-1 Characteristics of Culture

A WORLD OF DIFFERENCE

When one individual meets another individual, they may fail to understand each other because of differences in language, education, values, rules, understanding of health and illness, gestures, emotional expressions, body language, cultural norms, family backgrounds, age-related norms, religious or family rituals, gender expectations, and previous life experiences. Here are some common characteristics of what society considers to be *culture*:

- A *way of life* for a group of individuals
- The sum of *socially inherited* characteristics, handed down from generation to generation
- A group's *design for living*—socially transmitted assumptions about the physical and social world
- *Learned* from birth
- *Roles change* with an individual's age, sex, and family position
- Influenced by social groups not genetics
- *Unique* to each ethnic group
- *Shared by members* of the same group who *identify* with each other
- *Complex* and all-encompassing
- Often an *unconscious process*
- An *adaptation* to various conditions, such as environment, educational background, and available resources
- *Dynamic* and always changing

Adapted from Merriam-Webster online dictionary (http://www.merriam-webster.com/dictionary/culture).

population will greatly increase; older adult populations will increase from about 49 million in 2016 to nearly 85 million in 2060 (Johnson, 2020). Nursing students also comprise a subculture because of the unique experiences and growth process that are universal components of all student nursing populations. There are many subcultures that exist in the United States.

Definitions of Race

The term **"race"** is used to differentiate large groups of humankind that share common biological and sociological characteristics (Merriam-Webster, n.d.). *Race* implies physical characteristics associated with having ancestors from a specific part of the world. Race should not be confused with ethnicity or culture. The nurse must be aware that obvious physical attributes, such as skin, hair, or eye color, are not accurate indicators of race. Genetic diseases are not limited to individuals who physically appear to be of a particular race. Physical and cultural characteristics of a group may differ from those of the predominant group of a particular region.

For statistics and data gathering purposes, the U.S. Census Bureau (the Bureau) looks at the American population in term of basic racial characteristics. These data are compiled and used for legislative purposes, to distribute funds, and to provide services to the individual. Box 8-2 summarizes the mission and uses of population data.

The Bureau is also aware that individuals often identify with more than one race or, as stated by the Bureau, "in combination with one or more races." Many individuals have more than two races within their ancestry. The racial groups and their generally federally accepted definitions, listed alphabetically by race alone or in combination, are as follows:

- American Indian and Alaska Native—origins in any of the original peoples of North and South America, including Central America, and who maintain tribal affiliation or community attachment
- Asian—origins in any of the original peoples of the Far East, Southeast Asia, or the Indian subcontinent
- Black or African American—origins in any of the Black racial groups of Africa
- Hispanic or Latino—individuals of Cuban, Mexican, Puerto Rican, South or Central American, or other Spanish culture or origin *regardless of race*
- Native Hawaiian and other Pacific Islander—origins in any of the original peoples of Hawaii, Guam, Samoa, or other Pacific Islands
- White—origins in any of the original peoples of Europe, the Middle East, or North Africa
- Combinations
- Multiracial—origins in two or more of the federally designated racial categories

Racial and Ethnic Underrepresented Groups

Racial and ethnic **underrepresented** populations are groups whose numbers are less than half the total amount of a total group. According to the 2020 U.S. Census, over 40% of the population currently belongs to a racial or ethnic underrepresented group. The U.S. Census Bureau looks at the American population in terms of basic racial characteristics. The primary groups that are considered racial-ethnic underrepresented groups in America include American Indian or Alaska Native, Asian American, Black or African American, Hispanic or Latino, and Native Hawaiian or other Pacific Islander. Each group has specific and distinctive features. These groups can be divided into smaller groups; for example, Hispanic, also referred to as Latino, includes people of Mexican, Puerto Rican, Cuban, and Guatemalan descent, among others. Racial-ethnic underrepresented groups can also be identified according to religion, occupation, sexual orientation, or gender.

Nursing considerations for people who belong to underrepresented populations may differ from the majority or white population. Health indicators, such as life expectancy and infant mortality, have improved for most Americans, but some populations continue to experience a disproportionate burden of preventable disease, death, and disability (Centers for Disease Control, 2020).

> **SPECIAL CONSIDERATIONS** **Culture and Ethnicity**
>
> Cultures and subcultures are not stagnant or unchanging. Race and ethnicity are also words with evolving definitions. Economics, migrations of populations, and politics influence these concepts.

Ethnicity is the common heritage shared by a specific culture (Merriam-Webster, n.d.). Many people work hard to

> **Box 8-2 The U.S. Census Bureau: Mission and Goals**
>
> The purpose of gathering these data are to properly represent citizens and to monitor the needs of the citizens as changes do occur.
>
> - *Mission of the U.S. Census Bureau*
>   To serve as the leading source of quality data about the nation's people and economy
> - *Goal of the U.S. Census Bureau*
>   To provide the best mix of timeliness, relevancy, quality, and cost for the data we collect and services we provide
> - *Uses of data*
>   - To determine the distribution of Congressional seats to states
>   - Mandated by the U.S. Constitution
>   - Used to apportion seats in the U.S. House of Representatives
>   - Used to define legislature districts, school district assignment areas, and other important functional areas of government
> - To make decisions about what community services to provide. Changes in your community are crucial to many planning decisions, such as where to
>   - Provide services for the elderly
>   - Build new roads and schools
>   - Locate job training centers
> - To distribute more than $400 billion in federal funds to local, state, and tribal governments each year. Census data affect how funding is allocated to communities for many services, such as
>   - Neighborhood improvements
>   - Public health
>   - Education
>   - Transportation
> - To provide specific information
>   - Qualifying for Social Security and other retirement benefits
>   - Passport applications
>   - Proving relationship in settling estates
>   - Researching family history or an historical topic

U.S. Census Bureau. (2019). *What we do*. https://www.census.gov/about/what.html

retain their cultural and ethnic identification. This is demonstrated in Scandinavian celebrations; Hispanic celebrations of Cinco de Mayo; traditional Mardi Gras celebrations; Native American Pow Wows; and Lunar New Year celebrations. Many ethnic groups celebrate special occasions, such as weddings, with traditional activities and foods. Some people strongly identify with their culture of origin and make an effort to pass traditions along to their children. Cultures are often associated with religious beliefs, and religion may be a strong factor in a person's ethnicity.

Groups show ethnic pride in various ways. For example, a celebration of religious and cultural heritage is demonstrated by the St. Patrick's Day Parade in New York City. Some ethnic groups retain links to their country of origin by wearing specific items, such as a sari (India), clothing, or Native American jewelry. Your nursing care needs to demonstrate an understanding of the unique ethnic celebrations of your geographic area.

Cultural Diversity and Cultural Competence

Cultures have become so interwoven that specific identification of cultural groups can be difficult. The concept of **cultural diversity** reflects the fact that most societies are made up of a multitude of different cultures. According to the CDC and the U.S. Census Bureau, the Hispanic community is the fastest-growing group in the United States. The Asian/Pacific Islander group is also expanding rapidly. To date, as many as 150 different ethnic groups and more than 500 tribes of Native Americans have been identified in the United States. In addition to expanding birth rates among specific ethnic groups, immigrants from many countries are entering the United States in large numbers. Migrations of populations worldwide are influencing demographics, culture, and economics in many countries.

As you can see from your own experience, cultural diversity has become part of our world. Individuals will meet people of many ethnic groups, both as citizens and as nurses. **Cultural competence** refers to the ability to respect the beliefs, language, interpersonal styles, and behaviors of individuals, families, and staff receiving or providing services. It is likely that nurses will understand the language, values, and beliefs of clients from their own culture. When a nurse encounters clients from unfamiliar cultures, however, understanding and communication may become difficult. To be effective, the nurse must transcend cultural barriers and approach every client with patience, empathy, concern, and competence. A high level of self-awareness is also important. Before you can understand another person's culture, you must first understand and accept your own.

> **NCLEX Alert**
>
> Components of test questions may include a variety of cultural concerns. For example, you may be asked to identify common cultural food needs (pork, alcohol, vegetarian) as well as nursing concerns related to diseases that may be found in certain racial and ethnic groups (hypertension, diabetes, genetic disorders).

Barriers to Culturally Competent Care

Prejudice is a belief based on preconceived notions about certain groups of people. Many people have been the victims of prejudice based on a variety of factors, including weight, sexual orientation, or their ethnicity and race. Prejudice may exist in subtler forms, for example, having a fixed negative opinion against authority figures. Many individuals are prejudiced without realizing it. For example, you may be prejudiced against people with beards or individuals with high IQs. It is important for the nurse to keep an open mind in dealing with clients regardless of their race, culture, or ethnicity.

> **Key Concept**
>
> Some individuals may be sensitive to a comment that involves a cultural reference and perceive it as a form of prejudice. For example, if you hear or use the word Mexican, Filipino, or Muslim in a sentence, does that mean that the statement reflects prejudice? If your instructor states that country XYZ has a high mortality rate of tuberculosis, is that a statement of fact or is the statement considered derogatory?

Ethnocentrism is the belief that one's own culture is the best and only acceptable culture, which shows an inability to understand, appreciate, and work with other cultures. As a nurse, seeing beyond your own particular ethnic/cultural group is important for effective communication and understanding of your client's individual needs.

The term **"stereotype"** refers to classifying or categorizing people and believing that all those belonging to a certain group are alike. In the movies, the villain is often stereotyped as wearing the black hat, whereas the hero wears the white hat. Stereotyping implies preconceived, but often incorrect, negative notions. It is inappropriate to assign derogatory characteristics (e.g., lacking work ethic, dishonest, or unintelligent) to groups. In addition, individuals will always maintain some uniqueness within a group.

CULTURAL SENSITIVITY

Cultural sensitivity is the understanding and tolerance of all cultures and lifestyles. It is crucial in the delivery of competent nursing care. You should develop cultural sensitivity when working with individuals from every ethnic/cultural group. Cultural sensitivity allows the nurse to understand more accurately and to accept the behavior of others. Nurses are better able to deliver care when they are sensitive to cultural factors involved in the client's health or illness.

No culture is better or worse than another. In addition, cultures are ever changing; they evolve over many generations. Box 8-3 lists many nursing considerations that can be used as part of cultural assessments.

CULTURALLY INFLUENCED COMPONENTS

Being a member of a cultural group means that certain components of that culture are common to many of its members. Common cultural components can be classified in terms of *values and beliefs, taboos and rituals*, concepts of *health and illness, language and communication, diet and nutrition* practices, *elimination* patterns, *personal space* and *eye contact customs*, and attitudes toward *death and dying*. These factors are discussed throughout this text. Remember that you can learn much more about all aspects of ethnicity and culture than can be presented here.

Beliefs and Values

Each ethnic/cultural group has **beliefs** or concepts the members hold as true. Beliefs can be based on fact, fiction, or a combination of both. Beliefs can be difficult to change. A change in belief systems can be a milestone in an individual's life. For example, the recognition of the reality or fantasy of Santa Claus usually denotes a change in a child's belief system. Historical belief systems can change, leading to new beliefs, such as the change from a monarchy to a democracy.

A group lives by **values**, which shape how an individual perceives right or wrong and what is desirable or valuable. Values influence a person's responses to the world and to others. People's values define who they are, their identity, and their views of the world. Each person's values are unique and influence behavior and self-esteem. From values evolve **norms**, which become rules for behavior in a group. Society develops sanctions or laws that serve to enforce norms.

Nurses must recognize that different beliefs and values exist. The issues of life and death are value-laden concepts that affect nursing. For example, the decision to terminate life support, have an abortion, or refuse blood products may be related to the client's cultural, ethnic, and/or religious beliefs and values. Even if nurses do not always agree with client decisions, they must respect that individuals have the right and responsibility for their own beliefs and values.

Taboos and Rituals

Every culture has **taboos** that its members cannot violate without discomfort and risk of separation from the group. A taboo is a social, religious, or cultural custom that forbids discussion or practice of a particular person, place, or thing. For example, most adults avoid the use of profane language in the presence of children. Each culture also has **rituals**. Rituals are formal ceremonies consisting of prescribed actions in a specific order often done by respected leaders of a group. Members are often required to include rituals as part of cultural and/or religious practices. Some Native Americans may use the healing knowledge, skills, and rituals of a **shaman** (traditional healer). Latinos may have **curandero/a** (folk healers) who assist a client with herbs and counseling. Moslems (Muslims) may follow the guidance of a **mullah** (specially educated Muslim trained in religious law and beliefs). Christians may have **ministers** or **priests**, and those who are Jewish may have **rabbis** who are also specially educated in their religious laws and beliefs. Often, taboos and rituals are associated with religious or spiritual services pertaining to healing, death, or dying. Nurses need to be aware that these are important components of the client's system of health beliefs.

> **Key Concept**
>
> People may be more tied to their cultural and ethnic beliefs when ill than when feeling well, following familiar taboos and rituals. Illness is stressful and may lead individuals to revert to what is known and comfortable.

Box 8-3 Transcultural Nursing Considerations and Cultural Assessment

Transcultural nursing stresses that many subgroups exist within each culture. Not all members of a group share the same beliefs or traditions.

Consider your responses to the following questions as you work with others:

- What is your own cultural background?
- How are you different from or similar to other individuals?
- What is the definition of health and illness accepted by another's ethnic group?
- What place does religion have in another's culture?
- What is the importance of religion, religious beliefs, and religious practices?
- What are the concepts and beliefs of another's culture relating to the causes of illness and injury?
- What ethnic or folk medicine practices are used (i.e., the use of special clothing, amulets, or rituals)?
- What are the attitudes toward various types and models of healthcare (e.g., holistic, biomedical, spiritual) of the culture?
- What are the relationships, responsibilities, and roles of different genders in the culture?
- Who makes the financial decisions? Who makes the healthcare decisions? Are the decisions made by the same person?
- What considerations must be made relating to the socioeconomic status of the client and the family?
- Are there any environmental factors that could pose related disorders such as hanta virus or lead poisoning?
- What are the general rules of verbal and nonverbal communication patterns, such as personal space, touching, and eye contact?
- What are the language differences between the healthcare staff and the client/family?
- What cultural beliefs exist about the relationship between a person's gender and modesty, machismo, and the concept of the human body?
- What are cultural reactions to pain, birth, and death?
- How does an individual react to an older generation and the care of older adults?
- What are the resources for, and sources of, support persons, such as family, friends, or religious groups?
- How does a cultural group feel about mental illness or intellectual disability?
- What are the food restrictions or preferences, if any?
- What are the individual and the group attitudes about factors such as physical appearance, amputation, obesity, and adaptation to prescribed therapeutic diets?
- What is known about group identity; the importance and type of family structure; the cohesiveness within the group; and the traditional roles of different genders?
- What are the concepts related to the physical visibility of an ethnic background (e.g., Black or African American, or Asian American)?
- Are there any specific disorders genetically integrated into a group, such as Tay–Sachs or sickle cell anemia?
- What are the attitudes about education, time, and authority?
- What are the predominant occupations within the group; role models?
- What are the effects of "Westernization" of the younger members of a culture?
- How does Westernization of a culture affect traditional roles of a family?
- What are the effects of a large number of people belonging to a cultural group in the same geographic area as the healthcare facility?
- What are the predominant prejudices within a cultural group relating to other members of the same group; stereotypes of and prejudices against other particular groups?
- What are the attitudes toward individuals with mixed races, religions, or cultural backgrounds?

Adapted from Timby, B. K., & Smith, N. E. (2018). *Introductory medical-surgical nursing* (12th ed.). Wolters Kluwer.

Health and Illness

Culture greatly influences an individual's concepts of health, illness, and death. Such beliefs can affect a person's recovery from illness or injury. Each society has norms relating to the meaning of illness, how an ill person should behave, and what means should be used to assist the individual through periods of illness as well as during times of approaching death. Strive to accommodate each client's healthcare beliefs and practices (as long as they are safe), even if you do not fully understand or agree with them. Traditional religious beliefs and practices, related to death, are summarized in Chapter 14, Box 14-1.

Health Belief Systems

Several health belief systems exist. Among these systems are the following:

Magico-religious: The belief that supernatural forces dominate. For example, the Christian Scientist religion believes in healing by prayer alone. Many people believe we are influenced by spirits, gods, or demons. Some cultures believe fate decides life, in that things happen for a purpose designed by a higher spiritual being. It is often not necessary that the individual understand the event. Other groups believe that illness and adversity serve as punishment for sins. Some people believe that trouble or pain is God's will.

Scientific/biomedical: The belief that physical and biomedical processes can be studied and manipulated to control life. For example, the Shintoist religion believes that people are inherently good; illness is caused when the person comes into contact with pollutants. Western medicine often takes the approach that the body has individual body systems (e.g., pulmonary, integumentary, endocrine). Therefore, specialists are hired to address the specific concerns of diseased or injured parts of the human body.

Holistic medicine: The belief that the forces of nature must be kept balanced. This holistic approach combines the physical, psychological, and spiritual health or illness of an individual. Health is defined in terms of the person's relationship with nature and the universe (wholeness). Life is considered as only one aspect of nature. From this belief system come holistic medicine, herbal medicine, and concepts of Mother Earth. Many individuals who are Native American or Asian may follow the holistic approach. Native Americans often follow three holistic concepts: *prevention, treatment,* and *health maintenance.*

Yin/yang and hot–cold theories: The belief that illness develops when life forces are out of balance. Many cultures believe in the yin/yang theory or hot–cold aspects of wellness and illness, as summarized in Box 8-4.

Many people also believe in a complex system of five basic energies/elements/substances in nature (wood, fire, earth, metal, water). This theory is an expansion of yin/yang theory and is also involved in the healing process. Many Filipino and Hispanic groups believe that heat, cold, wetness, and dryness must be balanced for health. Certain illnesses are considered hot or cold, wet or dry. Foods, activities, medications, and herbal substances, classified as hot or cold, are added or subtracted to bring about balance. Other ethnic groups that use parts of the yin/yang or hot–cold theories include Asian, Black or African American, Arab, Muslim, and Caribbean peoples. An important point is that various ethnic groups have differing beliefs as to which illnesses and which treatments are hot or cold.

Healthcare systems are constantly evolving and incorporating elements from many different belief systems. Be aware of popular and folk practices among members of your community. By doing so, you will better appreciate the range of services available for use by clients. Chapter 3 introduces some complementary therapies, many of which are based on elements of the above systems.

Treatment and Healing Beliefs and Practices

Cultural/ethnic groups have many beliefs and practices for times of illness. Use caution when learning concepts of culture because it is possible to stereotype individuals based on perceived cultural generalizations. Clients are often happy to explain their beliefs to you, so you can better understand and care for them.

Attitudes Toward Mental Illness

Mental illness is not accepted in all cultures as a consequence of biological disease. Western medicine and psychiatry and their approaches to mental illness are based on the accepted findings of late 20th-century science. The belief that chemical changes in the brain can cause mental disorders is a relatively new concept for many cultures. Some cultures consider mental disorders a disgrace to the individual and to the family.

In contrast to the biological, scientific approach of Western medicine is the belief in the spirit world. Science may consider a person's behavior to be abnormal or even psychotic if spirits, angels, or a deity is involved. Members of that culture may hear the spirits talking. Some individuals believe in a curse or "evil eye." Western medicine traditionally considers this type of belief a deviation, whereas it may be an accepted belief in a client's culture.

Some may consider behavior to be deviant because an individual chooses not to follow cultural norms (e.g., length of hair, type of dress, type of lifestyle).

Language and Communication

Nurses and clients may speak different languages. In addition, a person may speak the English language in everyday life, but may be uncomfortable trying to use medical terms in their second language. *Clients will be appreciative if you learn a few words in their language.* Also, many people find it difficult to speak in a second language when they are ill. Difficulties arise when no one is available to translate. Such situations may interfere with client care. Accurate interpretation of verbal and nonverbal communication is particularly important in an area such as the mental health unit, where these factors are integral to diagnosis and treatment.

Box 8-4 Yin/Yang Theory

Yin and yang represent "unified opposites" that are interrelated. A yin condition requires a yang treatment and vice versa. The forces of nature are balanced to provide harmony and homeostasis.

Yin	Yang
Matter	Energy
Female	Male
Negative	Positive
Darkness/night	Light/day
Cold	Warmth
Emptiness	Fullness
Weak	Strong
Expansion	Contraction
Hypofunction	Hyperfunction

> **Key Concept**
> At least half of communication takes place using the multitude of nonverbal cues seen in body language, facial expression, or eye contact. Remember that a smile is understood in almost any language.

Ways to Facilitate Communication

Methods are available to facilitate transcultural communication. Chapter 44 discusses therapeutic communication in more detail. Box 8-5 gives some practical solutions to English language barriers. The following paragraphs provide various ways to facilitate communication:

Professional interpreter: If possible, obtain the services of a trained interpreter, either in person or by telephone. An interpreter can help set up a list of common terms or a photo board for routine requests. In addition to providing the client with comfort and safety, a trained interpreter often understands the culture of the person, as well as the language. The skilled interpreter can explain nonverbal cues, in addition to what the client says. The objective interpreter is an invaluable staff resource, as illustrated in Figure 8-1.

Family as interpreter: If a trained interpreter is not possible, sometimes, a family member or significant other can act as an interpreter. Having a member of

---

Box 8-5   Communicating With Clients

Below are some nursing considerations that may be helpful when working with non-English speaking clients or with clients who do not speak English as their primary language.

DETERMINING UNDERSTANDING
- Consider the client's and the family's body language, which can be very informative (e.g., pain, fear, grief, confusion).
- Determine if the client speaks or reads English, or both.
- Ask the client to "read this line," to determine the client's ability to follow written instructions, which are provided in English.
- Speak words or phrases in the client's language, even if it is not possible to carry on a conversation.
- Learn a second language, especially one spoken by a large ethnic population serviced by the healthcare agency.

BASIC COMMUNICATION
- Avoid using technical terms, slang, or phrases with a double or colloquial meaning, such as: "Do you have to use the john?"
- Ask questions that can be answered by a "yes" or "no."
- Repeat the question without changing the words, if the client appears confused.
- Give the client sufficient time to process the question from English to the native language, and respond back in English.
- Construct a loose-leaf folder or file cards with words in one or more languages spoken by clients in the community.
- Provide the client with written information in their primary language for wound care, diabetes care, and so forth. Translators in your community can help build standardized lists for the most commonly heard languages in your community.
- Provide the client with questionnaires written in their primary language so that these can be kept in the client/family's medical information and taken to all future healthcare visits. Questions should include allergies, a listing of all medications, over-the-counter healthcare treatments, cultural healthcare treatments, previous surgeries, previous medical problems, memory loss, acute/chronic pain, and depression.
- Rely on nonverbal communication, and pantomime if necessary.
- Avoid displaying impatience.
- Be aware that you may not be aware of a culture's etiquette and may, unintentionally, be insensitive.
- Speak slowly, not loudly, using simple words and short sentences.
- Consider avoiding eye contact.

TRANSLATING
- Refer to an English/foreign language dictionary for bilingual vocabulary words; many medical dictionaries contain words and phrases in languages such as Spanish, French, or German. Appendix A, has common English–Spanish healthcare phrases.
- Several healthcare dictionaries have appendices that assist with translations of common healthcare concerns.
- Develop a list of employees or individuals to contact in the community who speak a second language and are willing to act as translators; in an extreme emergency, international telephone operators may be able to provide assistance.
- Select a translator who is the same gender as the client and approximately the same age, if possible.
- Tell the translator to ask the client/family not to withhold any information and to inform the provider if there are objections to the form of treatment or something that the provider says.
- Look at the client, not the translator, when asking questions and listening to the client's response.

Adapted from Timby, B. K., & Smith, N. E. (2018). *Introductory medical-surgical nursing* (12th ed.). Wolters Kluwer.

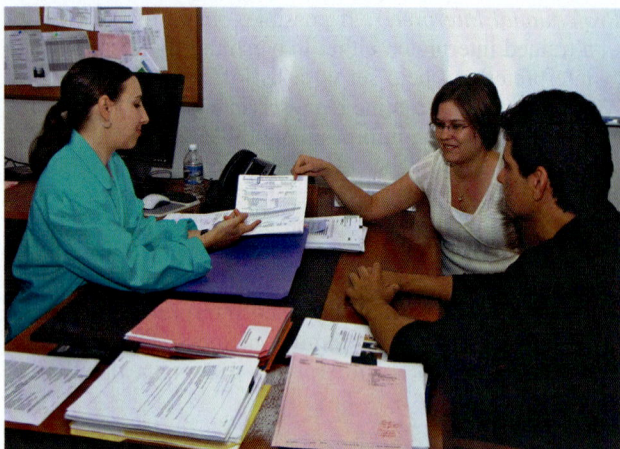

Figure 8-1 Interpreters are important components of the healthcare team. An interpreter used in healthcare settings should have several qualities: (1) the interpreter should know and understand the nuances of medical language; (2) the interpreter should know the formal, slang, and conversational levels of the language that they are interpreting; and (3) the interpreter should be able to communicate without inferring judgment, bias, or personal opinions.

the family translate may be inappropriate, however, because it may compromise the client's confidentiality. Translations may be inaccurate if family members are unfamiliar with healthcare terminology. They may unintentionally change the meaning of what is said or may omit information, not realizing the importance of every word. Mistakes may also be intentional, to avoid embarrassment. Gender differences may increase translation difficulties. People may not be comfortable discussing reproductive system concerns or anatomy with someone of a different gender.

Nurse as interpreter: In some cases, a nurse or other healthcare worker who is bilingual can assist with translating; however, problems may arise with this method as well. The bilingual healthcare worker may not know medical terminology in the native language and may not have time available to leave their own clients to translate for others.

Personal Space and Touching

Personal space refers to a person's comfort zone. Types of personal space include *intimate space* (reserved for close family members) and *personal space* (for contact with the general public). Americans, Canadians, and the British have the largest personal space zone of all cultures, requiring several feet for comfort. In many cultures, such as those of Latin America, Japan, and the Middle East, maintaining such a large space would be considered rejecting and insulting.

Touching is often culture-related. Nurses must touch clients to perform treatments; however, they need to remain aware that taboos are also involved. For example, Europeans often pat children on the head as a sign of affection. In some Asian cultures, however, touching a child on the head is a sign of disrespect and is believed to cause illness. A safer approach is to touch children on the hand or arm when talking to or looking at them, but not to touch them on the head without permission.

Individuals who are Hispanic and those from Mediterranean regions frequently touch each other. Individuals may kiss each other when meeting, regardless of gender, or hold hands while walking. When meeting clients, offer to shake hands, but do not be offended if they decline. Many cultures consider touching a member of a different gender or making the first move to offer the hand to a superior to be improper. For example, some Middle Eastern cultures teach that women may not touch any man other than their husbands.

A nurse may be in a particular dilemma if they need to undress a client from particular cultures. For example, a young female nurse may ask an older adult gentleman to remove his shirt for an x-ray. The client may resist the request for two reasons. It may not be appropriate in his culture for a younger person to give commands to an older person. In addition, it may not be appropriate for a male to undress when requested by a stranger, especially if the stranger is female. If you were the nurse, what would you do?

> **NCLEX Alert**
>
> Cultural questions may include components of critical thinking and activities of daily living. For example, what should the nurse do when the client's cultural habits (e.g., undressing) are contrary to Western-style healthcare?

Eye Contact

Eye contact can give important cues about clients. This action is culturally influenced. In most European-based cultures, direct eye contact is considered normal. If not part of the total body language, lack of eye contact in that culture may imply lack of respect, inattention, and avoidance of the truth.

In Native American, Arab, and some Southeast Asian cultures, members believe that looking a person in the eye during conversation is improper and impolite. It may also be interpreted as challenging or hostile. Some individuals may stare at the floor and hesitate before answering, a sign that they are concentrating on what is being said. Others are taught to respect their elders and authority figures. They often expect nurses to make eye contact with them, but do not reciprocate. A Muslim-Arab woman may avoid eye contact, especially with men, as a sign of modesty. Facial expressions may be totally absent. Take care not to misinterpret these nonverbal cues. Consider the possibility of cultural influences.

Diet and Nutrition

Cultural eating rituals vary. In some cultures, adults of different genders do not eat together or do not eat with children.

In others, eating is a family event, and all family members eat together. Eating utensils vary from the knife, fork, and spoon of Western cultures to the chopsticks of many Asian cultures.

Some religions maintain strict dietary practices. For example, those who practice Orthodox Judaism and Islam do not eat pork and will not eat meat and dairy products together. They also keep separate dishes for these foods. People within the Islamic culture may strictly observe religious holidays, keeping a long fast that is often followed by a large feast. In the Church of Jesus Christ of Latter-day Saints and Seventh-day Adventist religions, diet also plays an important part. Most followers eliminate tea, coffee, alcohol, and strong spices. Some religious groups are vegetarians. Most ethnic groups have special food customs and rituals surrounding holidays and special events, such as weddings. Because nutrition and dietary customs play such a large part in health and treatment of illness, a separate chapter (Chapter 31) is devoted to this subject.

Elimination

People of various cultures treat the elimination of bodily wastes (voiding and defecation) differently. Many cultures consider elimination to be a private function. Some people are unable to void or to use a bedpan or commode unless they have complete privacy, which may be difficult in a healthcare facility. People of Arab cultures may consider the left hand dirty and use it only to clean themselves after elimination.

Death and Dying

Each cultural group has an attitude or series of beliefs about death and dying. Some cultural groups consider death a natural part of life that is not to be feared. For example, many Asian cultures consider death to be preordained, believing that when a person's time to die has come, nothing can stop it. Traditional Western culture tries to prevent death and to prolong life at all costs. Ways of mourning also differ. Some cultural groups believe that the person is happier or better off and rejoice; others cry and mourn loudly. In some cultures, survivors formally mourn for a designated period of time. Others isolate children from death, not allowing them to see a dead body. In some cultures, a pregnant woman is not allowed to see a dead body, fearing danger to the fetus. Many cultures forbid suicide. In some cultures, the person who commits suicide may not be allowed a funeral or traditional burial.

RELIGIOUS/SPIRITUAL CUSTOMS AND TRADITIONS

Religion is a vital part of many people's lives. Because nurses will be caring for clients of different faiths, they should learn about major religious differences. By doing so, nurses, with the help of clients, will be better equipped to determine sources of spiritual and religious support.

Those who are injured or ill need reassurance, and they may talk to a nurse about their illness and spiritual beliefs. Respect their confidences. Maintain a nonjudgmental attitude. Suggest a visit from a spiritual leader, but do not contact such a person without first asking if the client wants such counsel.

> **Key Concept**
>
> Although members of a religious, ethnic, or cultural group may share similarities, each person is different. Remember not to stereotype individuals. All members of a group do not behave or believe alike.

Christianity

Christians worship God and his son, Jesus Christ. Sunday is the major day of worship in most Christian sects. Easter (Christ's resurrection) and Christmas (the day of Christ's birth) are the most important holidays, but Christians also observe other holy days. Bible reading and prayer are important aspects of faith.

Judaism

The term *Jewish* refers to the total culture, religion, history, and philosophy of life shared by a group of people whose origins trace back to the prophet Abraham. Their religious beliefs are called Judaism. Judaism is practiced at three major levels: Reform, Orthodox, and Conservative. Reform Jews are the most liberal in their beliefs; Orthodox Jews adhere strictly to their traditions; Conservatives fall in the middle. Within the Orthodox group are various branches, including a sect called Hasidism. Hasidic Jews live and work only within their own community and wear traditional clothing. Some of the strictest groups select only specific healthcare providers.

Within the Jewish faith, circumcision of male infants is considered a religious ceremony. The spiritual leader is called a rabbi. The Jewish day of worship, or Sabbath, is from sundown Friday to sundown Saturday. Other than the Sabbath, the most important Jewish holidays are Yom Kippur, Rosh Hashanah, and Passover. Elective procedures, such as diagnostic tests, are not performed on the Sabbath or holy days.

Kosher laws govern dietary practices for Orthodox Jews. This custom is often difficult for Jews to follow during illness. Although nonsectarian healthcare facilities do not prepare kosher meals, frozen kosher meals are available. The person's family can also bring in food. Not all Jews observe kosher dietary laws. Ask your clients and notify the dietary department accordingly. Practicing Jews generally do not eat pork or shellfish, even if they do not follow kosher laws otherwise.

Islam

Muslims (Moslems) are believers in Islam, the religion founded by Mohammed. Islam contains many divisions of varying strictness. Be sensitive to what type of Muslim a client is because many variations exist within the religion. They generally follow the teachings of the Koran, which influences diet, attitudes about gender, and death. Muslims pray five times a day, facing Mecca. The Sabbath is Friday. Pork and alcohol are prohibited. Muslims do not believe in faith healing and do not baptize infants. In death, prescribed procedures for washing and shrouding the body are followed by the religious leader, also called the **imam**. A mullah is an official who is trained in Muslim religious law and doctrines.

Eastern Religions

Many people from China, Korea, Japan, India, and Southeast Asia practice various forms of religions, and numerous people of non-Asian descent are becoming followers as well. North America is increasingly accepting of traditional Asian therapies, such as acupuncture, yoga, and biofeedback. Transcendental meditation influences hypnotherapy and relaxation practices.

Two main branches of the Buddhist religion exist: the northern (*Mahayana*) and southern (*Hinayana*). Based on the teachings of Gautama Buddha, Buddhists believe that hard work and right living enable people to attain **nirvana**, a state in which the soul no longer lives in a body and is free from desire and pain. On many holy days, Buddhists may decline surgery or other treatment. Baptism is performed after a child is mature. Life is preserved; life support is acceptable. If a Buddhist dies, the family will usually send for a Buddhist priest, who performs last rites and chanting rituals. Buddhists are often cremated.

Often considered the oldest religion in the world, Hinduism has many different divisions. Hindus in the United States generally follow a scripture (the *Vedas*) and believe that Brahman is the center and source of the universe. Reincarnation is a central belief. Life is governed by the law of **karma**, stating that rebirth (reincarnation) depends on behavior in life. Karma is also significant in promoting health or causing disease. The goal of life is to attain nirvana, as in Buddhism. Some Hindus believe in faith healing; others believe illness is punishment for sins. Hindus often do not eat meat, but the religion does not dictate this practice. Some religious practices are dictated by the caste system (hierarchy of society); others are based on race or skin color. There are many spiritualists in some Hindu sects.

Confucianists have a high appreciation of life. Their desire to keep the body from untimely death results in an emphasis on public health and preventive medicine. *Taoism* teaches that good health results from harmony of the universe with proper balancing of internal and external forces. Following Tao is to know and to live a natural life.

> **Key Concept**
> No matter how different your beliefs might be from those of your clients, respect each person's values. Respond in a nonjudgmental manner.

IMPLEMENTING CULTURALLY COMPETENT CARE

This chapter has presented a great deal of information about various cultural, ethnic, and religious groups. Remember to consider all aspects of the total person. **Transcultural nursing** is defined as caring for clients while taking into consideration their religious and sociocultural backgrounds. Many culturally related considerations and procedures are integrated throughout this text.

Cultural Influences on Individual Clients

Determine cultural influences that might have an impact on the client's progress through the healthcare system. The registered nurse will perform a thorough nursing assessment that includes a cultural assessment. The nursing plan of care is written by the team with cultural assessment in mind. This assessment is one component in the information gathering and planning phases of the nursing process. The licensed practical nurse will assist in performing culturally competent nursing care, based on the nursing care plan. The client may be involved in the development of the plan. Client and family compliance with the plan of care depends largely on whether or not that plan is acceptable within the client's particular culture. Help to make sure that the client understands what is to be done and why. Figure 8-2 provides examples of common cultural concerns.

The Culturally Diverse Healthcare Team

As seen in Figure 8-3, diversity within the healthcare team is common. The critical shortage of registered nurses in the United States has led to increased recruiting of nurses who were born and trained in other countries. It may be difficult for these nurses to work in the United States because of differences in educational background, difficulties in becoming licensed, and language barriers.

All nurses bring cultural, ethnic, and religious backgrounds to nursing. Learn from cultural diversity, whether from clients or coworkers. Nurses should capitalize on and appreciate the heritage of all peoples, including their own.

CHAPTER 8 Transcultural Healthcare   93

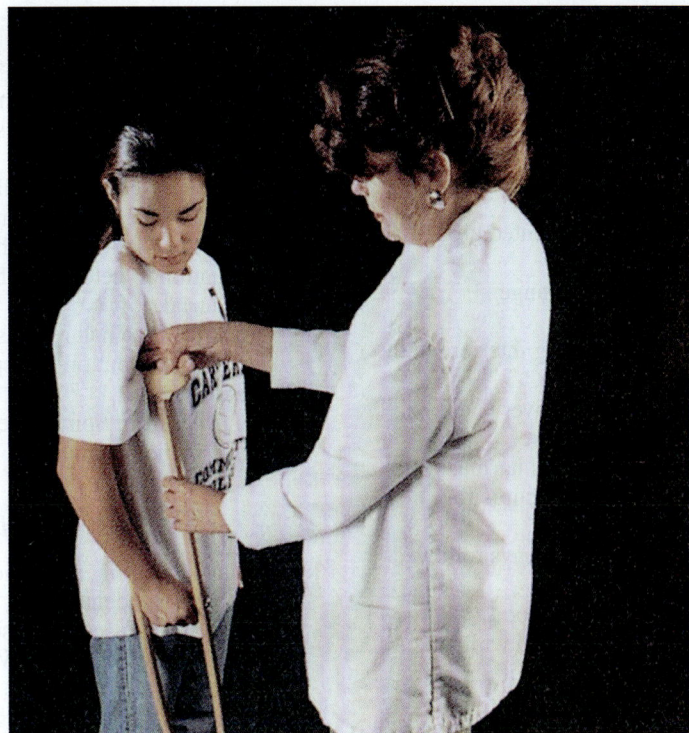

Figure 8-2 In the healthcare environment, nurses must communicate with clients of different ages, genders, races, and cultures. A nurse needs to remain sensitive to the needs of the client. In this example, imagine that the client being fitted for crutches has been told one of the following scenarios: (1) they will not be able to go to the school prom; (2) they will need to have their leg removed to save their life from the cancer in the leg; or (3) they will not be able to lift their 2-year-old child until the injury is healed. Consider that there are differences in age, race, gender, or culture between the nurse and the client. How would these differences affect your approach to this client?

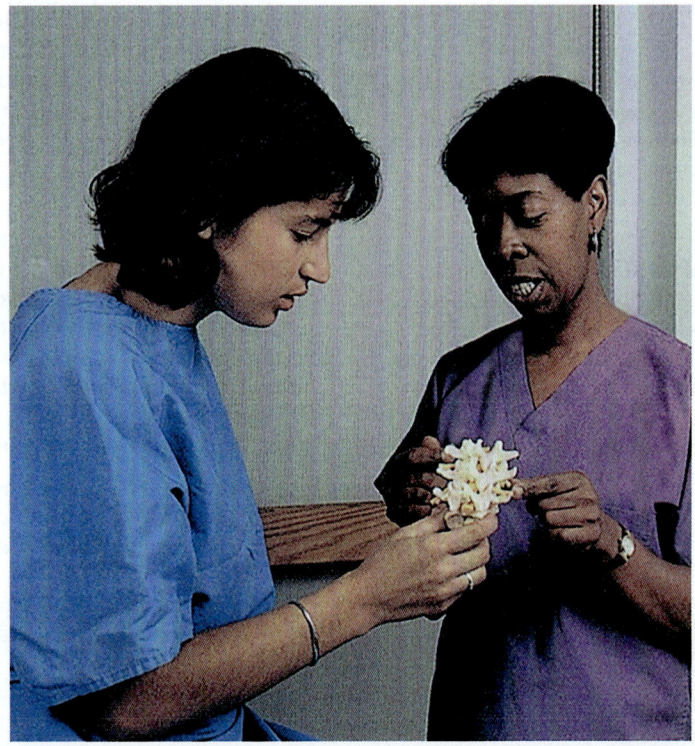

Figure 8-3 Within a culturally diverse healthcare system, communication is the key. Individuals communicate verbally, with the types of language that they use, with their body language, and with silence. Here, a nurse is communicating using a model of the spine. The nurse uses lay terms for body parts and frequently asks the client to restate or explain what has been taught to her.

STUDENT SYNTHESIS

KEY POINTS

- Many definitions are possible for *culture*. *Culture* refers to a shared set of beliefs and values among a specific group of people.
- Subcultures and racial-ethnic underrepresented groups are components of cultural heritage.
- The ethnic groups in the United States change continually.
- Prejudice, ethnocentrism, and stereotyping interfere with providing culturally sensitive nursing care.
- Many ethnic/cultural factors affect the delivery and acceptance of traditional Western healthcare.
- Many cultures subscribe to beliefs such as karma, yin/yang theory, spirits, or fate as causes and cures for illness.
- Cultural and religious traditions are not always followed by every member of a group.
- To facilitate communication and promote good nursing care, the nurse should be acquainted with the predominant cultural and religious groups within the community.
- The nurse may suggest a visit from a spiritual leader, but should not call one without first asking the client.
- Transcultural nursing is nursing that considers the religious and sociocultural backgrounds of all clients.

CRITICAL THINKING EXERCISES

1. Consider the beliefs of at least three cultures regarding illness and health. How do they compare with your personal beliefs?
2. Your nursing instructor uses the word "Mexican" in a sentence when describing a client. Would the use of a word such as Mexican, Filipino, Polish, Arab, Russian, or Black or African American be discriminative? What is the difference between descriptive and discriminative?
3. Quickly write your initial and immediate reactions to each of the following situations. Do not change or amend your initial answer after writing it. After you have responded to all the situations, evaluate and discuss your responses in terms of the transcultural nursing concepts presented in this chapter. How might any of the following situations be modified to be more comfortable for the client, you, and the healthcare staff?
   - A Native American client wants to burn herbs in their room and wants to see a healer from their tribe while in the facility.
   - A lesbian is at your clinic for intrauterine insemination, accompanied by her female partner.
   - A client who is a Jehovah's Witness is seriously hemorrhaging and refuses to have a blood transfusion.
   - A client is accused of child abuse after performing religious healing rites that left bruises on their child; the client is in the hospital for mental health evaluation to determine if they will be competent to stand trial.
   - An Amish woman refuses to take off her customary clothing and put on a hospital gown before a diagnostic test.
   - A family from Somalia refuses to leave their child alone in the hospital.

NCLEX-STYLE REVIEW QUESTIONS

1. The nurse is caring for a client with acute blood loss from a duodenal ulcer. The client is a Jehovah's Witness and refuses to consent for blood administration ordered by the physician. Which action by the nurse is appropriate?
   a. Sedate the client and assist with the blood administration.
   b. Inform the client that death is probable without the blood.
   c. Respect the client's wishes and continue to monitor the client's condition.
   d. Have the client sign out of the hospital against medical advice.

2. The nurse is attempting to obtain data from a client who only speaks Spanish. Which action by the nurse is best?
   a. Obtain a professional interpreter.
   b. Ask a family member to interpret.
   c. Ask a bilingual nurse to assist.
   d. Use a translation application on a smartphone.

3. A Muslim-Arab female client is in the clinic for a gynecologic procedure. The client does not directly look at the nurse or physician in the eye when speaking. Which statement is correct regarding the nurse's interpretation regarding this behavior?
   a. The client does not trust the caregivers.
   b. The client is demonstrating modesty.
   c. The client believes she has a sexually transmitted infection.
   d. The client has been sexually abused.

4. A client who practices Orthodox Judaism is hospitalized. Which food item may need to be eliminated from this client's diet?
   a. A slice of ham
   b. Fruit cup with mandarin oranges and pineapple
   c. A tossed salad with lettuce, tomato, and cucumber
   d. A roll with butter

5. To be culturally sensitive, which area should the nurse avoid touching when working with children who are Asian?
   a. Back
   b. Hand
   c. Arm
   d. Head

CHAPTER RESOURCES

Enhance your learning with additional resources on thePoint!

Student Resources related to this chapter can be found at **thePoint.lww.com/Rosdahl12e**.

Development Throughout the Life Cycle

UNIT 3

9 The Family

Learning Objectives

1. Define the concept of family.
2. List the functions and tasks of families.
3. Describe various types of family structures.
4. Explain the influences of culture, ethnicity, and religion on the family.
5. Discuss the stages of the family life cycle and important milestones and tasks of these stages.
6. Identify common stressors on today's family.
7. Differentiate between effective and ineffective family coping patterns.

Important Terminology

binuclear family
blended family
cohabitation
communal family
commuter family
dual-career/dual-earner family
dysfunctional family
extended family
foster family
functional family
gay or lesbian family
nuclear dyad
nuclear family
siblings
single-adult household
single-parent family
stepfamily

The family has traditionally been a central focus of caregiving and nursing. As the basic unit of society, the family profoundly influences its individual members. All nursing care should involve the family. When giving care, nurses must consider the particular needs, circumstances, goals, and priorities of each family and the members within it.

Key Concept
Understanding concepts related to the family and its influence over individuals is essential for providing appropriate nursing care.

CHARACTERISTICS OF THE FAMILY

What is a **family**? This question may seem simple, but the answer constantly evolves, reflecting changes that occur within society. The names of the types of families may be different, too, depending on the circumstances. A basic definition of family may be a group of two or more individuals who are related to each other by blood, marriage, or adoption and who usually live together. A broader definition, which reflects societal changes, is that a family consists of two or more people who are joined together by legal, genetic, and/or emotional bonds. A family can also be considered to be any group of people living together for mutual emotional, spiritual, and financial support.

Historically, the meaning of family has centered around childbearing and childrearing. As a cultural unit of society, the primary purpose of a family unit or group is to provide for the physical survival of the unit and to instill the cultural knowledge, customs, values, and spiritual beliefs of the group. The family unit provides the structure for a dependent individual to become an independent person.

Key Concept
A client's family includes any person that they identify as a family member.

The Family as a Social System

The family is a living social system. Although it is a basic unit of society, it is also complex. The family is a group of individuals who are interdependent; the choices and actions of one family member often influence other family members. For example, when one family member is ill, the entire family is affected. Likewise when a parent returns to full-time outside employment after several years of staying at home to care for children, ramifications abound for all members of the immediate, and perhaps the extended, family.

The roles people play within a family may be many and varied. The parent–child relationship is one major example; another is the relationship between siblings.

Parenting

Parenting is the ability of one or more people to help a child meet their needs and to guide that young person through developmental tasks. Parenting styles differ in each family. Some families are strict in discipline, whereas others are lenient or

97

even indifferent. A person's own upbringing may guide their parenting style. Other parents learn their styles by watching role models, by reading, or by following moral or religious teachings.

Parenting is an enormous responsibility and brings rewards and challenges. Although essential parental tasks include providing children with food, shelter, and safety, the ability to help children develop their own identity, self-confidence, and creativity is also of fundamental importance. You will often need to communicate to parents and other family caregivers the importance of encouraging their children and helping them to meet their needs. In Practice: Educating the Client 9-1, you will find suggestions for helping families to build their children's self-esteem and independence.

> **Key Concept**
>
> The lack of adequate self-esteem may play a role in the development of problems later in life, including chemical dependency, eating disorders, and depression.

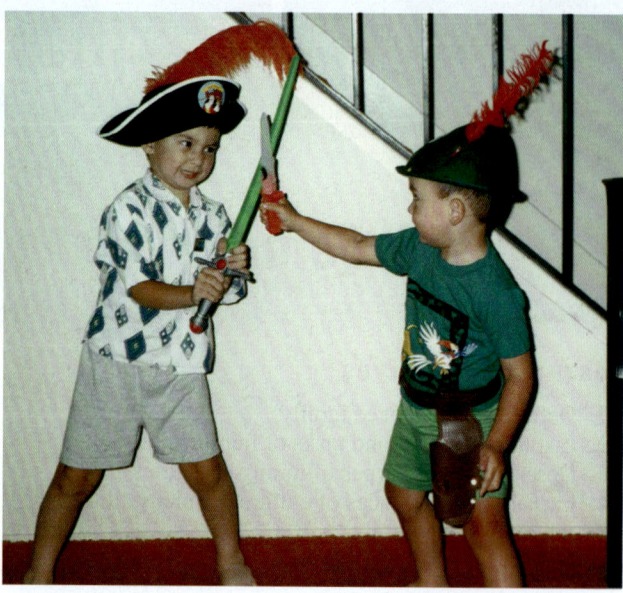

Figure 9-1 The sibling relationship is extremely influential. Siblings fulfill many roles for one another, including companion, teacher, and friend. They also like to compete in games and for the affection of their parents. (Photo courtesy of Mary T. Kowalski.)

Siblings

Because of continued interaction over many years, **siblings** (brothers and sisters) exert powerful influences on one another. The sibling relationship is the first peer relationship that many people experience. It is longstanding, often lasting for 6 decades or more.

Siblings can fulfill many roles for each other: protector, supporter, comforter, teacher, social planner, friend, and disciplinarian (Fig. 9-1). Although siblings share many experiences, each one has a different perspective on those experiences. Birth order often plays a role in shaping the experiences of siblings. For example, the firstborn in a family usually recalls experiences differently than the youngest child. Many other factors, including the time between each child's birth, are as influential on sibling relationships as birth position.

Family Functions and Tasks

The family is organized as a unit for the achievement of certain functions. Five basic family functions can be identified:

1. Providing for physical health
2. Providing for mental and spiritual health
3. Socializing members
4. Reproducing
5. Providing economic well-being

The reproductive function is obviously significant for society because it is necessary for maintaining human life on earth. Supporting individuals in their physical, emotional, economic, and social growth, however, is also vital to family and societal well-being.

The family performs many tasks that encompass these five functions and that are critical for survival and continuity. Notice how the essential family tasks relate to Maslow's hierarchy of basic human needs, which are discussed in Chapter 5:

1. Physiologic needs = Providing food, shelter, and clothing
2. Security and safety = Providing safety, healthcare, financial resources

---

IN PRACTICE
EDUCATING THE CLIENT — Ways to Promote Children's Self-Esteem and Independence

- Spend quality time with children, including playtime and instruction.
- Communicate with children, using eye contact and listening attentively to their questions and responses.
- Establish and maintain routines.
- Encourage children in their endeavors, and express pleasure, enthusiasm, and interest over their achievements and activities.
- Offer constructive criticism when necessary.
- Recognize the difference between normal incidents of misbehavior and continued patterns of behavioral problems.
- Adapt expectations to children's level of maturity and age group.
- Give children room to make their own decisions, while providing supportive guidance.
- Act as a role model for appropriate behaviors.
- Use discipline with logic and consistency.
- Apologize for mistakes, but never apologize for fair punishments.
- Read to children.
- Tell children that they are loved and special, and reinforce these words with actions.

3. Love, affection, and belonging = Establishing emotional bonds with individuals in the family unit and delegating societal responsibilities outside of the family structure
4. Self-esteem = Forming lifelong views of oneself and instilling philosophical connections to other groups, families, or cultural backgrounds
5. Self-actualization = Developing insight, affection, and abilities to meet life's challenges

> **NCLEX Alert**
>
> Clinical situations on an NCLEX might discuss a variety of family healthcare issues. You need to consider what issues are being disclosed. The correct option could relate to a variety of concerns, including preventive care, topics that need be taught to family members, cultural issues, or socioeconomic concerns. The correct response will be realistic and within the Nurse Practice Act of your license.

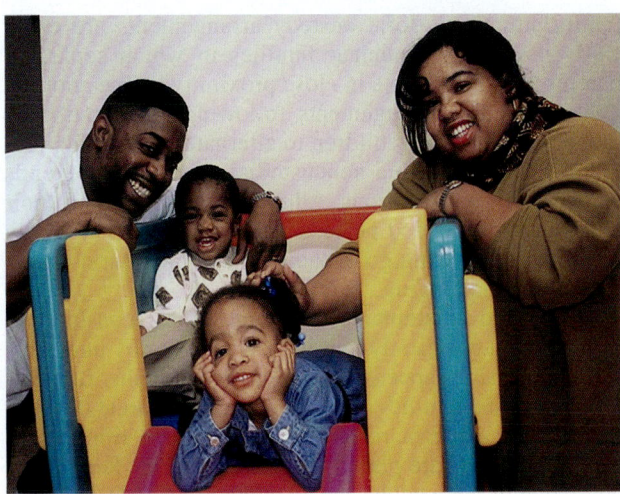

Figure 9-2 The nuclear family consists of a married couple with one or more children, living together in one household.

FAMILY STRUCTURE

Many different types of families exist in today's society. When working with clients, nurses will encounter many variations. No type of family structure is inherently better than another. Rather, it is the quality of interactions among individuals that dictates the family's ability to cope, adapt, and thrive. Although the family structures of clients may differ from the nurse's own personal experience, understanding and appreciating various family forms is critical for providing culturally sensitive and culturally competent care, that is to say nonjudgmental and informed nursing care.

A **single-adult household** consists of an adult living alone. No children are involved. This scenario is common for young adults before entering into other types of family structures or for older individuals who have lost a partner through separation, divorce, or death. Some people also make a lifetime commitment not to marry, cohabitate with a romantic partner, or to have children. Individuals may focus on their careers in lieu of the traditional family lifestyle. Friends, coworkers, and/or relatives supply social interactions and emotional bonds.

A **nuclear dyad** is a married couple that lives together without children. Couples with no children, or couples with children who reside elsewhere, are examples of nuclear dyads.

Nurses must be aware of the family structure. The ability to care for children or adults within these societal units is commonly a major financial, emotional, or organizational concern for healthcare interventions.

Nuclear Families

The most familiar family form is the **nuclear family**: a two-generation unit consisting of a husband, wife, and their immediate children—biologic, adopted, or both—living within one household (Fig. 9-2). A **dual-career** or *dual-earner family* is a nuclear family in which both parents work outside the home. Outside employment for both partners in a family may necessitate careful structuring of household tasks. Childcare arrangements often become a major issue for working parents. In the **commuter family**, adults are employed outside the home. Often the adults in this type of family both work at a distance from the home. The decision to commute to work involves many family dynamics such as childcare after school, financial costs of commuting, or a sacrifice of time away from the family unit.

Extended Families

The **extended family** consists of the nuclear family and other related people, such as grandparents, aunts, uncles, and cousins. These family members may live together in one house or in close proximity to one another. Various members may share babysitting and disciplining of children. Members of the extended family may also influence parental decisions regarding childrearing.

The family in which grandparents assume responsibility for raising children is becoming increasingly common for a number of reasons. An adolescent parent may be in school or at work during the day and may need the assistance of a parent or grandparent in order to complete specific goals such as employment or schooling. Some parents are unable to care for their children because of divorce, drug abuse, mental illness, or imprisonment. Although family involvement is often an asset, older grandparents may have difficulties meeting basic needs for the family because of financial difficulties or illness.

Single-Parent Families

The **single-parent family** involves an adult head of the house with dependent children. The adult may be single as a result of separation, divorce, death, or never being married. Divorce and births to unmarried women have contributed to the continual shifts from the two-parent family to the single-parent family.

Binuclear and Stepfamilies

A **binuclear family** is one in which a separation or divorce of the adult partners occurs, but both parents continue to assume a high level of childrearing responsibilities. Divorce has contributed greatly to changes in common family situations. Joint custody arrangements are especially useful for binuclear families in which separated parents continue to live in close proximity to one another. Other custodial arrangements following a separation or divorce may require children to alternate households regularly or to live with a noncustodial parent on weekends or over summer vacations. Adults who live without their children for extended periods often find that continually resuming and letting go of their hands-on parental role is especially challenging.

A **blended or stepfamily** is literally the reconstruction of more than one family unit into a single family unit. This situation often happens when divorced adults remarry. Blended or stepfamilies also occur when one parent dies and the remaining parent remarries. Any children from previous relationships are placed together into a new family unit consisting of these adults and all children. In addition, these families may include infants born into such an arrangement.

Alternative Families

The term "**cohabitation**" refers to unmarried individuals in a committed partnership living together, with or without children. People may live in cohabitation arrangements before, in between, or as an alternative to marriage.

In a **gay or lesbian family**, partners of the same sex may live together in a familiar relationship. One or both of the homosexual partners may have children from a previous heterosexual relationship, or the couple may adopt children together. Artificial insemination is an option for lesbian couples who wish to bear and raise children. A gay couple may use a surrogate mother. Surrogate mothers carry a pregnancy for intended couples. Various types of reproductive technologies are discussed in Chapter 70.

In a **communal family**, several people live together. They often strive to be self-sufficient and minimize contact with the outside society. Members share financial resources, work, and childcare responsibilities.

In a **foster family**, children live in temporary arrangements with paid caregivers. Theoretically, these children are meant to return to their family of origin when conditions permit or otherwise to be placed for adoption. In some cases, the children remain in the foster home until adulthood.

INFLUENCE OF CULTURE, ETHNICITY, AND RELIGION

Families develop a culture that is reflected both internally and externally. Family members use their accumulated group experiences to interpret and to define acceptable behaviors and actions based on prevailing family belief systems. The internal beliefs of the elder family members are taught to younger members. Externally, family members may interact with society differently, reflecting the belief systems of a particular age group. For example, an adolescent may reject family beliefs in order to be perceived as more popular in school.

Each culture or ethnic group sets standards for its members (Chapter 8), and people in general tend to live in communities of like-minded people or people of similar ethnic background. This network gives its members support and helps

Box 9-1 | Cultural, Ethnic, and Religious Considerations That May Influence Family Choices

- Choice of marriage partner (who chooses the spouse)
- Dating customs
- How many spouses a person may have
- Living arrangements
- Status of different genders
- Family decision-makers
- Roles of various family members
- Attitudes toward children
- Type of discipline
- Family disciplinarian
- Attitudes toward older adults in the family
- Choice of vocation or occupation
- How to deal with crises and emotions: anger, grief, sadness, use of defense mechanisms
- Attitudes toward education, birth control, abortion, and sexual practices

Adapted from Hatfield, N. T. (2017). *Introductory maternity & pediatric nursing* (4th ed.). Wolters Kluwer.

them maintain their ethnic ideals. Families may move outside the ethnic community by geographic relocation, or younger members may move to attend a school or college. As these changes occur, some individuals' ethnic ideals may evolve.

In past centuries, families married within their own ethnic, racial, or religious groups. Today, families with partners from different ethnic groups and racial heritages are common. A family may represent two very different religious or spiritual groups. Each person brings into the family cultural factors reflecting their background. Adjustments must be made to acknowledge and accept each other's differences. Box 9-1 lists various examples of cultural factors related to family.

FAMILY STAGES

In the following chapters, you will learn about developmental stages and tasks for individuals to achieve. The family also develops through various stages and tasks. Table 9-1 summarizes the important features of these stages, which revolve around the processes of childbirth and childrearing and are most reflective of nuclear families. Other types of families may skip or overlap certain stages or may never experience them.

Transitional Stage

The transitional stage refers to the period when single young adults, usually in their 20s or early 30s, are financially independent from their family of origin and live outside the family home. This stage has evolved as a norm as young adults delay marriage, often choosing to live alone or with others of a similar age first. During the transitional stage, individuals usually develop intimate relationships, perhaps leading to cohabitation or marriage. Different genders experience this stage differently, depending on their goals, which may be family and children, career success, or both.

CHAPTER 9 The Family

TABLE 9-1 Stages of the Family Life Cycle and Associated Developmental Tasks

STAGE	SPECIFIC TASKS
Transitional	• Separating from one's family of origin • Developing intimate relationships • Establishing independence in work and finances
Expanding Family	
• Establishment	• Building a mutually satisfying relationship • Incorporating spouse/partner into relationships with extended family • Setting up a household and delineating household responsibilities for each partner • Planning for own family
• Childbearing	• Integrating an infant into the family • Maintaining a satisfying couple relationship • Expanding relationships with extended family by adding the parenting and grandparenting roles
• Childrearing	• Meeting basic physical needs of all family members • Socializing children (peers, school, community) • Integrating new child members while meeting needs of other children • Maintaining a satisfying couple relationship
Contracting Family	
• Child launching	• Releasing young adults to work, college, military service, and marriage with appropriate assistance • Adjusting the couple relationship as children leave the family home • Expanding the family circle with the marriage or relationships of children
• Postparenting	• Assisting older adult parents • Maintaining a healthy lifestyle • Continuing relationships with children and parents • Adjusting to retirement • Strengthening the couple relationship
• Aging	• Finding a satisfactory living arrangement • Maintaining a satisfying couple relationship • Coping with the loss of a life partner • Keeping intergenerational family connections open • Accepting one's own mortality

Expanding Family Stage

In the expanding family stage, families are created, new members are added, and roles and relationships increase. This stage begins when an individual selects a partner with whom they make a commitment and ends when the first child leaves the home to begin their own transitional stage.

Establishment

Single adults move into the establishment phase when they choose a partner and set up a household. Establishing a household may or may not involve marriage. Building a mutually satisfying relationship, maintaining relations with an extended family, and deciding whether or not to have children are developmental tasks associated with establishment. This phase often contains its own transitions, as individuals shift from living independently to learning to share and maintain an interdependent relationship.

Childbearing

A family enters the childbearing phase with the birth or adoption of its first child. No matter how an individual or couple may initially feel about a pregnancy, the arrival of a first child is usually an occasion of wonder and joy. Individuals, finished with waiting, are ready for their new role as parents. The transition to parenthood, however, is often difficult. Although new parents are now faced with childcare responsibilities, they also need to maintain a mutually satisfying relationship as a couple during this period.

An enormously important issue that dual-earner families must confront during this time is adequate childcare arrangements. Regardless of whether both parents work out of financial necessity or by choice, they need to develop and adjust to a plan that leaves young children in the care of another. Sometimes parents can arrange different work schedules for childcare purposes. Although children may benefit from always being with one parent or the other, the relationship between the adults may suffer because of inadequate time for each other.

Childrearing

Families in the childrearing phase include those with preschoolers, school-age children, and adolescents. Once children arrive, family life forever changes. The members of the family must continually adjust to one another.

Socialization of children is a major task of childrearing. Along with peer relationships and school activities, parents often encourage participation in community activities. Family transportation may seem never ending, as children are taken to and from their activities. Childrearing families often are pressured for time. Children's schedules must be considered as part of the family timetable. The parents' mealtimes and sleep patterns must change when children arrive. As children grow older, the scheduling of family members may become more hectic. Arrangements must first be made for babysitters, then often for carpools and attendance at school functions. The adults' responsibilities and community contacts may also increase during this active time. However, it is beneficial to encourage the growth tasks of all members of the family and combine them into a family design or plan (Fig. 9-3).

At this point in the family cycle, communication is a developmental task for all members. Communication between partners, including sexual relations, may be sharply displaced as the family grows. Private conversation is difficult because children are omnipresent. Adults need to plan times when they can be alone together without children, to maintain a mutually gratifying relationship. They also need to encourage communication for the entire family and keep the channels open for children to share their daily experiences, thoughts, ambitions, and ideas.

Contracting Family Stage

During the contracting family stage, the family becomes smaller. Children who have grown into adults leave to begin lives and families of their own. Parents must adjust to new roles as individuals. A couple may begin to rediscover one another or to reevaluate their relationship and individual paths.

Child Launching

In the child-launching phase, the family has reached its maximum size. Child launching begins when the first child leaves home to live independently and ends when the last child leaves home. This phase represents the outcome of preparing children for adult life. As each child leaves home, the parental task is to reorganize the family from a home with children to a home again occupied only by adults. The length of this period varies. In past generations, adults were involved in childrearing until old age. With a longer lifespan and smaller families, parents may now launch children 20 years before they retire. In some families, children live at home until their 30s or return to the family home after college—usually for financial reasons—lengthening the child-launching phase of the family. An important developmental task at this time is to accept and to appreciate, even if one does not always approve of, the differences in ideals, habits, and philosophies of the new generation.

Postparenting

Postparenting begins when the youngest child leaves the home and continues until the retirement or death of a partner. Once associated with middle years (approximately ages 40–60 years), this phase may occur later, as couples delay starting their families and adult children continue to live in the parental home. Many people find their middle years a comfortable and serene period. Fewer demands allow more time to enjoy life. Financial burdens related to children are fewer, and time for shared activities increases. Readjustment to a period in which children figure somewhat less prominently is necessary. Couples who share common goals and interests are likely to enjoy this period. An important task is maintaining relationships with aging parents and grown children. During this

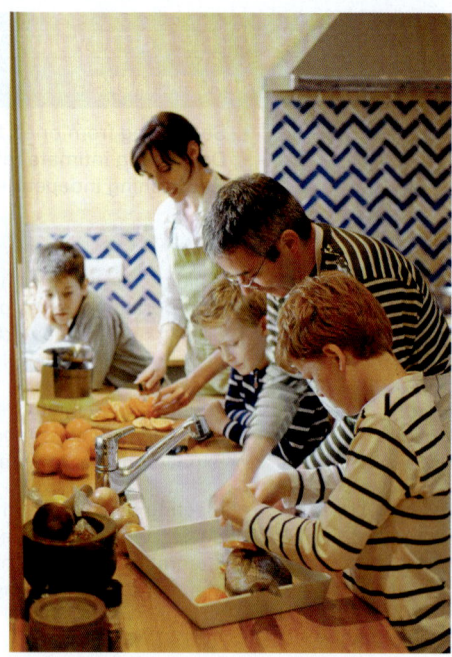

Figure 9-3 The family in the childrearing stage focuses much attention on socializing children and on spending time communicating and sharing activity. (Bowden, 2010.)

Key Concept

Adjustment to retirement may be difficult if careful financial planning is not done or if hobbies and activities were not developed in earlier years.

phase, individuals may take on a new role—grandparent. The middle-aged couple finds that the rewards of time allow both of them to come to terms with themselves and to gain satisfaction in opportunities still available. Planning for financial security in later years is essential. The expense of raising children has been lifted, and family income is usually at its peak.

Aging

As partners get older, they face several challenges. Many older adults decide to relocate. Deciding where to live is difficult for many older people. Often they have lived in the same home for 20 or 30 years or more. The place holds many memories, and it is hard to let go. Sometimes, the need for one partner to go to a nursing home makes the decision more difficult.

Fixed retirement income is insufficient for many people because of inflation. Even though costs go up, the income stays the same. Many older people have saved what they once thought would be enough money to take care of themselves in their retirement years; however, even one short illness can wipe out a modest savings account. Older adults then may be forced to sell their home or seek financial assistance.

As people get older, they may experience a decline in their physical faculties. A good sense of humor is probably the greatest asset in dealing with this deterioration. Older adults must get some sort of exercise, maintain an adequate diet, and get sufficient rest. Single adults may experience difficulty with proper nutritional habits. Individuals who lose a partner may not know how to cook or may not want to bother to cook just for themselves. A regular physical examination is important to detect minor difficulties before they become major problems.

Older adults must accept death as another stage of life. They need to plan their legal affairs and to discuss finances for the future. If they have not yet made a will, they should do so now. Many people will live alone at least part of their lives because of divorce or death of a partner.

STRESS AND FAMILY COPING

Every family encounters stress, which is inevitable but can be faced and handled appropriately. In addition to the normal changes, adaptations, and pressures of the family cycle, financial, physical, and emotional stresses may occur at any time. Often, stressors are interrelated, contribute to, and exacerbate one another.

Family stress is different from other types of stress because of the interdependent relationships that exist in families. When one member is under stress, the entire family is affected. Many families are able to develop socially acceptable means of dealing with stress. These **functional families** use resources to cope and often become stronger as a result of the stressful experience. Other families cannot cope. The result is that, as stressors build, coping systems disintegrate. The latter type of family is called a **dysfunctional family** or *at-risk family*.

> **NCLEX Alert**
>
> An NCLEX clinical situation may discuss types, functions, or dysfunctions of a family. Knowing the specific defined name of the "family" (e.g., single, nuclear, extended) may not be as important as knowing how to assist the individuals when needed in times of stress. Keep in mind that stress can involve survival, psychosocial, or financial needs. The priorities of these needs often vary between families, individuals, and cultural/religious/ethnic groups. Prioritization of needs is critical.

Socioeconomic Stressors

Socioeconomic circumstances can greatly influence families. Income determines recreational pursuits. One family may be able to afford a vacation, whereas another family finds recreational opportunities in picnics and free community offerings. A family's income level often influences choices such as housing, education, daycare facilities, material goods, and nutrition.

Because of economic constraints, adults may have to work two jobs or several part-time jobs to provide for the family, which affects the amount of time they can spend with partners or children. Older siblings may be required to take on more household or childcare responsibilities. Daycare may replace home care for children. In extended families, grandparents, aunts, or uncles may provide childcare. All these circumstances can place significant levels of stress on the entire family unit.

Poverty knows no boundaries. Families whose income is below the federal poverty threshold may face a variety of health and social challenges, including homelessness, high rates of infant mortality, malnutrition, anemia, lead poisoning, inability to earn a high school diploma or equivalent, and shortened lifespan. Individuals whose income is below the poverty threshold may include those experiencing homelessness, undocumented workers, residents of low-employment areas (including rural, mountain, and urban communities), and many older adults. Women living alone or with their children represent a significant percentage of people living in poverty. Further difficulties can arise when a parent fails to pay needed child support.

Divorce and Remarriage

A family's coping ability may be significantly compromised during a divorce. Adults who are facing separation from their partners—and a return to single life—may feel overwhelmed. They may become preoccupied with their own feelings, thereby limiting their ability to handle the situation effectively or to be strong for their children. The breakdown of the family system may require a restructuring of responsibilities, employment, childcare, and housing arrangements. Animosity between adults may expose children to uncontrolled emotions, arguments, anger, and depression.

Children may feel guilt and anxiety over their parents' divorce, believing the situation to be their fault. They may be unable to channel their conflicting emotions effectively. Their school performance may suffer, or they may engage in misbehavior. Even when a divorce is handled amicably, children may experience conflicts about their loyalties and may have difficulties making the transition from one household to another during visitation periods.

The arrival of a stepparent in the home presents additional stressors for children. Adapting to new rules of behavior, adjusting to a new person's habits, and sharing parents with new family members can cause resentment and anger. When families blend children, rivalries and competition for parental attention can lead to repeated conflicts.

Violence and Abuse

Violence in a family is a concern of all ages—from infants to older adults. Abuse of children, partners, siblings, and older adults usually manifests itself in physical, emotional, or sexual mistreatment, exploitation, and neglect. Other, less blatant forms of abusive behavior include interfering with another family member's outside social networks; misusing money and other resources; displaying inappropriate jealousy; monopolizing another person's time; and blocking a person from receiving needed healthcare. Cultural and economic pressures may contribute to such situations because abused individuals may be afraid to expose the situation to outsiders or may be financially or emotionally dependent on their abuser. Survivors of violence and abuse often retain lifelong physical and emotional scars.

Abusive situations and other dysfunctional patterns of coping can have a negative impact on children. Children model their behaviors and develop their attitudes by watching the adults they love and trust. Children who were abused or who witnessed abuse in their families may grow up to be abusive as well, continuing a cycle of family violence. Child abuse is discussed in more detail in Unit 11.

Addictions

The family in which one or more members have an addictive disorder faces continual pressure and stress. Addictions may be in the form of drug or alcohol abuse, gambling disorders, sexual compulsions, or "workaholism." In all such cases, the addiction begins to replace the family as a wellspring of support and a source for social interaction. The entire family suffers as it begins to focus on ways to accommodate and incorporate the addictive behavior, while hiding it from those outside the family circle. Partners and children are often neglected, and financial resources often begin to dwindle as addicted individuals continue their behavior. Chapter 95 presents a detailed discussion of issues related to substance abuse and other addictions.

Acute or Chronic Illness

Illness can strike anyone at any time. Some illnesses are acute, whereas others become chronic. In either case, the family must deal with an enormous amount of pressure when one of its members faces illness. Financial issues may become a great concern, even if the family has good insurance coverage. Employment issues may need to be reconsidered, along with adjustments in schedules and social activities. Worry, anxiety, concern, and fear may be issues for the family witnessing a loved one's compromised or declining condition.

> *Key Concept*
> As a nurse, you are likely to work with many families who are dealing with acute and chronic illnesses. It is important to identify key issues or problems.

> **Box 9-2 Phases of a Family's Response to Major Stress**
>
> **ADJUSTMENT PHASE**
> 1. The family tries to maintain the status quo with minimal disruption to the family unit.
> 2. The family may deny or ignore the stressor.
> 3. The family may remove the demands of the stressor.
> 4. The family may accept the demands created by the stressor.
>
> **ADAPTATION PHASE**
> 1. The family realizes that regaining stability will involve changes in the family structure.
> 2. Friends and community provide assistance with the problem-solving process during the stressful period.
> 3. Roles, rules, boundaries, and patterns of behavior within the family are altered as needed in order to regain stability.

Effective and Ineffective Coping Strategies

Individuals and families respond to both everyday and more severe stressors in many ways. The response to major stressors can be depicted in two phases: adjustment and adaptation. During each phase, a family will employ different coping strategies. Box 9-2 highlights the two phases of a family's response to stress.

STUDENT SYNTHESIS

KEY POINTS

- The family is the basic unit of society, but it is a complex unit.
- All nursing care should involve clients and their families.
- Each family is a unique structure with cultural values and rules. Families move through life cycle stages.
- Roles and relationships within a family are many and varied; the primary ones include parent–child and sibling relationships.
- The functions and tasks of the family help individuals to meet their basic human needs.
- Although many different family structures exist, all can be efficient, supportive, and satisfying.
- Cultural, ethnic, and religious factors influence family outcomes.
- Family development progresses through predictable stages, with important developmental tasks.
- The family that can cope with stress is functional; families that cannot cope are dysfunctional or at risk.

CRITICAL THINKING EXERCISES

1. This chapter presents the stages of family development, based primarily on the nuclear family. Consider how family structure might influence the family life cycle in the following situations: a single-parent family, a family in which grandparents are raising grandchildren, a blended family, and a binuclear family.

2. S.H., a sophomore in high school, is pregnant with her first child. She lives with her mother (who works full time), grandmother, and younger brother. Her parents have been divorced for several years, and she has limited contact with her father. Her boyfriend wants to help raise the child. Based on this information, identify potential stressors for S.H. and her family. Assess possible ways the family can best handle her pregnancy. What effects will the new baby have on the family's structure and stages?

3. Consider special needs for the following individuals and ways families can identify and meet those needs: children of a blended family, adopted children, older parents living with their grown children, a widow with no children, a single father, a gay couple considering adoption, and a couple who must live apart for 6 months because of employment considerations.

NCLEX-STYLE REVIEW QUESTIONS

1. A 10-year-old child is brought to the school nurse with a black eye, after being involved in an altercation with another child. Which statement by the child would be of greatest concern to the nurse?
   a. "It is my fault my parents are getting a divorce."
   b. "I want to be their friend, but they don't like me."
   c. "I got angry when they said my clothes aren't nice."
   d. "I'm just not having a good day today."

2. When obtaining data from a client, the nurse asks "Who do you live with?" The client states, "I live with my parents, brother, and grandparents." Which documentation is appropriate to describe the family structure?
   a. Nuclear dyad
   b. Extended family
   c. Binuclear family
   d. Blended family

3. The nurse is discussing the family tasks that are critical for survival and continuity. Which task, identified by a family member, would take priority?
   a. Providing financial support for healthcare needs
   b. Establishing emotional bonds
   c. Developing recognition for achievements
   d. Providing food, shelter, and clothing

4. A client's 16-year-old child is addicted to heroin. The client tells the nurse that friends of the family are assisting with helping them cope. The nurse documents that the client and family are in which phase of response to major stress?
   a. Acceptance phase
   b. Adjustment phase
   c. Adaptation phase
   d. Transitional phase

5. When the client is in the establishment stage of life, which issues might the client discuss with the nurse?
   a. Whether to enter into parenthood
   b. Sleep patterns of their child
   c. Concerns about living alone since the last child left home
   d. Financial decisions regarding retirement

CHAPTER RESOURCES

Enhance your learning with additional resources on thePoint*!*

Student Resources related to this chapter can be found at **thePoint.lww.com/Rosdahl12e.**

10 Infancy and Childhood

Learning Objectives

1. List the characteristics and sequence of human growth and development.
2. Explain developmental milestones, developmental delays, and regression.
3. Discuss the importance of anticipatory guidance for caregivers.
4. Describe Erikson's stages of psychosocial development, including the challenges and virtues of each stage.
5. Explain the four stages of human cognitive development as described by Piaget.
6. Describe the role of play in childhood development.
7. Discuss growth and development for infants, toddlers, preschoolers, and school-aged children, highlighting key areas of concern.

Important Terminology

anticipatory guidance
bonding
bottle mouth
cephalocaudal
cognitive
development
developmental delays
developmental milestones
developmental tasks
encopresis
enuresis
environment
genetics
growth
heredity
infancy
interdependent
masturbation
newborn (neonate)
nutrition
object permanence
parallel play
pincer grasp
proximodistal
regression
separation anxiety
solitary play
stranger anxiety
temperament
toddler

The preceding chapter discusses the importance of the family: its functions, types, and stages. Individuals also move through developmental stages. The study of individual growth and development begins with this chapter on infancy and childhood.

Chapter 5 discusses basic human needs. An understanding of these basic needs is necessary before attempting to study growth and development across the lifespan. For example, infants require assistance to meet their most basic survival needs, such as food, water, and elimination. When these needs are met, toddlers begin to develop needs for safety, security, and socialization. As children become adolescents and eventually adults, they begin to meet their higher-level needs and to assist members of the younger generation in meeting these needs.

Children are a country's future—its citizens of tomorrow. As a nurse, you are likely to care for healthy as well as acutely ill and chronically ill children.

CONCEPTS OF GROWTH AND DEVELOPMENT

Growth and development occurs in an orderly sequence; a person must accomplish a simple developmental task before they can progress to attempt another, more complex task. Most children are able to perform certain tasks at about the same age, although normal variations exist.

In relation to the body, the process of growth and development follows cephalocaudal and proximodistal directions (Fig. 10-1). **Cephalocaudal** means from head to tail; babies lift their heads before they sit up; they make sounds before they walk. **Proximodistal** means from the center to the outside; babies roll over before they grasp small objects.

Growth progresses from simple to complex; the baby learns to sit before learning to walk, and to babble before learning to speak. Normal development involves several fundamental skills. The multifaceted aspects of growth and development are inclusive and holistic, involving the child and family, plus the physical, social, and emotional, or psychosocial environments.

In this text, physical growth, psychosocial (i.e., emotional and social) development, and cognitive and motor development are discussed in relation to specific age groups. These three categories combine to cover the basic developmental skills:

- **Physical growth**—a change in body size and structure
- **Psychosocial development**—the ability to interact with others and to form relationships, to cooperate, and to respond to the feelings of others
- **Cognitive and motor abilities**
  - *Cognitive:* the ability to think, learn, understand, solve problems, and remember
  - *Language:* the ability to communicate by speech (verbal language) and body gestures (nonverbal language)
  - *Gross motor:* the use of the large muscle groups in activities such as maintaining balance, sitting, standing, or running
  - *Fine motor:* the use of smaller muscles in conjunction with large muscle groups in activities, such as holding a cup, using a fork, buttoning a shirt, or drawing a picture

CHAPTER 10 Infancy and Childhood

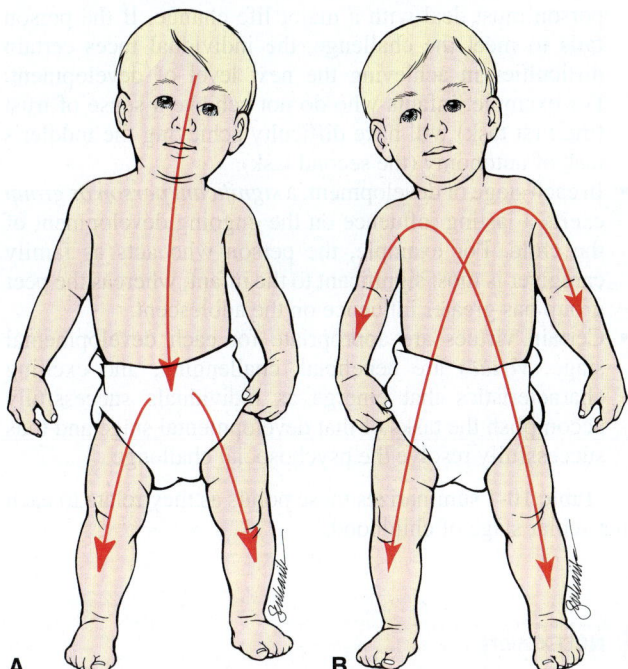

Figure 10-1 Principles of growth and development. **A.** Cephalocaudal growth and development proceed from head to toe or tail. **B.** Proximodistal growth and development proceed from the center outward.

All aspects of growth and development are influenced by each other, or are **interdependent**. For example, children cannot learn to control their bowel movements (development) until their muscles are strong enough (growth) and until they can understand what is expected of them (development). Each age has its developmental milestones related to growth.

> **Key Concept**
>
> Growth is a change in body size and structure; development is a change in body function. The process of growth and development has the following characteristics:
>
> - Orderly sequence
> - Simple to complex
> - Cephalocaudal
> - Inclusive
> - Proximodistal
> - Interdependent

DEVELOPMENTAL MILESTONES AND DEVELOPMENTAL DELAYS

Understanding normal patterns is an important factor in caring for children. They accomplish skills and abilities in predictable patterns and within general age-specific timeframes called **developmental milestones** or **developmental tasks**. Examples of developmental milestones include smiling for the first time, taking a first step, or learning the words of a language. The timing of the achievements or milestones is unique to each child. Problems arise when one or more milestones are delayed.

Developmental delays occur when a child does not achieve the predicted developmental milestones within acceptable patterns. By knowing how most children can be expected to behave at particular stages, you will be better prepared to care for any child. An understanding of normal behavior is also necessary before you can recognize abnormal behavior. For example, it is helpful to know that regression may occur during illness. During **regression**, a child's behavior may go backward to that of an earlier stage of development—for example, during an acute illness, a child who has not needed diapers for a long time may have episodes of incontinence (wetting the bed).

GROWTH AND DEVELOPMENT

Growth and development, often considered a single process, continues throughout childhood and into adulthood. **Growth** is defined as a change in body size and structure; **development** is a change in body function.

Anticipatory Guidance

During each stage of childhood, growth and developmental issues will be of concern to caregivers. The nurse provides examples of growth and development and the many variations involved within these concepts to caregivers. Many caregivers express worries that their children are not behaving like other children of similar age. The caregivers need to be able to recognize each child's unique natural abilities. The nurse must educate caregivers about expected changes; this is called **anticipatory guidance**. Children's instinctive curiosity and physical growth carry them to new fields to conquer. The challenge of parenting is to help children develop in such a way that they maintain their eagerness to learn throughout their lives. Many parenting education and support groups are available in the community health system or through a hospital education program.

Influences on Growth and Development

Heredity, nutrition, and environment are three major influences on a child's growth and development. **Heredity** is the biological process responsible for transferring physical traits from one generation to another. Characteristics of heredity, or the biological traits within genes, are inherited from parents and passed on to another generation. **Genetics** is the study of heredity in biology. Sex, skin color, eye color, and body build are examples of hereditary characteristics. Some disorders are genetically transmitted, for example, Huntington disease and some forms of breast cancer. Personality and temperament are also influenced by heredity. **Temperament** is the combination of an individual's characteristics, the way the person thinks, behaves, and reacts to the environment.

Nutrition is the selection, preparation, ingestion, and assimilation of foods by the body. By maintaining a healthy diet, many known health issues can be avoided. For example, nutrition is a major factor in the body's ability to resist infection and combat diseases. Motor skill development is affected by both inadequate and excessive food intake. Eating habits are established early in childhood and are carried to adulthood. Nutrition affects the growth, development, and health of the individual throughout his or her lifetime.

Environment is the sum of all the conditions and factors surrounding the child. Housing, neighborhood, number of siblings, placement in sibling order, and amount of healthcare available are examples of environmental elements. A baby born into a large family may develop differently from one born into a small family. Religious practices, ethnicity, and location of birth also influence a child's development. Socioeconomic levels of the family, availability for child care and healthcare, and parental use of alcohol or drugs also affect the child's developmental environment. Exposure to water pollution and air contamination such as tobacco smoke are known environmental risks (CDC, 2019). Chapter 7 discusses environmental hazards in more detail.

Growth and Development Theories

A number of theories exist that can be used to understand, explain, and predict human development as a series of overlapping states occurring in predictable patterns. No one theory covers the whole spectrum of behavior, so it is wise to consider each person from a combination of viewpoints. Two especially important theories include Erik Erikson's psychosocial development theory and Jean Piaget's cognitive theory.

Erikson: Psychosocial Development

Erikson's theory of human development focuses on the psychosocial and environmental aspects of personality as the person progresses from birth to death. Erikson stresses that each individual is the product of interactions among heredity, environment, and culture. He emphasizes that the rate of development varies. The main points of Erikson's theory are:

- Each stage of development contains a psychosocial task or crisis. This *challenge* is a critical period during which the person must deal with a major life change. If the person fails to meet the challenge, the individual faces certain difficulties in achieving the next level of development. For example, infants who do not achieve a sense of trust (the first task) will have difficulty achieving the toddler's task of autonomy (the second task).
- In each stage of development, a *significant person or group* exerts a lasting influence on the ongoing development of the child. For example, the person who acts as family caregiver is most significant to the infant, whereas the peer group has greater influence on the adolescent.
- Certain virtues are appropriate for each developmental stage. *Virtues* are beneficial, challenging, and exciting characteristics that emerge as individuals successfully accomplish the tasks of that developmental stage and thus successfully resolve the psychosocial challenge.

Table 10-1 summarizes these points as they relate to each particular stage of childhood.

> **NCLEX Alert**
>
> The concepts of psychosocial development as presented by Erikson may be found in a variety of NCLEX questions. Erickson's "ages and stages" must be understood to answer these growth and development questions.

Piaget: Cognitive Development

The term **cognitive** refers to knowledge, understanding, perception, or intellectual development. Thus, cognitive development is the development of the thinking process. Piaget stated that cognitive development is a continuous progression of four principal stages. The first stage begins with the spontaneous and automatic reflexes of the newborn and uses the five senses (sight, smell, hearing, taste, touch). The infant progresses to acquired habits. The child then goes on to acquire knowledge and develop intelligence.

TABLE 10-1 Erikson's Theory of Psychosocial Development—Childhood

CONCEPT	INFANCY (1–12 MONTHS)	TODDLERHOOD (1–3 YEARS)	PRESCHOOL (3–6 YEARS)	SCHOOL AGE (6–12 YEARS)
Challenge	Trust vs. mistrust	Autonomy vs. shame and doubt	Initiative vs. guilt	Industry vs. inferiority
Significant other	Family caregivers	Family	Family	School and neighborhood
Necessary accomplishment	Develop trust	Learn appropriate behaviors; learn right from wrong	Learn rules and regulations; establish independence	Learn to get along with others; learn school subjects
Virtues	Hope	Self-control; will-power	Direction; purpose	Self-esteem; competence
Ways to help the child succeed	Establish routines; satisfy basic needs	Set limits; let child make simple choices; encourage curiosity; give gentle guidance	Consistent discipline; explain things; praise	Manage sibling rivalry; give responsibility; recognize accomplishments away from home

Bowden, V. R., & Greenberg, C. S. (2014). *Children and their families: The continuum of nursing care* (3rd ed.). Wolters Kluwer Health/Lippincott Williams & Wilkins; Hatfield, N. T., & Kincheloe, C. A. (2018). *Introductory maternity & pediatric nursing* (4th ed.). Wolters Kluwer; and McLeod, S. A. (2018). *Erik Erikson's stages of psychosocial development.* Simply Psychology. https://www.simplypsychology.org/Erik-Erikson.html

Cognitive development is cumulative; that is, what is learned is based on what has been known before. An example of cumulative cognitive development could be the curriculum of your nursing program. Information is presented to you in a progression from simple to complex. For example, you learn normal body structure and function and normal development before you study deviations from those parameters.

Piaget's four major levels of cognitive development are:

1. *Sensorimotor.* Up to age 2, children learn by touching, tasting, and feeling. They learn to control body movement. They begin to associate cause and effect; for example, touching a toy can cause it to move. They develop an understanding of **object permanence**, the knowledge that an object seen in a particular spot, but temporarily hidden from view under a blanket, continues to exist and will return to view when it is uncovered.
2. *Preoperational.* From the ages of 2–7, children investigate and explore the environment and look at things from their own egocentric point of view. A child interprets experiences from his or her own perception. As children experience more things, their point of view changes. In this early phase, they have only a minimal concept of time and their concept of quantity is distorted. For example, four ounces (120 mL) of juice in a small glass seems like less than four ounces of juice in a large glass.
3. *Concrete operations.* Between ages 7 and 11, children develop the ability to think in the abstract. They can solve problems, classify, and organize information within their environment. They can understand the difference between different volumes and weights. They are beginning to consider another person's point of view.
4. *Formal operations.* After age 12, children can think in the abstract. Complex problem-solving includes the ability to understand double meanings of words and jokes. The adolescent can discuss theories, and philosophy, and then develop conclusions from the facts provided.

Role of Play in Child Development

Play is important to child development. Children learn about the world through play. Experimentation, exploration, success, and failure are a part of maturation. Play with other children encourages peer cooperation, interaction, and sharing. Children learn about their environment using all five senses. Play promotes fine and large muscle coordination and strengthens muscles. It enhances the child's awareness of fairness, and of the rules and regulations of social situations. The attention span of infants and toddlers lasts for only a few minutes, so a need to change activities is necessary. Language becomes an important part of play as the child grows and develops.

Solitary play occurs in infancy when children play alone with their own toys in the same area as others but without interaction. Toddlers exhibit **parallel play**, which occurs when two children play side-by-side with the same or similar toys but do not interact with each other or the other's toy (Fig. 10-2). Preschoolers begin to play directly with other

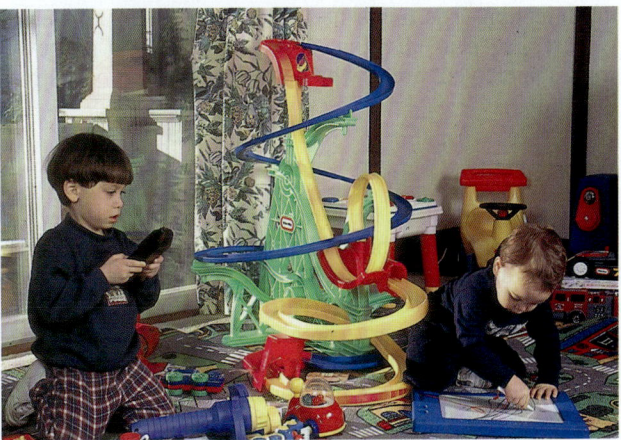

Figure 10-2 Toddlers show their growing interest in peers through parallel (side-by-side) play. (Weber & Kelley, 2003.)

children. Young school-aged children engage in cooperative and interactive play and may expand the playgroup from two or three children to an entire classroom. Older school-aged children play structured games with defined roles, rules, and ways to win. They learn to take turns, play fairly, and accept losses graciously.

Communicating with Infants and Young Children

Communication is the ability to exchange information between individuals. The process of communicating can consist of the use of one or all of the following: *verbal exchange* (language), *sounds* (alarms or cries), *writing* (handwritten or manufactured), *symbols* (signs), *colors (red, orange, green), body language* (behaviors), or *smells* (pheromones). Children communicate by using an accumulated series of abilities associated with their age. Chapter 44 discusses therapeutic communication in more detail.

Infants communicate with others using sensory cues, for example, the volume of voice and the feel of touch. The nurse needs to establish a sense of security, safety, and comfort by talking in a calm, soothing voice, cuddling the infant, and avoiding a hurried, rushed, or abrupt manner.

Young children retain an egocentric view of their surroundings; they cannot understand the complex concept of "another's point of view." Therefore, communication should only pertain to how a child's experience will affect their own environment. Language is limited to short sentences with words that are familiar. The nurse communicating with a young child needs to know that child's stage of development. Nursing implications related to communication involve knowing the developmental milestones associated with the child's age. For example, provide toddlers with a choice, such as "Do you want the yellow or the blue cup for your medicine?" rather than asking them "Will you drink the medicine now?" The use of positive reinforcement and nonthreatening gestures is important. Avoid statements like "the shot feels like a bee sting" because young children process words literally (concrete thinking). The child could be more afraid of bees than of the injection. The nurse needs to be aware of nonverbal gestures, such as clinging, crying, or trying to get away from a perceived threat, which are typical signs of distress in children.

Anxiety

Stranger anxiety is a form of distress related to survival instincts that occur when children are exposed to individuals who are unfamiliar to them. The child may get very quiet or become loud and verbally object to the stranger or hide behind the primary caregivers. Infant stranger anxiety typically starts between 7 and 9 months, which is when the child becomes aware of people other than the primary caregivers. By this age, infants first begin to move (roll, scoot, crawl) away from their security base, that is, the caregivers. Infants may have stranger anxiety for only a few months as they get accustomed to new variables within their environment.

A different aspect of stranger anxiety is seen between the ages of 12 and 24 months. Stranger anxiety at this stage occurs when children face new environments or circumstances. Anxiety is a natural part of development but not experienced by every infant or young child. Numerous factors influence the development of stranger anxiety. These factors are very relevant to a child who is being exposed to the newness of a healthcare environment, such as a doctor's office or a hospital. The following list presents possible issues that promote anxiety:

- *Temperament*—Some infants are generally more fearful or shy than others.
- *Past experiences with strangers*—Some infants do not want to be picked up by anyone other than their primary caregivers.
- *New environments*—Most infants become accustomed to routines and physical surroundings.
- *Presence of primary caregiver*—Some infants tolerate the unknown better if the primary caregivers are present.
- *Interaction of stranger*—An infant can be sensitive to a stranger's verbal and nonverbal behaviors, such as having a calm demeanor, smiling, or working with the child when the child has a familiar toy.
- *Numbers of caregivers*—If an infant is used to being cared for by a limited number of individuals, rather than a number of caregivers, the infant may have more anxiety with a wider circle of people.
- *Age*—As children begin to have cognitive development and are able to assert their own independence, they can discriminate more effectively between threatening and nonthreatening environments.

Separation anxiety is a behavior that is also a normal developmental milestone, beginning at about 7–9 months and resolving by 24 months. The child may be fussy, scream, have tantrums, or cling to their caregiver. The concept of time and ability to remember is lacking in an infant. As the child matures and develops memory skills, these episodes typically disappear. If separation anxiety is severe and lasts longer than the child's second birthday, a healthcare professional should be consulted. Separation anxiety is not uncommon in toddlers, as discussed later in the chapter.

> **Key Concept**
>
> It is common for young children to protest being with people other than their primary caregivers. Consider the factors of the child's circumstances and support the child by providing familiar items such as a blanket or toy, having a caregiver present during treatment and examinations, and adapting nonthreatening body language and verbal tones.

THE NEWBORN

A baby is called a **newborn** or neonate for the first 28 days, sometimes stated as the first month. The newborn's reactions to internal and external stimuli help to shape the child physically, intellectually, emotionally, and socially. The newborn is extremely vulnerable, tender, and delicate. Both healthcare professionals and caregivers must take many precautionary measures to help ensure the newborn's safety and ability to thrive. Chapters 67 and 69 discuss newborn care in more detail. Healthcare workers and caregivers can access a variety of Websites, such as www.cdc.gov/parents/infants/milestones.html, that will provide educational information relating to growth and development at each age. Anticipatory guidance and providing access to educational sources is an important aspect of pediatric nursing.

INFANCY: 1–12 MONTHS

The period from 1 to 12 months of age is called **infancy**. During this stage, the person matures both physically and emotionally with greater speed than at any other time of the lifespan. Individual patterns of growth and development vary for each infant. A protective, loving environment in a nurturing, responsive family contributes enormously to an infant's ability to thrive and adapt.

Physical Growth

Important milestones of an infant's first year pertain to weight, height, body circumferences, and closure of fontanels. By the age of 6 months, most infants have doubled their birth weight. By the end of 1 year, they weigh about three times their birth weight. Initially, most weight gain is fat, then muscle, and then bone density. Height increases about 6 in during the first 6 months. At a year of age, the infant has grown 10–12 in. (25.4–35 cm).

At birth, the infant's head circumference is usually slightly larger than that of the chest, which is about the same as the abdominal circumference. The chest circumference starts to exceed the head circumference between the fifth and seventh months. The space between the cranial bones is called the *fontanels* or soft spots. They are made up of strong fibrous, elastic tissues. The posterior fontanel usually closes by the end of the second or third month. The anterior fontanel closes between the ages of 12 and 18 months. Keep in mind that the cranial bones do not ossify (become bone) until later in childhood.

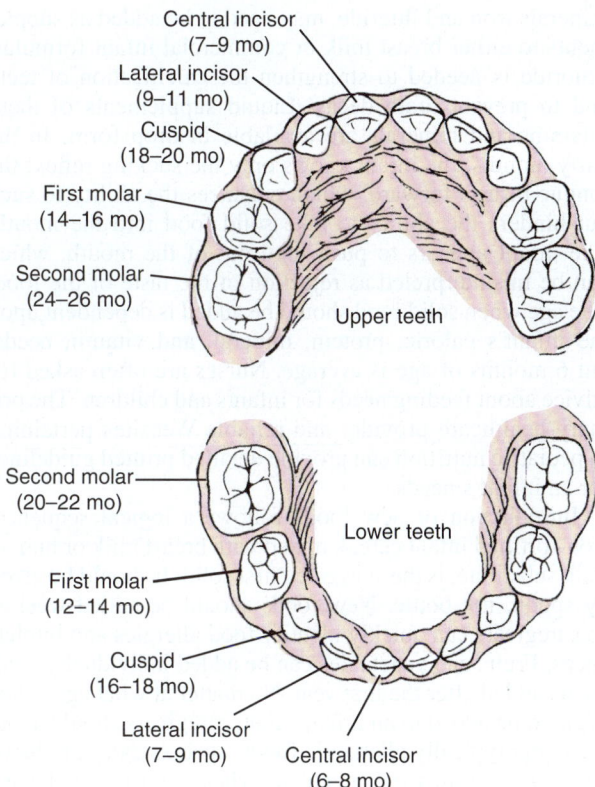

Figure 10-3 Approximate ages of eruption and locations of deciduous (baby) teeth.

Teeth begin to erupt at 6–9 months of age. The first teeth to erupt generally are the two lower central incisors, followed by the four top central incisors. By age 1 year, most babies have six to eight teeth (Fig. 10-3). Because tooth eruption patterns vary greatly, however, caregivers should not be alarmed if an infant does not follow the usual pattern.

The first teeth are known as deciduous teeth. The term *deciduous* literally means "falling off" or "subject to being shed." Like the leaves shed by deciduous trees, children eventually lose their deciduous or baby teeth, which the permanent teeth replace.

> **NCLEX Alert**
>
> Critical concepts for the NCLEX include knowing the normal major physical growth patterns, especially those of the child's first year.

Psychosocial Development

Infants are helpless beings, entirely trusting others to meet their basic needs. If trust is not established, the later challenges of autonomy and initiative will be delayed.

Accomplishing Tasks

Being totally dependent on others for care, infants must learn to develop trust—the feeling that caregivers will meet their needs. Refer to Table 10-1 for a review of Erikson's developmental concept of *trust versus mistrust* for the infant.

Needs of the infant include safety, holding, cuddling, feeding, stroking, and sucking (breast-feeding, bottle, pacifier). Infants are able to tolerate frustration in small amounts only. They expect their needs to be met immediately.

Caregivers must assist infants in the establishment of a system of routines. This system should include items such as feeding, playtime, rest, and sleep. Routines help infants to establish feelings of trust because they begin to learn what to expect.

Bonding

Bonding, which is the attachment to parents, family, or other caregivers, is of vital importance for infants. The feeling of love, nurturing, and connection to other people is one of the most important aspects of being human. Bonding between mother and child begins before birth. The process of attachment between mother and baby continues during infancy and truly begins to develop between father and child at this time. Skin-to-skin contact is important because touch contributes to a baby's ability to thrive. Babies bond with others as well, whether they act in place of or in conjunction with parents. Attachment is an interactive process, relying on participation from both adult and baby to be successful.

Changing Families and the Role of Caregivers

Children in today's world often have a variety of caregivers. Some parents are leaving their jobs or working from home to stay with their children while the other parent continues their career outside the home. Many children are growing up with a variety of caregivers, such as grandparents, aunts and uncles, or other relatives, because of family circumstances (e.g., custody/divorce situations), or the inability of parents to care for their children (e.g., due to parental incarceration or substance abuse). Foster parents can be a temporary or an off-and-on situation in which strangers act as the primary nurturers. Remember, however, that most women still carry the main responsibility for childcare. Many women are also the main providers for their families, adding to increased role expectations, family stressors, and a need for outside support systems (Pew Research, 2015).

Cognitive and Motor Development

During infancy, as throughout the entire lifespan, the rate of each infant's development varies, depending on his or her physical maturity and environmental factors. The aspects of a healthy life are closely related to nutrition.

1–3 Months

During the first 3 months of life, an infant's progress can be witnessed almost daily. When babies are 6 weeks old, they begin to make purposeful movements and stop crying when picked up; they are beginning to expect that someone will comfort them. As they become aware of their surroundings and by 8 weeks, they can stare directly ahead for a short time. The lack of head control is still marked. Babies smile, babble when spoken to, and follow lights within view. They turn their head toward sounds and can differentiate between pleasant and unpleasant noises. They pay attention to their parents' voices. Babies cry to signal needs and stop crying when they are comforted and satisfied. Although sleeping habits vary widely, infants at this stage will probably sleep from 18 to 20 hours a day.

By 3 months, babies can reach for and grasp objects. They laugh, squeal, and look at items for several seconds. They can follow a moving object with their eyes. Between 2 and 3 months, infants develop a social smile and respond to pleasurable interactions with expressions of happiness.

4–8 Months

Between 4 and 8 months, a baby's motor skills involve sitting with support and, for a short time, without support. They learn to recognize people; stranger anxiety may be noticed. Development of fine motor skills begins with the appearance of the **pincer grasp**, which is the ability to use the forefinger and thumb to hold small objects. Touching various textures, shapes, and objects, infants learn about the world. They put objects into their mouths, especially their toes. Gross motor abilities include the ability to hold the head steady, pull up to a sitting position, and hold their bottles by themselves. Babies can turn over in bed and can splash in the bath. Language skills involve the ability to coo and babble, especially when someone talks to them. Babies can distinguish between good and bad voices and will listen for tones of approval. They can smile at their reflection in the mirror. Physical changes include the development of lacrimal glands (tear glands) and they can shed tears. Sleeping patterns include the ability to sleep all night in addition to taking two or three naps during the day.

9–12 Months

As infants near completion of the first year, they have learned to crawl and can be very curious, exploring their world. Babies of this age respond when called by name, can copy movements, and know the meaning of the word "no." By 10 months, babies can usually pull up to a standing position while holding onto something and can walk with both hands held. They then learn to walk around furniture and stand alone. At 1 year, most children can take a few steps alone. They can walk if someone else holds one hand.

One-year-olds hold their bottles and drink out of cups without difficulty. They have strong pincer grasps, and pick up small objects, such as raisins, from the table. They say two or three simple words, such as "baby" and "bye-bye." They laugh aloud. These babies imitate a variety of speech sounds, and begin to say "mama" and "dada," referring specifically to each. They love games such as simplified hide-and-seek. They distinguish between people they recognize and strangers, clinging to familiar persons and pulling away from strangers.

Areas of Concern

Feedings

Breast milk or infant formula offers nearly complete nutrition in the first 4–6 months. Vitamins C and D, plus the minerals iron and fluoride, may need to be added as supplements to either breast milk or commercial infant formulas. Fluoride is needed to strengthen the calcification of teeth and to prevent tooth decay. Liquid supplements of these vitamins and minerals are available in drop form. In the early months, the infant knows only the sucking reflex; the tongue thrusts forward, which enhances the ability to suck but hinders the ability to take solid food into the mouth. The infant appears to push food out of the mouth, which can be misinterpreted as rejection of the taste of the food. The age when solid food should be added is dependent upon the infant's caloric, protein, mineral, and vitamin needs, but 6 months of age is average. Nurses are often asked for advice about feeding needs for infants and children. The primary healthcare provider and reliable Websites pertaining to pediatric nutrition can provide detailed printed guidelines for an infant's needs.

Introduction of new foods follows a logical sequence. Iron-fortified infant cereal, mixed with breast milk or human milk substitute, is the suggested first solid. It should be given by spoon, not bottle. New foods should be added weekly, so caregivers can quickly identify food allergies and intolerances. Fruits and vegetables can be added individually, with meats added after the first year. No matter at what age solids begin to be added to an infant's diet, caregivers should avoid including typically allergenic foods, such as dairy products, citrus fruits, tomatoes, chocolate, wheat, seafood, and eggs, until after age 1 year. Although formula or breast milk may still be used, many infants drink whole milk starting at age 1 year.

The feeding process is nurturing and pleasurable for infants. Babies grow and thrive when they receive affection, tactile stimulation, and a feeling of satiety (fullness) during feedings. Skin-to-skin contact and vocal responses from caregivers are important at these times. For breast-fed infants, bottle feedings are a convenient method for fathers and other family members to bond with infants and show them attention. Both breast-fed and bottle-fed babies need to be held closely, stroked, sung to, and rocked during feedings.

Bottle Mouth

Nursing **bottle mouth** is a serious dental condition that results when infants are placed in bed with a bottle of breast milk, formula, or juice that is propped on a blanket or towel. Also known as *bottle caries*, bottle mouth causes erosion of tooth enamel, deep cavities, and tooth loss result from the prolonged contact of milk and juice sugars with emerging teeth. Lost deciduous teeth cannot maintain needed space for the incoming permanent teeth. In some instances, these early childhood caries may cause the permanent teeth to erupt decayed. Nursing bottle mouth may affect appearance, chewing, eating habits, and speech development.

Weaning

Weaning, the change from feeding infants exclusively breast milk or formula to incorporating a variety of solid foods, should begin when babies can sit upright on their own, support their own head and neck, and grasp objects in their fingers and put them in their mouths. The ability to take sips from a cup when it is offered is one of the early signs of an infant's readiness to take foods in ways other than from a bottle. Later, introduce a spoon and a bowl. Sucking is pleasurable for an infant, so it can be traumatic to the child to cease using the breast or bottle. Weaning is a process that occurs according to each child's internal schedule. A bottle at nighttime may be helpful in the weaning process. To avoid bottle mouth, do not allow the child to take the bottle to bed.

Sucking

Infants need to develop their sucking reflexes. They will suck on their thumbs, fists, and fingers when they are not feeding. Sucking provides comfort and relieves tension and anxiety. Some babies use a pacifier for sucking when they are tired or fussy. Thumb sucking may begin at around 3 or 4 months of age. Most infants pop everything into their mouth by the time they reach 7 months, and the thumb is a handy object.

Childcare

Selecting appropriate childcare is a difficult decision that many caregivers must consider. Various options are available, including daycare centers, preschool learning centers, family daycare homes, or daycare providers (e.g., nannies) in the home. Many states require childcare providers to be licensed and to meet certain requirements, such as provider training, health and safety laws, and home or center inspection. Studies have supported the idea that children thrive in daycare centers where each child is given a high level of individualized attention. One of the most important factors for caregivers to consider when making the decision is the ratio of daycare personnel to children. Cost is also a factor. Safety is vital.

TODDLERHOOD: 1–3 YEARS

The **toddler** phase encompasses approximately ages 1–3 years. Although physical growth is not as rapid as in infancy, communication and mobility abilities accelerate. Psychosocial and cognitive development accompanies the motor skills and the child learns new words. Toddlerhood is a period of great learning, and children's personalities begin to emerge more distinctly during these years. Growing independence, however, may lead to increased conflicts and difficulties with family caregivers. Caregivers must reevaluate the child's environment and institute safety measures. Refer to In Practice: Educating the Client 10-1 for more detailed accident prevention and safety measures. Nursing care includes educating caregivers about the importance of accepting each child's individual timetable of physical growth and psychosocial development.

Physical Growth

The physical growth of toddlers is slower than that of infants. Between 1 and 4 years of age, children usually gain about 5–10 lb (2.3–4.5 kg) per year. The toddler gains about 3 in. (7.6 cm) in height. By their second birthday, children can usually stand alone and have the ability to walk without assistance. Fine motor skills continue to develop. For example, they fit simple objects into appropriate holes and build towers of three or four blocks or more. Toddlers drink easily from a cup with a spout. Potty training is partially or totally complete during this stage. Most children have 20 deciduous teeth by age 2.5 years and readily self-feed table foods. See Figure 10-3, which shows approximate ages of eruption of deciduous teeth.

IN PRACTICE
EDUCATING THE CLIENT 10-1 — Accident Prevention for Children

Motor Vehicle
- Restrain child in a safety seat for all car trips.
- Place child in the back seat of the car, away from air bags.
- Closely supervise the child outdoors.
- Provide fenced-in play areas.
- Teach child never to run into the street.

Drowning
- Supervise the child near all water—bathtubs, toilets, pools, sinks, small basins, and so forth. A small child can drown in a very small amount of water.
- Empty small pools after use. Fence in pools.
- Teach child not to run near bodies of water.

Fire and Burns
- Turn handles of pans toward center of stove.
- Keep child away from stoves, fire, matches, electrical cords, sockets, and so forth.
- Set hot water heater temperature at 120–130 °F.
- Test water temperature before immersion.
- Use safety covers on electrical outlets.

Falls
- Gate stairways; teach child to hold railings.
- Open windows from top. Use window guards.
- Move furniture away from upstairs windows.

Ingestion and Aspiration
- Avoid feeding the child nuts, grapes, popcorn, raisins, hard candy, or lollipops.
- Childproof the home for coins, pins, balloons—especially near the crib.
- Teach child not to run with objects in the mouth and not to open things with teeth.

Poisoning
- Keep child-proof caps on toxic products.
- Store and lock all medications and vitamins, out of children's reach.
- Read labels carefully before using any drugs.
- Keep poison control center number on all phones.
- Inspect homes you are visiting for safety hazards.

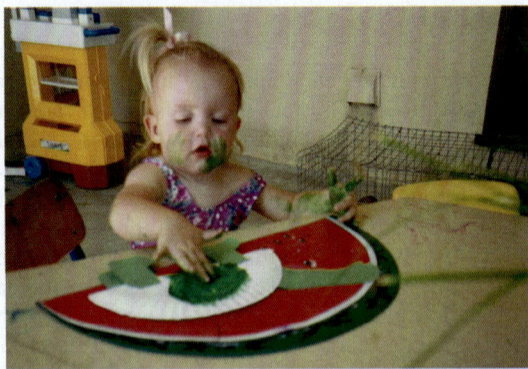

Figure 10-4 Toddlers enter a stage of autonomy, promoting exploration. (Photo courtesy of M.T. Kowalski.)

Psychosocial Development

According to Erikson's model, the child's psychosocial task during the toddler years is to develop autonomy (independence). The opposing psychosocial consequence is shame and doubt (see Table 10-1). The active and very mobile toddler begins to establish independence by walking, self-feeding, playing, and speaking.

During this stage, the need for consistent guidance and discipline is important. The toddler varies in his or her ability to maintain self-control and willpower. Caregivers can foster the development of self-control and willpower by allowing toddlers to make simple choices, thereby reinforcing independence. This process also enhances the development of self-pride and the beginnings of positive self-esteem.

Cognitive and Motor Development

Intellectual and social development becomes more evident as toddlers grow physically. Children moving into toddlerhood have passed through several peak stages of accomplishment (*equilibrium*) and several stages of frustration (*disequilibrium*). New skills continue to appear. For example, creeping 1-year-olds become dashing, climbing explorers at 15 months (Fig. 10-4). Peak periods of accomplishment, however, are farther apart.

Verbal skills improve. By age 18 months, toddlers have a vocabulary of about 20–30 words, although they understand many more, as shown by their ability to follow directions. Social contacts begin to broaden, as toddlers share playtime with other children. Toddlers play next to their playmates rather than with them. This parallel play continues until social skills develop further.

By 18 months of age, children begin to sense that they can control certain aspects of their environment. They start to take advantage of their ability to exert control to the fullest. Toddlers may sometimes seem to take the greatest pleasure from always opposing others. Responding in a negative manner or *negativism* is typical of this age. Caregivers need to understand that this behavior is a method of asserting individuality rather than of opposition to the caregiver. Young toddlers climb up the stairs without help but often crawl. Generally, 18-month-old children cannot go down the stairs. They run on level ground, seldom fall, and pull along toys.

They throw a ball to another person without falling and turn pages in a book two or three at a time. Eighteen-month-olds identify certain items in a book, and indicate their own nose, eyes, and ears.

As mid-toddlers learn to move with more sureness, they explore their surroundings with interest. Because these children have untrained fine and gross muscular abilities, accidents are common; definite limits are necessary. By age 2, neuromuscular coordination increases. *Ritualism* is common. This behavior includes the repetition of activities that involve gestures (brushing teeth), words (directions to get dressed), or objects (reading a book at bedtime). Children now put on and take off simple items of clothing, such as slip-on shirts. They climb upstairs without crawling and throw or kick a large ball. Most toddlers love to build towers of blocks then knock it over and set it up again. These toddlers string large beads, scribble with crayons, turn a doorknob, put on socks and pants, wash their hands, and turn book pages one at a time.

Typical 2-year-olds like riding toys. These children become frustrated with toys they cannot manage or with things they cannot do. Emotions are close to the surface—extremely happy or very sad. Children at this age love activity, noise, water, animals, and other people, as long as they get their own way. At the same time, they want acceptance from their families. Their favorite word is "no."

By age 3 years, toddlers begin to reach a stage of happy, conforming equilibrium. "No" changes to "yes," and routines become more flexible. Increased motor and language skills enable 3-year-olds to accomplish the developmental tasks required as they head into the preschool years.

> **NCLEX Alert**
> Knowing what toy is appropriate for each stage of development is important. Safety issues are always a priority.

Areas of Concern

Toilet Training

Toilet training is a major developmental accomplishment and a learning process that requires patience and family encouragement. Toddlers are ready for toilet training when they can control their anal and urethral sphincter muscles, which typically occurs between the ages of 18 and 24 months. Anal sphincter control usually develops first. The child's own behavioral and emotional readiness must align with his or her physical development. A child may be physically ready by 24 months but not psychologically ready until age 3 years. Caregivers need to be role models for the desired behaviors and to respond to accidents with re-teaching, not punishment.

Bowel training is usually accomplished with less effort than bladder training, but this is not true for all children, especially boys. Some perfectly normal children still do not have total conscious control by 5 years of age. Most family caregivers are relieved to find that toilet training, barring

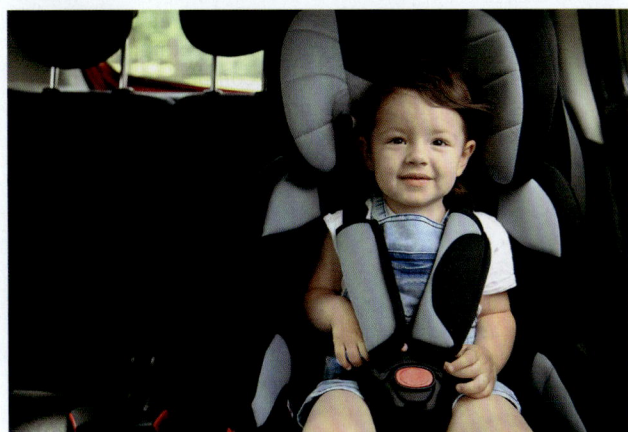

Figure 10-5 Safety considerations are of vital importance for all children. Child safety seats are an important measure in the prevention of injury or death from motor vehicle accidents. The legislation of child restraints in vehicles may differ between states. Check the state's individual Department of Motor Vehicle's Website for current rules and regulations.

occasional accidents, is well under way by 3 years of age. Accidents, however, are likely during illness, emotional upsets, or schedule changes. Hospitalization of a child is a common cause of regression to an earlier phase of bowel and bladder training.

Accident Prevention

Safety issues are important concerns for children of all ages. During the toddler stage, children begin to explore more often and with greater recklessness. They require constant supervision from family caregivers to prevent all sorts of accidents, ranging from minor scrapes and bruises to life-threatening tragedies. Accidents involving motor vehicles top the list, followed by drowning, burning, poisoning, and falling.

> **Key Concept**
> Accidents are the leading cause of death for children between the ages of 1 and 4 years. Safety education for all children is a high priority.

Along with continual supervision, family caregivers can take many measures to prevent accidents for toddlers and older children as well (Fig. 10-5). In Practice: Educating the Client 10-1 contains several tips for preventing minor problems and major catastrophes. Chapter 72 also discusses safety precautions for children.

Setting Limits

Although families should encourage the endless curiosity of toddlers, they must begin to establish limits for children during this stage. At this young age, simple, consistent guidance is important. Toddlers must know exactly what behaviors are expected and what behaviors are unacceptable. Such guidance enables toddlers to learn right from wrong. It also sets a pattern for later years, when rules and regulations evolve into discipline.

Nonnutritive Sucking

Nonnutritive sucking is the repetitive action of sucking and swallowing followed by breathing; it does not include sucking used for feedings. Nonnutritive sucking includes behaviors that vary from sucking at a mother's breast or sucking on the nipple of a bottle without the ingestion of breast milk or formula. The infant also sucks part of the hand or may use a pacifier. Physically, sucking stimulates secretion of digestive enzymes and hormones. Emotionally, infants receive comfort and gratification through nonnutritive sucking. Hunger, fatigue, or stress may trigger sucking.

Typically, the infant's urge for nonnutritive sucking decreases between the ages of 15 and 18 months. An infant who continues this behavior beyond the age of 3 years should be referred to a pediatrician. The long-term effects of the habit depend on factors such as frequency, duration, and intensity. Most dental authorities agree that thumb sucking can cause long-term dental problems. The more frequent the sucking and the greater the percentage of time it is practiced, the higher the potential for permanent damage to mouth structure. Prolonged pacifier use has been associated with otitis media (middle ear infection). The caregivers should discuss the benefits and risks of nonnutritive sucking for a child who uses it long term.

Peer pressure may eventually embarrass children and cause thumb sucking to stop. Helping children to stop thumb sucking is difficult. Suggestions include:

- Substitute a pacifier for the thumb. Pacifiers are softer and less damaging to the teeth.
- Try to redirect behavior into other activities.
- Praise children when they avoid sucking the thumb for a period of time.
- Give these children a little extra attention: thumb sucking may reflect insecurity or loneliness (Healthwise, 2019; Bowden & Greenberg, 2014).

Temperamental Behaviors

The "terrible twos" is a familiar term given to the behaviors that toddlers are apt to display during their second and third years. As their sense of independence broadens, *dawdling* and *temper tantrums* are seen. Dawdling occurs when the child cannot seem to follow the instructions of the caregiver. The child has periods of stubborn inactivity. Temper tantrums are not uncommon and can include excessive crying, screaming, throwing themselves on the floor, hitting, kicking, biting, throwing things, yelling, head banging, and breath holding. These behaviors need to be recognized as normal stages of psychosocial development. Tantrums are outbursts of anger and frustration. Tantrums are more common when children are hungry, tired, frustrated, or feeling neglected.

When dawdling or tantrums occur, caregivers need to realize that reasoning, scolding, and punishment are nonproductive; the child is not yet equipped to understand that this behavior is unacceptable. During these episodes, the child needs to be monitored and the adult needs to remain calm; in other words, ignore the tantrum but not the child. Caregivers should avoid giving in to children's demands during these outbursts because doing so can encourage future instances of such behavior. When children throw tantrums in public, they should be physically removed from the situation and alerted that such behavior is unacceptable. Family caregivers must discipline with love and confidence without getting caught up in the toddler's out-of-control emotions. Caregivers can try diverting the child's attention and removing the child from the causative situation.

Sleep Habits and the Family Bed

Regular sleep restores energy, heals the body, and helps to organize the thoughts of the day. Most toddlers sleep 12 hours overnight and take naps during the day. Sometimes children resist sleep because they think that they are missing out on family activity. When overly tired, toddlers may actually have an extra burst of energy and want to run, jump, and play. Promoting regular sleep habits is essential. Bedtime rituals to relax a child include dimming the lights, reading a story, or singing a song while rubbing the child's back gently. Warm milk promotes relaxation and sleep because it contains the enzyme tyramine.

Some children fear darkness. Insisting on sleep at sleep times may be impossible occasionally; family caregivers may need to settle for children taking some quiet rest time alone instead.

Many family caregivers struggle with the decision to bring children into their bed when they cry in the middle of the night. Some authorities believe that this "family bed" prevents children from learning to fall asleep on their own and leads to children exerting control over adults. Other authorities promote the idea of the family bed as comforting to the child. The alternative is allowing children to cry themselves to sleep, which may upset and disturb many families, leading to frustration and mistrust. Each family must resolve this dilemma for itself according to the caregivers' beliefs about childcare. What works for one family may not work for others.

Separation Anxiety

As stated earlier regarding infants, toddlers may also display signs of anxiety when confronted with strangers or separated from the caregiver. When separated from loved ones, children may cry, scream, lash out physically at others, and call for the missed person. Separation is a necessary component of socialization and emotional development. Family caregivers need to provide reassurance that they will return. The child should be given a reasonable and understandable timeframe for when to expect the return of the parents or other caregivers. Any time a child is expected to begin spending time in a new place (e.g., a daycare center or the pediatric care unit of a hospital), it is beneficial for the child and caregivers to visit the new place together a few days before the actual event. Being introduced to the new environment ahead of time will lessen the child's stress. In general, either separation or stranger anxiety can peak and recur, depending on the occasion (e.g., having a new babysitter or going to a dentist for the first time). Because these anxieties are fear responses, they can recur when there is a major developmental shift in abilities and cognition. For example, 7- or 8-year-old children are beginning to be more independent of parents, so they will be more comfortable

in most strange environments. Therefore, a first- or second-grade student typically will not resist meeting strangers in a familiar shopping center when accompanied by a parent. However, it would not be uncommon for children in this age group to become shy around new children and adults when changing schools.

> **Key Concept**
>
> Safety and security concerns dictate that children must be taught how to react when approached by people they do not know. Remember that because a school ground, grocery store, or shopping center is a familiar environment, children may feel safe when approached by someone they do not know.

PRESCHOOL: 3–6 YEARS

Between the ages of 3 and 6 years, the preschool stage, children assume greater responsibility in their daily activities and exhibit more mature levels of interaction with others. Their enhanced ability to communicate gives preschoolers confidence, which contributes to their willingness to cooperate with caregivers and to express needs and frustrations. Curiosity is rampant and imagination is vivid during these years. Preschoolers pretend and experiment; however, they may exhibit aggressive behavior and develop minor fears due to enhanced levels of activity and imagination.

Physical Growth

Preschoolers weigh about 30–35 lb (13.6–15.6 kg) and are 30–36 in. (76–91 cm) tall. Although by age 3 years, children achieve about half of their eventual adult height, physical development slows. Proportionally, height increases greater than weight. A 3-year-old retains some of chubby, baby-faced look while the 5-year-old child appears leaner and taller. Typically, boys are thinner than girls. Preschoolers will probably gain about 3–5 lb (1.4–2.3 kg) per year and about 3 in. (7.6 cm) in height annually until entering school.

Dentition is the development and arrangement of teeth. The first set of teeth, the deciduous teeth, have grown in and are getting ready to fall out. By about 5–6 years of age, the central incisors are ready to be replaced by the permanent teeth.

Psychosocial Development

According to Erikson, preschoolers love to make things; they acquire the initiative to do new things without having to be told. If caregivers habitually scold, criticize, or correct the child, a sense of guilt will prevail. Later in life the individual's learned guilt at not succeeding could result in that adult's learned insecurity (see Table 10-1).

The family unit functions as the primary relationship in the life of preschoolers. However, their social circle now includes friends and adults. Individual independence continues to be important. Constant talking and questioning allow preschoolers to learn. Favorite words are "why" and "how."

Generally, these children try hard to do what is expected and to be obedient and helpful. They are sensitive to social interactions, and scolding may easily hurt their feelings. Socially, preschoolers play with other children, as well as next to them. They make up simple games by age 3. They learn to share and wait their turn. When quarreling, boys of this age often engage in physical fighting, including hitting, kicking, and biting. Girls are more likely to yell at each other in their disagreements.

Preschoolers begin to learn sexual roles through playing with toys, watching television, and observing adults. They also become aware of, and are sometimes anxious about, body differences between males and females. Sigmund Freud termed this stage the *oedipal stage, also known as the phallic or genital phase*. During these years, children focus attention and interest on the parent of the opposite sex. Children may feel competitive and jealous toward the same-sex parent; boys talk of marrying their mother and girls of marrying their father. Caregivers need to be aware that this phase is normal and not related to the more mature emotions that occur with the hormonal influences of puberty. Children may also mimic the actions of their same-sex caregivers who are their role models. The concepts of "good touch" and "bad touch" should be introduced to the child. Preschoolers should know that no one should touch them, or suggest that they touch another person, in a manner that makes them feel uncomfortable or is unpleasant.

Cognitive and Motor Development

Preschoolers show increased gross and fine motor skills by age 3 years. Most children now dress and undress almost completely, manage large buttons and zippers, form objects with clay, and use a crayon to draw recognizable forms, such as a square or a person. They climb up stairs, now alternating feet. They must put both feet on each step while coming down, jumping off the bottom step. They can stand on one foot and ride tricycles; they build towers with 9 or 10 blocks and can copy a circle on paper. Intellectually, development progresses to the point where children count to three or higher, identify objects in pictures, and tell which of several objects are alike. Their vocabulary numbers about 1,000 words, which 3-year-olds use in incessant talk. Four-year-olds now have a speaking vocabulary of at least 2,000 words and can probably count to 15 or 20. The ability to use words also reflects their growing ability to reason; these children ask questions constantly.

Preschoolers have a great desire to accomplish goals. They like to be independent and to do things on their own. However, parental supervision is essential, for example, with brushing teeth. Safety issues must be part of everyday concern.

By age 5 years, many caregivers will find that preschoolers are comfortable with themselves and their relationships with others. They are satisfied with the world of home and family. They know their full address and telephone number. Many may learn with computers. *Magical thinking* is a normal intellectual development. The child can think or image something without actually seeing it. Magical thinking includes hearing a statement like, "Summer is just around the corner"; the child might actually to look "around a corner" to see the event. Television or storybook characters are real to a preschooler and they become upset or cry when a storybook character is sad or injured. Imaginary playmates and having make-believe adventures are parts of normal childhood development.

Areas of Concern

Sibling Rivalry

A preschooler may be the only child in a family's life. Many preschoolers must eventually handle the arrival of a new and younger sibling. Siblings may be the result of changing circumstances such as divorce or remarriage. The child then becomes part of a blended family. These situations require adjustment for all family members, but they may present special problems and stressors for preschoolers. Children may fear that they are loved less than the others. Rivalry for the caregiver's attention may cause ongoing conflicts and unhappiness. Jealousy, regression, or acting-out behaviors are not uncommon. For example, the preschooler may feel jealous of the attention given to the new baby, may crawl instead or walk, or have temper tantrums. Children need to be appreciated for themselves and feel that they are loved and welcome. Nursing care requires making sure that caregivers are aware of each child's emotional coping skills. Reassure the family that adjustment phases are normal. Awareness of the needs-related changes in family structure allows the caregiver to learn that individualized attention and interest in each child will help promote adjustment and transition.

Phobias and Nightmares

Preschoolers develop thought processes in less sheltered environments and have more exposure to new situations than do infants and toddlers. For example, they watch TV, go to the movies, or go grocery shopping. Activities occurring during new events cannot be completely or accurately understood by the immature mind. Using their developing imaginations, preschoolers create internal views about how situations may affect them. Aggression and arguments in the home are frightening to a child, who commonly thinks that he or she is the cause of the problem. As these thought processes and memories develop, children may experience *phobias* (fear) of the dark or that a monster lives under their bed. *Nightmares* (frightening dreams) are not uncommon. Caregivers need to be aware of the preschooler's thought processes as well as of the need to minimize a child's exposure to situations and images that may be perceived as threatening. Nursing care includes providing reassurance, helping caregivers understand the differences between an adult's and a child's thought processes, and discovering and discussing the causes of fears and nightmares.

Masturbation

Masturbation is the word given to the handling and self-stimulation of the genital organs. Children like to touch and handle things. Early in life, they may discover that touching certain parts of the body gives them pleasant sensations. A preschooler may find that handling the genitals relieves stress. Teaching a child that masturbation should be practiced in private is a more effective approach to the behavior than shaming, threatening, or punishing the child.

Enuresis and Encopresis

Enuresis is more commonly known as repeated episodes of bed-wetting. It is common in children but not diagnosed as a disorder until the age of 5 or older. *Nocturnal enuresis* is wetting the bed at night; daytime bed-wetting is called *diurnal enuresis*. Some children have one or both forms. Enuresis may be a result of a physical or emotional disorder. There may be a hereditary component to the behavior. Typically, it relates to one of more of the following problems: a small bladder, numerous urinary tract infections, developmental delays that interfere with toilet training, and persistent, severe stress. A child with enuresis may be a heavy sleeper and may not waken at night to void. Some children may outgrow the disorder but others may require medical intervention. Treatment of nocturnal enuresis may consist of restricting fluids before bedtime, waking the child during the night, and, sometimes, medications that may decrease bladder irritability. Treatment for diurnal enuresis includes teaching the child to voluntarily hold urine for increased lengths of time, which may increase the bladder's size or capacity to retain urine.

Encopresis is the repeated defecation of feces in places other than a toilet, such as in underwear, the floor, or in bed. It may be due to physical problems, such as long-term constipation, or emotional problems, such as any form of stress. Treatment depends upon the cause. Since constipation is a common cause, the following actions can be helpful: maintaining regular bowel habits (using the bathroom at regular times of the day), monitoring nutritional intake (providing adequate fiber and fluids), and toilet training (in ways that avoid stressful expectations from caregivers).

SCHOOL AGE: 6–10 YEARS

Achievements youngsters make during infancy, toddlerhood, and preschool prepare them for going to school. In the sixth year, the child, who physically still resembles the toddler, is very active, and has a limited attention span. By the 10th year, the child has begun to have the physical appearance of an adult, has different attitudes about others, and enjoys solitary activities. School-aged children embark on a period of rapid learning, not only in the educational setting, but through increased encounters with people outside the family circle, and expanded awareness of the world around them. As they complete this stage, children approach physical maturity and head into the emotional, social, and intellectual challenges of adolescence (see Chapter 11).

Physical Growth

As they approach age 6 years, children begin to lose their deciduous teeth. Permanent teeth usually start to erupt in the early school years. From the time children enter school, a slow, steady period of growth begins. School-aged children gain about 5–6 lb (2–3 kg) and grow about 2.5 in. (6 cm) a year until puberty (sexual maturity), at which time they experience a growth spurt. Growth rate involves a wide range of variations.

Psychosocial Development

During the school years, the significant person for children changes from the family to people from the school or neighborhood, such as teachers, schoolmates, or best friends. Independence is important. Learning to produce things (schoolwork, projects) takes precedence. These children explore their ever-expanding world and begin to collect pets, dolls, rocks, baseball cards, video games, books, and other objects. School-aged children enjoy personal activities such as playing a musical instrument, or group activities such as membership in school clubs. Cooperative participation in groups, such as the Girl or Boy Scouts, 4 H, or a sport, encourages interpersonal skills that will be important in a work or career environment. Being a member of a sports team develops gross and fine motor skills and physical coordination and teaches the importance of rules and fair play.

Erikson's psychosocial task for the school-aged child is to develop a sense of *industry*. Success in the completion of group or individual activities helps the child's self-esteem and promotes a feeling of self-confidence. If the child cannot complete projects or fails at personal and group activities, a feeling of *inferiority* results. Recognition of achievements is an important aspect of developing a sense of self-worth. This recognition leads to a sense of belonging and a feeling of being able to succeed, and promotes the individual's concept of self-worth. Encourage families to recognize that self-development and reaching out beyond the family are signs of maturation.

Cognitive and Motor Development

Because school occupies so many waking hours, events there play a large part in the lives of school-aged children. As they explore this new world beyond home, children become increasingly independent. Fitting in is very important to school success. The influence of peers takes on more acceptance and importance than does that of the primary caregivers. Family values continue to affect standards of conduct and conscience. The child of this age is beginning to see the world from another person's point of view. The process of intellectual development gradually encompasses the ability to think in the abstract. The child can think in terms of *reversibility*, that is, the ability to recognize that numbers, directions, or objects can be changed and returned to their original condition. For example, the child can return home from school by

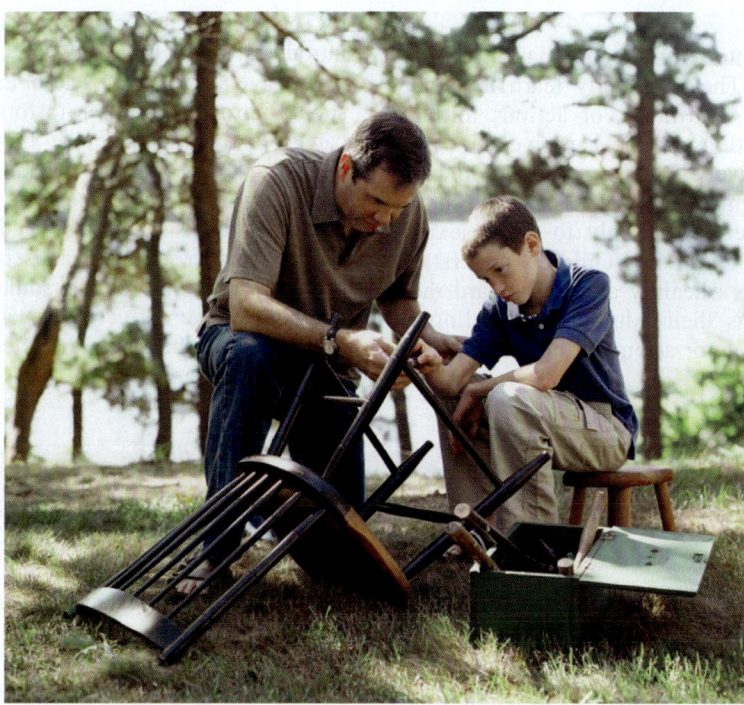

Figure 10-6 Assisting a caregiver helps a child develop a sense of belonging and accomplishment.

traveling the route taken to school, but in the reverse order. Children begin to learn that they must abide by rules, not only at home but in school and other outside settings as well.

Reasoning and conceptual powers expand. By age 6 years, most children can tell time and count to at least 40 or 50; typically, they recognize the letters of the alphabet, numbers from 1 to 10, and their own name. At 7 years of age, they produce all language sounds, use simple logic, and grasp basics of mathematics. Printing becomes clearer.

During the early school years, many children express the desire for a special private place of their own. Boys and girls of this age are aware of each other, but typically prefer not to play together. In fact, they are usually antagonistic and may fight and call each other unkind names. Classrooms of children may break up into several distinct play groups. Friends begin to occupy an important place in children's lives. The members of the clique usually share secrets, including a favorite hangout. Boys and girls may fight openly at times.

Between the ages of 8 and 10 years, children learn to write in cursive. By age 9 years, most children spend much of their time with friends, clubs, and groups. Despite evidence of self-reliance, children may begin to worry and complain about tasks that involve responsibility, such as schoolwork and home chores. At the completion of this stage, well-adjusted 10-year-olds are friendly and realistic, accepting themselves and life as it comes.

Areas of Concern

Sibling Rivalry

As discussed in the previous section on preschoolers, sibling rivalry, the competition among brothers and sisters, may lead to jealousy, trauma, verbal arguments, and sometimes physical fights. This rivalry is natural; brothers and sisters compete, whether as preschoolers or as schoolchildren. Adults may become referees in an attempt to maintain a calm family atmosphere. Caregivers must treat each child equally and fairly. As siblings progress through the school years, they should become responsible for resolving their own differences. Families should be aware of the inevitability of sibling rivalry, and adults should intervene only when absolutely necessary. However, adults must be sure to set definite ground rules for siblings (e.g., no physical or emotional harm). In dealing with this issue, families can teach and learn the importance of mutual respect, forgiveness, and appreciation of individual talents.

Responsibilities

The school-aged child should have some responsibilities in the home (Fig. 10-6). Age-appropriate activities in real-life situations are enjoyed by the active, project-oriented child. Responsibilities may be as simple as cleaning the bedroom, setting and clearing the table, washing dishes or loading the dishwasher, taking out the trash, or walking the family pet. These tasks allow the child to acquire a sense of responsibility (see Table 10-1).

Sex Education

Children are socialized into feminine and masculine gender roles from infancy. They gradually learn to understand expected behaviors, attitudes, or actions initially by watching the interactions of the caregivers in their life. Some societies actively focus on sexual topics in their television programming, movies, songs, and clothing. Sexual education refers not only to adult sexuality and reproduction; it also helps children understand sexual roles and develop a healthy attitude toward their own bodies, and informs their adult understanding of what it means to be a male or a female in contemporary society.

The question arises of when and where should a child be introduced to the topics of sex. Controversy exists over the proper age at which the school and/or the family caregivers should introduce children to formal sex education. Family caregivers must realize the importance of being able to explain sexual issues and questions to their children outside the classroom. Adults who feel uncomfortable or awkward talking to their school-aged children about such matters should consider setting up a discussion between a healthcare provider or another reliable adult and the child. In this way, children receive correct information from trusted individuals, rather than believing the often inaccurate stories passed along from peers.

STUDENT SYNTHESIS

KEY POINTS

- Growth and development is an ongoing process throughout childhood and is affected by heredity, nutrition, and the environment.
- Growth and development progresses in a particular sequence (cephalocaudal: head to toe; and proximodistal: center outward).
- Developmental milestones (tasks) are unique to each child; a child who has significant problems accomplishing development skills may be experiencing developmental delays.
- Theorists, including Erikson and Piaget, have identified specific tasks to accomplish and stages to pass through to become a mature, fully functional person.
- Play is an important element of growth and development that helps prepare children for more mature levels of functioning.
- A neonate or newborn is a baby in the first 28 days of life.
- Infancy, which ends at age 1 year, is the period of fastest growth and development over the entire lifespan.
- Toddlerhood (1–3 years) is a time marked by exploration, growing independence, and conflicting emotions.
- Children during the preschool years (3–6 years) exhibit imagination, improved communication skills, and curiosity.
- School greatly influences children aged 6–10 years as they branch away from the family home. They develop relationships with peers, participate in school and community activities, and learn more about the world around them.

CRITICAL THINKING EXERCISES

1. Based on Erikson's psychosocial theory, discuss why children with parents who are too lenient or who are overprotective may experience difficulties with issues of trust and autonomy.

2. A mother, who has just given birth to a newborn boy, is facing difficulty with her 3-year-old daughter, C.J. C.J. has been stealing and hiding the baby's toys, crawling around the house, and having emotional outbursts more often. Considering C.J.'s age and stage of development, explain what is happening and ways for C.J.'s mother to handle the situation.

3. A.K., who is 10 years old, lives with her father D.K., a single parent. She has not received much information about sex and body development from D.K. because he feels very awkward discussing such issues with her. A.K. has just started her first menstrual cycle. How can D.K. handle the situation, ensuring that his daughter receives accurate information?

NCLEX-STYLE REVIEW QUESTIONS

1. According to Erikson, what intervention provided by the nurse caring for a 9-month-old infant during a hospitalization can assist the infant in mastering the developmental task of trust versus mistrust?
   a. Satisfy the basic needs of the infant without delay.
   b. Teach the infant right from wrong.
   c. Let the baby cry so the infant will learn patience.
   d. Teach the infant self-control.

2. The parent informs the nurse that their toddler is toilet trained but since being in the hospital has begun soiling. What nursing action is appropriate at this time?
   a. Inform the parent that the child has regressed to an earlier stage due to the stress of hospitalization.
   b. Inform the parent that the child was probably not fully toilet trained prior to the hospitalization.
   c. Inform the parent that the child most likely is developmentally delayed.
   d. Inform the parent that the child did not master the developmental task of toileting.

3. The nurse is observing two toddlers in the pediatric play room, playing side-by-side but not interacting with each other. What type of play does the nurse determine this is?
   a. Cooperative play
   b. Fantasy play
   c. Solitary play
   d. Parallel play

4. The parent of a 1-month-old infant states a concern that the "soft spots" on the baby's head have not yet closed. What is the best response by the nurse?
   a. "The anterior fontanels should be closed by now and the posterior fontanels should close next month."
   b. "The anterior fontanels may not close until 12–18 months and the posterior at 2–3 months."
   c. "The anterior fontanel may not close until 6–8 months and the posterior by 8–10 months."
   d. "The anterior fontanel may not close until 2–3 months and the posterior at 12–18 months."

5. What priority teaching should occur for a toddler well child exam?
   a. Setting limits
   b. Stages of play
   c. Safety
   d. Behavior

CHAPTER RESOURCES

Enhance your learning with additional resources on thePoint*!*

Student Resources related to this chapter can be found at **thePoint.lww.com/Rosdahl12e.**

11 Adolescence

Learning Objectives

1. Explain the term *puberty* and its relationship to adolescence.
2. Relate the theories of Erikson and Piaget to adolescent growth and development.
3. Discuss the three major stages of adolescence.
4. Describe the specific physical changes that occur between the ages of 11 and 20 years.
5. Discuss sexual development that occurs during adolescence.
6. Describe the cognitive, emotional, and moral development that occurs during adolescence.
7. Design a plan for presenting information about human sexuality to adolescents.

Important Terminology

adolescence
menarche
nocturnal emission
peer group
preadolescence
puberty

Puberty (from the Latin word meaning *adulthood* or *maturity*) is the period when a person becomes able to reproduce sexually. **Adolescence** is the developmental period between puberty and maturity that can be divided into distinct stages. Generally, it spans the ages between 10 and 20 years, after which a person enters early adulthood.

A rapid growth spurt marks adolescence, by the end of which individuals achieve adult height. Although tremendous physical growth occurs, emotional needs predominate during this period; adolescents spend much of their time searching for meaning in life and for a sense of identity. Adolescents are required to make critical choices that may help to determine the shape of their lives. Such choices include the use of alcohol and other substances, moral obligations and respect for others, school attendance, relationships (family, friends, and sexuality), education after high school, and career alternatives. The Internet has been shown to be both a positive and negative influence on behaviors of this age group.

Skill development is part of cognitive growth and is also preparation for the future. Skill development includes activities such as gymnastics, photography, writing, carpentry, auto mechanics, and dancing. Many skills developed during the teen years help adolescents make educational and career choices. Teens enhance their leadership and diplomatic abilities by participating in student government, debate, and other school programs. During these years, moral judgments and thinking are no longer egocentric. Rules involve a sense of circumstances. Religious groups geared for teenagers often hold many activities that attempt to provide a sense of moral instruction as well. Sports often become a primary interest. Cooking may appeal to many adolescents. Today's adolescents have never known life without computers and may develop a keen interest in experimenting with them. Adult encouragement and guidance are needed for skill development.

GROWTH AND DEVELOPMENT THEORIES

The theories of Erikson and Piaget continue to apply to individuals as they enter the adolescent stage. Both theories stress the adolescent's burgeoning maturity and expanding abilities.

Erikson: Psychosocial Development

According to Erikson's psychosocial developmental theory, the major challenge of adolescence is the achievement of *identity:* Who am I? Where am I going? With whom? How am I going to get there? If this phase is not resolved, the result is *role confusion* (Table 11-1). As individuals go through the various stages of adolescence, they confront many difficult decisions. Personal identity merges with psychosocial developments. That is, individuals' unique perspectives of self—the thoughts, goals, and ideas of independence—merge with their acquired ability to confront challenges, such as the concepts of good and bad or psychosocial developments that occurred earlier in life. Adolescents must learn through experience that success and failure are the results of their own actions. Caregivers foster personal growth by understanding that they can and should no longer take total responsibility for the activities, thoughts, and actions of their children. Granting independence is an important phase for both the adolescent and the caregivers. It is not uncommon for the adolescent to break rules in support of his or her own feelings of independence. Role confusion is a normal aspect of the hormonal and philosophical changes occurring during this age range. However, when young adults emerge from this decade of emotional and physical changes, they should be able to identify their own personal, unique traits.

The **peer group** is the significant group for the adolescent. Peers consist of contemporaries or a group of people

CHAPTER 11 Adolescence

TABLE 11-1	Erikson's Theory of Psychosocial Development—Adolescence
CONCEPT	**ADOLESCENCE**
Challenge	Identity vs role confusion
Significant others	Peer group, romantic relationships, family
Necessary accomplishments	Make life decisions; achieve personal identity; accept responsibility
Virtues	Independence; self-esteem; self-reliance; self-control; devotion; fidelity
Ways to help the adolescent succeed	Provide privacy; encourage activities; support decisions; allow independence; give recognition and acceptance; maintain a good family atmosphere; facilitate information gathering

Bowden, V. R., & Greenberg, C. S. (2014). *Children and their families: the continuum of nursing care* (3rd ed.). Wolters Kluwer Health/Lippincott Williams & Wilkins; Hatfield, N. T., & Kincheloe, C. A. (2018). *Introductory maternity & pediatric nursing* (4th ed.). Wolters Kluwer; https://www.simplypsychology.org/Erik-Erikson.html.

that the individual has sufficient cognitive development to sort through different plans and to devise different solutions to situations before acting upon them. Past experiences, present conditions, and future consequences are now part of the individual's way of thinking.

ADOLESCENT GROWTH AND DEVELOPMENT

Adolescence can be divided into stages categorized as *early*, *middle*, and *late* adolescence. During these stages, young people complete their transition into adulthood. The developmental changes of adolescence prepare them to exhibit the independence and responsibility that they will need in future adult roles. Adolescents have an increased need for energy supplies due to alterations in body chemistry, developmental challenges, and growth spurts. The need for increased amounts of nutrition provides challenges to the adolescent as well as to the family or caregivers. As with all the years of growth and development, the ages for each individual are unique; stages range according to the individual's heredity, nutrition, and environment.

Characteristics of Developmental Stages

Early Adolescence (Ages 11–14 years)

Also known as **preadolescence** or pubescence, early adolescence ranges from ages 11 to 14 years. Girls often mature earlier than boys. This time is sometimes referred to as an "awkward stage," as the person teeters between childish and mature ways of appearing, thinking, and behaving. Young people often waver between a desire for independence and trust from their families and silliness, playfulness, and a need for regular approval. Rebellion against authority figures, noisy and fault-finding quarrels with siblings, and evasion of household tasks can be sources of conflict. Patience is essential. As early adolescents attempt new undertakings to test independence and self-reliance, they need strong familial support and guidance. As they get older, adolescents become more controlled emotionally and better able to see situations in perspective. Psychological awareness and objectivity begin to broaden beyond the self to an ability to understand the feelings and behavior of others. A growing sense of humor helps to make family relationships more pleasant. Because young adolescents are usually enthusiastic, they bring spirit and buoyancy to their undertakings. Involvement in extensive projects in school shows initiative and effort. Planned parties and social events require adult supervision.

As they head toward middle adolescence, young teenagers may display tendencies to seclusion and moodiness. Emerging reasoning leads to reflection on themselves and others and assessment of new experiences. Appraisals of interaction between self and the world require a place and time, so young teenagers may begin to spend more time alone. Because adolescents have long associations with the mirror, they will use the mirror as a prop for role-playing and for testing and measuring themselves in imagined situations. As they develop their own perspective of family structure and roles, their criticisms and withdrawals often become

with whom the teen associates (Fig. 11-1). The peer group is often more important than the family and can influence adolescents in many ways. Peers can be of great influence on the individual's present and future lifestyle choices. For example, is it more important to study for good grades needed for college or to attend social events? Should the individual decide on a military career or focus on getting employment after high school? Peer pressure to try cigarettes, alcohol, or drugs can be the first step to substance abuse.

Piaget: Cognitive Development

According to Piaget, the person from about 12 to 15 years of age enters stage 4 of cognitive development: *formal operations*. In earlier stages of development, the child solved problems by using trial and error. Formal operations mean

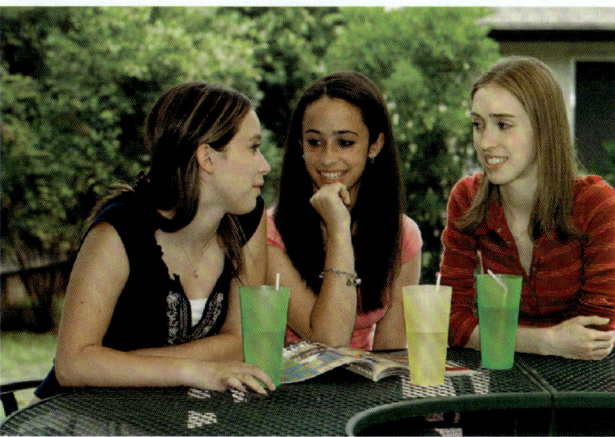

Figure 11-1 Throughout adolescence into young adulthood, peer relationships influence psychosocial development.

a source of puzzlement and hurt to family members. The maturing adolescent takes frequent flights of independence but has a strong need to return to the "nest" for guidance and encouragement.

By the age of 14 years, adolescents are becoming more accepting of other people, and more conscious of what makes their own personality unique from others. They may begin to develop better relationships with siblings, finding that they like their brothers and sisters more than they thought. Some authorities state that verbalizing ideas is a true growth characteristic and a developmental achievement. Teenagers show maturity as they have acquired a natural ability to perceive many sides of a situation. They are able to express ideas, debate concepts, and verbalize opinions.

Middle Adolescence (Ages 15–17 years)

Middle adolescence lasts from ages 15 to 17 years. Individuals of these ages are most likely to exhibit behavior considered "typical" of the adolescent. Introspection and fluctuations in self-assurance mark the middle adolescent years, which can baffle many families. Physical alterations, loud self-assertion, self-preoccupation, rapid shifts between dependent and independent attitudes, blithe spirit, and mood swings are challenges for even the most supportive families. Teenagers are pulling away from childhood in a quest for self-reliance (see Table 11-1). Although they value the ability to depend on home and school, these teenagers need to counterbalance security with independence. As they are searching for balance, immaturity frequently results in withdrawal, belligerence, or defiance. They may begin to believe that any advice from family caregivers is an effort to control them completely. Adolescents may seek guidance away from home.

By the age of 15 or 16 years, most adolescents begin to form some ideas about the future and to plan for more than present interests and activities. Vague ideas about courtship, marriage, career, and families of their own result in scrutiny of the family of origin. Family members may sometimes feel rejected because they fail to meet the perfectionist standards of middle teenagers.

Increased independence and interest in romantic relationships now cause many young people to take more responsibility for self-care and personal cleanliness. They like to choose their own clothing. Many adolescents of this age group seek part-time employment because a job provides money.

By the time they are about 17 years of age, most middle teenagers are beginning to exhibit true attitudes of maturity. In interpersonal relationships, they show an interest in others and an awareness and acceptance of social responsibilities. As they head into late adolescence and young adulthood, they tend to have friendships with many people of both sexes.

Late Adolescence (Ages 18–20 years)

The late adolescent stage lasts about from ages 18 to 20 years. Older adolescents begin to grapple with typically adult or mature issues. They physically move away from familiar people, places, and things. Graduation from high school leads many teens to colleges and universities far from home, where they become responsible for themselves. Those attending school who remain close to home or at home still find their social circles expanded and their intellectual horizons challenged, as they take courses of particular interest and importance to them. Some late teens enter the workforce or join the military after finishing school. Branching into such worlds necessitates increased maturity and improved social and professional skills. During these years, moral questions and issues involving ethical decision-making gain relevance. Increased knowledge and awareness may lead to reflection and internal reevaluation. Exposure to different peoples and other ways of thinking may lead young people to question previously accepted values and ideas.

Relationships are usually important during these years. Young men and women may enjoy dating a variety of individuals. Long-term romantic relationships and friendships that lasted throughout high school may be tested or come to an end, as social circles expand and interests change. As teenagers move into the adult world and are expected to behave maturely, previously critical adolescents may come to appreciate and develop better relationships with parents and other family members.

Physical Growth

Physical changes characterize adolescence. Similar to the childhood periods of growth and development, outward signs of maturity vary. By the age of 11 years, all adolescents have reached one half of their adult weight, but girls have achieved 90% of their adult height while boys achieve 80% of adult height. Full height is achieved around the age of 21 years. Permanent teeth are present, by the age of 12 years, except for the second and third molars. Hormonal changes control growth and many other physical aspects. Starting as early as 9 years of age, the secondary sexual characteristics develop. Increased glandular activity causes an increase in sweat and contributes to the development of body odors. Glandular changes also are partly responsible for the development of acne in some adolescents. Body hair grows in previously hairless areas: the pubic area, under the arms, and for boys, on the face and chest. Hair on other areas such as the arms and legs becomes thicker and coarser.

At the end of the adolescent stages, a person has reached full height, reproductive organs are adult size, and secondary sex characteristics are developed.

Sexual Development

Development in Boys

Some boys at the age of 11 years do not yet show the changes of puberty. Others have started to grow rapidly again, and yet others may already have a heavy or defined skeletal structure. Physical growth varies markedly in 12-year-old boys as well. The average boy shows some pubertal changes by the end of this year. The testicles and penis enlarge, and changes occur in the appearance of the scrotum. Pubic hair begins to appear. Spontaneous erections and occasional ejaculations without external cause may be confusing. Young boys should understand that the involuntary discharge of semen while sleeping (**nocturnal emission**) is a normal part of reproductive health. Other natural developments of puberty are a change in voice and the appearance of chin whiskers.

Most boys grow more at the age of 14 years than at any other age. A strong, muscular appearance and continued deepening of the voice add to the impression of maturity. By the age of 16 years, most young men are close to their adult height.

Development in Girls

Girls also show great variation in sexual development even as early as 9 years of age. The average 11-year-old girl has begun a period of rapid growth and shows signs of approaching sexual maturity. Breast and hip development may be noticeable during these years. Pubic hair starts to grow. By the age of 13 years, many girls have experienced **menarche**, the onset of menstruation. Early periods frequently are irregular, and normal cycles may not be established for a few years.

By the age of 14 years, many girls have the physical appearance of young women. Breasts and other secondary sex characteristics are those of an adult. By the age of 16 years, the menstrual cycle has become regular and the young woman generally accepts menstruation as part of adult life.

Sexual Identity and Orientation

Exploring sexual orientation is a typical part of adolescence. Many LGBTQ+ individuals first come to realize their sexual orientation during the teen years. Most people discover their sexual orientation during the teen years due to the onset of puberty. However, affirmation of sexual orientation, ambiguous feelings regarding sexual orientation, and renegotiating sexual orientation and identity are all possible throughout the life course of an individual.

Mainstream culture in the United States subscribes to the idea of heteronormativity. Heteronormativity supports a gender binary by assuming that men and women are attracted to members of the "opposite sex" while homosexual people are attracted to members of the "same sex." In a period marked by the need for self-acceptance and a sense of belonging, LGBTQ+ adolescents are at risk for alienation, doubt, and depression in a culture that only accommodates for the categories of man, woman, heterosexual, or homosexual.

Sex Education

Most adolescents are naturally curious about sex, sexuality, and changes in their bodies. If adults provide information with sensitivity, adolescents can form healthy sexual attitudes. If parents, teachers, and counselors do not give such information, adolescents will seek answers elsewhere. Attitudes and belief systems may develop from inadequate or biased information they receive from peers and older adolescents. It is normal for the adolescent to feel stigmatized or to be confused and uncomfortable talking about romantic and sexual relationships.

Sexual activity during middle and late adolescence is not uncommon. The young adult may fear pregnancy but fail to recognize the risks of sexually transmitted infections (STIs) such as gonorrhea, syphilis, genital warts, and HIV/AIDS. Many young people fail or refuse to use birth control because of embarrassment or feelings of insecurity. They may lack the technical understanding of how to use a birth control device such as a condom. The topics of pregnancy and transmission of STIs should be included in discussions with the young adult. The nurse may be considered a confidential, reliable source of information.

> **Nursing Alert** Adolescents must understand that all forms of birth control contain some risk of failure. Only abstinence is 100% effective against pregnancy and STIs.

Psychosocial Development

The major task of adolescence is to form a sense of identity. Group conformity and "fitting in" with peers is of great importance to most adolescents. At the same time, outward expressions of rebellion against parents, teachers, and other authority figures are common. The individual develops a sense of uniqueness of self through interactions with others.

Family Relationships

Family relationships may be delicate throughout adolescence. Attitudes toward younger siblings may alternate between protectiveness and annoyance. Attitudes toward family caregivers range from harsh criticism and displeasure to genuine understanding and great love. During adolescence, solid family relationships can influence lifetime interpersonal success because they foster self-esteem and respect for and from others. Respect from others is essential for adolescents to maintain psychological and emotional health. Such respect includes recognizing the need for self-assertion, privacy, information, acceptance, experimentation, and growth in all developmental areas.

Peer Relationships

During adolescence, close friendships and first romantic relationships become important factors in the development of a young person's identity as a future adult. These relationships also influence feelings of acceptance and belonging.

Friendship

Adolescence is a time of forming friendships, with members of both the same and different genders. Social activities are usually with the same selected groups of individuals. School cliques are common. Many adolescents also have one or two best friends of the same gender during these years with whom they spend large amounts of time. These friendships are often important emotional preparation for more intimate and romantic relationships with others as the person matures.

Dating

Dating becomes a significant issue during these years (Fig. 11-2). Early teen dates usually consist of large groups of adolescents going on group outings together, such as going to the movies. As adolescents get older, they begin to pair off into couples. Many people experience their first

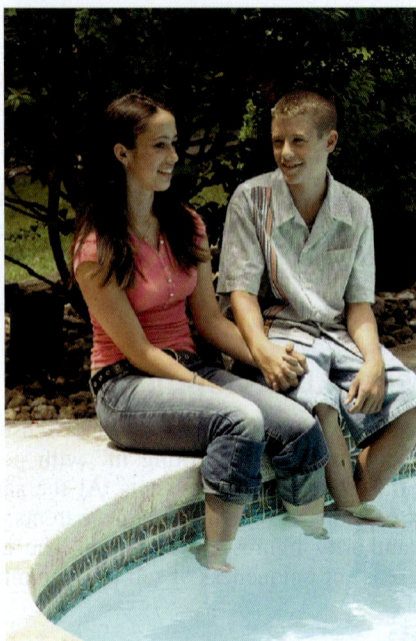

Figure 11-2 A primary developmental task of adolescence is to achieve new and more mature relationships.

consequences of their actions, or they may insist that they do not care. They are especially vulnerable to unsafe situations because of natural immaturity and the pressure for acceptance. Many adolescents feel a sense of immortality, assuming that nothing bad can happen to them. They are often competitive, with a desire to set themselves apart from the crowd.

Families can help adolescents to overcome peer pressure by modeling safe habits and practices. When dealing with the adolescent, active, nonjudgmental listening is often more productive than dictating the hazards of risky behaviors. When individuals feel judged or pressured, it is not uncommon for them to reject the conclusions and judgments of others. An effective approach is to make the teenager feel part of the solution. Positive reinforcement is often an effective approach for long-term change. A nurse's job includes active listening and encouraging the adolescent to seek well-informed sources for guidance.

Food and Eating Habits

Adolescents have special nutritional needs that are important for optimum health. Multiple nutritional information sources are available online. For example, www.cdc.gov and www.ChooseMyPlate.gov provide nutritional insight for a variety of ages and developmental stages. Young people may indulge in a diet composed primarily of "junk food" that is high in fat, sugar, and empty calories. Bad nutritional habits combined with inadequate exercise can lead to a susceptibility to illness such as diabetes.

Teenage boys normally have huge appetites. Some boys become concerned with achieving a muscular appearance, consuming protein drinks and spending time at a gym in an effort to build muscle. Teenagers are often very concerned about appearance. Anorectic or bulimic patterns of eating may emerge during these years in any adolescent, regardless of gender. Anorexia is marked by eating minimal amounts of food. Bulimia is characterized by a pattern of binge eating, followed by induced vomiting or the use of laxatives. Chapters 73 and 88 discuss both disorders.

Body Image

Adolescents develop physically and socially at various rates. A young person's body image will be a reflection of their upbringing and environment throughout childhood. The degree of affection, and mutual respect between caregivers and adolescents are key factors in the development of a positive body image. As a nurse, you need to be prepared for questions related to these areas. In Practice: Educating the Client 11-1 lists tips for providing guidance.

steady relationship during these years. First love brings many complicated feelings. A breakup with a first romantic partner can be extremely difficult for the adolescent to handle emotionally.

> **NCLEX Alert**
>
> Questions relating to adolescents may include nutrition (e.g., overeating, anorexia) or risky behaviors (e.g., driving habits, sexual explorations). Peer pressure issues may be included as part of the scenarios or the options.

Areas of Concern

Peer Pressure and Risk Taking

To define their identity, exert their independence, and "prove" to peers that they are maturing, adolescents may take significant risks with their health and well-being, school success, and relationships. Such risk-taking behavior includes noncompliance with a medical regimen, school truancy, sexual promiscuity, dangerous activities, such as skydiving or car racing, drinking, and using drugs. Adolescents may not be fully knowledgeable of the possible

---

IN PRACTICE
EDUCATING THE CLIENT 11-1 — Adolescent Concerns About Growth and Development

- Development of healthy habits: cleanliness, balanced nutrition, sleep and rest, activity and exercise
- Safety measures with motor vehicles and bikes
- Importance of scholastic and skill achievement
- Importance and development of self-respect
- Selection of peers as friends
- Wise counseling about sex and sexuality
- Responsibilities resulting from sexual activity
- Problems that arise from substance use and abuse (cigarette smoking, alcohol, recreational drugs)

IN PRACTICE

Adolescents are learning to make decisions and to assume responsibility for their decisions. Home support is invaluable. Adults must remember that many fluctuations in adolescent behavior are a normal part of growing up. Adolescents who are loved, accorded a measure of freedom and responsibility, disciplined sensibly and respectfully, and encouraged to grow and to achieve personal identity usually respond with love and respect for their family and the community in general. The future family life of young people, when they raise their own children, will probably be patterned after these positive family experiences.

Key Concept

Parents need help in accepting their "child" as an "adult."

STUDENT SYNTHESIS

KEY POINTS

- Adolescence is a turbulent time, marked by rapid physical growth and frequent emotional upheavals.
- Puberty is the time when a person matures sexually and becomes able to reproduce.
- The developmental tasks of adolescence involve identity versus role confusion, which include the formation of a self-image, establishment of goals for the future, and building relationships with others.
- Adolescence can be divided into stages categorized as early, middle, and late adolescence.
- Caregivers need to be positive role models for adolescents who are trying to withstand peer pressure, which often accompanies risk-taking behaviors.
- Nutritional discussions for the adolescent should include the interrelationships between obesity, diabetes, and personal well-being.
- Sex education from trusted adults helps teenagers avoid unplanned pregnancies and STIs.

CRITICAL THINKING EXERCISES

1. Twelve-year-old L.G. comes to the healthcare facility upset. He is the shortest boy in his class. While other boys have begun to show some facial hair, L.G. is still waiting for his voice to change. Explain how you would address L.G.'s concerns. What information would you give him?
2. P.D. is 15 years old and has been dating J.M. for a few months. They are not sexually active, but many of their friends are. P.D. is afraid to have sex, believing he and J.M. are too young. He is becoming increasingly anxious, however, under the pressure and scrutiny of his friends. He is afraid to talk to his parents about the situation; however, when sorting the laundry, his parent found a condom in his pocket that a friend had given to him "just in case." P.D.'s parent consults you for healthcare advice. Based on your knowledge of peer pressure and adolescent sexuality, what advice would you provide P.D. and his parent?
3. D.W. is 17 years old and a junior in high school. She has many friends and is mature for her age. Recently, a friend's older brother, a college junior, has taken an interest in D.W. and asked her out on a date. D.W. is excited by the prospect of seeing someone who is older, but she is worried about his expectations. What is your reaction to this situation? What questions might she have?

NCLEX-STYLE REVIEW QUESTIONS

1. Parents of a 15-year-old child are concerned about the influences of peers on their child's behavior. What suggestion can the nurse make to help the parents encourage the child to overcome these pressures? Select all that apply.
   a. Model safe habits and practices.
   b. Listen without judgment.
   c. Limit the time allowed to spend with peers.
   d. Give positive reinforcement for good behaviors.
   e. Have the child make decisions without parental input.
2. Parents inform the nurse that they found laxatives in their daughter's room and have heard her vomiting in the bathroom with the door locked after eating. What should the nurse provide information to the parents regarding?
   a. Pregnancy
   b. Bulimia
   c. Gastric ulcers
   d. Diabetes
3. The nurse obtains a 24-hour food recall from a 14-year-old child and determines that the majority of the food consumed is "junk food" or empty calories. What education should be provided to the adolescent?
   a. Teach the client how to shop for food.
   b. Inform the client that junk food should be eliminated and replaced with only healthy food.
   c. Tell the client there is nothing to worry about at this time but the child will need to be careful when older.
   d. Provide information and suggestions for improvements in diet choices and portions.
4. The nurse is talking to a 15-year-old client with diabetes type 1. What statement made by the client demonstrates further instruction regarding risky behaviors is required?
   a. "I need to check my blood sugar before and after I play football."
   b. "If I begin to feel like my blood sugar is low, I will eat a fast-acting carbohydrate."
   c. "I am going to eat what I want. It won't hurt me."
   d. "I will let my parents know if I have an injury."

5. A 16-year-old states to the nurse, "Don't worry about me, nothing bad will happen. It's just sex and doesn't mean anything." What is the best response by the nurse?
   a. "I wouldn't be so cavalier about sex if I were you."
   b. "Do you want to get a sexually transmitted infection?"
   c. "I would like to talk with you about the consequences of sexual activity."
   d. "I am going to have to tell your parents about your behaviors."

CHAPTER RESOURCES

Enhance your learning with additional resources on thePoint!
Student Resources related to this chapter can be found at **thePoint.lww.com/Rosdahl12e.**

12 Early and Middle Adulthood

Learning Objectives

1. Describe and differentiate between Erikson's two psychosocial developmental stages: intimacy versus isolation and generativity versus stagnation.
2. Discuss the typical developmental path of early adulthood.
3. Identify issues that women need to face during early adulthood.
4. Identify the transitions of adulthood necessitated by current demographics.
5. Discuss the typical developmental path of middle adulthood.

Important Terminology

demographics
emerging adulthood
generativity
intimacy
isolation
midlife transition (midlife crisis)
presbycusis
presbyopia
stagnation

This chapter examines the development of the individual throughout early and middle adulthood and the transitions between these stages. The variety of ages in demographics has become part of the definition of the developmental ages and stages. Certain aspects of late adolescence, the beginning of adulthood, and middle adulthood are interrelated and may overlap. Adults achieve tasks individually depending upon personal circumstances. The term **emerging adulthood** may be applied to the very diverse and unique period of life that ranges from the later teens to the mid-40s.

ERIKSON'S ADULT GROWTH AND DEVELOPMENT THEORY

Adult Challenges

As discussed in Chapters 10 and 11, Erikson's theory examines the psychosocial development of various age groups. Table 12-1 shows his theory for early and middle adulthood.

Remember that Erikson focuses on the *psychosocial challenges* that individuals face in the various life stages. People must meet and master these challenges before moving successfully to the next stage. As with children and adolescents, adults continue to face challenges as sets of positive versus negative outcomes. A younger individual may follow the motto, "Do now, worry about the consequences later." As people mature, however, challenges become choices over which adults exert control. Adulthood implies that individuals are no longer simply confronted with a challenge to conquer. Rather, adults consider issues and make judgments that directly affect outcomes. Consequences of decisions are thought out before choices are made. In addition, adults revise their choices as circumstances change throughout life.

Early Adulthood: Intimacy Versus Isolation

In early adulthood, people confront choices about their occupation, education, relationships, living environment, and independence. Young adults often work hard to achieve financial and emotional independence from their families of origin. They begin to establish life goals and values, although their attitudes may change later in life. *Intimacy versus isolation* is the challenge of this stage. Individuals choose to establish relationships with others (**intimacy**) or to remain detached (**isolation**) from others. Related choices include such options as entering a serious relationship or remaining single, or working in a people-oriented occupation (e.g., nursing) versus a quieter occupation (e.g., freelance work in one's home).

Middle Adulthood: Generativity Versus Stagnation

The tasks of **generativity** occur when adults decide to pass on learning and share skills with younger generations. The adult will accept and adjust to physiological changes such as loss of physical abilities or prowess. Erikson's theory suggests that **stagnation** involves adults who focus on personal pursuits and interests. The welfare of future generations and contributions to others are not of major concern to an individual in the phase of stagnation. Examples of the opposing choices of generativity versus stagnation include the following:

- Climbing the corporate ladder as part of a team or working as an individual pursuing personal goals

TABLE 12-1 Erikson's Theory of Psychosocial Development—Early and Middle Adulthood

CONCEPT	EARLY ADULTHOOD	MIDDLE ADULTHOOD
Challenge	Intimacy vs. isolation	Generativity versus self-absorption
Necessary accomplishments	Choose relationship style; select occupation; build independence	Develop self; plan retirement; raise family; enhance relationships
Virtues	Affiliation; love	Production; caring; cooperation

Taylor, C., Lynn, P., & Barlett, J. (2018). *Fundamentals of nursing: The art and science of nursing care* (9th ed.). Wolters Kluwer and McLeod, S. A. (2018). *Erik Erikson's stages of psychosocial development*. Simply Psychology. https://www.simplypsychology.org/Erik-Erikson.html

- Developing a lifestyle that includes a significant other or pursuing solitary interests
- Learning new activities or participating in events developed for self-satisfaction

Nurses need to have knowledge of expected developmental stages. When tasks are not accomplished during the stage in which they usually occur, an individual will have to deal with these tasks within the framework of the next stage. For example, a 29-year-old who is diagnosed with a severe illness may need to reevaluate their options for starting a family or making career choices. Transitions into the next phase (e.g., generativity) depend upon successful completion of prior challenges (e.g., intimacy). Illness can interfere with the successful transition from one phase to another.

> *Key Concept*
> Establishing intimacy is a key challenge for young adults. Cultural patterns and societal expectations greatly influence romantic relationships and their forms.

EARLY ADULTHOOD

Emerging Adulthood

Early adulthood encompasses the conversion from adolescence to adulthood. This transition period can be referred to as *emerging adulthood*. Individual circumstances differ, and exact age ranges are difficult to quantify but may range from the later teens to well within the fourth decade. Commonly, the emerging adult faces ongoing lifestyle changes and choices in areas including occupation, marriage, children, living situation, and education past high school. Many young people become employed full time after high school and may continue employment in the same or similar trades for many decades. In contrast, other young adults whose career choices require specialized training or advanced education after high school tend to focus on educational needs rather than the standardized steps of transitioning from a young adult to a mature adult. For example, individuals planning a career in cardiovascular surgery or pediatric oncology may not complete the required years of training until their mid-30s. After schooling, such specialists must establish a medical practice or clinic before their career is stabilized. For highly trained individuals, personal life (e.g., spouse, children, and finances) often must be sacrificed in lieu of educational and professional requirements.

Areas of Concern: Early Adulthood Transitions

Leaving Home

One of the first concerns of early adulthood is the transition of moving away from a home of origin, which typically is the home of a parent or guardian, to go to a new environment, location, or lifestyle. Leaving home involves changes of emotional attachments as well as new financial and security issues. Each person has different approaches to the issues involved in leaving home. Sometimes the individual returns home intermittently, for example, going off to college and returning for breaks. Others may get married. Some breaks are abrupt and difficult. Some young people face financial problems that force them to return to their family homes. Leaving home can follow any of several patterns:

- A person leaves home and does not move back.
- A person stays at home until he or she is forced to leave by family members.
- A person leaves, returns, leaves, returns, and continues a cycle of moving in and out.
- A person leaves, but remains within close proximity to the family of origin by moving nearby.

Choosing a Career

Occupational choices are closely tied to education and financial independence from the family caregivers. Careers involve other important tasks of adulthood, such as coping with stress, responding to authority, and getting along with others. Stress is part of any career. Individuals feel less stress, however, when they enjoy their work, believe they are doing the best with their abilities, and feel they are contributing to the society. Sometimes, circumstances prevent individuals from achieving a specific goal that was part of a childhood desire. Transitioning typically means some sort of change, and change can be stressful. Adaptability to change can define an individual's ability to achieve happiness and the feeling of accomplishing tasks that benefit others. Success in the work environment affects a person's sense of pride and self-worth. The choice of a career often increases social connections—a necessary component of adulthood.

Establishing an Adult Identification: Seeking Oneself

Families, peers, and surrounding cultural attitudes influence an individual's sense of personal identity. Maturation involves development of a sense of self-worth, self-esteem, and sense of purpose. Self-identity can be a component of personal relationships or of the choice to avoid relationships. Individual choices can be irreversible; often a person's life cannot be changed, or a decision settles an issue forever. Consider, for example, the decision to remain married or single, or the choice to have children or not to have children. Marriage and parenting are significant choices, which may change a person's lifestyle permanently even if the marriage dissolves or partners change at some point in the future. A sense of freedom can be lost when lifestyle choices are made.

Establishing Adult Relationships

Early adult relationships involve geographical or online social networks and, commonly, both. Belonging to a group for social support can be a challenge but creates a sense of security and well-being. Social connections are developed in a variety of environments, such as the workplace, online, or by an activity of joint interest (e.g., religion, politics, or sports). Another important source of early adult relationships is the college campus, where students are commonly surrounded by similar-aged and like-minded individuals. With time, they form new friendships and intimate relationships that provide support and understanding. Later in life, relationships include coworkers, housemates, intimate partnerships, marriage, and children.

Couples in their early adulthood who cohabitate (live together) may prefer to postpone marriage until after completing college, establishing a career, and building up adequate financial resources. Others do not want to commit to a long-term relationship until later in life, if at all. Some adults cohabitate for the same reasons that others choose to marry—for protection, to share expenses, or to escape the parental home.

Starting a Family

In general, societies maintain traditional home-based behaviors or traditions. Many adults marry and establish a family and home (Fig. 12-1). It is not uncommon for some adults to postpone marriage or children until they are in their 30s or 40s, preferring to establish careers and to become financially secure first. Both partners can be the providers, caregivers, and protectors, regardless of gender. As a result, the two-income family has had to adjust and redistribute family roles. For many couples, division of labor includes sharing childcare responsibilities. Participation of both parents in household tasks and childrearing can be a focus of stress. Shared roles of dual parenting can contribute to close parent–child relationships and a strong family unit.

Reappraising Commitments

As adults transition into their 30s, restlessness, confusion, and doubt become common. Adults may find themselves asking, "Now that I am where I wanted to be, what do I want out of this life?" The 20s and 30s are ages when individuals often make new choices and reappraise previous commitments. Adults who are married may question staying with their partners. They may consider a career change. Some

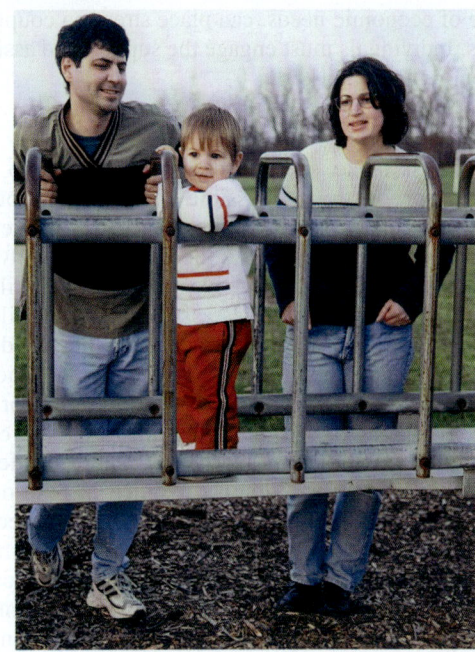

Figure 12-1 Starting and shaping a family are significant aspects of the young adult period.

adults now realize that they can make their own decisions based on their own feelings and not the beliefs of others.

Settling In

In their late second to fourth decade, adults begin to settle. If personal economics are favorable, many adults purchase a home. They are usually established in a lifestyle and career. They become more comfortable with their family, intimate friends, and other adult relationships. When compared with youth, life becomes more rational and orderly.

Making Career Decisions

Career issues are important and exist as part of adult transitioning. Developmental transitions occur as the adult adjusts to the unique needs required of a working life and a home or family situation. Personal desires may conflict with family circumstances. A couple working different hours or shifts can develop difficulty with marital interaction time, family time, and childrearing responsibilities in their relationship. Employment issues are interrelated with available finances and issues of personal growth.

Those who desire upward mobility in their work environments need to follow the rules of the corporate culture. Advanced degrees or training may be part of a career decision. Companies may require individuals to transfer from one city to another. For dual-career families, conflicts may arise. For example, if one partner receives a desirable job offer in another state, the couple must choose to stay together and continue with the present employment, to move and have the other partner seek a suitable job in the new state, or to live apart and have a commuting relationship.

Adults at any age may find themselves without a job. Some adults decide to embark on a new career path or to return to school. Changes in career status, either voluntary or because of economic needs, can place stress on couples and families. Individuals must engage the support and assistance of the entire family.

Women's Issues

Women must make specific decisions related to childbearing. Reproduction is possible any time after puberty. The majority of American women give birth in their second and early third decade. As the third decade advances, women may feel pressured to give birth to a first child. The differences and the difficulties associated with childbearing and childbirth are known to increase with each decade. Career goals and motherhood can conflict. Adoption and assisted reproductive technologies are options for some women (Chapter 70). Women who have children outside a committed relationship face the responsibilities and challenges of single parenthood. Women in relationships who have delayed pregnancy may face difficult decisions about employment, childcare arrangements, and financial responsibilities. Childbearing for women during or after the fourth decade is possible due to advances in medical knowledge and techniques. However, childbearing and childbirth difficulties can magnify problems with permanent consequences for the mother, child, and family members.

MIDDLE ADULTHOOD

Demographics is the study of characteristics and changes in a population. Changing demographics reflect a significant broadening of the age range for middle adulthood because of the trends in recent years toward a longer period of early adulthood, increased life expectancy, and the improved health and functioning of older adults. Middle adulthood may now be considered to encompass a broad age range. The period from the mid-30s to age 79 years can be considered the time between early adulthood and late adulthood. A more focused definition of aging can place the middle range of adulthood beginning around age 40 years and transitioning into late adulthood in the mid-60s. As the demographics show, individual circumstances and evolving societal changes help differentiate between young, middle, and late adulthood.

Areas of Concern: Middle Adulthood Transitions

Many developmental and psychosocial changes have occurred and continue to occur as adults face middle adulthood. Growing children spend more time away from home and are more interested in being with their own peers. Images of significant others also change in middle adulthood. As they look at partners, siblings, and friends of similar ages, adults recognize that they too are getting older. Individuals become concerned with guiding future generations. Middle adulthood is a time of realization. Adults in this phase of life have a great deal to offer in the way of experience and advice. They can view younger generations with a softer, less critical eye.

Adults responsible for childrearing may experience feelings of loss and loneliness, wondering what they will do when children leave home. Career changes, unemployment, and transfers to other cities may make home life and intimacy less stable.

As their children leave home, parents begin to examine their own intimate relationships. Marital and relationship status sometimes changes during this phase. Couples may develop a new depth of intimacy. In even the most stable and long-lasting marriages and partnerships, fluctuations are common. Some individuals divorce or separate; spouses or significant others die. In any case, adults must adapt to new roles and expectations. A divorced adult may face the challenges of dating and financial instability, as well as redefining the relationship with the ex-partner and children of that marriage. As adults transition and confront their own issues, they must acclimate to new situations and adjust to the many faceted role changes.

Some people at this stage are unable to accept aging and may feel frustrated and unfulfilled. They may feel that they have failed to achieve the goals of their youth. Theorists call these circumstances a **midlife crisis** or a **midlife transition**. Anxiety and panic are not uncommon. They may believe other people their age have achieved more than they and that they must do something creative or impressive before it is too late. A midlife transition can involve a sense of failure in the chosen profession, feelings of sexual inadequacy, fear of inevitable death, or frustration with aging parents or grown children. Sometimes, individuals feel an incredible desire to escape. They may act out temporarily in inappropriate or unexpected ways. Problems that may ensue if individuals fail to resolve this stage include brooding, physical illness, suicide, chemical dependency, and depression.

> **NCLEX Alert**
>
> Health concerns and priorities for an adult are commonly very different from those of the younger population. In the scenario, several issues may be suggested, such as financial problems or chronic health conditions. When responding to NCLEX questions, it is important to identify the priority issue. The priority issue will have pertinent, health-related situations that can be addressed by the LVN/LPN.

Adjusting to Role Changes

At some unidentified point in time, an individual can no longer be categorized as young or youthful but is not yet considered old. Self and family perceptions and roles begin to change. For example, as children grow, the realization becomes apparent that children are becoming adults. The adult's role as a parent changes, often adjusting to the needs of the grown child who might need financial support for school, or a place to live, or assistance with the next generation of children.

Adults often face the health issues, economics, and aging of their own parents. Arrangements may be necessary for placement in a nursing home or for home care. Sometimes people are caught between caring for both aging parents and their own growing children. Such adults have been referred to as the "sandwich generation." Personal needs and goals are often replaced, giving priority to the new needs of a changing family situation. Commonly, roles are reversed, with adults becoming the caregiver for their parents while maintaining their role as the main caregiver of their own children.

Physical Aspects of Aging

Physical changes related to aging are generally among the first become noticeable by the late third or fourth decade. Physical changes associated with aging become more prominent during each subsequent decade. Adults in this age range exhibit a loss of physical fitness when compared with those in their 20s and early 30s. By the end of the fourth decade, an individual typically gains about 10–20 lb (5–10 kg). By the fifth decade, muscle strength and flexibility decrease. Gray hair and hair loss become more noticeable. Wrinkles are due to a loss of skin elasticity. *Age spots, senile lentigines, or solar lentigines* are harmless flat, oval, or round spots on the surface of the skin. Their pigmentation is tan, brown, or black. They typically occur on the skin's surface that has been exposed to the sun and are harmless, unlike other skin eruptions that can be cancerous. Age spots are not related to any liver problem but are sometimes referred to as liver spots.

Changes in hearing (*presbycusis*) and vision (*presbyopia*) are two normal changes of aging that are not signs of illness and cannot be prevented. **Presbycusis** is the gradual loss of hearing in both ears that occurs gradually starting in middle age and becoming very noticeable by the mid-60s. Hearing loss interferes with daily life, making the spoken word hard to understand and alarms, phones, and doorbells difficult to hear. **Presbyopia** is the loss of flexibility of the lenses of both eyes, making it difficult to see close objects. The individual typically begins to use "reading glasses," which magnify the printed word and make it easier to read (Fig. 12-2). Both of these conditions may be exacerbated (worsened) by other conditions such as structural abnormalities (e.g., nearsightedness or farsightedness). Hearing problems are also commonly caused by long-term exposure to sounds, known as *noise-induced hearing loss*. The structures in the ear are very delicate and can be damaged by sounds that are too loud or last too long. Loud music and other noises (e.g., loud engines), which occurred in adolescence or young adulthood, are common causes of hearing loss that occur before the onset of presbycusis. Hearing protection for many occupations is mandatory.

Nursing implications for age-related changes include educating the client regarding normal changes versus abnormal conditions. The nurse must understand, as well as educate caregivers, that accommodations for the loss of hearing and vision include taking safety measures, speaking in a clear voice while facing the client, and providing reading materials in larger print. Many Websites allow text to be converted to a larger font (e.g., A, A, or A). Other nursing interventions include the discussion of nutrition and diet. As a person enters the third decade, metabolism changes. By the fourth decade, a person cannot eat the same amount of calories as the adolescent or young adult without gaining unwanted

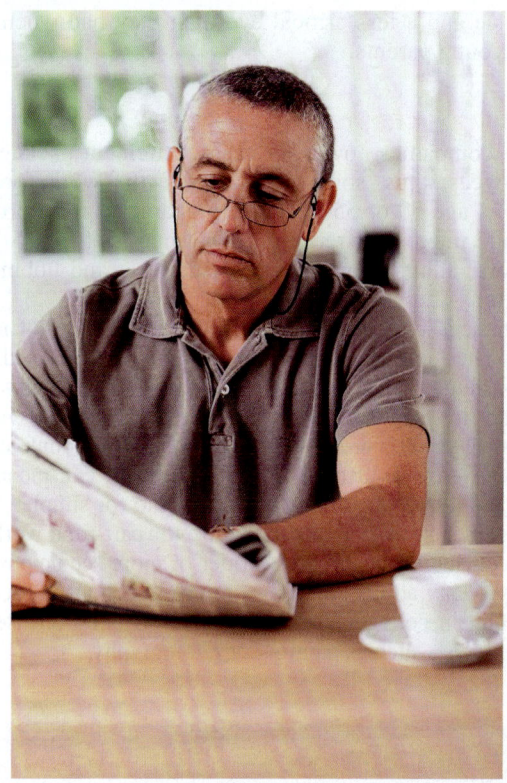

Figure 12-2 Presbyopia occurs typically in the fourth decade when vision changes due to aging. Wearing reading glasses to see the fine print of a newspaper becomes necessary.

weight. The possibility of obesity and diabetes increases due to a slower metabolism. Excessive caloric consumption hastens the weight gain, which tends to be insidious (sneaky), and it is typically very difficult to lose weight.

Perceiving One's Own Mortality

As individuals approach age 50 years, death becomes more of a reality. Often, initial concepts of death and dying occur after a relative or friend of the same age dies unexpectedly. Adults start to conceive the possibility of their own mortality. They may become frightened by the prospect of death. As one ages, it is not uncommon to reevaluate one's religious beliefs. A spiritual revival may occur and the individual becomes more comfortable with death's inevitability.

Reestablishing Equilibrium

As they head toward their 60s, adults look forward to new challenges. They often accept life with a degree of complacency and contentment. Plans for retirement begin to take shape. Personal equilibrium is reestablished.

As children move into their own homes and raise their own families, adults realize that life has achieved a point of comfortable habituation. Personal feelings tend to be less anxious or frantic when compared with earlier decades. Grandchildren may arrive and provide excitement and renewal. As grandparents, many adults can spend more time with their grandchildren than they did with their own children. The passage of time and a different perspective help many adults to view grandchildren with more patience and a less critical eye than they had when they were young parents.

Planning for Retirement

Some companies now offer early retirement packages to employees; thus, some people leave the work force as early as age 50 or 55 years. In preparation for a productive and interesting retirement that may last for 25 years or more, adults should develop interests and hobbies in midlife.

Financial planning is an important component of retirement. The money available for pensions has declined or is nonexistent in many places of employment. Adults need to start to plan their own retirement funds and investments when they are young when a small amount of savings can grow as decades pass. Retirement can mean that large family-oriented houses may be sold for simpler living arrangements. Individuals may look for part-time work and may consider relocating to warmer or more scenic environments. Many adults consider a return to school at this age, enrolling in colleges and universities or taking classes for new interests such as painting or photography.

TRANSITION FROM MIDDLE ADULT TO OLDER ADULT

The transitioning of the roles of adulthood is ongoing. If *middle age* or *middle adulthood* refers to the span of years beyond young adulthood but before old age, then a new, broadened concept of middle adulthood must take into account the more active role of older adults between the ages of 50 and 79 years. People in this age range are highly individualistic and assume multiple roles, as parents, grandparents, and employees. Actual age ranges may be defined according to the roles or actions of the individual, rather than the calendar age of the person. The terms *middle adult* and *older adult* may coexist in a practical, everyday sense. The generation known as the "baby boomers," born between 1946 and 1964, have now passed 50 years and are continuing to be an active part of the society while advancing into their 60s, 70s, and 80s. For the purposes of this text, middle to older adults ranging in age from 50 to 79 years will be termed *older adults*, in a category of their own. The issues facing older adults at this stage of life, as well as the concerns of the *oldest adults*, older than 80 years, will be discussed in detail in Chapter 13.

STUDENT SYNTHESIS

KEY POINTS

- Erikson's psychosocial developmental stage of intimacy versus isolation is the challenge of early adulthood.
- Generativity versus stagnation is Erikson's challenge of middle adulthood.
- Early adulthood's tasks include leaving the home of origin, choosing a career, seeking one's own identity, establishing adult relationships, and organizing long-term lifestyle commitments.
- Middle adulthood is concerned with transitions of lifestyle, adjusting to role changes, adapting to physical changes, and perceiving mortality.

CRITICAL THINKING EXERCISES

1. Based on the developmental stages as outlined in this chapter, explain how a serious illness, such as a heart attack, can affect the achievement of developmental tasks for the following clients: a 35-year-old; a 45-year-old; and a 55-year-old.
2. Describe how developmental stages for men and women may differ, based on gender roles in the society.
3. Consider your own developmental stage. What developmental task is the highest priority for you right now?

NCLEX-STYLE REVIEW QUESTIONS

1. The nurse is providing care for a client with presbycusis. Which nursing action should the nurse perform to accommodate the client's condition?
   a. Speak in a clear voice while facing the client.
   b. Provide educational brochures in large print.
   c. Speak very loudly so that the client can hear.
   d. Have the walkways to the client's bed clear from obstruction.

2. A middle-aged client informs the nurse of a 15-lb weight gain without changing any eating habits or level of activity. Which response by the nurse is the best?
   a. "You are going to have to go on a diet."
   b. "That's what happens when you don't exercise and eat junk food."
   c. "This occurs from excessive calorie intake and decreased metabolism."
   d. "I wouldn't worry about 15 lb. That isn't so bad."

3. A middle-aged client is experiencing some age-related skin changes. Which action is a priority by the nurse related to these changes?
   a. Tell the client to be checked every 3 months for skin changes.
   b. Inform the client that there are no problems related to these changes.
   c. Discuss with the client normal versus abnormal changes.
   d. Inform the client that the age spots on the hands can be cancerous.

4. A middle-aged client informs the nurse of an increasing weight gain. Which screening should the nurse prepare the client for to assess for potential complications of the weight gain?
   a. Glucose level to screen for diabetes
   b. White blood count to screen for infection
   c. Hemoglobin and hematocrit to screen for anemia
   d. Urine specimen to screen for ketones

5. A client asks the nurse why so many wrinkles have developed on the client's face. Which response by the nurse is the best?
   a. "This is related to problems with your liver."
   b. "The wrinkles are caused by stress."
   c. "Wrinkles are the result of a loss of elasticity."
   d. "The wrinkles are caused by an increase in pigmentation."

CHAPTER RESOURCES

Enhance your learning with additional resources on thePoint!

Student Resources related to this chapter can be found at thePoint.lww.com/Rosdahl12e.

13 Older Adulthood and Aging

Learning Objectives

1. Identify the demographic trends for individuals aged 50–100 years.
2. Define the following words: ageism, geriatrics, gerontology, oldest adult, and young-old adult, and provide examples of the process of senescence.
3. Differentiate between Erikson's developmental states of generativity versus stagnation and integrity versus despair.
4. Discuss the physical and mental health challenges of the adult that typically occur between the ages of 50 and 79 years.
5. Identify the interactions between the development of chronic conditions that occur as part of the aging process and the influences of medical technology.
6. Discuss the benefits and risks related to individuals in the workplace for the ages between 50 and 79 years.
7. Discuss the physical and mental health challenges of individuals greater than age 80 years.
8. Discuss five types of losses that occur as a result of aging.

Important Terminology

ageism, gerontology, proprioception, stagnation
generativity, oldest adult, reminiscence, young-old
geriatrics, polypharmacy, senescence

Acronyms

ADL, IADLs

Individuals reaching age 65 years have an average life expectancy of an additional 19.5 years. Females are expected to live an additional 20.6 years and males 18.1 years. "A child born in 2017 can expect to live 78.6 years, which is more than 30 years longer than a child born in 1900 who only lived 47.3 years" (Administration for Community Living, 2018). As a result of this expansion in life expectancy, the demographic definitions of "old" are in transition and have not been standardized. As described in Chapter 12, for the purpose of this text, middle to older adult individuals ranging in age from 50 to 79 years are termed *young-old adult individuals*. The young-old adult begins to notice and to live with the majority of physical, psychosocial, and economic trends of biological aging. The term *oldest adult individuals* describes those individuals who range in age from 80 to 100+ years. The oldest adult individuals have typically experienced the majority of the biological symptoms and physical effects of aging, which tend to increase in intensity rather than in number at this stage of life. The oldest adult individuals include the fastest growing segment of current generations. The number of people over 100 years old is increasing proportionally and should continue to grow.

The economics of healthcare and an understanding of how to provide competent healthcare for the older adult are major considerations for the LVN/LPN. As a nurse, you may practice in a hospital, extended care facility, ambulatory care clinic, or in home-based nursing, where you will need specific knowledge related to the normal and abnormal physical and mental changes that accompany aging.

Knowledge of the normal aging process enables you to help clients understand and adapt to normal changes in function. By knowing and recognizing normal changes that accompany aging, you are prepared to identify abnormal, pathologic developments. Unit 13 provides more detail about gerontologic nursing.

WORDS RELATED TO AGING

The study of the aging process in all its dimensions (physical, psychological, economic, sociologic, and spiritual) is called **gerontology**. **Geriatrics** is the study of medical and social problems and care associated with older adult individuals. The term gerontology is a more holistic and all-inclusive term, but either term refers to the study of the older adult. Nurses who specialize in the care of the older adult use the term *gerontologic nursing* for their specialty. The term older adult has many implications, which can be either complimentary or offensive, depending on its usage. Generally, older adult is a term applied to an individual who is past age 50 years and is approaching the later years of life. It often implies that a person is old and frail, but can also connote an older person who is respected and dignified. **Senescence** is the process of becoming old or can refer to the characteristics of old age. The term young-old may refer to an individual 50 years of age and older or to a group of individuals who share the mutual experience of age. The *young-old* phase includes those who share the aging experience of other adults ranging in age from about 50 to 79 years; however, this group may differ in many other aspects such as race, religion, or ethnicity. The *oldest adult* phase includes those individuals 80 years and older who are experiencing the accumulated effects of physical and psychological aging and are coping with functional changes that affect health and lifestyle.

Ageism refers to labeling and discriminating against older adult individuals. It is prejudice based on chronological age. Examples of ageism are the assumption that older people are incapable of thinking for themselves, uninformed, and dependent upon others for care or that they are grumpy, rigid, or stingy. Even healthcare providers may show ageism by, for example, calling older people names that define them by their age, such as "grandpa," or by using inappropriate and disrespectful terms, such as "sweetie," "honey," or "sweetheart." In some healthcare facilities (e.g., long-term care nursing facilities), the use of inappropriate words may be reported to the facility's licensing agency and can result in significant monetary sanctions. To develop a better relationship with older adult individuals, nurses need to be respectful of each individual and avoid language, attitudes, and behaviors of ageism.

> *Key Concept*
>
> Tasks of older adulthood are important challenges for development. Remember that each older person, because of their life history, will experience aging uniquely.

ERIKSON'S ADULT GROWTH AND DEVELOPMENT THEORY

Growth and development occur naturally as the older adult biologically and psychologically matures. These processes are identified by developmental theorists. As discussed in previous chapters, the developmental psychologist Erik Erikson identifies eight stages that are separated by age-related tasks and challenges.

Erikson: Psychosocial Development for the Older Adult

Erikson's definitions are influenced by an individual's ability to function in society and to maintain self-esteem and are not necessarily related to a calendar age. Individuals living longer may continue to work either full or part time. Since many individuals are working past age 65 years, the defined age of retirement for the 20th century developmental theory based on age is in transition.

Adult Challenges: The Young-Old Adult

Stage 7 of Erikson's psychosocial developmental stages for the middle to the young-old adult is **generativity** versus *stagnation*. As discussed in Chapter 12, the tasks of generativity occur when adults decide to pass on learning and share skills with younger generations. Erikson's theory suggests that **stagnation** applies to adults who focus on personal pursuits and interests without concern for the welfare of future generations or contributions to others. Review the discussion of generativity versus stagnation in Chapter 12, as it applies to individuals from the mid-30s to around age 50 years.

Adult Challenges: The Oldest Adult

Stage 8, Erikson's final developmental stage, pertaining to late adulthood, is *integrity* (or *ego integrity*) *versus despair*, which pertains to human development in the most advanced stages of adulthood. Table 13-1 reviews the basic challenges, accomplishments, and virtues of this age. Young-old adult individuals and the oldest adult individuals reflect on the events and decisions of their lives. Individuals achieve integrity, or acceptance of self, when they sense that their lives have meaning and have been worthwhile. They are comfortable with past resolutions and do not regret past decisions. If older adult individuals do not meet the challenges of aging, they are likely to feel that life is unfulfilled. A self-review or life review can help older clients avoid feelings of failure, depression, and despair. If an individual's state of mind includes overwhelming regrets, feelings of failure may envelop them. By reviewing life's events, older adult individuals can gain a positive perspective on the conflicts of earlier stages. When working with older clients in healthcare practice, you can encourage **reminiscence**, the act of discussing, thinking, or writing about things that happened in the past.

> **NCLEX** *Alert*
>
> In real-life practice, the nurse is presented with many situations related to the physical, the psychological, and the social concepts of aging. Concepts such as *integrity* and *despair* may be integrated into NCLEX questions. Therefore, you must be able to identify and differentiate all of Erikson's stages.

TABLE 13-1	Erikson's Theory of Psychosocial Development—Late Adulthood
CONCEPT	**LATE ADULTHOOD**
Challenge	Integrity (or ego integrity) versus despair
Necessary accomplishments	Balance choices, achieve stability, retire, evaluate life, accept life choices
Virtues	Renunciation, wisdom, dignity

DEVELOPMENT IN OLDER ADULTHOOD

The older adult of the 21st century is more educated and aware of personal healthcare issues and responsibilities when compared to the same age groups of the last century. The majority of people between the ages of 64–74 years are married and live with a spouse (CDC, 2013). The majority of young-old adult individuals who live alone function independently with the capacity to perform important and essential activities, also called the *instrumental activities of daily living* (**IADLs**). For example, they are able to manage money, prepare meals, take medications, and physically care for themselves. Many of the oldest adult individuals retain some or most of their IADLs; however, many older adult individuals become increasingly dependent upon others and need assistance with some, if not all, of their *activities of daily living* (**ADLs**). Eventually, support may be provided by professional healthcare workers for survival needs.

The physical changes of senescence, which begin around the start of the fourth or fifth decade and continue through to death, are a major influence on an individual's thoughts of retirement. For the aging individual, physical changes interrelate and coexist with financial resources and lifestyle decisions, such as when to set the date to retire.

The Young-Old Adult

Biological age and chronological (calendar) age are among the factors that have had major impact upon use of the term "middle-age or older adult." The *young-old adult* can be defined as the person whose age ranges approximately between 50 and 79 years, based on the biological effects of aging and the individual's functional capacity. The baby boomer generation, born from 1946 to 1964, has now reached this age range (Chapter 12).

An individual's functional age may be very different from their chronological age, biological age, or psychosocial age. The World Health Organization (WHO) notes that age classification varies between countries and reflects instances of social class differences and functional ability related to the workforce. The WHO also points out that the definition of old and older adult is often a reflection of political and economic situations as well as having a strong link to an arbitrarily delineated retirement age (WHO, 2015).

Areas of Concern: Young-Old Adult Transitions

Physical Health

The biological aspects of aging typically are associated with the numerous physical changes that are noticeable as early as the third decade and interfere with lifestyle activities by the late 40s. Aging is associated with having one or more chronic medical conditions that can interfere with lifestyle but not necessarily prohibit activities needed for work or recreation. For example, the pain and limitations of arthritis commonly start in the late 30s or early 40s, but the individual can generally continue some type of work.

Box 13-1 Major Physical Changes Related to Normal Aging Processes

- Loss of strength, flexibility, and endurance
- Decrease in functioning of organs
- Changes in visual acuity; cataracts
- Auditory changes; hearing loss in upper frequencies
- Decreased reaction time
- Unsteady gait, decreased sense of balance
- Decrease in tactile sensations
- Diminished sense of smell and taste
- Loss of bone density
- Less restful sleep; more frequent naps
- Stiff joints
- Increased emotional and physical losses
- Decreased capacity for recovery from injury or illness

Common physical changes that come with aging include changes in vision, hearing, muscle strength, and reproductive functioning. Examples of functional changes that occur throughout adulthood include use of reading glasses and needing assistance with physical tasks (e.g., opening jars or lifting objects). Young-old adult individuals may notice that they need more time for some cognitive functions. While not designated as impaired, they may need more time to process information, identify sensations, remember facts, solve complex problems, or retrieve information. It is not uncommon for a young-old adult individual to ask for information to be repeated. The nurse should speak clearly and look directly at the individual. While many concerns of the young-old adult individual need to be referred to the primary healthcare provider, good nursing care may involve active listening skills and reassurance that a stated concern is a normal phenomenon of aging. Physical changes due to aging are reviewed in Box 13-1 and are discussed in more detail in Chapter 92.

The quality of life for the young adult client in recent decades has been influenced by access to improved healthcare, especially in the field of pharmacology. Medications such as NSAIDs (nonsteroidal anti-inflammatory drugs) for muscle aches and arthritis pain have had a significant effect on quality of life. Education about the hazards of smoking, obesity, an unhealthy diet, and inactivity has multiple beneficial effects that support a healthy population.

The Centers for Disease Control and Prevention (CDC) notes that preventative services are a key public health strategy. However, many life-saving services are used by less than half of adults aged 50 years and above. Preventive health screening and early detection practices provide significant benefits for the individual and are cost-effective uses of the healthcare system. Clinical preventative services can prevent or detect disease in its early stages when treatment outcomes are more beneficial and, thus, more cost effective. These

Box 13-2 Lifestyle Changes in the Aging Population

- General change in physiologic, psychological, and sociologic functions and roles
- Change in most body functions and abilities
- Adaptation to chronic physical or emotional disorders
- Change in employee or employer role
- Greater amount of leisure time
- Reduction of income
- Change of residence
- Change in parenting roles (sometimes a reversal)
- Adaptation to loss of spouse or partner, friends, and family members
- Development of coping mechanisms to deal with accumulated changes
- Adaptation to possible changes in sexuality
- Reevaluation of self-worth
- Maintenance of self-esteem and independence
- More time for meditation and contemplation of life
- Adaptation to prospect of death

services include screenings for chronic conditions, immunizations, for example, influenza and pneumonia, and counseling about personal health behaviors. Prevention is less expensive and more effective than treatment. Individuals should be encouraged to have colorectal screening, schedule a mammogram and a bone density test, and be evaluated for depression.

Psychosocial changes happen in collaboration with the physical changes because the individual learns to function within new limitations that affect mobility, self-care, and attitude. Box 13-2 reviews the major adjustments needed for lifestyle changes in the aging. Refer to Chapter 12 for a more thorough discussion of the challenges of becoming an adult such as leaving home, choosing a career, seeking personal identity, having relationships, developing a family and career, dealing with the changes associated with aging, and contemplating mortality.

Chronic Conditions

A chronic condition is defined as an ongoing illness lasting a year or more that requires continual medical attention. Eighty percent of young-old adult individuals have at least one chronic condition, and more than half of all adults have several (National Council on Aging, 2020) (Fig. 13-1).

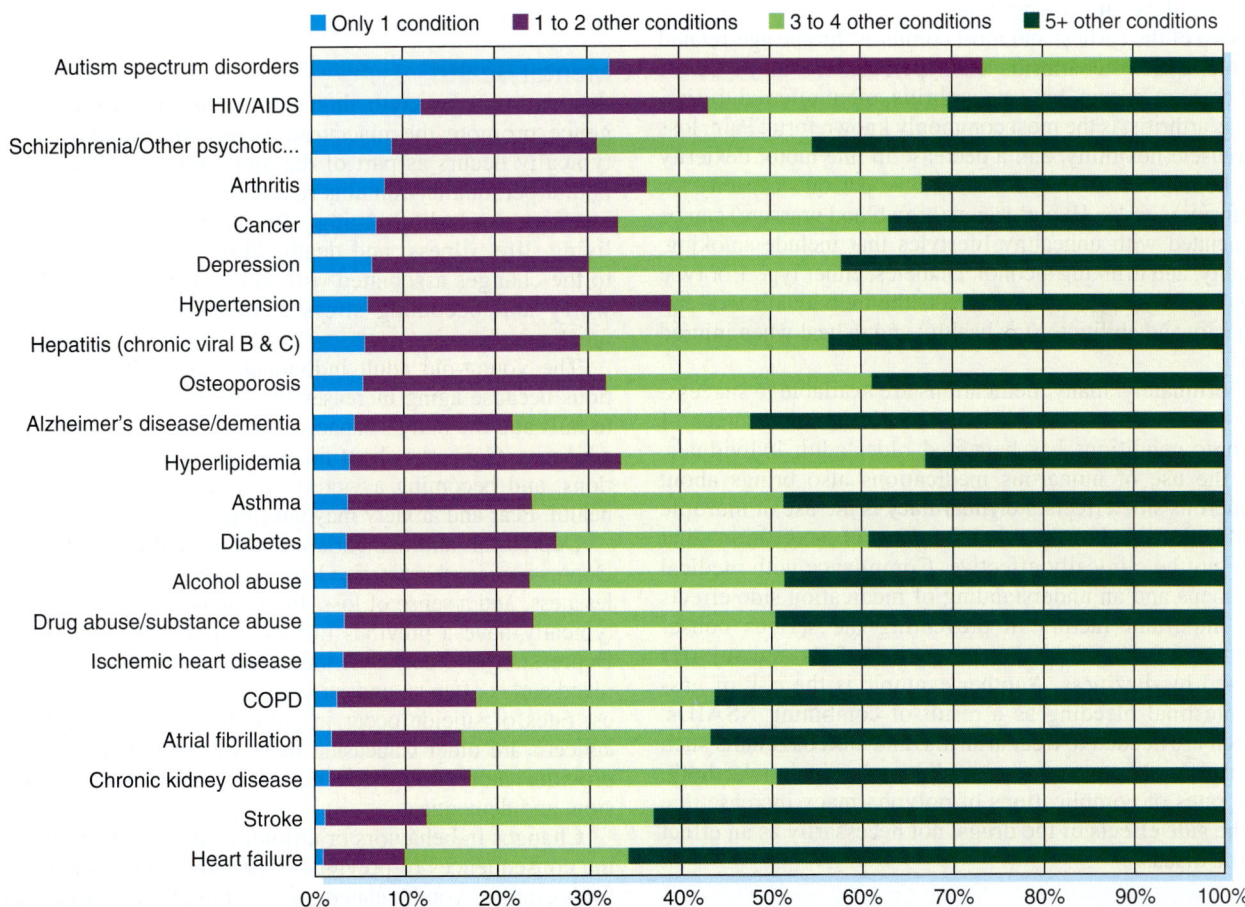

Figure 13-1 Multiple chronic conditions among Medicare fee-for-service beneficiaries: 2017. This graph compares the percentages of single chronic illnesses (blue) to the percentages of individuals with multiple chronic diseases (violet, green, orange). This emphasizes that most young-old/oldest adult individuals have three or more long-term disorders. (Centers for Medicare & Medicaid Services. [2017]. *Chronic Conditions Charts*. https://www.cms.gov/Research-Statistics-Data-and-Systems/Statistics-Trends-and-Reports/Chronic-Conditions/Downloads/cc_charts.zip)

The care and cost of treating chronic conditions are major concerns to both the individual and to those engaged in the finances of healthcare in any society. For example, in 2017, older adult individuals spent more of their total budget on healthcare related expenses than other consumer groups (roughly 13.4% of their total budget compared to 8.2% among all consumers) (Administration for Community Living, 2018).

The number of individuals with chronic conditions will continue to rise due to the demographics and population trends of the older generation. These conditions require healthcare from a professional healthcare provider and may need additional home care support from a family member or caretaker. Chronic conditions are the leading causes of death among U.S. adults aged 65 years or older. The trend of increased longevity is greatly influenced by the ability of healthcare providers to successfully treat diseases and disorders that, in previous generations, were often life threatening.

The aging population's physical problems are commonly related to avoidable diseases or disorders. Examples of avoidable risk factors include the use of tobacco products, being in environments containing secondhand smoke, lack of effective exercise, and poor eating habits. Risk factors often lead to acute and chronic conditions, such as, but certainly not limited to, cardiovascular diseases, diabetes, kidney disorders, and emphysema.

Two of the earliest and most common chronic age-related problems are osteoarthritis and hypertension. Many types of arthritis are known, but osteoarthritis, often referred to simply as arthritis, is the most commonly known form. Pain, loss of muscle flexibility, and a decrease in fine motor dexterity can be minor or major influences on a person's capacity for performing tasks. Hypertension (high blood pressure) can be associated with unhealthy lifestyles that include smoking, obesity, and drinking alcohol. Diabetes, either type 1 or type 2, is a costly condition that effects the individual's working capacity and ability to stay healthy and to heal when injured or ill.

Fortunately, many medications are available to successfully treat chronic conditions. Medical management of chronic conditions has benefited older adult individuals, but the use of numerous medications also brings about numerous side effects. **Polypharmacy** is the use of multiple medications and/or the administration of medications that may not be clinically effective. Compliance with medical regimens and an understanding of medication side effects are important factors in preventing the serious consequences of drug interactions, such as falls and injuries caused by dizziness. Another example is the risk of gastrointestinal bleeding as a result of combining NSAIDs, which are needed to treat arthritis, and anticoagulants such as aspirin. Many young-old adult individuals take both. The rates of complications of polypharmacy increase due to the side effects of the drugs, not necessarily as an effect of the disease.

Influences of Medical Technology

Advances in available treatment options and the availability of effective medications that treat and/or cure diseases or disorders affect a multigenerational population. Multiple and specific improvements in diagnostic technology and the capability to successfully manage chronic disorders have fundamentally changed population demographics. For example, radiographic imaging (e.g., mammogram) has been noted to be a successful intervention in the early diagnosis and eventual treatment of breast cancer. Similarly, the categories of medications that treat cardiovascular diseases have had a positive impact on the prevention of two major causes of death in the United States, myocardial infarction (heart attack) and stroke.

Costs of Healthcare

The longevity of current and future generations has a direct effect on the costs of healthcare. As individuals are living longer, they are also living with one or more chronic conditions. The social and personal influences of these facts are immense. Medicare, the main supplemental healthcare financial support for ages 65 years and up, becomes the primary healthcare financial resource but, typically, does not cover all of the costs of healthcare (e.g., medications). The costs of daily medications can severely deplete the individual's available retirement income. As individuals age, their personal finances are proportionally affected by the costs of healthcare.

Mental Health

Ageism and the myth that aging interferes with intelligence promote the inaccurate belief that mental illness typically occurs as part of the aging process. The reality is that personality remains relatively unchanged throughout a person's life. Aging affects one's perceptions of living, life, illness, and death. Most aging adults adjust to the changes associated with aging, having learned that worry and becoming stressed are not effective coping mechanisms.

The young-old adult individual is typically more cautious because aging increases the chances of injury related to falls and the body's capacity for healing decreases as age advances. Concerns about finances, evolving health restrictions, and becoming a victim of crime may affect mental health. Fear and anxiety may develop.

Depression and dementia are not normal parts of aging. Depression is characterized by sadness, feelings of helplessness, and a sense of loss. Individuals who are depressed typically have a previous history of psychiatric problems. Depression in older adult individuals is not readily recognized and is often an undertreated medical illness. The highest rates of suicide occur in the older adult. Of particular concern are older Caucasian men who live alone. Unit 13 provides more discussion regarding gerontology, depression, and dementia.

Changes in behaviors or attitudes can often be traced to the consequences of previous or new traumas to the brain, for example, youth-related sports injuries or cerebrovascular attacks related to blood vessel disorders. It is not uncommon for depression to co-occur with other serious physical illnesses such as heart disease, cancer, or diabetes. Major illness may be the instigating factor of depression.

Nursing considerations include recognition of mood and behavior changes.

> **Key Concept**
>
> Severe depression is not a normal consequence of aging. As a nurse, you need to notify the healthcare provider of signs or symptoms of depression. Depression can often be effectively treated by medications and/or counseling.

The Older Adult in the Workplace

The fact that people are living longer lives has influenced the likelihood that an employee will be working past the age of 65 years. On-the-job injuries are not directly associated with aging. The older worker has more experience, tends to be more cautious, and is typically more aware of physical limitations. Safety regulations in the workplace, such as adequate light, ergonomic environments, and safety awareness programs, have limited injuries of the older worker. Aging does increase the overall likelihood of falls, however, and when older workers are injured, they are more likely to be more seriously injured and require more recuperative time.

An age-friendly workplace has many benefits. Studies by the National Institutes of Health and Safety document that the older worker benefits the employer in several ways (CDC, 2018). The older worker tends to have greater institutional knowledge and usually more experience; thus, they do not need expensive employee-sponsored training programs. In general, they have learned productive work habits, communicate better with coworkers, and bring less stress to the job than do younger workers. Proactive employers are willing to be more flexible with the work schedule and find that ergonomic interventions are often inexpensive and easily implemented. Work supervisors who focus on preventative safety-oriented approaches to the work environment achieve positive outcomes with a multigenerational workplace.

The Oldest Adult

Age is more than an accumulation of years. The aging process affects people in different ways. Some people age faster than others. Some people seem never to age. The various aspects of aging—physical, psychosocial, and spiritual—do not occur at the same rate for all individuals. Heredity, congenital conditions, altered use of nutrients by the body, changes in hormone production, electrolyte imbalance, physical demands, environment, lifestyle (e.g., smoking and exercise), and lifetime nutritional habits contribute to the way individuals age. To fully adapt to aging and to be able to thrive in this new stage, the oldest adult individuals must confront and adapt to lifestyle changes. Some of the oldest adult individuals no longer have the capability to care for themselves and many are dependent upon others for some level of assistance. When a person can no longer perform ADLs, support from caregivers such as family, friends, or professional healthcare workers becomes the priority. Examples of ADLs for the frail older adult include personal hygiene, nutritional needs (e.g., food preparation) and possibly feeding, and assistance with physical activities, such as moving from bed to chair, chair to commode, or exercise of muscles.

Areas of Concern: The Oldest Adult

Physical Health

The oldest adult individuals are the generation most vulnerable to the physical and psychosocial aspects related to normal aging. Senescence changes are unique, proceeding on an unpredictable biological schedule from a vaguely known genetic inheritance. The consequences of healthy and unhealthy lifestyle factors that were present during the individual's growth and development and current access to dental, mental, and physical healthcare will also become more apparent in the oldest adult. In addition, the overall aging process varies from person to person. Optimal function for each individual's age is the goal.

The oldest adult individuals have typically felt the majority of the effects of biological aging. They most commonly have multiple chronic conditions. In earlier life, as young-old adult individuals, they were able to adapt to the normal physical changes that were occurring gradually. As oldest adult individuals, however, they are more vulnerable to the pathological changes that have been accumulating over time, as part of the aging process. For example, osteoarthritis typically begins in the young-old adult, but, with time, arthritic changes cause joint disorders, and loss of calcium in the bone affects bone density. Joint deformity and thinning bones can result in fractures, particularly hip fractures. Scientists and healthcare providers are continually learning more about ways to limit disabilities and to promote optimum functioning in advancing years.

Chapter 92 continues the discussion of aging and the nursing care needed for the individual who needs assistance to meet daily needs. In Unit 4, each chapter covers a particular body system. These chapters conclude with the effects of aging on each particular system and a table that reviews such changes.

Psychosocial Considerations

The oldest adult individuals usually want to remain independent for as long as possible. Independence does not necessarily mean living alone. However, it does mean retaining control over the major aspects of life. The three key elements of maintaining independence are healthcare, financial stability, and social resources. Transportation opportunities are part of these concerns. A loss of functional ability may make self-care difficult. Financial losses may prevent the maintenance of living quarters.

Participation in social activities is important for the oldest adult individuals. Family and friends may be unavailable for social support. Such factors place oldest adult individuals in danger of losing their independence. Older individuals and their families can strive to promote independence in every area possible. See Special Considerations: Culture and Ethnicity.

SPECIAL CONSIDERATIONS — **Culture and Ethnicity**

Independence
Remember that in many cultural groups, it is considered unthinkable for older relatives to live alone or in nursing homes. In these situations, independence is linked with maintaining a pivotal role as part of an extended family.

Loss of Independence and Mobility

The vast majority of the oldest adult individuals are active, healthy adults. Sometimes, people mistakenly consider normal aging processes to be signs of illness. Loss of independence due to changes in mobility is one of the greater losses of aging for most people. For the oldest adult individual, coping skills and attitudes toward life will, in part, determine if individuals can accept these losses.

At some point, individuals may have to give up driving, which is a major component of independence. The oldest adult individual may live in an area that is unsafe for walking alone, eliminating walking as a mode of transportation. Getting on and off a bus may be difficult and hazardous. Taxicabs can be costly. The need for transportation creates a need for assistance from others. As individuals need increasing help getting to grocery stores, banks, healthcare facilities, and places of worship, they become more dependent on support persons among their relatives and friends. Taking advantage of community resources will help lessen this dependence on family and friends.

Falls are a major consideration for both young-old adult individuals and oldest adult individuals. Falls are a leading cause of hospital admissions (National Council on Aging, 2020). Most fractures, traumatic brain injuries, and the majority of fatal injuries occur due to changes of mobility. As people age, muscle flexibility, bone strength, and the sense of *proprioception* are diminished. **Proprioception** is the unconscious awareness of how one's body is positioned when standing, sitting, or moving in a space, that is, *spatial orientation*. This awareness is due to multiple neurological factors, including the receptors in the inner ear, which govern balance and spatial orientation. Problems with proprioception plus changes in vision can result in hazardous outcomes, such as injuries related to falls. For example, when the older adult goes up or down stairs or reaches to lift items out of a cupboard (stimulating the receptors in the inner ear as the head tilts back), the body is not as quick to balance itself. Chapters 92 and 93 discuss safety issues in more detail.

The Social Environment and Loss

The oldest adult individuals realize that social activity is necessary for life. They should choose and plan activities that will bring them joy and happiness. Some enjoy working long past a retirement age. Others spend time with spouses, romantic partners, grandchildren, and other loved ones. Participation in volunteer work is rewarding for many older individuals. Some begin to renew interests in hobbies or develop interests in new fields (Fig. 13-2). Educational opportunities are available for both the young-old adult and the oldest adult. They may go back to school to finish a college or graduate degree or complete individual courses in subjects such as art or music, managing finances, acting, and computers. Agencies that offer opportunities for study and travel that are geared to the needs of older persons are available.

Finances and Loss of Income

Most people have to adjust to a fixed income after retirement. The oldest adult individuals are extremely vulnerable to loss of income. After 80 years of age, healthcare costs increase significantly while income tends to decrease, and healthcare may become a significant burden. Simultaneously, food, shelter, clothing, and traveling expenses may increase. Basic needs, such as payment for food and shelter, often compete with the cost of medications. Some older adult individuals have little or no income when a financially supportive spouse or family member dies. They may live at a distance from family and other persons who could be of assistance if they lived closer. A few key facts relating to financial issues and the older adult population are listed in Box 13-3.

Stress and Loss

The word "loss" can be considered the one word that summarizes the aging process. Stress is a result of the many

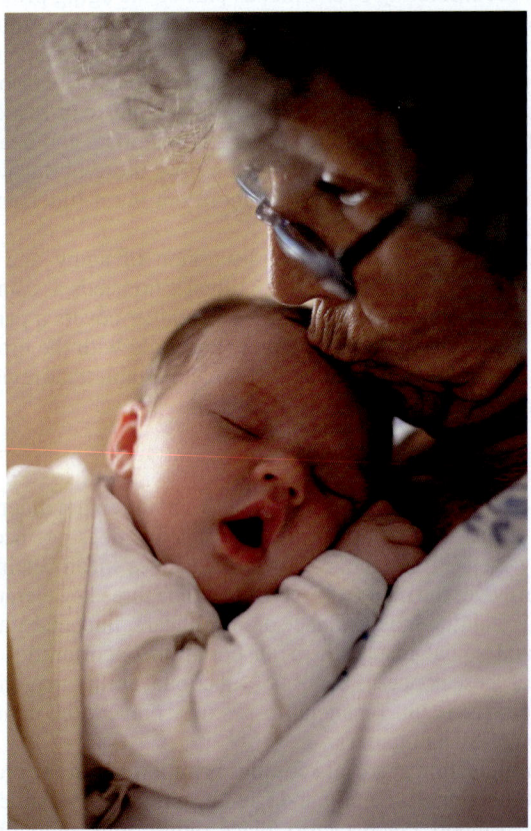

Figure 13-2 Volunteers are sometimes used in hospitals to hold infants who need long-term care. Physical touch for the infant is essential for growth and development. Young-old adult individuals offer companionship and gain a sense of usefulness.

Box 13-3 Financial Issues and Socioeconomic Issues Facing the Older Adult Population

- Many older adult individuals live on a fixed income, which often represents a reduction in financial resources that were available in earlier life.
- Income is from savings, investments, and retirement.
- Some individuals continue to work full or part time past the age of 65 years for financial reasons or personal fulfillment.
- A majority rely on Social Security Income, originally designed as a *supplement* to other retirement income.
- Many widowed individuals are living at a much lower income level than they did when their partner was alive.
- Most older adult individuals own their own homes; many do not move after retirement.
- Most older adult individuals live in urban areas. Trends in housing are toward group housing, shared housing, or retirement communities.
- Older ethnic minority populations are more likely to face health problems because they are more likely to live below the poverty level.
- Healthcare needs for the older adult female are often different than for an older adult male; healthcare workers may not be aware of these differences.
- About one third of prescription medications are taken by young-old adult individuals.
- The cost of medications may be a financial burden to many young-old adult individuals.
- Adverse drug reactions are more likely to occur in older adult individuals.
- Multiple drugs (polypharmacy) are often taken by one person.
- Older adult individuals typically have at least one chronic condition and, as they age, may have several.
- Each chronic condition adds to the total cost of healthcare for the individual and for agencies that pay for healthcare.
- Health problems and disabilities increase with advancing age, thus adding costs for healthcare.
- Health problems and disabilities increase with advancing age.
- Children of aging parents are frequently faced with responsibility for partial or total care of their parents.
- Difficulties arise because many family caretakers are themselves over the age of 65 years and are experiencing disabilities due to aging.

losses that the oldest adult individuals encounter; adapting to stress and loss is a normal life cycle requirement of getting older. Losses can be subtle or catastrophic. They are often cumulative. As they age, individuals experience loss in physical appearance and physical abilities, loss of roles (parent, employer), and loss of a spouse and other peers. Isolation from family, society, or friends involves significant stress and loss.

The ability to adapt to change is important. Individuals who try to adapt, as they did in the past, may find that many of the options of youth are no longer available. People with fixed habits and attitudes may face difficulty adjusting to change. The accumulation of stressors can be stressful in itself. For example, the loss of a spouse is traumatic, but to lose a spouse who had been the major source of income and the supplier of transportation can be overwhelming.

Generally, experience with past crises influences the response of older adult individuals to stress. An active lifestyle helps. Choosing and maintaining social and civic activities and functions appropriate to health, energy level, income, and personal interests can help individuals to cope and even to thrive.

Mortality and Loss

Death of spouses and peers causes adults to reflect on their own death or mortality. Religious or spiritual beliefs may strongly influence their attitudes. People prepare for death in different ways. They may systematically talk about the past and be especially interested in sharing family history and experiences with their offspring. Some wish to take a life inventory. They may draw up a family tree, create a scrapbook, organize photograph albums, or create an audiotape or videotape to share memories with grandchildren (Fig. 13-3). They may plan for their funeral, choosing music and scripture to be used. Funeral planning should not be considered morbid but a part of a person's ability to maintain control over the organization of life. Technology and advanced life support capabilities should be considered and be part of the planning process. An advanced directive may need to be revised or developed. Nursing considerations during periods of loss include active listening skills.

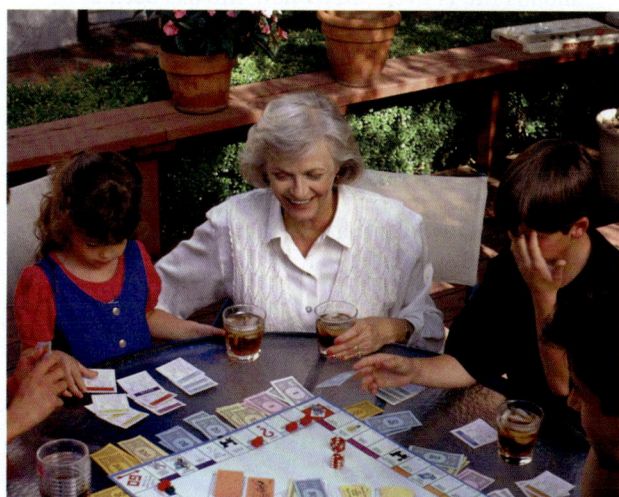

Figure 13-3 Social relationships provide an opportunity to share past experiences.

STUDENT SYNTHESIS

KEY POINTS

- Demographics related to the current aging population have shown that the aging generation has greatly affected the industrial sector, housing, social agencies, and the healthcare system.
- Erikson's developmental stages of generativity versus stagnation and integrity versus despair present challenges associated with productive aging.
- Physical, financial, and social aspects of life are in major transition due to the number of older adult individuals, the prevalence of those living with one or more chronic health conditions, and the longevity of this generation.
- The insights of demographic data have shown that young-old adult individuals have at least one chronic condition and the majority of the oldest adult individuals have multiple chronic conditions.
- Potentially life-saving preventative services are available but are not effectively utilized by the majority of the young-old adult population.
- Many young-old adult individuals continue to work past the age of 65 years.
- Safety issues in the workplaces of the older adult include adequate lighting, ergonomic working stations, and proactive safety regulations to prevent falls and injuries.
- Loss and change are key issues of the aging process; the ability to adapt to change facilitates one's ability to deal with loss.

CRITICAL THINKING EXERCISES

1. L.C., a 70-year-old man, comes in for a regular checkup to the healthcare facility where you work. He is in good health. During the past few visits, he has made remarks indicating that he feels useless and his life is over. "My whole life has been a disappointment," he said sadly on his last visit. L.C.'s wife died about a year ago. His children live close by. Though he is lonely, he wants to maintain independence and "not be a burden" on them. Based on your reading contained in this chapter, how would you respond to L.C.? How can you help him to realize his self-worth and integrity? What suggestions would you give him to help him conquer loneliness?

2. Consider the lifestyle you hope to enjoy as an older adult. What measures can you take now to help ensure the possibility of such a lifestyle? Explain the importance of good nutritional practices and preventive healthcare measures in your plan.

3. Think about your reactions when you see older people in the grocery store, in the bank line, or driving in traffic ahead of you. Are any of your reactions examples of ageism? Are your ideas about the behavior of older people proven correct or incorrect most of the time? As a nurse, what measures can you take to avoid treating clients with prejudices based on age and other factors?

NCLEX-STYLE REVIEW QUESTIONS

1. A young-old adult nurse wishes to mentor the younger new nurse and asks the supervisor for permission to be a mentor. According to Erikson, which developmental stage is the young-old adult nurse experiencing?
   a. Stagnation
   b. Generativity
   c. Integrity
   d. Despair

2. The nurse is talking with an oldest adult client and the client states, "I have done so many things in life and was able to achieve my goals." Which developmental stage has this client achieved?
   a. Ego integrity
   b. Despair
   c. Stagnation
   d. Generativity

3. The nurse overhears an oldest adult client saying to another client, "I feel depressed because I have so many regrets about my life." Which activity can the nurse provide to help this client gain a positive perspective?
   a. Provide a craft project
   b. Encourage ambulation
   c. Provide a game such as Bingo
   d. Encourage reminiscence

4. Which client should the nurse monitor more closely for signs of developing depression?
   a. A 58-year-old Hispanic female raising a grandchild
   b. A 70-year-old married African American male
   c. A 68-year-old Caucasian male who lives alone
   d. A 46-year-old married mother of three

5. A young-old adult client informs the nurse, "I want to remain independent and not have to depend on my children." What key elements does the nurse recognize will allow this to occur? Select all that apply.
   a. Healthcare
   b. Financial stability
   c. Number of adult children
   d. Social resources
   e. Psychological integrity

CHAPTER RESOURCES

Enhance your learning with additional resources on thePoint!

Student Resources related to this chapter can be found at thePoint.lww.com/Rosdahl12e.

14 The End of Life: Death, Dying, Grief, and Loss

Learning Objectives

1. Discuss the progression of experiences and general patterns related to death and dying.
2. Differentiate between the types of care needed for a curable illness versus a terminal illness and state why palliative care is acceptable for both.
3. Identify at least five processes found in the dying client and provide nursing considerations for each.
4. Discuss the economic needs and financial impact of death on the caregivers.
5. Identify the difference between physical care and emotional care of a dying client.
6. Discuss Kübler-Ross philosophy of grief, loss, and death.
7. Define each of the following stages: denial, anger, bargaining, depression, and acceptance.

Important Terminology

acceptance, anger, bargaining, Cheyne–Stokes, cyanosis, denial, depression, grief, impaction, incontinence, infarction, loss, mottling, palliative care, terminal illness

Acronyms

DABDA, VS

Understanding death as a normal part of life is a fundamental concept. Despite great advances in technology, medicine cannot cure every illness, and science has yet to be able to stop the aging process. All people eventually deal with the death of a loved one. As humans age, they also must face their own impending mortality. Nurses are likely to find themselves caring for dying individuals in many situations, including emergency rooms, acute care, in a hospice program, in a nursing home, or in a client's home. This chapter examines death as the final stage of growth and development. Chapter 59 discusses specific nursing care for dying individuals and their families.

THE DYING PROCESS

Dying is an intimate and unique process for each individual. The progression of experiences often follows a general pattern, but events do not always proceed in a predictable sequence. Table 14-1 provides an overview of the normal processes, the effects on the client and caregivers, and offers considerations for care of the dying client.

> **Key Concept**
> Death is one of the most profound emotional experiences humans encounter. Fear and anxiety are natural. A continuing challenge for many individuals is to resolve personal feelings about the processes of dying and the finality of death. As a nurse, you can become more comfortable with the concept of death by confronting your personal feelings.

End-of-Life Care

Specific acute situations, illnesses, or trauma affect the events related to the dying process. **Terminal illness** is a state in which an individual faces a medical condition that will end in death within a relatively limited period. During the months, days, or hours that occur during a terminal condition, *palliative care* is often incorporated into the treatment plan. **Palliative care** is a collaboration of client, caregiver, and family care focused on the treatment of symptoms for clients with serious illnesses, usually, but not always, associated with a terminal illness. Palliative care is appropriate for situations when death is the expected outcome of the disease or disorder. The goal of palliative care is to improve the quality of life by providing for relief of symptoms such as pain, nausea, anxiety, and depression. In contrast, curative treatments focus on recovery from one or more physical or emotional issues with the expectation of lengthening the lifespan. Palliative care is appropriate for many illnesses and can be provided simultaneously with curative care. Hospice care and palliative care are discussed in Chapter 100.

As natural death approaches, in a period called *active dying*, the role of the long-term caregiver changes. Previously, caregivers may have focused on medicines or treatments related to healing and recovery of specific disease-related issues. As the client enters the last phases of life, a steady decline toward death becomes notable, and the care given to the client must adjust to changing needs. The needs of the dying client vary according to the individual's condition. For example, a client with advanced cancer tends to show a steady decline toward death, whereas an individual who has had serious, chronic illnesses may have peaks and valleys of health that can give the inaccurate impression of recovery or cure.

TABLE 14-1 Nursing Considerations: Care of the Dying Client[a]

ASPECTS OF THE NORMAL PROCESSES OF DYING	NOTATIONS FOR CAREGIVERS	CONSIDERATIONS FOR CARE
Withdrawal from the external environment *Rationale:* Social withdrawal is common due to the fact that bodily functions, e.g., brain and organs, cease to function. Dying clients can lose interest in others. Some clients have a slow, steady decline toward death; others tend to have peaks and valleys giving the inaccurate impression of recovery.	• Clients may be less communicative • Conversation may be unintelligible • Many clients have an alert period preceding death that can last for an hour or up to a day • Dying processes are unique and not everyone follows a predictable sequence of events	• Always identify yourself • Speak clearly • Do not shout • Allow time for silence • Use gentle touch • Provide reassurance • Be aware that alertness periods are typically of short duration
Visions and hallucinations *Rationale:* Blood flow decreases to the brain and levels of consciousness change.	• Normal for the dying person to talk to someone that caregiver cannot see or hear • Often, not always, part of the dying experience • Commonly seem to talk to and to see loved ones who have died • Not necessary to reorient to "reality," which can cause emotional distress	• Do not judge or be prejudicial • Identify self or others in room • Remain supportive to client's comments • Caregivers can become more distressed than client
Loss of appetite *Rationale:* Blood flow decreases to organs which are shutting down. Nutrients are not required.	• Normal for the client to lose interest in food and drink • Ability to swallow becomes impaired • Choking, aspiration, or "clenched jaw" may be a result of forcing foods and fluid • Difficult for client to take oral meds	• Provide ice chips • Do not force food or fluids • Consider treatments for dry mouth (Biotene® gel, lozenges, spray, moisturizing liquids, etc.) • Use lip balm on chapped lips
Changes in bowel and bladder function *Rationale:* Normal for muscles to relax and release contents of bowel or bladder. It may not occur until late in the active dying process.	• **Incontinence** (loss of bowel or bladder control) and constipation not uncommon due to inactivity, decreased intake, and pain meds • Complications of bowel or bladder retention (**impaction**, infarction, and **incontinence**) can cause severe abdominal pain, vascular obstruction to colon, and death • Urine concentrates and becomes dark or tea-colored • Urinary catheter or use of protection (diapers) may be helpful	• Keep areas clean and dry • Monitor client for signs or symptoms of incontinence constipation, impaction, or infarction • Discuss care options with healthcare professional
Changes in vital signs (VS) *Rationale:* Blood is shunted away from extremities and organs. Blood pressure decreases to organs. VS change.	• Temperature fluctuations • Skin feels feverish, cool, warm, or moist to touch • Blood pressure, respiratory rate, and heart rate change • VS become irregular • VS rates decline; may be difficult to obtain or detect • Eyes may become glazed or tear	• Do not panic • Expect more changes • Avoid routine VS since they can cause unnecessary worry/concern • Ask the client if they want/need a blanket • Position client for comfort • Gently wipe the face and hands with moist cloth • Apply eye drops if needed for dry eyes
Changes in mental acuity *Rationale:* Causes may include reduced oxygen to the brain, side effects of medications, metabolic changes, or dehydration.	• Confusion, restlessness, and agitation are common • Client may be trying to obtain a sense of completion or resolve unsettled issues	• Provide a sense of security • Allow family, friends, and significant others to talk to client • Consider light massage or soothing music • Consider medical intervention for pain or anxiety

(Continued)

TABLE 14-1 Nursing Considerations: Care of the Dying Client[a] (Continued)

ASPECTS OF THE NORMAL PROCESSES OF DYING	NOTATIONS FOR CAREGIVERS	CONSIDERATIONS FOR CARE
Fatigue and sleep *Rationale:* Sleeping during most of the day and night is normal because metabolism slows. The body has less need for food or water, and dehydration occurs.	• Constant fatigue normal	• Allow client to sleep • Avoid abrupt noise or movement • Consider possibility that client is in pain
Changes in sleep–wake patterns *Rationale:* Higher brain functioning (thinking, reasoning) is shutting down. Client develops an increasing detachment from the physical world.	• Sleeps more • Fewer and shorter periods of being awake • May drift into and out of consciousness • May hear words and feel touch of hand • Unconsciousness tends to occur in the last hours	• Continue talking to client • Continue to hold client's hand • Keep room casually lit but not with bright light
Pain *Rationale:* Depending on the cause of death, pain may be severe or excruciating. Pain relief is beneficial and is commonly associated with a client who becomes more awake and alert after medication is given. Fatigue or withdrawal can be a result of unrelieved pain.	• May be seen as grimace, groans, yelling when touched, or a restless sleep • Client may not present any physical symptoms of pain but still have significant pain	• Ask client's perception of pain on 1–10 scale • Watch for signs of pain • Do not be prejudicial regarding treating pain • Use comfort measures (positioning, hot/cold packs, etc.) in addition to medication • Medicate for pain according to 1–10 pain scale • Notify healthcare provider if pain is not managed
Congestion in the lungs or throat *Rationale:* Secretions buildup in the back of throat as client has difficulty coughing or swallowing. Less oxygen is available to the brain and breathing centers.	• Normal phenomena • Can cause concern, distress in caretakers as it is associated with "death rattle" • May see **Cheyne–Stokes** breathing (repeating breathing patterns that are shallow and quick, to deeper and rapid, to periods of apnea)	• Do not panic • Raise head of bed (or use pillows) • Position body for better drainage from mouth • Wipe mouth using soft, moist cloth • Notify healthcare provider if secretions are severe or Cheyne–Stokes breathing occurs
Skin changes *Rationale:* Skin and organs receiving less blood and oxygen. Cyanosis and mottling occur as blood flow decreases. Changes start to occur in distal extremities and progress to proximal extremities. Gravity affects pooling of blood. Body core temperature fluctuates.	• **Cyanosis** (bluish coloring) and **mottling** (purplish-bluish blotches) noted • Skin on back, knees, hands, and feet become purple or deep blue • Near death, the skin may appear yellowish or waxen • Skin color changes may indicate that death is imminent	• Maintain physical comfort • Use light coverings • Consider a fan to circulate air (not directly onto client) • Use damp, cool washcloth when client is too warm or hot • Do not use electric blankets

[a]As death approaches, the role of the caregiver changes. Previously, the caregivers provide much physical assistance with activities of daily living (ADLs). As death approaches, more emotional care is needed, such as reassurance. Provide dignity and soothing actions.
Content of this table is adapted from WebMD, (2020). *What to Expect with Your Loved One Is Dying.* www.webmd.com/palliative-care/journeys-end-active-dying; Stanford School of Medicine. (n.d.). *Signs of impending death.* https://palliative.stanford.edu/transition-to-death/signs-of-impending-death/

The needs of each client typically vary from day to day. As death approaches, emotional support, reassurance, and pain relief become the caregiver's priorities. Table 14-1 reviews these processes.

> **Key Concept**
> Physical care and emotional care are two very different types of care. Physical care, usually some form of treatment, can be observed and quantified. Emotional care relates to psychological support; its effects cannot be measured and may seem less immediately obvious than those of physical care, but it is equally important to the well-being of the client.

Impact of the Dying Process

Often families and caregivers are coping with deep feelings of anticipated loss. The stress of the caregivers or the family should not be overlooked as it can be overwhelming. They are coping with deep feelings of anticipated loss and may not know how to approach their dying loved one. Efforts to appear hopeful and cheerful may appear nonsupportive or insincere. Be aware that not all family members can cope with death and the dying process. Each family member or caregiver will progress through the grieving and loss process, as discussed in the next section.

End-of-life Discussions and Advanced Directives

End-of-life discussions should take place as a routine, practical adult responsibility. If not discussed earlier, end-of-life plans should occur as soon as possible after a terminal diagnosis has been given. Thoughtful discussions need to include the goals of care and clarification of treatment options. For example, include issues regarding the goals of care and treatment options, which range from an overview of the needs for basic nutritional supplementation to the use of advanced life support.

The utilization of advance directives can be of great assistance to the dying client and their family. The wishes of the client are more likely to be followed if that individual has considered their own desires and ensured that these wishes are given in writing to physicians, family, and significant others. Without an advance directive, the healthcare provider or a family member may be given the responsibility to dictate life or death decisions. Often these decisions can result in feelings of guilt, self-doubt about making the "right" decision, and hostility among family members.

Relief of Pain

Caregivers want to be supportive, but they may not know the actions to take that will be of help. The relief of pain is an important palliative treatment. The use of opioid analgesics, narcotic pain medications such as morphine, are known interventions of palliative care. However, caregivers may be afraid to give medications that could be beneficial because of a rumored fear of addicting the client or causing the client's premature death due to medication overdose. Research in palliative and hospice care has documented the benefits of narcotics for pain relief for the terminal client (Lowey, 2020). Providing adequate pain medication can result in a client who has improved alertness because their physical body is not fighting pain. When the client is able to swallow, oral pain medications can be used. However, as the dying process evolves, the client may not be able to swallow; injections or intravenous medications are given.

> **Key Concept**
> The family should realize that crying or sadness in front of dying loved ones is acceptable. Such behavior can be therapeutic because otherwise the dying individual may feel that nobody cares.

Finances and Economic Concerns

Many aspects of caring for the dying client are related to the economics of healthcare. Financial concerns, such as cost of medications or specialized equipment, may become an increasing source of worry and stress. Daily events and routine concerns contain economic considerations. For example, groceries and food needs must be met for the client as well as other family members. Medical expenses, transportation to appointments, or temporary housing for out-of-town visitors may need to be addressed. Funeral or commemorative services can be costly. Some individuals prepay for finances related to funeral and burial services so that these costs do not affect the personal finances of caregivers or family members. Occasionally, accumulated stress becomes difficult for families to handle, resulting in increased conflicts and outbursts of emotion or domestic violence. Support from friends, neighbors, and coworkers can be helpful (Fig. 14-1).

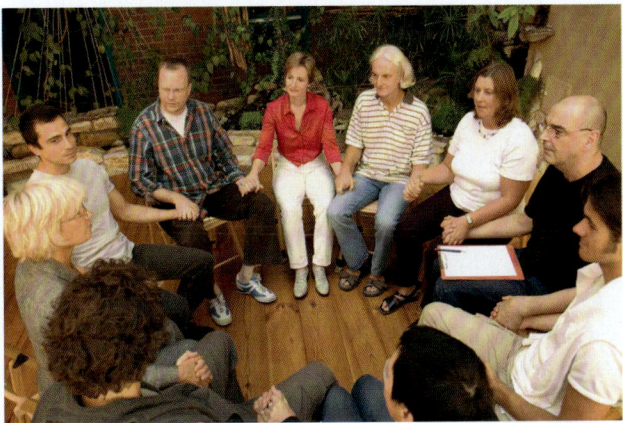

Figure 14-1 Support groups can help people work through their feelings of grief. (Craven & Hirnle, 2009.)

Children and Their Concerns

Families question how to handle death when children are in the family. Although very young children may be unable to express their thoughts clearly, they do grieve and need to be part of the family's mourning. Adults should talk honestly and clearly with children about illness and death when it occurs. Children should be allowed to see the body or attend the funeral (or both) if they wish to do so. Children who are dying should be told the truth and be allowed to ask questions.

> **SPECIAL CONSIDERATIONS** **Culture and Ethnicity**
>
> Cultural, ethnic, and religious beliefs help to shape people's attitudes toward death. The cultural context often determines the procedures related to death, dying, and after death care. Some cultures view death as an intensely personal experience, with families keeping most of their emotions and feelings within a private circle. Other cultures grieve openly. Box 14-1 lists the common practices of a number of cultures and religions.

KÜBLER-ROSS STAGES OF GRIEF AND LOSS

Dr. Elisabeth Kübler-Ross, a psychiatrist, has described certain phases through which a person may pass in an attempt to cope with impending death. Formerly referred to as the stages of death and dying, Kübler-Ross's traditional stages are more commonly associated with the stages of grief and loss. This is because the idea that grief, loss, and death have been identified as separate topics having similar phases of human behavior. In her development of the theories of grief and loss, Kübler-Ross is well known for her initiation of the terms *death, anger, bargaining, depression, and acceptance* (**DABDA**) which are discussed below. Table 14-2 reviews the stages of dealing with grief and loss.

Box 14-1 Traditional Religious Beliefs and Practices Related to Death

RELIGION	PRACTICES
Amish and Mennonite	Family cares for the body; funeral is often at home
Baptist	Prayer; communion; call pastor
Buddhist	Priest performs last rites and chanting rituals; cremation is common
Christian Science	Reader is called; no last rites; autopsy is forbidden
Episcopal	Prayer; communion; confession; sacrament of the sick
Friends (Quakers)	Individual communicates with God; no belief in afterlife
Greek Orthodox	Prayer; communion; sacrament of the sick; mandatory baptism
Hindu	Priest performs ritual of thread around neck or wrist; water is put in mouth; family cares for the body; cremation is common
Judaism	After death, a rabbi or designate cleanses the body
LDS/Mormon	Baptism required (adults); body is dressed in temple garments; call bishop/elder
Lutheran	Prayer; communion; call pastor
Muslim	Imam performs specific procedures for washing and shrouding body, with assistance of the family; body is buried facing Mecca
Pentecostal	Prayer; communion; call pastor
Presbyterian	Prayer; communion; call pastor
Roman Catholic	Prayer; sacrament of the sick; communion; mandatory baptism
Russian Orthodox	Prayer; communion; sacrament of the sick; mandatory baptism
Scientologist	Confession; visit with pastoral counselor
Seventh-Day Adventist	Baptism; communion
Unitarian	Prayer; cremation is common

Nursing Alert A key nursing intervention for the dying client is to be aware that physical care is enhanced by understanding the grieving process and augmented by providing emotional support during these phases.

Grief is common to all individuals; however, not all individuals experience grief in the same way. Nurses must be aware that there is no correct or right way to grieve; that is, there is no right or wrong way to experience the pain of grief, loss, or death. Nurses must also be aware that coping with the physical and psychological pain of this experience has the potential to be healing and to strengthen those going through this process.

Loss can include grief but does not necessarily have to include death. Loss can be related to any emotional suffering, such as the loss of health, the breakup of a relationship, or the loss of employment. Loss also includes the realization that one's personal ambitions will not or cannot be achieved. Maslow hierarchy of needs discusses the stages of life and potential losses. Chronic illness, such as depression, unrelieved pain, or diseases, such as Alzheimer's, are also associated with grief and loss.

All terminally ill people pass through some of these stages, unless death is instantaneous or the person is unable to resolve conflicts. The family also may pass through the same basic stages. These stages can overlap, and a person can go back and forth from one stage to another.

Key Concept
The Kübler-Ross stages of grief and loss typically also occur in individuals who are close to the person who has died or is expected to die. These stages have also been identified and used for many of life's situations.

Denial

Denial, the preliminary stage, occurs when the person does not believe that the diagnosis is correct: *This can't be happening to me.* During the stage of denial, the individual may seek advice from several doctors, hoping that one of them will offer a more acceptable prognosis. Because hope is maintained, the client is susceptible to unorthodox, illegal, or harmful ways of coping with a diagnosis.

Nursing Alert In caring for an older adult client who is dying, it is important to use the client's statements as clues to the client's stage of grief. A statement of "Why did this happen to me?" indicates that the client is in the anger stage of grief. In anger, the client asks "Why?" Conversely, a statement of "No, not me!" reflects the denial stage of grief.

Anger

In the **anger** stage, the individual is angry and may have periods of acting-out or rage. They may ask: *Why did this happen to me? Why now? Who is to blame?* Often, the individual envies the person who is young and healthy; they may lash out at family members or healthcare personnel. Sometimes, the person facing terminal illness is young, which brings

TABLE 14-2 Stages of Dealing With Grief and Loss

STAGE	TYPICAL TYPE OF GRIEF AND LOSS RESPONSE	SUGGESTIONS FOR CAREGIVERS
Denial Shock, statements of disbelief, often followed by a feeling of isolation	*No, not me!*	• Answer questions honestly • Allow the person to talk to physician • Do not argue
Anger Rage, acting out physically or verbally against family or health professionals	*Why me?*	• Listen • Do not take the client's anger personally • Do not get let yourself become angry
Bargaining Guilt and developing awareness of diagnosis	*Yes me, but...* *If I could just live until...*	• Try to assist in client's wishes • Encourage family support • Offer spiritual assistance from clergy or support groups
Depression Grief, sadness, and loneliness	*Yes, me.*	• Be there as sign of support • Listen • Only offer counseling or social service assistance if client requests assistance • Allow person to rest
Acceptance Self-reliance and a feeling of peace	*My time is close, and it's OK.*	• Provide physical care • Provide emotional support • Do not criticize or be judgmental • Keep room lighted if OK with client • Support family members

additional stress. The anger that the person is expressing generally is related to the feelings of hopelessness and of helplessness involved with the situation and not the actions of you, the nurse, or of others who are trying to help. When dealing with an individual who is facing terminal illness and seems angry, upset, or argumentative, it is helpful to understand that the person is probably reacting within the normal stages of death and dying.

Bargaining

Bargaining is a stage of developing awareness of the situation. An individual makes deals or bargains with God or with themselves: For example, *If I live just 2 more weeks, I can see my son get married.* The timeframe for this stage may be relatively short. When the bargained for time has passed, the person may make another such bargain, in the hopes of postponing death indefinitely.

Depression

Depression has been reached when the person realizes that they are going to die and that nothing can be done to stop it. The sentiment of this phase would be *I am so sad, I have no hope of recovery.* Unlike some forms of psychologically diagnosed depression, this stage and form of depression is considered a normal, healthy phase.

However, it may be beneficial for the client and, occasionally, family members to receive psychological therapy, including medication.

> **NCLEX Alert**
>
> Questions found on nursing examinations may include the definitions and concepts of Kübler-Ross. It is imperative that you learn to identify the stages, apply appropriate nursing interventions, and use effective therapeutic communication.

Nursing considerations related to depression include recognizing that the individual concentrates on past losses. You may assist by listening actively and making sure that pain is relieved. Beware of citing commonplace phrases such as *everything will be OK* or *the universe works in mysterious ways*. A touch of the hand is commonly helpful. Some people find comfort in remaining active, writing the story of their lives, or reminiscing on past experiences. False hope or encouragement are generally not meaningful or helpful nursing actions.

Acceptance

Acceptance, rather than depression, is demonstrated when the client wishes to plan for life after death or for their family after they die. The feeling could be summarized as saying *I am at peace with the diagnosis*. As an individual resolves emotional conflicts about death, they enter the stage of realization and acceptance of the inevitability of death. To reach this point, a person usually must have had time and assistance in working through the earlier stages. As dying persons resign themselves to death, they may seem devoid of all feeling. This time is particularly difficult for the family, who may interpret an individual's acceptance of death as a rejection of life and of them. The family must come to understand that the person will be unable to die comfortably unless the family helps the individual to give up everything associated with life. Although the dying person may be unable or unwilling to communicate, they usually will appreciate short visits or the presence of a family member.

Key Concept

Examining Kübler-Ross stages of grief and loss can help you understand a person's reactions to illness, stress, loss, or death. The stages of *denial*, *anger*, *bargaining*, *depression*, and *acceptance* are a range of normal reactions that clients may express. Never assume that a person should be in any one stage at a particular time. Individuals work through their grief in their own ways, moving back and forth from one stage to another and even skipping some stages. Your role is to be understanding and supportive.

STUDENT SYNTHESIS

KEY POINTS

- The physical and emotional progression of dying tends to follow a general pattern, but these events do not always proceed in a predictable sequence.
- Physical needs change as the client goes through the processes related to dying.
- Palliative care involves meeting emotional needs in a client with a terminal illness.
- Caregivers want to be supportive and to provide appropriate care but may need the nurse's assistance to show them how to relieve pain or to show emotional support.
- Kübler-Ross has developed a model showing five stages of grief and loss, which are common emotions seen during periods of significant life-changing events.
- The five stages of grief and loss include denial, anger, bargaining, depression, and acceptance.
- The client, caregiver, or family member may process these five major stages in any order and may revolve through these stages more than once.

CRITICAL THINKING EXERCISES

1. You are working with a person who is terminally ill. Discuss what you might observe in each of Kübler-Ross stages. How would you modify your behaviors and expectations for each of these stages?

2. Consider experiences that you have had with death among your family members or friends. Examine these experiences as closely as you can remember, and compare them with the stages that Kübler-Ross describes. What did others say that was helpful to you? Determine how you can build on your experiences to help others during your nursing career.

3. Describe how your spiritual beliefs would affect your responses in the following situations: a client who asks you to pray with them; a person who questions angrily why God allows them to suffer; an ill family member who asks you to help them to "end it all."

NCLEX-STYLE REVIEW QUESTIONS

1. A client diagnosed with terminal lung cancer states to the nurse, "I am okay with this. I have had a wonderful life and my family will be with me." Which stage of grief does the nurse recognize the client is experiencing?
   a. Denial
   b. Anger
   c. Bargaining
   d. Acceptance

2. The nurse enters the room of a client who was just informed of having an inoperable brain tumor by the physician. The client is throwing items off of the bedside table and yelling. Which action is the priority by the nurse?
   a. Inform the client that this behavior is not making the situation better.
   b. Inform the client that it would be best to get a second opinion.
   c. Understand that the client is reacting in the anger stage of grief.
   d. Call security and have the client restrained.

3. A terminally ill dying client begins to have visual hallucinations. Which nursing action is appropriate at this time?
   a. Orient the client to reality.
   b. Tell the client "You are hallucinating."
   c. Identify self and others in the room.
   d. Administer a sedative.

4. A dying client is not eating and only drinks small sips of fluid occasionally. Which action by the nurse is appropriate?
   a. Use a syringe to feed the client.
   b. Obtain an order for a nasogastric tube.
   c. Inform the client that life cannot be sustained without food and fluids.
   d. Do not force food or fluids.

5. The nurse hears a CNA talking with a client who is in the end stage of pancreatic cancer and depressed. Which statement made by the CNA does the nurse recognize as nontherapeutic?
   a. "Everything happens for a reason; it will be okay."
   b. "I will stay with you for a while."
   c. "What can I do for you?"
   d. "Is there anyone you would like me to call for you?"

CHAPTER RESOURCES

Enhance your learning with additional resources on thePoint!

Student Resources related to this chapter can be found at **thePoint.lww.com/Rosdahl12e.**

Structure and Function | UNIT 4

15 Organization of the Human Body

Learning Objectives

1. Define *homeostasis*; relate this to the study of anatomy/physiology.
2. Define *chemistry, physics,* and *matter.* State how these relate to homeostasis.
3. State the three types of matter and describe each of them.
4. Describe the basic organization of atoms, elements, compounds, and mixtures.
5. Differentiate between protons, neutrons, and electrons and their relationship to forming compounds.
6. Describe how an isotope differs from a normal atom.
7. Explain the difference between physical and chemical changes.
8. Demonstrate the ability to break down medical terms into the root, prefix, and suffix.
9. Define and differentiate among anatomy, physiology, and pathophysiology.
10. Demonstrate the anatomic position, describing its importance in healthcare. Differentiate among the sagittal, transverse, and frontal planes.
11. Define the following terms: superior, inferior, anterior, posterior, proximal, distal, ventral, and dorsal.
12. Describe the body's four basic structural levels, differentiating between them.
13. Identify the basic structural elements of the human cell, describing the functions of each.
14. Differentiate between RNA and DNA.
15. Compare and contrast mitosis and meiosis.
16. List four major types of tissue; give an example of each.
17. Identify the major organs in each body system.

Important Terminology

anabolism	compound	inferior	nucleus	quadrant	
anatomic position	cytoplasm	isotope	organ	sagittal	
anatomy	diaphragm	lateral	pathophysiology	superior	
anterior	distal	medial	physical change	system	
atom	dorsal	medical	physiology	tissue	
body cavity	electron	terminology	plane	transverse	
catabolism	element	meiosis	plasma membrane	ventral	
cell	enzyme	membrane	platelet	viscera	
cell membrane	eponym	metabolism	posterior		
chemical change	frontal	mitosis	proton		
chromosome	gene	mixture	protoplasm		
cilia	homeostasis	neutron	proximal		

Acronyms

DNA
ER
LLQ
LUQ
RBCs
RLQ
RNA
RUQ
WBCs

Normal anatomy and physiology are presented as a basis for your nursing course. By becoming familiar with these normals, you will learn to recognize abnormal deviations. The human body is a precisely structured arrangement of liquids, gases, and solids. The body is made up of atoms, molecules, and chemicals and is approximately 45%–75% water, depending on age and sex (Table 17-1). The body's chemical reactions result in specific independent, yet interrelated, actions, essential for normal body function. Nurses must be knowledgeable about these concepts because caring for clients involves recognizing deviations from normal. Also, the nurse must be able to recognize how alterations in one system affect other systems. Most healthcare is *interdisciplinary* in nature. Individuals working in some areas, such as the laboratory or pharmacy, use information related to the cellular, molecular, and chemical aspects of the body. Other individuals, including physicians, nurses, and therapists, focus more on body structures and normal and abnormal functioning of complete body systems. All healthcare professionals share a basic understanding of body structure and function and use common terminology when communicating. This chapter briefly introduces medical terminology, chemistry, and anatomy and physiology.

CHEMISTRY AND LIFE

Before beginning any course in life science, a basic knowledge of chemistry and physics is important. *Chemistry* is the science concerned with the structure and composition of matter and the chemical reactions these substances can produce. *Physics* is the science of the laws of matter and their interactions with energy (*Energy* = the capacity to perform work—potential [stored] or kinetic [active]). Types of energy include *chemical, electrical*, and *radiant*.

Chemistry is the basis for **homeostasis**, the dynamic interactions between anatomy and physiology. Homeostasis means physical and emotional *equilibrium* (balance) and involves an individual's cumulative chemical reactions, physical condition, and emotional status.

The discussion of chemistry begins with the description of matter. *Matter* is anything that occupies space and has weight. The three *types* of matter are elements, compounds, and mixtures. The three *states* of matter are solids, liquids, and gases.

Elements, Compounds, and Mixtures

All matter, living and nonliving, can be broken down into 92 natural and 20 manufactured elements. An **element** is a pure, simple chemical. Twenty-three elements are found in the human body. All elements have specific letter abbreviations, some of which are used in healthcare. Seven elements compose approximately 99% of human body weight. These elements are oxygen (O)—65%, carbon (C)—18.5%, hydrogen (H)—9.5%, nitrogen (N)—3.3%, calcium (Ca)—1.5%, phosphorus (P)—1%, and potassium (K)—0.4%. Elements found in very small amounts, but which are vital to human life, are sulfur (S)—0.3%, sodium (Na)—0.2%, chlorine (Cl)—0.2%, magnesium (Mg)—0.1%, iron (Fe)—0.004%, and iodine (I)—0.00,004%. Other elements found in trace amounts in the body are fluorine (F), chromium (Cr), manganese (Mn), cobalt (Co), copper (Cu), zinc (Zn), silicon (Si), selenium (Se), boron (B), and molybdenum (Mo) (Willis, 2018).

An **atom** is the smallest part of any element. Atoms are composed of *subatomic* (smaller than an atom) particles or structures. The main subatomic particles are protons, neutrons, and electrons. **Protons** (carrying a positive electrical charge) and uncharged **neutrons** or *nucleons* (carrying no charge—"neutral") are located in the nucleus (center) of atoms (with the exception of hydrogen). **Electrons** (negative charge) are much smaller than protons and whirl around the nucleus like a cloud. An atom of one element differs from that of another element due to the arrangement of its subatomic particles. A normal, electrically stable atom has an equal number of electrons, neutrons, and protons. It is considered to be electrically neutral. For instance, a hydrogen atom has one proton and one neutron within the nucleus, with one electron whirling around it in a random path. An oxygen atom has a nucleus containing eight protons and eight neutrons, with eight electrons whirling around it (Fig. 15-1). The number of protons plus neutrons determines the approximate *atomic mass* of the element. Thus, the atomic mass of oxygen is approximately 16. Each element has a distinct number of protons in its nucleus; this number is the *atomic number*. For example, hydrogen (H) has one proton in its nucleus; thus, its atomic number is 1. Carbon (C) is 6, nitrogen (N) is 7, and oxygen (O) is 8.

Each atom of an element always has the same number of protons. Since neutrons are neutral, they do not carry an electrical charge. However, the number of neutrons can be altered, changing the atomic mass and forming an **isotope**. Isotopes are important in nuclear medicine, for example, in treatment of cancer or diagnosis of disorders. (Since the atomic mass of an atom is its atomic weight, this number is altered in an isotope.)

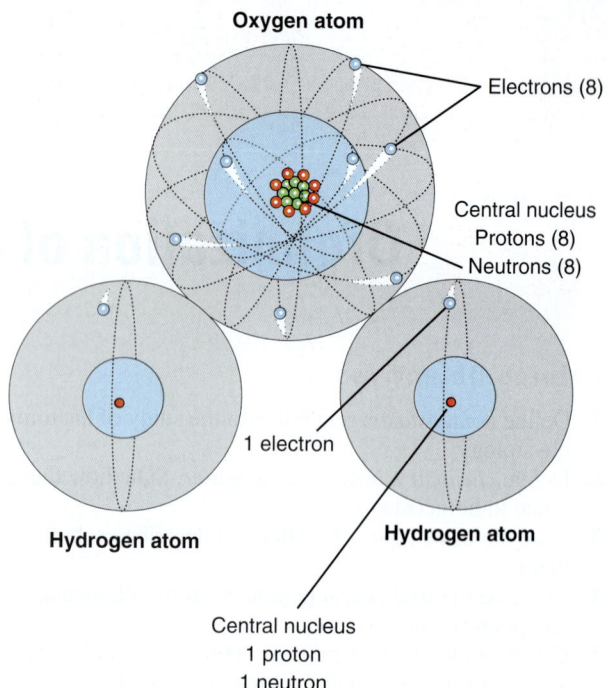

Figure 15-1 The compound water (H_2O). Note the structure of the oxygen and hydrogen atoms.

Atoms of one element are able to interact only with atoms of certain other elements. When atoms of two or more elements react *chemically* with one another, they form a substance called a **compound**. In every compound, elements combine in specific proportions. For example, the most common compound found on earth and in the human body is *water*. Water forms when two hydrogen atoms combine with one oxygen atom. The two hydrogen atoms each have one electron and one proton. The oxygen atom has eight electrons and eight protons, which because of its specific electrical charge, can combine with only two hydrogen atoms. In chemical shorthand, water is expressed as H_2O (two parts hydrogen to one part oxygen). Water is considered to be an *inorganic* (not derived from living matter) compound. *Organic* compounds are those that contain carbon or carbon–hydrogen combinations. They include carbohydrates (CHO), fats, and proteins. Most common in the body are sugars and starches (see Chapter 30).

Chemical reactions involve unpaired electrons in the outer ring of atoms. An element's *valence* refers to the number of unpaired electrons in its outer ring or shell. The valence allows this atom to combine with other elements in a precise order. Several types of chemical bonds exist (e.g., hydrogen, ionic, and covalent bonds), which are beyond the scope of this book. Several types of chemical reactions can occur. The formation of water is an example of a *synthesis* reaction (anabolism or "building up"). Other chemical reactions may break down a compound into its components: a *decomposition* reaction (catabolism—"breaking down"). An *exchange* reaction is a combination of synthesis and decomposition. Two compounds break down, and the resulting atoms reunite to form two new compounds. In a *reversible* reaction, a compound is reduced to its original elements, usually requiring an external force, such as heat (Willis, 2018). Not all elements or compounds combine chemically when brought together. A **mixture** is a blend of two or more substances that have been mixed together *without forming a new compound*.

Salt water (*saline*) is an example of a mixture. Both the salt (the *solute*) and the water (the *solvent*) remain as separate compounds. Their chemical composition is not changed. They can be brought together in any proportion, and they can be easily separated. (When water is used as the solvent in a mixture, this is an *aqueous* solution.)

Physical and Chemical Changes

If you lower the temperature of water (normally a liquid) so it freezes, it changes to a solid (ice); if you raise the temperature of the water so it boils, it becomes water vapor (steam, a gaseous state). The water has undergone a **physical change**, that is, a change in its outward properties. However, the chemical composition is still H_2O in any of the three states. *Its chemical structure remains unchanged.*

If you pass a direct electric current through a sample of water, however, a different change occurs. The water gradually disappears because electricity causes water to break down into its two invisible gaseous elements: hydrogen and oxygen. A **chemical change** has occurred. Familiar types of chemical changes are burning (combustion), rusting of iron (oxidation), and digestion of food in the body (a decomposition reaction). In chemical reactions, substances change into substances that now have different chemical structures. Completely rusted iron no longer has the characteristics of iron; burned wood is no longer wood, but ashes and gases.

> **Key Concept**
>
> *Physical change.* Outward properties change, but chemical properties remain the same (e.g., changes in temperature convert water into ice or steam).
>
> *Chemical change.* One substance changes to another, or the compound breaks down into atoms of elements, and its energy is transferred (e.g., an electric current breaks down water into hydrogen, oxygen, and heat).

MEDICAL TERMINOLOGY

To study body structure and function, an understanding of the vocabulary used in healthcare, **medical terminology**, is necessary. Because medical terminology is complex, it may be studied as a separate course.

Sources of Medical Terms

Determining the meaning of a medical term is easier when it is broken down into its components. Many medical terms have Greek or Latin roots. Common usage is another source of medical words. Some terms are *acronyms*, which are words formed by combining letters of a word or phrase. For instance, MASH stands for "mobile army surgical hospital." AIDS is an acronym for "acquired immunodeficiency syndrome." Many acronyms used in healthcare are listed in Appendix B (available online). **Eponyms** are words based on the names of people—for example, Parkinson disease or Alzheimer's syndrome.

Parts of Words

Most medical terms consist of two or three parts: prefix, root, and/or suffix. The *prefix* begins the word; and may or may not be present. The *root* of a medical term is the word's foundation. All medical terms have at least one root, which may begin the word. Appendix C, available online, lists prefixes and roots *followed* by a dash (e.g., intra-, hypo-, or sub-). The *suffix* is the word's ending. Most medical terms have a suffix. Appendix C lists suffixes *beginning* with a dash (e.g., -itis, -ic, or -pathy).

A combining vowel (usually o) joins a root to another root or to a suffix, for example, thermometer (therm = heat; meter = measuring device). Medical terminology texts list roots combined with a vowel; this form is known as the *combining form*. Examples of combining forms are *hepat-o* (pertaining to the liver), *oste-o* (pertaining to bone), and *neur-o* (pertaining to nerves).

Although the root is the core of the word, a prefix or suffix can totally change its meaning. A prefix introduces another thought or explains the root. For example, epigastric means "on the stomach," whereas hypogastric means "below the stomach." The suffix is added to clarify, to make a new word, or to change the meaning of the root. For example, tonsillitis means "inflammation of the tonsils," and tonsillectomy means "removal of the tonsils."

Prefixes, roots, and suffixes may be used in various combinations. Some words are a combination of two or three roots and connecting vowels. For example, electrocardiogram breaks down as follows: a record (suffix: -gram) of electricity (root: electr-) of the heart (root: cardi-). Note the two uses of o as a combining vowel: joining two roots, and joining a root and suffix. Therefore, electrocardiogram means "a record of the electrical activity of the heart." In comparison, an *electroencephalogram* is "a record of the electrical activity of the brain" because *cephal-o* means head or brain.

Medical terms are analyzed by breaking them into components. Start with the suffix, then the prefix, then the root. For example, *intravenous*: -ous (suffix) means "pertaining to"; *intra-* (prefix) means "within"; *ven* (root) means "vein." Thus, the word intravenous means "pertaining to within a vein."

> **Key Concept**
>
> Healthcare professionals use medical terminology to communicate assessment findings, diagnostic test results, and other pertinent information.

> **NCLEX Alert**
>
> Understanding medical terminology is important when answering NCLEX questions. Appropriate and effective communication, as well as coordination of client care, is demonstrated by correct knowledge of the language of medicine.

ANATOMY AND PHYSIOLOGY

The study of body *structure* is called **anatomy**. (Gross anatomy relates to structures that can be observed with the naked eye. Microscopic anatomy requires the use of a microscope or other device.) The study of how the body *functions* is called **physiology**. Nursing requires knowledge of body structure and of how these structures relate to and function with one another. Awareness of normal anatomy and physiology is essential to understanding abnormal conditions, such as disease or injury. The study of disorders in body function is called **pathophysiology**.

BODY DIRECTIONS, AREAS, AND REGIONS

Using the science of medical terminology, these terms can be applied to body structure and function. Areas and directions of the body are described in several ways. Using medical terminology helps to accurately specify the location of an organ or system and helps healthcare professionals to communicate with each other.

Anatomic Position

Medical texts often present the body from a standard reference point known as **anatomic position**. The body is pictured standing erect as shown in Figure 15-2. When viewing anatomic pictures or diagrams, the right side of the body is on the left side of the drawing (as when looking at a person facing you).

Body Planes

A body **plane** is an imaginary flat surface that divides the body into sections (see Fig. 15-2). The following are examples of body planes (imagined in the center or at another position):

- **Frontal** (*coronal plane*): the vertical plane that passes through the body longitudinally from head to toe, dividing it into front (**anterior**) and back (**posterior**) parts.
- **Sagittal**: the *vertical plane* passing through the body lengthwise. This divides the body into right or left sides; the *midsagittal* (median) plane passes through the midline from top to bottom, dividing the body into equal right and left halves. (Other sagittal planes may be parallel to the median plane and divide the body into unequal parts.)
- **Transverse**: the *horizontal plane* passing through the body at right angles to the **frontal** and sagittal planes, dividing it into upper (**superior**) and lower (**inferior**) parts. (This plane may also be referred to as the *transaxial* or *axial* plane.)

Body Position

In addition to viewing the body in terms of planes, the body is also described by the relationship of one body part to another. These are *body positions* or *body directions* (Fig. 15-3A and B). Body directions help describe locations of organs or body positions. Table 15-1 lists and describes body directions and positions.

Body Cavities

A **body cavity** is a space within the body that contains internal organs (**viscera**). The two groups of body cavities are the **dorsal** (posterior, back) and the **ventral** (anterior, front) (Fig. 15-4).

Subdivisions

The dorsal cavity is subdivided into cranial and spinal (vertebral) cavities. The ventral cavity is subdivided into thoracic and abdominal cavities. The thoracic cavity can be subdivided again into the pleural cavity (containing the lungs), the pericardial (containing the heart), and the mediastinum (containing large blood vessels and other structures). The **diaphragm** is a large muscle that separates the ventral cavities. Often, the abdominal cavity is subdivided again into the abdominal and pelvic portions or is referred to as the *abdominopelvic* cavity. (No specific anatomic division exists between the abdominal and pelvic areas.) Table 15-2 lists the contents of each body cavity.

The abdominal cavity can be divided into more precise areas containing specific organs by two different methods. The first method divides the abdomen into four **quadrants**,

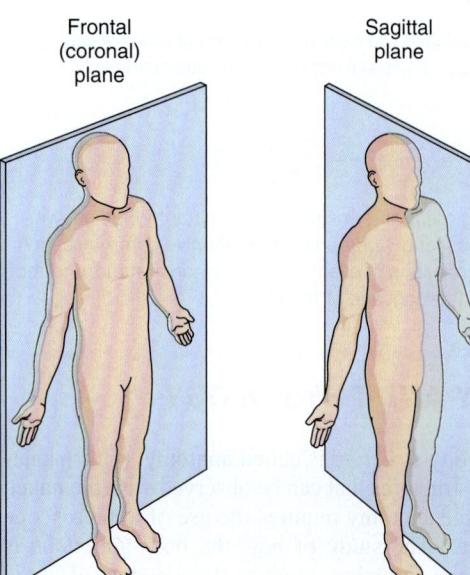
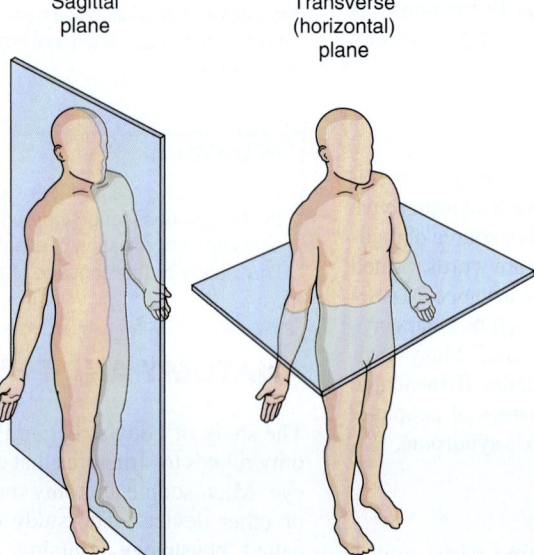

Figure 15-2 Body planes. The body is shown here in anatomic position.

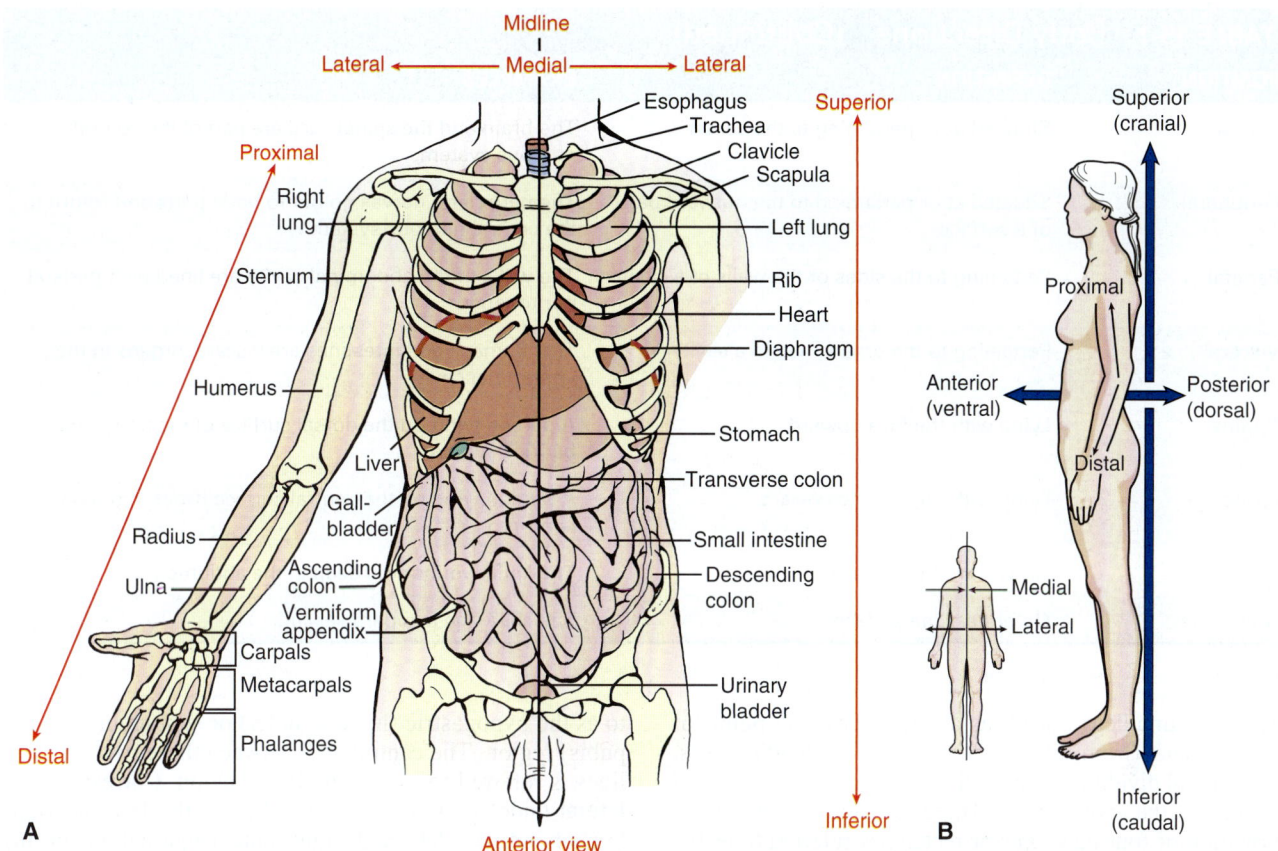

Figure 15-3 **A.** Body directions assist in describing the location of organs or body positions. **B.** Directional terms.

TABLE 15-1	Body Directions	
POSITION	DEFINITION	EXAMPLES
Superior	"Above" or in a higher position	The knee is superior to the toes, but inferior to the femur.
Inferior	"Below" or in a lower position	The lips are inferior to the nose, but superior to the chin.
Cranial	In or near the head	The brain is in the cranial cavity.
Caudal	Near the lower end of the body (i.e., near the end of the spine), "tail"	The buttocks are located in the caudal area.
Anterior (ventral)	Toward the front or "belly" surface of the body	The nose is on the anterior, or ventral, surface of the head. The palm of the hand is considered anterior when one is in the anatomic position.
Posterior (dorsal)	Toward the back of the body	The calf is on the posterior, or dorsal, surface of the leg.
Medial Inferomedial	Nearer the midline Nearer the feet, closer to the median	The nose is medial to the eyes. The medial malleolus of the ankle is inferomedial to the scapula.
Lateral Superolateral	Farther from the midline, toward the side Nearer the head, further from the median	The ears are lateral to the nose. The scapula is superolateral to the ribs.
Internal	Deeper within the body	The stomach is an internal body organ.
External	Toward the outer surface of the body	The skin covers the external surface of the body.
Proximal	Nearer the origin of a part	The area above the elbow is proximal to the forearm below.
Distal	Farther from the origin of a part	The area below the knee is distal to the thigh.

(Continued)

UNIT 4 Structure and Function

TABLE 15-1 Body Directions (Continued)

POSITION	DEFINITION	EXAMPLES
Central	Situated at or pertaining to the center	The brain and the spinal cord are part of the central nervous system.
Peripheral	Situated at or pertaining to the outward part of a surface	The peripheral nerves go out to body parts and return to the central nervous system.
Parietal	Pertaining to the sides or the walls of a cavity	The walls of the abdominal cavity are lined with parietal peritoneum.
Visceral	Pertaining to the organs within a cavity	The stomach and intestines are visceral organs in the abdominal cavity.
Supine	Lying with the face upward	A person lying on the dorsal surface of the body (the back) is supine.
Prone	Lying with the face downward	A person lying on the ventral surface (front of the body), is prone.
Deep	Away from the surface	The knife wound was deep in the abdomen.
Superficial	On or near the surface	The child had a superficial cut.

using the umbilicus (navel) as a central crossing point for the horizontal (from side to side) and vertical dividing lines. The vertical dividing line extends from the tip of the xiphoid process to the mons pubis. These divisions result in the formation of four quadrants or rectangles referred to as the right upper quadrant (**RUQ**), right lower quadrant (**RLQ**), left upper quadrant (**LUQ**), and left lower quadrant (**LLQ**) (Fig. 15-5).

The second method uses the costal (rib) margins and pubic bones as horizontal dividing lines for three major regions. The central area above the costal margins is referred to as the epigastric (epi = above; gastr = stomach) region. The central area below the pubic bones is referred to as the hypogastric (hypo = under) or suprapubic (on the pubis) region. The central area between these two dividing lines is referred to as the umbilical region. Corresponding **lateral** (side) regions are referred to as the left and right hypochondriac; left and right iliac (inguinal or groin) regions; and between these, the left and right lumbar (lateral or loin) regions (Fig. 15-6).

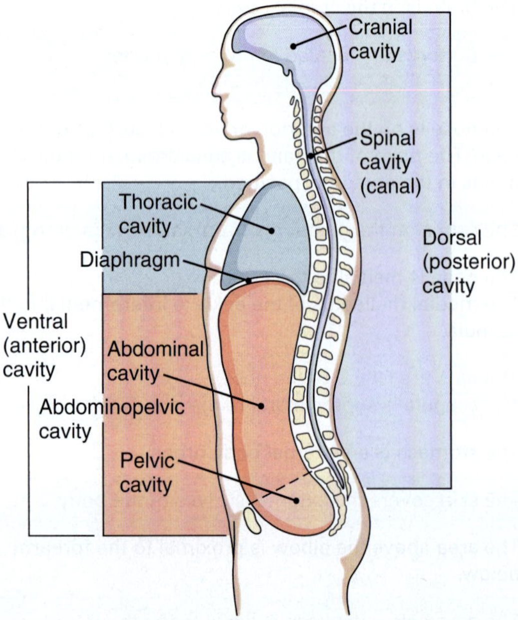

TABLE 15-2 Body Cavities and Their Contents

CAVITY	CONTENTS
Dorsal (Posterior) Cavity	
Cranial cavity • Oral cavity • Nasal cavity • Orbital cavity	Brain Mouth Nose Eyes
Vertebral (spinal) cavity	Spinal cord
Ventral (Anterior) Cavity (See Fig. 15-3A and B)	
Thoracic cavity • Pericardial cavity • Two pleural cavities Mediastinum	Heart Each contains a lung Large blood vessels, trachea, esophagus, and thymus gland
Abdominal (Abdominopelvic) Cavity	
• Upper abdominal cavity	Stomach, most of the intestines, liver, gallbladder, pancreas, spleen, kidneys, adrenal glands, and ureter
• Pelvic cavity	Urinary bladder, remaining part of intestines, rectum, and internal reproductive organs

Figure 15-4 Side view of the body cavities.

CHAPTER 15   Organization of the Human Body   161

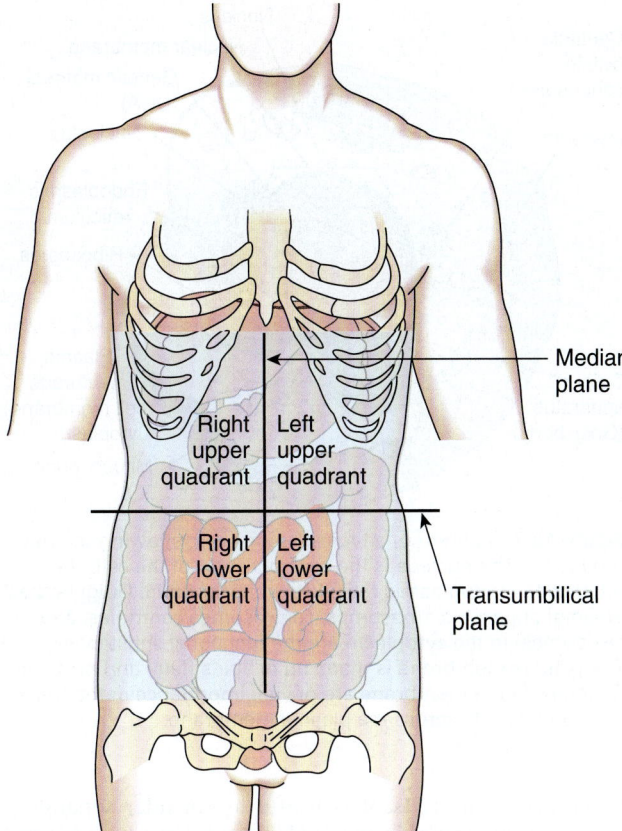

Figure 15-5 Quadrants of the abdomen, showing some of the organs within each quadrant.

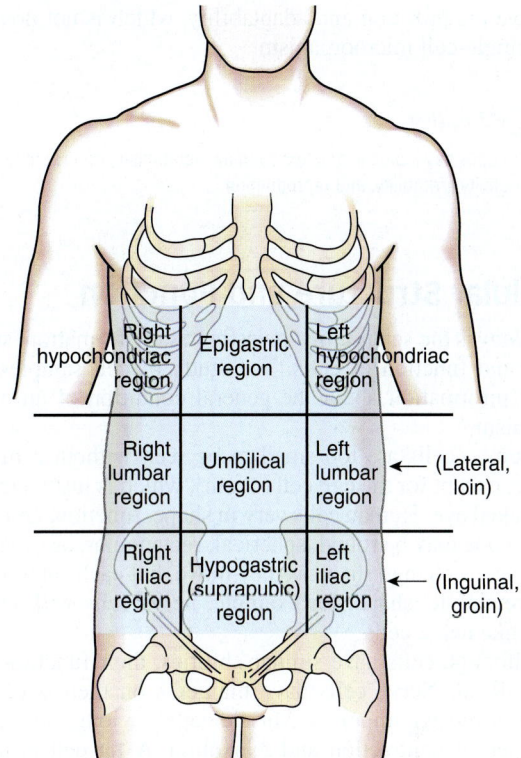

Figure 15-6 The nine regions of the abdomen (anterior view).

Laterality

Several terms relate to the sides of the body. *Bilateral* refers to both sides—for example, the kidneys and ears are bilateral. *Unilateral* refers to one side—the heart is unilateral. *Ipsilateral* means on the same side—the right leg and right arm are ipsilateral. *Contralateral* refers to opposite sides—for example, when using a cane, the cane is held in the hand contralateral to an injury.

STRUCTURAL LEVELS IN THE BODY

Four basic structural levels exist within the body:

Cells—the basic units
Tissues—made up of cells
Organs—made up of tissues
Systems—made up of organs

CELLS

The **cell** is the basic unit of structure and function in all living things. Each cell is alive and carries out specific activities. The smallest forms of life, such as bacteria, are composed of a single cell. The human body, on the other hand, is made up of trillions of cells. Although the human body has many different types of cells, all cells contain the same basic chemicals and similar structural features. Despite being the smallest living subunit of the human body, the cell functions as a member of a highly organized team.

> **Key Concept**
>
> The cell is the basic unit of structure and function for all living things.

Special Properties

As team members, cells are specialized in anatomic structure and physiologic function. Some cells have highly developed abilities for **metabolism**—the ability to process the chemicals found in foods to obtain energy and create new products. The two phases of metabolism are anabolism and catabolism. **Anabolism** is the building up, assimilation, or conversion of ingested substances. **Catabolism** is the breaking down, disintegrating, or tearing of substances into simpler substances. By virtue of the breakdown of substances, particularly food, energy is released.

Cells have other specialized properties:

- *Contractility:* Muscle cells can stretch or contract.
- *Conductivity:* Nerve cells are specialized to send and receive impulses.
- *Irritability:* Cells respond to stimuli.
- *Reproduction:* Cells duplicate themselves.

The properties of metabolism, contractility, conductivity, irritability, and reproduction are present to some degree in all human cells. However, an individual cell does not function independently. Rather, it develops specialties, interrelated with other cells. This teamwork permits the organism to have organization and adaptability, which is not possible in a single-cell microorganism.

> **Key Concept**
>
> Human cells have special abilities such as metabolism, contractility, conductivity, irritability, and reproduction.

Cellular Structure and Function

Cytology is the science that investigates the formation, structure, and function of cells. The study of cell samples can yield information about the general condition of an entire organism.

Human cells are too small to be seen without a microscope, except for the egg cell (ovum), which is just visible to the naked eye. Human cells vary in shape, function, and size. Cell shape may be round, spherical, rectangular, or irregular. Some cells change shape as they move, but each category of cell retains its shape; for example, nerve cells will always look like nerve cells.

Although cells have similar abilities, their functions are specialized. Nerve cells have filaments on their ends that carry or receive impulses. Muscle cells are long, thin fibers that permit contraction and relaxation. A fat cell is large, with empty spaces for storing lipids (fats).

Most cells vary in size from 1 to 100 micrometers (commonly referred to as a micron, abbreviated μ). A micron is one millionth of a meter or one thousandth of a millimeter (1 micron = 1/25,000 of an inch). Ten to 1,000 cells fit on the head of a pin, depending on the cell type.

Although minute in size, the complexity of cell structure is amazing, as shown in Figure 15-7. Collectively, all parts that make up a cell are called **protoplasm**. The cell parts can be divided into those in the nucleus and those in the cytoplasm (outside the nucleus). The cell's **nucleus** is its control center, responsible for reproduction and coordination of other cellular activities. The nucleus contains nucleoplasm and is surrounded by the *nuclear membrane* and houses the chromosomes and the nucleolus. Nuclear pores provide a means for the nucleus to communicate with the cytoplasm and to transport substances.

Cytoplasm is gel-like fluid inside the cell that is not located in the nucleus. It contains *cytosol*, a semitransparent liquid made up mostly of water and containing some salts and sugars. Structures in the cytoplasm are *inclusions*, such as melanin and glycogen, and distinct structures called *organelles*. Organelles include *mitochondria* (which produce adenosine triphosphate, an enzyme used for cellular energy), the *Golgi apparatus* (Golgi bodies, which process and package carbohydrate and protein), *lysosomes* (containing digestive enzymes), and *endoplasmic reticulum* (ER). **ER** is a network of tubules enclosed in a membrane and is made up of "rough ER" (which produces some proteins) and "smooth ER" (which contains enzymes to synthesize lipids [fats]). Also contained in the cytoplasm are *ribosomes* (sites of protein synthesis) and *centrosomes* (which contain centrioles and are active in cell division) (Table 15-3). Cytoplasm is the medium for chemical reactions; all functions for cell reproduction occur here. To simplify the study of the cell and the functions of its parts, it is useful to consider separately the structures found in the nucleus and those found in the cytoplasm.

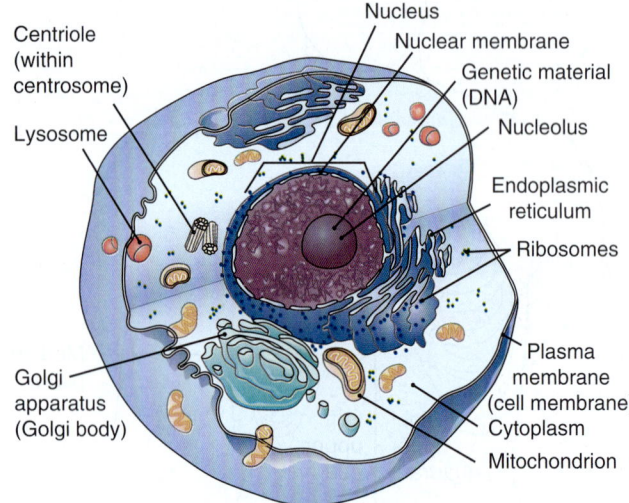

Figure 15-7 Diagram of a typical animal cell, showing the main organelles. The nucleus is the control center of the cell. The organelles (endoplasmic reticulum, mitochondria, Golgi bodies or Golgi apparatus, ribosomes, centrosomes/centrioles, and lysosomes) in the cytoplasm are the functional substances. The plasma membrane is made up of lipids (fats) and proteins. Channels in the membrane are of vital importance in the transport of materials across the plasma membrane.

Inside the nucleus is a structure called the *nucleolus* (plural: nucleoli). The nucleolus is composed of protein and threads of chromatin containing deoxyribonucleic acid (**DNA**, a double-stranded molecule), as well as ribonucleic acid (**RNA**, a single-stranded molecule). The nucleolus' function is not well understood, but it is involved in transfer of genetic material to ribosomes in the formation of chromosomes.

DNA is made up of nucleotides, which are linked to a sugar joined to a base (see Chapter 17). DNA bases include double-ring bases or *purines* (adenine and guanine) and single-ring bases or *pyrimidines* (thymine and cytosine). Purines bond only with pyrimidines. RNA transfers genetic information needed for protein synthesis to the ribosomes. Three types of RNA exist. *Ribosomal RNA* makes ribosomes in the ER, where the cell makes proteins. *Messenger RNA* directs the arrangement of amino acids to make protein after passing from the nucleus into the cytoplasm and attaching to ribosomes. (Messenger RNA is complementary to DNA, which has the instructions for synthesizing protein.) *Transfer RNA* is made up of short nucleotide chains, each specific to one amino acid. Genetic codes are transferred by transfer RNA from messenger RNA to the ribosomes to produce amino acids (Willis, 2018).

Chromosomes are made up of a complex of DNA, RNA, and protein and contain genetic material called genes. **Genes** contain information about inherited characteristics. These genes are carried on the chromosomes in single file. The human cell has 46 chromosomes. Therefore, as described above, DNA (Fig. 15-8) and RNA are key to the reproductive process. Cell reproduction will be discussed briefly later in this chapter.

TABLE 15-3 Cellular Parts and Their Functions

PART	FUNCTION
Parts Found in the Nucleus	
Chromosome	Carries genetic factors
Gene	Contains hereditary information found on the chromosome
Nucleoli	Globules that contain RNA and DNA
DNA	Stores and transfers genetic information
RNA	Chemical messenger that facilitates duplication of genes by DNA
Parts Found in the Cytoplasm	
Mitochondria (source of aerobic respiration)	Powerhouse of the cell—a double membrane; the *matrix* contains enzymes of the Krebs cycle to make energy (ATP); the *cristae cutis* (crista = sing) on the membrane's surface contain enzymes of the electron transport system
Golgi apparatus (Golgi body)	Synthesizes carbohydrates; modifies, concentrates, and transports proteins out of cell within round vesicles
Lysosomes	Sacs containing digestive enzymes to break down biologic materials (DNA, RNA, proteins, and some fats, as well as bacteria, damaged cells and worn-out organelles. Separated by membrane from rest of cytoplasm)
Endoplasmic reticulum (ER)	Extensive tubule network—*rough ER* synthesizes/transports proteins (mostly in liver and pancreas); *smooth ER* synthesizes and transports lipids and steroids
Ribosomes	Site of protein synthesis: some in endoplasmic reticulum and some free floating in cytoplasm
Centrosome	Plays role in cellular reproduction (mitosis) (The centrioles are contained *within the centrosome*)
Cell membrane	Maintains cell shape, protects cell, and regulates what enters and leaves the cell

The **cell membrane** or **plasma membrane** is the external wall of the cell and is a double layer of phospholipid cells with proteins randomly embedded. Substances soluble in lipids (fats) easily pass through (e.g., alcohol). Water passes through the protein-lined pores. The cell membrane surrounds the cell's outer boundary, provides shape, maintains the integrity of the cell, and is capable of selective permeability, meaning that it can regulate what enters and leaves the cell. (Chapter 17 addresses cellular transport, which is the movement of substances across membranes.) Some cells have **cilia**: hair-like threads that sweep materials across the cell surface. Refer to Table 15-3 for functions of cellular parts and to Figure 15-7 for their locations.

Cell Reproduction

Mitosis

Through a complicated process called **mitosis**, cells divide into two parts to reproduce themselves. Each "daughter cell" is an exact genetic duplicate of the original or "mother" cell. The human or animal body is a group of cells, and mitosis is responsible for growth, repair, and replacement of injured and dead tissues.

The amazing process of mitosis occurs as a result of a rearrangement of particles in the nucleus (Fig. 15-9). Briefly, two clusters of cytoplasm located near the nucleus separate and are drawn toward opposite ends of the cell (*metaphase*). The clusters split, and half of each moves toward opposite ends of the cell. The cell then begins to elongate, thinning in

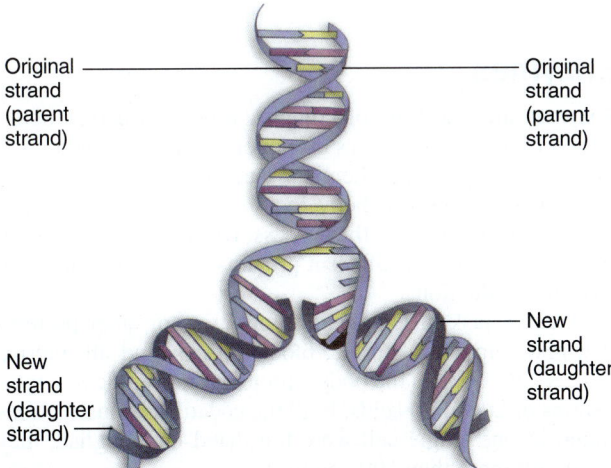

Figure 15-8 A DNA molecule (simplified), showing the double strands (double helix). Deoxyribose and phosphate groups make up the outer shell, and the nitrogen pairs (adenine and thymine, guanine and cytosine) make up the horizontal bars. When the cell divides, the double strands duplicate the original strands. (Willis, 2012.)

Interphase
During *interphase*, the nucleus and nuclear membrane are well defined, and the nucleolus is visible. As chromosomes replicate, each forms a double strand that remains attached at the center by a centromere.

Prophase
In *prophase*, the nucleolus disappears and the chromosomes become distinct. *Chromatids*, halves of each duplicated chromosome, remain attached by the centromere. Centrioles move to opposite sides of the cell and radiate spindle fibers.

Metaphase
Metaphase occurs when chromosomes line up randomly in the center of the cell between the spindles, along the *metaphase plate*. The centromere of each chromosome then replicates.

Anaphase
Anaphase is characterized by centromeres moving apart, pulling the separate chromatids (now called *chromosomes*) to opposite ends of the cell. The number of chromosomes at each end of the cell equals the original number.

Telophase
During *telophase*, the final stage of mitosis, a nuclear membrane forms around each nucleus and spindle fibers disappear. The cytoplasm compresses and divides the cell in half. Each new cell contains the diploid (46) number of chromosomes.

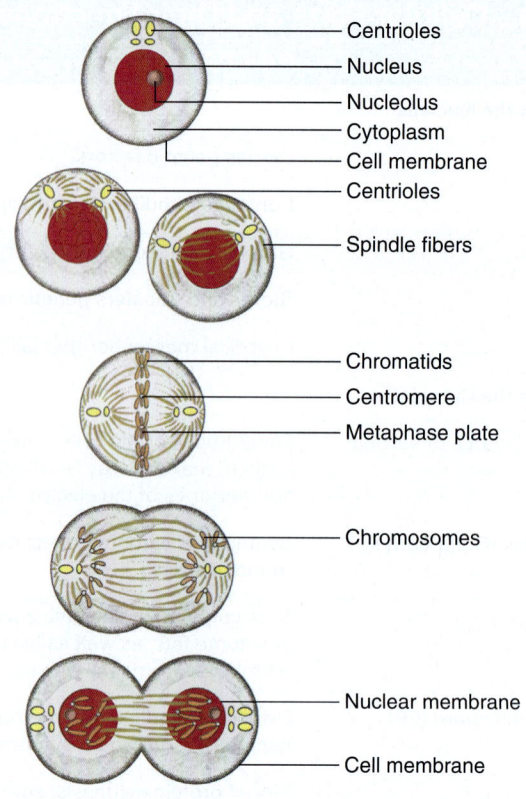

Figure 15-9 Stages of mitosis, through which the nuclear content of all body cells (except gametes) reproduces and divides. Two new daughter cells are formed, each containing the diploid (46) number of chromosomes. (The cell shown here is not a human cell.) (Willis, 2012.)

the middle with the plasma (cell) membrane following the same shape (*anaphase*). The cell finally splits into two parts, with half of the cytoplasm, nuclear material, and cell membrane in each new cell. Because of the genes, each new cell is identical to the original from which it was formed. This process is more complex in human reproduction. Mitosis is essential for the following:

- Growth of a single fertilized egg; after conception, the fertilized egg grows into trillions of cells and becomes an individual person or animal
- Repair of wounds by replacing damaged or dead cells
- Tumor formation in which abnormal cells, dividing by mitosis, result in more abnormal cells

Certain cells in the body cannot reproduce in an adult. Muscle cells or neurons (nerve cells) that die lose their functions. Loss of muscle cells in the heart due to a heart attack may damage the heart so severely that it loses the ability to contract effectively. Destroyed spinal cord neurons cannot reproduce, often causing paralysis and loss of sensation below the level of the injury.

Meiosis

Human sperm cells and ova reproduce by meiosis, a more complex process of cell division. In **meiosis**, cell division produces eggs or sperm that contain half the total number (23) of chromosomes (called a *gamete* or *germ cell*). Upon fertilization, the nuclei of an egg (ovum) and a sperm cell fuse, forming a *zygote* or fertilized ovum. This zygote now has the full complement of chromosomes (46 chromosomes) and continues to divide to create a human individual (see Chapter 65).

Enzymes

Enzymes are one type of complex protein structure determined by DNA. (Enzymes do not enter into chemical compounds, but speed up chemical reactions.) Every chemical reaction in the human body requires a specific enzyme to speed it up or facilitate the process. DNA directs the formation of thousands of different proteins to meet the needs of enzyme production.

Another task of DNA is the formation of other proteins that make up skin, muscle, blood vessels, and all internal organs. DNA builds the body's proteins from endless combinations of 20 amino acids. If all the coded DNA instructions found in one single cell were translated into English, they would fill more than 100 volumes.

> **Key Concept**
> Enzymes are complex proteins that speed up chemical reactions.

TISSUES

Cells of the same type and structure form **tissues**, each of which has a special function. The list below identifies the four principal types of human body tissues and their basic functions:

- *Epithelial tissue* protects body parts and produces secretions (see Chapter 16 and Box 16-1).
- *Connective tissue* anchors and supports other body structures (see Chapter 18). *Blood* is a special type of connective tissue that brings food and oxygen to the cells and carries wastes away (see Chapter 23).
- *Muscle tissue* provides movement of the body (see Chapter 18).
- *Nerve tissue* conducts impulses to and from all parts of the body (see Chapter 19 and Fig. 19-1).

Epithelial Tissue

Functions
The following are the main functions of epithelial tissue:

- Covers and protects all body surfaces (e.g., skin), cavities, and lumina (hollow portions of blood vessels or body tubes)
- Absorbs and secretes substances from the digestive tract
- Secretes substances from glands
- Provides filtration in the kidneys
- Forms highly specialized epithelial tissues in the taste buds and nose
- Transports particles contained in mucus away from the lungs

Generally, epithelial tissue is *avascular* (without blood vessels). To receive nourishment, this tissue must receive nutrients from underlying tissue, such as connective tissue, through a process called *diffusion* (see Chapter 17).

In places where epithelium is subject to much destruction, the tissue is modified to provide greater protection. For example, calluses form on the bottom of the feet or on the palms of the hands to withstand greater wear and tear. Because the outer layers of epithelial cells are constantly being worn off at the body's surface, the underlying layers of epithelium are continually producing new cells. Therefore, epithelium is in a continuous state of regeneration.

Types
Several types of cells make up epithelial tissue. Each type of cell has a characteristic shape and may be found in single or multiple layers (Table 15-4). *Simple* epithelium is made up of a single layer of cells. *Stratified* epithelium consists of several layers of cells. For example, simple squamous (scaly) epithelium can be found in single layers, as in the alveoli (air sacs) of the lungs, or can be stratified, as in the mouth and esophagus.

Transitional epithelium is a type of stratified squamous epithelium that can change shape (e.g., it enables the bladder to fill and stretch without damaging its walls).

Ciliated epithelium is a type of columnar epithelium containing cilia (hair-like threads). In a very effective protective mechanism, specialized cilia sweep mucus with trapped dust and bacteria away from sterile areas, such as the lungs, toward nonsterile areas, such as the trachea and mouth. Cilia are also found in the oviducts (uterine tubes) and help move the ovum toward the uterus.

Goblet-shaped epithelial cells (glandular epithelium) are able to form secretions. These cells are *glands* (see Chapter 20).

Connective Tissue

Different types of connective tissue vary greatly in structure and function. The main functions of connective tissue are:

- Support, bind, or connect other tissues
- Provide nutrients to all body organs and remove waste

TABLE 15-4 Types of Epithelial Tissue

DESCRIPTION	ILLUSTRATION
Simple squamous (basement membrane) tissue is found in the lungs.	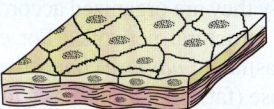
Simple cuboidal tissue is found in the ovaries, thyroid, sweat glands, and salivary glands.	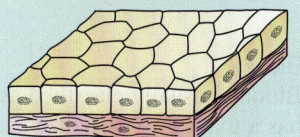
Simple columnar tissue is found in the stomach and intestines and in ducts of glands.	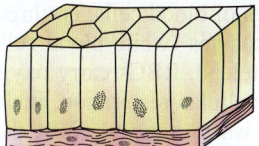
Pseudostratified columnar tissue (ciliated shown) is found in the mucous membranes of respiratory passages and eustachian tubes. It also exists in nonciliated form, which is found in the ducts of some glands, such as the parotid salivary gland and the male urethra.	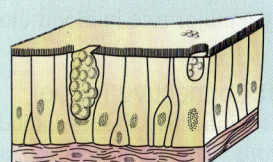
Transitional tissue lines the urinary bladder. It varies in shape, depending on whether the bladder is full or empty; when full, the cells slide and stretch.	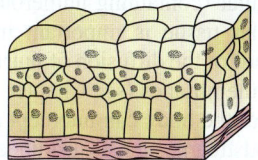
Stratified squamous tissue makes up the epidermis of the skin and the lining of the mouth, pharynx, ovaries, and vagina.	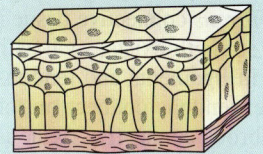

Types of epithelial tissue not shown include stratified columnar, which is found in the epiglottis, parts of the pharynx and anal canal, and the male urethra; and simple ciliated columnar, which is found in the lining of bronchi, the nasal cavity, the oviducts, and in the lining of the uterus.

- Store vital nutrients (e.g., fat or calcium)
- Provide protection for organs

The classification of connective tissues varies, but generally they are organized according to their specific *matrix* (type of structural network). For example, the matrix of *blood* is plasma; of *adipose* connective tissue, collagen fibers, and adipose (fat) cells. Bone has a matrix of tightly packed cells, rich in calcium. Cartilage is also considered a connective tissue.

Blood

Blood is usually classified as a connective tissue because it has a matrix of specialized cells, *plasma*, the liquid portion of blood. The major formed elements of plasma are the three types of blood cells: erythrocytes (red blood cells or **RBCs**), leukocytes (white blood cells or **WBCs**), and thrombocytes (platelets). RBCs carry oxygen and carbon dioxide needed for cellular respiration, including the formation of energy and waste removal. WBCs destroy pathogens and develop immunity to some diseases. **Platelets** are cell fragments that play a major role in blood-clotting (see Chapter 23).

Soft Connective Tissue

Soft connective tissues include *areolar* (loosely structured), *fibrous* (densely structured), and *adipose* (fatty).

Areolar tissue (loose connective tissue) is the body's most abundant connective tissue. It resembles packing material, holding structures in place. It provides support for body parts and allows for some stretching in all directions. It is highly vascular (containing numerous blood vessels) and therefore, areolar tissue is important in cell nutrition. It is perfectly suited for the diffusion of nutrients and waste materials across cell membranes (see Chapter 17). Areolar tissues are located where the body can intercept pathogens before they enter the bloodstream, such as just underneath the skin and beneath the epithelial tissue lining the digestive and respiratory tracts.

Fibrous connective tissue is found where a need for flexible strength exists, such as in the dermis layer of the skin and in ligaments and tendons. (Ligaments connect bone to bone; tendons connect muscle to bone.) The blood supply to fibrous connective tissue is poor; thus, it heals relatively slowly (see Chapter 18). *Elastic* connective tissue can stretch to one and one half times its original size. As with a rubber band, it snaps back to its original size. It is found in areas that are stretched on a regular basis, such as large arteries, the larynx (voice box), alveoli (air sacs), and external ear.

Adipose tissue is fatty. Located throughout the body, it stores fats (lipids) as a food reserve and serves as padding to protect body structures, such as the eyeballs and kidneys. It insulates against heat loss. Researchers state that most of our body's adipose tissue is formed prenatally (before birth) and during the first year of life. Although dieting and exercise may eliminate stored fat within adipose tissue, the adipose tissue itself remains, waiting to be restocked with new energy stores (i.e., new fat). Adipose tissue also secretes the hormone leptin, which reduces appetite.

Hard Connective Tissue

Hard connective tissue includes *bone* (the hardest connective tissue) and cartilage. Bone gives the entire body structure, support, mobility, and protection. Being well supplied with blood vessels (vascular), bone is the site of numerous metabolic activities, such as calcium storage. Some bones contain red bone marrow, which produces RBCs.

Cartilage is tough, elastic tissue found between segments of the spinal cord (vertebrae) and between the ends of long bones. Cartilage gives shape to the nose, larynx, and external ear. Between bones, cartilage serves as a shock absorber and reduces friction between moving parts. (Formation of most bones begins in the fetus with cartilage that later converts into bone [*ossification*].) Cartilage is poorly supplied with blood vessels; therefore, injured cartilaginous tissue heals slowly, if at all.

Muscle Tissue

Muscle tissues contain unique fibers that can contract (shorten) and relax, bringing about movement. Chemicals sent as stimuli to muscles from the nervous system supply the stimulus to contract.

Muscle tissue may be classified in several ways. It may be classified according to the following:

- Function—skeletal, smooth, and cardiac
- Appearance—striated (striped) and nonstriated
- What controls its action—voluntary or involuntary (Chapter 18 describes muscle tissue and its function in more detail.)

Nerve Tissue

Nerve tissue is composed of neurons and neuroglia. Its major characteristics are irritability and conductivity. *Neurons* are the actual working nerve cells that respond to stimuli. There are several types of neurons, but the two main types are *sensory* (afferent—toward the brain) nerves and *motor* (efferent—away from the brain) nerves. They send impulses to, and receive impulses from, all parts of the body (see Chapter 19).

> **NCLEX Alert**
>
> An understanding of the structure, composition, and functions of various tissues in the human body will help you choose the correct clinical nursing actions. The NCLEX requires you to differentiate between normal and abnormal anatomy and physiology.

Membranes

Membranes are sheets of epithelial or connective tissue that act together to cover surfaces, line surfaces, or separate organs or lobes (such as in the lungs). Some membranes produce secretions.

Epithelial membranes are subdivided into mucous and serous membranes. Connective tissue membranes are subdivided into skeletal and fascial membranes.

Epithelial Membranes

Mucous membranes (*mucosa*) secrete a substance called *mucus*. Mucosa line body cavities that open to the outside of the body. The mucus secreted by epithelial membranes lubricates and protects against bacterial invasion and other foreign particles.

Serous membranes (*serosa*) line body cavities that do not open to the exterior. These membranes secrete serous fluid, which is thinner than mucus. Serous fluid prevents friction when organs are in contact with one another. Serous membranes are divided into two layers: parietal and visceral. The *parietal* layer is attached to the body cavity wall; the *visceral* layer covers internal organs.

Connective Tissue Membranes

Skeletal membranes are connective tissue membranes that cover bones and cartilage. They act chiefly to support body structures. *Synovial* membrane lines freely moveable joint cavities and secretes *synovial fluid*, a lubricant that provides for smoother motion of bone, reducing friction between moving parts.

Fascial membranes are sheets of tissues that hold organs in place. The superficial fascia is a layer that connects the skin to underlying structures. Deep fascia binds muscles to tendons in order to anchor bones and separates muscles into functional groups.

ORGANS AND SYSTEMS

An **organ** is a group of different types of tissues that form in a specific manner to perform a definite function. For example, the heart is a combination of muscle, nerve, connective (blood), and epithelial tissues. Organs do not work independently, but are associated with other organs. Organs have many functions.

Groups of organs are called **systems**. Each organ contributes its share to the function of the whole. Systems do specialized work in the body, but all systems depend on one another. This book is organized in relationship to body systems (the *systemic* approach). An understanding of structure and function of body systems is the basis for all healthcare, including nursing. The remainder of this Unit discusses normal structure and function of body systems and their organs. Unit 11 describes and discusses deviations from this normal structure and function in children (pathophysiology) and disorders of adults are discussed in Unit 12. Table 15-5 lists body systems and their components.

> **Key Concept**
>
> Chapter 47 introduces the "head-to-toe" approach in data collection.
>
> It is important to remember that body organs and systems are *interdependent*. That is, they depend on each other for proper functioning. In general, a malfunction of one system of the body often causes malfunctions in other systems as well.

> **Key Concept**
>
> The body operates as an integrated whole. The optimum functioning of one body system usually depends on the functioning of other systems.

TABLE 15-5 Major Body Systems and Their Components

SYSTEM	COMPONENTS
Integumentary	Skin and its appendages (hair, nails, and sweat and oil glands)
Musculoskeletal	Bones, joints, and muscles that enable the body to move and give it shape
Nervous	Brain, spinal cord, and nerves that carry impulses and interpret them
Endocrine	Organs (thyroid, pituitary, adrenal, pancreas, ovary, testis) that produce hormones that regulate body functions
Sensory	Organs (eyes, ears, tongue, nose, skin) that supply the body with information
Cardiovascular	The heart, along with blood vessels and tissues that transport blood to and from all parts of the body
Hematologic and lymphatic	Blood and its components (including erythrocytes, leukocytes, platelets, and plasma) that carry oxygen, nutrients, and wastes to and from all parts of the body
Immunologic	Specific blood cells and lymphatic organs that help to prevent disease
Respiratory	Lungs and passages leading to the lungs that take part in oxygen and carbon dioxide exchange
Digestive	Organs (mouth, esophagus, stomach, intestines, liver, gallbladder, pancreas) involved in taking in and converting food to substances the body can use
Urinary	Organs (kidneys, ureter, bladder, and urethra) that rid the body of waste and water
Male reproductive	External sex organs and all related internal structures (penis, testes, vas deferens, epididymis)
Female reproductive	External sex organs and all related internal structures (vagina, oviducts, ovaries, uterus, vulva)

STUDENT SYNTHESIS

KEY POINTS

- The human body is made up of solids, liquids, and gases that function independently, but are interrelated.
- The study of the human body can be subdivided into the studies of anatomy (structure), physiology (function), and pathophysiology (disorders of body structure and/or function).
- Medicine has developed a sophisticated system of describing anatomy and physiology called *medical terminology*. To assist the learner, much of this terminology can be broken down into prefixes, suffixes, and root words.
- The body is described in terms of superior, inferior, dorsal, and ventral directions. It is also described in terms of transverse, frontal, and sagittal planes, and specific cavities containing viscera.
- An individual's physical and mental functioning is kept in equilibrium through dynamic interactions between anatomy and physiology (homeostasis).
- Substances are capable of undergoing physical changes in outward appearance or chemical changes with the transfer of energy and change in structure.
- The body can be described in terms of a single cell, which collaborates with similar cells in groups called tissues.
- Each cell is composed of many complex structures. Each structure has a specific duty that relates to the body as a whole. These include metabolism, contractility, conductivity, and irritability.
- Genes, the controllers of heredity, are found on chromosomes. Human cells have 46 chromosomes.
- Body cells replicate (reproduce) through mitosis. Sex cells (eggs and sperm) replicate through meiosis.
- The body is made up of four basic kinds of tissue: epithelial, connective, muscle, and nerve.
- The body is organized according to systems (groups of organs) that work together to perform certain functions that contribute to the overall workings of the body.

CRITICAL THINKING EXERCISES

1. Pick one body system and explain how its failure may affect other systems.
2. After listing the functions of the four types of body tissue, explain how these tissues complement each other.
3. A classmate is having trouble understanding the functions, structure, and properties of cells. How could you help this person to understand?
4. Using medical terminology, break down the following terms, determining their meaning: *myocarditis, atrioseptoplasty, bradycardia, mastectomy,* and *dermatitis.*

NCLEX-STYLE REVIEW QUESTIONS

1. The nurse is scheduling a tonsillectomy for a 10-year-old child. When explaining the procedure to the child and parents, which information should the nurse include?
   a. "The surgeon will be removing the tonsils."
   b. "The surgeon will make an incision and drain fluid from the tonsils."
   c. "The surgeon will incise the tonsils and pack them with antibiotic solution and gauze."
   d. "The surgeon will place a tube in the eustachian tube."

2. A client is diagnosed with a disorder that prevents impulses from transmitting to other parts of the body. The nurse may suspect the client has which disorder?
   a. Connective tissue disorder
   b. Nerve tissue disorder
   c. Muscle tissue disorder
   d. Epithelial tissue disorder

3. The nurse is caring for a client with a low platelet count. The nurse should monitor the client closely for which clinical manifestation?
   a. Inability for the blood to clot
   b. Infection
   c. Difficulty breathing
   d. Lethargy and weakness

4. A client is taking a medication that will suppress the immune response and decrease white blood cell production. The nurse should include which information in client teaching?
   a. Use an electric razor versus a straight blade.
   b. Stay away from crowds during cold and flu season.
   c. Hold direct pressure to the area if a cut or laceration is sustained.
   d. Report difficulty with daily activities and shortness of breath.

5. A client states to the nurse, "I can't get rid of the fat around my abdomen." Which response by the nurse is best?
   a. "Diet and exercise may eliminate stored fat but fat tissue will still remain."
   b. "You should try targeting the abdominal muscles when you exercise."
   c. "You may be on the wrong type of diet plan."
   d. "Intermittent fasting will help eliminate the stored fat."

CHAPTER RESOURCES

Enhance your learning with additional resources on thePoint!

Student Resources related to this chapter can be found at thePoint.lww.com/Rosdahl12e.

16 The Integumentary System

Learning Objectives

1. Describe the structures and main functions of the skin.
2. Explain the functions of keratin and melanin.
3. Identify the structures and functions of a fingernail or toenail.
4. Compare and contrast the functions of sudoriferous and sebaceous glands.
5. Define radiation, convection, evaporation, and conduction; give an example of each.
6. Explain the mechanism and purpose of "goose bumps" ("goose flesh").
7. Discuss the skin's role in sensory awareness.
8. Name five changes that occur in aging skin.
9. Describe four ways to protect the skin from damage.

Important Terminology

alopecia, carotene, cerumen, collagen, conduction, convection, corium, cutaneous, dermis, desquamation, diaphoresis, epidermis, evaporation, freckles, friable, hair follicle, hemoglobin, hypodermis, integument, integumentary, keratin, melanin, nevus, pores, radiation, sebaceous glands, sebum, skin turgor, squamous, subcutaneous tissue, sudoriferous glands, thermoregulation, transdermal, vitiligo

Acronyms

Hb or Hgb, SPF, UV

The skin (*integument*) and its accessory structures form the body's **integumentary** (covering) system. Because skin covers the entire outside of the body, it is the *body's largest organ*. The skin of an average adult covers 1.5–2.0 m^2 (16.1–21.5 sq ft) and is about 2–3 mm (0.1 in.) thick. The skin is an *organ* because it is composed of a variety of tissues, each of which has a specific purpose. (Tooth enamel is considered part of the integumentary system and is discussed in Chapter 26.)

The skin contains several types of epithelial tissue, partially responsible for its protective and absorptive functions. Epithelial tissues not only cover the surface of the body; they line body cavities and form some glands. For example, a single layer of squamous epithelial cells attached to a membrane lines the heart and lymphatic and blood vessels.

Glands in the skin provide internal secretions to the external world. Other types of related tissues include connective tissues (attach skin to underlying muscle) and nervous tissue, integrated throughout the skin to help the body react to the world around it (sensations of heat, cold, pain, touch, vibration, and pressure). In addition, the integumentary system depends on other tissues, organs, and systems. The skin and its accessory structures create a dynamic surface for communication between internal and external forces.

> **Key Concept**
> The integumentary (covering) system is composed of the skin and its accessory structures: hair, nails, and glands. Cutaneous means "of the skin."

STRUCTURE AND FUNCTION

Primary functions of the integumentary system are *protection*, *thermoregulation* (temperature regulation), *metabolism*, *sensation*, *communication*, and *storage* (Box 16-1). The skin produces substances that aid in protection and metabolism. Secreted oil provides waterproofing and protects the skin from drying and cracking. Perspiration helps eliminate waste products and helps in cooling. The skin has some absorptive powers, the basis for **transdermal** (through the skin) medications (see Chapter 63). Certain skin cells are also important components of the immune system, which helps fight off foreign invaders (see Chapter 24). A skin specialist is a dermatologist.

SKIN

The skin is divided into layers. The **epidermis** is the skin's thin, superficial outer layer. Below the epidermis lies a thicker layer, the **dermis**, which contains important structures: hair, glands, blood vessels, and nerves. The **hypodermis** (*subcutaneous [under the skin] tissue*), a single *fatty layer*, lies directly below the dermis. It is not actually part of the skin but is discussed here because it cushions, supports, nourishes, and insulates the skin and anchors skin to underlying tissues and organs (Fig. 16-1).

The Epidermis

The **epidermis** is the outermost, protective layer of the skin ("epi-" means over or upon). It is composed of **squamous** (scaly) epithelium, stratified into several layers (see Tables 15-4 and 16-1). The layers of the epidermis (from outside down) are the *corneum* (horny layer), *granulosum* (granular layer), *spinosum* (spinous layer), and *basale* (basal layer or *germinativum*) (see Fig. 16-1). In the palms and soles,

Box 16-1 Functions of the Integumentary System

PROTECTION
- Provides a physical barrier against microorganisms and foreign materials
- Helps prevent absorption of harmful substances from outside the body
- Defends against many chemicals
- Protects against water loss or gain
- Protects underlying structures, such as fragile organs
- Protects against excessive sun exposure (ultraviolet rays)
- Cushions internal organs against trauma
- Produces secretions for protection and water regulation
- Absorbs helpful medicines
- Prevents nutrients from being washed out of the body
- Serves as a containment structure to give shape and form to the body

THERMOREGULATION
- Controls body temperature by convection, evaporation, conduction, and radiation, as well as changes in size of superficial blood vessels
- Helps body adjust to external changes in temperature
- Helps dissipate heat during exercise
- Produces shivering and "goose flesh" to keep body warm in cool temperatures

METABOLISM
- Provides insulation (skin hairs, subcutaneous fat)
- Helps produce and use vitamin D
- Helps the body eliminate certain waste products
- Contributes to changes in cardiac output and blood pressure
- Absorbs gases; some oxygen, nitrogen

SENSATION
- Perceives stimuli: heat, cold, pain, pressure, touch, vibration, injury
- Provides social and sexual communication
- Allows for physical intimacy

COMMUNICATION
- Communicates feelings and moods through facial expressions
- Portrays feelings of anger, embarrassment, or fear (e.g., flushing, sweating, pallor)
- Communicates cultural and sexual differences through skin and hair color
- Portrays body image via skin's general appearance

STORAGE
- Stores water
- Stores fat
- Stores vitamin D

there is an outer layer called the lucidum or "clear layer." The outer layer of the epidermis, the *stratum corneum*, is relatively waterproof and provides a barrier against light, heat, bacteria, and other foreign substances. This layer is much thicker in some parts of the body, such as the soles of the feet, and thinnest in the eyelids. It contains all the dead cells from layers below. These cells are rubbed off constantly through washing and friction (**desquamation**).

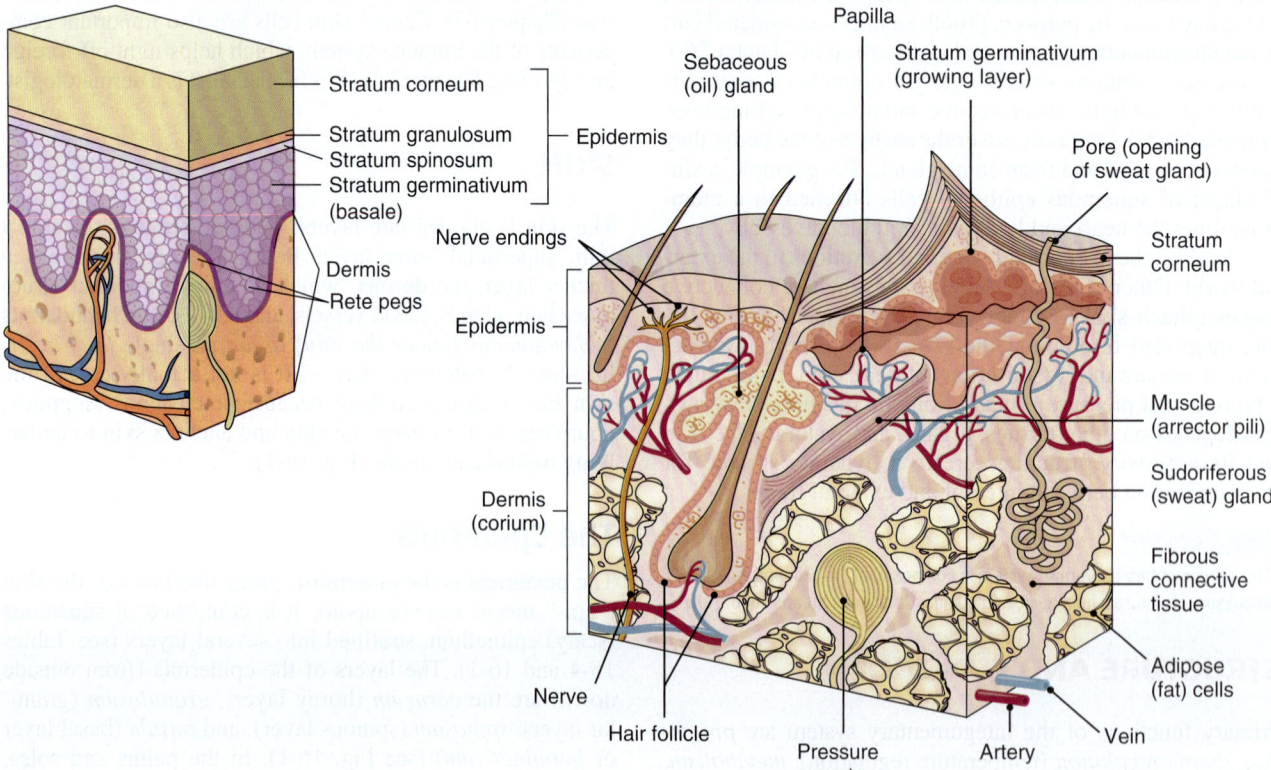

Figure 16-1 Cross section of skin structures.

TABLE 16-1	Principal Cells of the Epidermis
TYPE	FUNCTION
Keratinocyte	Produces keratin, which waterproofs and protects the skin
Melanocyte	Produces the pigment melanin
Langerhans cells (also called *nonpigmented granular dendrocyte*)	Provides immune response Participates in allergy response
Merkel cells	Promotes sensation of touch

Key Concept
Every minute, the human body loses 30,000–40,000 cells (about 9 lb per year)!

All that is left of skin cells after desquamation is a fibrous protein, **keratin**, which creates a waterproof barrier and is the body's true protector. It prevents most microorganisms from penetrating unbroken skin.

The innermost layer of the epidermis, composed of living cells, is the *basal layer, stratum basale*, or *stratum germinativum*, indicating its role in germinating new cells. Here in the deepest level of the epidermis, mitosis (division/replication of cells) occurs. Most epidermal cells are *keratinocytes* (Table 16-1), which divide in the basale and push older cells toward the body's surface. Thus, the living inner epidermal cells continually replace the outer cells. It takes between 2 and 6 weeks for the outer layer to be totally replaced. (Other epidermal cells are *Merkel cells* [Merkel discs], involved in the sense of touch; and melanocytes and Langerhans cells, both of which are discussed below.)

Melanocytes are cells within the epidermis that, through a

Key Concept
Damage through the basale, extending to the dermis (such as in a second- or third-degree burn), takes longer to heal because the damaged skin has lost its mitotic (reproductive) structures.

complex process, create the pigment melanin. **Melanin** gives color to hair, skin, and other structures. Also within the epidermis are *Langerhans cells*, part of the skin's immune system. They help detect foreign substances, in order to defend against infection and are also involved in skin allergies.

The epidermis has no nerves or blood supply (avascular) and does not receive nourishment directly from the circulatory system but receives nutrients and oxygen by diffusion from the underlying dermis, via tiny finger-like projections called *rete pegs*. The epidermis and dermis do not lie flat on one another. The rete pegs extend down from the epidermis and up from the dermis, increasing the contact between these layers. The projections cause ripples or ridges on the skin surface, particularly visible on the tips of the fingers (fingerprints, see Fig. 16-1). These ridges help provide some friction, in order to grasp objects.

Sometimes external friction causes a separation between the epidermis and dermis, leading to tissue fluid accumulation (blister). Areas of greater friction, such as the soles of the feet and palms of the hands, cause the epidermis to thicken and develop *calluses* (lucidum).

Key Concept
A callus can also develop from repeated use, such as the fingertip calluses that form after repeatedly playing a steel-stringed guitar.

SPECIAL CONSIDERATIONS Lifespan

Wrinkling of Skin
Wrinkles occur due to loss of elastic fibers and collagen in the skin, thinning dermis, and loss of oil (sebum). Oilier skin wrinkles less. Cigarette smoking causes faster destruction of elastic fibers and can lead to wrinkle development at a younger age. Exposure to sun and genetics are other factors causing wrinkling.

The Dermis

The dermis, the **corium**, is the "true skin." It is the thickest skin layer, composed entirely of live cells. The dermis nourishes the evolving epidermis via blood and lymphatic vessels. The dermis also contains loose connective tissue, to cushion and protect the delicate nerve endings and blood vessels within it. Like the epidermis, the dermis is layered, with the upper layer (*papillary layer*) containing blood and lymph vessels, nerve endings, and apocrine glands. Deeper in the dermis are hair follicles, sweat (sudoriferous) glands, and oil (sebaceous) glands. The dermis also contains elastic tissue (elastin) as well as fat, collagen, and fibrin. The *reticular layer*, deep within the dermis, is much thicker and is attached to the subcutaneous tissue.

Key Concept
Mechanoreceptor nerve endings provide the senses of touch and heat.

Several types of connective tissue (matrix) are found in the dermis. The major one is **collagen** ("colla" means glue), a tough, resistant, and flexible fibrous protein. The dermis also contains elastic fibers. In youth, collagen is loose and elastic. Collagen hardens and loses elasticity with age.

The Subcutaneous Tissue

The **subcutaneous tissue** (*hypodermis*, *fatty layer*, or *superficial fascia*) lies beneath the dermis and above a layer of muscle. Its purpose is to attach the epidermal and dermal layers to underlying organs and help cushion, protect, and hold these structures in place. It is a heat insulator and specializes in the formation and storage of *lipocytes* (fat cells). The amount of fat stored depends on the body region and an individual's age, sex, and nutritional state.

Key Concept
Since fat is stored in subcutaneous tissue, the thickness of the tissue is greatly influenced by a person's nutritional status.

Skin ligaments extend through the subcutaneous tissues and attach the dermis to deep fascia, which does not contain fat. It forms bundles that envelop and divide muscles into groups or compartments (*intermuscular septa*). An injury can cause dangerous swelling and compression within this intermuscular space (compartmental syndrome) (see Chapter 77). The deep fascia also contains other structures that support tendons and allow structures to move by preventing friction.

Skin Color

A combination of three pigments produces normal skin coloration: melanin, carotene, and hemoglobin.

Melanin is the brown–black pigment produced by *melanocytes*, found mostly in the stratum basale. People of all races have the same number of melanocytes. Individual differences in skin color depend on the amount of pigment the melanocytes produce. This is a reflection of genetics and exposure to ultraviolet (**UV**) light. Sun exposure causes extra melanin production, helping to protect the body from damaging effects of UV light and causing the skin to darken (tan). The skin also contains DNA-repair enzymes that help reverse UV damage. If the genes for these enzymes are absent, or if the DNA is damaged, a person is more susceptible to skin cancer, the most dangerous form of which is malignant melanoma.

Albino individuals are born without the ability to produce melanin. A person with true albinism has totally white hair and skin. This person's eyes look red due to the absence of pigment in the iris and the reflection of blood vessels in the eyes.

> **SPECIAL CONSIDERATIONS** **Culture and Ethnicity**
>
> The skin of black people has more variation between parts of the body than does the skin of people of other racial groups. This is partially due to variations in skin thickness. In addition, darker skin can hinder penetration of UV rays and may lead to a deficiency of vitamins, including vitamin D.

Freckles are patches of melanin clustered together. "Liver spots" (age spots) are also clusters of melanin, forming flat, brown-to-black, freckle-like patches as a person ages. **Vitiligo** is a skin condition in which the melanocytes stop making melanin, causing distinct, localized areas of white on the skin. A *mole* (**nevus**) is a circumscribed area on the skin; it may be raised. Moles may be dark or flesh-colored. Moles usually do not represent an abnormality, but any changes that occur to an existing mole should be brought to the attention of a healthcare professional.

> **Key Concept**
>
> Damaged skin often forms a scar. This area is often depigmented or discolored.

Carotene is a yellowish pigment found in parts of the epidermis and dermis. It is the precursor to vitamin A, which helps maintain epithelial tissues, promotes proper growth of skeletal and soft tissues, and is necessary for night vision. Carotene tends to be more abundant in the skin of Asian people.

Hemoglobin is the pigment in red blood cells. Oxygen binds to hemoglobin (**Hb, Hgb**) and is carried by the red blood cells. Although hemoglobin is not a pigment in the skin, the bright-red color of oxygenated blood flowing throughout the dermis gives a pinkish tone to the skin, which is more noticeable in light-skinned people.

ACCESSORY STRUCTURES

The hair, nails, sebaceous (oil) glands, sudoriferous (sweat) glands, and ceruminous glands are the main accessory structures (appendages) of the skin.

Hair

Hair derives from the subcutaneous fatty layer and covers almost all the skin except for a few areas, such as the lips, palms, soles of the feet, and penis. Dense hair covers the scalp, axilla, and pubis in adults. Male hormones are responsible for the greater density of hair on men's entire bodies and influence their ability to grow facial and chest hair.

Hair is composed of keratinized cells. The visible, but dead, portion of hair above the skin is the *shaft*. The part lying below the skin is the *root*. Each hair grows from a tiny sac or bulb within a **hair follicle** (see Fig. 16-1). The dermal layer provides nutrients for growing hair. Sebaceous glands provide a substance, *sebum*, which gives hair its shine and provides some waterproofing. (Topical hair care products do not affect hair growth, only the general appearance of visible hair.) Hair grows slowly (approximately 1 mm every 3 days). Each follicle contains a single hair root, which, as long as it is alive, will continue to grow a hair. Normally, there are about 100,000 hair follicles on the adult human head.

Baldness (**alopecia**) is related to disease, high fever, emotional stress, surgery, pregnancy, starvation, chemotherapy, radiation, or heredity. The male hormone, testosterone, contributes to *male pattern baldness* in men. Healthy women rarely become totally bald, although they may experience thinning hair with age. (Hair loss in chemotherapy is related to hormonal influences and interference with DNA synthesis.)

> **Key Concept**
>
> The adult human has about 5 million hairs, about the same number as a gorilla, although human hair is finer and shorter. All humans lose about 50–100 hairs daily; each hair is pushed out by the growth of a new hair.

Hair color is due to the type and amount of melanin in a layer of hair. The greater the amount of melanin, the darker the hair. Red hair is due to an iron-based pigment, *trichosiderin*. Curliness of hair depends on the shape of the hair follicle. Straight hair is round, growing out of a round follicle. Curly hair bends—its cross-section is oval, and it grows out of an oval follicle.

Surrounding each hair follicle are small, smooth muscles called *arrector pili* (singular: *arrectores pilorum*). Stimulated by cold or fear, these involuntary muscles contract, making the hairs stand erect. This phenomenon gives the skin the appearance of "goose flesh" or "goose bumps"—the *pilomotor reflex*. These erect hairs provide an "air cushion" for the skin—a protective, insulating body mechanism. (In animals, this makes the animal look larger and more threatening.)

 SPECIAL CONSIDERATIONS **Lifespan**

Melanin in Hair
As people age, they lose melanin, and their hair appears gray; with a total loss of melanin, hair appears white.

> **Box 16-2 Functions of Hair**
>
> - Helps regulate body temperature
> - Provides protection in various areas
> - Enhances sensation
> - Contributes to regrowth of damaged epidermis through stem cells in a portion of the hair follicle
> - Can reveal facts about the condition of the body
> - Can be used for identification: the DNA in hair is unique to an individual

The primary function of hair is protection (Box 16-2). Scalp hair protects against sunlight and insulates against cold. Eyelashes and eyebrows have the distinctive purpose of keeping dust particles and perspiration out of the eyes. Nostril hair protects against inhaling objects, such as foreign particles or insects. Hair in the ear canal serves a similar purpose.

Clinically, hair can reveal several adverse conditions. A hair sample can reveal environmental exposure to heavy metals, some drugs, or poisons much more accurately than a blood specimen. Hair texture can also reveal an individual's nutritional status. A sample containing hair follicles or roots yields DNA and therefore can be used for identification purposes.

SPECIAL CONSIDERATIONS Culture and Ethnicity

There are ethnic variations in the normal amount of body hair a person has, with people of Mediterranean descent, for example, having more body hair and people of Scandinavian and Asian descent having less.

Nails

Nails are tightly packed cells of the horny layer of the epidermis and help protect the sensitive tips of fingers and toes. They also help a person grab and pick up objects. The nail is made up of keratinized dead cells (Fig. 16-2).

Nail growth occurs in the nail matrix. New cells push older cells away from the nail bed at a rate of approximately 1 mm per week. A fingernail lost through trauma takes about 3–5 months to regrow, and a toenail takes about 12–18 months to regrow. A nail will continue to regrow as long as the live cells in the nail bed remain undamaged. Abnormalities in nails are shown in Figure 47-11.

SPECIAL CONSIDERATIONS Nutrition

Effects of Diet on Skin, Hair, and Nails
Healthy skin, hair, and nails depend on a well-balanced diet. Protein and vitamin deficiencies cause skin and hair to become dull, dry, and flaky. Minerals such as iron, copper, and zinc are necessary for prevention of abnormal skin pigmentation and changes in hair and nails (DiBaise & Tarleton, 2019). Starvation can cause excessive hair loss and nail deformities.

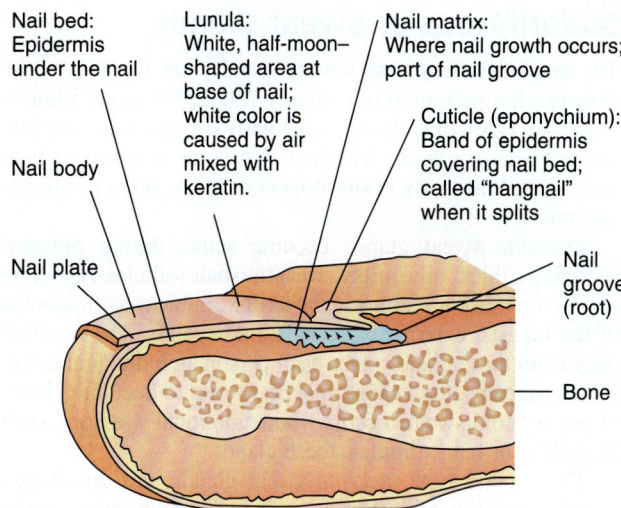

Figure 16-2 Parts of a fingernail.

Nails normally reflect a pinkish tone because of rich vascular areas in the fingers. When gentle pressure is applied and released, the nail becomes lighter white but quickly returns to a pink color. Unhealthy nails or slow blood return may point to poor circulatory status, several nutritional deficiencies, and emotional conditions.

> **Nursing Alert** Nail-biting is often a nervous habit. Caution clients against nail-biting, because it can lead to serious infections.

Sebaceous or Oil Glands

The **sebaceous glands** (oil glands) lie close to the hair follicles, into which they usually drain (see Fig. 16-1). **Sebum** is the oily secretion of these glands; it travels to the surface of the skin through hair follicles. Sebum helps make the skin soft and hair glossy. Sebum prevents drying of the skin, thereby protecting it from cracking. Cracked skin can lead to infection and can allow foreign substances to be absorbed. Sebum also helps waterproof the top layer of the epidermis (*stratum corneum*). Sebaceous secretions increase at puberty. Sebum may trap bacteria in the pores, causing inflammation or infection ("pimples" or acne).

> **Key Concept**
>
> When the arrector muscles cause the "hair to stand on end," this compresses sebaceous glands, increasing sebum production.

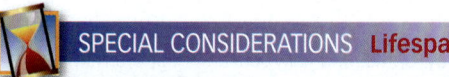
SPECIAL CONSIDERATIONS Lifespan

Sebaceous Glands
Aging decreases sebum production; therefore, older skin is transparent, dryer than youthful skin, and more fragile (**friable**). This is due to flattening of epidermal and dermal skin layers and thinning of dermal layers, which predisposes an older adult to skin damage.

Sudoriferous or Sweat Glands

The **sudoriferous glands** (sweat glands) are located in the dermis. One inch of skin contains 750–2,000 sweat glands. The three types of sudoriferous glands are apocrine, eccrine, and mammary glands. The first two types respond to heat and stress. Your body is sweating constantly, often in minute amounts.

Apocrine sweat glands become active during puberty, secreting a thick, oily, milky sweat into hair follicles. Apocrine glands are most numerous in the axillae, pubic region, areolae of the breasts, external ear canals, and eyelids. The nominal odor from these glands gives each person an individual scent. Skin surface bacteria cause apocrine sweat to become odoriferous. A "cold sweat" occurs when emotional stressors, such as anxiety or fear, stimulate these glands.

The second type, *eccrine* sweat glands, are distributed widely over the body but are especially numerous on the upper lip, forehead, back, palms, and soles. (There are no eccrine glands on the lips themselves or on the glans penis.) Eccrine glands secrete sweat into numerous ducts that empty into **pores** (tiny holes in the skin) and respond to external and internal heat. Perspiration (sweat) is nearly 100% water, with trace amounts of urea, uric acid, salts, and other elements. The primary function of perspiration is to assist in body temperature regulation by providing a cooling effect. Perspiration also moisturizes the skin and excretes wastes through the pores. In some diseases, the skin increases its capacity as an excretory organ, which may be a sign of pathology. (**Diaphoresis** refers to excessive perspiration.)

> *Key Concept*
> When sweat joins with sebum, the secretion is a thick, sticky, protective film. This film on the fingers helps a person to pick up items.

Mammary glands secrete milk and are a third, specialized type of sudoriferous gland. Chapter 29 discusses these glands in greater detail.

Ceruminous Glands

Ceruminous glands secrete **cerumen** (ear wax) and are specialized glands found only in the skin of the external auditory meatus, the passage leading into the ear. They function to protect the tympanic membrane (eardrum), which is essential to hearing. Excessive cerumen may impair hearing and promote infection in the ear canal. The moisture content of cerumen varies somewhat among people of different ethnic backgrounds.

SPECIAL CONSIDERATIONS   Culture and Ethnicity

Cerumen
Dry cerumen (gray, brittle, and flaky) occurs most often in Native Americans (84%), Alaska Natives, and people of Asian descent. The remaining populations have wet cerumen (dark brown, moist, and sticky). This occurs most often in people of African (99%) and European descent (97%). Do not confuse these differences with physical disorders. For example, flakes of cerumen can be mistaken for the dry lesions of eczema or psoriasis (Andrews, Boyle, and Collins, 2020).

SYSTEM PHYSIOLOGY

Although the integumentary system has many functions, protection is very important.

PROTECTION

The skin and accessory structures guard the body from invasions by pathogens and other foreign substances. It also protects the body by retarding body fluid loss, assisting in heat regulation, and excreting waste products. The Langerhans cells are a component of the adaptive immune system.

THERMOREGULATION

The integumentary system, in combination with the lungs, is also responsible for regulating and balancing the body's internal temperature, a process called **thermoregulation**. The body's temperature must remain fairly constant (around 98.6 °F [37 °C]) for all other systems to function properly. Body temperature is an indicator of the physiologic status of a person's body. An important nursing technique is accurate body temperature measurement. Body heat is lost through four processes: radiation, convection, evaporation, and conduction (Table 16-2). The skin conserves heat through shivering and "goose flesh" and gives off heat via the sweat glands. All of these thermoregulation mechanisms are the body's attempt to maintain homeostasis (balance).

SPECIAL CONSIDERATIONS   Lifespan

Preventing Heat Loss in Infants and Newborns
Very young infants do not have the ability to shiver in order to produce heat. They are also susceptible to heat loss via all four mechanisms of heat transfer, particularly evaporation, because of their large body surface area in proportion to size. This is most true immediately after birth. To prevent excessive newborn heat loss, keep the infant away from drafts, and place him or her in a temperature-regulated environment. Keep the infant dry and add clothing, especially a hat.

Mechanisms of Heat Loss

If the body becomes too warm, a message is sent from the hypothalamus in the brain. The dermal capillaries dilate (widen), and more blood flows to the skin surface. Because of the added surface blood, body heat is lost to the surrounding air by radiation, convection, evaporation, or conduction.

Radiation
People and animals give off infrared heat rays through **radiation**. A large percentage of a person's body heat is lost through uncovered skin.

Convection
In **convection**, heat is transferred and given off from the skin to the air. For example, an air current (e.g., a fan) can move warm air away from the skin's surface. (The body attempts to equalize its temperature with that of the environment.)

TABLE 16-2 Mechanisms of Heat Transfer

	RADIATION	CONVECTION	EVAPORATION	CONDUCTION
Definition	The diffusion or dissemination of heat by electromagnetic waves.	The dissemination of heat by motion between areas of unequal intensity.	The conversion of a liquid to a vapor.	The transfer of heat to another object during direct contact.
Example	The body gives off waves of heat from uncovered surfaces.	An oscillating fan blows currents of cool air across the surface of a warm body.	Body fluid in the form of perspiration and insensible loss is vaporized from the skin.	The body transfers heat to an ice pack, causing the ice to melt.

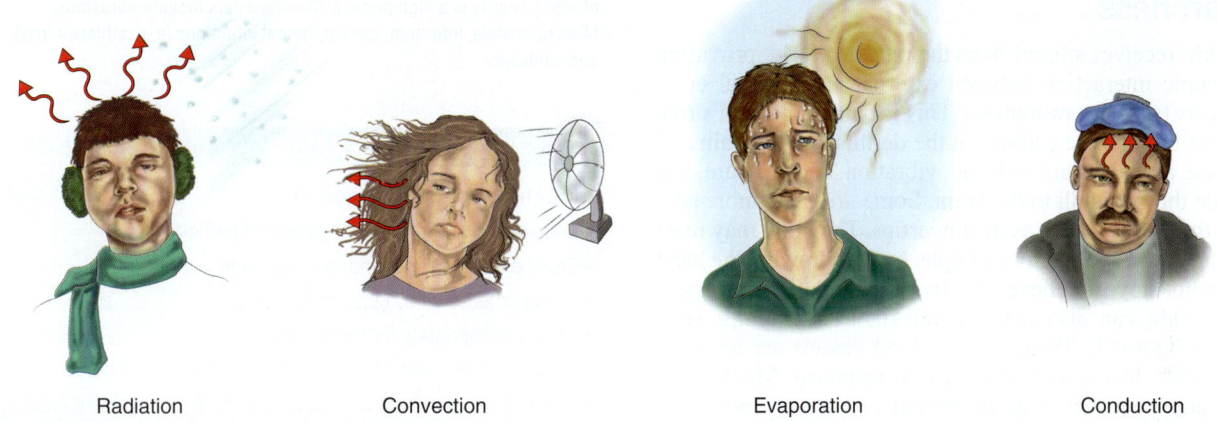

Radiation   Convection   Evaporation   Conduction

From Taylor, C., Lillis, C., LeMone, P., & Lynn, P. (2008). *Fundamentals of nursing: the art and science of nursing care* (6th ed.). Wolters Kluwer Health/Lippincott Williams & Wilkins.

Evaporation

Evaporation is the returning of water to the air through vapor, which causes cooling. Water on the body's surface can be perspiration or water from an outside source, such as a shower. The body normally loses about 500 mL of water per day due to insensible (unnoticed) evaporation. Too much water loss can lead to dehydration.

> **Key Concept**
> In a burn, the skin's control of evaporation is lost, causing excessive fluid loss.

Conduction

Conduction, the transfer of heat from one object to another by direct contact, is the least important mechanism in the transfer of heat away from the body; however, within the body, a large amount of internal heat is transmitted by conduction to the skin via blood vessels. When the body comes in contact with a cooler object, it transfers heat away from itself. For example, a cool cloth on the forehead can help a person feel cooler on a hot day. Table 16-2 summarizes the mechanisms of heat transfer.

Mechanisms of Heat Production and Conservation

Blood vessel constriction, shivering, and "goose flesh" are thermoregulation processes that help warm the body. When the body becomes too cool, dermal capillaries constrict (narrow), reducing the amount of heat lost through the skin. This constriction of superficial capillaries also causes the skin color to change from its normal color to a more pale color. The reflex action of shivering helps produce added heat, and goose flesh raises the hairs in the skin to provide insulation (see Fig. 16-1). The more subcutaneous fat a person has, the better the body's ability to insulate itself. If a person has excess subcutaneous fat, it will be more difficult for that person to remain cool in a hot environment.

> **Nursing Alert** Vasoconstriction in the extremities can cause pallor (whiteness) and coolness of the skin. *Cyanosis* (red–blue coloring) is a condition caused by *hypoxia* (lack of oxygen in the tissues) or *hypothermia* (severe decrease in body temperature).

VITAMIN D PRODUCTION

The skin plays a role in the body's production of vitamin D, important for bone growth and repair. It facilitates calcium and phosphorus absorption from the small intestine. Vitamin D is produced in the skin when stimulated by sunlight (UV light); then, via enzymes in the body, it is changed into *calcitriol* (*calciferol*), which plays a role in calcium absorption. Vitamin D also assists in retention of certain other vitamins. Chapter 30 describes the role of vitamin D in nutrition.

SPECIAL CONSIDERATIONS Lifespan

Vitamin D Deficiency

Lactase, the enzyme needed to break down the milk sugar lactose, decreases with advancing age, resulting in milk intolerance (lactose intolerance) for some older adults. Decreased intake of irradiated milk (milk into which vitamin D has been forced) accompanied by limited sun exposure increases the risk of vitamin D deficiency in older adults. Bone loss (due to inability to metabolize calcium) is one consequence of vitamin D deficiency.

Communication and Sensory Awareness

The skin receives stimuli from the outside world, providing a dynamic interaction between external and internal environments (sensory awareness). This is part of the skin's role in protection. Nerve endings in the dermis register pain and pleasure, as well as hot and cold, vibration, and pressure, and provide these stimuli to the brain. Some areas are more sensitive than others, such as the fingertips. The body may react with a reflex response, for example, by withdrawing the hand from a hot stove. (Reflexes are discussed in later chapters.)

The skin can also detect comfortable sensations, such as a loving touch. The skin and blood vessels are involved in foreplay, lovemaking, and sexual response. Much communication between a newborn and its parents comes via touch. Nurses also use therapeutic touch in client care. Communication also occurs through facial movements and changes in skin color. For example, blushing usually changes the skin color to a redder or darker hue. A smile is understood by all people. Disorders of the skin and other structures of the integumentary system are discussed in Chapter 75.

> **Key Concept**
> The average square inch of the skin contains about 1,000 sweat glands, 20 blood vessels, 60,000 melanocytes, and more than 1,000 nerve endings.

> **NCLEX Alert**
> You should be aware of the primary functions of the integumentary system as they commonly relate to nursing care or actions, client safety, and infection control. The NCLEX may include scenarios related to the hazards of immobility, illness, or injury of one or more anatomical systems.

> **NCLEX Alert**
> Be alert to normal differences in the integumentary system. Changes throughout the lifespan will relate to the actions you take regarding safe and effective care.

SPECIAL CONSIDERATIONS Lifespan

The aging process produces significant effects on the integumentary system. Normal changes are influenced by heredity, dietary habits, drug or alcohol abuse, sun exposure, smoking, hydration level, and general health. See Table 16-3.

MAINTENANCE OF HEALTHY SKIN

The various functions of the skin (and related structures) make it a very important organ of the body. The skin requires nutrients and hydration to keep it functioning well. Sun exposure can be dangerous; excess exposure can cause burns, premature aging of the skin, or skin cancer. Recommendations for limiting exposure are given in the display below. Sunscreen with an **SPF** (sun protection factor) of at least 15 is helpful (see Educating the Client 16-1).

> *Key Concept*
> Skin is the first line of defense against infection. Therefore, maintenance of skin integrity is a high priority. Skin disorders include abrasions, blisters, rashes, infection, cancer, fungal infections (e.g., athlete's foot), and sunburn.

SPECIAL CONSIDERATIONS Lifestyle

- It is important to protect your skin.
- Keep skin clean, to prevent growth of pathogens.
- Clean and cover cuts and open wounds.
- Use cosmetics sparingly; remove daily.
- Dress appropriately for the weather.
- Eat a balanced diet; drink plenty of water and other fluids.
- Protect your skin from excessive sun; wear long-sleeved clothing and a hat, and stay in the shade. Skin cancer has been related to excessive UV exposure.

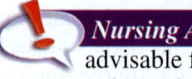 *Nursing Alert* The use of sunscreens is not advisable for infants younger than 6 months due to excess absorption.

IN PRACTICE
EDUCATING THE CLIENT 16-1 Sunscreens

Sunscreens are used to protect skin from the sun's UV rays. They can assist in prevention of skin cancers caused by sun exposure. The SPF determines the amount of UV rays reaching the skin. Most often, SPF 15 or 30 is used. Apply sunscreen thoroughly and evenly; cover completely. Reapply after sweating or swimming. Remember, even if the SPF factor is high, the amount of exposure time to the sun should be limited, to prevent sunburn. Read and follow the directions.

Consider allergies to sunscreen ingredients and consult a physician if taking medications. Sunscreen may cause problems for people with skin conditions, such as skin cancer, psoriasis, or lupus or for people undergoing radiation or chemotherapy.

It is important not to block all UV rays; cases of vitamin D deficiency have been reported in people who have no exposure to the sun.

TABLE 16-3 Effects of Aging on the Integumentary System

FACTORS	EXAMPLES OF RESULTS	NURSING IMPLICATIONS
Melanin is either lost or migrates and clusters in the epidermal layer	"Age spots" or "liver spots" (senile lentigo) result White areas (vitiligo) may appear	Reinforce self-esteem Discuss available makeup
Epidermal and dermal layers flatten. Skin becomes thinner. Glandular secretion decreases	Skin tends to tear ("fragile" or friable skin). More susceptible to skin breakdown and infection. Slower healing	Assess for skin tears Use caution in handling the older person
Capillary bed in dermis becomes more friable (fragile)—blood can ooze into dermis	Dark red patches in the skin (purpura) are commonly seen on arms of older adults Person may bruise easily	Be careful when handling the arms of clients with purpura Protect from bruising
Capillaries leak small amounts of blood into tissues	Petechiae occur (small red dots on the skin [senile angioma])	Explain to the person that makeup may be used
Individual may have loss of sensation	Person is unable to detect or treat the cause of ulcerated areas; pressure wounds may develop more quickly May be more susceptible to falls. May not sense heat or cold	Inspect skin frequently, especially bony prominences, arms, and feet Protect from falling Teach protective measures
Loss of elasticity in dermis, loss of subcutaneous layer of fat, and loss of collagen fibers	Wrinkles. Decreased strength of skin layer. Women's skin is thinner and dryer; thus, wrinkles appear earlier. Skin may sag	Discourage smoking and exposure to the sun Reinforce self-esteem
Skin turgor (tension or fullness) is lost	Wrinkles Pinched skin does not return to normal position. "Tenting" on some areas can give false-positive (for dehydration) results	Avoid using areas of skin that normally develop wrinkles for assessing turgor. (Do not use the back of hand; OK to use arm or leg.)
Some insulating function is lost with loss of subcutaneous fat	Heat is lost more rapidly. Older person may be chilly	Provide extra blankets or sweater Avoid chilling during treatments
Dermal layer thins	Skin becomes transparent and less elastic	Explain to client. Prevent injury
Changes occur in hair distribution, influenced by heredity and other factors. General loss of body hair occurs. Hair pigment (melanin) decreases	Axillary, pubic, and scalp hair thins Men may develop thicker hair in nose, ears, and eyebrows; hair on head becomes thinner Hair appears white or gray	Be careful when giving hair care Excess hair in nose or ears may be clipped carefully
Female and male hormones are lost	Women may develop facial hair (hirsutism) Males have decrease in beard and scalp hair (male pattern baldness)	Assist in removal of facial hair. Prevent injury
Nails grow more slowly and become thicker	Nails, especially toenails, become thick and brittle. May be malformed or discolored	Refer to podiatrist as needed Foot soaks may be needed
Glands in skin decrease secretions	Less perspiration and less oily skin than before; skin may become very dry (may appear scaly [senile keratosis]). Hair becomes coarser	Advise that daily shower or bath may not be needed (bath may dry skin more). Be sure skin is clean because skin is more fragile and more subject to breakdown. Use lotion as needed
Thermoregulation abilities lost	More susceptible to heatstroke or chilling	Teach individual to avoid overheating Observe in hot weather; encourage intake of adequate fluids
Circulation reduced Mucous membranes dryer; decreased number and output of sweat glands	Wound healing takes longer—old or damaged cells not readily replaced More difficult to maintain body temperature; painful intercourse (dyspareunia); dry eyes; dry mouth	Provide careful wound care. Prevent further injury. Refer to physician as needed Treat symptomatically

STUDENT SYNTHESIS

KEY POINTS

- The skin and its accessory structures (hair, nails, and glands) make up the integumentary system.
- The primary functions of the integumentary system are protection, thermoregulation, metabolism, sensation, and communication.
- The skin, the largest organ in the body, is vital for survival. The principal layers of the skin are the superficial epidermis and the deep dermis.
- The subcutaneous tissue (hypodermis) lies below the dermis and binds the skin to underlying muscle tissue. It is made up mostly of fat cells that insulate and protect underlying tissue.
- The epidermis is the outermost protective skin layer. It contains keratin, which protects the body from excessive water loss or gain, and melanin, which protects the body from ultraviolet rays and influences skin tone.
- The dermis underlies the epidermis and contains nerves, hair follicles, blood and lymph vessels, and glands. It is composed of tough connective tissue containing collagen, which contributes to the skin's elasticity.
- Skin color is due to the presence or absence of melanin, carotene, and hemoglobin.
- Glands are unicellular or multicellular structures of epithelial tissue that produce secretions. The functions of integumentary system glands are protection and thermoregulation.
- The skin regulates and balances body temperature via radiation, convection, evaporation, conduction, shivering, dilation or contraction of blood vessels, and "goose flesh."
- Infants and the elderly have a higher risk of heat loss than do other age groups.
- Through sensory awareness, the skin provides a dynamic interaction between external and internal environments.
- Effects of aging include wrinkling, loss of subcutaneous fat, atrophy of glands, and a decreased number of protective cells. Skin problems are often more common for older adults.
- To protect the skin, one should eat a healthy diet and drink an adequate amount of daily fluids. Additional protection is required when in the sun.

CRITICAL THINKING EXERCISES

1. Describe the skin's role in vitamin D synthesis. Identify two groups of individuals at risk for vitamin D deficiency. Explain why they are at risk.
2. Why would you not expect an epidermal wound to bleed?
3. Explain why it hurts to have a hair plucked out, but does not hurt to have a haircut.
4. Identify differences in skin and hair that you would expect to see in a 25-year-old versus a 75-year-old client.

NCLEX-STYLE REVIEW QUESTIONS

1. The nurse is gathering data from a client with a loss of melanin production from age-related changes. What observation made by the nurse correlates with this change?
   a. White hair
   b. Freckles on the nose and cheeks
   c. Ridges on the skin surface
   d. Thickened areas on the palms and heels

2. The nurse observes facial wrinkling on a 35-year-old client. What questions should the nurse ask pertaining to this finding? Select all that apply.
   a. What type of moisturizer do you use?
   b. Do you smoke?
   c. Do you spend a lot of time outdoors?
   d. Did either of your parents wrinkle pr
   e. Do you drink alcohol?

3. A client lacks the DNA-repair enzyme that helps reverse UV damage. Which information related to this lack of enzyme would the nurse include when teaching the client?
   a. Wear sunglasses when outdoors.
   b. Avoid any activities that involve the outdoors.
   c. Apply aloe vera after a sunburn.
   d. Closely check the skin for new or changes in moles.

4. A client informs the nurse that a bookshelf fell on the client's toe and the toenail fell off. The client asks the nurse when to expect the toenail to regrow. Which response by the nurse is best?
   a. "You will not have regrowth of that toenail."
   b. "You should have a new nail in about 3 months."
   c. "You should have a new nail in about 12 to 18 months."
   d. "The nail will be back in about 2 weeks."

5. What nursing action is essential in order to prevent heat loss through evaporation?
   a. Apply blankets.
   b. Move a space heater closer to the client.
   c. Dry the client with a towel when perspiring.
   d. Apply a warm cloth to the forehead.

CHAPTER RESOURCES

Enhance your learning with additional resources on thePoint!

Student Resources related to this chapter can be found at **thePoint.lww.com/Rosdahl12e.**

17 Fluid and Electrolyte Balance

Learning Objectives

1. Define homeostasis in fluid/electrolyte balance. Define negative and positive feedback.
2. Describe intracellular and extracellular fluid compartments, including their components, the total percentage of body weight, and the major cation and anion of each.
3. Describe how the thirst center, ANP, and the RAA system help regulate fluid balance.
4. Explain "third-spacing"; describe four ways edema can occur. Describe client teaching to decrease/prevent edema.
5. Identify four functions of water.
6. Name three major electrolytes necessary for neuronal and muscular function; describe two nursing actions to help maintain electrolyte balance.
7. Differentiate between freely permeable and selectively permeable membranes; state factors affecting permeability.
8. Contrast transportation of fluids and other molecules by diffusion, osmosis, filtration, and active transport.
9. List normal sources of water gain and the mechanism of water loss. Identify normal daily intake and output for an average adult.
10. Describe major components and actions to maintain acid–base balance, including the significance of arterial blood gas values.
11. Explain why infants, young children, and the elderly are at risk for fluid/electrolyte imbalance. Describe two nursing actions to assist seniors to maintain homeostasis.

Important Terminology

acid
active transport
anasarca
anion
ascites
base
buffer
cation
dehydration
diffusion
edema
electrolyte
endocytosis
feedback
filtration
hypertonic
hypotonic
insensible
interstitial
intravascular
ion
isotonic
osmosis
permeable
salt
solute
solvent
third-space (fluid)

Acronyms

ABGs
ADH
ANP
ATP
Ca^{++}
$Ca_3[PO_4]_2$
$CaCl_2$
$CaCO_3$
Cl^-
CSF
ECF
Fe^{++}
GI
H^+
HCl
HCO_3^-
H_2O, HOH
HPO_4^-, $H_2PO_4^-$
ICF
IVF
K^+
KCl
mEq
Mg^{++}
ml
Na^+
NaCl
NaOH
Na_2SO_4
NS
O^{--}, O_2
OH^-
$PaCO_2$
PaO_2
pH
RAA
SO_4^-

Every body tissue and organ has an active role in maintaining the body's *homeostasis* (equilibrium, balance, stability). Body fluids, composed of water and substances dissolved and suspended in it, form the environment of each body cell. Fluids move into and out of cells, bringing with them enzymes, hormones, and nutrients, as well as removing waste products (end products of metabolism). This continual movement of fluids is necessary to maintain homeostasis. This chapter reviews the importance of water and selected electrolytes and major systems of fluid transport within the body.

HOMEOSTASIS

Homeostasis is the dynamic process through which the body maintains balance; it constantly adjusts to internal and external stimuli. (*Home/o* means constant or sameness and the suffix, *-stasis*, means controlling; therefore, *homeostasis* means "controlling sameness.") This provides temperature regulation and stability, regulation of body glucose (sugars), timing of sleep cycles, and other life-sustaining processes. The concept of homeostasis is fundamental in understanding most physiologic processes. To maintain homeostasis, the body must be able to sense minute (tiny) changes and react appropriately. To do so, the body has sensors and integrating centers involving all body cells and systems.

> **Key Concept**
> Homeostasis is maintained by balancing fluids, electrolytes, acids, and bases.

Negative and Positive Feedback

All components of the body constantly send tiny signals, causing responses. **Feedback** is the relaying of information to the appropriate organ or system.

> **Key Concept**
> Receptor (sensing component) → control center (brain) → appropriate response (effector—muscles, organs, hormones) → change (positive or negative feedback) = homeostasis.

Negative feedback occurs when the body reverses an original stimulus to regain physiologic balance (homeostasis). Body systems resist deviations, normally allowing for small variations only. Blood pressure control and maintenance of normal body temperature are negative feedback systems. Illness interrupts negative feedback; healthcare measures attempt to restore and maintain homeostasis (*equilibrium*) as much as possible.

In *positive feedback*, the body enhances or intensifies an original stimulus. The body senses deviations, but positive feedback generally is not homeostatic. In fact, the body often responds by increasing the deviation. An example of helpful positive feedback is blood clotting following an injury. Another normal example is a woman in labor. When labor begins, impulses are sent to cause the release of the hormone, oxytocin, which stimulates uterine contractions. An example of dangerous positive feedback is a very high fever. Therefore, in some situations, positive feedback can lead to greater instability or death.

Systems Involved in Feedback

The major systems involved in feedback are the nervous and endocrine systems, which are discussed in Chapters 19 and 20. The nervous system regulates homeostasis by sensing system deviations and sending nerve impulses to appropriate organs; the endocrine system uses the release and action of hormones to restore and maintain homeostasis.

> **Key Concept**
> An individual must maintain homeostasis to maintain health.

BODY FLUIDS

Fluids make up a large portion of the body (50%–60% of total body weight). Body fluids are composed of water and dissolved substances, including glucose, amino acids, electrolytes, and other nutrients.

Location of Fluids

Body fluids are divided between two main compartments: *intracellular fluid* (ICF) and *extracellular fluid* (ECF). ICF, the fluid inside cells, constitutes one half to two thirds of total body fluid in adults. ECF, the fluid outside cells, constitutes about one third of total body fluid in adults. Fluids continuously move between compartments (Fig. 17-1). The compartments contain slightly different components, and several homeostatic mechanisms maintain the correct balance of fluid versus solids within each compartment.

Intracellular Fluid

Intracellular fluid functions as a stabilizer for the parts of the cell and helps maintain cell shape. ICF also assists with transport of nutrients across the cell membrane, in and

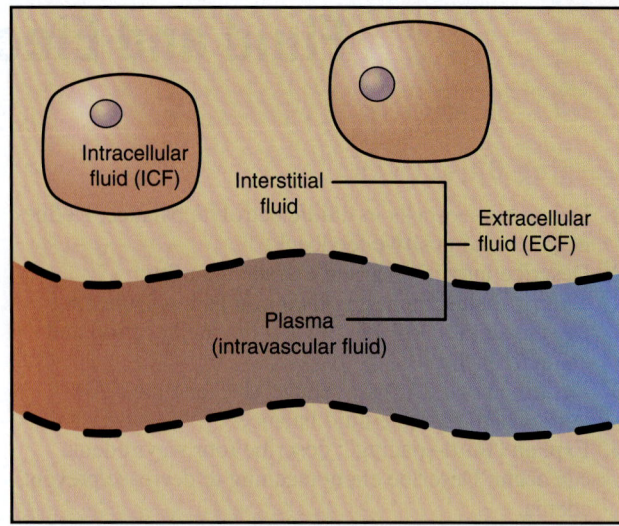

Figure 17-1 Major fluid compartments. Intracellular fluid (ICF) is fluid within cells. Extracellular fluid (ECF) is fluid outside of cells. The ECF includes interstitial fluid surrounding the cells, and plasma, the fluid component of blood. (In addition, specialized ECF includes synovial fluid, CSF, aqueous fluid in the eye, and some specialized GI secretions.) Fluid continually moves between the major compartments.

out of the cell. The liquid portion of cytoplasm is *cytosol*. Cells vary in water content. Skeletal muscle contains about 75% water; fatty tissue contains about 10% water (with the remainder being lipids [fats]). The adult body is about 60% water; therefore, ICF is 40% of total body weight (approximately 28 L). The major ions in ICF are potassium, magnesium, and phosphate (in addition to proteins).

Extracellular Fluid

ECF appears mostly as *interstitial* (tissue) fluid and *intravascular fluid* (**IVF**—within blood and lymphatic vessels). **Interstitial** fluid is found *between cells* and accounts for about 15% of body weight (approximately 3.5 L). **Intravascular** fluid is the watery fluid in blood (*plasma*). Specialized ECFs, *transcellular fluids*, are usually within epithelial-lined spaces; these include synovial fluid in joint cavities, cerebral spinal fluid (**CSF**) in the brain and spinal cord, and aqueous (ocular) fluid in the eyes. Some additional ECFs are located in the gastrointestinal (**GI**) tract, liver, biliary tract, and lymphatic vessels. Bladder urine is also considered a transcellular fluid. Major ions in ECF are sodium, chlorine, and carbonate.

The volume of ECF is the most important regulated aspect of body fluid balance. Without adequate ECF, the body cannot maintain normal blood pressure. A significant loss of ECF volume can drop blood pressure to a life-threatening point where cells can no longer function, due to a lack of oxygen and nutrients. This condition is known as *hypovolemic shock* (see Chapter 43). Too much ECF can place a person in a state of fluid overload, leading to high blood pressure and at risk for conditions such as heart failure.

> **Key Concept**
> ECF is the most important fluid in regulation of fluid balance.

The body monitors ECF volumes closely and sends messages to the brain, kidneys, and pituitary gland to maintain control. Primary mechanisms involved in regulation include actions of the thirst center in the hypothalamus; release of antidiuretic hormone (vasopressin—**ADH**) from the pituitary; effects of the renin–angiotensin–aldosterone (**RAA**) system; and release of atrial natriuretic peptide (**ANP**) hormone by the heart (Fig. 17-2). This mechanism is described in Chapter 27.

The Thirst Center
The thirst center in the hypothalamus stimulates or inhibits the desire for a person to drink. (Excessive fluid intake [*polydipsia*], particularly of plain water, can cause severe electrolyte imbalance.)

Antidiuretic Hormone
ADH (vasopressin) is released from storage in the posterior pituitary gland as part of the negative feedback mechanism, in response to conditions within the cardiovascular system. ADH regulates the amount of water kidney tubules absorb (reabsorption) and is released in response to low blood volume (e.g., in low blood pressure or hemorrhage) or in response to an increase in concentration of sodium and other solutes (increased plasma osmolarity) in intravascular fluid (plasma). When ADH is released, urine production is decreased and water reabsorption is increased.

The RAA System
The RAA system controls fluid volume. When blood volume decreases, blood flow to the renal (kidneys') juxtaglomerular apparatus is reduced, activating the RAA system. Renin is released by the kidneys, causing secretion of angiotensin I, which is converted to angiotensin II (by an enzyme) in the lungs. Angiotensin II causes both vasoconstriction (increasing blood pressure) and secretion of aldosterone by the adrenal cortex. Aldosterone causes increased reabsorption of

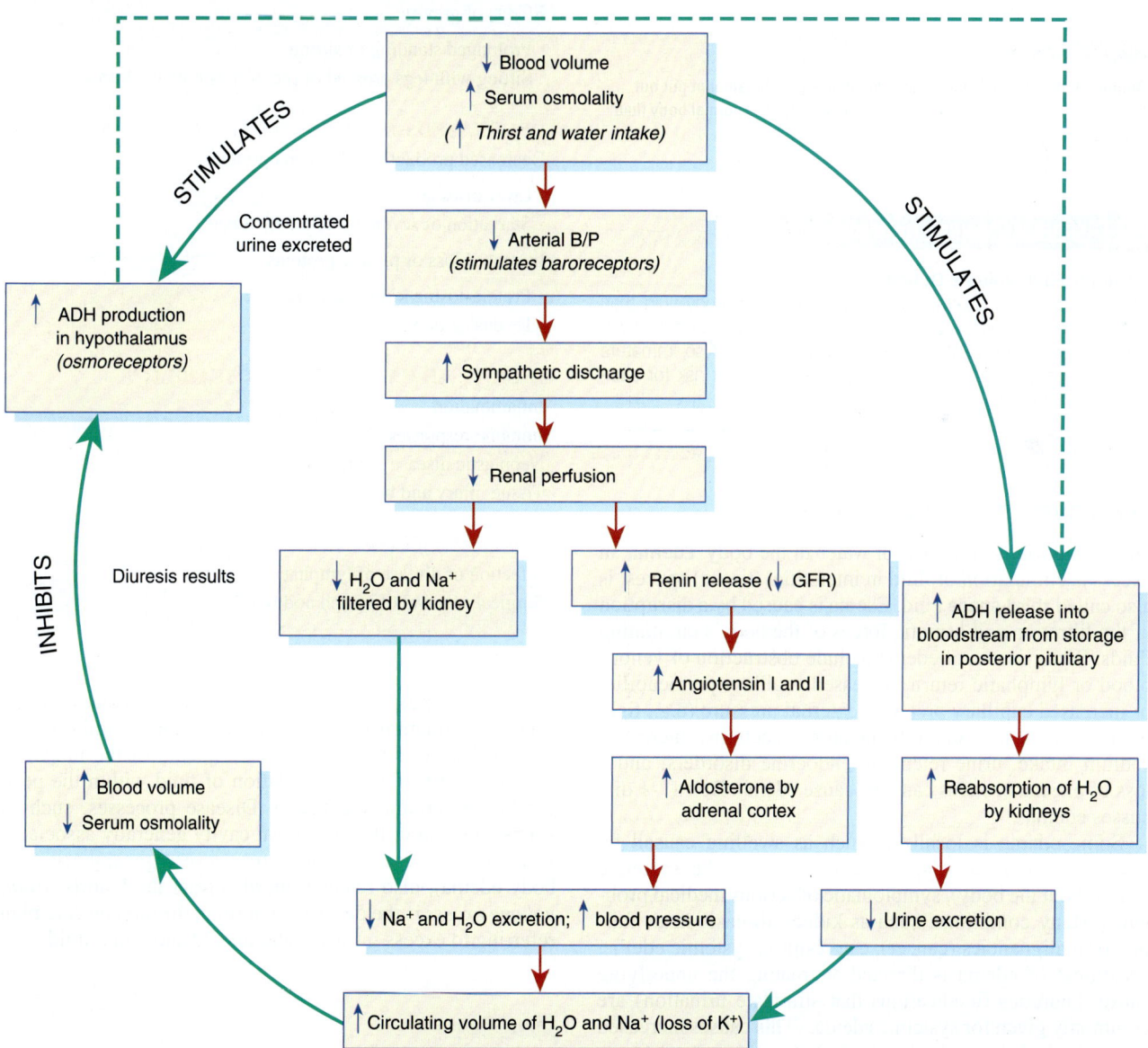

Figure 17-2 Fluid regulation cycle, including antidiuretic hormone (ADH) and the renin–angiotensin–aldosterone (RAA) system. GFR, glomerular filtration rate.

sodium and water by the kidneys in an attempt to increase blood volume. (Water "follows" sodium [salt], explained later in this chapter.) Excretion of potassium is also increased in an attempt to restore homeostasis (see Fig. 17-2).

Atrial Natriuretic Peptide

The heart also plays a role in correcting overload imbalances, by releasing ANP from the right atrium. ANP promotes renal diuresis (kidney excretion) of sodium and water (see Chapter 27).

Normal Intake and Output

An adult human at rest takes in approximately 2,500 mL of fluid daily. Approximate levels of intake include fluids 1,200 mL, foods 1,000 mL, and metabolic products 300 mL. Daily output should approximately equal intake. Normal output occurs as urine, breathing, perspiration, feces, and in minute amounts in vaginal secretions.

> **Key Concept**
>
> Amount of fluid taken in must approximately equal the amount put out, to maintain homeostasis. The term *euvolemic* refers to normal body fluid volume.

SPECIAL CONSIDERATIONS *Lifespan*

Risk for Fluid Volume Deficit
Infants have a considerably higher percentage of body fluid than adults, most of which is ECF. They are at increased risk for fluid volume deficit because ECF is lost more easily than ICF. Also, immature kidney function places infants and young children at risk for alterations in fluid and electrolyte levels.

Overhydration and Edema

Overhydration is an excess of water in the body. **Edema**, an excess accumulation of fluid in interstitial (tissue) spaces, is also called **third-space** fluid. Edema is caused by a disruption of the filtration and osmotic forces of the body's circulating fluids. Some causes of edema include obstruction of venous blood or lymphatic return, increased capillary permeability or increased capillary pressure, external pressure (e.g., tight binders or casts), and inflammatory reactions. Increased sodium intake, urine retention, endocrine disorders, and a loss of plasma proteins can also cause edema. Box 17-1 discusses edema.

Some edema is localized, such as swelling caused by inflammation in an injury. Edema can also be systemic (throughout the body), symptomatic of serious medical problems. Many conditions, such as kidney disease, heart failure, or malignancies (cancer), can result in systemic edema. Treatment of edema is directed at treating the underlying cause. Diuretics (medications that stimulate urination) are commonly given for systemic edema. (This causes increased loss of body fluids and salts via the kidneys.)

Some body fluids are not available for functional use. These are ECFs occurring within interstitial spaces in the body. Excess fluid accumulation in interstitial spaces is often caused by inflammation. Examples include pleural effusion (accumulation of fluid between the pleura of the lungs) or pericardial effusion (accumulation of fluid within the pericardial sac around the heart). Disease processes, such as **ascites** (edema in the peritoneal cavity generally associated with liver damage) and **anasarca** (severe generalized total body edema), also result from abnormal fluid shifts. *Fluid volume excess* is the descriptive term in the nursing care plan referring to excess intravascular and/or interstitial fluid.

Box 17-1   Sample Causes of Edema

INCREASED CAPILLARY PRESSURE

Arteriolar dilation

- Allergic responses (e.g., hives, angioneurotic edema)
- Inflammation

Venous obstruction

- Hepatic obstruction
- Heart failure
- Thrombophlebitis
- External pressure

Increased vascular volume

- Increased levels of adrenocortical hormones
- Premenstrual sodium retention
- Pregnancy
- Environmental heat stress

Effects of gravity

- Prolonged standing or sitting
- Sitting with legs crossed or pressure behind the knees

DECREASED COLLOIDAL OSMOTIC PRESSURE

Decreased production of plasma proteins

- Liver disease
- Starvation or severe protein deficiency

Increased loss of plasma proteins

- Protein-losing kidney diseases
- Extensive burns

INCREASED CAPILLARY PERMEABILITY

Inflammation
Immune responses
Neoplastic disease (cancers)
Tissue injury and burns

OBSTRUCTION OF LYMPHATIC FLOW

Infection or disease of lymphatic structures
Surgical removal of lymph nodes

> **Key Concept**
>
> In edema, the body attempts to restore homeostasis by increased secretion of natriuretic ("salt-losing") peptides, decreased ADH, increased urine output, and reduced thirst.

Dehydration (Impaired Fluid Homeostasis)

Many disorders result in a deficiency of body water or excessive loss of water (**dehydration**). In dehydration, water output is greater than intake. Dehydration can be associated with sodium loss or disturbance of another electrolyte, such as potassium. External causes of dehydration include prolonged sun exposure and excessive exercise, as well as diarrhea, vomiting, and burns. In some cases, inappropriate use of diuretics, malnutrition, excessive fasting, anorexia, or bulimia causes dehydration. Decreased fluid intake, fever, GI suction, certain medications, and hemorrhage may also contribute to dehydration, as well as stimulant or alcohol abuse. Disorders such as electrolyte dysfunction and Addison disease can also be causes. Diabetes (both mellitus and insipidus) and related factors, such as hyperglycemia and glycosuria, may also cause a fluid deficiency.

Early in dehydration, the person feels thirsty and drinks more fluid. If fluid intake cannot keep up with fluid loss, dehydration increases in severity. The body compensates by reducing both urine output and sweating. Water moves from ICF compartments into intravascular fluids. If dehydration is not corrected, body tissues dry out and malfunction. Brain cells are particularly susceptible to dehydration; one early sign of severe dehydration is mental confusion. Untreated, this can progress to coma. Dehydration can also cause severe damage to organs such as the kidneys and liver, due to low blood pressure caused by reduced circulating blood volume. As in edema, treatment of dehydration is first directed at the underlying cause. Supplemental fluids and electrolytes are often administered. *Fluid volume deficit* is the descriptive term for dehydration. Disorders related to fluid and electrolyte balance are discussed in Chapter 76.

> **Nursing Alert** Thirst is a primary indicator of hydration status. Therefore, be aware that thirst is an early symptom of dehydration.

Water

Water is vital for life and composes the greatest percentage of body weight; the human body consists of 45%–77% water (Table 17-1). It provides an efficient medium for delivery of nutrients to and export of waste products from body cells, and helps regulate many body processes and pressures. It protects and lubricates body surfaces. It is especially important in regulation of blood pressure and fluid and electrolyte balance (Box 17-2).

> **Key Concept**
> Water (H_2O) is vital to human life. The body cannot carry on most of its activities without it.

Age, sex, and individual body composition cause variations in total body percentage of water. Children can be composed of more than 75% body water; adult men about 60%. Fat cells contain the least water of any cells, thus adult women normally have the lowest water content (about 50%), because of the presence of greater amounts of subcutaneous fat. Table 17-1 summarizes the breakdown of body water by individual and by water compartment.

TABLE 17-1 Water as a Percentage of Body Weight

WATER COMPARTMENT	INFANT (%)	ADULT (%)		ELDERLY PERSON (%)
		MAN	WOMAN	
Extracellular				
Intravascular	4	4	5	5
Interstitial	25	11	10	15
Intracellular	48	45	35	25
Total body water	77	60	50	45

> **NCLEX Alert**
> The NCLEX includes terminology found in this chapter, including concepts such as homeostasis, ECF, body fluid balance, and fluid volume excess or deficit. These concepts are basic to understanding your role in providing nursing interventions, use of medications, and prevention of complications.

Special Characteristics of Water

Specific properties of water make it important in body chemistry. This will aid in understanding of rationales underlying nursing interventions.

- *A great temperature difference is needed to cause a physical change (to solid or gas) in water—which is normally liquid* (see Chapter 15). Water boils at 212 °F (100 °C) and freezes at 32 °F (0 °C). This temperature

Box 17-2 Functions of Water

- Primary solvent within the body
- Primary compound in all body fluids
- Suspension agent
- Helps regulate body temperature, body pH, and fluid pressures inside and outside cells
- Assists or participates in chemical reactions
- May be end product of chemical reactions

WATER IN SOLUTION WITH OTHER SUBSTANCES

- Transports nutrients and oxygen to cells
- Transports waste products away from cells
- Acts as "bumper" to protect cells and organs
- Lubricates to prevent outer walls (parietal) from rubbing against inner walls (visceral) of organs
- Participates in maintenance of blood pressure
- Helps regulate acid–base and fluid–electrolyte balance
- Facilitates the use of water-soluble vitamins (C and B complex)

span is sufficient to cause physical changes that do not affect the chemical composition of water. However, this change is difficult and relatively slow to occur. Heat is needed to change water from liquid to gas, but water can absorb much heat before increasing its temperature. (The evaporation process [change from liquid to gas] removes heat from the body.)

- *Water directly and indirectly participates in all chemical reactions in the body.* Chemically, each water molecule (H_2O) is made up of two elements, hydrogen (2 atoms) and oxygen (1 atom). During metabolism, numerous chemical changes separate water molecules into their component elements for use elsewhere. Hydrogen is the main component of the pH system of the body (described later). Oxidation is the process through which the body uses oxygen to form needed new substances. Indirectly, water acts as the solution in which other chemicals ionize (dissociate). When substances change into ions, also discussed later, they become available to participate in other chemical reactions.

- *Water is a good solvent.* A **solvent** is a liquid that dissolves substances; a **solute** is the substance dissolved. Many compounds, such as salts and sugars, dissolve easily in water. This is known as a solution. (A solution does not involve a chemical change in the composition of either solvent or solute.) Nutrients and wastes are transported as solutes in water. Body water contains two main types of solutes: nonelectrolytes and electrolytes. Nonelectrolytes include proteins, glucose, carbon dioxide, oxygen, and organic acids. Electrolytes are solutes that generate an electrical charge when dissolved in water. They are discussed in the next section.

- *Water functions as a suspension agent.* Many larger molecules, such as lipids and proteins, are easily suspended in water. (A suspension is not the same as a solution.) Suspensions must be kept in motion, or larger molecules will settle to the bottom. For example, red blood cells (RBCs) settle out of suspension unless kept in motion in the watery medium of blood. An individual's blood pressure partially depends on intravascular water as a suspension agent, with specific amounts of proteins, electrolytes, and minerals as solutes.

- *Water exerts pressure against the walls of vessels that contain it—hydrostatic pressure.* This occurs because water has weight and volume. The amount of hydrostatic pressure depends on the depth of the liquid. (Regardless of the amount, water in a tall, thin container exerts more hydrostatic pressure than water in a shallow container.)

- *Osmotic pressure* develops when a semipermeable membrane separates two solutions containing different concentrations of solutes. The amount of solutes in water affects the pressure that can be exerted against surrounding membranes. The greater the amount of solutes, the greater the amount of pressure. The body's osmotic pressure is normally maintained within very narrow limits. For example, body cells have an osmotic pressure nearly equal to that of the circulating fluid of the blood. Solutions exerting equal pressures on opposite sides of a membrane are said to be **isotonic** (of equal tension). Stronger (more concentrated) solutions, compared with those on the opposing side of a membrane, are said to be **hypertonic** (increased tension). Immersion in a hypertonic solution will result in shrinkage of blood cells because osmosis (discussed later) will draw fluid out of the cells. Weaker solutions, compared with an opposing solution, are called **hypotonic** (reduced tension). Immersion in a hypotonic solution will result in swelling of blood cells (see Fig. 17-3).

SPECIAL CONSIDERATIONS Lifespan

Risk for Fluid Volume Imbalances in Older Adults
Loss of thirst sensation in older adults often leads to decreased consumption of fluids; therefore, these clients are at increased risk for fluid volume deficit. Cardiovascular disorders, renal disorders, and poor nutritional habits may cause sodium and water retention, leading to fluid overload.

Electrolytes

An **electrolyte** is a substance that will dissociate into *ions* (see discussion below) when dissolved in water. An ion is

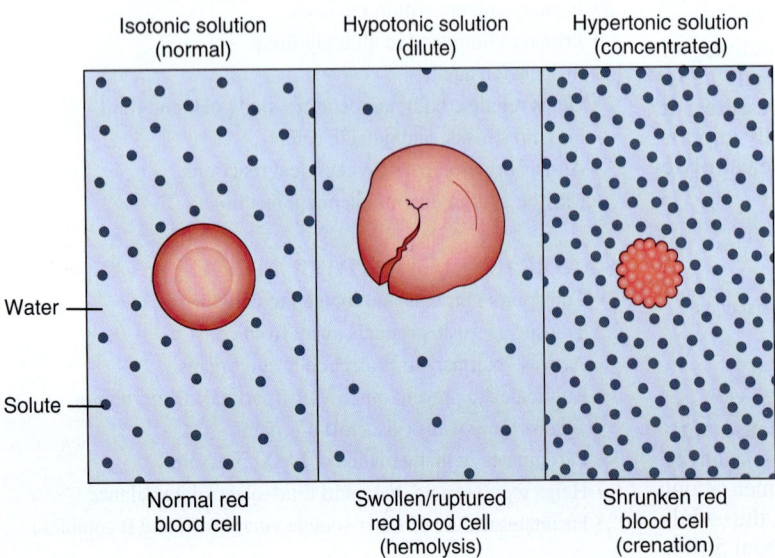

Figure 17-3 Osmosis and red blood cells, showing water moving through a red blood cell membrane in solutions with three different concentrations of solute. All these actions have the goal of equalizing the solute concentration on both sides of the cell membrane. **Left:** Isotonic (normal) solution has the same concentration as the cell, and the water moves into and out of the cell at the same rate. **Center:** Hypotonic (diluted) solution causes the cell to swell and eventually hemolyze (burst) because of the large amount of water moving into the cell. **Right:** Hypertonic (concentrated) solution draws water out of the cell, causing it to shrink (crenation).

able to conduct a weak electric current. Electrolytes are found in all body fluids and are found as inorganic salts, acids, and bases. Specific electrolytes and their concentrations vary. Because electrolytes are active chemicals, their concentrations are measured according to their chemical activity and expressed as milliequivalents (**mEq**). Laboratory tests are done to determine blood levels of electrolytes. Electrolyte concentration affects fluid balance and specific electrolytes affect various body functions. An excess or deficiency of key electrolytes can cause serious physical disorders.

Ions

Each chemical element has an electrical charge, either positive (+) or negative (−). An element usually is able to connect or "bond" to another element. The bonding ability or attraction between chemicals is determined by the electrical charge and specific characteristics of each element.

Many elements are able to gain or lose electrons that circle around them, as introduced in Chapter 15. An atom that has gained or lost one or more electrons is called an **ion**; it has acquired an electrical charge and bonding ability. Ions are atoms or groups of atoms in search of a bonding partner. Some ions are able to bond with only one other ion; others can bond with two or more. This ability is expressed in terms of a positive ($^+$) or negative ($^-$) value, the *valence*. Thus, the valence represents the combining power of an element in a chemical compound, the result of a chemical change. This is also known as the "oxidation number." For example, sodium has a valence of +1 (Na^+); chlorine has a valence of −1 (Cl^-); sulfate (a combination of sulfur and oxygen) has a valence of −2 (SO_4^{--}). The number of plus or minus signs in the valence indicates the number of ions with which a particular ion is able to bind. Therefore, sodium (Na^+) can bind with only one negatively charged ion that has a valence of −1, such as chlorine (Cl^-). This compound would then be **NaCl**, which is *sodium chloride* (common table salt). If hydrogen (H^+) combines with sulfate, two hydrogen ions would be required to fill the two minus bonds of the sulfate, yielding sulfuric acid (H_2SO_4). Water is composed of two hydrogen (H^+) ions and one oxygen ion (O_2, O^{--}) and is expressed as H_2O.

> **Key Concept**
> A salt is any compound composed of a base and an acid. Common table salt is the compound yielded when sodium and chlorine chemically combine. (Some elements have more than one valence value and, thus, can combine with ions that have various valence values.)

A positively charged ion is known as a **cation**. A negatively charged ion is known as an **anion**. Examples of cations include sodium (Na^+), potassium (K^+), calcium (Ca^{++}), magnesium (Mg^{++}), iron (Fe^{++}), and hydrogen (H^+). Examples of anions include chlorine (Cl^-), bicarbonate (HCO_3^-), sulfate (SO_4^{--}), oxygen (O^{--}), and phosphate (HPO_4^-). (Use this memory helper for cation: [ca + ion]. This denotes the positive charge, thereby identifying which substances are cations and which are anions.) The cation, because it has a positive charge, is attracted by a negatively charged ion. The anion, because it is negatively charged, is drawn toward the positive charge. *Opposites attract.* The normal situation in which the charges are equal is known as electroneutrality.

Ionization

The process of *ionization* (osmolarity) involves dissociation of compounds into their respective free-standing ions. This separation of chemical compounds into ions releases them for use in other chemical reactions. Ionization of water (H_2O, **HOH**) releases two hydrogen ions (H^+) and one hydroxyl ion (OH^-). Each of these ions is now free to combine with another substance to form an acid, base, or salt. The ionization of table salt, sodium chloride (NaCl), releases a sodium ion (Na^+) and a chlorine ion (Cl^-). Each of these ions can recombine with other ions into new substances, such as the combination of hydrogen and chlorine, hydrochloric acid (**HCl**).

Important Electrolytes

The major *intracellular* (inside cells) electrolytes are potassium (K^+), magnesium (Mg^{++}), sulfate (SO_4^{++}), and phosphate (HPO_4^-). The major *extracellular* electrolytes are sodium (Na^+), chlorine (Cl^-), calcium (Ca^{++}), and bicarbonate (HCO_3^-). Sodium is the most important extracellular *cation* (positive charge). Chlorine is the most important extracellular *anion* (negative charge). These ions can combine to form sodium chloride or NaCl (salt), one of the most common compounds in the body. "Normal" (isotonic) saline (**NS**) is a salt solution (0.9% NaCl); it is commonly administered IV (intravenously) to augment body fluids. NS is isotonic because it has the same NaCl concentration as normal body fluids.

> **Key Concept**
> Remember that NaCl (salt) is a compound; a chemical change has taken place to form it. Saline solution (salt and water) is a mixture, because it can be separated without a chemical reaction. A compound combines elements in exact proportions, which are the same each time. A mixture can mix components in different proportions. Therefore, a saline solution can be isotonic (0.9%), or it can be in any other proportion and still be a saline solution, such as half-normal saline (0.45% NaCl), also a common IV solution.
>
> A gain or loss of sodium is the cause of most common electrolyte disorders. This is based on factors such as food content, urine excretion, vomiting, perspiration, and specific disorders.

The most dominant cation intracellularly (inside cells) is potassium (K^+). The most dominant anion is phosphate (HPO_4^-). ICF also contains sodium, but in much smaller amounts than outside the cell. The balance between intracellular potassium and extracellular sodium is an extremely important aspect of energy production.

The body needs all these electrolytes and more for normal functioning of nerves and muscles, developing body cells, blood clotting, and coordinating all body activities. Table 17-2 summarizes major electrolyte functions and their dietary sources. Organs involved in homeostatic mechanisms to maintain electrolyte balance include the kidneys and the adrenal, parathyroid, and thyroid glands. In the clinical setting, *electrolyte balance* refers to the maintenance of normal

TABLE 17-2   Major Functions and Food Sources of Electrolytes (Dissolved in Body Fluids)

ELECTROLYTE	MAJOR FUNCTIONS	FOOD SOURCES
Cations		
Sodium (Na^+) (major ion in extracellular fluid [ECF])	Maintenance of osmotic pressure; thus, maintains body fluid balance Assists with normal functioning of neurons and muscle cells Essential for buffer system (acid–base balance)	Table salt, meat, dairy foods, eggs; many processed and preserved foods including bacon, pickles, and ketchup
Potassium (K^+) (major ion in intracellular fluid [ICF])	Maintenance of osmotic pressure; thus, maintains body fluid balance Normal functioning of neurons and muscle cells, including the heart Essential for buffer system (acid–base balance)	Dry fruits, nuts, many vegetables, meat
Calcium (Ca^{++})	Assists with normal functioning of neurons and muscle cells, including the heart Essential for neurotransmitter release Maintenance of bones; bone formation Essential for blood clotting	Milk and other dairy products, broccoli and other green leafy vegetables, sardines
Magnesium (Mg^{++}) (mainly in ICF)	Assists with normal functioning of neurons and muscle cells, including the heart; required for ATP use; enzyme production Maintenance and formation of bones	Green leafy vegetables, legumes, chocolate, peanut butter, whole grains
Anions		
Chloride (Cl^-) (mostly in ECF, combined with Na^+)	Maintenance of osmotic pressure; thus, maintains body fluid balance Essential for buffer system (acid–base balance) Maintains acidity of gastric juice (stomach acid–HCl)	Cheese, milk, fish An excess of chloride ions is called acidosis (NaCl = table salt)
Bicarbonate (HCO_3^-) (most important in ICF)	Maintenance of osmotic pressure; thus, maintains body fluid balance Essential for buffer system (acid–base balance)	Does not need to be specifically included in the diet Excess bicarbonate ions can result from overuse of antacids, such as sodium bicarbonate ($NaHCO_3$, baking soda). The body also can lose acids as a result of illness. An excess of bicarbonate ions is called alkalosis
Phosphate (HPO_4^-) (mostly occurs in ICF)	Maintenance of bones and teeth Assists with normal functioning of nerves and muscle cells Assists with formation of ATP (adenosine triphosphate); energy storage Assists with metabolism of nutrients	Whole grains, milk and other dairy foods, meat, fish, poultry
Sulfate (SO_4^{--}) Proteins	Important in protein metabolism; amino acids Maintenance of osmotic pressure; organic acids	Protein-rich foods Meat, fish, legumes, eggs, nuts, dairy products

serum concentrations of electrolytes. Measuring electrolyte concentration in the ICF is difficult; therefore, serum concentrations (ECF: intravascular) are used to assess and manage clients with imbalances. Table 17-3 provides normal serum electrolyte ranges for adults. Chapter 76 describes disorders occurring when electrolytes are out of the normal range.

FLUID AND ELECTROLYTE TRANSPORT

Total electrolyte concentration affects the body's fluid balance. Nutrients and oxygen must enter body cells, whereas waste products must exit. During this exchange, substances pass through various fluid compartments and cellular membranes (plasma membranes). Each ion or molecule has a specific way or ways in which it can be transported across membranes. The cell membrane separates the intracellular environment from the extracellular environment. The composition of these two environments is very different. These differences must be maintained for the cell (and thus, the organism) to survive. Cell membranes allow some molecules to pass through, while resisting or preventing others from entering (or leaving) the cell.

There are several means of fluid and electrolyte transport (moving substances between cells and body fluids). These include diffusion, osmosis, active transport, and endocytosis. Filtration also functions to move dissolved substances into the interstitial fluid (between cells and tissues).

TABLE 17-3	Normal Serum Electrolyte Values
ELECTROLYTE	SERUM VALUE
Cations	
Sodium (Na+)	135–145 mEq/L
Potassium (K+)	3.5–5.0 mEq/L
Calcium (Ca++)	4.3–5.3 mEq/L (8.9–10.1 mg/dl)
Magnesium (Mg++)	1.5–1.9 mEq/L (1.8–2.3 mg/dl)
Anions	
Chloride (Cl−)	95–108 mEq/L
Bicarbonate (HCO$_3$−)	22–26 mEq/L
Phosphate (HPO$_4$−, H$_2$PO$_4$-)	1.7–2.6 mEq/L (2.5–4.5 mg/dl)

Normal value ranges may vary slightly between laboratories.

The ability of a membrane to allow molecules to pass through is known as **permeability**. Factors that affect permeability include:

- Size of pores in the membrane (which can be altered in response to pressures or hormones)
- External and internal pressures exerted on the molecules (*osmotic pressure*)
- Pressure of fluid against the membrane (*hydrostatic pressure*)
- Electrical charges of the molecule, the plasma membrane, or the body fluid
- Solubility of the molecules
- Size of the molecules

Permeability of Membranes

Freely permeable membranes allow almost any food or waste substance to pass through. Freely permeable walls allow easy transfer of fluid and substances from intravascular fluid to interstitial fluid. After substances arrive in the interstitial fluid around the cells, they must still penetrate the cellular membrane to reach the ICF, where the majority of the body's work occurs.

The cellular membrane is *selectively permeable*, meaning that each cell's membrane allows only certain substances to pass through. Movement across the cellular membrane occurs in one of four ways:

- Molecules move through the cell membrane itself (including oxygen, carbon dioxide, and steroids).
- Substances pass through membrane channels. These channels are of various sizes and allow only a certain size range and electrical charge to cross.
- Carrier molecules in the membrane assist substances across the barrier.
- A vesicle (membrane-bound sac) transports large molecules or whole cells across the plasma membrane.

Some molecules move passively through the membrane; thus, they do not require energy output. *Passive transport* mechanisms include diffusion, osmosis, and filtration. Another form of transport (**active transport**) uses energy and requires assistance. Active transport is used when molecules are too large or too specialized to pass through membranes without assistance.

Passive Transport
Diffusion

Diffusion, or the process of "being widely spread," is the random movement of molecules from an area of higher concentration to an area of lower concentration. Molecules constantly move and bombard each other at random, with the goal of *equalization*—the molecular equivalent of seeking homeostasis. If molecules are highly concentrated, they collide often and attempt to move to a place with fewer collisions. Following total diffusion, equilibrium is reached, with no further exchange of molecules. The molecules continue to move, but the number in each area or on each side of a membrane stays the same. (Heat speeds up diffusion because heat makes molecules move faster.) Diffusion commonly occurs in liquids and gases. For example, when cream is added to coffee it spreads out (diffuses). Smoke or perfume diffuses in a room.

Factors affecting the rate of diffusion include:

- The concentration gradient (greater concentration = faster diffusion)
- Particle size (smaller particles diffuse faster)
- Lipid (fat) solubility (more soluble fats diffuse faster)

Diffusion is the most important mechanism by which nutrients and wastes pass across the cell membrane. In the body, oxygen and carbon dioxide diffuse across cell membranes of the alveoli in the lungs, as shown in Figure 17-4A. When a person takes in air, more oxygen (O_2) molecules are drawn into the alveoli. These oxygen molecules are pushed passively toward the pulmonary (lung) capillaries where the O_2 level is lower. This difference in pressures forces oxygen to cross the cell membrane out of the lungs (diffuse) into the pulmonary capillaries. The *oxygenated* (oxygen-rich) blood then is transported to various parts of the body. Carbon dioxide (CO_2) gas is exchanged in the same manner, except in the reverse direction, because of the pressure. The designation "Pa" or "P" indicates the "pressure" or "potential" of oxygen (PaO_2) or carbon dioxide ($PaCO_2$).

> **Key Concept**
>
> Dialysis is an example of diffusion. An isotonic solution on one side of a membrane causes body wastes to flow into it (due to higher pressure), in an effort to equalize pressures.

Osmosis

The homeostatic mechanism of **osmosis** equalizes concentrations of nondiffusible solutes within the body. Thus, osmosis is the diffusion of a pure solvent, such as water, *across a semipermeable membrane* in response to a concentration gradient, in situations where molecules of the higher concentration are nondiffusible. In other words, water molecules move passively from an area where the water molecules are higher in number (more dilute solution, with fewer nondiffusible solutes) to an area where they are lower in number (more concentrated, with more nondiffusible solutes; see Fig. 17-4B). Water moves from

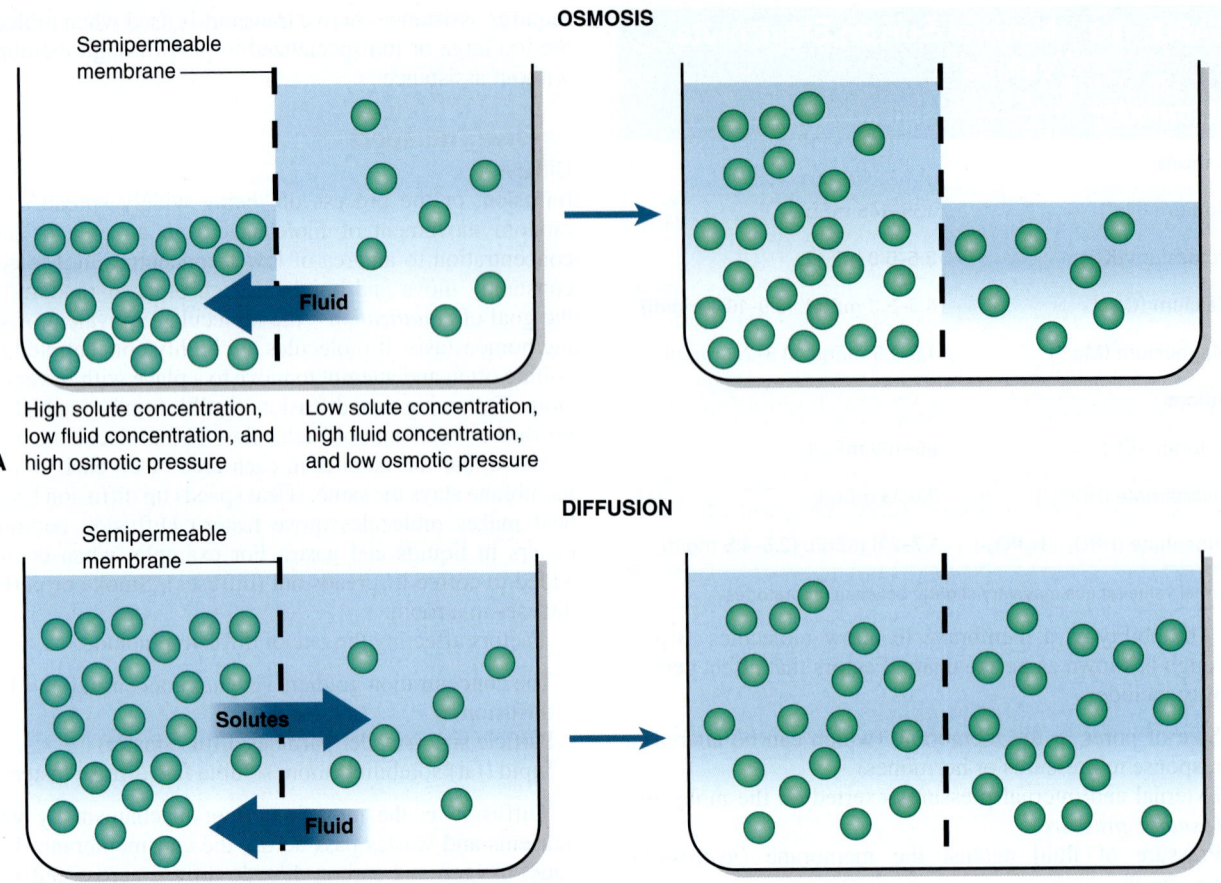

Figure 17-4 **A.** The process of osmosis, showing the flow of water, in an attempt to equalize concentrations of solute on both sides of a semipermeable membrane. (Water flows from the dilute solution into a more concentrated solution.) The level of the fluid column is maintained by osmotic pressure. **B.** The process of diffusion, showing gas exchange in the alveoli. Oxygen is transported across the alveolar–capillary membrane from the alveoli of the lungs to the capillaries, to add oxygen to the unoxygenated blood returning from the systemic circulation. Carbon dioxide in the capillaries (area of greater concentration) moves into the alveoli (area of lesser concentration). This simple diffusion is an example of passive transport.

a *hypotonic solution* (dilute solution with fewer solutes) to a *hypertonic solution* (concentrated solution with more solutes). As stated before and as shown in Figure 17-3, if water from a less-concentrated solution is moving into an RBC, the RBC becomes swollen and may rupture (*hemolysis*) because of this influx of water. An RBC will shrink (*crenation*) if it is losing water to a surrounding hypertonic solution (a concentrated solution with a solute level higher than that found in the RBC).

Although there are many possible solutes, a common one is salt (NaCl). Therefore, when thinking about osmosis, think of salt as the solute and think about the phrase "water follows salt." This will help you remember which direction the water moves. Osmosis can be thought of as "pulling pressure," pulling water in to equalize or dilute the concentrated solution.

Key Concept
The term osmotic pressure refers to pressure exerted to stop the flow of water across a membrane. Osmosis stops when the solute concentration is equal on both sides of a membrane.

Filtration
Filtration is the transport of water and dissolved materials through a membrane from an area of higher pressure to an area of lower pressure and is very common in the body. It operates somewhat like a sieve. *Filtration requires mechanical pressure.* Liquids and solutes are passed through holes in a membrane. The size of the holes and differences in pressures (mechanical force) on each side determine the amount of filtration. Filtration can be thought of as "pushing pressure" because it pushes water and solutes through a membrane from a higher pressure area to a lower pressure area. Figure 17-5 shows filtration through an arteriole and a venule. The rate of filtration depends on the amount of pressure applied. Blood pressure (mechanical force) pushes water and small dissolved particles, such as sugars and salts, through capillary walls into interstitial fluid. Larger blood cells and proteins are too large to be pushed through and remain inside the capillaries.

Active Transport
Active transport mechanisms require specific enzymes and energy expenditure, as adenosine triphosphate (ATP). Adenosine is a combination of adenine, containing nitrogen,

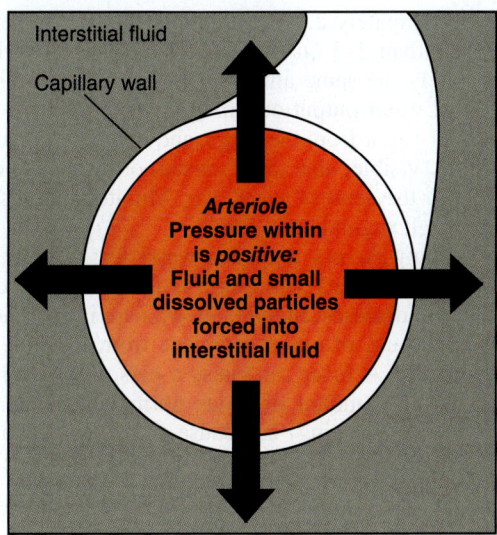 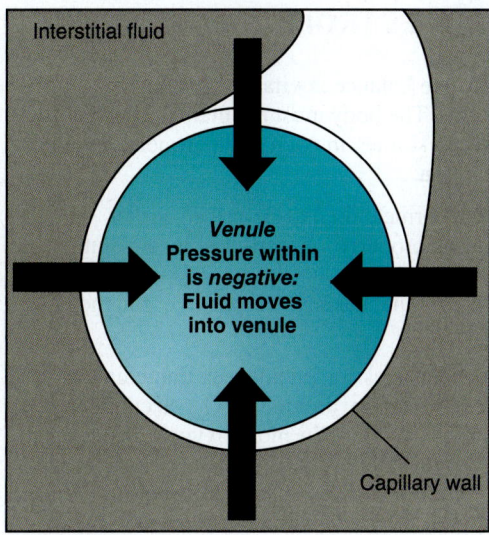

Figure 17-5 Filtration.

and ribose, a 5-carbon sugar. Adenosine plus three phosphate groups makes up ATP. ATP must be converted to ADP in order to produce energy. In this complex process, energy is released using nutrients and assisting ADP to convert back to ATP, to be reused. Active transport processes can move solutes "uphill," against normal rules of concentration and pressure. Specific molecules outside a cell, even if they are fewer in number, can be assisted into the cell, even though a greater concentration already exists in the cell.

The best example of active transport is the *sodium–potassium pump*. More sodium ions exist outside the cell than inside. The natural tendency would be for sodium to diffuse across the cellular membrane into the cell. If this process continued unchecked, however, the homeostatic mechanism (which governs nerve transmissions and muscle contractions) would go berserk. Active transport mechanisms figuratively "pump out" sodium ions from inside the cell, while transporting potassium into the cell. Another example of active transport involves the transport of glucose and amino acids (proteins) into cells lining the small intestine. The intestinal cells use ATP to create active transport, even if the concentration of solutes would seem to require transport in the opposite direction (Fig. 17-6A).

In another form of passive transport, **endocytosis**, particles or fluids are actively transported through the cell membrane into the cytoplasm of a cell in two ways. In *phagocytosis*, particles too large to pass through the cell wall are engulfed and carried into the cell. In *pinocytosis*, ECFs or dissolved substances are engulfed and carried into the cell (Fig. 17-6B). Both of these processes are considered active transport because they utilize ATP for energy (see Fig. 17-6A and B and Chapter 27).

Key Concept

Passive transport does not need energy; active transport requires energy. Hydrostatic pressure is pressure exerted by a stationary liquid or fluid in a state of equilibrium. Hydrostatic mechanisms respond to changes in ECF; *gains must equal losses.*

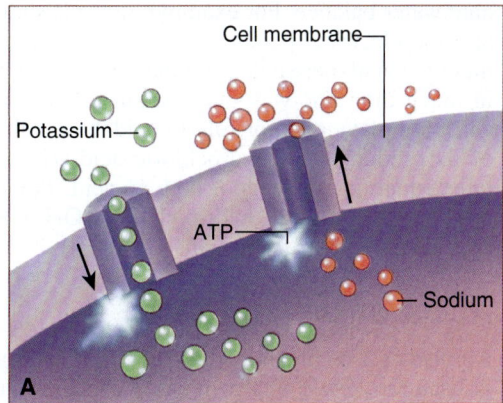 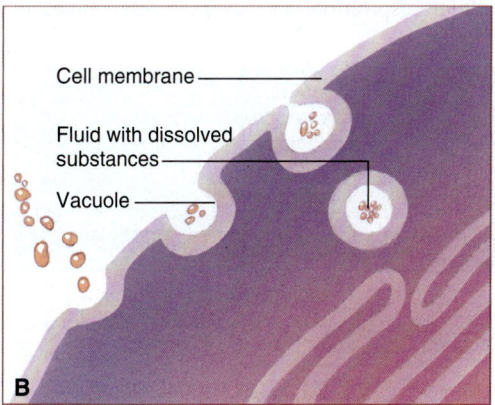

Figure 17-6 **A.** The sodium–potassium pump. This active transport mechanism "pumps" excess sodium ions out of the cells while potassium ions are pumped into the cell. This mechanism goes against the natural tendency (which would be to diffuse these substances in the opposite direction). **B.** Pinocytosis is a form of phagocytosis. Extracellular fluids or small particles of dissolved substances that would ordinarily be too large to pass through the cell wall are engulfed and carried in by special cells called pinocytes. (A&P Made Incredibly Easy, 2013, p. 18.)

FLUID AND ELECTROLYTE BALANCE

Fluid and electrolyte balance is vital for proper functioning of all body systems. The body must maintain the correct proportion of fluids to solutes in each compartment. This balance is dependent on:

- Cell membrane permeability, as described earlier
- Osmolarity—the property of particles in a solution to dissociate into ions
- Electroneutrality—the balance of positive and negative charges

The body compensates for imbalances immediately. For example, if excess carbon dioxide (CO_2) accumulates, a person breathes faster to take in more oxygen. If the respiratory system cannot handle the imbalance, chemical buffers attempt to achieve a balance. In addition, the kidneys can adjust the pH of the ECF. Numerous hormones also act to influence fluid and electrolyte retention and excretion. Electrolytes may be lost through vomiting, diarrhea, or hemorrhage, thus upsetting the body's fluid and electrolyte balance. Tests to determine disorders in electrolyte balance include blood tests, such as blood urea nitrogen (BUN), complete blood count (CBC), and evaluation of arterial blood gases (ABGs), as well as urinalysis (UA).

Water Intake and Output

The body conserves and reuses water as much as possible. The kidneys, and to some extent the intestines, continuously filter and recycle water. Each day, a person must take in approximately the same amount of fluid as is lost. The body can survive many days without food, but only a few days without water. The term health professionals use as an external monitor of fluid balance is *intake and output*. Accurate intake and output records and daily weights are vital when caring for clients with fluid deficits or excesses. Table 17-4 gives sources and approximate amounts for human intake and output. Chapter 52 describes the procedure for determining intake and output.

Intake refers to water and other fluids taken into the body. Water is obtained from: liquid intake (by mouth or a method such as IV), metabolism of food, and as the end product of cellular respiration. The average adult takes in approximately 2,000–3,000 mL (milliliters) per day (a little more than 2–3 quarts). To avoid a water overload, approximately the same amount that is taken in must be put out. Most water output occurs through the kidneys, in sweat, as water vapor from the lungs, and in feces. Sweat may be sensible (visible, able to be sensed) or insensible (not perceptible to the senses) water loss. Minute amounts are also lost through vaginal secretions.

Many factors influence water loss. For example, water output increases with exercise, fever, some medications, and certain diseases. Individuals who are ill may need more fluids because of excess drainage from wounds, vomiting, or bleeding. A fever can cause a person to require about four times the amount of fluids normally needed. *Diaphoresis* (profuse sweating) can cause considerable fluid loss. Each form of fluid loss will also alter the body's electrolyte concentrations.

SPECIAL CONSIDERATIONS   Lifespan

Adolescents

Adolescents are at risk for fluid and electrolyte imbalances due to excessive exercise, poor fluid intake during or after exercise, excessive use of salt and high-sodium foods and soft drinks, and following fad diets or diets lacking important nutrients—especially iron and calcium. Bulimia and anorexia are also considerations.

Key Concept

In special situations, a much greater volume of fluids must be consumed, such as in the case of the nursing client, who must offset the amount of fluid output in breast milk.

ACID–BASE BALANCE

Acid–base balance is another important aspect of homeostasis. In the discussion on ionization, you learned that chemical compounds that break up into ions are called electrolytes and that electrolytes can combine and recombine to form acids, bases, and salts. The body needs many of these substances to regulate acid–base levels and coordinate water balance. For example, it needs sodium to maintain the electrical potential across cell membranes and to maintain acid–base balance. Potassium acts within the cells in much the same way that sodium acts outside the cells. Chlorine plays a major role in acid–base balance because of its production of hydrochloric acid (HCl). Water contains equal components of both an acid (the hydrogen ion or H^+) and a base (the hydroxyl ion or OH^-). Pure water is considered a *neutral solution*.

Acids, Bases, and Salts

An **acid** is a compound containing the hydrogen ion (H^+). A **base** (an *alkali*) is a compound containing the hydroxyl ion (OH^-). A **salt** is a combination of a base and an acid and is created when the positive ions (usually a mineral) of a base replace the positive hydrogen ions of an acid. A salt is an electrolyte made up of a cation (other than hydrogen) and an anion (other than hydroxyl). For example,

TABLE 17-4	Normal Water Balances (Intake and Output)		
INTAKE		**OUTPUT**	
SOURCE	AMOUNT (ML)	SOURCE	AMOUNT (ML)
Liquids	1,200	Urine	1,500
Foods	1,000	Skin[a]	500
Metabolism	300	Lungs[a]	300
		Feces	200
Total	2,500	Total	2,500

[a]Often referred to as "insensible water losses."

hydrochloric acid (HCl) can combine with the base sodium hydroxide (**NaOH**) to yield water and table salt. Thus, HCl + NaOH = HOH + NaCl. (Or an acid plus a base yields water [HOH, H_2O] and a salt.)

The body contains several important salts: sodium chloride (NaCl), potassium chloride (**KCl**), calcium chloride (**CaCl$_2$**), calcium carbonate (**CaCO$_3$**), calcium phosphate (**Ca$_3$[PO$_4$]$_2$**), and sodium sulfate (**Na$_2$SO$_4$**).

Potential of Hydrogen (pH)

The symbol **pH** refers to the potential or power (p) of hydrogen ion (H^+) concentration within a solution. The pH scale ranges from 0 to 14. Pure water, which is *neutral*, has a pH of 7. If the pH number is lower than 7, the solution is an acid. Vinegar (pH 2–3.5), lemon juice (pH 2.3), wine (pH 3.5), black coffee (pH 5.0), and tomato juice (pH 4.1) are common household acids. Acids contain more hydrogen ions than bases.

If the pH is greater than 7, a solution is basic (alkaline). The pH of ICF is approximately 6.8–7.0; the pH of ECF is 7.35–7.45. Baking soda (pH 12), toothpaste (pH 9.9), milk of magnesia (pH 10.5), detergents, and oven cleaners are common alkaline products. Basic solutions contain more hydroxyl (OH^-) ions than acids.

Key Concept

A common remedy for excess stomach acid is baking soda (sodium bicarbonate), which is alkaline (a base).

Fluids outside the body may be strongly acidic or alkaline and not harm the body. For example, lemon juice is highly acidic (pH = 2.3) and sodium bicarbonate (baking soda) is highly alkaline (pH = 12), but they are not harmful to the body. On the other hand, some substances, either in the environment or in the body, such as hydrochloric acid (HCl, pH 0.0) could be very harmful. Figure 17-7 shows the pH of some body fluids.

Key Concept

Low pH = high number of hydrogen ions; high pH = low number of hydrogen ions. Correct body fluid pH is vital because pH affects both the composition and function of proteins.

A change in the pH of a solution by one pH unit means a 10-fold change in hydrogen ion concentration. For example, a substance with a pH of 5 contains 10 times more hydrogen ions than a substance with a pH of 6 (1 unit = 10^1). A pH of 5 means that a substance has 100 times more hydrogen ions than a substance with a pH of 7 (2 units = 10^2). Understanding the impact of changes in pH on the body is extremely important. For example, the pH of blood and lymph (ECF) is normally slightly alkaline, about 7.35–7.45. The body must maintain the slightly alkaline pH of blood within this narrow range because a decrease or increase of only one pH unit would result in chemical disaster. One of the body's normal negative feedback mechanisms is continually correcting the body's tendency to develop acidosis (too many hydrogen atoms) by returning the serum pH back into its alkaline state. The lungs and kidneys are the organs of the body most involved in H^+ regulation.

Key Concept

Regulation of H^+ levels in the body is a function of kidney excretion, buffer systems, and respiration effectiveness.

Buffers

Chemical reactions occurring constantly in the body release many acidic or basic ions. Because of constant changes in this mixture, a buffering or stabilizing system must exist to prevent pH imbalance. A **buffer** is a chemical system set up to resist changes, particularly in hydrogen ion levels. Buffering reactions, which can occur in less than a second, constantly alter acids and bases, to maintain a correct ratio. The body has many buffer systems related to maintaining homeostasis. Some buffer systems use phosphates;

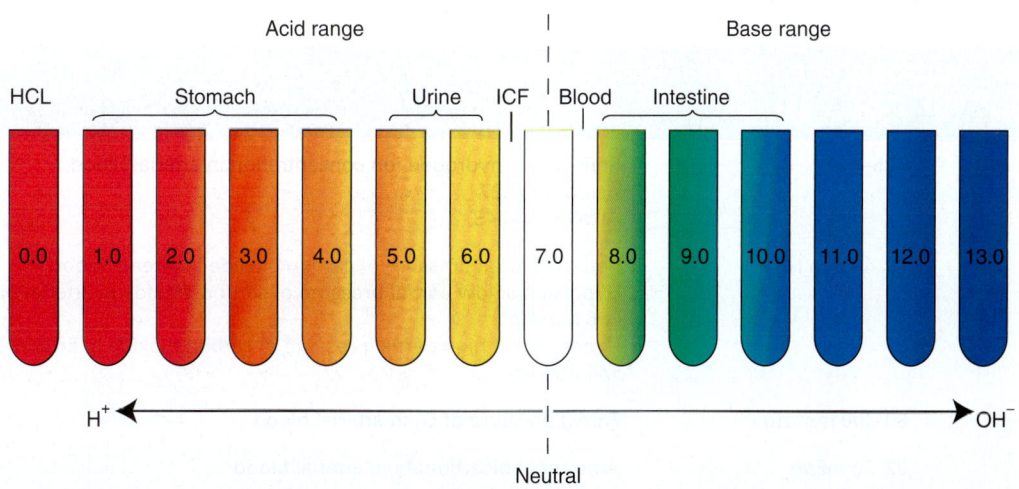

Figure 17-7 The pH scale measures degree of acidity (H^+ ion concentration) or alkalinity (OH^- ion concentration).

for example, phosphates in the kidneys buffer urine. Protein buffers can release H^+ in hemoglobin; other special amino acids also serve as buffers. One of the major buffer systems is the bicarbonate buffer system discussed below.

The Bicarbonate Buffer System

The body's major chemical buffers are sodium bicarbonate, a base (pH = 8.4; $NaHCO_3$ [baking soda]) and a weak acid, carbonic acid (H_2CO_3). Because of its tendency toward acidosis, the body has a greater need for sodium bicarbonate. (The body contains 20 times more sodium bicarbonate than carbonic acid.)

Carbon Dioxide

Chemical buffers are clinically significant, particularly in respiratory illnesses. Carbon dioxide (CO_2) is a potential acid because, once dissolved in water, it becomes carbonic acid, H_2CO_3 ($CO_2 + H_2O = H_2CO_3$). When CO_2 increases (as in a client with chronic obstructive pulmonary disease [COPD]), the carbonic acid content also increases. The opposite can occur in hyperventilation—CO_2 decreases, resulting in a decrease of carbonic acid. Therefore, much of the body's acid is controlled by the respiratory system, specifically the lungs. The major compound controlled by the lungs is CO_2. The respiratory system can very rapidly compensate for too much acid or too little acid by increasing or decreasing the respiratory rate, thereby altering the level of CO_2. When considering respiratory acidosis or alkalosis, think about the lungs and how they compensate for imbalances, using carbon dioxide (CO_2) dissolved in the blood.

Bicarbonate

The kidneys regulate the bicarbonate level in the ECF by conserving or excreting bicarbonate ions within the renal tubules. Bicarbonate levels are vital in maintaining acid–base balance. Bicarbonate ions (HCO_3^-) are basic (alkaline), and the kidneys are key in regulating the amount of bicarbonate in the body. If there is too much or too little base in the body, one way the body compensates is by excreting more or fewer bicarbonate ions via the kidneys. When considering acid–base balance, remember the utilization of bicarbonate ions by the kidneys. When pH drops, bicarbonate ions *accept* H^+ ions, forming carbonic acid (H_2CO_3); when pH rises, carbonic acid *donates* H^+ ions, creating a base (HCO_3^-). These are vital factors in preventing severe acidosis or alkalosis.

> **Key Concept**
>
> Consider:
>
> Lungs—Acid—$CO_2 \rightarrow H_2CO_3$
>
> Kidneys—Base—HCO_3^- ions
>
> Major mechanisms to control acid–base balance:
>
> - The kidneys excrete ammonia (NH_3) in the form of ammonium (NH_4^-), in an effort to balance hydrogen ions
> - pH buffers: bicarbonate—base; carbon dioxide—acid
> - Excretion of CO_2 (constantly produced by cells)
> - Hydrogen ions are making constant chemical changes

Measurement of ABGs

ABGs are measured to determine the extent of compensation by the buffer system. The pH level and amounts of specific gases in the blood indicate if there is more acid or base and their associated values. The normal range for ABGs is used as a guide, and determination of disorders is often based on blood pH. If the blood is basic, the HCO_3^- level is considered because the kidneys regulate bicarbonate ion levels. If the blood is acidic, the **PaCO₂** (partial pressure of carbon dioxide in arterial blood) is assessed because the lungs regulate the majority of acid. Table 17-5 shows normal ABG values. Table 17-6 illustrates acidosis and alkalosis in relationship to pH, CO_2, and HCO_3^- values and the distinction between metabolic and respiratory states.

Respiratory acidosis occurs when breathing is inadequate and $PaCO_2$ (respiratory acid) builds up. The extra CO_2 combines with water to form carbonic acid, causing acidosis. This is common in emphysema. *Respiratory alkalosis* (low blood $PaCO_2$) can occur as a result of hyperventilation or excess aspirin intake.

In *metabolic acidosis*, normal metabolism is impaired, causing a decrease in bicarbonates and a buildup of lactic acid. This can occur in diarrhea, ketosis, and kidney disorders. *Metabolic alkalosis* occurs when bicarbonate ion concentration increases,

TABLE 17-5	Approximate Normal Arterial Blood Gas Values (ABGs)	
ABBREVIATION	NORMAL RANGE	DEFINITION
pH	7.35–7.45	Reflects the hydrogen ion concentration in arterial blood Acidosis: <7.37 Alkalosis: >7.43
$PaCO_2$	35–45 mm Hg	Reflects partial pressure of carbon dioxide in arterial blood Hypocapnia: low partial pressure of carbon dioxide in arterial blood, <36 mm Hg[a] Hypercapnia: high partial pressure of carbon dioxide in arterial blood, >44 mm Hg
PaO_2	80–100 mm Hg	Partial pressure of O_2 in arterial blood
HCO_3^-	22–26 mEq/L	Amount of bicarbonate in arterial blood

[a]Hg, mercury (as a measurement indicator).

CHAPTER 17 Fluid and Electrolyte Balance

TABLE 17-6 A Comparison of Respiratory and Metabolic Acidosis and Alkalosis

ACIDOSIS				ALKALOSIS
Respiratory	↓ pH	Normal	↑ pH	Respiratory
	↑ CO_2	Serum pH	↓ CO_2	
Metabolic	↓ pH	7.35–7.45	↑ pH	Metabolic
	↓ HCO_3^-		↑ HCO_3^-	

The primary difference between these respiratory conditions is a variation in pH that is influenced by changes in CO_2 levels. The primary difference between metabolic acidosis and alkalosis is a variation in pH that is influenced by changes in bicarbonate ion concentration (HCO_3^-).

causing an elevation in blood pH. This can occur in excessive vomiting, dehydration, and endocrine disorders.

To make blood gas values easier to remember, it is common to use the pH range of 7.35–7.45 and a $PaCO_2$ range of 35–45 as an *approximate* guideline. Chapter 76 describes disorders in fluid balance; Chapter 86 discusses respiratory disorders.

Key Concept
Electrolytes are vital in maintenance of homeostasis. This includes regulation of heart, muscle, and nerve function, as well as acid–base balance. Disorders related to imbalance of homeostasis include cardiac arrhythmias, diabetes, dehydration, edema, and gout. One of the most common causes of problems in homeostasis is renal failure.

SPECIAL CONSIDERATIONS Lifespan

The Aging Process
The aging process can produce significant effects on fluid and electrolyte balance. See Table 17-7.

NCLEX Alert
During the NCLEX examination, be aware of the importance of aging on the body's ability to restore or maintain homeostasis. The function of specific body organs, such as lungs and kidneys, is related to the nurse's ability to solve clinical situations. The NCLEX may require judgment regarding methods of documenting nursing actions or client and family teaching.

TABLE 17-7 Effects of Aging on Fluid and Electrolyte Balance

FACTOR	RESULT	NURSING IMPLICATIONS
Intracellular fluid levels decrease (about 8%); muscle tissue changes to fat; thirst sensation declines	Dehydration is common and a serious problem in aging	Encourage intake of foods and fluids; regulate temperature control
Muscle tissue turns to fat	Older adults may gain weight	Encourage exercise, activity, and a balanced diet
Many medications cause fluid loss	Medications may contribute to dehydration	Be sure that the client on certain medications drinks enough water
Certain medications commonly taken by older adults cause loss of electrolytes (e.g., potassium) Laxative use is common Bones may lose calcium in an effort to maintain serum calcium levels	Severe deficiency disorders may develop Reduced absorption of fluid and electrolytes Osteoporosis is common	Administer supplements as ordered. Monitor blood electrolyte levels. Observe for overt signs of electrolyte imbalances Counsel regarding use of over-the-counter medications Client may be more likely to fall or may sustain spontaneous fractures
Circulatory (heart disorders) and renal disorders (e.g., renal failure) may cause fluid and electrolyte imbalances Poor eating patterns and lack of exercise can influence body fluid levels	Edema may develop Inefficiency of control systems	Monitor client's sodium intake and blood pressure; encourage intake of foods with potassium; administer medications as ordered

STUDENT SYNTHESIS

KEY POINTS

- Homeostasis is a state of dynamic equilibrium, balance; the body constantly adjusts to external and internal stimuli to maintain homeostasis.
- Feedback is the relaying of information to and from organ systems (especially nervous and endocrine systems). Feedback keeps the body's functioning capacity within normal boundaries.
- The body has two main fluid compartments: intracellular (within cells) and extracellular. Extracellular fluid is located in blood vessels (plasma) and tissues (interstitial fluid).
- Homeostatic mechanisms involved in regulation of ECF include actions of the thirst center, antidiuretic hormone (ADH), renin–angiotensin–aldosterone system (RAA), and atrial natriuretic peptide (ANP).
- Water acts as a solvent and suspension agent. It helps regulate body temperature, pH, and fluid pressures inside and outside cells. It assists and participates in chemical reactions.

- Electrolytes are substances that dissociate in water into ions, electrically charged particles that circulate in body fluids and take part in the body's chemical reactions.
- Normal saline (0.9% NaCl) is an *isotonic* solution. Stronger (more concentrated) solutions are hypertonic; weaker solutions are hypotonic.
- Fluids and other substances are transported into and out of cells passively (without ATP energy) or actively (with ATP energy).
- A person's intake and output must be balanced to avoid a fluid deficit (dehydration) or a fluid excess (edema).
- The body has buffer systems that help maintain serum pH in the narrow range between approximately 7.35 and 7.45 (actually 7.37 and 7.43). Acids and bases are important components of this system.
- The lungs retain or excrete carbon dioxide and the kidneys retain or excrete bicarbonate, as part of the buffer system, to regulate pH. Arterial blood gases indicate the status of the body's acid–base balance.
- Minute fluid and electrolyte and acid–base changes occur constantly throughout the body, but the overall status in the healthy person is stability and equilibrium. The healthy person's body must be maintained within very close tolerances.
- The three major regulatory systems of body pH are *chemical* (buffers), *biologic* (blood and cellular activities), and *physiologic* (lungs and kidneys).

CRITICAL THINKING EXERCISES

1. Considering the importance of maintaining ECF volume in the body, identify how an excessive dietary intake of table salt can be dangerous.
2. Explain why a person with heartburn or upset stomach may take an over-the-counter antacid for symptom relief without causing fluid and electrolyte imbalance.
3. Older adults are at increased risk for fluid and electrolyte imbalances, partially due to decreased thirst. Discuss why extreme outdoor temperatures can place seniors at significant risk.

NCLEX-STYLE REVIEW QUESTIONS

1. The nurse is reinforcing education for a breast-feeding mother. Which statement made by the client demonstrates an understanding of adequate fluid intake?
   a. "If my mouth is dry, I will drink more fluids."
   b. "As long as I am eating food, I don't need to increase fluids."
   c. "I won't lose fluid when my baby is breast feeding."
   d. "I will drink more fluid than I did when I was not breast-feeding to replace lost fluids."

2. The nurse is caring for a client with dehydration. Which observation made by the nurse should be reported immediately?
   a. The client is drinking water frequently.
   b. Urine output of 30 mL/hr.
   c. The client has become confused.
   d. The client's mucous membranes are dry.

3. An older adult client is at risk for fluid volume deficit. Which action by the nurse could prevent this event?
   a. Offer fluids frequently.
   b. Withhold fluids after bedtime.
   c. Increase the amount of sodium in the diet.
   d. Insert an indwelling urinary catheter.

4. A client had severe diarrhea for 3 days. When arterial blood gases (ABGs) are obtained, which acid–base disturbance does the nurse anticipate observing?
   a. Metabolic acidosis
   b. Metabolic alkalosis
   c. Respiratory acidosis
   d. Respiratory alkalosis

5. The nurse obtains the blood gas results for a client experiencing respiratory difficulty. Which blood gas result would require immediate intervention by the nurse?
   a. pH 7.35, paCO$_2$ 37, HCO$_3$ 23
   b. pH 7.28, paCO$_2$ 58, HCO$_3$ 26
   c. pH 7.42, paCO$_2$ 44, HCO$_3$ 22
   d. pH 7.45, paCO$_2$ 39, HCO$_3$ 25

CHAPTER RESOURCES

Enhance your learning with additional resources on thePoint*!*

Student Resources related to this chapter can be found at thePoint.lww.com/Rosdahl12e.

18 The Musculoskeletal System

Learning Objectives

1. List the four classifications of bones, according to shape.
2. Locate and name the major bones of the body; describe their functions.
3. Explain the function of red bone marrow.
4. Name four types of joints; give an example of each.
5. Differentiate between the axial and appendicular skeletons.
6. List the five divisions of the vertebral column and the number of vertebrae in each division.
7. Differentiate between the adult and infant skull; identify the anterior and posterior fontanels on a newborn, explaining their functions.
8. Compare and contrast skeletal, smooth, and cardiac muscles and their functions.
9. Identify major muscle groups in the body, including the functions of each group.
10. Discuss factors influencing bone growth.
11. Describe the process by which muscles produce heat.
12. Differentiate between types of exercise; give examples; state the purpose of each.
13. Differentiate between tendons and ligaments.

Important Terminology

acetabulum, articulation, atrophy, bursae, calcaneus, carpal, cartilage, clavicle, coccyx, contractility, diaphysis, elasticity, epiphysis, extensibility, extension, facet, femur, fibula, flexion, hematopoiesis, humerus, ilium, irritability, isometric, isotonic, joint, ligament, malleolus, mandible, marrow, maxilla, muscle tone, ossification, osteoblast, osteoclast, osteocyte, patella, pelvis, periosteum, phalanges, pubic arch, radius, range of motion, reabsorption, sacrum, scapula, sinus, sternum, symphysis pubis, tendon, thorax, tibia, ulna, vertebral column

Acronym

IV (disc)

Most people take for granted the fact that their bodies can move. By working in harmony, the components of the *musculoskeletal* system provide movement. This system can also be called the *locomotor* system. It includes the skeleton, joints, ligaments, muscles, tendons, and accessory structures. The skeleton provides the bony framework for the human body, and the muscles assist the body to move. The musculoskeletal system works in coordination with other systems of the body, including the nervous and cardiovascular systems.

Key Concept

Skeletal system = bones and cartilage—offer support and protection
Articular system = joints and ligaments—provide movement sites
Muscular system = muscles and tendons—act to move the bones.

Structure and Function

A systematic way to study the structure and function of the musculoskeletal system is to study the skeleton, the muscles, and how they work together. Although each component is distinct and unique, the system overall cannot function without cooperative action between the separate parts. An examination of the musculoskeletal system must consider both the *skeleton and the muscles*.

THE SKELETON

The functions of the skeleton are support (structure), protection, movement, *hematopoiesis* (blood formation), and storage (Box 18-1). Movement is possible because many of the bones are used as *levers*. Not only is the skeleton the framework of the body, it is also a living structure. Although bone itself is hard and filled with calcium deposits, the cells of the bone (*osteocytes*) are living organisms. Each bone is made up of several types of tissue; therefore, bones are considered organs.

Bones

Bones are living, highly specialized connective tissue. The adult human body has 206 bones (Fig. 18-1). More than half

Box 18-1 Functions of the Skeleton

SUPPORT
- Supports the body
- Provides framework for the body
- Gives shape to the body

PROTECTION
- Protects vital organs
- Protects soft tissues

MOVEMENT
- Provides locomotion (walking, movement) by attachment of muscles, tendons, and ligaments

HEMATOPOIESIS
- Produces red blood cells
- Produces white blood cells
- Produces platelets

STORAGE
- Provides calcium
- Provides phosphorus

of the bones in the body are found in the hands, wrists, feet, and ankles. Bones, the marrow within certain bones, and the minerals of which bones are made (primarily calcium and phosphorus) contribute to the homeostatic functioning of the body.

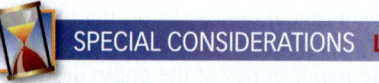

SPECIAL CONSIDERATIONS Lifespan

Infants
A baby has approximately 300 bones at birth. Fusion of some of them takes place and the process is complete by about age of 25 years.

> **Key Concept**
> Bones are living tissue and contain blood and lymphatic vessels and nerves. They may shrink (atrophy) if unused or may enlarge (hypertrophy) with excess weight-bearing.

Classification

Bones are classified according to shape: long, short, flat, or irregular. *Long bones* have an extended shape and provide the body with support and strength. *Short bones* are approximately cube shaped. *Flat bones* are shaped exactly as the name suggests and provide broad surfaces for muscle attachments. *Irregular bones* are similar to short bones, but are irregular in shape. The irregular bone classification includes small, rounded bones, the *sesamoid bones*, which develop within joints and tendons. The patella (kneecap) is the largest sesamoid bone. Other special irregular bones are those in the middle ear. The smallest bone in the body is the stapes (stirrup) in the middle ear. Table 18-1 lists the classifications of bones, their functions, and examples.

Structure

Bone tissue comprises two types. *Compact bone* is hard and dense and forms the shaft of long bones and the outer layer of other bones. *Spongy bone* (*cancellous bone*) is composed of small bony plates, resembles a sponge, and contains more spaces than compact bone.

The hollow inner part of most bones, the *medullary cavity*, is lined with *endosteum* and contains a soft substance called **marrow**. There are two types of bone marrow. Yellow marrow (as seen in soup bones) is in the medullary cavity of long bones and is mostly fat. Red marrow is found in the ends of long bones, in the bodies of vertebrae, and in flat bones. Red bone marrow is responsible for manufacturing red blood cells, white blood cells, and platelets. This process is called **hematopoiesis**.

The **periosteum** is a thin, hard, fibrous, dense connective tissue membrane that covers the outside of most bones. It often merges with tendons and ligaments (Fig. 18-2B). The periosteum contains blood vessels that supply oxygen and nutrients to bone cells (osteocytes), keeping them alive. The circulation also supplies minerals and other bone-building substances that fill intercellular spaces. This is particularly important in the healing of fractures.

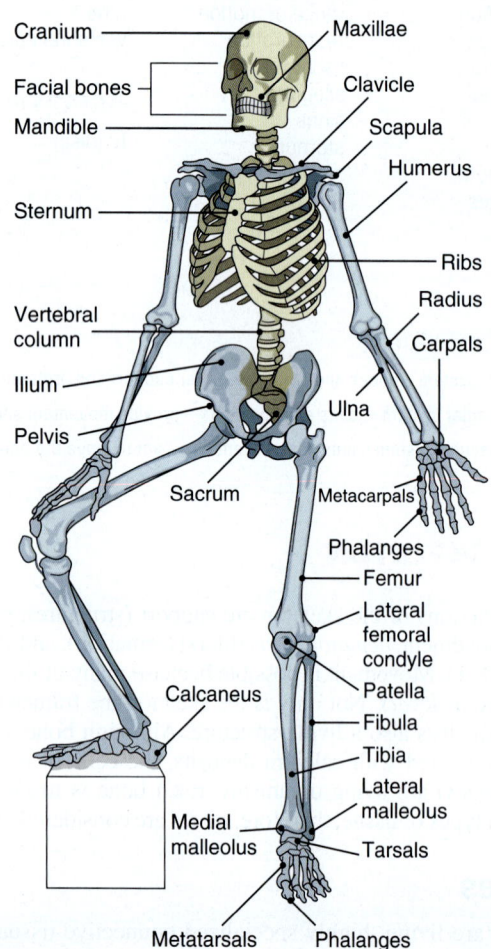

Figure 18-1 The skeleton.

CHAPTER 18 The Musculoskeletal System   197

TABLE 18-1 Classification of Bones

CLASSIFICATION	FUNCTIONS	LOCATIONS	EXAMPLES
Long (tubular)	Act as levers; support frame	Arms, legs	Femur, tibia, radius
Short (cuboidal)	Facilitate movement; transfer forces	Wrists, ankles	Tarsals, carpals
Flat	Serve as muscle attachment; protection	Head, chest, shoulders, hips	Cranial, ribs, pelvis, ilium, sternum
Irregular Sesamoid (spongy or cancellous)	For attachment of other structures or articulations or for special functions Protect tendons from wear; change tendon angle	Face, back, middle ear Knee, foot	Facial, vertebrae, bones of middle ear (malleus, incus, stapes) Patella, first metatarsal

The construction of long bones of the extremities involves two types of *osseous* (bony) tissue. The **diaphysis**, or shaft of the long bone, is *hard and compact*. The end of the long bone, the **epiphysis**, is *spongelike* and is covered by a shell of harder bone (compact bone; Fig. 18-3). The diaphysis and epiphysis do not fuse until adulthood. The diaphysis and epiphysis meet at the *epiphyseal growth plate*.

> **Key Concept**
>
> The layers of a bone are, from the outside in, periosteum, compact bone (on the epiphysis), cancellous bone (spongy bone), endosteum (tissue lining the medullary cavity), and bone marrow within the cavity (thick, jellylike; makes blood cells).

There are several recognizable contours on bones that have structural significance. A **facet** (fah-set') is a small plane or smooth area. The vertebrae of the spinal column contain facets, which are the locations for articulation (joints) with the heads of the ribs. A line (*linea*) can show up as an elevation, as on the tibia. The **malleolus** is a rounded prominence, as the medial and lateral malleoli of the tibia and fibula (Fig. 18-1). A *protuberance* is a projection of bone, as in the cranium (Fig. 18-4).

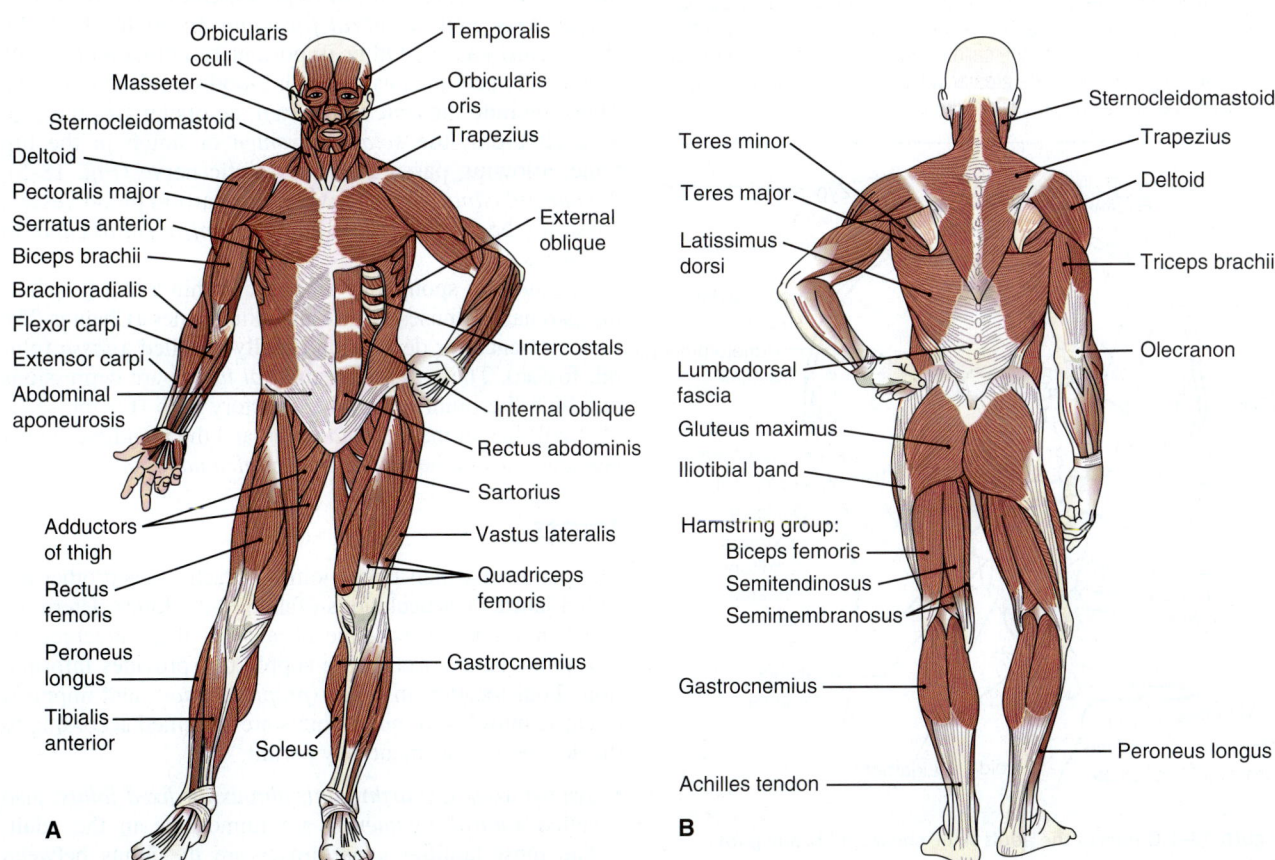

Figure 18-2 Selected muscles of the body. **A.** Anterior view. **B.** Posterior view.

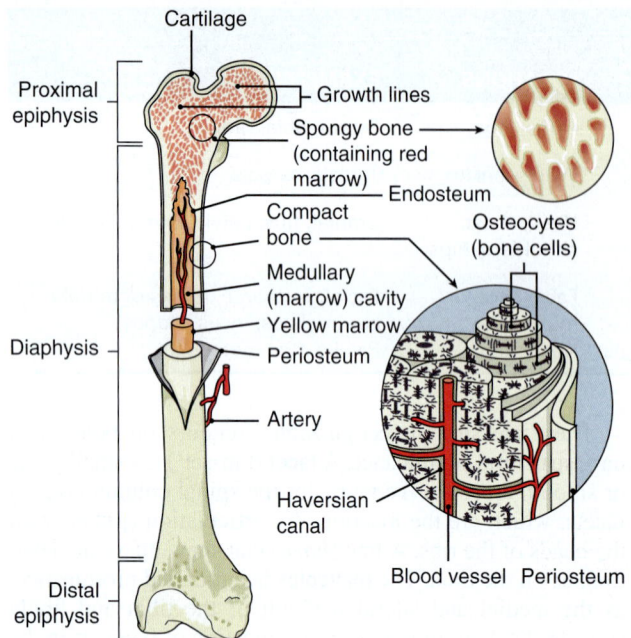

Figure 18-3 The structure of a long bone; the composition of compact bone. (Nerve tissue is also present, near blood vessels.)

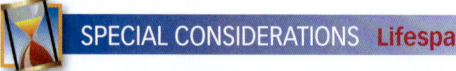

Damage to the Epiphyseal Growth Plate

Damage to the epiphyseal growth plate by trauma usually causes cessation of growth in long bones and results in shortening of the limb involved. The younger the child is when injured and the greater the severity of the injury, the greater will be the final deficit in length between the injured and uninjured limb.

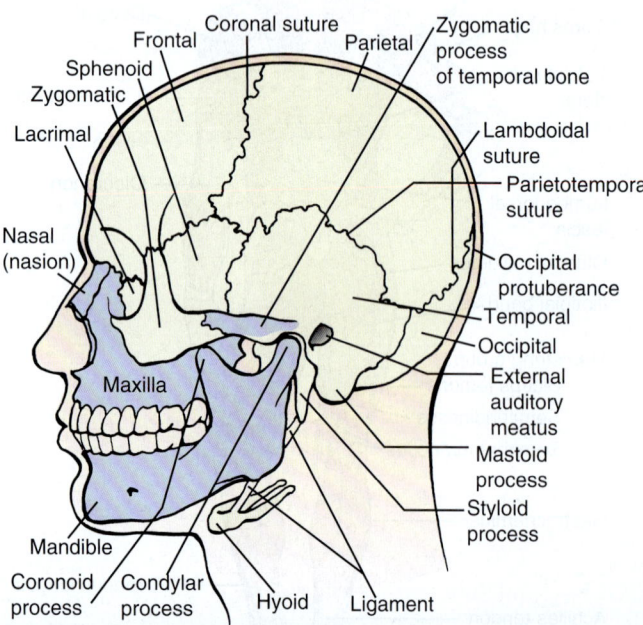

Figure 18-4 Bones of the adult skull, showing fibrous joints (sutures).

A *condyle* (e.g., the head of the femur) is a large, rounded projection, usually for articulation with another bone. (An *epicondyle* is a structure above a condyle.) A *tuberosity* is a large, elevated, knoblike projection, usually for muscle attachment. A *tubercle* is a small, rounded knob or nodule, usually for attachment of a tendon or ligament. The tibia has condyles and tuberosities on both ends, where it articulates with the thigh and ankle bones and connects with muscles and tendons (Fig. 18-1).

A flat projection or area is called a *plate*. The dental plate (dorsal or roof plate) composes the roof of the mouth. The footplate is the flat portion of the stapes bone in the middle ear (Chapter 21).

Any prominence or projection of bone is called a *bony process*. A spine (spina) is a *sharp process* (thornlike, as on the vertebrae); a ridge or crest is a *thin* or *narrow process*. (A distinct border or ridge, usually on the superior aspect of a bone, is most commonly called a *crest*.) The great (greater) *trochanter* of the femur is a large bony process. A familiar crest in the body is the iliac crest, which lies at the top of the ileum, or iliac bone of the pelvis. Each bone of the vertebral column also contains several processes, including the spinous process and the transverse process. The *pedicle* is another process that forms part of the vertebral arch of the vertebral column.

Bones also have recognizable structural openings (holes or open areas). A hole through which blood vessels, ligaments, and/or nerves pass is a *foramen* (plural: foramina). A long, tubelike hole is sometimes called a *canal*. Within the bones of the spinal column are found the *transverse foramina*, through which blood vessels and nerves pass, and *vertebral foramina*, through which the spinal cord passes. Other important foramina and canals in the body provide passages for blood vessels and nerves. These include the *apical foramen*, an opening in the root of each tooth; the *sciatic foramen* or notch in the hip bone, allowing passage of the sciatic nerve (Fig. 18-5); the *carotid canal*, through which the carotid blood vessels pass into the cranium (head); and the *infraorbital canal* in the eye socket.

A **sinus** is a spongelike air space within a bone, such as the paranasal sinuses within the skull bones (Chapter 25). A dent, trench, or depression usually is called a *fossa* (plural: fossae). The *cranial* or *cerebral fossae* are depressions in which the brain rests. The olfactory bulb (for the sense of smell) lies in the *ethmoid fossa*, and the mandible (lower jawbone) lies in the *mandibular* or *glenoid fossa*.

Joints

The points at which bones join or attach to each other are called **joints** or **articulations** (Table 18-2). Joints determine which motions are possible because of their attachments. The joints have a rich nerve supply that provides information about location in space (*proprioception*) and impulses to cause muscles to move. Joints are classified according to the degree of movement they permit:

- *Synarthroses* (*synarthrodial*, *fibrous*, or *fixed joints*; also called *sutural ligaments*) are immovable in the adult. The most familiar synarthroses are the joints between

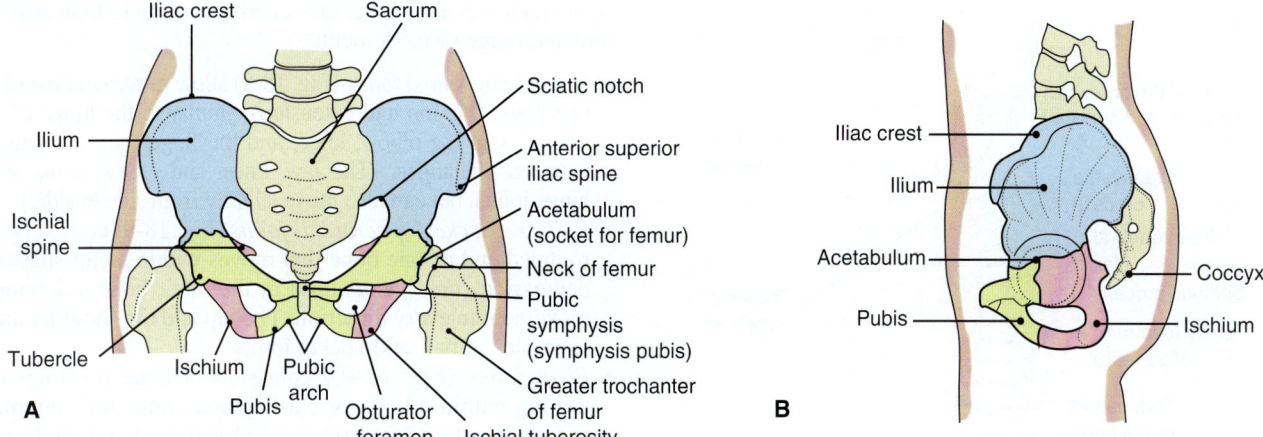

Figure 18-5 The pelvic bones. **A.** Anterior view. **B.** Lateral view.

skull bones. These joints are not firmly fixed in infants, but become fused by adulthood, because of interlocking projections and fibrous connective tissue growth. They are also called *sutures* because they are so tightly bound, as if they are sewn together. A *gomphosis* is a fibrous joint in which a conical process is inserted into a socket, as is a tooth in its bony socket.

- *Amphiarthroses* (*amphiarthrodial* or *cartilaginous joints*) are slightly movable. Examples are the symphysis pubis and articulations between the ribs and spinal column. Here, cartilage lies between articulating bones. A *synchondrosis* is a joint in which cartilage is converted to bone by adulthood, as in the coccyx.

- *Diarthroses* (*synovial joints*) are freely movable, allowing movement in various directions, as at the ends of long bones; they are the most common joints in the body. These joints also contain ligaments and cartilage (discussed later). A thin, smooth layer of articular cartilage covers and pads synovial joints, and an articular capsule encloses the ends of the bones. The capsules are lined with synovial membrane, which secretes *synovial fluid*, a lubricating and nutrient-bearing material. Some synovial joints, notably knees, shoulders, elbows, and hips, also contain **bursae**, fluid-filled sacs that cushion the movements of muscles and tendons.

TABLE 18-2	Classification of Joints	
TYPE OF JOINT	ACTIONS	EXAMPLES
Synarthroses: immovable, fibrous	No motion	Bones of the skull fitted together with interlocking notches (in adults) (see Fig. 18-4)
Amphiarthroses: slightly movable, cartilaginous	Slight degree of motion or flexibility	Vertebral column (see Figs. 18-6 and 18-7) Symphysis pubis
Diarthroses: freely movable (synovial)		
Hinge joints	Motion like a door on hinges	Finger, elbow, and knee joints (Fig. 18-8)
Ball-and-socket joints	Rotation	Shoulders and hips (Fig. 18-9)
Pivot joints	Motion like that of turning a doorknob	Wrist (turns forearm) (Fig. 18-10)
Gliding joints	Gliding motion	Wrist
Condyloid joints	Allow motions in two planes at right angles	Wrist, foot, hand
Saddle joints	Opposing surfaces are concavo-convex (fit together like two saddles with riding surfaces together); allow a wide range of movements	Thumb

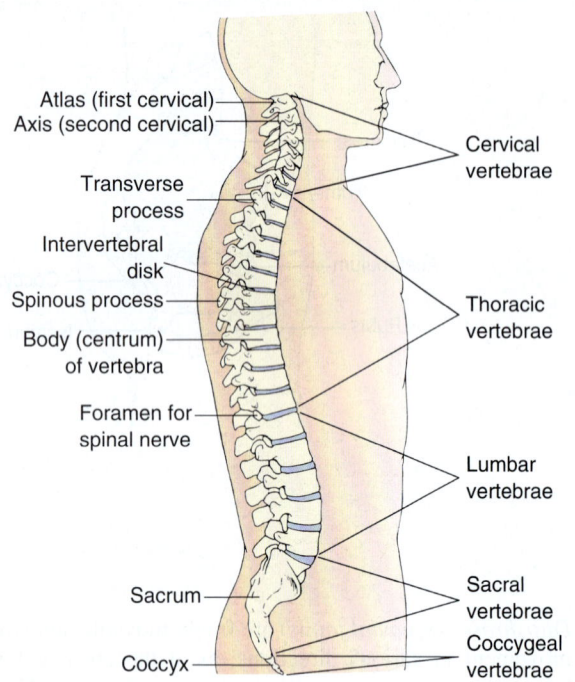

Figure 18-6 A normal spine. Note the several curvatures of the adult spine. (The normal infant's spine is shown in Chapter 47.)

Synovial joints are further classified according to their structure and range of movement:

- *Hinge (ginglymus) joints* (Fig. 18-8) allow movement in only one plane (flexion and extension), similar to the hinge of a door—as in the elbow, knee, and the finger and toe joints between phalanges. (The jaw, knee, and elbow joints are hinge joints, but can also move slightly from side to side.)
- *Ball-and-socket (spheroidal) joints* (Fig. 18-9) consist of a rounded end of one bone that moves within a cup-shaped depression (*the acetabulum*) in the other bone, allowing movement in every direction. The hip and the shoulder are examples of ball-and-socket joints.
- *Pivot joints* (Fig. 18-10) consist of a bone pivoting or turning within a bony or cartilaginous ring. An example is found in the atlas (first cervical vertebra) and the head rotating on the axis (second cervical vertebra). Another example is the wrist joint.
- *Gliding (arthrodial, plane) joints* are those in which bones slide against each other, as in intervertebral joints and parts of the wrist and ankle joints.
- *Condyloid joints* involve the oval-shaped head of one bone moving within an elliptical cavity in another, permitting all movements except axial rotation. Examples are the wrist (between radius and carpal bones) and at the base of the index finger (Fig. 18-11A).

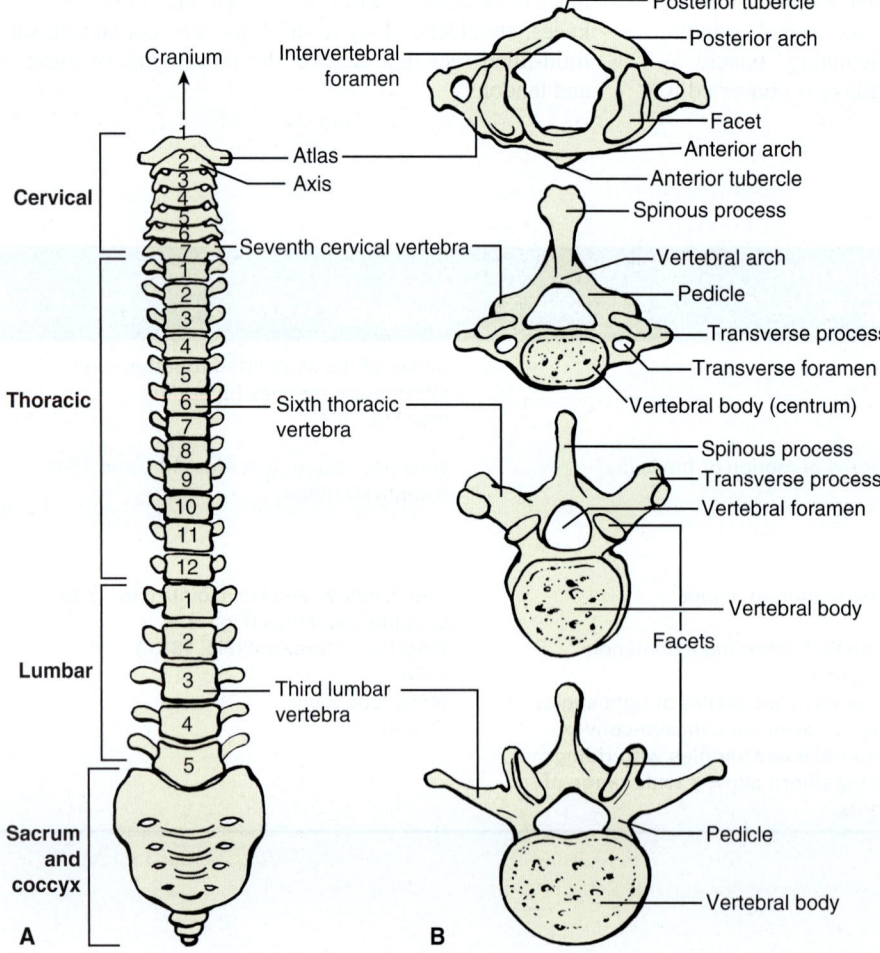

Figure 18-7 A. Front view of the vertebral column. The *atlas* is number 1 and is above the *axis*, which is number 2. (This is a synovial joint, specifically, a pivot joint.) B. Vertebrae from above.

CHAPTER 18   The Musculoskeletal System   201

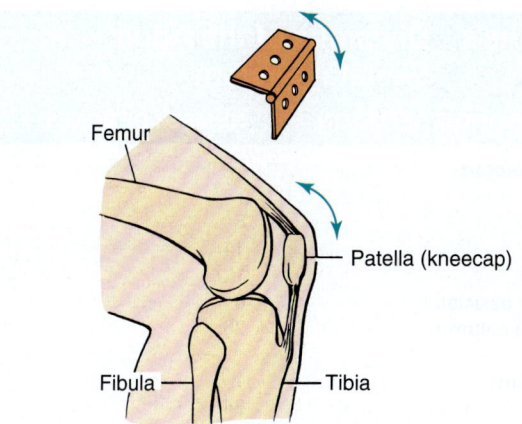

Figure 18-8 Hinge joint (knee).

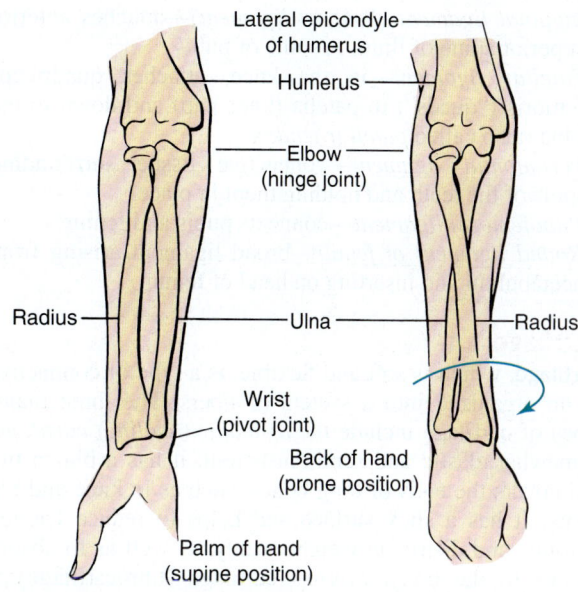

Figure 18-10 Pivot joint (wrist) and hinge joint (elbow). The pivot joint permits a wide range of motion, while the hinge joint only allows flexion and extension.

- *Saddle joints* allow movements that can be shifted in several directions, as in the base of the thumb (carpometacarpal joints). These joints allow humans to perform movements not present in most animals, such as the ability to pick up a very small object (Fig. 18-11B).

Ligaments

Strong fibrous bands called **ligaments** hold bones together. Some ligaments, the *accessory ligaments*, do not move or stretch, but strengthen or support other ligaments, to produce stability in a joint. Some ligaments connect bones to muscles or cartilage. Ligaments also support internal organs and other structures. Many ligaments allow for great flexibility, stretching, and movement. A ligament is said to *arise* or originate in the bone or structure that is more stationary. It is said to *insert* into the bone that does most of the movement.

There are hundreds of ligaments in the body. Common examples include the following:

- *Arcuate ligament*—connects the diaphragm with the lowest ribs and first lumbar vertebrae
- *Broad ligament* of uterus—arising in the peritoneum; supports the uterus, connecting it to the pelvic wall
- *Broad ligament* of liver (*falciform ligament*)—fold of peritoneum; helps attach liver to the diaphragm; also separates right and left lobes of the liver
- *Cruciate* ("cross-shaped") *ligaments* of knee—one anterior, one posterior—arise from the femur and attach to the tibia at the knee (frequent site of football injury)
- *Henle ligament*—attaches rectus abdominus muscle to pubic bone

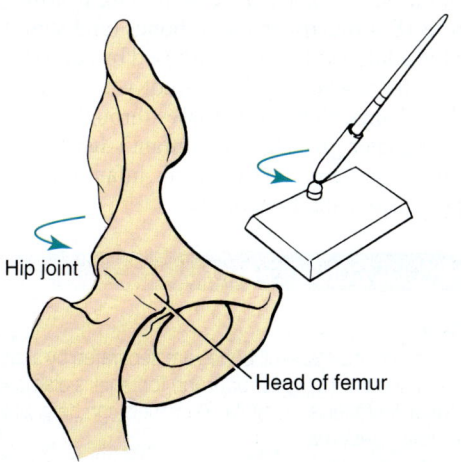

Figure 18-9 Ball-and-socket joint (hip). This joint permits movement in many directions.

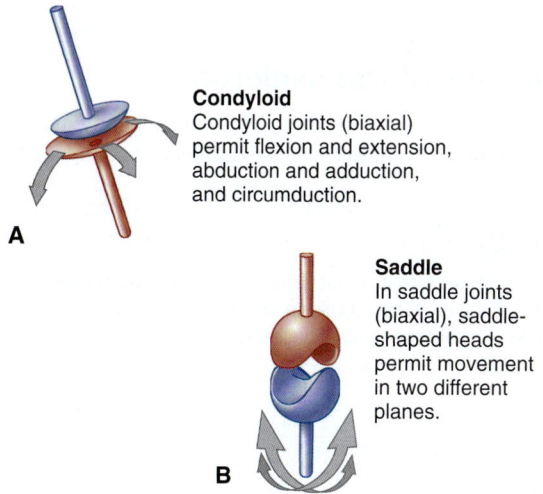

Figure 18-11 **A.** Condyloid joint—biaxial (permits flexion–extension, abduction–adduction, and circumduction—as in proximal phalanx of metacarpal). **B.** Saddle joint (carpometacarpal joints; allows movements in several directions and in two planes, allowing humans movements not available to most animals—as in base of thumb). (Moore K. L., Agur A. M., & Dalley A. F. [2014]. *Essential clinical anatomy* [5th ed.]. Wolters Kluwer Health.)

- *Inguinal ligament* (*Poupart ligament*)—attaches anterior superior spine of ilium to spine of pubis
- *Patellar ligament*—in the knee, attaches quadriceps femoris ("quads") to patella (knee cap) and down to the tibia (also called *patellar tendon*)
- *Periodontal ligament*—connective tissue surrounding roots of the teeth and holding them in place
- *Pubofemoral ligament*—connects pubis and femur
- *Round ligament of femur*—broad ligament arising from acetabulum and inserting on head of femur

Cartilage

Cartilage, which is soft and flexible, is a type of connective tissue organized into a system of fibers. The three major types of cartilage include the *articular (hyaline) cartilage*. Somewhat elastic and semitransparent, it has a bluish tint and covers the ends of long bones, such as in knee and hip joints. It has a slick surface and helps to reduce friction in joints and distribute weight evenly, as well as to absorb shocks to the body. *Fibrous* cartilage (fibrocartilage) is strong and rigid, as in the symphysis pubis. *Elastic* (reticular) cartilage is opaque and has a yellowish tint and is the most pliable, as in the auditory canal. Cartilage has no blood supply and receives oxygen and nutrients by diffusion. The fibrous connective tissue surrounding cartilage (except in joints) is called *perichondrium*.

SPECIAL CONSIDERATIONS — Lifespan

Pliability of Bones

Children's bones are more pliable than those of adults. Some infant bones at birth are entirely cartilage and some are a combination of bone and cartilage. Children's bones can bend more easily for this reason, helping to prevent fractures. (The cartilage is slowly replaced by bone as the child matures.)

Divisions of the Skeleton

The skeleton has two divisions: axial and appendicular. Table 18-3 summarizes major bones and divisions of the skeleton.

> **Key Concept**
>
> The axial skeleton contains the bones in the center (axis) of the body, such as the skull, vertebral column, and rib cage. The appendicular skeleton contains the bones of the pelvic girdle, extremities, and appendages.

The Axial Skeleton

Skull

Twenty-eight separate bones comprise the skull (Box 18-2). The dome-shaped roof protecting the superior aspect of the brain, the *calvaria*, is made up of the parietal bones and the posterior occipital bone. The eight flat bones of the cranium protect the brain, eyes, and internal ear structures. The 14 facial bones protect the face; they are lightweight, irregularly shaped, and generally small. The three pairs of bones of the middle ear (ossicles) are essential for hearing (Chapter 21). Figure 18-4 illustrates major bones (and sutures) of the skull. In the adult, skull bones are fused by sutures and so do not move. The newborn's skull is not yet fused, permitting the skull to change shape as it passes through the birth canal and allowing later growth of the infant's head (Fig. 18-12). The membranous areas between an infant's cranial bones ("soft spots") are called *fontanels*.

TABLE 18-3 Divisions of the Adult Skeletal System

REGIONS OF THE SKELETON	NUMBER OF BONES
Axial Skeleton	
Skull	
Cranium	8
Face	14
Hyoid	1
Auditory ossicles	6
Vertebral column	26
Thorax	
Sternum	1
Ribs	24
	Subtotal = 80
Appendicular Skeleton	
Pectoral (shoulder) girdles	
Clavicle	2
Scapula	2
Upper limbs (extremities)	
Humerus	2
Ulna	2
Radius	2
Carpals	16
Metacarpals	10
Phalanges	28
Pelvic (hip) girdle	
Hip, pelvic, or coxal bone	2
Lower limbs (extremities)	
Femur	2
Fibula	2
Tibia	2
Patella	2
Tarsals	14
Metatarsals	10
Phalanges	28
	Subtotal = 126
	Total = 206

SPECIAL CONSIDERATIONS — Lifespan

Fontanels

In newborns and infants, skull bones are separated by spaces (fontanels or "soft spots"). The anterior (front) fontanel is diamond shaped; the posterior fontanel is triangular. Fontanels can be gently palpated on all healthy newborns.

Box 18-2 The 28 Bones of the Adult Skull

BONES OF THE CRANIUM (8)
Two parietal: top and sides of head
One occipital: back and base of head
One frontal: forehead, roof of skull, and nasal cavities
Two temporal: sides and base of skull (contain ear cavities); mastoid cells in tip
One sphenoid: center of base of skull
One ethmoid: roof of nasal cavity, base of cranium, upper part of nasal septum (also includes the paired and fused superior and middle conchae)

BONES OF THE FACE (14)
Two nasal: bridge of nose
One vomer: divides nasal cavity, as part of nasal septum
Two inferior turbinates (conchae): in the nostrils
Two lacrimal (orbitals): front part of eye sockets
Two zygomatic: prominent part of cheeks; base of eye sockets
Two palate (palatines): back of hard palate
Two maxillae: upper jaw, front of hard palate
One mandible: lower jaw—only movable bone in skull

AUDITORY OSSICLES (6) IN THE EAR
One pair malleus (hammer)
One pair incus (anvil)
One pair stapes (stirrup)

The skull is covered by the *true scalp*, made up of three layers. Outermost is a thin skin, made up of sweat and sebaceous glands and hair follicles. The scalp has good blood supply and lymphatic drainage. (This is why open head wounds bleed profusely.) The middle layer of the true scalp consists of loose connective tissues, including vascular and cutaneous nerves. The inner layer, the *aponeurosis*, a tendinous sheet, is also called the *epicranius*.

Under the true scalp is a layer of loose connective tissue, made up of spongelike spaces, allowing limited movement of the scalp proper. The *pericranium* is the dense connective tissue which is the external periosteum of the cranium. A memory guide for the layers of the scalp is SCALP: S—skin; C—connective tissue; A—aponeurosis; L—loose connective tissue; P—periosteum. Chapter 19 describes the structure and function of the brain, and Figure 19-4 illustrates the meninges, structures under the scalp.

Although the basic shape and arrangement of cranial and facial bones are universal, subtle variations contribute to each person's unique face. There are two *maxillae* (singular: maxilla) that fuse to create the upper jawbone. The lower jawbone, the mandible, is the only movable facial bone. The mandible can move up, down, and sideways, as well as forward (*protraction*) and backward (*retraction*).

A small horseshoe-shaped bone, the *hyoid*, lies just behind and below the mandible, directly above the larynx. The hyoid is not directly attached to any skull bone; it is attached by muscles and ligaments and seems to float. Tongue muscles are attached to the hyoid bone, to assist in swallowing and speaking.

Four pairs of cavities (sinuses) in the cranial bones make the skull lighter and enhance vocal sounds. The sinuses are named for the bones in which they lie: *frontal, ethmoid, sphenoid,* and *maxillary*. Sinuses are lined with mucous membrane continuous with nasal mucosa and drain into the nasal cavity.

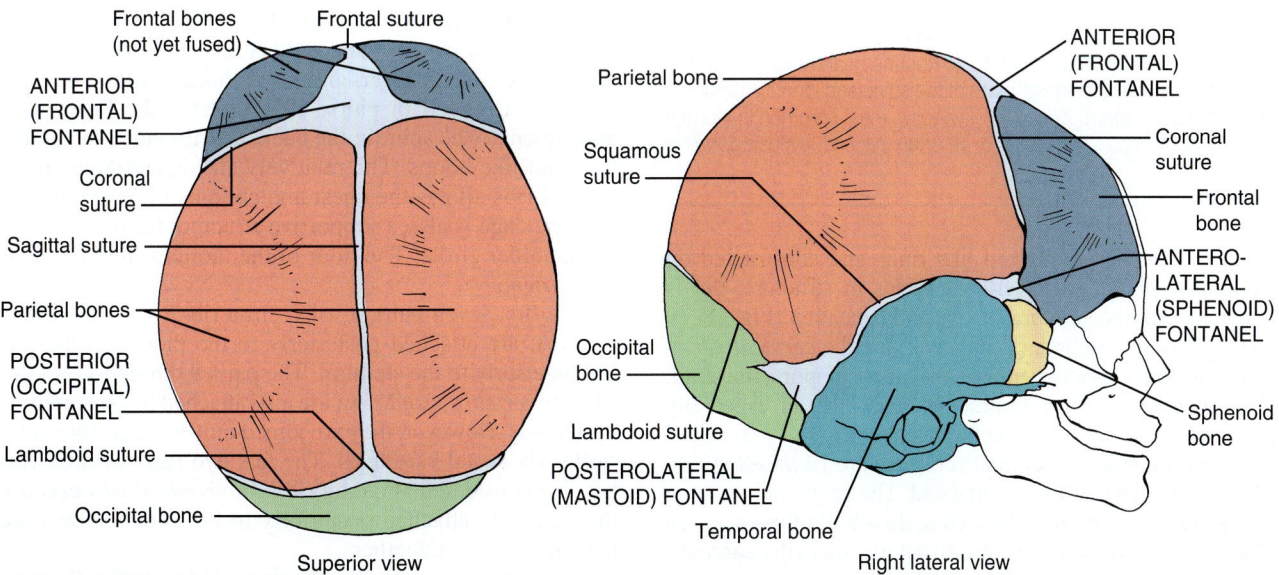

Figure 18-12 Fontanels of the skull at birth.

SPECIAL CONSIDERATIONS   Lifespan

Protection of Skeletal Structures

It is important to protect skeletal structures:
- Wear a helmet and other protective equipment when skateboarding, skiing, or riding a bicycle, motorcycle, or snowmobile.
- Make sure to get enough calcium by consuming milk and dairy products or appropriate substitutes.
- Get enough activity to keep bones strong.

VERTEBRAL COLUMN

The **vertebral column** (spine) holds the head, allows twisting and bending, stiffens and supports the middle portion of the body and holds it upright, and provides attachments for the ribs and pelvic bones (Fig. 18-6). The spine also protects the spinal cord, which passes from the brain down through the vertebral foramina (Fig. 18-7). In children, the vertebral column consists of 33 or 34 bones. Fusions of these bones occur; therefore, most adults have 26 vertebrae. The normal spine has four curves that help balance the body (Fig. 18-6). Disease, injury, and poor posture distort these curves.

The vertebral column is served by many blood vessels and nerves. Two major ligaments stabilize the vertebral column and help prevent spinal injuries. One extends from the pelvic surface of the sacrum to the first cervical vertebra (C_1, the atlas) and the occipital (skull) bone. Another weaker ligament runs within the vertebral canal and is attached mainly to the intervertebral discs.

SPECIAL CONSIDERATIONS   Lifespan

Spine Abnormalities

Scoliosis is an abnormal lateral (sideways) spinal curvature. It occurs most commonly during adolescence and is most frequently found in girls. *Lordosis* ("swayback") is an exaggeration of the normal lumbar spine curve in the small of the back. Routine health examinations in children evaluate the straightness of the spine and identify abnormal curvatures (Chapters 72 and 73). *Kyphosis*, most common in women ("widow's hump," "humpback"), is often caused by osteoporosis (Chapter 92).

The vertebrae are shaped like rings and constructed on a common plane; each vertebra varies in structure, but is designed to fit the vertebrae above and beneath it (Fig. 18-7). The top seven vertebrae (in the neck) are the *cervical vertebrae*. The first cervical vertebra, the *atlas*, supports the skull. The second cervical vertebra, the *axis*, has an especially wide surface so the head can turn freely.

Directly below the cervical vertebrae are 12 *thoracic vertebrae*, to which the ribs are attached. The next five vertebrae are the *lumbar vertebrae*, located in the small of the back. In adults, the *sacral vertebrae* are fused together (the **sacrum**), which anchors the pelvis. The spinal column ends in a single bone in adults, the **coccyx**, commonly called the *tailbone*.

SPECIAL CONSIDERATIONS   Lifespan

Sacral Vertebrae in Children

Children have five sacral vertebrae that fuse to form the sacrum. The last four vertebrae, the coccygeal vertebrae, are small and incomplete and later fuse to form the coccyx.

Rounded plates of cartilage, intervertebral (**IV**) discs (disks), separate the vertebrae anteriorly from one another (Fig. 18-13). Each IV disc is composed of an outer fibrous material and inner gelatinous material. These act as "shock absorbers" during walking, jumping, or falling and are called *cartilaginous* (gliding) joints. A "slipped" disc refers to an IV disc that has shifted out of position. A "ruptured" disc occurs when pressure forces less dense tissue sideways, causing a protrusion in the disc walls (like a squashed grape). Either situation can place pressure on a nerve, causing great discomfort.

On the inner side of each vertebra is a bony structure, the *arch*, forming the spinal (intervertebral, vertebral) foramen, the opening through which the spinal cord passes. Jutting from the arch are several bony processes or extensions, to which ligaments and tendons of the back muscles are anchored. The muscles, ligaments, and cartilage discs help make the vertebral column strong, yet flexible. They enable the person to comfortably bend forward, backward, and side to side and to rotate the central portion of the body.

The ribs articulate with the vertebrae at *facet joints*. These joints are lined with cartilage, but may become misaligned. Many cases of back pain, particularly in the lower back, involve misalignment of facet joints (Fig. 18-7).

THORACIC (RIB) CAGE

The **thorax** (chest) cavity is formed by 12 pairs of flat, narrowed bones, the *ribs* (*costae*) (Fig. 18-14). The ribs form the thoracic or rib cage and protect internal structures such as the heart, lungs, liver, and great thoracic blood vessels. Ribs are arranged in pairs, 12 on each side. From their attachment to the spine at the back, the ribs curve out and to the front like hoops. The relatively elastic cartilage on the ends of ribs allows the chest and abdomen to expand. The thoracic cage is also a supportive structure for the bones of the shoulder girdle. The floor of the thorax is the muscular *diaphragm*.

The first seven pairs of ribs, "true ribs" or *vertebrosternal ribs*, are attached posteriorly to the thoracic vertebrae and anteriorly to the sternum. The pairs 8 through 12, "false ribs" or *vertebrocostal ribs*, are also attached to the vertebrae posteriorly. However, they are joined only to each other anteriorly, via costal cartilages. The last two pairs of false ribs are also considered "floating ribs" or *vertebral ribs* because they are only attached posteriorly to the vertebrae and are not attached to each other.

The front boundary of the upper thorax is the **sternum** (*breastbone*), a flat, sword-shaped bone in the center chest

CHAPTER 18 The Musculoskeletal System   205

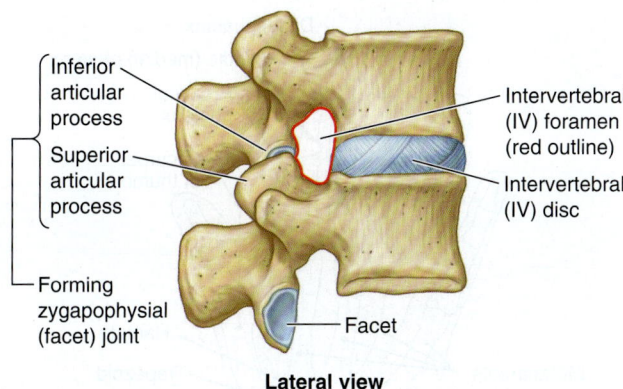

Figure 18-13 Side view of two lumbar vertebrae, showing the intervertebral (IV) disc, spinous processes, and inferior facet joint. (Moore K. L., Agur A. M., & Dalley A. F. [2014]. *Essential clinical anatomy* [5th ed.]. Wolters Kluwer Health.)

opposite the thoracic vertebrae in the back. The sternum consists of three sections: the *manubrium* at the top; the *body* in the middle; and the *xiphoid process* projecting out at the bottom.

The Appendicular Skeleton

The appendicular skeleton is composed of the bones of the upper and lower extremities and pelvic girdle (Fig. 18-1).

Upper Extremities

The upper extremities include the shoulders and arms. Four bones form the *shoulder girdle*, which anchors the arms. Two long, thin bones, the **clavicles** (collar bones), are attached to the sternum and extend outward at a right angle to it on either side. Opposite the clavicles on each side of the back is a **scapula** or shoulder blade. A scapula is a flat, triangular bone attached to the outer end of the clavicle on the skeleton. It attaches to the trunk of the body medially with the manubrium of the sternum. The structure of the scapula gives the body free movement of the shoulders and arms.

The **humerus** is the long bone in the upper arm. The upper end is attached to the scapula, and the lower end meets the two forearm bones to form the elbow joint. (Each long bone is wider at the ends and thinner in the middle, providing strength where it meets another bone.)

The forearm has two bones that lie beside one another. The larger is the **ulna** and the smaller is the **radius**. Two hollows, or depressions, in the upper end of the ulna provide positioning for other bones. One depression holds the lower end of the humerus; the other holds the upper end of the radius. Both radius and ulna are attached to wrist bones to form the wrist joint. The arrangement of these bones allows the palm to be turned forward (*supine position, supination*) or backward (*prone position, pronation*). The radius and ulna move so freely with the wrist bones and each other that when the palm turns down, the radius crosses the ulna (Fig. 18-10).

The many small bones in the hands and wrists allow for great range of motion (ROM), such as twisting and grasping. These bones enable human beings to perform activities such as playing musical instruments, writing, and picking up minute objects with thumb and forefinger.

> **Key Concept**
>
> More than one quarter of the bones in the body are in the hands and wrists.

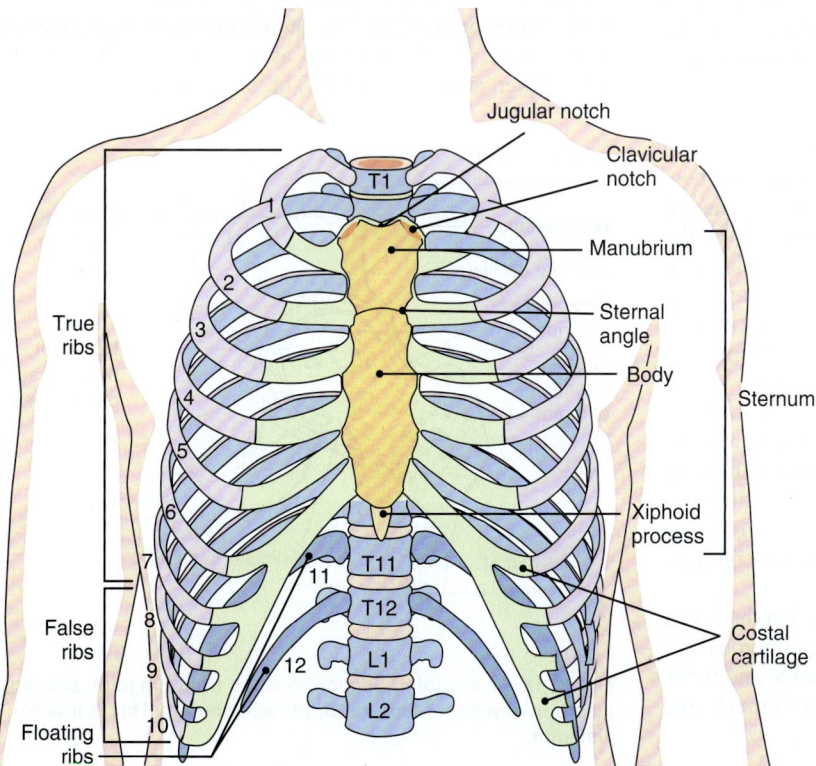

Figure 18-14 Bones of the thorax (anterior view). The first seven pairs of ribs—true ribs; pairs 8 through 12—false ribs (the last two pairs are floating ribs). The sternum is the structure shown in yellow. The thoracic vertebrae are indicated here and numbered as T_1, T_{11}, and T_{12}. L_1 and L_2 are lumbar vertebrae.

Figure 18-15 depicts the bones of the hand. The eight **carpal** bones, wrist bones, are small, irregular bones that support the base of the palm. They are attached to the radius, the ulna, and five long, slender, and slightly curved metacarpal bones forming the palm of the hand. The other ends of the metacarpals attach to the *phalanges*, or finger bones. Three phalanges are in each finger and two in each thumb, with joints between each phalanx. (Any bone of either a finger or a toe is called a **phalanx**.)

Lower Extremities

The **femur** (thigh bone) is the bone in the upper leg. Being the body's longest and strongest bone, it supports the weight of body. The lower end of the femur is attached to the tibia of the lower leg at the knee joint. The upper end of the femur, the head, is attached to the pelvic bone in a ball-and-socket joint, where its rounded head fits into a depression, the **acetabulum** (Fig. 18-16). The head of the femur joins the shaft of the femur by a short length of bone, the *neck*. (This is a common site of fractures, particularly in seniors.) Elevations on either side of the junction of the shaft and the neck, called *trochanters*, serve as points of muscle attachment.

There are two bones in the lower leg: the **tibia** (shin bone) and **fibula**. The tibia is the long weight-bearing bone of the lower leg. The upper end of the tibia is attached to the lower end of the femur at the knee joint (Fig. 18-17). A sesamoid bone, the **patella** (kneecap), protects the front of the knee joint and is buried in a tendon passing over the joint. The lower end of the tibia meets the bones of the ankle and the fibula to form the ankle joint. A protrusion on the lower end of the tibia can be felt on the medial side of the ankle. This is the *medial malleolus*.

The fibula, smaller than the tibia, is attached to the tibia at its upper end. The fibula is not a weight-bearing bone and not part of the knee joint. The lower end of the fibula is part of the ankle joint. Similar to the medial malleolus of the tibia, another projection called the *lateral* (side) *malleolus* is located where the distal end of the fibula meets the ankle bones.

The foot is constructed to support the weight of the entire body and still to provide flexibility and resilience. The ankle's seven *tarsal* bones are compact and shaped irregularly; the largest of which (the **calcaneus**) is in the heel. (The others are the talus, navicular, cuboid, and three cuneiforms [Fig. 18-18].) The tarsal bones join the five *metatarsal* bones (instep bones) to form two arches: the *longitudinal arch*, which extends from heel to toe, and the *transverse* or *metatarsal arch*, which extends across the foot. The weight of the body falls on these arches, and the many joints spring and give during walking. Weak muscles lessen this spring, and high spiky heels and poor posture upset the body balance, flattening the arches. The 14 bones of the toes, the *phalanges*, are attached to the metatarsals. The big toe has two phalanges; each of the other toes has three.

In general, the hands and feet are built alike, but the bones of the hands are finer and the joints more numerous (27 bones are in each wrist and hand, 26 in each ankle and foot). The hands are designed for fine and flexible movements and the feet for support.

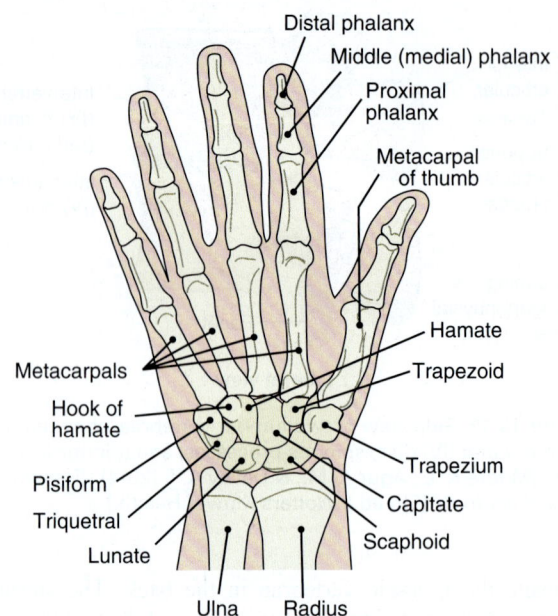

Figure 18-15 Bones of the right hand, anterior (palmar) view. The wrist contains eight carpal bones. The hand contains 5 metacarpals, and 14 phalanges. The total number of bones in both hands is 54. The joint at the base of the thumb is a saddle joint, permitting almost unlimited mobility. The joints between the hand and fingers are *condyloid* joints (biaxial) and permit movement in several directions. The joints between the phalanges are hinge joints.

The Pelvic Girdle

Two large, irregularly shaped innominate *hip bones* (*os coxae*) attach posteriorly to the sacrum (Fig. 18-5) to form the *pelvic girdle* or **pelvis**. The pelvis supports the spinal column and protects parts of the digestive, urinary, and reproductive systems. The pelvic bones spread outward at the top and become narrow at their front lower edges. The **ilium** is the upper flaring portion of the pelvis, usually identified as the hip bone. The *ischium* is the lower, stronger portion. The pubic bones meet in front

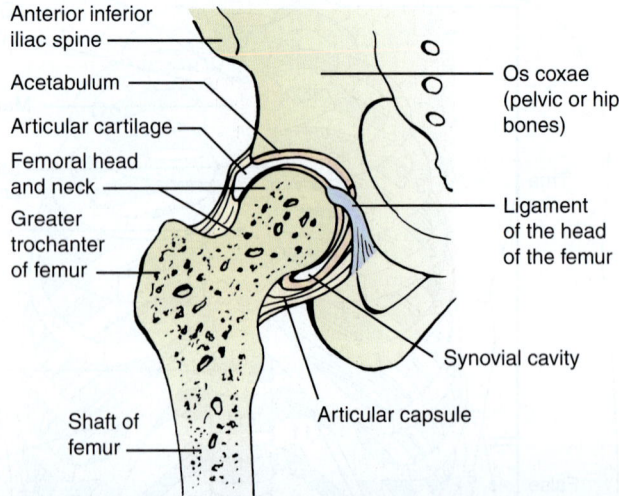

Figure 18-16 Hip joint. Section through right hip joint, showing insertion of head of femur into the acetabulum. This is a synovial joint.

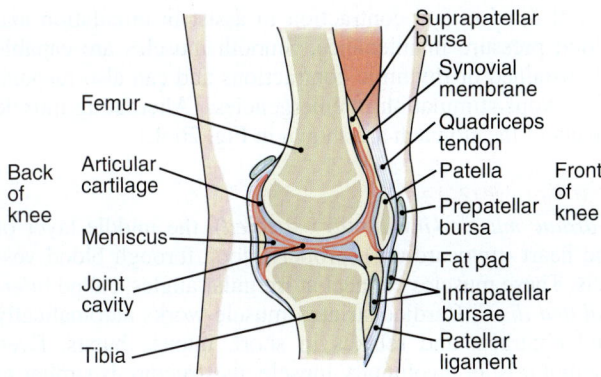

Figure 18-17 Knee joint (sagittal section).

and are joined by a pad of cartilage called the **symphysis pubis**. Connected to the sacrum and coccyx posteriorly, these bones form the *pelvic cavity*, which houses the urinary bladder, the rectum, and in women, the uterus and ovaries. In men, the prostate and some glands are within the pelvis. A woman's pelvis is larger and wider than a man's, which provides room for development and vaginal delivery of the fetus (Chapters 29 and 66). The angle of the pelvic opening (**pubic arch**) is less than 90° in men and greater than 90° in women.

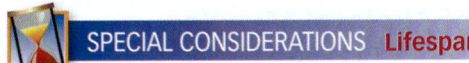

Pelvic Bones

In the fetus, pelvic bones develop as three separate bones known as the ilium, ischium, and pubis, which usually fuse by about age 25 years.

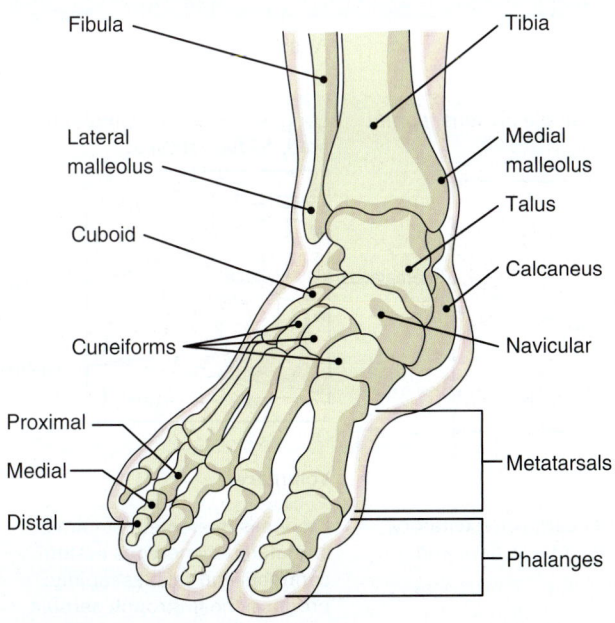

Figure 18-18 Bones of the right foot.

NCLEX Alert

The NCLEX not only requires knowledge of the structures and functions of muscles and bones, it also requires that you know the differences in nursing care between injuries, illness, or inherited disorders of muscles or bones.

THE MUSCLES

Functions of the skeleton include providing the body shape and mobility, using bones as levers. Without muscles, the body would be immobile. Although the skeleton determines the size of the body's framework, muscle and fat determine body shape. Functions of muscles are body movement, blood circulation, and heat production (Box 18-3). All muscle tissues have specific characteristics (contractility, extensibility, elasticity, and irritability), as described later.

Key Concept

Without muscles, the bones would be unable to move.

Muscle Classification

Chapter 15 lists three types of muscle tissue by function: skeletal, smooth, and cardiac. Each is also identified by appearance. Skeletal and cardiac muscles are *striated*, consisting of fibers marked by bands and appearing striped. Smooth muscle is *nonstriated*. Muscles are further described as *voluntary* or *involuntary*. Table 18-4 presents muscle types. (Muscle tissue is approximately 15% denser than adipose [fat] tissue.)

Skeletal Muscles

Skeletal (voluntary striated) muscles control skeletal movements and are under voluntary (conscious) control. There are more than 630 skeletal muscles in the human body, constituting approximately 40% of body weight (Fig. 18-2A). Their functions include locomotion, facial expression, and posture. The two types of voluntary muscles are *fast-twitch*—those which contract quickly and powerfully, but encounter rapid fatigue—and *slow-twitch*—those which can sustain a contraction, but do not exert great force.

Key Concept

The masseter (jaw) muscle is considered the body's strongest muscle by volume, exerting great bite strength. The tongue is actually made up of 16 muscles and is also a strong muscle.

Smooth Muscles

Smooth muscle forms part of the walls of blood vessels and hollow internal organs (*viscera*). It controls involuntary motions and is also known as *involuntary* or *visceral muscle*. Smooth muscle is responsible for actions such as propelling urine through the urinary tract, moving food in the digestive tract, dilating the pupils of the eyes (Fig. 21-1), and activating arrector pili in the skin (Fig. 16-1). It also controls blood

Box 18-3 Functions of Muscles

VOLUNTARY MOVEMENT
- Enable walking, standing, sitting, chewing, and other movements
- Maintain body in upright position
- Participate in body balance

INVOLUNTARY MUSCLE ACTION
- Maintain heartbeat to pump blood
- Provide arterial blood flow
- Promote lymphatic and venous blood return to heart
- Dilate and contract blood vessels to control blood flow
- Maintain respiration—the largest muscle of respiration is the diaphragm
- Perform digestion processes
- Perform elimination processes
- Participate in reflexes
- Enable all other involuntary actions of body

PROTECTION
- Protect body in emergency by reflex action
- Cover, surround, and protect internal organs (viscera)
- Support internal organs

MISCELLANEOUS
- Produce heat
- Assist in maintaining stable body temperature (in shivering, "goose flesh," and muscles give off heat)
- Provide shape to body

vessel dilation and contraction to assist in circulation and blood pressure maintenance. Smooth muscles are capable of sustained or rhythmic contractions and can also respond to nervous stimulation in emergencies. (Alternating muscle layers of the stomach are shown in Fig. 26-4.)

Cardiac Muscle

Cardiac muscle (*involuntary striated*), the middle layer of the heart (myocardium), propels blood through blood vessels. These muscles connect at irregular angles, called *intercalated discs*. Cardiac striated muscle works automatically and contracts and relaxes in short, intense bursts. Even though it is an involuntary muscle, its structure is similar to skeletal muscle (Chapter 22).

> **Key Concept**
> - Skeletal muscles, responsible for locomotion, facial expression, and posture, are under voluntary control.
> - Smooth muscle controls involuntary motion inside body organs and structures.
> - Cardiac muscle, which is involuntary, is responsible for propelling blood through blood vessels. The heart muscle is the longest working muscle, pumping continually for life.

Structure of Skeletal Muscles

Skeletal muscles are considered organs. They possess multinucleated cells and a connective tissue framework. Several layers of this connective tissue lie in sheets and cords beneath the skin, covering the bones. Each muscle fiber is comparable in size to a human hair and can hold about 1000 times

TABLE 18-4 Comparison of Different Types of Muscle Tissue

	SMOOTH	CARDIAC (INVOLUNTARY STRIATED)	SKELETAL (VOLUNTARY STRIATED)
Location	Wall of hollow organs, vessels, respiratory passageways	Wall of heart	Attached to bones
Cell characteristics	Tapered at each end, single nucleus, *nonstriated*	Branching networks, single nucleus, *lightly striated*	Long and cylindrical, multinucleated, *heavily striated*
Control	Involuntary	Involuntary	Voluntary
Action	Produces peristalsis; contracts and relaxes slowly; may sustain contraction; helps maintain blood pressure by regulating size of arteries	Pumps blood out of heart; self-excitatory, but influenced by nervous system and hormones	Produces movement at joints; stimulated by nervous system; contracts and relaxes rapidly; produces heat through aerobic production of energy; assists in blood return to heart

its own weight. Muscle fibers are made up of many thin elongated threads called *myofilaments* (*myofibrils*). The contractile unit of the myofibril is the *sarcomere*, many of which make up one myofibril. *Myosin* and *actin* are the contractile elements of muscle fibers, the basic functional unit of the muscle. (Myosin, the principal muscle protein, combines with actin to form *actomyosin*, to create the contractile property of the muscle. This process is facilitated by ATP.)

Each muscle fiber is covered by a cell membrane, the *sarcolemma*. This is covered by *endomysium*. Individual muscle fibers are bound together by *perimysium* into bundles called *fascicles*; a number of fascicles form a single muscle. The total muscle is covered by *epimysium*. (In many cases, epimysium extends beyond the muscle as a tendon, which is then attached to a bone [Fig. 18-19].)

> **Key Concept**
>
> A cross section of a muscle reveals the number of sarcomeres operating in parallel. This determines the amount of force of an individual muscle.

Each muscle is covered by a sheath of connective tissue (*fascia*), which separates individual muscles or surrounds muscle groups, forming *compartments*. Most muscles attach one bone to another or extend from one part to another.

One end of the muscle, the *origin*, is relatively immobile and is attached to the more stationary of two bones. The *insertion* is the part of the muscle attached to the more mobile bone. Bones act as levers, to facilitate movement with a prying action. The leverage strength depends on the origin and insertion of the muscles. The longer the lever in proportion to the part being moved, the greater the mechanical advantage. The main part of the muscle is the *belly*. The fibrous connective tissue that covers bone is *periosteum*, which is continuous with collagen fibers, forming tendons and ligaments.

> **Key Concept**
>
> In percentage of body mass, the average adult male is 40%–50% skeletal muscle and the average female is 30%–40% skeletal muscle.

Tendons

The ends of muscle fascia lengthen into tough cords called **tendons**, attaching muscles to bones. Tendons have sheaths lined with synovial membrane, permitting smooth, gliding movement. To understand the anatomy of a muscle and its tendon, place the hand on the thick muscle at the calf. Some of the strongest muscles in the body are located here. Move the hand toward the ankle. As both the leg and the muscles become narrower, the tissues become tough, fibrous, and ropelike. This occurs because approximately halfway to the ankle, the muscle is attached to the *Achilles tendon*, which extends down to the heel (Fig. 18-2B).

Major Muscles of the Body

Table 18-5 lists the body's important muscles, also identified in Figure 18-2. Most are named in relation to function, shape, body attachment, location, size, or number of attachments (e.g., biceps). Muscles may also be classified by appearance. Examples include pinnate (featherlike); fusiform (spindle-shaped); parallel (fascicles parallel to long axis of muscle); convergent (broad attachment, then fascicles converge to a single tendon); circular (muscle surrounding an opening—sphincter); or digastric (two muscle bellies in series with intermediate tendon).

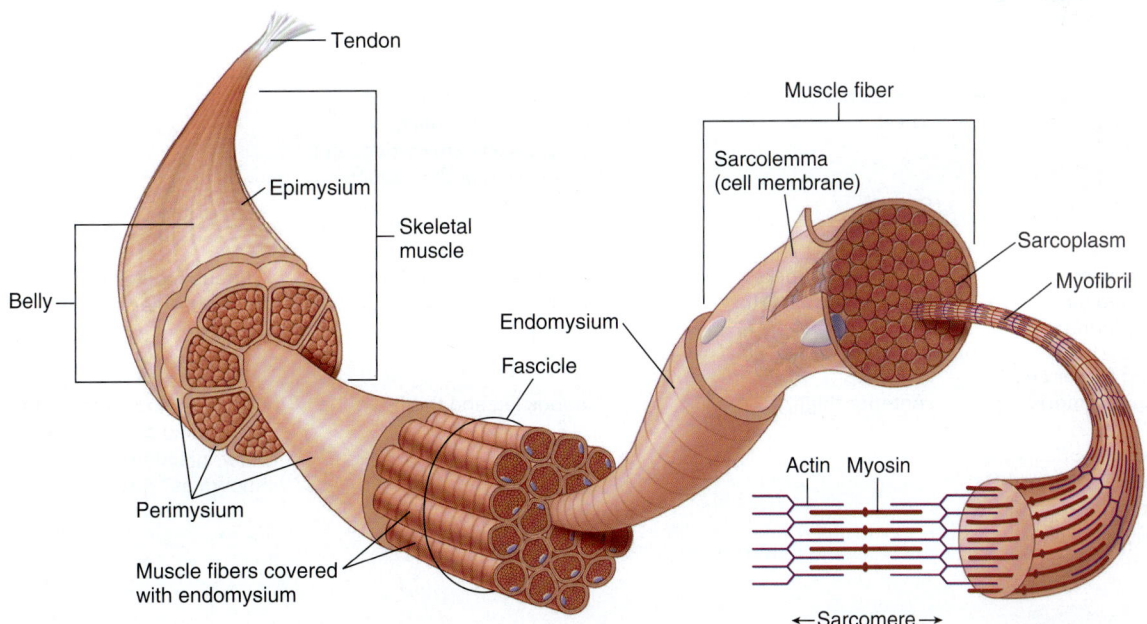

Figure 18-19 Structure of a skeletal muscle, showing a motor unit. The motor neuron and muscle fibers innervated by it are shown. Actin (thin) and myosin (thick) use ATP as a power source and are the contractile elements in the muscle fiber. (Moore K. L., Agur A. M., & Dalley A. F. [2014]. *Essential clinical anatomy* [5th ed.]. Wolters Kluwer Health.)

TABLE 18-5 Important Muscles of the Body

MUSCLE	LOCATION[a]	ACTION	NOTES
Neck and Shoulders			
Sternocleidomastoid	Side of neck	Helps keep head erect	If diseased or injured, head is permanently drawn to one side (torticollis)
Deltoid	Shoulder	Moves upper arm outward from body	Site for intramuscular injections
Arm and Anterior Chest			
Biceps	Front of upper arms	Flexes forearm	
Triceps	Posterior to biceps	Extends forearm	
Pectoralis major Pectoralis minor Serratus anterior	Anterior upper portion of chest Anterior chest, arising from ribs	Helps to bring arms across chest	Known as "pecs"
Respiration			
Diaphragm (Figs. 25-1 and 25-4)	Between the abdominal and thoracic cavities	Assists in process of breathing	When diaphragm contracts, it moves downward, making chest cavity larger, forming a partial vacuum around lungs, and causing air to rush into them. When it relaxes, it pushes upward, and air is forced out of lungs
Intercostal	Between the ribs	Helps to enlarge the chest cavity (side to side and back to front)	Same actions as above
Abdomen			
Internal oblique External oblique Transversus abdominis \Rectus abdominis	Flat bands that stretch from ribs to pelvis, overlapping in layers from various angles	Supports abdominal organs	An opening in muscle creates weakness where a hernia (rupture) may occur Common is an inguinal hernia; known as "abs"
Back and Posterior Chest			
Trapezius dorsi	Across back and posterior chest	Helps to lift shoulder	
Latissimus dorsi and other back muscles	Across back and posterior chest	Works in groups; helps body to stand erect, balance when heavy objects are carried, and turn or bend body; adducts upper arm	
Gluteal			
Gluteus maximus Gluteus medius Gluteus minimus	Form the buttocks	Helps change from sitting to standing positions; helps in walking	Gluteus medius used as site for intramuscular injections
Thigh and Lower Leg			
Quadriceps femoris group Rectus femoris Vastus lateralis Vastus intermedius Vastus medialis	Anterior thigh	Extends leg and thigh	Rectus femoris and vastus lateralis used as sites of intramuscular injection Known as "quads"

TABLE 18-5 Important Muscles of the Body (Continued)

MUSCLE	LOCATION[a]	ACTION	NOTES

Hamstring group
    Biceps femoris
    Semimembranosus
    Semitendinosus
	Posterior thigh	Flexes and extends leg and thigh	

Gracilis	Thigh	Flexes and adducts leg; adducts thigh	
Sartorius	Thigh	Flexes and rotates thigh and leg	Called "tailor muscle" because it allows sitting in cross-legged position
Tibialis anterior Gastrocnemius Soleus Peroneus longus	Anterior lower leg Calf Calf Calf	Elevates and flexes foot Flexes foot and leg Extends and rotates foot Extends, abducts, and everts foot	Gives calf rounded appearance
Achilles tendon	Attaches calf muscles to heel bone	Allows extension of foot and gives "spring" to walk	Term derived from Greek mythology
Head Orbicularis oculi+	Head	Moves eyes and wrinkles forehead	Disorder may cause strabismus ("cross-eye")
Orbicularis oris	Head	Moves mouth and surrounding facial structures	
Masseter temporalis, lateral and medial pterygoid	Jaw	Chewing (strongest body muscle)	Masseter temporalis is considered the strongest muscle in the body, in relationship to size
Buccinator	Head	Moves fleshy portion of cheek for smiling	

[a]For location of many of these muscles, see Figure 18-2.

Diaphragm and Intercostals

The *diaphragm* is one of the body's most vital muscles (Fig. 15-3A). The *intercostal muscles* lie between the ribs. The diaphragm and intercostals are the primary muscles of respiration (Chapter 25). They are partially under conscious control.

Muscles of the Hands and Feet

The muscles and tendons of the hands and feet are arranged in a slightly different manner from other muscles in the body. Many of these structures, including bones, are necessary to provide movement of these complex body parts. Because bulky muscles would be clumsy, the larger muscles used to move the hands and feet are located in the forearms and lower legs. For example, when you flex your fingers to clench your fist, you can feel the muscles move and tighten in your forearm. Other muscles begin at the wrist and extend into long, thin tendons that attach to the bones of the fingers. This placement permits accuracy and a variety of movements, without great bulk.

System Physiology

FORMATION OF BONE TISSUE

Bones develop from embryonic connective tissue called *mesenchyme*, either directly or via cartilage derived from mesenchyme. Long bones grow by ossifying the shaft (diaphysis) of the bone. During bone growth, *epiphyseal plates* exist between the diaphysis and epiphyses. These plates are gradually replaced by bone on both sides. When bone growth is complete, the ends of the bone fuse with the shaft and the seam is shown on x-ray as the epiphyseal line.

Bones are active, living organs, changing greatly during the lifetime. The small, mostly cartilaginous bones of the baby grow in diameter and length and continue to harden and/or fuse together until growth is complete. Although bone structure and size alter primarily to accommodate growth, change also continues into later life. Bone cells multiply rapidly in the growing years. When growth spurts have stopped, new cells form only to replace dead or injured ones and to repair breaks. With age, bones may become harder and more brittle, breaking more easily.

Although bone tissue hardens due to deposits of calcium and phosphorus, bones are made up of living cells. Bone-building cells are called **osteoblasts**. **Ossification** is the formation of bone by osteoblasts and is the process by which bones become hardened, due to an increase in calcified tissue. Ossification progresses from the middle of the shaft outward. The hardened, mature bone cell is the **osteocyte**. Other cells, **osteoclasts**, assist in resorption (**reabsorption**, removal by absorption) or breakdown of bone. Resorption allows bones to grow and change shape; bones continue building up and resorbing throughout life.

SPECIAL CONSIDERATIONS Lifespan

Bone Growth
Bone growth is rapid during infancy, steady in childhood, and has a rapid spurt in adolescence before the epiphyseal growth plate hardens and growth ceases.

The following factors affect bone growth and maintenance:

- *Heredity:* genes, genetic (inherited) tendencies
- *Nutrition:* protein, vitamins (especially A, D, C), and minerals (calcium, phosphorus) (Chapter 30)
- *Exercise:* weight-bearing (provides stress to strengthen bones)
- *Hormones:* affect rate of bone growth, calcium metabolism, energy production, and overall maintenance (Chapter 20)

SPECIAL CONSIDERATIONS Nutrition

Lack of Vitamin D
Lack of vitamin D causes a bone malformation in children called *rickets*; in adults, the disorder is called *osteomalacia*.

NCLEX Alert
The healing of tissues, muscles, and bones can be the basis of many NCLEX clinical situations. The correct option can also require that you understand the nursing care and pharmaceutical concepts of pain management.

MUSCLE CONTRACTIONS

Specific characteristics of muscles are similar to those of a heavy rubber band when stretched. Contractile filaments of muscles move past each other and change the shape and size of the muscle. Muscle tissue has the following special characteristics:

- **Contractility**: ability to shorten and become thicker
- **Extensibility**: ability to stretch
- **Elasticity**: ability to return to normal length after stretching
- **Irritability**: ability to respond to a stimulus (nerve impulses)

Muscles operate under an all-or-none principle. *An individual muscle fiber cannot partially contract.* If a stimulus is strong enough to cause contraction, each stimulated fiber will contract as much as it can. If the stimulus is not strong enough, the fiber will not contract. The nervous system responds to a stimulus and directs muscle action (Chapter 29). Muscles do not respond without stimuli.

Key Concept
Skeletal muscle contraction is stimulated by electrical impulses transmitted by nerves, particularly motor neurons. Cardiac and smooth muscle contractions are caused by internal cells, which stimulate regular contractions. All skeletal muscle contractions and many smooth muscle contractions are facilitated by the neurotransmitter acetylcholine.

Contraction and Relaxation

Elasticity of muscles allows them to work in pairs, having opposite actions. When one muscle of the pair contracts, the other relaxes. A single muscle or set of muscles, the *prime mover*, initiates movement. When an opposite movement is to be made, another set of muscles, the *antagonist*, takes over. Muscles that assist one another in movement are called *synergic* or *synergistic* muscles. When the elbow bends, the muscle in the upper arm contracts, hardens, and thickens as muscle fibers shorten to raise the forearm (**flexion**). At the same time, muscles on the back of the upper arm relax, lengthen, and pull against the front muscles. They will then pull the forearm straight (**extension**) in the opposing movement. The related muscles are referred to as flexors and extensors. *Abductors* facilitate movement away from the body's midline; *adductors* enable movement toward the midline. Specific ROM movements are described and illustrated in Chapter 48. Some muscles are attached to organs such as the skin or eyeball or to mucous membranes. The muscles of respiration are illustrated in Chapter 25.

Power Source

The major function of muscles is to produce force and cause motion. This requires energy. In fact, most of the body's energy resources are used in muscle actions. Foods furnish carbon, hydrogen, and oxygen from which the body makes *glycogen* (sugar), a special form of stored glucose the body uses for fuel. The glucose molecule is metabolized in an anaerobic process (without oxygen), *glycolysis*, into materials, including lactic acid (lactate) and ATP *(adenosine triphosphate)*, that can be stored and used for energy. In addition, an aerobic process (using oxygen) yields even more ATP. The aerobic process also yields pyruvate, but no lactic acid. Muscles break down fatty acids and conserve energy as *creatine phosphate*, generated from ATP. (ATP can also be regenerated in the body, using creatine kinase.) Muscle fibers also use the proteins *myosin* and *actin* and other substances to carry out muscle contraction. (ATP powers the myosin.) The reaction between these substances creates a contraction (Fig. 18-19).

Blood brings oxygen and ATP, which react with one another (oxidation), to the muscle cells. The result of this oxidation (aerobic) is energy and heat. (Most of the body's heat originates from muscle activity.) When muscles are very active, they draw on stored glycogen. When the body is cold, muscles can automatically produce heat by general muscle action (*shivering*). To produce a great amount of heat in an emergency, the body produces the more violent action of *total body chilling*.

> **Key Concept**
> Cardiac muscle can easily use any of the nutrients, protein, glucose, or fat in an aerobic process. This does not require a warm-up period and yields maximum ATP.

In addition to energy and heat, oxidation produces waste products, carbon dioxide, and lactic acid. The blood carries carbon dioxide to the lungs, where it is removed in breathing. The urinary system and sweat glands remove the lactic acid. Vigorous or prolonged muscle action quickly depletes oxygen. Because they are fast-twitch muscles, skeletal muscles cannot remain contracted for a long time. Gradually, due to the lack of oxygen, a muscle becomes fatigued and painful. Consequently, after exercise or prolonged use, muscles may ache. Aerobic muscle action in summary:

$$\text{muscle cell + fuel and oxygen}$$
$$\downarrow$$
$$\text{heat and energy}$$
$$\downarrow$$
$$\text{by-products: lactic acid and carbon dioxide } (CO_2)$$

> **Key Concept**
> Soreness occurring after exercise is usually the result of tiny tears (microtears) in muscle fibers and oxygen depletion.

Muscle Tone

Because humans stand erect against gravity's constant pull, many muscles remain in a mild state of contraction, to help maintain balance. These are slow-twitch muscles. Even relaxed muscles are ready to act, if they are in good condition. This state of slight contraction and the ability to spring into action is called **muscle tone** (*tonus*). Physical exercise improves muscle tone and increases muscle size. An idle muscle loses tone and wastes away. If a person does not use muscles or uses them very little, they become flabby and weak (atonic) and may **atrophy** (waste away).

> **Nursing Alert** Inactivity and pressure on muscles causes pain and skin breakdown. People on bedrest require frequent repositioning and may require support when getting out of bed. A client who must remain in bed for any length of time should be positioned as if they were standing. If this position is not ensured, the muscles may become shortened due to lack of gravitational pull (resulting in a *contracture*).

EXERCISE

Isometric and Isotonic Contractions

In addition to constant muscle contractions causing muscle tone, two other types of contractions are important. **Isometric** contractions do not increase the length of a muscle, but do increase muscle tension. For example, if you push against an unmovable object or tense the muscles in your upper arm, your muscles tighten. This is an isometric contraction or exercise. Bedridden clients are encouraged to do isometric exercises, even if they cannot be out of bed. **Isotonic** contractions shorten and thicken the muscle, causing movement. Exercises such as swimming, jogging, or bicycling are examples, but a person in bed also can move the extremities and move about in bed to exercise the muscles. It is important to vary the exercise program; different exercises use different muscles.

Aerobic and Anaerobic Exercise

Aerobic exercise (using oxygen) involves a long period of less-than-maximum exertion. Muscles are used for a longer time, but not maximally contracted. These exercises use a greater percentage of slow-twitch muscles; fat, carbohydrate, and protein are all used for energy. In addition, a great deal of oxygen is used and very little, if any, lactic acid is produced. Running a marathon is an aerobic exercise.

In anaerobic exercise (without oxygen), mostly fast-twitch muscle fibers are used, at close to maximum contraction strength. In this case, ATP and glucose are the main energy sources, little oxygen is used, and a great deal of lactic acid is produced. The lactic acid inhibits ATP production. As a result, anaerobic exercise cannot be sustained for a long time. Examples include fast sprints or weight lifting. Training increases the ability to eliminate waste products and to sustain contractions. In addition, lactic acid can be used for energy or converted back to pyruvate by the liver, depending on the level of training.

> **Key Concept**
> Exercise does not increase the number of muscle fibers. The existing fibers just enlarge.

Rehabilitation

Except for the simplest movements, muscles work in groups. An injured or inactive muscle can be retrained or another muscle can be trained to take over its function Therefore, rehabilitation requires working a number of muscles in order to recover function. Rehabilitation is usually performed with the guidance of physical and occupational therapists, but nurses often carry out prescribed exercises. Reeducating muscles is sometimes a long and painful process, and clients need a great deal of encouragement.

MOBILITY

Body mechanics is the term used to denote the efficient movement of the body (Chapter 48). Chapter 10 describes growth and development patterns of infants and children. Increased mobility allows for increased independence. An adult *gait pattern* (manner of walking) develops between ages 3 and 5 years. Infants have a wide-based gait, and, as children mature, the base narrows. They swing their arms in coordination. Stride and walking speed increase, and movements become smooth. Normal changes of aging may cause the gait of older adults to widen again.

Range of motion (ROM) is the total amount of motion of which a joint is capable (Chapter 48). ROM exercises are important for prevention and rehabilitation of musculoskeletal conditions (Chapters 48, 77, and 97). Lack of mobility can result in changes in most organ systems. Musculoskeletal changes include decreased joint flexibility, decreased muscle tone and strength, and blood clots in the legs (as a result of muscle inactivity, needed to move blood). Tests of muscle function and/or disorders include the blood level of creatine kinase, electromyogram (measurement of electrical activity of muscle tissue), and muscle biopsy. Disorders of the musculoskeletal system are discussed in Chapter 77.

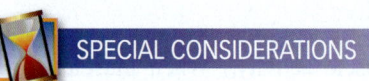

SPECIAL CONSIDERATIONS Lifespan

Older Adults

Nursing care for older adults must adapt to changes related to aging. The aging process produces significant effects on the musculoskeletal system (Table 18-6).

NCLEX Alert

The effects of aging are particularly noticeable with muscles and bones. Common NCLEX questions relate to osteoporosis, arthritis, or muscle atrophy, among others. The situations may require integration of aging issues, safety, communication, and client/family teaching.

SPECIAL CONSIDERATIONS Lifespan

Fractures

Fractures in older adults heal more slowly because of a decrease in bone metabolism. Calcium and vitamin D supplements may reduce the risk of fractures.

TABLE 18-6 Effects of Aging on the Musculoskeletal System

FACTOR	RESULT	NURSING IMPLICATIONS
Bones		
Bone mass and strength lost; body posture may change	Osteoporosis, fractures	Prevent falls; assess for fractures (particularly of the hip)
Calcium is lost (greater in postmenopausal women); bone tissue not replaced quickly	Hunched posture (kyphosis: humpback; lordosis: swayback) Back pain Brittle bones	Encourage vitamin D and calcium supplements Advise exercise to minimize bone loss Teach safety and prevention of falls; medications may be helpful Hormone replacement therapy may be prescribed
Vertebral column shortens	Decrease in height (demineralization of bones)	Encourage preventive diet (protein, minerals, especially calcium) and vitamin D Encourage exercise
Joints		
Joint degeneration	Arthritis (degenerative joint disease) Osteoarthropathy Joint stiffness, muscle aches, back pain	Encourage to increase mobility with active and passive range of motion exercises Hydrotherapy and external heat often helpful
Muscles		
Muscle cells are lost or atrophy Muscle cells replaced by fat Elasticity of fibers is lost	Loss of muscle strength Gain of fat tissue (and weight) Loss of flexibility Easy fatigability Resting tremors may occur	Give suggestions on carrying items (e,g., groceries) safely Encourage to control weight Suggest walking and swimming (good exercise for older adults); physical activity reduces loss of muscle, tissue, tone, and elasticity; increases flexibility Advise that exercise promotes psychological stimulation Encourage proper nutrition

STUDENT SYNTHESIS

KEY POINTS

- The skeleton is the living framework of the human body.
- The four main types of bone are long, short, flat, and irregular.
- Red bone marrow is found in the ends of long bones, in the bodies of vertebrae, and in flat bones. This bone marrow is responsible for hematopoiesis, the manufacture of red blood cells, white blood cells, and platelets.
- Joints, bursae, ligaments, tendons, and cartilage are responsible for connecting skeletal parts, enabling movement, and protecting the skeleton from injury.
- The two divisions of the skeleton are the axial skeleton, containing bones of the body's center, and the appendicular skeleton, containing bones of the extremities.
- Types of muscle tissue are skeletal or heavily striated (voluntary), smooth or nonstriated (involuntary), and cardiac.
- Muscle movements are voluntary (controlled by the person) or involuntary.
- Ossification is the process by which bones become hardened because of an increase in calcified tissue. Bones change in size and composition during one's lifetime.
- Muscles work in groups that have opposing actions. When one paired muscle contracts, the other relaxes.
- Most body heat is generated from the cellular muscle activity of ATP and oxygen.
- The musculoskeletal system often loses flexibility and strength as people age.

CRITICAL THINKING EXERCISES

1. If a hip joint becomes immobilized, what bones and muscles could potentially be affected? What bones and muscles could be affected if the shoulder is immobilized?
2. Give examples of and demonstrate complex tasks (other than those in the text) that human beings can perform, which are partly due to the arrangement of bones and muscles in the wrists and hands.
3. Darren, who has stopped his exercise routine, reports that during the past 6 months, he has become flabby and less toned and feels weaker. He asks you to explain why this has happened and what he can do to correct it.
4. Based on your knowledge of the musculoskeletal system, explain why differences exist in the way fractured bones and injured muscles are treated.

NCLEX-STYLE REVIEW QUESTIONS

1. The nurse is discussing preventative interventions to avoid musculoskeletal injuries. Which should the nurse encourage the client to take with calcium to help metabolize the calcium?
   a. Vitamin B_6
   b. Magnesium
   c. Vitamin D
   d. Potassium

2. An older adult client is admitted to the acute care facility. Which nursing action is a priority to help with the prevention of falls?
   a. Perform a fall risk assessment.
   b. Have restraints in the room if the client tries to get out of bed.
   c. Obtain a walker for ambulation.
   d. Inform the client not to get out of bed without assistance.

3. The nurse is caring for a client who states, "My knees are so stiff this morning." Which nursing action may the healthcare provider order to alleviate the discomfort?
   a. Apply cool compresses to the knees.
   b. Encourage adequate nutrition.
   c. Apply moist heat to the knees.
   d. Administer a narcotic analgesic.

4. A client suffered a stroke that affected the left side of the body. Which nursing action will assist with the prevention of contractures of the lower extremities?
   a. Apply heat to the extremities.
   b. Position the client as if standing.
   c. Apply sequential compression devices to the lower extremities.
   d. Stand the client on both feet several times a day.

5. A client is having symptoms associated with an alteration in muscle function. Which diagnostic tests should the nurse prepare the client for? Select all that apply.
   a. Creatine kinase
   b. Electromyogram
   c. Lumbar puncture
   d. Muscle biopsy
   e. Electrocardiogram

CHAPTER RESOURCES

Enhance your learning with additional resources on thePoint*!*

Student Resources related to this chapter can be found at thePoint.lww.com/Rosdahl12e.

19 The Nervous System

Learning Objectives

1. Name and describe parts of a neuron and how neurons transmit impulses.
2. Give an example of a sensory, motor, and interneuron impulse.
3. List primary functions of each of the brain's four cerebral lobes.
4. Explain how an injury to the cerebellum might manifest itself in an individual.
5. Identify the role of the limbic system in maintaining a person's level of awareness.
6. State functions of the medulla, pons, and midbrain. Describe two nursing considerations appropriate for a client with brainstem dysfunction.
7. Identify the three meninges, and explain the functions of the spinal cord and cerebrospinal fluid.
8. List the 12 cranial nerves and function of each. Describe the functions of spinal nerves.
9. Compare and contrast the functions of the parasympathetic and sympathetic nervous systems.
10. Explain nerve transmission, including definitions for resting potential, action potential, and neurotransmitter.

Important Terminology

action potential	effectors	midbrain	parasympathetic	synapse	CHT
afferent	efferent	myelin (myelin	parietal lobe	temporal lobe	CNS
axon	frontal lobe	sheath)	plexus	thalamus	CSF
brainstem	ganglion	nerve	pons	ventricle	EEG
cerebellum	hypothalamus	neuroglia	receptors		ICP
cerebrum	interneuron	neurology	reflex	**Acronyms**	LP
cranial nerves	limbic system	neuron	spinal cord	ANS	PNS
decussation	medulla	neurotransmitter	spinal nerves	BBB	RAS
dendrites	meninges	occipital lobe	sympathetic		SNS

In this chapter, one of the body's major control systems is presented. The nervous system coordinates and rapidly responds to external and internal stimuli. In Chapter 20, the endocrine system is presented; it controls slower, longer lasting responses to internal stimuli. The functions of these two systems are closely interrelated and have major influence on all other body systems. The nervous system is responsible for much of the communication between body systems.

The *nervous system* receives and stores information from the outside world (*external stimuli*) and uses it for future application. It also coordinates messages from internal body systems (*internal stimuli*), enabling the body to readjust constantly to changing internal and external environments. The nervous system may be compared to a complex hardwired computer network. Through a system of wires (**nerves**), messages enter a central processor (brain and **spinal cord**), where connections are made, and messages are transmitted to the body via outgoing nerves. **Neurology** is the study of the nervous system. The basic functions of the nervous system are to receive sensory input (stimuli), to integrate and interpret stimuli, and to respond to the stimuli. The nervous system is vital in total organ system functioning.

STRUCTURE AND FUNCTION

The functions of the nervous system are communication and control (Box 19-1). Basic to understanding these functions is information regarding the specialized cells of the nervous system (*neurons* and *neuroglia*) and structures composed of these cells.

CELLS OF THE NERVOUS SYSTEM

The nervous system is made up of neurons (nerve cells) and neuroglia (glial cells). The **neuron** is the *basic structural and functional cell* of the nervous system. Neurons are specialized to respond to electrical, chemical, and physical stimuli (e.g., pain, pressure, hot/cold), and messages are conducted and transferred through them (*neurotransmission*). The human brain regulates more than 10 billion neurons throughout the body at all times. **Neuroglia** (described later) outnumber neurons by a ratio of ten to one; they support and connect nervous tissue but do not transmit impulses.

Neurons

Neurons perform many functions. In the brain, they influence thinking, affect memory, and regulate other organs and glands. Although neurons are microscopic, they vary greatly in size and length. A neuron has only one *cell body*, containing the nucleus, mitochondria, and other organelles. In addition, each neuron contains two *processes* (one *axon* and numerous *dendrites*) (Fig. 19-1). The cell body may be relatively far away from its axon or dendrites.

Box 19-1 Functions of the Nervous System

COMMUNICATION
- Monitors impressions and information from external stimuli
- Monitors information from internal stimuli
- Responds to danger, pain, and other situations
- Responds to internal and external changes
- Helps maintain homeostasis
- Responds to conscious decisions and thoughts
- Coordinates processing of new learning
- Stores and retrieves memories, including previous learning
- Facilitates judgment, reasoning, and decision making

CONTROL
- Directs all body activities
- Maintains blood pressure, respiration, and other vital functions
- Regulates body systems (in coordination with endocrine system)
- Coordinates reflex actions
- Controls instinctual behaviors
- Controls conscious movement and activities
- Stores unconscious thoughts

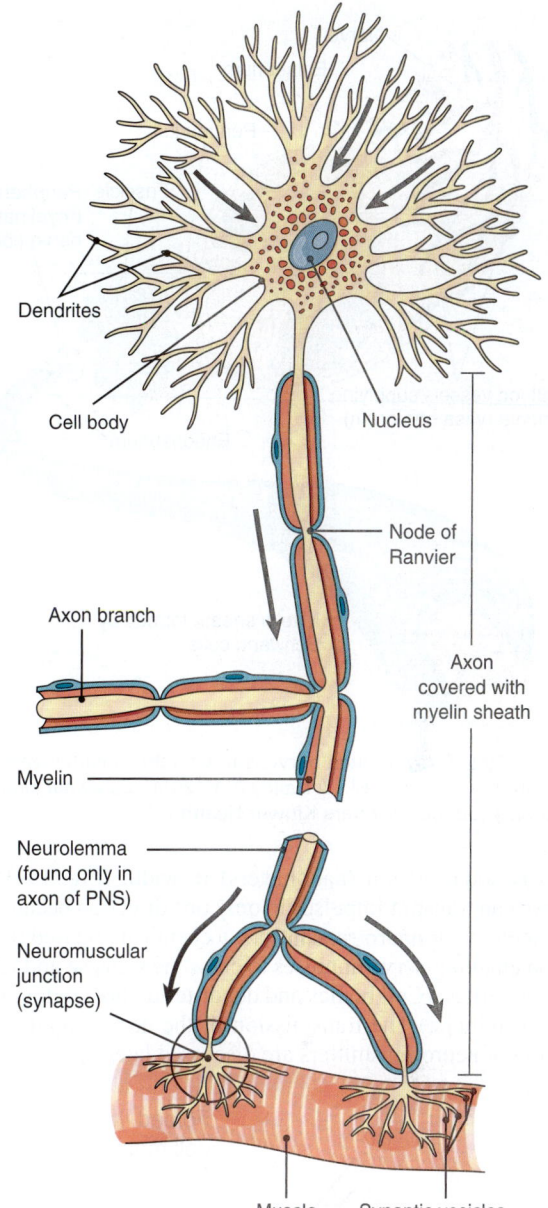

Figure 19-1 A myelinated motor neuron. In the center is the cell body containing the nucleus, surrounded by mitochondria and other organelles. The tips of the dendrites receive messages from the axons of other cell bodies across the synapse. The axon transmits messages from the cell body to the next cell body. (The break in the axon shows that the axon is longer than pictured.) The *arrows* show the direction of the nerve impulse.

Many neurons make up a *nerve*, which contains axons bundled into groups (*fascicles*). A nerve resembles a muscle cell, with many branches becoming smaller and smaller and forming the *axon*. Connective tissue, the *epineurium*, surrounds each entire nerve. Fat tissue and blood vessels surround nerve fascicles (groups of axons), wrapped in *perineurium*. The innermost layer, the *endoneurium*, wraps individual axons. Neurons do not divide and reproduce by mitosis, as do other body cells. If a nerve cell body is destroyed, it is lost forever. Protein synthesis occurs within the cell body in specialized organelles, the *Nissl bodies (chromatophilic substance)*, unique to the neuron.

Axons
An **axon** is an extension that carries impulses *away from the neuron cell body*. An axon may be as short as a few millimeters, or it may be longer than a meter. It may be myelinated (covered in a protective layer), or it may be bare. This structural difference is important.

> **Key Concept**
> All neurons have the same basic structure but differ in size and shape, depending on their function.

An axon surrounded by *myelin* (a fatty covering) is said to be *myelinated*. This **myelin sheath** electrically insulates one nerve cell from another. Without this sheath, these particular nerve cells would short circuit. Myelin is formed by the plasma membranes of specialized glial (neuroglial) cells, the *Schwann cells*, which provide nutrition and support. The gap between Schwann cells is called the *node of Ranvier* (Fig. 19-2). These nodes provide points along a neuron where a signal is generated. Signals jumping between these nodes travel hundreds of times faster than signals traveling on axons with a bare surface (nonmyelinated).

Thus, myelinated axons conduct impulses faster than nonmyelinated axons. The axons within a nerve fiber lie in bundles and are surrounded by connective tissue and blood vessels.

Dendrites
Dendrites are short, often highly branched extensions of the cell body. They *receive* impulses from axons of other neurons and transmit these impulses *toward the cell body*. Dendrites respond to chemical messages sent across the **synapse** (the *synaptic cleft* or *myoneural junction*), the tiny space separating neurons from each other. This very narrow

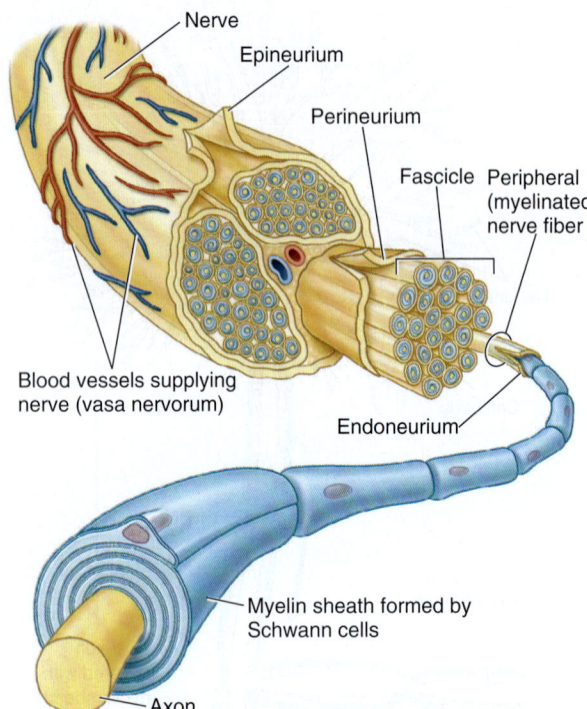

Figure 19-2 A myelinated nerve, showing the sheath layers. (Moore K. L., Agur A. M., & Dalley A. F. [2014]. *Essential clinical anatomy* [5th ed.]. Wolters Kluwer Health.)

gap is about 20 nm (nanometers) in width (Fig. 19-3). A nerve can transmit impulses in only one direction because of the location of **neurotransmitters**, a chemical released by the axon enabling nerve impulses to cross the synapse and reach the dendrites. (Cell bodies and dendrites do not contain neurotransmitters.) The transmission of the nerve impulse and action of neurotransmitters are discussed later.

Classification of Neurons

Neurons can be classified according to shape but are more commonly associated with their functions: sensory, motor, or as **interneurons**.

- *Sensory* (**afferent**) neurons receive messages from all parts of the body and transmit these messages (about hormone levels, blood pH, touch, sound, light, and pressure) *to the central nervous system*. Sensory neurons usually have long dendrites and a short axon.
- *Motor* (**efferent**) neurons receive messages *from the central nervous system* (*CNS*) and transmit them, as *motor output*, causing an action, to muscles and glands in all parts of the body. Signals carried by these neurons alter muscle activity or cause glands to secrete. Motor neurons usually have short dendrites and a long axon.
- *Interneurons* (*connectory, association neurons,* or *integrators*) function as a link between the two other types of neurons. They are *interconnecting* neurons and are located only within the central nervous system.

> **Key Concept**
>
> The three types of neurons are sensory, motor, and interneurons.

Sensory neurons compose *sensory (afferent) nerves*. Motor neurons compose *motor (efferent) nerves*. Mixed nerves, discussed later, contain both sensory and motor neurons.

Neuroglia

Neuroglia (*glial cells*) are more numerous than neurons (10:1) and can multiply to fill spaces previously occupied by neurons. (Some brain tumors, *gliomas*, are caused by rapid growth of glial cells.)

Neuroglia in the *CNS* are composed of several types of cells, with specific functions:

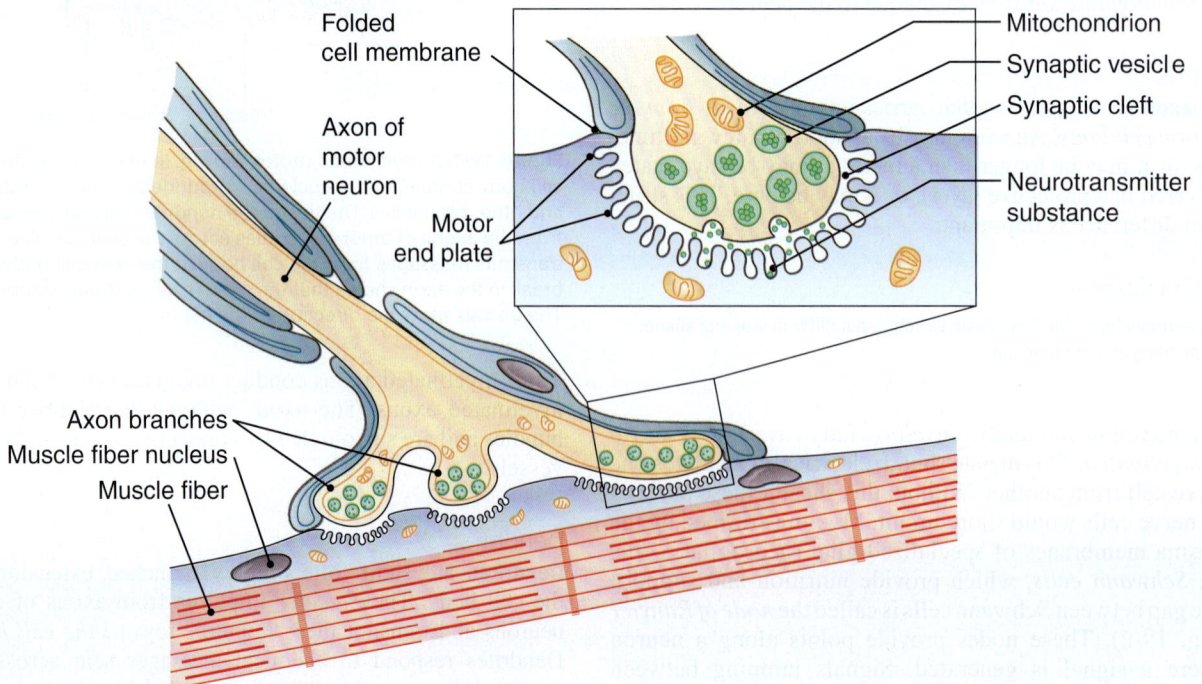

Figure 19-3 The synapse (myoneural junction).

- Astrocytes (astroglia)—supply nutrients to the neurons and form part of the blood–brain barrier (BBB), to keep harmful materials out of the brain
- Microglia—ingest and destroy microorganisms and wastes; they are phagocytes
- Oligodendrocytes (oligodendroglia)—surround and insulate axons
- Ependymal cells form the lining of the brain's ventricles and participate in the production of cerebrospinal fluid (**CSF**)

The two types of neuroglia in the *peripheral nervous system* (*PNS*) are satellite cells and Schwann cells. The neuroglia also help form the CSF and myelin sheath. Neuroglia obtain nutrients (specifically, glucose and oxygen) for the neurons; they support and protect the CNS and PNS by maintaining homeostasis; surround and insulate neurons and hold them in place; destroy pathogens; and remove dead neurons.

SPECIAL CONSIDERATIONS Lifespan

Infant Blood–Brain Barrier
Infants have an immature blood–brain barrier, allowing substances to pass into the infant's brain that would not normally enter an adult's brain.

DIVISIONS OF THE NERVOUS SYSTEM

The nervous system is divided into two major parts: the **CNS** and the **PNS**. The CNS, the largest part of the nervous system, consists of the brain and spinal cord. The PNS consists of the cranial nerves, spinal nerves, and the autonomic (automatic) nervous system. The CNS is protected by the CSF and meninges (Fig. 19-4).

Central Nervous System

The CNS encompasses the brain, spinal cord, and accessory structures. The *spinal cord* is the major communication pathway between the body and the brain. The *brain* interprets this information and directs body responses.

The Brain

The human brain contains approximately 100 billion neurons, as well as innumerable synapses. It weighs approximately 1.36 kg (kilograms) (3 lb), about 2% of the body's weight. However, the brain requires approximately 20% of the body's circulating blood flow (about 750 mL/min). The adult human brain, spread out, would be about the size of a pillowcase. (An infant's brain triples in size during the first year of life.) The brain is also referred to as the *encephalon*; the word element pertaining to the brain is *encephal(o)*.

The brain has an extensive, specialized vascular (blood vessel) supply, with a higher metabolic rate than the rest of the body; this rate remains constant during physical or mental exercise. The brain requires a constant flow of oxygen and nutrients, particularly glucose, and is very sensitive to toxins and/or drugs. A loss of blood flow for as little as 10 seconds causes unconsciousness. (See Chapter 23 for brain circulation.) Although the brain has many parts, it functions as an integrated whole. Its major divisions are the **cerebrum**, **cerebellum**, and **medulla** oblongata (Table 19-1).

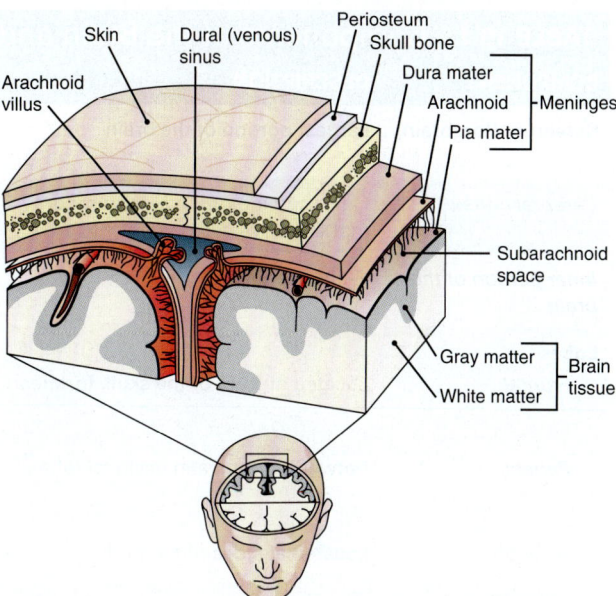

Figure 19-4 Frontal (coronal) section of the top of the head, showing meninges and related structures.

Cerebrum

The **cerebrum** composes 80% of the brain's volume (Fig. 19-5) and fills the upper part of the *cranium* (skull cavity). It is sometimes called "the seat of consciousness" because it coordinates sensory data and motor functioning and governs intelligence, reasoning, learning, memory, and other complex behaviors. The cerebrum is divided into two *layers* and two *halves (hemispheres)*. The *longitudinal fissure*, or cleft, runs from the front of the brain to the back, thus forming the hemispheres. Each portion of the cerebrum has specialized functions, but all are integrated, and many areas overlap.

Cerebral Cortex

The adjective, *cerebral*, pertains to unique human abilities of learning, intelligent reasoning, and judgment. The *cerebral cortex* is the thin (1–4 mm) outside layer of the brain, composed of soft *gray matter*, mostly nerve cell bodies. It is not covered with myelin, and thus it appears gray. The cortex is wrinkled and folded back on itself many times in folds called *convolutions* or *gyri* (singular: *gyrus*), with crevices between the folds, the *fissures*, or *sulci* (singular: *sulcus*). Because of the folds, the cortex has a large surface area and therefore is able to contain its millions of neurons. The cerebral cortex is divided into four lobes, with the same names as the overlying cranial bones: *frontal, parietal, temporal,* and *occipital*.

- The **frontal lobe** is large and contains the areas for *written* and *motor speech*. It is largely responsible for the ability of humans to achieve higher levels of mental functioning, including conception, judgment, abstract reasoning, social behavior, speech, and communication, and is also involved with motor functions.
- The *sensory area* is located in the **parietal lobe**, where sensations such as touch, taste, pressure, temperature, and pain are received from the skin and interpreted. Spatial ability (ability to recognize shapes and sizes) is also located in this area. (The parietal lobe on the person's nondominant side is concerned with awareness of body shape.)

TABLE 19-1 Components of the Brain and Their Functions

COMPONENT	DESCRIPTION	FUNCTION
Cerebrum (forebrain)	Largest portion of the brain	Center of conscious thought and higher mental functioning (intelligence, learning, and memory)
Cerebral cortex	Outer coating of the cerebrum; gray matter (nerve cell bodies)	Contains convolutions (grooves) and elevations (gyri) that increase brain's surface area
Inner portion of the brain	White matter	Location of billions of connections, due to presence of dendrites and myelinated axons
Lobes		
Frontal	Located at front of the skull, forehead	Location of higher mental processes (intelligence, motivation, mood, aggression, and planning); site for verbal communication and voluntary control of skeletal muscles
Parietal	Between frontal and occipital lobes	Location of skin, taste, and muscle sensations; speech center; enables formation of words to express thoughts and emotions; interprets textures and shapes
Temporal	Located at sides of the skull	Location of sense of smell and auditory interpretation; stores auditory and visual experiences; forms thoughts that precede speech
Occipital	Located at back of the skull	Location of eye movements; integrates visual experiences
Hemispheres	Longitudinal fissure divides the brain into right and left halves	
Corpus callosum	Connects hemispheres internally	
Diencephalon (Interbrain)	Located between cerebral hemispheres and brainstem	
Thalamus	Located within cerebral hemispheres	Central relay point for incoming nerve messages ("switching center")—consolidates sensory input (especially extremes and pain); influences mood and body movements; associated with strong emotions
Hypothalamus	Located below thalamus, at base of cerebrum	Regulates homeostasis—center for body temperature regulation, hunger, peristalsis, thirst and water balance, sexual response, and sleep–wake cycle; controls heart rate and blood vessel diameter; influences pituitary gland secretions; controls muscles of swallowing, shivering, and urine release; links nervous and endocrine systems; associated with emotions
Limbic system	Consists of hippocampus and reticular formation	Screens sensory messages to the cortex; responsible for learning, long-term memory, wakefulness, and sleep; basic drives, such as hunger and sexual arousal
Cerebellum ("little brain")	Second largest part of the brain (part of hindbrain); attached to back of brainstem, below the curve of cerebrum. Connected, via midbrain, to the spinal cord and motor area of the cortex	Location of involuntary movement, coordination, muscle tone, balance, and equilibrium (semicircular canals); coordinates some voluntary muscles
Brainstem		
Midbrain (mesencephalon)	Smallest and most primitive part of the brain	Connects cerebral hemispheres with spinal cord
	Located at top of brainstem, below thalamus	Acts as visual and auditory reflex center; righting reflex located here
Pons (bridge)	Between cerebrum and medulla	Carries messages between cerebrum and medulla; acts as respiratory center to produce normal breathing patterns
Medulla (oblongata)	Located at floor of the skull below midbrain; connects brain to spinal cord	Vital for life; descending nerve tracts from the brain cross here to the opposite side; contains centers for many body functions (cardiac, vasomotor, and respiratory center; swallowing, coughing, and sneezing reflexes)

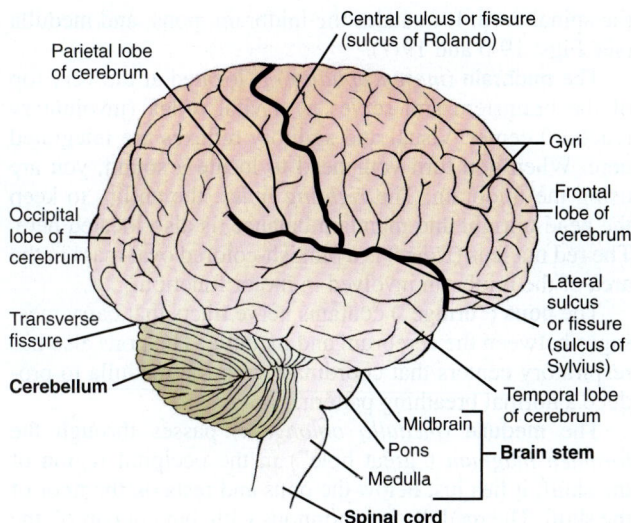

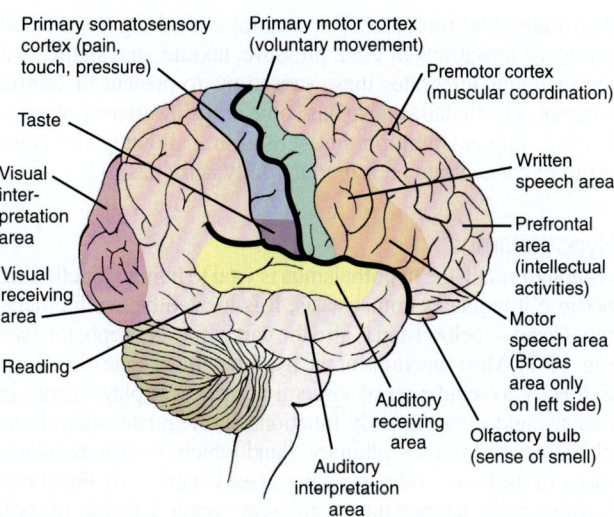

Figure 19-5 Lateral view (right side) of the external surface of the brain, indicating lobes of the cerebrum, as well as the cerebellum and brain stem. Major sulci are also shown.

Figure 19-6 Lateral view of the brain, indicating major functional areas.

- The **temporal lobe** receives and interprets auditory signals and processes language, and controls the sensations of hearing, auditory interpretation, and smell. Memories are stored here, as well as in other areas of the brain.
- Visual transmissions and interpretation occur in the *visual* areas of the **occipital lobe**.

White Matter
The interior of the brain lies under the cerebral cortex and consists of *white matter*. It contains billions of synapses between axons and dendrites. This area is white due to the presence of myelinated axons connecting the cerebral lobes to each other and to all other parts of the brain.

Cerebral Hemispheres
The right cerebral hemisphere (right half) controls the muscles and receives sensory information from the left side of the body. The left hemisphere is the opposite. This phenomenon is a result of **decussation** (crossing) of nerve tracts within the brain's medulla. The functional areas of the cerebrum are shown in Figure 19-6. However, the brain's two hemispheres process information differently. The right hemisphere relates to spatial perception, art, and musical ability; the left controls analytic and verbal skills (e.g., reading, writing, symbols, mathematics, and speech) in addition to walking.

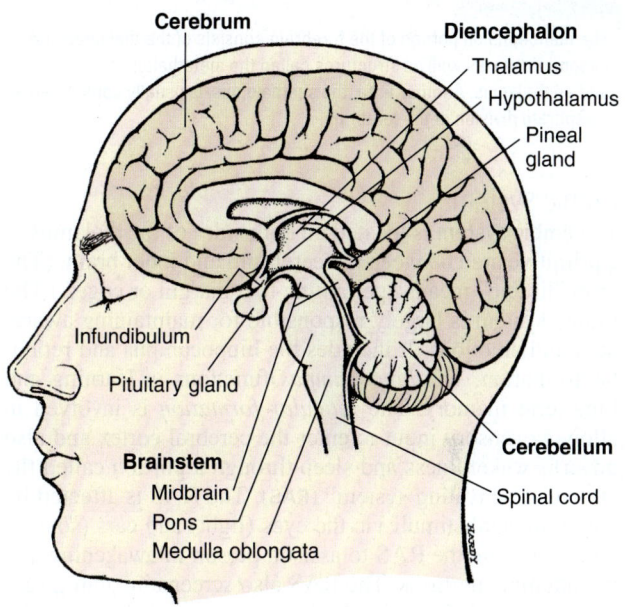

Figure 19-7 Brain, midline cross-section, showing the thalamus, hypothalamus, and pituitary.

The *corpus callosum* resembles a band of matted white fibers and contains approximately 200 million neurons. It lies between and interconnects the right and left cerebral hemispheres, deep within the longitudinal fissure, and allows one cerebral hemisphere to share information with the other. If this structure is severed, the right hand will literally not know what the left hand is doing.

Thalamus
The **thalamus** is located in the posterior area of the forebrain, the *diencephalon* portion of the brain, between the hemispheres and **brainstem** (Fig. 19-7). The thalamus lies just superior and posterior to the **hypothalamus** and is the relay station between cutaneous (skin) **receptors** and the cerebral cortex for all sensory impulses (except smell). The thalamus integrates sensations; thus, the person perceives a whole experience rather

> **Key Concept**
>
> Individuals who have had a cerebrovascular accident (e.g., CVA, "stroke") affecting one brain hemisphere show external symptoms on the opposite side of the body. Since language and speech are usually processed in the left hemisphere, a left-sided stroke often causes speech and language impairment, although physical symptoms (e.g., paralysis) often are on the right side of the body.
> - Language comprehension (Wernicke area)—damage impairs the ability to comprehend written and spoken language, but the person can still speak
> - Speaking ability (Broca area)—damage causes speech impairment but does not affect language comprehension

than individual impulses. For example, touching a snowball produces sensations of cold, pressure, texture, and shape, and the thalamus integrates these sensations to present the entire concept. The thalamus also has some crude awareness of pain. It may suppress unimportant sensations, allowing the cerebrum to concentrate on important daily activities.

Hypothalamus

Although small, the **hypothalamus** is vital to human functioning because it regulates homeostasis. It is located below the thalamus (*hypo-* = below) and is also the part of the diencephalon (see Fig. 19-7). Most functions of the hypothalamus relate directly or indirectly to regulation of visceral activities. It plays a role in increasing/decreasing body functions and regulates the release of hormones from the pituitary gland which, in turn, regulates many of the body's other hormones (see Chapter 20). Functions include body temperature regulation, water balance (thirst), sleep, hunger, sexual urges, and emotions. The hypothalamus is a *major link between the nervous and endocrine systems.*

> **Key Concept**
> The diencephalon portion of the forebrain consists of the thalamus and hypothalamus, as well as structures called the metathalamus and epithalamus. Another area, the subthalamus, is usually considered as a separate division of the forebrain.

Limbic System

The **limbic system** is located on both sides of the thalamus in a primitive area between the cerebrum and inner brain. (The term "limbic" means "pertaining to a margin or edge.") The limbic system is largely responsible for maintaining awareness and emotions. It includes the hippocampus and reticular formation. The *hippocampus* functions in learning and long-term memory. The *reticular formation* is involved in allowing sensory input to enter the cerebral cortex and also governs wakefulness and sleep through a portion called the "reticular activating system" (**RAS**). The RAS is affected by environmental stimuli via the eyes (light) and ears (sound), which activate the RAS to assist a person in awakening and maintaining alertness. The RAS also screens incoming sensory input and channels it to specific areas of the brain. An area called the *cingulated gyrus* coordinates smells and sights with pleasant memories and helps to regulate aggression.

Cerebellum

The **cerebellum**, the second-largest portion of the brain, also has two hemispheres (see Fig. 19-5). Its functions are concerned with movement: muscle tone, coordination, posture, and equilibrium. It coordinates the actions of voluntary muscles and adjusts to impulses from proprioceptors within muscles, joints, and sense organs. (*Proprioceptors* relay information about balance and body position.) Adjustments made in the cerebellum help a person to maintain balance and to make coordinated movements such as participating in sports or other activities (e.g., inline skating).

Brainstem

The **brainstem**, the smallest portion of the brain, continuous with the spinal cord, connects the cerebral hemispheres and the spinal cord. It includes the midbrain, pons, and medulla (see Figs. 19-5 and 19-7).

The **midbrain** (*mesencephalon*) is located at the very top of the brainstem and serves as a vital **reflex** (involuntary reaction) center. Visual and auditory reflexes are integrated here. When you turn your head to locate a sound, you are using the midbrain. The *righting reflex*, the ability to keep the head upright and maintain balance, is also located here. The red nucleus (*ruber*) is a pinkish-colored oval mass in the area of the midbrain involved in motor function.

The **pons** ("bridge") contains nerve tracts that carry messages between the cerebrum and medulla. The pons also has respiratory centers that coordinate with the medulla to produce a normal breathing pattern.

The **medulla** (*medulla oblongata*) passes through the *foramen magnum* ("great hole") in the occipital region of the skull; it lies just below the pons and rests on the floor of the skull. The medulla is continuous with, but not part of, the spinal cord. Nerve tracts descending from the brain cross to the opposite side here (decussation). The medulla contains centers for many vital body functions, including the *cardiac center* (regulates heart rate), *vasomotor center* (regulates blood vessel diameter, thereby regulating blood pressure), and *respiratory center* (regulates breathing). Other activities of the medulla are concerned with reflexes, such as swallowing, coughing, sneezing, hiccupping, and vomiting. Because the medulla is responsible for regulating so many vital body processes, any injury to the occipital bone at the base of the skull can be instantly fatal because of its proximity to the medulla.

The Spinal Cord

The **spinal cord** is a long mass of nerve cells and fibers extending through a central canal on the *dorsal* side (back) of the body. It contains two dorsal (*posterior*) horns, relaying sensations such as pain and temperature and two ventral (*anterior*) horns, assisting in voluntary motor activities and reflexes (Fig. 19-8). The spinal cord contains gray matter, mostly composed of cell bodies and dendrites, surrounded by white matter, composed of interneuronal axons (tracts), arranged in bundles. Some nerve tracts are *ascending* (to the brain)–*sensory* tracts; others descending (from the brain) are *motor* tracts. The spinal cord extends from the medulla to the approximate level of the first or second lumbar vertebra (see Chapter 18). Its position within the vertebral column helps protect it from shocks and injuries. This protection is essential since nerve fibers of the spinal cord cannot regenerate if they are destroyed. The spinal cord has two main functions: to conduct impulses to the brain (afferent) and from the brain (efferent) and to act as a *reflex center*. The reflex center in the spinal cord receives and instantly sends messages through nerve fibers without entering the brain. This "circle" is known as a *reflex arc* (see Fig. 19-8). The reflex center acts as a substation for messages and relieves the brain of routine work. The reflex arc is a protective mechanism, initiating rapid responses to dangerous stimuli.

> **Key Concept**
> The CNS is protected by the skull and the vertebrae of the spinal column.

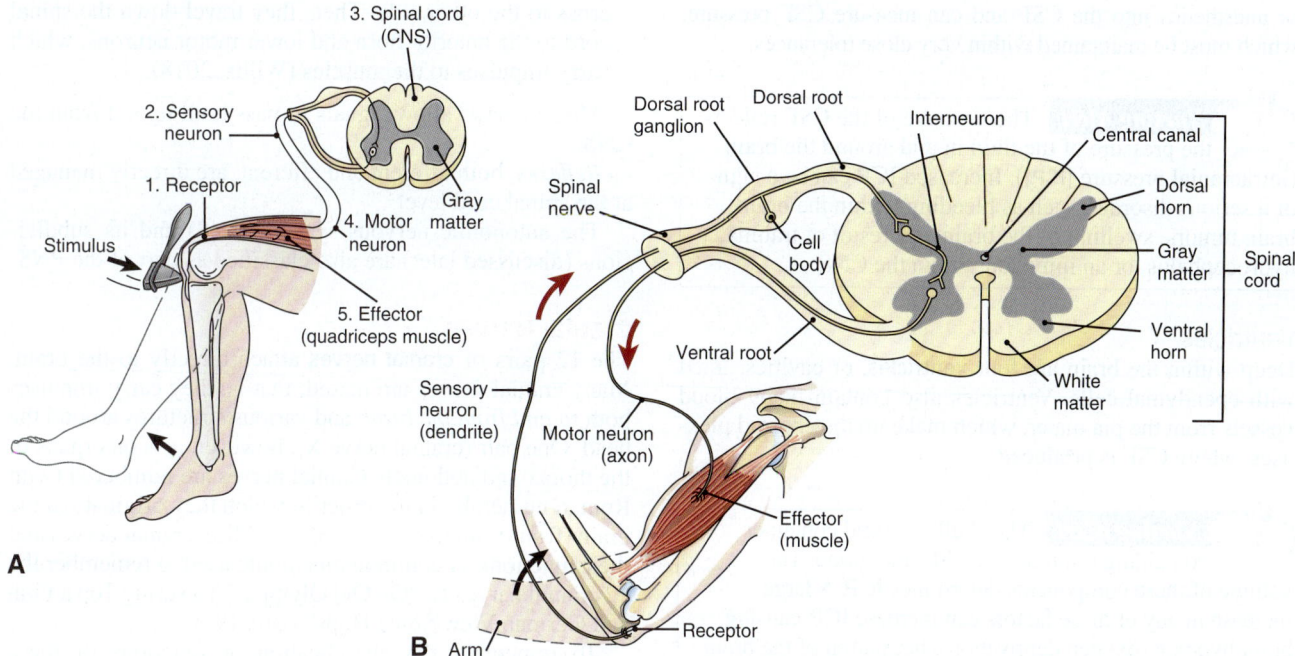

Figure 19-8 Reflex arcs, showing pathways of impulses in response to a stimulus. **A.** The cross-section of the spinal cord shows the simplest reflex, the patellar (knee-jerk) reflex, which involves only sensory and motor neurons. **B.** The response to a painful stimulus, such as a flame, also involves a central neuron. This is a three-neuron reflex arc.

Accessory Structures

The three major accessory structures of the CNS are the meninges, CSF, and ventricles.

Meninges

The brain and spinal cord (CNS) are covered with three protective membranes, the **meninges** (see Fig. 19-4). The dura mater, the outer layer, is a tough, fibrous covering that adheres to the skull bones. (The layers of the dura are the *endosteal periosteum* of the skull, continuous with the lining of the vertebral canal, and the *meningeal layer*, covering the brain.) The dura provides protection and support for the brain. The middle layer of protective membrane is a delicate web of tissue, the *arachnoid membrane*. The inner layer, the pia mater, lies closely over the brain and spinal cord. It is thin and vascular, containing many blood vessels that bring oxygen and nutrients to nervous tissue. The space between the dura mater and the arachnoid membrane is called the *subdural space*. The space between the arachnoid membrane and the pia mater is the *subarachnoid space*. (The subarachnoid space contains CSF, the tissue fluid of the CNS.)

Cerebrospinal Fluid

CSF is a lymph-like fluid composed of water and traces of protein, glucose, and electrolytes that forms a protective cushion around and within the CNS (Box 19-2). CSF allows the brain to "float" within the cranial vault, which changes the *effective weight* of the brain from about 1,500 g (grams) to about 50 g. The CSF removes cellular waste from nerve tissue and lessens damage caused by impact trauma by spreading out the force of trauma. It is produced in specialized capillary networks (*choroid plexuses*) in the brain's ventricles. About 800 mL of CSF are produced each day, although only 150–200 mL circulate at any one time. Arachnoid villi reabsorb some CSF into the blood, where it returns to blood plasma.

> **Nursing Alert** If fluid is leaking from the ears or nose following head trauma, the fluid is tested for glucose, a component of CSF. If the glucose test is positive, this indicates a life-threatening situation.

A small amount of CSF may be withdrawn through the space between two vertebrae, a *lumbar puncture* (**LP**) or *spinal tap*. Laboratory studies of CSF can reveal many situations, such as bleeding into the CNS or infections of the brain or its meninges. An LP can also introduce medications such as antibiotics

> **Key Concept**
> Closed head trauma (**CHT**) can result in intracranial (within the skull) bleeding, with blood accumulating under the meninges: under the dura mater (subdural) or under the arachnoid mater (subarachnoid). This causes increased and potentially dangerous intracranial (within the skull) pressure. Disorders can also result when the brain is smashed against the skull bones by a blow to the head (coup-contrecoup). Parkinson disease is the result of a deficiency of the neurotransmitter, dopamine. Alzheimer's dementia indicates an accumulation of protein plaques in the brain. Many drugs, such as methamphetamine, cocaine, LSD, heroin, marijuana, alcohol, caffeine, and insecticides, are known to interfere with conduction of impulses across synapses, causing related dysfunction or disorders (see Chapter 78).

> **Box 19-2   Functions of Cerebrospinal Fluid**
> - Acts as shock absorber for the brain and spinal cord
> - Carries nutrients to the brain
> - Carries wastes away from the brain
> - Keeps the brain and spinal cord moist, thus preventing friction
> - Can be tested to determine the presence of some disorders
> - Can be used to transmit medications

or anesthetics into the CSF and can measure CSF pressure, which must be maintained within very close tolerances.

> **Nursing Alert** The pressure of the CSF reflects the pressure of the fluid in and around the brain (intracranial pressure [ICP]). Increased ICP can be a sign of a serious disorder, such as bleeding within the brain, brain tumors, swelling of the brain as a result of trauma, hydrocephalus, or an infection within the CNS.

Ventricles

Deep within the brain are four **ventricles**, or cavities, lined with ependymal cells. Ventricles also contain many blood vessels from the pia mater, which make up the choroid plexuses, where CSF is produced.

> **Nursing Alert** The skull is a rigid container containing brain tissue, CSF, and blood. The volume of these components determines ICP. A large increase in any of these factors can increase ICP, causing brain hypoxia (oxygen deprivation), herniation of the brain (brain pushed through an opening), brain compression (brain crushed against the rigid skull), necrosis (death) of brain tissue in a specific area, or death of the individual.

Peripheral Nervous System

The PNS consists of bundles of neurons connecting the brain and spinal cord (CNS) to the rest of the body. The PNS consists of two nerve groups: cranial nerves (originating in the brain) and spinal nerves (originating in the spinal cord). The nerves of the PNS are sensory, motor, or mixed.

The *afferent (sensory) division* of the PNS conveys information *to the brain*, primarily from sensory organs, such as the skin. Muscle spindles convey information regarding posture and joint position. The sense of *proprioception* conveys awareness of where parts of the body are, in relation to space. (If you close your eyes and wave your hand, you still know where your hand is.) Several areas of the brain (the cerebellum and red nucleus) coordinate movements and positioning, using this proprioceptive feedback. Deeper muscles, such as those controlling posture, are controlled by nuclei in the brainstem and basal ganglia. (Much sensory input of the PNS remains below conscious awareness. However, some can be brought into consciousness.)

The *efferent (motor, descending) division* of the PNS sends voluntary and involuntary commands *from the CNS* to muscles and stimulates glands to secrete hormones. Signals to muscles nearly always originate in the primary motor cortex of the frontal lobe, just in front of the central sulcus, dividing the brain's frontal and parietal lobes.

Motor neurons form two major systems:

- **Pyramidal** (*corticospinal tract*)—relates to fine, skilled movements of skeletal muscle. Impulses travel from the motor cortex through the internal capsule to the medulla, where they cross to the other side and continue down the spinal cord.
- **Extrapyramidal** (*extracorticospinal system*)—controls gross motor movements. Impulses originate in the premotor area of the frontal lobes and travel to the pons, where they cross to the other side. Then, they travel down the spinal cord to the anterior horn and lower motor neurons, which carry impulses to the muscles (Willis, 2018).

Mixed nerves allow signals to pass both to and from the CNS.

Reflexes, both afferent and efferent, are directly managed at the spinal cord level.

The autonomic nervous system (ANS) and its subdivisions (discussed later) are also classified as part of the PNS.

Cranial Nerves

The 12 pairs of **cranial nerves** attach directly to the brain. Many cranial nerves are mixed; that is, they carry impulses both *to and from the brain* and various structures around the head. One pair (cranial nerve X), however, acts on organs of the thorax and abdomen. Cranial nerves are numbered (with Roman numerals) in the order in which they originate in the brain (from front to back). Table 19-2 lists cranial nerves and their functions. A common mnemonic used to remember the 12 cranial nerves is: "On Old Olympus' Towering Top a Finn and German View Some Hops" (Box 19-3).

To remember the classification of functions of these nerves, use the mnemonic: "Some Say Marry Money But My Brother Says Bad Business Marry Money" (Box 19-4). The S represents *sensory* nerves, M represents *motor* nerves, and B denotes that the corresponding nerve has *both* sensory and motor functions (a *mixed nerve*). The oculomotor, trochlear, abducens, accessory, and hypoglossal are actually mixed nerves; however, they are *primarily motor*. Therefore, this mnemonic reflects these nerves' primary function (motor).

Although all cranial nerves are important, one deserves special attention. The *vagus nerve* (cranial nerve X) serves a much larger portion of the body than the others. It affects many body functions that are beyond conscious control. Branches of the vagus nerve innervate muscles of the pharynx, larynx, respiratory tract, heart, esophagus, and parts of the abdominal viscera. Therefore, the vagus nerve has reflex control of heart rate, sneezing, hunger, secretions from stomach glands, and constrictions within the respiratory tract. It is also involved in *sympathetic* and *parasympathetic* responses. For this reason, it is called "the wanderer."

Box 19-3	Mnemonic for Names of Cranial Nerves	
On	I	Olfactory
Old	II	Optic
Olympus	III	Oculomotor
Towering	IV	Trochlear
Top	V	Trigeminal
A	VI	Abducens
Finn	VII	Facial
And	VIII	(Acoustic) Vestibulocochlear
German	IX	Glossopharyngeal
View	X	Vagus
Some	XI	(Spinal) Accessory
Hops	XII	Hypoglossal

TABLE 19-2 The Cranial Nerves and Their Functions

NUMBER	NAME	MAIN FUNCTION	DISTRIBUTION
I	**O**lfactory	Smell (**S**ensory)	Nasal mucous membrane
II	**O**ptic	Vision (**S**ensory)	Retina
III	**O**culomotor	Eye movements (**M**otor)	Most ocular muscles
IV	**T**rochlear (smallest cranial nerves)	Voluntary eye movements (**M**otor)	Superior oblique muscle of eye
V	**T**rigeminal (largest cranial nerves)	Sensations of head and face; movement of mandible (**B**oth)	Skin of face; tongue; teeth; muscles of mastication (chewing)
	Ophthalmic branch	Sensations from front of head and face, eye sockets, and upper nose (**S**ensory)	
	Maxillary branch	Sensations from nose, mouth, upper jaw, cheek, and upper lip (**S**ensory)	
	Mandibular branch	Sensations of tongue, lower teeth, chin, clenched teeth, chewing (**B**oth)	
VI	**A**bducent (Abducens)	Eye movements (**M**otor)	Lateral rectus muscle of eye
VII	**F**acial	Taste; facial expressions (**B**oth)	Muscles of expression; taste buds
VIII	Vestibulocochlear (**A**coustic)	Hearing and balance	Internal auditory meatus
	Cochlear division	Conduct impulses related to hearing (**S**ensory)	
	Vestibular division	Conduct impulses related to equilibrium (balance) (**S**ensory)	Inner ear
IX	**G**lossopharyngeal	Controls swallowing; gives information on pressure and oxygen tension of blood; taste (**B**oth)	Pharynx, posterior third of tongue, parotid
X	**V**agus ("wanderer") (the only cranial nerve not restricted to head and neck)	Somatic motor function; parasympathetic functions; speech; swallowing; gag reflex (**B**oth)	Pharynx, larynx, heart, lungs, esophagus, stomach, abdominal viscera
XI	Accessory (**S**pinal accessory)	Rotation of head; raising of shoulder (**M**otor)	Arising from medulla and spinal cord
XII	**H**ypoglossal	Movement of tongue (**M**otor)	Intrinsic muscle of tongue

BOX 19-4 Mnemonic for Functions of Cranial Nerves

Some	Sensory	I	Olfactory
Say	Sensory	II	Optic
Marry	Motor	III	Oculomotor
Money	Motor	IV	Trochlear
But	Both	V	Trigeminal
My	Motor	VI	Abducens
Brother	Both	VII	Facial
Says	Sensory	VIII	(Acoustic) Vestibulocochlear
Bad	Both	IX	Glossopharyngeal
Business	Both	X	Vagus
Marry	Motor	XI	(Spinal) Accessory
Money	Motor	XII	Hypoglossal

The gross functioning of most cranial nerves can be assessed with simple actions, such as asking the client to clench the jaw (assessing cranial nerve V: mandibular branch of the trigeminal nerve). See In Practice: Data Gathering in Nursing 47-1 in Chapter 47.

Spinal Nerves

The 31 pairs of **spinal nerves** attach to the spinal cord. Each group of spinal nerves is named for its corresponding attachment site on the spinal cord: cervical (8 pairs), thoracic (12 pairs), lumbar (5 pairs), sacral (5 pairs), and coccygeal (1 pair). Each spinal nerve contains a dorsal (posterior) root that receives sensory information and a ventral (anterior) root that carries motor impulses to muscles and glands. The spinal nerves carry impulses such as temperature, touch, pain, muscle tone, and balance. They also transport motor impulses to skeletal muscles. (In some situations, medication is injected to block these nerves, reducing pain or discomfort.) On the dorsal root of each spinal nerve is a collection of knot-like nerve cell bodies, the *dorsal root* ganglion (plural: ganglia).

(There are many ganglia in the body, nearly all of which are located outside the CNS.) The **ganglia** here serve as relay stations for impulses such as touch, pressure, vibration, and pain, which are transmitted via the thalamus to the sensory cortex in the brain.

A group of spinal nerves forms a **plexus** (plural: plexus or plexuses). Examples include the cervical plexus, where the phrenic nerve (which controls the diaphragm) arises; the brachial plexus, where the nerves to the upper arms (e.g., radial and ulnar nerves) arise; the lumbosacral plexus, from which the sciatic nerve arises; and the pudendal plexus, from which nerves to the perineum arise. An injury to any of these could cause nerve damage, resulting in weakness, numbness, or diminished movement in the affected area. The cervical plexus and phrenic nerve have an important role in respiration; if the cervical plexus is damaged above the area of the phrenic nerve, respiratory arrest will occur.

> ### Key Concept
> **Spinal Nerves**
> Cervical: 8 pairs: (cervical plexus—phrenic nerves—diaphragm)
> Thoracic: 12 pairs
> Lumbar: 5 pairs: (lumbosacral plexus—sciatic nerve)
> Sacral: 5 pairs
> Coccygeal: 1 pair

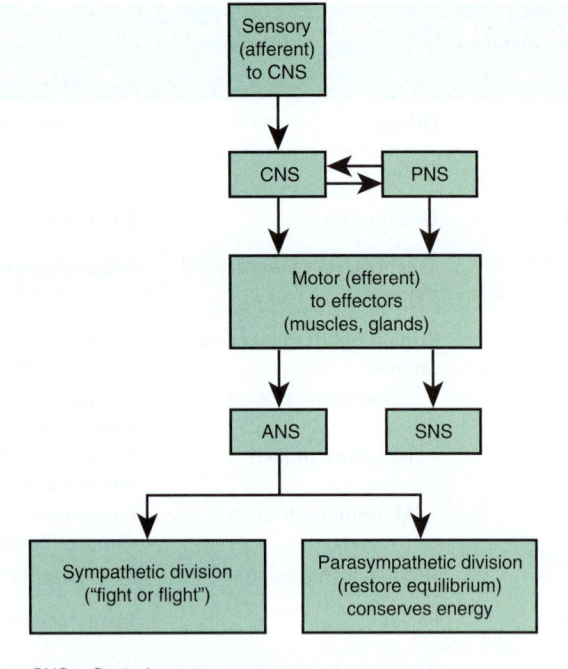

Figure 19-9 Organization of the nervous system.

Spinal Cord Injuries

Injury to the spinal cord causes swelling, which can result in temporary paralysis. If the spinal cord is cut through completely (*transection*), paralysis below the level of injury is permanent because nerves cannot regenerate and nerve impulses are interrupted. Research continues in an effort to assist persons with cord transaction to be able to walk. If an injury is close to the junction of the brain and spinal cord, damage to respiratory and other vital centers can result in death (see Chapter 78).

Autonomic Nervous System

The **ANS** is composed of portions of the CNS and PNS (Fig. 19-9). It is generally classified as part of the PNS; however, the ANS is highly specialized. The ANS functions independently, without conscious effort, innervating organs not under voluntary control, particularly cardiac muscle, glands, and smooth (visceral) muscles, such as those in the intestine, bladder, and uterus. The ANS contains *visceral motor neurons* to these areas (Fig. 19-10). The body's ability to maintain homeostasis is largely due to the ANS.

The ANS has two divisions: *sympathetic* and *parasympathetic*. As shown in Figure 19-10, stimuli to the structures originate in both divisions, but they often function in opposition to each other (*antagonistic reactions*). For instance, sympathetic nerves increase heart rate and dilate the pupil of the eye; parasympathetic nerves slow heart rate and constrict the pupil. Table 19-3 summarizes the effects of both divisions of the ANS on selected organs.

Many chemicals are produced by the ANS that also function in a similar manner as do the autonomic nerves. Some chemical substances "turn on" or mimic either the sympathetic or parasympathetic nervous system. Other drugs "turn off" or "lyse" the sympathetic or parasympathetic subdivisions of the ANS.

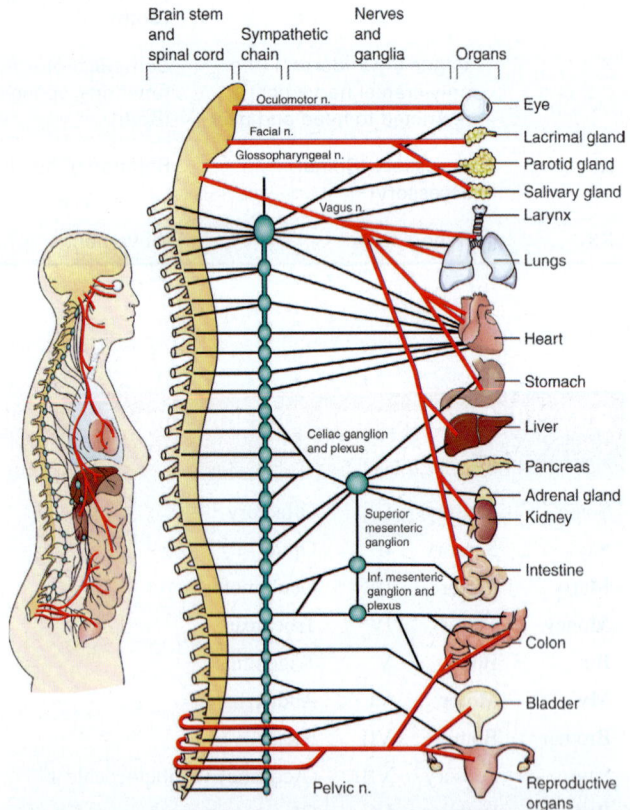

Figure 19-10 Anatomy of the autonomic nervous system. The *red lines* represent the parasympathetic nervous system (craniosacral division). The *black lines* represent the sympathetic nervous system (thoracolumbar division). (The oculomotor, facial, glossopharyngeal, and vagus nerves are cranial nerves, shown here to illustrate their autonomic functions.)

TABLE 19-3 Effects of the Sympathetic and Parasympathetic Systems on Selected Organs

EFFECTOR	SYMPATHETIC SYSTEM	PARASYMPATHETIC SYSTEM
Pupils of eye	Dilation	Constriction
Sweat glands	Stimulation	None
Digestive glands	Inhibition	Stimulation
Heart	Increased rate and strength of beat	Decreased rate and strength of beat
Bronchi of lungs	Dilation	Constriction
Muscles of digestive system	Decreased contraction	Increased contraction (peristalsis)
Kidneys	Decreased activity	None
Urinary bladder	Relaxation	Contraction and voluntary emptying
Liver	Increased release of glucose	None
Penis	Ejaculation or relaxation	Erection
Adrenal medulla	Stimulation	None
Blood vessels		
Skeletal muscles	Dilation	Constriction
Skin	Constriction	None
Respiratory system	Dilation	Constriction
Digestive organs	Constriction	Dilation

Sympathetic Division

The **sympathetic** division of the ANS produces a response that prepares individuals for an emergency, extreme stress, or danger. This "fight or flight" response readies people to defend themselves or flee from danger. During an emergency, the heart beats faster and the breathing rate and blood pressure increase. The skin becomes pale, secondary to the diversion of blood flow to more vital organs. Blood flow also decreases to structures such as external genitalia and abdominal organs. Thus, body processes such as digestion slow or stop, allowing more blood to flow to the brain, lungs, and large muscles that move the body during an emergency. Involuntary defecation or urination can occur. Obviously, the body can sustain an emergency reaction for only a limited time. The homeostatic mechanism that balances the sympathetic nervous system (**SNS**) is the parasympathetic nervous system (PNS).

Parasympathetic Division

The **parasympathetic** division of the ANS is involved in *relaxation*. The parasympathetic division generally produces responses that are normal functions of the body while at rest or not under unusual or extreme stress. The effects are usually opposite to the effects of the SNS. Unlike the sympathetic division, however, the parasympathetic system does not normally activate in a way that affects the total body. For example, it can decrease the body's heart rate without affecting other organs. To return to homeostasis after a "fight or flight" episode, the parasympathetic nerves return the heart rate to normal, resume digestive processes, and restore blood flow to the skin, abdominal organs, and genitalia. Previously normal patterns of defecation and urination return.

Key Concept

The ANS functions independently, without conscious effort, to innervate cardiac muscle and smooth visceral muscle and glands. The sympathetic division prepares the body for an emergency; the parasympathetic division maintains normal body functions and returns a person's body to normal after a stressful situation. These opposing reactions (antagonism) maintain homeostasis.

System Physiology

TRANSMISSION OF NERVE IMPULSES

Messages from one part of the body to another can take several possible nerve pathways. The body is thrifty in its use of resources and in patterns of automatic activities. Generally, it uses the quickest route to send a message. The body builds patterns (reflexes) and habits by using the same nerve pathways repeatedly. The same kind of message tends to follow the same path every time. Repeated motions become more or less automatic.

Resting Potential and Action Potential

Electrical and chemical influences enable nerve impulses to occur. An unequal distribution of ions (electrically charged particles) exists between the inside and outside of the neuron's cellular membrane. Outside the membrane are sodium (Na^+) and some potassium (K^+) ions. Inside the nerve cell are a number of negatively charged ions. This charge difference is called the *resting potential*.

A stimulus, or *nerve impulse*, causes an organized, rapid shift of sodium and potassium ions across the cell membrane (called "firing," as in firing a gun), instantly reversing the polarity (ionization or electrical charge) of the cell. (Sodium crosses first, then potassium.) The impulse is an electrical charge that can be measured; it spreads like an electric current along the membrane, beginning at one spot and spreading the length of the nerve cell. (The movement of ions and regulation of the process is a result of *active transport* [against concentration gradients], the *sodium–potassium pump*—see Chapter 17.) The changed polarity of the neuron's plasma membrane and the electrical impulse generated by ion movement is called **action potential**. An action potential takes only milliseconds (1 ms = 1/1,000 s). Thus, many neurons can transmit impulses more than several meters per second.

After this, a *refractory period*, during which the membrane cannot be stimulated, prevents nerve impulses from going backward. The potassium channels open to allow the potassium to again pass to the outside of the membrane. This reversal of the cell's polarity, back to its original state, occurs instantly (within 0.1–1.0 ms). Therefore, as quickly as polarity occurs, it reverses itself to bring the cell back to its resting state. This alternating depolarization and repolarization moves as a wave along the length of the neuron and becomes a transmitted message.

Neurotransmitters

> **Key Concept**
>
> Nerve cell at rest = *resting potential* (plasma membrane more positive on outside).
>
> Nerve stimulus—Sodium moves inside the membrane, followed by potassium = **action potential** (membrane now more positive on inside) → *nerve impulse*.
>
> Potassium ions flow out of nerve cell, followed by sodium = *refractory period* (resting potential restored).

For nerve impulses to cross the synaptic cleft, *neurotransmitters* are required. There are more than 30 known neurotransmitters. These chemicals are stored in small *synaptic or neurotransmitter vesicles*, clustered at the tip of the axon (see Fig. 19-3). When an action potential arrives at a neuron, some of the vesicles move to the end of the axon and discharge their neurotransmitters into the synaptic cleft. These substances diffuse across the cleft and bind to receptors on the next cell's membrane, causing ion channels to open and enabling the desired action. This allows nerve impulses to cross the synapse and transmit an impulse, which either excites or inhibits the target cell. After the action, neurotransmitters are immediately destroyed by enzymes in the synaptic cleft, diffuse out, or are reabsorbed by the cell, preventing a continuous impulse.

An example of a neurotransmitter is *acetylcholine*, inactivated by the enzyme *cholinesterase*. *Dopamine*, *norepinephrine*, and *serotonin*, as well as specific hormones, are also neurotransmitters. These names are familiar because many have been developed into useful pharmacologic products.

The All-or-None Law

Either a nerve impulse is transmitted across a particular synapse or it is not—with no exceptions. Because an impulse cannot be partially transmitted, this law is known as the *all-or-none* response of nerve tissue.

Electroencephalogram

An electroencephalogram (**EEG**) is a visual record of the electrical activity of the millions of neurons in the brain. Brain wave activity helps diagnose neurologic problems, and in many states, cessation of brain wave activity is an important legal consideration in the confirmation of biologic death.

Actions of Three Types of Neurons

Sensory Neurons

The sensory neurons (neurons of sensation) are *afferent* neurons because they carry impulses *to* the brain or spinal cord from the periphery of the body by means of **receptors**, end organs that initially receive stimuli from outside or within the body (Fig. 19-11). Receptors are classified in three ways. *Exteroceptors* (related to the external environment) are involved in touch, cutaneous (skin) pain, heat, cold, smell, vision, and hearing. *Proprioceptors* carry sensations of position and balance or location of the body in space. *Interoceptors* (related to the body's internal environment) respond to changes in the internal organs (viscera), such as visceral pain, hunger, or thirst. After the receptors receive an impulse, fibers of sensory neurons carry the sensation to the CNS. Here, interneurons analyze and distribute the impulses. Some interneurons act as integrators, and the impulse is carried directly to a motor neuron.

Motor Neurons

If an action is required after receiving a stimulus, the CNS sends an impulse via motor (efferent) neurons to a muscle or gland to cause the proper response. Motor neurons carry impulses *away* from the CNS to structures that carry out activity, **effectors**. Effector neurons are classified as *somatic–voluntary* or *visceral–involuntary*. To understand the difference between the types of effector neurons, consider an insect bite. A sensory (afferent) neuron makes the

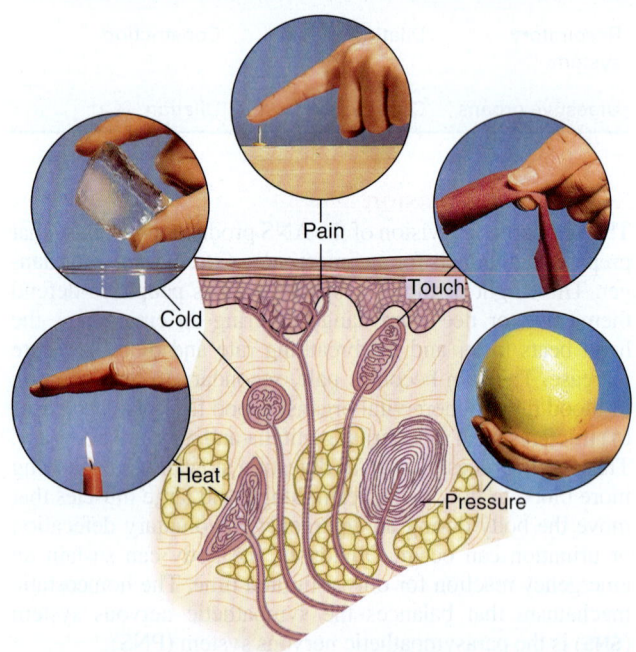

Figure 19-11 The receptors (exteroceptors) in the skin receive stimuli related to temperature, pain, touch, and pressure. These neurons are sensory (afferent) neurons, which carry stimuli via the sensory pathways to the central nervous system for interpretation.

initial sting known to the brain. The brain interprets the sensation and sends a message via *somatic–voluntary* (efferent) neurons to appropriate muscles. A person manifests a response by slapping the insect. This action is *voluntary*, in that it can be controlled. An example of a *visceral–involuntary* response is the peristaltic movement of food through the digestive system. Such movement is not under a person's voluntary control; rather, it depends on the nervous system's ability to process information and relay appropriate messages.

Interneurons

Neurons that integrate signals between neurons of various parts of the CNS are *interneurons* and are found only in the CNS (see Fig. 19-8B). They carry out or integrate sensory or motor impulses and assist with thinking, learning, and memory. They can be thought of as a link between sensory and motor neurons.

REFLEXES

A **reflex** is an automatic or involuntary response to a stimulus; a reflex occurs without conscious thought. Reflexes are homeostatic; they attempt to maintain balance. They move the body from danger, keep the body from falling, and maintain a relatively constant blood pressure, pH, and level of water reabsorption. Some reflexes are more complex than others. Reflexes do not operate as isolated parts of the nervous system but are integrated into the CNS as a reflex arc; the brain may inhibit or exaggerate a reflex when it receives a stimulus. For example, a person reflexively blinks the eyes when danger approaches, but after the brain realizes the danger, the person acts as a whole unit and moves the body away. Other reflexes include constriction of the pupil of the eye when exposed to light, automatic increase in heart rate when the body senses a lowering of blood pressure, and the patellar (knee-jerk) reflex that occurs when an examiner taps the patellar tendon just below the kneecap. Deep-tendon reflexes are often tested as part of a clinical assessment to determine if the nervous system is functioning properly. Figure 19-7 illustrates simple reflexes. Special education is required to gain competency in reflex testing.

> **SPECIAL CONSIDERATIONS** Lifespan
>
> **Reflexes**
>
> Infants and small children have slower reflexes due to the immaturity of their nervous system. The myelin sheath is still forming during infancy; therefore, an infant's response to stimuli is not as rapid as an older child's or an adult's. Some reflexes are present in infants and disappear by adulthood. These include the Moro, rooting, sucking, Babinski, and stepping reflexes. If any of these reflexes occur in an adult, this is an indication of serious brain damage or improper development (see Chapter 47 and Fig. 67-4).

> **NCLEX Alert**
>
> The NCLEX requires knowledge of the nervous system and its ability to receive and send messages in the body. An NCLEX clinical situation can describe an individual with paraplegia, quadriplegia, or hemiplegia. Depending on the described situation, the most appropriate response can relate to hazards of long-term paraplegia or basic functions of the nervous system.

> **Key Concept**
>
> It is important to teach people to use helmets, infant car seats, seat belts, and other protective equipment to prevent traumatic brain injuries. In addition, some conditions, such as tetanus, encephalitis, and clostridium food poisoning, as well as drugs, such as methamphetamine, can permanently affect neurologic functioning.

> **SPECIAL CONSIDERATIONS** Lifespan
>
> Nursing care for older adults must adapt to changes related to aging. The aging process produces significant effects on the nervous system. See Table 19-4.

> **NCLEX Alert**
>
> Two of the most common problems in older adults are hypertension and strokes. The NCLEX may provide clinical situations that require you to respond with appropriate nursing interventions, use of medications, and long-term rehabilitation. Safety and preventive measures may be components of client/family teaching concepts.

TABLE 19-4 Effects of Aging on the Nervous System

FACTOR	RESULT	NURSING IMPLICATIONS
Thought processes and ability to learn or reason should be retained. (Genetics, environmental conditions, and physical changes may influence thought processes.)	Losses in the thought process, reasoning, or learning are not normal.	Treat older adults as normal, intelligent people. Evaluate any changes in personality or thought processes. Encourage reading and learning new things; working puzzles; social activities. If underlying pathology exists, understand the disease and its progression. Adjust environment to provide safety and security for client.

(Continued)

TABLE 19-4 Effects of Aging on the Nervous System (Continued)

FACTOR	RESULT	NURSING IMPLICATIONS
Sleep patterns may change; however, amount of sleep needed often is relatively unchanged. Less rapid eye movement (dream) sleep occurs.	Person feels less rested; wakefulness periods at night are common. Older individuals may start using sleeping aids.	Watch for behavioral changes caused by prescription and over-the-counter drugs. Caution against excess use of sleep aids. Be aware of client's stressors; clinical depression secondary to cumulative losses is common. Encourage exercise during the day and eating a light meal in the evening. Reassure client that shorter periods of sleep are common. Treat frequent voiding and/or incontinence at night.
Number of neurons decreases.	Person exhibits decrease in voluntary movements.	Allow for longer response time.
Rate and spread of nerve transmission decrease.	Persons may be startled more easily. Reflexes may be slowed. Decision making may be slower.	Prevent accidents. Teach safe driving and defensive driving techniques.
Thermoregulation abilities often are reduced.	Older adults are more susceptible to heatstroke or effects of cold. Skin may remain pink, even if client is cold (may not become pale or blue).	Increase layers of clothing in all weather. Teach signs of heat-related disorders. Tell client foot protection is important because of decreased sensation and slowed circulation.
Some short-term memory loss may be normal.	Person may be disoriented as to time and date.	Reorient client as needed.
Long-term memory usually is retained.		Initiate opportunities to reminisce; reminiscing is beneficial. Assess and treat situations that may cause confusion—electrolyte imbalance, hypoxia, small strokes (TIA), drugs, pain, stress, infection, anemia.
Motor skills may be affected by physiologic changes in other systems.	Person may lack dexterity. Falls may occur.	Encourage maintenance of abilities by daily exercise (walking is excellent). Encourage use of cane or walker for stability, if needed. Remove obstacles, such as scatter rugs, to prevent falls.
Brain or nerve cells may be damaged and cannot regenerate. Conditions such as shingles (inflammation of nerve endings) may be very painful.	Assess for CVA, Alzheimer's disease, and conditions related to atherosclerosis ("hardening of the arteries"). Encourage older clients to get shingles immunization.	Provide adequate lighting. Treat symptomatically.

CVA, cerebrovascular accident; TIA, transient ischemic attack.

STUDENT SYNTHESIS

KEY POINTS

- The primary functions of the nervous system are communication and control.
- The primary nerve cell is the neuron, supported by neuroglia.
- A neuron consists of a cell body, axon, and dendrites.
- The functions of the neuroglia are to protect and support the central nervous system (CNS) and peripheral nervous system (PNS).
- The central nervous system consists of the brain, spinal cord, and accessory structures.
- The four cerebral lobes—frontal, parietal, temporal, and occipital—are located in both hemispheres of the brain. The frontal lobe is responsible for higher mental processes. The parietal lobe is responsible for speech and some sensory input. The temporal lobe is responsible for smell, hearing, and some memory. The occipital lobe is responsible for vision.

- The hypothalamus regulates many body functions, such as temperature, thirst, hunger, urination, swallowing, and the sleep–wake cycle. It also secretes some hormones and influences release of hormones from the pituitary, thereby influencing the metabolism of nutrients and regulation of fluid balance and general homeostasis.
- The cerebellum is responsible for muscle control.
- The brainstem is made up of the midbrain, pons, and medulla. The midbrain functions as a reflex center. The pons contains nerve tracts and carries messages between the cerebrum and medulla and is also responsible for respiration. The medulla contains centers for vital body functions, such as heart rate, vasomotor tone, and respirations.
- The spinal cord conducts impulses to and from the brain and acts as a reflex center.
- The meninges cover the brain and spinal cord and include the dura mater, arachnoid mater, and pia mater.
- Twelve pairs of cranial nerves arise from the brain. Most of these convey impulses to and from the brain and the structures of the head.
- The spinal nerves are attached to the spinal cord. They are divided into 8 cervical pairs, 12 thoracic pairs, 5 lumbar pairs, 5 sacral pairs, and 1 coccygeal pair.
- The autonomic nervous system is divided into the sympathetic and parasympathetic divisions. The sympathetic system prepares individuals for emergencies. The parasympathetic system maintains body functions under normal conditions.
- The three types of neurons are sensory (afferent), motor (efferent), and interneurons (integrators). Sensory neurons carry information to the brain. Motor neurons carry information away from the brain. Interneurons integrate signals between the two.

CRITICAL THINKING EXERCISES

1. Discuss how an injury to each of the following areas of the brain might manifest itself in an individual: frontal lobe, parietal lobe, temporal lobe, and occipital lobe. Differentiate between these in terms of signs and symptoms and if they occur on the right side versus the left side of the brain.
2. Explain why a person who suffers an injury to the spinal cord that results in physical paralysis can still retain brain functioning, but a person who suffers a brain injury may experience limited or no movement.
3. Describe at least three physical adaptations that might be required for a client with a brain injury. Relate these to the area of the brain that has been injured.
4. Demonstrate the following actions with your *eyes closed:* quickly touch the tip of your nose with your extended forefinger and then point at the wall and repeat, stand still on one foot, and clap your hands together. Describe what part of the nervous system is involved, and state what makes it possible to perform these actions without the sense of vision.
5. Using the Data Gathering in Nursing Display 47-1, discuss the functions of at least six cranial nerves and the simple determination of their adequate functioning.

NCLEX-STYLE REVIEW QUESTIONS

1. A client sustains a head trauma after falling from a roof. The nurse observes clear fluid leaking from the nose. What priority action should the nurse take?
   a. Use a Q-tip to gently clean the nasal passages.
   b. Pack the nose with nasal packing.
   c. Instruct the client to blow their nose to clear the passages.
   d. Have the fluid checked for glucose.
2. A client suffers a stroke located in the medulla. Which is the priority action by the nurse?
   a. Support the client's respiratory function.
   b. Assist the client with ambulation.
   c. Orient the client to surroundings frequently.
   d. Monitor the client for swallowing food and fluid.
3. A client with chronic alcoholism and late-stage cirrhosis of the liver has significant damage to Wernicke area. Which data obtained by the nurse are indicative of this damage?
   a. The client is unable to ambulate independently.
   b. The client does not comprehend written and spoken language but speaks.
   c. The client has speech impairment but is able to comprehend language.
   d. The client's left hand is experiencing paralysis.
4. A client who sustained head trauma in a motor vehicle crash is determined to have an increase in intracranial pressure (ICP). Which complications related to an increase in ICP should the nurse be aware of? Select all that apply.
   a. Brain hypoxia
   b. Herniation of the brain
   c. Brain compression
   d. Paralysis of the lower extremities
   e. Urinary retention
5. A client is having a colonoscopy, and suddenly the client's heart rate drops from 72 beats per minute (BPM) to 52 BPM. Which cranial nerve does the nurse determine has been stimulated?
   a. Cranial nerve I (olfactory)
   b. Cranial nerve V (trigeminal)
   c. Cranial nerve IX (glossopharyngeal)
   d. Cranial nerve X (vagus)

CHAPTER RESOURCES

Enhance your learning with additional resources on **thePoint**!

Student Resources related to this chapter can be found at **thePoint.lww.com/Rosdahl12e**.

20 The Endocrine System

Learning Objectives

1. Differentiate between exocrine and endocrine glands.
2. Describe the general functions of the endocrine system and the actions related to each.
3. Describe the relationship between the hypothalamus and the pituitary gland.
4. Identify major hormones released by the anterior, middle, and posterior divisions of the pituitary; describe the functions of each.
5. Describe the actions of hormones responsible for calcium balance.
6. Describe the relationships between "releasing" hormones and "inhibiting" hormones.
7. Describe the hormones involved in "fight or flight"; give examples of their effects and body's responses during an emergency.
8. Explain the functions of the thyroid hormones.
9. Describe the functions of mineralocorticoids and glucocorticoids secreted by the adrenals.
10. Discuss the location of insulin secretion; explain how insulin and glucagon regulate blood sugar levels.
11. Discuss the role of the thymus as an endocrine organ and its relationship to the body's immune response.
12. Briefly identify male and female sex hormones and functions of each.
13. Name the hormones secreted by nonendocrine glands or organs; state the function of each.
14. Discuss negative and positive feedback as they relate to the endocrine system.
15. Explain the role of prostaglandins.
16. Describe four effects of aging on the endocrine system.

Important Terminology

adenohypophysis
adrenal gland
corticosteroid
endocrine gland
endocrinology
erythropoietin
exocrine gland
glucagon
glucocorticoid
goiter
gonadotropin
hormone
hypothalamus
insulin
islets of Langerhans
mineralocorticoid
neurohypophysis
parathyroid
pineal gland
pituitary gland
prostaglandin
thymus
thyroid

Acronyms

ACTH
ANf
ANP
CRH
CT
FSH
GH
GHIH
GHRH
GnRH
GRH
HCG
hGH
ICSH
LH
LT
MIF
MSH
PIH/DA
PRH
PRL
PTH
T_3
T_4
TRH
TSH

The *endocrine system* controls body processes via chemical substances. Most of these substances are secreted in glands. *Endocrine glands* are located throughout the body, and each contains a group of specialized cells that secrete *hormones*, chemicals that regulate body processes, in response to body signals. *Endocrinology* is the specialty that studies endocrine glands, their secretions, and related disorders.

Exocrine glands secrete special substances (hormones and/or other materials) into ducts that open onto the body's external or internal surfaces. Exocrine glands include sweat, mammary, and salivary glands, as well as mucous membranes and lacrimal (tear) glands. Examples of exocrine secretions are sweat, milk, bile, tears, and pancreatic fluid. Unlike exocrine glands, **endocrine glands** (*ductless glands*, glands of internal secretion) secrete hormones directly into the bloodstream, where they are transported throughout the body. These hormones act on remote tissues (*target tissues*) via *endocrine signaling*. Certain glands can perform both endocrine and exocrine functions. Table 20-1 compares endocrine and exocrine glands.

Hormones are chemical messengers that unlock, initiate, regulate, integrate, and/or coordinate body activities. They speed up or slow down activities of entire body organs or systems. Some hormones affect the rate of activities of individual cells. Hormones also affect one another. Too much or too little of a particular hormone interferes with or counteracts actions of other hormones. Some glandular secretions signal each other in sequence. This is known as a *hormonal axis*. An example of a hormonal axis is the hypothalamic → pituitary → adrenal axis.

Hormones may be produced in response to nervous stimulation, the level of specific substances in the blood, or other hormones.

There are several hormone categories. S*teroid hormones* are fat soluble. *Nonsteroid hormones* (polypeptides) exist as whole proteins or amino acids and function via a second-messenger system. Amines are derived from tyrosine. Prostaglandins (*tissue hormones*) affect only nearby cells. See discussion below.

TABLE 20-1	Comparison of Endocrine and Exocrine Glands			
GLAND	DEFINITION	ACTION	FUNCTIONS OF SECRETIONS	EXAMPLES
Endocrine	Ductless glands; glands of internal secretion; vascular; usually contain vacuoles or granules to store hormones	Secrete hormones into circulation	Regulatory	Insulin, adrenocorticotropic hormone (ACTH)
Exocrine	Secrete into a duct; glands of external secretion; less vascular than endocrine glands	Secrete substances directly into duct or body opening	Protective, functional	Digestive juices, tears, sweat, saliva

Key Concept

Endocrine glands work in conjunction with the nervous system. The nervous system causes fast responses and reactions. The endocrine system causes slower and more long-lasting responses.

STRUCTURE AND FUNCTION

The endocrine system provides a mechanism for regulation, integration, and coordination of all body cells, organs, and systems. The main functions of the endocrine system are regulation of growth, maturation, metabolism, and reproduction (Box 20-1).

The glands of the endocrine system include the pituitary, thyroid, parathyroid, adrenal, and pineal. In addition, several organs that are not exclusively endocrine glands also contain cells that secrete hormones. (Four such organs are the hypothalamus, gonads, pancreas, and thymus.) Figure 20-1 illustrates shapes and locations of specific endocrine structures. In addition, specialized hormones are secreted in such diverse organs as the gastrointestinal tract, kidneys, and heart. Following are descriptions of glandular locations, their hormones, and hormonal actions.

Key Concept

Functions of the endocrine system include regulation of growth and maturation, metabolism, and reproduction. Genetics determine the basis of a person's body structure and function. Hormones carry out these genetic instructions. The ultimate goal is homeostasis.

Several types of hormones and hormone-like substances include

- *Steroids*—derived from cholesterol (e.g., aldosterone and cortisol). Steroid hormones are lipid (fat) soluble and can pass directly through the plasma membrane of a target cell. They move through the cell into the nucleus and bind with the appropriate receptor (hormone-receptor complex). This complex acts on DNA and causes formation of new proteins—specific effects. Steroid hormone responses are usually slower than those of nonsteroid hormones (Patton & Thibodeau, 2019).
- *Polypeptides*—protein compound, made up of amino acids. These include many hormones of the anterior pituitary (e.g., growth hormone, corticotrophin, and prolactin), posterior pituitary (e.g., oxytocin), parathyroid hormones, and pancreatic hormones (e.g., insulin and glucagon). These nonsteroid hormones exist as whole proteins or amino acids and function via a second-messenger system. The protein hormone message is sent to cells of the endocrine gland (target cell)—"first messenger." Then, the information works inside the cell to regulate cellular activity—"second messenger" (Willis, 2018).
- *Amines*—derived from tyrosine, an amino acid in proteins, include thyroxine, epinephrine, norepinephrine, and dopamine. (Amines are also precursors of melanin, the pigment in skin.)
- *Prostaglandins* are not actually hormones, but have some hormonal actions. They are lipid-based fatty acids and act as messenger molecules. Sometimes called *tissue hormones*, they can diffuse only short distances to affect nearby cells (often in the same tissue). For example, prostaglandins induce labor at the end of pregnancy.

Receptors are protein molecules within body cells that bind with hormones to initiate specific physiologic processes.

Pituitary Gland

The **pituitary gland**, also called the *hypophysis*, is about the size of a pea. It is located in a saddle-shaped hollow in the sphenoid bone, the *sella turcica*. (The sphenoid bone is

Box 20-1 Functions of the Endocrine System

GROWTH AND MATURATION
- Regulates growth and maturation
- Regulates body's response to stress

METABOLISM
- Regulates metabolism
- Regulates absorption of nutrients
- Regulates use of glucose in cellular respiration
- Maintains body pH by maintaining fluid and electrolyte concentrations

REPRODUCTION
- Produces sexual characteristics
- Controls reproductive and birth processes
- Promotes normal growth and development
- Activates lactation
- Influences sexual response

234 UNIT 4 Structure and Function

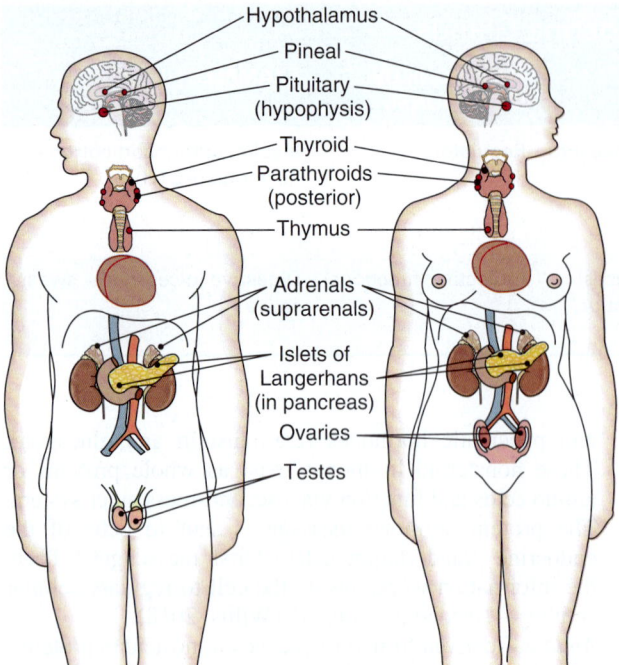

Figure 20-1 Location of major endocrine glands in the body.

located at the base of the brain's frontal lobe.) Two parts make up the pituitary gland: the anterior and posterior lobes. These lobes are sometimes classified as two separate glands, because their functions and embryonic development are very different. The pituitary body is adjacent to the hypothalamus.

Role of the Hypothalamus

The **hypothalamus** is a tiny but complex portion of the brain, attached to the pituitary by means of the *infundibular (hypophyseal) stalk*. The hypothalamus is considered to be the "master controller" or "integrator." Specialized cells in the hypothalamus release hormones that either inhibit or promote release of other hormones from the anterior lobe of the pituitary. These hypothalamic hormones are described as *releasing hormones (RH)* or *inhibiting hormones (IH)* (Table 20-2). Figure 20-2 illustrates the role of the hypothalamus in regard to the pituitary gland and the influence of its hormones.

Anterior Lobe

The anterior (largest) pituitary lobe, the **adenohypophysis**, releases several hormones (Table 20-3). (The prefix *adeno-* means gland.) Many are *glycoproteins*, made up of carbohydrates and proteins. The hypothalamus controls the adenohypophysis; therefore, neural commands release these hormones. Five of these hormones (the tropic hormones) control the growth, development, and proper functioning of other endocrine glands.

Tropic Hormones

Tropic hormones stimulate another endocrine gland to secrete hormones. Corticotropin-releasing hormone (**CRH**) from the parvocellular neurosecretory neurons (corticotropes) of the hypothalamus causes release of adrenocorticotropic hormone (**ACTH** or *corticotropin*) from the anterior pituitary. ACTH stimulates the adrenal cortex to produce glucocorticoids and androgens (corticosteroids)—such as cortisol—which are vital in metabolizing carbohydrates. ACTH also has melanocyte-stimulating properties that can increase skin pigmentation.

Thyrotropin-releasing hormone (**TRH**), also from the parvocellular neurosecretory neurons (thyrotropes) of the hypothalamus, causes release of thyroid-stimulating hormone (**TSH** or *thyrotropin*) from the pituitary, as well as the release of prolactin. TSH stimulates the thyroid gland to produce and to secrete thyroxine (T_4) and triiodothyronine (T_3) (discussed later). The hypothalamus also functions to inhibit TSH and GH, by releasing growth hormone-inhibiting hormone (**GHIH**).

The hormone known as growth hormone (**GH**), human growth hormone (**hGH**), or *somatotropin* is produced by somatotropic cells and released from the anterior pituitary. This hormone is stimulated by the release of growth

TABLE 20-2	Major Hypothalamus Hormones Affecting Hormone Secretion From the Pituitary Gland	
RELEASING HORMONES (STIMULATING HORMONES) FROM HYPOTHALAMUS	**INHIBITING HORMONES FROM HYPOTHALAMUS**	**PITUITARY HORMONES STIMULATED OR INHIBITED**
Corticotropin-releasing hormone (CRH)	Melanocyte-inhibiting factor (MIF)	Adrenocorticotropic hormone (ACTH) Melanocyte-stimulating hormone (MSH)
Growth hormone-releasing hormone (GRH or GHRH)	Growth hormone-inhibiting hormone (GHIH) or somatostatin (SS)	Growth hormone (GH) or human growth hormone (hGH) or somatotropin
Thyrotropin-releasing hormone (TRH)	Growth hormone-inhibiting hormone (GHIH) or somatostatin (SS)	Growth hormone (GH), thyroid-stimulating hormone (TSH) or thyrotropin; (minor effect—stimulates prolactin release)
Prolactin-releasing hormone (PRH)	Prolactin-inhibiting hormone (PIH) or dopamine (DA)	Inhibits release of prolactin (PRL) and thyroid-stimulating hormone (TSH)
Gonadotropin-releasing hormone (GnRH)		Interstitial cell-stimulating hormone (ICSH) in men or luteinizing hormone (LH) in women Follicle-stimulating hormone (FSH)

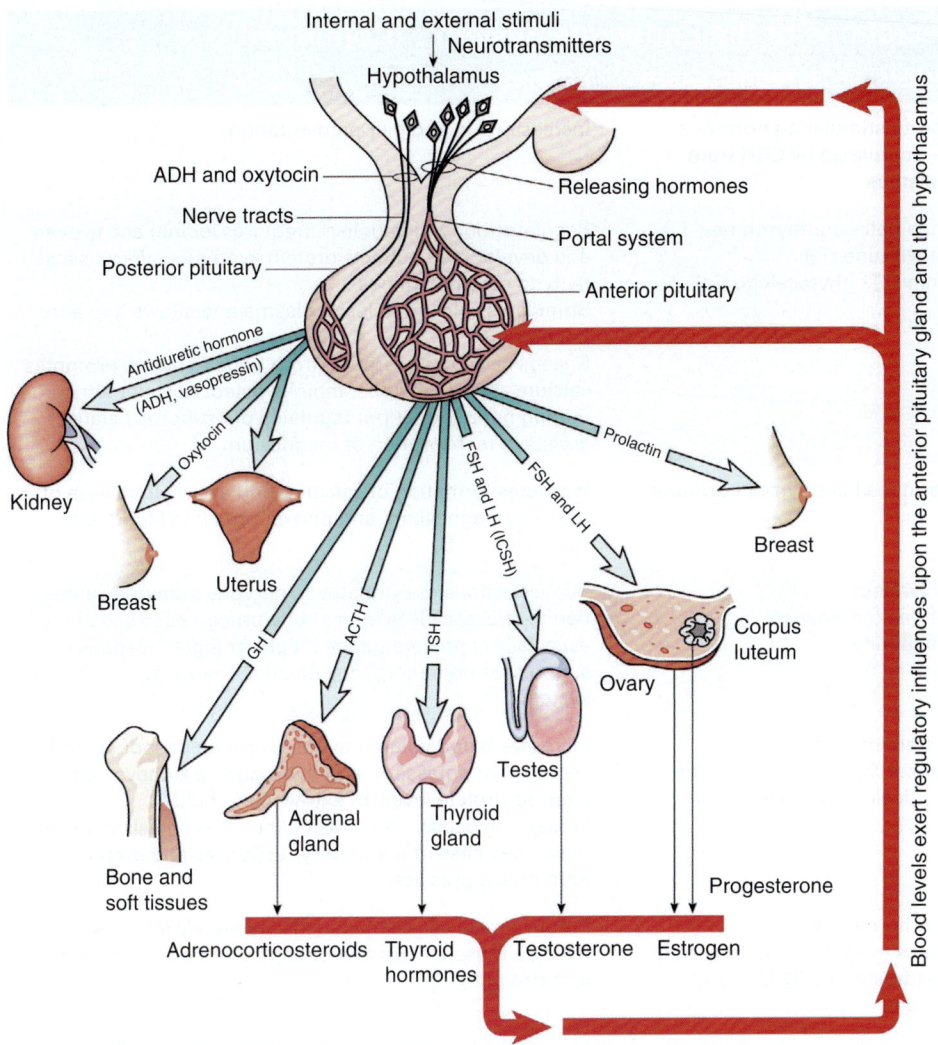

Figure 20-2 The pituitary gland, the relationship of the hypothalamus to pituitary action, and the hormones secreted by the anterior, middle, and posterior pituitary lobes.

TABLE 20-3 Important Secretions of the Endocrine System

GLAND/ORGAN	HORMONE(S) SECRETED/RELEASED	ACTIONS
Pituitary Anterior lobe (adenohypophysis)	Adrenocorticotropic hormone (ACTH, corticotropin)—stimulated by CRH from hypothalamus Growth hormone (GH or hGH), somatotropic hormone—stimulated by GRH, GHRH from hypothalamus Thyroid-stimulating hormone (TSH), thyrotropin—stimulated by TRH from hypothalamus Follicle-stimulating hormone (FSH)—stimulated by GnRH Luteinizing hormone (LH) (in females) Prolactin, lactogenic hormone (PRL)—stimulated by PRH from hypothalamus LH (in males) Interstitial cell-stimulating hormone (ICSH) (males) Lipotropin	Stimulates adrenal cortex to produce cortisol, corticosteroids, and androgens; can stimulate melanocytes Controls bone and tissue growth and regulates metabolism (influences secretion of insulin-like growth factor I from liver) Regulates thyroid hormone (via secretion of thyroxine [T_4] and triiodothyronine [T_3]) Stimulates growth and secretion of eggs in ovaries (female) and sperm in testes (male) Helps control ovulation and menstruation; important in sustaining pregnancy Stimulates mammary glands to produce milk (after pregnancy); influences sexual gratification Stimulates Leydig cells to produce testosterone; stimulates secretion of male hormones (androgens) Influences breakdown of lipids (fats), production of steroids, and melanin production
Posterior lobe (neurohypophysis) Stores hormones only— no production	Oxytocin Vasopressin (antidiuretic hormone—ADH)	Causes uterine contractions; contractions of cervix and vagina; influences orgasm; stimulates milk production; Raises blood pressure (some vasoconstriction); promotes water reabsorption in kidney tubules; influences uterus

(Continued)

TABLE 20-3 Important Secretions of the Endocrine System (Continued)

GLAND/ORGAN	HORMONE(S) SECRETED/RELEASED	ACTIONS
Middle lobe (intermediate pituitary lobe)	Melanocyte-stimulating hormone (MSH)—stimulated by CRH from hypothalamus	Increases skin and hair pigmentation
Thyroid	Thyroxine (tetraiodothyronine—T_4) Triiodothyronine (T_3) Calcitonin (CT—thyrocalcitonin)	Regulates body metabolism (requires iodine) and growth and development; affects protein synthesis; affects sensitivity to catecholamines Stimulates calcium to leave plasma and allows it to enter bones Speeds calcium absorption from bone to blood; promotes calcium storage in bone; inhibits osteoclasts, thereby promoting bone formation; regulates phosphorus balance; assists in reabsorption of magnesium
Parathyroid	Parathormone/Parathyroid hormone (PTH)	Promotes formation of calcitriol and assists in release of calcium, magnesium, and phosphorus into blood; activates vitamin D
Adrenals (Suprarenals) Adrenal medulla	Catecholamines Epinephrine (adrenaline) Norepinephrine	Mimics actions of sympathetic nervous system, adaptation to stress; causes many body processes to speed up, especially in an emergency ("fight or flight" response); suppresses nonemergency functions; suppresses immune system
Adrenal cortex	Corticosteroids/corticoids Mineralocorticoids (mainly aldosterone) Glucocorticoids (mostly cortisol)	Increases blood volume by reabsorption of sodium and secretion of potassium and hydrogen by kidneys; regulates electrolyte levels in extracellular fluid Influence glucose, amino acid, and fat synthesis in metabolism; decrease inflammatory responses and promote immunosuppression
	Male sex hormones Androgens (males)—including dehydroepiandrosterone (DHEA) and testosterone	Produce male sex characteristics (anabolic steroids—develop muscle mass and strength, increase bone mass and strength)
	Female sex hormones (estrogens)—very small amount Dopamine Enkephalins	Produce female sex characteristics, Increases heart rate and blood pressure, Regulate pain, mood, behavior; serve as neurotransmitters
Gonads Testes (male)	Testosterone	Develops male sex characteristics (also influenced by androgens)
Ovaries (female)—from ovarian follicle of corpus luteum	Estrogen and progestins (progesterone is the primary progestin)	Regulate female sex characteristics, functions, menstruation, allow sperm penetration, maintain pregnancy (inhibit premature onset of labor, suppress lactation, inhibit immune response toward embryo, anti-inflammatory)
	Progesterone	Reduces gall bladder activity, regulates levels of certain minerals, assists thyroid function, promotes healing, promotes nerve functioning, prevents endometrial cancer in women
	Estradiol	Prevents apoptosis (destruction) of germ cells, increases liver function, promotes blood coagulation, assists in fluid and electrolyte balance
	Inhibin	Inhibits FSH production
Pancreas Alpha cells (islets)	Glucagon	Speeds glycogenolysis; raises blood sugar; stimulates breakdown of fats and proteins

TABLE 20-3	Important Secretions of the Endocrine System (Continued)	
GLAND/ORGAN	HORMONE(S) SECRETED/RELEASED	ACTIONS
Beta cells (islets)	Insulin	Regulator of carbohydrate, protein, and fat metabolism. Enables cells to use glucose; lowers blood sugar; facilitates synthesis of triglycerides; suppresses exocrine secretions of pancreas
	Amylin	Helps regulate glucose balance; sends satiety signals to brain
Delta cells (islets)	Somatostatin	Inhibits release of insulin and glucagon; lowers rate of gastric emptying, reduces smooth muscle contractions and intestinal blood flow
F cells (islets—"PP cells")	Pancreatic polypeptide	Inhibits secretion of somatostatin and pancreatic digestive enzymes
Thymus	Thymosin (thymic hormone)	Stimulates production of T cells for cellular immunity
Pineal body	Melatonin (an antioxidant)	Regulates sleep–wake cycles; may play a role in influencing reproductive processes
Heart	Atrial-natriuretic peptide (ANP), atrial-natriuretic factor (ANf)	Reduces blood pressure by decreasing vascular resistance and fluid volume; influences balance of sodium and fats in blood
	Brain-natriuretic peptide (BNP)	Influences lowering of blood pressure
Liver	Thrombopoietin	Stimulates platelet production
	Insulin-like growth factor (somatomedin)	Regulates cell growth and development; also has insulin-like effects
	Angiotensin and angiotensinogen	Vasoconstriction; influence release of aldosterone from adrenal cortex
Kidney	Renin	Activates renin-angiotensin system by stimulating production of angiotensin I and angiotensinogen
	Erythropoietin (EPO)	Stimulates production of erythrocytes (red blood cells [RBCs])
	Calcitriol	Increases calcium and phosphate absorption, inhibits release of parathyroid hormone (PTH)
	Thrombopoietin	Stimulates platelet production by the megakaryocytes
Stomach and small intestine	Gastrin and histamine	Stimulate secretion of gastric acid
	Ghrelin	Secreted by cells in stomach lining—slows metabolism and fat burning, may contribute to obesity; stimulates appetite; stimulates secretion of GH
	Leptin	Secreted by fat-storing cells—regulates hunger and fat metabolism
	Neuropeptide Y (NPY)	Increases food intake; decreases physical activity; decreases secretion of bicarbonate
	Secretin and pancreozymin	Enhance effects of cholecystokinin (CCK); stop production of gastric juice; stimulate pancreas to release pancreatic juice. Stimulate secretion of bicarbonate from liver, pancreas, and duodenum (Brunner glands)
	Somatostatin	Suppresses release of gastrin, cholecystokinin (CCK), secretin, and other substances; reduces rate of gastric emptying; reduces smooth muscle contractions and intestinal blood flow
	Histamine	Stimulates gastric acid secretion
	Endothelin	Influences smooth muscle contractions in stomach

(Continued)

TABLE 20-3 Important Secretions of the Endocrine System   (Continued)

GLAND/ORGAN	HORMONE(S) SECRETED/RELEASED	ACTIONS
Duodenum	Cholecystokinin (CCK)	Stimulates release of digestive enzymes from pancreas, release of bile from gall bladder; suppresses hunger
Ilium and colon	Human incretin hormone (glucagon-like peptide-I)	Influences secretion of insulin by pancreas
Striated muscle	Thrombopoietin	Stimulates megakaryocytes to produce platelets

The placenta serves as an endocrine gland during pregnancy—see Chapter 65.

hormone-releasing hormone (**GRH** or **GHRH**) by the hypothalamus. GH stimulates growth and cell reproduction in all body tissues. It assists with movement of amino acids into tissue cells and transformation of amino acids into needed proteins. It aids in the release of fatty acids from adipose (fat) tissue to be used for energy. GH helps regulate blood nutrient levels after eating and during fasting. GH also stimulates the release of insulin-like *growth factor 1* from the liver. When sufficient amounts of GH and TSH have been released, the hypothalamus secretes GHIH (discussed previously) to inhibit further release of GH.

> **Key Concept**
>
> Hormone balance depends on "feedback loops." If a hormone level is too low, endocrine glands are stimulated to secrete more hormone and vice versa. For example, growth hormone and insulin have opposite effects on glucose metabolism. A balance must be maintained between opposing hormones.

Gonadotropin-releasing hormone (**GnRH**) secreted in the neuroendocrine cells of the preoptic area causes the anterior pituitary to secrete two hormones, **gonadotropins**, which stimulate the sex glands (gonads). These two hormones are follicle-stimulating hormone (FSH) and luteinizing hormone (LH):

- **FSH**, produced in gonadotropic cells, stimulates both the growth and secretion of ovarian follicles in women and the production of sperm in men.
- **LH**, also produced in gonadotropic cells, in women stimulates ovulation and the formulation of the corpus luteum (luteinization), which then produces progesterone. In men, LH stimulates the production of sex hormones, including testosterone, in specialized areas of the testes and is also called interstitial cell-stimulating hormone (**ICSH**). LH/ICSH and FSH are known as *gonadotropic* hormones because they influence the gonads (reproductive organs).

Prolactin
Prolactin (**PRL**), stimulated by prolactin-releasing hormone (**PRH**), and secreted by lactotropic cells, is secreted by the anterior pituitary and stimulates breast development and milk production in women following pregnancy. (PRL also exists in men, but its function is not known.) Inhibition of prolactin and TSH occurs when the hypothalamus' arcuate nucleus secretes prolactin-inhibiting hormone or dopamine (**PIH/DA**).

Lipotropin
Lipotropin (also produced by corticotropes) influences lipolysis (breaking down of fats) and steroidogenesis (production of steroids, as in the adrenals) and stimulates melanocytes to produce melanin.

Middle Lobe
The most important hormone secreted by the pituitary's middle lobe (pars intermedia) is melanocyte-stimulating hormone (**MSH**), stimulated by CRH from the hypothalamus. MSH influences skin pigmentation and is chemically similar to ACTH (produced in the anterior lobe). The hypothalamus *inhibits* secretion of MSH by secreting melanocyte-inhibiting factor (**MIF**).

Posterior Lobe
The pituitary's posterior lobe, the **neurohypophysis**, is actually an outgrowth of the hypothalamus and is embryonically derived from the nervous system. Its makeup is similar to nervous tissue, and it comprises about one quarter of the pituitary. Hormones are not secreted there but are stored and released. The hypothalamus and pituitary gland are close to each other. The two hormones released by the posterior lobe, oxytocin and vasopressin, are secreted *in the hypothalamus* by neurosecretory cells and then *released* by the neurohypophysis (see Fig. 20-2).

Oxytocin (from neurosecretory cells) stimulates the uterus to contract during delivery and helps to keep it contracted after delivery (to prevent hemorrhage). It also stimulates the release of milk from a new mother's breasts and is involved in orgasm and circadian homeostasis (body temperature, wakefulness, and activity level).

Vasopressin or *antidiuretic hormone* (ADH or AVP) functions in several ways. It stimulates contraction of blood vessels to raise blood pressure; affects the uterus; and influences reabsorption (resorption) of water by the kidney tubules (see Chapter 27 and Table 20-3).

> **Key Concept**
>
> Although there are subtle differences in the definitions of reabsorption (the term used in this book) and resorption, these terms are often used interchangeably to mean the reuse of materials, such as proteins, glucose, and electrolytes, to restore essential components to the body. An example is the selective reabsorption of extracellular fluid in the kidney tubules.

Thyroid Gland

The **thyroid gland**, the largest endocrine gland, lies in the anterior neck, just below the larynx, with a wing (lobe) on either side of the trachea, separated by the *isthmus* (Fig. 20-3). The thyroid stores an iodine-based hormone precursor, colloidal iodinated thyroglobulin, which is stimulated by TSH to form thyroid hormones. The epithelial cells of the thyroid synthesize two hormones: thyroxine (tetraiodothyronine or T_4) and triiodothyronine (T_3) from the iodine. T_4 is the less potent form of thyroid hormone. More T_4 (90%) is found in the blood, compared with T_3. It is believed that T_4 is converted to T_3 before it is effective. Thyroid hormones regulate body metabolism, controlling the rate at which cells function. Protein synthesis relies on these hormones, and they also affect sensitivity to catecholamines (important in stress responses) and sympathetic amines (e.g., dopamine and epinephrine). Because the thyroid requires iodine to form T_4, a person's diet must supply iodine.

SPECIAL CONSIDERATIONS Nutrition
Iodine food sources include ocean shellfish and iodized salt. A lack of iodine in the body could cause a decrease in thyroid function over time. Common symptoms of decreased thyroid function are fatigue, weight gain, and chills.

A lack of dietary iodine may cause an enlarged thyroid gland (**goiter**). In this case, the hypothalamus secretes excess TSH, causing the thyroid gland to enlarge.

Another hormone, secreted in the parafollicular cells of the thyroid, is *calcitonin* (**CT**) or *thyrocalcitonin*. CT (and parathyroid hormone) are involved in the maintenance of calcium levels. When the circulating calcium level is high, calcitonin responds by promoting increased storage of calcium in bones and increased renal excretion of calcium, resulting in lowered serum calcium.

Parathyroids

The **parathyroids** are the smallest known endocrine glands, each about the size of a pea, that lie embedded on either side of the undersurface of the thyroid gland (see Fig. 20-3). Usually, there are four, in two pairs. Despite their relatively small size, the parathyroids are essential to life.

The chief cells of the parathyroids secrete a hormone, *parathormone* or *parathyroid hormone* (**PTH**), that regulates the amounts of calcium and phosphorus in the blood, which in turn affects nerve and muscle irritability. When the blood calcium level is too low, PTH is secreted, increasing the number and size of osteoclasts (large cells associated with reabsorption of bone). Therefore, PTH causes calcium to leave the bones and also enhances reabsorption of calcium and magnesium and excretion of phosphorus in the kidneys. PTH also affects the kidneys by promoting *calcitriol* formation. This is a hormone synthesized from vitamin D, which increases the rate of calcium, magnesium, and phosphorus absorption from the gastrointestinal tract into the blood. (Therefore, PTH and calcitonin have opposite actions.)

> **Nursing Alert** Calcium levels must be maintained within very small tolerances, or death can result. A client with severe calcium deficiency may exhibit muscle twitching and spasms (*tetany*), and sometimes, seizures.

Adrenal Glands

The two **adrenal glands**, also known as *suprarenal glands*, sit like hats, one atop each kidney (see Fig. 20-1). As with the pituitary, the adrenals each have two parts; each part producing different hormones.

Adrenal Cortex

The zona glomerulosa, zona fasciculata, and zona reticularis, cells of the outer part of the adrenals (the adrenal cortex), secrete many compounds called **corticosteroids** or *corticoids*; all derived from cholesterol. The outermost area, the glomerulosa, secretes mineralocorticoids, especially aldosterone. The middle and largest area, the fasciculata, secretes glucocorticoids, such as cortisol (hydrocortisone), corticosterone, cortisone, and some sex hormones—androgen (testosterone, male) and estrogen (dehydroepiandrosterone [DHEA], female). The innermost area, the zona reticularis, secretes some sex hormones.

Mineralocorticoids regulate the body's electrolytes. *Aldosterone*, the most important mineralocorticoid, stimulates reabsorption of sodium into plasma and secretion of potassium and hydrogen in the kidney, resulting in increased water reabsorption and, therefore, an increase in blood volume.

Glucocorticoids have an important influence on the synthesis of glucose, amino acids, and fats during metabolism. They also depress the immune response, decrease the inflammatory response, and contribute to the maintenance of normal blood pressure. Corticosteroid production is normally increased during stress. *Hydrocortisone* (*cortisol*) is the predominant glucocorticoid.

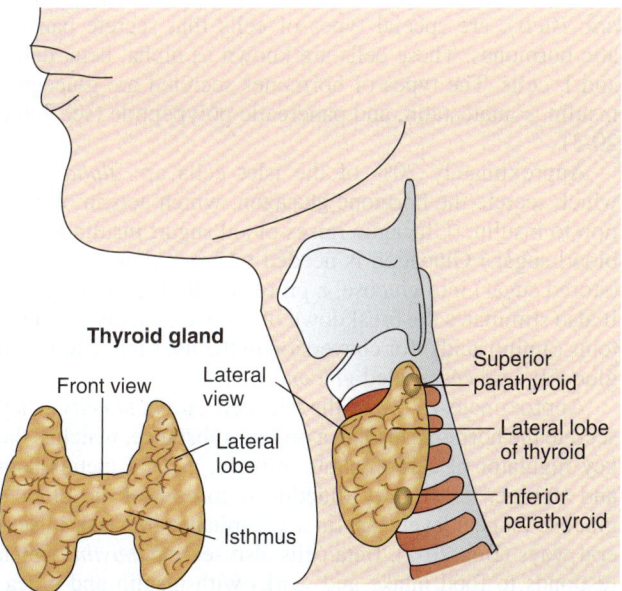

Figure 20-3 The thyroid gland as viewed frontally and laterally. The lateral view also shows the location of the parathyroid glands. The thyroid gland is made up of follicles, each containing an outer wall of follicular cells, with colloid material inside.

> **Nursing Alert** Clients taking glucocorticoids often experience lengthened healing times and may have a decreased response to infections due to the drug's anti-inflammatory and immunosuppressive actions. Therefore, consider a small rise in temperature significant in these clients.

Sex hormones of the adrenal cortex (*androgens, estrogens*, and *progestins*) supplement the sex hormones of the gonads. The adrenals primarily produce androgens, with only minute amounts of estrogen and progesterone secretion (see Table 20-3). Recently, abuse of anabolic steroids (synthetic derivatives of testosterone) has increased, particularly in relation to sports (see Chapter 95).

> **Nursing Alert** Look for classic signs in clients taking glucocorticoids, the result of fat redistribution, giving the client an appearance of being overweight. Signs include a round face ("moon face"), large abdomen, and a hump on the back ("buffalo hump").

Adrenal Medulla

The central portion of the adrenal gland, the *medulla*, is considered a neuroendocrine structure, and is actually part of the sympathetic nervous system (see Chapter 19). The medulla secretes *catecholamines*, hormones synthesized from amino acids. Examples include epinephrine and norepinephrine, produced in the chromaffin cells. *Epinephrine* (adrenaline) constitutes about 80% of the medulla's total secretion and is important in managing and adapting to stress. Epinephrine causes an increase in pulse rate, blood vessel contraction, a rise in blood pressure, and increased muscle power, by causing the liver to release glucose for energy. The hormone *norepinephrine* has some—but not all—actions of epinephrine. These two hormones mimic the action of the sympathetic nervous system and are active in emergencies; fright, anger, love, and grief stimulate them. They are said to enable "fight or flight" reactions. If the adrenal medulla is absent, the sympathetic nervous system can take over its activities.

> **Key Concept**
> Epinephrine and norepinephrine are major catecholamines and are involved in the "fight or flight" response.

Dopamine, also produced in the chromaffin cells, increases heart rate and blood pressure. Another type of substance from the same cells, the *enkephalins*, helps regulate pain. These substances also function as neurotransmitters, are involved in movement, mood, and behavior, and are found in a number of locations in the body.

Pineal Gland

The **pineal gland** (pineal body) is a small, cone-shaped structure located near the top of the brain's third ventricle (see Fig. 20-1). It produces *melatonin* in cells called pinealocytes. Melatonin functioning is not completely understood but is related to exposure to environmental light. It is an antioxidant and is thought to participate in the maintenance of the sleep–wake cycle. In sunlight, sympathetic nerve fibers release norepinephrine, inhibiting melatonin secretion and resulting in wakefulness. In darkness, the lack of norepinephrine stimulates melatonin secretion, resulting in sleepiness. The pineal gland is sometimes referred to as "the third eye," receiving sensory information from the optic nerves regarding circadian cycles. The pineal gland is also believed to influence body temperature and cardiovascular function and may influence reproductive functions.

Gonads

The *gonads* are the glands of reproduction: the male testes and female ovaries (see Fig. 20-1). In addition to producing sperm, the Leydig cells of the testes produce *testosterone*, the male sex hormone. Other steroid hormones, the *androgens*, produce masculinizing effects.

The female ovaries produce *estrogen* (primarily estradion) and *progesterone*, which, in addition to regulating female sex characteristics, are responsible for menstruation; they also influence pregnancy, labor, and lactation. In addition, progesterone has an influence on many body functions, including blood clotting, thyroid and nerve function, and the gall bladder. Chapters 28 and 29 describe these hormones in more detail.

Pancreas

The *pancreas* is a triangular structure located behind the stomach, between the duodenum and spleen (Fig. 20-4). It is both an endocrine (hormone-secreting) and exocrine gland. As an exocrine gland, it releases digestive enzymes into the duct system leading to the small intestine (see Chapter 26).

The endocrine portion of the pancreas exists in the 1–2 million small islands (*islets*) scattered throughout its body and tail. Within these islets, **islets of Langerhans** (*pancreatic islets*), are special types of cells that secrete pancreatic hormones. These cells are known as alpha, beta, delta, and F cells. The types of hormones secreted are glucagon, insulin, somatostatin, and pancreatic polypeptide (see Table 20-3).

Approximately 20% of the islet cells are *alpha cells*, which secrete the hormone **glucagon**, which acts in opposition to insulin. (Glucagon raises blood sugar; insulin lowers blood sugar.) Glucagon is needed to break down glycogen (stored sugar) into glucose, a process called *glycogenolysis*. It also stimulates the breakdown of fats (fatty acids) and proteins (amino acids) for conversion in the liver into additional glucose, a process called *gluconeogenesis*.

Approximately 70% of the islet cells are *beta cells*. They secrete the hormone **insulin**, a protein substance, which is the key regulator of carbohydrate, protein, and fat metabolism and storage. Its primary function is to control the blood's glucose (sugar) level. Insulin accomplishes this task in several ways (Box 20-2). Beta cells also secrete *amylin*, which responds to food intake and works with insulin and glucagon to help regulate glucose balance. Amylin acts especially during the few hours immediately after eating (postprandial period) by slowing the production of glucose to the liver.

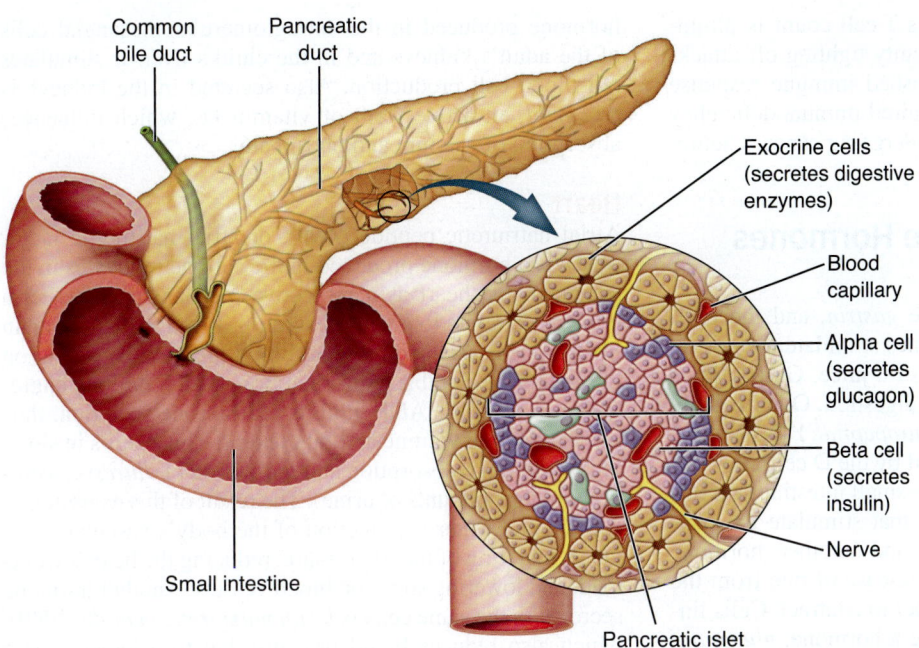

Figure 20-4 Pancreas.

This helps the person feel full or satisfied (satiety) by sending a signal across the blood–brain barrier. (In type 1 diabetes, both insulin and amylin are not secreted. In type 2 diabetes, both hormones are produced, but in insufficient amounts.) Endocrine disorders are discussed in Chapter 79.

> **Key Concept**
>
> Stages of insulin production in the islets of Langerhans:
> - Neuron stimulation—(hormone precursor) = preproinsulin
> - Preproinsulin converted to proinsulin in the endoplasmic reticulum
> - Proinsulin converted into insulin in the Golgi apparatus
> - Insulin is excreted into the blood stream by exocytosis

Box 20-2 Actions of Insulin to Control Glucose Level

- The major stimulus for synthesis and secretion of insulin is elevated blood glucose.
- Insulin increases the cell membrane's permeability to glucose. After it is in the cell, glucose is used in cellular respiration to produce energy.
- Insulin stimulates the liver to convert extra glucose into glycogen (*glycogenesis*) and helps the liver and muscles to store glycogen. Glycogen is stored as body sugar, commonly referred to as *animal starch*.
- Insulin increases the transfer of amino acids across muscle membranes for synthesis into proteins.
- Insulin speeds fatty acid synthesis (*lipogenesis*) for fat storage.
- Insulin slows *glycogenolysis* (glycogen breakdown) and *gluconeogenesis* (formation of glucose from noncarbohydrate sources).

Approximately 5% of the islet cells are *delta cells*. Delta cells secrete *somatostatin*, which is identical to the GHIH secreted by the hypothalamus. Somatostatin inhibits release of insulin and glucagon; the control mechanism is unknown. (Somatostatin is also secreted by the "D" cells of the stomach.) It suppresses the release of gastrin, cholecystokinin (CCK), secretin, motilin, vasoactive intestinal peptide (VIP), gastric inhibitory polypeptide (GIP), and enteroglucagon. Thus, it lowers the rate of gastric emptying and reduces smooth muscle contractions and blood flow in the intestines.

The remaining 5% of the islet cells are *F cells or PP cells*. F cells secrete *pancreatic polypeptide*, believed to inhibit secretion of somatostatin and pancreatic digestive enzymes.

> **Key Concept**
>
> Insulin is a hormone needed to transport glucose into cells, to enable cells to function. A lack or incorrect functioning of insulin will cause an increased blood glucose level (hyperglycemia). Diabetes mellitus results from inadequate glucose oxidation or utilization (often the result of beta cell malfunction). Because insulin is necessary for adequate body functioning, medical intervention is necessary to manage this disorder.

Thymus

The single, unpaired **thymus** consists of lymphatic tissue and lies behind the sternum (breast bone). It also consists of an outer cortex and inner medulla. In infants and children, the thymus is relatively large; after puberty, it becomes smaller. The thymus is the lymphatic system's primary controlling gland. It produces *thymosin* (thymic hormone), a protein that promotes growth of lymphatic tissue, and a naturally occurring immunologic hormone, *thymopoietin*. Thymosin stimulates production of small lymphocytes called *T-cells* (also called *T lymphocytes, T-helper cells*, or *thymus-dependent cells*) and also secretes other hormones believed to assist in maturation of T-cells. T-cells are essential for the development of cellular immunity and the body's response to invading organisms. If a person's T-cell count is diminished, that person would have difficulty fighting off attacking pathogens. This type of diminished immune response may be seen in the person with acquired immunodeficiency syndrome (AIDS) or in the client undergoing cancer chemotherapy (see Chapters 24 and 85).

Other Sites That Secrete Hormones

Gastrointestinal Tract

The G cells of the *stomach* secrete *gastrin*, and the ECL cells secrete *histamine*; both hormones stimulate the gastric glands (parietal cells) to secrete gastric juice. Gastric juice contains gastric acid, which aids in digestion. Other cells in the stomach produce *ghrelin* and *neuropeptide Y* (NPY) (see Table 20-3). *Somatostatin* is secreted by the D cells.

The lining of the upper part of the small intestine secretes hormones (*pancreozymin, secretin*) that stimulate the pancreas to release pancreatic juice and another hormone (*cholecystokinin*) that regulates the release of bile from the gallbladder and causes the gallbladder to contract. Cells lining the ilium and colon also secrete a hormone, *glucagon-like peptide*-I (GLP-I), which acts as a satiety signal, slowing emptying of the stomach and stimulating the pancreas to release insulin (see Chapter 26).

Liver

The hepatocytes of the liver produce several hormones. These include *insulin-like growth factor* (IGF, somatomedin), which has insulin-like effects in regulating cell growth and development. These cells also produce *angiotensinogen*, which, on hydrolysis by renin, gives rise to *angiotensin-converting enzyme* (ACE), causing vasoconstriction, rising blood pressure, and the release of aldosterone from the adrenal cortex. The actions of these hormones in the kidney are discussed below and in more detail in Chapter 27. Another hormone produced by the hepatocytes is *thrombopoietin*, which stimulates the production of platelets. This hormone is also present in the kidneys and striated muscles.

Placenta and Uterus

The placenta is a temporary endocrine gland that secretes hormones to assist in maintaining pregnancy (see Chapter 65). These hormones include estrogen and progesterone (see Chapter 29) and human chorionic gonadotropin (**HCG**). The pregnant uterus also secretes *prolactin*, which influences the production of milk after delivery.

> **Key Concept**
>
> The presence of elevated levels of HCG in a woman's body provides the basis for commonly used tests to determine pregnancy.

Kidneys

A structure within the kidney called the *juxtaglomerular apparatus* produces a hormone called *renin* (part of the renin–angiotensin–aldosterone [RAA] mechanism), which acts on the vascular system to assist in blood pressure control (see Fig. 27-5). **Erythropoietin** (renal erythropoietic factor) is a glycoprotein (protein and carbohydrate combination) hormone produced in the extraglomerular mesangial cells of the adult's kidneys and in the child's liver. It stimulates red blood cell production. Also secreted in the kidneys is *calcitriol*, an active form of vitamin D_3, which influences absorption of calcium and phosphate.

Heart

Atrial natriuretic peptide (**ANP**), or atrial natriuretic factor (**ANf**), is a hormone produced in the cardiac myocytes in the atrium of the heart as a protective mechanism. (The term *natriuretic* refers to sodium excretion.) ANP helps maintain fluid homeostasis and regulate blood pressure by acting on the kidneys to inhibit renin secretion, which inhibits angiotensin production. ANP inhibits aldosterone secretion, thus lowering blood volume and fat content. This results in slowing of sodium reabsorption and promotion of *diuresis* (secretion of large amounts of urine). The result of this excretion of sodium and water is reduction of the body's vascular resistance, lowering of blood pressure, reducing the heart's workload, and lowering stress on blood vessels. Another hormone secreted in the same cells is *brain natriuretic peptide* (BNP), which also reduces blood pressure, but to a lesser degree than does ANP.

> **Key Concept**
>
> ANP acts as an antagonist to aldosterone to regulate kidney function.

Other Specific Hormone Production

In addition to cells in the liver, myocytes in voluntary (striated) muscles secrete *thrombopoietin*, which stimulates platelet production. Adipocytes in fatty tissue produce *leptin*, which causes a decrease in appetite and increased metabolism (see Table 20-3).

Most Tissues

Leukotrienes

Leukotrienes (**LTs**) are hormones involved in the body's inflammatory process. This process can cause bronchoconstriction and anaphylaxis (similar to the effect of histamine, except leukotrienes are released at a slower rate). Drugs (*leukotriene inhibitors*) have been developed to decrease the amount of leukotrienes in the body; they are used to prevent asthma attacks.

Prostaglandins

The **prostaglandins** ("*tissue hormones*") are specialized fatty acids first isolated in the seminal fluid of the prostate, from which their name is derived. They diffuse over short distances to affect nearby cells, often in the same tissue. Since they are produced in many body tissues, they are widespread in the body. The three most common prostaglandins are prostaglandins A (PGA), E (PGE), and F (PGF). Prostaglandins are not hormones, but rather are hormone-like substances sharing characteristics with hormones and neurotransmitters. They can cause pain, perform a role in platelet function, and stimulate either contraction or relaxation in smooth muscle. The prostaglandins influence blood pressure, respiration, digestion, reproduction, and inflammatory responses—and in some cases actually can have opposite effects on these functions. For example, one prostaglandin may cause dilation of the bronchioles, whereas another may cause constriction. Prostaglandin research continues. Many disorders may be treated in the future by the administration of substances that control prostaglandin secretion. A current over-the-counter pain-reducing medication called *ibuprofen* works primarily as an anti-inflammatory agent by inhibiting prostaglandin production.

SYSTEM PHYSIOLOGY

> **NCLEX Alert**
>
> The NCLEX requires understanding of the interdependence of normal and abnormal functioning of the body's systems. The correct option will most commonly reflect a priority of needs for the body as a whole.

System Relationships

The endocrine system is closely related to other body systems. One prominent relationship is that with the nervous system. These two systems cannot be separated; each needs the other for optimum performance. Therefore, they are *interdependent* (each relies on the other). For example, parts of the nervous system stimulate or inhibit hormonal release. Likewise, hormones promote or inhibit nerve impulse generation. Both systems function to stimulate and control body actions. Generally, the effect of nerve stimuli is immediate and lasts only as long as the stimulation is present. The action of a hormone is slower, with more prolonged stimulation or regulation. Table 20-4 identifies signaling within the endocrine system.

The endocrine and circulatory systems are also interdependent because hormones travel from the glands through blood and lymph. The endocrine and digestive systems also rely on one another; for example, insulin is secreted by the endocrine system and enables the digestive system to use glucose and glycogen from foods.

> *Key Concept*
>
> Remember that glands can secrete too much or too little of a hormone. Hypersecretion (overproduction) and hyposecretion (underproduction) can result in serious physical disorders. Homeostasis must be maintained.

Information Relay to Target Cells

The hypothalamus and anterior and middle pituitary are components of a unit that functions as an "information relay system." Specialized cells in the hypothalamus respond to internal and external changes and respond by secreting hormones (see Table 20-2). These directly stimulate or block the release of hormones from the anterior pituitary (e.g., CRH stimulates the release of ACTH; MIF blocks the release of MSH). The hormones secreted by the hypothalamus and released from the anterior and middle pituitary then circulate to certain target tissues. These hormones usually bind to receptors on the target tissues in a "lock-and-key" fashion. (There is only one location and only one way possible for them to fit together.) The response of target cells to the hormone then involves acceleration or inhibition of certain biochemical processes.

> *Key Concept*
>
> A hormone can only cause a response from a cell that has a specific receptor for that hormone (a *target cell*).

Negative and Positive Feedback

The fine balance within the endocrine system called *feedback* regulates the rate and quantity of hormone secretion.

As discussed in Chapter 17, *negative feedback* signals the controller (the specific gland) to correct a deviation from normal. Negative feedback receptors (e.g., glands) require close monitoring by body cells in order to maintain the desired hormone level. After the desired effect is achieved, information is sent to the gland to halt hormonal secretion. This is a *negative feedback system* or *loop*, because the body has again achieved homeostasis. This situation will now cause an inhibited glandular response. An example is the secretion of insulin to correct the situation of excess blood sugar.

A *positive feedback system* or *loop* can also occur. For example, if a hormone is needed to meet the body's needs, a message is carried to the appropriate gland (as in the negative feedback system). The result is increased hormone production. Hormone secretion does not cease (as in negative feedback), but instead continues and intensifies. An example of a positive feedback system is the hormone oxytocin, produced during labor. Oxytocin intensifies uterine contractions and enables the uterus to expel the fetus.

Most body systems utilize both negative and positive feedback. The goal of feedback systems in the body is to help promote *homeostasis*. The basic mechanisms controlling hormonal release include stimulation by other hormones, chemical signals, and nerve stimulation.

TABLE 20-4	Signaling Within the Endocrine System
TYPE OF SIGNALING	**EFFECT**
Endocrine	Hormone carries the signal.
Paracrine	Hormone binds to nearby receptor—target cell—and affects their function.
Autocrine	Hormone affects the same cell that produced it; targets the same cell.
Neuroendocrine	Interaction occurs between nervous and endocrine systems in response to stimulus from both systems.
Neurocrine	Signaling occurs between neurons within the nervous system; endocrine influence on or by the nerves (neurosecretion).
Juxtacrine	Signals transmitted along cell membranes via proteins or lipids; can affect adjacent cell or same cell.

TABLE 20-5 Effects of Aging on the Endocrine System

FACTORS	RESULT	NURSING IMPLICATIONS
Overall effects of aging vary Decreased production of and receptivity to hormones at cellular level	Individualized changes	Monitor changes in metabolism or blood sugar levels; identify hormone level changes Be alert to symptoms of diabetes and thyroid disorders Notify physician of abnormal laboratory values
No generalized decreases occur, except in estrogen and testosterone levels	Decreased bone mass; decalcification	Monitor for problems related to osteoporosis
Reproductive hormones decrease	Onset of menopause in middle age Sexual organs shrink; women lose ability to become pregnant Hirsutism in women Atrophy of subcutaneous breast tissue; fat replaces glandular tissue; breasts sag Decreased sperm production; impotence may occur (but is not universal)	Monitor for heart disease, which increases in women after menopause, with loss of estrogens Advise about facial hair removal Sexual counseling may be suggested; medications available to assist in erection
Sexual tissue atrophies	Loss of pubic hair Longer time needed for sexual orgasm Lessened amount of vaginal secretion	Explain that libido is essentially unchanged Lubricant may aid in comfortable intercourse; estrogen cream may be helpful
Decrease in thyroid hormones	Decreased metabolic clearance rate Thinning hair; male pattern baldness Dry skin	It may take longer to do daily activities Be alert for complaints of feeling cold Offer skin lotions
Decrease in pancreatic secretions	Decreased ability to metabolize glucose	Monitor weight. Counsel on exercise and proper nutrition

SPECIAL CONSIDERATIONS Lifespan

Nursing care for older adults must adapt to changes related to aging. The aging process produces significant effects on the endocrine system. See Table 20-5.

Key Concept

Endocrine disorders may be related to
- Unregulated release of hormones
- Inappropriate response to hormonal signals
- Damage to an endocrine gland; absence of a gland
- Hypofunction or hyperfunction of a gland
- Dysfunction of the hypothalamus (which controls secretion and release of many hormones)
- Malignancy (see Chapter 79)

STUDENT SYNTHESIS

KEY POINTS

- Endocrine glands secrete hormones directly into the bloodstream; exocrine glands secrete hormones into ducts.
- Hormones are chemicals that regulate, integrate, and coordinate body systems and functions.
- Many hormones are secreted in the hypothalamus; they, in turn, control the release of hormones by the pituitary.
- The many hormones released by the anterior, middle, and posterior pituitary have widespread effects on the body.
- The thyroid is responsible for controlling the body's rate of metabolism, and it affects calcium storage.
- The parathyroid glands regulate the amount of calcium and phosphorus in the blood, and they activate vitamin D.
- The adrenal medulla secretes hormones that mimic the action of the sympathetic nervous system. Adrenal hormones are active in emergencies or in stressful situations.
- The adrenal cortex makes three types of steroid compounds from cholesterol: mineralocorticoids, glucocorticoids, and sex hormones. (These sex hormones supplement those secreted by the gonads, the glands of reproduction.)
- As an endocrine gland, the pancreas secretes insulin, which facilitates lowering of blood sugar, and glucagon,

causing blood sugar to rise. These substances also influence fat and protein metabolism.
- The thymus secretes hormones that play a role in cellular immunity.
- Melatonin, secreted by the pineal gland, helps regulate the sleep–wake cycle.
- Prostaglandins are hormone-like substances. Their effects are localized to the area in which they are produced. They influence blood pressure, respiration, digestion, and reproduction.
- The endocrine system has close interrelationships with other body systems.
- Negative and positive feedback mechanisms influence hormonal blood levels.
- Hormones are specific to target tissues and often act in a "lock-and-key" fashion.
- Other structures in the body, such as the heart, liver, kidneys, and digestive system, also produce specific hormones.
- During pregnancy, the placenta and uterus secrete hormones.
- Reduced hormonal production occurs as part of the normal aging process.

CRITICAL THINKING EXERCISES

1. Determine which hormones are working in the following scenarios: a woman who is ovulating; a woman in labor; a mother nursing their newborn; a firefighter in a life-or-death situation; a pubescent boy.
2. Explain how melatonin levels may contribute to sleep disorders. Relate this to the nurse who works night shifts and the nurse who works rotating shifts.
3. What special situations for older individuals are related to the endocrine system? Suggest possible preventive measures.

NCLEX-STYLE REVIEW QUESTIONS

1. A client states to the nurse, "I feel cold all of the time, have gained 20 lb, and I'm always tired." Which laboratory studies will the nurse likely need to review?
   a. 24-hour catecholamine study
   b. T_3 and T_4
   c. Prolactin levels
   d. Luteinizing hormone levels

2. The nurse observes facial twitching and spasms of the hand when the blood pressure cuff is inflated on a client after surgical removal of the thyroid gland. Which action is the priority by the nurse?
   a. Administer a calcium supplement such as calcium gluconate as ordered.
   b. Administer a glass of water with a tablespoon of salt by mouth.
   c. Administer oral potassium chloride as ordered.
   d. Administer a diuretic such as furosemide (Lasix) as ordered.

3. A client is taking oral glucocorticoids for the treatment of asthma. Which finding by the nurse would be a significant concern?
   a. A respiratory rate of 22
   b. A blood pressure of 140/60 mm Hg
   c. A heart rate of 92
   d. A temperature of 100 °F

4. The nurse is obtaining objective data from a client taking long-term oral glucocorticoids. Which findings obtained by the nurse correlate with glucocorticoid therapy? Select all that apply.
   a. Round or "moon" face
   b. Hypoactive bowel sounds
   c. A large abdomen
   d. Ridges on the fingernails
   e. "Buffalo" hump on back

5. A client has been prescribed a leukotriene inhibitor. Which positive client outcome does the nurse monitor for?
   a. The client will have a decrease in fever.
   b. The client will not report chest pain.
   c. The client will have clear lung fields.
   d. The client will have active bowel sounds.

CHAPTER RESOURCES

Enhance your learning with additional resources on thePoint!

Student Resources related to this chapter can be found at thePoint.lww.com/Rosdahl12e.

21 The Sensory System

Learning Objectives

1. Identify the location of receptors for each of the five senses; explain how these stimuli are interpreted in the brain.
2. Describe major structures of the eye and functions of each; differentiate between aqueous and vitreous humor.
3. Identify which cranial nerves are responsible for the blink reflex, pupillary changes, visualization, and pain sensation in the eye.
4. Differentiate between myopia, hyperopia, and astigmatism.
5. Identify structures and dividing lines between the outer, middle, and inner ear.
6. Trace the path of light rays as they enter the eye and focus on the retina; describe transmission to the brain.
7. Trace the path of sound waves through the external, middle, and inner ear. Describe amplification and interpretation of sound waves.
8. Explain how cerumen, ossicles, and eustachian tubes protect the ear.
9. Discuss how the organs of the inner ear provide a sense of balance.
10. Describe locations and functions of taste buds; identify the associated flavors of each.
11. Identify the structures related to the sense of smell; describe how they function.
12. Describe the effects of aging on the sensory system.

Important Terminology

accommodation	conjunctiva	lacrimal gland	ophthalmology	presbyopia	stapes
aqueous humor	cornea	lens	optic disk	proprioception	tinnitus
astigmatism	eustachian tube	macula	orbit	ptosis	tympanic membrane
audiology	gustation	malleus	organ of Corti	pupil	
auricle	hyperopia	membranous labyrinth	ossicle	retina	vertigo
cataract	incus		otology	rods	vitreous humor
cochlea	iris	myopia	pinna	sclera	
cones	labyrinth	olfaction	presbycusis	semicircular canals	

Without the sensory system, you would know nothing about your surroundings. Sensory perceptions are those of seeing, hearing, tasting, smelling, and touching. Humans also receive impressions of warmth, softness, pressure, vibration, and pain through the sensory system. Another important function of the sensory system is equilibrium, that is, knowing whether or not the body is moving and sensing the body's posture and position in space. By detecting environmental changes, the sensory system provides humans with protection and with mechanisms for experiencing the world.

STRUCTURE AND FUNCTION

From the study of the nervous system (Chapter 19), it is apparent that in order to be aware of information from the world, a person must possess the following:

- Receptors to receive a stimulus
- Nerve routes to carry the stimulus to the brain
- Centers in the brain to interpret the stimulus

(Note: In some cases, emergency reflexive responses occur in the spinal cord.)

The principles of stimulus reception and transmission apply to the sensory system, as well as the nervous system. Sensory structures must be able to detect a stimulus or *change* in stimulus. The stimulus must be transformed into an electrical signal (nerve impulse) and must be transmitted to the brain or spinal cord for interpretation and/or immediate action.

General sense organs include microscopic sensors, widely distributed in muscles, tendons, joints, and internal organs. They detect stimuli such as pain, all types of touch (e.g., light, persistent, vibration), temperature, pressure, itching, and proprioception (awareness of the body in space). *Special sensory organs* are the eyes, ears, tongue, nose, and skin. The functions of the special sensory organs are vision, hearing, taste, smell, and touch and will be discussed in this chapter. Without information related to environmental changes, your body would not be able to achieve and maintain homeostasis. Box 21-1 outlines sensory system functions.

The senses of taste, smell, and touch are as interesting and useful as are sight and hearing. Although they are not as often involved in illness as are sight and hearing, alterations in these other senses can pose safety hazards. For example, an altered sense of taste presents the risk of ingesting spoiled food or poison. An altered sense of smell would not allow

> **Box 21-1 Functions of the Sensory System**
>
> - Visual sense receives images (light).
> - Hearing receptors process sound waves (auditory sense).
> - Through proprioceptors and the inner ear, the system helps to maintain a sense of balance, equilibrium, and position in space.
> - Chemoreceptors in the mouth obtain information about tastes (gustatory sense).
> - Chemoreceptors in the nose receive sensations of odors (olfactory sense).
> - Touch receptors receive information about the surrounding world (e.g., touch, pressure, hot, cold, pain).
> - Internal organs receive sensations of pain, pressure, fullness, and vibration.
> - The brain interprets most of these sensations.

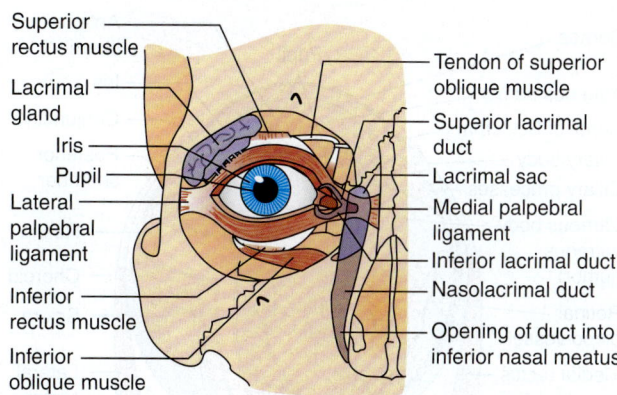

Figure 21-1 The right eye and its appendages (anterior view).

a person to smell smoke. Alteration in the sense of touch presents the risk of burns. The tongue's role in digestion is discussed in Chapter 26; the nose and breathing in Chapter 25; and the sense of touch in Chapter 16 (the integumentary system [Fig. 16-1]).

> **Key Concept**
>
> Sight and hearing are most frequently involved in illness; however, alterations in taste, smell, and touch can present safety hazards. These senses also provide pleasurable sensations.

THE EYE

The eye (denoted by the prefix *ophthalm[o]-*) is the organ of vision. It lies in a ball-shaped cavity of the skull, the **orbit**. Figure 21-1 illustrates major eye structures. The medical specialty related to the study of the eye and vision is **ophthalmology**.

> **Key Concept**
>
> The human eye contains more than 65% of the body's sensory receptors. It has a 200-degree viewing angle, can see 2.7 million different colors (including over 500 shades of gray), and can see a candle flicker 14 miles away.

The eyelids, *palpebrae*, are retractable covers for the eye's anterior surface. (The prefix for eyelid is *blephar[o]-*.) The oval opening between upper and lower eyelids is called the *palpebral fissure*. Several types of glands are in the eyelids, secreting sebum and sweat. Also covering and protecting the anterior eye, beneath and lining the eyelids (the cornea and sclera), is a thin, transparent mucous membrane, the **conjunctiva**, which is supplied with blood vessels and nerve endings.

The **lacrimal glands** produce tears (lacrimal fluid), about 1 mL/day, to moisten and lubricate the eye's surface (Fig. 21-2). Lacrimal glands are located at the outer corner (*lateral canthus*) of each eye. Tears drain from the eye through a small opening, the *punctum*, into the *nasolacrimal duct*, located in the inner corner of the eye (*medial canthus*). The nasolacrimal ducts drain tears into the nose. Tears contain an enzyme that helps protect the eyes from bacterial infections. Chemical and mechanical irritants (e.g., onions or dust) or foreign objects cause oversecretion by the lacrimal glands to wash irritants away. Humans are the only species that form tears in response to emotions.

Eyeball

The eyeball is a hollow sphere about 1 in. (2.54 cm) in diameter, with only the anterior surface being visible. The eyeball consists of three layers of tissue, the *tunics:* the sclera and cornea, choroid layer, and retina. The lens is another important eye structure, illustrated in Figure 21-3.

Sclera and Cornea

The tough, fibrous, protective outer layer of the eyeball is the sclera (the "white" of the eye). The sclera helps maintain the eyeball's shape. It is continuous with the transparent, yet tough, section over the front of the eyeball, the cornea, which permits light rays to enter the eye. The junction between the

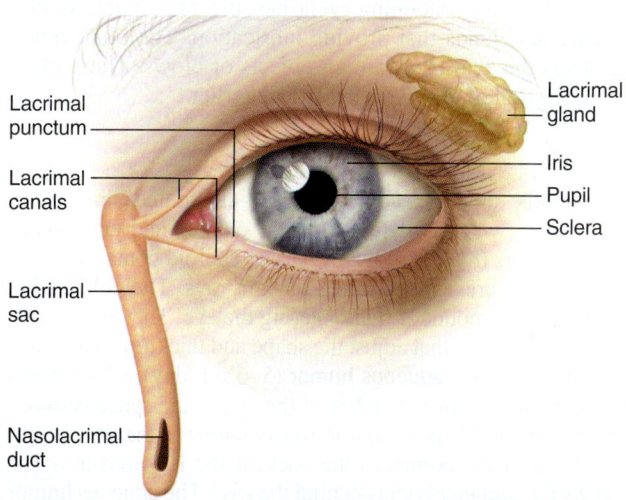

Figure 21-2 Tears are secreted by the lacrimal gland and lubricate the eye. They then drain through the nasolacrimal duct into the nose. (Anatomy & Physiology Made Incredibly Easy, 2012.)

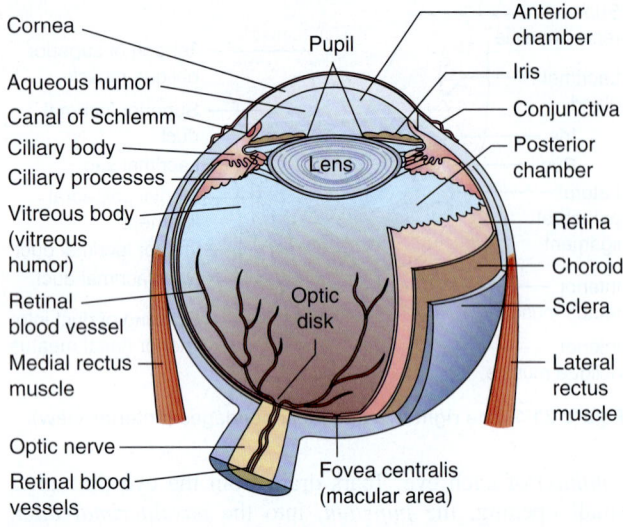

Figure 21-3 Transverse section of the eyeball.

cornea and sclera is the limbus. The cornea, which is covered with a protective coating of stratified squamous epithelium, influences visual acuity by refracting light rays. The cornea is very sensitive to touch and pain; even minor irritations will stimulate pain and the blinking reflex.

The cornea is often removed after death as a tissue for *corneal transplantation*. The absence of corneal blood vessels facilitates this procedure, which restores vision to thousands of people with defective or diseased corneas. Other procedures are performed to *change the shape of the eyeball*, to improve vision. These include radial keratotomy (RK), a series of laser slits to flatten a misshapen cornea, and astigmatic keratotomy (AK), laser cuts made across the cornea. A laser-assisted procedure (LASIK) is used to correct nearsightedness.

Protection

The eye is protected by the surrounding bony eye socket, which also includes a cushioning fat layer. The eyebrows, eyelids, and eyelashes provide further protection. In addition to hair follicles containing eyelashes, the lid margins contain sebaceous glands that provide lubrication. The blink reflex protects the eye from foreign objects or blows. The protective function of tears was described earlier.

Choroid Layer

The middle tunic, the *choroid*, contains the iris and ciliary body. This layer, which is vascular, brings oxygen and nutrients to all the layers (tunics) of the eyes. The choroid contains a dark pigment, to prevent scattering of light rays. The colored iris controls the amount of light entering the eye. The *ciliary body* contains muscles that adjust the shape and thickness of the lens and also secretes **aqueous humor** (5–6 mL/day), which flows through the anterior chamber of the eye in the space between the cornea and lens. (The *anterior chamber* is the space from the front of the cornea to the back of the lens and iris. The *posterior chamber* begins behind the iris.) The aqueous humor maintains *intraocular* (within the eye) *pressure* (normal is about 24 mm Hg). It also provides nutrients and oxygen to the avascular (without blood vessels) lens and cornea.

Over the front of the eyeball, the choroid develops into a pigmented section, the **iris**, which gives the eye its specific color. The amount of pigment in the iris determines eye color. Smooth and radial muscles in the iris control the size of the pupillary opening (Fig. 21-2). The **pupil** is the black center opening within the eye that allows light to enter. In strong light, iris muscles constrict the pupil, to allow less light to enter. The reverse occurs under low-light situations (the Purkinje effect). When a bright light is suddenly shined into the eye, the pupil should contract quickly, as a protective mechanism. This pupillary reflex is tested in a routine eye examination and to determine cerebral function (Chapter 47).

> **Key Concept**
>
> The anterior chamber of the eye contains aqueous humor. Aqueous humor is thin and is produced by the ciliary body and supplies oxygen, glucose, and proteins to the eye. The posterior chamber contains vitreous humor, a thicker, clear gel.

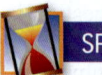 **SPECIAL CONSIDERATIONS   Lifespan**

Eye Color
The iris is normally blue or slate gray in light-skinned infants and brown in dark-skinned infants. Permanent eye color differentiates by age 6–9 months.

Lens

The **lens** is an opening controlled by ciliary body muscles (including the iris and three auxiliary muscles). It is located immediately behind the pupil and iris and has a major role in focusing light rays on the retina. The space behind the lens (posterior chamber) is filled with a transparent gelatin-like material called **vitreous humor**, which helps maintain the eyeball's shape and contributes to *intraocular* (within the eye) pressure. Loss of the vitreous humor causes blindness.

Retina

The eyeball's inner layer, the **retina**, is an incredible light-sensitive membrane. The retina's pigmented layer is composed of simple cuboidal epithelium and contains the optic nerve receptors. The *optic disk*, sometimes called the "blind spot," is an oval area on the posterior retina that allows the optic nerve to enter at the *nerve head*. The *physiologic cup* is a depression within the optic disk. The retina also contains specialized neurons, rods and cones (photoreceptor cells), which permit the perception of light, dark, and color. Each retina contains between 100 and 120 million **rods**, dispersed over the retina. They receive sensations of *black and white* and can register shapes, but not colors. Because the pupil dilates in dim light, the light strikes all parts of the retina, thereby activating the rods. Therefore, rods are useful in night vision (*scotopic vision*). Each retina also contains approximately 6–7 million **cones**, on which color vision depends. They are concentrated in the retina's center and function in daylight and bright light (*photopic vision*). The majority of cones are concentrated around the *fovea* *centralis* (about 5% of the retina), the *fovea lutea* (Fig. 21-3). The cones are of three individual classes; each receives red, blue, or green light waves, combined to form colors. Cones also add to visual acuity (visual sharpness) but require a significant amount of light. Thus, you see shades of gray, rather than color, in dim light because only the rods are receiving stimuli (Table 21-1). If you look slightly to the side of an object in dimmer light, you will focus on the edge of the retina where there are more rods.

> *Key Concept*
>
> The adaptation to darkness (Purkinje effect) depends on good blood flow to the eye. Blood flow is inhibited by vasoconstrictors, including tobacco and alcohol.

"Color blindness" is an error in production of photopigments in the cones. It causes difficulty in distinguishing between colors, particularly red and green, and affects 1 in 30 people, most often men (Chapter 47). The **macula** is in the center of the retina, lateral to the optic disk, and surrounding the fovea centralis (Fig. 21-3). Since this area contains the most cones, it is the major receptor for vision and color. The macula is considered the region of greatest visual acuity. A disruption, macular degeneration, results in visual difficulties and can lead to blindness.

Nerves and Muscles

The *optic nerve* (CN II) carries visual stimuli from each eye. Stimuli are transmitted from the optic nerve of one eye and meet the optic nerve of the other eye at the *optic chiasm*. Here, half the optic nerves cross, continue as the *optic tract*, and then are conducted to the brain's occipital lobe, where the nerve tracts reunite. The left side of the brain's occipital lobe receives visual images from the right side of an object, and vice versa. In addition, images presented to the brain are made up of millions of tiny portions of raw data, which the occipital lobe must translate into a seamless, meaningful total image. The *ophthalmic nerve*, a branch of the *trigeminal nerve* (CN V), carries sensations of eye pain (e.g., from a foreign object) and temperature to the brain.

Smooth muscles control pupil size and lens action. Three pairs of *extraocular* (outside the eye) muscles, attached to the sclera, move the eyeball. Another muscle, attached to the upper eyelid, holds the eye open; when this muscle relaxes, the eyelid shuts. The *oculomotor nerve* (CN III) innervates some of the voluntary muscles that move the eyeball and eyelid. This cranial nerve is also involved in some autonomic eye reactions, such as pupil *accommodation* to varying degrees of light. The *trochlear nerve* (CN IV) assists with some voluntary eyeball movements. The *abducens nerve* (CN VI) coordinates with cranial nerves III and IV to move the eyes (Table 21-2).

> *Key Concept*
>
> Both sides of the brain's occipital lobe interpret visual images. Smooth (involuntary) muscles control pupil size and lens accommodation.

THE EAR

The ear is the organ of hearing (auditory sense) and equilibrium (proprioception). It has three parts: external, middle, and inner ear (Fig. 21-4). The human auditory system can distinguish between over 300,000 sounds. The medical specialty concerned with disorders of the ear is **otology**; **audiology** is related to hearing and measurement of hearing acuity.

External Ear

The *external ear*, the **pinna** or **auricle**, is the only readily visible part of the ear. It is composed mostly of cartilage and is funnel shaped, to gather and guide sound waves into its small opening, which extends into the *auditory canal*. This opening is the *external auditory meatus*. This canal is covered with tiny hairs and contains *ceruminous glands*, which

TABLE 21-1 Functions and Placements of Rods and Cones

	PLACEMENT	FUNCTION: COLOR	FUNCTION: VISION
Rods	Widespread over retina	Receive black and white and shapes	Scotopic (night) vision
Cones	Center of retina	Receive color	Photopic (bright light) vision

TABLE 21-2 Nerves and Muscles of the Eye

CRANIAL NERVE	FUNCTION
II Optic	Carries visual images to the brain
III Oculomotor	Constricts and dilates pupil; elevates eyelid; innervates superior, inferior, and medial rectus and inferior oblique muscles
IV Trochlear	Voluntary eye movement
V Trigeminal (ophthalmic branch)	Carries sensations of eye pain and temperature
VI Abducens	Innervates the lateral rectus muscle
VII Facial	Controls blinking reflex
MUSCLE	**FUNCTION RELATED TO EYEBALL**
Superior rectus	Controls upward movement
Inferior rectus	Controls downward movement
Lateral rectus	Controls outward movement
Medial rectus	Controls inward movement
Superior oblique	Controls upward and outward movement
Inferior oblique	Controls downward and inward movement

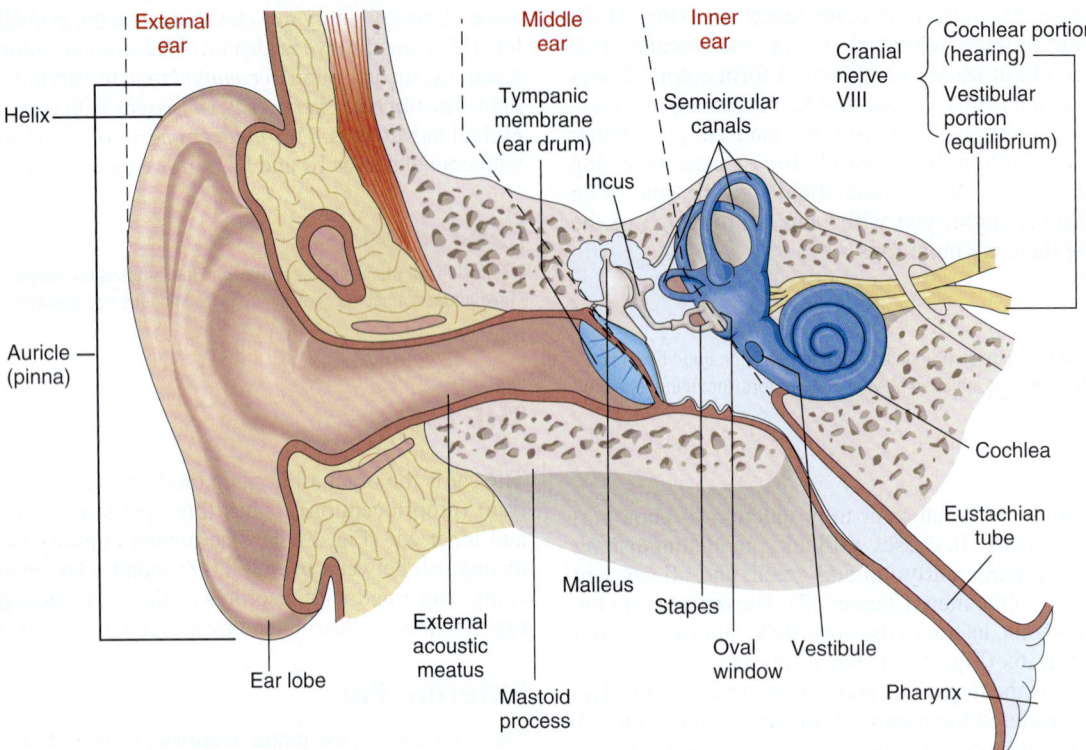

Figure 21-4 The ear, with its external, middle, and inner subdivisions.

secrete a waxy substance, *cerumen* or ear wax. The hairs and wax aid in protecting the ear from foreign objects. The auditory canal is very short, approximately 1 in. (2.54 cm) in an adult, and extends to a thin membrane, the *eardrum* (**tympanic membrane**). The tympanic membrane contains fibrous tissue and mucous membrane; it separates the external from the middle ear. (When reacting to sound, the eardrum moves less than the diameter of a hydrogen molecule.) The external auditory meatus is angled differently in a child, which has implications for administration of ear drops (Chapter 63).

Middle Ear

On the other side of the tympanic membrane is the *middle ear* (tympanic cavity), a small air-filled cavity in the temporal bone, which is lined with mucosa (Fig. 21-4). Within this cavity are three tiny bones. The **malleus** (hammer) has a long process, the *manubrium* (handle), attached to the movable section of the eardrum. The **incus** (anvil) is the bridge between the malleus and stapes. The **stapes** (stirrup) is the smallest bone in the body (0.1–0.3 in.; 2.5–3.3 mm); the stapes transmit sound vibrations to the fluid-filled inner ear at the *oval window*, which separates the middle ear from the inner ear. These three bones, collectively called **ossicles**, are so small that sound waves can set them in motion (Fig. 21-5).

Two small muscles attach to the stapes and malleus. These muscles reflexively contract at sudden, loud noises. This reflex stops the ossicles' vibration, thereby protecting the vital internal organs of the middle and inner ear from injury.

Key Concept

Hearing in the external and middle ear is accomplished by *air conduction*. The inner ear utilizes *bone conduction*.

Extending from the middle ear are two openings. One leads into the mastoid cells behind it, and the other leads downward into the **eustachian tube**, or auditory tube, which communicates with the nasopharynx. To function properly, the middle ear pressure must equal to the external atmospheric pressure. The eustachian tube opens during swallowing or yawning to equalize the pressure in the middle ear with the atmospheric pressure. Thus, pressures on both sides of the tympanic membrane are equal, allowing the eardrum to vibrate freely. (Otherwise, hearing is impaired.) For this reason, people are instructed to chew gum (to promote swallowing) or yawn frequently when flying or deep-sea diving—to equalize pressures. Unequal pressures will cause pain, which may be severe and may cause the eardrum to rupture. The eustachian tube also helps drain the middle ear. The middle ear, eustachian tube, nasopharynx, and the passage to the mastoid cells are lined with a continuous coating of mucous membrane. Clenching the jaw inhibits eardrum movement and impairs hearing.

SPECIAL CONSIDERATIONS Lifespan

Ninety percent of a young child's learning is facilitated by hearing. Hearing loss must be treated very early to prevent a lag in learning. In infants and children, the eustachian tube is shorter, wider, and positioned at a different angle than in adults. This predisposes children to inner ear infections because it is easier for pathogens to migrate into the ear. The child's eustachian tubes can also be blocked more easily by allergies, enlarged adenoids, or inflammation of the nose and throat. If the eustachian tubes are chronically blocked, a tiny PE tube may be inserted to drain fluid and allow air to enter the middle ear and equalize pressure.

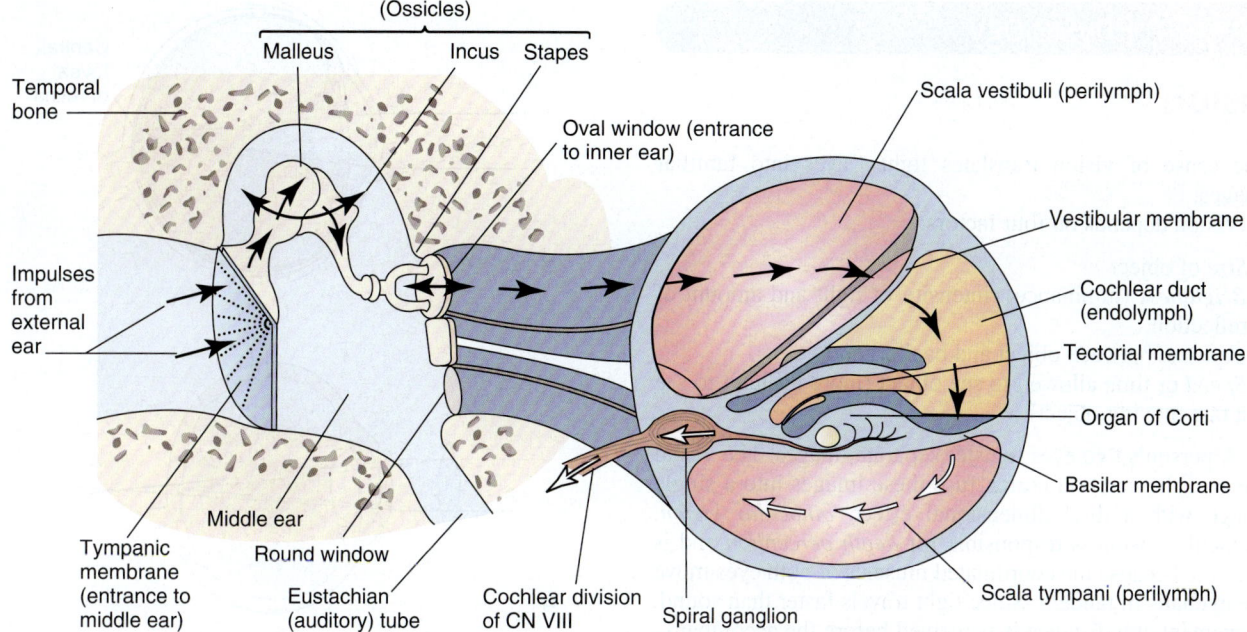

Figure 21-5 Path taken by sound waves reaching the inner ear. Sound travels from the external environment → external auditory canal → tympanic membrane, where vibrations begin. The vibrations travel through the middle ear → oval window into the inner ear, where they travel through the cochlear fluid (perilymph and endolymph) → receptors (hair cells) of organ of Corti. From here, the vibrations are transmitted to auditory nerve fibers → vestibulocochlear nerve → cerebral cortex, where they are interpreted.

Inner Ear

The division between the middle ear and inner ear is the *oval window* (fenestra ovalis). The *inner ear* is embedded in the temporal bone, the densest bone in the body. Here, the *bony labyrinth* contains the **membranous labyrinth** (or just **labyrinth**). Both labyrinths are filled with fluid similar to cerebrospinal fluid. (The fluid in the bony labyrinth [*perilymph*] is thinner and that in the membranous labyrinth is thicker [*endolymph*].) The labyrinths are important in sound wave transmission and in determination of body balance and positional changes. The three sections of the inner ear are the cochlea, vestibule, and semicircular canals (Fig. 21-4).

Cochlea

The **cochlea** is shaped like a hollow snail shell. Inside the bony cochlea lies the cochlear duct, containing the **organ of Corti**, a very small but very intricate structure. It is approximately 1.5 in. (3.75 cm) long and contains approximately 7,500 separate parts. This organ is referred to as the "true organ of hearing" because transmission of nerve stimuli related to sound begins here.

Vestibule

The *vestibule*, between the cochlea and semicircular canals, contains two membranous sacs, the *utricle* and *saccule*, suspended in perilymph. The utricle and saccule have specialized areas of hair cells, *maculae*, which send sensory information to the cerebellum and midbrain. These areas of the brain relay changes in body position, primarily when at rest (static balance).

Semicircular Canals

Another section of the inner ear includes the **semicircular canals**. Shaped like horseshoes, they lie behind the cochlea and are primarily concerned with balance when the body is moving (acceleration/deceleration or head movements). At the end (ampulla) of each semicircular canal is a receptor, the *crista* (crista ampullaris), which contains sensory hairs. Movement activates endolymph within the canals, which sets in motion the tiny hairs of the crista, transmitting information about the body's position to the brain. Each semicircular canal is on a different plane, or angle, in space (superior, posterior, and lateral) (Fig. 21-4). Thus, the endolymph in these canals flows in various directions and senses more types of motion than if all the canals were on the same plane. Sensory receptors for equilibrium (balance) in the moving body are on nerve endings in the semicircular canals (active balance). The sensations are transmitted to the brain via the vestibular division of CN VIII. Proprioception is primarily managed in the cerebral cortex.

Nerves

Sound is conducted via the pinna and middle ear to the inner ear's auditory nerves. The nerve receptors for hearing are within the cochlea in the organ of Corti. These hairlike receptors connect to the *cochlear nerve*, a division of the *acoustic* or *auditory nerve* (CN VIII). Sound is conducted to the center for hearing, in the temporal lobe of the brain's cerebral cortex. The acoustic nerve has two divisions, the cochlear nerve (for transmission of sound) and vestibular nerve (for transmission relating to balance and position). Thus, CN VIII is sometimes called the *vestibulocochlear nerve*.

System Physiology

VISION

The sense of vision translates light waves into familiar images.

Vision depends on four factors:

- *Size* of object
- *Brightness* (luminance): intensity of light and amount of reflection
- *Contrast* between object and background
- *Speed* or time allowed to see object (more difficult to see a fast-moving object)

A person's two eyes register separate images. The visual areas of the cerebral cortex fuse these images into a single image with a three-dimensional effect, *binocular vision*. Binocular vision is responsible for *depth perception* and is possible because the coordinated muscles of both eyes move the eyeballs in tandem. Since light travels faster than sound, movement at a distance is perceived before the accompanying sound is heard (e.g., lightning and thunder).

> **Key Concept**
> The vestibuloocular reflex (VOR) stabilizes images on the retina when the head moves.

A phenomenon called *smooth pursuit movement* (SPM) allows the eyes to follow a moving object, usually requiring conscious effort. *Vergence movement* causes the eyes to converge (move toward each other) when viewing a close object or diverge for far away objects. This is closely related to accommodation. When you look at a distant object, the ciliary muscles around the lens relax and the lens flattens. Looking at a nearby object causes the muscles to contract, pulling the choroid coat forward and causing the lens to bulge.

Light rays enter the eye through the cornea and pass through the aqueous humor, pupil opening, lens, and vitreous humor before focusing on the retina (Fig. 21-3). *Refraction* (bending of light rays) occurs within these components.

> **Key Concept**
> When light rays converge on the retina, the image is upside down. In the visual cortex of the brain, the image is corrected and perceived as upright.

Within the lens, parallel light rays are *refracted* (bent) so they focus directly on the retina (Fig. 21-6), making the image clear. Ciliary muscles of the eye also play a role in clear image formation. As the eye moves, the exposure is adjusted by the iris and also as a result of a chemical reaction. The formed image is reflected on the retina, the nerve center of the eye. The *central fovea (fovea centralis)* is responsible for the sharpest vision. The goal is to have light rays fall precisely on this central fovea. The lens plays the major role in this process by adjusting light rays. This lens adjustment

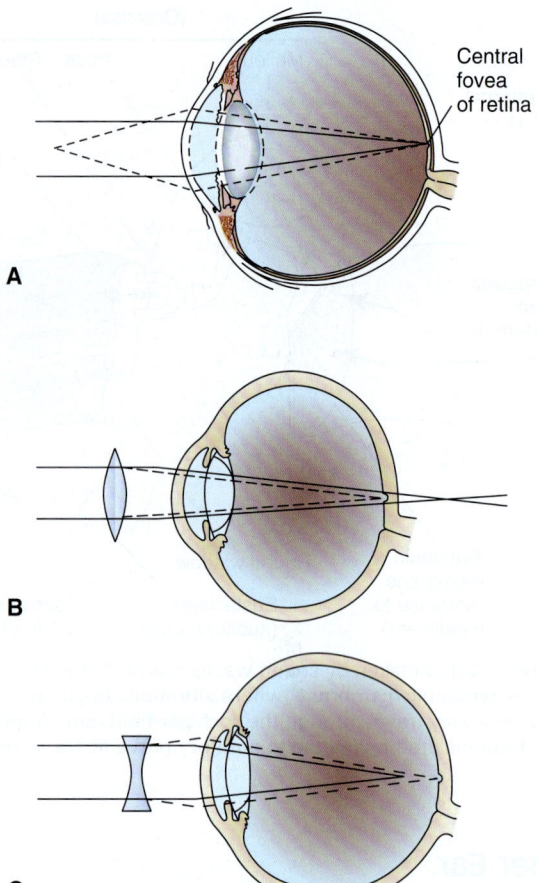

Figure 21-6 A. Accommodation. The *solid lines* represent rays of light from a distant object, and the *dotted lines* represent rays from a near object. The lens is flatter for the former and more convex for the latter. In each case, the rays of light focus on the retina. **B.** Hyperopia, corrected by a biconvex lens, as shown by the *dotted lines*. **C.** Myopia, corrected by a biconcave lens, as shown by the *dotted lines*. In each illustration, the goal is to focus light rays exactly at the central fovea.

to cause a clear image, **accommodation**, is controlled by the autonomic nervous system. If the eyeball is too short, the light rays land behind the retina, causing farsightedness (**hyperopia** or hypermetropia). In this instance, the refracted light rays do not come together directly on the retina but are absorbed by it. Therefore, the farsighted person cannot see close objects clearly.

In nearsightedness (**myopia**), light rays are focused in front of the retina because the lens muscles contract too tightly, not allowing enough light to enter the eye, or because the eyeball is too long. The nearsighted person sees close objects clearly, but distant objects are blurry.

Astigmatism is caused by irregularities in the curvature of the cornea and lens. The eye cannot bring horizontal and vertical lines into focus at the same time, causing blurry vision.

> **Key Concept**
> Farsightedness, hyperopia, is caused when light rays focus behind the retina. Nearsightedness, myopia, occurs when light rays focus in front of the retina.

The retina's receptors send visual impulses through the nerve fibers to the *optic nerve* (CN II), which meets the retina at the **optic disk** (Fig. 21-3). (The optic disk, the "blind spot," is not light sensitive.) The *optic nerve* carries the information to the cerebral cortex of the brain's occipital lobe for interpretation. The brain must differentiate between foreground and background, as well as edges, shapes, and symbols. Box 21-2 summarizes the pathway of light transmission. Chapter 80 describes visual disorders and their treatment.

> **Key Concept**
>
> Many vision problems can be corrected with prescription eyeglass lenses, contact lenses, or surgery.

The *field of vision* is the entire area visible when the eyes are fixed in one position. *Peripheral vision* (side vision) is that which the eyes see on the side when they are looking straight ahead; all that is visible *outside* the central area of focus. About 95% of the retinal area is concerned with peripheral vision. Peripheral vision can detect large objects and movement, although the images are not clear. The total field of vision is an important concept in vision testing. For example, if a person's peripheral vision is impaired, it may be difficult to safely drive a car (see visual field testing in Chapter 47).

HEARING

Sound is energy that moves in waves of pressure; sound waves are perceived by the brain via firing of auditory nerve cells. The perception of sound is *audition*; hearing is measured by *audiometer*. Sound waves enter through the ear's external auditory canal and strike the tympanic membrane (eardrum), which vibrates at various speeds in response to various pitches of sounds. The ossicles within the middle ear contact each other and act as a movable bridge to transmit vibrations to the oval window.

Because the oval window is so much smaller than the tympanic membrane, sound waves are concentrated, thereby amplifying them (*hydraulic* principle). The base of the stapes fits into the oval window. When stimulated, the stapes vibrates against this membrane, setting cochlear fluid (in the inner ear) in motion. This wavelike action transmits vibrations onto tiny hairlike nerve endings (receptors) in the organ of Corti. These microscopic protein filaments ("hair cells") are *mechanoreceptors* that release a chemical neurotransmitter when stimulated. (The sound waves bend the filaments, causing them to fire.) The stimuli from the organ of Corti are sent to the *vestibulocochlear nerve* (a portion of CN VIII) and then to the temporal lobe in the cerebral cortex, where sounds are interpreted.

Sound Amplification

Figure 21-5 shows the pathway of sound transmission. Sound waves are amplified in three ways:

- The ear canal is open, and resonance there approximately doubles sound waves.
- The ossicles (hammer, anvil, and stirrups) act as *levers*. This mechanical advantage amplifies sound approximately threefold. (This, when multiplied by amplification in the ear canal, now equals a total of a sixfold amplification.)
- The relative sizes between the eardrum and oval window amplify or increase sound waves approximately 30 times more, as depicted here.

Relationships Between Hearing Structures and Sound Amplification

External ear → Ossicles of middle ear → Relative sizes between eardrum and oval window → Amplification × 2   × 3 (= 6 × total)   × 30 (= 180 × final total)

Hearing can be damaged by extremely loud sounds or music (*noise trauma*), by certain drugs (e.g., aminoglycosides—streptomycin, loop diuretics—furosemide, or aspirin—*ototoxicity*), blast injuries, foreign objects, or specific illnesses. The ensuing hearing loss can be temporary or permanent. Chapter 80 describes hearing disorders and their treatment.

> **Key Concept**
>
> A process of localizing the direction from which a sound originates is called "Echo Positioning." The central nervous system analyzes sounds from each ear to locate the source.

BALANCE AND EQUILIBRIUM

The sense of *static balance* (the person at rest) is centered in the *utricle* and *saccule* of the inner ear. Balance with movement (*active balance*) is associated with the semicircular canals. CN VIII (vestibulocochlear nerve) plays an important role in both balance and hearing. This nerve transmits impulses to other cranial nerves responsible for control of

---

Box 21-2 Light Transmission Through the Eye to the Brain

Cornea (refraction)
Anterior chamber and aqueous humor (refraction)
Pupil (constriction and dilation)
Lens (accommodation)
Vitreous chamber and vitreous humor (refraction)
Retina—rods and cones (receiving images of black/white and color)
Central fovea (light rays focus for sharpest vision)
} Eyeball anatomy

Optic disk (nerve fibers converge, called the *blind spot*)
Optic nerve (cranial nerve II)
Optic chiasm (cranial nerves cross)
Thalamus
Cerebral cortex (interprets impulses)
} Optic nerve pathway

head and neck movement. It also sends and receives information (about the body's static and active positions) from inner ear structures, including the semicircular canals, so the body can maintain positional balance and equilibrium.

Balance is a complex process. In addition to receptors in the ears, proprioceptors exist in muscles. Visual input and tactile skin receptors also contribute to our sense of position in space. Sometimes, the motion of fluid in the ears without accompanying visual reference can confuse the sensory system. For example, consider the sensation felt on a carnival ride if your eyes are closed. This dizzy—sometimes ill—feeling or sense of being rotated, **vertigo**, differs from dizziness. True vertigo is the sensation that either you or the room is spinning; *dizziness* is a sensation of light-headedness. Inner ear diseases or defects in conductive pathways and/or the central nervous system cause true vertigo. Nausea often accompanies vertigo, as does **tinnitus**, a high-pitched buzzing or "ringing in the ears." Tinnitus, which affects about 15% of people, may also occur without vertigo.

TASTE

The sense of taste (**gustation**) is based on perceptions of sweet, salty, sour, bitter, metallic, and fatty or meaty (*umami*) flavors and their combinations. Over 10,000 taste receptors, the *taste buds*, are located in the mouth. *Chemoreceptors* (gustatory cells) in taste buds detect chemicals in solution in the mouth. Basic tastes are perceived by taste buds on the tongue, as well as in the lining of the cheek and roof of the mouth (Fig. 21-7). Most foods have a combination of taste sensations. In addition, many characteristic tastes are greatly influenced by the sense of smell, such as the taste of an onion. Two cranial nerves carry the sensation of taste to the brain: the *facial nerve* (CN VII) and the *glossopharyngeal nerve* (CN IX). The sense of taste is interpreted in the parietal and temporal lobes of the cerebral cortex (the anterior cingulate).

> **Key Concept**
> Some people can taste more acutely than others. Some people have a dulled sense of taste and can tolerate more spicy foods. Smoking damages taste buds.

SMELL

The nerve of smell, **olfaction**, is the *olfactory nerve* (CN I). Odors are tiny chemical molecules in the air, which may be mixed together. These molecules enter the nose and rise in the upper nasal cavity to the sensory area (olfactory epithelial tissue), about the size of a postage stamp (Fig. 21-8). Specific receptors for different odors interact in a "lock-and-key" fashion with the nerves; millions of sensory receptors in the olfactory nerve receive and transmit these impulses. Interpretation occurs in the olfactory center of the temporal lobe (the same area of the brain as the center for emotions). In order for odors to be detected, chemicals must be dissolved in the watery mucus lining the nasal cavity.

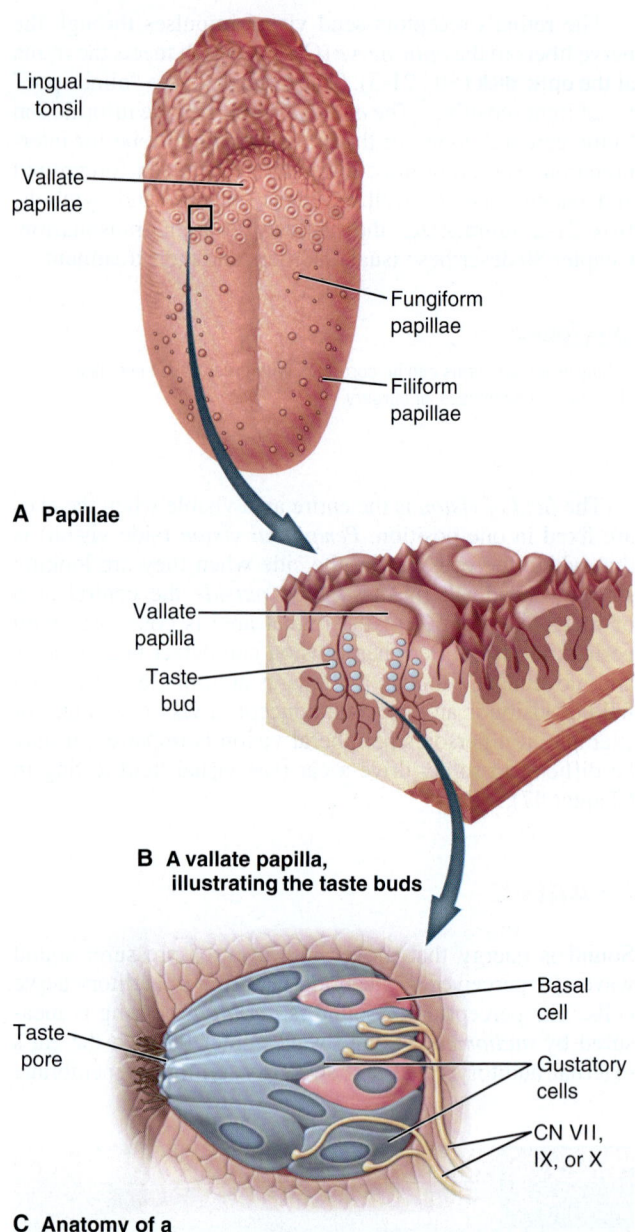

Figure 21-7 The tongue and tonsils. **A.** The dorsal surface of the tongue, showing locations of papillae. **B.** Individual taste buds are located within the papillae. **C.** Cross section of a single taste bud. The facial nerve (CN VII) carries most gustatory sensations to the brain.

> **Key Concept**
> Humans can differentiate between 5,000 and 10,000 different odors. Women generally have a more sensitive sense of smell than men, due to estrogen production, especially during pregnancy. The sense of smell is most acute when a person is hungry. Some medications, including antibiotics, statins, and blood pressure medications, may impair the sense of smell. The olfactory sensory receptors can become fatigued, so after prolonged exposure to an intense odor, we cease to be aware of it ("nose blind").

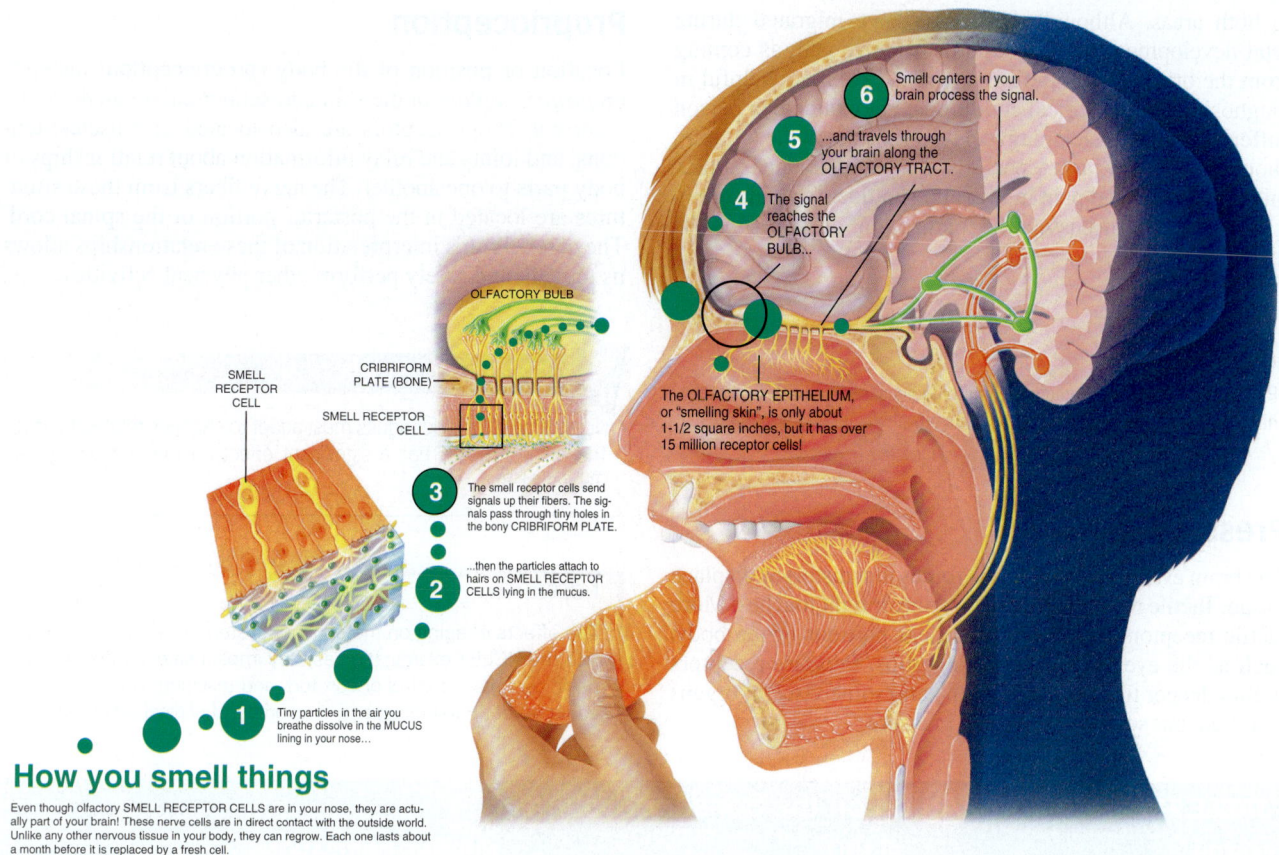

Figure 21-8 How your sense of smell works (Anatomical Chart Company chart ISBN 9781587797477).

TOUCH/TACTILE SENSE

The sense of touch is developed in utero, the first sense to appear. The body receives tactile signals constantly. Tactile (touch) *receptors* or *corpuscles* are found mostly in the skin, which has more than 4 million sensory receptors, the majority of which are for pain. Sensory receptors are constantly receiving nerve impulses, transmitting pressure, vibration, pain, or the pleasures of softness and warmth. They signal the dangers of too much heat or cold. A greater number of touch receptors are located in some areas, including the fingertips, back of the neck, soles of the feet, and around the lips. The midback has fewer sensory receptors (Chapter 19, Fig. 19-11, and Chapter 16, Fig. 16-1). The brain's parietal lobe interprets most tactile stimuli. Some sensory signals are relayed immediately to the spinal cord and brain stem. Temperature, pain, pressure, and proprioception are internal tactile stimuli described below.

> **Key Concept**
> Being touched can reduce stress. This has implications for nursing.

OTHER SENSATIONS

Temperature

Two types of temperature receptors (*thermoreceptors*) are widespread in the body: *heat receptors* and *cold receptors*. The ratio between these receptors varies in different locations. For example, 10–15 times more cold receptors than heat receptors exist in the skin. Both types are abundant in the lips and mucous membranes of the oral and anal regions. The temperature sense protects the body, for example, by preventing burns or by causing sweating or shivering in response to hot or cold stimuli. One definition of comfort is "no conscious sensation of heat or cold."

> **Key Concept**
> Thermoreceptors stop functioning at about 40 °F (4.4 °C). At this point, the skin feels numb. At a temperature of more than 113 °F (45 °C), pain receptors take over.

Pain

Pain is usually protective, a warning system. It causes people to move away from a painful stimulus or to seek medical attention for an internal disorder. Pain receptors are sensory nerve endings stimulated by chemicals such as histamine, released when tissues are damaged. Pain may trigger release of endorphins, to block pain. Different types of pain can occur, depending on its location. Pain in an external location, such as the skin, is considered *superficial pain*. Pain in an internal organ system is described as *visceral pain*. Pain receptors also respond to extremes in temperature, such as when an ice cube touches a decayed tooth.

Pain originating in an internal organ and perceived in another location is called *referred pain*. This type of pain is felt at the site where the organ was originally located during fetal development; the same part of the spinal cord connects to both areas. Although the organs have migrated during fetal development, the nerves still perceive pain as coming from the original site. Referred pain is extremely helpful in diagnosing many medical conditions. For example, a person suffering a heart attack may feel referred pain in the left arm, shoulder, neck, or jaw. A person having a gallbladder attack might have referred pain in the right shoulder (scapula area).

Chapter 55 discusses the perception of pain and its management.

Key Concept

Pain may be blocked by medications. Analgesics, such as aspirin, block histamine production; narcotics, such as morphine, imitate endorphins.

Pressure

The brain evaluates mechanical forces that distort or displace tissue. Tactile receptors can detect fine or light touches. More tactile receptors are found in hairless portions of the body, such as the eyelids, lips, and fingertips. Pressure receptors within deeper tissues, some joints, and some visceral organs also transmit sensations of deep pressure.

Proprioception

Location or position of the body (**proprioception**) depends on *proprioceptors* in the skin and semicircular canals of the inner ear. Proprioceptors are also located in muscles, tendons, and joints and relay information about relationships of body parts to one another. The nerve fibers from these structures are located in the posterior portion of the spinal cord. The cerebellum's interpretation of these relationships allows us to walk and safely perform other physical activities.

SPECIAL CONSIDERATIONS Lifespan

Nursing care for older adults must adapt to changes related to aging. The aging process has a significant effect on the sensory system (Tables 21-3).

NCLEX Alert

The effects of aging on the sensory system may be integrated into the NCLEX examination as they impact safety, effective basic care, pain control or comfort, and teaching. The options could reflect nursing actions in a variety of clinical settings.

TABLE 21-3 Effects of Aging on the Sensory System

FACTOR	RESULT	NURSING IMPLICATIONS
Vision/Eye Changes Lens accommodation decreases; lens loses elasticity	Presbyopia (farsighted); difficulty seeing close objects or reading	Corrective lenses helpful, especially for reading (bifocals or trifocals)
Depth perception decreases	Difficulty judging height of curbs and steps Falls common	Encourage use of hand rails, canes, and walkers Advise to avoid fast moves or turns Make client aware of dangers
Peripheral vision decreases	Driving may be dangerous	Encourage a defensive driving class Avoid standing at client's side
Pupil size decreases; ability to react to darkness and bright light decreases; night vision decreases	Takes longer for eyes to adjust when entering a dark room or bright sunlight May require additional light for reading	Advise use of a night light Advise person to avoid night driving if possible Reading glasses may be needed Wear sunglasses (especially amber, orange, or brown lenses) when outside
Color perception decreases Depth perception decreases Clouding of lens	Difficulty discerning hues of blue, green, and violet and distances Cataract (may occur at any age)	Use yellow, red, and black for signs Surgical removal and replacement with artificial lens
Grayish white ring (*arcus senilis*) forms around iris due to deposits of calcium and cholesterol salts Vitreous gel liquefies	May lower self-esteem and body image (does not affect vision) Posterior visual detachment (*PVD*), causing "floaters" in eyeball	Enhance client's self-esteem Usually not treated
Tear formation decreases	Dry, itchy eyes More susceptible to infections	Advise about medication ("artificial tears") Advise against rubbing eyes
Fluid circulation in eye decreases	Increased risk for glaucoma	Encourage regular visual examinations, including intraocular pressure measurement
Debris builds up in eyes Color changes in sclera	Result of long exposure to sunlight (UV rays), dust, wind—("flashers" and "floaters") Yellowing or browning (more common in dark-skinned people); bluish hue (thinning of sclera)	Counseling—usually not treated Counseling—support client's self-esteem

TABLE 21-3	Effects of Aging on the Sensory System (Continued)	
FACTOR	RESULT	NURSING IMPLICATIONS
Weakening of eyelid muscles Macular degeneration Retinal detachment Diabetic retinopathy	Upper lids droop (ptosis); lower lids droop (ectropion) Loss of central vision; peripheral vision maintained longer; may lead to blindness Separation of retina from back of eye, eventual loss of vision Eye changes caused by diabetes; may lead to blindness	Surgical correction if vision is affected; advise against contact lenses Laser treatment and injections in some cases; special vitamins (AREDS formula) may be helpful Prompt surgery to repair hole and prevent leakage of vitreous humor (may be done by laser, heat, or cold) Control blood sugar levels
Hearing/Ear Changes Functional and structural changes in ear structures, especially deterioration of cochlea (flattening and loss of hair cells), and fusing of ossicles (impairing their movement)	Presbycusis; progressive hearing loss (highest pitches lost first); certain consonants difficult to hear (K, T, S, P)	Discuss hearing aid evaluation Person may benefit from "helper" dog, telephone volume controls, or computerized phone messaging
Causes include injury; illnesses such as diabetes, otitis media, and Meniere syndrome; bone formation around oval window; decalcification of skull (interferes with bone conduction); nerve disorder; perception disorder; side effects of certain medications	Loss of perception of sound location, tracking sounds, normal conversation Increased incidence of dizziness and tinnitus	Face person when talking to them Speak clearly but not too loudly Advise against driving, if hearing compromised Advise use of hand rails and to avoid sudden movements
Calcium sludge forms in semicircular canals	Benign positional paroxysmal vertigo (BPPV, BPV)	Vertigo may be relieved by specific exercises (Epley maneuver)
Structural changes affect balance and equilibrium	Increased incidence of falls Dizziness on change of position	Advise use of hand rails and other fall prevention Advise person to change positions slowly
Increased cerumen buildup	Hearing loss	Frequent ear examinations and cerumen removal
Long exposure to loud noises, destroys hair cells in cochlea	Hearing loss	Ear protection required in industry, rock bands, etc.; advise people not to play loud music in autos or when using ear buds
Taste Changes Taste sensation decreases; may be caused by lack of sensation transmission to brain; decreased number and function of taste buds (may be related to decreased sense of smell)	Decreased appetite; less enjoyment of food May try to compensate by increasing salt and sugar intake, aggravating conditions such as hypertension and diabetes; risk for consuming spoiled foods	Monitor nutritional status Teach proper nutrition Client may require dietary supplements, such as Ensure or boost Teach client to check expiration dates on containers
Smell Changes Smell perception decreases	May not smell smoke or poisonous substances (e.g., gas leak) Affects sense of taste	Teach client to install smoke and CO_2 detectors and preventive safety measures Teach safe dietary modifications
Tactile Changes Efficiency and the number of sensory nerve endings (all sensations affected) decrease	Stronger stimuli needed for person to perceive sensations; pain may not be perceived	Monitor client's overall condition; do not ignore complaints; observe for body language signs of pain

STUDENT SYNTHESIS

KEY POINTS

- The five senses are seeing, hearing, tasting, smelling, and touching.
- The eye is the organ of vision. It has many protective mechanisms. Light rays travel through several eye structures before focusing on the retina.
- The eyeball has three major tissues: sclera and cornea, choroid, and retina.
- Several cranial nerves are involved in vision.
- Three sets of extraocular muscles control eye movements.
- The occipital lobe of the brain receives and interprets visual stimuli.
- The three parts of the ear are the external, middle, and inner ear.
- The external ear protects internal ear structures from foreign substances and catches and carries sound waves to the middle ear. The middle ear is responsible for sound transmission. The inner ear transmits sound waves and information about body position to the brain.
- The semicircular canals of the inner ear determine one's position in space. Many factors contribute to the achievement of body balance.
- Taste buds are responsible for perceptions of sweet, salty, sour, bitter, metallic, and meaty.
- Receptors for the sense of smell (olfactory receptors) are in the upper nasal cavity.
- Receptors for the sense of touch (tactile receptors) are located throughout most areas of the body.
- Proprioceptors are located in muscles, tendons, and joints and contribute to the sense of balance.
- Referred pain is perceived in a place other than where it originates.
- The temporal lobe of the brain interprets sounds transmitted via the vestibulocochlear nerve from the inner ear. The parietal and temporal lobes interpret tastes. The occipital lobe receives visual information via the optic nerve. The cerebellum is responsible for maintaining equilibrium and coordination.

CRITICAL THINKING EXERCISES

1. What anatomic structure of the eye does a contact lens come in contact with? Why is meticulous care of contact lenses necessary?
2. Referring to Table 21-1, explain how injury to each of the listed cranial nerves would affect vision.
3. Explain why your ears plug in an airplane, especially when you have a cold.
4. Explain to a client why taking a sour liquid medication through a straw helps minimize the unpleasant taste.

NCLEX-STYLE REVIEW QUESTIONS

1. A client informs the nurse that he is color blind. Which colors does the nurse determine the client will likely have difficulty distinguishing?
   a. White and black
   b. Red and green
   c. Blue and purple
   d. Orange and pink

2. The nurse asks a client to use the eyes to follow finger movements to the left and right and then to close and open the eyes. Which cranial nerve will the nurse document as intact if the client is able to perform these movements?
   a. Cranial nerve I
   b. Cranial nerve II
   c. Cranial nerve III
   d. Cranial nerve IV

3. A client states to the nurse, "I am taking a trip by plane and the last time I flew, the problems with my ears were awful!" Which suggestion would the nurse provide to alleviate discomfort?
   a. Use a Q-tip to remove impacted wax to decrease pressure when flying.
   b. Insert saline drips into both ears every hour while flying.
   c. Irrigate the ear prior to the trip to remove wax and decrease pressure.
   d. Chew gum to promote swallowing.

4. Which information would the nurse provide to the client about prevention of cataract formation? Select all that apply.
   a. Wear sunglasses when outside with amber, orange, or brown lenses.
   b. Do not stare at a computer screen for prolonged periods of time.
   c. Instill saline drops twice daily into both eyes.
   d. Make sure eyeglasses fit well.
   e. Wear contact lenses rather than glasses.

5. An older adult client informs the nurse of a "terrible ringing in the ears." Which question would be a priority for the nurse to ask the client?
   a. "Do you irrigate your ears?"
   b. "When was the last time you had an ear examination?"
   c. "Does anyone in your family have this problem?"
   d. "What medications do you take?"

CHAPTER RESOURCES

Enhance your learning with additional resources on thePoint!

Student Resources related to this chapter can be found at **thePoint.lww.com/Rosdahl12e**.

22 The Cardiovascular System

Learning Objectives

1. Describe the three major layers of the heart wall and how they relate to the pericardium; identify the three layers of arteries and veins.
2. Identify and describe the function of the heart chambers, major vessels that enter and exit each chamber, and the atrioventricular valves, semilunar valves, chordae tendineae, and papillary muscles.
3. Trace the path of blood through both sides of the heart; identify the coronary arteries supplying the myocardium; define collateral circulation.
4. Compare and contrast the structure and function of arteries, capillaries, and veins.
5. Describe the path of an electrical impulse through the heart's conduction system; describe the purpose of this electrical activity.
6. Explain the events associated with S_1 and S_2 heart sounds, indicating where each of these sounds is best heard.
7. Describe cardiac output, including factors involved in its regulation.
8. Differentiate between systolic and diastolic blood pressure, explaining the actions occurring during each. Identify major factors that affect blood pressure regulation.
9. State changes in the cardiovascular system caused by aging. Discuss related nursing implications.

Important Terminology

afterload, aorta, aortic valve, apex, atria (atrium), baroreceptor, bicuspid valve, collateral circulation, coronary sinus, diastole, electrocardiogram, endocardium, epicardium, ischemia, mediastinum, microcirculation, mitral valve, myocardium, perfusion, pericardial fluid, pericardium, preload, pulmonic valve, pulse, pulse pressure, semilunar valve, septum, systole, tricuspid valve, ventricle

Acronyms

AV, BP, CO, CO_2, dBP, ECG, HR, IVC, LAD, LCA, LCX, LMCA, MI, O_2, PDA, RCA, S_1, S_2, SA node, sBP, SV, SVC, SVR

The cardiovascular (heart and blood vessel) system is designed for transportation and communication throughout the body. In approximately 1 minute, a drop of blood travels through the right side of the heart, lungs, left side of the heart, and the systemic circulation, completing its circuit by returning to the right side of the heart. In this brief time, all body cells, even those located at the tips of the toes and fingers, receive oxygen (O_2) from the lungs and nutrients from the intestines. They simultaneously send carbon dioxide (CO_2) and other wastes to be excreted. Thus, the cardiovascular system is vital in maintaining homeostasis within the body. (The lymphatic system is also concerned with transportation of substances important to life, and with waste removal; this system is discussed in Chapter 23.)

Key Concept

In an average lifetime of 65–70 years, the human heart will beat approximately 2.5 billion times (about 100,000 times each day). The embryonic heartbeat is detectable about 23 days after conception and the nurse will learn to listen to and count these *fetal heart tones*.

STRUCTURE AND FUNCTION

The cardiovascular system consists of the heart and blood vessels. Its functions include pumping blood and transporting gases, nutrients, hormones, and wastes (Box 22-1). The term "**perfusion**" refers to the delivery of blood to a capillary bed.

HEART

The human *heart* is a strong, muscular double pump about three quarters the size of a clenched fist and weighs less than 1 lb (approximately 250–350 g). It lies in the thoracic cavity in the mediastinal space or **mediastinum** (a mass of tissues and organs lying behind the sternum, between the lungs, and in front of the vertebral column, between the second and sixth ribs). The heart is shaped like an irregular and slightly flattened cone. The inferior (lower) point is the **apex**, which is formed by the tip of the left ventricle. The apex is referred to as the *point of maximal impulse* because heart sounds are loudest here. The *apical pulse* is counted here. The wide superior (top) margin, called the *base*, lies opposite the apex and is formed mostly by the left atrium. The heart wall has three layers: endocardium, myocardium, and epicardium (Fig. 22-1).

- The **endocardium** (inner heart) is a membrane lining the heart's interior wall. It is made up of endothelial tissue, small blood vessels, and some smooth muscles.

Box 22-1 Functions of the Cardiovascular System

FUNCTIONS OF THE HEART
Pumping Action
- Pumps blood to body and lungs
- Receives blood from body and lungs
- Influences blood pressure

FUNCTIONS OF THE BLOOD VESSELS
Transportation
- Provides channels through which blood and lymph travel
- Provides areas (capillaries) where transfer of gases, nutrients, fluids, electrolytes, and wastes can occur

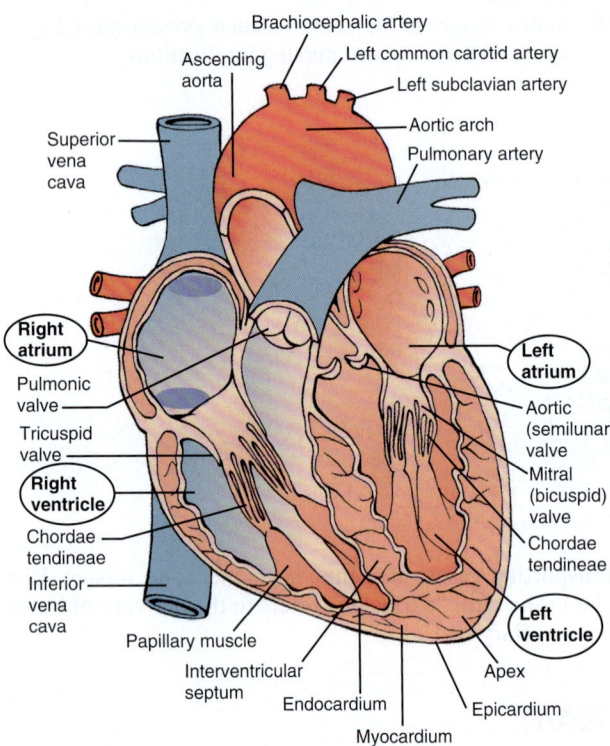

Figure 22-1 Heart and great vessels (anterior view). The heart is enclosed in the pericardial sac, the innermost layer of which is the epicardium.

- Thick, strong muscles make up the **myocardium** (*myo* = muscle), the middle and thickest layer. Cardiac muscle (Chapter 18) is a unique type of *involuntary* muscle with lightly striated cells, found only in the heart.
- The **epicardium** (*epi* = upon) is the thin, outer layer of the cardiac wall (also called the visceral layer of the serous pericardium). It is composed of squamous epithelial cells over connective tissue.

  The **pericardium** (*pericardial sac*) is a sac that surrounds and protects the heart. It is also made up of three layers:

- The *epicardium* portion of the heart wall, which also makes up the pericardium's visceral layer, adheres to the heart's surface. (A space between the visceral and parietal layers is the *pericardial space* or *cavity*. It houses a small amount of serous fluid, **pericardial fluid**, which acts as a

lubricant and reduces friction between the layers as the heart contracts and relaxes.)
- The parietal layer is the *inner serous pericardium*.
- The outermost layer is the *fibrous pericardium* (composed of dense fibrous connective tissue). This tissue protects and anchors the heart in the mediastinum and prevents overfilling.

Heart Chambers and Valves

A complete muscular wall, the **septum**, divides the heart into right and left sides. The two sides are completely separated, with no communication from right to left. Each side is a separate pump.

 SPECIAL CONSIDERATIONS Lifespan

Congenital Heart Defects
If a child is born with a hole in the cardiac septum, surgical correction is usually necessary.

Chambers
The interior of the heart is divided into four chambers (Fig. 22-1).

Atria
The two upper chambers are the right and left **atria** (singular: atrium). These thin-walled, low-pressure chambers are receiving centers for blood.

Ventricles
The two lower chambers are right and left **ventricles**. Ventricles are high-pressure chambers; they pump blood out of the heart. The left ventricle must contract with sufficient force to send blood to the entire body; therefore, its muscle walls are thickest and its internal pressures the highest. The right ventricle needs only to pump blood into the low-pressure lungs; therefore, it is a thinner walled chamber.

> **Key Concept**
> The left ventricle contains the heart's thickest muscles and must pump strongly enough to send blood out to the entire body. The right ventricle also has thick muscles; the muscles in the atria are thinner than those of either ventricle.

Valves
As each heart chamber contracts, it pushes blood either into a ventricle or out of the heart to the lungs or body. Cardiac valves are one-way tissue flaps that open and close in response to pressure changes within the chambers. These unidirectional (one-way) valves allow blood to flow in one direction only, preventing backflow.

Atrioventricular Valves
The atrioventricular (**AV**) valves lie between the atria and ventricles (Fig. 22-2A). The valve between the right atrium and right ventricle, the **tricuspid valve**, is formed of three flaps (cusps) of tissue. The valve between the

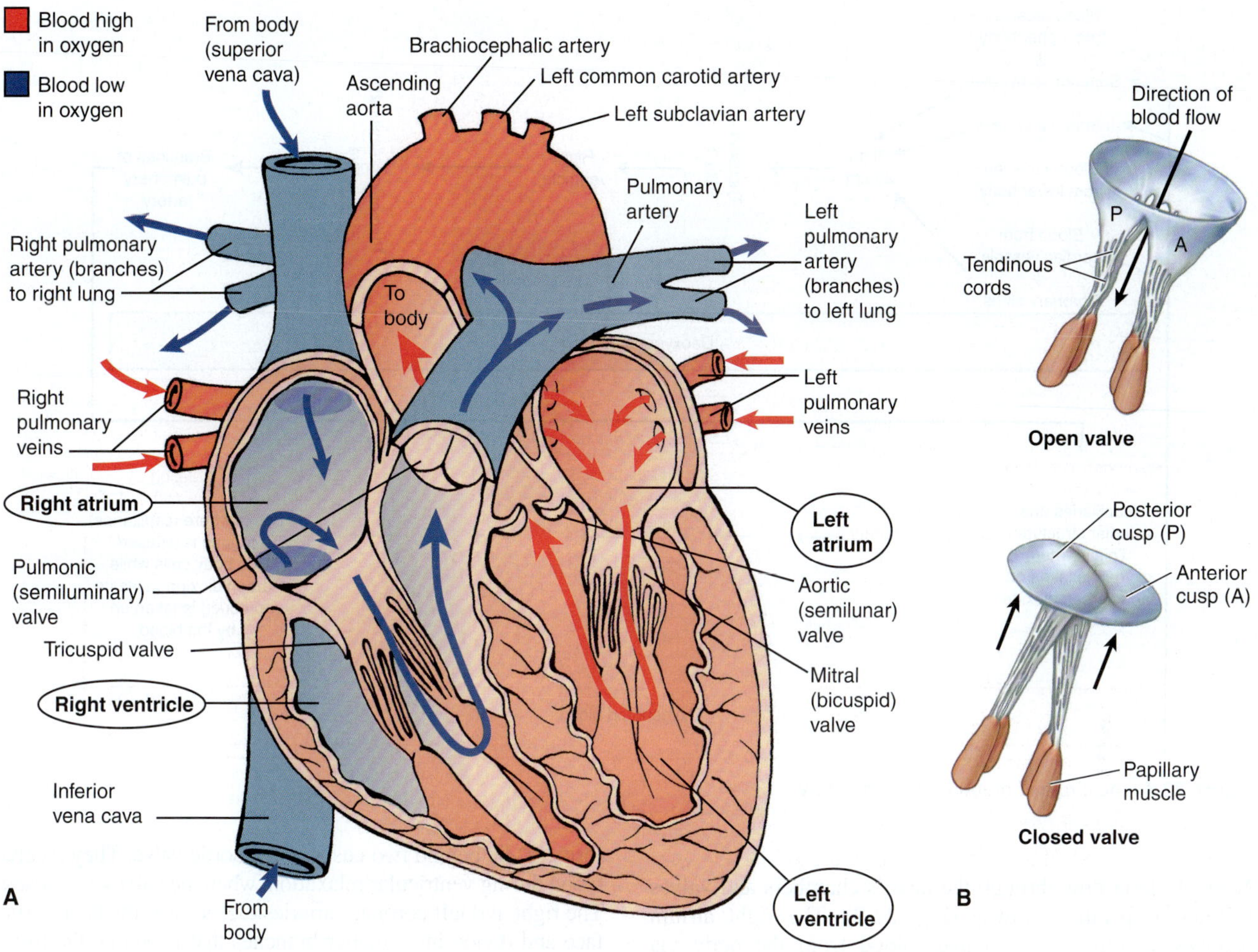

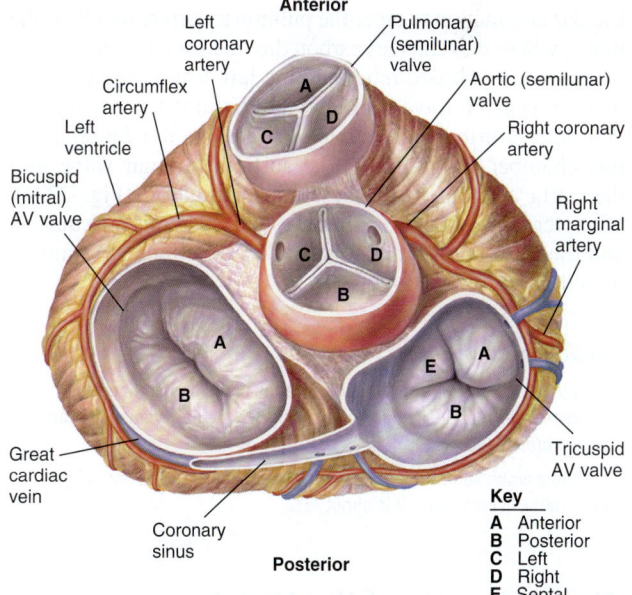

Figure 22-2 **A.** Blood flow through the heart. **B.** Illustration of open and closed mitral (bicuspid) valve.

left atrium and left ventricle, the **mitral** or **bicuspid valve**, has only two flaps of tissue (Fig. 22-2B). The tissue flaps of these valves attach to tendon-like strands, the *chordae tendineae* (tendinous cords), which are anchored to papillary muscles located on the inner surface of the ventricles.

Blood flows from the atria to the ventricles through open AV valves when ventricular pressure is lower than atrial pressure. During this time, the papillary muscles and chordae tendineae relax.

As the ventricles contract, increased pressure causes the AV valves to close. The papillary muscles also contract at this time, tightening the chordae tendineae, to prevent the valve cusps from everting (turning inside out). If the AV valves, chordae tendineae, or papillary muscles become damaged, backflow of blood (*regurgitation*) into the atria can occur with ventricular contraction.

Overflow Valves

Each ventricle empties through a valve with three crescent-shaped (half-moon) cusps, the **semilunar valves** (Fig. 22-3). The *pulmonary semilunar valve* (**pulmonic valve**) separates the right ventricle from the pulmonary artery. The **aortic** (semilunar) **valve** separates the left ventricle from the aorta, the body's largest artery. Increased ventricular pressure, as when the ventricles contract, opens the semilunar valves. As the ventricles relax, blood begins to flow backward

Figure 22-3 Valves of the heart.

toward the ventricles. Blood fills the semilunar cusps and causes the valves to close. Therefore, semilunar valves prevent backflow from their respective arteries into their ventricles.

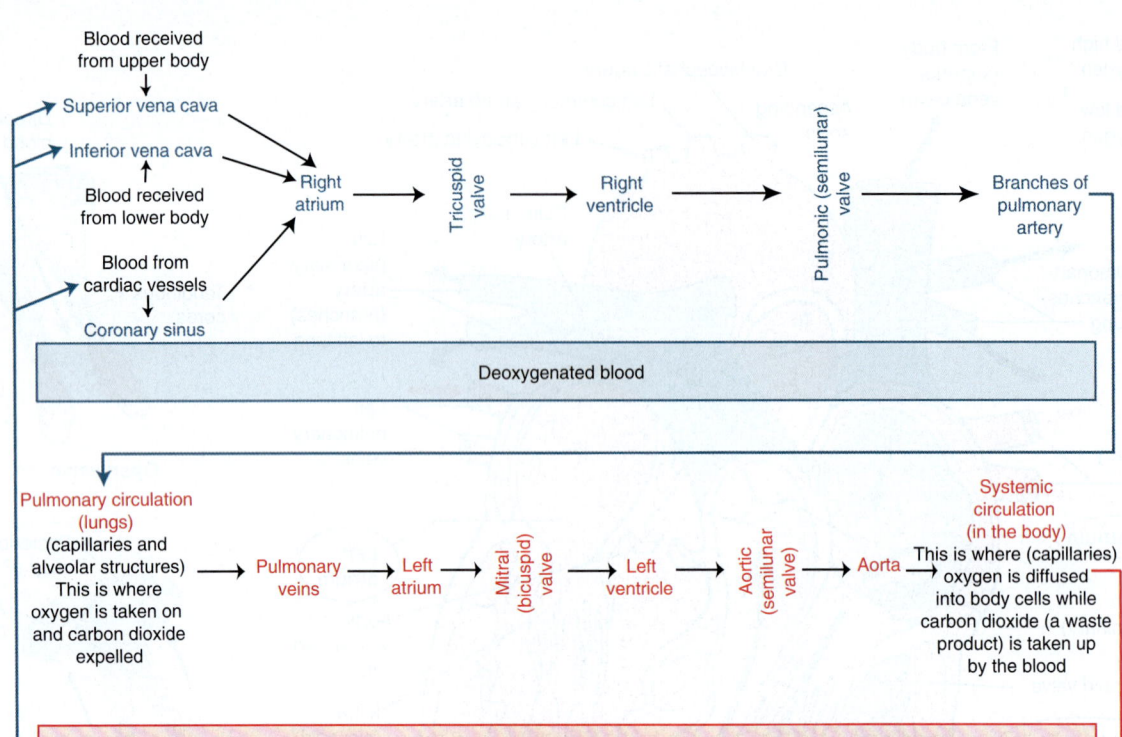

Figure 22-4 The circle of blood flow in the body.

Route of Blood Flow Through the Heart

Normal blood flow through the heart's chambers and valves follows a specific pathway (Fig. 22-2). The right atrium receives venous (*deoxygenated*) blood from the body via the superior and inferior vena cavae and the coronary sinus. Blood then passes through the tricuspid valve into the right ventricle. It moves on through the pulmonic valve during ventricular contraction to enter the pulmonary artery and then the lungs, where it exchanges carbon dioxide for oxygen.

Oxygenated blood returns to the left atrium via four pulmonary veins. It travels through the mitral valve into the left ventricle. During ventricular contraction, the blood from this chamber exits through the aortic semilunar valve into the aorta and out to the systemic circulation (Fig. 22-4). (Chapter 23 describes pulmonic and systemic circulation and the makeup of blood. Chapter 25 describes gas transfer in and out of blood vessels.)

> **Key Concept**
>
> The pulmonary arteries are the only arteries in the body that carry *deoxygenated* blood. The pulmonary veins are the only veins that carry *oxygenated* blood.
>
> The oxygen saturation of hemoglobin within arteries is normally 95%–100%. Within veins, it is about 75%.

Blood Vessels of the Heart

Coronary Arteries

Heart muscle requires its own blood supply because heart tissue does not absorb blood from its chambers. Therefore, two *coronary arteries* (right and left) branch off the ascending aorta to provide blood to heart muscle (Fig. 22-5). Their openings (orifices) lie behind two cusps of the aortic valve. They receive blood during ventricular relaxation, when the valves are closed. The right and left coronary arteries extend over the heart's surface and divide into smaller branches that penetrate the myocardium to supply heart tissue with oxygen and nourishment. They are called *coronary* arteries because they fit over the heart like a crown (*corona*). Their patterns and branches vary among individuals more than any other cardiovascular anatomy.

Left Coronary Artery

The left coronary artery (**LCA**), also known as the left main coronary artery (**LMCA**), passes along the left atrium and divides into two branches: the anterior interventricular branch or left anterior descending (**LAD**) artery and the left circumflex (**LCX**) artery. The LAD artery descends along the anterior intraventricular groove to provide blood to most of the ventricular septum and anterior portion of the left ventricle. The LAD artery and its branches also supply blood to the anterior papillary muscles, the apex of the left ventricle, and the right and left bundle branches. The LCX artery extends around the left side of the heart, along the groove between the left atrium and left ventricle, to supply blood to the left atrium and the lateral and posterior portions of the left ventricle. It supplies blood to the sinoatrial (SA) node in approximately 40% of the population and to the AV node in approximately 10% of the population.

Right Coronary Artery

The right coronary artery (**RCA**) branches out along the right AV groove to supply blood to the right atrium and right ventricle. It also supplies the SA node when not supplied by the LCX artery. The main branch of the RCA, the *marginal branch*, supplies the right heart. In most people, a second branch travels down the posterior intraventricular septum to supply blood

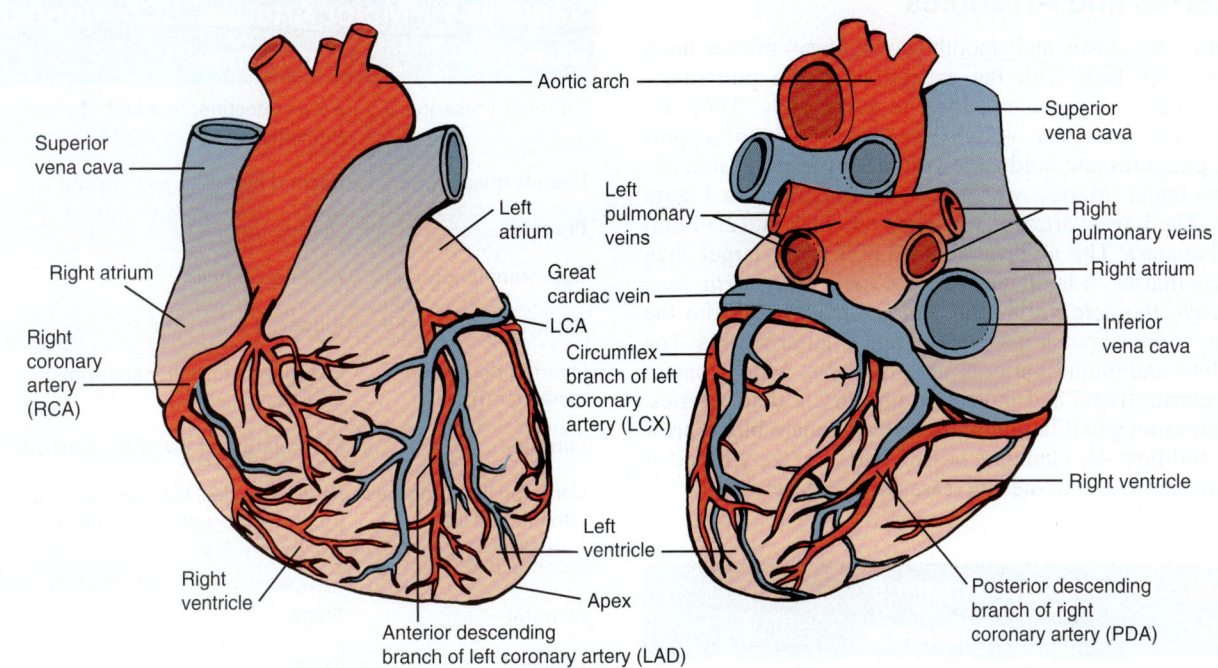

Figure 22-5 Coronary arteries and veins. **Left.** Anterior view. **Right.** Posterior view. It is important to note that coronary circulation patterns vary among people. The apex is the "point of maximal impulse."

to the posterior septum, the inferior and posterior portions of the left ventricle, and the posterior left papillary muscle. This branch is called the posterior descending artery (**PDA**). In some people, the PDA branches off the LCX artery to supply blood to these areas (known as "left coronary dominance").

Collateral Circulation

An important factor in heart physiology is that the large coronary arteries join in very few places. Consequently, if one of these arteries becomes plugged, the blood cannot detour. Coronary artery blockage causes either myocardial insufficiency, **ischemia** (reversible cell injury due to decreased blood/oxygen supply), or myocardial infarction (**MI**), a localized area of dead tissue (commonly known as a "heart attack"). Over time, **collateral circulation** may take over (two vessels interconnect to supply the same area). This helps supply blood to "at risk" tissue. Very small interconnections are normally found among microscopic branches of coronary arteries. When coronary obstruction occurs gradually (e.g., atherosclerosis), these vessels can enlarge to supply endangered heart muscle.

> **Key Concept**
> If a significant portion of the heart is deprived of circulation, surgical intervention is necessary. This may restore circulation by coronary artery bypass or placement of a stent. Anatomic variations among individuals make these procedures extremely challenging for the surgeon. Chapter 81 describes selected cardiovascular procedures.

Coronary Veins

The coronary arteries drain into capillaries in the myocardium, where delivery of oxygen and nutrients occurs, along with waste removal. Blood then leaves the capillaries, and most of it enters the venous system via two principal veins: the *great cardiac vein*, which drains blood from the anterior heart surface, and the *middle cardiac vein*, which drains the heart's posterior surface. These vessels transport blood into an opening, the **coronary sinus**, which returns blood to the right atrium (Fig. 22-4).

SYSTEMIC BLOOD VESSELS

Blood is carried through the body by arteries, arterioles, capillaries, venules, and veins. The arteries carry blood *away* from the heart, the capillaries serve as "in-between" channels, and the veins carry blood *toward* the heart. (The maintenance of cerebral [brain] circulation is vital to life. This is discussed in Chapter 23; also see Fig. 23-8.)

> **Key Concept**
> Arteries carry oxygenated blood away from the heart. Veins carry deoxygenated blood toward the heart. (This is opposite only in the pulmonary circuit.)

 SPECIAL CONSIDERATIONS   Lifespan

Physiologic Differences and Coronary Artery Disease
Anatomic and physiologic differences make coronary heart disease potentially more dangerous for women than men. Women's hearts are, on average, 10% smaller than men's hearts, with corresponding smaller coronary arteries. Smaller vessel size leads to decreased perfusion (circulation), especially in the presence of atherosclerosis. Clots can form more easily in women's coronary arteries due to higher fibrinogen levels and greater fibrinolytic activity with advancing age. Increased clot formation, coupled with decreased coronary artery size, can increase the risk of vessel occlusion. Female hormones also appear to influence the development of coronary artery disease.

Arteries and Arterioles

Arteries are elastic and smooth (involuntary) thicker muscular tubes that, with the exception of the pulmonary artery, carry oxygenated blood to body cells. They are known as "resistance vessels" because they can support high pressures and hold large volumes of blood. Table 22-1 lists major arteries, which are also illustrated in Figure 22-6. The largest artery is the aorta (about 1 in. (2.54 cm) in diameter). The aorta is about 3,000 times larger than the capillaries. It is divided into the *ascending aorta, aortic arch, thoracic aorta,* and *abdominal aorta.* From the aorta, arteries branch into smaller and smaller vessels. The smallest and thinnest arteries are *arterioles,* which contain less elastic tissue and more smooth muscle than arteries. Constriction and dilation of arterioles regulate blood pressure and flow. By changing vessel diameter, the volume of blood supplied to tissues increases or decreases.

TABLE 22-1 Major Arteries

NAME	DISTRIBUTION
Branches of the Ascending Aorta	
Left and right coronary arteries	Heart muscle
Branches of the Aortic Arch	
Brachiocephalic (innominate) branches into	
Right subclavian	Right upper extremity
Right common carotid	Right side of head and neck
Left common carotid	Left side of head and neck
Left subclavian	Left upper extremity
Each subclavian artery extends into	
Axillary	Axilla
Brachial	Arm proper
Radial	Thumb side of forearm and wrist
Ulnar	Medial side of hand
Branches of the Thoracic Aorta	
Bronchial	Lungs
Esophageal	Esophagus
Intercostals	Muscles and other structures of chest wall
Superior phrenic	Posterior and superior surfaces of diaphragm
Branches of Abdominal Aorta	
Celiac trunk branches into	
Left gastric	Stomach
Splenic	Spleen
Hepatic	Liver

TABLE 22-1 Major Arteries (Continued)

NAME	DISTRIBUTION
Superior mesenteric	Small intestine, first half of large intestine
Inferior mesenteric	Second half of large intestine
Phrenic	Diaphragm
Suprarenal (adrenal)	Adrenal glands
Renal	Kidneys
Ovarian (female) or testicular (male)	Sex glands formerly spermatic arteries
Lumbar	Musculature of the abdominal wall
Common iliac branches into internal iliac	Pelvic muscles, bladder, rectum, prostate, reproductive organs
External iliac branches into	
Femoral	Thigh
Popliteal	Knee
Tibial	Leg, ankle, heel
Dorsalis pedis	Foot

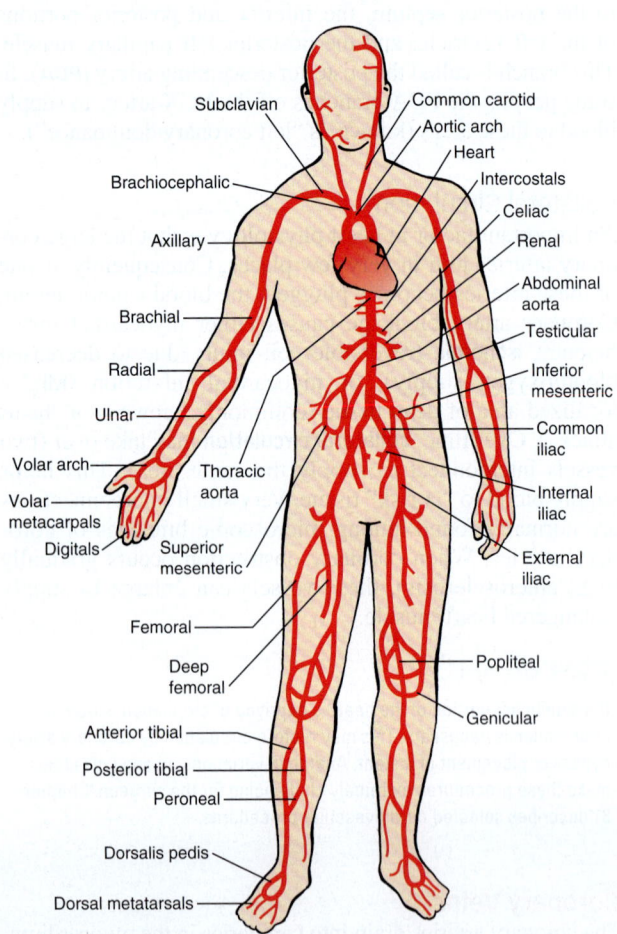

Figure 22-6 Principal systemic arteries. The arterial system carries blood away from the heart. Major pressure points (pulse points) are used to count the pulse or to stop hemorrhage.

Capillaries

From arterioles, blood flows into the smallest vessels, the *capillaries*. A capillary is microscopic, about 8 μm (micrometers—1/8 millionth of a meter). Blood flow through capillaries is known as **microcirculation**. Capillaries are composed of a single layer of endothelial cells. They are so small that tiny red blood cells must pass through them in single file. Capillaries make up most of the great length of the body's blood vessels. In the capillaries, overall resistance is very low, so blood flows very slowly, allowing time for oxygen and nutrients to leave blood vessels and enter body tissues. (See Chapter 17 for information regarding transport of nutrients, salts, gases, and wastes across cell membranes and through capillary walls; diffusion and filtration.) The relatively high osmotic pressure of albumin (a plasma protein) within capillaries pulls interstitial fluid into them. The fluid pulled back into capillaries contains cellular waste products to be taken to the kidneys for excretion. *Ecchymotic* areas (black and blue marks) result from ruptured capillaries.

> **Key Concept**
> The capillaries are very important. They are known as "exchange vessels" because here the exchange of nutrients and wastes occurs.

Veins and Venules

At the same time blood is delivering materials to cells, it is picking up waste products. From capillaries, blood starts back toward the heart through *venules*, the smallest veins. Venous branches grow larger and become fewer as they near the heart, until finally blood reaches the body's largest veins, the *superior vena cava* (**SVC**) and *inferior vena cava* (**IVC**) (plural: cavae). These two large veins return blood to the right atrium. The SVC returns blood from the head, neck, and arms, and the IVC returns blood from the lower body. Venous blood is dark red because oxygen has been replaced with carbon dioxide and other wastes. (*The exception occurs within pulmonary veins.*) Table 22-2 lists major veins, illustrated in Figure 22-7.

Venous Blood Return

Venous valves contribute to efficient venous blood flow from the extremities; they also permit blood flow in one direction only. Also contributing to venous return is the location of veins between skeletal muscles, where contractions squeeze blood toward the heart. (Exercise can increase blood flow to skeletal muscles.) Because of its slow journey through capillaries, blood loses the original heartbeat force by the time it reaches veins. Therefore, veins do not pulsate.

> **Key Concept**
> When a vein is cut, muscles in the wall constrict, and blood flows in a steady stream (arterial blood pulsates).

Systemic veins and venules are also called "blood reservoirs" or "*capacitance vessels*." They house approximately 60%–70% of the body's blood volume at rest and have the capacity to expand and store more blood when needed. Healthcare professionals often administer medications that promote *vasodilation*, which results in increased venous storage capacity, thereby decreasing the blood volume returning to a failing heart and lowering blood pressure. The venous system can tolerate fairly large volume changes without major effect on blood pressure. The venous "reservoir" system also serves as a depot for blood that can quickly be diverted to other vessels if needed. For example, *vasoconstriction* (contraction) of veins helps compensate for blood loss during hemorrhage. Therefore, if blood pressure

TABLE 22-2 Major Veins

NAME	DRAINAGE AREAS
Superficial Veins	
Cephalic, basilic, median cubital	Hand, forearm, elbow
Saphenous	Lower extremities
Temporal	Skull
Deep Veins	
Axillary, brachial, subclavian	Arms
Radial, ulnar	Hands
Femoral, popliteal, tibial	Thigh, knee, leg
Iliac, internal and external	Pelvis, legs
Jugular	Face, neck
Brachiocephalic	Union of subclavian and jugular veins
Superior Vena Cava	Upper half of body; formed by union of both brachiocephalic veins
Azygos vein	Chest wall into superior vena cava
Inferior Vena Cava	Lower half of body; begins with union of two common iliac veins
Receives venous blood from	
Iliac veins	Pelvis, legs
Lumbar veins	Dorsal part of trunk, spinal cord
Testicular/ovarian veins	Sex organs
Renal veins	Kidneys
Suprarenal veins	Adrenal glands
Hepatic veins	Liver
Hepatic Portal Vein	Abdominal organs to the liver
Receives venous blood from	
Mesenteric veins	Intestines
Splenic vein	Spleen
Gastric vein	Stomach
Pancreatic vein	Pancreas

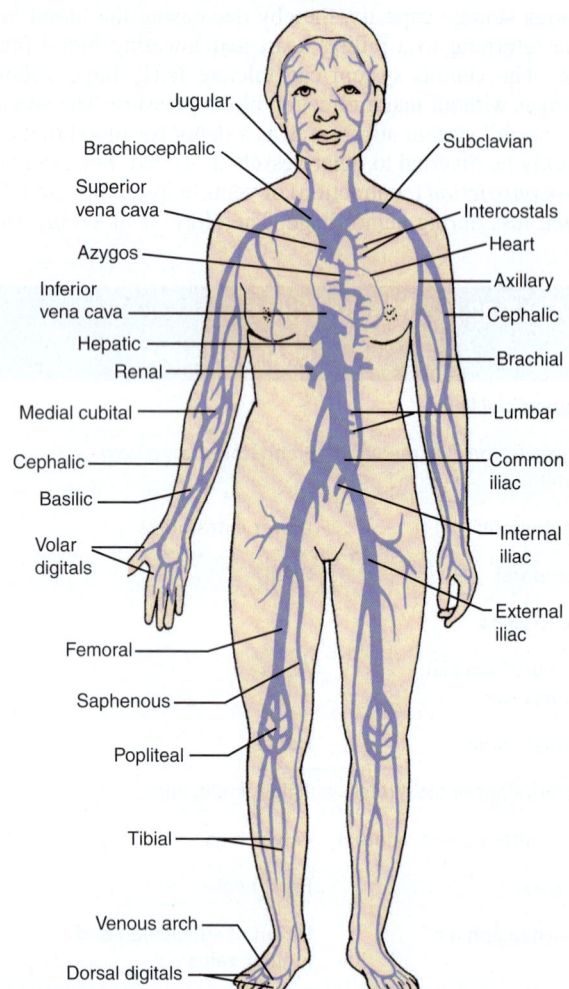

Figure 22-7 Principal systemic veins. The veins carry blood toward the heart.

is falling, specific veins constrict, rerouting blood to vital organs, such as the brain.

Key Concept

If placed end-to-end, the blood vessels in an average human body would measure about 96,500 km (60,000 miles)—about 2.5 times around the earth!

Some blood vessels are modified to serve specific functions. Examples include the sinusoids (terminal blood channels or cavities) of the liver and spleen and the choroid plexuses that project into the ventricles of the brain and secrete cerebrospinal fluid.

NCLEX Alert

The cardiovascular system includes structures commonly involved in clinical healthcare issues. To best succeed on the NCLEX, you should know the pathology of cardiovascular disorders such as heart failure, hypertension, and myocardial infarction. Often, the rationales of disorders, treatments, and nursing care relate directly to understanding the structures and functions of a system.

Tissue Layers Within Blood Vessels

Arteries and veins are composed of three layers. Layers of the arteries are thicker and more flexible because they contain stronger muscle fibers. All blood vessels are lined with endothelium, which assists in regulation of constriction and dilation. Arteries and veins all contain elastic fibers, collagen fibers, and smooth muscle fibers. The veins also contain special one-way valves.

The layers within arteries and veins are as follows:

- *Tunica adventitia*, the outermost layer, is composed of connective tissues and nerve cells, as well as nutrient capillaries in larger vessels. This layer protects the outside of the vessel.
- *Tunica media*, the middle layer, contains the thickest elastic fibers, as well as connective tissue composed of polysaccharides. This layer is covered by a thick elastic band (the *external elastic lamina*) and smooth muscle fibers, which control vessel's caliber (size).
- *Tunica intima*, the innermost layer, is the thinnest, a single layer of simple squamous endothelium (Fig. 15-10), held together by an intercellular matrix. This layer is surrounded by connective tissue interlaced with elastic bands (*internal elastic lamina*).

Capillaries are one cell layer thick, made up of endothelium (and occasionally, connective tissue).

Key Concept

The blood vessels do not pump blood, but they can regulate their diameter (especially arteries). This helps change blood flow to specific organs, regulate blood pressure, and regulate body temperature (thermoregulation).

System Physiology

CARDIAC CONDUCTION

Special bundles of unique tissue in the heart transmit and coordinate electrical impulses to stimulate the heart to beat and pump blood (Fig. 22-8). The first of these bundles, the *sinoatrial node* (**SA node** or *sinus node*), is embedded in the endocardial wall of the right atrium where it is joined by the SVC. It is also considered the heart's "pacemaker." Normal heartbeat originates in the SA node (electrical coil systole—the QRS impulse), typically at a rate of 60–80 beats per minute. The normal sinus impulse is transmitted over the myocardial electrical tree within the heart, via specialized fibers, the *conduction system* or *syncytium*. (A syncytium is a merging of cells interconnected by cytoplasmic bundles. This meshwork allows an electrical stimulus in one cell to spread through the network to the other cells.) These impulses stimulate the heart's chambers to contract. The SA node sets the pace, and the rest of the heart follows. This swift message is first sent out over the internodal pathways to the muscular tissue of the atria, which causes the atria to contract. The person with a poorly functioning SA node usually requires the implant of an electronic pacemaker.

The pacemaker cells of the heart have specific characteristics:

- *Automaticity*—the cells contract automatically and continuously without neural input—they can independently generate an electrical impulse.

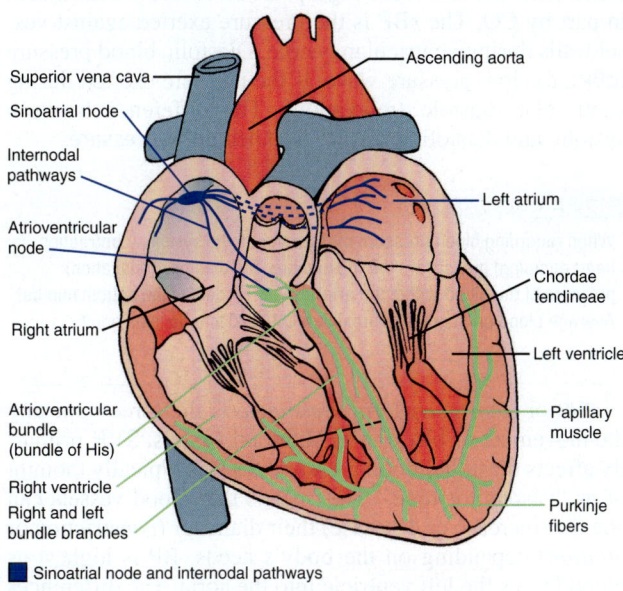

Figure 22-8 The conduction system of the heart.

- *Conductivity*—each cell passes the signal on to the next cell.
- *Contractility*—the cells have the ability to shorten fibers in the heart to pump blood in response to an impulse/signal.

The next bundle, the *atrioventricular node (AV node)*, is in the lower part of the right atrium near the ventricle. The AV node picks up the message from the SA node like a receiving station and holds onto it until the atria have contracted and emptied blood into the ventricles. When the ventricles are ready to receive the impulse, the AV node transmits it through the AV bundle (the *bundle of His*—pronounced *hiss*) and down the interventricular septum to the *right* and *left bundle branches*. From there, the fibers penetrate the ventricular muscle and terminate in the subendocardial branches (*Purkinje fibers*), which fan out across the ventricles and conduct the impulse, causing the ventricles to contract. The heart then rests for a short period and begins the process again.

> **Key Concept**
> The electrical activity of the heart must occur before mechanical, pumping, activity of the heart can respond with a heartbeat.

Should the SA node fail to fire an impulse, escape beats from other pacemaker cells within the AV node or ventricles will usually take over to keep the heart beating. Thus, the heartbeat becomes slower. If the SA node *and* AV node fail to fire an impulse, the ventricles must fire an impulse to maintain heartbeat. Ventricular contraction in this case will only occur about 20–40 beats per minute; a heart rate this slow (bradycardia) might not support life. If the ventricles do not fire a backup impulse, cardiac arrest (heart stoppage) will occur.

The conduction system of the heart is as follows:

- SA (sinoatrial) node (pacemaker) →
- AV (atrioventricular) node →
- Bundle of His (AV bundle) →
- Right and left bundle branches →
- Purkinje fibers to muscles of ventricles

CHAPTER 22 The Cardiovascular System

An **electrocardiogram (ECG)** is a graphic record of minute electrical currents generated within the heart's conduction system. Major characteristics of the ECG are the P wave, QRS complex, and T wave. These tracings indicate the *depolarization* and *repolarization* as the heart beats (Fig. 81-2).

If the heart can no longer be regulated by the normal functions of the body, other interventions (e.g., medications or pacemaker insertion) would be required to reestablish homeostasis. To maintain homeostasis in individual situations, such as an emergency, the autonomic nerves send input from cardiac centers in the brain's medulla to the heart. These cardiac centers have both accelerating and braking devices. Together, they permit accurate and delicate control of heart rate in response to internal and external stimuli. (See Chapter 19 related to the autonomic nervous system.)

CARDIAC CYCLE

In less than 1 second, both atria contract as both ventricles relax. Immediately, both ventricles contract as both atria relax. This process is considered one *cardiac cycle* or one heartbeat. This sequence of dual contractions, the atria followed by the ventricles, is called **systole**. Systole takes up one-third of the cardiac cycle. Atrial relaxation, followed by ventricular relaxation, is called **diastole**. Diastole takes up two-thirds of the cardiac cycle, allowing time for the chambers to fill adequately with blood. One cardiac cycle is made up of systole of the atria and ventricles and diastole of the atria and ventricles. These contraction and relaxation processes occur almost simultaneously on the left and right sides of the heart.

> **Key Concept**
> The contraction that pumps blood *from the heart* is systole; the period of *heart relaxation* is diastole. The heart is actually in systole twice, once for the atria (atrial systole) and once for the ventricles (ventricular systole).
>
> In addition, both atria and ventricles have periods of diastole. Systole + diastole = one cardiac cycle. The autonomic nervous system can respond to changes, such as increased exercise, and speed up the cardiac cycle.

Heart Sounds

Events in the cardiac cycle produce sounds that can be *auscultated* (heard) with a stethoscope. These sounds include normal heart sounds and might also include abnormal heart sounds.

Normal Heart Sounds

The first normal heart sound (S_1) is called the "lub" and is produced by closure of the AV valves when the ventricles contract. The second heart sound (S_2) is called the "dub" or "dup" and is produced by the closure of the aortic and pulmonary semilunar valves when the ventricles relax. Thus, S_1 occurs at the beginning of systole and S_2 occurs at the beginning of diastole. The first sound is loudest and longest. It can be heard over the entire pericardium but is usually loudest at the apex of the heart. S_2 is more easily heard at the base of the heart. (Some abnormal heart sounds are gallops, rubs, and murmurs and are discussed in Chapter 46.)

Pulse

Arterial walls are strong and elastic and they expand with each heartbeat. This rhythmic expansion is the **pulse** (an average of 72 beats per minute in an adult). The pulse can be felt where arteries are close to the surface. Pulse assessment locations are named for the artery in each area: *radial* (wrist), *carotid* (neck), *popliteal* (back of knee), *femoral* (groin), *tibial* (ankle), *pedal* (foot), *axillary* (armpit), and *temporal* (temple). These points are called *pressure points* or *pulse points* and may also be used to arrest severe bleeding (Fig. 43-5).

CARDIAC OUTPUT

Cardiac output (**CO**), the amount of blood pumped by the ventricles in 1 minute, is normally from 4 to 6 L in the resting adult. Stroke volume (**SV**), the volume of blood ejected by the left ventricle with each heartbeat, is only about two-thirds of the blood contained in the left ventricle. CO is related to SV and beats per minute (heart rate—**HR**). Therefore, changes in the amount of blood leaving the heart or changes in heart rate will affect cardiac output. Increases in SV or HR will result in increased CO. This can occur during exercise to increase blood volume to the rest of the body. *Low* cardiac output can result in decreased blood supply to the body and, thus, decreased oxygen and nutrients to the cells. (*Do not confuse CO, as used here, with the symbol for carbon monoxide.*)

Factors Affecting Cardiac Output

To adapt to the body's metabolic needs, the heart can alter its CO. In addition, the autonomic nervous system can influence HR. For example, in a dangerous situation, the heart rate increases, increasing cardiac output.

Factors called *preload* and *afterload* can affect SV. **Preload** is the amount of pressure or "stretching force" against the ventricular wall at end diastole (maximum relaxation of the heart). When more blood volume is returned to the ventricles, the muscle fibers in the ventricles stretch to accommodate the excess. *Starling law* states that the greater the stretch, the greater the following force of contraction (*contractility*). The greater the contraction, the more volume ejected, resulting in increased SV. **Afterload**, the amount of pressure or resistance the ventricles must overcome to empty their contents, must be powerful enough to overcome resistance in the aorta and other arteries. A decrease in this resistance would make it easier for the ventricles to empty, resulting again in an increase in SV. Norepinephrine and epinephrine, released by the sympathetic nervous system, also improve the ability of the ventricles to overcome resistance and empty, by increasing the strength of contractions.

BLOOD PRESSURE

Blood pressure (**BP**), a function of CO and *systemic vascular resistance* (SVR) (resistance in blood vessels), is the force that blood exerts against blood vessel walls. (Blood pressure is stated in millimeters [mm] of mercury [Hg], although mercury is no longer used in the measuring instrument.) Systolic blood pressure (**sBP**), the high-pressure wave, is determined in part by CO. The sBP is the pressure exerted against vessel walls during ventricular systole. Diastolic blood pressure (**dBP**), the low-pressure wave, is the pressure exerted during ventricular diastole (relaxation). The difference between systolic and diastolic pressure is called **pulse pressure**.

> ### Key Concept
> When recording blood pressure measurement, the systolic (contraction, heart pumping) pressure is the top number. The diastolic (relaxation) pressure of the blood within the arteries is recorded as the bottom number. Average blood pressure is approximately 120/80 mm Hg in an adult.

SVR or *total peripheral resistance* is the force opposing the movement of blood through blood vessels. SVR primarily affects diastolic blood pressure. SVR is typically thought of as "vasomotor tone." This means that blood vessels can change (increase or decrease) their diameter (*constriction* or *dilation*) depending on the body's needs. BP is highest as blood leaves the left ventricle into the aorta. The differences in BP as blood flows through the systemic circulation are necessary for filtration of nutrients through capillaries.

> ### Key Concept
> Blood flows from high pressure to low pressure.
> Continuous capillary flow is a result of the following:
> - Minimal resistance in large vessels
> - Ability of large vessels to expand and contract
> - Resistance provided by arterioles to even out the intermittent pressure caused by heartbeats

Blood Pressure Regulation

Many factors other than the force and rate of the pumping heart help maintain or regulate blood pressure. BP is mainly determined by the small arteries and arterioles. The arterioles have very thick walls in proportion to their bore and are primarily made up of smooth muscle, which has an inherent tonus, helping to regulate the blood flow within. They can quickly dilate and contract, to regulate blood pressure. In addition, the greatest pressure drop occurs within the arterioles.

Blood pressure regulating systems include the nervous, endocrine, cardiovascular, and urinary systems. Factors affecting BP are those that affect CO, SVR, or both. These factors may include the amount and contents of circulating blood, elasticity and ability of smooth muscles in arterial walls to dilate and constrict, plaque buildup on arterial walls, kidney functioning, and hormones. Special sensory receptors in blood vessel walls, **baroreceptors**, are stimulated by blood pressure changes. They send signals causing body reactions to help maintain normal BP. Other factors also influence BP including diet, physical and emotional status, smoking, and heredity. It is very important to maintain BP within normal limits; many medications are available to help in BP maintenance. Measurement of pulse and blood pressure are described in Chapter 46. Disorders of the cardiovascular system are presented in Chapter 81. Box 22-2 lists factors that have an effect on the cardiovascular system.

Box 22-2 Factors Influencing the Cardiovascular System

CLIENT-CONTROLLED LIFESTYLE FACTORS
- Amount, type, and regularity of exercise
- Quality of rest and sleep
- Weight, in relation to optimal weight
- Stress factors
- Salt intake, particularly in non-Caucasian people
- Fat intake and cholesterol levels
- Carbohydrate intake
- Medication compliance
- Oral contraceptives and other hormone-based medications
- Use of OTC (over-the-counter) cold remedies, particularly those containing pseudoephedrine
- Use of moderate to large amounts of OTC aspirin, ibuprofen, and other related medications
- Smoking and smokeless tobacco use
- Use of street drugs
- Anorexia/bulimia and other eating disorders

OTHER FACTORS
- Diabetes
- Hypertension
- Other chronic illnesses
- Previously unknown heart or blood vessel disorders or defects
- Lung disorders
- Heredity/genetics
- Kidney disorders
- Decreased blood clotting time
- Water retention/edema
- Systemic infection
- Hemorrhage
- Disorders of the blood and lymph, including hemophilia, leukemia, sickle cell disease, lupus erythematous, anemia
- Streptococcal infections
- Electrolyte imbalance
- Sex (males and postmenopausal females = higher risk)

Key Concept
Vasoconstriction can be induced by hormones, such as vasopressin and angiotensin, as well as neurotransmitters, such as epinephrine. Vasodilation is caused by antagonists, the most important of which is nitric oxide, which increases the force of the blood within vessels, causing vasodilation.

Key Concept
Smoking is a major contributor to heart and blood vessel disease. The nurse can assist the client to stop smoking by counseling and by administration of smoking cessation items such as nicotine patches, inhalers, gum, and lozenges. In addition, there are medications that help reduce the desire to smoke.

NCLEX Alert
The heart has fundamental structures for survival. The NCLEX may incorporate these structures (e.g., myocardium, coronary arteries, cardiac conduction, etc.) into clinical situations that may need specific medications, unique physical care, or awareness of emergency resuscitation measures.

SPECIAL CONSIDERATIONS Lifespan
Nursing care for older adults must adapt to changes related to aging. The cardiovascular system often shows structural and functional losses associated with aging (Table 22-3).

TABLE 22-3 Effects of Aging on the Cardiovascular System

FACTOR	RESULT	NURSING IMPLICATIONS
Blood Vessels		
Increased rigidity of blood vessels (decreased elasticity and calcification—arteriosclerosis) Fat and cholesterol deposits in arteries (atherosclerosis)	Increased blood pressure (BP) Left ventricle (LV) hypertrophy (dilation) Widened pulse pressure Myocardial fibers less elastic (less distensible) Narrowed arteries, reduced/slowed blood flow	Advise to decrease fat and sodium intake Counsel clients not to smoke Assess client on antihypertensive and diuretic medications for hypotension (low BP) and diabetes Teach client to monitor own blood pressure and report abnormalities
Dilation of blood vessels, due to weakening muscle tone; blood vessel damage	Risk for varicose vein formation	Prevent venous stasis and pressure wounds; encourage exercise Check venous return with nail bed pressure and release
Heart Valves and Conduction System		
Reduced coronary artery blood flow Blood vessel occlusion Malfunction of venous valves	Interference with heart pumping action and perfusion "Downstream ischemia," leading to tissue necrosis Varicose veins, blood flow obstruction	Administer medications Assist with exercise programs; observe for blockages. Treat pain Promote exercise; monitor symptoms

(Continued)

TABLE 22-3 Effects of Aging on the Cardiovascular System (Continued)

FACTOR	RESULT	NURSING IMPLICATIONS
Fibrosis in heart conduction system; fewer pacemaker cells; decrease in AV bundle fibers Calcification and fatty accumulation in heart valves	Changes on ECG; heart block; extra heartbeats Bradycardia or irregular heartbeat Heart valve stenosis (narrowing); often aortic valve	Pace activities; provide rest periods Teach client to take own pulse rate and recognize abnormalities Symptomatic treatment Surgery may be required
Heart valves may not close completely	Systolic heart murmurs	
Increased size of myocardium and atria	Fatigue Signs/symptoms of heart failure possible Abnormal heart sounds	Assess dizziness Advise client to sit up slowly, to avoid dizziness and falls Medications as ordered; treat symptomatically Oxygen may be needed
Heart slightly smaller	Heart is less efficient; cardiac output decreases	Adjust work and exercise accordingly
Cells		
Decreased ability of cells to absorb oxygen	Heart rate takes longer to return to normal after exercise	Encourage rest periods Measure oxygen saturation of blood Some clients require supplemental oxygen
Baroreceptor Responses in Arteries		
Decreased sensitivity to stimuli	Dizziness, fainting possible; postural hypotension can occur	Teach client to get up and move slowly. Assess all client medications. Assess electrolyte levels Encourage exercise, healthy diet, and normal cholesterol and weight maintenance Counsel client not to smoke
Other		
Lifestyle and habits (diet, smoking, obesity, stress)	Poor habits accentuate cardiac abnormalities	Appropriate medications may be available
Heredity	Some cardiac disorders unavoidable	May need fluid restriction or diuretic medications
Vasculitis (blood vessel inflammation)	May be autoimmune or caused by infection	
Edema	Imbalance between intake and output	

STUDENT SYNTHESIS

KEY POINTS

- The cardiovascular system consists of the heart and blood vessels.
- The heart is a strong, muscular pump that lies between the lungs in the mediastinum.
- The heart wall has three layers: endocardium, myocardium, and epicardium. The epicardium is also considered to be the *innermost layer* of the pericardium that surrounds the heart to cushion and protect it.
- Arteries and veins consist of three layers: tunica intima, tunica media, and tunica adventitia. Capillaries are one cell layer thick.
- The septum divides the heart into right and left halves. The heart is further divided into four chambers: two superior atria and two inferior ventricles.
- The valves of the heart allow unidirectional blood flow through the heart.
- The principal arteries that supply the heart muscle itself with blood are the right and left coronary arteries.
- Arteries, capillaries, and veins carry blood throughout the body.
- The conduction system of the heart consists of unique tissue specializing in the formation, transmission, and coordination of electrical impulses that stimulate the heart to beat.
- The normal "pacemaker" of the heart is the SA node.
- A cardiac cycle normally lasts less than 1 second and consists of the contraction (systole) and relaxation (diastole) of both atria, followed immediately by both ventricles.

- Events in the cardiac cycle create recognizable heart sounds.
- Cardiac output is the amount of blood the ventricles pump out in 1 minute (normally 4–6 L/min).
- Blood pressure is the force exerted by the blood against the walls of the blood vessels. Systolic blood pressure is the force during ventricular contraction. Diastolic blood pressure is the force during ventricular relaxation.
- The nervous, endocrine, cardiovascular, and urinary systems work together to regulate blood pressure.
- Separating normal physiologic changes of the cardiovascular system in older adults is difficult because changes are often interrelated with heredity, lifestyle habits, and coexisting diseases or disorders.
- The nurse can assist the client to stop smoking by various means, as prescribed by the medical provider.

CRITICAL THINKING EXERCISES

1. Explain why a client with coronary artery disease is at high risk for developing a venous disorder.
2. Discuss the ways that you think electrolyte and acid–base imbalances would affect the cardiovascular system. Give a rationale for your answer.
3. Based on your knowledge of cardiovascular anatomy and physiology, identify some reasons the following factors could adversely affect cardiovascular functioning: high levels of stress, smoking, lack of exercise, poor diet, and diabetes.

NCLEX-STYLE REVIEW QUESTIONS

1. When auscultating the heart of a client with pericarditis, which finding should the nurse anticipate reporting?
   a. A rub
   b. Murmur
   c. Gallop
   d. Second heart sound

2. The nurse is obtaining data from an older adult client. Which finding would the nurse recognize as consistent with "stiffening" of the large arteries?
   a. Respiratory rate of 18 breaths per minute
   b. Heart rate of 64 beats per minute
   c. Blood pressure of 100/60 mm Hg
   d. Blood pressure of 160/72 mm Hg

3. The nurse is determining the location of the point of maximal impulse for a client during an examination. Where will the nurse place the stethoscope?
   a. The mediastinum
   b. The apex of the heart
   c. The right lower sternal border
   d. The left upper sternal border

4. The nurse observes a client with a heart rate of 76 beats per minute. Where does the nurse identify the heartbeat originates?
   a. Sinoatrial node (SA)
   b. Atrioventricular node (AV)
   c. Bundle of His
   d. Purkinje fibers

5. A client states to the nurse, "I want to quit smoking. My father had a heart attack and he was a heavy smoker." Which action by the nurse is appropriate?
   a. Inform the client it would be best to stop immediately without aids.
   b. Provide information regarding counseling and smoking cessation aids.
   c. Encourage the client to quit because quitting is the only way to avoid a heart attack.
   d. Inform the client to get a prescription for anxiety before trying to stop.

CHAPTER RESOURCES

Enhance your learning with additional resources on thePoint!

Student Resources related to this chapter can be found at **thePoint.lww.com/Rosdahl12e**.

23 The Hematologic and Lymphatic Systems

Learning Objectives

1. Describe the principal functions of blood and its homeostatic mechanisms.
2. Identify the plasma proteins and their chief functions.
3. Describe the structure and function of red blood cells, white blood cells, and platelets.
4. Discuss the importance of chemotaxis and phagocytosis in fighting invading organisms and other foreign materials.
5. Briefly describe the mechanism of blood clotting.
6. Identify the four blood groups and define the term Rh factor. Explain the concept of universal donor and universal recipient.
7. Describe lymphatic circulation and the filtration role of lymph nodes.
8. Describe the circle of Willis and the blood–brain barrier, including the function of each.
9. Explain the process of hepatic portal circulation.
10. Discuss changes in the hematologic and lymphatic systems related to aging.

Important Terminology

agglutination
albumin
anastomose
coagulation
embolus
endocytosis
erythrocyte
fibrin
fibrinogen
globulin
hematocrit
hematopoiesis
hemorrhage
hemostasis
leukocyte
lymph
lymph node
lymphocyte
macrophage
monocyte
phagocytosis
pinocytosis
plasma
platelet
prothrombin

Acronyms

Rh factor
spleen
thrombin
thrombocyte
thrombus
tonsil
type and crossmatch
APC
BBB
Hb
Hgb
MABP
RBC
Rh+
Rh−
WBC

The hematologic system consists of blood (i.e., plasma and formed elements) and bone marrow, the primary organ that manufactures blood cells. The lymphatic system consists of the lymphatic vessels and tissues and lymph. Other organs and structures, such as the spleen, liver, and kidneys, also perform specific related functions.

> **Key Concept**
>
> The hematologic and lymphatic systems have transportation and protective functions in the body. Also, blood functions in regulatory processes, and lymph functions in the manufacture of formed elements, removal of foreign substances, and absorption and storage of specific substances.

Structure and Function

The functions of the *hematologic system* are transportation, regulation, and protection. These functions involve delivery of nutrients and oxygen, as well as immune substances and hormones to the cells. This system also removes wastes and regulates blood volume, blood cell and antibody production, and blood coagulation. The *lymphatic system* transports dietary fats, drains interstitial fluid (ISF), and provides immunity against infection. It also recycles and returns excess proteins that may escape from blood vessels back into the systemic circulation. Box 23-1 lists some functions of the hematologic and lymphatic systems.

BLOOD

Blood is a versatile vascular fluid, heavier, thicker, and more viscous than water. Although it is a liquid, its unique qualities allow it to form solid clots. The primary purpose of blood is to maintain a constant environment for all body tissues. It maintains this *homeostasis* via its viscosity (thickness) and by its ability to carry dissolved substances to all body parts. Blood is responsible for transportation of oxygen, carbon dioxide, nutrients, heat, waste products, disease-fighting substances, and hormones to and from the cells. It also helps regulate pH, body temperature, and cellular water content. It contributes protection from blood loss and foreign body invasion.

Blood is considered a *connective tissue* because it shares many characteristics with other connective tissues, in terms of origin and development (Huether et al., 2020). However,

Box 23-1 Functions of the Hematologic and Lymphatic Systems

BLOOD

Transportation
- Transports oxygen to body cells and carbon dioxide away from body cells
- Exchanges oxygen for carbon dioxide at cellular level
- Transports water, nutrients, and other needed substances, such as salts (electrolytes) and vitamins, to body cells
- Aids in body heat transfer
- Transports waste products from cells to be removed from the circulation (e.g., kidney removes excess water, electrolytes, and urea; liver removes bile pigments and drugs; lungs remove carbon dioxide)
- Transports hormones from sites of origin to organs they affect
- Transports enzymes

Regulation
- Contributes to regulation of body temperature
- Assists in maintenance of acid–base balance
- Assists in maintenance of fluid–electrolyte balance

Protection
- Fights disease and infection (leukocytes)
- Promotes clotting of blood (platelets and specialized factors)
- Provides immunity due to antibodies and antitoxins (specialized cells)

LYMPH

Transportation
- Carries fluid away from tissues
- Carries wastes away from tissues

Absorption
- Absorbs fats and transports fats to blood (lacteals)
- Stores blood (spleen)
- Destroys worn-out erythrocytes

Protection
- Filters waste products out of blood
- Filters foreign substances out of blood (including dead blood cells, bacteria, smoke by-products, cancer cells)
- Destroys bacteria
- Participates in antibody production to fight foreign invasion

Manufacture
- Manufactures lymphocytes and monocytes
- Manufactures erythrocytes (spleen in fetus)

---

it differs from other connective tissues because its cells are not fixed, but move freely *to all body cells*.

Hematopoiesis (hemopoiesis) refers to production, multiplication, maturation, and specialization of blood cells in the bone marrow. The red bone marrow manufactures blood cells, or "formed elements," of blood. (In the embryo, red blood cells [**RBCs**] are produced in the liver and spleen as well.) Other tissues, such as lymph nodes, spleen, and thymus, contribute to additional production and maturation of agranular white blood cells. *Erythropoiesis* refers to the formation of RBCs (erythrocytes). A glycoprotein-type hormone, *erythropoietin*, is secreted by the kidneys in adults; this stimulates stem cells in bone marrow to produce RBCs. Dietary elements such as iron, cobalt, copper, amino acids, and certain vitamins are also required for erythropoiesis. The bone marrow releases immature RBCs (e.g., reticulocytes), which mature in about a day.

> **Key Concept**
>
> A form of erythropoietin, derived in DNA technology, may be used to treat the type of anemia caused by insufficient or ineffective RBCs. This is called *recombinant human erythropoietin* (RHE) or epoetin alfa.

Blood is composed of both plasma and formed elements. It is carried through a closed system of vessels pumped by the heart (Chapter 22). The volume of circulating blood differs with individual body size; however, the average adult body contains approximately 4–6 L of blood. Table 23-1 lists some normal laboratory values for blood components.

Plasma

Blood **plasma**, the fluid portion of circulating blood, constitutes 55% of blood volume. Plasma is 90% water. Its remaining 10% consists primarily of plasma proteins, but it also includes salts (electrolytes), nutrients, nitrogenous waste products, gases, hormones, and enzymes. Plasma absorbs salts from food for use by body cells. The maintenance of these salts within the plasma controls the chemical and acid–base balance of the blood and contributes to the entire body's homeostasis. Electrolytes contained in plasma are sodium (Na^+), calcium (Ca^+), potassium (K^+), and magnesium (Mg^{++}). Plasma also contains ions of other elements such as bicarbonates, sulfates, chlorides, and phosphates (Chapter 17).

Plasma Proteins

Four groups of plasma proteins are manufactured in the liver. **Albumin,** the largest group, accounts for 50%–60% of plasma proteins. Its important function is to provide thickness to the circulating blood volume, thus maintaining *osmotic pressure*. (Osmotic pressure draws water from surrounding tissue fluid into capillaries and, thus, maintains fluid volume and blood pressure.) Loss of albumin can result in dramatic fluid shifts, edema, hypotension, and even death (Chapter 17). **Fibrinogen** and **prothrombin** are two other plasma proteins, essential for blood clotting.

Globulin is the fourth type of plasma protein. Two types of globulin (*alpha* and *beta*) are formulated in the liver and act as carriers for molecules, such as fats. *Gamma* globulins (immunoglobulins [Ig]) are antibodies, materials synthesized by the body in response to antigens (foreign invaders), thus providing immunity against infection and disease (Chapter 24).

UNIT 4 Structure and Function

TABLE 23-1 Selected Approximate Normal Laboratory Values[a]

	MALE	FEMALE	NEWBORN
Hemoglobin (Hgb)	14–18 g/dL	12–16 g/dL	16.5–19.5 g/dL
			Children vary by age.
Cell Counts			
Erythrocytes (red blood cells [RBCs])	4.6–6.2 million/mm^3	4.2–5.4 million/mm^3	Children vary by age.
Leukocytes (total) (white blood cells [WBCs])	(All adults) 5,000–9,000 million/mm^3		
Differential (Diff) in percentages (all adults)			
Band neutrophils	3–5		
Segmented neutrophils	54–62		
Lymphocytes	25–33		
Monocytes	3–7		
Eosinophils	1–3		
Basophils	0–1		
Platelets	150,000–400,000/mm^3		

[a]Values vary slightly by laboratory.

> **Key Concept**
> Albumin, the largest group of plasma proteins, helps maintain blood pressure and circulating fluid volume. The three other circulatory plasma proteins are fibrinogen, prothrombin, and globulin.

Formed Elements

The remaining blood volume consists of formed elements. These elements are RBCs, white blood cells (**WBCs**), and platelets. Figure 23-1 illustrates the types of WBCs and RBCs.

Red Blood Cells

RBCs, also called **erythrocytes** (*erythro* = red; *cyte* = cell) or *red corpuscles*, are flattened, biconcave disks. (*Biconcave* means that both faces of the cell are thinner in the center than at the edges. In cross section, the RBC is shaped like a dumbbell.) When RBCs mature, they have no nucleus (and therefore, no DNA; so RNA cannot be synthesized). Thus, they cannot reproduce and are also unable to synthesize protein. RBCs consist mainly of hemoglobin, in a surrounding medium, the *stroma*. Each cell is enclosed in a cell wall.

Erythrocytes are the most numerous blood cells, about 25 trillion in the human body. Approximately 3,000 RBCs could be placed side by side within a 1-inch space. They are made from stem cells in red bone marrow, mostly in large bones. The RBCs are fragile and wear out quickly.

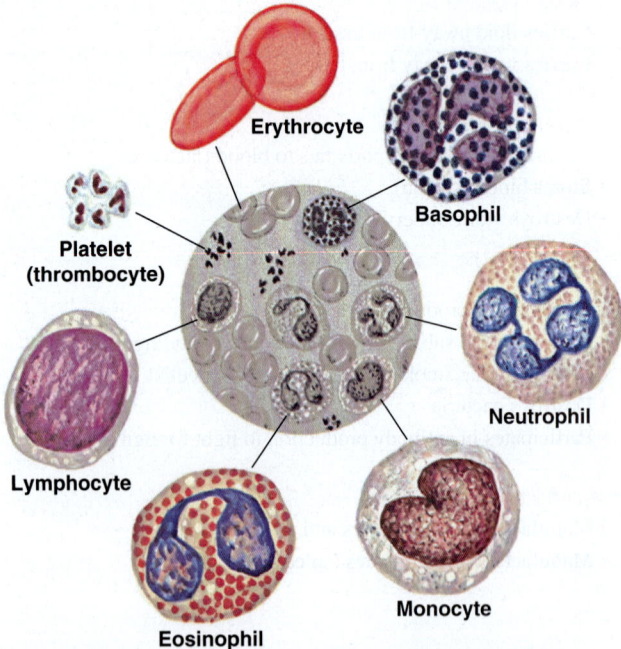

Figure 23-1 Normal blood cell types. Erythrocytes are red blood cells. Also shown are platelets (thrombocytes). All the other cells shown are types of white blood cells (leukocytes). Granulocytes (granular leukocytes) are basophils, neutrophils, and eosinophils. Agranulocytes (agranular leukocytes) are monocytes and lymphocytes.

Macrophages in the liver and spleen ingest old, used RBCs and salvage iron, which is transported to bone marrow to make new RBCs. The life of an individual RBC is about 120 days. (Every second, about 2+ million RBCs die and are replaced. The body manufactures about 120–180 million RBCs every minute!) Erythropoiesis begins in kidney cells, stimulated by decreased oxygen levels to release the hormone, erythropoietin, which stimulates red bone marrow to produce RBCs.

Each RBC contains more than 250 million molecules of the compound, hemoglobin (**Hgb** or **Hb**). Hemoglobin is composed of the iron-containing pigment *heme* and a protein, *globin*. (Iron is the pigment that makes RBCs appear red.) As blood circulates through the lungs, the iron in hemoglobin attracts and binds to oxygen in a loose combination. (Hemoglobin allows blood to carry 60 times more oxygen than would plasma.) Hemoglobin saturated with oxygen, *oxyhemoglobin*, causes blood to appear bright red. As blood circulates through the capillaries, hemoglobin gives its oxygen to the body cells. Although RBCs are smaller than most other human cells, they are larger in diameter than the smallest capillaries. This forces oxygen transfer from RBCs into individual body tissues. Most carbon dioxide waste is carried away from cells as bicarbonate, dissolved in plasma. Deoxygenated blood is much darker (almost maroon) in color. (Some RBCs may be stored in the spleen and dumped into the blood during exertion or stress, increasing the oxygen-carrying capacity of the blood.) In addition to the transportation of oxygen, RBCs have several other functions (Box 23-2).

Hyperbaric oxygenation (high-pressure oxygenation) involves high-concentration oxygen administration while the total body is subjected to greater than normal atmospheric pressure. This forces oxygen into the body and allows it to be carried, not only by hemoglobin but also by other portions of the blood, such as plasma. It is used in treating disorders such as carbon monoxide poisoning, diver's hypoxia, and gas gangrene (caused by the anaerobic organism, *Clostridium*), as well as the performance of some surgeries.

> **Key Concept**
> - Iron in hemoglobin picks up oxygen in the lungs. This oxygen is exchanged for carbon dioxide at the cellular level, which is returned to the lungs in plasma, to complete the cycle. (RBCs do not use any of the oxygen they transport.)
> - The average female has fewer RBCs than males.
> - A deficiency of RBCs is one form of anemia.
> - During inflammation, RBCs may "stack up" due to elevation of specific serum proteins (a "rouleaux formation").
> - People living in high altitudes have more RBCs because each RBC carries less oxygen.
> - RBCs must be in an isotonic solution to survive (Fig. 17-3).

Pulse oximetry indirectly measures arterial oxygen content. This is based on the color variations between oxygenated and deoxygenated blood (colorimetric technique). Specific blood tests include the RBC count (number of RBCs per volume of blood); **hematocrit** (percentage of blood volume occupied by RBCs); and Hgb (hemoglobin) level. Glycosylated (glycated) Hgb (HbA1C, HA1C, A1C) is an average of blood sugar levels over time, which is important in diabetes management.

White Blood Cells

About 1% of blood volume in the healthy adult consists of WBCs, also known as **leukocytes** (*leuko* = white; *cyte* = cell), because they do not contain hemoglobin. All leukocytes are derived from a cell in the bone marrow, the *hematopoietic stem cell*. WBCs are widespread throughout the body, in both the blood and lymphatic systems. WBCs defend the body against disease organisms, toxins, irritants, and other foreign materials. They differ greatly from RBCs. WBCs are larger than RBCs, contain nuclei, and can move independently in an ameboid fashion. WBCs also assist in repairing damaged tissues; sometimes they die during this activity and collect with bacteria to form *pus*. Other characteristics of WBCs are presented in Box 23-3. The two types of WBCs are granular and agranular.

> **NCLEX Alert**
> Basic knowledge of the hematologic and lymphatic systems will facilitate your understanding of diagnostic tests and laboratory values that may be included throughout the NCLEX.

Granular Leukocytes (Granulocytes)

Granular leukocytes are also called *polymorphonuclear leukocytes* (PMNs) or *segmented neutrophils* (segs) because their nuclei have so many lobes or the lobes are so divided as to look like more than one nucleus. In granulocytes, membrane-bound enzymes aid in digestion of

---

Box 23-2 Functions of Red Blood Cells

In addition to transportation of oxygen, red blood cells (RBCs) have the following functions:
- If RBCs experience stress because blood vessels are constricted, they release adenosine triphosphate (ATP), which causes vessel walls to relax and dilate.
- RBCs also produce ATP (the energy carrier) by fermentation.
- When hemoglobin is deoxygenated, RBCs release substances that assist in dilation of blood vessels and facilitate blood flow to oxygen-poor areas.
- RBCs store iron in the body; RBCs themselves are stored in the spleen.
- RBCs are involved in the immune response. If RBCs are lysed by pathogens, the hemoglobin releases free radicals that break down cell walls of the pathogens.
- Myoglobin, a compound related to hemoglobin, stores oxygen in muscle cells.
- RBCs are important in acid–base balance and have an influence on specific gravity of blood because they contribute viscosity (thickness) to the blood.

Box 23-3 White Blood Cells

- An abnormal number or character of leukocytes often indicates disease. For example, in leukemia, there is an increase in leukocytes or they are immature.
- The pus that forms in wounds contains an abnormally large number of leukocytes.
- A reduced number of leukocytes, leukopenia (leukocytopenia), may be caused by disease or as an unwanted side effect of medications, such as chemotherapy for cancer or clozapine.
- Some leukocytes migrate to specific tissues and remain there, fixed leukocytes. These include Kupffer cells (in the hepatic [liver] system), histiocytes (large macrophages), mast cells (in connective tissue), and microglia (which attack waste products in the nervous system).

foreign particles in a process called endocytosis (Fig. 23-2). Granulocytes are divided into three subgroups: neutrophils, eosinophils, and basophils, based on their staining properties.

- *Neutrophils*, the most numerous WBCs (50%–75%), are phagocytes. These are the granulocytes most commonly called PMNs. Because they are segmented (containing multiple lobes), they are also called *segs*. Neutrophils are colorless, unless they are stained to be visible under a microscope. They are considered to be a first line of defense against bacteria and also defend against fungi, in some measure. Neutrophils can move away from blood vessels and travel directly to sites of infection or damaged tissues because of their attraction to specific chemicals (*chemotaxis*). They push or squeeze through the capillary wall (*diapedesis*) and rush to the threatened spot, where they increase in number and engulf and devour invaders (*endocytosis*). The term **endocytosis** involves both **phagocytosis** (engulfing of particulate matter) and **pinocytosis** (engulfing of extracellular *fluid* materials). Neutrophils increase in number during bacterial infections, burns, or inflammation. Because they have a short lifespan (approximately 10 hr), they need to be replaced frequently. When an infection occurs, more neutrophils are released from bone marrow. When the demand for these granulocytes is very high, the bone marrow releases immature neutrophils called *bands*. When looking at WBC counts, *an increased number of bands signifies an infection*; this may also be described as a "shift to the left."

> **Key Concept**
>
> Neutrophils are the first cells to arrive at the site of an injury. They devour invading organisms and extracellular fluids and are the major component of pus.

- *Eosinophils* make up 0.3%–7% of circulating WBCs. They are characterized by speckled or grainy cytoplasm and survive only about 12 hr to 3 days. They increase in number during allergic reactions and parasitic infections and are believed to release chemicals to assist the body in detoxifying foreign proteins or engulfing and devouring invaders, including antigens and antibodies. They are also able to squeeze through capillary walls and usually respond to allergens. They collect in loose connective tissue and may also have a role in decreasing the release of chemical mediators during allergic reactions.
- *Basophils* are not phagocytes. They make up less than 2% of WBCs and are involved in allergic and inflammatory reactions. They contain heparin (an anticoagulant) and release histamine, in response to inflammation or another immune stimulus. Histamine, in particular, increases the permeability of blood vessels. It, along with other substances, acts on foreign invaders in the body. These

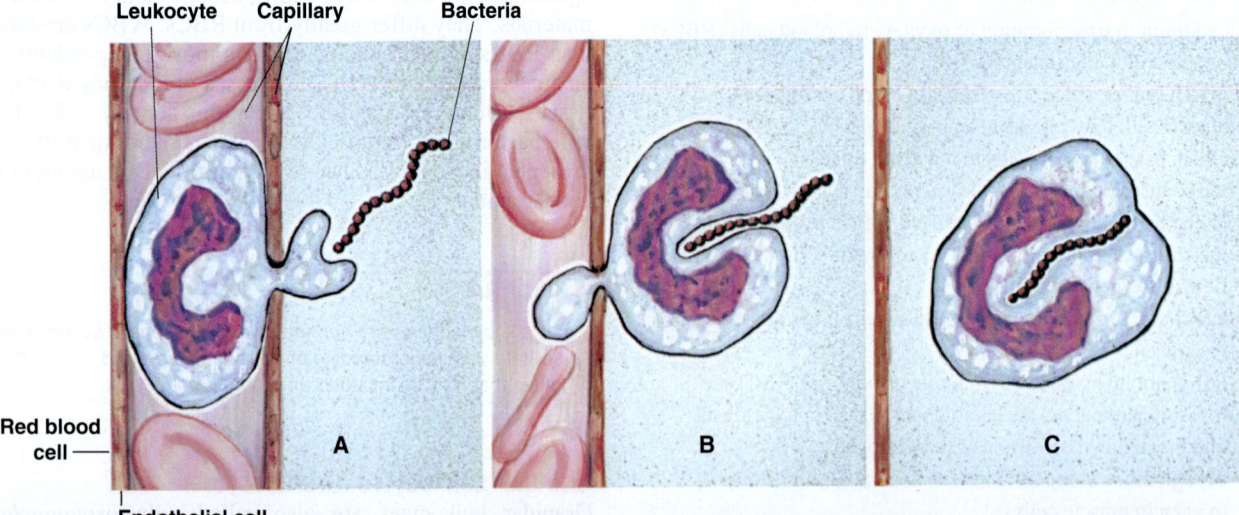

Figure 23-2 Phagocytosis. **A.** Leukocytes squeeze out of blood vessels and rush to the site of an invading organism. **B.** When foreign matter (e.g., bacteria or dead tissue [shown here as a streptococcus]) comes in contact with the cell membrane of the neutrophil, the cell membrane surrounds and pinches off the area, leaving the membrane intact. **C.** Consequently, the engulfed material is enclosed in a membranous vesicle within the neutrophil, where enzymes within the cell destroy the foreign material.

substances cause a hypersensitivity reaction, resulting in vasodilation and edema, itching, and possibly bronchial constriction, an allergic or inflammatory response.

Agranular Leukocytes (Agranulocytes)

The nuclei of these WBCs do not contain lobes. The two subgroups are **lymphocytes** and **monocytes** (mononuclear leukocytes). Under normal conditions, agranular leukocytes are functional for about 100–300 days. They are produced in the lymphatic tissue of the spleen, lymph nodes, and thymus and in hemopoietic tissues in red bone marrow.

- **Lymphocytes** are the smallest and most numerous of the agranular WBCs (20%–43%). They mature in bone marrow and can be differentiated into several types. The most important types are *B-lymphocytes* (*B-cells*) and *T-lymphocytes* (*T-cells*). B-cells make antibodies that bind to pathogens so they can be destroyed. T-cells are of several types. CD_4, or "T-helper cells," coordinate the immune response. CD_8 cells are *cytotoxic* (cell-destroying) and can kill viruses, infected cells, and tumor cells. *Natural killer cells* can kill special cells that are displaying a unique signal (after having been invaded by a virus or becoming cancerous). Other T-cells also exist. The B- and T-lymphocytes play an important role in the immune response and are discussed in greater detail in Chapter 24. Lymphocytes increase in number during infectious processes, particularly those caused by viral infections or immune disorders.
- **Monocytes** are the largest WBCs and are characterized by the absence of granules in their cytoplasm, except for lysosomes. They comprise about 1%–9% of the WBCs and play a role in acute and chronic inflammatory processes. They move from the bloodstream to other tissues, where they are transformed into macrophages or dendritic cells (*histiocytes*). (Dendritic cells function to activate T-lymphocytes.) The monocytes also "clean up" after phagocytosis by ingesting cellular debris and dead tissue, as well as presenting fragments of pathogens to the T-cells so they can be killed or so antibodies can be formed. A high monocyte count may be caused by a viral or fungal infection, tuberculosis, or certain chronic diseases.
- **Macrophages** are phagocytic cells, as are neutrophils. Macrophages collect in body structures such as the spleen, liver, and lymph nodes, where large amounts of fluids are processed. Here, they defend against invading microorganisms and promote wound healing. They engulf and digest cellular debris and pathogens after phagocytosis. They also stimulate lymphocytes and other immune cells to function.

> **Key Concept**
>
> Blood cells have a short lifespan and are constantly being manufactured in the body. The average lifespan for specific cells is as follows:
>
> - RBCs: 120 days
> - Neutrophils: 10 hr
> - Eosinophils: 12 hr to 3 days
> - Monocytes and lymphocytes: 100–300 days

Platelets

Platelets, or **thrombocytes** (*thrombo* = clot; *cyte* = cell), exist in the billions and are formed in red bone marrow by megakaryocytes. They are the smallest formed elements in the blood and are essential in blood clotting. They stimulate contraction of injured blood vessels and also can form a hemostatic plug, to stop or slow bleeding by clumping of many platelets together (*aggregation*). They also combine with plasma to speed blood coagulation. Platelets are not whole cells, but rather fragments of larger cells. They lack nuclei but are capable of ameboid movement.

Blood Clotting and Hemorrhage

Hemostasis refers to cessation of bleeding (*heme* is commonly used to denote blood; *stasi* = stopping). When blood vessels are damaged or ruptured, the hemostatic response must be quick and carefully controlled, to stop excessive blood loss. The hemostatic *initial response* includes vascular spasm (vasoconstriction), platelet plug formation, and blood clotting (i.e., the **coagulation** process that forms a fibrin clot) (Garmo et al., 2020).

Blood Clotting

Blood clotting protects the body from losing vital plasma and blood cells by sealing off broken blood vessels; without clotting, individuals would not survive even minor cuts and wounds. The process of clot formation involves a number of complex activities in a chain reaction within the blood, some of which are not totally understood. A brief description of blood clotting follows.

When a blood vessel is disrupted, subendothelium proteins (mostly collagen) are exposed, causing circulating platelets to break down almost instantly and release the chemical, *thromboplastin* (tissue factor). Thromboplastin binds collagen with specific glycoprotein receptors, other circulating proteins, and calcium ions to form *prothrombin activator*. When this activates platelets, granules of adenosine diphosphate (ADP), serotonin, platelet-activating factor (PAF), and other substances are released into the plasma. This activates more platelets and causes a chain reaction, the *coagulation cascade of secondary hemostasis*. During this process, calcium ions are introduced and the plasma protein, *prothrombin*, is converted to **thrombin**. Thrombin then activates various amino acid factors and specifically converts the soluble plasma protein, *fibrinogen*, into insoluble threads of **fibrin** (the "building block" of the hemostatic plug). The threads of fibrin form a net to entrap RBCs and platelets to form a clot, which acts like a plug in a hole and tends to draw injured edges together. As the clot shrinks, a clear yellow liquid, *serum*, is squeezed out. Serum is like plasma, except that fibrinogen and other clotting elements are now absent.

Coagulation is a complicated mechanism that cannot occur if any necessary elements are missing. Vitamin K is necessary for the formation of prothrombin and other clotting factors. (Bacteria in the colon produce most vitamin K.) Figure 23-3 briefly introduces the human clotting mechanism. A **thrombus** is a stationary clot. An **embolus** is a clot that circulates. Both of these clots can lead to death if they plug arteries to the heart, lungs, or brain. Several medications are available to treat blood clots (Unit 9).

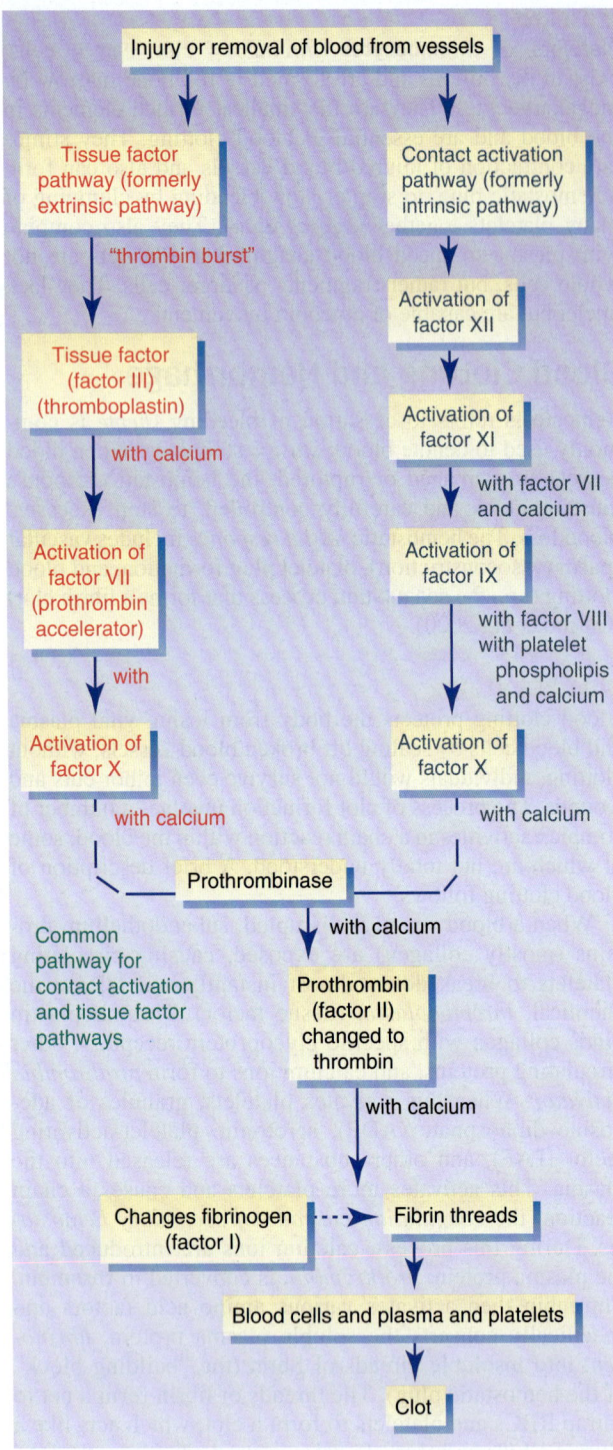

Figure 23-3 The coagulation cascade of secondary hemostasis (blood clot formation). Most coagulation factors are enzymes; some are glycoproteins (e.g., transglutaminase).

> **Key Concept**
>
> The initial response to disruption in a blood vessel includes vascular spasm (vasospasm), platelet plug formation, and the coagulation process that forms a fibrin clot. Platelets, calcium ions, and vitamin K are important elements in this complex coagulation process. A scab is the evidence of a fibrin clot.

Hemorrhage

The literal definition of **hemorrhage** is escape of blood from blood vessels; however, hemorrhage is usually thought of as the loss of a considerable amount of blood after injury. Hemostatic mechanisms, such as clotting, help prevent hemorrhage in smaller vessels, but extensive hemorrhage from larger vessels requires medical intervention. Severe hemorrhage is life threatening because the body loses so much fluid and oxygen-carrying RBCs. Inability to clot in extensive hemorrhage may be caused by several factors: force of blood flow, size of wound, volume of blood lost, or deficiency in any of the coagulant components. Severe hemorrhage must be stopped; the person often receives blood replacement, using blood or blood components from another person (*transfusion*).

> **Key Concept**
>
> Often, more blood is lost from a torn or nicked blood vessel than from a vessel that is cleanly cut through. The muscles in a blood vessel contract as a protective measure. If the muscles are cut unevenly, they cannot effectively close the vessel.
>
> Hemorrhage from an artery comes in spurts, hemorrhage from a vein in a steady flow.
>
> Hemophilia, a medical condition in which the blood clotting ability is severely reduced, causes the person to bleed severely from even a slight wound (Chapter 82).

Blood Groups

Human blood falls into one of four inherited (genetic) groups (blood types): A, B, AB, and O (Table 23-2). Combinations of antigens and antibodies, glycoproteins, including glycophorin C, exist on the surface membranes of RBCs. Blood types are due to variations in these surface glycoproteins. The **type and crossmatch** test compares donor and recipient cells to check for dangerous **agglutination** (cell clumping). If an incompatible type of blood is given to a person, a fatal transfusion reaction may result. Except for blood types, no differences exist in the blood of healthy people of different races or genders. Blood does not carry or transmit mental, emotional, or physical characteristics.

Rh Factors

Just as with a blood group, **Rh factors** are inherited *antigens*. (The Rh system is named after the rhesus monkey used in early experiments.) Of the several types of antigens that may be found on the surface of RBCs, more than 90 are loosely connected to the Rh system. The most commonly found Rh factor and the one most likely to cause a transfusion reaction is abbreviated D (Duffy). Blood is tested for the presence of D antigen. If the blood contains D factor, the person is said to be Rh-positive (**Rh+** or D+); if this factor is absent, the person is Rh-negative (**Rh−**). The percentage of Rh-negative people is lower within some ethnic groups; approximately 2%–7% of African Americans and 1% of Asians and Native Americans are Rh-negative, whereas more than 10% of Caucasians are Rh-negative. When an Rh-negative person receives Rh-positive blood, he or she develops antibodies that could cause a severe reaction to subsequent blood transfusions. This can also occur with an Rh-positive pregnancy in an Rh-negative mother. (Unit 10 discusses the Rh factor, as related to pregnancy.)

TABLE 23-2 Blood Groups and Compatibilities

BLOOD GROUP	PERCENT OF POPULATION	ANTIGEN ON ERYTHROCYTES	ANTIBODY IN PLASMA	CAN DONATE RED BLOOD CELLS TO	CAN RECEIVE RED BLOOD CELLS FROM
A	41%	A	Anti-B (reacts against B antigen)	A or AB	A or O
B	10%	B	Anti-A (reacts against A antigen)	B or AB	B or O
AB ("universal recipient")	4%	A and B	None	AB	A, B, AB, or O[a]
O ("universal donor")	45%	None	Anti-A and Anti-B (reacts against both A and B factors)	A, B, AB, or O[b]	O

[a]Blood group AB is known as the universal recipient because people of this group may receive red blood cells from donors of any ABO group in an extreme emergency. NOTE: It is also important to consider the Rh factor of donor and recipient when preparing blood for transfusion.
[b]Blood group O is known as the universal donor because these red blood cells may be given to people of any ABO group in an extreme emergency.

LYMPH

The lymphatic system is related to, yet separate from, the hematologic system (Fig. 23-4). The lymphatic system also functions as part of the body's immune system and is sometimes referred to as the *secondary circulatory system*. It includes the lymphatic conduits and specialized lymphoid tissue. Lymphoid follicles are regions of specialized lymphoid tissue densely packed with lymphocytes and some other WBCs, enmeshed in connective tissue. (As lymph passes through this tissue, damaged cells and waste materials are filtered out.) Lymphoid tissue may be organized into lymph nodes or may be loosely organized tissue known as *mucosa-associated lymphoid tissue* (MALT).

The *primary lymphatic system* consists of the thymus gland and bone marrow (involved in production and early selection of lymphocytes). The *secondary lymphatic system* consists of encapsulated tissue (the spleen and lymph nodes,

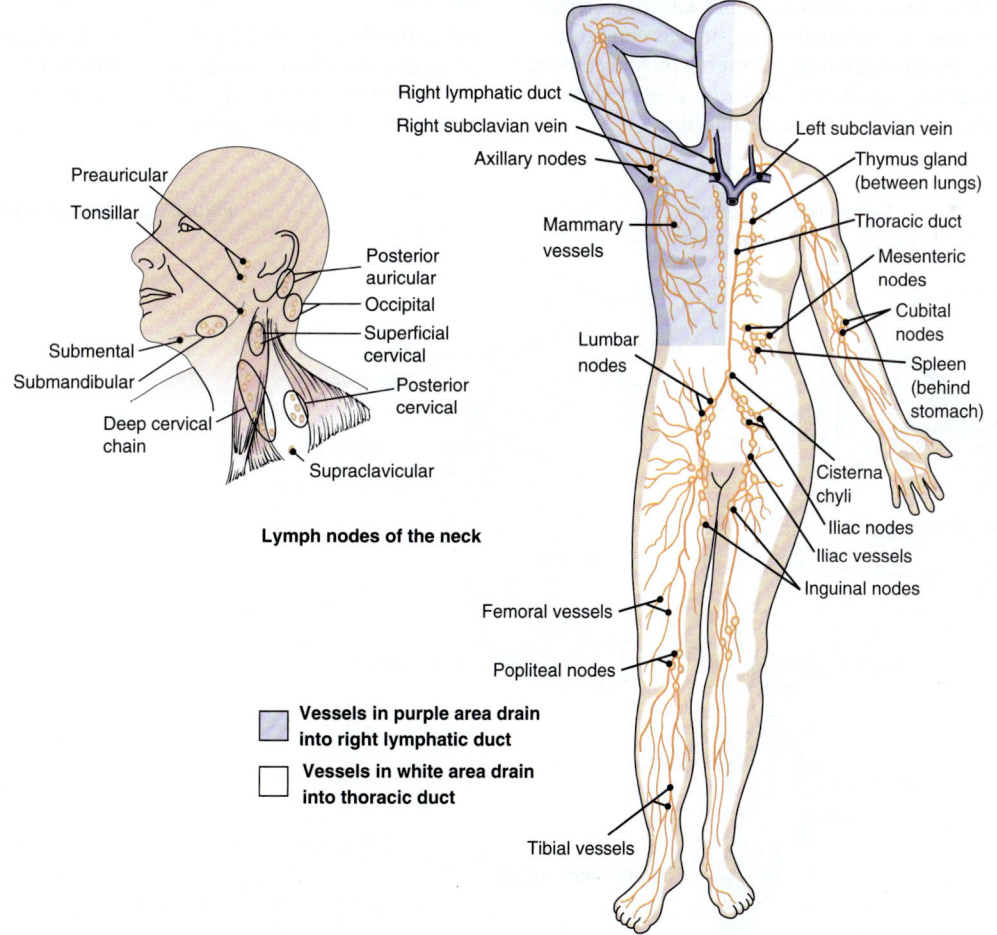

Figure 23-4 The lymphatic system. (Weber & Kelley, 2007.)

covered with connective tissue) and nonencapsulated tissue (intestinal lymphoid tissue and tonsils). The lymph nodes and lymphoid follicles of the tonsils provide an environment for antigens to interact with lymphocytes. *Peyer patches* are MALT areas in the digestive system. Researchers have identified a tertiary lymphoid system, which must import lymphocytes and only functions when antigens cause inflammation.

Functions of the lymphatic system include the following:

- Immune response—defense against infection and prevention of metastasis (spreading) of malignancies
- Removal of excess ISF from tissues
- Absorption and transport of fatty acids and fats (as chyle) to the circulatory system
- Transport of antigen-presenting cells (**APC**), such as dendritic cells, to lymph nodes, to activate an immune response.

Formation of Lymph

Body cells normally are bathed in tissue fluid, some of which drains into blood capillaries and flows directly into veins. Another group of vessels, the *lymphatic vessels*, also drains this fluid. The lymphatic vessels begin as a network of tiny closed-ended lymphatic capillaries, slightly larger than blood capillaries, in spaces between cells. Their unique structure allows ISF to flow into them but not out. (Of the body's ISF, 10%–20% enters lymph capillaries.) As ISF comes into contact with blood, it accumulates more lymphocytes, other cells, proteins, and certain waste products. When ISF enters lymphatic conduits, it becomes the thin, watery, colorless liquid known as **lymph**. Because lymph originally derives from plasma, its composition is much the same, except that lymph is lower in protein content. (Specialized lymphatic capillaries, *lacteals*, absorb digested fats and fat-soluble vitamins in the small intestine.)

Movement of Lymph

Lymphatic vessels contain one-way semilunar valves that prevent backflow of lymphatic fluid into the ISF. The functional unit of larger lymph vessels is the *lymphangion* (the segment between two valves), which can move or stop the flow of lymph. Lymphatic vessels are located both superficially (near the skin surface) and deeper in the body. The larger lymphatic vessels are lined with a single layer of flattened endothelial cells surrounded by smooth muscles encircling the endothelium. (These muscles only change the size of the vessel's lumen.) The outer layer, the adventitia, consists of fibrous tissue. The smallest lymphatic capillaries have only the single layer of endothelial cells.

Most lymphatic vessels are located near the venous system and are named accordingly. For example, *femoral* lymphatic vessels are in the thighs. Lymphatic vessels carrying fluid eventually form a network of vessels in specific areas of the body, *regional nodes*. After the fluid moves through the nodes, it is transported by other lymphatic vessels to either the right lymphatic duct or the thoracic duct. Lymphatic fluid is propelled through the body by rhythmic contractions that occur because of changes in abdominal and thoracic pressure during breathing and because of skeletal muscle contractions. The pulsation of arteries also aids in movement of lymph. All of these promote the return of venous blood—and subsequently lymphatic fluid—to the heart.

Lymph Nodes and Nodules

Small bundles of special lymphoid tissue termed **lymph nodes** are situated in clusters along the lymphatic vessels (Fig. 23-5). A lymph node, consisting of three layers, is encapsulated or enclosed in a fibrous capsule. The outer area, the superficial

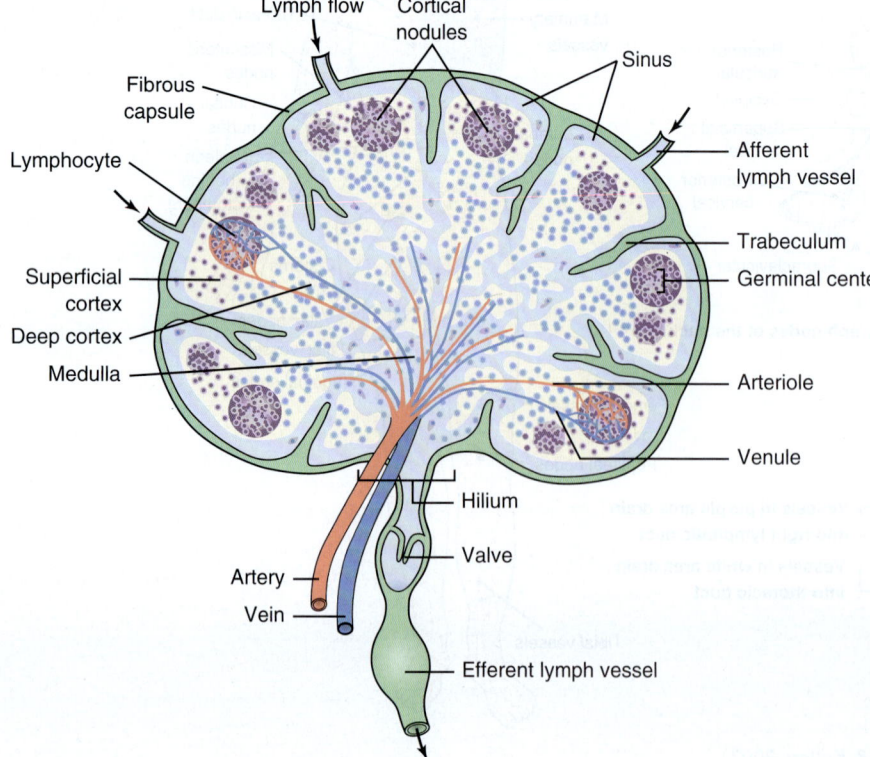

Figure 23-5 Lymph node construction.

cortex, contains lymphoid follicles; the deep cortex and interfollicular areas contain mostly T-cells; and the inner portion, the *medulla*, is made up of plasma cells that secrete immunoglobulins. An area called the *hilum* provides a portal for efferent lymph vessels and for arteries and veins. Many lymph nodes appear in the neck (*cervical*), groin (*inguinal*), and armpits (*axillary*) (Fig. 23-4). Before lymph reaches the veins or lymphatics, it passes through these nodes.

Lymph nodes perform several vital functions. The most important is that of filtering out and destroying pathogens. The "swollen glands" that may appear in a person's cervical, inguinal, and axillary regions during illness are lymph nodes at work. The nodes have enlarged as their macrophages (phagocytic cells) eat and destroy invaders. When palpated, these enlarged, nonmalignant nodes are soft and tender and may become painful.

Lymph nodules are small masses of nonencapsulated lymphatic tissues that stand guard in all mucous membranes. Because membranes line cavities that open to the external environment, these nodules are in strategic locations to filter substances that enter the body. Mucous membranes line the respiratory, gastrointestinal, urinary, and reproductive tracts.

Lymph Nodes and Cancer

Cancer cells can travel from the primary site of invasion to distant sites via the lymphatic circulation and lymph nodes. Lymph nodes may either function to filter out cancer cells or may inadvertently spread cancer to other body sites. For this reason, when cancer surgery is performed, lymph nodes in the area are tested. If no cancer cells are present in adjoining lymph nodes, the cancer was most likely localized to its original site. If cancer is found in the lymph nodes, it is said to be *spreading* or *metastasizing*. Adjoining lymph nodes may be removed, either as a precautionary measure or because the nodes already contain cancer cells. Palpable cancerous lymph nodes may be enlarged and, unlike nodes fighting infection, feel firm and nontender. Chapter 83 discusses cancer in more detail.

Lymphatic Organs

The lymphatic organs are the tonsils, spleen, and thymus, masses of lymphatic tissue with somewhat different functions than those of lymph vessels or nodes. The tonsils and spleen are designed to filter tissue fluid, although not necessarily lymph. The thymus plays a role in development of the immune system.

Tonsils

Tonsils form a ring of lymphatic tissue around the pharynx (Fig. 23-6). This tissue forms a protective barrier for substances entering the oral and respiratory passages. The tonsils may become so infected that removal (tonsillectomy) is advisable. A slight enlargement, however, is not an indication for surgery.

> **Key Concept**
>
> In the past, children often had tonsils removed at the first sign of infection (tonsillitis). Today, it is known that tonsils (because they are lymphatic material) provide filtration and protection; they are removed only if absolutely necessary.

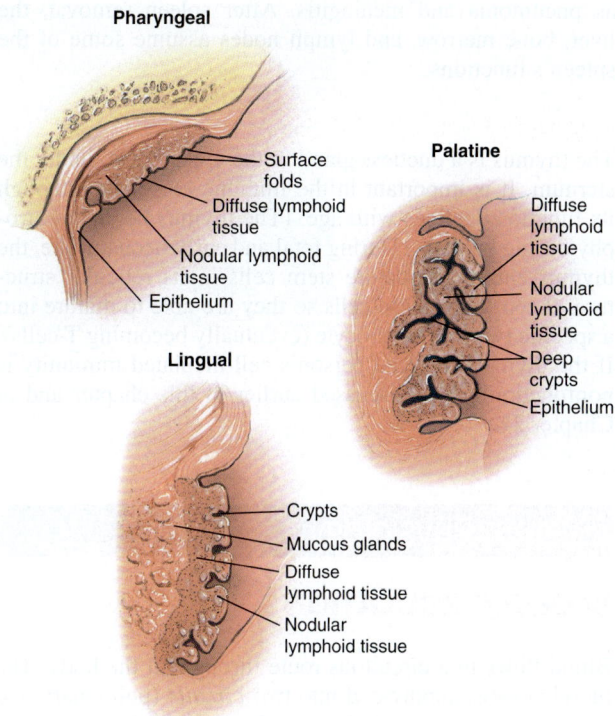

Figure 23-6 The tonsils are lymphatic tissue. They form a protective ring around the pharynx. (See also Fig. 26-2.)

Spleen

The **spleen** is the largest lymphatic organ and is located directly below the diaphragm, above the left kidney, and behind the stomach. It contains lymphoid tissue designed to filter blood. It is a somewhat flattened, dark purple organ about 6 in. (15.24 cm) long and 3 in. (7.62 cm) wide. The interior of the spleen contains splenic pulp consisting of *red pulp*, blood-filled sinusoids that fill the interspaces of the spleen's sinuses. The sinusoids of red pulp are surrounded by reticular fibers, mononuclear phagocytes, lymphocytes, plasma cells, and monocytes. Also within the red pulp is the *white pulp*, sheaths of lymphatic tissue surrounding the arteries of the spleen, particularly the splenic artery.

The spleen has several functions. In the fetus, the spleen (along with the liver) has a role in blood cell formation (a role later assumed by red bone marrow). In an adult, the spleen destroys old RBCs and forms *bilirubin* from hemoglobin. It acts as a reservoir for blood, which can be released to the body quickly in an emergency, such as hemorrhage. Twenty percent to 30% of the body's platelets are stored here. (In bone marrow failure, the spleen may also produce some RBCs.) The spleen filters and destroys pathogens and other foreign materials from the blood. It also contains specially treated B-lymphocytes that produce antibodies against foreign antigens and T-lymphocytes that attach to invading viruses or foreign entities. Both of these lymphocytes have an active role in the immune system (Chapter 24). The monocytes in the spleen become macrophages, which fight infection by phagocytosis. As described earlier in this chapter, all of these agranulocytes help the body fight infection in different ways.

Although its functions are important, the spleen can be removed without ill effects. An adult without a spleen, however, is more susceptible to some bacterial infections, such as pneumonia and meningitis. After spleen removal, the liver, bone marrow, and lymph nodes assume some of the spleen's functions.

Thymus

The thymus is a ductless gland in the upper chest, under the sternum. It is important in the immune response, although its function declines with age. (The thymus begins to atrophy during puberty.) During fetal and early neonatal life, the thymus entraps immature stem cells in its reticular structure. It sensitizes these cells so they are able to mature into a specific type of lymphocyte (eventually becoming T-cells). If the thymus fails, the person's cell-mediated immunity is nonfunctioning, as discussed earlier in this chapter and in Chapter 24.

System Physiology

BLOOD CIRCULATION

Blood flows in a circuitous route throughout the body. The blood vessels, subdivided into two *circuits* (pulmonary and systemic), together with the four chambers of the heart, form the closed system for the flow of blood (Chapter 22).

Pulmonary Circulation

The phase of circulation in which blood is pumped through the lungs to eliminate waste products (particularly CO_2) and pick up oxygen (O_2) is the *pulmonary circulation*. Blood is pumped out of the heart into the lungs by the *right ventricle*. It enters the *pulmonary artery* (the only artery that carries deoxygenated blood) and continues to capillaries in the lungs. Here, carbon dioxide is exchanged for oxygen. Small veins collect oxygenated blood from the capillaries. These veins combine eventually into four *pulmonary veins*, which pour oxygenated blood into the *left atrium* of the heart. (These veins are the only veins carrying oxygenated blood.) From here, the blood is pumped to the rest of the body (systemic circulation). Figure 23-7 illustrates pulmonary and systemic circulation.

Systemic Circulation

From the left atrium, oxygenated blood enters the *left ventricle*. The left ventricle pumps blood out of the left side of the heart into the general or *systemic circulation to* carry nutrients and oxygen to body cells and return with accumulated waste products. As blood leaves the left ventricle, it surges into the largest artery of the body, the *aorta*. The aorta is further divided into the *ascending aorta, aortic arch, thoracic aorta*, and *abdominal aorta*, which is divided into smaller arteries. The blood travels through smaller and smaller arterial branches. From the smallest arteries, the *arterioles*, the blood enters capillaries, where oxygen and nutrients are exchanged for wastes (Chapter 17). The blood then returns from the capillaries to the heart via *venules*, then larger *veins*, and finally through the *inferior* and *superior vena cavae* to the right atrium, thereby completing the circuitous route.

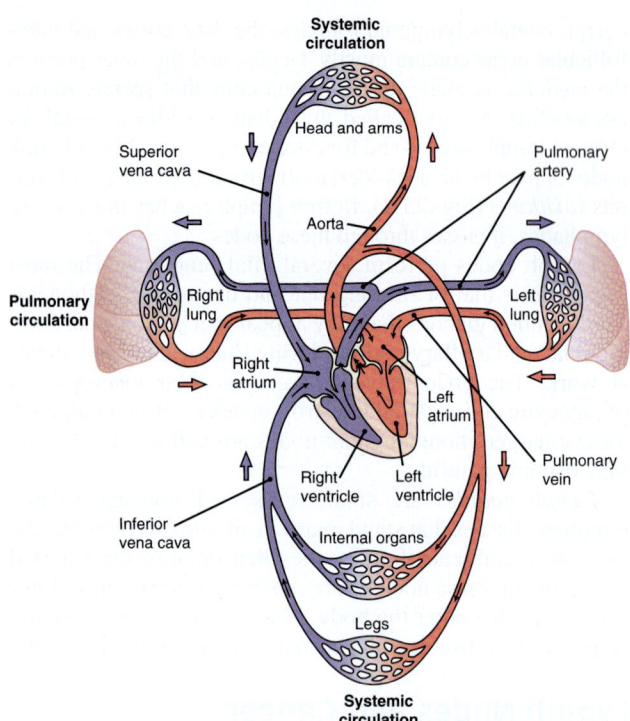

Figure 23-7 The heart is a double pump. The *pulmonary circuit* carries blood to the lungs to be oxygenated; the *systemic circuit* carries blood to all other parts of the body.

Hepatic Portal Circulation

The hepatic portal circulation is a subdivision of systemic circulation. It is an efficient detour in venous return, directed at transporting raw materials (carbohydrates, fats, and proteins) from the digestive organs and spleen to the liver. The hepatic portal circulation is unique because it begins and ends with capillaries (Fig. 23-8). The capillaries from the

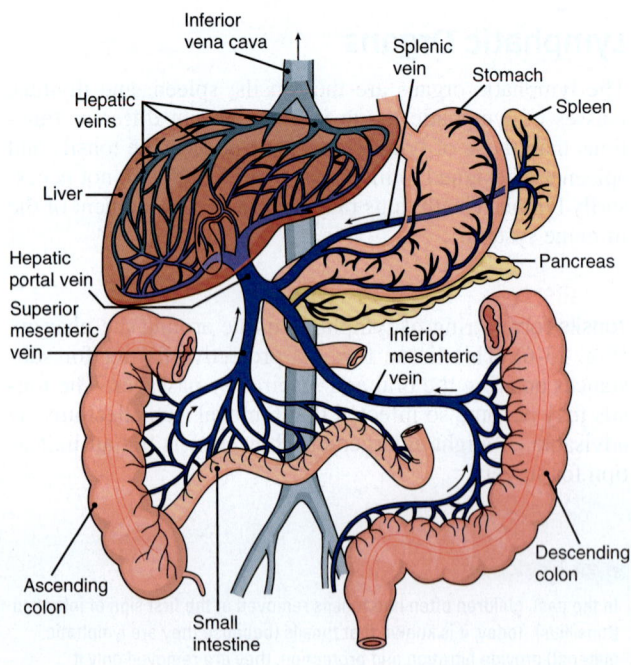

Figure 23-8 Hepatic portal circulation.

stomach, intestine, spleen, and pancreas empty into veins. These veins drain into a common vessel, the *portal vein*, which leads into the liver.

In the liver, blood again enters capillaries, called *sinusoids*. Here, the liver extracts appropriate materials and chemically modifies them. The liver synthesizes, stores, detoxifies, regulates, and transforms these raw materials into useful substances to meet body needs. The useful substances and blood then empty into the *hepatic vein* that leads to the *inferior vena cava*. Chapter 26 further describes digestion and liver functions.

Cerebral Circulation

Circulation to the brain is vital in maintaining life and functioning ability. Anteriorly, one branch of the *common carotid artery* is the *internal carotid artery*. The internal carotid **anastomoses** (connects) with the circle of Willis, thus providing oxygenated blood to the brain. The *right vertebral artery* and *left vertebral artery* branch from the *subclavian artery* at the posterior aspect of the brain and join at the brain stem to create the *basilar artery*. From here, blood is also transported to the circle of Willis. The *circle of Willis* (*cerebral arterial circle*) is formed by the *anterior communicating artery, posterior communicating artery, anterior cerebral artery, posterior cerebral artery*, and *internal carotid artery*. Figure 23-9 shows the arteries that supply the brain, including the arteries of the circle of Willis. All these arteries supply different areas of the brain with blood. Blood returns to the heart via venous sinuses that transport blood to the internal jugular veins and back to the heart.

Cerebral blood flow is 10%–15% of total cardiac output. Blood pressure is one factor that has an impact on blood flow. Adequate *cerebral perfusion* (blood flow to the brain) is required. The mean arterial blood pressure (**MABP**) is calculated based on the relationship between the systolic and diastolic BP. The brain requires a continuous flow of blood because it requires a constant supply of oxygen and nutrients (specifically glucose) to survive. The brain does not have the ability to create a collateral circulation, as the heart does in some cases.

The circle of Willis is important because it allows blood to continue to flow in the brain if one of the arteries supplying the brain is blocked. (An *embolus* is a clot that can lodge in an artery, thereby causing a blockage, a cerebral vascular accident [CVA] or stroke.) In the brain, the *middle cerebral artery* branch is the most likely location for emboli (Slater, 2020). A disruption of blood flow for any reason, for even a short period of time, can cause unconsciousness. Brain damage or death can occur if the disruption lasts for more than a few minutes (due to brain cell death).

Blood–Brain Barrier

The blood–brain barrier (**BBB**) is an "adaptation of the circulation" that protects the brain. Specialized cells in brain capillaries allow only certain substances from the blood to enter the brain. Capillaries in the brain are less permeable and much tighter than other capillaries in the body, thus limiting what substances are admitted into the cerebral circulation and to brain tissue. Also, specialized brain neuroglia, *astrocytes*, assist in creating selective permeability in the brain.

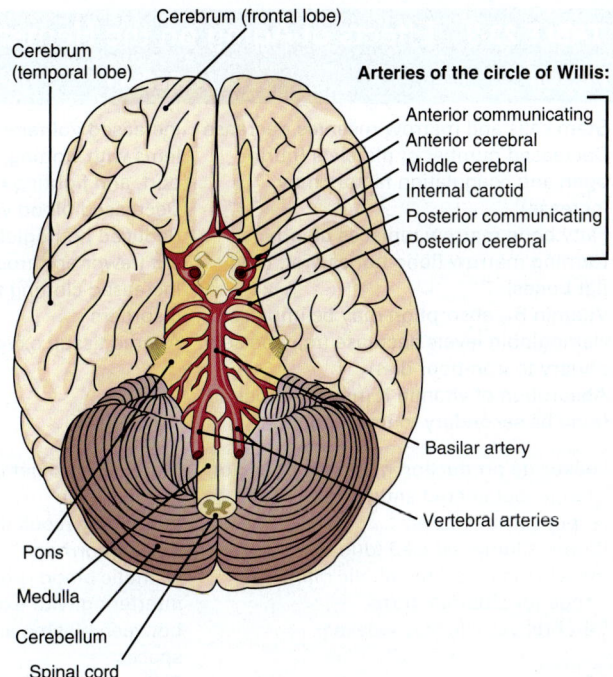

Figure 23-9 Arteries that supply the brain, viewed from behind. The arteries that make up the circle of Willis are shown in the center of the brain.

> **Key Concept**
> The circle of Willis helps provide uninterrupted blood supply to the brain. The blood–brain barrier protects the brain from harmful substances.

LYMPHATIC CIRCULATION

Lymph only carries fluid *away* from tissues. The initial lymphatics (prelymphatics, lymph capillaries) drain into larger lymph vessels. As discussed, the lymphatic system does not have an internal pumping system. The lymph from the upper right quadrant of the body drains into the *right lymphatic duct*. The remainder of the lymph drains into the left lymphatic duct, commonly known as the *thoracic duct*. The right lymphatic duct and thoracic duct then drain into the *left subclavian vein* at the base of the neck, where lymph mixes with blood plasma and becomes part of the general circulation.

Lymph enters lymph nodes through several *afferent* ("bringing toward") lymph vessels. The lymph nodes filter out dangerous substances (e.g., cancer cells and bacteria), dead RBCs, and foreign matter (e.g., smoke by-products) that become trapped in the nodes. The lymph then continues to flow away from the node through one or two *efferent* ("taking away") lymph vessels into the bloodstream. Plasma cells and lymphocytes that have reproduced within a lymph node can also be added to lymph for transportation to the blood.

Disorders of the blood and lymph can be quickly life threatening. Chapter 81 discusses heart and blood vessel disorders; Chapter 82 describes blood and lymph disorders; and Chapter 83 discusses cancer, which is often spread via the lymphatic system.

TABLE 23-3 Effects of Aging on the Hematologic and Lymphatic Systems

FACTOR	RESULT	NURSING IMPLICATIONS
Stem cells and marrow reserves decrease Decreased number of platelets (fibrinogen and coagulation factors may increase) Fatty bone marrow replaces blood-forming marrow (long bones first, then flat bones) Vitamin B_{12} absorption may be impaired Hemoglobin levels decrease (may be secondary to iron-poor diet) Absorption of vitamin K may be impaired (may be secondary to iron-poor diet)	Increased vulnerability to problems with clotting, oxygen transport, and fighting infection Decreased blood volume Reduced hemoglobin and hematocrit (fewer erythrocytes) Increased clotting time, bleeding disorders Altered tissue oxygenation	Assess the aging adult for weakened ability to compensate for illness or injury Decreased oxygen transport; client may require supplemental oxygen, especially during stress Monitor oxygen levels Discourage smoking Assess for evidence of gastrointestinal or other internal bleeding Ensure adequate dietary intake Encourage regular medical checkups, including colon and bladder examinations Assess prostate-specific antigen (PSA) in men
Leukocyte production generally does not change, but altered antigen–antibody responses may occur Blood volume reduced (due to decreased muscle mass and metabolic rate) Range for albumin drops Cerebral vessels may weaken	More likely to get infections; may feel less pain Injury may result in more dangerous hemorrhage Osmotic blood pressure drops, interfering with exchange of fluids between plasma and interstitial spaces CVA possible	Monitor closely for early signs of infection (e.g., increased fatigue, anorexia, confusion); fever or elevated leukocyte count may not be present Treat injuries immediately Observe for hemorrhage Take steps to maintain homeostasis Observe for signs of CVA and treat immediately

SPECIAL CONSIDERATIONS Lifespan

Nursing care for the older adult must adapt to changes related to aging. The aging process can have a significant effect on the hematologic and lymphatic systems (Table 23-3).

NCLEX Alert

Variations of growth and development across the lifespan are common NCLEX clinical concepts. Issues related to aging may involve prenatal, infant, young adult, mature adult, or older adult concerns.

STUDENT SYNTHESIS

KEY POINTS

- The functions of the hematologic system include transportation, regulation, and protection.
- Hematopoiesis, the formation of blood cells, originates in stem cells in red bone marrow.
- Blood is composed of plasma and formed elements, including RBCs, WBCs, and platelets.
- Plasma is 90% water. The remaining 10% is composed of proteins, salts, nutrients, wastes, gases, hormones, and enzymes.
- Erythrocytes (RBCs) are the most numerous blood cells. Each RBC contains hemoglobin, responsible for carrying oxygen.
- WBCs fight infection. Each type (basophil, eosinophil, neutrophil, lymphocyte, monocyte) has different mechanisms for this function.
- Platelets and numerous clotting factors must react in sequence before blood clotting can occur.
- Hemorrhage is usually thought of as the loss of a considerable amount of blood. Hemostasis refers to the stoppage of bleeding.
- ABO and Rh blood groups are inherited combinations of antigens and antibodies.
- Lymph tissues filter blood, destroy pathogens, and develop antibodies against antigens.
- Lymphatic organs include the tonsils, spleen, and thymus.
- Pulmonary circulation allows blood to be oxygenated for distribution in the systemic circulation.
- The largest circulatory route is the systemic circulation, which transports oxygen, nutrients, and wastes to and from all body cells.
- Several arteries come together in the brain to form the circle of Willis. This arterial circle helps maintain and protect cerebral blood flow.
- The blood–brain barrier selectively determines what substances will enter the brain from the blood, to prevent harmful substances from entering the brain.
- The hepatic portal circulation moves venous blood from abdominal organs (gastrointestinal [GI] system, pancreas, spleen) to the liver via the portal vein. The blood travels through the liver, where it undergoes a variety of changes before entering the hepatic vein and then the inferior vena cava for transport back to the heart.
- The lymph system drains interstitial fluid into lymphatic vessels, which empty into the veins.

CRITICAL THINKING EXERCISES

1. Explain how blood, interstitial fluid, and lymph are related to maintenance of homeostasis.
2. Explain why some people choose to have some of their own blood removed and stored for possible future use in an emergency.
3. Discuss how inhalation promotes or inhibits the flow of lymphatic fluid.

NCLEX-STYLE REVIEW QUESTIONS

1. A client sustained a partial thickness burn to the chest and neck. Which laboratory test will the nurse monitor for elevated levels?
   a. Neutrophils
   b. Eosinophils
   c. Lymphocytes
   d. Monocytes
2. The nurse reviews a client's laboratory studies and observes a hemoglobin level of 9.6 g/dl. Which data collected by the nurse would be significant related to this laboratory result?
   a. The client has a blood pressure of 110/78 mmHg.
   b. The client has a temperature of 99.6 °F.
   c. The client has expiratory wheezes.
   d. The client has rectal bleeding.
3. An older adult client is suspected to have impaired absorption of vitamin B_{12} due to lack of intrinsic factor. Which nursing intervention is appropriate for this client?
   a. Monitor the stools for blood.
   b. Monitor the client's temperature.
   c. Monitor the oxygen saturation.
   d. Prepare the client to receive a blood transfusion.
4. The older adult client has a decrease in stem cells and marrow reserves. Which nursing action would the nurse perform to decrease the occurrence of complications?
   a. Monitor for weakened ability to compensate for illness or injury.
   b. Administer vitamin K as prescribed.
   c. Encourage the intake of fiber-rich foods.
   d. Monitor closely for early signs of dementia.
5. A client with chronic kidney failure has a hemoglobin level of 8.6 g/dL and is chronically fatigued. Which nursing action would the nurse prepare to administer?
   a. IV gamma globulinl
   b. Subcutaneous heparin
   c. Recombinant human erythropoietin
   d. Vitamin K

CHAPTER RESOURCES

Enhance your learning with additional resources on thePoint!

Student Resources related to this chapter can be found at
thePoint.lww.com/Rosdahl12e.

24 The Immune System

Learning Objectives

1. Describe lymphocytes, their functions, and where they are produced.
2. Differentiate between B cells and T cells (lymphocytes).
3. Describe nursing implications related to the absence of or a deficiency in antibody production.
4. Differentiate between nonspecific and specific immunity. Compare and contrast naturally acquired and artificially acquired active and passive immunities.
5. Describe the process of antibody-mediated immunity. Explain how the "lock-and-key" concept applies to the antigen–antibody complex.
6. Explain mechanisms antibodies use to destroy antigens.
7. Describe effects of aging on the immune system.

Important Terminology

acquired (adaptive) immunity
antibody-mediated immunity
artificially acquired immunity
B cells/B lymphocytes
cell-mediated immunity
complement fixation
cytokine
gamma globulin
humoral immunity
immunization
inborn immunity
naturally acquired immunity
nonspecific immunity
specific immunity

Acronyms

T cells/T lymphocytes
thymus
vaccine
Ab
Ag
GG
Ig
IgA
IgD
IgE
IgG
IgM

The human body must always protect itself against foreign invaders. It does so using a "layered defense" system, which includes the skin and chemical barriers, as well as innate and adaptive immune systems (immunity). This chapter is primarily concerned with the latter. Remember that pathogens are able to mutate rapidly, thus avoiding the immune system's defenses.

Immunity is the body's ability to recognize and destroy specific pathogens, such as bacteria, viruses, fungi, and also parasites, and to prevent infectious diseases. The immune system also recognizes some tumor cells. When the immune system is compromised, immunodeficiency diseases may occur. When the immune system is overreactive, disorders such as allergies and autoimmune disorders may result.

Key Concept
The immune system must distinguish between "self" (normal components of the body) and "nonself" (foreign tissues or substances). In some cases, this mechanism is faulty and the body destroys its own cells.

STRUCTURE AND FUNCTION

The body's *immune system* includes *bone marrow, lymphoid organs,* and the *mononuclear phagocyte system* (the *reticuloendothelial system*). This system is closely related to the circulatory system, which assists by transporting immune components. Primary functions of the immune system include defense, homeostasis, and surveillance. Box 24-1 describes these functions. Figure 24-1 shows many specific organs and tissues in the immune system.

BONE MARROW AND LYMPHOCYTE PRODUCTION

Cells in bone marrow can develop into any of three types of blood cells: erythrocytes (RBCs), leukocytes (WBCs), or thrombocytes (platelets). WBCs defend against disease organisms, toxins, and irritants. The two types of WBCs are granular (neutrophils, basophils, and eosinophils) and agranular (monocytes and lymphocytes). Lymphocytes are found in blood, lymph, and lymphoid tissues, such as lymph nodes and tonsils. They form immune cells and their precursors and are the focus of this chapter. (Chapter 23 described the other blood cells in more detail.)

- Lymphocytes are the "cornerstone" of the immune system; they alone have the ability to recognize foreign substances in the body.
- Differentiation of lymphocytes into special lymphocytes called **B cells** (**B lymphocytes**) and **T cells** (**T lymphocytes**) must occur before detection of foreign invaders begins. T lymphocytes can recognize invaders and certain cancer cells. They help protect against viral infections and destroy recognized cancer cells. B lymphocytes develop into cells that produce antibodies (plasma cells).

Figure 24-2 illustrates the development of immune system cells.

Key Concept
Lymphocytes formed in bone marrow and lymphatic tissues can transform into specialized cells, B cells and T cells. B cells provide humoral immunity by reacting to antigens and producing antibodies. (The term *antigen* is an abbreviation for "*antibody generator*.") Antibodies then target antigens for destruction. T cells, which proliferate at the direction of thymic hormones, attack infected cells and provide cell-mediated (cellular) immunity.

CHAPTER 24   The Immune System   287

> **Box 24-1   Functions of the Immune System**
>
> **DEFENSE**
> - Resists invasion by foreign microorganisms, including viruses and intracellular parasites
> - Attacks some pathogens directly
> - Attacks foreign antigens—usually proteins (including transplanted organs)
> - Helps body to fight cancer cells
> - Produces antibodies and immunoglobulins
> - Produces inflammatory response
> - Produces memory cells
>
> **HOMEOSTASIS**
> - Digests and removes damaged cellular substances
> - Kills diseased cells (especially those infected with viruses)
>
> **SURVEILLANCE**
> - Recognizes and destroys cellular mutations
> - Recognizes and destroys foreign cells
> - Monitors for presence of antigens

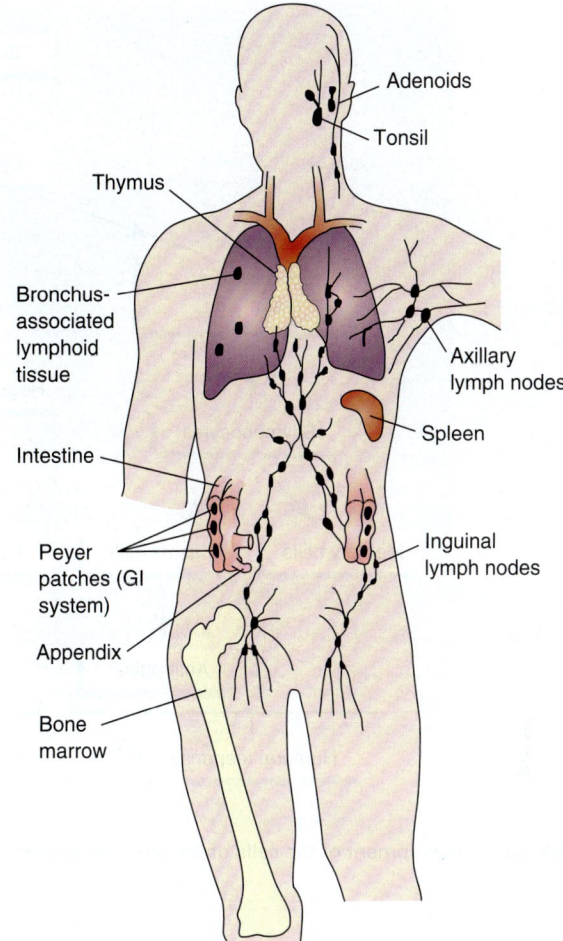

Figure 24-1 Central and peripheral lymphoid organs and tissues involved in the immune system.

B Lymphocytes

Stem cells in bone marrow are responsible both for production of B lymphocytes and for their maturation. After maturing, B cells can produce antibodies. Exposure to an antigen causes B cells to enlarge, rapidly multiply, and produce colonies of clones, although B cells do not respond to all pathogens. Most of these clones become plasma cells, which produce specific *antibodies* to circulate in the blood. These antibodies provide humoral immunity (*humoral* = body fluid). In **humoral immunity**, *macrophages* (large cells) engulf and destroy antigens after antibodies have identified them for destruction.

Those clones that do not become plasma cells remain in the body as *memory cells*. On repeated exposure to an antigen, memory cells can immediately produce antibodies. This "immunologic memory," in many cases, makes a person immune to *reinfection* after having had a disease, but this is not true for all diseases.

> **Key Concept**
>
> The second exposure to an antigen can cause a quicker and more dramatic response than the first because of "immunologic memory." (The first exposure causes a more delayed reaction because it takes time to form antibodies, which are ready for the second exposure and act quickly.) This is an important concept when related to allergic reactions.

B lymphocytes are found predominantly in organized lymphoid tissues, such as the spleen. They constitute only about 10%–20% of circulating lymphocytes in the blood. Even fewer B cells are found in lymph. The B cell recognizes whole pathogens without antigen processing. Each specific B cell recognizes a specific antigen.

Antigens and Antibodies

An antigen (**Ag**) is any foreign substance or molecule entering the body that stimulates an immune response (the activity of B or T lymphocytes). Most antigens are large protein molecules found on the surface of foreign organisms, RBCs, or tissue cells; on pollen; and in toxins and foods. Some carbohydrates and lipids also act as antigens.

An antibody (**Ab**) is a protein substance the body produces in response to an antigen. *B lymphocytes* are responsible for antibody production. All antibodies are contained in the *gamma globulin fraction* of blood plasma. Therefore, antibodies are commonly called **gamma globulins** (**GG**) or immunoglobulins (**Ig**). The five basic groups of immunoglobulins are as follows:

- **IgM**: Antibody produced on initial exposure to an antigen (e.g., after a first tetanus immunization); stimulates complement activity. IgM is abundant in blood, but not usually present in organs and tissues; not transferred across the placenta.
- **IgG**: The only antibody transferred from mother to fetus across the placenta; protects fetus against antitoxins, viruses, and bacteria and protects the newborn for the first few months. IgG is the most common antibody and is produced on second and future exposures to an antigen (e.g., after a tetanus *booster*). It is present in the blood (intravascular) and in the tissues (extravascular); often

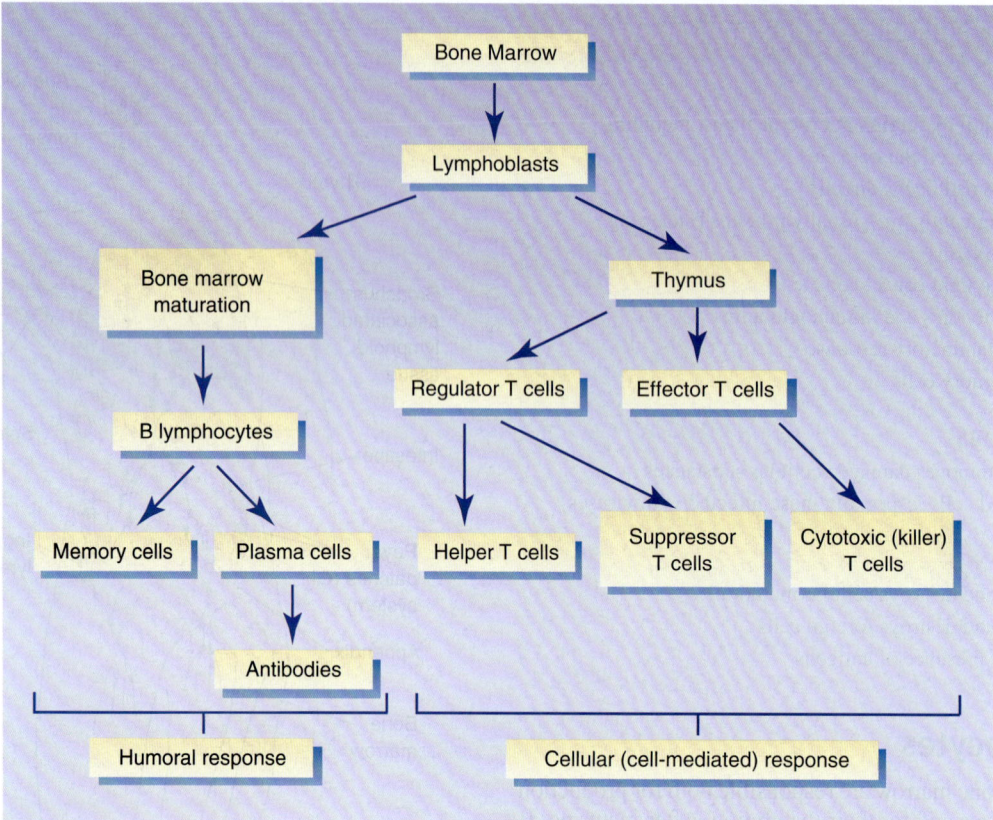

Figure 24-2 Development of the cells of the immune system.

called gamma globulin, it is the main component of commercial immunoglobulin.
- **IgA**: The major component of secretions such as saliva, tears, and bronchial fluids, IgA is transported across mucous membranes and protects mucosal surfaces. It is important in defense against invasion of microbes via the nose, eyes, lungs, and intestines. IgA is found in blood, in gastrointestinal (GI) and mucosal secretions, and in breast milk.
- **IgE**: Responsible for immediate-type allergic reactions, including latex allergies, which can cause many problems for healthcare personnel (ranging from hives to anaphylaxis and death). Although this antibody causes problems in developed countries, it is helpful in the developing world in fighting against parasitic infections, such as river blindness.
- **IgD**: Believed to function as an antigen receptor, it is present in the blood in very small amounts.

Each *antigen* (foreign invader) stimulates production of its own specific *antibody*. The human body can make about one million individual antibodies. Antibodies do not destroy antigens themselves, but label antigens for destruction by other substances.

Key Concept
Functions of immunoglobulins vary, depending on the antigen. Immunoglobulins disable bacteria (antitoxins), *opsonize* (coat) bacteria so they become targets for phagocytes, and/or link to antigens to create enzymes (complement action).

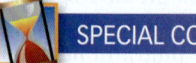 SPECIAL CONSIDERATIONS Lifespan

A child with spina bifida (congenital spinal column defect) is at increased risk for latex allergies because the mucous membranes of bladder and rectum are exposed to latex during frequent examinations and procedures, such as urinary catheterization. Nonlatex gloves and equipment should be used when possible for all children, particularly those with this disorder. (This would help prevent development of latex allergy in healthcare workers as well.)

T Lymphocytes

Some immature stem cells produced in the bone marrow migrate to the thymus gland to become T cells (thymus-derived lymphocytes), an action primarily stimulated by the hormone *thymosin*. T cells make up 80%–90% of lymphocytes found in circulating blood. While in the thymus, T cells proliferate and become sensitized (capable of combining with specific foreign antigens, to produce an immunity called **cell-mediated immunity**).

T lymphocytes are generally responsible for fighting cancer cells, viruses, and intracellular parasites. They are particularly important in dealing with viruses because they kill the host cell and prevent replication. T cells enable the body to differentiate between "self" and "nonself," which is usually helpful to the body. However, this function can cause problems, for example, when T cells cause tissue or organ rejection after transplantation, by recognizing these tissues

TABLE 24-1 Lymphocytes Involved in Immune Responses

CELL TYPE	FUNCTION	TYPE OF IMMUNE RESPONSE
B cell	Produces antibodies or immunoglobulins (IgA, IgD, IgE, IgG, IgM)	Humoral
T cell		Cellular (cell-mediated)
Helper T$_4$	Attacks foreign invaders (antigens) directly	
	Initiates and augments inflammatory response	
Helper T$_1$	Increases activated cytotoxic T cells	
Helper T$_2$	Increases B-cell antibody production	
Suppressor T	Suppresses the immune response	
Memory T	Remembers contact with an antigen and on subsequent exposures mounts an immune response	
Cytotoxic T (killer T)	Lyses cells infected with virus; plays a role in graft rejection	
Non-T or B lymphocytes		Nonspecific
Null cells	Destroys antigens already coated with antibody	
Natural killer (NK) (granular lymphocyte)	Defends against microorganisms and some types of malignant cells; produces cytokines	

From Hinkle, J., & Cheever, K. (2018). *Brunner & Suddarth's textbook of medical-surgical nursing* (14th ed.). Wolters Kluwer.

as "nonself" and working to eliminate them. (Specific antirejection medications must be given to neutralize this rejection response in recipients of most transplants.)

Several types of T lymphocytes exist, each having its own function. For a T cell to react with a specific antigen, the antigen must first be presented to the T cell on the surface of a macrophage. Macrophages, when combined with T cells, release substances called *interleukins*, which stimulate T-cell growth. Table 24-1 identifies types and associated functions of B lymphocytes and T lymphocytes.

One type of T cell is the *helper T cell*, which has several subtypes. These cells often have no cytotoxic (cell-killing) function per se. They help regulate innate and adaptive immune responses by instructing other cells to kill infected cells or pathogens. Many receptors on the helper T cell must be bound by specific antigens to activate the helper cell; this requires a longer time of exposure. They also release *cytokines*, which help macrophages and help activate antibody-producing B cells.

Killer T cells (cytotoxic T cells) are another subgroup of T cells that kill cells infected with pathogens or are otherwise damaged or defective. Killer T cells search for cells where receptors possess a specific antigen and then release a specific cytotoxin, such as perforin. (Perforin allows pores [holes] to form in the plasma membranes of target cells, allowing cellular contents to flow out and substances to enter these cells [osmotic lysis] and kill them.) Unlike helper T cells, killer T cells can be activated when bound to a single antigen molecule.

Key Concept

T cells recognize a "nonself" target only after antigens have been processed and presented, combined with a "self-receptor" called a major histocompatibility (MHC) molecule, which coats the molecule with an antibody.

B cells are involved in humoral immune response. T cells provide cell-mediated (cellular) immune response. Both B cells and T cells have receptor molecules that recognize specific target cells.

Other Lymphocytes

A *natural killer (NK) cell* is slightly larger than a B or a T cell and is considered "nonspecific" in immune response. These specialized lymphocytes secrete some cytokines and kill certain microbes (particularly viruses) and cancer cells. They are called *natural* because they do not require maturation and "education" as do B and T cells but are ready to target specific cells as soon as they are produced. Thus, they are part of the body's natural defense against cancer.

Cytokines are proteins that act as messengers to help regulate some functions of lymphocytes and macrophages during the immune response and some are given by injection to treat specific diseases.

Types of cytokines include the following:

- *Interferon-alpha:* used to treat certain cancers, such as hairy cell leukemia
- *Interferon-beta:* believed to be helpful in multiple sclerosis
- *Interleukin-1:* produced by macrophages, mobilizes T lymphocytes
- *Interleukin-2:* produced by T cells, stimulates production of interferon. Used to treat many solid cancers, such as malignant melanoma and kidney cancer (also has adverse effects)
- *Interleukin-3:* required for differentiation of certain T cells
- *Interleukin-8:* guides neutrophils to the source of an antigen
- *Interleukin-12:* stimulates natural killer cells
- *Granulocyte colony-stimulating factor:* helps increase neutrophils in clients who are undergoing chemotherapy
- *Lymphokines:* secreted by lymphocytes

Key Concept

When NK cells are incubated with interleukin-2, they are called lymphokine-activated killer T cells. They then function even more effectively than do NK cells as a biologic treatment for cancer.

LYMPHOID ORGANS

Primary (Central) Lymphoid Organs/Tissues

In addition to bone marrow, the **thymus** gland is considered a *central* or *primary* lymphoid organ. This small gland weighs 1 oz at most and is located in the mediastinum of the upper chest. It is most active early in life and begins to shrink at puberty. (Premature involution of the thymus may be caused by starvation or disease.) T lymphocytes mature in the thymus in children (and also in other lymphoid tissues in adults) before they can perform their immune functions. The thymus produces the hormones *thymosin, thymic humoral factor* (*THF*), *thymic factor* (*TF*), and *thymopoietin*, which promote proliferation and maturation of T cells.

Peripheral (Secondary) Lymphoid Organs

The *peripheral* or *secondary* lymphoid organs of the immune system include lymphoid structures scattered in submucosal layers of the respiratory, gastrointestinal (Peyer patches), and genitourinary tracts. In addition, accessory tissues include the tonsils, adenoids, lymph nodes, and spleen. The defense functions of these organs are primarily related to filtration of tissue fluid or lymph for foreign particles and external microorganisms (Chapter 23).

THE MONONUCLEAR PHAGOCYTE SYSTEM

The *mononuclear phagocyte system*, or *reticuloendothelial system*, consists of specialized cells throughout the body that can ingest foreign particulate matter. These cells begin as monocytes and transform into macrophages (*phagocytic* or *endocytic* cells) after entering other tissues via the bloodstream. This system is concerned with destruction of worn-out blood cells, bacteria, cancer cells, and other dangerous foreign substances. Some macrophages have special names, such as *Kupffer cells* in the liver sinusoids and *dust cells* in the lungs.

Mononuclear phagocytes play a very important role in both specific and nonspecific immunity. In specific immunity, they are responsible for capturing (via phagocytosis), processing, and presenting antigens to lymphocytes for destruction. The macrophage-bound antigen, when presented to the B or T lymphocyte, triggers the humoral or cell-mediated immune response.

System Physiology

NONSPECIFIC DEFENSE MECHANISMS

The body possesses several defense systems. *Nonspecific defense mechanisms* (sometimes called **nonspecific immunity**) fight a variety of foreign invaders. Examples of nonspecific defense mechanisms include the following:

- The *skin* provides a physical barrier and secretes enzymes that kill or reduce virulence of bacteria.
- Mechanical reactions, such as coughing or sneezing, help remove pathogenic material.
- Chemical barriers, such as normal flora (microorganisms) of the GI system, neutralize or kill microorganisms.
- *Tears* dilute and wash away irritating substances and microbes.
- *Neutrophils, dendritic cells*, and *monocytes* (cellular barriers) ingest and destroy bacteria and toxins and remove cellular debris. They "patrol" the body for pathogens or can be called in by cytokines. Macrophages live in tissues and produce enzymes and other chemicals; neutrophils are the most common. They go to the site of inflammation (by *chemotaxis*) and are the first to arrive. They are antigen-presenting cells and activate the adaptive immune system, as well as clean out debris from the infection.
- *Interferon*, a protein made by several types of cells, inhibits virus production and infection.
- *Fever* and *inflammation* intensify the effects of interferons, inhibit the growth of some microbes, and speed up body reactions, aiding in tissue repair.
- *Cilia* and *macrophages* (phagocytic cells) in the mucous membrane of the respiratory tract trap and remove microbes and dust. Tiny hairs in the nose and the turbulent air flow there also serve as mechanical barriers to dust and other foreign particles.
- *Hydrochloric acid* in the stomach destroys pathogens taken in with foods.
- Other substances, such as earwax, mucus, vaginal secretions, prostatic fluid, and semen, provide protection against pathogens.
- *Vomiting, defecation*, and *urination* expel microbes from the body, along with normal waste products.

SPECIFIC DEFENSE MECHANISMS

Specific defense mechanisms (**specific immunity**), the final line of defense against disease, allows the body to recognize and respond to foreign substances. Cellular defenses include *humoral immunity*, which occurs quickly when lymphocytes recognize a foreign substance. *Cell-mediated immunity* occurs more slowly and depends on T lymphocytes. Both types are considered specific defense mechanisms because they act against specific, individual harmful substances. Specific immunity can be classified into two main categories: inborn and acquired, both based on antigen–antibody response (Fig. 24-3).

Inborn Immunity

Inborn immunity is inherited or genetic. This inherited, natural, or innate immunity may be common to all members of a species (e.g., humans have specific immunity to many diseases of animals). Inborn immunity may also be common to a specific population, sex, or ethnic group or to an individual person.

Acquired (Adaptive) Immunity

Acquired or adaptive immunity is attained through natural or artificial sources. Both *naturally* and *artificially* acquired immunity can be attained either *actively* or *passively* (Fig. 24-3).

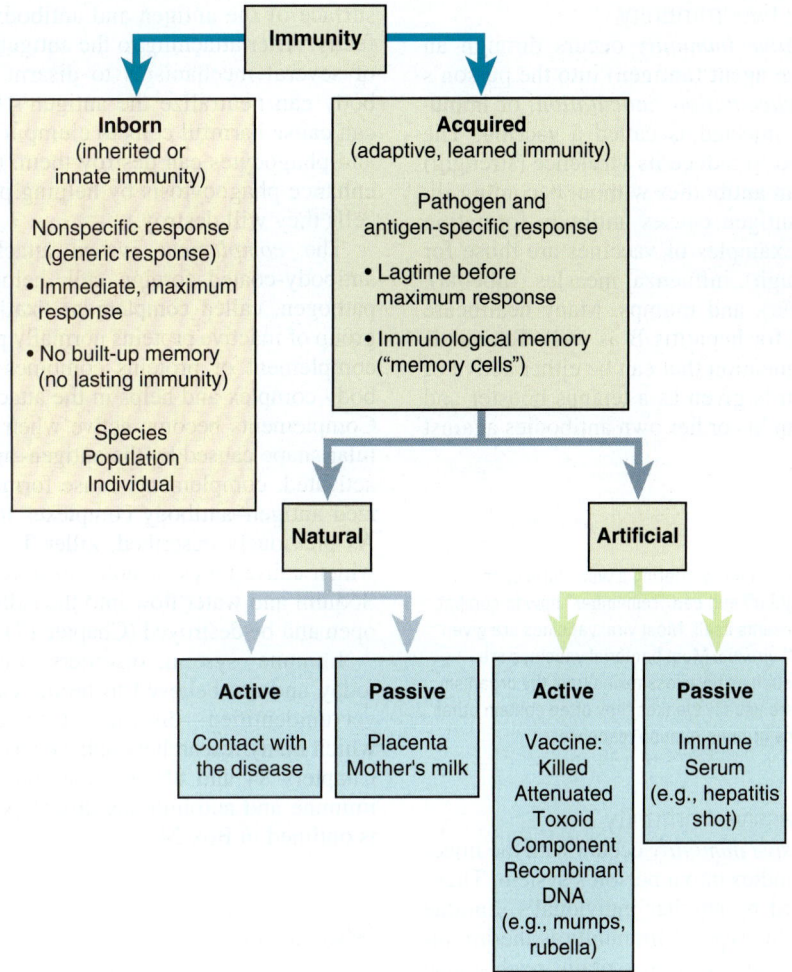

Figure 24-3 Types of specific immunity.

Naturally Acquired Immunity

Naturally acquired immunity occurs when a person is not deliberately exposed to a causative agent. This immunity can occur both *actively* and *passively*.

Naturally Acquired Active Immunity

Naturally acquired active immunity results when a child is exposed to and develops a disease (e.g., measles or chickenpox) and subsequently builds up antibodies (immunity) to infections caused by the same organism. Individuals can also develop acquired immunity during their lives as they are exposed to disease-causing organisms. They do not necessarily have to become ill with the disease; they may build up immunity slowly. In other words, acquired immunity is built on lifetime exposures. Remember that the body manufactures not only cells that target the infecting antigen but also memory cells. Each time the person is exposed to a disease, the memory cells activate a response that produces antibodies to the offending antigen. Usually, the response is faster with each exposure, as the "memory" increases. Naturally acquired active immunity can last a few years or a lifetime.

> **Key Concept**
>
> Exposure to disease-causing organisms during one's life stimulates the process of naturally acquired active immunity.

Naturally Acquired Passive Immunity

Naturally acquired passive immunity occurs between mothers and infants. Immunity is transferred from mother to fetus during pregnancy via the placental circulation exchange. If the baby is breastfed, the baby also receives protection after birth through the mother's breast milk. Naturally acquired passive immunity can last to about 6 months of age, when the infant's own immune system begins to take over. (The infant does not synthesize antibodies; they are "borrowed" from the mother.)

Artificially Acquired Immunity

Artificially acquired immunity occurs when a person is deliberately exposed to a causative agent and can also be acquired through *active* or *passive* means.

Artificially Acquired Active Immunity

Artificially acquired active immunity occurs through an injection of the causative agent (antigen) into the person's system. This is called *vaccination, inoculation,* or **immunization**; the substance injected is called a **vaccine**. The causative agent is diluted to reduce its virulence (strength) so the recipient will form antibodies without becoming ill. (The presence of the antigen causes antibody formation in the person's body.) Examples of vaccines are those for pertussis (whooping cough), influenza, measles (rubeola), German measles (rubella), and mumps. Many healthcare workers are immunized for hepatitis B as well. Tetanus is an example of an immunization that can be either active or passive. The active form is given as a tetanus booster and causes the person to form his or her own antibodies against tetanus.

> **Key Concept**
>
> A vaccine boosts the immune system by offering a weak form of an infection that the body can fight off and can "remember" how to combat when a more virulent form presents itself. Most viral vaccines are given as live attenuated (weakened) viruses. Most bacterial vaccines are based on other components, such as harmless toxins from the organism. Because bacterial vaccines are usually weaker, they often contain other substances designed to induce greater immune response.

Artificially Acquired Passive Immunity

Artificially acquired passive immunity occurs with the injection of ready-made antibodies into a person's system. These antibodies were produced by another individual's immune system. An example of this type of immunity is the immunization for rabies. This immunization contains ready-made anti-rabies antibodies and is given in the event of a bite by a rabid animal or if the animal cannot be located and tested. Tetanus toxoid can also be given in the passive form if a person has become ill with tetanus.

Another type of artificially acquired passive immunity is instituted with the injection of immunoglobulin IgG (gamma globulin). This immunization is given after disease exposure and results in only short-term immunity.

ANTIGEN–ANTIBODY REACTION

Antigen–antibody reactions begin with B lymphocytes, whose job is to produce humoral immunity. *Humoral immunity* is the body's resistance to circulating disease-producing antigens and bacteria. B cells become plasma cells and then work to produce antibodies.

Antibody-mediated immunity changes an antigen, rendering it harmless to the body. The antibody accomplishes this by binding to the antigen, forming an antigen–antibody complex. This binding can be compared to a "lock-and-key" mechanism; an antibody forms in response to only one specific antigen. The patterns on the membrane surface of the antigen and antibody must fit together perfectly. After attaching to the antigen, the antibody uses one of several mechanisms to disarm the antigen. The antibody can neutralize the antigen's toxins, or the antibody can cause harmful cells to clump together so macrophages and phagocytes can destroy them. (Antibodies promote or enhance phagocytosis by helping phagocytes attach to the cells they will destroy.)

The *complement system* attacks the surface of an antibody-coated foreign cell, helping antibodies kill the pathogen, called **complement fixation**. A *complement* is a group of inactive proteins normally present in the blood. The complement of proteins combines with the antigen–antibody complex and helps in the attack on invading antigens. Complements become active when exposed to altered cellular shape caused by the antigen–antibody complex. When activated, complements cause formation of highly specialized antigen–antibody complexes that target specific cells. As previously described, killer T cells release cytotoxins, which cause pores or holes to develop in cell membranes. Sodium and water flow into the cells, causing them to burst open and be destroyed (Chapter 17).

Immune system disorders are identified frequently today and are believed to be the cause of many other—as yet unidentified—disorders. Chapter 83 describes cancer, which many researchers believe has an immune component. Chapters 84 and 85 describe some of the more common immune and autoimmune disorders. The immune response is outlined in Box 24-2.

> **Key Concept**
>
> Some researchers have found that if a person remains calm and unstressed, they are less likely to sustain an autoimmune disorder. This is because the immune system "panics" under stress, believing that something is attacking the body from within.

SPECIAL CONSIDERATIONS Lifespan

Nursing care for older adults must adapt to changes related to aging. The aging process can produce a significant effect on the immune system (Table 24-2).

> **NCLEX Alert**
>
> The nurse should know terminology related to immunity, as well as processes related to the development of immunity. Be alert to the needs of the immune system across the lifespan. Nursing actions can involve client safety, prevention of infection, and concepts related to client teaching. Appropriate actions can involve multiple concepts that are intertwined in the NCLEX clinical situations.

CHAPTER 24 The Immune System

Box 24-2 Description of the Immune Response

- Recognition (of antigen) via antigen processing: Mostly by macrophages. Antigens ingested, broken up, packaged, carried to the surface of cell membrane, and assigned to T-cell receptor.
- Basophils and eosinophils secrete chemicals to defend against parasites. They also play a role in allergic reactions in asthma.
- Mobilization (of immune system): Cytokines released, other lymphocytes activated, and natural killer cells stimulated to secrete interferon. Interleukin-8 acts as signal to guide neutrophils to antigen (chemotaxis).
- Attack (killing or eliminating microbes): By macrophages, neutrophils, and natural killer cells. If invading microbe cannot be eliminated, it can be encapsulated or imprisoned by special cells (granuloma); for example, granuloma (tubercle) encloses the bacteria causing tuberculosis, rendering it unable to make the person ill.

HYPERSENSITIVITY DISORDERS
- Type I: anaphylaxis, hay fever, allergy
- Type II: cytotoxic, autoimmune hemolytic anemia, transfusion reactions
- Type III: immune complex disease reaction to Hepatitis B, some cancers
- Type IV: delayed (cell-mediated) hypersensitivity, PPD reactions, latex allergy, sarcoidosis

AUTOIMMUNE REACTION
- Malfunctioning or misinterpretation by immune system of body's own tissues (e.g., rheumatoid arthritis, scleroderma, myasthenia gravis [MG], pernicious anemia, systemic lupus erythematosis [SLE], type I diabetes mellitus, ankylosing spondylitis, Sjogren syndrome, multiple sclerosis [MS]).
- Mast cells are formed in connective tissue and mucous membranes. They help regulate the inflammatory response (mostly in allergy and anaphylactic reactions). They contain histamine, heparin, and other substances.

IMMUNODEFICIENCY DISORDERS (ABNORMAL RESPONSE TO ONE'S OWN TISSUES)
- Immune system is compromised and does not function adequately to prevent infections. Some immune disorders, such as HIV and AIDS, take advantage of the immune system's weaknesses and make themselves appear to be a normal part of the body.
- The innate (biologic) immune system (immediate nonspecific reactions), such as phagocytosis and the normal flora (microbes) of the GI system—does not require previous exposure to the antigen—is closely related to the nervous and sensory systems.
- The adaptive (acquired) immune system adapts to specific infection and improves the recognition of the invader (immunologic memory, humoral and cell-mediated immunity), producing a faster and stronger reaction—requires prior exposure to the antigen—and develops to recognize specific pathogens ("immunologic memory"), due to T cells and B cells.
- "Herd immunity" is the phenomenon of organisms living closely together and sharing minor infections all the time.

TABLE 24-2 Effects of Aging on the Immune System

FACTOR	RESULT	NURSING IMPLICATIONS
Numbers of T and B cells decrease, those remaining function poorly as stem cells Decreased antibody response Accessory lymphatic areas decrease (e.g., tonsils, thymus—become small islets of tissue)	Slowed or muted immune system reaction Increased incidence of tumors Greater susceptibility to infections	Assess regularly for signs of infection. Blood tests for even small rise in temperature or any signs of infection.
Baseline body temperature is lower	Absence of febrile response to infection Infection not obvious Organisms may not killed	Observe clients closely for clinical signs or symptoms of infection. Offer warmed blankets and keep room warm. *Change* in temperature is often more significant than actual temperature.
Body loses ability to differentiate between self and nonself	Autoimmune disorders increase	Mostly symptomatic treatment and specific procedures.
Immune system cannot recognize and destroy mutant cells In unrecognized infection, cardiovascular system cannot keep up with metabolic demands, causing cerebral hypoxia	Greater likelihood of cancers Change in mental status, delirium, confusion Susceptibility to bacteremia, septic shock, which can lead to death	Administer chemotherapy and other medications as ordered. Routine screening recommended. Any change in mental status should be assessed for possible infection first before other treatment initiated.

STUDENT SYNTHESIS

KEY POINTS

- Immunity is the specific resistance to disease involving production of a specific lymphocyte or antibody against a specific antigen.
- Both B cells and T cells derive from stem cells in the bone marrow.
- B cells go on to mature in the bone marrow, whereas T cells complete their maturation and develop immunocompetence in the thymus gland.
- Antigens (antibody generators) are substances (usually proteins) the immune system recognizes as foreign.
- An antibody is a protein that reacts specifically with the antigen that triggers its production.
- Humoral immunity refers to destruction of antigens by antibodies.
- Immunity can be inborn or acquired. Both naturally and artificially acquired immunity can be actively or passively acquired.
- Cell-mediated immunity refers to destruction of antigens by T cells.
- Exposure to disease-causing organisms over one's lifetime stimulates the process of acquired immunity.
- Humoral or antibody-mediated immunity protects against circulating disease-producing antigens and bacteria.
- Antibodies use several mechanisms to destroy antigens: neutralizing toxins, facilitating phagocytosis, imprisoning invader cells (granuloma), and complement fixation.

CRITICAL THINKING EXERCISES

1. Disease-producing organisms are all around you. Brainstorm how these organisms could contaminate the food supply. Which widespread effects could such an occurrence have on a population? Which defenses does your body employ to counteract microorganisms in food?
2. The mother of a newborn visits your facility. She has been reading about vaccines but does not understand how they work or why they are so important. How would you address this issue? Which information and explanations would you give to the mother to promote her understanding?
3. Based on the information above, what advantages in terms of immunity might an infant who is breastfed have over an infant who is formula fed?
4. Describe the relationship between immunity and the medical condition AIDS.

NCLEX-STYLE REVIEW QUESTIONS

1. The nurse is assigned to care for a child with spina bifida that requires routine urinary catheterization. Which priority action by the nurse is important to prevent complications caused by an IgE-mediated reaction?
   a. The use of nonlatex gloves for all procedures.
   b. Administer epinephrine prior to performing the procedure.
   c. Administer diphenhydramine (Benadryl) every 4 hour to prevent an allergic reaction.
   d. Ensure that the child does not receive antibiotics.

2. An older adult client has a decrease in the number of T cells and B cells. Which nursing action is a high priority for this client?
   a. Monitor for signs of infection.
   b. Give warm blankets and keep the room warm.
   c. Encourage the client to eat six small meals a day.
   d. Obtain strict intake and output.

3. A client has a decrease in T cells and B cells. The nurse would monitor the client for which complication?
   a. Altered kidney function
   b. Blood loss
   c. Joint swelling and tenderness
   d. Signs of infection

4. A client arrives in the emergency department after being bitten by a raccoon that wandered into the yard. The nurse should anticipate administering a rabies vaccine to provide which type of immunity?
   a. Naturally acquired active immunity
   b. Artificially acquired passive immunity
   c. Antibody-mediated immunity
   d. Naturally acquired passive immunity

5. The nurse is discussing the benefits of breastfeeding to a pregnant mother. Which statement made by the client demonstrates understanding of the benefits?
   a. The infant will receive artificially acquired active immunity to protect the infant from viruses.
   b. The infant will receive artificially acquired passive immunity to protect them from diseases such as multiple sclerosis.
   c. The infant will receive naturally acquired passive immunity to last approximately 6 months.
   d. The infant will receive antibody-mediated immunity to prevent the child from acquiring respiratory disorders for 1 year.

CHAPTER RESOURCES

Enhance your learning with additional resources on **thePoint**!

Student Resources related to this chapter can be found at **thePoint.lww.com/Rosdahl12e**.

25 The Respiratory System

Learning Objectives

1. Differentiate between internal and external respiration.
2. Describe anatomic relationships between the larynx, trachea, and esophagus.
3. Name and describe ways in which the respiratory system is protected.
4. State the function of surfactant.
5. Diagram the path of air flow in and out of the lungs, identifying structures involved and their functions.
6. Explain how the mechanisms of inspiration and expiration occur.
7. Describe the pleura and its function.
8. Describe two regulators of breathing and how they function.
9. Describe how the exchange of gases takes place in the alveoli of the lungs.
10. Describe effects of aging on the respiratory system and their nursing implications.

Important Terminology

alveolar duct	epiglottis	larynx	pleura	visceral pleura	IRV
alveolar sac	eupnea	lung	pleural cavity/	vocal cord	O_2
bronchi	expiration	mediastinum	pleural space		RV
bronchiole	external respiration	nares	respiration	**Acronyms**	TLC
cellular respiration	inspiration	nasopharynx	sinus	CO_2	TV
cilia	intercostal muscles	oropharynx	surfactant	ERV	URI
diaphragm	internal respiration	parietal pleura	trachea	FRC	VC
dyspnea	laryngopharynx	pharynx	ventilation	IC	V_T

The *respiratory system* is responsible for drawing air (containing oxygen) into the lungs, exchanging oxygen (O_2) for carbon dioxide (CO_2), and removing CO2 and other gaseous wastes. The lungs depend on the cardiovascular system to contribute to the gas exchange and deliver oxygen to body's cells. Remember: a person can live a few weeks without food, a few days without water, but only a few minutes without oxygen.

Respiration is the exchange of gases between the external environment and body cells. Respiration involves three processes: *ventilation* (breathing), *gas exchange* (in the alveoli of the lungs and body cells), and oxygen and carbon dioxide *transportation* (for metabolism, body processes, and waste removal). The air a person breathes in contains approximately 21% O_2 and 0.4% CO_2: normally, this provides ample oxygen for a person's needs. Exhaled air still contains approximately 16% O_2, but contains increased CO_2 (approximately 4.5%). The flow of air in the respiratory system also produces speech.

STRUCTURE AND FUNCTION

Respiratory system functions (Box 25-1) include taking oxygen from the atmosphere, exchanging it for carbon dioxide from the body, and assisting with regulation of body pH. (The circulatory system transports gases and the nervous system receives chemical and nervous stimuli at the brain's respiratory centers to initiate and control respirations.) Figure 25-1 illustrates the respiratory system. Its structures include air passages, pulmonary blood vessels, lungs, and muscles of breathing. Within these structures, atmospheric air is filtered, warmed, humidified, and gases are exchanged.

> **NCLEX Alert**
>
> The respiratory system involves the life-sustaining priorities of Airway and Breathing. Be alert to the terminology of normal and abnormal respiratory functioning.

UPPER RESPIRATORY TRACT

The upper respiratory tract (Fig. 25-2) consists of the nose, sinuses, pharynx, and larynx, which serve as pathways for air to enter and exit the lungs, where exchange of gases takes place.

Nose

Air enters the body through the right and left external **nares** (*nostrils*). If the nares become occluded (e.g., packing of the nose, a foreign object, swelling), breathing can occur through the mouth. The *nasal septum*, consisting of bone and cartilage, divides the internal nose into two sides or *cavities*. Nerve endings in the septum and nasal passages are responsible for the sense of smell. The olfactory nerve (CN I) transmits these nerve impulses to the brain (Chapter 21).

Mucous membrane, richly supplied with blood vessels, lines the nasal cavity. These blood vessels aid in warming and moistening air before it reaches the lungs. Sticky mucus

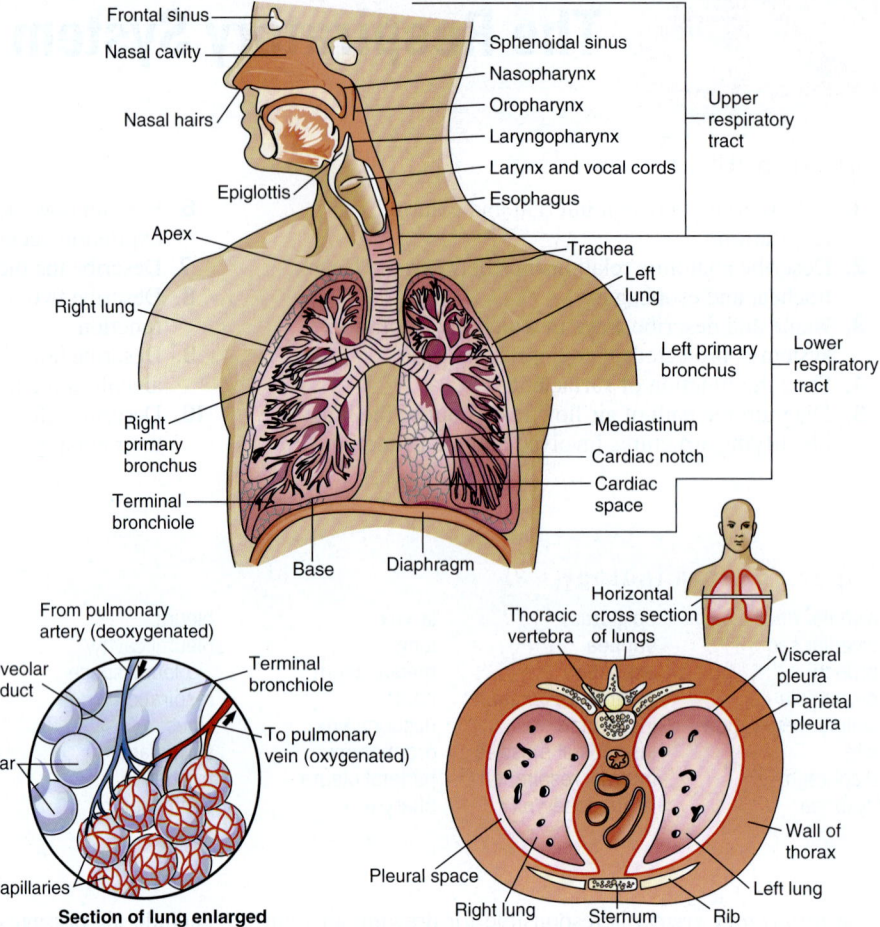

Figure 25-1 The respiratory system. **Top.** Upper respiratory structures and the structures of the thorax. **Bottom left.** An enlarged section of the lung showing the alveoli and capillary exchange. (The alveoli on the far left are shown without blood vessels.) **Bottom right.** A horizontal cross section of both lungs indicating the visceral and parietal pleurae and surrounding bones. The center portion is the mediastinum, containing the heart, esophagus, and major blood vessels.

Box 25-1 Functions of the Respiratory System

OXYGEN–CARBON DIOXIDE EXCHANGE
- Takes in oxygen from outside air
- Exchanges carbon dioxide for oxygen in lungs
- Exchanges oxygen for carbon dioxide at the cellular level
- Eliminates carbon dioxide from body

ACID–BASE BALANCE
- Assists in regulating body's pH
- Eliminates some water

PROTECTION
- Warms and moistens air before it enters lungs
- Mucus in nose traps foreign particles
- Coughing and sneezing dislodge foreign particles
- Yawning and swallowing help equalize pressures between inner ear and atmosphere

SPEECH PRODUCTION
- Air passes over vocal cords to produce sound

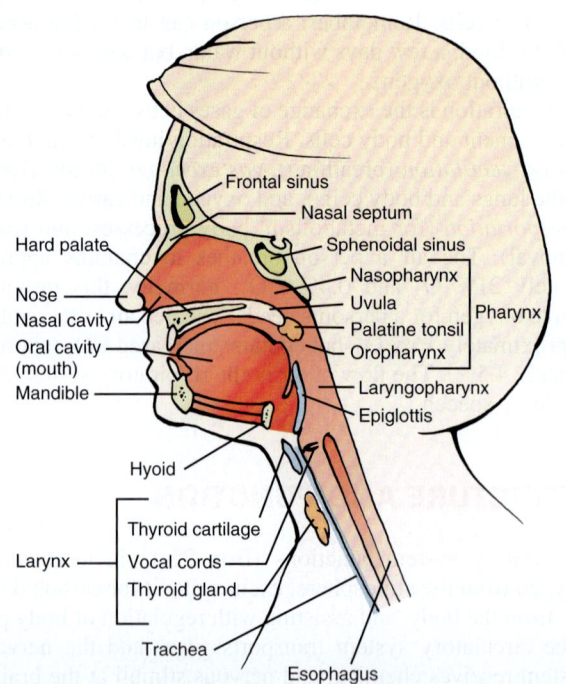

Figure 25-2 Anatomy of the upper respiratory tract.

(about 125 mL per day) traps dust particles, dirt, and microorganisms from the air. Hairs at the entrance of the nostrils and *cilia* (tiny hairlike projections) on the membranes serve as filters to remove some foreign particles that otherwise might be carried to the lungs. The cilia all beat in one direction, channeling mucus from the upper respiratory tract into the throat (known as the *mucociliary escalator*). Most secreted mucus is swallowed, where hydrochloric acid from the stomach destroys many pathogens. Three small bones, the *turbinates* or *conchae*, project into the nasal cavity to increase the surface area of the mucous membrane. This increased surface area helps warm and filter room air. The *nasolacrimal ducts* (*tear ducts* from the eyes) open into the upper nasal cavities, adding lubrication and also causing the "runny nose" that accompanies crying. (Cartilage is also present in the system from the nose to the small bronchi.)

Sinuses

Four cavities (**sinuses**) are located on each side of the nasal area (a total of eight). Mucosa, continuous with nasal mucosa, lines these sinuses and the entire respiratory system (called the *mucous blanket*). Sinuses lighten the skull and provide resonance for the voice, as well as enhancing the sense of smell. The names of the sinuses correspond with the facial bones in which they are situated. The largest are the *frontal sinuses* (one on each side above the eye socket) and the *maxillary sinuses* (one on each side of the nose, in conjunction with the maxillary bone). The *ethmoidal sinuses* lie between the eyes, and the *sphenoidal sinuses* lie on each side of the nasal cavity in the area of the orbit (eye socket). Figures 25-1 and 25-2 show several sinus cavities.

> **Nursing Alert** Sinuses drain directly into the nasal cavities, which drain into the throat. Because of the direct connection between the sinus cavities and the nasal mucosa, infection in one area can easily spread to the other. An infection in this area, an *upper respiratory infection* (URI), is very common and often causes excess sinus secretions.

Pharynx

Air travels from the nose to the **pharynx**, a tube-shaped passage for air and food. Refer to Figures 25-1 and 25-2 as you read the following descriptions.

Nasopharynx

The section of the pharynx extending from the nares to the uvula is the **nasopharynx**, a passageway for air only. In childhood, it contains the *adenoids (pharyngeal tonsils)* (not shown in the adult pictured). The adenoids are located in the posterior wall of the nasopharynx and, along with the palatine tonsils, assist the body in its immune response to foreign invaders (Chapter 24). Enlargement of adenoids can cause snoring or upper airway obstruction. When an individual approaches adulthood, the adenoids usually atrophy (waste away). During swallowing, the soft palate and uvula elevate to block the nasal cavity, preventing food from entering the respiratory system. The auditory (*eustachian*) tubes connect the nasopharynx with the middle ear (Fig. 21-3). These tubes allow air to enter or leave the middle ear cavities, permitting proper functioning of the tympanic membranes (eardrums) and equalizing pressures between the external environment and the middle ear.

Oropharynx

The **oropharynx** is the part of the pharynx extending from the uvula to the epiglottis. Commonly called the "throat," the oropharynx carries food to the esophagus and air to the trachea. Two sets of tonsils are in the oropharynx: the two *palatine tonsils* are located posteriorly, on each side of the oral cavity, and the *lingual tonsils* are at the base of the tongue. The palatine tonsils are those commonly removed by tonsillectomy (Fig. 25-2). These two sets of tonsils encircle the throat and are involved in the immune response (in addition to the adenoids). They function to collect and destroy foreign substances that are inhaled or ingested.

> **Key Concept**
> Tonsils are not removed unless absolutely necessary because of their lymphatic functions.

Laryngopharynx

The **laryngopharynx** is the lowest portion of the pharynx. It extends from the epiglottis to its division into two separate passageways, the larynx (for air) and esophagus (for food).

Larynx (Voice Box)

From the pharynx, air passes into the **larynx**, a boxlike structure in the midline of the neck, composed of cartilages held together by ligaments. The function of the cartilages in the larynx is to keep the airway open at all times. (The largest and most prominent cartilage, particularly in males, is the *thyroid cartilage* or *laryngeal prominence*, commonly known as the "Adam apple.")

The larynx serves as an air passageway between the pharynx and the trachea. Although the pharynx acts as a dual passageway for air and food, only air is allowed to pass into the larynx. A lid or cover of cartilage, the **epiglottis** ("trap door cartilage"), guards the entrance to the larynx. The epiglottis automatically closes when swallowing, preventing food from entering the lower respiratory passage. In this area, a small pair of bands—the false vocal cords—do not produce sound. They move together during swallowing, to help close the larynx and prevent choking. The *glottis* is the vocal structure of the larynx, consisting of the true vocal cords and their related openings.

> **Nursing Alert** If a portion of food accidentally becomes lodged in the larynx, coughing can usually dislodge it. If not, the air passage may be blocked; such a blockage can be fatal unless immediate emergency treatment is given. (Nurses are trained in treating obstructed airways and cardiopulmonary resuscitation.) Accidental choking and suffocation kill many people each year.

Vocal Cords

At the base of the larynx are the **vocal cords** (*vocal folds*), two thin, triangle-shaped reedlike folds or fibrous bands

(Fig. 25-2). One end of each is attached to the trachea's front wall; the other end is attached to a tiny cartilage near the trachea's back wall. These cartilages can move to produce many sounds or can be spread apart to allow silent breathing. When the vocal cords are close together, air passing over them causes them to vibrate, producing sound, similar to a reed organ. The size of the vocal cords and larynx varies, accounting for differences in people's voices. A man usually has a larger larynx—and therefore a deeper voice—than most women. The voice becomes louder and stronger when a great deal of air is forced out rapidly.

LOWER RESPIRATORY TRACT

The lower respiratory tract consists of the trachea, bronchi, and lungs (Fig. 25-3).

Trachea (Windpipe)

Air passes from the larynx into the **trachea**, a tube approximately 4.5 in. (11 cm) long and 1 in. diameter in adults. It consists of C-shaped hyaline cartilage and connective tissue and extends from the lower end of the larynx into the chest cavity behind the heart. The trachea transports air to and from the lungs when an individual breathes. Immediately posterior to the larynx and trachea is the tube, the *esophagus*, which transports food from the pharynx to the stomach (Chapter 26). The trachea's 15–20 horseshoe-shaped cartilaginous rings provide sufficient rigidity to keep it open at all times, allowing air to pass through. The rings are flexible enough, however, to permit bending of the neck. At the bottom of the trachea, the single tubular system begins to branch into the bronchi (Fig. 25-1). By the time the tubes reach the alveoli in the lungs, they have branched 20–23 times. Ciliated mucous membrane lines the trachea. As in the nose, mucus in the trachea traps inhaled foreign particles, which waves of cilia carry out of the respiratory tract through the pharynx.

> **Nursing Alert** In the event of a blocked airway, a tracheotomy may be needed. This is an artificial opening from the outside, either temporary or permanent, into the trachea.

Bronchi

As the trachea enters the chest cavity, it divides into two smaller tubes, the **bronchi**. In an indented area, the *hilum*, each bronchus enters the lung and branches off. The arteries, veins, and nerves also enter the lungs at the hilum. One (primary) bronchus enters each lung. The right bronchus is straighter, more vertical, and wider than the left. The cartilage in the small bronchi within the lungs exists as interspersed plates, rather than rings. There is more elastic tissue here as well. The bronchi and bronchioles are encircled by smooth muscles.

> **Nursing Alert** Because the right bronchus is straighter down and wider than the left, it is more susceptible to aspiration of fluids or foreign objects.

The Tracheobronchial Tree

Each bronchus continues to divide into smaller branches to form the *bronchial tree* or *tracheobronchial tree* (which looks like an upside-down tree). Each main bronchus divides into *secondary lobar bronchi* (three on the right and two on the left). These divide into *segmental (tertiary) bronchi* in each segment of the lungs. As the bronchi become smaller, their walls become thinner, the amount of cartilage decreases, and they become known as **bronchioles**. The bronchi and

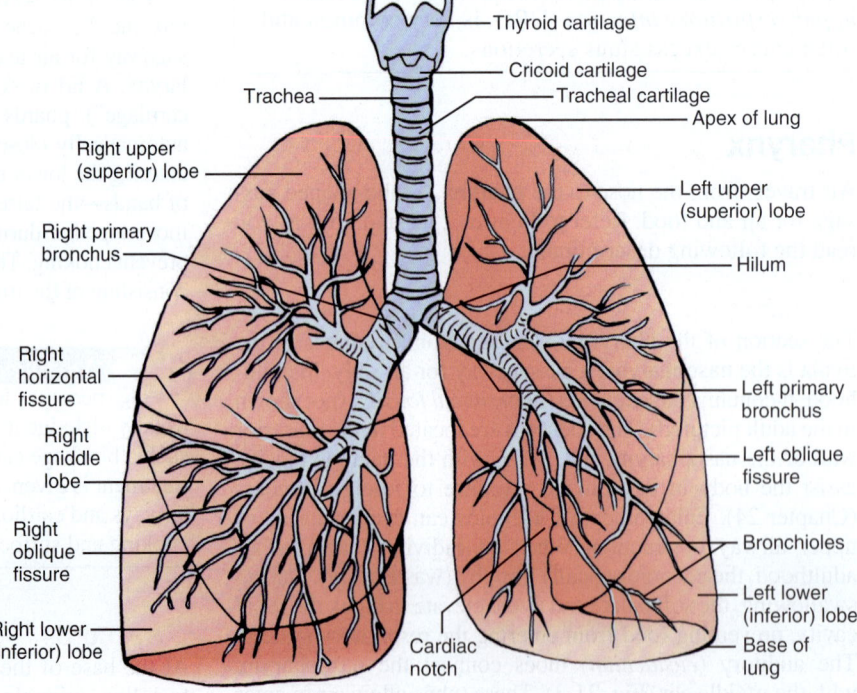

Figure 25-3 The lower respiratory tract viewed from the front (anterior view). The lungs consist of five lobes. The right lung has three lobes (upper, middle, lower); the left has two (upper and lower). The left lung has an indentation called the cardiac notch, which provides space for the heart. The pulmonary lobes are further subdivided by fissures. The bronchial tree inflates with air to fill the lobes.

bronchioles continue to be lined with ciliated mucous membrane. The bronchioles branch first into **alveolar ducts**, which look like stems, and end in many **alveolar sacs**, which look like clusters of grapes (Fig. 25-1). Each lung contains millions of alveoli. These microscopic "balloons" give the lungs their spongy appearance. The alveolar walls are composed of a single layer of simple squamous cells and are lined with a chemical called *surfactant*, which helps prevent the alveolar walls from collapsing between breaths. (The alveoli are the basic structural units of gas exchange.)

Surfactant

Surfactant (surface active agent) is secreted by the great alveolar (type II) cells of the lungs and is a mixture of phospholipids (a special type of fat, containing phosphorus). The main phospholipids in surfactant are *lecithin* and *sphingomyelin* (L-S). Surfactant acts to break up surface tension in the pulmonary (lung) fluids. This reduces friction and preserves the elasticity of lung tissue, thus preventing collapse of the alveoli (*atelectasis*) between breaths.

SPECIAL CONSIDERATIONS Lifespan

Fetal Lung Development
During pregnancy, the fetal respiratory system is dormant, although the lungs are developing. At birth, exposure to air causes the system to begin functioning. The alveolar type II cells do not begin functioning until about the seventh gestational month, causing surfactant deficiency in the preterm infant. This premature newborn often has *respiratory distress syndrome* (RDS or *hyaline membrane disease*) and must exert tremendous energy to breathe. The infant with RDS may die due to atelectasis, fatigue of respiratory muscles, and/or inadequate ventilation. Treatment involves mechanical ventilation and administration of synthetic surfactant. Steroid injections during pregnancy may help prevent this condition. A test of amniotic fluid, the *L-S ratio*, helps determine lung maturity in a fetus (Chapter 69).

Lungs

Humans have two cone-shaped **lungs** that fill the chest cavity. They are the stations where oxygen is delivered from outside air and carbon dioxide is removed. The top (*apex*) and the lower, wide portion of the lungs over the diaphragm (*base*) are illustrated in Figures 25-1 and 25-3. The *cardiac notch* or *cardiac impression* is much larger and deeper on the left in order to allow space for the heart. The lungs are spongy tissues filled with alveoli, nerves, and many blood and lymph vessels. They are separated by the heart, the large blood vessels, the esophagus, and other contents of the **mediastinum**, the area lying between the lungs in the thorax (chest). The lungs are divided into sections called *lobes*. The right lung has three lobes, and the left has two.

Pleura

The lower respiratory tract contains a smooth double-layered sac of serous membrane called **pleura** (Fig. 25-1). The inner layer covers the lungs (**visceral pleura**), and the outer layer (**parietal pleura**) lines the chest cavity. Their surfaces are in constant contact and are moist because they secrete serous lubricating fluid. The pleura allow the lungs to move without causing pain or friction against the chest wall. The space between the two layers of pleura, the **pleural cavity or pleural space**, normally is a vacuum. This vacuum changes in intensity during breathing.

> **Key Concept**
>
> *Pleurisy*, inflammation of the pleura, causes a "sticking" pain on inspiration (breathing in). Causes include lung tumors, tuberculosis, lung abscess, and pneumonia.

The respiratory tract is lined with epithelium, the type of which depends on location. Most of the tube system, from the nose to the bronchi, is covered by pseudostratified columnar-ciliated epithelium (respiratory epithelium). In the bronchioles, the epithelial cells become more cuboidal in shape, but continue to be ciliated.

> **Nursing Alert** Air or fluid accumulation in the pleural space can cause lung collapse, an airless situation (atelectasis). The collapse may involve all or part of a lobe or an entire lung; atelectasis may be acute or chronic and may be life-threatening.

System Physiology

VENTILATION

Ventilation (breathing) is the mechanical process of respiration that moves air to and from alveoli. Ventilation is divided into inhalation and exhalation. Breathing air in is called *inhalation* or **inspiration**; breathing out is called *exhalation* or **expiration**. One ventilation or respiration takes about 2 seconds. Adults usually average between 12 and 20 respirations per minute; the rate is higher in children, lowering as the child becomes older. Normal respiration is called **eupnea**; difficult breathing is **dyspnea**. *Orthopnea* denotes dyspnea that is relieved when the person sits up. Chapter 46 describes assessment of breathing in more detail.

Normal breathing occurs as a result of nervous stimulation of the respiratory center in the brain's medulla. Because the lungs cannot move by themselves, actions of the surrounding muscles inflate and deflate them. The medulla sends impulses to the diaphragm and the intercostal muscles. The **diaphragm** is a dome-shaped muscle separating the thoracic and abdominal cavities, which contracts and flattens to increase both chest (pleural) space and pleural vacuum (Fig. 25-4). The **intercostal muscles** (between the ribs) contract to lift and spread the ribs during inhalation, adding to the vacuum. Other muscles assist in breathing, including the mastoid (raises the sternum), trapezium (helps raise the thoracic cage), pectorals (raise the chest), and abdominis rectus (pulls down the lower chest).

The actual movement of air from external to internal environments occurs due to differences in existing pressures between the atmosphere and chest cavity. On inspiration, the chest cavity increases in size, creating an internal vacuum. Air goes into the lungs when the *intrathoracic* (within the thoracic cavity) *pressure* is below that of the surrounding atmosphere (*subatmospheric*). If breathing becomes difficult, accessory muscles (e.g., the sternocleidomastoid

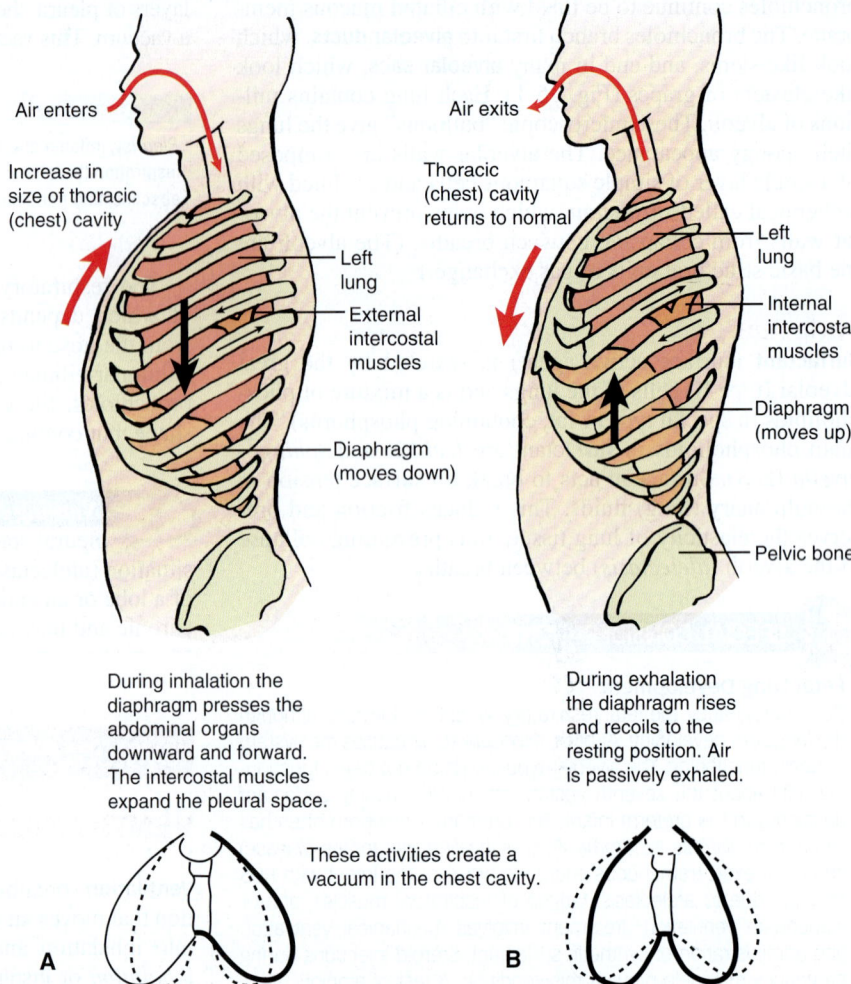

Figure 25-4 Pulmonary ventilation. **A.** Inhalation (inspiration). **B.** Exhalation (expiration).

and neck muscles) assist. Movement of these muscles can be visualized. This movement is particularly diagnostic of respiratory distress in infants and small children.

> **Nursing Alert** Any interruption in the closed chest can be immediately life-threatening because it disrupts the vacuum necessary for inspiration. Therefore, a puncture wound or other opening into the chest must be immediately plugged, to prevent death.

Expiration is passive. The muscles of the chest wall and lungs relax. Movements of the diaphragm and intercostal muscles decrease the volume of the thoracic cavity. Air rushes out when pressures within the thoracic cavity rise above that of the atmosphere. In addition, the reduced size of the thoracic cavity and natural elasticity (rebound action) of the lungs force air out.

> **Key Concept**
> During forced exhalation, such as when blowing up a balloon or playing a musical instrument, abdominal and thoracic pressure is consciously generated by muscle movement, including the diaphragm, controlling air flow out of the lungs. The neck muscles also contract.

Regulation of Respirations

The medulla's respiratory center automatically controls the depth and rate of respirations without requiring conscious thought. The pons works with the medulla to produce a normal breathing rhythm. The cerebral cortex allows some voluntary control over breathing when talking, singing, eating, or changing the rate of breathing. You can stop breathing for a short time by holding your breath, but the medulla will assume control eventually. Chemoreceptors in the medulla stimulate the muscles of respiration in response to changes in carbon dioxide levels. Therefore, *carbon dioxide* (CO_2)—not oxygen—is the major regulator of respiration. (The infant's neurologic system is particularly sensitive; shaking or dropping a baby can destroy breathing controls and cause death.)

> **Key Concept**
> An excess of CO_2 in the blood of a healthy person lowers the blood's pH. This stimulates the medulla to increase respirations, blowing off excess CO_2.

Lung Volumes and Capacities

Lung capacity varies with sex, size, physical condition, and age. Pulmonary diseases and other diseases that limit expansion of the chest greatly influence a person's comfort

TABLE 25-1 Lung Volumes and Lung Capacities

TERM	SYMBOL	DESCRIPTION	NORMAL VALUE[a]	SIGNIFICANCE
Lung Volumes				
Tidal volume	V_T or TV	The volume of air inhaled and exhaled with each breath	500 mL or 5–10 mL/kg	The tidal volume may not vary, even with severe disease.
Inspiratory reserve volume	IRV	The maximum volume of air that can be inhaled after a normal inhalation	3,000 mL	A sigh takes advantage of the IRV potential.
Expiratory reserve volume	ERV	The maximum volume of air that can be exhaled forcibly after a normal exhalation	1,100 mL	Expiratory reserve volume is decreased in restrictive disorders, such as obesity, ascites, and pregnancy.
Residual volume	RV	The volume of air remaining in the lungs after a maximum exhalation	1,200 mL	Residual volume may be increased in obstructive disease.
Lung Capacities				
Vital capacity	VC	The maximum volume of air exhaled from the point of maximum inspiration VC = TV + IRV + ERV	4,600 mL	A decrease in vital capacity may be found in neuromuscular disease, generalized fatigue, atelectasis, pulmonary edema, and COPD.
Inspiratory capacity	IC	The maximum volume of air inhaled after normal expiration IC = TV + IRV	3,500 mL	A decrease in inspiratory capacity may indicate restrictive disease.
Functional residual capacity	FRC	The volume of air remaining in the lungs after a normal expiration FRC = ERV + RV	2,300 mL	Functional residual capacity may be increased in COPD and decreased in ARDS.
Total lung capacity	TLC	The volume of air in the lungs after a maximum inspiration TLC = TV + IRV + ERV + RV	5,800 mL	Total lung capacity may be decreased in restrictive disease (atelectasis, pneumonia) and increased in COPD.

From Hinkle, J., & Cheever, K. (2018). *Brunner & Suddarth's textbook of medical-surgical nursing* (14th ed.). Wolters Kluwer.
ARDS, acute respiratory distress syndrome; COPD, chronic obstructive pulmonary disease.
[a]Values for healthy men; values for women are 20%–25% less.

and ability to survive. The ability of the lungs and thorax to expand also influences lung volumes and capacities. Table 25-1 contains key terms, descriptions, and normal values for a healthy male adult. (Values for women are 20%–25% lower.)

> *Key Concept*
> It is important to note that, even after expiration, some air (residual) remains in the lungs. This is the basis for the Heimlich maneuver used in choking victims.

EXTERNAL (PULMONARY) AND INTERNAL (TISSUE) RESPIRATION

The two types of **respiration** (gas exchange) are external and internal. The exchange of oxygen (O_2) for carbon dioxide (CO_2) *within the alveoli of the lungs* (by diffusion—passive transport) is called **external respiration** (*pulmonary respiration*) because it is involved with the external environment (Fig. 17-3). Notice the difference in pressures between nonoxygenated and oxygenated blood. After oxygen is brought into the body, it attaches to hemoglobin for transport to tissues and cells. The exchange of O_2 for CO_2 *within the cells* is called *tissue respiration*, **internal respiration**, or **cellular respiration** (*cell breathing*). An increase in CO_2 levels stimulates respiration. CO_2 and water are the waste products of respiration. Some water is excreted as waste; some is recycled for use in the body.

> *Key Concept*
> Respiration is the exchange of gases between a person's external environment and internal cells. The alveoli are the functional structures of the lungs.
>
> External respiration is gas exchange at the lung level. Internal respiration is gas exchange at the cellular level.
>
> For the respiratory system to function, it must remain moist (to dissolve gases), its cells must be thin (to allow for gas transfer), there must be a source of oxygen, and the respiratory system must communicate with the circulatory system.

Gas Exchange

Chapters 22 and 23 introduce the concept of pulmonary circulation. Nearly all the blood in the body travels through the lungs every minute. Figure 22-2 illustrates the branching of pulmonary blood vessels to and from the heart. The pulmonary artery exits the right ventricle of the heart, carrying *deoxygenated* blood, and splits into the right and left pulmonary arteries. These arteries branch into pulmonary and bronchial capillaries in the lungs where the exchange of O_2 and CO_2 occurs. Alveolar walls are one cell layer of *epithelial* cells thick (approximately 0.1 μm). Alveoli are surrounded by equally thin capillaries, a single *endothelial* cell thick. Extensive branching of pulmonary blood vessels leads to very low pressure within the vessels, facilitating gas exchange (Fig. 25-1). At the capillary level, oxygen diffuses into the capillaries and most of it is bound to hemoglobin (in red blood cells) in capillary blood (*oxyhemoglobin*). Small veins collect the now-oxygenated blood from the lung capillaries. These veins combine eventually into four pulmonary veins (two left, two right), which pour *oxygenated* blood into the heart's left atrium. (Remember: these are the only veins in the body that carry oxygenated blood.) This blood is pumped by the left ventricle through the aorta to the rest of the body. Oxygenated blood travels to tissues where the oxygen–hemoglobin bond is broken easily and oxygen is released into tissues. (A small amount of oxygen is carried in plasma and is measured as the partial pressure of oxygen in arterial blood [PaO_2].) This is the basis for hyperbaric oxygenation (Chapter 87).

In the lungs, at the same time oxygen is diffusing from outside air via the alveoli into the capillaries, the capillaries are giving up carbon dioxide (a waste product of metabolism) back into the alveoli. (In the average resting adult, 250 mL of oxygen is taken in per minute; about 200 mL of carbon dioxide is expelled.) CO_2 is transported by the blood from the body's cells to pulmonary capillaries in three main forms: dissolution in plasma, in combination with proteins, and by formation into bicarbonate (HCO_3^-) ions in the blood. The bicarbonate ions undergo a chemical change that yields CO_2 and water (H_2O). During exhalation, CO_2 and some of the water are released from the lungs into the air. (Chemical messengers, such as hormones, are also deleted and added in the lungs. Small blood clots are removed by the fine capillaries in the lungs.) This cycle then begins again and continues to maintain homeostasis and electrolyte balance in the body.

Nursing Alert Many factors can cause a decrease in gas exchange, including immobility, thoracic/pulmonary surgery, or pneumonia. Encouraging frequent coughing and deep breathing should assist in improving oxygen delivery to the lungs and tissues. Supplemental oxygen may also be ordered to improve arterial oxygen levels (O_2 saturation).

REGULATION OF ACID–BASE BALANCE

Although the primary function of the respiratory system is gas exchange, it is also vital in the regulation of the pH of all body fluids. The respiratory and renal systems interact to maintain *homeostasis*. CO_2 can alter pH because it reacts with water to form carbonic acid (H_2CO_3). Carbonic acid can break down to form the H^+ and HCO_3^- ions (hydrogen and bicarbonate). These ions are important to the buffer system (the respiratory process is part of the buffer system), which helps the body maintain proper pH levels (Chapter 17). The hydrogen ion often combines to form acids, such as hydrochloric acid (HCl). The bicarbonate ion often combines to form basic compounds, which counteract acids. One such base compound is sodium bicarbonate ($NaHCO_3$), which outside the body is known as baking soda.

> **Key Concept**
>
> The respiratory system is the major mechanism for excretion and elimination of CO_2 from the body. (CO_2 is constantly being produced by the body as a by-product of metabolism.) If a person has a breathing disorder, CO_2 can build up, forming excess carbonic acid and dangerously lowering blood pH. This condition, *respiratory acidosis*, can be caused by airway obstruction in disorders such as emphysema, severe pneumonia, asthma, and pulmonary edema, as well as in drug overdose. Untreated respiratory acidosis is life threatening. Too little CO_2 in the blood, *respiratory alkalosis*, is most commonly caused by hyperventilation (excessively rapid, deep breathing) but can also be caused by overuse of antacids or can be related to early pulmonary edema or pulmonary embolism.

RESPIRATORY REFLEXES

Coughing and sneezing are protective reflexes needed to dislodge materials from respiratory passages. The bronchi and trachea have sensory receptors that initiate a cough in response to foreign particles or irritating substances. The sneezing reflex is similar to coughing, except that the irritation is in the nasal passages. Yawning is another respiratory reflex. Theorists conjecture that yawning is a response to a lack of oxygen or an accumulation of carbon dioxide. Yawning also equalizes pressure between the middle ear and the outside atmosphere, helping a person to maintain balance and reducing discomfort when flying or deep-sea diving.

A deep breath, a *sigh*, can be taken on occasion. Mechanical ventilators are often programmed to deliver a sigh breath regularly to increase the client's comfort.

Respiratory disorders are very common. They are aggravated by such things as pollutants in the air and cigarette smoking. Chapter 86 describes respiratory disorders in more detail, and Chapter 87 outlines steps in administering supplemental oxygen.

Nursing Alert Smoking can decrease the efficiency of the respiratory system. Nicotine causes a decrease in bronchial diameter, constriction of blood vessels, and paralysis of cilia (which assist in moving foreign particles out of the respiratory tract), and it can destroy lung tissue itself over time. These factors can all result in decreased gas exchange. In addition, many tobacco products contain substances (e.g., tars) that can build up in the lungs. It is also known that smoking causes lung and mouth cancer.

VOCALIZATION

The movement of gases through the mouth, larynx, and pharynx allows a person to speak (*phonate*) or sing. Phonation is caused by the passage of air over the vocal cords in the larynx, causing vibrations, which are modulated by the person into speech or singing.

TABLE 25-2 Effects of Aging on the Respiratory System

FACTOR	RESULT	NURSING IMPLICATIONS
Functional capacity decreases because of:		
• Increased rigidity of thorax and diaphragm; chest wall loses mobility	More energy needed to breathe Decreased ability of lungs to expand Less air exchange—altered ratio of O_2 and CO_2, impairing gas exchange at cellular level	Encourage good ventilation with daily exercise, such as walking. Pulmonary exercises may be helpful.
• Decreased numbers of alveoli and diffusion ability; lungs more rigid	Less ability to compensate for respiratory needs in stress or illness Changes in pulmonary pressures; may lead to acid–base imbalance	Advise older person to avoid contact with children or others with respiratory tract infections. Supplemental oxygen may be needed. Encourage client not to smoke.
• Decreased strength in breathing and coughing; reduced muscle strength	Hypoventilation leading to respiratory problems and pneumonia Possible dyspnea (shortness of breath) with exertion Morning cough common (decreased ability to eliminate secretions) Reduced vital capacity	Advise client to see physician early if symptoms occur. Encourage changing position slowly to avoid orthostatic vital sign changes. Advise to change position at least every 2 h during the night. Postural drainage may be prescribed. Discourage excessive use of antihistamines. Encourage client not to smoke.
• Size of chest wall decreases, as a result of kyphosis and osteoporosis.	Difficulty breathing deeply Trachea may deviate	Help client know their own ability. Encourage supplemental calcium or other medications to prevent/treat osteoporosis.
• Immobility is common Decreased elasticity of lungs and bronchioles, decreased ciliary action, decreased mucus secretion, decreased numbers of alveoli, pain	Increased risk for pneumonia and circulatory disorders	Encourage client to receive pneumonia immunization. Encourage moving, coughing, and deep breathing. Encourage adequate fluid intake. Encourage client not to smoke.
The client may be overweight or extremely inactive • Atrophy of tonsils or removal of tonsils as a child; reduced mucous production • Deviated septum, enlargement of nasal septum, excess cartilage growth, nasal enlargement	Obstructive sleep apnea may occur Decreased ability to combat infections Difficulty in breathing; abnormal appearance	The use of a continuous positive airway pressure machine at night often relieves symptoms and facilitates better and safer sleep. Encourage client to elevate head of bed at night. Treat infections early. Surgery may be helpful. Enhance client self-esteem.

NCLEX Alert

Homeostasis relates to the integration and balance of body systems. The NCLEX may provide clinical situations that describe relationships of the respiratory system to other systems, especially the circulatory and renal systems. You also need to know normal versus abnormal changes in aging.

Key Concept

Disorders of the respiratory system include obstructive disorders (asthma, emphysema), restrictive disorders (alveolar damage, pleural effusion, fibrosis), vascular and circulatory disorders (pulmonary embolism, pulmonary edema), and infections or environmental disorders (pneumonia, tuberculosis, asbestosis, pollution-related disorders).

The respiratory system has many mechanisms to protect itself from diseases.

SPECIAL CONSIDERATIONS Lifespan

Nursing care for older adults must adapt to changes related to aging. The aging process can produce a significant effect on the respiratory system (Table 25-2).

STUDENT SYNTHESIS

KEY POINTS

- The pathway for external breathing is nose → pharynx → larynx → trachea → bronchi → bronchioles → alveoli (oxygen exchanged for carbon dioxide) → bronchi → external environment (carbon dioxide exhaled).
- The pathway for oxygen distribution and carbon dioxide return (internal breathing) is alveoli → capillaries (hemoglobin combines with oxygen) → cells → capillaries (carbon dioxide exchange) → alveoli. Deoxygenated blood moves to the lungs via general circulation and pulmonary circuit. In the alveoli, carbon dioxide is exchanged for O_2 and CO_2 is exhaled.
- The pharynx is divided into nasopharynx, oropharynx, and laryngopharynx.
- The trachea and esophagus are both located in the pharynx. The epiglottis is a protective flap covering the trachea during swallowing, to prevent foreign matter from entering the respiratory system.
- The pleura have two layers. One covers the lung; the other lines the chest wall. Serous fluid secreted by the pleura enables the lungs to move without pain or friction.
- External respiration is exchange of gases (oxygen and carbon dioxide) at the lung level. Internal respiration is exchange of gases at the cellular level.
- Various lung volumes and capacities describe the volume of air in the lungs in relation to inspiration or expiration. These amounts can vary depending on sex and size of the client and on existing respiratory disorders.
- Nasal hair, mucus, and cilia are protective structures of the respiratory system. Sneezing, coughing, and yawning are protective reflexes of the respiratory system.

CRITICAL THINKING EXERCISES

1. Alterations in systems other than the respiratory system can affect the process of breathing and gas exchange. List systems that may be involved and describe types of alterations that might cause such problems.
2. Based on information in this chapter, explain why you think a person with a cold sometimes experiences changes in their voice.
3. Explain the relationship between aerobic exercise and optimum pulmonary functioning. Provide support for your answer.
4. Define each of the following acronyms. Discuss a possible medical cause and two nursing implications for each:

    decreased ERV

    decreased TLC

    increased FRC

    decreased FRC

    increased RV

NCLEX-STYLE REVIEW QUESTIONS

1. A client has a defective cranial nerve I. Which data would the nurse gather in order to determine function?
    a. Use a tuning fork to determine bone conduction.
    b. Instruct the client to smell and identify a variety of scents.
    c. Ask the client to open and close the eyes.
    d. Request the client to stick the tongue out and say "ah."
2. A client is eating supper and begins coughing. Which action should the nurse take first?
    a. Insert fingers into the mouth to do a blind sweep and remove object.
    b. Lay the client flat and perform chest thrusts.
    c. Pat the client on the back to assist with dislodging the foreign body.
    d. Do nothing. Coughing will usually dislodge the foreign body.
3. The rescue squad brings into the emergency department a client who has a blocked airway after choking on a piece of steak. The client is unresponsive, and resuscitation efforts are continued with a bag valve mask. Which action by the nurse is a priority?
    a. Gather equipment for an emergency tracheotomy.
    b. Intubate the client.
    c. Start an intravenous infusion.
    d. Perform a blind finger sweep.
4. The nurse is caring for a client with left lower lobe pneumonia. Which nursing action would assist in improving oxygen delivery to the lungs and tissues?
    a. Encourage frequent coughing and deep breathing.
    b. Position the client with the head of the bed slightly elevated.
    c. Provide deep endotracheal suctioning.
    d. Use a bag valve mask to ventilate the client.
5. Which intervention provided by the nurse would assist the client with early chronic obstructive lung disease to improve efficiency of lung function?
    a. Administer breathing treatment with a bronchodilator.
    b. Provide smoking cessation information.
    c. Perform chest physiotherapy.
    d. Encourage coughing and deep breathing.

CHAPTER RESOURCES

Enhance your learning with additional resources on thePoint*!*

Student Resources related to this chapter can be found at **thePoint.lww.com/Rosdahl12e**.

26 The Digestive System

Learning Objectives

1. On a chart, trace the digestive pathway, naming major organs of the gastrointestinal (GI) system and the function of each.
2. Define the following terms and processes: mastication, deglutition, and peristalsis.
3. Explain the actions of hydrochloric acid (HCl), gastrin, intrinsic factor, cholecystokinin, and pancreatic juice in the process of digestion.
4. Explain two functions of the pancreas and gallbladder as they relate to digestion.
5. Describe the functions of the liver related to digestion.
6. Describe the physiology of digestion and absorption, including how carbohydrates, fats, and proteins are broken down; describe absorption in the small intestine.
7. Identify and describe two major categories of metabolism.
8. Explain how the large intestine changes its contents into fecal material.
9. List the effects of aging on the digestive system.

Important Terminology

absorption, alimentary canal, anus, appendix, bile, bolus, cardiac sphincter, cecum, chyme, colon, defecation, deglutition, dentin, digestion, duodenum, dysphagia, egestion, emesis, esophagus, feces, gallbladder, gingival, ileum, ingestion, jejunum, lacteal, liver, mastication, micelle, peristalsis, peritoneum, pyloric sphincter, rectum, rugae, saliva, salivation, tongue, villi

Acronyms

ATP, CCK, CHO, GERD, HCl, LES

The body needs a constant supply of energy to perform its many tasks and to maintain life. These actions are possible because the digestive system converts food eaten into fuel for the body's energy demands. In a lifetime, the human digestive system will process about 50 tons of food! Food is taken into the body (*ingestion*), mechanically broken down by chewing (*mastication*), swallowed (*deglutition*), *digested* in the stomach and intestines, *absorbed* into the bloodstream, and wastes are eliminated (*defecation, egestion*). This entire mechanical and chemical process is often called **digestion**. Food is broken down into smaller elements—*catabolism*. These food elements are transported via the circulation and passed into the body's cells—*absorption*. Here, the elements are used for energy and building cells—*anabolism*—and wastes are eliminated.

SPECIAL CONSIDERATIONS Culture and Ethnicity

Regional, ethnic, and financial factors are involved in dietary choices of groups of people. Although specific foods chosen may vary, all people require the same types and amounts of nutrients to maintain health (Chapter 30).

The efficient food processing machine responsible for digestion and absorption, the digestive tract, is also called the **alimentary canal**, *gastrointestinal (GI) tract*, or *GI system*. (The related medical specialty is *gastroenterology*.) The GI tract or canal is a tube, approximately 28–30 ft (9.1 m) long, running through the body and open to the outside at both ends (mouth and anus—Fig. 26-1). Food travels through the GI tract in about 24–36 hours. The digestive system is controlled by the nervous and endocrine systems. Compounds broken down by digestion to provide fuel for the body (*nutrients*) are carbohydrates, proteins, and fats. They consist of carbon, hydrogen, and oxygen; proteins also contain nitrogen.

Key Concept

Because the GI tract is open to the outside, and because nonsterile material (food) is introduced into it, it is not considered sterile.

STRUCTURE AND FUNCTION

Figure 26-1 shows major organs of the digestive system. The main function of the overall GI system (Box 26-1) is to break down food into simpler forms that circulatory vessels can carry and pass through cell membranes to the cells, to be used for energy and to build, maintain, and repair body tissues.

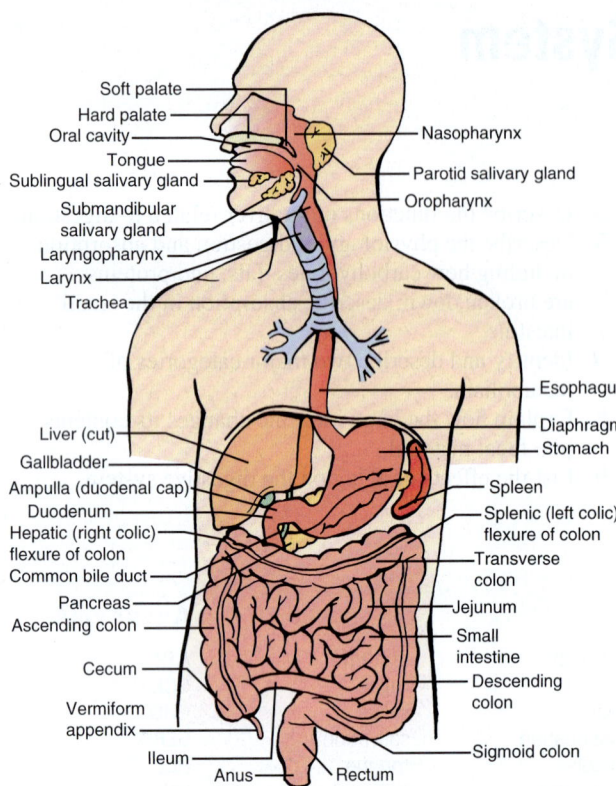

Figure 26-1 The digestive system.

> **Box 26-1 Functions of the Digestive System**
>
> **FOOD PROCESSING AND STORAGE**
> - Breaks down food into smaller particles (mechanical digestion)
> - Converts food into substances that can be absorbed (chemical digestion)
> - Moves food materials through the gastrointestinal tract (peristalsis)
> - Stores nutrients until needed
>
> **MANUFACTURE**
> - Manufactures enzymes, hydrochloric acid, intrinsic factor, mucus, and other materials to assist in digestion
> - Manufactures regulatory hormones in stomach
> - Manufactures vitamin K and some B-complex vitamins in large intestine
>
> **ABSORPTION**
> - Provides absorption of nutrients, mainly from small intestine, into capillaries
>
> **REABSORPTION AND ELIMINATION**
> - Reabsorbs water for reuse by the body
> - Reabsorbs minerals and vitamins
> - Forms feces from remaining waste products
> - Produces defecation

MOUTH

The mouth (*oral cavity, buccal cavity*) takes in food, where digestion begins (the *cephalic phase* of digestion). Here, teeth cut, chop, and grind food, so food particles become smaller (*mechanical process*), exposing additional food surfaces to actions of digestive juices and enzymes (*chemical process*). The mouth's chief digestive functions are to receive food via **ingestion** ("to take in"), prepare food for digestion, and begin digestion of starch/carbohydrates.

Palate

The roof of the mouth is composed of hard and soft palates. The *hard palate,* close to the front of the mouth, consists of the palatine bones and parts of the maxillary bones. The *soft palate,* mostly muscle tissue, separates the mouth from the nasopharynx. Shaped like an arch in the back of the mouth, it opens onto the oropharynx. The small structure, seen suspended in the back of the open mouth (when you say "ahhh"), is the *uvula.* The soft palate and uvula prevent foods from entering nasal cavities above the mouth. The *tongue* covers the floor of the mouth; the walls are the *cheeks* and *teeth.*

Salivary Glands

When one sees or thinks about food, the salivary glands begin to function, making the "mouth water." Three pairs of salivary glands pour 1–1.5 L of saliva into the mouth daily. These glands are *exocrine* glands (their secretions are not released directly into the circulation); saliva is released into the oral cavity. Two types of **saliva** exist. One is thin and watery; it wets food to facilitate swallowing. The other is a thicker, mucous secretion containing *mucin,* which lubricates and causes food particles to stick together to form a **bolus** (ball or lump) of food. Saliva contains *ptyalin* (*salivary amylase*), as well as water, mucus, and salts. Salivary glands are named by location. *Sublinguals,* the smallest, located under the tongue, secrete only mucus-type saliva; their ducts open onto the floor of the mouth. *Parotids,* the largest, are located in the cheek; they secrete serous saliva, containing enzymes, but no mucus. *Submandibulars,* under the lower jaw, are compound glands, secreting a combination of serous and mucus-containing saliva. The nervous system controls the secretion of saliva (**salivation**). Through the action of ptyalin, saliva begins to break down starch (polysaccharides) into smaller sugar molecules and helps reduce friction when chewing. Saliva helps prevent oral infections because it contains *lysozymes* (bacteriocidal enzymes) and immunoglobulins (IgA). The pH of saliva is normally about 6.8 (weak acid). Saliva also assists with speech and taste.

 SPECIAL CONSIDERATIONS Lifespan

Prolapsed Glands
Submandibular gland prolapse may occur in older adults and could be mistaken for a tumor. Unlike tumors, however, these drooping submandibular glands feel soft and are seen on both sides of the neck.

Teeth

The teeth are set in spaces (*sockets*) in the upper and lower jaw bones—*maxilla* and *mandible*. Their chief function is to break food into smaller particles, accomplished through **mastication**, chewing. Humans have two sets of teeth: *deciduous* ("falling out," "baby teeth") and a *permanent* or adult set (Fig. 26-2). A baby's deciduous teeth usually begin to erupt between 6 and 8 months of age, and the 20 teeth are usually complete by 30 months of age (Fig. 10-3). At the age of about 6 years, children's permanent teeth begin to appear. As the permanent teeth grow in, they push out the deciduous teeth, replace them, and fill in the spaces in the jaw. The permanent set has 32 teeth.

Types and Locations
The teeth are named and located as follows:

- The sharp, flat *incisors,* front teeth, cut and tear food.
- The pointed *canines (cuspids),* side teeth, hold, pierce, and tear food.
- The *bicuspids* (premolars) and *tricuspids* (molars) crush and grind food.
- The last permanent teeth, the third molars ("*wisdom teeth*"), located far back in the mouth, sometimes do not appear before adulthood. If jaw space is limited, wisdom teeth may become *impacted* in the bone or tissue and require surgical removal.

Parts
A tooth has three parts: crown, neck, and root (Fig. 26-3). The *crown* is the enamel-covered part of the tooth, visible in the mouth. (Tooth enamel is the hardest structure in the body and is considered part of the integumentary system.) The tooth narrows into a *neck* at the gum (**gingival**) line. The *root* is in the bony socket lined with fibrous periodontal membrane, which helps anchor the tooth to the bone. A bonelike connective tissue, *cement (cementum),* covers the root and holds the tooth in place. Beneath the enamel and cementum is another bonelike material, **dentin**, providing the bulk of tooth material. In the center, the *pulp cavity (pulp chamber)* contains connective tissue, as well as many nerve endings and blood and lymphatic vessels, which enter through the roots (via the root canal) from tooth sockets. Teeth are embedded in and nourished by the bone.

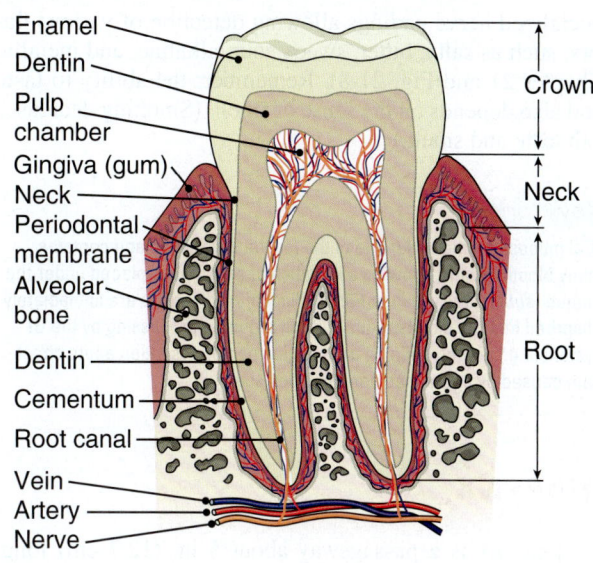

Figure 26-3 A tooth.

> **Key Concept**
>
> When tooth decay is so advanced that it permanently damages the pulp, a root canal procedure or removal of the tooth (*extraction*) is required.

Tongue

The **tongue** (*lingua*) is a tough skeletal muscle, covered with smooth mucous membrane. Attached to four bones, the mandible, two temporal bones, and the hyoid, it is believed to be the only muscle in the body only attached at one end. On the bottom of the tongue is a fold of mucous membrane, the *frenulum,* which helps attach the tongue to the floor of the mouth. In some cases, the frenulum is short or too tightly attached, making speech difficult; the person is said to be "tongue-tied," a situation that can easily be surgically corrected.

The tongue has several functions, in addition to speech. It senses the temperature and texture of food, mixes food with saliva, and moves food into position to be chewed. Voluntary movement of the tongue begins the swallowing process (**deglutition**), by lifting and pushing the bolus of food, mixed with saliva, into the pharynx, the next portion of the digestive tube. The upper surface of the tongue appears rough because of visible indentations (*fissures*) and projections (*papillae*). The taste buds are microscopic nipple-like projections located on the sides of the papillae. They are

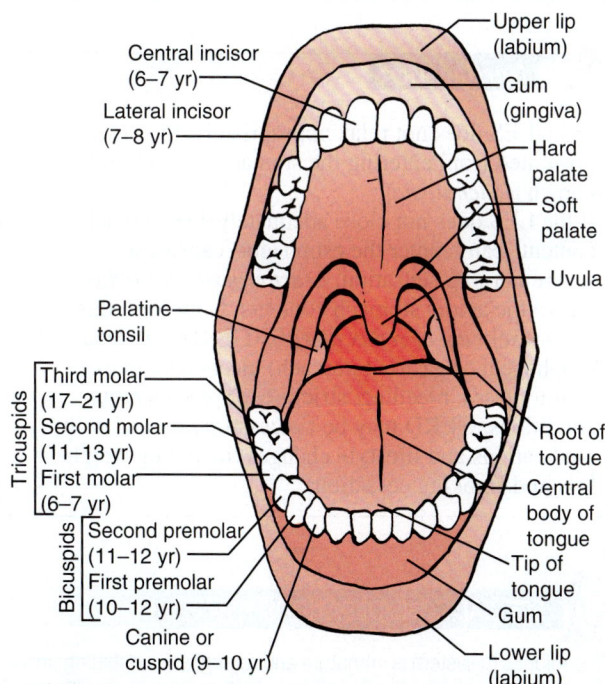

Figure 26-2 The adult mouth, showing the teeth and tonsils. Approximate ages for eruption of permanent teeth are shown.

specialized nerve endings allowing detection of various flavors, such as salty, bitter, sweet, sour, alkaline, and metallic (Chapter 21 and Fig. 21-8). Remember: the ability to taste food also depends on the sense of smell. (Smoking decreases both taste and smell.)

> **Key Concept**
>
> Oral mucosa on the underside of the tongue is very thin and contains many blood vessels, allowing absorption of substances placed under the tongue (*sublingual*) (Chapter 63). Sublingual medications are immediately absorbed into the bloodstream, without requiring processing by the GI system (e.g., nitroglycerin, to treat angina pectoris [sudden acute chest pain caused by decreased cardiac blood supply]).

PHARYNX

The pharynx is a passageway about 5 in. (12.7 cm) long, used for both food and air (Fig. 25-1). Its areas relate to location. The *nasopharynx,* behind the nasal cavity, is lined with ciliated columnar pseudostratified epithelium. The *oropharynx,* behind the oral cavity (mouth), and the *laryngopharynx* (hypopharynx), situated just below the epiglottis, are both lined with stratified squamous epithelium. In this area, the respiratory and digestive tubes divide. (The larynx is located directly in front of the pharynx and is the structure through which air passes into the lungs.) Because the larynx and pharynx are so close, a special structure, the *epiglottis,* prevents aspiration of food and fluids into the lungs during swallowing. This flap of tissue drops down to cover the larynx and trachea (windpipe) during swallowing. (Food has the "right of way" over air here.) Initial swallowing of food is voluntary, but when the food bolus enters the pharynx, swallowing becomes involuntary, as the medulla's swallowing center takes over. Contractions of the pharynx push food into the muscular *esophagus.* The smooth (involuntary) muscles pass food through the entire GI tube by waves of contractions, **peristalsis**, an alternating muscular relaxation and contraction, without which digestion cannot occur.

> **Key Concept**
>
> The medical term for difficulty in swallowing is **dysphagia**.

ESOPHAGUS

The **esophagus**, *gullet,* is approximately 10 in. (25.4 cm) in length and approximately 2 cm in diameter, following the curvature of the vertebral column and lying between the lower border of the laryngeal part of the pharynx and cardia of the stomach. The mucosa of the esophagus consists of stratified abrasion-resistant epithelium. The remainder of the digestive tract consists of simple columnar epithelium. The entire digestive tract is lined with mucous membrane, producing mucus to coat the lumen of the canal and facilitate the passage of food. The esophagus extends from the pharynx down the neck and thorax and, through an opening in the diaphragm, the *esophageal hiatus,* to the stomach. The role of the esophagus in digestion is to serve only as a passageway; no digestion takes place here—food passes through in 5–10 seconds. Two

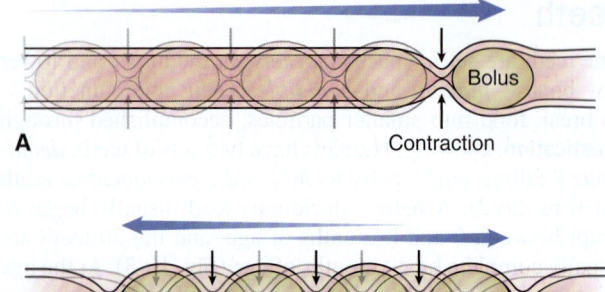

Figure 26-4 **A.** Peristalsis entails progressive movements that move food onward in the digestive tract in a wavelike motion. **B.** Segmentation involves back and forth movements that break food apart and mix it with digestive fluids.

layers of smooth (involuntary) muscles facilitate peristalsis. The outer layer runs up and down (*longitudinal*); the inner layer lies in *concentric circles*. This provides alternating contraction and relaxation, resulting in peristalsis. In addition to peristalsis, a process called *segmentation* assists in breaking up food particles (Fig. 26-4).

A strong circular muscle, the **cardiac sphincter** (*lower esophageal sphincter* [LES] or *gastroesophageal sphincter*) lies between the esophagus and stomach. This sphincter prevents food from backing up into the esophagus. As waves of peristalsis push food through the lower esophagus, the LES opens (allowing food to enter) and immediately closes (to keep food in the stomach). At this junction, there is an abrupt change from esophageal to gastric mucosa known as the Z-line (Fig. 26-5). Just above the Z-line is the *physiologic inferior esophageal sphincter.* Food and liquid may be stopped here momentarily, to allow the stomach to prepare for the influx of food substances.

> **Nursing Alert**
>
> - If the LES does not relax appropriately, food can be prevented from entering the stomach, a condition known as *achalasia*.
> - If the LES does not close adequately, the stomach contents can reenter the esophagus, causing a severe burning sensation, *heartburn* or *acid reflux,* due to the acidic stomach contents. Untreated, this *gastroesophageal reflux disease* (GERD) can lead to esophageal or gastric (stomach) ulcers and, in more serious cases, bleeding, stricture, or precancerous conditions. GERD may be successfully treated with medications and lifestyle changes (including weight loss and smoking cessation).

> **SPECIAL CONSIDERATIONS** **Lifespan**
>
> The infant's GI system is immature and regurgitation ("spitting up") of feedings is common, usually resolving by 3 months of age. "Burping" or "bubbling" the baby helps remove excess air and gas from the stomach.

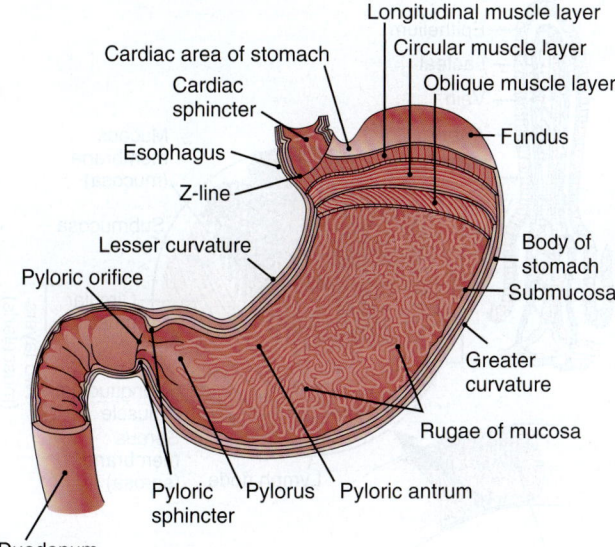

Figure 26-5 Longitudinal section of the stomach and a portion of the duodenum. Rugae and the three muscle layers are shown.

STOMACH

The stomach (*gaster*), located in the upper left side of the abdominal cavity, functions as a reservoir and "food blender." The *gastric or peptic phase* of digestion is initiated here. The stomach is a C-shaped muscular, collapsible pouch or sac capable of being greatly distended (expanded); its abundant blood supply derives from the celiac artery. Stomach volume is approximately 1/5 cup when empty, but it can expand to hold more than 8 cups after a meal (Fig. 26-5). The walnut-sized *pyloric sphincter* controls the opening between the lower stomach and duodenal portion of the small intestine. (The prefix referring to the stomach is *gastr[o]-*.)

SPECIAL CONSIDERATIONS   Lifespan

In infants, projectile vomiting (vomiting with great force) can be a sign of *pyloric stenosis* (narrowing of the pyloric sphincter) and can be life-threatening.

The outside of the stomach is covered by *serous membrane*. Next is a thick pad of *muscles*, lying in three layers. The outermost longitudinal layer contains muscle fibers going from top to bottom, central muscle fibers encircle the stomach, and innermost, the oblique muscles are on a slant or angle. The spread and action of these muscles stir and churn food, break it into small particles, and move it through the system. When the stomach is empty, it collapses and lies in folds called **rugae**, which allow the stomach to distend greatly when food is eaten.

Key Concept

The entire digestive tract, from pharynx to anus, contains longitudinal and circular muscle fibers. Only the stomach contains an oblique muscle layer.

Under the stomach's muscular layers lies the *submucosa*, containing connective tissues that contain nerves, as well as blood and lymph vessels. The innermost stomach layer is the extensively folded *mucosa*, connective tissue covered with gastric glands. Hydrochloric acid (HCl, gastric acid) and pepsinogen (precursor to the enzyme, pepsin) are secreted here. In addition, this layer secretes mucus, which lubricates food and protects the stomach lining from acids and other gastric juices.

Key Concept

Layers of the stomach wall:

- Serous membrane (outer wall)
- Muscles—longitudinal, horizontal, oblique
- Submucosa—containing nerves, blood/lymph vessels
- Mucosa (mucous membrane)—with gastric glands that secrete mucus, HCl, hormones, and precursors to digestive enzymes

In the stomach, foods mix with mucus and gastric acid, as well as pepsin and other digestive enzymes (about 3 quarts—2.8 L a day). These substances churn until they are in a semiliquid, milky form called **chyme** (pronounced "kime"), a process usually taking 3–5 hours. (The stomach's parietal cells also secrete *intrinsic factor,* enabling the body to absorb vitamin B_{12}.) Peristalsis of stomach muscles moves food toward the pyloric outlet. The **pyloric sphincter** at the lower opening of the stomach contracts to keep food in the stomach until it is thoroughly mixed. It then relaxes so that peristaltic waves can squirt food in small amounts into the small intestine. (Although most nutrients move as chyme into the small intestine, some small molecules, such as alcohol, are directly absorbed into the bloodstream from the stomach.) If the stomach is irritated or too full, the direction of peristaltic waves may reverse and force material back into the lower end of the esophagus. This reverse peristalsis, combined with contractions of abdominal muscles and the diaphragm, forces food back through the esophagus and out through the mouth, vomiting (**emesis**).

Key Concept

Stomach acid does not break down food particles. It provides the proper acid–base environment, allowing digestive enzymes to act on food. It prepares proteins for digestion and also kills unwanted microorganisms ingested with food.

SMALL INTESTINE

The *intestinal phase* of digestion begins with the small intestine, the longest portion of the digestive tract (Fig. 26-1). It is approximately 20 ft (6.1 m) long and 1.5 in. (3.81 cm) in diameter (about 18 ft longer than the large intestine). It lies in circular folds, *plicae circularis,* greatly increasing the surface area to allow for nutrient absorption, and it is coiled on itself, to allow it to fit into the abdominal cavity. (The prefix referring to the intestines is *enter[o]-*.) The areas of the small intestine are the *duodenum, jejunum* (midsection), and *ileum* (terminal section). As food elements move through the small intestine, they are altered by several secretions and enzymes. The smooth (involuntary) longitudinal and circular muscles here are antagonistic; when one contracts, the other relaxes. The wavelike contractions of circular muscles narrow the lumen of the intestine, squeezing food onward. When the longitudinal muscles contract, the circular muscles relax, increasing the size of the lumen and allowing food to pass. These rhythmic waves constitute intestinal peristalsis and *segmentation* (Fig. 26-4), which helps break up food particles. (Peristalsis is weaker in the jejunum and ilium unless an obstruction is present.) In addition to muscles, the intestinal wall contains loose connective tissue, the submucosa (tunica mucosa), rich in blood and lymphatic vessels, and the Meissner plexus, which is a network of nerves (Fig. 26-6).

Most digestive processes occur in the small intestine. Intestinal glands in the mucous membrane secrete enzymes, proteins that act as *catalysts,* promoting and speeding up chemical reactions (not undergoing changes themselves). These enzymes break carbohydrates, proteins, and fats into materials the cells can use. To be absorbed by blood and lymph capillaries, carbohydrates must be broken down to simple sugars—monosaccharides: glucose, fructose, and galactose. Proteins must be converted to their simplest state, amino acids; fats must be converted to fatty acids and glycerol.

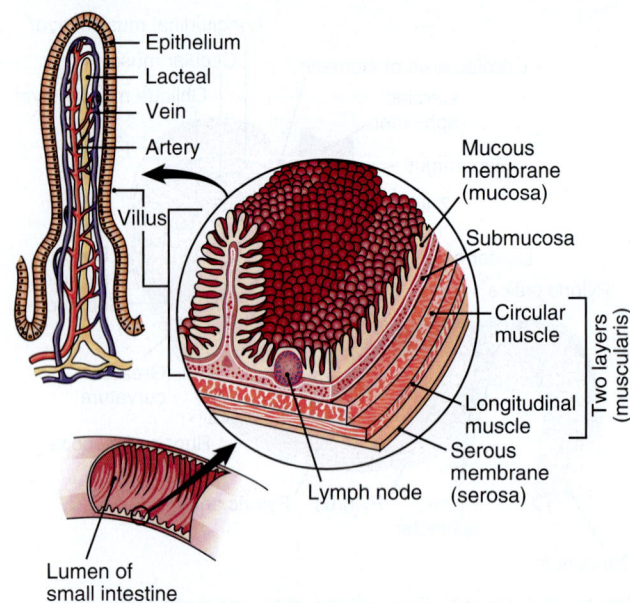

Figure 26-6 The wall of the small intestine, showing numerous villi. At the left is an enlarged drawing of a single villus.

Key Concept
Very few chemical reactions in the body can occur without catalysts. Each enzyme facilitates specific chemical reactions. For example: • Maltase—maltose into glucose • Lactase—lactose into galactose and glucose • Sucrase—sucrose into fructose and glucose • Pepsin, trypsin, chymotrypsin, carboxypeptidase, aminopeptidase, dipeptidase—proteins into amino acids

The small intestine also creates other secretions. *Mucus,* secreted by *Brunner glands,* lubricates and protects the intestinal lining from the highly acidic chyme and digestive enzymes. *Cholecystokinin,* a hormone, stimulates the pancreas to secrete pancreatic juice and the gallbladder to contract, resulting in the release of *bile,* which is secreted in the liver and acts to digest fats—lipids. *Secretin,* another hormone, influences the pancreas to secrete pancreatic juice, containing bicarbonate ions (HCO_3^-) to combine with sodium ions (Na^+) and form sodium bicarbonate ($NaHCO_3$), a basic (alkali) substance to neutralize the very acidic chyme (Table 26-1).

DUODENUM

The first portion of the small intestine is the 10- to 12-in. C-shaped **duodenum** (Figs. 26-1, 26-5, and 26-7). The duodenal wall contains specialized cells and glands to secrete mucus, to protect the small intestine from chyme. As chyme enters the duodenum, more digestive juices are added. **Bile**, a greenish brown liquid manufactured by the liver and stored in the gallbladder, pours in through the *bile duct* to emulsify fats in preparation for further digestive action. The duodenum has several distinct areas and joins the jejunum at the duodenojejunal flexure.

JEJUNUM AND ILEUM

Chyme travels through the remaining portions of the small intestine, the **jejunum** (about 8 ft long), and the terminal **ileum** (about 11 ft long). (The word *jejunum* derives from a Latin word meaning "fasting intestine," so named because it is almost always empty. The word ileum means "flank" or "groin.") The entire small intestine is lined with mucous membrane. Numerous lymph nodules are in the ileum's submucosa, solitary and grouped (called *aggregated lymphatic follicles, Peyer patches*). A sphincter-like muscle, the *ileocecal valve,* located where the large and small intestines meet (the ileum and cecum), acts to prevent backflow of material to the small intestine and also regulates forward flow.

Key Concept
As acidic chyme passes through the digestive tract, it becomes more basic (less acidic). This allows enzymes to function more effectively to break down nutrients into their simplest forms and facilitate absorption into the bloodstream.

LARGE INTESTINE

The large intestine is lined with mucous membrane, as is the entire GI tract. It is much wider than the small intestine (approximately 2.5 in. [6.35 cm] in diameter), but it is only about 5 ft (1.5 m) long. It does not coil, but lies in folds, and

TABLE 26-1 Digestive System Secretions and Their Actions

AREA OF DIGESTIVE SYSTEM	SECRETION	ENZYME	ACTION
Mouth			
Salivary glands	Saliva (also contains water, mucus, and salts)	Salivary amylase (ptyalin)	Begins to break down starch into simpler carbohydrates, such as dextrin Assists swallowing Softens and lubricates food Dissolves some food components
Stomach			
Stomach lining	Mucus Mucin		Protects lining Stimulates secretion of gastric acid (HCl) and pepsin
Specialized cells of pyloric glands	Gastrin (regulatory hormone)		Weakly stimulates secretion of pancreatic enzymes and HCl Stimulates contraction of gallbladder Stimulated by arrival of food in stomach; inhibited by low pH (acids)
Parietal cells	Hydrochloric acid (HCl)		Hydrolyzes some CHO into glucose and fructose Destroys microorganisms Changes pepsinogen to pepsin
	Intrinsic factor		Needed for absorption of vitamin B_{12}, needed for development of RBCs (also requires folate)
Chief cells	Pepsinogen	Pepsin	Begins digestion of proteins into polypeptides
	Gastric lipase	Lipase	Begins digestion of fats by breaking down triglycerides (very little occurs in stomach); acts only on emulsified fats
Liver	Bile		Emulsifies fat to fatty acids, so they can be absorbed Helps neutralize acidic chyme; provides proper pH for enzyme function Excretes bilin and bile acids
Pancreas			
Acinar cells (exocrine function)	Pancreatic juice	Amylase Lipase Trypsin Chymotrypsin Carboxypeptidase Aminopeptidase Dipeptidase Bicarbonate ions	Breaks down dextrin into maltose Breaks down fats into monoglycerides and fatty acids Breaks proteins into amino acids Helps neutralize acids, to facilitate enzyme action
Pancreas (endocrine function)	Insulin (hormone) Glucagon (hormone) Somatostatin (hormone)		Enables cells to use glucose Elevates blood sugar levels Inhibits release of glucagon and insulin

(Continued)

TABLE 26-1 Digestive System Secretions and Their Actions (Continued)

AREA OF DIGESTIVE SYSTEM	SECRETION	ENZYME	ACTION
Small Intestine			
Duodenum and jejunum	Cholecystokinin—CCK (hormone secreted in response to presence of fat)		Activates gallbladder to release bile Stimulates pancreas to secrete pancreatic juice
	Secretin (hormone)		Stimulates secretion of pancreatic juice and some bile Stimulates secretion of bicarbonate ions from pancreas (responds to acid in chyme)
	Bile *from* gallbladder		Breaks fats into tiny droplets (emulsification)
	Pancreatic juice *from* pancreas	Pancreatic protease (trypsin)	Splits proteins into amino acids
		Chymotrypsin	More complex proteins broken down in intestine and at brush border
		Carboxypeptidase	Stimulates release of water and HCO_3^- (bicarbonate) from pancreas
		Pancreatic amylase (and intestinal amylase)	Converts complex CHO into maltose and isomaltose
		Pancreatic lipase	Breaks down emulsified fat into fatty acids, glycerol, and monoglycerides
		Intestinal lipase	Completes digestion of monoglycerides
		Sucrase	Breaks sucrose into fructose[a] and glucose[a] Decreases churning of stomach to slow stomach emptying—in duodenum
	Gastric inhibitory peptide (GIP)		Induces insulin secretion
Intestinal wall mucosa		Maltase	Breaks maltose into glucose
		Lactase	Breaks lactose into glucose and galactose[a]
		Protein enzymes (peptidases)	Assists in digestion of proteins

[a]Complex carbohydrates must be broken down into monosaccharides (simple sugars) before they can be absorbed through the intestinal mucosa. The monosaccharides are glucose, fructose, and galactose. Fiber is mostly excreted undigested.

is divided into areas, the *cecum, colon, rectum,* and *anus.* Water reabsorption is the large intestine's main function. Intestinal bacteria inhibit growth of pathogens here; some produce vitamin K, necessary for blood clotting. Absorption of vitamins and minerals and formation and defecation (egestion) of feces also occur here.

CECUM AND APPENDIX

The proximal portion of the large intestine is the **cecum**, a blind pouch about 2–3 in. (5–7.6 cm) long. A small finger-like projection of the cecum is the *vermiform* (worm-shaped) **appendix**, known simply as the appendix, with no known function. (*Appendix* derives from Latin, meaning "appendage.") It has the same lymphoid tissue as tonsils, and as with tonsils, it frequently becomes infected (*appendicitis* because fecal material cannot always drain out. The body can survive without the appendix, removed by *appendectomy*. The cecum and appendix are located in the right lower quadrant of the abdominal cavity (Fig. 26-1).

COLON

The next and longest portion of the large intestine is the **colon**, a continuous tube classified into three areas, named for the course they follow (Fig. 26-1). The *ascending* (going up) *colon* travels up the right side of the abdominal cavity and is narrower than the cecum; the *transverse* (going across) *colon* crosses to the left side in the upper part of the cavity and is the largest and most mobile portion of the colon; and the *descending* (going down) *colon* goes down the left side into the pelvis. The first two portions absorb fluids, salts, and vitamins; the descending colon holds resulting wastes. The next and last portion, the *sigmoid* (*sigma* is the Greek letter S) *colon*, follows the curve of the sacrum and coccyx and ends at the rectum. It stores feces until defecation occurs via the anus.

RECTUM AND ANUS

The **rectum** is about 5 in. (12.7 cm) in length and terminates at the anal canal, the terminal (end) portion of the large intestine, which is about 1–1.5 in. long (2.54–3.8 cm). Waste products are excreted (**egestion**, defecation) via the opening to the outside (**anus**), which is guarded by internal and external sphincters. The external sphincter can be consciously contracted and relaxed. (Rectal examination yields information about the prostate and seminal glands in males, cervix in females, and other lower pelvic internal structures.)

> **Key Concept**
>
> The pathway of food through the body: mouth → pharynx → esophagus → (cardiac sphincter) → stomach → (pyloric sphincter) → small intestine (duodenum → jejunum → ileum) → (ileocecal valve) → large intestine (cecum → colon: ascending, transverse, descending, sigmoid) → rectum → anus.

ACCESSORY ORGANS

Accessory organs of the digestive system include the liver, gallbladder, pancreas, and peritoneum. Figure 26-7 shows accessory organs of digestion.

Liver and Spleen

The **liver**, the body's largest glandular organ, lies just below the diaphragm in the upper right quadrant of the abdominal cavity, behind the lesser omentum, a fold of the peritoneum. It receives blood supply from the hepatic artery and is divided into two major and two minor lobes. Its functional unit is the *lobule*. (The prefix referring to the liver is *hepat[o]-*.) In humans, the liver weighs about 3 lb (1.36 kg) and resembles calf liver in color and texture.

The liver plays such an important part in overall bodily function that severe disease or injury is life threatening. *Only the brain is capable of more functions than the liver.* Some of the liver's major functions include the following:

- Secretion of bile
- Absorption of bilirubin after destruction of old red blood cells (RBCs)
- Detoxification of blood (removal of toxins or poisons)
- Storage of fat-soluble vitamins (A, D, E, K)
- Formation of vitamin A and some nonessential amino acids; storage of vitamin B complex and iron
- Formation of plasma proteins (albumin, prothrombin, globulins)
- Synthesis of urea, a waste product from protein anabolism
- Storage of glucose as *glycogen* (helps regulate glucose levels)
- Synthesis of clotting factors (fibrinogen; prothrombin; factors V, VII, IX, X)

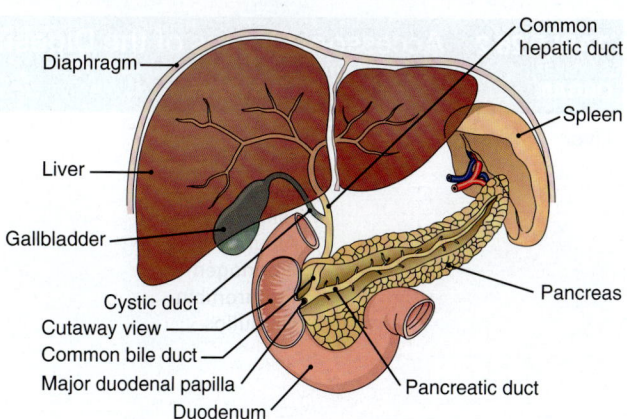

Figure 26-7 Accessory organs of digestion.

- Formation of triglycerides and cholesterol
- Secretion of heparin (anticoagulant)
- Synthesis of immunoglobulins
- Breaking down of fats (lipids)
- Metabolism of carbohydrates; storage of fats and carbohydrates
- Regulation of amino acids
- Production of body heat
- Storage of minerals
- Production of lymph

Table 26-2 lists digestive system accessory organs and functions. The liver's major digestive function is bile production, which aids in fat digestion and absorption of fat and fat-soluble vitamins from the small intestine. The salts in bile *emulsify* fat (break fat into small droplets, like a detergent) so digestive enzymes can act on fat more effectively. The spleen is the body's largest lymphoid organ, lying near the liver. It produces antibodies and filters out damaged red blood cells; it is discussed in Chapter 23.

> **Nursing Alert** Rupture of the liver can occur if a fractured rib penetrates the diaphragm. Since the liver is so vascular, this is an emergency situation.

> **NCLEX Alert**
>
> The digestive system has many structures and functions. To correctly respond to an NCLEX situation, you may need to identify correct nursing actions, appropriate medications, or normal laboratory values.

Gallbladder

The **gallbladder** is a muscular pear-shaped sac 3–4 in. long (7.5–10 cm) located under the liver. It is sometimes considered to be an enlargement of the *cystic duct* through which it drains. (The prefix relating to gallbladder is *chole-*.) Its major functions are storage and release of bile, as needed in the small intestine for fat emulsification. It also concentrates bile by absorbing water and salts. Removal of the

TABLE 26-2 Accessory Organs of the Digestive System and Their Functions

ORGAN	SECRETIONS	FUNCTIONS
Liver	Bile	Emulsifies fats
		Stores glucose (as glycogen)
	Heparin	Anticoagulant
	Plasma proteins	
	Albumin	Provides osmotic pressure for blood pressure
	Fibrinogen	Necessary for blood clotting
	Prothrombin	Necessary for blood clotting
	Globulins	Forms immunoglobulins (antibodies)
		Other Functions of the Liver
		Filters blood; removes toxins
		Breaks down fat and protein
		Stores protein, fat, carbohydrates, and minerals, including iron
		Prepares waste (urea); absorbs bilirubin
		Regulates amino acids
		Produces body heat
		Detoxifies poisons
		Forms vitamin A; stores vitamins A, D, E, K, and B complex
		Forms triglycerides and cholesterol
Gallbladder		Stores and releases bile
Pancreas (exocrine function)	Bicarbonate ions	Helps neutralize HCl (hydrochloric acid)
Acinar cells	Pancreatic juice (pancreatic amylase)	Digests starch (carbohydrates)
	Trypsin	Digests protein
	Pancreatic peptidase	Digests fats (triglycerides)
Pancreas (endocrine function)—islets of Langerhans	Alpha cells—glucagon	Helps regulate blood glucose levels
	Beta cells—insulin	Helps regulate blood glucose levels
	Delta cells—somatostatin	Helps control release of glucagon and insulin

gallbladder (*cholecystectomy*) is a common surgical procedure, after which other structures, particularly the liver, assume its functions.

The system of passageways for bile transport from the liver to the gallbladder to the intestine is complex; it is known as the *biliary apparatus*. First, liver cells manufacture bile and small ducts emerge from these cells and join to form the *hepatic duct*. As bile is produced in the liver, it flows down the hepatic duct and up *into* the cystic duct to the gallbladder for storage. As part of digestion in the small intestine, *cholecystokinin* activates the gallbladder to release bile, which flows *from* the gallbladder down through the cystic duct, which is about 4 cm long. The cystic duct then joins the hepatic duct to create the *bile duct* (formerly known as common bile duct or common hepatic duct). The bile duct, in combination with the pancreatic duct, then empties bile into the duodenum at the *major duodenal papilla* (just beyond the pyloric portion of the stomach).

Pancreas

The pancreas is a long, fish-shaped glandular organ about 6 in. (15 cm) long, located behind the stomach. It has both endocrine and exocrine functions. As an endocrine gland, it secretes the hormones *insulin, glucagon,* and *somatostatin* into the bloodstream, to help regulate blood sugar levels (Chapter 20). Its exocrine function is to produce pancreatic juice, which is necessary for life, because it is vital in digestion. It is produced by the *acinar cells*. The acinar cells secrete three main enzymes that assist in digestion of specific nutrients:

- Pancreatic amylase: starch/carbohydrates
- Trypsin: protein
- Pancreatic lipase: fats—lipids (into triglycerides)

Most pancreatic enzymes are produced in inactive forms and are activated in the small intestine. (The inactive forms help minimize the risk of pancreatic self-digestion.) In addition to the wide variety of digestive enzymes in pancreatic juice, bicarbonate and water are also present. Bicarbonate ions (HCO_3^-) are secreted from small ductules in the pancreas and combine with hydrogen ions to neutralize the hydrochloric acid in chyme. (Enzymes work best in a solution with a pH between 5 and 8.) The potent pancreatic juice enters the duodenum through the *pancreatic duct*.

Peritoneum

The **peritoneum** is a large sheet of serous membrane covering and protecting many abdominal organs. It also secretes the thin *peritoneal fluid*, providing lubrication between its *visceral* (next to organs) and *parietal* (next to abdominal wall) layers. The peritoneal peritoneum attaches the jejunum and ileum to the posterior abdominal wall, to prevent twisting. The peritoneal folds providing support and protection are called *mesenteries,* sheets of connective tissue. Some have names (e.g., the *greater* and *lesser omentum*). Some body structures, such as the kidneys, lie behind the peritoneum (*retroperitoneal*), allowing kidney surgery to be performed from the back.

TABLE 26-3	Human Digestive Process
Chewing of food	5–10 s
Swallowing	10–15 s
Food mixing in stomach	3–5 hr
Movement through small intestine	3–4 hr
Movement through large intestine	18–48 hr

SYSTEM PHYSIOLOGY

Processes of Digestion

For nutrients to reach individual cells, food first must be broken down. After this, **absorption** (passage of nutrients into body cells) can occur (Chapter 30). The body performs two types of digestion: mechanical and chemical. Table 26-3 summarizes the digestive process.

- *Mechanical digestion* is the physical breakdown of food caused by chewing and the movement of food in the digestive tract. Breaking food into smaller pieces exposes more food surface area to the effects of enzymes, acids, and other chemicals.
- *Chemical digestion* is the breakdown of chemical bonds in food, with the addition of enzymes, acids, and water. Some digestive processes begin in the mouth, pharynx, and stomach, but most digestion occurs in the duodenum.

Enzymes

As described previously, enzymes are the driving force behind chemical digestion. They are secreted by salivary glands, the stomach, small and large intestines, liver, and pancreas. Enzymes often derive their names from the substances on which they act and each enzyme is effective only on a specific nutrient (Table 26-1).

Mucus and Water

The GI tract requires fluids to lubricate, liquefy, and digest food. Mucus, formulated by the mucous membrane lining of the entire GI tract, lubricates food and protects the GI tract's lining from mechanical or chemical injury (from stomach acids). Water liquefies food, making it easier to digest and absorb. Water also participates in chemical reactions and is the solvent that follows electrolytes (osmosis) across the intestinal wall in either direction (Chapter 17).

Digestion in the Stomach

The fundus and body of the stomach act mostly for storage; the pylorus is the primary site of stomach digestion. Both mechanical digestion and chemical digestion occur in the stomach. Saliva from the oral cavity continues starch digestion in the stomach, but carbohydrates are not fully digested there. Fat digestion continues in the stomach, due to lingual lipase, but only a very small amount is broken down there. Pepsin begins protein digestion in the stomach, but it is not completed there either. In addition to mucous membrane, the stomach lining also contains secretory cells: *chief cell*s and *parietal cells.*

- *Chief cells* secrete pepsinogen and gastric lipase. *Pepsinogen* is a precursor of pepsin, the enzyme needed to break down proteins. *Gastric lipase* breaks down triglycerides in butterfat (found in milk and dairy products).
- *Parietal cells* secrete *hydrochloric acid* (HCl), which functions to activate pepsinogen and kill most stomach microorganisms. When activated, pepsinogen changes into the enzyme *pepsin,* which begins to break down proteins. Another secretion of parietal cells is *intrinsic factor,* essential for life, because it is required for vitamin B_{12} absorption, needed to develop red blood cells in bone marrow. Vitamin B_{12} deficiency results in pernicious anemia.

The stomach also produces regulatory hormones, such as *gastrin,* which stimulates HCl secretion, and pepsinogen. It also weakly stimulates the pancreas to secrete enzymes and the gallbladder to release some bile.

Digestion in the Small Intestine

Most digestion occurs in the small intestine. Here, *cholecystokinin* (CCK), a hormone, is secreted by the duodenum and jejunum in response to the presence of fat in the duodenum. CCK activates the gallbladder to release bile, which flows through the *cystic duct* into the *bile duct* and is deposited in the duodenum. There, the action of bile breaks fat droplets into smaller particles. Bile also helps neutralize the acidic chyme and facilitates excretion of waste products, including bilin and bile acids. CCK also stimulates the pancreas to secrete pancreatic juice, which is then changed into an active form in the small intestine. Specific enzymes (amylase, trypsin, and lipase) in pancreatic juice digest starch, protein, and triglycerides (fats), respectively. CCK also assists in inhibition of digestive processes in the stomach when appropriate.

The balance of acidity and alkalinity is vital. The pH in the upper digestive tract is weakly acidic, beginning the breakdown of carbohydrates (CHO). Most digestive enzymes cannot function in the stomach because it is too acidic; thus, CHO digestion is inhibited there. However, the low pH (acid) in the stomach begins protein breakdown. In the small intestine, the pH rises (becomes more basic/alkaline), due to the addition of bicarbonates. Enzymes can now function and CHO digestion resumes, along with fat and protein breakdown. Sucrase, maltase, and lactase—enzymes secreted by the intestinal mucosa—assist in digestion of CHO. Several protein enzymes, *peptidases,* also assist in digestion of proteins. When digestion is completed, the *simplest form* of all nutrients remains and these substances are ready to be transferred into the bloodstream for use by the body (absorption). Table 26-1 summarizes the actions of enzymes, hormones, and other substances in digestion.

> **Key Concept**
>
> Digestion is accomplished by the following processes:
>
> - Physical breakdown (mastication)
> - Churning
> - Diluting
> - Chemical breakdown
> - Dissolving
>
>   To be absorbed, foods must be broken into their simplest form:
>
> - Carbohydrate to monosaccharides (simple sugars): glucose, galactose, fructose
> - Protein to amino acids (and some dipeptides)
> - Fat to fatty acids (lipids) and glycerol

> **NCLEX Alert**
>
> The digestive system's physiology is important. Concepts such as liver disease, nutrition, ulcer formation, or malignancies may be included in scenarios. The NCLEX commonly provides scenarios that integrate the body's normal anatomical functions with abnormal situations.

Absorption in the Small Intestine

Absorption of approximately 85% of nutrients used by the body occurs across the **villi**, small finger-like projections on the mucosa of the small intestine, into the capillary network (Fig. 26-6). To increase surface area, villi contain *microvilli,* microscopic folds on the surface of epithelial cells in the cell membrane. (Unfolded and straightened out, one person's villi and microvilli could completely cover more than 2,000 square feet, half a basketball court.) Villi wave to keep food molecules thoroughly mixed with digestive juices. Amino acids are absorbed in the duodenum and jejunum; most fats are absorbed in the jejunum. Because villi are so important in absorption, they are heavily supplied with capillaries, which carry nutrients, via hepatic portal circulation, to the liver for further processing. Recall that *active and passive transport* (Chapter 17) are the means by which nutrients are absorbed into the circulation and then to the body's cells.

> **Key Concept**
>
> Absorption of nutrients into the bloodstream occurs via the small intestine. The body cannot use these food materials, however, until the bloodstream delivers them to the cells by transporting the particles across each cell's membrane.

Fat Absorption

Bile salts are important in forming micelles, colloid (glue-like) particles, most often arranged in a parallel chain, which transport digested fats to intestinal villi for absorption. Most fatty acids (long-chain) are transported this way, then absorbed into **lacteals** (dead-end lymph capillaries within each villus that absorb fat-soluble nutrients), and carried by the lymphatic system to be used by the body. Because of the fat content in lacteals, their contents, called *chyle* (pronounced kile), appear milky. Fats eventually reach the bloodstream via the thoracic and right lymphatic ducts.

> **Key Concept**
>
> Digestion of one substance can occur in several locations as food passes through the digestive system. For example, starch, a complex carbohydrate, is broken down as follows:
>
> *STARCH* (mouth—salivary amylase, chewing) → *DEXTRIN* (small intestine—pancreatic amylase) → *MALTOSE* (intestinal wall mucosa—maltase) → *GLUCOSE* → absorbed into body.

Absorption in the Large Intestine

After "food" has been in the small intestine for about 4–6 hours, it passes into the large intestine. All that remains is water, electrolytes, and waste products. This represents about 1,500 mL of chyme per day. As chyme travels through the large intestine, intestinal walls of the *proximal* (first section) colon reabsorb about 80% of remaining water back into the circulation, helping prevent dehydration. Water travels by osmosis, following absorption of mineral salts, mainly sodium (Chapter 17). After reabsorption, only wastes remain, which are concentrated in the terminal portions of the colon. When wastes reach the end of the colon (*distal colon*), the **feces** are excreted out of the body as stool (defecation).

METABOLISM

Metabolism is defined as "biotransformation," the total of all physical/chemical changes occurring within the body to maintain life. Physical conversions include chewing and breaking down food into smaller particles. Chemical conversions include actions of enzymes, which alter food into chemically smaller substances. The liver is vital for metabolism. The two major categories of metabolism are catabolism and anabolism:

- *Catabolism* (destruction, catabolic phase) is the breakdown of larger molecules into smaller ones, releasing energy. *Cellular respiration* is a series of catabolic reactions. The end products of catabolism resulting from cellular respiration are carbon dioxide, water, and energy.
- *Anabolism* (construction, anabolic phase) is the synthesis of simpler substances into new, organized substances to be used by body cells. Examples of anabolism include synthesis of glycogen, triglycerides, or proteins.

Energy Synthesis and Release

During catabolism, energy is released, which is synthesized into a vital compound, adenosine triphosphate (ATP), without which anabolism cannot occur. ATP stores energy and uses it to drive all related cellular processes, including transport of ions and molecules across cell membranes, contraction of muscle fibers, and synthesis of many other compounds. The term *basal metabolism* refers to the minimum amount of energy (calories) the body requires to maintain baseline vegetative vital functions, such as breathing, body temperature, and circulation.

> *Key Concept*
> **Metabolism**
> - Catabolism (destructive metabolism): breaking down foods into useable substances (generates heat, carbon dioxide, water, and ATP)
> - Anabolism (constructive metabolism): using products of catabolism to build and repair body cells and maintain life

ELIMINATION

Since there are no enzymes in the colon, minimal digestion occurs there. Whatever nutrients are not reabsorbed and sent to the portal (liver) circulation are eliminated as solid intestinal wastes (**defecation**, *bowel movement, egestion*). After water reabsorption, a plant fiber, *cellulose,* other undigested material, living and dead bacteria, and mucus remain. These mass together and pass into the rectum as *solid or semisolid waste* or *feces (excrement, excreta),* where they stimulate sensory nerve endings, causing a sensation of accumulating bulk and initiate the defecation (evacuation) reflex. Peristaltic waves push feces against the anal muscle as a signal for emptying the rectum (the *defecation reflex*), and parasympathetic-controlled nervous activity causes strong contractions. The internal sphincter relaxes and pressure from peristalsis, along with pressure *consciously* exerted by the diaphragm and abdominal muscles, brings about defecation. To expel feces, the external anal sphincter, a skeletal muscle, relaxes voluntarily. If the defecation reflex is ignored routinely, the impulse tends to die and constipation often occurs. This can become life threatening if it results in bowel obstruction.

Chapter 20 describes endocrine influences on digestive processes. Chapter 30 introduces the science of nutrition, and transcultural and social aspects of nutrition are discussed in Chapter 31. The application of nutrition to nursing and diet therapy and special diets is described in Chapter 32. Some digestive disorders are genetic; others are acquired. Chapter 88 describes many digestive disorders and their treatment in more detail.

> *Key Concept*
> The stages of digestion are as follows:
> - Ingestion—taking in of food
> - Breakdown—mechanical and chemical conversion of food into useable molecules
> - Absorption—transfer of nutrients into circulatory/lymphatic systems for use by the body
> - Egestion—elimination of waste products by defecation

SPECIAL CONSIDERATIONS   Lifespan

Nursing care for the older adult client must adapt to changes related to aging. The aging process has a significant effect on the digestive system (Table 26-4).

TABLE 26-4 Effects of Aging on the Digestive System

FACTOR	RESULT	NURSING IMPLICATIONS
Saliva production decreases	More difficulty swallowing	Provide adequate fluids
Decreased gag reflex	Choking	Observe carefully for choking Provide liquid with medications. May need to crush medications or place in applesauce
Bony structures decrease around the mouth	Mouth discomfort Poor eating habits Difficulty chewing Sunken appearance of mouth Low self-esteem, less desire for social contact	May need softer foods or ground foods Monitor for adequate intake Assess fit and comfort of dentures Reinforce self-esteem
Loss of teeth. Tooth loss is not a normal function of aging; usually the effect of poor nutrition and hygiene	Loose teeth, ill-fitting dentures, difficulty eating; reduced biting strength Mouth discomfort Periodontal disease	Monitor nutrient intake Encourage high protein supplements Puree or chop food, as needed Promote good oral hygiene and dental care

(Continued)

TABLE 26-4	Effects of Aging on the Digestive System (Continued)	
FACTOR	RESULT	NURSING IMPLICATIONS
Taste decreases, especially sweet and sour tastes. Sense of smell decreases	Food not enjoyed Increased amounts of salt and sugar eaten Less desire to eat, leading to poor nutrient intake	Assess for eating patterns Explain the harm of excess calories and salt Teach about a balanced diet Encourage use of programs such as Meals on Wheels
Cardiac sphincter relaxes	Reflux of undigested food into esophagus (heartburn common) May lead to excess use of over-the-counter (OTC) antacids	Discourage overuse of OTC antacids. Can lead to electrolyte imbalance and reduced absorption of fat-soluble vitamins
Gastric mucosa atrophies and secretions such as HCl, intrinsic factor, and enzymes may decrease	Digestion usually adequate May have decreased absorption of some vitamins and calcium	Monitor nutrient intake Watch for signs of pernicious anemia
Food stays in stomach longer	Indigestion Bloating Excess gas	Tell client to limit foods that cause problems, such as spicy foods and foods that form gas (e.g., nuts, beans)
Peristalsis decreases Reduced secretion of digestive juices Ignoring the need to defecate	Constipation Slowed defecation Some food left undigested; may lead to insufficient food or nutrients Use of OTC laxatives or enemas	Encourage fluid and fiber intake Encourage exercise Do not expect daily bowel movement Monitor laxative and enema use Teach about fluid and fiber use; may need stool softeners (e.g., Colace) Check for impaction or bowel obstruction
Occurrence of gallstones may increase	May need gallbladder removal	Provide surgical care Ensure lower fat intake postoperatively
Lower tolerance to some foods Ignoring hunger or thirst Decreases in absorptive surfaces in intestines, due to decreased villi height and decreased intestinal motility Fat tissue replaces muscle tissue Reduced exercise; poor diet Caloric needs decrease Physical inactivity Difficulty swallowing (may be due to disease process such as stroke, Huntington disease, etc.) Dementia—may forget to eat or may repeats meals Financial factors—cannot afford nutritious diet Unable to properly prepare foods Anal sphincter insufficiency	Increased stomach upset, heartburn, nausea, diarrhea Inadequate intake of food or fluids Inadequate digestion Weight gain; flabby body tissues May be influenced by reduced efficiency of digestive system Afraid to eat because afraid of choking Fecal incontinence	Select foods carefully Encourage intake of varied fluids Encourage safe exercise program Monitor intake Encourage exercise program and dietary adjustments Encourage use of food shelf, meal programs Advise use of diaper items Reorient as needed Counsel regarding high-quality but inexpensive foods; encourage use of food bank Suggest "Meals on Wheels" Provide with pads, bedside commode, barrier creams

STUDENT SYNTHESIS

KEY POINTS

- Primary functions of the digestive system include digestion, absorption, and elimination.
- The digestive (gastrointestinal—GI) tract is a continuous tube beginning at the mouth and ending at the anus. It is open to the outside on both ends and is not sterile.
- Accessory organs of the digestive system include the liver, gallbladder, pancreas, and peritoneum.
- The two types of digestion are mechanical (chewing, peristalsis) and chemical (breakdown of food into a useable form).
- The breaking down of food into smaller molecules is digestion, utilizing enzymes, acids, and ATP. Absorption is the passage of these molecules into the circulation.
- Most nutrient absorption occurs in the small intestine.
- The large intestine mainly reabsorbs water, produces vitamin K and some B-complex vitamins, and prepares wastes for elimination.
- Metabolism is the total of all physical and chemical changes that occur in the body. It includes catabolism and anabolism.
- A variety of digestive changes in older adults can place them at risk for fluid and electrolyte imbalance, dehydration, constipation, malnutrition, and inappropriate weight.

CRITICAL THINKING EXERCISES

1. Based on this chapter, anticipate types of digestive problems that might occur if the following organs or structures were to malfunction: the teeth, esophagus, stomach, liver, gallbladder, small intestine, or large intestine.
2. An older adult man comes to the healthcare facility complaining of constipation. He has been using laxatives often to help alleviate this problem. What is your reaction? What advice would you give this client? What lifestyle changes could he make to help his situation?
3. A client has had a cholecystectomy. Explain to them the function of the gallbladder and why its removal is not life threatening.

NCLEX-STYLE REVIEW QUESTIONS

1. A client is scheduled for a cholecystectomy. Prior to the procedure, the client asks the nurse, "what will happen without my gallbladder?" Which response by the nurse is the best?
   a. "Another structure such as the liver will take over its function."
   b. "When you have a bowel movement, you will not have solid stools."
   c. "Since you have an inability to process glucose you will have to take insulin."
   d. "You will have to take medication to help your blood clot."

2. A client informs the nurse that due to a busy work schedule, the need to defecate is often ignored and he then often feels constipated. Which action should the nurse take first?
   a. Give the client a soapsuds enema
   b. Auscultate for bowel sounds
   c. Administer a laxative
   d. Instruct the client to defecate when the urge is present

3. The nurse is caring for a client with anal sphincter insufficiency who is bed confined and requires ADL (activities of daily living) assistance. Which nursing actions should be included when caring for this client? Select all that apply.
   a. Turn the client every 2 hours
   b. Insert a rectal tube
   c. Provide pads on the bed
   d. Ensure a bedside commode is readily accessible for the client
   e. Use barrier cream to protect the skin

4. A client is experiencing indigestion, bloating, excess gas, and constipation due to delayed gastric emptying. Which suggestion offered by the nurse may help alleviate these symptoms?
   a. Limit the amount of fluid intake
   b. Increase the amount of dairy in the diet
   c. Limit spicy and gas forming foods
   d. Decrease the amount of fiber ingested

5. A client has a diagnosis of pernicious anemia due to a loss of intrinsic factor. An order has been issued. Which treatment will the nurse most likely need to prepare to administer to the client?
   a. Vitamin B_{12} injection
   b. A blood transfusion
   c. A dose of heparin subcutaneously
   d. Intravenous fluids

CHAPTER RESOURCES

Enhance your learning with additional resources on thePoint*!*

Student Resources related to this chapter can be found at thePoint.lww.com/Rosdahl12e.

27 The Urinary System

Learning Objectives

1. Identify the organs of the urinary system on an anatomical chart or model.
2. Describe the anatomy and physiology of the nephron.
3. Explain how the urinary system influences homeostasis.
4. Describe the functions of the two hormones secreted by the kidneys.
5. Explain how the kidney, ANP, and the RAA system impact red blood cells, blood pressure, water and electrolyte balance, acid–base balance, and vitamin D synthesis.
6. Describe blood supply to, within, and from the kidneys.
7. Illustrate the pathway of waste products from the blood to the external environment.
8. Describe the formation of urine. Include concepts of glomerular filtration, tubular reabsorption, and tubular secretion.
9. Describe chemical differences between plasma, glomerular filtrate, and urine.
10. Compare and contrast normal micturition and incontinence.
11. List characteristics and usual components of normal urine.
12. Describe effects of aging on the urinary system and related nursing implications.

Important Terminology

bladder, Bowman capsule, calyx (calyces), convoluted tubule, erythropoietin, glomerulus, incontinence, kidney, loop of Henle, micturition, nephron, nocturia, renal cortex, renal medulla, renal threshold, renin, retention (urinary), ureter, urethra, urination, urology, void

Acronyms

DCT, GFR, JGA, PCT, TM

As the body builds and repairs tissues and produces energy for life processes, waste products form and must be removed. By perspiring and breathing, the integumentary and respiratory systems remove some water, carbon dioxide, and nitrogenous wastes. Through defecation, the digestive system removes solid wastes. Another system, the *urinary* or *excretory system*, is also involved in waste removal, the body's "filtration and removal plant." (When combined with the male reproductive system, it is known as the *genitourinary* system—GUS.) Circulating blood carries wastes from the cells to the kidneys for urinary elimination. Much material removed by the kidneys is water, although solid wastes are also dissolved or in suspension in urine. *Uro-* is the word element referring to urine. A specialist who deals with the female urinary system and the male genitourinary system is the *urologist*; the related science is **urology**. Although the anatomy of the urinary system is relatively simple, it is vital in maintenance of homeostasis.

Structure and Function

The major structures of the urinary system are as follows:

- Two *kidneys* extract wastes from the blood, balance body fluids, and form urine.
- Two *ureters* conduct urine from the kidneys to the urinary bladder.
- The *urinary bladder* serves as a reservoir for urine.
- The *urethra* conducts urine from the bladder to the outside of the body for elimination.

The urinary system is able to adapt to wide variations in dietary and fluid intake and also adjusts and maintains the composition of blood, tissue fluids, and interstitial fluids; in addition, the volume of circulating fluids in the blood affects blood pressure. The urinary system helps control blood volume by excreting or conserving water. (An accumulation of water in tissues is *edema* [see Fig. 76-2]; an abnormal decrease is *dehydration*.) By excreting or conserving minerals (especially sodium and chlorine), the urinary system regulates specific levels of electrolytes in body tissues and fluids. Box 27-1 summarizes functions of the urinary system.

KIDNEYS

The **kidneys** are two reddish-brown, bean-shaped organs in the small of the back, at the lower edge of the ribs on either side of the vertebral column (Fig. 27-1). They are each about the size of a human fist (about 4 in. [10 cm] long, 2 in. [5 cm] wide, and 1 in. [2.5 cm] thick). On top of each kidney lies an *adrenal* (suprarenal) gland (ad = near,

Box 27-1 Functions of the Urinary System

MAINTENANCE OF HOMEOSTASIS
- Controls water and blood volume
- Maintains blood pressure
- Regulates electrolyte levels; reabsorbs some electrolytes
- Maintains pH balance
- Helps maintain acid/base balance
- Activates vitamin D (for bone calcification)

MANUFACTURE
- Secretes renin and erythropoietin

PROCESSING OF WASTES
- Filters blood
- Forms urine (kidneys)
- Stores urine (bladder)

ELIMINATION
- Eliminates protein wastes, excess salts, and toxic materials

A person can easily live with one kidney. *Ren-* is the prefix related to kidneys; the descriptive term is *renal*. The word element referring to the kidney is *nephr(o-)*.

The kidneys are extremely *vascular* (heavily supplied with blood vessels), to provide blood supply for filtering and waste removal. Approximately 10% of the body's blood circulates through the kidneys daily. Each kidney is surrounded by *perinephric* (around the kidney) fat and is surrounded by a fibrous capsule, which continues downward, forming the outer layer of the ureter covering. The fatty pads, plus renal fascia, anchored to surrounding tissues, help hold the kidneys in place. On the medial surface of each kidney (toward the middle of the body) is an indented area called the *hilum*, a notch through which blood vessels, nerves, and the ureter enter. The kidneys can precisely regulate and adjust electrolyte levels. Body fluid volume is regulated by management of sodium chloride (NaCl) levels. The kidneys balance pH in the blood, the body fluids, and within body tissues by eliminating acids directly into the urine or by excreting acids bound to chemical buffers. These buffers change strong acids into weaker acids, enabling the kidneys to excrete large amounts of acid without dramatically altering (or lowering) urine pH. (However, urine is still 1,000 times more acidic than blood.) Other major functions of the kidneys include hormonal secretion of renin and erythropoietin and activation of vitamin D.

SPECIAL CONSIDERATIONS Nutrition

Urine Acidity and Alkalinity
Urine is normally acidic, with a pH of about 6 (pH range: 4.5–8). Foods ingested can alter the acidity or alkalinity of urine. Foods that will acidify urine are cranberries, meat, and a high-protein diet. Foods that will alkalinize urine are citrus fruits, dairy products, and legumes. Foods ingested can also alter the odor of urine. Certain foods and medications alter the color of urine.

If the kidney is cut in half longitudinally, it is clearly divided into two parts: the outside, the *cortex*, and the inner portion, the *medulla* ("middle"). The **renal cortex** is the outer reddish-brown part of the kidney that extends from the outside of the kidney (renal capsule) to the bases of the renal pyramids and into the spaces between them (Fig. 27-2). The renal corpuscles (glomeruli and Bowman capsules) and the proximal and distal portions of the convoluted tubules make up the major portion of the renal cortex (see "Nephrons" section and Fig. 27-3).

The **renal medulla** contains the remainder of the renal tubules, loops of Henle, and collecting tubules. These tubules form a number of cone-shaped structures, the *renal pyramids*. These 8–12 pyramids are arranged so their bases are on the outside near the renal cortex. The tips (*renal papillae*) of the renal pyramids point medially toward the *renal pelvis*, a funnel-shaped basin at the upper end of the ureter. Urine flows from the collecting tubules through the pyramids and into cup-like extensions of the renal pelvis, the *calyces* (singular: **calyx**). Table 27-1 summarizes key information.

over); these influence blood pressure, as well as sodium and water retention in the kidneys. (See Chapter 20 for endocrine functions.)

The kidneys are *retroperitoneal* (behind the peritoneum), allowing kidney surgery to be performed from the back, without entering the abdominal cavity. The right kidney is slightly lower than the left, making space for the liver.

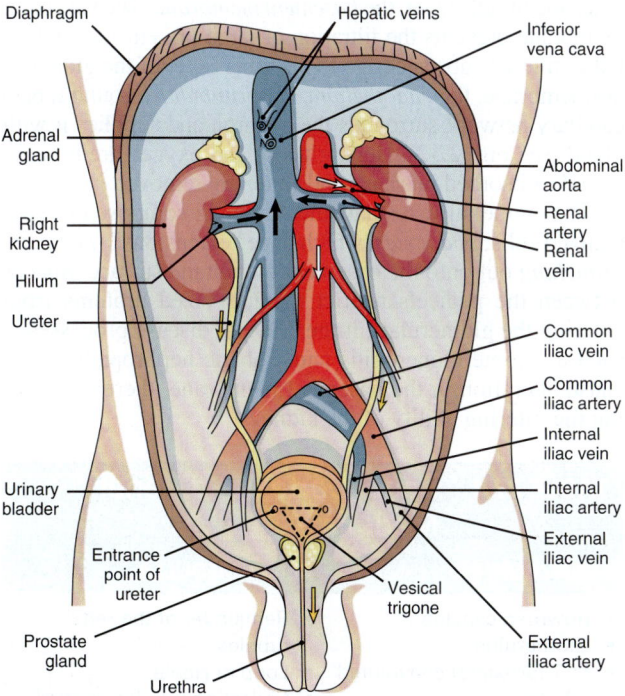

Figure 27-1 The male urinary system, with blood vessels, as viewed from the front. *Yellow arrows* indicate direction of urine flow. *White and black arrows* indicate direction of blood flow into and out of the kidney. The renal artery branches directly off the aorta.

Nephrons

The major role of the kidneys is the filtration of water-soluble wastes out of the blood. **Nephrons** (from Greek: *nephros* = kidney) are the functional units of the kidney.

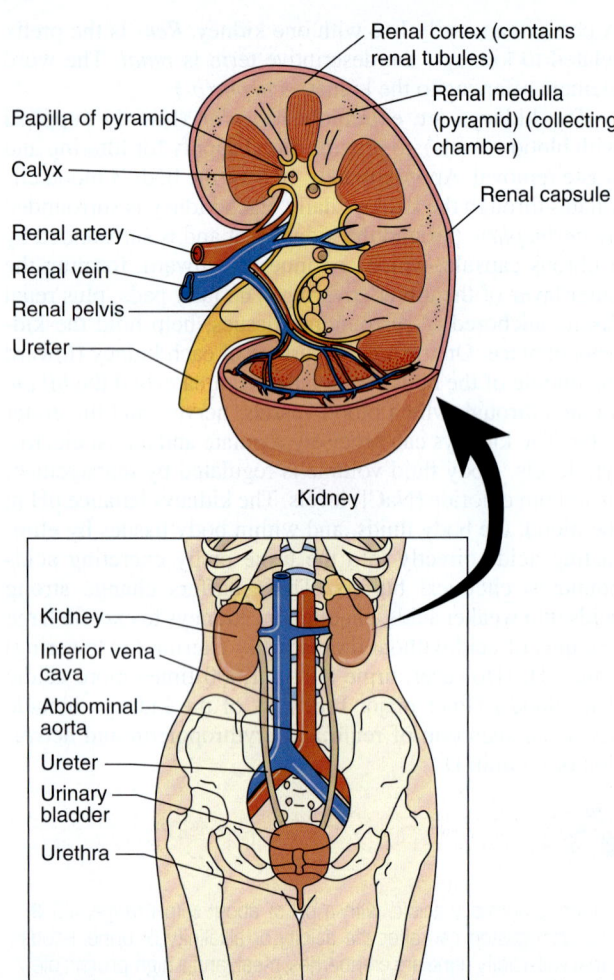

Figure 27-2 Internal structure of the kidney and blood vessels and location in the female body.

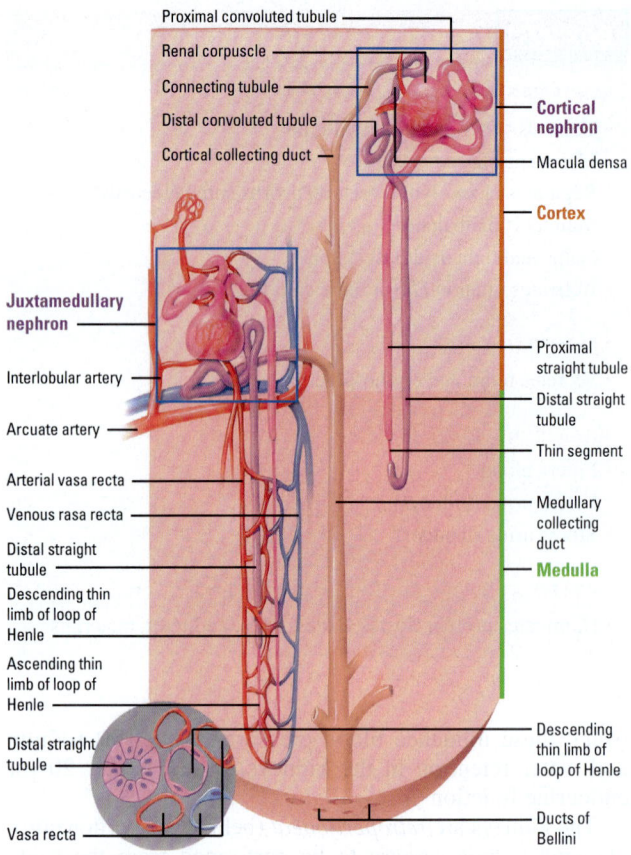

Figure 27-3 A nephron. (Anatomy and Physiology Made Incredibly Easy.)

Nephrons *form* urine; the other structures of the urinary system *expel* urine. More than 1 million microscopic nephrons are in each kidney, but humans can survive using only one third of their nephrons.

Most of each nephron is in the renal cortex (superficial and midcortical nephrons), except for a small tube in the medulla. *Juxtamedullary nephrons* are those near the medulla. At one end of each microscopic nephron is a knotted cluster, tuft, or loop of capillaries, the **glomerulus** (plural: glomeruli; from Latin *glomus* = ball), which are supported by a thin membrane, the *mesangium* (see Fig. 27-4B). The glomerulus is partially enclosed in a funnel-shaped structure, **Bowman capsule** (*Bowman space, glomerular capsule*) (see Fig. 27-3), which pressure-filters small solutes out of the blood through pores. The glomerulus and Bowman capsule together are known as the *renal corpuscle* (or *malpighian corpuscle*), which is the beginning of the nephron. Because the efferent arteriole (leaving the glomerulus) is smaller in diameter than the afferent arteriole, the pressure in the glomerulus is increased, assisting in pressure filtration of molecules out of plasma.

The glomerular walls contain three layers that filter blood (Fig. 27-4B,C). The outside layer of the glomerular membrane, the *epithelium* or *capsular membrane*, is a thin, porous membrane which has large openings (pores) that allow all blood components, except RBCs, to pass through until they reach the middle layer, the *basement membrane*. The basement membrane prevents the filtration of large proteins through it. Other filtered substances go to the inner layer of the glomerular membrane, the *endothelium*. A *peritubular* (around tubes) capillary network surrounds the nephron and supplies it with blood (see Fig. 27-3). Here, glucose and oxygen are brought in and reabsorbed nutrients and water are removed.

The epithelial (capsular) membrane is composed of specialized cells, *podocytes*, which have "extensions" (*pedicels*) branching out onto the basement membrane surface. Spaces between the pedicels restrict medium-sized proteins from entering the glomerular filtrate. Several disease processes—such as glomerulonephritis and diabetic nephropathy—can cause alteration in the basement membrane, thereby reducing the filtering ability of the kidneys.

TABLE 27-1	Renal Cortex and Renal Medulla
RENAL CORTEX	**RENAL MEDULLA**
• Bowman capsule • Glomerulus • PCT (proximal convoluted tubule) • DCT (distal convoluted tubule) • Largest part of each nephron	• Remainder of the renal tubules • Loop of Henle • Collecting tubules (ducts) (make up renal pyramids) • Renal pyramids

CHAPTER 27   The Urinary System   323

in a dilute solution. The capillaries of the glomerulus unite to form the *efferent arteriole*, which carries away remaining blood. Extending from Bowman capsule is a long twisted tube, the **convoluted tubule** (*renal tubule*) (see Fig. 27-3), consisting of freely permeable cell membranes. The first portion is the *proximal convoluted tubule* (**PCT**). Here, glucose, amino acids, and salts (electrolytes) are actively transported across membranes and returned to the blood. The PCT accomplishes the process of selective reabsorption because it contains a "brush border," with many villi. Adenosine triphosphate (*ATP*) is also produced by mitochondria here, to assist in active transport. The next portion of the convoluted tubule is the **loop of Henle** (*nephron loop*), the major function of which is to concentrate salts by reabsorbing water (by osmosis). The final portion (the end of the nephron unit) is the *distal convoluted tubule* (**DCT**), the site of tubular secretion. Molecules secreted here include creatinine and hydrogen ions. Fluids filtered through the glomerulus, with their dissolved contents, travel the length of these renal tubules. (Nephrons contain straight tubules as well.) The juxtaglomerular apparatus (JGA) or juxtaglomerulus, consisting of specialized glandular cells responsible for maintaining blood pressure (discussed later), lies at the point where the DCT contacts the afferent arteriole.

After blood leaves the DCT, it moves to the *collecting tubule* or duct system (*medullary collecting duct, collecting duct*), where antidiuretic hormone (ADH) exerts its effects to allow the tubule to become partially permeable to water (see next section). Therefore, the collecting tubule is an important regulator in concentration/dilution of urine. The peritubular capillaries reabsorb much of the water and salts and all of the glucose. The urine, containing wastes, then continues through the renal pyramid to the renal pelvis and onward to the ureter and bladder. Table 27-2 summarizes nephron structures and their functions.

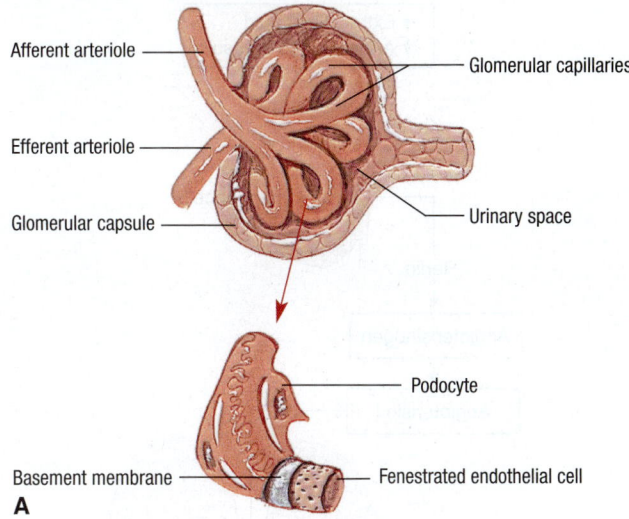
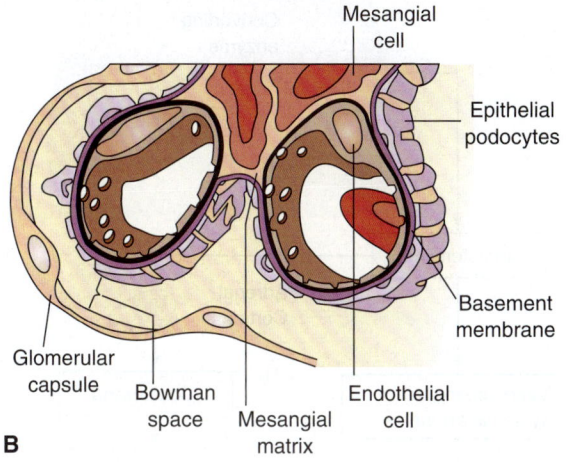
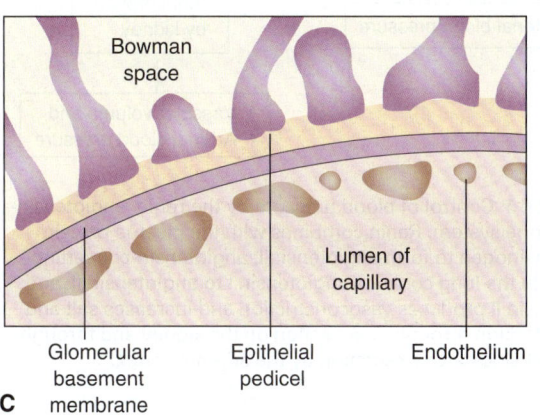

Figure 27-4 Renal corpuscle. **A.** Structures of the glomerulus. (Atlas of Human Anatomy, 2001.) **B.** Position of the mesangial cells in relation to the capillary loops and Bowman capsule. **C.** Cross-section of the glomerular membrane, showing the position of the epithelium (with epithelial pedicels), basement membrane, and endothelium.

Blood, with its filterable wastes and food products, enters the glomerulus through the *afferent arteriole*, which divides to form the capillary loop (Fig. 27-4A). Water, wastes, glucose, and salts filter through the thin walls of the glomerulus, as described above, and then enter Bowman capsule

> **Key Concept**
>
> Pathway of urine in the kidney:
>
> Afferent arteriole → glomerulus and Bowman capsule → PCT → loop of Henle (descending limb, *permeable to water and impermeable to salts;* ascending limb, *impermeable to water and pumps sodium out of filtrate*) → distal convoluted tubule (*with parathyroid hormone, reabsorbs calcium, excretes phosphate; with aldosterone, reabsorbs sodium, excretes potassium; also regulates pH with hydrogen and ammonium*) → JGA (end of nephron) → collecting duct system.

Role of Hormones and Other Substances

The kidneys secrete two hormones: renin and erythropoietin.

Renin and the RAA Mechanism

Renin is very important in blood pressure regulation. If blood pressure or circulating blood volume falls too low, cells of the JGA secrete renin into the bloodstream. This activates the *renin–angiotensin–aldosterone* (RAA) *mechanism*, to raise blood pressure (Fig. 27-5). Renin stimulates the formation of angiotensin I, which, in the presence of a converting enzyme, converts to angiotensin II. Angiotensin II causes blood vessel constriction, directly raising blood pressure,

TABLE 27-2 Nephron Structures and Their Functions

STRUCTURE	FUNCTION
Glomerulus and Bowman capsule	Filters water, wastes (urea), glucose, and salts (electrolytes) out of blood (filtrate consists of water plus all non-protein components of the plasma)
Convoluted tubules	
Proximal convoluted tubule	Reabsorbs some needed electrolytes (potassium, chlorine), water, and glucose, as well as some amino acids and bicarbonate
Loop of Henle	Reabsorbs water and additional electrolytes
Distal convoluted tubule	Reabsorbs sodium, water, and remainder of glucose

and stimulates the adrenal cortex to secrete *aldosterone*. (The adrenal cortex secretes corticosteroids and androgens; the medulla secretes epinephrine [adrenalin] and norepinephrine.) Angiotensin II also stimulates the thirst center in the hypothalamus, encouraging a person to increase fluid intake, resulting in an increase in blood volume and, subsequently, a rise in blood pressure. (See also Chapter 17 and Fig. 17-2.)

Aldosterone promotes sodium and water retention, increasing blood volume, again elevating blood pressure. A mineralocorticoid hormone, aldosterone responds to blood levels high in potassium or low in sodium. In these cases, aldosterone stimulates excretion of potassium ions and reabsorption of sodium ions. Sodium ions return to the blood, water follows the salt via osmosis, and potassium ions are excreted in urine.

Antidiuretic Hormone

In response to angiotensin II and low fluid levels, the posterior pituitary secretes ADH. ADH increases reabsorption of water by kidney tubules, thereby decreasing the amount and increasing the concentration of urine. The result is maintenance of circulating blood volume and blood pressure and, therefore, homeostasis.

Atrial Natriuretic Peptide

Atrial natriuretic peptide (ANP), a hormone secreted by cells in the atria of the heart, increases kidney filtration and blood flow when blood volume increases. This causes the kidneys to excrete water and sodium and suppresses the ADH and aldosterone secretion. The result is reduced strain on the heart, because it does not need to pump as hard.

Erythropoietin

The second hormone produced by the kidneys, **erythropoietin** (EPO), stimulates the stem cells in red bone marrow to increase formation of red blood cells (RBCs, erythrocytes). This is known as *erythropoiesis*. EPO is secreted when *hypoxia* (impaired oxygenation) is recognized,

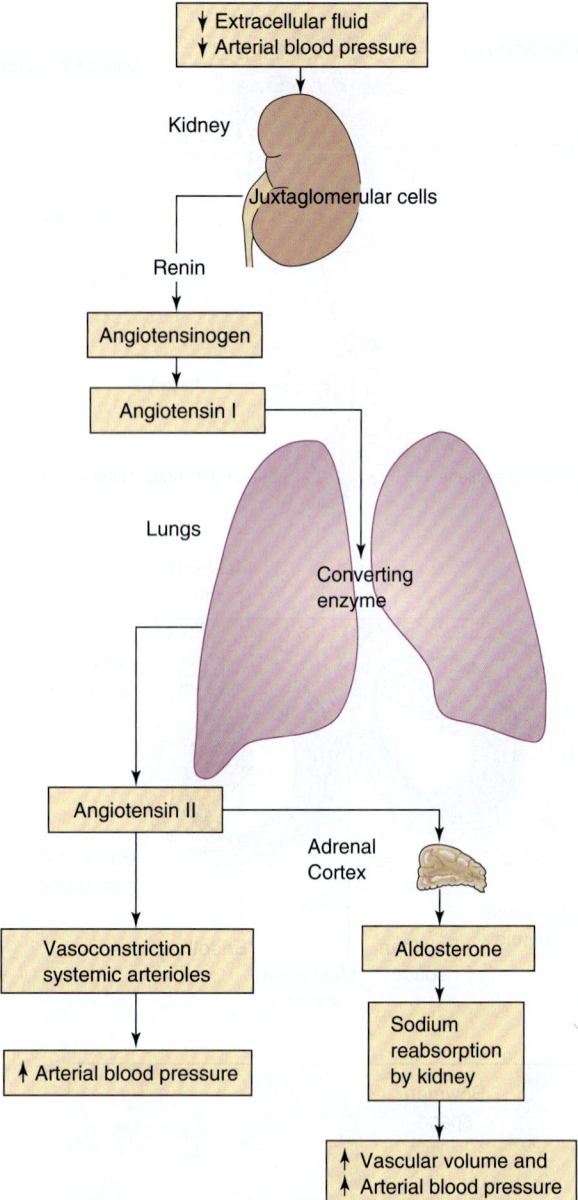

Figure 27-5 Control of blood pressure by the renin–angiotensin–aldosterone system. Renin combines with the plasma protein angiotensinogen to form angiotensin I; angiotensin-converting enzyme in the lung converts angiotensin I to angiotensin II; and angiotensin II produces vasoconstriction and increases salt and water retention through direct action on the kidney and through increased aldosterone secretion by the adrenal cortex.

usually the result of injury or cardiac or pulmonary disorders. (Erythropoietin is produced in the liver in the fetus.) This process is discussed in Chapter 23.

> **Nursing Alert** In chronic renal failure, *end-stage renal disease* (ESRD), the kidneys do not function properly, resulting in inadequate erythropoietin production, usually resulting in anemia. Synthetic erythropoietin (epoetin alfa) is often given to alleviate this anemia.

Vitamin D

Vitamin D is another substance that must be supplied in active form to the client with ESRD, because these kidneys cannot synthesize it. Vitamin D from diet and sunlight is in an inactive form and cannot be directly absorbed. For it to become metabolically active, conversion must first occur in the liver and then in the kidneys. If the body cannot synthesize vitamin D, bone demineralization will occur, because calcium cannot be absorbed from the GI tract.

Renal Blood Flow

The kidneys receive their generous blood supply from the renal arteries, and because they branch directly from the abdominal aorta, renal blood is highly oxygenated (see Fig. 22-4). The renal arteries diverge, forming smaller arteries, until they become the *afferent arterioles* supplying blood to the glomeruli (see Fig. 27-3). Glomerular blood pressure is higher than in most capillaries (60 mmHg vs. 30 mmHg), necessary for the formation of glomerular filtrate (discussed later). *Efferent arterioles* carry blood away from glomeruli. First, they branch off to form peritubular capillaries, surrounding the convoluted tubules (see Fig. 27-3). These capillaries drain into a system of veins (the *interlobular, arcuate,* and *interlobar veins*), ending at the *renal vein*, which empties into the *inferior vena cava* to return blood to the heart (Fig. 27-6). The two sites of capillary exchange in the kidneys are the glomeruli and peritubular capillaries. The glomeruli begin urine formation; peritubular capillaries carry substances from the kidneys back to the circulatory system for reuse and also nourish the renal tissue itself.

> **Key Concept**
>
> Functions of the kidneys
> - Waste removal (e.g., urea)
> - Regulation of electrolytes by excretion and reabsorption (particularly sodium, potassium, calcium)
> - Secretion of specific hormones
> - Maintenance of acid–base, fluid, and electrolyte balance
> - Conversion of vitamin D to a useful form

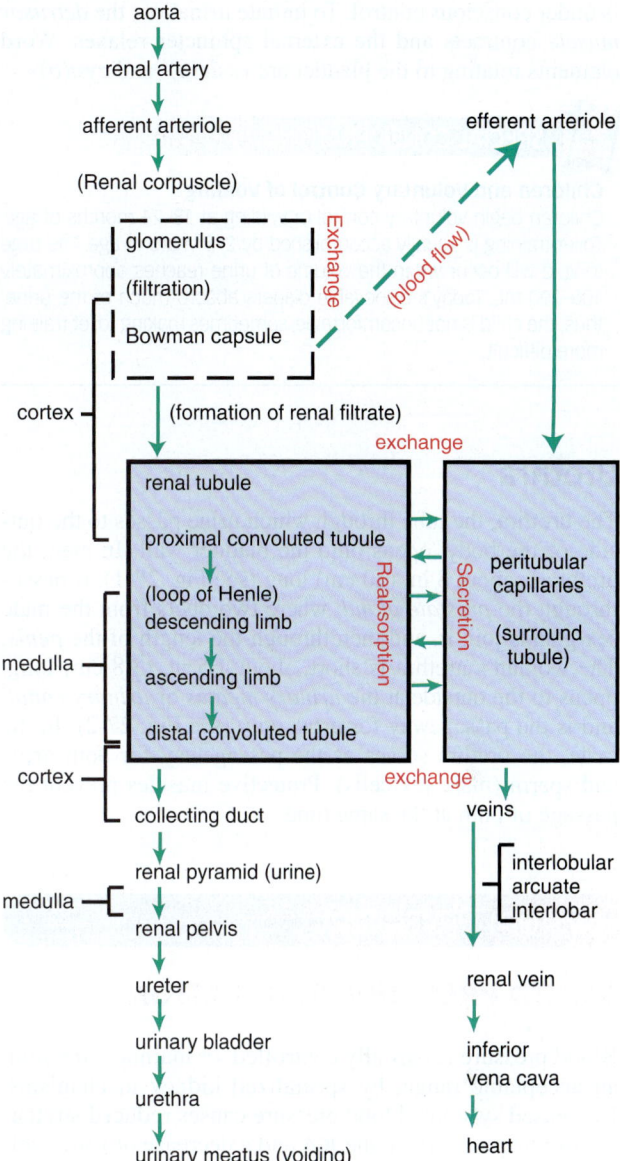

Figure 27-6 Formation of urine, with renal blood flow.

ORGANS OF URINE STORAGE AND ELIMINATION

Ureters

Urine travels from the renal pelvis into the fibromuscular **ureters**, narrow tubes about one-fifth inch (0.5 cm) in diameter and about 10–12 in. (25–30 cm) long (see Fig. 27-1). The left ureter is slightly longer. The ureters attach to the kidneys at the renal pelvis (see Fig. 27-2) and carry urine from the kidneys down to the urinary bladder for storage. Ureters consist of three layers. Innermost is the *mucosa*, made up of transitional epithelium; in the middle, the *muscularis* (smooth muscles) contract in peristaltic waves, to carry urine, drop by drop, to the urinary bladder. The outer *fibrous coat* protects and holds tissues in place. The ureters also contain many sensory nerves.

Bladder

The urinary **bladder** (*vesica*) is normally sterile; it is a hollow muscular sac which, when empty, lies behind the symphysis pubis and stores urine (see Fig. 27-1). When full, the bladder may extend well up into the abdominal cavity. The bladder is composed of transitional epithelium and lined with mucous membrane. The *trigone* (vesical trigone) is a triangular area on the floor of the bladder that does not expand. The three points of this triangle are the attachments of the two ureters and the urethra. Bladder capacity varies, but most people experience the desire to **void** (empty the bladder) when it fills to 200–400 ml (in 2–5 hr), although the maximum capacity is about 1,000 mL. Inability to void is called (urinary) **retention**. The muscles in the bladder walls distend (stretch and expand) as it fills with urine; they contract as the bladder empties. An involuntary *internal* sphincter (circular muscle) relaxes as it senses the impulse to void, an *external* sphincter is under conscious control. To initiate urination, the *detrusor muscle* contracts and the external sphincter relaxes. Word elements relating to the bladder are *vesic(o)-* and *cyst(o)-*.

SPECIAL CONSIDERATIONS Lifespan

Children and Voluntary Control of Voiding
Children begin voluntary control of voiding at 18–24 months of age. Toilet training is usually accomplished by 2–5 years of age. The urge to void will occur when the volume of urine reaches approximately 100–200 mL. Today's disposable diapers absorb much of the urine; thus, the child is not uncomfortable, sometimes making toilet training more difficult.

Urethra

The **urethra**, the tube through which urine passes to the outside of the body, opens onto the bladder wall. In men, the urethra is about 8 in. (20 cm) long (see Fig. 27-1). It passes through the *prostate gland,* where two ducts from the male sex glands join it, and then through the length of the *penis*. The woman's urethra is short, about 1.5 in. (3.8 cm) long, opens to the outside at the *urinary meatus* or *urinary canal*, and is the passageway for urine only (see Fig. 27-2). In the male, the urethra serves as the passageway for both urine and sperm (male sex cells). Protective muscles prevent the passage of both at the same time.

System Physiology

BLOOD PRESSURE REGULATION

Blood pressure is partially controlled, or maintained within an acceptable range, by specialized kidney mechanisms. Decreased systemic blood pressure causes reduced stretching of receptor cells in the **JGA** and a decrease of water volume in the kidneys. This causes the JGA to secrete renin, which in turn initiates the RAA mechanism (see Fig. 17-2). This causes blood pressure to return into a safe range by vasoconstriction of peripheral arterioles, increasing glomerular filtration rate, and preventing water and salt from being excreted, thus increasing blood volume. In addition, when blood pressure is decreased, the afferent arterioles constrict, causing decreased kidney blood flow and channeling blood to other vital areas, including the heart and brain. (Decreased renal blood flow results in reduced urinary output.)

URINE FORMATION

Normally, about 750–2,000 ml of urine is formed daily. Urine is formed in the nephron by glomerular filtration, tubular reabsorption, and tubular secretion. A fourth process allows additional water reabsorption via hormonal control (ADH). This is often considered to be an integral part of the regulatory processes in urine formation. These four steps are closely interrelated. Figure 27-7 illustrates the process of urine formation.

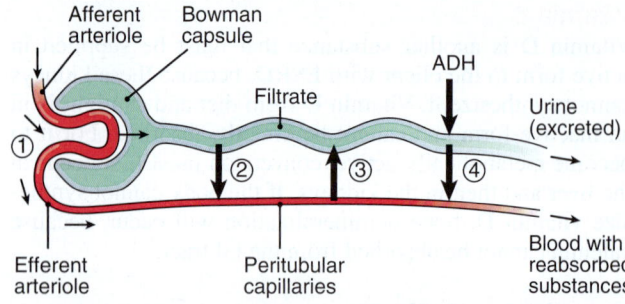

① Filtration from blood into nephron (glomerular filtration)
② Reabsorption from filtrate into blood (tubular reabsorption)
③ Tubular secretion from blood into filtrate
④ Reabsorption of water under effects of ADH

Figure 27-7 Summary of urine formation in the nephron. ADH, antidiuretic hormone.

Glomerular Filtration

Filtration removes particles from a solution by allowing the solvent to pass across a barrier, much like a sieve. The barrier allows certain solutes, which are small enough, to pass through. Larger solutes remain in the original solution, because they are too large to pass through the barrier (see Chapter 17). *Glomerular filtration* denotes the movement of wastes across glomeruli into Bowman capsule (see Fig. 27-6). Blood enters the glomerulus and flows through smaller and smaller vessels. This increases the pressure (described below) within the vessels and forces a fluid (*glomerular filtrate*) out of the glomerulus into Bowman capsule. This fluid resembles plasma, but it contains no blood cells and almost no protein. (Large protein molecules and RBCs are filtered out and cannot pass into the glomerulus.) Glomerular filtrate contains water, glucose, urea, creatinine, and numerous electrolytes. The amount of filtrate formed in all glomeruli of both kidneys per minute is called the *glomerular filtration rate* (**GFR**). Normal GFR in an adult is about 125 mL/min (about 180 L/day). Glomerular filtration depends on relative pressures. The diameter of the *afferent* (entering) arteriole is greater than that of the *efferent* (leaving) arteriole, making it easier for blood to enter the glomerulus than to leave it. Glomerular blood pressure is much higher than that of other body capillaries. Consequently, the high pressure continually filters (squeezes) wastes from the glomerulus into Bowman capsule. In the kidneys, specific forces promote, and other forces resist, filtration of waste products into the kidneys. In a healthy person, forces enabling filtration of blood to occur in the glomerulus will win by a small margin, the *net filtration pressure*; usually about 10 mmHg.

Tubular Reabsorption

Tubular reabsorption occurs via several processes. As glomerular filtrate leaves the renal corpuscles and flows through the convoluted tubules, 99% of the filtrate is reabsorbed back into circulation (see Fig. 27-7) via the efferent arteriole and peritubular capillaries. Useful substances, such as water, salts, and organic molecules, enter the interstitial fluid. Eventually, reabsorbed fluid enters renal veins, thereby returning to the general circulation. The remaining 1% becomes urine, about 750–2,000 mL/day in the adult.

Reabsorption is accomplished by active and passive transport (see Chapter 17). Water is reabsorbed by *osmosis* via the highly permeable convoluted tubules. The proximal tubules reabsorb most (approximately 65%–80%) of the electrolytes that the body retains. Sodium ions (Na^+) are carried by *active transport*, and transport of all solutes is tied to *transport* of sodium ions; thus, excess sodium intake causes water retention. Following reabsorption of positive sodium ions, many negative ions also return to the blood because of the opposing ionic charges. (Positive sodium ions attract negative ions.) Potassium ions and glucose are also absorbed. *Pinocytosis* (a process in which a cell ingests substances) is responsible for reabsorption of most small proteins and peptides. Specialized areas of the kidney tubules are permeable to specific sizes, shapes, and types of molecules. Therefore, certain substances, including water, can be reabsorbed only in certain portions of the kidney.

The kidneys have a limit (*threshold*) of reabsorption to many substances. The tubules have an upper limit of the amount of each substance that can be reabsorbed into the general circulation (the **renal threshold**). When tubules reach that threshold, the excess amount of each substance is excreted into urine. Time is also a factor in determining renal threshold. When the renal threshold for a given substance is reached within a given time period, the *transport maximum* (**TM**) has been reached.

Key Concept

Nephrons function to reabsorb and secrete various solutes:
- Ions (e.g., sodium)
- Carbohydrates (e.g., glucose)
- Amino acids (e.g., glutamate)

Tubular Secretion

Tubular secretion, the process by which substances move from blood into the urine (opposite of reabsorption), occurs by active or passive transport (see Fig. 27-7). Molecules secreted in *peritubular capillaries* (see Figs. 27-3 and 27-6) move into tubular cells and then into the tubular lumen. Secretions into urine include end products of metabolism and other body processes, such as ammonia (NH_3), bile pigments, and urea, along with metabolites (end products) of drugs. Ions, such as hydrogen (H^+) and potassium (K^+), are also subject to tubular secretion. (Acid–base regulation by the kidneys depends on tubular secretion of hydrogen ions.)

Key Concept

In tubular reabsorption, substances move: URINE → BLOOD.
In tubular secretion (opposite), substances move: BLOOD → URINE.

Water Reabsorption Under the Influence of ADH

In addition to water reabsorption via osmosis, some water (about 10%) is reabsorbed when ADH is secreted. ADH allows water to be reabsorbed from the distal convoluted tubule and collecting duct back into the blood (see Fig. 27-7). Therefore, less water is excreted and urine is more concentrated. The secretion of ADH depends on the amount of water in the blood. The lower the concentration of water in the blood, the more concentrated the blood is (*elevated osmotic pressure*). High osmotic pressure causes more ADH to be secreted, allowing additional water reabsorption back into the blood. The reverse effect also occurs. This regulatory mechanism helps maintain the body's homeostasis.

Key Concept

Urine production is influenced by
- Kidney functioning (glomerular filtration rate)
- Renal blood flow
- Hormonal balances
- Changes in the body's fluid/electrolyte status
- Salt intake
- General physical condition, illnesses, exercise
- Some medications

NCLEX Alert

Multiple factors affect urine production. These may be incorporated throughout the examination due to the impact on many diseases and conditions (e.g., hypertension or renal failure). Be able to identify normal laboratory values.

CHARACTERISTICS AND COMPOSITION OF URINE

The kidneys secrete fluids and dissolved substances, which are stored in the urinary bladder and excreted as urine through the urethra. Many factors influence the quantity of urine, including the amount of fluid and salt a person takes in, perspiration, hemorrhage, blood pressure, vomiting, external temperature, drugs, fever, and various diseases. Urine is initially a clear yellow liquid, with a characteristic odor. Several factors influence urine color. Amber or dark yellow urine may indicate a decrease in water and dehydration; some foods and drugs influence urine color. Urine may become cloudy (*turbid*) or have an ammonia-like odor, if left sitting. Normally, urine has an acidic pH, but this can vary.

Chapter 52 discusses the concept of *specific gravity* (the relationship between that urine and pure water) and its measurement. The specific gravity of pure water is 1.000; normal urine is only slightly concentrated, with a specific gravity of about 1.010–1.025. A higher specific gravity indicates concentrated urine, the result of dehydration or urinary retention. Lower specific gravity indicates dilute urine, secondary to overhydration or a physical disorder. When the kidneys are diseased, they are often unable to concentrate urine; therefore, specific gravity remains dilute.

Certain wastes are always present in urine, but analysis indicates the presence of abnormal substances. The composition of normal urine is about 95% water (a solvent) and 5% solutes. Solutes may be composed of the following:

- *Nitrogenous waste products* from breakdown of proteins; common protein wastes are urea, uric acid, and creatinine
- *Excess minerals* from the diet, such as sodium, potassium, chloride, calcium, sulfur, magnesium, ammonium, and phosphate
- *Toxins* and certain *drug metabolites*
- *Hormones* (especially those related to the person's sex); male *sperm cells*
- *Pigments* caused by certain foods or drugs may also appear; urobilinogen

In case of disease or malfunction, abnormal products, such as blood, glucose, pus, large amounts of bacteria, casts, ketone bodies, bile, and albumin (protein), may be present. Urine is normally *sterile* (free from microorganisms); nonsterile urine implies disease or infection.

> **Key Concept**
> Kidney transplants are the most frequently performed type of organ transplant. They were also the first organ transplant to be successful, with many recipients surviving 35 years or more.

MICTURITION

The release of urine (**urination**) from the body is also called *voiding*, or **micturition**. Involuntary micturition is called *urinary* **incontinence**; inability to void is *urinary* **retention**. The verb "to void" means "to vacate" or "make empty." Urine flows from the collecting tubules into the renal pelvis, down the ureters, and collects in the bladder. As urine distends the bladder, nerve endings in the bladder walls are stimulated. The brain interprets the message of fullness, and the nervous system stimulates the *internal* and *external sphincter muscles* controlling the urethral opening to relax. Since the external sphincter is controlled voluntarily, the person can control voiding. Many conditions can cause urinary incontinence. Chapter 89 describes urinary disorders, and Chapter 90 describes male urinary disorders, in conjunction with reproductive disorders.

SPECIAL CONSIDERATIONS Lifespan

Nursing care for the older adult must adapt to changes related to aging. The aging process has a significant effect on the urinary system. See Table 27-3.

> **NCLEX Alert**
> When reading an NCLEX scenario or situation, note possible changes relative to the aging process of the anatomical systems. The urinary system has normal as well as abnormal changes; either can impact effective nursing actions.

TABLE 27-3 Effects of Aging on the Urinary System

FACTOR	RESULT	NURSING IMPLICATIONS
20% loss in kidney weight and 30%–50% decrease in the number and size of functioning nephrons by the age of 80 years	Lessened ability to concentrate urine and to form urine (reduced GFR—decreased clearance of protein wastes) Lessened ability to remove ammonia and other wastes	Be aware of intake and output Assess laboratory values Assess for dehydration and edema Assess blood pressure Weigh daily, as necessary Measure intake and output as needed
Nephron membranes thicken	Decrease in rate of filtration, excretion, and reabsorption	Be aware that foreign substances will concentrate in the blood Assess for toxic levels of electrolytes (either high or low levels)
	Rise in blood urea nitrogen (BUN), creatinine, and uric acid May be more susceptible to gout	Watch laboratory reports for abnormal levels of BUN, creatinine, and uric acid
Blood flow to kidney decreases	Lessened urine formation	Watch intake and output Check for urinary retention Check for edema or dehydration Offer fluids throughout day (maintain minimum of 2,000 mL/day) Administer medications, such as Lasix, carefully and observe output

TABLE 27-3 Effects of Aging on the Urinary System (Continued)

FACTOR	RESULT	NURSING IMPLICATIONS
Some medications, such as blood pressure preparations, are "potassium wasters"	Tetany and other disorders may occur. This might be life-threatening	Administer supplemental medications, such as potassium, as required
Bladder lining may become fibrotic	Decreased capacity of bladder Incontinence	Allow for frequent bathroom visits
Client may have decreased ability to control bladder contractions	Loss of muscle tone may occur, causing nocturia (waking at night to void) or incontinence Urinary frequency Dribbling, stress incontinence	Make available devices or pads to absorb leaks for ambulatory clients Make sure sufficient bed pads are in place. Use cloth pads Provide a bedside commode for easy access
Reduced bladder sensation	May not completely empty bladder (residual urine). May not feel the urge to void Urinary retention	Watch for bladder infection and urinary retention Allow 3 hour between administration of last evening fluids and bedtime
		Advise clients: in the evening, do not drink fluids that stimulate voiding (e.g., coffee, tea, colas, alcohol) Make bathroom and bedroom safe for nighttime visits—move obstacles, keep a night light on. A bedside commode may be needed
Cancer or benign hypertrophy of the prostate is common in men	Frequent urge to void Retention of urine Sexual dysfunction	Encourage frequent testicular self-examination. Evaluate for possible prostate or testicular cancer Encourage medical evaluation Treat symptomatically
Pelvic muscles may weaken and relax or atrophy in women, owing to decreased levels of estrogen and perineal trauma from childbirth	Incontinence Uterine or bladder prolapse Bladder infections common	Instruct in pelvic exercises Do not use paper incontinence pads for clients confined to bed (to prevent ulcers); use cloth pads Offer bedpan or assist client to bathroom every 2 hour Provide adult incontinence pads or diapers for ambulatory clients Assess symptoms of bladder infections Teach proper feminine hygiene
Reduced creatinine clearance in some people Lower thresholds for glucose Reduced aldosterone and renin Decreased renal reserve, due to kidney trauma, infection, obstruction	Indicates impaired kidney function Urea, creatinine, uric acid in urine Increased blood sugar levels—may indicate diabetes Kidneys less responsive to ADH—reduced ability to clear drugs—may reach toxic levels (not adequately processed) Kidneys have lessened ability to return to normal after abrupt blood volume change or change in acid–base balance	Monitor laboratory values Treat as ordered Observe for signs of overdose, even with normal dosages of medications

GFR, glomerular filtration rate.

STUDENT SYNTHESIS

KEY POINTS

- The urinary system eliminates wastes, controls water volume, regulates electrolyte levels, maintains pH balance, activates vitamin D, secretes renin and erythropoietin, and helps to regulate blood pressure.
- The kidneys lie behind the peritoneum (retroperitoneal).
- Nephrons, the functional units of kidneys, form urine, which is eliminated by the rest of the urinary system.
- Nephrons consist of renal corpuscles (glomerulus, Bowman capsule) and renal tubules (proximal convoluted tubule, loop of Henle, distal convoluted tubule).
- Urine is 95% water and 5% solutes (salts, nitrogenous waste products, metabolites, hormones, toxins).
- Urine is formed by three processes: glomerular filtration, tubular reabsorption, and tubular secretion. In addition, ADH assists in regulation of water balance in the kidneys, to maintain the body's homeostasis.

- Micturition (voiding) is the release of urine; involuntary voiding is called urinary incontinence; inability to void is urinary retention.
- As the body ages, the number of functional nephrons decreases.

CRITICAL THINKING EXERCISES

1. Based on the discussion of anatomy in this chapter, explain whether you believe men or women have a higher incidence of urinary tract infections. Give reasons for your answer.
2. Annie, a 65-year-old woman, comes to the healthcare facility concerned. She has noticed that she is waking up during the night to urinate. A few times she has been unable to control her bladder. What information would you give Annie to address her concerns?
3. Discuss why an adequate intake of water is essential to proper functioning of the urinary system.

NCLEX-STYLE REVIEW QUESTIONS

1. The nurse is caring for a client who has been vomiting for 2 days and is receiving intravenous fluids at 75 mL/hr. Which finding would indicate that the nurse should request an increase in fluid rate?
   a. A specific gravity of 1.014
   b. Ammonia-smelling urine
   c. Amber-colored urine
   d. Clear light yellow urine
2. The nurse is caring for an older adult client with bladder incontinence due to decreased bladder capacity. Which intervention should the nurse provide that would best protect the client's dignity?
   a. Insert an indwelling urethral catheter
   b. Allow for frequent bathroom visits
   c. Apply an adult brief
   d. Place paper pads on the bed
3. A male client comes to the clinic and informs the nurse that he has a frequent urge to void and is having difficulty sustaining an erection at times. After collecting data, which procedure should the nurse prepare the client for?
   a. A testicular and prostate examination
   b. A cystoscopy
   c. An electrocardiogram
   d. An arterial blood gas test
4. A client is diagnosed with chronic kidney failure and is unable to excrete the nitrogenous waste products that build up. Which diagnostic test results would the nurse expect to observe related to the waste build up? Select all that apply.
   a. Low potassium level
   b. Elevated BUN (blood urea nitrogen)
   c. Elevated uric acid levels
   d. Elevated creatinine levels
   e. Elevated hemoglobin
5. Parents are attempting to toilet train their 2½-year-old child and are having a difficult time. The parents state, "Our child doesn't seem to care about wet diapers." Which response by the nurse is best?
   a. "The child cannot feel the wetness from the diaper. Try putting the child in underwear."
   b. "You should stop trying to toilet train. The child is probably just getting frustrated."
   c. "Children are not ready to be toilet trained until age 3. Wait until then."
   d. "We should test the child for a urinary tract infection."

CHAPTER RESOURCES

Enhance your learning with additional resources on thePoint!
Student Resources related to this chapter can be found at **thePoint.lww.com/Rosdahl12e.**

28 The Male Reproductive System

Learning Objectives

1. Identify the three major classifications of hormones that influence the male reproductive system and the functions of each classification.
2. Describe the structures of the male reproductive system and their functions.
3. Discuss the specific roles of the epididymis, ductus deferens, and ejaculatory duct.
4. Describe how sperm migrate through the reproductive system.
5. Describe the components of ejaculatory fluid and their sources.
6. Explain the process of the male sex act.
7. State three effects of aging on the male reproductive system.

Important Terminology

androgen
bulbourethral (Cowper) gland
circumcision
climacteric
copulation
ductus deferens
ejaculation
epididymis
erection
foreskin (prepuce)
gamete
glans penis
gonad
interstitial cells
nocturnal emission
orgasm
penis
perineum
prostate
puberty (male)
scrotum
semen
seminal vesicle
seminiferous tubule
spermatozoa
testes
testosterone

The previous systems studied have focused on sustaining the individual. The *reproductive systems* work distinctly to continue the species and pass genetic information from parents to child. Unlike other body systems that are generally similar for both sexes, the reproductive systems in adult males and females are different. This chapter examines the male reproductive system. Chapter 29 discusses the female reproductive system.

Sexual reproduction involves the combined effort of both internal and external structures. Sexual reproduction is a dependent process involving reproductive systems of both a man and a woman.

Structure and Function

The organs of the male reproductive system produce and transport sperm (Box 28-1). A man's reproductive capacity is directly associated with sexual excitement, penile erection, and ejaculation. (A woman's ability to reproduce does not depend on sexual excitement, and conception can occur through mechanical means [e.g., artificial insemination].) Sexual gratification, however, is equally important for both sexes.

The *male reproductive system* consists of the testes (produce sperm), ductal system and seminal vesicles (transport and store sperm), scrotum (holds testes and regulates their temperature), penis (deposits sperm in female), and accessory glands (produce male hormones and other secretions). The area between the scrotum and anus is the male **perineum**. Figure 28-1 illustrates male reproductive structures.

TESTES

The paired **testes** (singular: testis), *testicles*, reproductive organs, or sex organs, produce sex hormones in addition to **spermatozoa** (sperm cells), through the process of *spermatogenesis* (Fig. 28-2). (The combining forms for testis are *orcho/o-, orchi/o-,* and *orchid/o-*.)

SPECIAL CONSIDERATIONS Lifespan

Nocturnal Emissions
Pubescent boys may experience penile erection and spontaneous ejaculation of semen during sleep. These **nocturnal emissions** are normal and are thought to be caused by hormonal changes.

In the adult man, the testes are two small almond-shaped glands (approximately 1.5–2 in. [3.7–5 cm] long and 1 in. [2.5 cm] wide and thick), one in each side of the scrotum. Usually, one testis hangs lower than the other. Each testis is suspended from the ductus deferens, the beginning portion of the spermatic cord. Tissue layers cover each testis, one of which partitions the testis into 250–300 wedge-shaped lobules, each containing the **seminiferous tubules**, the functional units of the testes. Most of this tubule is tightly convoluted, although one portion is straight (Fig. 28-2). The combined length of a man's seminiferous tubules is about half a mile! Within the tubules and the cells lining them, sperm cells are produced and mature almost completely. Between the tubules are small clusters of specialized endocrine cells, **interstitial cells**, which secrete *testosterone* and other *androgens* (male hormones).

332   **UNIT 4**   Structure and Function

> **Box 28-1**   **Functions of the Male Reproductive System**
>
> **DEVELOPMENT OF SEXUAL CHARACTERISTICS**
> - Secretes hormones that initiate puberty
> - Maintains specific male characteristics
> - Secretes mucus, spermatic fluid, and other substances
>
> **REPRODUCTION**
> - Produces sperm
> - Passes genetic information to offspring
> - Participates in copulation and fertilization

THE DUCTAL SYSTEM

The male reproductive organs have an extensive system of ducts that store and transport sperm from the testicles to the urethra, including the paired epididymides (singular: *epididymis*), ductus deferentia (singular: *ductus deferens*), and *ejaculatory ducts*.

Epididymis

The **epididymis** is a long, comma-shaped organ attached to the posterior surface of the testis that stores sperm cells. This tightly coiled tube is approximately 20 ft (6 m) long, but is so tiny it can barely be seen with the naked eye. Also, within the epididymis, millions of sperm cells are in final stages of maturation. Here, they develop a tail and gain motility (ability to move). (Sperm cells are unable to fertilize an egg unless they mature in the epididymis.) Smooth muscles propel mature sperm into the ductus deferens.

Ductus Deferens

The sperm are transported by peristaltic waves from the epididymis to the ejaculatory duct through the paired *vas deferens* (**ductus deferens**—Latin: "carrying-away vessel"), which are about 11.5–18 in (30–45 cm) long. Each ductus deferens passes upward behind the testis, into the abdomen, over and down the

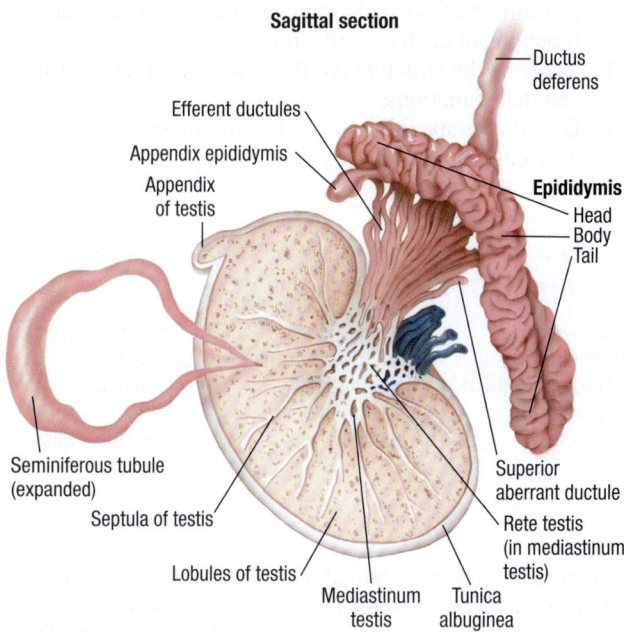

Figure 28-2 The testis is the site of sperm production in the male. The rete testis (network of channels formed by the seminiferous tubules) contains concentrated sperm and fluid. It helps the epididymis to absorb this fluid; otherwise, the man would be infertile.

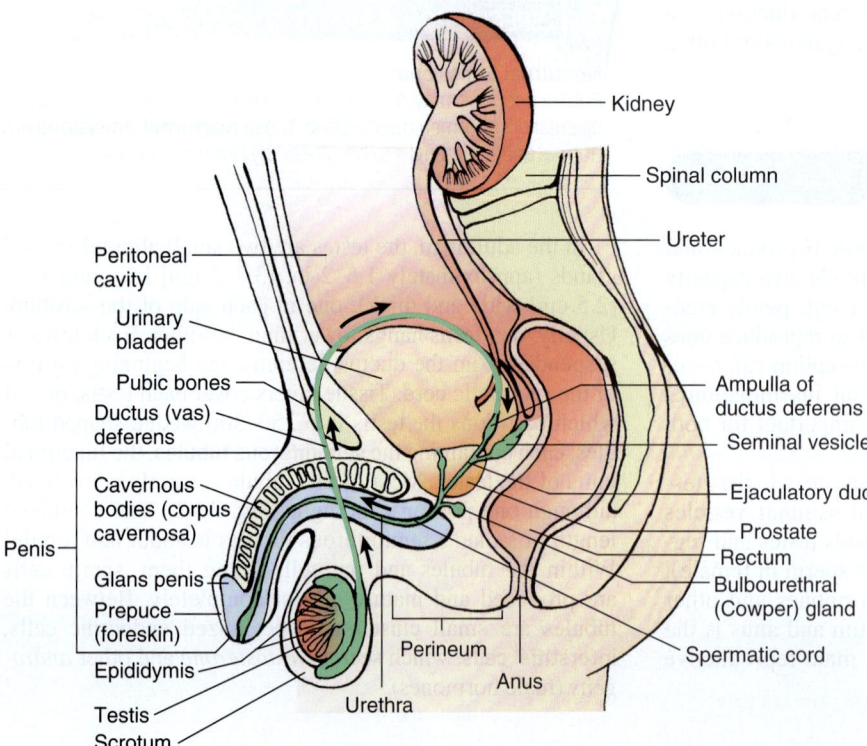

Figure 28-1 Organs of the male reproductive system, showing one testis. The *arrows* indicate the course of sperm cells through the system.

posterior surface of the urinary bladder, and into the pelvic cavity (Fig. 28-1). Each ductus then joins a duct from the seminal vesicles; these ducts, together with blood vessels, lymphatic vessels, nerves, and connective tissue coverings, comprise the *spermatic cord*, which is covered with connective tissue. The spermatic cord passes through an opening in the muscular abdominal wall, the *inguinal canal*. Normally, the inguinal canal firmly encloses the spermatic cord, but it is a weak spot and a common site for herniation in men (*inguinal hernia*). (This is also where the testicles descend into the scrotum before birth.)

> **Key Concept**
> The two vas deferens or ductus deferentia are ligated (tied) and cut in the male sterilization procedure, *vasectomy*. This operation does not affect erection or ejaculation; it just prevents sperm from passing.

Ejaculatory Ducts

The *ejaculatory ducts* are about 1 in. (2 cm) long, each originating where the ampulla of the ductus deferens joins the duct from the seminal vesicle (Fig. 28-1). The ejaculatory ducts receive secretions from the prostate gland, to make up semen and empty into the urethra. (The semen, mixed with various secretions, is now ejaculatory fluid.)

SCROTUM

The two testes are supported and protected in a saclike structure, the **scrotum**, suspended behind the base of the penis. The external appearance of the scrotum varies, depending on environmental conditions and muscle contraction. The scrotum regulates the temperature of the testes; the *cremasteric muscles* involuntarily contract and tighten the spermatic cord to bring the testicles closer to the body as external temperature lowers (the *cremasteric reflex*). This reflex may also occur in response to severe danger or during sexual intercourse. The temperature of the testes (35 °C or 95 °F) is lower than internal body temperature (normally 37 °C or 98.6 °F) to facilitate sperm production. Exposure to increased temperature over a period of time can impair *spermatogenesis* (sperm production) in the testes. Tight-fitting clothing also can cause decreased sperm production, due to increased heat.

SPECIAL CONSIDERATIONS Lifespan

Undescended Testes
Undescended testes (*cryptorchidism*), failure of the testes to move down into the scrotal sac, can occur in infants. This occurs more often in premature infants, but may also occur in some full-term infants. Cryptorchidism increases the temperature within the testes, resulting in decreased sperm production. Therefore, documentation of the location of the testes is important for all male infants. Immediate corrective surgery may be required.

PENIS

The **penis**, a cylindrical organ between the upper thighs immediately in front of the scrotum, is composed of three masses of cavernous (*erectile*) tissue. Each contains smooth muscle, connective tissue, and blood sinuses (large vascular channels). The *corpus cavernosum* is on either side, with the *corpus spongiosum* in the center. When blood flow through these sinuses is minimal, the penis is soft and flaccid. At the time of sexual excitement, blood fills the sinuses and the penis becomes firm and raises up, an **erection**. During sexual intercourse, the erect penis is capable of penetrating the vagina to deposit sperm.

> **Key Concept**
> Route of sperm: testes (seminiferous tubules; produce sperm and male hormones, begin maturation of sperm cells) → *epididymis* (sperm storage, final sperm maturation, sperm become motile) → *ductus deferens* (up past testis into abdomen; up front, over top, and down back of urinary bladder) → joins seminal vesicle → *ejaculatory duct* → through prostate → through *inguinal canal* → *urethra* → expelled to outside.

The smooth, sensitive cap of the penis, the **glans penis**, or head of the penis, surrounds the corpus spongiosum. It is covered by a fold of loose skin, forming the hoodlike **foreskin** (**prepuce**)—Figure 28-3. The foreskin protects and lubricates the penis. The outside of the foreskin looks like other external skin, whereas the inside is a membrane like the inside of the eyelid. It is attached to the penis by a sensitive, stretchy band, the *frenulum* (frenulum preputii penis), which extends under the glans penis and connects to the mucosa of the shaft of the penis. The frenulum helps contract the prepuce over the glans and prevents it from being retracted too far. Surgical removal of the foreskin, **circumcision**, is sometimes performed on male babies (Chapter 67).

The urethra within the penis serves as a common passageway for the urinary and reproductive systems, although urine and ejaculatory fluid do not pass simultaneously. The opening is at the distal tip of the penis. An involuntary sphincter at the base of the bladder and prostate gland automatically inhibits micturition (voiding) during semen ejaculation.

> **NCLEX Alert**
> The close proximity of the urinary and reproductive systems may be relevant for your consideration in client teaching, preparing a client for a procedure, or for the client's self-care after the procedure.

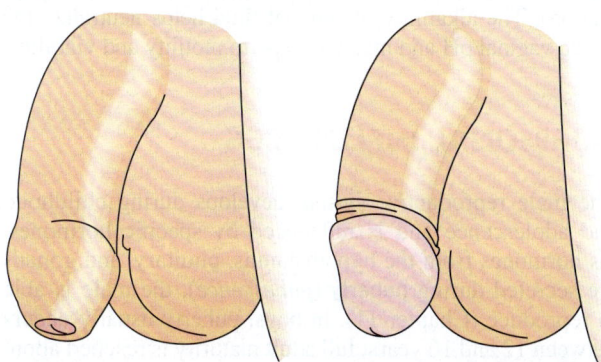

Figure 28-3 **Left.** The foreskin or prepuce of an uncircumcised male covers and protects the glans penis. The frenulum underneath helps contract the foreskin around the glans. **Right.** The foreskin can be manually retracted to expose the glans. (From Pilletteri, 2014.)

ACCESSORY GLANDS

Seminal Vesicles

The two **seminal vesicles**, convoluted, sac-shaped glands about 2 in. (5 cm) long, are located posterior to the urinary bladder and secrete a sticky, alkaline, yellowish substance, **semen**, the fluid medium for sperm. They secrete about 60% of all of a man's semen.

Prostate Gland

The **prostate**, a donut-shaped muscular structure just larger than a walnut, lies below the bladder and surrounds the neck of the urethra as it emerges from the bladder (Fig. 28-1). Glandular prostate tissue adds an alkaline secretion to semen, which increases sperm motility. Prostatic contractions during ejaculation expel semen from the urethra.

> **SPECIAL CONSIDERATIONS Lifespan**
>
> **Prostate Removal**
> Some men are unable to have an erection after prostate removal, but recently a "nerve-sparing" surgical procedure has been developed and is sometimes successful in maintaining potency. Medications may also be helpful (Chapter 90).

> **NCLEX Alert**
> Several changes in the reproductive system are normal as the individual ages. You should be aware of both normal and abnormal conditions of the reproductive system, which may be integrated into a clinical scenario on the NCLEX.

Bulbourethral Glands

The **bulbourethral (Cowper) glands** are located between two layers of fascia just below the prostate. Approximately the size of a pea, they are composed of several lobules held together by fibers and secrete alkaline mucus into tiny ducts, which empty into the urethra. This mucus coats the urethra to neutralize the pH of urine residue; it also lubricates the penis. A woman's vagina is acidic, due to its normal flora (natural bacterial population). The alkalinity of seminal fluid helps neutralize the acidic vaginal pH and maintains sperm motility and viability.

HORMONAL INFLUENCES

The male reproductive system develops during childhood and adolescence and is influenced by specific hormones. As hormones from the hypothalamus, pituitary, and gonads are secreted during **puberty** (*pubescence*), the male is able to reproduce (Chapter 11). In boys, puberty usually occurs between 12 and 16 years; full adult maturity is reached about age 20 years. Before puberty (*prepubescence*), blood concentrations of **androgens** (male hormones) and *estrogens* (female hormones) are the same in every person.

The fetal precursor of specific male gonads is the *Wolffian duct*, which develops into the epididymis, vas deferens, ductus deferens, ejaculatory duct, and seminal vesicles. When a boy reaches puberty, the hypothalamus stimulates the secretion of both interstitial cell-stimulating hormone (*ICSH*) and follicle-stimulating hormone (*FSH*) from the anterior pituitary (Chapter 20); both are gonadotropic hormones. In the man, these hormones have two main effects:

- They stimulate the **gonads** (sex glands) to secrete specific male hormones (androgens).
- FSH stimulates the formation of sperm.

The major androgen is **testosterone**; its production is stimulated by ICSH. During puberty, male glandular development becomes very active and also influences the development of *secondary sexual characteristics*, including the typical male beard, pubic, and axillary hair, as well as increased body hair. Unique musculature develops; the shoulders become broader and the hips remain narrow. The voice deepens, and the "Adam apple" (unique to the male) develops in the anterior throat. Testosterone also maintains the functioning of male accessory organs and stimulates protein anabolism. As a result, a man usually has larger and stronger musculature than a woman.

> **Key Concept**
> If a man receives testosterone replacement therapy, the testes will shrink, since they no longer need to manufacture testosterone. Pituitary gonadotropin drugs will cause testes enlargement. Testicular disorders include undescended testicles, injury, orchitis (inflammation), cancer, hydrocele (fluid around the testis), and spermatic cord torsion (twisting), any of which can influence sperm production and fertility. Removal or failure of both testes, *castration*, renders the man sterile and will require external testosterone to maintain male characteristics.

System Physiology

SPERM CELLS AND SPERMATOGENESIS

Beginning at about 12–13 years and continuing throughout life, the seminiferous tubules of the testes (male gonads), stimulated by testosterone, form sperm cells. The sperm cell (plural is also sperm) is the male **gamete**, one of two cells (containing 23 chromosomes) that must unite to initiate development of a new individual. This formation of mature, functional spermatozoa is called *spermatogenesis*. Normal spermatogenesis does not occur if the testes are too warm or too cold (above or below 35 °C [95 °F]), as described above.

> **Nursing Alert** Mumps (parotitis) can be dangerous to adult males, leading to *orchitis* (inflammation of the testes) and resulting in sterility, emphasizing the need for infant immunization.

Sperm cells develop from stem cells, *spermatogonia (singular: spermatogonium)*. A "mother cell" helps create spermatogonia and a specific cell, the Sertoli cell, facilitates spermatogenesis. Spermatogonia divide by mitosis and then meiosis to form *spermatocytes* (Chapter 15). In the next stage, the cells are *spermatids*, which eventually develop into *spermatozoa (singular: spermatozoon)*, a total process requiring about 2 months. (Each primary

CHAPTER 28 The Male Reproductive System

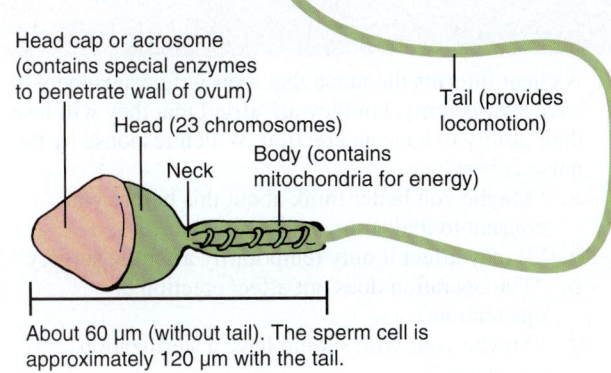

Figure 28-4 A human sperm cell.

spermatocyte forms four functional gametes.) The testes produce millions of spermatozoa each day, and they are stored in the ductus deferens. Sperm cells are highly specialized and are have several divisions (Fig. 28-4). The *head* contains 23 chromosomes (half of the human genetic material), and the tip of the head, the *acrosome*, contains enzymes that can dissolve the tough cell wall of the ovum (female sex cell). The *body* (center sections) contains mitochondria, providing energy for locomotion. The whiplike *tail* is a flagellum that propels the sperm with a lashing motion.

After sperm and semen combine in the ejaculatory duct, the *ejaculatory fluid* contains about 60–100 million sperm cells per milliliter. (Semen with a sperm count of less than 10–20 million per milliliter may have difficulty fertilizing an ovum.) The amount of semen ejaculated (expelled) varies from 2 to 5 mL. After ejaculation into a woman's vagina, a sperm cell *can survive up to 3 days*. Of the average 250 million sperm cells ejaculated, only about 100 survive to contact the ovum in the oviduct, although usually only one sperm fertilizes the ovum.

COPULATION

Sexual intercourse or sexual union between a man and a woman is called **copulation**, *intercourse*, or *coitus*. The man inserts his erect penis into the vaginal canal and deposits semen containing sperm when he ejaculates. Other substances in semen include citric acid, fructose, enzymes, coagulation proteins, lipids (fats), prostaglandins, and other secretions from the seminal vesicles and prostate. During sexual arousal, the bulbourethral glands secrete a clear liquid, preejaculate, which helps lubricate the urethra so sperm can pass; it also cleans out any urine or foreign matter. The male sex act is a complex series of reflexes consisting of several components: erection, secretion, emission, and ejaculation. *Erection* occurs when nervous impulses from the spinal cord and brain cause vasodilation of the arteries of the penis. When this occurs, venous return is obstructed and the cavernous tissue in the penis becomes engorged with blood. This blood can only leave via a system of veins around the outside of the corpus cavernosum. The expanding tissue constricts these veins and contains the blood until orgasm is achieved. *Emission* is the accumulation of sperm cells and secretions in the urethra. **Ejaculation** is the forceful expulsion of semen from the ejaculatory ducts, through the urethra. **Orgasm** is the physical, emotional, and pleasurable sensation that occurs at the climax of sexual intercourse; in men, it is accompanied by ejaculation. Inability to achieve erection is called *impotence*. Difficulty in achieving orgasm is called *anorgasmia*. Low sperm count is called *oligospermia*. Disorders of the male reproductive system are discussed in Chapter 90. Sexually transmitted infections and infertility are described in Chapter 70.

 SPECIAL CONSIDERATIONS Lifespan

Nursing care for the older adult must adapt to changes related to aging. The aging process has a significant effect on the male reproductive system (Table 28-1).

TABLE 28-1 Effects of Aging on the Male Reproductive System

FACTOR	RESULT	NURSING IMPLICATIONS
No sharp cessation of reproductive ability, as in women. Testosterone levels decrease (may be called andropause or male **climacteric**)	Degeneration of testicles; reduction in size Decrease in sperm production Difficulty in achieving and maintaining an erection; longer refractory period after orgasm Frequency of erection decreases May result in weight gain or changes in body shape More susceptible to atherosclerosis and/or osteoporosis	Educate client that these changes are normal Refer client to counseling, if needed Counsel client in healthy dietary patterns
Enlargement of prostate gland (hypertrophy or hyperplasia) Prostatectomy or other surgery	May be benign or malignant (prostate cancer); may have difficulty voiding (retention) or urinary incontinence or difficulty in attaining erection May be sexually impotent	Encourage testicular self-examination Encourage medical examination and PSA test to catch early prostate cancer Counsel about alternative means of sexual expression; use of medications, aids to intercourse
Fibrosis, sclerosis, and vascular changes occur in penis Bulbourethral glands become smaller; reduced volume and thinner secretions	Decrease in frequency and strength of erection May require additional lubrication for intercourse	Encourage medical examination Refer client to counseling, if needed Medications may be helpful; surgical procedures are available Educate client in types of lubrication

STUDENT SYNTHESIS

KEY POINTS

- Internal organs of the male reproductive system include the testes (containing the seminiferous tubules), ducts, and glands (seminal vesicles, prostate, bulbourethral).
- External structures of the male reproductive system are the scrotum (a sac supporting and protecting the testes) and the penis, a common passageway for the urinary and reproductive systems.
- Ducts of the male reproductive system include the epididymis, ductus deferens, and ejaculatory duct. Sperm mature in the epididymis, travel through the ductus deferens, and join other secretions in the ejaculatory duct before exiting the body.
- The male reproductive system is under the influence of hormones from the hypothalamus, pituitary, and gonads.
- Male hormones are androgens. Testosterone is the major male androgen.
- In men, gonadotropic hormones stimulate the formation of sperm and the secretion of hormones from the sex glands.
- Ejaculatory fluid contains semen from the seminal vesicles, sperm from the vas deferens, alkaline secretions from the prostate, nutrients, and mucus from the bulbourethral glands.
- Sperm cells, spermatozoa, are stored in the ductus deferens.
- During copulation, the penis becomes firm in order to penetrate the vagina. The urethra within the penis serves as a passageway for sperm and semen during ejaculation. (No urine is able to pass during sexual intercourse.)

CRITICAL THINKING EXERCISES

1. Sperm cannot survive in conditions that are too warm or too cold. Discuss circumstances in which a man's sperm count might be lowered.
2. A 50-year-old man comes to the facility where you work. He is marrying a woman of childbearing age. The couple plans to try to have a baby. The man is worried about his chances for conception because of his age. What information would you give this man?

NCLEX-STYLE REVIEW QUESTIONS

1. A parent brings their 13-year-old son into the clinic and informs the nurse that they think something is wrong with their son. The parent states, "Every morning when I make his bed, there is a large wet spot on the sheet." What should the nurse discuss with the parent?
   a. The child is having normal nocturnal emissions caused most likely by hormone changes.
   b. The child may have regressed to a previous stage of development and started wetting the bed again.
   c. The child may have a urinary tract infection and should be checked.
   d. There may be some type of penile dysfunction that the physician will check.

2. A client informs the nurse that their wife wants them to have a vasectomy, but they are afraid that they will lose their ability to have an erection. Which response by the nurse is best?
   a. "Maybe you better think about this before you consent to major surgery."
   b. "It may affect it only temporarily after the surgery."
   c. "The operation does not affect erection or ejaculation."
   d. "Maybe your wife should have a sterilization procedure."

3. The nurse is caring for an infant in the newborn nursery and observes that the right testicle appears to be undescended. Which nursing action is appropriate at this time?
   a. No action is required; this is a normal finding.
   b. Document the finding and report it to the physician.
   c. Inform the parents that the baby may not be able to have children.
   d. Do not apply a diaper.

4. A client is scheduled to have a prostatectomy in 1 week. The client informs the nurse that they realize that their sexual life is over. Which information should the nurse provide to the client? Select all that apply.
   a. Alternative means of sexual expression
   b. Use of medications prescribed by the physician
   c. Strategies for how to accept the loss of a sexual life
   d. Aids to intercourse
   e. Prevention of infection

5. A client tells the nurse that they are having trouble with sexual intercourse since they have had atrophy of the bulbourethral glands. Which suggestions can the nurse make to alleviate the discomfort for them and their partner?
   a. Use additional lubrication such as water-soluble gel.
   b. Take warm baths prior to intercourse.
   c. Use medication to sustain erections.
   d. Use aids to intercourse.

CHAPTER RESOURCES

Enhance your learning with additional resources on thePoint!

Student Resources related to this chapter can be found at thePoint.lww.com/Rosdahl12e.

29 The Female Reproductive System

Learning Objectives

1. Name the major hormones that influence the female reproductive system.
2. Describe the functions of the ovaries, uterus, clitoris, and vagina.
3. Explain the role of the mammary glands in the reproductive process.
4. Describe the functions of LH, FSH, estrogens, and progesterone in the female reproductive system.
5. Discuss the process of oocyte maturation and ovulation.
6. Explain the three phases of the ovarian cycle, including what occurs during each phase.
7. Describe the three phases of the uterine cycle, including what occurs during each phase.
8. Discuss menopause (climacteric) and the physical changes that accompany it.
9. Identify two effects of aging on the female reproductive system (other than menopause) and list related nursing implications.

Important Terminology

Bartholin gland, cervix, clitoris, embryo, endometrium, estrogen, fimbriae, gonadotropic hormone, hymen, labia majora, labia minora, mammary gland, menarche, menopause, menstruation, mons pubis, oocyte, ova, ovaries, oviduct, ovulation, perineum, progesterone, uterus, vagina, vulva, zygote

Acronyms

ERT
HRT

The male and female reproductive systems are responsible for the continuation of the human species. Human reproduction normally occurs by internal fertilization, via sexual intercourse. The erect penis of the male is inserted into the female vagina; ejaculation (forceful expulsion) of semen containing the male sperm is deposited in the vagina. The female system produces eggs (ova). Sperm can fertilize ova, thereby beginning the reproductive process. The female reproductive system also has the amazing added function of providing an environment necessary for growth and development of a *fetus* (a developing infant in the uterus). The word element *gyn-* or *gyneco-* means woman. (A healthcare provider specializing in treating disorders unique to women is a *gynecologist.*)

Development of the reproductive and urinary systems is closely related. A structure, the Müllerian duct in fetal life, develops to form a number of female structures. In addition, a number of fetal structures are the same in male and female but develop differently as a result of hormones and are differentiated between the sexes in adult life. These are *homologous* structures. Examples include the following:

- Cowper gland in male; Bartholin glands in female—secrete lubricants
- Penis in male; clitoris in female—contain erectile tissue and contribute to sensation
- Testes in male; ovaries in female—produce gametes
- Prostate gland in male; Skene gland in female—produce ejaculatory and lubricating fluid and sensation

Although men begin to produce sperm during puberty and continue to do so for the rest of their lives, a woman's reproductive capacity is limited, beginning with the first menstrual period and ending during menopause. The menstrual cycle is extremely important in understanding the female reproductive system and is explained later.

Structure and Function

The *female reproductive system* consists of paired ovaries and oviducts and the uterus, vagina, and external genital structures. The *internal organs*—uterus, vagina, and ovaries—are located within the pelvis between the urinary bladder and rectum and are held in place by a group of ligaments. The *external structures* make up the *vulva*. The *mammary glands* (breasts) are also considered female reproductive organs. Figures 29-1 and 29-2 illustrate the female reproductive system. Box 29-1 reviews its primary functions.

REPRODUCTIVE ORGANS

Ovaries

The gonads (sex organs) in women are the **ovaries**, which produce female gametes or **ova** (singular: ovum) and secrete female sex hormones (estrogens). Although several estrogens exist (the primary one is *estradiol*), the entire classification, **estrogen**, commonly refers to all female sex hormones

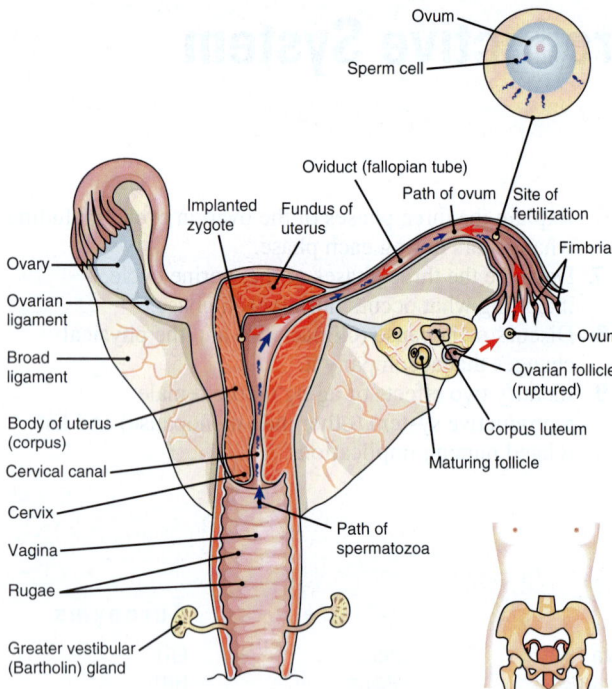

Figure 29-1 The female reproductive system (interior view), illustrating the location of fertilization of the ovum. *Red arrows* indicate the path of the ovum to the site of fertilization. *Blue arrows* indicate the path of spermatozoa. (The fertilized ovum then continues down into the uterus.)

collectively. The ovaries are two almond-shaped glands, each about 1.5 in. (3.8 cm) in length, located within the brim of the pelvis, one on either side of the uterus (Fig. 29-1). (The combining form relating to ovary is *oophor/o-*.)

Oviducts

Sometimes called *uterine tubes, ovarian tubes,* or *fallopian tubes,* the **oviducts** are the passageway for the ovum between the ovary and the uterus (Fig. 29-1). The oviducts are 4–5 in. (10–12.5 cm) long. One oviduct is associated with each ovary and is connected to each side of the uterus.

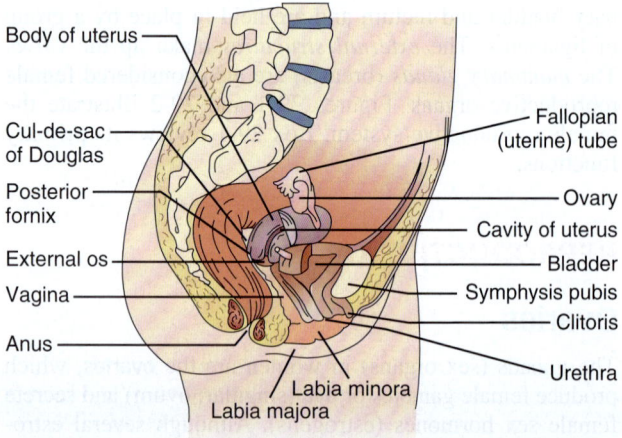

Figure 29-2 Female reproductive organs, as seen in sagittal section.

Box 29-1 Functions of the Female Reproductive System

DEVELOPMENT OF SEXUAL CHARACTERISTICS
- Secrete hormones that initiate puberty
- Maintain specific female sexual characteristics
- Secrete mucus, vaginal fluids, and other substances

REPRODUCTION
- Produce ova
- Pass genetic information to offspring
- Participate in copulation and fertilization
- Maintain and nourish fetus until birth

INFANT NOURISHMENT
- Produce breast milk

Ova

The human ovum consists of protoplasm enclosed within a two-layered cell wall. The outer layer is the *zona pellucida*; the inner layer is the *vitelline membrane*. The ovum cell contains a large nucleus, within which is the nucleolus, the germinal spot. The ovum is larger than the sperm cell (and is the only human cell normally visible to the naked eye).

As the ovum bursts from the ovary into the pelvic cavity, the oviduct catches it in structures called **fimbriae**, fringe-like ends of the oviducts. Cilia on the inner surfaces of the fimbriae, and the lining of the oviducts, as well as peristaltic waves of the oviducts' smooth muscles, help move the ovum toward the uterus. The inner layer of the oviducts contains mucus-secreting cells that lubricate the oviducts and may also provide nutrients for the ovum. (The transit of the ovum from ovary to uterus may occur in a few hours or may take several days.) *Fertilization* of the ovum (the meeting of sperm and ovum) normally occurs about midway in the oviduct (discussed later). If fertilization does not occur, the ovum dissolves. Because no closed connection exists between the ovary and the oviduct, it is possible for the ovum to "escape" into the abdominal cavity. (It is the oviduct that is ligated [tied] and cut in the female sterilization procedure, *tubal ligation*.)

> **Nursing Alert** An *ectopic* (outside the uterus) pregnancy within the oviduct is an emergency situation, endangering the life of the mother. In this situation, the fertilized ovum becomes lodged in the oviduct; this can lead to ductal rupture and hemorrhage (Chapter 68).

Uterus

The **uterus** (*womb*) is a hollow, muscular, upside-down pear-shaped organ in the center of the pelvic cavity above and behind the urinary bladder (Fig. 29-2). The uterus is considered to be the major female sex organ, even though the gonads are the ovaries. The nonpregnant uterus is about 3 in.

(7.5 cm) long, 2 in. (5 cm) wide, and 1 in. (2.5 cm) thick. The zygote matures into a full-term fetus in the uterus. The uterus normally is tipped forward (*anteverted*), but in some women, it is tipped posteriorly (*retroverted*). Although it is movable, the uterus is held in position by strong structures, the *broad ligament* (Fig. 29-1) and the *round ligament*. During pregnancy, the uterus increases in size about 16 times (from about 60 g to about 950 g); its capacity increases from about 2.5 to 5,000 mL. After a term pregnancy, the uterus shrinks considerably, but never returns to its original size.

The uterus contains several areas (Fig. 29-1). The *fundus* is the round upper surface; the oviducts enter here. The body (*corpus*) is the broad, large central portion. The cylindrical or conical cervix is the narrow lower end, which opens into the vagina at the *external cervical os* (mouth of the cervix). The normal size of the cervical os is about the diameter of the graphite in a pencil. The nonpregnant cervix feels like the end of your nose. About half of the cervix can be visualized during vaginal examination. (The combining form relating to uterus is *hystero-*. Removal of the uterus is called hysterectomy.) The uterus has three layers: serous, muscular, and mucous. The *serous* (outer) *layer*, the *perimetrium*, is a fold of the peritoneum. The *muscular layer*, the *myometrium*, is the smooth muscle that increases in size during pregnancy and contracts during labor and delivery. The *mucous layer*, the endometrium, forms the maternal portion of the placenta during pregnancy. The uterus receives the fertilized ovum and provides housing and nourishment for a fetus. At the end of gestation, the uterus expels the fetus (*delivery*). Pregnancy, labor, and delivery are discussed in Unit 10. In some cases, a couple has difficulty conceiving a child. Fertility and fertility control are discussed in Chapter 70.

Vagina

The cervix projects into a fibromuscular canal, about 4 in. (10 cm) long, the vagina (Fig. 29-1). The vagina is attached to the uterus through the cervix and meets the external organs at the vulva. The vagina's superior, domed portion has deep recesses, *fornices* (singular: fornix), around the portion of the cervix extending into the vagina. Glandular secretions from *Bartholin glands* (greater vestibular glands) and the mucous membrane lining its walls moisten the vagina. The mucus is acidic and retards microbial growth. (The alkaline semen can temporarily neutralize the vagina's acidic environment.) *Rugae*, expandable folds within the vaginal walls, accommodate insertion of the penis and passage of the fetus during childbirth. The vagina's functions are to receive sperm, provide an exit for menstrual flow, and serve as the birth canal.

The hymen is a thin membrane over the vaginal opening. It may close the vaginal orifice completely, or it may be absent from birth. More commonly, it has one or more perforations. A woman can injure the hymen in various ways (e.g., during normal exercise, horseback riding, by using tampons, or during the first sexual intercourse). The presence or absence of a hymen is *not a reliable indicator of a woman's virginity*.

External Genitalia

The external genitalia are collectively called the vulva (*pudendum*), including the vestibule and surrounding

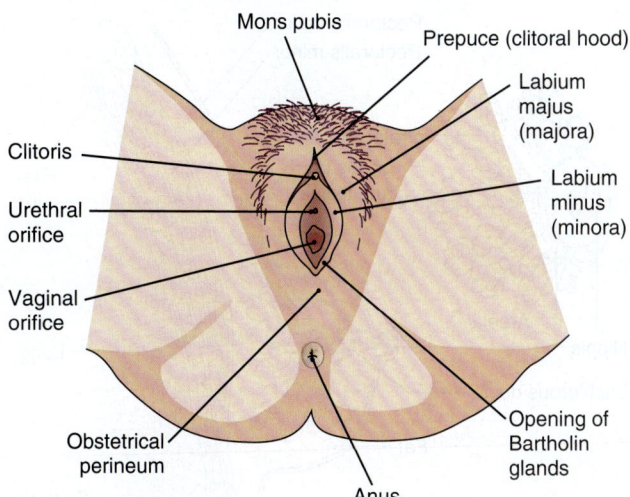

Figure 29-3 External female genitalia, seen from below. The area lying between the orifice of the vagina and the anus is the *obstetrical perineum*. Note the location of the urethral (urinary) orifice (meatus, opening).

structures. The *vestibule* contains the openings of the urethra, vagina, and Bartholin glands (Fig. 29-1). The external structures also include the mons pubis, labia majora, labia minora, clitoris, and prepuce (Fig. 29-3).

The mons pubis is a fatty pad over the symphysis pubis (Fig. 29-3). Posterior to the mons pubis extend two rounded folds of skin, the labia majora (*labium majus*). After puberty, the mons pubis and labia majora are covered with coarse pubic hair. A thin pair of skin folds medial to the labia majora are the labia minora (*labium minus*), which unite just above and with the clitoris to form the *prepuce of the clitoris* or *clitoral hood*. The labia minora skin folds enclose the vaginal opening and can be spread apart or "opened" to expose the vestibule floor. The vestibule floor contains Bartholin glands (greater vestibular glands), which lubricate the vagina. (If the openings of these glands become obstructed, Bartholin cysts can result.) The clitoris is a small erectile structure that responds to sexual stimulation. The structure of the clitoris is similar to that of the penis. Both become engorged with blood as a result of sexual excitement, and stimulation of either structure often leads to orgasm. The female (obstetrical) perineum is the space between the vaginal orifice and the anus. It is made up of strong muscles that act as sling-like supports for pelvic organs.

> ### Key Concept
> During childbirth, the skin and muscles of the perineal area may be torn. To prevent such tearing, an incision, an *episiotomy*, is often made. (A clean, straight incision heals better than an irregular skin and muscle tear.) Slow stretching of the perineum during delivery may prevent tearing and make an episiotomy unnecessary.

BREASTS

The breasts are not involved in gestation; however, they are hormonally influenced and are directly linked to the reproductive process, providing nutrition for babies following childbirth. Before puberty, breast structure in boys and girls

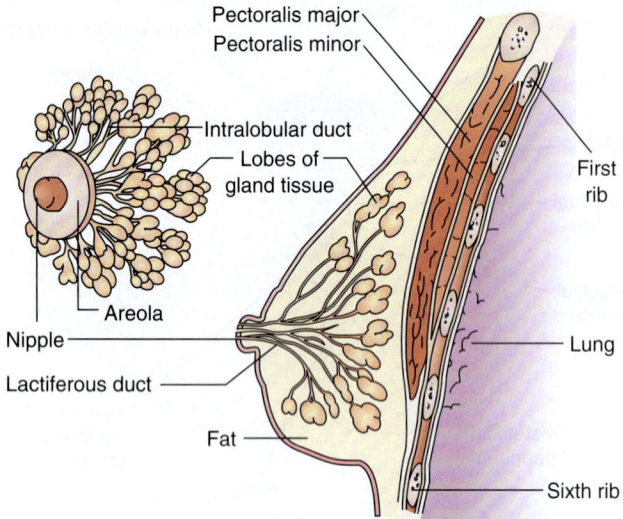

Figure 29-4 The breast, showing the glandular tissue and ducts of the mammary glands.

is similar. Both have rudimentary glandular systems. With the onset of puberty, *estrogens* and *progesterone* in girls lead to breast enlargement. Both boys and girls may have some breast sensitivity in early puberty. Boys may develop slight swellings as well, but this is usually temporary.

Within the breasts are **mammary glands**. They are modified sweat glands (Fig. 29-4) and are located anterior to the *pectoralis major* muscles. Hormones (*prolactin* and *oxytocin*) stimulate them to produce and release milk after childbirth. Each breast is divided into 15–20 *lobes* of glandular tissue, covered by adipose (fat) tissue, which gives the breast its shape. The lobes are made up of *lobules,* which consist of milk-secreting cells in glandular alveoli. From the alveoli, small *lactiferous ducts* converge toward each nipple like the spokes of a wheel. Each lactiferous duct forms a small reservoir for milk. The structures of the breast include the nipple, the areola, and the areolar glands. The *nipple* is a circular projection containing some erectile tissue and surrounded by the pigmented *areola. Areolar glands,* close to the skin's surface, make the areola appear rough. The secretions of areolar glands keep the nipples from drying out, particularly during *lactation* (milk production). Hormonal release of estrogen and progesterone during pregnancy causes the breasts to enlarge. The areolae become more heavily pigmented (and do not totally return to their previous color after pregnancy).

> **Nursing Alert** NCLEX questions may require knowledge of the terminology of the structures and functions of the female reproductive system. Be sure you can differentiate between appropriate and inappropriate nursing care, laboratory results, or diagnostic procedures.

HORMONAL INFLUENCES

The hypothalamus, pituitary, and gonads all contribute to hormonal regulation of the female reproductive system. (Remember that before puberty, androgens [male hormones] and estrogens [female hormones] are at similar levels in both boys and girls.) The hypothalamus stimulates the secretion of **gonadotropic hormones**, which include luteinizing hormone (LH) and follicle-stimulating hormone (FSH) in women. The main effects of LH and FSH include stimulating both the formation of ova and the secretion of hormones from sex organs. Gonadotropic hormones also stimulate development of secondary female sexual characteristics. The ovaries begin to secrete *estrogens,* including estradiol, estriol, and estrone. After puberty, the corpus luteum of the ovary produces another hormone, **progesterone**, which functions primarily during pregnancy. The pubescent girl exhibits many changes as a result of estrogen production. Characteristic secondary sexual characteristics of the female include a smaller stature, higher percentage of body fat, pubic and axillary hair, and development of breasts. The female pubic arch (subpubic angle) of the pelvis and hip structure is wider than that of the male, to facilitate childbirth. Sweat glands become more active. Although voice changes are not as marked as those in a boy, the voice does deepen and mature in tone and quality. As glands of reproduction become active, menstruation occurs. All female secondary sex characteristics depend on secretion of *estrogens* and *progesterone.*

System Physiology

EGG CELLS AND OOGENESIS

In humans, all the *ova* (egg cells) that an individual woman will produce in their lifetime are present as **oocytes** at their birth. Each oocyte develops in different stages throughout a woman's life. About 5–7 million begin as *oogonia* in the female fetus' fourth to fifth gestational month. Before birth, most oogonia (singular: oogonium) either degenerate or begin the very complex process of *meiosis* (cell division). At the start of meiosis, the oogonium is a *primary oocyte;* a newborn girl has about two million primary oocytes. Then, between birth and puberty, the number of primary oocytes decreases to 300,000–400,000; of these, only 300–400 eventually develop into mature egg cells. Eventually after puberty, the oocyte (*gamete*) contains half the genetic material required to form a new individual (23 chromosomes) and is called a *haploid cell.* (Only if fertilized by a male sex cell, the spermatozoa, does the gamete develop into an embryo and fetus.)

At puberty, hormones stimulate the primary follicle to continue developing and to become a *secondary follicle.* The secondary follicle enlarges and forms a bump on the ovary. When the secondary follicle matures, it is called the *Graafian follicle.* From the time of puberty until menstruation ceases during menopause, at approximately monthly intervals, a mature Graafian follicle ruptures the surface of the ovary. Now known as the *ovum,* it is expelled into the pelvic cavity near the oviduct (leading to the uterus). This ovum will live up to 24 hour before it begins to degenerate, unless *fertilized* by a sperm in the oviduct. The fertilized ovum, the **zygote**, travels to the uterus, where it becomes embedded in the uterine lining, in preparation for further growth. Once the zygote becomes completely embedded in the lining, it is called an **embryo**. When the fetus is developed enough to survive outside the uterus, the cervix dilates and uterine contractions cause the fetus to be expelled through the vagina (childbirth). Chapter 65 describes this process.

MENSTRUAL CYCLE

The *menstrual cycle* is actually two interrelated continuous cycles: the *ovarian cycle* and the *uterine cycle* (Fig. 29-5). The anterior pituitary releases secretions that control both cycles. These changes occur in sexually mature, nonpregnant women and culminate in **menstruation**, the flow of blood and other materials from the uterus through the vagina. The first menstrual period, **menarche**, marks the onset of female puberty. This rhythmical series of changes (the *menstrual period, menses,* or *period*) then occurs about every 28 days. Great variation occurs, however, among women and also within one woman's month-to-month cycle. Menstrual cycles continue as long as ovarian hormones stimulate the uterine lining. Between approximately 40 and 55 years of age, the ovaries become less active because they no longer respond to FSH. Thus, eggs no longer mature, and the ovaries stop producing estrogens. This decrease in ovarian function occurs gradually. The result is the lack of ability to become pregnant and the onset of **menopause** (*climacteric*, cessation of menstruation). Menopause, a normal process, sometimes occurs abruptly. Usually, however, it is so gradual that the woman's body adjusts without difficulty. Because many hormonal changes are involved, however, menopausal women may experience some unpleasant symptoms, such as headaches, irritability, insomnia, anxiety, or depression. One of the most common symptoms is the sensation of sudden heat (*hot flashes*). Hormonal imbalances affect the diameter of blood vessels, causing their abrupt dilation or contraction. External indicators of menopause include a tendency to gain weight, thinning of hair, growth of hair on the upper lip and chin, and dry, itchy skin.

> **Key Concept**
> The onset of menopause can begin as early as 35–40 years. It is defined as the cessation of menses for more than a year. It is possible to become pregnant during developing menopause.

Ovarian Cycle

During the ovarian cycle, the ovum matures and is expelled from the ovary into the oviduct. The maturation of another ovum is then withheld until the next cycle. The three phases of the ovarian cycle are the *follicular phase, ovulation,* and the *luteal phase* (Fig. 29-5). Table 29-1 discusses the hormones and phases of the ovarian cycle.

Follicular Phase

The *follicular phase* lasts from about day 4 to about day 14. During this time, under the influence of FSH, several follicles begin to ripen and the ovum within each begins to mature. One follicle, the *Graafian follicle*, will become dominant. The other follicles stop growing.

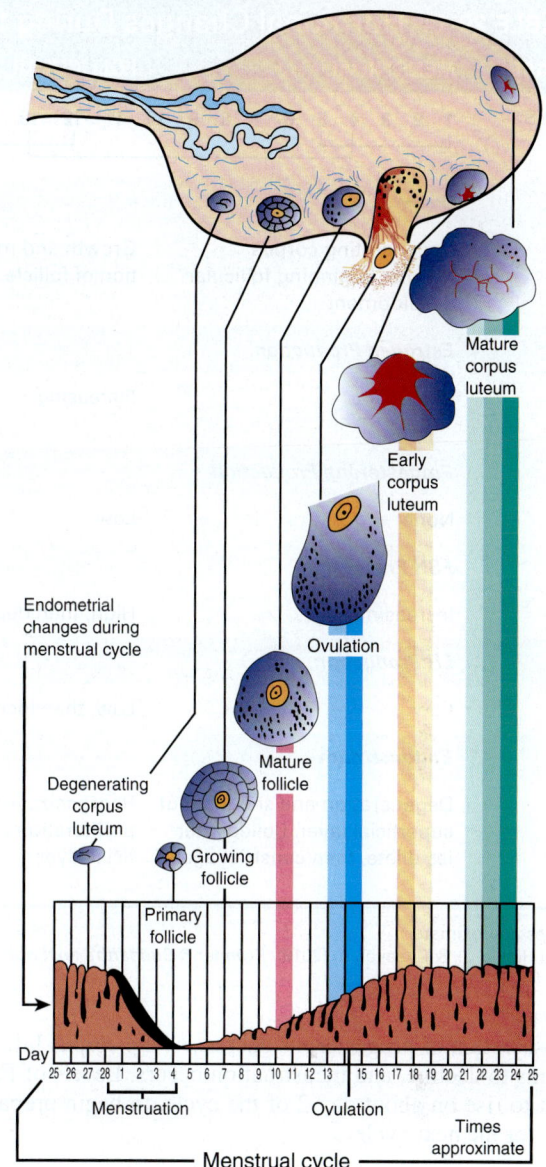

Figure 29-5 One menstrual cycle and the corresponding changes in the endometrium (if the ovum is not fertilized).

Ovulation

About day 14, a surge of hormones causes the ovum to burst through the ovary, **ovulation**. It usually occurs in the middle of the 28-day menstrual cycle (about 14 days before the onset of the next menses). Some fertility control and fertility enhancement methods are based on calculation of the time of ovulation. Some women experience sharp pains or cramps when ovulation occurs. This is known as *mittelschmerz* (meaning "middle pain" in German).

Luteal Phase

During the *luteal phase,* the empty, ruptured Graafian follicle becomes the *corpus luteum* and begins to secrete *progesterone* and *estrogen*. These hormones cause the *endometrium* (the endometrial lining of the uterus) to become greatly thickened and vascular (engorged). If the ovum is fertilized, it becomes embedded in the *endometrium* and becomes a fetus. If the ovum is not fertilized,

TABLE 29-1 Hormonal Changes During the Menstrual Cycle

PHASE	MENSTRUAL	FOLLICULAR	OVULATION	LUTEAL	PREMENSTRUAL
DAYS[a]	1 2 3 4 5 6 7 8 9	10 11 12 13 14	15 16	17 18 19 20 21 22 23 24 25	26 27 28 1 2
Ovary	Degenerating corpus luteum; beginning follicular development	Growth and maturation of follicle	Ovulation	Active corpus luteum	Degenerating corpus luteum
Estrogen Production	Low	Increasing	High	Declining, then a secondary rise	Decreasing
Progesterone Production	None	Low	Low	Increasing	Decreasing
FSH Production	Increasing	High, then declining	Low	Low	Increasing
LH Production	Low	Low, then increasing	High	High	Decreasing
Endometrium	Degeneration and shedding of superficial layer. Coiled arteries dilate, then constrict again	Reorganization and proliferation of superficial layer	Continued growth	Active secretion and glandular dilation; highly vascular; edematous	Vasoconstriction of coiled arteries; beginning degeneration

[a]Times approximate.
From Hinkle, J., & Cheever, K. (2018). *Brunner & Suddarth's textbook of medical-surgical nursing* (14th ed.). Wolters Kluwer.

the secretion of progesterone decreases, the corpus luteum begins to decline, and menstruation occurs. Levels of FSH start to rise on about day 2 of the cycle, to begin preparation for the next cycle.

Uterine Cycle

The endometrium of the uterus has a similar cycle (Fig. 29-5), the *uterine cycle* or *endometrial cycle*. This process prepares the uterus for implantation of an ovum (egg). The uterine cycle is controlled by the ovarian cycle and will vary, depending on whether or not fertilization of the ovum occurs. The three phases of the uterine cycle are the *proliferative phase*, the *secretory phase*, and the *menstrual (menstruation) phase*.

Proliferative (Buildup) Phase
While the ovarian follicles are producing increased amounts of estrogen, the endometrium prepares for possible fertilization with pronounced growth. It thickens from about day 4 to about day 14, as shown at the bottom of Figure 29-5.

Secretory Phase
If fertilization does not occur, the corpus luteum degenerates and hormonal levels fall. Withdrawal of hormones causes the endometrial cells to change, and menstruation begins.

Menstruation
The sloughing off of the endometrium and unfertilized ovum causes *menstruation*. Menstruation averages 3–5 days but may last 2–8 days. During menstruation, FSH levels rise and several ovarian follicles begin to develop again. Thus begins the next endometrial cycle. Hormonal changes during menstruation are shown in Table 29-1. The changes that take place if the ovum is fertilized and pregnancy is established are described and illustrated in Chapter 65. Disorders of the female reproductive system are discussed in Chapter 91.

> **Key Concept**
> Maturation of an ovum occurs during the ovarian cycle; growth of the lining (endometrium) of the uterus occurs during the uterine cycle. Together, these cycles are known as the menstrual cycle.

FEMALE SEXUAL RESPONSE

Female neural pathways involved in controlling the sexual response are the same as those found in the male. During sexual excitement, the erectile tissues within the clitoris and around the vaginal opening become engorged with blood. The vestibular glands secrete mucus before and during coitus (sexual intercourse). If the clitoris is stimulated with sufficient intensity and duration, the woman will feel the physical and psychological release of orgasm. The nipples of the breasts also contain erectile tissues that respond to sexual excitement and orgasm. Unlike a man, a woman can experience successive orgasms with minimal rest.

> ### Key Concept
> Many disorders can be spread by sexual contact and are generally known as sexually transmitted diseases (STDs) or sexually transmitted infections (STIs). These disorders are discussed in Chapter 70.

SPECIAL CONSIDERATIONS Lifespan

Nursing care for the older adult must adapt to changes related to aging. The aging process has significant effects on the female reproductive system (Table 29-2).

> ### NCLEX Alert
> The reproductive system has multiple normal changes throughout the lifespan. The changes that occur during pregnancy, childbirth, and postpartum care are very important. You may be expected to demonstrate knowledge of these changes as they relate to effective client care, client teaching, and preparation for procedures.

TABLE 29-2 Effects of Aging on the Woman's Reproductive System

FACTOR	RESULT	NURSING IMPLICATIONS
Ovaries reduce secretion and eventually stop producing estrogen and progesterone (female *climacteric, menopause*)	Lose ability to become pregnant Menstruation ceases—woman may have hot flashes, headaches, dizziness, or heart palpitations	Watch for signs of depression Refer for medical evaluation Refer for counseling, if needed Treat symptomatically
	May need estrogen (hormone) replacement therapy (**ERT** or **HRT**) Uterus and ovaries get smaller Vaginal mucosal wall shortens and thins Vaginal secretions decrease; intercourse may become painful (dyspareunia) More susceptible to vaginal infections	Controversy surrounds HRT. Women should seek medical advice Counsel client to use water-soluble lubricant, if needed for comfort Hormone-based lubricant may be prescribed Assess for and treat infections promptly
	Breasts get smaller and softer; fatty tissue increases Hair thins on scalp, axillae, and external genitalia	Advise client to wear a good support bra The client may wish to wear a wig
	Hair may grow on upper lip or chin Muscles of upper arms and legs may lose tone Weight gain around midline often occurs	Discuss removal by electrolysis or waxing Educate client about an exercise program Discuss need for fewer calories to maintain weight Stress exercise
	Skin dries; skin may itch; client may develop psoriasis or excessive dandruff	Advise client to use a lotion or moisturizer. Dandruff shampoo may be helpful
Estrogen production decreases After menopause, rate of heart and vascular disease equal between men and women Damage to vaginal and urinary structures as a result of aging and childbirth	Risk of atherosclerosis increases *Osteoporosis* risk increases; bones become subject to fractures if they demineralize and become porous and brittle; spontaneous fractures are possible Genital structures may sag; may fall (prolapse) into vagina Incontinence may occur	Educate client about a low-fat, low-salt diet Educate about increased calcium intake Encourage exercise and weight maintenance Refer for physical examination and possible estrogen therapy Bone density test is often done. Supplemental calcium is often recommended Educate about symptoms of heart disease that differ between men and women Surgery may be necessary Treat symptomatically

STUDENT SYNTHESIS

KEY POINTS

- The internal organs of the female reproductive system include the ovaries, oviducts, uterus, and vagina.
- The external organs of the female reproductive system are the vulva and breasts.
- The egg cell is called an oocyte. Maturation of egg cells begins in the fourth or fifth month of a female fetus' gestation and ends with menopause. A mature oocyte is called an ovum.
- Fertilization of the ovum usually occurs in the oviduct. A fertilized ovum, the zygote, becomes embedded in the uterine lining. Once embedded, it is called an embryo.
- The mammary glands function to produce and release milk and other substances after childbirth.
- Hormones from the hypothalamus, anterior pituitary gland, and gonads influence the female reproductive system.
- Female hormones are called estrogens.
- In women, gonadotropic hormones stimulate the formation of ova and secretion of hormones from sex organs.
- Menarche is the first menstrual period and marks the onset of puberty.
- Menstruation is the monthly flow of blood and other materials from the uterus.
- Menopause is the time when menstrual periods cease and the woman can no longer reproduce.
- The three phases of the ovarian cycle are the follicular phase, ovulation, and the luteal phase.
- The three phases of the uterine cycle are the proliferative phase, secretory phase, and menstruation.

CRITICAL THINKING EXERCISES

1. Explain why a 32-year-old woman who had their uterus and ovaries removed might want to consider hormone replacement therapy.
2. A 12-year-old girl is experiencing their first menstrual period. Their parent brings them to the healthcare facility for you to explain the physical process that is occurring. What information would you give the client? How would you explain menstruation to them?

NCLEX-STYLE REVIEW QUESTIONS

1. A 45-year-old client informs the nurse that they think the signs of menopause have started and would like to know if they can stop their birth control pills. Which response by the nurse is best?
   a. "It is possible for you to become pregnant during developing menopause."
   b. "That would be fine. You should not take the pills during menopause."
   c. "You cannot become pregnant during this time due to decreased ovarian function."
   d. "Your symptoms are probably related to some other disorder."

2. The nurse is obtaining a menstrual history from a female client. The client states that at times, they experiences cramps about 2 weeks after their menstrual cycle ends. Which information would the nurse provide the client?
   a. The client will have to have a biopsy to determine cancerous ovaries.
   b. The cramps may occur due to ruptured ovarian cysts.
   c. The cramps usually indicate ovulation.
   d. No education is required since there is nothing wrong with the client.

3. Which nursing action would be provided to a client who has a decrease in estrogen production?
   a. Discuss the necessity for hormone replacement.
   b. Discuss the need for a low-fat, low-salt diet.
   c. Discuss the increase in hair growth on the scalp, axillae, and external genitalia.
   d. Discuss the likelihood of an increase in musculature of upper arms and legs.

4. A client and their partner have been trying to conceive without results over the past 3 months. Which suggestion can the nurse make that is noninvasive and may increase the probability of success?
   a. Medications can be taken.
   b. It has only been 3 months, let nature take its course.
   c. Determine time of ovulation by checking basal body temperature.
   d. It is time to seek the advice of a fertility specialist.

5. A 13-year-old girl arrives in the clinic and informs the nurse that they just had their first menstrual period on April 23. Which documentation for this event is accurate?
   a. Onset of menstruation on April 23
   b. Onset of menarche on April 23
   c. Onset of menopause on April 23
   d. Onset of puberty on April 23

CHAPTER RESOURCES

Enhance your learning with additional resources on thePoint!

Student Resources related to this chapter can be found at thePoint.lww.com/Rosdahl12e.

Nutrition and Diet Therapy | UNIT 5

30 Basic Nutrition

Learning Objectives

1. Define nutrition and explain the functions of each of the six classes of major nutrients.
2. Discuss the concepts of the MyPlate Food Guidance System and the Nutrition Facts Label.
3. List the major dietary sources of carbohydrates and differentiate among monosaccharides, disaccharides, and polysaccharides.
4. Differentiate between saturated and unsaturated fatty acids. Explain cholesterol, LDL, and HDL.
5. Define amino acid. Differentiate between complete and incomplete proteins.
6. Explain the body's need for water and describe at least four functions of water.
7. List six major minerals and four trace minerals and state their functions.
8. Name the fat-soluble and water-soluble vitamins and list their main functions and food sources.
9. Discuss BMI, obesity, and malnutrition and how they relate to a healthy diet.
10. Identify common special nutritional considerations related to infancy, childhood, adolescence, early and middle adulthood, and older adults.

Important Terminology

amino acid	kwashiorkor	nutrient density	scurvy	DV	MUFA
beriberi	linoleic acid	nutrition	trans fat, trans-	EAR	PCM
cholesterol	linolenic acid	pellagra	fatty acids	EER	PKU
disaccharide	lipid	phytochemical	triglyceride	FDA	PUFA
enzyme	macronutrient	plaque		GDM	RBC
essential nutrient	malnutrition	polysaccharide	**Acronyms**	HCl	RDA
glucose	marasmus	prebiotics	AI	HDL	REE
glycogen	micronutrient	probiotics	BMI	HFCS	UL
hydrogenated	mineral	protein	CHO	IBW	USDA
hyperglycemia	monosaccharide	rickets	DRI	kcal	USP
hypoglycemia	nutrient	saturated fat		LDL	

Food is vital to life. Humans eat to stay alive and to be healthy. In fact, food is one of the most important items in Maslow hierarchy of human needs (see Chapter 5). Food is also enjoyable and brings pleasure to life.

Nutrition is the study of nutrients and how the body utilizes the nutrients in food. Nutrition has a great impact on human well-being, behavior, and the environment.

The science of nutrition continues to evolve as our understanding of its role has shifted from simply preventing dietary deficiencies to reducing the risk of chronic diseases, including osteoporosis, cancer, and heart disease. For instance, before the U.S. Food and Drug Administration (FDA) initiated the Nutrition Labeling and Education Act of 1993. At that time, food labels were required to list the B vitamins thiamine, riboflavin, and niacin because deficiencies in these nutrients were once common. Public health trends are monitored by the FDA and changes are made to the nutrition labels that will be nutrients of public health significance (FDA, 2020). Current public health concerns are reflected in the order in which mandatory dietary components must appear on food labels: serving sizes, total calories, calories from fat, total fat, saturated fat, trans fat, cholesterol, and sodium.

Results from many research studies have indicated that nutrients and other compounds found in food may increase optimal health and even prevent specific health problems. New discoveries about previously unidentified components in plant foods, known as **phytochemicals**, suggest that thousands of naturally occurring chemicals in foods may help protect against disease. Future recommendations for daily nutrient intakes will likely be made from the perspective of optimizing health, rather than simply preventing deficiencies.

This chapter begins with the concept of basic nutrition and information about the functions and sources of nutrients.

Nutrient digestion is included where appropriate. With this knowledge as a foundation, characteristics of a healthy diet are presented and common nutritional problems are discussed. The chapter concludes with a discussion of nutritional concerns across the lifespan.

NUTRIENTS

Nutrients are substances needed for growth, maintenance, and repair of the body. The body can make some nutrients if adequate amounts of necessary precursors (building blocks) are available. **Essential nutrients** are those that a person must obtain through food because the body cannot make them in sufficient quantities to meet its needs. The six classes of nutrients are carbohydrate, fat, protein, water, minerals, and vitamins. Carbohydrate, fat, and protein provide energy and are called **macronutrients**. Vitamins and minerals regulate body processes and are called **micronutrients**. Water is necessary for virtually every bodily function (see Chapter 17).

The MyPlate guidelines initiated in June 2011 and the Dietary Guidelines for Americans of 2020 provide specific recommendations for making food choices that will improve the quality of an average American diet. This nutritional framework provides practical health, activity, and nutritional guidance for the client. Guidelines for pregnant and breastfeeding women, children, adolescents, adults, and other specific audiences are included in the overall concepts of the plan.

The official government Website is a comprehensive source of information and is useful for teaching nutritional concepts to clients. For more information, go directly to *ChooseMyPlate.gov*. The Nutrition Facts Label found on food products should be used as a complementary guide to the MyPlate Framework. Figure 30-1 shows the MyPlate diagram and its relevant content. Food groups are listed in Table 30-1. Table 30-2 reviews nutrient content. Serving sizes are viewed on the ChooseMyPlate Website's Food Gallery. The Nutrition Facts Label is discussed later in this chapter. You may also search for United States Department of Agriculture (**USDA**) food and nutrition information for an extensive list of resources and general nutritional data.

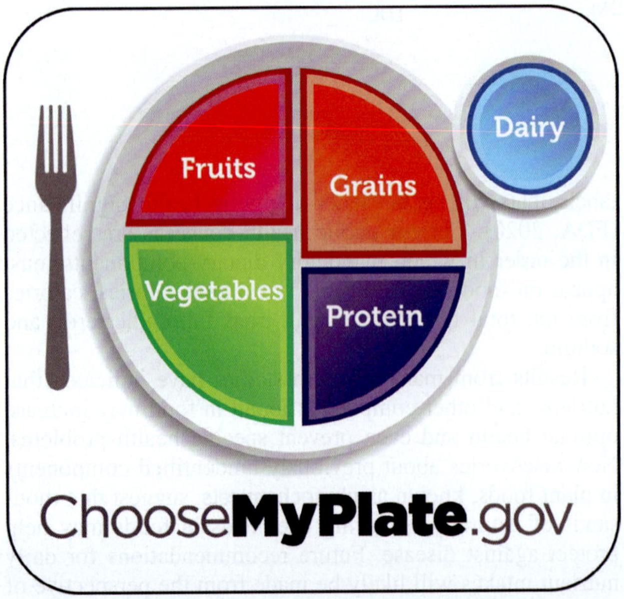

From the nurse's perspective, the MyPlate concept is of benefit when teaching clients about the interrelationships among nutrition, activity, and diet therapy. In general, the concepts review balancing caloric intake, using appropriate amounts of fruits and vegetables, whole grains, and fat-free or low-fat milk, and reducing the amounts of foods containing higher amounts of sodium and sugar. More specifically, these recommendations suggest that the individual

- Eat more of some foods, such as fruits, vegetables, whole grains, and fat-free or low-fat milk products that contain essential nutrients.
- Eat less of other foods, such as foods high in saturated or trans fats, added sugars, cholesterol, salt, and alcohol.
- Provide variety in the diet—eat foods from all food groups and subgroups.
- Balance calorie intake with energy needs to prevent weight gain and/or promote a healthy weight.
- Eat in moderation.
- Be physically active everyday.

Additional concepts are found in Chapter 31; see In Practice 31-1: Guidelines for Healthier Eating Across All Cultures.

> **Key Concept**
>
> Healthy diet—a diet that
> - Emphasizes fruits, vegetables, whole grains, and fat-free or low-fat milk and milk products.
> - Includes lean meats, poultry, fish, beans and peas, eggs, and nuts.
> - Is low in saturated fats, trans fats, cholesterol, salt (sodium), and added sugars.

> **Key Concept**
>
> Eat a variety of foods. No single food supplies all essential nutrients in amounts needed. Variety also helps to reduce the risk of nutrient toxicity and accidental contamination.

Dietary References and Terminology

In 1941, the Food and Nutrition Board of the National Academy of Sciences published the first Recommended Dietary Allowances (RDAs) that set a standard for the intake of specific nutrients to meet the needs of healthy Americans. Continued research has shown that the RDA levels have limited value and are often misrepresented and misused. The focus of RDAs has traditionally been the prevention of deficiency disorders. The Food and Nutrition Board of the National Academy of Sciences changed its approach to setting nutrient reference levels. The study of nutrition has expanded to include the role of nutrients in preventing chronic diseases.

Figure 30-1 MyPlate. The proportions of food content and food groups are suggested by the MyPlate diagram. (United States Department of Agriculture [USDA], n.d., www.choosemyplate.gov.)

TABLE 30-1 ChooseMyPlate.gov Food Groups

GRAINS	VEGETABLES	FRUIT	DAIRY	PROTEIN
Goal				
• Whole grains should be at least 1/2 of total grain intake.	• Make 1/2 of plate fruits and vegetables. • Include fresh, frozen, canned, or dried.		• Include calcium-rich foods. • Use fat-free (skim) or low-fat (1%) milk.	• Include lean protein foods. • Include seafood that is rich in omega-3 fatty acids.

EXAMPLES
Serving sizes: See Food Gallery examples at ChooseMyPlate.gov.

GRAINS	VEGETABLES	FRUIT	DAIRY	PROTEIN

Whole Grains[a]
• Whole-wheat flour
• Bulgur (cracked wheat)
• Oatmeal
• Whole cornmeal
• Brown rice
• Millet
• Popcorn
• Amaranth
• Some ready-to-eat breakfast cereals
Refined Grains[b]
• White flour
• White bread
• Crackers
• Grits
• Noodles
• Pasta
• White rice
• Cornbread
• Some ready-to-eat breakfast cereals
	Dark Green
	• Bok choy
	• Broccoli
	• Collard greens
	• Dark green lettuce
	• Kale
	• Romaine lettuce
	• Spinach
	• Turnip greens
	• Watercress
	Red and Orange
	• Acorn squash
	• Butternut squash
	• Carrots
	• Hubbard squash
	• Pumpkin
	• Red peppers
	• Sweet potatoes
	• Tomatoes
	• Tomato juice
	Starchy
	• Cassava
	• Corn
	• Fresh cowpeas, field peas, or black-eyed peas (not dry)
	• Green bananas
	• Green peas
	• Green lima beans
	• Plantains
	• Potatoes
	• Taro
	• Water chestnuts
	Beans and Peas[c]
	• Black beans
	• Black-eyed peas (mature, dry)
	• Garbanzo beans (chickpeas)
	• Kidney beans
	• Lentils
	• Navy beans
	• Pinto beans
	• Soy beans
	• Split peas
	• White beans
		• Apples
		• Apricots
		• Bananas
		• Berries:
		  • Strawberries
		  • Blueberries
		  • Raspberries
		• Cherries
		• Grapefruit
		• Grapes
		• Kiwi fruit
		• Lemons
		• Limes
		• Mangoes
		• Melons:
		  • Cantaloupe
		  • Honeydew
		  • Watermelon
		• Mixed fruits (fruit cocktail)
		• Nectarines
		• Oranges
		• Peaches
		• Pears
		• Papaya
		• Pineapple
		• Plums
		• Prunes
		• Raisins
		• Tangerines
		• 100% fruit juice:
		  • Orange
		  • Apple
		  • Grape
		  • Grapefruit
			Milk
			• Fat free (skim)
			• Low fat (1%)
			• Reduced fat (2%)
			• Whole milk
			• Lactose reduced
			• Lactose free
			• Flavored milk
			• Milk-based desserts:
			  • Puddings
			  • Ice milk
			  • Frozen yogurt
			  • Ice cream
			• Calcium-fortified soy-milk/soy beverage
			Cheese
			Hard natural cheeses:
			• Cheddar
			• Mozzarella
			• Swiss
			• Parmesan
			Soft cheese:
			• Ricotta
			• Cottage
			Processed cheeses:
			• American
			Yogurt
			• Fat free
			• Low fat
			• Reduced fat
			• Whole milk yogurt
				Meats
				Lean cuts of:
				• Beef
				• Ham
				• Lamb
				• Pork
				• Veal
				Game meats:
				• Bison
				• Rabbit
				• Venison
				Lean ground meats:
				• Beef
				• Pork
				• Lamb
				Lean luncheon or deli meat
				Organ meats:
				• Liver
				• Giblets
				Poultry
				• Chicken
				• Duck
				• Goose
				• Turkey
				• Ground chicken and turkey
				Beans and Peas[c]
				• Black beans
				• Black-eyed peas
				• Chickpeas (garbanzo beans)
				• Falafel
				• Kidney beans
				• Lentils
				• Lima beans (mature)
				• Navy beans
				• Pinto beans
				• Soy beans
				• Split peas
				Nuts and seeds
				• Almonds
				• Cashews
				• Hazelnuts (filberts)
				• Mixed nuts
				• Peanuts
				• Peanut butter
				• Pecans
				• Pistachios
				• Pumpkin seeds
				• Sesame seeds
				• Sunflower seeds
				• Walnuts

(Continued)

TABLE 30-1 ChooseMyPlate.gov Food Groups (Continued)

GRAINS	VEGETABLES	FRUIT	DAIRY	PROTEIN
	Other • Artichokes • Asparagus • Avocado • Bean sprouts • Beets • Brussels sprouts • Cabbage • Cauliflower • Celery • Cucumbers • Eggplant • Green beans • Green peppers • Iceberg (head) lettuce • Okra • Onions • Parsnips • Turnips • Wax beans • Zucchini			*Seafood* Finfish such as: • Catfish • Cod • Flounder • Haddock • Halibut • Herring • Mackerel • Pollock • Porgy • Salmon • Sea bass • Snapper • Swordfish • Trout • Tuna Shellfish such as: • Clams • Crab • Crayfish • Lobster • Mussels • Octopus • Oysters • Scallops • Squid (calamari) • Shrimp Canned fish such as: • Anchovies • Clams • Tuna • Sardines *Eggs* • Chicken eggs • Duck eggs

[a]**Whole grains** contain the entire grain kernel (e.g., the bran, the germ, and the endosperm).
[b]**Refined grains** have been milled which is a process that removes the bran and the germ. Refined grains have a longer shelf life and a finer texture but are often lacking in dietary fiber, iron, and many B vitamins. Most refined grains are *enriched* which means that some B vitamins (e.g., thiamin, riboflavin, niacin, folic acid) and iron are added back into the processed product.
[c]**Beans and peas** are considered unique foods because they are a good source of plant proteins, minerals such as zinc and iron, and many B vitamins.
Adapted from http://www.choosemyplate.gov (2020) and http://www.fda.gov (2020).

A combination of experts in several food and nutrition organizations had instituted an expanded system called the Dietary Reference Intakes (**DRIs**). This system includes four standards that list reference intake levels of essential nutrients for most healthy population groups. The DRIs consist of RDAs, adequate intake, tolerable upper intake level, and estimated average requirement. These standards are described below.

- **RDAs**: Recommendations for average daily dietary intake level that is sufficient to meet the nutrient requirement of nearly all healthy individuals (97%–98%) in a particular life stage and gender group.
- Adequate intake (**AI**): Recommended nutrient intake that is assumed to be adequate. It is based on observed or estimated nutrient intake by a group (or groups) of healthy people and is used when an RDA cannot be determined.
- Tolerable upper intake level (**UL**): The highest level of daily nutrient intake that is likely to pose no risk of adverse health effects for almost all individuals in the general population.
- Estimated average requirement (**EAR**): A daily nutrient intake value that is estimated to meet the requirement of half the healthy individuals in a life stage and gender group.

Food Pattern and Food Group Terms

The use of nutrition, as a basis of health and disease prevention, has grown to include concepts related to daily

TABLE 30-2 Food Groups With Vitamin and Mineral Content

FOOD GROUP	MAJOR VITAMINS PROVIDED WITHIN THIS FOOD GROUP	MAJOR MINERALS PROVIDED WITHIN THIS FOOD GROUP
Grains	• Thiamine • Riboflavin • Niacin • Folate • Pyridoxine • Vitamin E	• Magnesium • Potassium • Selenium • Zinc • Iodine • Iron • Chromium
Vegetables	• Beta-carotene • Vitamin C • Vitamin K • Folate	• Magnesium • Potassium • Calcium • Iron
Fruits	• Beta-carotene • Vitamin C	• Potassium
Dairy	• Vitamin A • Vitamin D • Pyridoxine • Cobalamin • Riboflavin	• Phosphorus • Potassium • Calcium • Iodine
Protein	• Pyridoxine • Cobalamin • Niacin • Riboflavin	• Phosphorus • Selenium • Copper • Zinc • Iron • Potassium
Oils*	Vitamin E	No minerals

*
- Not a food group
- To be used with discretion
- Are a major source of polyunsaturated fatty acids, including the essential fatty acids

Adapted from http://www.choosemyplate.gov (2020) and http://www.fda.gov (2020).

food patterns, caloric intake, and other terms presented below.

- **Daily food intake pattern:** Identifies the types and amounts of foods that are recommended to be eaten each day and that meet specific nutritional goals.
- **Estimated energy requirement (EER):** Represents the average dietary energy intake that will maintain energy balance in a healthy person of a given gender, age, weight, height, and physical activity level. The calorie levels for the food intake patterns were matched to age/sex groups using EERs for a person of average height, healthy weight, and sedentary activity level in each age/sex group.
- **Discretionary calorie allowance:** The balance of calories remaining in a person's energy allowance, or EER, after accounting for the number of calories needed to meet recommended nutrient intakes through consumption of foods in low-fat or no-added-sugar forms.
- **Nutrient-dense foods:** Those foods that provide substantial amounts of vitamins and minerals and relatively fewer calories.
- **Ounce-equivalent:** In the grains food group, the amount of a food counted as equal to a 1-oz slice of bread. In the meat, poultry, fish, dry beans, eggs, and nuts food group, the amount of food counted as equal to 1 oz of cooked meat, poultry, or fish.

> **Key Concept**
>
> Choose a diet with plenty of whole-grain products, vegetables, and fruits. Plant foods provide fiber, complex carbohydrates, vitamins, minerals, and other substances important for good health. They are also generally low in fat.

Kilocalories and Energy

The unit of measurement that specifies the heat energy in a particular amount of food is called a kilocalorie (**kcal**). A *kilocalorie* is defined as the amount of heat required to raise the temperature of 1 kg of water 1 °C. The caloric value of foods can be determined in the laboratory. In this process, the heat that is given off by the burning of the test food raises the temperature of a known amount of water. Calorie charts stating the number of kilocalories in an average serving of various foods are available without cost from a number of sources.

The 4–9–4 kilocaloric values of energy nutrients follow:

- 1 g carbohydrate → 4 kcal
- 1 g fat → 9 kcal
- 1 g protein → 4 kcal

> **NCLEX Alert**
>
> Nutritional concepts and terminology are very important nursing considerations for clients. On the NCLEX, a clinical scenario may include topics related to the kcal yields of 4-9-4, different populations, such as children, older adults, or during pregnancy. The client may need to learn new dietary habits, have specific teaching concerns (e.g., diabetes or cardiovascular disease), or have existing knowledge reinforced or updated.

Requirements

From a nutrition standpoint, calories are synonymous with energy. The amount of energy (calories) a healthy individual needs depends on their age, sex, weight, body composition, and activity level. The energy requirements of an individual are the total calories needed to maintain body processes or resting energy expenditure (**REE**). For most adults, REE accounts for most of the energy used in a typical day. REE is higher for men than for women because men have more muscle mass; likewise, younger adults have a higher REE than older adults because people lose muscle mass as they age. Growth, pregnancy, lactation, and fever increase REE.

In adults, activity typically accounts for 25%–30% of total energy used. The actual amount of energy used for physical activity depends on the duration and intensity of the activity. For instance, people at desk jobs need fewer kilocalories than do laborers who use their muscles a great deal. Also, heavier people use more energy than do lighter people when performing the same activity because they move a greater amount of weight.

Empty Calories

The term *empty calories* is an imprecise term applied to foods that supply calories with few or no nutrients. Examples of empty calorie foods are candy, soft drinks, alcohol, and sugar. Empty calorie foods can contribute to nutrient deficiencies if they take the place of other nutrient-rich foods, such as substituting soft drinks for milk or alcohol for food. Although not considered a nutrient, 1 g of alcohol provides 7 kcal.

Activity Levels

An integral part of the MyPlate concept is the individual's ability to use their nutrients. In other words, activity levels influence the amount of calories/energy that an individual needs. Moderate and vigorous intensity levels are used toward meeting physical activity needs. The following are definitions used to delineate activity lifestyles.

- Sedentary: A lifestyle characterized by little or no physical activity during leisure time. Activities include only the physical activity of independent living.
- Light intensity: A lifestyle that includes some physical exercise that does not typically raise the heart or respiratory rates. Examples include casual walking, grocery shopping, or doing light housework.
- Moderate physical activity: A lifestyle that includes exercise that promotes some exertion but in which the individual has a minimal increase in heart and respiratory rates. Examples of moderate physical activity include walking briskly, general gardening, golf, water aerobics, canoeing, tennis (doubles), dancing, or bicycling on level terrain.
- Vigorous physical activity: A lifestyle that includes exercise that promotes a noticeable increase in heart and respiratory rates. Vigorous physical activity may be sufficiently intense to represent a substantial challenge to an individual, and it results in a significant increase in heart and breathing rates. Examples include running or jogging, heavy yard work, aerobics, swimming continuous laps, basketball (competitive), or tennis (singles).

> **Key Concept**
>
> Balance the foods you eat with physical activity to maintain or improve your weight. Excess weight increases the risk of numerous chronic diseases, such as hypertension, heart disease, and diabetes.

Enzymes and Digestion

Thousands of chemical reactions occur daily in the body. Without enzymes, these reactions would take much more time and use excessive energy. **Enzymes** are biologic catalysts made of proteins. With the exception of pepsin and trypsin, all enzymes end in the suffix -ase. Each enzyme has a specific three-dimensional form that works only with matching shapes of other chemicals in a lock-and-key manner; each enzyme will catalyze only one specific reaction. Enzymes temporarily bond with the other chemicals until they form a new compound, at which point the enzyme is released. Several factors affect enzyme action. For example, each enzyme works best in a particular pH and temperature. Temperatures greater than 106 °F (41 °C) destroy most enzymes; thus, the body generally cannot survive sustained high temperatures.

A major area of enzyme action is digestion. The salivary glands in the mouth make enzymes that begin starch digestion. Enzymes found in pancreatic secretions and in the intestinal wall brush border villi break food into particles that can be absorbed. More information about enzymes is included in the following discussions of specific nutrients.

Carbohydrates

Carbohydrates (**CHO**), commonly referred to as "carbs," are made of carbon, hydrogen, and oxygen; they are classified as either simple or complex, based on the number of sugar molecules present. The major function of carbohydrates is to provide energy. Carbohydrates are the most widely used energy source in the world. For the people of many countries, 80% of their total daily calories come from complex carbohydrates. All carbohydrates, with the exception of

TABLE 30-3 Summary of Nutrients: Carbohydrates, Fats, and Proteins

NUTRIENT	RECOMMENDED % OF TOTAL CALORIES	SOURCES	FUNCTIONS
Carbohydrate	45%–65%	• Bread and cereals • Pasta and rice • Potato, lima beans, corn • Dried beans and peas • Fruits, vegetables, milk • Sugar, syrup, jelly, jam, honey	• Major source of energy (glucose) • Provides fiber • Spares protein • Excess is stored as fat
Fat	20%–35%	• Butter and cream • Salad oils and dressings • Cooking and table fats • Fat in meats • Olives, avocados • Fried foods	• Supplies large amount of energy in a small amount of food • Excess fat stored as adipose tissue • Conserves body heat • Helps keep skin healthy by supplying essential fatty acids • Carries vitamins A, D, E, and K • Important in structure of nerve tissue; protects and insulates body parts
Protein	10%–35%	• Meat, fish, poultry, eggs • Milk and cheese • Dried beans and peas • Peanut butter and nuts • Fortified bread and cereals	• Builds and repairs all tissues • Helps build blood and forms antibodies to fight infections • Supplies energy; excess stored as fat • Assists in acid–base and fluid balance

fiber, provide 4 kcal per gram. (Fiber is not truly digested, and therefore provides no energy.) The simple carbohydrate *glucose* is the body's major source of energy.

Another important function of carbohydrates is the ability "to spare protein"; that is to say, to save protein for body repair, not energy production. If inadequate carbohydrate is available, however, the body burns protein for energy. This protein comes from food and from the body's own muscle tissue. Therefore, in cases of inadequate carbohydrate and protein intake, not only would muscle wasting occur but also adequate protein would not be available to repair body tissues.

All plant foods, except plant oils (e.g., corn, soy, and olive), contain carbohydrates. Milk is the only nonplant source of carbohydrate. Rich sources of carbohydrate include breads and cereals, legumes and dried beans, fruits, and vegetables. Sugar and "sweets" also provide noncomplex carbohydrates. Table 30-3 summarizes facts about carbohydrates.

Digestion
Digestion of carbohydrates begins in the mouth. In this process, the action of salivary amylase or ptyalin, enzymes present in saliva, begins breaking down starch into smaller carbohydrates, known as dextrins. Some carbohydrates may be hydrolyzed into units of glucose and fructose when subjected to the stomach's hydrochloric acid (HCl).

In the small intestine, an enzyme from the pancreas called "pancreatic amylase" converts complex carbohydrates into maltose, a disaccharide (double sugar). In the intestinal wall, the enzymes sucrase, maltase, and lactase are available to complete the digestion process. The end products of carbohydrate digestion—*glucose, fructose,* and *galactose*—are absorbed through the intestinal mucosa. The liver converts fructose and galactose to **glucose**, which can be used for immediate energy or stored in the liver and muscle as **glycogen**. Glucose that remains after energy and glycogen needs are met is converted to fat and stored. The only form of sugar that the body can use is glucose.

Fiber in the diet is acted on by digestive enzymes but passes out of the body virtually undigested.

Simple Carbohydrates
Monosaccharides and **disaccharides** contain one (mono-) or two (di-) sugar (-saccharide) molecules; they are classified as *simple carbohydrates* or *simple sugars*. Simple carbohydrates may or may not taste sweet. Glucose, fructose, and galactose are monosaccharides. Sucrose, lactose, and maltose are disaccharides.

Monosaccharides
Glucose, also called *blood sugar or dextrose*, is the most commonly occurring sugar in the body. Terms such as **hyperglycemia**, which means abnormally high blood sugar, or **hypoglycemia**, which means abnormally low blood sugar, refer to the blood's level of glucose. The body must change other forms of sugar into glucose before it can use these sugars. Sources of natural glucose are honey, fruits, and some vegetables.

Fructose, also called *levulose* or *fruit sugar*, is the sweetest simple sugar; it is found naturally in honey, fruits, and saps. Commercial forms of fructose, namely crystalline fructose and high-fructose corn syrup (**HFCS**), are widely used in sweetened processed foods and soft drinks.

Galactose is not usually found free in nature, but it is found combined with glucose in the disaccharide lactose (milk sugar). Few other significant sources of galactose exist.

Disaccharides
Sucrose, commonly known as table sugar, is composed of fructose and glucose. The most common sweetener in the diet, it is used on the table and in cooking. Although it goes

> **Box 30-1 Added Sugars**
>
> - Sugars and syrups are added to foods during processing or preparation.
> - Limiting simple sugar intake (monosaccharides or disaccharides) can reduce overall calories, decrease or maintain weight, and decrease dental caries.
> - Read the Nutrition Facts Label on food products for sugar content.
> - Read the Total Carbohydrates "sugar" section of the Nutrition Facts Label for *naturally occurring sugars* such as those found in milk, yogurt, and fruit.
> - *Note that added sugars in processed foods may be listed as various names:*
>
> | | |
> |---|---|
> | • Beet sugar | • Lactose |
> | • Brown sugar | • Levulose |
> | • Cane sugar | • Maltose |
> | • Confectioner's sugar | • Malt syrup |
> | • Corn sweetener | • Maple syrup |
> | • Corn syrup | • Molasses |
> | • Dextrose | • Powdered sugar |
> | • Fructose | • Raw sugar |
> | • Fruit juice concentrates | • Sucrose |
> | • Glucose | • Sugar |
> | • High-fructose corn syrup | • Sugar cane syrup |
> | • Honey | • Syrup |
> | • Invert sugar | • Table sugar |
> | • Turbinado sugar | |
>
> Adapted from materials at www.choosemyplate.gov (2020) and www.fda.gov (2020).

by many different names (*crystallized sugar, raw sugar, turbinado sugar, brown sugar, powdered sugar, molasses*), no caloric or nutritional difference exists among its many forms. Sources of sucrose are sugar beets, sugar cane, maple syrup, and some fruits. See Box 30-1.

Lactose is the sugar found in milk. It is neither as soluble nor as sweet as sucrose. It is not found in plants; it is formed only in the mammary glands. The enzyme lactase splits lactose into galactose and glucose. Most infants can tolerate lactose, but many adults cannot. If a person lacks the enzyme lactase, bloating, gas, and diarrhea can occur when milk products are ingested. This condition, known as *lactose intolerance*, is different from an actual milk allergy caused by an immune reaction to protein in milk. Many people with lactose intolerance can tolerate hard cheese, yogurt, and lactase-containing milk, although individual tolerances vary greatly. Commercial products are available over the counter that provide the enzymes needed to digest lactose.

Maltose is not found freely in food but is produced as an intermediate in starch digestion. It is also produced through the process of malting (malted milk) and brewing (beer). Because it is readily soluble and easily changed into glucose, it is often used in infant formulas in the form of maltodextrin.

Sugar has been blamed for causing obesity, diabetes, heart disease, and hyperactivity in children. Sugar, like other fermentable carbohydrates, can increase a person's risk of dental cavities. Sugar is considered "empty-calorie" food because it contains no nutrients (honey contains some trace nutrients), and its consumption often displaces nutrient-dense foods in the diet. Box 30-1 provides information about sugar in the diet.

Complex Carbohydrates

Complex carbohydrates or **polysaccharides** are made of long chains of many sugar molecules arranged in such a way that they do not taste sweet. They are usually insoluble in water. Starch, dextrin, glycogen, and fiber are complex carbohydrates.

Starch

Starch, the form of carbohydrate stored in plants, is the chief source of carbohydrates in the diet. Starch is made up of many glucose units linked together. The main sources of starch are grains, roots, bulbs, legumes, tubers, and seeds (Fig. 30-2). Starch grains are encased in a tough covering that is broken down in the process of digestion. Cooking starch-containing foods speeds up their digestion because enzymes in saliva can act on cooked starch but have little effect on raw starch. Starch must be broken down into glucose before the body can use it.

Dextrin

Dextrin is formed as an intermediate in starch digestion by the action of enzymes or heat (e.g., cooking and toasting). Dextrin is a gummy material that forms as a part of starch's digestive process.

Fructans

Fructans are a group of naturally occurring carbohydrates (saccharides) found in onions, bananas, wheat, artichokes, garlic, and other whole foods. A nurse may see these saccharides (namely, oligosaccharide and fructooligosaccharide) in liquid nutritional supplements, such as Ensure, for clients who need an increase in caloric intake. Used as a probiotic, fructans are also extracted from chicory or manufactured from sucrose for use in the food industry. Prebiotics and probiotics are discussed later in this chapter.

Glycogen

Glycogen is not a significant form of carbohydrate in the diet, but it is the body's storage form of carbohydrate. After the body meets its energy needs, the liver and muscle cells convert excess glucose to glycogen and store it for later use. On average, adult glycogen storage is limited to slightly more than 1 lb. Athletes may practice *carbohydrate loading* to maximize their glycogen storage for long-distance events.

Dietary Fiber

Dietary fiber, commonly known as *roughage*, is a group name for the portion of plants resistant to digestion by human enzymes. Although they are not truly digested, some

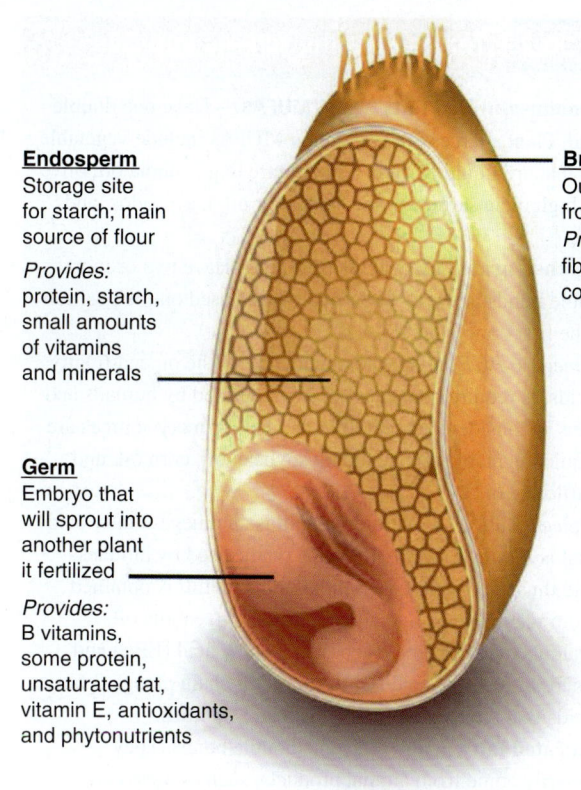

Figure 30-2 A whole wheat kernel. The compartments of the whole wheat kernel are the bran, the germ, and the endosperm. (From Dudek, S. [2017]. *Nutritional essentials for nursing practice* [8th ed.]. Wolters Kluwer.)

types of fiber are broken down by colonic bacteria to produce fatty acids and gas. Most plant foods are composed of various amounts and types of both water-insoluble and water-soluble fiber (see Box 32-2, Source of Fiber).

Cellulose, lignin, and some hemicelluloses are the framework of plants and are water insoluble (cannot be broken down with water). They are most abundant in wheat bran and other whole-grain bread and cereals. The skin, stalks, leaves, and pulp of vegetables and the skin and pulp of fruits are all good fiber sources. Insoluble fiber holds water, increases stool bulk, decreases transit time of food through the intestines, and helps prevent constipation.

Pectin, gums, mucilages, and some hemicelluloses are water-soluble fibers that absorb water to form a gel. They slow gastric emptying time, improve glucose tolerance in people with diabetes, and bind bile acids (which helps to lower some forms of elevated cholesterol levels). Water-soluble fibers are found in oats, legumes, apples, and citrus fruits.

Dietary fiber plays a role in preventing constipation, lowering serum glucose and cholesterol levels, and possibly aiding in weight reduction by promoting a feeling of fullness. Experts recommend that Americans eat more fiber of all types, increasing total daily intake to at least 20–35 g. People can obtain this amount of fiber each day by eating at least five servings of fruits and vegetables and at least six servings of breads and cereals that are identified as good or excellent sources of fiber.

Fats (Lipids)

Fats or **lipids** give flavor and texture to food. Fat is a concentrated energy source that the body can easily store. Most fat in food is in the form of **triglycerides**, which are composed of three fatty acids (tri-) and one glycerol (-glyceride). Like carbohydrates, triglycerides are made of carbon, hydrogen, and oxygen. The body also stores fat in the form of triglycerides, which it can make in the liver from an excess of carbohydrate, protein, and fat.

The major function of fat is to provide energy. Fat provides 9 kcal per gram—more than twice the calories of carbohydrate or protein. At rest, fat normally supplies about 40% of the body's energy needs. Fat also carries fat-soluble vitamins in the body and provides essential fatty acids that play a role in cholesterol metabolism. It helps maintain the function and integrity of capillaries and cell membranes and is a precursor of the hormones known as *prostaglandins* and the phospholipids in cell membranes. Fat cushions major organs to protect them from injury and insulates the body from extreme temperatures. Dietary fat provides *satiety* (satisfaction) because fat leaves the stomach more slowly than carbohydrate or protein.

Fat comes from animals and plant oils. Fat that can be easily identified in foods that appear fatty, such as ground meat and butter, is known as *visible fat*. Fat hidden in foods that do not appear fatty, such as milk, cheese, egg yolks, nuts, desserts, and meat that is marbled with fat, is called *invisible fat*. Table 30-3 summarizes information about fats.

Digestion

Because fats do not dissolve in water, no fat digestion occurs in the mouth and very little occurs in the stomach. When fat reaches the small intestine, bile released from the gallbladder breaks the fat into tiny droplets. In the small intestine, pancreatic lipase breaks down these droplets of emulsified fat into fatty acids, glycerol, and monoglycerides. Once these are inside the mucosal cells of the small intestine, intestinal lipase completes the digestion of monoglycerides into fatty acids and glycerol. Most fatty acids are absorbed via the lacteals in the small intestine of the lymph system; only glycerol and certain fatty acids can be absorbed directly into the bloodstream.

Fatty Acids

Based on the number of double bonds between carbon atoms, fatty acids are classified as either *saturated* (no double bonds) or *unsaturated* (one or more double bonds). The two types of unsaturated fatty acids are *monounsaturated* (one double bond) and *polyunsaturated* (two or more double bonds). Most food fats contain all three types of fatty acids; the type present in the greatest proportion determines whether a food is considered unsaturated or saturated.

Saturated Fatty Acids

Generally, foods that are high in **saturated fat** content are solid at room temperature because they already contain their full complement of hydrogen. Except for the fat found in poultry and many fish, all animal fats are high in saturated fat. Coconut, palm, and palm kernel oils are the only plant sources naturally high in saturated fat. Because a high saturated fat intake raises serum cholesterol levels, Americans are advised to lower their intake of total fat and saturated fat. Many terms exist relating to fats and oils, and these are defined in Box 30-2.

A trans-fatty acid is created when a polyunsaturated fatty acid, such as vegetable oil, is hydrogenated to make it solid at room temperature (as in margarine). In this process, known as *hydrogenation*, manufacturers add hydrogen to liquid oils—such as corn, cottonseed, soybean, and coconut oils—to make them more stable and to decrease the chance of rancidity. The degree of hydrogenation determines the saturation and firmness of the resultant product. **Hydrogenated** fats have fewer essential fatty acids than the original oil because the unsaturated fat content is lowered. Additionally, trans-fatty acids are associated with adversely altering serum levels of some specialized proteins called *lipoproteins*. Lipoproteins are discussed later in this chapter.

Unsaturated Fatty Acids

Unsaturated fatty acids are capable of adding more hydrogen to their molecular structure because one or more double bonds exist between carbon atoms. Unsaturated fats tend to be soft or liquid at room temperature and are susceptible to rancidity when exposed to light and oxygen over a long period. Poultry, freshwater fish, and all plant oils (except coconut, palm, and palm kernel oils) are high in unsaturated fat. Olive, canola, and peanut oils are high in monounsaturated fats. Safflower, sunflower, soybean, and corn oils are rich sources of polyunsaturated fats. Both monounsaturated and polyunsaturated fats help lower blood cholesterol levels when used in place of saturated fats.

Linoleic acid and linolenic acid are polyunsaturated fatty acids considered essential fatty acids because people lack the enzymes needed to synthesize them. Because arachidonic acid is made from linoleic acid, arachidonic acid becomes an essential fatty acid when linoleic acid intake is deficient. Each essential fatty acid has a distinct role in cell

---

Box 30-2 Terms Relating to Fats and Oils[a]

- **Monounsaturated fatty acids (MUFAs)**—Have one double bond. Plant sources that are rich in MUFAs include vegetable oils that are liquid at room temperature (e.g., canola oil, olive oil, high oleic safflower and sunflower oils), avocados, and nuts.
- **Polyunsaturated fatty acids (PUFAs)**—Have two or more double bonds and may be of two types, based on the position of the first double bond.
  - *Omega-6 PUFAs*—**Linoleic acid**, one of the omega-6 fatty acids, is required but cannot be synthesized by humans and thus is considered essential in the diet. Primary sources are liquid vegetable oils including soybean oil, corn oil, and safflower oil.
  - *Omega-3 PUFAs*—**Linolenic acid** is an omega-3 fatty acid that is required because it is not synthesized by humans and thus is considered essential in the diet. It is obtained from plant sources including soybean oil, canola oil, walnuts, and flaxseed. Eicosapentaenoic acid (EPA) and docosahexaenoic acid (DHA) are long-chain omega-3 fatty acids that are contained in all fish and shellfish.
- **Saturated fatty acids**—Have no double bonds. They primarily come from animal products, such as meat and dairy products. In general, animal fats are solid at room temperature.
- *Trans-fatty acids or trans fats*—Unsaturated fatty acids that contain at least one nonconjugated double bond in the trans configuration. Sources of trans-fatty acids include hydrogenated/partially hydrogenated vegetable oils that are used to make shortening and commercially prepared baked goods, snack foods, fried foods, and margarine. Trans-fatty acids also are present in foods that come from ruminant animals (e.g., cattle and sheep). Such foods include dairy products, beef, and lamb.
- **Solid fats**—Fats that are solid at room temperature, such as butter, lard, and shortening. These fats may be visible or may be a constituent of foods such as milk, cheese, meats, or baked products. Solid fats come from many animal foods and can be made from vegetable oils through *hydrogenation*. Solid fats are generally higher than oils in saturated and/or trans-fatty acids.
- **Oils**—Fats that are liquid at room temperature, such as the vegetable oils used in cooking. Oils come from many different plants and from fish. Some common oils are corn, soybean, canola, cottonseed, olive, safflower, sunflower, walnut, and sesame. Some foods are naturally high in oils, such as nuts, olives, some fish, and avocados. Most oils are high in monounsaturated or polyunsaturated fats and low in saturated fats. *A few plant oils, including coconut oil and palm kernel oil, are high in saturated fats and, for nutritional purposes, should be considered to be the same as solid fats.*

[a]The words or phrases emphasized in bold and/or italics are the ones that would most likely be on the NCLEX.

Adapted from materials at http://www.choosemyplate.gov (2020) and http://www.fda.gov (2020).

structure and function and is important in normal development. Vegetable oils, leafy vegetables, meat, and fatty fish are sources of essential fatty acids. Because dietary sources are common and the body stores them, essential fatty acid deficiency is extremely rare. Infants given formulas deficient in linoleic acid and hospitalized clients receiving prolonged lipid-free parenteral nutrition are among the few groups of individuals at risk for fatty acid deficiency. A fatty acid deficiency causes, among other symptoms, a rash or dermatitis.

Cholesterol

Cholesterol is a member of a large group of compounds called *sterols*. Cholesterol is found only in animal tissues, and the body supplies it in the amounts needed to produce substances such as hormones, vitamin D, and bile acids. Cholesterol is a component of all cell membranes and also a major part of the brain and nerve tissue. Cholesterol does not need to be added to the individual's diet. The body makes cholesterol from metabolites produced during the metabolism of energy, that is, the breakdown of food into calories. Foods high in cholesterol include organ meats (e.g., liver, kidneys, and brains) and egg yolk. Lesser amounts of cholesterol are found in whole milk products and meats. Excess amounts of cholesterol, typically found in individuals who consume food containing high amounts of cholesterol, are known to be hazardous to a person's health. The development of atherosclerosis, arteriosclerosis, plaques, and emboli, which lead to strokes, are side effects of high cholesterol levels. The estimated cholesterol content of foods is found on the Nutrition Facts Label (discussed later).

Cholesterol is transported by lipoprotein molecules, which are found in the blood. High-density lipoproteins (**HDL**), the "good cholesterol," function to transport cholesterol from the tissues back to the liver and, in doing so, help lower serum cholesterol levels and the risk of heart disease. HDL levels can be increased by exercise, weight loss, smoking cessation, and moderate alcohol consumption. Low-density lipoproteins (**LDL**), the "bad cholesterol," transport cholesterol from the liver to the tissues. They are implicated in the development of atherosclerosis and coronary artery disease. A diet that is high in saturated fat increases serum LDL levels. Theorists believe that the ratio between these HDL and LDL levels is more significant for assessing health risk than is total cholesterol count. Trans-fatty acids are known to increase serum levels of LDL, while decreasing serum levels of HDL.

> **NCLEX Alert**
>
> Clinical situations commonly require knowledge of the uses and nutritional requirements for carbohydrates, fats, proteins, vitamins, minerals, and water. General nutritional concerns as well as specific concepts such as diabetes or atherosclerosis/arteriosclerosis could be the focus of the scenario. Options often require nursing actions and client/family teaching.

Protein

Protein is the foundation of every cell in the body and is the only nutrient that builds and repairs tissue. In the absence of dietary protein, the body begins to use protein from the bloodstream, muscles, and organs to carry on daily activities. Every major organ, except the brain, will shrink during a prolonged dietary deficiency of protein. Proteins are made up of amino acids, which consist of carbon, hydrogen, oxygen, and nitrogen. Some amino acids also contain phosphorus, sulfur, cobalt, and iron. A small pool of amino acids is stored throughout the body for use in building proteins.

Proteins produce and repair all major body constituents. They are needed for the formation of muscles, connective tissue, glands, organs, skin, and blood clotting factors. Every cell in the body contains some protein. Proteins also help maintain the body's fluid balance; blood proteins called *albumins* and *globulins* help keep intracellular and extracellular fluids where they belong. If a person has a low-protein intake, fluid balance may not be controlled, and edema may develop in the lower extremities. Another important function of protein is its contribution to the body's acid–base balance (see Chapter 17).

Hormones such as *thyroid hormone* and *insulin* are made from protein; all enzymes are proteins. *Antibodies* are also made from protein; therefore, proteins are a key component of the body's immune system (see Chapter 24). Proteins can be converted to glucose and burned for energy. The protein that remains after the body's protein needs are met may be converted to triglycerides in the liver and stored as fat. The body cannot store excess protein as protein.

Protein comes from both animal and plant sources (see Tables 30-1 and 30-3).

Digestion

Chemical digestion of protein starts in the stomach. An enzyme (pepsin) breaks down the basic structure of the protein into polypeptides. In the small intestine, pancreatic juices containing enzymes (e.g., pancreatic protease [or trypsin] and chymotrypsin) split some of the proteins into amino acids. These amino acids are absorbed directly into the blood and used by the body.

The remaining *dipeptides* (two amino acids linked together) and *tripeptides* (three amino acids linked together) are further broken down into amino acids in the intestine and at the brush border villi of the intestinal walls.

Amino Acids

Proteins are complex molecules composed of at least 100 individual units known as **amino acids**. The variations in physical characteristics and functions of individual proteins are caused by the difference in the amounts and types of individual amino acids present and the order in which they are arranged.

Of the 22 known amino acids, nine are considered essential because the body cannot make them at a rate sufficient to meet its needs for growth and maintenance. Therefore, they must be supplied by the diet. The essential amino acids are valine, leucine, isoleucine, phenylalanine, threonine, methionine, lysine, tryptophan, and histidine.

The body can synthesize nonessential amino acids if the diet contains enough nitrogen and energy. Nonessential amino acids are no less important than essential amino acids, but a dietary intake of them is unnecessary. The more common nonessential amino acids are alanine, cystine, glutamine, glycine, and serine.

> **Key Concept**
> Essential and nonessential amino acids are needed to maintain life and normal growth; essential amino acids must be consumed through the diet.

Complete and Incomplete Proteins

"Complete" and "incomplete" are simplistic, imprecise terms used to indicate the quality of a protein. *Complete proteins,* or *high-quality proteins,* provide all essential amino acids in sufficient quantities and proportions for growth and maintenance. All animal proteins, except gelatin, are complete proteins. Some plant proteins, such as processed soy protein, are also complete. *Incomplete proteins* lack sufficient amounts of one or more essential amino acids. Plant proteins are generally considered incomplete, although the actual quality of protein varies considerably among different plant sources. Fortunately, different plants are missing different essential amino acids. By eating a variety of plant proteins over the course of the day, a person can obtain all essential amino acids.

Water

With the exception of oxygen, nothing is more essential to life than water. Human beings can survive for weeks without food but only days without water.

About 60% of an adult's body weight and up to 80% of an infant's body weight is water. Additionally, an adult loses about 2.5 quarts (2.37 L) of water per day by perspiring, urinating, and exhaling. To maintain fluid balance in body cells, lost fluid must be replaced. Food provides some fluid, but it must be supplemented by drinking water and other liquids. Most authorities agree that the average adult needs six to eight glasses of fluid per day.

Water composes a large percentage of cellular makeup. Blood distributes nutrients to the cells; water is one of blood's essential components. Water is the solvent in which vital chemical changes occur in the body, and it is also necessary for controlling body temperature. No organ of the body can function without water. Water is so necessary to life that nature has provided human beings with an inborn warning device: thirst is our strongest appetite.

Minerals

Minerals are vital for building bones and teeth. They help maintain muscle tone, regulate body processes, and maintain acid–base balance. Tables 30-4 to 30-6 summarize information on minerals. The body absorbs some minerals more readily than others, and foods vary considerably in the amount of minerals they contain. Some minerals are lost in cooking, and some are lost in body wastes.

TABLE 30-4 Summary of Major Electrolytes

ELECTROLYTE AND SOURCES	FUNCTIONS	DEFICIENCY/TOXICITY SIGNS AND SYMPTOMS

Sodium (Na)
Adult
• 1 tsp salt = 2,400 mg Na
• 75% of Na intake is from processed foods
• Canned soups, meats, or vegetables
  • Convenience foods
  • Restaurant foods
  • Pizza
  • Processed meats
	• Fluid and electrolyte balance
	• Acid–base balance
	• Maintains muscle irritability
	• Regulates cell membrane permeability and nerve impulse transmission
		Deficiency
		• Can occur with:
		  • Chronic diarrhea
		  • Excessive vomiting
		  • Renal disorders
		  • Nausea
		  • Dizziness
		  • Muscle cramps
		  • Apathy
		Toxicity
		• Hypertension
		• Edema

Potassium (K) • Fruits and vegetables • Dried peas and beans • Whole grains • Milk • Meats	• Fluid and electrolyte balance • Acid–base balance • Nerve impulse transmission • Catalyst for many metabolic reactions • Involved in skeletal and cardiac muscle activity	*Deficiency* • Muscular weakness • Paralysis • Anorexia • Confusion (occurs with dehydration) *Toxicity (from supplements/drugs):* • Muscular weakness • Vomiting
Chloride (Cl) • 1 tsp salt ≈ 3,600 mg Cl • Same sources as sodium	• Fluid and electrolyte balance • Acid–base balance • Component of hydrochloric acid in stomach	*Deficiency* (Rare) • May occur secondary to chronic diarrhea or vomiting and certain renal disorders • Muscle cramps • Anorexia • Apathy *Toxicity* • Normally harmless • Can cause vomiting

From Dudek, S. (2017). *Nutritional essentials for nursing practice* (8th ed.). Wolters Kluwer.

TABLE 30-5 Summary of Major Minerals

MINERAL AND SOURCES	FUNCTIONS	DEFICIENCY/TOXICITY SIGNS AND SYMPTOMS
Calcium (Ca) • Milk and milk products • Fortified orange juice • Green leafy vegetables • Dried peas and beans	• Bone and teeth formation and maintenance • Blood clotting • Nerve transmission • Muscle contraction and relaxation • Cell membrane permeability • Blood pressure	*Deficiency* • Children: impaired growth • Adults: osteoporosis *Toxicity* • Constipation • Increased risk of renal stone formation • Impaired absorption of iron and other minerals
Phosphorus (P) • All animal products (meat, poultry, eggs, milk) • Bread • Ready-to-eat cereal	• Bone and teeth formation and maintenance • Acid–base balance • Energy metabolism • Cell membrane structure • Regulation of hormone and coenzyme activity	*Deficiency* • Unknown *Toxicity* • Low blood calcium
Magnesium (Mg) • Green leafy vegetables • Nuts • Dried peas and beans • Whole grains • Seafood • Chocolate, cocoa	• Bone formation • Nerve transmission • Smooth muscle relaxation • Protein synthesis • CHO metabolism • Enzyme activity	*Deficiency* • Weakness • Confusion • Growth failure in children • Severe deficiency: convulsions, hallucinations, tetany *Toxicity* • No toxicity demonstrated from food • Supplemental Mg can cause diarrhea, nausea, and cramping • Excessive Mg in Epsom salts causes diarrhea
Sulfur (S) • All protein foods	• Component of disulfide bridges in proteins • Component of biotin, thiamin, and insulin	*Deficiency* • Unknown *Toxicity* • In animals, excessive intake of sulfur-containing amino acids impairs growth

From Dudek, S. (2017). *Nutritional essentials for nursing practice* (8th ed.). Wolters Kluwer.

Electrolytes

Electrolytes consist of minerals in the form of salts, acids, and bases. A more detailed discussion of electrolytes may be found in Chapter 17. Sodium (Na^+), potassium (K^+), chloride (Cl^-), and magnesium (Mg^+) work together in a close electrolyte relationship and have many similar functions. They are essential for maintaining the osmotic pressure balance between a cell and its surrounding fluids, for helping to maintain normal acid–base balance, and for normal nerve and muscle functioning. Major electrolytes are summarized in Table 30-4.

Sodium

Sodium (Na) is the major ion in extracellular fluids. The body's actual requirement for sodium is very small; most North Americans consume many times more sodium (table salt) than necessary. Usually, the greater a person's sodium intake, the greater the amount of sodium they excrete in the urine. Some individuals retain sodium, which can result in edema and hypertension. Because research shows that populations who have a high intake of sodium are at greater risk for hypertension and cardiovascular disease, individuals should choose a diet moderate in salt and sodium. High sodium intake may also increase the risk of osteoporosis by promoting increased urinary calcium excretion. Although meat, milk, and some vegetables provide sodium, approximately 75% of consumed sodium in the United States comes from processed and convenience or "fast" foods. Box 30-3 provides information pertinent to sodium and potassium.

Potassium

Potassium (K) is the major ion in intracellular fluid (fluid inside the cells). Potassium is widespread in foods and is especially abundant in fruit (bananas particularly), bran, fresh meats, and many vegetables. Salt substitutes often contain potassium in place of sodium. People are advised to eat more fruits and vegetables to boost their potassium intake, which may help reduce blood pressure.

Chloride

Chloride (Cl) is needed for the production of HCl in the stomach. It is also one of the ions involved in the body's complex buffering system. Most chloride in the average Western diet comes from salt (60% of salt is chloride).

Magnesium

Magnesium (Mg) has many functions, including bone formation and maintenance of homeostasis. Magnesium combines with calcium and phosphorus in the bones (50%–60% of the body's magnesium is in the bones). Magnesium is also an activator of enzymes and is involved with RNA in protein synthesis.

TABLE 30-6 Summary of Trace Minerals

MINERAL AND SOURCES	FUNCTIONS	DEFICIENCY/TOXICITY SIGNS AND SYMPTOMS
Iron (Fe) • Beef liver • Red meats • Fish • Poultry • Clams • Tofu • Dried peas and beans • Fortified cereals • Bread • Dried fruit	• Oxygen transport via hemoglobin and myoglobin • Constituent of enzyme systems	*Deficiency* • Impaired immune function • Decreased work capacity • Apathy • Lethargy • Fatigue • Itchy skin • Pale nail beds and eye membranes • Impaired wound healing • Intolerance to cold temperatures *Toxicity* • Increased risk of infections • Apathy • Fatigue • Lethargy • Joint disease • Hair loss • Organ damage • Enlarged liver • Amenorrhea • Impotence • Accidental poisoning in children causes death
Zinc (Zn) • Oysters • Red meat • Poultry • Dried peas and beans • Certain seafood • Nuts • Whole grains • Fortified breakfast cereals • Dairy products	• Tissue growth • Wound healing • Sexual maturation and reproduction • Constituent of many enzymes in energy and nucleic acid metabolism • Immune function • Vitamin A transport • Taste perception	*Deficiency* • Growth retardation • Hair loss • Diarrhea • Delayed sexual maturation • Impotence • Eye and skin lesions • Anorexia • Delayed wound healing • Taste abnormality • Mental lethargy *Toxicity* • Anemia • Elevated low-density lipoprotein (LDL) • Lowered high-density lipoprotein (HDL) • Diarrhea • Vomiting • Dizziness • Fever • Impaired calcium absorption • Renal failure • Muscle pain • Reproductive failure
Iodine (I) • Iodized salt • Seafood • Bread • Dairy products	Component of: • Thyroid hormones that regulate growth, development, and metabolic rate	*Deficiency* • Goiter • Weight gain • Lethargy • During pregnancy may cause severe and irreversible mental and physical retardation (cretinism) in fetus *Toxicity* • Enlarged thyroid gland • Decreased thyroid activity

TABLE 30-6 Summary of Trace Minerals (Continued)

MINERAL AND SOURCES	FUNCTIONS	DEFICIENCY/TOXICITY SIGNS AND SYMPTOMS
Selenium (Se) • Seafood • Liver • Kidney • Other meats • Grains grown in selenium-rich soil • Brazil nuts • Walnuts	Component of: • Antioxidant enzymes • Immune system functioning • Thyroid gland activity	*Deficiency* • Enlarged heart • Poor heart function • Impaired thyroid activity *Toxicity* (Rare) • Nausea • Vomiting • Abdominal pain • Diarrhea • Hair and nail changes • Nerve damage • Fatigue
Copper (Cu) • Organ meats • Seafood • Nuts and seeds • Whole grains • Drinking water	• Used in the production of hemoglobin • Component of several enzymes • Used in energy metabolism	*Deficiency* (Rare) • Anemia • Bone abnormalities *Toxicity* • Vomiting • Diarrhea • Liver damage
Manganese (Mn) • Widely distributed **Best sources:** • Whole grains • Tea • Pineapple • Kale • Strawberries	Component of: • Enzymes involved in the metabolism of carbohydrates, protein, and fat • Bone formation	*Deficiency* (Rare) *Toxicity* (Rare) • Nervous system disorders
Fluoride (Fl) • Fluoridated water • Water that naturally contains fluoride • Tea • Seafood	• Formation and maintenance of tooth enamel • Promotes resistance to dental decay • Bone formation and integrity	*Deficiency* • Susceptibility to dental decay • May increase risk of osteoporosis *Toxicity* • Fluorosis (mottling of teeth) • Nausea • Vomiting • Diarrhea • Chest pain • Itching
Chromium (Cr) • Meat • Whole grains • Nuts • Cheese	• Cofactor for insulin	*Deficiency* • Insulin resistance • Impaired glucose tolerance *Toxicity* • Dietary toxicity unknown • Occupational exposure to chromium dust damages skin and kidneys
Molybdenum (Mo) • Milk • Legumes • Bread • Grains	• Component of many enzymes • Works with riboflavin to incorporate iron into hemoglobin	*Deficiency* • Unknown *Toxicity* • Occupational exposure to molybdenum dust causes gout-like symptoms

From Dudek, S. (2017). *Nutritional essentials for nursing practice* (8th ed.). Wolters Kluwer.

> **Box 30-3 Sodium and Potassium**
>
> - Individuals with hypertension, African Americans, and middle-aged and older adults are often more sensitive to table salt (NaCl) than others.
> - Increasing the dietary intake of potassium can lower blood pressure and blunt the effects of salt on blood pressure in some individuals.
> - Salt substitutes containing potassium chloride (KCl) may be useful for some individuals who want to limit sodium intake, but the increase in potassium can be harmful. A healthcare professional needs to be consulted before using salt substitutes.

Adapted from materials at http://www.choosemyplate.gov (2020) and http://www.fda.gov (2020).

Calcium

Calcium (Ca) is the mineral most likely to be deficient in a typical adult diet. Calcium makes up about 2% of the adult human body; 99% of the body's calcium is in the bones and teeth. It also has other important uses, such as keeping the body fluids balanced, helping blood clot, and regulating heart and other muscle activity and nerve responses. Normal blood levels of calcium are maintained (even when calcium intake is inadequate) through the action of hormones. These hormones influence calcium absorption, urinary calcium excretion, and the movement of calcium into and out of bones. Because bone gives up calcium at its own expense when calcium intake is inadequate, a chronic calcium deficiency increases the risk of *osteoporosis* (thinning of the bone). Altered blood calcium levels occur secondary to other disorders or from hormonal abnormalities, not from a dietary deficiency.

The best sources of dietary calcium are cow's milk, yogurt, hard cheese, and calcium-fortified orange juice. The vitamin D, phosphorus, and lactose content of milk also promote calcium absorption. Good sources of calcium include calcium-fortified soy and almond milk, cereals, kale, broccoli, and canned salmon with bones. The most recent DRI for calcium was increased to 1,000–1,200 mg for most adults to maximize bone density and to reduce the risk of osteoporosis for women and men.

If normal dietary intake does not supply the DRI, supplementation may be indicated. Calcium carbonate is an excellent form of calcium for people up to the age of 50 years. Calcium citrate is a more readily absorbable form of calcium due to decreased release of **HCl** in the stomach, and it is recommended for people older than 50 years.

Phosphorus

Every cell in the body contains phosphorus (P), which accounts for about 1% of adult body weight. Of the phosphorus in the human body, 80% is found in the bones and teeth. Phosphorus has more functions than any other mineral in the body. It helps the cells use carbohydrates, fats, and proteins and regulates acid–base balance. It is also important for normal nerve and muscle functioning. Almost all foods contain phosphorus, especially those rich in protein (meat, fish, poultry, nuts, legumes, milk, and milk products).

Trace Minerals

Some minerals are present in, and needed by, the body in very small amounts; they are nevertheless important in body processes. These minerals are called *trace minerals*. Table 30-6 summarizes some of the trace minerals utilized by the body.

Iron

Iron (Fe) is an essential part of every body cell and is also a constituent of hemoglobin (Hgb), a substance in the red blood cells (**RBCs**) that carries oxygen. The body is thrifty with its supply of iron and continually reuses it by salvaging the iron from worn-out RBCs. Young children, teenagers, and women require more iron than do men. Iron-deficient anemia is the most common deficiency disorder in the United States.

Iodine

Iodine (I), which is needed for production of the hormone thyroxine, is essential for normal thyroid gland functioning. Some parts of the United States, especially areas near the Great Lakes and the Rocky Mountains, have almost no iodine in the soil; consequently, food products from these regions contain no natural sources of iodine. Goiter, an enlargement of the thyroid gland, was common in these areas before the use of iodized salt, which has virtually eliminated goiter in the United States.

Other Trace Minerals

Other trace minerals include chromium (Cr), which plays a role in the function of insulin; copper (Cu), which helps form hemoglobin; and zinc (Zn), which is important in producing hormones and RNA, and which can enhance or depress the immune system depending on whether intake exceeds or fails to meet requirements. Selenium (Se) is a component of an antioxidant and is being studied for its role in cancer prevention. The following trace minerals may be essential for humans in very small amounts: arsenic, boron, bromine, cadmium, fluorine, lead, lithium, manganese, molybdenum, nickel, silicon, tin, and vanadium (see Table 30-6).

Vitamins

"Vita" is the Latin word for "life." The word "vitamin" signifies the importance of vitamins to humans. *Vitamins* consist of carbon, oxygen, hydrogen, and sometimes nitrogen or other elements. When first discovered, vitamins were given alphabetical names such as vitamin A, vitamin B, and so on. Research has shown that vitamins belong to groups. Because they are organic substances, vitamins can be converted to other forms and are susceptible to oxidation and destruction. They may also be precursors to other chemicals. As a result of the increasing awareness of individual vitamins, vitamins are more accurately referred to by a group name or a specific name such as "ascorbic acid" for vitamin C. Tables 30-7 and 30-8 contain both common and specific names of most known vitamins.

TABLE 30-7 Summary of Fat-Soluble Vitamins		
VITAMIN AND SOURCES	**FUNCTIONS**	**DEFICIENCY/TOXICITY SIGNS AND SYMPTOMS**
Vitamin A *RETINOL* • Liver • Dairy products • Egg yolk • Ready-to-eat cereals *BETA-CAROTENE* • Green leafy vegetables • Broccoli • Carrots • Peaches • Pumpkin • Red peppers • Sweet potatoes • Winter squash • Mango • Watermelon • Apricots • Cantaloupe	• Enables the eye to adapt to dim light • Normal growth and development of bones and teeth • Formation and maintenance of mucosal epithelium to maintain healthy functioning of skin and membranes, hair, gums, and various glands • Important role in immune function	*Deficiency* • Night blindness • Slow recovery of vision after flashes of bright light at night • Bone growth ceases • Bone shape changes • Enamel-forming cells in the teeth malfunction • Teeth crack and tend to decay • Skin becomes dry, scaly, rough, and cracked • Keratinization or hyperkeratosis develops • Mucous membrane cells flatten and harden • Xerosis (eyes become dry) • Irreversible drying and hardening of the cornea can result in blindness • Decreased saliva secretion → difficulty chewing, swallowing → anorexia • Decreased mucous secretion of the stomach and intestines → impaired digestion and absorption → diarrhea, increased excretion of nutrients • Susceptibility to respiratory, urinary tract, and vaginal infections increases *Toxicity* • Headaches • Vomiting • Double vision • Hair loss • Bone abnormalities • Liver damage • Can cause birth defects during pregnancy
Vitamin D • Sunlight on the skin • Liver • Some fish • Egg yolks • Fortified milk • Some ready-to-eat cereals • Margarine	• Maintains serum calcium concentrations by: • Stimulating gastrointestinal (GI) absorption • Stimulating the release of calcium from the bones • Stimulating calcium reabsorption from the kidneys	*Deficiency* • Rickets (in infants and children) • Retarded bone growth • Bone malformations (bowed legs) • Enlargement of ends of long bones (knock-knees) • Deformities of the ribs (bowed, with beads or knobs) • Delayed closing of the fontanel → rapid enlargement of the head • Decreased serum calcium and/or phosphorus • Malformed teeth; decayed teeth • Protrusion of the abdomen related to relaxation of the abdominal muscles • Increased secretion of parathyroid hormone • Osteomalacia (in adults) • Softening of the bones → deformities, pain, and easy fracture • Decreased serum calcium and/or phosphorus, increased alkaline phosphatase • Involuntary muscle twitching and spasms *Toxicity* • Kidney stones • Irreversible kidney damage • Muscle and bone weakness • Excessive bleeding • Loss of appetite • Headache • Excessive thirst • Calcification of soft tissues (blood vessels, kidneys, heart, lungs) • Death

(Continued)

TABLE 30-7 Summary of Fat-Soluble Vitamins (Continued)

VITAMIN AND SOURCES	FUNCTIONS	DEFICIENCY/TOXICITY SIGNS AND SYMPTOMS
Vitamin E • Vegetable oils • Margarine • Salad dressing • Foods made with vegetable oil • Nuts and seeds • Wheat germ • Dark green vegetables • Whole grains • Enriched cereals	• Acts as an antioxidant to protect vitamin A and polyunsaturated fatty acid (PUFA) from being destroyed • Protects cell membranes	*Deficiency* • Increased red blood cell (RBC) hemolysis • In infants: anemia, edema, and skin lesions *Toxicity* • Relatively nontoxic • High doses enhance action of anticoagulant medications
Vitamin K • Bacterial synthesis • Green leafy vegetables • Liver • Eggs • Cabbage-related vegetables	• Synthesis of blood-clotting proteins • Synthesis of a bone protein that regulates blood calcium	*Deficiency* • Hemorrhaging *Toxicity* • No symptoms have been observed from excessive vitamin K

From Dudek, S. (2017). *Nutritional essentials for nursing practice* (8th ed.). Wolters Kluwer.

TABLE 30-8 Summary of Water-Soluble Vitamins

VITAMIN AND SOURCES	FUNCTIONS	DEFICIENCY/TOXICITY SIGNS AND SYMPTOMS
Thiamin (Vitamin B_1) • Whole grain • Enriched breads and cereals • Liver • Nuts • Wheat germ • Pork • Dried peas and beans	• Coenzyme in energy metabolism • Promotes normal appetite • Promotes nervous system functioning	*Deficiency* • Beriberi • Mental confusion • Decrease in short-term memory • Fatigue • Apathy • Peripheral paralysis • Muscle weakness and wasting • Painful calf muscles • Anorexia, weight loss • Edema • Enlarged heart • Sudden death from heart failure *Toxicity* • No toxicity symptoms reported
Riboflavin (Vitamin B_2) • Milk and other dairy products • Whole grain • Enriched breads and cereals • Eggs • Meat • Green leafy vegetables	• Coenzyme in energy metabolism • Aids in the conversion of tryptophan into niacin	*Deficiency* • Dermatitis • Cheilosis • Glossitis • Photophobia • Reddening of the cornea *Toxicity* • No toxicity symptoms reported

Niacin (Vitamin B_3)
• All protein foods
• Whole grain
• Enriched breads and cereals
	• Coenzyme in energy metabolism
	• Promotes normal nervous system functioning
		Deficiency
		• Pellagra (four Ds)
		  • Dermatitis and glossitis
		  • Diarrhea
		  • Dementia, irritability, mental confusion → psychosis
		  • Death, if untreated
		Toxicity (from supplements/drugs)
		• Flushing
		• Liver damage
		• Gastric ulcers
		• Low blood pressure
		• Diarrhea
		• Nausea
		• Vomiting

TABLE 30-8 Summary of Water-Soluble Vitamins (Continued)

VITAMIN AND SOURCES	FUNCTIONS	DEFICIENCY/TOXICITY SIGNS AND SYMPTOMS

Vitamin B_6
• Meats
• Fish
• Poultry
• Fruits
• Green leafy vegetables
• Whole grains
• Nuts
• Dried peas and beans
	• Coenzyme in amino acid and fatty acid metabolism
	• Helps convert tryptophan to niacin
	• Helps produce
	  • Insulin
	  • Hemoglobin
	  • Myelin sheaths
	  • Antibodies
		Deficiency
		• Dermatitis
		• Cheilosis
		• Glossitis
		• Abnormal brain wave pattern
		• Convulsions
		• Anemia
		Toxicity
		• Depression
		• Fatigue
		• Irritability
		• Headaches
		• Sensory neuropathy characteristic

Folate • Leafy vegetables • Dried peas and beans • Seeds • Liver • Orange juice • Some fruits • Breads • Cereals and other grains fortified with folic acid	• Coenzyme in DNA synthesis, therefore vital for new cell synthesis and the transmission of inherited characteristics	*Deficiency* • Glossitis • Diarrhea • Macrocytic anemia • Depression • Mental confusion • Fainting • Fatigue *Toxicity* • Too much can mask B_{12} deficiency

Vitamin B_{12}
• Meat
• Fish
• Poultry
• Shellfish
• Milk and dairy products
• Eggs
• Some enriched foods
	• Coenzyme in the synthesis of new cells
	• Activates folate
	• Maintains nerve cells
	• Helps metabolize some fatty acids and amino acids
		Deficiency
		• GI changes
		• Glossitis
		• Anorexia
		• Indigestion
		• Recurring diarrhea or constipation
		• Weight loss
		• Anemia
		  • Pallor
		  • Dyspnea
		  • Weakness
		  • Fatigue
		  • Palpitations
		• Neurologic changes
		  • Paresthesia of the hands and feet
		  • Decreased sense of position
		  • Poor muscle coordination
		  • Poor memory
		  • Irritability
		  • Depression
		  • Paranoia
		  • Delirium
		  • Hallucinations
		Toxicity
		• No toxicity symptoms reported

Pantothenic Acid Widespread in foods • Meat • Poultry • Fish • Whole-grain cereals • Dried peas and beans	• Part of coenzyme A used in energy metabolism	*Deficiency* (Rare) • General failure of all body systems *Toxicity* • No toxicity symptoms reported, although large doses may cause diarrhea

(Continued)

TABLE 30-8 Summary of Water-Soluble Vitamins (Continued)

VITAMIN AND SOURCES	FUNCTIONS	DEFICIENCY/TOXICITY SIGNS AND SYMPTOMS
Biotin Widespread in foods • Eggs • Liver • Milk • Dark green vegetables • Synthesized by GI flora	Coenzyme in: • Energy metabolism • Fatty acid synthesis • Amino acid metabolism • Glycogen formation	*Deficiency* (Rare) • Anorexia • Fatigue • Depression • Dry skin • Heart abnormalities *Toxicity* • No toxicity symptoms reported

Vitamin C
• Citrus fruits and juices
• Red and green peppers
• Broccoli
• Cauliflower
• Brussels sprouts
• Cantaloupe
• Kiwi fruit
• Mustard greens
• Strawberries
• Tomatoes
	• Collagen synthesis
	• Antioxidant
	• Promotes iron absorption
	• Involved in the metabolism of certain amino acids
	• Thyroxin synthesis
	• Immune system functioning
		Deficiency
		• Bleeding gums
		• Pinpoint hemorrhages under the skin
		• Scurvy, characterized by:
		  • Hemorrhaging
		  • Muscle degeneration
		  • Skin changes
		• Delayed wound healing
		• Reopening of wounds
		• Softening of the bones → malformations, pain, easy fractures
		• Soft, loose teeth
		• Anemia
		• Increased susceptibility to infection
		• Hysteria and depression
		Toxicity
		• Diarrhea
		• Abdominal cramps
		• Nausea
		• Headache
		• Insomnia
		• Fatigue
		• Hot flashes
		• Aggravation of gout symptoms

From Dudek, S. (2017). *Nutritional essentials for nursing practice* (8th ed.). Wolters Kluwer.

Small amounts of vitamins are necessary to help regulate body processes, including synthesizing body compounds, such as bone and blood, and extracting energy from carbohydrates, fat, and protein. Most vitamins work in the form of a coenzyme that promotes the action of enzymes. Without vitamins, thousands of chemical reactions cannot occur. The body, with a few exceptions, cannot produce vitamins; therefore, vitamins are an essential component of a healthy diet. Box 30-4 provides some general principles related to vitamins.

Foods are the natural sources of vitamins and should supply daily vitamin needs. Foods differ greatly in the amount and number of vitamins they contain. Tables 30-7 and 30-8 identify the major vitamins, their sources, their functions, and deficiency disorders that occur when the body does not get enough of a particular nutrient.

Vitamins are available in commercial, over-the-counter forms. Some vitamins are available by prescription because healthcare providers may want to prescribe high dosages for certain marked deficiencies. Vitamins vary in their solubility, which influences how they are absorbed, transported through the blood, stored, and excreted. Vitamins with the United States Pharmacopoeia (**USP**) seal on the label are guaranteed to meet set purity and solubility standards.

> *Key Concept*
>
> A, D, E, and K are fat-soluble vitamins; C and B complex are water-soluble vitamins.

Many healthy individuals choose to take commercial vitamins as a safeguard against less-than-optimal food choices. Those who take supplements should select a balanced multivitamin that does not exceed the UL for any nutrient. It is important to note that nutrients in foods, namely phytochemicals, are still being discovered today. Therefore, people should strive to meet their vitamin and mineral needs through diet. See In Practice: Educating the Client 30-1 for more information about vitamin supplements.

Fat-Soluble Vitamins

Fat-soluble vitamins (see Table 30-7) are absorbed into the lymphatic circulation with fat and must attach to a protein carrier to be transported through the blood. The body stores fat-soluble vitamins primarily in the liver and in fat tissue. Because they are stored, deficiency symptoms are slow to develop. Vitamins A and D are toxic when consumed in excess of need over a prolonged period. Cooking does not easily destroy fat-soluble vitamins.

Box 30-4 General Principles Related to Vitamins

- **Some vitamins are lost by exposure to air or during food storage.** Fresh foods retain most vitamins when properly stored. Frozen foods are second, although their vitamin C content may be higher than that of improperly handled fresh food. Canned foods are third. (Canned foods should be processed carefully and not stored too long.)
- **Some vitamins are fat soluble and are stored in the body in this form.** The diet must include sufficient fat to carry an adequate supply of these vitamins (15–20 g).
- **Some vitamins are water soluble.** Cook foods in a small amount of water and use the cooking water, if possible, in gravies, sauces, and soups.
- **High temperatures destroy vitamins.** Do not overcook food, and serve it at once.
- **Avoid discarding the high-nutrient portion of some foods.** The highest concentration of some vitamins may be found in the outer leaves of lettuce and vegetable peels.
- **A clinical condition called *hypervitaminosis* can occur as a result of an excess of a particular vitamin or vitamins.** Hypervitaminosis occurs almost exclusively from supplement use, not from dietary intake.

Adapted from materials at http://www.choosemyplate.gov (2020) and http://www.fda.gov (2020).

Vitamin A

Retinol or vitamin A is a group of related substances that promote growth, sustain normal vision, support normal reproduction, and maintain healthy skin and mucous membranes (thereby increasing the body's resistance to infection). Preformed vitamin A is found only in animal sources, such as liver, butter, and egg yolk; fortified milk is also a good source. Carotene is a precursor of vitamin A; that is, the body converts carotene to vitamin A, but not quickly enough to be toxic. Excellent food sources of carotene are deep orange and deep green fruits and vegetables, such as sweet potatoes, winter squash, carrots, broccoli, spinach, green leafy vegetables, and cantaloupe.

Vitamin D

Calciferol or vitamin D is a group of sterols essential in regulating the body's use of calcium and phosphorus. A marked deficiency of vitamin D hampers growth and affects bone hardness. This deficiency causes a childhood condition known as **rickets**, in which the bones do not harden as they should, but instead bend into deformed positions, such as bowlegs. Pregnant and lactating women must provide themselves with sufficient vitamin D to prevent rickets from developing in the child and to preserve their own bones and teeth. Sunlight on the skin plays a role in the conversion of vitamin D to its active form, as does the functioning of the liver and kidneys. The best food sources of vitamin D are fish liver oils and fortified milk.

Groups at the highest risk for vitamin D deficiency are totally breast-fed infants, vegetarians who consume no dairy products (see Chapter 31), and people who get little sunshine (e.g., institutionalized or homebound individuals). Secondary vitamin D deficiency can occur in people with liver disease, kidney disease, or fat malabsorption syndromes. Because excess vitamin D is toxic, it should be supplemented only with healthcare provider's approval.

Vitamin E

Although the role of *alpha-tocopherol* or vitamin E is not fully understood, it has been proven to be a powerful antioxidant. In this role, it protects vitamins A and C, as well as some fatty acids and phospholipids in the cell membrane, from destruction by oxidation. Vitamin E deficiency is rare, except in malabsorption disorders, such as cystic fibrosis and pancreatic disorders. Vitamin E is found in plant fat and vegetable oils, products made with vegetable oils (e.g., margarine and shortening), wheat germ, nuts, and green leafy vegetables.

IN PRACTICE
EDUCATING THE CLIENT 30-1 — Vitamins

Encourage people who take vitamin supplements to consider the following:
- *Freshness:* Vitamin pills can lose their potency over time, especially when stored in a bathroom medicine cabinet. Look for pills with an expiration date on the label. Do not use after the expired date.
- *Price:* In most cases, cost has little to do with vitamin quality.
- Supplements should provide no more than 100% Daily Value because more is not necessarily better and in some instances is toxic.
- Supplements should contain no unnecessary ingredients. The average diet supplies enough biotin, pantothenic acid, phosphorus, iodine, and chloride. Trace minerals, such as nickel, silicon, and zinc may be unnecessary. Sugar in vitamins is safe because the small amount contained within a vitamin pill is not harmful.

Vitamin K

Menadione or vitamin K is essential in the formation of prothrombin and at least five other proteins that are required for the clotting of blood. Because vitamin K is found in a variety of foods, the average diet supplies an adequate amount. Good sources are liver, egg yolk, cauliflower, cabbage, spinach, and other green leafy vegetables. Intestinal bacteria synthesize vitamin K in insufficient quantities to meet the total vitamin K requirement. The limited amount the body stores is found in the liver. A dietary deficiency is unlikely. Intake of foods that contain high amounts of vitamin K should be monitored when taking anticoagulants, such as warfarin (Coumadin), because vitamin K can interfere with the effectiveness of warfarin. Some clients' diets may routinely contain these vegetables; therefore, the dosage of warfarin needs to be adjusted to include the routine intake of these vitamin K–rich foods. Signs of hemorrhaging may be due to a vitamin K deficiency, which is treated in adults with either oral or intramuscular administration of vitamin K.

Water-Soluble Vitamins

Water-soluble vitamins (see Table 30-8) include vitamins C and B complex. They are absorbed directly through the intestinal walls into the bloodstream. They are also easily absorbed and excreted in urine when consumed in excess. Water-soluble vitamins are considered nontoxic because the body generally does not store them. Deficiencies develop more quickly with them than with fat-soluble vitamins because water-soluble vitamins are not readily stored and are excreted rapidly. Food, light, heat, acids, and alkaline solutions can easily destroy water-soluble vitamins.

Vitamin C

Vitamin C is probably equally well known by its chemical name, *ascorbic acid*. Over the years, experts have recognized its many functions but continue to discover further uses. One of the functions of vitamin C in vital body processes is to aid in the formation of collagen, the most important protein in connective tissue. By holding cells together, collagen contributes to healthy tissue and to the proper functioning of blood vessels, skin, gums, bones, joints, and muscles—essentially, all body tissues and organs. Vitamin C is also involved in reactions involving numerous other compounds, such as folic acid, histamine, neurotransmitters, bile acids, leukocytes, and corticosteroids. Vitamin C enhances the absorption of the form of iron that is predominant in plants and is an effective antioxidant. Individuals who have had surgery or who have suffered extensive burns frequently receive large supplemental doses of ascorbic acid; it is essential to wound healing.

The classic disease of vitamin C deficiency, **scurvy**, is rare in the United States. Symptoms of scurvy include bleeding gums, loose teeth, sore and stiff joints, tiny hemorrhages, and great weight loss. Lesser vitamin C deficiencies affect health by causing listlessness, irritability, and lowered resistance to disease.

Vitamin C is probably the most unstable of all the vitamins. Exposure to air, drying, heating, and storing destroy it. As an acid, it survives longer in acidic surroundings; therefore, baking soda (the alkali, sodium bicarbonate) should not be added to food sources of vitamin C during cooking. Tomatoes retain vitamin C better than other vegetables because they contain acid. Freezing fruits and vegetables helps to preserve their vitamin C content, but they should be used immediately after thawing. Carefully canned fruits and vegetables also retain this vitamin because air is excluded during the canning process.

Because vitamin C is destroyed by heat and is water soluble, cooking should be done in as little water as possible, and overcooking should be avoided. Many raw fruits and vegetables, especially citrus fruits, are high in vitamin C. For instance, one cup of orange juice provides more than the RDA for vitamin C. Research has yet to confirm Linus Pauling's theory that vitamin C can prevent or cure the common cold. Because of its antioxidant properties, vitamin C may play an important role in cancer prevention. However, some studies have shown that mega doses of vitamin C may increase the resistance of cancer cells to chemotherapy treatment. Doses greater than the DRI may increase the risk of kidney stones in some people.

Populations at risk for vitamin C deficiency include people who do not eat fruits and vegetables, alcoholics, and people of low socioeconomic status. Smokers require extra vitamin C because nicotine inhibits its absorption.

Vitamin B Complex

The B complex vitamins are generally known as thiamine, riboflavin, niacin, folate or folic acid, cobalamin, pyridoxine, biotin, and pantothenic acid. Most B complex vitamins have numbers such as B_1, B_{12}, and so on. However, the trend is to identify the vitamin by its proper name instead of a number (see Table 30-8).

The following B complex vitamins are all widely distributed in foods. Although each one is chemically distinct, they share many similar functions, dietary sources, and deficiency symptoms.

Thiamine (B_1): Thiamine promotes general body efficiency. It plays a role in growth, cell metabolism, appetite, neurologic functioning, RNA and DNA formation, and normal muscle tone in cardiac and digestive tissues. As part of a coenzyme, thiamine is essential for the metabolism of carbohydrate and certain amino acids. Signs of a deficiency of thiamine are poor appetite, fatigue, irritability, general lethargy, nausea, vomiting, loss of weight and strength, depression, mental confusion, and poor intestinal tone. A severe deficiency causes **beriberi**, a disease of the nervous system that leads to paralysis and death from heart failure.

The best food sources of thiamine are pork, whole-grain and enriched breads and cereals, legumes, peas, organ meats, and dried yeast. The body does not store thiamine to any great extent. Thiamine is lost during cooking, especially when cooking is prolonged or at high temperatures. Alkalis also destroy thiamine. In the United States, thiamine deficiency occurs most frequently in persons who abuse alcohol because they "waste" thiamine in the metabolism of alcohol. A thiamine supplement is usually prescribed for these clients.

Riboflavin (B_2): Riboflavin functions primarily as a component of two coenzymes that catalyze many reactions, including the metabolism of carbohydrate, fat, and protein. It is essential for growth. Riboflavin deficiency is rare in the United States; people at the greatest risk for deficiency are those who take in large amounts of alcohol, older adults, people on low-calorie diets, and people with malabsorption syndromes. Signs of a riboflavin deficiency include *cheilosis* (cracking and sores at the corners of the mouth), *glossitis* (inflammation of the tongue, with a smooth texture and purplish-red color), and *stomatitis* (inflammation of the lining of the mouth). The body does not store riboflavin to any extent; therefore, a person's diet must provide a steady supply.

Riboflavin is available in a wide variety of foods but only in small quantities. The best sources are milk and milk products, meat, poultry, fish, and whole-grain or enriched breads and cereals. Exposure of riboflavin to light while in solution destroys it.

Niacin (B_3): Niacin exists as *nicotinic acid* and *nicotinamide*. It plays a vital role in the release of energy from carbohydrate, fat, and protein. It is also needed for the production of fatty acids, cholesterol, and steroid hormones.

The best sources of niacin are lean meat, liver, kidney, yeast, peanut butter, whole-grain and enriched products, and dried peas and beans. Niacin is not readily destroyed by heat, light, acids, or alkalis. The body stores only a small amount of niacin.

- A marked niacin deficiency leads to the disease **pellagra**. The mucous membranes of the mouth and digestive tract become red and inflamed, and lesions appear on the skin. Symptoms of severe deficiency progress through the four Ds: dermatitis, diarrhea, dementia, and death. Niacin deficiency is rare, except in persons who abuse alcohol. Healthcare providers sometimes prescribe nicotinic acid in gram quantities to help lower blood cholesterol levels; however, side effects are common. These possible side effects include flushing of the skin, hot flashes, headache, hypotension, tachycardia, hypoglycemia, and liver damage.

Folate/folic acid (B_9): Folate is the group name for this B complex vitamin. Folate plays a major role in the synthesis of DNA and RNA and in the formation of red and white blood cells. Folic acid is the form of folate used in vitamin supplements. It is also involved in the synthesis of certain enzymes and in amino acid metabolism. Folate is available in many foods. Excellent sources include enriched cereals, liver, organ meats, milk, eggs, asparagus, broccoli, green leafy vegetables, dried peas and beans, and orange juice. Cereals and breads are now required by the FDA to be fortified with folic acid.

- Deficiency results in megaloblastic (macrocytic) anemia, glossitis, diarrhea, poor growth, impaired nerve function, and increased risk of heart attack. Intake of high amounts of folate masks vitamin B_{12} deficiency (*pernicious anemia*), which, when left untreated, can cause irreversible neurologic damage or death. Folic acid deficiency is common in all parts of the world. In the United States, folic acid deficiency is most common among older adults, pregnant women, alcoholics, fad dieters, and women taking oral contraceptives. A folate supplement is usually prescribed for these individuals. New research has proved that folate, given before conception and during early pregnancy, helps prevent neural tube defects, such as spina bifida.

Cobalamin (B_{12}): Cobalamin is a family of compounds, all of which contain cobalt. It is important in folate metabolism and in blood cell formation. It is also involved in maintaining the myelin sheath covering certain nerves. Cobalamin and folate are needed to activate each other.

- For the intestine to absorb vitamin B_{12}, intrinsic factor must be present. *Intrinsic factor* is a protein-containing compound the stomach produces in the presence of HCl. Conditions that impair the secretion of intrinsic factor, such as gastric surgery or gastric cancer, cause B_{12} malabsorption and pernicious anemia, an anemia characterized by abnormal RBCs known as *megaloblasts*. Vitamin B_{12} deficiency in the United States is due to impaired absorption, not an inadequate dietary intake.
- Vitamin B_{12} deficiency leads to anemia, neurologic symptoms, increased risk of heart attack, and other generalized symptoms. Because the body stores vitamin B_{12}, it may take years for symptoms to develop.
- Vitamin B_{12} is found exclusively in animal sources; therefore, pure vegetarians who consume no animal products are at risk of vitamin B_{12} deficiency. Bacteria in the small intestine may produce small amounts of absorbable vitamin B_{12}.

Pyridoxine (B_6): Vitamin B_6 is a family of compounds—*pyridoxal, pyridoxine,* and *pyridoxamine.* The official name is pyridoxine, but it is commonly interchanged with the more common term vitamin B_6. Pyridoxine is needed for enzyme activity in the metabolism of protein, carbohydrate, and fat. It is especially important in protein metabolism. Other functions include forming heme for hemoglobin, metabolizing neurotransmitters, synthesizing myelin sheaths, and maintaining cellular immunity.

- Rich sources of pyridoxine (B_6) are meat, fish, poultry, and eggs. Whole wheat products, nuts, and oats are also good sources. Most diets contain adequate amounts of this vitamin.
- A deficiency of vitamin B_6 is most likely to occur secondary to malabsorption syndromes, alcoholism, or certain drug therapies and is most likely to develop in people with multiple B vitamin deficiencies. Symptoms may include retarded growth, confusion, headaches, and seizures. A deficiency of pyridoxine may also increase the risk of heart attack. Large quantities of vitamin B_6 taken for months or years can cause neurologic problems, such as difficulty walking, numbness of the feet and hands, clumsiness, and nerve degeneration. Symptoms gradually improve after the vitamin is discontinued.

Biotin: Biotin (rarely seen as vitamin H) is essential in the functioning of many enzymes. It acts as a coenzyme in the metabolism of carbohydrate and fat and aids in the removal of certain nitrogen groups from amino acids.

- Biotin is found in almost all foods. Liver, egg yolks, soy flour, cereals, and yeast are the best sources of biotin.
- Biotin deficiency is rare except when a person consumes large amounts of raw egg whites. A substance in the egg white, avidin, binds biotin and keeps it from being absorbed.

Pantothenic acid: Pantothenic acid is involved in a number of metabolic processes in humans, especially in the metabolism of protein, carbohydrates, and fats. Because of its central role in energy metabolism, it is vital to all energy-requiring body processes. The average diet supplies a sufficient amount; no RDA has been established. The word pantothenic means "widespread," and pantothenic acid is found in many foods. Good sources include liver, organ meats, egg yolk, dried peas and beans, broccoli, whole grains, lean meats, and poultry.

Prebiotics and Probiotics

Based on emerging science, prebiotics and probiotics are now believed to benefit both the well and the ailing client. **Prebiotics** are nondigestible food ingredients that selectively feed probiotic bacteria. **Probiotics**, on the other hand, are healthy live bacteria. Together, prebiotics and probiotics work to maintain a healthy digestive system and may boost immune function. Both prebiotics and probiotics are also available in supplement form.

Probiotics may be found in some whole foods and specialized food products. The biggest category of foods in the United States that contains live and active cultures is fermented dairy products, such as kefir, yogurt, and cheeses.

Specialized food products containing probiotics are increasingly found on store shelves. Currently, the major group of prebiotics in use in the United States food supply is the *fructans*, which are discussed in the carbohydrate section.

Resistant starch is another category of prebiotics that are found naturally in raw potatoes and unripe fruit, such as bananas. Commonly manufactured for use by the food industry, it may be difficult to recognize on food labels; therefore, look for claims on the label such as high fiber, reduced-energy, or reduced-carbohydrate.

CREATING THE HEALTHY DIET

A healthy diet is one that provides an adequate amount of each essential nutrient needed to support growth and development, perform physical activity, and maintain health. In addition to meeting physiologic requirements, diet is also used to satisfy a variety of personal, social, and cultural needs. These factors must be considered in diet planning. The diets of all individuals must consist of foods that are easily attainable and affordable. People can use an infinite variety and combination of foods to form a healthy diet. The current philosophy of a healthy diet is that foods should be enjoyed in moderation.

Although ensuring that the diet provides sufficient nutrients is important, of greater concern for most Americans today is avoiding dietary excesses, particularly of calories, fat, cholesterol, and sodium, which are associated with the development of several chronic diseases. Many Americans can achieve risk reduction by implementing dietary and lifestyle changes.

How can you choose a diet that provides sufficient amounts of essential nutrients but not excessive amounts of others and help your clients do the same? Where is the line between adequate nutrition and "over"-nutrition? As a nurse, you are often in a position to promote wellness by counseling clients and their families on the "why" and "how to" of food choices. Today's most important nutritional concepts are *variety, moderation,* and *balance.* The FDA has provided several resources that assist in creating a healthy diet for an individual. The *Nutrition Facts Label,* the *ingredients list,* and MyPlate.com provide extensive information for the consumer. Nurses should be able to incorporate these resources when they discuss healthy eating. A wide variety of people can benefit from this information, including the growing child, the adult, or the person with diabetes, heart disease, or a gastrointestinal disorder.

> **Key Concept**
> The purpose of food is to be ingested, broken down, assimilated, and reformed into the ingredients that the body needs to make and repair biochemical substances, such as enzymes, blood, bone, tissue, and urine.

The Nutrition Facts Label

The Nutrition Facts Label was introduced 2 decades ago to educate the American public about food choices and how to select foods based on nutritional facts. The FDA requires that this label be placed on most food packages in the United States. Since its inception, the label has been periodically modified to include new information that reflects the results of research in the area of *nutrition science*. The goal of the Nutrition Facts Label is to help the public be more aware of the nutritional value of a food product. Since the introduction of this informational tool, consumers have increasingly used this label as a guideline for their purchase of food products. As healthcare providers, nurses must be aware of the contents of the label, comprehend the uses of the individual nutrients, and incorporate the label in teaching sessions with the client.

> **Key Concept**
> Food is divided into nutritional categories consisting of six major nutrients: carbohydrates ("carbs"), fats, proteins, water, vitamins, and minerals. Excesses or deficits of these biochemical ingredients, called nutrients, often result in unhealthy disorders.

The Nutrition Facts Label shows an overview of the *percent daily value* (**%DV**) or the percentage of total fats, total carbs, proteins, and some vitamins or minerals in one serving of food. The listed %DV is for a healthy adult on a 2,000-calorie per day diet. The %DV helps the consumer make healthy food choices by determining if the nutritional value of a food is high or low. Specific information about some nutrients of *public health significance* are listed on the label, such as saturated fats, trans fats, cholesterol, sodium, dietary fiber, sugars, added sugars, vitamin D, calcium, iron, and potassium. The label is required to list some elements, while the listing of other nutrients, such as calcium, is voluntary. Figure 30-3 illustrates the Nutrition Facts Label and highlights the priority nutrition-related concepts that help the average person understand and use this resource as a guide for appropriate serving sizes, caloric intake, and nutrient contents per serving. The choice of healthier foods will be beneficial for the consumer. For example, choosing foods that are low in saturated fats, trans fats, and cholesterol will minimize effects on the cardiovascular system. It is the consumer's responsibility to purchase the healthier product.

Reading the Nutrition Facts Label

To obtain information from the Nutrition Facts Label, begin by looking at the product-specific information: *serving size, calories,* and *nutrients.* Serving sizes are listed in household (cups, pieces) and metric measurements (milligrams, grams). The amounts of some nutrients should be limited, such as saturated fat, trans fats, and sodium. Other nutrients are not always eaten in adequate amounts (e.g., fiber, calcium, or iron), and these are listed separately. Look at the percentage of total fat, total carbs, and proteins. (For more information, refer to www.ChooseMyPlate.gov.) A balance of nutrients is of critical importance for overall health.

> **Key Concept**
> Refer to *MyPlate Dietary Guidelines for Americans 2020–2025* at the Website www.ChooseMyPlate.gov, which contains specific nutrient information. This commentary is designed to help maintain healthy eating conditions during the ages and stages of the general population as well as to assist the healthcare community in their understanding of nutrients.

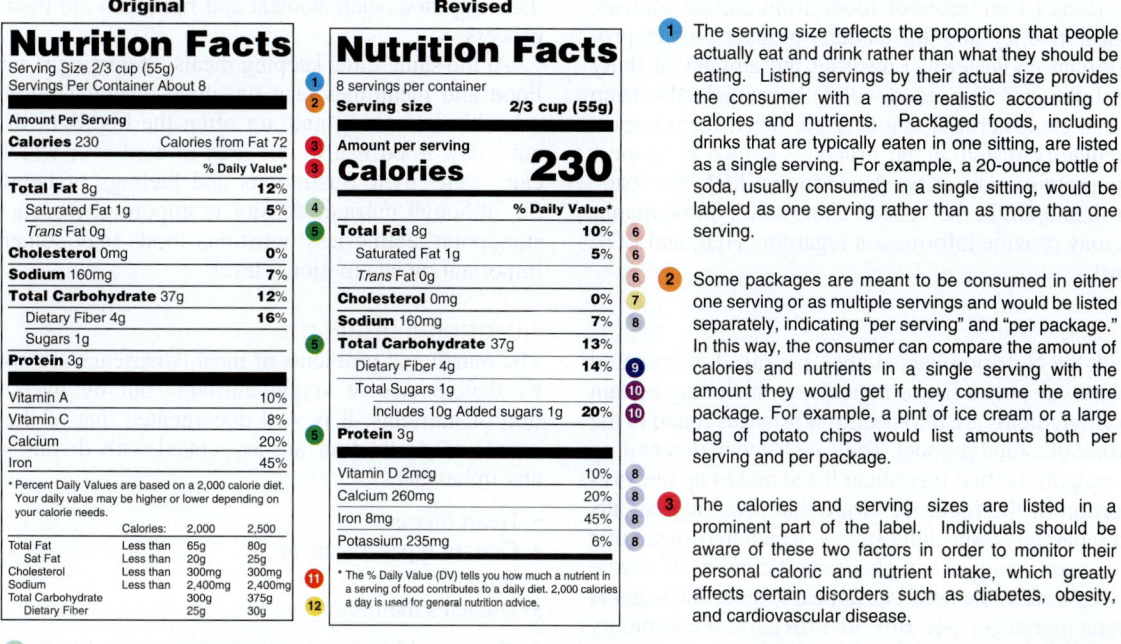

Figure 30-3 Comparison of original and revised Nutrition Facts Label. Match colored numbers in list to the same color and number beside the Nutrition Facts label for a full understanding of the revised label. Free nutritional information, provided on various government websites, is available for a variety of ages and conditions. These useful and practical data are suitable for students, instructors, and as a resource for client teaching sessions. Instructional videos and Fact Sheets are often provided. For further information go to: www.fda.gov, www.MyPlate.gov, and www.cdc.gov. (United States Food and Drug Administration, 2020.)

The next section of the Nutrient Facts Label concerns the fats: *saturated fat, trans fat,* and *cholesterol.* These potentially unhealthy substances are precursors to many disorders, for example, atherosclerosis, blood clots, and strokes. Try to minimize these items. The amount of *sodium, dietary fiber, sugars,* and *added sugars* will tell you how much of the nutrient is being consumed in one serving. It is better to have more dietary fiber (roughage) than sugar or added sugars, which add calories but not necessarily useful nutrients. The levels of some vitamins and minerals are listed (e.g., vitamin C and sodium). Sodium levels tend to be higher in processed foods than in fresh or frozen foods. Figure 30-3 provides additional information about the details of the Nutrition Facts Label.

Cholesterol

Cholesterol is not a nutrient, nor is it essential for the body to obtain it through food intake. Cholesterol is made by the body in adequate amounts. It is a waxy, fat-like substance that can form clumps between arterial walls, forming deposits known as **plaque**. Plaque can lead to gradual or sudden closure of circulation, which leads to emboli that block blood vessels in the brain and heart. When using the

Nutrition Facts Label, monitor foods from animal sources, such as meat, poultry, and full-fat dairy products, which provide additional cholesterol. Lowering the amount of daily cholesterol obtained from food will be beneficial. Also keep in mind that cholesterol is uniquely packaged for transport in the circulatory system in the structures known as *lipoproteins*. Lipoproteins exist as two basic forms: *LDL*, the "bad" cholesterol, and *HDL*, the "good" cholesterol. Some manufacturers may provide information regarding HDL and LDL cholesterol.

Ingredients

Along with the Nutrition Facts Label, packaged or prepared foods need to display a list of ingredients, including certain additives. Ingredients are the specific substances found in the total mixture of a food product. They are listed in descending order by weight; the first ingredient listed makes up the largest proportion of the food. Be aware that some ingredients are listed separately, especially sugars, which may mean that the total content of sugar is higher than it appears. If sugars are listed separately, the label can appear to state that sugar is not the main ingredient. See Box 30-1 for a list of commonly used sugar ingredients.

On the ingredient list, also look for foods to avoid, such as coconut oil or palm oil, which are high in unhealthy saturated fat. Avoid foods that are hydrogenated, which are high in trans fat. Healthy ingredients include soy and monounsaturated fats, such as olive, canola, or peanut oils, or whole grains, such as whole wheat flour and oats. Foods high in fiber are recommended. These include dried beans, fruits, vegetables, and grains.

The Nutrition Facts Label, the ingredients list, and the MyPlate nutritional guidelines are free and readily available to help the consumer understand the various aspects of nutrition science. These nutritional resources provide information of public health significance for the client with certain heart diseases, diabetes, and obesity. Used as part of teaching sessions, healthcare providers, especially nurses, can educate both children and adults about healthy versus unhealthy eating. Individuals can access additional information from the Internet and make personal choices. The nurse can highlight the effects of excesses or deficits of nutrients on an individual's health. Control of the intake of specific nutrients, such as various types of fats, sodium, or sugars, is ultimately the responsibility of the adult.

Diet Planning

In the hospital or other healthcare facility, a dietitian will most likely plan menus. As a nurse, you will need to understand dietary requirements to teach clients effectively. Emphasize foods with **nutrient density** (i.e., foods that provide significant amounts of key nutrients per volume consumed). Nutrient density, as well as caloric density, becomes increasingly important for those with diminished appetites owing to nausea, pain, inactivity, boredom, or anxiety. For instance, hospitalized individuals often have increased protein requirements to promote healing. However, for the protein to be used for healing and not for energy, adequate calories need to be consumed. Encouraging clients with high protein requirements to consume the higher calorie foods on their tray first, such as meat and milk, can aid their healing process.

At the same time, keeping meals interesting is important. Food and mealtimes take on much greater significance in a healthcare setting and are often the highlight of the client's day. Food is also one area of care over which clients can "vent" their frustrations and feelings of helplessness. So, although nutrient density is important from a medical standpoint, eating less nutritious foods may sometimes be important on an emotional level.

Nutritional Problems

The nutritional problems of most Americans are not caused by deficiencies of single nutrients but by overconsumption of nutrients. It is well documented that of the leading causes of death, four are associated with dietary excesses and imbalances:

- Heart disease
- Certain types of cancer
- Stroke
- Diabetes mellitus

Overnutrition also contributes to such conditions as hypertension, osteoporosis, dental caries (decay), gastrointestinal diseases, and obesity. Although no one can say for certain exactly what proportion of these disorders is caused by diet, evidence suggests that a diet high in calories, fat (especially saturated fat), cholesterol, and sodium, but low in complex carbohydrates and fiber, contributes significantly to the high rates of chronic diseases among many North Americans.

Health and Body Weight

Body Weight Assessment

In the past, *ideal body weight* (*IBW*) was used to describe optimal weight for optimal health. Newer standards for weight replace "ideal" with "healthy" because "ideal" is difficult to define.

Body mass index (*BMI*) is used more frequently than IBW. BMI measures weight in relation to height. Defined as weight in kilograms divided by height in meters squared, BMI allows comparison of weights among people of differing heights. BMI nomograms (graphs) have eliminated the need to perform calculations, and these are readily available on the Internet. The classification "obese BMI" is generally 30–40, with very obese BMI considered to be >40. Clients in these BMI categories may be more susceptible to numerous physical disorders. Bariatric (weight loss) surgery may be considered (see Chapter 88).

Also, consider the concept that some people may be above their "healthy weight" according to their BMI but not be "overweight." Neither IBW nor BMI takes into account the body composition of people who are muscular (e.g., athletes) or who have greater bone density and therefore may weigh more than their "healthy weight."

Overweight and Obesity

The percentage of Americans who fall into the "overweight" and "obese" categories has increased dramatically over the past few decades and is now considered to be at epidemic levels. Overweight individuals are individuals who weigh 10%–20% more than the "ideal" weight per height. *Obesity* refers to an excessive amount of fat on the body. Adolescent obesity is of special concern because these individuals are much more likely to develop lifelong complications such as diabetes or cardiovascular disease at a relatively younger age. Overweight or obese people do not necessarily consume adequate amounts of all nutrients, although they tend to consume more calories than are needed for metabolism.

Malnutrition

Malnutrition literally means "bad nutrition." Too much or too little of one or more nutrients may cause poor nutrition; however, malnutrition most commonly refers to *under*nutrition. Inadequate food intake may cause malnutrition, or it may occur secondary to alterations in digestion, absorption, or metabolism of nutrients.

Although certain population groups are at risk for vitamin and mineral deficiencies (e.g., alcoholics, adolescent girls, pregnant and lactating women, people of low socioeconomic status, and people with certain chronic diseases), severe deficiencies are rare in the United States. The prevalence of mild deficiencies, which may not produce obvious physical symptoms but can be detected through blood analysis, varies among nutrients. Ironically, hospitalized clients are at risk for protein–calorie malnutrition (**PCM**), which is seen in diets that are low in calories and protein. Clients with PCM, which is often unrecognized and not diagnosed, have prolonged hospitalizations. They do not heal well because there is not enough protein to make or repair new tissue, and they have a lowered resistance to infection.

Two other types of protein deficiencies are identified but not commonly found in the United States or Canada: **marasmus** and **kwashiorkor**. *Marasmus* is extreme malnutrition and emaciation that occurs chiefly in young children as a result of inadequate calories and proteins. It may be seen in starvation or in the child with failure to thrive, as described in Chapter 72. The child has progressive wasting of subcutaneous tissue and muscle. Slow and gradual addition of foods and maintenance of fluid and electrolyte balance are keys to survival and growth.

Kwashiorkor is also a form of severe malnutrition found primarily in children; it is caused by severe protein deficiencies. Typically, the child with kwashiorkor has access to some calories and does not lose weight as drastically as does the child with marasmus (who has an inadequate intake of protein *and* an inadequate amount of calories). Kwashiorkor commonly occurs as a child is weaned from the breast because a new sibling has been born. The infant receives the mother's breast milk, while the older child receives some nutrients and calories from the food sources available, but does not receive adequate proteins. Eventually, the malnourished child experiences mental and physical retardation, dermatoses, necrosis, and fibroses. The child may also experience nervous system irritability, edema, anemia, and fatty degeneration of the liver, often visualized as an edematous or distended abdomen, which is a result of liver necrosis and ascites. Mental retardation is permanent, but with adequate nutritional interventions, physical growth can resume. Box 30-5 summarizes major dietary guidelines and key recommendations for the general population.

NUTRITION ACROSS THE LIFESPAN

Eating a balanced diet throughout life is the basis of good health. Because cultural and family background often influences diet, educating women during pregnancy and family caregivers during child-rearing years has the potential to have a positive impact on the nutritional health of future generations.

> **NCLEX Alert**
>
> Lifespan differences in nutrition are of great importance. You may need to identify the significant nutritional concerns and differences, especially of the basic six nutrients, for these population groups on an NCLEX clinical scenario.

Pregnancy

Women who consume an adequate diet during pregnancy provide the fetus, placenta, and maternal tissues with the nutrients necessary for growth and development. A good diet cannot guarantee a successful pregnancy, but it can optimize the chance of delivering a healthy full-term infant. Although the requirements for almost all nutrients increase during pregnancy, adequate intake of protein, iron, calcium, vitamin D, and folic acid is especially important. Calorie needs generally need to be increased by only 300 kcal/day during the second and third trimesters for a total caloric intake of about 2,000–2,500 per day and not at all during the first trimester if prepregnancy weight is adequate. Therefore, nutrient density is necessary to avoid overeating. Most healthcare providers prescribe prenatal vitamin and mineral supplements.

Pregnant women with a family history of diabetes are at increased risk for gestational diabetes mellitus (**GDM**). All women should be screened for GDM between weeks 24 and 28 of their pregnancy. If a woman tests positive for GDM, they must be monitored closely, and they should see a dietitian to be placed on a special diet to control their blood sugar. GDM places the baby at higher risk for pre- and postnatal complications. Women who are diagnosed with GDM are at high risk for developing type 2 diabetes later in life. Achieving a healthy body weight after pregnancy lowers this risk.

Infancy

The first year of life is marked by the most rapid growth outside the mother's womb. Infants double their birth weight in 6 months and triple it in a year. This rapid growth explains an infant's high use of energy.

The American Academy of Pediatrics recommends exclusive breastfeeding for the first 5–6 months of life. Breast milk provides all essential nutrients in optimal amounts and in a form that the infant can easily tolerate and digest, without artificial colorings, flavorings, or preservatives. Overfeeding is unlikely. Breastfeeding is associated with a significant decrease in the incidence and duration of both gastrointestinal and nongastrointestinal infections, and it protects against food allergies. Breastfeeding may also decrease the risk of certain chronic diseases later in life, such as type 2 diabetes and Crohn disease.

Formula feeding is an acceptable alternative if breastfeeding is contraindicated or the mother is unable or unwilling to

Box 30-5 Dietary Guidelines and Key Recommendations for the General Population

NUTRIENTS AND CALORIC NEEDS
- Consume a variety of nutrient-dense foods and beverages within and among the basic food groups while choosing foods that limit the intake of saturated and trans fats, cholesterol, added sugars, salt, and alcohol.
- Adopt a balanced eating pattern such as that recommended by the United States Department of Agriculture (USDA) and the MyPlate.gov guidelines.
- Maintain a body weight in a healthy range.
- Balance calories from foods and beverages with the amount of calories expended.
- To prevent gradual weight gain over time, make small decreases in food and beverage calories and increase physical activity.
- Engage in regular physical activity.
- Promote physical fitness by including cardiovascular conditioning, stretching exercises for flexibility, and resistance exercises or calisthenics for muscle strength and endurance.
- Consume a sufficient amount of fruits and vegetables while staying within calorie/energy needs.
- Choose a variety of fruits and vegetables each day.
- Include all five vegetable subgroups (dark green, orange, legumes, starchy vegetables, and others).
- Consume three or more ounce-equivalents of whole-grain products per day.
- The remaining grains should come from enriched or whole-grain products.
- At least half of the grains per day should come from whole grains.
- Consume three cups per day of fat-free or low-fat milk or equivalent milk products.
- Consult and use the Nutrition Facts Label found on food products.

FATS
- Consume less than 10% of calories from saturated fatty acids.
- Keep total fat intake between 20% and 35% of calories, with most fats coming from sources of polyunsaturated and monounsaturated fatty acids, such as fish, nuts, and vegetable oils.
- Minimize daily intake of cholesterol (<300 mg/day) and trans-fatty acids.
- Select meat, poultry, dry beans, milk and milk products that are lean, low fat, or fat free.
- Limit intake of fats and oils that are high in saturated or trans-fatty acids.

CARBOHYDRATES
- Choose fiber-rich fruits, vegetables, and whole grains often.
- Choose and prepare foods and beverages with little added sugars or caloric sweeteners.
- Reduce the incidence of dental caries by practicing good oral hygiene and reducing the consumption of sugar- and starch-containing foods.

SODIUM AND POTASSIUM
- Consume less than 2,300 mg (about 1 teaspoon of table salt) of sodium per day.
- Choose and prepare foods with little salt.
- About 75% of salt consumption in the American diet is derived from salt added by manufacturers.
- Natural salt (sodium) content in food accounts for only about 10% of total intake.
- Consume foods that are rich in potassium, such as fruits and vegetables, including leafy green vegetables, fruit from vines, and root vegetables.

ALCOHOLIC BEVERAGES
- Individuals who drink alcoholic beverages should do so in moderation and sensibly, which is defined as up to one drink per day for women and up to two drinks per day for men.
- Certain individuals should abstain from any alcoholic beverages, including women of childbearing age who may become pregnant, pregnant and lactating women, children and adolescents, individuals taking medications that can interact with alcohol, and those with specific medical conditions.

FOOD SAFETY
- To avoid microbial foodborne illnesses.
- Clean hands, food contact surfaces, and fruits and vegetables.
- Wash or rinse meat and poultry.
- Separate raw, cooked, and ready-to-eat foods while shopping, preparing, or storing foods.
- Cook foods to a safe temperature to kill microorganisms.
- Refrigerate perishable food promptly and defrost foods properly.
- Avoid raw (unpasteurized) milk or any products made from unpasteurized milk, raw or partially cooked eggs or foods containing raw eggs, raw or undercooked meat and poultry, unpasteurized juices, and raw sprouts.

Adapted from http://www.choosemyplate.gov (2020).

---

breastfeed. Infant formulas designed to resemble breast milk provide comparable nutritional benefits, although they lack some of the unique qualities of breast milk. Cow's milk and whey-adjusted formulas are available for full-term infants; formulas made from soy isolates or casein may be given to infants intolerant to routine formulas. A variety of formulas are also available for infants with special needs, such as premature infants and infants with specific metabolic disorders such as phenylketonuria (**PKU**) (see Chapter 72). Because cow's milk is a poor source of iron, may cause intestinal bleeding, and provides unsuitably high levels of protein, phosphorus, and electrolytes, it should not be given until after the age of 1 year. Whole milk should be used between ages 1 and 2 years.

Feeding infants on demand (when they are hungry) is preferable. If an infant is hungry, cries, and is then fed and satisfied, the caregiver creates a sense of trust and prevents frustration. Holding the infant while feeding is important, even if using a bottle. Mealtime should be pleasurable and comforting because infants react to their caregivers' emotions.

Generally, infants are not developmentally ready for solid foods until 6 months of age. Iron-fortified infant rice cereal is recommended as the first solid food because it is unlikely to cause an allergic reaction (it is *hypoallergenic*). Caregivers should introduce plain new foods one at a time for 5–7 days; if the infant is allergic, the caregiver can easily identify the offending food. As the intake of solid food increases, the intake of breast milk or formula should decrease to avoid displacing the intake of other nutrient-rich foods. By 12 months of age, milk intake should total 16–24 oz per day, all by cup. Because of the risk of botulism, infants should not be given honey until after the age of 1 year.

Supplement use for infants is controversial. From birth to the age of 6 months, breastfed infants may be given supplemental fluoride and vitamin D, with iron added after 4 months of age. Formula-fed infants may be given iron if the formula is not fortified and fluoride if the local water supply is not fluoridated. Infants usually do not need supplements during the second 6 months of life if they are fed iron-fortified infant cereal and their diet is adequate in vitamins C and D. High-risk infants may be given a multivitamin or multimineral supplement.

Childhood

Caregivers with healthy eating habits set a good nutritional example for children. Permanent eating habits usually develop during childhood.

> **Key Concept**
> Children should not be forced to eat. Usually, children eat as much as needed.

Appetite fluctuates widely because of erratic growth patterns. Children should be allowed to eat to satisfy hunger. Generally, for young children a serving size equals 1 tablespoon of food per year of age; thus, the serving size for a 2-year-old child is 2 tablespoons. Offering seconds is better than overwhelming the child with too much food. Young children eat an average of five to seven times a day; well-planned snacks can significantly contribute to total nutrient intake.

A child's food preferences may change. Small amounts of new foods can be introduced with familiar favorites. Adults should encourage children to taste new foods but respect their individual likes and dislikes. It is not important if children refuse to eat a particular food (e.g., squash), as long as they have a reasonable intake from each of the major food groups. Small children usually prefer mildly flavored foods and finger foods.

Children should not be required to clean their plates but should stop eating when they are no longer hungry. Nutritious desserts, pudding, fruit, and low-fat yogurt should be part of the meal, not bribes or rewards for eating other foods. To decrease the risk of choking in young children, supervised eating and avoidance of foods that most often cause choking (e.g., hot dogs, candy, nuts, grapes, popcorn, celery, and tough meat) are necessary.

Minimizing distractions and noise promotes enjoyable meals. Family caregivers should eat with children, allowing 20–30 minutes per meal. Food should never be used to reward, punish, bribe, or convey love. Occasional table accidents should be expected. A high chair, infant seat, booster chair, or child's table and chairs next to the adult's table may encourage eating and make children more comfortable. Children should be encouraged to participate in food preparation and clean-up.

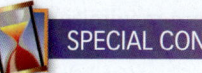

SPECIAL CONSIDERATIONS Lifespan

Children and Fat

Fat is an important energy source for children because they have small stomachs and high-energy needs. Children, especially those younger than 2 years, need fat in their diets for growth and brain development. Children between the ages of 1 and 2 years should consume whole milk. Children older than 2 years should drink low-fat milk. Failure to thrive has been seen in children whose families are overly concerned about avoiding obesity in children and therefore severely restrict fat in the child's diet.

Common nutritional problems during childhood are iron deficiency anemia and obesity. Iron deficiency anemia is often caused by children drinking too much milk, which displaces iron-rich foods. Dietary changes, combined with prescribed supplements, can usually correct anemia. Obesity is harder to treat. Although obese infants do not necessarily grow up to be fat adults, an overweight 5-year-old may be on the road to lifelong weight problems. Childhood obesity has increased dramatically in recent years and has been linked to a sedentary lifestyle, which includes long hours of television viewing and playing computer games. Treatment for childhood obesity is not food restriction but changes in dietary practices (e.g., less junk food and fast food, and smaller servings) and an increase in physical activity.

Adolescence

A period of rapid growth, accompanied by an enormous appetite, characterizes the adolescent years. The teenager needs extra food to meet the needs of growth and body development. Enjoyment, along with peer and social pressures, often influences adolescent food choices more than nutritional and health considerations. Snacking may constitute 30% or more of an adolescent's total calorie intake each day. Unfortunately, snacks are often high in fat, sugar, or sodium. Adolescents must be encouraged to select nutritious snacks. Meal skipping—especially breakfast—is a common nutritional concern, as is the frequent use of fast foods. Eating disorders are described in Chapter 73.

> **Key Concept**
> Caregivers of adolescents need to be alert to disorders such as obesity, anorexia, and bulimia and should seek appropriate assistance for these disorders as soon as possible.

Caregivers should allow adolescents to make choices. Sometimes, the foods they choose are not very harmful. A slice of cold pizza for breakfast is better than no breakfast at all. Generally, nagging is ineffective.

IN PRACTICE
EDUCATING THE CLIENT 30-2 Iron

Iron deficiency is the most common nutritional deficiency in the United States. Groups at risk are infants younger than 2 years, adolescents, menstruating women, older adults, members of underrepresented ethnic groups, and people with low incomes. Preventive measures are maximizing iron intake and iron absorption. Dietary components do not affect the absorption of heme iron (mainly in meat) but greatly affect the absorption of nonheme iron (mainly in plants).

Measures to prevent iron deficiency include the following:
- Choosing iron-fortified cereals over nonfortified varieties.
- Using whole-grain products.
- Cooking in iron pots whenever possible.
- Consuming a rich source of ascorbic acid (vitamin C), such as orange juice or tomatoes at every meal. **Rationale:** *Ascorbic acid enhances absorption of iron.*
- Eating meat with every meal, if possible.
- Avoiding coffee and tea immediately before and after meals (both interfere with iron absorption).
- Avoid taking calcium and iron supplements at the same time. **Rationale:** *Calcium interferes with the absorption of iron.*

Iron deficiency anemia may be a problem for girls after the onset of menses and in boys during their growth spurt. Iron deficiency anemia can lead to fatigue and decreased ability to concentrate and to learn. Although an iron-rich diet can help to prevent iron deficiency, it usually cannot treat iron deficiency anemia after it is established. Iron supplements are then used in conjunction with diet. See In Practice: Educating the Client 30-2 for more information about iron deficiency.

SPECIAL CONSIDERATIONS Lifespan

Considerations for Specific Populations
- Adults older than 50 years may have inadequate intake of vitamin B_{12}; it is suggested that B_{12} be consumed in its crystalline form (i.e., fortified foods or supplements).
- Adults may consume adequate calories but still have deficiencies of calcium, potassium, fiber, magnesium, and vitamins A (as carotenoids), C, and E.
- Children and adolescents may have insufficient intake of calcium, potassium, fiber, magnesium, and vitamin E.
- Women of childbearing age who may become pregnant should eat foods high in heme-iron and/or consume iron-rich plant foods or iron-fortified foods with an enhancer or iron absorption, such as vitamin C-rich foods.
- Women of childbearing age who may become pregnant and those in the first trimester of pregnancy should consume adequate synthetic folic acid daily, which is found in fortified foods or supplements in addition to folate from foods found in a varied diet.
- Older adults, people with dark skin, and people exposed to insufficient ultraviolet band radiation (i.e., sunlight) should consume extra vitamin D from vitamin D–fortified foods or supplements.

Early and Middle Adulthood

During this period, calorie requirements may decrease because the person is no longer growing and is less active. Using the MyPlate guidelines and choosing a wide variety of foods will add interest to menu planning.

> **Key Concept**
> Good nutritional habits should be practiced throughout a lifetime. Education is the cornerstone to good nutrition; good nutrition is the cornerstone to good health.

Beginning in young adulthood, muscle and bone mass decline and the proportion of fat increases, resulting in a decrease in REE. Physical activity may also decline. These two factors result in a decrease in calorie requirements. Being overweight can become a problem during this stage of life. Suggestions for managing weight-related problems and developing an active exercise program can be found in the MyPlate guidelines for specific audiences. The need for most other nutrients, with the exception of iron, stays the same or increases in late adulthood. Thus, nutrient density is important to avoid overeating.

Older Adulthood and Aging

Throughout the life cycle, nutrition significantly affects health and the quality of life. Studies show that a lifetime of good eating habits promotes health maintenance in old age. Poor lifelong eating habits contribute to many degenerative disorders associated with aging, such as diabetes, osteoporosis, hypertension, and atherosclerosis.

As a group, older adults are at risk for nutritional problems because of physiologic, economic, and psychosocial changes. Some nutrient requirements, such as vitamin B_{12}, become greater with age because of a decreased ability to absorb nutrients.

> **Key Concept**
> Older adults should choose a diet low in fat, saturated fat, trans fat, and cholesterol. High-fat diets increase the risk of obesity and its health complications, heart disease, and certain types of cancer.

Many factors can negatively affect the food intake of older adults. Difficulty chewing, which is related to loss of teeth and periodontal disease, places many individuals at risk of poor intake. Changes in taste and smell cause food to be less flavorful and less enjoyable. Social isolation, impaired mobility, and depression are other factors that may influence food intake. Many older adults may have lower incomes; the lower the income, the greater the likelihood the diet will be inadequate. Also, multiple and chronic use of medications can impair intake by altering appetite, the ability to taste, or nutrient digestion, absorption, or utilization.

Constipation is common among older individuals. It is related to decreased abdominal muscle tone, decreased physical activity, and inadequate fluid and fiber intake. Constipation is also a common side effect of many drugs. Wheat bran and fresh fruits and vegetables (if chewing is not impaired) may help alleviate constipation. A decreased thirst sensation makes

CHAPTER 30 Basic Nutrition

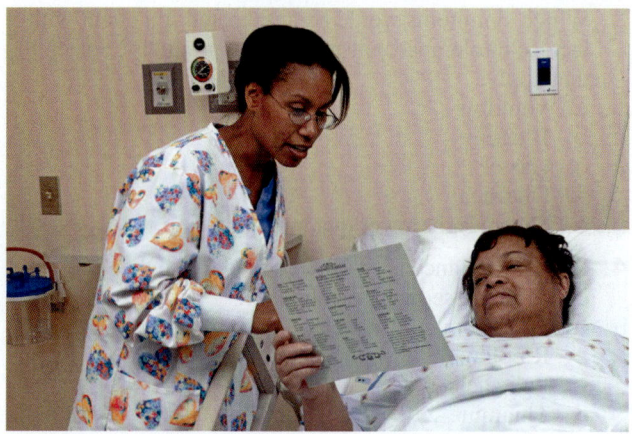

Figure 30-4 The nurse's role is to respect individual choices while also encouraging healthy eating. (Carter, P. & Lewsen, S. [2005]. *Textbook for nursing assistants: A humanistic approach to caregiving.* Lippincott Williams & Wilkins.)

older adults more susceptible to dehydration; they should be encouraged to drink even if they do not feel thirsty. As with younger people, variety, balance, and moderation are the keys to a good diet. Empty-calorie foods should be limited. Small, frequent meals may help maximize intake if appetite is impaired. Assistive devices are available for people whose physical impairments make eating or preparing food difficult.

Depression, common among the older population, can have a negative impact on eating behavior and may lead to malnutrition. Individuals who live alone or in long-term care facilities are at especially high risk. Positive socialization can improve their emotional state and food intake. Congregate dining programs provide a hot, balanced midday meal and the opportunity to socialize at low or no cost. Nurses working in long-term care facilities can have a tremendous impact on the emotional and physical well-being of these vulnerable individuals by providing them with compassionate and quality care (Fig. 30-4).

SPECIAL CONSIDERATIONS Lifespan

Calcium and Osteoporosis

Estrogen-deficient osteoporosis, a disease characterized by a decrease in total bone mass and deterioration of bone tissue, affects women. Although symptoms may not appear until old age, osteoporosis begins to develop much earlier in life. Although an adequate calcium intake is important throughout life, many researchers believe that the biggest impact on preventing osteoporosis is made between 4 and 20 years of age, when calcium retention in girls is at its peak.

Consuming an adequate calcium intake before and after puberty helps maximize peak bone mass, which is the greatest amount of bone mass an individual will ever have. Then, after the age of 35 years when bone loss exceeds bone gain, the body is better equipped to withstand the loss without adverse side effects. Unfortunately, few women consume the current RDA for calcium. Many women feel they do not want to add the extra calories in milk to their diet. Without milk or milk products in the diet, calcium needs are unlikely to be met. Encourage women to drink skim milk, to use skim milk yogurt for dessert, and to use calcium-fortified orange juice and calcium supplements, all excellent sources of calcium that the body absorbs well. Other types of osteoporosis affect men.

Calcium supplements should be considered in people older than 35 years. There are several types of calcium supplements, each with advantages and indications for use.

SPECIAL CONSIDERATIONS Lifespan

Salts and Sugar

Older adults may have a decreased ability to differentiate tastes, especially salts and sugars. Some adults compensate for this loss by increasing their intake of salts and sugar, which can be detrimental to their health. Too much salt can promote hypertension. Too much sugar can lead to dental caries, displacement of nutrient-dense foods, and weight gain.

STUDENT SYNTHESIS

KEY POINTS

- The guidelines of the MyPlate Framework and the Nutrition Facts Label provide the client and healthcare professionals with essential information that can be used to promote and maintain health.
- Essential nutrients (carbohydrates, fat, protein, water, minerals, and vitamins) provide energy, build and repair tissues, and regulate body processes.
- Kilocalories or calories provide the body with needed energy.
- Carbohydrates provide energy, fiber, and sweetness. They spare protein.
- Fats supply energy, essential fatty acids, satiety, and flavor. They carry fat-soluble vitamins, protect organs, and regulate body temperature.
- Proteins repair and build body tissues, contribute to fluid and acid–base balance, form hormones and enzymes, and provide immune functions.
- Fat-soluble vitamins are vitamins A, D, E, and K; water-soluble vitamins are vitamin C and B complex.
- In healthy people, vitamins and minerals should not be supplemented in excess of the DRIs.
- The key concepts in diet planning are variety, balance, and moderation.
- Four of the 10 leading causes of death are related to an overconsumption of nutrients.
- No one food or food group can supply all necessary nutrients.
- Calcium, iron, and protein are important nutrients in the diets of infants, children, adolescents, and pregnant and lactating women.
- Nutritional needs and patterns of intake vary with age.
- The Nutrition Facts Label on packages can be of great assistance when teaching clients how to improve, change, and understand their food intake.

CRITICAL THINKING EXERCISES

1. Demonstrate an understanding of the MyPlate Framework by planning a day's diet for yourself.
2. Consider the nutritional problems of Americans as they relate to leading causes of death. Would you recommend a low-fat diet to someone whose weight and cholesterol levels are normal?
3. Explain why you, as a nurse, should be familiar with nutrition and nutrients for yourself and your clients.
4. Describe the dietary challenges faced by the homeless person. How can this person be assisted?

NCLEX-STYLE REVIEW QUESTIONS

1. When discussing present physical activity, the client tells the nurse "I do casual walking 3 to 5 times per week and light housework." Which description fits the activity level of this client?
    a. Sedentary lifestyle
    b. Light intensity
    c. Moderate physical activity
    d. Vigorous physical activity
2. Which breakfast has the least amount of carbohydrates?
    a. Bacon and eggs
    b. A banana and toast with butter
    c. Waffles and an orange
    d. Oatmeal and blueberries
3. Which symptoms would be anticipated if a client with lactose intolerance consumes dairy products? Select all that apply.
    a. Vomiting
    b. Bloating
    c. Gas
    d. Diarrhea
    e. Severe right lower quadrant pain
4. Which substance is typically added to the diet of a client diagnosed with alcoholism?
    a. Potassium
    b. Riboflavin
    c. Folic acid
    d. Thiamine
5. Which symptoms may the nurse observe in a client who has a low-protein intake?
    a. Nosebleeds
    b. Diminished peripheral pulses
    c. Dry, scaly skin
    d. Edema in the lower extremities

CHAPTER RESOURCES

Enhance your learning with additional resources on thePoint!

Student Resources related to this chapter can be found at thePoint.lww.com/Rosdahl12e.

31 Transcultural and Social Aspects of Nutrition

Learning Objectives

1. Explain the common influences of geographical regions on food choices.
2. Identify common dietary practices of selected ethnic groups.
3. Define and discuss acculturation as it relates to nutrition for people from diverse and similar ethnic groups.
4. Identify dietary practices commonly associated with each of the following religions: Islam, Judaism, Mormonism, and Roman Catholicism.
5. Name the general types of vegetarian diets and identify what types of foods are typically eaten within each type of diet.
6. Relate the following factors to food choice: financial status, emotional state, social and physical factors, and ethnic heritage.

Important Terminology

acculturation   halal   kosher   vegan   vegetarian

There are many factors, including cultural background, ethnic heritage, and religious beliefs, that may, to a certain degree, influence food preparation and eating patterns. Because eating supplies food for the soul as well as the body, the science of nutrition is also an art. Although many Americans believe what they eat affects their health, nutritional considerations have a lesser impact on most people's food choices than do personal food preferences and aversions, which may be influenced by many different factors, including region, ethnic heritage, religious beliefs, and other sociocultural factors. Ignoring the significance of these factors in a client's food choices can undermine diet planning and nutritional counseling. This chapter explores how these factors may influence a client's food choices and the type of nutritional care the nurse may need to consider. Cultural, ethnic, and religious practices in general are discussed in Chapter 8.

Remember that each client is unique. Just because a client may be a member of a certain ethnic group or practice a particular religion does not automatically mean they adhere to each of the items discussed in this chapter. This chapter is meant as an introduction to common dietary variations based on a variety of factors to help broaden your awareness of nutritional variations and to help guide conversations you may have with clients. You should *never* make assumptions about a client's dietary preferences based solely on commonly occurring trends. The best way to help clients meet their nutritional needs is by having discussions with them.

There are an infinite variety and combination of foods. Many types of "diets" and foods can promote good health. Realizing the emotional value that some foods have for an individual is extremely important. For example, Figure 31-1 shows families celebrating special events with food.

REGIONAL PREFERENCES

Various regions of the United States developed unique eating patterns, based initially on the availability of certain foods and on the concentration of people of a similar ethnic background in the region. Many of these customs have carried through to the present day, despite the global marketplace and its ability to provide foods in places where they are not naturally available. However, the influence of fast-food and other types of restaurant chains have led to regional dietary customs becoming much less defined. Furthermore, grocery stores in many states offer ethnic foods that may be purchased by a variety of cultural groups. In Practice: Educating the Client 31-1 provides the student with many teaching concepts that are useful for clients living in our multicultural environment.

> **Key Concept**
> The nurse cannot change the dietary beliefs of clients. However, you can help clients to adjust their diet within their belief structures.

ETHNIC HERITAGE

Culture affects the way a person thinks, feels, and behaves. It also influences eating habits. Food preferences may become particularly important during illness. When illness necessitates dietary changes, healthcare professionals should attempt to integrate the person's ethnic and religious food preferences when possible. Understanding these preferences will enable you to assist clients in reaching optimum nutritional health. Some clients may refuse to eat hospital food. A dietary consultation and permission for the family to bring food from home can be helpful.

When people first immigrate to North America, they usually continue to eat their native foods as long as they can buy or grow the ingredients. Eventually, they may adopt Western food habits. The second generation, especially, may adapt to local foods and habits; they may observe traditional customs only on special occasions and holidays. With food changes, many people develop "Western" diseases. Box 31-1 lists how ethnic diets may affect health and illness.

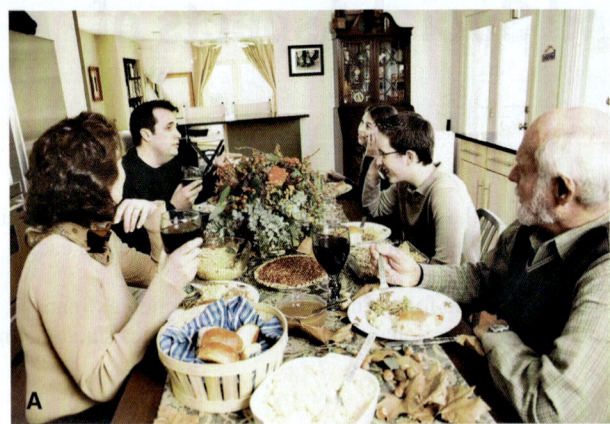
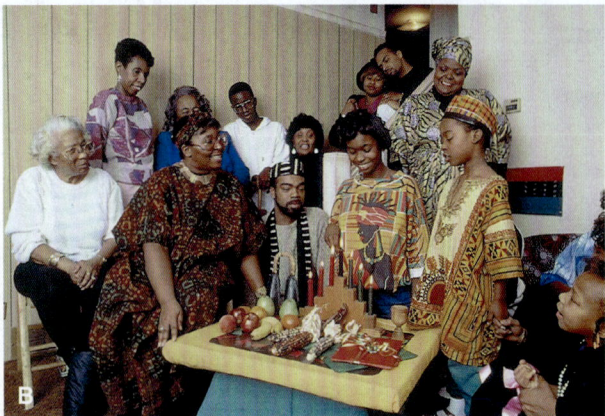
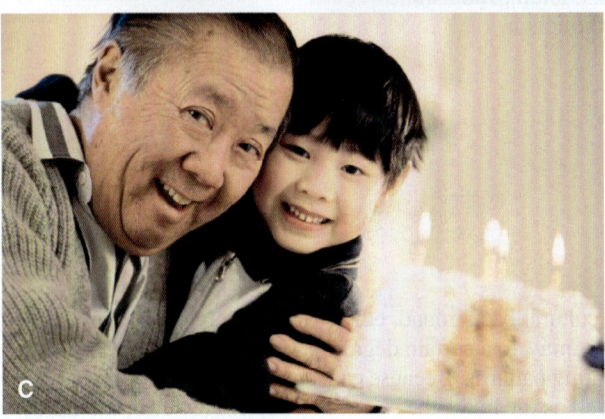

Figure 31-1 **A.** Many cultures celebrate social, cultural, and religious events by sharing food. **B.** Ceremonies can be elaborate or simple. **C.** Group gatherings with many generations attending allow individuals to share and to pass on their belief systems to others in the family or social unit. Often, special foods are prepared and play a central role at these events. (Carter, P., & Lewsen, S. [2005]. *Textbook for nursing assistants: A humanistic approach to caregiving.* Lippincott Williams & Wilkins.)

IN PRACTICE
EDUCATING THE CLIENT 31-1 — Guidelines for Healthier Eating Across all Cultures

Calorie Intake
Consume foods and drinks to meet, not exceed, total daily calorie needs.
- Plan ahead to make better food choices.
- Pay attention to feelings of hunger. Eat only until you are satisfied, not full.
- Limit calorie intake from solid fats and added sugars.
- Reduce portions, especially of high-calorie foods.
- Monitor the use of sauces that can add extra calories.
- Know your calorie needs. Weigh yourself and adjust what and how much you eat and/or your physical activity based on your weight change over time.
- Use smaller plates. Portion out small amounts of food.
- When preparing meals, include vegetables, fruits, whole grains, fat-free or low-fat dairy products, and protein foods that provide fewer calories and more nutrients.
- When eating out, choose a vegetable as a side dish.
- Request that cooked vegetables be prepared with little or no fat and salt.
- Keep salad dressing on the side to monitor portion size.
- When adding sauces, condiments, or dressings to vegetables, use small amounts and look for lower calorie options (reduced-fat cheese sauce or fat-free dressing).
- Experiment with healthy recipes and ingredient substitutions.
- Cut back on foods and drinks with added sugars or caloric sweeteners (sugar-sweetened beverages).
- Consider fruit in place of high-calorie desserts.
- Drink few or no regular sodas, sports drinks, or energy drinks.
- Prepare and pack healthy meals at home for children and/or adults to eat at school or work.
- Have healthy snacks available at home and bring nutrient-dense snacks to eat when on the go.
- Cook and eat more meals at home, instead of eating out, preferably as a family.
- Think about choosing healthy options when eating out.
- Think ahead before attending parties: Eat a small, healthy snack before heading out. Plan to take small portions and focus on healthy options. Consider whether you are hungry before going back for more. Choose a place to talk with friends that is some distance from the food table.

EDUCATING THE CLIENT 31-1 Guidelines for Healthier Eating Across all Cultures (Continued)

- If you tend to overeat, be aware of time of day, place, and your mood while eating so you can better control the amount you eat.
- Limit eating while watching television (or other "screen" times), which can result in overeating.
- If eating while watching television, portion out a small serving.
- Use the ingredients list on Nutrition Facts Label (Fig. 30-3) to choose foods with little or no added sugars (breakfast cereals and other packaged foods).
- Track what you eat using a food journal or an online food planner. Sites on www.ChooseMyPlate.gov can be helpful and educational.
- Identify the amount of calories from added sugars and solid fats contained in foods and drinks.

Vegetables
Increase vegetable intake.
- Eat recommended amounts of vegetables and include a variety of vegetables, especially dark-green vegetables, red and orange vegetables, beans, and peas.
- Include fresh, frozen, or canned vegetables in meals and in snacks.
- Add dark-green, red, and orange vegetables to soups, stews, casseroles, stir-fries, and other main and side dishes.
- Use dark leafy greens (kale and spinach) to make salads.
- Focus on dietary fiber (kidney, pinto, or garbanzo beans; split peas; lentils).
- Add beans or peas to salads, soups, and side dishes.
- Keep raw, cut-up vegetables handy for quick snacks.
- Choose lower calorie options for dips (yogurt-based dressings or hummus) instead of sour cream or cream cheese–based dips.

Fruits
Increase fruit intake.
- Eat recommended amounts of fruits and choose a variety of fruits.
- Choose whole or cut-up fruits more often than fruit juice.
- Use fruit as snacks, salads, or desserts.
- Use fruit to top foods (cereals or pancakes) instead of sugars, syrups, or other sweet toppings.
- Enjoy a wide variety of fruits, and maximize taste and freshness by adapting your choices to what is in season.
- Keep rinsed and cut-up fruit handy for quick snacks.
- Use canned, frozen, and dried fruits, as well as fresh fruits.
- Use unsweetened fruit or fruit canned in 100% juice as a lower calorie option.

Milk and Milk Products (Dairy Products)
Note: Approximately 65% of the world's adult population has some degree of lactose intolerance.

Drink fat-free (skim) or low-fat (1%) milk products (milk, yogurt, cheese).
- Switch gradually from whole milk to lower fat versions.
- Use fat-free or low-fat milk on cereal, oatmeal, or fruit salads.
- Substitute plain, fat-free, or low-fat yogurt for dips calling for sour cream.
- Use low-fat or reduced-fat cheese options.

Protein Foods
Choose a variety of foods from the protein foods group.
- Increase the variety of protein foods consumed by choosing fish, beans, nuts, and soy products in place of some meat and poultry.

Grains

Whole Grains
Increase whole-grain intake. Consume at least half of all grains as whole grains.
- Substitute refined grains with whole-grain choices (100% whole-grain breads; cereals, oatmeal, crackers, and pasta; brown rice).
- Check the ingredients list on product labels for the words "whole" or "whole grain" before the grain ingredient's name.
- Avoid foods labeled with the words "multi-grain," "stone-ground," "100% wheat," "cracked wheat," "seven-grain," or "bran," which may not contain any whole grains.
- Use the Nutrition Facts Label and the ingredients list to choose whole grains that are a good source of dietary fiber.

Refined Grains
Whenever possible, replace refined grains with whole grains.
- Avoid refined grain products (cakes, cookies, other desserts, and pizza).
- Replace white bread, rolls, bagels, muffins, pasta, and rice with whole-grain versions.

Oils and Solid Fats
Use oils instead of solid fats, when possible.
- Eat fewer foods that contain solid fats, such as cakes, cookies, pizza, cheese, processed meats (sausages, hot dogs, bacon, or ribs), and ice cream.
- Select lean meats and poultry and fat-free or low-fat milk and milk products.
- Limit saturated fat intake and partially hydrogenated oils and keep trans fat intake as low as possible.
- Replace solid fats (butter, beef fat, chicken fat, lard, stick margarine, or shortening) with nonsolid fats (liquid vegetable oil or soft spread margarines).
- Choose baked, steamed, or broiled rather than fried foods most often.
- Try grilling, broiling, poaching, or roasting.

EDUCATING THE CLIENT 31-1: Guidelines for Healthier Eating Across all Cultures (Continued)

- Use vegetable oils (olive, canola, corn, safflower, or sunflower oil) for cooking.
- Eat seafood in place of meat or poultry twice a week.
- Select from seafood that is higher in oils and lower in mercury (salmon, trout, and herring).
- Select lean meats and poultry.
- Trim or drain fat from meat and remove poultry skin before cooking or eating.
- Use the ingredients list to choose foods that contain oils with more unsaturated fats.
- Use the Nutrition Facts label to choose foods that contain less or no saturated fat and no trans fat.

Sodium
Reduce sodium intake.
- Reduce gradually the amount of high sodium foods.
- Trade in the salt shaker for the pepper shaker.
- Use spices, herbs, and lemon juice as alternatives to salt to season foods.
- Choose foods low in sodium and prepare foods with little salt.
- Increase potassium intake (potatoes, cantaloupe, bananas, beans, and yogurt).
- Select canned foods labeled as "reduced sodium," "low sodium," or "no salt added."
- Use the Nutrition Facts label to choose foods lower in sodium.

Alcohol
For adults of legal drinking age who choose to drink alcohol, consume it in moderation.

- Avoid alcohol if you are pregnant or may become pregnant; if under the legal drinking age; or if you are on medication that can interact with alcohol.
- Avoid alcohol if you have medical conditions that could be worsened by drinking and if planning to drive or operate machinery that could put you or others at risk.

Physical Activity
Limit screen time (television, computer games).
- Increase physical activity.
- Choose moderate- or vigorous-intensity physical activities.
- Avoid inactivity. Some physical activity is better than none.
- Slowly build up the amount of physical activity you choose.

Food Safety
- Warnings about food safety in restaurants need to be posted in the language(s) spoken/read by the workers employed.
- Wash hands, utensils, and cutting boards before and after contact with raw meat, poultry, seafood, and eggs.
- Keep raw meat and poultry apart from foods that will not be cooked.
- Use a food thermometer; the appearance of food is not an indicator of food safety.
- Chill leftovers and takeout foods within 2 hours and keep the refrigerator at 40 °F or below.

Adapted from U.S. Department of Agriculture. (2015). *2015-2020 Dietary guidelines for Americans* (8th ed.). https://health.gov/our-work/food-nutrition/2015-2020-dietary-guidelines/guidelines/

Box 31-1: Various Dietary Practices and General Relationships to Health and Illness

- People of all ethnic groups tend to have a source of starch or carbohydrate (e.g., pasta, potatoes, bread, rice).
- Low intake of milk and dairy products may predispose individuals to bone disorders, such as rickets or osteoporosis.
- Individuals with lactose intolerance must meet their calcium needs through other foods, such as soy or almond milk fortified with calcium.
- High sodium (salt) intake is often a factor in hypertension and cardiac disease.
- High caloric intake often causes people to be overweight. Obesity is a status symbol in some cultures.
- Intake of high amounts of fried foods and fats may predispose people to atherosclerosis, gallbladder disease, and obesity.
- Long cooking of vegetables causes a loss of water-soluble vitamins.
- High sugar intake may predispose individuals to dental caries or diabetes. A high sugar intake can increase the risk of nutrient deficiencies if empty-calorie foods (e.g., soft drinks) take the place of nutritious foods (e.g., skim milk). High intake of empty calories also increases the risk of obesity.
- Many people find comfort in traditional ethnic foods when ill, even if they do not follow these traditions when well.
- The family or client may insist on following religious or cultural practices during illness.
- Some Asian and Latino cultural groups ascribe certain foods as "hot" or "cold," according to properties unrelated to temperature. Individuals within these groups may eat specific foods to combat certain illnesses that are "hot" or "cold."
- Some cultural groups believe that specific foods cause illness. They believe other foods may cure or prevent illness.
- Food provided in a healthcare facility may be unacceptable to some people because it violates a cultural or religious practice. In some cases, the ill person is exempt from following religious food practices during illness.

> **NCLEX Alert**
>
> NCLEX clinical scenarios may include or describe religious or ethnic-related situations. The correct option may relate to how the client's health or illness is interrelated with food choices. For example, diabetes mellitus, hypertension, and cardiovascular or renal diseases can be greatly affected by cultural dietary choices (e.g., salt intake). Options for teaching the client how to change food habits may also be part of the NCLEX's options (In Practice: Educating the Client 31-1).

Acculturation is the process that occurs as individuals adopt the beliefs, values, attitudes, and behaviors of the dominant culture. Because of acculturation, dietary practices are changing rapidly among younger people. Acculturation is common in the United States and Canada, especially when buying food products. The main food groups and examples of these groups are found in Table 30-1. Often individuals are more influenced by the region in which they live and the availability of food products in that region than by their own specific ethnic or cultural background.

CULTURAL GROUPS

The following sections identify and describe cultural groups with significant representation in the United States. In this discussion related to ethnic heritage, generalizations are made based on commonly occurring habits. As previously stated, it is important to remember that each client is a unique individual. Not all members of a group observe these particular practices. Habits of some members of each particular group are described, and much blending of cultures and foods occurs. A balanced approach toward nutrition should be taught based on the diet identified by the client. These concepts should be considered and applied within the context of clients' cultural beliefs. They could help clients from various ethnic backgrounds with chronic illnesses, such as diabetes, assess and understand their own food usage.

> **SPECIAL CONSIDERATIONS** **Culture and Ethnicity**
>
> Global cultural and ethnic migrations are continuously in process. Keep in mind that one individual's beliefs and diets may mimic or be highly different from a traditional cultural or ethnic background. Always be sure to understand each specific client's needs rather than making assumptions based on generalizations.

People of European Origin

Anglo-European American, Anglo-Saxon, and White American are ethnic groups with European ancestors. Their diets many tend to show influences from British, French, Greek, Spanish, Italian, German, and Russian cultures, and so forth. Anglo-American foods are more typically categorized by specific familial lineage and cooking preferences. The expression of *westernizing* foods has become a global phenomenon of consuming excess amounts of simple sugars, fried foods, and calories (e.g., super-sized amounts). Obesity, hypertension, and diabetes are serious complications of unguarded dietary intake.

People of African Origin

People with African ancestry comprise many different cultural groups. Their food habits may be based on West Indian/Caribbean, African, or regional American influences.

Food preparation techniques used by individuals who are members of this group may emphasize common practices in the Southeastern United States, which include frying or barbecuing foods. Foods historically included in this diet are collards, kale, cress, mustard, black-eyed peas, and pokeweed. Recipes may include the use of lard, cornmeal, and offal. Cooking methods may call for the addition of onions, garlic, thyme, and bay leaf as flavor enhancers. This diet may be high in fat (fatty meats, fried foods), sodium (salted meats), and sugar and inadequate in calcium, vitamin D, and potassium.

Hypertension, heart disease, and obesity are common health problems for individuals consuming this diet. Alterations in diet, specifically reducing the high intake of sodium, fat, and sugar, may help prevent or minimize the effects of these chronic diseases. Careful increases of potassium intake in lieu of salt (sodium) intake have been shown to be beneficial for sodium-sensitive individuals. Lactose intolerance occurs in approximately 65% of the world's adult populations. Calcium and vitamin D intake may be inadequate in clients when milk products are avoided.

People of Latino or Hispanic Origin

Latino heritage represents the fastest-growing segment of the U.S. population. Latino Americans are a varied group, speaking over 20 different dialects of Spanish and other languages. Their food habits may vary as well. This population may include individuals who descend from Mexico, Central and South America, the Caribbean, Cuba, and Puerto Rico.

Throughout Latin America, foods may be viewed as being either "hot" or "cold," although neither term refers to a food's actual temperature. This is tied to the belief that a balance of hot and cold is needed to maintain health. Although this theory may affect food choices during illness, there are not rigid guidelines that classify foods or illnesses as hot or cold.

Mexico

Mexican Americans may use many varieties of beans, steamed rice, corn products such as tortillas, chili peppers, stewed tomatoes and tomato puree, potatoes, meat and sausages, fish, and poultry. Tortillas made from corn and treated with limewater are an important source of calcium and therefore are more nutritious than flour tortillas (which are becoming more common). Meats may be marinated or heavily spiced and may often chopped or ground. Chorizo, a Mexican sausage, is a popular food choice. Fried Mexican foods are common. Adults may use limited amounts of milk and milk products, except in popular sweet baked desserts. Mexican Americans may also enjoy eggs, milk custards and bread puddings, sweet chocolate and café con leche (coffee with milk), carbonated drinks, cakes, and pastries. They often consume beer with meals. Incidences of obesity and diabetes may be high.

Foods traditionally considered to be hot or cold should be balanced. Vegetables may be cooked to the point that they lose most of their nutritional value. The diet tends to be high in fiber and starch, and lard may frequently be added to food preparation. Because intake of milk, green leafy vegetables, and fruit may be low, this diet may be inadequate in calcium, iron, vitamin A, and vitamin C. Intake of fruits and vegetables may not match the Dietary Guidelines for Americans 2015–2020 and the nutritional information found at the ChooseMyPlate.gov Website. The main meal is usually served at lunchtime.

Caribbean

The term *Caribbean* primarily is related to the general geographical location and political history of islands south of Florida and east or north of Central and South America, also known as the West Indies. Many governments and ethnicities are found in this area, including those of Cuba, Puerto Rico, and the island of Hispaniola, which is divided into two countries: Haiti and the Dominican Republic. Caribbean ethnic background, history, languages, and cuisine can be traced to a multiplicity of cultural influences. Ethnic foods of this varied area consist of a fusion of dishes including those of Spanish, Native Americans, British, French, Dutch, Indian, and Chinese cultures.

Eating patterns reflect those of the country from which a person originated. Those who have emigrated from the Caribbean may rely on rice and bean combinations and may consume cooked starchy tubers, such as cassava, yams, and plantains, and tropical fruits such as mango and papaya. Nutritional and health-related concerns should, as with any client, be individualized based on the client's state preferences.

Cuba

Cuban Americans may reflect a predominantly Spanish influence in their cooking styles. This diet may incorporate rice and beans extensively as well as serve meat. Stews and casseroles may often be flavored with sage, parsley, bay leaf, thyme, cinnamon, curry, capers, onion, cloves, garlic, and saffron; soup may be served daily. Other common foods may include fried foods, especially fish, poultry, and eggs; rice; and many varieties of beans. Adults may use limited amounts of milk; therefore, calcium levels may be deficient. Food is not as highly spiced as in some other Hispanic cultures. Fried foods are popular. Traditionally, the main meal is served at noon.

> **Key Concept**
>
> Healthcare providers, including doctors and pharmacists, in many countries have and continue to use herbs and other plants for treatment of disease and other ailments. Nurses and medical providers should recognize that such remedies may be used as part of family traditions or as holistic-type treatments.

> **Nursing Alert** The use of home-based or herbal remedies by any culture can delay the search for specifically needed medical attention. Holistic herbs, hot–cold remedies, or over-the-counter treatments may be contraindicated with Western-style pharmaceuticals. For example, dark green leafy vegetables, such as collards or kale, are contraindicated with products such as aspirin (salicylates) or ibuprofen, and they can interfere with the effectiveness of blood-thinning medications such as warfarin (Coumadin).

Puerto Rico

Puerto Rico is also considered part of the geopolitical area of the Caribbean. Steamed white rice and many bean varieties may be served; eggs (omelets) may frequently be a main dish; other foods may include wheat breads; starchy fruits and vegetables, such as cassavas, yams, breadfruit, plantains, and green bananas; green peppers; tomatoes; garlic; dried, salted fish; salt pork; bacon; lard; olive oil; sugar; jams and jellies; sweet pastries; sugared fruit juices; and café con leche (coffee and hot milk).

There may be limited use of meats; most food may be cooked for long periods or fried. Some individuals belonging to this group may view malt beer as nutritious and, as such, may advocate it be given to children and people who are breastfeeding. This diet provides almost all essential nutrients but may be low in calcium.

The traditional Puerto Rican diet may be important, especially during illness. Traditionally, breakfast and lunch may be light, with dinner served later in the evening. Hospitalized clients may require adaptation of meal schedules. Soup made from homegrown chicken may be seen as a healing food. For some clients, foods considered "hot" in the stomach cannot be eaten during certain illnesses. "Hot" refers to believed reactions in the stomach rather than the temperature of food. Some women may not consume certain foods considered "sour" during menses, pregnancy, or immediately after childbirth.

People of East and Southeast Asian Origin

Asian American individuals represent a diverse group of more than 30 cultures. Rice tends to be a staple food for many Asian and Pacific Island cultures. For some individuals, rice may symbolize life and fertility. Asian foods found in the Philippines, Japan, Korea, and the Southeast Asian peninsula are commonly influenced by Chinese origins. Lactose intolerance is common in many Asian individuals. Limiting sodium can be difficult because of an extensive use of soy sauce and other high sodium seasonings.

The diet commonly consumed by Asian Americans has changed from one featuring low-fat, high-fiber foods to one characterized by higher fat animal protein, low fiber, and high levels of saturated fat. Studies have found that second-generation Asian individuals who have adapted American and Western food and lifestyle have health issues similar to those of European Americans. Cardiac diseases, hypertension, diabetes, cancer, and obesity risk are higher compared with those of first-generation immigrants.

China

Eating habits and cooking techniques of Chinese individuals may vary by geographic region. Some Chinese individuals may believe in the theory of yin–yang. Yin conditions are treated with Yang foods, and vice versa, to achieve a balance between positive and negative energy (Chapter 8). Yin foods are typically raw, soothing, cooked at low temperatures, and white or light green in color. Yang foods are high in calories, cooked in high heat, spicy, and red-orange-yellow in color.

This diet may tend to be low in fat and high in starch. Chinese Americans may use meats more as a condiment than as an entrée; therefore, quantities are small. Dinner may not have a main course. Stir-frying and steaming are common cooking methods; ovens may be rarely used.

Rice, rice gruel, and wheat noodles may be dietary staples. The diet may tend to be high in fiber and many nutrients. It may be low in fat and protein but high in sodium. Common ingredients include corn; green vegetables, especially from the cabbage family; squashes; cucumbers; eggplant; leafy vegetables; various shoots, including bamboo, mung, and soy; sweet potatoes; radishes; onions; peas and pods; mushrooms; roots; many local, seasonal vegetables; pickled vegetables; sea vegetables; plums; peaches; tangerines; kumquats and other citrus fruits; litchis; longans; mangoes; papayas; pomegranates; soybean products, such as tofu (soybean curd), soy sauces, bean noodles, and soy milk; small portions of pork, chicken, duck, and lamb; and sugar as seasoning. Obesity tends to be rare among individuals consuming this diet. Regional differences in food choices exist.

Chinese Americans may observe the yin–yang balance, especially during illness. For instance, ginger is used in cooking as well as a remedy to treat cold or any cold/yin illness, such as arthritis. Many Chinese dishes may add herbs for treatment, healing, or prevention of diseases and illness. Because of commonly used herbs and ingredients in Chinese dishes, it is important for the nurse to consider drug interactions. Although Chinese foods may contain high starch and sodium contents, hypertension might not be a common health issue; instead, health threats may be more tied to lifestyle instead of diet. Lifestyle-related health threats may include liver problems, hepatitis, and lung cancer.

Japan

Japanese American individuals may carefully prepare food and enjoy it for its simplicity, purity, and beauty. The arrangement of food, color contrast, and shape may be important elements of meals, which are light and use little animal fat. A good protein and calcium source is tofu (soybean curd).

Japanese American individuals may use many vegetables (including seaweed, bamboo shoots, and bean sprouts). Commonly, meals in this diet may contain fish, soup, fresh or pickled vegetables, and tea.

Common ingredients in this diet include rice; vegetables; pickled vegetables; soy as miso (soup), tofu, bean paste, and soy sauce; fruits; salads; fish with bones; sugar as seasoning; sea vegetables; seafood; ginseng; green tea; and fruit for dessert. Common preparation methods include broiling, steaming, boiling, and stir-frying. Meat portions may be small. Milk may be rarely used by adults. Raw fish (sashimi) and sushi may be a common meal.

As with the Chinese diet, a Japanese diet may be very health conscious in food preparation and dietary selection. Those consuming a Japanese diet may also advocate for natural food cures.

Korea

The Korean American diet may be similar in some respects to Japanese and Chinese diets. Rice, often mixed with other grains or red beans, may be served at most meals. Food tends to be well seasoned, and all three meals may be relatively the same size. Seafood may account for a large portion of this diet's animal protein, and it may be eaten raw, steamed, or salted and dried. Beef may be a common food choice as well. Kimchi, a spicy fermented cabbage, may also be commonly served as a side dish to many meals. Korean foods may include bean curd and soy milk. Garlic is a very common ingredient in many Korean dishes. Korean individuals may also use garlic as a natural food cure. Ginseng may also be used for healing and maintaining health. Sodium levels in the diet can lead to health risk factors, such as hypertension.

Philippines

Filipino foods have been influenced by Indian, Chinese, Arabian, Spanish, Mexican, and American foods. The traditional foods are rice, pork, fish, chicken adobo, pancit, panakbet (mixed vegetables), and lumpia (similar to Chinese egg roll). Adobo is the preparation of certain meats, such as pork or chicken, marinated in vinegar, garlic, soy sauce, bay leaf, and ground pepper. Rice may be consumed daily because it is believed to provide energy. Bagoong (fermented fish) and patis (fish extract) may be used daily as spices in food. Pancit (similar to Chinese chow fan) is rice pasta cooked with chicken, shrimp, or pork in soy sauce and garlic. Garlic and onions are commonly used because it is believed that they thin the blood and lower blood pressure. The Filipino diet is traditionally considered nutritionally complete because their basic staples are vegetables, fruits, and fish. Similar to other Asian diets, a high sodium content is the major risk factor of hypertension.

In Filipino culture, food may be used as gifts and to express appreciation, love, and gratitude. Guests may be offered merienda (snacks) when they arrive. These snacks often consist of high carbohydrate and/or sweet foods served with beverages high in sugar. Filipino cooking may use garlic, ginger, fish, and onions. Similar to other Asian cultures, individuals may adhere to the "hot-and-cold" food principle.

Southeast Asia

Rice (in large quantities) may be eaten at every meal, including rice noodles, rice sticks, and rice papers. Fish, soybean products, a wide variety of fruits and vegetables, and soft drinks and sweets may also be consumed regularly. Milk may be rarely used after childhood.

Cooking styles differ among regions in Cambodia, Vietnam, and Laos due to the variety of cultures influencing each area. The influence of India on Cambodian cooking is evidenced by the abundance of dishes with curry. Chinese and French culinary influences may be seen in Vietnam. Individuals may tend not to adhere to formal mealtimes; family members may serve themselves over a 1–3 hours period. The most important meal may be at midday.

Cambodian Americans may use plates, forks, and spoons but may consider knives at the table to be barbaric. Raw vegetable salads may be common, as are pungent sauces with meats and fish. Traditionally, Cambodian individuals may rarely snack between meals. Hot water may be a beverage of choice.

The diet of Vietnamese Americans may consist of poultry and cheaper cuts of pork, with beef used on rare occasions. Fermented fish (high in sodium) may often be used to make sauce that is added to most cooked dishes. Rice may be served separately, not mixed with other foods. Tea may be a common beverage. Stir-frying is common, and food may be quite spicy.

Laotian cooking may be similar to Cambodian, except food may be more highly spiced, often with lemon grass and curries of pepper and coriander. The eating utensils are the same as those used by Cambodian individuals; however, eating with the fingers may also be common. Meals may rely on fresh ingredients or on long cooking times. Bananas and other fruits are commonly eaten. Coffee and tea are the beverages of choice.

People of South Asian Origin

India

Individuals from India comprise a diverse community. Individuals belonging to this group may be influenced by the region of origin within India and the form of religion practiced. The followers of these different religions may observe different dietary laws and codes for fasting and feasting that influence their eating patterns. Hinduism is the predominant religion, followed by Islam, Buddhism, Jainism, Sikhism, Zoroastrianism, Christianity, and Judaism. Therefore, hospital food can present a problem for individuals, particularly those who strictly observe religious dietary restrictions. Hospital meals may be viewed as too bland for some Indian individuals.

Rice remains a dietary staple for Hindu individuals from Southern India and wheat for those from Northern India. A large majority of older Hindu individuals may be vegetarians or vegans, while some Hindu individuals may be lacto or lacto-ovo vegetarians. Chicken, mutton (lamb), and fish are consumed by Hindu individuals who are not vegetarians. Traditionally, those who are Hindu rarely eat beef. However, traditionally, those who are Muslim do not eat pork. Because gelatin is manufactured by processing the collagen in cow or pig bones, hooves, and connective tissues, traditional Indian individuals (especially those who are Hindu) may refrain from eating gelatin-based products like Jell-O, certain yogurts that are stabilized using gelatin, and marshmallows. Similar to **kosher** dietary laws, **halal** denotes foods that are religiously acceptable according to Islam. Those who are Muslim may consume halal yogurt and other halal meats. Fasting frequently is a common practice among older women and vegetarians. Healthcare providers should inquire about these practices and help clients practice their religious customs while working with them to mitigate adverse effects on their health.

The Indian diet may result in protein deficiency, iron deficiency, and vitamin A deficiency. Health issues facing the Indian immigrant population may include diabetes, hypertension, cardiovascular disease, cancer, osteoporosis for women, respiratory infections, intestinal infections, anemia, protein–energy malnutrition, and the associated complications from these conditions.

People of Middle Eastern Origin

As with other cultural groups, Middle Eastern origin includes traditions from several countries, including Iran, Iraq, Egypt, Lebanon, and Israel. Traditions for each Middle Eastern cultural group vary, but food staples tend to be similar. Some Middle Eastern cultural groups take a mouthful of food along with a bite of bread. Vegetables and legumes often may be an entrée; all forms of pork are customarily forbidden. Women may traditionally eat only after men and children are fed.

Common ingredients and dishes include lamb and goat, bread, rice, beans, lentils, yogurt, feta cheese, olives, tomatoes, and olive oil. Calcium and protein intake may be inadequate among individuals consuming this diet. Meals also may commonly include a large quantity of fat.

People of Native American Origin

Dietary practices vary among the nearly 600 Native American tribes in the United States, depending on their geographic location and the availability of food. Several chronic disorders are common, including obesity and diabetes. Many Native American individuals are lactose intolerant, and, as such, their diets may be calcium-deficient. Deficiencies of riboflavin and vitamins A and C are also common. Native American individuals may use many spices, including green chili (which contains vitamin C). Effects of vitamin and mineral deficiencies are discussed in Chapter 30.

Traditional ingredients and dishes vary by geography:

- *Southeast:* corn and cornmeal, coontie (flour from a palmlike plant), fried breads, pumpkins, squashes, papayas, alligator, snake, wild hog, duck, fish, and shellfish.
- *Northeast:* blueberries, cranberries, beans, corn, pumpkins, fish, lobster, wild game, and maple syrup.
- *Midwest:* bison, beans, corn, melons, squash, and tomatoes.
- *Southwest:* corn (many colors and varieties), beans, squash, pumpkins, chili peppers, melons, pine nuts, and cactus.
- *Northeast and Alaska:* salmon, caviar, other fish, otter, seal, whale, bear, elk, other game, wild fruits, acorns (and other wild nuts), and wild greens.

Food may have great religious and social significance. Corn may be seen as a status food for individuals from some tribes. Milk may be seldom used, so calcium intake may be low. As with all clients, a thorough understanding of a client's specific diet is important, as diets among some groups may be considered poor. High rates of obesity may also be seen.

RELIGIOUS BELIEFS AND PRACTICES

Many people eat specific foods in certain combinations or refrain from eating certain foods because of their religious beliefs. Cultural and religious practices are often intertwined. Box 31-2 identifies some major religious customs relating to diet. Particularly when ill, individuals are often unwilling to deviate from their religious dietary customs. The nurse will need to know this information when caring for clients. Foods that must be prepared using special equipment or under certain conditions can usually be ordered in advance or prepared by the client's family. Some clients may refuse to eat hospital food. A dietary consultation and permission for the family to bring all food from home can be helpful. As shown in Figure 31-1, special foods are often prepared when celebrating specific events.

VEGETARIAN DIETS

Many types of **vegetarian** diets exist, all of which have the common characteristic of being based mainly on plant foods. People choose a vegetarian diet for a variety of reasons: religious, ethnic, ecological, economic, philosophical, or ethical. Potential health benefits are another consideration. Four main types of vegetarian diets exist:

- **Vegans** are strict vegetarians and exclude all animal products (meat, fish, poultry, eggs, milk, and dairy products) from their diet.
- *Lacto-vegetarians* eat plant foods, plus dairy products (no eggs).
- *Ovo-vegetarians* eat plant foods, plus eggs (no dairy products).
- *Lacto-ovo vegetarians* eat plant foods, dairy products, and eggs.

Box 31-2 Dietary Practices Based on Traditional Religious Beliefs

The nurse needs to keep in mind that the concepts noted here are meant as a preliminary introduction to different dietary practices. Individual choices may differ from specific traditional religious, cultural, or ethnic beliefs.

JEWISH
Because of differences in interpretation, individuals who are Jewish vary in how strictly they follow dietary laws. Those who practice Reform Judaism may practice minimal observance of general dietary laws. Those who practice Conservative Judaism may follow dietary laws only at home. Individuals who practice Orthodox Judaism may adhere strictly to dietary laws. *Kosher* eating requires the following:
- Separate dishes, pans, and silverware are used to prepare and to serve meat and dairy foods.
- Meat and dairy may not be eaten at the same meal.
- Meats must be slaughtered by a ritual method and only the front quarter of the animal may be eaten.
- Only some parts of beef, veal, lamb, mutton, goat, venison, chicken, turkey, goose, and pheasant are eaten.
- Pork products, rabbit, shellfish, and scavenger fish are not allowed.
- Food must be prepared ahead of time for the Sabbath, which is sundown Friday to sundown Saturday.
- Certain days of fasting are observed, but a rabbi may excuse older or ill clients.

CHURCH OF JESUS CHRIST OF LATTER-DAY SAINTS (MORMON)
Mormons may not use stimulants (e.g., coffee, tea, or caffeine-containing carbonated beverages) and abstain from consuming alcoholic beverages. Members may observe "fast offerings," giving up two meals on the first Sunday of each month. Mormons live by a health code and the Word of Wisdom; they are to preserve their bodies and maintain the best possible health. Meat is eaten sparingly and "in season" (winter).

ROMAN CATHOLIC
Dietary and fasting regulations are mostly voluntary. Some Catholics may abstain from eating meat on Fridays. Those aged 14–59 years may fast and abstain from meat on Fridays during Lent. Ash Wednesday and Good Friday may be observed as days of fast and abstinence (a priest may excuse older or ill adults). Catholics may not eat or drink (except water) for 1 hour before taking Holy Communion.

SEVENTH-DAY ADVENTIST
Seventh-day Adventists may be lacto-ovo vegetarians or vegans. They may not use stimulants (coffee, tobacco) and may avoid pork, shellfish, and alcohol. In-between meal snacking may be discouraged. Many practices may be similar to those who are Jewish, such as food must be prepared ahead of time for the Sabbath, which is sundown Friday to sundown Saturday.

HINDU
Hindus may believe that all life forms are sacred because they might be the reincarnation of an ancestor. Most Hindus are vegetarian, while some are lacto or lacto-ovo vegetarians, and they may not use alcohol. Coffee, tea, and chocolate are widely used.

ISLAM (MUSLIM)
In Islam, alcoholic beverages and pork may be avoided. Muslims may observe Ramadan for 1 month each year, where they fast from dawn until after dark. Foods considered healthy are honey, dates, milk, meat, seafood, and olive oil.

Even among these broad classifications, variations are found to the extent in which vegetarians avoid animal products. For instance, some people call themselves vegetarians just because they do not eat red meat. More frequently, people declare they are "mostly" vegetarian, usually meaning that they are mostly lacto-ovo vegetarian, with meat products included in their diet from once per week to once per day. When caring for clients who consume a vegetarian diet, it is important to understand their specific dietary restrictions rather than assuming products they will consume based on generalizations.

Benefits of the Vegetarian Diet

Compared with nonvegetarians, vegetarians have lower rates of coronary artery disease, hypertension, non–insulin-dependent diabetes, and obesity. Studies have shown that Seventh-day Adventist vegetarians have lower mortality rates from colon cancer than does the general population. Vegetarian diets may also offer some protection against both lung and breast cancers.

Balancing the Vegetarian Diet

Many people mistakenly assume that consuming an adequate protein intake is impossible if they exclude animal products from their diet. They may think that they must give special attention to combining ("complementing") plant proteins at each meal, to ensure that all essential amino acids are present at the same time. In truth, plant sources of protein alone can provide sufficient amounts of essential and nonessential amino acids, if calorie intake is adequate and the types of plant proteins eaten are reasonably varied over the course of the day.

Although vegetarians often consume less protein than nonvegetarians, most vegetarian diets meet or exceed the Dietary Recommended Intakes (DRIs) for protein. Vegetarians who include some type of animal product in their diet are likely to consume an adequate amount of each nutrient, as long as they meet their calorie needs. Pure vegans (no animal products) need a reliable source of cobalamin (vitamin B_{12}), such as vitamin supplements or fortified foods like some breakfast cereals, soy beverages, and some brands of nutritional yeast. (Vitamin B_{12} is found naturally only in animal products.) If their exposure to sunlight is limited, vegetarians may require supplements of vitamin D. Calcium, iron, and zinc intake is usually adequate (even for children) when the diet is varied and contains adequate calories. Specific dietary recommendations for vegetarians are available in the Dietary Guidelines for Americans at www.ChooseMyPlate.gov. These guidelines are beneficial when teaching clients and promoting good health using nutritional concepts. In Practice: Educating the Client 31-2 gives general recommendations for a balanced vegetarian diet.

IN PRACTICE
EDUCATING THE CLIENT 31-2: Vegetarian Diets

Inform clients that vegetarian diets can meet all the recommendations for nutrients. The key is to consume a variety of foods and the right amount of foods to meet their calorie needs. Clients need to follow the food group recommendations for their age, sex, and activity level to get the right amount of food and the variety of foods needed for nutrient adequacy. Nutrients that vegetarians may need to focus on include protein, iron, calcium, zinc, and vitamin B_{12}.

Nutrients to Focus on for Vegetarians

- *Protein* has many important functions in the body and is essential for growth and maintenance. Protein needs can easily be met by eating a variety of plant-based foods. Combining different protein sources in the same meal is not necessary. Sources of protein for vegetarians include beans, nuts, nut butters, peas, and soy products (tofu, tempeh, veggie burgers). Milk products and eggs are also good protein sources for lacto-ovo vegetarians.
- *Iron* functions primarily as a carrier of oxygen in the blood. Iron sources for vegetarians include iron-fortified breakfast cereals, spinach, kidney beans, black-eyed peas, lentils, turnip greens, molasses, whole wheat breads, peas, and some dried fruits (dried apricots, prunes, raisins).
- *Calcium* is used for building bones and teeth and in maintaining bone strength. Sources of calcium for vegetarians include fortified breakfast cereals, soy products (tofu, soy-based beverages), calcium-fortified orange juice, and some dark green leafy vegetables (collard greens, turnip greens, bok choy, mustard greens). Milk products are excellent calcium sources for lacto-vegetarians.
- *Zinc* is necessary for many biochemical reactions, and it also helps the immune system function properly. Sources of zinc for vegetarians include many types of beans (white beans, kidney beans, chickpeas), zinc-fortified breakfast cereals, wheat germ, and pumpkin seeds. Milk products are a zinc source for lacto-vegetarians.
- *Vitamin B_{12}* is found in animal products and some fortified foods. Sources of vitamin B_{12} for vegetarians include milk products, eggs, and foods that have been fortified with vitamin B_{12} (breakfast cereals, soy-based beverages, veggie burgers, nutritional yeast).

Tips for Vegetarians

- Build meals around protein sources that are naturally low in fat, such as beans and lentils. Do not overload meals with high-fat cheeses to replace the meat.
- Calcium-fortified soy-based beverages can provide calcium in amounts similar to milk. They are usually low in fat and do not contain cholesterol.
- Many foods that typically contain meat or poultry can be made vegetarian. This can increase vegetable intake and cut saturated fat and cholesterol intake (e.g., pasta primavera or pasta with marinara or pesto sauce, vegetable lasagna, bean burritos, or tacos).
- A variety of vegetarian products look (and may taste) like their nonvegetarian counterparts but are usually lower in saturated fat and contain no cholesterol.
- For breakfast, try soy-based sausage patties or links.
- Rather than hamburgers, try veggie burgers. A variety of kinds are available, made with soy beans, vegetables, and/or rice. Make bean burgers, lentil burgers, or falafel (spicy ground chickpea patties).
- For barbecues, try veggie burgers, soy hot dogs, marinated tofu or tempeh, or veggie kabobs.
- Most restaurants can accommodate vegetarian modifications to menu items by substituting meatless sauces, omitting meat from stir-fries, and adding vegetables or pasta in place of meat. Some restaurants offer soy options (textured vegetable protein) as a substitute for meat and soy cheese as a substitute for regular cheese. Many Asian and Indian restaurants offer a varied selection of vegetarian dishes.

U.S. Department of Agriculture. (n.d.). *Tips for vegetarians*. Retrieved September 23, 2020, from https://www.choosemyplate.gov/node/5635

SOCIOCULTURAL FACTORS

In addition to religious practices and ethnic traditions, several other sociocultural factors influence people and their eating patterns, such as the following:

- Social aspects of eating
- Emotional attitudes about food
- Food fads and fallacies
- Economic conditions
- Physical status

> **NCLEX Alert**
>
> NCLEX questions may ask what factors contribute to the best or the least healthy diets. Be aware that socioeconomic factors, as well as nutritional contents, are pertinent to the correct answer. Teaching concepts for clients with health- and diet-related conditions can be integrated into NCLEX clinical situations.

Social Factors

Most people prefer to eat with others, rather than alone, and are probably used to eating their meals with family or coworkers. When people are admitted to a healthcare facility, they may suddenly find themselves alone in a room with a dinner tray. They may have limited input regarding what foods they are served. Illness and feelings of loneliness often result in poor nutritional intake. Following are some guidelines to provide a sense of social involvement for clients during meals:

- Visit the client for a few minutes.
- Allow two clients to eat together.
- In a double room, open the curtain.
- Let clients meet in a common lounge for meals.
- Encourage family members to visit at mealtime.
- Turn on the television or radio.
- Place flowers nearby.

Emotional Factors

Emotional factors influence nutritional behavior and total health. These factors may affect the eating patterns of the client in a healthcare facility. Food may become a reward. Purees of certain foods may be considered "for babies." A client may feel guilty for not eating all the food on the tray or may overeat just because the food is there. Clients who are sad, lonely, or depressed may overeat or refuse to eat. Trust, comfort, security, and love are concepts that integrate food and emotions starting during infancy. Having a parent hold an infant, in lieu of placing the infant in a crib, promotes family bonds. Sit-down meals at regular times of the day promote consistency and regular eating habits. Snacking leads to poor nutrition and can be a sign of eating for emotional comfort.

Food Fads and Fallacies

From quick weight loss schemes to home remedies for almost any ailment, food fads are big business in the United States. Sometimes, the claims behind food fads directly oppose scientific understanding of nutrition and health. Other claims capitalize on legitimate studies to exploit public interest. Either way, wasted money is only one consequence of following food fads. Direct toxicity and failure to seek legitimate healthcare are other possible outcomes that can significantly affect health.

The best protection against food frauds is to become a better-educated consumer. The *Dietary Guidelines for Americans* and the MyPlate framework provide an excellent foundation for basic nutritional principles and advice. In Practice: Educating the Client 31-3 gives pointers for the nurse to help clients evaluate a food fad or quick weight loss scheme. Clients, with specific concerns about food fads or who may be at risk for health problems because of them, should be directed to a dietitian.

Economic Conditions

A family's financial status may influence a person's eating habits. Food is relatively inexpensive in the United States. More affluent people may tend to eat at restaurants more often. They may generally consume more vegetables and fruits, but also eat more fat due to a higher intake of cheese, meat, fish, and poultry. Diets higher in fat are associated with heart disease, cancer, and other disorders. When income rises, people tend to eat fewer eggs, rice, and beans. People with lower incomes may skip meals. The homeless or "street people" may beg or look through trash for food.

Nursing Alert If you encounter a client who does not have enough money for food, initiate a referral for the client to social services.

IN PRACTICE
EDUCATING THE CLIENT 31-3 — Food Fads and Fallacies

Fad diets and quick weight loss schemes add up to a multimillion-dollar industry in the United States. Credentials are blurred, claims are exaggerated, and the consumer is bewildered. Because fad diets are often here today and gone tomorrow, it is hard to keep up with what is hot and what is not. Advise clients to look for the following criteria before they jump on the latest diet bandwagon:

- The plan is realistic and flexible, not a collection of rigid menus, a one-size-fits-all approach, or "must-have" food combinations.
- It suggests consultation with a healthcare provider.
- The plan uses food, not pills or potions, to meet nutritional requirements.
- It uses food from each of the major food groups, not eliminating any as "bad," unhealthy, or dangerous. The number of servings recommended from each food group compares with the suggestions in the MyPlate framework.
- It adequately supplies all nutrients.
- It is founded on sound nutritional principles, not unsubstantiated claims.
- It recommends exercise.
- It does not promote more than 1–2 lb of weight loss per week (greater amounts equate with loss of lean tissue and water, not true loss of fat, which is the actual goal).
- It is safe indefinitely. There are no time limits for discontinuation of the diet.
- It allows nutritious snacking.
- It emphasizes portion control.
- It recognizes the importance of behavior modification for long-term success.
- It offers a maintenance plan.
- It is reasonably priced.

Physical Condition

Clients experiencing illness may not be well or strong enough to eat. When caring for clients who are not strong enough to eat on their own, the nurse must take time to feed them. Feeding is an excellent time to make a physical and psychological assessment of the client. Consider absence of teeth, ill-fitting dentures, or difficulty swallowing when planning meals. When nutritional needs are increased, such as after major surgery to promote healing, obtaining an adequate amount of nutrients to treat acute illness takes precedence over following a low-fat or low-calorie diet for chronic disease prevention. Malnutrition is common among those with acquired immunodeficiency syndrome (AIDS); therefore, increased calorie and protein intake is required to replenish losses. Other diet modifications may be necessary to alleviate symptoms or complications, such as limiting fat for malabsorption, increasing fluid for diarrhea or fever, and providing small, frequent meals for anorexia or fatigue.

STUDENT SYNTHESIS

KEY POINTS

- Nurses play an important role in helping clients meet nutritional needs.
- To provide optimal care, understand the transcultural aspects of food and eating and work within a person's unique context and dietary requirements to promote optimal nutrition.
- Diets of any culture can magnify health concerns because of ingredients such as salt, sugar, or fats.
- Monitor dietary risk factors for hypertension, diabetes, or cardiovascular disease.
- Ethnic and religious factors may play an important part in food acceptance, especially during illness. Be sure to understand specific client needs rather than making assumptions based on generalizations.
- Vegetarian diets are healthy and contain adequate protein if a wide variety of foods are eaten and calorie intake is sufficient.
- Pure vegans may need vitamin B_{12} and vitamin D supplements.
- Cultural and socioeconomic factors and beliefs about food compound the individual's concepts of healthy eating.

CRITICAL THINKING EXERCISES

1. Some cultures use soy sauce and fish sauce extensively in food. Describe possible problems this practice may entail and what solutions may be culturally and nutritionally appropriate.
2. Give examples of cultures and religious groups and the common prohibited foods and beverages. Describe how this could affect your nursing care related to diet planning.
3. Your client is a lacto-ovo vegetarian. Outline particulars of a diet that would provide the client with a nutritionally adequate intake.

NCLEX-STYLE REVIEW QUESTIONS

1. The nurse is caring for a client who is on a regular diet but has not eaten any food from the tray for 2 days. Which nursing action would be appropriate at this time?
   a. Tell the client "You have to eat this or you will become even more ill."
   b. Obtain a dietary consult and permission to have food brought in by the family.
   c. Inform the client "If you don't eat, you will not be able to take your medication."
   d. Place a nasogastric tube in and feed the client through there.

2. A client says, "I have been using home remedies to thin my blood." Which food items should the nurse caution the client about ingesting while taking warfarin (Coumadin)?
   a. Dark, green, leafy vegetables
   b. Milk and milk products
   c. Berries
   d. Whole grains

3. The nurse is caring for a client who does not speak English. The family member present with the client informs the nurse that foods must be Yin since the client has a Yang condition. Which type of food would adhere to this request?
   a. High in calories
   b. Cooked at low temperatures
   c. Spicy
   d. Red-orange in color

4. A client who practices Orthodox Judaism and follows a kosher diet receives a tray for supper and requests that it be taken away. Which item on the tray would the nurse recognize that the client is unable to consume?
   a. Green salad with oil and vinegar dressing
   b. Cookies and a carton of milk
   c. Baked pork chop with gravy
   d. A cheese sandwich

5. The nurse is caring for a client who is Muslim in the acute care facility during the month of Ramadan. How will the client's eating patterns alter during this time period?
   a. "Hot" foods will be given for "hot" illness and "cold" foods given for "cold" illness.
   b. Yin foods will be given for Yang illness.
   c. No meat products will be consumed.
   d. A breakfast tray will be brought prior to dawn and a supper tray after dark.

CHAPTER RESOURCES

Enhance your learning with additional resources on thePoint!

Student Resources related to this chapter can be found at thePoint.lww.com/Rosdahl12e.

32 Diet Therapy and Special Diets

Learning Objectives

1. Describe several roles of the nurse in providing nutritional support to a client in an acute care hospital, a long-term care facility, and a home care setting.
2. Identify the rationale for offering meal supplements, increasing fluids, or decreasing fluids.
3. Identify specific reasons a client may need assistance with eating. State two nursing interventions for each type of circumstance.
4. Differentiate between the following types of diets: house diet, modified diet, and therapeutic diet.
5. State several methods of modifying diets in terms of nutrients, consistency, or energy value.
6. Differentiate between a clear liquid and a full liquid diet. State the rationale and the limitations for the use of each diet.
7. Differentiate between a digestive soft diet and a mechanical soft diet. State the rationale and the limitations for the use of these diets.
8. Differentiate between a high-fiber diet and a low-fiber diet. State the rationale and the limitations for the use of these diets.
9. Differentiate among the following diets: fat controlled, low cholesterol, and limited saturated fats.
10. Explain the two main uses of low- and high-protein diets.
11. Identify the components of a mild, moderate, and severe sodium-restricted diet.
12. Demonstrate the procedure for the insertion of a nasogastric tube.
13. Differentiate between TPN and PPN.

Important Terminology

anorexia
bland diet
carbohydrate-
    controlled diet
dysphagia
edentulous
    (edentia)
fat-controlled diet
hyperlipidemia
infusion
ketogenic diet
liquid diet
low-residue diet
modified diet
polydipsia
soft diet
stoma
therapeutic diet
tube feeding

Acronyms

DAT
G tube
GERD
IV
J tube
NG tube
PEG
PPN
TPN

Nutrition is a vital component of therapy for many disorders. For example, in any condition involving the healing of body tissues (e.g., after a burn or surgery), a high protein intake is essential to help rebuild and repair those tissues. A client who is hemorrhaging, vomiting, perspiring profusely because of a high fever, or suffering from diarrhea needs fluids and electrolytes to replace what is being lost.

Some disorders necessitate a special diet, either during acute illness or throughout life. Nutrition therapy is the cornerstone of treatment for diabetes mellitus. Persons with coronary or vascular disorders often must limit or modify their fat and sodium intake. People who are ill may need help fulfilling their nutritional requirements.

This chapter discusses some means that can be used to assist clients to meet their basic needs for adequate nutrition. As a nurse, you can perform specific activities to help clients, such as serving food attractively and providing assistance at mealtimes. Mealtime is an excellent time to introduce or to reinforce diet teaching. By observing clients during these times, you can help identify those at nutritional risk and communicate findings to appropriate team members (Fig. 32-1).

This chapter also discusses modified diets and nutritional support accomplished through alternative types of feeding.

HELPING THE CLIENT MEET NUTRITIONAL NEEDS

Eating is an event in the client's long day and should be as pleasant as possible. Keep in mind that some people revert to eating behaviors and food preferences of childhood during times of illness and stress. Nurses help clients meet nutritional needs in various healthcare settings.

SERVING FOOD

Train yourself to check each tray with the diet order.

- If you have a client who must be fed, serve trays first to the other clients who can feed themselves.
- Keep servings small. The sight of large quantities of food may take away the client's appetite.
- Serve hot foods hot and cold foods cold. Cover hot dishes.
- Avoid dribbles of food on the edges of dishes.
- Fill cups and glasses about three quarters full to avoid spilling the contents.
- Be sure that all foods on the tray are allowed for the person on a special diet.
- Observe whether a napkin, a spoon, or a glass is missing before you carry the tray to the client.

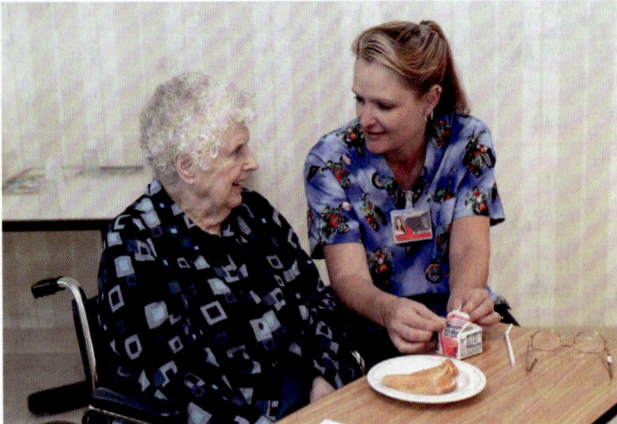

Figure 32-1 The nurse has a critical role in the nutritional health of the client. It is important to make observations related to consumption of food and the client's ability to prepare and eat food and to monitor and teach good dietary habits. Note that in this picture, the nurse is opening the food products. (Carter, 2012.)

- Remove any damaged silverware or chipped glasses.
- Be pleasant. Take a minute to chat.

Every healthcare facility has its own system of food service. Trays are usually brought to the nursing station on a cart in the hospital. Each tray is labeled with the client's name, room number, bed number, and appropriate diet. This information should be checked against the posted diet list before giving a tray to a client. Make sure that the client's name band matches the name on the food tray before serving the food (Fig. 32-2). In Practice: Nursing Care Guidelines 32-1 gives suggestions for helping to make hospital mealtimes more pleasant.

In an extended care setting, such as a nursing home or mental health unit, residents may sit together at dining tables, where food is served either by tray or family style. Although strict diet adherence may be sacrificed, family-style dining promotes better eating, an important consideration for a group that is often susceptible to poor food intake and nutritional problems.

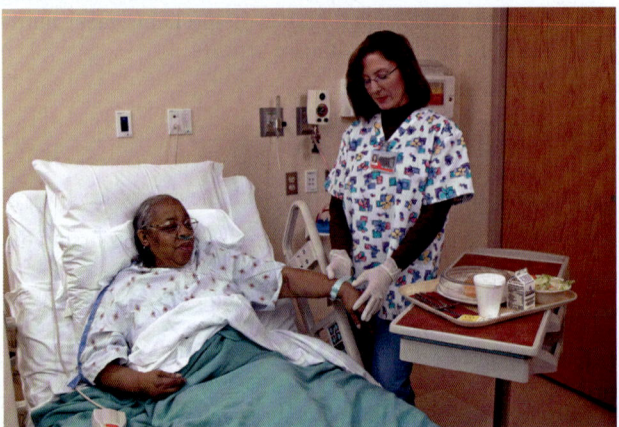

Figure 32-2 When serving food, always check the tray for the correct diet and check the client's identification to ensure that the food is going to the right client. Be especially aware of clients who can have nothing by mouth (NPO); be sure that food and drink are withheld during that time. (Carter, 2012.)

IN PRACTICE
NURSING CARE GUIDELINES 32-1 — Helping at Hospital Mealtimes

Preparing the Client for Meals
Give the person a chance to use the bathroom or bedpan before the meal.
- Assist the person to wash their hands and face and perhaps to rinse the mouth or brush the teeth.
- Help the client into as normal a position as possible: sitting in a chair, on the edge of the bed, or with the head of the bed elevated.
- Check the client's ID band to be sure that it matches the name on the tray.
- Put the overbed table in place; clear it of unnecessary items.
- Bring the tray promptly when the client is ready, to prevent overtiring the client.
- Avoid unpleasant or painful treatments just before or after a meal.
- Try not to give unpleasant-tasting medications before or during a meal.
- If possible, give any prescribed pain medication 30 min before a meal, which may provide some relief and allow the person to eat more comfortably.
- Remove unpleasant odors (bedpan, commode) and litter (dressings, linens).
- Cover unpleasant things (wounds, blood, intravenous bags).
- Change linens and gown, as needed.
- Give the person as much time as is needed.
- Offer assistance, as needed.
- Encourage the client to fill out the selective menu so that preferred foods will be served.
- Explain special diets and their purposes.
- Consider cultural aspects.
- Arrange the tray attractively.
- Arrange foods for easy access. Help as needed.
- Help arrange a towel or napkin so the client does not worry about spilling.
- Help the client to get some exercise during the day.
- Depending on the type of diet, the family can bring small amounts of favorite foods.

In home care settings, nurses are sometimes responsible for all aspects of routine nutritional care, from preparing and serving food to conducting nutritional screenings and counseling (Fig. 32-3). An advantage of the home setting is that the client is not subject to rigid meal schedules and limited food choices, as in other healthcare settings. Clients tend to eat better in the comfort of their own home, and nurses can use the time spent with them to reinforce diet principles. Clients, however, may be less cooperative with following diet plans at home, where they are used to being in charge. The home care nurse should consult a dietitian regarding a client with actual or potential nutritional problems.

Serving Food

Food should be presented in as attractive and appetizing a manner as possible. Because your attitudes can influence

CHAPTER 32 Diet Therapy and Special Diets

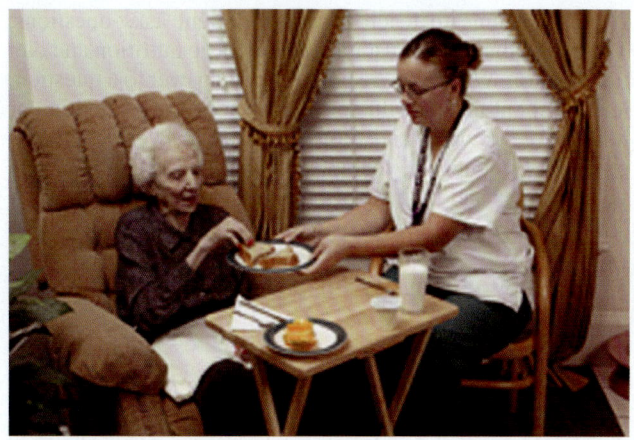

Figure 32-3 The observations for the home care nurse include noting that the client has the capabilities of getting and preparing food and is maintaining adequate weight. Home visits are an excellent time to listen to clients' concerns about their diets and to provide educational support about their nutritional needs. (Carter, 2012.)

the client's, refrain from negative comments or gestures pertaining to the food. Encourage clients to eat and to feed themselves, if possible, so they do not feel helpless. In Practice: Nursing Care Guidelines 32-2 has several mealtime guidelines.

In the acute or extended care facility, remove tray covers just before placing the tray on the overbed table to allow diffusion of food odors that intensify while collecting under the cover. Strong odors may destroy the client's appetite. Do not remove the cover too soon or the food will get cold. If a client is not hungry, remove the items from the tray and set the overbed table as you would a regular table, with napkin, utensils, and plate. This action simulates the home environment and makes meals more appealing. The time used in serving food is a good time for talking with the client. Answer questions about the meal and make the person feel comfortable before you leave the room.

Providing Between-Meal Supplements and Snacks

Between-meal and bedtime supplements are often given to clients who have high nutritional needs or poor appetites. These supplements may be ordered by healthcare providers or initiated by dietitians. Supplemental nourishment must be served on time. If supplements are given too early, the client may still feel full from the previous meal. If given too late, the nourishment may ruin the client's appetite for the next meal. Encourage the client to consume the nourishment and solicit flavor preferences if appropriate. Documentation of nourishment intake or refusal by the client is required, as is the client's intake of meals.

Encouraging Fluid Intake

Often, the healthcare provider gives orders to *force fluids* or *encourage fluids*, which means that you must encourage the client to take as much fluid as possible. Whenever you enter the client's room, offer a small amount of fluid. The client will find fluids more tolerable if they are cold, varied, and given in small amounts. Depending on the client's diet, you may occasionally offer ice cream, ice pops, frozen fruit juices, regular or diet soda, thin cereals, gelatin, coffee, or other fluids.

Promote increased fluid intake for any client who is in bed a great deal or who has difficulty moving. Adequate fluid intake helps prevent such complications as pressure wounds, renal calculi, bladder infections, constipation, and dehydration. Adequate fluid intake also helps establish a bladder and bowel routine. See Box 32-1 for tips on encouraging adequate fluid intake.

Restricting Fluid

In some cases, the healthcare provider orders a fluid restriction (e.g., *restrict fluids to 1,500 mL/day*). This order may be prescribed for the psychiatric client who has **polydipsia** (drinks excessive amounts of water) or for the person with end-stage renal disease. Managing this restriction may be easier if the client takes about half the fluids during the day and half in the evening. Intake of other substances (e.g., caffeine) may also be restricted. *Fluids* include all foods and beverages that are in fluid form at room temperature (e.g., ice cream, gelatin).

IN PRACTICE
NURSING CARE GUIDELINES 32-2 | Feeding Clients

- Wash your hands first.
- Make the person comfortable.
- Arrange a napkin or towel to avoid spills.
- Arrange the tray conveniently.
- Do not rush.
- Sit down; take time to make the meal relaxing.
- Visit with the person (be careful that the client does not choke).
- Use usual utensils (fork, spoon).
- Feed a small amount at a time.
- Ask the client how they like to eat; some people eat all of one food first, others rotate foods.
- Tell the person if something is very hot or cold; warn the person to test the food first.
- A straw or drinking cup may be helpful for sipping soup. Be very careful with hot liquids! Clients with impaired swallowing should not use straws.
- Wipe the chin and face, as needed.
- Let the person hold bread or otherwise help as much as possible.
- After the person has finished the meal, record intake and make the person comfortable.

Note: In some states or facilities, the nurse is required to wear gloves when feeding clients.

> **Key Concept**
> Persons who are encouraged to take fluids or who are on a fluid-restriction diet are usually being monitored for intake and output (I&O).

Box 32-1 Tips to Encourage Adequate Fluid Intake

Drink before you become thirsty. People who are thirsty need to drink to satisfy thirst plus a little extra.

Choose liquids with appealing taste. Clients who dislike their tap water should be urged to consider buying a water filter or bottled water. Refrigeration usually improves the taste of tap water.

Keep a water bottle at your desk. Iced water in a sports bottle enables "sippers" to drink at their leisure.

Make water part of your meals. Served with a meal, water does not seem like a troublesome extra that requires thought and planning.

Drink a glass of water before each meal, especially if weight control is a concern. Water can blunt appetite and help people eat less. Weight management programs often urge participants to drink adequate water as a means to control appetite.

Use water in place of carbonated beverages. It is better on the teeth, better at quenching thirst, and does not provide empty calories.

Pack bottled water in your lunch. This tactic eliminates the need to visit the soda machine.

Drink enough low-fat milk. Fluid, calcium, vitamin D, and protein are provided in one package.

Try sparkling water with a wedge of lemon or lime, for a little variety. Seltzer is pure, calorie-free, and loaded with bubbles.

Eat enough fruits and vegetables. Fruits and vegetables are generally high in water, even though the water they provide is usually not counted when fluid intake is calculated. Six ounces of 100% fruit juice counts as a serving from the fruit group.

Drink extra fluids before, during, and after exercise, especially in hot weather. General guidelines are to drink
- At least 16 oz of beverages up to 2 hr before a competitive event.
- 4–8 oz or more of water or sports drink 5–10 min before your workout or competition.
- 8–10 oz every 15–20 min during strenuous exercise.

Try using herbal tea, decaffeinated tea, or decaffeinated coffee in place of some or all caffeinated beverages.

From Dudek, S. (2017). *Nutritional essentials for nursing practice* (8th ed.). Wolters Kluwer.

Teaching

Clients and their families want to know how they can achieve good health. Although a dietitian usually performs diet counseling for clients, as a nurse you can reinforce diet teaching and identify counseling needs for further examination. Educating clients and families is an essential part of your provision of nursing care. Diet counseling is generally most effective when you provide both verbal and written instructions. Food models and pictures may be effective tools for teaching portion sizes. With any diet, advise clients to eliminate individual intolerances and alert the healthcare provider if a conflict exists between the prescribed diet and the client's religious beliefs or cultural practices. Report any adverse reaction to the diet. Clients should be able to repeat diet information to ensure their understanding of it.

A good time to teach is when a client asks questions. Therefore, the nurse must understand basic nutrition and diet information. When you do not know an answer to a question, tell the client that you do not know, speak to the dietitian or healthcare provider, and return with an answer as soon as possible. By doing so, you help the client build confidence in your abilities and in those of other staff members.

THE CLIENT WHO NEEDS ASSISTANCE WITH EATING

Encouraging independence in clients whenever possible is important. In some situations, however, you must feed clients their entire meal. In such cases, take the time to make your clients comfortable and encourage them to eat as much as they desire. A family member may wish to feed a client. This practice is relaxing for the client and makes the family member feel that they are helping to provide care. You are responsible, however, for ensuring that eating is easy and safe. If this is not the case, you must take over or supervise the feeding.

Feeding the Client

Even clients who can feed themselves may need assistance in spreading butter on bread, cutting meat, opening milk cartons, or pouring beverages. Always warn a client about extremely hot foods to prevent burns, especially if the client is using a straw. Encourage the person to do as much as possible to develop self-confidence and a sense of progress. Part of your responsibility in promoting good nutrition is to note any discomfort or digestive complaints the client expresses during feeding or afterward.

Very young, helpless, or confused individuals require special attention. You may have to feed them to make sure they ingest enough nutrients. Protecting them from possible injuries or accidents may also be necessary.

Use your judgment about how much a client can do—sometimes the person can hold a piece of bread but cannot manage other foods (see Nursing Care Guidelines 32-2).

The Visually Impaired Person

Most people with visual impairments can learn to eat without assistance if they are encouraged to be independent. When a client is blinded only temporarily (e.g., after eye surgery), you may need to feed the client every meal. The visually impaired person needs to learn to locate the food on the plate. You can help this process by describing the location of foods as if they were on the face of a clock (e.g., *the meat is at 6 o'clock*). In extended care facilities, consistent place settings promote independence. Always be sure to warn the client about very hot foods. Cut food into small pieces.

The Person With a Swallowing Disorder

Some clients have difficulty swallowing as a result of a neurologic or other disorder. **Dysphagia** is the medical term for a swallowing disorder. A speech therapist is often consulted to determine the appropriate diet consistency for the client with dysphagia; diets range from thick liquids only to solid foods and thick liquids. Fluids are thickened with a thickening agent. Thickened fluids slow the swallowing process so that clients are less likely to choke. Consult a dietitian to ensure that such diets are nutritionally adequate. Elevate the head of the bed, feed the client very slowly, and encourage swallowing after each portion of food. Progress the diet to the next level as the client's ability to swallow improves.

The Person Who Cannot Chew

Some people have trouble chewing because of poor dental health, missing teeth, or poorly fitting dentures. These clients will need the consistency of their diet modified. Assess each client's ability to chew and to swallow. Give this information to the team leader or healthcare provider.

Documenting and Reporting

If a client has a poor appetite, refuses food, has difficulty swallowing, or complains of nausea, you are responsible for recognizing and documenting these observations and calling them to the attention of the team leader. That person and the healthcare provider should then give you directions about how to provide the client with needed nourishment. A dietitian is also a valuable resource to consult whenever problems with diet, nutrition, or food preferences appear. Document other relevant observations in the client's health record, including fluid intake, caloric intake, or the amount of a tube feeding taken.

> **Key Concept**
>
> Diet is an integral part of the client's total treatment plan. Correct food must be served and, more importantly, consumed. Food presentation and the healthcare provider's attitude can greatly affect how well a client accepts food.

HOUSE DIETS

A normal diet in acute or extended care facilities is called a *house diet* or *regular diet*. The house diet is the one most frequently ordered, and it is served to clients whose condition does not require a special diet. You may also hear it called a *general diet, regular diet,* or *full diet*. It allows a wide choice of foods and includes almost everything. In many facilities, clients receive a menu and may select their meals for the next day, within the parameters of their diet orders. This may be called a *select diet* or *client's select diet*. A *regular diet as tolerated* (**DAT**) may be ordered. It is interpreted according to the client's appetite and ability to eat and to tolerate food.

MODIFIED DIETS

A **modified diet** is an important part of therapy for many diseases. When planning a special diet, the healthcare provider and dietitian consider the disease process and the client's general condition. Always follow dietary orders carefully. When in doubt regarding a diet, or when questions arise, consult the dietitian and the healthcare facility diet manual.

A **therapeutic diet** may be prescribed as part of the treatment of more than one disease or condition. For example, a client with a heart condition may also be overweight; a convalescent client may also have diabetes. Following are general reasons for therapeutic diets and common examples of associated disorders:

- Regulating the amount of certain nutrients in disorders of metabolism (*diabetes*)
- Increasing or decreasing body weight by adding or limiting calories and fat (*underweight* or *overweight*)
- Reducing or preventing edema by controlling the level of sodium (*cardiac conditions*)
- Aiding digestion by avoiding foods that irritate the gastrointestinal tract or interfere with stomach action (*ulcer, diverticulitis*)
- Helping an overburdened organ regain normal function (*nephritis*)
- Eliminating a food that the body is unable to tolerate (*allergies, phenylketonuria*)
- Slowing overactive intestinal motility (*colitis*)

Clients are more likely to comply with diet restrictions if they are not constantly reminded of their disease by having the diet classified according to a disease name. For instance, referring to a diabetic diet as a "controlled-carbohydrate" diet deemphasizes diabetes and focuses attention on nutritional habits the client should develop.

The following classifications indicate how diets are modified in treatment:

- Consistency and texture (liquid, soft, mechanical, high fiber, low fiber)
- Energy value (high or low calorie)
- Nutrients (controlled carbohydrate, high or low fat or protein, sodium, calcium, phosphorus, or potassium controlled)
- Amount (e.g., six small feedings)
- Specific allergens (e.g., eggs, dairy, nuts)

These categories indicate the kind of diet prescribed, although the amounts of specific nutrients will vary for clients, according to a healthcare provider's orders. If restrictions or special requirements are unnecessary, the client may have any of the foods listed for that type of diet. You must have a general knowledge of what kinds of foods are allowed for specific diets.

Consistency Modifications

The consistency and texture of the diet may be modified as clear liquid, full liquid, soft, mechanical soft, pureed, low fiber, and high fiber. Tube feedings are a form of modified diet discussed at the end of this chapter. Table 32-1 summarizes important concepts about clear liquid, full liquid, and soft diets.

Liquid Diets

A **liquid diet**, as the name suggests, consists entirely of liquids. (A liquid is described as a food that is fluid at room temperature or that becomes fluid at body temperature.) Liquid diets are prescribed after surgery as a person's first step toward taking solid foods. They may be used during an acute illness or for certain body disturbances, such as irritation of the intestinal

TABLE 32-1 Characteristics, Indications, and Contraindications for Liquid and Soft Diets

CHARACTERISTICS	FOODS ALLOWED	INDICATIONS	CONTRAINDICATIONS
Clear Liquid Diet A short-term, highly restrictive diet composed only of clear fluids or foods that are fluid at body temperature. It requires minimal digestion and leaves a minimum of residue. Although it provides some electrolytes and carbohydrates, clear liquid diets are inadequate in calories and all nutrients except vitamin C.	Bouillon; fat-free broth Carbonated beverages; coffee, regular and decaf; tea Fruit juices, strained and clear (apple, cranberry, grape) Gelatin; popsicles Sugar, honey, hard candy	Initial feeding after surgery or parenteral nutrition; in preparation for surgery and various diagnostic tests of the bowel	Long-term use
Full Liquid Diet Composed of foods that are liquid or liquefy at body temperature. Full liquid diets can be carefully planned or supplemented to approximate the nutritional value of a regular or high-calorie–high-protein diet, making it suitable for long-term use. Full liquid diets may be inadequate in folic acid, iron, vitamin B_6, and fiber. If the diet is used for longer than 2–3 days, modifications may be needed to increase calories and protein. Pureed or blenderized foods can be given as a form of liquid diet that is suitable for long-term use (e.g., when a fractured jaw is wired and the client cannot chew).	All the above plus: All milk and milk drinks, puddings, custards, and desserts All vegetable and fruit juices Refined or strained cereals Eggs in custard Butter, margarine, cream Dietary supplements, such as Ensure	Used as a transitional diet between a clear diet and a soft diet, and by clients who have difficulty chewing or swallowing	Severe lactose intolerance (diet relies heavily on milk and dairy products for protein and calories) Unless modified to decrease the cholesterol content, a liquid diet is not suitable for long-term use by clients with hypercholesterolemia
Soft Diet An adequate diet low in fiber, connective tissue, and fat. Restrictions vary considerably among institutions: Individual tolerances should determine the content of the diet.	All the above plus: Cooked vegetables, as tolerated Lettuce in small amounts Cooked or canned fruit Avocado, banana; grapefruit and orange sections without membranes Whole grain or enriched breads and cereals Potatoes Enriched rice, barley, pasta All lean and tender meats, fish, poultry Eggs, mild cheese, smooth peanut butter Butter, margarine, mild salad dressings	Diet can be used for clients who have difficulty chewing or swallowing. A *regular soft diet* is used as a transition between liquids and a regular diet. A *digestive soft diet* is low in fiber, connective tissue, and fats. It avoids gas-forming foods and irritating seasonings, which may be individual to the client. A *mechanical soft diet* is used primarily by clients who have difficulty chewing because they are edentulous (without teeth) or have ill-fitting dentures.	None

tract. Liquids are easily absorbed and do not overstimulate the digestive tract. According to a client's needs, liquid diets may be clear, full, or limited and are often progressive from clear liquids to full liquids to a regular diet. Feedings may be given every 2, 3, or 4 hr, as prescribed. For clients with diabetes, little, if any, changes need to be made to the regular liquid diets. Since clients with diabetes will continue their medications and have no other source of carbohydrates, they may have liquids with sugar. The American Diabetes Association recommends 30 g of carbohydrate every 2 hr.

Clear Liquid Diet

The clear liquid diet is inadequate in calories, protein, and most other nutrients. It should not be used for more than 3 days, unless the client is receiving nutritional support (nasogastric [NG] tube feedings or intravenous [IV] feedings) or other nutritional supplements. NG and IV feedings are discussed later in this chapter.

Full Liquid Diet

If a full liquid diet is to be used for a long time, nutritional supplements (e.g., Ensure, Glucerna) should be added. Be aware of any side effects of these supplements, such as diarrhea, constipation, gas, and bloating.

Soft Diet

A **soft diet** may vary from one facility to another. The terminology is sometimes nebulous, and the nurse must often clarify the healthcare provider's order regarding which type of soft diet is ordered. Knowing the rationale or purpose of the diet will help differentiate which type of soft diet is needed: regular, digestive, or mechanical. A soft diet may also be considered the same as a bland diet or a low-fiber diet.

One form of soft diet is the *digestive soft diet*. It is a nutritionally adequate diet that is low in fiber, connective tissue, and fat. Gas-forming foods are eliminated, and mild seasonings are used. In the postsurgical client, this diet acts as a transition between a liquid diet and the full or general diet. In the digestive soft diet, the healthcare provider may order modifications to the soft diet that eliminate some listed foods (see Table 32-1).

> **Key Concept**
> The progression of diets should be as follows: clear liquid, full liquid, soft, regular diet. A client's diet should progress as soon as possible to ensure an adequate nutritional intake and to increase the client's sense of well-being.

The *mechanical soft diet*, or dental soft diet, is used for the person who has difficulty chewing or swallowing, such as a client who is **edentulous** (without teeth), has oral problems, or has had a stroke. It is also a nutritionally adequate diet, and meats, fruits, and vegetables may be chopped, ground, or pureed, depending on the client's ability to chew and swallow. If necessary, the diet may be ordered as a pureed, mechanical soft diet.

High-Fiber Diet

A high-fiber diet has an increased amount of both insoluble and soluble fiber. *Insoluble fiber* helps increase stool bulk and stimulates peristalsis. *Soluble fiber* helps lower the serum cholesterol level and improves glucose tolerance in diabetes. A high-fiber diet is often ordered as part of the treatment for constipation and diverticulosis. Potential problems with a high-fiber diet are cramping, diarrhea, and gas, especially if fiber is added to a diet too quickly or in excessive amounts. To achieve a high-fiber diet, foods high in fiber are substituted for those low in fiber. Increased fluid intake is important in following a high-fiber diet. Box 32-2 lists good sources of fiber.

Low-Fiber Diet

The **low-fiber diet** is composed of foods that the body can absorb completely, so that little residue is left for the formation of feces. Chapter 30 discussed the value of fiber.

Box 32-2 Sources of Fiber

RICH IN INSOLUBLE FIBER
- Wheat and corn bran
- Whole wheat bread and cereals
- Brown rice
- Bananas
- Cauliflower
- Nuts
- Lentils
- Green beans
- Green peas

RICH IN SOLUBLE FIBER
- Citrus fruits
- Pectin

RICH IN BOTH INSOLUBLE AND SOLUBLE FIBER
- Oat bran
- Barley
- Navy beans
- Kidney beans
- Apples
- Broccoli
- Carrots

Some clients cannot or should not ingest fiber. *Low-fiber* diets are also known as "**low-residue**" diets. The wording is evolving because there is no scientifically acceptable definition of residue, and thus, the amount of residue produced by digestion of various foods cannot be accurately measured. *Low fiber* is considered the more accurate term. These diets are often utilized with tube feeding, which is discussed at the end of this chapter. Table 32-1 summarizes important concepts about clear liquid, full liquid, and soft diets. It may be prescribed for severe diarrhea, colitis, diverticulitis, other gastrointestinal disorders, intestinal obstruction, and before and after intestinal surgery. This diet may be inadequate in iron, calcium, and some vitamins and minerals because of limited food choices and overprocessing of fruits and vegetables. Suitable foods on the low-residue diet include

- Ground and well-cooked meats, chicken, and fish
- Seafood
- Eggs (not fried) and mild cheese
- Fruit and vegetable juices without pulp
- Pureed or strained vegetables
- Canned fruit and firm bananas
- White rice, plain noodles, plain pasta, and potatoes
- Refined white or seedless rye breads and crackers
- Two cups of milk or the equivalent (e.g., yogurt)
- Bouillon, broth, strained or cream soups made from allowed foods
- Plain desserts in moderation

Foods to be avoided on the low-residue diet include

- Whole-grain breads and whole-grain cereals
- Nuts, seeds, coconut, and anything containing them

- Potato skins, peanut butter, and popcorn
- Whole-grain pasta and wild or brown rice
- Raw vegetables and gas-producing vegetables
- All other fresh fruits and all dried fruits
- Tough, fibrous meats and dried peas and beans
- Spicy foods

Bland Diet

The **bland diet** has often been prescribed for those with ulcers, esophagitis, gastroesophageal reflux disease (**GERD**) or heartburn, gastritis, hiatal hernia, or other disorders of the gastrointestinal tract. The goal of this diet is to limit foods that stimulate the production of gastric acid. The impact of a bland diet may or may not be effective in treating a digestive disorder. Many prescriptions and over-the-counter medications are currently available to treat and/or cure GERD and stomach ulcers.

The following foods should be avoided on the bland diet:

- Alcohol
- Caffeine (including chocolate and cola drinks) and decaffeinated coffee and tea
- Red and black pepper
- Chili powder
- Fried foods and foods high in fat
- Peppermint and spearmint oils
- Citrus fruits and juices
- Tomato products

Individuals following a bland diet should be encouraged to avoid other foods that may cause them discomfort because intolerances are often individual. Instruct clients not to lie down for an hour after meals; to maintain ideal weight; and to eat smaller, more frequent meals. If they smoke, advise them to cut down or stop. Discourage milk-based diets—the stomach must secrete additional gastric acid to help neutralize milk's alkaline nature.

Energy Value Modifications

Diets modified for energy include high- and low-calorie diets.

High-Calorie Diet

Underweight occurs frequently in persons with prolonged illness. Symptoms such as lack of appetite, vomiting, diarrhea, and high fever can cause severe weight loss. A high-calorie diet may also be used for hyperthyroidism, undernutrition, and general malnutrition. The person who has been severely burned needs a large amount of protein to rebuild lost tissue and carbohydrate to spare protein. A high-calorie diet generally contains over 3,000 calories and 130 g protein.

The successful high-calorie diet accounts for individual food preferences and eating habits. The high-calorie diet is high in protein, carbohydrate, fat, vitamins, and minerals. Clients with a depressed appetite may need smaller and more frequent meals. Unless a definite reason exists for excluding solid foods, clients are allowed to have solids if they can chew and digest them easily.

Reduced-Calorie Diet

A reduced-calorie diet is used to promote weight loss in those with, or at risk for, complications related to obesity. A reduced-calorie diet that includes healthy carbohydrates, lean proteins, and healthy fats is the best way to achieve and maintain weight loss for the long term. The American Diabetes Association and the Academy of Nutrition and Dietetics have materials to provide guidance for clients desiring weight loss. See In Practice: Educating the client for more information on a reduced-calorie diet.

IN PRACTICE

EDUCATING THE CLIENT 32-1 — Reduced-Calorie Diet

To decrease calorie intake, encourage clients and families to practice the following dietary habits:

- Eat slowly and concentrate on the smell, taste, and texture of food.
- Eat a variety of foods that are low in calories and high in nutrients—check the Nutrition Facts Labels on packaged foods.
- Eat less fat and fewer high-fat foods.
- Eat smaller portions and limit second helpings of foods high in fat and calories.
- Eat more fruits and vegetables that do not have added fat or sugar.
- Eat pasta, rice, breads, and cereals without added fats and sugars used in preparation or at the table.
- Eat fewer sugars and sweets (e.g., candy, cookies, cake, and soda).
- Drink less or no alcohol.

Fad diets are dangerous because they are almost always unbalanced. Any diet that eliminates a food group should be avoided. Restricting calories to below 1,200 a day does not allow a client to meet all of their nutritional needs. A balanced reducing diet provides enough calories to supply body needs, while allowing for a safe weight reduction of 1–2 lb/week. To lose 1 lb/week of fat, a person needs to achieve a daily calorie deficit of 500 calories. A 1,000-calorie/day deficit is needed to lose 2 lb/week. This calorie deficit can be achieved with a combination of reduced intake and increased output from exercise. Experts advise limiting sustained weight loss to no more than 2 lb/week. Because fat can only be metabolized at a certain rate, weight loss beyond 2 lb/week consists of water and muscle. Guidelines for reducing calorie intake can be found in In Practice: Educating the Client 32-1.

NCLEX Alert

Questions on the NCLEX commonly require that the nurse be aware of therapeutic and modified diets. Modifications to diets may be instituted by the primary healthcare provider at the request of the nurse because it is the nurse who typically assists with meals and modified feedings.

Nutrient Modifications

Modification of certain nutrients is necessary for some conditions. Your knowledge of the nutrients contained in various foods will help you to explain these diets to your clients. Diets may be altered in their content of carbohydrate, fat, protein, minerals, or electrolytes. Nurses are often responsible for consumer education regarding various manufacturer statements related to food products.

Refer to Table 32-2 for nutritional content claims and nursing implications.

Carbohydrate-Controlled Diets
Diabetic Diet

The goals of diabetes mellitus treatment are to maintain blood sugar and fat levels as near to normal as possible and to prevent or delay the onset of complications. Nutrition therapy is the cornerstone of diabetes management, regardless of the affected person's weight, blood glucose levels, or use of medications. A variety of methods can be used for diet planning.

The American Diabetes Association and the Academy of Nutrition and Dietetics publish a series of booklets to assist clients in learning how to plan meals. One method is the "plate" model, which introduces foods as groups, and tips are included for using a plate to plan meals and snacks. Another method uses picture cues for portion sizes and color codes for food types. The **carbohydrate-controlled diet** uses carbohydrate counting. Common carbohydrate foods, such as cereals, rice, pasta, dairy, fruit, and vegetables, are assigned serving sizes that provide approximately 15 g of carbohydrate per serving. The Nutrition Facts Label is used to find the amount of carbohydrate in packaged foods. Typically, the dietician determines how many grams of carbohydrate to eat at each meal, and the client can choose any carbohydrate foods while staying within their limits. The last way to assist people with meal planning is using food groups. This method can be used for diabetes or weight management. Foods are grouped together based on their calorie, carbohydrate, protein, and fat content. The carbohydrate group contains starches, fruits, milk, other carbohydrates (sweets), and nonstarchy vegetables. The protein group includes both animal and vegetable proteins. The fat group lists added fats such as mayonnaise and salad dressing. Working with the client, a healthcare provider sets up an individualized meal plan containing specified numbers of choices from each group for the desired calorie level. This system provides the client with a simplified meal plan and a wide variety of foods from which to choose.

In hospitals and other healthcare facilities, the primary healthcare provider often orders a specific calorie-level diet for clients with diabetes. Most people with type 1 diabetes are of normal weight or underweight, and, therefore, their calorie level should be sufficient to maintain weight or to gain weight as needed. Of clients with type 2 diabetes, 80%–90% are obese. Reduced-calorie diets and weight loss can lower their blood glucose and fat levels and improve insulin action. Unfortunately, these clients seldom achieve long-term weight loss. Older residents of extended care facilities may follow a more liberal diet, often called a *consistent carbohydrate diet*, that simply limits the use of foods high in sugar and provides about the same amount of carbohydrates at each meal.

Clients with diabetes do not need special foods. Clients should eat foods in their natural form (whole fruits instead of juices, brown rice instead of white) to increase fiber intake. Fiber helps regulate blood glucose levels by slowing gastric (stomach) emptying time. Concentrated sweets (sugar, honey, molasses, jams, jellies, and desserts) are not prohibited, but they must be counted to maintain consistent carbohydrate intake. Also, because they provide few nutrients except calories, they should be limited if weight loss is desired. Alcohol should be used only with a healthcare provider's approval because it can cause hypoglycemic reactions, especially when combined with diabetes medication. Individualizing the diet according to the client's likes and dislikes and usual pattern of intake improves the chance of long-term compliance. Encourage the client to follow the treatment plan to minimize the possibility of complications.

Lactose-Restricted Diet

People with *lactose intolerance* lack sufficient amounts of the enzyme *lactase*, which is needed to digest the sugar (lactose) in dairy products. As a result, they develop cramping, gas, and diarrhea after ingesting lactose. Because individual tolerance to lactose varies greatly and lactose intolerance secondary to various gastrointestinal disorders may be temporary, these clients should be urged to include small amounts of milk in their diets to determine their level of tolerance. Often, individuals who are unable to tolerate a glass of milk between meals can tolerate yogurt, aged cheeses, lactose-reduced milk, or milk consumed with food. Milk in cooked breads and other foods is omitted for clients with severe lactose intolerance. Lactose-free milk and over-the-counter medications (e.g., Lactaid) may be helpful for lactose-intolerant clients.

High- and Low-Fat Diets
Fat-Controlled Diet

A **fat-controlled diet** is often the first step in treating individuals with elevated blood lipids or fats (**hyperlipidemia**). These clients may have a high cholesterol level, a high triglyceride level, or both. Untreated, hyperlipidemia can contribute to coronary artery disease, which often has such serious consequences as heart attack, stroke, or death. Heredity or improper diet may cause hyperlipidemia, or it may have a secondary cause, such as diabetes mellitus, hypothyroidism, nephrotic syndrome, or renal failure. In secondary hyperlipidemia, the primary goal is to treat the underlying disease.

The diet for hyperlipidemia is altered in both the total amount of fat and saturated fat provided. Overweight individuals should also lose weight. Diets of clients with hyperlipidemia may have calorie restrictions as well.

Low-Fat Diet

Low-fat diets are used for clients with malabsorption syndromes, pancreatitis, and gallbladder disease. When fat is not being absorbed properly, such as in end-stage liver disease, it causes or aggravates diarrhea and promotes nutrient losses. In all of these cases, total fat, including saturated and unsaturated, is limited to 25%–30% of total calories.

High-Fat Diet

High-fat diets are prescribed for children with seizure disorders when anticonvulsant drugs and a balanced diet have failed to control seizures. This **ketogenic diet** is extremely low in carbohydrates and is sometimes as high as 80%–90% fat. This diet is difficult to follow and must be supplemented with vitamins and minerals. It may lose its effectiveness over time.

Protein-Controlled Diets
High-Protein Diet

A high-protein diet encompasses a range of protein intakes depending on the severity of depletion and causative factors. Protein requirements increase whenever metabolism increases or when tissue needs to be replaced, such as following burns,

TABLE 32-2 Terminology Relating to Nutrient Content Claims and Nursing Implications

CLAIMS BY MANUFACTURER	SERVINGS OR INGREDIENT SIZES OR SERVINGS	CLIENT TEACHING AND NURSING CONSIDERATIONS
Claims for Calories—A "typical" caloric range is 2,000–2,500 calories per day, but this amount does not include considerations for individual needs and lifestyles.		
Calorie-free Low calorie	Less than 5 calories per serving 40 calories or less per serving	Suggestions include food or beverages of less than 20 calories and 5 g of carbohydrates per serving (e.g., diet soft drinks, sugar-free ice pops, sugarless gum, and sugar-free syrup).
Claims for Fat—A teaspoon of margarine weighs about 5 g.		
Fat-free Saturated fat-free Low fat Low saturated fat Reduced fat or less fat	Less than 0.5 g of fat or saturated fat per serving Less than 0.5 g of saturated fat and less than 0.5 g of trans fatty acids 3 g or less of total fat 1 g or less of saturated fat At least 25% less fat than the regular serving	Low-fat foods can be higher in carbohydrates and contain about the same calorie content of foods they replace (e.g., fat-free cookies are high-calorie, high-carbohydrate items). Trans fats are hydrogenated fats; they are produced when liquid oils are made into a solid fat. Avoid high-fat products, such as whole or 2% milk, high-fat meats, sausage, bacon, lard, butter, cream sauces, chocolate, palm oil, palm kernel oil, coconut and coconut oil, and poultry skin.
Claims for Sodium—Consume less than 2,300 mg sodium per day (1 tsp of table salt).		
Sodium-free or salt-free Very low sodium Low sodium Reduced sodium or less sodium Light in sodium Unsalted or no added salt	Less than 5 mg of sodium per serving 35 mg of sodium or less 140 mg of sodium or less At least 25% less sodium than the regular version 50% less sodium than the traditional serving or food No salt added during processing (does not necessarily mean that the food is sodium free)	Individuals with hypertension, African Americans (especially males), and middle-aged and older adults should consume no more than 1,500 mg sodium per day. Encourage foods that are high in potassium, such as leafy green vegetables, fruit from vines, and root vegetables. Adults should get about 4,700 mg of potassium per day, which is readily available in a healthy diet. Salt substitutes (NaCl) often contain potassium (KCl) and are not indicated for many medical conditions; consult the healthcare provider and/or dietitian. Individual products often vary widely as to their sodium content (e.g., reconstituted tomato soup can have a range of 700–1,260 mg of sodium per serving)
Claims for Cholesterol—Eat less than 300 mg cholesterol per day.		
Cholesterol-free Low cholesterol Reduced cholesterol or less cholesterol	Less than 2 mg per serving 20 mg or less At least 25% less cholesterol than the regular version	Include mono- and polyunsaturated fats in your diet. Saturated and trans fat can raise blood cholesterol and increase chances of heart disease. High-cholesterol products include high-fat dairy products (whole milk, ice cream), egg yolks, liver and other organ meats, high-fat meat, and poultry skin. The body makes cholesterol; the remainder of cholesterol comes from consumed foods.
Claims for Sugar—The recommendation is about 45–60 g per meal.		
Sugar free Reduced sugar No sugar added	Less than 0.5 g of sugar per serving At least 25% less sugar per serving than the regular version No sugar added during processing	Use nutrition labels to identify carbohydrates which break down to sugar. Monitor serving size on nutrition label. Does not mean that the product is carbohydrate-free Does not contain high-sugar ingredients, but it still may be high in carbohydrates
Claims for Fiber—The recommendation is 25–30 g of fiber per day.		
High fiber Good source of fiber	5 g or more of fiber per serving 2.5–5 g of fiber per serving	Western societies typically do not consume enough fiber. Encourage the use of dried beans, such as kidney or pinto beans, fruits, vegetables, and whole grains.

American Diabetes Association. (n.d.) *Get to know carbs.* https://www.diabetes.org/nutrition/understanding-carbs/get-to-know-carbs and Dudek, S. (2017). *Nutritional essentials for nursing practice* (8th ed.). Wolters Kluwer.

major trauma, surgery, multiple fractures, hepatitis, and sepsis. Malabsorption syndromes that waste protein, such as diseases of the gastrointestinal tract and the acute phases of inflammatory bowel disease and celiac disease, also elevate protein needs. Protein-losing hemodialysis and peritoneal dialysis clients are treated with a high-protein diet. Clients on dialysis must limit dairy products because of the high phosphorus and potassium content.

Sources of high-quality protein (i.e., protein that contains all the essential amino acids) include eggs (highest quality), meats, poultry, fish, cheeses, and milk. Commercial liquid protein supplements often boost protein intake. To ensure that protein is used for protein synthesis and not for energy needs, a high-protein diet should also be high in carbohydrates.

Protein-Restricted Diet

Kidney and end-stage liver disorders are treated with a controlled-protein diet. The amount of protein allowed may be based on the client's weight (e.g., 0.6–0.8 g/kg body weight) or may be ordered as a total amount per day (e.g., 40 or 60 g). Again, to ensure that dietary protein is used for protein needs, not energy requirements, nonprotein calorie intake should be high. Most protein should be of high quality and should be spread evenly over the day's meals. Other restrictions, such as sodium and fluid, may also be necessary. Because a low-protein diet differs dramatically from the typical American diet, long-term compliance is difficult for many to achieve.

Gluten-Restricted Diet

Celiac disease, a hereditary disorder, is a malabsorption syndrome caused by sensitivity to *gluten*, a protein found in wheat, rye, oats, and barley. A portion of gluten causes the intestinal villi to atrophy and flatten, which severely reduces the absorptive surface of the intestines and impairs brush-border enzyme activity. Consequently, the absorption of many nutrients is impaired. Permanent elimination of gluten from the diet quickly and almost completely reverses the intestinal changes, although lactose intolerance may persist. The gluten-free diet eliminates many foods, including numerous breads and cereals, beer, ale, commercial chocolate milk, anything with malt, cakes, cookies, commercial salad dressing (gluten is a stabilizer), and meat substitutes, such as textured protein products. Breads, cereals, and desserts made with rice, rice flour, corn, cornmeal, potato flour, arrowroot, soybean flour, and tapioca are acceptable. Oats do not contain gluten but may be exposed to gluten products during processing and packaging. Some people with celiac disease choose to avoid oats, and others do not. Special gluten-free products are commercially available, but they are expensive.

Diets With Controlled Minerals and Electrolytes

Sodium-Controlled Diets

The sodium-controlled diet has different levels of restriction, depending on the client's disease and the amount of edema present. *Edema* is an excess accumulation of water and salts in tissues, especially in the lower extremities, which can sometimes be controlled by limiting sodium intake. A sodium-controlled diet is often prescribed for those with cardiac, vascular, and some kidney diseases. Box 32-3 lists substances to avoid in sodium-restricted diets.

> **Box 32-3** Dietary Substances to Avoid or Omit in Sodium Restriction[a]
>
> Examples are given in parentheses.
> - Table salt
> - Vegetable salts (onion, celery, garlic salt); vegetable flakes (parsley, celery)
> - Any smoked, processed, or cured meat or fish (ham, smoked fish, bacon, corned beef, cold cuts, frankfurters, sausage, tongue, salt pork, chipped beef, anchovies, pickled herring)
> - Meat extracts, bouillon cubes, and meat sauces
> - Salty foods (potato chips, popcorn)
> - Prepared condiments (relish, Worcestershire sauce, steak sauces, catsup, pickles, mustard, olives, soy sauce)
> - Prepackaged frozen foods, packaged sauce mixes, packaged gravy mix, and soup mix; frozen peas and lima beans
> - Prepackaged noodle, rice, or potato dishes
> - Canned soups, chili, and beef stews
> - Prepared flour mixes (coating for frying chicken or fish)
> - Packaged baking mixes (cake mix, frosting, pancakes)
> - Frozen fish fillets and shellfish, except oysters
> - Sauerkraut
> - Canned meats, canned vegetables, and ready-made spaghetti sauces
> - Butter, cheeses, and peanut butter
>
> [a]Some foods are permissible if prepared without salt. Consult the label for dietary information.

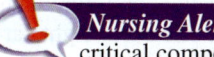

Nursing Alert Minerals and electrolytes are critical components of the body's natural chemistry. Caution must be used when restricting these important substances.

The tolerable upper intake level for adults is less than 2,300 mg or about 1 teaspoon of table salt. Figure 32-4 shows the ranges of healthy and unhealthy sodium in diets (CDC, 2018). The healthcare provider may recommend a *mild sodium restriction* called a *no-added-salt diet* or less than 4,000 mg/day. Salt, and seasonings containing salt, may not be added in cooking or at the table. Overtly salty foods, such as canned soups, beef stew, chili, pickles, olives, potato chips, soy sauce, and cured meats, are discouraged. This diet is used when a person suffers from mild hypertension and stable kidney or heart disease.

A *moderate sodium restriction* of 1,500 mg/day is used in cases of severe edema, hypertension, and heart disease. This diet omits the foods listed in Box 32-3. Salt is not used in cooking or at the table. Milk and milk products are limited to the equivalent of two cups of milk daily, and the use of regular bread may be restricted.

Strict and *severe sodium restrictions* of 500 and 250 mg/day, respectively, are unpalatable and hard to follow. They are used only in severe conditions and for short periods (usually only in a hospital setting). These diets eliminate virtually all foods with added salt and allow only limited quantities of meat, milk, and regular bread. The use of distilled water is necessary.

Salt substitutes are available but should be used only with a healthcare provider's approval. Salt substitutes often contain other electrolytes, such as potassium, which may also be restricted (especially in individuals with kidney disease).

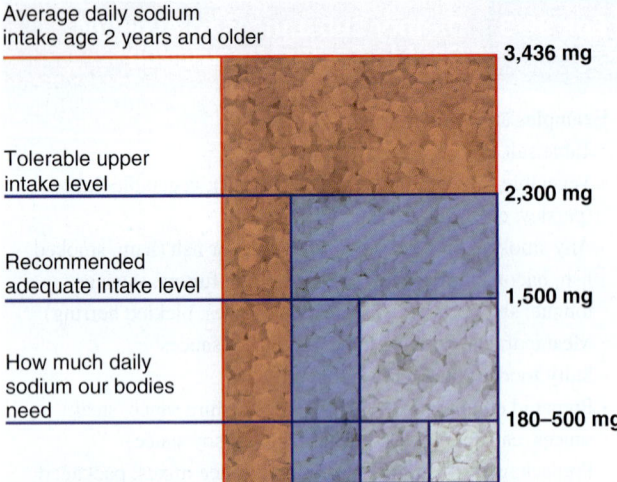

Decreasing sodium intake could prevent thousands of deaths annually because nearly 400,000 deaths each year are attributed to high blood pressure.

Figure 32-4 Ranges of sodium intake. Decreasing sodium intake can be one effective dietary measure in the management of hypertension—weight loss is another. It is important that the client take responsibility for risk factors that can be monitored at home. (Adapted from https://www.cdc.gov/heartdisease/sodium.htm)

Clients may use sodium-free blends of herbs and spices in place of salt to season foods.

The diet for clients with acute heart disease is sometimes divided into five or six small meals daily. Gas-forming foods, foods that are hard to chew or swallow, and stimulants such as coffee and tea may be avoided. The overweight cardiac or hypertensive individual is usually also on a calorie-controlled diet because extra weight adds to the burden on the heart. Sodium is usually restricted as well. These clients should be encouraged to quit smoking and to avoid alcohol.

Calcium- or Phosphorus-Modified Diets

A high calcium intake is indicated for both the prevention and treatment of osteoporosis. Excellent sources of calcium include milk, yogurt, and cheese. A low-phosphorus diet may be indicated for the person with kidney failure. Because protein foods are high in phosphorus, predialysis clients suffering from renal disorders *and* following a low-protein diet are automatically restricting their phosphorus.

Potassium-Modified Diet

A high-potassium diet is given to clients who are taking diuretics. Diuretics flush excess salt and water out of the body but also cause a loss of potassium. Potassium is widespread in the diet; excellent sources include milk, fresh or dried fruits (especially bananas), fresh vegetables, dried peas and beans, whole-grain bread and cereals, fruit juices such as orange and prune, sunflower seeds, watermelon, nuts, molasses, cocoa beans, fresh fish, beef, ham, and poultry. Potassium intake may be limited during end-stage renal failure.

> **Key Concept**
>
> Sodium and potassium restrictions are often needed for specific high-risk populations. No more than 1,500 mg of sodium per day and 4,700 mg/day of potassium are recommended for individuals who are 51 years of age or older, are African American, and have high blood pressure, diabetes, and/or chronic kidney disease (CDC, 2018).

Diets Modified by Serving Size

Often, small frequent feedings help maximize food intake in clients with high nutritional needs or **anorexia** (loss of appetite or refusal to eat). Clients who have recently undergone gastric surgery can usually tolerate frequent small meals. Six small feedings are common, although the number can vary. Any diet can be divided into six meals. Liquid supplements often replace one or more meals because they are nutritionally dense, are easily consumed, and tend to leave the stomach quickly, making them less likely to interfere with the next meal.

Diets Modified for Allergens

Sometimes people have an allergic reaction to certain food substances. This reaction is caused by an autoimmune response to specific proteins called *allergens* in these foods. Allergies to milk, eggs, chocolate, grains, peanuts, and specific fruits are common. Although fruits are not considered protein foods, they contain trace amounts of protein that can cause an allergic reaction. When necessary, these foods are eliminated from the diet. Depending on the number of allergens and how widespread they are in the diet, vitamin and mineral supplements may be necessary to ensure a nutritionally adequate intake.

> **Key Concept**
>
> The optimal modified diet in theory may not be practical for an individual in either the home or clinical setting. The practicality of a diet depends on the person's prognosis, level of intelligence and motivation, support systems, financial status, religious or ethnic background, and coexisting medical conditions.

NUTRITIONAL SUPPORT

Nutritional support is instituted when a person is unable to meet nutritional needs orally. Nutritional support can be short- or long-term. Hospitals often discharge clients who are still receiving nutritional support. Tube feedings are sometimes maintained indefinitely. Nutritional support includes tube feedings, total parenteral nutrition, and administration of intravenous fluids. See Chapter 88 for additional information.

Tube Feedings

A **tube feeding** is a means of providing liquid nourishment through a tube into the gastrointestinal (GI) tract. Tube feedings may also be called *enteral feedings* because they involve the GI tract. This type of feeding may be necessary in certain conditions that prohibit the person from taking adequate oral nourishment. Examples include loss of consciousness, inability to swallow, esophageal or gastric cancer or trauma, oral trauma, mouth surgery, or anorexia. Those suffering from conditions with increased nutritional requirements, such as burns, infection, surgery, or fractures, may also need supplemental nutrition. In some cases, tube feeding is necessary to supply or to maintain adequate nutritional status. A client with any type of enteral tube feeding *must* have a functioning GI tract (see In Practice: Nursing Procedure 32-1).

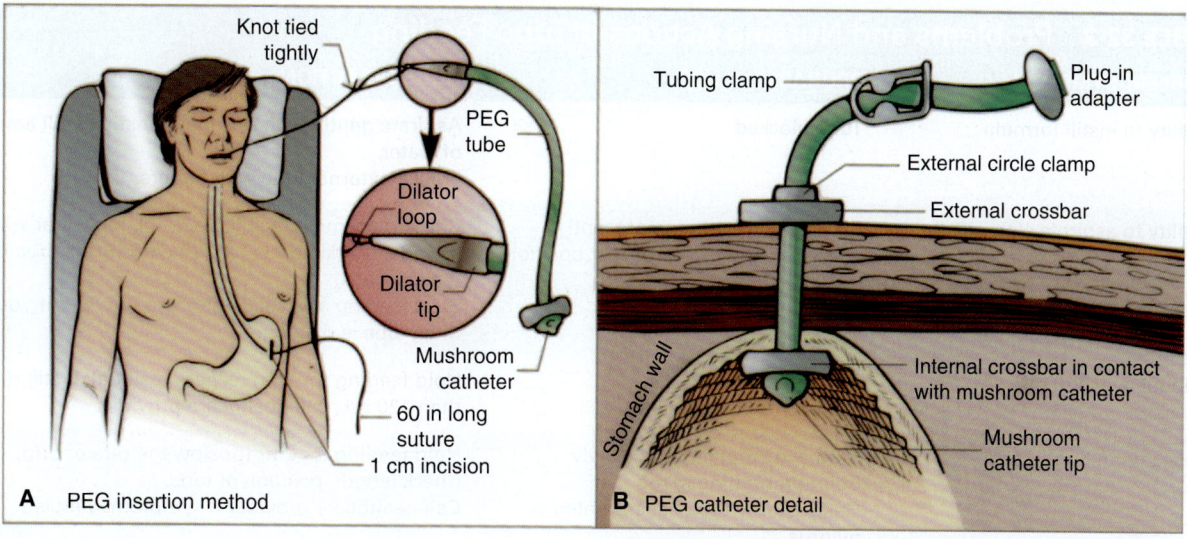

Figure 32-5 **A.** Percutaneous endoscopic gastrostomy (PEG). **B.** A detail of the abdomen and the PEG tube, showing catheter fixation.

Types of Formulas

The liquid formulas for tube feedings contain adequate amounts of protein, fat, carbohydrate, vitamins, and minerals to maintain good nutrition. Routine formulas generally provide about 1 calorie per milliliter. They are lactose free, low in fiber, and 14%–16% protein. Routine formulas are also available in high-calorie, high-protein, and high-fiber varieties. Specialized formulas marketed specifically for stress, renal failure, liver failure, diabetes, acquired immunodeficiency syndrome (AIDS), and other disorders are available.

A dietitian can help the healthcare provider to choose the right formula for an individual. Ready-mixed formulas are available in cans; powdered formulas are also available. Table foods pureed in a blender are often used in the home. Major considerations in choosing a formula are the type and amount of formula and the amount of extra water needed. The cost of different formulas varies.

Placement Sites

Sites of access to the GI tract may differ. If the tube is passed through the client's nose and into the stomach, it is called a nasogastric tube (**NG tube**). This method is uncomfortable and is not used for long-term administration. A tube called a gastrostomy tube (**G tube**) may be placed directly into the stomach through the abdominal wall, or a jejunal tube (**J tube**) may be inserted into the jejunum of the small intestine.

Tubes and Terminology

The name that is given to an enteral tube feeding device may be derived from a particular device, the type of procedure used, or the placement of the tube. Additional information regarding tubes and nursing care of specific tubes is found in Chapter 88. The following are common types of tubes:

- *Nasogastric:* through the nose into the stomach
- *Percutaneous:* percutaneous endoscopic gastrostomy (**PEG**): placed through the skin (Fig. 32-5)
- *Endoscopic:* placed with an instrument called an *endoscope*
- *Gastrostomy:* inserted into the stomach
- *Button feeding device:* a small silicone device used in place of a gastrostomy tube

Each tube has its own equipment, but the means of formula instillation is similar for all types of tubes.

The PEG tube extends 12–15 in. beyond the skin and has a cap covering the end. A short crosspiece (bolster) is placed near the opening through the skin (**stoma**). The nurse must note on the tube the level at which the tube enters the skin and report any change immediately.

A button may replace the PEG-type G tube, especially if long-term administration is anticipated. The function of the button is the same as for the PEG tube; however, the button is level with the skin. It is less cumbersome and more difficult for the confused or agitated adult client or the child to pull out.

Nursing Considerations

In Practice: Nursing Procedure 32-2 outlines steps in tube feeding. The nurse is also responsible for washing or replacing the feeding bag, as per hospital policy, and documenting care. Nursing considerations are also found in Chapter 88; In Practice Nursing Procedure 88-1, Irrigating an NG Tube.

Clients receiving tube feedings may continue to eat or drink by mouth, if the healthcare provider allows. The client may need an extra water ("free water") allowance, administered with or in-between feedings. Water is especially important if the person has a fever or if signs of inadequate hydration develop. Document findings and alert the healthcare provider if untoward signs develop: dry mouth, poor skin turgor (tone), complaints of thirst, illness, fever, or physical complaints (see In Practice: Educating the Client 32-2).

Table 32-3 summarizes problems in tube feeding and nursing actions to be taken.

> **Nursing Alert** The head of the bed must be elevated about 30° whenever a client is receiving a tube feeding. If the bed is put flat, even for a short period of time, such as for changing bed linens, the client has a chance of aspirating stomach contents. Serious complications, such as aspiration pneumonia, may lead to client morbidity or mortality.

TABLE 32-3 Problems and Nursing Actions in Tube Feeding

PROBLEM/SYMPTOM	PROBABLE CAUSE	NURSING ACTION
Inability to instill formula	Tube blocked	Aspirate gently with syringe or instill small amount of water. "Milk" external tube with fingers.
Inability to aspirate stomach fluid from tube	May be normal (none present) Tube dislodged from proper position	Check placement. Instill 10–20-mL tap water with syringe; quickly draw back (if discolored, tube is in the stomach). Stop feeding and call healthcare provider if you think tube is dislodged.
Residual over 120 mL	Feeding too fast Stomach slow to empty	Hold feeding for 2 hr, recheck residual; if still more than 120 mL, call healthcare provider.
Nausea, vomiting	Stomach emptying too slowly Solution running in too fast Gastrostomy tube has migrated to pylorus	Hold feeding for 2 hr (or slow the rate of drip). Check length, position of tube. Call healthcare provider if symptoms persist.
Abdominal cramps, diarrhea	Formula too high in fat Concentrated formula running too fast Formula cold Formula spoiled Change in formula or medications	Request/switch to lower-fat formula. Hold feeding for 2 hr (or slow drip rate). Call healthcare provider if symptoms persist (healthcare provider may order formula to be diluted or changed). Give canned formulas at room temperature; warm refrigerated formulas to room temperature in hot water. Refrigerate mixed formula; discard after 24 hr.
Gas	Too much air in the stomach	Decompress as ordered.
Stoma bleeding (more than few drops), red, irritated	Gastric leakage	Call healthcare provider STAT if blood mixed with stomach contents, or fever, odor. If persists, call healthcare provider.
Red, irritated skin around stoma	Improper skin care	Provide good skin care.
Thirst, weakness, fever (>100 °F), reduced urine output (normal is >1.5 L/day)	Infection Dehydration (body lacks fluids) Formula intolerance	Call healthcare provider (may increase amount of free fluids with or between feedings).
Change in skin color (to pale or dusky), cough, noisy breathing, wheeze, restlessness, agitation, fever >100 °F	Aspiration (backup of water or feeding into lungs)	Position the client with the head/upper body elevated 40°, keep elevated for 30 min after feedings. Add small amount of food coloring to formula (to determine if sputum coughed up is mixed with formula). Encourage person to cough and clear lungs. Call healthcare provider for further instructions.
Severe constipation (decrease in number of bowel movements expected because less residue in feeding formulas)	Lack of fluids in body Low-fiber formula Inactivity Change in formula or medications	Check for adequate fluid intake. Notify healthcare provider if continues more than 3 days. Request/switch to higher-fiber formula.
Formula will not drip with gravity system	Bag height too low Residue buildup in bag Residue buildup in tube	Raise bag to 3 ft above stomach level. Wash feeding bag and flush tubing with vinegar water (or replace). Flush tube with 50-mL warm water, diet soda, or cranberry juice. Use a small syringe (≤3 mL) to provide greater pressure and unclog tube.
Gastrostomy tube becomes dislodged from stomach	Malfunction of balloon or device holding tube in place	Notify team leader or healthcare provider immediately for instructions (tract may close off).
Gastrostomy tube is longer or shorter than usual	Tube has become dislodged or migrated down into the stomach or pylorus	Gently pull, push, or rotate tube to original position. Call healthcare provider if unable to relocate.

IN PRACTICE
EDUCATING THE CLIENT 32-2 — Tube Feedings

Many clients go home with tube feedings. Teaching the client and family how to mix formula, run the pump or use the gravity system, and care for equipment is an important teaching responsibility. Many home care interventions involve teaching appropriate tube feeding administration and maintenance.

Intravenous Therapy

Intravenous (**IV**) therapy or *parenteral therapy* involves injecting into a vein any number of sterile solutions that the body needs, including drugs and electrolytes. Simple IV solutions, infused through a peripheral vein, contain water with low concentrations of dextrose, electrolytes, or both. IV solutions are used on a short-term basis to restore or maintain fluid and electrolyte balance. Because it is nutritionally inadequate, simple IV therapy is not used for more than a few days without some sort of supplementation. Parenteral nutrition is used when the client cannot take sufficient amounts of nutrients via the enteral route (GI tract). These clients include those with severe burns or a disorder of the GI tract (e.g., surgical removal of parts of the GI tract) that may inhibit absorption of nutrients.

Total and Peripheral Parenteral Nutrition

Total parenteral nutrition (**TPN**) is a specifically formulated and calculated solution that is nutritionally complete to meet a specific individual's needs. Sometimes TPN is called *hyperalimentation*, although this term is not completely accurate.

Total parenteral nutrition is used when the GI tract is functioning improperly, such as in stomach cancer, or when a person has multiple trauma, severe infection, burns, or multiorgan failure. TPN is infused directly into the blood circulation and bypasses the digestive tract. TPN contains only carbohydrate and protein. Lipids are given separately to prevent an essential fatty acid deficiency. Several types of catheters (tubes) are used. The large catheter is surgically placed into the central vein near the heart to allow the concentrated solution to be diffused quickly into the circulation. TPN has grown in acceptance as both a short- and long-term therapy modality.

Chapter 88 introduces the care of central line catheters and nursing implications of TPN. One of the most important considerations is prevention of infection at the catheter insertion site.

Peripheral parenteral nutrition (**PPN**) contains lesser concentrations of the same ingredients found in central vein TPN, administered into a peripheral vein. It is used to provide temporary nutritional support and to promote protein synthesis

TABLE 32-4 Common Food–Drug Interactions

FOOD	DRUG	EFFECT
Grapefruit Grapefruit juice (Furanocoumarins)	Some statins: atorvastatin (Lipitor), simvastatin (Zocor), pravastatin (Pravachol) Some antihistamines: fexofenadine (Allegra) Some blood pressure meds: nifedipine (Procardia XL) Some antianxiety meds: buspirone (BuSpar) Some antiarrhythmia meds: amiodarone (Pacerone) Some thyroid replacement drugs Some birth control meds	Higher than normal amounts of the drug in the blood may become toxic.
Green leafy vegetables	Warfarin (Coumadin)	Vitamin K in the food reduces the effectiveness of the drug.
Natural black licorice (Glycyrrhiza)	Lanoxin (Digoxin) Hypertension meds: Hydrochlorothiazide (Microzide), spironolactone (Aldactone), and warfarin (Coumadin)	Enhanced effect from digoxin can result in altered heart rate. Decreases effectiveness.
Salt substitutes	Lanoxin (Digoxin) ACE inhibitors	Decreases effectiveness. Elevates blood potassium levels.
Tyramine-containing foods: • Aged cheese • Wine • Chocolate • Smoked meats • Aged/fermented meats • Hot dogs • Fermented soy products • Draft beer	MAO inhibitors	Increases blood pressure.

ACE, angiotensin-converting enzyme; MAO, monoamine oxidase.
National Consumers League and U.S. Food and Drug Administration (2017). *Avoid food and drug interactions: A guide from the National Consumers League and U.S. Food and Drug Administration* [Brochure].

and weight gain when oral intake is inadequate or contraindicated. **Infusions** given peripherally must be hypotonic or isotonic (to prevent dehydration and electrolyte imbalance). Therefore, PPN provides fewer calories than TPN.

> **Nursing Alert** The prolonged use of nothing by mouth (NPO) is a serious problem. A client may be NPO for tests, after surgery, or because of vomiting. A client who has been NPO for 3 or more days and is not receiving nutritional support is at serious nutritional risk. Bring this client to the attention of the team leader or healthcare provider.

FOOD AND MEDICATION INTERACTIONS

Occasionally, medications and foods mix poorly or cause unwanted side effects. Some foods render medications ineffective. Some medications should be taken with food or water, and some should be given between meals. A few medications react negatively with dairy products or alcohol. You should know the reactions of therapeutic medications when given with certain foods or liquids. Table 32-4 and Box 62-3 contain some of the most common food–drug interactions. Chapter 9 expands the discussion of specific medications and food interactions.

STUDENT SYNTHESIS

KEY POINTS

- As a nurse, you play an important role in helping clients to meet their nutritional needs.
- Fluid is required to maintain homeostasis; too much plain water can lead to electrolyte imbalance.
- Documenting food and fluid intake is an important part of nursing care.
- Some individuals need special assistance to eat because of their age or a physical disorder.
- Modified diets may include changes in consistency, nutrient content, or energy (calorie) value.
- The treatment and daily maintenance of diabetes depends greatly on the types and amounts of nutrients consumed.
- Tube feeding is a commonly used means of providing nourishment and nutritional support.
- Total parenteral nutrition (TPN) may be used in clients who have limited capacities or disorders of the gastrointestinal tract. TPN has many complications and nursing considerations.

CRITICAL THINKING EXERCISES

1. Your client is not eating the meals served in the hospital. Describe the skills you can use to help the client regain strength by eating.
2. Discuss persons who need special assistance with meals. Describe why they need such assistance and what help you can give.

NCLEX-STYLE REVIEW QUESTIONS

1. The nurse is assisting a client, who is visually impaired, with the meal tray. Which nursing action can promote independence in self-feeding?
   a. Feed the client if the client begins spilling items.
   b. Place the food on the utensil and give it to the client.
   c. Describe the location of the foods as if they are on the face of a clock.
   d. Only give finger food such as sandwiches.

2. The nurse is caring for a group of clients at an extended-care facility. Which clients would require documentation and reporting to the team leader?
   a. A client who is eating only 25% of the meal trays for 3 days.
   b. A client who states, "I feel nauseated and don't want to eat."
   c. A client who states, "I am having a hard time swallowing your food."
   d. A client who states, "Your food doesn't taste very good."
   e. A client who states, "I'm eating better here than I was at home."

3. The nurse is caring for a client who is edentulous and has difficulty chewing. Which therapeutic diet should the nurse suggest that would be helpful and nutritious?
   a. Mechanical soft diet
   b. Low-fiber diet
   c. Bland diet
   d. High-calorie diet

4. The nurse is discussing a client's concern regarding recent weight gain. About which type of diet should the nurse educate the client?
   a. Bland diet
   b. Reduced-calorie diet
   c. Mechanical soft diet
   d. Low-fiber diet

5. Which information should the nurse provide to a client regarding the ketogenic diet?
   a. Very low in carbohydrates and high in fat
   b. Allows for unlimited fruits and vegetables
   c. Low in protein and high in carbohydrates
   d. Reduced in calories

CHAPTER 32 Diet Therapy and Special Diets

Welcome Steps

Look at healthcare provider's orders.

Protocol for procedure.

Necessary equipment/supplies.

Wash hands using proper hand hygiene; put on gloves.

Explain the procedure and reassure the client.

Locate two identifiers to confirm correct client.

Comfortable and efficient position for nurse and client.

Obtain privacy.

Make sure to follow correct steps and body mechanics with good technique.

Ensure safety and observe deviations from normal.

End Steps

Ensure comfort and safety.

Note questions or concerns from client or nurse; note significant data.

Dispose of materials properly.

Disinfect the area and your hands.

Document and report the procedure and your findings.

IN PRACTICE

NURSING PROCEDURE 32-1 Inserting a Nasogastric (NG) Tube (Nasogastric Intubation)

Supplies and Equipment
Gloves
Additional PPE, as indicated
Nasogastric tube
Water-soluble substance (K–Y jelly)
Protective towel covering for client
Emesis basin
Nonallergenic tape for marking placement and securing tube, skin barrier
Normal saline or sterile water, for irrigation, per facility policy
Flashlight
Tongue blade
Irrigation set
Tissues
Clamp
pH paper
Glass of water (if allowed)
Straw for glass of water
Stethoscope
60-ml catheter tip syringe
Rubber band and safety pin
Suction equipment or tube feeding equipment

Note: Occasionally, two people may be needed for insertion. One person assists the client with positioning, holding the glass of water (if allowed), and encouragement.

Steps
Follow LPN welcome steps and then

1. Check the healthcare provider's order and determine the type, size, and purpose of the NG tube. *Rationale:* If the healthcare provider did not order a specific size, it is generally acceptable to insert a size 16 or 18 French, which are standard adult sizes. Sizes suitable for children vary from a very small size 5 French for children to size 12 French for older children. Larger NG (size 20–30 French) or enteric tubes, such as an Ewald tube (which is used for gastric lavage of toxins) and the Cantor tube or Miller–Abbott tube, may require insertion by a healthcare provider. The Cantor and Miller–Abbott tubes are quite large and have mercury-, air-, or fluid-filled bags attached to the distal end of the tube. The purpose of the bag is to advance the tube with peristaltic waves, with the therapeutic intent of breaking up intestinal blockages.

2. Check the client's identification band. *Rationale:* Be sure that the procedure is being done on the correct client, with the appropriate type of tube.

3. Set up tube-feeding equipment or suction equipment and test to make sure it functions properly. *Rationale:* Be sure that the equipment is functioning properly and is at the right rate of flow or strength of suction before using it on the client. The healthcare provider may order a specific type of NG tube, such as a Levin, for short-term use for gavage or lavage; or a Salem sump with its two lumens, generally used for lavage and gastric suctioning; or a silicone type tube, used for long-term placement for tube feedings.

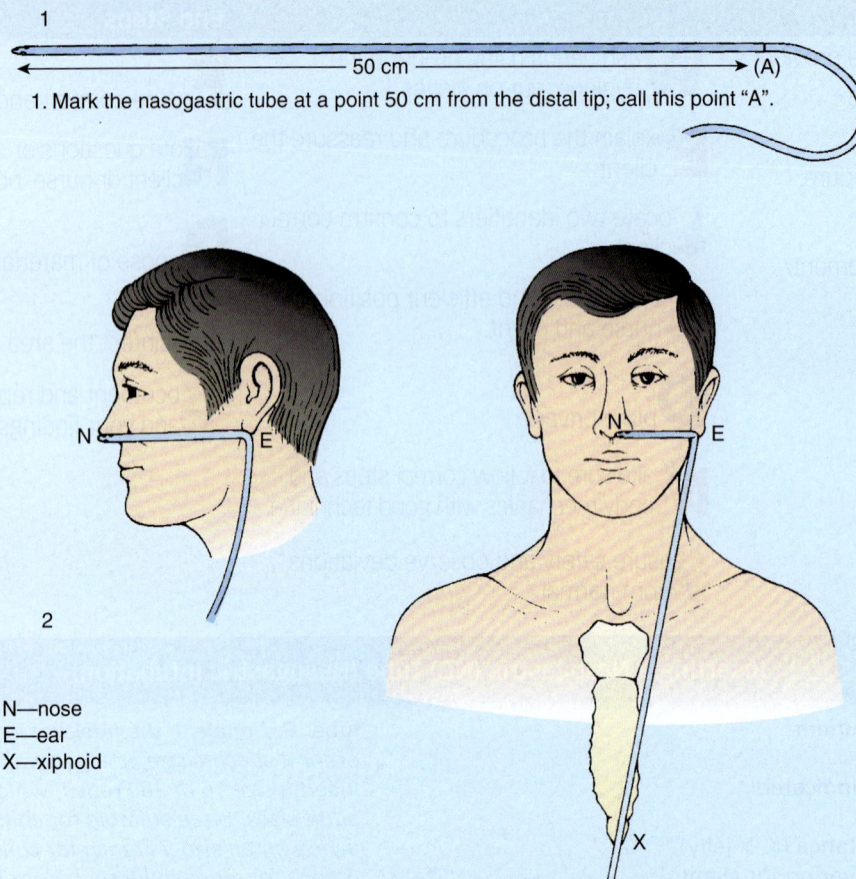

N—nose
E—ear
X—xiphoid

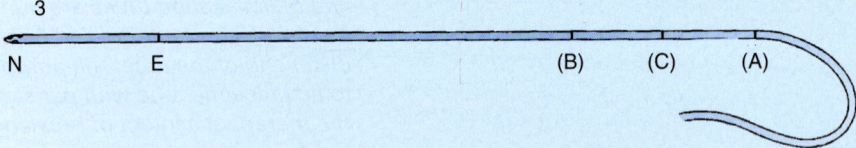

Measuring length of nasogastric tube for placement into stomach.

4. Instruct the client in the procedure and assess their capability of cooperating with the procedure. *Rationale: It is not advisable to explain the procedure too far in advance because the client's anxiety about the procedure may interfere with its success. It is important that the client relax, swallow, and cooperate during the procedure.*

5. Wash your hands. Put on gloves. *Rationale: Clean, not sterile, technique is necessary because the gastrointestinal (GI) tract is not sterile.*

6. Position client in full Fowler position if possible (see Chapter 48). Place a clean towel over the client's chest as a bib-type protection. *Rationale: Full Fowler position assists the client to swallow and promotes peristalsis. A towel is used as a covering to protect bed linens and the client's gown.*

7. Measure the length of the tube that will be needed to reach the stomach. The first measurement is made from the tip of the client's nose to the earlobe, and the second measurement is made from that point at the earlobe to the xiphoid process. Mark this spot with a small piece of temporary tape. *Rationale: Each client will have a slightly different terminal insertion point. Measurements must be made for each individual's anatomy.*

8. With a damp washcloth, wipe the client's face and nose. Do not use soap. It may be necessary to wipe the outside of the nose with an alcohol wipe. Be sure to cover the eyes with a small, dry towel or washcloth when wiping down the exterior of the nose with an alcohol wipe. *Rationale: The NG tube will stay more secure if taped on a clean,*

nonoily nose. If the nose has been cleaned with an alcohol wipe, the tape will stay more secure and the tube will not move in the throat—causing gagging or discomfort later.

9. Cover the client's eyes with a cloth. *Rationale:* This protects the client's eyes from any alcohol fumes from the alcohol wipe.

10. Ask the client if they have difficulty breathing out of one nostril. You may test for nares obstructions by closing one nostril and then the other and asking the client to breathe through the nose for each attempt. If the client has difficulty breathing out of one nostril, try to insert the NG tube in that one. *Rationale:* Many individuals have nasal obstructions or blocked nasal passages. After the procedure, the client may breathe more comfortably if the "good" nostril remains patent. The blocked nasal passage may not be totally occluded, and thus, you may still be able to pass an NG tube. It may be necessary to use the more patent nostril for insertion.

11. Apply water-soluble lubricant to 4–8 in. of the tube. *Rationale:* The tube slides in more easily if well lubricated. The mucosa is less likely to be damaged during insertion. The healthcare provider may numb the nose and nasopharynx with a numbing solution to ease client comfort and suppress the gag reflex. Sometimes, having the client hold ice chips in the mouth for a few minutes before the procedure can also have a numbing effect that can minimize the gag reflex.

12. With the client sitting up, flex the head forward. Tilt the tip of the nose upward and insert the tube gently into the nose to as far as the back of the throat. Guide the tube straight back. *Rationale:* Flexing the head aids in the anatomic insertion of the tube. The tube is less likely to pass into the trachea.

13. When the tube reaches the nasopharynx, stop briefly and have the client lower their head slightly. Have the client or the assistant hold the glass of water with the straw. Keep an emesis basin and tissues handy. *Rationale:* The positioning helps the passage of the NG to follow anatomic landmarks. Swallowing water, if allowed, helps the passage of the NG tube.

14. Ask the client to swallow as the tube is advanced. Advance the tube several times as the client swallows until the correct marked position on the tube is reached. Encourage the client to breathe through their mouth. *Rationale:* When the client swallows, the tube has a better chance of passing into the stomach instead of the trachea. Stimulating the gag reflex is normal, but swallowing while gently advancing the tube will minimize the gag reflex.

15. If coughing, persistent gagging, cyanosis, or dyspnea occurs, remove the tube immediately. *Rationale:* The tube may be in the trachea.

16. If obstruction is felt, pull out the tube and try the other nostril. *Rationale:* The client's nostril may deflect the NG into an inappropriate position. Let the client rest a moment and retry on the other side.

17. Insert the tube as far as the marked insertion point. Place a temporary piece of tape across the nose and tube. *Rationale:* In this way, you can check for placement before securing the tube. If you do not secure the tube before checking for placement, the tube may move out of position.

18. Check the back of the client's throat to make sure that the tube is not curled in the back of the throat. *Rationale:* On occasion, the NG will curl up in the back of the throat instead of passing down to the stomach. You will need visual inspection to see if this has happened. Remove the entire NG and start again if this has happened.

19. Check the tube for correct placement by at least two and preferably three of the following methods:

    A. Aspirate stomach contents. Stomach aspirate will appear cloudy, green, tan, off-white, bloody, or brown. It is not always visually possible to distinguish between stomach and respiratory aspirates. *Special note:* The small diameters of some NG tubes make aspiration problematic. The tubes themselves collapse when suction is applied via the syringe. Thus, contents cannot be aspirated.

    B. Check pH of aspirate. Measuring the pH of stomach aspirate is considered more accurate than visual inspection. Stomach aspirate generally has a pH range of 0–4, commonly less than 4. The aspirate of respiratory contents is generally more alkaline, with a pH of 7 or more.

    C. Inject 30 mL of air into the stomach and listen with the stethoscope for the "whoosh" of air into the stomach. The small diameter of some NG tubes may make it difficult to hear air entering the stomach.

    D. Confirm by x-ray placement. X-ray visualization is the only method that is considered positive.

20. Once stomach placement has been confirmed, tape the tube using your prepared tape strips or a commercial NG securing tape. *Rationale:* It is vital to ensure that the NG is in its correct place within the stomach because, if by accident the NG is within the trachea, serious complications related to the lungs would result. The goal of securing the tube in place is to prevent peristaltic movement from advancing the tube or from the tube accidentally being pulled out.

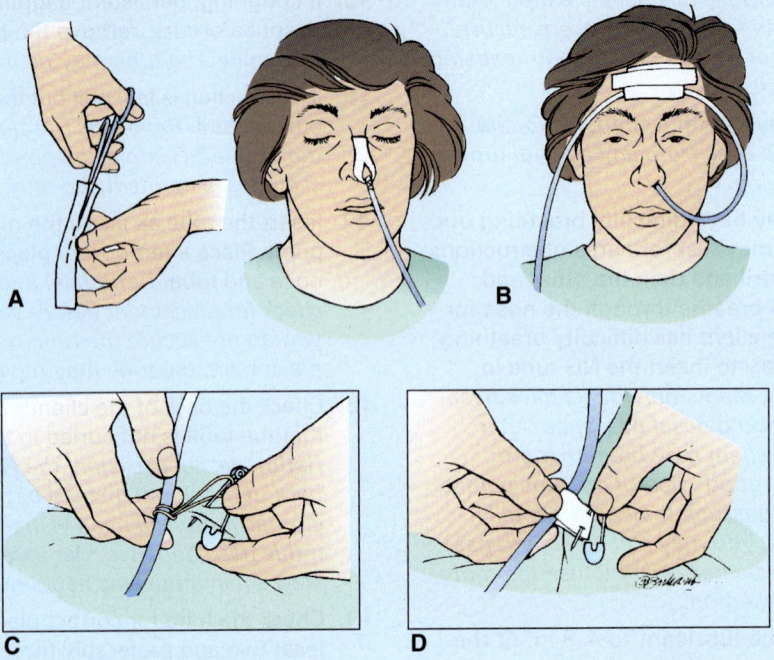

Securing nasogastric and nasoenteric tubes. **A.** The nasogastric tube is secured to the nose with tape to prevent injury to the nasopharyngeal passages; the cheek may also be used. **B.** Tape is placed on the forehead, and the nasoenteric tube is taped to it, thereby allowing the tube to be advanced until the desired placement is achieved. **C, D.** Secure tubing to the client's gown with an elastic band or tape attached to a safety pin to prevent tension on the line during movement.

Follow ENDDD steps.

Special Reminders
- Chart the procedure, stating the date, time, type, and size of NG tube used; left or right nostril used; amount and type of aspirate; suction or feeding started; and client response to the procedure (e.g., *16 French Levin tube inserted into right nostril with minimal difficulty and set to low intermittent suction at 25 mmHg per Gomco*).
- It is not uncommon to have slight bleeding from irritation of the mucosa in the nose. Any trauma or difficulty during the procedure needs to be charted, documented, and observed.
- After the procedure, chart and monitor the type of suction used and the amount of suction. During each shift, monitor and record the suction in millimeters of mercury (mmHg) and the amount and type of aspirate.
- Institute monitoring of intake and output (I&O).
- Always confirm placement of the NG tube before insertion of medications, application of suction, or instillation of tube feedings. *Rationale: It is possible for the tube to become dislodged between treatments.*
- To prevent aspiration of stomach contents during NG tube feedings, the head of the bed must remain elevated at 30° or more at all times.

IN PRACTICE
NURSING PROCEDURE 32-2: Administering a Tube Feeding

Supplies and Equipment
Gloves
Feeding pump (if ordered), IV pole
Clamp (optional)
Feeding solution at room temperature
Large catheter tip syringe (30 mL or larger)
Feeding bag with tubing
Water
Measuring cup
Other optional equipment (disposable pad, pH indicator strips, water-soluble lubricant, paper towels)

Steps
Follow LPN welcome steps and then

1. Prepare formula:
   A. Shake can thoroughly. Check expiration date. *Rationale: Feeding solution may settle and requires mixing before administration. Outdated formula may be contaminated or have lessened nutritional value.*
   B. If formula is in powdered form, mix according to the instructions on the package. Prepare enough for 24 hr only. Use a large-enough container for the mixed amount and refrigerate any unused formula. Label and date the container. Allow formula to reach room temperature before using. *Rationale: Formula loses its nutritional value and can harbor microorganisms if kept more than 24 hr. Cold formulas can cause abdominal discomfort.*

2. Explain the procedure to the client. *Rationale: Providing information fosters the client's cooperation and understanding.*

3. Check the position of the client. The position of the client with a tube feeding should always remain with the head of the bed elevated at least 30°–40°. Do not place the client in a supine position; this may lead to aspiration pneumonia and death from pulmonary complications. *Rationale: This position discourages aspiration of feeding solution that is already in the stomach back into the lungs.*

4. Determine placement of feeding tube by:

   Intermittent or bolus feeding
   a. Aspirating stomach secretions. *Rationale: Aspiration of gastric fluid indicates that the tube is correctly placed in the stomach. The amount of residual reflects gastric emptying time and indicates whether the feeding should continue. Residual contents are returned to the stomach because they contain valuable electrolytes and digestive enzymes.*
   - Attach syringe to end of feeding tube.
   - Gently pull back on plunger.
   - Measure amount of residual fluid (clamp tube if it is necessary to remove the syringe).
   - Return residual to stomach via tube and continue with feeding if amount does not exceed agency protocol or healthcare provider's orders (if greater than 120 mL or no return is obtained, refer to "problem list" in Table 32-3).

   b. Injecting 10–20 mL of air into tube (3–5 mL for children). *Rationale: A whooshing or gurgling sound usually indicates that the tube is in the stomach. This method may not be a reliable indicator with small-bore feeding tubes.*
   - Attach syringe filled with air to tube.
   - Inject air while listening with stethoscope over left upper quadrant.

   c. Measuring the pH of aspirated gastric secretions. *Rationale: Gastric contents are acidic, and a pH indicator strip should reflect a range of 1–4. Pleural fluid and intestinal fluid are slightly basic in nature.*

   d. Taking an x-ray or ultrasound (may be needed to determine tube placement).

5. **If using a feeding bag**:
   a. Hang the feeding bag setup 12–18 in. above the stomach. Clamp the tubing. Fill the bag with prescribed formula and prime the tubing by opening the clamp, allowing the feeding to flow through the tubing. Reclamp the tube. *Rationale: Formula clears air from the tubing and prevents it from entering the stomach.*
   b. Attach end of the setup to the gastric tube and open the clamp. Adjust flow according to the healthcare provider's order. *Rationale: Rapid feeding may cause nausea and abdominal cramping.*
   c. Add 30–60 mL of water to the feeding bag as feeding is completed. Clamp the tube and disconnect the feeding setup. *Rationale: Water clears the tube, keeping it patent. Clamping after feeding is completed prevents air from entering the stomach.*

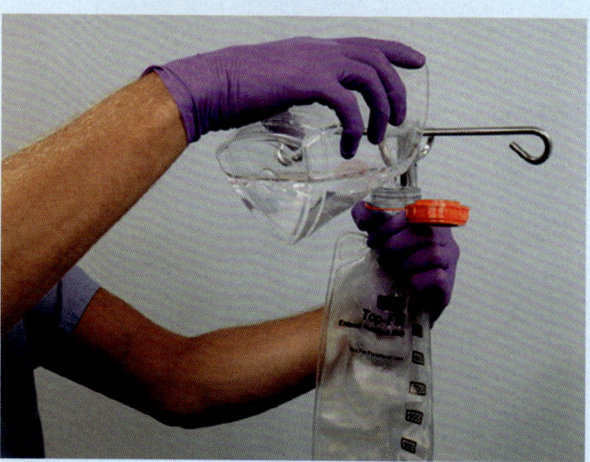

Adding water to rinse feeding tube. (Lynn, 2011.)

6. **If using a syringe:**
   Continuous feeding
   a. Clamp the gastric tube. Insert the tip of the large syringe, with the plunger or bulb removed, into the gastric tube. Pour feeding into the syringe. Raise the syringe 12–18 in. above the stomach. Open the clamp. *Rationale: Gravity promotes movement of feeding into the stomach.*
   b. Allow feeding solution to flow slowly into the stomach. Raise and lower the syringe to control the rate of flow. Add additional formula to the syringe as it empties until feeding is complete. *Rationale: Controlling administration and flow rate of feeding solution prevents air from entering the stomach and nausea and abdominal cramping from developing.*

7. **If using a feeding pump:**
   a. Clamp the feeding setup and hang on pole. Add feeding solution to the bag. Open the clamp and prime the tubing. *Rationale: Formula clears air from the tubing and prevents it from entering the stomach.*
   b. Thread the tubing through or load tubing into the pump, according to the manufacturer's specifications.
   c. Attach the end of the setup to the gastric tube. Set the prescribed rate and volume according to the manufacturer's directions. Open the clamp and turn on the pump. *Rationale: Pump controls the rate of administration and volume of formula.*
   d. Stop the feeding every 4–8 hr and assess the residual. Flush the tube every 6–8 hr. *Rationale: The amount of residual reflects gastric emptying time and indicates whether the feeding should continue. Flushing the tube keeps it patent.*

8. Terminate feeding when completed. Instill prescribed amount of water. Keep the client's head elevated for 20–30 min. *Rationale: Elevated position discourages aspiration of feeding solution into the lungs.*

9. Assess the skin around the injection site of surgically placed tubes. Cleanse skin with mild soap and water and dry thoroughly. Check site for redness, swelling, pain, or additional signs of inflammation. *Rationale: Careful assessment and care can prevent infection and skin breakdown.*

10. Provide mouth care by brushing teeth, offering mouthwash, and keeping the lips moist. *Rationale: These activities promote oral hygiene and improve comfort.*

Follow ENDDD steps.

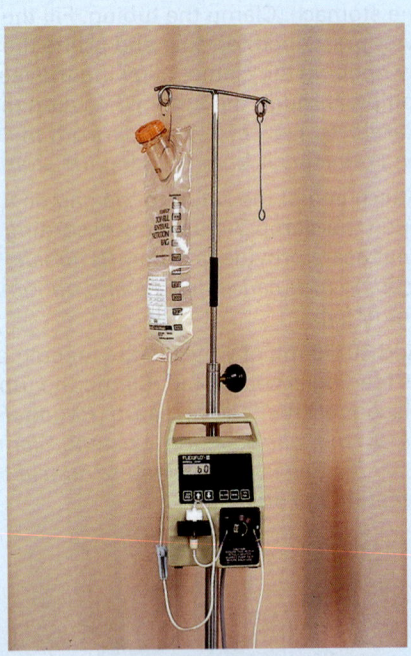

Feeding pump.

The Nursing Process | UNIT 6

33 Introduction to the Nursing Process

Learning Objectives

1. Define and discuss the process of problem-solving.
2. Differentiate between trial and error problem-solving and scientific problem-solving.
3. State the characteristics of critical thinking.
4. Identify how critical thinking is used in the problem-solving process.
5. Define the nursing process and relate it to the critical thinking method of solving problems.
6. Define the following steps of the nursing process: nursing assessment, nursing diagnosis, planning, implementation, and evaluation.
7. Discuss the following terms relating to the nursing process: *systematic, client-oriented, goal-oriented, continuous,* and *dynamic.*
8. Discuss how the nursing process is an important tool for providing measurable and observable quality nursing care for clients.

Important Terminology

client-oriented
critical thinking
evaluation
goal-oriented
implementation
long-term goal
nursing
assessment
nursing care plan
nursing diagnosis
nursing process
planning
potential needs
prioritization;
prioritizing
scientific
problem-solving
short-term goal
trial and error
problem-solving

Acronyms

NCP
UAP

A primary goal of nursing is to help individuals meet their basic and higher level needs. Meeting with clients leads to specific interactions, including communication, observation, support, education, and provision of care. Nurses support and encourage individuals in their healthy habits and help clients solve health problems. They provide care to clients by combining scientific problem-solving methods with critical thinking skills to provide care through the **nursing process**.

Key Concept

The nursing process is a fundamentally unique problem-solving process that highlights the differences in roles between licensed personnel (RN and LVN/LPN) and nonlicensed personnel (CNA, NA, UAP). The nursing process not only includes the actions involved in tasks but also integrates critical thinking. In other words, unlicensed personnel are required to know *how* to take vital signs. In addition to *how,* the licensed nurse must also know *why* the vital signs are important and *what* the relationship is between the numbers obtained and the condition of the client.

PROBLEM-SOLVING

Problem-solving is the basic skill of identifying a problem and taking steps to resolve it. Common sense is helpful in solving many problems. However, when a problem is complex or challenging to define, you may need to use other—more formal—methods of problem-solving.

Trial and Error

Trial and error problem-solving is an experimental approach that tests ideas to decide which methods work and which do not. Usually, the results are completely unknown until tried because the experimenter simply does not have sufficient information to anticipate results. Sometimes, you use trial and error to solve problems in your everyday life. Consider your dilemma if you have an allergy to an unknown substance in hand lotion but also have a problem with dry skin and wish to soften your hands. You try one brand, but develop a rash. You try another brand with the same results. These trials result in errors: The lotions continue to cause an allergic response. Eventually, you find a brand that works without causing a rash, and your trial is successful.

A form of trial and error experimentation is used in laboratory studies when testing several solutions to a problem. Solutions that are harmful or ineffective are discarded until helpful solutions are found. In other situations, trial and error is used when unexpected results occur that could possibly have beneficial outcomes for another problem. For example, minoxidil (Rogaine) was first marketed as an antihypertensive drug. However, the unexpected result of hair growth led to experimentation and development of drug forms for the treatment of hair loss.

Many advances in modern healthcare have resulted from this type of experimentation; however, trial and error must be used carefully when working with people because of the possible harmful results. Researchers develop strict guidelines to protect the safety and well-being of individuals and proceed with trial and error experimentation only with the permission and understanding of the individual involved.

Scientific Problem-Solving

Today's society prefers that only safe and proven effective treatments be given to those who are ill. Therefore, healthcare providers rely on previously proven facts to determine which treatments are safe. Scientists and healthcare researchers use a precise method to investigate problems and arrive at solutions. This method, called **scientific problem-solving**, allows researchers to discover the best possible safe and effective treatments for disease or dysfunction. The seven steps of scientific problem-solving are as follows:

1. Identify the problem.
2. Gather information relative to the problem.
3. Formulate tentative solutions (hypotheses); choose preferred solution.
4. Plan action to test suggested solution.
5. Experiment and observe the results.
6. Interpret the results (draw conclusions); understand what the results mean.
7. Evaluate the solution, either concluding or revising the study to test the solution again if results are unsatisfactory.

Scientific problem-solving requires both logical thought and imagination. When you use scientific problem-solving, you combine what you have learned from your own experience with facts previously proven through scientific study.

CRITICAL THINKING

Unless you have already been educated as a scientist, you probably confront problems and find solutions without using trial and error or scientific problem-solving. You may use a complicated mix of inquiry, knowledge, intuition, logic, experience, and common sense called **critical thinking**. This kind of thinking enables you to grasp the meaning of multiple clues and to find quick answers when facing difficult problems. Critical thinking is neither trial and error nor a structured scientific problem-solving system.

Critical thinking has some characteristics that are important for solving problems in healthcare. When you think critically, you examine facts and compare these facts with information you already know, thereby being actively curious

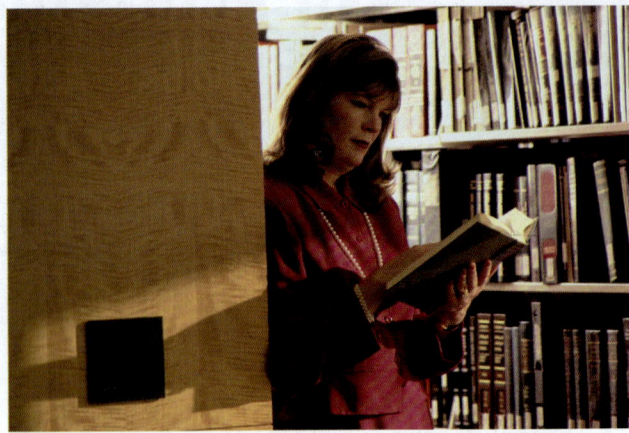

Figure 33-1 Critical thinking utilizes previous knowledge, research, and analysis, as well as common sense, to solve problems.

and critiquing ideas for reasonableness. You form ideas or concepts that are mental pictures of reality. You are reasonable and rational, continuously searching to understand the entire situation. You may think randomly, without a particular method or pattern; however, you do not jump to conclusions. As a critical thinker, you form your own beliefs or ideas rather than automatically accepting the thoughts or ideas of others. You become an open-minded person, flexible to alternatives. You also use your imagination and creativity systematically to gather information and draw conclusions (Fig. 33-1).

Consider a simple example of how you use critical thinking when confronted with a problem. Early one morning your car keys are not in their usual location. You have only 30 min to get to class for a required examination. What do you do first? You probably search frantically again, but then stop to think about where else you may have left your keys. Perhaps you retrace your steps of the previous day when you last had your keys. You ask yourself, "Where was I? What was I doing? Did I leave them in a pocket? What was I wearing?" By asking yourself logical questions, remembering the facts, creating a mental image of your activities, and perhaps following a hunch about where the keys are, you may solve your problem quickly and find your keys. If you do not find them within a reasonable time, you begin to think about other ways of handling the problem of getting to the required examination. This process is called critical thinking: remembering facts, using logic, asking key questions, forming a mental image, and analyzing all information.

Most client care problems have many possible causes and many probable solutions. When you think critically, you can grasp the nature and extent of problems more quickly and easily. You can make decisions that are logical, suitable for a particular client, and effective for solving a specific problem. This entire book presents exercises to help you develop your critical thinking skills as you continue to learn about nursing practice.

THE NURSING PROCESS

Although you will use critical thinking during your nursing career, it alone does not give you a framework for solving problems purposefully and methodically, a necessary safeguard in healthcare. As a nurse, you combine critical thinking skills with a scientific problem-solving method to identify client problems and to provide care in a structured, purposeful, and effective way. This framework for thinking and acting is called the *nursing process*. The nursing process is a special way of thinking about how to care for clients. The nursing process is also described as a systematic method that directs the nurse and client as they together (1) determine the need for nursing care, (2) plan and implement the care, and (3) evaluate the results.

You will use the nursing process framework throughout your nursing practice, but particularly as you learn to become a nurse. The nursing process is the method you use to identify and to treat client care problems. To ensure consistency among all nursing staff, use the nursing process to develop guidelines when caring for each client. Traditionally, these guidelines are developed into a format referred to as a **nursing care plan (NCP)**. Contemporary, clinical nursing units may use other terms in lieu of the nursing care plan, such as critical pathways, concept mapping, or clinical pathways, but the process of thinking through the nursing process remains basically unchanged whatever phrase is used. The nursing process framework enables you to develop plans of care individualized for each client, identifying what is suitable and desirable for that particular person. In Practice: Nursing Care Plan 33-1 presents a clinical scenario about an older adult woman with pneumonia. The accompanying photo display depicts the steps of the nursing process in action. You will need to review Nursing Care Plan 33-1 because it is a reference point for further discussion of the nursing process in the remaining chapters of Unit 6. The care plan helps you manage your time more effectively as you provide care. The nursing process also enables you to determine if your nursing care helped the client. Because the nursing care plan is available for other nurses to use as well, it provides consistency and focus in care.

IN PRACTICE
NURSING CARE PLAN 33-1 — An Older Adult Woman Hospitalized With Pneumonia

Note to Student: This is an example for a basic format and content of a simplified nursing care plan (NCP). See how the nursing process is formulated or put together, starting with basic data and information. In this sample NCP, the five steps of the nursing process are numbered to facilitate understanding of the nursing process (see Fig. 33-2).

Medical History: MT, a 78-year-old woman with a history of mild heart failure treated with diuretic therapy and sodium restriction, was brought to the emergency **department** by her daughter. Oxygen saturation (SaO_2) via pulse oximetry is 93%. Supplemental oxygen is ordered via nasal cannula at 4 L/min. Chest x-ray reveals patchy areas of consolidation in the right middle and lower lobes. White blood cell count reveals leukocytosis (increased white blood cells). Her daughter states, "I just thought that she had a bad cold, but now she's been coughing up some thick yellow mucus and says that it is hard to breathe." A sputum culture obtained was positive for *Streptococcus*. The client is admitted to the hospital.

Medical Diagnosis: Streptococcal pneumonia.

1. **DATA COLLECTION/NURSING ASSESSMENT**

   Note to Student: All NCPs are based on subjective and objective data. These data are collected and documented as an initial component of the nursing process.

   Client is diaphoretic (sweating profusely) and pale with complaint of shortness of breath. Temperature, 102.6 °F (39.2 °C) orally; pulse, 126 beats per minute (bpm); respirations, 38 breaths per minute, use of accessory muscles noted; blood pressure (BP), 100/60. Lungs with scattered coarse crackles (moist bubbling sounds as inhaled air comes in contact with secretions) and decreased breath sounds, especially in the right middle and lower lobes. Client describes a productive cough with thick, purulent sputum several times in the last hour. Daughter states, "I've tried to get her to drink some fluids, but she just seems so tired, coughing all the time."

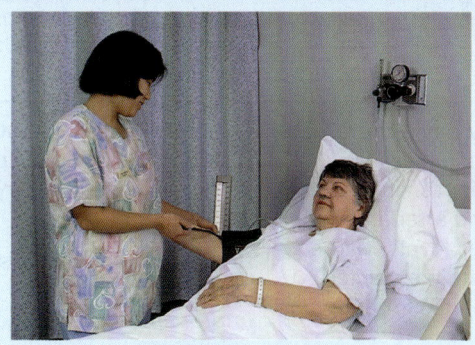

2. **NURSING DIAGNOSIS**

   Note to Student: One or many nursing diagnoses are inserted into the nursing care plan after the client's data are collected. The nurse obtains the wording from the standardized list of nursing diagnoses. These diagnoses are then quantified (made specific) to match the observations and data collected in the first phase of the NCP.

   - Ineffective airway clearance related to physiologic effects of pneumonia as evidenced by increased sputum, coughing, abnormal breath sounds, tachypnea, and dyspnea.

3. PLANNING	4. IMPLEMENTATION	5. EVALUATION
Short-Term Goals		
Note to Student: PLANNING is the thinking phase derived from the information from the client and the client's history and your nursing observations. The planning phase will be unique to each client. GOALS (outcomes) are defined, depending on the client's immediate and subsequent needs. The actual timeframe for short- or long-term goals will depend on the success of the initial actions or IMPLEMENTATIONS, also referred to as interventions. EVALUATIONS of the effects of a nurse's actions/interventions are provided.		
A. Within 4–6 hr, oxygen saturation will be maintained at 95% or greater with the use of supplemental oxygen.	• Administer supplemental, humidified oxygen via nasal cannula at the prescribed flow rate. **Note to Student: Rationales for implementations are given in this example care plan but are not typically part of the official care plan.** *Rationale: Supplemental, humidified oxygen aids in improving ventilation, thereby minimizing the risk for hypoxemia without drying the mucous membranes.*	Day 1–1,445 hr • SaO$_2$ at 95% via pulse oximetry; ABGs results confirm oxygen saturation at 95% and PaO$_2$ at 92 mmHg with supplemental oxygen therapy. ***Goal 1 met.***
B. Within 24 hr, client will state that breathing is easier.	• Monitor oxygen saturation levels via pulse oximetry; assist with obtaining arterial blood gases (ABGs) as ordered. *Rationale: Oxygen saturation levels and ABGs provide objective evidence of the client's tissue oxygenation.* • Assist client to assume semi-Fowler to high Fowler position and reposition frequently. *Rationale: Elevating the head of the bed facilitates breathing by permitting expansion of the lungs. Frequent repositioning prevents pooling and stasis of secretions. When in a sitting position, gravity lessens the weight of abdominal contents which push against the diaphragm.*	Day 2–0745 hr • Decreased use of accessory muscles; client reporting a decrease in shortness of breath and decrease in difficulty breathing. ***Goal 2 met.***
C. By day 2 of hospitalization, client's vital signs and arterial blood gas levels will be within expected ranges for age.	• Assess vital signs and respiratory status, including auscultation of lung sounds, initially every 1–2 hr and then as indicated. *Rationale: Frequent assessment of the client's status provides evidence of improvement or deterioration in the client's condition.*	Day 2–0900 hr • Temperature 100.4 °F (38.0 °C) orally; pulse, 100 bpm; respirations, 30 breaths per minute; BP, 110/64. Continued progress to meeting Goal 3. Day 2–2,100 hr • Mucous membranes pale but moist; IV site clean, dry, and intact, running at prescribed rate; IV antibiotic being administered without problems; vital signs within expected ranges. ***Goal 3 met.***

6. PLANNING	7. IMPLEMENTATION	8. EVALUATION

Long-Term Goals

A. By discharge, client's lungs will be clear to auscultation, and oxygen saturation will remain at greater than 95% without the use of supplemental oxygen.

- Instruct client in coughing and deep breathing and use of incentive spirometer.

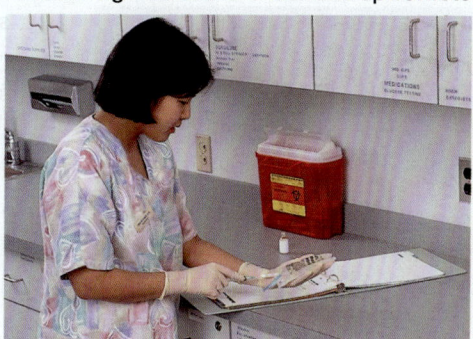

- Assist with prescribed nebulizer therapy as necessary.

Rationale: Coughing, deep breathing, and use of incentive spirometer aid in maximizing ventilatory capacity and mobilizing and expectorating secretions. Nebulizer therapy helps to open airways and keep membranes moist, facilitating expectoration.

- Continue monitoring vital signs and respiratory status every 4 hr, or as indicated, noting need for oxygen based on oxygen saturation levels.

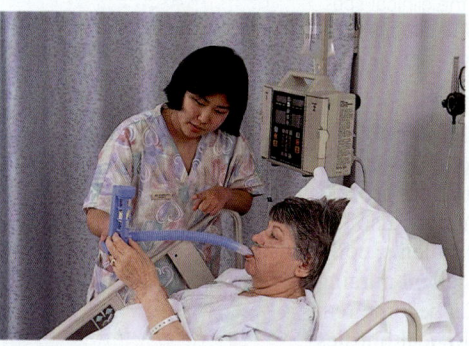

Rationale: Changes in the client's conditions will be observed and documented when timely VS are obtained.

Day 3–1,020 hr

- Client out of bed to chair for 20 min with supplemental oxygen in place; SaO$_2$ 98%.
- Afebrile; pulse, 84 bpm; respirations, 22 breaths per minute; BP, 116/70; lungs clear to auscultation except for small portion of right lower lobe.

Continued progress to meeting Goal 4.

- Vital signs remaining in expected range for age; afebrile. Lungs clear to auscultation.

Goal 4 met.

6. PLANNING	7. IMPLEMENTATION	8. EVALUATION
B. At the time of discharge, client and daughter will verbalize measures for continued therapy and follow-up to prevent a recurrence.	• Instruct client and daughter in measures for continued therapy and follow-up after discharge. 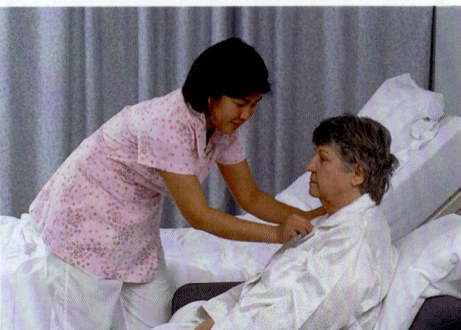 • Written discharge instructions given. *Rationale:* Knowledge about necessary therapy and follow-up aid in decreasing the risk for recurrence.	Day 3–1,745 hr • Daughter reporting return visit to primary care provider scheduled. • Client and daughter able to state signs and symptoms that might occur if problems occur. **Goal 5 met.**

> **NCLEX Alert**
>
> It is vital that the graduate understands the components of the nursing process. NCLEX questions take into account the individual components of the process, such as assessment/data collection, goal setting, appropriate actions, and reasonable evaluations using an effective communication technique. The correct response is commonly related to prioritization of the clinical scenario. Prioritization of needs begin with *Airway*, *Breathing*, and *Circulation* also referred to as the ABCs of nursing.

Potential needs or *potential problems* are those problems that might be prevented or problems that the client is at risk for developing. The effective use of the nursing process allows you to identify not only actual problems but also situations that might be avoided. Prevention of problems, complications, or impediments to care requires excellent nursing observations and interventions. Potential needs become real problems as a result of numerous events. Biological hurdles caused by a disease process or by hindrances to healing are common. For example, stasis ulcers, pneumonia, or infections are some of the more common potential but often preventable problems that nurses need to address before they have a chance to develop. The ability to foresee problems may avert painful, as well as costly, complications.

You can develop critical thinking and problem-solving skills by working through the nursing process framework repeatedly as you learn to identify and treat client needs. Often, you will practice the steps of the nursing process as you prepare nursing care plans. Keep in mind that every time you prepare a care plan, you are developing your critical thinking skills and expanding your nursing knowledge. Also, remember that every time you carry through with your plan, you are carrying out the work of nursing. Eventually this process of thinking and doing becomes automatic.

The nursing process framework has been a traditional aspect of nursing throughout the United States and Canada as a guide for identifying needs and treating clients. How it is used varies from one area to another. Its format varies among types of healthcare facilities and may be related to the differing roles of the RN and LVN/LPN. In some areas of practice, RNs are more likely to provide nursing assessments and nursing diagnoses for clients and set overall goals or plans of care. In other areas, LVN/LPNs may be responsible for the assessment, which may be referred to as data collection, the nursing diagnosis, and the plans or goals of the process. A fundamental aspect of obtaining and keeping your nursing license is to accurately function within your professional role based on the licensure of your facility, your responsibilities in that facility, and the mandated regulations of your licensing agency, also known as the Board of Nursing. Chapter 6 discusses the Nursing Process in detail. Chapter 2 discusses the written regulations for your license which can be accessed via your Board's online Website or by contacting the Board of Nursing for your state. Be sure that you know the differences between the regulations for LVN/LPNs and those for RNs.

> **Nursing Alert** It is also important to understand that individual states and clinical facilities will provide regulations, rules, and guidelines that are unique for the LVN/LPN and the RN. Each State's Nursing Board may define the roles of LVN/LPNs and RNs differently, especially when discussing the initiation and utilization of the nursing process. You will need to know the Nurse Practice Act and the local regulations for your location and situation.

Steps in the Nursing Process

The nursing process has specific steps in which you work with the client to plan and to carry out effective nursing care:

1. Nursing assessment: the systematic and continuous collection of data (Fig. 33-2)
2. Nursing diagnosis: the statement (or label) of the client's actual or potential problem
3. Planning: the development of goals for care and possible activities to meet them

4. Implementation: the giving of actual nursing care
5. Evaluation: the measurement of the effectiveness of nursing care

The next three chapters expand on these steps of the nursing process.

Characteristics of the Nursing Process

The steps in the nursing process lead to specific results. The characteristics of the nursing process, as discussed in the following sections, are critical to its effectiveness.

The five steps of the nursing process closely parallel the steps of scientific problem-solving. Table 33-1 shows the relationship between the steps of the nursing process and the concepts of the scientific problem-solving method.

Systematic

The nursing process is systematic. The nurse follows specific, orderly, and logical steps based on the client's most important and often most vital needs, also known as **prioritization** or **prioritizing**. By following the logical progression of steps to identify the client's needs, the nurse can plan activities to meet them.

Client-Oriented
The Nursing Process Is **Client-Oriented**

The needs of the client are identified, not the needs of the nurse, family, or other healthcare providers. The client and, if appropriate, the family or significant others become the nurse's partner in determining the goals for care.

You, as the nurse, focus on meeting individualized client needs, rather than on performing specific skills. A major difference between licensed nurses and nurse aides or unlicensed assistive personnel (**UAP**) is that nurses focus on the *rationale* of tasks, rather than just the completion of tasks. For example, a nurse must know when to take vital signs, what the data reveal, and how this information is related to the client's needs. The nurse aide or UAP may know the skill of taking vital signs but is not responsible for knowing *why specific actions are done.*

Goal-Oriented
The Nursing Process Is Goal-Oriented

Goals, objectives, or expected outcomes are established as an early part of the nursing process. The client, family, and significant others help to determine the goals. The healthcare team provides guidance for the establishment of goals. Goals can be short-term or long-term and are ranked according to the client's priority needs and preferences. **Short-term goals** are measurable outcomes that can be achieved in hours, days, or weeks, depending on the individual problem. **Long-term goals** take the short-term goals into consideration but also provide guidance for the days, weeks, or months during and after the time a client is seen by a health provider. See In Practice: Nursing Care Plan 33-1 for examples of short-term and long-term goals and how these goals interrelate with the other steps of the nursing process.

Continuous
The Nursing Process Is Continuous

Because the life and health of individuals change, reassessment of the client's needs is done frequently, sometimes hourly (or more frequently in critical care settings). Therefore, the existing nursing process must be redesigned spontaneously to fit the most current and highest priority needs. The nurse must continually reassess, make new goals, implement new plans, insert new interventions, and reevaluate the success of the overall process (see Fig. 33-2). A nursing care plan is revised as new needs are identified, changes in status occur, or when it is recognized that the

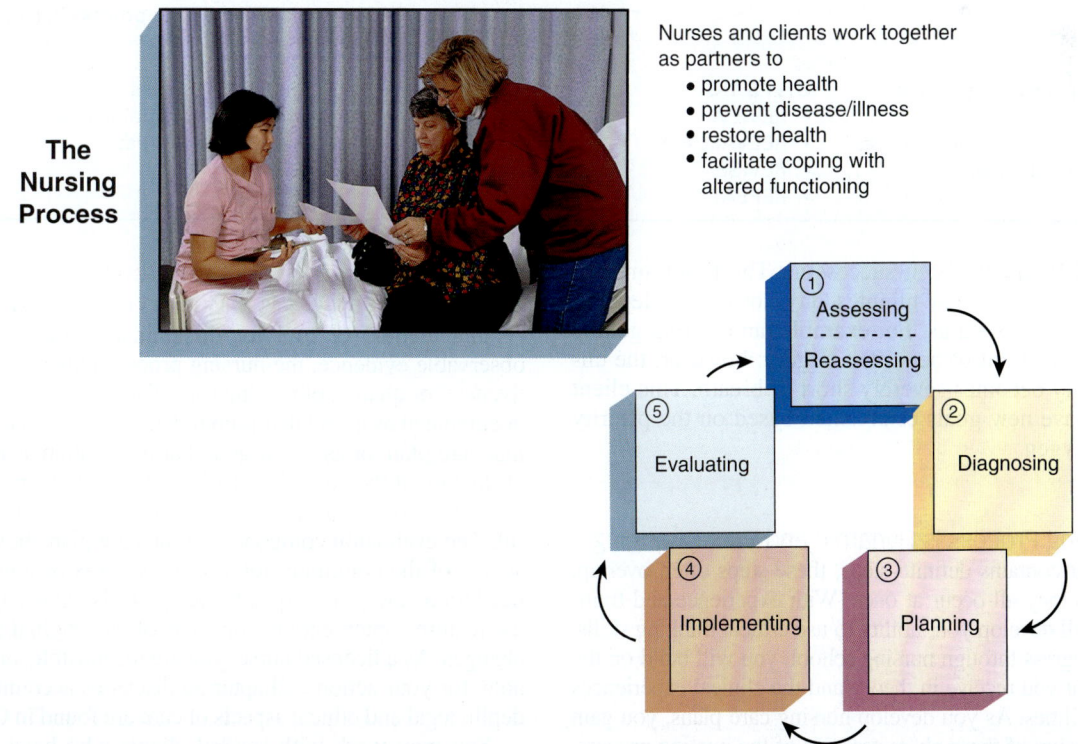

Figure 33-2 The nursing process is a continuous, scientific, systematic, client-oriented, and goal-oriented approach where the nurse and client work together to ensure quality care.

TABLE 33-1 The Nursing Process Compared With Scientific Problem-Solving

STEPS IN SCIENTIFIC PROBLEM-SOLVING	RELATED STEPS IN THE NURSING PROCESS	ACTIVITIES TO PERFORM
• Gather information relative to the problem.	1. NURSING ASSESSMENT	• Identify priorities (e.g., airway, breathing, circulation). • Collect data. • Update data when conditions change.
• Identify problem.	2. NURSING DIAGNOSIS	• Recognize and label significant data. • Recognize patterns or clusters. • Identify strengths and problems. • Reach conclusions. • Validate observations. • Write diagnostic statements.
• Formulate solutions. • Describe solutions for actual and potential problems. • Choose priority solutions. • Implement or initiate action toward solution.	3. PLANNING	• Identify priorities. • Establish expected outcomes or goals. • Anticipate nursing interventions. • Set short-term and long-term goals to suit the needs of the client. • Document specific actions for outcomes/goals by stating specific timeframes for actions of the plan.
• Test solutions.	4. IMPLEMENTATION—INTERVENTIONS	• Take actions that are necessary to achieve goals. • Adjust actions as conditions change. • Monitor and report results of assessment, goals, and interventions to other healthcare team members.
• Evaluate the results of actions. • Evaluate the goals that meet solution.	5. EVALUATION	• Analyze the client's responses to the problem. • Use critical thinking skills. • Determine success or need for change of goals and actions. • Identify factors that contributed to success or failure of the nursing care plan's outcomes or goals. • Continue with nursing process in a cyclic manner.
• Revise goals as conditions change. • Revise actions/interventions as conditions change.	STEPS 1–5 • REVIEW • REEVALUATE • REVISE • REPEAT	• Reevaluate and reassess. • Revise plan for future nursing care based on new assessments and data.

current NCP has not been successful. The timeframe for this entire process can be minutes, days, or longer, depending on the client's status. For example, an existing goal is to get the client out of bed after surgery; however, the client suddenly becomes severely short of breath. This client needs to have new goals established based on the priority need of oxygen.

Dynamic
The Nursing Process Is Dynamic and Ever-Changing
Although it contains definite steps, these steps often overlap. Sometimes they all occur at once. With experience and training, you will develop your ability to use critical thinking skills. As you progress through nursing school, you will build on the training that you receive in theory and the clinical experiences at your facilities. As you develop nursing care plans, you gain comprehension of these characteristics of the nursing process. Nursing care plans often reflect your growth in comprehension of the client's needs.

Communication and Quality Care
The Nursing Process Is a Method of Communication
As the method or tool for disseminating measurable and observable evidence, the nursing process indicates the effectiveness, or quality, of nursing care. The quality of care can be documented as a goal that is completed, as written in the original care plan, or as a new goal that is rewritten as a result of evaluation of the goals. Due to the individual nature of healthcare, it is not possible for all proposed goals to be successful. The evaluation component of the care plan should be the source of the communication of the success of a goal or the need for a new goal. A quality care plan also may suggest that the features, interventions, or goals of the original plan need changes. As a licensed nurse, you are responsible, or accountable, for your actions. Chapter 36 discusses accountability in depth; legal and ethical aspects of care are found in Chapter 4.

You may work with several clients who have the same medical problem; however, each person will have special considerations. Let's say, for example, that you have two clients, Mrs. M. and Ms. R., who have just learned they have diabetes type 1. Both clients must learn to give themselves insulin by injection to manage the disease. Mrs. M. has no prior knowledge of diabetes, but Ms. R. cared for her diabetic mother and administered insulin by injection for a number of years. Thus, you will develop care plans for both clients that consider their specific learning needs. Because all the nurses providing care for a client refer to the same care plan, consistency of care is ensured. You can measure how the client is progressing according to the plan. If goals are not being met, a reevaluation will indicate what further needs must be identified.

> **Key Concept**
>
> The nursing process is scientific, systematic, client oriented, goal oriented, continuous, and dynamic. The nursing process consists of the following steps:
> - Nursing assessment
> - Nursing diagnosis
> - Planning
> - Implementation
> - Evaluation
>
> The steps may overlap, change, repeat themselves, or happen all at once.

STUDENT SYNTHESIS

KEY POINTS

- Scientists have used scientific problem-solving for many years to systematize their research.
- Critical thinking is an important nursing strategy for problem-solving.
- The nursing process is a framework of scientific problem-solving combined with critical thinking skills.
- The nursing process provides individualized care that is accountable.
- Steps in the nursing process include nursing assessment/data collection, nursing diagnosis, planning, implementation, and evaluation.
- The nursing process can be used to identify not only the client's actual problems, but also potential needs or problems.
- The client and the family are involved in developing the nursing care plan.
- The steps of the nursing process, that is, the nursing care plan, may overlap, change, repeat, or need total revision due to potential needs becoming actual problems. These steps can even in some cases happen simultaneously.

CRITICAL THINKING EXERCISES

1. Your client, 21-year-old Tiffany, delivered a baby girl 3 hr ago and has just told you that she feels nauseated. This is the first time she has reported this symptom. What additional information would you ask her, or seek from other sources, before reporting this information to your team leader? Which observations would you make? Explain the rationale for your choice of questions and observations.

2. You are currently working with two clients who have had a stroke. Both clients are paralyzed on the right side. Based on your understanding of holistic nursing and of individualized client care, describe factors that you would expect to consider when working with each client to design a plan of care.

NCLEX-STYLE REVIEW QUESTIONS

1. In which situation would the nurse revise the nursing care plan?
   a. The client is losing weight and only eating small amounts of food.
   b. The wound care provided by the nurse is demonstrating healing of the wound.
   c. The client's urine in a catheter bag is clear yellow.
   d. The client's blood pressure has increased from 90/60 to 120/72 mmHg.

2. The charge nurse requests that the nurse provide oral hygiene every 2 hr for a client with a nasogastric tube. Which part of the nursing care plan does this describe?
   a. Assessment
   b. Planning
   c. Implementation
   d. Evaluation

3. A client is being treated for an infected sacral pressure wounds. The nurse has performed prescribed wound care twice a day for 5 days. Which part of the nursing process should be performed next?
   a. Development of the nursing diagnosis
   b. Development of goals
   c. Implementation of nursing care
   d. Evaluation of the care provided

4. The nurse is assisting the nursing team in developing a plan of care for a client in the long-term care facility. After data collection, which step of the nursing process should then be initiated?
   a. The development of a nursing diagnosis
   b. The development of goals for care
   c. Implementation of care for the client
   d. Ensuring that the care was effective

5. The nurse is caring for a client who has been involved in a motor vehicle crash. Which symptom displayed by the client is the highest priority for the nurse?
   a. The client is having difficulty breathing.
   b. The client is bleeding from a laceration on the leg.
   c. The client states "I have pain in the lower back."
   d. The client states "I voided on the stretcher."

CHAPTER RESOURCES

Enhance your learning with additional resources on **thePoint**!

Student Resources related to this chapter can be found at thePoint.lww.com/Rosdahl12e.

34 Nursing Assessment

Learning Objectives

1. Identify the rationale for performing a nursing assessment.
2. Differentiate between objective data and subjective data. Give examples of each.
3. Identify sources of observation that the nurse uses when developing a plan of care for a client. Give examples of each source.
4. Differentiate between the terms *nursing history* and *medical history*.
5. Identify methods of organizing data for use in a nursing care plan.

Important Terminology

congruence
data analysis
health interview
nursing assessment
nursing history
nursing progress notes (nurses' notes)
objective data
observation
subjective data

Acronyms

BCP
CC
HRT
LMP
PSA
STI

All steps of the nursing process depend on complete and accurate information about the client. The nurse carefully collects this information, also called *data*, during the first step of the nursing process. This chapter discusses this first step of the nursing process: assessment.

NURSING ASSESSMENT

The nursing process begins as soon as you enter a nurse–client relationship. **Nursing assessment** is the systematic and continuous collection and analysis of information about a client (Fig. 34-1). The assessment begins with collecting data and putting the data into an organized format. Prioritization of data is very important. During the data-collection assessment phase, the nurse begins to perceive and identify existing problems or needs. *Existing needs* often are the priority over *potential needs*, which are often listed as *at risk for*. For example, the goals and needs for a client recovering from a stroke have priority over a potential need, such as *at risk for infection*. However, the risk for infection is still a priority concern because the client may be at risk for infection of the lungs (pneumonia), which is a hazard of immobility.

Data Collection

The best sources of information about the client are the client and family. You also consult other members of the healthcare team for their information and analysis of the client. In addition, you learn information from the client's previous and present health records, laboratory reports, and reference books dealing with the client's medical diagnosis or condition. Nurses should be alert to the *congruence* of information. **Congruence** occurs when two or more sources of data are compatible or consistent, having the same or very similar descriptions. For example, the nursing staff should confirm that the client's statements are congruent with the laboratory findings.

The physical examination also yields important data. See Chapter 47 for a detailed description of the physical examination. Data to be gathered from the client also are identified in Chapter 45 and throughout this book.

> **Key Concept**
>
> Many sources provide the healthcare team with information. In spite of the source, HIPAA's confidentiality regulations (Chapter 4) mandate that information about the client can be shared only with the client. The healthcare team is allowed to review data but is not approved to share this information with family or caretakers unless the client specifically designates the others as acceptable recipients of the information.

Data collected about a client generally fall into one of two categories: *objective* or *subjective*.

Objective Data

Objective data include all the measurable and observable pieces of information about the client and his or her overall state of health. The term *objective* means that only precise, accurate measurements or quantifiable descriptions are used. Therefore, other healthcare providers can verify objective data. Judgments, opinions, or client statements are not considered objective data.

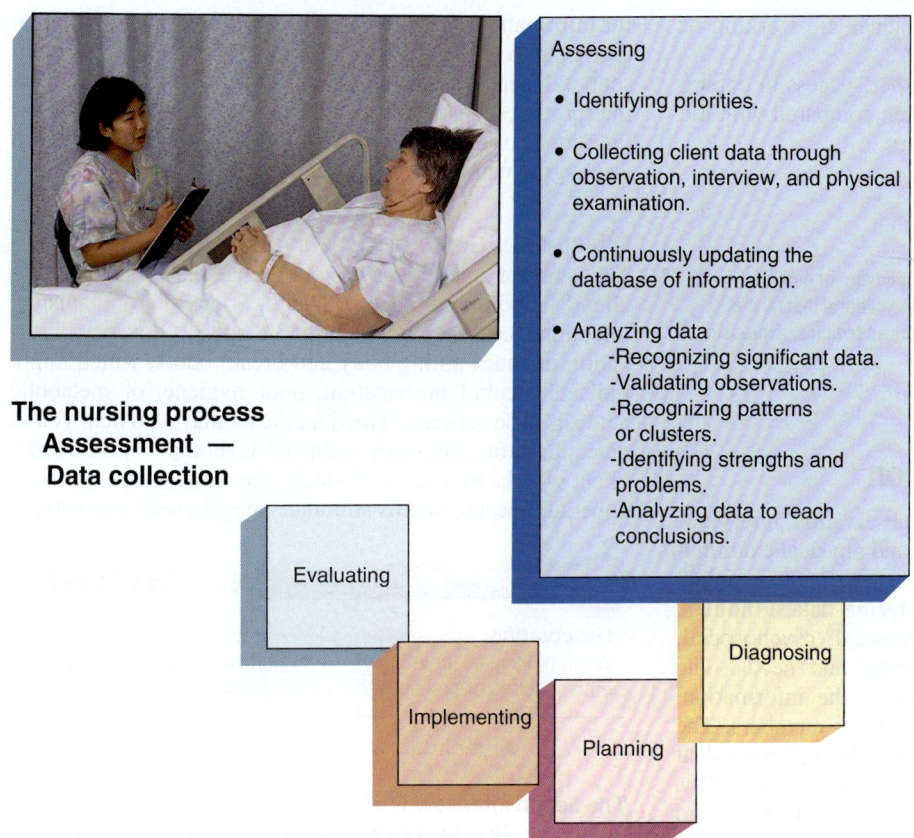

Figure 34-1 The nursing process begins with the assessment or collection of facts. The nurse collects as much objective and subjective data about the client as possible.

As a nurse, you measure the client's vital signs, height, weight, and urine volume. You use specific descriptions about the size and color of a wound. Measurements of body structure and function that involve extent, rate, rhythm, amount, and size are usually made with instruments—such as a stethoscope or sphygmomanometer—or are the results of laboratory tests or radiologic diagnostic tools. Laboratory tests also measure the chemical makeup of the blood and urine.

The critical thinking skills that you use while collecting objective data about the client involve asking key questions. What are the client's vital signs? What can you directly observe? Have you read the physician's history and progress notes? What do the other members of the healthcare team have to say about the client? What do laboratory reports tell you about the client's condition?

Subjective Data

Subjective data consist of the client's opinions or feelings about what is happening. Only the client can tell you that he or she is afraid or has pain. Sometimes the client communicates through body language: gestures, facial expressions, and body posture. Both spoken and written words and body language tell you the client's opinions and feelings. Often this information cannot be confirmed through any other source (Fig. 34-2). To obtain subjective data, you need sharp interviewing, listening, and observing skills. Always be sure to consider cultural factors, such as specific body postures and use of eye contact, the client's beliefs about health and illness, or the use of special amulets or folk remedies (see Chapter 8 for more information about culture). Chapter 44 discusses therapeutic communication and interviewing in more detail.

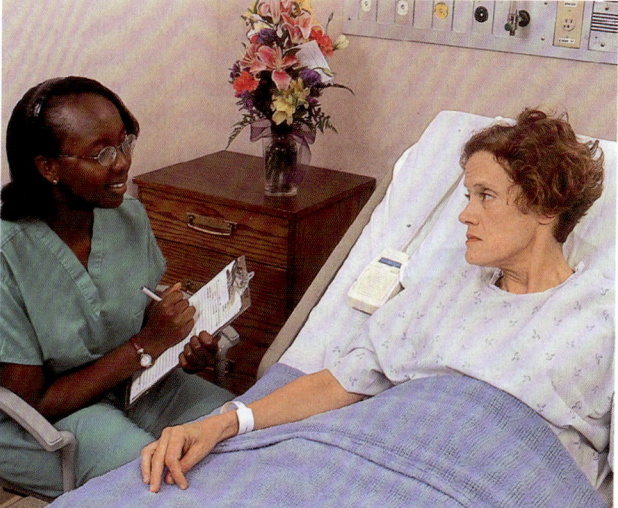

Figure 34-2 Effective communication is a key component in obtaining subjective data about the client. The nurse must take into consideration the client's body language, including posture, gestures, and facial expressions, as well as what the client says.

The following considerations are critical thinking questions to ask yourself when obtaining subjective data about the client:

- What is the client saying about how he or she is feeling? (*subjective data*)
- Do the client's words and behaviors say the same thing? (*congruence*)
- What does the client say is the reason for coming to the healthcare facility? (*subjective data*)

- According to the client, what techniques are working or are not working? (*subjective data*)
- How does the client describe his or her success in coping with the healthcare environment when compared with the home environment? (*subjective data*)

> **Key Concept**
>
> *Objective data* are obtained from *objects* that measure or quantify information. *Subjective data* are gained from the client's, that is, the *subject's*, verbal or nonverbal point of view such as feelings, expressions, or sensations of pain.

Methods of Data Collection

Methods used to collect data include observation, interview, laboratory and other diagnostic tests, and physical examination. By using all of these methods, you can obtain complete and accurate information. When analyzing data, a holistic picture emerges that may include physical, psychosocial, and socioeconomic problems, concerns, and needs. The nurse individualizes the data, prioritizes the information, and shares this information with other team members. The confidentiality of this information must be maintained at all times. See Chapter 4 for a discussion of confidentiality. Remember, data must be factual, unbiased, impartial, and updated continuously.

Observation

Observation is an assessment tool that relies on the use of the five senses (sight, touch, hearing, smell, and taste) to discover information about the client. This information relates to characteristics of the client's appearance, functioning, primary relationships, and environment.

Visual Observation

The sight provides an abundance of clues that you must continually process when assessing the client. A few examples to consider are body movements, general appearance, mannerisms, facial expressions, mode of dress, nonverbal communication, interaction with others, use of space, skin color and appearance, and cleanliness. You use visual observation to collect subjective data, such as when noting the client's facial expression and body language. You also use visual observation to collect objective data, such as when you inspect the client's skin for rashes or irritation and note the cleanliness and level of safety of the client's immediate environment.

Tactile Observation

The sense of touch provides valuable information about the client. For example, touch or *palpation* of the skin assesses factors such as muscle strength, temperature, moisture, edema, rash, or swelling.

Auditory Observation

Hearing allows you to listen actively to the client and family as they interact with you and other members of the healthcare team. You may also use specialized equipment to listen for information. For example, data collected by auscultation (listening to the heart, lung, or bowel sounds with a stethoscope) depend on your sense of hearing and level of skill in interpreting such sounds. Similarly, you must be able to hear the sounds of the pulse when measuring blood pressure with a sphygmomanometer and stethoscope.

Olfactory or Gustatory Observation

The sense of smell identifies odors that can be specific to a client's condition or state of health. Some microorganisms' infections have specific, identifiable odors. Olfactory observation includes noting body and breath odors, which might indicate alcohol intoxication, poor hygiene, or metabolic acidosis. The senses of smell and taste may also help you to detect harmful chemicals in the air. It should be noted that a client who lacks a sense of smell often is anorexic (lacks an appetite) because smells stimulate specific taste sensations.

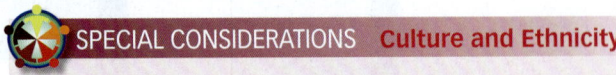

> **SPECIAL CONSIDERATIONS** Culture and Ethnicity
>
> **Observation**
> When making observations, be sure that you consider cultural and ethnic factors or practices that may influence your findings.

The Health Interview

The **health interview** is a way of soliciting information from the client. This interview may also be called a **nursing history**. If the interview is conducted when a client is admitted to a healthcare facility, it may be called an *admission interview*. When a healthcare provider obtains this information, it is called a *medical history*. In some areas, RNs take the nursing history, with a nursing student or LVN/LPN assisting with the process. In other healthcare settings, the practical/vocational nurse may conduct the health interview. The RN assesses the data and works with the team to formulate a nursing diagnosis and plan of care.

Each facility has its own health forms for you to complete in partnership with the client and the other members of the healthcare team. Prewritten forms may target the specific needs of the client (e.g., rehabilitation after a hip replacement) or may be organized according to body system (e.g., integumentary, digestive, cardiovascular). Long-term care, home healthcare, hospice care, rehabilitative care, postpartum care, and other specific areas may have forms that suit the specific needs of their clients. When you go to your clinical facilities, you should make a note of how each facility, and sometimes a specific unit within that facility (e.g., critical care units, obstetrics, outpatient), uses the nursing interview and documents the information onto the nursing progress notes. The **nursing progress notes** are commonly referred to as the **nurses' notes**. Chapter 37 discusses charting in more detail.

During the health interview, you may guide the conversation with direct questions or the client may direct the dialogue by discussing health problems, symptoms, or feelings about his or her needs. For maximum effectiveness and efficiency, plan for the interview before meeting the client. When you greet the client, tell the individual that the purpose of the interview is to enable the nursing staff to plan effective and personalized care that will meet his or her individual needs.

When gathering information, all methods of communication should be used. Data collection and assessment are combinations of open-ended questions, detailed questions (often closed-ended), plus observational and tactile skills. It is also important to consider factors, such as the client's level of pain, comfort, exhaustion, or physical situation (e.g., post trauma). Most facilities and/or departments provide their own form to use for the purposes of interviewing, gathering data, and assisting with the assessment process.

Remember, clients have the right to refuse to answer questions that they believe are too personal. In some cases, you may need to talk with family members because some clients are too ill or confused to respond or too young to speak for themselves. Even when the client can respond, family members may give you additional information. Keep in mind that you must protect the confidentiality of the client, never revealing any information previously unknown to the family without the client's permission.

Components of the Nursing History

A complete health history helps you develop an effective plan of care for the client. Table 34-1 gives sample questions to ask during an initial interview. This table provides an overview of the contents related to basic data-gathering questions and is not intended to be an all-inclusive interview. Typically, the following information is obtained:

Biographical data: Includes name, age, birth date, spouse, support person, children, address, phone number, occupation, financial status, insurance, and so forth.

Reason for coming to the healthcare facility: Addresses the *primary* reason, also described as the client's chief complaint (CC) or perception of the illness. What does the client expect to happen in the healthcare facility?

Recent health history: Includes symptoms of recent disease treated with medications and/or surgery and exposure to communicable diseases.

Important medical history: Includes family history of disease, allergies, immunizations, medications, and use of alternative/complementary therapies and herbal supplements.

Pertinent psychosocial information: Addresses family relationships, employment, living conditions, emotional stability, sexual relationships, substance use or abuse, medications, and so forth.

Activities of daily living (ADLs): Involves how well the client is able to meet basic needs, such as eating, drinking, bathing, dressing, and toileting. Does the client get adequate exercise, food, rest, and sleep?

The Physical Examination

Chapter 47 discusses how to assist with the physical examination. You also will learn some basic skills of physical examination so that you may continually monitor the condition of your clients as you care for them.

> **Key Concept**
> You will use the following methods to collect data:
> - Observation (use of the five senses)
> - Interview (the nursing history)
> - Physical examination (general survey and specific examinations)

DATA ANALYSIS

During and after data collection, you must critically examine each piece of information to determine its relevance to the client's health problems and its relationship to other pieces of information. Through systematic **data analysis**, you can draw conclusions about the client's health problems. During data analysis, you also use critical thinking skills to ponder other questions that might be important or to develop a visual image of what the client is telling you.

Recognizing Significant Data

The information itself may pose difficulty when interpreting data. You may find that you have too much information or not enough information. When preparing to analyze data, ask yourself which items are pertinent to client care and which are not. By doing so, you are thinking critically. As a nursing student, you must discuss your assessments with your team leader or instructor. Once you have gained experience, you will make more decisions on your own.

> **NCLEX Alert**
> The correct response to an NCLEX test question may require that the graduate relate and prioritize data, such as noting which one of several given situations has the most significance to the client at that time. For example, oxygen saturation levels are connected with two of the three prioritization ABCs, that is, airway and breathing. Remember, the correct first response typically is *not* to "notify the physician," but rather to perform a bedside nursing action, such as apply oxygen, and *then* to notify the appropriate nursing supervisor and/or healthcare provider.

Validating Observations

One way to validate observations is to "check them out" with the client. Do your observations agree with what the client is experiencing or are they only your interpretations? Sometimes, thinking of clients as "team leaders" who are directing the members of the healthcare team is helpful. You may also consult with your nursing team leader or colleagues to validate your observations.

Recognizing Patterns or Clusters

Some data are similar or have a pattern or connection and are identified as symptoms. Patterns may occur at a particular time of day or night, after eating, after walking, or when the client is in a certain position. These symptoms can be grouped together in clusters for further analysis. For example, you will see a relationship among symptoms when a client reports pain and bloating in the abdomen and no bowel movement for 3 days. Recognizing data clusters helps you determine relevant information.

> **Key Concept**
> Nurses must be able to connect basic laboratory results with client symptoms. For example, a decreased red blood cell count may present the symptom of shortness of breath. Another common example occurs when the client has an elevated white blood cell count, which may be reflected as a client's elevated temperature and rapid pulse.

TABLE 34-1 Samples of Questions to Ask at the Initial Client Interview

ESSENTIAL, INTRODUCTORY QUESTIONS	FOLLOW-UP QUESTIONS FOR ADDITIONAL DETAIL
Background Information	
What is your primary language?	What language do you speak at home?
Do you need a translator for assistance with conversations or with reading?	What language would be most beneficial for you? Would you like a translator?
Why did you come to this facility today? Did you have an accident and injury, or do you have a history of previous medical problems?	How long have you had this problem? Have you had this problem before? Where does it hurt?
By what means did you come to the healthcare facility?	Who, if anyone, was with you?
Are you under the care of a physician or healthcare provider?	If so, what is the physician's name? Where do you usually go for healthcare treatment?
Do you use other types of healthcare providers or healers?	If so, what types of treatment are provided? Are you taking any medications, teas, or herbs suggested by the healers?
Did you come from home, an acute care facility, a hospital, a long-term care facility, or another type of healthcare facility? Do you feel safe at home? Have you recently been camping, traveled out of the country, or had visitors from outside the country?	For what condition(s) are you being treated? What situations occur that make you feel unsafe? When did these events occur? Did any of your current health problems occur during or after your travels?
Do you smoke or chew any tobacco products?	For how long? How many packs per day?
Do you drink alcoholic beverages?	For how long? How many drinks per day?
Have you been hospitalized before?	Have you had surgery? For what? How long ago? Where?
Do you have an advance directive or other type of healthcare living will?	If not, do you need help in preparing one?
Allergies and Sensitivities	
Are you allergic to any prescription or nonprescription medications?	What happens when you take these medications?
Have you ever had a problem or reaction such as rash or difficulty breathing after taking any medication?	What is the problem or reaction? When was the last time you had this problem?
Are you allergic or sensitive to any foods?	What happens when you eat these foods?
Are you sensitive or allergic to latex? Are you sensitive to bananas, avocados, kiwis, tropical fruits, potatoes, or chestnuts?	What happens when you are in contact with latex products? What type of problem or reaction do you have when eating any of these items?
Medications	
What prescription medications do you currently take? Do you have a list of medications with you?	What is the dosage for these medications? Do you take these medications as prescribed? Do you miss dosages?
What over-the-counter medications or nutritional supplements do you currently take?	How long have you been taking these products/medications?
Do you have a current list of all of your medications and supplements?	What nutritional supplements do you take? Do you take iron or calcium supplements? If so, why?
Do you take medications regularly for headaches, anemia, stomach problems, menstrual problems, diarrhea, constipation, earaches, congestion, or any other reason?	Is your current problem related to or similar to any conditions that you have had previously?

TABLE 34-1   Samples of Questions to Ask at the Initial Client Interview   (Continued)

ESSENTIAL, INTRODUCTORY QUESTIONS	FOLLOW-UP QUESTIONS FOR ADDITIONAL DETAIL
Do you have financial concerns about paying for your medications?	Do you avoid getting any prescriptions filled because of the cost of the drug?
Do you take recreational drugs?	What recreational drugs do you take?
Detailed Health History	
What significant illnesses have you had in the past? What surgeries have you had in the past?	When? Please provide details of these illnesses or surgeries.
Have you ever had a blood transfusion or received a blood-related product?	Have you been tested for HIV or AIDS? Would you like to be tested for HIV or AIDS?
Have you ever had a broken bone?	For what bone? What happened? Did you have any problems recuperating?
What types of food do you typically eat? What type of diet do you follow at home?	Are you on any special type of diet? If so, why? Does your religion prohibit you from eating any particular foods? Do you avoid meat, eggs, or cheese? Do you have any definite food likes or dislikes?
What do you do for exercise?	Would you consider your physical activities as sedentary, mild, moderate, or athletic exercise?
Have you had a recent, sudden, or unexplained weight loss or gain?	Why do you think you have lost or gained weight?
Do you have any trouble chewing or swallowing?	What problems or sensitivity do you have with your teeth? Do you wear dentures?
Do you have difficulty speaking?	Are you supposed to wear dentures? Why do you not wear your dentures?
Do you wear contact lenses, glasses, or a hearing aid?	Why do you use these items? Are they helpful?
Do you wear any prosthesis such as an artificial limb?	What problems, if any, do you have with these items?
Do you use a cane, crutches, or a walker?	Why do you use these items?
Describe your home environment.	Do you need to climb stairs?
Describe your work environment.	Are you exposed to cigarette smoke, toxins, fumes, pesticides, chemicals, infectious diseases, or other environmental substances?
How would you describe your stress level at work?	What do you do to manage your stress levels?
Do you have a history of problems with any of the following? (Only a brief review of systems is provided below.) Heart disease? Diabetes? Lung problems? Seizures? Cancer? Stomach problems?	How long have you had this problem? What is the treatment for this problem? Does anyone else in your family have a history of these or similar problems? Please describe the details of these issues.
Describe your normal bowel routine.	Are you constipated, or have diarrhea, or take laxatives? Do you pass blood in your stool?
Describe your normal bladder functioning.	How many times a day do you void? At night? Do you pass blood in your urine?

(Continued)

TABLE 34-1 Samples of Questions to Ask at the Initial Client Interview (Continued)	
ESSENTIAL, INTRODUCTORY QUESTIONS	**FOLLOW-UP QUESTIONS FOR ADDITIONAL DETAIL**
Activities of Daily Living	
What assistance, if any, do you need in caring for yourself at home?	Can you dress yourself? Can you prepare your own meals? Can you clean your living space? Can you get groceries on your own?
Describe your support system.	Do you have family? Can they care for you if you are ill? Does your family depend on you for financial or physical support? Do you depend on your friends or family for care?
Does your religious belief system provide a source of spiritual or physical support?	Can you call on friends or religious group members for assistance, if needed?
Social services and other resources may be available for your assistance. Would you like to talk with someone from the Social Services Department?	What type of assistance you think that would be of most benefit to you? Examples include: day care, assistance with meals, bathing, finances, or hospice?
Women's issues	
When was your last menstrual period (**LMP**)?	Do you think that you might be pregnant?
How many children do you have?	How many times have you been pregnant?
Could you have a sexually transmitted infection (STI) or a genital infection? Do you take birth control pills (**BCP**)?	Have you previously been treated for any STIs? Did you complete your course of therapy/medications as ordered? How long have you been taking BCPs? Have you had any problems with clots (emboli)?
Do you or have you in the past been on hormone replacement therapy (**HRT**)?	How long have you been on HRT?
When was your last Pap smear?	What were the results of your Pap smear?
For men	
When was your last prostate/testicular examination?	Have you ever had a prostate-specific antigen (**PSA**) examination? If so, what was the result?
In Conclusion	
What do you expect from the nurses and doctors at this facility?	Is there anything else that you would like to share with us?
What are your most important concerns?	What else should we know about you?

Identifying Strengths and Problems

While assessing the client, look for strengths the client has that he or she can use in coping with problems. Through careful analysis of data clusters, you may identify actual or potential problems.

Reaching Conclusions

After initiating the preceding steps, you are ready to reach a conclusion. Four conclusions are possible:

1. The client has no problem. No further nursing care is needed; you reinforce the client's current health habits and recommend other health-promotion activities.
2. The client may have a problem. You need to gather more information.
3. The client is at risk for a problem. This finding indicates a potential nursing diagnosis. You continue through the nursing process by planning, implementing, and evaluating. The client may deny that a problem exists or may refuse treatment.
4. The client has a clinical problem. The client has a nursing diagnosis or medical diagnosis.

The problem is a *nursing diagnosis* if it falls in the domain of nursing, and nursing staff may treat it without consulting a physician (see Chapter 35 for further discussion). If the problem requires medical treatment (*medical diagnosis*), you have identified a collaborative problem. When this occurs, you must consult a physician and work together to resolve the problem.

> **Key Concept**
>
> Nursing assessment is the systematic and continuous collection of data about a client. It includes the following steps:
>
> - Identifying assessment priorities related to the purpose of the interview
> - Collecting data about the client from observation, interview, and physical examination
> - Continuously updating the database of information
> - Recognizing significant data
> - Validating observations
> - Recognizing patterns or clusters
> - Identifying strengths and problems
> - Analyzing data to reach conclusions

> **NCLEX Alert**
>
> Be sure to read all responses given in a multiple-choice question. The responses may contain more than one correct answer, but there is only one *best correct answer* for that particular clinical scenario.

STUDENT SYNTHESIS

KEY POINTS

- Nursing assessment is the systematic and continuous gathering and analysis of data about the client.
- Assessment includes use of the senses and observation, the interview, and the physical examination.
- Data collected include objective data (factual, measurable; what you can directly observe) and subjective (what the client tells you; the client's opinions and feelings).
- Data analysis requires recognizing significant data, validating observations, recognizing patterns or clusters, identifying strengths and problems, and reaching conclusions.

CRITICAL THINKING EXERCISES

1. Your client has just reported to you that he has the following symptoms: ringing in his ears, swelling of his right ankle, difficulty swallowing, pain in his right knee, a tingling sensation in his right toes, a toothache, and numbness in his right calf. Which symptoms might be related? Do you find more than one cluster? Which additional information would help you understand his problem(s)?

2. Identify ways that you can target your assessments to meet the specific needs of clients. What particular methods would you use for a client who comes from a background different than your own? How would you work with a client who presents with various conditions? How would you handle a situation in which a client appeared noncompliant or did not want to participate in care planning?

NCLEX-STYLE REVIEW QUESTIONS

1. The nurse is collecting data from a client in the clinic. Which observation documented by the nurse is an olfactory observation?
   a. The client's skin is warm and dry.
   b. The client has cyanosis around the lips.
   c. The client's breath has a fruity odor.
   d. The client wheezes bilaterally when the chest is auscultated.

2. A client is admitted to the hospital, and the nurse prepares to collect data. Which methods will the nurse use in order to obtain necessary information? Select all that apply.
   a. Ask another nurse "What do you think is wrong with the client?"
   b. Look through the client's personal belongings to find indications of the problem.
   c. Observe the client.
   d. Interview the client.
   e. Perform a physical examination of the client.

3. The nurse is interviewing a client with a rash over the face, arms, and trunk. Which question asked by the nurse takes priority?
   a. "Are you allergic to any foods, medicines, or topical creams?"
   b. "How many children do you have?"
   c. "Do you get adequate exercise?"
   d. "Do you have money to pay for this visit?"

4. A client has a fever, foul-smelling drainage from a leg wound, and erythema around the wound. Which diagnostic test is a priority for the nurse to observe?
   a. Chest x-ray
   b. White blood cell count
   c. Liver function tests
   d. Cholesterol levels

5. A family member of a client in the hospital asks the nurse what the physician thinks is wrong with the client. Which response by the nurse is best?
   a. "I am not able to discuss the client's condition with anyone without the client's consent."
   b. "I am not really sure what is wrong with the client, let me let you look at the chart."
   c. "Let's go talk with the physician and find out."
   d. "Why do you need to know about the client?"

CHAPTER RESOURCES

Enhance your learning with additional resources on thePoint!

Student Resources related to this chapter can be found at
thePoint.lww.com/Rosdahl12e.

35 Nursing Diagnosis and Planning

Learning Objectives

1. Define and identify the purposes of a nursing diagnosis. Differentiate the legal, licensing, and appropriateness of a registered nurse (RN) initiating a nursing diagnosis for the nursing care plan.
2. Differentiate a nursing diagnosis from a medical diagnosis.
3. Discuss the rationale for use of nursing diagnoses.
4. Identify the three segments of a diagnostic statement and give examples of a comprehensive diagnostic statement.
5. Discuss the following components of planning nursing care: setting priorities, establishing outcomes, and implementing nursing interventions.
6. Define and discuss the rationale for using both short-term goals and long-term goals in the development of a nursing care plan.
7. Discuss the uses for each method of care plan development and how all of these methods can be used collaboratively to plan nursing care of a client.
8. Demonstrate examples of written or electronic nursing care plans using the computer printout method, standardized care plan, and a formal written, individualized care plan.

Important Terminology

collaborative problem
expected outcome
long-term goal (objective)
medical diagnosis
nursing diagnosis
planning
prognosis
short-term goal (objective)

Acronyms

AEB
CMS
ICD-10-DM, ICD-10
NANDA-I
NCHS
R/T

The first step of the nursing process is *data collection*, which is the collection of objective and subjective information for the *nursing assessment*. Standing alone, the data gathered are useless until you determine what they mean. The second step of the nursing process is identifying the nursing care problem—otherwise called the *nursing diagnosis*—based on your analysis of the data. Only then can you move on to the third step of the nursing process, which is *planning* client care based on the problems or diagnoses you have identified.

NURSING DIAGNOSIS

A nursing diagnosis is a statement about the actual or potential health concerns of the client that can be managed through independent nursing interventions (Fig. 35-1). Nursing diagnoses are concise, clear, client-centered, and client-specific statements.

In some geographic areas, practical/vocational nurses do not make nursing diagnoses; it is considered the duty of the RN. Keep in mind that a nursing diagnosis is an approved label that identifies the client's problems in nursing terminology. Whether or not you make a nursing diagnosis yourself or this step is considered the providence of the RN, all nurses must understand the meaning of a nursing diagnosis and how it is used to plan and to implement nursing care.

History of Nursing Diagnoses

Since 1973, a group of nurse researchers and educators formulated plans to standardize communication and categories of nursing care. Before this standardization, descriptions of nursing care differed both between hospitals and also within one hospital because nurses literally invented their own descriptions of nursing-related concerns for clients. In 1982, with members from Canada and the United States, the group became the organization known as the North American Nursing Diagnosis Association (NANDA). In 2002, the organization was revised and became NANDA International, written as NANDA-I, using an updated model of health called Taxonomy II.

Standardization of nursing terminology has become a highly effective nursing tool for communication of clients' problems and concerns. The nomenclature, criteria, and categories developed by this organization are commonly referred to as *nursing diagnoses*. Subjective and objective data, which nurses collect to communicate effective nursing care for all types of clients, became more understandable as it was adapted by all nursing units at the various types of clinical facilities. Nursing diagnoses are a required facet of nursing care by multiple accrediting agencies.

The words, phrases, and/or terms of nursing diagnoses are actually the diagnostic labels or categories on which an evidence-based, client-oriented nursing diagnosis statement is built. The wording of the phrases is divided into three specific components. These components start with a general concept and add clarification of the concept to individualize

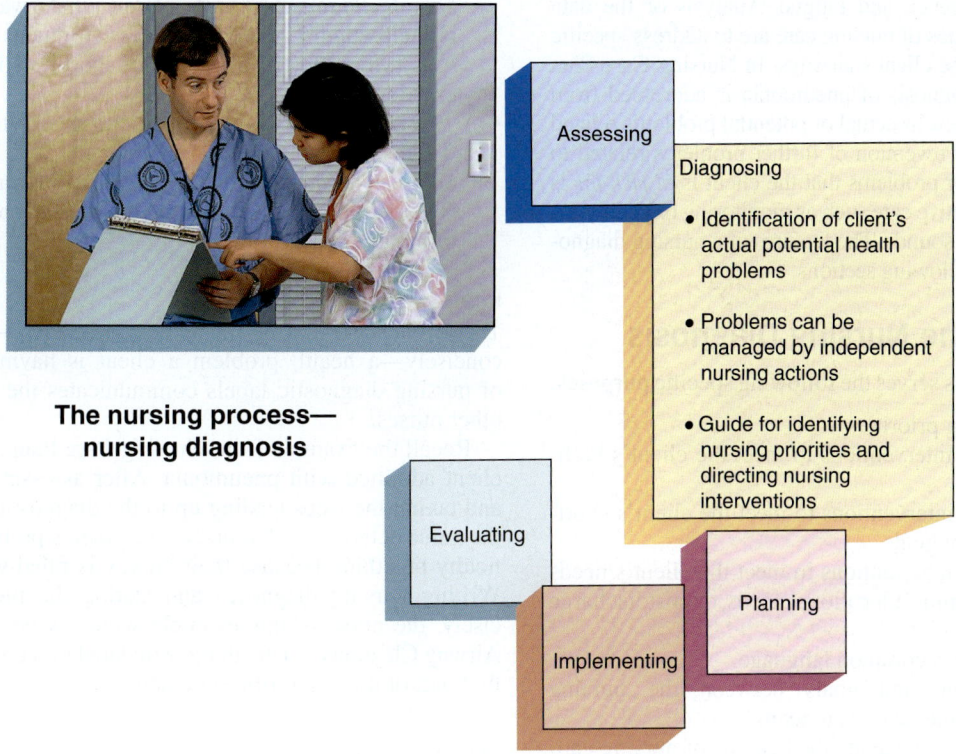

Figure 35-1 In the second step of the nursing process, nursing diagnoses are developed based on analysis of the data collected during nursing assessment.

the total phrase. The result is standardized, generalized communication, which also becomes a unique description of a client's problem or concern. The nursing process uses these nursing diagnoses as part of the fundamental steps involved in the concepts of critical thinking.

Healthcare facilities have their specific version of nursing diagnoses list posted in a central location or in the medical information system for all nurses to use. Nursing diagnoses remain a basic component and a foundation for prioritization of a nursing care plan.

Medical Diagnosis Versus Nursing Diagnosis

Medical diagnoses are not to be confused with nursing diagnoses. Medicine emphasizes the disease process or the etiology of the disorder. A **medical diagnosis** is obtained from a list of accepted medical problems compiled in a major database known as the International Statistical Classification of Diseases and Related Health Problems. It is more commonly known as the International Classification of Diseases, 10th Revision (**ICD-10**) and commonly shortened to *ICD-10*. The list is compiled by the National Center for Health Statistics (**NCHS**) and the Centers for Medicare & Medicaid Services (**CMS**). The medical diagnoses are listed by body system, such as diseases of the nervous system, or by general commonalities, such as injury and poisoning (CMS, 2020). Examples of medical diagnoses include hypertension, pneumonia, diabetes mellitus, and renal failure.

Remember these facts about a *medical diagnosis*:

- A medical diagnosis identifies the disease a person has or is believed to have.
- Physicians arrive at a medical diagnosis by studying the physiologic manifestations of the illness and establishing its cause and nature.
- A medical diagnosis provides a basis for **prognosis** (projected client outcome) and medical treatment decisions.

Nursing diagnoses focus on the client—the individual's physical and psychological responses to an existing or potential condition. Nursing diagnoses look at nursing observations and actions and how nursing care can affect the needs of the client, such as an individual's ability to function, to cope with specific problems, or to learn how to care for a problem (self-care).

Remember these general concepts relating to the *nursing diagnosis:*

- A nursing diagnosis is based on nursing observations and data collection.
- A nursing diagnosis suggests nursing actions or nursing interventions.
- A nursing diagnosis recognizes the client's ability for self-care, to cope with specific problems, or to respond to existing or potential conditions.

Recall the client described in the Nursing Care Plan 33-1. Their medical diagnosis is pneumonia. When you look at the data that have been obtained about the client, you are concerned about their ability to function and what you, as the nurse, can do to help them to improve their physical condition or to prevent other problems from occurring. From the nursing assessment data, you determine that the client has abnormal breath sounds, a cough with thick yellow sputum, increased respirations, difficulty breathing, fever, and fatigue. Analysis of the data reveals that the priorities of nursing care are to address specific problems related to the client's airways. In Nursing Care Plan 33-1, the medical diagnosis of pneumonia is addressed from the nurse's point of view as actual or potential problems related to airway clearance. Prevention of further problems related to the respiratory tract or problems that the client is *at risk for* is addressed by preventative care such as monitoring oxygen saturation levels and lung sounds. The features of a nursing diagnosis are found in the following sections.

Purposes of the Nursing Diagnosis

The nursing diagnosis serves the following specific purposes:

- Identifying nursing priorities
- Directing nursing interventions to meet the client's high-priority needs
- Directing nursing interventions to meet the client's short-term and long-term goals
- Directing nursing interventions to meet the client's needs for discharge planning, educational needs, or postdischarge follow-up
- Communicating in a common language
- Integrating actions and goals between the nursing professionals and the healthcare team
- Forming a process to evaluate the benefits of nursing care
- Providing assistance when determining the client's acuity level or the client's needs for nursing care

The Diagnostic Statement

This section provides an overall look at two ways of writing the diagnostic statement. A more detailed description of each component follows. During the assessment/data collection component of the nursing process, it is likely that the client will present with more than one problem. Therefore, the nursing care plan may be made up of multiple *diagnostic statements*. Each diagnostic statement has two or three parts.

The three-part nursing diagnostic statement consists of the following components:

- *Problem:* General label (e.g., airway clearance, ineffective). Notice that the nursing diagnosis is written alphabetically with the descriptive noun (*airway clearance*) followed by a *comma*, followed by the specific problem of airway clearance (*ineffective*).
- *Etiology:* Specific, related factors such as excessive mucus or foreign body obstruction. Note that the etiology is obtained from a nursing observation (excessive mucus).
- *Signs and symptoms:* Specific, defining characteristics (signs or symptoms) written in the following format: *as evidenced by* (**AEB**) or *as manifested by* objective or subjective data such as shortness of breath on exertion, or abnormal lung sounds (crackles, wheezes, rhonchi), or ineffective cough. Note that the signs and symptoms are specific events or issues that have developed from the basic etiology.

The following examples separate each of the three compartments of the diagnostic statement for the purpose of definition and demonstration:

- A three-part diagnostic statement consists of the problem, etiology, and signs and symptoms.

- *Sample nursing diagnostic statement*: Airway clearance is ineffective // related to excessive mucus production // as evidenced (manifested) by shortness of breath on exertion.
- A two-part diagnostic statement consists of the problem and signs and symptoms.
- *Sample nursing diagnostic statement*: Airway clearance // is ineffective as evidenced (manifested) by shortness of breath on exertion.

Problem

The *problem* portion of a statement describes—clearly and concisely—a health problem a client is having. The use of nursing diagnostic labels communicates the problem to other nurses.

Recall the example from Nursing Care Plan 33-1 for the client admitted with pneumonia. After assessing the client and taking the steps leading up to the diagnostic statement, the nurse determines that one of the client's problems is difficulty breathing because their airway is filled with mucus. Writing nursing diagnoses and stating the problem concisely, the nurse in this example would write "Ineffective Airway Clearance." This diagnostic label of a problem is the first part of the diagnostic statement.

> **Key Concept**
>
> Writing nursing care plans is a process that continually evolves. It is important that the contemporary nurse document according to their licensure limitations and within the guidelines of the employing institution.

Etiology

The *etiology* part of the diagnostic statement is the *cause* of the problem. Etiology may be physiologic, pathophysiologic, psychological, sociologic, spiritual, or environmental. For the client with pneumonia, the etiology for the problem "Ineffective Airway Clearance" consists of the physiologic effects of pneumonia. As a nurse, you will know the pathophysiology, that is, the disease process, of pneumonia.

Signs and Symptoms

Data collected during the nursing assessment delineate the nursing diagnosis. The third part of the diagnostic statement summarizes these data. You may need to include several *signs and symptoms*. For instance, the client with pneumonia had cough with thick sputum, abnormal breath sounds, increased respirations (tachypnea), and difficulty breathing (dyspnea). For them, the third part of the statement would be "increased sputum, coughing, abnormal breath sounds, tachypnea, and dyspnea." Refer to In Practice: Nursing Care Plan 33-1.

> **Key Concept**
>
> A nursing diagnosis has three components:
> P—Problem (diagnostic label)
> E—Etiology (cause)
> S—Signs and symptoms (the objective and subjective information observed and documented)

Writing the Diagnostic Statement

The diagnostic statement connects problem, etiology, and signs and symptoms. The first two parts of the statement are linked by *related to*, sometimes abbreviated R/T. The last two parts are linked by *as evidenced by*, sometimes abbreviated AEB. Therefore, the statement for the client with pneumonia described in Nursing Care Plan 33-1 would read as follows:

- Ineffective Airway Clearance *related to* physiologic effects of pneumonia *as evidenced by* increased sputum, coughing, abnormal breath sounds, tachypnea, and dyspnea.

When formulating a nursing diagnosis, make sure that it is something the nursing staff and the client can treat without orders from the physician. Such actions are called *independent nursing actions*. If treatment requires something you cannot do, such as prescribe medication for the cough, the problem is a collaborative problem. A **collaborative problem** means that you will work together with the physician or other healthcare providers. For instance, the physician will prescribe the medication, but the nurse will decide whether or not to administer a PRN (as needed) medication at bedtime.

> **Key Concept**
>
> The nursing diagnosis is a statement about the client's actual or potential health concerns that can be managed through independent nursing interventions. It contains the following steps:
> - Establishing significant data
> - Writing a two- or three-part diagnostic statement

PLANNING CARE

After identifying the nursing diagnoses, you begin planning nursing care. **Planning** is the development of goals to prevent, reduce, or eliminate problems and to identify nursing interventions that will assist clients in meeting these goals. Setting priorities, establishing expected outcomes, and selecting nursing interventions result in a plan of nursing care (Fig. 35-2).

> **NCLEX Alert**
>
> Nursing priorities on NCLEX-PN and NCLEX-RN questions are written using the form of the diagnostic statement (i.e., problem, etiology, and signs and symptoms). LVN/LPNs and RNs must be aware of these concepts as they are used throughout their nursing careers.

Setting Priorities

The assessment or data collection component of the nursing process reveals situations that are concerned with immediate or critical needs. These are called the priority needs. The nursing diagnoses associated with these situations are given a higher priority than those not connected to survival needs. The most important, that is, priority needs must be identified and addressed first. On the nursing care plan, nursing diagnoses are prioritized, that is, nursing diagnoses, goals, and actions must be listed in order of importance. Survival needs or imminent life-threatening problems take the highest priority. For example, the needs for air, water, and food are survival needs (refer to Maslow's hierarchy of human needs in Chapter 5). Nursing diagnostic categories that reflect these high-priority needs include ineffective airway clearance and dehydration. Safety needs are the next priority, with nursing diagnostic categories such as safety or fall risk. At a lower level of priority are the social and psychological needs for love, self-esteem, companionship, and fulfillment; some possible nursing diagnostic categories are caregiver fatigue, acute anxiety, and depression. The client's specific situation, as observed and documented, will guide the prioritization of actions.

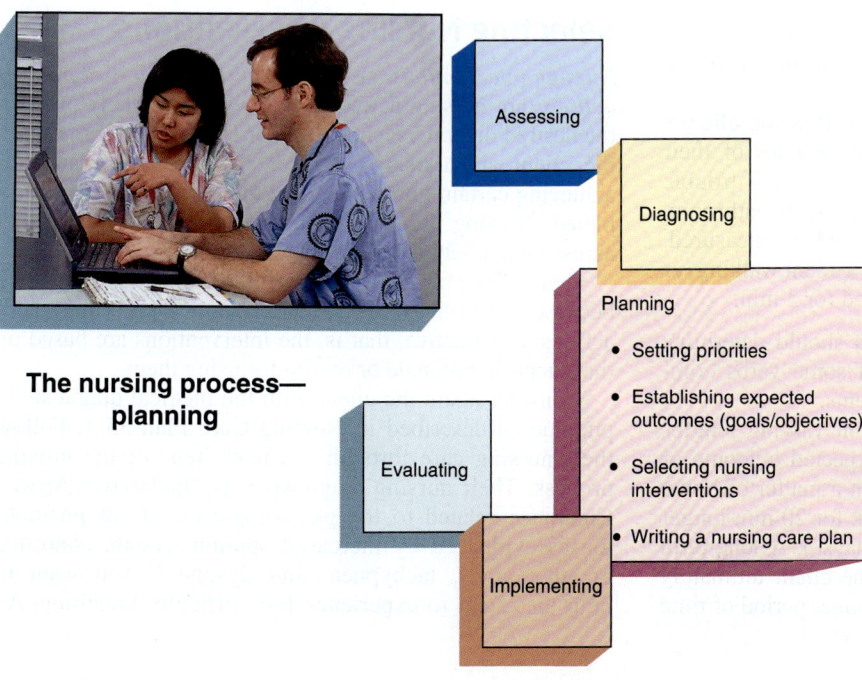

Figure 35-2 During planning, the third step of the nursing process, goals are established and interventions are identified to assist the client in meeting the goals.

The medical diagnosis may be the legal reason for admission to your facility. However, the medical diagnosis may not be the priority nursing concern at any given moment. For example, the medical diagnosis of "right hip fracture" will involve many aspects of nursing care, immediate, rehabilitative, and long term. During the hospital stay, the client will have a number of nursing diagnoses that are indirectly involved with the primary medical problem. Nursing care will involve relief of pain, prevention of complications due to immobility, or psychosocial concerns. Attempts to address nonpriority problems may be unsuccessful because the client has more urgent, immediate needs. Even though some problems can be deferred until a later time, the nurse must simultaneously keep in mind the care needed for future problems.

In addition, materials and human resources availability, as well as time limitations, affect the order of priority. Equipment, supplies, and staff must be available. Keep in mind that you might not be able to actively address every nursing diagnosis a client may have. The client also determines the priority of health concerns. For example, a client who smokes may be fully aware of the health risks of smoking, but may choose to continue. In this case, plans to help the client quit smoking will fail, even though the need for oxygen is a requirement for survival, and thus, is a high priority.

Establishing Expected Outcomes

You are familiar with learning objectives or behavioral objectives in your nursing program. A similar type of objective or outcome is established for the client. An **expected outcome** is a *measurable* client behavior that indicates whether the person has achieved the expected benefit of nursing care. It may also be called a *goal* or *objective*. An expected outcome has the following characteristics:

- *Client oriented:* The client, not the nurse, is expected to meet this outcome. For instance, "the client will walk around the room at least once per shift."
- *Specific:* Everyone, including the client, knows what is to occur. For instance, "the client will walk up and down the hall for 5 min."
- *Reasonable:* The outcome should be within the client's capacity and abilities, considering the confines of their condition. For example, if the client is having trouble breathing, walking may be limited to trips to the bathroom.
- *Measurable:* The behavior can be observed and measured. For example, nursing staff can observe a client walking, or the client can state that he or she walked for 5 min.

Working together, you and the client should determine outcomes. Box 35-1 gives examples of some verbs commonly used in expected outcome statements.

Expect clients to achieve outcomes in varying lengths of time. A **short-term objective** is an expected outcome or goal that a client can reasonably meet in a matter of hours or a few days (e.g., "The client will walk for 20 min longer each day for the first 3 postoperative days"). A **long-term goal, or objective,** is an outcome that the client ultimately hopes to achieve, but which requires a longer period of time

---

Box 35-1 Examples of Verbs Used in Expected Outcome Statements

- Cough
- Demonstrate
- Describe
- Discuss
- Express
- Has a decrease in
- Has an absence of
- Has an increase in
- Identify
- List
- Perform
- Relate
- Share
- Sit
- Stand
- State
- Use
- Verbalize
- Walk

---

to accomplish. Sometimes, the longer period means that the client will not still be in the healthcare facility when the objective is achieved. You can help the client put this objective in writing. Then, while working toward self-care, the client can probably identify the desired long-term goal or objective. They can learn how to measure the progress toward achieving the objective. For example, the client's long-term goal may be "to return to college" after self-care is achieved.

Key Concept
Expected outcomes are client oriented, specific, reasonable, and measurable.

NCLEX Alert
The correct response on an NCLEX multiple-choice question may relate to the ability to know which option is the most specific, measurable, and realistic for the given clinical scenario.

Selecting Nursing Interventions

Nursing interventions, also called *nursing orders* or *nursing actions*, are nursing activities that will most likely produce the desired outcomes (short-term or long-term). Sometimes, the client and nursing staff set specific target dates for achieving certain goals, checking them off as they are completed. Nursing orders may include such things as further assessment, client teaching, or referral.

Generally, specific nursing interventions are selected because scientific research has demonstrated that these actions are effective, that is, the interventions are based on the scientific rationale or reason for using them.

Consider again the client with the medical diagnosis of pneumonia described in Nursing Care Plan 33-1. Follow their nursing care through the next steps of the nursing process. Their nursing diagnosis was "Ineffective Airway Clearance related to the physiologic effects of pneumonia as evidenced by increased sputum, cough, abnormal breath sounds, tachypnea, and dyspnea." You want to help the client to experience less difficulty breathing. An expected outcome could be "Within 24 hr, the client will state that breathing is easier." To achieve this outcome, you would select nursing interventions such as the following examples:

- Offering fluids frequently
- Positioning the client with the head of the bed elevated for optimum breathing
- Teaching the client deep-breathing exercises
- Monitoring vital signs frequently
- Encouraging correct use of the incentive spirometer
- Administering oxygen as ordered by the physician
- Ensuring that respiratory therapy is administering nebulizer treatments as ordered

Writing a Nursing Care Plan

The nursing care plan is the formal guideline for directing the nursing staff to provide client care. Ideally, the entire nursing team formulates the nursing care plan at a meeting called a *nursing care conference* or *team conference* (Fig. 35-3). Sometimes one or two nurses may create the care plan. The initial care plans are written to provide instructions and guidelines for the total healthcare team to use for direction and communication.

The nursing care plan usually includes nursing diagnoses or client problems (according to priorities), expected outcomes (short- and long-term objectives or goals), and nursing orders (activities nurses carry out to help the client achieve goals). Nurses develop the care plan shortly after a client is admitted to the facility. However, the plan is an ever-changing guide, which is updated regularly as the client's condition changes. Because each healthcare facility develops its own format according to the particular health needs of its clients, the content and the structure of the written nursing care plan vary. Be sure to familiarize yourself with the format used in your facility and for the specific needs of the department of the facility (e.g., medical/surgical unit or intensive care unit).

The written care plan is kept in several ways. Most handwritten information systems concerning clients have been replaced with computerized versions, also known as computerized medical information systems. As medical and nursing data are inputs into the system, the nursing care plan is developed, often automatically, as part of a client's computerized health record. Changes to the client's status will instigate updates within the care plan.

Regardless of the manner in which the care plan is developed, it becomes part of the client's permanent health record. Documentation of a nursing care plan is a requirement of agencies such as the Joint Commission, nursing home regulators, and Medicare. Personnel from such organizations review health records during site visits to the facility. If a nursing care plan does not exist within 12–24 hr of the client's admission, the healthcare facility will be cited for noncompliance. Penalties can be severe.

The ideal nursing care plan is individualized for each client. Many facilities, however, use a standardized nursing care plan and incorporate the usual and expected outcomes for a particular type of nursing care problem or nursing diagnosis. These standardized care plans allow for additions or substitutions so that the care plan can be individualized to the specific client. The standardized care plan is efficient and a welcome aid when you must work with many clients.

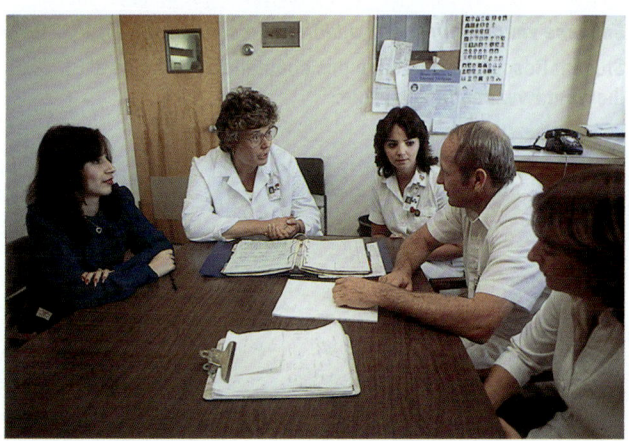

Figure 35-3 The nursing team often holds a nursing care conference to develop a nursing care plan for a client with complex healthcare needs.

Key Concept

Planning is the development of goals to prevent, reduce, or eliminate problems and to identify nursing interventions that will assist clients in meeting these goals. Remember the following steps involved in planning:

- Setting priorities
- Establishing expected outcomes
- Selecting nursing interventions
- Writing a nursing care plan

STUDENT SYNTHESIS

KEY POINTS

- Nursing diagnosis is a statement about the client's actual or potential health concerns that can be managed through independent nursing interventions.
- Medical diagnoses are concerned with the disease process. Nursing diagnoses are concerned with the client and how the disease affects that person's ability to function.
- Nursing diagnoses help identify nursing priorities and the goals that are established to maintain quality and continuity of care.
- A nursing diagnosis is stated in terms of a problem, its etiology, and signs and symptoms.
- After establishing the nursing diagnosis, the planning of nursing care begins. A nursing care plan is written based on priorities, expected outcomes, and selected nursing interventions.

CRITICAL THINKING EXERCISES

1. Compare a written nursing care plan for a client in a long-term care facility (e.g., nursing home) with that of a client in an acute care facility (e.g., hospital). What are the similarities and differences? Because all people have similar needs, why do you think these differences exist?

2. Practice making a nursing diagnosis. From the following data, write a three-part nursing diagnostic statement: A male client, age 69 years, complains that he has difficulty swallowing because of a severe sore throat. He complains of having a dry tongue and feeling thirsty and light-headed. He has not urinated in 5 hr and does not feel the urge to urinate now.

NCLEX-STYLE REVIEW QUESTIONS

1. The nurse is caring for a client admitted to the hospital with aspiration pneumonia. Which diagnostic label is a priority for this client?
   a. Impaired gas exchange
   b. Aspiration risk
   c. Decreased mobility
   d. Anxiety

2. Which nursing diagnostic category is the highest priority for an older adult client who is dehydrated, has a 3 × 2 cm wound on the lower extremity, and is anxious about living alone?
   a. Depression
   b. Acute anxiety
   c. Altered skin integrity
   d. Dehydration

3. Which does the nurse determine is the first step in the planning process?
   a. Establish expected outcomes.
   b. Select the nursing intervention.
   c. Set priorities.
   d. Write the care plan.

4. Which priority nursing intervention will assist the client confined to bed with meeting the goal of prevent contractures?
   a. Turn the client every 2 hr.
   b. Perform passive range of motion exercises every 2 hr.
   c. Assist the client with activities of daily living.
   d. Encourage fluid intake every 2 hr.

5. The nursing care team is setting short-term goals for a client with end-stage chronic obstructive pulmonary disease. Which short-term goal is the most realistic for this client?
   a. The client will ambulate 10 ft with 2 L/min of oxygen via nasal cannula without a decrease in oxygen saturation by day 3.
   b. The client will be able to perform all activities of daily living without dependency on oxygen.
   c. The client will be able to live independently without assistance.
   d. The client will be free of shortness of breath.

CHAPTER RESOURCES

Enhance your learning with additional resources on **thePoint**!

Student Resources related to this chapter can be found at **thePoint.lww.com/Rosdahl12e**.

36 Implementing and Evaluating Care

Learning Objectives

1. Define the process of nursing implementation. Consider the concepts of nursing interventions and nursing actions as the mechanisms or tools of nursing implementation.
2. Differentiate between dependent action and interdependent action.
3. Define accountability. Discuss the legal implications of nursing accountability and responsibility.
4. Identify the three main skills used in implementing nursing care.
5. Discuss the rationale for this statement: *A key to nursing care is communication*.
6. Identify the component of evaluation in the nursing process. Describe methods of evaluation.
7. Discuss the statement: *Discharge planning begins on admission of the client into a facility*.

Important Terminology

accountability	evaluation	independent actions	interdependent actions	nursing action	technical skills
dependent actions	implementation			nursing	
discharge planning		intellectual skills	interpersonal skills	intervention	

After collecting data, identifying nursing diagnoses, developing goals, and writing a nursing care plan, your next step is to implement, that is, to carry out, the care plan. **Implementation** of a nursing care plan may also be referred to as providing **nursing interventions** or **nursing actions** (Fig. 36-1).

IMPLEMENTING NURSING CARE

"Do it," "share it," and "write it down" are the action phrases of implementation. You "do" nursing care with and for the client. You "share" the results by communicating with the client and other members of the healthcare team, individually or in a planning conference. You "write" information by documenting it so that the next healthcare provider can act with purpose and understanding. Always remember that adequate communication and documentation facilitate the continuity of care (Fig. 36-2).

Dependent, Interdependent, and Independent Actions—"Do It"

When implementing care, you will do things, or as nursing prefers to say, intervene on behalf of the client. The nursing actions that are done may be *dependent, interdependent, or independent*. A nurse intervenes, that is, gets involved, by providing actions that carry out the healthcare provider's orders.

Dependent actions are based on orders or specific directions from the healthcare provider, such as providing medication or treatments. The nurse is given explicit instructions. For example, the nurse is ordered to administer medications or perform certain treatments. Remember that your licensing (regulatory) requirements as an LVN/LPN provide guidance as to whether you are permitted to complete these orders.

Interdependent actions are those that you perform collaboratively with other care providers; the healthcare provider may write orders for some of these actions. These actions are interventions for collaborative problems. For example, the healthcare provider may write an order to give a pain medication to a client when necessary. You use your nursing observational skills and nursing judgment to determine when to give the pain medication. Nursing observations include the client's stated level of pain, for example, a 7 on the 1–10 pain scale. Another nursing action will be to determine that the interval of time that the pain medication starts to be effective and remains effective is appropriate. The healthcare provider will prescribe the type of medication and its dosage. Before giving the medication, you will affirm, by nursing actions, the client's name and allergy status. If the client is allergic (or has previously had an unexpected reaction) to the pain medication, you will withhold the medication and notify the healthcare provider so that a different medication can be ordered. Together, you have collaborated to provide client care.

Independent actions are nursing actions that do not require a healthcare provider's orders. Only you—as a member of the nursing staff—perform independent nursing actions, which are based on your judgment. Independent actions are those actions that you take to assist the client with activities of daily living (e.g., bathing, toileting) or to help reduce stress (e.g., using therapeutic listening or providing a warm blanket).

To understand the different types of nursing actions, consider the example of the woman with pneumonia described in Nursing Care Plan 33-1. The healthcare provider writes an order for supplemental oxygen at a specified flow rate.

435

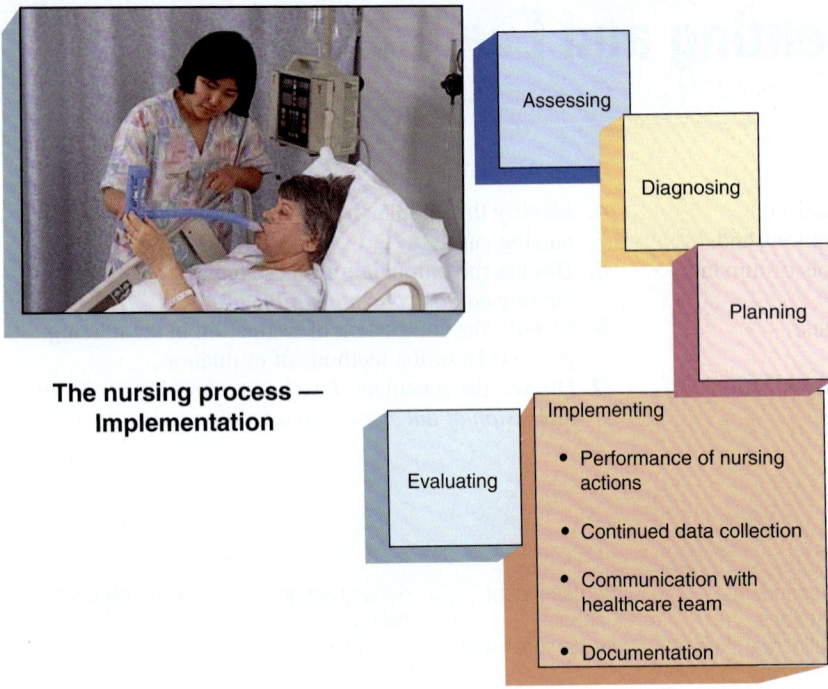

The nursing process — Implementation

Figure 36-1 During implementation or interventions, the fourth step of the nursing process, you put the client's plan of care into action.

You may choose, however, to give the antipyretic medication based on the client's temperature, for example, when the client's temperature is greater than 100.4 °F (38.0 °C). This action is *interdependent:* you are following the healthcare provider's orders, but you are making a decision based on your judgment about timing and effective treatment. Additionally, you may decide *independently* to apply cool compresses to aid in reducing the client's fever. Independent actions may be written as nursing orders, such as "assist with getting out of bed to chair at least once daily," "encourage frequent sips of fluid," "assist client to assume semi-Fowler to high-Fowler position and reposition frequently," "monitor vital signs and respiratory status every 1 to 2 hours." Ask your instructor or team leader if you are unsure about any nursing actions.

Key Concept

Nursing actions involve the use of *common sense* and *critical thinking*. For example, you may take vital signs (VS) or use a pulse oximeter whenever you observe changes in the client. In everyday practice, you need to obtain pertinent information such as VS *before* calling the healthcare provider.

You are responsible for all actions you perform, whether they are dependent, interdependent, or independent. This responsibility is also called **accountability**, an important aspect of the legal requirements of nursing practice. Using critical thinking skills will greatly assist you to make the safest and most helpful choices for each of your clients.

NCLEX Alert

NCLEX questions commonly seek the answer to questions such as "Which of the following is the *most appropriate nursing* action?" It is vital for you to understand the difference between nursing actions and healthcare provider's actions. Look for a correct response to the clinical scenario that is the priority *nursing* action.

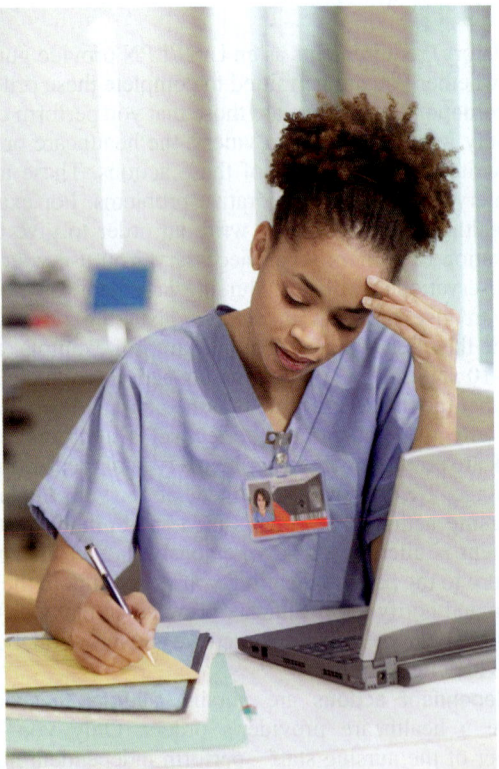

Figure 36-2 The nurse may use the computer to document care, print out a nursing care plan, or retrieve data (e.g., laboratory or x-ray) about the client. The healthcare providers may also input orders for a client to be carried out by the nurses. Nursing students and graduates will also find a wealth of healthcare information on the Internet.

Administering oxygen, which is considered a medication, is a *dependent action*, as is administering the client's intravenous (IV) fluid and antibiotic therapy. The healthcare provider also writes an order for an antipyretic as needed (PRN). Administering the medication is a *dependent action*.

Skills Used in Implementing Nursing Care

Certain skills influence the implementation of the nursing care plan. These skills include your ability to perform intellectual, interpersonal, and technical skills. **Intellectual skills** involve knowing and understanding essential information (e.g., basic sciences, nursing procedures, and their underlying rationale) before caring for clients. Critical thinking is one type of intellectual skill essential for making quick decisions and taking swift action. **Interpersonal skills** involve believing, behaving, and relating to others. Solid communication techniques and client encounters that promote the development of a trusting relationship (rapport) are interpersonal skills (see Chapter 44 for more information about therapeutic communication). Behaving professionally also involves interpersonal skills. **Technical skills** involve the ability to manually perform a task. Nursing has a vast array of procedures, which include changing a sterile dressing, inserting a urinary catheter, or administering an injection. To safely and competently perform manual tasks, the student and, later, the licensed nurse need ongoing training in techniques, adequate practice, and confidence.

The Nursing Care Plan in Action

The nursing team determines if the plan, as written, makes sense. Using critical thinking, ask yourself the following questions when reviewing a care plan:

- Does this plan protect the client's safety?
- Has the plan been developed according to a scientific problem-solving approach? Is it based on sound nursing knowledge?
- Do the nursing orders logically achieve the desired results? Are the orders arranged in an appropriate sequence?
- Do the nursing orders enhance and facilitate the client's care and progress to recovery and goal achievement?
- Did the client have active involvement in this plan, and can the client give some ideas about whether it is appropriate?

How you manage your time, the client's time, and your activities are important concepts in determining what you and the client accomplish during the day. Prepare a timetable so the client can see the schedule of activities for a full day. Encourage client participation in planning the timetable. Remember to include both the client and the family in this process.

Continuing Collection of Data

As you care for clients, observe them carefully. Listen to what clients say; watch what they do; check their VS. Use critical thinking continually to determine if the nursing orders are effective in moving clients toward meeting their specified goals.

Communication With the Healthcare Team—"Share It"

Periodically, a *client planning conference* is held in which information about the client is shared among the various members of the healthcare team, for example, nurses, physical therapists, and diabetes educators. If the client is to be discharged from healthcare services, this conference serves as a *discharge planning conference*. Interdisciplinary planning conferences offer an excellent way to coordinate your nursing care and to interact with other health disciplines. If you do not personally attend the conference regarding a client for whom you are providing care, you are responsible for giving both verbal and written information to those attending. By doing so, you help ensure that the plan of care is not only coordinated with those of other healthcare providers but also is evaluated by them.

Written Communication With the Healthcare Team—"Write It Down"

You also will document all care given to your client. Documentation, whether written by hand or by computer, is an extremely important aspect of accountability and responsibility of nursing care. Verbal communication, unless audio recorded, is temporary. Written documentation, such as a printout of discharge instructions, can be taken home for the client and the client's caregivers to review later. There are many legal considerations related to written communication. Consider the phrase: *If it is not written, it was not done.* Chapter 37 presents a detailed discussion about documentation and reporting.

> **Key Concept**
>
> Nursing implementation means the carrying out of the nursing care plan. It includes the following steps:
> - Putting the nursing care plan into action
> - Continuing the collection of data
> - Communicating care with the healthcare team
> - Documenting care

EVALUATING NURSING CARE

Evaluation is measuring the effectiveness of assessing, diagnosing, planning, and implementing. The client is the focus of the evaluation. Steps in the evaluation of nursing care are *analyzing the client's responses, identifying factors contributing to success or failure,* and *planning for future care* (Fig. 36-3).

You can use several means to evaluate the effectiveness of nursing care:

Client: The primary source of evaluation criteria is the client. The family may also be helpful in determining if care given was effective.

Team conference: A conference is helpful not only to plan nursing care but also to evaluate the effectiveness of care and design a discharge plan.

Community health agencies: Another way of evaluating outcomes of care is to contact healthcare providers in community agencies who are in touch with clients after they leave your facility. Such care providers include public health nurses, school health nurses, social workers, and receptionists and nurses who work in healthcare provider's offices.

Analyzing the Client's Response

The previously established goals and objectives of the nursing care plan become the standards or criteria by which to measure the client's progress. Evaluation of care is based

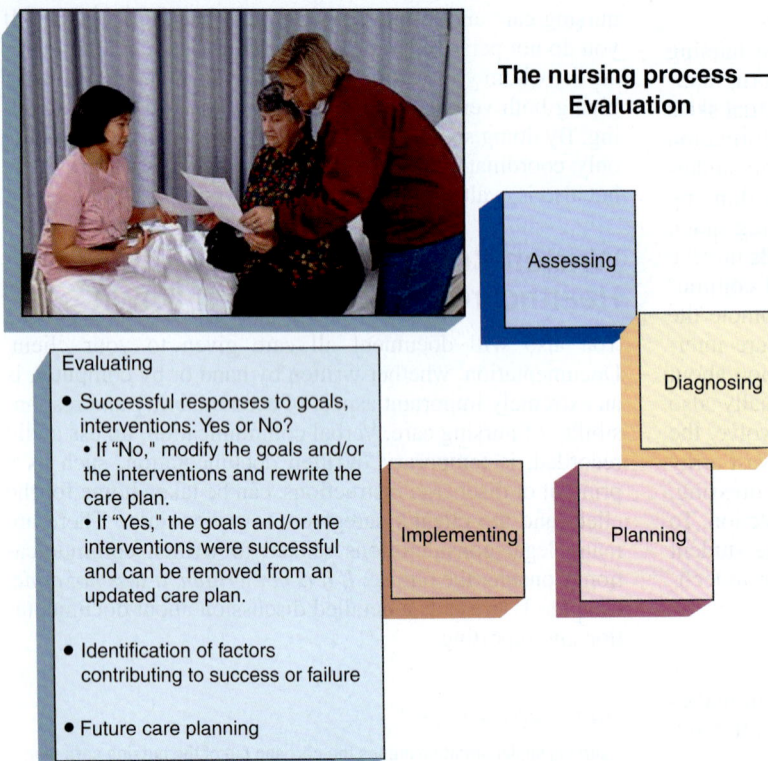

Figure 36-3 During evaluation, the last step of the nursing process, the nurse and client jointly measure how well the client has achieved the goals that were specified in the plan of care. Any factors that contributed to the client's success or failure are identified, and the plan of care is revised as necessary. The client's responses to the plan of care determine whether the plan continues as is, is modified, or is ended.

on these criteria. Was each goal met? The evaluation criteria should also consider whether nursing care has helped the client realize self-care goals. For example, for the woman with pneumonia described in Nursing Care Plan 33-1, resolution of fever, decreased use of accessory muscles, decreased shortness of breath and easier breathing, changes in sputum color, clearer lungs on auscultation, and increased activity level without supplementary oxygen provide evidence that the goals identified on the nursing care plan were being met.

Identifying Factors Contributing to Success or Failure

The evaluation process is not intended as a positive or negative response to nursing care. Various factors contribute to the achievement of goals. Evaluations are based on the client's overall responses to nursing care, medical interventions, and physiologic reactions. Ideally, the client's condition will improve. However, each client's responses to care will be unique. The client may have unexpected consequences, such as an ineffective or allergic response to medications. The client may be too sick to follow the initial plans. The client's condition may worsen in spite of all healthcare interventions. During the evaluation phase of the nursing process, the nurse needs to be objective when reviewing data, focus observations on factors related to goals, and combine common sense with critical thinking skills in order that new goals match the client's condition.

Sometimes you, the nurse, may be a factor. For example, you may lack knowledge about how to perform certain actions or may be thinking about personal problems and therefore perform a procedure incorrectly. *Remember:* You are responsible for ensuring that your knowledge and skills are always of the highest quality.

NCLEX Alert

When an NCLEX question asks you *Which of the following would represent a valid evaluation?* be sure to review the initial written plan or goal for that client. The evaluation should reflect achievement or revision of a stated goal.

Discharge Planning

The nursing process is dynamic and cyclical. Problems may resolve or change. Resolved problems are noted on the care plan or care path as "resolved." As clients meet their goals, new goals are set. If goals remain unmet, you must consider the reasons these goals are not being achieved and suggest revisions to the nursing care plan.

For the woman with pneumonia described in Chapter 33, one goal is to acknowledge the need for follow-up to prevent a recurrence of problems. By the time of discharge, both the client and the daughter are able to identify signs and symptoms that would indicate a recurrence. However, if this evidence was lacking, the plan of care would need to be modified to address additional teaching for the client and the daughter.

Key Concept

Nursing evaluation is the measurement of the effectiveness of assessing, diagnosing, planning, and implementing. Evaluation includes the following steps:

- Analyzing the client's responses
- Identifying factors that contributed to the success or failure of the care plan
- Planning for future nursing care

Box 36-1 Examples of Components of Discharge Planning

A discharge plan includes specific components of client teaching, with documentation of exactly what was taught, who did the teaching and when, who was present (members of the healthcare team, client, and/or family), and the client's reaction or expressed level of understanding. Examples of specific components include the following.

EQUIPMENT NEEDED AT HOME
- Documentation that the family has obtained equipment or knows where to get it
- Documentation of instruction and return demonstration in the use of any special equipment
- Documentation of ability to understand instructions

DIETARY NEEDS: SPECIAL DIET
- Documentation by the dietitian as to teaching the client and family
- Document their level of expressed understanding

MEDICATIONS OR PROCEDURES
- Explanation of reason for use of new medications
- Demonstration of method needed for use of medications (e.g., inhalers, insulin, injections, skin lotions)
- Documentation of instructions and special precautions
- Demonstration of procedures, such as a dressing change or insertion of catheters
- Demonstration and return demonstration until client can complete task satisfactorily
- Documentation of ability of the client or significant other to do the procedure

RESOURCES
- Written contact numbers and addresses of resources
- Referral to public health or home care services
- Documentation of expected first date of service
- Documentation of contact numbers
- Documentation for follow-up care

EMERGENCY RESPONSE: DANGER SIGNS
- Documentation of specific urgent problems that may develop
- Documentation of emergency numbers and healthcare provider's numbers

ACTIVITY
- Documentation that instructions were given and understood
- Examples of activities allowed or not allowed

SUMMARY
- Documentation of verbal teaching, demonstrations, and return demonstrations
- Documentation that a copy of the written instruction sheet was given to the client and/or significant others
- Description of each specific concept or task that was taught
- Documentation ability of the client or significant other to comprehend instruction
- Documentation of planned follow-up by facility or healthcare provider

---

Discharge planning is the process by which the client is prepared for continued care outside the healthcare facility or for independent living at home. Clients, family, or other healthcare workers may provide continuing care. Planning for discharge begins when a client is admitted to the healthcare system and is ongoing throughout the client's plan of care. Because clients achieve different levels of care at different times, the discharge plan must be individualized. Some facilities incorporate the discharge plan into the nursing care plan or clinical care path.

Ideally, before the client is ready for discharge from the facility, the healthcare team holds a conference with the client, the client's family, and caregivers, if possible. The purpose of this conference is to identify long-term goals that are still unresolved and to plan for continued assistance to the client.

Working together, the healthcare team and client may set new goals at the discharge conference. The caregivers learn to help the client to meet new and to review former goals. The primary nurse, or team leader, is responsible for seeing that the client, family, or caregivers have the necessary discharge instructions. Each client will have a unique situation, for example, follow-up phone numbers or dates for the next visit. Discharge from any healthcare environment can be stressful; the anxiety involved in these situations often limits the client's ability to absorb instructions, especially detailed instructions. Therefore, verbal instructions are given along with documented follow-up information. All information is individualized. Standardized printouts are commonly used, but individualized written information needs to be added. Box 36-1 and Chapter 37 discuss components of documentation in the nurse's notes of the client's hospital record.

Key Concept

Discharge teaching begins on admission and continues throughout the client's care. The client and family cannot be expected to remember a large amount of teaching at one time, especially just as the client is leaving the facility.

NCLEX Alert

Discharge planning may include written instruction, skills demonstration, and/or verbal teaching. The client, the family, and one or more significant persons may be included in the discharge planning. Always consider the uniqueness of the client and the client's situation when providing an NCLEX answer. Although it is generally preferable that the family participate in the client's care after discharge, this is not always possible.

STUDENT SYNTHESIS

KEY POINTS

- Implementation involves dependent, interdependent, and independent actions.
- Nurses use intellectual, interpersonal, and technical skills to implement care plans.
- During implementation, nurses collect further data and communicate information with other members of the healthcare team.
- During evaluation, client responses are analyzed, factors contributing to the success or failure of the plan are identified, and planning for future care occurs.
- Discharge planning and future planning are based on nursing care plans.

CRITICAL THINKING EXERCISES

1. Describe various skills a nurse needs to implement care. Give examples of these skills and determine which skills you perform best. Draw up a plan to become more proficient in your weaker skills.
2. Your client has had a complicated recovery from surgery, including wound infection, increased length of hospital stay, and a lack of supportive significant others. Discuss how this client's initial preoperative nursing care plan had to be changed and reevaluated after surgery. What specific concerns would you want to include in discharge planning?

NCLEX-STYLE REVIEW QUESTIONS

1. The nurse is caring for a client who states, "I am having discomfort in my lower back from lying in bed." Which independent nursing action can the nurse provide?
   a. Administer Tylenol 650 mg PO.
   b. Reposition the client in bed for comfort.
   c. Apply a medicated patch to the lower back.
   d. Administer an opioid analgesic.
2. A client states, "I feel nauseous," after a surgical procedure. Which is an appropriate dependent nurse action to implement for this client?
   a. Place an emesis basin where the client can reach it.
   b. Elevate the head of the bed to 45°.
   c. Apply a cool, damp cloth to the forehead.
   d. Administer an antiemetic as ordered.
3. A client reports shortness of breath and wheezing and is given a nebulizer treatment with a bronchodilator. Which evaluation recorded by the nurse indicates a positive outcome of the treatment?
   a. The client has decreased wheezing with no shortness of breath.
   b. The client requires oxygen at 4 L/m by nasal cannula.
   c. The client requires transport to a higher level of care unit.
   d. The client states the need for another treatment.
4. The nurse is planning for discharge of a client with diabetes. When would the nurse begin the discharge planning of this client?
   a. When the client is admitted to the healthcare system
   b. The day the client is to be discharged
   c. The day before the client is to be discharged
   d. Before the client is escorted out of the facility
5. Which methods would be optimal to be sure the client has an understanding of the discharge instructions? Select all that apply.
   a. Written instructions
   b. Skill demonstration
   c. Verbal teaching
   d. A webinar when the client goes home
   e. A message delivered via secure patient portal

CHAPTER RESOURCES

Enhance your learning with additional resources on **thePoint**!

Student Resources related to this chapter can be found at thePoint.lww.com/Rosdahl12e.

37 Documenting and Reporting

Learning Objectives

1. State the reasons for maintaining a written and continuous health record.
2. List the categories of information that are included in the health record.
3. Discuss the advantages and disadvantages of both manual and computerized documentation.
4. Discuss the rationale for use of accountability (core) measures, how these measures are integrated with the documentation of interventions, and outcomes of client care standards.
5. Differentiate among the following types of charting in progress notes: narrative, SOAP, SOAPIER, APIE, PIE, DAPE, DARP, DARE, and CBE.
6. State the advantages and disadvantages of the following types of documentation: narrative, problem-oriented, discipline area, charting by exception, case management, critical pathways, and medication administration records.
7. Identify the data that are commonly found on a flow sheet.
8. State eight guidelines that are generally accepted for documentation.
9. Practice using descriptive terms, abbreviations, and acronyms commonly used in charting.
10. Identify and differentiate the regulations and method of documenting for the following: an error in charting, a late entry, and an error that occurred regarding care for a client.
11. Describe the process and content of reporting information to nurses. Discuss how this type of report differs from communicating to other members of the healthcare team.

Important Terminology

accountability measures
case management
change-of-shift reporting
charting by exception
core measures
discipline area (multidisciplinary) documentation
electronic medical records
evidence-based practice
focus charting
graphic flow sheet
medication administration record
narrative charting
nurses' notes
problem-oriented medical records
progress notes
walking rounds

Acronyms

APIE
CBE
DAPE
DARE
DARP
EMR
MAR
MDS
MIS
PIE
POMR
RAP
RIE
SOAP
SOAPIER

DOCUMENTATION

The *health record* is a manual (handwritten) or electronic (computer) account of a client's relationship with a healthcare facility. Healthcare providers chronologically and systematically record all information regarding the client's health, past and current problems, diagnostic tests, treatments, responses to treatments, and discharge planning through handwritten or keyboard entries. Because you, the nurse, are usually a primary caregiver, the information that you put in the record is very important to inform other caregivers of the client's appearance, behavior, and responses. You must record such information clearly, accurately, and frequently. The commonly used term for documentation is "charting." The client's health record is usually called the "chart."

Purposes of the Health Record

Accurate and complete documentation in the client's health record is an essential communication tool. It is used

- To maintain effective communication among all caregivers
- To provide written evidence of accountability
- To meet legal, regulatory, and financial requirements
- To provide data for research and educational purposes

Communication

Because the goal of the healthcare team is to work together to provide the best possible care for the client, the health record is a communication tool that all caregivers use to exchange information with one another. Each caregiver enters information about the client's condition, treatments, responses to treatments, and plans. Instructions for treatment of the client (e.g., healthcare provider orders, care plans, or care paths) are also included in the health record. Together, these data, notes, and instructions provide a way for healthcare providers to remain in touch about the nature of the client's health problems, possible treatments, treatments given, and client responses.

Think of the health record as a bank where information is deposited, stored, and made available to all who need it. This central resource for information ensures that a client's care is consistent and effective.

Another aspect of communication that is important to the client is the documentation and verification of their own health status. A client may require this record of information for specific reasons, such as employment or for a disability application.

See Box 37-1 for some thoughts on how nurses help facilitate communication.

> **Key Concept**
>
> When communicating with others, it is important to consider each person's age, sex, ethnic and religious background, state of health, life experiences, body image, feelings about being in the healthcare facility, language preference, and other personal factors.

Accountability

As you learned in Chapter 36, accountability means responsibility for actions. The health record is *documented evidence* that the healthcare agency and providers have acted responsibly and effectively. Such evidence of accountability is required for legal, regulatory, and financial reasons.

Accountability for documentation, as well as initiation of appropriate actions, is a component of the nursing process and nursing regulations. The Joint Commission, in conjunction with the Centers for Medicare and Medicaid Services (CMS), has developed **core measures** that provide standards of care. Reclassified as **accountability measures**, their goal is to delineate criteria that produce the greatest positive impact on the outcomes of client care. Each healthcare facility associated with the Joint Commission and CMS is required to meet the standards set by these measures. Financial incentives and improved client outcomes provide a stimulant for compliance with this system. The measures can be found in the Specifications Manual for National Hospital Inpatient Quality Measures. Nursing care and documentation are very important in the record keeping for these measures. Facilities may provide specific checklists that ensure documentation of the accountability measures.

The following list outlines the major issues involved with compliance and accountability:

- *Legal Requirements and Protection.* The healthcare record fulfills a legal requirement mandating all businesses and corporations that provide public services keep records of their interactions with clients. Thus, the health record is a *legal document*. The health record is an important piece of evidence when questions of inadequate, incorrect, or poor healthcare arise. If a client, family member, or attorney questions the quality of care given, the well-written and comprehensive health record is the best source of information describing what actually occurred. Accurate, precise, and timely entries into the health record are your protection against accusations of inadequate or poor nursing care.

> **NCLEX Alert**
>
> If your health records are audited or if you go to court, the basic legal concept is: if it was not documented, it was not done.

> **Box 37-1 Facilitating Communication in Healthcare**
>
> Nurses facilitate communication between clients and members of the nursing team in various ways, including:
> - Maintaining the confidentiality of all information about clients
> - Skillfully interviewing clients to determine their healthcare needs
> - Listening attentively to what the client is saying
> - Teaching clients and their families certain aspects of care
> - Documenting information on the nursing care plan and in the client's record
> - Reporting the condition of the client to other members of the healthcare team
> - Participating in team conferences and client care conferences
> - Treating each client as a unique individual
> - Using both verbal and nonverbal means of communication and observing client's verbal and nonverbal reactions
> - Using touch as a therapeutic modality, while not invading the client's personal space or threatening the client

- *Documentation Criteria.* All healthcare agencies must meet certain *standards of care* established by governmental or voluntary regulatory agencies. Written documentation that demonstrates compliance with a standard of care has a relationship to, or has a proximal connection to, the outcome. That is, standards of care connect the accuracy of the evidence-based process with the outcome. Accountability measures are designed to minimize or eliminate unintended adverse effects. Complete and accurate healthcare records recognize the implementation of safe and effective healthcare.
- *Financial Accountability.* Just as payment for your groceries requires a receipt listing the items you selected, clients and third-party payers depend on a complete list of services and products provided before paying for healthcare. To facilitate this process, you must record all treatments given, examinations administered, and special equipment used (e.g., an air mattress). Third-party payers will not reimburse the healthcare facility unless billed for services and supplies are recorded in the health record. Thus, you must enter every aspect of your care to tell the third-party payer what has been done. Failure to do so may result in a loss of payment to the employing agency, ultimately leading to higher costs for clients and consumers.
- *Research and Education.* Strong scientific evidence or **evidence-based practice** demonstrates the rationales for medical care and nursing interventions. Research is implemented by major healthcare universities and by the various branches of the National Institutes of Health such as the National Institute for Nursing Research (NINR). Healthcare planners examine health records of individuals and groups to determine patterns of illness, trends, or effective treatment strategies. This research is necessary to select the best treatment for an individual

or to search for better treatments and medications for specific health problems. Health records, particularly those kept in computer databases, provide excellent research opportunities in healthcare.

The health record is also an excellent educational tool. Students in healthcare vocations benefit from reading and comparing the data of various clients as they enlarge their knowledge of health, illnesses, treatments, and responses.

Documentation Systems

The health record is either a manual (paper) document, an electronic document, or a combination of both. Electronic documents are located in a *medical information system* (**MIS**), which is housed in a computer network. The MIS may contain only specific medical information. Another documentation system is referred to as **electronic medical records** (**EMRs**). As MISs and EMRs become more user-friendly and cost-effective, healthcare facilities have commonly converted from manual to electronic formats because of the advantages of simplified and rapid data management (see Fig. 36-2).

Manual Records

The *manual health record* is a collection of various forms and documents. You may keep some of the forms in a client's record at the bedside for your practical convenience—for example, a fluid intake and output sheet or a flow sheet. The nurse is held legally responsible for the legibility, thoroughness, and timeliness of documentation. As computer systems have become bedside tools, manual records may be phased out or eliminated. Table 37-1 lists the purposes of the various forms included in the health record.

> **NCLEX Alert**
>
> Questions on any NCLEX might include the proper way to document information. Using your skills at definition of the stages of the nursing process including assessment/documentation gathering, implementation/interventions, appropriate goal setting, and evaluation will help you answer the question correctly.

Computer Records

Initially, computer access allowed healthcare facilities to use electronic medical record keeping for data entry such as laboratory results, dietary information, standardized pharmacy requests, or healthcare provider orders, plus medical billing and statistical data entry. Sophistication of computer software had evolved to enable the bedside practitioners to store, process, and transmit client data. Nursing care plans, treatment strategies, discharge instruction, and medication administration are only a few of the available areas that are centered in a healthcare computer network. EMR systems use networks of terminals attached to a satellite of terminals that handle the actual storing and processing of information. Usually, individual computer sites consist of a monitor and keyboard that are located in every client room, nursing care station or unit, as well as in other key places throughout the healthcare facility. Mobile stations are also known as computer on wheels (COW) or workstation on wheels (WOW). The healthcare provider can enter information via a keyboard, a light pen, a mouse, or by touching the screen. Healthcare providers can often retrieve an individual's data using a variety of devices that have Internet access.

Usually, the type of electronic documentation is designed for a healthcare agency's specific needs or needs delineated by accrediting agencies, such as The Joint Commission. Although requirements for documentation are basically the same for all healthcare facilities, each agency's requirements and, thus, their system, are unique. For example, an outpatient surgical clinic will have different needs than a long-term care facility or a newborn unit in an acute care hospital. They will all utilize various methods to record assessment data, care plans, nursing information, client responses, and changes in the client's condition.

Training for these systems is traditionally done during a new-hire's orientation with updates or refresher courses available according to the facility's protocol. The employee maybe required to successfully complete mandated instruction. Additionally, it is the employee's responsibility to ask for continued or advanced training using any computerized system. Commonly the employer assumes that the new employee will have had basic knowledge of computers and keyboard systems.

Direct transfer of electronic information from one hand-held machine (e.g., blood glucose monitor) to another machine (e.g., the client's computerized record) has many advantages. Additionally, electronic data can simultaneously be transmitted to a healthcare provider's office or be transmitted to a distant location for interpretation by an expert (e.g., the radiologist). Computers have become standard equipment within each client's unit; electronic charting at the bedside has replaced most pen and paper documentation.

> **Key Concept**
>
> If the healthcare facility where you work uses an electronic system, you will need to take orientation classes to learn how to use the system correctly. NEVER share your access code(s) to a facility's electronic documentation system.

Contents of the Health Record

The health record contains four general *categories of information:* assessment documents, plans for care and treatment, progress records, and plans for continuity of care.

> **Key Concept**
>
> Confidentiality is a major concern. It is imperative that a client's healthcare information be protected. Never share electronic information unless documentation protocols provide for the transmitting of data from one person or place to another person or place.

Assessment Documents

Assessment documents record all information about the client obtained through interview, examination, diagnostic procedures, or consultation. These documents include the healthcare provider's history and physical examination, the nursing admission history, and other records that list or describe related aspects of information about the client. All caregivers contribute to this bank of information. For examples of some specific forms, purposes, and responsible caregivers, see Table 37-1. The actual formats of the various records and forms vary among agencies. You will acquaint yourself with the forms of your facility as part of your orientation with any healthcare employer. Long-term care and some home care agencies use a standard form called a *minimum data set* (**MDS**) as part of the admitting nursing history. This form is sometimes called a *resident assessment protocol* (**RAP**). This form measures a client's ability to perform the activities of daily living (ADLs) and identifies functional losses that affect this ability. Several other assessment forms are available to aid the nursing care team in developing an individualized plan of care for each client. Federal and state regulatory agencies require these forms. You must answer all the questions asked on the form to ensure that your employer is complying with regulatory requirements.

The MDS helps to ensure that all clients are assessed in the same way. Because these forms are the same in all agencies, you will find them easy to use if you move from one agency to another.

Plans for Care and Treatment

The purpose of the *plans for care* is to ensure that all caregivers provide cohesive, coordinated care and treatments for the client. The healthcare provider's plan of care contains goals for treating the client and specific instructions called *orders* to guide the nursing staff. Some Nurse Practice Acts require that the nursing care plan be developed by the registered nurse after a thorough assessment of the client's health status. Commonly a team approach is used. The development of a plan of care uses both LVNs/LPNs and RNs. When discussing initiation and assessment of a care plan, the legal role of the LVN/LPN differs from state to state. Additionally, each type of clinical facility will have in-house guidelines and regulations for the nursing plans of care. State regulating agencies for acute versus long-term care will also mandate specific approaches for the development of nursing care plans. Discussed later in this chapter, another version, called the *clinical care path*, is a plan that specifies expected outcomes and treatments at specified times for all members of the healthcare team.

As stated previously, numerous formats and versions of plans of care are fundamentally based on the traditional nursing care plan. The needs of the client, the facility, and the nurse commonly dictate which format will be chosen. It is not uncommon to have several versions within one facility. For example, the care plan format in an emergency department will differ from that of a critical care unit, a maternal-child unit, or a medical-surgical unit. The graduate will be oriented to the appropriate version of documentation after he/she has been hired as an employee.

Formats of Documentation

Many formats for charting or documenting the client's progress exist. These formats use various versions of the nursing process. Charting is based on the nursing process: assessment, nursing diagnosis, planning and goal setting, implementation/interventions, and evaluation. Reasons to use a progress note entry are to

- Establish a baseline of data
- Document the accountability (core) measures of admission
- Enter data at regular intervals
- Summarize the client's condition
- Document changes in the client's condition
- Document a response to treatment

Several systems of data entry are used. To know what type of charting, record keeping, and documenting that you need to use, you should first consult your instructor and the institution's policy and procedure manuals. As part of orientation to your student experiences and later, when you are employed as a nurse, you will be informed of the facility's needs, forms, and formats. Each format has advantages and disadvantages.

Typical documentation formats include

- Narrative–chronological
- Problem-oriented (focus)
- Discipline area (multidisciplinary) documentation
- Charting by exception
- System flow sheet
- Case management
- Critical pathway
- Collaborative pathway
- Care mapping
- Graphic flow sheet
- Medication administration record

Narrative–Chronological

Progress notes are written in several formats, often using specific forms, which usually are designed by each institution. A progress note essentially summarizes the progress of the client toward achieving their care plan goals. Typically written in a narrative, chronological format, a progress note can be a summary or narration of an event, conversation, assessment, or activity. This narrative format is kept chronologically. Charting can be done hourly, every 2 hour, per event, or more often.

When nurses chart on a progress note, the form is commonly called the **nurses' notes**. Some facilities use a team approach where all documentation is continuous on one general progress note. Most hospitals use separate progress notes for healthcare providers, nurses, physical therapy, respiratory therapy, and other healthcare specialties. Additional information about discipline area (multidisciplinary) documentation is provided in this chapter.

Narrative charting is a type of nurses' notes that essentially documents what is occurring throughout the day in a chronological manner. Appendix D Figure 1 demonstrates narrative–chronological charting. The usual opening note on charts that use narrative style is the nurse's first assessment

TABLE 37-1 Contents of the Health Record

GENERAL CATEGORY	SPECIFIC FORM OR SCREEN	PURPOSE	RESPONSIBLE CAREGIVER
Assessment documents: forms/screens	Admission record	Lists client's name, address, sex, age, healthcare provider, insurance company, reason for admission	Admitting staff
	Medical history and physical examination	Records healthcare provider's history and physical examination findings	Healthcare provider
	Nursing admission history	Records nurse's history	Usually RN, but may be LVN/LPN in some facilities
	Minimum data set (MDS)	Records information that identifies the client's ability to perform activities of daily living and functional losses that affect this ability	Admitting RN, but may be LVN/LPN in some facilities
	Laboratory record	Records results of blood, urine, stool, or other body substance analysis	Laboratory personnel: healthcare providers, technicians
	Consultation	Records findings and opinions from consults requested by primary caregivers	Consulting healthcare provider or other care provider
Plans for care and treatment	Problem list	Describes healthcare provider's goals for treatment	Healthcare provider
	Healthcare provider's orders	List instructions to nurses or technicians to implement client's diagnostic tests, treatments, or medications	Healthcare provider
	Nursing care plan	Lists client's expected outcomes of nursing care Lists nursing actions to achieve outcome	Usually RN, but may be an LPN in some facilities
	Teaching plan	Identifies client's teaching needs Lists teaching strategies	Nursing staff
	Clinical care path	Lists diagnostic tests, treatments, and expected client outcomes on a timeline; usually designates responsible caregiver	All caregivers
	Consents for treatment	Explains expected and possible adverse outcomes for treatments; contains client's signature	Admitting personnel; healthcare provider; nursing staff
Progress records: forms/screens	Flow sheet	Documents large amounts of information briefly and concisely by a timeline. Includes intake and output sheets, graphic sheets for vital signs, anesthesia sheets during surgery, routine nursing care sheets, intensive care unit records. Efficient records	Depending on purpose of flow sheet, all care providers but particularly RN, LPN, and perhaps aides
	Medication administration record	Lists ordered medications, amount, route, and ordered time of administration for noting the time of actual administration and response to medication	Depending on facility's system, may be prepared by pharmacy via computer printout; medication administration documented by RN, LPN
	Progress note	Describes client's treatment, responses to treatment, and unusual events; documents progress toward achieving outcomes. Can be a general form or format for all team members or individual formats used by specialty areas, such as nursing, healthcare providers, respiratory, and physical therapy	All care providers
Plans for continuity of care form/screen	Teaching record	Lists times and teaching strategies used; client's responses	Usually RN, but may be LVN/LPN in some facilities
	Transfer form/screen	Summarizes client's condition and responses to treatment to prepare for transfer to another unit, facility, or community health agency	Usually RN, but may be LVN/LPN in some facilities
	Discharge/transfer summary	Summarizes client's condition on discharge from the healthcare facility	Healthcare provider and RN or LPN

after assuming responsibility for that client. The nurse may do a body system assessment starting with general observation, then assessments of the neurologic, integumentary, cardiovascular, gastrointestinal, and genitourinary systems and others. This is often referred to as "head-to-toe" charting. The framework of an assessment will include the accountability or core measures; those concerns that are considered a medical or nursing priority. Subsequent entries add to the assessment, note changes in condition, or record facts. For example:

08:30 Reports pain of 8 on a 0–10 pain scale.—*M. Garcia, LVN*
08:45 Medicated with 50 mg Demerol IM as per order in LUOQ.—*M. Garcia, LVN*
09:30 States, "I feel so much better; the pain is only a 3 now."—*M. Garcia, LVN*
10:15 Dr. E. Jones removed and replaced abdominal dressing. —*M. Garcia, LVN*

Narrative charting is very thorough and detailed. It is also time-consuming. Narrative, chronological charting is useful and popular with nurses who need to document complex descriptions with thorough assessments.

Area Charting

Some formats of charting focus on a specific problem rather than on general assessment data. When **problem-oriented medical records** (**POMR**) charting is used, the whole healthcare team works collaboratively to identify priority problems and they work collectively to solve these problems. This type of charting focuses on specific problems and is sometimes called **focus charting**.

Several shorter versions of narrative charting have been devised and are used for POMR, which have the benefit of greater time efficiency, but may not include pertinent data that would be included in narrative formats. Acronyms provide memory aides on what to include in charting. Types of charting include **SOAP, SOAPIER, APIE, PIE, DAPE, DARP,** and **DARE**. These acronyms are identified in Table 37-2. In general, these acronyms delineate the following terms: subjective, objective, approach, analysis, plan, interventions, response, education, and evaluation. Figures 2 (SOAP) and 3 (APIE) in Appendix D, available online, are examples of problem area (focus) charting.

Discipline Area (Multidisciplinary) Documentation

Documentation by discipline area would include separate notes for healthcare providers, nurses, and other healthcare team members, such as dietary, respiratory therapy, physical therapy, occupational therapy, or home health providers. Each specialty may have specific formats or forms used to chart about that particular field. Forms and formats used include narrative or a version of SOAP.

The main advantage of this type of record keeping is that providers in each subspecialty can find their own forms quickly and follow the progress of their therapies without having to read notes from other disciplines. However, it can be difficult to monitor data as a holistic view of the client. The data can appear separate and fragmented, which might not be seen as related to other subspecialties. For example, respiratory therapy may chart that the client did not tolerate the breathing treatment. The nurse may not read the individual entries of the healthcare team and may be unaware that the client is not benefiting from respiratory treatment.

Charting by Exception

Charting by exception (**CBE**) is a type of narrative charting that usually uses a flow sheet listing body systems and their typical findings, such as lung sounds: clear, crackles, or rhonchi. The nurse checks off the correct assessment findings on the preprinted sheet. Flow sheets have the advantage of listing the most common normal and abnormal findings, so the chance of leaving out important documentation is decreased.

After charting or checking off normal findings, the next step of CBE is making a notation about the abnormal findings on a separate nurses' note. In other words, normal findings are given a check on a box on the flow sheet; abnormal findings and the care for these findings are more thoroughly documented in separate nurses' notes. CBE could be considered a short-hand version of narrative charting and may be considered more efficient, especially for the client who is physically stable with an uncomplicated care plan. However, it may be a disadvantage when a legal defense claim, such as negligence, is necessary. When CBE is used, the nurse must be sure that all charting is thorough and complete. Charting by exception is seen in Appendix D, Figure 4, which is available online. Also, note in Appendix D that Figures 4 (Charting by Exception) and 5 (Graphic Flow Sheet) show a collaborative method of documentation.

> **Key Concept**
>
> In some areas, "reporting by exception" is practiced. In this case, not all recurring client information is repeated. The nurse only reports changes in the client's condition, new orders, upcoming procedures, and unusual or changing behavior.

Case Management

Case management is popular in situations in which the emphasis is on quality care that is delivered in the most cost-effective manner. The client is considered the focus of a case study, and the goal is to achieve specific outcomes that are identified in a multidisciplinary team approach. This type of record keeping is also known as *case studies, care mapping, collaborative pathways*, or *critical pathways*. The team shares information and priorities. It is often used in a "typical" stable client and may be seen in home care organizations, such as in the provision of postoperative wound care. Case management may not be suitable for a client with special or complex individual needs.

TABLE 37-2 Commonly Used Nursing Note Formats

ACRONYM	CATEGORY	CONTENT
POMR (Specific problems are identified)		
SOAP	**S** Subjective	Subjective client data; usually direct quotes from client
Or	**O** Objective	Objective client data identified through observation, examination, or interview
SOAPE	**A** Assessment or analysis	Conclusions drawn from data; often stated as a nursing diagnosis or client care problem
Or		
SOAPIE	**P** Plan	Expected outcome; if an SOAP note, this states nursing strategies to treat the nursing diagnosis or client care problem
Or	**I** Intervention	Nursing strategies to treat the nursing diagnosis or client care problem
SOAPIER	**E** Evaluation **R** Revision	Outcomes of nursing care; reassessment of client New plans for treatment of care problem based on client outcomes or responses
APIE	**A** Assessment	Objective and subjective data about the client; may include a conclusion in the form of nursing diagnosis or client care problem. (If system is PIE, A is recorded on a flow sheet at regular intervals)
Or	**P** Plan	Expected outcome listed or
PIE		Planned strategies to treat the nursing diagnosis or client care problem
	I Intervention	Nursing care given
	E Evaluation	Outcomes of nursing care; responses of client; reassessment information
Focus (Problem stated as nursing diagnosis or client care problem)		
DAPE	**D** Data	Objective and subjective data about client obtained through observation, interview, and examination
	A Assessment	Conclusions drawn from data; may be nursing diagnosis or client care problem
	P Plan	Expected outcomes listed or planned strategies to treat the nursing diagnosis or care problem
	E Evaluation	Outcomes of nursing care; responses of the client; reassessment information
DARE	**D** Data **A** Action **R** Response **E** Education	Objective and subjective assessment data that support the Focus Nursing interventions to treat the problem Outcomes of interventions; reassessment data Client education
DARP	**D** Data	Subjective data per client (e.g., pain) followed by assessment or action taken (pain medication needed or given). Response to assessment or action charted (pain relieved by pain medication). A plan is formed for further evaluation (provide medication per orders)
	A Assessment or Action **R** Response **P** Plan	
Charting by exception (CBE)	Uses an SOAPIER or a system flow sheet format for progress notes where abnormal signs or symptoms (the "exception" to normal status) are specifically identified, assessed, and interventions are documented.	See above for SOAPIER content. A system flow sheet provides routine assessment/data collection at intervals. Normal or expected data are checked or initialed. Abnormalities or unexpected findings are referred to progress notes for further discussion

Graphic Flow Sheet

A **graphic flow sheet** is a graph, form, or picture that records large amounts of information collected at intervals over a specified period in brief, concise entries.

> **NCLEX Alert**
>
> Because of the wide variety of specific documentation methods, NCLEX questions tend to relate specific clinical situations. From these situations, the graduate must choose the most appropriate, clear, and effective response. More than one response may be correct, but there is only one, best correct answer to the given situation.

The **medication administration record** (**MAR**) lists all medications that the healthcare provider has ordered for the client, with spaces for the caregiver to mark when medications are given. Injection site locations are also documented. A facility may separate the MARs from the bulk of the client's health record for convenience so that the nurse has rapid access to a listing of all current medications, can document medications immediately after they are given, and can administer medications according to the healthcare provider's orders.

In addition to the MAR, other examples of information that is kept on a graphic flow sheet include

- Vital signs
- Intake and output
- ADLs
- Dietary or eating patterns
- Neurologic checks ("neuro checks")
- Restraint observation and documentation
- Frequent blood sugar monitoring
- Postoperative records
- Wound care and monitoring

As stated, these forms often include some form of graphic representation that will help care providers see visual representations of trends or clusters of information. This type of form is commonly used by nonlicensed personnel as well as licensed nurses.

Both manual and MIS records have flow sheets. The flow sheet in the manual records is a page in the client's record or a separate sheet kept near the client's bedside. A computerized flow sheet may be a screen that has a simple "yes" or "no" response that can be completed quickly and efficiently using a light pen or keyboard. The flow sheet may have highlighted blanks for data entry similar to recording intake and output on paper.

Sometimes the data on the flow sheet are summarized elsewhere in the health records so that not all data or forms are kept. An EMR system is particularly useful for data compilation and storage. If the record is a manual paper chart, the flow sheet itself may be discarded by the primary care nurse or team leader because the formal, summary entry is recorded elsewhere. For example, data from a bedside intake and output flow sheet may be discarded at the end of each shift because the data are summarized and placed in the MIS.

Plans for Continuity of Care

The length of a client's admission to the healthcare agency varies from a few days to a few years, depending on the nature of the illness or disability. During admission, transfer, or discharge from the agency, healthcare personnel use specific forms to ensure that the client's care is continuous, consistent, and effective. Teaching plans, transfer notes, and discharge summaries contain information that enables other caregivers to ensure continuity of care.

Guidelines for Documentation

The quality of your documentation says much about the kind of care you give. *Accurate* and *complete* documentation is important for effective communication and accountability. Regardless of the particular format your agency uses, always practice the following skills in documentation.

Document What You See

Describe exactly what you observe, and document what you see. Describe your assessments objectively; do not give your opinions or interpretations. Be specific. For example, when you observe bleeding, indicate how much blood there is; its color; whether it is gushing, oozing, or running; and its source. When you are describing a client's response, describe the client's activity, not what you think it means. For example, "client crying and rocking back and forth in chair" is an objective and descriptive statement. If you try to interpret the client's actions, however, you may come to several subjective conclusions, with no guarantee that any of them are correct. One interpretation might be "client lonely"; another might be "client out of touch with reality"; and still another might be "client in pain." Such interpretations may be incorrect and serve only to confuse issues and to distract care providers from treating the client's primary problems.

Is the client having trouble moving? Does the client stumble? Can the person stand in a normal fashion? Is speech coherent? Is speech clear and appropriate? Does urine or stool smell foul? Does the client's breath have a foul odor? These are the types of questions to ask yourself so that your assessments are accurate and your documentation is informative.

Identify the client's reaction to your actions, whether it is to a medication given, client teaching, or nursing interventions. Record the client's response, as well as the time, dosage, description, and any adverse effects. Check the health record for previous adverse reactions to this medication or treatment.

Be Specific

Avoid ambiguous statements and generalizations. For example, "had an uncomfortable night" does not say anything specific, whereas "client was up 10 times with diarrhea during the night" tells *why* the client had an uncomfortable night and *why* sleep was interrupted. Avoid judgmental words such as *well, fair, poor,* or *good.*

Use Direct Quotes

Directly quote the client, and differentiate the client's words from your observations. Enclose the client's statements in quotation marks so others will know exactly what the client said. The following statement serves as an example:

Mrs. C. stated, "I have a throbbing pain in my head."
Note that this documented statement is specific, describing how the client interprets the pain.
Do not chart hearsay, such as what someone else has told you about the client, unless you quote it. For example:
Mrs. R.'s husband said, "My wife does not like the food here."

Be Prompt

Document immediately after giving all care, medications, and treatments. The health record does not have memory lapses, although you may. Always document *after* you give a medication or perform a treatment, *never before*. If you forget to document a pertinent fact and add it after you have entered other documentation in the health record, you must identify your entry as a "late entry."

Be Clear and Consistent

Correct spelling, punctuation, and sentence structure are essential. "Bathed in wheelchair in hall" is not a clear statement. "Client had a bed bath given by the nurse and is now sitting in a wheelchair in the hallway" is clear and accurate.

On manual records, write or print neatly in black ink. Make sure the record is continuous and *legible*. Use the format specified by that particular agency. Indicate the date and time of each entry. Be aware that most facilities use the 24-hour clock (Table 37-3).

Use only standard abbreviations. Table 37-4 lists some common abbreviations and acronyms. There are literally thousands of medical abbreviations, acronyms, and symbols. To decrease the chances of misreading or misinterpreting, prevent medication errors, and promote safety for the client, the Joint Commission has compiled a "do not use" list, shown in Table 37-5. Other possible future additions to this list are shown in Table 37-6. Each healthcare facility has a list of acceptable abbreviations, acronyms, and symbols; the list usually is located in the policy and procedure manuals. Boxes 37-2 and 37-3 list some symbols and acronyms that are commonly used in documentation.

Sign the chart with your first initial or full first name and full last name and classification (e.g., *C. Jacobs, LVN,* or *Carol Jacobs, LVN*). Your facility will dictate the form of signature that is required for documentation.

Do not leave vacant lines in the health record. Using every line maintains the chronology of charting. If you continue on the back of a sheet or on a new page, again write the date, time, and "(continued)" before continuing your entry. If a vacant line is left between entries, draw a line through it, to indicate that the documentation is chronological.

TABLE 37-3 Comparison of Features of 12 and 24-Hour Clocks With Acceptable Wording and Configuration Variations

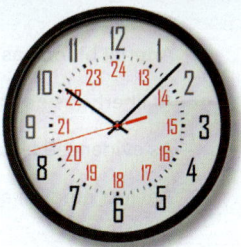

Standard clock showing 12- and 24-hour settings. note the large black numbers near the outer edge signify a 12-hour cycle. The red numbers within the inner circle conform to the 24-hour clock.

12-HOUR CLOCK	24-HOUR CLOCK OR MILITARY TIME
12 Midnight (end of day)	24:00 (end of a day)
12:00 (start of a day)	00:00 Midnight (start of a day)
12:01 AM	00:01 (read as zero, zero, zero, one hours)
6:15 AM	06:15 (read as zero six fifteen hours)
7:30 AM	07:30 (read as zero seven thirty hours)
12 PM (noon)	12:00 (middle of day for 24-hour clock)
1 PM	13:00 (read as thirteen hundred hours)
8:30 PM	20:30 (read as twenty thirty hours)
10 PM	22:00 (read as twenty-two hundred hours)
11 PM	23:00 (read as twenty-three hundred hours)
11:59 PM (last minute of a day)	23:59 (last minute of a day)

Adapted from materials found: http://militarytimechart.com/ and http://en.wikipedia.org/w/index.php?title=24-hour_clock

Always replace the health record where it belongs. Do not remove it from the nursing station unless you have consulted the charge nurse or team leader.

Record All Relevant Information

Read the healthcare provider's notes. If you have any questions or concerns, bring them to the healthcare provider's attention. Document all communications with other members of the healthcare team. Other departments also have policies and procedures that you must follow to protect the

TABLE 37-4 Abbreviations and Acronyms Commonly Used in Documentation

ā	Before	ML (also seen: ml, Ml, mL)	Milliliter (metric unit of measurement)
AC, ac	Before meals	Mm	Millimeter (metric unit of measurement)
ABG	Arterial blood gas	NG	Nasogastric
Ad lib	At liberty, as desired	NKA	No known allergies
AEB, AMB	As evidenced by, as manifested by	NPO, npo	Nothing by mouth
AMA	Against medical advice	NS	Normal saline
Amb	Ambulate	N/V, N/V/D	Nausea and vomiting; nausea, vomiting, and diarrhea
BM	Bowel movement	O	Oral
BID, bid	Twice per day	O_2	Oxygen
BRP	Bathroom privileges	p̄	After
c̄	With	PC, pc	After meals
c/o	Complains of	Per, per	By
CO_2	Carbon dioxide	PO, po	By mouth
CPR	Cardiopulmonary resuscitation	PR	Per rectum, rectally
DNR	Do not resuscitate	PRN, prn	As needed, when required
DSG, dsg	Dressing	Pt, pt	Patient, pint
DX, Dx, dx	Diagnosis	Pulse Ox	Pulse oximetry
FOB	Foot of bed	QH, qh	Every hour
Fx, fx	Fracture	QID, qid	Four times per day
g (also seen: Gm, gm, G)	Gram (metric unit of measurement)	R, r	Respiration, rectum
Gr	Grain (apothecary unit of measurement)	®, rt	Right
Gtt	Drop, drops	R/O, r/o	Rule out, eliminate
HOB	Head of bed	ROM	Range of motion
Hx, hx	History	ROS	Review of systems
I&O	Intake and output	R/T, r/t	Related to
IM	Intramuscular	RX, Rx	Prescription, take, treatment
IV	Intravenous	s̄	Without
KVO, TKO	Keep vein open, to keep open (an IV infusion)	S/P, s/p	Status post, after
L, lt	Left	STAT, stat	Immediately
L (also seen: l)	Liter (metric unit of measurement)	Subq, subq, sc, sq	Subcutaneous
LMP	Last menstrual period	Supp, supp	Suppository
mEq	Milliequivalents (metric unit of measurement)	Susp	Suspension
Mg (also seen: mg)	Milligram (metric unit of measurement)	S&S	Signs and symptoms

TABLE 37-4 Abbreviations and Acronyms Commonly Used in Documentation (Continued)

Sx	Symptom(s)	TPN	Total parenteral nutrition
TID, tid	Three times per day	TPR	Temperature, pulse, respiration
t, tsp	Teaspoon (household unit of measurement)	TX, Tx	Treatment
T, Tbsp	Tablespoon (household unit of measurement)	Ungt, ung	Ointment
TF	Tube feeding	VS	Vital signs

Some abbreviations are identical, but have different meanings. It is always best to write out the whole word rather than be unclear. Each facility has a list of approved abbreviations, which should be your main guide for documentation and use of acronyms and abbreviations. For additional information, see Table 60-1 and Box 60-1 for common abbreviations of measurement. The Joint Commission has delineated that some common abbreviations, symbols, and acronyms should no longer be used in healthcare settings. See Table 37-5.

client. If, for example, the care plan notes that the call light must be within client's reach, document that you have followed this guideline. If you do not carry out this order, you must state the reason in the documentation.

Respect Confidentiality

Confidentiality means that conversations with clients and nursing observations and assessments are shared only with the appropriate caregivers in the proper setting. What you record and show to the client and other health professionals is never to be shared with anyone else. Do not discuss clients "over coffee"; your conversation may be overheard. Remember to maintain confidentiality during telephone conversations, taking care that a bystander does not hear confidential information and that you do not violate client confidentiality through telephone conversations with the client's family or friends. Do not allow clients to see the computer screen. Be careful to maintain client confidentiality in the home care setting as well, when family or friends are present and eager to learn about your client. Keep in mind that you may be held liable in court for "breach of confidentiality" (see Chapter 4).

Record Documentation Errors

Erasures and the use of correction fluid on a client's manually written health record are *illegal*. Such measures could be considered as an attempt to hide poor nursing care or an error made in client care. If you make an *error in documenting*, cross out the incorrect statement with a single line, enclose it in parentheses, and write ERROR and your initials next to it. Your original note must be readable (see Appendix D, 1B). Some agencies recommend using *recorded in error* (**RIE**) instead. Other agencies use the term "mistaken entry." After filling in the term that your agency uses, record the correct statement. *(An error in client care is an entirely different matter that you must report to your instructor or team leader at once.)*

You may also make an error in the electronic chart. The EMR has a mechanism by which you may review your

TABLE 37-5 Official "Do Not Use" List[a]

DO NOT USE	POTENTIAL PROBLEM	USE INSTEAD
U (unit)	Mistaken for "0" (zero), the number "4" (four), or "cc"	Write "unit"
IU (International Unit)	Mistaken for IV (intravenous) or the number 10 (ten)	Write "International Unit"
MS	Can mean morphine sulfate or magnesium sulfate	Write "morphine sulfate"
MSO_4 and $MgSO_4$	Confused for one another	Write "magnesium sulfate"
Q.D., QD, q.d., qd (daily)	Mistaken for each other	Write "daily"
Q.O.D., QOD, q.o.d., qod (every other day)	Period after the Q mistaken for "I" and the "O" mistaken for "I"	Write "every other day"
Trailing zero (X.0 mg)[b] Lack of leading zero (.X mg)	Decimal point is missed	Write X mg Write 0.X mg

[a] Applies to all orders and all medication-related documentation that is handwritten (including free-text computer entry) or on preprinted forms.
© Joint Commission Resources. Official "Do Not Use List". Oakbrook Terrace, IL: Joint Commission on Accreditation of Healthcare Organizations, 2020. Reprinted with permission. https://www.jointcommission.org/-/media/tjc/documents/fact-sheets/do-not-use-list-8-3-20.pdf
[b] **Exception:** A "trailing zero" may be used only where required to demonstrate the level of precision of the value being reported, such as for laboratory results, imaging studies, that report size of lesions, or catheter/tube sizes. It may not be used in medication orders or other medication-related documentation.

TABLE 37-6 Additional Abbreviations, Acronyms, and Symbols (for Possible Future Inclusion in the Official "Do Not Use" List)

DO NOT USE	POTENTIAL PROBLEM	USE INSTEAD
> (greater than)	Misinterpreted as the number "7" (seven) or the letter "L"	Write "greater than"
< (less than)	Confused for one another	Write "less than"
Abbreviations for drug names	Misinterpreted due to similar abbreviations for multiple drugs	Write drug names in full
Apothecary units	Unfamiliar to many practitioners Confused with metric units	Use metric units
@	Mistaken for the number "2" (two)	Write "at"
Cc	Mistaken for U (units) when poorly written	Write "ml" or "milliliters"
Mg	Mistaken for mg (milligrams) resulting in one thousand-fold overdose	Write "mcg" or "micrograms"

© Joint Commission Resources. Official "Do Not Use List". Oakbrook Terrace, IL: Joint Commission on Accreditation of Healthcare Organizations, 2020. Reprinted with permission. https://www.jointcommission.org/-/media/tjc/documents/fact-sheets/do-not-use-list-8-3-20.pdf

entries and make an immediate change before final approval of the information. If you later recognize your error and wish to make a change, the EMR has a mechanism for "late entries," in which you may identify your earlier error. Be sure you learn about the methods for making both an immediate change and a late change in the electronic chart during your agency's orientation.

Box 37-2 Commonly Used Symbols

>	Greater than (See Table 37-5)
<	less than (see Table 37-5)
↑	Increase
↓	Decrease
Δ	Change
=	equal to
≠	not equal to
→	leads to, results in
1°	primary, first degree
2°	secondary, second degree
3°	tertiary, third degree
!	Female
#	Male

Box 37-3 Commonly Used Acronyms for Diseases or Disorders

Acronym	Disease or Disorder
AMI	Acute myocardial infarction
ASCVD	Arteriosclerotic cardiovascular disease
ASHD	Arteriosclerotic heart disease
BPH	Benign prostatic hypertrophy
CA	Cancer
CABG	Coronary artery bypass graft
CAD	Coronary artery disease
CHF	Heart failure, congestive heart failure
COPD	Chronic obstructive pulmonary disease
CVA	Stroke, cerebrovascular accident
DM, IDDM, NIDDM	Diabetes mellitus, insulin-dependent diabetes mellitus (type 1), non–insulin-dependent diabetes mellitus (type 2)
HTN, ↑BP	Hypertension, high blood pressure
MI	Myocardial infarction
PE	Pulmonary emboli, pulmonary edema
PVD	Peripheral vascular disease
STD	Sexually transmitted disease
URI	Upper respiratory infection
UTI	Urinary tract infection

> **Key Concept**
>
> The importance of careful documentation in healthcare cannot be overstated. You must make sure to document all nursing assessments and actions completely and accurately.

> **NCLEX Alert**
>
> Documentation is a fundamentally important concept for the nurse. Therefore, NCLEX questions and scenarios may seek the correct wording of charting and are commonly integrated into the question's scenarios and response options.

REPORTING

Several times during the day the nurse must "report off" to another nurse. The first nurse summarizes the activities and conditions of assigned clients because he or she is leaving the unit for a break or at the end of a shift. The report may be very brief or quite detailed, depending on the purpose of the report and each client's condition. These reports must be efficient and accurate to make effective use of nursing time and to ensure continuity of client care.

Change-of-shift reporting is a means of exchanging information between the outgoing and incoming staff on each shift (Fig. 37-1). In Practice: Nursing Care Guidelines 37-1 gives pointers for change-of-shift reporting. The team leader may report to the entire incoming shift, or reports may be given from caregiver to caregiver. The report may be recorded on a tape recorder or may be given in walking rounds. In **walking rounds**, caregivers move from client to client, discussing pertinent information. Walking rounds encourages client participation and enables the oncoming staff to view equipment, dressings, and other treatments with the previous nurse. The outgoing nurse introduces the incoming nurse to the client. This technique personalizes client care and helps to establish rapport.

> **Key Concept**
>
> This change-of-shift report may be given in person, in writing, or by tape recorder. If the report is verbal, make sure it is given in a location where clients or visitors cannot overhear you.

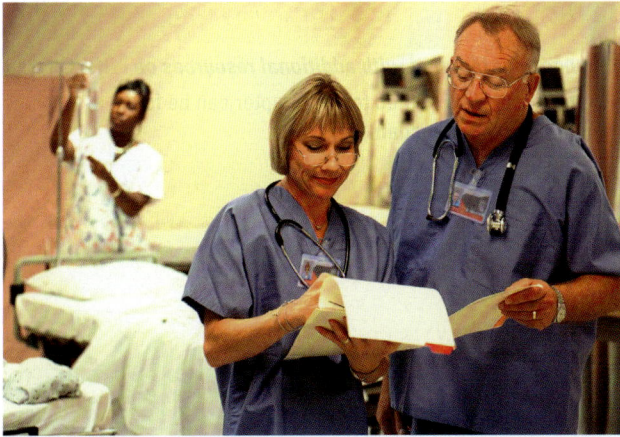

Figure 37-1 By reporting to one another, nurses ensure that clients have continuity of care around the clock. This report may be face-to-face, by tape recorder, or in a "walk-around" format.

Nursing students will practice reporting-off. Reports may be given to the instructor, team leader, or nurse who is coassigned to the care of clients while students are in the clinical facility. As a student or in the role of the nurse, in addition to reporting as one goes off duty, the nurse reports whenever going off duty even if this includes going on a short break, to a pharmacy or laboratory, or to lunch.

Information commonly included in the change-of-shift report may include the information in In Practice: Nursing Care Guidelines 37-1 (more or less maybe required).

IN PRACTICE
NURSING CARE GUIDELINES 37-1 — Change-of-Shift Reporting

Identify Basic Information
- Client's room number (*Rationale:* Many shift reports are given according to room assignments for the staff, thus the beginning of a report tends to begin with a room number.)
- Client's name
- Client's age
- Diagnosis on admission
- Primary healthcare provider name/s
- Primary nurse or case manager, if applicable
- Past medical or surgical history
- Significant changes in medical history

Include Updated Information and Pertinent Events
- Related nursing and medical orders
- Recent diagnostic, laboratory test, procedural results *with significant changes emphasized*
- Scheduled diagnostic or laboratory tests, procedures, or surgery
- Healthcare provider visits or treatments
- Vital signs
- Activity level
- Diets and nutritional supplements
- Pain level and what relieves the pain
- Dressing care and other treatments
- Intravenous (IV) sites, antibiotics, types of infusions
- Blood or blood product infusions
- Medications and side effects
- Advance Directive/Do Not Resuscitate (DNR) status
- Significant psychosocial events (e.g., social workers, discharge planners, family events and interventions)
- Teaching plan with comprehension levels
- Discharge plans
- Prepare a written summary if this is a protocol of your agency
- Any other data or relevant information

Use Facility's Interstaff Protocol (e.g., Nursing Care Plan)
- State each nursing diagnosis or listed problem
- Report on significant, observed accountability (core) measures, or assessed data
- Identify interventions and changes for each nursing diagnosis or goal; corelate with specified accountability (core) measures
- Identify if short- or long-term goals achieved

STUDENT SYNTHESIS

KEY POINTS

- The primary purposes of the health record are to facilitate communication among caregivers, provide evidence of accountability, and facilitate health research and education.
- Healthcare records use sundry versions of medical information systems (MIS) to enter, store, process, and retrieve client data.
- Assessment documents record all client information.
- Minimum data sets and resident assessment protocols guide nurses to develop individualized care plans, especially in long-term facilities and home care.
- Plans for treatment of the client include the healthcare provider's orders and the nursing care plan.
- Progress records describe the treatment and responses of the client.
- Healthcare facilities use various formats to organize nursing progress notes in the health record.
- Plans for the continuity of care include teaching plans, transfer notes, and discharge summaries.
- Accurate and complete documentation ensures effective communication and accountability.
- Confidentiality means a client's right to privacy that healthcare personnel safeguard in both documentation and reporting.
- Reporting is an oral method of communicating that is timely, precise, and accurate.

CRITICAL THINKING EXERCISES

1. Compare the various progress notes formats found in Table 37-2 with the nursing process. Which phase of the nursing process does each format represent?
2. Confidentiality is an important client right. List ways in which you can ensure confidentiality in both manual and electronic charting.

NCLEX-STYLE REVIEW QUESTIONS

1. An older adult client is admitted to the hospital with intact skin. Prior to discharge, the nurse observes a decubitus ulcer on the sacrum but no documentation describes its presence or preventative measures taken. Which outcome does the nurse anticipate?
   a. The client will be discharged home with instructions for the family to dress the wound.
   b. The nurses that have been assigned to care for the client will be terminated.
   c. Payment for care may be denied by third-party payers.
   d. There is no penalty since skin impairment occurs in all older adults.

2. The nurse is documenting the care provided to a client. Which statements would the nurse need to consider when documenting? Select all that apply.
   a. The nurse should only document if there is a change in the client's condition.
   b. The nurse should document the information clearly and legibly.
   c. The nurse should only document accurate information and not assumptions.
   d. The nurse should document frequently.
   e. The nurse should use a black pen if manual entry is required.

3. The nurse is changing a dressing for a client with a burn to the back of the left leg. Which information should the nurse avoid documenting in the chart?
   a. The wound is pink around the edges.
   b. The wound has no drainage or odor.
   c. The client must not have felt the hot object burning the leg.
   d. The client states, "My pain is a 3 on a 1–10 scale."

4. The nurse is observing a new graduate documenting care for a client. Which documentation error by the graduate requires the nurse to intervene?
   a. A nurse is documenting on the nurse's notes with a green pen.
   b. A nurse uses the approved facility abbreviation, "NPO."
   c. A nurse indicates the time and date of documentation entry.
   d. The note is signed using the nurse's first and last name and title.

5. The nurse is documenting in the nurses' notes and realizes the entry is incorrect. Which is the appropriate action by the nurse?
   a. Use "white-out" to block out the entry.
   b. Draw one line through the entry, enclose it in parentheses, and document the error in charting.
   c. Draw a large X throughout the entire entry.
   d. Take out the paper the entry was written on and rewrite it.

CHAPTER RESOURCES

Enhance your learning with additional resources on thePoint!

Student Resources related to this chapter can be found at thePoint.lww.com/Rosdahl12e.

UNIT 7
Safety in the Healthcare Facility

38 The Healthcare Facility Environment

Learning Objectives

1. List and describe components included in the basic client unit.
2. Compare and contrast the basic client unit in the hospital, long-term care, and home care settings.
3. Discuss the relationship between housekeeping procedures and client safety.
4. Summarize the guidelines for all nursing procedures.
5. Describe direct client care departments in hospitals.
6. Describe the functions of at least four hospital support departments.

Important Terminology

autopsy	tele-	CP	GERI	OB	QI
client unit	communications	CQI	GU	OPD	REHAB
commode	telehealth	CRU	GYN	OR	RPT
intercom		CSR	HIM	ORTHO	RR
morgue	**Acronyms**	CSS	ICU	OT	RRA
neurodiagnostic		CT	IV	OTR	RRT
nuclear medicine	ADL	DERM	LTC	PACU	RT
nursing unit	ART	DSM	MH, MHU	PARR	SDSU
ophthalmoscope	ASU	ECF	MICU	PEDS	SICU
otoscope	CCU	ECG/EKG	MIS	PICU	TICU
pathologist/	CD	ED	MRI	PM&R	UAP
pathology	CDU	EEG	NEURO	PSYCH	UROL
protocols	COTA	EHR	NICU	PT	US
rationale	COW	EMG	NMR	PTA	

Client needs include the *basic needs* of all human beings (Chapter 5) and *special needs connected with illness or injury*. Essential physiologic needs are oxygen, water, nutrients, waste elimination, sleep and rest, activity, and exercise. Higher level needs include safety, shelter, emotional and spiritual support, and meaningful relationships. The highest level needs address self-esteem and a feeling of self-fulfillment. It is important to note that some people do not progress beyond the most basic of needs, particularly if they are ill. These healthcare clients have special needs, including essential medical and nursing care, assistance to return to normal or baseline functioning, and diversion. The client's progress toward recovery, comfort, and satisfaction relates to the extent to which these needs can be satisfied. Meeting special client needs involves teamwork among many people, including the client and their family.

Traditionally, most nursing care was provided in a hospital or extended care facility (**ECF**), sometimes known as a long-term care (**LTC**) facility. Changes in the delivery of healthcare have greatly expanded nursing into the community, including a number of nonhospital settings (Fig. 38-1) (Unit 15).

Your experience with clients may be in a hospital or ECF, but it may also be in a community health agency, in the client's home, or perhaps in an urgent care center such as a Minute clinic. This type of clinic, where clients with noncritical conditions are treated, may be located in a pharmacy, shopping center, or other community facility (Chapter 99).

Wherever you practice, it is important to be familiar with basic healthcare equipment. It is also important to know about specialized departments and support services found in many healthcare facilities. You will then be able to obtain appropriate services for clients and to explain the functions of various healthcare personnel to clients and families.

THE CLIENT UNIT

The **client unit** is the area where most client care is provided. This area may be around the client's bed in a hospital, ECF, or in the person's home. The unit usually includes a bed, as well as other furniture and equipment used in the client's

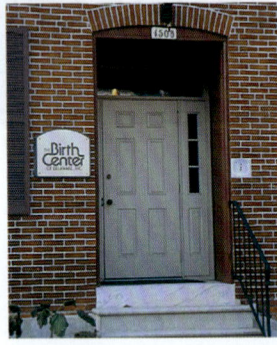 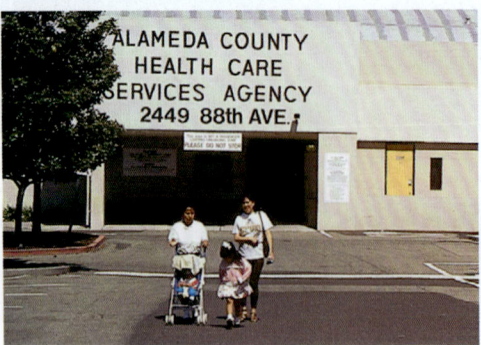 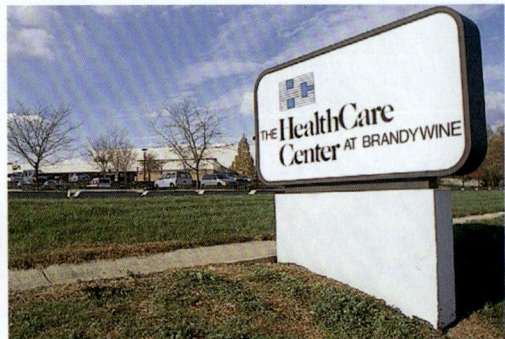

Figure 38-1 Traditionally, most nursing care was provided in a hospital or extended care facility. Today, a great deal of our health care has moved into the community, including the client's home.

daily care (Fig. 38-2). In the hospital or ECF, the client may be in a private or semiprivate room or in a *ward* containing three or more beds. Consider each bed and the accompanying furniture as one client unit. In the home, the client unit is the primary area where the client receives care. It may be the bedroom or main living area—where the person is most comfortable and where adequate room is available for essential equipment such as a hospital bed, oxygen, intravenous (**IV**) pole, or commode. Today, facilities strive to provide clients with surroundings that are homey and pleasant, as well as practical. The **nursing unit** is an area containing several client units, usually with a centralized desk or office. Several "substations" may be distributed throughout the unit, each providing access to several client rooms/units. Usually, in acute care, each client unit has a bedside computer or a computer on wheels (**COW**) is moved from room to room.

Components of the Basic Client Unit

The following components make up the basic client unit in hospital, ECF, and home care settings:

Furniture: Bed, bedside stand, chair, lamp, and overbed table. Most hospital beds have built-in side rails, containing TV controls, telephone, and nurse call signals (Fig. 38-2B). Regular beds in the home do not have attached side rails, and require additional safety considerations. In the home, clients may use a sofa, recliner, or bed, or may rent a hospital bed. Some clients bring a favorite chair to the LTC facility.

Linens: Mattress pad, sheets, pillowcases, blankets, bedspread, bath blanket, face towel, washcloth, bedpan cover, bathrobe, gown, or pajamas. In some facilities, each client unit has an individual covered linen hamper. In the home, personal preferences, living conditions, and limited resources may affect the type and amount of linens available for use.

Toilet equipment: Washbasin, soap dish and soap, lotion, toothbrush and container, toothpaste, mouthwash, denture cup (if needed), disposable tissues, emesis basin, comb/hair pick, bedpan, and a urinal for male clients. A portable **commode**, or toilet, is lightweight and sturdy and may be placed next to the bed. Home care clients may adapt the bathroom with safety equipment to ease toileting and bathing (Fig. 97-1). Chapter 98 provides an overview of nursing care in the client's home.

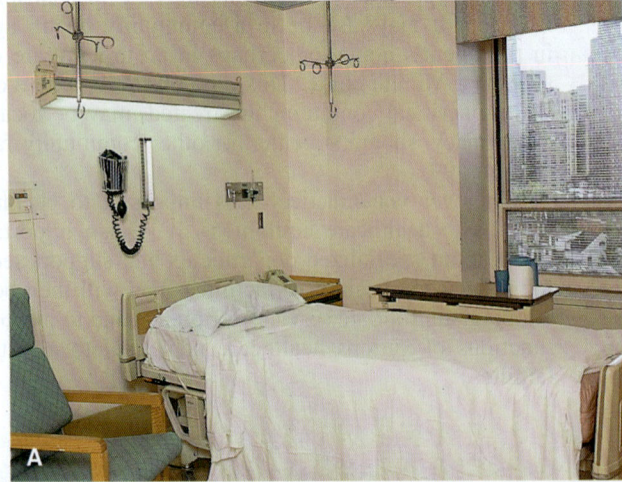 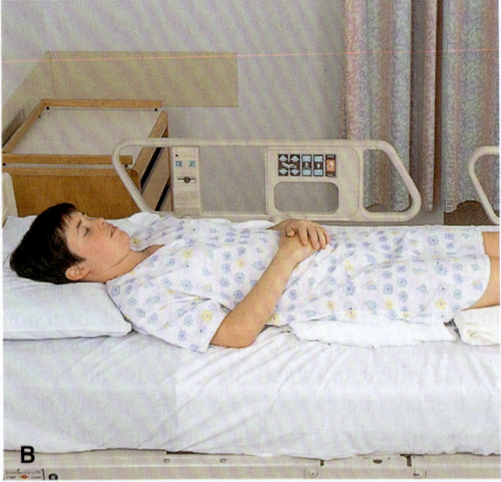

Figure 38-2 A. Typical hospital room furnishings. Notice the built-in side rails, as well as the blood pressure apparatus and ports for suction and oxygen on the wall. Hangers above the bed can hold intravenous (IV) or tube feeding bags. The foot of the bed is removable to be used for emergency CPR. The bedside stand and overbed table are near the window. On the table is an individual water pitcher and drinking glass, as well as a private telephone. A safe, comfortable chair with arms is next to the bed, to be used when the client gets up, as well as for visitors. The window shows a pleasant view of the city. **B.** The side rails are integrated into the basic gatch bed; they contain controls to raise and lower the head and foot of the bed, as well as the bed itself. (These may be locked, if moving would endanger the client.) Also contained are the nurse call signal and controls for the TV. (Photos by B. Proud.)

Other articles: Water pitcher and drinking glass or insulated mug and straw, call signal, screen or curtain, TV, DVD player, and telephone. A trash container is necessary for safe disposal of tissues and other items. Hospital units often have built-in blood pressure equipment, nasogastric (*NG*) suction, and oxygen, as well as an intercommunication (**intercom**) system. The intercom allows clients to communicate with healthcare providers at the nursing station. In some situations, the client is also monitored by camera and/or other electronic monitors.

Equipment for nursing treatments is kept in each client's room; new items are in a storeroom. The client unit should always be complete and ready for use, to save steps and prevent delays. Home care nurses may bring blood pressure equipment and other essential items to the home on each visit. Medical equipment supply companies deliver beds, oxygen, infusion pumps, and other supplies directly to the client's home.

> **Key Concept**
> Nearly all equipment and supplies used in health care are disposable and used for only one client, in an effort to prevent the spread of infection between clients and to protect healthcare workers. Occasionally, items are used for more than one client; if so, they must be carefully disinfected between uses.

Furniture
Hospital Bed
The hospital bed is specially constructed and equipped to provide maximum safety and comfort for clients and caregivers. Chapter 49 describes the bed, its attachments, and bed-making skills, as well as special beds. Many home care clients rent a hospital bed because the entire bed can be raised and lowered, making care easier for nurses and family caregivers. To enhance client comfort, the head and foot of the bed can also be raised.

Overbed Table
The overbed table can be moved over the bed and can be raised or lowered. It is useful when the client is eating, reading, or grooming. The table can be opened, revealing a mirror and space for small articles. The top is adjustable, permitting a book to be held at a comfortable angle for reading.

Bedside Stand
The bedside stand is durable and easy to clean. Bedside stands include a drawer and an enclosed storage space containing shelves for bedpan or urinal. Some facilities have lockers or closets, so clients can store clothing and other personal items. Although healthcare facilities usually have a central vault, clients are generally encouraged to leave valuables at home, particularly for short stays.

In the home, TV stands, end tables, dressers, or coffee tables may serve as the bedside stand. Often, personal items and mementos surround the home care client. It is important to realize that the nurse is a visitor in the client's home and must consider the client's physical surroundings and ethnic/cultural practices.

Other Components
When orienting the client and family to the healthcare facility, demonstrate how to operate equipment. The client needs to know how to obtain assistance. Teach the client the use of the nurse call button; allow them to practice using the intercom. Assure the client that a healthcare worker will either respond in person or from the nursing station via intercom.

Home care clients may use a bell or other device to attract the caregiver's attention. They may also choose to install a self-activated alert system, transmitting a signal to a hospital or other facility in an emergency. Personnel then respond by telephone or through video surveillance. The client at home may also transmit vital data, such as an *ECG* (electrocardiogram) or blood pressure reading, by phone to the healthcare provider for interpretation.

Safety and Nursing Care Equipment
When special equipment is built into the client unit, it is important to explain that it exists in all units, in case it is needed. If it is a multibed room, a curtain will hang around each client's area for privacy. This curtain usually runs in a track on the ceiling and can be pushed out of the way when not needed.

Ventilation and Air Quality
With concern for air quality, healthcare facilities work prevent pollution. National accreditation regulations prohibit smoking, either in healthcare facilities or on the grounds. Usually heating and cooling are centrally controlled and windows are sealed. However, it is important to ensure each client's comfort, particularly in relation to temperature. There must be a balance between heat lost and heat produced. The room temperature that most effectively maintains a comfortable balance is between 68 °F and 72 °F (20 °C and 22.2 °C). Protect your client from becoming chilled; illness or injury may predispose the client to feeling chilly. Offer extra blankets to the client; often a *blanket warmer* is available. Protect an ambulating client with a warm blanket over the shoulders, a bathrobe, and sturdy slippers. Place chairs away from drafts. Cover the client with a bath blanket when giving a bed bath or performing other treatments (for warmth and privacy).

Odors
Illness may make a person extremely sensitive to odors. Remove bedpans, urinals, and soiled dressings from the client's bedside immediately after use. Most healthcare facilities do not permit staff to wear scents, such as perfume or aftershave lotion. The smell of smoke is very offensive, particularly to the person who is ill. If you smoke, be sure that your breath is clean and your clothes do not smell of smoke. You may need to explain the facility's smoke-free policy to the client and visitors. (You are also expected to abide by this policy.)

Noise
Noise can overstimulate or frighten the client and produce fatigue. Therefore, attempt to minimize or eliminate noise as much as possible. Slamming doors or dropping equipment startles clients and may cause restlessness and irritation. Turn radios and TVs to low volume; headphones or under-the-pillow speakers may be available. Assist clients to be respectful and avoid annoying other clients. *Be especially aware of the noise level at night.* Even two nurses talking can

irritate the client who is having difficulty sleeping. Overhead music is often played softly to help make the environment more pleasant and comfortable and to provide "white noise," to mask other sounds.

Privacy

You are obligated to respect and preserve the privacy of all clients. Be sure to use screens, curtains, bath blankets, or drapes to keep the person covered as much as possible during treatments. Shut the client's door during procedures. (A sign may be placed on the door, for additional privacy.) If a client is confused and pulls off covers, pajamas may be more practical than a hospital gown. Respect the client's privacy when visitors are present. It may be necessary to enforce the facility's visiting policy, to protect the privacy and ensure comfort of other clients. Many facilities permit only one or two visitors at a time. This is sometimes difficult to enforce when a crisis occurs and cultural practices require the presence of many relatives, spiritual leaders, and significant others (sometimes overnight).

> **Key Concept**
>
> It is vital to protect the client's privacy relating to personal medical information. Never give out any information about a client without specific written permission. Be sure to log off your computer whenever you leave it and keep the screen turned, so information cannot be read by anyone else. You are not allowed to access any client's information without a valid reason to do so. Violation of this policy is cause for *termination of employment*.

Neatness of the Unit

Always keep the unit neat and orderly. Good housekeeping helps prevent accidents and infections and helps to carry out effective nursing care. Arrange equipment and supplies so all personnel can locate items easily and quickly. Consistency from room to room helps maintain order. These measures help clients feel secure and make falls and other accidents less likely.

Restocking the Unit

Replace used supplies promptly. Check equipment and inspect for breaks, cracks, or defects that might be harmful. Inspect electrical cords to ensure that they are intact. Remove and replace broken or damaged equipment and report any damage immediately. Many facilities maintain an ongoing inventory of equipment as a basis for ordering new articles or replacing damaged ones. Some facilities have an automated system for tracking supplies and order new supplies as they are used.

> **Key Concept**
>
> Never use a broken or damaged piece of equipment. If unsure, remove and replace it.

Cleaning the Unit After Use

Housekeeping personnel are usually responsible for cleaning client units in hospitals and ECFs. However, in an emergency, all nurses should know how to clean a unit, according to their facility's policies and the principles of medical asepsis (Chapter 41). In some situations, you will supervise such procedures. Always make sure the unit is cleaned after a client has been discharged or transferred to another room and before another client uses the room. In the hospital or ECF, everything in the unit is considered contaminated and must be discarded or disinfected before it can be used by another client. Such measures help prevent the spread of infection. Cleanliness is just as important in the home, although it may be more difficult to attain. If you work in home care, you will need to teach clients and their families measures for maintaining sanitary and safe conditions. Many of these measures are discussed throughout this unit of this book.

The Examination Room

The examination room on the nursing unit or in the healthcare clinic includes the following items:

- *Furniture:* Examination table (with attached stirrups), Mayo stand (holds equipment for the examination), examination light, and rolling stool. A covered trash container and sharps container are necessary. Most examination rooms have a sink and cabinets for supplies.
- *Linens:* Sheets, disposable paper to cover the examination table, small pillow, paper towels, tissues, disposable or cloth gown, and drapes or small towels for privacy.
- *Other articles:* An **ophthalmoscope** (instrument used for examining eyes) and an **otoscope** (instrument used to examine inside ears, nose, and throat), often mounted on the wall, and a scale, with height measure, to weigh clients and determine height. Also available are blood pressure apparatus, a thermometer, and disposable supplies, such as tongue blades, Q-tips, and disposable otoscope tips of varying sizes. (A new tip is used for each client.) If needed, equipment for gynecologic (female) examinations (a speculum) and for obtaining various smears and cultures is provided. Equipment for drawing blood or starting IVs is usually provided as well.

PROVISION OF NURSING CARE

The nurse will provide most nursing care directly in the client unit. Healthcare facilities and agencies have specific policies outlining standards for care. Procedures or **protocols** are available to employees and students in that healthcare setting. Usually, these are provided online; copies can be printed for personal use. All students and staff are expected to follow the caregiving procedures of the facility. (Even though specific procedures may vary slightly between facilities, underlying *rationales*, detailing why an action is taken, remain constant.) In Practice: Nursing Care Guidelines 38-1 describes general steps to follow for all procedures, regardless of the setting.

In acute care facilities and ECFs, you are likely to perform several specific procedures together for efficiency. These skills may be grouped because they are associated with the same time of day or with a special kind of treatment. Many nurses know these blocks of nursing care by group names. In Practice: Nursing Care Guidelines 38-2 provides some examples of specific types of care, according to time of day. Usually, you will have more than one client to care for and you will need to consider your facility's routines when planning each

IN PRACTICE
NURSING CARE GUIDELINES 38-1 — General Guidelines for Performing Nursing Procedures

- Check the healthcare provider's orders; review the IP (inpatient) snapshot on the computer, the nursing care plan, care map, or critical pathway.
- Review the protocol for the procedure, as performed in that facility. Follow all steps carefully, considering underlying rationales.
- Identify the client in at least two ways. Make sure you have the correct person. (Ask the client to tell you their name. Check or scan the ID band.)
- Perform all procedures on time.
- Follow standard precautions (Chapter 41).
- Thoroughly wash your hands or use hand sanitizer before and after every procedure.
- Wear gloves for most procedures (follow your facility's protocol).
- Assemble all necessary equipment so you can carry out the procedure easily, quickly, and efficiently. Ensure client safety at all times.
- Introduce yourself and state your role (e.g., nursing student, LPN). Explain the procedure to the client, to allay fears of pain or discomfort. (Clients may be apprehensive about such things as machines, sharp instruments, hot or cold applications, or equipment that covers the face.)
- Avoid using the words "hurt" or "painful." Say instead, "You may feel some discomfort," or "You will have to lie in one position, but I will help make you comfortable."
- Emphasize positive aspects and reassure the client: "The procedure won't take long," or "It will make you feel better." A client will usually be more cooperative if they know what to expect. Try to let the client know how long a procedure will take, if more than a few minutes. Never tell a client "There's nothing to it," when you know that a procedure has some painful or uncomfortable aspects.
- Make sure the client is as comfortable as possible. Also, position yourself as comfortably as possible. Use good body mechanics (Chapter 48).
- Offer prescribed pain medication before uncomfortable procedures or before the client gets out of bed soon after surgery.
- Ensure the client's privacy.
- Stay with the client during examinations and procedures. Explain and answer questions promptly.
- Disinfect the area as necessary.
- Care for equipment, as required by the facility's policies (e.g., discard or return to central supply department).
- Discard all dressings and disposable equipment, following facility protocol.
- Discard all sharps in the designated container.
- Discard all medication packages as specified by the facility. Consider appropriate "hazardous to handle" medication disposal.
- Make sure to identify all hazardous waste, including anything containing body fluids, and dispose of it properly.
- Document procedures, the time they are performed, results noted, and any client deviations from normal. Report any pertinent symptoms or observations to the appropriate person. Report emergencies immediately.
- Answer any client questions. Offer to obtain further information, if necessary.

client's care. When preparing your work plan, consider meal hours, healthcare provider rounds, and appointments for surgery, x-ray examinations, therapy, and laboratory procedures. You may be asked to assist temporarily with emergencies. In all situations, your clients are your first responsibility.

Key Concept

It is vital to identify each client correctly in at least two ways before any care is given. Be aware of similar names. You may have two clients named Michael or two clients named Ng. Identification is done by

- Checking or scanning the client's arm ID band (Fig. 38-3). (If the client refuses to wear a name band, this must be documented. In some cases, the name band is applied to the client's ankle, so it cannot be easily removed.)
- Asking the client their name and birth date. (Do not ask the client if they are "Mr. Smith." Some clients will answer "yes" to anything and you could have the wrong client. This is particularly true if the client does not speak the predominant language or if the client has dementia, a mental health condition, or a hearing disorder.)
- In an emergency, ask another staff person to identify the client.
   Remember: "Check two for safety."

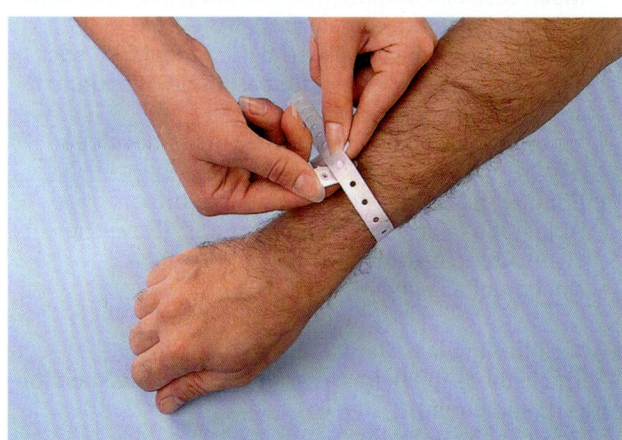

Figure 38-3 Each client must have an identification (ID) band. Always check or scan this, ask the client their name and birth date, and compare these data to the client record or medication sheet before performing any procedure or giving any medication. Here, the nurse is shown applying an ID band for a new client or replacing an unreadable band. Before the band can be applied, the client must state their name and birth date; these data must agree with the name band. (Timby, 2005.)

IN PRACTICE
NURSING CARE GUIDELINES 38-2 — Guidelines for Performing Grouped Procedures

You will conduct most of the following procedures when working in acute or extended care settings, where clients receive a great deal of round-the-clock attention. Times for some of the following procedures may vary, according to facility policies. As often as possible, perform these procedures at the time most comfortable and therapeutic for the client, not necessarily for your convenience. For example, a client might be accustomed to bathing at night, rather than in the morning. It may be possible to accommodate such a preference. Do any painful procedures first, then give a back rub and perform other comfort measures, so the client is better able to rest after the procedure. Also, offer the client a bedpan, urinal, or assist them to the bathroom before washing their hands. Give medications after you have given other care, unless pain control is needed before the procedure or the medications are otherwise ordered.

Early Morning (AM) Care
Perform these measures before breakfast for the client's health and comfort:
- Offer a bedpan or urinal, or assist the client to the bathroom. Empty catheter bag, if present.
- Wash or assist the client to wash face and hands.
- Brush or assist the client to brush their teeth.
- Adjust the bed and bedclothes.
- Take the client's temperature, pulse, respiration, pulse oximetry, and blood pressure. (If performing orthostatic blood pressure measurement, do the first reading before the client gets out of bed.)
- Ask about pain each time other vital signs are measured, or as needed. Offer PRN medications as needed.
- Give AM medications as ordered.
- Make sure all equipment is operating properly (e.g., IV pump, oxygen, catheter).
- Perform procedures needed before breakfast, such as blood glucose testing, first AM urine or sputum specimen, or daily weight.
- Make sure all fasting blood specimens have been drawn.
- Change the client's position for comfort.
- Adjust the table for the breakfast tray. (Have the client sitting up, if possible.)
- Document as needed.

Later Morning (AM) Care
Perform these measures after the client's breakfast for health and comfort:
- Remove the breakfast tray.
- Offer a bedpan or urinal or assist the client to the bathroom. Empty catheter bag, if present.
- Obtain vital signs, as ordered or if needed.
- Give the client a bath or assist with bathing (bed bath, tub, or shower, depending on the client's condition). At least, allow the client to wash the hands and face and brush the teeth.
- Change the client's position or help them to sit in the chair or ambulate.
- Make the client's bed. Change linens according to your facility's policies. Help the client put on a clean gown.
- Comb hair or assist the client to comb their hair.
- Care for the client's nails.
- Perform any AM treatments and give noon or other medications, as ordered.
- Perform blood glucose testing before lunch.
- Give the client a back rub or hand massage.
- Tidy the unit. Ready the overbed table for the lunch tray or assist the client into the chair.
- Document as needed.

Afternoon Care
Perform these measures to relax the client in preparation for visitors:
- Make sure all equipment is operating properly.
- Obtain vital signs as ordered or if needed.
- Change the client's position or help the client to ambulate.
- Offer the client a bedpan or urinal or assist them to the bathroom. Empty the catheter bag, if present.
- Wash or assist the client to wash face and hands.
- Perform afternoon treatments and give medications, as ordered.
- Give the client a back rub or hand massage.
- Check the client's blood glucose before dinner, as ordered.
- Document as needed.

Evening (HS or "Hour of Sleep" Care)
Perform these measures for health, comfort, and to prepare the client for sleep:
- Complete evening treatments. Make sure all equipment is operating properly.
- Obtain vital signs as ordered or if needed. Check blood glucose, as ordered.
- Offer a bedpan or urinal or assist the client to the bathroom. Empty catheter bag, if present.
- Wash or assist the client to wash face and hands.
- Brush or assist the client to brush their teeth.
- Comb and tidy the client's hair.
- Change the client's position or assist the client to ambulate.
- Adjust the bed and bedclothes.
- Give the client a back rub.
- Give HS medications as ordered or PRNs as requested.
- Tidy up the client unit. Be sure all obstacles are out of the way, so healthcare team members and the client do not fall over them during the night. Turn on the night light.
- Document as needed.

Each nursing procedure is complete in itself. There is a reason, or **rationale**, for each step in every nursing procedure. These reasons guide you in making the procedure safe and effective. Although individual steps may vary among healthcare facilities, your nursing care will be safe if you *do not violate basic underlying principles*. As skills are presented in this book, underlying rationales for steps are given to guide you in adapting your care to individual situations after graduation. As a student, follow procedures exactly as taught by your instructors until you have a firm grasp on nursing's underlying principles.

The 24-Hour Clock

Most hospitals and many other healthcare facilities today use the 24-hour clock (also called *military time*) to time and record procedures and medication administration. This helps prevent errors and misunderstandings. For example, 7 o'clock in the morning is 0700, 7 o'clock in the evening is 1,900, and midnight is 2,400. One minute after midnight is 0001. Written in military time, these times will not be confused with each other; this increases the accuracy of recording (Table 37-3).

HEALTHCARE PERSONNEL AND SERVICES

Healthcare facilities offer a variety of services; therefore, they are staffed with people experienced in many different areas. Many of the following services are provided in—or linked to—ECFs or LTC facilities, clinics, surgery centers, and home care agencies as well as hospitals. It is important to have a general understanding of many departments and services because you will work with people from many of these disciplines (Fig. 38-4). You will also need to explain services to clients and families. Many abbreviations and acronyms are commonly used in healthcare facilities. They are listed at the beginning of this chapter and defined throughout the chapter (Appendix B).

Diagnostic and Treatment Departments

Clinical diagnostic *laboratories* perform numerous tests to assist providers in diagnosing disorders. **Pathologists**, laboratory technologists, and their associates determine the underlying nature of diseases through examination and study of tissue and body fluid specimens, including blood, sputum, feces, and biopsied tissues. Pathologists also perform **autopsies** (examinations after death [*postmortem*]). The *morgue* is under a pathologist's direction; bodies are kept there until identified and released to a funeral home or family. Autopsies may take place in the hospital or in an outside facility. Some large teaching hospitals also include a *research laboratory*, where studies and experiments are conducted to understand, cure, or prevent disease.

The *radiology department* performs diagnostic x-ray studies to aid healthcare providers in determining the exact location and nature of disorders. *Radiation therapy* is also given, to treat disorders, such as cancer. Sometimes, this entire department is called **nuclear medicine**. Other procedures performed by this department include computed tomography (**CT**) scans, xerography and mammography (breast studies), magnetic resonance imaging (**MRI**) or nuclear magnetic

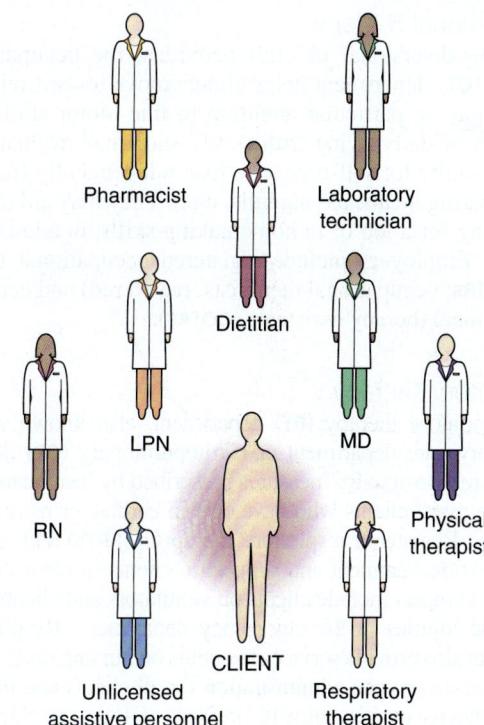

Figure 38-4 Many people with specialized skills or knowledge are involved either directly or indirectly with the client's healthcare. (There are a number of other possibilities, such as translators, nurse practitioners, and physician's assistants.) Note that the client is at the center and is an active participant in their care. (Timby, 2005.)

resonance (**NMR**), and ultrasound (**US**) studies. This department also supervises and performs the implantation and injection of radioactive and opaque materials for treatments and examinations. In some cases, voiding studies and other urologic examinations are done in this department.

The *electroencephalography* (**EEG**) department, also known as the **neurodiagnostic** department, records results of the "brain wave" test, which determines electrical activity within a client's brain. The EEG department also administers evoked-potential examinations, does specialized sleep studies, and monitors clients who have seizures. (An EEG is one of the specific diagnostic tools used to determine biologic death.)

The electrocardiogram (**ECG/EKG**), a recording of the heart's electrical activity, may be done by a specialized department or by the intensive care unit (ICU) or EEG department. The electromyogram (**EMG**), a record of minute electrical impulses within muscles, may be done by the EEG, ECG, physical therapy, or respiratory care department or in the clinical laboratory.

Direct Client Care Departments

Therapies
Physical Therapy
The physical therapy (**PT**) department directs its efforts toward preventing physical disability. PT staff members assist clients to regain the best possible function of affected body parts through individually planned programs of exercise and activity, with emphasis on gross (large) motor muscle activity. PT employees include registered physical therapists (**RPTs**) and physical therapist assistants (**PTAs**).

Occupational Therapy

By using diversional or craft activities, the occupational therapy (**OT**) department helps clients move toward rehabilitation, paying particular attention to fine motor skills and activities of daily living (**ADLs**). OT staff may evaluate the client's ability for self-care or to live independently (including preparing meals, paying bills, etc.). They may aid clients in training for a job or in homemaking skills, in addition to therapy. Employees include registered occupational therapists (**OTRS**: occupational therapists, registered) and certified occupational therapy assistants (**COTAs**).

Respiratory Therapy

The respiratory therapy (**RT**) department, also known as the respiratory care department or cardiopulmonary (**CP**) department, is responsible for measures prescribed by healthcare providers to assist clients who have certain cardiac or respiratory disorders. Registered respiratory therapists (**RRTs**) and technicians provide treatment and support to clients in other departments. Examples include clients on ventilators and clients with traumatic injuries in the emergency department. Respiratory therapists also provide services to clients on nursing units. They often oversee oxygen administration for all clients and the use of continuous positive airway pressure (CPAP) machines to assist clients with nighttime breathing. The RT department may administer nebulizer treatments, draw blood for blood gas analysis, and perform special tests, including pulmonary function, vital capacity, and cardiac stress tests.

Other Therapies

Some facilities also provide therapies such as music therapy, recreational therapy, and play therapy. These services are most common in facilities that contain rehabilitation, psychiatric, chemical dependency, and children's therapy units and those that work with people who have an intellectual impairment or dementia.

Surgery

The staff members in the operating room (**OR**) and the postanesthesia care unit (**PACU**)—also called the recovery room (**RR**) or the postanesthesia recovery room (**PARR**)—are concerned with care of surgical clients immediately before, during, and after surgery. They may also manage a same-day surgery unit (**SDSU**) or ambulatory surgery unit (**ASU**). Freestanding surgery centers in the community provide similar services (Chapter 56).

Nursing Care Units

The person responsible for management of one or more nursing units (stations) may have various titles, such as head nurse, clinical care supervisor (CCS), or nurse manager. Their responsibility is the day-to-day unit functioning and monitoring of quality of care. Others, such as charge nurses, provide direct supervision during their assigned shift. Other nursing personnel include team leaders, primary nurses, and staff nurses or clinical nurses, as well as nursing assistants or other unlicensed assistive personnel (**UAP**). Clinical nurse specialists and case managers are often part of the nursing team. Many units also have a *secretary*.

In larger facilities, nursing care units are often designated to care for clients within specific groups or with specific disorders or needs. In many cases, nursing staff members are required to obtain specialized in-service education in order to practice in a specialized area.

Pediatrics Unit

The *pediatric* (**PEDS**) unit is responsible for the care of children. In large hospitals, the PEDS department may be subdivided according to children's ages.

Obstetrics Department

The *obstetrics* (**OB**) department, sometimes called a "birthing center," provides care to mothers and newborns. Traditionally, the OB department was divided into a labor room, delivery room, newborn nursery, and postpartum unit (where women received care after delivery). Many hospitals now provide birthing center rooms where women go through labor, deliver their newborns, and remain with their babies throughout the postpartum period. In the current healthcare climate, the length of stay in birthing centers is short, often 24–48 hour (Unit 10).

Medical/Surgical Care Units

The *medical* unit cares for adults with medical conditions or disorders that do not require surgery. The *surgical* unit cares for clients before and after surgery. In a large facility, basic medical–surgical care may be subdivided. Divisions include *orthopedics* (**ORTHO**) for musculoskeletal disorders; *urology* (**UROL**) or genitourinary (**GU**) for disorders of the kidneys, bladder, liver, and male reproductive system; *neurology* (**NEURO**) for central or peripheral nervous system disorders, including disorders of the brain and head trauma; *dermatology* (**DERM**) for skin disorders; *oncology* for clients with cancer; and *gynecology* (**GYN**) for female reproductive disorders.

Burn Center

The *burn center* provides care for clients with frostbite and serious wounds, as well as those who have been burned.

Geriatric Units

Older clients are cared for in the *geriatric* (**GERI**) unit; those with dementia and related disorders are often in a *memory care* unit.

Dialysis Unit

The dialysis unit provides care for clients who need chronic renal (kidney) dialysis.

Mental Health Unit

The mental health (**MHU, MH**) or psychiatry unit (**PSYCH**) serves clients with emotional or psychiatric disorders. Severely disturbed clients may be in a Psych ICU. A special mental health emergency room or *crisis center* (Acute Psychiatric Services—APS) is usually available in a large hospital, and a call-in crisis phone line may be managed by this department. In addition, psychiatric staff often responds to behavioral emergencies throughout the facility.

Chemical Dependency Unit

The chemical dependency (**CD**) unit serves persons with chemical abuse issues and their significant others on an inpatient and outpatient basis.

Rehabilitation Unit
The rehabilitation (**REHAB**) unit, also called physical medicine and rehabilitation (**PM&R**), provides psychosocial support and rehabilitative services to people with physical disabilities and who need assistance to regain as much capacity for activity as possible. Many clients in REHAB have experienced trauma, strokes, head injuries, or brain damage related to drugs.

Outpatient Department
The outpatient department (**OPD**) provides ongoing care for clients who do not need to be admitted to the facility.

Specialized Client Care Departments
Specialized departments and units are designed to give care for different degrees of illness.

Emergency Department
The emergency department (**ED**; emergency room—ER) gives care to those whose condition requires immediate attention. Clients may arrive on their own, by ambulance, or by air transport. A *triage* specialist identifies client acuity and determines which clients need to be seen first (Chapter 39). ED staff is specially trained and prepared to manage traumatic injuries, provide cardiopulmonary resuscitation, and care for clients with a variety of critical and urgent conditions. In some facilities, social workers, chaplains, and crisis teams also provide services in EDs.

Intensive Care Unit
The intensive care unit (**ICU**) provides inpatient care for critically ill clients. Larger facilities have specialized ICUs, such as neonatal/newborn (**NICU**), pediatric (**PICU**), surgical (**SICU**), medical (**MICU**), trauma (**TICU**), and neurologic ICU. Nurses in ICUs are usually required to obtain critical care certification.

Coronary Care Unit
The coronary care unit (**CCU**) cares for clients with serious heart disorders. Nurses here are specially prepared in cardiac care and interpretation of ECGs. After their conditions have stabilized, these clients may move into a coronary step-down unit or a coronary rehabilitation unit (**CRU**).

Clinical Decision Unit/Observation Unit
The clinical decision unit (**CDU**) provides care for clients who need additional observation, diagnostic testing, or treatment before hospital admission or discharge. Stays in this unit are usually less than 24 hour. Many facilities use this area as a chest pain center and treat and observe stable chest pain clients here.

Intermediate Care Unit
The intermediate care unit provides care for clients requiring a moderate amount of skilled nursing care.

Self-Care Unit
The self-care unit provides care for clients who are transitioning from the hospital or skilled nursing facility to home. Clients care for themselves as much as possible; staff members provide assistance as needed.

Hospice Care Unit
Hospice, also called *palliative care*, gives physical and emotional care to dying individuals. Hospice staff provides clients and families with support and assistance in dealing with terminal illness and death (Chapter 100).

Urgent Care
The urgent care department provides care to clients who can be treated without being admitted to the hospital and who are not considered to have emergency conditions.

Hyperbaric Chamber
A large facility may also maintain a hyperbaric chamber for use in specialized situations where high-concentration oxygen is required. This may include infections with anaerobic organisms (e.g., gas gangrene), the deep-sea diver who has surfaced too rapidly ("the bends"), or clients with some specific medical conditions. Some types of surgery may also be done in the chamber. Special training is required to work in the chamber; these people are often former Navy divers (Chapters 87 and 102).

Support Services
Administration
The facility's *administration* oversees all departments. The administrative team may include several executives responsible for different functions, such as nursing, clinical services, human resources, financial services, or physician services.

Dietary Department
The *dietary* department (*nutritional therapy*) prepares meals for clients, in accordance with instructions given by healthcare providers and ethnic requirements of clients. *Dietitians* evaluate client needs and teach clients and families about special diets. This department also may prepare meals for staff and visitors.

Client Education
The client education department provides educational services for staff, clients, and the community. Educators teach complex procedures to clients and their family caregivers. This department is often responsible for staff development and community wellness programs.

Pharmacy
The pharmacy dispenses medications ordered by healthcare providers. Pharmacists may instruct clients on the use and side effects of prescribed medications. A consulting *pharmacologist* may also be available for intensive instruction or to advise clinicians regarding suggested medication regimens.

Housekeeping
The housekeeping department (*environmental services*) provides cleaning services to client units and common areas. Housekeeping staff usually cleans client units after clients leave.

Laundry
The laundry provides clean bed linens, client gowns and robes, and other items, such as drapes used in surgery, scrub suits for specific areas (such as OR), and staff laboratory coats.

Building Maintenance
Building maintenance maintains the buildings and grounds, including heating and cooling, lawn mowing and snow shoveling, and repairs. This department often maintains fire extinguishers, elevators, bathrooms, and sprinkler systems.

Central Service Supply
The central service supply (**CSS**) or central supply room (**CSR**) cleans and sterilizes equipment and instruments for use throughout the facility.

Admissions and Business
The admissions department determines the client's identity and assigns clients to units when they enter the facility. The business office processes bills and insurance claims.

Medical Records
The medical records (MR) department maintains records for all clients who have ever been in the facility (inpatient or outpatient). This department is responsible for ensuring that all information is entered into the client's record. The MR staff assigns **DSM** (*Diagnostic and Statistical Manual for Mental Disorders* [Chapter 94]) or DRG/RUG (diagnosis-related group/Resource Utilization Group) codes (Chapter 3). They check to ensure that the client's record is complete. The accredited record technician (**ART**) or registered record administrator (**RRA**) may be called to testify regarding a client's record. The MR department must be able to access any client record quickly and may collect research data. In nearly all healthcare facilities, medical records are stored electronically.

Volunteer Services
Volunteers provide many services; they may operate a gift shop; deliver mail, flowers, magazines, toys, and books to clients; operate an information desk; maintain a historical museum, or run a coffee shop. They often transport clients to the nursing unit from the admitting department and throughout the facility for tests or discharge. Volunteers often assist families of clients who are having surgery or are in the ICU or remain with new fathers during and immediately after delivery ("a daddy sitter").

Chaplaincy
The chaplaincy staff provides spiritual support to clients and families during illness, surgery, or death and assists with specific ethnic religious rituals. A Bible, Koran (Quran), or other religious item is often available from the Chaplain. Many facilities have a chapel, with scheduled services.

Translation Services
Many facilities serve clients from various countries. Specially trained and certified translators are required, and strict requirements are followed, to ensure privacy and accuracy in the transmission of information to and from clients. It is *not appropriate* for the client's family members to interpret for the client. Electronic interpretation is available 24 hour a day.

Social Services
The social services department provides counseling and assistance to clients and families in matters of finance, home care, discharge planning, and living arrangements. *Social workers* refer clients to community agencies (e.g., public health nursing) for special assistance, arrange transportation and housing, and facilitate support groups and family team meetings.

Management Information
The management information services (**MIS**) or health information management (**HIM**) department provides computer support for the organization. This includes maintenance of all *electronic health records* (**EHR**), computers, scanners, and related activities. Many hospitals, clinics, and outpatient services are linked through a network and can communicate with one another. Automated services may include documentation in client records, billing, reporting laboratory and x-ray results, records of clinic visits, medications and treatments given in the past, and other pertinent information regarding the client's care, whether inpatient or outpatient. This department often trains new employees to use the facility's computerized systems and assists in troubleshooting computer problems. This department is also responsible for merging paper charts and other documents into the electronic record.

Telecommunications
The telecommunication department facilitates distance communication, allowing healthcare providers to communicate with clients and other specialists in faraway locations via telephone and computer. Providers can review images, tests, laboratory values, and ECGs; examine skin conditions; and diagnose medical conditions without requiring clients to come to the facility. This service is particularly important in areas with limited medical and transportation resources and allows consultation with specialists in other countries. This department may also conduct webinars and conference calls.

Biomedical Electronics
The biomedical electronics department purchases and maintains items such as computers, cardiac monitors, IV pumps, ECG machines, and other electronic equipment.

Case Management
Case management provides service coordination, health assessment, education, and discharge planning for clients, particularly those at high risk for readmission. After discharge, case managers follow up with clients in the community to maximize wellness and coordinate services.

Quality Improvement
The quality improvement (**QI**) department, also called *continuous quality improvement* (**CQI**), promotes the organization's efforts toward ensuring quality care by continually improving systems, services, and processes. QI staff also participates in the safety committee (Chapter 39). Clients and families are asked to evaluate care during and after hospitalization in an ongoing effort to meet and exceed customer expectations, improve performance throughout the organization, and remove barriers to excellent service.

Consulting Nurse Service
The consulting nurse service (**telehealth**) provides telephone advice to callers who need assistance in deciding

if and when to seek medical attention. Based on the severity of a caller's symptoms, the service advises callers to seek care immediately, to make an appointment, or to try home care measures. Nurses use preapproved, computerized *protocols* to assess the problem and provide advice. In many organizations, this service is combined with physician referral services and community health and wellness education services.

Outreach
Some facilities have an outreach department, particularly in an area such as psychiatry. Outreach staff visit clients at home, often on an emergency basis, to help determine what action should be taken. The facility may also maintain a *crisis line* or *suicide prevention center* as part of the outreach.

Poison Control
Some large facilities maintain a poison control center for the state or region.

STUDENT SYNTHESIS

KEY POINTS
- The needs of clients include the basic needs of all humans, plus special needs connected with illness or injury.
- The client unit is the area in which the nurse delivers most nursing care.
- A clean and orderly unit helps prevent accidents and infections and maximizes efficiency.
- Certain guidelines are common for all nursing procedures. Some procedures are grouped according to time of day.
- Healthcare facilities offer a wide variety of services and are often staffed with personnel with special education/training. Direct client care departments, specialized client care departments, and support services are available in most facilities.
- Many services provided in the hospital can also be provided in ECFs, clinics, and the home.

CRITICAL THINKING EXERCISES
1. Your acute care client is spending the first full day in your care. Describe the basic activities for that day. Discuss your responsibilities. How will your coordination and organization of activities help your client?
2. Your client is a right-handed 35-year-old homemaker and single mother of three small children. They have fractured their right arm and is soon to be discharged. Describe hospital and community support services that they may use while in the facility and after discharge.
3. How would your role and degree of autonomy change in the following settings: hospital, ECF, clinic, home care.
4. Discuss how telecommunications, consulting nurse services (telehealth), and case management can help to provide cost-effective care for the client outside the hospital setting. How does this care reduce healthcare costs?
5. Describe the role of housekeeping in providing safer client care. (Consider the roles of both housekeeping and nursing staff.)

NCLEX-STYLE REVIEW QUESTIONS
1. The nurse enters a client's hospital room to administer medication. Which observation made by the nurse would be of greatest concern?
   a. The overbed table has a telephone on it.
   b. The call light is attached to the bed within the client's reach.
   c. The head of the bed is elevated to 45°.
   d. The bed is elevated to a high position and the side rails are down.

2. The nurse hears a client crying out, "Someone please help!" After meeting the client's immediate needs, which nursing action should be provided?
   a. Instruct and have the client demonstrate use of the call bell.
   b. Inform the client that the call bell must be used in order for someone to come.
   c. Place the client in the chair at the nurse's station.
   d. Sedate the client with medication.

3. The nurse smells cigarette smoke coming from a client's hospital bathroom. Which action by the nurse is the priority?
   a. Inform the client discharge from the hospital is likely.
   b. Inform the client that the hospital has a no-smoking policy.
   c. Call the security officer to handle the situation.
   d. Do nothing because the client has the right to smoke.

4. A client requests that the nurse increase the heat in the room. The temperature is presently 72 °F. Which is the priority action by the nurse?
   a. Tell the client to put more clothing on.
   b. Inform the client that it is warm in the room.
   c. Tell the client that you cannot comply with that request.
   d. Bring the client a blanket from the warmer.

5. The CNA informs the nurse that a confused client keeps removing the covers and exposing themselves. Which intervention can the nurse suggest to the CNA to protect the client's privacy?
   a. Use soft wrist restraints so the client cannot remove the covers.
   b. Use safety pins to fasten the gown to the bed sheets.
   c. Obtain pajamas for the client to wear.
   d. Tie the covers to the side rails.

CHAPTER RESOURCES

Enhance your learning with additional resources on thePoint!

Student Resources related to this chapter can be found at thePoint.lww.com/Rosdahl12e.

39 Emergency Preparedness

Learning Objectives

1. List 10 nursing measures that help prevent accidents.
2. Identify five potentially hazardous materials used in healthcare.
3. Describe the use of a Safety Data Sheet (SDS).
4. Describe at least five safety tips for using, storing, disposing of, and cleaning up hazardous substances.
5. Explain the use of the emergency bathroom signal.
6. Describe evaluation of client fall risk.
7. Identify possible methods of communication during an emergency.
8. List considerations in developing a personal emergency preparedness plan.
9. Discuss the differences between an internal and external disaster.
10. Describe procedures if a bomb threat occurs.
11. Define emergency triage.
12. List three important considerations when client evacuation is necessary.
13. List steps taken in the event of an infant or child abduction.
14. Explain the acronyms RACE and PASS and their relationship to the fire plan.
15. List four classes of fire extinguishers and their uses.

Important Terminology

command center
crash cart
employee right-to-know laws
external disaster
internal disaster
triage

Acronyms

AED
CPR
DMAT
JSA
OSHA
PASS
RACE
SDS
START

Safety promotion and accident prevention are vital in the healthcare facility, community, and at home. A safe environment is one in which a minimum of risk for illness or injury exists. Every person in a healthcare organization is responsible for safety.

The disastrous events of September 11, 2001, the bridge collapse in Minneapolis in 2007, and several hurricanes in the Gulf Coast have graphically illustrated the need for emergency preparedness by all healthcare facilities. In addition, each staff member and student must understand the necessity for safety and emergency preparedness, the facility's disaster plan, and each person's role in emergencies. It is also important to consider your personal safety at work and in your daily life. This knowledge helps you perform competently and confidently if an emergency occurs.

SAFETY AND PREPAREDNESS

Safety in the healthcare facility extends to clients, employees, students, and visitors. The goal is twofold: to prevent accidents and to be prepared for emergencies. *Prevention is the key.* Nurses are important providers of safety and emergency care. As a nurse, you will be exposed to safety hazards and emergency conditions in healthcare facilities and in the community. In addition to prevention, you must know where emergency equipment is kept in your facility or in the client's home and how and whom to call in an emergency.

The Safety Committee

Every healthcare facility is required to have a designated safety committee, whose goal is to provide a safe environment for everyone in the facility. Some committee responsibilities include providing security services, establishing principles of worker safety and occupational health, analyzing job safety, investigating accidents, and tracking injury and illness rates. The committee is also responsible for preparing disaster plans, safety policies and procedures, procedures for handling hazardous substances, and information regarding these substances. Committee representatives include administration, infection control, quality improvement, industrial hygiene, fire/safety, engineering, environmental management, human resources, medicine, and nursing.

Client Safety

A client has the right to expect a healthcare facility to protect against injury and disease. Facility safety measures include precautions such as general emergency preparedness, plans for specific emergencies (e.g., fire), plans for evacuation, policies for resuscitation, and accurate administration of medications and treatments. Many procedures aim to prevent the spread of infection. For example, hand sanitizer is located throughout your facility and in public places, such as supermarkets. A more subtle aspect of safety is proper waste disposal, to prevent both environmental contamination and exposure to infectious materials or injury from discarded needles.

In addition, many clients and healthcare providers are allergic to latex; reactions can range from mild irritation to anaphylactic shock and death. Latex is contained in many items, including balloons, envelope glue, erasers, condoms, and some medical supplies such as catheters and other tubes, surgical gloves, elastic bandages, and heating pads. Healthcare organizations have plans for providing safety for latex-sensitive individuals, and many items formerly made of latex are now made of substitute materials (Chapter 42 discusses treatment of allergies in greater detail).

Accident Prevention

Most accidents are preventable with knowledge and attention to safety. All staff must work together to prevent accidents. It is your responsibility to take action in potentially hazardous situations. For example, if you notice a piece of chipped glass on a client's food tray or a spilled substance on the floor, take immediate corrective action. If an accident does occur, follow your facility's procedure for documenting the circumstances in an official incident report. In Practice: Nursing Care Guidelines 39-1 provides accident prevention information.

The Left-Handed Client

Most people are right handed; the typical client environment is arranged for them. However, when the client is left handed, modifications are necessary to provide comfort and safety. Ask if the client is right or left handed. If the client is left handed, rearrange items appropriately. For example, place the telephone and bedside stand and, if possible, the call signal and television controls on the client's left side. These principles also apply to the client who has the use of only one arm or hand or who has one eye patched. Remember that the left-handed client is often also "left footed" and consider this when assisting the client out of bed and when the client is ambulating.

> **Key Concept**
> Most healthcare facilities require all staff to attend regular safety training sessions. Topics often include fire safety, handling of hazardous materials, and code or disaster procedures.

Fall Risk Assessment

A major goal in all healthcare is fall prevention. Routine fall prevention includes factors such as making sure wheelchairs are locked when the client is transferring, assisting with ambulation when needed, and making sure all spills are cleaned up immediately. In addition, falls are the most common cause of injury for disabled, sedated, confused, and older adults. All clients in the healthcare facility (except those in active labor [automatic high risk] or in the newborn ICU) and all clients in home care are assessed regularly for fall risk. Fall Risk Assessment must be documented on the client's record at least once every 24 hours and more frequently, if necessary. Many healthcare facilities provide a checklist for this purpose. Box 39-1 is an example of a Fall Risk Assessment checklist used for adults. (Special checklists exist for children.)

IN PRACTICE
NURSING CARE GUIDELINES 39-1 — Preventing Accidents in the Healthcare Facility or Client's Home

- Keep floors dry and clean, to prevent falls. Follow proper, safe methods for spill cleanup.
- Keep halls and client rooms free of obstacles; promote good room order.
- Double-lock medicine carts and medicine rooms; do not leave them unattended. If keys are used, keep them on your person at all times. In the home, be sure all medications are kept out of the reach of children.
- Get adequate assistance to move and walk clients. Use a transfer belt or walker when necessary.
- Always use two objective means to identify each client before performing any procedure or giving medication.
- Administer medications carefully; ask for clarification if you have a question. Know how to access drug references.
- Provide adequate lighting. Encourage use of a night light.
- Place the client's necessary items within reach, particularly the call light or bell.
- Check the temperature of any liquid or solution (including water) before giving it to the client.
- Raise the height of the client's bed, to prevent back strain, when working with a client. Keep the bed in low position at other times.
- Raise side rails as ordered. When the side rails are down, do not leave the client unattended.
- Do not perform unfamiliar procedures without proper supervision. You are responsible for learning your facility's protocols and their underlying rationales.
- Check all equipment routinely, to ensure proper functioning. Check electric cords for tangles, loose plugs, or fraying. Remove any defective equipment from the area immediately.
- Make sure sterile packages are dry and unopened and that medications have not expired or are otherwise unfit for use.
- Check all clients frequently, to make sure they are comfortable and safe.
- Always be aware of safety rules. Think before you act.
- Be sure any item heated in a microwave is safe for microwave use and monitor the oven while it is running. Make sure items are not too hot when giving them to clients.
- Know how to call "codes" in your facility. Know code procedures to follow.
- Know the location of fire extinguishers on your unit or in the home and how to use them. (*You must know the location of these wherever you work.*)
- Keep up to date on CPR training and nursing continuing education (CEUs).

Box 39-1 Fall Risk Evaluation

Clients are evaluated on a regular basis for fall risk. One evaluation tool used is the Hendrich Fall Risk Tool. (Additional items have been added to this basic questionnaire.) The client is scored on each risk factor. If a factor is absent in the client, the score for that factor is 0. If the *total score* is 5 or greater, the client has a high risk of falling and requires special observation by staff. Usually, this client also wears a special yellow name band and socks and has special room identification warning of fall risk. High-risk clients may require 1:1 supervision.

Risk Factor	Risk Points	Discussion/Examples
Confusion/disorientation (level of awareness; ability to communicate and understand)	+4	Disorganized, unable to follow instructions; poor judgment; forgets limitations
Depression insomnia, fatigue, high score on depression test	+2	Hopelessness, sad affect, lethargy, suicidal thoughts
Altered elimination (4+ times a night), urgency, needs assistance with toileting, severe diarrhea or constipation	+1	Urinary/bowel incontinence, frequency, nocturia
Dizziness, vertigo, unsteady	+1	Orthostatic change on rising, complaints of dizziness
Gender (male)	+1	Men more likely to take risks or not ask for help
Prescribed anticonvulsants (might alter sensorium)	+2	Includes carbamazepine (Tegretol), divalproex sodium (Depakote), gabapentin (Neurontin), lamotrigine (Lamictal), phenobarbital (Luminal), topiramate (Topamax), phenytoin (Dilantin)
Prescribed benzodiazepines (might alter sensorium) (Other drugs, such as opiates, antihypertensives, diuretics, or laxatives are included in the JH[a] scale.)	+1	Includes alprazolam (Xanax), buspirone (Buspar), chlordiazepoxide (Librium), clonazepam (Klonopin), diazepam (Valium), flurazepam (Dalmane), lorazepam (Ativan), midazolam (Versed), oxazepam (Serax), temazepam (Restoril), triazolam (Halcion)
Get-up-and-go test (rise from chair). Includes safe use of mobility devices, such as canes/walkers	0	Able to rise in single movement
	+1	Pushes up, successful in one try
	+3	Multiple attempts, but successful
	+4	Unable to rise without assistance

[a]Johns Hopkins Medical Center (JH) has developed a similar rating scale that identifies the client as "automatic low risk" (client completely paralyzed/immobilized), "automatic high risk" (history of a fall within 6 months, or as determined by healthcare personnel), or not meeting automatic criteria. The JH rating scale addresses most of the criteria of the Hendrich scale, plus client age (the older the client, the higher the score), impulsivity, and mobility (independent, with assist, unsteady, and visual/auditory impairment). It also considers equipment that "tethers" the client (e.g., IV, chest tube, catheter). Another factor is a sedated procedure within 24 hours.

Adapted from Hartford Institute for Geriatric Nursing, New York University College of Nursing, n.d. and Johns Hopkins, n.d..

The client at risk for falling is often identified by a distinctive wristband, colored slippers (usually yellow), and/or a special identifying sign on their room (Fig. 39-1). In addition, a special alert is displayed in the electronic health record. This client will have a specific "high fall risk" care plan, including frequent observation, special attention to room lighting and placement of furniture, and other measures, such as side rails or a "wander guard," as determined by the team. In the event of a fall, immediate action is taken to determine if any injury occurred and to make sure the client is protected from future falls, and an "incident report" is filed.

Additional factors are considered in home care. These include the following:

- Placement of furniture and avoidance of loose scatter rugs
- Level of lighting
- Presence of small animals/pets in the home
- Availability of caregivers
- Stairs
- Other factors, such as age, substance abuse, and specific disorders (pulmonary, cardiovascular, seizures), are considered on an individual basis
- Fall risk interventions to be documented for all high-risk clients, whether in the home or a healthcare facility, include the following:
  - Call signal within easy reach and client able to use it
  - Bed in low position, brakes locked
  - Room neat; no clutter
- Evaluation of medications, to determine possible danger
- Side rails up as needed
- Assistance with elimination as needed; bedpan/urinal/commode easily available

CHAPTER 39 Emergency Preparedness

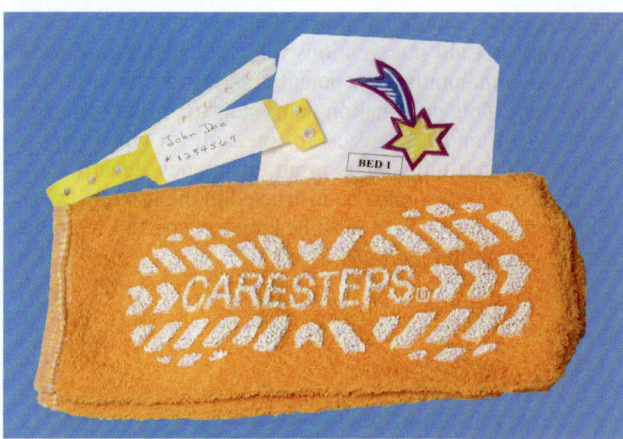

Figure 39-1 The client at risk for falling is often identified by a special yellow wristband, yellow slipper socks, and a "falling star" or other sign outside the room. (Photo courtesy of Keith Bunker Rosdahl.)

- Nonslip footwear
- Night light in use
- Bed alarm/wander guard in use
- Restraints used as needed
- Client reorientation

This information is given to the client and caregivers in the home or "sitters" in the healthcare facility. Any additional risk factors or interventions are also documented in the client record.

> **Nursing Alert** Fall risk must be documented at least every 24 hours on every inpatient client.

Electrical Safety

Electric shocks are preventable. Impurities in water (particularly salt) conduct electricity. Dry your hands before inserting a plug into or removing it from an electric outlet. Never turn appliances on or off when in contact with water. Always disconnect equipment by grasping the plug; *do not pull on the cord.* Frayed or worn cords must be repaired to prevent fires, short circuits, and blown circuit breakers. Disconnect and turn off electrical equipment as soon as you are finished using it. Teach clients and family members to follow the same safety measures. If you are working in a healthcare facility, notify the maintenance or biomedical electronics department of any malfunction, including excess heat or burning odors from a running motor. Notify your supervisor when you identify safety hazards. In the client's home, discuss safety with the client and caregivers.

> **Key Concept**
> Before you do anything else, immediately remove or otherwise address any source of imminent danger. *Do not try to repair* any piece of equipment yourself.

Other Considerations

Factors such as air quality and management of piped-in medical gases (e.g., oxygen) are managed by building maintenance. If a leak occurs in the system, an alarm will be activated and it may be necessary to evacuate clients. Nurses are responsible for immediately reporting any problem. Report the location and describe the display on the alarm panel. If there is a problem with air quality, heating, or air conditioning, the nurse will most likely be the first person to become aware of the problem. Usually, the situation can be easily corrected. If a client or visitor is smoking, make the individual aware of the no-smoking regulations and explain the dangers of smoking in the facility. *Do not allow anyone to continue smoking; notify security, if assistance is necessary.*

Reporting of Incidents

All adverse events (critical incidents) must be reported, whether they cause injury or death. Preventable adverse events include pressure wounds; medication errors; any client fall; injuries from faulty medical equipment; blood transfusion reactions; and surgical errors. Injuries to staff (e.g., a needle stick or assault by a client) also must be reported. The event is described, listing probable causes, ways to prevent recurrence, action taken and notifications made, and severity of the result.

Employee Safety

In 1991, the Occupational Safety and Health Administration (**OSHA**) mandated that each workplace (including healthcare facilities) must establish plans for reducing accidents and injuries. In addition, OSHA requires a job safety analysis (**JSA**) for each position. Individual states have enacted **employee right-to-know laws** (*ERTK*), with the legislation enforced by OSHA. These laws state that employees have the right to know about all dangers associated with hazardous substances, infectious agents, or dangerous physical situations they might encounter in the workplace (Table 39-1). (In addition to chemicals, hazards also include noise [employer must provide hearing protection], injection [e.g., needle stick], radiation, and extreme temperatures [e.g., cryogenic liquids used to treat by freezing, blanket warmers].) The Safe Medical Device Act of 1990 provides for monitoring device malfunction and death/serious injury caused by medical devices.

TABLE 39-1	Occupational Hazards
HAZARD	**EXAMPLE**
Flammables	Oxygen
Poisons	Chlorosorb
Skin or eye irritants	Hibiclens
Carcinogens	Formalin
Biological agents	Blood, body fluids, infectious organisms
Radiation	X-rays, radioactive implants
Chemical agents/medicinal agents	Some chemotherapy drugs; some other medications, such as divalproex (Depakote)

Each facility must have on file a Safety Data Sheet (**SDS**) describing any substance considered hazardous. Routes of entry for hazardous substances include absorption (skin, eyes), inhalation (lungs), and ingestion (foods, liquids). The SDS provides information about a substance's contents and potential dangers. Manufacturers of commercial products are required to supply a description of the product, its ingredients, physical properties, fire or explosion hazards, and reactivity. The SDS also gives information on protective equipment required, safe handling information (in case of a spill or leak), and first aid interventions for accidental exposure. An SDS is also maintained for potential industrial hazards in the community. This information helps staff to provide appropriate treatment and take necessary precautions when exposed to contaminated individuals in an emergency department or ambulance. All staff must be instructed in the use of SDS and protective gear; any SDS must be kept for a period of not less than 30 years (Fig. 39-2 and Box 39-2).

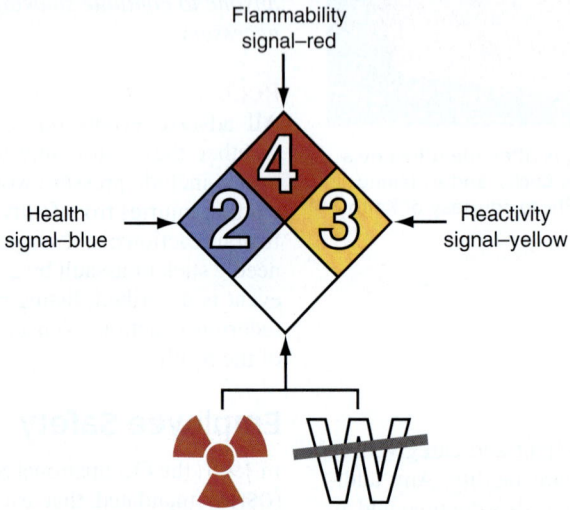

	Identification of Health Hazard Color Code: **BLUE**		Identification of Flammability Color Code: **RED**		Identification of Reactivity (Stability) Color Code: **YELLOW**
	Type of possible injury		Susceptibility of materials to burning		Susceptibility to release of energy
SIGNAL		**SIGNAL**		**SIGNAL**	
4	Materials that on very short exposure could cause death or major residual injury even though prompt medical treatment was given.	4	Materials that will rapidly or completely vaporize at atmospheric pressure and normal ambient temperature, or that are readily dispersed in air and that will burn readily.	4	Materials that in themselves are readily capable of detonation or of explosive decomposition or reaction at normal temperatures and pressures.
3	Materials that on short exposure could cause serious temporary or residual injury even though prompt medical treatment was given.	3	Liquids and solids that can be ignited under almost all ambient temperature conditions.	3	Materials that in themselves are capable of detonation or explosive reaction but require a strong initiating source or that must be heated under confinement before initiation or that react explosively with water.
2	Materials that on intense or continued exposure could cause temporary incapacitation or possible residual injury unless prompt medical treatment is given.	2	Materials that must be moderately heated or exposed to relatively high ambient temperatures before ignition can occur.	2	Materials that in themselves are normally unstable and readily undergo violent chemical change but do not detonate. Also materials that may react violently with water or that may form potentially explosive mixtures with water.
1	Materials that on exposure would cause irritation but only minor residual injury even if no treatment is given.	1	Materials that must be preheated before ignition can occur.	1	Materials that in themselves are normally stable, but that can become unstable at elevated temperatures and pressures or that may react with water with some release of energy, but not violently.
0	Materials that on exposure under fire conditions would offer no hazard beyond that of ordinary combustible material.	0	Materials that will not burn.	0	Materials that in themselves are normally stable, even under fire exposure conditions, and that are not reactive with water.

Figure 39-2 Rating system and criteria for classifying hazardous materials. (McCall, 2003.)

> **Box 39-2 Description of a Safety Data Sheet (SDS)**
>
> Any hazardous material in the facility must have an SDS on file. The criteria shown in Figure 39-2 illustrate the basis for the SDS, which includes the following:
>
> | Material | Selected Examples |
> |---|---|
> | Name, synonyms | Acetone, dimethyl formaldehyde |
> | Chemical formula | C_3H_6O |
> | Molecular weight | 58.08 |
> | Chemical class | Ketone |
> | Physical description | Colorless liquid, with fragrant, fruity odor |
> | Boiling point | 56.1 °C, 133 °F |
> | Melting point, flash point, auto ignition, vapor pressure | Flash point: −17 °C (closed cup), −9 °C (open cup) |
> | Specific gravity | 0.791 @ 20 °C |
> | Water solubility | Miscible |
> | Incompatibilities | Oxygen, acids |
> | DOT hazard class | Flammable liquid |
> | Categories | 1. Fire hazard, flammable 2. Acute toxicity: adverse effects to target organs |
> | Health hazard | Slightly hazardous to health. As a precaution, wear self-contained breathing apparatus. |
> | Flammability | This material can be ignited under almost all temperature conditions. |
>
> The SDS also lists target organs, symptoms, human toxicity data, first aid for exposure, and other pertinent data. If there are questions about any material, consult the SDS.

Guidelines for Using Hazardous Substances

Hazardous substances are used daily in healthcare facilities and in the home. Remember the following safety tips when using and storing hazardous substances:

- Have the phone number of the local poison control center available (Chapter 43, Nursing Care Guidelines 43-7).
- Read labels carefully; note emergency information.
- Follow instructions for use, storage, and disposal of all materials.
- Avoid spills; use proper procedures for cleaning up spills.
- Use protective equipment as recommended.
- Never use any unlabeled or outdated substance.
- Never store hazardous materials in alternate containers.
- Do not use or store gasoline, paint, or turpentine indoors.
- Do not mix substances.
- Do not use hairspray or other aerosol products around an open flame, eyeglasses, or contact lenses.
- Avoid breathing mists or vapors; keep areas well ventilated (Chapter 43 for first-aid measures).

- Follow radiation prevention guidelines closely; radiation has a potential for danger.

Cleanup of Hazardous Wastes

There are many hazardous materials in the healthcare facility, including chemicals such as those identified in Table 39-1. Biological materials (e.g., blood and body fluids) are also considered hazardous. If any hazardous substance is spilled, consult facility or home care agency procedures for the approved method of cleanup (Fig. 39-3). Always wear gloves and carefully wash hands when cleaning up spills; wear other protective gear as needed. Major spills must be cleaned up by specially trained personnel. Subsequent chapters in this book describe protective gear, isolation methods, and disposal of hazardous wastes in more detail.

> **Key Concept**
>
> Every staff member in a facility should participate in accident prevention and in client and employee safety.

Considerations Affecting Client and Employee Safety

Weapons, Narcotics, and Other Contraband

Clients, staff, and visitors must be protected at all times. Weapons, such as guns or knives, may be brought into the facility and pose an immediate threat to all concerned. (A weapon is defined as *any object that can be used to threaten or injure another person*.) This situation is particularly dangerous in areas such as psychiatry or chemical dependency units, where clients may attempt to escape or obtain drugs, or in the obstetrical department, where infant abduction may occur. Local and federal laws prohibit carrying a firearm into a healthcare facility, except by a police officer. If you suspect that a client or visitor has a weapon, report it to your security department immediately. *Nurses should never attempt to handle this situation without assistance.* A "security code" will be called, and security personnel or police officers will

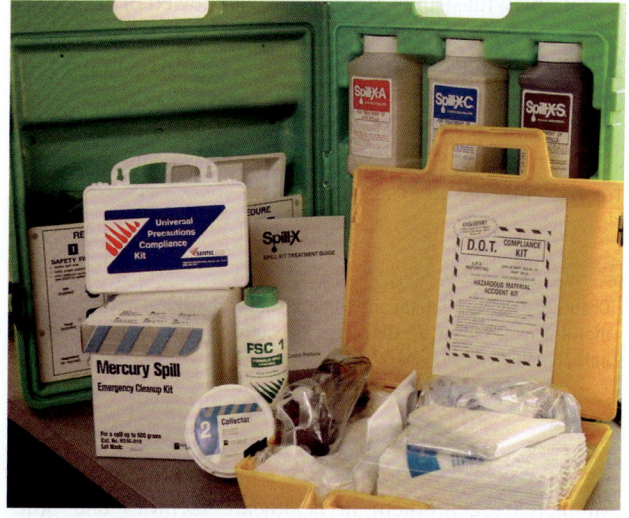

Figure 39-3 Kits used for cleanup of biohazardous materials. (McCall, 2003.)

manage the situation. Illegal weapons are confiscated and usually not returned. In some situations, alcohol, narcotics, or other drugs are brought into the hospital; much the same action is taken as that regarding a weapon. In either case, it is possible that the person may be arrested. Nurses must carefully document any dangerous situation. Be sure to include a complete description of the problem involved, description of the incident, and any actions taken and by whom. The healthcare provider may request that a client involved in illegal activities be discharged against medical advice (AMA) or, if the person is dangerous, that they be jailed or confined in a locked area of the facility. Many facilities have a "package inspection" policy; packages brought into the facility may be searched if it is believed they contain contraband. Most facilities also reserve the right to search outgoing packages (carried by clients, visitors, or staff), in an effort to deter theft. In some facilities, everyone must pass through a metal detector on entering. Use of cell phones is prohibited in client areas because of client privacy.

> **Nursing Alert** If there is any danger in the healthcare facility, the nurse should never attempt to manage the situation without assistance.

Flowers and Gifts

Flowers and other gifts can pose a threat to clients. For example:

- Live plants or cut flowers cannot be brought into areas such as a Burn Unit or Bone Marrow Transplant Unit (because of infection danger).
- Certain items, such as plants with natural moss, can be dangerous to immunocompromised clients.
- In most facilities, latex balloons are not permitted because of latex allergies. (Mylar balloons are usually allowed, except in psychiatry and other special areas.)
- Some materials have a high potential for fire. These include straw, dry vines, and celluloid and usually are not allowed.
- Glass or porcelain items, soda cans, and certain clothing that may be dangerous, such as neckties, heavy boots, or clothing with strings, usually are not allowed in psychiatry or chemical dependency units.
- Tools and other sharp items usually are not allowed.
- Cigarettes, lighters, and smokeless tobacco usually must be checked in at the desk by visitors.

If you have a question about the appropriateness of a gift for a client, consult your supervisor.

> **Key Concept**
> Clients with a "no information" status do not wish to have anyone know they are in the facility. These clients do not receive gifts, visitors, phone calls, or mail.

Workplace Violence

An increasing problem in healthcare facilities and other places of employment is that of workplace violence. Some of this can be attributed to the increasing use of drugs. If a client or visitor becomes threatening, you must take immediate action. Protect other clients and yourself by speaking calmly, moving those threatened to a safer area, and notifying security immediately. *Remember, a weapon does not only mean a gun; it can be a knife, club, mace, or any other item that can be used to inflict harm.*

Emergency Preparedness

Nurse Call Light and Intercom

Place the nurse call light button within reach of the client at all times, demonstrate its use, and remind the client to use it whenever necessary. Explain how to use the intercom; explain that this will help the healthcare staff to respond appropriately. Check clients frequently if they are sedated, confused, or physically unable to use the call light. A tap bell may be used in certain situations, such as when oxygen is being used or cords are not allowed.

Emergency Signal

In most facilities, the call signal in the client's bathroom causes an additional light to flash or a buzzer to sound at the central nursing station. This emergency signal may be used by the client when experiencing difficulty while in the bathroom or by staff to request immediate assistance, for example, if the client falls or experiences cardiac arrest. Staff must respond immediately to the emergency signal. If the client is in a multibed room, another client can help by activating the bathroom alarm and using the intercom to explain the nature of the emergency.

Many home care clients can activate an alert system when they are having difficulty or feel they have an emergency. The signal is carried by the client and activates an alarm in a designated location, such as an emergency or police department. The client is then contacted by telephone, a neighbor is alerted to check on the client, or local emergency medical response providers are contacted and directed to the client's residence.

Emergency Resuscitation

Knowing the location and use of emergency resuscitation equipment is essential. In the hospital and skilled nursing facility (SNF), each area generally has a locked emergency cart (**crash cart**) stocked with emergency medications and equipment (Fig. 43-6). Check this cart regularly according to the facility's protocol, to make sure all items are there and equipment, such as suction, the defibrillator, and oxygen tanks, are operating properly.

Know the procedure for calling the cardiopulmonary resuscitation (**CPR**) team in the facility ("calling a code") or the emergency response service in the community health setting (usually 911 in the United States). It is important to know where the *automated external defibrillator* (**AED**) is located in community facilities. Healthcare facilities have specific codes for emergencies (e.g., "code blue" or "Dr. Blue" commonly designates a cardiopulmonary arrest). Clinics and dental offices also have resuscitative equipment and emergency plans. Most healthcare organizations require regular CPR certification for all healthcare personnel.

Key Concept

Each emergency has a specific code name in the facility's public address system. All healthcare providers must learn how to initiate this code system(s); in some facilities, 911 is used. When calling a code, be sure to give your location, the nature of the code, and your name and phone number. (Your facility may have additional requirements.)

Personal Preparedness

Preparing for emergencies is important in the home, workplace, and community. Unexpected emergencies, such as an earthquake, hurricane, blizzard, tornado, or flood, can disrupt your personal life. Home care nurses must be prepared for travel through a weather emergency, disaster area, or other emergency situation. You may be asked to help during an emergency and provide care in a variety of settings including shelters, clinics, or other healthcare facilities. You may also be asked to return to your facility to assist. This may involve working long hours away from your home and family. Taking the time to develop a *personal emergency preparedness plan* will help you cope with such a situation; making good decisions and coping with disruptions are facilitated when you are well prepared. Box 39-3 offers pointers for developing your personal emergency preparedness plan.

THE DISASTER PLAN

A facility's *disaster plan* describes actions to take in a disaster. This plan is activated when an incident produces so many casualties that routine methods for client care must be altered. All employees must know how to access the facility's disaster plan. Healthcare facilities are required to have regular, periodic fire and disaster drills to allow their staff to practice emergency skills. Each facility must have a plan for natural disasters common to its area of the country. These disasters may include tornadoes, blizzards, hurricanes, earthquakes, avalanches, floods, or mudslides. Facilities also have plans for bomb threats and hazardous material spills. It is important to know the local disaster plans, so you will be prepared and able to protect yourself and your clients if a disaster occurs. Box 39-4 is an example of a disaster plan for a bomb threat. In any disaster, staff may be required to work extended hours or to return to the facility.

> **Nursing Alert** With any threat, notify the facility's security personnel or the local police immediately. Do not attempt to decide if the threat is real or how to handle it. Trained personnel must decide what action to take.

Internal Versus External Disasters

Two basic types of disaster alerts are used in healthcare facilities. An **internal disaster** is one in which the facility itself is in danger or damaged and/or function is impaired. An internal disaster may be caused by a fire, explosion, terrorist activity, radiation, a biological spill, or a storm. An **external disaster** occurs outside the facility and has an

---

Box 39-3 Personal Emergency Preparedness

- Plan for prolonged power outages. Keep flashlights, battery-powered lamps, portable radio, and extra batteries handy.
- Keep a first-aid kit stocked and on hand.
- Store 1 gallon of water, per person in your household, per day, and adequate food supplies to last 4 days. Store additional water and food for pets.
- In an area with frequent power outages, it is helpful to have a portable generator.
- Maintain sufficient gas in your car and have cash on hand to last several days. During power outages, gas pumps, cash machines, banks, and most retail stores are closed.
- Store prescriptions, glasses, dentures, hearing aids, and other essential items in a secure and accessible area.
- Develop a family plan. Identify safe areas in the home during different types of disasters. Establish a nearby meeting place for emergencies, such as fire. Also establish a place away from the home in case you are unable to return because of floods or blocked roadways.
- Select someone outside your area as a contact for your family to call and with whom to leave messages. Write down addresses and telephone numbers for family members to keep in their wallets. Enter emergency numbers under "ICE" on your cell phone. Knowing your loved ones are safe will help you focus on your work.
- Carry an emergency kit in your car, including walking shoes, flashlight, batteries, maps, water, extra clothing, blankets, flares, jumper cables, wire, duct tape, and clothing appropriate for conditions in your area.
- Plan ahead and write down what you would take if you had to evacuate your home. Decisions are more difficult to make during a crisis.
- Have a plan for child care when school closures occur.
- Identify potential hazards that might block your usual travel route. Identify alternate routes that would be free from water, debris, or other roadway disruption.
- Carry a charged cell phone with you at all times; have a car charger.
- Carry an emergency "hammer" in your car. This contains a cutting tool to cut seat belts and a hammer to break windows, in case of emergency.

---

impact on normal operations. The organization must activate the disaster plan to prepare to receive a large number of casualties or to evacuate. It may require existing clients to be moved or discharged, to make room for incoming casualties. Earthquakes, floods, hurricanes, explosions, airplane crashes, or large chemical spills are examples of external disasters. Specific plans are executed for each type of disaster. (The severity of the disaster may be rated. Level 1 = facility resources adequate; level 2 = outside assistance required; level 3 = all outside resources required [disaster].) In some situations, such as an earthquake or tornado, the facility may be required to prepare for both an internal and an external disaster. A facility that has sustained significant

Box 39-4 Sample Bomb Threat Disaster Plan

If you receive any bomb threat, immediately notify your supervisor and security personnel. If you receive the threat over the phone:
- Immediately check the "caller ID," to determine the origin of the call.

ASK THESE QUESTIONS AND WRITE DOWN THE CALLER'S ANSWERS WORD FOR WORD
- Where is the bomb, exactly?
- What does it look like?
- What will make it explode? When will it explode?
- How can we stop it from exploding?
- Why was it put there?
- Did you put it there or did someone help you?
- Who are you? (Ask last, to encourage answers to the other questions)

LISTEN TO OTHER CUES AND NOTE THE THINGS YOU HEAR
- Voice characteristics: loud, pleasant, intoxicated
- Speech: fast, slow, slurred
- Location: did the caller seem familiar with the building?
- Language: foul, use of scientific terms
- Accent: local, foreign, male or female
- Manner: calm, angry, incoherent
- Background noises: machines, airplanes, street traffic, voices, music

GENERAL GUIDELINES
- Do not touch or move any suspicious object. In nearly all situations, a search will be conducted by the bomb squad.
- You must report anything unusual and follow the instructions of the professionals.
- Protect your clients as much as possible. Give clear, firm directions.
- A bomb threat is usually not assigned a code name and is not paged overhead. Communication is done by phone.
- Stay away from windows or large glass objects during the search.
- Do not use elevators until cleared.
- Carefully document the incident after the danger has passed.

When telephone service is disrupted, several other means of communicating with healthcare providers are available, including the following:
- Amateur radio ham operators
- Television or radio broadcasts
- Automatic email
- Contacts outside the affected area
- Pagers
- Portable or handheld radios
- Police

Implementation

The healthcare facility's disaster plan describes duties and responsibilities of staff in a disaster. Nursing staff are asked to report to their usual nursing area or to a centrally designated area for assignment. Persons working at the time of the disaster may be asked to assist in another area or location. Specific duties are assigned. The disaster plan will identify the location of the **command center**, which provides overall direction of the facility's activities. Additional responsibilities include communicating with areas receiving those affected, assigning personnel to areas needing assistance, releasing information to the press, and monitoring the extent of the disaster and its potential effect on the facility and the community.

Triage

You may be assigned to assist in **triage**, the process of *sorting and classifying injured persons to determine priority of needs*. All injured people are identified, if possible, along with names of next of kin. Triage assigns victims for treatment; in the event of a major disaster, people with minimal injuries may be asked to assist with those who are in more critical condition. When a disaster involving many injuries occurs, how people are triaged can mean the difference between life and death. The simple triage and rapid treatment (**START**) system identifies people who will die quickly if they do not receive immediate medical care and is used by first responders trained in advanced first aid (Chapter 43).

Disaster Medical Assistance Team

A disaster medical assistance team (**DMAT**), consisting of healthcare provider, nurses, and emergency personnel, provides assistance and support in many environments, both in and out of healthcare facilities. The DMAT team may set up a temporary hospital or may be called on to relieve facility staff during a major disaster. During a disaster, staff often work long hours and may be stressed physically and emotionally. Healthcare personnel often provide care for injured clients when they may have suffered personal losses. The DMAT can provide relief during a shortage of workers and can relieve workers who need to rest.

Evacuation

Sometimes the threat of fire or disaster is sufficiently severe to require evacuation of the facility or a portion thereof. The extent and nature of the emergency will affect the decision to evacuate. Clients who can walk or use wheelchairs are usually evacuated first. Others may

---

damage may require evacuation of portions of the building, while continuing to provide emergency care from another location, including the establishment of a satellite treatment center in a distant location.

Staff Notification

Healthcare facilities often use an emergency staff notification system during a disaster. One such method is a cell phone text alert. This system is a means of notifying both on- and off-duty staff that their assistance is needed immediately. A text message is sent to all staff, and personnel are expected to arrive at the facility, if at all possible, within 30 minutes.

CHAPTER 39 Emergency Preparedness 475

must be carefully identified. You may be asked to help relocate essential equipment, such as crash carts and IV pumps and solutions, for use in another area. Each client should be wearing an ID band; preferably two name bands are used. Take the client's personal items, such as glasses, dentures, and hearing aids, if time permits. Consider taking your personal belongings as well. Sometimes long delays exist before anyone can reenter an evacuated area. In most cases, *elevators cannot be used*.

During times of disaster, home care agencies usually try to involve family members or friends in evacuating clients. If this is not possible, local emergency preparedness agencies must help with transport. These agencies need to know locations of clients and their specific needs to ensure fast and safe evacuation. If the home care client cannot be moved to the home of family or friends outside the area, they may be admitted to a hospital or ECF. Most shelters are not equipped to deal with clients with special needs, particularly during a disaster.

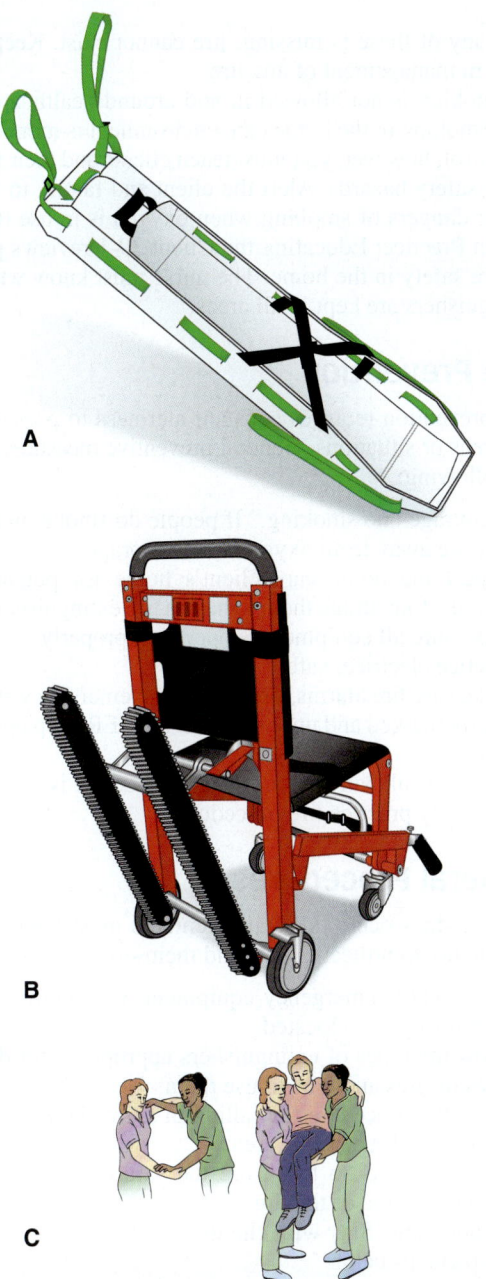

> ### Key Concept
> If only a portion of a facility is to be evacuated, clients are moved "horizontally"—that is, on the same level of the facility—to speed up the process and avoid using stairs. If clients must be moved to another level, they are moved down, if possible. In any evacuation, clients are grouped, and staff must make sure all are accounted for. Someone is also assigned to check all rooms after evacuation, to make sure everyone has left. Each room is marked with a dropped pillow or towel, to denote that it has been searched and is empty.

Special Situations

Bomb Threat
It is possible that someone may call in a bomb threat. Box 39-4 describes steps taken in this event. It is vital that you act quickly and calmly.

Infant/Child Abduction
The abduction of a baby or small child in a healthcare facility involves special procedures. Most hospitals do not allow any hospitalized baby or small child to be carried—they must be in a rolling bassinet or crib. If you see a baby in hospital garb being carried, call a "code" and alert security. Many hospitals use the term "code pink" or "alert pink" to denote a missing baby. In the event of such a code, all entrances in the immediate area and to the facility are immediately locked and guarded, and the facility is thoroughly searched until the child is found. All unauthorized people are denied entrance, and no one is allowed to leave. In many facilities, an electronic bracelet is placed on all children in the newborn nursery and pediatric units. An alarm will sound if any child is taken out of the area.

If you believe there has been a child abduction, notify the appropriate person(s) immediately.

- Give a full description of the child and the suspect, including what they were wearing.

Figure 39-4 In an extreme emergency, clients may need to be evacuated. **A.** The rescue sled or slide provides a means of moving an immobile client. The sled can be carried by two or more staff members or can be dragged by a single person (only for a horizontal evacuation). **B.** The rescue chair is used for a horizontal or vertical evacuation. The client is securely strapped into the chair. Two staff members are required to lower the chair down the stairs. One member holds the handles in the front of the chair and the other member holds the back of the chair. The gripper mechanism on the back of the chair allows control while lowering the chair down the stairs. **C.** Chair/seat carry is used in an extreme emergency only. Two rescuers interlock their arms to carry the client.

require transporting on stretchers, dragging on sheets or special "sleds," and the use of a stair-climbing device (Fig. 39-4). Nursery and pediatric nurses may wear large aprons that can hold several babies at one time. New mothers may be asked to transport their own babies; babies

- Tell other parents to stay with their children in their rooms.
- Move the parents of the abducted child to a private area; a person (often a chaplain or social worker) is assigned to stay with them.
- Be prepared with as much of the following information as is available about the abducted child for law enforcement personnel:
  - Infant footprints
  - Full written description
  - Photos
  - Blood samples
  - Condition of the child
  - Any special health problems of the child, such as diabetes or seizures

Nursing Alert If a parent/caretaker is the suspected abductor, legal action can be taken to access medical records and any other pertinent information. In a stranger abduction, parents must give consent.

Remember that the above emergency instructions are *general guidelines*. If you recognize a clear and imminent danger to clients or others, you must take immediate steps to provide safety to all concerned.

Work Stoppages

Work stoppages can involve nurses and other healthcare personnel. If there is a strike in your facility, you must decide whether to cross the picket line if you are a part of the involved bargaining unit. If you are not on strike, you will usually be expected to work. You may also be asked to work in an area of the facility that is different from your regular assignment.

THE FIRE PLAN

Fire is a major hazard that can be caused by improper management of flammable materials or gases, careless smoking, frayed electrical wiring, or faulty equipment. It is important to remember the three factors that must be present in order to create fire:

- Source of heat
- Source of fuel
- Oxygen

If any of these is missing, fire cannot exist. Keep this is mind in management of any fire.

Smoking is not allowed in and around healthcare facilities. Smoking in the home care environment is more difficult to control; however, you must teach clients and their families about safety hazards. Alert the client and family to the particular dangers of smoking when oxygen is in use (Chapter 87). In Practice: Educating the Client 39-1 reviews pointers for fire safety in the home. The nurse must know where fire extinguishers are kept in all areas.

Fire Prevention

Fire prevention requires constant alertness to possible danger areas or situations. General preventive measures include the following:

- Encourage "no smoking." If people do smoke, make sure they are away from oxygen use or storage.
- Inspect the home care client's home for potential fire hazards. Encourage them to have a fire extinguisher handy.
- Make sure all equipment is operating properly.
- Practice electrical safety.
- Make sure fire alarms, fire doors, and emergency stairs are clearly marked and unobstructed. NEVER prop open a fire door!
- Make sure all hallways are clear and nothing is stored there.
- Regularly practice fire procedures.

General Procedures

If a fire does occur, all staff members must know exactly what to do, to protect clients and themselves:

- Know where emergency equipment, fire alarms, and fire extinguishers are located.
- Know the types of extinguishers appropriate for different types of fires and how to use them.
- Know the procedure for calling in a fire alarm. Note your location and secure the area.
- Know what to do to ensure the safety of clients in the immediate area of the fire.
- Do not panic. Stay with clients.
- Keep clients calm.
- Know how to protect clients from injury.
- Use common sense.

IN PRACTICE
EDUCATING THE CLIENT 39-1 — Ways to Promote Fire Safety in the Home

- Check for frayed or cracked electrical cords and do not allow them to be placed under rugs or to be in the flow of traffic. Make sure extension cords are used properly and there are no three-prong adapters or "cluster plugs."
- Make sure there are smoke detectors and they are working properly and have fresh batteries.
- Assist the family to develop an emergency exit plan.
- Check space heaters and keep them out of the flow of traffic and away from flammable materials. Make sure they will turn off if tipped over. (Make sure gas heaters are not emitting carbon monoxide.)
- Assess the kitchen for adequate ventilation. Make sure no flammable materials are near the stove.
- Make sure potential fire sources are cleared away from the bed. Do not allow the client to smoke in bed.
- Observe storage areas for flammable liquids.

- Know the code name for "fire" in your facility. "Mr. Red," "Dr. Red," and "code red" are common names used.
- Keep yourself and your client between the exit and any fire.

Key Concept
Remember: Any fire in a healthcare facility *must* be reported, even if it has been extinguished. Any indication that there has been a fire must be reported. This includes the automatic activation of the sprinkler system, a smoke alarm, or the smell of smoke. (Be sure to indicate a "fire-out" when calling in this case.)

RACE is an acronym that may help you to remember the general order of procedures for a fire:

R = *Rescue:* Remove clients from the general area.
A = *Alarm/Alert:* Sound alarm.
C = *Confine:* Contain fire (close doors and windows, make sure fire doors close).
E = *Extinguish* fire (if possible).

Various facilities may use different acronyms, but the intent is the same.

Rescue
Rescue the client and others from immediate danger before doing anything else. Lead the client who can walk into the hall. Close the door to the room, and then sound the alarm. Assist the client who cannot walk into a chair and remove it from the room, or drag the client out of the room on a sheet. (Do not try to carry a client, other than small children.) If the client is involved in the fire, call aloud for help.

Alarm/Alert
Use your facility's procedure to get help. Usually you will pull a fire alarm and call the switchboard operator or 911. When you make the call, be sure to state the fire's exact nature and location and your name and title. Make sure all clients are in a safe place. Notify other staff and assign someone to stay with clients.

Confine/Contain
After calling in the alarm, close all doors, including fire and room doors. Check to make sure "automatic" doors fully close. Close open windows. (These procedures help to confine fire and smoke.) *Do not lock any doors. Do not use elevators.* Do not use the telephone unnecessarily. Turn off or unplug unnecessary electrical appliances. Report to the charge nurse for further instructions.

Extinguish
Attempt to put out a fire *only if you are sure you can do it safely*. Different types of fire extinguishers are available for different types of fires (Table 39-2). Be sure you know the type of extinguisher to use on a particular fire. (Use an "ABC" extinguisher, if unsure.) Putting out a fire is the *last* thing to do after you have protected others and notified the authorities. *Do not* try to put out a fire yourself without first calling for help. Again, use common sense. It is your responsibility to know the location and operation of all fire extinguishers. Remove the extinguisher from its enclosure. Avoid contact with the contents of the extinguisher. If you must put out a fire, remember the letters **PASS**:

P: Pull the pin (on the fire extinguisher).
A: Aim at the base of the fire, near the edge.
S: Squeeze the handles together.
S: Sweep across the *base of the fire*, with a back and forth motion.

After use, the extinguisher must be refilled or replaced.

Key Concept
Remember: Notification is made for any suspected fire or fire-out, including the smell of smoke, the activation of a fire alarm or sprinkler, or the presence of any charred material.

NCLEX Alert
NCLEX situations can require responses to the nurse's responsibility in implementing emergency actions and ensuring client safety. You will need to be aware of common emergency acronyms (e.g., CPR, RACE, PASS, etc.).

TABLE 39-2 Fire Extinguishers and Their Uses

TYPE	SYMBOL	CONTENTS	USE	MEMORY TIP
A	A	Water under pressure	Burning paper, wood, cloth	Burns to **Ash**
B	B	Carbon dioxide	Fires caused by gasoline, oil, paint, grease, and other flammable liquids, chemicals, and other flammable liquids, chemicals, gases, anesthetics	**Boiling** chemicals
C	C	Dry chemicals	Electrical fires	Electric **Current**
ABC	A B C	Graphite	Any type of fire	

STUDENT SYNTHESIS

KEY POINTS

- The safety committee functions in evaluating accidents that occur and in planning to prevent future accidents.
- All clients are evaluated regularly for fall risk.
- Nurses must not only prevent accidents but also know what to do if an accident occurs.
- Staff members must be able to identify potentially hazardous substances and describe what to do if exposed to them.
- A personal emergency preparedness plan will help you to cope personally with the disruption caused by a disaster, allowing you to focus on caring for clients.
- A facility's disaster plan is established to deal with both internal and external emergencies.
- Every staff member in a healthcare facility or community setting must be knowledgeable about fire safety.

CRITICAL THINKING EXERCISES

1. If a fire occurred in your work area, describe the steps you would take to address the situation safely.
2. You arrive at your client's home to change a dressing and find the client in bed, sleeping, and barely holding onto a burning cigarette. Describe how you might handle this situation. What things are important to consider when assessing the home for safety?
3. A large earthquake occurs in the middle of the night. You are at work in the healthcare facility, which sustains damage. What type of disaster is this? How would you handle this situation? What factors are important to consider? How would you handle communications if the phones were out? How would you check on the safety of your family?
4. How might a disaster or emergency affect your ability to provide care in the community or home?

NCLEX-STYLE REVIEW QUESTIONS

1. The nurse reports a small fire in a trash can located in the break room. After obtaining a fire extinguisher, what is the initial action in using the extinguisher?
   a. Sweep across the base of the fire.
   b. Squeeze the handles together.
   c. Aim at the base of the fire, near the edge.
   d. Pull the pin of the fire extinguisher.

2. The smoke alarm sounds on the unit at the long-term care facility. Which acronym will guide the nurse's actions in the situation?
   a. RACE
   b. PASS
   c. CARE
   d. ACRE

3. The nurse is working at the acute care facility and has been informed that there is a bus and multiple vehicle crash with 75 people seriously injured. Which action should the nurse take first?
   a. Perform CPR.
   b. Initiate the disaster plan.
   c. Call everyone in the hospital to help.
   d. Immediately have the provider discharge clients in preparation.

4. The nurse splashes a chemical used for disinfecting surgical instruments on both hands. Which resource will provide information regarding the contents of the chemical?
   a. Disaster plan
   b. Physician's Desk Reference
   c. Safety Data Sheet
   d. Poison control

5. The nurse observes a large amount of smoke and some flames coming from an unoccupied room in the hospital. After calling in the alarm, which action does the nurse take?
   a. Lock all of the doors so people cannot enter rooms.
   b. Open windows to let the smoke out of the room.
   c. Close all doors to confine smoke and fire.
   d. Take the elevator to the lowest floor in the hospital.

CHAPTER RESOURCES

Enhance your learning with additional resources on thePoint*!*

Student Resources related to this chapter can be found at thePoint.lww.com/Rosdahl12e.

40 Introduction to Microbiology

Learning Objectives

1. Define the term *microorganism*; state why an understanding of them is vital for healthcare workers.
2. Identify basic characteristics of the five main types of microorganisms.
3. Name and describe essential factors influencing microbial growth.
4. Describe how culture and sensitivity (C&S) procedures and staining aid in identification and treatment of infectious diseases.
5. Describe classifications of bacteria.
6. Discuss practices used to help prevent development of drug-resistant microorganisms.
7. Describe factors that help determine the virulence of a pathogen.
8. Describe effects of toxins on the body.
9. Explain three basic means by which infectious diseases are transmitted to people.
10. Name the components of the "chain of infection"; suggest ways to stop the spread of infection at each point in the chain.

Important Terminology

aerobe	endotoxin	mycology	spore
anaerobe	epidemic	mycosis	sterile
bacillus	etiology	opportunistic	suppurative/
bacteria	eukaryote	parasite	suppuration
bacteriology	exotoxin	pathogen	toxin
coccus	flagella/flagellum	prodromal	vector
communicable	Gram stain	prokaryote	virology
disease	incubation period	reservoir	virulence
contagious	microbe	saprophyte	virus
culture	microbiology	sensitivity	
endemic	microorganism	spirillum	

Acronyms

ABR	MRSA
AMR	NDM
C&S	pH
CDC	RNA
CRKP	SARS
DNA	TB
EMRSA	VRE
ESBL	
EVD	
HA-MRSA	
HAI	

A **microorganism** or **microbe** is an individual living animal or plant that is so small; it can be seen only with the aid of a microscope. Microorganisms are found literally everywhere in the environment. Most do not cause disease, under normal conditions. Organisms present all or most of the time in and on the body are said to be **endemic**. The scientific study of microorganisms is **microbiology**. For purposes of this chapter, selected algae, fungi, and protozoa, as well as bacteria and viruses, will be discussed.

Billions of species of microorganisms exist. Most, such as those adding flavor and character to cheeses and yogurt or fermenting beer, are beneficial. Microorganisms also help revitalize the soil by decomposition of animal and plant wastes. However, some microorganisms cause disease. In the study of nursing, many of these harmful microorganisms are discussed. Disease-producing agents, the **pathogens**, are the focus of this chapter. This chapter is an introduction to basic facts about microorganisms (their characteristics, capacity for harm, and growth). Each of these topics in microbiology is a separate course of detailed study and is beyond the scope of this book. In many cases, the category of microbes called *bacteria* will be used to illustrate a point that may apply to other microbes as well.

Improvements in microscopic technology have facilitated new discoveries regarding microorganisms, both pathogenic and nonpathogenic. The study of pathogens allows scientists to improve the identification, treatment, and prevention of disease transmission. As a result, means to facilitate delivery of safer healthcare have been developed. You, as a nurse, are responsible for taking steps to prevent disease transmission. This chapter discusses types and characteristics of pathogenic organisms, methods of studying them, and the chain of infectious disease transmission. Emphasis is on breaking this chain of transmission, thus preventing the spread of infection.

MICROORGANISMS

Microorganisms possess many characteristics of larger cells. In most microorganisms, these characteristics include the following:

- Metabolism—ability to utilize nutrients
- Reproduction—ability to group together to form colonies or of individual cells to become larger
- Irritability—response to the environment
- Motion—ability to move from place to place
- Protection—including spores, mutation, and development of drug-resistant strains

These topics are discussed throughout this chapter.

METABOLISM AND GROWTH

Microorganisms are said to "grow" when the number at an individual site increases. At the beginning of a bacterial infection, a group of bacterial cells may number only a few hundred. As the bacteria reproduce, they form groups of many millions of individual cells, collectively called *colonies*. Certain environmental factors affect the metabolism of microorganisms.

Oxygen

Most microorganisms require oxygen for growth; these are called *obligate* aerobes. Some, called *obligate* anaerobes, cannot survive in the presence of oxygen. Other microorganisms can live in either the *presence or absence of oxygen* (*facultative anaerobes*). Some bacilli are divided into those that use oxygen to metabolize sugars (*oxidizers*) and those that metabolize sugars in the absence of oxygen (*fermenters*).

Nutrients

A key ingredient for microbial growth is the presence of organic (carbon-containing) nutrients. Microorganisms also require other chemical elements, such as nitrogen for the manufacture of protein and sulfur for protein and vitamin synthesis. Some microorganisms make their own food from raw materials, such as carbon dioxide. Others must find their nutrition ready-made.

Parasites are microorganisms that live on or within another living being (the host). Saprophytes live off the organic remains of dead plants and animals.

Temperature

The temperature at which a specific microorganism grows best is its *optimal temperature*. Most pathogenic microorganisms flourish at normal body temperature. Some types of microorganisms prefer either extremely cold or hot environments. Cold temperatures often significantly slow the growth of microorganisms, the reason refrigeration is used to control bacterial growth in food. High temperatures usually kill most microorganisms. Steam sterilization and boiling water are two common techniques used to kill pathogenic microorganisms.

Moisture

All microorganisms require water or moisture to grow. The matter in or on which they grow must contain available moisture (e.g., jellies) or may be liquid (e.g., milk or blood).

pH

A substance's pH (hydrogen ion concentration; *acidity or alkalinity*) also affects growth. Generally, microorganisms survive only in environments with a pH that is neither too acidic nor too alkaline (Chapter 17).

Light

Some microorganisms need light for growth. Other microorganisms, however, flourish in darkness. Many microorganisms die when exposed to the sun's ultraviolet rays, although moderately diffused light does not affect them.

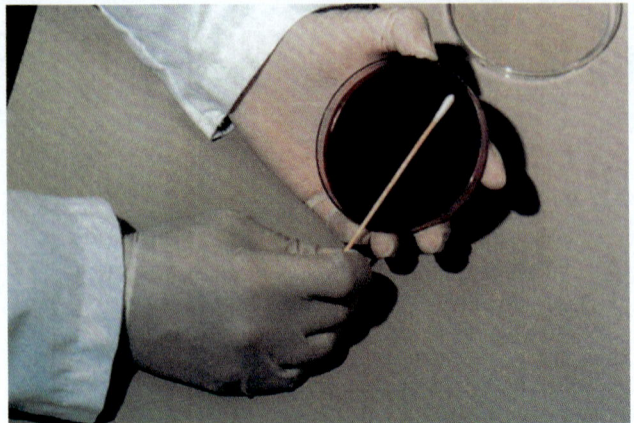

Figure 40-1 Inoculating a sterile agar plate (Petri dish) with a small amount of material from a client's infected wound. This *culture* will be used to determine the causative organism, as well as which antibiotics will kill or arrest the growth of the organism (*sensitivity*), a *culture and sensitivity* (C&S) test. (Molle, E. A., & Kronenberger, J. [2005]. *Comprehensive medical assisting* [2nd ed.]. Lippincott Williams & Wilkins.)

Cultures of Organisms

Microbiologists can grow microbes under controlled conditions in the laboratory in order to study them. These cultures are used to identify the organism and, in the case of a pathogen, to then determine ways in which to arrest its growth. Cultures are usually grown in test tubes or on small, flat, covered plastic plates called *Petri dishes*. The material in or on which the microorganisms are placed is the *culture medium*. Various types of culture media (plural) serve different purposes. Solid media contain *agar*, which is obtained from a form of seaweed. Liquid media are called *nutrient broths*. All culture media contain specific nutrients designed to promote the growth of one or more types of microorganisms. Culture media must start out sterile (free from microbial contamination) for a valid study (Fig. 40-1).

To see and study individual characteristics of microorganisms grown in cultures, a small amount of material to be examined is placed on a clean rectangular piece of glass, a *slide*, which is prepared for observation of the microorganisms. Here, the microorganisms can be viewed in their living, moving state in a drop of liquid culture. Identifying a specific disease-causing microorganism is important in disease treatment. After a pathogenic microorganism is *cultured* (grown), a *sensitivity* test is ordered. This culture and sensitivity (C&S) test serves the following purposes:

- Identifies the pathogenic microorganism (culture)
- Determines which treatment will eliminate the microorganism (sensitivity)
- Monitors the microorganism's response to the treatment

The C&S report will indicate the type of specimen (e.g., blood, urine, sputum), type of report (preliminary [within 24 hr] or final [usually within 48 hr]), colony count, type of microorganism (may be several), and susceptibility (sensitivity) testing. The report will indicate the antibiotics (if any) to which the organism is sensitive. It is important that specimens for culture be collected before antibiotic therapy is initiated. Antibiotics can reduce the number of pathogens in the person's bloodstream, masking signs of infection and making the culture inaccurate. Chapter 52 describes methods of specimen collection.

Types

Microorganisms, like all living creatures, are categorized based on a variety of physical and biologic characteristics. There are several main levels (taxa) of identification or *taxonomy*; these are the kingdom, phylum, class, order, family, genus, and species. The two used in bacteriology are genus and species. The *genus* refers to the general grouping; the *species* defines a biologically unique category. For example, the common bacterium, *Escherichia coli* (*E. coli*) is found in the colon. (*Escherichia* denotes a family of gram-negative, rod-shaped, facultative anaerobes; *coli* denotes the colon.) Microorganisms fall into a number of large groups: these include some algae and fungi, as well as protozoa, bacteria, and viruses.

Organisms with a true nucleus enclosed by a nuclear membrane and containing chromosomes that divide by mitosis are called **eukaryotes**. Their cells also contain structures such as mitochondria, lysosomes, and the Golgi apparatus. Plants, animals, protozoa, fungi, and most algae are eukaryotes. (Other organisms, such as bacteria, are *prokaryotes*.)

Algae

The many types of algae resemble plant cells. Algae are often found on sunlit water, appearing as green scum or green cloudy water. They are an important part of the environmental food chain and rarely cause human disease.

Fungi

Fungi include single-celled yeasts and multicellular molds. They are not in the same cellular domain as bacteria and are considered *eukaryotes*. An infection caused by a fungus is called a **mycosis**. Common *mycoses* (plural) include types of tinea ("ringworm," causing ring-shaped lesions). One type of ringworm, *tinea capitis*, causes a lesion of the scalp; another, *tinea pedis*, causes "athlete's foot." **Mycology** is the study of fungi.

Yeasts

Yeast cells reproduce by a process called *budding*. Each parent cell produces a "daughter cell" or bud that eventually breaks off and grows in the same manner as the parent cell. Yeasts require sugars in solution as their food. When yeasts metabolize sugars in the absence of oxygen (anaerobic), a chemical change, *fermentation*, occurs, producing alcohol and carbon dioxide. Controlled fermentation is used to manufacture products such as beer and bread.

An example of a pathogenic yeast is *Candida albicans*, which causes *thrush*, a white growth in a person's mouth and on the tongue (Fig. 40-2). *C. albicans* also causes approximately one third of cases of vaginitis ("vaginal yeast infection").

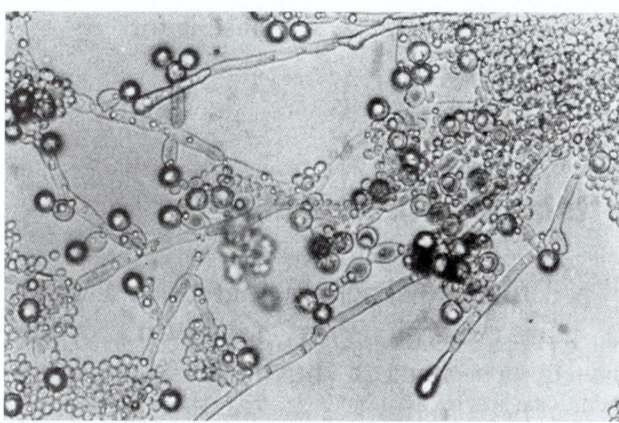

Figure 40-2 The pathogenic fungus *Candida albicans*, which causes thrush and a specific type of vaginitis (inflammation of the vagina). (Molle, E. A., & Kronenberger, J. [2005]. *Comprehensive medical assisting* [2nd ed.]. Lippincott Williams & Wilkins.)

Molds

Multicellular molds are common in the environment. Some familiar molds appear as fuzzy patches on jelly, greenish growth on spoiled breads, and blue veins in some cheeses. Many molds grow best at room temperature or with some cooling and have a characteristic musty smell. They send threads or branches, *hyphae*, throughout the material on or in which they grow. Some hyphae extend beyond the surface of the host material and, when mature, produce rounded capsules, containing spores, at their tips. **Spores** give molds their characteristic colors. The slightest air current wafts spores about; when they find a suitable surface, they attach themselves and reproduce to form another colony.

Infections caused by molds include *coccidioidomycosis* ("desert fever," common in hot, dry regions, such as the American Southwest) and *histoplasmosis*, which affects the lungs. A more virulent form may spread throughout the body.

Protozoa

Protozoa are single-celled microorganisms visible under an ordinary laboratory microscope. As with fungi, protozoa are not in the same cellular domain as bacteria, but are eukaryotes. Two common protozoa are the ameba and paramecium. Protozoa are able to take in nutrients and excrete wastes, reproduce sexually, and generally live in a moisture-rich environment. Some protozoa capture and engulf their food and even feed on bacteria.

Although most protozoa are nonpathogenic, there are some notable exceptions. Amebic dysentery is caused by *Entamoeba histolytica*, which forms ulcers in the colon and attacks red blood cells. This ameba produces a capsule (cyst) to protect itself and then infects people through their contact with contaminated food or water. Malaria is caused by one or more species of the protozoan genus, the most common of which is *Plasmodium malariae*. It reproduces in the *Anopheles* mosquito and is transmitted to people through bites. It can also be spread from monkeys to humans. Malaria causes thousands of deaths each year and the incidence is increasing, partially because of resistant strains of the organism. *Trichomonas vaginalis* ("trik") causes vaginal infection in women and urinary tract infection in men. It is commonly transmitted by sexual intercourse.

Bacteria/Prokaryotes

Many microbes studied in relation to illness are scientifically categorized as **prokaryotes**. The term *prokaryote*, any member of the kingdom Monera, includes bacteria and blue-green bacteria (formerly known as blue-green algae). Prokaryotes are the most abundant form of life on the planet and were the first cells to appear on earth, approximately 4 billion years ago. About 3,000 species of prokaryotes have been discovered, but it is believed that many thousands of additional species exist.

Prokaryotes are divided into two distinct categories: the *archaea* and the **bacteria**. Bacteria are primarily *unicellular* (containing one distinct cell), although certain other forms do exist. The study of bacteria is **bacteriology**. Much of the remainder of this chapter focuses on bacteria, particularly those that cause disease.

Prokaryotes have specific characteristics, distinguishing them from eukaryotes. In all prokaryotes, except the genus *mycoplasma*, there is a rigid cell wall, but no true nucleus; the DNA is unbound. (This is unlike the human cells studied in Chapter 15 and the protozoa presented in this chapter, both of which are *eukaryotes*.) Some prokaryotic cells appear in groups, but each cell is identical and can exist independently; there is no specific communication between them. Prokaryotes can live in environments in which eukaryotes cannot live. Prokaryotes that can live at very cold temperatures are *psychrophiles*; at room temperature or body temperature *mesophiles*; and at a very high-temperature *thermophiles*. They all need water in its liquid form but can live in very dry conditions. These factors add to the disease-producing potential of these organisms.

Prokaryotes are very diverse and can perform some forms of metabolism rare in eukaryotes. For example, prokaryotes assist in nitrogen fixation, the production of nitrogen gas and ammonia. They also assist in photosynthesis, which produces carbohydrate and adds oxygen to the environment.

> **Key Concept**
>
> Eukaryotes: plants, animals, fungi, protozoa, and most algae. Cells of these organisms have a true nucleus enclosed within a cell membrane, with chromosomes that divide by mitosis.
>
> Prokaryotes: archaea and bacteria. Each cell is individual. The DNA is unbound; there is no nuclear membrane.

Structure and Function

The structure of prokaryotes will be discussed in terms of the bacteria. Many specific characteristics assist pathogenic bacteria to cause disease.

Prokaryotes are very small and consist of three architectural regions:

- Cell envelope (capsule, cell wall, and plasma membrane)
- Appendages (flagella and pili)
- Cytoplasmic region (containing the cell genome—DNA, ribosomes, and various inclusions)

Cell Envelope

Prokaryotes have a continuous cell wall that protects the cell from lysis by osmosis (Chapter 17).

- *Capsule:* Most bacteria have a polysaccharide layer outside the cell envelope (or outer membrane) known as the *capsule* or *glycocalyx*. The capsule or "slime layer" can help bacterial cells attach to surfaces. The capsules also protect bacteria from engulfment by white blood cells—phagocytes (the body's protective cells)—and from attack by antimicrobial agents (used to kill microbes). These characteristics allow pathogenic bacteria to cause disease.
- *Surface components:* The surface components of the bacterial cell help to "sense" the surrounding environment. They provide a selective permeability barrier, adhesive qualities, enzymes (to mediate various reactions), and sensing proteins (to respond to environmental conditions, such as light, oxygen, temperature, and pH).
- *Cell wall and staining:* The cell envelope of the organism is the structure that either allows a stain (the **Gram stain**) to be retained or not. In *gram-positive* bacteria, the cell envelope is a thick layer of murein, and it retains the stain, turning purple.
- In *gram-negative* bacteria, the murein layer is thin and is surrounded by an outer membrane. In this case, the stain is not retained, and the organism looks light pink. (The primary means by which microbes in the archaea category are distinguished from those in the bacteria category is the absence of murein in the archaea.) The cell envelope of a gram-negative organism also contains a substance called lipopolysaccharide (LPS), or endotoxin, which is toxic to animals.
- *Plasma membrane:* Although they do not have specific structures for this, many species can perform specialized functions in their plasma membrane. These functions include synthesis of substances such as adenosine triphosphate (ATP), which provides energy to the organism. The plasma membrane also serves as a permeability barrier, selectively allowing only certain materials to pass into or out of the cell (Chapter 17).

Surface Projections/Appendages

Flagella

Flagella (singular: flagellum) are fairly long protein filaments on the cell surface. They provide the cell with the ability to move by a "swimming" motion, *motility*, or spontaneous movement (Fig. 40-3). The flagella of bacteria are powered by a different source than the flagella of eukaryotic cells. The distribution patterns of flagella are illustrated in Figure 40-3. The attachment of flagella at one or both ends of the organism is called *polar distribution*. If the flagella are distributed over the entire surface of the organism, this is *peritrichous distribution*. The distribution of flagella is one means used to differentiate between types of bacteria.

- *Tactic behavior:* Prokaryotes demonstrate specific *tactic* behavior. They can swim in response to specific environmental stimuli. For example, they can move toward or away from light (*phototaxis*); in response to oxygen (*aerotaxis*); or to a magnetic field (*magnetotaxis*). *Chemotaxis* refers to the ability to swim to a useful food source or nutrient or to swim away from harmful substances.

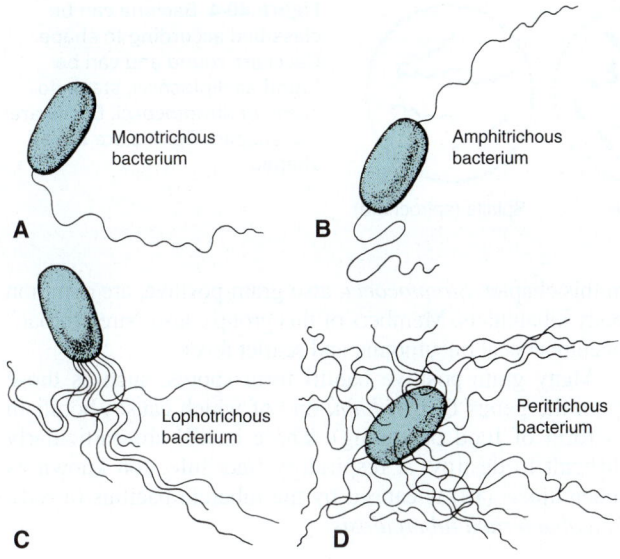

Figure 40-3 Four basic types of flagella on bacteria: **(A)** one flagellum at one end; **(B)** one flagellum at each end; **(C)** a tuft of flagella at one end; and **(D)** flagella spread over the entire surface. (Adapted from Burton, G. R. W., & Engelkirk, P. G. [1999]. *Microbiology for the health sciences* [6th ed.]. Lippincott Williams & Wilkins.)

Fimbriae/common pili: Pili are short, hairlike projections on the surface of the cell consisting of protein. They are shorter and stiffer and of smaller diameter than flagella. The "sex pili" mediate the transfer of DNA between mating bacteria. The more numerous common pili, usually called *fimbriae*, provide adherence to the surface of the cell. This is a major factor in bacterial virulence, which allows pathogens to attach to body tissues and colonize into groups. It also allows bacteria to resist attack by the body's defensive white blood cells (phagocytes).

Cytoplasm

Chromosomes (DNA): Bacterial cells contain a large, naked, double-stranded, round module of **DNA** (genetic material) floating free within the cytoplasm. The cells may also contain pieces of DNA called *plasmids*. The total of all DNA is called the *genome*. Bacterial cells do not undergo meiosis or mitosis as do eukaryotic cells; replication and segregation into two identical cells are coordinated by the cell membrane.

Ribosomes: Ribosomes are involved in protein synthesis (in a different way than in eukaryotes); they give the granular appearance to cytoplasm.

Inclusions: Inclusions are usually materials being reserved for future use by the organism, such as glycogen or fats.

Classification of Bacteria by Shape

As stated, bacteria can be identified by their flagella, how they move, Gram stain reaction, and their relationship to oxygen. In addition, bacteria are identified by their shape. Most bacteria fall into one of three categories based on shape (Figs. 40-4 and 40-5). A round or spherical bacterium is a **coccus** (plural: cocci); rod shaped, a **bacillus** (plural: bacilli); and spiral shaped, a **spirillum** (plural: spirilla or spirochete).

The cells of cocci do not always separate when they reproduce. Sometimes, they form pairs (*diplococci*), clusters (*staphylococci*), or chains (*streptococci*). Likewise, *diplobacilli* are paired bacilli and *streptobacilli* are chains of bacilli. Bacilli may have tapered ends (*fusiform* bacilli) or may be shaped like long threads (*filamentous* bacilli).

> **Key Concept**
>
> Bacteria may be classified according to their flagella, motility, Gram stain result, and relationship to oxygen, as well as their shape.

Reproduction and Survival

Unlike eukaryotes, such as protozoa, bacteria do not reproduce by binary fission. In bacterial cell division, genetic material is duplicated and distributed loosely to "daughter" cells, a process (*genetic recombination*) coordinated by the cellular membrane.

There are three means by which bacteria exchange genetic material:

- *Conjugation*—DNA crosses a sex pilus to the new cell by cell-to-cell contact.
- *Transduction*—genes are transferred by a virus.
- *Transformation*—DNA is acquired from the environment after being released by another cell.

The implication for disease control relates to the fact that bacteria usually develop genes for drug resistance (*resistance transfer factors* [RTF]) on structures called *plasmids*. The plasmids are often the vehicle for cell-to-cell DNA transfer and are able to pass drug resistance to other duplicate cells, other strains of bacteria, and even to other species during the exchange process.

Protective *spores* are formed by certain bacteria. Examples are *Clostridium tetani*, which causes tetanus, and *Bacillus anthracis*, which causes anthrax. When conditions are unfavorable to their survival or growth, spore-forming bacilli develop a protective covering (spore) and go into a nonactive (dormant) phase. The spore is resistant to the environment and can survive extreme conditions of light, drying, boiling, and many chemicals. When more favorable conditions return, the spore germinates and the bacteria cell reactivates. Spore-forming bacteria are the most difficult bacteria to control and destroy. All pathogenic bacteria die at water's boiling point (100 °C or 212 °F) *except the sporeformers*.

Common Pathogenic Bacteria

Many bacteria are able to cause disease (*pathogenicity*). To be pathogenic, bacteria must possess the following characteristics:

- Ability to colonize and invade the host
- Ability to resist or endure the antibacterial defenses of the host
- Ability to form substances that are toxic to the host

Table 40-1 lists important pathogenic bacteria.

Neisseria are diplococci and cause gonorrhea, upper respiratory infections, and infectious meningitis. The bacillus *Pseudomonas* is responsible for **suppurative** (pus-forming)

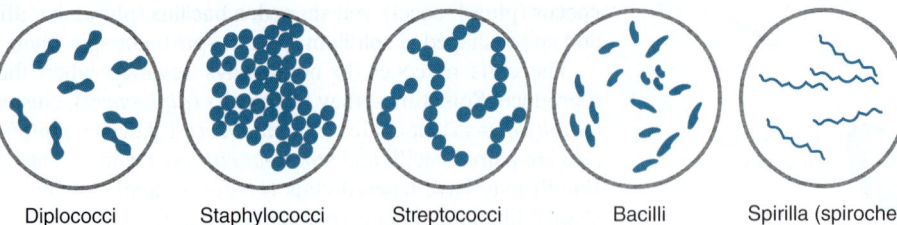

Figure 40-4 Bacteria can be classified according to shape. Cocci are round and can be found as diplococci, staphylococci, or streptococci. Bacilli are rod shaped. Spirilla are spiral shaped.

infections. Bacteria from the genus *Legionella* cause the infamous, pneumonia-like Legionnaires disease (legionellosis).

Rickettsiae are a special form of bacteria. Some are bacilli; others are cocci. They can grow only within the cell of a host organism. Rickettsiae are transmitted to people through the bite of an infected insect or tick, resulting in infections ranging from mild to fatal. One form of rickettsiae causes Rocky Mountain spotted fever. Members of the typhus group cause epidemic and endemic typhus.

Staphylococci are gram-positive bacteria always present in the environment; they are normal inhabitants of the skin and respiratory tract. *Staphylococcus aureus* is the most dangerous of this group; it produces poisons (*toxins*) and frequently resists antibiotics. The antibiotic-resistant form is *methicillin-resistant Staphylococcus aureus* (**MRSA**) and is discussed later in this chapter. *Streptococci*, also gram-positive, are common body inhabitants. Members of this group cause "strep throat," pneumococcal pneumonia, and scarlet fever.

Many gram-positive bacilli form spores, such as those from the genus *Clostridium*, one of which causes botulism (a form of food poisoning). These bacilli are particularly difficult to destroy. A respiratory tract infection known as tuberculosis (**TB**) is caused by the tubercle bacillus (a rod), *Mycobacterium tuberculosis*.

Viruses

Although scientists long suspected the existence of microorganisms smaller than bacteria, it was not until 1935 that the first **virus** was discovered. Since then, advances in electron and x-ray microscopy and biochemical technology

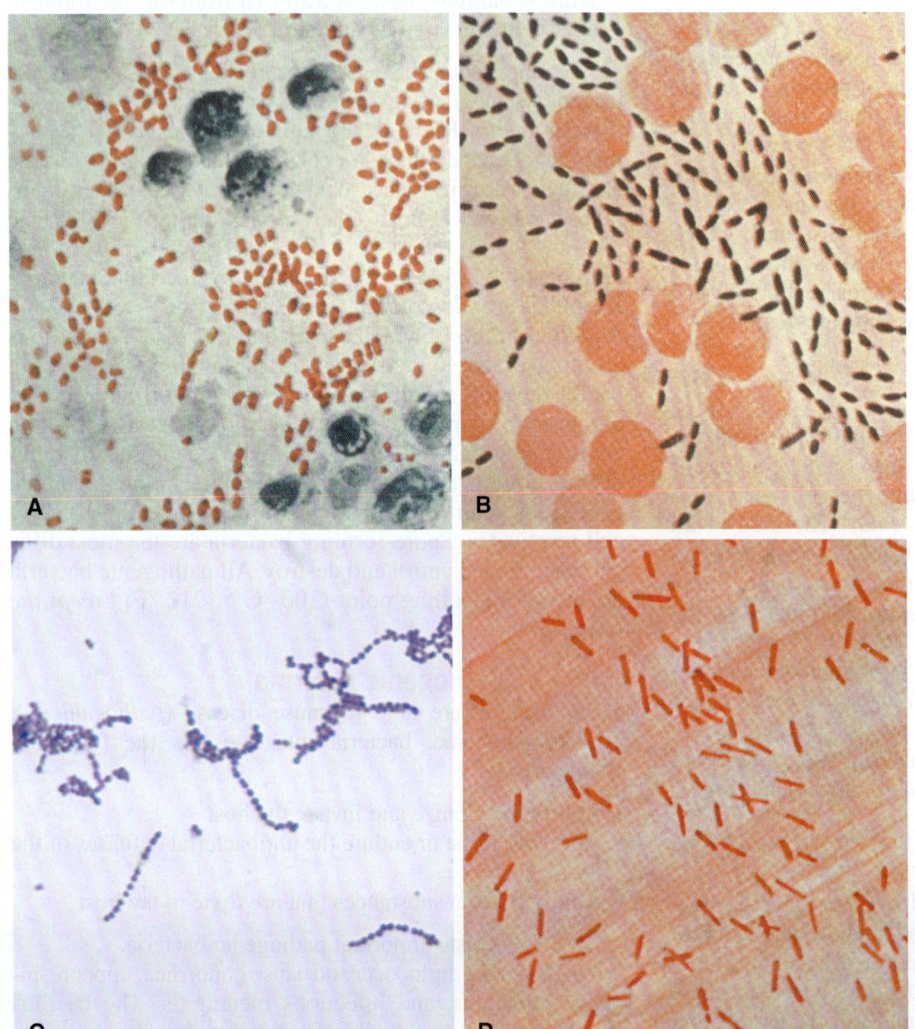

Figure 40-5 A sampling of microscopic bacteria demonstrating a variety of shapes and sizes: **(A)** bacilli known as *Vibrio cholerae*, which causes cholera; **(B)** diplococci known as *Streptococci pneumoniae*, which causes pneumonia; **(C)** diplococci identified with Gram stain; and (D) bacilli known as *Escherichia coli*. (From Public Images Library, Centers for Disease Control and Prevention. Available at: http://phil.cdc.gov.)

TABLE 40-1 Some Important Pathogenic Bacteria

BACTERIUM	DISEASES	TYPE	GRAM STAIN REACTION[a]
Bacillus anthracis	Anthrax	Spore-forming rod	+
Bordetella pertussis	Whooping cough	Rod	−
Borrelia burgdorferi	Lyme disease	Spirochete	−
Brucella abortus and Brucella melitensis	Brucellosis, undulant fever	Rod	−
Chlamydia trachomatis	Lymphogranuloma venereum, trachoma	Coccoid	−
Clostridium botulinum	Botulism (food poisoning), also produces the toxin Botox	Spore-forming rod	+
Clostridium difficile	Enterocolitis, especially in persons receiving antibiotics (developing resistance to antibiotics-VRE)	Spore-forming anaerobic bacteria	+
Clostridium perfringens	Gas gangrene, wound infections	Spore-forming rod	+
Clostridium tetani	Tetanus (lockjaw)	Spore-forming rod	+
Corynebacterium diphtheriae	Diphtheria	Rod	+
Escherichia coli	Urinary tract infections	Rod	−
Francisella tularensis	Tularemia	Rod	−
Haemophilus ducreyi	Chancroid	Rod	−
Haemophilus influenzae	Meningitis, pneumonia	Rod	−
Klebsiella pneumoniae	Pneumonia	Rod	−
Mycobacterium leprae	Leprosy	Rod	±
Mycobacterium tuberculosis	Tuberculosis	Rod	±
Neisseria gonorrhoeae	Gonorrhea	Diplococcus	−
Neisseria meningitidis	Nasopharyngitis, meningitis	Diplococcus	−
Proteus vulgaris and P. morgani	Gastroenteritis, urinary tract infections	Rod	−
Pseudomonas aeruginosa	Respiratory and urogenital infections	Rod	−
Rickettsia rickettsii	Rocky Mountain spotted fever	Rod	−
Salmonella typhi	Typhoid fever	Rod	−
Salmonella species	Gastroenteritis	Rod	−
Shigella species	Shigellosis (bacillary dysentery)	Rod	−
Staphylococcus aureus	Boils, carbuncles, pneumonia, septicemia	Cocci in clusters	+
Streptococcus pyogenes	Strep throat, scarlet fever, rheumatic fever, septicemia	Cocci in chains	+
Streptococcus pneumoniae	Pneumonia	Diplococcus	+
Treponema pallidum	Syphilis	Spirochete	−
Vibrio cholerae	Cholera	Curved rod	−
Yersinia pestis	Plague	Rod	−

[a]+, gram positive; −, gram negative; ±, gram variable.
From Fader, R., Engelkirk, P., & Duben-Engelkirk, J. (2019). *Burton's microbiology for the health sciences* (11th ed.). Wolters Kluwer.

have provided a clearer picture of these elusive structures. Scientists are now able to culture specific viruses, which they can maintain in the laboratory indefinitely. The study of viruses and related diseases is **virology**.

Viruses are protein-covered sacs containing genetic material of either DNA or ribonucleic acid (**RNA**) and other organic materials. They lack most characteristics of living organisms. However, when a virus enters the cell of a living organism, the virus's nuclear material is activated and the host cell becomes a culture medium for viral reproduction. A virus must use the host's ability to make protein and energy because the virus itself lacks the capacity to carry on metabolism.

Viruses cause a wide range of diseases. Table 40-2 summarizes common pathogenic viruses, most of which cannot be easily controlled or destroyed. Immunization is the

TABLE 40-2 Common Pathogenic Viruses

DISORDER GROUP	NAME	COMMON DISORDERS CAUSED	COMMENTS
Internal disorder producers	Picornavirus (enteric group)		
	Poliovirus	Poliomyelitis	At least three types
			Vaccine available
	Echovirus	ECHO syndrome (*e*nteric *c*ytopathogenic *h*uman *o*rphan), aseptic meningitis, diarrhea neonatorum, paralytic disease	At least 30 types
			No vaccine
	Picornavirus (rhinovirus group)	Common cold, upper respiratory infections	No vaccine
	Coxsackievirus	Aseptic meningitis, myocarditis, pericarditis	At least 30 types
			No vaccine
Rash producers	Poxvirus	Smallpox	Possibly eradicated in the United States; may be used as a bioterrorism weapon
			Vaccine available
	Rubella virus	German measles (rubella)	Can cause birth defects
			Vaccine available
	Rubeola virus	"Red" measles (rubeola), encephalomyelitis	No vaccine
	Erythema infectiosum	"Fifth" disease	Vaccine available
	Varicella zoster (herpes zoster)	Chickenpox (varicella), shingles (herpes zoster)	
	Herpes simplex virus	Cold sores (herpes simplex)	No vaccine
	Herpes simplex virus type II	Herpes labialis (genital herpes), encephalitis, vulvovaginitis	Two types
			No vaccine
	Roseola infantum virus	Roseola infantum ("rose rash," exanthem subitum)	
Genital warts	Condylomata acuminata	Human papillomavirus (HPV) infection	Vaccine available
Respiratory disorder producers	Influenza virus (myxovirus types A, B, C)	Influenza ("flu," grippe), croup, pneumonia	Three types
			Vaccine available (moderate effectiveness)
	Mumps virus (paramyxovirus)	Parotitis (mumps), orchitis (inflammation of testes), meningoencephalitis	Vaccine available
	Infectious mononucleosis virus (Epstein–Barr virus)	Infectious "mono"	No vaccine
	Adenovirus	Conjunctivitis	

TABLE 40-2	Common Pathogenic Viruses	(Continued)	
DISORDER GROUP	NAME	COMMON DISORDERS CAUSED	COMMENTS
Chronic (latent) disorder producers	Hepatitis		
	Type A	Type A hepatitis (formerly called infectious hepatitis)	Vaccine available
	Type B ("Dane particle")	Type B hepatitis (formerly called serum hepatitis)	Vaccine available
	Type C (non-A, non-B)	Type C hepatitis (parenterally transmitted)	No vaccine
	Type D	Type D hepatitis (can be coinfection with type B)	
	Type E	Type E (transmitted by fecal–oral route)	
	Papovavirus	Warts (verrucae)	
	Arbovirus		
	Group A	Equine encephalitis	Vaccine possible
	Group B	Yellow fever	Vaccine possible
	Diplovirus	Colorado tick fever	No vaccine
	Rabies virus (rhabdovirus)	Rabies (hydrophobia)	Vaccine available
Autoimmune disorder producers	Human immunodeficiency virus (HIV)	Opportunistic infections, such as *Pneumocystis* pneumonia and Kaposi sarcoma. Can develop into full-blown acquired immunodeficiency syndrome (AIDS)	Virus has been identified. No vaccine available. Transmitted via body fluids, especially blood and semen

most effective means of preventing viral infections, such as measles and polio. In 2015, an outbreak of measles at Disneyland emphasized the need for immunizations. Viruses affect every system and tissue of the body. A well-known virus, the human immunodeficiency virus (HIV), causes acquired immunodeficiency syndrome (AIDS).

An outbreak of *Ebola hemorrhagic fever* in West Africa caused worldwide concern, although the virus was originally discovered in 1976. This virus, Filoviridae, genus *Ebolavirus*, includes several species, most named for their region of origin (e.g., Zaire, Sudan, Taï Forest). Ebolavirus disease (**EVD**) causes high fever, severe headache, muscle pain and weakness, diarrhea and vomiting, and unexplained hemorrhage and may be fatal. A vaccine is not yet available. Special isolation procedures are used to care for these clients (CDC, 2015b).

Antimicrobial-Resistant Microorganisms

Effective antimicrobial drug therapy normally destroys or significantly reduces the number of pathogenic microorganisms. Specific medications target them and allow the body's natural defenses to take over and eliminate them. However, certain microorganisms, including bacteria, viruses, fungi, and parasites, are able to evolve into strains resistant to existing medications (**ABR**-antibiotic resistant; or more general, **AMR**-antimicrobial resistant). The development of these microorganisms occurs most often if antimicrobial therapy is unnecessary or incomplete, allowing some pathogens to survive. These microorganisms then are able to transfer their resistance to future generations, rendering future antimicrobial therapy ineffective. AMR microorganisms continue to develop. Individuals at greatest risk are people with *compromised* immune systems, whose bodies are unable to fight off infections and destroy AMR pathogens. To help prevent development of drug-resistant microorganisms, several procedures should be in place for nurses and clients:

- Take antimicrobial drugs only as prescribed and only if absolutely necessary, not for mild infections.
- Take antimicrobial drugs for the entire period prescribed, even if symptoms of illness disappear.
- Do not share these drugs with others or take "leftover medications."
- Do not use antibiotics for viral infections.

> **NCLEX Alert**
>
> Factors leading to development of antimicrobial-resistant microorganisms may be included in the examination. You may be required to know which medications are being considered, topics regarding client and family teaching, use of personal protective equipment, or methods of wound care.

S. aureus is an organism normally found on the skin of all people; it is not normally pathogenic. However, in certain situations, it is considered **opportunistic** and becomes pathogenic. That is, it will cause illness in a person with a compromised immune system or open wound. (The organism is "pathogenic" only to that person.) In addition, this organism produces a substance called β-lactamase, which degrades penicillin-type medications. MRSA is known as "golden staph" and has become resistant to many antibiotics, including methicillin, as well as more common antibiotics, such as penicillin, amoxicillin, ampicillin, erythromycin, and ciprofloxacin. "Staph" infections, including MRSA, occur most frequently in healthcare facilities, thus the name **HA-MRSA** (hospital or healthcare-acquired MRSA). *The major route of MRSA transmission is via contaminated hands of healthcare workers.* (People with MRSA who have not been hospitalized or who have not had an invasive medical procedure within the past year are said to have *CA-MRSA* [community-associated or acquired MRSA].)

MRSA can be responsible for serious or fatal infections in newborns and postsurgical clients and can also cause food poisoning. Most cases involve skin or soft tissue infections, such as an abscess or cellulitis. This client is isolated and personnel follow special procedures (Chapters 41 and 42). An outbreak of "staph" in a healthcare facility is so serious that healthcare facilities are usually required to report outbreaks.

> **Key Concept**
>
> The most important factor in preventing the spread of MRSA and other healthcare-associated infections is careful handwashing. Other means are also used, such as wearing gloves and, in some cases, isolation (Chapter 42). Wash or sanitize your hands often.

Risk factors for clients in healthcare facilities include the following:

- A compromised immune system due to conditions/situations such as AIDS, cancer, aplastic anemia, chemotherapy, radiation, and injection of or overproduction of corticosteroids (Cushing disease)
- A break in the skin following situations such as surgery or a burn
- Presence of a central or peripheral intravenous catheter
- Invasive medical procedures, such as urinary catheterization, dialysis, tracheostomy, or colonoscopy
- Serious underlying disorders, such as chronic kidney disease, diabetes, peripheral vascular disease, and dermatitis or other skin lesions
- Previous exposure to antimicrobial drugs, reducing the body's normal flora, giving the opportunistic organism an advantage
- Repeated hospitalizations, thus increasing exposure
- Very old or very young age, increasing vulnerability
- Previous infections by multi–drug-resistant organisms

Organisms and situation that cause healthcare-associated infections include the following:

- MRSA—methicillin-resistant *S. aureus* ("golden staph"), HA-MRSA, and **EMRSA** (epidemic MRSA)
- **VRE**—vancomycin-resistant enterococci (e.g., *Clostridium difficile*, also known as *C. difficile*)
- PRSP—penicillin-resistant *Streptococcus pneumoniae*, which causes pneumonia, often in older people
- The virus causing **SARS**—severe acute respiratory syndrome, believed to be a strain of *coronavirus*
- **ESBLs**—extended-spectrum β-lactamases (resistant to cephalosporins)
- **NDM**—*New Delhi metallo-beta-lactamase* is made by gram-negative organisms, such as *E. coli* and *Klebsiella pneumoniae*, and renders bacteria resistant to many antibiotics of the carbapenem family (often used to treat antibiotic-resistant bacterial infections)
- **CRKP**—carbapenem-resistant *K. pneumoniae*, normally present in the GI system but can lead to infections, such as pneumonia, in older adult or debilitated clients, particularly those receiving treatments with invasive devices, such as ventilators or central venous catheters

Prevention of transmission of NDM organisms and CRKP is especially important because of their extensive drug resistance. Healthcare-associated infections (**HAI**) are a serious concern in today's healthcare. HA-MRSA and VRE are today's most prevalent HAIs (both are antimicrobial resistant).

INFECTIOUS DISEASE

An *infection* is a condition in which pathogens invade the body. Diseases caused by pathogenic microorganisms are *infectious diseases*. The pathogens increase in number and produce symptoms of illness. The term **etiology** describes specific causes of disease. Many diseases caused by microorganisms are **communicable**; they can spread from person to person. **Contagious** diseases are communicable diseases transmitted to many individuals quickly and easily. When a large number of people in the same area are infected in a relatively short time, the disease is said to be **epidemic** (such as the Ebola outbreak in West Africa).

Chain of Infection

Communicable diseases spread easily. Scientists and healthcare workers use knowledge gained in *epidemiology* (the study of disease transmission) to develop methods for preventing the spread of microbial infections. The Centers for Disease Control and Prevention (**CDC**) in Atlanta, Georgia, is dedicated to the study of pathogens and communicable disease control. Diseases will spread if the *chain of infection* is unbroken (Fig. 40-6). The chain of infection contains the following elements:

- *Causative agent* (pathogenic microorganisms)
- *Reservoir* in which pathogenic microorganisms can live and grow
- *Portal of exit* from which microorganisms can leave the reservoir
- *Vehicle* to transmit organisms
- *Portal of entry* through which microorganisms can enter a host
- *Susceptible host* in which microorganisms can find a new reservoir

Some of these elements are controllable and some are not. The following sections discuss each component of the chain of infection and measures that can be taken at each stage to break the chain.

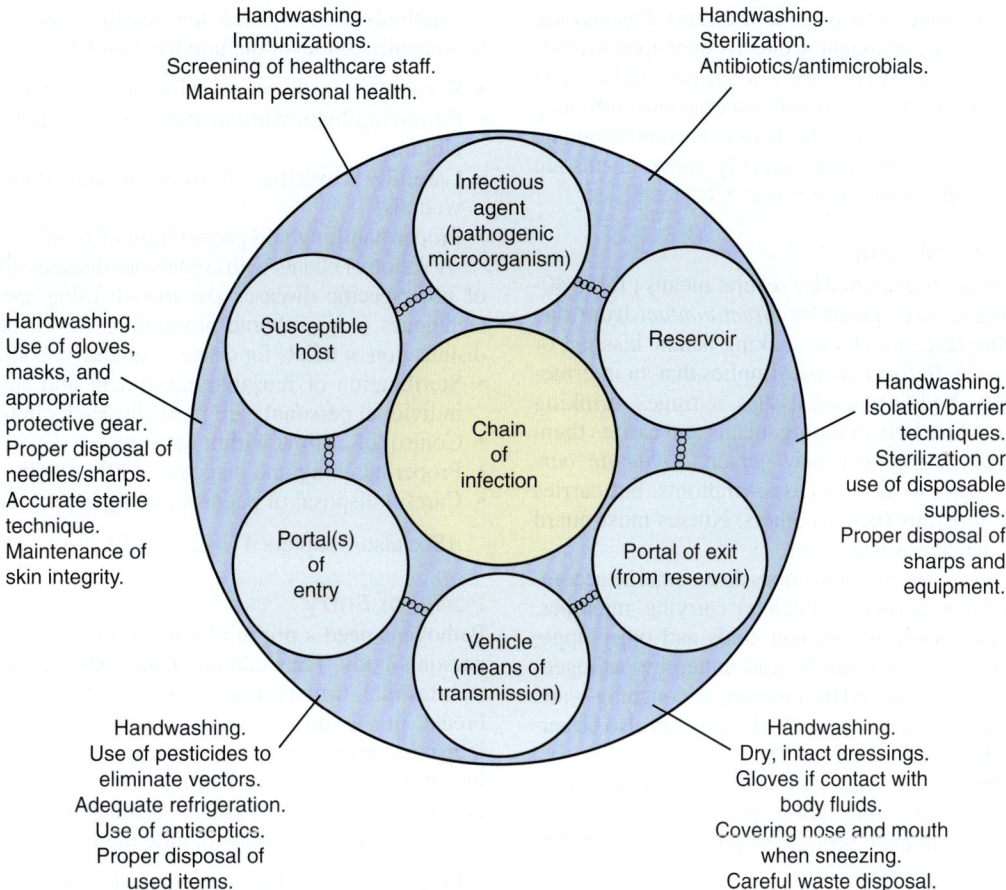

Figure 40-6 The cyclic process through which an infection occurs. To prevent a disease from spreading, the chain of infection must be broken by means such as those listed here.

Causative Agent (Pathogenic Microorganisms) and Reservoir

Because pathogenic microorganisms exist everywhere, the **reservoir** is any place where a pathogen can survive before moving to another place where it can multiply. Reservoirs may be living beings (e.g., people, domesticated or wild animals, or insects) or inanimate objects (e.g., air, soil, food, fluids, bedding, and utensils).

Healthcare personnel can break the chain at this point by destroying the microorganism or retarding its growth through the following measures:

- Following *Standard Precautions* at all times (Chapter 41)
- Sterilizing instruments and dressings used in the operating room and elsewhere
- Disinfecting floors and equipment; promptly cleaning up spills, particularly body fluids
- Using bedpans or other personal items for one client only
- Discarding disposable equipment (e.g., thermometer probe covers, catheters) and trash (e.g., medication packages) in appropriate receptacles after use; discarding other equipment, such as bedpans, urinals, and water pitchers, when the client is discharged
- Giving baths using soap and water or a special disinfectant solution, to remove drainage and dried secretions
- Changing dressings promptly when they become wet or as per provider's order
- Placing contaminated articles (e.g., dressings, tissues, or linen) in moisture-proof bags; using red, specially labeled biohazard bags when indicated
- Discarding contaminated needles and syringes and other sharps in appropriate moisture-resistant, puncture-proof "sharps" containers—never throw them in the trash or put your fingers inside the container!
- Making sure drainage tubes and collection bags drain properly; emptying them according to agency policy
- Never using any sterile package that is wet or has a broken seal
- Using personal protective equipment as needed (Chapters 41 and 42)
- *Most importantly*, performing frequent and thorough handwashing or sanitizing
- In addition, healthcare personnel should not work when they might be a source of infection

Portal of Exit

Microorganisms must be able to escape from their reservoir. Portals of exit include all body orifices (openings), as well as any natural body fluids (e.g., sweat, mucus, semen, sputum, saliva, urine, or feces, as well as vomitus, drainage, or blood from breaks in the skin).

The chain of infection can be broken here by preventing microorganisms from escaping with thorough handwashing, appropriate waste disposal, and careful management of secretions and drainage. Always use Standard Precautions. Avoid talking, sneezing, or coughing directly over open wounds or a sterile field. Always wear gloves when potential contact with body secretions exists. Clients with airborne infections may wear masks or receive ordered medications to prevent coughing. Follow infection control protocols carefully. Some clients are isolated, to prevent the spread of infection (Chapter 42).

Vehicle of Transmission

Microorganisms are transmitted by several means (Table 40-3). Many pathogens are spread by *direct contact* from one person to another (e.g., touching, shaking hands, kissing, or sexual intercourse). *Indirect contact* implies that an intermediary object (e.g., bedding, used tissues, syringes, drinking cups, or dressings) harbors microorganisms and carries them from an infected person to a new person. A *human carrier* usually does not exhibit disease symptoms, but carries pathogens and transmits them to others. Nurses must guard against being a carrier of pathogens.

Airborne transmission of an infectious disease can be accomplished by moisture particles (droplets) carrying microbes. Infectious diseases, such as common colds and other upper respiratory infections (URI), can be transmitted by pathogen-containing droplets—produced by sneezing or coughing—and can be propelled far from the carrier. Pathogens can also be carried by dust particles (e.g., desert fever).

Contaminated public water supplies will produce *waterborne disease transmission*. Food poisoning can result from eating foods that have been improperly refrigerated or cooked (*foodborne transmission*).

Living carriers of pathogens to humans are called **vectors**, the most common of which are mosquitoes, flies, fleas, ticks, and lice. Vectors spread disease by transferring microorganisms from their feet, wings, or bodies to food, which a person eats, unaware that the food is contaminated. Another method of disease spread occurs when vectors become infected and bite or sting a victim, who then also becomes infected. (Ebola is believed to have been initially spread by infected bats.)

Methods used to break the infection chain at the vehicle of transmission level include the following:

- Burning all trash in nonresidue incinerators
- Removing linen without shaking it or allowing it to touch clothing
- Carefully covering all infected and some noninfected wounds
- Proper handling and preparation of food

Isolation of clients with contagious diseases and being aware of how specific diseases are spread; using specific isolation techniques (e.g., airborne precautions for clients with **TB**, or disinfection of toilets for diseases spread by body excretions)

- Sterilization of reusable equipment and supplies; use of individual personal care items for each client
- Control of airflow within facilities
- Proper handling and disposal of all body fluids
- Careful disposal of needles and syringes

(See also Chapters 41, 42, and 64.)

Portal of Entry

Pathogens need a portal of entry (place) to gain access to a person's body. They can enter through the respiratory, gastrointestinal, urinary, and reproductive systems and through breaks in the skin or mucous membranes. Open wounds, incisions, puncture sites from injections, or body orifices into which catheters (tubes) or similar devices are inserted are common portals of entry. Methods to prevent pathogens from entering a new host include the following:

- Follow Standard Precautions at all times.
- Keep the client's skin clean and dry. Apply moisturizers to dry skin or lips, to prevent cracking.
- Be very careful if clipping a client's nails; instruct clients not to bite the fingernails or cuticles and not to pull on hangnails.
- Avoid positioning clients against tubes or objects that could cause skin breaks.
- Frequently reposition clients with impaired mobility.
- Provide clean, dry, wrinkle-free linen.
- Make sure urine collection bags are lower than the client.
- Disinfect drainage tubes and IV ports before collecting specimens.
- Cover draining wounds and skin breaks.
- Use sterile technique when performing invasive procedures, such as injections (Chapter 57).

As a healthcare worker, you are also at risk for infection. Wear gloves to protect yourself when handling any blood or body fluids or other potential pathogenic reservoirs (i.e., contaminated equipment). Wear protective eyewear, masks, gowns, and shoe covers if any danger exists of splashing or spraying body substances (Chapters 41 and 42). Procedures such as careful handwashing and proper wound and catheter care also help break the chain of infection.

Susceptible Host

Normally, healthy people have many defenses against infection, both nonspecific (e.g., skin as a barrier, fever) and specific (e.g., immunity, phagocytosis). Ill or inactive people, however, are more susceptible to infections. Their immune systems may be compromised. Chronic fatigue, poor nutrition, injury, shock, and trauma weaken the body's ability to respond fully. Side effects of some medications also

TABLE 40-3 Transmission of Infectious Disease

TYPE OF TRANSMISSION	EXAMPLES OF METHODS
Direct or indirect contact	Touching, kissing, shaking hands, sexual intercourse
Airborne	Dust particles and spores in the air, droplets from sneezing
Foodborne	Spoiled and uncooked food, food contaminated with feces or soil
Waterborne	Feces-contaminated water supply
Vectors	Bites by infected insects, dogs, cats, rodents
Contaminated articles	Dishes, bedding, needles, syringes
Bloodborne	Transfusions, kidney dialysis, injections, accidental needle stick

contribute to susceptibility. Emotional factors, such as anxiety, may alter body defenses. Infants, young children, and older adults are especially vulnerable.

Help reduce each client's susceptibility to infection by treating underlying conditions. Provide adequate rest and skin care. Give nutritional support. Help reduce anxiety. Encourage adequate fluid intake. Help with coughing and deep breathing for the immobilized client. Encourage proper immunization of children and adults at high risk of acquiring communicable diseases. Practice infection control measures. Preventing infection is the daily job of every healthcare worker.

> 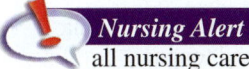 **Nursing Alert** Observe Standard Precautions in all nursing care. Chapter 41 details this concept. *Assume that all clients have an infection* and act accordingly.

Actions of Pathogens in the Body

Pathogenic microorganisms can cause two damaging effects: local destruction of tissue or production of poisonous substances (toxins).

Toxins

Although some pathogens destroy tissues in which they live, many organisms cause damage to host tissues far from the infection site, due to the action of poisonous **toxins** produced by pathogenic microorganisms. Toxins cause harmful effects and varying symptoms by traveling through the circulatory system to damage body cells. The wide variety of their cellular effects includes interrupting cellular metabolism, stopping protein synthesis, and destroying cell membranes. Microorganisms produce two types of toxins. **Endotoxins** are part of the cell walls of gram-negative bacteria. When a microorganism dies, the cell wall decays and releases the toxins. **Exotoxins** are toxins manufactured by the microorganism and excreted into the surrounding tissue. They are released into host blood vessels, where they are carried to other body parts.

RESPONSE TO INFECTION

Whether or not a pathogen produces an active infection depends on both the organism and the host. A healthy individual often has appropriate physical defense mechanisms to ward off disease. Persistent and effective pathogens, however, can overwhelm even the healthiest person.

Normal Course of Infection

When an infection occurs, it usually follows a progressive course. The first stage is the **incubation period**, the time from when the pathogen enters the body to the appearance of the first symptoms of illness. For example, after the *Varicella zoster* virus (which causes chickenpox) enters the body, it takes 2–3 weeks before any lesions appear. The second phase is the **prodromal** stage, the period from the onset of initial symptoms (e.g., fatigue or low-grade fever) to more severe symptoms. Many illnesses are the most contagious during the prodromal stage. The third phase is the full stage of *illness*. During this period, the symptoms are acute and specific to the type of infection, such as a high fever, nausea, lesions, cough, headache, or congestion. The final stage is the *convalescence* stage. During this period, the acute symptoms of the infection subside and the person recovers.

Factors That Influence the Development of Infection

Normally, the body has many defense mechanisms that contribute to resistance to pathogenic infection. Although the individual is unaware of it, the body is almost constantly defending itself against foreign invaders. Chapter 24 discusses nonspecific mechanisms that fight disease, as well as the crucial role of the immune system. Review that chapter for a better understanding of the human body's natural defenses against pathogenic microorganisms.

Several factors other than the strength of the body's natural defenses help determine whether or not disease-causing microorganisms will ultimately cause an infection in an individual.

Specific Portal of Entry

In general, microorganisms cause disease only if they gain access to the body through a specific portal of entry. For example, *S. pneumoniae* (a gram-positive diplococcus) causes pneumococcal pneumonia only when it enters the respiratory system; entry via any other portal of entry does not result in infection. Likewise, the typhoid bacillus (*Salmonella typhi*, a gram-negative rod) must enter the digestive tract. Meningococcus (*Neisseria meningitidis*), causing some types of meningitis, uses the nose as its chief portal of entry.

Number of Microorganisms

Usually, large numbers of microorganisms are needed to cause infection. If the number of pathogens entering the body is small, the body's natural defenses can easily overcome them. The greater the number of pathogens, the greater the opportunity to cause disease.

Virulence

A pathogen's *strength to cause disease* is called **virulence**. Some bacteria form protective capsules that increase their virulence by making them less likely to be destroyed by the host's white blood cells. Other bacteria produce enzymes that destroy blood cells, stop normal blood clotting, or consume muscle fibers. Each of these enzymes increases the virulence of the particular species that produces them.

As previously described, some pathogens are able to mutate so they are not susceptible to certain antibiotics. These organisms are more virulent just because commonly used antibiotics will not destroy them.

Host Resistance

Naturally occurring microorganisms in the body do not cause disease in healthy people. In fact, some play a necessary role in disease resistance and maintenance of health and body functioning. The ability of some species of microorganisms to live together is called *symbiosis*. An association in which one species of microorganism prevents the growth or actually destroys members of another species is called *antibiosis*. (The term *antibiotic* is derived from this term.) Some naturally occurring body flora have an antibiotic relationship with pathogens and contribute to an individual's overall health.

UNIT 7 Safety in the Healthcare Facility

If a person is *immunocompromised* (decreased immune system functioning), they will not be able to fight off disease. Examples include people with AIDS or agammaglobulinemia (congenital absence of normal gamma globulin), people undergoing some forms of cancer chemotherapy, persons receiving certain corticosteroid injections, or people recovering from a bone marrow transplant. In these cases, even normally occurring microorganisms can cause disease (*opportunistic infections*).

STUDENT SYNTHESIS

KEY POINTS

- Some microorganisms are beneficial. Others (pathogens) cause disease in human beings.
- All microorganisms, except viruses, engage in the same general life functions as do other plant and animal cells. These functions may occur in a modified form.
- The reproductive processes and spread of infection caused by pathogens depends on the proper set of conditions.
- Culture and sensitivity reports and staining identify pathogens and suggest appropriate treatment for them.
- Microorganisms are classified by physical and biologic characteristics into basic groups, each with distinguishing means of reproducing and, if they are pathogens, of causing infections.
- With the number of drug-resistant and multi–drug-resistant microorganisms increasing, appropriate antibiotic use is essential.
- Viruses cause disease by taking over the host cell's metabolism and genetic material and by reproducing in extremely large numbers.
- Most common microbial diseases are communicable and are spread by direct or indirect contact; via contaminated air, water, or food; or through vectors.
- Healthcare professionals who practice antiseptic techniques and Standard Precautions can help break the chain of infection.
- Infections follow a progressive course. Many factors contribute to a pathogen's ability to cause disease.

CRITICAL THINKING EXERCISES

1. Discuss methods of teaching clients and families about disease transmission. What suggestions would you make to control infection and break the chain of infection in the home, clinic, and school setting?
2. What suggestions would you make to a homeless person who comes to your clinic seeking treatment for a severe wound infection on the leg?

NCLEX-STYLE REVIEW QUESTIONS

1. The nurse is preparing to perform a dressing change for a client who has an open surgical wound of the abdomen. Which action by the nurse is most appropriate when finding the seal on the sterile 4 × 4-dressing package is broken?
   a. Discard the 4 × 4 closest to the broken seal and use the others.
   b. Proceed with using the 4 × 4s.
   c. Discard them and obtain a new package.
   d. Use them for the outside of the dressing only.

2. A client is infected with the fungal infection *tinea capitus*. Which objective data would the nurse document for this client?
   a. Green, foul-smelling discharge from the vagina
   b. A white patch on the mouth and tongue
   c. Lesions on the scalp
   d. Lesions on the feet

3. A client has been prescribed an antibiotic for a bacterial infection. Which information is important for the nurse to tell the client?
   a. "Be sure to complete the drug for the entire period prescribed even if symptoms are better."
   b. "It is advisable to take any 'leftover' medications if another type of infection develops."
   c. "The antibiotics can also be used if you develop a virus."
   d. "The medication may be given to a family member if they develop the same symptoms."

4. A hospitalized client has been taking antibiotics for several days and develops *C. difficile*. Which symptom of this infection should the nurse expect to provide care for?
   a. Cough
   b. Diarrhea
   c. Vomiting
   d. Vaginal discharge

5. A client is suspected of having a urinary tract infection. Which specimen does the nurse obtain to determine which bacteria is present as well as which antibiotic to use?
   a. White blood cell count
   b. Urinalysis
   c. Urine for culture and sensitivity
   d. Hemoglobin

CHAPTER RESOURCES

Enhance your learning with additional resources on thePoint!

Student Resources related to this chapter can be found at thePoint.lww.com/Rosdahl12e.

41 Medical Asepsis

Learning Objectives

1. Describe basic procedures in Standard Precautions; state why they are used.
2. Differentiate between endogenous and exogenous organisms.
3. Identify factors that predispose clients to nosocomial infections.
4. Describe the elements of medical asepsis. Explain how antimicrobial agents and environmental controls contribute to medical asepsis.
5. State the single most effective nursing measure in preventing spread of disease.
6. In the laboratory, demonstrate proper handwashing technique after routine client care, before contact with a severely immunocompromised client, and after performing an invasive procedure. State when hand sanitizers may safely be used.
7. Describe the most commonly used personal protective equipment.
8. In the laboratory, demonstrate the use of barrier techniques.
9. Demonstrate teaching of infection control to a client or family member.
10. Describe the nurse's role in disposal of biohazardous waste and in cleaning up biohazardous materials.
11. List the functions of the Infection Committee.

Important Terminology

antimicrobial agent
asepsis
bacteremia
endogenous
exogenous
invasive
medical asepsis
Standard Precautions

Acronyms

PPD
PPE
TST

In Chapter 40, information was presented about pathogenic microorganisms and how they contribute to the spread of infectious disease. Preventing infections is vital to any healthcare facility's operation and to the provision of healthcare in the community and the home. Practicing techniques of *medical asepsis* will help protect you, your clients, and your coworkers.

STANDARD PRECAUTIONS

Because it is impossible to know which clients may be carrying communicable diseases, the Centers for Disease Control and Prevention (CDC) established a set of guidelines *to be used in delivery of all healthcare*. These guidelines are called "**Standard Precautions**"—Tier 1 (Fig. 41-1). Standard Precautions are to be followed at all times by all healthcare personnel when delivering any care or performing any procedures. This includes healthcare workers outside the hospital, such as dentists, acupuncturists, home care workers, and clinic nurses. Because a client's infectious status is never definitely known, all clients are treated as though they could be infectious. Clients may not know they have an infection or may not divulge the fact. All exposures to blood or any other body fluids have potential to cause infection. It is vital to protect nurses, other clients, and visitors. (Specific Transmission-Based Precautions—Tier 2—are discussed in Chapter 42.) If you have questions, consult your facility's protocols. Every nurse must be thoroughly familiar with these guidelines (In Practice: Nursing Care Guidelines 41-1).

IN PRACTICE
NURSING CARE GUIDELINES 41-1 Implementing Standard Precautions

- Wear gloves when in contact with any body fluid, including blood, secretions, and excretions, as well as nonintact skin, mucous membranes, or contaminated items, and when performing any invasive procedure, including administering injections. *Rationale: Body fluids contain microorganisms. Nurses may be at risk or could spread disease.*
- Change gloves before and after each client contact or if gloves become perforated or soiled. Double gloves may be worn if needed. *Rationale: Gloves must be replaced if there is any possibility of contamination.*
- Wash/sanitize hands and skin immediately and thoroughly if they become contaminated with blood

UNIT 7 Safety in the Healthcare Facility

IN PRACTICE
NURSING CARE GUIDELINES 41-1 Implementing Standard Precautions (Continued)

or body fluids; after each client contact; and after removing gloves. *Rationale: This helps prevent transfer of microorganisms. Proper handwashing/sanitization helps stop the spread of infection.*
- Wear a gown or apron when your clothing could become soiled. *Rationale: This helps prevent the spread of infection.*
- Wear a mask, eye protection, and face shield if splashing or spraying of blood or body fluids is possible. Healthcare facility protocol determines the type of protection required. *Rationale: Infection could enter your body through the mucous membranes of your mouth or nose or through your eyes.*
- Do not recap or break needles. Place all sharp objects (needles, glass, scalpels) in a special, puncture-resistant sharps container. Never reach into this container. Use the needleless system or safety syringes when available. Otherwise, protective caps must be used to cover needles after use (Chapter 64). *Rationale: Recapping (even with the "scoop" method) or breaking a needle promotes accidental finger sticks. Protect yourself and housekeeping personnel.*
- Report any exposure to blood or body fluids to your supervisor or facility health service immediately. *Rationale: Occupational Safety and Health Administration (OSHA) requires initial screening and follow-up of the accident. Reporting also protects your safety (Chapter 39).*
- Clean or process equipment after client use. Discard disposable, single-use items. Discard soiled and designated items in red biohazard disposal bags or bins. *Rationale: Proper cleaning and disposal help prevent transmission of infectious microorganisms.*
- Do not allow client linens to touch your clothing and do not place linens on the floor. Place all linens in designated containers. *Rationale: This helps prevent spreading microorganisms to staff and others.*
- Wipe down all surfaces (e.g., tables, chairs, telephones) frequently with an antimicrobial agent. *Rationale: Even if soil is not visible, it is important to provide as clean an environment as possible.*
- If an item is used by multiple clients, such as a blood pressure cuff, it must be disinfected between uses. *Rationale: This helps prevent cross contamination.*
- Assume all clients have an infectious disease. *Rationale: It is not possible to determine all sources of infection or contamination. Standard Precautions apply to care of ALL clients.*
- With the advent of antimicrobial-resistant microorganisms, following Standard Precautions is particularly important (Chapter 40).

Adapted from Centers for Disease Control and Prevention. (2019). *Isolation precautions*. https://www.cdc.gov/infectioncontrol/guidelines/isolation/index.html

Standard Precautions include the following:
- Maintenance of the nurse's personal immunizations; do not work if you are ill
- Frequent, thorough handwashing or sanitizing (*hand hygiene*), with soap and water or antibacterial solution
- Wearing gloves and other protective equipment as needed
- Respiratory hygiene/cough etiquette
- Educating clients and visitors regarding *respiratory hygiene*/cough etiquette
- Safely administering injections and disposing of all sharps (never recap or break off a needle; dispose of sharps in designated containers [Chapter 64])
- Proper handling/disposal/cleanup of all linens, used equipment, medication packages, and biohazardous materials, such as laboratory specimens
- Surface disinfection as needed, including spill cleanup
- Maintenance of sterility of needles, catheters, and other equipment
- Use of Ambu bags or mouthpieces for resuscitation
- Private rooms for infectious clients
- Wearing mask and other PPE for lumbar punctures

These topics are introduced in this and the next chapter and will be referred to throughout this book.

MEDICAL ASEPSIS

Asepsis refers to practices that *minimize* or *eliminate* pathogenic organisms. The two categories of asepsis are medical and surgical. **Medical asepsis** (*clean technique*) is discussed in this chapter and is used in all client care. The goal is to *reduce numbers of microorganisms and* prevent transmission

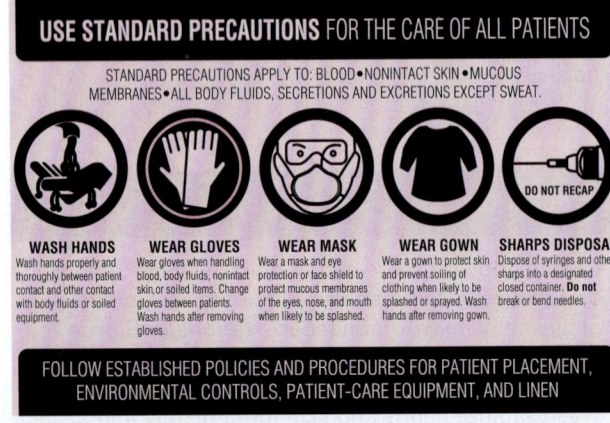

Figure 41-1 Signs reminding all healthcare personnel to use Standard Precautions are posted in prominent places throughout any healthcare facility. All personnel are expected to follow these guidelines when giving any client care. (From Timby, B. K. (2005). *Fundamental nursing skills and concepts* (8th ed.). Lippincott Williams & Wilkins.)

of microorganisms from one person (or source) to another. *Surgical asepsis* (sterile technique) aims to *destroy all organisms* and is used only in certain situations (Chapter 57).

Nurses and Healthcare-Associated Infections

As described in Chapter 40, *healthcare-associated infections* (*HAIs*), those acquired in a healthcare facility, are a serious problem. A person's risk of acquiring such infections is high for several reasons. Healthcare personnel may contribute to development of HAIs. For example:

- Failure to follow Standard Precautions, particularly adequate hand sanitization; the chain of infection is not interrupted (Chapter 40)
- Inadequate use of protective equipment
- Inaccurate performance of procedures, such as injections, and caring for IVs or catheters, possibly introducing pathogens
- Multiple personnel provide client care, thus increasing the client's possible exposure to pathogens
- Healthcare personnel care for multiple clients, increasing possible cross contamination

> **Key Concept**
> HAIs can lengthen the person's stay in the healthcare facility, increase the cost of treatment, and even cause death. Many HAIs are easily preventable.

> **NCLEX Alert**
> Infection prevention and client teaching are common NCLEX concepts. You may be given situations in which nurses could contribute to or prevent the spread of HAIs.

Common Healthcare-Associated Infections

According to the Department of Health and Human Services (2020), the most common HAIs include the following:

- Catheter-associated urinary tract infections
- Surgical site infections
- Bloodstream infections
- Pneumonia
- *Clostridium difficile*

Other types of HAIs are presented in Chapter 42.

In some cases, **endogenous** (always present) microorganisms cause infection (Table 41-1). In other cases, **exogenous** (from outside the body) microorganisms are responsible. The *Salmonella*, *Clostridium*, and *Aspergillus* genera are examples of exogenous microorganisms that cause HAIs. Gram-negative organisms cause most of today's HAIs. However, it is predicted that lesser-known pathogens and new strains will cause more infections in the future. It is also predicted that the number of antibiotic-resistant pathogens will increase.

Clients and Healthcare-Associated Infections

> **NCLEX Alert**
> First or priority actions are common correct NCLEX responses to a clinical scenario. Actions such as "wash your hands," "provide for privacy," or "put on gloves" may be the correct response. The nurse is responsible for protecting the client from complications.

Infections can occur when a *person's resistance (ability to fight off pathogens) is lowered*. Many factors can contribute to this:

- *Trauma and illness:* Injury or illness lowers the body's resistance. Illness requires energy, and trauma can cause breaks in skin; nonintact skin provides avenues for infection. Examples include burns, compound fractures (bone exposed), stab wounds, and lacerations (cuts).
- *Preexisting disease, generally poor health, or frequent illness:* The client may have an infection or chronic condition that has lowered body defenses.
- *Age:* The very young and very old often have reduced defenses. Immunity transmitted by breastfeeding lasts for a short time and does not protect against all diseases. Older adults may be poorly nourished, chronically ill, have fragile skin, or be inactive, causing impaired resistance.
- *Inactivity:* The postoperative client or person who is ill usually does not exercise, weakening the body's defenses. Conditions promoted by inactivity include pneumonia and thrombophlebitis (blood clots).

TABLE 41-1 Examples of Endogenous Microorganisms

SITE OF NORMAL GROWTH	ENDOGENOUS ORGANISM	POSSIBLE INFECTION
Skin	*Staphylococcus aureus*	Impetigo, wound infection
	Staphylococcus epidermidis	Acne
Respiratory tract	*Streptococcus pneumoniae*	Bacterial pneumonia
	Neisseria species	Meningitis (inflammation of meninges of nervous system)
Colon	*Escherichia coli*	Urinary tract infection
	Pseudomonas species	Wound infection
Vagina	*Clostridium perfringens*	Diarrhea, gas gangrene
	Yeasts	Moniliasis, pneumonia

The central nervous system, bladder, and blood are normally sterile and do not contain endogenous organisms.

- *Poor nutrition/inadequate hydration:* Malnutrition, dehydration (not enough fluid in tissues or circulation), or overhydration (too much fluid, fluid retention) can lead to illness. Inadequate protein hinders tissue repair and production of antibodies. Impaired skin integrity is often present, as well as inadequate circulation. People experiencing homelessness, people with substance abuse disorders, or people with eating disorders (such as anorexia) may be in this group.
- *Stress or emotional shock:* Increased stress increases cortisone levels, reducing resistance to disease (sometimes by immunosuppression). Prolonged stress may result in physical exhaustion. Examples include physical stress caused by trauma, such as a motor vehicle accident, or emotional stress, such as the death of a spouse or divorce.
- *Fatigue:* The sleep-deprived person cannot effectively fight off disease. Included are people who are fighting illness or injury, family trauma, or those who have had surgery. Older adults often have difficulty sleeping as well.
- *Invasive therapy:* The term "**invasive**" means any procedure that enters or *invades* the body (by a means other than normal), either through a skin break or incision or through an instrument that enters an otherwise sterile area. Examples of invasive therapy include surgery, injections, intravenous or central line therapy, urinary catheterization, and tracheostomies (inserted into the trachea to open an airway).
- *Frequent use of broad-spectrum antibiotics:* Microorganisms in a person's body may develop *resistance* to antibiotic therapy after repeated exposure to the same antibiotic. In this case, these antibiotics are later ineffective against the resistant pathogen.
- *Inappropriate use of antibiotics:* The client may stop taking an antibiotic before the full course of therapy is completed, may take left-over antibiotics, or antibiotics may be unnecessarily prescribed. These practices often lead to antibiotic-resistant strains of pathogens, making effective therapy difficult later.
- *Inadequate primary and secondary defenses:* The body's primary defenses may be altered because of a break in the skin, low white blood cell count, an autoimmune disorder, or diminished lung function.
- *Immunosuppressive situations:* The client's immune system may be inadequate as a result of chemotherapy, bone marrow transplant, administration of steroids to reduce inflammation, radiation, or an autoimmune disorder such as AIDS or agammaglobulinemia.

Breaking the Chain of Infection

As emphasized previously, following Standard Precautions in all nursing care is vital in controlling the spread of infection. In addition, many nursing procedures are aimed at breaking the "chain of infection" (Chapter 40). Possibilities of infection can be interrupted at several points. Following is a brief review:

- *Causative agent:* Reduction in numbers and/or virulence of pathogens involves procedures such as antibiotic administration and careful handwashing/sanitization.
- *Reservoir for growth of pathogens:* Procedures such as proper disposal of contaminated dressings, body fluids, outdated IV solutions or medications, as well as of disposable materials, and broken sterile packages remove possible reservoirs. Other procedures include proper spill cleanup; sterilization; personal immunizations; not wearing jewelry or artificial fingernails (because they may harbor pathogens); and careful handwashing/sanitization.
- *Portal of exit:* Special attention is given to handling any body fluids. This includes covering wounds, encouraging safer sex, following prescribed isolation protocols, and handwashing/sanitization.
- *Vehicle of transmission:* Transmission of pathogens is arrested by correct use of personal protective equipment (PPE); careful disposal of any body fluids, including soiled dressings, diapers, or tubing; sterile injection technique; sterile catheterization and maintenance of urinary drainage equipment (Chapter 57); and careful handwashing/sanitization.
- *Portal of entry:* Helping prevent pathogens from entering a client's system involves protective isolation (Chapter 42); cleansing from clean to dirty when performing procedures such as perineal care or injections; using correct sterile technique; and careful handwashing/sanitization.
- *Susceptible host:* Nursing actions aimed at increasing client resistance include promoting adequate nutrition, hydration, exercise, and rest; careful monitoring and maintenance of skin integrity; properly administering prescribed medications, including antibiotics; and carefully caring for the immunocompromised client.
- *Client history:* A careful history is obtained on admission to a healthcare facility. Addressed are factors such as recent surgery or major illness; new conditions, such as diabetes; any undiagnosed symptoms; knowledge of current infection; past related infections; allergies; and immunization status.

> **Nursing Alert** Maintenance of intact skin is of utmost importance because the skin is the first and best barrier to pathogens.

Risks for the Nurse

Just as clients are at risk, nurses too are at risk as the result of repeated contact with infectious materials and exposure to communicable diseases. Risks for infection in nurses after exposure to diseases such as tuberculosis or hepatitis are of concern. It is important for the nurse to take protective preventive measures, including appropriate immunizations. Box 41-1 lists immunization recommendations for healthcare personnel. In many facilities, a yearly influenza immunization ("flu shot") and other immunizations are required; if the nurse has a valid reason for refusing, a mask is worn when caring for clients. A yearly purified protein derivative (**PPD**), **TST** (tuberculin skin test) test (for TB) is usually required, with a chest x-ray for positive PPD/TST. In some states and provinces (e.g., Manitoba), healthcare workers must report if they have an infection that might cause an HAI. Careful hand sanitization and Standard Precautions are vital in protecting the nurse. In Practice: Nursing Care Guidelines 41-2 lists additional preventive measures.

IN PRACTICE
NURSING CARE GUIDELINES 41-2 — Preventing Infection for Nursing Staff and Clients

- Get plenty of sleep and exercise. Eat nutritious foods. Practice safer sex.
- Practice good personal hygiene. Keep immunizations up to date.
- Use sanitizer on community-based objects, such as shopping carts.
- Follow facility protocols for mandatory and voluntary immunization and routine PPD/TST or chest x-ray.
- Keep up to date in infection control protocols and specific related nursing skills.
- Report needlesticks or any breaks in the skin.
- Do not use nonprescribed medications.
- Stay home from work when ill.
- Practice meticulous hand sanitization, at work and at home.
- Do not wear artificial nails, nail polish, or jewelry with prongs or protruding stones.
- Wear gloves when in contact with any body fluids or if in doubt.
- Wear appropriate PPE (masks, goggles, etc.) when performing care.
- Isolate infected clients and carefully follow isolation protocols (Chapter 42).
- Use sterile techniques for procedures such as catheterization, catheter care, injections, or dressing changes (Chapter 57).
- Do not use sterile packages if the seal is broken, the wrapper is torn or wet, or if the sterilization monitor has not registered. Do not use a sterile package or medication if it is past the expiration date.
- Store sterile and clean supplies separately and keep cupboards closed where sterile materials are stored.
- Change clothes immediately if they become soiled with any body fluids. (Scrub clothing is usually available.)
- Teach clients hygiene and good techniques for self-care.
- Do not shake linens, place linens on the floor, or allow them to touch your clothing. Use covered linen hampers.
- Make sure sitz baths, bathtubs, showers, lounge chairs, tables, kitchens, or other common areas are carefully disinfected between clients.
- Do not store client trays; some foods will spoil.
- Ensure that a new electronic temperature probe cover is used for each client and covers are disposed of appropriately.
- Sanitize items, such as blood pressure cuffs and stethoscopes, between clients. Change items such as examination table paper, and otoscope or ophthalmoscope tips, between clients.
- Use disposable equipment and supplies whenever possible; appropriately dispose of all used items.
- Dispose of large amounts of blood or other body fluids in designated "Biohazard" waste containers or red bags.

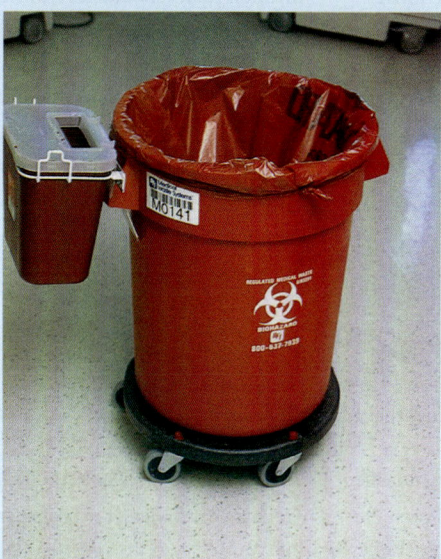

Biohazardous waste containers and bags are red. Note the universal symbol for biohazardous waste on the barrel. Attached to this bucket is a container for sharps disposal. (Photo by B. Proud.)

- Follow procedures carefully for pre- and postoperative clients (Chapter 56).
- Use gloves and waterproof bags to send heavily soiled or moist linens to the laundry.
- Send items to be sterilized to central supply room per facility protocol.
- Ensure that all trash is collected in heavy-duty plastic or coated paper bags. Most facility trash is incinerated.
- Make sure that any spilled body substances are cleaned up immediately, using prescribed protocols. Carefully handle any specimens, such as blood tubes and urine or stool samples.
- Report any personal or client infection *immediately*.
- Follow careful procedures when caring for the client in their home or elsewhere in the community.
- Monitor and encourage other healthcare personnel to comply with infection control practices.
- Ask questions if you are not sure of a procedure or protocol.

Box 41-1 Recommended Immunizations for Healthcare Personnel

Hepatitis B	Initial injection; next in 1 month; again in 6 months; may require booster
Measles/mumps/rubella (MMR)	Adults with any question of immunization status should have MMR series; rubella titer determines level of protection
Poliovirus	Once for life
Tetanus	Booster every 10 years for adults; booster in event of invasive injury
Diphtheria	Given with initial tetanus immunization
Influenza	Yearly immunization, using prevailing strains of virus
Pneumococcal disease	Once for life
Meningococcal disease	Once for life
Shingles vaccine	Adults older than 50 years, one time
Purified protein derivative (PPD/TST) test for tuberculosis (TB)	Once a year to detect exposure or active TB

The Infection Control Committee

Healthcare facilities are required to establish an Infection Control Committee to monitor HAIs and other safety practices. Committee functions include the following:

- Watchfulness for any HAIs
- Investigation of any infections
- Compiling statistics regarding HAI events
- Teaching staff, clients, and families infection prevention
- Serving as a liaison between the facility and the community
- Identifying and monitoring community or worldwide infections, assisting in their management, and planning for possible local cases

You may be asked to serve as a member of this important committee.

Handwashing

Handwashing or sanitization is the single most effective measure to reduce the risk of transmitting disease. In general, the frequency and products for handwashing relate to the duration, type, sequence, and intensity of your activities. For example, touching an item that is sterile does not require handwashing; touching something contaminated with blood or body fluids requires thorough handwashing with soap and water. In many instances, using hand sanitizer is adequate. The type of cleaning agent and handwash depends on several factors. Box 41-2 describes handwashing in different healthcare situations. In Practice: Nursing Procedure 41-1 outlines basic steps in handwashing. Follow your facility's guidelines if you have any questions.

The "long wash" involves a thorough washing of the hands, with lathering of the hands at least twice, and careful cleaning of the fingernails (Nursing Procedure 41-1). It is used:

- At the beginning and end of each shift and after using the rest room or taking a meal break
- When hands are visibly soiled
- If you have touched blood or body fluids with or without gloves

The "short wash" is required at all other times. The CDC recommends routine handwashing for at least 20 s (20 s is approximately the length of time to sing "Happy Birthday" from beginning to end twice).

Reasons for handwashing include the following:

- Reducing flora on the nurse's skin
- Protecting nurses, in case their skin is not intact
- Reducing risk, if gloves break or are punctured
- Reducing chances of disease transmission

The CDC recommends handwashing in the following situations:

- When hands are visibly soiled
- Before and after contacts with all clients

Box 41-2 Handwashing Guidelines

Handwash with soap or detergent, to remove soil and transient microorganisms:

- At beginning and end of work shift; when returning from breaks; whenever leaving unit
- Routine client care; before and after client contact
- When hands are visibly soiled
- If any possibility of fecal or body fluid contact, even if not visible
- After contact with any source of microorganisms
- After removing gloves

Perform *hand antisepsis*, using antimicrobial soap or alcohol-based handrub, to remove or destroy transient microorganisms:

- Before contact with severely immunocompromised clients and all newborns
- After caring for an infected client or one likely to be colonized with microorganisms of epidemiologic concern
- Before and after contact with clients in high-risk units

Perform *surgical hand scrub* (variation of the long scrub) using antimicrobial soap or detergent to remove/destroy transient microorganisms and reduce resident flora:

- Before and after client contact when performing invasive procedures (Chapter 56 describes the surgical hand scrub.)
- If assisting with a surgical procedure, such as suture removal, dental extraction, or in the operating room.

- After contact with a source of microorganisms (e.g., blood/body fluids [including specimens], or mucous membrane, nonintact skin, or contaminated objects)
- Before and after performing invasive procedures
- Before removing gloves if they are visibly soiled and *each time* after removing gloves

Hand Sanitization

Hand sanitizers are conveniently located and commonly used in healthcare facilities and elsewhere. They are easy and fast to use. Everyone (including visitors) is urged to "foam in/foam out" whenever entering/leaving a nursing unit or having any contact with a client. Hand sanitization is adequate if there is no visible soil on the hands and no body fluids are present. *Remember to do thorough handwashing if you have questions and any time you have left the unit and/or returned.*

> **Nursing Alert** If any visible soil is present or after contact with fecal material or body fluids, a thorough handwashing must be done. Hand sanitizer is not adequate. *If in doubt, wash your hands.*

> **Key Concept**
> Handwashing is the single most important procedure for protecting yourself and your clients against disease transmission.

Barrier Techniques

Barrier techniques include the use of **PPE**: gloves, eye protection, gowns, and masks (Fig. 41-2). Reasons for PPE use are to keep organisms from entering or leaving the nurse or client's respiratory tract, eyes, or breaks in the skin. They also help protect nurses from the client's body fluids.

Gloves

Gloves are the most commonly used protective item and must be worn for any client care with potential exposure to body fluids. Gloves greatly reduce hand contamination and provide a protective barrier when touching any body fluids. (If blood or body fluids are visible, it is a good idea to double-glove.) Gloves help provide protection from microorganisms and help prevent the spread of pathogens from one person to another. Disposable, clean gloves are available in all healthcare facilities, including community-based settings. The nurse must always wear gloves if there are any breaks in the skin of the hands. Gloves must be discarded appropriately, whether in the acute care facility or the community. (Chapter 57 describes use of sterile gloves.) In Practice: Nursing Procedure 41-2 outlines the procedure for putting on and removing gloves. Special nitrile gloves are available for use when working with "hazardous to handle" substances (Chapter 63).

> **Nursing Alert** If gloves are not intact (e.g., ripped or punctured), they must be immediately discarded, hands washed, and gloves replaced. If in doubt, wear gloves for any procedure and change the gloves as needed. *Remember:* Using gloves *does not eliminate* the need for frequent, careful handwashing.

Latex Allergies

Formerly, one component of all healthcare gloves was latex (rubber). Latex allergies are increasing among healthcare workers and the general public. Be alert for latex sensitivity in clients. *Allergic* or *sensitivity reactions* may occur from direct contact and may also occur because cornstarch powder on gloves is dispersed into the air. Latex proteins attach to the powder and cause reactions through contact or breathing. Overall latex sensitivity has increased since 1987 when Standard Precautions were introduced and glove use became universal. Most healthcare organizations use gloves made of a product other than latex because sensitivity is increasing in healthcare workers and clients. Repeated latex exposure heightens sensitivity reactions.

Latex sensitivity includes varying levels of

- Skin irritation

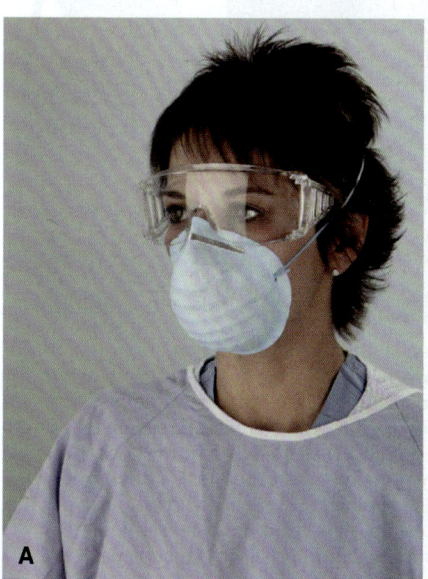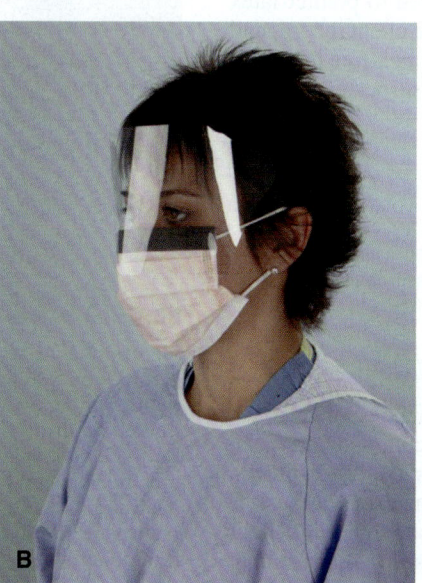

Figure 41-2 Simple mask and eye protection. The nurse must also wear gloves if there is any possibility of exposure to blood or body fluids or if they have a cut or nonintact skin. Other personal protective equipment (PPE) may also be needed. This nurse is wearing a protective gown over regular clothing. **A.** Goggles are put on after gown, gloves, and mask. **B.** A mask with a solid eye shield. (From Evans-Smith, P. [2005]. *Taylor's clinical nursing skills: A nursing process approach.* Lippincott Williams & Wilkins.)

- Contact dermatitis and/or
- Generalized anaphylaxis

Only a simple skin reaction may occur. However, sensitivity may progress to localized contact dermatitis, the most common allergic reaction to latex. Other localized symptoms of latex sensitivity include hives or rash (which may become crusty), itching, cracking, scaling, or weeping of the skin. A localized allergic reaction in the lungs may also occur when sensitized individuals are exposed. These individuals may develop facial swelling; itchy, red eyes; excessive sneezing or a runny, stuffy nose; an itchy nose or palate; and asthma or hay fever, with difficulty breathing. The third and most serious latex reaction is a systemic reaction that may quickly progress to *general anaphylaxis*, which is life threatening. (Anaphylaxis is discussed in more detail in Chapter 43 and Box 43-2.)

Some people are more likely to develop latex sensitivity than others. Be particularly watchful of the person with a history of the following:

- Asthma
- Multiple surgeries and other invasive procedures
- Spina bifida
- Genitourinary birth defects
- Daily catheterizations
- Allergies to certain foods (rich fruits such as bananas, kiwi, and avocados; other fruits such as peaches, pears, cherries, and pineapple; and chestnuts)
- Frequent use of gloves (e.g., by food service or medical personnel)

Although latex-free gloves are commonly used, it is important to remember that other items in the healthcare facility and community may also contain latex. These include catheters, rubber binders, elastic waistbands, condoms, scuba gear, balloons, and many other items. (Latex paint does not cause sensitivity because it contains synthetic latex.) Substitute latex-free items may be made of vinyl or plastic.

On admission, clients are asked about latex sensitivity, including difficulty with balloons, elastic waistbands, or condoms, or if they work with rubber. A careful medical history and specific blood test can be used to predict latex sensitivity. Latex sensitivity is noted in the client record, and the client must wear an allergy ID band. Latex-free materials are used for this client's care. Report any suspected personal or client latex sensitivity immediately.

Key Concept

A healthcare worker with a severe latex allergy should carry a self-injectable epinephrine syringe ("EpiPen") to be used in an emergency. This should also be available in the facility for the sensitized client.

Masks

Masks help protect clients and healthcare personnel from upper respiratory infections and certain communicable diseases. A mask is used for clients with respiratory disorders. For example, if a client is coughing or sneezing, a mask is worn by the nurse; the client may also be required to wear a mask. Healthcare facilities have established policies about the use of masks. In some cases, everyone coming in contact with a client, including visitors, wears a mask, or the client may wear a mask when outside their room. In the operating room, newborn nursery, and protective isolation, simple masks help protect clients from possible infection by staff members (Fig. 41-2).

Simple masks only screen out larger particles. In some situations, a *particulate mask* or *respirator mask* is used. This mask is fitted specifically to each nurse and is designed to filter out very small particles, such as the tubercle bacillus. The particulate mask is denser and fitted tighter to the face than the simple masks more commonly used (Fig. 41-3). Considerations in mask use:

- Put on mask before gloves.
- Do not touch mask until it is to be removed.
- Masks must be changed when moist or soiled.
- Wash hands and remove gloves before removing masks.
- Handle masks by strings or elastic only.
- Dispose of a used mask immediately.
- Never leave a mask dangling around the neck.

In Practice: Nursing Procedure 41-3 describes other general considerations in using a mask.

Eye Protection

Wear goggles with side and forehead shields if there is any danger that body fluids may splash or spray (or if the client spits). The nurse may wear personal glasses with side shields or goggles that fit over glasses. In some types of isolation, disposable goggles are worn (Chapter 42). In situations when extra protection is needed, such as in the operating room, emergency department, or morgue, full-face shields are used. These protect the eyes and forehead, as well as the mouth. The situation dictates the type of PPE used.

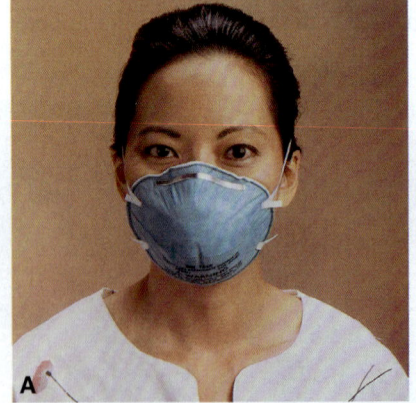 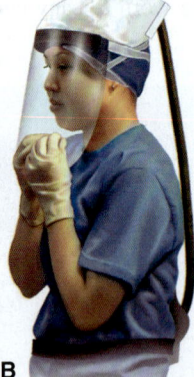

Figure 41-3 **A.** A special high-filtration particulate or respirator mask (Type N95) is worn when caring for clients with active pulmonary tuberculosis and certain other conditions. These masks are disposable or with replaceable filters. They are fitted for the individual to obtain a face seal. The nurse's respirations may be visualized by movements of the mask. Other types of special masks are also available. **B.** A powered air purifying respirator (PAPR) uses a blower to remove contaminated air though a filter and supplies purified air to a facepiece.

Gowns or Aprons

A fluid-resistant gown or protective apron is worn to protect the nurse's clothing when body fluids might splash. When using gowns or aprons:

- The inside of the garment is clean; the outside is contaminated.
- The garment must be long enough to cover the nurse's clothing. The apron covers the front and sides, but not the sleeves. The gown or apron opens in the back and must be full enough to overlap at the back. A tie around the waist keeps the garment in place.
- The neck of the garment is considered clean because the nurse does not touch it with contaminated hands.
- If the nurse is wearing long sleeves, the sleeves are rolled up above the elbows before putting on the garment.
- A supply of clean garments is kept outside the client's room.
- After use, remove the garment and dispose of it inside out (contaminated side in). The garment is placed in the receptacle for contaminated material or the specific linen hamper. (DO NOT hang and reuse this garment; it is contaminated.)
- After removing any protective garment, wash the hands thoroughly. (Chapter 42 further describes isolation procedures.)

Removal of Personal Protective Equipment

PPE must be removed in the following specified sequence, to minimize the potential for disease transmission:

- Wash hands.
- Remove gloves (Nursing Procedure 41-2).
- Remove mask by touching only the string tied behind the head.
- Remove eye protection, without touching the face.
- Wash hands.
- Remove protective garment, touching only the inside; turn it inside out, to contain contamination; and place in laundry hamper.
- Properly dispose of all PPE.
- Wash hands.

Accidental Needlesticks or Other Contamination

Unfortunately, the nurse may sustain an accidental stick with a contaminated needle. If this occurs, follow these procedures:

- Immediately wash the area thoroughly with germicidal soap and water.
- Encourage bleeding from a puncture wound, if possible.
- Report immediately to the employee health service, emergency department, or safety officer. An exposure risk assessment will be done.
- File an incident report.
- Blood tests of the client and nurse will usually be performed.
- The nurse may be required to take medication as postexposure prophylaxis.

If material is splashed into the eyes, nose, or mouth, wash with copious amounts of water. Use an eyewash station, if available (Nursing Care Guidelines 43-4) and report, as above.

Clean and Controlled Environment

Using Antimicrobial Agents

Chemicals that decrease the number of pathogens are **antimicrobial agents** (Table 41-2). They limit and eliminate pathogens by suppressing and/or destroying their growth. Some agents are used to clean equipment; others to clean skin. Examples of common antimicrobial agents include *disinfectants* and *antiseptics*.

Cleaning Up Spills

It is important to immediately and properly clean up spilled biohazardous or biomedical wastes. These include any body fluids or discharge (blood, urine, feces, sputum, wound drainage, emesis, and items such as used tissues and soiled laundry). Each facility has written protocols and materials for safely cleaning up such spills (Fig. 39-3). Because biohazardous materials are highly contaminated, it is important to

- Wear gloves.
- Follow facility protocols for cleaning and sanitizing the area.
- Dispose of contaminated material and supplies immediately.
- Carefully wash your hands with soap and water.
- Call in specialists to clean up spills on carpeting or upholstery.

Table 41-3 lists typical nursing procedures, with recommendations for decreasing the risk of exposure to bloodborne pathogens.

Disposing of Biohazardous Wastes

After cleaning up a spill, the nurse is responsible for properly disposing of all materials. In addition to spilled body fluids, other biohazardous wastes include soiled dressings, used blood tubes, syringes, catheters, IVs, and certain medications and their packages. Follow your facility protocols. Some items are placed in red "biohazard" bags for disposal (Nursing Care Guidelines 41-2). These bags are handled in a specific manner by housekeeping staff. (Use these bags only for specifically identified materials; disposal is expensive.) Remember to put all sharps, needles, lancets, razor blades or disposable razors, suture removal scissors, scalpel blades, or glass, in the designated "sharps" container. Ask if you have any questions.

The nurse in a community-based setting or in home care is responsible for disposal of biohazardous wastes and for teaching clients and families how to dispose of them as well. Consult agency protocols for specific procedures.

Leaving a Client's Room

When leaving a client's room, take special care not to spread infection.

Keep in mind:

- Use prescribed handwashing techniques, keeping fingertips down, as detailed in Nursing Procedure 41-1.
- Do not touch any part of the sink or faucets with the hands. Use foot or knee controls or automatic electronic controls, as well as a foot-controlled soap dispenser, if possible. Scrub hands thoroughly.
- Use paper towels and discard them appropriately.
- Use a dry towel to turn off faucets.

TABLE 41-2 Antimicrobial Agents

TYPE	MECHANISM	EXAMPLE	USE	CAUTIONS
Antibacterial soap	Lowers surface tension of oil on skin, which holds microorganisms; facilitates removal during rinsing	Dial, Safeguard	Hygiene	Common bar of soap, easily contaminated; use foot pedal.
Detergent	Same as soap, except detergents do not form precipitate with water	Dreft, Tide	Sanitizing eating utensils, laundry	Allergies possible; do not inhale powder.
Alcohol wipes	70% concentration injures protein and lipid structures in inner cellular membrane of some microorganisms	Isopropanol, ethanol	Cleansing skin, instruments	Dries quickly; disinfects as it dries. Must be dry before venipuncture or injection. Not usually used with Accu-Chek for blood sugar.
Alcohol-based hand sanitizers (must be at least 60%–90% alcohol)	Penetrates bacteria cell membrane; denatures it (makes membrane inert—proteins cannot fold properly); strips outer layer of oil off hands, creating inhospitable environment for bacteria. Makes skin surface less hospitable for viruses	Isopropanol alcohol (many brand names—foam, wipes, gel)	Cleansing skin, if no visible soil; does not kill viruses	Use dime-sized dollop; must last 30 s. Do not use if visible soil or fecal matter present. Not substitute for good hand-washing—adjunct only.
Iodine	Damages inner cell membrane of microorganisms; disrupts their enzyme functions; not effective against *Pseudomonas*, a common wound pathogen	Betadine	Cleansing skin	Question client about allergy to shellfish or iodine products.
Chlorine	Interferes with microbial enzyme systems; inhibits some viruses	Bleach, Clorox	Disinfection of surfaces, utensils; blood spills. Some effectiveness against HIV virus	Must be diluted in water for most uses. Do not use on skin or inhale fumes; wear gloves.
Chlorhexidine	Damages inner cell membrane of microorganisms; ineffective against spores and most viruses	Hibiclens	Cleansing skin and equipment	Skin irritation possible.
Mercury	Alters microbial cellular proteins	Merthiolate, Mercurochrome	Disinfecting skin	Must be carefully disposed of, according to agency protocol.
Glutaraldehyde	Inactivates cellular proteins of bacteria, viruses, and microbes that form spores	Cidex	Sterilizing some equipment	Irritating to skin, wear gloves.

Adapted from Timby, B. K. (2005). *Fundamental nursing skills and concepts* (8th ed.). Lippincott Williams & Wilkins.

> **Nursing Alert** All discarded materials used by both nurses and clients are considered contaminated.

Terminal Disinfection

Terminal disinfection refers to cleaning the client unit after the client moves to another room, is discharged, or dies. In acute care facilities, this procedure is usually done by housekeeping personnel, but nurses must understand the underlying principles. The nurse may be required to supervise or teach procedures to other staff or family members or to clean a unit in an emergency. Procedures must be sufficiently thorough to destroy disease-causing organisms. Some organisms are more difficult to destroy than others and some can live up to 6 months on furniture and other surfaces, if these surfaces are not properly cleaned. Terminal disinfection considers all the links in the chain of infection. *It is a vital step in the prevention of HAIs.*

TABLE 41-3 Nursing Activities and Required PPE to Decrease Blood-Borne Pathogen Exposure

PROCEDURE	HANDWASHING	GLOVES	GOWNS	MASK	EYEWEAR
Talking with client					
Hygienic care	■				
Feeding a client	■	■			
Adjusting IV rate or noninvasive equipment	■	■ (preferred)			
Examining client without touching blood, body fluids, or mucous membranes	■				
Examining client with contact to blood, body fluids, or mucous membranes	■	■	Eyewear, if possible to splash		
Drawing blood	■	■	Same as above		
Inserting arterial or venous access devices	■	■	Gown, mask, and eyewear usually required		
Handling soiled waste, linen, or other materials	■	■	Use gown, mask, and eyewear if splattering is likely		
Operative and other procedures that produce extensive splattering of blood or body fluids	■	■	■	■	■
Handling laboratory specimens	■	■	Use gown, mask, and eyewear if splattering is likely		

Nursing Alert Anything that touches the client is contaminated and must be decontaminated or sterilized if used for another client. Most personal care items are discarded. Think before doing any nursing care, to prevent contamination or spreading microorganisms. *One break in technique is all it takes to spread infection!* Remember, good handwashing is vital. *If in doubt, wash your hands!*

CLIENT AND FAMILY TEACHING

Preventing and controlling the spread of infection is a vital part of nursing. However, family caregivers and visitors in healthcare facilities may be unfamiliar with appropriate aseptic techniques. Teach clients, families, and visitors about infection, modes of disease transmission, and methods of prevention. Client teaching includes the following:

- Handwashing technique
- Hygienic practices to reduce pathogenic growth and spread, including use of disinfectants, proper mouth care, and maintenance of skin integrity (prevention of skin breakdown)
- Proper methods of food handling, preparation, and storage
- Aseptic techniques for self-care activities, such as urethral catheterization, medication administration, and wound care
- Proper methods for handling and disposing of contaminated material
- Importance of adequate fluid and food intake and exercise
- Importance of following instructions regarding medications, including taking all of an antibiotic prescription, even if symptoms have improved
- Special procedures or individual precautions
- Remember to document any client/family teaching. (If it is not documented, it is considered not done!)

Be sure to encourage the client and family to ask if they have questions.

STUDENT SYNTHESIS
KEY POINTS

- Standard Precautions assume that every client's blood and body fluids are potentially infectious; thus, Standard Precautions are used in care of all clients.
- Healthcare-associated infections are those acquired by clients in the healthcare facility.
- Clients are more susceptible to infections in healthcare facilities, because their resistance to disease is often lowered, and facilities house many pathogens.
- Medical asepsis helps lower the number of microorganisms in the environment and reduces their transmission.

- Handwashing is the single most important measure to prevent disease spread.
- Commonly used protective barriers include gloves, eye protection, gowns, and masks.
- Keeping a clean and controlled environment is essential in maintaining medical asepsis.
- Antimicrobial agents, such as antiseptics and disinfectants, limit and destroy pathogens.
- Following proper methods of leaving a client's room; use of proper handwashing technique; use of PPE; and terminal disinfection help prevent the spread of microorganisms.
- Teaching aseptic practices to clients, families, and visitors is essential for protection against disease, particularly because clients often leave the healthcare facility before they are completely well.

CRITICAL THINKING EXERCISES

1. Discuss possible differences and similarities in practicing medical asepsis in the healthcare facility, the clinic, and the client's home.
2. Review steps in the chain of infection. Describe the role of medical asepsis in interrupting this chain.
3. Discuss why clients in healthcare facilities are more likely to contract infections than people in the community. Give reasons.
4. Develop a teaching plan for clients and other nurses regarding asepsis in home care.

NCLEX-STYLE REVIEW QUESTIONS

1. The nurse is preparing to irrigate a draining wound. Which personal protective equipment should be donned because of a risk for splashing? Select all that apply.
   a. Shoe protectors
   b. Particulate filter mask
   c. Face shield
   d. Gloves
   e. Mask

2. Which observation made by the charge nurse requires that the LVN/LPN receive further education?
   a. Recapping a needle after injecting a client.
   b. Placing the safety lock on the needle after injecting a client.
   c. Washing their hands after injecting a client with medication.
   d. Placing a syringe and needle in the sharps container.

3. A nurse is providing care to a client when the client's IV becomes dislodged and blood splatters in the nurse's eye. After using the eyewash, which is the next appropriate action?
   a. Call the physician to see if another IV should be started.
   b. Report the incident to the supervisor.
   c. Apply Neosporin ophthalmic ointment.
   d. No further action is required at this time.

4. The nurse observes the CNA provide assistance to a client. Which observation made by the nurse regarding the care administered by the CNA requires intervention?
   a. Wearing gloves when providing perineal care.
   b. Cleaning a water spill from the floor.
   c. Wiping the bedside table with antimicrobial wipes.
   d. Placing linens on the floor after taking them off of the bed.

5. The nurse is providing care to a group of clients. Which priority action by the nurse can help decrease the spread of infection to this client group?
   a. Have the client wear a mask whenever care is delivered.
   b. Administer prophylactic antibiotics to all clients.
   c. Wash hands when entering and leaving client rooms.
   d. Wear gloves whenever delivering client care.

CHAPTER RESOURCES

Enhance your learning with additional resources on thePoint!

Student Resources related to this chapter can be found at thePoint.lww.com/Rosdahl12e.

CHAPTER 41 Medical Asepsis 505

Welcome Steps

Look at healthcare provider's orders.

Protocol for procedure.

Necessary equipment/ supplies.

Wash hands using proper hand hygiene; put on gloves.

Explain the procedure and reassure the client.

Locate two identifiers to confirm correct client.

Comfortable and efficient position for nurse and client.

Obtain privacy.

Make sure to follow correct steps and body mechanics with good technique.

Ensure safety and observe deviations from normal.

End Steps

Ensure comfort and safety.

Note questions or concerns from client or nurse; note significant data.

Dispose of materials properly.

Disinfect the area and your hands.

Document and report the procedure and your findings.

IN PRACTICE
NURSING PROCEDURE 41-1 — Handwashing

Supplies and Equipment
Liquid soap, with foot pedal
Paper towels

Steps

1. Remove jewelry. A plain wedding band may remain in place. *Rationale: Rough places or prongs in jewelry can harbor microorganisms.*

2. Stand in front of sink; avoid leaning against it. *Rationale: This avoids transfer of contamination from sink to nurse's uniform.*

3. Turn on water and regulate its flow and temperature. Knee or foot pedals are most appropriate and safest. In some facilities, water automatically flows when placing hands under the faucet. *Rationale: Controlling the force of flow limits splashing. Warm water is more comfortable and less irritating to the skin. It is much safer not to touch faucet handles.*

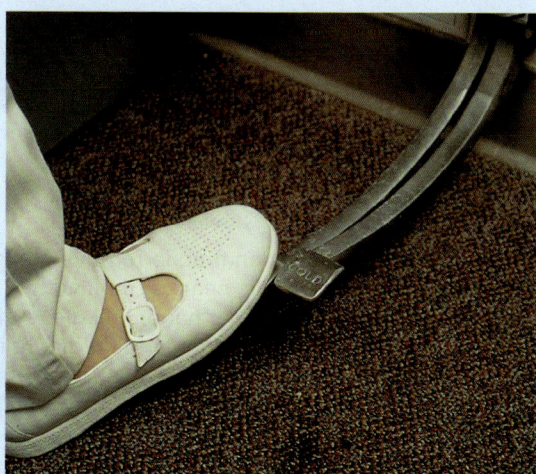

Use of a foot control eliminates the need for the nurse to touch contaminated sink faucets. (Timby, 2005.)

4. Wet hands and forearms with water, keeping hands lower than elbows. *Rationale: This allows water to flow from least contaminated area toward the hands, which are the most contaminated area.*

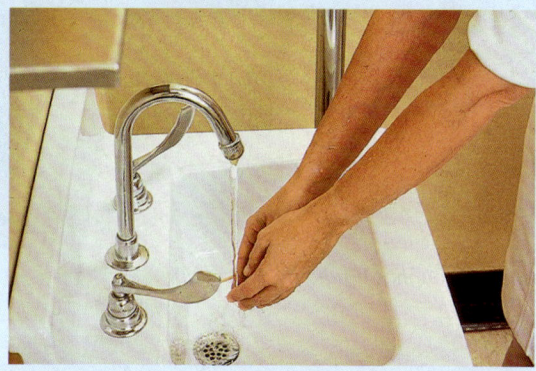

Wetting hands, keeping the most contaminated area lower. (Photo by B. Proud.)

5. Apply antibacterial liquid soap. If you must press a lever to dispense soap, do so with a paper towel. Liquid soap with foot- or knee-operated dispenser is the most sanitary. *Rationale: The dispenser may be contaminated. Using a paper towel or foot-operated dispenser is important, to prevent further contamination.*

6. Wash your hands, wrists, and lower forearms for a minimum of 20 s (about the length of time it takes to sing "Happy Birthday twice"), using a scrubbing motion. Interlace fingers and rub back and forth. *Rationale: Friction loosens dirt and bacteria on all surfaces.*

506 UNIT 7 Safety in the Healthcare Facility

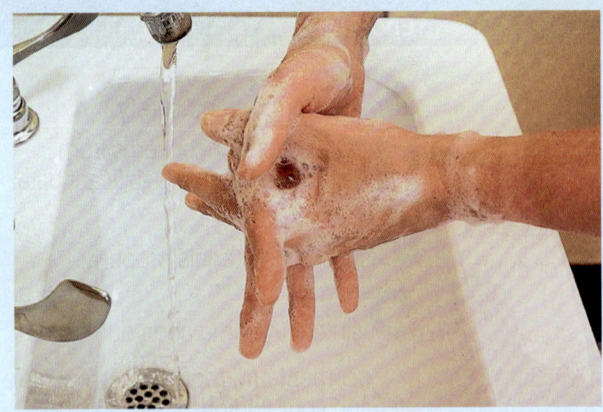

Using scrubbing motion to wash hands. (Photo by B. Proud.)

7. Insert fingernails from one hand under those of the other hand, using a sweeping motion to clean them or use a disposable brush. Repeat with other hand. *Rationale: Bacteria accumulate under fingernails.*

8. Rinse thoroughly for at least 10 s, keeping hands lower than forearms. *Rationale: Keeping hands lower than forearms prevents soap lather from recontaminating clean areas.*

9. Repeat procedure if hands are very soiled. *Rationale: This ensures a thorough cleaning.*

10. Dry hands thoroughly with a paper towel. Discard towel. *Rationale: Drying thoroughly prevents chapping. Using paper towels helps prevent spread of microorganisms.*

11. Use the foot pedal or a clean paper towel to turn off faucets. *Rationale: A dry, clean towel prevents recontamination of hands with organisms on faucets and helps keep faucets clean. A wet towel would allow passage of microorganisms back to the hands.*

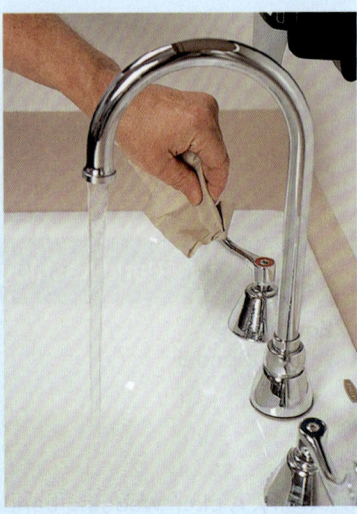

Using a clean paper towel to turn off faucets. (Photo by B. Proud.)

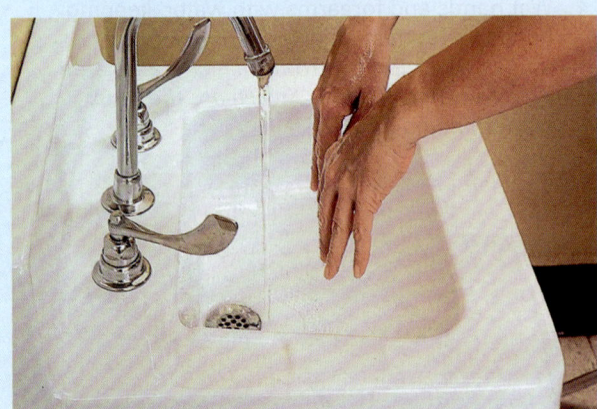

Rinsing thoroughly. (Photo by B. Proud.)

IN PRACTICE
NURSING PROCEDURE 41-2 — Using Clean (Nonsterile) Gloves

Supplies and Equipment
Appropriate-sized gloves

Donning Gloves

1. Wash hands and dry thoroughly. *Rationale: The nurse's hands must be as clean as possible. Gloves may be sticky if hands are damp.*

2. Choose correct size glove. *Rationale: Gloves must fit properly to be effective and comfortable.*

3. Bunch one glove up and pull onto hand; ease fingers into glove. Repeat for other hand. Adjust from the outside, not the cuff. *Rationale: Bunching up allows for ease in pulling gloves on.*

Removing and Disposing of Gloves

1. Wash hands with gloves on first. To remove gloves, grasp *outside* of one glove, near the cuff, with thumb and forefinger of other hand. Pull glove off, turning it inside out while pulling and holding it in the hand that is still gloved. *Rationale: Remove as much contamination as possible before removing gloves. Turning the glove inside out during removal confines contamination to the gloves.*

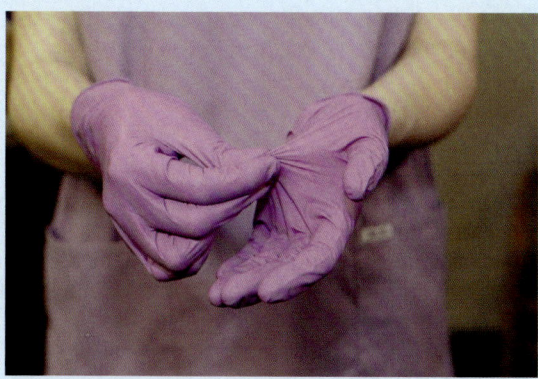

Removing first glove (glove to glove). (Carter, 2012.)

2. Hook bare thumb or finger inside other glove and pull it off, turning it inside out and over the already-removed glove. **Rationale:** *Hooking the finger on the inside of the other glove prevents contamination of ungloved hand, while confining contamination to the gloves.*

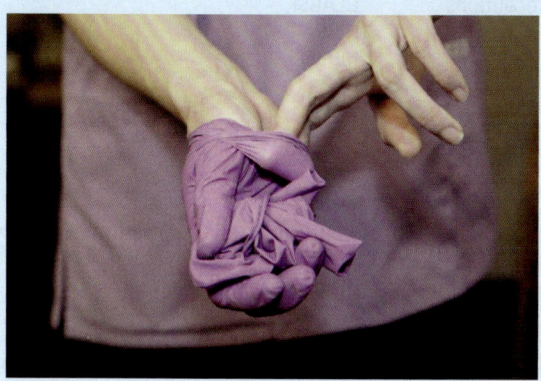

Pulling off second glove (skin to skin). (Carter, 2012.)

3. Roll the two gloves together, with the side that was nearest nurse's hands on outside. The side of glove that touched the client was contaminated to the client. The inside of glove that touched the nurse's hand is considered clean, but not sterile, because it touched the nurse's hands. **Rationale:** *This action confines contamination by covering the glove surface that came into contact with the client with the glove surface that was in contact with the nurse's clean hands.*

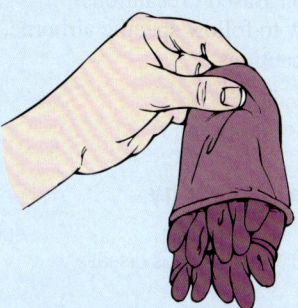

Roll the two gloves together.

1. Drop gloves into appropriate waste receptacle. **Rationale:** *Proper disposal assists in preventing the spread of infection.*
2. Wash hands again. **Rationale:** *Handwashing further assists in preventing the spread of infection.*

IN PRACTICE
NURSING PROCEDURE 41-3 Using a Mask

Supplies and Equipment
Mask in container

Putting on a Mask

1. Wash hands. **Rationale:** *The nurse's hands must be clean, to prevent contaminating the mask.*
2. Remove mask from container or package, handling it as little as possible and by strings only. **Rationale:** *Too much handling will reduce the mask's efficiency to screen out microorganisms.*
3. Place mask so it completely covers your mouth and nose. Bend strip at the top of mask so it fits tightly around nose. **Rationale:** *Mouth and nose must be completely covered to prevent transfer of microorganisms. If nurse wears glasses and the strip is not tight over the bridge of nose, glasses will fog.*
4. To tie mask, loop top ties over ears and tie under your chin in a bow, not a knot. **Rationale:** *Tying is necessary to secure mask in place; a bow is easiest to untie. It is difficult to safely remove mask if both strings are tied behind the head.*
5. Tie bottom ties behind the neck in a bow. **Rationale:** *By tying mask in this manner, only one bow needs to be untied to take off the mask. In addition, if top bow is tied behind your head, it may slip down and cause mask to fall off.*
6. Change mask if it becomes damp. **Rationale:** *A moist mask harbors and transmits organisms.*

Removing a Mask

1. To remove mask, untie the tie behind neck. Touch mask by strings only. Be careful not to let mask drop onto your clothes. **Rationale:** *The mask is now considered contaminated.*
2. Discard mask in proper receptacle. **Rationale:** *Proper disposal helps prevent infection spread.*
3. Wash hands. **Rationale:** *Handwashing after mask removal further helps prevent spread of infection.*

42 Infection Control

Learning Objectives

1. Explain the relationship between Standard Precautions (Tier 1) and Transmission-Based Precautions/Isolation (Tier 2), as related to infection control.
2. Explain the purpose, use, and components of Transmission-Based Precautions.
3. Identify how to follow specific airborne, droplet, and contact precautions.
4. Describe how to set up a client's room for isolation, including appropriate barrier techniques.
5. Demonstrate precautions to take during medication administration, vital sign monitoring, and transport of a client who is potentially infectious.
6. Explain what is meant by protective (neutropenic/reverse) isolation.

Important Terminology

airborne precautions
colonization
contact precautions
droplet precautions
infection
infectious disease
isolation
neutropenic isolation
protective isolation
special respiratory precautions (special respiratory isolation)
Transmission-Based Precautions

Acronyms

BBP
CAUTI
CLABSI
HICPAC
MDRO
PRP
VAE
VRE

The risks to clients of healthcare-associated infections were presented in Chapters 40 and 41, as have the risks of infection for healthcare workers. An **infection** is described as an invasion and multiplication of pathogenic organisms in body tissues, particularly those causing injury to the host. The chain of infection was introduced in Chapter 40. An **infectious disease** occurs if the chain of infection remains intact; it is not interrupted. The goal of all healthcare is to *break this chain of infection*.

Today, a number of organisms are developing resistance to antibiotics, and new organisms are surfacing. Sometimes there is a need for measures in addition to Standard Precautions, as presented in Chapter 41. This chapter discusses *special precautions and isolation procedures*.

INFECTION CONTROL

The best method of infection control is prevention, successful only when the chain of infection is successfully broken. A number of methods accomplish this, including Standard Precautions, as discussed in Chapter 41. The Joint Commission requires healthcare facilities to have an effective infection control plan in order to qualify for accreditation. The plan must include these elements:

- An infection control committee
- Surveillance and reporting of healthcare-associated infections
- An employee health program
- Isolation policies and procedures
- Infection control in-service education for employees
- Procedures for environmental sanitation and waste disposal
- An available microbiology laboratory

The Centers for Disease Control and Prevention (CDC) and Hospital Infection Control Practices Advisory Committee (**HICPAC**) continually update the guidelines for isolation precautions in healthcare facilities, in an attempt to reduce the risk of transmission of pathogens. The guidelines include two tiers of precautions. The first and most important are Standard Precautions, designed for the care of *all clients, regardless of diagnosis or infection status* (Chapter 41). The second tier of precautions, Transmission-Based Precautions, is designed for clients with specific infections or diagnoses and is discussed in this chapter.

The Infection Control Committee

As described in Chapter 41, each accredited healthcare facility must have an infection control committee that monitors and evaluates any infection occurring in the facility. If a break in technique is identified, the committee will determine alternate procedures, develop new protocols, evaluate their effectiveness, and plan related in-service education. This committee will also maintain statistics related to infections, report to governmental agencies, identify antimicrobial-resistant organisms, evaluate new products related to infection control, and assist in employee health and wellness programs.

Standard Precautions

As described in Chapter 41, Standard Precautions have been developed to reduce the risk of transmitting blood-borne pathogens (**BBP**) and those from moist body substances.

These precautions apply to blood; all body fluids, secretions, and excretions (except sweat); nonintact skin; and mucous membranes. They are designed to reduce the risk of pathogen transmission from *both known and unknown* sources of infection.

The Occupational Safety and Health Administration (OSHA) has implemented standards for client care. These standards require and enforce the implementation of policies, procedures, and control measures that will prevent employee exposure to blood and/or body fluids of clients (Standard Precautions). Violations of Standard Precautions carry a severe fine to the healthcare facility. OSHA regulations require that healthcare employers must

- develop an infection control policy, conforming to OSHA guidelines, that identifies when personal protective equipment (PPE) is required, how to clean up spills of blood or body fluids, how to take or send laboratory specimens, and how to dispose of infectious waste.
- educate staff about the policies.
- provide free hepatitis B immunizations to staff who might be exposed to blood or body fluids.
- provide follow-up care to staff members who are accidentally exposed to splashes of blood or body fluids or needlesticks.
- supply rapidly accessible PPE.
- provide proper sharps disposal containers and replace them regularly.

Standard Precautions stress the use of handwashing and PPE to protect against contracting diseases. You must report unusual exposure to potential infection (e.g., a needlestick or body fluid splash into your eyes) immediately. OSHA requires initial screening and follow-up care.

> **Key Concept**
>
> In most cities, blood and body fluids can be flushed down the client's toilet or a central hopper. Most sewage treatment systems are able to decontaminate this material. Protective gear against splashing must be worn when emptying these materials. If the amount of fluid or tissue is too large or bulky to be flushed, it must be bagged in a red biohazard bag and placed in the identified biohazard container (Fig. 41-3).
>
> Cleaning up spills of biohazardous materials requires special supplies and equipment (see Fig. 39-3 and facility protocols).
>
> Handling of materials and equipment, such as suction containers, chest tubes, blood infusion fluids, or dialysis fluids, requires specific in-service education.
>
> Cytotoxic wastes (e.g., materials used in cancer chemotherapy or body fluids of these clients) require special handling and disposal, and their staff and family caregivers also require specific in-service education.

Transmission-Based Precautions

Standard Precautions are used when caring for all clients. **Transmission-Based Precautions** are implemented when caring for clients with a suspected or known infectious disease. Specific precautions are based on the disease's route of transmission. Transmission-Based Precautions are designed to interrupt the transmission of epidemiologically important pathogens, to break the "chain of infection." Specific barrier methods are employed for either the client and/or healthcare worker. These precautions are grouped into three categories: *airborne, droplet,* and *contact precautions.* When treating clients who require any of these precautions, they are used *in addition to Standard Precautions.* Table 42-1 presents an overview of Transmission-Based Precautions and the types of diseases for which they are used.

> **Key Concept**
>
> - Standard Precautions—Treat blood and all body fluids (except sweat) from all clients as infectious.
> - Transmission-Based Precautions—Use barrier precautions for clients with suspected or diagnosed infections.
> - The combination of Standard Precautions and Transmission-Based Precautions minimizes the risk of exposure from known infectious agents, as well as undiagnosed infectious agents.
> - Special situations—Use PPE as needed (e.g., for a violent client who spits or bites). Goggles or a face shield are often recommended (Figs. 41-2 and 42-1).
> - In some cases, reverse (protective) isolation is needed, to protect the client.
> - All isolation rooms have a sign posted outside the door alerting staff and visitors that this client is being isolated (Fig. 42-2).

Airborne Precautions

Airborne transmission occurs when microorganisms from evaporated droplets remain suspended in the air or are carried on dust particles. Air currents disperse the microorganisms, which a susceptible host can easily inhale. Special air handling and ventilation are required to prevent this type of disease transmission. Tuberculosis (TB), measles, and chickenpox are examples of airborne-transmitted infections.

Clients requiring **airborne precautions** are placed in a private room with special, monitored air flow requirements (Table 42-1). The facility may have a special portable air-filtering machine for use in this situation. The door to the room is kept closed and nurses caring for this client must wear a mask.

Special Respiratory Precautions

Clients are screened for tuberculosis (TB) on admission to the facility (Chapter 47). Because of the recent resurgence of TB and other conditions that can transmit infection over long distances, healthcare facilities require **special respiratory precautions** (SRP) or special respiratory isolation (SRI) as protection for healthcare staff and visitors, if the client is still considered communicable. *Personal respiratory protection* (**PRP**) in this case consists of a special *high-filtration particulate respirator* (N95 or HEPA-filtered) (Fig. 41-3) or a *powered (positive) air-purified respirator* (PAPR), as per CDC recommendations. The N95 respirator is fitted to the individual nurse. It fits the face more tightly than does the typical surgical mask and can filter out 95% of particulates (0.3 μm or larger) in the air, providing the mask is fitted properly. The PAPR covers the head and face and incorporates a blower to remove contaminated

TABLE 42-1 Transmission-Based Precautions

CLIENT PLACEMENT	PROTECTION	EXAMPLES OF DISEASES
Airborne[a]		
• Private room • Negative air flow pressure[b] • Discharge of room air to environment or filtered before circulation	• Follow Standard Precautions • Confine client to room • Wear mask or particulate air filter respirator (N95 or higher level respirator for healthcare personnel) • Client wears a mask if transport required • Keep door closed	• Pulmonary tuberculosis • Measles (rubeola) • Chickenpox (varicella) • SARS • Smallpox (variola), COVID-19, and SARS require both airborne and contact precautions • EVD
Droplet[a]		
• Private room or room with similarly infected client(s) preferred • If no private room, use one in which there is at least 3 ft between other client(s) and visitors	• Follow Standard Precautions • Wear a mask when entering the room, but especially when within 3 ft of infected client • Place mask on client if transport is required • Door may be open or closed	• Influenza • Measles (rubella) • Mumps (epidemic/infectious parotitis) • Meningococcal meningitis • Streptococcal pneumonia/pharyngitis • Whooping cough (pertussis) • Chickenpox (varicella) • EVD
Contact[a]		
• Private room or room with similarly infected client(s), or • Consult with infection control professional if above options are unavailable	• Follow Standard Precautions • Don gloves before entering room • Mask may be required • Remove gloves before leaving room • Change gloves during care, after contact with any infective material • Perform hand sanitization immediately after removing gloves • Do not touch potentially contaminated surfaces or client after removing gloves and sanitizing hands • Wear gown when entering room, if you or your clothing will touch client or items in the room • Wear gown if client is incontinent, has diarrhea, has underwent an ileostomy, has underwent colostomy, or has wound drainage not totally contained by dressing • Remove gown before leaving room • Avoid transporting client; if required, use special precautions • Clean bedside equipment and client care items daily • Use items such as stethoscope, blood pressure apparatus, and other assessment tools exclusively for infected client and terminally disinfect when precautions are no longer necessary • Door may be open or closed	• Gastrointestinal, respiratory, skin, or wound infections, especially those that are drug-resistant (including PRSP and CRKP) • Any draining wound • MRSA • Acute diarrhea/gastroenteritis • Draining abscess • Impetigo or scabies • Pediculosis • VRE • Herpes simplex virus • Gas gangrene • Acute viral conjunctivitis • Hepatitis A • Smallpox and SARS require both airborne and contact isolation • EVD

CRKP, carbapenem-resistant *Klebsiella pneumoniae*; PAPR, powered (positive) air-purifying respirator; PRSP, penicillin-resistant *Streptococcus pneumoniae*; SARS, severe acute respiratory syndrome; VRE, vancomycin-resistant enterococcus—often *Clostridium difficile*.
[a]Special precautions are used in EVD (Ebola virus disease). They involve combinations of the above isolation procedures and are being perfected at the time of this writing (CDC, 2019).
[b]Negative air pressure (with 6–12 air changes per hour) pulls air from the hall into the room when the door is opened, as opposed to positive air pressure, which pulls room air into the hall. Room air is exhausted to outside of building or is specially filtered. Daily monitoring is required.
Adapted from Garner & HICPAC, 2001; Timby and Smith, 2018; Centers for Disease Control and Prevention, 2019.

air, which is replaced with purified air. This device is used when an adequate fit cannot be obtained with the N95 respirator (e.g., the nurse with facial hair or injury) and can also be used for victims exposed to hazardous chemicals or materials of terrorism. These devices provide the greatest respiratory protection available. The client with special respiratory precautions must be assigned to a room with the same air-filtering equipment and nursing procedures as in airborne precautions. In-service education is usually required for nurses.

Key Concept

A high-filtration particulate respirator must be discarded at the end of the shift, and also if it

- becomes contaminated with body fluids
- has a damaged filter
- loses its shape
- becomes difficult to breathe through
- cannot maintain the face seal

CHAPTER 42 Infection Control   511

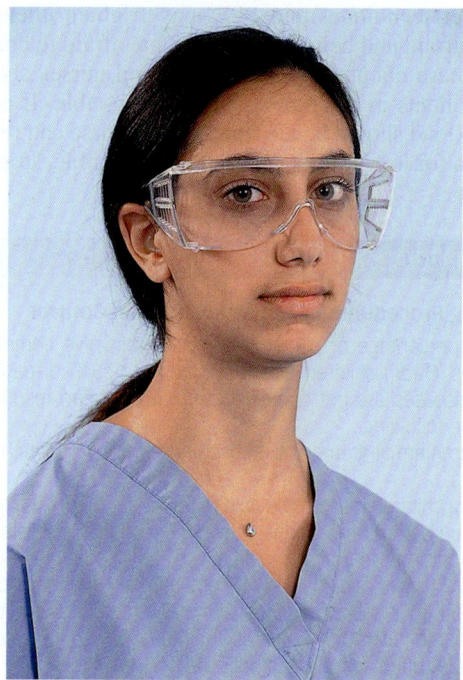

Figure 42-1 Protective eyewear is worn to protect the mucous membranes of the nurse's eyes from accidental splashing of clients' body fluids. (Photo by B. Proud.)

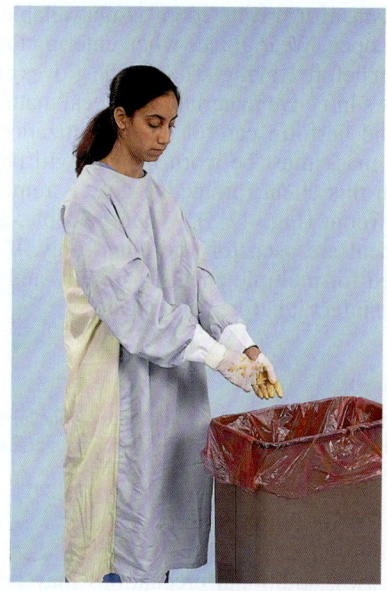

Figure 42-3 When using personal protective equipment (PPE), the nurse removes and disposes of the most contaminated items first. Gloves are removed before the gown. (Photo by B. Proud.)

Most facilities also require all direct client care staff to have either a negative purified protein derivative (PPD—"Mantoux test"; TST—tuberculin skin test) or negative blood testing and system survey, including a chest x-ray, when they are hired and yearly.

Droplet Precautions

Droplet transmission occurs when droplets containing microorganisms are propelled through the air from an infected person and deposited on another person's eyes, nose, or mouth. Transmission can occur through sneezing, coughing, talking, or during certain procedures such as suctioning or bronchoscopy. Examples of illnesses spread by droplets include meningococcal meningitis, streptococcal pharyngitis (in infants and young children), pertussis, influenza, mumps, and rubella. Airborne precautions are not effective in these clients because the droplets do not remain suspended in the air.

A client requiring **droplet precautions** is placed in a private room. However, if a private room is unavailable, they can share a room with another client with the same infectious disease. The room's door may remain open. Wear a mask when working within 3 ft of the client. The client must wear a mask if they are transported outside the room.

Contact Precautions

Contact transmission is the most frequent mode of disease transmission in healthcare. Transmission can occur as a result of *direct contact* between a susceptible host's body surface and an infected or colonized person. (**Colonization** occurs when a microorganism is present in a client, but they show no clinical signs or symptoms of infection.) *Indirect contact* occurs when a susceptible host comes into contact with an intermediate contaminated object (e.g., dirty instrument, needle, or hands). Examples of illnesses spread by contact transmission include gastroenteritis and respiratory, skin, and wound infections, as well as hepatitis A, herpes simplex virus, impetigo, scabies, and pediculosis (infestation with lice). Precautions are particularly important in cases caused by drug-resistant organisms, such as MRSA or VRE.

A client who requires **contact precautions** can be placed in a room with other clients who are infected with the same

---

Visitors—Report to Nurses' Station Before Entering Room

1. Masks are indicated for all persons entering room.
2. Gowns are indicated for all persons entering room.
3. Gloves are indicated for all persons entering room.
4. HANDS MUST BE WASHED AFTER TOUCHING THE PATIENT OR POTENTIALLY CONTAMINATED ARTICLES AND BEFORE TAKING CARE OF ANOTHER PATIENT.
5. Articles contaminated with infective material should be discarded or bagged and labeled before being sent for decontamination and reprocessing.

Figure 42-2 An instructional card is placed on the door of the room of a client in isolation. Wraparound gowns that do not require ties are available. (Timby, 2005.)

microorganism, if a private room is unavailable. The door may remain open. Wear gloves when entering the room and remove them before leaving. Change the gloves after contact with a client's infective material (e.g., fecal matter or wound drainage) and perform careful hand sanitization. A gown, gloves, and mask must be worn if there will be any direct contact with this client; protective gear is removed before leaving the room (Fig. 42-3). When possible, all supplies and equipment are used for one client only. If equipment must be used for multiple clients, carefully and thoroughly clean and disinfect it before using again.

> **Key Concept**
>
> Certain infectious diseases such as chickenpox (varicella), smallpox (variola), and SARS require both airborne and contact precautions.

Additional Transmission-Based Precautions

In special cases, additional precautions may be necessary. The infection control committee will usually be involved in making this decision and determining what precautions are needed. In-service education is required before caring for these clients. Each healthcare organization has specific local protocols for clients requiring additional Transmission-Based Precautions.

ISOLATION

Standard Precautions and Transmission-Based Precautions are the currently followed isolation guidelines. Historically, other systems were used; some facilities may use these, in addition to Standard and Transmission-Based Precautions. In *category-specific isolation*, specific types of isolation are based on the client's diagnosis (e.g., respiratory, contact, enteric, wound). Color-coded cards are posted outside the client's room; visitors must check with nurses before entering. *Disease-specific isolation* uses a single all-purpose sign. Nurses select the items on the card appropriate for the client's specific disease.

Nursing Measures in Isolation

Setting Up a Client's Room for Isolation

Clients who require isolation usually are confined to their rooms. The goal is to protect other clients, staff, and visitors and to restrict contamination only to the client's immediate environment. This also facilitates concurrent and terminal disinfection. All healthcare facilities have specific protocols for isolation and designate the use of specific PPE. These protocols also identify specific measures if the client needs to be taken out of the room for a treatment or test.

Education and Preparation

When setting up the isolation room, explain the precautions to the client and family. If they understand reasons for preventive procedures, they will be more likely to cooperate and not to break technique. Children are often not allowed to visit a client in isolation; children are susceptible to infection and may not be able to follow the specific instructions.

Barrier techniques and PPE may frighten clients, who may be afraid and believe that others are afraid to come near them. These clients are often lonely and nurses should try to visit clients in isolation as much as possible. If possible, the workload should be arranged, so the nurse can remain in the room for longer periods. Whenever possible, stop by and say hello.

SPECIAL CONSIDERATIONS   Lifespan

Nursing Procedures in Pediatric Infection Control

A high percentage of pediatric admissions involve communicable diseases. Often, children are not immune to such diseases and if these diseases are not contained, an outbreak can result. Keep in mind the following:

- Children are at greater risk of acquiring viral infections than are adults.
- Young children may not be able to understand good handwashing and barrier precautions; they require adult supervision.
- Environmental surfaces must be as clean as possible because children may have physical and oral contact with them. Children also put toys and other objects into their mouths. Some toys may be shared in facility playrooms; they must have cleanable surfaces. (Stuffed animals and dolls are not permitted in the facility because they cannot be adequately disinfected.) In some cases, books and magazines are also not permitted.
- Barrier techniques are important to employees who care for children because children require close contact (e.g., rocking, cuddling, and feeding).

> **Nursing Alert**   If you will be working with children, determine your immune status regarding childhood communicable diseases; you may require immunization (Chapter 72). Some isolation procedures may be slightly different in pediatrics.

Supplies for Isolation

The client's room is equipped with standard supplies and equipment and personal items needed by the client. (Disposal of these items is usually necessary on the client's discharge.) Provide a telephone and television, if possible. Additional items include paper towels; plastic or coated paper bags for trash disposal; washable blankets and bedspreads; and impervious laundry bags, as well as the usual linens needed for a client unit. (Pillows are usually discarded on discharge and/or as needed.) The room should have a sink with foot or knee control and a covered linen bag and stand; this client should have a private bathroom and shower.

Items to place outside the client's room or in an anteroom include a bedside stand or cabinet stocked with PPE, as required for the client's condition. A sink should be available or nearby for handwashing, as well as hand sanitization materials. Other items include clean laundry bags, large trash bags, biohazard bags, a sharps container, and tape or tags and marking pens for marking contaminated bags. Healthcare facilities require a sign for the door; the sign will vary depending on the specific precautions being followed.

Administering Medications in Isolation

Follow Standard Precautions when administering medications. Use and dispose of materials in the client's room. General pointers for medication administration include the following:

- Unwrap medications, but take the packages with you into the client's room.
- If you will need juice or applesauce in which to mix medications, take it with you into the room. If using a medication tray, be sure it is disposable.
- Do not take scanners or original MARs (medication administration records) into the client's room. Scan the medications outside the room and (if allowed) enter them as "given," after leaving the room. Print out a copy of the MAR, take it into the client's room to use for reference, and dispose of it there after giving the medications.
- If you are not going to touch the client or any item in the room, you may only need to wear gloves and a mask. Be sure to scrub carefully on leaving the room.
- If giving an injection, wear gloves (per Standard Precautions). Wear other PPE as per protocol. Place needles and syringes into the sharps container in the room. Avoid accidental needlesticks; use a safety syringe or needle cap and the sharps container (Figs. 64-3 and 64-4A and B).
- Use disposable medication cups.
- Use and discard intravenous (IV) solution bags in the client's room.
- Generally, glass items are not used in isolation. If they must be used, dispose of small items in the sharps container and larger items in a separate bag, clearly marked "glass." This must be double-bagged out of the room (see discussion later).
- Dispose of all materials in the client's room. The trash and laundry will be double-bagged out of the room and properly handled by the facility's housekeeping department.

Sending a Specimen to the Laboratory

Before collecting a specimen, label the container. After collection, place the container on a clean paper towel in the anteroom. Remove gloves and do a thorough handwash. Put on clean gloves and carefully scrub the outside of the container and place the specimen into a sealable biohazard bag (see illustration in Nursing Care Guidelines 41-2). (It may also be necessary to inform laboratory personnel of specific suspected microorganisms, such as MRSA or VRE.) Wash your hands again. In some cases, the specimen must be double-bagged. Make sure the laboratory receives the specimen as soon as possible. Remember to touch the request cards or sheets and the outside of the bag only with clean hands.

Taking Vital Signs

Necessary equipment for vital signs should be kept in the client's room; it is thoroughly disinfected when the client is no longer infectious or is discharged. When taking vital signs of a client in isolation:

- Use the equipment in the room.
- Wear gloves and whatever other PPE is indicated.
- Usually there is a clock on the wall, so you do not need a watch. If you must bring a watch, place it on a paper towel and touch only the bottom of the towel with contaminated hands, or seal the watch in a plastic bag. Open the bag on leaving the room. Pick up the watch or take it out of the bag after you have scrubbed outside the room.
- Use disposable thermometers, cuffs, and stethoscopes, if available. Many facilities use temperature indicator dots or other disposable systems for measuring temperature. A blood pressure apparatus is usually on the wall. The cuff and stethoscope are disinfected or discarded when the client is discharged.

> **Nursing Alert** If a drug-resistant organism such as VRE or MRSA is present, all equipment remains in the isolated client's room.

- If checking the client's blood sugar, use the client's own machine or obtain a separate machine to be used while that client is in isolation. When the client comes out of isolation, the machine must be thoroughly disinfected.

Using Double-Bagging

Although refuse and linen from all clients are considered contaminated, in some types of isolation, these items are "double-bagged" out of the room. Two nurses must carry out the procedure. The nurse inside the room is considered "contaminated"; the nurse outside is considered "clean." Both nurses wear gloves and, if specified, gowns and/or masks. The contaminated nurse places dirty items into a bag and closes the top. This entire bag, inside and out, is "contaminated." The clean nurse, outside the room, has a second bag that is considered "clean." The top of the clean bag is folded down on the outside to make a cuff. The clean nurse keeps the hands protected by this cuff. The contaminated nurse then places the contaminated bag inside the clean bag, while the clean nurse holds the clean bag (Fig. 42-4).

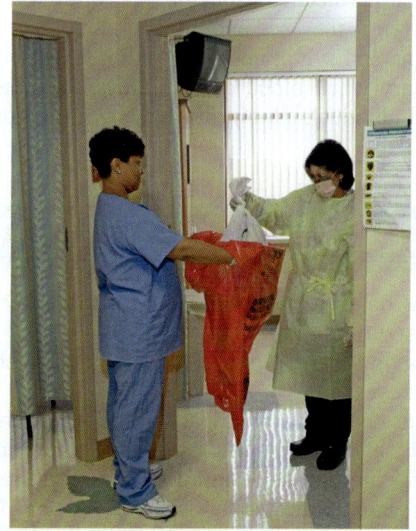

Figure 42-4 Double-bagging laundry out of an isolation room. The nurse in blue is considered to be the "clean" nurse. The "contaminated" nurse in the room wears gown, gloves, and a mask. (Carter, 2005.)

The contaminated nurse touches only the *inside* of the clean bag; the clean nurse touches only the *outside* of the clean bag and does not touch the contaminated bag. The clean nurse folds over the top of the clean bag, seals it carefully, and labels it, touching only the outside of the bag. After this is completed, both nurses wash their hands thoroughly.

Transporting the Client to Other Departments

In rare cases, transporting the client to a new room or for a special procedure or x-ray is necessary. Follow these precautions when transporting an isolated client to another area:

- Wear PPE as needed.
- The client must also wear appropriate PPE.
- Control and contain any drainage.
- Drape the wheelchair or stretcher with a clean sheet or bath blanket. Wrap the client with the clean material. (The inside is now considered contaminated.)
- Escort the ambulatory client to any other area.
- Notify the other department, so personnel there can prepare and perform accordingly.
- Carefully disinfect the wheelchair or stretcher after use.

Caring for the Client's Body After Death

If a client in isolation dies, special precautions are necessary, to prevent the spread of infection. Follow facility protocols. Many healthcare facilities follow these precautions for all clients who die. In Practice: Nursing Care Guidelines 42-1 describes care of the body of the person who was in isolation.

Protective (Reverse or Neutropenic) Isolation

Sometimes, the client must be protected from the outside environment. In this case, isolation procedures are reversed: other people's microorganisms are kept away from the client. This **protective**, reverse, or **neutropenic isolation** attempts to keep harmful microorganisms away from the client. Box 42-1 lists general procedures in protective isolation.

Clients in protective isolation are often immunosuppressed. Even if they become infected, they may not show classic signs and symptoms of infection because they lack the necessary white blood cells to create an inflammatory response. Individuals placed in protective isolation include those who have experienced burns or bone marrow transplants. Clients with AIDS, who are undergoing chemotherapy, who have received large doses of corticosteroids, or who are experiencing low resistance from another cause (e.g., agammaglobulinemia), may also require protective isolation.

ANTIBIOTIC-RESISTANT ORGANISMS AND SPECIAL INFECTIONS

A number of antimicrobial-resistant organisms have emerged. As stated, the two most common are MRSA and VRE. Other multidrug-resistant organisms (**MDRO**) also exist

---

Box 42-1　General Procedures in Protective/Neutropenic Isolation

- The client requires a private room or total neutropenic unit, such as a burn unit.
- Healthcare workers and visitors may not enter if they have a cold, influenza, or other communicable disease.
- Anyone entering the room must wear a mask and practice strict handwashing before coming into contact with the client. In some cases, such as in the burn unit, all staff and visitors may be required to wear gowns and gloves.
- The client cannot receive fresh fruit, vegetables, or flowers.
- Rectal temperatures, enemas, suppositories, intravenous and intramuscular injections, and other invasive procedures are to be avoided, if possible.
- The tympanic ear probe or forehead sensor is used to monitor the client's temperature, which is done at least every 4 hr.
- A blood culture is done if any reason exists to suspect infection.
- In most cases, sterile linens and specially laundered scrub suits and shoe covers are used. Some facilities require special hair covering. Staff members working in these units often wear laboratory coats when leaving the units.
- Special air purification measures are used.

IN PRACTICE
NURSING CARE GUIDELINES 42-1　Caring for the Body of a Deceased Person Who Was in Isolation

- Follow the measures for caring for the body of any deceased person in Chapter 59.
- Wear a gown and gloves. A mask may be required in some cases.
- Wrap the body while you are in the isolation room. Usually, it will be placed in a plastic zippered bag.
- Transfer the body to a cart that has been draped with a clean bath blanket or sheet. A "clean" person outside the room will wrap the clean blanket around the body.
- Environmental services (housekeeping) personnel will decontaminate the room, according to facility protocol.
- The person caring for the body inside the room is considered contaminated. It is important to do a thorough handwash and to properly dispose of gloves, gown, and mask when leaving the room. Afterward, you may touch only the *outside* of the wrapping or shroud.
- Label the body, stating the type of isolation or causative disease. (The pathologist treats all bodies as if they have an infectious disease but must know if a specific infection is present.)
- Check your healthcare facility for special procedures.

and are becoming more common (Chapters 40 and 41). Because these organisms are not easily treated by antibiotics, they are becoming more dangerous to healthcare clients and staff.

Special terms relate to infections acquired in specific ways. *Catheter-associated urinary tract infections* (**CAUTI**) are infections caused by urinary catheters; a client on a ventilator may contract *ventilator-associated enterococcus* (**VAE**). The client with a central venous catheter may contract a *central line associated blood stream infection* (**CLABSI**), usually the most serious of these specific infections. Facilities have specific protocols for nursing care of these clients.

Methicillin-Resistant *Staphylococcus aureus*
Clients with MRSA are placed on contact precautions. Newborns of mothers with MRSA are usually roomed-in with the mother. Staff and visitors must follow the protocols for contact precautions. Surveillance cultures are done at least 7 days apart and at least 7 days after completion of clinical treatment. Cultures are taken in nares (nostril) and/or specific wound or drainage sites. Usual procedures state that cultures must be negative three times in order to discontinue isolation. Some isolated clients must remain in isolation while in the hospital. These clients include residents of long-term care facilities; those with chronic skin breakdown (e.g., pressure wounds) or open wounds, wound drainage; and clients with long-term invasive devices, such as percutaneous endoscopic gastrostomy (PEG) tubes.

Vancomycin-Resistant Enterococcus
Most of the procedures for clients with VRE are similar to those for MRSA. These cultures are obtained from the peri-rectal (around the rectum) area and/or an open wound or drainage site.

Nursing Alert If there is an outbreak of MRSA or VRE within a facility, special measures are followed, as prescribed by the facility, under the guidance of the state or province. In some cases, healthcare workers must be screened, as well as clients.

STUDENT SYNTHESIS

KEY POINTS
- Infection is best controlled by prevention—breaking the links in the chain of infection.
- The Joint Commission requires every healthcare facility to have an infection control plan.
- The Infection Control Committee monitors and evaluates infections in clients or in staff who have been exposed.
- Transmission-Based Precautions are designed to prevent the spread of specific infections: airborne, droplet, and contact precautions. The specific type of Precautions for any client is used in conjunction with Standard Precautions.
- Barrier techniques are designed to prevent microorganisms from leaving a client's room.
- Before entering a client's room, choose all necessary PPE and equipment.
- Special filtered respirator masks are required when caring for a client with active or suspected pulmonary TB.
- Isolation procedures may vary among facilities; it is important to be aware of local protocols.
- Protective isolation helps prevent organisms from coming into contact with clients.
- Isolation is often frightening and misunderstood by clients and families.

CRITICAL THINKING EXERCISES
1. Identify the appropriate PPE you would use in the following situations. Give your rationale for each.
   a. Discontinuing an IV for a client with no known or suspected infection
   b. Giving intramuscular medications to a client with no known or suspected infection
   c. Measuring the vital signs of a client with hepatitis
   d. Changing a bloody dressing on a client with TB
   e. Changing bed linen for an incontinent client with MRSA
   f. Giving a bath to a client who is HIV positive
   g. Assisting with wound irrigation for a client with no known or suspected infection

2. Explain how you would expect to use Standard and Transmission-Based Precautions in a variety of settings (e.g., schools, clinics, industry, and home care). How would implementation of care change from place to place? How would the need for these precautions be taught to clients and families?

3. You are providing care for a homeless client in a clinic. You learn that the client has been diagnosed with TB but is not taking the prescribed medication. How would you handle this situation?

NCLEX-STYLE REVIEW QUESTIONS
1. Which of these clients need to be placed in protective isolation? Select all that apply.
   a. A client with severe burns over 50% of the body
   b. A client taking antibiotics for an infection
   c. A client receiving large doses of corticosteroids
   d. A client with bronchitis
   e. A client receiving a bone marrow transplant

2. A client is suspected to be infected with methicillin-resistant *Staphylococcus aureus* (MRSA) in a sacral wound. Which precautions would the nurse follow during wound care?
   a. Droplet
   b. Contact
   c. Airborne
   d. Standard

3. The nurse is preparing to administer medication to a client who is in isolation. What action would the nurse take?
   a. Take the original medication administration record (MAR) into the room.
   b. Obtain a computer for documentation and take it into the room.
   c. Unwrap medications and take them into the room in their packages.
   d. Take needles and syringes out of the room and dispose of them in the medication room.

4. A client is placed on neutropenic precautions. Which observation made by the nurse requires immediate intervention?
   a. Housekeeping personnel don a mask before entering the client's room.
   b. The physician uses strict handwashing prior to entering the room.
   c. Dietary dons gown, mask, and gloves when bringing in the lunch tray.
   d. A family member brings a basket of fresh fruit into the client's room.

5. Which client requires a negative pressure room?
   a. A client with pneumonia
   b. A client with pharyngitis
   c. A client with a draining leg wound
   d. A client with pulmonary tuberculosis

CHAPTER RESOURCES

Enhance your learning with additional resources on thePoint*!*

Student Resources related to this chapter can be found at **thePoint.lww.com/Rosdahl12e.**

43 Emergency Care and First Aid

Learning Objectives

1. Discuss the importance of assessing safety at an emergency scene.
2. Describe how *triage* applies to emergency care.
3. Describe the medical identification tag and its purpose.
4. Describe, in order, steps for assessing an ill or injured person in an emergency.
5. Identify early, common, and progressive signs of shock. Describe common types of shock, including hypovolemic shock, identifying nursing actions in emergency-induced shock.
6. Describe general emergency actions for chest, neck, back, and head injuries.
7. Demonstrate in the laboratory, emergency actions for a chest puncture wound.
8. Discuss first aid for musculoskeletal injuries, including a fracture, demonstrating the ability to splint an ulnar or radial fracture safely, using common household materials.
9. Describe signs of increasing intracranial pressure.
10. Describe emergency care for hemorrhage in different areas of the body.
11. Explain symptoms and first aid for injuries caused by exposure to cold, including frostbite and hypothermia.
12. Describe symptoms and immediate first aid for heat-related illnesses and injuries, including heat exhaustion and severe burns. List signs of an inhalation injury following a fire.
13. Describe immediate rescuer actions in suspected heart attack.
14. Describe causes, symptoms, and treatment of anaphylaxis.
15. Identify precautions when a client has been exposed to hazardous materials. List immediate actions when a person is suspected of being poisoned.
16. List factors that identify a psychiatric emergency or potential for suicide.
17. State and demonstrate the procedure for calling a code in your healthcare facility or agency.
18. Describe steps in basic cardiac life support, including cardiopulmonary resuscitation (CPR).

Important Terminology

AMBU-bag	epistaxis	mediastinal shift	thrombolytic therapy	AED	HAZMAT
anaphylaxis	extrication	near drowning	tourniquet	AVPU	ICP
antidote	fracture	pneumothorax	toxin	BCLS	LOC
avulsion injury	frostbite	poison	trauma	BLS	MI
bandage	heat cramps	rabies	triage	CMS	MVA
biological death	heat exhaustion	shock	wind chill factor	CPR	PERRLA+C
café coronary	heat index	splint		CVA	PTSD
caustic	heat stroke	sprain	**Acronyms**	DNI	RICE
clinical death	hemorrhage	strain		DNR	SIRES
code	hypothermia	stridor	ABCDE	EMS	SIRS
debridement	intrusion injury	sudden death	ACLS	EMT	TIA
dislocation	intubation	syncope		FAST	

Trauma refers to a wound or injury caused by an outside force. Thousands of people die yearly as a result of trauma and sudden illness. Traumatic injuries are caused by events such as motor vehicle accidents (**MVAs**), poisonings, burns, responses to temperature extremes, obstructed airways, and gunshot wounds. Sudden disasters emphasize the need for first-aid training for all healthcare workers, emergency and rescue personnel, law enforcement officers, and the general public. This chapter describes actions to assist someone who has experienced sudden illness or trauma. Cardiopulmonary resuscitation (**CPR**) and basic life support (BLS) are not described in detail in this chapter. To learn the detailed methods of CPR and removal of airway obstruction, the nurse *must* take a specific course. Healthcare organizations require all employees to have current CPR certification, and each healthcare provider must take responsibility for obtaining this training and for getting recertification as needed. This chapter briefly outlines measures in administering basic first aid for selected injuries and accidents.

PRINCIPLES OF EMERGENCY CARE

Simply because you are a nurse, people will expect you to be able to deal with emergencies. Good Samaritan Laws (Box 43-1) in most states and provinces require the nurse

> **Box 43-1 Good Samaritan Laws**
>
> - Most states have a law that protects emergency care rescuers from legal liability, provided that the rescuers give *reasonable assistance* to the extent of training, without danger or peril to the person or themselves.
> - Some states consider rescuers guilty of violating the law if they do not give aid to someone who needs it. In general, if emergency rescue personnel are already on the scene, you are not required to assist, unless you are specifically asked to do so.
> - Nurses are required to assist in an emergency only *to the level of first-aid training*. Do only what you are trained to do in an emergency. Become familiar with the laws in the areas in which you work, live, and travel.

to assist at the scene of an accident up to the level of their training. Each nurse must be able to meet this obligation. Basic emergency care principles provide the foundation to act appropriately when first aid is needed. In an emergency, the first responder must decide *quickly* what to do. For example, a person's brain cells begin to die within 4 to 6 min without adequate oxygen. Therefore, emergency care must be administered quickly. The nurse's stress level is high during an emergency, so having a predetermined, orderly plan of action and method of assessment is critical. It is also important to be able to reassure victims and onlookers, and in many cases to enlist the assistance of others. In many cases, it is best to call 911 before doing anything else.

Assess Safety

First, be sure that the scene is safe before rushing to assist in an emergency. Is there any danger of fire, explosion, or building collapse? Is there danger of being caught in traffic or being hit by a car? Are there electrical hazards, downed live wires, or other hazardous materials? Is the person in danger of drowning? If the scene is unsafe, the first responder should call for additional help *before assisting injured persons*. In a dangerous situation, it may be necessary to move victims before starting first-aid care. However, never move an injured person if the area is safe. *Rationale: Unnecessary movement can compound or cause additional problems.*

> **Nursing Alert** If the person is a victim of an automobile accident, remember to assign someone to direct traffic, to prevent further injuries.

Summon Assistance

Summoning help is an important part of emergency care. A victim's life may depend on rapid response. In most communities in the United States and Canada, the fastest way to summon the emergency medical service (**EMS**) is by telephoning 911. *Be sure to know the local emergency number if it is not 911.* If possible, send someone to call, but make sure the person has all necessary information, including the exact location and nature of the emergency.

Identify Problems

Is there anything unusual about the situation? Are containers lying about that suggest attempted suicide or poisoning? Do medications give a clue to a medical problem (e.g., diabetes, epilepsy)? Are there signs of alcohol or drug abuse? Is there any indication of foul play? Is the person wearing a medical information tag?

> **Key Concept**
> If there is any indication of foul play, treat the victim without disturbing what has now become a crime scene.

When reporting an MVA, note the vehicle's condition. Is the vehicle upside down, on its side, or in a ditch? Is the vehicle in the water? Is there a gasoline spill? Note areas of intrusion: the driver's side, passenger's side, roof, front end, or back end. Were victims wearing seat belts? Were airbags deployed? Was anyone thrown from the vehicle; if so, how far? If the victim was riding a bicycle or motorcycle, were they wearing a helmet and protective clothing? This information can help emergency personnel anticipate equipment and treatment required.

MedicAlert Tag and Alert System

It is important to check any nonresponsive victim for a medical identification (ID) tag or billfold insert. A commonly used ID tag is the MedicAlert tag, used by more than 4 million people worldwide. This tag is worn as a necklace, bracelet, or boot tag and has an easily recognized symbol on the front (Fig. 43-1). Many of the tags contain condition-related information, such as diabetes, epilepsy, or high blood pressure, as well as allergies, and a small number identify implanted devices, such as pacemakers. A 24-hr emergency number allows rescue personnel to access vital medical information immediately, as well as an unidentified person's identity, address, and next of kin. In some states, a "do not resuscitate" (**DNR**) order can be engraved on the emblem and serves as an actual DNR order. It is also possible to call the MedicAlert Foundation to verify the client's DNR status and obtain a faxed copy of a signed DNR order or other advance directives. A release for organ or tissue donation is also available by this means and may be specified on the person's driver's license. This information should be reported as soon as possible. (However, remember that if a person dies, the next of kin may veto permission for organ and/or tissue donation, even if the person has chosen to be a donor.) MedicAlert also has an alarm option, managed by a base unit, with a wrist signal or emergency button pendant. A built-in battery back-up runs the system for 72 hr in a power failure. If the emergency button battery gets low, MedicAlert is automatically notified and the unit is replaced (www.medicalert.org).

Critical Access Standards

In 2005, The Joint Commission instituted Critical Access Standards for all rescue personnel. These standards state that healthcare facilities are required to store all critical client-provided information in the permanent client record. In addition, if a person is wearing emergency identification,

CHAPTER 43 Emergency Care and First Aid

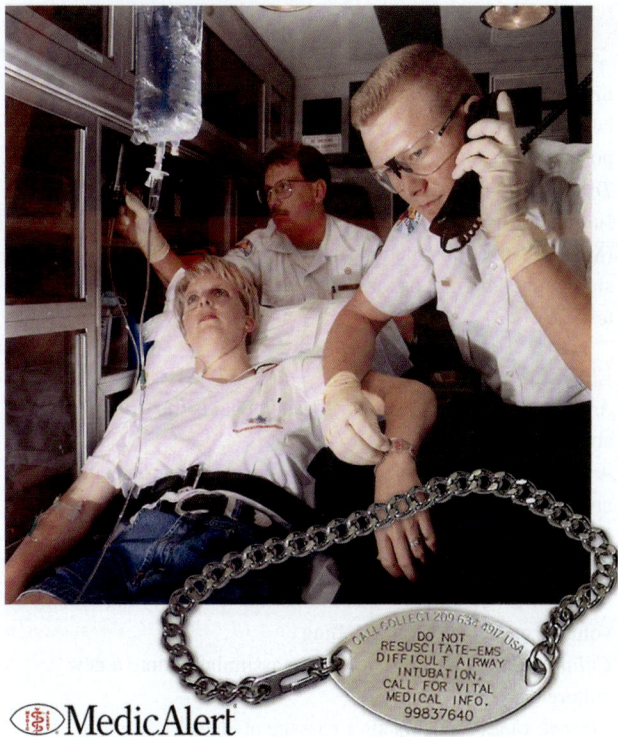

Figure 43-1 Emergency responders are required by law to check for MedicAlert or other emergency identifiers as an indication of a nonresponsive victim's identity and past medical history. This is a *client directive* that legally allows EMS to access the person's stored medical information by calling the MedicAlert Foundation's 24-Hour Emergency Response Center (1-800-625-3780 or the collect number on the tag). Each MedicAlert member has a unique secure client identifier on the emblem, as well as other vital information. Additional information is on file at MedicAlert. Shown at left is the MedicAlert symbol, which appears on the front of the tag. In addition to specific medical information, signed documents, such as a living will, can be faxed immediately to emergency staff. (Photo by MedicAlert Foundation, Turlock, CA.)

healthcare and rescue workers are obligated by law to call for information if the client is unable to respond. (If this system is not activated by the healthcare facility in an emergency, this constitutes a *sentinel event* or critical incident and must be reported.)

> **Key Concept**
> You, as a nurse, can encourage your friends, family, and clients to wear a medical identification tag. This may save their lives if they are in a serious accident or other life-threatening situation.

Perform Triage

Triage, the process of sorting and classifying to determine priority of needs, involves determining life-threatening situations and assisting those clients first (see Chapter 39). If there are many victims, less seriously injured people may be able to assist others. It is also important to *identify* victims and their next of kin whenever possible. The person doing triage must determine whom to assist first, when and how to call for help, and how untrained bystanders can assist. After an event, bystanders may be enlisted to help move victims to safety. If there are numerous victims, the local hospital(s) must be notified, so they can activate disaster plans. Nurses also use triage in emergency departments (EDs) and clinics, whether through telephone screening or on a walk-in basis.

Assess and Treat for Shock

Shock, often the first phase of the body's "alarm reaction" to trauma or severe tissue damage, occurs because the body loses its ability to circulate an adequate supply of oxygenated blood, particularly to the brain. After an accident, many conditions can lead to shock; however, shock most commonly is the result of inadequate circulation (see Chapter 22). The body attempts to compensate for any trauma. Because the central nervous system (CNS) controls all body functions, it monitors changes and immediately implements *compensatory circulation* to maintain an adequate blood supply to vital organs (e.g., the brain and heart) in an emergency. This action quickly adjusts the rate and strength of heart contractions and blood vessel tone and shuts down blood flow to the skin, digestive system, and kidneys. Blood that would normally go to these areas is *shunted* (transferred) instead to the heart and brain. Compensatory circulation is a basic survival mechanism that ensures that the body's most vital organs are adequately perfused with blood until the last possible moment.

The symptoms of shock are largely related to this compensatory mechanism. In severe injury, the body cannot compensate or adjust, and shock develops. Shock may develop rapidly following trauma (or more slowly in other situations). Consequently, *every injured person* should receive preventive and precautionary treatment for shock. Anything that could cause increased blood loss or otherwise contribute to shock should be avoided. Therefore, never handle or move injured persons unnecessarily and make every attempt to keep them calm. Shock is classified into three major categories: *primary*, the nervous system's response immediately after a severe injury or other traumatic event; *secondary*, one or more hours after an injury, perhaps up to 24 hr later (*delayed* or *deferred shock*); and *hemorrhagic*, caused by blood loss. The major types of shock, along with less commonly known types, are listed in Box 43-2.

Hypovolemic Shock

Trauma resulting in excessive blood loss decreases the amount of blood volume available for the heart to pump, leading to *hypovolemic shock*. The loss of about one fifth of the body's total blood volume can cause this type of hypovolemic shock. In addition to hemorrhage, hypovolemic shock may result from the following: severe dehydration (lowered *intravascular* [within blood vessels] fluid volume); possibly, hyperthermia, *diaphoresis* (excessive sweating) or diseases, such as diabetes insipidus and, in some cases, diabetes mellitus; severe diarrhea; protracted vomiting (over a long period of time); intestinal obstruction; *peritonitis* (inflammation of the peritoneum); acute *pancreatitis* (inflammation of the pancreas); and severe burns. Postpartum hemorrhage, which can cause hypovolemic shock, can occur with the delivery of the placenta, but can also occur up to 12 weeks after delivery.

Box 43-2 Types of Shock

MAJOR TYPES OF SHOCK

- *Cardiogenic (cardiac) shock*—primarily failure of the heart to adequately pump. The heart muscle is severely compromised. Possible causes include failure or stenosis (narrowing) of heart valves, cardiomyopathy (primary heart disease), or rhythm disturbances. Low cardiac output often results from an acute MI (heart attack) or heart failure.
- *Hypovolemic shock (hemorrhagic shock, traumatic hemorrhagic shock)*—most often a result of hemorrhage either due to acute bleeding, or bleeding due to soft tissue damage and release of immune system activators. The body has insufficient blood volume to maintain adequate cardiac output, blood pressure, and tissue perfusion. Hypovolemic shock and traumatic hypovolemic shock are caused by insufficiency of circulating plasma volume.
- *Distributive shock*—marked decrease in peripheral vascular resistance, causing hypotension. Results from a lack of regulation of vascular tone, with volume being shifted within the vascular system or being shifted into the interstitium (spaces between tissues and organs). Three types of distributive shock are as follows:
  - *Anaphylactic (allergic) shock*—severe, life-threatening reaction to a substance to which the client is allergic. (See Data Gathering in Nursing 43-1 for a list of symptoms of anaphylaxis.)
  - *Neurogenic shock*—vasodilation (blood vessel enlargement) secondary to cerebral trauma, spinal cord injury, very deep general or spinal anesthesia, or central nervous system (CNS) depression caused by toxins or drugs, such as "downers." The major mechanism is decreased peripheral vascular resistance.
  - *Septic shock (endotoxic shock, endotoxin shock, toxic shock)*—results from overwhelming infection throughout the body, secondary to release of toxins, usually by gram-negative bacteria (particularly *Escherichia coli*) and by cytokines (see Chapter 24). Viruses can also cause septic shock. Endotoxins, stimulated by infection, cause excess blood to be held in capillaries and veins and, therefore, to not be available to the general circulation; causing dangerous hypotension. Other symptoms include chills, fever, warm and flushed skin, increased cardiac output, and hypotension (less than in hypovolemic shock). If therapy is ineffective, symptoms resemble those of hypovolemic shock. Septic or toxic shock is one stage in the systemic inflammatory response syndrome (**SIRS**), most common in newborns or people older than 50 years, and in persons with diabetes, cirrhosis of the liver, or compromised immune systems (e.g., due to AIDS, cancer chemotherapy, bone marrow transplant).
- *Toxic shock syndrome*—specific type of shock caused by infection, usually by a *Staphylococcus* or *Streptococcus* organism (has been associated with tampon use); can progress to untreatable (irreversible) shock. Bacteria produce a toxin that enters the bloodstream and causes sepsis. Treatment involves removal of the tampon and vigorous antibiotic administration. May also occur in anyone with a skin wound or post-surgery.
- *Traumatic shock*—any shock caused by trauma, injury, or surgery, or heart damage following a myocardial infarction (MI); intestinal obstruction; perforation/rupture of viscera; strangulated hernia; or torsion of viscera (including ovary or testicle).

LESS COMMONLY KNOWN TYPES OF SHOCK

- *Anaphylactoid reaction*—pseudoanaphylaxis (not true anaphylaxis)
- *Anesthesia shock*—from overdose of or reaction to general anesthetic
- *Burn shock*—caused by loss of plasma
- *Chronic shock*—due to peripheral circulatory insufficiency in seniors with debilitating diseases, or due to subnormal blood volume, caused by slow bleeding
- *Cultural shock*—distress related to assimilation into a new culture or country
- *Electric shock*—occurs after passage of electric current through the body. This usually results from accidental contact with electric circuits or wires but may be caused by lightning. Damage depends on the pathway of the current, the amount of current, and the skin's resistance.
- *Epigastric shock*—caused by an abdominal blow or extensive abdominal surgery
- *Hypoglycemic shock (is not a medical term but is used by lay people to describe severe hypoglycemia)*—secondary to low blood glucose (<40 mg/dL). Frequently caused by administration of too much insulin.
- *Irreversible shock*—is the final category of shock when changes produced cannot be corrected by treatment; death is inevitable.
- *Osmotic shock*—rupture of plasma membrane/loss of cellular contents due to exposure to a hypotonic environment (see Chapter 17), causing sudden change in intracellular osmotic pressure
- *Pleural shock*—hypotension secondary to *thoracentesis* (withdrawing excessive fluid from lung cavity). Symptoms include cyanosis (blueness of skin and mucous membranes), pallor (paleness), dilated pupils, and disturbances of pulse and respiration.
- *Postoperative shock*—shock occurring after surgery
- *Protein shock*—secondary to central arterial line protein administration
- *Psychic (mental) shock*—secondary to emotional stress, manifested by excessive fear, joy, anger, or grief
- *Serum shock*—anaphylactic shock secondary to administration of foreign serum to sensitized person
- *Shock lung*—(acute respiratory distress syndrome [ARDS])—pulmonary damage occurring early in shock. Symptoms include acute respiratory distress and pulmonary edema.

> **Box 43-2 Types of Shock** (continued)
>
> Pulmonary vessels may plug with blood cells and platelets, leading to anoxia, damage to alveoli and capillaries, and generalized tissue hypoxia. Decreased surfactant (lubricating substance allowing lung expansion) may lead to *atelectasis* (collapsed lung).
> - *Shell shock (battle fatigue)*—mental disorder identified in World War I. Now known as *posttraumatic stress disorder* (**PTSD**).
> - *Spinal shock*—loss of spinal reflexes after acute transverse spinal cord injury. Flaccid paralysis below the level of injury and loss of reflexes and sensation occur.
> - *Surgical shock*—occurring during/after surgery.
> - *Testicular shock*—results from sharp blow to testes.
> - *Vasogenic shock*—shock secondary to marked vasodilation (loss of vascular tone), usually resulting from damage to vasomotor centers in the brain stem or medulla.

The signs of hypovolemic shock, caused by a critical drop in cardiac preload that causes negative consequences in tissue metabolism and triggers an inflammatory reaction, include:

- Hypotension (lowered blood pressure, after a slight increase)
- Weak, thready pulse
- Cool, clammy skin
- Tachycardia (increased pulse)
- Tachypnea (increased respiratory rate)
- Hyperpnea (very deep breathing, gasping)
- Restlessness, anxiety (caused by decreased blood flow to the brain)
- Weakness
- Decreased urinary output

Remember, most of these signs and symptoms are related to the compensatory mechanisms of the body.

In the healthcare facility, additional information is obtained by diagnostic procedures such as monitoring of central venous pressure, pulmonary wedge pressure, and cardiac output; ECG; serum electrolyte levels; urine volume and specific gravity; arterial blood gases; and complete blood count. In hypovolemic shock, many of these values are abnormal.

Distributive Shock

This is the most commonly occurring type of shock, technically referred to as *distributive shock*. It is caused by widespread *vasodilation* (enlargement of the blood vessels). Distributive hypovolemic shock is divided into three types: *septic shock* (a life-threatening response to an infection); *anaphylactic shock* (a massive histamine-mediated vasodilation and shift of fluids); and *neurogenic shock* (common in spinal injuries). In distributive shock, blood volume is normal, but it cannot adequately supply tissues with oxygen, because of the enlarged size of the blood vessels. The symptoms are largely the same as those seen in hypovolemic shock.

The other two types of shock classified by the National Institute of Health are *cardiogenic shock* (primarily a disorder of cardiac function leading to decreased cardiac output) and *obstructive shock* (caused by an obstruction of the large vessels or events that occur prior to or after the heart, as in a thromboembolism).

Late Signs of Hypovolemic Shock

Late signs of hypovolemic shock include lowered body temperature, shallow respirations, and a narrowed *pulse pressure* (the difference between the systolic and diastolic blood pressure readings). If the shock is not successfully treated, *decompensated shock* occurs late in the process. The client in decompensated shock is extremely hypotensive; this situation is particularly life threatening.

Hypovolemic Shock Sequel

Hypovolemic shock can lead to serious and life-threatening conditions, such as *metabolic acidosis* (resulting from increased lactic acid), or irreversible cerebral (brain), hepatic (liver), and renal (kidney) damage. A condition known as *disseminated intravascular coagulation* (widespread blood clots, mostly in the capillaries) can also occur and is life threatening.

Treatment of Shock

Shock is present in most serious injuries or illnesses, even though the classic signs may not be apparent. Compensatory action may keep a person responsive, and in some cases alert even when massive blood loss has occurred. Continue to assess for signs of a change in the person's level of consciousness (**LOC**) (see Chapter 78). Progressive deterioration in LOC indicates that cerebral circulation (blood circulation to the brain) is inadequate. Falling blood pressure is a *late sign* of shock.

Treatment of hypovolemic shock is symptomatic, aimed at correcting imbalances and removing the underlying cause of the shock. The treatment of most types of shock is approximately the same. In a first-aid situation:

- Efforts are made to increase blood supply to the brain. In many cases, this involves elevating the feet or lowering the head.
- Bleeding sites are identified. If there is bleeding, it is controlled. Methods of controlling bleeding are discussed later.

Advanced procedures for treating shock include:

- Replacing fluid loss
- Administering blood and blood components
- Supporting blood pressure with medications, such as dopamine or norepinephrine

- Administering intravenous (IV) antibiotics, if the cause is an infection (after a culture and sensitivity [C&S] test)
- Treating an infection: draining abscesses, debriding (removing necrosed dead tissue), removing other possible sources of infection (e.g., catheters, IV, drainage tubes, tampons)

In all cases, the underlying causes of shock are treated. In any emergency, *if in doubt, treat for shock*. In Practice: Nursing Care Guidelines 43-1 gives further pointers in recognition and treatment of shock.

> **Key Concept**
>
> Look for all signs of shock. Falling blood pressure is a late sign of shock and is ominous. Remember, shock may be caused by many things other than blood loss. Regardless of the cause, symptoms and treatment are similar in the early stages.

ASSESSING THE PERSON IN AN EMERGENCY

The *primary assessment* is performed as soon as rescuers arrive at an emergency scene. During this assessment, life-threatening problems or injuries are identified and handled. If there are no life-threatening problems to correct, the primary assessment usually can be completed within 60 s.

The *secondary assessment* involves taking and recording the victim's vital signs (see Chapter 46) and continues with a head-to-toe assessment. This secondary assessment should take from 1 to 2 min, unless injuries requiring immediate intervention are identified. If the person has life-threatening problems, the secondary assessment may be delayed until the person is being transported. *Keep in mind that the assessments of the nurse acting as a first-aid person can be performed only to the level of the individual nurse's skills and training.*

Whenever assessing a person in an emergency, use the acronym **ABCDE** to help you remember the order for assessment:

A = Airway and cervical spine
B = Breathing
C = Circulation and bleeding
D = Disability
E = Expose and examine

IN PRACTICE
NURSING CARE GUIDELINES 43-1 — Treating Shock in an Emergency

- Keep the person lying down and as calm as possible; reassure both the person and bystanders. Have someone call for assistance. Handle the injured person gently. *Rationale: If the injured person becomes excited, the body's oxygen needs will increase, thus increasing shock. The person may need advanced life support.*
- Establish, maintain, and monitor airway, breathing, and circulation. *Rationale: These functions are vital to life.*
- Administer a high concentration of oxygen, if available. Assist breathing as needed. *Rationale: Administration of external oxygen increases the oxygen available in the blood and helps the person to breathe with less effort.*
- Control bleeding. *Rationale: Additional bleeding leads to more blood loss and adds to shock.*
- Maintain body temperature; many people become chilled after an accident. Cover with a blanket or coats, if necessary. Do not overheat the person. *Rationale: The parasympathetic nervous system takes over in an emergency and reroutes blood to vital organs and away from the skin. Excessively low or high body temperature causes the heart to work harder.*
- Try to put something under the person. *Rationale: The ground is usually colder than the person; this will cause heat loss by drawing heat from the body.*
- Keep the person dry. *Rationale: If a person becomes wet, chilling occurs much more quickly.*
- Give nothing by mouth. *Rationale: The person could aspirate, choke, or vomit.*
- Elevate the lower extremities, unless contraindicated. *Rationale: Elevating the legs helps blood to flow toward the brain where it is needed. Some people may need to have the head elevated, to breathe. In head injury, the body is kept level.*
- Use the position most comfortable for the person, within medical limits for the injury. *Rationale: Proper positioning maintains client comfort and prevents further injury.*
- Immobilize fractures. *Rationale: Immobilization prevents further injury.*
- Monitor level of consciousness. Take and record vital signs at least every 5 min. *Rationale: LOC and vital signs provide important information about the client's status. Emergency and medical personnel must know the person's reactions to the injury.*

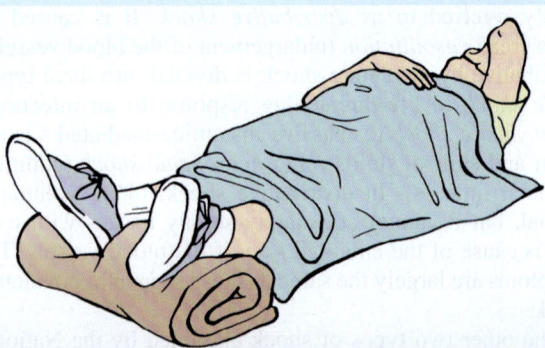

In many emergencies and injuries, the person must be treated for shock. Keep the person lying down. Maintain body temperature with blankets or coats. Elevate the feet and legs unless contraindicated.

A: Airway and Cervical Spine

Evaluate the airway to determine whether it is *patent* (open). While doing so, keep in mind the injury's mechanism, location, and scope. The person must be able to breathe before other first-aid measures can be instituted.

If a possibility of spinal injury exists, *stabilize the person's cervical spine* before attempting other activities. If proper equipment is not available, wait for emergency rescue personnel to arrive. Unless there is an immediate danger, such as of explosion or fire, *do not move the person!*

B: Breathing

Assess breathing by listening for breath sounds, watching for chest movements, and feeling for breath against your cheek and ear.

Maintain the Airway

Maintain the person's airway, even if breathing is present. Blood, body fluids, and vomitus may accumulate in the person's mouth and should be removed. Be sure the person's tongue is out of the way; the tongue can occlude the airway in even a minor event, such as fainting. Position the person on the side if vomiting is imminent, while maintaining cervical spine alignment.

> **Nursing Alert** The most common airway obstruction in an unconscious person is caused by the tongue falling back and occluding the airway.

Observe Respirations

As you assess breathing, note if *respirations* appear to be of normal rate and depth (see Chapter 46). Examine the person's mouth, gums, lips, and nail beds for color and moisture. Blueness (*cyanosis*) or duskiness in the skin, nail beds, or mucous membranes indicates a lack of oxygen.

Look for Life-Threatening Chest Injuries

If indicated by the injury's mechanism, examine the person's chest for life-threatening injuries. Chest injuries may cause internal bleeding and injury to the heart and lungs. If the body's ability to exchange oxygen and circulate oxygenated blood diminishes, permanent brain damage or death will occur, if left uncorrected. Immediately care for injuries such as rib fractures, punctured lung, stab wounds, gunshot wounds, compression injuries that result in a caved-in or open chest wall, and cardiac contusions.

> **Nursing Alert** If the chest wall is not intact, *plug the hole at once*. This is an emergency, life-threatening situation. If this is not done, the chest vacuum will be lost, and the victim's lungs will collapse.

A serious situation in a crushing injury is *flail chest*, loss of chest wall stability, caused by several fractured ribs or detachment of the ribs from the sternum. The loose portion of the chest moves opposite its normal direction when the person breathes (*paradoxical respiration*). In other words, the chest *rises on expiration and falls on inspiration.* It is important to stabilize the chest wall as much as possible with whatever is available. For example, apply an all-cotton elastic roller bandage and have the person lie on the affected side, to apply pressure to the chest wall. Transport the person immediately.

Be alert for important signs of chest injuries, which include:

- Pain at the site of injury and on breathing
- Shortness of breath, gasping
- Failure of the chest to expand
- Coughing up blood
- Rapid, weak pulse and low blood pressure
- Cyanotic (bluish/greyish) lips, gums, fingernails, or fingertips
- Panic, agitation, nasal flaring
- Abnormal breathing sounds, such as wheezing or stridor (see Chapters 46 and 47)
- Abnormal chest movements on breathing

C: Circulation and Bleeding

The heart must be pumping effectively for oxygen to be carried to the cells. There also must be sufficient blood volume to carry needed oxygen. Therefore, any disruption in the pumping action of the heart, blood pressure, or the amount of blood available can compromise the person's condition.

Palpate the Pulse

Palpate the victim's pulse, using the carotid artery in the neck, for 5 to 10 s (Fig. 43-2). If no pulse is present, ask bystanders to call for assistance; *this person needs advanced life support as soon as possible.* Begin cardiac compressions immediately, if qualified. (This technique should be learned in a special CPR course.)

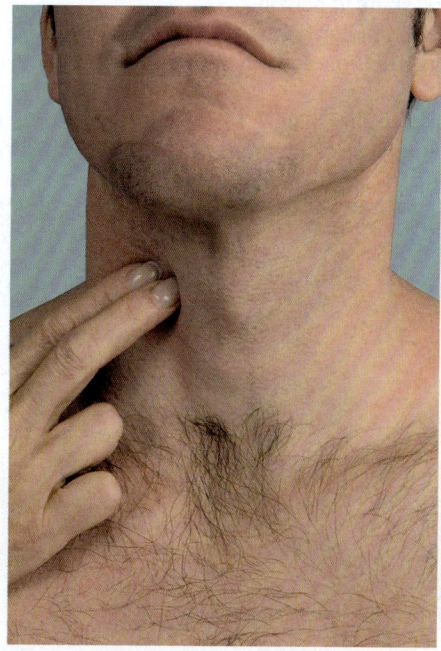

Figure 43-2 Palpating the carotid pulse on the same side as the rescuer. (Photo by B. Proud.)

> **Nursing Alert** Do not reach across the person's neck to feel the pulse. Feel it on the side nearest you. **Rationale:** Reaching across might accidentally cut off the airway.

Observe the Pulse

If a pulse is present, note its rate and regularity. Does it seem normal? Do *not* count the pulse at this time; just try to get a sense of its quality. While palpating the pulse, also observe skin color, temperature, and neck veins (for distention).

Reassess Breathing

A person may have a heartbeat without having respirations; therefore, reassess breathing. If the person is not breathing, begin rescue breathing immediately. (This technique is also learned in a special CPR course.)

> **Nursing Alert** Use a one-way filtered breathing mask for CPR, whenever possible, to protect the rescuer.

When the EMS personnel arrive, they can "bag" the person with an 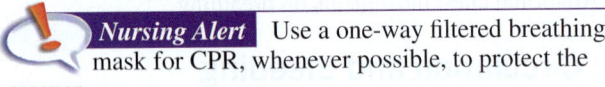-bag (Fig. 43-3). This is a bag attached to a face mask, used to "breathe for" the person. This method is safer, more effective, and less tiring for the rescuer than rescue breathing. Supplemental oxygen can also be delivered via AMBU-bag.

Assess for Progressing Shock

Always consider the possibility of shock in any injury. Use the *capillary refill test* to evaluate for shock, as follows:

- Press a finger into the middle of the person's forehead until the spot being pressed turns white or a lighter color in a dark-skinned person.
- Remove the finger. Count the seconds it takes for color to return. (Count: one-one thousand; two-one thousand, and so on.)
- If it takes more than 2 s for color to return, *shock is progressing* (see discussion earlier in this chapter).

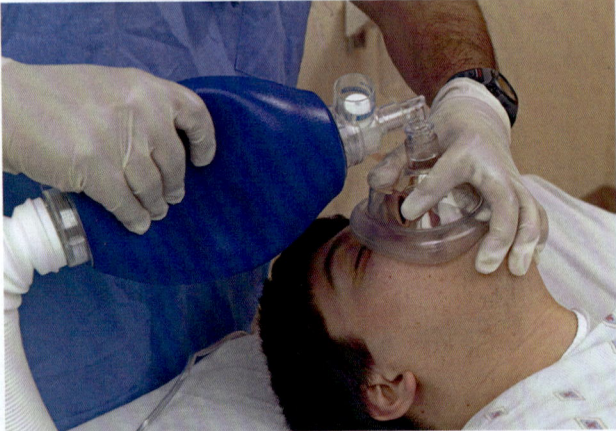

Figure 43-3 The use of an AMBU-bag replaces mouth-to-mouth resuscitation. Wear gloves whenever possible (Evans-Smith, 2005).

Assess and Control Hemorrhage

The presence of a palpable pulse indicates that the person's heart is beating. However, you must also assess for major bleeding (*hemorrhage*).

Control hemorrhage *immediately* or the person will die from blood loss. With gloved hands, place sterile compresses over wounds and apply pressure. If blood seeps through the compresses, *do not remove them*, but place additional compresses over the top of those already in place. As necessary, apply additional pressure over the wound.

> **Key Concept**
> Follow Standard Precautions whenever possible in administering first aid.

Measures used to stop bleeding include:

- Apply direct pressure; this should be done first. (If no sterile compresses are available, use the cleanest item, such as a clean towel.)
- Elevate a bleeding limb.
- Apply an ice or cold pack, if available (CAUTION: place ice over several layers of dressings to avoid freezing body tissues).
- Apply *indirect pressure:* press the blood vessel at a pressure point against a bone (see Fig. 43-4).
- If severe bleeding continues, reach into the wound and try to grasp the bleeding vessel with your fingers.
- If a woman has delivered a baby within the past few weeks, consider postpartum hemorrhage. This is most often caused by relaxation of the uterus (*uterine atony*). Immediate first aid is to have the woman empty her bladder and then to massage the uterus in an attempt to cause uterine contraction and stop the hemorrhage. Then, apply gentle, firm pressure to expel clots. She should be transported to an ED immediately.
- Apply a tourniquet *as a last resort* (see procedure later). Mark the tourniquet with the time it was applied. Also put a "T" on the client's forehead, so rescue workers know a tourniquet is in place. *Do not release* a tourniquet after it is applied.

D: Disability

Neurologic Assessment

Conducting a neurologic assessment at an accident scene will help receiving medical personnel in the ED. Identify levels of consciousness. The acronym **AVPU** will help in remembering these levels.

A = Alert: Speaks and moves spontaneously; answers questions about name, place, and date correctly
V = Responsive to *verbal stimuli* only; answers when directly addressed
P = Responsive to *painful stimuli* only (e.g., rubbing the sternum or pressure on nail beds)
U = *Unresponsive*

Eye Signs

Assess the person's pupillary responses. The pupils of both eyes should be *round* and the same size (*equal*). They should

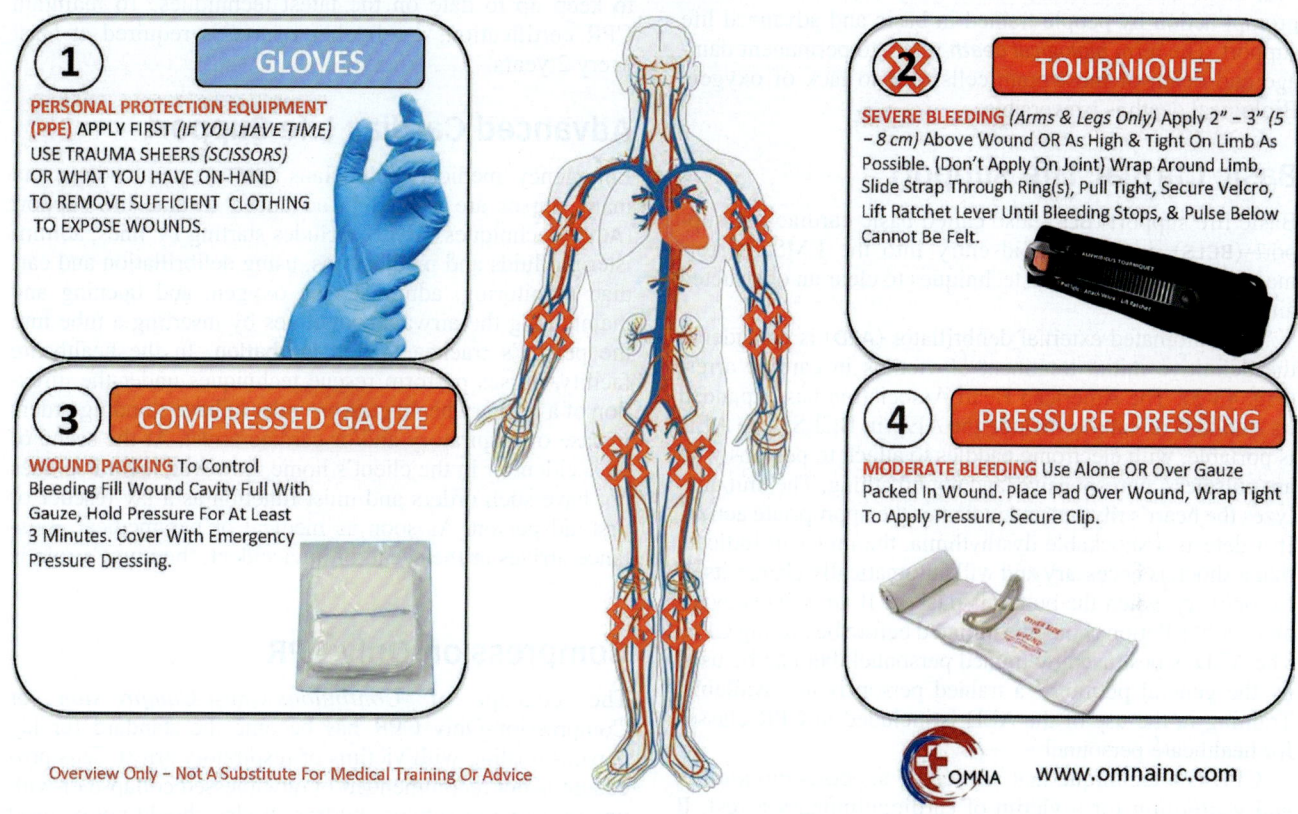

Figure 43-4 When hemorrhage occurs, be sure to correctly use pressure on wounds and use tourniquets, when necessary, to control bleeding. (Courtesy of Omna Inc. https://www.omnainc.com/blogs/news/bleeding-control-tools-an-overview)

constrict when a bright light quickly shines into them (*react to light*). The pupils should change size between close and far vision (*accommodation*). Reactions should be the same in both eyes, and they should move together when following a moving object (eyes *coordinated*). Remember this procedure by following **PERRLA+C** (see Chapter 78):

PE = Pupils Equal
R = Round
RL = React to Light
A = Accommodation OK
C = Coordinated

E: Expose and Examine

Expose and examine any site of possible injury or any area that the person complains about, even if the area was examined previously. After having controlled immediately life-threatening problems, obtain the person's medical history, including any illnesses or allergies, if possible. Sources include the person, a MedicAlert tag, the family, or bystanders. Try to find out what happened. If equipment is available, take vital signs (temperature, pulse, respiration, blood pressure) and ask about pain every 5 min after life-threatening problems are under control (see Chapter 46). Count pulse and respirations for at least 30 s. This recording establishes a baseline for further treatment. Report findings to rescue personnel when they arrive.

SUDDEN DEATH AND LIFE SUPPORT

Sudden death occurs any time breathing and heartbeat stop abruptly or unexpectedly (*cardiopulmonary arrest*). It is required that all nursing students and graduate nurses maintain current certification in CPR, to be able to assist in a sudden death emergency.

Causes of sudden death include the following:

- Electrocution and severe electric shock
- Drowning and near drowning
- Anaphylaxis (severe allergic reaction)
- Drug overdose
- Poisoning
- Shock
- Myocardial infarction (heart attack)
- Cerebrovascular accident (CVA), stroke
- Total airway obstruction or suffocation
- Smoke inhalation, carbon monoxide poisoning, inhalation of other gases

- Severe trauma
- Adverse reaction to general anesthesia

Two definitions for death exist: clinical and biological. **Clinical death** occurs when a person's breathing and heartbeat stop. Sudden clinical death may be reversible, with prompt action by people trained in basic and advanced life support. The term **biological death** refers to permanent damage and death of most brain cells, due to lack of oxygen. Biological death is irreversible.

Basic Cardiac Life Support

Basic life support (**BLS**), also called basic cardiac life support (**BCLS**), includes rapid entry into the EMS, performance of CPR, and use of techniques to clear an obstructed airway.

The automated external defibrillator (**AED**) is considered the definitive initial treatment of victims in cardiac arrest (Fig. 43-5). The American Heart Association has expanded its standard of care to include the AED in BCLS. The AED is portable, with electronic paddles to attach to persons who are pulseless, unresponsive, and not breathing. The unit analyzes the heart's rhythm and indicates the appropriate action. If it detects a shockable dysrhythmia, the unit will indicate that a shock is necessary and will automatically charge itself for delivery, when the button is pushed. If an AED is available, defibrillation should be initiated before beginning CPR. The AED is best used by trained personnel, but can be used by the general public, if a trained person is not available. Training in the use of the AED is included in CPR classes for healthcare personnel.

CPR is a technique that artificially supports *circulation* and *ventilation* for a victim of cardiopulmonary arrest. It helps provide oxygen to the brain, heart, lungs, and other organs until advanced life support can be given. CPR must be performed immediately after cardiac and respiratory arrest, or it will not reverse clinical death and biological death will follow. The American Heart Association and the American Red Cross have established guidelines for CPR. They make changes as new medical and emergency techniques are developed. All healthcare workers are expected to keep up to date on the latest techniques. To maintain CPR certification, a refresher course is required at least every 2 years.

Advanced Cardiac Life Support

Emergency medical technicians (**EMTs**), paramedics, and many nurses are trained in advanced cardiac life support (**ACLS**) techniques. ACLS includes starting IV lines, administering fluids and medications, using defibrillation and cardiac monitoring, administering oxygen, and opening and maintaining the airway, sometimes by inserting a tube into the person's trachea, called **intubation**. In the healthcare facility, nurses perform rescue techniques under the direction of a primary healthcare provider or have standing orders in case of respiratory and/or cardiac arrest. At the scene of an accident or in the client's home, however, the nurse does not have such orders and must function as a lay rescuer or first-aid person. As soon as medical or paramedical assistance arrives at the scene of an accident, the nurse's role is to assist.

Compression-Only CPR

The concept of *Continuous-Chest-Compression* or Compression-Only CPR has become the standard for lay persons dealing with victims of respiratory arrest. This procedure is not recommended in unwitnessed collapse or with unresponsive infants or children. It also should not be used if the collapse appears not to be related to a heart disorder; this would include choking, drowning, or drug overdose. If an adult is seen to collapse, the EMS system is activated first. Then, if the victim is not responsive and not breathing, an airway is established, and continuous chest compressions are given at about 100 per minute until a trained person can take over. In this case, rescue breathing is not done. (The rate of CPR is approximately the pace of the song, "Staying Alive.")

The Client at Home

When providing care to a client at home, plans for emergencies are included in the client's initial plan of care. Keep in mind the following:

- Know the client's DNR and **DNI** (do not intubate) status before beginning care. If the client is DNR/DNI, a copy of the documentation must be in the home-care records.
- Review plans for resuscitation with the client and family before administering any care. The client's family must be comfortable with the DNR/DNI status if this is the case.
- Carry a pocket mask and gloves at all times, in case of emergency.
- Encourage the family to be trained in CPR if the client is "full code" (not DNR/DNI). This is a helpful skill for all people.

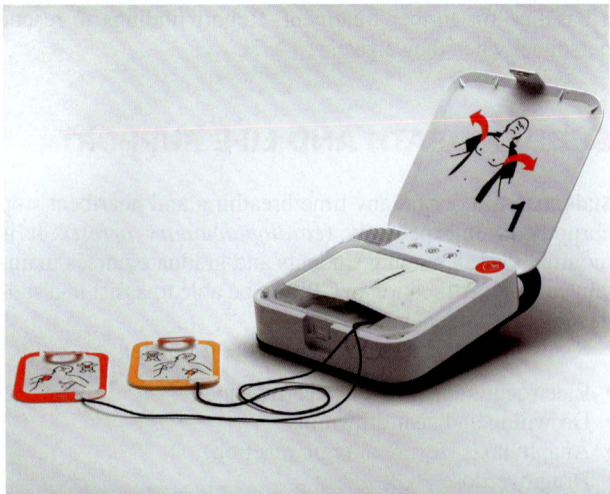

Figure 43-5 Many people in the community, such as police officers, school employees, and the general public, have been trained to use the automated external defibrillator (AED). The paddles are applied, and the machine gives prompts to the rescuer as to what to do. Many public places have an AED onsite. (Courtesy of Stryker Corporation.)

Unless specified as DNR, the client receiving home care is to be resuscitated. In this case, if the client goes into cardiac or respiratory arrest while you are in the home, do the following:

- Have a family member call 911.
- Begin CPR immediately. (It is important for all home care personnel to have this training.)
- Before the ambulance arrives, have a family member turn on the porch light and watch for the ambulance.
- Ask the family to move furniture to clear a pathway to the client.
- Reassure the family after the event.
- Document the event and its outcome.

Code in a Healthcare Facility

When an emergency occurs in a healthcare facility, the nurse must activate the agency's signal for a **code**. ("Code Blue" or "Dr. Blue" are common signals for a cardiopulmonary emergency [see Chapter 39].) In some facilities, a "rapid response" code is called for an emergency, other than cardiopulmonary arrest (e.g., the client who is unresponsive as a result of very low blood sugar, who has a grand mal seizure, or who tries to commit suicide).

Assisting With a Cardiopulmonary Emergency

When a "Code Blue" is called, obtain necessary emergency equipment: crash cart; back board; manual breathing bag; emergency medications; heart monitor; stethoscope; blood pressure and oxygen apparatus; pulse oximeter; IV lines, fluids, and poles; suctioning equipment; oral airways; and a computer-on-wheels. Crash carts are usually standardized throughout a facility, so everyone is familiar with the setup (Fig. 43-6). The carts may be equipped with color-coded resuscitation tape (Broselow tape) for pediatric emergencies; this system identifies equipment sizes, drug doses, and defibrillation settings, based on height and body build. During resuscitation attempts, the nurse assists the code team. Duties include locating emergency medications and administering them as ordered; helping set up emergency IV, suction, or oxygen equipment; obtaining vital signs; keeping records of medications and treatments given; and calling in other personnel as needed.

If resuscitation measures are successful, the person's pulse will resume, pupils will constrict, color will improve, and breathing will begin. The person may cough, move, or vomit. If assisting a code team and suction is available, turn the client's head to the side and suction the mouth. Do not place fingers in the client's mouth. If it is necessary to open the client's mouth, use an instrument, such as a tongue depressor or spoon. *Always wear gloves.* After the person is resuscitated, a mechanical ventilator, IV therapy, or vasopressor drugs may be needed for maintenance. Until it is determined that the person is out of danger, the person needs close observation in the ED or intensive care unit in case another emergency resuscitation is required.

Whatever the outcome, the entire procedure is carefully documented on the computer-on-wheels, if possible, including the time the arrest was discovered and the primary provider's estimate of when the arrest occurred; emergency measures taken by the first person on the scene; the time the code team arrived; procedures performed from that time on and by whom; medications given, stating dosages and times; the victim's responses to medications and treatment; and laboratory work, electrocardiograms, x-rays, and other tests done. Finally, the outcome of the resuscitation efforts and subsequent nursing care, if appropriate, are noted. A code constitutes a "sentinel event" and must be reported. Chapter 39 describes codes other than cardiopulmonary codes that may occur in the healthcare facility.

FIRST-AID MEASURES

All nurses are expected to know basic first-aid measures; this will also prove beneficial in the role of parent, sports coach, or neighbor. Injury or sudden illness can occur at any time and the nurse may be called on to assist.

> **Key Concept**
> Remember: The nurse can legally perform first aid only to the level of their training and local laws.

Chest, Back, Neck, and Head Injuries

Do not attempt to move or transport any injured person, particularly a person with a chest, back, neck, or head injury, until the EMS team arrives, except in very unusual situations. If the person must be moved, only those who have special instruction and equipment should do so. The *only time* unqualified people should attempt extrication is if the person's life would be in great danger if they are not moved. This would apply, for example, to a person on a canoe trip or mountain climbing in the wilderness without available

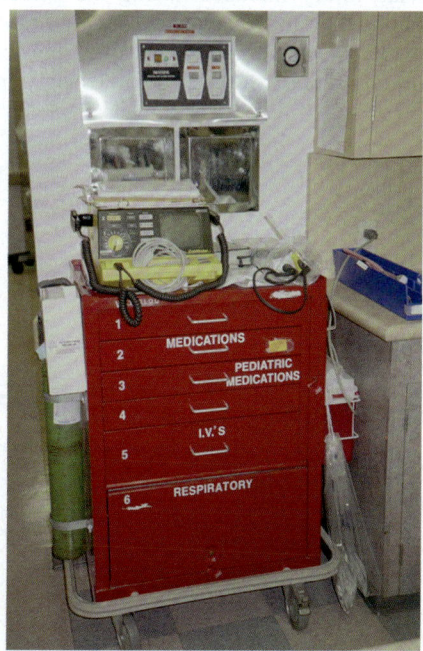

Figure 43-6 The crash cart contains emergency medications and equipment. A backboard is often attached to the cart or hanging nearby. (Photo by M. Kowalski.)

EMS assistance, or a person in a dangerous situation such as a burning building, a car under water, or a car that may explode. In extreme cases, the person must be moved with the utmost care, even though moving might aggravate the injuries. In cases such as these, you may be required to supervise the cautious **extrication** (emergency removal) of the victim. When moving a person with a neck injury to a stretcher, it is vital to immobilize the neck and back first, then keep the body straight. Sometimes a person who is lying in an abnormal position can be placed on a stretcher in the same position. *Rationale: Careful transfer protects both the injured person and the rescuer* (see Chapter 48).

Chest Injuries

Stabbings, shootings, and MVAs are the most common causes of chest injuries. CPR may also cause fractured ribs, which may injure soft tissues by puncturing a lung or tearing blood vessels. When such complications are not present, fractured ribs are treated by immobilizing the person's chest with an elastic bandage.

If a lung is ruptured, death from hemorrhage or suffocation is a very real threat. A wound that penetrates the chest requires immediate first aid because air can enter the chest cavity, which can disrupt the normal vacuum within the chest and collapse the lungs. In some cases, the lungs cannot adequately expand, a condition called **pneumothorax**. Signs of pneumothorax include difficult breathing, weak and rapid pulse, restlessness, distended neck veins, hypotension, chest and shoulder pain, and cyanosis. If pneumothorax is present, seal the open wound on three sides in any way possible: use Vaseline gauze, plastic wrap, or a rolled-up occlusive dressing or towel. Placing an air/water-tight dressing over a sucking chest wound is necessary until medical assistance is obtained. Specific dressings for this are available in most emergency kits. When transporting a person whose chest has been punctured by a foreign object, make sure that the *object remains in place.*

Rationale: Removing the object could increase the size of the hole and could do more tissue damage, thus increasing the amount of bleeding. Hold the dressing in place with a gloved hand. Oxygen is helpful, and mask-to-mouth or manual breathing bag resuscitation may be needed. Sealing will help the lungs reexpand. Tape a dressing on all sides. If the person's condition seems to worsen, loosen the dressing to let out air that is building up in the chest, to prevent a tension pneumothorax (described below); then reseal the wound. After the client arrives at a healthcare facility, chest tubes will be inserted for continuous, closed drainage.

A *tension pneumothorax* is particularly dangerous. This situation occurs when air leaks out of the lung or bronchus into the chest cavity and cannot escape, causing air to collect and pressure to build in the chest. The lung on the same side of the chest as the leak collapses because of excess pressure. In this case, breath sounds will be greatly diminished or absent on the *affected side*. A tension pneumothorax that remains uncorrected will worsen, resulting in a **mediastinal shift**. The heart, great vessels, and trachea shift to the side opposite the injury, the *unaffected side*, as a result of building air pressure on the affected side. This then prevents the unaffected lung from expanding. In addition, the amount of blood returning to the heart to be pumped to the body will diminish, as will the ability of the heart to pump, resulting in rapid progression toward death. A primary healthcare provider or paramedic may place a large-bore IV needle or chest tube through the chest wall to release excess air.

> **Nursing Alert** Never remove an item puncturing the chest. Stabilize the item with gauze and tape if possible prior to transfer. *Rationale: The article will help seal the hole; its removal may cause added damage. Surgical removal is necessary under controlled conditions.*

Back and Neck Injuries

When a person is a victim of an MVA or fall, suspect a neck or back injury. Great danger exists for further injury, particularly to the spinal cord, by moving the person without proper preparation. Always treat this person as though they have a back or neck injury until such is proved otherwise. Immobilizing devices, such as the cervical collar, head blocks, or the back board, are applied by EMS personnel before the person is moved (Fig. 43-7). It is better to be too careful than to risk causing further injury. Only specially trained personnel should apply immobilizing devices, except in extreme circumstances when assistance is not available.

Head Injuries

Because the scalp is very vascular, scalp lacerations cause profuse bleeding, making even the smallest wound appear serious. Determining the extent and cause of the injury is important. A blow to the head that causes a laceration may also cause injury to the skull or brain. Observe for blood or fluid draining from the nose or ears (with no known injury to the nose), bruising behind the ears or under the eyes, persistent bleeding, or a change in behavior since the accident. *These are all serious danger signs.* Emergency care for a potential head injury includes having the person *lie flat*, while restricting their movements. *Do not lower the person's head!* Keep the person warm and check for signs of increasing *intracranial pressure* (**ICP**; see below). Apply an ice pack

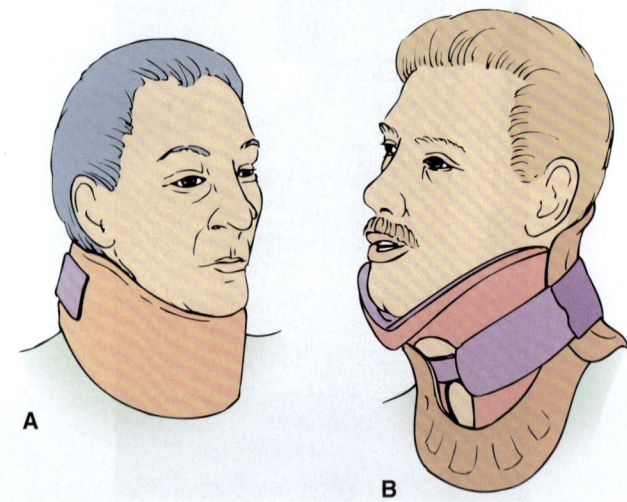

Figure 43-7 A, A foam cervical collar. **B,** A rigid cervical collar. Untrained personnel should not attempt to apply a cervical collar, except in an extreme emergency (Timby, 2005).

to the area of injury. Instruct family to watch for signs of complications every 2 hr for at least 24 hr. Always advise the client to see a physician after *any* head injury.

> **Nursing Alert** Any person who has a head injury, no matter how minor, should be observed carefully for at least 24 hr. Late complications can occur.

Monitoring for signs of increased ICP is crucial. The following are serious signs of increasing ICP:

- Confusion, disorientation, or agitation
- Loss of memory
- Any change in vision, such as blurred or double vision
- Decreased LOC or difficulty arousing; extreme lethargy
- Numbness, tingling, or weakness in an arm or leg
- Persistent vomiting (sometimes projectile)
- Severe headache
- Speech problems
- Seizures

If the person with a head injury must be moved, their head must be stabilized in a neutral position and in line with the back. Emergency personnel provide immobilizing equipment, such as cervical collars, head blocks, and short and long spine boards, which they will use to prepare the person for transport. Stabilize the person without moving them, until proper equipment and assistance arrive.

Cold-Related Injuries

Severe injuries, even death, can result from exposure to cold, even if the temperature is not extreme. Cold injuries can occur if body parts are exposed, because the body automatically cuts down blood flow to peripheral structures and redirects it to the vital organs (heart and brain) if it becomes too cold.

Factors influencing cold-related injuries include the following:

- Temperature
- Wind chill factor
- Wetness
- Length of exposure time
- Part of the body exposed
- Other injury or irritation, such as blisters on the feet or tight shoes
- Person's age and mental status
- Circulatory status
- Nutritional and hydration status
- General physical condition
- Drug or alcohol use

Frostbite

If you work in a public healthcare facility in a cold climate, you will likely see frostbite, especially among people who are experiencing homelessness, those who have mental illness, people who are inebriated, older adults, or physically debilitated. **Frostbite** is the freezing of body tissues resulting from exposure to cold temperatures. The body part becomes so cold that ice crystals form in the spaces surrounding the cells; the cells then die. The body is most vulnerable to frostbite when there is a high wind, because blood rushes to the skin to warm it, then cools quickly, due to rapid heat loss. The mathematical calculation of temperature and wind speed is called the **wind chill factor**. Skin can freeze when the wind chill factor is below the freezing point, even if actual air temperature is considerably higher. If the person is wet, this increases the possibility of frostbite. Frostbite is most likely to affect hands, feet, noses, ears, and cheeks. Noses, ears, and cheeks are vulnerable because they are exposed; hands and feet are vulnerable because circulation to these areas is slowest. However, larger body surface areas can be affected as well.

When a body part becomes frostbitten, the area is first painful and then numb. The frostbitten part is pale and cool to the touch and feels like a block of wood or marble. These symptoms exist initially, regardless of how mild or severe the frostbite. In late stages, hemorrhage may occur and the part may swell. In severe frostbite, blisters form quickly (and should not be broken). The skin may slough off. In general, frostbite looks like a burn. A person suffering from frostbite needs immediate medical attention. *Do not rub* a frostbitten part to restore circulation; rubbing, particularly with snow, will only *increase* the damage and can contribute to gangrene. Protect frozen body parts and handle them gently. Loosen tight clothing. Do not allow the person to walk on a frostbitten foot. Separate frozen fingers and toes with soft cotton wedges; however, do not use bandages, ointments, or salves. Place frozen parts in water between 98°F and 104°F (36.6°C and 40°C); if no thermometer is available, the water should feel *tepid* (lukewarm) to the wrist. Rewarming the affected part will take 20 to 45 min. The person may experience some pain as the part warms. The part will turn pink or bright red as circulation resumes. Protect the part against refreezing. It sometimes takes providers several days to assess the extent of frostbite damage. If hypothermia accompanies frostbite (see next section), this is a *medical emergency*. Box 43-3 presents degrees of frostbite. Frostbite is often treated like a burn, with treatment provided in a burn unit. If treatment is unsuccessful, the area may become gangrenous, turning black and crusty. In this case, amputation may be necessary.

Box 43-3 Degrees of Frostbite

- **First degree** (*superficial*): Temporary tenderness, reddened skin, some peeling may occur—usually no permanent damage. Sometimes called *frostnip*.
- **Second degree** (*partial-thickness*): Blisters and some tissue and nerve damage—can result in permanent hypersensitivity to cold and increased risk of future frostbite. Subsequent exposure to even mild cold can cause *chilblains* (painful chilling and burning sensations). Sometimes called *pernio*; may persist for years.
- **Third degree** (*full-thickness*): Tissue death—often includes nerve and bone damage. Often leads to *gangrene*, even if treated. Usually requires skin grafting or amputation. Often treated in a burn center in the same manner as a burn.

Adapted from Frostbite—the Big Chill. Burn Center, Hennepin County Medical Center, Minneapolis, Minnesota.

Immersion Foot

Immersion foot occurs most often in hikers and canoers when the feet are in moist, cold boots for several days. It can also occur in military personnel who spend several days in the field. In rare cases, this condition can affect the hands. The feet (or hands) should be gently warmed, cleaned, dried, and elevated. Because infection often occurs, antibiotics are given, as well as a tetanus booster.

Hypothermia

Hypothermia occurs when the body loses heat faster than it can burn food (fuel) to replace it. Hypothermia is caused when a person is exposed to extreme cold or is chilled sufficiently long to lower their *core* (internal) *body temperature* to a dangerous level. A critical level of hypothermia can lower the core temperature to as low as 94°F (35°C) or lower. Profuse sweating over time can also cause hypothermia. Windy or wet conditions greatly accelerate the onset of hypothermia. Hypothermia caused by such external forces is known as *accidental hypothermia*. Hypothermia also occurs when the body's temperature regulation malfunctions. In addition, temperature is sometimes intentionally lowered to make surgery safer. This procedure is called *induced* or *surgical hypothermia*. Induced hypothermia confined to one body part is called *local hypothermia*.

Accidentally lowering the body's core temperature even a few degrees can result in serious symptoms and death. Symptoms of hypothermia include sleepiness, slow and clumsy movements, shaking, cardiac dysrhythmia, loss of reflexes and slowed reaction times, impaired judgment, confusion, and respiratory failure. Hallucinations may occur. If the person is in water, drowning is very possible, as a result of weakness and confusion. In a first-aid situation, the initial warning signs are *confusion*, disorientation, slurred speech, obvious shivering, and lethargy. The person may also complain of blurred vision, dizziness, tiredness, or feeling very cold. Definitive diagnosis of hypothermia is based on an accurate measurement of core temperature. Special monitoring equipment is necessary, because normal clinical thermometers often do not register low enough to measure core temperature accurately.

> **Key Concept**
>
> Preventing hypothermia is important, especially for individuals engaged in strenuous outdoor activities. Because major heat loss occurs via the uncovered head (which acts like a chimney), *wearing a hat is important.* Wool clothing helps, because it is warm, even when wet. Wearing layered clothing also is beneficial because the air pockets between layers serve as insulation. Eating enough food and obtaining adequate fluids are also important. Warn campers and hikers to remain dry and to avoid sitting on wet surfaces, cold ground, rocks, or cold metal surfaces. Snow should not be eaten for fluid. It should be melted and warmed first.

Treatment of Hypothermia

Gradual rewarming is necessary. *Rationale: When the body is rewarmed too quickly, cold blood returns to the heart, causing severe dysrhythmia and sometimes cardiac arrest.* The person's cardiac status is continually monitored during rewarming. When providing first aid, remove wet clothing and dress the person in warm, dry clothing, particularly covering their head, hands, and feet. Have them lie or sit on a ground cover, which provides a barrier against moisture and insulates against cold. Keep the person *awake* until medical assistance arrives. Warm, not hot, beverages also help, if the person is alert and can safely swallow. If the person is unconscious, immediate transfer to a healthcare facility is vital. There, the body is warmed until the core temperature is approximately 94°F (35°C). *Then*, the extremities are warmed. Warmed blankets and warming lights (and sometimes, warm water) are used. In addition, warmed oxygen and warmed IV infusions may be given. Blood may be circulated through a pump oxygenator and warmed before returning it to the body's core circulation. Warm fluids may be instilled into the gastrointestinal (GI) system. Treatment continues until the body's core temperature is near normal (98.6°F; 37°C).

Nursing Considerations

The client with severe hypothermia must be moved very carefully, to prevent cardiac dysrhythmia or arrest. During the rewarming process, nursing care includes careful monitoring of vital signs and IV infusion, close observation of skin condition, special mouth and eye care, and measurement of oral and IV intake and urine output (I&O). The body's core temperature is carefully monitored, using a special electronic thermometer. (Complications in the person receiving an IV include bleeding and gastric distention.)

> **Nursing Alert** Give *immediate* emergency care in any case of hypothermia, particularly if accompanied by frostbite. Note that the person with severe hypothermia is not considered dead until they have been rewarmed and still shows no signs of life. CPR is not usually recommended for this person until they are in the ED. *Rationale: There is an increased risk of cardiac standstill (cardiac arrest).* Remember that *air temperature does not need to be extremely cold for hypothermia to occur.*

Heat-Related Injuries

Heat-related injuries are most likely to occur on days of high humidity, with temperatures from 95°F to over 100°F (35°C-37.8°C and over), and no breeze. *Rationale: The body's major defense against heat accumulation is sweating; evaporation of sweat cools the body. When humidity exceeds 75%, particularly without a breeze, evaporation decreases.* The **heat index** is expressed in terms of "the temperature feels like," which is a combination of heat and humidity. The higher the heat index, the more likely are heat-related injuries to occur. Heat injuries typically occur in early summer before people have acclimated themselves to high temperatures. Such injuries can also occur inside enclosed areas, when the outside temperature is low, but other heat sources increase a person's internal heat load. For example, on a bright day, a parked car can quickly become a *fatal* enclosed area for children and pets because of the radiant heat produced by the sun. Heat produced in some work areas also can cause illness. Any enclosed area where equipment and lighting produce a large amount of accumulated heat has the potential to cause heat-related illness. Although sensitivity to heat varies among individuals, certain groups are particularly susceptible. High-risk people include infants, older adults, those who are very obese, people who chronically abuse drugs or alcohol, and persons with underlying illnesses. Military personnel and athletes are also vulnerable, because of the tendency to overexercise in the heat, sometimes in heavy clothing.

Heat Cramps

Heat cramps, severe muscle spasms, usually occur after hard exertion and are frequently found in physically fit young people, who have been sweating profusely and drinking plain water. Heat cramps can occur in cool environments, as well as hot ones, and are usually located in the legs, arms, or abdomen. The person may show signs of heat exhaustion (see next section) in addition to heat cramps. Heat cramps are relieved by drinking very dilute salt solutions. Give the person a mixture of up to one-fourth teaspoon of salt per quart of water or another balanced salt solution. Commercial products, such as "sports drinks" (e.g., Gatorade), also contain extra sodium and other electrolytes. If symptoms continue longer than an hour, seek medical advice. Salt tablets are *not recommended*, because they are gastric irritants. Moving the person to a cooler environment is helpful, but make sure the person's head is uncovered (to allow heat escape) and keep them calm. Explain what is happening and advise the person to avoid exertion for at least 12 hr. Teach the person to add a small amount of salt to food before exertion, to drink adequate liquids (*not just plain water*), and to stop exercising if they feel ill. Misting the skin with water and using a handheld fan also helps.

> **Key Concept**
>
> Persons in cooler climates, such as mountain climbers or competition skiers, may experience heat cramps because they are dressed too warmly, causing excessive sweating. Massaging cramped muscles will *not* cure heat cramps and, in fact, may increase the pain.

Heat Exhaustion

Heat exhaustion may occur in physically fit people who are exerting themselves in a hot environment over a length of time. Under such conditions, when people do not take in sufficient water and sodium to replace lost fluids and electrolytes, a serious blood flow disturbance results, similar to shock. Pure forms of heat exhaustion are rare. Heat exhaustion that occurs quickly is likely to be related to *water depletion*. Another type of heat exhaustion, called *salt-depletion heat exhaustion*, develops over time. True heat exhaustion is rarely life threatening. As a person loses large amounts of water and salt through sweating, blood flow decreases, if water is not replaced. Decreased blood flow affects brain, heart, and lung functioning. When a person loses salt as well as water, heat cramps may occur, along with headache, dizziness, anxiety, nausea, and weakness. Other symptoms of heat exhaustion include excessive sweating, faintness, hypotension, loss of appetite, and unconsciousness (usually brief). Fainting or unconsciousness is most common when the person is standing, because blood pools in the legs, interfering with blood flow to the brain. Skin is pale, cool, and usually sweaty; body temperature may be subnormal, and blood pressure is low. The person's eyes are dilated, breathing is rapid and shallow, and pulse is slow and weak. The person may have difficulty walking.

Treatment for heat exhaustion includes cooling the person, without chilling. Move the person to a cool place, remove and loosen as much clothing as possible, and apply cold, wet compresses to the skin. Fanning is helpful. Have the person lie down with the head about 8 to 12 in. below the feet. *Rationale: The goal is to increase circulation to the brain.* Water replacement and rest will usually relieve symptoms of heat exhaustion caused by *water depletion*. However, the *salt-depleted* person will usually need sips of a salt solution, given slowly over a period of time. With any doubts about the person's condition, transport them to a healthcare facility immediately. *Rationale: Differentiating between heat exhaustion and heat stroke may be difficult.* If blood pressure and pulse remain low for more than a half hour, suspect heat stroke.

Heat Stroke

Heat stroke is a potentially *life-threatening condition* that often develops rapidly and requires immediate treatment. *Classic heat stroke* occurs when the body's heat-regulating mechanisms fail and core temperature soars. When a person's core temperature reaches 105°F to 110°F, sweating stops, brain cells become damaged or destroyed, and death results. Classic heat stroke usually occurs during a summer heat wave, with high temperatures and humidity. It most often affects the poor, homeless or those living in poorly ventilated housing and without air conditioning, older individuals who do not take in enough water, and chronically ill persons, who often are taking medications that contribute to heat stress. However, the recent deaths of athletes in excellent physical condition emphasize the dangers of extreme heat and humidity for all people, regardless of age or physical conditioning.

Exertional heat stroke develops from an increased internal heat load, due to muscular exertion, along with high external temperature and humidity. It usually occurs rapidly (within a few hours) in young, healthy, athletic individuals, simply because their heat-regulating systems become overwhelmed. In about half the cases of exertional heat stroke, the person is sweating.

Persons with *classic heat stroke* usually are brought to the healthcare facility because of hypotension, fever, and coma. Persons with *exertional heat stroke* are usually brought in because of bizarre behavior, confusion, or collapse. Both forms of heat stroke can be life threatening and require immediate medical care. *Rationale: The longer a person goes without treatment, the greater the danger.* Persons suffering from either form of heat stroke share many of the symptoms of heat exhaustion. However, some distinct differences exist (Table 43-1). Persons suffering from heat stroke have hot skin, and usually a high body temperature—above 106°F (41.1°C). Persons suffering from heat exhaustion have cool skin and normal or even slightly below normal body temperature.

TABLE 43-1 Heat Exhaustion Versus Heat Stroke

ELEMENT	HEAT EXHAUSTION	HEAT STROKE
Skin	Cool	Hot
Sweat	Person may or may not sweat.	*Classic heat stroke*—person is usually dry. *Exertional heat stroke*—person is usually sweating.
Body temperature	Normal or below normal	High (often >106°F)
Symptoms	Headache, nausea, dizziness, weakness, faintness, pale skin, weak pulse, tachycardia, anorexia, hypotension, brief periods of unconsciousness, rapid breathing	*Classic heat stroke*—hypotension, fever, coma *Exertional heat stroke*—confusion, bizarre behavior, collapse
Treatment	Cool the person without chilling; elevate their feet.	Cool person rapidly, monitor airway and circulation, observe seizure precautions.
	Water depletion—give water.	
	Salt depletion—give salt solution.	
Medical attention	Seek medical attention if in doubt.	Seek medical attention immediately in all cases.

After activating the EMS, first-aid treatment for heat stroke includes rapidly cooling the person to at least a temperature of 101°F. Place the person in a cool, shady place and remove their clothing. Wrap the person in cold, wet sheets or spray the body with a cold mist of water. Place ice packs on the person's forehead, under the armpits, and at the neck and groin. *Rationale: These areas access the circulation fastest.* If the person is conscious, give sips of cold liquids containing a dilute salt solution. Tell the person not to drink too quickly (to prevent nausea). Prevent shivering. Monitor the person's airway, breathing, and circulation. If necessary, begin CPR. Watch for seizures. *Immediately transport the person for emergency care.*

Nursing Alert If the person suffering from any type of heat-related illness vomits, *stop giving fluids immediately*. The person needs IV fluid replacement. This is usually the only time a person with *heat exhaustion* needs to be hospitalized. Any person with *heat stroke* needs immediate medical attention. Certain illnesses, such as cystic fibrosis and scleroderma, restrict the client's ability to sweat. These individuals are more susceptible to heat stroke.

Burns

Burns occur from many heat sources. (See Chapter 75 for further discussion, including classifications, area calculations, and treatment.) The most common emergency cases of burns are caused by thermal, electrical, chemical, and radiation sources. Flames, steam, hot liquids, and hot objects may cause *thermal burns*. Electrical power sources or lightning may cause *electrical burns*. Strong chemicals can cause severe *chemical burns* to the skin, respiratory system, or eyes. Radiation sources (e.g., power plants, nuclear sources) may cause *radiation burns*; sunburns also fall in this category.

First Aid for Sunburn

Too much exposure to the ultraviolet rays of the sun or a sun lamp causes *sunburn*. A person of any skin tone can be sunburned, but the effects vary with the person's skin tone and previous levels of sun exposure. It is important to apply sun block before spending any length of time in the sun, particularly if the person is susceptible to sunburn. Excessive exposure to the sun is also known to cause certain types of skin cancer.

The person who is sunburned will have reddened skin and may have a fever; blisters and peeling may develop later. First aid involves neutralizing the burning with vinegar, milk, or certain commercial preparations. The sooner these measures are applied, the less chance exists for long-term damage to result. In cases of severe sunburn or if the person develops a fever, they should receive emergency medical care.

First Aid for Other Types of Burns

The seriousness of a burn is estimated by its depth, percentage of the body burned, location, age of the victim, and any underlying complications (see Chapter 75). The following are examples of special considerations:

- A burn that involves more than 10% of the body's surface is extremely serious.
- Any second- or third-degree burn is serious.
- Burns to the hands, feet, mouth, throat, and perineum are serious.
- Full-thickness, circumferential burns to the limbs or chest are particularly dangerous, because they can restrict circulation or breathing.
- Diabetic persons of any age have more difficulty recovering from burns, because their healing is slowed; they may also have underlying circulatory, kidney, or other difficulties.
- Any underlying injury can affect a person's recovery after a burn.
- A person with a compromised immune system is at a particularly high risk for infection, especially if the skin is broken.

In Practice: Nursing Care Guidelines 43-2 summarizes immediate first-aid measures for burns.

IN PRACTICE
NURSING CARE GUIDELINES 43-2 — Providing Emergency First Aid for Burns

- Stop the burning process by removing the heat source. Make sure burning clothing is *cooled*. Do not remove burning fabric or other materials, unless they fall off. **Rationale:** *Some synthetic materials continue to smolder or melt and must be neutralized; however, removing the clothing could tear the person's skin and damage it further.*
- Remove as much clothing in the burned area as possible if it is not stuck to the skin. Tight clothing can be especially dangerous later. **Rationale:** *Often, swelling occurs. Tight clothing contributes to swelling by hampering circulation. Removal of clothing also helps to cool the person. (Make sure the person does not become chilled.)*
- Always check a chemical container for directions on emergency treatment. **Rationale:** *Some chemicals react adversely when in contact with water.*
- Unless contraindicated, flood the area with cool water. Do not apply ice. **Rationale:** *The goal is to cool the area to stop the burning and reduce the incidence of scarring. Ice may further irritate the burned area by cooling it too quickly.*
- Continue to flood the area with cool water. **Rationale:** *Cool water helps control pain; discontinuation may increase pain temporarily, because of damaged nerve endings.*
- Flood most chemical burns with a gentle, continuous flow of plain water until emergency help arrives. **Rationale:** *Flooding with water will help stop the burning process and cool the area. It will also help dilute and wash away caustic chemicals.*
- Watch for shivering, if you are using water to cool a burn covering more than 10% of the body. Change to dry, sterile dressings if shivering occurs. **Rationale:** *Exposure to cold may cause hypothermia.*
- Do not put anything other than water or a specifically prescribed substance on a burn. **Rationale:** *Materials such as salves, ointments, or butter occlude the burn, so it becomes difficult to examine. These substances promote infection and pain on removal.*
- Remove the injured person's jewelry. Put it in a safe place. **Rationale:** *It can remain hot and continue the burning process. Swelling usually occurs later, making it impossible to remove rings or other jewelry; if left on, jewelry can cut off circulation.*
- Monitor the person's airway, breathing, and circulation. Be prepared to initiate CPR. **Rationale:** *Respiratory or cardiac arrest (or both) can occur from shock.*
- If the burn is extensive, cover it with a dry, nonstick, sterile dressing. Do not use gauze. **Rationale:** *Gauze will peel off additional tissue and cause more damage.* For all large burns, use only a dry, sterile dressing, following removal of the heat source and cooling down period. **Rationale:** *The dressing will help prevent infection.*
- Keep dressings cool and dry. Be sure to keep person warm and monitor for hypothermia. **Rationale:** *Wet dressings may promote hypothermia.*
- Prevent contamination of the wound as much as possible. **Rationale:** *Infection is a major hazard with burns.*
- Treat for shock. **Rationale:** *Pain, loss of body fluids, and anxiety contribute to shock.*
- Determine what first-aid measures others have already given. **Rationale:** *Some of these measures may be dangerous. Emergency and medical personnel need to be aware of what has been done prior to their arrival.*

Associated problems often cause more harm than the burn itself. Be alert for *inhalation injuries and breathing problems*, as well as for broken bones or other injuries. Check for the following signs of possible inhalation injury:

- Burned or singed nasal hairs or burns in or around the mouth
- Flecks of soot in the client's saliva
- Smell of smoke on the client's breath
- Hoarse voice

Remember, a person can experience a burn *internally*, such as from inhaling hot air or smoke or from swallowing a caustic substance. These injuries can be life threatening. The trachea and lungs can be burned or severely eroded. The gases in smoke can replace the air in the lungs, rendering the person unable to oxygenate their blood. In any case of suspected inhalation injury, immediately transport the person for emergency care.

Nursing Alert If a burned person was trapped in a confined space and exposed to chemicals or smoke, suspect smoke or heat inhalation injury.

Inflicted Burns
In certain mental disorders, such as borderline personality disorder, a burn may be self-inflicted by the person. Also, a common method of child abuse is to inflict a burn on a child, often in a location that is covered by clothing. Figure 43-8 illustrates some suspicious burn patterns. Any such burn pattern should be immediately investigated and reported to the authorities, particularly in the case of a child or vulnerable adult (e.g., intellectual disability, mentally ill, older adult).

Near Drowning

Drowning is suffocation from submersion in liquid. **Near drowning** implies that recovery has occurred after submersion. Most drownings occur in swimming pools, lakes, rivers, and oceans. However, children can drown in the toilet, bathtub, wading pool, or a bucket. Assess victims of near drowning for associated injuries or illnesses, such as cardiac arrest, airway obstruction, head injury, spinal injury, and internal injuries. Long-term brain damage may result from extended *anoxia* (absence of oxygen). Submersion in cold water may also cause hypothermia; however,

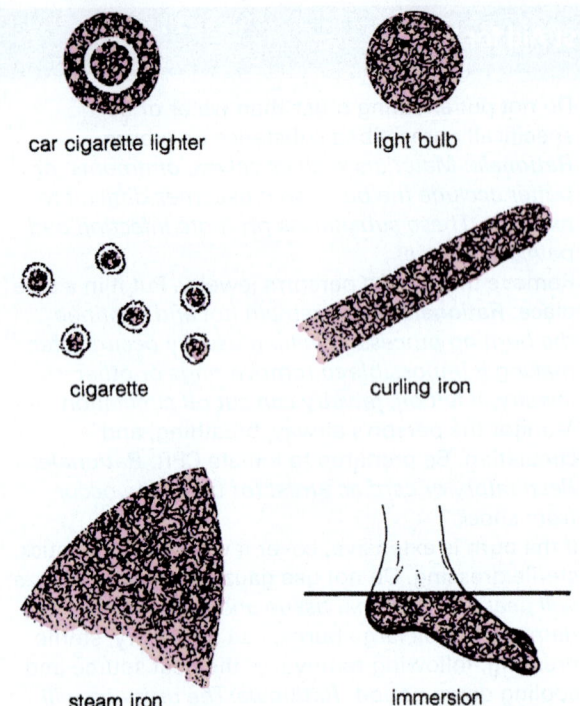

Figure 43-8 Look for specific patterns in burns, some of which indicate they are self-inflicted or inflicted by an abuser. All instances of suspected abuse must be reported (Klossner & Hatfield, 2010).

individuals submerged in cold water *may survive* because when body temperature is lowered, metabolism slows, which decreases the brain's need for oxygen. Victims of near drowning may appear dead because of reduced brain and cardiovascular function. However, rescuers should initiate and continue lifesaving measures, including CPR, until the person can be evaluated by electroencephalogram. People, particularly children, may respond to prolonged resuscitation efforts without sustaining brain damage after near drowning. Treat all near drowning victims for hypothermia and shock; maintain circulation and respiration until the person is cleared medically.

Musculoskeletal Injuries

Musculoskeletal injuries are those involving bones, muscles, or joints.

Fractures, Sprains, and Dislocations

When a person has been involved in an MVA or fall, examine for possible injuries:

- **Fracture**: broken bone
- **Sprain**: twisting of a joint, with rupture of ligaments and other possible damage
- **Strain**: twisting or stretching that damages a muscle or tendon
- **Dislocation**: displacement of a bone from a joint

Sometimes, determining the difference between a sprain and a fracture is difficult. If in doubt, assume that a fracture has occurred and treat the person accordingly. Apply ice and seek medical treatment. Usually, the person will have pain on movement after sustaining a fracture. *Do not have the person stand or walk on a suspected fracture to check for pain. Rationale: Doing so is likely to aggravate the injury.* The cardinal rule is *do not move the person.* Get emergency help. Question the person if they are conscious. Observe for obviously deformed limbs; cover them with a blanket until you can obtain adequate help. If the person must be moved, the injury must be immobilized. *Never attempt to reposition the bones,* whether or not the skin is broken. (If fractured ends of bone protrude through the skin, this is a *compound fracture.* If the skin is not broken, this is a *simple fracture.*) Cover any open wounds with a sterile dressing and control excessive bleeding by direct or indirect pressure.

Remember the acronym **RICE** in emergency procedures for sprains and strains:

R = Rest
I = Ice
C = Compression (such as with a roller bandage)
E = Elevation (keep the part above the level of the heart, if possible)

Splinting

Do not attempt to splint a fracture or sprain if the EMS has been activated. However, if the person must be transported, a **splint** is applied. This device *immobilizes* a fracture or sprain. You can use any hard, straight item. A good emergency splint for an arm is a thick magazine wrapped around the arm and tied. Any long, straight item can be used as a temporary splint for a leg (Fig. 43-9). Be careful not to tie the splint so tightly as to cut off circulation. Numerous commercial splints are available. Traction splints are best for most major leg fractures and should be applied only by EMS personnel. Inflatable splints may also be used. If a fracture of a wrist, knee, or elbow is suspected, splint the joint in its existing position. **Rationale:** *Because of the joint's close proximity to arteries, veins, and nerves, straightening the joint can put pressure on blood vessels, cutting off circulation or sensation to the extremity's distal portion.* An effective splint for a fractured toe is the adjacent toe; tape the digits together ("buddy taping"). The same is true for fingers; an ice cream stick or tongue blade is a handy item to use for a finger splint.

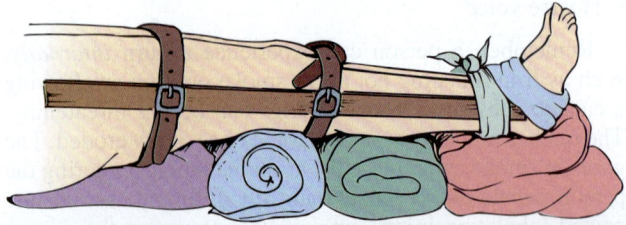

Figure 43-9 An emergency leg splint immobilizes the injured leg to the uninjured leg. The makeshift splint can be made of any rigid item, such as a board, broom handle, or golf club, and tied with neckties or belts. The legs are kept elevated (Timby, 2005).

> **Nursing Alert** When splinting a fracture, check the person's distal pulse *before and after* splinting. An *absent* pulse is a medical emergency. Obtain medical attention *immediately*.

Dressing a Wound

If emergency assistance is unavailable, it may be necessary to apply a dressing to an open wound, such as that which accompanies a compound fracture. Although many articles can be used as a dressing in an emergency, use a sterile dressing whenever possible. If a sterile dressing is unavailable, use the cleanest material at hand. A clean handkerchief or ironed dishtowel is suitable. Unused newspaper also can be used, because it is clean. *Remember to wear gloves, if at all possible.*

Using Bandages

A **bandage** is a piece of material used to hold a dressing or splint in place, to give support, or to apply pressure. When applying a bandage in an emergency:

- Apply the bandage firmly, but not so tightly that circulation is restricted. Watch for evidence of tightness—blanching of skin, loss of sensation, and absent pulse. Loosen the bandage, if necessary.
- If a knot is used, always tie a square knot, because it will not slip and can be easily untied.
- If possible, leave the tips of the person's toes and fingers exposed. *Rationale: Checking for impaired circulation is necessary to ensure adequate tissue perfusion.* Assess for pallor, lack of pulse, pain on passive motion, paresthesia (burning, tingling), or paralysis. (This assessment is known as **CMS**: color, motion, and sensitivity or sensation; see Chapter 77.) Chapter 53 discusses the application of bandages in more detail (see Table 53-1).

Applying Cravat Bandages and Slings

A *triangular* or *handkerchief bandage* can be made from a square of cloth or dishtowel and secured without tape or pins, if necessary. Fold the cloth several times to make a *strip* or *cravat bandage*. A triangular bandage also may be used to make a sling for arm support. Applying a sling is described in In Practice: Nursing Procedure 43-1.

Dental Injuries and Missing Teeth

Teeth may be displaced or knocked out accidentally. A tooth that is pushed up into the socket is an **intrusion injury**; a tooth that is knocked out is an **avulsion injury**. In either event, *immediate dental care* is necessary. In an avulsion injury, a dentist may be able to reimplant and reposition the tooth. An avulsed tooth that is reimplanted within 30 min has a 90% chance of being saved. It *may* be saved if reimplanted within 2 hr. First aid for avulsed teeth is outlined at In Practice: Nursing Care Guidelines 43-3.

Foreign Objects

A *foreign object* is any abnormal object or substance lodged in a body orifice or structure.

Foreign Objects in the Eyes

Foreign objects in the eye can be particles of dust or soot or an eyelash resting on the eyelid's lining or cornea. Anything that lodges on the cornea irritates it, especially when the eyelid opens and closes; in addition, particles may become embedded. Any foreign object can scratch or permanently damage the cornea. Irritation of the cornea causes tears to flow, a natural body defense mechanism. Often, tears will wash out the foreign object and no treatment is needed.

Most contact lenses used today can remain in the person's eyes for several hours, or even overnight, without incident. If lenses are left in place following an accident, the medical team must be aware of this fact. The person's corneas can become ulcerated if they do not blink. Hard or gas-permeable contact lenses are more likely to cause corneal ulcers than soft lenses. In some cases, removal of contact lenses at the scene of an accident is necessary; a special suction cup is available for this purpose.

Caustic substances are those that burn or destroy flesh. A caustic substance in the eye is extremely irritating and very dangerous. If chemicals enter a person's eye, immediate action must be taken to flush the eye with water. In Practice: Nursing Care Guidelines 43-4 summarizes emergency care of eye injuries. If any question exists about the injury's severity, seek medical assistance as soon as possible.

IN PRACTICE

NURSING CARE GUIDELINES 43-3 — First Aid for Avulsed Teeth

- Ask bystanders to look for the missing tooth. Instruct them to pick it up with a sterile piece of gauze by the crown and not to touch the root. *Rationale: Touching the root may damage important structures of the root.*
- Call a dentist immediately. The person must see a dentist or go to an emergency department as soon as possible. *Rationale: The sooner a tooth is repositioned, the more likely it is to be saved.*
- Clean the person's mouth with gauze. Using sterile gauze, have the client gently bite down. *Rationale: Doing so will restrict bleeding and reduce pain.*
- Instruct the person not to put pressure on adjacent teeth. *Rationale: The accident may have loosened adjacent teeth.*
- If possible, have the person bite gently on a dry tea bag. *Rationale: Tannin in tea acts as a natural coagulant and helps to stop bleeding.*
- Do not allow the client to suck on a straw or smoke. *Rationale: The sucking action may loosen a blood clot and cause more bleeding.*
- Place the tooth on sterile gauze. You may clean it by dipping it in milk, while holding the crown. Keep the tooth under the person's tongue or in milk until arriving at the dentist. *Rationale: Using water or any solution other than milk or the person's own saliva may damage the root. The person's saliva or milk will help preserve the tooth's root system.*

UNIT 7 Safety in the Healthcare Facility

IN PRACTICE

NURSING CARE GUIDELINES 43-4 — Giving First Aid for Eye Injuries

First Aid for Foreign Objects in the Eye
- Instruct the person not to rub the eye. Have the person keep the eye closed and avoid blinking. *Rationale: Rubbing or blinking may drive a foreign object deeper into the eye.*
- Never use an instrument, toothpick, or match to remove a foreign object. *Rationale: These items are unsterile and may introduce pathogens into the eye and scratch the cornea.*
- Never attempt to remove a foreign object if the slightest possibility exists that it is embedded in the cornea. *Rationale: You could drive the object deeper into the eye and cause more damage.*
- Remove contact lenses, if possible. *Rationale: Contact lenses can contribute to further aggravation and injury.*
- Treat both eyes even if only one is injured. *Rationale: A sympathetic injury can occur.*

When the Object Is Not Embedded
- Pull down the person's lower eyelid to see whether the object is on the eyelid membrane. *Rationale: If the object is on the inside of the eyelid, you may be able to lift it off by touching it gently with the corner of a clean handkerchief or with a cotton-tipped applicator moistened in water.*
- Always moisten the cotton tip of an applicator before touching it to the eye. *Rationale: Small particles of dry cotton can become lodged in the eye.*
- If the object is under the person's upper eyelid, grasp the lashes of the upper eyelid with your forefinger and thumb; ask the person to look upward; gently pull the lid forward and downward over the lower eyelid. *Rationale: Usually the eyelash movement dislodges the foreign body and tears wash it away.*
- Flush the eye with plain water. *Rationale: Sometimes the pressure of the water will flush an object out of the eye.*

First Aid for Caustic Materials in the Eye
- Flush the eye with large amounts of water or normal saline solution. *Rationale: Eyes are sensitive to chemical or thermal burns. It is vital to use a large amount of fluid to cleanse the eye.* You can use a sterile medicine dropper or a small sterile bulb syringe. Do not use an unsterile eye cup. *Rationale: Eye cups may introduce pathogens into the eye.*
- Use an eyewash sink, if possible. Have the person stand over the sink, with the eyes close to the jets. Encourage the person to keep the eyes open as much as possible. When the water is turned on, the jets direct a continuous stream of water into the eyes. *Rationale: Large amounts of water are necessary, which are easily provided with an eyewash sink.*

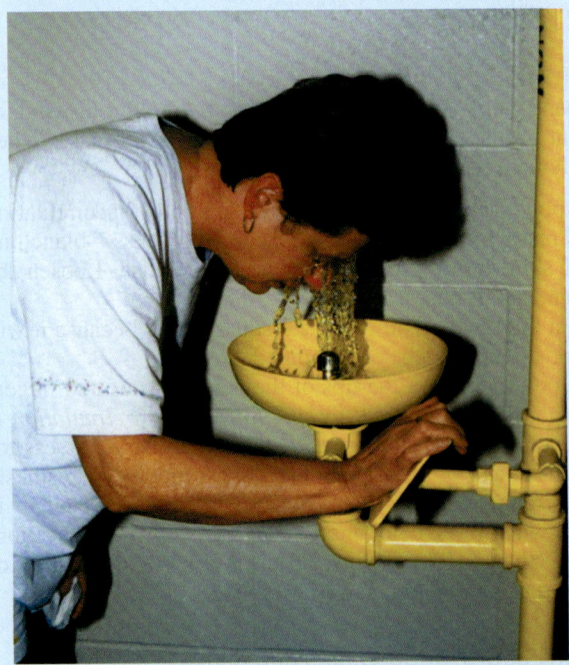

If any caustic material splashes into the eye, immediately flush the eye with large amounts of water. (Photo Copyright Kimberly Malcolm Rosdahl.)

- Do not instill another substance into the eye in an attempt to neutralize a caustic substance. *Rationale: Putting another substance into the eye could do more damage.*
- Have the person see a physician immediately. *Rationale: Prompt action is necessary to prevent permanent eye damage.*

Foreign Objects in the Nose or Ears

Children often insert small objects into their noses or ears. To remove an object from a child's nose, have the child blow the nose gently with *both* nostrils open. Unless the object is clearly visible and at the edge of the nostril, do not attempt to remove it with a finger or instrument. Call for medical assistance. If a foreign object lodges in a person's ear, do not attempt to remove it. Instead, transport the person to a healthcare facility.

> **Nursing Alert** Be aware that an object such as a bean or a dried pea will swell when moistened. This makes these objects difficult to remove, especially from the nose.

Airway Obstruction

Foreign objects often become lodged in the throat. If the foreign object is not visible, but the victim is able to breathe adequately, call for emergency medical assistance or take the person to an ED. If the person is not exchanging air and shows signs of respiratory distress, call 911 and use appropriate obstructed-airway techniques if you have been properly trained. (All nursing students should have current CPR and obstructed airway training.) An airway obstructed by a foreign body will quickly cause respiratory arrest. Anytime a person (particularly a child) becomes cyanotic, stops breathing, and collapses for no apparent reason, suspect an obstructed airway.

In an adult, foreign-body obstruction is usually caused by a large piece of food (usually meat) becoming lodged in the airway. Poorly fitting dentures, alcohol ingestion, and certain medical conditions, including a neuromuscular disease such as Huntington disease, strokes, cleft palate, brain injury, seizure disorders, heavy sedation, decreased saliva production, or a diminished or absent cough or gag reflex can increase the risk for choking. Older adults who cannot chew food well are also at risk for choking. Airway obstruction often occurs in restaurants. Suspect an obstructed airway when you see a person coughing and gasping, who looks frightened and suddenly leaves the table, heading for the restroom. Follow the person to ask if they are choking. If this person goes off alone, they may die of an apparent heart attack but they are really experiencing a choking death. In the 1980s, a physician coined the term **café coronary** to describe this sudden death during a meal, but this term is misleading.

The person who has a *partially obstructed airway* with good air exchange will cough forcefully. Wheezing may be present, but air exchange is obvious. Encourage the person to cough. *Do not interfere* with attempts to expel the obstruction, and do not leave the person. Offer encouragement and continue to monitor them. If the person's condition does not rapidly improve, activate the EMS. Poor air exchange may be identified by ineffective coughing and sometimes by high-pitched wheezing sounds, **stridor**. The person often experiences increasing respiratory difficulty and may become cyanotic. In *complete airway obstruction*, the person is unable to talk, breathe, or cough, and may indicate the condition by using the universal signal for choking, clutching the neck between the fingers and thumbs of both hands (Fig. 43-10). In complete airway obstruction, no oxygen enters the lungs. The person will soon become unconscious unless the obstruction is removed. Use the *Heimlich maneuver*, also called *abdominal thrusts*, in the case of complete airway obstruction. (This maneuver is learned in a CPR class.) All nurses should be able to perform this skill.

Cardiovascular Emergencies

Fainting

Fainting (**syncope**) is caused by an insufficient supply of blood and oxygen to the brain. Extreme hunger, tiredness, heat, being in an oxygen-deprived environment, or severe emotional shock can cause fainting. Severe hemorrhage, excruciating pain, and standing in one place for a prolonged period, especially with the knees locked, are other causes. The symptoms of imminent fainting include dizziness, blackness or spots before the eyes, pallor, and excessive perspiration. The person loses consciousness; the pulse is weak and breathing is shallow. In Practice: Nursing Care Guidelines 43-5 may be used for the person who has fainted or who feels faint.

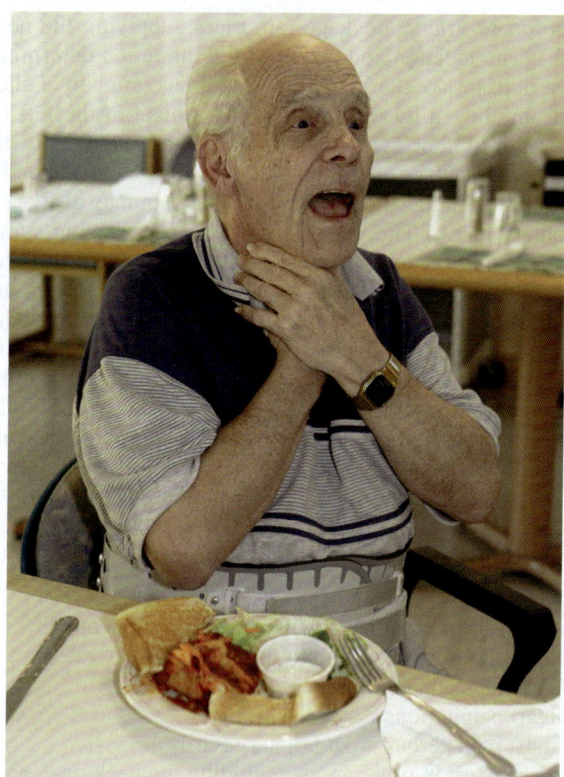

Figure 43-10 Grasping the throat is the universal sign for choking. Emergency first aid must be instituted immediately (Carter, 2005).

Suspected Heart Attack

Chapter 81 discusses cardiovascular conditions, including myocardial infarction (**MI**), commonly known as *heart attack*. In an MI, some of the heart's blood supply is cut off, causing heart muscle tissue to die. This is usually the result

---

IN PRACTICE

NURSING CARE GUIDELINES 43-5 — Assisting the Client Who Feels Faint

- When someone complains of feeling faint, have them sit or lie down and bend their head forward between the knees. Maintain the person in this position. *Rationale: When the head is lower than the heart, more blood is carried to the brain.*
- Loosen tight clothing. *Rationale: Tight clothing can constrict breathing, further reducing the amount of oxygen carried to the brain.*
- If the person is unconscious, assess for respirations and pulse. Start CPR if necessary. *Rationale: A life-threatening condition may be the cause of unconsciousness.*
- When the person regains consciousness, help them to rise slowly, first to a sitting position. *Rationale: The person may feel weak and could fall.*
- Do not allow the person to move until they have fully regained consciousness. *Rationale: The person's altered level of consciousness may be due to a serious condition, such as a skull fracture, concussion, stroke, cerebral hemorrhage, or shock.*

of coronary artery blockage (an artery supplying the heart itself). The location and extent of the infarction determines the seriousness of the MI. Men most often complain of chest pain, unrelieved by rest, which may radiate to the left (or right) arm. Other symptoms include pain radiating to the back, neck, jaw, or teeth; the pain may also be mistaken for heartburn or indigestion. (Be aware that pain may also occur in other places.) The person may have been having symptoms off and on for several days (*unstable angina*). Other common symptoms of MI include restlessness, panic, and a sense of impending doom; difficulty breathing and other signs of respiratory distress; and changes in pulse quality and rate. The skin is cold and clammy, and the person may be cyanotic (indicating lack of oxygen to the tissues). If a person has any of these symptoms, suspect a heart attack and call for help *immediately*.

Since most MI research has been done on men, and the symptoms may be different, an MI may not be recognized in a woman. Heart attack (MI) symptoms in women often include the following:

- Shortness of breath, difficulty in catching the breath
- Nausea and flu-like symptoms, chills, cold sweat
- Light-headedness, faintness
- Heart palpitations
- Chest pain perhaps, but not necessarily
- Discomfort in other areas, including the neck, jaw, back, and arms (most often the left arm); a common location of pain is the shoulder blades or between the shoulder blades
- Heartburn and stomach pains
- Extreme fatigue

Prompt action is the most important factor in whether a person lives or dies following an MI. **Thrombolytic** medications dissolve the clot and clear the blocked blood vessel. Plain aspirin is often chewed as an immediate emergency first-aid measure, to help thin the blood. (Aspirin has improved the success rate in saving lives when administered within 1 hr of the attack.) In Practice: Nursing Care Guidelines 43-6 presents first aid for the person with a suspected heart attack.

> **Nursing Alert** The most frequent common denominator in MI is *denial*. The person cannot believe they are having a heart attack.

Suspected Cerebrovascular Accident

A **CVA**, stroke, or "brain attack" is more likely to occur in an older person, although the victim may be any age. A CVA is the occlusion or rupture of a blood vessel in the brain, causing anoxia, with varying results, including paralysis and/or death. Immediate action is vital. If any of the following warning signs are observed, activate the EMS system immediately. Medications, such as tPA (tissue plasminogen activator), may be able to stop or reverse the symptoms (see also Chapter 81). These are truly "clot busters."

For signs and symptoms of a CVA, remember the acronym **FAST**:

- **F**: Face drooping, especially on one side
- **A**: Arm weakness
- **S**: Speech difficulties
- **T**: Time to call EMS

Other symptoms include any sudden numbness or tingling, confusion, inability to understand, inability to walk, dizziness, loss of balance, and "the worst headache" ever experienced. "Small strokes," called transient ischemic attacks (**TIA**), may also occur and should be treated immediately (American Heart Association, n.d.).

Bleeding

Nosebleed (Epistaxis)

The medical term for *nosebleed* is *epistaxis*. In Practice: Nursing Procedure 43-2 gives the basic steps for treating a nosebleed.

> **Nursing Alert** If the person with a nosebleed has a fractured skull, *do not attempt to stop the bleeding*. **Rationale:** *Doing so could increase intracranial pressure.* In severe hypertension, a nosebleed may be the body's safety valve against a CVA (stroke).

IN PRACTICE
NURSING CARE GUIDELINES 43-6 — Giving First Aid in Suspected Heart Attack (MI)

- Have someone call 911. **Rationale:** *Prompt treatment is vital.*
- Keep the person completely quiet. Do not allow the person to move, no matter how much better they claim to feel. **Rationale:** *Most people say they feel better. This is part of denial.*
- Loosen any tight clothing. **Rationale:** *Loosening clothing helps to make breathing easier.*
- Cover the person with a blanket or coat. Put a ground cover under the person, if possible. **Rationale:** *Keeping the person covered helps to prevent chilling and shock. These complications add exertion to the already stressed heart.*
- Place something under the person's head and upper back. If necessary, assist the person to sit up to breathe. **Rationale:** *The person usually finds it easier to breathe if the head is elevated.*
- If the person shows signs of shock, keep them flat, unless this inhibits breathing. **Rationale:** *Lying flat helps to control shock. However, the person will become more panicky if they cannot breathe.*
- Be prepared to initiate CPR. **Rationale:** *Cardiopulmonary arrest is a relatively common complication of heart attack. If the person can be maintained until arrival at the healthcare facility, there is an increased chance for a positive outcome.*

Minor Wounds

Place a sterile pad directly over a minor bleeding wound. A commercial adhesive bandage strip (e.g., Band-Aid) is an adequate dressing for a small cut or scratch. These are packaged individually in various sizes and should be in every home and automobile first-aid kit. Do not touch the part of the sterile dressing that covers the wound. Put the dressing exactly where it is to stay; it cannot be moved afterward, without contaminating it. Be sure the bandage is firmly applied, yet not so tight as to cut off circulation. Telfa (nonstick) pads are much less irritating on removal than conventional gauze bandages. Band-Aids impregnated with antibiotic are available and often enhance healing.

If a sterile dressing is not readily available, use a clean handkerchief (not tissue) or cloth. Press the dressing firmly on the bleeding area; then apply a firm bandage to hold the dressing in place. The dressing should stop minor bleeding. If bleeding is more severe, apply an inflated blood pressure cuff or air splint, or insert a firmly rolled sterile pad under the dressing. *Rationale: A rolled pad applies more pressure than a flat pad.* Fasten the bandage securely in place. Fasten a dressing on an arm or leg with an all-cotton elastic–type roller bandage, but be sure not to shut off circulation. A roller bandage placed over the dressing may also help to control bleeding. Skinned or scraped areas, with scant bleeding or not at all, can be sprayed with a "liquid bandage," such as Nu-Skin, to protect the wound.

Hemorrhage

When a blood vessel is cut or torn, bleeding occurs. The amount of bleeding depends on the number and size of injured blood vessels. A person can lose a great deal of blood if bleeding is excessive before clotting occurs.

> **Key Concept**
>
> If a person loses a large amount of blood, the hemoglobin reading will not show an immediate drop. The decreased laboratory value will occur in 24 to 48 hr.

Bleeding that is abundant or uncontrollable is called **hemorrhage**. A severe injury to one large blood vessel can cause a serious hemorrhage; however, an injury to many small vessels or capillaries can cause an equally life-threatening hemorrhage. In an emergency involving bleeding, the first and most important step is to stop the bleeding. The second step is to treat the shock that accompanies hemorrhage (see earlier discussion). Because blood is the chief means of transmission of many diseases, be sure to follow Standard Precautions.

When you are faced with a situation involving bleeding, quickly assess for the type of bleeding:

- In *capillary bleeding*, blood oozes slowly out of the wound.
- In *arterial bleeding*, blood comes in spurts with each heartbeat and is bright red or pink. Arterial bleeding is usually the most severe type of hemorrhage. (Note: If an artery is nicked, it is likely to bleed profusely. If it is cut across [transected], it may bleed very little, because the ends of the vessel draw together. Arterial bleeding is a *serious medical emergency.*)
- In *venous bleeding*, blood flows steadily and is dark in color. Usually, venous bleeding is minor and stops by itself, unless the person has a bleeding disorder.

In any case of hemorrhage, place the person on a flat surface and slightly elevate their feet (unless the person has a head injury or nosebleed).

Applying Direct Pressure

In external hemorrhage, cut the person's clothes away from the site to reveal the site and amount of bleeding. Apply direct, firm pressure at the site, which will control bleeding in most injuries. Elevate the injured part unless the possibility of fracture or other trauma to the area exists. Direct pressure on a wound for at least 10 min is successful the majority of the time.

Applying Indirect Pressure

If direct pressure does not control hemorrhage, you may need to apply *indirect pressure.* This means that you do not apply pressure directly to the wound, but to an artery at a pressure point between the wound and the heart (see Fig. 43-4). You will need a firm surface to press against, to cut off the blood flow from the heart to the wound. Therefore, choose a pressure point in which the supplying artery lies close to a bone. If bleeding is severe enough to require the use of a pressure point, maintain the pressure until medical assistance arrives. If you release pressure, the clot that formed may dislodge and bleeding will resume. Danger of embolism also exists.

> **Nursing Alert** Never wipe a blood clot from a wound. The clot acts as a plug for ruptured blood vessels. If the clot breaks loose, death may result from *external hemorrhage* or from *embolism.*

Using a Tourniquet

A **tourniquet** is a tie used on an extremity over a pressure point to stop hemorrhage. Use a tourniquet *only in catastrophic situations with life-threatening bleeding.* The tourniquet must be tight enough to cut off the blood flow in the artery completely. If it is too loose, it will only prevent the blood from flowing back through the veins, and thus will increase bleeding. Many states are implementing programs to train everyone in appropriate tourniquet use and make them available in all schools. In Practice: Nursing Procedure 43-3 outlines the steps for applying a tourniquet.

> **Nursing Alert** Using a tourniquet may mean that the person will lose the limb as a result if left on too long.

Internal Bleeding

A person experiencing *internal bleeding* can develop life-threatening shock before the bleeding is discovered.

Consider internal bleeding in all cases of trauma, especially in older clients. Possible causes of internal bleeding include blunt trauma, fractures, GI bleeding, and vaginal bleeding. A fracture is the most common cause of internal bleeding. A fractured pelvis is the most severe fracture, as related to blood loss. Signs of upper GI bleeding may include vomiting bright red blood or passing bloody or black stools. Coffee ground–like emesis or rectal bleeding usually indicates bleeding in the lower GI tract. A person with GI bleeding can deteriorate very quickly. Treatment is aimed at stopping bleeding and replacing blood and fluids lost. Report the following observations to the EMTs or physician immediately if you see them in any person, regardless if the person is in a healthcare facility or not:

- Large or unexplained bruises and contusions
- Bleeding from the mouth, rectum, ears, or other body opening
- Dizziness when rising from a lying to a standing position, without a known cause
- Cold, clammy skin
- Profuse sweating
- Restlessness, anxiety, unexplained combative behavior
- Confusion, without other known causes
- Weak, rapid pulse
- Shallow, rapid breathing
- Extreme thirst
- Unexplained weakness
- Falling blood pressure
- Altered LOC

Anaphylaxis

Normally, when the body senses the presence of an antigen, an antigen–antibody reaction occurs, to protect the person from foreign toxins (see Chapter 24). In anaphylaxis, the antigen–antibody reaction works to the person's detriment because it is so severe. The release of chemicals, such as histamine, causes systemic reactions, affecting several body systems. **Anaphylaxis** (anaphylactic shock) is a type I allergic, life-threatening reaction to a substance. A severe type I reaction occurs within minutes of exposure and is immediately *life-threatening.*

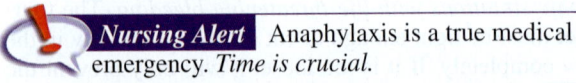

Nursing Alert Anaphylaxis is a true medical emergency. *Time is crucial.*

Anaphylaxis is highly individualized; people can be hypersensitive to almost any substance. Common triggers include the following:

- Bee stings
- Certain foods (e.g., peanuts, cow's milk, shellfish)
- Food additives or preservatives (e.g., sulfite, MSG)
- Medications (e.g., antibiotics, aspirin)
- Chemicals
- Inhaled substances

In Practice: Data Gathering 43-1 lists signs and symptoms of anaphylactic shock. The person's LOC is especially significant; they will be restless and panicky and may faint or have a seizure. Loss of consciousness often occurs early in severe anaphylaxis. The time range for an allergic reaction is from a few seconds to several hours. Reactions are often generalized and violent. *Each occurrence is more serious than the last.* People who have severe allergies should carry medication such as subcutaneous epinephrine (e.g., an "Epi-pen") with them at all times, and family and friends as well as the person should learn how to administer this medication. This person should always wear a MedicAlert tag. Common medications for anaphylaxis are listed at In Practice: Important Medications 43-1.

Remember the acronym **SIRES** when faced with an allergic or anaphylactic situation:

S = Stabilize
I = Identify the toxin
R = Reverse the effect of the toxin
E = Eliminate the toxin
S = Support (respiration, circulation)

First-aid care begins with creating an open airway. Activate the EMS system immediately. Ask the person if appropriate medication is available. If so, the person may need assistance in administering this.

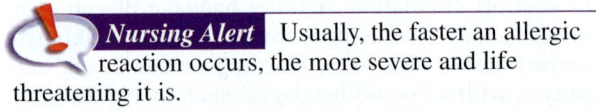

Nursing Alert Usually, the faster an allergic reaction occurs, the more severe and life threatening it is.

Animal Bites and Scratches

Animal bites and scratches are a common problem, particularly among children. Most often, the child is bitten by a household pet. **Rabies**, a communicable disease transmitted through animal bites, is caused by the *rhabdovirus*, which follows the person's nerves to the CNS. Untreated rabies is almost always fatal. A specific **antidote** (substance that neutralizes poisons) for rabies is available but is painful and expensive.

Animal bites and scratches can also cause an infection, which may become serious. Cat bites or scratches are usually more likely to become infected than dog bites. Cat and dog infections include *cat-scratch disease (fever)*, which is usually mild, resulting only in swelling of regional lymph nodes. *Cat-bite disease* can be more serious. Usually, the cat does not show any signs of disease in either case. A dog bite can be serious and disfiguring, especially if it involves the face. Some dog attacks can result in death, particularly in children. When a person is bitten, cleanse the wound with warm, soapy water and rinse the area thoroughly. Swab the area with Zephiran or alcohol. If a puncture wound is present, flush the area with sterile normal saline. *Do not delay in obtaining medical care.* Follow the physician's orders for further care. Usually, the nurse or physician will **debride** (cut away) any loose tissue. A tetanus injection or antibiotics to prevent or treat infection may be administered. One commonly used in animal-related injuries is amoxicillin/clavulanate (Bactrim). If a rabies antiserum is required, the manufacturer will include specific instructions and these instructions must be followed exactly.

IN PRACTICE
DATA GATHERING IN NURSING 43-1: Signs and Symptoms of Anaphylaxis

Skin
- Raised hive-like patches (*urticaria*)
- Reddening of the skin
- Severe itching (*pruritus*)
- Pallor
- Perspiration
- Cold, clammy skin or flushed skin
- Blueness (*cyanosis*) around the lips and nails

Neurologic System
- Dizziness, fainting
- Weakness, confusion
- Restlessness
- Throbbing headache
- Tingling and numbness
- Seizures or stroke
- Coma

Circulatory System
- Dilation of blood vessels
- Blood volume loss
- Decreased cardiac stroke volume
- Decreased cardiac output
- Lowering of blood pressure
- Weak, rapid, or slow pulse
- Irregular pulse
- Circulatory collapse
- Cardiac standstill

Respiratory System
- Difficulty breathing
- Coughing, sneezing, wheezing
- Itching nose
- Swelling of face, tongue, throat (angioedema)
- Chest tightness
- Dyspnea
- Choking sensation
- Respiratory arrest

Gastrointestinal System
- Nausea and vomiting (especially if trigger was eaten)
- Abdominal cramping
- Diarrhea

Other
- Watery, itching eyes
- Metallic taste
- Swelling of eyes, hands, and feet
- Throbbing in the ears
- Incontinence

Key Concept

In an animal bite, the animal is captured and observed, whenever possible. If it cannot be located or captured, obtain an accurate description of the animal and the circumstances. Do not destroy the animal; sometimes quarantine is needed to determine if it is diseased or not. In the case of a household pet, the animal will be subject to an enforced quarantine. If a wild animal is not available for observation, the person usually must undergo antirabies treatment. A fine may be assessed if a pet has bitten someone previously. Any animal bite must be reported immediately. (Human bites may also cause infection.)

Exposure to Hazardous Materials

Hazardous materials (**HAZMATs**) are used in production of many common products including fuel, medications, plastics, and home cleaning agents. These materials are normally stored, used, and transported safely. However, when they are improperly handled, they pose environmental hazards and can cause poisoning, burns, toxic fumes, groundwater contamination, and explosions. Other environmental emergencies are chemical or oil spills and gas leaks. The oil spill in the Gulf of Mexico in 2010 is an example of a major environmental emergency. *Primary exposure* occurs when a person is exposed directly to a hazardous substance, for example, by breathing fumes from evaporating liquids. *Secondary exposure* occurs when the rescuer or healthcare provider is exposed to a contaminated person. To prevent exposure, follow these safety measures:

- Do not walk into or touch spilled material.
- Avoid inhalation of gases, fumes, and smoke.
- Do not assume that gases or vapors are harmless because they are odorless.
- Do not go near accident victims if you cannot identify the hazardous material.
- Do not walk into or drive into a gas cloud. If you are accidentally caught in one and are unable to drive out, roll up your car windows, close the vents, turn off the fan, unlock the doors, and wait for assistance.

Emergency personnel specially trained in the management of hazardous materials will respond, to eliminate and prevent contamination. Clients exposed to hazardous materials require specialized care. Complete the process as quickly as possible, and then treat the victim's injuries.

IN PRACTICE
IMPORTANT MEDICATIONS 43-1: To Treat Anaphylaxis

For severe anaphylaxis, the following drugs may be used:
- Epinephrine (adrenaline)
- Corticosteroids
- Histamine-1 receptor antagonists (antihistamines)

For milder forms of anaphylaxis, medications such as diphenhydramine hydrochloride (Benadryl) or hydroxyzine (Vistaril, Atarax) may be used.

If life-saving procedures are necessary before decontamination is possible, personnel must wear appropriate protective barriers to avoid contamination. Take these additional precautions:

- Wear personal protective equipment, to help prevent secondary exposure.
- Decontaminate the victim by washing off the chemical. (Most EDs have showers for this purpose. This may be a special room with an outside entrance or a portable self-contained shower.)
- Remove the person's clothing and store in a designated hazard bag.
- Use a special decontamination stretcher for the client who cannot shower independently.

If a contaminated person presents to the ED or clinic, avoid exposing the entire department to the hazard. (After a hazardous chemical enters a building, the area may require evacuation and decontamination.)

Poisoning

Any substance that threatens a person's health when absorbed or makes contact with the body is defined as a poison. Poisons are in such common substances as household cleaning agents, insecticides, antifreeze, furniture polish, kerosene, nail polish remover, and nail polish. Accidental poisoning is a particular danger for children. In Practice: Nursing Care Guidelines 43-7 outlines first-aid care for poisoning. In Practice: Important Medications 43-2 lists common antidotes for poisoning.

In any case of poisoning or drug overdose, call the Poison Control Center (1-800-222-1222) *immediately*. They will advise you what to do; in nearly all cases, the victim should be transported to an ED for treatment. The recommendations for treatment have changed recently; *gastric lavage* ("pumping the stomach") is not often used, except in cases of certain drugs, such as a large dose of aspirin (which tends to clump), or in an overdose of drugs, such as lithium, iron, or calcium channel blockers. Induced vomiting is not recommended. The National Poison Control Center organization gives the following tips for prevention of poisoning:

- Keep all potential poisons locked up or high and out of sight.
- Keep all poisons in their original containers.
- Know the current weights of all children younger than 6 years.

IN PRACTICE
NURSING CARE GUIDELINES 43-7 — Giving First Aid in Poisoning or Overdose

- Call for help: 911. *Rationale: Treatment for poisoning depends on the poison ingested. Expert assistance is needed.*
- After calling 911, contact the Poison Control Center (800-222-1222). In some EMS areas, 911 dispatchers can connect the call to the Poison Control Center and monitor the call. *Rationale: The Poison Control Center can instruct the caller in proper treatment. Usually, the person needs to be transported to an emergency department. Vomiting is almost never recommended.*

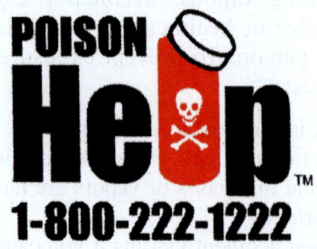

- Attempt to identify the poison. Question the person, if possible. Save all vomitus, urine, or stools and remains of food or drugs that may have been responsible. Look for medication bottles or other containers. Bring all these materials to the medical facility with the person. *Rationale: This information is necessary to determine the nature and amount of poison or drug taken.*

- Use the sense of smell to detect the odor of alcohol or other chemicals on the person's breath. *Rationale: Many drugs are more dangerous when combined with alcohol.*
- In cases of suspected overdose, ask questions of the person and the family. Was this a suicide attempt or an accident? Was there a suicide note? Was the person depressed or despondent? How many pills or how much alcohol was taken? *Rationale: This information will be important to the medical team in planning emergency treatment and continuing medical care.*
- Give supportive care. Keep the person warm. Use artificial ventilation, if the person is having difficulty breathing. Maintain the heartbeat. If possible, keep the person awake. Follow basic life support procedures if CPR is needed. *Rationale: Poisoning or overdose is a medical emergency. Load and go as quickly as possible. Maintain the person in the most stable condition possible until arrival at the healthcare facility.*
- Follow the instructions of the Poison Control Center. *Rationale: They are experts in treatment of poisoning or overdose.*
- Do not give anything to eat or drink or any medications without specific instructions to do so. *Rationale: This could be dangerous and cause additional complications.*
- Remember the acronym SIRES (**S**tabilize victim, **I**dentify poison, **R**everse effects, **E**liminate poison, **S**upport vital functions). *Rationale: This acronym will help to guide your actions.*

IN PRACTICE
IMPORTANT MEDICATIONS 43-2 For Poisoning and Drug Overdose

The following medications are commonly used for treating poisoning or overdose:
- All-purpose antidote: activated charcoal (Actidose-Aqua, CharcoCaps)
- Acetaminophen overdose: acetylcysteine (Mucomyst)
- Heroin and other painkillers (fentanyl, methadone) overdose: naloxone (Narcan)

When caring for the person receiving any of these medications, keep in mind the following:
- Never combine these medications.
- Be sure that activated charcoal is available to all first-aid personnel and in the home medicine cabinet, if help will not be readily available.
- Assess the first bowel movement after activated charcoal is given. It should appear black. Watch for constipation; bowel obstruction may occur. Push fluids.
- Do *not* give syrup of ipecac.
- Keep monitoring after administering naloxone. It has a short half-life; the client could become unconscious again.

- Do not take medications while children are watching—they may copy you.
- Never refer to medication as "candy," and do not use fun-shaped medications (even vitamins).
- Syrup of ipecac (an *emetic*, which causes vomiting) is no longer recommended for the home or day-care provider's medicine cabinet.
- Keep activated charcoal in the home medicine cabinet if the home is far from an ED.
- Always call the Poison Control Center (1-800-222-1222) for any questions or incidents.
- Keep the number of the Poison Control Center by each phone in the house.

Key Concept
The treatment of choice in nearly all poisoning or overdose situations is *activated charcoal.* An emetic is no longer recommended because of the following reasons:
- Research shows that the outcome of serious overdose or poisoning has not been altered by induced vomiting.
- Ipecac can be abused by persons with an eating disorder, such as bulimia.
- A serious potential for aspiration exists during vomiting, particularly if the person does not have a gag reflex or is sedated, inebriated, having seizures, in severe shock, or unconscious.
- Vomiting after ingestion of a caustic substance, such as gasoline, will cause more damage because of the second exposure to the poison in the throat and lungs when the person vomits.

Medication Poisoning
All medications are potentially poisonous, but many do not have such effects because they are given in small doses. Accidental drug poisoning may result from misreading a label or taking medicine from an unlabeled bottle or in the dark. Older persons may take extra doses of medications, because they forgot that they have already taken them. A drug overdose may be accidental or intentional (e.g., a suicide attempt). Care in a suicide attempt is discussed in Chapter 94.

Food Poisoning
Food poisoning is almost always caused by eating contaminated food. Bacteria's normal action on food causes *decomposition*, which forms **toxins** (poisonous substances). Another cause of food poisoning is the accidental eating of poisonous fruits, berries, or vegetables (e.g., toadstools or poisonous mushrooms). Symptoms of food poisoning include abdominal pain, nausea, vomiting, and diarrhea. Onset is acute (within a few hours after eating the contaminated food). The sooner the symptoms occur, the more serious the poisoning is. Symptoms usually disappear in 1 to 2 days, after the person has excreted the toxins. One form of food poisoning may be caused by the bacteria *Salmonella*. *Salmonella* lives in the intestines of humans and animals. It is excreted in feces. It causes infection when the bacteria finds its way into food or drinking water and is consumed. It can cause severe diarrhea, fever, and stomach cramps for 8 to 72 hr. Another severe form of food poisoning, *botulism*, is caused by the organism *Clostridium botulinum*. It occurs rarely and results in death in approximately 5% to 10% of cases. Home-canned foods that have been improperly sterilized or have lost their seal are a common cause. Symptoms, which are progressive, include weakness, headache, paralysis of the eye and throat muscles, and finally, respiratory paralysis. Specific antitoxins are effective, if given early. Rescue breathing may be required until EMS personnel arrive. The person may need to be maintained via endotracheal tube on a mechanical ventilator until the antitoxin takes effect and spontaneous respirations resume.

Nursing Alert Warn clients never to use a home-canned or commercially canned item if the top is bulging, if there is dark leakage around the seams, or if there is any discoloration in the contents of jarred foods. *If there is any doubt, throw it out!*

Psychiatric Emergencies
Psychiatric emergencies affect people of all ages and can occur at any time. A person requires medical attention when severe anxiety results in hallucinations, paranoia, confusion, or suicidal or homicidal threats or gestures. *Anxiety* or "panic attack" may cause the person's heart to race and respirations to become rapid. Sometimes the fingers and hands become numb and tingly. The person may feel incapable of functioning. Assess for suicidal tendencies and potential risk for harming self or others. The nurse working in home care or community-based nursing may be the first and only healthcare person to encounter this client and to recognize

the symptoms of a psychiatric emergency. Call for assistance when any of these factors are present:

- Threat to harm self or others
- Suicidal thoughts (ask specifically if the person has a plan or not. Always have them identify the plan if they have one, e.g., weapons, pills, jumping.)
- Refusal to talk further when a psychiatric emergency is suspected
- History of prior suicide attempts
- Severe depression
- Intoxication or drug abuse, combined with suicidal or violent thoughts or actions
- Self-injurious behavior (e.g., burning or cutting oneself)
- Out-of-control or bizarre behavior, causing major disturbances in the community
- Evidence of self-harm (e.g., empty pill bottles, unresponsiveness, suicide attempt)
- Evidence of not caring for one's self, such as not eating, not sleeping, living in a trash-strewn house, or not taking prescribed medications
- Reports of any of the above by family or neighbors

Assist emotionally disturbed people by remaining calm. Show them respect and offer to help. Ask questions that allow them to explain the situation. Avoid close-ended questions, those that elicit yes or no answers; encourage the person to talk. Help generate a positive plan of action. Communicate on the client's level. Listen attentively. Obtain medical assistance as soon as possible. (The police may be required to assist in taking the person to the hospital.) Chapter 94 describes psychiatric emergencies in more detail.

Key Concept

When dealing with an emotionally disturbed person, remain calm and speak softly, slowly, and clearly. Maintain a nonthreatening posture and tone of voice. Do not allow the person to get between you and the door—maintain an "escape route" for yourself. Prevent the person from injuring themself or anyone else, but keep yourself safe. Seek assistance as soon as possible.

STUDENT SYNTHESIS

KEY POINTS

- Nurses are with clients much of the time in the healthcare facility. Therefore, the nurse may be in the position to recognize and alert the appropriate staff to deal with cardiopulmonary arrest and other emergencies.
- Nurses must use Standard Precautions when administering first aid (to whatever extent possible).
- In emergencies, nurses and nursing students function *only at their level of first-aid training*. Quick evaluation of the scene and planning for action are crucial.
- Calling 911 will summon the EMS system in almost all areas of the United States and Canada. The nurse must know how to summon assistance in an emergency.
- When assessing an emergency, the most important considerations are to make sure the person is breathing, that their heart is beating, and no major bleeding is present.
- Be sure to treat the injured person for shock.
- Do not move an injured person, unless the situation is life threatening. Take precautions to prevent further injury.
- All healthcare workers, including nurses, should know how to perform CPR and remove an airway obstruction in an emergency. Maintain current CPR certification.
- The nurse may be called on to provide first-aid assistance in a community. Each nurse has the responsibility to be knowledgeable in basic first-aid techniques.
- Chest injuries can result in inadequate air exchange and are immediately life threatening. Ensure that the chest wall is intact. Plug any open wound of the chest. Do not remove any penetrating objects.
- Be aware of the possibility of injury from excessive heat or cold. Take prompt action in life-threatening situations.
- A person who is having a heart attack is often in denial. EMS personnel may need to be very persuasive to get the victim to appropriate medical care.
- The first-aid person must be knowledgeable in methods used to stop bleeding.
- Anaphylaxis is a medical emergency that requires immediate treatment.
- Follow the instructions of the Poison Control Center in the event of poisoning or overdose.
- Remain calm when dealing with an emotionally upset client. Be alert for the possibility of suicide.

CRITICAL THINKING EXERCISES

1. A motorcyclist has been hit by a car and thrown from the bike. What actions should people on the scene take? What should you do if you are there? Discuss Standard Precautions in relation to the accident scene.

2. You notice a pregnant woman choking and coughing in a restaurant. She runs to the bathroom. What actions would you take and why?

3. You are caring for a client in their home who tells you they want to die. You believe they have the means and are serious about harming themself. How would you handle this situation?

4. Your neighbor is mowing their lawn when they suddenly fall to the ground. Describe what actions you should take and why.

5. State the reporting procedure in your facility if you suspect child abuse.

NCLEX-STYLE REVIEW QUESTIONS

1. A client is being treated for frostbite of the toes of both feet after exposure to severe cold. The provider has issued orders. What are the likely actions that the nurse will take in caring for this client? Select all that apply.
   a. Rubbing the client's toes to rewarm
   b. Loosening tight clothing from the client
   c. Separating the toes with cotton wedges
   d. Rewarming the toes with tepid water
   e. Covering the feet with hot towels

2. A client has been camping in the woods in cold temperatures and is brought to the Emergency Department with suspected hypothermia. What ordered action is important at this time?
   a. Warm the client rapidly to a body temperature of 98.6°F.
   b. Apply hot packs to the skin.
   c. Give the client hot coffee or tea.
   d. Gradually rewarm the client.

3. The nurse is caring for a client involved in a house fire with burns to the chest and upper arms. What signs observed by the nurse indicate the client may have also sustained inhalation injuries? Select all that apply.
   a. Fever
   b. Neck pain
   c. Flecks of soot in the saliva
   d. Hoarse voice
   e. Singed nasal hairs

4. When a client has sustained a serious burn, what is the immediate action by the nurse?
   a. Apply burn cream to the area.
   b. Apply ice to the burned area.
   c. Stop the burning process.
   d. Remove burning fabric or other material from the skin.

5. A client is brought to the urgent care center with an injury to the left ankle sustained from a fall. X-ray interpretation determined that there is no fracture present, but the client does have a sprain. What education will the nurse reinforce to the client?
   a. PASS
   b. RICE
   c. RACE
   d. CPR

CHAPTER RESOURCES

Enhance your learning with additional resources on thePoint!

Student Resources related to this chapter can be found at **thePoint.lww.com/Rosdahl12e**.

UNIT 7 Safety in the Healthcare Facility

Welcome Steps

Look at healthcare provider's orders.

Protocol for procedure.

Necessary equipment/supplies.

Wash hands using proper hand hygiene; put on gloves.

Explain the procedure and reassure the client.

Locate two identifiers to confirm correct client.

Comfortable and efficient position for nurse and client.

Obtain privacy.

Make sure to follow correct steps and body mechanics with good technique.

Ensure safety and observe deviations from normal.

End Steps

Ensure comfort and safety.

Note questions or concerns from client or nurse; note significant data.

Dispose of materials properly.

Disinfect the area and your hands.

Document and report the procedure and your findings.

IN PRACTICE

NURSING PROCEDURE 43-1   Applying a Sling

Supplies and Equipment
36- to 40-inch cloth square or triangular bandage
Pins (if tying is not possible).

Steps
Follow LPN WELCOME Steps and Then

1. Put one triangle end over the person's shoulder on the *uninjured* side. The point of the triangle should point toward the elbow of the injured arm and be placed under it. *Rationale: Placing the sling around the person's neck will support the injured arm.*

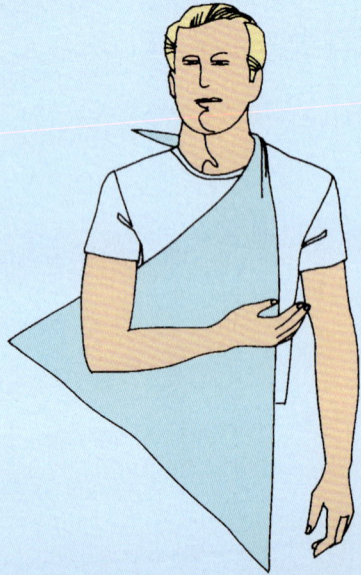

2. Bring the other end of the triangle over the person's shoulder on the *injured* side. Tie the two ends of the triangle together in a square knot at the side of the neck. *Rationale: Tying the knot on the side of the injury will pull the knot away from the neck, preventing discomfort. A square knot is easier to untie.*

   If the nature of the injury or another situation makes this impractical, place some sort of padding beneath the knot. *Rationale: Padding the area minimizes pressure on the neck.*

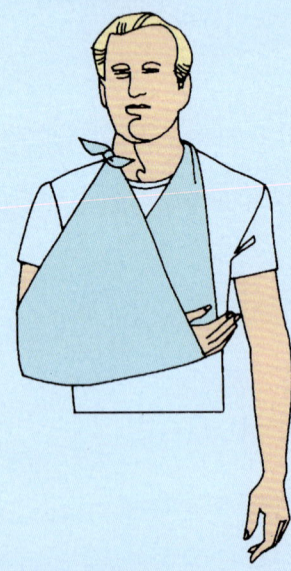

3. Bring the point of the triangle backward around the person's elbow and pin it to the back of the sling. You can adjust the sling by adjusting the knot or by pinning a tuck in the front of the sling above the person's hand. Elevate the hand 4 to 5 in. above elbow level. *Rationale: Elevation helps to prevent swelling and pain.*

Follow ENDDD Steps

IN PRACTICE
NURSING PROCEDURE 43-2: Assisting the Client Who Has a Nosebleed

Supplies and Equipment
Gloves
Gauze
Cold compresses
Basin

Steps
Follow LPN WELCOME Steps and Then

1. Have the person sit and lean forward slightly, to allow the blood to run into the basin. If this position is impossible because of other injuries, have the person lie down, keeping their head and shoulders elevated. Turn head to the side. *Rationale: The head should be above the heart to reduce pressure. Large amounts of blood should be allowed to run out, or the person may aspirate and will most likely vomit later.*

2. Apply pressure to the nostrils or the bridge of the nose with thumb and forefinger for 5 to 10 min, without releasing the pressure. *Rationale: This location will place pressure on some of the blood vessels supplying the nose. Releasing the pressure too soon will allow a clot to break loose, and bleeding will resume.*

3. Place cold compresses on the person's nose and face. *Rationale: Cold causes vasoconstriction and slows blood circulation to the area.*

4. If bleeding continues for more than 5 min, pinch the nose again. If bleeding continues for more than 20 min, activate the EMS system. Unless rescue services are not available, do not place anything in the nose. *Rationale: Placing anything in the nose could cause further irritation and its removal could release a clot, causing further bleeding.*

5. Apply pressure above the person's upper lip if they are conscious. *Rationale: Applying pressure helps cut off some of the blood supply to the area.*

6. Seek medical assistance if bleeding is uncontrollable or occurs several times a week. *Rationale: Continued bleeding may be a symptom of a more serious disorder and may also become life threatening. An inflatable balloon packing may be needed.*

7. Tell the person that they probably will have black stools for a day or two because of swallowed blood. *Rationale: If the person is not told this, they might be very concerned by the first stools.*

Follow ENDDD Steps

IN PRACTICE
NURSING PROCEDURE 43-3: Applying a Tourniquet

Supplies and Equipment
Gloves
Small object such as a pencil or stick
Piece of cloth—at least 2 to 3 in. wide and 3 to 4 feet long
Tightly rolled, firm pad

Steps
Follow LPN WELCOME Steps and Then

1. Try all other methods of controlling severe hemorrhage (direct pressure) first. If this method fails, apply a tourniquet. *Rationale: Use of a tourniquet may necessitate later limb amputation. However, a life may be saved.*

2. Place a compact, rolled piece of material over the artery's pressure point, controlling blood flow to the injury. Wind the tourniquet over this pad. *Rationale: This measure applies pressure over the blood vessel.*

3. Tie a half knot at the side of the injured limb. Place a stick or similar object over it and tie a square knot over the stick. Twist the stick tightly enough to control bleeding. *Rationale: The tourniquet must be tight enough to inhibit bleeding.*

4. Secure the stick firmly. *Rationale: The tourniquet may loosen if not secure.*

5. Do not cover the tourniquet; it should be in full view. *Rationale: Medical personnel have to know it is there. If not, it could remain in place too long, causing severe limb damage.*

6. Do not loosen the tourniquet without a physician's order. *Rationale: Clots may form, which, if dislodged, could cause embolism.*

7. Tag the client with a note stating the location of the tourniquet and the time of application. It is also a good idea to print a "T" on the person's forehead with a marker or lipstick. *Rationale: Emergency and medical personnel must know that a tourniquet is in place. Prompt action may help to save the limb.*

8. Keep the bleeding part immobile and elevate it if possible. *Rationale: This action slows circulation.*

9. Treat the person for shock and observe for cardiac arrest. *Rationale: Clients with severe hemorrhage are at high risk for cardiac arrest.*

10. Transport the person to the nearest medical facility immediately. *Rationale: Medical care is needed to save the extremity and to treat shock or other cardiovascular problems.*

Follow ENDDD Steps

Client Care — UNIT 8

44 Therapeutic Communication Skills

Learning Objectives

1. Define communication; list the five components of communication.
2. Discuss the three parts of the communication process.
3. Explain rapport and its importance in nursing.
4. Differentiate between verbal and nonverbal communications. Give examples of each.
5. Discuss factors that influence the effectiveness of communication.
6. Demonstrate the interviewing and communication skills of questioning, therapeutic silence, and clarifying.
7. Demonstrate a teaching session for clients of different age levels, those with sensory problems, and clients who do not speak the same language as the nurse.
8. Describe relationships between communication and the nursing process.

Important Terminology

aphasia
assertiveness
body language
closed-ended question
communication
congruent communication
eye contact
interview
nonverbal communication
open-ended question
personal space
proxemics
rapport
therapeutic communication
verbal communication

Acronyms

NVC
ROI

Communication means giving, receiving, and interpreting information through any of the five senses by two or more interacting people. **Therapeutic communication** is an interaction that is helpful and healing for one or more of the participants; the client benefits from knowing that someone cares and understands, and the nurse derives satisfaction from knowing that they have been helpful. The nurse communicates in different ways: as a teacher, a caregiver, and a supporter. This requires self-awareness and interpersonal skills. Successful therapeutic communication encourages increased client coping skills and motivation toward self-care (Fig. 44-1). Effective communication is important, both in your nursing career and your personal life and is the foundation on which *interpersonal relationships* are built. The art of therapeutic communication does not necessarily come naturally, but can be learned. Therapeutic communication is described in In Practice: Nursing Care Guidelines 44-1.

COMMUNICATION

Communication and the Nursing Process

Without accurate and therapeutic communication, the nursing process cannot exist.

Communication is related to the nursing process in many ways:

- Problem-solving depends on individual and group communication.
- The nurse must be able to collect client data accurately by listening and paying attention to both verbal information and nonverbal cues.
- The nursing diagnosis and care plan must be clear and concise.
- Planning involves accurate communication among all members of the healthcare team, as well as the client and family.
- During implementation of the nursing care plan, the nurse communicates with the client and family and relates professional impressions and observations to other members of the healthcare team.
- Ongoing evaluation of the effectiveness of nursing interventions depends on clear and coherent communication among all concerned.
- Client teaching and preparation for discharge depend on accurate and empathic communication and client understanding.

Personal characteristics of genuineness, caring, trust, empathy, and respect promote understanding among individuals; this harmony and agreement is **rapport** (ra-pore'). Conveying these attitudes to another person creates a social

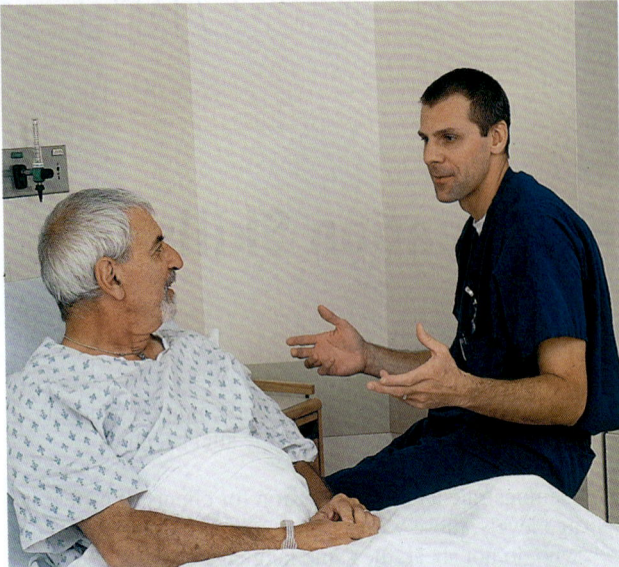

Figure 44-1 This nurse uses principles of therapeutic communication when interacting with his client. He uses appropriate positioning (eye level), does not invade the client's personal space, makes appropriate eye contact, and generally mirrors the client's body position. He speaks and then carefully listens to what the client says. (Timby, 2005.)

IN PRACTICE
NURSING CARE GUIDELINES 44-1 — Using Therapeutic Communication

The nurse successfully using therapeutic communication will:
- Put the client at ease and develop rapport.
- Provide privacy.
- Respect the client's rights.
- Respect the client's personal space.
- Try to be at eye level with the client.
- Use appropriate and congruent eye contact.
- Be a good listener.
- Keep information confidential, as appropriate.
- Begin the interview with general information and ask emotionally difficult questions after the client gains confidence and trust.
- Adjust language level, as appropriate, for the client. Do not use complex medical terms or "talk down" to the client.
- Ask an interpreter to assist, if the client speaks a language different from that of the staff or is hearing impaired. Utilize only certified interpreters. Guidelines for interpreter use are presented in later sections of this chapter.
- Establish a communication system if the client cannot speak or hear or if the client speaks a different language than the nurse (see Box 44-3).
- Be attentive; concentrate on what the person says. Show sincere interest.
- Try not to write or use a computer during the interview. Clarify details with the client later.
- Ask the client about his or her perceptions. Why did they come to the facility?
- Listen to the client's choice of words; any repetition; variations in tone of voice; silence; body language; assertiveness; repetitive behaviors; anxiety; and specific movements, such as tics or unusual speech patterns.
- Determine if the client is confused or not making sense. Are there hallucinations or delusions?
- Assess the client's attitudes or ask before touching the client. (Sometimes, it is necessary to touch the client [e.g., counting pulse]—*task-oriented touch*.)
- Include the family in conversations if the client prefers. Be aware of client confidentiality. If the client seems uncomfortable, ask to speak to the client alone.
- Consider the client's cultural background and life experiences in all interactions and assessments (see Chapter 8).

climate that communicates goodwill and empathy, even when fears or concerns cannot be fully expressed verbally. It is important to provide unbiased nursing care. To be most helpful, the nurse develops the ability to convey a nonjudgmental attitude, especially if another person's beliefs and values differ from the nurse's own. Clients must experience a feeling of rapport with the nurse in order to share personal, and sometimes embarrassing, information. The client and the nurse are working toward a *common goal*.

Key Concept

In some cases, the nurse has the right to request a different assignment if working with this client may cloud professional judgment. For example, a nurse whose religion forbids abortion may request not to assist with this procedure. The client has the right to his or her own beliefs and so does the nurse. In addition, it is not advisable to care for a family member or close friend.

NCLEX Alert

When reading NCLEX questions relating to communication, look for the best possible and most beneficial response for the client. Therapeutic communication options typically differ from conversations you have in a social setting.

Components of Communication

Communication requires several components (Fig. 44-2):

Sender: The originator or source of the idea
Message: The idea
Medium or *channel:* A means of transmitting the idea, which can be verbal or nonverbal
Receiver: The person who receives and interprets the message
Interaction: The receiver's response to the message through internal feelings and verbal and nonverbal feedback

Think of communication as a *reciprocal process* in which both the sender and the receiver of messages participate simultaneously. All the senses can be involved in communication. We see and hear other people through conversations. Nurses sometimes touch others to express concern or care. The sense of smell or taste can also convey information. Sometimes, a combination of factors affects communication.

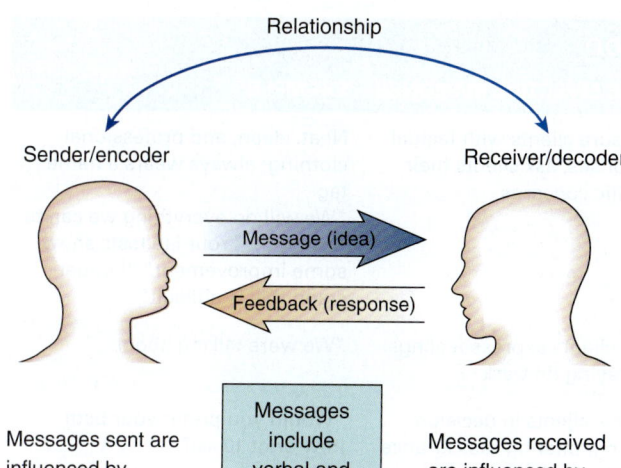

Figure 44-2 Components in the process of communication. Communication can be carried out in person or by telephone, or by texting, alpha paging, AudioVox, Vocera communication, or other electronic methods.

For example, noise, a TV playing, or other people talking in the background can distort interactions. Conducting therapeutic communication in private or in a quiet area helps avoid distractions that detract from its effectiveness.

NCLEX Alert
NCLEX options can provide examples of comments you might make when caring for a client. Therapeutic communication skills, such as listening, restating, and silence, might maximize client care.

Types of Communication

Nurses communicate with clients often and in various ways. Two types of communication are *verbal communication* (using words) and *nonverbal communication* (facial expressions, actions, and body position). Verbal communication is sometimes differentiated from oral communication as in written communication in charting. When a nurse is taking a phone call, it is good to verify the message, write down the message, and repeat the message. Effective communication occurs when words and actions convey the same message (*congruency*). This is essential for *therapeutic communication* to occur. When a "mixed message" is sent, communication is not effective or is confusing (Box 44-1).

Key Concept
In general, verbal communication is used to communicate information. Nonverbal communication conveys feelings and attitudes. Nonverbal communication occurs whether we want it to or not.

Box 44-1 Verbal and Nonverbal Communications

VERBAL COMMUNICATION
Use of words (e.g., speech, sign language, writing, slang)

ORAL COMMUNICATION
Vocal sounds (e.g., grunt, snort)

NONVERBAL COMMUNICATION
Personal space (*proxemics*)
Body characteristics: Body art, piercings, plastic surgery, scarification, weight, clothing (cultural differences in what is beautiful), grooming
Facial expression
Eye contact, eye gaze
Touch (*haptic* communication)
Body gestures and movement (*kinesics*): Posture, culturally related gestures, gang signals, as well as friendly, warning, or obscene gestures
Vocal characteristics: Geographic differences and accents, pronunciation, fluency/dysfluency, sarcasm
Gender differences: Relationships with those of different genders
Cultural mores: Behaviors specific to a cultural group or geographic location (how people behave and relate)

Verbal Communication

Verbal communication, sharing information through the written or spoken word, is used extensively in nursing. Nurses converse with clients, write care plans, document information and impressions, input data into the electronic record, and give oral or written change-of-shift reports (Fig. 44-3). Much information is related through vocabulary, sentence structure, spelling, and pronunciation. People reveal their education, intellectual skills, interests, and ethnic, regional, or national background

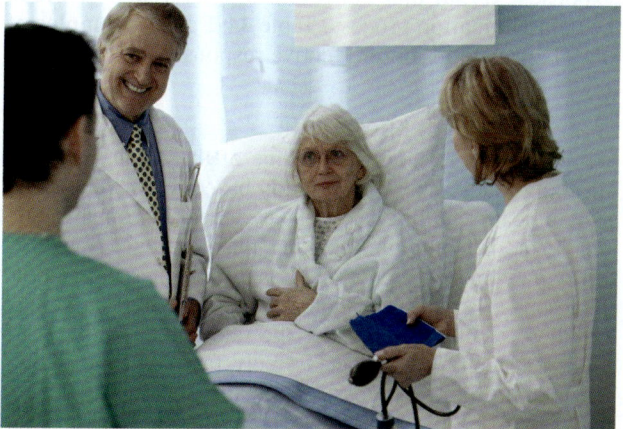

Figure 44-3 Walking bedside rounds allow face-to-face personal communication between the team and the client. This may be at change of shift or during the shift. (Timby, 2013.)

TABLE 44-1 Barriers to Effective Communication

BARRIER	EXAMPLE	MORE EFFECTIVE RESPONSE	EXAMPLE
Failing to look professional; not identifying self Offering empty reassurances	Unkempt, messy hair, long or dirty fingernails, unclean uniform, offensive body odor "Everything will be OK." "You will be alright."	Reassure clients with factual responses; ask clients their specific concerns	Neat, clean, and professional clothing; always wears a name tag "We will do everything we can to help you." "Your lab tests show some improvement." "I understand this is difficult."
Changing the subject	"The weather is really nice today."	Help clients express feelings by staying on track	"We were talking about…"
Using trite clichés	"The doctor knows best."	Involve clients in decision-making; offering reassurance and alternatives	"Would you prefer your bath now or at 10 AM?"
Imposing your ideas or values on clients and giving advice, according to your values	"You should…"	Help the client explore their own values when a decision or choice must be made	"What do you feel is best for you?" "How can we best help you?"
Disapproving of or judging the client; not respecting the client	"That is a dumb idea." "That won't work." Calling the client by inappropriate names (e.g., "Honey," "Gramps")	Accept each client as unique; consider ethnic and cultural practices; show respect	"Is there an alternative?" "How else might we…?" "How does this make you feel?" "Hello, Mr. McCarthy. My name is…"
Voicing personal experiences, especially those that are health-related	"I had that disease last year."	Allow clients to discuss their own concerns; answer questions factually; offer client-oriented reference material	"I would be happy to get some information about that disorder from the Internet for you."

through verbal communication. Voice inflections and sounds reveal messages. Although a client may say what the nurse wants to hear, his or her tone of voice may imply a totally different meaning, referred to as *noncongruent*, between verbal and nonverbal communications. *Congruent communication* is when the words, tone, and body language are all sending the same message. The person may make sounds or gestures that indicate true feelings. A snort, hiss, click, or rolling of the eyes, for example, may denote disgust. Be aware that some responses, *verbal and nonverbal barriers*, stop or block the communication process. Table 44-1 gives examples of these barriers and more effective responses.

Characteristics of Speech
It is important to note the volume of the client's speech. Speaking loudly may be culturally based. However, it may also indicate conditions, such as a hearing impairment, mania, or difficulty in speaking the language. Speaking softly may imply such things as nervousness, paranoia, shyness, or lack of self-confidence, or may also reflect the client's culture. Consider the rate and rhythm of the client's speech. Speaking extremely fast may imply anxiety, mania, flight of ideas, or impatience. Speaking very slowly may be the result of a brain disorder, mental illness, fear, or minimal knowledge of English. Medications can influence the client's speech. Hesitation in speaking, thought-blocking, difficulty in finding words, or total aphasia may indicate that the client does not speak English well, has a brain disorder, or is hallucinating (seeing or hearing things that others do not perceive). These are examples; many other factors may be involved (see Chapter 94 related to mental illness).

Aphasia is a defect in, or loss of, the ability to speak, write, or sign, or of the ability to comprehend speech and communication. Aphasia is usually caused by an injury or disorder of the brain's speech centers or by a mental illness. *Expressive aphasia* is difficulty in speaking or finding the correct word; *receptive aphasia* is a brain disorder that interferes with comprehension of language (see Chapter 92).

Listening
Thoughtful listening is a vital component of communication. The nurse learns a great deal about the client by careful listening and by paying attention to nonverbal cues (see Fig. 44-1).

Nonverbal Communication
Nonverbal communication (NVC) is sharing information without using words or language. NVC expresses emotions and attitudes, as well as enhancing what is being expressed verbally. NVC is one component of **body language** and is sometimes more powerful in conveying

CHAPTER 44 Therapeutic Communication Skills

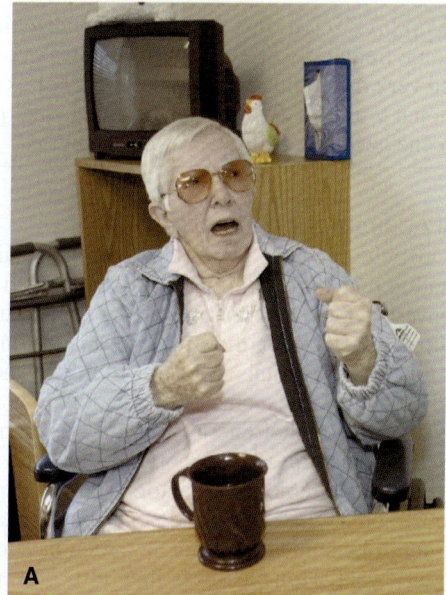

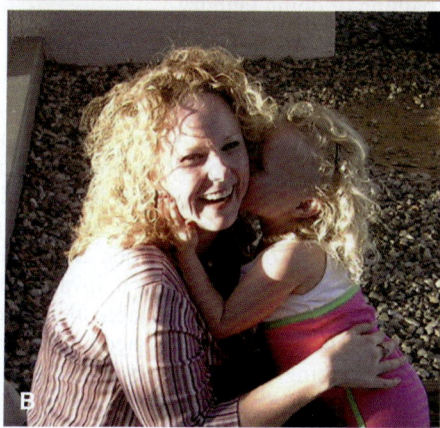

Figure 44-4 Nonverbal communication is powerful and conveys a strong message, whether you intend it to do so or not. **A and B.** What message is being conveyed nonverbally by the people in these pictures? (A: Carter, 2016; B: Photo by Mary Kowalski.)

a message than is verbal communication. If verbal and nonverbal messages are not congruent, the receiver usually believes the nonverbal cues (see Box 44-1). If body language and verbalizations are not congruent, confusion occurs. For example, Mr. H., a young client with diabetes, begins clenching and unclenching his fists when the nurse asks about his sexual activity. He says, "everything is fine," through gritted teeth. Later, when he trusts the nurse more, he admits that he has been impotent for the past 6 months. Often, body language (e.g., posture and movements, gestures, facial expressions) provides more powerful information than verbal language, because it points to the person's true feelings (Fig. 44-4). The study of body language is referred to as *kinesics*. It is important to be aware, however, that nonverbal behavior has different meanings in different situations, and it is important to clarify with clients the meaning of their body language before making assumptions. (Remember: NVC includes factors such as clothing, body ornamentation, body shape and size, as well as gestures.)

> **Key Concept**
> Be sure your verbal and nonverbal communications convey a congruent message to clients. When verbal and nonverbal messages conflict (are not congruent), others are most likely to believe the nonverbal message.

Proxemics and Personal Space

Human **proxemics** or *territoriality* (space, in relationship to communication) varies greatly among individuals and between cultures or ethnic groups. All people have an area around themselves called **personal space**, which is reserved for only close friends or intimates. This culturally learned behavior varies greatly across cultures, although it may also vary from person to person within an ethnic group. Other variables include sex and social status. In traditional Western cultures, personal space or communication zones divide approximately as follows:

- Intimate (less than 1.5 feet): behavior with loved ones, sharing secrets, physical assessment in healthcare
- Personal (1.5–4 ft): general conversation, interviews, teaching one-on-one, private conversation
- Social (4–12 ft): demonstrations, group interactions, parties
- Public (>12 ft): lectures, behavior with strangers

Although the concepts of proxemics are true for many Americans, they may differ between cultures. For example, in some cultures, the area of personal space is smaller. An action that would be considered an invasion of personal space by a person from one culture may be considered acceptable by a person from another culture. In nursing, it is important to consider the client's personal space boundaries. If the nurse comes too close, it is considered an invasion; if the nurse stays too far away, the client may feel isolated. Usually, it is possible to sense another person's personal boundaries. Unique to nursing, however, in many cases, the client's personal space must be invaded in order to provide care. Be sensitive to the discomfort this may cause. Always alert clients before coming too close. Touch clients gently on the arm or hand before further intruding into their personal space, to provide reassurance and help them feel safer. Often, an approach from the side, rather than directly from the front, is perceived as less confrontational.

Sometimes, the client's use of personal space is not cultural, but indicates a mental or physical disorder. For example, the psychiatric client who consistently invades the personal space of others is said to be *intrusive* and may be threatening. Another client who maintains a large personal space may be paranoid and afraid of contact with others. On the other hand, the client with a hearing or visual disorder may need to be close to the speaker, in order to determine what is being said. It is important to consider the reasons for variations in expected personal space boundaries when giving nursing care.

> **Nursing Alert** Remember: nursing care often involves invasion of a client's traditional personal space. Be aware that some clients may react in an assaultive manner when touched, particularly those with psychiatric conditions or dementia. Always be alert to this possibility. In addition, some clients may invade your personal space; it is important to set limits and to seek assistance if this behavior continues.

Eye Contact

Eye contact or *eye gaze* means looking directly into the eyes of the other person. Lack of direct eye contact has various meanings among cultures. Sometimes indirect eye contact means that a person is nervous, shy, or lying. However, it may also signify respect, as in Southeast Asian, Hispanic American, and Native American cultures. (In these cultures, direct eye contact may signify hostility.) Staring may be interpreted as defiance, rudeness, or as a threat. Rolling the eyes is often interpreted as disgust. On the other hand, cultures such as those of the Middle East and Eastern European consider a lack of direct eye contact as inattention, lack of concern, or even rudeness. Eye contact also varies depending on gender in some cultures. For example, in some cultures, those of the same gender can have direct eye contact with each other, whereas it is expected to avoid direct eye contact when speaking to someone of a different gender. In Western cultures, direct eye contact or a wink between people may be a part of dating behavior.

Facial Expressions

Facial expressions convey messages of many emotions: for example, joy, sadness, anger, and fear. Some people mask their feelings, making understanding what they are thinking difficult. Nurses learn to control facial expressions when experiencing emotions that may offend the client or block effective communication. For example, the nurse remains calm, with a neutral expression, when viewing wounds or smelling body secretions.

Body Movements and Posture

A twitching or bouncing foot may indicate anger, impatience, boredom, or nervousness. A slouched appearance may indicate depression or pain. Wringing of hands may indicate fear, pain, or worry. Shrugging the shoulders implies, "I don't know," in many cultures. Pacing, rocking, and other repetitive movements may be a side effect of medications or may indicate fear or discomfort. It is important to avoid making assumptions about body language messages; ask clients what they are feeling.

Gestures and Rituals

We use several gestures as a matter of course in daily life. Waving may indicate a greeting or "goodbye" or may be used to send someone away. A wink may indicate a mutual secret or may be a flirting gesture. In some countries, people greet each other by kissing on both cheeks. In Western culture, the "air kiss" is a common greeting.

> **Nursing Alert** It is important to realize that some frequently used Western gestures may be interpreted very differently in other cultures. For example, the traditional Western "thumbs up" gesture is interpreted as an obscene gesture in Middle Eastern countries.

Personal Appearance and Grooming

Personal hygiene, general appearance, clothing, and body ornamentation relate information about clients (and nurses). These nonverbal messages may convey people's true feelings about themselves, or they may be misleading, especially in illness. Individuals who are trying to meet their basic physiologic needs, such as oxygenation, may not have the physical or emotional energy to work on higher order needs, such as cleanliness or grooming. Lack of personal care may also reflect emotional factors, such as depression. In addition, people with severe and persistent mental illness or out-of-control chemical dependency often have difficulty managing self-care. Homelessness may also prevent a person from bathing or doing laundry.

Therapeutic Use of Touch

Touch, referred to as *haptic communication* or *affective touch*, can say "I care" (Fig. 44-5). A firm touch can discourage a child from doing something dangerous; a light touch can encourage a person to walk down the hall. Touch involves movements such as holding hands, a "high five," or a pat on the shoulder. Some people do not like to be touched, feeling that it invades their personal space, and can be uncomfortable if unnecessarily touched. Sometimes, the nurse may need to touch a client to carry out a nursing procedure; in this case, verbally prepare the client for the action and convey understanding of the client's discomfort.

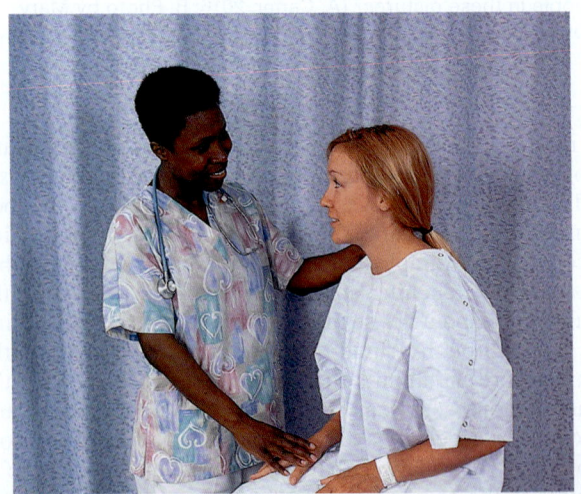

Figure 44-5 Therapeutic use of touch (affective touch) is the most potent nonverbal communication technique. A gentle, reassuring touch conveys that the nurse cares and is there to help. Be sure to touch clients *only if it is nonthreatening* to them. (Timby, 2005.)

CHAPTER 44 Therapeutic Communication Skills

> **Key Concept**
> Nursing care revolves around verbal and nonverbal communications: giving, receiving, and interpreting information. Listening is an essential communication tool.

Changes Due to COVID-19

Measures to prevent the spread of infectious disease during COVID-19 in 2020 affected our use of nonverbal communication. Social distancing describes what people learned to do when the threat of infection from COVID-19 emerged. It general, social distancing noted the acceptable and safe area of personal space was six feet or more. This change in acceptable distance between people led to urban areas being repurposed. Rather than standing directly next to someone when conversating, people began leaving larges spaces between themselves and others when conversating and socializing. Many areas required masks to be worn, especially when indoors within six feet of another person. This change in acceptable social space has shed light on social disparities, as many people live in neighborhoods with little access to green spaces outside where appropriately distanced socialization can occur. Others may live in areas with unsafe outdoor conditions due to crime or traffic, which limits their ability to get outside and socialize safely. COVID-19 greatly changed how the majority of healthcare professionals used nonverbal communication. Wearing masks in all interactions changes how one may use facial expressions and, in turn, how one might interpret facial expressions during communication. Changes in our ability to communicate as we normally would also affected clients. Clients could no longer see a friendly, caring smile from their healthcare teams. It increased the number of clients who experienced loneliness, anxiety, and stress, as family members who were usually allowed to accompany and support clients were not allowed to visit.

Factors Influencing Communication

Many factors influence the effectiveness of communication. Some factors enhance communication, and other, seemingly harmless factors create barriers.

Attention

Lack of concentration or selective listening may present a communication barrier. The listener hears only what he or she wants or expects to hear. The nurse may not pay attention or may not hear because of emotional responses to what the client is saying. Or, the nurse may be mentally framing the next question or thinking of something else. Sometimes, a client is experiencing pain or discomfort (physical or emotional) so great that he or she cannot listen or concentrate. The client may also be preoccupied with internal stimuli (e.g., auditory hallucinations). If both the sender and the receiver are not able to give full attention to the current communication, an effective nurse–client relationship cannot occur, and the interaction may need to be postponed.

> **SPECIAL CONSIDERATIONS** Culture and Ethnicity
>
> - The nurse objectively describes eye contact, rather than applying judgments. For example, "client looks at the floor when speaking" is descriptive and nonjudgmental. (A judgmental statement such as "good eye contact" implies that all clients should behave like most Western Europeans or European Americans.) The nurse might go on to state that (in the nurse's opinion) the client is "insecure and afraid." However, this assessment may be incorrect if the client is looking down as a sign of respect.
> - The nurse objectively describes behavior related to personal space, for example, "client maintains approximately 3 ft of personal space and moves away when approached." Inappropriately, the client might be described as "staff-avoidant," but this assessment may be incorrect, depending on the client's cultural background.
> - The nurse describes the tone and volume of the client's verbalizations in objective terms. An objective statement might be, "client speaks very loudly." The judgment that the client is "hostile" may be incorrect, however, when the nurse considers that in some cultures, all people speak very loudly. (On the other hand, the client may be hearing-impaired and may speak loudly as a result.)
> - A male nurse may write about a female client, "client refuses to speak." However, it might be incorrect to say that the client is "paranoid" or "aphasic." It is important for this nurse to remember that, in some cultures, women are not permitted to speak to men outside their families.
> - Objective documentation may be, "client speaks softly." However, rather than stating that client is "shy" or "afraid," it is important to remember that in some cultures, women are expected to speak softly at all times.
> - The use of profanity is common in some cultures and is considered part of everyday language. Documenting what the client says, in quotation marks, rather than making judgments, is objective.
> - Many people of the world consider folk medicine or mystical beliefs to be a normal part of life. Therefore, if a client talks about the "evil eye" or a "cold disease," documentation of the actual statement is appropriate and objective. A nurse might wrongly determine that this client is "delusional," for example, when these beliefs are common to most members of that client's culture.
> - Reaction to pain varies among cultures. Some groups are stoic, and others cry out. Document exactly what was said.
>
> The preceding are examples. The nurse uses the same general guidelines when documenting other nonverbal behaviors, such as body posture or general attitudes about health and illness. The nurse will be objective if the client's exact words and actions are presented in quotation marks, rather than making judgments based on the nurse's interpretation. (Formal nursing assessments are made using standardized guidelines. Unit 6 of this book, The Nursing Process, describes these guidelines in more detail.)

Age

Age can be an advantage or disadvantage to effective communication. Very young or very old clients may be unable to communicate fully, because of reduced physical or intellectual capacity. Some clients are uncomfortable with caregivers much younger or older than they are. A young nurse may have difficulty working with a client near the same age. On the other hand, age can be an advantage. An older client may prefer to receive care from an older nurse, or a younger client may be more willing to accept instructions from an older nurse. An older client may also be energized by the presence of a younger nurse.

Gender

Gender roles and stereotypes may influence nurse–client interactions. For example, a client who is accustomed to being in charge may resent being told what to do by a nurse of a different gender, particularly if the nurse is much younger. A nurse who believes men should be tough may find it difficult to see a client cry. A client may be embarrassed by a nurse of a different gender performing personal care procedures. It is also important to consider the client's ethnic background; in some cultures, interactions between people of different genders are specifically prescribed. Approaching a personal situation matter-of-factly or professionally may eliminate embarrassment.

Culture and Subculture

Cultural norms and traditions influence the behaviors and perceptions of all people, including nurses. Chapters 8 and 31 discuss transcultural aspects of nursing. Each nurse would be well advised to develop an awareness of his or her own personal beliefs and practices, based on culture and ethnicity, for example, in relation to concepts such as personal space, eye contact, and interactions between men and women. Understanding and accepting differences are keys to developing therapeutic communication. The effective nurse actively seeks and maintains the client's sense of self-worth by acting in a nonjudgmental manner.

> **Key Concept**
> Remember: A smile is part of the universal human language and is understood by all.

Difficult Client Behaviors

Inappropriate behavior on the part of clients creates a barrier to communication.

Sexual Harassment

Sexual harassment is defined as any unwanted sexual activity. This includes any inappropriate or unwanted touching, as well as sexual statements, or lewd jokes or comments. The use of profanity and name-calling is also included. If a client (or other staff member) sexually harasses you, consult with your supervisor to handle this inappropriate behavior correctly. If these inappropriate actions continue after the person is warned, the nurse may consider pressing charges. (It is important to consider the client's physical condition. For example, the client who has Alzheimer disease may not be totally responsible for their actions.)

> **Key Concept**
> A nurse is never required to allow inappropriate behavior from a client or other staff members. This includes verbal or physical abuse, as well as sexual harassment.

Aggressiveness

Some clients are very anxious or angry when admitted to a healthcare facility. They may respond with aggression, which may be directed toward the nurse or the situation in general. It is important to remain objective and practice **assertiveness** (confidence without aggression or passivity). Box 44-2 gives a brief description of aggressive and assertive behaviors and an introduction to assertiveness training for nurses. It is also important to maintain personal safety.

Box 44-2 Aggressive Versus Assertive Behavior

Clients may be upset or afraid on admission to the healthcare facility and may react in a manner that is unusual for them. Some clients may be aggressive or hostile by nature. Some personality traits may challenge the nurse's objectivity. (These suggestions may also be helpful in your daily life.)

CHARACTERISTIC

Passivity: This person does not seem to care what happens and may be forgetful and indifferent. (Example—shrugging the shoulders, looking the other way, saying "whatever.")

Aggressiveness: This person seems angry and hostile, argues, and disagrees with everything that is said, and displays angry body language. This person is often inflexible and argumentative and may be very intrusive.

Passive-aggressive: This person seems passive and pleasant on the surface but does things to undermine or sabotage care (or the work environment). Actions include intentional disregard for physicians' orders, intentional inefficiency, saying one thing and doing another or saying different things to different people, and engaging in other manipulative or obstructive behaviors.

Assertive behavior/assertiveness: This is an important skill for nurses. The assertive person can make statements without conveying either aggressiveness (overdominance) or passivity (submission). The assertive person makes confident statements of fact, without making judgments. *Assertiveness training* is a helpful tool in all interactions, whether with clients or peers. It teaches the nurse to express personal feelings freely, to speak up nonjudgmentally for his or her rights, to communicate comfortably and clearly, and to express a legitimate complaint appropriately and not aggressively. Using these techniques, all persons involved can negotiate mutually satisfying solutions to interpersonal situations.

SUGGESTED APPROACH

Involve the client and family in decisions about his or her care. Explain what is being done and answer questions thoughtfully. Ask the client to repeat back to you, in their own words, what was said, to make sure the teaching was understood.

Remain calm. Do not argue or become angry. Be assertive, not aggressive. Keep your voice low, although the client may be yelling at you. Reinforce what is expected of the client in a firm, nonjudgmental way. Repeat, as necessary ("broken-record approach"). Protect yourself from assaultive behavior.

Document instructions given to the client, along with the client's actions or exact words (in quotes). Give the client a written list of instructions or expectations, to avoid confusion and reinforce the care plan.

If you feel that a client is threatening you and you are in danger, seek immediate assistance. (Chapter 94 describes safety measures used in psychiatry; Chapter 98 discusses safety in home care.) If you are in doubt, withdraw from the situation and seek help.

> **Nursing Alert** Remember that any aggressive behavior toward clients by a nurse, whether physical or verbal, constitutes *assault on the part of the nurse.*

Social Factors
Social acceptance of a particular illness plays a role in a person's reaction to the illness. For example, a sexually transmitted infection or psychiatric disorder may be more difficult or embarrassing for the client than a disorder such as glaucoma or diabetes, because of society's attitudes. The person with an arm or leg amputation or colostomy may feel more self-conscious than the person who has had some type of surgery that is not visible to others.

Religion
Members of some religious groups do not utilize traditional Western medicine (e.g., Christian Scientists). Others do not believe in receiving blood transfusions or certain types of surgery. Some religions do not allow abortions. Some groups believe in faith healing or alternative medicine only. Such beliefs may directly conflict with procedures and goals of a healthcare facility. It is important for the nurse to be nonjudgmental. Chapter 8 describes the implications of religion and culture for healthcare in more detail.

History of Illness
People who have never been sick may feel threatened or incapacitated by loss of control and may react by becoming very fearful, depressed, hostile, or resistant. Chronic or continuing illness can affect coping skills and motivation toward self-care and independence.

Body Image
How clients feel about themselves and illness affects communication. For example, athletes who rely on exceptional physical conditioning may see illness as a threat to their self-image and their ability to function productively. A client who has had a mastectomy or who has become impotent may worry about their sexual appeal. The body part affected, its symbolic meaning, and the visibility of bodily changes may influence how the client relates to others.

Physical Disabilities
Clients often have health conditions that impair their ability to communicate. For example, the person with Alzheimer disease or who has had a stroke may have difficulty communicating verbally. This person may not be able to process what you are saying or may not be able to formulate a response (aphasia). Also, the client may not have brought his or her glasses or hearing aid to the healthcare facility or may have lost them. Thus, a client may not be able to see or hear you. Effective nursing care considers all these factors.

THERAPEUTIC COMMUNICATION TECHNIQUES

Therapeutic communication techniques build and maintain rapport and encourage clients to express their thoughts and feelings more effectively. Some techniques are verbal; others are nonverbal (Fig. 44-6). Nontherapeutic communication stops the communication process or is perceived as a threat by the client. Examples of nontherapeutic actions include the nurse who talks too much, uses only closed-ended questions, or demonstrates impatient or threatening body language.

Interviewing

An **interview** is a goal-directed conversation in which one person seeks information from another. In nursing, the interview is the communication technique used to evaluate the client's understanding of his or her health concerns and to acquire valuable information from and concerning the client. The effective interview depends on the selection of suitable questions for which the client can provide answers. Sometimes, questions require simple responses (e.g., "What medications are you taking?" or "Do you have children?"). This type of question is a **closed-ended question** because only brief and predictable responses are required. A question that elicits a "yes" or "no" answer is a closed-ended question. An **open-ended question** encourages longer and more thorough answers. Table 44-2 compares these two types of questions.

Nonverbal Therapeutic Techniques
Just as the client's body language provides cues in communication, the nurse's body language indicates a great deal about how the nurse is feeling. It is important for the nurse to use effective NVC techniques (e.g., maintaining an openly accepting facial expression, appropriate eye contact,

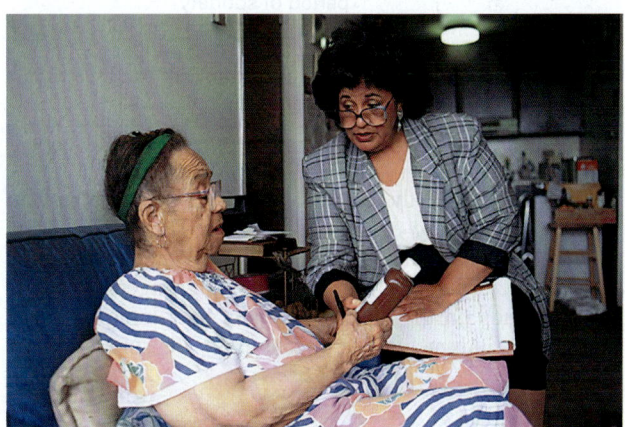

Figure 44-6 Therapeutic communication techniques are the tools for building and maintaining rapport. The client here is much more likely to learn what is being taught about her medications if she is comfortable in the interaction. Note that the home care nurse is displaying an open posture and appropriate eye contact and is sitting at eye level. She is leaning toward the client and allowing the client to handle and read the instructions on the medication bottle. The client is being encouraged to repeat instructions back, to avoid confusion. The client's questions are answered in a nonjudgmental way.

TABLE 44-2 Examples of Closed- and Open-Ended Questions

CLOSED-ENDED	OPEN-ENDED
(Allow "yes" or "no" answers)	(Promote discussion)
Do you sleep well?	Tell me about your usual sleep patterns
Do you like dairy products?	Do you eat milk and dairy products? If so, which ones, and how often? Describe any discomfort caused by dairy products. What are your food preferences?
How many children do you have?	Tell me about your family
Do you have a normal sex life?	Tell me about your means of sexual expression
Does your leg hurt often?	Describe the pain in your leg
Did you have a bowel movement today?	What is your usual pattern of bowel movements?
When was your last period?	Describe your menstrual history
Are you hearing voices?	Describe your hallucinations
Do you abuse alcohol? Street drugs?	Tell me about your alcohol and/or drug use. Describe any withdrawal symptoms. What street drugs do you use? How much and how often?
Have you ever had chemical dependency treatment?	Identify chemical dependency treatment you have had in the past. What was your longest period of sobriety?
Smoke? Chew?	Tell me about your tobacco, smokeless tobacco, and electronic cigarette use

and mirroring what the client says or does). It helps to lean toward the client, to express acceptance. The nurse who is an effective communicator learns to avoid gestures such as crossing the arms over the chest, pointing fingers, or holding the hands on the hips. (The client may interpret these gestures as judgmental or threatening.) Be sure to listen carefully.

Use of Silence

Silence gives the nurse and the client an opportunity to collect their thoughts and prepare to continue the conversation. Many people have difficulty coping with silence; they feel they must say something. Often, clients respond verbally to silence. If the nurse pauses for a few seconds, the client will often answer a question or make a statement that he or she would not have made before. Learning to use silence effectively is a valuable communication tool.

Key Concept

Practice waiting in silence for a client to speak. This is a very effective communication tool but is difficult for many nurses.

Clarification

Clarification is necessary if the client's answer is unclear or the nurse wants additional information. The nurse can ask the client to repeat what was said, or may say, "Tell me more about it" or "Explain that to me" or "What do you mean by…?".

Reflection

Reflection can be used in two ways. First, the nurse may echo the client's words, allowing the client to hear what he or she has just said. In this way, the client can reevaluate the words, to determine if they expressed what was meant.

CLIENT: "My life has been one frustration after another."
NURSE: "Your life has been full of frustrations?"
The second way to reflect is to point out the client's behavior or attitude that seems to be underlying his or her words.
CLIENT: "I'm just a worthless old man, and no one cares about me!"
NURSE: "You say that as if you were angry."
CLIENT: "I am angry. I raised six children and gave them the best years of my life. If they cared about me, they would come to visit me."

Paraphrasing

Use of paraphrasing helps the nurse to clarify the interpretation of the message by restating it in other words.
CLIENT: "It was really noisy here last night. It was like Grand Central Station."
NURSE: "You didn't get a good night's sleep? What can we do to help you sleep better?"

Summarizing

If the nurse tells the client what they heard, it helps the nurse to make sure it was what the client meant. Often the person adds more to the statement or clarifies the nurse's interpretation.

CLIENT: "I was in the hospital 2 years ago and I swore I would never come here again."
NURSE: "You were dissatisfied with your stay?"
CLIENT: "The food was so tasteless. I could not eat. My roommate died. The noise at night kept me from sleeping. I went home in worse shape than when I came in."
NURSE: "Sounds like you were very uncomfortable when you were here and are apprehensive about being admitted to the hospital again. How can we help improve the situation?"

Another example of summarizing is as follows:

CLIENT: "I don't eat meat. My son says I should, but I don't."
NURSE: "You don't eat meat?"
CLIENT: "That's right. I can't chew it anymore." Or,
CLIENT: "That's right. I can't afford meat." Or,
CLIENT: "That's right. I have become a vegetarian." Or,
CLIENT: "That's right. I'm afraid of the cholesterol." Or

CLIENT: "I don't eat meat on Fridays and on religious holidays." *Or*
CLIENT: "My religion forbids me to eat pork." *Or*
CLIENT: "I cannot eat the meat here because it is not Kosher."

By allowing the client to continue talking, the nurse can find the real reason that the client does not eat meat.

Using Unfinished Statements
Sometimes, if the nurse makes an unfinished statement, the client finishes it. For example:

NURSE: "You're going to live with your daughter…?"
CLIENT: "Well, I don't know. She really wants to put me in a nursing home, but I don't want to go!"

Communicating in Special Situations

Not all communication can be handled in the same way. Modifications to communication techniques are often necessary when working with children, older adults, mentally ill people, or people with special sensory or behavioral problems. Chapters 92 and 93 discuss communication with older clients and those with dementia; Chapter 94 describes special communication and listening techniques used in psychiatry.

Communicating With Different Age Levels
The Young Child
When working with small children, keep normal developmental stages in mind (see Chapter 10) and communicate at an appropriate level for the child's age. Remember: children often regress (revert) to an earlier stage of development when ill. Role-playing or drawing pictures may be helpful to determine what a child is feeling. Play is often the most effective means of communicating with a child (Fig. 44-7).

The Older Adult
It is important to respect and treat the older adult as you would expect to be treated. The effective nurse communicates with older adults at an appropriate level and is considerate of personal dignity. It is important not to "talk down to" any clients, whether younger or older. Show respect by addressing the person using an honorific ("Mr.", "Ms.", "Mx.") and adding the client's last name. It is disrespectful to refer to an older person by such names as "Grandpa" or "Sweetie." (If the client asks to be called by their first name, it may be acceptable to do so.) Think how you might feel if a younger person did not treat you with respect.

Communicating With the Client Who Has Sensory Problems
The Visually Impaired or Hearing-Impaired Person
Communication with sensory-impaired people is discussed in more detail in Chapter 80. Remember these important points:

- Do not frighten the person. The visually impaired person cannot see you coming; the hearing-impaired person cannot hear you. Make sure the person knows you are in the room before you touch them.
- Remember, the person with a sensory impairment is normal and has the same basic needs as all people. Take a little extra time to stop and communicate with this client.
- Utilize the services of a sign language interpreter if the client is able to communicate in this way. (Be aware that there are several sign languages, including American Sign Language [*ASL*], finger spell, and Signed English, Fig. 44-8.) ASL is *not universal*.

The Unconscious Client
Many people who have been unconscious for some time remember—when they recover—everything that occurred while they were unconscious. Use these guidelines for communicating with the unconscious client:

- Always assume the client can hear you.
- Introduce yourself.
- Explain what you are going to do.
- Talk *to* the client.
- Describe what the client can expect (cold, wet, pressure).
- Do not talk *about* the client in their presence. (Be sure the client's family does not do so as well.)

The Person With Aphasia
Aphasia commonly involves the inability to communicate verbally. However, aphasia may also include the client who cannot communicate via writing or by sign language or who cannot comprehend what is being said. Aphasia often results from a neurologic disorder or brain injury or a psychiatric disorder. Clients who have experienced a cerebrovascular accident (CVA), stroke, or traumatic brain injury (*TBI*) may have some level of aphasia. This is very frustrating for clients because their intelligence is usually unaffected. The client may take their frustration out on the nurse and family by showing anger, swearing, ignoring others, being argumentative, or assaultive and other disruptive behaviors. Develop some system or method of communication, to help prevent withdrawal and social isolation. See Box 44-3 for examples of helpful communication skills used with people who have speech or communication difficulties.

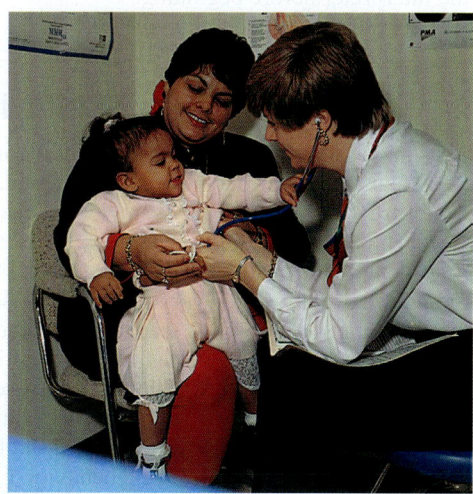

Figure 44-7 When working with small children, keep developmental stages in mind and communicate at an appropriate level for the child's age. Allow the child's caregiver to hold the child whenever as possible.

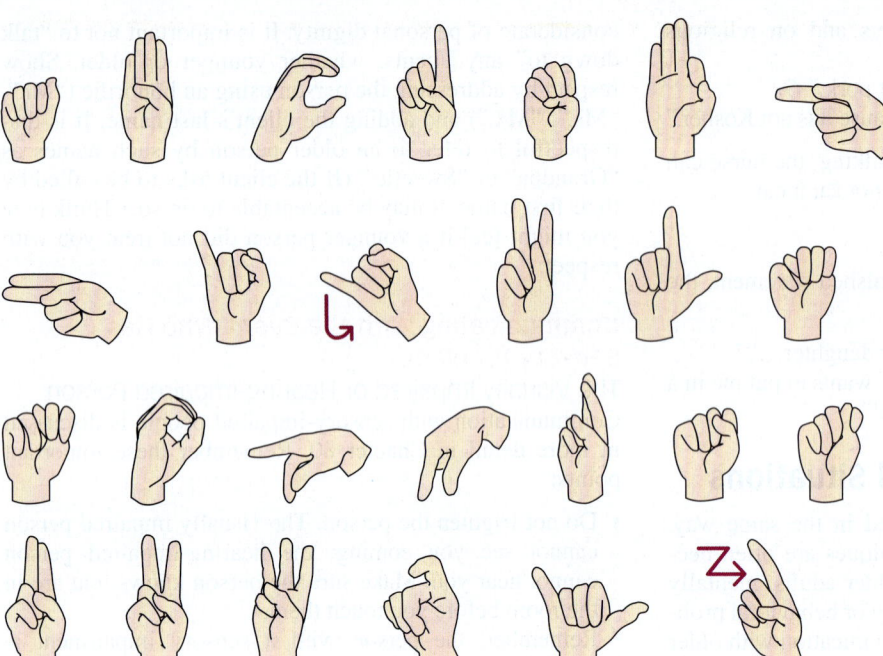

Figure 44-8 The alphabet in American Sign Language. (Timby, 2013.)

> **Key Concept**
> It is important to establish some sort of communication system for all clients.

Communicating With a Person Who Speaks a Language Different Than the Nurse's

Speaking different languages may make complete and effective communication difficult, but it need not prevent social interaction. A smile is understood in all cultures, and people can often use hand signals to communicate their needs. Drawings or photographs can help to explain or to ask something. For example, a drawing of a toilet or bedpan may ask the question, "Do you need to use the toilet?" when you cannot ask in the client's native language. A collection of drawings or photos may help the client to tell you when he or she is hungry, thirsty, cold, or in pain (see Fig. 44-9). Learn a few key words in the languages common in your area. Speaking a few words of another language often helps the client to appreciate the nurse's efforts. Appendix A, available online, provides a list of Spanish and English words to help in working with Spanish-speaking clients. For technical health-related communications, certified interpreters must be used. Using a friend or family member violates the client's privacy and may not provide accurate translation. Chapter 8 presents cultural considerations and Box 8-6 offers communication suggestions.

Guidelines for Use of Interpreters

The Health Insurance Portability and Accountability Act (HIPAA) regulations require special training and certification for interpreters. The interpreter and facility must have documentation of this training, and the person must be an approved volunteer or employee of the healthcare organization.

- Interpretation *must be offered* to all clients.
- Only the client can refuse interpreters, not the family, and must sign a release documenting refusal, with the aid of an interpreter. Even if the client refuses, the provider may request the interpreter to stay, particularly if the client is a minor or the family does not speak English.
- Interpretation via video or telephone is available 24 hr a day if a live interpreter is not available.
- All the above *must be documented*.
- Brief the interpreter before beginning.
- Speak in short segments and talk *to the client*.

Dealing With Specific Client Behaviors

Some clients may be anxious, or they may be afraid of being hospitalized, fear dying, or feel generally depressed. Some people do not trust anyone and are suspicious. Others will question everything the nurse does. Some clients regress and become dependent on the nursing staff, while others isolate themselves and reject everything the nurse tries to do. Some people may be very fearful, may react with false bravado, or may become threatening or assaultive. Be patient and open-minded with all clients. Reassure them while making sure that they are not a danger to themselves or others. Let all clients know you care, but do not allow them to display dangerous or threatening behavior. Chapter 94 further discusses some of these behaviors, along with suggested interventions.

Box 44-3 Special Communication Techniques

The nurse is obligated to establish a means of communication with each client. Suggestions are as follows.

THE CLIENT WHO IS NOT ABLE OR WHO REFUSES TO SPEAK

- Provide the client with a "magic slate," pencil and paper, or word and picture cards (Fig. 44-9). Encourage them to write or use a computer to indicate requests and comments.
- Establish hand signals or eye signals that are understood by both client and staff. It is most important to establish signals for "yes" and "no," if possible.
- Remember that most clients can hear and often understand, even if they are unable to speak or are not fluent in the language spoken.
- Treat each person with respect. Do not "talk down to" the client or talk about the client.
- Talk to the client, even if they are unable to answer.
- Many clients who cannot speak can use a computer. Assist the person to try this.
- Allow the client time to formulate words. Do not rush.
- Encourage the client to read. This may help the aphasic person to find more words.

THE CLIENT WHO SPEAKS A DIFFERENT LANGUAGE

- Provide a client's language-to-English language dictionary at the bedside.
- Schedule a certified interpreter for physician's visits, team conferences, and other meetings. (Telephone or video interpreters are available if an on-site interpreter is not.)
- Try to learn a few words of the client's language.
- Ask the client to repeat back what was said. Many people who do not speak the language being spoken will say they understood, even if they did not. It is important to make sure the client understands questions and instructions.
- Ask the client their name. Do not ask, "Are you Mr. Gonzalez?" Many clients will say "yes" to any question to cooperate.
- Computer programs and translation devices are available to assist people to communicate in a language other than their own.
- Try to assign staff who can speak some of the client's language. Introduce the client to others who speak the same language.
- Encourage family members and friends to visit. They can provide encouragement to the client and may be able to give information to the staff. *Do not use family members to interpret.*

BOTH THE CLIENT WHO IS UNABLE TO SPEAK AND THE CLIENT WHO SPEAKS A DIFFERENT LANGUAGE

- Design a picture board showing commonly requested items. The client can point to items requested. Put the English word with each picture (see Fig. 44-8).
- If a client is not English-speaking, try to add the corresponding word from the client's language with each photo.
- Remember: everyone understands a smile.
- Be conscious of body language. Make sure it is not misunderstood. Do not touch the client until you are sure the client understands what you are going to do.
- Consider cultural differences.
- Encourage the person to speak. Reinforce attempts to speak.
- Be patient. Give the person a chance to communicate.
- Remember that hesitation before speaking or avoiding direct eye contact may be a cultural sign of respect.
- Make liberal use of hand gestures. Be aware that some gestures used in the United States mean *something entirely different* in another country.
- Speak slowly and clearly.
- Avoid slang. Keep statements simple.
- Do not raise your voice—the person is not hearing-impaired. Saying something louder will not help the person to understand.
- Do not repeat the same thing over and over. Try to phrase it in a different way. Use simple language. Do not use slang.
- Remember that many clients can understand more than they can speak.

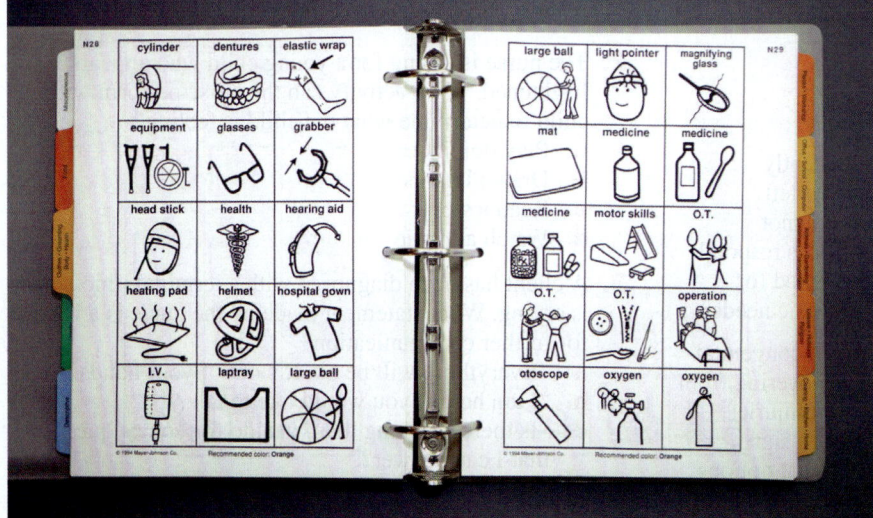

Figure 44-9 A word-and-picture card can assist in communicating with a person who has difficulty hearing or speaking or with one who speaks a language different than that of the nurse. Sometimes, each word is also written in the client's language. (Carter, 2016.)

FACILITATING COMMUNICATION IN HEALTHCARE

Nurses facilitate communication between clients and members of the nursing team in various ways, including the following:

- Skillfully interviewing clients, to determine their healthcare needs
- Listening attentively to what the client is saying
- Teaching clients and their family members certain aspects of care
- Documenting information on the nursing care plan and in the client's record
- Reporting the condition of the client to other members of the healthcare team
- Participating in team conferences and client care conferences
- Maintaining the confidentiality of information about clients. Be sure to have a signed release of information (ROI) before disclosing any information about a client to any unapproved person
- Treating each client as a unique individual; it is important to consider each person's age, sex, ethnic and religious background, state of health, life experiences, body image, feelings about being in the healthcare facility, language preference, and other personal factors
- Using both verbal and nonverbal means of communication and observing clients' verbal and nonverbal reactions
- Using touch as a therapeutic modality, but not invading the client's personal space or threatening the client

All aspects of communication influence the quality and effectiveness of client care. How the nurse handles this responsibility will directly influence the client's recovery. (See also Chapters 37 and 45 for discussion of specific aspects of communication in the healthcare setting.)

STUDENT SYNTHESIS

KEY POINTS

- Effective communication is the cornerstone to competent nursing care, no matter what the setting.
- Communication involves a sender, receiver, channel, message, and feedback.
- Developing rapport with the client is a basic ingredient of the nurse–client relationship.
- All communication has verbal and nonverbal components. NVC is powerful.
- The nurse must consider all personal and cultural factors about each client when communicating and providing care.
- Nurses conduct interviews to learn information about clients and to teach.
- Nurses can make many important observations, in addition to what the client says verbally.
- Nurses use techniques other than words to communicate with clients who have special communication needs.
- Competent nursing care requires caring, accurate, and ethical communication with clients and the healthcare team.
- It is critical to maintain each client's confidentiality when communicating, whether verbally, by computer, or in writing.

CRITICAL THINKING EXERCISES

1. Your client is Mr. J., 77 years old, who recently had a cerebrovascular accident (stroke) that left him with receptive aphasia. Although he cannot understand the meaning of language, he does respond to body language. What is an effective method for communicating so you can meet Mr. J.'s basic needs?

2. Your client is a 5-year-old child, who has a congenital hearing loss. The client is hospitalized, recovering from an accident in which they received internal injuries. Before the accident, they had begun to learn sign language, but you do not have this skill. What options do you have to communicate with this child?

3. A 43-year-old client from Somalia has been admitted to your unit. Neither the client nor anyone in their family speaks English. You do not speak Somali and an interpreter is not available. Describe ways in which you could establish a communication system with this woman. What orientation would you provide to your coworkers?

4. Review Chapter 8 and discuss therapeutic communication skills, as related to specific ethnic and religious beliefs about health and illness.

NCLEX-STYLE REVIEW QUESTIONS

1. The nurse is interviewing a client during admission to the hospital and the client gives information that is unclear to the nurse. What statement made by the nurse best demonstrates "seeking clarification?"
   a. "I don't know what you are talking about."
   b. "What did you say?"
   c. "We can move on to something else."
   d. "Would you please explain what you meant?"

2. The nurse is caring for a young child who appears frightened. What activity can the nurse perform with the child to determine what the child is feeling?
   a. Play dominoes
   b. Draw pictures
   c. Read a story
   d. Watch a movie

3. A client has been diagnosed with a terminal illness and is crying. What statement made by the nurse is a barrier for further communication?
   a. "Everything will be ok. It's out of your hands."
   b. "I am here if you would like to talk."
   c. "Is there anything that I can do for you or questions that I can answer?"
   d. "This must be difficult for you."

4. A client is having abdominal pain. What open-ended statement can the nurse use to find out more about the client's condition?
   a. "Tell me more about how you feel."
   b. "Rate your pain on a scale of 1–10."
   c. "Point with one finger to where your pain is located."
   d. "What medication are you taking?"

5. The nurse has provided discharge instructions to a client. What statement made by the nurse can best help determine if the client understood the instructions?
   a. "Reread the instructions that I gave you."
   b. "Did you understand the instructions?"
   c. "Please repeat back in your own words the instructions I gave you."
   d. "I am going to give you questions regarding the instructions and I want you to answer them."

CHAPTER RESOURCES

Enhance your learning with additional resources on thePoint!

Student Resources related to this chapter can be found at **thePoint.lww.com/Rosdahl12e**.

45 Admission, Transfer, and Discharge

Learning Objectives

1. Demonstrate in the skills laboratory how to orient a new client to the healthcare facility.
2. Discuss concepts related to caring for the client's clothing and valuable items on admission.
3. List client dehumanization and how it is avoided.
4. State nursing considerations related to admission of a client.
5. Identify information that the nursing student or practical nurse (LVN/LPN) should report to the registered nurse (RN).
6. In the skills laboratory, demonstrate the ability to transfer a client from one nursing unit to another safely and effectively.
7. Identify nursing considerations related to a client's discharge from the healthcare facility.
8. Explain teaching that should occur during hospitalization and at the time of a client's discharge.
9. Differentiate among the responsibilities of the healthcare facility, the healthcare provider, and the nurse when a client signs out of the facility against medical advice (AMA).
10. Describe how HIPAA legislation applies to the admission process and during a client's entire stay in the healthcare facility.
11. Describe effective nursing communication (Chapter 44), in relation to admission, transfer, and discharge.

Important Terminology

acuity
dehumanization
vital signs

Acronyms

AKA	BRP	kg	TPR
AMA	CXR	O_2 sat	VORB
AWOL	D/C	SBAR	VS
BIB/BIBA	DNR	S/P	W/C
BP	ID	TORB	

To provide effective nursing care, the nurse must be aware of client needs, attitudes, and emotions. Understanding the basic human needs of all people, as well as cultural considerations and the stages of human development, provides the foundation for planning and administering nursing care (see Chapter 5). By maintaining safety and drawing on communication and interviewing skills, nurses help clients and their families to express and work through their feelings about admission.

NCLEX Alert

Be alert during the NCLEX examination to concepts studied in previous chapters: maintaining client safety, understanding cultural differences, preventing the spread of infection, and communication and interviewing techniques and skills. In the examination, you may need to demonstrate your understanding of the implementation of nursing procedures related to the client's admission or transfer to another unit or care setting.

ADMISSION

Admission has more than one meaning in healthcare: Admission to the healthcare facility means the activities surrounding a client's arrival at the facility for the purpose of receiving healthcare. Also, each continuous period of time a client spends in a facility is considered *one admission*. Box 45-1 identifies sources of information about admission to specialized areas.

The Admitting Department

The first contact most clients have on arrival at the healthcare facility is with the Admitting Department or the admitting clerk in the Outpatient Department. (There are specific exceptions: The client may arrive by ambulance for an emergency admission and be taken immediately to surgery. Some clients are preregistered, including same-day surgery clients or women at the full term of pregnancy. These clients will often go directly to their receiving area.) In any event, the Admitting Department is responsible for necessary administrative activities, including assigning ICD—International Codes, related to the client's diagnosis. All HIPAA facilities were mandated to begin using these codes by the end of 2015. When the client enters the facility, it is important that all personnel make every effort to put the client at ease. Information about the client (e.g., name, address, age, sex, marital status, next of kin, employer, healthcare provider, and health insurance) is entered into the health record.

An identification band (**ID**) with the client's name (and **AKA**—"also known as," or alias, if applicable) and agency identification number (also called *medical record number* or *history number*) is applied to the client's wrist. Other information, such as birth date, date of admission, healthcare provider's name, and facility unit, may also be printed on the ID band. A separate wrist ID band is applied noting any client *allergies*. Check the facility protocol to determine what types of reactions are considered

CHAPTER 45 Admission, Transfer, and Discharge

> ### Box 45-1 Admission and Discharge in Various Facilities
>
> Much of the material in this chapter is geared toward admission and discharge of the client as related to the acute-care facility. Some specific procedures apply when the client is to be admitted to, or discharged from, other areas, such as the long-term care facility, home care, a hospice program, same-day surgery, or an outpatient department. These topics are considered in other chapters of this book:
>
> Chapter 66—the woman in labor and delivery
> Chapter 67—the newborn in the nursery
> Chapter 71—admission or discharge of a child
> Chapter 94—the mental health unit
> Chapter 95—the chemical dependency unit
> Chapter 97—rehabilitation facilities
> Chapter 98—home care nursing
> Chapter 99—ambulatory care
> Chapter 100—hospice care
>
> In addition, specific admission and discharge procedures are discussed in conjunction with particular disorders in Chapter 12.

true allergies. (If the client has no known allergies, a band must be worn stating this fact.) If the client is at risk for falling, a *fall risk* name band is applied as well (Fig. 45-1). (Specific procedures for assessing fall risk and identification of the client at risk are described in Chapter 39.) Seizure precautions may also be noted on the ID band. Each ID band is usually a specific color, according to facility policy. (Commonly, the name band is *white;* the allergy band, *red;* and the fall risk band, *yellow.*) The facility may also specify on which arm each band must be worn. In some facilities, the fact that a client is not to be resuscitated (DNR) is also noted on a special ID band. Because these ID bands are so important, they are waterproof and difficult for the client to remove.

> **Nursing Alert** Legally, the client cannot be allowed to receive treatment, undergo diagnostic tests or surgery, or receive medications without a legible ID band.

Diagnostic tests (e.g., x-ray examinations and blood tests) are often performed before the client is escorted to a nursing care unit. During admission, the client signs documents giving consent for treatments. The client or responsible person also signs documents accepting financial responsibility for costs not covered by insurance and designating insurance payments to be made directly to the facility. As described in Chapter 4, the Health Insurance Portability and Accountability Act (HIPAA) guidelines *must be followed,* to protect client privacy. The agency's privacy policies are reviewed with the client, the client is given a copy of the policy, and the client or responsible person signs a document confirming that these policies were discussed. Give the client an opportunity to ask questions, if needed (Fig. 45-2).

> **Key Concept**
>
> In many facilities, the entire admission process is carried out electronically. All data are immediately entered on the computer. The client's signature is required on some items, and this can be done electronically or on paper.

Advance Directives and Donor Status

Each client must be asked if they have a *living will* or other *advance directive.* The client who has any advance directive or living will submits a copy of the documentation for their record. (This may be in electronic form.) All clients must be advised of their right to create an advance directive while in the healthcare facility and must be offered assistance in

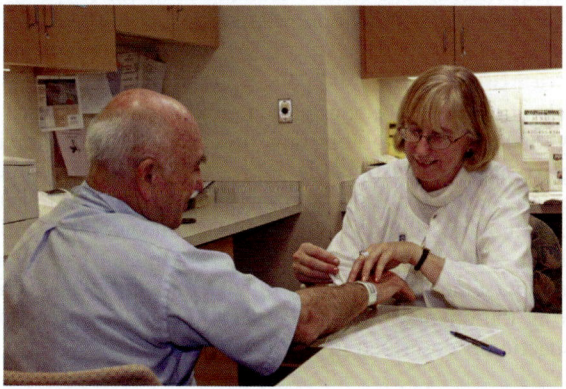

Figure 45-1 Proper identification of each client is vital. ID bands are used in all inpatient facilities, such as hospitals and long-term care facilities, as well as emergency departments and diagnostic treatment areas, such as dialysis, magnetic resonance imaging (MRI), and radiation therapy. In addition to the name band, the client wears an allergy band, whether or not they have allergies. (Carter, 2016.)

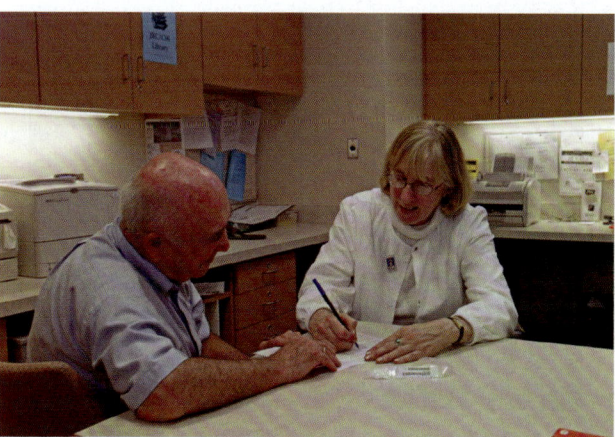

Figure 45-2 The client or new resident is assisted in filling out any necessary forms and signing permits and release of information requests. (Carter, 2016.)

preparing this. Whether or not the client has an advance directive, what type it is, and that the opportunity was given to prepare one, must be documented in the admission notes. (*Remember, if it is not documented, legally, it was not done.*)

In addition, each new client should be asked if they are an organ or tissue donor. Although the client's family must make the final decision, it is helpful for them to know the client's wishes in advance.

The Client's Arrival on the Nursing Unit

Before the client's arrival, check to be sure that the unit is completely equipped and the bed is available. The client may walk in or may arrive in a wheelchair or on a gurney. If possible, introduce the client to the staff before taking them to the room. If possible, give the client a tour of the unit. (If this is a scheduled admission, a tour may have been completed previously.) Remember: first impressions are very important; make the client as comfortable as possible. Routines, equipment, and procedures that are common for healthcare workers may seem frightening to the newly admitted person. Explain the purposes for all of these to the client, to ease discomfort (Fig. 45-3). Usually, the person is asked to wait in their room for the admission interview (see Chapter 34) and physical examination.

Removing the Client's Clothes

In many situations, the client will be asked to put on a hospital gown and robe, to facilitate the physical examination and any necessary treatments (discussed below). Some people may be allowed to wear their own pajamas, in which case, the family is responsible for this laundry. In some areas, such as chemical dependency, psychiatry (mental health), or long-term care, the client is encouraged to wear street clothes. Give the client whatever assistance is needed to undress. Sometimes a family member will assist, particularly if the client is immobile or is a child. ***Rationale:*** *A child may resist being undressed by a stranger or may not understand the need for wearing pajamas during the day*. Refer to In Practice: Nursing Procedure 45-1 when undressing the immobile client. The client's clothing and other property are inventoried and stored appropriately (Fig. 45-4).

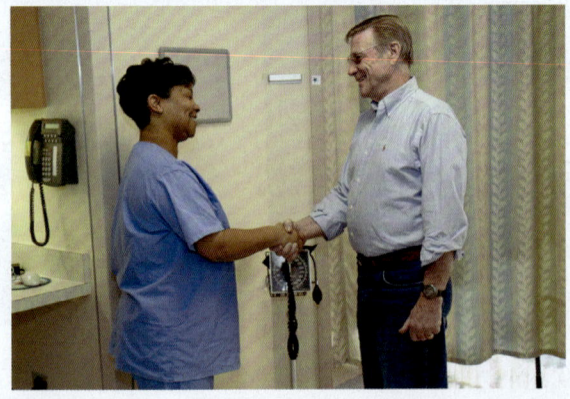

Figure 45-3 Greet the new client and make them feel welcome. Remember to orient them to the surroundings, pointing out the bathroom, and to demonstrate how to use equipment, such as bed controls, TV controls, and the nurse call/intercom system. (Carter, 2016.)

Inventory of Personal Effects

Resident ____________ Room No. ____________

Description :	
Bathrobe	Cane
Bed Jackets	Comb Brush
Belts	Crutches
Blouses	Dentures-Full Upper ( ) Lower ( )
Bras	Partial Upper ( ) Lower ( )
Coat	Furniture
Dresses	Glasses-Rimmed ( ) Rimless ( )
Girdles	Luggage
Hat	Other
Hose	Prosthesis
Nightgowns	Purse
Pajamas	Radio
Panties	Razors - Electric ( ) Safety ( )
Shirts	Rings
Shoes	Toothbrush
Skirts	Walker
Slips	Watch
Slippers	Wheelchair
Sweaters	
Ties	
Trousers	
Undershirts	
Undershorts	
Wallet	

I certify that the above is a correct list of my personal belongings.
I take full responsibility for retaining in my possession the articles listed above and any others brought to me while a resident in this facility.

ALL ITEMS BROUGHT FOR THE PERSONAL USE OF THE RESIDENT MUST BE PROPERLY MARKED AND LISTED AS ARE THE ABOVE. Please bring additional items to the Nurses' Station for proper handling.

Resident's washable clothing to be: ____________ taken home for laundering ____________ laundered here at the center.

I understand the Management will not be responsible for any valuables, money, or clothing left in the possession of the resident.__________ Date__________

Signature of Resident (or Relative) ____________ Date ________
Signature of Nurse ____________ Date ________

Disposition on Discharge *Upon Discharge, all personal items are sent with resident or picked up by responsible party. Upon transfer, all personal items are to be boxed and placed in designated storage area for safekeeping.

Signature of Nurse ____________ Signature of Resident/Relative ________
Date ____________ Date ____________

Figure 45-4 It is the responsibility of nursing staff to inventory all items brought by the client. In the acute-care facility, most valuable items are sent home with the family or placed in the vault, but in the long-term care setting, the client will usually bring more property. In some cases, the facility is responsible for helping safeguard client property. (Carter, 2016.)

Inspecting for Skin Integrity

Each client must be carefully checked on admission for any open wounds or existing pressure areas. Any existing wounds or questionable areas must be carefully documented when the client is admitted. If the client's skin is not intact on admission and this is not documented, the facility will most likely not be reimbursed for related care given. (Reimbursement is usually withheld for injuries occurring during the client's facility stay.) The procedure for wound inspection is described in Chapter 58.

Assisting the Client Into Bed

If a client is weak or tired when admitted, remove the client's shoes and outdoor clothing and help them to lie down immediately. Cover the client with a bath blanket or bedclothes. The client may have exerted considerable effort to get to the healthcare facility; lying down may help. As soon as possible, assist the client to put on a hospital gown or pajamas, if necessary, and explain why this is desirable. ***Rationale:** Wearing the hospital gown facilitates the physical examination and various treatments. It also prevents soiling of the client's clothes. (Remember that in some areas, street clothes are worn.)*

> **Key Concept**
>
> Nursing *data collection* begins immediately at the nurse's first contact with the client (see Chapter 47).

Orienting the Client to the Facility

The healthcare provider's admission orders will include the client's allowed activity status, such as bathroom privileges (**BRP**) or complete bed rest. If the client is able to be out of bed, indicate the location of the bathroom and closet. Check to see if the client is to give a urine specimen or is on intake and output (a recording of all fluids taken in and urine expelled). If so, give the client a urinal, toilet hat, or urine cup and explain what the client is to do and why. Ask the client not to void directly into the toilet until needed samples are obtained. (Chapter 52 describes methods for collecting specimens.)

Allow time for the client to unpack, if items have been brought to the facility. Encourage clients to send any unnecessary items home with the family. (In the long-term care facility, the client will often bring more clothing and personal items than are needed while in the acute-care facility.) Help the client, if necessary, and describe where you are putting items. Place the bathrobe and slippers in a handy spot. Arrange the client's personal belongings. Place special items, such as eyeglasses, on the bedside table or in the drawer. (Make sure all valuables, such as jewelry, credit cards, and cash, are either sent home with a family member or locked in the hospital vault for safekeeping.) Adjust the window shades, regulate ventilation, and position the head or foot of the bed for the client's comfort. Put the entire bed in the *low position,* regardless of whether or not the client can get in and out of bed without assistance. If the client is at risk for falls, the side rails are usually put up until a thorough evaluation is completed. Explain how the bed works and let the client know how to adjust it. (If the client would be endangered by adjusting the bed, the controls can be locked.) Teach the client how to work the TV, nurse call signal, and lights over the bed. Tell the client the hours of meal service and the procedure for ordering meals (usually a selective menu). Determine what the client may have to eat or drink and when. Make sure a meal is ordered for each new client, after checking the provider's orders to determine if the client is on a special diet or fluid restriction. Encourage the client to be patient with all the admission procedures. Explain that nurses function under the direction of a healthcare provider. Introduce the client to any roommates. Make sure that the client's questions have been answered and the person is comfortable and safe before leaving the room. Leave the door or curtains open or closed, as the client wishes.

Intercom System

Show the client how the communication system works, and place the nurse call signal within easy reach. Also show the client where the signal mechanism is located in the bathroom. ***Rationale:** Taking time to explain things to the client helps alleviate fear and anxiety in unfamiliar surroundings.*

> **Key Concept**
>
> Explain to the new client that the signal light in the bathroom is for emergencies only. Usually, there is both a button and a pull cord. Using either signal will probably ring an alarm and activate the nurse-call light. Ask clients not to use this signal unless they need emergency assistance.

Toilet Articles

The healthcare facility usually supplies such essential toilet articles as toothbrushes, toothpaste, mouthwash, deodorant, shampoo, combs or hair picks, tissues, lotion, and soap. (These supplies may be sold in a pharmacy or gift shop within the facility, or nearby, if the facility does not automatically provide them.) Many clients have personal preferences and like to choose these articles themselves. Many acute-care facilities provide new clients with a prepackaged set of supplies that contains the listed toiletries, as well as a plastic water cup, water carafe, and, if needed, a bedpan, urinal, bath basin, and emesis basin. Clients may use and discard these articles or take them home on discharge. Nurses may need to provide other items, such as denture cups, for individual clients; be sure these are labeled, *both on the container and the lid.* (If you handle the client's dentures or used tissues, *wear gloves;* see Chapter 50.) Some facilities also provide disposable blood pressure cuffs, thermometers, and telephones, to reduce the risk of cross-contamination.

Hospital Gown

As stated previously, the client is asked to don a hospital gown, in most cases. This is especially important if the client is bleeding, incontinent, vomiting, or having wound drainage. The facility laundry uses special methods to prevent cross-contamination. (In long-term facilities, clients may be charged a fee for laundry service.) In addition, the hospital gown allows easier access to suture lines, wounds, and equipment, such as intravenous (IV) lines, and facilitates special tests and procedures. Hospital gowns are easy to put on and remove. Explain that these gowns provide convenience, comfort, and safety. They usually open in the back and fasten with ties, Velcro, or snaps. The sleeves also may open to accommodate IV tubing. Be sure that a client's gown is long and large enough. Be sure the gown's ties are not uncomfortable when secured; tie with bows to the side. (Clients in psychiatry are usually not allowed gowns with ties.) Clients should also be provided with a robe and slippers, if they did not bring them.

> **Key Concept**
>
> Most hospitals provide extra-large gowns and robes. If a client is unusually large, it may be necessary to use two gowns, one opening in the front and one opening in the back. Some facilities allow very large clients to wear special scrub suits. In some cases, jail clothing must be worn.

Individual Equipment

Inform clients that equipment in their unit, such as suction machines, oxygen, and inhalation equipment is for only their use. In some cases, individual blood pressure cuffs and temperature probes are provided. Point out which closet and drawers are for each client's use. Generally, each client's towels will be hung on their own bedside stand or near their bed if a bathroom is shared. (In the acute-care area, shared bathrooms are rare.)

Client Identification

Be sure each client is wearing the proper ID bands, as described previously. Remember to check for allergies, fall precautions, seizure precautions, or resuscitation status. Check the information on all ID bands to make sure that it is correct. Ask the client or family also to verify the information, if possible.

A "care plan board" or "communication board" is often near the bed. This white board contains the date, the client's first name, the provider's name, social worker's name, and name of the nurse caring for the client during the current shift. The board often indicates the client privileges (e.g., "bedrest"); the diet; the client's goals for the day; and other pertinent information, such as orders for intake and output or seizure precautions. Regularly check this information and update it, as needed. A tag indicating the client's first name may be placed near the door of the room as well.

> **Key Concept**
>
> If white boards are used or if name tags identify clients' rooms, only the first name should be used (to protect client confidentiality). In addition, if a master board with all clients' names and room numbers is placed at the nursing station, it should be in such a position that passers-by cannot read the names.

Caring for the Client's Personal Belongings

Clothing

Each client in the acute-care facility has a place for a bathrobe and slippers and a drawer for other articles. Clients are encouraged to keep only essential items in the hospital. (In the long-term care facility, the client has more items and more storage space.) In same-day surgery, clothing is placed in a marked garment bag and returned to the client when they go home. Fill out a property sheet, including a description of every item of clothing. Follow the system the facility has established; doing so protects the client and the facility. Have the client sign the property sheet after they check the list (see Fig. 45-4).

Valuables

Valuables, such as jewelry, credit cards, and cash, should not be brought to the facility. If they are brought, they should be kept in the facility's vault. When clients learn they cannot keep these belongings with them, they may prefer to send them home with a person they designate. Clients usually keep a small amount of change to buy newspapers and other items from the coffee or gift shop.

> **Key Concept**
>
> In some situations, such as in a Memory Care unit or mental health unit, the facility does assume some responsibility for client belongings, because the client may not be competent to do so. In this case, your careful listing and description of the client's property becomes even more important. (The facility may be required to reimburse this client for lost items.) In these units, the client may not be allowed to keep any jewelry (other than a wedding ring) or any money at the bedside.

The client who is competent often keeps personal items, such as eyeglasses, dentures, a prosthesis, a watch, or wedding ring, at the bedside. These items are noted and described on the property sheet. Usually, the client signs a waiver verifying that these items are to remain at the bedside at *their own risk*. (In a long-term care facility, mental health unit, hospice unit, or chemical dependency unit, the client usually keeps more personal items. In this case, all items must be labeled with the client's name and room number; this usually includes all of the client's clothing in the long-term facility. Cloth name tags are usually recommended for clothing.) When labeling client belongings, be sure to use a label that can be easily removed without damaging the item when the client is discharged. Cell phones are usually not permitted in the facility, because they can take photos, which would violate other clients' privacy.

If the client goes to surgery or has a lengthy examination, items such as a watch or eyeglasses are given to the family for safekeeping or are sent to the hospital vault. The client must sign later to verify that the items have been returned.

> **Key Concept**
>
> It is very important to list the client's property carefully. Describe items as clearly as possible. For example, "blue Nike ski jacket" or "3 white T-shirts." When describing jewelry, do not make judgments about values. For example, it is best to say "clear stone" instead of "diamond" or "gold-colored bracelet" instead of "gold bracelet." If the client has valuable jewelry or an amount of money greater than about $20, these items should be sent to the facility's vault or home with the family. If the client chooses to keep a valuable item, such as a wedding ring, this must be noted on the property sheet, and the client assumes responsibility for it. (If the client is confused or unable to make decisions, the concept of property becomes a difficult legal question. Consult your supervisor if you have a question.)

Preventing Dehumanization

It is important to prevent **dehumanization**, depriving a person of personality, privacy, and other human qualities, and neglecting their individuality, ignoring their specific needs, and failing to allow them to have input about their care. Whenever possible, the nurse should develop rapport and trust with the client before delving into personal matters or procedures that may embarrass or threaten their individuality or privacy. This indicates that the nurse sees the client as an individual and an important person. The person admitted to the healthcare facility surrenders clothes, belongings, and loses personal decision-making. The client is expected to follow orders about what to eat, and when to eat, sleep, take a bath, and even when and where to go to the bathroom. A stranger asks when the client last had a menstrual period, sexual relations, or a bowel movement. All these personal factors must be handled carefully, in order to avoid dehumanizing the person.

Whether giving care in a hospital, extended-care facility, or in the home, the nurse can take many measures to prevent clients from feeling dehumanized. Handle questions and procedures with the utmost tact and respect for the individual. Always think of each client as a person whose need for physical and emotional support is greater than normal because of illness. Emphasize the client's strengths rather than weaknesses. This can promote the client's recovery. Always allow the client to maintain personal dignity.

> **Key Concept**
>
> Imagine how you would feel if a stranger expected you to answer personal questions about your toileting habits, your menstrual history, and your sex life. Consider the client's feelings when asking these questions. Remember: Treat the client as you would wish to be treated.

Anxiety or Apprehension

A person facing illness or surgery often feels very anxious. People may be worried about their family or about finances. What may concern one person, however, may have no effect on another. In addition, the degree of anxiety may be related to the severity of illness or the person's previous experiences. Anxiety may also aggravate the client's physical disorder or may affect the client's ability to cope. Consider Maslow's hierarchy of human needs (see Chapter 5). If a person's lower level needs (e.g., oxygen, food, etc.) are not met, they will have difficulty concentrating and learning. This person will probably not be able to remember and identify what medications are being given, learn self-care, or participate in the development of their care plan at such a time. Levels of anxiety or absence of anxiety range from the person who is calm to the person who is in a state of extreme agitation or panic.

> **Key Concept**
>
> The client's anxiety level may be estimated as follows:
>
> Calm = Not anxious
>
> +1 anxiety = Increasing uneasiness and apprehension
>
> +2 anxiety = Increasing uneasiness, apprehension, dread
>
> +3 anxiety = Increasing apprehension, dread, paranoia
>
> Panic = Symptoms may include a feeling of choking, difficulty breathing, inability to sit still, chest tightness or pain, trembling, sweating, increased pulse rate and blood pressure, or headache

Anxiety may be *rational* (logical or justified) or *irrational* (out of proportion, unrealistic, inappropriate to the situation). Anxiety differs from fear in that the person often *cannot identify a specific cause for anxiety.* (The source of fear can often be verbalized.) Anxiety and fear can be precipitated by factors such as fears of the unknown, of death, and of body image changes and threat to self-concept, loss of significant other, or financial concerns. Some of these factors may be realistic in the case of a serious illness or accidental trauma. Generalized anxiety or panic is often not realistic, in relationship to the situation. Severe anxiety or panic can interfere with medical care. For example, nonemergency surgery may be canceled if the client is extremely apprehensive.

Nursing interventions aimed at alleviating anxiety and fear include the following:

- *Assessment* of level of discomfort
- *Clear explanations* and clear answers to questions
- Offering the client an *opportunity to express feelings*
- Providing more helpful *coping mechanisms*
- Allowing the client to *make decisions* relating to their care

Fear of the Unknown

Perhaps the most intense fear is fear of the unknown. The client may be afraid of serious illness or death. People may be threatened by illness, especially if the treatment involves surgery. Some people feel that healthcare personnel are not telling the truth about their disease or condition, or that their condition is more serious than it actually is.

> **NCLEX Alert**
>
> It is important to recognize clients' communication abilities/difficulties. Your knowledge of how to support the emotional, mental, and social well-being of clients being admitted to a healthcare setting may be required in the examination.

Fear of Body Image Changes

Body image refers to the way an individual perceives themselves. People respond differently to a threat to body image. If upcoming surgery involves a procedure such as limb amputation or breast removal, the concern about disfigurement may very likely cause anxiety. The client may be concerned about the family's response to the surgery, the reaction of friends, or the possible loss of a job or mobility. Even if surgery does not cause a visible change in appearance, the client may be concerned. Life situations influence responses to changes in body image. Consider the situations of a fashion model, an Olympic-level skier, a parent of a toddler, an 80-year-old, or a construction worker about to have a leg amputated. Their reactions are likely to be very different.

Financial Concerns

Another concern of many clients is the fear of financial burden. Insurance coverage varies. Some people do not have adequate insurance to cover the costs of healthcare. Some clients cannot afford hospitalization or admission to extended-care facilities. They may be concerned about how their family will manage while they are away. Such preoccupation with financial and family concerns can affect the client's progress toward recovery.

Embarrassment

Many people are embarrassed when personal services, such as bathing or assistance in toileting, must be performed for them. Providing as much *privacy* as possible and *explaining* what is occurring during treatments are vital. Client discomfort during nursing care may be caused by superstitions, folk medicine beliefs, cultural beliefs about illness, or cultural practices regarding the roles of men and women. Lack of medical knowledge about the body can also cause client confusion and misunderstanding.

The Client Who Has Difficulty Hearing or Understanding English

The client who does not speak or understand English is much more likely to be uncomfortable in a healthcare facility where everyone else speaks only English. The person with a hearing or vision disorder is often in the same situation. These people do not understand what is happening, and staff members are unable to explain things, to lessen the client's discomfort. Obtain a certified interpreter for these people as soon as possible. Chapter 8 describes ways to communicate with people of different cultures, and Chapters 44 and 80 describe ways to communicate with the person with a visual or hearing impairment.

Data Gathering, Reporting, and Documentation

After orienting the client to the nursing unit and the room, the admissions interview and history are done, unless the client's health needs dictate that this must be done later. (In some situations, such as in a psychiatric or emergency department, the client may be too agitated, confused, sedated, or ill to participate; the interview may need to be postponed.)

Table 34-1 lists sample questions to ask during the admissions interview. In Practice: Nursing Care Guidelines 45-1 gives tips for performing the admissions interview.

The nurse takes vital signs (see Chapter 46), asks about pain, and measures pulse oximetry, height, and weight. In Practice: Nursing Care Guidelines 45-2 discusses the procedure for weighing clients and illustrates various types of scales that may be used. Urine, stool, or sputum specimens may also be collected at this time (see Chapter 52). A nurse may accompany the client to the Radiology Department or to a laboratory for tests. The admission notes and other data are entered into the computer data base.

During time with the client, the nurse must be observant. Report to the team leader if you observe any unusual signs or symptoms, or if the client complains of severe pain.

IN PRACTICE
NURSING CARE GUIDELINES 45-1 — Performing the Admissions Interview

- Gather necessary supplies (e.g., healthcare provider's orders; computer [or written] records; equipment for vital signs and oximetry; brochures regarding client privacy, client rights, advance directives, and unit procedures, such as visiting regulations).
- Become familiar with information from the Admitting Department before meeting the client.
- Introduce yourself; explain that you will be taking information and discussing routines of the facility.
- Verify the client's name and birth date, as printed on the ID band. Ask the client to state this information and check the name band to make sure it is correct. (Do not ask the client if he is "Mr. Johnson." Some clients will say yes, even if this is not the case.)
- Record pertinent information during the interview. Make sure to focus on the client and not on the computer (Fig. 45-5).
- Observe the client's general appearance (e.g., posture, ability to ambulate, mood, body language).
- Note the client's general condition (e.g., level of alertness, orientation to reality).
- Observe the client's skin condition (e.g., temperature, color, turgor, scars, lesions, abrasions, pressure areas, edema). Carefully describe any abnormalities or breaks in the skin on the admissions database, indicating their location, appearance, and size.
- Monitor the client's respiratory status (e.g., coughing, wheezing, shortness of breath, inability to breathe unless sitting up).
- Assess the client's psychological status, as evidenced by verbal and nonverbal responses.
- Measure weight and height.
- Measure vital signs (Chapter 46).
- Ask about pain (Chapter 55).
- Measure pulse oximetry (Chapter 46).
- Ask how the client got to the facility (**BIB** family, brought in by family; **BIBA**, brought in by ambulance).
- Maintain the client's privacy and confidentiality.
- Obtain health history and information regarding the following:
  - Next of kin, emergency contact person.
  - Reasons for admission.
  - Whether the client has been out of the country in the past 21 days.
  - Current medications: were they brought to the facility?
  - Allergies to medications, foods, and other substances (e.g., latex). Verify all allergies with the allergy name band and in the client record.
  - Use of tobacco, alcohol, or street drugs.
  - Daily eating, sleeping, elimination, and exercise routines.
  - Whether or not the client feels safe at home.
  - Use of appliances or prostheses (e.g., artificial limbs, hearing aids, contact lenses, dentures). Were they brought to the facility?
  - Family support (e.g., Will people visit regularly or stay in the facility with the client? Is someone available at mealtimes to help feed the client? Will they bring in food? Who should be contacted in an emergency?). Be sure to obtain home, work, cell phone numbers, and email address.
  - Employer or school.
  - Resuscitation or DNR (do not resuscitate) status.
  - Advance directives. Be sure a copy is in the record.
  - Payee or guardian.

(See Table 34-1 for sample questions to ask in the admissions interview.)

IN PRACTICE
NURSING CARE GUIDELINES 45-2 — Weighing the Client

- Calibrate the scale so it is at zero before weighing the client. (Chairs and slings will automatically deduct the weight of the equipment.) Determine the client's weight by using the weights and indicator on the free-moving balance arm or by using the digital readout.
- The client who is strong enough may stand on a transfer paper or paper towel on the *balance scales* or step-on scale. Assist client to step onto the scale (to prevent falls).

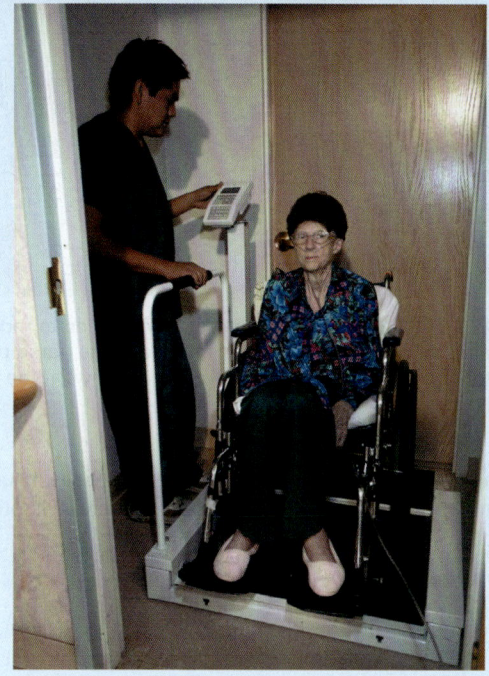

The sitting (chair) scale is used if the client has difficulty standing. The chair scale is available with a balance beam (as shown in Fig. 47-4) or with an electronic readout, as shown here. (Carter, 2016.)

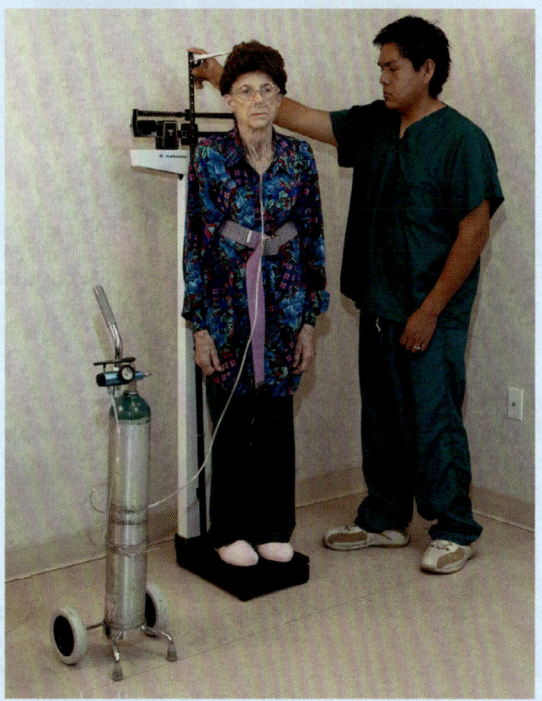

The standing (step-on) scale is used most often. Shown here is a balance-beam type, which is used in many healthcare settings, particularly in physician's offices. On the balance scale, the client's weight is determined by sliding the small and large weights along the balance bar until the pointer of the bar balances without touching. In this photo, the client's height is being measured at the same time. (Standing scales with attached handrails are also available.) Standing scales with electronic readouts are used most often in inpatient facilities. The electronic scale can convert between kilograms and pounds. (Carter, 2016.)

- Clients who are unable to stand are weighed on *chair scales* or on the bed itself, if it includes a scale. The chair scale resembles the step-on scale but is equipped with an armchair for the client's comfort. Assist the client to step up onto the platform under the chair and to be seated in the chair.

- An immobile client is weighed lying down on a sling scale (bed scale, litter scale), a sling-type apparatus that looks like a suspended hammock or a client hydraulic lift. Ask for assistance to place the client on this scale (for client safety). The machine raises the client from the bed's surface and then displays the weight.

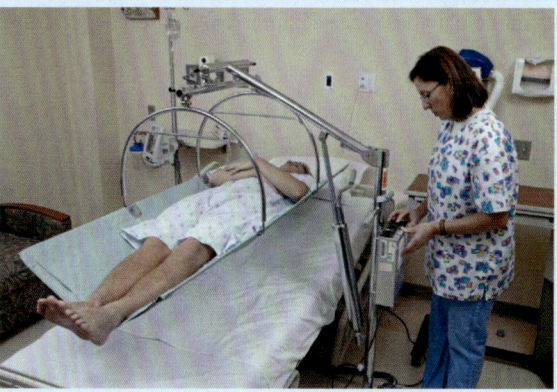

The sling scale (litter/bed scale), shown here, is used to weigh the client who has difficulty getting out of bed or who cannot sit or stand. Some special beds have a built-in scale (see Chapter 49). (Carter, 2016.)

- Weight is usually recorded in kilograms (**kg**), particularly if the client is to have surgery or if other medication doses will be based on weight. Electronic scales will convert kilograms to pounds, for the client's benefit.

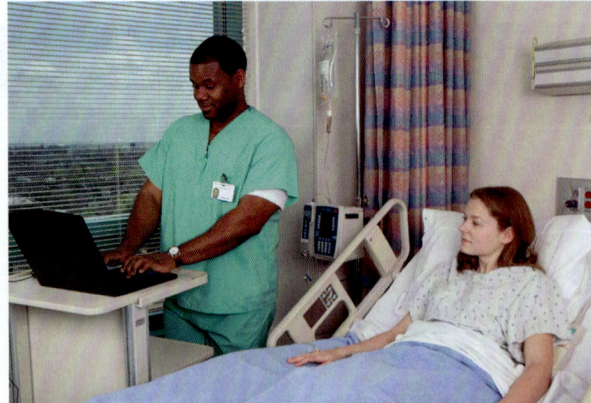

Figure 45-5 The computer-on-wheels (COW) is used to record pertinent data during the admission interview. The nurse pays close attention to the client's body language and what the client is saying. (Taylor et al., 2015.)

Knowing the client's diagnosis is helpful when observing signs and symptoms (see Chapter 47). Review Chapter 44 for specific interviewing techniques.

Weight

Measure and record the client's weight on admission. (Do not go by what the client says.) Fluctuating weight may indicate when the client is or is not retaining fluids. Recent changes in usual weight can also indicate situations, such as anorexia or binge eating. In addition, some medications encourage weight gain. The client may experience weight loss as a result of many factors, including illness, chemotherapy, and depression. The initial weight, compared with the client's height, helps determine if the client is overweight or underweight. The admission weight also establishes a baseline for further observations or calculations of medication doses or anesthesia. In Practice: Nursing Care Guidelines 45-2 describes the steps in weighing the client. Record weights in the data base (see Chapter 46) as soon as possible.

Height

Measure and record the client's height on admission. Ask the client to remove shoes and stand straight, with their back against the measuring bar. Lower the L-shaped sliding bar so that it lightly touches the top of the client's head. Record the height (usually in centimeters; not feet or meters) on the graphic sheet. If the client cannot stand, an approximate height is obtained while the client lies in bed. Have the client lie on the back and stretch out as much as possible. Place a mark on the sheet under the person's heel and at the top of the head. Then measure between these two marks on the taut bottom sheet. Record as "estimated" height (Fig. 45-6).

Vital Signs

Measure and record the client's **vital signs** (**VS**) during admission and as ordered while the client is in the healthcare facility (Chapter 46). Vital signs include body temperature, pulse (rate of heart beats), respiration (rate of breathing), and blood pressure (the pressure the blood exerts against the walls of the arteries). These readings are abbreviated as **TPR** (temperature, pulse, respiration) and **BP** (blood pressure). They are called *vital* signs because they must be present for

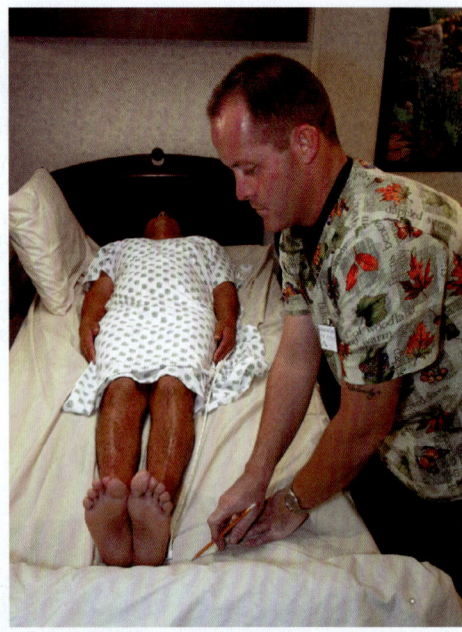

Figure 45-6 If it is necessary to determine the approximate height of a client confined to bed, mark on the sheet at the top of the head and at the heels and then measure between the marks. (Carter, 2016.)

a person's life to continue. Vital signs are an important factor in healthcare. Pain is considered to be the fifth vital sign. Chapter 46 describes and illustrates the measurement of vital signs; Chapter 55 describes evaluation of pain.

Pulse Oximetry

In many facilities, the client's baseline oxygen saturation is a standard component of the admission process and is entered in the electronic record, along with the vital signs. This procedure measures the percentage of oxygen in the client's blood, while breathing room air. Most clients test at 95%–99%. If the client's O_2 saturation (**O_2 sat**) is below 95%, this should be reported to the healthcare provider. The procedure for measuring the O_2 sat is outlined in Chapter 46.

Collecting Specimens

Often, a urine specimen will be ordered. Most often, a midstream or "clean-catch" specimen is to be collected; instruct the client on how it is done. Other specimens are not usually collected immediately on admission. However, if the physician requests other specimens, collect them per protocol (see Chapter 52).

Radiology and Laboratory Examinations

Some clients are given a chest x-ray (CXR) on admission. A chest x-ray provides basic baseline information about the heart and lung structure. It can be used to rule out some diseases, fractures, or abnormalities in size. Most clients will also require admission blood work to be done by the laboratory. If x-rays or laboratory work are ordered, the nurse may transport the client to the Radiology Department or Laboratory. Be sure to follow the guidelines in Chapter 48 for transporting a client by wheelchair or stretcher.

SPECIAL CONSIDERATIONS Lifespan

Admission Assessment for Children

- The child who is scheduled for surgery often tours the facility prior to admission, to relieve anxiety.
- Observe for signs of anxiety and fear, as evidenced by crying or temper tantrums.
- Be knowledgeable about developmental stages, to be better able to judge each child's physical and emotional needs (see Chapters 10 and 11).
- Determine if a parent or family member will stay with the child. Allow them to hold the child, if possible.
- Determine how much self-care the child can perform.
- Be aware that regression often occurs when a child is ill. (The child may revert to a previous level of functioning.)
- Check with the child, to determine how much they understand. You may need to find an alternate method for teaching the child. (Pictures, videos, role play, storybooks, or toys are often used.)
- Determine what special words the child uses for toileting needs (such as "potty," "tinkle," "poopoo"). Determine any other special words or signs used.

Reporting the Admission

The Joint Commission (JCAHO) requires that an RN perform formal admission assessments and formulate nursing diagnoses. When a nursing student or licensed vocational nurse/licensed practical nurse (LVN/LPN) has completed the client orientation and the assigned admission procedures, they can notify the admitting RN. The LVN/LPN reports their specific observations, along with other pertinent data, such as the client's vital signs, weight, and client-reported symptoms. The provider's orders are checked; the dietary order is transmitted to the Food Services Department; and other orders are sent to the laboratory, radiology, pharmacy, and other departments. The client is also logged into the computer; in most acute-care facilities, all orders are entered into the computer and automatically transmitted to other departments, such as the Laboratory or Radiology.

Head-to-toe observations are an important component of the admission process (see Chapter 47). Much of the data are collected by the admitting nurse and/or primary provider, but the LVN/LPN assists in the process. Initial observations provide a starting point for later development of a medical diagnosis and nursing care plan. The assigned RN is responsible for completing the admission assessments, formulating a problem list, and developing nursing diagnoses. The individualized nursing care plan is based on the identified problem list, and the entire team works to develop a multidisciplinary care plan. Box 45-2 lists pointers for admission documentation. In many units, each client unit has a computer; in other cases, a mobile computer, connected to the facility's network, is brought to the client's room for the admission. These computers are sometimes called "COWs"—computers on wheels (see Fig. 45-5).

Advance Directives

As stated previously, the law requires all clients to be informed about advance directives on admission to a healthcare facility. As discussed in Chapter 4, an advance directive is a written document that allows the individual to specify choices of healthcare treatment if they become so ill that

---

Box 45-2 Admission Documentation

In many facilities, it is the responsibility of the RN to document official interview assessments, but nursing students and licensed vocational nurses or licensed practical nurses (LVNs/LPNs) often record the following information:

- Weight and height
- Vital signs, including pain
- Pulse oximetry
- Whether any laboratory tests were done, blood drawn, or x-ray studies done
- Any other procedures
- Who is accompanying the client
- Specimens sent to the laboratory: note the amount of urine voided and its appearance, or the client's inability to void
- Any prostheses or appliances the client uses (e.g., dentures, contact lenses, glasses); note where these items were placed ("at bedside," "sent home with family," etc.)
- Listing and location of the client's property, including all clothing. List all items sent to the vault. Provide a receipt to the client and place one in the client record

Report any other information or symptoms directly to the charge nurse or team leader. Tag and send any dangerous items, such as knives or other weapons, to the Security Department for safekeeping until the client is discharged. Illegal weapons, street drugs, or other contraband, such as drug paraphernalia, may be confiscated and destroyed. It may also be necessary to notify the police. Refer any questions to the team leader or charge nurse. (See also Table 34-1.)

---

they are unable to make or to communicate healthcare decisions. It is important to explain and document that the client has received information regarding advance directives when admitted to the facility. If the client has an advance directive or a living will, be sure this is entered in the appropriate location on the computer. Sometimes, a paper copy is kept in a separate place. In some facilities, a special ID band is also worn.

> **Nursing Alert** A copy of any advance directive must be in an accessible location. If the client has an electronic form of medical information, such as the E-HealthKey (see Chapter 43), the pertinent data must be transferred to the facility's records, either in hard copy or electronically.

TRANSFER TO ANOTHER UNIT

The client may be transferred to another unit within the facility for several reasons:

- Assignment to a certain unit is temporary.
- A change in client **acuity** (level of illness) requires a different level of care.
- The client is becoming agitated by a very busy unit and requires a quieter environment.

- The client is disturbing others, for example, by snoring loudly, and needs a private room.
- The client's condition becomes serious enough to require transfer to an intensive care unit (ICU).
- Another condition is discovered than that for which the client was first admitted and a specialty unit is required.
- The client has delivered a baby and is being moved into a postpartum area.
- The client has had surgery and is being moved to postsurgical care.
- The client is recovering, for example, from an MI, and is moved to a step-down unit.
- The client is being moved from "observation" status to inpatient, or vice versa.
- The client is exhibiting behavior that is dangerous to self or others and requires transfer to a psychiatric or other secure unit.
- The client has some form of dementia and is moved to a locked unit for safety.

In Practice: Nursing Care Guidelines 45-3 outlines steps to follow when transferring a client.

Key Concept

The procedures for transfer to another area of the facility are carried out in much the same manner as if a client is to be transferred to another healthcare facility.

DISCHARGE

Planning for the client's discharge (**D/C**) begins at admission. The nursing care plan is updated and resolved throughout the client's stay. At discharge, nursing problems are either resolved or progress toward resolution and follow-up plans are described. The client and family are taught about the illness or surgery; they must have an opportunity to practice procedures and dressing changes, care of tubes and drains, administering medications, and to learn about special diets. The client is informed about what danger signs to look for and whom to call if any questions or problems arise. Plans for home care or Public Health Nursing visits can be made. The staff and client work on these activities throughout the client's hospitalization, but at discharge, final plans are made. Discharge from a rehabilitation center or extended-care facility is similar, with the goal of returning the client to self-care as soon as possible. (Chapter 96 reviews client transfer from one level of extended care to another.)

Chapter 36 introduces discharge planning and client teaching. The total nursing care team, client, and family are involved in discharge planning and organizing care at home. A discharge summary is printed out and given to the client/family on discharge. This includes the following:

- Ordered medications
- Specific treatments and instructions for performing them
- Activity restrictions
- Special diet instructions
- Signs of complications and where to call for assistance
- Date, time, and location of follow-up appointments
- Arrangements for home care
- Means of transportation to home

The nurse discharging the client must provide verbal instructions and must go over the written instructions. Often, the client is asked to sign a copy of the discharge instructions and this is placed in the permanent record. The client also signs a copy of their property sheet, verifying that all personal property brought to the facility is back in their possession.

Nursing students and LVNs/LPNs give suggestions and assist with discharge teaching. In Practice: Educating the Client 45-1 describes discharge education. Facility protocols identify specific staff members' roles in this process. To confirm that the client and family members understand, it is important that they are able to verbalize information and to perform return demonstrations of procedures (Fig. 45-7). Carefully document all discharge teaching and client responses. For example, "Client was shown how to change colostomy bag and was able to return demonstration accurately. Plan to have client change bag independently tomorrow."

Before the day arrives for the client to go home, discuss the best time for them to leave. Ask when the family will be available to pick up the client. Instruct the family to bring clothing, pillows, or blankets if they will be needed.

Key Concept

Remember that discharge planning begins on admission to the healthcare facility. All members of the healthcare team are responsible for a safe and efficient discharge.

The Day the Client Is Discharged

On the day of discharge, if their condition permits, the client can dress in street clothes and rest on the bed or chair until it is time to go. Make sure all discharge procedures have been completed before the client leaves the facility. In Practice: Nursing Care Guidelines 45-4 provides discharge guidelines.

Documentation

In some healthcare facilities, only RNs perform discharge documentation. A student or LVN/LPN may be asked to

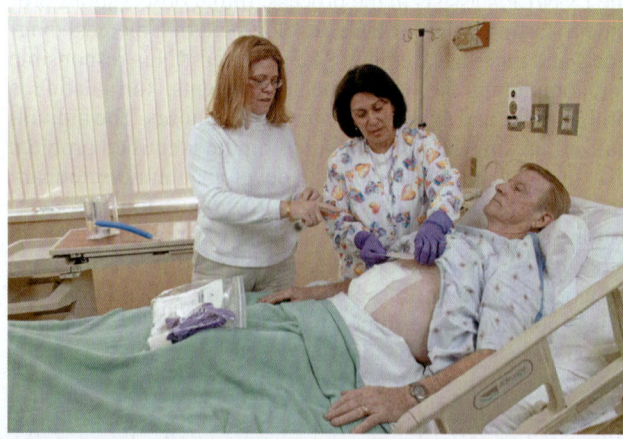

Figure 45-7 Discharge planning and teaching begin on admission. The client and caregiver are taught to care for the surgical wound, in preparation for discharge. A return demonstration allows the nurse to determine if teaching has been effective and to review points of concern. (Carter, 2016.)

IN PRACTICE
NURSING CARE GUIDELINES 45-3 — Transferring the Client to Another Unit

Preparation for the Transfer
- Explain reasons for the transfer and when it will occur to the client and family. *Rationale: Clients are less anxious if they are aware of what is happening.*
- Assemble all the client's personal belongings, as well as paper records, permits, and advance directives, Addressograph cards, name stickers, vault receipts, x-rays, and special reports. Be sure the client's information is transferred in the computer to the new location. Double-check for all clothes, flowers, and other articles. *Rationale: If items are left behind, the client's care may be compromised because the new unit does not have all pertinent information. In addition, it is more difficult to find items once they have been left behind. It causes more work and frustration for everyone.*
- Collect all the client's medications (including any brought from home), IV bags, and tube feedings, and take these to the new unit. Check the nursing flow sheet and medication administration record (MAR) for accuracy. *Rationale: All treatments performed and medications given must be documented, to prevent duplication or omission.*
- Determine how the client will be moved. *Rationale: You are responsible for safely moving the client. Type of transportation depends on the client's condition. Seldom is the client allowed to walk.*
- Provide for client safety. Take measures to accommodate IV bottles, drains, and catheters. Protect the client from drafts; cover the client with a blanket for warmth and privacy. *Rationale: It is important not to worsen the client's condition.*
- Review the client's health record and check for completeness.
- Write a transfer note stating the time, the unit to which the transfer occurs, type of transportation (wheelchair or stretcher), and the client's physical and psychosocial condition. A brief review of the client's history may also be required. For example, "1410: Client diagnosed with COPD transferred from Room 312B to Room 110A via **W/C** (wheelchair). Medication, chart, and belongings given to P. Johnson, RN. Client's VS (vital signs) stable, O_2 sat = 97% on room air, IV infusing in right hand via pump at 80 mL/hr. C. Bunker, PN student." *Rationale: It is important for the receiving unit to know as much about the client as possible. This will ensure continuity of care from staff on the new unit.*
- Make sure the receiving unit is ready. Usually a short verbal report is given to the receiving nurse. *Rationale: To provide immediate continuity of care on the new unit.*

Transporting the Client
- Keep the client safe during the move. *Rationale: Being moved is traumatic in itself. It is important not to further upset or endanger the client.*
- Introduce the client to the staff at the new nurses' station, if their condition permits. *Rationale: Make the client feel as much at home as possible.*
- Give a report to the staff on the new unit, if this was not done on the phone before the transfer.
- Leave medications and records with the receiving staff. Double-check to make sure the transfer records are completed. Notify all necessary departments of the transfer, if the facility is not computerized. *Rationale: To ensure that the client will continue to receive their treatments, tests, meals, medications, mail, visitors, and flowers. (The computer will automatically make the transfers.)*
- Take the client to their room and assist into bed, making sure the client is comfortable.
- In some cases, when a client is moved, they will require all new orders. *Rationale: Make sure no important procedures are missed because the client has been moved.*
- If the client is dangerous, under police custody, on a 72-hr hold, or an escape risk, request assistance from security personnel. *Rationale: This helps make sure the client arrives at the new unit safely.*
- Observe procedures for transporting a client who requires isolation or reverse isolation (see Chapter 42). This might include having the client wear a mask and/or gown. Be sure the receiving unit is aware of the isolation status in advance. *Rationale: This maintains client and public safety.*

---

assist. The observations of all staff members are important, whether they are written or input directly into the health record, or reported to another person. The nurse discharging the client completes all items in the health record, records the hour of discharge, and documents who accompanied the client and the means of transportation. The client's destination is noted, along with the address and phone number. A nursing summary, including identified nursing problems and their resolution or revision, may be required in the client record. For example, "42-year-old client admitted with diagnosis of coronary artery disease. Status/post (**S/P** [following]) placement of two stents. Client denies angina. BP 134/74; apical pulse 82, with normal rhythm; respirations even and unlabored; O_2 sat = 97%; skin color WNL (within normal limits). Client able to perform wound care independently; verbalize medications with doses, times, and side effects; and describe exercise and diet regimens. Client informed of time/date for postop examination. Postoperative course has been unremarkable. Client has phone numbers to call if problems" (nurse to sign and date).

IN PRACTICE
EDUCATING THE CLIENT 45-1 — Discharge Preparation

Remember that planning and teaching for discharge begins immediately upon the client's admission to the healthcare facility. Teaching while preparing the client for discharge includes the following:

- Explain the *safe change of dressings.* This includes how often dressings should be changed, the method for removal and safe disposal of used dressings, and safe application of new dressings. Allow the client and family to practice while you watch, to be sure they know how to do the procedure. Provide a list of needed supplies and, if these supplies are not immediately available, send some home with the client.
- Describe the amount of *rest* the client will need, permitted activities, and their duration. Describe and demonstrate suggested *exercises*, detail walking regimens, and have the client/family return demonstrations.
- Outline *dietary restrictions:* foods that should be eaten and their amounts; foods required daily; and foods that are not allowed on the prescribed diet. A dietitian should consult with the client and be available to answer questions. Explain carbohydrate counting if the client is diabetic.
- Show caregivers how to *provide personal care,* for example, how to make the bed, give a bed bath, move and turn the client, give and remove the bedpan, adjust pillows, and maintain body alignment and skin integrity for clients who will be confined to bed at home. Allow caregivers to practice and demonstrate back to you.
- Demonstrate the *operation of equipment* and care of tubes and ask caregivers to demonstrate back to you.
- Communicate to the family the *client's preferences* for how treatments are performed.
- Emphasize the importance of self-care and building the *client's independence and self-esteem.* Teach the family to encourage self-care by the client as much and as soon as possible.
- Provide information about *public health* and home nursing services, including phone numbers. If needed, help them to arrange services.
- Explain where to buy or rent *equipment,* including materials for dressing changes, oxygen supplies, special beds, walkers, or wheelchairs. Give this information to the client/family in writing.
- Advise the family if substitute pieces of *equipment* can be used (e.g., in some cases a regular bed placed on blocks can replace a special hospital bed. Make sure the client can safely get in and out of a higher bed.)
- Describe *medication administration,* such as how and when to take medications and undesirable side effects. Give the client/family written guidelines for medication administration and a list of possible side effects. Be sure the client and family understand the need for accuracy. A checklist, with administration times, is often included.
- Identify situations and possible adverse signs and symptoms that require the client to be seen by the *primary care provider.* Include situations that require immediate emergency attention. Write names and phone numbers of providers and instructions on obtaining emergency assistance.
- Write the phone number of the facility, so the client can call if there are any questions.
- Communicate the date, time, and location of the *next scheduled examination,* if known.
- Discuss with the physician the need for a public health nursing referral, if the team feels that the client and/or the family will not be able to manage the client's care safely at home.
- Make sure the client has all personal property. Retrieve items from the vault if the client or family will be unable to do so.
- Give the client/family a printed copy of all instructions and pertinent information, including appointment times, dates, and locations.
- Document all activities. Remember: if it is not documented, legally it was not done.

The primary healthcare provider is also required to write a discharge summary for the health record within 24 hr of discharge.

LEAVING THE HEALTHCARE FACILITY AGAINST MEDICAL ADVICE

The Client Who Signs Out AMA

Occasionally a client leaves the healthcare facility without permission. Such action is called against medical advice (AMA). Report to the team leader any client who says they are leaving the healthcare facility AMA. A client who leaves AMA is asked to sign a dated release form that absolves the providers and facility of all responsibility in the event of client complications. A licensed nurse witnesses the client's signature. The primary provider also writes a note documenting the AMA discharge. If the client refuses to sign, the refusal must be noted on the form and also signed by at least two licensed witnesses. The nursing student cannot legally witness any legal papers, including the AMA form.

The Client Who Leaves Without Permission

Sometimes, a client goes on a pass or walks off the unit and leaves the facility without being discharged. This client is

IN PRACTICE
NURSING CARE GUIDELINES 45-4 — Discharging the Client

- Verify the discharge order.
- Check for new orders.
- Check orders for take-home medications, special treatments, or special equipment.
- Check orders for last-minute procedures, laboratory tests, or x-ray examinations.
- Make sure the person has a place to go.
- Coordinate transportation if necessary. You may need to make a telephone call to request an ambulance or taxi service or to contact a neighbor. Social Services may assist.
- Determine what type of clothing the client should wear. (If they are being discharged to extended care, pajamas or a robe may be appropriate, rather than street clothes.)
- Assist the client with packing and dressing for discharge. Check the closet and bedside stand for personal items.
- Secure release of any valuables checked into the vault. Have the client sign the property sheet, verifying that they have all personal property.
- Arrange for a small utility cart for easy conveyance of belongings to the exit.
- Go over discharge orders and instructions, medication orders, and follow-up appointments with the client.
- If the client is leaving the facility with actual medications, go over them with the client to make sure the instructions are understood and the medications are correct. If generic names are on the bottles, make sure they are also on the discharge information.
- Have the client sign the discharge form and make sure they receive a copy.
- Notify necessary departments of the discharge. (This is often done electronically.)
- Escort the client from the clinical unit to the door. Use a wheelchair. Assist the client into the car or taxi. (Usually, clients are not allowed to walk on discharge.)
- Write or input a discharge note in the chart or the electronic record.

considered **AWOL** (absent without leave). In many facilities, this client would be officially discharged AMA at midnight. If the client who is AWOL returns after midnight, or the next day, they usually need to be readmitted, using the complete admission process, and may be denied admission. This is considered a new admission for the client. (In many cases, insurance will not cover the client who goes AWOL and then returns to the facility.)

Long-term facilities usually identify vulnerable clients who are likely to leave without permission. These clients wear a WanderGuard or other special transmitter (see Figs. 48-22B,C and 96-3). An alarm sounds if the client tries to leave without permission, so staff can intervene. This is important for safety, particularly if the client is confused or otherwise vulnerable. In addition, some areas are locked, to prevent vulnerable or dangerous clients from wandering away or going AWOL.

COMMUNICATIONS AMONG HEALTHCARE TEAM MEMBERS

In admission, transfer, and discharge, as in other areas, the nurse must know how to interact effectively with other members of the healthcare team. (See also Chapter 37.)

Primary Healthcare Providers' Orders

Orders from the primary healthcare provider are one form of communication among members of the healthcare team. The primary healthcare provider may be a physician, but may also be an osteopathic physician (DO), an advance practice nurse or nurse practitioner, or a physician's assistant. These orders are most often communicated via computer. The provider expects the nurse to interpret these orders correctly, to make accurate observations concerning the client, to document those observations, and to question any unclear orders. *The orders state what is to be done and nursing protocols specify methods to be used.* The provider may give verbal instructions to explain written ones. Some providers' orders are absolute; others may require nursing judgment. The nurse may need to decide when (or if) to give a PRN (as needed) medication, for example. Judgment is required to decide which nursing procedures may be safe to perform without an order and which procedures require clear and specific orders from the physician. For example, a nurse can place a client on fall precautions, but usually the provider must remove such an order. Protocol and agency procedures must be followed.

Verbal Orders

In rare situations, such as during a "code," it may be necessary for the provider to give verbal orders. These orders are legal but must be signed by the provider as soon as possible. If given in person, the verbal order is abbreviated **VORB**, which means "verbal order, read back." If given by telephone, a verbal order is called a telephone order and is abbreviated **TORB**, "telephone order, read back." (All orders are read or stated back to the provider, to make sure the nurse has heard and recorded the order accurately. This must then be documented as VORB or TORB, and the provider identified.) Verbal orders are very rare, because providers can enter orders into the electronic record from any computer. (Chapter 101 briefly presents the licensed nurse's role in taking verbal orders.)

> **Nursing Alert** The nursing student, nursing assistant, or unit secretary should never take verbal orders, whether in person or by telephone. Only a licensed nurse (usually an RN) has legal authority to take verbal orders.

Telephone Communication

Whenever a nurse telephones someone, the nurse should give their name and the name of the person being called. If the nurse calls a primary care provider, it may be necessary to explain to the office nurse what the call is about and whether or not it is an emergency. (Office nurses usually triage calls, for efficiency.) The **SBAR** (situation, background, assessment, recommendations—see Box 96-2) method of communication is used to organize information when calling a primary provider.

The nurse should not chew gum or eat while on duty or when conducting business by telephone. Do not cover the receiver and continue a conversation with someone else. If a caller must be put on hold, be sure to follow telephone etiquette as outlined below.

Answering the Telephone

Wherever you work as a nurse, one of the duties will be to answer the telephone. When doing so, give the name of the department, along with your name and position, so callers know to whom they are speaking. For example, you might answer the telephone as follows: "Station Main 2 West, (state your name), nursing student, speaking." The caller then knows if you can help or if someone else is needed.

The following are keys to proper telephone usage:

- Answer promptly—it may be an emergency.
- Ask "How may I help you?"
- Know how to use the telephone system, including transferring calls and placing the caller on hold.
- Ask callers if it is OK to put them on hold or if they would like to call back or leave a message.
- If someone is on hold, go back every minute to see if they still want to hold, if they want to leave a message, or if someone else can help.
- Do not give out any client information without a signed release and without knowing to whom you are speaking.
- Do not make personal calls or send personal emails from the nursing unit.

Taking Messages

Write down messages carefully. Do not try to remember them. Repeating the message to the caller helps clarify the message. Write the date, time, and your name on all messages you take. Deliver messages promptly.

Making Emergency Calls

Sometimes a nurse must make an emergency call (see Chapter 39). If so, give all necessary information. Remain calm. The prime responsibility of the caller in an emergency is to get assistance, but the call will not be effective unless all necessary information is conveyed.

> **Nursing Alert** Be sure you know emergency numbers and code names used in your facility. For example, "Mr. Red" is a common code name for fire; "code blue" or "Dr. Blue" is a common code name for cardiac arrest; and "Pink Alert" is often used for an infant abduction. When calling, give the exact location and nature of the emergency and your name.

Computer Use in the Healthcare Facility

In most facilities, all staff members document care in the electronic record. Thus, client information can be quickly and easily accessed by all authorized personnel. This includes admission information, medical history, progress notes, test results, physical examinations, care plans, medications ordered and given, and discharge planning. Information from clinic visits and previous hospitalizations is often available as well. It is vital for you to learn competent and safe operation of your facility's computer system.

Confidentiality about clients is vital. Make sure no unauthorized person can access client information. Remember that the chart (whether computerized or on paper) is a legal document. All information in the client record may be called into court, and nurses may be asked to testify. Think about this whenever you make an entry into the client's record. If you appropriately access information about another staff member, this is called "breaking the glass" and will be thoroughly scrutinized by administration.

> **Nursing Alert** Remember to guard client privacy. Always log off when completing documentation and keep the screen protected, so unauthorized people (including other clients) cannot read confidential information. Remember: a nurse may be discharged for inappropriately accessing a client's record.

STUDENT SYNTHESIS

KEY POINTS

- The admission process helps establish client feelings and potentially influences the effectiveness of admission and care in the facility.
- Measures are taken to preserve the client's privacy and maintain confidentiality.
- Clients may have serious concerns about their physical condition and about unfamiliar procedures in the healthcare facility.
- All clients must be carefully identified and must wear an ID band. In addition, special ID bands are worn for allergies, fall risk, and sometimes for other situations.

- Baseline vital signs, pulse oximetry, pain level, height, and weight are important components of the admission information.
- Nurses perform initial data gathering.
- No matter what type of healthcare facility or program will be serving the client, an admission procedure is required.
- Clients' belongings must be properly identified and listed; valuables are sent home or to the facility's vault.
- Careful documentation of admission is important, to establish a baseline and give information to other members of the healthcare team.
- Any existing wounds or pressure areas on admission must be carefully documented.
- When a client is transferred, the procedure must be explained to the client; belongings, records, gifts, and medications must be transferred with the client.
- Safety in transporting the client is essential.
- Continuity of care is enhanced when thorough and accurate reporting occurs between nursing shifts.
- Discharge teaching begins on admission. All teaching is individualized and must be documented.
- All client belongings and valuables must accompany the client at discharge.
- The client is escorted, usually in a wheelchair for safety, to the door.
- Some clients sign out of the healthcare facility against medical advice (AMA) or leave without permission (AWOL). This must be carefully documented.
- It is important to make a positive impression when answering the telephone.

CRITICAL THINKING EXERCISES

1. A 91-year-old client is admitted to the healthcare facility for stomach surgery. They are oriented to time, place, and person. Their verbalizations are logical. Describe what actions or skills you will use when they arrive on the unit, including assessments and reports.
2. Explain the causes, effects, and methods by which you can obtain necessary information while preventing feelings of dehumanization in your clients. Practice with your classmates.
3. Describe possible effects of illness and surgery on body image. How would you feel if you were suddenly faced with a body-altering disease, condition, or illness? Try to evaluate the reasons for your feelings.
4. Using information from Chapter 36 and this chapter, describe planning, teaching, and actual discharge procedures and the documentation that must be done when the client leaves the healthcare facility.

NCLEX-STYLE REVIEW QUESTIONS

1. A client is being prepared for surgery and states, "I am so scared and nervous." Which action by the nurse will help alleviate the anxiety felt by the client?
   a. Allow the client to express feelings.
   b. Inform the client there is no time to have second thoughts.
   c. Tell the client that there is nothing to worry about.
   d. Inform the client that if unable to calm down, the surgery will be canceled.

2. When asking a client sensitive personal questions related to admission, which action would the nurse take to avoid dehumanizing the client?
   a. Do not maintain eye contact with the client when asking the questions.
   b. Rapidly go through the questions so that the client doesn't have time to become embarrassed.
   c. Tell the client not to answer anything the client does not want to answer.
   d. Develop rapport and trust with the client prior to beginning the interview.

3. The nurse is updating the "communication board" in the client's room. Which information would the nurse include? Select all that apply.
   a. The date
   b. The nurse's name
   c. The diagnosis
   d. The provider's name
   e. Results of current laboratory studies

4. A client is scheduled for an invasive diagnostic procedure. The nurse observes that the client is unable to sit still, is sweating, has an elevated blood pressure and heart rate, and has trouble breathing. What anxiety level does the nurse notify the healthcare provider that the client is experiencing?
   a. +1
   b. +2
   c. +3
   d. Panic

5. The nurse is preparing to bathe a client. The client states, "I feel embarrassed that I can't do this myself." Which action by the nurse can assist with maintaining the client's dignity?
   a. Avoid bathing the client until a family member comes in to do it.
   b. Provide as much privacy as possible during the bath.
   c. Administer sedation prior to giving the client a bath.
   d. Inform the charge nurse the client refuses the bath.

CHAPTER RESOURCES

Enhance your learning with additional resources on thePoint!

Student Resources related to this chapter can be found at **thePoint.lww.com/Rosdahl12e**.

Welcome Steps

Look at healthcare provider's orders.

Protocol for procedure.

Necessary equipment/supplies.

Wash hands using proper hand hygiene; put on gloves.

Explain the procedure and reassure the client.

Locate two identifiers to confirm correct client.

Comfortable and efficient position for nurse and client.

Obtain privacy.

Make sure to follow correct steps and body mechanics with good technique.

Ensure safety and observe deviations from normal.

End Steps

Ensure comfort and safety.

Note questions or concerns from client or nurse; note significant data.

Dispose of materials properly.

Disinfect the area and your hands.

Document and report the procedure and your findings.

IN PRACTICE
NURSING PROCEDURE 45-1 — UNDRESSING THE IMMOBILE CLIENT

Supplies and Equipment
Healthcare facility gown
Slippers
Bath blanket

Steps
Follow LPN WELCOME Steps and Then

1. Push the client's blouse or shirt off one shoulder. *Rationale: This focuses on one side at a time.*
2. Roll the sleeve on the same side down to the wrist. *Rationale: This facilitates ease in removing the shirt.*
3. Slip off the sleeve. *Rationale: This removes the sleeve from one side.*
4. Repeat steps 1–3 on the other side. *Rationale: This avoids overtaxing the client.*
5. Put a gown on the client before removing the shirt. *Rationale: This avoids overexposing the client.*
6. Unfasten the waistband, and push all lower garments down as far as you can. *Rationale: This facilitates removal of lower garments.*
7. Ask the client to raise the hips while you pull down the clothes. *Rationale: This promotes client participation and eases clothing removal.*
8. If the client cannot raise their hips, request assistance from other healthcare personnel. *Rationale: This prevents overexertion and injury to client or nurse.*
9. If garments must come off over the head, slip the client's arms from the sleeves, push the clothing up to the hips, and ask the client to raise the hips. Pull the garments up to the shoulders. To get clothing over the shoulders more easily, turn the client's shoulders first to one side and then to the other. Remove the client's glasses and hearing aid, if necessary, while removing clothing over the head. *Rationale: This minimizes risk of exposure and prevents injury to the client or equipment, while quickly accomplishing the task.*
10. Slip garments over the face by raising the client's head and gathering the clothes together into a roll behind the head. Do not cover the client's face, and avoid dragging clothing over the face. *Rationale: This reduces the risk of frightening the client and prevents possible injury to the face.*
11. When putting the gown on the client, cover them with a bath blanket and work under it as much as possible. *Rationale: This avoids undue exposure or embarrassment and provides warmth.*

Follow ENDDD Steps

46 Vital Signs

Learning Objectives

1. Identify measurements that constitute vital signs. State why they are called vital signs. Describe the relationships among them.
2. Give examples of causes of body temperature variations. Describe related physiology.
3. State normal adult body temperature, as measured in four different body areas.
4. Differentiate among the terms *febrile, afebrile, intermittent and remittent fevers, crisis,* and *lysis*.
5. In the laboratory, demonstrate the ability to measure body temperature by various methods and with different types of equipment.
6. Describe measurement of radial, apical, and apical–radial pulse. In the laboratory, demonstrate the ability to measure each. Identify other pulse points on the body.
7. In the laboratory, demonstrate the ability to count and describe respirations.
8. In the laboratory, demonstrate the ability to accurately measure resting and orthostatic blood pressure, using the arm cuff and thigh cuff; demonstrate the use of the aneroid manometer and the electronic vital signs monitor.
9. State the normal adult ranges for pulse rate, respiration rate, and blood pressure.
10. Define pulse oximetry and demonstrate the ability to perform this procedure.

Important Terminology

apical pulse	diastole	lysis
apical–radial pulse	dyspnea	oral
apnea	eupnea	orthopnea
auscultation	Fahrenheit	oximeter
axillary	febrile	palpation
bradycardia	fever	pedal pulse
bradypnea	hypertension	popliteal pulse
Celsius	hypotension	pulse
Cheyne–Stokes respirations	Korotkoff sounds	pulse pressure
crisis	Kussmaul respirations	pyrexia
cyanosis		radial pulse

rectal		
sphygmomanometer		
stertorous breathing		
stethoscope		
systole		
tachycardia		
tachypnea		
temporal		
tympanic		

Acronyms

AP	O, PO
A-R	PMI
Ax	R
BP	SBP
BPM	TA
C	TM
DBP	TPR
F	VS
HR	
HTN	
MAP	

Body temperature, pulse, respiration (**TPR**), and blood pressure (**BP**) are basic client assessments. Taken and documented over time, these data demonstrate the course of a client's condition. TPR and BP are called *vital signs* (**VS**) or *cardinal symptoms* because these measurements are indicators of life-sustaining functions. They must all be within normal limits (WNL) to sustain life. In the 1990s, pain assessments were evaluated. At this time, the Joint Commission determined that pain was the fifth vital sign and noted that it should be assessed each time other vital signs were measured. However, rapid increases in pain medication usage in the early 2000s and the opioid prescription crisis began to have significant effects in healthcare by the mid 2010s. Further studies into pain management were conducted, and by 2016, the Joint Commission's statement designating pain as a vital sign were reversed. Chapter 55 describes assessment and management of pain in greater detail.

Temperature, pulse, respiration, and blood pressure are usually observed together. Many healthcare facilities require routine observation of TPR and BP at least every morning and afternoon or evening for all clients. For some illnesses, much more frequent observation of vital signs is necessary, to indicate a change in the client's condition. Often, variations occur in more than one vital sign. The healthcare provider determines frequency of VS assessments in the client with an unstable condition. The nurse also uses judgment, to determine if a client requires more frequent measurement of vital signs.

THE GRAPHIC RECORD

The *graphic record* is usually in the computer and easily documents the client's vital signs. It is possible to format this information into a chart or graph, visually showing changes and relationships from day to day. In addition to VS, oral food and fluid intake and output (I&O), parenteral (e.g., intravenous) fluid intake, weight, bowel movements, dressing changes, lesion descriptions, and other information may be added to the graphic record. Follow the format of your facility. In rare cases, a paper record is used. When complete, whether on paper or an electronic record, this information presents a picture of variations that occur throughout the client's illness.

Recording Vital Signs

Vital signs must be recorded accurately and promptly to assist the primary provider and nurses in planning and providing timely client care. Caregivers can easily access the information and quickly respond to the client's condition. Nurses must know the format for documenting vital signs in their facility. If a paper record is used, the facility will provide in-service education in its use. Briefly, the temperature is recorded with a dot parallel to the temperature value under the designated time and connected with the previous reading with a short line. The pulse rate is indicated in a similar manner. The respiratory rate, blood pressure, weight, and I&O are recorded, using numbers.

> **NCLEX Alert**
>
> You must be alert throughout the examination to integrate your knowledge of client safety, including the use of equipment and timeliness of procedures. Documentation must be timely, accurate, and appropriate. The NCLEX may suggest ways of recording your findings.

Frequent Vital Signs

Sometimes a client's condition is serious enough to require taking vital signs every 5, 10, or 15 min. The *frequent vital signs sheet* may be a paper document (most often in critical care areas, after surgery, or in the immediate postpartum period). Graph vital signs in the same way on the frequent vital signs sheet as you would on the regular record. In many cases, space is available to record other information, such as intravenous (IV) fluids, I&O, weight, medications, and notes. Frequent vital signs are entered on the computer in a similar manner. Alternatively, the client may be connected to a monitor which gathers and records vital signs, including oxygen saturation levels as often as the healthcare provider ordered.

ASSESSING BODY TEMPERATURE

Body temperature, the measure of heat inside a person's body (core temperature), is the balance between heat produced and heat lost (see Table 16-2). The body generates heat as it burns food and loses heat through the skin and lungs. Body temperature measured orally (in the mouth) (O; or per os, PO) normally remains at approximately 37 °C or 98.6 °F. However, variations may occur and still be considered "normal" for an individual. Temperature measurements significantly higher or lower indicate a dysfunction in the body's regulatory system. Signs of an elevated temperature include a flushed face, hot skin, unusually bright eyes, restlessness, chills, and thirst. A listless manner and pale, cold, clammy skin are often signs of subnormal temperature.

Temperature is measured on the **Celsius** (centigrade—**C**) or the **Fahrenheit** (**F**) scale. Most Americans are more familiar with Fahrenheit values. If a nurse works in an agency using Celsius measurements, it is important to learn

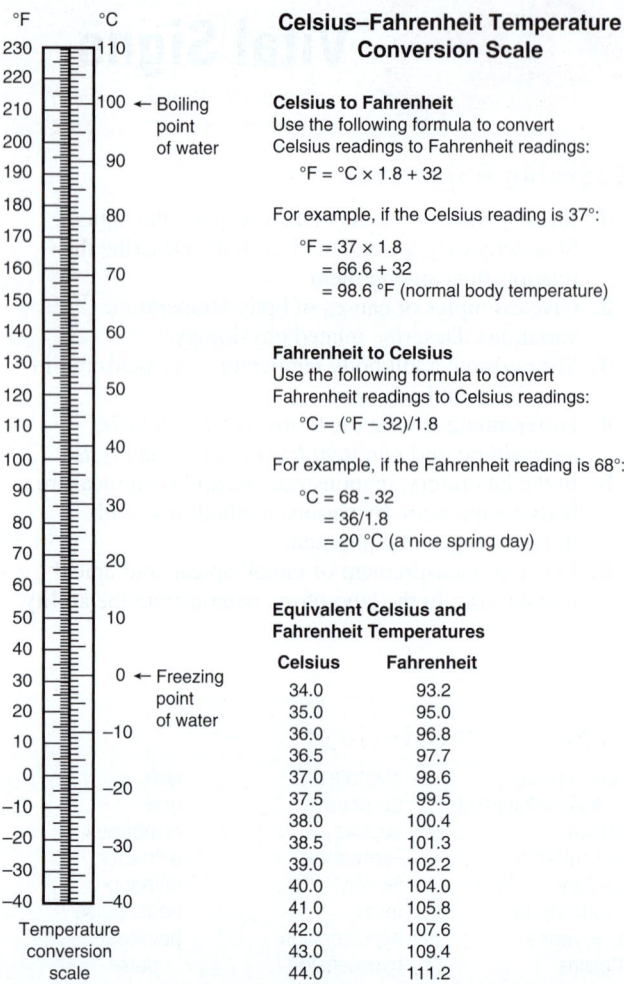

Figure 46-1 Celsius and Fahrenheit conversions and equivalents. (Molle & Kronenberger, 2005.)

Fahrenheit equivalents in order to translate measurements easily for clients and their family. Converting measurements from Celsius to Fahrenheit and vice versa is often necessary. Figure 46-1 explains conversions and gives equivalents.

Regulation of Body Temperature

The hypothalamus, the brain's heat-regulating center, controls body temperature by controlling blood temperature. Heat is a product of metabolism; activities of muscles and glands generate most of the body's heat. When the body is cold, exercising the muscles warms it; if a person is angry or excited, the adrenal glands become very active and they feel warm. Digestion increases body temperature, while cold, shock, and certain drugs depress the nervous system and decrease heat production. The hypothalamus senses these changes and makes appropriate adjustments.

Normal Body Temperature

Normal temperature variations in humans are quite small. A difference of a degree or more (Fahrenheit) is considered to be WNL, if the client is not showing symptoms of fever or hypothermia. The significant factor is the "normal" temperature for that individual. Most clients know when they have a fever or do not feel well. The key is to follow the temperature

TABLE 46-1	Range of Normal Temperatures	
ROUTE	TEMPERATURE RANGES	TIME
Oral (mouth)	35.5 °C–37.5 °C (95.9 °F–99.5 °F)	0.5–1.5 min
Rectal (anus)	36.6 °C–38 °C (97.9 °F–100.4 °F)	0.5–1.5 min
Axillary (armpit)	34.7 °C–37.3 °C (94.5 °F–99.1 °F)	1–3 min
Tympanic (auditory canal)[a]	35.8 °C–38 °C (96.4 °F–100.4 °F)	1–2 s
Temporal artery[a]	35.8 °C–38 °C (96.4 °F–100.4 °F)	1–2 s

[a]Temporal artery and tympanic: usually documented without conversion; possible to convert to rectal equivalent.

variations for *that person* and make sure these values do not significantly deviate from that person's *baseline*. Normal body temperature is often lowest in the morning and highest in late afternoon and evening. (Normal temperatures for newborns are higher than for adults. The body temperature gradually lowers to adult normal temperature as the child matures.) Other influences on normal body temperature include ovulation, childbirth, and individual metabolism. Table 46-1 gives average normal temperatures for adults (known as *afebrile*, or without fever). The length of time to keep the temperature sensor in place for an accurate reading in different body areas is also listed. (Times for electronic thermometers are shorter.)

> **Key Concept**
> In general, rectal temperatures are discouraged in infants, if the temperature must be taken frequently, due to the possibility of injury. Axillary temperatures are used instead.

Elevated Body Temperature
Temperature rises when the body's heat production increases or heat loss decreases; both may occur simultaneously. If the temperature is elevated, **fever** (**pyrexia**) is present, indicating a disorder within the body. The person is said to be **febrile**. Fever usually signifies that the body is fighting an infection. In some cases, a slightly above-normal temperature is useful for fighting microorganisms. For this reason, treating a fever may be delayed until a diagnosis is confirmed.

Oral temperatures in fever can range from 37.5 °C to 39.4 °C (100 °F to 103 °F) or greater. A very high temperature can be life-threatening. Figure 46-2 illustrates types of fevers related to their course.

- A temperature that alternates between a fever and a return to normal or subnormal reading each day is an *intermittent fever*.
- A temperature that rises several degrees above normal but does not return to normal or near normal is a *remittent fever*.
- A *constant/sustained/continuous fever* stays elevated.
- A sudden drop from fever to normal temperature (usually related to treatment) is called **crisis**.
- When an elevated temperature gradually returns to normal, it is called **lysis**.

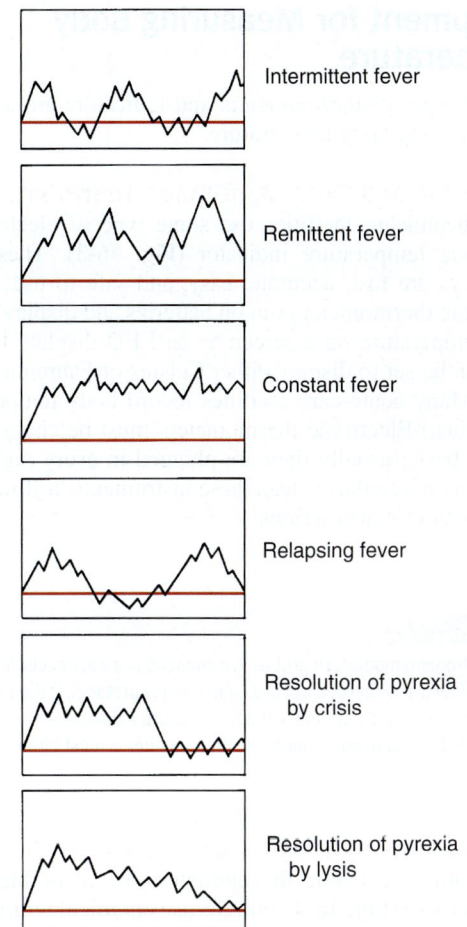

Figure 46-2 Common courses of fever and its resolution. The colored line represents average "normal" temperature (37 °C or 98.6 °F).

- A fever that is recurring and separated by periods with no fever is defined as a *relapsing fever*.

> **Key Concept**
> Remember, everyone has a "temperature," but not everyone has a "fever" (elevated temperature).

Lowered Body Temperature
A temperature significantly below normal is called *hypothermia*. A low body temperature may precede death or result from overexposure to the elements or cold water, as in near drowning. In some instances, body temperature slightly below normal is desirable: lowered body temperature slows metabolism and, thus, decreases the body's need for oxygen. *Clinical hypothermia* is induced to perform some surgical procedures; *accidental hypothermia* is life-threatening and requires immediate treatment. Hypothermia can also indicate impending death, a normal element in the dying process.

> **Nursing Alert** An extremely high temperature (*hyperthermia*) or low temperature (*hypothermia*) can be fatal. Survival is rare if the core temperature is above 108 °F (42.2 °C) or below 93.2 °F (34 °C).

Equipment for Measuring Body Temperature

Several types of thermometers and indicators are available for measuring body temperature.

Electronic and Other Automatic Thermometers

Many healthcare facilities use some type of electronic or automatic temperature indicator (Fig. 46-3). These thermometers are fast, accurate, easy, and safe to use. Digital electronic thermometers run on batteries and display the client's temperature on a screen as an LED display. Usually, they can be set to display either Celsius or Fahrenheit readings. (Many acute-care facilities record body temperatures in Celsius.) Electronic thermometers must be charged on a regular basis; usually they are plugged in every night. It is important to regularly clean these instruments, following the manufacturer's instructions.

> **Key Concept**
>
> All electronic temperature probes are encased in a new cover for each client. They are discarded according to agency protocol. If the client is in isolation or deemed infectious, the temperature indicator is not shared; in this case, the disposable single-use thermometer is most often used.

Disposable Single-Use Thermometer

Disposable electronic thermometers are available, often for home use (Fig. 46-4). Single-use chemical temperature indicators are available for one-time use. These indicators are often used in isolation units and are also inexpensive and convenient for home use. They are also convenient when traveling. To use, remove the wrapper and place the indicator under the client's tongue. Some types of indicators are designed to be held against the client's forehead (Fig. 46-5A,B). Follow the manufacturer's instructions.

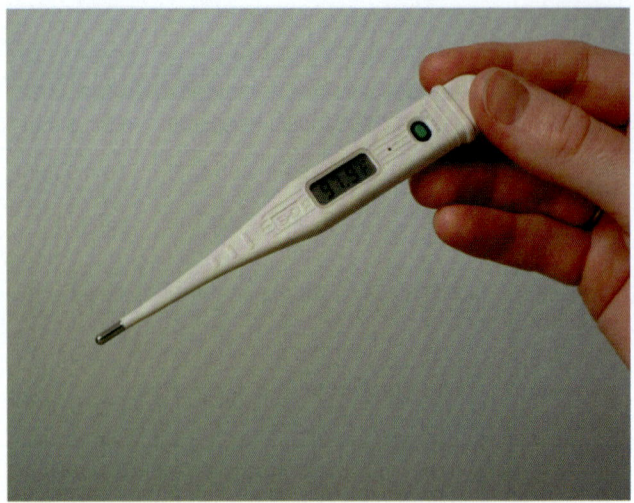

Figure 46-4 This battery-operated digital temperature sensor is discarded when no longer needed or when the battery is depleted. The temperature shown here (97.9 °F) is displayed digitally on the screen. (Timby, 2013.)

Measuring Body Temperature

Several locations are used to measure body temperature. They are as follows:

- **Oral (O, PO)**—mouth
- **Rectal (R)**—anus
- **Axillary (Ax)**—armpit
- **Tympanic**, aural, or otic (**TM**, tympanic membrane)—ear canal
- **Temporal** artery (**TA**)—forehead

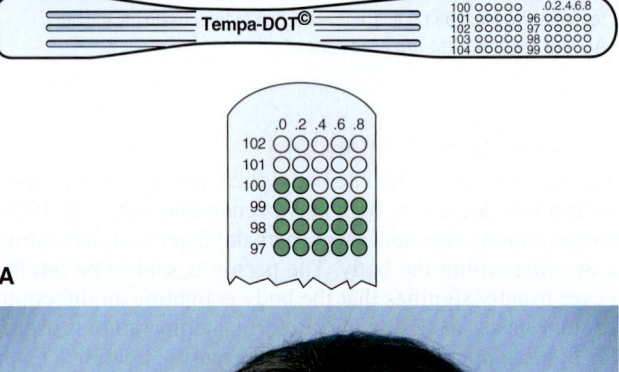

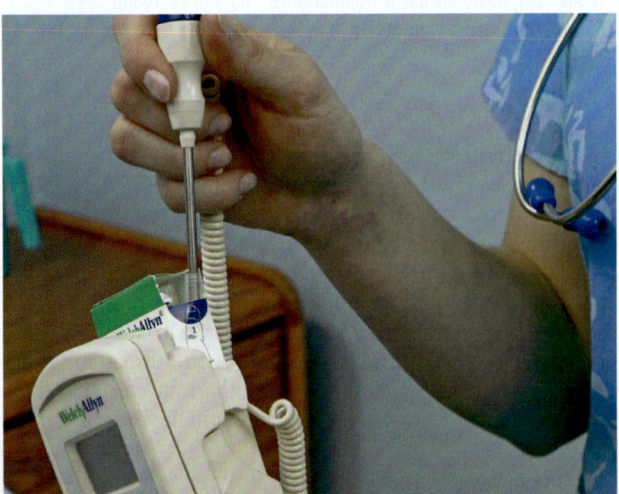

Figure 46-3 One type of electronic thermometer. A new probe cover must be used for each temperature measurement and discarded, according to facility protocol. (Timby, 2013; Photo copyright Rick Brady.)

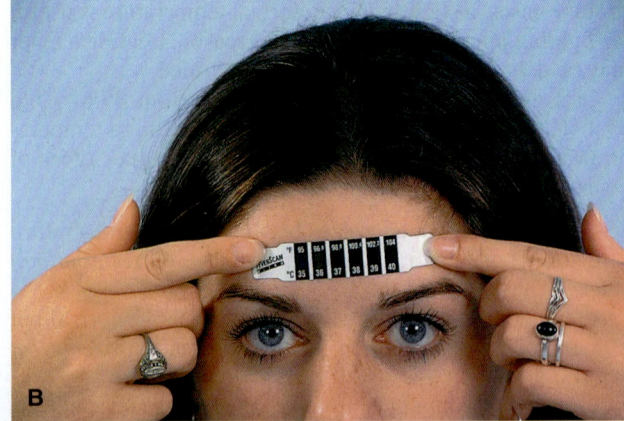

Figure 46-5 **A.** Chemical thermometer, showing a temperature reading of 100.2 °F. **B.** Applying a disposable chemical thermometer containing heat-sensitive liquid crystals. (A: Timby, 2005. B: Timby, 2013; Photo by B. Proud.)

For all these locations (except the temporal artery), the thermometer probe is covered with a paper or plastic cover, which is discarded after each use, or in the case of single-use thermometers, the entire device is discarded. The tip of the probe is surrounded by body tissues in these cases. The temporal artery temperature indicator is simply held over the forehead and discarded after use. Thermometer probes should be cleaned after use, according to the manufacturer's instructions. All these devices measure temperature quickly and indicate the reading in digital numbers. In Practice: Nursing Procedure 46-1 presents the methods for taking oral, rectal, axillary, tympanic, and temporal artery temperatures. Certain rules apply to using all types of thermometers and body areas:

- Every healthcare agency has an established protocol for measuring the client's temperature. Follow guidelines accordingly.
- Wash or sanitize your hands between clients.
- Place the bulb or probe so that body tissues completely surround it, except for temporal artery.
- When using the tympanic probe, surround it with the skin of the outer ear, rather than the mucous membrane, to minimize the risk of spreading infection.
- Cover temperature probes and multiuse thermometers during use. Slip the cover tightly over the thermometer, take the temperature, and then remove and discard the cover according to facility protocol.
- Prelubricated covers are available for rectal thermometers.
- Record the temperature on the client's graphic record. The electronic thermometer provides a digital readout to one-tenth of a degree. Some special electronic thermometers read the temperature to a more exact measurement.

Oral Temperature

The oral temperature measurement method is fairly easy and comfortable for the client and is frequently used. It measures the temperature within the *lingual* arteries under the tongue (*sublingual*) (Fig. 46-6). It is more accurate than axillary and less accurate than rectal measurement. If a client has had a hot or cold drink or has been smoking, wait 15 min before taking an oral temperature. Use of gum and smokeless tobacco can also affect oral temperature. Do not use the oral method for clients who are unconscious, confused, uncooperative, actively suicidal, or otherwise not responsible, or for clients with an active seizure disorder. This method is also not used with infants or young children. *Rationale: Any of these clients may accidently bite the thermometer.* The oral method is usually contraindicated in clients who have had oral surgery or injury to the nose or mouth; those with conditions in which they must breathe through the mouth; or those who are receiving oxygen. *Rationale: The person must be able to keep the sublingual space sealed while the temperature is measured.* Use another method to measure the temperature in these clients.

> **NCLEX Alert**
>
> During the examination, you need to be aware of different ways to obtain VS, as well as the differences in normal/abnormal values and ranges. These will vary for infants, children, adults, and the elderly as well as for different diseases or chronic conditions and injuries.

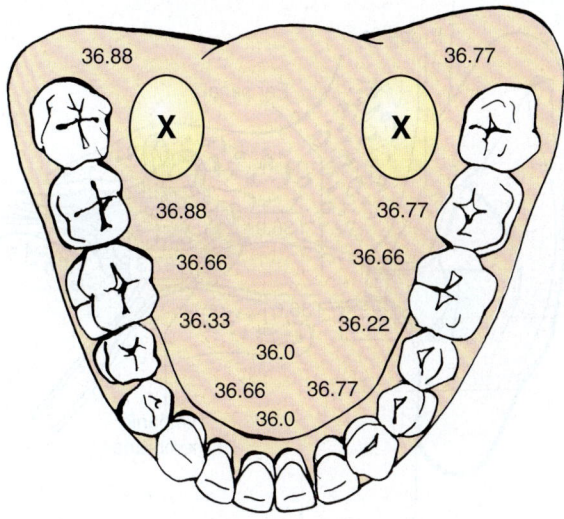

Figure 46-6 Oral temperature measurements vary with the placement of the probe. Placement in the rear sublingual pocket (shown by the "X") provides the most accurate measurement. (Measurements shown here are in Celsius.) (Timby, 2013.)

Rectal Temperature

The rectal temperature is highly accurate because the probe is placed in an enclosed cavity. If any question arises about the accuracy of an oral temperature, it can be checked against a rectal temperature. In some healthcare agencies, the policy is to recheck temperature by the rectal or temporal artery method when the oral reading is above a certain level. A rectal temperature may be used for the client who is unconscious or after mouth surgery. However, tympanic or temporal artery measurements are used more often. The rectal temperature is contraindicated after rectal surgery (and often after vaginal surgery) and in conditions such as diarrhea, colitis, or cancer of the rectum.

Axillary Temperature

The axillary (Ax) temperature is the least accurate measurement because the skin surfaces in the axillary space may not come together to form a tightly closed cavity around the probe tip. Hold the device tightly in place in the client's armpit when using this method. The axillary method is used frequently for taking the temperature of newborns (see Chapter 67). For other clients, axillary temperatures are used only when conditions negate the use of any other method.

Tympanic Temperature

The tympanic thermometer is placed snugly into the client's outer ear canal. It measures the thermal radiation given off by the tympanic membrane (TM; eardrum) and the ear canal. Because the temperature of the TM's blood supply is similar to that of the blood surrounding the thalamus (the body's thermoregulation center), this is an ideal site for measuring the body's core temperature (Fig. 46-7). The tympanic thermometer records temperature in 1–2 s. Many pediatric and intensive care units use this type of thermometer, because it records temperature so rapidly. Charge and care for this equipment as you would other electronic thermometers.

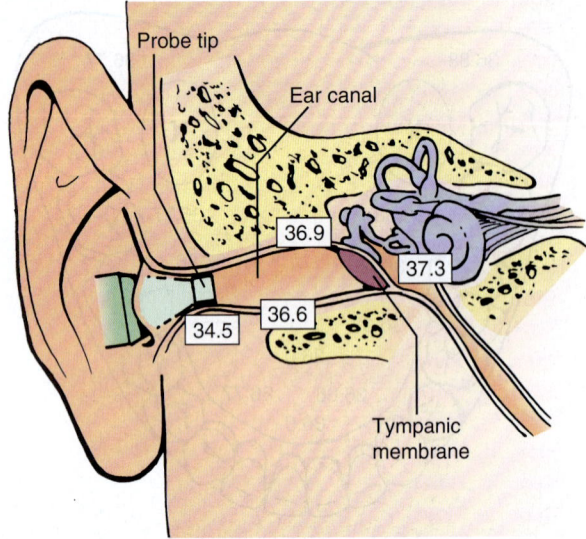

Figure 46-7 Obtain the most accurate tympanic temperature by aiming the probe toward the anterior inferior third of the ear canal (toward the jaw line). (Readings here are shown in Celsius.) (Timby, 2013.)

> **Key Concept**
>
> Crying, ear infections, and earwax do not affect tympanic temperature readings. Technique must be correct to obtain accurate results, particularly with the tympanic thermometer.

Temporal Artery Temperature

The temporal artery (TA) scanner calculates core body temperature or *peak body temperature.* The TA scanner is moved across the forehead, measuring the temperature of the blood in the temporal artery, via infrared technology (Fig. 46-8). This method is the quickest (almost instant) and most noninvasive method, because the device is not inserted into the body. The

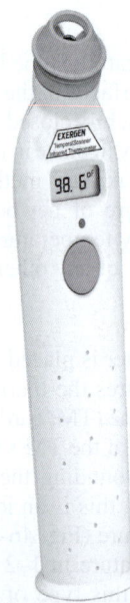

Figure 46-8 The temporal artery temperature sensor uses a special scanner to determine body temperature, using the temporal artery in the forehead. (Carter, 2005.)

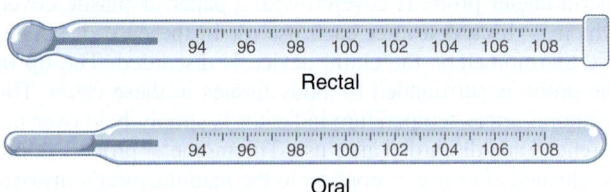

Figure 46-9 The glass thermometer may use alcohol to gauge temperature. Shown here are rectal and oral versions of the glass thermometer, calibrated in Fahrenheit measurements. (Adapted from Molle & Kronenberger, 2005.)

TA method can be used in many situations, such as with a sleeping child, an unconscious person, or a person with a hearing aid or an ear infection. It is helpful when working with clients with special needs or those who are assaultive or tactile defensive (unwilling to be touched). The TA method is being increasingly used in acute-care facilities and is said to be more accurate than the tympanic and at least as accurate as the rectal method. It is better tolerated than other methods. A probe cover is not necessary, although the device should be cleaned after each use.

Use of the Glass Thermometer

You may find a glass mercury-containing thermometer in a client's home. However, as of January 1, 2006, it has been illegal in the United States to sell or distribute thermometers, sphygmomanometers (for measuring blood pressure), or other items containing mercury. Considering this ban, the nurse should take the opportunity for client education and encourage individuals to dispose properly of any mercury-containing items in their homes.

> **Key Concept**
>
> Some pharmacies allow clients to trade mercury-containing thermometers for safer types. If this service is not available, each mercury-containing item should be sealed in a separate airtight plastic bag, securely wrapped in bubble wrap, and taken to a hazardous waste collection facility. (Call 1-800-RECYCLE to locate the nearest facility.)

You may also encounter another type of glass thermometer in a healthcare facility, perhaps an extended-care facility. These thermometers contain alcohol, rather than mercury. They are marked with a scale showing whole numbers from 93 °F or 94 °F to approximately 106 °F (or Celsius equivalents), scaled in increments of two-tenths (Fig. 46-9). These thermometers may be for oral use (with a slender-tipped end) or rectal use (with a bulb-shaped end). The glass thermometer is difficult to read. The fluid must be briskly shaken down after each reading. Glass thermometers must be rinsed in cool water; hot water will break them. If you encounter a glass thermometer, follow the protocol of your agency for use and disinfection. The use of glass thermometers is briefly discussed in In Practice: Nursing Procedure 46-1.

DETERMINING PULSE

Every heartbeat produces a wave of blood that causes pulsations through the arteries. This wave or vibration is called

CHAPTER 46 Vital Signs 587

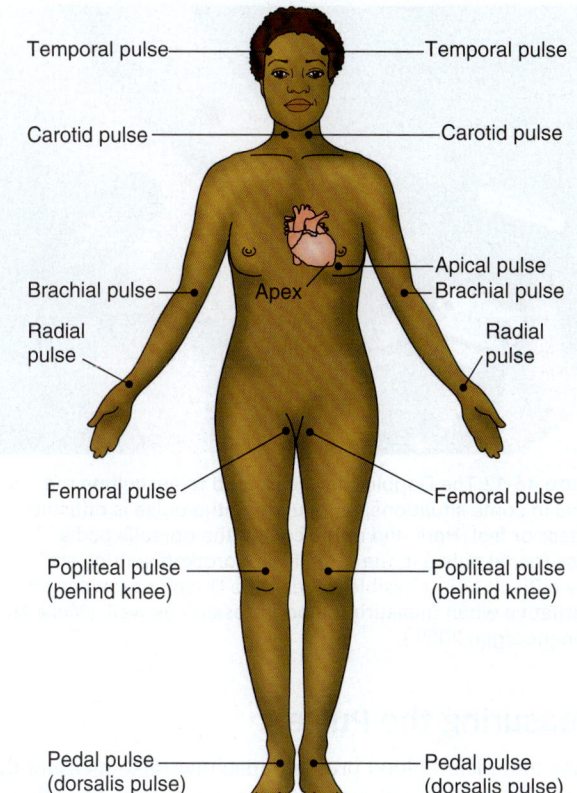

Figure 46-10 When counting a person's pulse, it is common to place your fingers on the radial artery (in the wrist). An apical pulse can be counted by placing a stethoscope on the person's chest, over the apex of the heart. Other pulse points are also shown here. (Carter, 2005.)

the **pulse**. The pulse can be felt through the nerves in the fingertips if the fingers are placed over one of the large arteries lying close to the skin, especially if the artery runs across a bone and has very little soft tissue around it. The pulse can be felt most distinctly over the:

- Temporal artery just in front of the ear (*temporal pulse*)
- Mandibular artery on the lower jawbone (*mandibular pulse*)
- Carotid artery on either side of the neck in front (*carotid pulse*)
- Femoral artery in the groin (*femoral pulse*)
- Radial artery in the wrist at the base of the thumb (**radial pulse**)

If a specific pulse location is not stated in documentation (Fig. 46-10), it is assumed that the pulse was a *radial pulse* (see Chapter 47).

Regulation of Pulse

Pulse Rate
The *pulse rate* tells how often a person's heart beats per minute (*heart rate*, **HR**). Pulse rate varies with the client's age, size, and weight. The normal adult pulse rate is 60–80 beats per minute (**BPM**). Women have a slightly higher average rate than men. The pulse of a newborn ranges from 120 to 140 BPM. Rates for children fall between those for adults and newborns, according to each child's size and age (see Chapter 71).

Activity affects pulse rate. The heart does not work as hard when a person sleeps; thus, pulse rate decreases. After running, vigorous exercise, or strenuous physical work and during disease, the heart beats faster; thus, the pulse rate increases. Excitement, anger, and fear increase the rate, as do some drugs. The pulse rate is faster in persons with a fever or an overactive thyroid gland. It increases in proportion to the body's temperature: pulse rate rises about 10 beats for every 1 °F (0.56 °C) increase in body temperature. A condition in which the pulse rate is consistently above normal (>100 BPM) is called **tachycardia**. Many of the previously mentioned conditions cause a temporarily rapid rate. An abnormally rapid rate that persists may signify a serious cardiac disorder such as heart disease, heart failure, or hemorrhage.

Sometimes, the pulse rate is continuously slow (<55–60 BPM). This condition is called **bradycardia**. Well-conditioned athletes often have a lower than normal pulse rate; otherwise, bradycardia often suggests an abnormality. Bradycardia may occur during convalescence from a long feverish illness, can signify cerebral hemorrhage, indicating increased pressure on the brain, or may be a sign of complete heart block (nonfunctioning of the heart's electrical conduction system; see Chapter 22). Certain medications also lower pulse rate.

Pulse Volume
Pulse volume varies with arterial blood volume, strength of heart contractions, and elasticity of blood vessels. When every beat is full and strong, a normal pulse can be felt with moderate finger pressure. Stronger finger pressure obliterates (or reduces the ability to count) the heart beats. If a pulse is difficult to obliterate, it is strong and is called *full* or *bounding*. In hemorrhage, when a considerable amount of blood has been lost, every pulse beat may be weak or *thready* and the pulse is easy to obliterate and difficult to feel.

Pulse Rhythm
Pulse rhythm denotes the spacing of the beats. With normal or *regular rhythm*, intervals between beats are the same. When the pulse occasionally skips a beat, this irregularity is described as an *intermittent* or *irregular pulse*. A pulse may be regular in rhythm, but irregular in force; that is, every other beat is weak; these beats may be so weak that they are not felt in the radial (wrist) pulse. This finding is serious, because it means the heart is actually beating twice as fast as the radial pulse rate indicates. This condition can be detected by measurement of the **apical–radial pulse** (simultaneous measurement of apical and radial pulses), discussed later in this chapter. Pulse may be irregular in force *and* rhythm (*dysrhythmia*), a sign of some forms of heart disease or of an overactive thyroid gland (see Chapter 81).

Methods and Equipment
Palpation
Palpation (feeling with the fingers) is used to assess the radial, temporal, mandibular, carotid, and femoral pulses. To locate the area of strongest pulsation, palpate the client's pulse with the first, second, and third fingers of one hand and

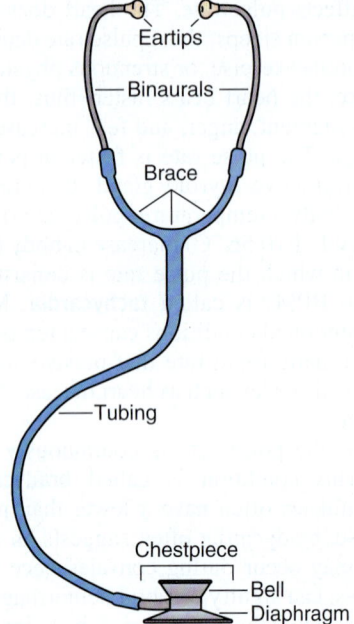

Figure 46-11 Parts of a stethoscope. (Timby, 2005.)

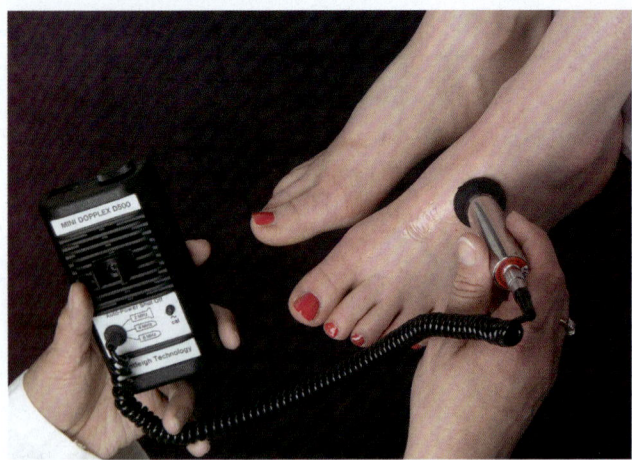

Figure 46-12 The Doppler device is used to auscultate the pulse in some situations, particularly if the pulse is difficult to hear or feel. Here, the nurse counts the dorsalis pedis pulse (pedal pulse) in the foot. If the Korotkoff sounds are very difficult or impossible to hear, the Doppler provides an alternative when measuring blood pressure as well. (Molle & Kronenberger, 2005.)

calculate the number of BPM. (Do not use the thumb, which has its own pulse.) Count the initial pulsation as zero.

Auscultation With a Stethoscope

Auscultation (listening to sounds) and counting the **apical pulse**, normally heard at the heart's apex, will usually give the most accurate assessment of pulse rate. For this assessment, one instrument, the **stethoscope** may be used; sounds received are amplified as they pass through the chestpiece and are heard in the earpieces (Fig. 46-11). Most stethoscopes have two parts in the chestpiece: the diaphragm and the bell. The flat diaphragm is pressed against the skin to test high-frequency sounds: breath, normal heart, and bowel sounds. The cup-shaped bell is pressed lightly on the skin to collect low-frequency sounds, such as abnormal heart sounds. (To change from one to the other, turn the chest piece until the desired receiver clicks into place and sounds can be heard.) The diaphragm of the stethoscope is placed over the heart's apex to assess apical pulse. (The apical pulse can be palpated with the fingers in about 50% of adults.) The apex of the heart is the point of maximal impulse (**PMI**) and is the location where the apical pulse is best heard. Each heartbeat consists of two sounds. S_1, the first sound, is caused by closure of the mitral and bicuspid valves, which separate the atria from the ventricles. S_2, the second sound, is caused by the closure of the pulmonic and aortic valves. The result is a muffled "lub-dub" sound, which constitutes one heartbeat (see Chapter 22).

Doppler

Another instrument used to auscultate heart sounds and peripheral pulses is the ultrasonic vascular Doppler device (Fig. 46-12). Apply a conductive gel and place the Doppler transmitter over the heart or artery being assessed. The earpieces or a special speaker attached to the Doppler amplify the sounds. They may also be recorded on a computer or on a special printout. The nurse will need special instruction in the use of this device.

Measuring the Pulse

Many automated blood pressure machines also measure the pulse. If this is not the case, the nurse counts the client's pulse (heart rate). There are a number of locations for doing this (see Fig. 46-10).

Radial Pulse

The radial artery in the wrist is most commonly used to count the pulse because of its convenient location. In Practice: Nursing Procedure 46-2 describes counting a radial pulse.

Apical Pulse

The apical pulse (**AP**) is more accurate than the radial pulse and is always the pulse taken for children younger than 2 years. It also provides a means of identifying abnormal heart rhythms and sounds in adults. In Practice: Nursing Procedure 46-3 outlines the steps in counting the apical pulse. Always measure the client's apical pulse if any question arises about the heart's rhythm or rate, if there are abnormal heart sounds, or if it appears that the heart has stopped. In some cases, the healthcare provider orders apical pulse measurement as a routine order.

Abnormal Heart Sounds

Abnormal heart sounds, sometimes called *extra sounds*, may be described as gallops, rubs, or murmurs and can be heard by apical auscultation. *Gallops* occur when ventricular filling creates audible vibrations during the normally silent diastolic phase. *Rubs* are heard when layers of the pericardium rub together, due to inflammation, as in pericarditis. *Murmurs* are extra heart sounds resulting from turbulent blood flow through the heart's chambers and valves. A heart murmur may be clinically significant, especially if related to a structural defect in heart valves or the walls separating the heart's chambers. In adults, murmurs are most typically caused by narrowing (*stenosis*) of a valve or by blood regurgitating through a valve that does not close properly. (The nurse requires special in-service education to recognize these abnormal sounds.) Many

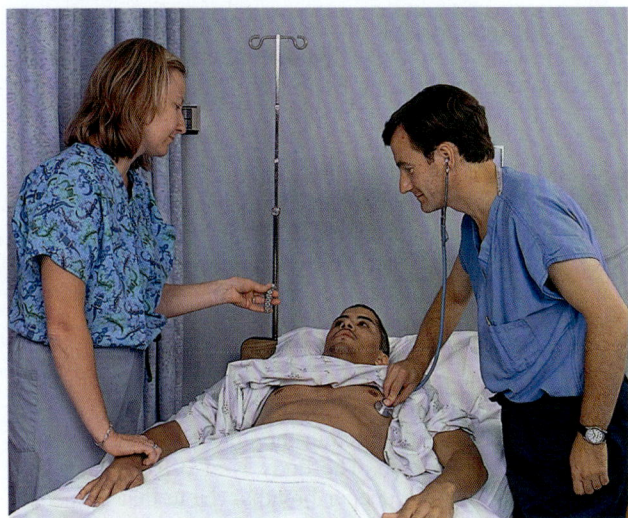

Figure 46-13 Apical–radial pulse. One nurse counts the radial pulse while the other counts the apical rate. Both use the same watch. The person counting the radial pulse calls the time. (Timby, 2013; Photo by B. Proud.)

children and 10% of adults have nonpathologic murmurs, called "functional murmurs." (See Chapter 81.)

Apical–Radial Pulse

An apical–radial pulse (A-R) measurement is ordered when it is suspected that the client's heart is not effectively pumping blood. If the apical and radial measurements are not the same, a *pulse deficit* exists. This must be reported to the healthcare provider. Two nurses are needed to carry out this procedure (Fig. 46-13). In Practice: Nursing Procedure 46-3 gives the steps for taking this measurement.

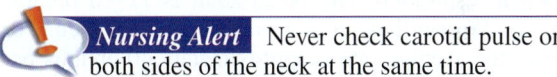 **Nursing Alert** It is impossible for the apical pulse to be lower than the radial. If this finding occurs, you have made a mistake. Take both pulses again.

Pedal Pulse

The **pedal pulse** (foot pulse) is felt over the dorsalis pedis artery or the posterior tibial artery of the foot. The pulse point is located on top of the foot, posterior to the toes (see Fig. 46-12). The status of blood circulation to the foot can be determined at these pulse points. A strong pulse indicates that circulation to the lower extremities is unrestricted, whereas a weak and irregular pulse suggests impaired or restricted blood flow. Use caution in palpating the pulse site, so the pulse is not completely obliterated with excessive pressure. Inspect the feet for color, temperature, and presence of edema (swelling). Also observe the condition of the client's toenails and cuticles. Always check pedal pulse bilaterally (in both feet) for comparison. If a pedal pulse cannot be detected, the documentation should state "pedal pulses not palpable" and indicate if this is in the right or left foot, or both. Avoid documenting "absent pedal pulses" because the pulses may actually be present but are not detectable manually; this is an instance in which the Doppler might be used. If pedal pulses cannot be detected, documentation also should include what was done, such as elevating the involved foot (feet). The nurse should also document findings such as "capillary refill less than 3 seconds (or more), skin color pink (or otherwise), and foot warm to touch (or not)." Any abnormalities should be reported immediately.

Popliteal Pulse

The **popliteal pulse** is located posterior to the knee. It is palpated by placing the fingers in the space behind the knee. Use this site to assess the status of circulation to the lower leg or as an alternative means of assessing blood pressure with a large leg cuff.

Carotid Pulse

The carotid pulse, on either side of the neck, can be located directly over the carotid artery. Palpate this pulse along the medial edge of the sternocleidomastoid muscle above the cricoid notch (see Fig. 47-36). The carotid artery is easily accessible for checking the peripheral pulse. Individuals who must do self-checks often use this method. It is also used in cases of shock when other pulses are not palpable and to determine the need for cardiopulmonary resuscitation (CPR).

The pulse is counted on either side of the neck. The client's head is positioned midline to the body. *Rationale: Such positioning provides easier access to the pulse, which is reduced when the head is turned to one side or the other.*

Nursing Alert Never check carotid pulse on both sides of the neck at the same time. *Rationale: Doing so could cut off circulation to the brain, possibly causing a CVA, "stroke."* Use the fingertips to palpate the carotid pulse. *Do not reach across the person's neck to count carotid pulse. Rationale: The client's airway could be occluded by the pressure of the examiner's arm.* Count the carotid pulses in the client's neck on the side closest to you.

ASSESSING RESPIRATION

Oxygen keeps body cells alive; accumulated carbon dioxide kills cells. Respiration is the process that brings oxygen into the body and removes carbon dioxide. This exchange takes place in the lungs (see Chapter 25). Observing respiration closely is necessary, to detect signs of interference with the breathing process.

Regulation of Respiration

Respiratory Control

The brain's respiratory center, stimulated by the proportion of carbon dioxide in the blood, controls and regulates respiration. Injury to the respiratory center or to the nerves connecting it with the lungs affects respiration; too little or too much carbon dioxide in the blood also affects breathing. Respiratory functioning may also be impaired by conditions (e.g., fractured ribs or thoracic surgery), causing pain on breathing, or by obstruction of the airway. The organs of respiration are the lungs, chest muscles, and diaphragm; injuries to these structures affect respiratory functioning. Respiration is automatic; people breathe without thinking about it. You can control your breathing to some extent by taking deeper or shallower breaths or even by holding your breath for a limited time. When the limit is reached, automatic control

TABLE 46-2 Normal Respiratory Rates at Various Ages

AGE	AVERAGE RANGE OF RESPIRATION (PER MINUTE)
Newborn	30–80
Early childhood	20–40
Late childhood	15–25
Adulthood	
Men	12–18
Women	16–20

Timby (2005).

takes over, and your chest muscles relax, despite your efforts. If this automatic resumption of breathing does not occur, a breathing disorder exists. An example is **apnea** (cessation of breathing), which occurs in sudden infant death syndrome (SIDS), sleep apnea, and other conditions.

Rate and Depth

The normal respiration rate for an adult is 12–18 breaths per minute. Women have a more rapid rate than men. For newborns, the average rate is approximately 40 breaths per minute; for children, the average rate varies from 25 to 35 breaths per minute (Table 46-2).

Nursing Alert In the adult, a respiration rate below 10 or above 24 breaths per minute is a sign of respiratory impairment. Report this situation promptly.

Normal breathing is called **eupnea**. Abnormally rapid breaths (>20–24 breaths per minute) signify **tachypnea**. Abnormally slow respirations, below 10 breaths per minute, signify **bradypnea**. Table 46-3 discusses abnormal breathing patterns. Excitement, exercise, pain, and fever increase respiratory rate. Rapid respiration is characteristic of lung diseases, such as pneumonia and emphysema. Heart disease, hemorrhage, and nephritis also increase the rate, as do some drugs. Rapid respiration indicates that the body is making an increased effort to maintain the correct balance of oxygen and carbon dioxide. The body is also trying to adjust the balance by taking deeper breaths. (Note that all people sigh or yawn occasionally to cleanse the lungs and physiologically expand the small airways and alveoli that are not used during ordinary respiration. This also helps equalize the pressure between the outside atmosphere and the middle ear, via the auditory (eustachian) tube. Do not confuse sighing with abnormal or difficult breathing.

Pressure on the brain's respiratory center or cerebral hemorrhage decreases the respiration rate. Some drugs, such as opium preparations, also depress the respiratory center. Poisons that accumulate in the body in uremia and diabetic coma increase the depth of respirations. Known as **Kussmaul respirations**, this breathing pattern is characterized by labored

TABLE 46-3 Adult Respiration Patterns

TYPE	DESCRIPTION	PATTERN/CLINICAL INDICATION
Normal	12–20/min and regular	Normal breathing pattern
Tachypnea	>24/min and shallow	May be a normal response to fever, anxiety, or exercise
		Can occur with respiratory insufficiency, alkalosis, pneumonia, or pleurisy
Bradypnea	<10/min and regular	May be normal in well-conditioned athletes
		Can occur with medication-induced depression of the respiratory center, diabetic coma, neurologic damage
Hyperventilation	Increased rate and increased depth	Usually occurs with extreme exercise, fear, or anxiety
		Kussmaul respirations are a type of hyperventilation associated with diabetic ketoacidosis. Other causes of hyperventilation include disorders of the central nervous system, an overdose of a salicylate drug, or severe anxiety
Hypoventilation	Decreased rate, decreased depth, irregular pattern	Usually associated with overdose of narcotics or anesthetics
Cheyne–Stokes respiration	Regular pattern characterized by alternating periods of deep, rapid breathing followed by periods of apnea	May result from severe heart failure, drug overdose, increased intracranial pressure, or renal failure. May be a sign of impending death
		May be noted in elderly persons during sleep, not related to any disease process
Biot respiration	Irregular pattern characterized by varying depth and rate of respirations followed by periods of apnea	May be seen with meningitis or severe brain damage

breathing; respirations are abnormally deep and gasping. Diabetic acidosis and diabetic ketoacidosis increase the total acid in the body, and the body compensates by trying to rid the body of the excess acid through deeper and faster respirations.

Respiration Sounds

Snoring occurs when the air passageway is partially blocked. It is common during sleep, when the person's tongue falls back, due to relaxation, particularly if the person is sleeping on the back. Snoring is a significant sign of sleep apnea. **Stertorous breathing** occurs when air passes through secretions present in the air passages. These bubbling noises or rattles are characteristic before death, when air passages fill with mucus. (Sometimes, very loud snoring is referred to as stertorous breathing. Obstruction near the glottis causes a hissing, crowing sound.)

Difficult Breathing (Dyspnea)

When a person is making a distinct effort to obtain oxygen and get rid of carbon dioxide, breathing becomes difficult. The term for difficult or painful breathing is **dyspnea**. This condition may be temporary, such as when a runner breathes in gasps at the end of a race, or when a person runs upstairs and pants to get their breath when reaching the top. Obesity also can cause dyspnea, especially on exertion. In some cases, breathing difficulty is constant, as in the acute stages of pneumonia or emphysema or in some types of heart disease. When the difficulty is so marked that the client can breathe only when in an upright position, it is called **orthopnea**. Obstructions of the air passages by secretions or foreign objects interfere with breathing. *Asthma* is a condition that causes difficult breathing because of spasms and edema of the bronchi (see Chapter 86).

Normally, the proportion of respirations to heartbeats is 1:5 in adults. Respirations usually increase if pulse rate increases, but not always in definite proportion. Usually, pulse rate increases faster than respiration rate. However, respiration rate increases faster than pulse rate in respiratory diseases.

Characteristic signs of breathing difficulty are heaving of the chest and abdomen, a distressed expression, distention of the neck veins, and **cyanosis** (bluish or grayish tinge) in the skin, especially in the lips (*circumoral cyanosis*) and mucous membranes of the mouth, due to an accumulation of carbon dioxide. In severe conditions, cyanosis spreads to the nail beds and extremities and eventually, becomes apparent over the entire body. Cyanosis also may result from a circulatory or blood disorder. It is easier to detect in people with lighter colored skin; cyanosis appears as a dusky gray color in persons with darker colored skin. **Cheyne–Stokes respirations** are slow and shallow at first, gradually growing faster and deeper, then tapering down until they stop entirely. Periods of apnea may last for several seconds and then the cycle is repeated. When observing a client with these respirations, document the length of the apnea period in seconds. Usually, the client experiencing Cheyne–Stokes respirations is not cyanotic. Cheyne–Stokes respirations are serious and usually precede death in cerebral hemorrhage, uremia, or heart disease.

Counting Respirations

Respirations are the easiest vital signs to determine. Each time such determinations are made, check them against the baseline information (see In Practice: Nursing Procedure 46-4).

ASSESSING BLOOD PRESSURE

Assessing blood pressure (BP) is especially important for clients with abnormally high or low readings, for postoperative clients, and for clients who have sustained serious injury or shock. The BP reading gives significant information about the client's status and is one of the most important parts of the nursing assessment. In routine client care, BP is usually assessed at least twice daily.

> **NCLEX Alert**
>
> Taking and recording of VS is used to help delineate or map out the course of a client's condition. As you read the scenarios in the NCLEX examination, it will be important for you to demonstrate your knowledge and understanding of correct technique in obtaining VS.

Regulation of Blood Pressure

As the heart forces blood through the arteries, the blood exerts pressure on the arterial walls. Blood pressure is determined by two major factors: *cardiac output* and *peripheral resistance*.

Cardiac output is a combination of the *heart rate* and the amount of blood pumped out of the heart with each contraction (*stroke volume*). These are measured over 1 min. Peripheral resistance is the resistance of blood vessels to the flow of blood (how much the vessels can stretch). Peripheral resistance affects both blood pressure and the work required of the heart to pump the blood. When peripheral resistance is increased, the heart must pump harder to push blood through the blood vessels. Factors increasing peripheral resistance include a loss of elasticity in the walls of the vessels (*arteriosclerosis*, "hardening of the arteries"), a buildup of plaque (*atherosclerosis*), or a combination of the two. The "hardened" arteries and plaque increase resistance to blood flow. The heart must work harder, and blood pressure is higher. Peripheral resistance can be lowered when the walls of the blood vessels become stretched (distended). If peripheral resistance is low, the heart does not have to pump as hard, and blood pressure lowers. However, the vessel walls must have a certain amount of elasticity for blood to circulate.

The amount of blood in the circulatory system also influences blood pressure. If the total amount of circulating blood decreases (e.g., in hemorrhage), the amount of blood available for the heart to pump out with each contraction decreases and blood pressure decreases. On the other hand, if the circulating volume is too high, the stroke volume increases, and blood pressure increases. High BP is called **hypertension** (**HTN**); low BP is called **hypotension**.

> **Key Concept**
>
> If heart rate, stroke volume, circulatory volume, or peripheral resistance increases, blood pressure increases. If there is a decrease in heart rate, stroke volume, circulatory volume, or peripheral resistance, blood pressure decreases.

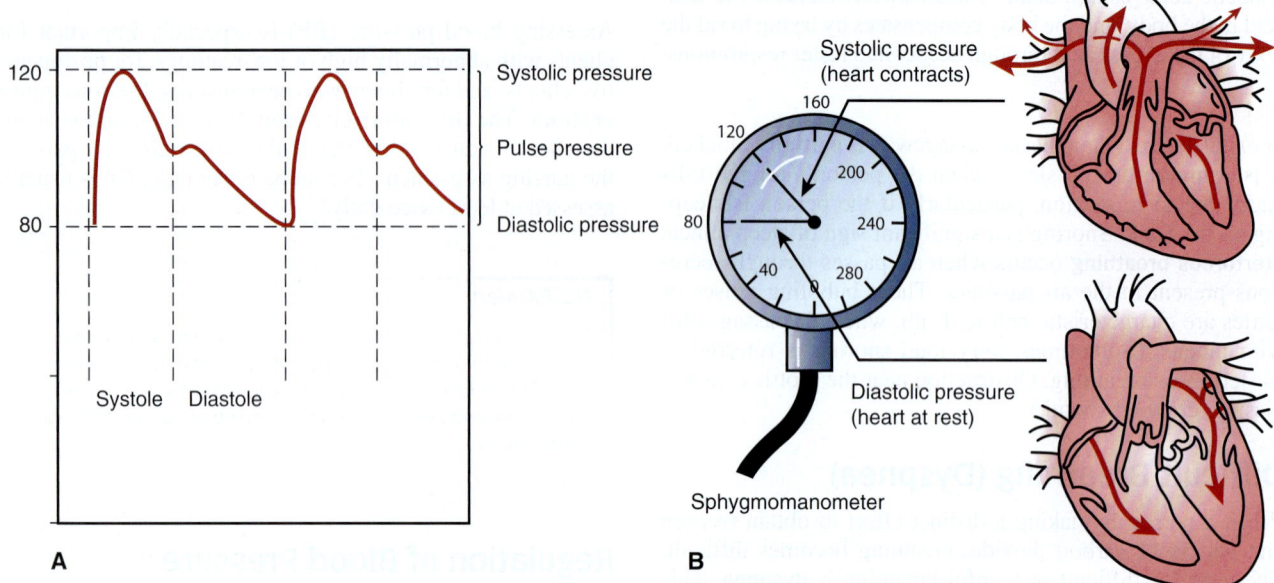

Figure 46-14 **A.** Blood pressure measurement identifies the amount of pressure in the arteries when the ventricles of the heart contract (systole) and when they relax (diastole). (Weber & Kelley, 2007.) **B.** The pressure of blood in the arteries is higher during systole (SBP) and is lower during diastole (DBP). (Timby, 2013.)

Systole and Diastole

The blood pressure is at its highest with each heartbeat during heart contraction or **systole**; this measure is the *systolic blood pressure* (**SBP**). Pressure diminishes as the heart relaxes. Pressure is lowest when the heart relaxes before it begins to contract again (**diastole**); this measure is the *diastolic blood pressure* (**DBP**) (Fig. 46-14). The difference between the systolic and diastolic readings is the **pulse pressure**. If the pulse pressure is narrow, this indicates that the arteries are not properly relaxing between heartbeats, due to a condition such as arteriosclerosis. If the pulse pressure is too wide, the vessels may not have enough elasticity or tension to sustain adequate blood flow.

A value called the *mean arterial pressure* (**MAP**) is calculated using a mathematical formula. The MAP denotes the average pressure within the arteries (Fig. 46-15). When using an electronic blood pressure monitor, the MAP is calculated and displayed. (Be aware that the MAP can sometimes be confused with the pulse rate, as it is displayed on some monitors.)

Normal Blood Pressure

Normally, the difference between the systolic pressure and the diastolic pressure (*pulse pressure*) is a number equal to one third to one half of the systolic pressure. Both readings give information; a very wide or very narrow difference between the two indicates a problem. Average systolic pressure for an adult aged 20 years is approximately 115–120, and average diastolic pressure is approximately 75–80. In the person with a BP of 120/80, the pulse pressure is 40, or one third (1/3) the systolic and one half (1/2) the diastolic. Some people have a naturally low BP; if it is around 100/60, this is still considered WNL. Blood pressure may increase gradually with age, although this is not considered desirable. Any increase results from aging of the heart and arteries. Any pressure significantly higher than recommended values (*hypertension*) is a sign of a circulatory problem. A low BP (*hypotension*) may indicate hemorrhage or shock. A systolic reading of 60 or less usually indicates serious difficulty. A diastolic reading greater than 90 is usually considered dangerously high. Medications can cause variations, and *antihypertensive* ("against high blood pressure") medications can be given to lower blood pressure. The normal blood pressure in a child, as with other vital signs, varies with age. Chapter 71 details normal ranges for children of various ages. Table 46-4 identifies recommendations regarding blood pressure parameters.

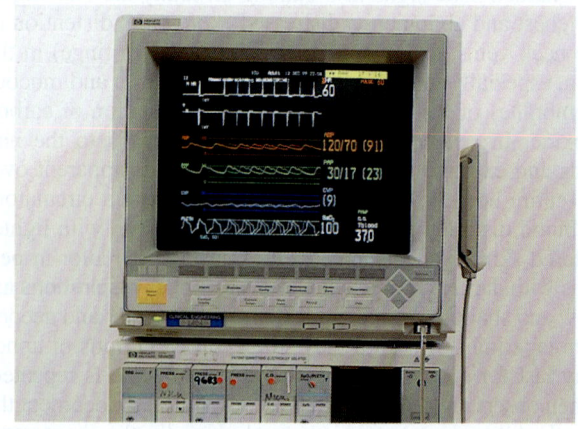

Figure 46-15 An automated vital signs monitor is often seen in intensive care units, coronary care units, and emergency departments. This machine not only shows a continuous readout of arterial blood pressure (120/70), pulse or heart rate (HR 60), and electrocardiogram (ECG), it can print an ECG strip at the push of a button. In addition, this monitor indicates more sophisticated measurements, such as mean arterial pressure (91), central venous pressure (9), venous blood pressure (30/17), and mean venous pressure (23). (Timby, 2013; Photo by B. Proud.)

TABLE 46-4	Recommendations for Normal Blood Pressure Parameters[a]	
AGE (YEARS)	SYSTOLIC (MM HG)	DIASTOLIC (MM HG)
Newborn	80	46
10	103	70
20	120	80
40	126	84
60	135	89
The American Heart Association (AHA) identifies the following categories in persons not receiving antihypertensive medications:		
Normal	<120	<80
High normal (prehypertension)	120–139	80–89
Stage I HTN	140–159	90–99
Stage II HTN	160+	100+
The AHA states that the risk of heart disease and stroke increases at the following rates:		
115/175	Normal	
135/85	×2	
155/95	×4	
175/105	×8	

HTN, hypertension.
[a]Note: These recommended classifications vary among references.

Methods and Equipment

Direct and Indirect Blood Pressure Measurement

Direct measurement of BP is accomplished by means of a probe or catheter inserted into the client's artery (arterial line). The tip of the catheter has special sensors that measure pressures and transmit this information electronically. The systolic and diastolic pressures are displayed in the form of a wave. Many critical care units use this type of measurement because constant monitoring is essential (see Fig. 46-15). Automated BP and VS monitoring can also be accomplished *indirectly*, using a traditional blood pressure cuff and a less sophisticated electronic machine. In this case, the cuff inflates and deflates periodically, and values are digitally displayed on the screen. Many of these machines can be set to keep a record of the readings. If the automatic machine is set to measure *indirect blood pressure*, fewer values are obtained.

Sphygmomanometer

Blood pressure can be measured indirectly with a **sphygmomanometer**. This device consists of an inflatable bladder, enclosed in a cuff, attached to a bulb or pump; the bladder also has a deflating mechanism. The BP is displayed on the monitor or obtained by using a stethoscope (Fig. 46-16).

The cuff is wrapped around the arm. Cuffs come in various sizes, as indicated in Table 46-5. If an incorrect size is used, accurate compression of the artery may not occur, and the measurement will be incorrect.

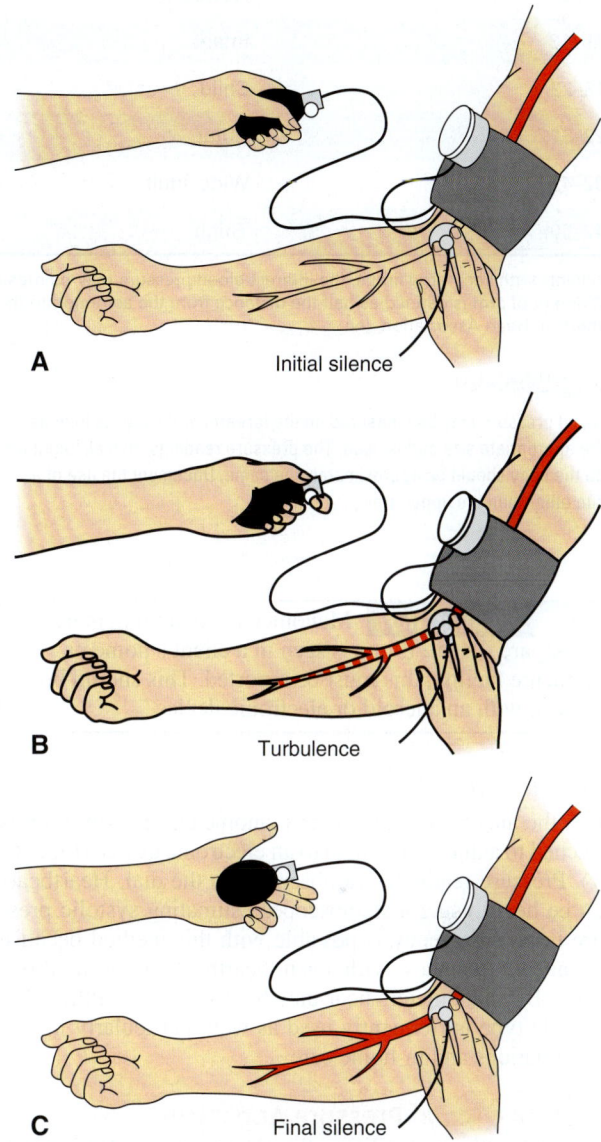

Figure 46-16 Korotkoff sounds, using an aneroid manometer and stethoscope. The readings here are approximate, based on a blood pressure (BP) of 120/80. **Phase I** (**A** and **B**) (following initial silence, turbulence begins): Characterized by first appearance of faint, but clear, tapping sounds that gradually increase in intensity. The first sound is recorded as the systolic pressure (about 120–110). **Phase II:** Characterized by blowing, muffled, or swishing sounds (about 109–100). These sounds may temporarily disappear, especially if the client is hypertensive. This absence of sound, the *auscultatory gap*, may be as great as 40 points. Failure to recognize this gap may result in error, overestimating the diastolic pressure. **Phase III:** Characterized by distinct, loud, sharp sounds as the blood flows relatively freely through the increasingly open artery (about 99–88). These sounds are softer than those in phase II. **Phase IV:** Characterized by a distinct, abrupt, muffling sound with a soft, blowing quality (about 87–80). The onset of this phase is the diastolic pressure in children. **Phase V** (**C**): The last sound heard before a period of silence (below 80). This point is recorded as the diastolic pressure in adults.

TABLE 46-5 Recommended Bladder Dimensions for Blood Pressure Cuff

ARM CIRCUMFERENCE AT MIDPOINT[a] (CM)	CUFF NAME	BLADDER WIDTH (CM)	BLADDER LENGTH (CM)
5–7.5	Newborn	3	5
7.5–13	Infant	5	8
13–22	Child	8	13
22–32	Adult	13	24
32–42	Wide adult	17	32
42–50+	Thigh	20	42

In clients with very large limbs, the indirect blood pressure may be measured in the leg or forearm. Be sure to use the correct size cuff.
[a]Midpoint of arm is defined as half the distance from the acromion to the olecranon.
American Heart Association, Inc.

> **Key Concept**
> Blood pressure may be measured on the forearm or the leg, as long as the appropriate size cuff is used. The pressure readings from all locations on the body should be approximately the same. Document the use of a site other than the upper arm.

> **Nursing Alert** Manometers containing mercury are illegal. If one is seen in a client's home or healthcare facility, this must be reported. This should be replaced with an aneroid or electronic device.

> **Nursing Alert** Do not use a client's arm for blood pressure measurement if it is compromised in any way. For example, *do not use the arm* if the client has
> - A vascular access for dialysis, a stent, or fistula
> - Had a recent mastectomy on that side
> - An arm injury or open wound
> - A splint or cast
> - An IV or saline lock in that arm
>
> If any of these situations exist, use the other arm. If both arms are unavailable, use of an alternate site, such as the leg, is necessary.

Aneroid Manometer

With the aneroid (spring-type) manometer, the arm wrap is attached to a dial, rather than to an electronic device (Fig. 46-17). Pressure readings are observed on the dial. Heartbeats can be heard using a stethoscope. Estimating systolic pressure in an emergency is possible with this method because the needle bounces with each heartbeat. Most facilities mount BP manometers near the client's bedside, although a portable type is frequently used as well, particularly in rescue situations and in-home care.

Electronic Blood Pressure Apparatus

In most healthcare facilities, the electronic monitor is used. This device does not require the use of a stethoscope. The electronic blood pressure apparatus measures the BP via a sensor or microphone in the cuff and provides a digital display of the client's BP. Many of these machines are automatic. The cuff is wrapped, a button is pushed, and the machine pumps up the cuff and displays the BP reading. The pulse and mean arterial pressure are usually displayed as well. The cuff for the electronic BP machine is applied in the same manner as for the aneroid manometer. An arrow on the cuff indicates where the artery should be, in relation to the cuff.

In some situations, an automatic blood pressure cuff cannot be used. For example, in the client with Huntington disease or another type of chorea or with severe tremors caused by medications, the automatic cuff reacts to client movement and either will not register or will be inaccurate. Some clients feel that the automatic cuff becomes too tight, and they cannot tolerate its use.

Palpation

When a stethoscope is unavailable, blood pressure can be estimated using the manometer. Palpate pulsations of the artery, as pressure is released from the cuff. Estimate the systolic pressure when the pulsation is first felt. You will also be able to visualize pulsations on an aneroid dial. It is possible only to estimate systolic pressure using this technique, because pulsations do not diminish as the cuff pressure is released. Palpation may be the only technique for estimating BP if the client is in hypovolemic shock caused by hemorrhage or another emergency. In this case, the nurse often cannot hear the sounds. Electronic BP measurement is usually more accurate, or a Doppler ultrasound may be used.

Doppler Ultrasound

If sounds are difficult to hear or indistinct, a Doppler ultrasound, instead of the stethoscope, may be used for amplification. Comparable to palpation, only the systolic pressure can be obtained using this method of determining blood pressure (see Fig. 46-12).

Measuring Blood Pressure

In Practice: Nursing Procedure 46-5 presents steps for measuring blood pressure using a manual or electronic device.

> **Key Concept**
> Measure BP and pulse initially in both arms, especially if the client has known vascular disease or if the reading is not within normal range. A difference of 5–10 points commonly exists between arms. A difference in readings of more than 10 points usually indicates arterial occlusion in the arm with the lower pressure.

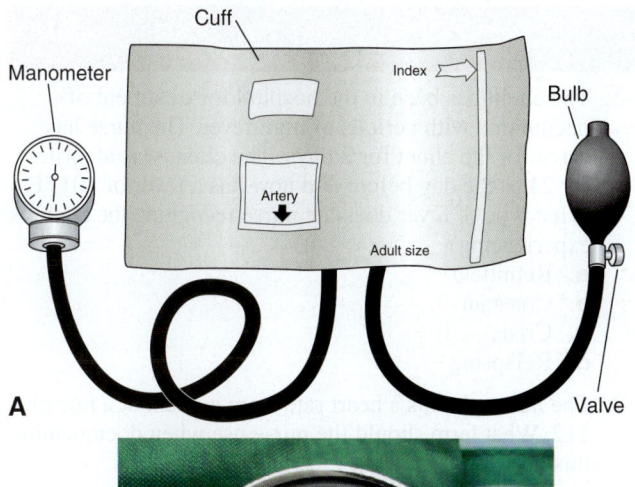

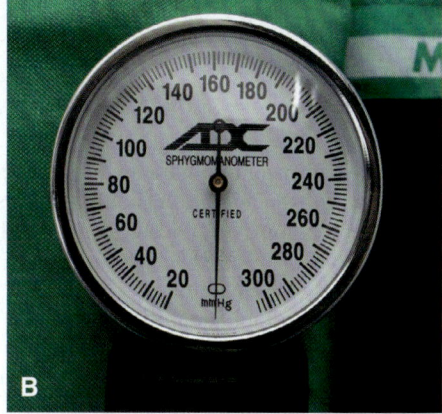

Figure 46-17 An aneroid manometer, attached to a blood pressure (BP) cuff (**A**, top). A close-up shows the indicator needle and numbers (**B**, bottom). (Carter, 2005.)

identified as a *thigh cuff*) is available. Wrap the cuff at mid-thigh with the cuff's bladder in the back. Be careful to use a cuff that is the correct width. Auscultate over the popliteal artery in the back of the knee if a stethoscope is used.

> *Key Concept*
>
> The lower arm also can be used, with auscultation over the radial artery in the wrist. If using an alternate site for taking BP, *identify it in the documentation* and use the same site continuously throughout the client's care, to maintain comparable data.

Orthostatic Blood Pressure Measurement

Some clients, particularly those who are older or taking certain medications, will experience a drastic drop in BP and/or an increase in pulse when changing from lying to sitting or from sitting to standing. A drop of as much as 25 points systolic or 10 points diastolic, as well as dizziness, must be reported. When a severe drop in BP occurs, the condition is known as *orthostatic* or *postural hypotension*. See In Practice: Nursing Procedure 46-5 for the steps involved in taking an orthostatic blood pressure measurement.

> *Key Concept*
>
> Certain medications, including many antiseizure medications and antipsychotics used in psychiatry, commonly cause orthostatic hypotension. Clients on these medications or those who are receiving treatment for anorexia (reduced food intake) often have routine daily orthostatic blood pressure readings. The client with postural hypotension must be careful when rising, due to the danger of fainting.

Whenever BP is measured with a manual manometer, listen to the heartbeat through the stethoscope and watch the manometer at the same time. When the cuff deflates, blood returns through the artery. **Korotkoff sounds** are heard in the stethoscope. There are five phases of Korotkoff sounds, as described in Figure 46-16. The onset of phase I is the recorded systolic pressure. The onset of phase IV indicates diastolic pressure in children, and phase V indicates diastolic pressure in adults. When using the electronic device, it is not necessary to listen to heart sounds; the systolic and diastolic pressures are indicated on the meter.

Measure BP when the client is resting and quiet. Physical exertion or emotional stress will affect BP. Prepare the client by explaining that the cuff on the arm may feel tight for a second or two; otherwise, the procedure is not bothersome and will take only a few minutes. The client should be sitting, with both feet on the floor. Sometimes, it will be impossible to measure BP in the client's arm (e.g., in the client with an IV or the client recovering from mastectomy). Use the thigh if a cuff that is sufficiently wide and long (specifically

PULSE OXIMETRY

In many situations, such as during the admission process or when the client is receiving supplemental oxygen, pulse **oximetry** is considered a component of baseline vital signs. Oximetry is a noninvasive procedure that uses a photoelectric impulse to measure the amount of light transmitted or reflected by deoxygenated, as opposed to oxygenated, hemoglobin. It yields a measurement of the oxygen saturation of functional hemoglobin in the blood, indicated as a percentage. The instrument used is called a *pulse oximeter* or transducer. A sensor is placed on a finger, toe, or earlobe. The healthcare provider orders the minimum acceptable level of oxygen saturation before using supplementary oxygen. (Chapter 87 describes means of delivering supplementary oxygen.) In Practice: Nursing Procedure 46-6 lists the steps in using a pulse oximeter.

STUDENT SYNTHESIS

KEY POINTS

- Temperature, pulse, respiration, and blood pressure are called vital signs (or cardinal symptoms) because they are indicators of functions of the body that are necessary to maintain life. Pulse oximetry is often included.
- Documentation of vital signs is essential to collecting information regarding the client's status and well-being.
- Temperature is the measurement of heat inside the body (core temperature). It is the balance between the heat the body produces and loses.
- Pulse is the vibration or waves of blood through the arteries as the heart beats. It is measured by rate and rhythm.
- Respiration is the process by which the lungs bring oxygen into the body and remove carbon dioxide.
- Blood pressure measures the pressure the blood exerts on the walls of the arteries. Rate and force of heartbeat, blood vessel condition, and blood volume determine the reading as the ventricles contract and rest.
- Pulse oximetry indicates the percentage of oxygen saturation in the hemoglobin.

CRITICAL THINKING EXERCISES

1. You are measuring a client's temperature by the oral method. You find a variation from normal. What steps do you take next? Why?
2. Using a wall-mounted aneroid sphygmomanometer, you begin wrapping the cuff around the client's upper arm when you realize the cuff is the wrong size. Why is this a problem? What do you do next to ensure an accurate measurement?
3. Your client, Mr. B., is sound asleep when you enter his room to take his vital signs. Should you measure any of his vital signs before waking him? If so, which ones and why? How will you measure them?
4. Mrs. P. has never taken her temperature using an electronic thermometer. She now must monitor her daily temperature because of a recurring infection. Explain what steps she must take to measure and record her body temperature accurately.
5. Describe how you would explain self-blood pressure measurement to a client who is being discharged from the hospital.

NCLEX-STYLE REVIEW QUESTIONS

1. The nurse is obtaining a temperature from a client. What symptoms exhibited by the client correlate with a temperature of 102.6 °F? Select all that apply.
   a. Flushed face
   b. Hot skin
   c. Pale skin
   d. Cold, clammy skin
   e. Restlessness and chills

2. The client has been in the hospital for treatment of pneumonia with periods of high fever. The nurse has cared for the client for 2 days. The client was afebrile for 24 hr the day before and now has a fever of 101 °F. What type of fever does the nurse recognize the client is experiencing?
   a. Remittent
   b. Constant
   c. Crisis
   d. Relapsing

3. The nurse obtains a heart rate from a client at a rate of 112. What term should the nurse use when documenting this heart rate?
   a. Tachycardia
   b. Bradycardia
   c. Irregular
   d. Palpitation

4. The nurse is preparing to obtain an oral temperature from a client. In what situation should the nurse delay taking the temperature for at least 15 min? Select all that apply.
   a. The client is chewing gum.
   b. The client just drank a cup of coffee.
   c. The client just had a chest x-ray.
   d. The client has just finished smoking a cigarette.
   e. The client is chewing tobacco.

5. The nurse observes that a client's respirations are slow and shallow, then gradually become faster and deeper, and then stop, with the cycle then repeating itself. How should the nurse document this type of respiration?
   a. Cheyne–Stokes respiration
   b. Eupneic respirations
   c. Orthopnea
   d. Dyspnea

CHAPTER RESOURCES

Enhance your learning with additional resources on thePoint!

Student Resources related to this chapter can be found at thePoint.lww.com/Rosdahl12e.

CHAPTER 46 Vital Signs

Welcome Steps

Look at healthcare provider's orders.

Protocol for procedure.

Necessary equipment/supplies.

Wash hands using proper hand hygiene; put on gloves.

Explain the procedure and reassure the client.

Locate two identifiers to confirm correct client.

Comfortable and efficient position for nurse and client.

Obtain privacy.

Make sure to follow correct steps and body mechanics with good technique.

Ensure safety and observe deviations from normal.

End Steps

Ensure comfort and safety.

Note questions or concerns from client or nurse; note significant data.

Dispose of materials properly.

Disinfect the area and your hands.

Document and report the procedure and your findings.

IN PRACTICE

NURSING PROCEDURE 46-1 Measuring Body Temperatures

Using the Electronic Temperature Probe

These steps are used to measure body temperature with the electronic temperature probe (thermometer), using the oral, rectal, tympanic, or axillary method. Perform *hand sanitization* before and after measuring temperature.

1. Turn on the thermometer. Usually, it will count down for about 5 s before it is ready for use. It may flash a "ready" sign or may beep. (The tympanic thermometer may be turned on after inserting into the ear canal, depending on the model.) *Rationale: Make sure the unit is ready to use, to ensure an accurate reading.*

2. Insert the probe into a new disposable cover and push gently until it clicks into place. *Rationale: The disposable sheath helps prevent the spread of infection.*

3. The probe is inserted into the appropriate body area, and body tissues are closed around it. *Rationale: The most accurate measurement is obtained if the space all the way around the probe is touched by body tissues.*

4. Remove the probe when the "beep" sounds, when the digital numbers stop flashing, or when the digital reading is displayed on the screen. *Rationale: It is important to wait until the correct temperature is displayed. The signal indicates that the reading has been recorded.*

5. Push the "eject" button on the probe to remove the probe cover. Discard the cover per agency protocol. *Rationale: The eject button allows you to dispose of the contaminated probe cover without touching it. Proper disposal helps prevent the spread of microorganisms to others. Sanitize hands.*

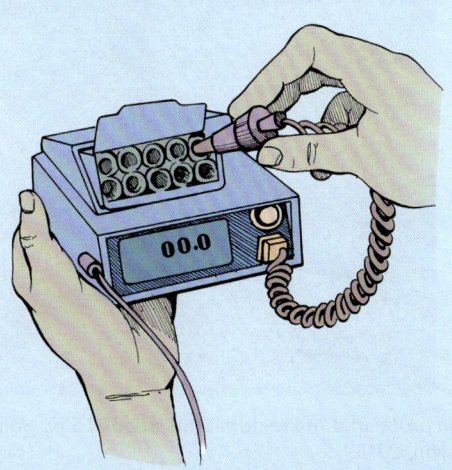

Insert the probe into a disposable cover. (Timby, 2005.)

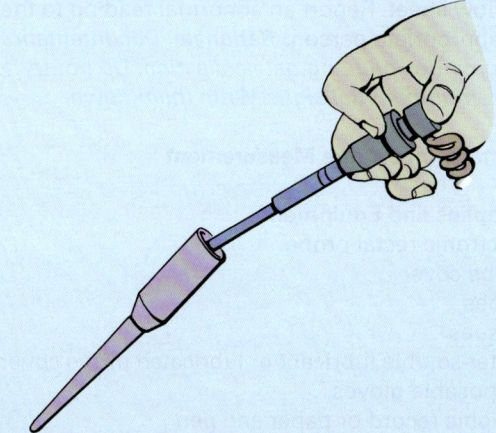

Push the button on the end of the probe to release the probe cover. (Timby, 2005.)

6. Record the temperature measurement in the designated manner. *Rationale: This ensures communication between members of the healthcare team.*

Note: A 15-second timer may be available on the handheld electronic thermometer. This can be used to count pulse or respirations. It is activated by pushing the "timer" or "T" button on the device.

Oral Temperature Measurement

Supplies and Equipment
Temperature sensor, with probe
Disposable probe covers
Disposable gloves (if required by agency protocol)
Paper or flow sheet
Pen

Steps
Follow LPN WELCOME steps and then

1. Place the probe under the client's tongue at the base of the sublingual pocket on either side (see Fig. 46-5). *Rationale: Heat from superficial blood vessels in the sublingual pocket produces the temperature reading.*

2. Instruct the client to close the lips (not the teeth) around the probe and lower the tongue. The client may wish to hold the probe in place. *Rationale: Closing the lips steadies and secures the thermometer. Lowering the tongue exposes more body tissues to the probe. Injury may occur if the client bites the probe. If the client holds the probe, it is usually more comfortable.*

3. Remove the probe from the client's mouth and read the displayed temperature. Eject the probe cover and discard per facility protocol. *Rationale: The electronic instrument will display the client's measured temperature. It is important to prevent spread of organisms.*

Follow ENDDD steps

Special Reminder
- Record the client's temperature on paper or the flow sheet. Report an abnormal reading to the appropriate person. *Rationale: Documentation provides ongoing data collection. Do not try to remember vital signs. Write them down.*

Rectal Temperature Measurement

Supplies and Equipment
Electronic rectal probe
Probe cover
Wipes
Tissues
Water-soluble lubricant or lubricated probe cover
Disposable gloves
Graphic record or paper and pen

Steps
Follow LPN WELCOME steps and then

1. Turn the client on one side, preferably the left side. *Rationale: This position exposes the client's rectal area for thermometer placement. Lying on the left side takes advantage of the normal anatomy of the rectum.*

2. Prepare the electronic probe. (Be sure to use only a probe designated for rectal use.) Lubricate the probe or use a prelubricated probe cover. You may wish to lubricate the external rectal area as well. *Rationale: Lubrication reduces friction and makes it easier to insert the probe without injuring body tissues. Applying lubricant with a wipe or from a single-use packet prevents contamination of the lubricant supply.*

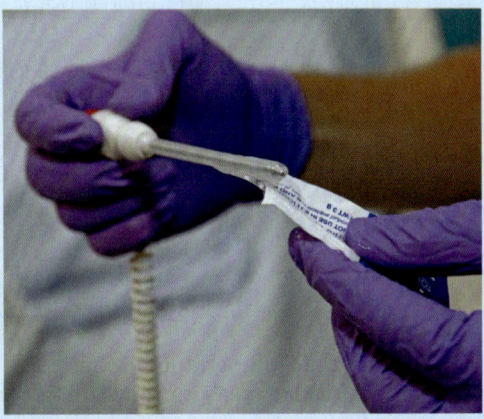

Lubricate the probe cover by inserting it into the single-use lubricant packet. (Use a wipe to apply the lubricant if a stock supply is used.) (Taylor et al., 2018.)

3. Fold back the bedclothes and separate the client's buttocks so the anal opening is clearly visible. Keep the client covered as much as possible. *Rationale: This allows for easy probe insertion. Provide privacy.*

4. Ask the client to take a slow, deep breath and insert the thermometer about 1.5 in. *Rationale: Deep, slow breaths allow the client to relax the anal area. Insertion depth is necessary for blood vessels in the rectum to surround the probe.*

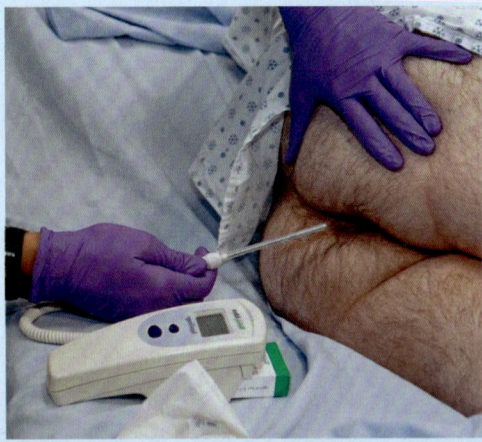

Insert the probe into the rectum/anus about 1.5 in. Hold it in place. (Lynn, 2015.)

5. Hold the probe in place until the machine beeps and the temperature is displayed. NEVER leave a client who has a rectal probe in place. *Rationale: The thermometer is held in place for safety and so it is not expelled. The probe is removed immediately if the client becomes combative or restless. The client could roll onto the probe, causing it to break or to be pushed too far into the rectum. Adequate time is needed for the temperature reading to register.*

6. Remove the probe and eject the probe cover. Dispose of the probe cover and your gloves, according to facility protocol. Note: If a probe is used for rectal temperatures, it should be used for that client only and carefully disinfected when the client is discharged. *Rationale: This helps prevent the spread of infection.*

Follow ENDDD steps

Special Reminder
- Document the temperature indicating that the temperature was taken rectally by putting "R" next to it or clicking the appropriate space in the electronic record. *Rationale: A difference in normal values exists between oral and rectal temperatures. (The electronic thermometer can often be set to automatically convert between rectal and oral equivalents.)*

Axillary Temperature Measurement

Supplies and Equipment
Electronic thermometer and probe
Probe cover
Disposable gloves (if required by agency protocol)
Graphic chart or computer
Pen and paper

Steps
Follow LPN WELCOME steps and then

1. Prepare the machine. Cover the probe. *Rationale: This ensures an accurate reading. The probe is covered to prevent transmission of organisms.*

2. Be sure the client's axilla is dry. If it is moist, pat it dry gently before inserting the probe. *Rationale: Moisture will alter the reading.*

3. Place the covered probe into the center of the axilla and bring the client's arm down against the body as tightly as possible, with the forearm resting across the chest. *Rationale: Close contact of the probe or bulb of the thermometer with superficial blood vessels in the axilla ensures a more accurate temperature registration.*

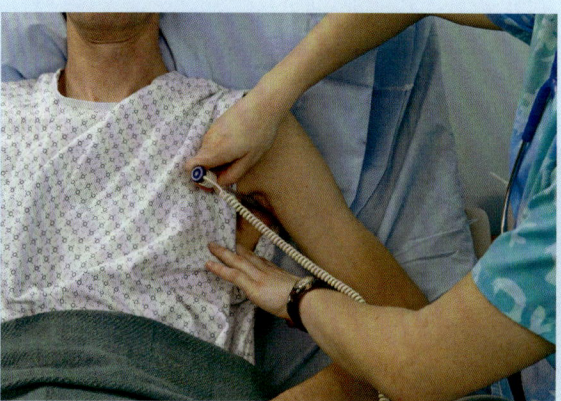
Place the probe in the center of the dry axilla. Then, move the arm down to close the space. (Taylor et al., 2018.)

4. Hold the electronic probe or thermometer in place until the machine beeps or the reading is displayed. Remove the probe, discard the probe cover, and read and record the temperature. *Rationale: This helps ensure an accurate reading.*

Follow ENDDD steps

Special Reminder
- Record the reading per agency procedures. Indicate that the axillary method was used: "(Ax)." *Rationale: Axillary temperature readings usually are lower than oral readings.*

Tympanic Temperature Measurement (Otic, Aural)

Supplies and Equipment
Tympanic thermometer
Disposable probe cover
Disposable gloves (if required by agency protocol)
Recording materials

Steps
Follow LPN WELCOME steps and then

1. Prepare the tympanic probe. (A special probe/cone sheath is used to cover this probe.) If the person wears a hearing aid, remove it carefully and wait 2 min before taking the temperature. *Rationale: This ensures a more accurate reading.*

2. Select the desired parameters. For a child younger than 3 years, rectal equivalents are often used. Most acute-care facilities use Celsius readings. *Rationale: Follow the protocol in your facility.*

3. Grasp the client's external ear at about the midpoint. For an adult, gently pull the external ear up and back. For a child aged 6 years and younger,

pull the ear down and back. *Rationale: You need to straighten the curved ear canal as much as possible to obtain optimum visualization by the equipment.*

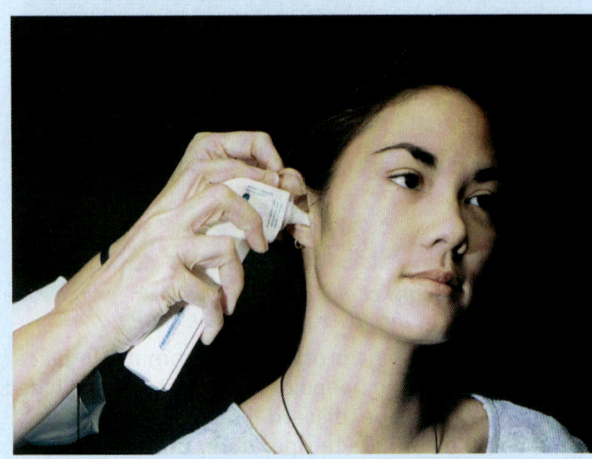

Gently pull the ear up and back for an adult. Seal the ear canal with the tympanic probe and hold it in place. (Molle & Kronenberger, 2005.)

4. Slowly advance the probe into the client's ear with a back and forth motion until it seals the ear canal (see Fig. 46-7). *Rationale: Sealing the tip of the probe confines radiated heat within the area being measured.*
5. Point the probe's tip in an imaginary line from the client's sideburns to their opposite eyebrow. *Rationale: Be sure to align the probe with the client's tympanic membrane.*
6. As soon as the instrument is in correct position, press the button to activate the thermometer. *Rationale: Initiate sensing within 2.5 s to ensure an accurate reading.*
7. Keep the probe in place until the thermometer makes a sound or flashes a light. *Rationale: Wait for the procedure to be completed.*
8. Read and record the temperature and discard the probe cover and gloves according to facility protocol. *Rationale: Limit the spread of microorganisms.*

Follow ENDDD steps

Temporal Artery Temperature Measurement

Supplies and Equipment
Temporal artery temperature device
Recording materials

Steps
Follow LPN WELCOME steps and then

1. Remove the protective cap. Be sure the lens is clean (see Fig. 46-8). (If it is not, clean it with a cotton swab and a *very small* amount of alcohol.) *Rationale: This helps ensure an accurate reading.*
2. Gently position the lens side of the probe flat on the center of the client's forehead halfway between the eyebrow and the normal hairline. Press and hold the "SCAN" button and lightly slide the scanner sideways across the forehead to the hairline just above the ear. You will hear a beep and a red light will blink. *Rationale: This verifies that the temperature is being scanned. Accurate procedure ensures accurate results.*
3. If the client is perspiring, hold the button down, lift the probe, and touch the neck just behind the earlobe. *Rationale: This supplies additional data for the machine's computations.*
4. Release the SCAN button, remove the scanner from the head, and read the temperature on the digital display. The thermometer will automatically shut off in 30 s. To turn it off immediately, press and release the SCAN button quickly. *Rationale: It is important to know how to operate the machine.*
5. Replace the protective cap. *Rationale: This helps protect the lens when the instrument is not in use.*
6. Clean the device according to manufacturer's instructions. Record the reading appropriately.

Follow ENDDD steps

> **Nursing Alert** Be sure to sanitize your hands between clients when measuring vital signs.

Temperature Measurement Using the Glass Thermometer

The mercury-filled glass thermometer is not legal in the United States. If you find that a home care client is using an alcohol-filled glass thermometer, you may need to teach the client or caregiver its proper use and handling. Follow the manufacturer's instructions for reading this thermometer. Remember that this thermometer cannot be exposed to hot water or other heat or it will break and must be shaken down each time it is.

The temperature is measured in the same manner as for any other oral, rectal, or axillary thermometer. Follow Standard Precautions and make sure to use only an oral thermometer for oral measurements and a rectal thermometer for only rectal measurements. *These two are never interchanged.* (You have the legal right to refuse to use a mercury-filled glass thermometer.)

CHAPTER 46 Vital Signs

IN PRACTICE
NURSING PROCEDURE 46-2: Measuring Radial Pulse Manually

Supplies and Equipment
Watch with a second hand
Paper or flow sheet
Pen

Steps
Follow LPN WELCOME Steps and Then

1. For manual counting of radial pulse, position the client's forearm comfortably with the wrist extended and palm down. *Rationale:* This position allows for easy assessment.
2. Place the tips of your first, second, and third fingers over the client's radial artery on the inside of the wrist on the thumb side. *Rationale:* The fingertips are sensitive and better able to feel the pulse. Do not use your thumb, because it has a strong pulse of its own.
3. Press *gently* against the client's radial artery to the point where pulsations can be felt distinctly. *Rationale:* Excessive pressure will obliterate the pulse.
4. Using a watch, count the pulse beats for 30 s and multiply by 2 to get the rate per minute. *Rationale:* Thirty seconds is sufficient time to assess the pulse rate when it is regular.
5. Count the radial pulse for 1 full minute or count the apical pulse, if you find any abnormality. *Rationale:* Counting 1 full minute permits a more accurate reading and allows assessment of pulse strength and rhythm. Apical pulse may be necessary to measure irregular or weak beats.

Follow ENDDD Steps

Special Reminders
- Use the second hand on the watch as a timer. You can also determine the character of and rate of respirations at the same time. Electronic temperature devices usually count the pulse and usually contain a timer.
- Report any irregular findings. Record the results appropriately.

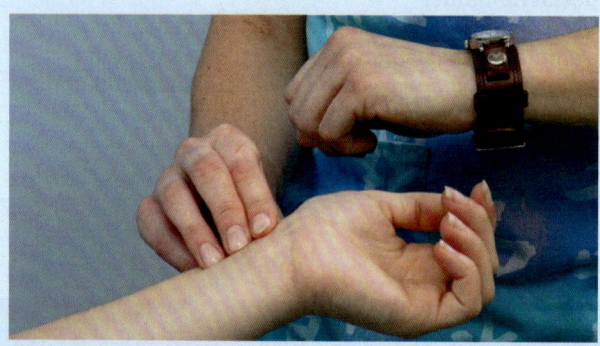

Measuring radial pulse. (Lynn, 2015.)

IN PRACTICE
NURSING PROCEDURE 46-3: Measuring Apical Pulse

Supplies and Equipment
Stethoscope
Pen and paper or flow sheet
Watch with second hand

Steps
Follow LPN WELCOME steps and then

1. Expose the client's left chest area. *Rationale:* Noise from clothing and bedclothes will distort pulse sound. Remember to respect the client's privacy.
2. Locate a point over the apex (the pointed bottom of the heart) in the upper left chest. This point is usually at the fifth intercostal space, approximately 3 inches left of the client's sternum (just below the left nipple). *Rationale:* Correct placement ensures that pulse will be heard.

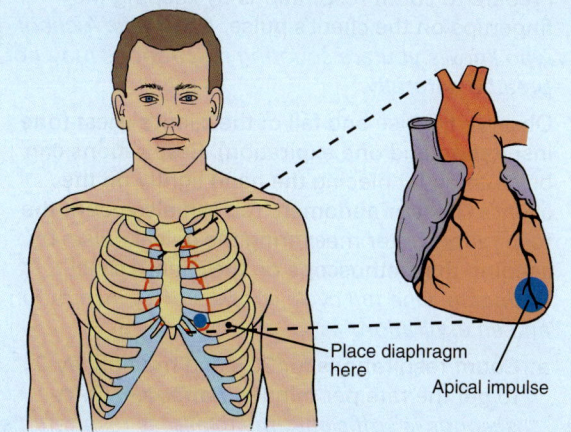

Place the diaphragm of the stethoscope over the apex of the heart, located just below the left nipple. (Evans-Smith, 2005.)

3. Warm the stethoscope's diaphragm in the palm of the hand. *Rationale: A cold metal diaphragm is uncomfortable.*
4. Place the diaphragm firmly over the PMI (point of maximal impulse) and auscultate (listen) for heart sounds. *Rationale: Lub-dub is the opening and closing of the heart valves to make one beat.*
5. Count for 1 full minute. *Rationale: This ensures accuracy.*
6. Determine regularity and abnormal heart sounds. (Abnormal heart sounds are briefly introduced earlier in this chapter.) *Rationale: Irregularity or abnormal sounds may indicate a need for further evaluation and should be reported and documented.*

Follow ENDDD steps

Measuring Apical–Radial Pulse

Supplies and Equipment
Stethoscope
Pen and paper or flow sheet
Watch with second hand
Two nurses

Steps
Follow LPN WELCOME steps and then
1. Using the same watch, one nurse counts the client's apical pulse for 1 min, while the other nurse counts the radial pulse. *Rationale: Using the same watch ensures that the times used will be the same, making the findings more accurate.*
2. Both nurses start counting at the same time. The nurse counting the radial pulse calls for the timing to start and stop and times 1 min with the second hand. *Rationale: The count must be done simultaneously for accuracy.*
3. Each nurse reports their count and documents the two figures at the end of 1 min (e.g., "A-R pulse 76/72"). *Rationale: Accurate documentation is important. A discrepancy between the apical and radial pulses may indicate serious circulatory disorders.*

Follow ENDDD steps

Special Reminder
- Normally, the two readings are the same. If a difference exists between them, it is called the *pulse deficit* and must be promptly recorded and reported. *The apical pulse must be the same or higher than the radial pulse.*

IN PRACTICE
NURSING PROCEDURE 46-4 Counting Respirations

Supplies and Equipment
Watch with second hand
Paper or flow sheet
Pen

Steps
Follow LPN WELCOME steps and then
1. Prepare to count respirations by keeping the fingertips on the client's pulse. *Rationale: A client who knows you are counting respirations may not breathe naturally.*
2. Observe the rise and fall of the client's chest (one inspiration and one expiration). Respirations can be counted by placing the hand lightly on the client's chest or abdomen. You can also count the respirations after measuring the apical pulse, by keeping the stethoscope on the client's chest. *Rationale: One full cycle consists of an inspiration and an expiration.*
   a. Count respirations for 30 s and multiply by 2 to get the rate per minute. *Rationale: Thirty seconds is sufficient time to assess respirations, when the rate is regular.*
   b. Count respirations for 1 full minute for an infant, a young child, or for an adult with an irregular, more rapid rate. *Rationale: Children normally have an irregular, more rapid rate. Adults with an irregular rate require more careful assessment, including depth and rhythm of respirations.*
   c. If the client has an irregular or abnormal breathing pattern, such as Cheyne–Stokes respirations, document the length of apnea and the number of breaths per minute. Usually, this is done for at least 3 min, counting the rate for each minute separately. These figures can then be compared.

Follow ENDDD steps

Special Reminder
- Record the rate, report any irregular findings to the appropriate person, and document the information, noting "A-R pulse."

CHAPTER 46 Vital Signs 603

IN PRACTICE
NURSING PROCEDURE 46-5 — Measuring Blood Pressure (Aneroid Manometer and Manual Cuff)

Supplies and Equipment
Stethoscope
Sphygmomanometer
Blood pressure cuff (appropriate size)
Alcohol wipe
Paper or flow sheet
Pen

Using a Manual Cuff for an Adult

Steps
Follow LPN WELCOME steps and then

1. Select a cuff that is the appropriate size for the client. Cleanse the stethoscope's earpieces and diaphragm with an alcohol wipe. **Rationale:** *Incorrect cuff size may give an inaccurate reading. Cleansing the stethoscope helps prevent the spread of infection.*

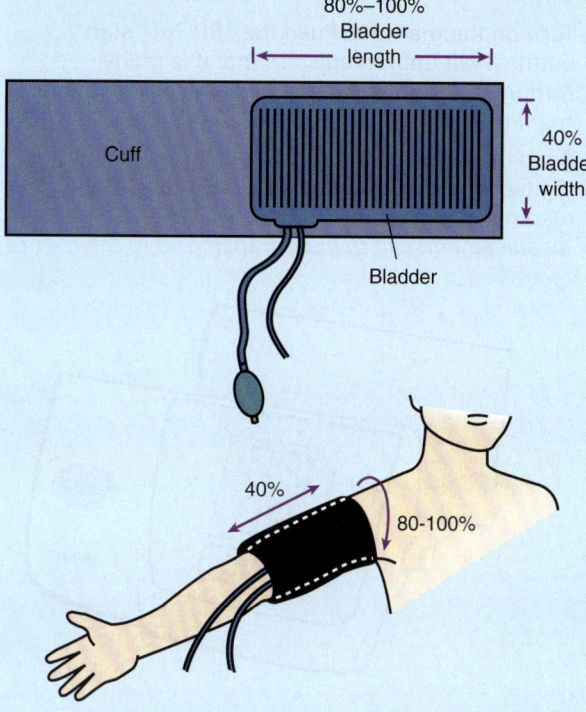

To determine the appropriate size of the blood pressure cuff, the width of the bladder should be 40% of the midarm circumference and the length should be at least 80%. (Timby, 2013.)

2. Assist the client to a comfortable position. Ask the client to sit or lie still for about 5 min. Support the selected arm; turn the palm upward. Remove any constrictive clothing. Instruct the client to relax the arm and place both feet flat on the floor when sitting. **Rationale:** *Ideally, the arm is at heart level for accurate measurement. Rotate it so the brachial pulse is easily accessible and not constricted by* clothing. Having the legs crossed obstructs blood flow.

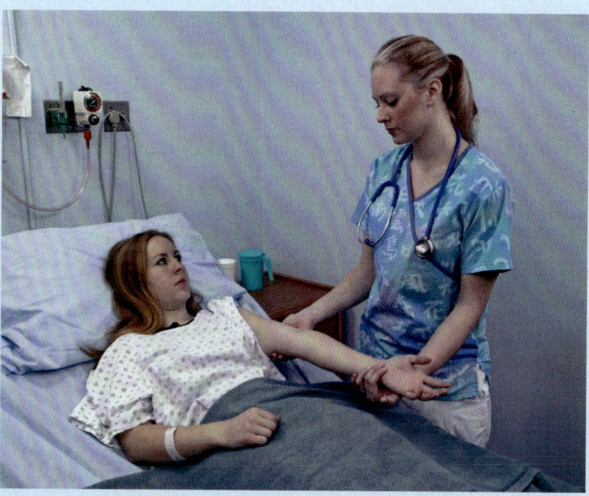

Assist the client to a comfortable position. (Evans-Smith, 2005.)

3. Palpate the brachial artery in the bend of the elbow. Center the cuff's bladder approximately 1 in. (2.5 cm) above the site where you palpated the brachial pulse. **Rationale:** *Centering the bladder ensures even cuff inflation over the brachial artery.*

4. Wrap the cuff snugly around the client's arm and secure the end appropriately. Make sure the reading on the aneroid manometer starts at zero. **Rationale:** *The blood pressure (BP) reading will be inaccurate if you apply the cuff too loosely. Starting at zero assures that the BP reading will be accurate.*

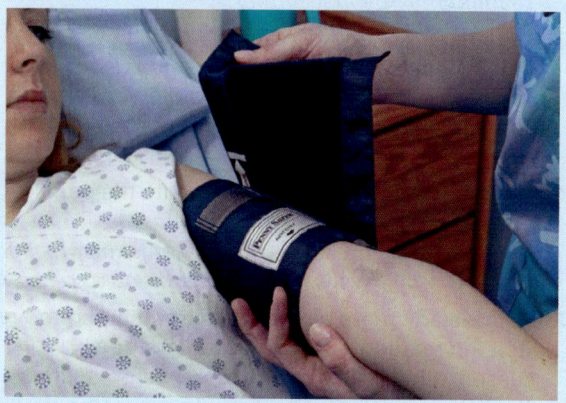

Wrap the cuff around the client's arm and secure the end. (Lynn, 2015.)

5. Palpate the radial or brachial pulse with one hand. Close the screw clamp on the bulb and inflate the cuff while still checking the pulse with the other hand. Observe the point where the pulse is no longer palpable. **Rationale:** *Palpation identifies the approximate systolic reading.*

6. Open the screw clamp, deflate the cuff, and wait 30 s. *Rationale: Short interval eases any venous congestion that may have occurred.*
7. Position the stethoscope's earpieces comfortably in your ears (turn tips slightly forward) and place the diaphragm portion of the chestpiece over the client's brachial artery. *Rationale: BP is easier to hear when you place the stethoscope directly over the artery.*

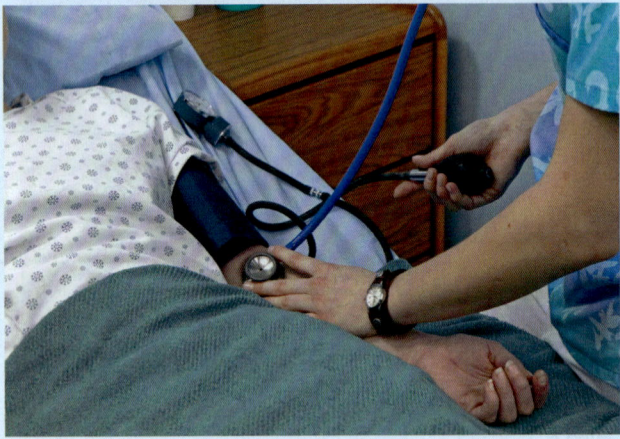

Place the diaphragm of the stethoscope over the brachial artery and inflate the cuff. (Lynn, 2015.)

8. Close the screw clamp on the bulb and inflate the cuff to a pressure of 30 points above the number where the pulse had disappeared. *Rationale: This ensures that the systolic reading is not underestimated.*
9. Open the clamp and allow the aneroid dial to fall at a rate of two to three points per second. *Rationale: If deflation occurs too rapidly, the reading may be inaccurate.*
10. Note the point on the column or dial at which you initially hear a distinct sound. *Rationale: The first sound heard represents the systolic pressure or the point where the heart is able to force blood into the brachial artery.*
11. Continue deflating the cuff and note the point where the sound disappears. *Rationale: This is the adult diastolic pressure. It represents the pressure that the artery walls exert on the blood at rest.*
12. Release any remaining air in the cuff and remove it. If the reading must be rechecked for any reason, allow a 1-minute interval before taking the BP again. *Rationale: This interval eases any venous congestion and provides for an accurate reading when you repeat the measurement. In some cases, it is advisable to use the other arm for a recheck.*
13. Assist the client to a comfortable position. Advise the client of the reading. *Rationale: This action shows your interest in the client's well-being and allows them to participate in care.*

Follow ENDDD steps

Special Reminder
- Record the systolic pressure over the diastolic (e.g., 120/70). Indicate the site where you took the BP if the brachial site was not used. Report any irregular findings.

Using an Automatic Cuff
Follow LPN WELCOME steps and then

1. Wrap the cuff in the same manner as above. Let the client know that the cuff will probably be quite tight, but it will not remain inflated. Ask the client to sit very still with both feet on the floor and relax the arm. *Rationale: The blood pressure will be determined in basically the same manner as for the aneroid manometer. The client may be uncomfortable; they need to know that you understand and that the procedure will be completed quickly. If the client moves or tenses the arm, the machine will start over or will register an "error."*
2. Turn on the machine. Push the "BP" or "start" button. Wait until it registers that it is ready. *Rationale: These steps ensure a more accurate reading.*
3. Read the blood pressure and pulse values on the digital screen. Most machines beep when the reading is completed. *Rationale: These values are displayed and can then be transferred to the client's record.*

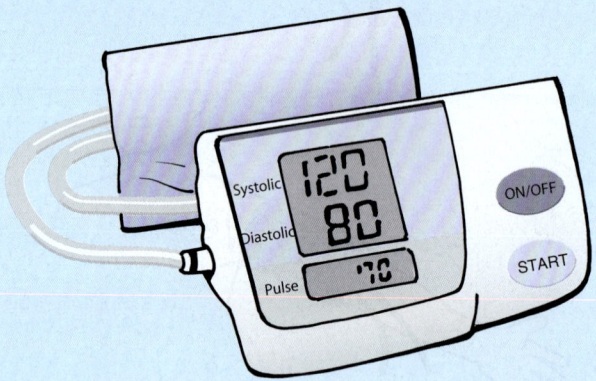

Read the BP and P values on the digital readout of the automatic electronic monitor. (Timby, 2005.)

Follow ENDDD steps

Measuring Thigh Blood Pressure
Use the same procedures as in measuring BP on the arm. The cuff must be designated as a "thigh" cuff and must be large enough to fit comfortably around the client's thigh. If a stethoscope is used, it is held behind the bend of the knee (the popliteal space).

CHAPTER 46 Vital Signs

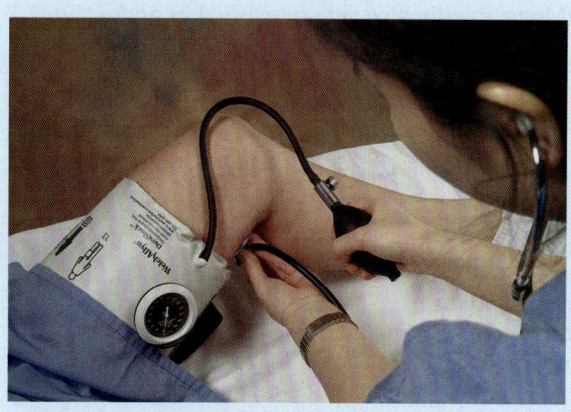

Application of blood pressure cuff to the thigh. (Timby, 2013.)

Measuring Orthostatic Blood Pressure

Supplies and Equipment
Blood pressure equipment
Alcohol wipe
Paper or flow sheet
Pen

Steps
Follow LPN WELCOME steps and then

1. Measure the client's blood pressure and pulse with the client lying down (or sitting). Wait at least 5 min.

2. Without removing the BP cuff, ask the client to stand. *Rationale: The cuff remains in place to ensure a more accurate measurement.*

3. Immediately measure the BP and pulse (P) again. Report a significant drop in blood pressure (25 points systolic or 10 points diastolic). A drop in BP may also affect the pulse rate. The pulse rate may decrease, but often it increases. Report a pulse rate increase of more than 12–15 beats per minute (BPM). *Rationale: A decrease in blood pressure with an accompanying rise in pulse may also indicate low circulating blood volume, as in hemorrhage.*

4. The client may feel dizzy or light-headed on standing and may be susceptible to falling or fainting. Carry out measures to ensure the client's safety. *Rationale: Instruct the client to rise slowly, to adjust to each new position in the future.*

5. In some cases, three readings are made: lying down, sitting, and standing. Allow at least 5 min between each measurement. *Rationale: This assures an accurate orthostatic reading.*

Follow ENDDD steps

Special Reminders
- Orthostatic blood pressure is recorded as follows, with appropriate times:
  - ↓150/80, P 76 (lying down or sitting)
  - ↑120/66, P 92 (standing)

IN PRACTICE
NURSING PROCEDURE 46-6 Using a Pulse Oximeter

Supplies and Equipment
Pulse oximeter device
Sensor; finger, toe, or ear clip (transducer)
Nail polish remover (if needed)
Alcohol wipe

Steps
Follow LPN WELCOME steps and then

1. Choose the sensor appropriate for the client's size and location to be used (finger, toe, ear). *Rationale: Inappropriate size or device may cause inaccurate results or pain.*

2. Remove any fingernail polish or acrylic nails on the fingers to be used, if possible. *Rationale: The sensor may be unable to provide an accurate reading through nail polish or acrylic nails.*

3. Before applying the sensor, use an alcohol wipe on the site. The sensor should also be cleansed. Allow the alcohol to dry. *Rationale: Using alcohol ensures that the site is clean and dry. Cleansing the device helps prevent the spread of infection. Alcohol cleans as it dries.*

4. Place the adhesive sensor or finger clip sensor for adults on the client's index, middle, or ring finger. Adhesive sensors also can be placed on a client's toe, unless the client has decreased circulation in the lower extremities. A small earlobe clip is available for use on small adults, children, and infants. If necessary, place the newborn adhesive sensor on the baby's toe. *Rationale: Appropriate location ensures accurate reading.*

5. With any doubts about the chosen site, check the client's proximal pulse and capillary refill. Check capillary refill by pressing on the client's skin. Normal color should return immediately when pressure is released. *Rationale: Decreased circulation could skew oxygen saturation readings.*

6. Check the sensor's markings to make sure the light-emitting diode and photo detector are correctly aligned; they should be opposite each other. *Rationale: If the sensors are not aligned, the sensor will give an inaccurate reading.*

7. Attach the sensor to the client cable and turn it on. The digital readout or light bar should show readings and alarm settings. The type will depend

on the specific monitor being used. *Rationale: A readout or light bar indicates that the machine is working.*

8. Obtain a one-time reading or keep the sensor in place and the monitor on continuous monitoring status, if ordered. If continuous monitoring is ordered, always make sure the alarms are on before leaving the client. The monitors have preset limits that can be changed, per provider's order or facility policy. (If the monitor is turned off, the alarm limits will default to the original settings.) The continuous pulse oximeter gives audible and visual alarms. The audible alarm can be silenced for 60 s at a time by pressing "audio alarm off." Most monitors will reset after 60 s. *Rationale: Setting the alarms ensures notification of the nurse if the client's values are out of the desired range, indicating a possible problem that requires intervention.*

9. Move an adhesive sensor every 4 hr and a clip-type sensor at least every 2 hr. Watch for signs of tissue breakdown or irritation from adhesives or clips. *Rationale: Moving the sensor helps to prevent tissue irritation and necrosis.*

10. Cleanse the sensor with an alcohol wipe when it is removed.

Follow ENDDD steps

Special Reminder

- *Documentation includes* each oximeter reading and location of the sensor (e.g., "O_2 sat 97%"). If the client is not receiving oxygen, the reading is documented "on room air." Document if the client is receiving supplemental oxygen and, if so, how much (e.g., O_2 @ 3 **LPM**—liters per minute). Report any downward changes in oxygen saturation of 3%–5%. The provider may order supplemental oxygen if O_2 saturation is too low.

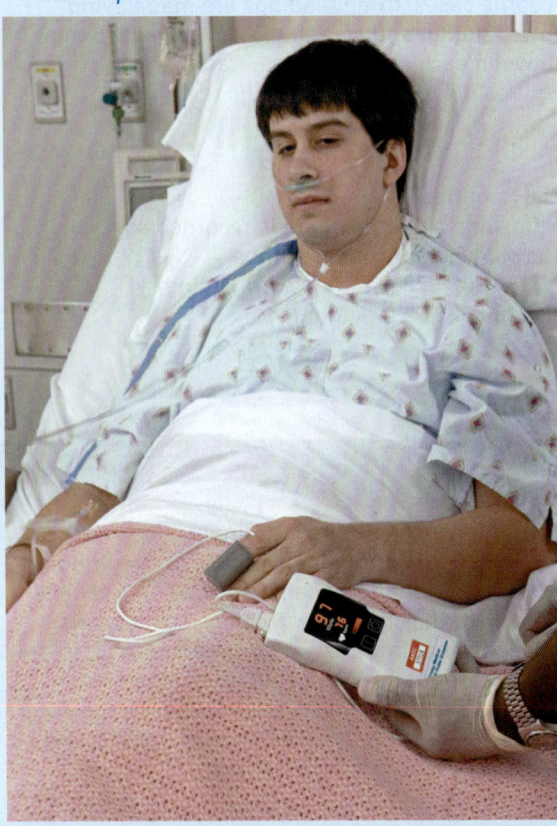

A portable pulse oximeter is used to determine the client's state of oxygenation. Connect the sensor probe to the oximeter unit. Make sure it turns on. The transducer sensor is placed on the client's finger. A toe or the earlobe may also be used. The top reading is the oxygen saturation as a percentage (97% oxygenation). The bottom reading is the client's pulse rate (76). (Carter, 2005.)

47 Data Collection in Client Care

Learning Objectives

1. Explain the role of the practical/vocational nurse in data collection.
2. Identify common risk factors for disease and illness.
3. Define and differentiate between acute and chronic, and between primary and secondary illnesses.
4. Describe the effects of inflammation and infection on the body.
5. State the rationale for obtaining a metabolic panel (profile), UA, CBC, UTox, or UPT.
6. List four types of tests and procedures that primary healthcare providers use to establish a medical diagnosis. Describe the information each test contributes to the medical diagnosis.
7. Discuss the purpose of the physical examination done by the primary healthcare provider and supporting data collected about the client by the registered or practical/vocational nurse.
8. Describe common examination techniques: observation, inspection, palpation, percussion, and auscultation. In the skills laboratory, demonstrate each technique.
9. Describe common formats used to organize the physical examination.
10. In the skills laboratory, perform a daily client data collection on sample client, distinguishing between normal and abnormal findings.
11. Recognize and describe common deviations from normal body structure and function, as described and illustrated in this chapter and throughout this book.
12. Discuss the importance of client and family teaching during the entire healthcare process.

Important Terminology

abscess, accommodation, acuity, acute disease, anasarca, auscultation, biopsy, chronic disease, cognitive function, complication, conjunctivitis, crackle, diplopia, dysphasia, ecchymosis, emaciation, endoscope, erythema, exudate, fistula, granulation tissue, guaiac, hemoccult, hemorrhage, herniation, Homans sign, induration, infection, inflammation, inspection, keloid, kyphosis, lordosis, macule, malaise, necrosis, nodule, observation, pain, pallor, palpation, papule, percussion, primary disease, purulent, pustule, rales, rhonchi, risk factor, scoliosis, secondary disease, sequela, serosanguineous, serous, sign, slough, spirometry, strabismus, striae, stridor, suppuration, symptom, thrombophlebitis, tumor, turgor, ulcer, vesicle, wheal, wheeze, wound sinus

Acronyms

ABG, BMD, CAM, CBC, CMG, C&S, CT/CAT, E-CAT, ECG, EEG, EKG, EMG, ENG, ERCP, IVP, KUB, LOC, LP, MRI, O&P, PERRLA + C, PET, PFT, PSA, SPECT, SXA, T&X, TST, UA, UPP, UPT, US, UTox

---

The process of collecting data about the client's condition, combined with the physical examination, identifies and clarifies a client's health status. It identifies health problems the client may be experiencing. When collecting health data about the client, it is important to consider the client's general state of health, specific risk factors, deviations from normal body structure and/or function, and changes since the last examination. (The client and family are the primary resources for much of this information.) In addition, it is important to consider the client's understanding of the healthcare system and previous experience, ability to cooperate with testing and examinations, and the client's ethnic and cultural background, as well as the client's age and developmental status. The nurse must also understand specific procedures and tests used to establish medical and nursing diagnoses. All healthcare providers must be able to distinguish between abnormal and normal physical findings. The mnemonic COLDSPA can help the nurse remember important data that need to be collected (Box 47-1). An organized format of data collection ensures thoroughness. It is also important to use correct language to describe findings, so all members of the team will understand.

MEDICAL AND NURSING DIAGNOSIS

It is important to understand the roles of all healthcare providers in data collection and diagnosis. Remember the distinction between medical diagnosis and nursing diagnosis, as discussed in Chapter 35.

> **Box 47-1 The COLDSPA Mnemonic**
>
> **COLDSPA**
> **CHARACTER:** Describe the sign or symptom. How does it feel, look, sound, smell?
> **ONSET:** When did it begin?
> **LOCATION:** Where is it? Can you identify a specific location? Does it radiate?
> **DURATION:** How long does it last? Does it recur?
> **SEVERITY:** How bad is it? Can you rate it on a scale of 1–10?
> **PATTERN:** What makes it better? What makes it worse?
> **ASSOCIATED FACTORS:** What other symptoms occur with it?

Medical Diagnosis

The *medical diagnosis* is determined by a primary healthcare provider—a person such as a physician, osteopathic physician, or advance practice nurse. The medical diagnosis emphasizes the disease process and includes identification of the specific disease or disorder, as well as an estimation of the course and outcome of the disease (*prognosis*). A diagnosis of *pneumonia* is a medical diagnosis. The medical diagnosis is based on both *objective* observations and *subjective* data. In the procedures in this chapter, the role of the nurse is to assist in this process by gathering as much information as possible about the client and their problems and by assisting the primary healthcare provider to collect additional data. Data gathered by nurses, in combination with the physical examination and specific diagnostic tests, assist the primary healthcare provider to formulate the medical diagnosis. The nurse needs a basic understanding of data collection and examination procedures to collaborate effectively in this process.

The Nursing History and Nursing Diagnosis

As discussed in Chapter 34, the initial *nursing history* is the interview in which the nurse asks questions and observes the client. This helps the nurse to obtain the client's understanding and perspective on their state of health and illness and is combined with what the nurse observes. The licensed practical nurse or licensed vocational nurse (LVN/LPN) assists in much of the data collection. The collection of specific physical findings about the client is another component required to formulate a nursing diagnosis. The interview and examination of the client assist all members of the healthcare team to make both medical and nursing diagnoses and develop and implement an effective total plan of care.

Once the nursing history and accompanying data collection have been completed, the nursing diagnosis can be formulated by the nursing team, under the direction of the registered nurse. The LVN/LPN is an integral member of this team. The *nursing diagnosis* focuses on the person and their needs in response to the disease, rather than on the disease itself. A nursing diagnosis is the concise problem-centered description of actual or potential health problems based on the nursing process and stated in terms of nursing diagnoses. Therefore, nursing diagnoses for the person with pneumonia might be "Ineffective *Airway Clearance*" and/or "Altered *Breathing Pattern*" because the person is coughing and needs assistance in breathing.

The Nursing Care Plan and Data Collection

Unit 6 describes how the *nursing care plan* is formulated, based on the nursing diagnosis. All members of the healthcare team participate in carrying out this plan. Data collection is ongoing throughout the client's contact with the healthcare system. Each time a healthcare worker contacts a client, data are collected. For example, as the nurse assists a woman to move from bed to chair, the nurse evaluates how the client is breathing, whether they are moving more or less stiffly than the day before, how much they are able to do for themselves, and whether they appear to be in pain. This information is documented in clear language that will be easily understood. Learning to assess breathing, movement, and pain and knowing accurate terms with which to describe these observations can be more readily done if the nurse understands the format and techniques of a systematic physical examination.

> *Key Concept*
>
> Remember to determine if clients use complementary and alternative medicine (**CAM**) treatments, such as vitamins, herbs, acupuncture, homeopathic remedies, or chiropractic care. Some forms of CAM have been proven to be helpful and safe; others pose serious health risks to the individual when used after self-diagnosis. In addition, some herbal supplements have negative interactions with prescribed medications (see Boxes 62-1 and 62-2). Some alternative treatments may cause harm or may mask symptoms, so timely medical treatment is not obtained. Remember to be accurate, but not judgmental when discussing CAM therapies.

FACTORS THAT INFLUENCE DATA COLLECTION

Many factors influence disease and the body's response to disease. Different people react in different ways to physical and emotional disorders. In addition, cultural and ethnic factors influence how an individual might respond to a disease process or its treatment.

Risk Factors for Disease and Illness

Chapter 6 discusses disease and illness in more detail. Some individuals are more susceptible to illness than others. They may have predisposing physical and emotional conditions, genetic predisposition, or lifestyle practices that increase the likelihood of developing a certain disease or disorder. These are called **risk factors**. Table 47-1 lists common risk factors with examples of diseases that may occur as a result of these risk factors. As part of the nursing history, the nurse asks the client if any of these risk factors are present.

TABLE 47-1 Risk Factors for Disease

RISK FACTOR	EXAMPLE/EXPLANATION	EXAMPLES OF POSSIBLE DISEASE OR DISORDER
Diet	Excess intake of fatty foods	Cholecystitis (inflammation of the gallbladder); weight gain, increased cholesterol and triglycerides
	Excess intake of sodium (salt)	Increased incidence of hypertension; edema and/or water retention
	Lack of vitamin C	Scurvy, slow wound healing
	Low intake of protein	Poor wound healing, breakdown of muscle tissue
	Low intake of calcium	Demineralization of bones, increased incidence of osteoporosis and/or fractures
Immobility, lack of exercise	Leg/arm immobilized in a cast secondary to fracture	Atrophy (tissue wasting) of muscles, decreased functionality
	Individual confined to bed rest	Increased incidence of pneumonia, constipation, thrombophlebitis, weight gain; pressure wounds on bony prominences
Age	Toddler	Accidental poisoning, swallowing of foreign objects, other accidents, drowning in toilet or bathtub
	Older adult	Chronic constipation; risk of falling, increased risk of fractures; increased incidence of chemical dependency, accidental overdose; enlarged prostate and/or sexual dysfunction, cataracts; osteoporosis; overweight and underweight; hearing and vision difficulties; depression and suicide; loss of satisfying relationships; financial difficulties
	Young adult	Auto accidents, drug abuse, unsafe sex, eating disorders, depression and suicide
Obesity	Decreased ability to perform usual physical activities	Shortness of breath, muscle atrophy (wasting); increased incidence of hypertension, diabetes mellitus, accidental injuries, coronary artery disease, certain cancers, gallbladder disease, sexual dysfunction
Smoking and use of smokeless tobacco	Constant irritation of lung tissue from smoke; systemic effects of nicotine; irritation of throat and mouth	Cancer of the mouth, larynx, bronchi, or lung; peripheral vascular disease; coronary artery disease, hypertension, chronic obstructive pulmonary disease (COPD; emphysema)
Excessive use of alcohol and other drugs	Predisposition to family and personal difficulties	Liver disorders, dysfunctional family and employment relationships, auto and other accidents, poor nutritional status, depression, coexisting drug abuse, risk of suicide, death
Heredity	Genetically transmitted disorders or predisposition	Coronary artery disease, diabetes mellitus, hypertension, hemophilia, sickle cell disease, Huntington disease
Race	Disorders specific to certain racial groups	Sickle cell disease, Tay-Sachs disease

Course of the Disease

An **acute disease** develops suddenly and runs its course in days or weeks. A **chronic disease** may continue for months, years, or life. **Acuity** refers to a disorder's level of severity. A **complication** is an unexpected event in the disease's course that often delays the client's recovery. Complications may occur at early, continuing, late, or terminal stages of a disease. A disease or injury may also be described as independent (*primary*) or dependent (*secondary*). A **primary disease** occurs independently (by itself), such as a streptococcal sore throat. A **secondary disease** directly results from, or depends on, another disorder. This is also known as a **sequela** (plural: sequelae). An example is rheumatic heart disease, secondary to rheumatic fever. Both of these conditions are secondary (*sequelae*) to a streptococcal infection in the throat and/or tonsils.

The Body's Response to Disease

When gathering data about a client, the examiner looks for evidence of health or illness. **Signs** are *objective evidence* (data) of disease that can be seen or measured, such as a rash, swelling, or change in vital signs. **Symptoms** are *subjective evidence* (data) of disease, sensations that only the client knows and can report, such as pain, itching, nausea, fear, or light-headedness. While collecting data on the client, the examiner looks for evidence of change or abnormalities and asks the client to describe previous signs and symptoms. To gather health data accurately, it is important to understand normal characteristics and use correct examination techniques. While determining objective physical findings in the client, the examiner also needs to ask pertinent questions to gather subjective information from the client. Together, objective and subjective information help clarify the client's

TABLE 47-2 Common Signs and Symptoms of Disease and Illness

SIGN	DEFINITION	SELECTED CAUSES
Anorexia	Loss of appetite; refusal to eat	Infection, gastrointestinal (GI) disorders, mental illness, poor dentition, mouth or throat cancer
Cough	Forceful expiratory effort	Abnormal substances in respiratory tract, noxious irritation to the respiratory mucous membranes, cancer, tuberculosis, allergies
Cyanosis	Bluish discoloration of skin and mucous membranes	Low oxygen levels in the blood, anemia, lung disorders, heart and circulatory disorders
Diarrhea	Frequent, watery stools	GI inflammation or obstruction, medication side effect, fecal impaction, bulimia
Dyspnea	Shortness of breath; difficult or painful breathing	Low blood oxygen levels due to respiratory disease or obstruction, chemical imbalances, pneumonia, lung cancer
Edema	Swelling of tissues; fluid retention	Circulatory disease, local inflammation or infection, malnutrition, electrolyte imbalance, kidney disorders, fluid retention; obesity
Emesis	Vomiting	GI inflammation, infection, or obstruction; irritation of GI lining; electrolyte imbalance; bulimia; medication side effect
Fatigue	Loss of energy	Sleep deprivation, poor nutrition, inflammation, infection, depression, circulatory disorders
Hemorrhage	Abnormal or unexpected bleeding	Trauma or injury to tissues, nutritional losses, blood clotting disorders, high blood pressure, cancers, certain medications and herbal supplements
Jaundice	Yellowish discoloration of skin and mucous membranes	Obstruction of bile pathways due to gallstones, inflammation, tumors; liver disorders
Malaise	Generalized discomfort	Infection, biochemical imbalances, various diseases, emotional difficulties
Pallor	Paleness; loss of normal skin color/tone	Acute or chronic blood loss, nutritional deficiencies (e.g., iron), hypothermia, panic, trauma, anemia
Pyrexia (fever)	Fever; elevated body temperature	Inflammation, infection, brain dysfunction, drug toxicity

health problems. Table 47-2 lists common signs and symptoms of illness and disease, with some possible causes.

Inflammation and Infection

One of the most common health problems is **inflammation** (heat, redness, often accompanied by swelling). Inflammation is the body's response to an injury, irritant, or foreign substance. Inflammation can affect nearly every body tissue, organ, or system. It results when white blood cells rush into an area in an attempt to fight off a foreign body, heal an injury, or prevent an infection from developing or spreading. The suffix *-itis* is used to designate inflammation in a body part (e.g., *appendicitis* is inflammation of the appendix, *cholecystitis* is inflammation of the gallbladder, *tendonitis* is inflammation of a tendon).

Infection is the invasion of cells, tissues, or organs by pathogens. Infection is harmful to the body and may result in inflammation, tissue destruction, tissue or organ dysfunction, or even cellular, tissue, or organ death. Diagnosis of infection is made when microorganisms are identified as present through microscopic examination and culture of tissues or drainage from the site of inflammation. An inflammation or infection may be *local* or *generalized*. A local inflammation or infection is confined to one body part, such as an organ or a limb. A generalized infection affects the entire body. The most common signs of local inflammation are redness, swelling or edema, heat, pain, and loss of function. Inflammation or infection may also be described as *acute*, *subacute*, or *chronic*. If an infection becomes generalized, the person may also experience some feelings of general discomfort, such as headache, fever, loss of appetite, and general **malaise** (an overall feeling of illness). A generalized infection is more likely to be life-threatening than is a localized infection. Generalized *septicemia* is an example of a life-threatening generalized infection.

In *acute inflammation*, an excess of fluid and cells (**exudate**) is usually present in, or oozing from, tissues. A *serous exudate* involves clear drainage from a wound (*serum*). An exudate may be mucoid, such as the discharge from a nasal cold (*coryza*) or *fibrinous*, which causes *adhesions* (abnormal joining of tissues) to form, as tissues are repaired. Bloody (*sanguineous*) exudate is the result of small **hemorrhages** (bleeding) in the area. **Serosanguineous** exudate contains a combination of serum and blood. An exudate described as **purulent** contains pus, caused by the presence of bacteria. (The formation of pus is called **suppuration**.) A collection of pus in a localized area is called an **abscess**. When bacteria grow within an inflammation site, the disorder has become an *infection*, in which pathogens release *toxins* (poisons) that destroy white blood cells and tissues. Tissue death is called **necrosis**. Destroyed tissue may be cast off (**sloughed**, pronounced "sluffed"), leaving behind an area that fills with new tissue (**granulation tissue**). Sometimes, a local unhealed area of epithelial tissue is left, called an **ulcer**. (A healed injury often leaves a *scar*—**keloid**.) A canal or passage leading to an abscess is called a **wound sinus**. An abnormal tube-like passage that connects two internal organs, or connects an internal organ to the surface of the body, is called a **fistula**. A fistula is often difficult to heal, the most common being an anal fistula in the rectal area. Evaluation and treatment of wounds, particularly those caused by pressure, are described in Chapter 58.

Chronic inflammation persists over a long period of time, often for the remainder of the individual's life, and does not follow the usual healing process. A *subacute inflammation* denotes inflammation midway between acute and chronic. The person may appear to be clinically well. However, laboratory tests, radiologic (x-ray) examinations, or computed tomography/computed axial tomography (**CT/CAT**) scans (also called emission-computed axial tomography—**E-CAT** scans) may diagnose the condition. For example, a person may be a carrier of a disease, such as hepatitis, but may not show any outward symptoms of the disease. (An *acute infection* is one that heals and leaves no aftermath or other related disorders [sequelae].)

Pain

Physical **pain** is a subjective symptom reported by the client. It is a feeling of distress, discomfort, or suffering caused by stimulation of specific nerve endings. Pain is usually protective, warning the person that tissues are being damaged. A number of pain rating scales are available to assist in quantifying reported pain. The topic of pain evaluation and its management is so important that its identification and treatment constitutes an entire chapter, Chapter 55, in this book.

Laboratory Tests

Laboratory tests are often done as part of the physical examination, and their results are used in planning the client's care. Some laboratory tests are a routine part of screening; others are specific for certain disorders. Many of these tests are discussed in relationship to disorders of specific body systems throughout the remainder of this book.

Examples of common laboratory tests include urinalysis (**UA**), complete blood count (**CBC**), stool examinations for blood (**guaiac** or **hemoccult**) or for ova and parasites (**O&P**), and blood tests for specific antibodies, electrolytes, chemicals, or abnormal blood components. The prostate-specific antigen (**PSA**) test is done to determine the likelihood of prostate cancer in the male. Tuberculin (purified protein derivative) skin testing (**TST**; **PPD**) screens for

> **Box 47-2 Admission Screening for Tuberculosis (TB) and/or Other Communicable Diseases**
>
> Ask the client if they have:
> - Had a new cough, greater than 2 weeks' duration
> - A chronic cough, which has changed in character
> - A cough associated with symptoms of TB (bloody sputum, unexplained weight loss, lethargy, weakness, night sweats, fever, loss of appetite)
> - Sputum smear positive for acid-fast bacilli
> - Traveled outside of the United States in the past 21 days.
>
> Screening includes TST (tuberculin skin testing, PPD), or blood tests (including interferon gamma release assay), chest x-ray, and careful evaluation of signs/symptoms of TB.
>
> This client is placed in special respiratory isolation until the absence of TB can be established.
>
> If active TB is diagnosed, the client's contacts may need to be treated with special medications.
>
> Adapted from https://www.cdc.gov/tb/default.htm

tuberculosis (Box 47-2). Various metabolic panels or profiles are often done and may include a wide variety of tests, as many as 40+, all done at the same time. Various laboratories have different lists of tests to be included in their basic panel. Other tests may be added, as needed. The panel may include blood and urine samples. Reasons for performing a metabolic panel include the following: to provide a baseline set of values for the client on admission or before surgery, to differentiate mental illness from other disorders, to evaluate clients with total-body situations (e.g., alcoholism or drug toxicity), and to assess a number of organs at once.

Specimens of body fluids may be cultured to isolate pathogens and determine the appropriate medication for treatment: culture and sensitivity (**C&S**). Arterial blood gas (**ABG**) analysis or analysis of a sputum specimen can help determine a client's respiratory status or diagnose a disorder, such as tuberculosis. Specific blood tests can help determine damage to heart (cardiac) muscle and other conditions. The client's blood may be typed and crossmatched (**T&X**) for later blood transfusions. Blood or urine may be tested for levels of various drugs (e.g., *urine toxicology* [**UTox**]) to evaluate situations, such as driving under the influence of alcohol, the amount and identification of a drug used in a suicide attempt, or presence of drugs of abuse. It may be necessary to determine the blood level of a therapeutic drug, in order to adjust dosages. It is common to perform a urine pregnancy test (**UPT**) before prescribing certain medications, because these medications can cause fetal damage. Chapter 52 describes procedures for specimen collection in detail.

> **Key Concept**
>
> If a C&S study is ordered, along with antibiotic therapy, the C&S must be done before antibiotic therapy is started or it will not be valid.

Special Types of Diagnostic Procedures

Many diagnostic procedures are done to determine abnormalities or disorders of various body systems. Preparation of the client and results obtained through many of these examinations are discussed throughout this text. Table 47-3 lists common diagnostic tests for several body systems. Some of these are discussed in more detail below. Table 48-7 illustrates positioning for many diagnostic tests.

> **Key Concept**
>
> It is important to remember that preparation for many diagnostic tests is done by the client at home. Be sure the client and family understand both the goals of the specific test and exactly what preparation is needed. It is vital to obtain the client's cooperation, or testing will not be accurate and diagnostic. Factors that may influence the client's ability to perform an adequate preparation include stress and fear, improper specimen collection, physical and mental disabilities, and communication deficits.

Client and Family Teaching

The nurse must remember at all times that the client and family are important members of the healthcare team. It is vital that they know what is to be done and what to expect. The nurse has the responsibility to teach the client about every procedure and to answer questions before any procedure is done.

> **Key Concept**
>
> It is important for the nurse to realize that medical procedures and terminology are all foreign to the client. It may be difficult to remember how much you have learned during your nursing program. Try to remember how you felt when you first heard medical language or observed medical and laboratory procedures. Explain terms to the client and the family so they can understand and have them repeat back to you. This will help the client to be more comfortable and will improve the accuracy of the test or procedure.

> **NCLEX Alert**
>
> An NCLEX situation commonly incorporates various new educational topics that a client must learn about to improve their health status. These topics are individualized and include areas such as nutritional or dietary concerns, observation of wounds after discharge, or demonstration of self-injection of insulin. Part of these lessons will include putting medical terminology into phrases, examples, or language that is understood by the client. You may be asked to choose the best response that addresses the client's needs for instruction.

Endoscopy

An **endoscope** is a long, slender, flexible tube with a fiberoptic scope (similar to a TV camera) on the end. The provider passes this tube through a body orifice to examine internal body areas. The use of endoscopes can help determine a client's digestive or respiratory structure and function. Specially trained providers examine areas such as the esophagus (*esophagoscopy*), stomach (*gastroscopy*), large intestine (*colonoscopy*), or rectum (*sigmoidoscopy*). A *bronchoscope* is used to examine the trachea, bronchi, and lungs (*bronchoscopy*). Minor surgical procedures, such as polyp removal and biopsy, are often performed via endoscopy. These procedures are minimally invasive, because they do not require an incision. Endoscopy is also used for surgery and tests of internal areas of the body, via a tiny incision. Abdominal surgery is done using the *laparoscope*; joint surgery uses the *arthroscope*. These procedures are invasive, but much less invasive than traditional incisional surgery. Chapter 99 describes ambulatory endoscopic surgery in more detail.

Biopsy

If a growth or body tissue appears questionable, a **biopsy** is performed to determine the presence of cancer or other disorders. The provider obtains a piece of tissue or a small amount of fluid and sends it to a laboratory, where it is examined microscopically. A biopsy specimen may be obtained with an endoscope or needle or by making an incision through the skin. A special syringe or cutting device may also be used to withdraw a specimen. The examiner may obtain a biopsy specimen of a woman's cervix during a pelvic examination.

X-ray and Other Examinations

Many tests not requiring surgery can yield valuable diagnostic information about the status of the body's internal organs and structures. They include x-ray and fluoroscopy examinations of all body areas (e.g., upper and lower gastrointestinal [GI] series, kidney films, or x-ray examinations of bones to determine fractures and other pathology); ultrasonography (ultrasound), CT scan, magnetic resonance imaging (**MRI**), and measurement of brain waves by electroencephalogram (**EEG**). The positron emission tomography (**PET**) scan combines intravenous (IV) administration of radioactive isotopes and the E-CAT scan to image tissues *and their functioning*. (Unlike MRI and CT imaging, the PET scan can provide data regarding body structure and function, as well as biochemical information, such as utilization of fatty acids, glucose, oxygen, and protein. PET imaging can also differentiate between new tumor growth and dead tissue.)

Spirometry and pulmonary function tests help determine a client's respiratory status. Tests such as the electrocardiogram (**ECG/EKG**) and the stress test help evaluate a client's cardiovascular status. These procedures are for the most part noninvasive, requiring no incisions or injections. However, some procedures require a very small incision (a "stab wound") or the injection of dye (*contrast media*). Some dyes are radioactive. Box 47-3 describes necessary precautions when dye is used.

Lumbar Puncture

A lumbar puncture (**LP**), also called a *spinal tap*, may be done to determine the status of the client's nervous system. Lumbar puncture can determine intracranial pressure—ICP (within the head and spinal cord) and the presence of abnormal components, such as blood, pathogens, or pus in the cerebrospinal fluid, or it can be done to inject drugs or spinal anesthesia. Chapter 78 discusses this test in more detail.

Arteriography

An arteriogram is a procedure in which a catheter is inserted into a blood vessel in order to visualize a particular area,

TABLE 47-3 Selected Diagnostic Tests

TYPE OF TEST	PURPOSE	PROCEDURE
Skin Tests		
Biopsy	Identifies tissue abnormalities (often to determine presence of cancer)	Provider surgically removes a portion of tissue, which is examined microscopically
Intradermal test	Identifies client's previous exposure to an allergen; controls may be used to determine if client is anergic (unable to formulate antibodies); test for exposure to tuberculosis	Provider or nurse injects an amount of the allergen intradermally and later examines the area to identify changes in color (e.g., *erythema*—redness) or temperature or the presence and size of *induration* (hardened tissue, lump). Frequently used to test for tuberculosis (tuberculin skin test [TST]) or allergies
Patch or scratch test	Identifies allergies	*Patch:* Filter paper or gauze impregnated with allergen is applied to skin. *Scratch:* Minute amount of allergen is applied to tiny scratch. These tests are read in a manner similar to that used for the intradermal test
Transdermal testing (transdermal iontophoresis)	Used most commonly to diagnose cystic fibrosis; also to monitor drug therapy (e.g., lithium levels), or to detect abnormal concentrations of electrolytes (e.g., sodium), or glucose	Collects substances such as sweat, using a patch on intact skin
Musculoskeletal Tests		
Electromyogram (**EMG**)	Diagnoses conditions such as amyotrophic lateral sclerosis (ALS), poliomyelitis, and other muscle disorders	Measures electrical activity of skeletal muscles. Recordings are obtained while muscles are relaxed, when contracted voluntarily, and when contraction is electrically stimulated
Rectal EMG	Identifies abnormal voiding patterns, dysuria, enuresis, caused by sensory deficits in bladder muscles or sphincters	Identifies bladder sensations (e.g., fullness, bladder capacity)
Radiography (x-ray)	Identifies disorders such as bone fractures. Also used in combination with dyes, radioactive materials, and other equipment to evaluate condition of most internal structures of the body	Film pictures of internal structures—procedure depends on x-ray being done. Often combined with computer analysis
Bone marrow biopsy (aspiration)	Identifies hemolytic blood disorders and certain malignancies; helps evaluate effectiveness of chemotherapy	Specimen of bone marrow is obtained via needle or aspiration
Bone mineral density (**BMD**), bone densitometry. DEXA/DXA, dual-energy absorptiometry; pDXA, peripheral DXA; **SXA**, single-energy x-ray absorptiometry; RA, radiographic absorptiometry	Measures density of bone minerals to diagnose osteoporosis. DEXA/DXA measures spine, hip, and forearm density; pDXA, forearm; SXA, heel and forearm; RA, phalanges	Special radiographic procedures used to evaluate bone strength. Early treatment can be provided to help prevent fractures in osteoporosis
Bone scan	Most often used to detect primary or metastatic cancers in bony tissue	Dye is injected and the total skeleton is visualized, using x-ray and computerization

(Continued)

TABLE 47-3 Selected Diagnostic Tests (Continued)

TYPE OF TEST	PURPOSE	PROCEDURE
Neurologic Tests		
Cerebrospinal fluid analysis—Lumbar puncture (LP) (spinal tap)	Measures pressure of cerebrospinal fluid; collects specimen to determine organisms causing disorders, such as encephalitis, and to measure drug levels and levels of substances, such as chloride, glucose, protein, and to locate tumor markers. Also to inject contrast media, drugs, or spinal anesthetics for spinal block	Client positioned on left side. Hollow needle is introduced into subarachnoid space (lumbar sac) between L4 and L5 (because using this area is least likely to cause injury)
Electroencephalogram (EEG)	Diagnoses disorders such as seizure disorders (epilepsy), brain tumors, or other brain disorders; sleep studies. Also, one of the criteria for establishing brain death (cerebral death). Can measure *evoked potentials* (induced responses) or brain activity at rest	Recording of electrical potentials in different areas of the brain. Electrodes applied to head with gel or needles. May be done with client awake or asleep, depending on purpose
Electroneurography (**ENG**)	Detection of neuromuscular abnormalities; to differentiate between nerve and muscle disorders	Electrodes placed and testing done when at rest and when exercising, to determine disorders such as spinal cord lesions or ALS
Neuropsychiatric testing	Determines level of functioning, ability to care for oneself, presence of intellectual impairment; measures intelligence and ability to learn, presence of some psychiatric disorders; determines ability to think and to reason	Battery of various tests, including intelligence tests, motor tests; tests of reasoning, verbal ability and thought processes; spatial abilities, and personality tests (e.g., Minnesota Multiphasic Personality Inventory [MMPI]) (see Chapter 94)
Sleep studies—sleep-disordered breathing study (SDB)	To determine the presence of sleep apnea (temporary cessation of breathing during sleep) or sleep disordered breathing. To evaluate heart rate and rhythm during sleep. Done preoperatively in bariatric surgery	The client is studied during normal sleeping time. Simultaneous ECG, pulse oximetry, chest wall movement, and oral/nasal airflow are measured. EEG may also be done
Cardiovascular Tests		
Electrocardiogram (ECG) (formerly known as EKG)	Graphically records electrical impulses of cardiac musculature, to identify dysrhythmias or tissue damage	Electrodes attached to client's chest wall and limbs to record electrical impulses within cardiac muscles
Stress testing (exercise test, graded exercise tolerance test, submaximal effort test)	Identifies changes during cardiovascular stress	Client walks on a treadmill or rides stationary bike (ergometer) with ECG, blood pressure (BP), oxygen saturation, and pulse recordings. Recovery stages also recorded. (May also be done by injection of a specific drug, without exercise)
Echocardiogram	Measures heart size and thickness; identifies valve function; measures cardiac output; identifies structural deformities, cardiac lesions, and aneurysms	External probe (Doppler transducer) sends high-frequency sound waves through the chest wall, creating "echoes" that can determine depth and size of tissue. External ECG often done simultaneously
Angiography	Outlines blood flow through cardiac vasculature to identify blockages, deformities, or aneurysms	Small catheter is threaded through a vein or artery into the heart vessels; dye is injected and radiographs are taken
Cardiac catheterization (usually combined with angiography)	Measures pressures within heart chambers to determine muscular strength, valve function, cardiac output, and fluid volume	Catheters are threaded through veins or arteries into heart chambers; catheters have devices to measure pressure. Interior of heart and vessels can be visualized via fiberoptics. Client will be placed in various positions

TABLE 47-3 Selected Diagnostic Tests (Continued)

TYPE OF TEST	PURPOSE	PROCEDURE
MUGA (multigated acquisition) scan	Evaluates ventricular function of the heart at rest and during stress. Contraction and relaxation of the heart can be visualized	A sample of the client's blood is tagged with special material and reinjected. An ECG is run simultaneously with the scanning equipment. All results are combined and computerized, to obtain results
Myocardial perfusion (nuclear medicine scan, cardiac imaging)	To diagnose ischemia of the heart and to differentiate myocardial infarction from other causes of ischemia. To assess effectiveness of coronary artery bypass and angioplasty	Testing is done at rest and under stress. Radioactive material is injected, and **SPECT** (single-photon emission computed tomography) imaging is done
Cardiac flow studies (nuclear medicine scan, cardiac imaging)	To evaluate blood flow through the great vessels and after vessel surgery	Dye is injected, and a computerized camera documents blood flow
Respiratory Tests		
Chest radiograph (x-ray)	Provides images of structures of the chest cavity, particularly lungs and heart; identifies tissue changes, fluid collection, narrowed airways, collapsed alveolar tissue, enlarged heart, tuberculosis; also used to determine deformities of mediastinum, diaphragm, and thyroid gland	A flat-plate radiograph is taken. Dye may be used
Pulmonary function tests (**PFTs**)	Measures lung size and airway patency; identifies lung volumes and airflow and pulmonary disease	Using a spirometer, client takes in maximal inhalation and then exhales forcefully and as rapidly as possible. Room air, helium, or 100% oxygen may be used
Pulse oximetry	Estimates percentage of oxygenated blood flow through a body part (see Nursing Procedure 46-6)	Sensor is attached to the client's finger or earlobe and light is used to determine the amount of oxygen attached to circulating hemoglobin in the blood
Bronchoscopy	Allows direct visualization of the airways to diagnose disorders; foreign bodies may be removed and airway stents placed	Flexible fiberoptic scope with a tiny camera is inserted into airways; an image is projected on a viewing screen. Specimens may be collected for biopsy or culture
Arterial blood gases (ABGs)	Identifies blood levels of oxygen, carbon dioxide, and alkalinity (provides fast evaluation of lung function)	A sample of arterial blood is withdrawn through arterial puncture
Gastrointestinal Tests		
Oral endoscopy	Allows direct visualization of the esophagus, stomach, duodenum; samples taken of gastric fluids and other contents; assesses gastric bleeding	Flexible fiberoptic scope with a tiny camera is inserted into upper GI system through the mouth and projects an image on a screen. Samples may be taken for microscopic analysis or culture
Gastric analysis/tube gastric analysis	Stomach contents are examined for abnormal substances and to determine gastric acidity	Specimens are collected via nasogastric tube
Magnetic resonance imaging (MRI, MR—spatial imaging)	Allows visualization of body tissues through a series of images recorded in layers (can be used in any body area); differentiates between normal and abnormal tissue. Yields detailed sectional images	Client is positioned in scanner; images obtained by superconducting magnet and radio frequencies; contrast media is frequently used. (The machine's noise may be frightening to clients)
Computed (axial) tomography (CT, CAT) scan or emission-computed axial tomography (E-CAT) scan	Used for head, body, or abdomen to assess abnormalities, tumors, aneurysms, and many other disorders. Entire body scan may be done	Client lies on motorized table which moves through the CT gantry (open CT is also available). Contrast media used. Thin beam of x-ray reveals images in layers (not obscured by other structures)

(Continued)

TABLE 47-3 Selected Diagnostic Tests (Continued)

TYPE OF TEST	PURPOSE	PROCEDURE
Endoscopic retrograde cholangiopancreatography (ERCP) and manometry	Provides radiologic visualization of the gallbladder and common bile duct; obtains pressure readings. Evaluates disorders of the entire hepatobiliary system	Combines endoscopy with x-ray imaging, using contrast media
Proctoscopy or colonoscopy	Allows direct visualization of the colon or rectum to identify abnormalities and obtain biopsies; small polyps can be removed	Flexible fiberoptic scope with a tiny camera is inserted into lower GI system through the rectum and projects an image on a viewing screen
Barium enema	Allows x-ray visualization of large intestine	Client is given a retention enema containing barium, a radio-opaque substance. A postevacuation x-ray is often taken
Urologic Tests (Urodynamic Studies) and Tests of Male Genitourinary System		
Uroflowmetry (flow study, urine flow study)	Provides graphic representation of urinary flow (urodynamic studies) to evaluate sphincter competence, voiding problems, or incontinence	Bladder is quite full at start of test. Client voids during test
Cystoscopy/cystourethroscopy	Allows visualization of the lower urinary tract, including the urinary bladder, urethra, ureters, and male prostate gland, via endoscope. Can diagnose malignancies, infections, and bladder/voiding disorders	Scope is inserted through the urethra. Usually, fluid is instilled to distend the bladder. The area is directly visualized through the scope and minor procedures can be performed
Cystometrography, cystometrogram (CMG)	Provides graphic recording of pressures in the bladder during filling and emptying; also measures residual after voiding	Amount of fluid instilled into bladder and client's sensations of fullness and urge to void are recorded and compared with measured pressures
Urinalysis (UA)	Detects presence of bladder/urinary infections, pregnancy, drug use, generalized physical disorders, presence of abnormal components of urine; aids in diagnosis of many disorders, bleeding, fluid retention, or dehydration	Urine sample is obtained and tested in various ways. Culture and sensitivity may be done, to determine best antibiotic to prescribe
Testicular and rectal examination	Aids in diagnosis of male genitourinary (GU) system, such as prostatic hypertrophy, testicular or prostate cancer	Examiner inserts gloved finger into rectum and palpates prostate; external examination of testes; combined with prostate-specific antigen (PSA) blood test and biopsy, to diagnose prostate cancer
Urethral pressure profile (UPP)	Records urethral pressures, to evaluate incontinence and other abnormal voiding patterns	Specially designed catheter, coupled with a transducer, records urethral pressures as it is withdrawn
Cystourethrogram	Diagnosis of voiding abnormalities, including incontinence; visualization of urethra	X-ray contrast medium is instilled into the bladder and various x-rays are taken. Studies also done after catheter is removed, as contrast medium is voided
Intravenous pyelogram (IVP) and KUB (kidney, ureter, bladder) x-rays	To evaluate the anatomy of urinary system structures. Can rule out ascites, organ enlargement, rupture, stone formation, and foreign bodies	KUB is a simple x-ray. For IVP, a contrast medium is injected
Gynecologic Tests		
Pelvic examination	Provides opportunity to assess general condition of vagina, cervix, vaginal secretions; obtain cultures, Pap test for cervical cancer; determines state and stage of pregnancy and progress of labor	Female client placed in lithotomy position; vaginal speculum inserted. Examiner visualizes structures, obtains samples of secretions for laboratory tests or biopsy, or performs procedures, such as conization or cervical biopsy

TABLE 47-3 Selected Diagnostic Tests (Continued)

TYPE OF TEST	PURPOSE	PROCEDURE
Film mammography, xerography (xeroradiography); digital mammography	Allows breast examination to determine presence of cystitis/mastitis, breast tumors, or breast malignancy. Film mammography uses x-rays; digital mammography stores images electronically (areas can be magnified)	Client's breasts are visualized from various angles. Breasts are compressed. Powder and deodorant should not be worn. Digital process often used for very dense breasts
Miscellaneous		
Ultrasonography (**US**)	Allows visualization of many deep body structures by recording the echoes of ultrasonic waves. Used to diagnose disorders of the thyroid, prostate, testicles, breast, gallbladder, kidney, and many other structures. Used to visualize fetus in pregnancy and to place or locate an IUD (intrauterine device) for fertility control	Bladder often full for abdominal and pregnancy examinations. Preparation depends on area of body to be studied. Uses a transducer-gel/cream applied to skin first—transducer moved about on the skin

via fiberoptics. Contrast media may be used, in combination with x-ray. Many areas of the body are examined and treated using arteriography, particularly the heart and large blood vessels. This procedure is often used to place a stent (a device that expands and keeps a vessel open), to perform angioplasty (a procedure to enlarge the lumen of a blood vessel), place tubes or filters, embolize tumors (introduction of a substance to occlude a vessel or obstruct a tumor), or drain an abscess.

Ultrasound Imaging (Sonography)

Ultrasound (very high-frequency sound) is used to examine nearly every structure in the body. Ultrasonic waves are produced by a *transducer*, which creates "echoes." These echoes are directed at body tissues, and some are relayed back to the transducer, depending on their density. The computer converts these echoes to a "picture," used to visualize structures in the body and determine abnormalities (see Fig. 46-12). Ultrasonography is particularly useful in obstetrics, to visualize the fetus and to determine size and diagnose a multiple pregnancy. It is used to diagnose tumors in many areas of the body, including heart and blood vessels, abdominopelvic organs, and eyes. Ultrasonography can visualize kidney stones, gallstones, or bladder stones.

Preparing the Client for Diagnostic Procedures

Clients must completely understand what is to be done. *Informed consent* is required for most procedures. This means that the client has had a full explanation of the test, the reasons for the test, preparation, what to expect during the procedure, and possible adverse effects of the test, before signing the permission form. Clients who know what to expect are likely to be less apprehensive and more relaxed during the examination. Chapter 4 discusses informed consent in more detail.

When assisting with all tests and examinations, follow Standard Precautions to protect yourself, clients, and other healthcare staff. In areas of high radiation exposure (e.g., Radiology Department), *healthcare workers and clients* wear lead shields to protect vital organs from overexposure to radiation. (Radiology staff will give instructions on specific precautions.) Many diagnostic tests are discussed throughout this book in connection with specific body disorders.

> **Key Concept**
> Remember that before and after any interaction with a client, including data collection, it is important to wash or sanitize your hands. This helps prevent the spread of infection. Be sure to carefully document all instruction given and preparations carried out.

Nursing Responsibilities in Diagnostic Examinations

There are many nurse-specific responsibilities before and during special diagnostic examinations. These include assisting the client to maintain NPO (nothing by mouth) status or to eat a special meal before the examination; giving special medications before the examination; and reassuring the client and answering questions. The nurse may transport the client to the area where tests are to be done. Make sure the client's record is up to date before the test; sometimes, a special checklist is used. The nurse assists the client to dress properly (usually in a hospital gown) and assures that the client either voids or does not void before the test, as ordered. The nurse often helps to position and drape the client (see Table 48-1) and may remain during the test. In some cases, frequent vital sign monitoring and other special nursing care is required after the test.

THE PHYSICAL EXAMINATION

The *physical examination* is a tool that healthcare providers use to distinguish between normal and abnormal body structure and function. Each provider, however, has different goals when performing the examination. A primary provider

> **Box 47-3 Precautions When Tests Are Performed Using Dye**
>
> In any procedure in which a dye or contrast medium is used, a skin test may be done first, to determine if the client is sensitive to that dye. Ask if the client is allergic to shellfish or iodine. (If so, notify the healthcare provider immediately. *Many dyes contain iodine or similar chemicals.*)
>
> During, and for about one half hour after the test, be alert for signs of *anaphylaxis* (an exaggerated and life-threatening allergic reaction). Data collection includes noting untoward signs such as:
>
> - Restlessness, apprehension, agitation
> - Weakness
> - Perspiration; cold, clammy skin
> - Tingling sensations, numbness
> - Sneezing, nose itching
> - Rash, generalized pruritus (itching)
> - Watery, itchy eyes
> - Throbbing in the ears
> - Difficult breathing, wheezing, choking sensation, coughing
> - Rapid, thready, or irregular pulse; heart palpitations
> - Lowered blood pressure
> - Swelling or edema
> - Flushed skin
> - Incontinence
> - Seizure or stroke
> - Coma
>
> Usually an anaphylactic reaction involves either respiratory or cardiovascular symptoms but not both. If you observe any of these symptoms, notify the primary provider immediately. Death can result very quickly (within 1–2 min) if the allergy is severe and not treated at once.
>
> In addition, after the use of dye, the nurse should do the following:
>
> - Encourage fluid intake—the client should drink 2–3 L of fluid within the next 24 hr (to help the body excrete the dye).
> - Monitor urine output—report output of less than 30 ml/hr (because the dye can be harmful to the kidneys and may impair kidney function).
> - Report any untoward symptoms or severe client complaints.

will look for abnormalities to establish a medical diagnosis, monitor disease progression, or evaluate changes in the client's condition. This examination may be extensive and thorough, or it may focus on a particular body area. A physical therapist will examine the client's functional abilities and ability to move, develop a therapy plan, and monitor the client's progress. A dentist or dental hygienist will examine only the client's mouth structures. Occupational therapists often determine the client's level of functioning in self-care.

Nurses have several goals when examining clients. The primary purpose is to determine the client's physical status, and to identify potential or actual problems that can be prevented or treated. Because nurses assess physical, emotional, psychological, developmental, and spiritual aspects, data gathered can help determine how a client's physical condition affects overall health and functioning. This information lays the groundwork for nursing diagnosis and then for developing a nursing care plan to meet client needs. The LVN/LPN helps collect data needed to develop the care plan.

If a client complains of physical symptoms, the affected body area is examined for signs that might explain the symptoms. For example, if the client complains of constipation and gas pains, the nurse will inspect and then auscultate (listen to) the abdomen in all four quadrants with a stethoscope. The nurse will also lightly palpate the abdomen, to determine physical clues about the source of the pain. (Deep palpation requires specific training.) Another important purpose of the examination is to evaluate the outcomes of nursing and medical treatments, such as the client's response to medications or physical therapy.

> **Key Concept**
>
> Palpation is done only after inspection and auscultation, to prevent pockets of gas from moving in the intestines and being mistaken for normal bowel sounds.

Because nurses collaborate with other healthcare professionals to provide care, each healthcare worker must report and record continuing assessments promptly, so other providers may act as needed. Carefully documented data about physical findings portrays a picture of the client's condition over time.

The goals of data gathering and physical assessment performed by nurses are to

- Distinguish between normal and abnormal
- Identify potential problems
- Promptly report changes and unusual or abnormal findings to the appropriate person
- Deliver client care within the prescribed scope of practice

In collaboration with the primary provider, nurses examine the client's entire body regularly to determine changes or may focus on a particular body part when the client has a complaint. For example, the nurse may examine only the abdomen when the client complains of constipation.

Examination Abilities and Techniques

Effective oral and written communication skills are essential to successfully interview the client and accurately document findings. Knowledge of the body's normal structure and function (see Unit 4) is crucial, in order to discover abnormal findings. Objectivity ensures that all examiners approach the physical examination without previously set expectations.

The healthcare examiner uses five techniques to find information:

- **Observation**: looking at the client or watching for *general characteristics*, such as overall appearance, skin color, grooming, body posture, gait, mood, interactions with others, and other factors that do not require closer scrutiny or the use of measurement aids (e.g., a stethoscope).
- **Inspection**: careful, close, and detailed visual examination of a body part (Fig. 47-1A).

- **Auscultation**: listening for sounds from within the body, usually with the aid of a stethoscope or an ultrasound (Doppler) (Fig. 47-1B).
- **Palpation**: feeling body tissues or parts with the hands or fingers (Fig. 47-1C).
- **Percussion**: tapping or striking the fingers or a special "percussion hammer" against the body; the resulting sounds indicate the location and density of body tissues or organs. Percussion requires a high level of expertise, developed with experience.

Appendix B lists and describes many descriptive terms used in the documentation of physical findings. Common abbreviations used in documentation are listed in Table 37-4. A list of Joint Commission "Do Not Use" abbreviations appears in Table 37-5.

Examination Tools

Several tools are used during the physical examination. Although the examiner's own eyes, ears, hands, and nose may be the most important tools, the examiner also uses items such as the thermometer, stethoscope, sphygmomanometer, and tongue blade. For example, the client is asked to perform a number of activities to test the function of cranial nerves (see In Practice: Data Gathering in Nursing 47-1).

For more complex examinations, primary care providers use an *ophthalmoscope* (instrument to look at the retinas of the eyes through the pupils), an *otoscope* (instrument to examine the ear canals and eardrum), a *tuning fork* (for checking hearing), and a *reflex hammer* (to test deep tendon reflexes; see In Practice: Nursing Care Guidelines 47-1). A

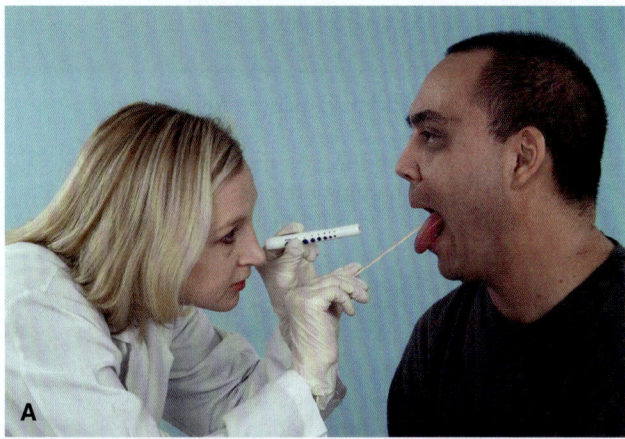
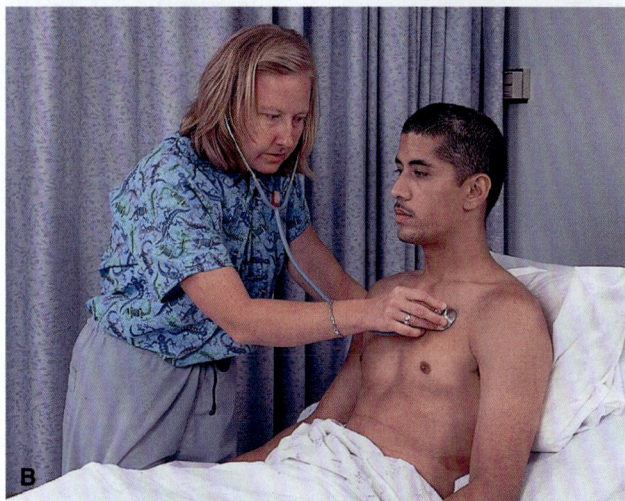
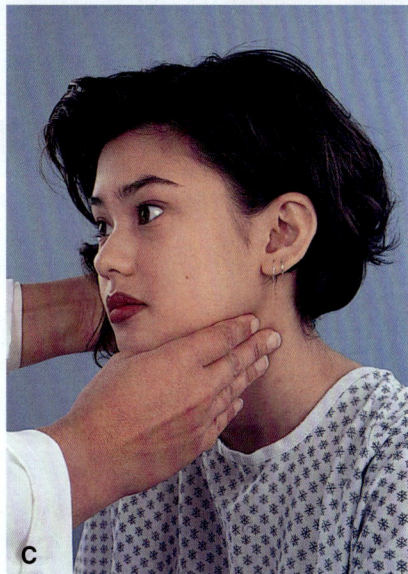

Figure 47-1 Techniques used in data collection. **A.** Inspecting the mouth using a tongue blade and penlight. The nurse wears gloves for this procedure. Note that this penlight contains measurement indicators for pupillary size or PPD readings. **B.** Auscultating the chest using the stethoscope. **C.** Lightly palpating the throat using the fingertips. (A, C: Photos by B. Proud; B: Evans-Smith, 2005.)

IN PRACTICE
DATA GATHERING IN NURSING 47-1 — Gross Functioning of Cranial Nerves

The gross functioning of most of the cranial nerves can be observed by simple actions. For example, the examiner asks the client:

Action	Cranial Nerve Evaluated
To follow a moving finger with the eyes (with or without moving the head)	III Oculomotor IV Trochlear VI Abducens
To move or clench the jaw	V Mandibular branch of the trigeminal
To smile or make a funny face	VII Facial
To stand with the eyes closed	VIII Vestibular division of the vestibulocochlear
To swallow	IX Glossopharyngeal
To shrug the shoulders and turn the head	XI Accessory
To stick out the tongue and move it from side to side	XII Hypoglossal

UNIT 8 Client Care

IN PRACTICE
NURSING CARE GUIDELINES 47-1 — Measuring Reflexes

Some reflexes can be observed because they occur spontaneously, such as automatic constriction of the pupil when a light is shined into the eye. Other reflexes must be specifically elicited.

To elicit deep tendon reflexes:

1. A reflex hammer is used in adults; a finger will work well to elicit most infant reflexes.
2. The hammer is held between thumb and index finger.
3. Extremity is positioned so the tendon is slightly stretched.
4. The client is asked to relax. (May require distraction techniques, to assist the client to relax.)
5. Tendon is struck briskly, using a full swinging motion.
6. This is repeated on the other side of the body.
7. Results from both sides are compared.
8. Normally, reflexes should be the same on both sides.
9. Reflexes are graded on a scale from 0 to 4+. A reflex graded 2+ is considered normal. Above this, reflexes are considered *hyperactive* (very brisk). Below this level, they are considered *hypoactive* (weak) or *absent* (written as "0").
10. All findings are documented.
11. The appropriate person is notified of abnormal findings or a change from previous readings.

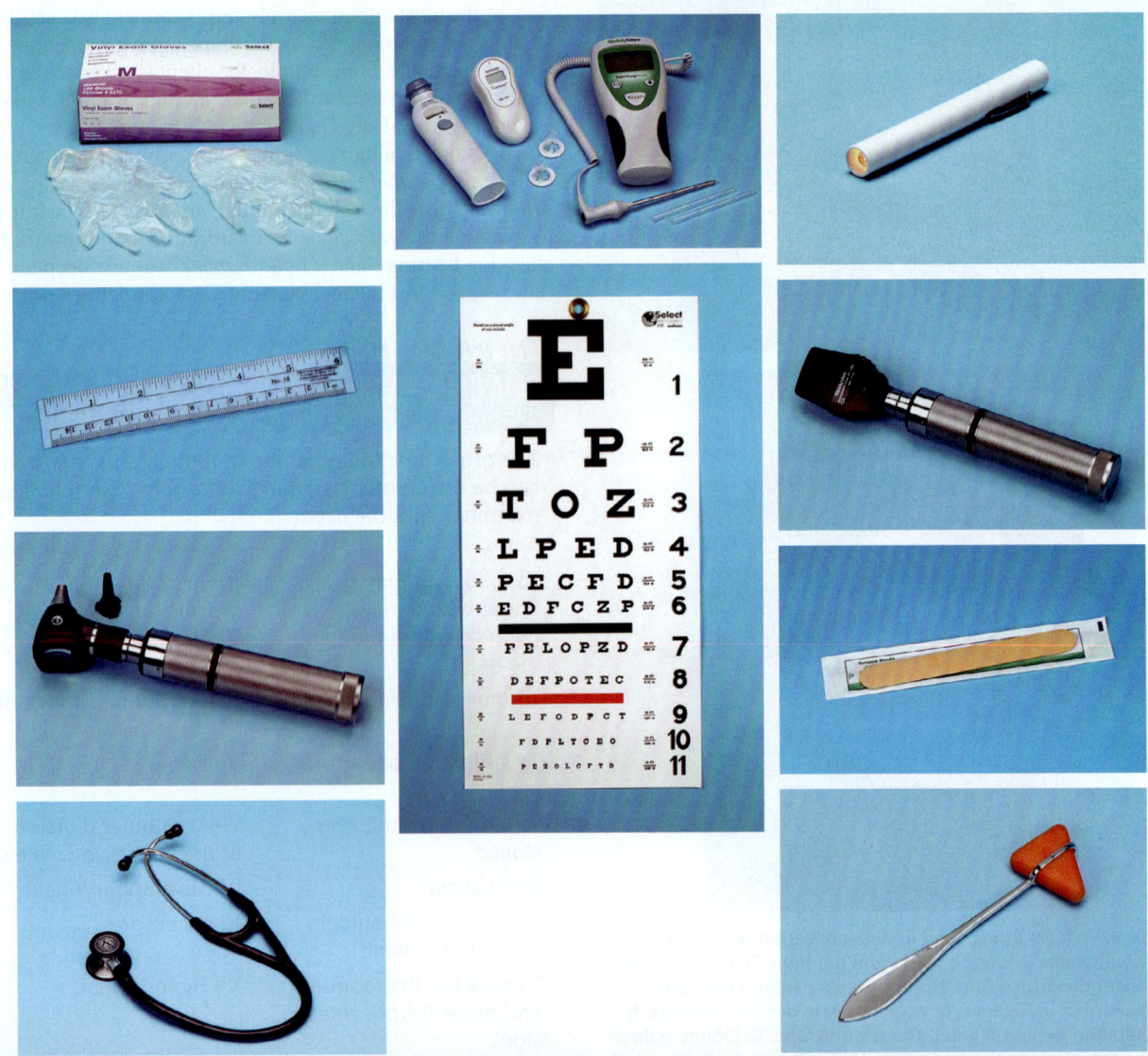

Figure 47-2 Basic equipment and supplies used for physical examination and data gathering. Clockwise, from bottom left: stethoscope (auscultation), otoscope (ear visualization), metric ruler, gloves, thermometers, penlight, ophthalmoscope (eye visualization), tongue blade, percussion hammer (eliciting reflexes); Snellen eye chart in center. (Weber, 2014.)

vaginal speculum and a *nasal speculum* are other instruments used for specialized examinations. Primary care providers may also use some type of device to test the tactile senses of sharp, soft, hot, or cold and use substances to test smell and taste. Figure 47-2 shows several instruments used in physical examinations.

Examination Format

A common format for the physical examination is the *head-to-toe method*. It begins with a general appearance examination, then moves to the head, and proceeds to the neck, chest, breasts, abdomen, arms, legs, back, and perineum. As the examiner moves to each area, the focus is not only on the *structures*, but also on the *functions* of these body areas. The head-to-toe method flows smoothly and provides the examiner with a mental road map of directions to follow while conducting the examination. The other common format used in the physical examination is similar to the head-to-toe but focuses instead on *body systems* (e.g., musculoskeletal, nervous, cardiovascular, respiratory, digestive). (This textbook is organized in relationship to body systems.)

A variation of this format is the *focused physical examination*, in which one body system is thoroughly examined because the client has a particular complaint or problem in that area. For example, the client admitted to the Emergency Department complaining of chest pain and severe shortness of breath will have a focused cardiovascular and respiratory examination. The examination of a pregnant woman will focus on her pregnancy and fetus. Table 47-4 compares the techniques.

Each examiner develops an examination method that is thorough but brief, accurate, and easy to use. When techniques are correct, findings agree among healthcare providers. The primary provider is expected to interpret the findings, based on data collected by all members of the team. As the nurse's expertise and knowledge grow, an understanding of the meaning of these findings will develop. Some healthcare agencies require all nurses to use the same method of data collection and provide documentation data sheets or electronic pages for recording these findings.

TABLE 47-4 Sequence of Major Methods of Physical Examination

ADULT HEAD-TO-TOE	INFANT AND CHILDREN HEAD-TO-TOE	SYSTEMS APPROACH
General survey	General survey	General survey
Vital signs	Vital signs	Integumentary system
Hair, scalp, cranium, face	Weight	Fluid and electrolyte balance
Eyes and vision	Skin	Musculoskeletal system
Ears and hearing	Heart sounds	Head and neck
Oral cavity	Lung sounds	Extremities
Cranial nerves	Head, scalp, cranium (including measurements)	Nervous system
Thyroid gland	Eyes	Endocrine system
Neck veins and nodes	Oral cavity	Sensory system
Upper extremities	Neck	Cardiovascular system
Nails	Ears	Immune system
Breasts	Musculoskeletal system and reflexes	Respiratory system
Precordium (heart and upper thorax)	Upper extremities	Digestive system
Anterior thorax	Chest and back	Urinary system
Abdomen	Abdomen	Reproductive system
Back	External genitals	
Internal and pelvis	Lower extremities	
Anus and rectum		
Lower extremities		

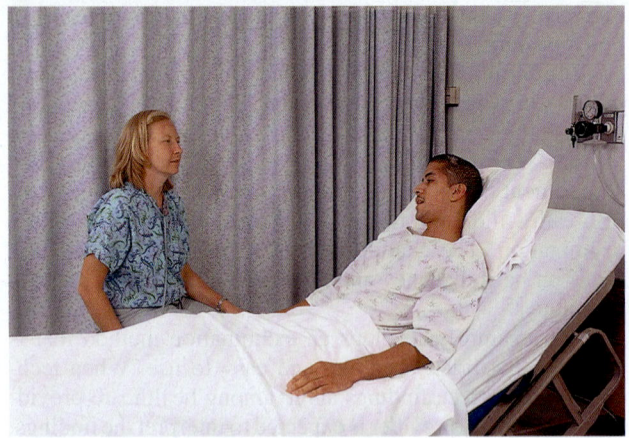

Figure 47-3 To begin the process of data collection, introduce yourself and explain what you are about to do and why. Continue to explain before each part of the examination. This helps alleviate anxiety and makes the client more comfortable. (Photo by B. Proud.)

Preparing for the Physical Examination

Before any examination, it is necessary to explain the purpose of it to the client (Fig. 47-3), answer questions, and provide privacy for the client. Ask the client to empty the bladder or bowel if necessary. (See Table 48-1 for examination positions.) Guidelines for performing the head-to-toe data collection of an adult and special considerations for the child can be found at the end of this chapter.

Care of the Client Following Any Examination or Testing

It is important to make the client comfortable following any test. Answer questions, ensure client safety, and follow agency protocols for posttest care. Tell the client when results may be available and be sure to follow up and ensure this information is given to the client. Carefully document any procedures that have been done and the client's response. Report any untoward responses immediately.

> **NCLEX Alert**
>
> Observation is one of the most important aspects of nursing. You must be able to detect any difference(s) between a client's normal physical and mental condition and any aspects that signify change (or abnormal) conditions. Some changes you observe may indicate improvement in the client's health status. The NCLEX scenario can describe a clinical situation, and you must be able to discern what observation, if anything, needs to be addressed by a *nursing* action.

DATA COLLECTION IN NURSING

Following are basic guidelines for data collection. These guidelines are not intended to teach the performance of a comprehensive physical examination.

General Examination—Observe overall body appearance.

Action/Rationale	Normal Findings	Changes From Normal
Introduce yourself to the client and explain what will be done (see Fig. 47-3). *(Not all procedures will be performed daily.)*		
Observe client for signs of distress. *(Alert the primary healthcare provider to immediate concerns. If serious distress is noted, the client may require healthcare interventions before the examination is continued.)* (See Chapter 45.)		The client shows labored breathing, wheezing, coughing, wincing, sweating, guarding of body part (suggests pain), nausea and/or vomiting, crying, anxious facial expression, or fidgety movements (see Chapter 86).
Note client's general appearance: posture, gait (manner of walking), and movement. *(Identify obvious changes.)*	Posture is upright. Gait is smooth and equal for the client's age and development. Limb movements are bilateral.	Posture is stooped or twisted. Limb movements are uneven or unilateral. Client is limping.
Observe client's facial expression. *(Facial expression suggests mood and mental status and pain.)*	Eyes are alert and in contact with the examiner, *as is culturally appropriate.* The client smiles or frowns appropriately and has a calm demeanor. The client is able to converse easily. Offer the client an interpreter and follow appropriate guidelines.	Eyes are closed or averted. (Consider cultural variances.) The client is frowning or grimacing. They are unable or unwilling to answer questions, avoids answering, or is fidgety, and appears anxious. Note if the client does not speak English. (See Chapter 44.)
Observe the client's general height/weight correlation. Measure height and weight if performing an admission examination (Fig. 47-4). *(Height/weight indicates nutritional status.)* (See Chapter 45 for height and weight procedures.)	Height and weight are in balance.	Obesity, **emaciation** (physical wasting of tissues), or uneven fat distribution over the client's trunk is observed. Client reports significant *unintentional* weight gain or loss in short time.
Evaluate grooming, hygiene, and dress. *(Personal appearance can indicate self-comfort. The client's grooming status may suggest their ability to perform self-care. The client may have family caregivers who can assist.)*	Clothing reflects gender, age, and climate. Hair, skin, and clothing are clean, groomed, and appropriate for the occasion. Body or mouth odor is absent.	The client wears unusual clothing for gender, age, or climate. Hair is unkempt. Excessive oil or perspiration is on the skin. Body odor is present. The client is unable to care for themselves due to factors such as age, mental illness, or intellectual status.
Measure vital signs. May include pulse oximetry. *(Vital signs provide baseline data.)* (See Chapter 46.)	Temperature, pulse, respirations, and blood pressure are within normal limits for the client's age. Oxygen saturation should be at least 94% on room air.	Abnormal findings include fever, hypothermia, dyspnea, tachypnea, orthopnea, tachycardia, bradycardia, dysrhythmia, hypertension, hypotension, postural hypotension, or low oxygen saturation of the blood. (See Chapter 46.)

Skin Observation—Observe integumentary structures (skin, hair, nails) and function.

Action/Rationale	Normal Findings	Changes From Normal
Examine the backs and palms of the client's hands (Fig. 47-5A). Compare right and left sides. Examine feet and toes, comparing right and left sides (Fig. 47-5B). *(Condition of extremities indicates peripheral cardiovascular function.)* (See Chapter 81.)	Hues range from pale white to deep brown, depending on the client's race and ethnicity. Color variations on dark, pigmented skin may be best seen in the mucous membranes, nail beds, sclera, or lips.	**Erythema** (redness), loss of pigmentation (vitiligo), cyanosis, **pallor**, or jaundice is noted (Table 47-5; Fig. 47-6). Abnormal skin color for race is noted.
Palpate skin over the sternum or forehead for moisture and texture. Gently pinch the skin on the forearm or upper chest (Fig. 47-7). *(Palpation and the pinch test indicate the skin's degree of hydration and* **turgor** *[skin resiliency and plumpness].)*	Plump, firm, elastic skin is slightly moist. Pinched skin that promptly or gently returns to position when released signifies normal turgor. (Return to position may be slower in the older person.)	The skin is excessively dry or flaking. Moisture, perspiration (*diaphoresis*), or oiliness is noticeable. Pinched skin is very slow to return to normal position. Slow return of skin to normal position often indicates dryness (dehydration).

(Continued)

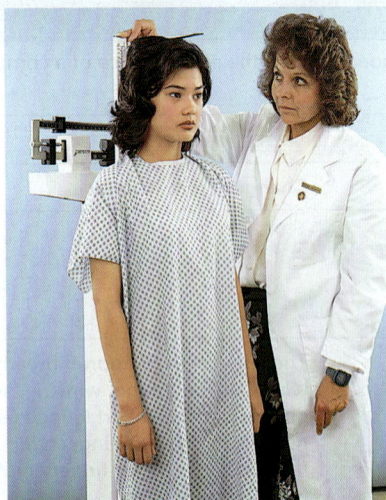

Figure 47-4 Using a balance scale or electronic scale for accurate measurement of weight. Height can be measured at the same time. (See Nursing Care Guidelines 45-2 for use of other types of scales.)

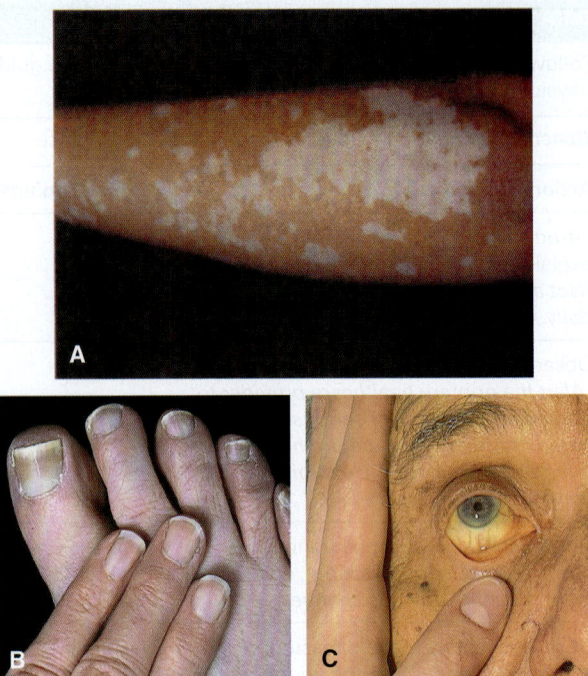

Figure 47-6 A. Loss of pigmentation (vitiligo), most evident in persons of color. **B.** Cyanosis (bluish in white skin; dusky color in dark skin). **C.** Jaundice (most evident in whites of eyes).

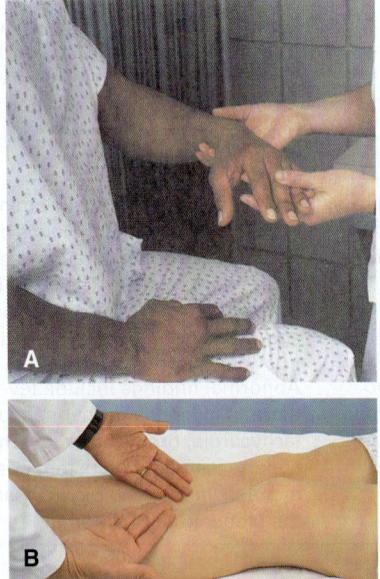

Figure 47-5 Inspection of the skin. **A.** Inspection of the hands and upper arms for skin color and warmth, as well as for any lesions. **B.** Palpation of the skin temperature in the legs and feet. Shown here is *simultaneous bilateral palpation*. B: Photo by B. Proud.

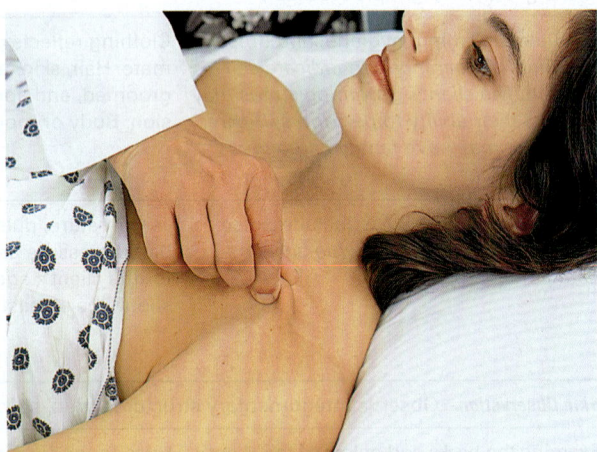

Figure 47-7 Checking skin turgor by pinching a fold of skin, releasing it, and watching the skin return to its natural shape. A slow return suggests loss of usual turgor.

DATA COLLECTION IN NURSING (Continued)

Skin Observation (Continued)

Action/Rationale	Normal Findings	Changes From Normal
Palpate skin temperature with the back of the hand, particularly noting and examining any reddened areas. Compare the client's left and right hands, arms, and feet (Fig. 47-8). *(Comparison indicates the bilateral status of peripheral circulation.)*	Skin is warm to touch; temperature may vary among body parts. Hands and feet may be cooler than head or trunk. Both hands and arms are the same; both legs and feet are the same.	Skin is very cool or warm to touch; reddened skin areas are warmer than other body parts. Extremities are much cooler, particularly the feet and toes. (Often, cool skin is very pale.) Swelling in the ankles, fingers, or over bony prominences, particularly the sacrum, is noted. *(Edema indicates fluid retention, a sign of circulatory disorders. Body prominences are prime sites for skin breakdown. Sacral edema may occur in the bedfast client, with no other edema noted.)* One hand, arm, or foot is noticeably different in temperature or size from the other.
Palpate and inspect for edema. (See Chapter 76.) Press the fingers against suspected edematous areas for 10 s; then, observe the area for indentations (Fig. 47-9).	No edema, no abnormal swelling. Skin and tissue return immediately to original shape (no *pitting* [denting] remains). Skin should resume shape in 2 s.	"Pits" or "dents" remain for >2 s after pressure is released (*pitting edema*); or edema is obviously present, but skin is shiny and hard and does not dent, even when pressed (*nonpitting edema*). Massive generalized edema is known as **anasarca**.
Press the tip of the nail until the flesh under the nail *blanches* (loses color). Release pressure quickly (Fig. 47-10). *(This checks capillary refill, an indicator of peripheral vascular function.)* Inspect nails and surrounding tissues for abnormalities and cleanliness.	Color returns immediately (<3 s) when pressure is released. Nails should have no discoloration, ridges, pitting, thickening, or separation from the base. Nails are clean and even.	Color returns to nail slowly. Client's nails are dirty, broken, or torn. Chewed or torn nails or cuticles. Nails are discolored. *Clubbing* of fingertips (bulb-type shape on ends of fingers) (Fig. 47-11).
Inspect skin for lesions throughout the remainder of the examination. Note appearance, size, and location of lesions, as well as the presence and appearance of any drainage. *(Note abnormal growths or trauma that suggests abnormal physiologic processes.)*	Skin is intact, without reddened areas, but with variations in pigmentation and texture, depending on the area's location and its exposure to light and pressure. (Freckles and moles are normal.) Moles should not change in size or darken in color; hairs may indicate abnormality.	Abnormal findings include *erythema* and **ecchymosis** (bruising or discoloration of the skin). Lesions include rashes, **macules**, **papules**, **vesicles**, **wheals**, **nodules**, **pustules**, **tumors**, warts, or ulcers (Table 47-6; Fig. 47-12). Wounds include incisions, abrasions, lacerations, pressure wounds (see Fig. 58-3).

TABLE 47-5 Skin Color Variations

COLOR	POSSIBLE CAUSE	CHANGES IN DARK-SKINNED PERSON
Redness (erythema)	Dilation of superficial blood vessels due to exposure to heat, increased body temperature, local inflammation, or hypertension.	Skin color darkens; may appear purple. Often, the skin is also warmer than other body areas; compare temperature with another body area.
Gray-blue around mucous membranes, nail beds, lips (cyanosis) (see Fig. 47-6B)	Constriction of superficial blood vessels due to exposure to cold, lowered body temperature; may result from low oxygen levels in blood (hypoxemia) due to heart or respiratory disease. Abnormal hemoglobin levels may be due to genetic disorders.	Color loss appears with tinges of blue or deepened color in mucous membranes of mouth and nail beds. Skin may appear dusky or gray.
Loss of color or pallor	Vasoconstriction due to lower body temperature; shock from loss of blood volume; decreased amount of hemoglobin in blood causing anemia.	Skin appears gray or ashen, particularly on palms or soles or around mouth.
Yellow (jaundice) (see Fig. 47-6C)	Destruction of red blood cells releasing bilirubin into skin; liver or kidney disease.	Sclerae of eyes are yellow; color changes in nail beds or palms.

(Continued)

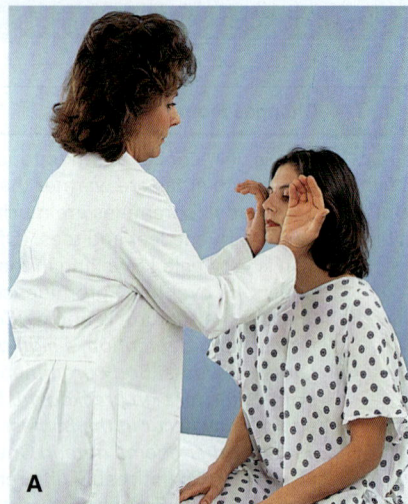

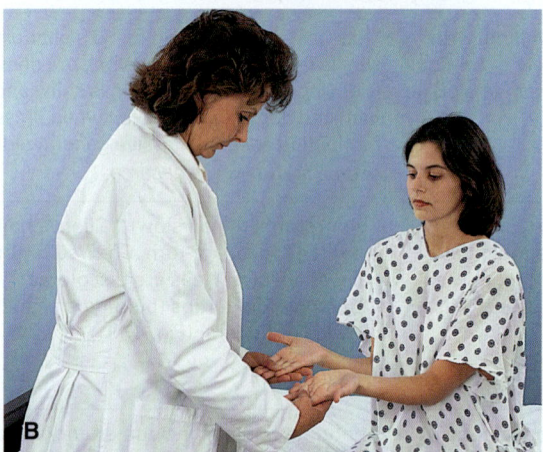

Figure 47-8 **A.** Palpation of the client's skin temperature with the back of the hands. **B.** Comparing the client's palms for bilateral status of peripheral circulation.

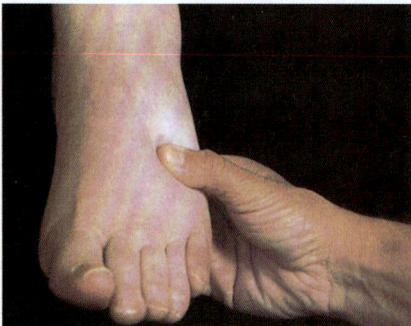

Figure 47-9 The skin over bony areas of the body, such as the feet and ankles, is gently pressed, to determine the presence of edema. In *pitting edema*, a dent will remain after release of pressure.

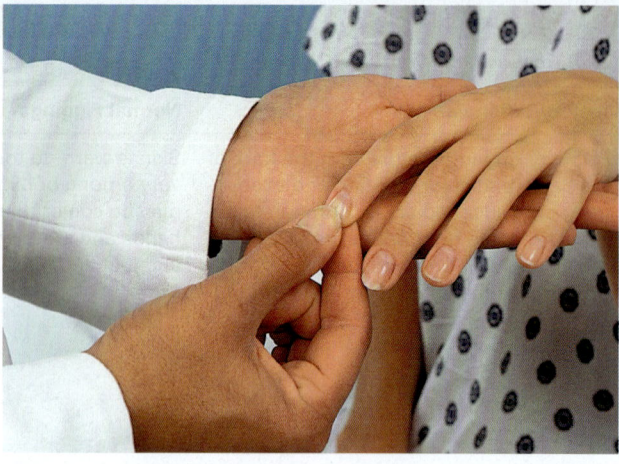

Figure 47-10 Checking capillary refill by pressing against the nail beds, releasing, and monitoring return of color.

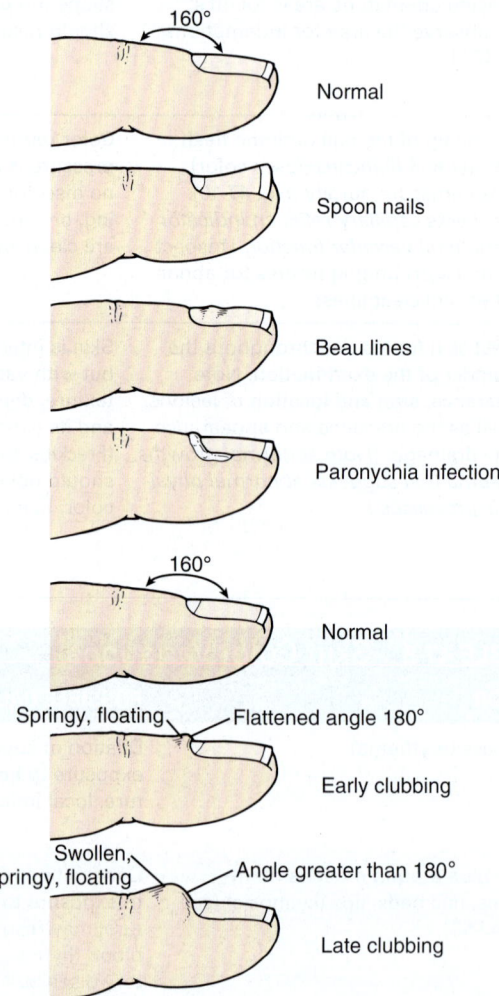

Figure 47-11 Normal and abnormal fingernails.

TABLE 47-6 Primary Skin Lesions

LESION	DESCRIPTION	EXAMPLE
Macule	Small (<1 cm in diameter); well-defined border; flat and nonpalpable on skin surface; no color change	Freckle, liver spots of aging, some skin rashes (Fig. 47-12A)
Papule	Small (<0.5 cm diameter); palpable; elevated solid tissue	Mole, wart (see Fig. 47-12E)
Wheal	Slightly irregular in shape; transient superficial elevated area of localized edema	Hive, insect bite (Fig. 47-12B)
Vesicle	Small (<0.5 cm diameter); well-defined border; elevated cavity filled with serous fluid	Blister, chickenpox, herpes simplex (see Fig. 47-12F)
Pustule	Well-defined border; elevated superficial cavity filled with pus	Acne lesion, impetigo, burn (Fig. 47-12C)
Fissure	Linear crack in skin	Chapped lips, fungal infection, such as athlete's foot (see Fig. 47-12G)
Ulcer	Loss of top layers of skin tissue	Pressure wound; Venous stasis ulcer (Fig. 47-12D)
Nodule	Small (<2 cm diameter); well-defined border; palpable elevated mass	Fatty tumor (lipoma), localized scar tissue, cyst
Tumor	>1–2 cm in diameter; irregular border; palpable elevated mass	Larger lipoma or malignancy

From Weber, J., & Kelley, J. (2018). *Health assessment in nursing* (6th ed.). Wolters Kluwer.

DATA COLLECTION IN NURSING (Continued)

Skin Observation (Continued)

Action/Rationale	Normal Findings	Changes From Normal
For PPD (tuberculin skin testing [TST]) skin tests given 48 or 72 hr previously: **Induration** (swelling) is measured and recorded in millimeters (mm). Redness (erythema) is usually not recorded unless it is unusually large. Consult agency protocols.	There should be no induration after a skin test (indicates a negative reaction).	Exudates from open wounds are present; they may be **serous** (contain clear fluid), purulent (contain pus), sanguineous (bloody), or serosanguineous (contain bloody and serous fluid). Changes in the size or color of moles and warts may be detected as compared with previous examinations. Malignant melanoma (Fig. 47-13) is a life-threatening skin lesion. (See Chapter 75.)
Inspect the hair for texture, uniform growth and distribution, infestation, and scalp lesions (Fig. 47-14). *(Identify abnormalities.)*	Texture varies from fine to coarse; hair should appear glossy with bilateral growth and distribution.	Hair is excessively dry or oily. The client has unilateral or excessive hair loss (alopecia—Fig. 47-15), dull sheen to the hair, excessive scalp scaliness, or raised lesions. There is evidence of lice (*pediculosis*) or another infestation or disorder, such as scabies or eczema.

Head and Neck Data Collection—Check central neurologic function, vision, hearing, and mouth structures.

Observe the face and head for size, shape, and symmetry.	The head is symmetrical, round, and erect in the midline. The eyes, nose, mouth, and ears are approximately symmetrical.	The skull is enlarged or irregularly shaped. Eyes, ears, or mouth are asymmetrical. One side of the face droops or sags abnormally. Unilateral or bilateral eyelid drooping (*ptosis*) seen. The client drools.
Note the client's ability to respond to verbal commands. *Responses indicate the client's speech and* **cognitive function** *(ability to think)*.	The client responds appropriately to commands.	The client has confused, disoriented, or inappropriate responses. The client does not understand the nurse's language or cannot hear. The client does not respond.

(Continued)

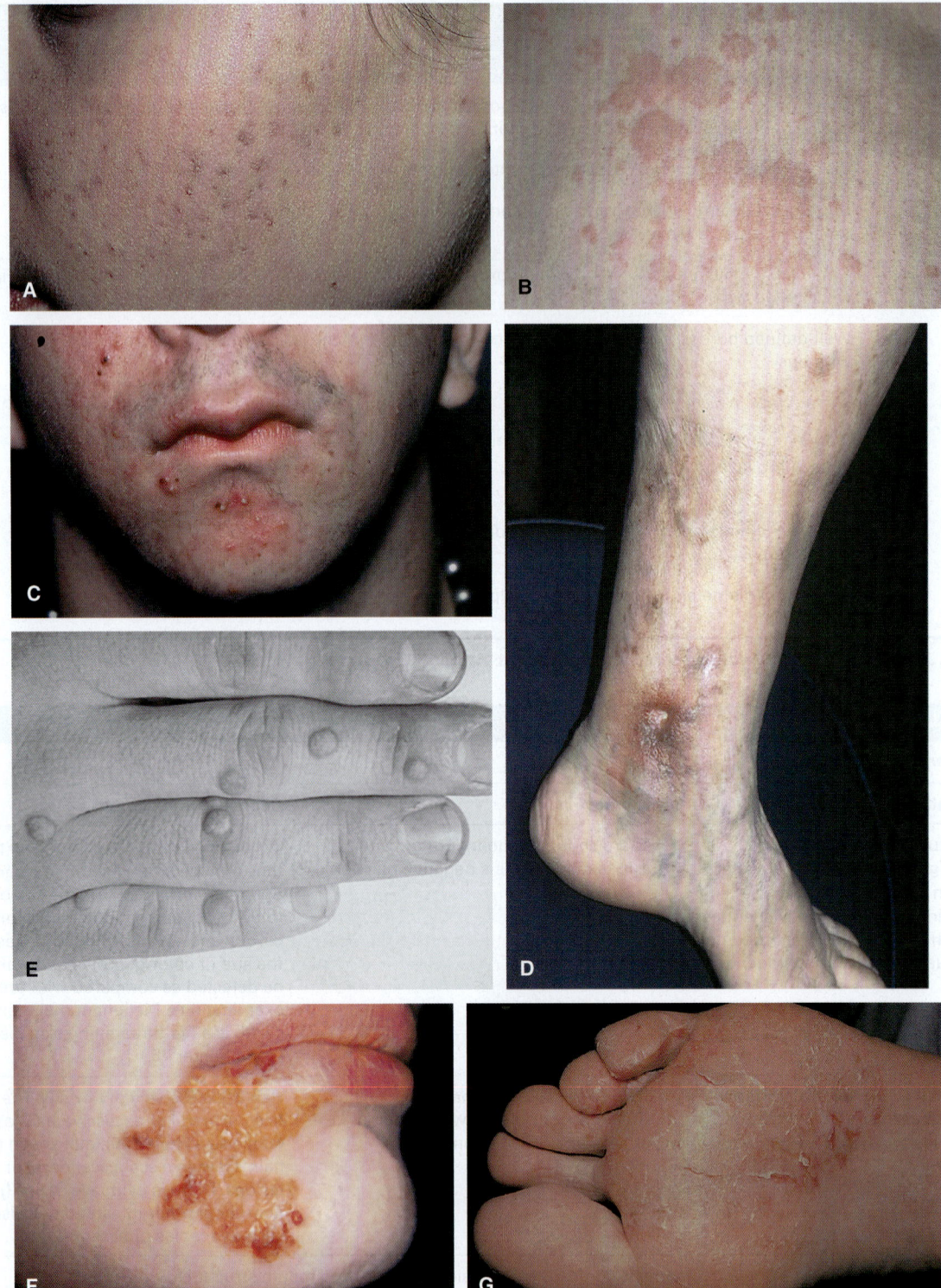

Figure 47-12 There are many different types of skin lesions. **A.** Macules are small, flat, reddened lesions. **B.** Wheals are raised transient lesions that generally last less than 24 hr. **C.** Pustules are vesicles that contain pus, a product of infection. Pustules are characteristic of acne vulgaris, shown here. **D.** An ulcer is an open sore caused when tissue dies. The dead tissue breaks down, leaving a crater behind. The ulcer shown here is a venous stasis ulcer. These ulcers develop as a result of poor blood flow through the veins in the legs. (Goodheart, 2003.) **E.** Warts (a firm papule), usually caused by a virus. Papules can be felt by lightly running the fingers over the area. **F.** Herpes simplex (a vesicle). Vesicles are small blister-like lesions that contain fluid. **G.** Athlete's foot (tinea pedis). A fissure is a crack in the skin, such as those associated with athlete's foot.

DATA COLLECTION IN NURSING (Continued)

Head and Neck Data Collection (Continued)

Action/Rationale	Normal Findings	Changes From Normal
Observe the client's level of consciousness (*LOC*)—degree of wakefulness, stages of response to stimuli; and orientation. Ask the client to state their own name, current location, and the approximate day, month, year, and time of day. Ask who the President of the United States is. (This is orientation to person, place, and surroundings.) *(Responses indicate the client's brain function. LOC is the degree of awareness to environmental stimuli. It varies from full wakefulness and alertness to coma. Orientation is a measure of cognitive function or the ability to think and reason.)* (See also Chapter 43.)	The client is fully awake and alert: eyes are open and follow people or objects. The client is attentive to questions and responds promptly and accurately to commands; they move willingly. If the client has been sleeping, they are easily awakened and responds to verbal or physical stimuli and demonstrates wakefulness and alertness. The client is "*alert and oriented × 4*"—aware of who they are (orientation to *person*), where they are (orientation to *place*), what time it is (orientation to *time*), and who the President is (orientation to *surroundings*).	Client has a lowered LOC and shows irritability, short attention span, or dulled perceptions. Client is uncooperative or unable to follow simple commands or answer simple questions. At a lowered LOC, they may respond to physical stimuli only (e.g., deep pain). The lowest extreme is deep coma, when the eyes are closed and the client fails to respond to verbal or physical stimuli, with no voluntary movements. The Glasgow Coma Scale is often used (see Table 78-2). The client's responses are carefully noted. (See Chapter 78.)
Observe the client's ability to think, remember, process information, follow directions, and communicate. *(These processes indicate cognitive functioning.)*	The client is able to follow commands and repeat and remember information. (The client is able to remember a list of three objects for at least 5 min and state them back to the examiner.) They are able to see and identify objects within the room.	Abnormal findings include **dysphasia** (difficulty in understanding or expressing language), **dysarthria** (inability to speak), memory loss, disorientation, or hallucinations (see Chapter 80). The client demonstrates thought-blocking or speech latency or may be voluntarily mute (as in psychiatry; see Chapter 94).
Observe the client's ability to see, hear, smell, and distinguish tactile sensations. Inspect the eyes, ears, and nose and check for symmetry and intactness. Special hearing and vision tests may be performed by the primary provider. *(These tests indicate the functional status of the client's vision, hearing, smell, and tactile sensation.)* Tests for color blindness, visual fields, or peripheral vision may be done.	The client can hear even though the speaker turns away. They identify objects or reads a clock in the room, and distinguishes between sharp and soft objects. The eyes are moist and symmetrical; the lids open and close together and on command. The client is able to see things moving to the side of the head (peripheral vision).	The client cannot hear low or very high tones and/or must look directly at the speaker to distinguish what is being said. They cannot read a clock or distinguish sharp from soft. Redness or swelling appears around the eyelids or eyes. Excessive tears, exudate (abnormal drainage from eyes or ears), or **conjunctivitis** (redness of eyes) is present. The eyelids itch. (See Chapter 80.)
Inspect the pupils to compare for size, shape, response to light, and ability to focus (*accommodation*) (Fig. 47-16). Check eye coordination (eyes moving together). *(Pupillary size, shape, and accommodation are indicators of the status of brain function and intracranial pressure. Coordination of eye movements indicates brain function and muscular attachments to eyes.)*	Pupils are equal, round, and responsive to light (pupils reduce size quickly when light is shined into them); client able to see objects both near and far away (*accommodation*). Eyes move together to view objects (*coordination*). This examination is abbreviated as **PERRLA + C** PE: pupils equal R: round RL: respond to light A: accommodation ok C: coordinated (move together)	Pupils are unequal and/or unresponsive or sluggishly responsive to light. **Strabismus** ("cross-eyes" or "wall-eyes") present, or eye movements asymmetrical. Client reports **diplopia** (double vision) or blurring of vision. Eyelids are drooping (*ptosis*) or have asymmetrical movements.
Ask the client to open the mouth and say "aah." With gloved hands, insert a tongue blade to open the lips and inspect the inside of the mouth. Check the lips, mouth, teeth, gums, and tongue (Fig. 47-17). *(Identify abnormalities of these structures.)*	Lips are smooth. Oral mucous membranes are pink, moist, and smooth. Teeth are firm, intact, and clean. The tongue is pink, moist, and symmetrical.	Lips are dry and cracked. Mucous membranes show abnormal color changes: pallor, cyanosis, jaundice. Lumps or ulcerations are visible in mucous membrane. Teeth are loose, absent, or show decay or are chipped; gums are receding, discolored, or bleeding. *Halitosis* (bad breath) is present (see Chapter 88). Client shows involuntary tongue or mouth movement (may signify medication side effects—see Chapter 94).

(Continued)

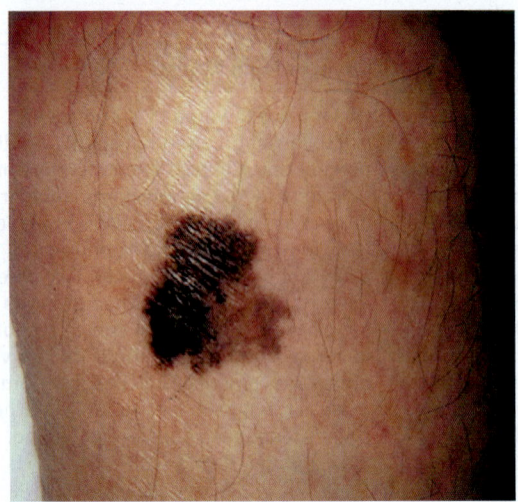

Figure 47-13 Malignant melanoma.

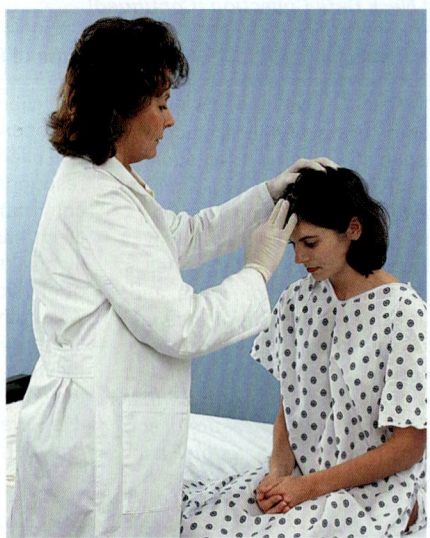

Figure 47-14 Inspection of the client's hair and scalp.

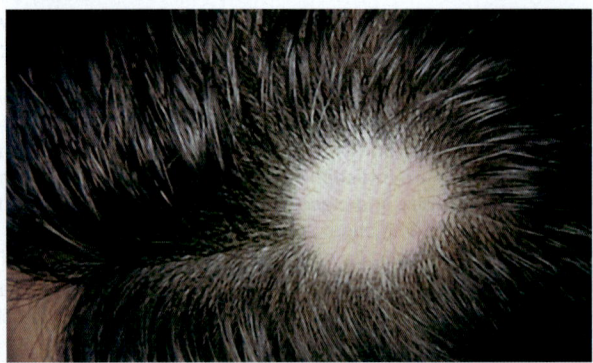

Figure 47-15 Excessive hair loss—abnormal *alopecia* (not the same as male pattern baldness).

DATA COLLECTION IN NURSING (Continued)

Action/Rationale	Normal Findings	Changes From Normal
Musculoskeletal Observation—Check muscles, joints, body movement, and neuromuscular function.		
Observe the client while they are raising both arms over the head, lowering them to a point outward from the shoulder, pointing them forward, then lowering them to the side. The right and left sides are compared. *(These movements demonstrate range of motion of the shoulder joint.)*	Client holds both arms straight above the head, lowers arms to right angles with the body, then lowers arms to rest at the side, with elbows slightly flexed. Movements are equal bilaterally.	Client reports pain or exhibits limitation in rotation, flexion, or extension on one or both sides.
Observe the client while they flex and extend the elbows. *(This movement demonstrates the range of motion of the elbows.)*	With flexion, the client completely closes the angle between the upper and lower arm; with extension, they hold the upper and lower arms in a straight line. Movements are equal bilaterally.	Client reports pain or exhibits limited flexion or extension in one or more joints.
Inspect the shape, size, and symmetry of both arms. *(Identify changes in muscle size.)*	Both arms are equal in size, shape, and symmetry.	Client shows asymmetry or a loss of muscle mass (atrophy).
Ask the client to squeeze one of your fingers with each of their own hands. *(Squeezing demonstrates strength in the client's hands.)*	The grasp is strong and equal.	Client shows unilateral weakness or loss of strength.
Ask the client to make a fist, and then to spread the fingers. Observe while the client rotates the hand from palm up to palm down; flexes the wrist up and down and sideways; and flexes the fingers up and down. *(These movements demonstrate range of motion of the finger joints and wrist.)*	Fingers and joints flex and extend completely. Movements of wrist rotation, flexion, and extension are smooth and free. Movements are equal bilaterally.	Client reports pain or exhibits limited flexion, extension, or rotation in one or both hands and fingers. Arthritic changes are evident in finger joints.
While the client lies on the bed or examining table, observe the client bending each knee up to the chest and pulling firmly toward the abdomen. *(This movement demonstrates range of motion of the knees and hips.)*	With complete knee and hip flexion, the top of the thigh rests on the abdomen, and the opposite leg rests fully extended. Joint range varies according to age and weight.	Client reports pain or exhibits incomplete flexion or extension in one or both hips and knees.
Ask the client to extend both legs on the bed; grasp one leg at the ankle and move it away from the midline; and then return it. Repeat movements on the other leg. Compare findings between right and left leg. *(These movements demonstrate range of motion of the hip joint.)* Movement away from the midline is *abduction;* movement toward the midline is *adduction.*	The client's leg can be moved to about a 40- to 50-degree angle from midline.	The client experiences pain, or limited abduction and adduction, on one or both sides.
Inspect the client's legs for size, shape, and symmetry. *(Abnormalities or changes in muscle size are identified.)*	Legs are equal in size, shape, and symmetry.	Legs show loss of muscle mass or asymmetry. (See Chapter 77.)
Ask the client to bend the foot so the toes point upward (*dorsiflexion*); downward (*plantar flexion*); to rotate the ankle from side to side; to curl and straighten the toes. Compare the movements of the right and left ankles and toes. *(These movements demonstrate the range of motion of the ankle and toes.)*	The foot dorsiflexes about 20° and plantar flexes about 45°. The ankle rotates slightly, laterally and medially.	The client experiences pain or limited joint movement in one or both sides. Pain in the calves on dorsiflexion is **Homans sign**, an early indicator of deep vein **thrombophlebitis** (blood clot formation within the vein). (See Chapter 81.)

(Continued)

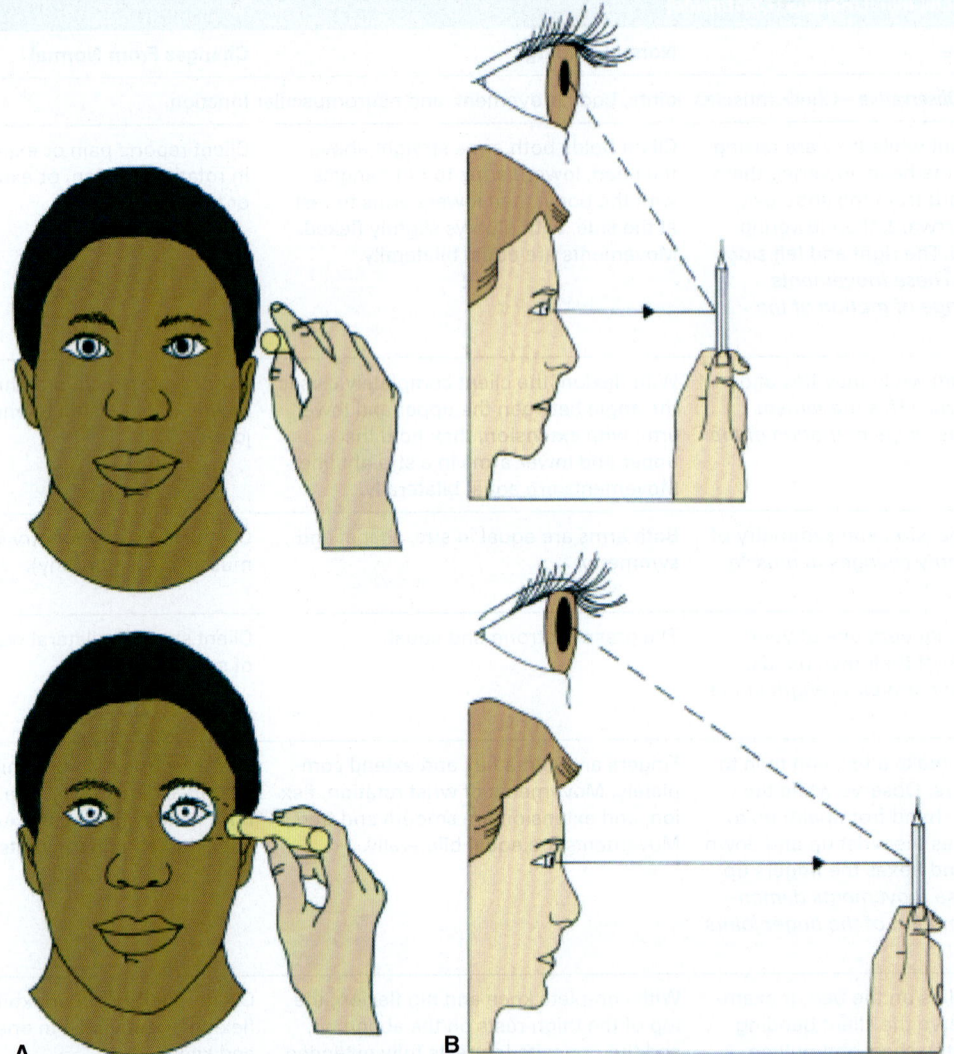

Figure 47-16 **A.** Checking the client's pupils for equality of size, reaction to light, and coordination. To test for reaction to light, a penlight is moved quickly from the side to shine on the client's pupil. The pupil should quickly constrict. Reporting of normal findings is expressed as PERRLA + C (pupils equal, round, react to light, accommodation OK, and eyes coordinated). **B.** Checking the ability to focus the eyes (accommodation).

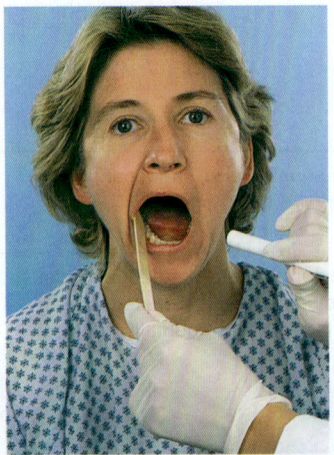

Figure 47-17 Wearing clean gloves when inspecting the mouth. A tongue blade and penlight are used.

DATA COLLECTION IN NURSING *(Continued)*		
Musculoskeletal Observation (Continued)		
Action/Rationale	Normal Findings	Changes From Normal
While the client is standing, ask them to bend forward as far as possible and backward as far as possible (Fig. 47-18). *(These movements indicate range of movement and flexibility of the lumbar spine.)*	Person should be able to bend about 90° forward (*flexion*) and about 30° backward (*extension*).	The client cannot bend or flex without pain or limited movement. The client cannot bend over without flexing the knees. The client has difficulty straightening up again after bending. Abnormal spinal curvatures are evident.
Ask the client to bend sideways as far as possible, both to the right and the left (Fig. 47-19). *(These movements check the lateral flexibility of the spine.)*	The person should be able to flex about 35° in each direction from the midline.	The client has limited movement or has pain on movement, either to one side or both sides. The client is not able to keep both feet on the floor while flexing the spine. The client loses their balance while doing this maneuver. (See Chapters 18 and 48.)
Hold the client's foot and ask them to push against your hand. Repeat with the other leg (Fig. 47-20). *(This checks and compares leg strength.)*	Strength is equal bilaterally.	One or both legs are weak; client unable to push against force. The client has pain on movement.
Observation of Chest—Observe respiratory and cardiovascular structures and functions.		
Open and remove the client's examination gown. Ask the client to sit on the side of the examining table or bed. (If the client cannot sit up alone, raise the bed to a high Fowler position). Observe the shape and movement of the anterior chest (Fig. 47-21). Compare the two sides. *(Asymmetric shape or movement is identified; respiratory movement is observed.)*	Shoulders are level; breasts and lower rib margins are symmetrical. Chest wall rises and falls slightly with inspiration and expiration.	Movement of the chest wall is asymmetrical on respiration; shoulders are uneven; breasts or lower rib margins are asymmetrical. Client has supraclavicular retractions or contractions of accessory muscles during inspiration (see Chapters 43, 46, and 86).
Palpate the anterior and posterior chest wall. *(This helps distinguish between normal and abnormal structures; painful areas are identified.)*	No tenderness, pain, abnormal swelling, or masses present.	Tenderness, pain, or masses are present. Client identifies tender or painful areas.
Stand behind the client and observe the posterior chest for shape and movement. *(Shape and movement are identified and respiratory movement is assessed.)*	Shoulders are even; scapulae are at the same level; spine is midline and straight. Posterior chest slightly rises and falls with respiration.	When the client stands, structural deformities or asymmetry are present: **scoliosis** (lateral curvature), **lordosis** (extreme lumbar curvature), or **kyphosis** (humpback or hunchback appearance). Breathing patterns are asymmetrical.
Auscultate the lungs by placing a stethoscope over the posterior intercostal spaces, beginning above the scapula and moving below the costal margin. Ask the client to breathe deeply through the mouth. Listen to both sides for lung (and heart) sounds (Fig. 47-22). *(The stethoscope amplifies lung sounds.)*	A low, soft-pitched, blowing sound is heard throughout all areas of the lungs. The client's inspiration is approximately two or three times longer than the expiration.	Abnormal breath sounds are **rales**, **rhonchi**, or **crackles**, **wheezes**, or **stridor** (Table 47-7). (See Chapter 86.)
Palpate radial pulses bilaterally (Fig. 47-23). Pulses should be palpated *only with the fingertips, not the thumbs*. Count pulse rate; note strength and regularity of the beats. *(This helps determine overall circulatory status.)*	Radial pulse should be easily felt. Pulsations are palpable, strong, and regular. Pulses are equal bilaterally.	Irregular pulse or regularly missed beats. Very weak or thready pulse. Very fast pulse (*tachycardia*) or very slow pulse (*bradycardia*).
Auscultate apical pulse (see Chapter 46). Count the rate and identify any abnormalities. *(This helps determine cardiac status.)*	The heart rate should be 60–80 BPM in most adults. The pulsations should be easily heard and regular in rhythm. The rate of apical and radial pulses should be the same.	Irregular rhythm, missed beats. Any abnormal sounds should be reported (may be heart murmurs). Difference between apical and radial pulses is abnormal.

(Continued)

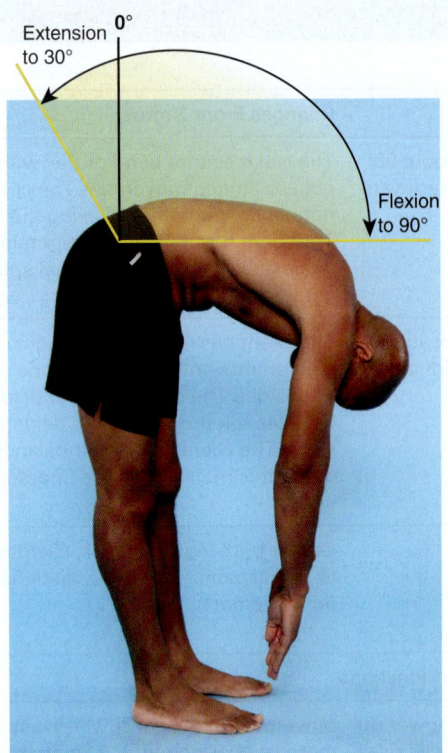

Figure 47-18 Range of motion of the spine—flexion and extension. (Weber, 2014.)

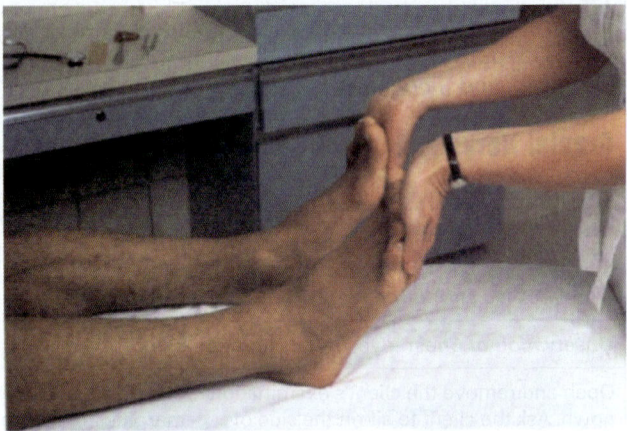

Figure 47-20 The client presses their legs against the examiner's hands to check bilateral leg strength.

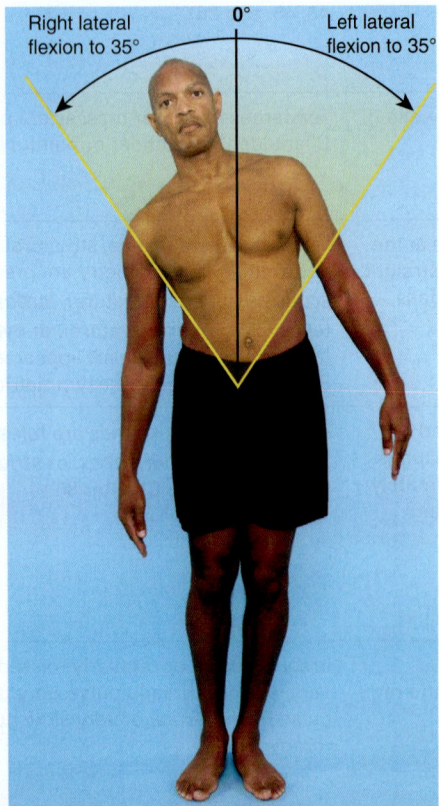

Figure 47-19 Range of motion of the spine—right and left lateral flexion. (Weber, 2014.)

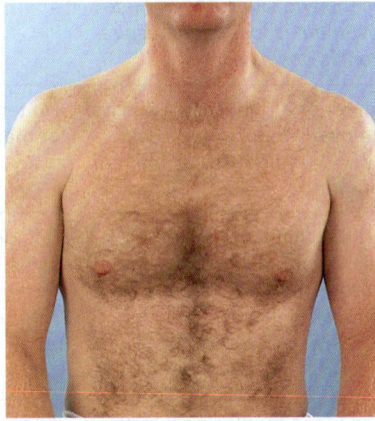

Figure 47-21 Normal appearance of the male's anterior chest.

TABLE 47-7 Abnormal (Adventitious) Lung Sounds

ABNORMAL SOUND	CHARACTERISTICS	POSSIBLE CAUSES
Fine crackles (formerly called rales) also called crepitus	High-pitched popping sounds during inspiration; simulated by rolling strand of hair near your ear; may be cleared by coughing	Fluid in air passages; sound occurs when air is drawn through small collapsed air passages Conditions: emphysema, bronchitis, asthma
Coarse crackles	Low-pitched bubbling, moist sounds throughout expiratory cycle; sounds like Velcro being pulled apart	Air drawn through fluid in large bronchi and trachea Conditions: pneumonia, pulmonary edema
Wheeze (sibilant stridor)	High-pitched continuous musical sound on inspiration and expiration (whistle)	Air drawn through constricted passages caused by swelling, secretions, or muscular spasm Conditions: asthma, chronic emphysema
Wheeze (sonorous) (rhonchi is lower pitched than wheeze)	Low-pitched moaning or grunting sound usually heard in expiration; may be cleared by coughing	Air drawn through constricted passages (as in sonorous wheeze) Condition: bronchitis, croup in children

From Weber, J., & Kelley, J. (2018). *Health assessment in nursing* (6th ed.). Wolters Kluwer.

DATA COLLECTION IN NURSING (Continued)

Observation of Chest (Continued)

Action/Rationale	Normal Findings	Changes From Normal
Locate and palpate other peripheral pulses (Fig. 47-24). The *carotid pulse* is located in the neck. This artery supplies the brain and is the pulse location used when performing CPR. (Palpate the carotid pulse *only on the side closest to the examiner.*) The *femoral pulse* is located in the groin and supplies the legs and feet on both sides. The *dorsalis pedis pulse* is palpated on the top of each foot and supplies the foot and toes in each foot. *(Pulses in these areas indicate overall peripheral circulatory status.)*	Pulses should be strong and regular in each location. The rate should approximate the apical heart rate. The ability to palpate bilateral pulses in the peripheral circulation indicates adequate circulation in these areas.	If unable to palpate a peripheral pulse, report this situation immediately. Note and report if there are irregular, weak, or missing beats as well (see Chapter 81).
Bilaterally examine the skin on the extremities (particularly the hands and feet) for color and warmth (Fig. 47-25). *(These findings also indicate status of peripheral circulation.)*	Color is appropriate for race and is pink on nail beds, palms, and soles bilaterally. Skin is warm and moist.	Pallor or cyanosis is observed on nails, palms, or soles bilaterally or unilaterally; temperature or color is different from one hand or foot to the other.
Observation of Breasts—Check breast structure.		
Visually inspect the nipples and breasts (Fig. 47-26). Ask the client to raise the arms above the head. (Note: *It may also be necessary to inspect male breasts.*)	The areola is darker than the breast; the nipple usually protrudes but may be inverted. The breasts should be approximately equal in size and shape, with arms down and with arms up.	Abnormal findings include rashes, ulcerations, nipple discharge, dimpling in one area, and asymmetry. Client reports pain, discomfort, or excessive itching.
Encourage the client to perform breast self-examination. The examiner may perform this procedure.	The client reports that they regularly examines their breasts. No abnormalities are found.	The client reports lumps or nodules in the breasts. Or, the client reports that they do not regularly examine their breasts. Teach as necessary (see Chapter 91).
Examination of the Male Genitalia—Assess the genitalia for abnormalities. Note: All males are encouraged to do a testicular self-examination on a regular basis. Any lumps, swelling, or tenderness should be reported to the healthcare provider immediately. Adult males 50 years of age and older are encouraged to have a blood test for prostate-specific antigen (PSA) yearly.		

(Continued)

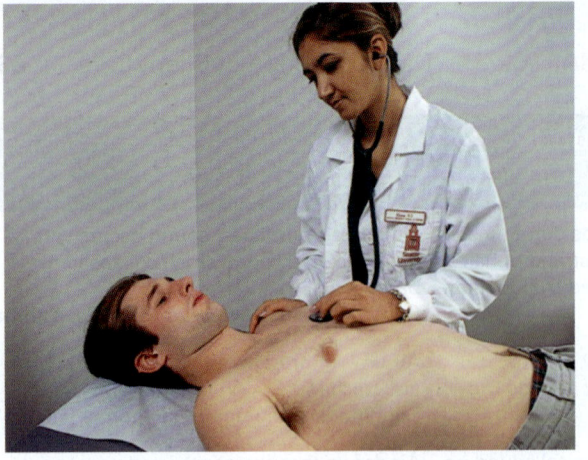

Figure 47-22 Auscultation of lung sounds in the chest.

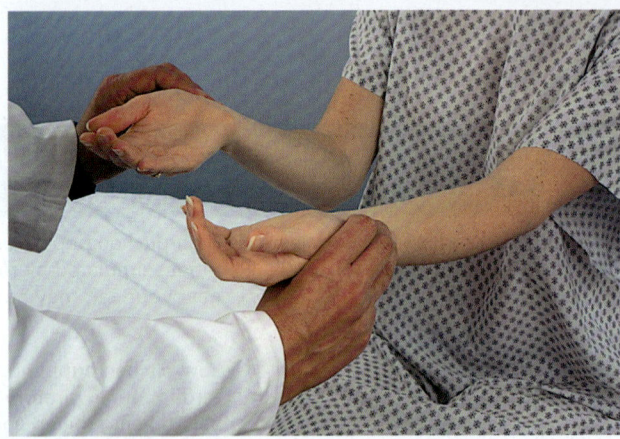

Figure 47-23 Palpation of radial pulse. The pulse in both wrists should be equal.

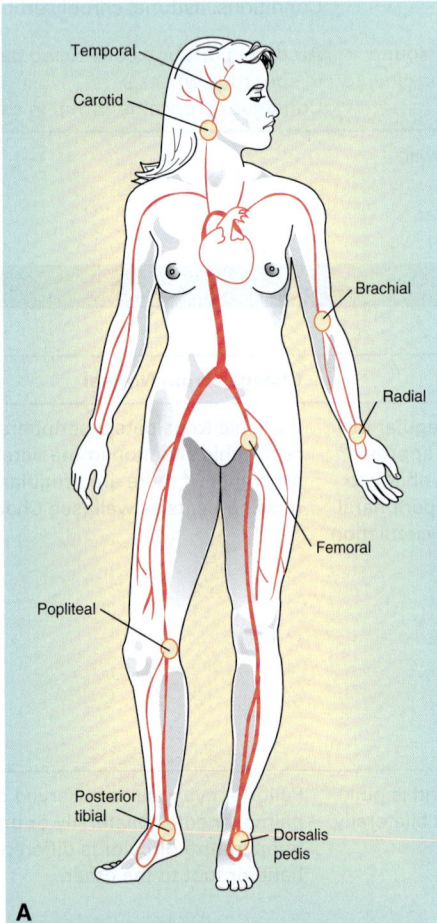

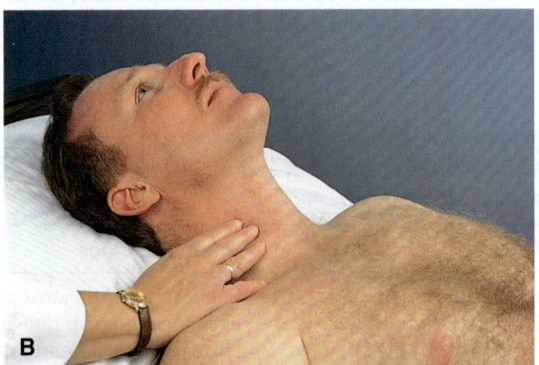

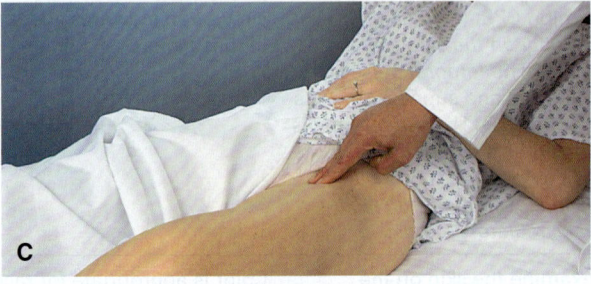

Figure 47-24 **A.** Sites of peripheral pulses (pressure points). **B.** Palpation of the carotid artery in the throat. *Do not reach over the client's neck.* **C.** Palpation of the femoral artery in the groin. (B, C: Photo by B. Proud.)

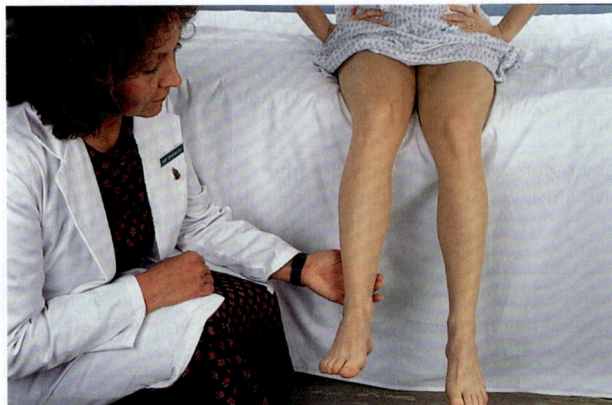

Figure 47-25 Inspection of both feet for color and warmth when they are dependent (hanging down).

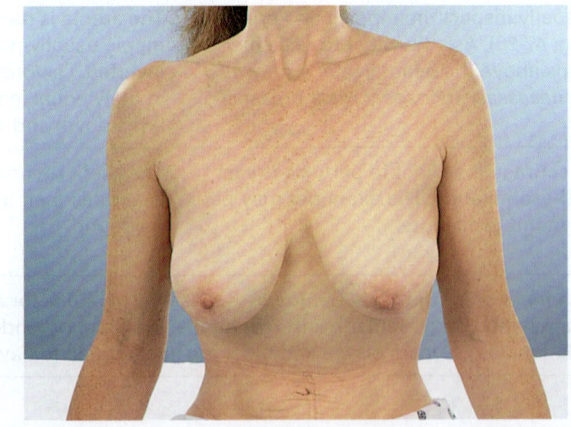

Figure 47-26 Observation of the breasts. They should be symmetrical.

DATA COLLECTION IN NURSING (Continued)

Observation of Breasts (Continued)

Action/Rationale	Normal Findings	Changes From Normal
To examine the male genitalia, sit while the client is standing. Note whether the client is circumcised or not. Retract the foreskin to expose the glans penis.	The scrotum is approximately symmetrical (Fig. 47-27).	It appears that one or both testes are not descended. Abnormal drainage; ulceration; evidence of infection or of lice or other infestation is noted.
Palpate the inguinal and groin areas.	The tissue in these areas is intact and no weakened areas are noted.	Weakened areas or hernias are discovered. Lumps, swelling, or masses are present. The client reports pain.
Ask the client if they have any pain, difficulty in urination, incontinence or sexual dysfunction.	The client identifies normal urination and sexual patterns.	The client complains of pain on urination, difficulty starting or maintaining the stream, urgency, hesitancy, frequency, incontinence, or inability to have an erection or ejaculation (see Chapter 90).

Abdominal Data Collection—Check gastrointestinal structures and function and kidney structure.

Action/Rationale	Normal Findings	Changes From Normal
With the client supine and arms resting at the sides, inspect the abdomen's skin surface. (See Table 48-1 for positioning.) The abdomen is divided into four quadrants: vertically, from xiphoid to pubis and laterally through the umbilicus. (See Chapter 15.) *(Identification of quadrants is necessary to locate changes when reporting information to other healthcare providers.)*	The abdomen is rounded, symmetrical, and smooth, with fairly even pigmentation. Umbilicus is centrally located and usually inverted, but can protrude; it may be darker than surrounding skin.	The presence of **striae** (stretch marks), scars, surgical incisions or other wounds at various levels of healing, exudates, or visible peristaltic waves is detected. **Herniation** (outpouching of tissue) appears around the umbilicus, at the inguinal line, or around incisions. Abdomen is *concave* (sunken in). This is typically seen in very thin or emaciated people (see Chapter 88).
Auscultate the abdomen over each of the four quadrants, using the diaphragm of the stethoscope (Fig. 47-28). *(To locate the position of bowel sounds heard on auscultation.)* Further examination by palpation may be performed by the primary provider.	The peristaltic action of the bowel produces between 5 and 34 clicks or gurgles per minute in each quadrant. Louder, prolonged gurgles or sounds (similar to "stomach growling") may occur.	Bowel sounds are diminished, absent, or excessively loud or active. The client reports excessive gas or flatus or pain when the abdomen is touched.

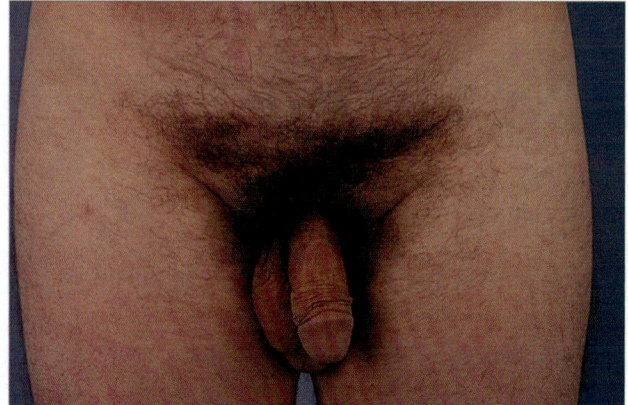

Figure 47-27 Appearance of the normal male genitalia. The foreskin is retracted, exposing the glans penis.

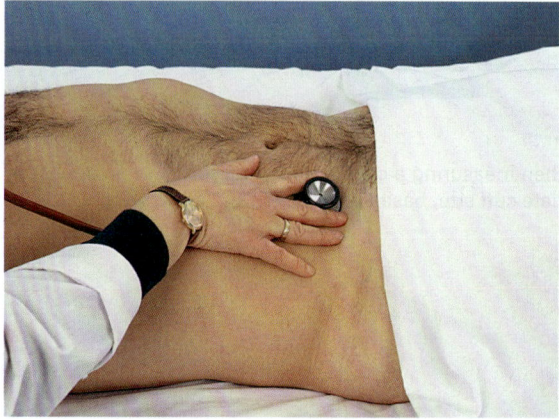

Figure 47-28 Listening to the abdomen in all four quadrants, using diaphragm side of stethoscope (auscultation).

DATA COLLECTION IN CHILDREN

General Examination

When collecting data from and about a young child, the examiner must build rapport with both the child and the caregiver. Encourage the caregiver to hold a small child.

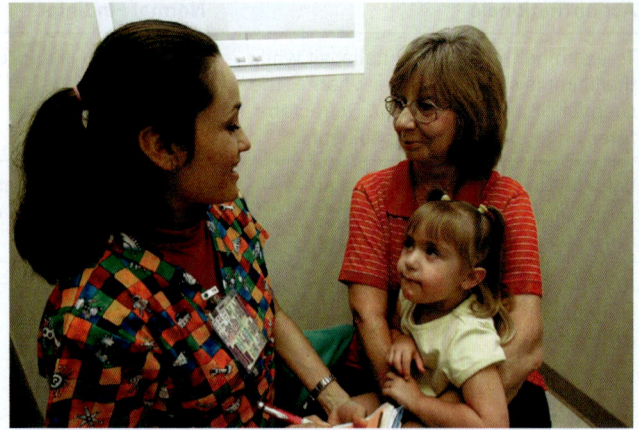

Older children and adolescents are treated with maturity to instill a sense of confidence and trust.

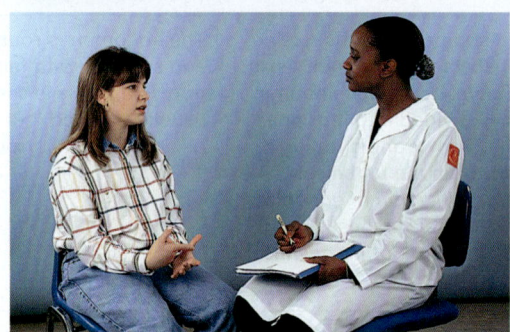

In children younger than 2 or 3 years, height is determined by measuring recumbent length. The child's head is held at the midline, and then, the knees are grasped and pushed downward until they are fully extended (see Chapter 45).

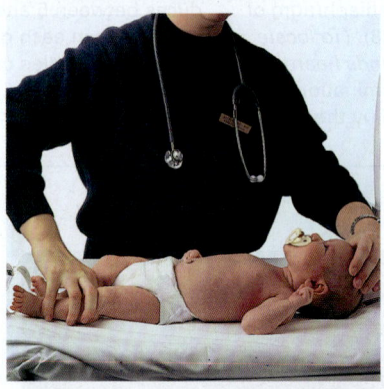

When measuring a child's blood pressure, use an appropriate cuff size, based on the child's size and weight.

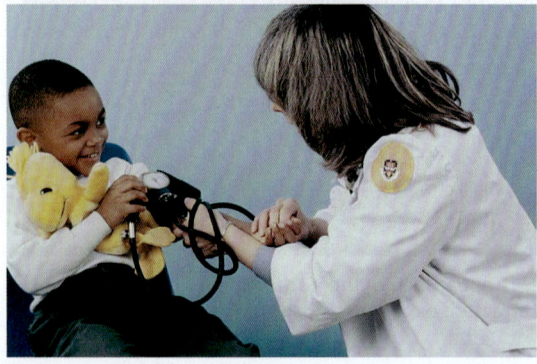

CHAPTER 47 Data Collection in Client Care

DATA COLLECTION IN CHILDREN (Continued)

Use simple toys and play to collect data about small children. Here, the nurse is evaluating the child's gross hearing acuity.

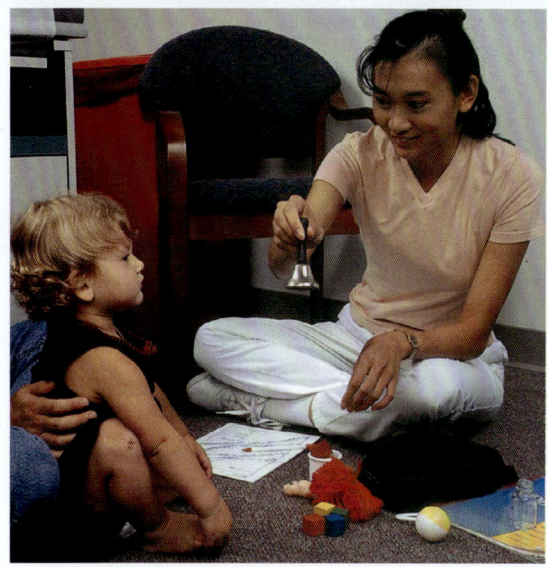

Skin Assessment

"Stork bite" is a normal finding on a newborn's skin. This red or pink birthmark will usually fade by the child's first birthday.

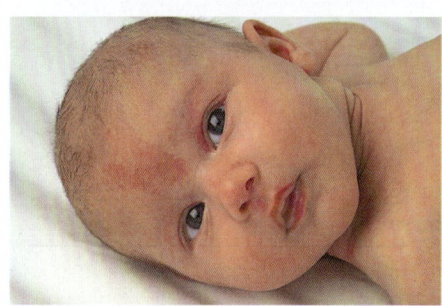

Slate gray nevi are common skin variations found in newborns. Common in newborns who are of Asian descent and/or those with darker skin.

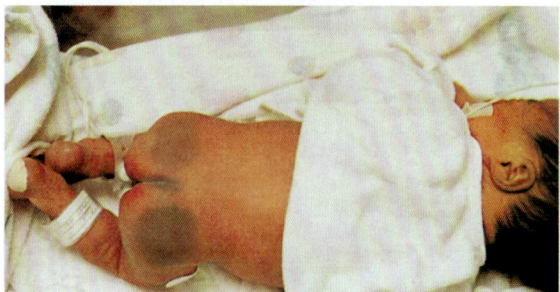

Head and Neck Assessment

Inspect the baby's *fontanelles* (soft spots) when assessing the head. These fontanelles should close between 12 and 18 months of age.

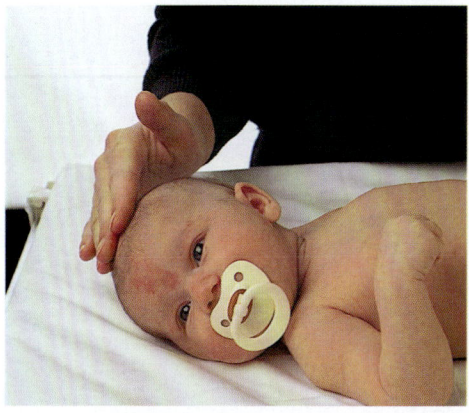

DATA COLLECTION IN CHILDREN (Continued)

Using a stuffed toy can help the child relax and actively participate in examinations.

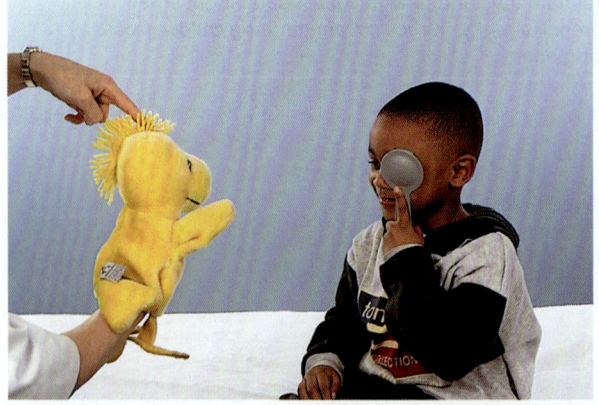

Check several cranial nerves of the face by asking the child to copy the funny faces made by the examiner (Evans-Smith, 2005).

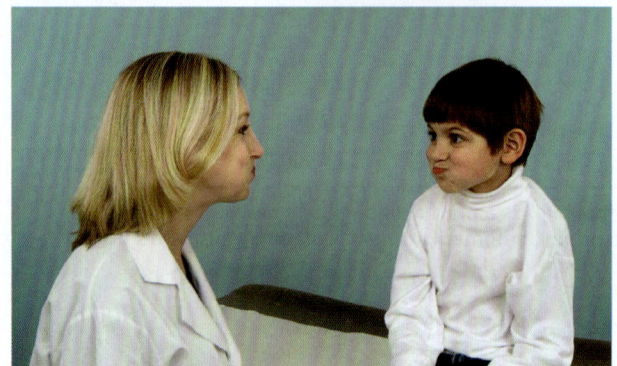

Musculoskeletal Assessment

Infants younger than 3 months have rounded spines.

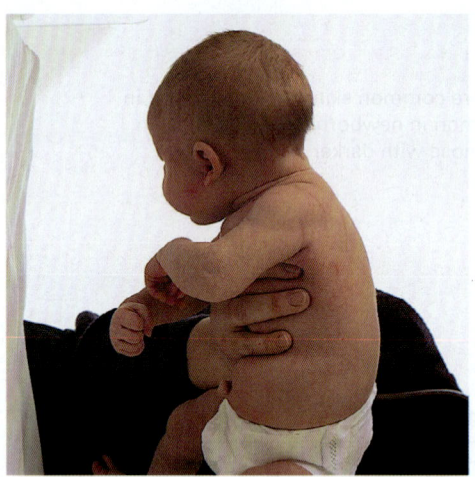

DATA COLLECTION IN CHILDREN (Continued)

An important musculoskeletal examination for preadolescents and adolescents is checking the spine for scoliosis (s-shaped curvature).

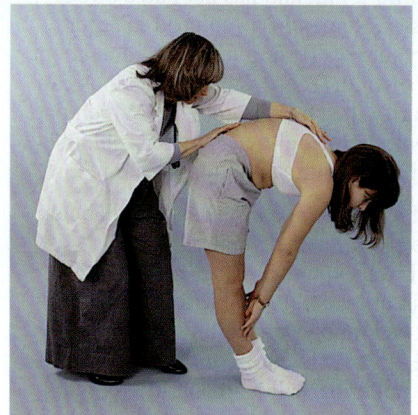

Assessment of Chest, Abdomen, and Pelvis

Diaper rash in infants is common, but must be treated.

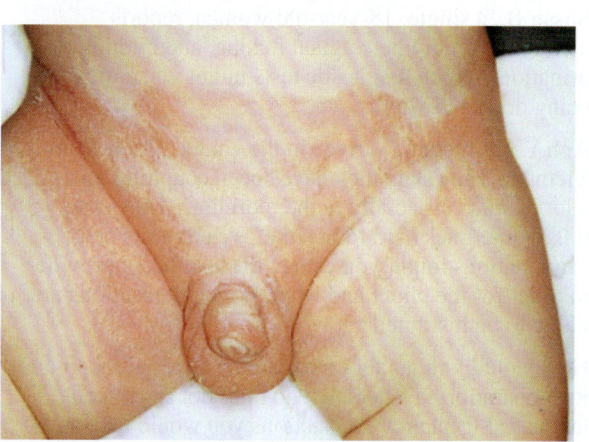

STUDENT SYNTHESIS

KEY POINTS

- Healthcare providers perform data collection and assessment and physical examination of clients for specific purposes. The primary purposes of nursing data gathering are to identify and report abnormal or unusual findings, identify potential problems, and provide needed care measures within the individual's scope of practice. This information provides the basis for the development of the nursing care plan.
- Disease is a change in body structure, a definite pathologic process. Illness is marked by a pronounced deviation from health.
- Lifestyle risk factors, such as obesity, smoking, or lack of exercise, can cause vulnerable people to develop some disorders.
- People may also have a genetic or hereditary predisposition to certain physical disorders or illnesses.
- Diseases are categorized in several ways according to etiology (effect on the person), such as acute versus chronic illness.
- Inflammation and infection can affect nearly every body system or part.
- Laboratory and diagnostic tests can help providers to establish medical diagnoses. Nurses need a basic understanding of such procedures to assist appropriately.
- The healthcare provider performs the physical examination with varying degrees of complexity and thoroughness, depending on the purpose of the examination.
- The most common formats for the physical examination are head-to-toe examination and examination done according to body systems.
- Teaching of the client and family is vital, to ensure the comfort and safety of the client and the accuracy of the test or examination.

CRITICAL THINKING EXERCISES

1. Your client, Mrs. F., is 83 years of age and has been residing in a long-term care facility for 2 years because of increasingly disabling arthritis. She requires assistance with her activities of daily living because of weakness, joint stiffness, and pain. She is very alert and is interested in many activities around her. On your

morning rounds, Mrs. F. tells you that she does not feel well, has not eaten for 24 hr, and has not had a bowel movement for 3 days. Remember, you need to report these concerns to your supervising nurse and document them in the client's health record. Which questions can you ask to help clarify the client's problem? Which part of data gathering will help you focus on the problem? Which findings will be significant to report and record?

2. Mr. T., 78 years of age, has insulin-dependent diabetes. His vision has been failing for several years. On your rounds, Mr. T. tells you that he has been having some "tightness" in chest and is unable to walk to the bathroom without becoming short of breath. Which questions can you ask to help clarify his problem? What part of data gathering will help you focus on his problem? What findings will be significant to report and record?

3. Susan B., a single, 18-year-old woman, reports abdominal cramping, vaginal itching, and burning on urination. Which diagnostic tests might you anticipate being done and why?

4. Anh Y. has recently arrived in the United States from Vietnam. They state they have "been coughing up a lot of stuff, especially in the morning." They state it is "sometimes hard to breathe." Which tests or examinations might you expect the healthcare provider to order for the client and why? Which precautions are likely to be instituted?

5. How would you go about explaining a colonoscopy and its preparation to a person who does not speak your language? Explain which actions you would take and why.

NCLEX-STYLE REVIEW QUESTIONS

1. The nurse is collecting data from a client admitted to the acute care facility. Which data obtained by the nurse would be documented as objective data?
   a. The client identifies severe itching on the leg.
   b. The client has a large sacral wound.
   c. A family member states that the client is confused.
   d. The client states, "I have been sick for 2 days."

2. A client states, "I feel bloated and have abdominal cramps." Which part of the assessment would the nurse perform first?
   a. Inspection
   b. Auscultation
   c. Percussion
   d. Palpation

3. The nurse is testing the function of a client's cranial nerves. Which statement made by the nurse would indicate testing of cranial nerve IX (glossopharyngeal)?
   a. "Shrug your shoulders and turn your head."
   b. "Move and clench your jaw."
   c. "Swallow."
   d. "Stand with your eyes closed."

4. The nurse is obtaining a pulse oximetry reading and vital signs for a client with pneumonia. Which finding would the nurse report immediately to the healthcare provider?
   a. Temperature of 98 °F
   b. Heart rate of 72
   c. Respiratory rate of 16
   d. Pulse oximetry of 89%

5. The nurse requests that a postoperative client dorsiflex the foot. While performing this task, the client reports having pain in the calf. Which potential complication of the immobility related to surgery does the nurse suspect has occurred?
   a. Deep vein thrombosis
   b. Fractured leg
   c. Muscle atrophy
   d. Dislocated hip

CHAPTER RESOURCES

Enhance your learning with additional resources on thePoint!

Student Resources related to this chapter can be found at **thePoint.lww.com/Rosdahl12e.**

48 Moving and Positioning Clients

Learning Objectives

1. Describe and demonstrate safely moving a client in and out of bed or chair, or onto a gurney, using a mechanical lift.
2. State the principles underlying proper body mechanics; identify instances when body mechanics are utilized in nursing.
3. Demonstrate safe, comfortable, and appropriate positioning for clients in bed.
4. State at least six client positions commonly used for examinations and treatments. In the skills laboratory, demonstrate the ability to assist a client to assume each of these positions, considering both client and nurse safety.
5. Differentiate between active and passive range of motion; state their purposes. Demonstrate the ability to perform passive range of motion exercises, to supervise active range of motion exercises, and to perform combinations of these.
6. With the assistance of another caregiver(s), demonstrate moving a client up in bed or to the side of the bed, using appropriate assistance devices.
7. Describe evaluation of fall risk; state its application to nursing care and client safety; identify components of fall prevention.
8. Describe and demonstrate the safe use of mobility devices (e.g., wheelchairs, canes, walkers).
9. Demonstrate the ability to use the powered and nonpowered wheeled stretcher (litter, gurney) safely.
10. Demonstrate the ability to teach each crutch-walking gait, including navigating up and down stairs with crutches, with or without a handrail.
11. Describe types of client protection devices; state precautions and nursing care for each; identify regulations and documentation for each; and state when each is used. Differentiate between client protection/reminder devices for client safety, for medical therapeutic reasons, and for the dangerous client in the mental health unit.

Important Terminology

abduction (abduct)
adduction (adduct)
base of support
body mechanics
center of gravity
circumduction
contracture
contralateral
dangling
dorsiflexion
eversion
extension
flexion
footdrop
Fowler position
gait
gait belt (transfer belt)
gravital plane
gurney
hemiplegia
hyperextension
inversion
isometric
lateral
line of gravity
lithotomy
litter
logroll turn
orthopneic position
paralysis
paraplegia
plantar flexion
pronation
prone
protective/reminder device
protraction
retraction
rotation
Sims position
supine
transfer board
Trendelenburg position
trochanter roll

Acronyms

AROM
CPM
OOB
PROM
ROM

Many nurses sustain back injuries as a result of lifting and moving clients. "Even if lifting is done correctly, the process places a great deal of strain on nurses' bodies." In addition, many clients are larger than in years past. A recent article states that "team lifting" is hazardous to the nurse; "there's still a chance of compression on disks in the back…and since each team member has different physical strength…force (can be) distributed unevenly." OSHA states that "mechanical lift assistance equipment is the only way to truly prevent nursing staff from being injured" (White, 2015). Most VA hospitals have installed lifts in all client rooms, according to National Public Media. One VA Safe Patient Handling and Mobility Coordinator stated that "nobody at that VA is allowed to move patients the traditional way anymore" (National Public Radio, 2015).

Correct procedures, including mechanical lifts, help prevent nursing injuries. In addition, nurses often teach clients procedures for safe walking and movement. The nurse must first understand the principles of body mechanics and safe methods of moving clients. People (clients and nurses alike) differ in weight, size, and ability to move. The nurse must understand when it is safe to assist a client to move and when a mechanical device must be used. The bottom line is to provide safety for both nurse and client.

BODY MECHANICS

Use of the safest and most efficient methods of moving and lifting is called **body mechanics**. This means *applying mechanical principles of movement to the human body.*

Box 48-1 Basic Principles of Body Mechanics

- It is easier to *pull, push,* or *roll* an object than it is to lift it. The movement should be smooth and continuous, rather than jerky.
- Often less energy or force is required to keep an object moving than it is to start and stop it.
- It takes less effort to lift an object if the nurse works as close to it as possible. Use the strong leg and arm muscles as much as possible. Use back muscles, which are not as strong, as little as possible. Avoid reaching.
- The nurse rocks backward or forward on the feet and with their body as a force for pulling or pushing.

Principles of Body Mechanics

Body mechanics, used alone, apply in some nursing situations. From the laws of physics, we derive general principles of body mechanics (Box 48-1). Remember, some ways of moving and carrying objects are more effective than others. Keep objects close to the body, do not bend at the waist, and avoid constant repetition of lifting. Principles underlying correct body mechanics involve major factors, including center of gravity, base of support, and line of gravity.

Center of Gravity

A person's **center of gravity** is in the pelvic area. Approximately half the body weight is distributed above this area, half below it, when thinking of the body divided horizontally (side to side). In addition, half the body weight is to each side, when thinking of the body divided vertically (up and down). When lifting an object, bend at the knees and hips and keep the back straight. By doing so, the center of gravity remains over the feet, giving extra stability. It is thus easier to maintain balance (Fig. 48-1).

Base of Support

A person's feet provide the **base of support**. The wider the base of support, the more stable the person, within limits (see Fig. 48-1). (If the feet are too wide apart, this causes instability.) The feet should be spread sidewise when lifting, to give side-to-side stability. One foot is placed slightly in front of the other, for back-to-front stability. The weight is distributed evenly between both feet, with the knees flexed slightly, to absorb jolts. The feet are moved to turn an object being moved. (*Do not twist the body.*)

Line of Gravity

Draw an imaginary vertical line through the top of the head, the center of gravity, and the base of support. This becomes the **line of gravity**, or **gravital plane** (Fig. 48-2). Gravitational pull runs from the top of the head to the feet. For highest efficiency, this line should be straight from the top of the head to the base of support, with equal weight on each side. Therefore, if a person stands with the back straight and the head erect, the line of gravity will be approximately through the center of the body.

Body Alignment

When lifting, walking, or performing any activity, proper *body alignment* is essential, to maintain balance. When the body is correctly aligned, the muscles work together for the safest and most efficient movement, without muscle strain. Stretching the body as tall as possible helps produce proper alignment, via correct posture (see Fig. 48-2). When standing, the weight is slightly forward and is supported on the outsides of the feet. Again, the head is erect, the back is straight, and the abdomen is tucked in. (Remember: the client in bed should be in approximately the same position as if they were standing [Fig. 48-3].)

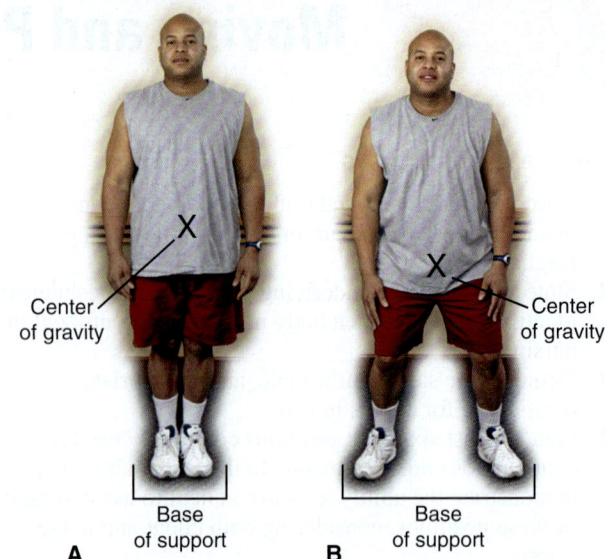

Figure 48-1 Maintaining balance. **A.** Poor body mechanics: the distance between this person's feet (*base of support*) is small, and the heaviest part of their body (*center of gravity*) is far away from the base of support, making them more likely to lose balance. **B.** Good body mechanics: by increasing the distance between their feet and lowering their body toward the ground, the person has increased ability to maintain side-to-side balance. The right foot is also slightly in front of the left, for back-to-front stability.

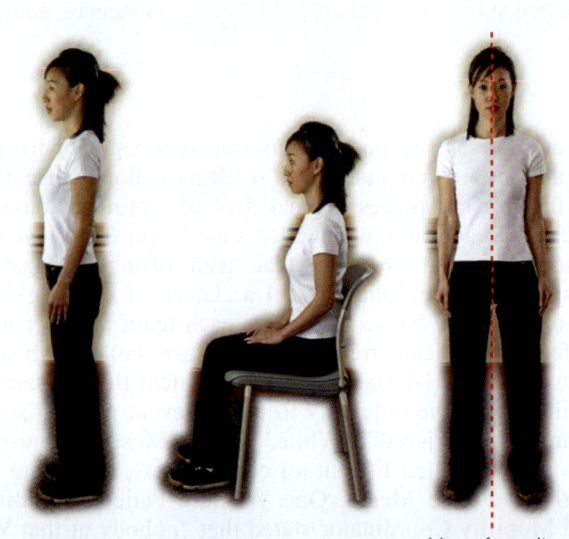

Figure 48-2 When the body is held in proper alignment, the back is in a "neutral" position, with the curve of the lower spine intact.

CHAPTER 48 Moving and Positioning Clients

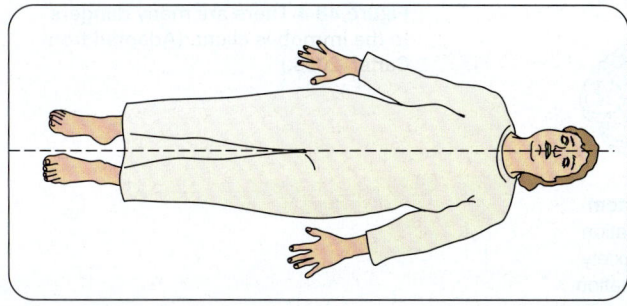

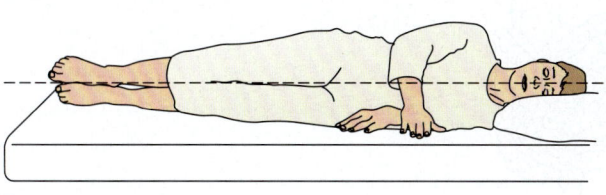

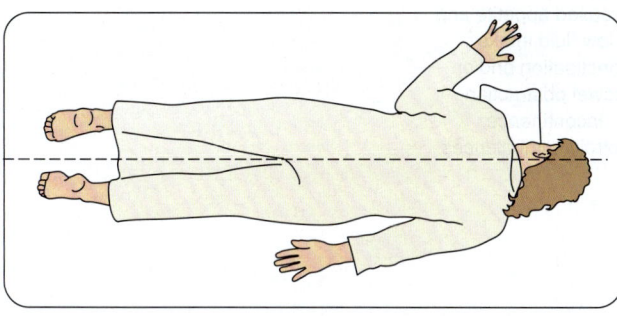

Figure 48-3 When a person is in proper alignment, an imaginary straight line can be drawn connecting the person's nose, breastbone (sternum), and pubic bone. Alignment in bed should be approximately the same as when standing. **A.** Proper body alignment for a person lying on the back (supine). **B.** Proper body alignment for a person lying on the side (lateral). **C.** Proper body alignment for a person lying on the stomach (prone). A small pillow or folded towel should be placed under the shoulder toward which the head is turned. (Adapted from Carter, 2008.)

POSITIONING THE CLIENT

Encouraging clients to move in bed, get out of bed, or walk, even though they are reluctant, accomplishes several positive goals. *Immobility* can contribute to a number of disorders, including pressure wounds, blood clots, constipation, muscle weakness and atrophy, pneumonia, joint deformities, urinary disorders, and depression. By assisting clients to maintain or regain mobility, you promote self-care practices and help prevent complications (Fig. 48-4). To prevent injuries to yourself or your clients, it is important to practice good body mechanics and use mechanical devices, when necessary, to lift and move clients or objects (Fig. 48-5).

Moving and Positioning Clients

There are many reasons to change the client's position, as illustrated previously. In addition, position changes restore function, relieve pressure, stimulate respiration and circulation, provide diversion, and enhance self-esteem. Clients are also assisted into specific positions for examinations and treatments. In Practice: Nursing Care Guidelines 48-1 gives tips on positioning clients.

> **Key Concept**
> An antifriction glide sheet may sometimes be used to help move clients. A mechanical lift should be used in most cases, however.

It is important to explain to the client the reasons for a position change and how it will be done. The knowledgeable client is more likely to maintain the new position. If the client can help, explain how. The client's cooperation will assist the nurse and give the client some exercise, increase independence and self-esteem, and instill a feeling of control. Sometimes, turning the client is an important part of treatment and the provider specifically orders it, particularly for older or immobile clients. Some conditions limit turning the client, such as the presence of traction or an unstabilized fracture. Otherwise, turning is encouraged. In some cases, the client is turned only to wash or rub the back; assess skin condition, wounds, or dressings; or change bed linens. Some clients may not be allowed or are not able to turn and must remain **supine**. In this case, the client may be instructed to do isometric exercises, if physically able, to pull up slightly on the overhead trapeze, and to allow back care and other interventions and get some exercise. Encourage the client to move as much as possible.

> **Key Concept**
> It is important to give meticulous skin care to the person who must remain on the back. If the person can use the trapeze, the nurse can wash and gently massage the back with the hand held flat. This helps prevent skin breakdown. In other situations, a special bed is used (see Chapter 49).

Special beds operate to relieve pressure and provide back support. Infrequently, the client who cannot turn is placed in a circle bed, which rotates the client from head to toe, or on a Stryker (wedge) turning frame, which rotates the client from side to side. More commonly, the client is placed in a rotating or oscillating bed (e.g., the Roto-Rest), a flotation bed, or other special type of bed, several of which are discussed and pictured in Chapter 49.

> **Nursing Alert** Be sure to request assistance to move clients. Use a mechanical lift, "HoverMatt," or other devices, and make sure you know how to safely operate this equipment.

Positioning for Examinations and Treatments

The client often must assume a special position as part of a treatment or test, an examination, or to obtain specimens. Because nurses assist clients into many of these positions and will see other positions used, it is important to know how to assist the client and to place necessary drapes.

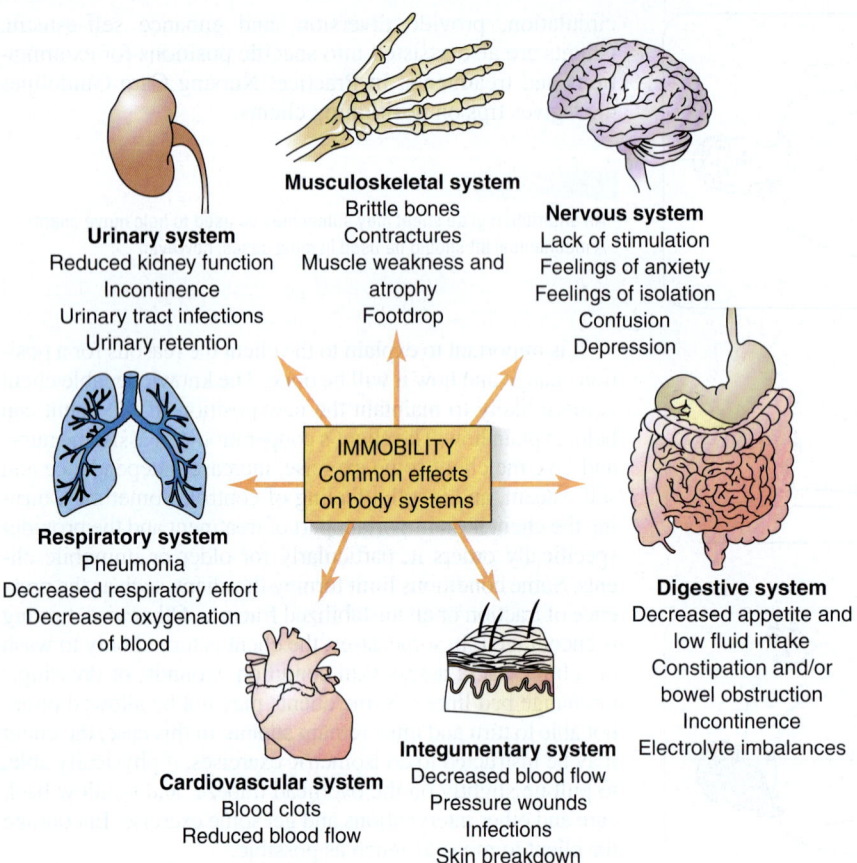

Figure 48-4 There are many dangers to the immobile client. (Adapted from Carter, 2008.)

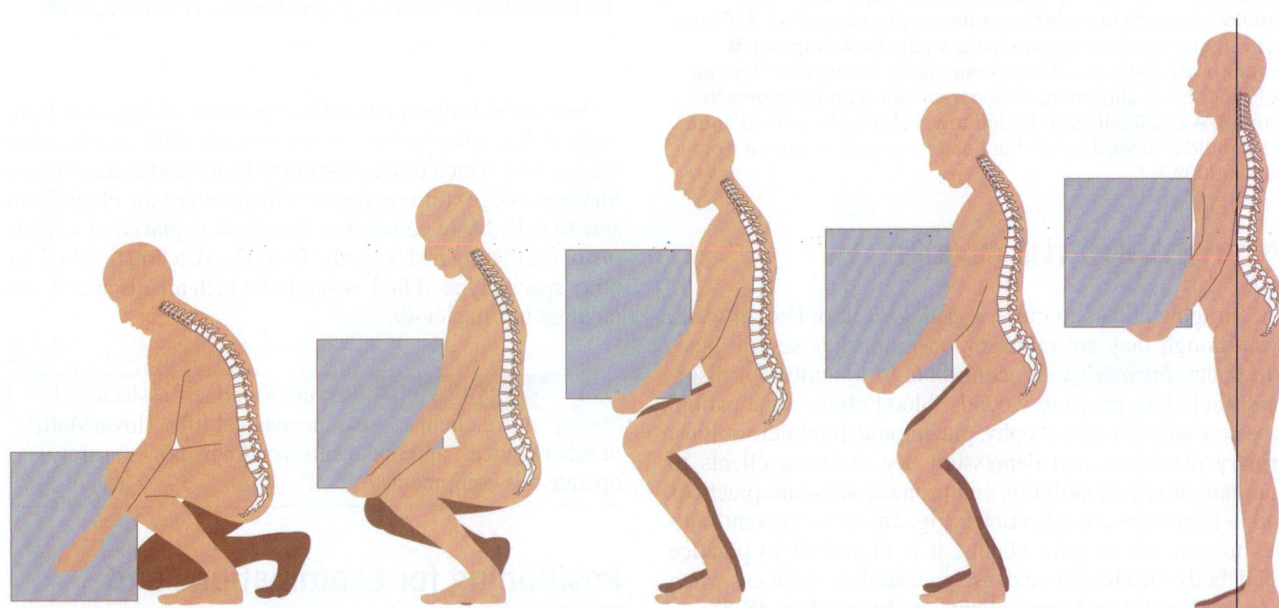

Figure 48-5 Lifting techniques, using good body mechanics. Use long, strong muscles of arms and legs. Hold the object so the line of gravity falls within the base of support. Keep the back straight and the load close to the body. Ask for assistance, if necessary. (Photo by Peter Gardiner/Science Source.)

IN PRACTICE
NURSING CARE GUIDELINES 48-1 — Positioning the Client for Comfort

- Maintain functional client body alignment. (Alignment is similar whether in bed or standing.)
- Maintain safety.
- Reassure the client, to promote comfort and cooperation.
- Properly handle the client's body, to prevent pain or injury.
- Follow proper body mechanics and standard precautions, to protect nurse and client.
- Use mechanical lifts or other devices whenever possible.
- Obtain assistance if needed.
- Follow specific provider's orders.
- Remember: a specific order is needed for a client to be out of bed.
- Do not use equipment such as splints, traction, or lifting equipment without specific in-service education.
- Make sure the client is comfortable and has the nurse signal cord available after positioning.

NOTE: Special turning and positioning systems are available to help prevent nurse injuries.

Commonly used positions are supine (*dorsal recumbent*, lying on the back), **prone** (on the abdomen), **Sims's** (semiprone, on the side [usually the left], with the upper knee flexed), **Fowler's** (on the back, with the head elevated), *knee-chest* or *genupectoral* (on the knees, with the chest resting on the bed), *dorsal* **lithotomy** (on the back, with feet in stirrups), and **lateral** (on the side). The supine position may be modified by bending the knees and placing the feet flat on the bed. **Trendelenburg's** (head-down, with the head lower than the feet) is used to treat shock, by promoting cerebral blood flow, and for some portions of postural drainage, to help drain secretions from particular segments of the lungs. Reverse Trendelenburg position may be used to enhance tube feeding and as an emergency procedure to help stop bleeding in a head injury (see Chapter 43). Two less commonly used positions are the *modified standing* position (standing while bending over forward) and the lumbar puncture position.

Special positioning is shown in Table 48-1. (Chapter 57 illustrates positioning for urinary catheterization. Chapter 47 described physical examination in more detail.)

The following measures are carried out before draping the client for examination:

- A signed release is obtained, if necessary.
- The client is asked to empty the bladder, unless contraindicated. *Rationale: This helps the person feel more relaxed and helps the examiner to better palpate the*

TABLE 48-1 Client Positions

POSITION	COMMENTS	USES
Supine (dorsal recumbent) 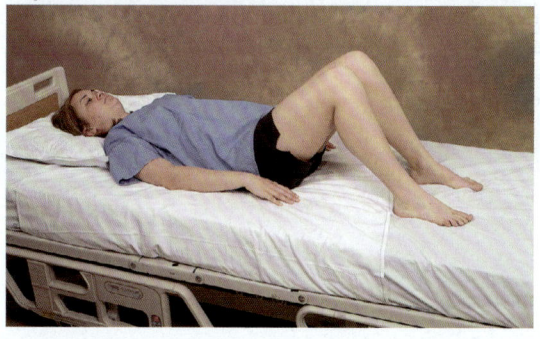	Back-lying, legs extended or slightly bent. Arms up or down. Small pillow allowed. May be uncomfortable for client with back problem.	General examination; examination of chest, abdomen, pelvic area.
Prone 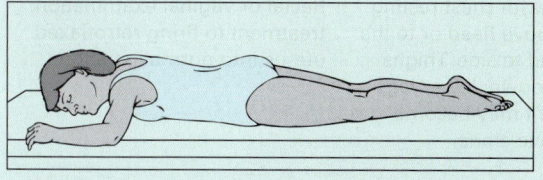	On abdomen, head to side. Arms above head or beside body. (Small pillow or folded towel may be placed under shoulder toward which head is turned.) Difficult for pregnant woman, obese client, or client with abdominal incision or breathing problem.	Examination of spine, back. (Long time in this position may cause neck strain and/or headache.)
Lateral, semiprone 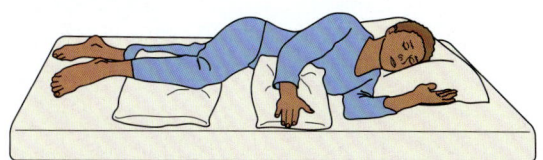	Side-lying, bottom arm behind or in front of client, not as extreme as Sims. Pillow placed under top leg for support. Comfortable for longer time than prone.	Client positioned for extended rest periods.

(Continued)

648 UNIT 8 Client Care

TABLE 48-1 Client Positions (Continued)

POSITION		COMMENTS	USES
Sims	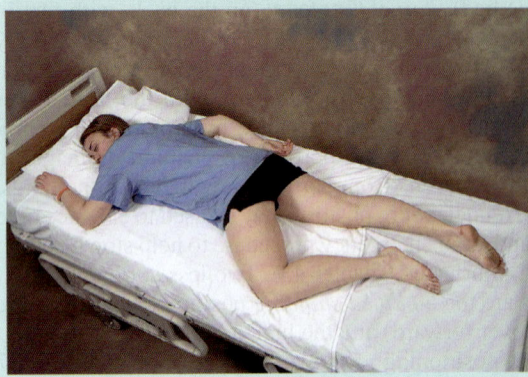	Side-lying (usually left side), upper knee flexed sharply, bottom arm behind body. Small pillow allowed under head. Pillow may be placed under top leg. Difficult for client with arthritis or leg injuries.	Rectal examination; procedures such as colonoscopy or enema.
Fowler	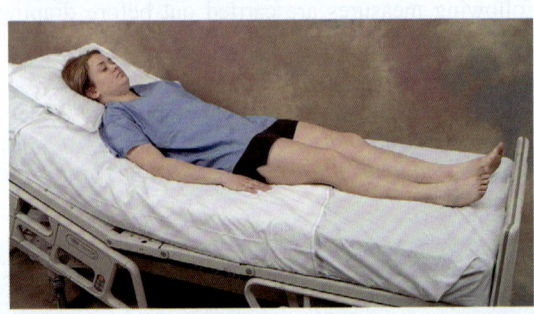	Supine, with head raised. Semi-Fowler (30°-45°); high Fowler (nearly vertical); often called orthopneic position, if required continuously. Knees elevated slightly. Watch for dizziness or faintness.	Promotes drainage; assists with breathing; preparation for dangling or walking.
Orthopneic	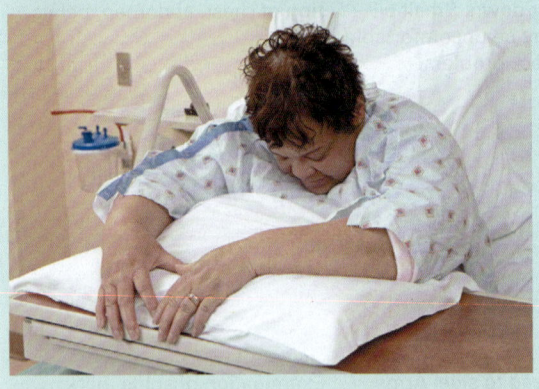	Client sitting fully upright; shown here leaning on overbed table, arms outstretched, head held up or turned to side on pillows. (Sometimes called "high Fowler" position.)	Facilitates breathing in client with severe cardiac or respiratory disorders. Can be used for an extended length of time.
Knee–chest (genupectoral)	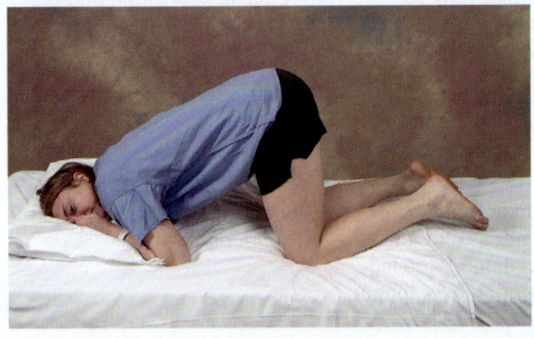	Client on knees with chest resting on bed. Arms above head or to the side; head turned to side. Thighs straight up and down; lower legs flat on bed. Client may become dizzy; do not leave alone.	Rectal or vaginal examination; treatment to bring retroflexed uterus into normal position.

TABLE 48-1 Client Positions (Continued)

POSITION	COMMENTS	USES
Lithotomy (dorsal lithotomy) 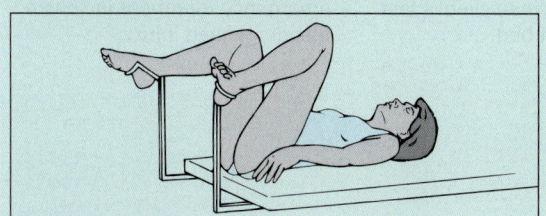	Supine, with legs separated, knees acutely flexed, hips at end of examination table, and feet in stirrups.	Pelvic or perineal examination.
Modified standing 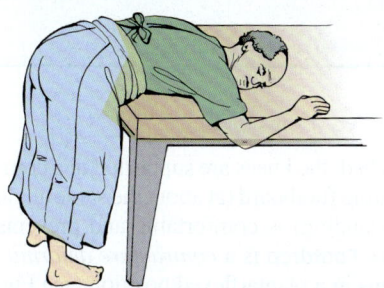	Standing, with chest, head, and arms on table.	Prostate examination.
Lumbar puncture 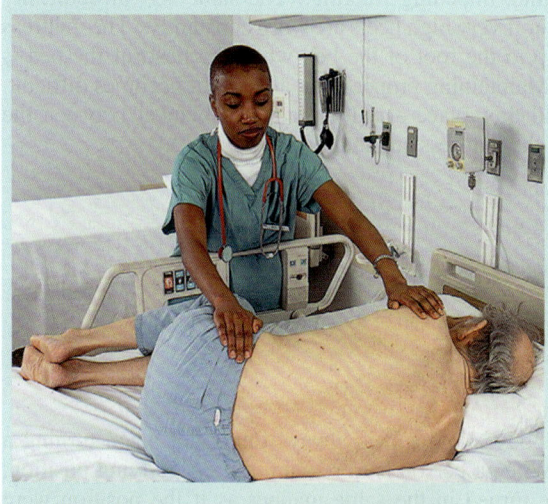	Lying on right side, knees and head flexed as sharply as possible; back exposed. Held in position by healthcare worker.	Lumbar puncture for examination of spinal fluid, spinal anesthesia, specific drug administration.
Trendelenburg position (head-down position) 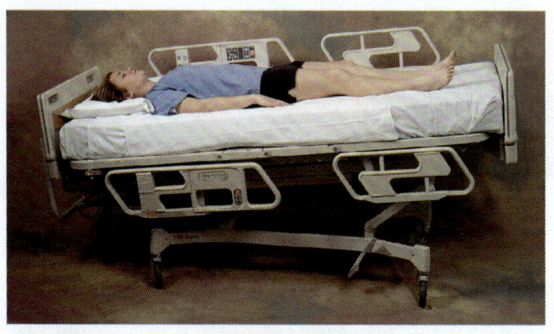	Head lower than feet. (May be simulated using pillows under feet in emergency.) Place pillow between client's head and headboard of bed.	Treatment of shock, promoting venous return.

(Continued)

TABLE 48-1 Client Positions (Continued)

POSITION	COMMENTS	USES
Reverse Trendelenburg (head elevated)	Head higher than feet. Place pillow between client's feet and footboard of bed.	To facilitate tube feedings, emergency treatment in severe bleeding, head injury.

area being examined. (In some cases, a full bladder aids in the examination.)

- A urine specimen is collected, as ordered.
- The client is encouraged to defecate before most examinations, particularly a rectal examination.
- The client is provided with an examination gown and/or bath towel to cover the chest and perineal area.
- A bath blanket or sheet is provided for warmth and privacy. In some cases, a small pillow is provided.
- The examination procedure is fully explained.
- The body is draped appropriately for client privacy and examiner's access.
- Appropriate lighting is provided.
- Necessary equipment and supplies are prepared.
- The nurse remains during the examination.
- The examiner and nurse wash or sanitize their hands before and after any examination.
- Gloves are worn in many cases.
- Other personal protective equipment is worn when needed.
- The nurse observes, in order to document the procedure, maintain client safety and confidentiality, provide client reassurance, and answer questions. It is important that the nurse understands the examination, to anticipate untoward events and accurately answer questions.
- After the examination, the nurse assists in disposing of equipment and supplies and readying the examination room for the next examination.

Turning and Moving Clients

As a nurse, you will be required to turn and move clients regularly, without endangering either the client or yourself.

Preventing Deformities

Any client who does not move the hands must have their hands supported in an open position, to prevent contractures (permanently shortened muscles). A hand roll is placed in both the client's hands, to support the wrists, keep the fingers bent slightly, and keep the thumb out in a grasping position (Fig. 48-6). The hand roll can be made by rolling a washcloth or small towel, or by using a commercially prepared hand roll. By using a hand roll, the client will later be able to functionally use the hand. Without this procedure, the muscles would pull the hand into a tight fist.

When the client is in bed, the knees are supported in a comfortable position. A slanting footboard (at about the same angle as if the person were standing) is comfortable and prevents footdrop (see Fig. 49-4). **Footdrop** is a *contracture deformity* in which the foot remains in a plantarflexed position (see Fig. 49-3). This deformity prevents the heel from being placed on the ground, impeding walking. (The same sort of deformity can occur if very high heels are worn constantly.) The mattress may slip to the foot of the bed when the head of the bed is raised. Maintaining proper body alignment becomes difficult. To avoid this, place a pillow or rolled blanket between the edge of the mattress and the foot of the bed.

> **NCLEX Alert**
>
> Appropriate body mechanics and positioning are commonly composites of situations that include client care, client and nurse safety, and prevention of the hazards of immobility.

Turning the Client to a Side-Lying Position

Proper body alignment is always important when turning a client. When a person is to remain in the side-lying position, they are turned in the same manner as if the position were

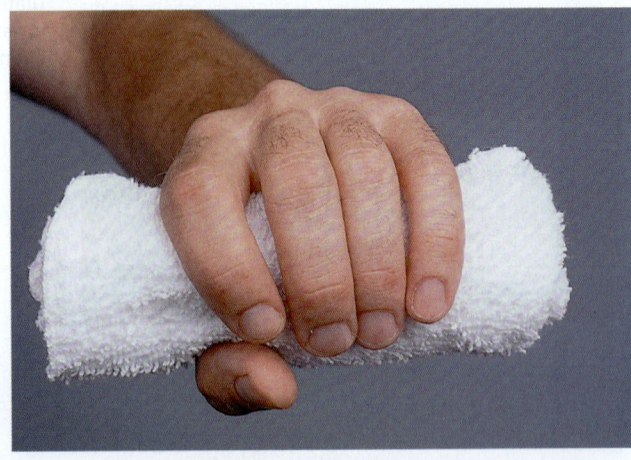

Figure 48-6 The hand roll (a rolled washcloth or commercially prepared hand roll) helps prevent contractures of the fingers (Timby, 2005).

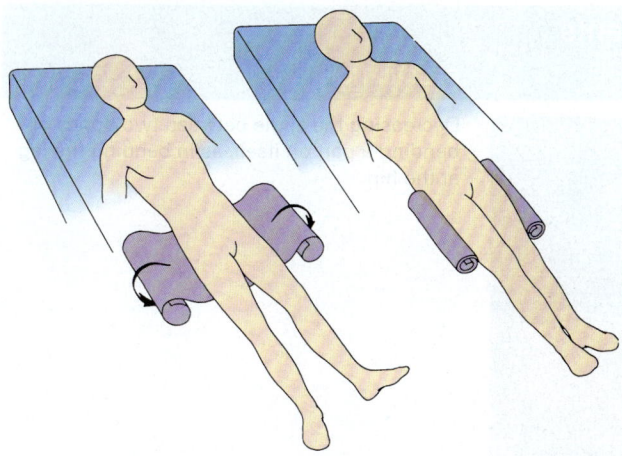

Figure 48-7 Placement of trochanter rolls, to prevent outward rotation of legs and hips. (Timby, 2005.)

temporary (e.g., to receive a backrub). Then, the client is propped into the new position. In Practice: Nursing Procedure 48-1 gives steps in turning the client to the side. Pillows may be placed as the client wishes, to add to their comfort.

Body Alignment With the Client on the Back (Supine Position)

Often clients prefer to lie on their backs most of the time, the *supine* or *dorsal recumbent position*. (They may return from side-lying to the back if they are not properly supported on the side.) When a client prefers this position, use pillows to support the head, neck, arms, and hands and a footboard to support the feet. This position allows digestive and respiratory organs to function, without being restricted. If the client's trunk must be flatter than the upper part of the body, only one pillow is needed to support the head and neck. A knee roll is placed under the knees, and a pad is placed under the ankles to prevent pressure on the heels. The footboard will be more nearly upright in this case. When the immobile client is to lie on the back for some time, **trochanter rolls** are placed on each side of the legs, to keep the legs and feet from rotating outward, causing later deformities (Fig. 48-7). Trochanter rolls are made by rolling a bath blanket or by using commercially prepared rolls.

Supporting the Client in a Sitting Position in Bed
Fowler Position

A client may sit up for a short time to eat meals, work at the overbed table, or change position, per the provider's order. The most commonly used position, the *Fowler position*, is a variation of the supine position, with the head of the bed raised (see Table 48-1). In *semi-Fowler* or *low Fowler*, the head of the bed is raised about 30° to 45°. In *high Fowler*, the head of the bed is raised to nearly vertical. High Fowler position is sometimes referred to as orthopneic position, particularly if required continuously.

The Orthopneic Position

Some clients with cardiac or respiratory conditions need to sit upright continuously, to ease breathing (*orthopnea*). This **orthopneic position** facilitates breathing and is achieved by placing the overbed table across the bed or in front of a chair with one or two pillows on top of the table. The client leans forward across the table with the arms on (or beside) the pillows and rests their head on the pillows. Pillows can also be placed behind the client's back, for additional support (see Table 48-1). In the alternative orthopneic position, the client sits up straight, with arms supported by pillows.

Prone Positions

The person may be positioned on the stomach (prone) for short periods, to provide variety (see Table 48-1). The full prone position, however, is uncomfortable for extended times, because having the head turned to the side can strain the neck and cause headache.

The Semiprone Position

The semiprone (*lateral*) position is a variation of the prone and side-lying positions. It is more comfortable than lying on the stomach, and breathing is easier than in the full prone position. To place a client into a semiprone position from back-lying, roll the person as in In Practice: Nursing Procedure 48-1. The major difference is that the bottom arm may be placed behind the client, rather than in front, and the client more on the stomach than on the side. The upper arm and leg are supported with pillows. (Usually, pillows are not needed behind the person.) The semiprone position is similar to the Sims position, but not as extreme. (See Table 48-1.)

> **Key Concept**
> The client's body alignment when lying down should be approximately the same as if the person were standing. If in doubt about moving any client, ask for assistance.

The Logroll Turn

The logroll turn is a method of turning the client that keeps the body in straight alignment (like a tree log) and may be used for linen changes, change of body position, or to give back care. This helps relieve pressure areas over bony prominences and generally adds to the client's comfort. The logroll turn is used for clients with spinal cord injuries or who have had back surgery. Because the goal is to turn the client's body as one intact unit, this method helps prevent further injuries to the back or spine. Two or three nurses are required to turn the client in logroll fashion. Only in an emergency, such as if the client is vomiting, can one nurse perform this procedure. The logroll turn is used *only with specific provider's orders and special in-service education*. This turn is introduced in In Practice: Nursing Procedure 48-2.

JOINT MOBILITY AND RANGE OF MOTION

Each body joint has a specific, but limited, opening and closing motion, its *range of motion* (**ROM**). Chapter 47 introduces this concept (see Figs. 47-18 and 47-19). The limit of a joint's range is between the points of resistance at which the joint will neither open nor close any further. Generally, all people have a similar ROM for major joints. Factors such as body development, genetics, presence/absence of disease or deformity, and amount of exercise obtained determine individual differences. The musculoskeletal system and its movements are introduced in Chapter 18; Table 48-2 reviews

TABLE 48-2 Range of Motion in Body Movements

MOVEMENT	ILLUSTRATION	DESCRIPTION
Flexion	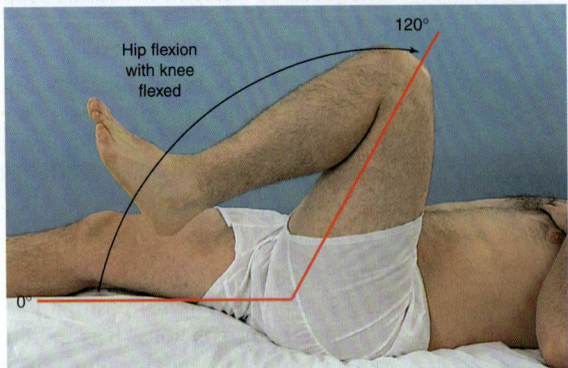	Decreasing the angle between two bones or bending a part on itself, as in bending the leg at the hip
Extension	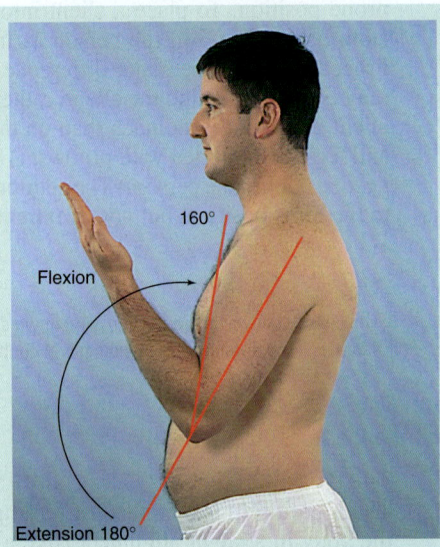	Increasing the angle between two bones, as in straightening the arm
Hyperextension	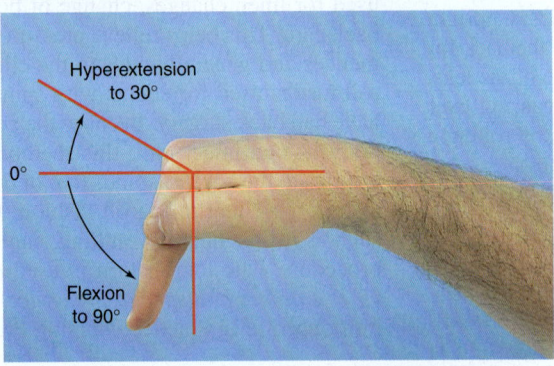	Increasing the angle of an extremity beyond normal, as in bending the head back to look at the ceiling or bending the fingers back
Dorsiflexion	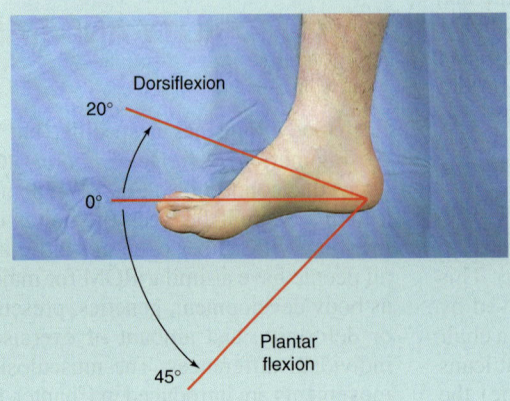	Bending a body part toward the dorsum (backward), as in moving the foot so the toes are pulled toward the knee and thus facing backward

CHAPTER 48 Moving and Positioning Clients

TABLE 48-2 Range of Motion in Body Movements (Continued)

MOVEMENT	ILLUSTRATION	DESCRIPTION
Plantar flexion	See previous	Bending the foot so that the toes are pointed downward
Abduction	(0° / 30° Adduction)	Moving a body part away from the midline of the body
Adduction	See previous	Moving a body part toward the midline of the body
Circumduction	Circumduction	Moving an extremity in circles; the extremity draws a cone, with the joint as the apex of the cone—as in swinging arms in circles
Rotation	Rotation	Moving a bone on a longitudinal axis (horizontally), as in shaking the head no, or moving in a circle from the waist
Supination	(90° Pronation / 90° Supination)	Inversion. Turing the palm upward

(Continued)

TABLE 48-2 Range of Motion in Body Movements (Continued)

MOVEMENT	ILLUSTRATION	DESCRIPTION
Pronation	See previous	Turning the hand so the palm faces downward or backward
Inversion	(see illustration below)	Turning a body part so that it faces medially or inside, such as turning the ankle so that the sole of the foot faces the opposite foot
Eversion	See previous	Turning the foot so the sole faces away from the other foot. (Both illustrations here show the *right foot*.)
Protraction	(see illustration below)	Moving forward or anteriorly, as in jutting out the jaw
Retraction	See previous	Moving backward or back into anatomic position

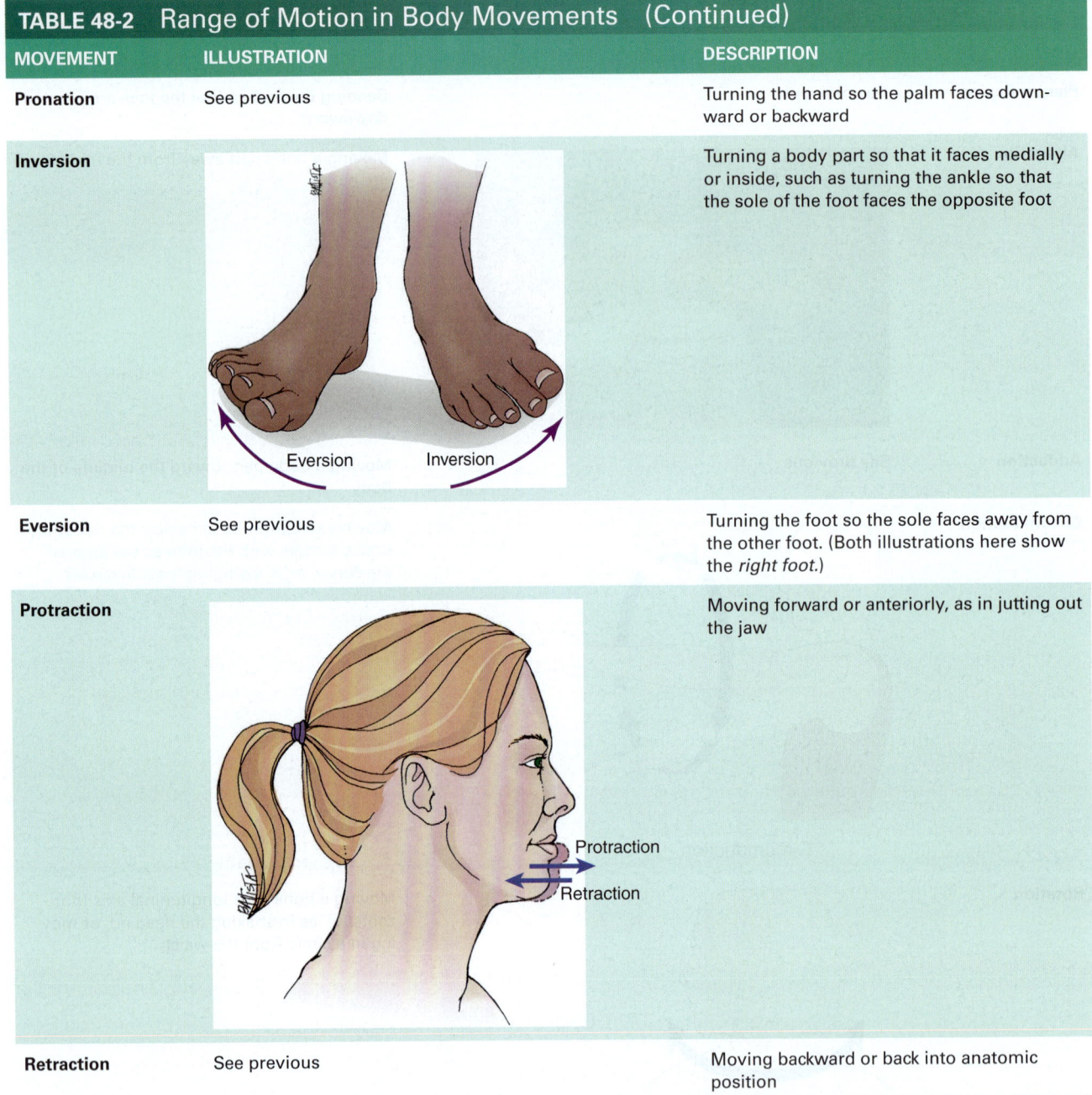

basic joint movements. Ligaments, muscles, and tendons connected to bones control joint movement; injuries/disorders of these structures often cause limited joint movement and pain. Every major joint (e.g., neck, shoulder, elbow, wrist, finger/thumb, hip, knee, ankle, and toe) must move regularly to prevent stiffness and deformities. For healthy, active people, this exercise occurs normally in everyday life. For the ill or immobilized person, however, joint movement may be limited or impaired. To avoid abnormalities, nurses assist clients to exercise all joints—several times daily—through ROM exercises.

Nursing and physical/occupational therapy share the responsibility for managing client ROM exercise programs, in order to prevent joint deformities. The most serious deformity is a **contracture**, the continuous, permanent contraction (shortening) of muscles. (Exercise also helps prevent conditions such as hypostatic pneumonia, thrombophlebitis, footdrop, circulatory difficulties, skin breakdown, urinary disorders, fecal impactions, and depression.) Attentive and frequent nursing care can help minimize these problems for the immobile client.

Passive Range of Motion

If a client is unable to move, the nurse performs *passive range of motion* (**PROM**) exercises. In PROM, the nurse

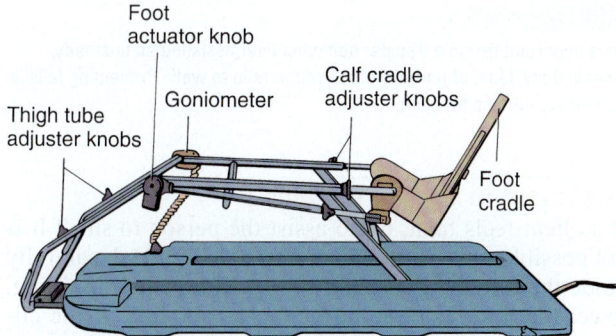

Figure 48-8 The continuous passive motion (CPM) machine. The goniometer measures the angle of the bend in the knee joint and controls the parameters of flexion and extension of the knee. Padding is added to protect the limb. (Timby, 2005.)

or therapist moves the client's joints and assists in assuming various positions. (If the client moves themselves, this is *active range of motion [AROM].*) In Practice: Nursing Procedure 48-3 gives information for providing PROM exercises. The physical therapist may draw up an exercise plan for a specific client and orient the client. Nurses help carry out this plan, particularly if exercises are repeated several times a day. Occupational therapy also provides exercises, often for smaller muscle groups.

Nursing Alert Do not force joint movement when doing PROM exercises. If the client complains of pain, stop and check with your supervisor.

Continuous Passive Motion

A mechanical device, the continuous passive motion (**CPM**) machine, may provide continuous motion to a specific joint, usually the knee or hip (Fig. 48-8). CPM machines are often used after joint replacement or arthroscopic joint repair. This machine automatically moves the client's leg, promoting joint mobility and speeding rehabilitation. The nurse must carefully explain the action and purpose of the machine, to avoid client anxiety. Some discomfort may also occur.

The electric CPM machine has a padded rack for the extremity, and the physical therapist or healthcare provider sets the machine's parameters (limits), including the number of movements per minute (speed) and the degree of joint flexion. The client's leg is secured in the rack, with the knee joint back far enough to allow flexing, without rubbing the skin. Be sure the call light is placed within the client's reach and the client is instructed to call if there is pain. It is often helpful to give a PRN (as needed) pain medication approximately 15 min before the intermittent CPM treatment begins, to relieve pain and allow greater joint movement during the treatment. In some cases, a client will return from surgery with the CPM machine already in place and moving. Many providers order CPM around the clock; others order the machine on only at night. The degree of flexion and speed of the CPM are gradually increased, per orders, helping build joint strength and mobility. (Be aware that some providers do not prescribe CPM, believing it does not promote healing and may increase inflammation.)

Active Range of Motion

The client doing individual self-directed exercises is performing **AROM**, although encouragement may be necessary, to ensure that the client moves all joints and muscles to the fullest extent possible. **Isometric** (*muscle-setting*) exercises are those the client performs by tightening and releasing certain muscle groups. Isometric exercises are helpful for strengthening abdominal, gluteal, and quadriceps muscles, those necessary for ambulation. Because these exercises only preserve muscle mass, they are *not useful in preventing contractures.* Isometrics are useful in preparing the client for crutch-walking or wheelchair use; maintaining muscle tone in a casted limb; or teaching bowel or bladder training. The routine that achieves the best results is a repetition of five sets of exercises, each lasting 5 s, with a 2-min rest period between "reps." (e.g., Tighten the abdominal muscles: count 1-1,000, 2-1,000, 3-1,000, 4-1,000, 5-1,000. Rest for 2 min. Repeat for five sets.) The client's thigh and leg muscles can be strengthened by *contracting the quadriceps femoris,* the large muscle on the anterior thigh; the client will feel as though they are pushing the popliteal space behind the knee downward into the mattress and pulling the foot upward. Other exercises are done while in bed or a wheelchair. The client lifts the hips by pushing the hands down into the mattress or the chair arms. For push-ups, the client lies face down with the hands placed flat on the mattress next to the shoulders, with elbows bent. The client extends the elbows stiffly to raise the head and chest off the bed. Some daily activities can be turned into useful exercise (e.g., reaching for objects on the bedside table; pulling the overbed table forward and pushing it away; brushing the hair). In addition, most beds contain an overhead trapeze (see Nursing Procedure 48-11). The client uses it to pull up in bed, thus exercising the arms. Frequent use strengthens muscles, and the client often creates individualized exercises when the importance of exercise is explained.

Assisting the Mobile and Partially Mobile Client

Some clients are allowed out of bed (**OOB**) for the entire day; others are up for specified lengths of time daily, as their conditions permit. Follow these basic principles when assisting clients out of bed:

- Check the provider's order to determine the client's allowed activities.
- Assist the client to put on bathrobe and slippers. Provide a bedpan, if necessary. Offer a blanket, to avoid chilling.
- Remind the client to tell you if they are becoming tired, faint, or weak.
- Offer PRN pain medication approximately 30 min before the client gets up. (This increases client comfort and may enable the client to be up longer.)
- Make sure the nurse call signal is within reach, if you leave the client while they are sitting up. (A client protective device may be necessary, to prevent the client from falling out of a chair.)
- Start with short periods out of bed and increase as the client is able.
- Help the client dangle on the edge of the bed before getting up.

Evaluating Fall Risk

It is everyone's duty in the healthcare facility to prevent client falls; a formal fall-risk evaluation is done on admission and throughout the client's stay. In the acute care facility, this evaluation is done twice a day; in long-term care, at least daily. Those clients who have difficulty moving or walking or who have had a recent fall are particularly vulnerable. Chapter 39 contains a discussion of fall-risk criteria (see Box 39-1). Although the formal Fall-Risk Assessment is done by an RN, the LVN/LPN plays a vital role in *observing* and reporting observations. All nurses are expected to assist and move clients in such a way as to prevent falling. Clients at risk for falling are often identified by special slippers (yellow), a yellow name band, and a special sign attached to the door of the room (see Fig. 39-1). Guidelines for fall prevention are given to clients on admission. These guidelines include calling for assistance, realizing that some medications and physical disorders cause dizziness, getting up slowly, and wearing proper footwear when up. Clients are reminded to use their glasses and hearing aids, *never to try to climb over side rails,* and to use handrails when needed. Family members may be encouraged to stay with high-risk clients and to make sure the client has a nurse call signal. A bed alarm may be needed, to warn staff if the client tries to get up (see Fig. 48-22) (Morgan et al, 2018).

Use of the Transfer Belt

The nurse can provide support to the weak or unsteady person by using a *transfer belt* (also called a **gait belt**). This belt is a sturdy webbed belt with a buckle, easily secured around the client's waist. Explain to the client that the belt provides safety and protection for both client and nurse. In Practice: Nursing Procedure 48-4 discusses use of a transfer belt.

> **Key Concept**
> It is important to use a transfer belt whenever assisting an unsteady, weak, dizzy, faint, or partially paralyzed person to walk. Preventing falls is a primary nursing function.

The Client in Danger of Falling

If a client feels faint, try to assist the person to sit. If it is not possible to assist the client into a chair or bed, carefully guide them to the floor (Fig. 48-9). If the client is sitting, lower the head as close to the lap as possible. If the client is on the floor, assist them to lie down. If help is not readily available, elevate the client's feet (see Nursing Care Guidelines 43-1).

> **NCLEX Alert**
> You should be alert to NCLEX situations or conditions that put clients of any age at risk for falls. It is the responsibility of all healthcare workers to prevent clients from falling. Teaching family members, visitors, or healthcare assistants may be part of your nursing responsibilities.

Dangling

Dangling refers to helping the client to sit on the edge of the bed, with the legs down and the feet supported on a footstool or the floor. This helps the client who has been in bed to prepare to sit in a chair and, eventually, to walk. *Be careful:* Allow the person to sit in the bed for a few minutes before assisting them out of bed. (It may be necessary to raise the head of the bed.) The client may experience light-headedness or weakness, due to a temporary fall in blood

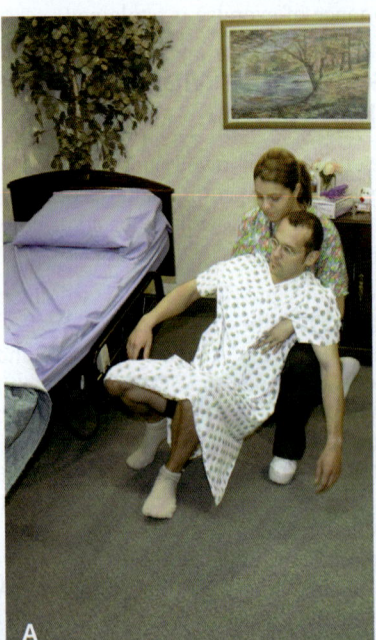
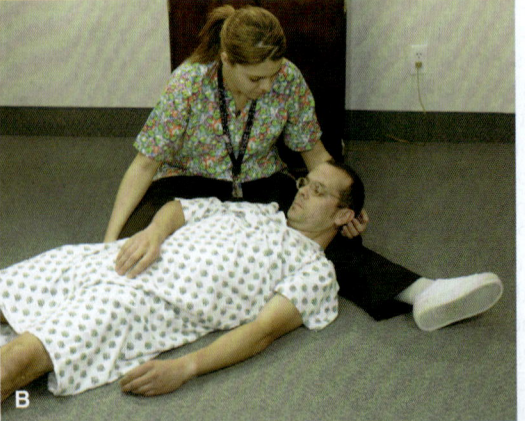

Figure 48-9 **A.** If a client feels faint and falling is inevitable, and you cannot turn them around to sit on the bed, gently ease them to the floor. Put your arms around their torso. (Grabbing the arm could cause more damage.) **B.** As the person slides down, lower yourself to the floor, cradling the client's head in your lap, to prevent injury. Stay with them and call for help. (Carter, 2008.)

pressure (*orthostatic* or *postural hypotension*). It is important to understand the client's limitations. They may only be strong enough to dangle and then lie down again. In Practice: Nursing Procedure 48-5 discusses the steps for dangling.

Helping the Mobile Client Out of Bed

Clients who are weak from long periods of bedrest or who are unsteady because of illness require assistance from bed. Take care to ensure that the client has a secure sense of balance before helping them out of bed. In Practice: Nursing Procedure 48-6 discusses the steps in helping the mobile client out of bed.

Helping a Client Move From Bed to Chair

Some clients have difficulty moving (transferring) from bed to chair or back again because of weakness or **paralysis** (inability to move a part of the body). The nurse can assist the mobile client, but if the client requires lifting, a mechanical lift should be used. In Practice: Nursing Procedure 48-6 outlines steps for assisting a mobile client to move from bed to chair or wheelchair. If a client is quite unsteady, heavy, or paralyzed, a mechanical lift is required. Use proper body mechanics as well.

> **Nursing Alert** Always request assistance if you are not sure whether you can transfer a client alone. Use a transfer belt or mechanical lift, if there is any question.

Helping the Client to Walk

Clients are usually encouraged to be up walking as soon as possible after surgery or serious illness. This helps prevent the serious complications of immobility (see Fig. 48-4). In many cases, the person needs some support, to prevent falling (Fig. 48-10). In Practice: Nursing Care Guidelines 48-2 provides guidelines on assisting the client to walk.

If the client feels dizzy or light-headed,

- Use a transfer belt the first time the client gets out of bed and each time after that, if needed. *Remember: the goal is to keep the client safe and injury free.*
- Help steady the person while they sit on the side of the bed. Return to the supine position (lying down) as soon as possible.
- If the client is in a chair, have them bend over at the waist and lower the head.
- If walking with a client who feels faint, help them to lean against a wall and bend over. If this does not help, and you are alone, ease them to the floor (see Fig. 48-9).

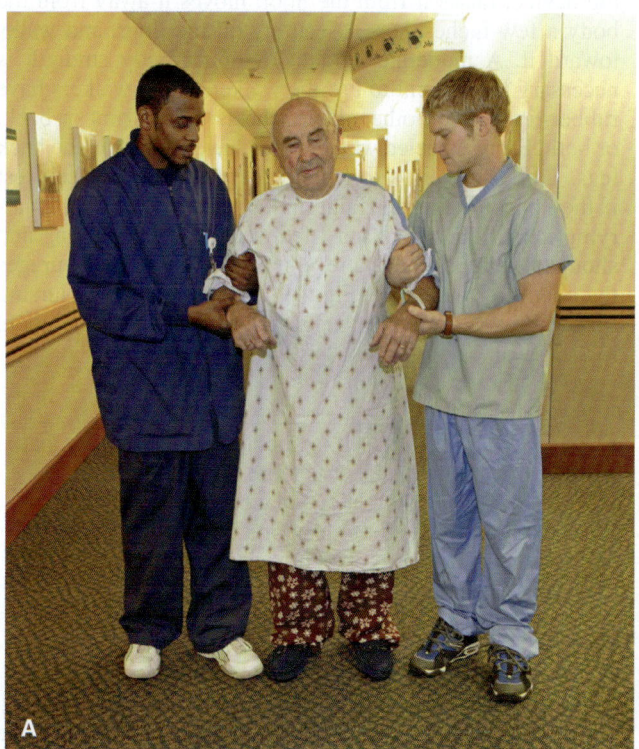
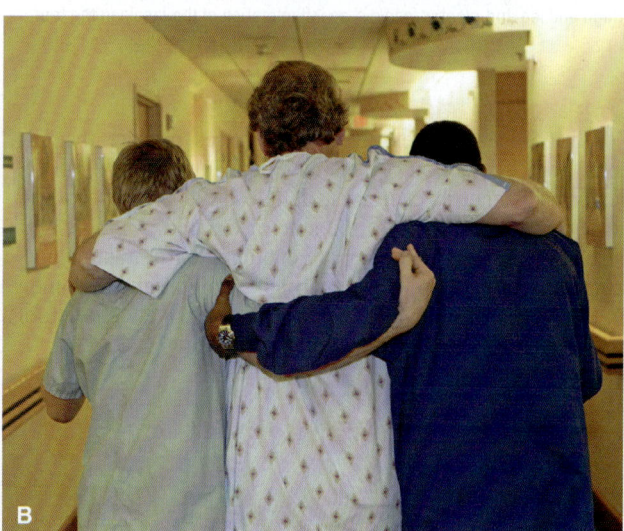

Figure 48-10 **A.** This client requires the support of two people to walk. **B.** Additional support is given by crossing the helpers' arms behind the client's back and having the client put the arms around their shoulders. A transfer belt is often used as well. (Evans-Smith, 2005.)

IN PRACTICE
NURSING CARE GUIDELINES 48-2: Assisting the Client to Walk

If the client is fully mobile,
- One nurse can assist.
- Have the client wear nonslip shoes with wide heels or firm slippers.
- Use a transfer belt for safety.
- Position yourself to the side and slightly behind the client.

If the client is more unsteady,
- Two assistants are required (see Fig. 48-10A). Often, one is a family member.
- Hold the client's arms and support the lower arms and hands.

If the client needs firm support,
- Two assistants are required.
- The assistants grasp each other's arms behind the client's back (see Fig. 48-10B).
- The client is asked to put their arms around the shoulders of the assistants.

Remember, in any case, if the client becomes faint and is going to fall, you can safely ease them to the floor, avoiding injury (see Fig. 48-9).

Key Concept

When the client gets up to walk, it is important that they wear sturdy shoes or slippers, with nonslippery soles. They should fit well and have low, broad heels. The client should not wear slipper socks, unless absolutely necessary, and never without gripper soles. (These factors help prevent falls. Slipper socks provide no arch support; extended use may cause serious damage to the feet, arches, and hips. The client may also step on something sharp and be injured.) Good arch support is important. This helps prevent conditions such as *sciatica*—pain along the sciatic nerve in the thigh and leg and *plantar fasciitis,* an inflammation of the fascia in the foot.

Conditioning and Strengthening Exercises

Conditioning and strengthening exercises prepare the client's body for action. The client pulls up on the trapeze, performs isometric exercises, dangles, sits in a chair, and practices standing next to the side of the bed. As the client performs these actions, they are encouraged to practice correct posture: head up, chest out, back straight, and abdomen in. Encourage the client to press the feet down on a footstool while sitting, to regain the feeling of standing.

USING MOBILITY DEVICES

Wheelchairs

A wheelchair is often used to move clients who cannot walk or who should be spared fatigue as much as possible (see In Practice: Nursing Procedure 48-6). After the client is in the wheelchair, make sure they are comfortable. If the client is to stay alone, secure the call signal within easy reach. If the client is unable to remain seated upright or may attempt to stand up alone, a *client reminder device* or *protective device* may be needed, to prevent them from falling. An order is required for the use of most protective devices (discussed later in this chapter). Check on the client frequently, because they may become faint or may have pain. Carefully assist the client back into bed. *Be sure to lock the wheels of the wheelchair for each transfer.* Sometimes, the client will be moved in a wheelchair to another area for examinations or tests. In Practice: Nursing Procedure 48-7 describes skills in pushing a wheelchair. (Many of these skills are also used when pushing a wheeled stretcher [a **litter** or **gurney**], used for moving people who cannot sit or walk.)

Canes and Walkers

A *cane* is a slender, handheld stick or device meant to provide support while walking. Three basic types of canes are shown in Figure 48-11A. The cane supports the client and assists in walking. It provides additional support when one side of a person's body is weak or if the client has pain in one hip or knee. The cane is held on the client's *strong side* and adjusted to the appropriate height. (This is the side **contralateral** to the weak or painful side.) In Practice: Nursing Procedure 48-8 describes additional considerations in using a cane. Chapter 97 describes many general principles of rehabilitation.

A *walker* is a four-legged tubular device with hand grips. It provides sturdy support for clients who are unable or too unstable to walk with a cane. The standard walker is made of lightweight aluminum (Fig. 48-11B). The client grips the device, raises it from the floor, moves it away from the body a few inches, sets it securely on the floor, and walks toward it. A moderate amount of upper body strength is necessary for a client to use the walker. Some walkers have rubber-tipped feet; others have wheels in the front or back, or both. Front wheeled walkers may have sliders on the back legs. Some walkers also have a seat so the client can rest if they become tired or faint and a basket, to facilitate carrying items. The client must feel secure when walking and should stand upright. The reverse walker further encourages the client to stand erect (Fig. 48-11C). In Practice: Nursing Procedure 48-9 provides suggestions for helping the client to use a walker.

> **Nursing Alert** It is important to remember that the wheeled walker is more difficult to use, because it does not stay in one place as easily. The client must be carefully taught to lean on this walker before shifting their weight, to prevent the walker from rolling away, causing a fall.

Crutches

Crutches are walking aids made of wood or metal in the form of a shaft (Fig. 48-12). They reach from the ground to the client's axillae (Fig. 48-13) or forearm. The Lofstrand crutch has a cuff that fits around the arm (Fig. 48-12B). People with a permanent or long-term disability often prefer this crutch. The person can drop the hand bar and grasp a handrail or do work, without losing the crutch. Although

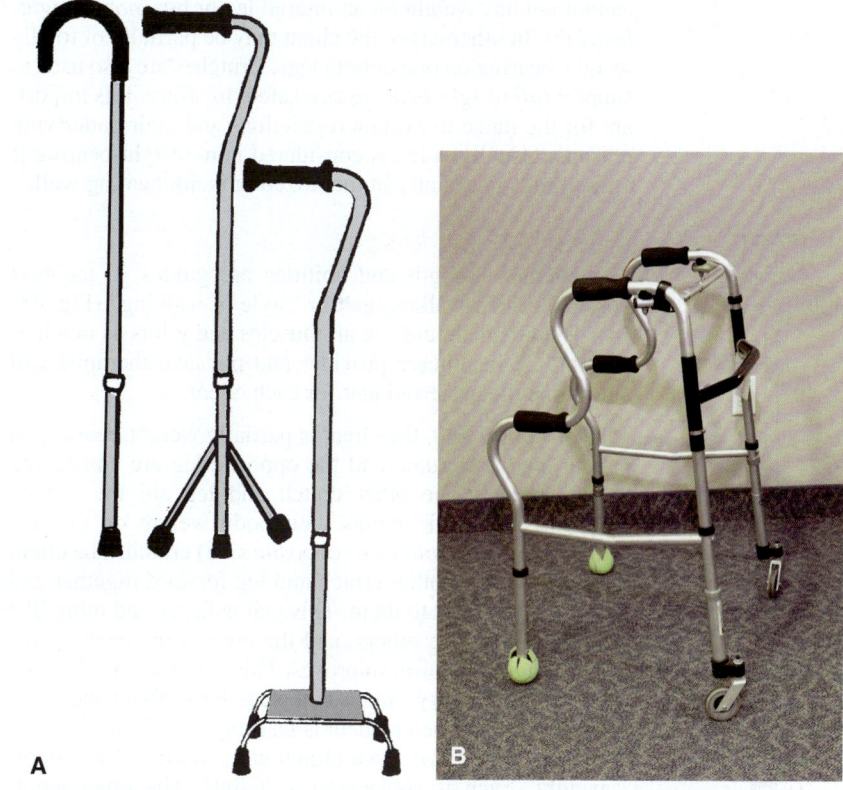

Figure 48-11 Canes and walkers. **A.** Three types of canes are the standard straight-legged cane, the tripod cane (three feet), and the quad cane (four feet). All canes should have a sturdy handle grip and rubber-tipped feet. (Ice grips are available for winter use.) **B.** This walker has lower handholds so the client can have support when getting up or sitting down. The higher handholds are used when the client is walking. Tennis balls can be placed on the back feet, to help the walker slide across the floor easier. **C.** The reverse walker is often recommended for long-term use, since it encourages the client to stand erect. The client stands inside the walker, facing forward. The walker is then moved behind the client. (This walker is often used for children.) (Carter & Lewsen, 2005.)

the Lofstrand crutch is more convenient than traditional crutches, it provides less stability. The platform crutch (Fig. 48-12C) is used in a similar manner. Another type of crutch is called a *rocker crutch*. This crutch has the two bars extending straight down to the floor, connected by a rounded end or rocker. The rocker end contains a rubber pad, to prevent slipping. This crutch gives more support, because it stays in contact with the floor while the client rocks on the crutch and swings the weight through.

Crutch Adjustment
To adjust crutches,

- Place the bottom of each crutch about 6 in. (15 cm) from the outside of the client's feet. The top of the crutch should be *two to three finger widths below the client's axillae* when their elbows are flexed approximately 30° (Fig. 48-13B).
- Adjust the hand bar so that the client can extend the arm almost completely when leaning on the palms. Even if crutches are the correct total length, the position of the hand bar may need to be adjusted. If crutches are shortened by more than 1 in., the position of the hand bar will most likely also need to be changed.

Crutches that fit properly and are used correctly are comfortable and do not create pressure under the arms. Rubber pads may be on the tops of the crutches to protect clothing. In many cases, the rubber pads are removed, to discourage clients from leaning on the tops of the crutches. The crutch tip is made of sturdy rubber that fits snugly. A large vacuum tip is a necessity, because it provides a firm base of support and prevents sliding. Ice grips are also available for slippery conditions.

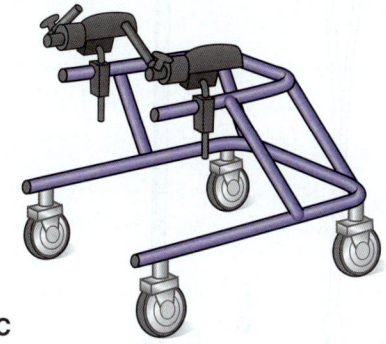

Nursing Alert Leaning on crutches in the axillae can cause a serious disorder (*brachial paralysis, crutch palsy*). To prevent this condition, the hands—not the axillae—should bear the weight of the client's body.

Preparation for Crutch-Walking
A number of things can be done in preparation for the use of crutches. The nurse can assist the client with various exercises aimed at strengthening and conditioning the upper body. Pull-ups can be done with a trapeze. The client can sit upright with arms extended downward and press the palms down on the bed to exercise the arm muscles. Push-ups can be done while lying on the stomach or while sitting in a wheelchair. Short crutches are available, so the client can practice and build strength while still in bed. Clients may be given instruction by Physical Therapy (PT) in the use of light hand weights and in various crutch-walking gaits. After initial teaching, nurses are often responsible for supervising the client's practice. In some situations, the nurse is also responsible for initial teaching in crutch-walking. This

660 UNIT 8 Client Care

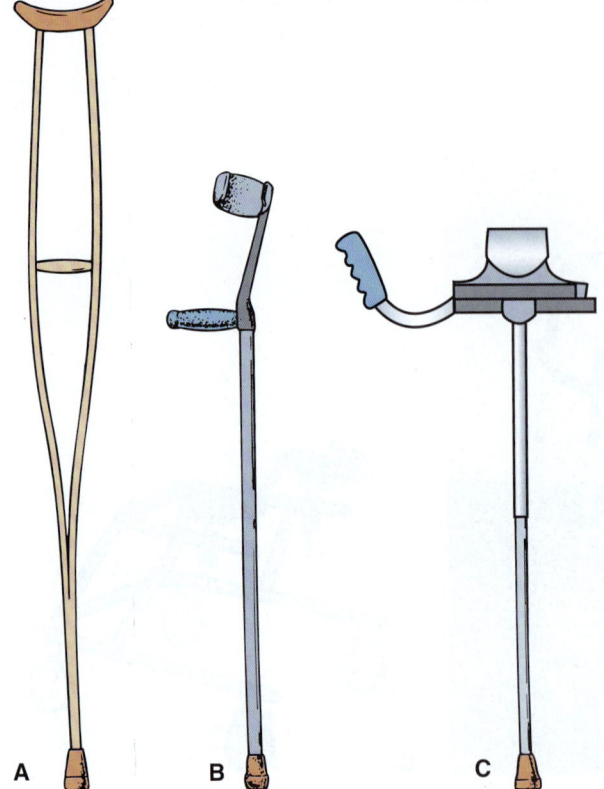

Figure 48-12 Three types of crutches. **A.** Axillary. **B.** Forearm (Lofstrand). **C.** Platform—the client's forearm is rested on the platform, while grasping the hand hold. (Timby, 2005.)

teaching includes learning a safe and comfortable crutch-walking gait, as well as learning how to go up and down stairs. Documentation of all client teaching is vital.

Weight-Bearing Restrictions

The primary provider determines how much weight the client can safely bear on the legs. In some cases, the client

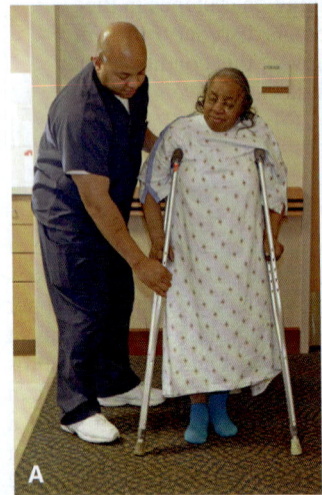
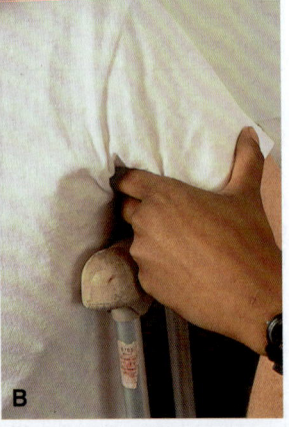

Figure 48-13 **A.** Teach the client to walk with crutches, using the safest crutch-walking gait. Support them until they are secure and safe in using crutches. **B.** Fitting crutches. They should be adjusted so the client's weight is borne on the hands. The top pads should not touch the axillae; no weight should be borne on the tops of the crutches (A: Evans-Smith, 2005.)

cannot put any weight on an injured leg or hip (*non–weight-bearing*). In other cases, the client may be partially or totally weight-bearing on one or both legs. Crutches are also used to support *full weight-bearing* as a safety measure. It is important for the nurse to explain restrictions and their underlying reasons. Usually, a leg is considered non–weight-bearing if a fracture is not totally immobilized or is not healing well.

Crutch-Walking Gaits

The client's strength and abilities are guides to the best possible crutch-walking **gait** or "style of walking" (Fig. 48-14). The client should use all muscles and joints as much as possible. A healthcare provider and physical therapist will determine the preferred gait for each client.

- In *two-point gait,* the client is partially weight-bearing on both legs. (A crutch and the opposite leg are considered one "point." The other crutch and leg are the second "point.") The client puts their body weight on one leg and on the *contralateral* (opposite side) crutch. The client then brings the other crutch and leg forward together and shifts the weight to them. This gait is faster and more like walking than the others, and the client can speed up the gait as muscle power improves. This gait is used following spinal cord injury; when both legs have about the same strength; and when a client is learning to walk again.

- In *three-point gait,* each crutch and only one leg support weight. Each is considered a "point." The other leg is *non–weight-bearing.* The person moves the non–weight-bearing leg and both crutches forward together, balancing the weight on the unaffected leg, while supporting the weight on the crutches. They then step forward with the weight-bearing leg. Steps should be of equal length and timed so no pauses occur. This gait is best when one leg is disabled and the other is strong enough to bear all of the client's weight. This gait keeps weight off the weak leg. Sometimes the client may place a small amount of weight on the weak leg, if partial weight-bearing is allowed. This gait is one means of strengthening the weak leg, without endangering the client.

- In *four-point gait,* each crutch and each leg move separately. Each of the four "points" supports weight. The client places one crutch forward, and then advances the contralateral foot; the client then brings the second crutch forward, and the other foot follows. Rhythmic, short, and equal steps are important. Counting helps develop rhythm: *one,* right crutch forward; *two,* advance left foot; *three,* left crutch forward; *four,* advance right foot. This gait is easiest and safest to use (the client always has three points of support). The client must be able to bring each leg forward and clear the floor with each foot. Those who are partially paralyzed, have fractures of both legs, or have arthritis often can safely use this gait.

- In *swing-through* or *tripod gait,* the client stands on the strong leg, moves both crutches forward the same distance, rests their weight on the palms, and swings forward slightly ahead of the crutches. The client then rests the weight again on the good leg and balances for the next step. Because this gait is fast, the client should learn to balance before attempting it. This gait is often used following a fracture, when no weight-bearing is allowed on one leg. It also is used following amputation, when the prosthesis is not in place (particularly for young people).

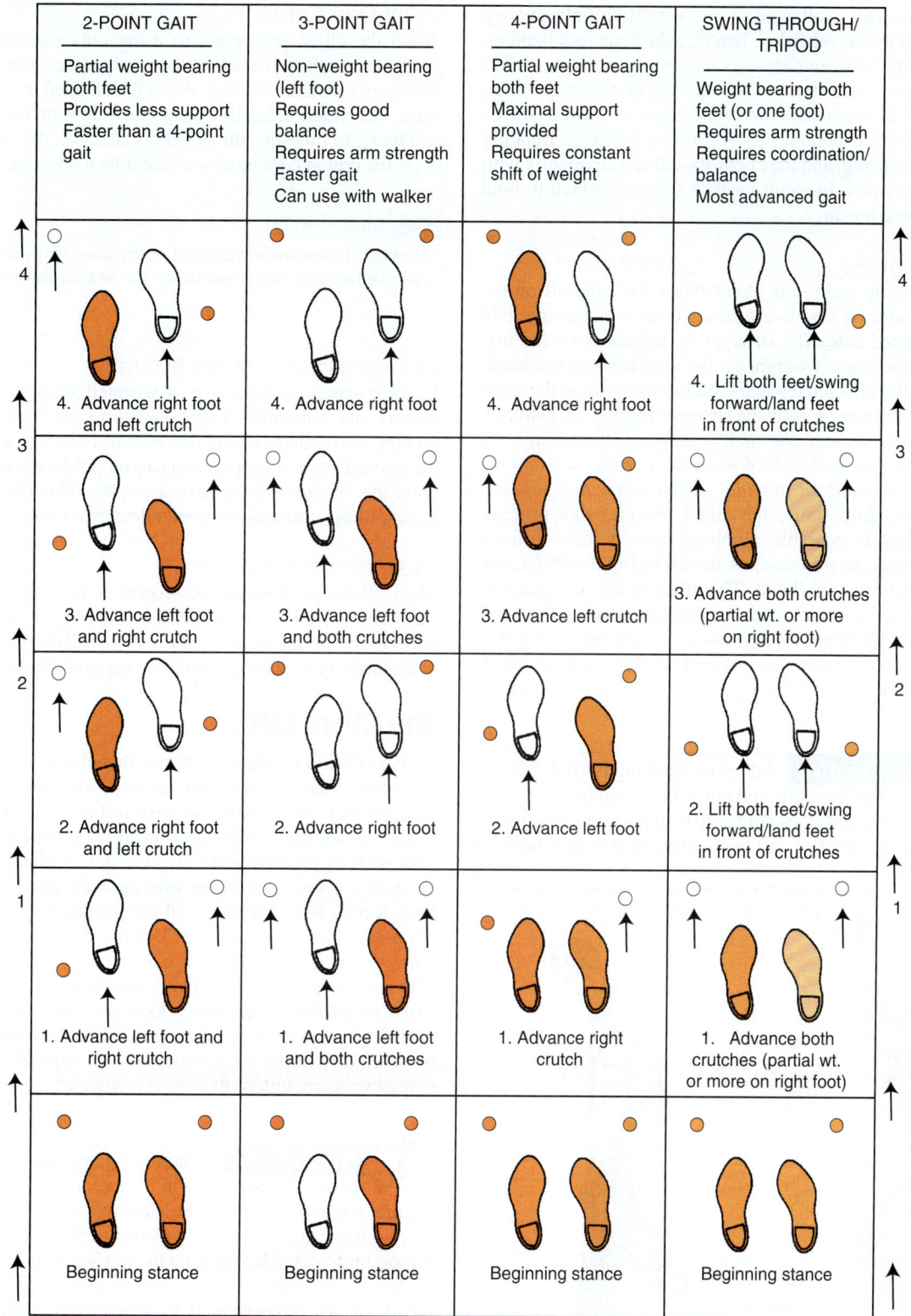

Figure 48-14 Crutch-walking gaits. *Shaded areas* indicate weight-bearing. *Arrow* indicates to advance foot or crutch. (*The illustration of each gait begins at the bottom of the picture.*) All gaits begin in the "tripod" position, with each crutch and both feet being the three points of the tripod.

The client who is allowed to put weight on only one leg must hold up the other leg, bending the knee (not bending at the hip). *Rationale: It is important to prevent hip contracture, an abnormal shortening of muscles, which can lead to permanent deformity and which can occur rapidly. This technique also improves balance.* Bending the knee is tiring, and the client should rest frequently with the leg elevated. In some cases, a strap is applied to hold the affected leg up.

Climbing Stairs

When going up stairs, the client holds the handrail on the unaffected side, if one is available. Both crutches are held on the affected side. The stronger leg advances up the first step, with the client's weight on the crutches and the handrail. Then, the affected leg and crutches move up to the same step, while the weight is on the stronger leg and the handrail. *Rationale: In this way, the client's weight is borne either by the crutches and the handrail or by the stronger leg and the handrail. The handrail provides added safety and support.* When descending stairs, the client reverses this process. If no handrail is available, climbing stairs is more difficult and dangerous. In this case, as shown in Figure 48-15, one crutch is held in each hand. The affected leg and crutches move together as a unit, with the strong leg doing the work of climbing. Excellent balance and a fair amount of strength are necessary to climb stairs using crutches when no handrail is available.

Nursing Alert Adequate teaching is vital. The physical therapist and nurse bear increased liability if the client does not receive adequate instruction and supervised practice. All instruction *must* be carefully documented.

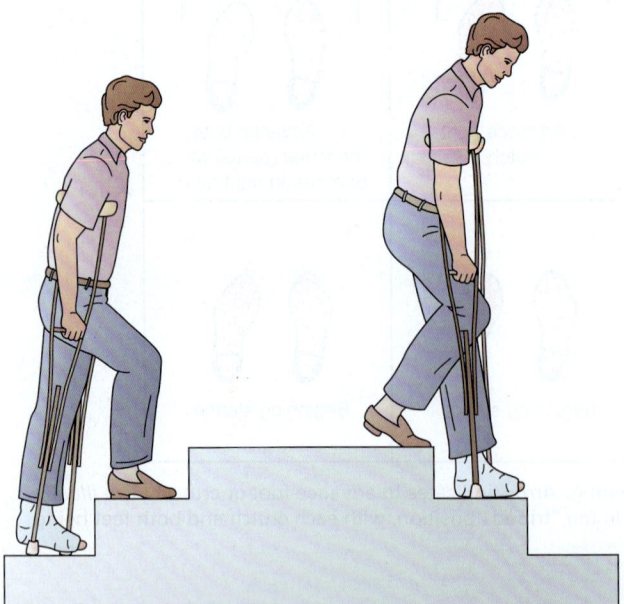

Figure 48-15 Stair climbing with crutches can be difficult, particularly if there is no handrail. Balance must be maintained to prevent falls. Step "up with the good"; step "down with the bad and support with crutches."

Using One Crutch

When the client progresses to using only one crutch, they place the crutch on the side of the stronger leg (contralateral to the injury or weakened leg). When the affected leg moves forward, the crutch naturally swings forward with the contralateral hand. In this way, the weight is either on the stronger leg or on the crutch combined with the affected leg, at all times.

> **Key Concept**
>
> A number of other special household modifications and pieces of special equipment are described in connection with rehabilitation in Chapter 97.

The Knee Walker (Knee Scooter)

In some cases, a client uses a wheeled support, with handlebars and sometimes a seat, called a knee walker or knee scooter, also called a *hands-free crutch*. The client kneels with the injured leg in a support and can propel forward, using the good leg, as you would drive a scooter. This device avoids having to use crutches or another device to move about.

The Motorized Scooter

Many clients use a motorized scooter to move about. In some cases, the scooter is used only when shopping or moving about out of the home. Other clients use a scooter all the time. This provides mobility to clients who otherwise would be homebound.

The Client Lift

A *client lift* is a mechanical device that elevates and transfers immobile clients to and from the bed, stretcher, wheelchair, tub, or toilet. Many hospitals have installed mechanical lifts in each client room. The mechanical lift assists in lifting clients, thereby protecting the nurse's back. A client lift *should be used to move any client who must be lifted.* Some lifts have a high load capacity and can handle bariatric clients. (Consider the client's weight. Usually, the weight limit of a bariatric lift is 500-550 lb [226.8-249.5 kg], although larger lifts may be available.) Lifts are attached to a swivel bar or to a hook on the ceiling and work much like a car jack or are electrically driven. Most floor-based lifts have legs that can be spread, to allow for a wider base of support and can be spread wide enough to fit around a wheelchair.

Nursing Alert When using any lift, be sure you have had instruction in its operation. If you are unsure, request assistance. At least two people should carry out a transfer using any mechanical lift. It is also important to consider equipment attached to the client, such as a cast, catheter, or IV, before attempting to move the client. All slings or mats must be disinfected between uses, kept for one client only, and discarded when no longer needed.

Types of Lifts

Several types of lifts are available (Fig. 48-16).

- The sling lift (often called the Hoyer lift) is equipped with a sturdy sling that is placed under the client and supports

the client's body in a sitting position when lifted (see Fig. 48-16D). When using this lift, be sure to support the client's head and any heavy casts or equipment.
- The *E-Z Lift* is a sling lift with a sling that is not totally placed under the client. This sling is placed behind the client's back, the client's legs are lifted one at a time, and the wings of the sling are placed under the legs. When the client is lifted, the client's buttocks are out of the sling. (This lift has a capacity of 600 lb [273 kg].) The *supine lift* (mechanical lateral-assist device) moves the client in a supine (lying down) position and keeps the client flat (Fig. 48-17). This provides support from head to foot. It is used for clients who cannot support their heads or for some clients with burns or other trauma who would be injured by sitting up.
- The *HoverMatt* provides for easy movement of clients from one horizontal surface to another and can also be used to move a client up in bed or onto a gurney. It has holes on the bottom surface and is inflated when needed. It then operates like an *airfoil*, creating a layer of air between the HoverMatt and the mattress or stretcher. This decreases the friction and reduces the amount of weight to be moved by 90%. The mat remains under the client and is inflated when the client is to be moved. Handles on the sides allow staff to easily move even very large clients from place to place.
- The *E-Z Stand* is a stand-assist lift that helps a partially weight-bearing client to stand or to be transferred (Fig. 48-18). It contains a harness that is placed behind the client's back and under the arms. It helps the client to

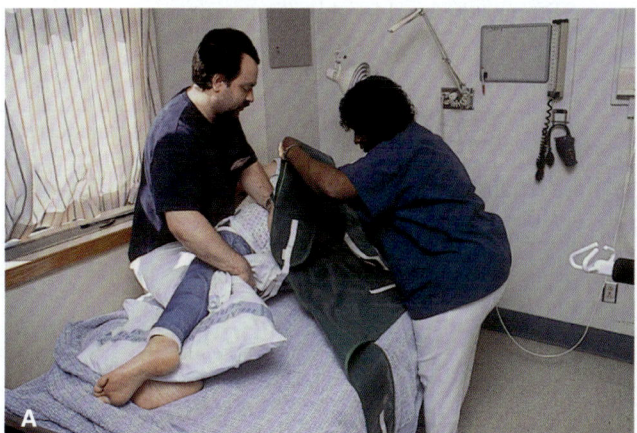
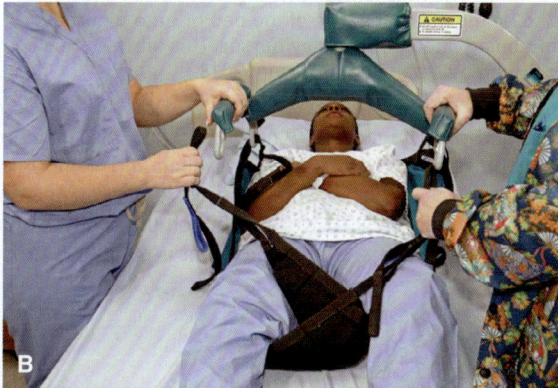
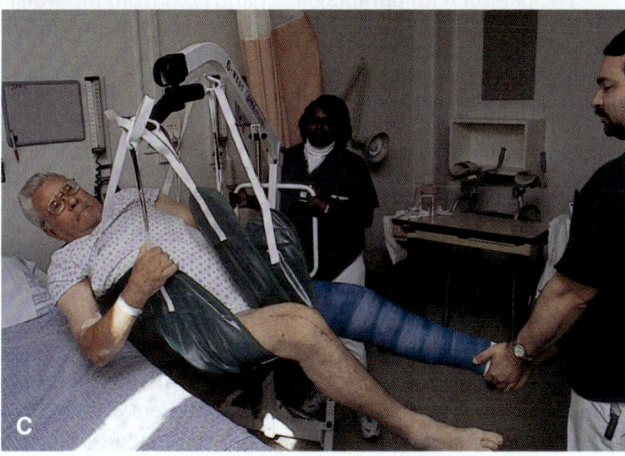
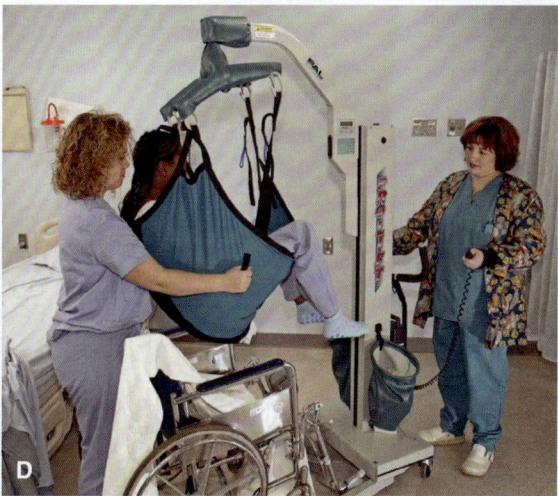

Figure 48-16 A hydraulic (mechanical) lift (two types are shown here). *At least two people should be in attendance when a client is to be moved using a lift.* The lift should be kept over the bed as much as possible (to provide safety, in case the sling releases accidently). **A.** This device is equipped with a special sling that supports the client's body while they are being moved. The client is rolled to the side to place the sling under their body. **B.** The straps of the sling are brought behind the client's back and between their legs. This sling holds the client's back and buttocks and is secured between their legs, to prevent them from slipping forward. (If the client cannot hold up their head, another sling is available to hold the head.) The ends of the straps are then attached to hooks on the swivel bar. (These hooks close with the pressure of the straps, so the straps cannot come out.) **C.** Some lifts are pressure driven and work much like a car jack, as the lever is pumped. Other lifts are electrical and are moved by pushing a button. (They must be kept charged.) As you lift the client from one surface to another, the sling holds their body securely. (The heavy leg cast is supported by a nurse during the transfer.) The sling is kept about 6 in. above the bed, whenever possible, for safety. **D.** The sling is swiveled over to above the wheelchair or chair. (Make sure all wheels are locked.) Then, the pressure is slowly released and the client lowered to the new surface. The client can assist by holding onto the sling. This also promotes the client's self-esteem and provides a feeling of security while being transferred. (In some facilities, the lift is attached to the ceiling.)

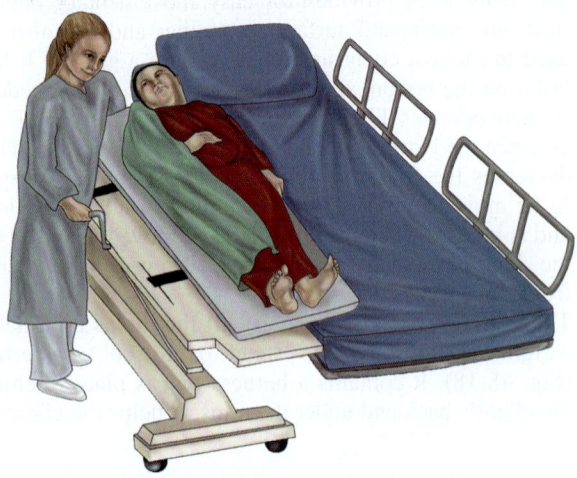

Figure 48-17 The mechanical lateral-assist device allows the client to be moved to the side of the bed or onto a gurney, without being lifted or pulled by nurses. This lift may be electrical or driven by a hand crank. (Lynn, 2018.)

stand and provide support when the client is standing. It can be moved to the bathroom or to a chair and, sometimes, contains a scale. It can also be used as a walker, after removing the footrest. It works in much the same manner as other types of lifts, except the client is standing.

> **Key Concept**
>
> Clients are often classified according to the amount of assistance required to transfer:

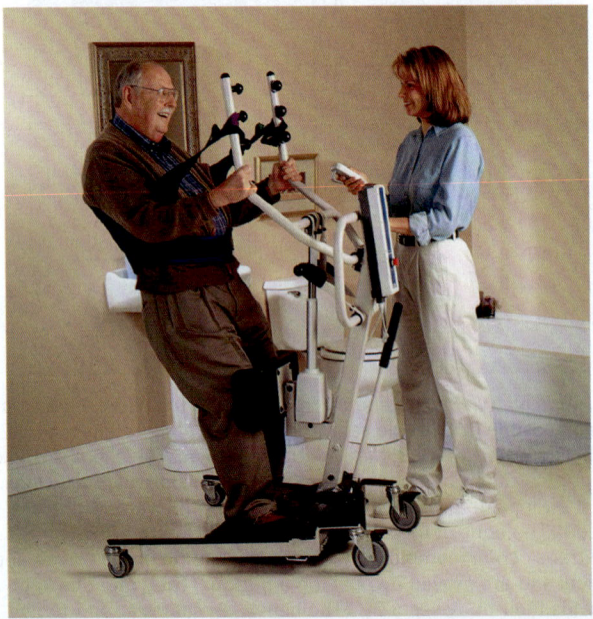

Figure 48-18 The powered stand-assist and repositioning lift. A sling is placed behind the client's back. While he holds the handles, the lift raises them to a standing position. He can then be moved to a chair or the bathroom. With the foot plate removed, this lift can also be used as a walker. (Lynn, 2018.)

- *Independent*—the client is able to transfer safely and move about without assistance. There is no recent history of falling, and the physical condition will not be endangered if the client moves about.
- *One-person assist*—the client is able to transfer or ambulate but may be confused at times or may require minimal assistance. The client is able to perform at least three-fourths of the task. A transfer belt is used in this case.
- *Two-or-more-person assist*—the client is able to bear some weight but is unsteady when walking. This person can follow simple instructions but is confused at times. This assist procedure is also used when the person's ability to transfer is unknown. A client lift is usually required, depending on the client's abilities.
- *Total lift*—this client is mentally or physically unable to safely transfer or ambulate without assistance or is unable to assist with transfer. This category also applies to any client who must be lifted from the floor. The mechanical lift must be used for this client.

> **Nursing Alert** If a client must be transferred from place to place in a hospital bed, two persons are required. If a large bariatric bed is used, at least three persons are required.

Moving the Client Who Is Partially Paralyzed

Paraplegia

The person with **paraplegia** is paralyzed from the waist area down. This person has limited or no ability to move the legs but is usually able to build up adequate arm strength. When assisting this person with a transfer, the nurse will need to help move the client's legs, but the client can help lift with the arms. The client can assist by grasping the arms of the chair (client's left hand—left arm of chair; client's right hand—right arm of chair). Usually, with minimal assistance, the client can use the arms to swing their buttocks into the chair. A transfer board may be used (see Fig. 48-19). The nurse moves the legs into position as the client moves the buttocks. If the client is not skilled enough or strong enough to move the upper part of the body, a mechanical lift must be used. If the client cannot stand steadily, the nurse braces the client's knees (see In Practice: Nursing Procedure 48-6) or a stand-assist device is used (see Fig. 48-18).

Hemiplegia

The person with **hemiplegia** is paralyzed on one side of the body, often the result of a "stroke." To help this client move into a chair, ask the client to move to the side of the bed. It is best to work on the client's strong side. The client is assisted to swing around, so the feet are on the floor. Then, the client is assisted to stand on the stronger leg, and pivot around into the chair. The client holds the arm of the chair corresponding to their stronger arm and gradually eases into the chair. If the client requires lifting, the mechanical lift should be used.

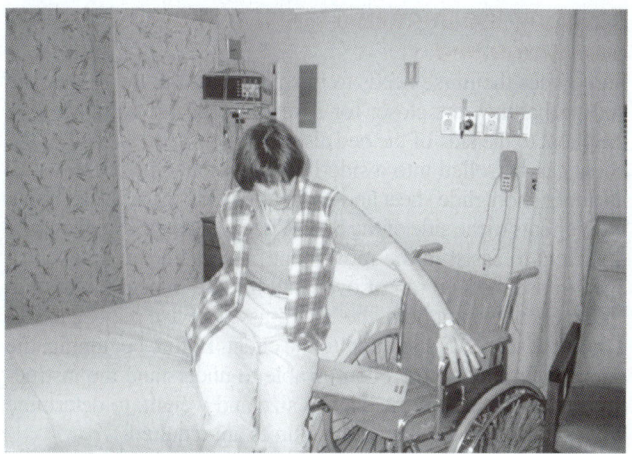

Figure 48-19 This client is able to transfer themselves independently from bed to chair and back with the use of a transfer board. The right arm rest is removed from the wheel chair, to facilitate transfer. (Timby, 2005.)

> **Key Concept**
> Make use of the client's abilities as much as possible. This protects the nurse and builds the client's strength, confidence, and self-esteem.

MOVING AN IMMOBILE CLIENT

Moving a totally immobile client is difficult and requires the use of a lift or HoverMatt and at least two to three people. It is important to use common sense in moving any client. If the nurse has any question or doubt, it is vital to seek assistance.

> **Nursing Alert** In many healthcare facilities, the staff is never allowed to lift clients. In this case, a mechanical device must be used for all transfers. Some facilities have a "lift team" consisting of staff members who assist in lifting clients throughout the facility, and they are required to use a mechanical lift as well. Check the requirements and protocols of your facility before assisting any clients to transfer.

Using the Transfer Board or Bridge (Sliding Board)

A **transfer board** (*transfer sled, sliding board,* or *bridge*) may be used by the client who is unable to stand. The board is made of hard plastic and is approximately 1/2 to 3/4 in. thick and long enough to reach from the side of the bed to a chair. It is about 1 to 1.5 ft wide. It is lightweight and has handholds on the sides, making it easy to handle. The board's surface is very smooth, allowing the person to slide easily. Using the board to transfer clients protects them from injury caused by stretching or pulling on their limbs or sliding them across the sheets and reduces their fall risk. It also conserves the nurse's energy and prevents nursing injuries. Explain to the client what will be done and how they can help.

> **Nursing Alert** Whenever you use a transfer/sliding board, make sure that there are linens between the client and the board. Many clients, particularly older people, have very friable (fragile) skin. If the skin is not protected, the client could be injured by shearing force.

Using the Transfer Board Without Assistance

In many cases, particularly if a client has been disabled for some time and has built up arm strength, the transfer between bed and chair can be made independently, by using a transfer board (see Fig. 48-19). This requires supervised practice. The nurse should supervise this client until it is evident that they can perform the transfer safely.

> **Nursing Alert** The transfer board can also be used as a backboard for emergency CPR. It provides a firm surface when placed under the client. (Transfer boards can also be used to move injured clients in an emergency evacuation or rescue situation, if emergency transfer sleds or chairs are not available [see Fig. 39-4].)

Moving the Client With a Lifting Sheet

In an emergency and if a client lift is not available, it is possible to transfer a client using a lifting sheet. If at all possible, an *anti-friction glide sheet* should be used. This procedure requires several people. The sheet is placed under the client, and the client is lifted a fraction of an inch off the bed and then moved into position. The lifting sheet can be used to move a client to the side of the bed, up in bed, or down in bed. This procedure may also be used to transfer a client to a gurney, in an emergency. (A client lift is required to move an immobile client into a chair.) Using a lifting sheet or glide sheet helps prevent injuries to nurses, as well as client injuries, such as sheet burns, shearing of tissue, or other skin breakdown caused by being pulled across bed linens. In addition, nurses should not pull on the client's shoulders or legs, or place their hands under the client's body. (Special care is necessary when working with older or very ill clients, to protect their friable skin.)

Moving the Client to and From a Stretcher

The wheeled stretcher (gurney) is used to move immobile clients who cannot sit up or who have appliances or casts that do not fit into a wheelchair.

Safety precautions to follow when using a wheeled stretcher:

- Be sure a waist strap and side rails are in place, to protect the client from falling.
- Be sure the stretcher covering is clean. Provide enough blankets to keep the client warm.
- Protect clients from injury when transferring them. Use a lateral-assist device (see Fig. 48-17) or HoverMatt if the client cannot transfer independently.
- Never leave a client alone on the stretcher.

Assisting the Client Confined to Bed

Clients confined to bed need exercise and regular changes in body position to preserve their skin integrity, muscle tone, normal body functions, and morale. A schedule is usually set up to turn such a client at regular intervals. Doing so helps prevent untoward events, such as musculoskeletal deformities, respiratory complications, circulatory disorders, constipation, and skin breakdown.

Adjusting the Backrest and Pillows

Raising and lowering the head of the bed is a simple, yet easy, way to change the client's body position. The nurse raises the client's head and shoulders to adjust the pillows.

Assisting the Immobile Client to Move Up in Bed

Gravity causes the immobile client to slide down in bed. This is uncomfortable and may interfere with breathing. The nurse will often need to adjust the client's position or move the client up in bed. In Practice: Nursing Procedure 48-11 discusses the moving of clients confined to bed. Before beginning, the nurse determines the client's ability to participate, encourages them to help as much as possible, and gives clear instructions on what the client is to do. The nurse must be aware of their own limitations and capabilities and ask for assistance if the client cannot be safely moved without more help. A mechanical device should be used whenever possible.

Assisting the Immobile Client to Move to the Side of the Bed

Sometimes the nurse needs to move the client to the side of the bed so that they are closer for a treatment or injection. Moving the client to the side of the bed also allows space in the bed so the client can be rolled into a side-lying position. One nurse, using an antifriction glide sheet and proper body mechanics, can move most clients to the side of the bed. Whenever possible, encourage the client to assist in the movement. The client can be encouraged to use the side rail or overhead trapeze to help in moving. (If the client cannot help, the lateral-assist device may be used.) The nurse serves as a support to the client. Before beginning, the nurse determines if the client is able to understand the instructions and also judges the client's size and weight, to determine what equipment and how many nurses are required.

USING CLIENT SAFETY DEVICES

A piece of equipment used to ensure the safety of the client and the healthcare environment is called a **protective device** or *client reminder device.* JCAHO (Joint Commission on Accreditation of Healthcare Organizations) and OBRA (Omnibus Reconciliation Act of 1987) have established firm standards for the use of any protective device or restraint. (The regulations are somewhat different for psychiatric situations than for other settings.) In Practice: Nursing Care Guidelines 48-3 includes important factors to consider before using any protective devices.

IN PRACTICE
NURSING CARE GUIDELINES 48-3 — Using Client Reminder or Protective (Safety) Devices

- Carefully verify the client's identity before using any client reminder/safety device.
- The client has the right to be free of any restraint applied for the convenience of staff or for disciplinary purposes.
- You must have special training before using any safety devices.
- Specific medical orders are required for the use of any safety device. (In an emergency, a device may be applied immediately, but the healthcare provider must interview the client *face-to-face* within 1 hr.)
- The legal requirements vary from one type of device to another.
- Provide privacy for the client.
- The procedure must be explained to the client and the family.
- In addition to gloves, you may require other personal protective equipment when applying safety devices.
- Apply the safety device *over a layer of clothing,* to protect the client's skin.
- Be sure to obtain enough help when applying any safety device.
- Documentation is vital; follow your facility's protocol. Documentation required depends on the reason for use and the type of device used, but evaluation must include vital signs, circulatory and respiratory status (including oxygen saturation, if ordered), skin condition, and client behavior, all of which must be monitored constantly.
- Skin care must be given.
- Some situations require one-to-one (arm's length) monitoring. In other situations, video monitoring is adequate.
- Any device must be released periodically (at least every 1-2 hr).
- The client must be given food, water, and the opportunity to void and defecate.
- Range of motion must be provided on a regular basis, and documented.
- Remove any device as soon as possible.
- The client is interviewed after the use of a safety device, to determine if other methods might have been used and if the client understands the need for the use of the device.

Explore all other alternatives before applying any safety device. Examples include

- Verbal intervention
- Diversion, such as television, craft projects, reading, puzzles. (It is often helpful to involve a family member.)
- Stress reduction, such as guided imagery, backrub, music
- Medications, as ordered
- Time out

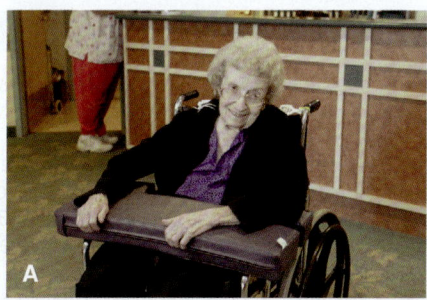
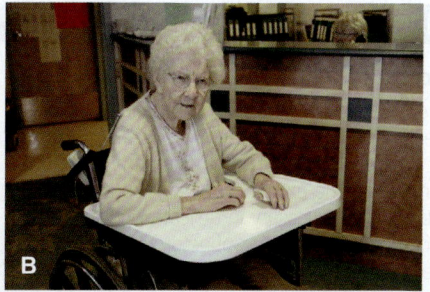
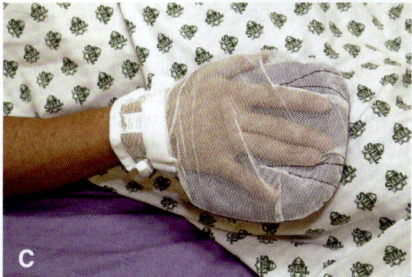
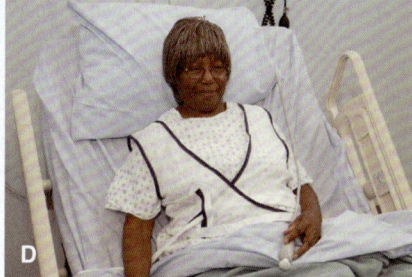
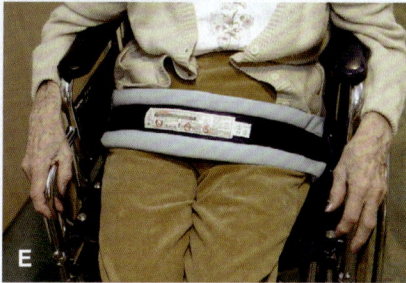

Figure 48-20 Types of commonly used safety devices (see also Nursing Procedure 48-12). The devices shown here limit client movement to various degrees and are used only if there is no alternative. (Other devices can be removed by the client and are only for client convenience.) **A.** Lap buddy. **B.** Chair with a tray table (Geri chair). **C.** Netted hand mitt. This device can be attached to the side of the bed, where it cannot be removed by the client. **D.** Criss-cross vest. This device may be safely used in bed. **E.** Lap belt, to support the client in a chair. (Carter, 2008.)

> **Key Concept**
> Any protective device, safety device, or restraint can only be used to provide safety to the client or to others. The regulations differ from one type of device and one healthcare setting to another. All staff must be thoroughly trained before using any safety device. The goal of all healthcare is to provide a *restraint-free* setting.

Types of Safety Devices

The client safety device is used when the client's behavior puts themselves at high risk for self-injury (or injury to others). The least restrictive method should always be used. Nursing Procedure 48-12 also illustrates some types of client safety/protective devices. Classifications of client safety devices or restraints include the following:

- The *medical healing device* is used to prevent the client from interfering with necessary medical care. For example, it may be necessary to use a netted hand mitt to prevent the pulling of tubes, catheters, or IV lines or to prevent a child from scratching an irritated area or suture line (Fig. 48-20C). Various means may also be used to prevent the client from slipping out of a chair or getting out of bed (Fig. 48-20A, B, D, and E). Sometimes, devices must be used in an emergency with a confused client who is unable to understand instructions, who is likely to wander away, or who may be unsafe if ambulating (see also Fig. 48-22B and C). In addition to tray tables, the most commonly used medical healing safety devices in the healthcare facility are vest safety devices. These include the Posey jacket and the criss-cross safety vest (Fig. 48-20D). The lap belt is commonly used to prevent a client from falling out of a chair or off a gurney (Fig. 48-20E).
- A *chemical restraint* is a drug, such as a benzodiazepine, used to calm or manage a client's dangerous behavior.
- The *behavioral health/behavioral management restraint* is used to prevent clients from harming themselves or others. If a client is extremely violent, assaultive, or out of control, locked restraints may be necessary. Many additional regulations apply to the use of these restraints. They are most often used in psychiatry, and their use and application are discussed in Chapter 94.

Be sure to check with your team leader or instructor before using any safety device. Improper application can be dangerous and could cause death from choking or suffocation. Figure 48-21 illustrates a quick-release knot that may be used to secure safety devices to the bed or the chair. It is important to create a knot that can be released quickly in an emergency. The restraint must be tied in a stationary location, to prevent it from accidently tightening (e.g., as the bed is raised). In Practice: Nursing Procedure 48-12 demonstrates the proper application of some protective devices.

> **Nursing Alert** A client using any safety device or restraint that they cannot release independently is considered to be *vulnerable* and must be carefully monitored. This helps protect the client from assault by other clients.

SPECIAL CONSIDERATIONS Lifespan

Client Reminder Devices for Children

If at all possible, *the nurse or caregiver should hold the child* if immobilization or control is necessary. In some extreme cases, a restraint or reminder device must be used, but only if no other means is available, because the child may become extremely frightened and agitated. A reminder device is often necessary in delicate procedures such as IV insertion, circumcision, or lumbar puncture. In addition, a child must be prevented from pulling on tubes or IVs, scratching a rash, or picking at a suture line. Since children often cannot understand explanations, some sort of restraint may be required. Nursing Care Guidelines 71-3 and Figure 71-6 illustrate several means of restraining a child. These methods include the following:

- Mummy restraint—the child is wrapped tightly in a blanket for a short time (see Nursing Care Guidelines 71-3C).
- Mitts—the hands are wrapped in Kerlix, or special mitts are used (to prevent scratching or pulling at tubes or sutures) (see Fig. 48-20C).
- Padded tongue blade reminder device—prevents bending the elbows (to protect suture line or tubes when mitts will not work, such as after cleft lip repair).
- Papoose board—the child is held tightly to a specially designed board for a very short time (for a surgical procedure, such as circumcision; see Nursing Care Guidelines 71-3, Fig. D).
- Bed net or bubble top—this is placed on the crib (to prevent child from jumping out).
- Jacket reminder device—similar to that for an adult, but smaller, placed (to keep child in a chair or bed; see Nursing Care Guidelines 71-3, Fig. A).
- Child can be held or secured in a rocking chair (which allows movement, but prevents scratching or picking at a suture line).
- Usually, children are not placed in arm, leg, or waist belts, because of the extreme danger of choking or suffocating. If these devices are necessary, one-to-one monitoring is essential. Chapter 71 describes child protective devices in more detail.

Alternatives to Client Safety Devices

Safety devices should be used only when there is no alternative. They are used solely to protect the safety of the client or others and never for staff convenience or retribution. It is important to attempt alternatives before using a physical or chemical restraint or safety device. Figure 48-22 illustrates some alternative ways to provide client safety. Additional ways include the following:

- Using a device that helps prevent slipping down in a chair, such as wedges, support pillows, nonslip materials, or a seat belt with a front release that the client can operate
- Providing gait training, exercise
- Providing reorientation, diversion
- Using a mild chemical agent to help the client to relax, within strict limits

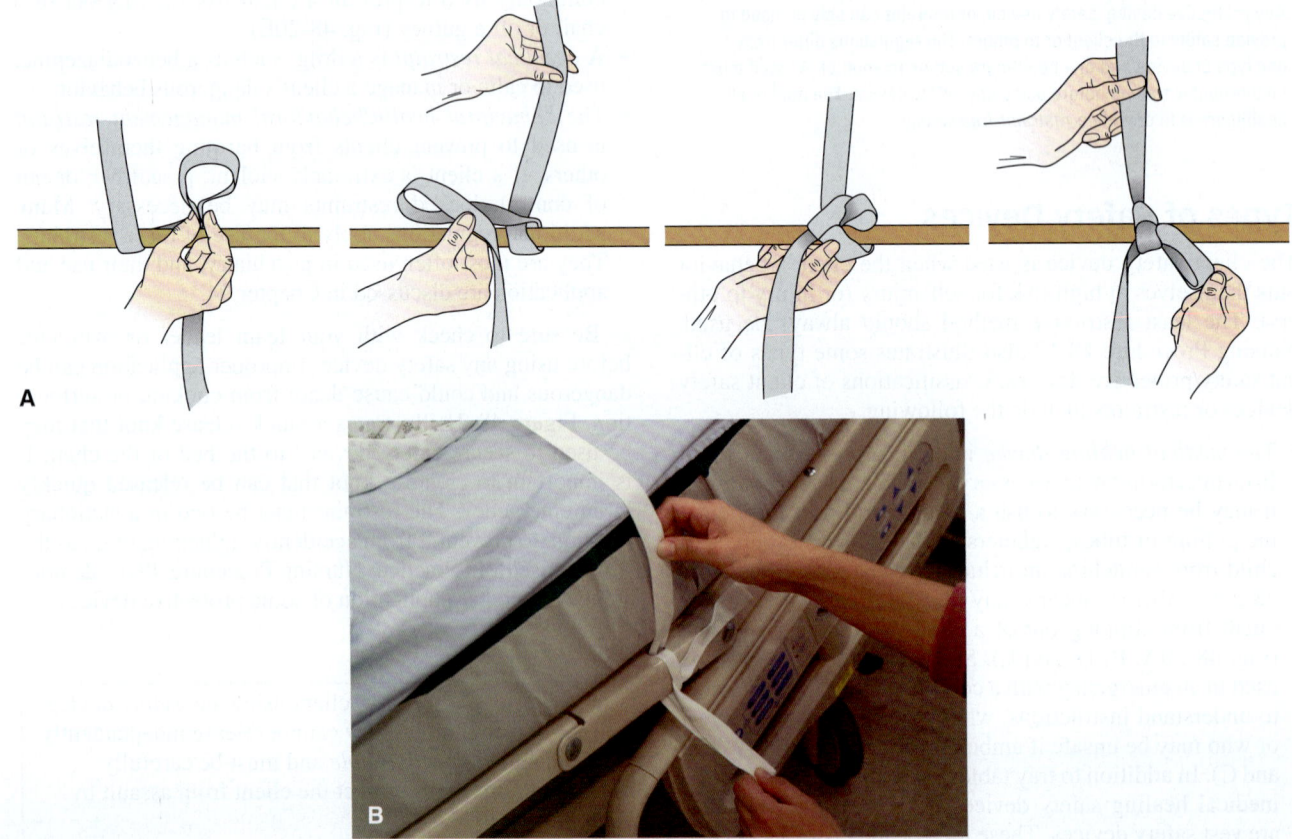

Figure 48-21 **A.** This quick-release tie is made using an overhand knot, but slipping a loop (instead of the end of the strap) through the first loop. This must be used when securing any client safety device, for quick release in an emergency. **B.** The straps are tied to the stationary portion of the bed frame, *never* to the side rails. (A: Carter, 2008; B: Evans-Smith, 2005.)

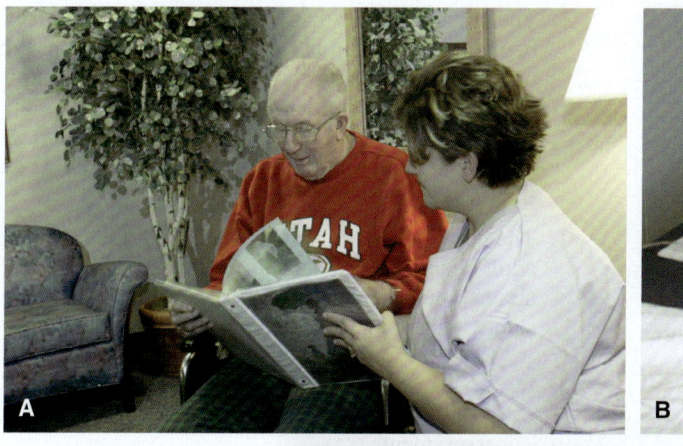
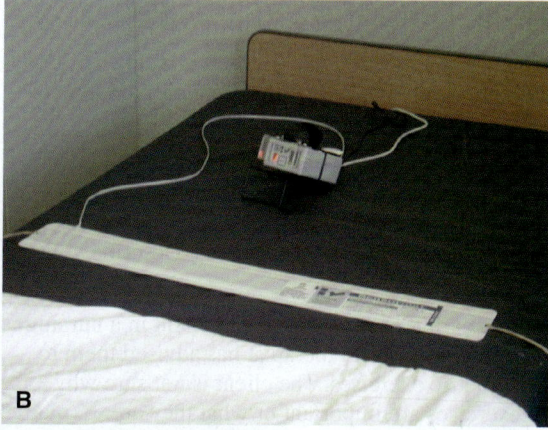
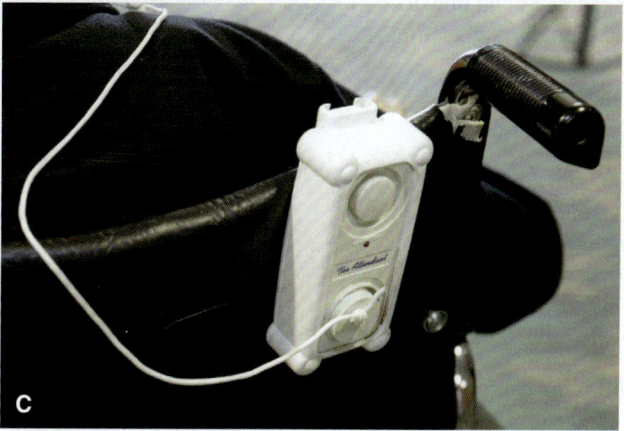

Figure 48-22 Always try to find an alternative before using a physical or chemical restraint. **A.** Allow the client to sit near the nurses' desk, or provide company and diversion. A family member or volunteer may assist. **B.** A pressure-sensing monitoring mat is located where the client's buttocks should be. The monitor, shown here on top of the mat, is hung from the headboard or back of the wheelchair, out of the person's reach and sight. If the person tries to get out of bed or chair, an alarm will sound, alerting the staff that the person needs help. (Some beds have built-in sensors.) **C.** A "wanderer" monitoring sensor is attached to the person's wheelchair or worn around the wrist or ankle. If the client tries to go through a door leading to an unsafe area, an alarm will sound, alerting the staff. This is useful for clients who are likely to stray away, such as those with dementia. (Courtesy of Bed-Check Corp., Tulsa, OK.)

STUDENT SYNTHESIS

KEY POINTS

- The mechanical lift is a vital piece of equipment, used to protect clients and nurses.
- The nurse can learn to transfer and position clients effectively for maximum safety and comfort for both nurse and client.
- Antifriction glide sheets, wedges, and other devices are available to help prevent nurses' back strain.
- Pulling, pushing, or rolling an object is easier than lifting it. Keeping an object moving requires less energy or force than starting and stopping it.
- The nurse must observe principles of good body mechanics whenever assisting clients.
- Rocking backward or forward on the feet uses the nurse's body weight as a force for assisting a client.
- A client may become dizzy or faint when first getting out of bed.
- The nurse should not allow the client to grab them around the neck; this force could seriously injure the nurse.
- Clients are assisted to move and walk using a number of devices, such as the hydraulic lift, the trapeze, and the wheelchair, walker, or crutches.
- The hospital bed should always be in low position, except when giving bedside care, to help prevent client falls.
- The client's body alignment when lying down should be approximately the same as if the person were standing.
- Joint movement is never forced during ROM.
- Safety for nurse and client is a priority when turning, moving, and transferring clients.
- Client reminder/protective devices must be used with caution and within agency and Federal guidelines.
- Alternatives should always be explored before using client protective devices or restraints.
- Special procedures may be required to assist children to remain still or not to interfere with equipment.

CRITICAL THINKING EXERCISES

1. Demonstrate how you would teach principles of body mechanics to the 30-year-old parent of a toddler.

2. Your client is a 25-year-old in traction, recovering following a femur fracture. They have been immobilized for several weeks. Now they are ready to begin walking, but will need assistance. They ask you about various kinds of walking aids. Describe your answer.

3. You are caring for an 88-year-old client in a nursing home. Their physical therapist has advised them to do isometric exercises. The client is not sure why the exercises are important or what they are. Explain to them the purposes of their exercises and how to do them. How would you lead them through some exercises?

NCLEX-STYLE REVIEW QUESTIONS

1. The nurse is caring for a client who is having difficulty with mobility. Which action taken by the nurse can assist the client with regaining mobility?
   a. Promote self-care activities.
   b. Perform tasks for the client.
   c. Reassure the client that they will not fall if they get up.
   d. Perform passive range of motion exercises every hour.

2. The nurse is preparing to transfer a client with obesity from the bed to the chair. Which action by the nurse is best to avoid injury to the nurse and the client?
   a. Use a team approach for lifting the client.
   b. Lift the client using a swivel and pivot motion.
   c. Leave the client in the bed because the client is too large to get up.
   d. Utilize a mechanical lift for the transfer.

3. The nurse observes that a bed-confined client's feet are beginning to remain in a plantar flexed position. Which nursing action is appropriate to correct this position?
   a. Place a pillow under the knees.
   b. Stand the client on the floor with assistance.
   c. Apply a slanting footboard to the end of the bed.
   d. Elevate the foot of the bed.

4. The nurse is assisting with the admission of an older adult client to the acute care facility. Which priority action would the nurse take to ensure promotion of safety and avoidance of falls?
   a. Place all four side rails up on the bed.
   b. Do not allow the client to walk unattended.
   c. Assist with the performance of a fall-risk assessment.
   d. Use restraints if the client is disoriented.

5. An ambulating client informs the nurse, "I feel faint." Which priority action would the nurse take?
   a. Assist the client to a sitting position.
   b. Have the client grab the nurse around the neck.
   c. Splash cold water on the client's face.
   d. Hold the client upright in a standing position.

CHAPTER RESOURCES

Enhance your learning with additional resources on **thePoint**!

Student Resources related to this chapter can be found at **thePoint.lww.com/Rosdahl12e**.

CHAPTER 48 Moving and Positioning Clients

Welcome Steps

Look at healthcare provider's orders.

Protocol for procedure.

Necessary equipment/supplies.

Wash hands using proper hand hygiene; put on gloves.

Explain the procedure and reassure the client.

Locate two identifiers to confirm correct client.

Comfortable and efficient position for nurse and client.

Obtain privacy.

Make sure to follow correct steps and body mechanics with good technique.

Ensure safety and observe deviations from normal.

End Steps

Ensure comfort and safety.

Note questions or concerns from client or nurse; note significant data.

Dispose of materials properly.

Disinfect the area and your hands.

Document and report the procedure and your findings.

IN PRACTICE
NURSING PROCEDURE 48-1 Turning the Client to a Side-Lying Position

Supplies and Equipment
Pillows
Side rails
Positioning support wedges or pillows
Lateral assist device (anti-friction glide sheet) with long straps, **or**
A turn-and-position system, with wedges
Microclimate body pads

Steps
Follow LPN WELCOME steps and then

1. Determine what type of turning/positioning system is used in your facility and read the manufacturer's instructions. It is most appropriate for at least two nurses to perform this procedure. Place the bed in high position, for your comfort, and lock the brakes. Lower the client's head to as flat a position as they can tolerate; then lower the side rail on the side away from the turn. Make sure all tubes and devices will not be caught or dislodged.
Rationale: A flat bed eliminates the need to pull against gravity. Catheters, drains, IVs, etc. must be protected. If two nurses perform this turn, it will not be necessary to go back and forth around the bed. This also reduces the risk of back injury.

2. The nurse on the side away from the turn moves the client close to the side of the bed opposite that which the client will face when the turn is complete, keeping the client's body in straight alignment and preventing the client's head and heels from dragging on the bed. Use an antifriction glide sheet or lateral-assist device, unless the client can move independently. The top of the glide sheet should be even with the client's shoulders. A microclimate body pad, if available, is placed under the client. Raise the side rail after moving the client.
Rationale: Positioning the client toward the side of the bed allows adequate room to place them in a side-lying position. Keeping the body straight promotes ease of turning and maintains a proper side-lying position. The microclimate pad helps control body heat and moisture. Raised side rails help keep the client safe.

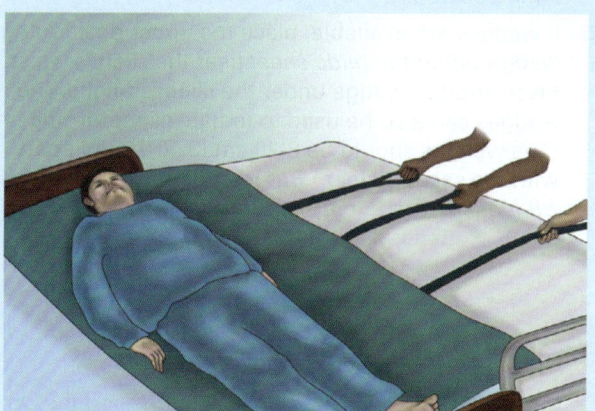

A lateral-assist (antifriction) glide sheet, with long handles, is kept under the client. This allows the client to be moved easily to the side of the bed, without reaching or lifting by the nurse. (Lynn, 2018.)

3. The client is asked to grasp the side rail and pull slightly, if able, to assist in turning. *Rationale: The side rail should remain up when rolling the client, to maintain safety. If the client can help, it promotes independence.*

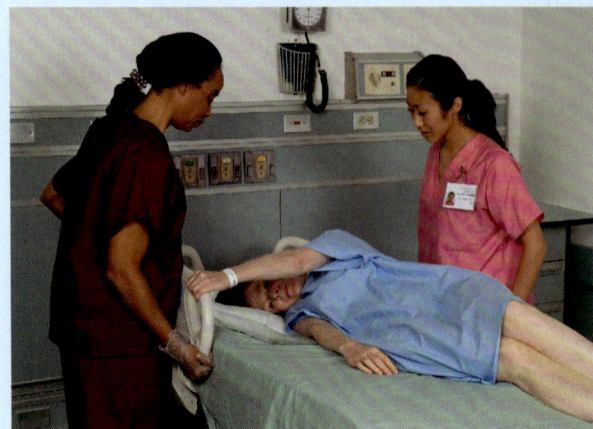

Ask the client to grasp the side rail and help pull onto their side. Keep client covered, as much as possible, to provide privacy (Lynn, 2018).

4. If the client cannot assist, the nurse on the side of the turn guides the client's shoulders and makes sure the client is safe. The nurse away from the turn assumes a broad stance (see Nursing Procedure 48-2, Step 2). This nurse's weight is shifted to the back foot, while tensing abdominal and gluteal muscles and pulling the antifriction glide sheet slightly. The "hip placement indicator" on the sheet serves as a guide. This turns the client and moves the client's buttocks slightly toward the side away from the turn. *Rationale: A broad stance provides a wide base of support and enables you to use large muscles to move the client. Shifting your weight uses the weight of your body to help roll the client. The glide sheet helps eliminate back strain for the nurse. If the client's buttocks are slightly behind the client's center, it will be easier to maintain a side-lying position.*

5. If wedges are available, place the upper positioning wedge *under the glide sheet* near the client's waist. Place another wedge under the client's thighs. The wedges can also be used to initiate client turning. (The wedges should be 8-20 cm [3.15-7.9 in.] apart, with the sacrum clear.) *Rationale: Keep the sacrum off-loaded, to prevent skin breakdown.*

6. If wedges are not used, roll and wedge a pillow behind the client's back, to maintain their position. Rolled blankets or towels may be added, for support.

7. Position the client's legs comfortably.
   a. Flex the client's lower knee and hip slightly.
   b. Bring their upper leg forward and place a pillow between the legs (see Table 48-1). *Rationale: This will prevent strain on the hip joint and minimize pressure on bony prominences.*

8. Adjust the client's arms.
   a. Shift their lower shoulder toward you slightly.
   b. Support their upper arm on a pillow. *Rationale: This serves to support the client's upper body and prevent pressure on bony prominences.*

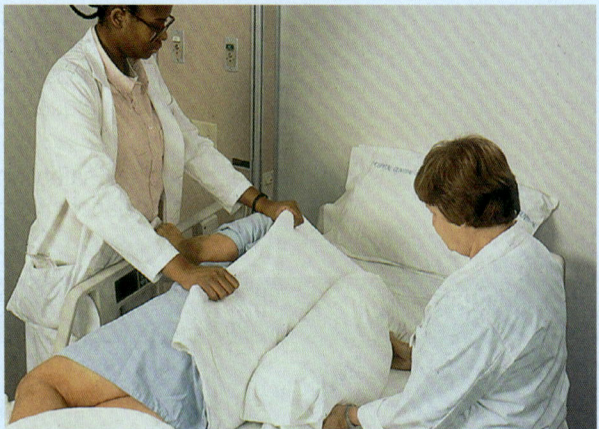

After the client is turned to the side, turning wedges or pillows will support the client in position. Pillows are also placed to support the upper leg and arm (Carter & Lewsen, 2005).

9. Lower the bed and elevate the head of the bed as much as the client can tolerate. Make sure all side rails are up. *Rationale: Repositioning provides for the client's comfort. Side rails help ensure safety.*

NOTE: Turning pads are discarded as needed. Glide sheets and wedges are used for one client only. They may be wiped with a damp cloth; do not launder them. If you are unfamiliar with any equipment, request in-service education.

Follow ENDDD steps

IN PRACTICE
NURSING PROCEDURE 48-2 Logroll Turn

Supplies and Equipment
Pillows
Lifting sheet

Steps
Follow LPN WELCOME steps and then

1. Determine the number of nurses needed. This turn requires at least two nurses to be accomplished safely. Raise the bed to a comfortable level for the nurses. Flatten the bed. Use a lateral-assist glide sheet, with long handles, or a turning and positioning system, if possible. *Rationale: Large clients require the use of a mechanical system and two or more nurses.*

2. Position yourselves on opposite sides of the bed. Nurses assume a broad-based stance, with one foot slightly ahead of the other. *Rationale: This provides access to the client and aids in distribution of the client's weight.*

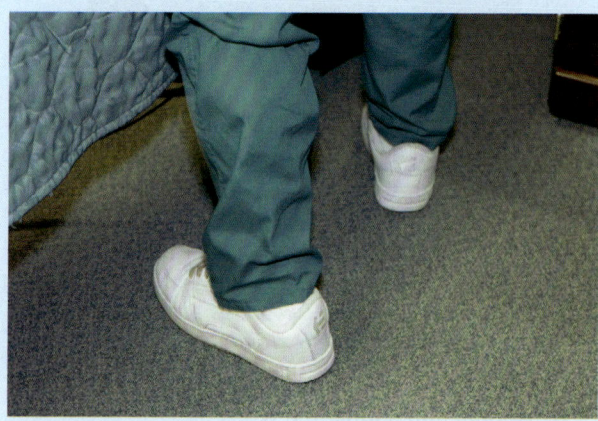

It is important to practice good body mechanics by using a broad-based stance (Carter & Lewsen, 2005).

3. Position the client's arms on their chest and make sure all tubes are out of the way. *Rationale: This prevents the client's arms from becoming entangled under the body during the turn. It is important to take equipment into consideration.*

4. The nurse(s) on the side away from which the client will be turned grasps the glide sheet or the handles on the turning sheet, near the client's shoulders and hips/knees (see Nursing Procedure 48-1). The nurse at the client's head calls the signals, and on the count of "3," the nurses shift the weight of their bodies, flexing their knees, thighs, and ankles, to move the client to the side of the bed where their back will be. The client's entire body is moved as a unit. DO NOT LIFT. If a friction-reducing sheet or turning wedges are used, it is possible for two nurses to turn a smaller client to the side. *Rationale: Calling signals ensure organization. The nurses use large muscle groups. The client's weight is evenly distributed, preventing injury to the client or nurses. Moving the client to the side of the bed allows room for turning. Be sure to maintain the client's body alignment.*

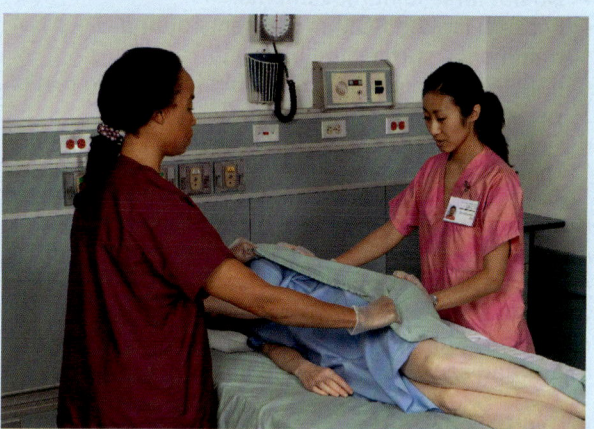

A small client can be turned to the side by two nurses, if using an antifriction turning sheet or turning wedges (Lynn, 2018).

5. The nurse on the side of the turn makes sure the client is safe. On the second count of three, that nurse, along with the other nurse(s), rolls and positions the client, as a unit, on their side, with the client's body ending up in the center of the bed. Take care to carry out all safety precautions in the turn. Position the client as in Nursing Procedure 48-1 and Table 48-1. *Rationale: This provides a safe and comfortable position change. The client is rolled as a unit, keeping the back straight. This prevents injury to the client with a previous back injury. Nurses roll the client, not lifting, protecting the nurses.*

6. The turning sheet remains under the client after the turn. *Rationale: This prevents having to replace the sheet. This allows for ease in turning the client.*

7. Lower the bed after the turn. Raise all side rails. Make sure the nurse call light is available. *Rationale: To provide safety for the client.*

Follow ENDDD steps

IN PRACTICE

NURSING PROCEDURE 48-3: Performing Passive ROM Exercises

Guidelines: Before Beginning These Exercises
- A provider's order may be needed for complete ROM exercises (either passive or active). The provider also may order ROM exercises for specific joints.
- Practice personal body mechanics, to prevent injury. For example, the nurse puts the bed in high position and moves the client close, to avoid stretching and bending.
- Work on one side at a time.
- *Do not force joint movements!*
- Perform limited ROM movements during treatments, such as the bed bath.
- If the client becomes tired, allow reasonable rest periods between exercises.
- Return the bed to low position before leaving the room.

Note: Joint movements are illustrated in Table 48-2. Although the movements illustrated there constitute *active range of motion* (movements the client makes without assistance), the procedures of *passive range of motion* simulate the same joint and limb movements and serve to protect the integrity of those joints.

Steps

Follow LPN WELCOME steps and then

1. Review the movements in range of motion presented in Table 48-2. Lower the side rail and raise the bed. Uncover only the limb to be exercised. *Rationale: This ensures warmth and protects the client's privacy. Raising the bed makes it more comfortable for the nurse.*
2. Support all joints during exercises. *Rationale: Cradling joints helps prevent injury and discomfort.*
3. Use slow, gentle movements. Repeat each exercise three times. Stop if the client complains of pain or discomfort. *Rationale: Repetitive motion maintains joint mobility. Discontinuing exercises, if they cause pain, prevents injury.*
4. Begin exercises with the client's neck and work downward. *Rationale: Performing procedures in a systematic manner ensures exercising all joints.*
5. Flex, extend, and rotate the client's neck very slowly. Support their head. *Rationale: This helps prevent flexion contracture of the neck.*
6. Exercise the client's shoulder and elbow. *Rationale: This maintains strength in the deltoid muscle and prevents contracture.*
    a. Support the client's elbow with one hand and grasp the client's wrist with your other hand.
    b. Raise the client's arm from the side to above the head.
    c. Perform internal rotation by moving the client's arm across their chest.
    d. Externally rotate the client's shoulder by moving the arm away from the client.
    e. Flex and extend the client's elbow.

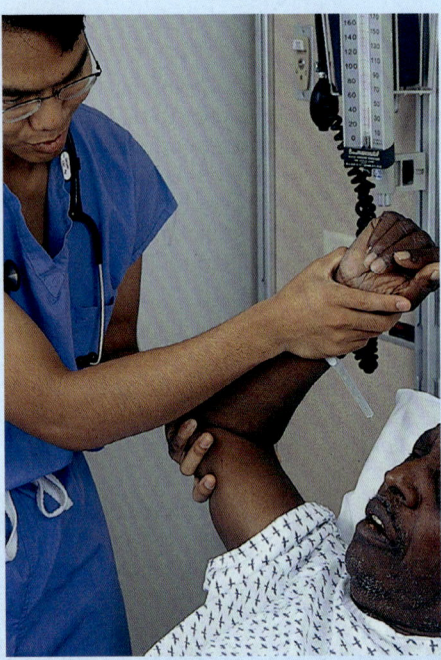

Exercise the elbow and shoulder joints, while supporting the elbow joint.

7. Perform all possible movements of the client's wrist and fingers. *Rationale: Exercises are needed to maintain strength and flexibility.*
    a. Flex and extend the wrist.
    b. Abduct and adduct the wrist.
    c. Rotate and pronate the wrist.
    d. Flex and extend the client's fingers.
    e. Abduct and adduct the fingers.
    f. Rotate the thumb.

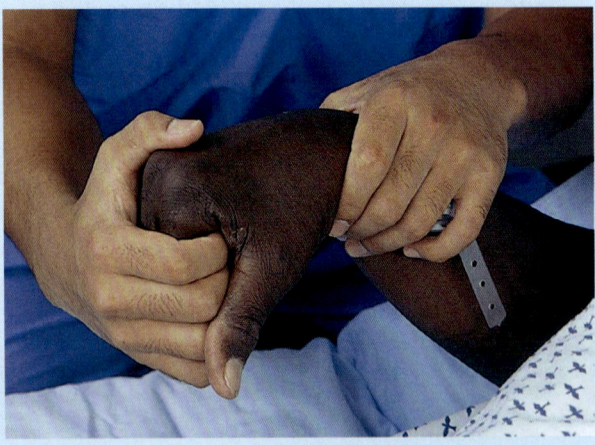

Flex and extend the wrist and each finger joint.

CHAPTER 48 Moving and Positioning Clients

8. Exercise the client's hip and leg. **Rationale:** *A contracted hip or fixed knee severely limits the client's ability to ambulate.*
   a. Flex and extend the hip and knee while supporting the leg.
   b. Abduct and adduct the hip by moving the client's straightened leg toward you and then back to median position.

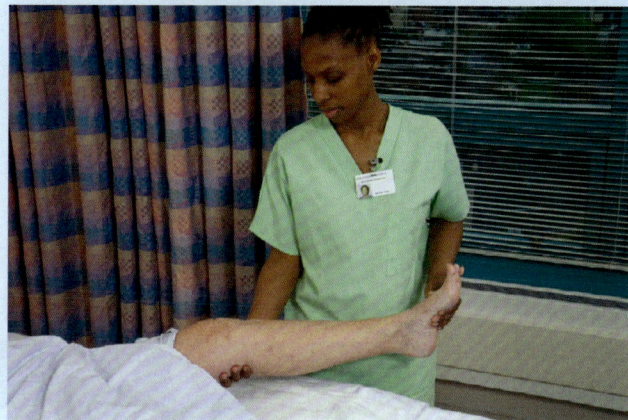

Exercise the hip joint by moving the client's straightened leg away from the body, and then extending it back past the midline, as much as possible (Lynn, 2018).

   c. Perform internal and external rotation of the hip joint by turning the leg inward and then outward.
9. Perform exercises on the ankle and foot. **Rationale:** *The feet must be maintained with adequate range of motion and positioning, to prepare for walking.*
   a. Dorsiflex and plantar flex the foot.
   b. Abduct and adduct the toes.
   c. Evert and invert the foot.

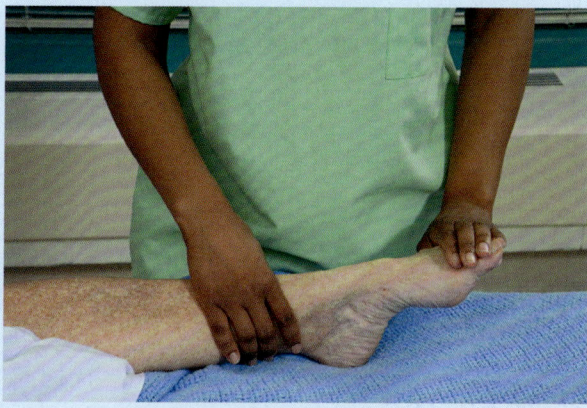

The foot is moved at the ankle into all possible positions. Then, all the toes are moved into all possible positions (Lynn, 2018).

10. Raise the side rails, move to the other side of the bed, and repeat exercises. **Rationale:** *Be sure that you exercise all joints.*
11. Reposition and cover the client. Return the bed to low position. Raise the side rails. **Rationale:** *Repositioning allows for the client's comfort. Lowering the bed and raising the side rails helps prevent falls.*

IN PRACTICE
NURSING PROCEDURE 48-4 Using a Transfer Belt, With Metal-Toothed Buckle

Steps
Follow LPN WELCOME steps and then

1. Place the belt around the client's waist, and over clothing, before they get up. It must be tight enough to support the client's weight and not slide down, but not so tight as to impair the client's circulation or breathing. Thread the end of the belt between the open slot and the gripper teeth on the hinged side of the buckle and out through the toothless side. Loop excess belt over and secure between the belt and the client. **Rationale:** *The belt provides confidence but must be able to support the client if they begin to fall. However, the belt must be loose enough for you to slip your hand into it. Clothing protects the client's skin from rubbing.*
2. Keep one hand inside the back of the belt at all times when transferring or walking with the client. Always insert your hand into the belt *from the bottom,* with your fingers pointing upward and the belt in the palm of your hand. **Rationale:** *If the client slumps or slips, you will be able to support the weight. If you grasp the belt from the top, it will slip out of your hand, due to the client's weight.*
3. Each client has a personal belt to keep in the room or in a designated location. (Label and store the belt outside the room if the client is depressed, is suicidal, or may assault someone.) The belt may be washed in warm water, without bleach, and air-dried or dried on low setting. **Rationale:** *The buckle could be used as a weapon. The belt could also be*

used for self-injury or suicide. The belt is labeled and used for only one client and discarded when no longer needed, to help prevent the spread of infection.

NOTE: A belt with a quick-release buckle is also available. This buckle is placed behind the client (Wintersgill, 2019).

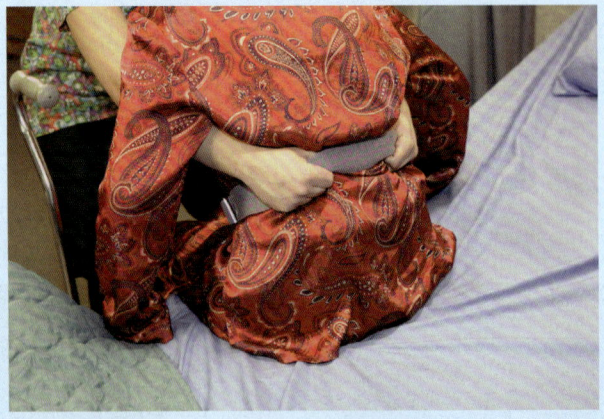

Use underhand grasp to hold the transfer belt (Carter, 2008).

Follow ENDDD steps

IN PRACTICE
NURSING PROCEDURE 48-5 Dangling

Supplies and Equipment
Blood pressure equipment
Bath blanket
Pillow
Footstool, if needed

Steps
Follow LPN WELCOME steps and then

1. Place the bed in low position. Explain the procedure. *Rationale: The client will be prepared to place their feet on the floor easily from the low position.*
2. Fan-fold the bedding to the foot of the bed, and cover the client with a bath blanket, if needed. *Rationale: This protects the client's privacy and prevents chilling.*
3. Measure and record the client's pulse and blood pressure. *Rationale: This provides a baseline to evaluate later how well the client tolerated being up.*
4. Check to see if the client has an IV, catheter, or other equipment and ensure that you know how to manage it before attempting to move the client. Obtain help if the client is dizzy or connected to multiple pieces of equipment. Elevate the head of the bed (Fowler or high Fowler position), unless the client can sit up without assistance. *Rationale: Prevents dislodging or twisting and tubing. Raises the client without manual lifting.*
5. Turn the client, using an easy-glide sheet or other lateral turning device (see Nursing Procedure 48-1). *Rationale: Turn the client's body as a unit.*
6. Assume a broad-based stance, as in Nursing Procedure 48-2. Shift your weight to turn the client toward you so their feet touch the floor. DO NOT LIFT. For shorter clients, provide a footstool. *Rationale: Practice good body mechanics. Supporting the client's feet is crucial, to prevent undue pressure on the backs of the knees. Pressure can contribute to falling, blood clots, nerve damage, and other disorders.*
7. If necessary, roll a pillow and tuck it firmly behind the client's back. *Rationale: This helps support the client in the sitting position.*
8. Dangle the client's legs for as long as ordered, if tolerated. Stay with the client. Help the client lie down, if they become light-headed or feels faint. *Rationale: When a person sits up for the first time, blood rushes into the legs. The client may feel faint, due to orthostatic (postural) hypotension.*

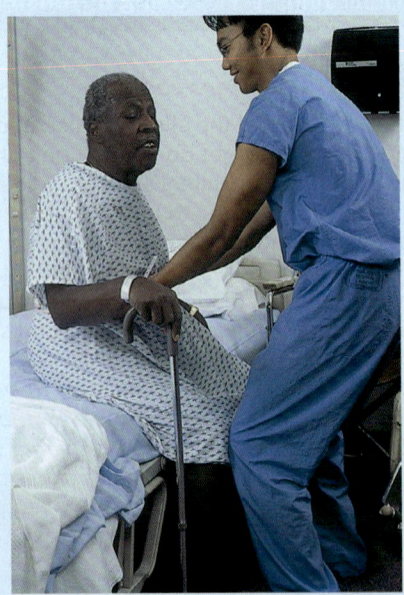

Stay with the client while their legs are dangling.

CHAPTER 48 Moving and Positioning Clients

9. After the prescribed time, help the client lie down, by supporting the shoulders and knees and turning the person around. Measure and record the client's pulse and blood pressure immediately. *Rationale: Make sure to prevent falls. These vital sign readings, compared against baseline measurements, help the provider determine how well the client tolerated the procedure.*

Follow ENDDD steps

Special Reminder
- Documentation should include how long the client's legs dangled, how they tolerated the procedure, vital signs before and after, and any unusual occurrences.

IN PRACTICE
NURSING PROCEDURE 48-6 Helping the Client From Bed and/or Into a Chair

Supplies and Equipment
Robe
Transfer belt
Nonskid footwear
Wheelchair or chair
Bath blanket

Steps
Follow LPN WELCOME steps and then

1. Remember: Most healthcare injuries are a result of falls. Get assistance if the client is unsteady. If the client is heavy or cannot stand easily, a mechanical lift must be used (see Fig. 48-16). *Rationale: Preventing falls and protecting your back are essential. Requesting assistance helps prevent accidents.*

2. Put a transfer belt around the client's waist in most cases (see Nursing Procedure 48-4). Make sure to protect all tubes and other equipment. *Rationale: If tubes or other equipment are not handled properly, the client could be injured. For example, tubes or catheters could become dislodged or pulled out. The transfer belt helps protect the client from falling.*

3. Position the client as for dangling (see Nursing Procedure 48-5). Choose a chair that will not move and place it next to the bed *or at a 45° angle to the bed.* (Use a chair with arms, if possible.) Lock the wheel brakes of both the bed and wheelchair and remove the wheelchair's footrests or place them in the "up" position. If the client has problems with weight-bearing on one leg, place the chair on the side of the client's stronger leg. For example, if the

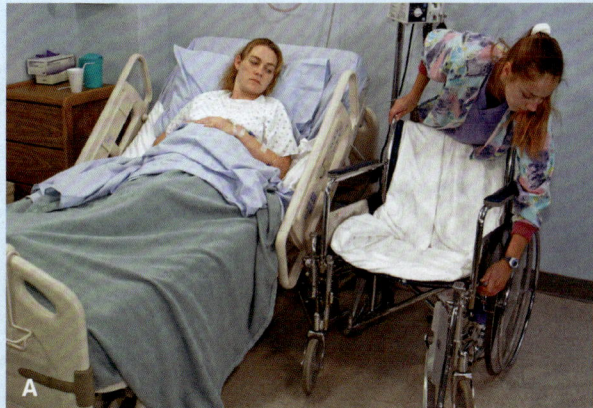

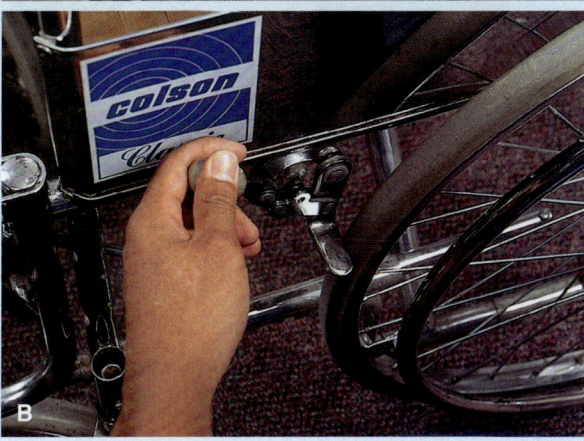

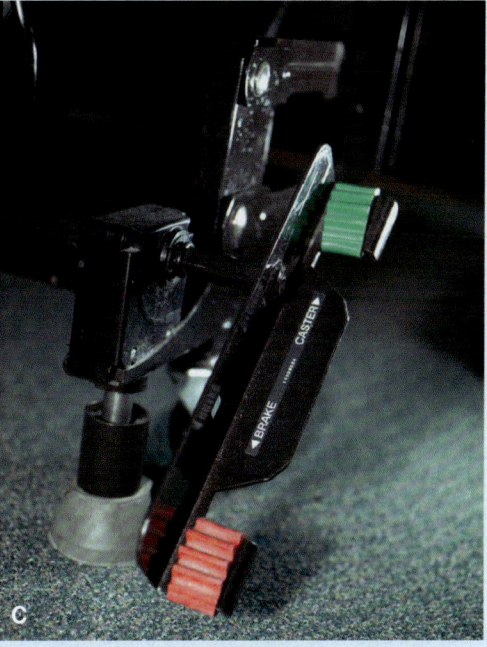

A. Position the chair next to the bed. B. Lock the wheels on both sides of the wheelchair, to prevent it from moving. C. On most beds, the red pedal locks the wheels and the green pedal unlocks them. (A: Photo by Rick Brady; B: Craven & Hirnle, 2007; C: Carter & Lewsen, 2005.)

client cannot bear weight on the right leg, place the chair on the left side of the bed. *Rationale: Starting with a sitting position facilitates movement out of bed. The other actions help prevent falls. Having the wheelchair on the client's strong side allows the use of the weight-bearing leg to lean and pivot into the chair.*

4. Help the client into clothing or a robe and appropriate footwear. Allow the client to dangle for a short time. *Rationale: This adds to the client's modesty, provides warmth, and helps prevent falls. It also adds to the feeling of normalcy. A gradual change in position lessens the chance of the client developing orthostatic hypotension.*

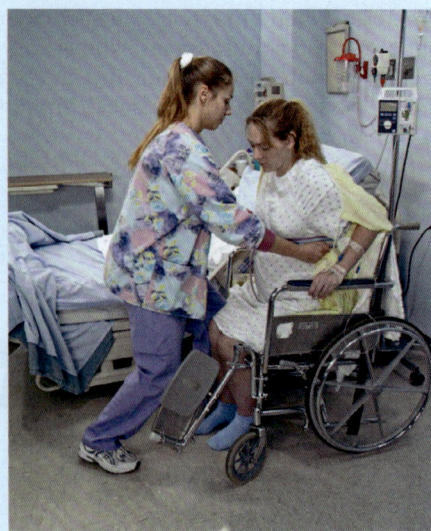

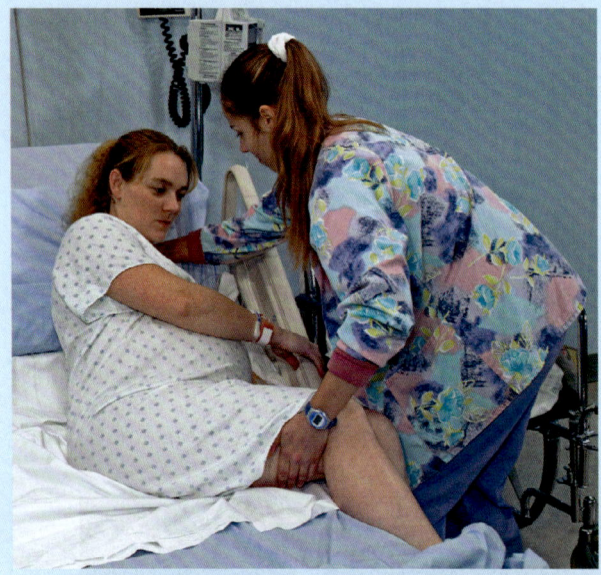

Support the client's legs, while helping them to turn and sit on the edge of the bed. (Photo by Rick Brady.)

The client can assist by grasping the arms of the chair or wheelchair and lowering themselves into the chair. The nurse steadies the client, to prevent them from falling. (Photo by Rick Brady.)

8. Make sure the client is correctly positioned in the chair and is comfortable. Reposition footrests or a footstool. Secure the client in a chair with a reminder device, if needed (see Nursing Procedure 48-12). Cover the client with a blanket. Provide the nurse call signal and any other items the client might need. *Rationale: It is important to ensure the safety and comfort of the client.*

5. Spread the client's feet and brace your knees against the outside of the client's knees. Prepare the client to stand. Bend your knees and not your back. If the client cannot stand independently, use a mechanical lift. *Rationale: By placing your knees on the outside of the client's knees in a cradling fashion, you can provide more support and control if the client becomes weak or loses balance. Practice good body mechanics, to prevent injury to yourself.*

6. Ask the client to push upward from the bed and stand. Use a wide stance, as illustrated in Nursing Procedure 48-2, Step 2. Do NOT lift the client. *Rationale: The nurse adds support while the client stands. The client gains confidence and independence and the nurse's back is protected.*

7. Instruct the client to reach for the arms of the wheelchair and pivot into the chair, while they supports their weight on the chair. Unlock the chair, if the client will be allowed to move about. *Rationale: This position supports and stabilizes the client as they move into the chair.*

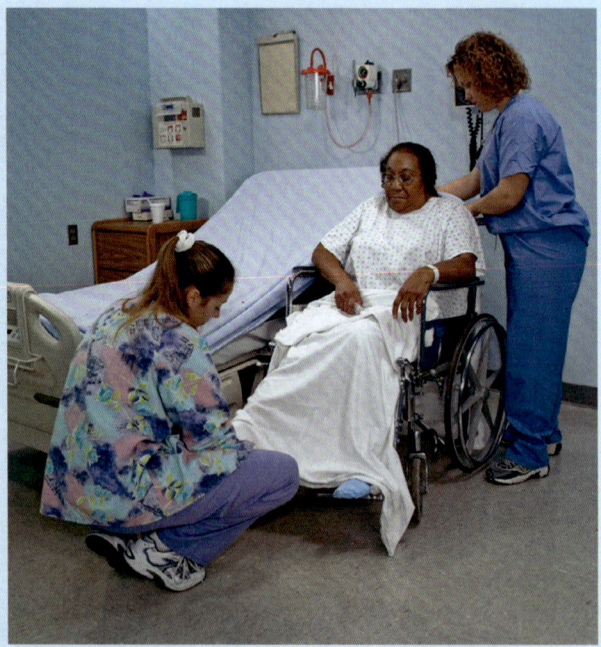

Make the client comfortable. Check with them frequently, to make sure they are OK (Evans-Smith, 2005).

9. To assist the client from a chair to standing or to a walker, ask the client to push up, using the chair arms. Then, steady the client, so the hands can be

moved to the handles of the walker. *Rationale: The transfer from chair to walker is an easy transition, and most clients can do it with minimal steadying by the nurse.*

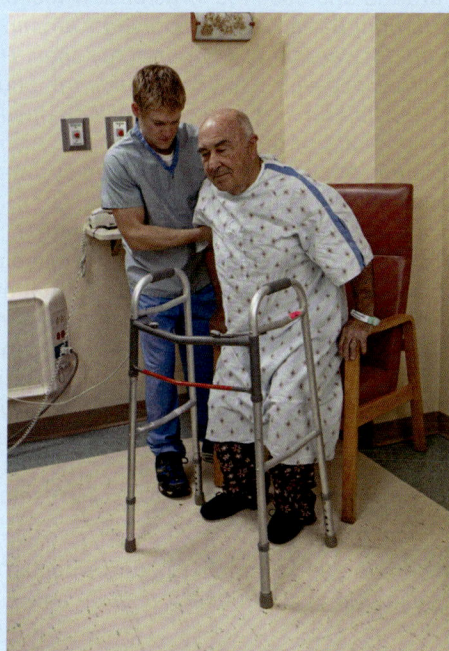

The client can use the arms of the chair to push up to standing. The nurse stands by to make sure the client is safe (Lynn, 2018).

Helping the Mobile Client to Walk to a Chair

1. Assist the client to a dangling position and help them to put on robe and sturdy shoes (see Nursing Procedure 48-5). Apply a transfer belt, as in Nursing Procedure 48-4.
2. When the client is stable, assist them to stand. Be sure to get assistance, if necessary. *Rationale: It is important to provide client and nurse safety.*
3. Assist the client to walk about the room or to the chair, while you are holding firmly to the transfer belt. Steady the client while they hold the chair arms and lowers into the chair. *Rationale: Make sure the client is safe.*

Follow ENDDD steps

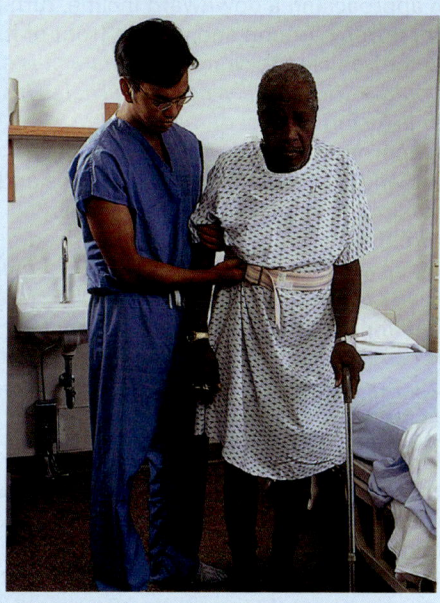

Walk with the client to the chair, using the gait belt. This client helps by using their cane. Note that the nurse's hand is placed under the bottom of the gait belt.

IN PRACTICE
NURSING PROCEDURE 48-7 — Pushing a Nonmotorized Wheelchair or Wheeled Stretcher/Gurney (Litter)

Steps
Follow LPN WELCOME steps and then General Guidelines
- Make sure to use a large enough wheelchair for the client's weight. The largest bariatric wheelchairs available usually have a weight limit of 550 lb (249.5 kg). *Rationale: Use of a wheelchair that is too small is dangerous and could break the chair and/or injure the client.*
- Take the client's chart (unless electronic data are available to all departments) when transporting from one area to another. Make sure the client is wearing appropriate ID bands at all times. This includes the name band, allergy information band, and, if the client is at fall risk, the fall-risk ID band. *Rationale: The chart or electronic record gives information about the client for the use of other departments. ID bands give vital information about the client that must be immediately accessible to all personnel. Treatments or tests will not be performed unless the client is properly identified.*
- Check to ensure that the wheels are intact. *Rationale: Prevent jarring the client.*
- Secure a safety belt, if needed. Some facilities require a safety belt whenever a client is transported. *Rationale: Prevent the client from falling.*
- Secure the client's equipment (e.g., IV stands, ventilatory machines, and drainage apparatus). *Rationale: This helps prevent injuries to client and nurse.*
- Push from the back; do not pull. *Rationale: This helps prevent back strain for the nurse.*

- Look for a clear traffic path ahead (e.g., avoid people approaching, equipment left in the hall, or wet floors). *Rationale: Always prevent accidents.*
- Negotiate corners slowly. (Often, a mirror is available, allowing visibility around corners.) *Rationale: This helps prevent client falls and prevents hitting someone coming the other way.*
- Use slow to moderate speed in pushing the gurney or chair. *Rationale: It is more difficult to stop a faster-moving object.*
- When approaching a downward incline, turn the chair or gurney around and walk in front of it. Wheel the vehicle backward. *Rationale: It is safer to be on the "downhill" side of the chair. This prevents losing control of the vehicle.*
- When approaching an upward incline, lean forward and use your strong leg muscles and body weight to propel the chair or gurney forward. If the incline is steep, a motorized gurney or wheelchair should be used. *Rationale: It is easier to push a vehicle up an incline (rather than pulling), because your leg muscles are better developed for forward motion. You put all your body weight into the motion and have better control of the chair.*

When Pushing a Wheelchair

Most states have laws preventing architectural barriers for wheelchairs and walkers. However, it may be necessary to negotiate a single stair or curb.

- When approaching a curb or single stair, tip the chair back and put the small wheels up on the curb or step. Move ahead by pushing the back wheels over the obstacle. *Rationale: This makes it easier to push and helps prevent jarring the client.*
- To go down a curb with a wheelchair, turn the chair around and *ease the large back wheel off the curb first*. *Rationale: This prevents lurching the client forward, possibly out of the chair. The large wheel is easier to roll over the curb, and if the wheelchair lurches, the client will be pushed against the back of the chair and not out. Also, the small front wheels may spin sideways and get stuck.*
- When entering or leaving an elevator with a wheelchair, use an elevator bridge, if available. (The bridge is a flat board, with a piece that fits into the slot between the elevator and the floor to which you are going.) This prevents the small wheels from getting stuck in the slot. If no bridge is available, always roll the *large back wheel into and out* of the elevator first. *Rationale: This keeps the small wheels going straight and prevents them from getting stuck, providing client safety.*

When Pushing a Wheeled Stretcher

- Steer from the end that has rotating wheels. *Rationale: This makes it easier to steer and control.*
- *Do not attempt* to go up or down a curb with a gurney. *Rationale: It is too difficult to control a gurney in this situation.*

Follow ENDDD steps

IN PRACTICE

NURSING PROCEDURE 48-8 Walking With a Cane

Steps
Follow LPN WELCOME steps and then

- Adjust the cane's height to allow for a slight bend in the client's elbow. The cane handle should be approximately at hip level. *Rationale: This position is the most comfortable and gives the client the most support.*
- As with one crutch, instruct the client to hold the cane on the strong side (*contralateral* to the injury), unless specifically contraindicated. *Rationale: This will allow the client to have a normal walking gait, including normal arm swing, while providing maximum support.*
- Check the client's balance. Assist the client by using a transfer belt, if necessary. *Rationale: It is important to prevent falls. Many clients using canes are older or debilitated and need extra practice.*
- Teach the client to move the stronger leg forward while carrying their weight on the weak side, combined with the cane. The cane and the weaker leg move together as a unit. *Rationale: The cane adds stability and support to the weaker leg. The stronger leg can support the client's weight without assistance.*
- Walk on the client's *affected* side when assisting and encourage the client to practice. *Rationale: It is important for you to be available, in case the client slips or stumbles, so you can support the client. If the client has weakness or instability, it will most likely be on the affected side. The client needs to achieve independence.*
- Make sure the client is not weak or dizzy before beginning to walk.

When teaching the client to use a cane, the following instructions should be given:

Using Stairs With a Cane

The procedure with a cane is similar to that for crutches; see earlier discussion.

- Use the handrail on the unaffected side for support. Hold the cane on the affected side.
- Use the stronger leg and handrail to step up, while supporting the weaker leg with the cane. Then, pull up the weaker leg, while holding the handrail.
- Reverse this process when going down stairs.
- If there is no handrail, hold the cane on the unaffected side and advance the unaffected leg up (or down) the stairs, then move the cane up (or down) the stairs first, and then bring up (or down) the weaker leg, while putting the weight on the stronger leg and the cane.

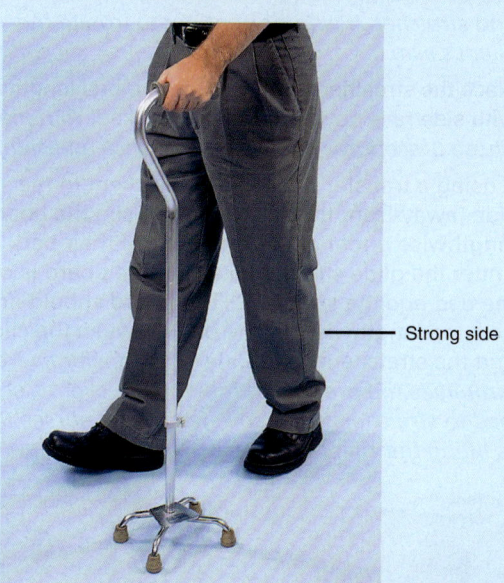

Walking with a quad cane. Note: The handle is parallel to the client's hip. (Photo by B. Proud.)

Sitting Down With a Cane

- Back up to a chair until it can be felt against the legs.
- Keep the cane handy.
- Grip both arms of the chair and ease down into the chair.

Rising From a Chair With a Cane

- Grip the arms of the chair, while holding the cane in the stronger hand.
- Put the stronger leg slightly forward and lean forward.
- Push up, using the arms of the chair.

Follow ENDDD steps

IN PRACTICE

NURSING PROCEDURE 48-9 Using a Walker

Steps

Follow LPN WELCOME steps and then

- Place a transfer belt on the client and keep it in place until the client is steady and safe in using the walker without assistance. *Rationale: Provide client safety.*
- Position the walker around the client and explain its use. *Rationale: The client must be comfortable with the use of the walker, in order to be willing and able to use it.*
- Have the client pick up the walker and move it ahead approximately 6 to 12 in. at a time, with weight equally distributed on both feet. *Rationale: It is important that the client learn to use the walker correctly, to prevent falls and instill confidence.*

When Both Sides Are Weak

- This client should have a walker with a seat. *Rationale: This will allow the client to safely sit, if becoming dizzy or weak.*
- Use the transfer belt, if necessary. Instruct the client to move the right foot forward, while shifting weight to the left side and the arms. You may need to gently assist, until the client can do this alone. *Rationale: Encourage the client to maximize their abilities. The client needs to learn their safe limits.*

- Next, reverse the process with the other foot. Continue helping the client to move forward in this manner. *Rationale: This will help the client learn how to use the walker most effectively.*

When One Side Is Weak
- Move the walker and the client's weak leg together, while carrying weight on the strong side. *Rationale: In this case, the walker is used in much the same manner as a cane or crutches.*
- Move the client's strong or unaffected side while the weight is carried on the weak side supported by the walker. Continue to assist the client to practice.
Remember: If the walker has wheels or sliders, the client must learn to maintain control of the walker and not let it slide or roll away.

Follow ENDDD steps

IN PRACTICE
NURSING PROCEDURE 48-10 — Moving the Client From Bed to Wheeled Stretcher/Gurney

Supplies and Equipment
Friction-free glide sheet or
Lateral-assist mechanical device
Bath blanket
Wheeled stretcher/gurney

Steps
NOTE: If the client is heavy and/or not able to assist, a mechanized lateral-assist transfer device should be used, to prevent nurse injury (see Fig. 48-17).

Follow LPN WELCOME steps and then

1. Lock the wheels of both bed and stretcher and raise the bed to the same height as the stretcher. Cover the client with a bath blanket and remove the top linens or fold them to the foot of the bed. *Rationale: The locked wheels keep the bed from moving. Having both at the same height makes the transfer easier and safer. The client should be covered, but bed linens should be out of the way.*
2. Ask the client to fold the arms across the chest. Make sure there is no equipment that could be dislodged. *Rationale: The client's arms and equipment need to be out of the way, to prevent injury.*
3. To insert an easy-glide sheet with long handles, roll the client to one side of the bed on their side and place the sheet next to the client's body, with the center seam at the client's back (see Nursing Procedure 48-1). Roll up the top layer of the sheet to the center seam and push the roll as close to the client's back as possible, with handles extended to the sides of the bed. Turn the client back over the rolled-up portion of the sheet and carefully pull out the end on the other side. A transfer board may also be used under the sheet. Keep linens between the client's skin and the sheet (and transfer board). *Rationale: The nurses should pull on the sheet's handles, if available, and not stretch to reach the client. The transfer board can provide an additional slippery surface, as well as a bridge between bed and stretcher. It is important not to irritate the client's skin.*
4. Place the stretcher firmly next to the bed lengthwise, with side rails down and wheels locked. *Rationale: These procedures ensure convenience and safety.*
5. If using a transfer board, turn the client to the side (away from the stretcher) and slip the board lengthwise under about one third of their back and under the glide sheet. Make sure the board is on the bed *and* the stretcher. (The board should now be lying lengthwise on the bed between the client and the stretcher.) *Rationale: The transfer board simplifies the process of moving the client from bed to stretcher. It is also safer for the nurses than is lifting the client.*

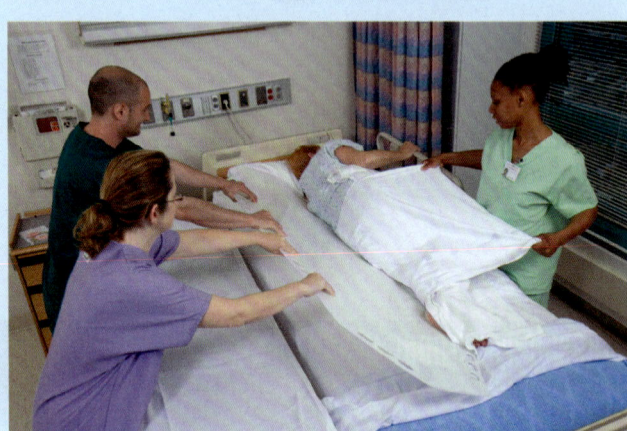

The transfer board is inserted under the transfer sheet. It should be half on the bed and half on the gurney (Lynn, 2018).

6. To move the client, two nurses stand on the side of the stretcher away from the bed and grasp the handles of the transfer sheet (or the sheet itself). One nurse stands next to the other side of the bed, grasps the transfer sheet, and calls the signals. On the count of three, the client is moved to the side of the bed near the stretcher with the glide

sheet. Pause. *Rationale: Distribute the load while moving a client. The handles on the glide sheet ensure a firm grip and prevent stretching. The sheet and transfer board provide easy movement of the client. One person calls signals, to avoid confusion. A slight pause ensures that everyone is ready to complete the transfer.*

7. In the next motion, the client is moved across the board onto the stretcher. Position the client and make sure they are comfortable. Put up the side rails of the stretcher and stay with the client. Most facilities require a safety belt whenever a client is on a gurney. *Rationale: It is important to ensure the safety and comfort of the client.*

Follow ENDDD steps

Special Reminders
- A minimum of three people is required to move most clients from bed to stretcher, unless the client is very small. Heavier clients should be moved with a mechanical lateral-transfer lift or HoverMatt transfer pad.
- If the client cannot hold up their head, another person is needed to hold the client's head during the transfer. In addition, another person may be needed to manage a cast or other special equipment.

IN PRACTICE
NURSING PROCEDURE 48-11 — Adjusting Pillows and Moving the Client Up in Bed

To Adjust Pillows

Supplies and Equipment
Overhead trapeze
Glide-free transfer sheet or
Mechanical device, such as a HoverMatt

Steps
Follow LPN WELCOME steps and then

1. Lock the wheels and raise the bed to a comfortable working level. Lower the side rails and the head of the bed, as much as possible. Remove the pillows, if the client can tolerate this. Fan-fold the top linens to the foot of the bed, but make sure the client is covered. *Rationale: These procedures add to the safety of the procedure. Lowering the head of the bed and removing pillows prevent working against gravity. Preserve the client's privacy.*

2. Ask the client to pull up on the trapeze, to raise their head and shoulders slightly. If this is not possible, request assistance. *Rationale: Prevent nurse injury.*

3. If the client needs to be assisted, ask them to fold the arms over the chest. Each nurse stands facing the client on opposite sides of the bed, assuming a broad-based stance (see Nursing Procedure 48-2, Step 2). With arms under the client's shoulders and the client's middle back, and on the count of 3, both nurses rock sideways toward the foot of the bed, helping the client to lift the head and upper back up off the bed. *Rationale: The client's arms need to be out of the way. It is important not to let the client grab you around the neck, which may cause injury to you. Using your body weight to move the client uses body mechanics. At least two persons are required, if the client cannot assist.*

4. The client is supported in a sitting position while pillows are adjusted. *Rationale: This will increase client comfort.*

Follow ENDDD steps

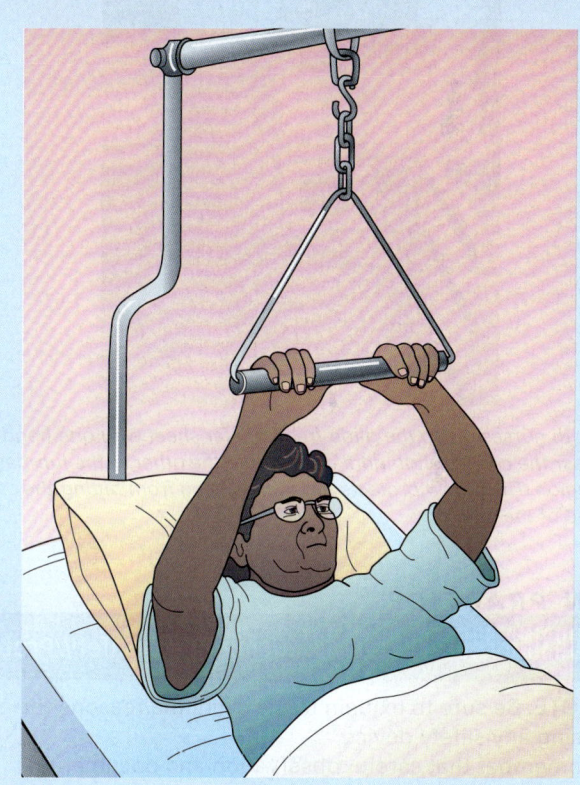

The client can pull up on the trapeze to assist in moving in bed (Timby, 2005).

To Move the Client Up in Bed

Steps
Follow LPN WELCOME steps and then

1. Remove the pillows, if the client can tolerate this. Place one pillow between the client's head and the head of the bed. Place a positioning glide sheet under the client, as described in In Practice: Nursing Procedure 48-10 and roll it fairly close to the client, or grasp the handles. Encourage the client to assist

by bending the knees and placing their feet flat on the bed. Encourage the client to grasp the overhead trapeze, or the client may be able to pull on the head of the bed. *Rationale: The pillow protects the client's head from being bumped on the head of the bed. The glide sheet serves as a handle to grasp on each side of the client and provides a slippery surface, to help move the client. The client will be able to assist by pushing with the feet and/or using the trapeze or the head of the bed, when instructed to do so. Allowing the client to assist fosters independence and assists the nurses.*

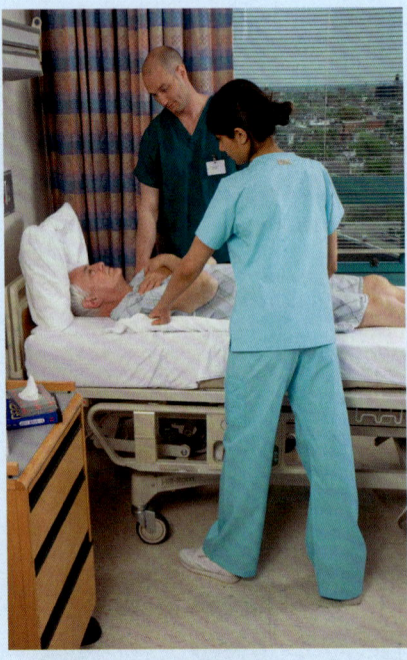

Both nurses grasp the glide-free transfer sheet with one hand near the client's shoulders or neck and the other in the lumbar region. The pillow protects the client's head from hitting the top of the bed.

2. Two nurses stand across the client's bed from each other and face each other. Both nurses assume a broad-based stance and bend the knees slightly. *Rationale: This widens the base of support and uses body mechanics.*

3. Both nurses grasp the transfer sheet, with one hand near the client's shoulders or neck and the other hand near the client's lumbar region. The palms and fingers are facing downward. *Rationale: Spreading the hands helps distribute the client's weight evenly. The placement of the palms and fingers helps increase the strength of the grip and enables the nurses to maintain their grip.* At a predetermined signal, both nurses rock carefully backward, away from the bed. *Rationale: This lifts the client's body off the bed.*

4. Then, moving together, both nurses rock onto their foot closest to the head of the bed, moving the client toward the head of the bed. *Rationale: The nurses' combined weight lifts the client off the bed and then moves the lifting sheet and the client up toward the head of the bed.*

A client may be moved to the side of the bed on their back, using the same procedures.
NOTE: If the client is heavy or totally unable to assist, a mechanical device such as the HoverMatt should be used, to prevent injury to the nurses.
Follow ENDDD steps

IN PRACTICE
NURSING PROCEDURE 48-12 Using Client Safety/Protective Devices

NOTE: Be sure to explain to the client the reasons for using any safety device.
Remember that careful observation and documentation are mandatory when using any safety device.

Criss-Cross Vest

Supplies and Equipment
Criss-cross vest of the correct size (see Fig. 48-20D).

Steps
Follow LPN WELCOME steps and then

1. This vest may be used in the bed or in a chair. Choose a vest of the proper size. *Rationale: A vest that is too small will restrict the client's breathing. A vest that is too large will not function correctly and may slip off or choke the client.*

2. Place the vest on the client, with the opening in the front, making a "V-neck." *Rationale: If the opening is placed in the back, the vest would be too high in the front and thus choke the client.*

3. Apply the vest over the client's clothing or hospital gown. Make sure the vest does not have any wrinkles. Pull the long tie on the end of the vest through the slit on the opposite side. *Rationale: Rubbing on the skin or wrinkles could contribute to skin breakdown.*

4. Cross over the client's abdomen. Be sure to cross the two sides of the vest in the front. Make sure the vest is not too tight. *Rationale: A vest that is too tight restricts the client's breathing.*

5. If the client is in bed, *the head of the bed must be raised. Rationale: This device is not safe if the client is flat in bed; they could slip down and choke.*

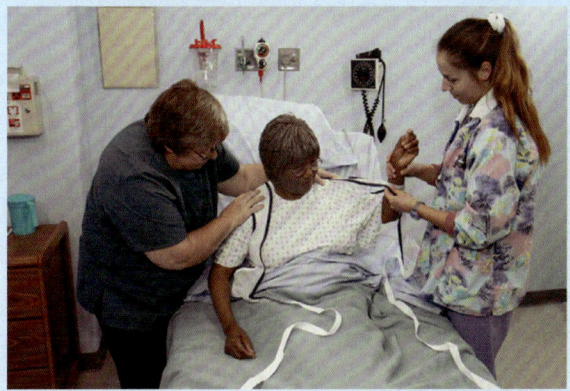

Support the client's back and shoulders while slipping their arms through the armholes of the vest (Carter & Lewsen, 2005).

6. Bring one tie down on each side and tie to the stationary part of the bed frame, NOT the side rails. (Thread the straps between the mattress and the side rails.) On the wheelchair, tie to the pegs on the lower back of the chair. (Thread the straps between the seat and arm rest or between the back of the seat and the back of the chair, according to manufacturer's instructions.) After making a quick-release tie (see Fig. 48-21A), tuck any extra length of strap out of the way. *Rationale: These actions help to provide safety for the client and help the client to remain in the chair.*

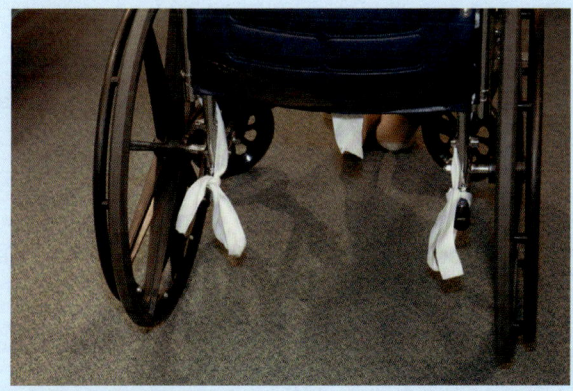

Use a quick-release tie to secure the lower straps of a client safety device to the posts at the back of the wheelchair (Evans-Smith, 2005).

Follow ENDDD steps

Posey Jacket Safety Device

Supplies and Equipment
Posey jacket of the correct size

Steps
Follow LPN WELCOME steps and then

1. This device can *only be used while the client is in a chair.* Put the jacket on with the opening in back. The side seams should be under the arms. (This jacket is also made so there is a "V-neck" in the front.) Close with zipper, ties, Velcro, or hooks. Some types have extra ties. *Rationale: Improper placement could be dangerous. Adjust for a snug fit.*

2. If the client is in bed, transfer them to a wheelchair. This jacket *cannot be safely used in bed.* Tie the upper shoulder loops around the push handles of the wheelchair. (Use only the loops to secure the jacket to the top of the chair.) Tie the lower waist straps to the posts at the bottom back of the wheelchair. *Never* tie anything around the client's neck. *Rationale: This device prevents the client from falling forward or sliding out of the chair. Also, the client could choke if ties are tied too high.*

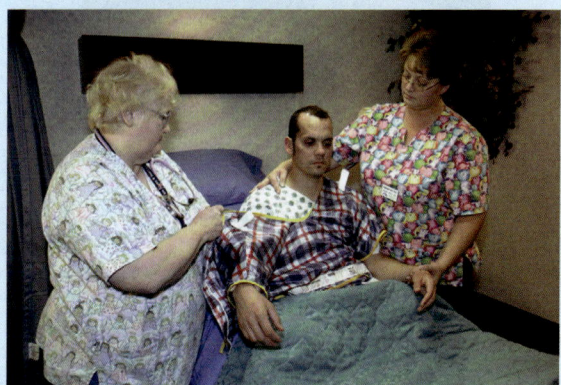

Jacket safety device. This may be applied in bed, but the client must then be transferred to a chair for safety (Carter & Lewsen, 2005).

3. Never leave a client wearing a safety jacket in bed. (However, the jacket may be easier to apply while the client is in bed. In this case, help the client to move into a chair after the jacket is on.) Be sure to check the client frequently while wearing a jacket. *Rationale: The jacket would not allow the client to turn in bed; they might aspirate or choke. Shoulder loops may choke the client who struggles in bed. This client must be carefully monitored.*

Follow ENDDD steps

Soft Wrist (Cloth) Protective Devices or Netted Mitts

Supplies and Equipment
Two soft wrist protective devices or netted mitts (see Fig. 48-20C).

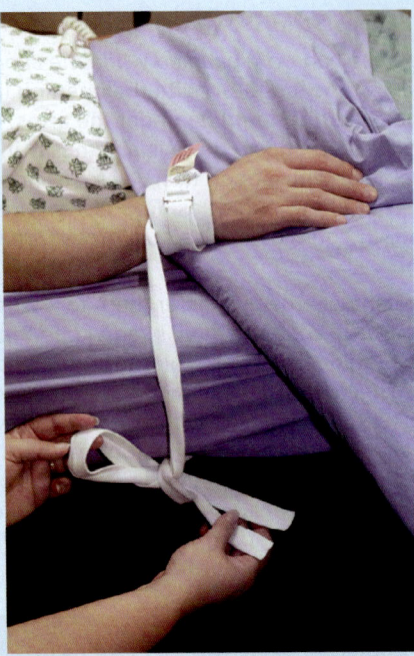

Wrist safety device, secured with a quick-release knot, and attached to the bed frame (Carter & Lewsen, 2005).

Steps
Note: These steps and precautions apply to wrist protective devices and netted hand mitts.

Follow LPN WELCOME steps and then

1. Secure both wrists. **Rationale:** *It is dangerous to secure only one wrist, in nearly all cases. The client could turn and fall out of bed or the chair or become entangled in the straps.*
2. Protect the wrist with clothing or padded dressing under the protective device, unless the device itself is well padded. **Rationale:** *This helps prevent skin breakdown.*
3. After applying the device, you must be able to slip two fingers between the device and the client's wrist. **Rationale:** *It is important to prevent circulatory impairment.*
4. Pull the long tie through the slit in the device; apply the Velcro, or close the buckle. **Rationale:** *This secures the device.*
5. Bring both ends of each long tie together and attach to the bed frame or to the lower chair parts with a quick-release tie. (*Never* tie straps to the side rails or wheels of a wheelchair.) Attach one set of straps on each side. **Rationale:** *This provides safety. If straps from both arms are tied on the same side, the client could turn, fall out of the chair, or be choked by the straps. If side rails are lowered or the chair moved, the client could be seriously injured.*
6. Measure the distance of the tie to allow for range of motion (ROM) of the arm while protecting tubes or equipment from hands. **Rationale:** *Total restraint is frightening and can add to a client's confusion, making the client combative. It helps to be able to move a little.*

Follow ENDDD steps

Lap Belt (Lap Strap)

Supplies and Equipment
Lap belt of the proper size

Steps
Follow LPN WELCOME steps and then

1. Choose a lap belt of the proper size. Lock the wheels if the client is in a wheelchair. Position the footrests or footstool comfortably. Assist the client into a comfortable sitting position, making sure the hips are as far back in the chair as possible. **Rationale:** *The client will probably be sitting in this position for some time. It is important to be comfortable and safe.*
2. Wrap the belt around the client's waist, adjusting the straps per manufacturer's instructions. Secure the straps to the posts on the lower back of the wheelchair, using a quick-release tie (see Fig. 48-21). Keep the belt at a 45-degree angle to the knees, holding the hips in the back of the chair (see Fig. 48-20E). **Rationale:** *This minimizes the risk of the belt sliding up toward the ribs and restricting breathing. It is important to consider safety and comfort at all times.*
3. A crotch strap may be used, if necessary. **Rationale:** *Some clients tend to slip forward. The crotch strap holds the client in the chair more securely.*

Follow ENDDD steps

49 Beds and Bed Making

Learning Objectives

1. State the purposes of bed making in the healthcare facility.
2. Demonstrate the ability to make an unoccupied, occupied, and postoperative bed.
3. Demonstrate the use of a bed cradle.
4. Explain the purpose of side rails and demonstrate the ability to adjust side rails safely.
5. Describe three devices that may be added to the basic hospital bed and their uses.
6. Identify the purposes of specialized hospital beds. Describe at least three specialized beds.

Important Terminology

bed cradle	flotation mattress	mitered (corners)	postoperative bed	unoccupied bed
closed bed	footboard	occupied bed	traction	
egg crate mattress	footdrop	open bed	trapeze	

Some clients are so ill they are totally or partially confined to bed. A bed should provide comfort and correct posture for the client, as well as proper height and accessibility for caregivers. The ideal bed is durable, lightweight, easy to move, and easy to clean. The most commonly used bed in healthcare facilities adjusts to different positions (the *Gatch bed*). This electric bed has controls incorporated into its side rails. The entire bed can be lowered, allowing the client to get in and out easily and raised to facilitate caregiving. The head and foot of the bed can be adjusted as well. The client and caregivers can use these controls to position the bed as desired. Usually, the controls for the TV, reading light, and nurse call are also incorporated into the bed controls. (In very old beds, the Gatch adjustments are operated with a hand crank.)

> **Key Concept**
> The bed controls can be locked so the client cannot make adjustments, if this could cause problems (e.g., if the client has a delicate suture line or unset fracture).

BED MAKING

Every client needs a smooth, clean bed for comfort and to prevent complications. In addition, a clean bed helps to decrease pathogens in the client's environment. Clean, dry, and wrinkle-free linens also help to reduce the potential for skin breakdown and can help to control odor. Necessary supplies for bed making include clean linens: a tight bottom sheet, to prevent wrinkles that might cause skin irritation and upper bed clothing that does not weigh on the client's body or restrict movements, but still covers their shoulders. It is very important to change linens that are soiled. One or more incontinence pads are added to the linens on the bed if the client is bleeding, incontinent, or vomiting. In some cases, a head-to-toe bed change is done daily. Adjustments in basic bed making may be necessary for comfort and to suit individual client conditions.

Schedules for changing beds vary among healthcare agencies. Usually the bed is changed after the client's bath or morning care. Make exceptions if the linen becomes soiled or if changing the bed may prove harmful to the client. For example, a client may be bleeding, receiving a special treatment, or feeling too weak or exhausted to be disturbed. *Change stained sheets immediately, however.* In some facilities, beds are not changed every day or are partially changed. Even if you do not change the bed, tuck in sheets and blankets, to get rid of wrinkles, make sure there are no crumbs, and fluff the pillows. Be sure to *follow the concepts of proper body mechanics,* to prevent injury to yourself (see Chapter 48).

Making an Unoccupied Bed

An **unoccupied bed** is one that is empty at the time it is made and is the easiest bed to make. The unoccupied bed can be made as either a closed bed or an open bed. When no client has been assigned to the bed, it is made as a *closed bed*. An *open bed* is a bed to which a client is already assigned. To make a **closed bed**, the top covers are pulled up to the head of the bed over the bottom covers. A pillow is placed on top of the linens or is covered with the bedspread, much as you would do in your home (Fig. 49-1A). To make the **open bed**, the top covers are fan-folded to the foot of the bed, so the client can get into bed easily (Fig. 49-1B). Steps in making an open bed and closed bed are shown in In Practice: Nursing Procedure 49-1. Figure 49-2 illustrates how to make a **mitered corner**. After making any bed, look to see if the linens are straight, firmly tucked under the mattress, smooth and without wrinkles, and hanging evenly on both sides.

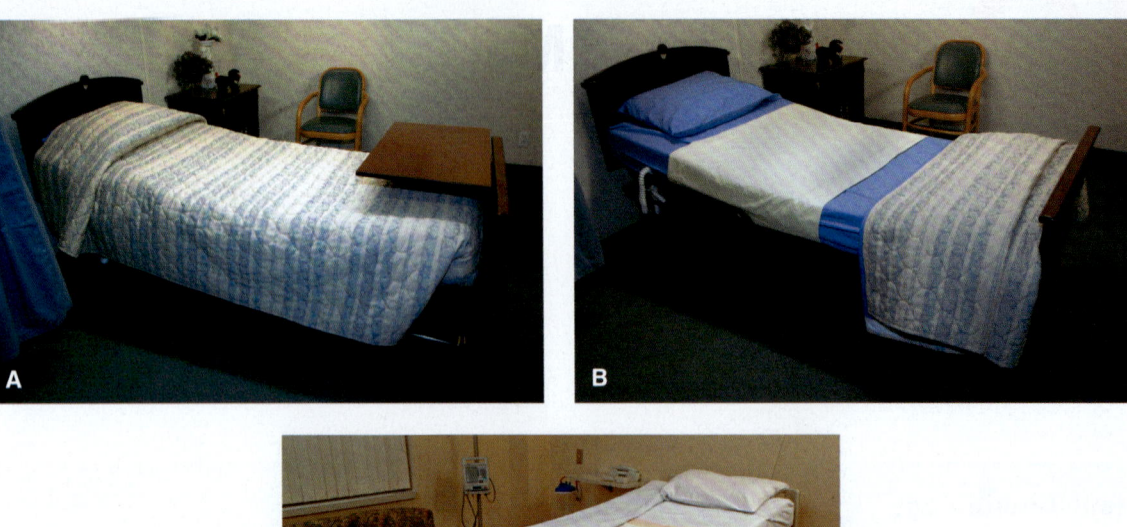

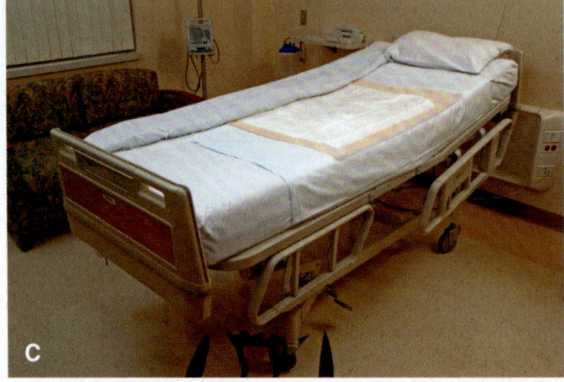

Figure 49-1 Methods of making beds. **A.** A closed bed is an unoccupied bed. **B.** When a closed bed is "opened," the top sheet, blanket, and bedspread are fan-folded to the foot of the bed, for easy entry by the client. Note that a draw sheet is in place, to help protect the bed and to facilitate turning the client. The bed is kept in low position for safety. **C.** A surgical or postoperative bed is a closed bed that has been "opened" to receive a person on a stretcher. The top linens are fan-folded to the side of the bed and out of the way. This bed is usually in high position, to conveniently receive the client from the stretcher. Clean linens should be used after surgery. (Carter, 2013.)

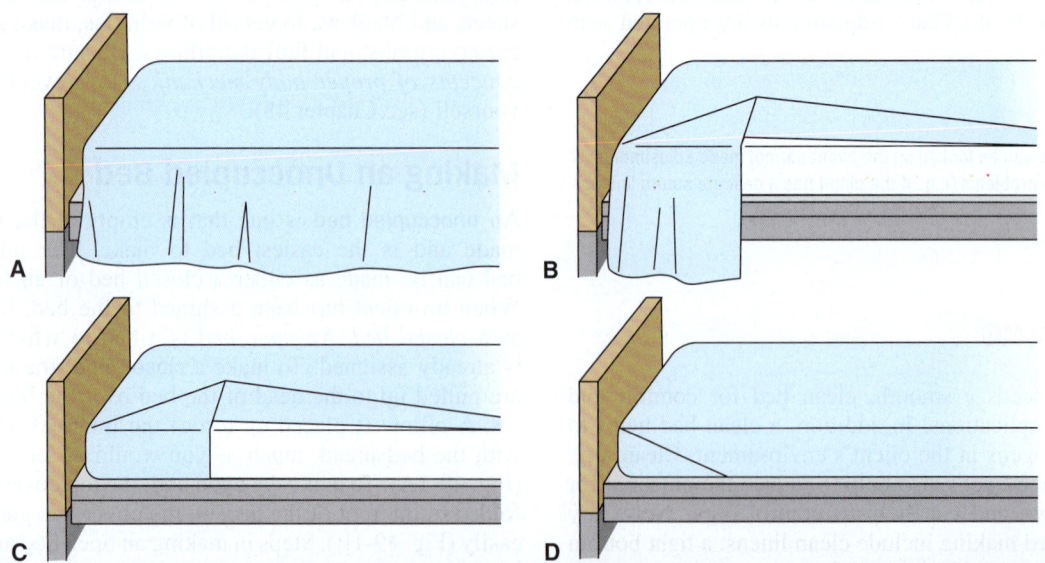

Figure 49-2 How to make a mitered corner. Here, a mitered corner is being made on a flat bottom sheet (if a fitted sheet is not used). **A.** The sheet is hanging over the sides of the bed. **B.** Grasp the edge of the sheet about 12 in. from the foot of the bed and lift it up, forming a triangle. Lay the triangular fold on top of the bed, and smooth the hanging portion of the sheet against the side of the mattress. **C.** Tuck the hanging portion of the sheet underneath the mattress, while holding the triangular fold taut against the top of the bed. **D.** Bring the triangular fold back down over the edge of the mattress, and tuck it underneath. This process is the same for the upper corners of the bottom sheet and for bottom end of the top sheet. (Adapted from Carter, 2016.)

Making an Occupied Bed

Some clients are unable to get out of bed, due to their specific condition or generalized weakness. Changing bed linens with the client in the bed is known as making an **occupied bed**. Work quickly and disturb the client as little as possible. (Remember: some clients must be moved in a particular way.) Making an occupied bed may be done by one nurse, especially if the client can help to turn over; however, if the client is large or their medical condition is unstable, ask a coworker to assist. It is vital to prevent back injury to yourself. In Practice: Nursing Procedure 49-2 gives steps in making an occupied bed. If done correctly, this procedure requires minimum exertion for both you and the client (see Chapter 48).

> *Nursing Alert* A client with an unstabilized fracture, tubing, or other special circumstances must be moved very carefully, to prevent complications.

Opening a Bed for a Client

The open bed has linens folded down, making it easier for the client to get into bed. Open a bed for a new client or leave it open when the client is out of bed for a short time. Follow these steps:

- With the bed in high position, turn the bedspread down from the top, and fold it around and over the top edge of the blanket. Then fold the sheet over the top of the blanket and spread. *Rationale: This protects the blanket, keeps the rougher blanket away from the client's skin, and makes it easier for the client to handle the bedclothes. Having the bed high helps protect your back.*
- Turn the top bedding down to the foot of the mattress and fold it back on itself. *Rationale: This shows the client that the bed is ready. Helping the person into bed is also easier when the bed is open.*

Always leave the bed in low position when you have completed caring for the client. *Rationale: This is vital to prevent falls.*

Making a Postoperative Bed

When a client is to return from the operating room or from another procedure that requires transfer into bed from a stretcher and sometimes from a wheelchair, a **postoperative bed** is prepared. The postoperative bed is made in such a way as to make it easy to transfer the client from a stretcher to the bed (Fig. 49-1C). In Practice: Nursing Procedure 49-3 outlines the steps in making this bed.

ATTACHMENTS AND ACCESSORIES

Bed Cradle

A **bed cradle**, a frame to prevent the bedclothes from touching all or part of the client's body, is used for clients with fractures, extensive burns, and open or painful wounds. A wide cradle fits across the entire width of the bed, lengthwise. A narrow cradle also fits along the bed lengthwise; it can be used over one extremity (see Nursing Procedure 49-4). Bed cradles may contain a low-level heating device. The bed linens are arranged over the cradle. In some instances, the linens are fastened to the cradle frame. Leave the linens long enough at the top to cover the client's shoulders comfortably. Place side rails up for safety. Instruct clients not to raise or lower their head or feet. *Rationale: Adjusting the bed could displace the cradle and cause injury to the client.* (It may be necessary to lock the bed controls.) In Practice: Nursing Procedure 49-4 describes how to make a bed that includes a bed cradle.

Side Rails

Side rails (*safety rails*) are built into most hospital beds. They not only prevent clients from falling out of bed, but also help them to change position in bed. TV controls and the nurse call signal are usually integrated into the side rails. Most facilities have standard protocols regarding side rail use. It is the nurse's responsibility to follow these protocols, always keeping the safety of your clients in mind.

> *Nursing Alert* In some cases, having the side rails up can be more dangerous than having them down. For example, an older, restless, or confused client may continually try to crawl out of bed. In this case, they might crawl over the side rails, making a fall more dangerous than if it were just from the bed at low level.

Some clients resent side rails, but this may be alleviated by the fact that everyone has side rails and also by the convenience of built-in TV and nurse-call controls. People may fear being shut in or may resent being treated as if they were irresponsible. Explain that side rails are for the client's protection. In some cases, additional protection is necessary; side rails may be cushioned with a mattress pad, bath blanket, or pillows. The client on "seizure precautions" has their side rails covered with special seizure pads.

Other Equipment

A **footboard** may be attached to the foot of the bed to prevent abnormal plantar flexion or a deformity called **footdrop**, which may occur when a client remains in bed for a prolonged length of time (Fig. 49-3) (see also Chapter 48). The footboard is set at a slight angle and is placed to support the client's feet in a *simulated standing position* (Fig. 49-4A).

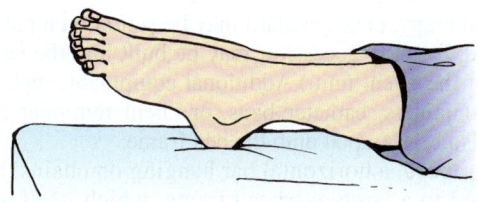

Figure 49-3 Abnormal plantar flexion, if not corrected, leads to a deformity called *footdrop*. (Taylor, Lillis, LeMone, & Lynn, 2015.)

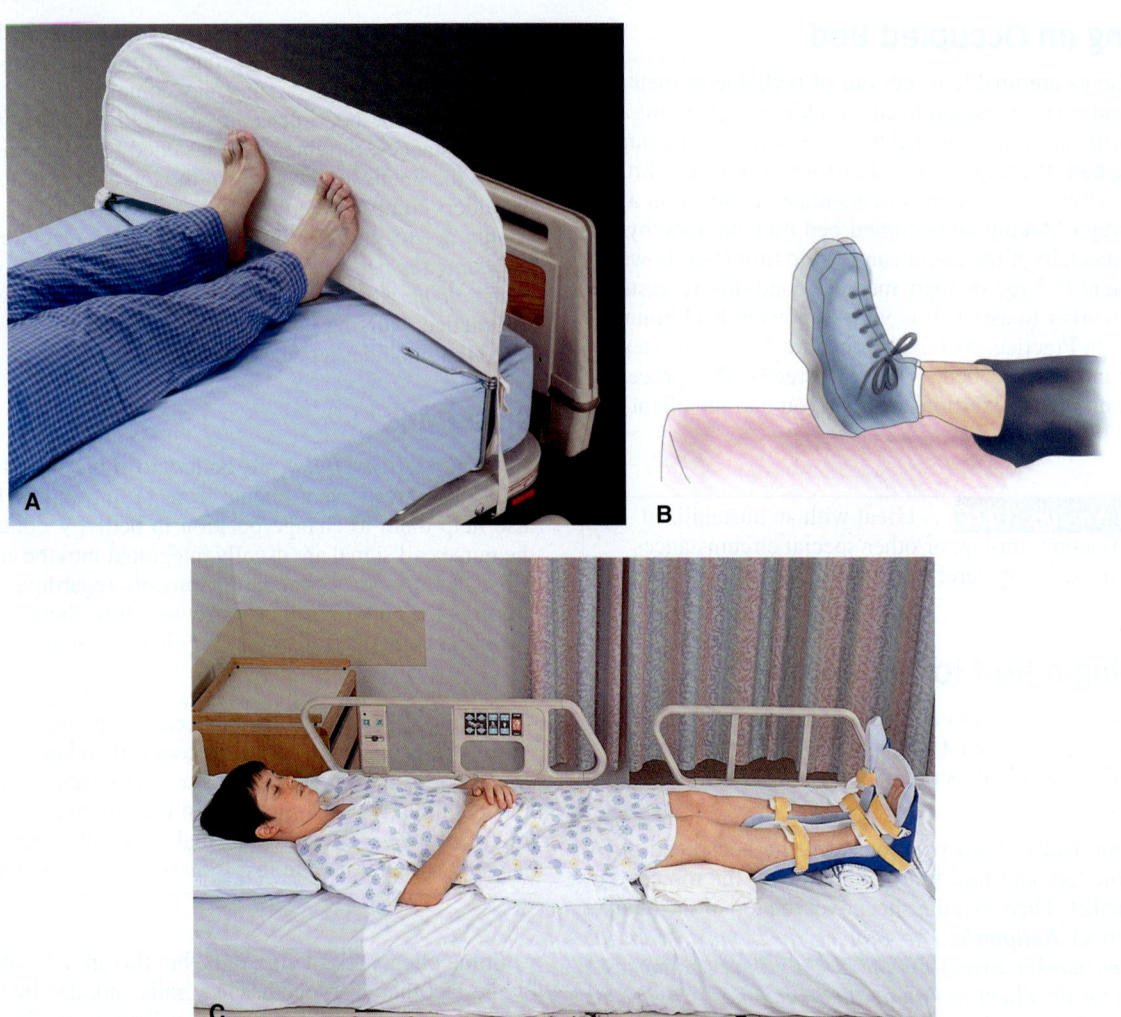

Figure 49-4 Prevention of footdrop. **A.** A padded footboard is placed at the foot of the bed. The padding helps prevent skin breakdown. When the feet are placed against the footboard, it keeps the feet in proper alignment (dorsiflexion). **B.** High-top shoes are an alternative to the footboard, particularly if the person moves about in bed a great deal. **C.** Protective boots (foot splints) are also available to prevent footdrop. (A: Photo courtesy of Posey Corporation; B: Taylor, Lillis, & Lynn, 2015; C: Timby, 2005.)

Several alternatives to the footboard, such as foot splints and high-top shoes, are also available (Fig. 49-4B,C).

A *bed board* may be placed under the mattress to support the body in correct alignment. A *CPR* (cardiopulmonary resuscitation) *headboard* is available on hospital beds and with crash carts (see Fig. 43-6). The headboard of the bed is easily removable, for placement under the client if CPR is needed (Fig. 49-5). A separate CPR board may be hung on the wall or a transfer board (see Chapter 48) may be used.

Hospital beds are also equipped with a means for attaching an *IV standard* that holds bags for intravenous (IV) or blood therapy. (The standard may be stored on a rack under the bed, for easy access, or may be built into the ceiling or wall of the client unit.) Additional equipment, such as suction containers, catheter bags, or client reminder devices, may also be clamped onto the bed frame.

A **trapeze**, a horizontal bar hanging on chains, is often attached to a large overhead frame, which itself attaches to the bed (see Nursing Procedure 48-11). The trapeze is used by the client to pull up to a sitting position or to lift the shoulders and hips off the bed. The trapeze is also used to exercise and strengthen the arms, particularly if the client will be using crutches or is a person with paraplegia (paralyzed from the waist down). The client may be placed in bed **traction**, a device consisting of a series of ropes, pulleys, and weights that serve to keep a body part, such as a fractured leg, in proper alignment. Generally, the bed of the client in traction is changed with the person in the bed (an occupied bed). However, in this case, used linens are removed and new linens brought down from head to toe. This client can assist by lifting the upper body using a trapeze. This differs from the method of making an occupied bed described earlier. (Chapter 77 describes care of clients in traction. The client may also have self-contained traction, in which case they can get out of bed.)

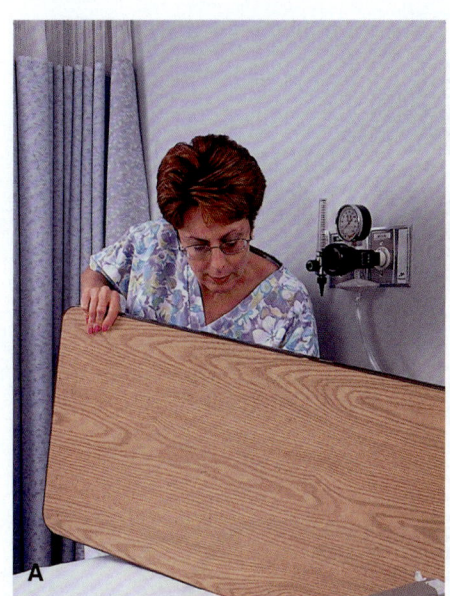
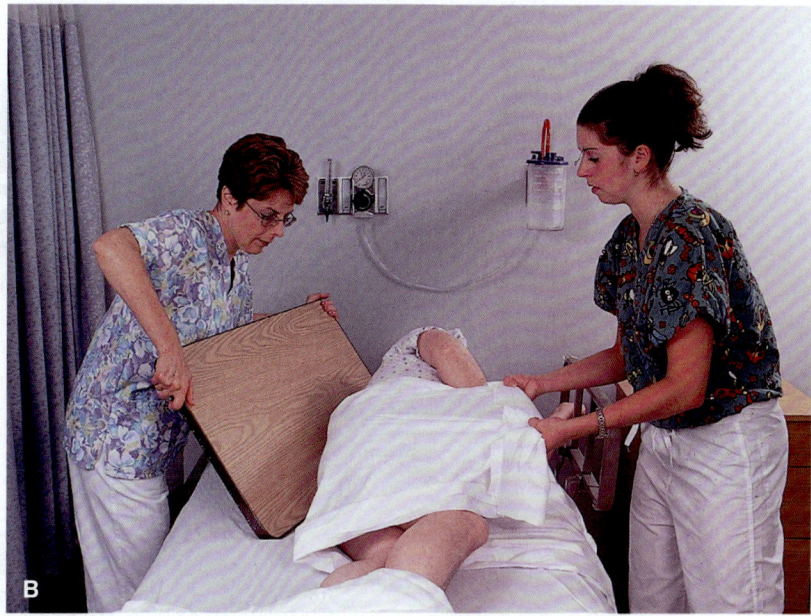

Figure 49-5 **A.** Removing the headboard for cardiopulmonary resuscitation. **B.** The headboard is placed under the client's upper body to provide a firm surface for resuscitation. A transfer board may also be used for this purpose. (Timby, 2005.)

> **Nursing Alert** Never remove traction weights without your specific instructions.

NCLEX Alert

Priority NCLEX concepts are the client safety, promotion of skin integrity, and prevention of infection. Client care may integrate these concepts. You need to choose the appropriate action or response.

SPECIAL BEDS AND MATTRESSES

Special mattress surfaces are used for clients on prolonged bed rest or for those with poor skin integrity. Examples include the **egg crate mattress**, a foam rubber pad with a surface shaped like an egg carton, and the **flotation mattress** or pad (usually used in a specific area of the body). The flotation mattress or pad contains a special gel-type material, which supports the body or body part in such a way as to avoid creating pressure points. Although egg crate mattresses and flotation pads provide client comfort, they do not necessarily prevent skin breakdown. Special skin care and measures for prevention of pressure wounds are described in Chapter 58.

Therapeutic beds are used to treat clients with severe joint contractures, prolonged immobility, or skin wounds such as pressure wounds or severe burns. These beds reduce or relieve the effects of pressure against the skin through various mechanisms. The surface of such beds often feels like a waterbed. These beds are more comfortable for clients who have severe contractures because their bodies float as if suspended in midair. Severe skin wounds are more likely to heal when the effects of pressure are reduced. Some special beds are pictured in Figure 49-6. Many special beds also are available in sizes that accommodate very large or heavy clients.

Special *orthopedic beds and frames* support clients who must remain immobilized. Although largely replaced by other computerized beds and overlay mattresses, the circle bed (Circ-O-Lectric bed) is still used in special situations (Fig. 49-6C). It functions to turn the client as a unit, keeping the body straight.

Key Concept

Bariatric beds are also available for very large clients. These beds are larger than regular hospital beds and of heavier construction. Usually three people are required to move a bariatric bed.

Throughout your nursing career, you will work with clients who need therapeutic beds, many of which are complex to use. Be sure to read carefully the instructions for use, paying particular attention to safety features. You are responsible for the safe and effective use of these therapeutic beds, as well as the safety and well-being of your clients.

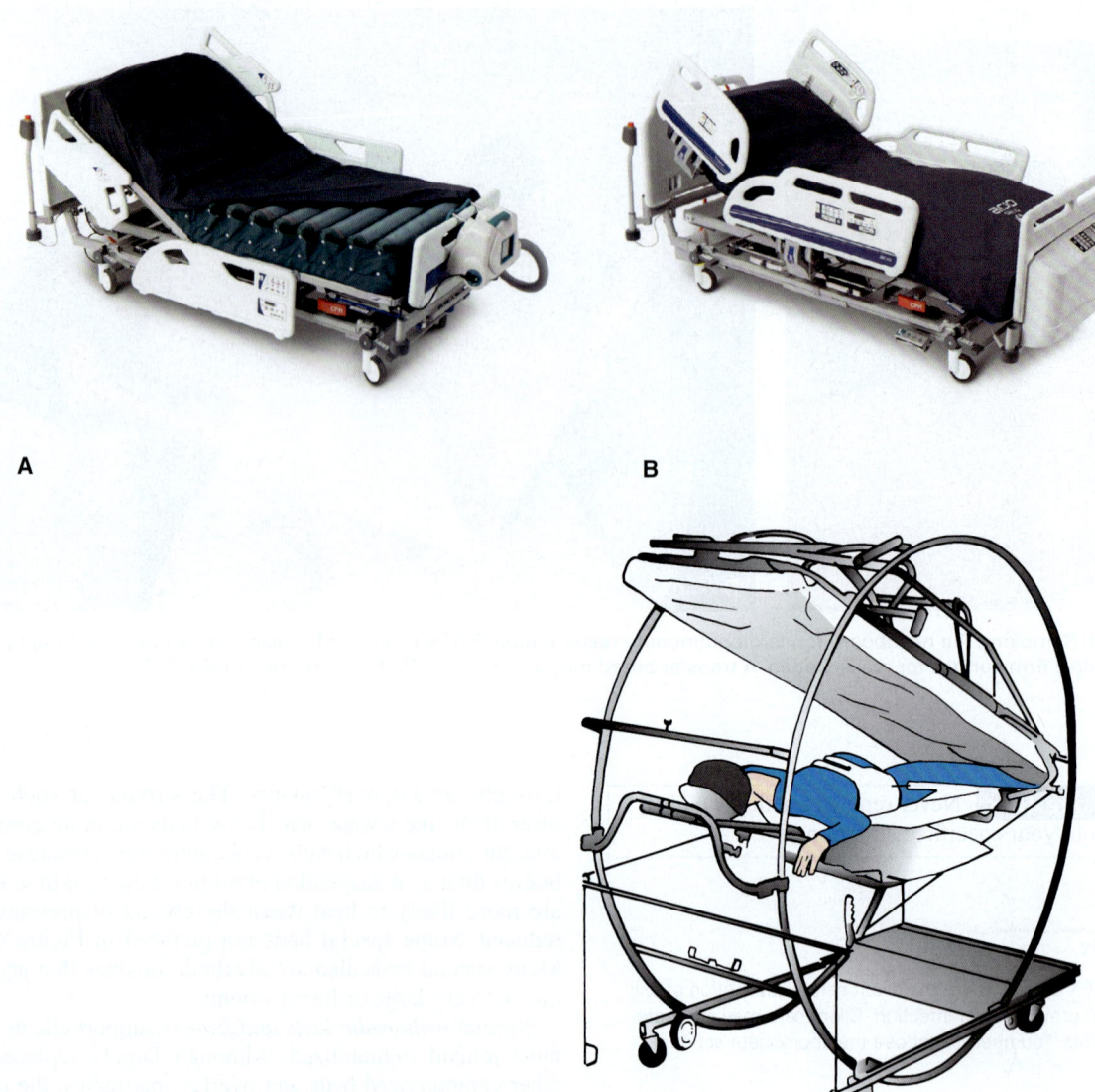

Figure 49-6 Many specialized beds are available to assist in client care, prevent deformities, and enhance client safety, particularly for the client who is very large, seriously ill, or disabled. In addition, these beds help prevent back injuries to nurses. **A.** TheraKair® Vizio - Advanced Low Air Loss (LAL) pressure relief with pulsation therapy. **B.** The TheraPulse ATP alternating pressure bed rotates air pockets, to reduce the possibility of developing pressure areas. The pump has a quick-release mechanism that expels the air, allowing a solid platform for cardiopulmonary resuscitation. **C.** The Circ-O-Lectric or circle bed is not often used, except in rehabilitation. It turns the client from front (prone) to back (supine), rotating around the feet. (B: Reprinted with kind permission of Arjo.)

STUDENT SYNTHESIS

KEY POINTS

- Organize work. Gather all supplies before making the bed. Strip and make one side of the bed at a time to conserve time and energy.
- To prevent the spread of microorganisms, never shake linen or put it on the floor and hold it away from your clothing.
- Keep each client's linens separate.
- Place soiled linen in a covered laundry hamper while continuing your work. Uncovered laundry bags are usually not used.
- Keep in mind that a well-made bed promotes comfort and rest, helps prevent skin breakdown, and provides safety for clients.
- Use special attachments and beds, as available, to meet a particular client's needs.

CRITICAL THINKING EXERCISES

1. Explain how to use correct body mechanics when you make an occupied bed.
2. A client's family member argues with you about side rails being placed in an up position. Describe your explanation of the use of side rails to the family member and to the client.
3. Do you agree or disagree with the statement that some people are safer with side rails down? Why or why not?
4. A client is returned to their room after surgery and the bed is as it was when they went for surgery. Describe and justify your concerns. What needs to be done?

NCLEX-STYLE REVIEW QUESTIONS

1. A client is lying in a hospital bed that is soiled with urine but states to the nurse, "Leave me alone right now." Which response by the nurse is best?
   a. "I can come back later when you are feeling better."
   b. "You will have to allow me to change the sheets because they smell terrible."
   c. "I need to make sure you are clean and dry to prevent irritation to your skin."
   d. "If you don't let me change your sheets, I will call your care provider."
2. The nurse is changing soiled sheets on a client's bed. Which action would the nurse take to avoid injury?
   a. Throw the soiled sheets on the floor to avoid having to turn to place them in a bag.
   b. Bend at the waist when moving the sheets under the client.
   c. Keep the bed in the lowest position while making the bed.
   d. Use proper body mechanics at all times when changing the sheets.
3. The nurse is attempting to make a bed occupied by a client who is obese and on bedrest. Which action is necessary to prevent injury to the nurse?
   a. Request assistance from a coworker to make the bed.
   b. Have the client sit in the chair while the nurse makes the bed.
   c. Avoid changing the sheets since it is difficult.
   d. Have the client assist with making the bed while in it.
4. A client has extensive burns and requires a bed cradle to keep the sheets off the body. Which instructions would the nurse provide the client?
   a. Leave the side rails down.
   b. Do not raise or lower the head or feet.
   c. Do not move at all while in the bed.
   d. No pillows may be used while the cradle is on the bed.
5. The nurse is caring for a group of clients. For which client would the bed rails be left down for safety?
   a. A confused, disoriented older adult client trying to get out of the bed
   b. A client who is unresponsive with a severe head injury
   c. An awake alert client who is ambulatory
   d. A client who has pneumonia and is able to use the bathroom

CHAPTER RESOURCES

Enhance your learning with additional resources on thePoint!

Student Resources related to this chapter can be found at thePoint.lww.com/Rosdahl12e.

Welcome Steps

Look at healthcare provider's orders.

Protocol for procedure.

Necessary equipment/supplies.

Wash hands using proper hand hygiene; put on gloves.

Explain the procedure and reassure the client.

Locate two identifiers to confirm correct client.

Comfortable and efficient position for nurse and client.

Obtain privacy.

Make sure to follow correct steps and body mechanics with good technique.

Ensure safety and observe deviations from normal.

End Steps

Ensure comfort and safety.

Note questions or concerns from client or nurse; note significant data.

Dispose of materials properly.

Disinfect the area and your hands.

Document and report the procedure and your findings.

IN PRACTICE

NURSING PROCEDURE 49-1 — Making an Unoccupied Bed

Supplies and Equipment
Gloves
Mattress pad
Sheets (either 2 flat sheets or 1 flat sheet and 1 contour [fitted] bottom sheet)
Draw sheet, used in most cases
Blankets, as needed
Bedspread
Pillowcases
Covered linen hamper
Chair or bag
Bedside table or chair

Steps

Follow LPN WELCOME Steps and Then

1. If the client is able to be out of bed while their linens are changed, use the following procedure. Adjust the bed to a comfortable working height for you. *Rationale: A bed at the proper height helps prevent back strain.*

2. Wear gloves to remove used linens. Loosen all used linens. Remove, roll up, and place in a covered linen hamper. Never place used linens on the floor or hold them against your clothing. Remove gloves and wash your hands after removing used linens. *Rationale: Linens may be soiled with body fluids. Many microorganisms are on the floor. Soiled linens from the bed or floor can contaminate your clothing, which may come in contact with other clients.*

Arrange and stack the linens needed to make the bed in the order in which they will be used. Hold the linens away from your body (to prevent contamination from your clothing). (Carter, 2016.)

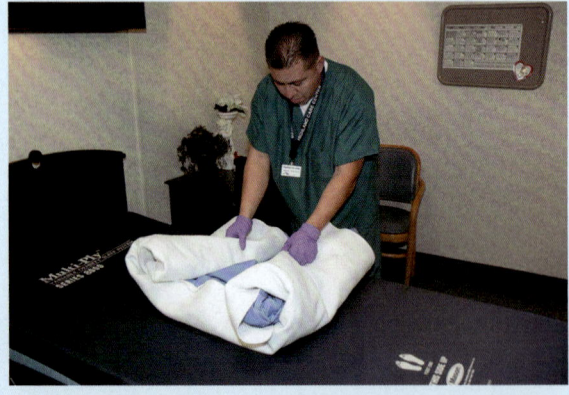

The area most soiled is rolled toward the center of the bed. The nurse wears gloves when removing used linens. (Carter, 2016.)

3. Refold the bedspread or any item that is to be reused. Place it on the back of the chair. *Rationale: Agency policy dictates which linens are to be reused, if they are not soiled.*

4. Remove used pillowcases and place them in the linen hamper. Move pillows to the chair. *Rationale: Removing pillows from the bed simplifies bed making.*

5. Slide the mattress toward the head of the bed. Place a mattress pad on the bed. *Rationale: Moving up the mattress provides more foot room for the client.*

6. If using a flat sheet, place it on the bed. Open it lengthwise, with the center fold along the bed's center. Unfold the upper layer of the sheet toward the opposite side of the bed. Slide the sheet upward over the top of the bed, leaving the bottom edge of the flat sheet even with the edge of the mattress. If using a fitted (contour) sheet, tuck it over the mattress at the upper and lower end of that side. *Rationale: Unfolding the sheet in this manner allows you to make the bed on one side.*

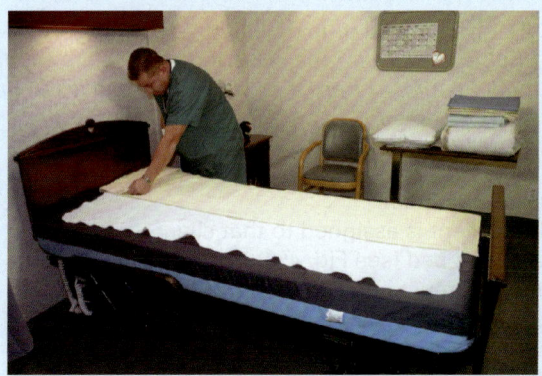

Place the bottom sheet so that only one vertical crease remains, down the center of the bed. (Carter, 2012.)

7. Tuck the sheet securely under the head of the mattress first. Make a diagonal or mitered (square) corner if the sheet is not fitted (see Fig. 49-2). *Rationale: A mitered corner has a neat appearance and keeps the sheet securely under the mattress.*

8. Tuck the sheet under the entire side of the bed. *Rationale: This secures the bottom sheet on one side of the bed.*

9. Place a draw sheet (if used) on the bed, folded in half, with the fold in the center of the bed. Lift the top half toward the other side of the bed. Tuck the draw sheet under the mattress. *Rationale: A draw sheet is an additional protection for the bed and serves as a lifting or turning sheet for an immobile client. Add incontinence pads, as necessary.*

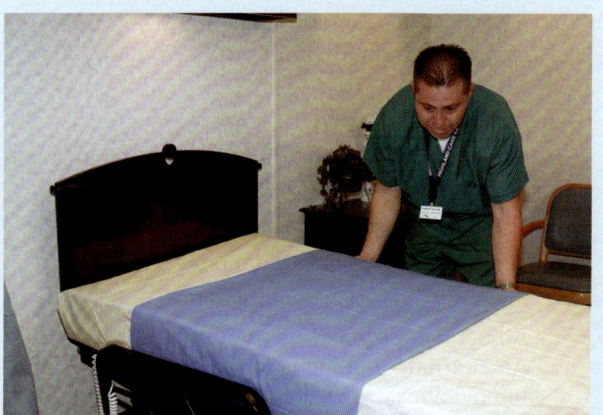

The draw sheet is placed over the bottom sheet. (One entire side is tucked in before moving to the other side. Then, the other side is tucked in.) (Carter, 2016.)

10. Place the top sheet on the bed, centering it in the same manner as the bottom sheet. Make sure the upper hem of the top sheet is level with the top of the mattress. Drop the lower end of the sheet over the end of the mattress. *Rationale: Staying on one side of the bed until it is completely made saves steps and time.*

11. Cover the top sheet with a blanket and/or bedspread. Tuck all these together under the bottom of the mattress. Miter the corner. *Rationale: A blanket provides warmth. A bedspread ensures a neat appearance. Tucking all these pieces together saves time and provides a neat appearance.*

12. Move to the other side of the bed. Tuck in the linens as in step 11. Fold back the cuff at the head of the bed with the sheet and bedspread if the client will be returning to bed. *Rationale: The cuff makes it easier to fold back the linens.*

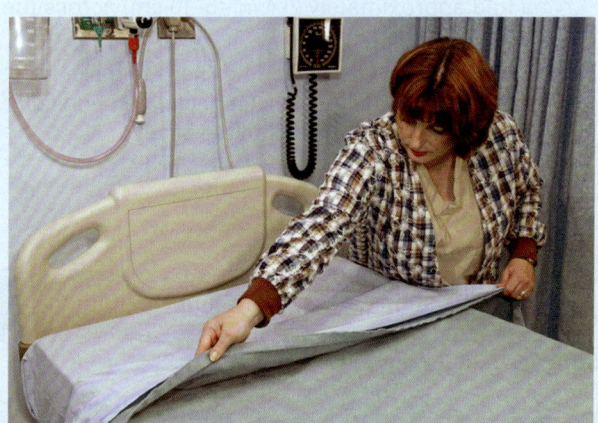

Fold back a cuff with the top linens if the client will be returning to bed. (Taylor, Lillis, & Lynn, 2015.)

13. Put a clean pillowcase on the pillow. *Rationale: Using this method minimizes shaking the pillow excessively:*
    a. Rest the pillow on a flat surface.
    b. Grasp the pillowcase in the center on the closed end.
    c. Turn the pillowcase back over your hand.
    d. Grasp the pillow through the pillowcase.
    e. Pull the pillowcase over the pillow.
    f. Adjust the pillowcase smoothly over the pillow. An alternate method is to put one hand inside the pillowcase and pull the pillow corners into the corners of the pillowcase.

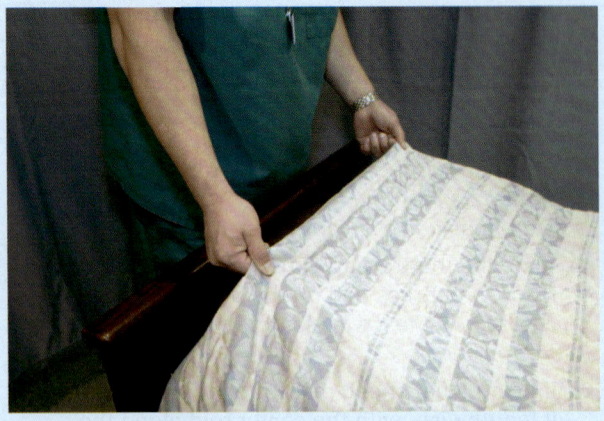

Make a toe pleat by pulling up on the top linens. This allows room for the client's feet when they are lying on the back (supine). (Carter, 2012.)

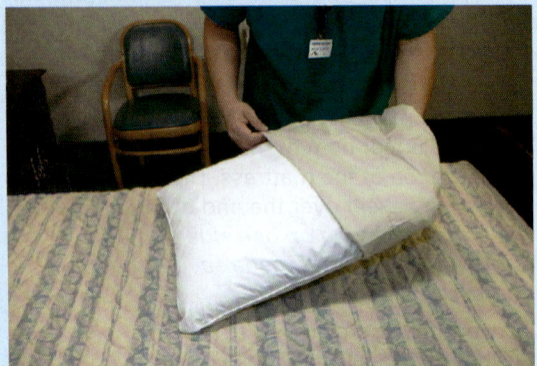

This shows one way to put the pillowcase on the pillow. Grasp the pillow through the closed end of the pillowcase and pull the pillowcase over the pillow. (Carter, 2012.)

14. Place a pillow at the top of the bed in the center, with the open end away from the door. *Rationale: A pillow is a comfort measure. The open end may collect dust or microorganisms.*
15. Make a toe pleat at the foot of the bed. *Rationale: Toe pleats allow freedom of foot movement.*
    a. For a horizontal pleat, gather the linens to make a fold approximately 2–4 in. (5–10 cm) across the foot of the bed.
    b. For a vertical pleat, gather the linens to make a fold approximately 2–4 in. (5–10 cm) perpendicular (up and down) to the foot of the bed.
16. Replace the call signal on the bed, secure it in place, and pull up the side rails on the far side, if needed. *Rationale: Provide safety for the client and the ability to call for help.*
17. Move the overbed table next to the bed. *Rationale: Bedside necessities will be within easy reach for the client.*
18. Return the bed to low position. *Rationale: This helps prepare for the client's return. (If the client will be moved from a stretcher, the bed is left in high position.)*

Follow ENDDD Steps

Special Reminder
- If no client is assigned to that client unit, make a closed bed (see Fig. 49-1A). Remember that the bed must have been thoroughly cleaned/sanitized before being made up. Pull the covers up to the head of the bed. Place the pillow on top or under the spread, if it is long enough. *Rationale: This keeps the bed clean and ready for the next occupant.*
- If a client is assigned to the bed, make an open bed (see Fig. 49-1B). Fan-fold the top of the linens to the bottom third of the bed. *Rationale: This allows the client easier entry into bed.*

IN PRACTICE
NURSING PROCEDURE 49-2 Making an Occupied Bed

Supplies and Equipment
Gloves
Mattress pad
Sheets (either 2 flat sheets or 1 flat sheet and 1 contour [fitted] bottom sheet)
Draw sheet (optional)
Blanket
Bedspread
Pillowcases
Covered linen hamper
Chair
Bath blanket

Steps
Follow LPN WELCOME Steps and Then

1. If the client is unable to get out of bed while linens are changed, use the following procedure. Adjust the bed to a comfortable working height for you. Wear gloves for this procedure. Remove the call bell if it is attached to linens. Lower the side rail on the near side, while keeping the other side rail raised. *Rationale: Proper bed height helps prevent back strain. The raised side rail provides more safety for the client.*

2. Lower the head of the bed if the client can tolerate it. *Rationale:* The bed is easier to make when it is flat.
3. Loosen the top bed linens. Remove the spread, refold it if it will be reused, and place it on the back of the chair. *Rationale:* Agency policy indicates which linens to reuse if not soiled.

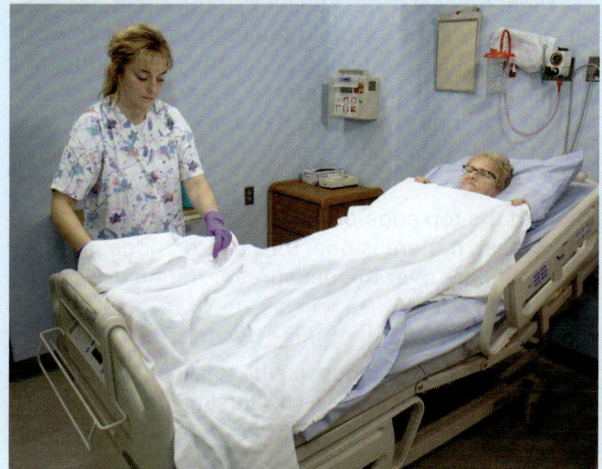

Remove the used top linens from under the bath blanket. (Taylor, Lillis, LeMone, & Lynn, 2008.)

4. Place a bath blanket over the top sheet and ask the client to hold onto the upper edge if they are able to do so. Remove the top sheet, and place it in the linen hamper. *Rationale:* The bath blanket keeps the client warm and protects their privacy.
5. Slide the mattress toward the head of the bed if necessary. Request assistance to do this. *Rationale:* Moving the mattress up provides more foot room for the client.
6. Assist the client to turn toward the other side of the bed. Adjust the pillow. The client can help by holding onto the side rail, if able. *Rationale:* Moving the client as close to the other side of the bed as possible gives you more room to make the bed.
7. Loosen bottom bed linens on your side. Fan-fold used linens from the side of the bed toward the middle and wedge them close to the client's back. Leave the mattress pad in place unless soiled. *Rationale:* Placing folded used linen close to the client allows more space to place the clean bottom sheets.
8. Place the clean bottom sheet on the bed, folded lengthwise; push it under the used sheet and under the client's back as far as possible. Roll the top half of the sheet under the client and under the used linens. Adjust the bottom sheet and miter the upper corner or tuck in the contour sheet at top and bottom. Place the draw sheet (optional) as in In Practice: Nursing Procedure 49-1. *Rationale:* Used linens can easily be removed. Clean linens are positioned to make the other side of the bed.

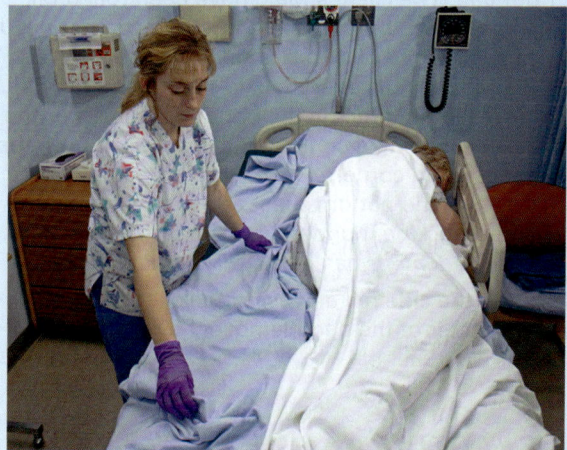

Place the clean bottom sheet on the bed, with the center fold close to the client's back. The clean linens are rolled close to the client, under the used linens. When the bottom of the bed is made, pull up the near side rail and ask the client to roll toward you as far over the rolled-up linens as possible.
(Taylor, Lillis, LeMone, & Lynn, 2008.)

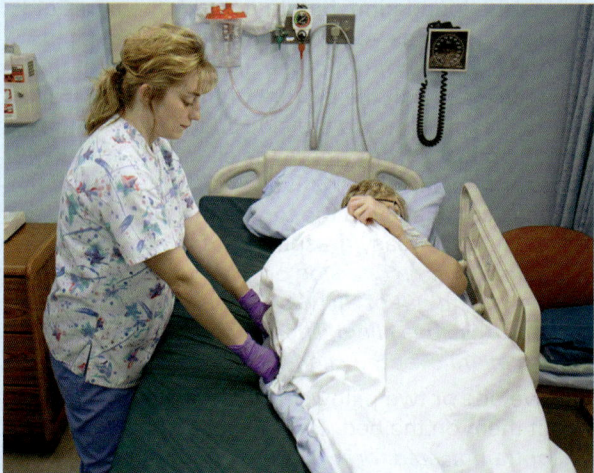

Fan-fold and wedge the used bottom linens as close to the client's back as possible. (Taylor, Lillis, LeMone, & Lynn, 2008.)

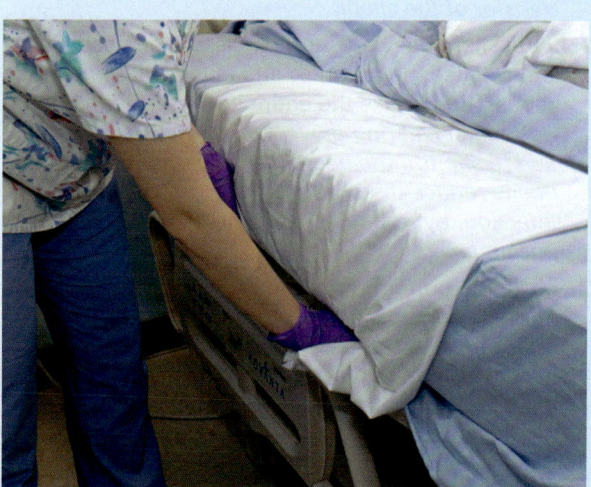

Tuck in all the bottom linens on your side of the bed before moving to the other side. (Taylor, Lillis, LeMone, & Lynn, 2008.)

9. Raise the side rail on your side. Help the client roll over the folded linen to your side of the bed. Ask the client to move as close to your side of the bed as possible. Ask the client to hold onto the side rail, if possible. *Rationale: Provides client safety and allows the client to assist.*

10. Move to the other side of the bed, lower the side rail, and *very carefully* ease the used bottom linens out of the bed. Hold them away from you. Place in the hamper or bag. Straighten the mattress pad. *Rationale: Used linens can contaminate your clothing. Make sure the base of the bed is flat, to prevent skin breakdown. Dragging linens out from under the client can cause shear damage to the skin.*

11. Grasp clean bottom linens and gently ease them out flat. (The client should have been rolled far enough over the clean linens so they do not need to be dragged out from under the client.) Spread the clean linens over the bed's unmade side. Pull them taut and tuck in the bottom sheet. Miter the corner. If using a contour sheet, tuck it in both top and bottom corners. Brace your knee against the bed. Pull the bottom sheet and draw sheet taut before tucking it under the mattress. *Rationale: Wrinkled linens can cause skin irritation.*

12. Raise the side rail and assist the client back to the center of the bed. Remove the pillow. Put on a clean pillowcase and place the pillow under the client's head. Adjust as desired by the client. *Rationale: The pillow is a client comfort measure.*

13. Place the top sheet over the bath blanket. Ask the client to hold onto the upper edge. Remove the bath blanket and place it in the linen hamper or client's closet. Add a blanket, if the client desires one for warmth. Unfold the bedspread over the top sheet and/or blanket. Tuck the lower ends securely under the mattress. Miter corners of all the top linens together. *Rationale: Tucking these pieces together saves time and provides neat, tight corners.*

14. Fold the top edge of the bedspread over the blanket, if there is one. Turn the top edge of the sheet back over the bedspread. *Rationale: This technique provides a neat appearance and keeps the blanket away from the client's face.*

15. Make a toe pleat or loosen the top linens over the client's feet (see In Practice: Nursing Procedure 49-1). *Rationale: Toe pleats allow for freedom of foot movement.*

16. Make sure side rails are raised. Lower the bed and adjust the head of the bed to a comfortable position. Replace the call signal on the bed. *Rationale: These measures provide for safety.*

Follow ENDDD Steps

IN PRACTICE

NURSING PROCEDURE 49-3 Making a Postoperative Bed

1. Wash your hands and put on gloves before beginning to make any bed that has been occupied. Leave side rails down. *Rationale: This helps prevent the spread of infection. The linens on the bed may be soiled. Side rails would be in the way for transfer of the client.*

2. If the client has had surgery, discard all used linens and cleanse the mattress and pillow with antiseptic wipes. Then, make the entire bed with clean linen. *Rationale: Wearing gloves to handle soiled linen and to sanitize the bed protects the nurse. Clean linens reduce the possibility of postoperative infection, by removing as much contamination as possible.*

3. Make the bottom (or foundation) of the bed as you normally would. The postoperative bed usually requires a draw sheet under the client's hips. You also may wish to place several disposable pads on the bed. These plastic-based pads should not be in direct contact with the client's skin. (Put them under the draw sheet.) If cloth incontinence pads are used, they may be placed on top of the draw sheet. A second draw sheet is placed under the client's head. *Rationale: By using a draw sheet and pads, changing the entire bed will be unnecessary if the client has an emesis or is incontinent. You can then change only the soiled articles. You may also use the draw sheet to lift the client.*

4. In some cases, top linens are fan-folded to the foot of the bed. In others, a full postoperative bed is made (see Fig. 49-1C). To do this, put the top linens over the foundation, but do not tuck them in. Fold down the top as you would for an occupied bed. Then fold the bottom of the linens up so that the fold is even with the bottom of the mattress. Fan-fold the top linens to the side so they are on the side opposite from where the client's stretcher will be for transfer. (Alternatively, you may fan-fold the linens completely to the foot of the bed.) Leave a tab on top for easy grasping. *Rationale: Placing the linens all to one side or folded to the bottom keeps them out of the way for easy transfer of the semiconscious client. The tab on top makes pulling the covers over the client easy after they are in bed.*

5. Have one or two pillows available, but do not put them on the bed. *Rationale: A pillow may be contraindicated for a client; usually the surgeon will determine when it is safe for the client to have one.*

6. Be sure all furniture is out of the way and side rails are down. *Rationale: You need to make room so the stretcher can be brought to the bedside easily.*

7. Be sure the call light is available, but keep it on the bedside stand until the client is in bed. *Rationale: It is important for the client to be able to summon help immediately if they have any postoperative complications. The call light cord is kept out of the way to facilitate the transfer of the client into bed.*

8. Determine what special equipment is needed, based on the client's surgery. For the client's convenience and safety, make the following items available: tissues, an emesis basin, a blood pressure cuff and stethoscope, temperature sensor, pulse oximeter, "frequent vital signs" flow sheet or computer, intake and output record, and an intravenous (IV) stand. Most clients will require a bedpan; males need a urinal. Often, a bath basin is also required for the first day or so after surgery. You will need to add other items, according to the client's specific requirements. Learn from the recovery room nurse's report whether your client needs such items as a suction machine, chest drainage setup, oxygen, cardiac monitor, or other special equipment. *Rationale: It is important to have all pieces of equipment available immediately upon the client's arrival. Omission of an important piece of equipment causes inconvenience and could be life-threatening.*

9. Report to your charge nurse when you have prepared the postoperative bed and assembled the necessary equipment. After the client is transferred, side rails will be up. *Rationale: The charge nurse will then know when it is safe to authorize the client's transfer from the recovery room.*

IN PRACTICE

NURSING PROCEDURE 49-4 Using a Bed Cradle

Supplies and Equipment
Gloves
Bed cradle
Linens used for changing a bed
Extra blanket
Bath blanket
Extra top sheet
Extra bedspread

Steps

Follow LPN WELCOME Steps and Then

1. Make the foundation of the bed as you would for any client. *Rationale: A smooth foundation is especially important for the client who spends a great deal of time in bed.*

2. Tuck the top sheet under the foot of the bed. *Rationale: This holds the sheet in place.*

3. Place the cradle. Draw the top sheet over the cradle. *Rationale: The cradle protects the client's limbs.*

4. Place another top sheet over the first top sheet, overlapping the two as much as is necessary. *Rationale: Make the linens long enough to cover the client's shoulders when the bed is completed.*

5. Hold the bottom of the second top sheet and the top of the first top sheet, with hems even, up off the bed. Roll them over each other, making a flat fold crosswise to the bed. Repeat this process as many times as is necessary to obtain the correct length of sheeting. *Rationale: The goal is to keep the client warm. The double fold will hold the sheets together, and they will seem like one long sheet.*

6. Tuck in the blanket at the bottom of the bed. Pull it up over the bed cradle. Add a second blanket, and fold it the same way as you did for the sheets. Follow the same procedure for the bedspread, folding the covers at the head of the bed as for an open bed. *Rationale: When all three layers of covers are folded together, they will be long enough to cover the client's shoulders and secure enough to pull up without separating.*

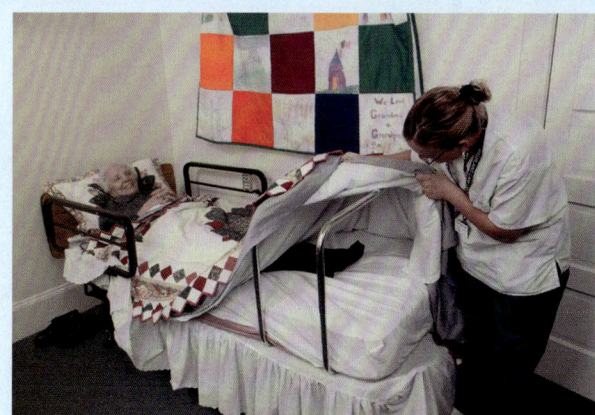

A bed cradle is used to keep the top linens off the client's extremities or off the entire body. Two sets of linens are folded together, to make them long enough to cover the client's shoulders. The linens are tucked in at the end of the bed and along the sides, to prevent chilling. A bath blanket may be added under the cradle for warmth. (Carter, 2008.)

7. Place a bath blanket under the cradle, covering the client as much as they desire.
Rationale: This prevents chilling or overheating the client.

8. Be sure the signal light is within the client's reach.
Rationale: The person needs to be able to call for help. The cradle restricts the client's movements, so they will need your assistance with daily needs.

This client often has a trapeze, to help in moving about in bed.

Follow ENDDD Steps

Special Reminder
- If you are using a cradle that applies heat, you will need specific instructions. *Rationale:* Burns must be prevented.

50 Personal Hygiene

Learning Objectives

1. State at least five therapeutic reasons for giving mouth care to a client.
2. In the skills laboratory, demonstrate assisting a client with oral care. Demonstrate cleaning and caring for dentures.
3. Identify steps involved in routine eye and ear care.
4. Demonstrate caring for the client's fingernails and toenails, addressing therapeutic reasons for attention to each area.
5. Describe how to assist clients to shave with an electric shaver and with a blade razor.
6. List at least three reasons for performing routine hair care and describe hair care for oily, dry, damaged, or very curly hair.
7. Describe and demonstrate giving a backrub, hand and foot massage, and foot soak.
8. State three types of cleansing baths and when each one is used. Demonstrate how to assist a client safely with each.
9. Describe reasons for careful assessment of the client's skin on admission and frequently thereafter.

Important Terminology

dental caries
friable
halitosis
nits
pediculosis
perineal care
periodontitis
pyorrhea
smegma
sordes

Feeling clean contributes to all people's sense of well-being, comfort, and dignity. In addition, cleanliness helps prevent diseases and disorders. This chapter describes how to assist clients to meet this need when they cannot do it alone.

MOUTH CARE

Frequent *mouth care* benefits everyone, but it is particularly beneficial to the ill person for several reasons:

- Food is not sterile and many disease-causing organisms enter the body through the mouth.
- Food particles lodged between teeth cause decay, breath odor (**halitosis**), and inflammation of tooth sockets (**pyorrhea**, **periodontitis**). (Untreated, pyorrhea can spread to the bone and cause loss of teeth.)
- Some illnesses cause irritation, dryness, or brownish deposits (**sordes**) on the tongue and the mouth's mucous membrane.
- Mouth breathing also causes dryness and irritation.
- Some gum infections can be transmitted from one person to another.
- A mouth condition may lessen a person's appetite and lead to nutritional deficiencies.
- Some oral conditions cause infection or pain locally or in other areas of the body.
- Breath odors or decayed teeth make people self-conscious and are often offensive to others.

Some clients may not have learned good oral health habits. Therefore, teaching them about effective oral hygiene is vital. The goal is to teach clients good oral hygiene, so they will continue to perform these procedures independently. Remind clients that this is beneficial because

- Appearance improves.
- Appetite improves and food tastes better.
- Healthy teeth and gums improve overall health.
- Discomfort and disorders are avoided.

Offer each client the opportunity to brush the teeth before and after each meal and at bedtime. When performing mouth care, observe the condition of the gums, tongue, mucous membranes, and teeth. If the client brushes the teeth, observe whether or not their procedures are correct. Document your observations, such as missing teeth, unusual tenderness, sensitivity to hot or cold, pain, bleeding, unusual redness, swelling, or odor. If the gums or teeth are unusually sensitive to touch or temperature changes, use "toothettes," or a tongue depressor wrapped in gauze, rather than a toothbrush, for oral hygiene. While assisting the client, teach and encourage future self-care. In Practice: Nursing Procedure 50-1 describes routine mouth care.

> **Key Concept**
>
> If brushing the teeth is impossible, encourage the client to rinse the mouth with water or mouthwash after eating.

Flossing the Teeth

It is important to floss between teeth, to promote healthy gums and remove debris that could cause tooth decay (**dental caries**) and offensive breath odor. If the client is not able to floss the teeth, the nurse can perform the procedure (In Practice: Nursing Procedure 50-2).

> **Nursing Alert** It is important to ensure that the client will cooperate with flossing the teeth before putting your fingers near the client's mouth. You could be seriously injured if the client bites down.

> **Nursing Alert** Remove dentures if a client is unresponsive, out of control, having frequent seizures, or going to have surgery or other anesthesia. If dentures are removed, document that fact, label them carefully, and store them safely.

The Client Who Wears Dentures

The client is asked on admission to the facility if they wear dentures (false teeth) or has a removable bridge or retainer. The presence of any of these should be recorded in the client's record. The client with dentures needs mouth care, similar to the client with natural teeth. Specially designed brushes and preparations for soaking dentures are available, to remove deposits. Brush dentures in the same manner as natural teeth. (Be sure to rinse them because denture cleaner may have a disagreeable taste.) See In Practice: Nursing Care Guidelines 50-1 and In Practice: Nursing Procedure 50-3. Be alert if the client refuses to wear their dentures or who removes them frequently. Ask the client why they are reluctant to wear the dentures. Also, inspect the client's mouth, looking for irritation or redness that may suggest a problem. The dentures may fit poorly or may cause irritation, which may also be the reason for refusal to eat and poor nutrition. Be particularly observant of the client who is experiencing confusion.

Special Mouth Care: The Dependent Client

In certain situations, clients need assistance with mouth care or require total care. For example, sordes that has collected on the tongue and teeth because of illness must be removed. In addition, special mouth care may be needed for clients who

- Breathe through the mouth.
- Are receiving supplemental oxygen or mechanical ventilation.
- Are unable to take fluids by mouth or have fluids restricted.
- Need to be encouraged to take food (cleansing the mouth before meals makes food more palatable).
- Are unresponsive or paralyzed.
- Are very young, confused, or otherwise unable to perform independent mouth care.

Oral cleansing sometimes removes secretions and thus helps prevent choking. In such cases, mouth care is

---

IN PRACTICE
NURSING CARE GUIDELINES 50-1 — Caring for a Client Who Wears Dentures or Other Mouth Appliances

It is vital to document the presence of any removable teeth or dental appliances, including dentures, removable bridges, retainers, bite guards, or nighttime appliances to whiten teeth, prevent grinding of the teeth, or to promote adequate breathing patterns. Some facilities require that removable oral appliances be removed when any client is unconscious, intubated, or being suctioned orally. *Rationale:* These items could be aspirated during surgery or other treatments, such as electroconvulsive shock therapy (ECT) or colonoscopy. In addition, insertion of an endotracheal tube (intubation) or suction apparatus could break an oral appliance or dislodge a false tooth. Any of these situations could cause serious complications, such as aspiration into the lungs, and could be fatal.

Most dentists encourage clients to wear their dentures all the time, especially in the daytime. *Rationale:* If dentures are removed for long periods, the gum lines change and dentures will no longer fit.

If the client must remove dentures or appliances, they should never be stored in cups or glasses used for drinking. *Rationale:* They may be accidentally swallowed, causing choking or aspiration, or may be thrown away.

Store all dentures and mouth appliances in specially marked opaque "denture cups." Both the container and lid must be clearly marked with the client's name and other pertinent information. Store dentures out of sight. *Rationale:* It is vital not to lose or mix up these items. The client may change rooms, but the facility ID number stays the same. Clients may be embarrassed and not want others to see their dentures. Safe storage in a drawer prevents them from being dropped or lost.

While dentures are being stored, they usually are kept in water. Ask the client who has some other type of appliance if fluid is required for storage. *Rationale:* Dentures usually must be kept moist to preserve their fit and general quality.

Take extra precautions to ensure that dentures or other oral appliances do not get lost. Be sure to check the client's food tray after meals and linens when the bed is changed. *Rationale:* Some clients remove dentures. They are expensive and may be very difficult for the client to replace.

Respect the client's privacy when cleaning their dentures. Wash your hands before and after handling dentures and wear gloves. Handle dentures carefully; they are slippery, fragile, and expensive. To avoid breakage, place a folded washcloth in the bottom of a basin of water or sink, holding the dentures over it. Do not hold them over a hard surface. In Practice: Nursing Procedure 50-3 reviews general steps associated with denture care. (The care of other dental appliances is usually similar to that of dentures.)

performed frequently. For the unresponsive client who is breathing through the mouth, oral hygiene is often ordered every hour because of the extreme dryness. (Some medications may also cause dry mouth and require the client to receive frequent oral care.) Follow the protocol in your facility. A basic procedure is given at In Practice: Nursing Procedure 50-4.

The mouth of the unresponsive client may become dry and cracked, creating a portal for harmful microorganisms. Keeping the mouth moist and intact is an important nursing action, to prevent infection. The unresponsive client is often kept in a side-lying position most of the time. If tolerated, the head of the bed can be lowered for special mouth care. *Rationale: In this position, gravity causes saliva to run out of the mouth and prevents the client from choking. This position also allows for the client to be suctioned (Nursing Procedure 86-1). While giving oral hygiene, inspect the gums and the mucosa of the mouth. Also inspect the lips for dryness and cracking. Apply petroleum jelly (Vaseline) or other ointment as ordered.*

Be gentle when giving mouth care. Use only a minimum of solution and make sure it is completely suctioned or drained out of the client's mouth. *Rationale: The oral mucosa is fragile and may be injured if mouth care is performed too vigorously. It is important to prevent aspiration in clients who are unable to swallow or spit out solutions.*

Extreme caution is required if giving mouth care to a client who has had oral surgery. The procedures to be used depend on the type of surgery that has been done. *Rationale: Inappropriate mouth care could cause damage to the suture line. If there is any question about procedures to use, consult the healthcare provider or team leader.*

NCLEX Alert

Be alert to the reasons for providing basic care to the client or assisting the client with personal hygiene, such as inspection for infection, providing comfort measures, identifying adaptive devices (e.g., dentures, hearing aids), and providing the nurse with opportunities for skin evaluation. This information may be integrated into the NCLEX examination.

ROUTINE EYE CARE

Normally, tears are produced by the *lacrimal glands*, situated at the top and outer portion of each eye. Tears help protect the eyes from bacteria, viruses, and other foreign matter and lubricate the eyes. With blinking, tears are washed across the eye and toward the *lacrimal ducts* located at the inner canthus of the eye (Chapter 21). Tears continually drain into the lacrimal ducts, which in turn drain into the nasopharynx. (This is why you get a runny nose when crying.) If a client has decreased tear production, does not blink, or has blocked lacrimal ducts, eye problems can occur. Infections may be caused by an accumulation of dried secretions on eyelids and eyelashes. Eye care should be done to remove secretions by applying a cotton ball or gauze square moistened with sterile water or normal saline to the eyelids. Some clients will also need supplemental moisture in the form of eye drops, as ordered. In Practice: Nursing Care Guidelines 50-2 describes routine eye care (Chapter 80). The administration of eye drops is covered in Chapter 63.

EAR CARE

A client's external ears are washed routinely during the bed bath. If excessive *cerumen* (earwax) is present, a special removal procedure may be necessary, to prevent hearing damage. (Medicated oil [e.g., Debrox] may be instilled by the nurse, to soften cerumen, or the outer ear canal may be irrigated with warm water by a specially trained practitioner, to remove excess cerumen.)

Nursing Alert Warn clients never to insert objects, such as cotton swabs ("Q-Tips"), toothpicks, or matches, into their ears to clean them. *Rationale: These objects can injure the ear canal, puncture the eardrum, or push earwax further into the ear canal, making removal more difficult.*

IN PRACTICE

NURSING CARE GUIDELINES 50-2 Caring for the Eyes

- Wash your hands and put on gloves. *Rationale: Handwashing and gloving help prevent the spread of infection.*
- Soak cotton balls or gauze squares in sterile water or normal saline. If eye care is being given as part of the bath and no infection is present, a clean, damp washcloth may be used. Wash the eye area before washing any other part of the body. *Rationale: It is important to avoid introducing harmful microorganisms into the sensitive eye tissues.*
- Wipe the client's eyelid from the inner (next to nose) to the outer canthus. *Rationale: Proper wiping technique moves debris away from the eye, prevents reinfection or contamination of the eye, and protects tear ducts.*

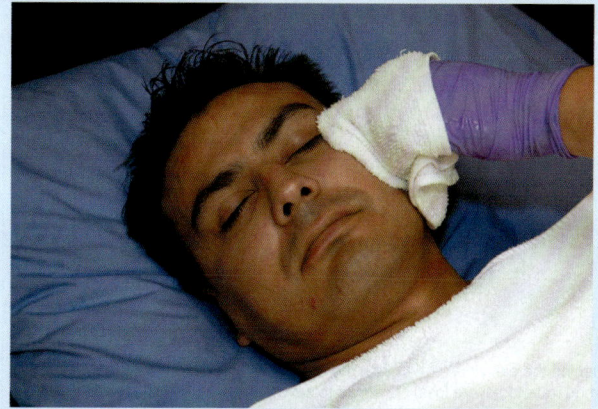

Wipe from inner canthus outward, using a separate part of the cloth for each eye (Carter, 2012).

NURSING CARE GUIDELINES 50-2 Caring for the Eyes (Continued)

- Repeat steps on the other eye, using clean supplies. *Rationale: It is important to use separate supplies for each eye. This helps prevent spreading infection between eyes.*

The Client Who Wears Contact Lenses
- Determine the type of contact lenses the client wears and the usual cleaning practices. *Rationale: Different types of lenses require different cleaning and storage techniques. Some contact lenses are disposable.*
- Encourage the client or a family member to remove the lenses and place them in cleansing or soaking solution. (Sterile normal saline can be substituted for lens soaking solution in an emergency.) *Rationale: It is important that hard or semipermeable lenses do not dry out. Proper storage is necessary to maintain the integrity of the lenses.*
- Be sure to label separate containers for each eye and include the client's name and facility identification number. *Rationale: Contacts have a separate prescription for each eye and can be easily switched. In some cases, a small dot indicates the right eye. The containers must be labeled carefully, to prevent loss.*
- Notify the practitioner if the client is unable to remove the lenses. *Rationale: A suction cup or other device is available for removal of contact lenses. This must be used by a specially trained person.*
- If lenses cannot be removed, notify the primary provider. *Rationale: Corneal damage may result if the client wears contact lenses for too long a time, particularly if the client's eyes are dry or if they cannot blink.*

Special Eye Care for the Client Who Cannot Blink
- Follow the steps for routine cleaning of the eyes.
- Instill lubricating drops in the eyes or ointment onto the lower lids, as ordered by the primary provider. *Rationale: Drops or ointment help keep eyes moist (Chapter 63).*
- Close the client's eyelids. If allowed by the facility, cover the eye with a sterile eye pad and secure with paper tape. (This procedure may vary; check the local protocol.) *Rationale: These procedures help maintain available moisture in the eye and help prevent corneal abrasions.*
- Document all procedures in the client's record. *Rationale: Documentation provides communication and coordination of care.*

Care of a Hearing Aid

Clients with a hearing impairment may use a *hearing aid*. A hearing aid is a battery-operated, sound-amplifying device consisting of an earpiece that fits into the ear and a power source. Hearing aids may be very small and may fit entirely into the outer ear (Fig. 50-1). They may also have a piece that fits behind the outer ear or may require a separate battery carried in a pocket and connected to the device by a cord or wireless system. The size of device depends in part on the type of hearing loss that exists. Some types of hearing aids have part of the device implanted within the person's body and a part worn externally. One example is a *cochlear implant* (Chapter 80), which requires surgery. Hearing aids also can be fitted with a "bluetooth" communication device. In Practice: Nursing Care Guidelines 50-3 provides information related to care of a hearing aid.

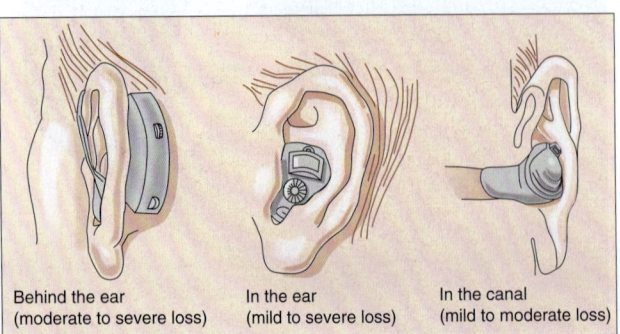

Figure 50-1 Several types of hearing aids. The general care and use are approximately the same for each (Taylor, Lillis, & LeMone, 2011).

> **Nursing Alert** It is important to teach clients and their families how to care for the teeth, mouth, eyes, and ears. They will be required to carry out this care when the client returns home.

> **NCLEX Alert**
> Be alert to the examples of client/family teaching regarding hygiene, especially skin care. As clients transfer to a home setting, family caregivers will assist in self-care and inspection for skin breakdown. Examination scenarios may include this information and you may be required to select your response, based on understanding of your role in client/family teaching.

CARE OF HANDS AND FEET

A client's general condition and health habits affect the condition of their fingernails and toenails. Brittle, broken, or discolored nails may be caused by improper diet, illness, infection, fever, or repeated bruising. Nail infections are fairly common. Some medical conditions cause ridges in the nails. In other cases, the nails become very thick, clubbed, or ingrown. Any unusual nail condition or complaint of pain in the hands or feet should be reported.

Caring for Fingernails

Stress may cause fingernail or cuticle biting. Some occupations cause fingernails to be stained or broken. Water, strong soaps, and washing powders make nails and cuticles dry. Nails that are well cared for are pleasing to look at and are a health protection measure. Conditions, such as torn cuticles

IN PRACTICE
NURSING CARE GUIDELINES 50-3: Caring for a Hearing Aid

- Clean the earpiece regularly with a Q-tip dipped in saline or the prescribed solution (to prevent cerumen buildup). Do not clean with alcohol. *Rationale: Alcohol may damage the delicate parts of the hearing aid. It may also be irritating to the client's ear canal.*
- Check and replace batteries regularly. Teach the client to have spare batteries on hand at all times. *Rationale: This avoids a gap in the client's ability to hear adequately.*
- Adjust the volume to meet the individual's needs.
- Turn off the aid when the client is not using it and remove the batteries if the client will not use it for an extended period. *Rationale: These procedures preserve battery life.*
- If a hearing aid is removed, place it in a plastic bag or other receptacle and carefully label it with the client's name and facility number and store it in a safe place. Be sure it is specified on the client's property list. *Rationale: Hearing aids are individualized and very expensive to replace.*
- Avoid exposing the aid to heat and moisture.
- Turn the volume down completely before inserting the aid into the client's ear. *Rationale: If it is too loud, it could be very irritating.*
- Evaluate client complaints about the hearing aid or repeated removal or refusal to use the aid. *Rationale: If a hearing aid is working properly, fits correctly, and does not hurt, the client usually will be willing to wear it. Refusal to use a hearing aid or its repeated removal usually indicates discomfort or device malfunction.*

(around nails), are an invitation to infection. Therefore, report reddened areas or breaks in cuticles. Dirty nails can spread infection. If a client's nails are torn or jagged, clip them with a sterile nail clipper and smooth with an emery board (if this is allowed in your facility). This helps prevent snagging on clothing or bed linens. (Scissors and metal nail files are not used. *Rationale: They may accidentally cut or nick the skin.*) Fingernail care is usually done after the client's hands have been in water. Soap and water, as well as cuticle oil or lotion, loosen dirt and temporarily soften cuticles. In Practice: Nursing Procedure 50-5 provides additional information about nail care.

> **Nursing Alert** Never give sharp items or scissors to a client who has unsteady hands or who is confused, depressed, or at risk for self-injury or injury to others.

The client going to surgery or who is experiencing respiratory distress usually is asked not to wear nail polish or artificial nails. This is also true for nurses in most facilities. *Rationale: Artificial nails can harbor pathogens, become infected, and/or spread infection. In addition, natural nails are usually "roughed up" when prepared for artificial nail application. This damages the nails and often causes difficulty when artificial nails are removed. Clients who have surgery or other procedures or who have serious respiratory disorders will have frequent oxygen saturation determination, and artificial nails interfere with this process.*

Hand Massage

Hand massage is valuable for soothing, relaxing, and calming clients and can help relieve pain. Circulation improves, as blood vessels dilate from the warmth of friction. In addition, muscle tone improves. A *hand massage* is an example of *therapeutic touch,* providing a connection between client and nurse. The nurse may perform hand massage, outlined in In Practice: Nursing Care Guidelines 50-4, but may also teach the client self-massage. The nurse can perform hand massage, with the client's permission, but without a provider's order, unless the client has an injury or has had recent hand or wrist surgery.

> **NCLEX Alert**
> This book emphasizes the importance of documentation of your observations as a means of communication with the healthcare team. This fosters continuity of care. Your understanding and awareness of this may impact your selection of nursing actions during the examination.

Caring for Toenails

Toenails need the same care as fingernails. Long toenails can scratch the client or catch on bedclothes and break. Soiled toenails can cause infection. However, cutting a client's toenails is an intervention that usually requires a provider's order. Never cut a newborn's toenails or those of a client with diabetes or hemophilia. (Chapter 79 describes special foot care for the client with diabetes.) Toenails are cut straight across. Cutting into the corners or rounding the corners contributes to the development of ingrown toenails. This condition is painful and may become serious enough to require surgical removal.

> **Nursing Alert** Do not cut a client's fingernails or toenails if you have any question about the condition of the nails. Special orders are required before cutting the toenails of any client, especially those with diabetes or hemophilia, or those with thickened nails, to avoid accidental injury. Ingrown toenails must be reported. (In some facilities, nurses are not authorized to cut toenails.) *Rationale: Wounds heal very slowly in clients with disorders such as diabetes or hemophilia. Thick nails often need to be cut by a specially trained person, using special equipment and techniques.*

When caring for toenails, follow the same procedure as for fingernails, with some exceptions. If the toenails tend to grow into the skin at the corners, place a wisp of cotton under the nail to move the nail up and prevent growth

IN PRACTICE
NURSING CARE GUIDELINES 50-4 — Performing Hand Massage

SPECIAL NOTE: The nurse must take into consideration how the client might interpret a hand massage. In some cases, it might be construed as a form of inappropriate touching or harassment and may cause discomfort or embarrassment to the client.

- Take either of the client's hands in both of the nurse's hands.
- Warmed lotion may be used.
- Gently shake out the client's hand. *Rationale: Gentle shaking relieves tiredness and assists the client to relax.*
- Rotate and twist each of the client's fingers, bending each finger back and forth. *Rationale: This motion redistributes synovial fluid around the finger joints and provides passive range of motion for the fingers.*
- Massage the palm of the client's hand with both thumbs, with fingers on top of the client's hand. Rotate in a circular motion. *Rationale: According to acupuncture theory, this motion relaxes the heart.*
- Massage the back (dorsum) of the client's hand with the thumbs, while the fingers are in the client's palm. Rotate in a circular motion. *Rationale: This action is soothing and relieves tension.*
- Massage the webbed area between the client's thumb and first finger. *Rationale: Pressure points for sinuses and intestines are located here. Massaging this area may also help to relieve headaches, constipation, or menstrual cramps.*
- Massage between each of the client's fingers. Massage each finger, from hand to tip. *Rationale: This helps encourage blood flow to the fingers.*
- Massage the client's wrist with an up-and-down stroke. *Rationale: This helps to increase circulation to the hand.*
- Gently pull on each finger and quietly place the hand on the table. *Rationale: This helps to maintain the relaxed feeling when the massage is completed.*
- Repeat the above steps on the client's other hand.
- Teach steps to the client for self-massage. *Rationale: The client can perform this massage whenever they feel stressed.*
- Document the procedure in the client's record. *Rationale: Documentation provides communication and promotes continuity of care.*

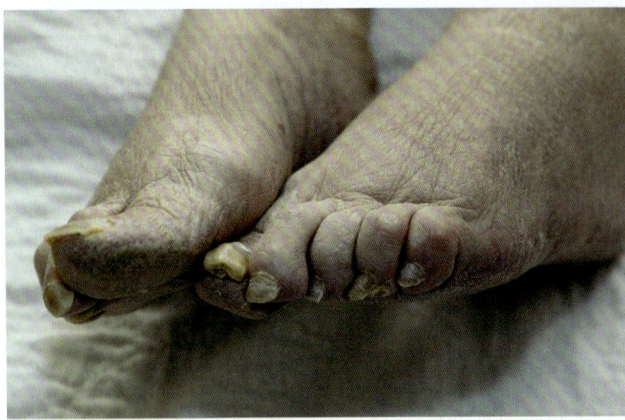

Figure 50-2 Observe the client's toenails for abnormalities. Do not cut toenails without a specific order or if you have any concerns or questions (Carter, 2012).

polish–like medication is available to treat fungal infections, as are creams and systemic medications.) While caring for toenails, observe whether corns or calluses are present on the client's feet. If so, apply oil or lotion to soften them, but nothing else. If the client is distressed by any abnormality of the feet (e.g., corns, ingrown toenails, bunions, thickened or yellowed nails, or hammer toes), report the condition (Fig. 50-2). Teach the client that corns and calluses may become infected if attempts are made to remove them by cutting or by using corn removers that contain salicylic acid. Cover an infected area with a sterile dressing and report this. Any additional treatment must be ordered by a primary provider. Be sure to document the procedure and document your observations. See In Practice: Nursing Procedure 50-5.

Foot Soak

A *foot soak* is of particular importance to the client who has edema, tenderness, or some form of foot infection. Soak the foot in warm water or in a variety of commercially prepared salts (e.g., Epsom salts) and solutions as ordered. Dreft or another mild detergent is often used. *Rationale: Warm water helps dilate blood vessels, to promote improved circulation, and relaxes the feet and legs. Salts and detergents contain medications or chemicals that the skin can absorb during soaking.*

The length of time ordered for a foot soak varies. In Practice: Nursing Procedure 50-6 lists the steps for giving a foot soak.

SHAVING

Many adults shave daily. (Some women have excessive facial hair [hirsutism] and may wish to shave. This may be embarrassing for them. Be sensitive to the client's feelings.) Clients who are unable to shave may feel or look untidy. Many healthcare facilities use electric razors because they are easier and safer to use than blade razors. If the client can shave without assistance, prepare the equipment, provide a mirror, and see that the room is well lighted. Allow as much privacy as possible for clients to carry out this part of their care. If the client cannot shave independently, the nurse

into the surrounding skin (ingrown toenail). The cotton must be changed at least daily. (If cotton cannot be inserted or removed safely, a strand of waxed dental floss may be used. Tape the loose ends, to ensure that the floss will remain in place.) A notch cut in the center of the toenail also will cause nails to grow toward the center. This will pull in edges and corners. People who jog or walk a great deal often have thickened toenails, especially on their great toes. Thickened and raised nails can also be a sign of fungal infection. (A nail needs to assist. Be sure to allow the client to do as much as possible. When using an electric razor, read the instructions carefully. Most healthcare facilities use a special shaver with a detachable head, to help prevent spread of microorganisms. Each client uses their individual shaver head. Clean the shaver head and razor after each use. Detach and label the shaver head with the client's name and keep in a safe place for the next use.

When shaving a client with a safety razor (blade razor), follow the facility's protocol. Be sure to follow Standard Precautions, to reduce the risk of exposure to the client's body fluids. Remember: the client's skin could be nicked accidentally during shaving. Follow the steps in In Practice: Nursing Procedure 50-7 for shaving clients. *All disposable shavers, shaver heads, and blades are disposed of in the sharps container.*

In some cases, the healthcare provider orders the client to be shaved before surgery or another procedure. This surgical scrub and shave is usually done in the operating room (OR) preparation area. If not, special instructions are required.

> **Nursing Alert** If your healthcare facility uses disposable blade razors, take extra precautions. Do not allow a client with unsteady hands or poor eyesight to shave with a blade razor. Also, closely supervise clients who are depressed, suicidal, or assaultive.

HAIR CARE

Hair care is part of daily care, whether the client is in the hospital, the long-term care facility, or their own home. It helps keep hair in good condition and improves morale. Encourage clients to do as much of their own hair care as possible. This provides exercise and diversion, helps the client achieve the desired hair style, and adds to the client's self-esteem. Daily hair care varies with the type of hair.

> **Key Concept**
> Some clients prefer to wear a wig, cap, or other head covering. If in a facility for some time, the hair should still be shampooed occasionally, the frequency depending on the type of hair.

Daily Hair Care

Some healthcare facilities, such as long-term care and rehabilitation facilities, have in-house beauty parlor and barber services. Although time is usually not available to provide elaborate hairstyles for clients in the healthcare setting, try to style the hair as becomingly as possible in the time allotted. The client's family will often assist.

Some clients prefer to shave their heads, especially when in the hospital for some time. It is important to shave very carefully, to prevent cutting or nicking the scalp. Some clients rub oil on their heads after shaving, to restore the natural scalp oils.

Some people have more oil on the shaft and ends of the hair than others. However, many people have very naturally curly, dry hair. In addition, hair that has been permed, relaxed, colored, or damaged in some other way is often very dry. Some illnesses also contribute to dry or damaged hair. Very dry hair is more susceptible to breakage than oily hair. The curliness and texture of certain types of hair make it difficult for natural scalp oils to work their way to the hair ends. These types of hair are also more likely to tangle. In Practice: Nursing Care Guidelines 50-5 includes a number of procedures performed when caring for a client's hair, as well as special considerations when caring for clients with oily, dry, or very curly hair.

Shampoo

A *shampoo* may be needed after lotions or other medications have been applied to the scalp; after an electroencephalogram for which a paste is used; or for cleanliness on admission or during a long-term illness. A shampoo may also be part of the treatment for lice (*pediculosis*) or dandruff (*seborrheic dermatitis*) or to remove foreign objects, such as glass or debris following a motor vehicle accident.

Giving a Shampoo to an Ambulatory Client

For an ambulatory client, the simplest method of shampooing is for the client to shampoo during a shower or bath. If a client cannot shampoo their own hair, but can ambulate or be moved in a wheelchair, a shampoo can be given in the bathroom, using the lavatory sink. Choose a chair at a level that allows the client's head to rest comfortably on the bowl's edge. Be sure to pad the edge of the bowl with towels. The person may prefer to sit facing the sink, resting the forehead on the edge and holding a folded towel over the eyes. If using a spray, adjust the water's temperature before beginning. If the client feels light-headed or faint, stop the procedure, wrap the client's head in a bath towel, and help them back to bed. The client who can be moved on a wheeled stretcher can be moved to a convenient sink for a shampoo. The shampoo is done while the client lies on the stretcher with the head near the edge of the sink. Use a trough to funnel the water back into the sink.

Providing Hair Care After an Accident

A client may come into the healthcare facility after an accident with dirt, blood, or glass in the hair. If no scalp wounds are apparent, the client's hair will usually be shampooed. *An order from the primary healthcare provider for the first shampoo is required.* If the client is able, a regular shampoo can be done in the shower or the bathroom basin. If the client cannot tolerate a regular shampoo, a product, such as the Shampoo Cap, is used (Nursing Procedure 50-8).

The shampoo removes debris from the hair and makes the client more comfortable. Performing a shampoo also provides the nurse with the opportunity to examine the client's hair and scalp further. Gloves must be worn until it is determined that no lesions, debris, or other conditions are present. Wear gloves if you have any question. Comb the hair carefully first. *Rationale: This allows removal of pieces of debris and careful inspection of the scalp.* If wounds or lesions are discovered, check with the team leader or primary provider before continuing.

IN PRACTICE
NURSING CARE GUIDELINES 50-5: Caring for Hair

General Procedures
- Ask each client about personal preferences and follow their instructions, as much as possible. *Rationale: The client can give you guidelines about how their hair should be cared for and styled.*
- The nurse provides daily hair care as a part of routine personal hygiene. *Rationale: This gives the nurse an opportunity to examine the client's hair and scalp.*
- Follow the direction of the client or general guidelines for the type of hair as to the daily or routine care to be given. *Rationale: It is important not to damage the hair.*
- Short hair should receive the same care as long hair.
- If the client has scalp lesions or cuts, pediculosis (lice), foreign objects in the hair (e.g., glass), or excessively dirty or matted hair, wear gloves. *Rationale: This helps prevent the transmission of pathogens and protects the nurse.*
- Be sure your fingernails are short and clean. *Rationale: It is important not to scratch the client or transmit pathogens.*
- Wash the client's comb, hair pick, or brush regularly. *Rationale: This helps keep the hair clean and prevents reinfection or reinfestation of the scalp in infectious conditions or pediculosis.*
- Comb one lock of hair at a time, holding the lock firmly near the scalp and leaving it slack between your hand and the client's head. *Rationale: This helps avoid pulling.*
- Avoid using hairpins or bobby pins. *Rationale: They may be uncomfortable and may injure the client's head while lying in bed. These items also may interfere with surgery and/or tests and treatments, such as electroconvulsive therapy (ECT), electroencephalograms (EEG), or magnetic resonance imaging (MRI).*
- Report and document any adverse condition, such as excessive dandruff, loss of hair, split ends or other damage, breaking hair, lice, crusts, or any lumps or lesions. *Rationale: Documentation and reporting provide communication and promote continuity of care.*

Care of Long Hair
- Long hair or very curly hair is often braided. *Rationale: This helps prevent tangles when the client lies on the hair and moves about in bed.*
- Start braids toward the front and keep them toward the side. *Rationale: This helps the braids to be more comfortable when the client lies in bed. If they are started in the back of the head, the client must lie on them.*
- Fasten braids with a "scrunchie" or short ribbon, instead of rubber bands. *Rationale: Rubber bands can pull or break hairs. Also, clients may be allergic to latex (rubber bands).*

Care of Oily or Semi-Oily Hair
- Daily brushing is helpful. *Rationale: This stimulates scalp circulation and distributes oil over the hair to give it sheen.*
- The hair is often shampooed every day or two. Sometimes, a special shampoo is available. *Rationale: This helps remove excess oils.*
- A client with long hair may wish to have a ponytail. This may be held to one side. *Rationale: This helps keep the hair from tangling. Placing the ponytail on the side makes it more comfortable when lying in bed.*
- A hat or scarf is usually not worn. *Rationale: This would increase oiliness.*

Care of Very Dry or Very Curly Hair
- Brushing is usually contraindicated. Use a wide-toothed comb or hair pick, with teeth rounded on the ends and without seams. *Rationale: The brush is likely to catch and break the hair. The specific comb (or hair pick) described here is least likely to damage the hair.*
- For the client in bed, or when preparing to go to bed, section off and braid the hair, tie it back, or wrap it. A ponytail is usually not advised. *Rationale: Braiding or wrapping helps retain oil and avoid tangles; tangled hair is more likely to break. The ponytail adds weight and can cause damage to dry hair.*
- Some clients wear woven braids or other hairstyles in which the hair is twisted or braided in very tight, small braids close to the scalp. These hairstyles are relatively easy to maintain and are left in place for a number of days. However, when these hairstyles are combed out and replaced, an effort should be made to vary the placement of braids. *Rationale: This helps to avoid constant pulling on the same sections of hair.*
- When in bed, the client may wish to wear a satin scarf, sleep cap, or to use a satin pillow case. *Rationale: This allows the head to move about (by sliding) without catching, helping to avoid tangles and breakage.*
- The client may wish to wear a hat, cap, scarf, head wrap, or other head covering when out of bed. *Rationale: This helps retain oils.*
- Wash the hair only about once a week or less often. Avoid alcohol-based products. Use little or no heat when drying the hair. *Rationale: It is important not to increase dryness of the hair.*
- Use a specific hair grooming product, such as shea (pronounced: shē) butter or jojoba oil, olive oil, or sunflower oil. Some sort of oil is usually added to the scalp between shampoos. A daily moisturizer is often used. Woven braids, cornrows, and dreadlocks require regular oil application. *Rationale: These products help moisturize the hair naturally and help to avoid breakage.*

NURSING CARE GUIDELINES 50-5 Caring for Hair (Continued)

- Avoid using petrolatum (Vaseline) or mineral oil to groom the hair, if possible. *Rationale: These products plug the pores of the scalp and restrict the release of natural oils.*
- If the client is perspiring, rinse the salt out with water, but do not use shampoo. *Rationale: This will cleanse the hair of salt and add moisture, without excessively drying the hair.*
- Use leave-in conditioner with each shampoo. Use specific shampoo for dry hair. *Rationale: These products help retain moisture.*
- Pat the hair dry; do not rub. *Rationale: Rubbing encourages hair breakage.*
- Massage the scalp daily. *Rationale: This encourages the release of oils.*

> **Nursing Alert** It is important to document carefully any debris found in the hair, particularly in the case of an assault, accident, or a police or insurance case. The order may include saving any debris removed from the hair. If in doubt, save the debris. Label any debris carefully and seal it in a plastic bag.

Using the Shampoo Cap

A product called a *Shampoo Cap* is helpful for the client who cannot get out of bed for a shampoo or for the uncooperative client or one who has severely matted or very dirty hair. (In some cases, a shampoo must be forced, for health reasons. In this case, it is much easier to use a Shampoo Cap than to try to force a shampoo with water.) The cap is safe for all types of hair because it contains conditioner, as well as shampoo. Following an accident, if there is glass or other debris in the hair, the Shampoo Cap can be used as a fairly safe means to clean the hair and head. A provider's order is required for this use, and the cap is usually left in place without the massage. In Practice: Nursing Procedure 50-8 describes the use of the Shampoo Cap.

> **Nursing Alert** If there is any debris in the client's hair, *do not massage* the Shampoo Cap. Leave it in place for a longer time and then gently comb the hair, to remove debris. *Rationale: If glass, rocks, or other debris is in the hair, massaging may damage the scalp.*

The Bed Shampoo

In most cases, the immobile client is given a shampoo using a product such as the Shampoo Cap or a dry shampoo that removes oil and can be brushed out. In very rare cases, or in home care, the client may require a shampoo in bed. In Practice: Nursing Procedure 50-9 briefly describes the process of a bed shampoo. Usually, a provider's order is not required for a bed shampoo. Consult the protocol of your facility.

SKIN CARE

The skin, the largest organ in the body, is the body's primary defense against disease and infection and helps regulate body heat. For these systems to be effective, the skin must remain unbroken (*intact*) and not irritated. When giving nursing care, observe for any signs of skin irritation or lack of skin integrity (breaks in the skin).

> **Nursing Alert** Skin breakdown is taken very seriously in the healthcare facility. If a client's skin breaks down after admission, the facility is considered to be responsible. In most cases, third-party payors *will not reimburse the facility* for costs incurred related to skin breakdown that was not present when the client was admitted. Therefore, it is vital to document carefully and completely any breaks or signs of irritation in the client's skin on admission to the facility (Chapter 45).

It is particularly important to check under breasts and any other skin folds for signs of inflammation or infection. Be particularly observant if the client complains of itching. *Rationale: These areas are susceptible to yeast infections. Itching may occur before the rash is evident. Early treatment with a cream, such as Ketoconazole, can prevent further spread of infection and discomfort.*

Once skin has broken down, it is very difficult to treat, particularly in the client with other health problems, such as diabetes. Frequent and effective *skin care* is essential to keep the skin intact and remove dirt, excess oil, and harmful bacteria. Feeling clean also enhances the client's self-esteem. If the skin is oily, regular cleansing is needed; if the skin is dry, a daily bath may be harmful. However, everyone's face, underarms, skin folds, and perineal area need daily cleansing. The Braden Scale for assessment of pressure wound risk is introduced and explained in Chapter 58 (Figure 58-5). Remember: Body fluids, such as perspiration, vomitus, urine, and feces, are generally acidic and are very irritating to the skin. They must be removed immediately. In addition, many older people, people confined to bed, and people who are ill have very fragile (**friable**) skin. These clients need special skin care, to prevent skin breakdown. Chapter 58 describes special skin and wound care.

> **Nursing Alert** If a client has been incontinent of urine or stool, avoid soap, cloth washcloths, Bag Bath, and shaving cream when cleansing the skin. *Rationale: These products and items do not provide protection if the client becomes incontinent again. Cleansing cloths containing special "barrier" skin cream are available.*

Protective Devices for the Skin

A number of protective devices, special products, and procedures are available to protect the skin. It is particularly important to protect bony and skin prominences (e.g., elbows,

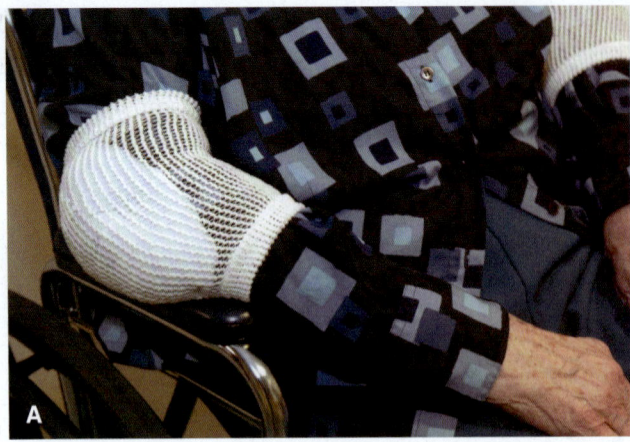
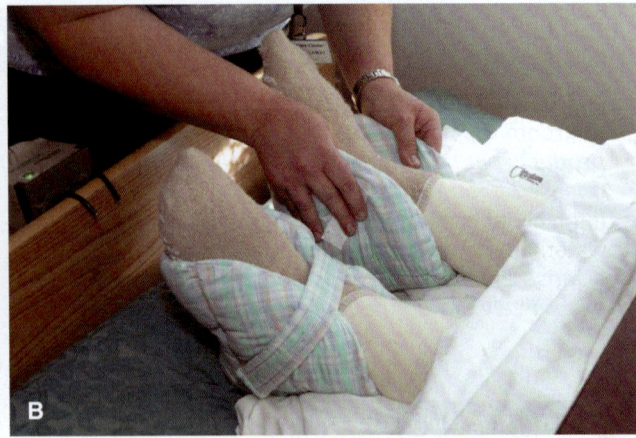

Figure 50-3 **A.** Elbow pads help protect the client while in a chair. **B.** Heel booties help prevent heels from rubbing against bed linens (Carter, 2012).

heels, coccyx, shoulder blades, backs of the ears, back of the head). This is vital for the immobile client. As presented in Chapter 49, a number of special beds and wheelchair pads are available to help prevent skin breakdown. Special elbow and heel pads are available and are used to further protect the client (Fig. 50-3). The bath, backrub, and careful skin care are also important factors in skin protection. (Special skin care and wound care is discussed in Chapter 58.)

> **Key Concept**
>
> It is the nurse's responsibility to inspect the skin during baths and other routine daily care. If any *reddened or irritated areas* are noted, they must be reported immediately. If these areas are treated quickly, actual skin breakdown can often be avoided.

Backrub

Although the nurse does not administer therapeutic body massage, the *backrub* provides relaxation and comfort. A backrub may be given as part of the bathing process or before bedtime. A backrub is soothing and relaxing for the immobile client and helps prevent skin breakdown. The backrub is often the highlight of the day for the bedfast client. It also allows the nurse direct observation of the client's skin condition. The patterns used in the backrub are as follows:

- *Stroking (effleurage)*: Stroke the large surfaces of the client's back in long, smooth strokes, with the palms of the hands. Stroke in the direction of venous circulation, toward the heart (upward in the middle [Fig. 50-4A], and downward on the sides, generally in a circular motion [Fig. 50-4B]). Use heavier pressure for the upward stroke. Use the thumb and fingers on smaller surfaces. Keep strokes and pressure even. Begin and end the backrub with effleurage.
- *Kneading (pétrissage or foulage)*: Press on muscle groups or single muscles, picking them up and squeezing them gently. Use the palms of the hands for large muscles and fingers and thumbs for single muscles. Use this movement for the outer and upper aspects of the back and for the neck. (See In Practice: Nursing Procedure 50-10 for illustration.)
- *Tapping (tapotement)*: Use a light tapping with the edge of the hands (the edge farthest from the thumb) to stimulate circulation.
- *Friction:* Rub around the bony prominences of the client's body, such as at the end of the spine and along each shoulder blade.

Other strokes that are sometimes used are as follows:

- Brushing (*frôlement*): Lightly touching the skin with the fingertips.
- Vibration: Rhythmically moving the skin, with cupped palms, causing it to shake or quiver.

Gloves are usually not needed for the backrub, unless the client has open lesions or body fluid drainage. Preparation steps in giving a backrub include the following:

- Reduce environmental stimuli. Keep the room quiet. Turn off bright lights. ***Rationale:*** *It is important to establish a relaxing environment.*
- Make sure the room is warm enough.
- Have the client go to the bathroom before the backrub. ***Rationale:*** *When the backrub is completed, the client may*

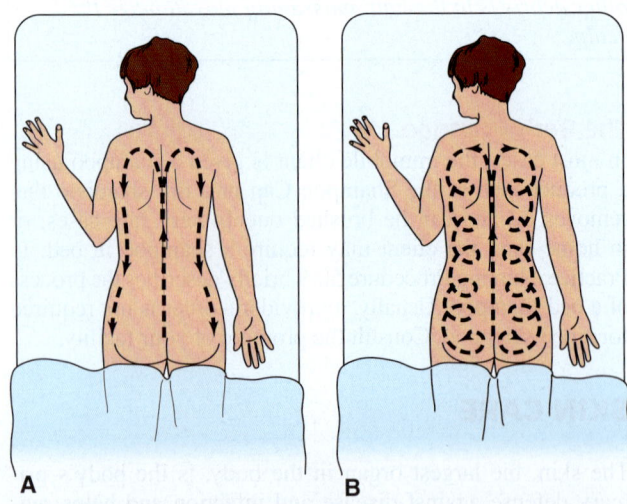

Figure 50-4 Effleurage follows the direction of venous flow. **A.** Upward stroke in the center is firmer. **B.** Downward stroke may be straight down or in a circular motion (Carter, 2012).

be able to rest or sleep. It is important that they not be disturbed.
- Provide privacy. *Rationale: A large portion of the client's body will be exposed.*
- Instruct the client to breathe slowly and deeply and to relax.
- Soft music may be helpful.
- Warm the hands and the lotion. Immerse a bottle of lotion in warm water for a few minutes to heat it. (The lotion bottle is often placed in the bath water during the bed bath.) *Rationale: This helps prevent chilling the client. Warm lotion is more soothing; cold lotion can be a shock.*

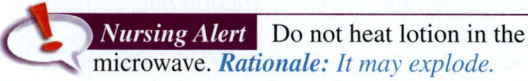

Nursing Alert Do not heat lotion in the microwave. *Rationale: It may explode.*

In Practice: Nursing Care Guidelines 50-6 includes some considerations when giving a backrub, and In Practice: Nursing Procedure 50-10 provides specific steps for the backrub.

Bathing

Baths remove waste products of perspiration and excretion, stimulate circulation, and refresh the client. A complete daily bath is not essential and often not advisable for every client. The client's personal bathing habits influence the frequency of healthcare agency baths. Consider the client's comfort and personal preferences, rather than agency routine. If a client had an uncomfortable, sleepless night, a rest after breakfast may be more appealing than a bath.

> **Key Concept**
>
> In some cases, a bath must be given, even if the client objects. For example, if the client has been incontinent or has bleeding or drainage, at least a partial bath is necessary, to prevent skin breakdown and infection. If a person comes into the facility with pediculosis (lice) or is very unclean, a bath/shower may need to be forced.

Three types of cleansing baths are the shower, tub bath, and complete or partial bed baths. (Partial baths most often include washing the client's face and hands and giving perineal care.) The client's condition determines which type of bath is safest and most appropriate. In some cases, the healthcare provider orders a specific type of bath. A bed bath is the least tiring for the client, but it is indicated only when the client is unable to leave the bed because of their condition or when the client is receiving specific treatments (e.g., continuous traction). Showers and bathtubs equipped with self-help devices allow clients to bathe themselves or to be bathed with nursing assistance. A hydraulic lift should be used when transferring clients with limited mobility from wheelchair or stretcher into a tub. A shower chair can allow the client to sit during the shower. *Rationale: It is vital to prevent injuries to nurses.* If a client is critically ill, a limited partial bath (bathing only the face, hands, and body parts that perspire or are soiled with body excretions) may be done. Remember to allow the client to perform as much of the bath as possible.

Washcloth Mitt
When washing a client's face and hands, giving perineal care, or giving a bed bath, a bath mitt is made of the washcloth (Fig. 50-5). This encloses your hand and is convenient. It also prevents dragging the ends of the washcloth across the client's face or body and helps prevent dripping.

Washing the Client's Face and Hands
The client's face and hands are washed before meals, during a bath, and at other times, for the client's comfort. Assist, if needed. In Practice: Nursing Care Guidelines 50-7 outlines steps in assisting the client to wash the face and hands. After the client's face and hands are washed, be sure to apply lotion to your own hands to prevent drying and cracking from repeated exposure to soap and water.

Nursing Alert Always teach clients to wash their hands after using a bedpan or urinal and before meals.

Assisting the Client With a Shower or Tub Bath
A shower or tub bath is the most refreshing type of bath. The client who has been ill usually welcomes it. Bathing the entire body and stimulating the skin is best accomplished with a soak in a tub or a shower. Avoid giving a bath or shower immediately after a meal because the warm water of the bath will draw blood to the skin and away from the client's digestive organs.

IN PRACTICE

NURSING CARE GUIDELINES 50-6 | Backrub

- Your fingernails must be short and smooth. Do not wear jewelry, other than a simple wedding ring. *Rationale: Long or artificial fingernails and jewelry can scratch the client. Both can collect lotion, skin debris, and microorganisms, causing transmission of pathogens.*
- Warmed lotion should be used.
- Apply appropriate pressure and friction. *Rationale: Light pressure is soothing; heavy pressure is stimulating.*
- Stroking, kneading, tapping, and friction are the simplest and most effective for the backrub given to stimulate circulation and relax contracted muscles. Perform all patterns at least three times.
- Give special attention to pressure-prone areas, such as bony prominences. *Rationale: This helps promote increased circulation and helps prevent skin breakdown.*
- Use long, firm strokes.
- Apply firmer pressure on the upstroke and lighter pressure on the downstroke. *Rationale: This aids blood return to the heart.*
- End with light strokes the length of the back.
- Use frôlement (light brushing) to prolong the sensation of relaxation.

IN PRACTICE
NURSING CARE GUIDELINES 50-7 — Washing the Client's Face and Hands

- Put on clean gloves. *Rationale: Using gloves helps to prevent the spread of infection.*
- Arrange equipment conveniently on the overbed table. Allow the client to do as much self-care as possible. *Rationale: Encouraging self-care promotes the client's self-esteem and enhances recovery.*
- Dip the washcloth in clear water and wring it out. *Rationale: This prevents dripping on the client.*
- If you are washing the client's face, wrap the washcloth around your hand and tuck in the ends to form a mitt (Fig. 50-5). *Rationale: Loose ends that remain exposed can drag over the client's face, or into the eyes, causing discomfort.*
- Avoid using soap on the face unless the client wants it. *Rationale: Soap is drying, especially to the face.*
- Carefully sponge the client's closed eyelids with clear water from inner to outer canthus, unless they are wearing contact lenses. (See In Practice: Nursing Care Guidelines 50-2.) *Rationale: Soap stings the eyes. If contact lenses are in place, the corneas are particularly sensitive to rubbing or pressure.*
- Wash carefully around the client's nose and ears. *Rationale: These areas collect perspiration, oil, and dirt.*
- Soak the client's hands for a few minutes in a basin of warm water. *Rationale: Soaking is very soothing and relaxing.*
- Ask the client to rub soap on the hands or do it for the client. *Rationale: Soap and friction help remove microorganisms.*
- Rinse the soap off the hands thoroughly. *Rationale: Soap remaining on the hands is drying and irritating.*
- Apply lotion to the hands. Also put lotion on the client's face, if desired. *Rationale: Lotion helps prevent drying and cracking of the skin.*
- Dispose of all equipment and your gloves. Wash your hands. Document any pertinent observations. *Rationale: This helps prevent the spread of infection. Documentation provides communication and promotes continuity of care.*

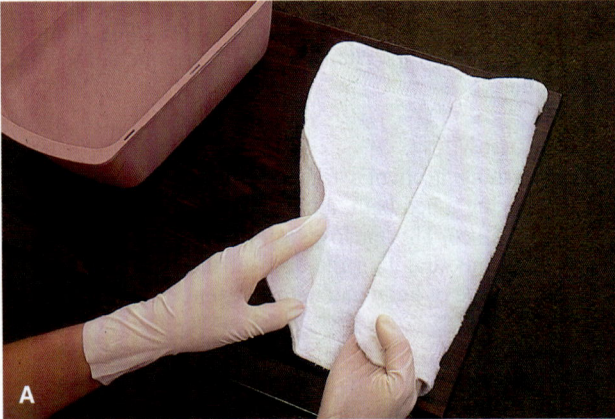

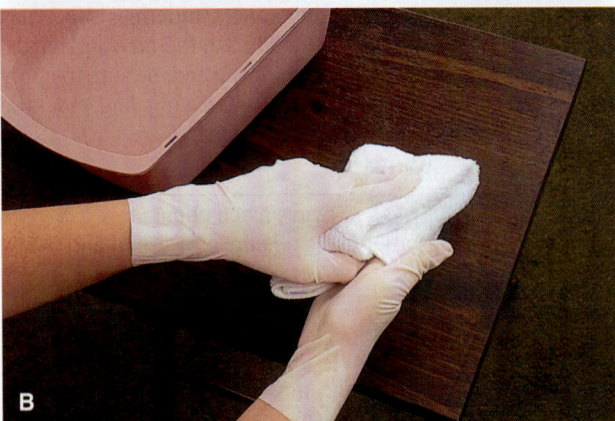

Figure 50-5 A neat bath mitt is formed using a washcloth. **A.** Fold the washcloth around the hand, with open ends on the palm side. Pull the washcloth out straight. **B.** Tuck the loose end in near the wrist, enclosing the fingers (Evans-Smith, 2005).

The Shower
Guide rails both inside and outside the shower stall are essential, for safety. Two sets of rails are needed. One set of rails is needed at a level the client can reach for support while sitting on a stool. The other set is needed higher up for support when standing. Some clients need to hold the guide rails with both hands. Be sure the shower has a non-skid surface. Carefully judge how much assistance the client needs in bathing. *Rationale: You are responsible for the client's comfort and safety.* Use a stool or a shower chair, so the weak client may sit while showering (Fig. 50-6). This promotes client independence and safety, while providing safety and minimizing the amount of energy required. No client who is weak, unsteady, or confused should be permitted to take a shower unattended.

The Tub Bath
Typically, bathtubs are low, to ease the process of getting in and out of the tub. However, some special tubs are available (Fig. 50-7). These are safer to use for the client who is weak or unsteady and much easier if staff assistance is needed. Guide rails and an emergency nurse call or pager are essential. Be sure to assist the client, as necessary and check the client frequently, for safety. In Practice: Nursing Procedure 50-11 gives tips for helping the client with a routine tub bath and illustrates another special type of tub.

> **Nursing Alert** The client who is suicidal, unsteady, or who may faint is *never* allowed to take a tub bath without an attendant present.

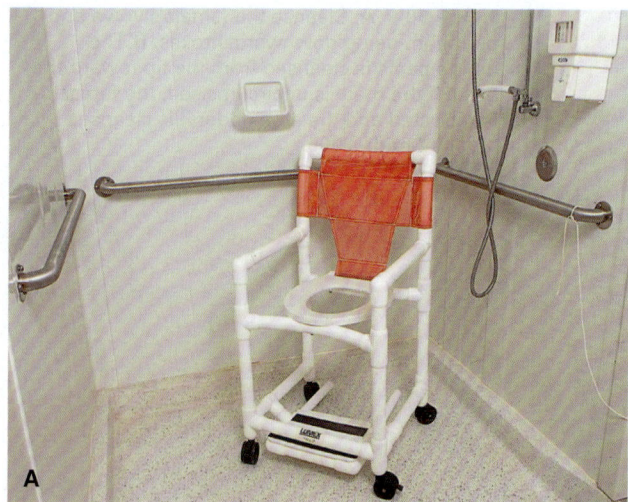

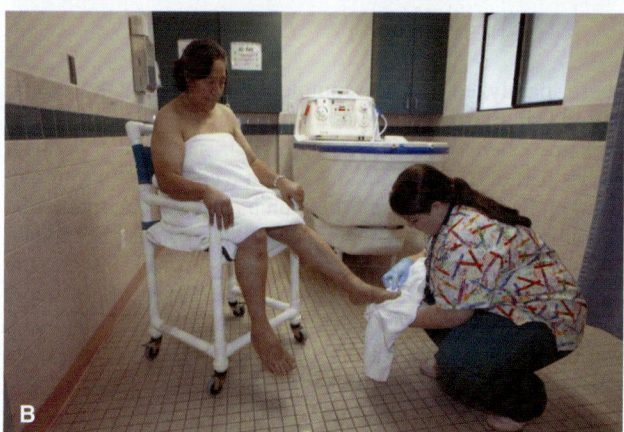

Figure 50-6 The shower chair has lockable wheels. **A.** The standard chair, with a back, provides more support than a stool. A hole in the seat allows water to drain and can also be used as a commode. **B.** After the shower or bath, assist the client to dry, giving special attention to areas where "skin meets skin," such as between toes and under skin folds and breasts (**A:** Timby, 2005; **B:** Carter, 2016).

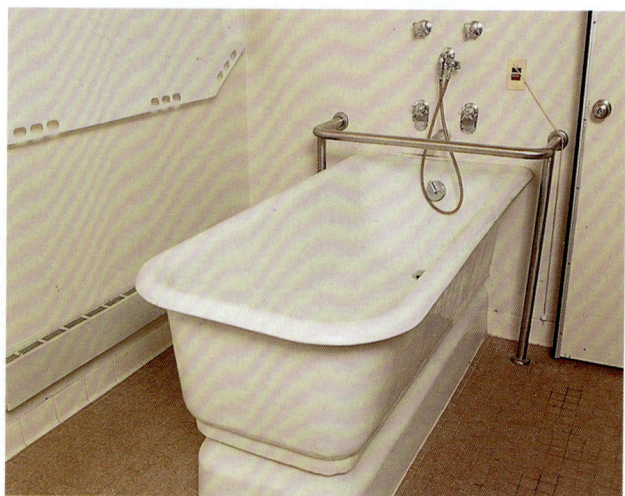

Figure 50-7 This facility bathtub has special features. Note the emergency signal cord and handrails. The shower attachment can be used to wash the client or shampoo hair. The transfer board on the wall can be used to move the client or for cardiopulmonary resuscitation. This tub is elevated, for easier access by staff. A hydraulic lift or sturdy stool may be required to assist the client into this tub (Timby, 2005).

restriction. Careful preparation and planning are essential. (You may not leave the unit for forgotten equipment after the bath is started.) If the bath is interrupted, the water will become cold, and the client may become chilled. In addition, the client is exposed, may fall out of bed, or may become overtired. The bed bath provides you an opportunity to closely inspect the client's body. Document the type of bath given and any significant observations. Follow the steps in In Practice: Nursing Procedure 50-12 for the client who cannot move without assistance and requires a *complete bed bath*.

Partial Bath or Sponge Bath

A *partial bath* consists of bathing the face, hands, axillae, back, buttocks, genital area, under any skin folds, and under the breasts of female clients. This bath may be given as a partial bed bath or may be performed by the client while sitting in the bed or the bathroom (Fig. 50-8). A partial bath is given when the client does not receive or cannot tolerate a complete bed bath. Encourage every client to do as much as possible for themselves; the person will exercise muscles, become more self-sufficient, and build self-esteem. The steps are similar to the complete bed bath, bathing only specific areas of the body. If the client is going to do the sponge bath, help set up needed equipment and supplies. Remember to include the nurse call signal or pager. Check frequently to make sure the client is not feeling faint or does not need anything. You can assist with washing the back, if the client desires this. The nurse can then assist the client to sit in the chair while the bed is being made.

Complete Bed Bath

Give complete *bed baths* for clients who are comatose, catatonic, or unable to leave their bed because of therapeutic

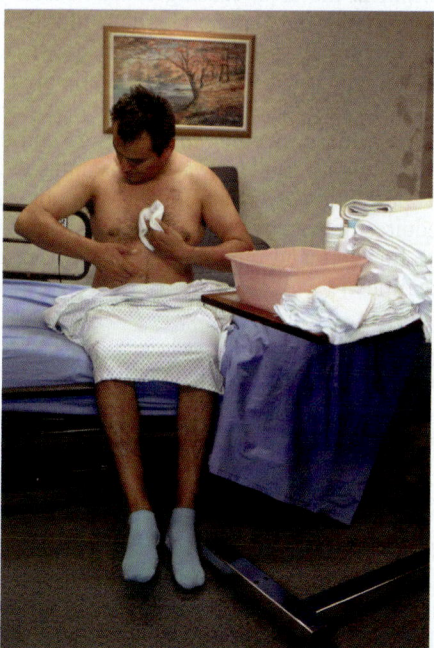

Figure 50-8 Some clients prefer to do their own partial bath at the bedside or in the bathroom. Assist, as needed (Carter, 2016).

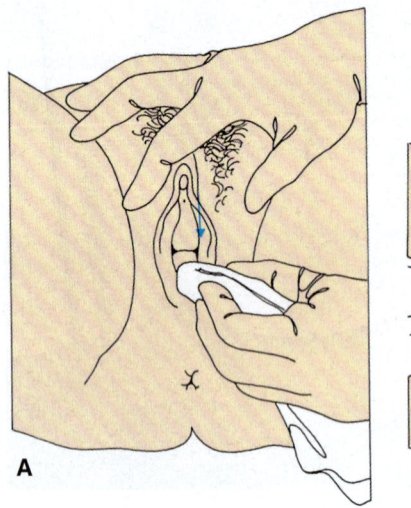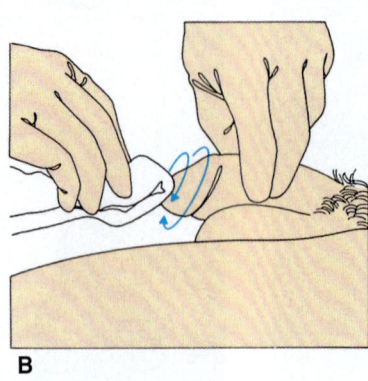

Figure 50-9 **A.** Cleanse the female's vulva and perineum using downward strokes. **B.** The male's penis is cleansed from the tip toward the base. If the male is uncircumcised, the foreskin is retracted and the area under it is cleansed (Evans-Smith, 2005).

Adjust this procedure to allow the person to do as much as possible, considering their condition.

Specialized Baths

The *sitz bath* is a special bath in which the client's buttocks are submerged in water. This is used after rectal surgery and sometimes after childbirth (Chapter 54). *Therapeutic baths* are frequently used to treat skin disorders. Medications or substances such as oatmeal are added to the water. Many times, these therapeutic baths are given in a whirlpool tub (Chapter 75). Another type of specialized bath is the *towel bath*. Gentle rubbing with a dry or damp towel helps improve circulation, offers some cleansing, and increases energy. In this procedure, a basin of water is not used. Instead, the nurse, wearing gloves, rubs a warm, dry or damp towel against the client's body, thereby creating friction. This produces warmth in the area, causing blood vessels to dilate, and thus improving circulation. Gentle to mild pressure in rubbing the body is all that is required. In some cases, lotion is used—then, it is called a *lotion bath*. While giving a towel or lotion bath, inspect the client's skin and bony prominences for irritation, redness, swelling, or discharge and document findings. If a quick, efficient way of cleaning the body is needed, a "*bath in a bag*" (Bag Bath) is available. This bath system requires no water or soap. (It is also handy for backpackers or travelers and others who do not have access to shower facilities.)

> **Nursing Alert** Certain conditions, such as hemorrhage, hemophilia, heart attack, or thrombophlebitis, *contraindicate* (negate the use of) friction or rubbing.

Giving Perineal Care

Perineal care, bathing the genitalia and surrounding area, is commonly referred to as "peri care" and is given to all clients. Those who have had perineal surgery, clients who have delivered a baby, and certain other clients will need *special perineal care*. These clients include persons who are psychotic and unable to care for themselves, confused, very obese, paralyzed, or in a complete body cast or those who have a urinary tract or vaginal infection.

Some clients may be embarrassed, but regular perineal care is part of total client care, even if a client is of a different sex than that of the nurse. Maintain a professional, matter-of-fact attitude. If the client can manage their own needs, provide a wet washcloth, soap, rinse water, and a towel. Instruct the client to bathe the genitalia. You may need to speak in simple terms so the client understands. For example, "I'll give you a washcloth so you can wash between your legs." Teach female clients to cleanse from front to back with tissue or sponges (Fig. 50-9A). A perineal bottle ("peribottle") is frequently used for women, although it may also be used for men. The peribottle is most commonly used in obstetrics and gynecology. This bottle is filled with warm tap water, sterile water, or saline, and the client thoroughly sprays the perineum, while sitting on the toilet or bedpan. This helps keep the perineal area free of infection. Sometimes, cotton balls or sponges moistened with an antiseptic agent are used. When working with a male client, teach them to cleanse from the tip of the penis toward the body (Fig. 50-9B). Remind the uncircumcised male to retract the foreskin to cleanse the penis. In Practice: Nursing Procedure 50-13 outlines steps in giving perineal care.

> **Nursing Alert** Teach the client to use each cotton ball or sponge only once. Teach the client to wipe the outside areas first, saving the last sponges for the urethral area.

SKIN INFESTATIONS

Care of the Client With Pediculosis

Pediculosis is the term for infestation by *lice,* tiny oval, gray insects that suck blood from the person they infest and spread disease. Pediculosis causes intense itching (*pruritus*) and the resulting scratches may become infected. Pediculosis usually involves hairy body parts. The tiny eggs, called **nits**, look like dandruff, but are solid specks, not flakes. They cling tightly to hair shafts and are hard to remove or destroy.

Head lice (*pediculosis capitis*) are found in the hair and on the scalp. Body lice (*pediculosis corporis*) are found on the body and clothing. "Crab lice" or "crabs" are found on other hairy body parts, especially in the pubic area or axillae (*pediculosis pubis*). A special fine-toothed pediculosis comb ("nitcomb") helps remove lice and nits. Lice spread via clothing, bedding, and combs and brushes. Look for signs of skin irritation, scratching, live lice, and nits on the body or in the hair when admitting any client to the healthcare facility.

Both nits and adult lice can be destroyed by a routine treatment, often with special shampoo or a shower with a specially medicated soap (called *licides*). Most licides are toxic and require at least a week before treatment can safely be repeated. If you observe lice in a client, isolate the person and report the situation immediately. The healthcare provider will order specific treatment. Chapters 72 and 75 further describe care of children and adults with lice, scabies, and other parasitic skin infestations.

Scabies

Scabies is a common contagious condition caused by the *itch mite*. It usually occurs in warm, protected areas of the body, such as skin folds. The skin lesions cause intense itching and are easily spread from person to person. Treatment is similar to that for pediculosis.

Bedbugs

Bedbugs (*Cimex lectularius*) may be carried into the facility by a client. Bedbugs are small, wingless insects, about the size of an apple seed; they feed on human blood at night. They do not spread disease but may cause severe allergic reactions or secondary skin infections related to scratching. If a client is admitted with unidentified bites and severe itching, they should be checked for bedbugs.

> **Nursing Alert** If you are treating a client with suspected pediculosis, scabies, or bedbugs, wear a gown, gloves, and shoe covers. If your hair is long, wear head protection. Do not touch the outside of your gown with bare hands.

If it is determined that a client has a parasitic skin infestation, it is vital to alert the family. They will need to consult the primary provider for instructions about elimination of the parasites from their home. In the case of a school child, the school must also be notified.

The nurse must be alert for any skin, hair, nail, or other disorders when giving routine daily care. Any unusual condition must be documented and reported immediately.

STUDENT SYNTHESIS

KEY POINTS

- The skin is one of the body's defenses against disease and infection. It must be kept clean and free of discharge or secretions.
- It is vital to inspect the client's skin carefully on admission to a facility, and daily, to discover any signs of irritation or skin breakdown.
- Careful documentation and reporting are vital if you observe any reddened areas or skin breakdown.
- Clients need some level of skin cleansing daily. Special skin care is required for clients with any evidence of skin irritation or breakdown.
- Certain conditions, such as hemorrhage, heart attack, hemophilia, and thrombophlebitis, contraindicate vigorous rubbing of the skin or scalp.
- Oral hygiene promotes comfort, cleanliness, and nutrition.
- Personal hygiene is important to the client's self-esteem and health. Encourage the client to provide as much self-care as possible.
- Shampooing the client's hair allows you to inspect the scalp for disease, parasitic infestation, or injury and to remove debris.
- Different types of hair require different methods of care.
- The backrub relaxes the client and provides an opportunity for you to observe the client's skin.
- The shower or tub bath provides cleansing and is relaxing for the client.
- The bed bath provides an opportunity for you to observe the condition of the client's skin.

CRITICAL THINKING EXERCISES

1. You are performing personal hygiene on a client. Describe information that can be obtained while giving a sponge or bed bath.

2. Your client is aged 78 years and is a different sex than you. They had a stroke that caused left-sided paralysis. The client responds only occasionally to your questions and does not move independently. Describe how you will explain what you are going to do for the client and what assistance you will provide.

3. Describe how you would care for the hair of a person confined to bed in the following instances.
    a. The client with very long hair
    b. The client with very curly, dry hair
    c. The client who is losing hair as a result of cancer treatment

NCLEX-STYLE REVIEW QUESTIONS

1. The nurse is assisting the client with removal of dentures prior to a surgical procedure and the client requests an explanation of why the dentures have to be removed. Which response by the nurse is best?
    a. "There is a risk of aspiration or damage to the dentures if they are left in."
    b. "We will put the teeth in your drinking cup so they won't get lost."
    c. "The teeth are dirty and a source of potential infection."
    d. "We have to do this for everyone, not just for you."

2. The nurse is providing mouth care for an unresponsive client. In which position would the nurse place the client to prevent complications?
   a. Prone position
   b. Side-lying position
   c. Supine with the head of bed elevated 90°
   d. Trendelenburg

3. A client requests the nurse to clean the earpieces of the hearing aid. Which action would the nurse take to be sure it is cleaned appropriately?
   a. Clean the earpieces with alcohol.
   b. Soak the earpieces in hydrogen peroxide.
   c. Wipe the earpieces with disinfectant wipes.
   d. Clean the earpieces with Q-tips dipped in saline.

4. A client who has diabetes states to the nurse, "I try to remove the calluses from my feet." Which information would the nurse be sure to discuss with the client to avoid complications?
   a. Use a sharp razor to remove the calluses.
   b. Use a salicylic acid solution to dissolve the calluses.
   c. Use a nail file to trim them.
   d. Use oil or a lotion to soften them only.

5. The nurse determines that a client requires a partial bath. In order to promote self-esteem, which action would the nurse take?
   a. Allow the client to rest while the nurse completes the full bath.
   b. Inform the client that they will need to complete the bath.
   c. Encourage the client to do as much of the bath as possible.
   d. Inform the client that if the bath cannot be completed, it can be done later.

CHAPTER RESOURCES

Enhance your learning with additional resources on thePoint*!*

Student Resources related to this chapter can be found at thePoint.lww.com/Rosdahl12e.

CHAPTER 50 Personal Hygiene 717

Welcome Steps	End Steps
Look at healthcare provider's orders. **P**rotocol for procedure. **N**ecessary equipment/supplies. **W**ash hands using proper hand hygiene; put on gloves. **E**xplain the procedure and reassure the client. **L**ocate two identifiers to confirm correct client. **C**omfortable and efficient position for nurse and client. **O**btain privacy. **M**ake sure to follow correct steps and body mechanics with good technique. **E**nsure safety and observe deviations from normal.	**E**nsure comfort and safety. **N**ote questions or concerns from client or nurse; note significant data. **D**ispose of materials properly. **D**isinfect the area and your hands. **D**ocument and report the procedure and your findings.

IN PRACTICE

NURSING PROCEDURE 50-1   Routine Daily Mouth Care

Supplies and Equipment
Gloves
Toothbrush
Toothpaste
Emesis basin or sink
Towels
Drinking water

Follow LPN WELCOME Steps and Then

1. Wear gloves. Assist the client to a comfortable upright position with an emesis basin in hand or assist the client to stand or sit near a sink. Protect the client's gown and bedclothes with a towel.
   Rationale: Organize materials so the client can do as much as possible for themselves.

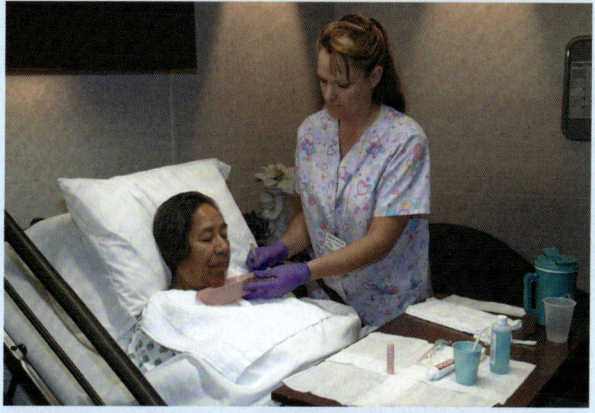

Place a towel on the client's chest; have an emesis basin handy. Wear gloves. (Carter, 2012.)

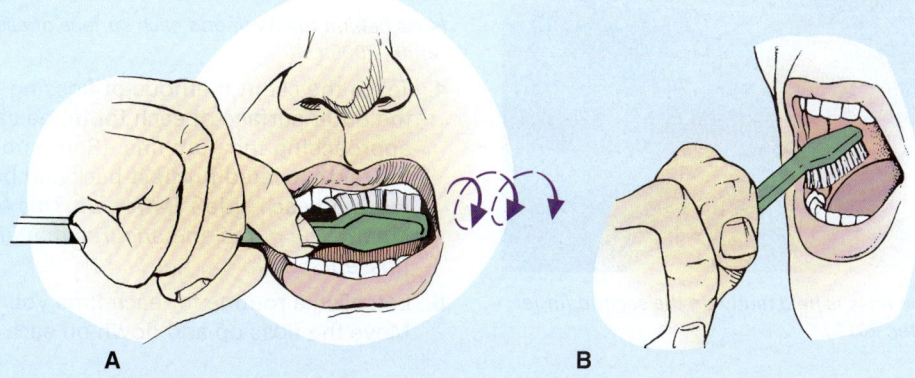

A   B

A. The client is taught to brush the inner and outer surfaces of the teeth with a rotating motion. **B.** Biting surfaces of the teeth and the tongue are brushed. (If the nurse performs this procedure, gloves are worn.) (Timby, 2005).

2. Encourage the client to floss the teeth, or assist in this procedure (In Practice: Nursing Procedure 50-2). *Rationale: This promotes good oral hygiene and helps prevent gum disease. Flossing before brushing loosens material between teeth, so it can be rinsed away.*

3. Use a soft or medium toothbrush, small enough to reach all teeth. Instruct the client to brush teeth by placing the bristles at a 45° angle against the teeth and direct the tips of the bristles under the gum line, using a rotating motion, following the direction of tooth growth. Continue until all outer and inner surfaces of the teeth and gums are clean. The client should then brush the tongue and biting surfaces of the teeth. If the client has an electric toothbrush, encourage its use. *Rationale: A very hard toothbrush can damage gums. The described motions clean all surfaces and stimulate the gums.* The electric toothbrush helps the weakened client to brush teeth more effectively.

4. Encourage the client to rinse with fresh water and spit into the emesis basin or sink. *Rationale: Rinsing removes debris that has been loosened by brushing.*

5. Observe the condition of the client's teeth, gums, and tongue. *Rationale: Observations should then be documented.*

6. Wipe the client's mouth and chin. Rinse the toothbrush and store it with bristles up. Do not store the toothbrush in the open air, particularly in the bathroom. Put away supplies. *Rationale: Having the bristles up helps promote drying of the toothbrush. Storing the toothbrush in the open unnecessarily exposes it to microorganisms.*

Follow ENDDD Steps

IN PRACTICE
NURSING PROCEDURE 50-2: Flossing the Teeth

Supplies and Equipment
Dental floss
Towels
Gloves

Steps
Follow LPN WELCOME Steps and Then

1. Break off about 1.5 ft of floss. *Rationale: This is an adequate amount to floss all teeth. Encourage the client to do as much as possible.*

2. Wrap the floss around the second finger of each hand and keep taut. Keep about 1.5 to 4 in. of floss between the fingers. *Rationale: Holding the floss taut facilitates debris removal and stimulates the client's gums.*

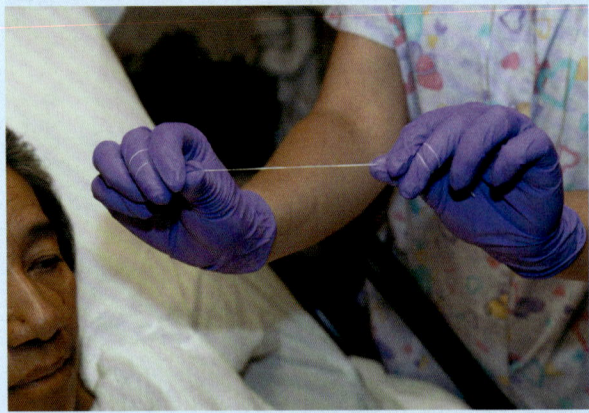

Wearing gloves, the floss is held tautly on the second finger of each hand. (Carter, 2012.)

3. Insert the floss gently behind the teeth, if possible, and then between each two teeth. It may be necessary to slide it back and forth to get between teeth. Do not force the floss. *Rationale: Forcing could cause pain and damage to teeth or gums.*

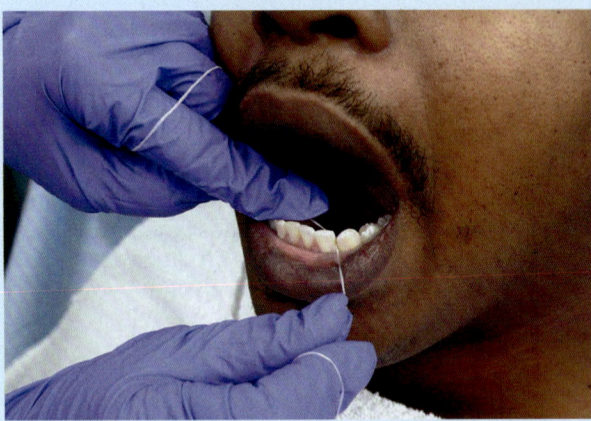

Floss behind the teeth and each surface of each tooth. (Evans-Smith, 2005.)

4. Teach the client methods of flossing, to include the outer surface of each tooth, be careful when approaching the gum line. (Remember to include the teeth located furthest back and behind the last tooth on each side.) *Rationale: This helps prevent cutting the gums and ensures that all surfaces are flossed.*

5. Establish a routine for each time you floss teeth. Move the floss up and down on each side of each

tooth. ***Rationale:*** *This will help avoid missing any spots.*

6. Advance the floss as it is used. ***Rationale:*** *Use fresh floss for best results.*

7. Wipe the client's mouth and chin. ***Rationale:*** *This ensures client comfort.*

8. Teach the client as you floss the teeth. ***Rationale:*** *This is important, to promote healthy gums. Encourage the client to continue flossing the teeth daily and to continue after discharge from the facility.*

Follow ENDDD Steps

IN PRACTICE
NURSING PROCEDURE 50-3 Caring for Dentures

Supplies and Equipment
Gloves
Gauze squares
Labeled denture container and lid
Washcloth
Denture toothbrush
Denture cleaner
Tap water
Mouthwash
Emesis basin
Towel

Steps
Follow LPN WELCOME Steps and Then

1. Position the client in an upright or side-lying position. ***Rationale:*** *Proper positioning maximizes efficiency and helps prevent aspiration.*

2. Label a denture container and the lid with the client's name and pertinent information. ***Rationale:*** *It is vital not to misplace the client's dentures. Use the client's facility ID and not the room number because the client may be moved to another room.*

3. Wear gloves. When possible, encourage the client to remove their own dentures. If the client is unable to do so, use a gauze square to grasp the upper plate with your thumb and index finger. Gently move the denture up and down or sideways. Try to grasp the gum area and not individual teeth. Put the denture in a labeled denture container. ***Rationale:*** *Moving the denture helps break suction and loosen the adhesive holding the denture in place. If pressure is put on the teeth, they may break off. The container helps protect the denture from breakage.*

4. Remove the lower plate by turning it at a slight angle and place it in the labeled container. ***Rationale:*** *Turning the plate at an angle breaks the suction and allows the denture to be removed. The container helps protect the dentures.*

5. Carry the container carefully to the sink or an emesis basin, into which a washcloth has been placed. Fill the basin with water or turn on cool water in the sink. Do not place dentures in a sink. ***Rationale:*** *The washcloth provides a cushion and prevents damage if dentures are dropped. The sink can contaminate the dentures.*

6. Pick up the dentures one plate at a time and scrub each with a denture cleaner on the toothbrush. A special denture toothbrush is best. Use the same motions as when brushing natural teeth. ***Rationale:*** *Using denture cleaner aids in removal of debris from the denture surface. The brush motions ensure that all surfaces are cleaned.*

Gloves are worn when caring for dentures. Use a dry gauze square to grasp the client's upper denture. (Evans-Smith, 2005.)

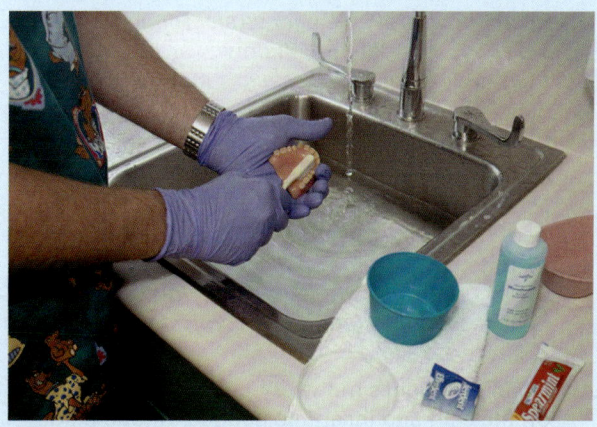

The dentures are scrubbed, using the same motions as with natural teeth. Note the running water, the washcloth in the bottom of the sink, and the denture container in a handy location. (Evans-Smith, 2005.)

7. Rinse the dentures with cool to lukewarm tap water. *Rationale: Rinsing removes food particles and denture cleaner. Using hot water may damage the dentures.*
8. Soak dentures in commercially prepared solution at the client's request. *Rationale: Soaking aids in further cleaning and maintaining moisture.*
9. Rinse with tap water. *Rationale: Rinsing removes the solution and any residual aftertaste.*
10. Inspect dentures for breaks, rough edges, missing teeth, and other damage. *Rationale: Inspection helps identify any potential problems that may cause injury.*
11. Inspect mucosa of the client's mouth for redness or irritation. *Rationale: Dentures may rub and cause irritation. Report irritation immediately.*
12. Assist the client to rinse the mouth with mouthwash. *Rationale: This is refreshing, helps control breath odor, and removes debris.*
13. Apply denture adhesive, if the client requests it. Use only a minimum of adhesive. Encourage the client to replace the dentures. If they are unable to do so, insert the dentures into the mouth, one plate at a time. Hold plate at a slight angle while inserting. Press gently to seat the plate in the adhesive. *Rationale: Proper insertion prevents injury to the lips and surrounding mucosa. Using too much adhesive makes dentures very difficult to remove.*
14. Wipe the client's mouth and chin with a towel. *Rationale: Keeping the client dry aids in comfort.*
15. If the client chooses not to wear the dentures or is unable to wear them, store the dentures covered with water in the labeled denture container. *Rationale: A covered denture container protects dentures from possible breakage and maintains the client's privacy. Moisture helps preserve dentures.*

Follow ENDDD Steps

IN PRACTICE

NURSING PROCEDURE 50-4 — Special Mouth Care: The Dependent Client

Supplies and Equipment
Gloves
Toothette mouth sponge or soft toothbrush
Tongue blade padded with 4 × 4 gauze sponge
Water, mouthwash, or hydrogen peroxide (H_2O_2)
Towel (and/or waterproof pad)
Water-soluble lubricant or petroleum jelly for lips
Suction catheter with suction apparatus (optional)
Emesis basin

Steps
Follow LPN WELCOME Steps and Then

1. Wear gloves. Raise the bed to a comfortable height for you. Lower the near side rail. Turn the client toward you, with side of the client's mouth tilted down toward the mattress. *Rationale: Proper positioning prevents back strain. Tilting the head sideways with the mouth downward encourages fluid to drain out of the client's mouth.*
2. Place a towel or waterproof pad and emesis basin under the client's chin. Have a suction catheter and apparatus available, if needed. *Rationale: The towel protects the client and the bed. The emesis basin and suction equipment are used to assist with removal of drainage from the client's mouth. In addition, suction equipment is necessary, if there is any chance of aspiration (Chapters 86 and 87).*
3. Open the client's mouth by pressing downward on the chin and insert the padded tongue blade between the client's back molars. *Never* insert your fingers into the client's mouth. *Rationale: The tongue blade assists in keeping the client's mouth open. Padding prevents lip and tooth injury. The client may reflexively bite down, if fingers are placed in their mouth.*

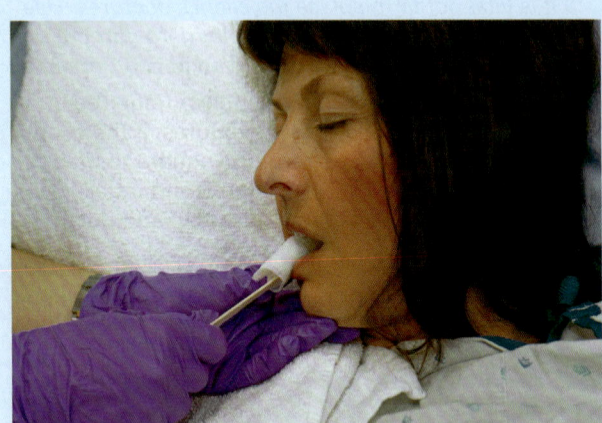

Carefully insert a padded tongue blade between the back molars. (Evans-Smith, 2005.)

4. Dip a toothette sponge, soft toothbrush, or another padded tongue blade in water, mouthwash, or diluted peroxide (H_2O_2). Mouthwash is most commonly used. (The peroxide can be diluted with mouthwash or water. The ratio is about four to six parts water or mouthwash to one part peroxide.) *Rationale: It is important to cleanse the mouth without injuring delicate tissues.*

5. Move the sponge, toothbrush, or padded tongue blade back and forth across all tooth surfaces and chewing areas. Cleanse the roof of the mouth and inner cheek area. Cleanse the gums and tongue. *Rationale: Friction cleanses the teeth. Cleaning solutions aid in removing residue on the client's teeth and in softening encrusted areas.*

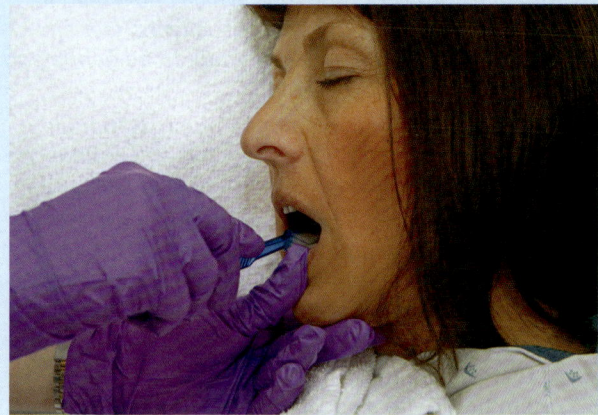

Brush all surfaces of the teeth. (Evans-Smith, 2005.)

6. Rinse the mouth, using a clean toothette or padded tongue blade moistened in water. Using an irrigating syringe, instill a small amount of water into the mouth. Suction the mouth if all fluid does not drain out. Wipe the client's mouth. *Rationale: Rinsing removes debris that might have been loosened. Suctioning is important, if any fluid or debris remains in the mouth; this helps prevent aspiration into the lungs.*

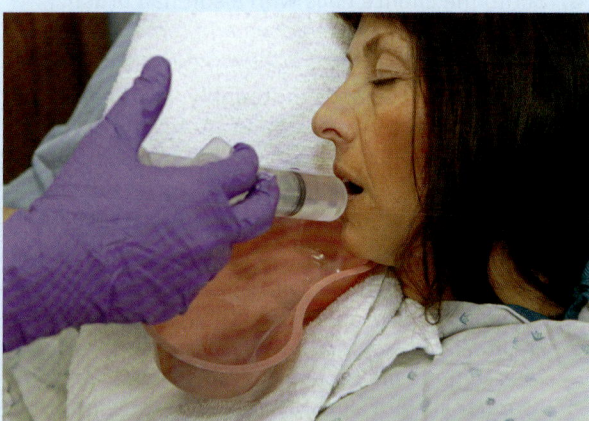

Irrigate the mouth. Make sure all fluid drains out or suction it out. (Evans-Smith, 2005.)

7. Apply petroleum jelly or water-soluble lubricant to the client's lips. *Rationale: This helps prevent lips from drying or cracking.*

8. Reposition the client on the side. Lower the bed and raise the side rail again. *Rationale: Repositioning with the bed at the proper height and side rails raised provides for the client's comfort and safety. The client should be placed on the side for a time after this procedure, to allow any excess saliva, secreted in response to the stimulation of brushing, to drain out of the mouth.*

Follow ENDDD Steps

IN PRACTICE

NURSING PROCEDURE 50-5 Caring for Fingernails and Toenails

Supplies and Equipment
Gloves
Basin half-full of warm water (gentle soap, such as Dreft, is often added)
Bath thermometer
Lotion
Towel
Nail brush
Nail polish remover (if needed)
Emery board
Nail clipper/toenail clipper
Orangewood stick
Manicure scissors and/or cuticle snips
The client may have other items, such as nail polish or cuticle oil.

Steps
Follow LPN WELCOME Steps and Then
Caring for Fingernails

1. Wearing gloves, assist the client to a comfortable upright position. *Rationale: The client often enjoys watching fingernail care. Encourage the client to assist as much as possible.*

2. Remove nail polish. *Rationale: This enables you to determine the true condition of the client's nails. It also aids in assessing the client's level of oxygenation (including with the pulse oximeter).*

3. Soak the client's fingers in a basin of warm water (approximately 35 °C-37 °C [95 °F-100 °F]) and mild soap. *Rationale: Soaking helps cleanse the nails and facilitates removal of dirt and debris. It also softens*

the nails for easier clipping and cleaning and softens the cuticle. Hot water can injure the client.

4. Scrub the client's nails with a soft nail brush. *Rationale: This helps loosen and remove dirt from under the nails. A stiff brush could cause injury.*
5. Dry the client's hands thoroughly. *Rationale: Wet hands are more likely to attract and spread microorganisms.*
6. Trim the client's fingernails straight across with nail clippers. *Rationale: This is a safe method of trimming.*
7. Shape the fingernails with an emery board, rounding the corners and smoothing the edges. *Rationale: The emery board is less dangerous than a metal file because of the sharp point and rougher surface. Rounded corners and smooth edges are less likely to catch and tear. Any break in the skin can be a site of infection.*
8. After softening in water, push the cuticle back with the blunt, smooth end of an orangewood stick. *Rationale: The stick is less likely to injure the nails than is a metal nail file.*
9. Clean under the client's nails with the more pointed end of an orangewood stick. *Rationale: This helps to get under the nail to remove debris.*
10. Clip hangnails with manicure scissors or the tip of the cuticle snips. Clip only dead portions of cuticle. *Rationale: Clipping hangnails helps keep them from tearing and discourages the client from picking or biting them. This helps prevent discomfort and infection. Clipping a live cuticle or using the entire blade of the snippers can cause it to tear, leaving a site for infection.*
11. Apply lotion to the client's hands and gently massage the hands and nails (In Practice: Nursing Care Guidelines 50-4). *Rationale: Scrubbing and soaking can dry the hands. Lotion helps prevent chafing and cracking, which can lead to infection. Hand massage helps relax the client.*

Caring for Toenails

1. Wear gloves. Assist the client to a sitting or lying position with the head of the bed elevated. *Rationale: This enables the client to soak the feet and is relaxing.*
2. Place the client's feet in a basin of warm water (approximately 35 °C-37 °C [95 °F-100 °F]) and soak them. *Rationale: This is soothing and helps soften nails, so they will be easier to trim.*
3. Gently dry the client's feet. *Rationale: Drying prevents areas of moisture, which could lead to irritation and breakdown. Most clients' feet are tender and ticklish. It is important to be gentle and to avoid tickling the client.*
4. Scrub toenails with a soft nail brush. *Rationale: This helps loosen and remove dirt and softens the nails. A stiff brush could injure delicate tissue.*
5. Trim toenails straight across with clippers (not scissors). *Rationale: Scissors often are not strong enough to cut toenails and also may cause injury. Trimming straight across helps prevent ingrown toenails.*
6. If toenails are thick and hard, you may need to cut them first (*with a specific order*) and then smooth them with a special file or emery board. *Rationale: These nails often chip and form rough edges when cut.*
7. Sometimes, very thick, hard toenails require the care of a podiatrist (foot specialist). *Rationale: Special equipment and techniques may be needed. Surgical removal may be necessary.*
8. Do not shape corners. *Rationale: Rounded toenail corners are much more likely to become ingrown.*
9. Clean under the client's nails with an orangewood stick. *Rationale: The orangewood stick is less irritating than a metal file to remove debris from under the nail.*
10. Apply lotion to the client's feet and gently massage them. *Rationale: The lotion helps to restore natural skin oils and prevents drying. Foot massage is very soothing.*

Note: If you have any difficulty cutting a client's toenails, stop and consult the primary practitioner.
Follow ENDDD Steps

IN PRACTICE
NURSING PROCEDURE 50-6 Giving a Foot Soak

Supplies and Equipment
Large basin
Warm water (approximately 35 °C-37 °C [95 °F-100 °F])
Towels
Protective pad for bed or floor
Gloves
Soap or detergent, such as Dreft (optional, or if ordered)
Commercially prepared salts, such as Epsom salts, oatmeal, or other solution, as ordered
Bath thermometer
Nurse call or pager

Steps
Follow LPN WELCOME Steps and Then

1. Wear gloves. Help the client to a comfortable upright position with the feet uncovered. If the client is too weak to sit in a chair, the client may recline in bed with the head of the bed elevated and the knees bent. *Rationale: Easy access to the feet is necessary and helps maximize efficiency and effectiveness.*

2. Place a protective pad on the bed or floor. *Rationale: A protective pad maintains safety and prevents water damage.*

3. Mix required solution of warm water in the basin and place the basin on the protected bed or floor. The client who is unable to cooperate may need to be supervised throughout the procedure. *Rationale: Proper positioning of the basin and supervision of the client prevent spilling. Make sure the client is comfortable and can tolerate the position.*

4. Place both feet in the wash basin, if the basin is large enough. Otherwise, soak one foot at a time, using fresh water or solution for each foot. Allow feet to soak for 10 to 20 min. Make sure the client has the call signal or pager handy. *Rationale: Soaking is comfortable. Medications must have time to act.*

5. Dry feet thoroughly with a blotting or patting motion. *Rationale: Adequate drying is important to prevent moisture retention, leading to skin breakdown. Harsh rubbing could damage tender or friable skin.*

6. Dry between each toe. *Rationale: Drying prevents cracking between toes and eliminates a growth medium for fungi.*

7. Check the condition of the client's toenails. Carefully observe skin integrity. Check for lesions, corns, calluses, or other abnormal conditions. Check pedal pulses, if ordered. *Rationale: Methodical drying of feet allows time for a thorough inspection.*

8. Apply lotion or creams, as ordered, and gently massage each foot. *Rationale: Lotion lubricates dry skin and provides comfort. A gentle foot massage is comforting.*

9. Apply foot powder if the client prefers. *Rationale: Foot powder is cooling and soothing and helps absorb moisture from perspiration. CAUTION: Foot powder may cake if it is exposed to excess moisture.*

Follow ENDDD Steps

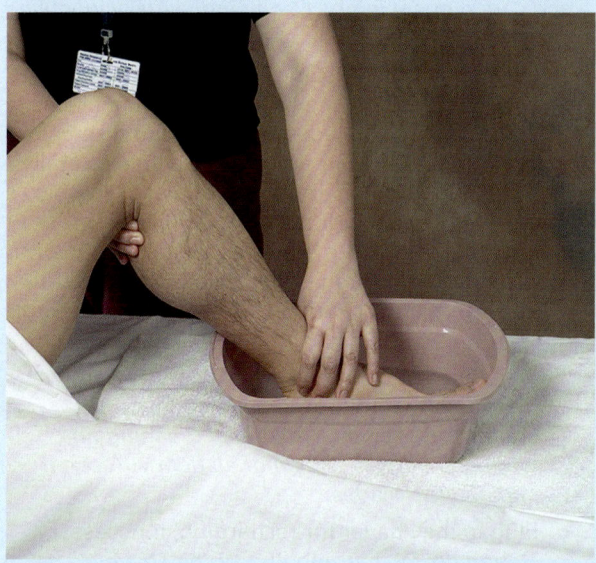

Make sure the client is in a comfortable position. Carefully examine the condition of the feet and toenails when giving a foot soak. (Ellis & Bentz, 2007.)

IN PRACTICE
NURSING PROCEDURE 50-7 Shaving a Client

Supplies and Equipment
Disposable safety razor or electric razor with disposable head (or the client's own razor)
Wash basin
Warm water
Gloves
Shaving cream or soap
Aftershave lotion, if desired
Moisturizer, if desired
Towels
(Some of these supplies may not be needed if an electric razor is used.)
Note: Some facilities do not allow the use of any scented material, such as aftershave lotion, scented moisturizer, or perfume.

Steps
Follow LPN WELCOME Steps and Then

1. Place a warm wet washcloth on the area to be shaved for 30 to 60 s. *Rationale: Moisture softens the beard.*
2. Apply shaving cream or soap to the area, if using a blade razor. *Rationale: Shaving cream or soap makes the hair easier to cut.*
3. Hold the skin taut while making strokes. *Rationale: Keeping the skin taut (especially with a blade razor) reduces the risk of cutting the skin.*
4. Holding the blade razor at a 45° angle to the skin, move it across the skin in short strokes in the direction the hair grows. If using an electric shaver, move it across the area as needed until all of the hair is cut. *Rationale: Moving the razor in the direction of hair growth helps to reduce skin irritation.*

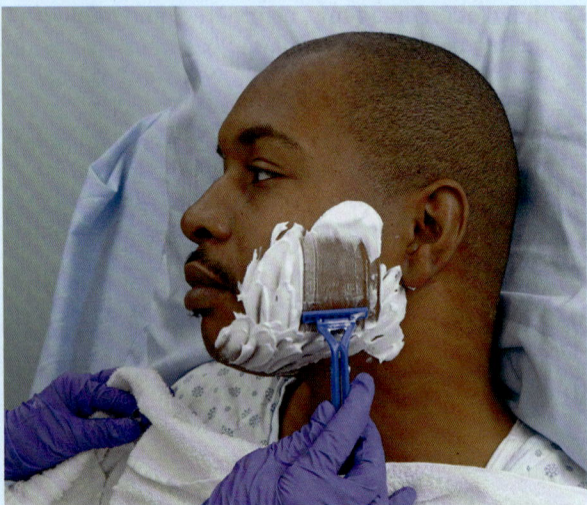

Shave in the direction of hair growth. (Evans-Smith, 2005.)

5. Wash the shaven area thoroughly with a clean, warm, moistened washcloth. *Rationale: This will remove any cream, soap, and stray hairs.*
6. Pat the area dry. *Rationale: Patting, rather than rubbing, prevents skin chafing.*
7. For men, apply aftershave lotion, if the client prefers. *Rationale: Aftershave stimulates and tones capillaries in the epidermis.*
8. If shaving a woman's legs or underarms, apply moisturizer if the client prefers and if allowed. *Rationale: Shaving may make skin dry. (Some facilities do not allow shaving of women's legs or underarms because of the danger of cuts. Often, hair removal creams are used instead.)*
9. If a disposable blade razor is used, discard it in the sharps container; if using the client's own razor, cover the blade and store it in a safe place, to prevent cuts and loss. If using a community electric shaver, use an individual electric shaver head, label it with the client's name, and keep it in a safe place with the client's grooming supplies or discard it in the sharps container. Clean the motorized portion of the community shaver carefully with an alcohol wipe after each use. *Rationale: Proper blade razor disposal and care prevent injury. Use of individually identified shaver heads helps prevent cross-contamination.*
   a. Clean the client's electric razor thoroughly after each use by removing the face plate and blades and cleaning the blades and surrounding areas with the small brush provided or with a carefully labeled toothbrush. Brush out all beard stubble and skin debris. *Rationale: Proper cleaning prevents damage to the razor, ensuring that it will be in proper working order for the next use. This also helps prevent the growth of microorganisms.*
   b. Then clean all surfaces around the blades with an alcohol wipe and allow to dry before reassembling. Try not to get alcohol on the blades themselves. *Rationale: Cleaning and wiping ensures removal of all debris. Alcohol can dull the blades.*
   c. Plug in the shaver for recharging, if necessary. *Rationale: Recharging allows the shaver to be ready for next use.*

Follow ENDDD Steps

IN PRACTICE
NURSING PROCEDURE 50-8 Using the Shampoo Cap

Supplies and Equipment
Shampoo cap
Microwave or very hot water
Gloves, if needed
Towel
Washcloth
Wide-toothed comb or hair pick

Follow LPN WELCOME Steps and Then

1. Check the cap. If the material in the cap is dry and crunchy, it is old and must be discarded. *Rationale: The shampoo material in the cap must be moist and pliable to be effective.*
2. Remove the cap from the outer package and heat it in the microwave for about 30 s or

place in hot water to heat. *Rationale: Heating activates the shampoo/conditioner. The bag must be removed promptly from the microwave, or it will explode.*

3. Make sure the cap is not too hot for the head. *Rationale: Remember: Gloves reduce sensitivity to heat. The head is very sensitive to heat.*

4. Place the cap on the client's head, covering all hair. *Rationale: All areas of the client's head should be cleansed.*

5. Very gently massage the scalp for 1 to 2 min if the hair is short; 2 to 3 min for long hair. If glass or debris is visible, *do not massage*. In this case, leave the cap in place for a longer period of time. *Rationale: It takes longer to process all the hair if the hair is long. Be very gentle in case some glass or debris is in the hair and not visible. Larger pieces of glass, rocks, or other debris can damage the scalp.*

6. If the hair is extremely tangled or matted, leave the cap on the head for several minutes and then massage. *Rationale: This will give the shampoo and conditioner time to work and help to dissolve and relieve tangling. (The cap can be reapplied if more time is needed.)*

7. If dirt, blood, or other nonsolid debris is in the hair, do not massage the head; leave the cap on longer. *Rationale: This will help dissolve dirt, blood, motor oil, or other debris. It can then be combed out, in most cases.*

8. Be extremely careful if glass is present. If glass is noted before application of the cap, gently comb it out. If debris remains when the cap is removed, gently comb out glass or other solid debris, such as rocks or pieces of metal, with a wide-toothed comb or hair pick. If nonsolid debris is still present, the cap may be reapplied or a new cap may be used for additional cleansing. *Rationale: It is important to protect yourself and the client from injury. If tiny shards of glass are still present, they could be pushed into the scalp and cut the client (or nurse). Reapplying the cap allows the chemicals a longer time to work.*

9. A washcloth may be needed to help remove blood, glass, or chunks of dirt or debris. *Rationale: Use the washcloth to pick out debris. This will help protect you and the client from injury.*

10. When all debris is gone and when the hair appears to be clean, remove the cap and towel dry the hair, using a patting motion. *Do not rub. Rationale: Rubbing tends to break hair and cause more tangles. In addition, if any debris remains, the client's head could be scratched.*

11. With the client's permission, comb out any tangles and style the hair. If severe matting or tangles remain in the hair, the client or caregiver may give permission to cut them out. If permission is not obtained, they must be left in place. *Rationale: Do not violate the client's basic rights. The client may not allow you to comb or style the hair.*

Follow ENDDD Steps

Special Reminder
- Wear gloves if the client has any infectious scalp condition, lesions, or debris in the hair. If you have any question, wear gloves. *Rationale: This helps protect yourself and others from pathogen transmission or injury.*

IN PRACTICE
NURSING PROCEDURE 50-9 The Bed Shampoo

Supplies and Equipment
Comb or hair pick
Gloves
Towels, washcloth, as needed
Waterproof pad
Pitcher
Pail or plastic wastebasket
Shampoo
Shampoo trough
Bath thermometer
Hair grooming supplies, as requested by the client

Steps
Follow LPN WELCOME Steps and Then

1. Wear gloves. Move the bed up to a comfortable height for you and lower the head to a flat position, if tolerated. Comb out the client's hair. Cover the client as needed. Lower the side rails on your side of the bed. Turn back the top covers. Place a waterproof pad under the client's head. Move the client's head and shoulders to your side of the bed. *Rationale: These procedures make the procedure as easy as possible for nurse and client and prepare the client for the shampoo.*

2. Pad the shampoo trough and gently place it under the client's neck, with the head above the trough. Direct the spout of the trough to the side of the bed and draining into the pail or wastebasket. If the client desires, gauze squares may be placed in the ears. The client may hold a towel or washcloth over the eyes, if desired. *Rationale: The trough allows*

water to be poured over the head and drained away. Make the client as comfortable as possible.

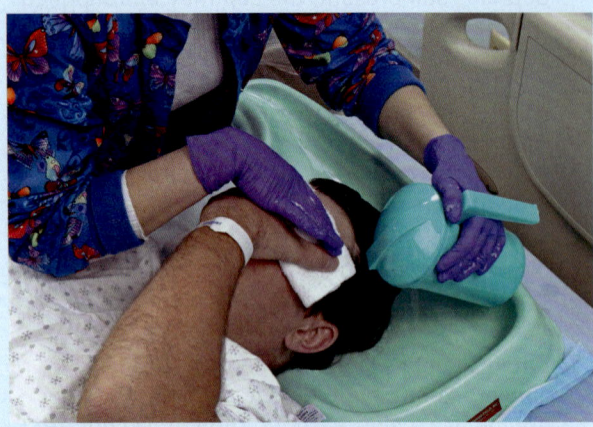

The client protects their eyes with a washcloth. Water is poured over the head and drains into a receptacle via the spout on the shampoo trough. (Evans-Smith, 2005.)

3. Wet hair thoroughly with warm water (about 35 °C–37.7 °C or 95 °F–100 °F). Apply shampoo, lather, and gently massage the scalp. Pour water from the pitcher to rinse. Repeat. Apply conditioner (leave-in conditioner is easiest). *Rationale: These procedures make the process as fast and easy for the client as possible. Scalp massage is very comforting.*
4. Squeeze excess water from hair and wrap a towel around the client's head. Gently pat hair dry. Comb out hair and style, as desired. *Rationale: Patting the hair dry reduces hair breakage.*
5. A hair dryer is usually not used by the nurse. The client may choose to use a personal hair dryer or curling iron, if allowed. *Rationale: Use of a hair dryer can dry the hair out too much and also presents the danger of burns. Special precautions are required with assaultive, depressed, or suicidal clients.*

Follow ENDDD Steps

IN PRACTICE
NURSING PROCEDURE 50-10 — Giving a Backrub

Supplies and Equipment
Unscented backrub lotion
Gloves, if indicated
Note: Alcohol and powder are not recommended because they are too drying to the skin.

Steps
Follow LPN WELCOME Steps and Then

1. Warm the lotion. Dim the lights and close the door. Provide privacy for the client. Raise the bed to a comfortable working level for yourself. Lower the side rail on your side of the bed. Position the client as close to your side of the bed as possible. Assist the client to lie on the side or prone, with the entire back and buttocks exposed. Apply warmed lotion all over the client's back. *Rationale: All of these actions help the client to relax and make the backrub comfortable for both client and nurse.*
2. Stand with your outside foot slightly forward and knees slightly bent. Rock on the feet while rubbing. *Rationale: Use good body mechanics, to avoid back strain.*
3. Rub up and down the client's back with a few long strokes (Fig. 50-4). Then, using the first three fingers of both hands, rub the neck under the client's hairline with a circular motion. *Rationale: This motion relaxes the client's neck, a frequent source of tension and headaches.*
4. Using the first three fingers of one hand, rub in the hollow at the back of the neck with a circular motion. *Rationale: This also helps to relax the client's neck.*
5. Separating the thumb and fingers of one hand, place the thumb on one side of the client's neck and the fingers on the other. Beginning at the hairline, rub the length of the neck, moving the fingers in a circular motion. *Rationale: Massaging in a circular motion helps relax the muscles.*
6. Using the first three fingers of both hands, continue the circular motion down each side of the spine to the coccyx, paying special attention to the coccyx. *Rationale: Tension builds along the spinal column. The coccyx is a bony prominence with very little fatty covering; thus, it is in great danger of skin breakdown. The rubbing motion stimulates circulation.*
7. With the palms of both hands, using light gliding strokes, stroke the length of the back up and down. (This is effleurage; Fig. 50-4A.) Apply more pressure when stroking toward the heart. *Rationale: This motion is soothing and assists in stimulating blood flow.*
8. Using the flat of both hands, with the fingers extended over the shoulders, rub the shoulders with a circular motion. Then, knead the client's skin by alternating grasping and compression motions (pétrissage). *Rationale: The shoulder blades are also bony prominences that need stimulation.*

CHAPTER 50 Personal Hygiene 727

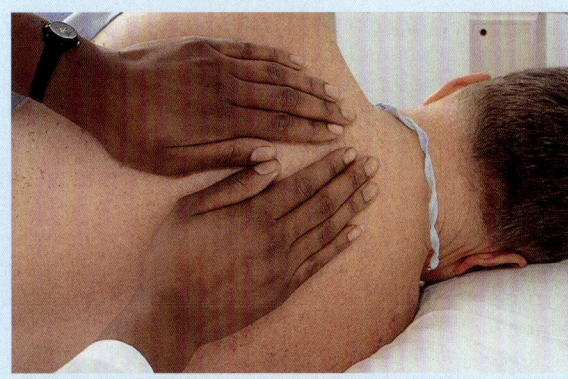

Using the flat of the hand, rub the shoulders with a circular motion.

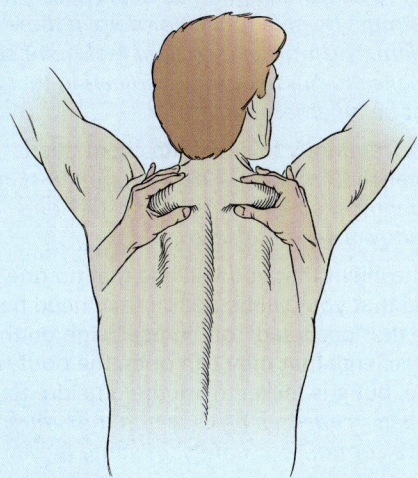

Pétrissage: Kneading the skin, particularly over shoulders and down the sides. (Evans-Smith, 2005.)

9. Continue the circular motion with the flat of the hands down the entire surface of the client's back and the buttocks (Fig. 50-4B). **Rationale:** *Using a circular motion is both stimulating and relaxing.*

10. Separating the first and second fingers of both hands, place them on either side of the client's spine and run them lightly up from the coccyx to the hairline and firmly down. **Rationale:** *This helps to relieve tension along the spinal column.*

11. Add any of the other techniques described in the text, as indicated. Most of the techniques are repeated three times. **Rationale:** *Various techniques are used to meet an individual client's needs and requests. Motions are repeated to increase effectiveness.*

12. The technique of frôlement (a very light touch with the fingertips) is often used last. **Rationale:** *This prolongs the sense of relaxation.*

13. Lightly cover the client, lower the bed, raise the side rail (if needed), and make sure the call light is within reach. Quietly leave the room. **Rationale:** *Leave the client in a comfortable position and avoid disturbing the client as much as possible. The client may now be able to sleep or rest.*

Follow ENDDD Steps

IN PRACTICE
NURSING PROCEDURE 50-11 Assisting With a Tub Bath

Supplies and Equipment
Bath blanket
Bath mat
Bath towels
Washcloths
Soap
Shampoo, if needed
Clean gown or pajamas
Clean hospital slipper socks or the client's slippers
Clean bed linen
Bath thermometer
Disinfectants for cleaning the tub
Gloves
Nurse call signal or pager

Steps
Follow LPN WELCOME Steps and Then

1. Check the bathroom's temperature, which should be warmer than normal room temperature. **Rationale:** *Doing so helps prevent the client from becoming chilled.*

2. Make sure the tub is clean. Scour it carefully with disinfectant. Unless using a long-handled swab, wear gloves when cleaning the tub. **Rationale:** *Proper cleaning helps prevent the spread of microorganisms.*

3. Rinse the tub well. **Rationale:** *Rinsing prevents harsh cleanser or disinfectant from coming into contact with the client's skin.*

4. Place a chair near the tub, with a bath blanket opened over it. If the chair has wheels, make sure they are locked. **Rationale:** *The bath blanket is convenient for the client to use to towel dry. It also allows the client to keep part of the body covered before and after getting out of the tub, to prevent chilling and exposure. If the chair accidentally moves, the client may be injured.*

5. Place towels, washcloth, soap, and shampoo where the client can reach them easily. *Rationale: Everything should be convenient for the client's use, to reduce the risk of injury.*

6. Fill the tub about halfway (less for a child). Never leave a child, a confused person, or a person who is suicidal or self-injurious alone. Make sure the tub has a nonskid bottom. In some facilities, a disposable tub liner is used. *Rationale: Limiting the amount of water in the tub helps prevent drowning, should the client slip or faint. It is not safe for some clients to bathe alone. It is important to prevent falls or self-injury.*

7. Test the water with a bath thermometer. Water temperature should be warm to very warm, but never more than 40.5 °C (105 °F). *Rationale: The bath thermometer is the only accurate way to measure water temperature.*

8. Place a bath mat in the front of the tub. *Rationale: The person needs a clean, dry, nonslippery place to stand.*

9. Bring the client to the bathroom. Help the client remove clothing and, if necessary, to get into the tub. Show the client how to use the handrails and nurse call or pager. To make getting into the tub easier, suggest that the client sit on the edge of the tub and swing their legs around, rather than to step over the edge of the tub. You may use a transfer belt if the client is unstable or weak. A special tub that opens is very helpful for older adults or clients with altered mobility. Place the client's used pajamas or gown into the laundry container. *Rationale: Assisting the client or using a transfer belt helps prevent falls by providing secure support. Providing suggestions for getting into the tub minimizes the risk for injury. When the used clothing is not available, the client will need to put on the clean clothing. Some clients will put soiled clothing back on, if it is available.*

10. Some clients prefer to shampoo hair while in the tub. In this case, you may need to help them rinse the shampoo out. *Rationale: It is dangerous for the client to rinse the hair in the tub, either under the faucet or by lying back in the water. Either of these activities might jeopardize the client's safety.*

11. Make sure the emergency call signal or pager is within reach, and explain its use. *Rationale: The client must be able to call for help, if there is a problem. This makes the client feel more secure and calls the nurse quickly, indicating that there might be an emergency.*

12. Check frequently to see if the client needs assistance. *Rationale: Checking on the client frequently ensures the client's safety and promotes a sense of security.*

13. Tell the client that you will see that no one comes in and that you will be near if they need help. Place the "occupied" or "in use" sign on the door. Show clients that they can open the door from the inside, but it is locked from the outside. *Rationale: This action ensures privacy and maximizes the client's comfort and safety. In some facilities, the*

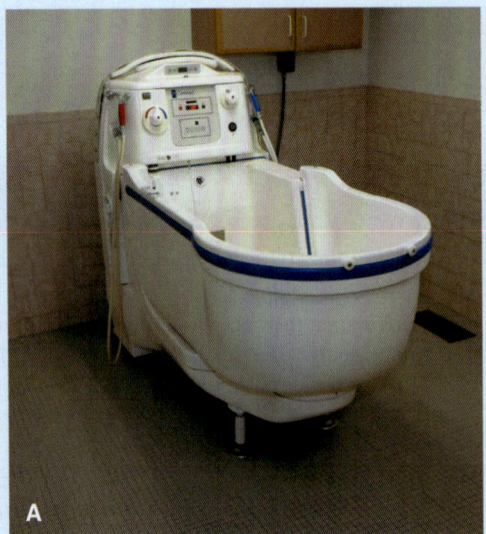 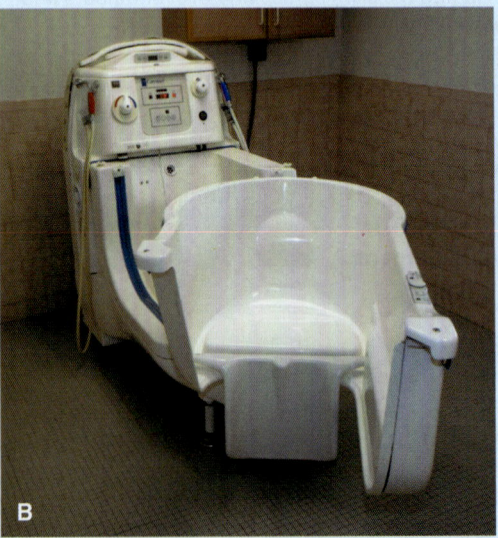

A special opening tub is used in long-term and rehabilitation facilities. It is high off the floor for staff comfort. This type of tub is available, with or without the whirlpool feature, for home use. **A.** *The whirlpool tub stimulates circulation, removes body wastes, cleans wounds, and gently massages the skin.* **B.** *The tub swings open for easy entry. (Carter, 2012.)*

CHAPTER 50 Personal Hygiene

client can lock the door from the inside. If this is the case, be sure to know how to open the locked door in an emergency.

14. When the client has finished bathing, help them out of the tub and to dry and dress, if assistance is needed. Assist the client back to their room. Have a wheelchair nearby, in case the client feels faint or weak. *Rationale: Assisting with drying off, dressing, and getting back to the room ensures* that the client remains safe and has available help if needed. Bathing can be tiring and may leave the client weak or light-headed.

15. Wearing gloves, carefully clean the tub after the client has completed the bath, following steps 2 and 3. *Rationale: Cleaning the tub ensures that it is ready for the next client.*

Follow ENDDD Steps

IN PRACTICE
NURSING PROCEDURE 50-12 Giving a Bed Bath

Supplies and Equipment
Gloves, 1 or 2 pairs, as needed
Bath blanket
Towels
Washcloths
Basin
Gown or pajamas
Personal items (deodorant, powder, and other requested items)
Bedpan or urinal
Clean bed linens
Covered linen hamper
Soap
Bath thermometer
Note: Change gloves and bath water whenever needed during this procedure. Also, ask the client about personal preferences regarding personal care items.

Steps
Follow LPN WELCOME Steps and Then

1. Assist the client to use a bedpan or urinal. *Rationale: Voiding before the bath prevents interruption of the procedure and promotes comfort.*

2. Assemble everything you will need for the bath. Raise the level of the bed. Remove the bedspread, fold it, and place it on a chair or table. Cover the client with a bath blanket. Remove the top sheet from under the bath blanket, while the client holds onto the bath blanket, if possible (Chapter 49). *Rationale: It is important to have everything you need, so the bath will not be interrupted. The level of the bed should be at a comfortable height for you. The bedspread may be reused, based on agency policy. The bath blanket provides warmth; use a top sheet, if a bath blanket is unavailable.*

3. Fill the basin about two-thirds full with hot water, at least 37.7 °C to 40.5 °C (100 °F-105 °F) and place it on the bedside table. It is acceptable to have quite hot water to start the procedure. *Rationale: Water at the proper temperature is relaxing and provides warmth. Water will cool during the procedure.*

4. Lower the near side rail. *Rationale: This allows access to the client, while using good body mechanics. Side rails may also be used to help the client turn in bed, even if the client does not need them at other times.*

5. Remove the client's gown, while keeping the bath blanket in place, covering the client. If the client has an intravenous line (IV), thread the tubing and bag through the sleeve of the used gown. (Gowns with sleeves that open on their entire length are also available for use with IVs.) Rehang the IV bag. Check the IV flow rate or pump activity. Properly manage any other equipment the client may have, such as a catheter drainage bag or continuous suction machine. *Rationale: It is important to safeguard any medical equipment being used. Removing the gown permits easier access when washing the client's upper body and allows a change of gown. Be sure all equipment is functioning and the IV is uninterrupted. Sterility of IVs, catheters, etc., must be maintained.*

6. Wear gloves. Assist the client to move toward the side of the bed nearest you. (Choose the side of the bed so your dominant hand is toward the foot of the bed.) Stand with your outside foot slightly ahead of the other foot. *Rationale: Most of the work will be completed with your dominant hand. Moving the client close to you limits reaching across the bed. This standing position will usually be the most comfortable for you and you can rock forward and back as you move up and down the client's body.*

7. Make a mitt with the washcloth (Fig. 50-5). Moisten the mitt with plain water and wash the client's eyes. Cleanse from the inner canthus (near the nose) to the outer canthus of each eye. Use a different section of the mitt to wash each eye (In Practice: Nursing Care Guidelines 50-2). *Rationale: Making a mitt prevents water from dripping*

across the client and gives better control. Washing from inner to outer canthus prevents sweeping foreign material or eye matter into the client's eyes. Using a separate portion of the mitt for each eye reduces the chance of spreading infection from one eye to the other.

8. Wash the client's face, neck, and ears. Use soap on these areas only if the client prefers. Dry carefully. *Rationale: Soap is particularly drying to the face.*

9. Uncover the client's far arm. Place a bath towel under it. Wash with long strokes, using the greatest pressure when moving toward the axilla. Rinse and dry the area. Pay special attention to the axilla. *Rationale: Washing the far side first prevents dripping bath water onto a clean area. Long strokes toward the heart improve circulation, by facilitating venous return. The axilla is a common site of body odor caused by perspiration.*

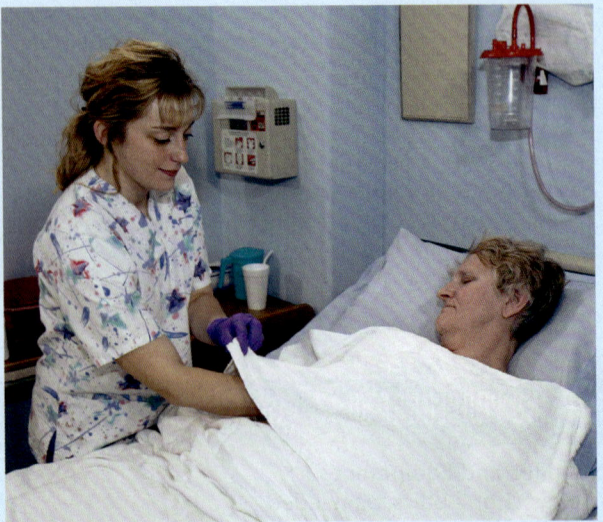

Wash the chest under a towel, exposing the client as little as possible. (Evans-Smith, 2005.)

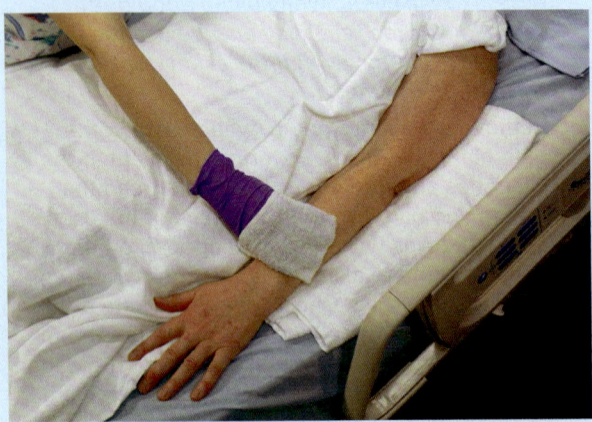

Expose the far arm and wash it, paying special attention to the axilla. Use the most pressure when moving the washcloth toward the heart. (Evans-Smith, 2005.)

10. Place the basin on a folded towel. Immerse the client's far hand in the water. Allow the hand to soak for a few minutes. Wash, rinse, and dry. Cover the client's arm with the bath blanket. Repeat these steps for the client's near arm and hand. *Rationale: Soaking the hand is comforting and aids in cleansing under the fingernails.*

11. Open a bath towel over the client's chest and fold the bath blanket back. Wash, rinse, and dry the client's chest. Wash, check, and carefully dry the skin under the breasts. You can also wash under the towel, without exposing the client's breasts, except to wash under them. Apply powder or cream, if the client desires. *Rationale: Moisture collects in the skin folds under the breasts and may cause irritation or infection. Powder is soothing and helps keep the area dry. Sometimes, special cream is applied, to prevent infection.*

12. Keeping the towel over the client's chest, lower the bath blanket to just above the pubic area. Wash, rinse, and dry the abdomen, paying special attention to the umbilicus or any skin folds. (You can also wash the abdomen under the towel.) Then, cover the client's chest and abdomen with the bath blanket and remove the towel. The client may put a gown on at this time, leaving it untied at the neck. *Rationale: The bath blanket continues to provide warmth and privacy. A client who is chilly may feel warmer if they wear a gown. This also provides privacy.*

13. You may need to change the water at this point. Then, uncover the client's far leg and place a towel under it. Wash with long strokes, rinse, and dry it. *Rationale: Washing the far side first prevents dripping bath water on a clean area. Long strokes improve circulation by facilitating venous return.*

14. Place the basin on a folded bath towel and carefully immerse the client's far foot in water. Allow the foot to soak for a few minutes. Wash, rinse, and dry the foot, paying particular attention to the area between the toes. Re-cover the leg and foot with the bath blanket. Repeat on the other side. *Rationale: Soaking the foot is comforting and aids in cleansing between the toes and beneath the toenails.*

15. Raise the side rail, if needed, and change bath water at this point, if necessary. Put the lotion bottle in the warm bath water and let it float there. *Rationale: If there is any chance that the client may fall out of bed, raise the side rail. Cool bath water is uncomfortable. The water is probably unclean by now. Change water earlier, if necessary, to maintain the proper temperature or if it becomes dirty. The lotion will be warming up for the backrub.*

16. Lower the near side rail, if it was raised. Change gloves, if needed. Assist the client to turn away from you onto their side. Uncover the client's back and buttocks. Fold a towel the long way and place it on the bed, parallel to the client's back. Wash, rinse, and dry the client's back and buttocks. Wash the rectal area. Change gloves again, as needed. Assess for reddened areas or skin breakdown. *Rationale: Skin breakdown usually occurs over bony prominences, and feces and urine are very caustic. Carefully observe the sacral area and back for any indications of skin breakdown or irritation and document any significant findings. Gloves are worn because the rectal area is contaminated.*

17. Give a backrub at this time (In Practice: Nursing Procedure 50-10). If the client's skin is intact, gloves may be removed for the backrub. Tie or snap the client's gown at the back or side of the neck. *Rationale: A backrub stimulates circulation and is a comfort measure. Contact with ungloved hands is more soothing and comfortable for the client.*

18. Return the client to their back and adjust the bath blanket so the client is covered. Use side rails for safety, and change bath water again. Wear gloves. Use a clean washcloth and towel to wash the client's perineal area, if the client is unable to do so (In Practice: Nursing Procedure 50-13). Otherwise, place necessary equipment within the client's reach and allow them to complete this care. Provide privacy. Re-cover the client with the bath blanket. Remove and discard gloves and wash your hands. *Rationale: Cleaning the perineal area helps prevent skin irritation and breakdown and decreases the potential for body odor. Self-care makes the client more comfortable and eliminates embarrassment. However, you must complete this step, if the client cannot do it.*

Gloves are needed, to prevent contact with feces or urine.

19. Assist the client with mouth care (In Practice: Nursing Procedure 50-1) or special mouth care (In Practice: Nursing Procedure 50-4), flossing the teeth (In Practice: Nursing Procedure 50-2), or caring for dentures (Nursing Procedure 50-3), as needed. Assist the client to shave, if needed (In Practice: Nursing Procedure 50-7). The client may also require a shampoo (In Practice: Nursing Procedure 50-9). *Rationale: The client who requires a bed bath will most likely need assistance with these procedures as well.*

20. Help the client put on a gown or pajamas. Assist with personal hygiene, such as deodorant and cologne, if permitted. Assist with hair care. Assist the client into a chair, if possible. The client may also require nail care (In Practice: Nursing Procedure 50-5). Encourage the client to do as much self-care as possible. *Rationale: A gown or pajamas provide warmth and privacy. Helping with specific hygiene needs personalizes the client's care. The bed is easier to make if it is unoccupied, and the client will get some exercise. Self-care promotes independence and enhances self-esteem.*

Note: Follow your facility protocols regarding scents. Many facilities do not allow any cologne, perfume, or scented lotions. *Rationale: Many people are allergic to scents, often more severe during illness.*

21. Make the bed with clean linens. Lower the bed and raise the side rails as ordered. Remember to wear gloves when removing used linens from the bed (In Practice: Nursing Procedure 49-1 lists steps in making an unoccupied bed; In Practice: Nursing Procedure 49-2, the occupied bed). *Rationale: These measures provide for comfort and safety for client and nurse.*

Follow ENDDD Steps

IN PRACTICE

NURSING PROCEDURE 50-13: Assisting With Perineal Care

Supplies and Equipment
Gloves
Washcloths (barrier cream washcloths are used if client is incontinent)
Basin
Waterproof pad
Towels
Soap
Shaving cream, if the client is not incontinent
Prescribed skin barrier ointment or cream, as ordered
Toilet tissue
Bath blanket

Steps
Follow LPN WELCOME Steps and Then

1. Wear gloves. Uncover the client's perineal area. Place a towel or waterproof pad under the client's hips. Place another towel over the perineal area. *Rationale: A towel or pad protects the bed. The towel can be used to dry the client's perineal and rectal areas. Provide as much privacy as possible.*

2. Make a mitt with the washcloth (Fig. 50-5). Cleanse the client's upper thighs and groin area with soap and water or shaving cream, if the client is continent. Use barrier cream prepared cloths, if the client is incontinent. Rinse and dry. Wash the genital area next. Work under the towel as much as possible. *Rationale: If the client's skin has the potential of breaking down, special skin care measures are required (Chapter 58). Provide privacy.*

Female Client

Unfold the mitt. Use a separate portion of the washcloth for each stroke, changing washcloths as necessary. Start from the outside and work toward the center. Separate the labia and cleanse downward from the pubic to the anal area (Fig. 50-9A). Wash between the labia, including the urethral meatus and vaginal area. Wash this area last. Rinse well and pat dry. Apply prescribed skin protection materials. *Rationale: Cleansing from the pubis toward the anus washes from a cleaner to a contaminated area, helping prevent contamination of the vaginal area and urinary meatus. Patting the area dry is more comfortable than rubbing.*

Male Client

Gently grasp the client's penis. Cleanse in a circular motion, moving from the tip of the penis downward toward the pubic area (Fig. 50-9B). In an uncircumcised male, carefully retract the foreskin before washing the penis. Remove any collected secretions (**smegma**). Rinse well and dry. Return the foreskin to its former position. Wash, rinse, and dry the perineum and scrotum carefully. *Rationale: Cleansing from the tip of the client's penis downward helps prevent transferring microorganisms from the anus to the urethra. Retracting the foreskin allows removal of collected secretions that can cause irritation and odor. Returning the foreskin to its normal position prevents discomfort and injury to tissue.*

Both Male and Female Clients

3. Assist the client to turn on the side. Separate the client's buttocks and use toilet tissue, if necessary, to remove fecal material. Use the prescribed product to remove feces, if the client has been incontinent. Disposable barrier cream cloths are handy and effective. If the client has not been incontinent, shaving cream may be used to clean the area because it is soothing to the skin. *Rationale: Removing fecal matter provides for easier cleaning. Remember that shaving cream and soap do not provide protection if the client is incontinent. (Chapter 58 describes special skin care.)*

4. Cleanse the anal area, rinse thoroughly, and dry with a towel. Change washcloths or barrier cream cloths, as necessary. *Rationale: Keeping the anal area clean minimizes the risk of skin irritation and breakdown, as well as helping prevent contamination of the urethra or vaginal area.*

5. Apply skin care products to the area, as ordered or per protocol. *Rationale: It is important to provide a moisture barrier, to prevent skin breakdown.*

Follow ENDDD Steps

51 Elimination

Learning Objectives

1. Describe the normal color, clarity, and odor of urine. Describe abnormal urination patterns.
2. Identify the normal color and consistency of feces. Explain deviations from normal feces.
3. Demonstrate techniques for assisting the client to the bathroom, giving and removing a bedpan or urinal, and transferring the client from bed to commode.
4. Explain the purpose and procedures for competent urinary catheter care.
5. Describe techniques for relieving urinary retention.
6. List purposes of cleansing, retention, and carminative enemas.
7. Demonstrate the technique for administering a self-contained (small-volume) disposable enema.
8. Describe the reasons and methods of manual disimpaction.
9. Describe the process of administering a bag-and-tubing enema.
10. Discuss nursing care for the client who is vomiting.

Important Terminology

anuria	dysuria	Kegel exercises	residual urine	voiding	
calculi	edema	melena	steatorrhea	vomitus	
constipation	emesis	micturition	urgency		
cystitis	enema	nocturia	urinary catheter		
defecation	enuresis	oliguria	urinary frequency		
dehydration	fecal impaction	polyuria	urinary retention		
diarrhea	flatus	projectile vomiting	urinary		
distention	incontinence	renal colic	suppression		

Acronyms

BM
BRP
BS
I&O
SP
TWE
UTI

The healthy human body smoothly and effectively eats, digests, absorbs, and metabolizes food to provide fuel and perform its many functions. Just as effectively, the healthy body rids itself of waste products to maintain homeostasis. Elimination of liquid and solid wastes is normally routine and uneventful, unless a change in habits or an illness occurs. Changes in bowel or bladder habits may be *signs* of illness, or they may *cause* illness. Assessing the client's products of elimination (urine and feces), observing their bladder and bowel function, and assisting with a disorder related to elimination are fundamental nursing responsibilities. The client may feel uncomfortable or embarrassed when discussing bladder or bowel elimination. Be sure to provide privacy and demonstrate understanding.

Nursing Alert Standard Precautions require the use of gloves and other protective devices when coming in contact with any bodily secretion or drainage. Basic protective gear always includes gloves and, in some cases, gowns or masks. A face shield or other protective eyewear is required if there is any danger of splashing fluids. Handwashing or hand sanitization is required before and after all client care. Long handwashing is required if your gloves become soiled.

Urine is the body's liquid waste product. Passing urine from the body is called *urination*, **micturition**, or **voiding**.

Feces, also called a *bowel movement* (**BM**) or *stool*, is the body's solid waste product. **Defecation** refers to excretion of feces. Urine and feces are the waste products of the urinary and digestive systems, respectively. Each has typical characteristics in the healthy client. However, abnormal urine and/or feces may indicate a bodily dysfunction (illness). Urine and stool specimens are frequently collected as part of nursing data collection (Chapter 52). Becoming familiar with the normal characteristics of these waste products and understanding the usual processes of elimination help identify variations or abnormalities.

NCLEX Alert

Throughout the chapter, you will see references to previously studied concepts such as client safety, prevention of falls, prevention of infection and complications, and use of standard precautions. To correctly respond to an NCLEX scenario, you may need to incorporate these into your selected nursing actions.

URINARY ELIMINATION

Urine, formed by the kidneys, consists of excess water from the body, carbon dioxide, a small amount of solid wastes, and abnormal substances filtered out of the blood. Urine is excreted from the kidneys into the bladder and out via the urethra (Chapter 27). The total adult urine output varies, according to the person's fluid intake and kidney efficiency. In addition, urine output is also influenced by normal processes, such as respiration, perspiration, salt intake, and the fluid contained in feces, although these cannot be specifically measured. (Fluids can also be lost through abnormal processes, such as vomiting and bleeding.) An adult of average size forms and excretes approximately 500–2400 mL of urine every 24 hr (about 1 mL of urine per kilogram of body weight, per hour). When the body freely perspires due to hot weather, exercise, or fever, urine volumes decrease. If the body retains water because of impaired circulation or kidney function, it forms and excretes less urine. In some disorders, such as diabetes mellitus and diabetes insipidus, more urine is excreted (Chapter 79).

> **Key Concept**
>
> An excess of body fluid collected in the tissues often causes puffiness called **edema** (overhydration; Fig. 47-9); a deficiency in body fluids leads to **dehydration**.

The urge to void (urinate) is triggered when approximately 250 mL of urine has collected in the bladder. However, the adult bladder can hold approximately 400–500 mL when moderately full. *Fluid output* is usually about equal to *fluid intake*. Encourage clients to drink adequate fluid. To maintain normal fluid balance, each adult needs six to eight 8-oz glasses of liquid daily. If ordered, the client's intake and output (**I&O**) is measured and documented every shift, to help monitor fluid balance (Chapter 52 describes the I&O monitoring procedure; In Practice: Nursing Procedure 52-1.).

Changes in the characteristics of urine or in usual urination patterns may be signs of urinary disorders and sometimes indicate disorders in other body systems as well. The nurse is in a unique position to observe the client's elimination patterns. Report and document any unusual or abnormal signs or symptoms.

Characteristics of Urine

Urine is observed for color, clarity, odor, and volume. Chapter 27 introduces the normal characteristics of urine. Any deviations may indicate an abnormality.

- *Color:* Freshly voided urine is light yellow or amber in color. *Overhydration* results in dilute urine that is nearly colorless. *Dehydration* results in concentrated urine that is dark amber or orange-brown. In addition, certain medications and foods can alter the color of urine (Table 51-1).
- *Clarity:* Freshly voided urine is clear or transparent. Abnormal substances, such as bacteria, blood, mucous shreds, or pus, or if it has been standing for a period of time can cause cloudiness.
- *Odor:* Freshly voided urine has a characteristic odor, sometimes called *aromatic*. Concentrated urine has a stronger odor and urine decomposes and emits a strong, ammonia-like odor when exposed to air for a time. Some foods or medications may alter the odor. Usually, a strongly offensive odor from freshly voided urine suggests an abnormality, such as a urinary tract infection.
- *Volume:* Typically, the adult voids from 250 to 400 mL at a time. Total output relates to each person's size, bladder condition, hydration level, and other fluid gains or losses.

TABLE 51-1 Color Variations in Urine

URINE COLOR	COMMON CAUSES OF VARIATION
Clear, colorless (dilute)	Large amount of liquid intake
	Abnormal conditions (e.g., diabetes insipidus [impaired tubular reabsorption], diabetes mellitus)
	Diuretic medications (particularly, if overused)
	Liver disorders (e.g., acute viral hepatitis, cirrhosis)
Bright, neon yellow	Vitamin supplements
Cloudy	Urine left standing, causing phosphates to precipitate out
	Pyuria (pus in the urine)
	Urinary tract infection, bacteriuria (bacteria in urine)
	Epithelial cells
	Blood
	Leukocytes (white blood cells)
	Kidney stones
Green	Pseudomonas infection
	Bile pigments
Dark yellow, gold	Low fluid intake
	Dehydration (concentrated urine)
	Inability of kidneys to dilute urine
	Bile
Pink, red	Hematuria—blood in urine (kidney or bladder infection, cancer)
	Some laxatives
	Some foods (red berries, food dye, beets, red gelatin, some red juices)
Orange, red brown	Some medications (e.g., sulfasalazine, phenazopyridine, doxorubicin, some laxatives, and some chemotherapy drugs)
	Some foods
	Some food coloring
	Dehydration
Blue, green	Some medications (e.g., amitriptyline, indomethacin, propofol)
	Some foods (e.g., asparagus)
	Some food dyes
	Some medical conditions

TABLE 51-1	Color Variations in Urine (Continued)
URINE COLOR	COMMON CAUSES OF VARIATION
Smoky, hazy	Hemoglobin (remnants of red blood cells)
	Chyle (product of digestion normally emptied into venous system)
	Prostatic fluid
	Yeast infection
Yellow brown	Bile
Dark brown, black	Methylene blue
	Typhus infection
	Some medications (e.g., iron)
	Some foods and food dyes
	Hematuria (blood in urine)
	Liver disorders (especially with light stools and jaundice)

Most changes in urine color are temporary. However, continuing and unexplained color changes should be followed up by physical examination.

- *Specific gravity:* Normal urine has a *specific gravity* of 1.010–1.025. (The specific gravity of pure water is 1.000.) Specific gravity may be measured by the laboratory as part of a routine urinalysis or the nurse may perform this test (Nursing Procedure 52-2).
- *Acidity:* Most body fluids are slightly alkaline (Chapter 17). A pH below 7 is acidic, a pH of 7 is neutral, and a pH above 7 is alkaline. Unlike many other body fluids, normal urine is slightly acidic, having a usual pH of about 4.5–6.5. This acidic condition helps control bacterial growth.
- *Abnormal components:* Abnormal components (e.g., microorganisms) in urine suggest dysfunction or disease. Sometimes, the urine's appearance is so changed that abnormalities are obvious; other times the urine appears normal to the naked eye. Many urine tests are performed in the laboratory. As a nurse, you will often be asked to obtain a urine specimen for urinalysis, drug screening, pregnancy tests, or urine culture. Obtaining a single voided specimen is described in In Practice: Nursing Procedure 52-3.

Key Concept
A urine dipstick can quickly measure pH, specific gravity, glucose, and ketones and indicates the presence of WBCs, blood, nitrites, protein, and urobilinogen. This provides quick diagnosis of urinary infections and other disorders.

Patterns of Urinary Elimination

Although observation of the client's urine can indicate renal (kidney) or urinary problems, a change in the usual pattern of urinary elimination is also a significant finding. Common signs and symptoms of abnormalities are as follows:

- **Urinary frequency:** Voiding more often than usual, without an increase in total urine volume, with a *decrease* in volume per voiding.
- **Urgency:** The desire or sensation of needing to void immediately. Often, the person is unable to delay voiding without some involuntary urine leakage (*incontinence*). Many definitions apply to different types of urgency (Chapter 89).
- **Dysuria:** A painful or burning sensation when passing urine (most commonly associated with infection). The person may also experience cramping or shooting pelvic pain.
- **Nocturia:** Frequent or repeated voiding during the night. (It may normally occur if the person drinks a large amount of liquid before bedtime.) Usually, frequency and urgency accompany abnormal nocturia.
- **Enuresis:** Involuntary voiding in bed (*bedwetting*). Enuresis is a common problem in children, but may also occur in adults. Enuresis also may be a side effect of medications.
- **Polyuria:** An increase in the expected amount of urine a person excretes over a period of time. It may occur when the person drinks a larger than usual amount of liquids, but it may also be a symptom of diabetes mellitus or certain types of kidney disease. A daily urine output greater than about 2,500 mL is considered polyuria.
- **Incontinence:** Involuntary loss of urine from the bladder or inability to hold urine. Loss of muscle tone, injury, or paralysis destroy the ability of urethral muscles to constrict enough to keep the urinary outlet closed; thus, urine dribbles, or the muscles relax without voluntary control. If nerve pathways to the brain's control center are injured, the person either does not feel the impulse to urinate or is unable to control the outlet muscles and voids involuntarily. If the cause is muscular weakness, bladder retraining may be effective (Chapter 89).
- **Urinary suppression:** The stopping or inhibition of urination. Several conditions fall into this category. It can denote suppression of *secretion* (urine is not formed) or of *excretion* (urine is not expelled).
- **Oliguria:** A decrease in the expected amount of urine a person secretes and excretes. A daily urine output of less than about 500 mL is considered to be oliguria, which may be caused by kidney disorders or urinary tract obstruction.
- **Anuria:** The absence of urine secreted by the kidneys (<100 mL/day). Anuria is a very serious sign of kidney dysfunction. Other signs of failing kidneys include headache, dizziness, edema, puffiness around the eyes, nausea, and dim vision.
- **Urinary retention:** Inability to empty the bladder fully, with attempts to void. (The nurse may gently palpate the lower abdomen for fullness—**distention**.) Urinary retention may have several causes. Sometimes, a person is unable to feel the urge to void or is unable to relax urethral muscles to allow urination. Certain medications and disorders, such as diabetes, Parkinson disease, or urinary tract infections, can contribute to retention. A common cause is trauma, particularly to the spinal cord. An obstruction may exist in the urinary tract, impeding the flow of urine as it exits the urinary bladder. Such obstructions may be caused by conditions such as kidney stones or cancer or may be a

result of an enlarged prostate gland in men. In the case of an obstruction, the bladder may empty, but not all urine is completely expelled. When an obstruction interferes with complete bladder emptying, the client may have dribbling of urine, due to *retention overflow* (the bladder expands until some urine flows out, due to increased pressure). *Temporary urine retention* may also follow abdominal surgery, any anesthesia, or for a short period of time following removal of an indwelling catheter. It is important to monitor urine output and watch for signs and symptoms of urinary retention, whether complete or incomplete. (See Nursing Care Guidelines 51-5 for bladder scanning to determine urinary retention.)

Report the following signs and symptoms:

- Retention of urine for 6–8 hr following catheter removal or sooner if the bladder is distended and the client complains of discomfort.
- Dribbling of small amounts of urine.
- Distended bladder following voiding.
- Urgency following voiding.

NCLEX Alert

It will be important for you to understand normal patterns of urination and defecation, as well as normal characteristics of urine and stool in order to identify and document abnormalities. Your observations and documentation aid healthcare providers to diagnose and treat the client's conditions. You will need to consider this as you select nursing actions in the NCLEX examination.

Urinary Tract Problems

Urinary Tract Infection

Urinary tract infections (**UTI**) are common, often occurring when microorganisms contaminate the usually sterile urinary tract through the urethral opening. UTIs are more common in women than in men because the female urethra is shorter and straighter. *Urethritis* technically means inflammation of the urethra; **cystitis** is an inflammation of the bladder; and *nephritis* and *pyelonephritis* refer to inflammation of the kidneys. Inflammation is most often caused by an infection, and the term *cystitis* is often used to denote any UTI. The person experiencing a UTI may complain of urgency, frequency, dysuria, chills, abdominal discomfort, and flank pain. The urine may appear cloudy, due to the presence of microorganisms or pus. Report these symptoms and encourage the client to drink 2–3 L of liquids each day. Water and juices are best; caffeinated drinks should be avoided because they irritate the bladder. A clean-catch urine specimen for culture may be ordered (Chapter 52). If antibiotics are ordered, obtain the culture specimen *before administering antibiotics*. Most UTIs respond quickly to specific antibiotics.

Urinary Calculi

Urinary **calculi** are *stones*. They may occur in the kidney (*renal calculi*) or bladder (*cystic calculi*). Calculi are formed from substances normally excreted by the body, such as calcium, or when certain conditions (e.g., infection, urinary

---

IN PRACTICE

NURSING CARE GUIDELINES 51-1 | Straining Urine for Calculi

Teach the client not to discard any urine until it has been examined. Each time the client voids:

- Wash your hands. Put on clean gloves. Prepare a graduated container with a fine wire strainer, in which clean gauze has been placed. *Rationale: Handwashing and using gloves help prevent the spread of infection, especially when handling body fluids. Measuring I&O is usually ordered when urine is being strained, so urine amount needs to be measured.*
- Pour urine through the strainer and gauze into the graduated container. Look for visible stones. *Rationale: This strains out any stones. You will need to report size, number, and appearance of any stones you recover.*
- Inspect any blood clots for the presence of stones by pressing them against the sides of the gauze in the strainer with a tongue blade. Report any blood clots or active bleeding. *Rationale: A blood clot could hide stones. Urinary hemorrhage may occur as a result of calculi. Bleeding may need to be treated, in addition to determining how to deal with the calculi.*
- Retrieve any stones and place them in a sterile specimen container to send to the laboratory for examination. *Rationale: Identification of stone composition is necessary, to determine the correct treatment and prevent future stone formation.*
- Discard gloves and wash your hands. Document findings. *Rationale: Proper glove disposal and handwashing reduce the risk of infection transmission. Documentation provides communication and enhances continuity of care.*

---

retention, or prolonged immobility) are present. In most cases, the specific cause of urinary calculi is unknown, but this condition may be familial (inherited). The stones may vary in size from tiny, microscopic pieces of sand to marble-sized accumulations. These stones may obstruct a client's normal urinary flow as they move within the urinary tract. If a stone becomes lodged in a ureter, the person usually experiences severe, penetrating pain in the lower back, called **renal colic**. If a stone moves to the urinary bladder, the client will often complain of dull, heavy, aching pain over the pubic area and across the lower back. In some cases, if the stone(s) move into the bladder, it/they can be passed in the urine without much difficulty (because the urethra is larger in diameter than the ureters). Calculi may also cause UTIs (Chapter 89). When caring for a client with possible kidney stones, the provider will most likely order the urine to be strained for calculi (In Practice: Nursing Care Guidelines 51-1). These stones may be analyzed, to determine their chemical makeup. Determination of calculi makeup may recommend the omission of specific foods, to help prevent recurrence.

BOWEL ELIMINATION

Similar to urinary elimination, changes in *bowel elimination* may occur because of gastrointestinal (GI) disorders or a disorder in another body system. The bowel responds to even the slightest changes in a person's usual eating or exercise habits. Bowel elimination can change quickly when a client is ill or immobilized. Daily data gathering includes noting the characteristics of a client's stools and any changes or difficulties that the client reports.

Characteristics of Feces

Feces (stool, bowel movement), the solid waste products of digestion, consist of the end products of metabolism and digestion of foods.

- *Color:* Normally, feces are yellowish brown (due to the presence of bile). A change in color suggests a change in (GI) functioning or stool contents. Gray- or clay-colored stools usually indicate that bile is missing, often a sign of gallbladder disease. Dark, black, or tarry stools usually indicate the presence of partially digested blood, called **melena**, indicating hemorrhage high in the GI tract or swallowed blood from a mouth, nose, or throat injury or disorder. Bright red blood in (or streaked on the outside of) stool indicates rectal or anal bleeding, often from hemorrhoids. Yellow or greenish stools indicate the abnormal presence of microorganisms, suggesting infection. Some medications or foods may alter stool color as well. Collection of a stool specimen is outlined in In Practice: Nursing Procedure 52-6.
- *Consistency:* Normal stools are soft and formed. Hard, dry stools (**constipation**) result when the rectum has not been emptied as needed and/or excess liquid has been absorbed by the body. Chronic constipation may occur if a person routinely ignores the impulse to empty the rectum. Constipation also results if the person has not taken enough fluids or has not had sufficient exercise to stimulate peristalsis. Constipation may also result from some types of medications (e.g., morphine and other narcotics or drugs to lower bladder motility) or may occur after surgery, as a result of immobility, anesthesia, surgical trauma, and drying agents (e.g., atropine).

  Diarrhea is the expulsion of loose, watery, unformed stools. Sometimes, the person has frequent, watery stools; in other cases, the diarrhea is explosive. Continuing diarrhea suggests chronic colon irritation, intestinal infection, food poisoning, or a parasitic infection. The person's emotional state may also affect stool consistency, causing either diarrhea or constipation. Diarrhea can also be a sign of **fecal impaction**, described below, with liquid stool passing around the impaction.
- *Shape:* Generally, stools have the same shape as the bowel's interior: round, oval, or cylindrical. Long, thin, pencillike stools suggest a narrowing of the rectum or anal opening, which could be caused by a mass or tumor. Stool that always assumes the same irregular shape is also suggestive of an abnormal growth in the rectum or anus.
- *Odor:* Stools have a characteristic odor. Note any unusual or very strong odors. Sometimes, medications, strong-flavored foods, or the presence of unusual microorganisms change the odor. The gaseous discharge (**flatus**) that occurs with or without a bowel movement can have a very strong odor.
- *Density:* Stool density is the weight concentration of feces, in relation to water. Normally, stools sink in water. Floating stools are less dense and suggest undigested fats, especially if they have a fatty or oily appearance. **Steatorrhea** is the term used to identify stools with a high fat content. Document if stools float; this may be an indication of gallbladder disease or cystic fibrosis.
- *Abnormal components:* The presence of pus or mucus in stool indicates an inflammation or infection in the GI system. The presence of undigested food products or medication tablets may also suggest GI malfunction. Abnormal stool color, described above, often suggests the presence of blood.
- *Fecal impaction:* The term *fecal impaction* denotes stool that is so hard and dry or puttylike that it cannot be expelled by the client, even after administration of laxatives and/or enemas. Fecal impaction is usually the result of chronic bowel problems, but can also be the result of immobility, paralysis, or dehydration. Some clients develop a fecal impaction following an x-ray procedure, the *barium enema;* this impaction results from retained barium. A client who has been treated with charcoal for poisoning may also develop an impaction (and will have black stools). Symptoms of fecal impaction include severe abdominal discomfort, hard abdomen, and a feeling of pressure. The person often feels the urge to defecate, but is unable to do so, or is unable to empty the bowel completely, and may have diarrhea. In fecal impaction, a rectal examination reveals a hard or puttylike mass. Digital removal of impacted stool (manual disimpaction) may be required. In Practice: Nursing Procedure 51-5 describes this procedure.

> **Key Concept**
> After manual disimpaction, the client may have several bouts of explosive diarrhea, before reestablishing a normal bowel elimination pattern.

Patterns of Bowel Elimination

Defecation usually occurs at regular intervals when the mass of feces moves into the colon because of the muscular action of the intestinal wall, *peristalsis*. The fecal mass causes pressure against the bowel walls, which signals to the person that they must defecate. Voluntary abdominal muscles help push stool from the rectum. Patterns of elimination are unique to each individual. Many people experience a bowel movement in the morning after breakfast; feces have accumulated during the night and food eaten stimulates peristalsis. Nursing data collection determines the *frequency* (how often) and *regularity* (intervals between stools) of an individual client's bowel movements. Document if the client reports a change in the frequency, regularity, or characteristics of stools. For example, a change in bowel habits is one of the warning signs of cancer. It is important to remember that not everyone has a bowel movement daily. If the person is symptom-free, bowel movements occurring less often are not a cause for concern, especially in older clients.

Flatus

Intestinal gas is called flatus (flay'-tus); the condition of expelling excess intestinal gas is *flatulence*. The normal intestine creates gas during the digestive process. Most flatus is reabsorbed through the vasculature of the intestinal wall; some is expelled with defecation. Some people develop and retain gas in uncomfortable amounts. Certain foods, such as broccoli, beans, cauliflower, and very spicy foods often cause excess gas to form and may accumulate and cause discomfort. Flatulence can often be avoided by use of a medication, such as simethicone.

Abdominal Signs and Symptoms

Data collection includes specific examination of the abdomen, particularly if the client reports pain or discomfort and/or changes in bowel habits.

- First, listen (*auscultate*) for bowel sounds (**BS**) in each quadrant of the abdomen. The action of peristalsis, which causes products of digestion to move through the intestine, creates distinctive sounds that can be heard with a stethoscope. *Diminished* or *absent* sounds indicate that the bowel is functioning improperly. Report and document such findings immediately. In Practice: Nursing Care Guidelines 51-2 describes listening for bowel sounds. Table 51-2 describes and identifies documentation of bowel sounds. *Rationale: Listen before doing anything else. Palpation can disturb bowel sounds.*
- After auscultating for bowel sounds, gently *palpate* the client's abdomen. Normally, the abdomen is soft and pliable. If the abdomen is hard, swollen, or tender, the client may have flatus, fecal impaction, or an intestinal obstruction.
- Document and report any changes or unusual discomfort that you observe or the client mentions.

ASSISTING WITH TOILETING

Elimination is a function included in "activities of daily living" when describing a client's independence level. Helping the client with elimination is a basic nursing

TABLE 51-2 Description of Bowel Sounds

WHAT IS HEARD	WHAT IS DOCUMENTED
Audible: Rate 4–32 times/min; no abnormal sounds	BS+ (audible bowel sounds in all quadrants; rate within normal limits)
Decreased and soft: hypoactive; occurs <4 times/min	BS↓ (decreased bowel sounds)
Increased and rapid: hyperactive; loud and high pitched; occurring >32 times/min	BS↑ (hyperactive bowel sounds)
Inaudible: no movement heard after listening for at least 5 min	BS− (bowel sounds absent or inaudible)

Bowel sounds are normally the same in all four quadrants of the abdomen. If this is not true, record the sound in each quadrant, e.g., BS↓ (left upper quadrant).

IN PRACTICE
NURSING CARE GUIDELINES 51-2 — Listening for Bowel Sounds

- Wash hands and position the client in a supine position (on the back). Gloves are usually not necessary. Expose the abdomen, but keep other areas of the client's body covered. *Rationale: This position allows access to the majority of the abdomen. Maintain the client's privacy, as much as possible.*
- Warm the stethoscope in your hands. *Rationale: The shock of a cold stethoscope can temporarily halt bowel sounds.*
- Place the flat side (diaphragm) of the stethoscope against the client's abdomen. Imagine the abdomen to be divided into four quadrants or regions (Fig. 15-5). Begin in a particular quadrant each time you do this procedure. Continue in a clockwise fashion around the abdomen.
- Always use the same pattern. *Rationale: The diaphragm offers coverage of a larger area than the bell and helps to detect high-pitched sounds. Following a specific pattern promotes efficiency and helps to remember to listen to each area. This improves your chances of hearing all bowel sounds.*
- Listen to peristalsis, which makes bubbling, gurgling, or clicking sounds that vary in intensity, frequency, and pitch. The sounds usually occur about every 5–20 s. (The normal range is approximately 4–32 sounds per minute.) One bowel sound may last for several seconds. Continue to listen. If sounds are difficult to hear, listen for at least 5 min before concluding that sounds are absent. *Rationale: Substances, including gas, are formed during normal digestion and peristalsis. The sounds are these substances (gases, wastes, and food substances) moving within the intestines via peristalsis. Sometimes, peristaltic movements pause or there is a minimum of gas for a short time.*
- Bowel sounds are described as *audible*, *hypoactive*, *hyperactive*, or *inaudible* (Table 51-2). If you are unable to hear bowel sounds or if they are very slow or very fast, this often indicates a serious condition and must be reported *immediately*. (Hyperactive bowel sounds may indicate diarrhea or early bowel obstruction. Hypoactive [or absent] bowel sounds often occur after abdominal surgery, in late bowel obstruction or paralytic ileus, and are often affected by spinal cord trauma.) Other sounds may be heard but are beyond the scope of this book. *Rationale: It is important to communicate clearly, so proper diagnosis and treatment can take place. A situation such as bowel obstruction can be life threatening.*
- Wash or sanitize your hands and document your findings. Report critical information to the provider. *Rationale: Documentation provides communication about the client's intestinal motility and enhances continuity of care.*

CHAPTER 51 Elimination

Giving and Removing a Bedpan or Urinal

Male clients confined to bed use a *bedpan* for defecation and a *urinal* for voiding. Female clients use the bedpan for both; a *female urinal* is also available, but not frequently used. Always wear gloves when working with bedpans or urinals. In Practice: Nursing Procedure 51-1 lists the steps for giving and removing a bedpan. Bedpans and urinals are disposable and discarded when the client no longer needs them. **Rationale:** *This helps prevent the spread of infection.*

> **Nursing Alert** Be sure to check whether a urine or stool specimen is required before assisting a client with a bedpan or urinal.

The Bedpan

A bedpan is a shallow disposable vessel of plastic or nylon resin, used for urination and defecation by clients confined to bed (Fig. 51-2). A child's bedpan is smaller than the standard size. Use a pediatric bedpan or fracture pan for an adult who requires complete assistance or who is unable to lie on the larger pan. A *fracture bedpan (fracture pan)* is smaller and shallower than a full size bedpan and has one flat end (Fig. 51-2B). This type of pan is intended for clients with fractured hips, those who are recovering from hip replacement or repair, or clients who are in skeletal traction or full body casts. However, this pan may be used for any client unable to raise the hips high enough or to roll over enough to get onto a standard-sized bedpan.

> **Nursing Alert** Remember that getting onto a bedpan in bed can be very difficult. Also remember that the fracture pan holds less and spills more easily than does the standard bedpan. Be sure to place a pad under the pan, to protect the bed.

Help the client as needed to get onto a bedpan. Provide as much privacy as possible; otherwise, the client may be unable to relax enough to void or defecate. If a client is confused or unable to follow directions, stay with the person. A full bladder is uncomfortable. Offer a bedpan or urinal to the client before meals and visiting hours and when they settle for the night. Avoid keeping a client waiting for a bedpan; holding urine or feces weakens sphincter tone and is physically and emotionally distressing. If a client does not have prompt attention before or after using the bedpan, they may try to walk to the bathroom alone and fall, may upset the bedpan, or may be incontinent in bed.

The Urinal

When the client asks to use the urinal, encourage them to position it themselves. If necessary, help the client to position the urinal (In Practice: Nursing Procedure 51-1). If allowed, the client may stand at the bedside to void.

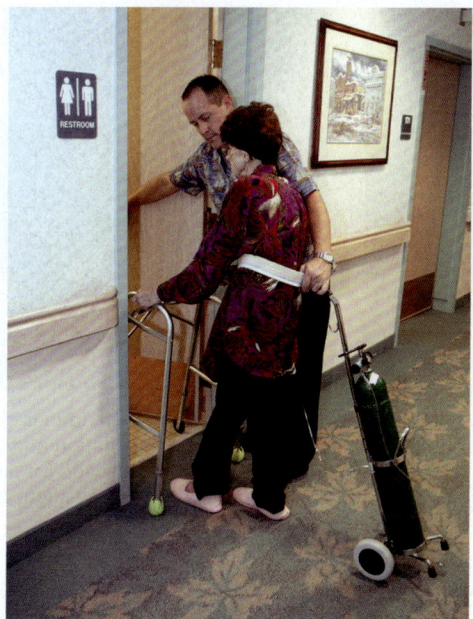

Figure 51-1 The client who is weak or who has several pieces of equipment will usually need help to walk to the bathroom. The nurse's fingers are firmly grasped under the bottom of the transfer belt. (Carter, 2016.)

responsibility. Various nursing interventions to assist the client with either bowel or bladder elimination may be called *toileting*.

Helping the Client to the Bathroom

The client who is weak, confused, sedated, extremely tired, or attached to medical equipment may require help getting to and from the bathroom (Fig. 51-1).

Important factors to remember are as follows:

- The client must have bathroom privileges (**BRPs**).
- Check to see if *I&O* are being recorded.
- Place a measuring "hat" under the toilet seat if urine is to be collected for measurement or testing (Chapter 52 and Fig. 52-2).
- Use a transfer belt if the client is at all unsteady.
- Help the client with locating the bathroom and opening the door.
- Move any apparatus, such as an oxygen tank, IV, or blood pressure monitor for the client. Make sure none of the equipment is tipped over or tangled.
- Encourage the client to use their own walker or cane.
- Make sure the client wears firm shoes with nonskid soles.
- Explain all procedures.
- Show the client how to use the signal light in the bathroom or give the client a signal pager, to call for help.
- Check back with the client frequently.

> **Nursing Alert** Be aware that some toilets, particularly wall-mounted toilets, have a weight restriction, often about 400 lb. If your client is heavier than this, an alternate (bariatric) toilet must be used.

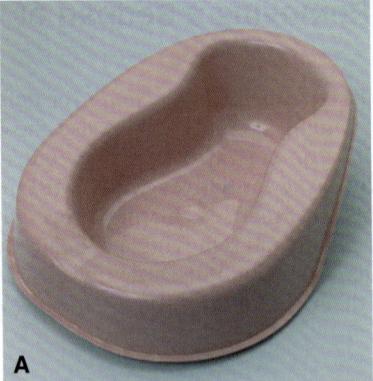 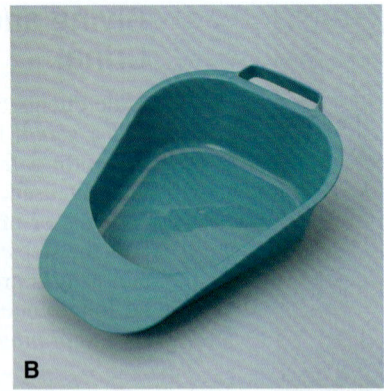 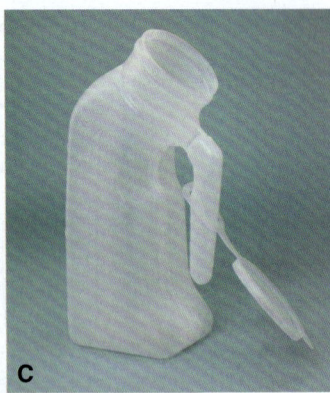

A **B** **C**

Figure 51-2 Bedpans are used for the client in bed (see Nursing Procedure 51-1). **A.** The standard (conventional) bedpan is similar to a toilet seat and is used when the client cannot get out of bed. It is used for defecation in men and for both urination and defecation in women. **B.** The fracture pan is small; it is used when the client cannot use a larger bedpan. It is sometimes used for a child as well. (A, B: Lynn, 2015.) **C.** Men who cannot go to the bathroom to urinate can use the urinal. It can be used while the client is standing or lying in bed (Nursing Procedure 51-1). (C: Carter, 2016.)

> **Key Concept**
> Rinse bedpans and urinals in cool to warm water. Hot water will cause the proteins in waste products to coagulate. Always wear gloves when handling bedpans or urinals. Make sure the client has an opportunity to wash their hands after elimination.

Helping the Client to Use a Commode

The Bedside Commode

The client may find it difficult to urinate or defecate when using a bedpan. This client may be able to use a bedside commode (Fig. 51-3B). Wear gloves when helping the client to the commode. Transfer the person from the bed to the commode as you would from the bed to any chair (Chapter 48). Stay with the client if there is any chance that they will become light-headed or dizzy. Be sure to provide privacy. The procedure for using and cleaning a commode is the same as that for a bedpan. Wash the client's hands, note the contents of the commode container, discard the urine or feces, rinse the commode container after use, properly dispose of gloves, and wash your hands. If the commode cannot be kept out of sight, it may be closed and kept at the bedside. However, it is best to keep it in the bathroom.

The Raised Toilet Seat or Over-Toilet Commode

Sometimes, it is difficult for the client to use a regular toilet. A raised commode can be placed over the toilet; therefore, the client does not have to bend as far and can use the handrails for support when sitting or standing (Fig. 51-3A). The toilet is then flushed, eliminating the need to clean a commode. Assist the client as necessary.

> **Key Concept**
> Make sure the client has the call signal or pager and toilet paper nearby when using the bedpan, commode, or bathroom. This will help protect the client from falling and help prevent spills.

> **NCLEX Alert**
> As you read the NCLEX clinical situations, you need to be aware of your role as a member of the healthcare team in teaching and assisting the client in their toileting activities.

ASSISTING WITH URINARY ELIMINATION

The Client Requiring a Urinary Catheter

A **urinary catheter** is a tube inserted in the bladder to drain urine. (Latex is not often used because of allergies.) It is approximately 24 in. long and is inserted into the bladder through the urethra, using sterile technique (Chapter 57). A *straight catheter* is inserted, urine drained, and the catheter removed and discarded (Fig. 51-4A). A *retention catheter* (*indwelling catheter*) is inserted, anchored in place, and continuously drains urine from the bladder. It is placed when a client is unable to void naturally or has had certain types of surgery. Several types of indwelling catheters are available, but the *Foley catheter* is most frequently used (Fig. 51-4B). This catheter usually has two tube-like *lumens* within it. One is connected to a balloon that is inflated inside the bladder and plugged, to anchor the catheter in place. Another lumen drains the urine. The distal end of the catheter is attached to a drainage bag for urine collection. Some catheters have a third lumen to provide a means for continuous bladder irrigation. (This may be used following bladder or prostate surgery.)

> **Nursing Alert** *Never remove a retention (indwelling) catheter without an order.* If it should fall out, report this immediately. A new, sterile catheter must be inserted, or the retention catheter may be discontinued if the client is now able to void. Be sure to report immediately if a client is pulling on a retention catheter.

The Suprapubic Catheter

In some cases, a catheter is inserted via a very small incision (a "stab wound") through the lower abdominal wall above the symphysis pubis and into the urinary bladder (Fig. 51-4C). This is called a *suprapubic* (**SP**) catheter ("supra" means above; "pubic" refers to the pubic bone in the pelvis). This catheter is held in place by a balloon, much like the Foley catheter, or by a hook-type device, or mushroom apparatus. A dressing or adhesive is often applied around the

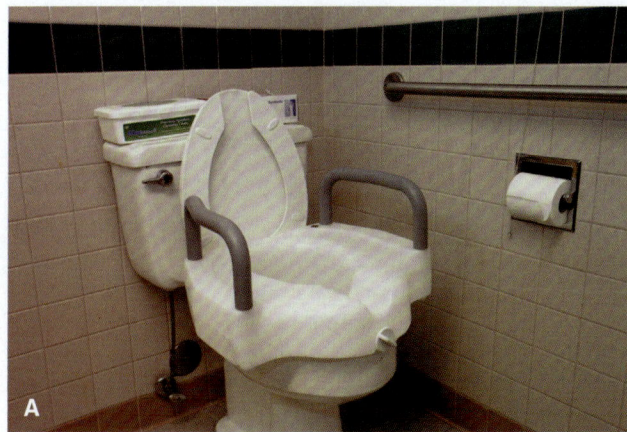
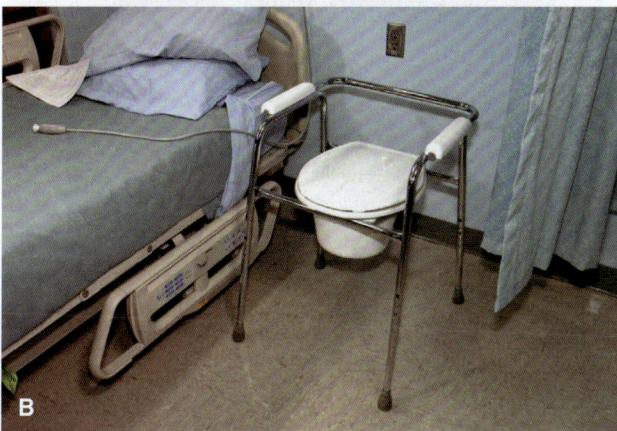

Figure 51-3 **A.** A commode seat fitted over a toilet. This apparatus makes it easier and safer to sit and stand up again because the seat is raised and handrails are attached. **B.** A bedside commode. In some cases, this type of commode is disguised inside a chair. (Carter, 2016.)

insertion site, to prevent leakage. A stitch may also be placed to secure the catheter to the skin and prevent it from migrating out or into the bladder. The SP catheter is connected to a urine drainage bag identical to the indwelling catheter bag (Fig. 51-5). The nurse cares for this catheter as well as the wound site. Indications for suprapubic catheter use include many types of gynecologic or urologic surgery when urine could contaminate the wound. In this case, the SP catheter is placed in the operating room. In the event of a spinal cord injury that prohibits normal bladder function, a permanent suprapubic catheter may be placed. When the postoperative client begins to regain bladder function, it is not unusual for normal voiding to take place with this catheter in place. This is often promoted in preparation for removal of the catheter (Chapter 89). This catheter may be clamped before removal, to ensure that the client will be able to void normally.

Inserting the Catheter

Chapter 57 describes the technique for inserting a catheter, a sterile procedure that must be performed with utmost care, to avoid introducing bacteria into the client's bladder. Indwelling catheters have been a major cause of hospital-acquired infections, and many protocols are in place to prevent these infections. Most retention catheters are packaged with a continuous tubing and drainage bag, to avoid contamination. The bag is lightweight and hung on the bed frame, but it can easily be

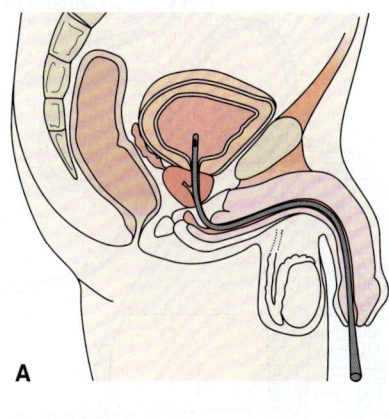
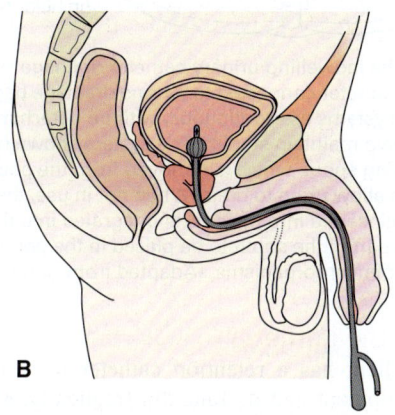
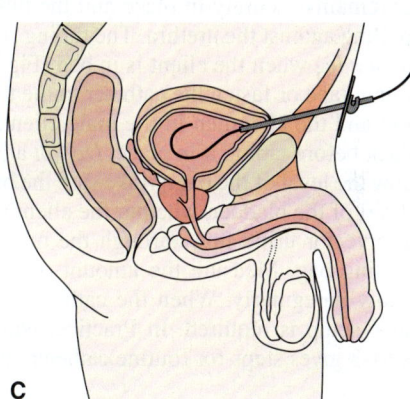

Figure 51-4 Types of catheters. **A.** Straight. **B.** Foley (retention or indwelling). Note the inflated balloon inside the bladder. **C.** Suprapubic. The client can be retrained to void normally with this catheter in place. (Adapted from Carter, 2016.)

fastened to an IV pole or wheelchair or held by the client while they are out of bed (Nursing Care Guidelines 51-3). Any closed urine drainage system collection bag must never be higher than the level of the client's bladder. *Rationale: Raising the bag could cause urine in the bag to flow back into the bladder, possibly leading to infection.*

Nursing Alert Many clients and healthcare workers are developing *latex sensitivity*. Be sure to ask about latex allergy before inserting a catheter. If the client is allergic to latex, use a vinyl or other latex-free catheter.

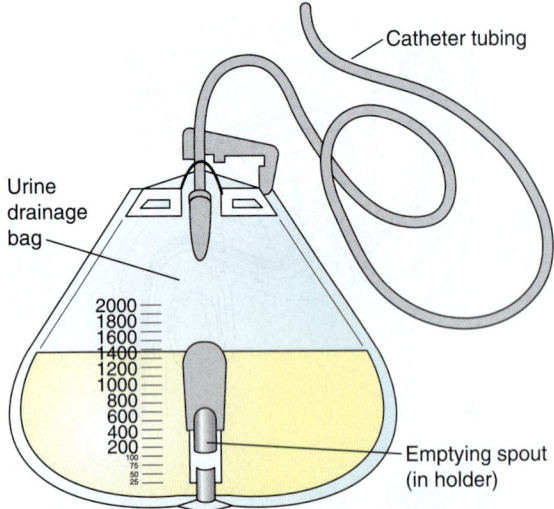

Figure 51-5 The indwelling urinary catheter drainage system consists of a catheter connected to a urine drainage bag by tubing. Most systems are continuous, with no detachable connections, to help maintain sterility. The system shown here has an emptying spout, which is removed from the pocket and unclamped to allow urine to drain. When not in use, the emptying spout is reinserted into the pocket integrated into the bag. Do not touch the part of the spout to be placed in the pocket, to minimize spread of microorganisms. (Adapted from Carter, 2016.)

Caring for the Catheter

When the client has a retention catheter in place, check both the equipment and its function frequently. Make sure the catheter remains securely in place and the tubing is not kinked or pulling against the urethra. The tubing should pass *over the client's leg* when the client is in bed (Fig. 51-6). To prevent pulling, tape or fasten the catheter to the thigh in the female client and the abdomen in the male client, allowing for some slack before taping it in place. *Do not* allow tubing to hang below the level of the bag. Make sure the bag is hung below the level of the bladder, whether the client is in or out of bed. Observe for urine flow through the tubing leading to the collecting bag. Measure the amount of urine in the bag and empty it regularly. When the catheter is changed, an entire new setup is required. In Practice: Nursing Care Guidelines 51-3 gives steps for routine catheter care.

Emptying the Urinary Drainage Bag

Emptying the drainage bag is done, while maintaining the sterility of the closed system. In Practice: Nursing Procedure 51-2 describes this procedure. (In Practice: Nursing Procedure 52-5 describes obtaining a specimen from a urinary catheter.)

Irrigating the Catheter

Catheters may be irrigated, to ensure patency and remove clots or debris that may obstruct free urinary flow. Irrigation is a sterile procedure and requires a *specific order* from the primary provider (Chapter 57).

> **Nursing Alert** Any catheter placed in the urinary bladder is a potential source of infection. The catheter must be inserted using sterile technique. In addition, care must be taken to maintain the integrity of the sterile system and prevent contamination.

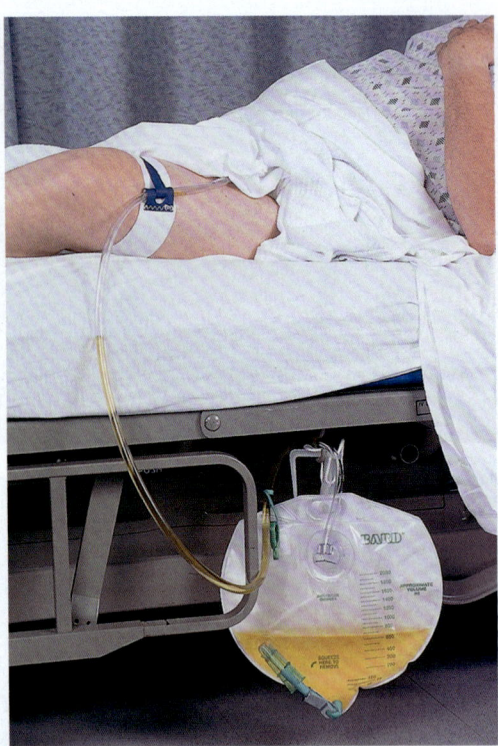

Figure 51-6 A urinary catheter in place. The drainage bag must be *below the level of the bladder*. The tubing above the bag is firmly anchored on the client's leg and should not be allowed to hang below the level of the bag. (Timby, 2005.)

Using External Catheter Systems

An *external catheter* or *condom catheter* is a noninvasive approach to managing urinary incontinence in the client. The elastic rubberized sheath is applied to the penis, much like a condom is applied. The sheath is attached to a urinary drainage bag and allows urine to flow out of the penis into the bag. The nurse should monitor the client closely for any associated complications. Some condom catheters are self-adhesive, and some require the application of elastic adhesive tape. Follow the manufacturer's instructions for application (In Practice: Nursing Care Guidelines 51-4). The drainage bag for the external catheter is either a large drainage bag similar to that used with a retention catheter or a small, supple plastic bag that the client wears strapped to the leg (Fig. 51-7). The smaller bags, called leg bags, have an outlet at the lower end, which is opened to drain urine. This drainage system is considered *clean*, not sterile. When caring for the client with a leg bag:

- Teach the client to care for the bag, if possible.
- Open the drainage port at the bottom to allow urine to drain out. Swab with antiseptic to limit transfer of microorganisms; this is done several times a day.
- Remove the catheter from the bag connection daily and swab the connections with antiseptic.
- At least once each day, disconnect the leg bag. Wash the bag in warm (not hot) soapy water, rinse it thoroughly, and hang it to dry. When dry, reattach it to the catheter. If the client is incontinent, two bags are often used, so one can be worn while the other is being cleaned. (Daily washing and rinsing are necessary, to remove urine and to avoid odor.)

IN PRACTICE
NURSING CARE GUIDELINES 51-3 — Performing Catheter Care

- A catheter is used only when absolutely necessary. Only trained personnel, using strict aseptic technique, should do the catheterization procedure. *Rationale: Catheterization is an invasive technique and is performed using sterile technique because the bladder and urinary system are considered sterile.*
- Ensure that the catheter drainage system is maintained as a closed sterile system. Be sure to maintain the integrity of the system. Do not disconnect any part of the system, except to drain urine from the bottom. *Rationale: It is important to make sure the bag and tubing are intact, to prevent infection. Disconnecting the tubing would break the integrity of the closed system.*
- Wash hands and wear gloves when working with catheters. *Rationale: Handwashing and using gloves help prevent the spread of infection, especially when working with body fluids.*
- Do not irrigate catheters, unless the provider specifically orders irrigation. *Rationale: Irrigation may introduce pathogens into the sterile system.*
- If the client ambulates, make sure the bag is taken along and is kept below the level of the bladder. *Rationale: Urine is produced continuously and must be collected. It is important to prevent urine backflow into the bladder, which could lead to infection.*
- Obtain sterile urine specimens from most catheter drainage systems by using a syringe and needleless cannula and aspirating from the designated specimen port. Be sure to cleanse the port with an antiseptic agent (In Practice: Nursing Procedure 52-5). Other specimens may be obtained from the bag-emptying plug at the bottom of the bag. However, this specimen is not as accurate and cannot be used for a urine culture. *Rationale: If a culture is to be done, all possible precautions should be taken to prevent contamination of the sample.*
- Secure the catheter externally to the thigh or leg. *Rationale: Properly securing the catheter prevents pressure and irritation (trauma) to the urethral meatus and prevents the catheter from being pulled out.*
- Cleanse the urethral meatus and the first 3–4 in. of exposed catheter twice a day with mild soap and water, or as ordered. When cleansing, wipe from the meatal opening outward. More frequent cleansing may be necessary to remove secretions. Also, cleanse the perineal area and be sure to rinse the area well. (Materials, such as powder, are usually not recommended because they may increase the risk of pathogenic growth, may damage the delicate skin, and may damage the catheter.) However, a specific perineal cleanser may be ordered (Chapter 58). *Rationale: Cleansing the meatal area and catheter helps prevent infection. Urine contains many microbes and is acidic. This may contribute to skin breakdown.*
- An antimicrobial ointment may be applied to the meatal area after the cleansing, per agency protocol. *Rationale: This can help prevent infection.*
- Check the drainage tubing for the presence of urine. Absence of draining urine can indicate obstruction or other serious problem. *Rationale: Observation of urine flow ensures proper functioning of the drainage system and allows for early identification of problems, should any arise. Urine retention or anuria is a sign of a serious disorder.*

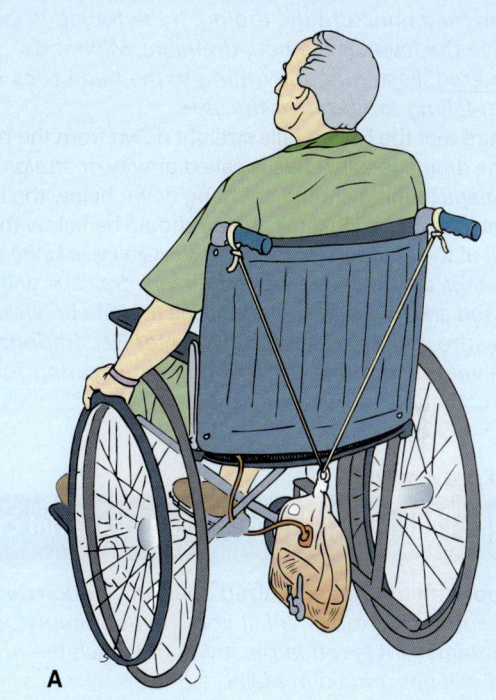

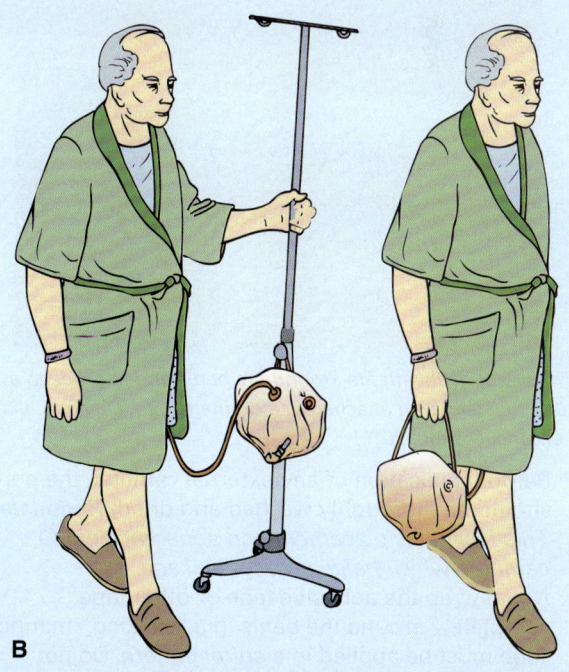

Techniques for suspending a drainage system below the bladder: **(A)** *wheelchair client;* **(B)** *ambulating client with and without an intravenous (IV) pole. (Timby, 2013.)*

NURSING CARE GUIDELINES 51-3 Performing Catheter Care (Continued)

- Position the tubing over the client's leg, not under it. *Rationale: The weight of the client's leg might slow or stop drainage.*
- Allow some slack in the tubing above the bed level. Fasten excess tubing to the bed. Do not use pins. Tape may be wrapped around the catheter, forming a tab, which can be pinned to the bed. *Rationale: Slack in the tubing allows the client to turn in bed. A pin may puncture the tubing. If the tubing is loose above the level of the bed, drainage will not be impaired. Fastening the tubing to the bed keeps it from falling too far over the side.*
- Ensure that the tubing falls straight down from the bed to the drainage bag. (This is called gravity or *straight drainage.*) Tubing should not hang down below the level of the bag, or be kinked. The bag should be below the level of the bladder. *Rationale: If the tubing is kinked or hangs down, or the bag is too high, drainage will be slowed and infection can occur due to urine backflow.*
- Measure and record output (Chapter 52). *Rationale: The volume of urine is important when caring for the catheterized person.*
- Observe the color, quality, and characteristics of the urine in the tubing and in the drainage bag. Report and document any significant findings. *Rationale: The freshly eliminated urine in the tubing has a truer color and more valid characteristics than does urine that may have been in the bag for some time. Sediments may have precipitated out while the urine was in the bag, and usually this urine will become cloudy or darker in color* (Table 51-1).
- Note the client's body temperature. *Rationale: Fever usually accompanies infection.*
- Dispose of gloves properly and wash hands after catheter care. *Rationale: Proper glove disposal and handwashing are important in reducing the risk for infection transmission.*
- Document all information properly. NOTE: Report any unusual findings, including severe pain or discomfort from the catheter, immediately. *Rationale: Documentation and prompt reporting ensure communication among healthcare team members and appropriate client care.*

IN PRACTICE
NURSING CARE GUIDELINES 51-4 Using External Catheter Systems

- Choose an appropriate-sized condom. *Rationale: If the condom is too small, it could cause circulatory problems; if it is too large, it will not catch the urine and will not remain in place.*

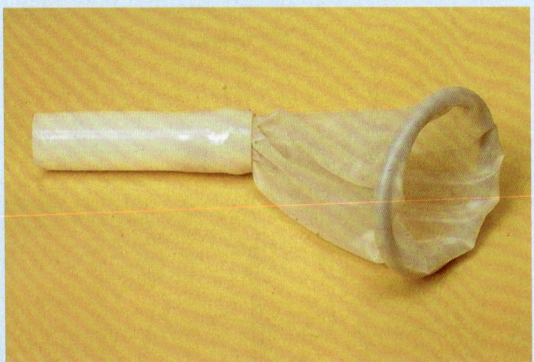

The condom sheath fits around the penis and attaches to a tube that is in turn attached to a drainage bag. (Taylor, Lillis, Lemone, & Lynn, 2011.)

- Before application of any external catheter, the penis should be thoroughly washed and dried. *Rationale: This facilitates placement and adherence of the catheter, which helps prevent leakage.*
- *Never* wrap the adhesive tape or other tape completely around the penis in a "choking" manner. Tape must be applied in a *spiral pattern*. Do not apply tape too tightly. *Rationale: These procedures help prevent circulatory problems.*
- Allow about 1 in. (2.5 cm) of space from the opening of the urethra to the end of the condom. *Rationale: This provides space to accommodate the flow of urine and to prevent it from backing up toward the base of the penis.*
- Check the catheter and the circulation in the penis at least every 4 hr. *Rationale: Look for leakage of urine and discomfort. Make sure the tape or the condom is not too tight.*
- Most facilities require that the catheter be changed every 24 hr. *Rationale: This helps prevent irritation and infection.*
- Inspect the skin thoroughly and provide perineal hygiene before the application of each new catheter. Be sure all old adhesive is removed. *Rationale: This provides for cleanliness, minimizes odor, and helps the new catheter to stay in place.*

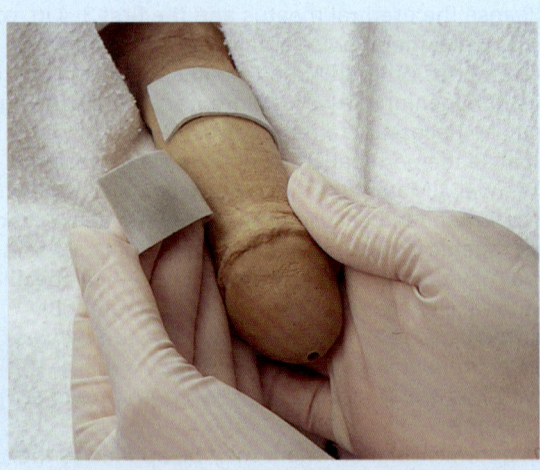

When wrapping adhesive or tape around the penis, always wrap in a spiral fashion, to prevent circulatory problems.

NURSING CARE GUIDELINES 51-4 Using External Catheter Systems (Continued)

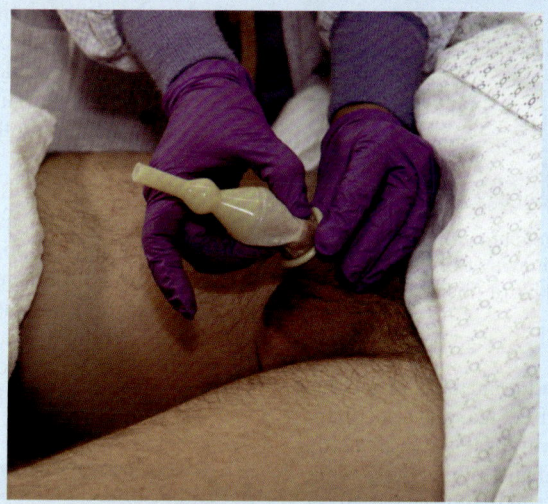

The condom is applied, leaving space between the tip of the penis and the end of the condom sheath. The outflow tubing is attached to a collection bag. (Evans-Smith, 2005.)

- If adhesive tape is used to hold the catheter in place, rotate the position of the strip. Be sure to use nonallergenic tape. **Rationale:** *This prevents irritation to areas where the tape was used before.*

Urinary Incontinence

Urinary incontinence (uncontrolled leakage) is a condition that may occur as people age, particularly in clients who have given birth as a result of childbirth trauma. Many other factors can contribute to incontinence. Unmanaged incontinence limits, in large part, the activities the client can participate in. The goal of treatment is to reduce or eliminate incontinent episodes and allow the client as normal a life as possible. The establishment of continence, or management of incontinence, is a key factor in determining where a client may be able to live. Managing bowel and bladder function can enable an individual to live independently. However, an individual who is unable to control this function may find it necessary to live in a long-term care facility.

Bladder incontinence is more difficult to control than bowel incontinence, but many clients can establish control. Plenty of fluids and exercise are important. Adequate fluid intake helps prevent urinary stasis and thus helps prevent infections. Incontinent episodes may occur during the training period. Reassure the client. Keep a careful record of I&O to maintain a balance and ensure that urine is not being retained. Complete bladder control is not achieved by every client, but many do accomplish it. Bladder control is important because a permanent catheter greatly increases the risk of bladder infection. In addition, urinary continence adds to self-esteem and enhances self-care. The goal is to keep the client as dry and comfortable as possible, while working toward bladder control (Chapter 89). For the male client who is incontinent, the external catheter can be used; a similar device is not available for women. However, women can wear a perineal pad or use a disposable incontinent brief, such as Depends (Fig. 51-8B). An external incontinence guard is also available for men (Fig. 51-8A). Change the pad or brief frequently, to minimize exposure of the skin to urine and reduce odor, gently washing and thoroughly rinsing the perineal area between changes. (Disposable wipes are available and are handy when the client is not home.) Check the skin frequently for signs of breakdown.

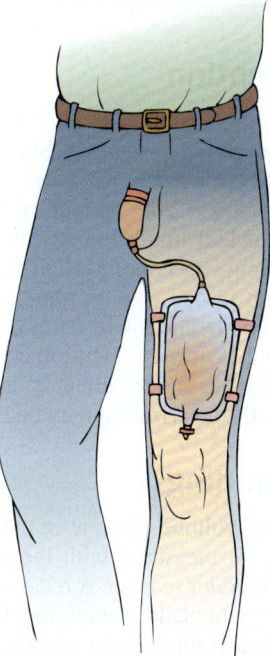

Figure 51-7 A leg bag may be used by male or female clients. It collects urine from a catheter, but it is concealed under clothing. This type of bag can be worn with either an external or indwelling catheter system. The bottom plug must be kept firmly closed, to prevent leakage.

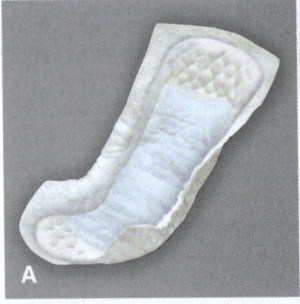 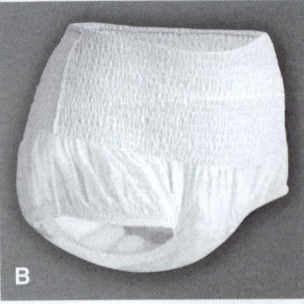

Figure 51-8 Incontinence pads and briefs are worn under clothing to absorb moisture and keep it away from the body. **A.** Depend Guards for men. **B.** Depend Extra Absorbency Underwear. (Carter, 2008.)

Foods that irritate the bladder and contribute to incontinence include caffeine (including coffee, tea, and chocolate), decaffeinated soda, carbonated beverages, alcohol, acidic fruits (e.g., oranges, lemons, grapefruit, pineapple), tomatoes and tomato-based products (e.g., barbeque sauce, pizza, red spaghetti sauce), spicy foods (e.g., Mexican, Indian, Thai, Cajun), milk products (e.g., cheese, yogurt, ice cream), sugar (including corn syrup, honey, and fructose), and artificial sweeteners (particularly aspartame).

> **Nursing Alert** Do not limit fluids for the client who is incontinent. This promotes concentrated urine, which is irritating to the bladder wall and the perineal area. This can cause more frequent urination and UTIs, increasing the incontinence.

Bladder Retraining

Some types of incontinence may be controlled by establishing a voiding routine (Chapter 89). The specific routine is determined by the primary provider or an incontinence specialist. Begin by documenting when the client's bladder empties, to determine if there is a pattern. Either give the client a bedpan or help them to the bathroom just before these times, to help establish a routine. Gradually increase the time between voidings, thus increasing the tone of the client's bladder muscles and increasing the bladder's capacity. The bladder eventually becomes trained to empty at regular intervals. The client may need to wear a disposable pad during the training period. If after 1 year, this conservative mode of treatment is not effective, corrective surgery may be available. Medications are also available to help control incontinence. An implanted electronic device is sometimes used. A newer procedure involves the injection of Botox into the bladder wall. This needs to be repeated periodically. **Kegel exercises** are often recommended, to increase sphincter tone. The client is taught to tighten the pelvic floor and urethral sphincter and to hold this tightening for as long as 10 s (Chapter 91, In Practice: Educating the Client 91-3).

> **Key Concept**
> Side effects of the medications include extreme dry mouth and constipation and may require discontinuation of the medication. The Botox procedure may cause urinary retention.

Bladder Retraining With a Closed Drainage System

Bladder retraining may be started while the catheter is connected to the closed drainage system. The goal is to help the client regain the sensation to void by allowing the bladder to refill, causing the bladder muscles to stretch and signal the brain. In Practice: Nursing Procedure 51-3 describes bladder retraining by clamping the catheter.

Self-Catheterization

In some cases, such as a client with paraplegia, normal voiding may not be possible. In this case, the client may be taught to self-catheterize on a regular basis, to prevent incontinence and establish a bladder routine. In this case, the catheter is usually considered to be clean, rather than sterile. Most clients become very adept at this procedure and are able to avoid wearing a leg bag or disposable pads.

> **Nursing Alert** Many clients are released from the healthcare facility without having overcome incontinence. This then becomes a family concern. Aggressive client and family teaching is necessary. Demonstrate to them how to keep the client dry without changing the entire bed. Absorbent pads, covered by a liner, can be placed next to the skin. The pads can be changed easily, and the liner helps prevent irritation. Disposable pads on the bed or chair are used, when possible. If the client has established a routine for voiding, teach the family the importance of maintaining this routine. Explain and demonstrate the use of disposable incontinent briefs or absorbent pads. Heavy cloth pads that may be laundered and reused are available. Emphasize the importance of fluids, diet, and cleanliness. Make sure they know how to prevent skin breakdown.

Urinary Retention

Sometimes, a client is unable to void. This is common for a short time after receiving anesthesia. Sometimes, the client on bedrest cannot sufficiently relax the urinary sphincters when using the bedpan. This temporary retention may be relieved through several simple nursing measures. These are described in Nursing Procedure 51-1. If the female client is permitted to sit up in bed or on a commode, they may be able to void. The male client will be more likely to void if he is able to stand. If urinary retention continues, the bladder becomes distended, and the client is uncomfortable; this must be reported. Catheterization may be necessary.

Bladder Scanning

The **residual urine** (volume of urine in the bladder after the client voids) can be measured with the noninvasive ultrasound (Doppler) bladder scanner. A residual less than 50 mL is considered adequate bladder emptying. Generally, a residual over 50 mL in a young person or more than 50–100 mL in an older adult is considered significant. Residual over 150 mL may require catheterization or other interventions. (A significant residual urine volume indicates a bladder outlet obstruction or deficient contractility in the detrusor

IN PRACTICE
NURSING CARE GUIDELINES 51-5 Using the Ultrasound Bladder Scanner

- You will need gloves, ultrasound gel or a gel pad, alcohol wipes or other sanitizer, paper towel or tissues, and the scanner. *Rationale: Have all supplies ready.*
- Sanitize hands. Wear gloves. Identify the client and explain the procedure. Provide privacy. Have the client void as much as possible. Perform the scan immediately *Rationale: Standard precautions are followed. The client needs to know what is being done. The bladder should be as empty as possible for accuracy. Delay would alter the results.*
- Move the bed to a convenient height. Lower the near side rail and ask the client to lie on the back. Turn on the scanner and program it to "male" or "female." (For the posthysterectomy female, use the male setting.) Clean the scanner head with sanitizer. *Rationale: Prepare the client and the scanner.*
- Expose the abdomen and apply gel or the gel pad just above the symphysis pubis. Place the scanner head on the gel, with the cord end pointing toward the client's head. Press and release the scan button. Read the bladder volume on the scanner; print, if ordered. Wipe off the gel and make the client comfortable. Lower the bed and raise side rails. Clean the scanner head again. Wash hands and document the results. File the printed result, if ordered. *Rationale: Proper procedure must be followed for accurate results. Client comfort and safety are important. Accurate documentation guides the provider, if further action is needed.*

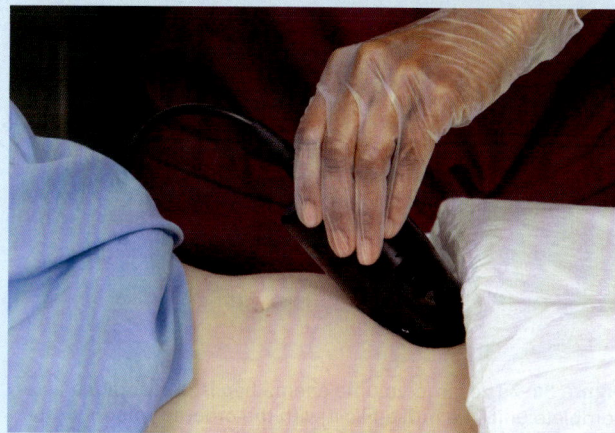

After applying gel, position the scanner just above the symphysis pubis, with the directional bladder icon pointing so the bladder image is centered on the crossbars of the scanner console. (Lynn, 2015.)

---

muscles—muscles that push down.) The amount of residual urine to be considered significant is determined by the healthcare provider. In Practice: Nursing Care Guidelines 51-5 briefly describe bladder scanning. In-service training is required for each specific scanner.

ASSISTING WITH BOWEL ELIMINATION

Changes in bowel function may result in fecal retention, either short term (*constipation*) or long term, resulting in *fecal impaction* or *bowel obstruction*. When monitoring bowel function, identify the client who has not had a recent bowel movement and determine if they require nursing intervention. The client's bowel movements are often documented. Normally, ingesting food creates peristaltic waves throughout the intestine that move feces from the colon into the rectum. The fecal mass stimulates rectal nerve endings, creating the urge to defecate. Ignoring this urge causes it to diminish and the feces become dry and hard, and defecation becomes difficult (constipation). The colon and rectum become distended and lose muscle tone as feces accumulate. This can lead to a bowel obstruction.

> **Nursing Alert** A bowel obstruction is life threatening and often requires surgery. It is most important to treat fecal impaction and/or constipation, to prevent obstruction.

Suppositories

Sometimes, the primary healthcare provider orders a rectal suppository to be given. The suppository is a bullet-shaped, soft waxlike mass inserted into a body opening for the purpose of administering a medication or lubricating the area. Suppositories can be administered rectally, vaginally, or into the urethra. The suppository melts after administration, releasing the medication or other substances. Sometimes, a suppository is given to soften stool and/or stimulate a bowel movement. Nursing Procedure 63-3 illustrates the procedure for administering a rectal suppository. (The procedure for administering a vaginal suppository is described in In Practice: Nursing Procedure 63-4.)

Enemas

An enema is the introduction of solution into the rectum and colon usually given to stimulate peristalsis, thereby causing elimination of stool. An enema may also be given to introduce medications or other therapeutic agents. In addition, enemas are often given before a procedure, such as colonoscopy or bowel surgery, to cleanse the bowel.

Two basic systems are used for most enema administration: the prepackaged disposable (small-volume) enema (e.g., Fleet enema) or a disposable (large-volume) enema bag with tubing (Fig. 51-9). Small-volume enemas generally contain 120–180 mL of a hypertonic solution. Large-volume bags may hold as much as 1,500 mL of solution. Both types

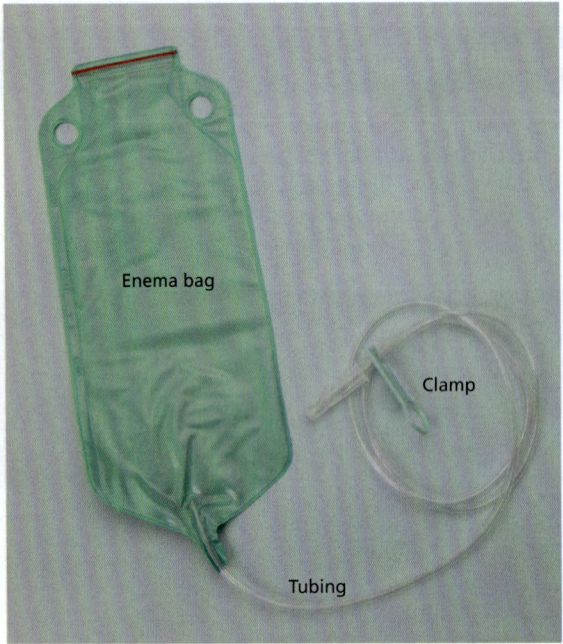

Figure 51-9 The large-volume enema bag is prepackaged as a complete unit. The nurse fills it with the ordered solution. After the enema is administered, the bag is discarded, per facility protocol. (Carter, 2016.)

have prelubricated tips, for ease and comfort of insertion; however, more lubricant may be added.

Nursing Alert Larger volumes of solution cause a forceful evacuation of the bowel or cause the client to strain and are contraindicated in conditions such as the follows:
- Increased intracranial pressure (ICP)
- Recent brain surgery or brain tumor
- Rectal prolapse (falling down of the rectum)
- Uterine prolapse
- Serious, unrepaired hernia
- Recent eye or ear surgery
- Recent rectal surgery
- Recent hemorrhage in any area of the body, including severe nosebleed
- Uncontrolled high blood pressure
- Other instances, as determined by the healthcare provider

Most commonly, an enema is given because the client is unable to empty the bowel naturally. The enema helps remove feces, but unless normal stimulation and regular defecation are established, the muscles could become weakened and the use of enemas could become necessary to achieve defecation. This situation should be avoided, if at all possible. A primary provider's order is required before giving an enema. The order states the type and frequency of enema administration. The order may be PRN (as needed) or scheduled. Before a surgical procedure or inspection of the rectum or lower colon (e.g., proctoscopy or colonoscopy), an order for "enemas until clear" may be written, if a colon-clearing laxative is not used. The small-volume Fleet-type enema is usually used in this case and may be safely and easily self-administered by the client or family.

Nursing Alert "Enemas until clear" indicates enema administration until the fluid returned is clear of fecal matter. Unless otherwise ordered, no more than 500 mL of solution should be administered at a time. In addition, no more than three consecutive enemas should be given. *Rationale: Too many enemas could cause severe fluid and/or electrolyte imbalance.*

Types of Enemas
Cleansing Enema
The *cleansing enema* is the instillation of enough fluid or of a specially formulated solution into the colon to help soften the feces, stimulate peristalsis, and provide lubrication in preparation for evacuation. The enema helps produce a bowel movement that empties the rectum and lower colon. The cleansing enema is given when the client is constipated or when the bowel must be emptied before surgery or a special procedure. Solutions most commonly used for the cleansing enema include tap water or normal saline. If other solutions are ordered, consult your facility protocol.

Nursing Alert When giving a tap water enema (TWE), be aware that tap water is hypotonic and may cause circulatory overload. Observe the client closely before administering the enema and monitor the client carefully for signs of circulatory overload (e.g., elevated blood pressure and/or bounding pulse) during and after the enema is given.

Commercially Prepared Small-Volume Enema (e.g., Fleet Enema)
This enema contains a small amount of hypertonic solution, usually saline, with 120 mL being the most common size. As a hypertonic solution, it pulls water from the colon tissue into the colon by osmosis. This adds liquid to soften hard stools and stimulates peristalsis and defecation. Effective evacuation usually results in approximately 10 min. This enema is useful for clients who are unable to retain larger quantities of fluid or who have anal incontinence. It also helps prevent fecal impaction in clients who must lie in one position or who are unable to sit. The Fleet enema is most frequently used as preparation for colon examinations or procedures. (Disposable Fleet-type enemas containing other special solutions are also available.)

Carminative Enema
The *carminative enema* is given to stimulate peristalsis so that flatus (gas) is expelled from the intestine, along with stool.

Anthelmintic Enema
Anthelmintic drugs help destroy intestinal parasites. Anthelmintic medications usually are given orally, but because they are toxic, some clients must have them administered rectally. In this instance, the solution containing the anthelmintic drug is usually instilled for *retention* (as long as the client is able to hold it).

IN PRACTICE
NURSING CARE GUIDELINES 51-6 Administering the Harris Flush

- Prepare the bag with the prescribed solution (usually warm tap water). *Rationale: A warm solution stimulates evacuation of gas.*
- Measure the client's abdominal girth before and after the procedure. *Rationale: This helps determine if gas was expelled and distention relieved.*
- Prepare and position the client as you would for any other enema; lubricate and insert the tube in the usual manner. (Be sure to clear the tubing of air, before inserting it into the rectum.) Wear gloves. *Rationale: Avoid adding air and increasing abdominal distention. Gloves help protect you from the highly contaminated feces.*
- Elevate the bag and instill a small amount of solution. Lower the bag, so that the solution flows back into the enema bag. Repeat several times. *Rationale: The in-and-out flow of fluid stimulates peristalsis.*
- If the solution becomes thickened with feces or if the tubing becomes clogged, replace the entire setup. *Rationale: It is important to allow free flow of the solution.*
- Be sure to dispose properly of gloves and wash your hands. *Rationale: Help prevent the spread of infection.*

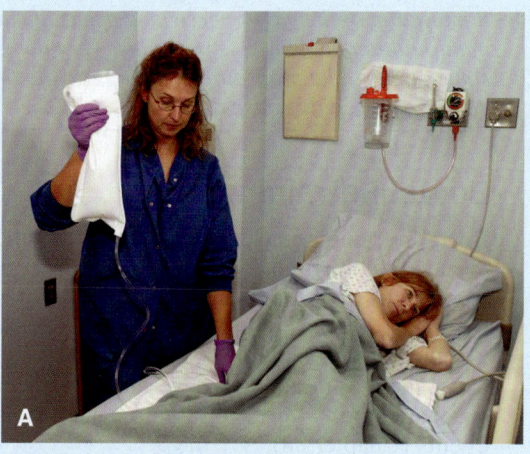
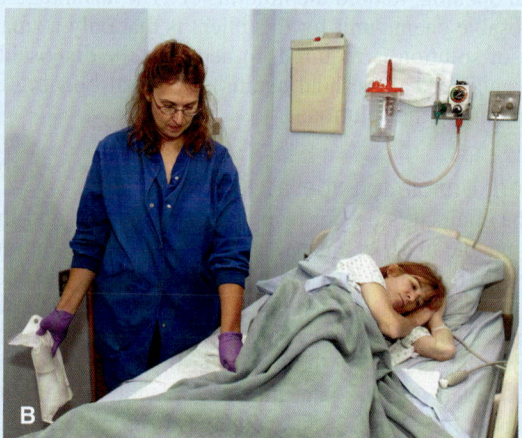

A. The bag is elevated above the client's hips and a small amount of fluid instilled into the colon. **B.** The bag is lowered, allowing the solution to run back into the bag. The process is repeated several times, stimulating peristalsis and allowing the client to expel flatus. (Evans-Smith, 2005.)

Emollient Enema
An *emollient enema* consists of a small amount of olive or cottonseed oil given to protect or soothe the mucous membrane of the colon. This enema is also to be retained.

Oil Retention Enema
The *oil retention enema* also contains a small amount of oil and is given in very small amounts because it must be retained to be effective. (Larger amounts stimulate bowel evacuation.) After retention, a bowel movement usually occurs. If this does not occur after several hours, it may be necessary to follow with a saline solution enema.

Medicated Enema
The *medicated enema* contains a drug to be administered rectally. Sometimes, this is the best way to give a medication to the client; the client may be vomiting, unconscious, or recovering from mouth or throat surgery. It may also be given rectally to cause immediate absorption; some drugs are rapidly absorbed by the colon's mucous membrane. Because this enema must be retained to ensure effective absorption, the drug is combined with a small amount of oil or saline, to reduce its irritating effect and to lessen the client's desire to expel it.

Key Concept
Encourage the client to hold an enema as long as possible before moving the bowels. Recommended times are as follows:
- Cleansing enema: 5–10 min
- Retention enema: 25–30 min
- Medicated enema: try not to expel

The Return-Flow Enema (Harris Flush)
The Harris flush is prescribed to relieve intestinal gas and distention, which causes pain. It is given with the bag-and-tubing equipment. The goal is to stimulate the expelling of flatus, thereby relieving abdominal distention and "gas pains." If the process is successful, the client will express relief from pain, and abdominal girth (distance around the abdomen) will be reduced. The process may cause the client to defecate as well. See In Practice: Nursing Care Guidelines 51-6 for the principles in administering the return-flow enema.

Administration of Enemas
See In Practice: Nursing Care Guidelines 51-7 for the principles underlying the administration of any type of enema. In Practice: Nursing Procedure 51-4 identifies specific steps to

use in administering an enema, using either a prepackaged small-volume enema or the bag-and-tubing method.

> **Nursing Alert** Never warm any enema in a microwave. *Rationale: It may explode, or the microwave may destroy the effectiveness of the solution.*

Special Circumstances

The Client Unable to Retain an Enema

If a client is unable to contract the anal sphincter muscles to hold a solution, place the client on the bedpan, commode, or toilet to administer the enema. If the client is in bed, elevate the head of the bed *slightly* and place a pillow in the lumbar region, to lessen back strain. In some cases, the enema tubing is passed through a ball, and the ball is held against the rectal opening, to hold the fluid inside. The advantage of the disposable enema unit for this client is that only a small quantity of solution is required. In addition, the disposable enema container can be held against the rectal opening to help in retaining the solution.

The Client Unable to Expel an Enema

When the sphincters do not respond to stimulation and the client is unable to expel an enema, the nurse must withdraw the solution. If using a bag-and-tubing setup, place the bedpan on a chair at the client's bedside, beneath the level of the rectum. (This procedure is performed in the same manner as lowering the bag in the Harris flush.) When the rectal tube is directed into the pan, the force of gravity helps to drain (siphon) the fluid. If an enema has been given with a Fleet-type enema, a rectal tube without a bag can be inserted into the rectum and the end of the rectal tube directed into a lowered bedpan. If this is not effective, consult the primary provider for further instructions.

Giving an Enema to a Client With Paralysis

Giving an enema requires a special approach if the person is paralyzed. Often, the client with paralysis is unable to retain the enema solution. If the client must have enemas regularly, give them at the same time every day. Later, a suppository at this time may be all that is necessary, to stimulate a bowel movement, until finally the client needs neither of these aids. Manual digital pressure to the abdomen or manual disimpaction may also be applied to assist this client with bowel evacuation (see following discussion).

Manual Removal of Impacted Feces

If a fecal impaction does not respond to an enema or if a client has paralysis, the provider may order manual or digital removal of the feces, a procedure known as *manual disimpaction* or *digital evacuation*. In Practice: Nursing Procedure 51-5 gives basic steps for digitally removing impacted feces. *Stop the procedure immediately* if the client complains of pain, faintness, or nausea, or if you note any untoward effect, such as bleeding. Usually, after the stool is broken into pieces, the client is able to expel it. The client may be given an enema for assistance. In some cases, you may remove the particles of feces after breaking up the stool. Remove the stool in as noninvasive a manner as possible.

> *Key Concept*
>
> In some cases, a client with paralysis is unable to establish a pattern of regular bowel evacuation, even after pursuing a bowel retraining program. In this case, the client performs their own manual disimpaction daily as a part of activities of daily living.

> **Nursing Alert** Digital removal of feces is contraindicated for most clients with cardiac conditions and after reproductive surgery, abdominoperineal repair, rectal surgery, colostomy, and genitourinary surgery. It is also contraindicated in clients who are receiving radioactive isotope therapy (especially in the abdominopelvic area) or perineal perfusion of anticancer drugs. Clients who have a bleeding tendency, especially in the rectal or vaginal area, should not receive this treatment, nor should pregnant women. *Rationale: Stimulation of the vagus nerve may occur during digital manipulation, making this procedure very dangerous for some clients. The procedure could aggravate an existing condition or could cause damage.*

Bowel Retraining

Bowel retraining may be necessary if the client is unable to have a bowel movement naturally or is incontinent of stool. This procedure is often used for the client with paralysis. Because the bowel responds to specific stimuli to function, natural means may be used to stimulate peristalsis. Some clients have an external colostomy, to evacuate stool. Bowel retraining can be helpful to these clients (Chapter 88).

These factors are helpful in bowel training:

Timing: The client is assisted with elimination at the same time each day.
Physical activity: The more exercise the client receives, the more likely it is that they will be able to achieve bowel control.
Fluid intake: A high oral fluid intake is recommended. The fluids should be varied, including water and fruit juices.
Diet: Recommended is a diet to assist in maintaining a fairly solid fecal consistency without causing constipation or diarrhea. Fruits and vegetables and foods high in fiber are often helpful. Probiotics may be helpful. Encourage the client to avoid foods that have caused loose stools and excess gas (flatus) in the past. If possible, assist the client to use the bathroom, rather than a bedpan or commode. *Rationale: Moving about helps stimulate a bowel movement, to achieve normalcy, and enhances the client's self-esteem.*

A successful bowel retraining program includes the steps listed in In Practice: Nursing Procedure 51-6. Always give the client positive reinforcement for any progress. Bowel retraining is a long process. However, some clients are never able to achieve full bowel continence.

Flatus

As stated previously, flatus is gas accumulated in the bowel, and expelling of gas is called flatulence. In some cases, the client is not able to expel flatus and the abdomen becomes

CHAPTER 51 Elimination

IN PRACTICE
NURSING CARE GUIDELINES 51-7 — Administering an Enema

The following guidelines apply, whether using the bag-and-tubing or the small-volume enema:

- Wash hands before and after giving an enema. Always wear gloves. A face shield may also be needed, if there is any chance of splashing fluids. *Rationale: Handwashing and wearing gloves, as well as other protective gear, help prevent the spread of microorganisms and protect the nurse. Feces are highly contaminated.*
- Check the package for the manufacturer's specific instructions for that type of enema. *Rationale: Each type of enema may have slightly different instructions.*
- Check to make sure the client does not have a latex allergy, or use a latex-free enema. *Rationale: If a latex-containing enema is used for a client with an allergy, a severe reaction may occur. (Most enemas are latex free.)*
- Know the correct *amount of solution* or size of enema to use, by reviewing the provider's order. If the client is a child, take the child's size into consideration (Nursing Procedure 51-4). *Rationale: Too much fluid could cause damage or discomfort.*
- Know what *type of enema solution* and type of enema to use. *Rationale: The client could be injured by receiving an incorrect type of enema or the wrong solution.*

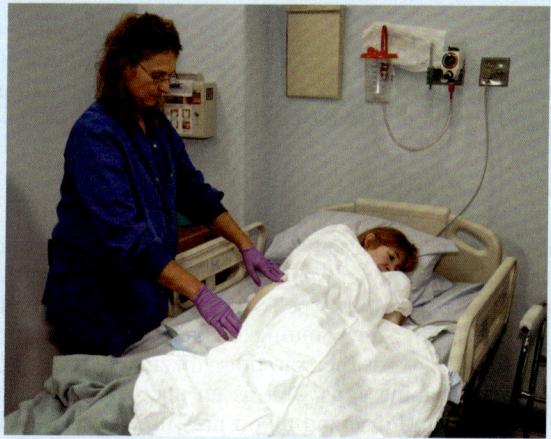

Ask the client to lie on the left side for most enemas. (Evans-Smith, 2005.)

- Store enemas and enema solutions at room temperature; never store them in a cold or hot place. Make sure the solution is just above body temperature before instillation. Use a thermometer, if possible. The temperature of the solution should not exceed 39 °C (102.2 °F). *A cold solution can cause intestinal cramping and could cause shock. It could also make it impossible for the client to relax enough to defecate. Excess heat could cause the solution to deteriorate and/or damage intestinal mucosa.*
- Ask the client to lie on the side (preferably the left—Sims position) for the cleansing enema, if possible. Place a waterproof pad under the client's buttocks. *Rationale: The colon's position within the body makes this position the most effective. A semi-Fowler position will cause solution leakage and the pad will protect the bed.*
- If the client is in traction or a cast, give the enema with the client supine (lying on the back). *Rationale: This is the next-best position for an enema. It is important not to injure this client by changing their position.*
- Place the client in a knee-chest (genupectoral) position for a retention enema (or rectal tube), if the client can tolerate this. *Rationale: This position encourages fluid retention for a longer period of time. (It is very difficult to give an enema effectively with the client sitting up.)*
- Drape the client, covering their body as much as possible. *Rationale: Preserves the client's privacy. This client will be more relaxed and more able to have good results from the enema.*
- Even though the tip of the enema or the tubing is prelubricated, lubricate it again. *Rationale: This will increase comfort for the client.*
- When using the bag-and-tubing method, clear the tube of air by opening the clamp until the solution flows. *Rationale: This avoids introduction of air into the colon, which could cause discomfort and reduce the amount of fluid the client can retain.*
- Use judgment to decide when to stop instilling fluid, based on the client's reactions. If the client complains of cramping, stop the instillation for a short time. *Rationale: Each person has a different limit for the amount of fluid they can retain.*
- Give the solution slowly. Instruct the client to retain the enema as long as possible. *Rationale: Both cleansing and retention enemas are held longer if given slowly. Longer retention enhances the enema's effectiveness.*
- Place a bedpan for the client or make sure they can get to the bedside commode or bathroom quickly. Make sure IVs and other equipment are out of the way. Be sure the signal cord or pager is within reach. Check back frequently with the client. *Rationale: Some clients may become weak or faint or may have difficulty getting to the bathroom. The client may need to get to the bathroom or commode quickly.*
- Offer the client the opportunity to wash their hands after the procedure is completed. Be sure to wash your hands thoroughly as well. Help the client to assume a comfortable position in bed or chair. *Rationale: Make the client comfortable and teach good hygiene habits.*
- Observe or ask the client about the results. *Rationale: It is important to determine if the enema was effective.*
- Document administration of the enema, the results, and the client's reactions. Document the type of solution used, its temperature, and the amount instilled. *Rationale: Documentation promotes communication and continuity of care.*

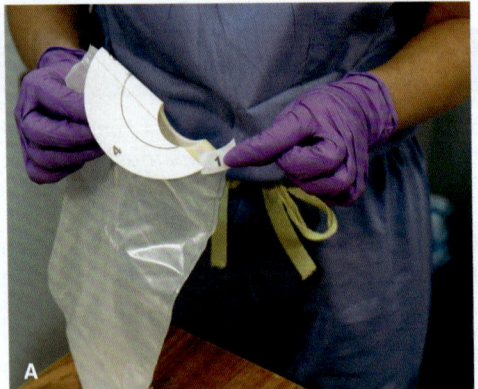
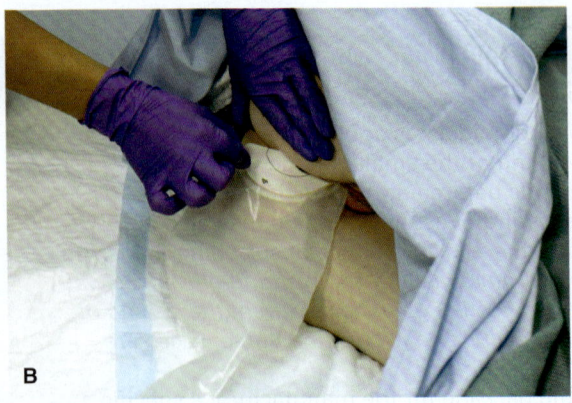
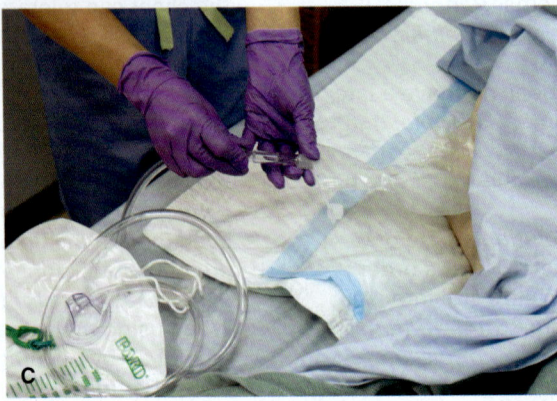

Figure 51-10 The fecal incontinence pouch protects the skin when the client is having frequent liquid stools. **A.** The paper backing is removed from the pouch's adhesive. **B.** The pouch is applied, covering the anal opening. **C.** The tube from the pouch is attached to the collection bag, positioned below the level of the client's buttocks and secured to the bed in the same manner as the urine collection bag. (Evans-Smith, 2005.)

distended. This can be very uncomfortable, particularly if the client has recently had abdominal surgery.

Some nursing measures to help relieve flatus include the following:

- Help the client to walk, if this is allowed.
- Help the client to dangle on the edge of the bed.
- Turn the client onto the left side.
- Avoid ice in drinking water and other fluids.
- Avoid the use of drinking straws.
- Apply a warm compress to the abdomen.

If these measures do not work, an order may be obtained for a rectal tube to be inserted into the rectum, to provide an outlet for accumulated gas and relieve distention. In Practice: Nursing Procedure 51-7 gives steps for helping to remove flatus. In addition, if distention is severe or threatens a suture line, an order may be obtained to perform a Harris flush (return-flow enema) (In Practice: Nursing Care Guidelines 51-6).

The Fecal Incontinence Pouch

In some cases, the client has very frequent liquid stools. This is very irritating to the skin, due to the acidic nature of the stool. To prevent the skin from becoming excoriated and raw, an incontinence pouch may be ordered. (If the skin is already excoriated, a skin barrier should be applied before applying the pouch.) Figure 51-10 shows the steps in applying the fecal incontinence pouch. It is important for the nurse to check the bag to determine if stool is being passed and frequently to check the condition of the client's perianal (around the anus) skin.

> **Key Concept**
> Chapter 58 describes special skin care and measures used to protect the skin. Also included are procedures for treating existing wounds.

NAUSEA AND VOMITING

Nausea is an unpleasant abdominal sensation, sometimes followed by vomiting. *Vomiting*, also called **emesis**, is an involuntary action that expels stomach contents. Symptoms of nausea leading to vomiting include weakness, frequent swallowing, profuse perspiration, dizziness, pallor (paleness), and shakiness, as well as an uncomfortable feeling in the stomach. Pulse and blood pressure may drop during vomiting. In some cases, vomiting is **projectile vomiting** (expelled with great force). This must be reported at once because projectile vomiting can be a sign of a serious condition, such as a brain tumor or brain trauma.

Vomitus means stomach contents. Its appearance and odor may indicate the cause of emesis. Assess for particles, color, odor, and consistency. Vomitus may contain bright red blood, a sign of gastric or esophageal bleeding or coffee-ground material, a sign of bleeding in the lower digestive tract. It may contain mucus or pus. Vomitus that contains bile is yellowish or greenish. Vomitus that has been forced back into the stomach from the intestine has a fecal odor.

Observe vomitus for the presence of undigested medications and specific foods. Observe the nature of vomiting. Was it violent or projectile? How does the client describe the episode? If you are monitoring the client's I&O, consider vomitus as output. Report the vomiting episode. Carefully document all observations. Always wear gloves when assisting the client who is vomiting or when taking a specimen of vomitus. **Rationale:** *Gloves must always be worn when working with any body fluids.* Measure and document the amount of vomitus, if possible. Always save any unusual vomitus for inspection. The primary provider may want the entire specimen sent to the laboratory for examination. As with any other specimen, be sure the container and lid are carefully labeled with the client's name and other identifiers. Place the specimen in a moisture-proof, covered container, and place the container in a biohazard bag. Make sure it gets to the laboratory immediately, along with the appropriate laboratory request.

The person who is nauseated or vomiting feels uncomfortable and helpless and usually does not want to talk. In some cases, vomiting is dangerous and should be prevented. For example, the client who has had recent abdominal surgery or delicate eye surgery may incur an injury as a result of the violent action of vomiting. The person who has ingested a caustic substance can experience additional injury by vomiting (the substance burns twice: once during ingestion and again in expulsion). Rather than ask questions, assist the person who is nauseated or vomiting with comfort measures. In Practice: Nursing Care Guidelines 51-8 describes nursing care of this client.

> **Key Concept**
> If the client vomits intact medication tablets, this should be reported immediately. Save the tablets for identification. The provider may order them to be repeated.

IN PRACTICE
NURSING CARE GUIDELINES 51-8 — Assisting the Client Who Is Nauseated or Vomiting

- Always wear gloves. If vomiting is projectile or any possibility exists that vomitus will splash, also wear eye goggles and gown. *Rationale: Using personal protective equipment helps prevent the spread of infection, especially when you are in contact with body fluids.*

The Client Who Is Nauseated

- Place a cool, damp washcloth on the client's forehead. *Rationale: This is soothing to the client and may help them to relax. Relaxation helps prevent vomiting.*
- Help the client to take slow, deep breaths through the nose. *Rationale: Deep breathing helps relax the client and distracts from the nauseated feeling. Adding oxygen to the blood, and thus the control center in the medulla of the brain, helps relieve nausea.*
- Have the client lie on the right side. *Rationale: This position moves gastric contents toward the stomach's bottom end and away from the cardiac sphincter, relieving irritation and stimulation of the cardiac sphincter.*
- Give antiemetic (antinausea) drugs by injection or rectally, as ordered. *Rationale: Antiemetics cannot be given by mouth because this might increase discomfort or cause vomiting.*
- Offer something dry, such as a bite of soda cracker or unbuttered toast. Do not give the food until the worst of the nausea subsides. Use only small amounts of food. *Rationale: Dry food may soak up some excess stomach acid and remove the disagreeable taste from the mouth. Food may cause further upset and irritation; it must be given cautiously.*

The Client Who Is Vomiting

- Hold an emesis basin (kidney basin) directly under the client's chin. Tell the client not to swallow vomitus. *Rationale: This basin can catch the emesis. Vomitus is very irritating; swallowing would irritate the stomach further.*
- If possible, have the client sit; if this is not possible, make sure the client lies on the side. *Rationale: Lying on the back while vomiting is dangerous because vomitus could be aspirated into the lungs.*
- Place a towel or incontinence pad under the basin. *Rationale: This protects the client's clothing and bed linens.*
- Carefully check the vomitus. Measure it, if possible. *Rationale: The appearance and nature of vomiting can be important to the provider in making a diagnosis. Vomitus is part of the client's daily output and is added to the input and output (I&O) sheet.*
- Immediately report if there is any blood or unusual material in the vomitus. *Rationale: Particularly with the client who has had recent surgery or who has stomach or esophageal ulcers, the presence of blood or partially digested (black) blood may be life threatening.*
- After vomiting has subsided, allow the client to rinse the mouth with mouthwash or a weak salt solution. Tell the client not to swallow any solution. *Rationale: Vomiting leaves a disagreeable taste in the mouth. Gastric contents are also irritating to the throat and mouth. Swallowing fluid could cause more nausea.*
- If the client has had recent surgery, carefully inspect the suture line. Report any abnormalities. *Rationale: Vomiting could disrupt new sutures, causing serious complications such as evisceration (protrusion of abdominal contents through the suture line) or disruption of delicate eye sutures.*
- Remove soiled linen and wash the client's face and hands. *Rationale: This action provides client comfort.*
- Empty the emesis basin promptly. *Rationale: The sight and smell of vomitus is very disagreeable.*
- Wash the emesis basin in cold water. Leave the clean basin close to the client, in case the nausea and vomiting return. *Rationale: Hot water will cause protein material to coagulate.*
- Check back with the client frequently. *Rationale: Determine if nausea and vomiting have returned.*

NURSING CARE GUIDELINES 51-8 Assisting the Client Who Is Nauseated or Vomiting   (Continued)

- Dispose of gloves and wash hands. *Rationale: Proper glove disposal and handwashing help to prevent spread of organisms.*
- Carefully document the event and pertinent observations. *Rationale: Documentation provides communication and continuity of care.*

STUDENT SYNTHESIS

KEY POINTS

- Adequate elimination is a basic function critical to health and life.
- Thorough handwashing and Standard Precautions are important when coming into contact with any body secretions or drainage from the client.
- It is vital to place the client in as comfortable a position as possible for elimination or when vomiting and to allow for privacy.
- In caring for the client with a retention catheter, precautions must be taken to prevent any source of infection from reaching the bladder.
- Diarrhea may be a symptom of impacted stool or a sign of another gastrointestinal disorder.
- Retraining of the bladder and bowel aids the client's health and self-esteem.
- Bladder and bowel continence or management can make the difference between independent living and the need for long-term care.
- Enemas may be used to assist in bowel elimination, to cleanse the bowel, or to instill medications.
- It is important to assist the client who is vomiting, to alleviate discomfort and prevent complications.

CRITICAL THINKING EXERCISES

1. You have been assigned to teach a client about the importance of proper bladder and bowel elimination. Describe how you would teach the importance of these self-care activities. Describe how you might assist the client who is incontinent of urine.
2. Your client, Mrs. R., is aged 87 years. They say they have not had a bowel movement for 2 days. They have asked for an enema. Their abdomen is soft and not distended; they deny pain. The healthcare provider has ordered TWE PRN or oil retention enema PRN. How would you assess this client to determine whether or not they need an enema and, if so, which type? Describe situations in which each type of enema might be used.

NCLEX-STYLE REVIEW QUESTIONS

1. A client is having urgency and frequency of urination with lower abdominal discomfort. The nurse observes that the urine is cloudy. After reporting this finding, which action is appropriate by the nurse at this time?
    a. Inform the client the symptoms will go away on their own.
    b. Encourage the client to drink 2–3 L of fluids.
    c. Recommend that the client drink caffeinated beverages.
    d. Administer antibiotics prior to obtaining a specimen.

2. The nurse removes an indwelling urinary catheter as ordered after a client has recovered from abdominal surgery. After removal of the catheter, which information would the nurse instruct the client to report? Select all that apply.
    a. Dribbling small amounts of urine
    b. Clear yellow urine output
    c. Voiding 1 hr after catheter removal
    d. Distention of the bladder after voiding
    e. Urgency after voiding

3. A client is having severe right flank pain and is suspected to have a kidney stone. The provider has issued orders. Which action will the nurse take during this time?
    a. Keep the client NPO.
    b. Strain the urine for passing of the stone.
    c. Give the client an enema.
    d. Insert an indwelling catheter.

4. A client has a bowel movement that is observed to be streaked with blood. Which action is a priority?
    a. Inspect the client for hemorrhoids.
    b. Administer an enema to see if the client is constipated.
    c. Check the client for a fecal impaction.
    d. Inform the client that too many iron supplements is causing this issue.

5. The nurse is auscultating bowel sounds from a client after abdominal surgery and hears few sounds. How would the nurse document this finding?
    a. Hyperactive bowel sounds
    b. Normal bowel sounds
    c. Hypoactive bowel sounds
    d. Inaudible bowel sounds

CHAPTER RESOURCES

Enhance your learning with additional resources on thePoint!

Student Resources related to this chapter can be found at thePoint.lww.com/Rosdahl12e.

CHAPTER 51 Elimination

Welcome Steps

Look at healthcare provider's orders.

Protocol for procedure.

Necessary equipment/supplies.

Wash hands using proper hand hygiene; put on gloves.

Explain the procedure and reassure the client.

Locate two identifiers to confirm correct client.

Comfortable and efficient position for nurse and client.

Obtain privacy.

Make sure to follow correct steps and body mechanics with good technique.

Ensure safety and observe deviations from normal.

End Steps

Ensure comfort and safety.

Note questions or concerns from client or nurse; note significant data.

Dispose of materials properly.

Disinfect the area and your hands.

Document and report the procedure and your findings.

IN PRACTICE

NURSING PROCEDURE 51.1 | Giving and Removing the Bedpan and Urinal

Supplies and Equipment
Gloves
Bedpan (regular or fracture pan)
Bedpan cover
Handwashing supplies for client
Toilet tissue
Air freshener (optional)
Waterproof pad (optional)

Steps
Follow LPN WELCOME Steps and Then

1. Obtain a bedpan or urinal or remove from the bedside cabinet. Use the appropriate type of bedpan. Make sure the equipment is labeled with the client's name or in their individual cabinet. *Rationale:* Each client has a separate bedpan or urinal, to avoid cross-contamination.

2. Lower the near side rail. Fold the bed linen away from the client, exposing as little of their body as possible. Place an incontinence pad on the bed if necessary or if using a fracture pan. *Rationale: Protect the client's privacy, while providing access for placing the bedpan. The incontinence pad protects the bed linens.*

3. Assist the client onto the bedpan. If possible, ask the client to flex the knees and lift the hips:

   a. Place the bedpan under the buttocks, with the wide, curved shelf end toward the client's back and the narrower open end toward the feet (Fig. 51-2A). *Rationale: Placing the pan in this position fits the contour of the body, alleviates discomfort, and prevents spilling of waste materials.*

   b. If a client is unable to use a regular bedpan, use a fracture pan. Place it under the buttocks with the flat end toward the client's back (Fig. 51-2B). *Rationale:* A fracture pan exerts less pressure on the hips and spine and is easier to place under the client. (It is more susceptible to spilling, however.)

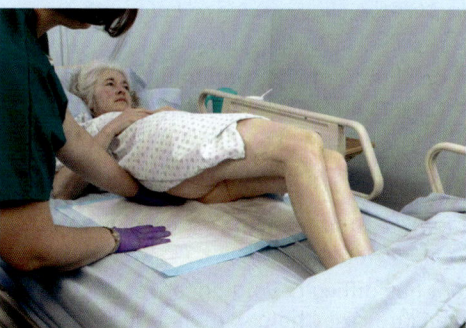

Place a waterproof pad under the client's buttocks. (Evans-Smith, 2005.)

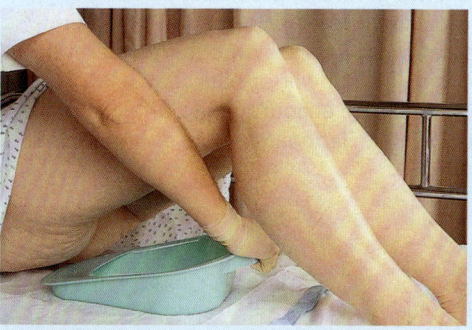

If the client cannot tolerate the larger bedpan, use a fracture pan.

4. If the client is immobile, roll the client onto their side away from you. Ask the client to help by pulling on the side rails, if possible. Position the bedpan against the client's buttocks, hold it firmly in place, and turn the client onto their back. Check the pan's location. *Rationale: Properly positioning the bedpan avoids spillage while ensuring the client's comfort.*

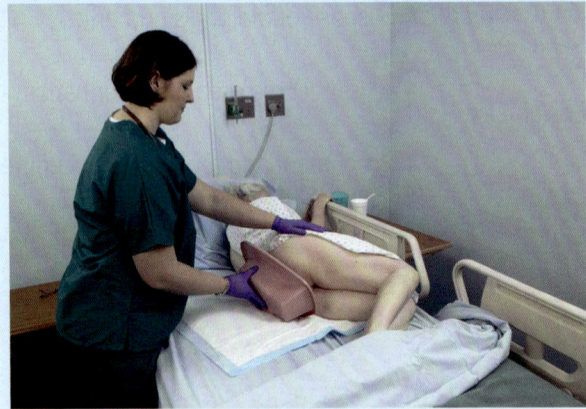

If the client is immobile, roll them away from you and place the pan against the buttocks. (Evans-Smith, 2005.)

5. Replace the bed linen back over the client. *Rationale: Protect the client's privacy.*

6. Elevate the head of the bed to a semi-Fowler position, if the client can tolerate it. Raise the side rail again. *Rationale: This position most closely resembles the normal position for elimination and uses gravity as an additional force. The raised side rail offers security to the client and provides something for the client to use to help with balance or to move.*

7. Place the call light or pager and toilet tissue within the client's reach and leave them alone if possible. Instruct the client to call when finished or if help is needed. If leaving the bedside, remove gloves and wash hands. *Rationale: The call signal provides for the client's comfort and security. Leaving the client alone allows for privacy.*

8. If the client has difficulty voiding, several simple measures may help stimulate the client's muscles to relax. These include the sound of running water or placing the client's hands in warm water, pouring warm water over the female client's genitalia, providing privacy, and relaxation techniques such as soothing music or visualization of a gentle mountain stream. If possible, a warm shower or bath may help. The client could also be encouraged to drink a small amount of water. *Rationale: These stimulate the urge to void.*

9. To remove the bedpan, wash hands and put on gloves. Lower the near side rail and the head of the bed. Uncover the client. Fold the toilet tissue and wipe from the front (pubic area) to the back (anus) if the client is unable to do so independently. *Rationale: Assist the client as needed.*

10. Steady the bedpan as the client either lifts the hips or is assisted to turn away from you. Place the bedpan on the chair and cover it. Cleanse the area with soap and water if necessary. If the client is not incontinent, you may use shaving cream. If the client is incontinent, special skin care products are used (Chapter 58). Dry carefully. *Rationale: Holding the bedpan steady and assisting the client off prevents spillage of contents. Keeping the client's skin clean and dry helps prevent skin breakdown.*

11. Offer handwashing supplies to the client. Return the client to a comfortable position. Lower the bed and raise the side rail. Use air freshener, if necessary. *Rationale: Handwashing helps prevent the spread of microorganisms and teaches good hygiene. Provide comfort and safety for the client.*

12. Measure output or obtain a stool sample, if ordered. Empty the pan into the toilet and rinse with cool water. Be sure to wash your hands carefully. *Rationale: Proper disposal and cleaning prevent the spread of infection.*

Follow ENDDD Steps

Special Reminder

Placing the Male Urinal

- The rationales for the procedure and care of the urinal are basically the same as for the bedpan. The urinal is rinsed after use, as is the bedpan.

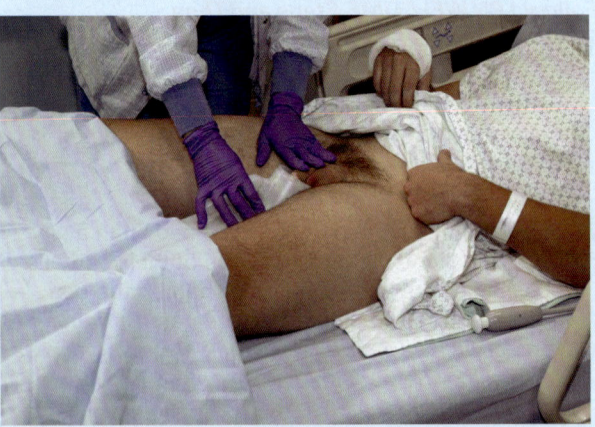

The male urinal is placed over the penis. The head of the bed is raised as much as possible. The provider's orders also may allow the client to stand next to the bed to void. Be sure that the client will not fall. (Evans-Smith, 2005.)

IN PRACTICE
NURSING PROCEDURE 51.2 — Emptying the Urinary Drainage Bag

Supplies and Equipment
Disposable gloves
Face shield
Measuring container (graduate)

Steps
Follow LPN WELCOME Steps and Then

1. Wash hands, put on gloves, and wear a face shield, according to agency protocol. *Rationale: Gloves are worn when handling any body fluids. A face shield protects against splashing urine.*
2. Carefully pull the drain tube (on the bottom of the bag) out of the storage pocket, without touching it below the level of the clamp. Hold the tube over the graduate and release the clamp, making sure that the drain tube does not touch anything. *Rationale: This helps prevent introducing pathogens into the bladder.*
3. When the urine has drained out, clamp the tube and carefully replace it in the storage pocket. Be sure the clamp is far enough up the tube to allow most of the tube to fit into the pocket. Do not move the clamp on the tube. *Rationale: These procedures help maintain the sterility of the catheter's closed drainage system.*
4. Measure the urine, if intake and output (I&O) is ordered. Observe the characteristics of the urine. *Rationale: I&O and observation of the urine provide information about the client's hydration status and kidney function. Possible significant changes may be identified.*

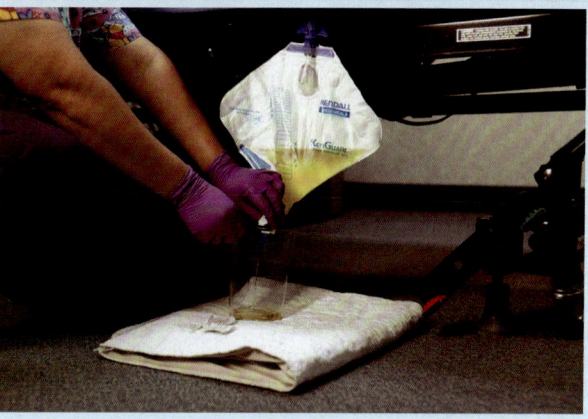

Pull the drainage tube out of the pocket on the bag and do not allow it to touch anything. Drain the urine into the measuring container. (Carter, 2012.)

1. Discard urine (unless a specimen is required) and rinse the graduated container with cool water. *Rationale: Hot water will coagulate proteins in urine and cause odor.*

Follow ENDDD Steps

Special Reminders
- If the client will be discharged from the facility with a catheter, explain each step of catheter use to the client and family. *Rationale: They need instruction about caring for the drainage system to prevent complications.*
- Ask the client or a family member to do a return demonstration after you have demonstrated the procedure. (They should practice several times.) Offer gloves to them. *Rationale: A return demonstration ensures that the client and family understand the procedure, so later they can do it themselves.*

IN PRACTICE
NURSING PROCEDURE 51.3 — Bladder Retraining With Closed Urinary Drainage

Supplies and Equipment
Protective pad for bed
Catheter clamp
Gloves

Steps
Follow LPN WELCOME Steps and Then

1. Position the client in a supine position with the head of the bed slightly elevated. *Rationale: Proper positioning prevents pressure on the bladder.*
2. Place a protective pad under the client. *Rationale: The pad protects the bed.*
3. Clamp the catheter tubing for the ordered amount of time, typically 1–2 hr. Monitor the client's tolerance when the tube is clamped. Document the client's reactions to the procedure when it is completed. *Rationale: Clamping allows time for the bladder to fill. The bladder gradually becomes accustomed to being full of urine.*
4. Open the clamp and allow the bladder to drain by gravity into the drainage bag. *Rationale: This measure empties the bladder and prevents urine stasis. Bladder emptying simulates normal voiding.*

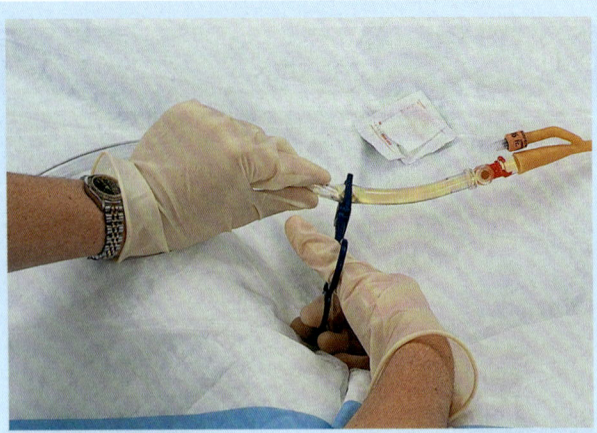

A special clamp that will not damage the catheter is used for this procedure. The catheter tubing is usually clamped for 1–2 hr at first; the time is gradually increased.

5. Repeat the procedure, as ordered. Increase the time the bladder is clamped off to 3 or 4 hr, as ordered. *Rationale: This continues the bladder retraining. Increasing the time for clamping aids in helping reestablish bladder control.*

Follow ENDDD Steps

IN PRACTICE
NURSING PROCEDURE 51.4 Giving an Enema

Supplies and Equipment
Gloves; face shield, if needed
Prescribed enema
Bedpan and cover, bedside commode, or easily available bathroom
Toilet tissue
Waterproof pad
Water-soluble lubricant
Bath blanket
Cleansing supplies; handwashing supplies for the client
IV pole, if bag-and-tubing method used

Using the Bag-and-Tubing Method

Steps

Follow LPN WELCOME Steps and Then

1. Follow the points in In Practice: Nursing Care Guidelines 51-7 that apply to the administration of any enema. Before beginning, if using an IV pole, make sure the pole is lowered to achieve the correct height of the bag—no more than 18 in. (45.7 cm) above the client's anus. *Rationale: Proper positioning prevents injury and overinflation of the colon.*

2. The cleansing enema for an adult, using the bag-and-tubing method, usually ranges from 500 to 1,000 mL. If using more than 500 mL, it often needs to be given in more than one session, giving the client time to defecate in between. (Amount given for an infant = 50–150 mL; for a toddler = 250–350 mL; and for a school-age child = 300–500 mL.) *Rationale: It may be uncomfortable or impossible for the client to retain a larger quantity of solution. By dividing the solution into smaller amounts, the client will tolerate the procedure better. A larger amount will stimulate rapid expulsion and reduce the effectiveness of the enema.*

3. Do not exceed three consecutive sessions of enema administration. *Rationale: This could cause serious fluid and electrolyte imbalance.*

4. The amount of fluid for a retention enema via the bag-and-tubing method is approximately 150–200 mL. *Rationale: A larger amount would usually not be retained.*

5. Unclamp the tube and run a small amount of the solution through the tube. Make sure the tube is well lubricated. *Rationale: This will prevent the introduction of air into the client's colon, causing abdominal distention from gas. Lubrication makes insertion more comfortable for the client.*

6. With the client in Sims position on the left side, separate the client's buttocks. Instruct the client to take a few short, panting breaths and relax while you are inserting the tube. *Rationale: Relaxation helps with insertion of the tube and helps the client retain the fluid longer, thus enhancing the effectiveness of the procedure.*

7. Insert the end of the tube carefully, paying attention to irritated skin, hemorrhoids, or resistance. If any resistance is met, the tube should not be forced. Pause briefly after entering the external sphincter (muscle), to allow the internal sphincter to relax. *Rationale: The anus has inside and outside sphincter muscles that together control the opening to the outside of the body. To be effective, the tube must be inserted*

carefully past both of these sphincters. Following these procedures makes the insertion of the tube more comfortable and effective and is safer for the client.

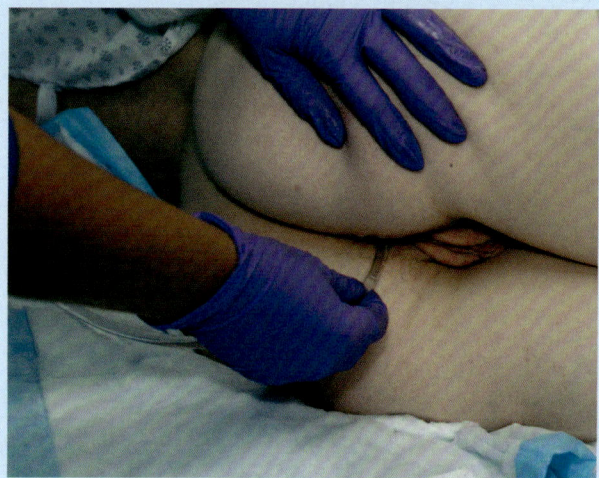

Insert the lubricated rectal tube into the anus, directing the tip toward the umbilicus. (Evans-Smith, 2005.)

8. The rectal tube is inserted approximately 3–4 in. (7.6–10.2 cm) toward the umbilicus (2–3 in. [5.1–7.6 cm] for a school-age child). *Rationale: It is important not to insert the tube too far, to prevent damage to the colon and discomfort for the client.*

9. If resistance is met, instill a small amount of solution and try to insert the tube further. *Rationale: This may help if hardened, dry stool is blocking the rectum.*

10. Regulate the speed and pressure by which any enema is given. Remember that the height of the bag affects the force and speed of the fluid flow. The higher the container is held, the greater the force of the flow. Never hold the container more than 18 in. (45 cm) above the client's anus (also In Practice: Nursing Care Guidelines 51-7). *Rationale: Proper positioning of the device and using appropriate pressure enhance the effectiveness of the enema and help to prevent injury.*

11. Consult In Practice: Nursing Care Guidelines 51-7 for steps to take following the administration of any enema.

Using the Small-Volume Enema

Steps
Follow LPN WELCOME Steps and Then

1. Choose the appropriate size enema. Children's sizes are available. *Rationale: Choosing the correct size is important, to prevent injury.*

2. Check to make sure you are using the correct solution. *Rationale: An incorrect solution could cause damage.*

3. Read and follow the manufacturer's instructions on the package. *Rationale: Each type of enema may be slightly different. It is important to administer the enema correctly.*

4. Store at room temperature. Warm the solution in a container of warm water. *Rationale: This makes the enema more comfortable for the client.*

5. Follow the points in In Practice: Nursing Care Guidelines 51-7, which apply to the administration of any enema. *Rationale: The general guidelines for administering any enema are the same.*

6. Position the client in the same manner as for the bag-and-tubing enema. The tube of the container is inserted in the same manner, using the same precautions. *Rationale: All enemas use the same body positioning.*

7. Roll up the small-volume (Fleet-type) enema container from the bottom as the solution is instilled. *Rationale: This helps push the fluid out of the container and avoids instilling air into the colon.*

8. Consult In Practice: Nursing Care Guidelines 51-7 for steps to take following the administration of the enema. *Rationale: It is important to observe and report the results.*

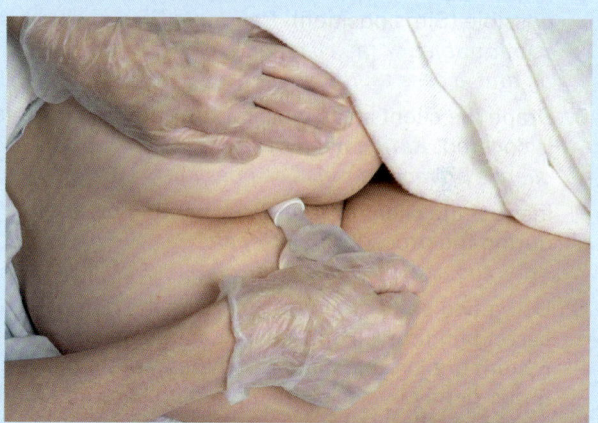

The compression technique demonstrated here is used to expel solution from the small-volume enema container. Note: The container is rolled from the bottom and compressed as the enema is being given. (Lynn, 2015.)

Follow ENDDD Steps

IN PRACTICE

NURSING PROCEDURE 51.5 Performing Manual Disimpaction

Supplies and Equipment
Gloves
Waterproof pad
Toilet tissue
Bedpan
Water-soluble lubricant

Steps
Follow LPN WELCOME Steps and Then

1. Check the provider's order. A specific order is required for this procedure. *Rationale:* This procedure carries a potential for vagal nerve stimulation, producing a lowered heart rate and blood pressure.
2. Take the client's vital signs. *Rationale:* Baseline vital signs are necessary for comparison, if the client shows signs of inappropriate vagal stimulation.
3. Wear two pairs of clean, disposable gloves for this procedure. *Rationale:* The feces are highly contaminated. Your gloved hands will be in direct contact with feces.
4. Place a disposable waterproof pad under the buttocks. *Rationale:* A pad helps to prevent soiling of the bed.
5. Position the client on the left side, with the knees (especially the upper knee) drawn up as far as possible (Sims position). *Rationale:* This position is comfortable for the client and allows an easy view of, and access to, the anal area.
6. Drape the client so as much of the body as possible is covered. *Rationale:* Proper draping preserves the client's privacy as much as possible.
7. Instruct the client to take short, panting breaths during the procedure. *Rationale:* Panting helps relax the anal sphincter.
8. Using two pairs of gloves, lubricate the first or second finger well and insert it *carefully* into the rectum until you feel the stool; then, rotate the finger gently in a scissors motion, to slice off small pieces of stool. *Rationale:* This helps break up the stool. Usually this procedure is all that is needed to assist the client to expel impacted feces.
9. Before removing your finger, gently stimulate the anal sphincter with a rotating motion. *Rationale:* This stimulation helps cause a natural response to defecate.

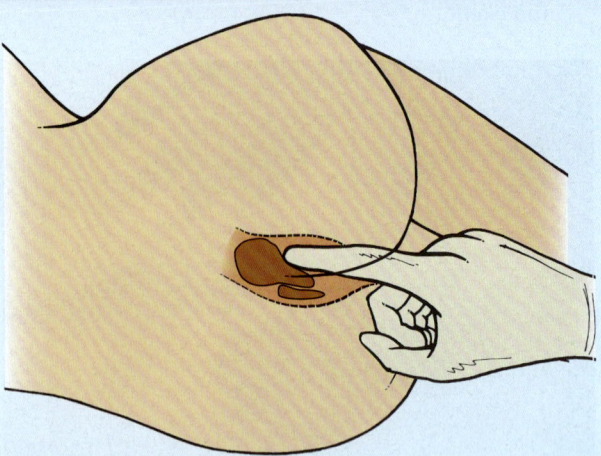

Insert the finger into the rectum until you feel the stool and then rotate the finger gently and slowly, to break up the stool. Gently stimulate the anal sphincter, which usually causes defecation.

1. Assist the client to the bathroom, commode, or bedpan as needed. *Rationale:* Client may be uncomfortable or weak and may need assistance.
2. Leave the client's signal cord or pager within reach. *Rationale:* The person may need the bedpan again in a short time. Diarrhea often occurs after nonroutine manual disimpaction.
3. Provide a washcloth and soap for the client to use for cleansing the rectal area, or clean the area if the client cannot. Leave the waterproof pad in place, to protect the bed. Dispose of gloves and wash hands. Provide handwashing supplies for the client to wash their hands. *Rationale:* Keeping the client and the bed area clean helps to prevent the spread of microorganisms.

Note: In some cases, the client will perform manual disimpaction on themselves on a daily basis.

Follow ENDDD Steps

Special Reminder
- Documentation of this procedure includes any particular client reactions, as well as the amount, color, consistency, and odor of any stool obtained or expelled. If the client is unable to expel impacted feces, report this immediately. *Rationale:* Documentation is important to provide continuity of care. Impacted stool must be reported immediately because it could become a bowel obstruction, which is life threatening.

IN PRACTICE
NURSING PROCEDURE 51.6 — Assisting With Bowel Retraining

Supplies and Equipment
Oral stool softeners or suppositories
Gloves
Bedpan or bedside commode, if needed

Steps
Follow LPN WELCOME Steps and Then

1. Choose a convenient time within the client's daily schedule. Use the same time each day. *Rationale: A daily routine will help to stimulate regular peristalsis and evacuation.*
2. Administer oral stool softeners daily or as ordered. Insert a prescribed suppository at least 30 min before the scheduled time for elimination (In Practice: Nursing Procedure 63-3). *Rationale: This action initiates retraining of the bowel to react to softeners or a suppository on a regular basis.*
3. Offer fruit juice or a cup of warm liquid. *Rationale: These liquids stimulate peristalsis.*
4. Assist the client to the toilet (or bedpan or bedside commode) at the designated time. Provide privacy. *Rationale: Assist the client as needed.*
5. Instruct the client to apply external pressure to the lower abdomen and bear down. *Rationale: This action stimulates the colon to empty.*
6. Apply clean gloves, if needed, to empty and cleanse the elimination receptacle. Discard gloves and wash hands. Assist client to wash their hands. *Rationale: Proper disposal and cleanup reduces the risk of infection transmission.*

Follow ENDDD Steps

Special Reminder
- The client may have a bowel retraining record. Follow the protocol of your facility in documenting the results of the procedure.

IN PRACTICE
NURSING PROCEDURE 51.7 — Helping to Relieve Flatus

Supplies and Equipment
Rectal tube
Evac-u-Sac, cardboard container or bag with tubing
Water-soluble lubricant
Gloves

Steps
Follow LPN WELCOME Steps and Then

1. Ask the client to lie on their side (preferably the left side) or in a knee-chest position, if tolerated. *Rationale: This position promotes client comfort and ease in inserting the tube. Flatus is lighter than stool and can be better expelled if not impeded.*
2. Lubricate the tube. If the client is allergic to latex, be sure to use a latex-free tube. *Rationale: Adequate lubrication eases the insertion.*
3. Insert the tube 3–4 in. (7.5–10 cm) into the rectum. *Rationale: The tube is inserted far enough to bypass the anal sphincters, as well as any stool in the lower rectum, and to reach gas above the stool.*
4. Determine the tube's patency. If the tube is patent (open), gas or feces will return. *Rationale: The tube can become plugged with stool; it must be kept open.*
5. Place the outer end of the tube in an Evac-u-Sac, cardboard container, or small bag. Activated charcoal or baking soda may be inserted into the container. Fasten the tubing to the client's leg. *Rationale: An Evac-u-Sac or cardboard container helps absorb odor and sound and helps minimize the client's embarrassment. Charcoal and baking soda absorb odors. It is important that the tube not fall out.*
6. Remove your gloves and wash your hands. Leave the tube in place for 15–20 min. *Rationale: After that time, pressure necrosis of mucosa can occur. Also, prolonged stimulation of the sphincter muscles cause loss of response and increase the difficulties.*

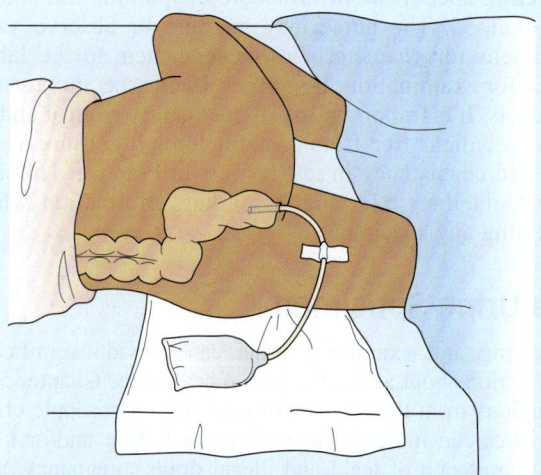

The rectal tube is placed into a container or Evac-u-Sac. This container helps absorb odors and collect any stool that might be discharged with the flatus. (Carter, 2012.)

7. After the allotted time, put on clean gloves and remove the tube. Observe the contents of the container. Document whether the client felt relief. *Rationale: Gloves protect your hands but need not be sterile. Documentation provides communication and continuity of care.*

Follow ENDDD Steps

52 Specimen Collection

Learning Objectives

1. Explain the purpose of monitoring a client's fluid intake and output (I&O). Describe and demonstrate how to accurately document I&O.
2. Demonstrate correct measurement of urine volume.
3. Describe what is meant by urine specific gravity (SG), listing one medical condition associated with high SG; one related to low SG.
4. Identify at least three reasons for laboratory examination of urine.
5. Describe and demonstrate correct collection of the following urine specimens: midstream, 24-hr, fractional, from an indwelling urinary catheter, and a specimen to initiate a kidney stone prevention program.
6. Identify and explain at least one reason for collecting specimens of stool and sputum.
7. Demonstrate correct collection of a stool specimen.
8. Demonstrate correct collection of a sputum specimen.
9. Briefly describe other types of specimens that nurses may collect and related procedures.

Important Terminology

expectorate (expectoration)
guaiac
Hemoccult
hydrometer
occult
specific gravity
urinalysis
urinometer

Acronyms

mL
NG
O&P

Collecting samples of body fluids and feces for laboratory study in one way in which healthcare providers and other members of the team learn information about the health status of clients. Nurses are often responsible for collecting specimens of urine, stool, sputum, and sometimes, blood. The nurse may measure or observe such specimens for characteristics or send them to the laboratory for examination. Be aware of your specific agency protocols. It is important to provide quality control and to keep specimens free from contamination, to ensure accuracy and consistency in test results. In Practice: Nursing Care Guidelines 52-1 highlights key information when collecting any specimen.

The Urine Specimen

Collecting and examining urine can provide significant information about a client's state of health (see Chapter 51). Deviations from the typical physical and microscopic characteristics can indicate factors such as kidney and/or liver status, presence of legal and illegal drugs, pregnancy, and identification of specific disease-causing organisms or disease conditions.

Keeping Intake and Output Records

The amount of fluids consumed and eliminated during a given period is an indicator of the client's nutritional and fluid balance. Over 24 hr, a person's normal fluid intake and urinary output (I&O: intake and output) will be approximately the same or *balanced*. Fluid I&O significantly out of balance because illness may be life-threatening. The client may be retaining fluid, have edema, or may be dehydrated. Records of the client's I&O help guide the provider's decision-making about increasing or restricting fluids or foods or prescribing medications. These records can also be used to assess specific elimination patterns. I&O fluids are documented and totaled automatically by the computer.

> **Nursing Alert** Always wear clean gloves when collecting specimens of urine, stool, sputum, wound drainage, blood, or any other body fluid. Thorough and consistent handwashing before and after any contact with clients and their specimens limits spread of pathogens and helps protect specimens from inadvertent contamination by the nurse.

Measuring Total Food and Fluid Intake

To measure *total* food and fluid intake, the order is given to "record food and fluid intake" or "I&O + calorie count." In this case, record exactly what the client ate, directly on the client menu, or as per agency protocol. (If the fluid content of solid foods is also being calculated, this will be done by the dietary department.) Each nurse is responsible for accurately documenting I&O as it is measured. If there is no bedside computer, a temporary worksheet at the bedside records I&O for each shift; a sample of this record is in Figure 52-1. If the facility has bedside computers, this information is entered immediately (and is in much the same format as the paper form). Otherwise, the bedside information is transferred to

IN PRACTICE
NURSING CARE GUIDELINES 52-1: Collecting Specimens and Samples

- Label specimen containers, including the lids, with the client's name and other data before collecting the specimen.
- Always observe all standard precautions, including careful handwashing and wearing gloves, before and after collecting any specimen. The need for masking and wearing eye protection should be anticipated in some cases, such as sputum collection. (In some facilities, eye protection is always worn when transferring a urine specimen from a bedpan, hat, or urinal into a graduate or specimen container.) *Rationale: All specimens are considered to be grossly contaminated.*
- Collect each sample according to the facility's protocols. Observe sterile technique for sample collection, even though the specimen is not always sterile. *Rationale: This helps ensure consistency and accuracy of results.*
- Place all specimens in biohazard bags. *Rationale: This alerts all staff to take special precautions and helps prevent spread of microorganisms.*
- Document the procedure. Check the client's record to determine if the provider needs to be notified of the results. *Rationale: Provide communication between members of the healthcare team.*

the 24-hr totals in the permanent record. Amounts recorded for I&O are measured in milliliters (**mL**). (The term *cc* [cubic centimeter] is rarely used today; 1 cc equals approximately 1 mL). **Remember:** *Fluid intake* includes items such as gelatin (Jello), ice, Popsicles, sherbet, thin cereal, broth, tube feedings, and intravenous (IV) fluids. *Count ice as 50% water* (e.g., 200 mL of ice would count as 100 mL of fluid intake). *Output* includes vomitus, bleeding, chest tube and other drainage, thoracentesis, paracentesis, and nasogastric (NG) suction, as well as urine. Also, document *diaphoresis* (excessive sweating).

Key Concept
Some normal situations can cause differences between fluid intake and output. As stated previously, fluid may be lost through perspiration or vomiting; extra salt may cause temporary tissue fluid retention.

Measuring Fluid Intake

Fluid *intake* includes all fluids consumed through the gastrointestinal (GI) system (by mouth or tube feeding) and fluids taken as part of IV therapy or total parenteral nutrition (TPN). When a client is on I&O, all fluid intake should be measured. Items such as those described above are all considered liquid intake, as are actual fluids. Each healthcare agency lists the quantities of liquid found in various containers (see Fig. 52-1). Use these amounts when recording I&O. Record all fluid the client takes in. If the client drinks from an unusual container, determine the volume by filling the same container with water. Then, pour the water into a measuring graduate and identify the volume.

DAILY INTAKE AND OUTPUT BEDSIDE WORKSHEET

DATE 5/15/17

Client Name: *Jane Doe*
Client Record Number: *3987624*
Physician: *Dr. Smith*
Unit/Room Number: *B763*

Record Shift totals on 24 Hr. Nurses Progress Notes

Approximate Measures in mL's	
1 oz.	30 ml
8 oz. water glass (tea)	240 ml
8 oz. glass of ice (melted)	120 ml
Soup bowl	150 ml
Jello (1 serving)	100 ml
Small milk carton	240 ml
8 oz. ice cream cup	90 ml
Small juice glass	120 ml
6 oz. hot styrofoam cup	180 ml
12 oz. tea glass	360 ml
Coca-cola paper cup	240 ml
Insulated coffee cup	220 ml
Canned 12 oz. drinks	360 ml

FOR ISOLATION PATIENTS

8 oz disposable cups (tea and water)	240 ml
6 oz. styrofoam cup	180 ml
5 oz. plastic glass	150 ml

INTAKE			OUTPUT			
ORAL/NG		I.V. FLUIDS	URINE Time/Amount	EMESIS	SUCTION	STOOLS
7-3 0700-1500	Juice 120 Milk 240 H₂O 120 H₂O 200 Jello 50 Coffee 100	D₅W 420	0830-200 1045-225 1300-300 1400-125	0930-50	Paracentesis 350 mL	
Shift Total	830	420	850	50	350	

Figure 52-1 A paper worksheet may be kept at the bedside, if bedside computers are not available. The information is transferred to the permanent chart regularly. (Form courtesy of AMI Nacogdoches Medical Center, Nacogdoches, TX.)

> **Nursing Alert** Be sure to determine the facility policy concerning recording of water intake from the bedside water pitcher. In some facilities, it is recorded when the pitcher is filled; in others, when it is empty. Do not fill a pitcher or empty one unless you are sure of the procedure.

Measuring Output

Fluid *output* includes all fluids excreted from the body by any means. Output includes wound drainage, emesis (vomiting), bleeding, watery diarrhea, and **NG** suction tube returns. When recording output other than urine, be sure to identify the output (e.g., NG drainage, watery stool). Wound drainage on dressings is measured by weighing the dressing after it is removed and comparing it with the dry weight of an identical dressing. Weights are done in milligrams and compared with a standardized chart to convert to milliliters.

Figure 52-2 shows the specimen hat (urinary hat, toilet hat, or half-pan). This device can be placed under the toilet seat to collect either urine or stool, without mixing them. (The collection receptacle is positioned to the front to collect urine and to the back to collect stool.) It has graduated volume marks on the inside to facilitate approximate measurement of urine. (If a more exact measurement is needed, the measuring graduate is used.) In Practice: Nursing Procedure 52-1 reviews how to measure urine volume. Do not empty a bedpan or urinal without first determining if the client's I&O is being recorded or if a urine specimen is required. Enlist the aid of the client or family, when possible, to assist with tracking I&O and reporting when the water pitcher is empty or when the client has voided.

> **Key Concept**
> The urinary output of an infant or incontinent adult can be determined in several ways:
> - A specimen collection bag can be used for infants (see Chapter 71). These are also available for adults but are rarely used.
> - The infant diaper, depend-type adult diaper, or sanitary napkin can be weighed and compared with the weight of the same item when dry. The weight can then be converted to urine volume, using a conversion chart. (One fluid ounce equals approximately 30 mL.)
> - Unsterile specimens can be collected by wringing out a diaper.

Maintaining the IV Fluids Record

The I&O record may be separate, but most often is integrated into a total I&O record. This record notes specific types of IV fluids, additives, amount of IV fluids absorbed, and amount remaining per shift. Make sure that all IV fluids are included in the 24-hr total (see Chapter 64).

Measuring Urine Specific Gravity

The urine **specific gravity** (SG) is an indicator of the concentration of urine, as compared with pure water. Usually, in acute care facilities, the SG is part of routine urinalysis, done in the laboratory. However, a nurse may perform this procedure if it is needed frequently or when working in home care or a healthcare clinic. Follow the protocol of your facility or agency. Urine SG is measured with a specialized instrument, the **urinometer** (**hydrometer**). The reading is expressed in decimal increments above 1.000, the reading for pure water.

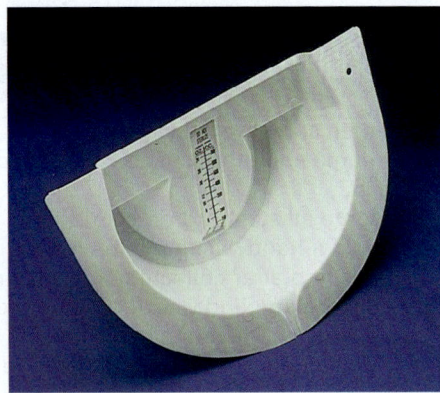

Figure 52-2 A specimen hat (toilet hat, half pan) is placed in the toilet or commode to obtain a stool specimen (receptacle to the back) or a clean-catch urine specimen (receptacle to the front). The approximate volume of urine can be measured.

Because the increments are in thousandths, be very accurate. The normal range of urine SG is from 1.010 (dilute) to 1.025 (highly concentrated). Test urine as soon as possible after obtaining it, for accuracy. In Practice: Nursing Procedure 52-2 outlines steps in measuring urine SG. Extremely concentrated urine (high SG, approximately 1.025) may indicate dehydration or tissue fluid retention (edema). Low SG (below 1.010) may indicate a disorder, such as diabetes insipidus, or excessive use of diuretic medications. A kidney disorder may cause either a high or low urine SG.

Collecting Urine Specimens for Examination

Urine specimens may be collected and sent to the laboratory for examination. **Urinalysis**, in which normal and abnormal components of urine are identified, is usually done on all clients at the beginning of treatment and as needed during an illness. In addition, urine is commonly collected to determine the presence of legal or illegal drugs, to determine pregnancy, and to assess for the presence of infection. Many other tests can be performed with urine samples, and some urine tests are significant in the diagnosis of physical disorders. In Practice: Nursing Care Guidelines 52-2 highlights important considerations in collecting urine specimens.

> **Nursing Alert** Place all specimens in prescribed leakproof containers. Keep the outside of these containers clean and dry. Place them in biohazard bags for transport to the laboratory. Label containers before use; if the container is wet, it will be difficult to label. In some facilities, you must also label the cover of the container and the biohazard bag. Be sure to include the appropriate laboratory request form or make sure the information is correctly programmed into the computer, so the laboratory staff knows which tests to complete.

Collecting a Single-Voided Urine Specimen

A *single-voided urine specimen* often is ordered. Tests are done to determine the efficiency of the kidneys or examine the urine for abnormalities. In Practice: Nursing Procedure 52-3 reviews steps for collecting urine specimens.

Nursing Alert In some cases, such as when doing drug testing, an *observed urine specimen* must be obtained. In this case, the nurse must actually observe the client voiding into the specimen container. (Be aware that there are a number of methods used to avoid detection when giving a false urine specimen.) To obtain accurate urine samples for drug testing, in-service education is required.

Collecting a Clean-Catch or Midstream Urine Specimen

By using the *clean-catch* or *midstream* method, a specimen is obtained with minimal contamination from external sources, without inserting a sterile catheter. Because the genital area and urethral opening are cleansed before the specimen is obtained, and the sample is taken after some urine has already been passed, any bacteria found in the laboratory tests are most likely from urine in the bladder. In

IN PRACTICE
NURSING CARE GUIDELINES 52-2 | Collecting Urine Specimens

- The amount and content of a urine specimen varies with time of day and with food and fluid intake. The provider may ask for specimens at different times of the day. The urine specimen collected for part of a day is called the *single fractional specimen*.
- Label specimen bottles with a waterproof label before the client voids. Include all required information. **Rationale:** *Doing so reduces handling after the bottle is contaminated and helps the label to adhere to the container.*

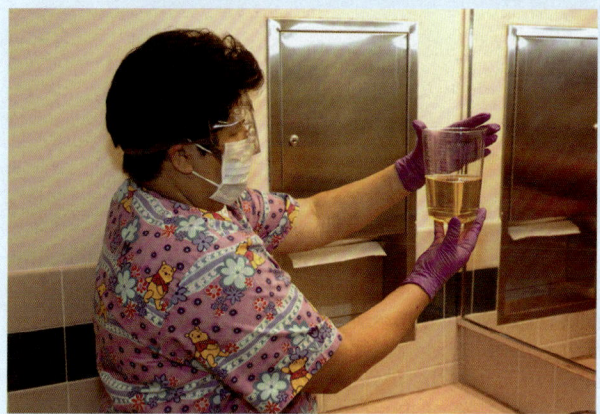

Label specimen containers before the client voids, using a waterproof label, if possible.

- Check the specimen after the client has voided, to make sure the label is still readable. If not, dry the outside of the bottle completely and apply a duplicate label. In some cases, the time and date of collection is also necessary. **Rationale:** *Proper labeling prevents errors. The label must be readable for the laboratory to do the test.*
- Wake a client in the morning to obtain a routine specimen. **Rationale:** *If all specimens are collected at the same time, the laboratory can establish a baseline. Also, this voided specimen usually represents urine that was collecting in the bladder all night—usually the longest period the client goes without voiding.*
- Note on the label if the female client is menstruating. **Rationale:** *One of the tests routinely performed is a test for blood. Menstruation can cause a false-positive reading for urinary blood.*

- To avoid contamination (and the necessity of collecting another specimen), encourage the client to wash their hands before and after collecting the urine specimen. **Rationale:** *It is important not to contaminate the specimen and to protect the client.*
- The client should wash the genital area with soap and water (or a special, prepackaged wipe) immediately before collecting the specimen. Instruct the female to wipe from front to back, the male to clean the tip of their penis, wiping from the urethra outward. **Rationale:** *It is important that the specimen be from the bladder and not be contaminated from external sources, particularly if a culture is ordered.*
- The nurse may need to assist the client in cleansing the perineum and obtaining the urine specimen. **Rationale:** *Some clients may be physically unable to cleanse the perineum adequately, because of serious illness, sedation, or conditions such as arthritis, Huntington disease, obesity, or Parkinsonism. In addition, the client may be confused or a child and not able to understand the instructions.*
- Use a clean specimen hat or half-pan in the toilet if the female client is ambulatory. Place the rounded end toward the front of the toilet, with the open end toward the back. **Rationale:** *Placing the toilet hat in this manner allows the client to have a bowel movement while collecting only urine.*
- If the client is confined to bed, use a clean bedpan. Ask the client to try not to have a bowel movement when using the bedpan. **Rationale:** *Feces would contaminate the specimen.*
- Give the male client a urinal to collect the urine specimen. He can use the toilet hat if he will also have a bowel movement. **Rationale:** *Most men are able to void comfortably into the urinal. Using the toilet hat will separate urine from feces.*
- Tell the client not to touch the inside of the container or its cover. The insides are considered sterile. **Rationale:** *Maintaining the sterility of the container helps ensure accurate results and prevents cross-contamination. Sterility must be carefully maintained, particularly if a culture is to be done.*
- Maintain standard precautions when collecting all types of urine specimens. **Rationale:** *Reduce the risk of infection transmission.*

766 UNIT 8 Client Care

NURSING CARE GUIDELINES 52-2 — Collecting Urine Specimens (Continued)

- To pour urine into the specimen container, hold the specimen hat or urinal over the toilet and fill the container about 3/4 full of urine. Be careful not to spill on the outside of the container or on your clean gloved hand. Your facility may require eye protection as well. *Rationale: This amount of urine is enough for most laboratory tests. (If more urine is needed, the laboratory should notify you in advance.) Keeping the outside of the container and your gloves dry preserves the label and reduces contamination.*

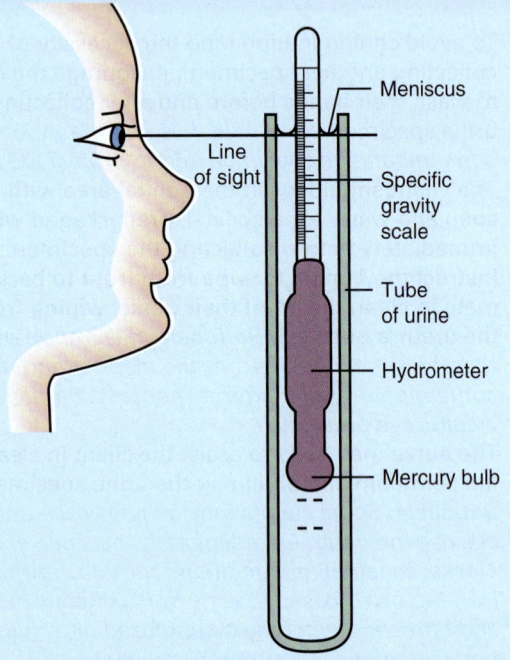

When pouring a specimen from a bedpan or specimen hat into the specimen container, hold the specimen cup over the toilet. Gloves are worn; eye protection may also be required (Carter, 2005).

- All specimens are placed in biohazard bags for transport to the laboratory. The outside of the bag is kept clean by using the clean gloved hand only. The contaminated hand touches only the specimen container and the *inside* of the bag. *Rationale: This prevents the sample from becoming contaminated and protects you and other healthcare workers.*

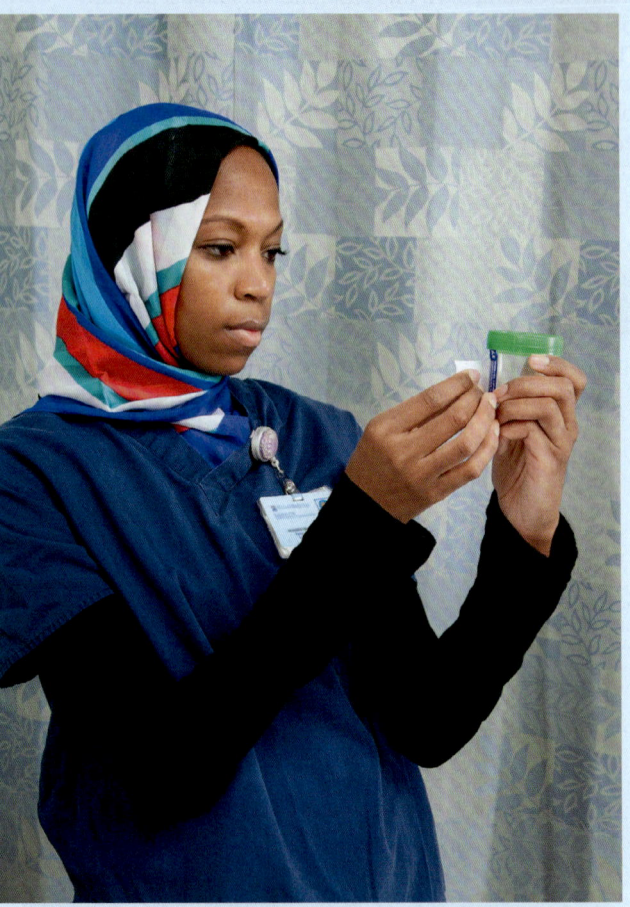

All specimens are considered to be biohazardous and are placed in a specially marked biohazard bag for transport to the laboratory. Touch the outside of the bag only with the clean glove. Touch the specimen container and the inside of the bag only with the contaminated glove (Evans-Smith, 2005).

- Wash your hands before and after the procedure and instruct the client to do the same. *Rationale: Handwashing helps prevent infection transmission and teaches good hygiene.*
- Document the procedure, to avoid duplication. *Rationale: Documentation provides communication and continuity of care.*

Practice: Nursing Care Guidelines 52-3 describes measures for collecting a clean-catch or midstream urine specimen.

Collecting a 24-hr Urine Specimen

An accumulated quantity of urine gives more detailed information than does a single specimen because the accumulated specimen better shows the type and quantity of wastes being excreted by the kidneys. The urine is usually collected for 24 hr or for some part of that period, depending on the specific order. In Practice: Nursing Procedure 52-4 describes the actions for collecting a *24-hr urine specimen* (see also Nursing Care Guidelines 52-3).

Collecting the Fractional Urine Specimen

A 24-hr *fractional* specimen is collected to determine amounts and characteristics of urine during various periods (fractions) of the day. Follow these actions in collecting the 24-hr fractional urine specimen:

- Follow all the steps as when collecting other urine specimens. Be sure to follow standard precautions. Depending on the order, determine how many bottles you will need. Usually, four specimen bottles are required. Label all bottles before you begin. Indicate times on each bottle. *Rationale: 6-hr segments are usually used. Specific times assist other staff members.*

IN PRACTICE
NURSING CARE GUIDELINES 52-3 Collecting Clean-Catch Midstream Urine Specimens

- As for all urine specimens, label the container before giving it to the client. Instruct the client to cleanse the urethral area thoroughly (see Nursing Procedure 52-3). Use prepackaged wipes, if available. *Rationale: Thorough cleansing limits external bacteria from entering the specimen. It is important to evaluate only bacteria that appear in the urine and not bacteria from the external genitalia. The wipes are sterile and convenient.*
- Instruct the female client to cleanse from front to back and to cleanse each side with a separate wipe or a separate area of the wipe, saving the last for the urethral area itself (see Fig. 50-9A). Instruct the male client to cleanse the penis, using a circular motion and going outward from the urethral meatus. The first wipe or portion of the wipe is used for the urethral meatus. The next wipe cleanses the end of the penis, and the last wipe again cleanses the urethral opening (see Fig. 50-9B). *Rationale: This avoids contaminating the urethral area with bacteria from the anal area, making the urethral area is as clean as possible.*
- Instruct clients to void a small amount into the toilet and hold the rest of their urine. Then, instruct the client to void into the sterile container, catching the *midstream urine*. Finally, instruct the client to void the last of the stream into the toilet. *Rationale: The first voided urine flushes the urethra and urethral meatus of external contaminants. The midstream urine is most characteristic of the urine produced by the kidney and is the best indicator of kidney function. The last part does not yield as much information.*
- Clients unable to stop the stream of urine once it has started may be instructed to slip the container into the stream shortly after beginning to urinate and remove the container before the bladder is emptied or when the necessary amount of urine has been collected. *Rationale: The nurse can help the client understand why it is important to obtain the specimen from the center of the stream (midstream).*
- Take or send the specimen to the laboratory immediately. *Rationale: Delay could cause a false-positive result, particularly in the case of a urine culture.*
- Follow standard precautions when dealing with any body substances. *Rationale: Reduce the risk of infection transmission.*

Collecting 24-hr Urine Specimens
- Store all specimens on ice or in a specimen refrigerator during the 24-hr collection period, unless instructed otherwise. *Rationale: Urine begins to decompose faster at room temperature. A specific refrigerator should be available. Be sure to prevent cross-contamination if samples from more than one client are in this refrigerator.*
- Take specimens to the laboratory immediately at the end of the 24-hr collection. Document: The total volume of urine collected, the time collection was completed, the time the specimen was sent to the laboratory, and special characteristics of the urine (e.g., abnormal color, presence of sediment, or a very strong odor). *Rationale: The laboratory testing is begun immediately before the urine decomposes. Your observations are very important as part of the testing process.*

- Ask the client to void and discard the first urine. Collect all urine from the first fraction of the day in bottle #1. Be sure to ask the client to void at the end of that period. *Rationale: Each new time slot begins and ends with an empty bladder. Each time slot must contain all the urine from that time slot. Each new time slot begins with an empty bladder. This ensures that all the urine from that specific time slot is in the collection bottle.*
- Continue for the other "fractions" of the day. The client should end the total day with an empty bladder. *Rationale: This ensures that all urine from the 24-hr period is being tested.*

Collecting a Urine Specimen for Kidney Stone Prevention

This 24-hr specimen may be obtained by the client at home, but the nurse will be required to provide instructions. This specimen is sent to a special diagnostic laboratory for analysis to determine components of urine that might lead to formation of kidney stones (lithiasis), which helps prevent further stone production. Equipment includes a large collection container, urine preservative, a small specimen tube, special labels and forms, the toilet hat, and a biohazard bag.

- The 24-hr collection is performed in the usual manner, starting with an empty bladder. At the first collected voiding, the preservative is poured into the large container, along with its lid and container. *Rationale: It is important to use all the preservative.*
- All subsequent urine for the collection period is poured into this large container, including the last voiding. This is the *stop time*. The total amount of urine is carefully measured and recorded on the provided form. *Rationale: This assists the laboratory with analysis.*
- The collection container is vigorously shaken, the small specimen tube filled about ¾ full with urine, and the rest of the urine discarded. The small tube is then submitted for testing (Litholink, 2017).

> **Nursing Alert** If urine is spilled or accidentally discarded during a 24-hr urine collection period or a specific fractional collection, report this error and anticipate that the collection may need to be restarted. Urine previously collected is discarded before beginning again and new containers used. *Remember:* All 24-hr collections begin with an empty bladder.

Collecting a Specimen From an Indwelling Catheter

Some clients have an indwelling catheter in the bladder, draining urine continuously (see Fig. 51-4). Clients are rarely catheterized simply to obtain a specimen, to prevent the possibility of contaminating the bladder. Contamination of any part of the catheter system can cause infection because microorganisms can travel up the catheter into the bladder. Therefore, be particularly careful not to endanger the client by contaminating the catheter system. *Never allow the collection bag to be above the level of the bladder or to touch the floor.* (See Chapter 51 for general catheter care.) In Practice: Nursing Procedure 52-5 describes steps in collecting a specimen from a urinary catheter. In acute healthcare facilities, usually a blunt-tipped cannula or needleless system is used. In some cases, a syringe and needle may be used. The procedure for both is basically the same.

> **Key Concept**
> The blunt-tipped cannula or needleless system is used to avoid accidental needle-stick injuries to client or staff. Follow the manufacturer's instructions.

Obtaining a One-Time Catheterized Urine Specimen

If a urine specimen cannot be obtained in any other way, catheterization may be ordered. This method may be used in the client who is unconscious, confused, or unable to void. However, this is rarely done only to obtain a specimen, because of the danger of infection. (If a retention catheter is inserted, a specimen is obtained at that time.) The urinary catheterization procedure is presented in Chapter 57. If the client has residual urine remaining in the bladder after voiding, the bladder scanner is used to measure the volume (see Chapter 51). An order for catheterization may specify that the catheter is to be left in place if the residual urine volume is significant (e.g., "100 mL or more"). In this case, the initial catheterization will be done with an indwelling type of catheter (e.g., Foley) in anticipation of this possibility. *Rationale: This would prevent catheterizing the client twice and further exposing them to the risk of infection.*

THE STOOL SPECIMEN

The stool specimen provides information about the functioning of the GI system and its accessory organs. The most common test is for the presence of **occult** (hidden) blood in stool, which indicates bleeding somewhere in the GI tract.

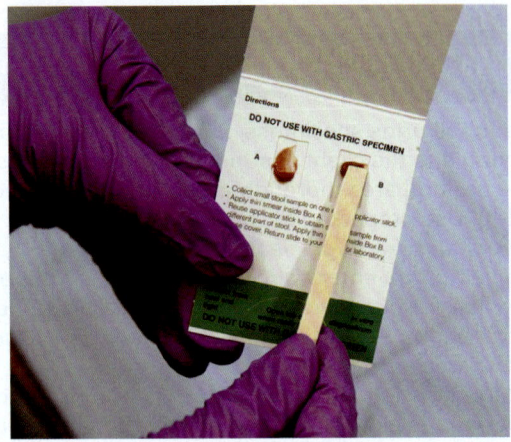

Figure 52-3 Collecting stool specimen for Hemoccult testing. The enclosed wooden applicator is used to apply stool sample to two places on the Hemoccult card. Sometimes, the nurse processes the test, according to the manufacturer's instructions, and sometimes, a sample is sent to the laboratory for analysis. (Lynn, 2015.)

Another common test is for ova and parasites (**O&P**), which indicates the presence of intestinal parasites or their eggs (ova). In Practice: Nursing Procedure 52-6 gives details for collecting stool specimens. In the ambulatory care setting or in the home, stools may be tested for occult blood using the **Hemoccult** brand method. Sometimes, the test is referred to as a **guaiac** test, named for the substance used to cause occult blood to change color (Fig. 52-3). In these tests, a smear of stool is placed on the testing card with a special stick and sent to the laboratory or tested according to the manufacturer's instructions. The test can be done by the client. Be sure to wear gloves when handling stool.

> **SPECIAL CONSIDERATIONS** *Lifespan*
>
> **Collecting a Stool Specimen From a Child**
> When an infant has diarrhea, the entire stool is often examined. Place the entire diaper in a biohazard bag, label it, and send to the laboratory immediately. If the stool is formed and a partial stool sample is required, remove a sample of the stool with a tongue blade and place in a specimen container, as for an adult.

> **Nursing Alert** False-positive results may occur with guaiac tests. These can be caused if the client has consumed large amounts of rare red meat or certain foods, such as radishes, tomatoes, beets, horseradish, or some melons. In addition, the client should not take more than 250 mg per day of vitamin C and should not take acetylsalicylic acid (Aspirin) or nonsteroidal anti-inflammatory drugs (NSAIDs) for 3 days before the test. Be sure to tell the client about the possibility of false-positive results. Usually, specimens are collected on 3 separate days before a determination of positive or negative is made. If test results are repeatedly positive, additional examinations, such as colonoscopy, are necessary.

THE SPUTUM SPECIMEN

For clients with some respiratory disorders, a sputum specimen may be ordered for examination or culture. This test is often used to rule out the presence of the tubercle bacillus, the causative organism for tuberculosis, as well as other bacterial, fungal, and viral infections. In addition, it may help in the diagnosis of malignancies. Sputum specimens are often collected for 3 days in a row. The best time to obtain a sputum specimen is immediately after the client awakens in the morning. (Sputum accumulates in the airways during the night and often, is more easily expelled by coughing in the early morning.) The first specimen of the morning is considered to be the most accurate. This specimen is obtained from deep within the bronchi, not saliva from the throat. Obtain the specimen before the client eats, uses mouthwash, or brushes the teeth.

Instruct the client to clear the nose and throat and rinse the mouth with water before beginning. Then, the client is instructed to breathe deeply several times and to cough with exhalation. Ask the client not to spit saliva into the container, but to **expectorate** (spit or cough up) the sputum from deep in the lungs (Fig. 52-4). Repeat as needed, to obtain a sample. A sputum specimen may also be obtained by nasotracheal suction. The nurse will require specific in-service instruction in this procedure.

As always, standard precautions are observed when collecting sputum specimens and the inside of the container is kept sterile. Keep the container covered as much as possible, to prevent contamination of the specimen or the surroundings. When the cover is removed, place the cover on the counter or table with the inside up. (Only the outside of the cover should touch the table.) You should touch only the *outside* of the container and its cover. *Rationale: The inside of the container is considered to be sterile; the outside is contaminated.*

Consuming adequate amounts of fluid and breathing humidified air or aerosolized medications often help to loosen and liquefy secretions, making it easier for the client to expectorate secretions. If the client has used aerosolized medications, document this in the health record, along with the fact that a specimen has been collected. In Practice: Nursing Procedure 52-7 describes collecting a sputum specimen.

The provider may write an order to *measure sputum*. If so, do this in one of two ways:

1. If enough sputum is collected in a graduated specimen container, read the amount directly or
2. Pour an equal amount of water into an identical container and measure the water.

In addition, do the following:

- Weigh the specimen, if ordered. Do so on a balance scale, subtracting the initial weight of the container.
- Take the specimen to the laboratory immediately after collection. *Rationale: A delay may alter the result of a culture.*
- Label the container appropriately and notify laboratory personnel that this is a sputum specimen. Make sure the proper requests are in place.
- Document the sputum's amount (copious, moderate, or small), color, odor, and consistency.

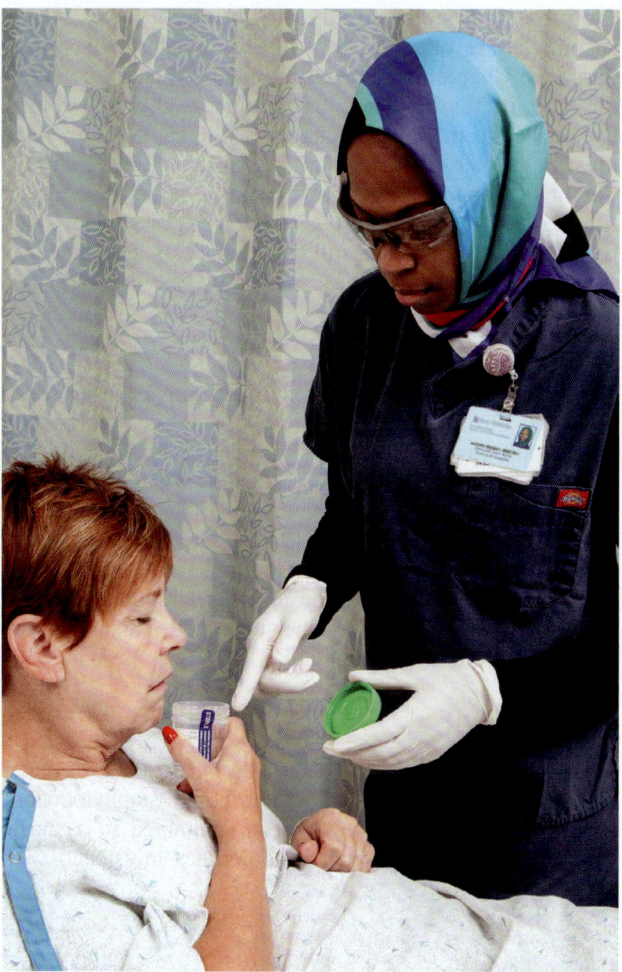

Figure 52-4 Wearing gloves and goggles, the nurse instructs the client to expectorate the sputum specimen into the sterile specimen container, without touching the inside of the container. The container is carefully labeled, inserted into a biohazard bag, and immediately sent to the laboratory. (Lynn, 2015.)

Nursing Alert

- The sputum specimen is considered highly contaminated. Treat it with caution.
- Tissues used by any client also are considered contaminated. Dispose of them properly, as per agency protocol.
- Wear gloves when handling tissues and sputum specimens and when providing any nursing care, if the client is coughing up sputum.
- Goggles and a mask or a full face shield may be necessary to protect the nurse from droplet secretions, particularly if the client is coughing or spitting. (A "spit shield" is also available. This is a net-type device placed over the client's head so they cannot spit at others.)

COLLECTING OTHER SPECIMENS

The nurse may be asked to obtain other specimens. Remember to observe *standard precautions* when working with any bodily fluid or drainage. Often, face and eye protection are required, in addition to gloves. Many specimens are obtained for culture, using sterile procedure (see Chapter 57). If culture medium is contained in the tube, it may be necessary to squeeze the tube gently, to release the medium. Sometimes, the stick of the swab must be broken off, making it possible to tightly replace the tube stopper. The nurse will require in-service education before obtaining these specimens. (The vaginal swab for sexually transmitted infections such as gonorrhea, is illustrated in Fig. 70-2.)

Throat Culture

This procedure is usually done to determine the presence of "strep throat." Make sure the client has not recently used mouthwash or antiseptic gargle. The throat culture is obtained using a sterile cotton-tipped swab, contained in a sterile tube. A tongue blade is used to depress the tongue and the swab moved around the tonsil area, without touching the tongue or teeth. The material obtained is smeared on a microscope slide and sealed in a sterile container or the swab is replaced within the tube and sealed. This procedure is briefly introduced in Chapter 86.

Nasal Swab

A nasal swab is cultured to determine the presence of respiratory infections, such as influenza and staphylococcus infections. A cotton-tipped swab is contained in a sterile capped test tube. The swab is sometimes moistened with sterile water before being inserted about 2 cm into one naris and rotated for 3 s (or five rotations), then held in place for 15 s. The procedure is repeated in the second nares, using the same swab.

Nasopharyngeal Swab

A nasopharyngeal swab is obtained to diagnose infections, primarily those caused by viruses. These include pertussis, diphtheria, meningitis, influenza, and respiratory syncytial virus (RSV). In some cases, antibiotic-resistant organisms (e.g., MRSA) or persons who are carriers may be identified. A sterile swab on a flexible wire is inserted deep into the nares and sent to the laboratory for culture (Lynn, 2018).

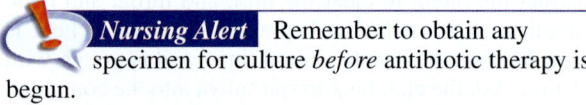

Nursing Alert Remember to obtain any specimen for culture *before* antibiotic therapy is begun.

NCLEX Alert

NCLEX concepts include the principles of standard precautions and transmission-based precautions. Situations may require knowledge of the principles of infection prevention and avoidance of cross-contamination.

STUDENT SYNTHESIS

KEY POINTS

- Standard precautions are used when collecting specimens involving any body fluids. All specimens and body fluids are considered biohazardous.
- Careful handwashing limits the transfer of microorganisms from one person to another and retards the spread of disease.
- Fluid intake includes all fluids consumed through the GI system (by mouth or tube feeding) and fluids taken as part of IV therapy or TPN.
- Output includes urine and all other fluids leaving the body by any means. This includes wound drainage, emesis (vomiting), watery diarrhea, bleeding, and NG or other suction returns.
- Routine specimen collection is usually scheduled for early in the morning.
- Any specimen collected should be transported or sent to the laboratory immediately, to ensure the most accurate results.
- Urine specimens collected include single-voided, clean-catch (or midstream), catheterized, 24-hr, and fractional urine specimens.
- Stool specimens are typically evaluated for occult blood and for O&P.
- Sputum specimen collection requires the client to expectorate or cough up secretions from the lower respiratory tract. The early morning specimen is the most accurate.
- A vital part of nursing function is to check the results of any test and notify the appropriate person if any abnormalities are noted.
- The nurse may collect other specimens, including throat cultures.

CRITICAL THINKING EXERCISES

1. Considering the reasons for accurate I&O records, identify possible client outcomes if I&O records are inaccurate.
2. If a 24-hr urine collection is not done accurately, how might the results be affected?
3. Describe how and why standard precautions apply to the collection of all specimens.

NCLEX-STYLE REVIEW QUESTIONS

1. A client is suspected of having tuberculosis. When would be the best time for the nurse to collect the sputum specimen?
   a. After the client brushes the teeth.
   b. Directly before the client goes to bed in the evening.
   c. Immediately after the client awakens in the morning.
   d. After the client eats a meal.

2. The nurse is to obtain a urine specimen from a client who is suspected of having a urinary tract infection. After collecting and labeling the specimen, which action would the nurse take to prevent contamination of the specimen?
   a. Place the specimen in a biohazard bag.
   b. Take the specimen and place it in the laboratory refrigerator.
   c. Call the laboratory to come and get the specimen.
   d. Inform the client that the results will be back soon.

3. A client has a dressing on a sacral wound that is saturated with drainage. How would the nurse obtain the output information from this dressing?
   a. Estimate the amount of liquid in the saturated dressing.
   b. The information cannot be obtained since it is not liquid.
   c. Weigh the dressing and document the results.
   d. Weigh the dressing and then weigh an identical dry dressing.

4. The nurse is obtaining a urine specimen from a client for a drug screen. Which is the appropriate action for the nurse to take?
   a. Have the client go into the bathroom and close the door to void.
   b. Have the client void in a urinal or bedpan and place the specimen in a container.
   c. Directly observe the client voiding in the specimen container.
   d. Give the client a cup of water to drink while in the bathroom to assist with voiding.

5. Prior to having a guaiac test performed, which instruction(s) would the nurse provide to the client? Select all that apply.
   a. Do not take more than 250 mg/day of vitamin C.
   b. Avoid taking acetylsalicylic acid (Aspirin) or NSAIDs 3 days before the test.
   c. Avoid eating rare red meat prior to testing.
   d. Do not take antihypertensive medication prior to testing.
   e. Avoid dairy products prior to testing.

CHAPTER RESOURCES

Enhance your learning with additional resources on thePoint*!*

Student Resources related to this chapter can be found at thePoint.lww.com/Rosdahl12e.

Welcome Steps

Look at healthcare provider's orders.

Protocol for procedure.

Necessary equipment/supplies.

Wash hands using proper hand hygiene; put on gloves.

Explain the procedure and reassure the client.

Locate two identifiers to confirm correct client.

Comfortable and efficient position for nurse and client.

Obtain privacy.

Make sure to follow correct steps and body mechanics with good technique.

Ensure safety and observe deviations from normal.

End Steps

Ensure comfort and safety.

Note questions or concerns from client or nurse; note significant data.

Dispose of materials properly.

Disinfect the area and your hands.

Document and report the procedure and your findings.

IN PRACTICE

NURSING PROCEDURE 52-1 — Measuring Urinary Output

Supplies and Equipment
Gloves
Eye protection, if necessary
Measuring graduate
Bedpan, urinal, or specimen hat (half-pan)

Steps

Follow LPN WELCOME steps and then

1. Label the specimen receptacle with the client's name. Figure 51-2 illustrates the urinal and two types of bedpans; Figure 52-2 illustrates the specimen hat. *Rationale: Labeling prevents cross-contamination. The client may move to another room and the equipment should move also.*

2. If using a specimen hat, position it in the toilet, with the collecting receptacle toward the front and the open end toward the back. *Rationale: Placing the hat in this manner acts as a reminder to the client and allows collection of urine without stool, if the client has a bowel movement.*

3. Ask the client to void in the receptacle. Tell the client to put toilet paper into the toilet or waste receptacle and *not in the collecting receptacle*. *Rationale: To be accurate, all urine output is measured. Toilet paper would alter the accuracy of the measurement.*

4. Pour the urine into the graduate, hold it at eye level, and read the urine volume in milliliters (see In Practice: Nursing Procedure 52-2). *Rationale: Using a graduated container ensures accurate measurement. Holding at eye level takes the volume of the meniscus into consideration.*

5. Pour the urine into the toilet and flush, unless the urine is to be saved. *Rationale: Sometimes more than one test is made from one urine sample.*

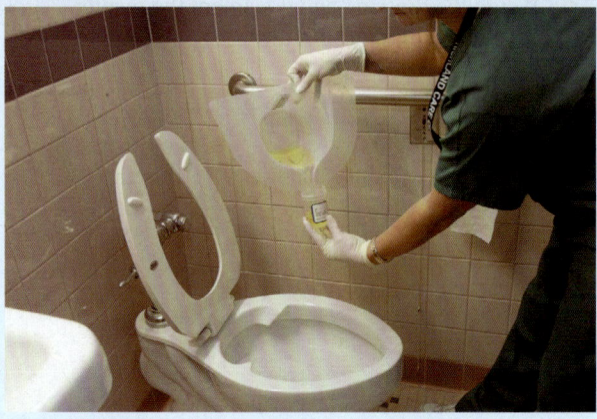

The graduate is held at eye level to properly determine the amount of fluid it contains. The volume is read at the bottom of the meniscus. A face shield may be required to protect against splashing. (Carter, 2005.)

6. Rinse the collecting receptacle and the graduate in cool water. Many facilities have a "showerhead" attachment on the toilet, which pulls down. This then sprays when the toilet is flushed and is used to rinse the specimen hat or bedpan. *Rationale: Hot water will cause proteins to coagulate and will break down the urine faster, releasing ammonia. The spray attachment is a convenient way to rinse bedpans and urinals.*

7. Encourage the client to wash their hands. *Rationale: Handwashing reinforces proper hygiene and reduces the risk of infection.*

Follow ENDDD steps.

Special Reminder
- The urine volume is documented, per facility protocol. Note also any abnormalities.

IN PRACTICE

NURSING PROCEDURE 52-2 Measuring Urine Specific Gravity

Supplies and Equipment
Specific-gravity beaker
Gloves
Eye protection, if needed
Hydrometer (urinometer)
Bedpan, urinal, or specimen hat

Steps
Follow LPN WELCOME steps and then

1. Collect urine and measure, if ordered (see In Practice: Nursing Procedure 52-1). Fill the specific-gravity beaker with urine to approximately 1 in. from the top. Gently drop in the measuring instrument, the *hydrometer (urinometer),* while spinning it gently. Be sure the hydrometer is floating freely and not touching the side of the beaker. *Rationale:* Volume measurements are completed before any other testing is done. A rotating hydrometer is easier to keep away from the side of the beaker. Handling the hydrometer gently avoids breakage. If the hydrometer touches anything, the reading will not be accurate.

2. Hold the beaker at eye level and obtain the SG reading at the bottom of the meniscus (the downward curve of the liquid's surface). *Rationale:* Liquids are always measured in this way for accuracy and consistency.

3. Properly dispose of urine and rinse the beaker and hydrometer in cool water. *Rationale:* In addition to coagulating the protein, hot water can break the instrument.

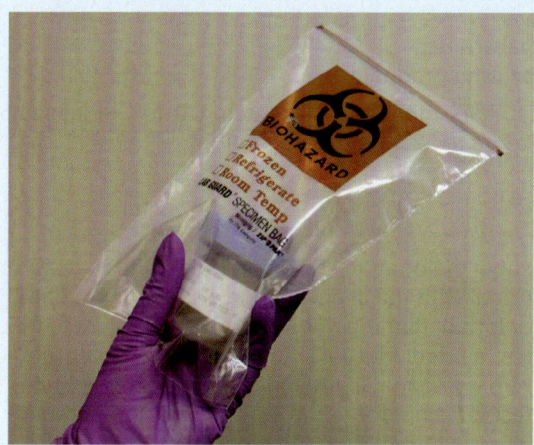

Measure urine SG at eye level for accuracy. Read at the bottom of the meniscus, which is the slight downward bulge or curve seen on the liquid's surface.

Follow ENDDD steps

IN PRACTICE

NURSING PROCEDURE 52-3 Collecting a Single-Voided Specimen

Supplies and Equipment
Covered specimen bottle or container (wide-mouthed)
Label
Clean bedpan, specimen hat, or urinal
Gloves
Eye protection, if needed
Biohazard bag

Note: Refer to In Practice: Nursing Care Guidelines 52-1 and 52-2 before beginning. For most tests, a midstream sample, rather than a catheterized specimen, is best if the client can cooperate (see In Practice: Nursing Care Guidelines 52-3).

Steps
Follow LPN WELCOME steps and then

1. Label the specimen container and the lid, if possible. Include the client's name and all pertinent identifiers. Apply the label before the client voids. *Rationale:* Proper labeling ensures correct identification and avoids mistakes. The laboratory will not test unlabeled specimens. The label may not stick if the container becomes wet.

2. Instruct the client to clean the genital area with soap and water or a specially prepared antiseptic towelette and then to obtain a midstream sample. The client should void a small amount, then collect the sample, and then finish voiding. Nursing Care Guidelines 52-3 describes the method of cleaning the genital area. A sterile specimen container or clean toilet hat or bedpan is used. *Rationale: Cleansing the genital area helps remove potential sources of contamination. The midstream specimen is the most accurate. Voiding into a clean receptacle prevents most cross-contamination.*

3. Remove the specimen as soon as possible after the client has voided. *Rationale:* Substances in urine decompose when exposed to air. Decomposition may alter test results and it causes odor.

4. Pour about 90–120 mL of urine into the labeled specimen container (unless the client has voided directly into the container). Cover the container. Place the container in a biohazard bag and send it to the laboratory immediately. *Rationale:* An adequate amount of urine is needed for the tests. Covering the bottle retards decomposition and prevents added contamination. All body substances must be transported in a biohazard bag to alert the laboratory staff and provide protection for anyone handling specimens.

Follow ENDDD steps

IN PRACTICE

NURSING PROCEDURE 52-4 Collecting a 24-hr Urine Specimen

Supplies and Equipment
Opaque 2-L collection bottle with lid (additional bottle may be needed)
Label(s) for container(s)
Container of ice or refrigerator for storage
Towel
Bedpan, urinal, or specimen hat
Gloves
Biohazard bag
Measuring graduate

Note: Refer to In Practice: Nursing Care Guidelines 52-1, 52-2, and 52-3 before beginning.

Steps
Follow LPN WELCOME steps and then

1. Label the opaque collecting bottle and bedpan or urinal with the client's name and pertinent data before beginning. Indicate the time and date the test started. Place a sign in the client's bathroom reminding the client and others that the 24-hr test is being done. The sign should state that no urine is to be discarded without contacting the nurse. *Rationale: Opaque bottles help prevent decomposition caused by exposure to light. Proper labeling ensures correct identification of the urine specimen by the laboratory. (The laboratory will not test unlabeled specimens.) It is important to obtain a full 24-hr specimen for this test.*

2. Instruct the client to void. If a bedpan or urinal must be used, discard it after this voiding. Also, *discard* this urine and record the time as the beginning time for the test in the client's chart and the collection bottle. *Rationale: Collection always begins with an empty bladder. If this collection is made from an indwelling catheter, proceed following the same timetable (see In Practice: Nursing Procedure 52-5).*

3. Use a new urinal or bedpan. After the collection period begins, measure each specimen of urine voided, and pour into the collecting bottle that is placed on ice or being cooled; record each amount. *Rationale: Measuring each voiding ensures that all urine is collected and available for analysis. Cooling helps retard decomposition of the urine.*

4. If the client has an indwelling catheter, the provider may order a new catheter setup inserted before the collection begins. A disposable cooler with ice is kept at the bedside and the catheter bag rests in the cooler. The collection bag still must be emptied at regular intervals. *Rationale: The ice keeps urine in the catheter bag "fresh" during the intervals between emptying. The urine is then placed in cool storage as the collection continues.*

5. Keep the collecting bottle opening covered. *Rationale: Urine decomposes into ammonia when exposed to air; limiting exposure to the air controls odor.*

6. Continue collection for 24 hr from the time the first urine was discarded. At exactly 24 hr after beginning the collection, instruct the client to void. Pour this voided amount into the bottle. *Rationale: Complete collection of all urine produced in 24 hr ensures accurate test results. The last voiding completes the 24-hr total; collection ends with an empty bladder.*

7. Note the exact time and amount of the last urine specimen collected on the bottle label. Cover the bottle tightly, place in a biohazard bag, and label as a 24-hr urine collection with the client's identification information. Maintain cleanliness on the outside of the bag. *Rationale: Proper labeling and timing ensures accurate results. Keeping the outside clean helps protect healthcare workers.*

Follow ENDDD steps

Special Reminders
- Be sure that the client voids before beginning the collection. Start with an empty bladder.
- Be sure to document start and stop times and total amount collected.
- Ensure that the specimen is sent to the laboratory immediately.
- If a "fractional collection" is ordered, a bottle must be prepared and labeled for each fraction of the 24 hr. (Most often, the fractional collection is timed in 6-hr segments.) In this case, the client is asked to start with an empty bladder and void at the end of each time segment. The urine collected is poured into the appropriate bottle for each time segment.

IN PRACTICE

NURSING PROCEDURE 52-5 Collecting a Urine Specimen From an Indwelling Catheter

Supplies and Equipment
Gloves
Clamp or rubber band
Container with label
Syringe (10- to 20-mL) with 21- to 25-gauge blunt-tipped (needleless) cannula; catheter must have needleless port
Biohazard bag
Alcohol prep or disinfectant swab

Steps
Follow LPN WELCOME steps and then

1. Label the sterile specimen container. *Rationale: Accuracy is vital; a mix-up between clients could be life-threatening. The laboratory will not perform tests on unlabeled specimens.*

2. Clamp the drainage tubing or fold the tubing over once and secure it with a rubber band below

the collection (aspiration) port. Allow adequate time for urine collection but *no longer than 15 min*. **Rationale:** *Collecting urine from the tubing guarantees a fresh specimen.*

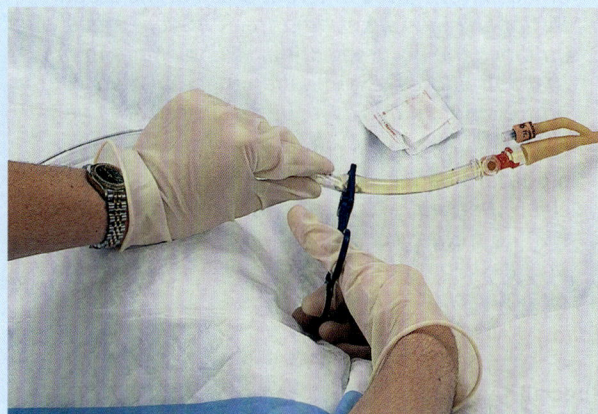

Clamp the drainage tubing below the collection port.

3. Cleanse the aspiration port with an antiseptic swab, such as an alcohol. **Rationale:** *Disinfecting the port deters microorganisms from entering the catheter.*
4. Open the syringe package, maintaining the sterility of the syringe and needleless hub or blunt-tipped needle (cannula). Insert the blunt-tipped needle into the aspiration port and withdraw urine into the syringe. The laboratory test required determines the amount of urine to collect. **Rationale:** *This technique provides an uncontaminated urine specimen while preventing contamination of the client's bladder. The blunt-tipped cannula helps prevent accidental needle sticks.*

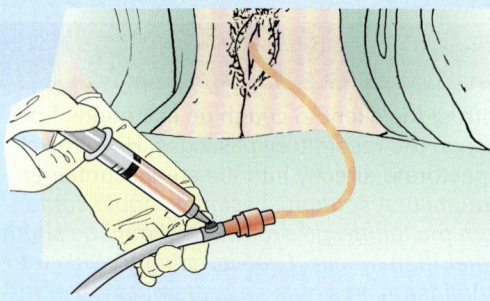

Insert the blunt-tipped cannula into the port and withdraw the required amount of urine for the specimen. (Evans-Smith, 2005.)

5. Transfer the urine to the sterile labeled specimen container and attach the cover. The container must be *sterile* for a culture and *clean* for a routine urinalysis. Dispose of the blunt-tipped needle in the sharps container. **Rationale:** *Careful labeling prevents confusion. Careful transfer of the specimen prevents contamination or confusion of the urine specimen. Correct disposal of sharps prevents injury to the nurse and others.*
6. Unclamp the catheter. **Rationale:** *This allows free urinary flow and prevents urinary stasis.*
7. Prepare the container and place in a biohazard bag, keeping the outside of the bag clean. Send the container to the laboratory immediately, with the proper documentation. **Rationale:** *Proper packaging ensures that the specimen is not an infection risk. Prevent microorganisms from growing in the specimen.*

Follow ENDDD steps

Special Reminder

- If a needleless system is not available in your facility, a syringe and needle are used. The urine specimen is collected in the same manner, using the collection port on the catheter system. *Do not pierce the catheter tubing with the needle.*

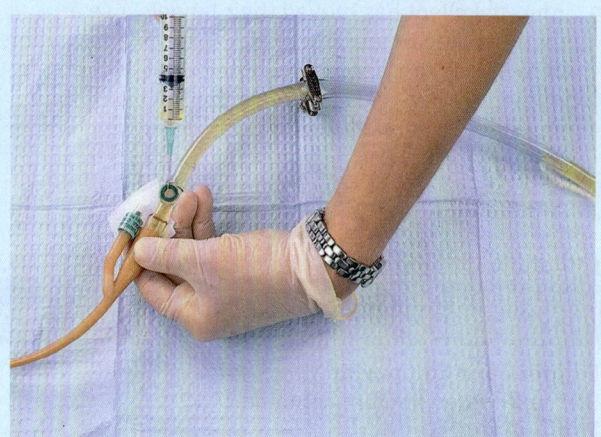

A specimen is obtained with a syringe and small sterile needle in the same manner as one obtained with a blunt-tipped cannula. Always use the collection port. (Timby, 2005.)

IN PRACTICE

NURSING PROCEDURE 52-6: Collecting a Stool Specimen

Supplies and Equipment
Gloves
Clean bedpan and cover or specimen hat
Closed specimen container and cover
Label
Wooden tongue blades or specimen sticks
Biohazard bag

Steps
Follow LPN WELCOME steps and then

1. Ask the client to tell you when they feel the urge to have a bowel movement. *Rationale: Most people cannot have a bowel movement on command.*
2. Label the container. *Rationale: Proper labeling ensures correct identification of the specimen by the laboratory.*
3. Give the client the bedpan when they are ready. If the client will be using the toilet, place the specimen hat turned toward the back of the toilet. *Rationale: It is most likely to obtain a useable specimen at this time. The specimen hat allows stool to be collected free of urine.*
4. After the client has moved their bowels, use a tongue blade or specimen stick to transfer a portion of the feces to a specimen container or to the Hemoccult card (see Fig. 52-3). Do not touch the specimen. *Rationale: It is grossly contaminated.*
5. If a specimen container is to be used, take a portion of feces from three different areas of the stool. *Rationale: Samples from three different areas will enhance the accuracy of the results. Keep in mind that sometimes, examination must be made of the entire stool. In this case, use a larger container.*
6. Cover the specimen container. Place it in a biohazard bag, keeping the outside of the bag clean. *Rationale: Covering the container ensures that no further contamination of the specimen will occur. Keeping the bag clean protects laboratory and other personnel.*

Follow ENDDD steps

Special Reminder
- Remember to take or send the container *immediately* to the laboratory with the appropriate request slip or computer entry. *Rationale: Examinations for parasites, eggs (ova), and organisms must be made when the stool is warm.*
- If testing for occult blood is to be done by nursing staff, use the Hemocult or other test kit, as described previously in this chapter and illustrated in Figure 52-3.

IN PRACTICE

NURSING PROCEDURE 52-7: Collecting a Sputum Specimen

Supplies and Equipment
Sterile, covered sputum container
Tissues
Labels
Gloves
Mask or face shield
Biohazard bag

Steps
Follow LPN WELCOME steps and then

1. Label the container, with two client identifiers, in presence of client (Joint Commission, 2020). *Rationale: Careful labeling ensures accuracy of the report and alerts laboratory personnel to the presence of a contaminated specimen.*
2. Collect the specimen as early as possible in the morning. *Rationale: The early morning specimen is most accurate and free of contaminants, such as food, toothpaste, etc. The client is most likely to be able to cough up secretions first thing in the morning.*
3. Instruct the client to cough up secretions from deep in the respiratory passages. Have the client expectorate directly into the sterile container. *Rationale: A sputum specimen should come from the lungs and bronchi. It should be sputum, rather than mucus. Expectorating directly into the container avoids outside contamination of the specimen or contamination of other objects.*
4. Cover the specimen immediately. Place in a biohazard bag, keeping the outside of the bag clean. *Rationale: Covering the specimen helps prevent contamination. Keeping the bag clean protects laboratory personnel.*

Follow ENDDD steps

Special Reminder
- Remember to transport the specimen to the laboratory *immediately* to ensure greater accuracy of test results and prevent inappropriate proliferation of organisms.

53 Bandages and Binders

Learning Objectives

1. State at least three purposes of bandages and binders.
2. State the most common indications for using the roller bandage.
3. Explain evaluation of the client's extremity when a bandage or antiembolism stocking is applied.
4. Identify the most common use of the T-binder; describe the differences between that used for a male and a female.
5. Explain the rationale for using Montgomery straps.
6. In the skills laboratory, demonstrate the ability to apply roller bandages and antiembolism stockings, and change a dressing using Montgomery straps.

Important Terminology

antiembolism stockings
bandage
Kerlix
maceration
Montgomery straps
peripheral neurovascular assessment

Acronyms

ACE
CMS-ET
PCD
PNA
SCD
TED sox

When the client's condition requires application of bandages or binders, understanding the reasons for their use and performing correct, safe application techniques are important. Bandages and binders exist in a number of forms. They may be elasticized or may be firmer. A **bandage** is a long strip, wrapped around a body part, such as the elasticized ACE bandage. (A dressing applied over a wound is sometimes called a bandage as well.) A *binder* may be applied to support a body part. Purposes and therapeutic benefits of bandages, binders, and other support devices include the following:

- Supporting a joint while allowing it to move (e.g., an ACE bandage or a knee brace—Fig. 97-5).
- Supporting a limb, to relieve pressure and pain (e.g., the sling—Nursing Procedure 43-1)
- Immobilizing a joint or limb or maintaining it in a specific position (e.g., with a cast or leg immobilizer—Chapter 77)
- Supporting a wound or incision, to prevent *dehiscence* (wound rupture) and *evisceration* (protrusion of internal contents through a wound)
- Holding dressings in place (Chapter 58)
- Holding a pad to absorb drainage (e.g., the T-binder)
- Holding a splint in place, particularly in an emergency (Fig. 43-9)
- Holding a cold pack or warm pack in place
- Providing compression, to promote venous return, as in venous insufficiency or postoperatively (e.g., the pneumatic compression device [PCD]—Fig. 53-2)
- Supporting circulation following hemorrhage (e.g., MAST trousers)
- Preventing edema and fluid loss after a burn (Fig. 75-5)
- Providing compression, to prevent contractures, as in a burn
- Shaping a stump before fitting a prosthesis

BANDAGES

Bandages are available in various widths and sizes. Some are rolled, to provide easy application. They may be clean or sterile. Table 53-1 provides examples of patterns used when wrapping bandages. Often, elasticized bandages are wrapped around a client's limbs to provide muscle or joint support or to increase or support circulation. This gentle pressure stimulates blood return to the heart and prevents blood from pooling in the extremity. Application that is too tight, however, can squeeze blood vessels and nerves (*constriction*), resulting in tissue damage. It is vital to determine carefully and frequently the status of circulation and nerve function in the client's fingers or toes, to ensure that a bandage or cast is not too tight. (Chapter 77 addresses general care of the client who has a cast.)

Evaluating Extremity Status

The descriptive term for evaluating the status of an extremity encased in a bandage or a cast is *peripheral neurovascular assessment* (**PNA**). (See In Practice: Data Gathering in Nursing 53-1.) The final assessment is done by an RN, but the LVN/LPN assists in making and reporting observations. Examples of observations related to the distal portion of the extremity (furthest from the heart) are listed here:

- Skin color
- Finger or toe motion
- Sensation in fingers or toes
- Distal pulses
- Capillary refill (Chapter 47)
- Edema or swelling (Fig. 47-9)
- Pain
- Severe pressure or tightness
- Skin temperature

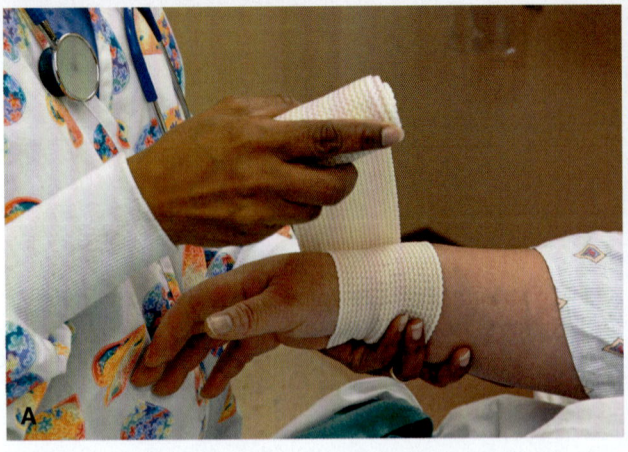 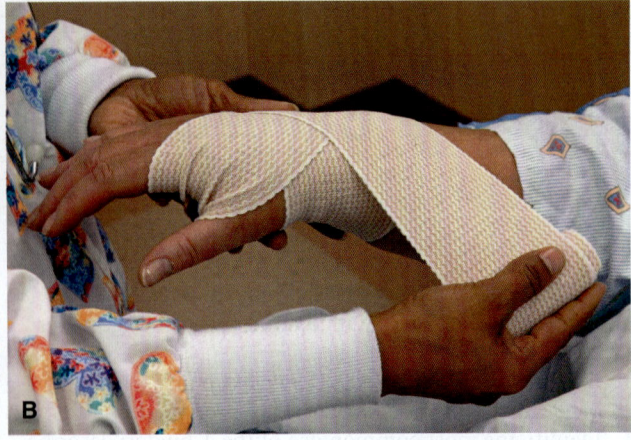

Figure 53-1 Wrapping the all cotton elastic (ACE) roller bandage on the client's arm. **A.** Wrap the bandage around the client's limb twice, below the joint, to anchor it. **B.** Use alternating ascending and descending turns to form a figure eight. Overlap each turn of the bandage by one half to two thirds the width of the strip. Fasten the end securely. Gloves are worn if the client has an open wound. (Evans-Smith, 2005.)

TABLE 53-1 Wrapping of Bandages

TYPE OF APPLICATION	DESCRIPTION	USES
Figure 8	Overlapping application: alternating with ascending and descending wrapping, with each pass of the bandage crossing over previous wrapping, as in a figure 8.	Stabilizes joints, such as wrist or ankle, and helps maintain immobilization.
Spiral	Wrapping a limb in ascending path, partially covering previous wrapping while moving up the limb.	Promotes venous return. Effective when a bandage needs to be applied around an arm, leg, or wrist. May be used to hold dressings in place.
Spiral reverse	Similar to spiral, except the bandage is folded back (distally) halfway through each pass. The appearance of a basket weave is produced.	May be more stable on arms, legs, thighs (extremities that are wider at one end than the other—cone shape) than spiral alone. Promotes venous return. Holds dressings in place.
Circular	Wrapping with continuous application in same place, such as a wrist.	Stabilizes ankle, wrist, fingers, and toes.
Recurrent	Anchored at the top with several spiral wraps, then back and forth across the end of the extremity or head. Finish with spiral reverse or figure 8.	Binds amputation stump in preparation for prosthesis fitting. Holds dressings on the head.

Figures from Timby (2013).

CHAPTER 53   Bandages and Binders   779

> **IN PRACTICE**
> **DATA GATHERING IN NURSING 53-1**   **The Client's Circulation When Using Bandages ("CMS-ET")**
>
> **Color of Toes or Fingers**
> - The toes or fingers should be a color appropriate for the client's normal skin tone. They should not be pale, white, dusky, cyanotic, or mottled.
> - Digits (toes, fingers) are checked by pressing them lightly. Skin tone should return to normal immediately after the pressure is removed (capillary refill). If the area that was touched remains lighter, the skin is *blanched* (indicating impaired circulation).
>
> **Motion or Mobility**
> - The client should be able to move the toes or fingers freely.
>
> **Sensitivity or Sensation**
> - The client should be able to feel your touch on the digits. This should be equal on both sides.
> - The client's subjective feelings—tingling, numbness, itching, or tightness (extreme tightness is a significant complication)—should be discussed, to obtain additional information.
> - The client's complaints of severe or excessive pain are significant.
>
> **Edema and Swelling**
> - When you press the client's hand or foot, an indentation should not remain. An imprint indicates pitting edema (Fig. 47-9). Nonpitting (brawny) edema is also possible.
>
> **Temperature**
> - The client's toes or fingers should be warm, with temperature equal on both sides and the same as the rest of the body.
>
> *NOTE:* These data gathering should be repeated at least every 2 hr (or more often, if necessary) for the client who has a cast, bandage, binder, or any other immobilization device in place. The acronym, **CMS-ET**, color, motion, sensitivity, edema, temperature, is used to denote this evaluation. Document and report any significant findings immediately.

When making these observations, note any abnormal findings and report them immediately. Often, a checklist is available to report frequent neurovascular observations. Follow your facility's protocol. It is also important to determine if bandages have loosened, particularly if the client is mobile or restless. Loose bandages are not therapeutic. Just as the client is checked frequently to determine if a bandage is too tight, you must also check to see if it is too loose.

> **NCLEX ALERT**
>
> You should be aware of the purposes and therapeutic benefits of bandages/binders and how they relate to nursing care. Examples in this chapter include the support of a limb/joint or wound/incision and holding a splint or warm/cold pack in place. Consider this as you select nursing actions in the NCLEX examination scenarios.

Roller Bandages

A commonly used bandage is an elastic roller bandage called the *all cotton elastic* (**ACE**) bandage (Fig. 53-1). (ACE is a brand name.) Although usually wrapped around a limb to give support, the ACE bandage may also be used to hold a dressing on an extremity or on the body's trunk. In first aid, an ACE bandage may be wrapped around a body part to exert pressure over a bleeding point.

Kerlix

In other cases, a type of stretchy gauze in a long roll, with the brand name **Kerlix**, is used to hold dressings in place. The steps for applying an ACE- or Kerlix-type bandage are described in In Practice: Nursing Care Guidelines 53-1.

Stretch-Net Bandages

Another bandage, called tube gauze, is frequently used. It consists of a very stretchy net or mesh-type material. These bandages come in assorted sizes, ranging from finger size to a size large enough to go around a person's body. They are often used to hold a wound dressing in place and are frequently used in first aid and burn care. This bandage is convenient to apply and comfortable for the client. Tape is not always required to hold this bandage in place. This dressing is used frequently in the healthcare practitioner's office or in the school or industrial setting, to dress a small wound or hold a small dressing in place. In Practice: Nursing Care Guidelines 53-2 describes the steps used to apply this dressing. The larger sizes of stretch-net dressings cover an arm or leg and are applied in a manner similar to the procedure outlined for dressing a finger. They are simply stretched and placed over the extremity. The body-size material is stretched and moved over the head and arms, to position it over the torso.

> **Nursing Alert**   When applying a large stretch-net bandage to the torso, be sure to explain the procedure to the client beforehand, to help alleviate surprise and apprehension.

IN PRACTICE
NURSING CARE GUIDELINES 53-1 — Applying a Roller Bandage (Arm or Leg)

- Wear gloves if the client has any nonintact skin or a rash. Consult your team leader if you are not sure. *Rationale: It is important to protect yourself and others from the spread of infection.*
- Follow your facility's protocol regarding dressings and dressing changes. The provider's orders indicate the specific part to wrap. A wound care specialist may order the frequency and specific instructions for dressing changes, if needed (Chapter 58). All instructions should be in the nursing care plan. *Rationale: The dressings will usually be changed when the bandage is rewrapped. It is important to follow all instructions; these are part of wound treatment or of the client's disorder. Complete instructions in the nursing care plan are available to all staff.*
- In many cases, a roller (ACE) bandage will be applied to support a body part (Fig. 53-1). A wound may or may not be present. *Rationale: The basic wrapping of the roller bandage is the same, whether or not a wound exists.*
- Use the correct bandage width, which is determined by the part to be wrapped. Generally, a bandage wider than 7.5 cm (3 in.) is difficult to keep in place on an arm or leg. (Wider bandages may be used on the chest or abdomen.) More than one roller bandage may be used, if necessary. Simply overlap ends. *Rationale: If a bandage is too narrow, it will pinch and bind. If too wide, it will fold over. In either case, the effectiveness of the bandage will be compromised.*
- Explain to the client what you plan to do and provide privacy. Wear gloves, if necessary. *Rationale: Ensure the client's cooperation and follow Standard Precautions.*
- Elevate the extremity to just above the level of the client's body if the client is recumbent. If the client has been sitting or walking and the foot or leg is to be wrapped, ask the client to lie down for at least 15 minutes before wrapping the bandage. If an arm is to be wrapped, elevate it above the client's heart level. Support the limb while wrapping. *Rationale: Elevation helps prevent congestion of blood and lymph in the area to be wrapped. Blood that may have pooled in the legs needs to be returned to the circulation. Otherwise, edema could interfere with the effectiveness of the bandage or cause pain and/or damage the limb.*
- Make sure the bandage is rolled before beginning to wrap. *Rationale: This helps ensure that even pressure is applied and will be more convenient for you.*
- Begin wrapping the bandage at the client's toes or fingers and move toward the hip or shoulder. *Rationale: Wrapping toward the heart enhances venous return.*
- Wrap the bandage firmly, but not too tightly. Stretch the bandage *very slightly* while wrapping. *Rationale: This gives support, but helps prevent the bandage from being wrapped too tightly and cutting off circulation.*
- Overlap each layer about half the width of the previous strip. Do not allow any gaps between strips. Keep the bandage free of wrinkles or folds. *Rationale: Overlapping ensures more even pressure. Wrinkles can quickly cause skin irritation and/or breakdown.*
- Anchor the top with hypoallergenic tape or the attached Velcro strips (located at each end of the ACE bandage). Clips or pins are no longer used. *Rationale: Pins or clips may scratch the client.*
- Check the circulation of the client's toes or fingers after applying the bandage. (See this procedure [CMS-ET] in Data Gathering in Nursing 53-1.) *Rationale: A bandage that is too tight can cut off circulation and quickly cause tissue damage. If too loose, it will not provide support and will usually fall down.*
- Dispose of soiled dressings and gloves appropriately. Wash or sanitize your hands. *Rationale: Used dressings are grossly contaminated.*
- Check the client's peripheral neurovascular status within 1 hr and at least every 2 hr after that. Rewrap, if necessary. *Rationale: It is important to make sure the bandage is applied appropriately.*
- Document the procedure, noting the client's reactions. *Rationale: Provide communication and ensure continuity of care.*
- Release the bandage at least every 4 hr, unless ordered otherwise. At this time, help the client exercise the extremity and give skin care. *Rationale: Releasing the bandage allows skin inspection; exercise and skin care increase circulation and help prevent deformities and discomfort.*

Antiembolism Stockings

Many physicians routinely order **antiembolism stockings** (also called thromboembolic disease stockings [TED sox]) for all postoperative clients. TED sox cover the foot (not the toes) and the leg, up to the knee or mid-thigh. A firmly wrapped ACE bandage may also be applied, but stockings provide firmer and more even pressure against the leg's blood vessels. TED sox help ensure adequate return circulation (*venous circulation*) to the heart and may help prevent blood clots (*emboli* or *thromboemboli*). To give proper support, the stockings fit tightly without binding the leg or cutting off circulation. Stockings are available in various sizes. Measure the client's thigh or calf, according to the manufacturer's instructions, and select the appropriate size. Apply the stockings before the client gets out of bed or after the client has remained *recumbent* (lying down) for at least 15 min. *Rationale: Doing so prevents pooling of fluid or blood in*

IN PRACTICE
NURSING CARE GUIDELINES 53-2 Applying a Stretch-Net Dressing to a Finger

- Read the manufacturer's instructions before beginning. **Rationale:** *There may be small variations between brands.*
- Wear gloves, if the client's skin is not intact. Place the ordered dressing over the wound. **Rationale:** *Help prevent microorganism spread.*
- Cut a length of netting about 2.5–3 times the length of the finger and bunch the netting over the supplied metal tubing (applicator). **Rationale:** *Extra length is required to complete the dressing and make sure it stays in place. The applicator facilitates placement of the netting, and safely secures the dressing.*
- Place the tubing, with netting on the outside, over the finger. Hold the end of the netting in place at the base of the finger and gently pull the applicator tube, with the excess gauze netting, toward the end of the finger with the free hand. **Rationale:** *This places the first layer of netting on the finger.*
- Gently pull the applicator tube about ½ in. away from the end of the finger, while still holding the base; you now have some extra netting. Twist the applicator and netting, to cover the end of the finger. **Rationale:** *This completes the first layer of the dressing and encloses the end of the finger.*
- Push the applicator gently back toward the base of the finger, gradually releasing the remainder of the netting, forming a double layer of netting on the finger, like a stocking cap. Repeat this process if a thicker dressing is required (remember to cut a longer strip before beginning). **Rationale:** *This encloses the entire finger in a double layer of gauze. The gauze stretches and will usually stay in place. It may be taped in place, if necessary. You can use as many layers as necessary.*
- Change the dressing as needed. **Rationale:** *It is important to keep wounds as clean as possible.*
- Dispose of your gloves and document the procedure, including any pertinent observations. **Rationale:** *Documentation is important, to provide continuity of care and safety for the client.*

---

the leg, thus increasing pressure and altering the effect of the TED sox. In Practice: Nursing Procedure 53-1 describes the application of elastic stockings. Unlike ACE bandages, these stockings do not loosen; thus, check the client's PNA at least every 2 hr. Remove them at least every 4–8 hr and examine the leg carefully for redness, pitting edema, or skin discoloration. Document your findings and report deviations from normal. Wash the client's legs gently each day; apply lotion if the skin is dry, and apply clean stockings.

> **Nursing Alert** Some antiembolism stockings are designed to leave a hole in the top, for examination of the toes (Nursing Procedure 53-1). Other types have the hole in the bottom (Fig. 53-2). Check the package to determine which type you are using. Be sure to *fit the client's heel firmly into the heel pocket* of the stocking.

The PCD Machine

Another type of device, called a *pneumatic compression device* (**PCD**), *sequential compression device* (**SCD**), or *intermittent sequential compression device* (ISCD), provides alternating pressure to the legs (Fig. 53-2). This device, used to support circulation, is used primarily for clients immediately after surgery and those with circulatory disorders. The sleeves around the person's lower legs contain multiple chambers, which alternately inflate and deflate, pushing blood through the veins. The inflation begins at the foot and moves up the leg, pushing blood toward the heart. When the top chamber is reached, the sleeve deflates and the cycle begins again.

BINDERS

A *binder* is a flat piece of fabric applied to support a specific body part or hold a dressing in place. Commonly used binders include the *arm sling* (Nursing Procedure 43-1) and occasionally, the *T-binder*, a T-shaped strap used to hold a vaginal, groin, or anal dressing in place (Fig. 53-3). Montgomery straps are also considered to be binders (Fig. 53-4). Rarely, a breast binder will be ordered for a woman after childbirth. However, usually the client is instructed to wear a good support bra instead. Most binders use hook-and-loop fasteners (Velcro).

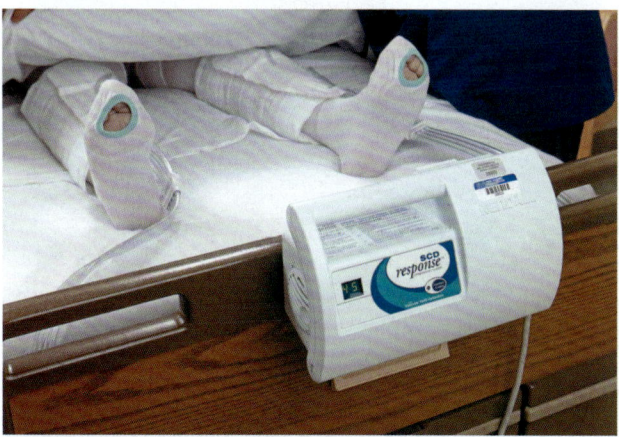

Figure 53-2 The pneumatic compression device (PCD) or sequential compression device (SCD) is frequently used following surgery to support the circulation. Note that the toe holes are on the bottom of these sleeves. (Carter, 2016.)

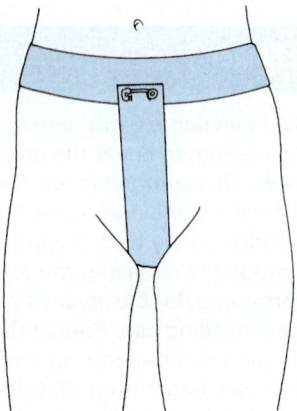

Figure 53-3 The T-binder comes in two configurations. Shown here is the female version. (The perineal strap is split in the middle [a "double T-binder"], to accommodate the male anatomy.).

T-Binder

T-binders are named for their shape. They come in a female and male design (Fig. 53-3). Although not used frequently in acute facilities, the nurse may see a T-binder used in home care. A T-binder can also be fabricated as a first aid measure, to hold rectal, perineal, or groin dressings in place. It may also be used to hold a perineal pad in place for the incontinent or menstruating female client, but adhesive sanitary

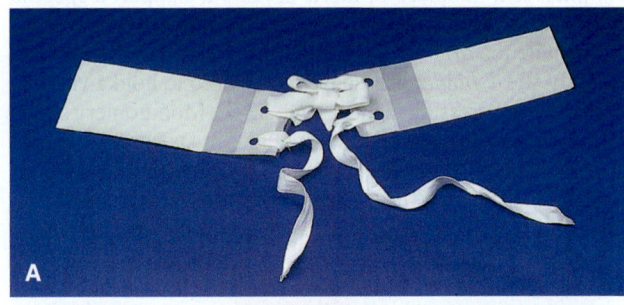

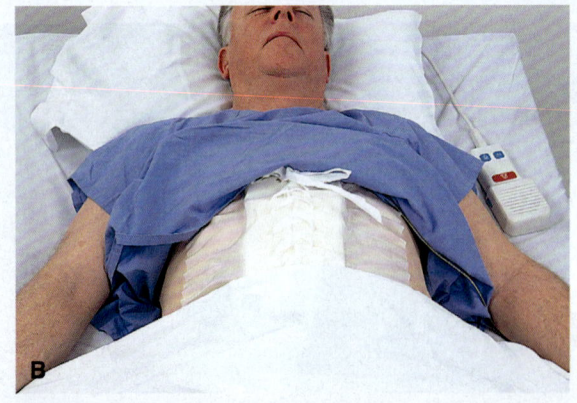

Figure 53-4 Montgomery straps are often used when dressings must be changed frequently. **A.** A short, single Montgomery strap is used for a small dressing. **B.** More than one strap is used for a larger dressing. This client's skin will be protected because it is not necessary to remove the tape for each dressing change. (Timby, 2013.)

IN PRACTICE
NURSING CARE GUIDELINES 53-3 — Applying a T-Binder

- Wash the hands before and after applying or adjusting a binder. Use Standard Precautions. If the client's skin is intact, gloves are not necessary.
- Be sure the T-binder is a size appropriate for the client. Apply the binder firmly enough to hold a dressing in place, but not too tightly. *Rationale: Using an incorrect size will not be effective and may constrict circulation or cause other damage. If the dressing is not applied firmly in place, bleeding could occur, support will not be effective, or the dressing's movement could irritate and/or contaminate the area.*
- Rewrap the binder every 2–4 hr and check the dressing. *Rationale: The client's movements tend to loosen the binder. When rewrapping the binder, assess the client's skin and check the dressing for amount and character of drainage. Check the wound at the same time.*

pads and underwear are usually used. The top longer band of the T-binder is placed around the client's waist and the perineal strap is brought between the legs (In Practice: Nursing Care Guidelines 53-3). It is fastened with Velcro or may be pinned in place in an emergency. (*Be very careful not to stick the client or yourself with the pins.*)

Abdominal Binder

An *abdominal binder*, very rarely used, supports the abdomen or large abdominal dressings. It may be used after cesarean delivery. The binder is applied from the bottom-up, to give the most support. If one is ordered, check your facility's protocol. Nursing Care Guidelines 53-4 gives general guidelines for nursing care of the client with a bandage or binder.

Tape

Instead of bandages and binders, strips of *hypoallergenic tape* sometimes are used to hold dressings in place. Tape may also be used to give support, as for sprained ankles, fractured ribs, or fractured toes. There are several kinds of tape that allow ventilation and help to prevent skin **maceration** (skin softening and breakdown, due to moisture accumulation and lack of circulation). To provide comfort, clip the client's hair close to the skin (particularly on hairy body areas) before applying large tape dressings because hairs stick to tape and make removal painful. Always remove tape in the direction of hair growth, for less discomfort. If tape is difficult to remove, carefully apply acetone to the skin at the edge of the applied strip. Keep moistening the skin close to the adhesive, as you gently peel off the tape. *Rationale: The acetone will help release the adhesion. (Nail polish remover can also be used.)*

IN PRACTICE
NURSING CARE GUIDELINES 53-4 — General Nursing Care of the Client With a Bandage or Binder

- Wear gloves, if the client's skin is not intact. *Rationale: Help prevent the spread of infection.*
- Perform peripheral neurovascular assessment (PNA) on a limb distal to any bandage or binder at least every 2 hr (or more frequently, as ordered). Danger signs include complaints of severe pain or tightness, as well as cyanosis or mottling of the skin, pallor, duskiness, coldness, numbness, swelling, tingling, or loss of sensation, and pulses that are difficult or impossible to palpate. *Rationale: Bandages or binders may compress nerves and/or blood vessels, if applied too tightly. They may also become too tight, if swelling occurs. Checking the PNA helps prevent permanent injury to tissue or the limb, due to loss of circulation or compression.*
- If the original application of a bandage or binder was performed by a nurse at the direction of a primary provider, the nurse may readjust or loosen it, if it becomes too tight. (If the provider placed the original device on the client, a specific order is needed to remove, adjust, or loosen it.) *Rationale: The nurse must practice within the scope of practice. It is important not to injure the client.*
- Remove bandages, as ordered, to periodically observe the skin, dressings, or wounds. Usually, this is done every 4 hr, but more frequent observations may be ordered, and a dressing change must be done if there is excessive drainage. *Rationale: The nurse should inspect the skin and wound area for irritation, breakdown, infection, irritation, or drainage. Provide skin care and dressing changes, as needed and ordered. Careful documentation about all aspects of the wound is vital (Chapter 58). Report any adverse signs immediately.*
- Elastic bandages should be applied with the greatest compression on the most distal point of the limb, with pressure gradually decreasing as the bandage is applied, moving up the limb toward the heart. *Rationale: This promotes venous return. Incorrectly applied elastic bandages can lead to edema and impaired circulation. Compartmental syndrome can also occur and may cause permanent nerve damage (Chapter 77).*
- Replace soiled bandages. *Rationale: A clean bandage helps prevent the spread of microorganisms and makes the client more comfortable.*
- Instruct the client or caregiver how to apply bandages and how to assess for impaired circulation, if the client will continue to use these after discharge. *Rationale: Client education facilitates compliance and helps prevent complications.*

Nursing Alert Make sure the client is not allergic to acetone or to the tape used. Also, be very careful with acetone and other substances used to remove tape adhesive. *Never* use these substances near an open flame, the client's eyes, or on an open wound! Also, remember that acetone will remove nail polish and paint from surfaces and may damage other surfaces, such as latex or plastic.

Montgomery Straps

Tape straps (**Montgomery straps**) may be used if frequent dressing changes are needed (Fig. 53-4A). They are available in different sizes, depending on the size of the client and the dressing. These straps are taped to the skin at the distal ends, leaving enough room in the center for the dressing; the ties are left free. This allows dressings to be changed, without removing tape from the client's skin. To change dressings, the ties are untied, wound care given and the dressing changed, and the ties retied (or buckled, or fastened with Velcro). This helps prevent skin irritation or injury (Fig. 53-4B). Gloves are worn for any wound care. Usually, hydrocolloidal or nonhydrocolloidal skin barrier is applied before application of the tapes (Chapter 58). The straps can remain in place unless there is skin irritation or they become soiled. Change the dressing as often as needed, without removing the tape from the skin each time. See In Practice: Nursing Procedure 53-2.

Nursing Alert If the client complains of pain or itching while any bandage is in place, assess the area immediately for bleeding, exudates, swelling, or changes in skin color. Report abnormalities immediately. Many people today are allergic to tape (Chapter 58).

NCLEX Alert

It will be important during the examination to show you understand your role in observing for and documenting abnormal findings in a client with a bandage or binder, as this relates to nursing actions that prevent complications.

STUDENT SYNTHESIS

KEY POINTS

- Elastic roller bandages may be used to encourage and support circulation after surgery. They are often used to support joints.
- Because elastic roller bandages apply direct pressure, they may be used to help control bleeding.
- When used, binders and bandages should be rewrapped every 2–4 hr. The client's skin should be observed and cleansed at this time.
- Antiembolism stockings should never be allowed to bunch or roll up. This could lead to constricting circulation in the leg. Be sure to seat the client's heel in the heel pocket of the stocking.
- When applying antiembolism stockings or an elastic roller bandage to an extremity, apply even pressure over the extremity. They are applied from the toes or fingers upward toward the heart.
- Peripheral vascular status is checked frequently, at least every 2 hr, when bandages or binders are used.
- Binders are used to supply support for specific body parts. Types of binders include T-binders and abdominal binders. Check circulation when binders are used.
- When a client requires frequent dressing changes, Montgomery straps or large binders can be used to avoid repeated tape removal and subsequent skin irritation with each dressing change.

CRITICAL THINKING EXERCISES

1. Describe five important elements for checking circulation when using bandages. Describe the significance of each element.
2. A client has TED stockings in place. The client has had a number of complaints during the stay in the facility and is now complaining that the TED stockings are "too tight." Describe your actions and reasoning. Which complications could occur?

NCLEX-STYLE REVIEW QUESTIONS

1. The nurse is preparing to apply an ACE bandage to a client's left ankle after the client has been walking. Which action would the nurse prioritize?
   a. Instruct the client to lie down for 15 min before wrapping.
   b. Have the client sit in a chair with the foot dangling before wrapping.
   c. Apply warm compresses to the ankle before wrapping.
   d. Begin wrapping from the knee to the toes.

2. After applying a bandage to the upper right extremity, which action would the nurse take next?
   a. Administer medication for pain.
   b. Check the circulation of the client's fingers.
   c. Provide instructions for care.
   d. Document the application of the bandage.

3. The nurse is preparing to apply a large stretch-net bandage to a client's torso. Which action would the nurse perform first?
   a. Clean the client's skin with an alcohol-based solution to remove dead skin.
   b. Obtain pins or clips in order to attach the dressing.
   c. Explain the procedure to the client.
   d. Apply the bandage tightly to the torso.

4. The nurse is collecting data from a client with a bandage on the lower extremity. Which observations made by the nurse should be immediately reported to the charge nurse or provider?
   a. Toes are cold to touch.
   b. Toes are cyanotic.
   c. Toes are pink and warm.
   d. Edema is present in the foot and toes.
   e. Diminished pulses distal to the bandage.

5. The client's bandage has become soiled. Which action would the nurse take to avoid spreading microorganisms?
   a. Place a dressing under the bandage.
   b. Wash the bandage to remove the drainage.
   c. Reinforce the bandage with another.
   d. Replace the bandage with a new one.

CHAPTER RESOURCES

Enhance your learning with additional resources on **thePoint**!

Student Resources related to this chapter can be found at **thePoint.lww.com/Rosdahl12e**.

CHAPTER 53 Bandages and Binders

Welcome Steps

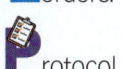ook at healthcare provider's orders.

Protocol for procedure.

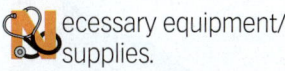ecessary equipment/supplies.

Wash hands using proper hand hygiene; put on gloves.

Explain the procedure and reassure the client.

Locate two identifiers to confirm correct client.

Comfortable and efficient position for nurse and client.

Obtain privacy.

Make sure to follow correct steps and body mechanics with good technique.

Ensure safety and observe deviations from normal.

End Steps

nsure comfort and safety.

Note questions or concerns from client or nurse; note significant data.

Dispose of materials properly.

Disinfect the area and your hands.

Document and report the procedure and your findings.

IN PRACTICE
NURSING PROCEDURE 53-1 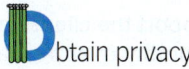 Applying Antiembolism Stockings (TED sox)

Supplies and Equipment
Stockings in the correct size
Talcum powder or baby powder
Tape measure
Gloves, if necessary

Steps
Follow LPN WELCOME Steps and Then

1. If the client's skin is intact, gloves are not needed. Measure the client's extremity to determine the proper stocking size. *Rationale: Stockings that are too tight may interfere with circulation. Stockings that are too loose do not encourage venous return.*

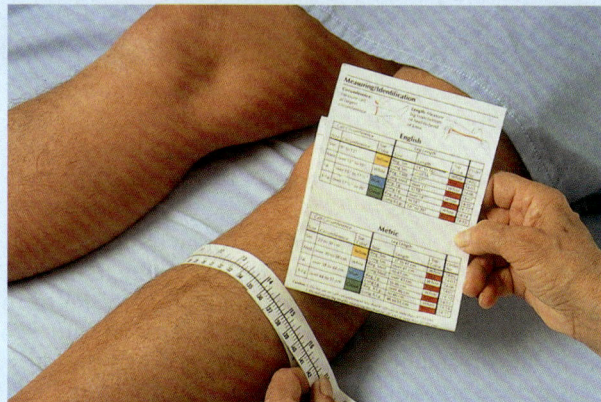

Use a tape measure and the package chart to determine proper stocking size for the client.

2. Assist the client to a supine position. Allow at least 15 minutes before applying stockings, if the legs have been down. *Rationale: Stockings are best applied early in the morning before the client gets out of bed; otherwise, the veins become distended and edema often occurs.*

3. Apply a small amount of powder to the client's feet and legs, if not contraindicated. *Rationale: Powder reduces friction and allows easier application of stockings.*

4. Grasp the stocking's heel and turn the stocking inside out. Slip the client's foot, toes, and heel into the stocking. Center the heel in the stocking's heel pocket; *be sure the heel is seated in this pocket.* Slip the stocking opening over (or under) the toes, so the toes are mostly exposed. Slide the stocking over the client's foot. *Rationale: This action allows application without bunching of the stocking on the client's foot, which constricts circulation.*

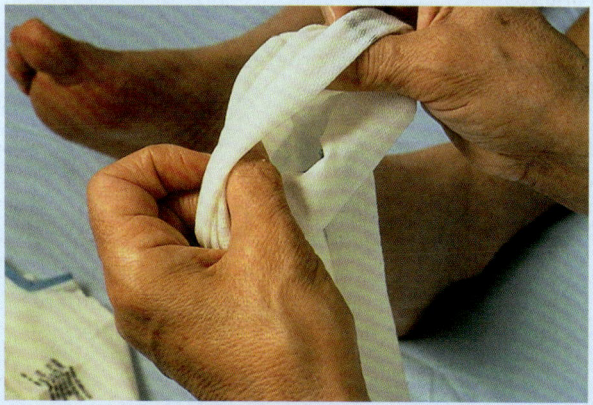

Grasp the stocking's heel and turn it inside out.

786 UNIT 8 Client Care

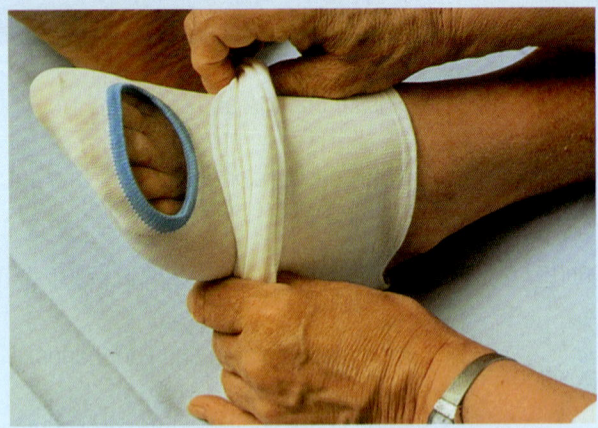

Put the client's toes, foot, and heel into the stocking. Proper positioning of the stocking on the client's foot prevents injury. The heel pocket is the guide as to whether the toe hole should be on the top or the bottom of the foot.

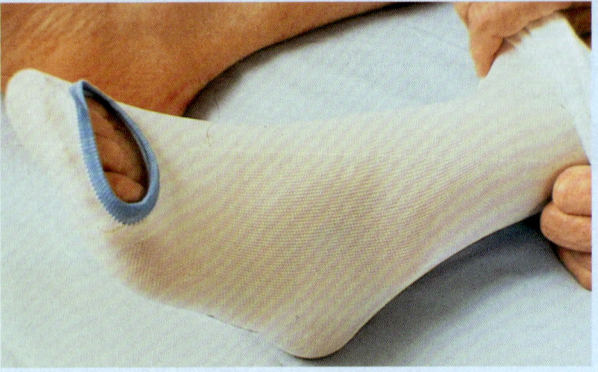

Ease the stocking over the calf and leg.

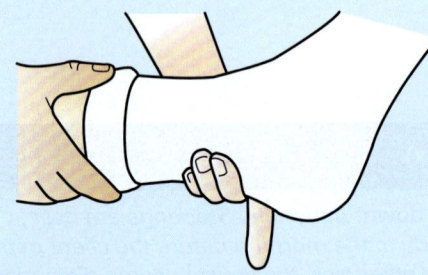

Adjust the stocking, making sure the heel is firmly seated in the heel pocket. (Craven & Hirnle, 2007.)

5. Support the client's ankle and ease the stocking smoothly over the calf and the remainder of the leg. *Rationale:* Smooth application prevents the formation of wrinkles, which can impede circulation.
6. Pull forward slightly on the stocking's toe section. Note that the toe holes are on the top of these stockings. *Rationale:* This eases pressure on the client's toes and nails.
7. Instruct the client to report any extreme discomfort. *Rationale:* Early reporting of complaints aids in preventing complications.

Follow ENDDD Steps

Special Reminders
- Check with the client at least every 4 hr, to make sure the stockings are not too tight. Check PNA regularly.
- The stockings must be removed at least every 8 hr and the legs washed and inspected. Sometimes, the client may leave the stockings off when they are in bed (depending on the specific order). *Rationale:* It is important to observe the condition of the skin and check the circulation in the legs. The stockings may be too tight, thus restricting circulation.

IN PRACTICE
NURSING PROCEDURE 53-2 — Applying Montgomery Straps

Supplies
Gloves
Dressing
Wound care supplies, as ordered
Montgomery straps

Steps
Follow LPN WELCOME Steps and Then

1. Choose Montgomery straps (Fig. 53-4) of the appropriate length. Two or more sets may be required for a very large dressing. Assist the client into a supine position. Position the Montgomery straps and open each to one side. *Rationale:* The straps must be spaced far enough apart to accommodate the dressing to be applied. They are opened out of the way to facilitate wound care and the application of the new dressing. Use as many sets of straps as needed.

2. To perform a dressing change, open the straps without removing the tape from the skin. Remove the old dressing and dispose of it properly. Perform prescribed wound care. Cover the incision with a new dressing. *Rationale:* Wound care must be performed correctly, as ordered. Covering the incision helps keep the incision free of microorganisms.

CHAPTER 53 Bandages and Binders 787

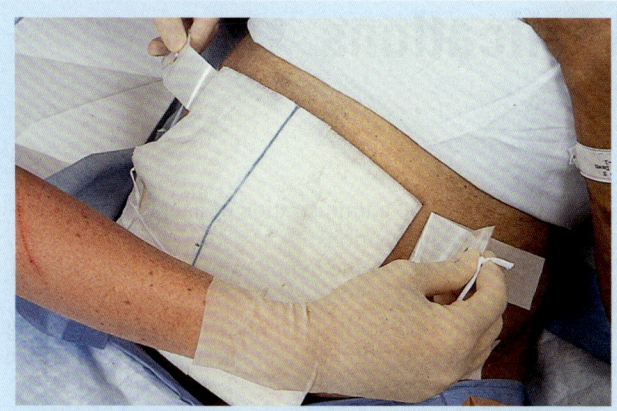

Use two or more sets of straps to secure a large, bulky dressing.

3. Secure the ends of the straps across the dressing with ties, buckles, or the Velcro closures. **Rationale:** *Make sure the dressing is securely supported.*
4. Leave straps in place until they become soiled or need to be changed or removed. Then, carefully remove the tape (see previous discussion related to tape). **Rationale:** *The straps should be removed very carefully and only when necessary, to preserve the integrity of the skin and to avoid further irritation or possible skin breakdown.*

Follow ENDDD Steps

Special Reminder
- Documentation is particularly vital when doing dressing changes. Factors to be included in documentation are presented in Data Gathering in Nursing 58-1. It is important to address all these factors in your documentation. Usually, the computer will provide a checklist for this purpose. Note also if the client complains of severe pain. In some cases, a line is drawn around a wound, so it can be determined if it is becoming smaller or larger each day. **Rationale:** *Because the wound is covered, the observations of the nurse are vital (Data Gathering in Nursing 58-1).*

54 Heat and Cold Applications

Learning Objectives

1. State indications for applying heat to the body; for applying cold.
2. Describe the rationale for maintaining normothermia.
3. Explain specific precautions when applying heat; when applying cold.
4. Demonstrate the administration of a leg or arm soak and of a sitz bath.
5. Demonstrate the use of the aquathermia pad.
6. Demonstrate the administration of a tepid sponge and state related precautions.
7. Describe the use of the hypothermia (cooling) blanket and indications for use.
8. Demonstrate the application of an ice collar or ice bag; describe the activation of a prepackaged single-use ice pack.

Important Terminology

aquathermia pad
hypothermia
hypothermia blanket
normothermia
sitz bath
tepid sponge bath
therapeutic soak

Acronyms

Aqua-K pad
SSI
WA

Some conditions benefit from heat and/or cold applications. However, these therapies are not without dangers; the nurse must follow all safety precautions carefully.

NORMOTHERMIA

Body temperature must be maintained within a fairly narrow range—**normothermia** (*normal body temperature*). This can be difficult during and after invasive procedures. It has been proven that normothermia during surgery helps prevent surgical site infections (**SSI**) and other postoperative complications. Surgical clients are particularly vulnerable to **hypothermia** (abnormally low body temperature). Special gowns and blankets are available to help maintain normothermia. Warmed IV fluids may be given, or a warming blanket may be used (Fig. 54-1). The nurse often helps manage this equipment.

HEAT THERAPY

Heat is a frequently used therapy, causing *vasodilation* (blood vessel enlargement), thus increasing blood flow. This increases the oxygen, nutrients, and blood cells delivered to specific body tissues and aids in waste removal from injured tissues (e.g., debris from phagocytosis).

Rationale for Heat Application

Heat application serves to

- Relieve local pain, stiffness, or aching, particularly of muscles and joints.
- Assist in wound healing.
- Reduce inflammation and infection.
- Make the chilly client more comfortable.
- Raise body temperature, to help maintain normothermia.
- Promote drainage (e.g., draw infected material out of wounds).

Because heat must be fairly intense to be effective, burns may result if heat is applied improperly. The application must be sufficiently hot to accomplish its purpose, but within a safe temperature range. Box 54-1 lists temperature ranges for hot (and cold) applications. Heat applied over a large area affords more warmth; however, the potential for injury is greater than that of heat applied over a small area. Make sure to observe all safety precautions. In Practice: Nursing Care Guidelines 54-1 outlines steps for applying heat therapy.

Both dry and moist heat provide local effects. Apply *dry heat* with a heating blanket or heating pad, a warmwater bag, heat lamp, water-filled heating pad (**aquathermia pad**), a forced-air warming blanket, or an electric heat cradle (Nursing Procedure 49-4). *Moist heat* warms the skin faster and is more penetrating than dry heat (water conducts heat better than air). Apply *moist heat* with compresses, packs, or soaks, including the sitz bath. Sometimes, wet compresses are used in combination with the aquathermia pad, to provide

CHAPTER 54   Heat and Cold Applications

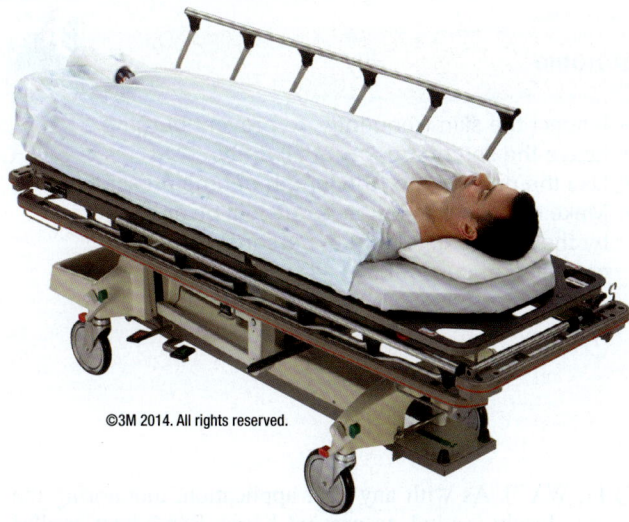

Figure 54-1 The forced-air warming blanket is used to maintain the core temperature of the client or raise the core temperature of a client who is hypothermic. It is important to prevent warming the client too much. The blanket is placed over the client, with plastic side up and the connecting air hose toward the foot of the bed. (Courtesy of 3M. © 2012, 3M. All rights reserved. 3M and the other marks shown are marks and/or registered marks. Unauthorized use prohibited.)

long-lasting moist heat. Because skin *maceration* (abnormal softening) may develop when moisture is applied directly to the skin, the client's skin may be protected by applying a thin layer of petroleum jelly (Vaseline), if ordered. The provider's order typically specifies the length of time for administration of heat applications. For example, the order may be "Moist compresses for 15 min every hour **WA** (while awake)."

> **Nursing Alert** Applying heat to a localized area of infection, such as an abscess or infected appendix, may cause rupture. *Heat application is contraindicated (should be avoided) in these cases.* A systemic infection (*generalized septicemia*) may occur and is life threatening.

> **NCLEX Alert**
>
> Heat therapies are commonly used in clinical settings, thus are likely to be integrated into an NCLEX clinical option. The nurse must understand and differentiate the effects of heat therapy versus cold therapy for the given situation. It is very important to understand *why* a particular therapy is chosen (i.e., the underlying rationale), *what* the goals of therapy are (e.g., assist muscle relaxation, improve circulation, encourage wound drainage, promote normothermia), and *how* to prevent complications of the therapy. Safety and client teaching regarding the equipment and monitoring for complications are also common NCLEX concerns.

Dry Heat Therapy

Aquathermia Pad

An aquathermia (**Aqua-K pad**), which produces dry heat, is used to treat muscle sprains and mild inflammations and for pain relief. Temperature-controlled, distilled water flows

Box 54-1 Approximate Range of Temperatures for Hot and Cold Applications

Hot	37.7 °C–40.5 °C	100 °F–105 °F
Warm	35 °C–37.7 °C	95 °F–100 °F
Tepid	26.6 °C–35 °C	80 °F–95 °F
Cool	18.3 °C–26.6 °C	65 °F–80 °F
Cold	10 °C–18.3 °C	50 °F–65 °F

To convert Fahrenheit to Celsius: $C = (F - 32) \times 5/9$

To convert Celsius to Fahrenheit: $F = (C \times 9/5) + 32$

IN PRACTICE
NURSING CARE GUIDELINES 54-1 Applying Heat Therapy

- Heat application must be ordered by a primary provider and applied with utmost caution. *Rationale:* Nerves in the skin are numbed easily. The client may not feel the pain of a burn, especially if heat has been applied often.
- Specific body parts, such as the eyelids, neck, and inside surface of the arm, are especially sensitive to heat. Each person has a personal sensitivity to heat. Apply the heat source slowly and ask the client for feedback. Infants, older people, and those with fair, thin skin have less heat resistance. Lowered body resistance because of illness also makes body tissues vulnerable. *Rationale:* It is important to determine how much heat is safe and for how long, considering each individual client.
- Clients who are unresponsive, anesthetized, paralyzed, or persons with any neurologic or mental disorder or dementia are at increased risk for heat-related injuries. *Rationale:* These clients may not realize or report when heat is too intense.
- Impaired circulation and some metabolic disorders make people more susceptible to burns (e.g., clients in shock or with a peripheral vascular disorder, or with diabetes). *Rationale:* Changes in body systems interfere with skin integrity and healing and may impair the client's ability to identify discomfort.
- Clients receiving radiation, chemotherapy, or certain medications are particularly susceptible to burns. *Rationale:* These clients often have compromised immune systems or skin integrity.
- Client complaints are very important. If the client complains of pain or discomfort, stop the treatment and consult the provider. *Rationale:* Each client is different. Only the client can state how the treatment feels.

through the waterproof pad. Follow the provider's orders. Make sure the pad is heating properly and not overheating; stop treatment and report malfunctions, if overheating occurs. In Practice: Nursing Procedure 54-1 describes the use of an aquathermia pad.

IN PRACTICE
EDUCATING THE CLIENT 54-1 Using Electric Heating Pads at Home

- Check to make sure the cord is intact. If there is any question, do not use the pad. Before applying the pad, plug it in and set the control on *high,* to see whether the pad heats promptly. Then turn it off and disconnect it.
- *Never* use safety pins or water near a heating pad.
- Make sure the pad is covered.
- After plugging it in, adjust the pad to *low* temperature and apply it *over* the body part; *do not allow the client to lie on it.*
- Inspect the skin frequently, to prevent burning.
- Leave the setting on *low* at all times.
- Use the pad only for the length of time prescribed.
- Make sure no one in the home will be endangered by the cord (e.g., children, persons who are confused or suicidal).

 **Nursing Alert** When disassembling the aquathermia pad after use:
- First, unplug the unit and clamp all tubing until over the sink.
- Empty the water out of the pump unit, the pad, and all tubes over a sink, to prevent leakage.
- Discard the pad (it is contaminated).
- Return only the heater/pump to the appropriate department.
- Carefully wash hands.

Forced-Air Warming Blanket
A forced-air warming blanket is placed over the client and circulates warm air around the client (Fig. 54-1). It is often used before, during, and after surgery, to assist the client in maintaining normothermia throughout the surgical process. It is important to monitor the client's body temperature and circulatory status during the treatment. Follow the manufacturer's instructions and facility protocol for use.

Heat Lamp Treatments and Ultrasound
Specially trained personnel give *heat lamp* and *ultrasound* treatments because the client's exposure to light rays must be carefully regulated, to prevent injury. The nurse in a provider's clinic may receive specific in-service education to administer *infrared* (*IR*), *ultraviolet* (*UV*), or *ultrasound* treatments. IR rays relax muscles, stimulate circulation, and relieve pain, as do other forms of dry heat. UV rays are not as penetrating as IR rays and are used to treat skin infections and wounds. Sunlight provides mild UV radiation; prolonged exposure will, however, burn sensitive skin. Ultrasound is a method of applying deep, penetrating heat to muscles and other tissues. Lubricating gel is applied to the client's skin, and the ultrasound paddle or wand is kept moving at all times during the treatment, to prevent burns. It is also important that the timer be set correctly. (Doppler ultrasound is also used to visualize and examine internal structures.)

The Heat Cradle
In rare instances, a *lamp* or special *heater* is mounted inside a bed cradle to provide dry heat (Nursing Procedure 49-4). The primary provider must clearly specify time limits; these orders must be followed exactly (e.g., "Heat cradle 20 min Q hr, WA."). As with any heat application, monitoring the client closely is vital, to prevent burns. Some heat cradles have an automatic timer that turns the lamp on and off at preset intervals.

Nursing Alert Do not perform any type of heat treatment without a specific order and special training in the use of the equipment.

Warmed Blankets
Clients are often chilly after anesthesia, after undergoing a treatment, or getting up for the first time. Most facilities have blanket warmers on the units and in treatment areas, to enhance client comfort. Bath blankets are warmed to about 130 °F (54.4 °C). Offer a warmed blanket whenever possible.

Electric Heating Pad
Acute care facilities rarely use the *electric heating pad,* but they may be used in extended care facilities or the client's home. This device is a covered network of wires that emit heat when electricity passes through them. Pads with a waterproof cover are safest. The client who is paralyzed, has very sensitive or *friable* (fragile) skin, or has a neurologic impairment is particularly vulnerable to a burn from the electric pad. These heating pads are also unsafe to use with young children; confused, irrational, or unresponsive persons; clients who are suicidal; or clients who have spinal cord injuries. In Practice: Educating the Client 54-1 describes the safest use of electric heating pads.

Nursing Alert *Never use pins with any heating pad.* They may puncture the Aqua-K pad, causing leaks, or may cause a shock if the pin touches a wire. If wires are bent or crushed, the pad can overheat, causing a fire.

Moist Heat Therapy
Warm, Moist Compresses and Packs
Warm, moist compresses and *packs* apply moist heat to an area to stimulate circulation, ease pain, promote wound drainage, and apply medications. The provider prescribes the type,

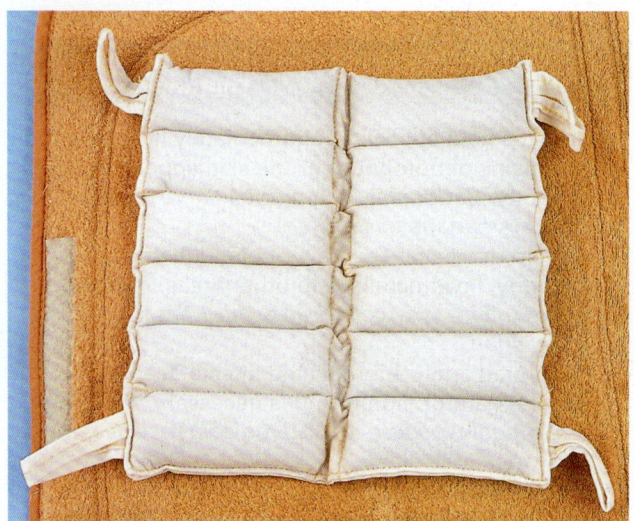

Figure 54-2 A commercial warm pack can be used to apply dry heat but is most often used as a moist heat application. Some of these packs can also be used as cold packs; follow the manufacturer's instructions. (Photo by B. Proud.)

location, and schedule of applications. The ordered solution is usually plain water, a mild antiseptic solution (e.g., 2% boric acid), or normal saline. Warm, moist compresses, such as 4 × 4 gauze or Telfa pads, are used to apply heat to a small area; large packs apply heat over a larger area. Commercially prepared packs are available and may be used to apply either dry or moist heat (Fig. 54-2). Covering any warm pack with heavy, dry material helps it retain heat longer. (Application of an Aqua-K pad over a pack enables the pack to remain heated almost indefinitely. However, remember to keep the temperature of the Aqua-K pad low.) Compresses and warm packs are usually not sterile. However, if there is a break in the client's skin, sterile dressings are used. The pack should be as warm as the client can comfortably tolerate. Apply it slowly, so the client can tell you how it feels. Only the client can judge the pack's comfort. During the procedure, the client may feel chilly, so make sure to keep the person warm and protected from drafts.

You may need to apply a warm compress to a client's eye. The eyelid and surrounding skin are thin and delicate, easily susceptible to injury. For an eye compress, use *tepid water only* (Box 54-1) and use extreme caution, to prevent injury.

Wash your hands carefully and wear clean gloves; the eye is highly susceptible to infection. If the eye is draining, discard each compress on removal. All reusable equipment is sterilized after the treatment. If applying compresses to both eyes, *use separate equipment* and wear new gloves for each eye, to prevent spreading infection from one eye to the other. *To apply warm,* moist compresses and packs to all body parts, follow the general rules as outlined in In Practice: Nursing Procedure 54-2.

Therapeutic Soaks

Moist heat may be applied by immersing the client's affected body part in warm water or medicated solution, a **therapeutic soak** or *warm soak* (Chapter 50). A therapeutic soak

- Improves circulation to a specific area.
- Provides comfort and pain relief.

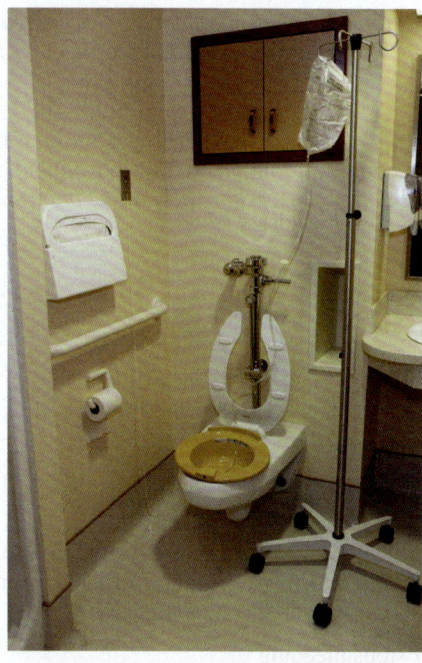

Figure 54-3 A disposable sitz bath fits inside a commode, with the toilet seat up. (This device is too small for an obese client.) (Evans-Smith, 2005).

- Assists in breaking down infected tissue.
- Applies medications.
- Cleans draining wounds.
- Loosens scabs and crusts from wounds.

Soaks may be done in a basin if the area is small (e.g., a foot or hand) or in a tub for a larger area. Often, a therapeutic soak may be combined with a whirlpool bath in the physical therapy department. The tub or whirlpool must be thoroughly disinfected between clients, per agency protocol. *Rationale: Persons receiving soaks often have open wounds. Thorough cleaning of the tub helps prevent the spread of infection between clients.* Nursing Procedure 54-3 describes the procedure for an arm or leg soak. A *foot soak* may also be ordered and is administered in much the same way. The client can often perform the foot soak independently. A foot massage may be given after completion of the foot soak. *Rationale: This adds to client comfort and helps the client relax.* (Administration of a foot soak is described in Nursing Procedure 50-6.) The foot soak can be continued at home, increasing the client's independence.

Sitz Bath

The purpose of a **sitz bath** (sitting in a tub of warm water) is to provide moist heat to the pelvic, perineal, and/or perianal area. Sitz baths are often used following childbirth or rectal/perineal surgery. Disposable sitz basins are preferable. They fit inside the toilet and are equipped with a bag, tubing, and nozzle, to allow water to flow freely to the affected area (Fig. 54-3). In the client's home, a bathtub with water covering the client's hips can be used. In Practice: Nursing Procedure 54-4 describes the use of the disposable sitz tub. Heat applications are usually contraindicated in clients with known cardiac conditions, those taking certain cardiac medications or antihypertensives, and always, if the client is actively bleeding. *Rationale: Heat application can increase blood flow and aggravate cardiac conditions or increase bleeding.*

> **Nursing Alert** Moist heat is *not used* if there is inadequate arterial blood flow to a wound area. *Rationale: In this case, eschar will protect the wound and must be kept dry (Chapter 58).*

COLD THERAPY

Cold causes *vasoconstriction* (shrinkage of blood vessels), decreasing blood flow, and slowing of the body's metabolism and its demand for oxygen.

Rationale for Cold Application

Cold application prevents escape of heat from the body by slowing circulation, also relieving congestion and muscle pain. Therapeutic goals of cold application:

- Slows or stops bleeding
- Slows bacterial activity in infection
- Relieves pain and swelling following surgery or injury (e.g., tooth extraction, headache, or muscle/joint injury, such as sprains)
- Reduces inflammation
- Blocks pain receptors
- Retards peristalsis in clients with abdominal inflammation
- Relieves pain in engorged breasts
- Controls pain and fluid loss in initial burn treatment
- Diminishes muscle contraction and muscle spasms
- Slows the basal metabolism for certain types of surgery

Cold application is more effective than heat for sprains or other soft-tissue injuries and is the preferred treatment within the first 48 hr after injury. Cold helps prevent swelling (*edema*); however, cold usually will not reduce preexisting edema. In Practice: Nursing Care Guidelines 54-2 lists important considerations when applying cold therapy.

> **Nursing Alert** The application of cold can cause *frostbite,* which can be very serious. It may require extensive débridement and surgery (including amputation) and/or cause infections (including gas gangrene).

> **NCLEX Alert**
>
> Cold therapies are often integrated into NCLEX situations and options. It is critical to understand when and why cold applications are more beneficial than heat (e.g., in the first hours after a bone fracture or muscle injury) and when and why it is hazardous to apply heat. It is important to understand *why* a particular cold therapy is chosen (i.e., the rationale for use), *what* the expectations are for cold therapy (e.g., vasoconstriction, decrease swelling, slow bleeding, etc.), and *how* to prevent complications (particularly frostbite) for the chosen version of cold therapy. Safety and client teaching regarding application of equipment and monitoring for complications are also common NCLEX concerns.

IN PRACTICE
NURSING CARE GUIDELINES 54-2 — Applying Cold Therapy

- Stop the cold application immediately if the client complains of numbness or the skin appears white or spotty. *Rationale: Cold numbs nerve endings and can damage tissues.*
- As cold decreases the flow of blood in one area of the body, flow increases to other areas. *Rationale: This explains why cold drafts cause nasal congestion.*
- Continued application of cold affects deeper tissues. Careful monitoring is necessary. *Rationale: Prolonged exposure to extreme cold may cause injury.*
- Cold is often applied to a sprain, strain, fracture, or burn. *Rationale: This helps remove blood and lymph congestion in the area and reduces pain.*

Cold Therapies

Cold, Moist Compresses

Cold, moist compresses are used to reduce swelling and inflammation in soft-tissue injuries or after tooth extraction. The size of the compress depends on the area to be treated. Gauze 4 × 4 pads are frequently used for tooth pain. They are applied directly to the tooth and are changed frequently because they warm rapidly, thereby losing their effectiveness. Medication (e.g., clove oil) may be added to the cold compress. In Practice: Nursing Care Guidelines 54-3 describes application of cold compresses. Figure 54-4 illustrates both moist and dry cold applications.

Icecap or Ice Collar

The flat icecap, used to apply *dry cold* to the head, has a wide opening that allows it to be filled easily with ice chips, as does the *ice collar,* a narrow bag curved to fit the neck. Disposable, single-use ice packs are frequently used. The provider may prescribe dry cold to treat a specific area of the body. However, an ice bag is often used for a headache or in an emergency, such as a sprain or nosebleed, without an order (see In Practice: Nursing Procedure 54-5).

Single-Use and Refreezable Ice Packs

Healthcare agencies and emergency services often provide ready-for-use ice packs, also used by sports teams, hikers, and campers. These ice packs release a chemical causing cooling of the bag when a capsule is broken or crystals are activated when the bag is shaken. It is usually not appropriate to refreeze these bags. *Rationale: The bag is contaminated and also may explode in the freezer.*

Some gel-filled packs that can be *frozen or heated* and used as either a cold or hot pack are available. These packs are used for *only one client,* to prevent cross-contamination. Follow the manufacturer's instructions carefully. The bag can explode in a freezer or microwave!

If the client complains of burning pain after application of a cold pack, treatment should be stopped immediately and

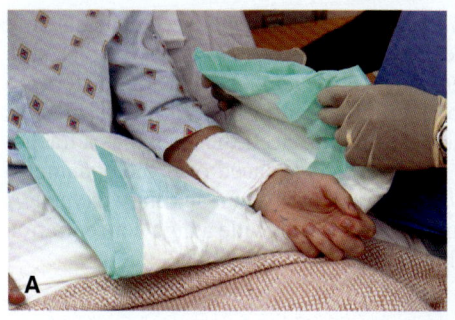 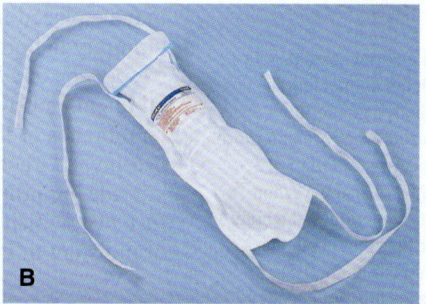

Figure 54-4 Cold applications are often used to reduce pain and swelling or arrest bleeding. **A.** The cold compress is a moist cold application (Timby, 2005). **B.** An ice pack or ice bag filled with crushed ice is a dry cold application. (The straps are removed for use in psychiatry or pediatrics.) (Photo by B. Proud.)

the provider notified. *Rationale: This indicates tissue ischemia (lack of blood supply) and may lead to tissue necrosis (tissue death). Untreated, this can lead to gangrene and necessitate amputation.*

> **Nursing Alert** Many single-use ice bags, particularly those with the capsule or crystals, become *very* cold and can cause frostbite rapidly. Therefore, use extreme caution when using them. If the client's skin becomes blanched or red, discontinue treatment immediately and check for further instructions.

IN PRACTICE
NURSING CARE GUIDELINES 54-3 Applying Cold Moist Compresses

- Wear gloves if the client has an open wound or has had surgery. *Rationale: This helps prevent infection transmission.*
- Put the compresses in a basin containing pieces of ice and a small amount of water. *Rationale: Ice water soaks and cools the compresses faster than does plain ice.*
- Explain that the treatment will relieve discomfort. *Rationale: If the client is relaxed, relief will be felt sooner.*
- Wring the compress thoroughly and apply. Add medication, if ordered. *Rationale: If ice water drips, it may startle the client. Medication may add to the effectiveness of the compress.*
- Change compresses frequently. *Rationale: Compresses warm rapidly, as they absorb body heat.*
- Continue the treatment, usually for 15 to 20 min, and repeat every 2 to 4 hr, as ordered. Clients may be able to apply the compresses themselves. *Rationale: Applying the cold application for the specified time promotes treatment effectiveness and helps prevent injury. Clients learn independence.*
- Properly dispose of gloves, if used, and wash the hands. Document the treatment, noting duration and the client's reaction. *Rationale: Help prevent infection transmission. Documentation promotes communication and continuity of care.*

Tepid Sponge

A **tepid sponge** (**bath**) is performed using moderately warm water (below body temperature), between 80 °F and 95 °F (26.6 °C and 35 °C). This sponge bath may be ordered to reduce a client's elevated temperature. The first effect of this water on the skin is blood vessel constriction. A tepid sponge may be temporarily soothing, but may not produce a marked temperature drop unless used for about 30 min. Tepid sponge baths are inadvisable for people with inelastic arteries (hardening of the arteries—arteriosclerosis), clients with arthritis or lowered resistance to disease (as a result of immunosuppression), and very young children. *Rationale: The water has the initial effect of depressing body systems.* See In Practice: Nursing Care Guidelines 54-4.

> **Nursing Alert** Constantly assess the client's temperature with an electronic thermometer during and about 15 and 30 min after the tepid sponge. If the client begins to shiver or if the temperature approaches the ordered level (approximately 38.7 °C [100 °F]), discontinue the treatment and report the findings immediately. Do not use alcohol. *Rationale: The temperature will usually continue to drop for a time after discontinuation of the tepid sponge. Alcohol evaporates very rapidly and causes excessive cooling.*

If hyperthermia (elevated temperature) becomes life threatening, other treatments are usually used to lower temperature more quickly and permanently. In these situations, an *ice mattress* or *hypothermia blanket* may be used.

Hypothermia Blanket

A **hypothermia blanket** (cooling blanket) is used cautiously to treat intractable (uncontrollable) hyperthermia (fever). It is a mattress pad through which cold water flows continuously. Hypothermia blankets may be used in surgery to slow body processes or elsewhere to lower dangerously high body temperatures. (*NOTE:* Today, it is more common to warm clients during surgery, to help prevent hypothermia and infections.) Hypothermia blankets can be preset to a desired temperature. It is important to follow the agency's protocol and the provider's orders. Check frequently to ensure that the client's core temperature does not fall too low. The client's body temperature is checked constantly when using the hypothermia blanket, as with the tepid sponge. The hypothermia blanket resembles the forced-air warming blanket (Fig. 54-1).

Key Concept
Risk occurs with the hypothermia blanket and, to a certain extent, with other cold therapies because cold interferes with the normal febrile (fever) response. Invading pathogens cause the body's temperature regulatory center (the hypothalamus) to produce a new body temperature set point in an effort to fight off the pathogen's negative effects. (Normally, the set point of body temperature is 37 °C or 98.6 °F.) When the hypothalamus raises this set point to a higher temperature, the body attempts to reach this new set point with mechanisms that begin the febrile response—shivering and peripheral vasoconstriction. Using a hypothermia blanket during this response decreases the actual body temperature, moving it further away from the set point. This may cause an even more severe febrile reaction. In addition, fever sometimes is helpful because it can help destroy pathogens.

Cold Humidity
Cold humidity is commonly ordered for clients with breathing disorders. In most facilities, air conditioning and heating systems provide a constant level of humidity. But if the humidity level is not high enough, an auxiliary humidifier may be placed in the room. Some clients need constant cold humidity in higher concentrations. A child may be placed in a *croupette* or a *humidity* (mist) *tent*. Oxygen administered to all clients must be humidified, to prevent drying of mucous membranes of the nose and throat. If the client has a tracheostomy, a "trach mask" may be placed over the opening to provide humidity, either with or without auxiliary oxygen. A *face tent*, which may be used to provide a high concentration of moisture in inhaled air, is also available.

> **Nursing Alert** When using any method for cooling the client's body, have bath blankets (preferably warmed) readily available for use in case of chilling. Be aware that body temperature can continue to fall after the treatment is discontinued. Stop the treatment and check with the provider when the client's temperature approaches the prescribed level (approximately 38.7 °C [100 °F]).

IN PRACTICE
NURSING CARE GUIDELINES 54-4 Giving a Tepid Sponge to Reduce Body Temperature

- Explain the procedure to the client. *Rationale: The tepid sponge is less likely to be effective if a client is nervous or fearful.*
- Encourage the client to void and/or defecate before the sponge. *Rationale: The client will be more comfortable. It is important to avoid having to stop during the sponge.*
- Record the client's baseline temperature and continuously monitor the temperature during the procedure. *Rationale: Temperature monitoring provides objective data about the effectiveness of the bath, thus helping to prevent reducing the client's core temperature too much. Remember, temperature will continue to drop after the bath. A continuous electronic thermometer is usually used.*
- Note whether the client has had an antipyretic (e.g., aspirin or ibuprofen) to reduce fever. *Rationale: Such medications may influence the sponge bath's effectiveness.*
- Add tepid water to the bath basin, 26.6 °C to 35 °C (80 °F-95 °F). Use a bath thermometer. *Rationale: These temperatures are below normal body temperature, so they will be effective in lowering the client's fever. However, they are not so cold as to be dangerous.*
- Place moist, cool cloths—wrung out just enough to prevent dripping—in the client's axillae and groin. *Rationale: The blood vessels here lie close to the skin and will cause rapid water evaporation.*
- The client's first reaction may be a sensation of chilliness, which disappears as the body adjusts. Therefore, continue the bath long enough to allow for this adjustment (at least 25-30 min).
- Sponge each limb for at least 5 min and the back and buttocks for at least 10 to 15 min. *Rationale: Sponging for this length of time is necessary for fever reduction.*
- Stop the procedure if the client becomes very chilled or begins to shiver. *Rationale: People respond to treatments differently. Stopping the procedure, due to complaints of chilling or evidence of shivering, prevents possible hypothermia.*
- Stop sponging immediately when the client's temperature is within 1.5 °F of normal (about 38.7 °C or 100 °F, orally). Give the client a bath blanket. *Rationale: The client's temperature will continue to drop after the sponge is completed. Stopping when the client's temperature is still above normal body temperature prevents it from dropping too low.*
- Wash the hands. Document the treatment, noting the client's reactions. Be sure to record the temperatures before, during, and after the procedure. *Rationale: Handwashing helps prevent infection transmission. Recording the client's responses to treatment is vital, especially if the procedure needs to be repeated.*
- Take the client's temperature 15 and 30 min after you complete the bath. Report the temperature immediately if it has fallen too low (below about 37.5 °C or 99.5 °F). *Rationale: The body takes about 25 to 30 min to fully respond to cold applications.*

STUDENT SYNTHESIS

KEY POINTS

- A major goal in healthcare is the maintenance of normothermia.
- Heat dilates surface blood vessels.
- Whenever heat is applied, take measures to prevent burns.
- Warm, moist applications heat the skin more quickly than dry heat applications.
- Water temperature for a soak should be no higher than 105 °F (41 °C).
- A sitz bath applies heat and water to the pelvic, perineal, and perianal area.
- Cold constricts surface blood vessels.
- Cold, moist compresses are applied to small body parts.
- A tepid sponge may be used to reduce body temperature temporarily.
- When cold is applied, it is important to prevent undue chilling and/or frostbite.
- Several methods may be used to administer heat or cold treatments.

CRITICAL THINKING EXERCISES

1. Describe how you would teach a client to use an electric heating pad at home.
2. Using heat or cold, how would you treat localized aching in an extremity? A muscle sprain? A headache? A fever? Why?

NCLEX-STYLE REVIEW QUESTIONS

1. The nurse is applying a moist heat compress to a client's lower extremity. Which action by the nurse is a priority in order to prevent skin maceration?
   a. Apply a thin layer of petroleum jelly prior to compress application.
   b. Wrap the moist compress with an occlusive dressing.
   c. Apply the moist dressing continuously for 24 hr.
   d. Place a warm blanket over the dressing.

2. Which primary care provider order would the nurse question prior to implementing?
   a. Use of a warm sitz bath for relief of discomfort related to a client's hemorrhoids
   b. Application of a warm compress to the lower back to relieve soreness after back strain
   c. Application of a warm compress to the abdomen of a client with suspected appendicitis
   d. Use of a warm compress to the lower abdomen of a woman with menstrual cramps

3. The nurse applies a cold pack to a client's wrist after a sprain. Which action by the nurse a priority when the client reports a burning pain at the site?
   a. Replace the compress with another cold compress.
   b. Place the wrist in hot water to reverse the cold.
   c. Administer an analgesic for the pain.
   d. Stop treatment and notify the primary care provider.

4. The nurse is providing a tepid sponge bath for a client with a fever. When the client begins to shiver, which action by the nurse is a priority?
   a. Pour isopropyl alcohol into the water.
   b. Discontinue the bath immediately and report findings.
   c. Increase the temperature of the water.
   d. Continue the bath since this is an expected reaction.

5. A client is scheduled for a surgical procedure. When assisting with implementation of the plan of care, which action can the nurse take to reduce surgical site infection?
   a. Administer oxygen during the preoperative phase.
   b. Wash the surgical site with soap and water prior to surgery.
   c. Apply warm blankets.
   d. Use antibiotic ointment before the incision is made.

CHAPTER RESOURCES

Enhance your learning with additional resources on thePoint*!*

Student Resources related to this chapter can be found at **thePoint.lww.com/Rosdahl12e**.

Welcome Steps

Look at healthcare provider's orders.

Protocol for procedure.

Necessary equipment/supplies.

Wash hands using proper hand hygiene; put on gloves.

Explain the procedure and reassure the client.

Locate two identifiers to confirm correct client.

Comfortable and efficient position for nurse and client.

Obtain privacy.

Make sure to follow correct steps and body mechanics with good technique.

Ensure safety and observe deviations from normal.

End Steps

Ensure comfort and safety.

Note questions or concerns from client or nurse; note significant data.

Dispose of materials properly.

Disinfect the area and your hands.

Document and report the procedure and your findings.

IN PRACTICE
NURSING PROCEDURE 54-1 — Using an Aquathermia (Aqua-K) Pad

Supplies and Equipment
Pad
Control unit
Cover for pad
Distilled water

Steps
Follow LPN WELCOME Steps and Then

1. Follow the manufacturer's instructions. Make sure the control unit is connected to the pad before any water is added or any clamps released. If the unit is empty, fill the receptacle to the indicated "fill" line with distilled water. *Rationale: If the control unit is not connected, the water will run out. Water is required for operation of the pad. Distilled water will not damage the unit, but tap water, which contains chemicals and minerals, might.*

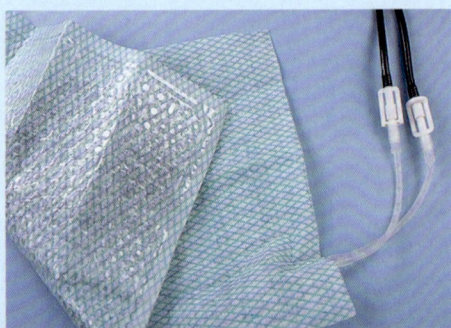

Connect the Aqua-K pad securely to the control unit before releasing any clamps or adding water (Timby, 2005).

1. Check the temperature setting; it should not exceed 40.6 °C (105 °F). *Rationale: This temperature delivers heat to the area without damaging tissue.*

2. Cover the pad with a pad cover, sheet, pillowcase, or towel. Plug in the control unit and place it on the bedside table. *Rationale: Covering the pad aids in protecting the client's skin. The pad must be preheated.*

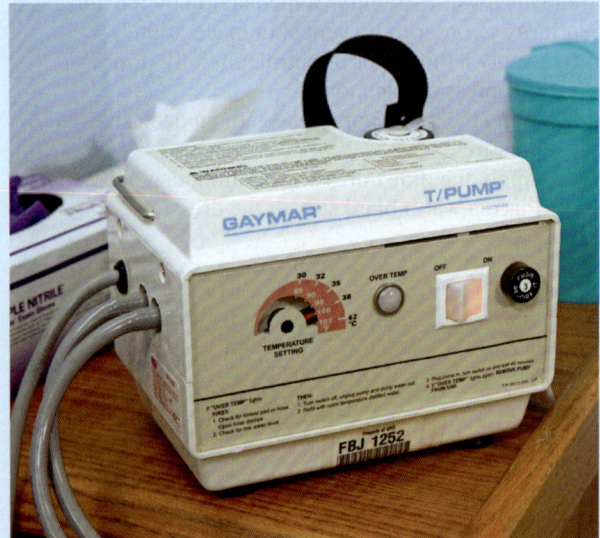

Place the control unit on the bedside table. It has been preset to the ordered temperature and must preheat (Evans-Smith, 2005).

1. When the pad is heated, apply it to the specific body part, as ordered. The pad should rest *on top of the body part,* unless specifically ordered otherwise. Instruct the client to avoid lying on the pad. *Rationale: Proper application ensures appropriate treatment. If the client lies on the pad, heat cannot escape, and burns are more likely.*

2. If the pad needs to be secured in place, use tape or a roller bandage. Never use safety pins. *Rationale: Pinpricks can cause the pad to leak and possibly to short circuit.*

3. Instruct the client that the correct temperature has been preset. (Usually, this cannot be changed.) *Rationale: Incorrect temperatures could cause burns (if too high) or cause an ineffective treatment (if too low).*

4. Place the call signal within the client's reach. *Rationale: The client must be able to obtain assistance.*

5. Check the area for redness after 5 min. *Rationale: Frequent evaluation reduces the risk of burns.*

6. Remove the pad after the specified treatment time. *Rationale: Following specific orders enhances the treatment's effectiveness. If the pad is in place too long, the treatment will not be effective and/or the client could be injured.*

7. The pad is stored in the client's unit and is used by only one client. When that client is finished using it, the pad is disconnected and discarded, and the pump returned to central supply for disinfection. Be sure all clamps or roller closures are *securely closed before disconnecting* the pad. *Rationale: Proper storage ensures ready availability. The pad is contaminated to that client. If clamps are open, the water will run out.*

Follow ENDDD Steps

Special Reminder
- In some facilities, the control unit is dispensed prefilled. Usually, the temperature is preset and cannot be altered.
- Be aware that any equipment with cords must be carefully monitored if the client is in danger of self-harm.

IN PRACTICE
NURSING PROCEDURE 54-2 Applying Warm, Moist Compresses and Packs

Supplies and Equipment
Compress or pack
Dry pack and moisture-proof cover, if ordered
Incontinence pad
Hot-pack machine and two forceps
Thermometer
Petroleum jelly (petrolatum, Vaseline)
Aquathermia pad, if ordered
Gloves

Steps
Follow LPN WELCOME Steps and Then

1. In most cases, start with sterile compresses. In most facilities, the electric hot-pack machine is no longer used. Use prewarmed compresses or immerse the compress or pack in hot tap water. (Microwaving is usually not recommended.) *Rationale: The hot-pack machine is cumbersome and can cause burns. The microwave is considered to be contaminated and hot packs can explode.*

2. Apply petroleum jelly to the client's skin before applying the pack. Place an incontinence pad under the area to be treated. *Rationale: Protect the client's skin from prolonged moisture. Protect the bed from moisture.*

3. Wring the compress or pack with forceps or by pressing it against a solid surface, removing as much water as possible. To wring out a pack with forceps, clamp one forceps onto each end of the pack and twist in opposite directions. *Rationale: Hot water dripping on the client's skin could cause a burn.*

4. Shake the pack lightly, and apply it to the area, gently at first, then gradually press it against the client's skin. *Rationale: Shaking the pack cools it a little. Because air is a poor heat conductor, eliminating air spaces between the compress or pack and skin makes the treatment more effective.*

5. Ask if the pack is too hot. If so, remove it and shake it again briefly, to lower its temperature. *Rationale: Applying a compress or pack that is too hot will cause a burn.*

6. Cover the moist compress or pack with a dry pack and moisture-proof cover or with the aquathermia pad. (Be sure the Aqua-K pad is set on low.) *Rationale: Covering the pack slows heat loss and moisture evaporation. The Aqua-K pad will keep the pack warm. Higher Aqua-K temperature can cause a burn because it maintains the pack's heat longer.*

7. Provide the client with blankets during and after the treatment. Offer warmed blankets. *Rationale: Moisture on the skin will evaporate quickly and may cause chilling. The client is especially susceptible to chilling following the removal of the warm pack or compress.*

8. Change the pack as often as necessary to keep the area heated. *Rationale: Keeping the pack warm for the specified time promotes the therapeutic effects. Small compresses cool more quickly than large packs.*

9. Assess the condition of the client's skin at least every 10 min. *Rationale: Continued exposure to heat and moisture can cause skin breakdown and/or maceration, as well as burns.*
10. Continue treatment for the prescribed time. *Rationale: This enhances the effectiveness of the treatment. The treatment will not be effective if left on too long or removed too soon.*
11. Use packs for one client only. Discard disposable supplies; disinfect and keep designated supplies to use again for that same client. *Rationale: Proper use, disposal, and cleaning of equipment minimize the risk for transmission of pathogens.*
12. Dry the skin and cover it, as ordered. Be sure to wipe off excess petroleum jelly. The client may appreciate a warmed blanket. *Rationale: Drying the skin and covering the area prevent chilling. Drying also helps reduce the risk of maceration caused by covering the skin. Prevent chilling the client.*

Follow ENDDD Steps

IN PRACTICE
NURSING PROCEDURE 54-3 Administering a Therapeutic Soak to an Arm or Leg

Supplies and Equipment
Towel
Gloves, per protocol
Bath thermometer
Sheet or bath blanket
Sterile dressing, if needed
Ordered medications for wound care
Detergent or other substance as ordered
Adequate size tub
Materials to clean tub

Steps
Follow LPN WELCOME Steps and Then

1. The disposable tub is used by only one client. Cover the tub with a bath towel. *Rationale: Prevent the spread of infection. The towel pads the tub, to help prevent pressure areas.*
2. Cover the client with a protective sheet or bath blanket. *Rationale: Protect the client's privacy and prevent chilling.*
3. Prepare the water in the tub at the specified temperature (usually 37.8 °C-40.6 °C or 100 °F-105 °F, for a small area). For a larger area, the water is usually warm, not hot (Box 54-1). Always use a bath thermometer. Use tap water or add ordered detergent (e.g., Dreft) or other substance (e.g., colloidal oatmeal, Epsom salts) and stir. *Rationale: Proper temperature prevents burns. Additives are ordered to treat specific conditions.*
4. Wear gloves if the client has an open wound or rash. Remove and dispose of dressings, per agency protocol. *Rationale: Help prevent cross-contamination and spread of infection. Some facilities require gloves in all cases.*
5. Gradually lower the client's affected body part into the water. *Rationale: This allows the arm or leg to adjust to the water temperature and avoids burns and discomfort.*
6. Adjust the padding on the edge of the tub for the knee or elbow to rest on; support the body part with a folded pillow, if necessary. *Rationale: Proper padding and support prevent injury to extremities.*
7. Test the water's temperature frequently with a bath thermometer. Add hot water slowly and carefully, as needed, and stir, to distribute the heat. *Rationale: This helps maintain the proper temperature, promoting vasodilation, without causing a burn.*
8. Usually a soak is given for 15 to 20 min. Remove the client's limb, as ordered, and towel dry. *Rationale: Adhering to the prescribed time limit enhances the treatment's effectiveness and reduces the risk of injury.*
9. Apply a sterile dressing (and medications) to the wound, as ordered. The tub should be thoroughly cleaned after each use and discarded when no longer needed. Properly dispose of gloves. *Rationale: Covering the wound and properly caring for equipment help prevent the spread of infection.*

Note: The foot soak is described and illustrated in Nursing Procedure 50-6.

Follow ENDDD Steps

IN PRACTICE
NURSING PROCEDURE 54-4   Using a Sitz Bath

Supplies and Equipment
Sitz bath toilet insert or large sitz bathtub
Bath towels
Cotton bath blanket
Bath thermometer

Steps
Follow LPN WELCOME Steps and Then

1. Put the toilet seat up. Place the sitz bath in the toilet and fill the reservoir with water at the *prescribed temperature.* This is often 37.7 °C to 40.5 °C (100 °F- 105 °F), as measured with a bath thermometer (Box 54-1). Do not exceed maximums. An obese client may not fit into this tub. *Rationale:* The correct temperature is necessary to ensure the desired therapeutic effect. If the aim of the sitz bath is to apply heat, the temperature is higher than if the goal is to cleanse and promote healing. Extremely hot temperatures may damage tissue, rather than promote healing. Consider the client's size in selecting the sitz tub.

2. Hang the water reservoir at a height that will allow water to flow from it through the tubing and into the basin. An IV pole is often used (Fig. 54-3). *Rationale:* The correct height is necessary. If the bag is too high, the water will flow too fast.

3. Assist the client to sit comfortably in the basin. Make sure the basin is filled to the correct depth. Place a folded towel in the lumbar area, if needed; a short client may need a stool under the feet. *Rationale:* The client's body will displace water in proportion to size. An adequate depth of water is needed to achieve therapeutic effect, but prevent overflowing. Promote client comfort when positioning. The stool prevents pressure on the legs' blood vessels and prevents complications.

4. Be sure the client has a robe or blankets to put over the shoulders. *Rationale:* Prevent chilling.

5. Place the call signal or bell within the client's reach. Watch the client closely for signs of fainting or weakness. *Rationale:* Heat promotes vasodilation, drawing blood away from the brain. The client should be instructed to call for help if they are uncomfortable or feel faint.

6. Instruct the client to remain in the tub for the prescribed length of time and return promptly. *Rationale:* Performing the sitz bath for the prescribed length of time promotes effectiveness of treatment. It is important not to leave the client alone for too long.

7. Assist the client out of the sitz bath and help them to dry the buttocks and return to bed. *Rationale:* Heat applied to a large body area causes vasodilation (and hypotension—low blood pressure). The client may feel weak or faint. Resting in bed allows the client's circulation to return to normal. It is vital to prevent injuries.

8. Label the sitz basin with the client's name and store in the client's room. *Rationale:* The tub/basin will be used for only one client.

Follow ENDDD Steps

IN PRACTICE

NURSING PROCEDURE 54-5: Applying an Icecap or Ice Collar

Supplies and Equipment
Icecap or ice collar
Basin of chipped ice (do not use whole ice cubes)
Small amount of cold water
Paper tape or cloth ties
Bath blanket (if needed)

Steps
Follow LPN WELCOME Steps and Then

1. Inspect the bag's stopper or closure and test the bag for leakage. *Rationale: Leaks cause the bedclothes to become wet, chilling the client and causing discomfort.*

2. Fill the icecap or collar about three-fourths full, using small pieces of ice. Pour a small amount of water over the ice. Flatten the bag on a hard surface and press, to expel as much air as possible. *Rationale: The bag will fit closely to the body and provide better cooling if the ice pieces are small and the bag is flat. Too much ice will be too heavy for comfort. Water melts the ice slightly, helps remove sharp edges, and enhances the coldness of the pack.*

3. Screw on the top, fold over the end, or secure the Velcro fasteners, making sure the seal is tight. Dry the icecap or collar and cover with a towel, securing the towel with tape. *Rationale: Proper closure prevents leakage as ice melts. Drying and the towel slow ice melt and help prevent moisture from condensing on the outside of the bag, which would cause discomfort.*

4. Adjust the bag or collar on the part of body to be treated and keep in place for 15 to 20 min (no longer). Wait 1 to 2 hr before reapplying it, unless directed otherwise. Document "on" and "off" periods. *Rationale: Prolonged application of cold reverses the full beneficial effects and may cause tissue damage. Ice melts in this time. The "off" time allows skin tissues to recover.*

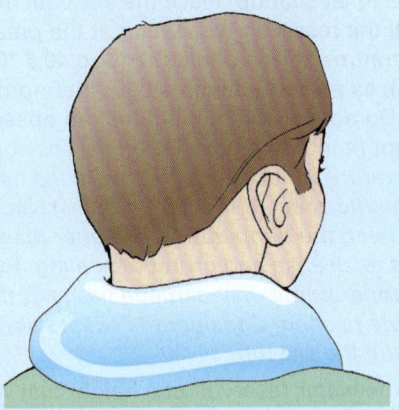

An ice collar applied to the neck.

Follow ENDDD Steps

Special Reminder
- If the skin becomes mottled or numb, or the client complains of increased pain, remove the ice pack. *Rationale: This indicates that the pack was too cold.*

55 Pain Management

Learning Objectives

1. Identify major underlying causes of pain.
2. Differentiate between the two major categories of pain.
3. Discuss the importance of regular pain assessment.
4. Identify important nursing considerations in data gathering regarding pain.
5. Discuss the impact of chronic pain on a person's life and on their significant others.
6. List and describe several tools used to quantify a client's pain.
7. Describe the relationships between endorphins and pain management.
8. Explain the role of analgesics in pain management; name classes of analgesics and specific uses for each.
9. Identify types/routes of analgesic administration.
10. Describe how surgery is used to provide pain relief.
11. List and describe physical, cognitive behavioral, and alternative therapy measures used to complement pharmacologic pain management.

Important Terminology

ablation	adjuvant	endorphin	nociception	referred pain	NCA
acute pain (nociceptive pain)	analgesic	guided imagery	pain		NSAIDs
	cancer pain	intractable pain	pain threshold	**Acronyms**	PCA
	chronic pain	neuropathic pain	pain tolerance	CCA	TENS

Pain, the body's distress signal, is difficult to ignore. It is one of the most common reasons for seeking healthcare. People try many remedies to relieve pain, often without success. Relieving pain and providing comfort are ongoing nursing challenges.

PAIN

Pain is difficult to define. It is a *subjective* symptom; only the client can describe it. It cannot be objectively measured by the practitioner. A noted pain theorist, Margo McCaffery, states in her classic writing that "Pain is whatever the experiencing person says it is, existing whenever he says it does" (McCaffery, 1968). In its clinical practice guidelines for acute pain management, the Agency for Healthcare Research and Quality (AHRQ) states that the "client's self-report is the single best indicator of pain." According to the International Association for the Study of Pain (IASP), pain is defined as "An unpleasant sensory and emotional experience associated with, or resembling that associated with, actual or potential tissue damage. Pain is always a personal experience…" (IASP, 2020, para 3). Acute pain and chronic pain are also identified as nursing diagnoses.

Causes of Pain

The person in pain seeks relief from discomfort. Determining the pain's cause is key, so effective treatment may be initiated. The causes of pain vary, and sometimes a definite cause may be difficult or impossible to determine. Nursing care is directed at *relieving pain*. Providing relief and comfort through medication administration and other interventions is an important nursing responsibility.

Several factors can initiate the pain response. Physical causes include mechanical stressors (e.g., trauma, surgical incision, tumor growth). The body responds with pain and discomfort to excesses in pressure, heat and cold, and certain chemicals (e.g., histamine, bradykinin, acetylcholine) released when tissues are damaged. Lack of oxygen (*oxygen deprivation*) and muscle spasms, resulting in decreased blood supply, can also cause pain. As discomfort increases, the body's natural response is to tighten muscles further, accentuating the problem. Fatigue, fear of the unknown, and lack of knowledge about pain management can cause further muscle tightening. Without intervention, a vicious cycle of pain can follow (Fig. 55-1). Pain receptors do not become less sensitive to adverse stimulation as the adverse stimulation continues, which makes it necessary to treat the pain or remove the cause.

Key Concept
Pain exists, even if no definite physical cause can be found. If the client feels pain, it is real to that person.

Pain Transmission

The term used to describe normal pain transmission and interpretation is **nociception**. It has four phases:

- *Transduction:* The nervous system changes painful stimuli in nerve endings to impulses.
- *Transmission:* The impulses travel from their original site to the brain.

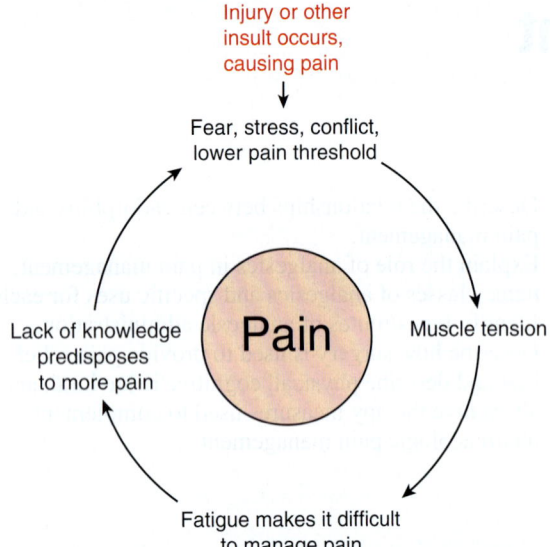

Figure 55-1 The pain cycle and some factors affecting it. Without intervention, the cycle continues and often worsens.

- *Perception:* The brain recognizes, defines, and responds to pain.
- *Modulation:* The body activates needed inhibitory responses to the effects of pain. If this modulation response is not successful, external intervention is required to manage pain. Some of these interventions are introduced in this chapter.

Types of Pain

The IASP has identified several categories of pain. Among these are acute pain, referred pain, cancer pain, and chronic pain.

Acute pain may range from mild to severe and usually occurs abruptly, most often in response to trauma. Common causes of acute pain are accidental trauma, infection, and surgery. It exists for only a short period of time, typically 6 months or less, and is usually intermittent, not constant. Acute pain results from the nervous system's normal processing of trauma to skin, muscles, and viscera (internal organs). Another term for acute pain is *nociceptive pain.* After the underlying cause is identified and successfully treated, acute pain disappears.

Referred pain is pain originating in one body part, but perceived elsewhere. It often originates within viscera and may be perceived in the skin, although it may also be perceived in another internal area.

Cancer pain results from malignancy. Often, cancer pain is very severe and may be considered *intractable* (untreatable) and chronic. Hospice nursing is often involved with the management of cancer pain (Chapter 100).

Chronic pain often has an unknown cause and is defined as discomfort that continues for a long period (6 months or longer); it may exist for life. Often, chronic pain interferes with the person's normal functioning and may be classified as *limited, intermittent,* or *persistent.* A variation of chronic pain, **neuropathic pain**, results from injury or malfunction of nerves, either in the central nervous system or in peripheral nerves. Neuropathic pain syndromes are very difficult to treat; the exact mechanisms involved are not fully understood. Chronic pain continues beyond what would be expected as a normal healing period for acute pain. Individuals with neuropathic pain typically report constant burning, tingling, and/or shooting pain. Customary interventions for relieving such pain may be ineffective; aggressive treatment is usually necessary. Chronic pain that resists therapeutic interventions is called **intractable pain**. In this case, a number of therapies have been tried, and none has relieved the pain. Intractable pain can have a known cause, such as an inoperable invasive tumor, or the cause may be unknown.

The effects of chronic pain can be destructive to a person's lifestyle and outlook, especially if the cause is unknown. The person's reaction may be frustration, anger, and/or depression; however, often expressing these feelings becomes difficult because family and friends do not seem to understand. The client may not want to worry loved ones, or the loved ones may have become tired of constantly "hearing about it." Thus, the client may avoid talking about it and internalize feelings. Often, the more anger, anxiety, and distancing the client feels, the more difficult the pain and frustration become. The client may begin to feel that no one believes the pain is real, and this may be true. When a person is not able to express feelings, suppressed anger may turn inward and result in *depression.* Symptoms of depression include inability to sleep or sleeping too much, lack of interest in surroundings or activities, hopelessness, lack of or excessive appetite, guilt feelings, and sexual impotence (Chapter 94). Persons with depression often suffer from lack of self-esteem and may feel worthless or burdensome to others. Severe depression, particularly when combined with chronic pain, *can contribute to substance abuse and dependency and presents a real danger of suicide or other self-injurious behavior.* Continued chronic pain often causes the person to withdraw socially and become physically inactive. Unfortunately, inactivity aggravates pain because muscles and joints stiffen and begin to deteriorate, causing the symptoms to intensify.

The nurse caring for the client with chronic pain faces special challenges. It is important to help the client understand the plan and realize that the healthcare team will take aggressive steps involving many different interventions. The client is assisted to identify factors that worsen pain because each of these intensifies and perpetuates the pain cycle and makes it more difficult to break (Table 55-1).

Interventions are aimed at interrupting this pain cycle. Symptoms surrounding the pain are treated because it may be difficult to identify the exact origin of the pain. Treatment is also focused on raising the client's self-esteem and helping the client to deal with feelings of anger, guilt, frustration, depression, and suicidal ideation. In Practice: Educating the Client 55-1 lists helpful tips for chronic pain management.

NCLEX Alert

You may be asked in examination scenarios to identify information you would include when teaching a client to manage chronic pain. Your basic understanding of pain (pain perception as a feeling of distress, and factors affecting this perception; causes, phases of pain transmission, and categories of pain) is essential to your ability to select nursing interventions for the specific scenarios in the NCLEX examination.

TABLE 55-1 Results of the Chronic Pain Experience

CHARACTERISTICS	SUGGESTED APPROACHES
Loss of control	Regain control over one part of life at a time; set intermediate goals with target dates; write out all goals and check off as they are accomplished
Decreased self-esteem	Participate in support groups, affirmations; build on abilities, not disabilities; find achievable recreational activities
Decreased communication (family members do not want to hear about pain any more)	Talk to others with chronic pain (who can relate); limit talking about pain with family; attend support group and individual therapy sessions; help family realize that many people experience chronic pain and it is very difficult; encourage family members to join a support group to enhance understanding
Inappropriate life goals	Try to control pain while resuming normal activities, trying for a longer period each day; prepare for possible job retraining if necessary; revise goals as necessary, take chronic pain into consideration
Change in relationships; lack of sexual activity; role changes within family	Attend marriage and family therapy; encourage expressions of love and caring, even though sexual activity may be difficult; seek financial counseling; explain to family why life is changed and what activities can continue; encourage family activities; assume leadership again gradually, one step at a time
Anger of family and friends over need to "take care of" client or do client's work	Participate in family therapy; receive vocational counseling; try to find appropriate job, within capabilities (start with volunteer work, if necessary)
Decreased activity	Find alternative activities, hobbies, entertainment; attempt to be active in something, such as a club, part-time job, volunteer work, visiting with grandchildren, or church
Decreased endurance	Build up strength gradually; find achievable activities, such as walking, riding stationary bicycle, swimming, low-impact aerobic exercise; participate in activities with other clients who have chronic pain; keep moving, to avoid further deterioration and depression

Factors Affecting Pain Perception

A person's **pain threshold** is the "the point at which a person becomes aware of pain." (National Cancer Institute, 2020, para 1). **Pain tolerance** denotes the point at which a person can no longer endure pain (Fig. 55-2). The body has internal mechanisms that help control pain perception. The central nervous system produces **endorphins**, naturally occurring substances that relieve pain. Endorphins are released with exercise and other forms of physical stimulation. Unfortunately, endorphins dissipate rapidly. Studies have shown that activities other than exercise, such as laughter, can also increase endorphin production. Intake of certain chemicals and foods, including caffeine, nicotine, alcohol, salt, and sugar, *decreases* endorphin production.

Key Concept

Remember: If a client feels pain, the pain is real. Medications and other interventions help increase the client's pain threshold and increase the client's pain tolerance.

IN PRACTICE
EDUCATING THE CLIENT 55-1 — Teaching the Client to Manage Chronic Pain

- *Medications:* Be sure to follow regular medication schedules exactly. This helps maintain an adequate blood level, rather than waiting until pain occurs.
- *Exercise:* Stay active. Exercise at a comfortable pace and level. Avoid competing with others; strive for your own personal best. Keep out of bed as much as possible. Walking is good exercise and is possible for most clients; this helps produce helpful endorphins and to maintain muscle strength and joint mobility.
- *Nutrition:* Maintain a healthy diet. Enjoy food and pleasant mealtimes. Drink plenty of water and other fluids, including fruit juices. Try to avoid salt, sugar, caffeine, alcohol, nicotine, and artificial sweeteners (particularly aspartame).
- *Recreation:* Have fun. Participate in enjoyable activities; spend recreational time with family and friends.
- *Relaxation:* Learn to relax, both *passively* (self-hypnosis, meditation, deep breathing) and *actively* (knit, sew, read, travel).
- *Support:* Join a support group. Learn how others manage chronic pain. Seek help from family and friends.
- *Hobbies:* Stay occupied. Try not to depend on others to entertain you. Develop hobbies compatible with physical abilities.
- *Rest/sleep:* Employ stress management techniques. Coping with pain is easier after rest. Be sure to get an adequate amount of sleep. Take naps during the day, if necessary.

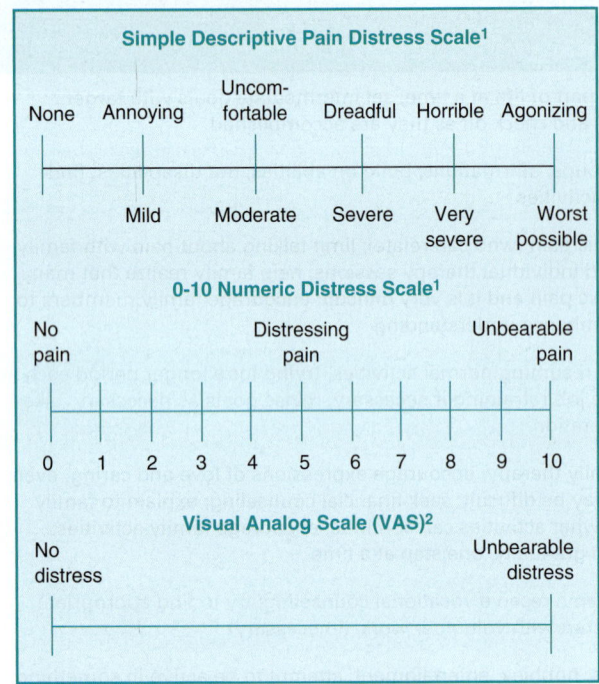

Figure 55-2 Sample Pain Distress Scales. These are called (**top**) *word scales* (using descriptive words); (**center**) *numeric scales* (using numbers); or (**bottom**) *linear scales* (drawn in a line) (Acute Pain Management Guide Panel, n.d.).

COLLECTION OF CLIENT DATA ABOUT PAIN

Since pain is *subjective,* it is vital to listen to clients' descriptions of their symptoms. Although it cannot be measured objectively, some manifestations of pain can be observed. Also consider your clients' culture; this may affect individual clients' reactions to their pain (Chapter 8). The nurse is in the best position to help collect information regarding pain.

SPECIAL CONSIDERATIONS Culture and Ethnicity

Expressions of Pain
The expression of pain is often related to cultural and ethnic factors. These factors may include, but are not limited to, the following:
- Beliefs about the causes of pain (e.g., evil spirits, "the evil eye," punishment from God, guilt)
- Manner of expressing pain in that culture (e.g., stoic vs very expressive)
- Perceived gender expectations (e.g., some genders should not express pain, while other should)
- Acceptance of traditional versus nontraditional medicine (e.g., healthcare providers vs healers, shamans)
- Belief that pain is related to imbalance of yin and yang or hot and cold
- Relationship between pain and immoral behavior
- Contribution of spiritual and religious beliefs to high pain tolerance

Importance of Pain Assessment

In the 1990s, pain assessments were evaluated. At this time, the Joint Commission determined that pain was the fifth vital sign and noted that it should be assessed each time other vital signs were measured. However, rapid increases in pain medication usage in the early 2000s and the opioid prescription crisis began to have significant effects in healthcare by mid 2010s. Further studies into pain management were conducted, and by 2016, the Joint Commission's statement designating pain as a vital sign was reversed. However, Joint Commission's regulations do state that clients are to be asked on a regular basis if they are experiencing pain. Evaluation of pain alerts healthcare providers to the necessity of addressing the client's pain. Relief of pain helps the client to be more comfortable and, therefore, to recover more quickly. The Joint Commission developed the following accreditation standards to go into effect in 2018 in an attempt to improve pain management (Joint Commission, 2017):

- Identifying a leader or leadership team that is responsible for pain management and safe opioid prescribing
- Involving patients in developing their treatment plans and setting realistic expectations and measurable goals
- Promoting safe opioid use by identifying high-risk patients
- Monitoring high-risk patients
- Facilitating clinician access to prescription drug monitoring program databases
- Conducting performance improvement activities focusing on pain assessment and management to increase safety and quality for patients

Key Concept
The documentation of pain includes the following:
- Level of pain
- Description of pain
- Action taken
- Response to interventions

Pain Rating Scales

The Joint Commission requires healthcare facilities to use pain scales to help clients determine their *level* of pain. Several pain scales to assist clients in quantifying pain are below. Clients rate their pain level, as compared with the choices on the scale. Rating scales, such as the Pain Intensity Scale or Pain Distress Scale, are usually reserved for children older than 7 years and for adults. The client is asked to rate their pain by choosing descriptive words, by choosing the appropriate number on a numerical scale from 0 (no pain) to 10 (unbearable pain), or by choosing a location on a linear scale (visual analog scale [VAS]) (Fig. 55-2). The person must understand what each number means. A child must be old enough to understand the concepts of "more than" and "less than" to use these scales. Another method of rating pain intensity uses a pain questionnaire, such as the McGill–Melzack Pain Questionnaire (Fig. 55-3).

McGill - Melzack Pain Questionnaire

Patient's Name ______ Date ______ Time ______ am/pm
Analgesic(s) ______ Dosage ______ Time Given ______ am/pm
______ Dosage ______ Time Given ______ am/pm

Analgesic Time Difference (hours): +4 +1 +2 +3

PRI: S ______ (1-10) A ______ (11-15) E ______ (16) M(S) ______ (17-19) M(AE) ______ (20) M(T) ______ (17-20) PRT(T) ______ (1-20)

1 FLICKERING, QUIVERING, PULSING, THROBBING, BEATING, POUNDING	11 TIRING, EXHAUSTING
2 JUMPING, FLASHING, SHOOTING	12 SICKENING, SUFFOCATING
3 PRICKING, BORING, DRILLING, STABBING, LANCINATING	13 FEARFUL, FRIGHTFUL, TERRIFYING
4 SHARP, CUTTING, LACERATING	14 PUNISHING, GRUELING, CRUEL, VICIOUS, KILLING
5 PINCHING, PRESSING, GNAWING, CRAMPING, CRUSHING	15 WRETCHED, BLINDING
6 TUGGING, PULLING, WRENCHING	16 ANNOYING, TROUBLESOME, MISERABLE, INTENSE, UNBEARABLE
7 HOT, BURNING, SCALDING, SEARING	17 SPREADING, RADIATING, PENETRATING, PIERCING
8 TINGLING, ITCHY, SMARTING, STINGING	18 TIGHT, NUMB, DRAWING, SQUEEZING, TEARING
9 DULL, SORE, HURTING, ACHING, HEAVY	19 COOL, COLD, FREEZING
10 TENDER, TAUT, RASPING, SPLITTING	20 NAGGING, NAUSEATING, AGONIZING, DREADFUL, TORTURING
	PPI: 0 No pain, 1 MILD, 2 DISCOMFORTING, 3 DISTRESSING, 4 HORRIBLE, 5 EXCRUCIATING

PPI ______ COMMENTS:

CONSTANT
PERIODIC
BRIEF

ACCOMPANYING SYMPTOMS: NAUSEA, HEADACHE, DIZZINESS, DROWSINESS, CONSTIPATION, DIARRHEA
COMMENTS:

SLEEP: GOOD, FITFUL, CAN'T SLEEP
COMMENTS:

FOOD INTAKE: GOOD, SOME, LITTLE, NONE
COMMENTS:

ACTIVITY: GOOD, SOME, LITTLE, NONE
COMMENTS:

Key:
PPI = present pain intensity
PRI = pain rating index
S = sensory components of pain
A = affective, or emotional, components of pain
E = evaluative terms
M = miscellaneous terms

Combinations of words can be identified: M(S) and M(AE) and the entire number totaled: PRI(T). (Copyright 1970. Ronald Melzack)

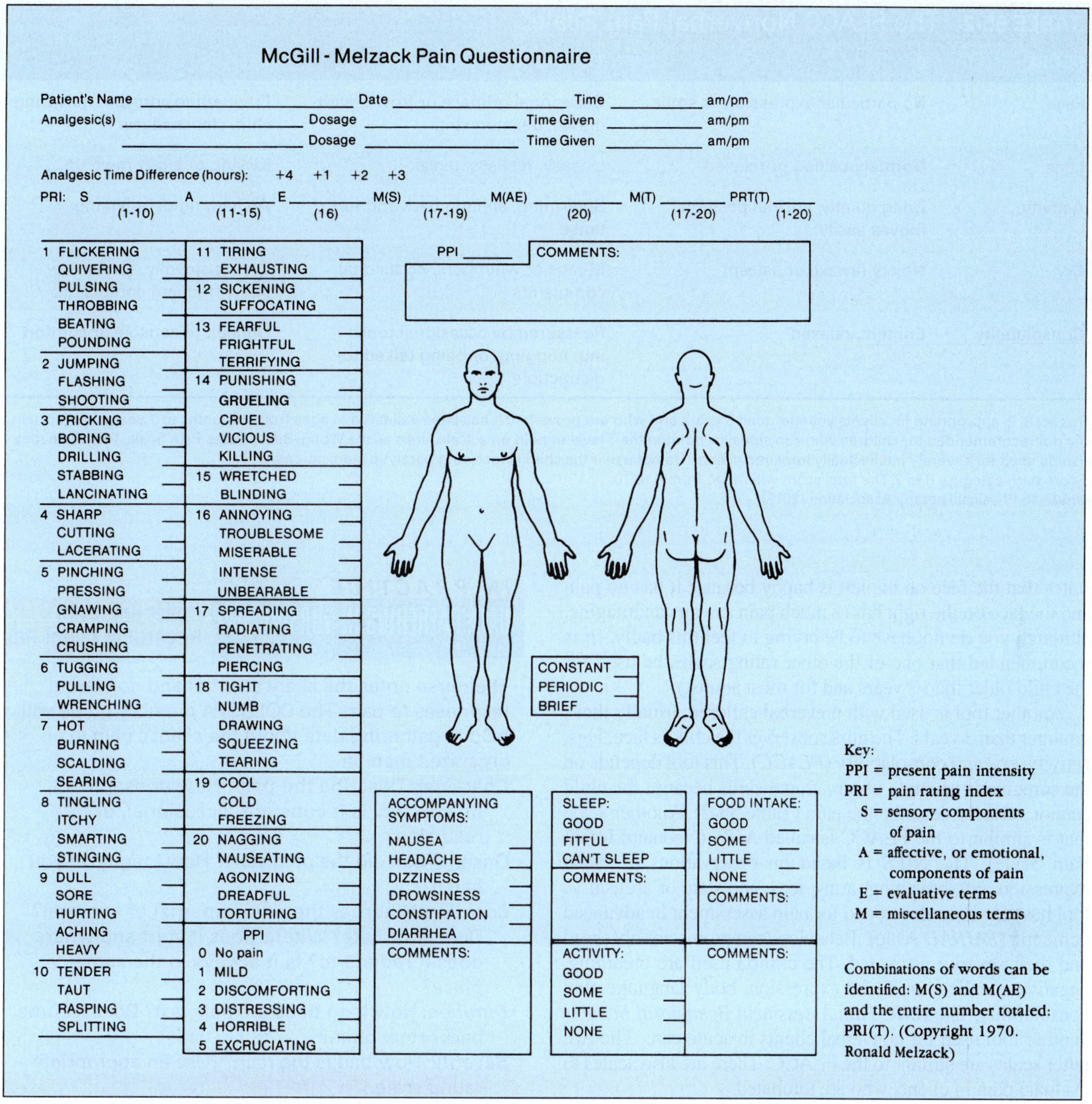

Figure 55-3 The McGill–Melzack Pain Questionnaire provides a comprehensive way to obtain information about a client's pain. (Adapted with permission from Katz, J., & Melzack, R. (1999). Measurement of pain. *The Surgical Clinics of North America, 79*(2), 231–252 and Melzack, R. (1975). The McGill Pain Questionnaire: major properties and scoring methods. *Pain, 1*(3), 277–299.)

The Wong–Baker Faces Pain Scale (a picture scale) was developed primarily for verbal children between the ages of 3 and 7 years. However, it can also be used for adults who have difficulty expressing themselves or people who do not speak the prevailing language in the facility. Figure 55-4 is an example of a picture scale that uses faces to express pain level. The client is asked to choose the face that best describes how they are feeling because of existing pain. The explanation given

Figure 55-4 An example of a *picture scale.* It is recommended for children aged 3 to 7 years. Point to each face, using the words to describe the pain intensity. Ask the child to choose the face that best describes their own pain and record the appropriate number. (Source: shutterstock.com/Oxy_gen.)

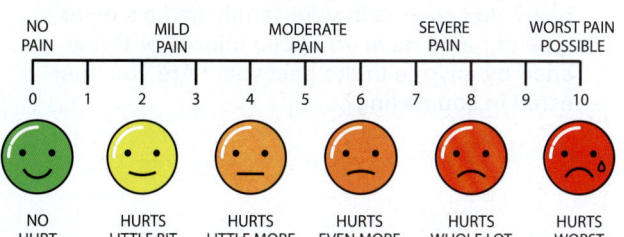

TABLE 55-2 The FLACC Nonverbal Pain Scale[a]

SCORE	0	1	2
Face	No particular expression or smile	Occasional grimace or frown, withdrawn, disinterested	Frequent to constant quivering chin, clenched jaw
Legs	Normal position or relaxed	Uneasy, restless, tense	Kicking or legs drawn up
Activity	Lying quietly, normal position, moves easily	Squirming, shifting back and forth, tense	Arched, rigid, or jerking
Cry	No cry (awake or asleep)	Moans or whimpers, occasional complaints	Crying steadily, screams or sobs, frequent complaints
Consolability	Content, relaxed	Reassured by occasional touching, hugging, or being talked to, distractible	Difficult to console or comfort

This scale is appropriate for clients younger than 3 years and who are preverbal. It has been validated at ages from 2 months to 7 years, but it is usually not recommended for children who can signal or point to their level of pain on a scale, such as the Wong–Baker Faces Pain Scale. This scale may also be used for severely intellectually impaired clients. Do not use if the child is receiving paralytic medications.
[a]Score each category 0 to 2. The total score will range from 0 to 10.
American Physical Therapy Association (2017).

---

states that the face on the left is happy because it has no pain and the face on the right has as much pain as you can imagine, although you do not have to be crying to feel this badly. (It is recommended that one of the other rating scales be used for the child older than 7 years and for most adults.)

Another tool is used with preverbal children, usually those younger than 3 years. The nurse observes the child's face, legs, activity, cry, and consolability (*FLACC*). This tool depends on the caregiver's accurate observational skills because the child cannot verbally describe the pain (Table 55-2). Another scale that is similar to the FLACC is called *NIPS* (Neonatal Infant Pain Scale). The NIPS is based on observations of facial expression, cry, breathing, arms, legs, and state of arousal. A tool has also been developed for pain assessment in advanced dementia (*PAINAD* scale). Behaviors/symptoms are observed and their severity estimated. The criteria used are breathing, negative vocalization, facial expression, body language, and consolability. The *DMC Pain Assessment Behavioral Scale* is another tool used for nonverbal clients in acute care. The two latter scales are similar to the FLACC. There are also scales to evaluate pain in clients who are intubated.

Description of Pain

In addition to determining the level of pain, other information must be obtained from the client, who alone can tell you this information. The memory guide, COLDSPA, is presented to help gather information about client symptoms, including pain. In Practice: Data Gathering in Nursing 55-1 provides detail in the use of this memory guide.

Many terms can be used to describe pain. Examples include the following:

- *Character*: The client may describe the *character* of pain with terms such as *aching, burning, cramping, crushing, dull, grinding, hammering, knifelike, penetrating, piercing, pounding, radiating, sharp, shooting, stabbing, tearing, throbbing, tingling,* or *undulating.*

IN PRACTICE
DATA GATHERING IN NURSING 55-1 — Collecting Data Regarding Client Pain

The nurse notes the client's verbal and nonverbal responses to pain. The COLDSPA memory guide will help in gathering data about the client's pain in an organized manner.

Character: Describe the pain. How does it feel? Be specific. Is it constant, occasional, or recurring?

Onset: When did the pain start? How long have you had it?

Location: Where is the pain? Internal or external? Does it radiate? Where does it start and where does it radiate to? Is it always in the same place?

Duration: How long does the pain last? Does it come back? How often?

Severity: How bad is the pain? (Use an appropriate rating scale.)

Pattern: Does anything relieve the pain? What? Does anything make it worse? Does anything specific seem to cause the pain?

Associated factors or related occurrences: Are other symptoms associated with the pain (headache, visual difficulties, sensitivity to light, nausea)? Are any obvious cultural factors involved? Have you had this same type of pain in the past? Is anything particularly stressful occurring in your life at this time? Have you had any recent injury or illness that might contribute to or cause this pain? Has anyone in your family had a similar type of pain? Have you been injured or threatened by anyone in the past year? Are you interested in counseling?

- *Duration*: The *duration* of pain may be described as *occasional, frequent, intermittent, spasmodic,* or *constant*.
- *Severity*: The intensity or severity of pain may be described as *mild, slight, moderate, severe,* or *excruciating*. (The client's descriptions of severity assist the provider to determine appropriate medication or other interventions.)
- *Associated factors*: Associated *sequelae* (consequences) *of unrelieved pain* may include *visual disturbances, nausea and vomiting, anorexia, fatigue, depression and suicidal thoughts, muscle spasms, anger and aggression, withdrawal, tearfulness,* or *regression*.

Key Concept
After pain is identified, focus nursing care and client and family teaching on breaking the cycle of chronic pain as soon as possible. Remember that some clients cannot rate or describe their pain because they cannot understand the instructions or because of factors such as dementia, mental illness, critical illness, intubation, or aphasia.

Special Note

Remember to check back with the client after giving medications or performing other pain interventions, to determine results. Document all interventions *and their results*.

PAIN MANAGEMENT

Successful management of pain is a primary goal of the healthcare team. Many interventions are available for pain management, which is unique to each individual; a successful intervention for one client may not work for another. Often, a number of interventions must be tried before one, or a combination, is successful. *Pharmacology,* the administration of medications, is often the cornerstone of successful pain management. A number of nursing interventions may also be helpful (e.g., backrub, hand massage, foot soak). In addition, the provider may order *alternative* or *complementary* interventions (e.g., acupuncture, guided imagery, yoga) provided by a specially trained person.

Pharmacologic Therapy

Analgesics are medications that relieve pain. Analgesia is usually most effective when given on a regular basis or at the very onset of pain. The *preventive approach* is recommended (e.g., give analgesics on a regular schedule around-the-clock, immediately after surgery, or before an uncomfortable treatment). If medication is given before pain occurs, pain control may be achieved. A needed analgesic that is withheld for too long may be ineffective when given. Some clients are allowed to administer their own analgesia through a *patient-controlled analgesia* (**PCA**) pump (Fig. 55-5). In some cases, a family caregiver is trained to manage the client's analgesia pump (*caregiver-controlled analgesia* [**CCA**]). During acute illness, the nurse may manage the pump (*nurse-controlled analgesia* [**NCA**]).

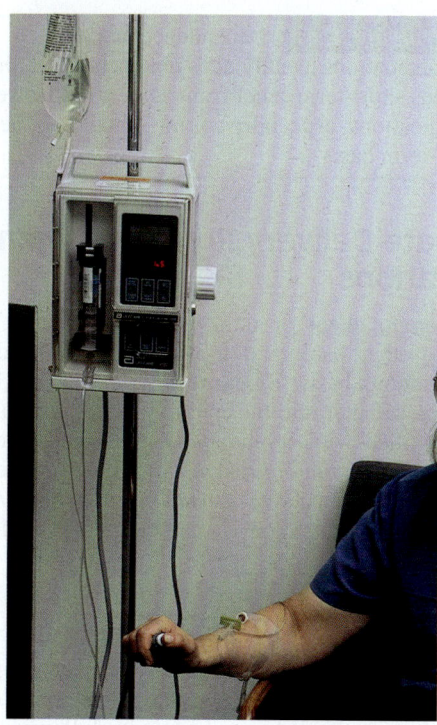

Figure 55-5 A patient-controlled analgesia pump allows clients to administer their own analgesia. Many are smaller and easier to carry, if the client is ambulatory.

Analgesics typically provide pain relief without causing a loss of consciousness (Lilley, Collins, & Snyder, 2020). Three classes of analgesics are commonly used for pain relief. These are as follows:

- *Nonopioid—nonsteroidal anti-inflammatory drugs* (NSAIDs): Examples of NSAIDs include *aspirin, ibuprofen (Motrin),* and *naproxen (Naprosyn, Aleve)*. These drugs are usually given to clients experiencing mild to moderate pain. Another *nonopioid analgesic* commonly used for mild pain is acetaminophen (Tylenol).
- *Opioids/narcotic analgesics:* The most commonly used example is *morphine* (and its derivatives). Opioids are usually used to manage pain in clients with moderate to severe pain.
- *Adjuvant drugs:* An **adjuvant** medication or treatment is one that enhances the effectiveness of another. The term may be applied to treatments or medications (e.g., *anticonvulsants, antidepressants,* or acupuncture). Adjuvant medications and treatments can help improve the client's mood, thus assisting in muscle relaxation. When muscles are relaxed, pain improves and endorphin production increases. *Ointments* and *liniments* that contain local anesthetics may provide pain relief. Such medications may also draw blood into the painful area, to increase temperature and improve circulation. Many other pharmacologic agents are used to manage pain; see Unit 9.

> **Nursing Alert** Dependence on pain medications usually does not occur when the client needs short-term relief from acute pain. However, these medications, especially opioids, should not be used on a long-term basis.

Alternate Delivery Routes for Pain Medications

In addition to client or nurse-controlled pumps and IM injections, other parenteral medications can be delivered on a continuous basis. *Epidural medications* are delivered by infusion catheter into the epidural space (just outside the dural sac, filled with cerebrospinal fluid, and surrounding nerve roots). *Continuous wound perfusion* delivers local analgesia to a surgical site. *Perineural administration* of a local anesthetic is instilled via catheter along the length of a wound.

Surgical Intervention

Surgery may be necessary to alleviate certain types of chronic pain. For example, when a herniated disk is the cause of lower back pain, the disk may be removed. Physical causes, such as tumors causing pressure, or pinched nerves, can be treated with surgery. In addition, the nerves transmitting the pain sensation may be cut (**ablation** surgery). However, with the advent of many less invasive techniques, this surgery is not often used.

Nursing Interventions

Empathic nursing can help provide pain relief. Independent *nursing interventions* include providing diversion, changing the client's position, bathing the client, giving a backrub, or massaging the client's hands. The provider may order the application of heat or cold (Chapter 54) or other treatments. These methods are usually used to complement, not replace, pharmacologic interventions. Some clients, particularly those with a terminal illness, may experience long-term and severe intractable pain, which is difficult to manage (Chapter 100). The Nursing Process section at the end of this chapter further outlines the application of the nursing process to pain management.

> **NCLEX Alert**
> Throughout the examination, you will be required to demonstrate your knowledge as you relate data to the selection of nursing actions to manage client pain. You must be able to describe documentation of pain—level, description, action taken, and results—and apply this information to your answers.

Comfort Measures

In addition to the nursing interventions mentioned above, the nurse can independently perform other comfort measures aimed at relieving pain. A clean bed, clean face and hands, restful music, a warm room, or a semi-lighted room may promote *relaxation*, which in turn may help lessen pain. Positional changes also help. The client is encouraged to eat

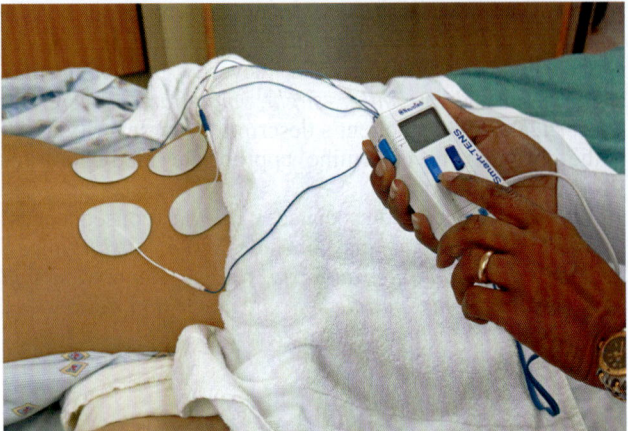

Figure 55-6 The transcutaneous electrical nerve stimulation unit relieves pain by providing physical stimulation. It can be controlled by the client or by healthcare personnel or family. (Evans-Smith, 2005.)

a nutritious diet and to obtain adequate fluids. Offer fluids often, including nutritional supplements, if ordered. It is important to assist with elimination by monitoring voiding and bowel patterns and by offering ordered medications to prevent constipation and diarrhea.

Physical Measures

Physical measures can be used in addition to pharmacologic pain management interventions.

Physical Stimulus (Cutaneous Stimulation)

Gentle massage or pressure may relieve congestion or promote circulation and oxygenation, and thus help relieve pain. This may be applied by gently massaging a painful area or more generally by giving a backrub. Specific and accurately directed stimulation is applied using the transcutaneous electrical nerve stimulation (**TENS**) unit (Fig. 55-6). TENS is a technique that allows the client to wear an electronic device and trigger an electrical stimulation when they feel pain. This gentle electrical shock blocks pain, allowing muscles to relax. The shock also stimulates the production of endorphins. (Similar units are commercially available.) The client will require assistance to begin operating the TENS unit. Other, more invasive, methods are also used, but are beyond the scope of this text.

Heat and Cold Application

The application of *heat* or *cold* (Chapter 54) is a nonpharmacologic technique that often helps control localized pain, by causing vasodilation (heat) or vasoconstriction (cold). Applying heat and cold is commonly used, both in nursing care and by clients at home.

Exercise

Actively *exercising* specific body parts, with a gradual, but steady, increase in activity levels, increases joint flexibility and muscle strength. Specific exercise is ordered by the primary provider or physical therapist and should be performed only to the body's tolerance. (Exercise is also required by all people to prevent loss of muscle tone and strength.) The client is taught to perform activities to prevent injury and, thus, lessen pain. Activities should vary and be enjoyable. Activities performed with others often are more enjoyable than those done alone. Encourage client participation in group programs; many health clubs have appropriate exercise programs. Exercise and activity programs are designed to increase endurance *gradually.* The activity level is increased a little each day, pushing just beyond discomfort. The client needs to understand that exercise might be uncomfortable; however, exercising to the point of severe pain is not recommended. Some discomfort often helps prevent further injury. Exercise helps stimulate endorphin production and increase endurance and strength. Teaching clients to monitor their own *body cues* (feelings one experiences by considering body rhythms) places the emphasis on self-care and self-monitoring.

Cognitive Behavioral Measures
Several *cognitive behavioral techniques* can also act as complementary pain control measures.

Distraction and Diversion
Activities, such as visiting, games, television, or craft projects, may help divert a client's attention from pain. Friends can often be helpful to each other by listening and offering support. It is often helpful for clients to realize they are not alone in a particular concern, such as pain.

Deep Relaxation and Guided Imagery
Deep relaxation techniques are often helpful. Many relaxation CDs are available. The client is taught to perform specific deep breathing/relaxation exercises. Next, the client concentrates on a pleasant and relaxing experience. Some clients learn through relaxation therapy to relax taut muscles, thereby relieving pain. **Guided imagery** is a process through which the client receives a suggestion to concentrate on an image to control pain or discomfort. Deep relaxation exercises are performed first, so the client is totally relaxed. Then the client is guided through specific images. For example, the suggestion may be that pain occurring over a large area of the body is moving down and out of the body. In this way, a smaller area can be involved; the eventual goal is to totally eliminate the pain. Another technique visualizes the destruction of the pain's origin. For example, this procedure is often used for individuals who have cancer. They visualize their defense cells as large and strong and the cancer cells as small and weak. People in pain also learn to visualize themselves as powerful and able to conquer their pain. In addition, they learn to change their pain perceptions, so discomfort is better tolerated.

Support Groups
Support groups and *group therapy sessions* can help individuals in pain by giving them an opportunity to express feelings and talk about pain with others who can relate. Group members often offer suggestions as to how they handled similar situations and concerns (Fig. 55-7). Some support groups provide information about financial assistance to help with medication costs, housing information, or vocational counseling to aid in maintaining functional abilities or job retraining. Usually, the client's family can also benefit from a support group. They learn to deal with the client's concerns, with their

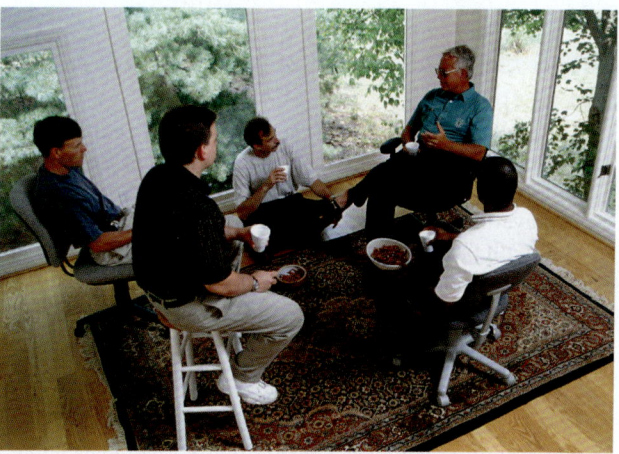

Figure 55-7 Support groups can be formal or informal. Friends can support each other over coffee. Or by sharing common experiences and concerns, members of a formal support group can enhance their coping skills, increase their ability to handle stress, and find a valuable avenue for understanding and encouragement. In many cases, they have become unable to talk about their pain to loved ones. (Photo by Will & Deni McIntyre/Science Source.)

own frustration, and how to be supportive. Some group therapists follow a program based on the 12 steps of Alcoholics Anonymous (Chapter 95). The first step is accepting that "I am powerless over this pain." If clients can accept feeling powerless, they can work on measures to regain control. Such programs have proved effective in many cases.

Stress Management
Stress may aggravate pain, and *stress management* techniques may be helpful in assisting the client to develop more effective coping mechanisms. Learning to be more assertive may help reduce stress. Other stress-reducing measures include physical activity, recreation, adequate fluids, and a well-balanced diet. Antidepressant medications also may be used (Chapter 94).

Alternative and Complementary Techniques
Clients have found many *nonpharmacologic measures* helpful in pain management. Some complementary therapies, such as *chiropractic care, acupuncture, acupressure, hypnosis, therapeutic massage,* and *biofeedback,* are being prescribed more frequently by healthcare providers (Chapter 3). These therapies are often integrated into the client's total pain control regimen. More nontraditional measures include *homeopathy, use of flower essences and aromatic oils,* and *herbal remedies.* All of the complementary therapies have proven helpful to many clients. Some of these allow clients to take personal ownership of their pain management.

> **Nursing Alert** The client with chronic pain is vulnerable to unscrupulous practitioners because the client is desperate and often willing to try anything to relieve the pain. Persons promoting "quack" cure-all schemes may take advantage of these clients.

NURSING PROCESS

DATA GATHERING
- The client's description of pain and the pain experience: the pain's *c*haracter, *o*nset, *l*ocation, *d*uration, *s*everity, *p*attern, and *a*ssociated factors. In addition, consider aggravating factors and any special phenomena associated with pain.
- What meaning, if any, the pain has for the client.
- The client's coping strategies and success or failure.
- Observation of behaviors in response to pain (e.g., moving away from the stimuli; grimacing, moaning, and crying; restlessness; protecting or massaging the painful area; isolation).
- Physiologic responses—*sympathetic responses when pain is moderate and superficial* (e.g., blood pressure, pulse rate, and respirations; pupil dilation; muscle tension and rigidity; pallor; increased adrenaline output and blood glucose level); *parasympathetic responses when pain is severe and deep* (e.g., nausea and vomiting; fainting or unconsciousness; decreased blood pressure and pulse rate; rapid and irregular breathing).
- Affective responses (e.g., weeping and restlessness, withdrawal, stoicism, anxiety, depression, fear, anger, anorexia, fatigue, hopelessness, powerlessness).
- Cultural aspects—how does this cultural group usually respond to pain?

POSSIBLE NURSING DIAGNOSES
- Acute pain
- Chronic pain
- Coping impairment
- Knowledge deficiency (of effective pain management program)
- Acute anxiety
- Compromised family coping

  Note: Initially, the nurse must view pain as a symptom and pursue its physical etiology. Interventions for pain performed before an accurate assessment may mask the true cause of pain, thus causing further suffering and possibly, death, by allowing the progression of signs, symptoms, and the disease process.

PLANNING
A plan of care is designed with the primary healthcare provider, the client, and family to achieve the following general goals:

- The client describes a gradual reduction of pain, using a scale of 0 (no pain) to 10 (pain as intense as it can get) or another evaluating device to quantify the pain.
- The client demonstrates competent execution of a successful pain management program.

For the client with chronic pain, appropriate goals may include the following:
- The client verbalizes (and demonstrates) the ability to control pain sufficiently to manage or enjoy everyday living.
- The client locates and attends an appropriate support group.
- The family relates the feeling of being better able to cope with the client's pain experience.

IMPLEMENTATION
- Establish a supportive and trusting nurse–client relationship.
- Teach about the function of pain and instill confidence that a successful pain management program can be developed.
- Remove or alter the cause of pain (whenever possible) and alter factors that decrease pain tolerance.
- Use appropriate noninvasive relief measures: distraction, imagery, relaxation, and cutaneous stimulation (massage, application of heat or cold, vibration, pressure).
- Administer prescribed analgesic; if a PCA unit is being used, instruct the client about its use.
- Learn about the client's use of other pain therapies, as appropriate: acupuncture, biofeedback, neurosurgery, electrical nerve stimulation, and others.

EVALUATION
Determine the adequacy of the plan of care by evaluating the client's achievement of the preceding goals. If the client is unable to meet key goals, modify the plan. Key evaluative criteria include the following:
- Client experiences and expresses adequate relief.
- Client demonstrates knowledge of pain relief measures.
- Client is satisfied with pain management program.
- Client feels sufficiently comfortable to attend to demands of everyday living.
- Client is able to return to work or recreational activities.
- Family members are able to recognize and report greater comfort for themselves and perceived relief for the client.

STUDENT SYNTHESIS

KEY POINTS
- Nociception (pain transmission) has four components: transduction, transmission, perception, and modulation.
- Acute pain (nociceptive pain) lasts less than 6 months and is relieved when its cause is identified and treated.
- Chronic pain (neuropathic pain) lasts for more than 6 months. Common treatment measures may fail to eliminate such pain.
- Factors that affect pain perception include a person's pain threshold and pain tolerance. Culture also influences the expression of pain.
- The body's naturally occurring endorphins help relieve pain.
- Early intervention in the cycle of pain may help control it.
- Nursing evaluation of the client in pain focuses on the client's self-report of the experience. A number of tools are available to assist the nurse in quantifying and rating the level of pain, with the assistance of the client.

- Pharmacology is the cornerstone of much pain management.
- Surgical intervention is sometimes necessary to relieve certain kinds of pain.
- Both physical and cognitive behavioral techniques are used to complement pharmacologic pain management.
- Pain must be assessed frequently. All nursing interventions should include gathering of information from the client about the presence or absence of pain. After medications or treatments for pain, the client should be asked if the intervention was helpful or not.

CRITICAL THINKING EXERCISES

1. You work in an extended care facility where many of your residents have chronic pain. Describe a basic plan and rationale for pain management for a resident with long-standing lower back pain who refuses to get out of bed.

2. A client is taking regular pain medications for intractable pain. They are interested in exploring alternative methods, in addition to medications. What recommendations would you make? How would you explain different therapies? If you were experiencing chronic pain, what alternative and complementary methods would be of most interest to you?

NCLEX-STYLE REVIEW QUESTIONS

1. A client is experiencing chronic pain related to a back injury. Which suggestions would the nurse make to help control pain perception? Select all that apply.
    a. Limit the intake of caffeine.
    b. Avoid smoking.
    c. Perform regular exercise.
    d. Increase sodium intake.
    e. Increase alcohol intake.

2. A client in chronic pain states that the pain medication does not work. Which response by the nurse is best?
    a. "You probably need a stronger narcotic."
    b. "Take your medications regularly, not waiting until pain occurs."
    c. "Do you think maybe the pain felt is exaggerated?"
    d. "The primary care provider has given you all you can have."

3. The nurse is gathering subjective data regarding pain from a client. Which information is important for the nurse to consider when gathering this information?
    a. Culture
    b. Physical symptoms
    c. Cause of pain
    d. Financial status

4. The nurse is gathering data regarding a 2-year-old child's pain level. Which scale would be most effective for obtaining this information?
    a. Pain Distress Scale
    b. Wong–Baker Faces Pain Scale
    c. McGill–Melzack Pain Questionnaire
    d. The FLACC scale

5. A client reports no relief of pain after administration of an opioid analgesic. Which nonpharmacologic action would the nurse provide to assist with relieving the pain?
    a. Give the client a backrub.
    b. Give another dose of the medication even though it may be too early.
    c. Administer an antiemetic with the medication.
    d. Ambulate the client in the hall.

CHAPTER RESOURCES

Enhance your learning with additional resources on thePoint!

Student Resources related to this chapter can be found at **thePoint.lww.com/Rosdahl12e**.

56 Preoperative and Postoperative Care

Learning Objectives

1. Discuss major categories that identify a surgical client as high risk.
2. List the two major classes/categories of anesthetics.
3. Describe the four stages of general anesthesia.
4. Explain the importance of client teaching, as related to surgery.
5. List the preoperative nursing steps.
6. State the function of a postanesthesia care unit and describe equipment found there.
7. Describe nursing measures taken upon client returning to the nursing unit from the postanesthesia recovery area.
8. Identify nursing actions used to alleviate postoperative pain, thirst, nausea, distention, and urinary retention, and possible immediate postoperative complications.
9. Outline reasons and procedures for turning the postoperative client, promoting respiratory function, and encouraging the client to be up as soon as possible.
10. Describe differences in pre- and postoperative care in same-day surgery, as opposed to the hospital.

Important Terminology

anesthesia
atelectasis
conduction block
dehiscence
elective surgery
embolus
evisceration
general anesthetics
hemorrhage
hypovolemic shock
hypoxemia
hypoxia
incentive spirometer
intraoperative
IV moderate sedation (conscious sedation)
local anesthesia
paralytic ileus
perioperative
pneumonia
postoperative
preoperative
regional anesthetics
spinal anesthetics
splinting (of wound)
surgery
suture
thrombolytic
thrombophlebitis
venous access lock

Acronyms

DAT
DVT
NPO
OR
PACU
PAR
PONV
TAC
TCDB

Surgery is performed when the best treatment for a client's disorder is repairing, removing, changing, or replacing body tissues or organs. **Surgery** is considered to be *invasive* because it usually involves an incision (cutting) into the body or removal of external structures. Careful and attentive nursing care often can differentiate between a negative or positive surgical experience, greatly affecting the client's recovery. (The client may understand the term "*operation*" rather than surgery.)

PERIOPERATIVE CARE

The term **perioperative** refers to the timespan that includes *preparation* for, the *process of*, and *recovery from* surgery (Fig. 56-1). Perioperative nursing consists of the following three phases:

- **Preoperative** nursing care—before surgery (preparation for surgery)
- **Intraoperative** nursing care—in the operating room (**OR**) and postanesthesia recovery (**PAR**) or postanesthesia care unit (**PACU**; the process of surgery)
- **Postoperative** nursing care—after surgery (recovery from surgery)

Factors in Surgery

Surgery is performed in several different types of healthcare facilities. If surgery is extensive or a person is classified as high risk, surgery will be performed in an acute care facility, such as a hospital. Less complex or less dangerous procedures, not requiring an overnight stay, are most often performed in a *walk-in* or *ambulatory* center, often called a *surgicenter, short-stay center,* or *same-day surgery center.* In these facilities, the client does the preparation at home, enters the facility, has the surgery, and goes home to recover the same day. This short-stay surgical center may be part of a healthcare provider's clinic, a department in a hospital, or a free-standing facility. The information in this chapter is important for the nurse, whether working in a surgical unit in a hospital or in an ambulatory surgery center. Pre- and postoperative care is basically the same, no matter where surgery is carried out. The surgeon or other provider will assess each client and determine where the surgery is to be performed. The surgeon also weighs the surgical risk against the need for surgery. In some cases, surgery must be done, despite the presence of risk factors (Tables 56-1).

CHAPTER 56 Preoperative and Postoperative Care

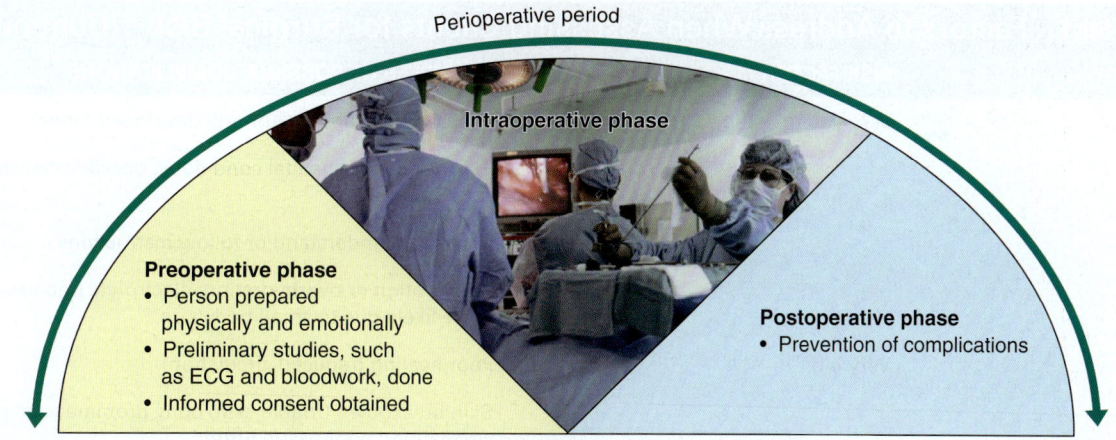

Figure 56-1 The perioperative period has three interrelated phases of care. (Carter, 2005.)

> **Key Concept**
> Only the immediate preoperative preparation and the surgery itself are completed in the same-day surgery center. In all cases, but perhaps even more so in same-day surgery, preoperative and postoperative teaching is vital. The client and/or caregiver must understand what needs to be done and what complications might occur. It is essential that the client receives written, as well as verbal, instructions.

Types of Surgery

Levels of client choice in surgery are as follows:

- *Optional/**elective surgery***: The condition is not life threatening. The client may choose whether or not to have the surgery. Examples include plastic surgery, removal of a nonmalignant birthmark, and tubal ligation or vasectomy for sterilization.
- *Required/nonelective:* The surgery is necessary at some time. The client has some choice as to when the procedure will be done. Examples are hernia repair, prolapsed uterus, or hip joint replacement.
- *Urgent/nonelective:* The surgery must be performed within a short time, to prevent further damage to the client. Examples are removal of a malignancy, repair of an aneurysm, or removal of an inflamed appendix.
- *Emergency:* The surgery must be performed immediately to save the client's life. Examples are ectopic pregnancy with threat of rupture, severe internal hemorrhage, ruptured appendix, and angioplasty after a heart attack.

Nursing Considerations

A variety of nursing diagnoses may be established for the perioperative client and their family. Examples may include the following:

TABLE 56-1 Factors to Address When Assessing Clients for Surgical Risk

CATEGORY	RISK FACTOR	EXAMPLES OF POSSIBLE COMPLICATIONS
Weight and eating disorders	Obesity	Poor healing (less circulation in fat tissue) Hypostatic pneumonia (less activity)
		More difficult surgery (more fat tissues to dissect)
		More underlying disorders likely (e.g., diabetes, poor lung function, cardiovascular conditions)
	Poor nutrition, malnutrition	Poor healing (lack of nutrients)
	Anorexia, bulimia, exercise bulimia	Skin breakdown (less padding over bony prominences, lack of protein)
		Associated conditions (electrolyte imbalance, esophageal lesions, poor dentition, bowel disorders)
Hydration status	Dehydration	Reduced circulation (lack of tissue fluid, electrolyte imbalance)
	Edema	Reduced circulation (retention of fluids, pressure within tissues)
Electrolyte balance	Imbalance	Many complications, depending on specific electrolyte

(Continued)

TABLE 56-1 Factors to Address When Assessing Clients for Surgical Risk (Continued)

CATEGORY	RISK FACTOR	EXAMPLES OF POSSIBLE COMPLICATIONS
Age	Very young	Respiratory problems (poorly developed lungs)
		Existence of congenital conditions, possibly causing complications
		Inability to understand or follow instructions
		Dehydration or overhydration, electrolyte imbalances more likely due to small body size
	Very old	Poor healing (reduced circulation)
		Skin breakdown (friable skin, bony prominences, poor circulation); poor tissue turgor
		Confusion (may be dementia or caused by anesthesia or change in routine)
		Hypostatic pneumonia (lack of activity, poor lung function, lung diseases)
		Dehydration or poor nutrition (poor eating habits, confusion)
		Poor muscle tone (lack of exercise, generalized disorders)
		Inadequate diet; lack of digestive enzymes
		Coexisting disorders more likely
Lifestyle factors	Smoking, use of chewing tobacco, vapor cigarettes	Lung disorders (inflammation, increased mucus production, diseased lung tissue, chronic bronchitis, lung or throat cancer)
		Circulatory disorders (e.g., blood clots or poor circulation, hypertension [nicotine constricts blood vessels])
	Caffeine	Cardiac disorders (atherosclerosis in heart vessels)
		Digestive disorders (e.g., peptic ulcer)
		Blood pressure disorders
		Withdrawal headaches, associated conditions (e.g., cystic conditions, hypertension)
Substance abuse	Abuse of chemicals, illegal drugs	Withdrawal symptoms (caused by removal of substance)
		Dependence (less resistance to dependency on prescribed medications because of abuse)
		High drug tolerance (requiring higher doses of pain medications to achieve comfort)
	Alcohol abuse	Lung disorders or circulatory disorders (general poor health)
		Poor nutrition, including vitamin deficiencies
		Withdrawal can be life threatening; medical team not always aware of alcoholism in client
Use of certain prescription drugs	Risk factors dependent on specific drug	Bleeding disorders, fluid retention, kidney damage, confusion, blood pressure disorders, and many other complications

TABLE 56-1	Factors to Address When Assessing Clients for Surgical Risk (Continued)	
CATEGORY	RISK FACTOR	EXAMPLES OF POSSIBLE COMPLICATIONS
Preexisting physical disorders	Risk factors dependent on disorder	Poor circulation, slowed healing, blood clotting disorders, pulse disorders, retention of fluids (heart disorders)
		Hypostatic pneumonia, poor oxygen exchange (lung disorders)
		Slowed healing, increased incidence of infections, insulin imbalances, inability to regulate blood sugar levels (diabetes mellitus)
		Allergic reactions to anesthesia or medications (allergies, asthma, anaphylaxis)
		Inability to control seizures (seizure disorders, epilepsy)
		Slowed healing, high incidence of infections (immune disorders, diabetes, cancer chemotherapy)
	Immune disorders; immunosuppression	Poor healing, inability to combat infections, contracting additional disorders
Psychological status	Excessive fear	Difficulty in understanding instructions, pulse disorders, cardiac arrest, difficulty in achieving anesthesia, panic attacks, postoperative disorders, lack of cooperation with regime
	Intellectual impairment	Inability to understand instructions, lack of follow through (psychiatric disorders, dementia, intellectual impairment)
	Depression	Lack of motivation to follow instructions
Physical activity status	Immobility, poor physical condition	Susceptible to thrombophlebitis, bowel obstruction or impaction, pressure wounds, orthostatic blood pressure changes, hypostatic and aspiration pneumonia, decreased stamina and strength, skin breakdown, other postoperative complications
Living situation	Lack of available caregivers	Difficulty in carrying out postoperative instructions, inability to care for oneself, inability to recognize complications, and inability to return for follow-up. Inadequate diet—inability to prepare meals
	Other factors	No telephone, inadequate sanitation, no plumbing, stairs, lack of food
		Inability to understand or speak the language spoken in the facility

- Fear
- Deficient knowledge
- Anticipatory grieving
- Disturbed body image
- Risk for aspiration, ineffective airway clearance
- Pain
- Hyperthermia, hypothermia
- Altered tissue perfusion (cerebral, peripheral)
- Deficient fluid volume
- Impaired tissue/skin integrity
- Impaired physical mobility

The following nursing interventions are common to all surgical procedures, regardless of the type:

- Providing emotional support to the client and family
- Preparing the client physically for surgery
- Ensuring that all legal matters, such as signing the surgical consent, have been carried out
- Ensuring that a physical examination and all required tests, such as electrocardiogram (ECG), ordered blood tests, and x-rays are done before surgery
- Providing client and family/caregiver teaching
- Providing routine preoperative and postoperative care

The time available for each nursing intervention related to surgery depends mainly on where the surgery is performed and whether or not it is an emergency. For example, if the surgery is an elective procedure and the person is a hospital inpatient, preparation and teaching time will be considerably longer than if the person is brought in by ambulance and must receive immediate emergency surgery. Older adults require some special care during the perioperative period. Box 56-1 lists special considerations for the older adult having surgery. For special considerations regarding children, see Chapter 71.

> **Key Concept**
>
> Clients and families usually experience some concern about surgery, which may be aggravated by the very short postoperative stay. It is vital to teach the client and family before surgery as much as possible about the procedure and what to expect. The better-informed client is less likely to be anxious. If a client is very anxious, the procedure may even need to be postponed.

Sedation

In some cases, procedures can be done with sedation alone. If sedation is not sufficient for the procedure that is to be done, the client will receive anesthesia. Sedation is progressive as the client moves through the stages of sedation identified below:

- *Minimal sedation:* client can respond to commands.
- *Moderate sedation:* depressed level of consciousness; client can breathe without assistance, responds to pain, and can follow some commands. Protective reflexes are maintained.
- *Deep sedation:* client cannot be easily aroused, but can respond after repeated stimulation. Respiration may need to be supported.

IV Moderate Sedation

In **IV moderate sedation**, formerly known as *conscious sedation*, intravenous (IV) sedative medications are used alone or in conjunction with local anesthetics. A client receiving moderate sedation has a depressed level of consciousness, but continues to breathe and is able to respond to verbal stimuli. Midazolam HCl (Versed) or another short-acting benzodiazepine, frequently used to induce sleepiness and relieve anxiety, is commonly used for moderate sedation, in procedures such as endoscopy or extensive dental procedures. This drug often results in amnesia about the procedure.

Anesthesia

Anesthesia is the complete or partial loss of sensation. *Surgical anesthesia* is defined as the degree of anesthesia at which an operation can safely be done and tolerated by the client. Medications called *anesthetics* induce anesthesia. The discipline of medicine that administers anesthetics is

---

Box 56-1 Perioperative Care in the Older Client

- Accurate height and weight are required, in order to calculate exact dosages of narcotics and anesthetics. Older clients are susceptible to overdose.
- Baseline respiratory assessment is required, in order to evaluate the possibility of aspiration and hypostatic pneumonia.
- Early mobility helps prevent complications secondary to immobility. Although this is important in all postoperative care, it is a greater concern for the older client.
- Older adults may be more susceptible to falls, so fall risk must be evaluated. Anyone older than 65 years is automatically placed on "fall precautions."
- Assess skin and body fat. Color, turgor, and temperature may not yield accurate observations in the older person.
- Skin breakdown is a particular danger because skin may be more *friable* (fragile) in seniors. A pressure wound evaluation scale, such as the Braden Scale, should be used (Chapter 58).
- Closely monitor blood pressure. Older adults are more susceptible to hypertension and/or postural hypotension.
- Closely monitor oxygen saturation. Older clients may have decreased lung function and/or circulation.
- Many older adults have diminished kidney function. Parenteral fluids may overload the circulation.
- Carefully monitor intake and output and electrolyte levels. Fluid and electrolyte balance may change quickly in older adults.
- Surgery is a greater risk for older people because they may have coexisting diseases or disorders that present risks (e.g., diabetes, kidney failure, cardiac disorders).
- Older clients may be less able to combat postoperative infection, due to diminished immune response.
- Encourage clients to wear their hearing aids and glasses, if possible, and provide good lighting. This provides security and helps to prevent confusion.
- Older clients may have poor vision and/or peripheral vision and may startle easily.
- Watch for unexpected medication reactions. Older clients may have an exaggerated or more rapid response or may react differently than expected. A reaction opposite to the expected effect, a *paradoxical reaction*, may occur.
- Medications may have a longer or more extreme effect, due to slower processing or excretion time (e.g., due to decreased kidney function).
- Older clients may be reluctant to complain of pain or may have decreased sensory input, expressive aphasia, or dementia; they may not feel or may not be able to express that they have pain.
- Older clients are more susceptible to postoperative lung disorders, urinary retention, and constipation and may have more difficulty ambulating postoperatively.
- Teach in brief periods and remember to include family/caregivers. Even a minor infection can cause confusion in the otherwise lucid older person. Apprehension may also cause confusion. Family members can assist.
- Teach and provide as much postoperative care as possible during the day. Older clients often become more confused in the evening ("sundowner effect") and may also tire more easily and go to sleep earlier.
- Include family members whenever possible to provide support and help avoid confusion. It is important for family caregivers to hear the instructions, so they can effectively assist postoperatively. In addition, some older clients would rather accept assistance from family than from nursing staff.

called *anesthesiology*. A healthcare provider trained in anesthesiology is an *anesthesiologist;* a registered nurse trained in anesthesiology is a *registered nurse anesthetist* (RNA). A visit from the anesthesiologist or nurse anesthetist before surgery enables a client to ask questions and allows the anesthesia professional to assess the client. The client often feels more comfortable if someone in the OR is familiar. In Practice: Nursing Care Guidelines 56-1 describes general nursing care for the client receiving anesthetics.

Types of Anesthesia

Anesthetics are divided into two main classes. **General anesthetics** block all body sensations and cause unconsciousness, relaxation, and loss of reflexes. **Local**, **regional**, **conduction blocks**, or **spinal anesthetics** disrupt sensation to specific body areas or parts, without causing unconsciousness (Box 56-2).

Key Concept

Clients receiving a local anesthetic are often given some type of sedation as well.

Methods of Administering Anesthesia

General anesthetics are most often administered IV, rectally, or by inhalation. They may also be administered by other routes. Abdominal or chest surgery is most often performed under general anesthesia, as are some orthopedic and many genitourinary procedures. The lesser the anesthetic used, the safer it is for the client; thus, *local, regional, or spinal anesthesia* is preferred whenever possible.

A *local anesthetic* may be administered topically, by injection, and, less commonly, by freezing with special substances, such as ethyl chloride. Commonly used local anesthetics include lidocaine (Xylocaine), procaine (Novocaine),

---

IN PRACTICE
NURSING CARE GUIDELINES 56-1 — Caring for the Client Who Is Receiving Anesthesia

- Check for allergies before any client has surgery and before administering any pre- or postoperative drug. An allergy wrist band must be worn by all clients, whether they have allergies or not, to ensure that the question of allergies has been addressed.
- Make sure the client is wearing an ID band and has been carefully identified by at least two staff persons. Often, two wrist bands are required.
- Make sure the client has verified the exact type of surgery that is to be done.
- Make sure the operative permit has been signed *before any premedication is administered*.
- Bring any abnormal laboratory results pre- or postoperatively to the surgeon's attention immediately. All laboratory results must be in the client's record for preoperative review by the surgeon and anesthesia personnel.
- Notify the surgeon immediately about any extreme apprehension, either before or after the administration of preoperative medication.
- After surgery using spinal anesthetics, keep the client flat until the anesthetic has worn off (sometimes as long as 12 hr, or as ordered).
- Postoperatively, check all vital signs, including pain, frequently as ordered. Report any deviations.
- Postoperatively, observe the client's urine output very carefully. Watch for bladder distention.
- Observe carefully for signs of respiratory distress following the use of neuromuscular blockers or any type of general anesthetic. Be cautious in administering postoperative narcotics because of the client's already-decreased respiratory drive following anesthesia.
- Watch carefully for signs of circulatory depression following the use of neuromuscular blockers or any general anesthetic.
- Observe the client's gastrointestinal (GI) status; listen for bowel sounds and monitor the presence or absence of a bowel movement. Do not give any oral fluids or food until bowel sounds are present.
- Keep in mind that neuromuscular blockers may *potentiate* (increase) effects of anesthesia when used with other central nervous system depressants, including alcohol. Anticipate the possibility of unexpected alcohol withdrawal.
- When epidural or spinal anesthetics or narcotics have been used, keep naloxone (Narcan) easily accessible, for reversal of untoward effects. Watch for respiratory depression, and safeguard the IV injection site. Almost always, the client has a running IV or a heparin/saline lock in place. Make sure it remains patent (open). The same principles apply when the client receives *postoperative pain medications* via spinal or epidural routes.
- When topical anesthetics have been used, watch for skin irritation.
- When eye anesthetics have been used, the eye-blink reflex may be slowed, causing the eyes to become dry. Administer eye medications, as ordered.
- Anticipate the need for pain medication early after recovery from anesthesia. Many new anesthetics are of short duration. This allows clients to leave surgery more alert. Because the anesthesia may wear off more quickly, clients require pain medication sooner. Often pain medications are given very early, in an attempt to block pain before it occurs (Chapter 55).
- Always be alert for adverse effects of any medication, even with short-acting pain medications or anesthesia.
- Report any unusual findings immediately.

Adapted from Kathleen McCullough RN, Surgical Department, Hennepin County Medical Center, Minneapolis, Minnesota, updated 2015.

Box 56-2 Types of Anesthesia

General: Unconsciousness (severe nervous system depression, narcosis) is induced by anesthetic agents. This causes absence of pain (*analgesia*) and sensation over the entire body and muscle relaxation, with loss of reflexes. The client cannot be aroused, and breathing must be maintained mechanically. General anesthesia is used for invasive procedures, such as open-heart surgery, hysterectomy, and appendectomy. It is also used when surgery is anticipated to take several hours, such as repair of multiple injuries due to trauma.

LOCAL (INFILTRATION AND TOPICAL ANESTHESIA)

Pain and sensation are blocked in a limited area, most often by injection of an anesthetic agent into a small (local) area or by topical application to the area. Dental work often involves topical application of anesthetic followed by injection of an anesthetic, such as procaine (Novocain), into terminal nerve endings, rendering a small area sensation-free. Insertion of stitches into a traumatic wound is also usually done using local anesthesia.

REGIONAL

Regional anesthesia is local anesthesia induced in a particular area (region), such as part of an extremity, by interruption of sensory nerve conductivity.

CONDUCTION BLOCK

There are many types of conduction blocks, depending on the nerve group affected by anesthetic injection. The *field block* encircles the operative area with several injections. A *nerve block* is done by injecting the anesthetic near the nerves supplying the area. These are commonly used in obstetrics. (A nerve block may also be done for management of chronic pain, most often back pain.)

SPINAL

Spinal anesthesia is an extensive conduction nerve block induced by injecting an anesthetic agent into the subarachnoid space of the spinal cord. It must usually be administered by an anesthesiologist (not an anesthetist), and the effect is achieved more slowly and resolves more slowly than with general anesthesia. Spinal anesthesia can be used for many types of surgery.

---

and tetracaine (Pontocaine). In some cases, epinephrine is combined with the local anesthetic. This constricts blood vessels, prolonging absorption of the anesthetic and reducing the amount of anesthetic required. Common procedures performed under local or regional anesthesia include dental work, many types of plastic surgery and skin suturing (stitching), and some types of eye surgery. Much brain surgery is also done using local anesthesia, allowing the client to respond to commands. Spinal anesthesia may be used for surgery of the lower extremities, perineum, and lower abdomen.

General anesthetics, most often given by inhalation, are volatile liquids such as halothane (Fluothane), enflurane (Ethrane), isoflurane (Forane), sevoflurane (Ultane), desflurane (Suprane), and methoxyflurane (Penthrane) and the gas, nitrous oxide (N_2O). Some of these are chemically related to ether, which currently is rarely used in the United States.

In many cases, the client is prepared for inhalation anesthesia with an IV injection of a barbiturate, such as thiopental sodium (Pentothal), or another agent, such as ketamine HCl (Ketalar, a dissociative agent). A combination of fentanyl citrate (Sublimaze, Actiq, a short-acting synthetic opioid) and droperidol (Inapsine) is called a *neuroleptanalgesic* and produces profound analgesia. With these agents, the client falls asleep or is unaware of the surroundings, after which they are intubated (an endotracheal tube placed in the throat) and then maintained during surgery on an inhalation anesthetic.

Stages of General Anesthesia

If sedation is not sufficient for the surgical procedure to be performed, the client receives general anesthesia. *The client under general anesthesia cannot be aroused and cannot breathe without assistance. A patent (open) airway must be artificially maintained. In some cases, cardiovascular function is also impaired.*

If a slow-acting anesthetic is used, the client passes through three recognizable stages of general anesthesia, listed below. As the client wakes up from the anesthesia, these stages are reversed. When narcotics and muscle relaxant medications are administered, some of these stages are passed through very quickly or are absent. The goal is smooth progression in and out of the stages, with no definite demarcation between them, and to provide anesthesia without progressing into stage IV. *The administration of a local anesthetic or sedation does not induce these stages.*

Stage I: *Beginning anesthesia* (analgesia and amnesia): Reflexes present, heart rate normal, slower rate and increased depth of respiration, normal blood pressure (BP), some dilation of eyes, with reaction to light.
Stage II: *Dreams and excitement* (delirium): Active reflexes, increased heart rate, irregular breathing, increased blood pressure, pupils widely dilated and divergent.
Stage III: *Surgical anesthesia*: Four planes, ranging from *light* to *deep*, with third or fourth plane usually best for most types of surgery. Progressive loss of reflexes, decreased heart rate, progressively depressed respirations until apneic (not breathing), normal to decreased BP, constricted to slightly dilated and centrally fixed pupils.
Stage IV: *Danger stage* (respiratory paralysis, toxic or extreme medullary depression)—DANGER stage: Too much anesthesia has been administered. No reflexes, weak and thready pulse, respiration completely flaccid, decreased BP, widely dilated pupils. *Prompt intervention is required* to prevent respiratory arrest, irreversible coma, and death.

> **Key Concept**
>
> The client under general anesthesia is completely dependent on others; they cannot control the most basic body functions, including breathing and maintenance of a patent airway. This person must be observed and monitored carefully at all times by specially trained anesthesia personnel.

PREOPERATIVE NURSING CARE

Before surgery, the surgeon or anesthesia personnel write orders indicating exactly what medications and physical preparation the client needs. Most preoperative preparation is carried out at home. It is important to teach the client to carry out preoperative orders exactly, including the underlying rationales, because preoperative preparation affects the surgery's success. Remember to consider the feelings of the client and family and provide reassurance. Many clients are admitted to the healthcare facility the day of surgery; usually they will not arrive on a nursing unit until the surgery is completed. In emergency surgery, the preoperative period may be very short. Within these constraints, remember to provide emotional support to clients, and their family members.

The client is usually instructed to discontinue aspirin, ibuprofen (Advil), and other nonsteroidal anti-inflammatory drugs (NSAIDs), or any specific agents affecting blood coagulation for at least 7–14 days before surgery, to reduce the risk of excessive bleeding. Certain herbal supplements are mild anticoagulants and can also contribute to the risk of bleeding. These include chamomile, cat's claw, feverfew, garlic, ginger, ginkgo, ginseng, goldenseal, grape seed extract, green tea leaf, horse chestnut seed, and turmeric. The preoperative client usually is advised to stop taking these herbal supplements as well.

Key Concept
It is important to remember the hierarchy of basic human needs, as defined by Maslow (Chapter 5), when performing pre- and postoperative nursing care. The physiologic needs (e.g., oxygen, food, water, elimination, sleep) must be met first, to sustain life. Most immediate postoperative care is concerned with these physiologic needs. Later in the perioperative period, the nurse can help the client feel safe and secure, with empathic teaching and support. The client's loved ones can also assist. Finally, the client is encouraged to participate in self-care as much as possible, to enhance self-esteem and self-actualization.

Preoperative Checklist

Each healthcare facility has a preoperative checklist to use for all clients requiring surgery. This checklist identifies assessments, medications, and other physical preparations that must be completed before the client is anesthetized. Preoperative care must be performed correctly and completely, and checklist items must be documented accurately. Each of the steps in preoperative preparation is purposeful. If any steps are omitted, the client's safety is jeopardized. Be sure that all items have been done and are checked off *before the client is transported to the surgical suite.* The list may be shortened if ambulatory surgery is done or if the client is to have a local anesthetic. In Practice: Nursing Care Guidelines 56-2 discusses the organization of preoperative nursing care and lists items regularly included in the checklist. Figure 56-2 shows an example of a paper preoperative checklist. This checklist can also be a part of the computerized client record. The goal for the client is to be in the best possible physical and emotional condition for surgery. A well-prepared client is more likely to have successful surgery and an uneventful course of recovery, leading to optimum rehabilitation. It is a nursing responsibility to interview the preoperative client, to make sure all steps in the preoperative preparation have been completed.

All clients coming to a short-stay (ambulatory or day surgery) unit must provide a responsible adult escort or driver to take them home. If this is not done, most types of surgery will be canceled. **Rationale:** *It is not safe for a person to drive for at least 24 hr after anesthesia. Judgment and reaction times are impaired by the medication.*

IN PRACTICE
NURSING CARE GUIDELINES 56-2 — Organizing Preoperative Nursing Care

General Measures
- Explain all procedures and their underlying rationales to the client/family as they are performed (In Practice: Educating the Client 56-1 and Box 56-3).
- Check the client's record and note preoperative orders.
- Verify the client has completed at-home preparation.
- Verify that the client has remained **NPO** (nothing by mouth) for the designated time, usually at least 8 hr.
- Ensure that the client has signed the surgical permit and it has been witnessed. (Nursing students should not witness legal papers of any type.)
- Determine if the client has an advance directive, such as a living will. If so, a copy of this document must be in the client's record.
- Review the client's medical record chart for indications of a special situation, such as the client who refuses to receive blood; the client must sign a disclaimer to that effect, and this must be in the client's record.
- Prepare the operative area, as ordered. Usually, nursing staff members in the preoperative area are responsible only for supervising a shower with a prescribed antimicrobial scrub. The actual surgical preparations and hair removal are usually done in the OR.
- If the client is having brain surgery, the head will probably be shaved. Make sure the client and family are aware of this. Ask them if they want the hair to be saved to make a wig. Let the client know if the eyebrows will be shaved or the eyelashes cut.
- Check the client's medical history for any essential respiratory, cardiac, blood pressure, or other drugs they take routinely. Notify the surgeon of these medications. The client may need to take these drugs on the morning of surgery, despite NPO status.
- See that all specimens and blood samples have been collected and sent to the laboratory.
- Verify that the history and preoperative physical examination are recorded in the client's record.
- Verify that results of all testing are on the chart; this includes laboratory tests, ECG, and sometimes a chest x-ray.

NURSING CARE GUIDELINES 56-2 — Organizing Preoperative Nursing Care (Continued)

- Give a sedative, if ordered. (Make sure all permits are signed first.)
- Withhold fluids and foods, as directed.
- Verify that client allergies are noted and the client is wearing an "allergy" ID band, whether or not they have allergies. The client must also wear a facility identification band, usually on both wrists, to ensure proper identification.
- Give preoperative instructions and provide emotional support to the client and family.

Immediately Before the Operation

- Check to make sure that the client is wearing the wrist bands. Ask the client their name and date of birth, to verify you have the correct client. Surgery will be canceled if the client is not properly identified.
- Record the client's temperature, pulse, and respiration (TPR), blood pressure (BP), and the existence or absence of pain (Chapter 55). Report immediately any deviation to the surgeon.
- Determine and document the client's *fall risk status*. If the client is a fall risk, a specific ID band must be worn; this must be noted in the client's record.
- Check that the client is wearing two special blood identification tags if the client has any possibility of receiving blood. The client's blood must be typed and crossmatched before surgery, and this information must be in the client's record.
- Make sure the client's weight is recorded on the chart in pounds and kilograms. This helps determine drug dosages.
- Help the client with bathing and other hygiene measures. Be sure the client removes all clothes before going to surgery and wears only a clean gown provided by the facility. (In some cases involving local anesthesia, the client may continue to wear street clothes.) If clothes have been removed, carefully label them and store in a safe place. If the client is to be admitted to the facility, transfer the clothing to the new room.
- Ask the client to remove any prostheses, braces, splints, wigs, barrettes, bobby pins or hair pins, hair scrunchies, contact lenses, hearing aids, false eyelashes, and glasses. Make sure to check for jewelry in any body piercings; these items must be removed. If the client will be expected to participate, such as in brain or eye surgery, hearing aids are usually left in place.
- Remove the client's jewelry and valuables, itemize them, and put them in the vault or give them to the client's family. Be sure to include the client's wedding band. If the client does not want to remove the wedding band, be sure to tape the ring securely to the client's hand. Carefully document what has been done with the valuables. If the client's family takes valuables home, have them sign for the items.
- Assist the client with putting on antiembolism stockings, if ordered.
- Provide the opportunity for the client to void immediately before going to the OR. If the client is unable to void, report this and document it on the record.
- Pull the hair back and cover it with a surgical cap. Hair should be washed the evening before surgery, if possible.
- Remove any complete or partial dentures and place them in a denture cup with clear water. Include removable bridges, retainers, and other dental appliances. Label the cup *and its cover* and put it in a safe place.
- Remove the client's lipstick, makeup, and nail polish. Remove artificial nails, if possible. The oximeter sensor may not register properly if nail polish or artificial nails are present. If the artificial nails are not removed, the surgical team can find another location on the body to monitor oxygen levels.
- Account for all items on the preparation checklist. Verify that the list is signed and attached to the client's chart or entered into the computerized record. If a paper chart is used, be sure it is sent with the client to the OR. (This checklist must be completed by 6:00 AM if the client is first on the OR schedule.) The nurse can carry out some procedures the evening before if the client is scheduled for early surgery and is in the facility overnight. In most cases, a nursing student is not allowed to do the final sign-off on the chart; follow the protocol of the facility.
- Ensure the client's safety by giving preoperative medications, as ordered, *after* completing all personal care and making sure that the checklist is completed and signed. The client must not be active or sign anything after taking a sedative.
- Verify that the side rails are up and the bed is in low position.
- Verify that all preoperative charting is up to date and signed before the client goes to the OR.
- After the client goes to the OR, notify the inpatient unit, so personnel there can begin to prepare the unit for their postoperative return. If the client will recover in a short-stay unit, prepare the recovery area.

Note: Some of the above procedures are done in the operating suite, if the client is admitted to the facility the morning of surgery. Many of these procedures are carried out by the client at home if the client will not be admitted to the hospital or if the client will be reporting directly to the surgery department on the day of surgery. It is important to note that the time constraints are severe in preoperative nursing. The nurse must be efficient, but thorough.

> **Nursing Alert** Be sure the client has signed the operative permit *before giving any presedation medications.* The client is not considered to be responsible after being medicated and cannot legally sign the operative permit. If the permit is not appropriately signed, the surgery must be postponed. Obtaining the client's permission for surgery is the responsibility of the surgeon; the nurse verifies this has been done. Remember the concept of *informed consent*; the client must *understand* what is being done and why. The client and/or family must be able to verbalize the type of surgery being done, and this statement must agree with the records and consent forms. If surgery must be canceled because of an error, such as inappropriate or incorrect signing of the operative permit or the absence of ID name bands, this is considered a *sentinel event* and must be reported and investigated.

Client and Family Support

The client facing surgery may be apprehensive. Most people fear pain. Some are concerned about losing consciousness; others are afraid they will die. Some are fearful of cancer or of being disabled. The client who has had previous surgery may compare the previous experience with this one. If the previous experience was difficult, the client may be particularly frightened. In addition to the anesthesia personnel, the client and family usually meet with the surgeon immediately before surgery and may wish to speak with their spiritual advisor or with a facility chaplain. Help to arrange this meeting, if requested. Make sure a certified interpreter is present for all interviews, if the client does not speak the language of the facility.

Preoperative Teaching

As stated previously, if the client and family understand pre- and postoperative procedures, they are usually more relaxed and cooperative. They need to know what to expect when the client returns from the OR (Box 56-3). Explain about any equipment (e.g., a catheter, chest tubes, IV lines) or suction that might be present after surgery. Teach the client how to perform breathing exercises (Fig. 56-3) and how to use equipment such as the incentive spirometer (Fig. 56-4; see Nursing Care Guidelines 56-3 for related procedure). Offer to tape the client's wedding ring in place, if it is not to be removed. All other jewelry is given to the family (make sure they sign a receipt) or locked in the vault. In Practice: Educating the Client 56-1 outlines the major points that are most commonly covered in preoperative teaching.

> **Nursing Alert** If a client will be on a ventilator or otherwise unable to speak after surgery, make arrangements for a communication system. Allow the client to practice this system preoperatively.

To help prepare the family, explain that the client will be taken to surgery 30–60 min before the scheduled procedure. In some cases, a family member can stay with the client in the preparation area until they are taken into the OR. Inform the family that after surgery the client will be taken to the PACU/PAR area, where specially trained personnel will observe the client until vital signs (VS) are stable and consciousness returns. If the family understands these procedures, they will be less upset by the length of time the client is gone. Inform the family where they may wait for news about the procedure. Usually, the surgeon speaks with the family immediately after surgery. The family must know where the client will be after surgery.

Gathering Data Preoperatively

Prompt, accurate gathering of information about the client before surgery helps ensure a successful outcome.

IN PRACTICE
EDUCATING THE CLIENT AND FAMILY 56-1 — Preoperative Instruction

In the time available, perform as much preoperative teaching as possible. Remember that all teaching must be carefully documented.
- Explain the reasons for special equipment at the bedside.
- Describe what equipment is likely to be present for the client postoperatively.
- Describe and allow the client to practice how to turn in bed without assistance.
- Allow the client to practice all procedures, as needed.
- Describe possible discomforts and how to alleviate them. Emphasize the use of medications to *prevent pain*, rather than waiting until pain exists.
- Show and practice with the client how to splint the incisional area.
- Demonstrate and allow the client to practice deep breathing exercises (Fig. 56-3).
- Explain the use of the incentive spirometer and allow the client to practice (Fig. 56-4).
- Demonstrate and practice other exercises to be performed postoperatively.
- Describe the amount and kind of ambulation allowed or expected after surgery. Explain the reasons for early ambulation.
- Provide a description of the OR and the postanesthesia care unit. (Sometimes, especially for children, a preoperative tour of these areas is helpful.)
- Describe appropriate wound care and show the client the supplies that will be used.
- Discuss optimum nutrition.
- Explain the importance of communication.
- Provide the client with written instructions to supplement the verbal instruction.
- Explain to the client and family where the family lounge is located. Make sure they know where to find food, coffee or soda, newspapers, computer access, and telephones. Suggest that they bring along something to do while they are waiting.
- Make sure there is a driver to take the client home from same-day surgery.

FORM 71.25A R6/98

UNIVERSITY OF CHICAGO HOSPITALS
PRE-OPERATIVE CHECK LIST
CHECK YES, NO OR NA FOR ITEMS 1 THRU 20 AND RECORD INITIALS

ADDRESSOGRAPH

	YES	NO	N/A	INITIALS
1. 2 ID bands applied (different extremities)				
2. 2 Blood bands applied #_____ Autologous/donor directed blood avail. (different extremities)				
3. Blood consent signed and witnessed and on chart				
4. If no blood consent, blood refusal form signed and on chart				
5. Advance directives signed and on chart				
6. Consent signed and witnessed and on chart				
7. Laterality identified on the consent form. Surgery will be on the (circle one) Right Left Bilateral Midline				
8. Laterality on the consent form is consistent with the patient's response				
9. Allergies NKA Latex _____ _____				
10. NPO since _____				
11. Pre-op medication Time:_____ Medication _____				
* 12. Vital Signs BP____ HR____ Temp____ Resp____				
13. Voided Time _____				
14. Height____ Wt.____				
* 15. Patient personal belongings dentures____ corrective lenses____ hearing aid____ jewelry____ clothing____ other _____ Disposition ☐ Admission Services ☐ Family Member (____name____) ☐ Remains w/Patient ☐ Other _____				
16. Nail Polish Removed				
17. Isolation *See Isolation Guidelines on opposite side. Type _____				
18. H & P on chart				
19. Previous Medical record with chart				
20. Addressograph plate on chart				

*Signature_____ Initials:_____

* If admit assessment form (54.41) is completed in DCAM pre-op or GOR pre-op, mark NA.

O.R. PRE-OPERATIVE CHECK LIST
CHECK YES, NO OR NA FOR ITEMS 1 THRU 4 AND RECORD INITIALS

	YES	NO	N/A	INITIALS
1. Wearing two I.D. Bands that are legible (one on wrist, one on ankle)				
2. Blood Bank two I.D. Bands in place (one on wrist, one on ankle)				
3. Consent Signed and Witnessed				
4. Laterality on the consent form is consistent with: - the OR schedule - patient response - the pre-op checklist				

5. Allergies _____
_____

6. Time Arrived in Pre-op Holding _____

7. Chart Checked for Completeness

8. IV Fluids   Amount _____

Signature:_____ Initials:_____

NOTE: _____
_____
_____

STATEMENT OF PATIENT COMPLIANCE
I AM AWARE OF THE DANGER TO ME OF FOOD OR LIQUID (INCLUDING WATER, COFFEE, OR TEA) IN MY STOMACH DURING ANESTHESIA AND I CERTIFY THAT I HAVE HAD NOTHING TO EAT OR DRINK SINCE _____

EXCEPTIONS:_____

I CERTIFY THAT I HAVE AN ESCORT HOME WHOSE NAME IS:
_____

PATIENT:_____

WITNESS:_____ DATE:_____

Isolation Precautions Guidelines		
	May go to Pre-op	May go to PACU
Airborne	No	No
Respiratory (Droplet)	No	No
Strict	No	No
Contact	No	Yes (in isolation room)
Special Handling (CJD)	Yes	Yes
Protective	No	No

Figure 56-2 An example of a preoperative checklist. This form may be provided on paper or in the computer. (Courtesy of University of Chicago Hospitals, Chicago, Illinois.)

Box 56-3 Steps in Teaching a Client

- Organize your teaching.
- Explain what you are going to do.
- Demonstrate the procedure.
- Have the client and/or family caregiver return the demonstration.
- Supervise the client's practice until the client/caregiver can accurately perform it independently.
- Reinforce successful behavior.
- Review the procedure.
- Provide written instructions, to reinforce the learning.
- Document that teaching has been done.

If you cannot answer a client's questions or do not understand equipment that will be used, request assistance.

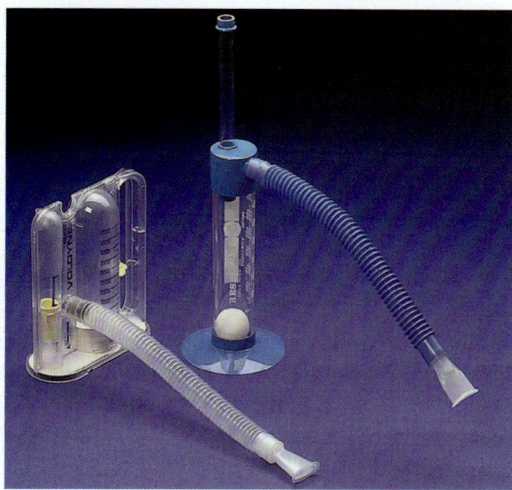

Figure 56-4 Two types of incentive spirometers, volume-activated (**left**) and flow-activated (**right**).

Observation

Observe the client carefully during preparation for surgery. Record any unusual reactions, including extreme anxiety, or observations in the client's record and report them to the charge nurse or surgeon at once.

Physical Examination and Laboratory Tests

As stated previously, the client undergoes a complete physical examination, including laboratory tests, about a week before the procedure in nonemergency surgery. Routine, preoperative tests often include a chest x-ray, complete blood count (CBC), urinalysis (UA), and ECG. A metabolic panel is often done, as well as a toxicology screen, to rule out alcohol or drug abuse. A pregnancy test may be done, to determine what, if any, medication can be used. A type and crossmatch is done, if any possibility of a blood transfusion exists. In this case, two blood ID bands must be worn, in addition to regular ID bands. A bleeding–clotting test, such as the prothrombin time, is often ordered. Vital signs recorded during the physical examination are used as baseline data for comparison during and immediately after surgery. The client's weight is documented because dosages of medications, including anesthetics, are usually calculated on the basis of the client's kilogram weight. Notify the surgeon about routine medications the client takes. Information about allergies and the wearing of an allergy ID band are necessary for all clients. If the client has no allergies, an allergy band stating this fact is worn. An allergy to latex is particularly important because some materials used in surgery and after surgery (e.g., catheters, chest tubes, gastric drains) are latex, unless a substitute is required. See the Nursing Process display at the end of this section.

Key Concept

The physical examination, laboratory tests, and other tests are all done before the client comes to the facility for surgery, unless the surgery is an emergency.

Skin Preparation

The skin, which is normally oily, harbors bacteria and must be thoroughly cleansed before surgery, to help prevent wound contamination and subsequent infection. Usually, the client is required to shower with antibacterial soap at home the evening before and/or in the hospital several hours before surgery. The operative site is further prepared just before or after the client is anesthetized. The skin is cleaned with an anti-infective agent and hair may be removed because microorganisms adhere to hair. These procedures are known as a surgical preparation or "prep." Most often, the prep and hair removal are performed in the OR, to further reduce the risk of infection. If the nurse is expected to perform this procedure, specific instructions will be needed.

Intestinal Preparation

The surgery, anesthetic, and client's condition determine if intestinal preparation is needed and, if so, what type. In many surgical procedures and examinations, such as colonoscopy, the intestinal tract should be as empty of feces as possible. If surgery is in the abdomen or pelvis, and in some other cases, the client will likely receive one or more enemas to empty the bowel (Chapter 51). Be sure the client expels the entire enema because an anesthetized client may expel the remainder on the operating table, contaminating the operative site. Enemas are

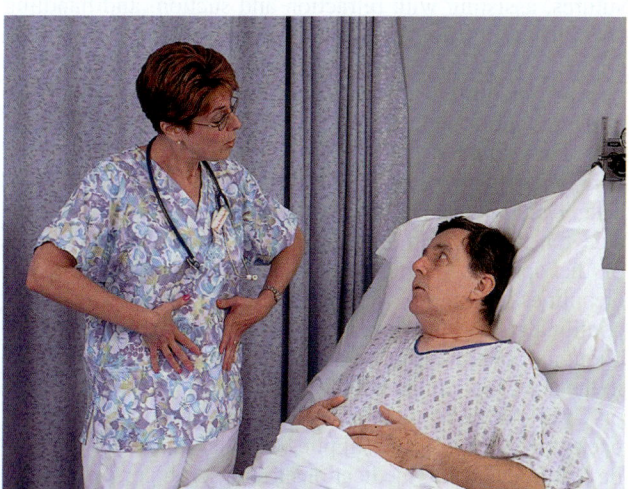

Figure 56-3 Preoperative teaching is vital and is often done before the client checks into the facility. Teaching deep breathing. (Photo by B. Proud.)

often done at home. A self-contained enema, such as the Fleet, is easy for the client to self-administer. The client may also be required to drink a cathartic solution, such as magnesium citrate or MiraLax, to cleanse the bowel. In some cases, the client must take a large amount, as much as several quarts, of a polyethylene glycol–electrolyte solution (GoLYTELY) or another bowel preparation called HalfLytely. The client needs encouragement and positive reinforcement to complete this task. If the client is to have spinal or general anesthesia or moderate sedation, they are asked to remain NPO (nothing by mouth) for at least 8–10 hr before surgery, to minimize the possibility of nausea and vomiting during anesthesia. In some cases involving extensive local anesthesia, or if there is any chance of an emergency requiring general anesthesia, maintaining NPO status is also needed. If vomiting does occur, aspiration is less likely if the client's stomach is empty.

Preoperative Medications

Four types of medications commonly are used preoperatively: sedatives, antibiotics, narcotics, and drying agents.

Because the client should have as much rest as possible before surgery, a *sedative* is usually ordered the evening before surgery, so that the client can sleep. This is a one-time-only order. Sedation also helps stabilize BP and pulse. Most surgeons prescribe *antibiotics* before surgery, to help prevent postoperative infections. These are usually taken for several days preoperatively.

On the morning of surgery, a preoperative *narcotic* is given to relax the client and enhance the anesthesia's effects. It may be ordered for a specific time of day or "on call to OR." In the latter case, the medication is taken when the OR is ready for the client. A *drying agent*/anticholinergic, such as atropine sulfate (AtroPen, Sal-Tropine), is given to help inhibit body secretions, so the client produces less mucus, reducing the likelihood of aspiration and *atelectasis* (collapse of the tiny air sacs in the lungs). Production of gastric and intestinal secretions is also reduced, so there is less abdominal distention postoperatively. (Atropine may contribute to postoperative constipation and other gastrointestinal [GI] complications.) Before giving preoperative medications, ask the client to go to the bathroom. Explain the purpose of any drug and its probable effects. Ask again about any drug allergies before giving medications. Explain to the client that after the narcotic or other presedation medication has been given, the side rails will be raised, they must remain in bed, or they must request assistance to go to the bathroom. Explain to family members that the client has received sedative medication and that, although they may sometimes stay in the room, they should allow the client to rest and not carry on a conversation. Be sure to offer a bedpan or urinal to the client immediately before they are taken to the OR. The client should not get up to go to the bathroom at that time. In Practice: Important Medications 56-1 provides additional information.

Client Transport

If the client was in the hospital preoperatively, prepare the client's room. (This procedure is described later in this chapter.) Make the client as comfortable as possible. Make sure all consent forms and the checklist are in the client's health record; the record will accompany the client to the OR or it will be entered into the computer where it will be available to personnel in the OR. Note in the record if the client has drug allergies or is taking cortisone, insulin, blood pressure medication, an anticonvulsant, or an anticoagulant. Make sure the client is wearing all the appropriate ID bands. Send a clean bath blanket with the client.

> **Nursing Alert** To prevent errors, always be certain the client is properly identified before transfer to the OR. *No* client is allowed to go to the OR without an identification bracelet! (This would cause the surgery to be canceled.) Some facilities require an ID bracelet on both of the client's wrists. The client also must be wearing an allergy band, stating existing allergies or stating that the client has no known allergies. If the client is a fall risk, a fall risk ID band is worn as well. Two blood ID bands also must be worn if the client might receive blood transfusions. *The ID bands of the client going to surgery must be checked by at least two staff people and verified by the client/family before the client enters the OR.* The client/family also must verify the type of surgery to be done. A procedure called a "time out" is taken when the client arrives in the OR, pausing to ensure they have the correct client, procedure, and surgical site.

INTRAOPERATIVE NURSING CARE

Observing a client undergoing surgery may be a component of a nursing student's experience. If this is possible, take advantage of the opportunity. Doing so will give you a better idea of surgical procedures and the atmosphere of the OR. Observation will help you understand the client's feelings and apprehensions and the reasons for postoperative pain and discomfort. Nurses and surgical technicians assist in the OR. The categories of staff working with the surgeon include the sterile assistant(s) (scrub assistant) and the circulating nurse(s). The *sterile assistant*, an RN, a specially trained LVN/LPN, or an *OR technician* is scrubbed, gowned, and gloved. They function within the sterile field. Duties include positioning and draping the client, handing instruments and medications to the surgeon, threading needles, cutting sutures, assisting with retraction and suction, and handling specimens (Fig. 56-5). Another person who may work in the OR may be the registered nurse first assistant (RNFA). This person functions under the supervision of the surgeon and performs more complex duties than the sterile scrub assistant. For example, the RNFA may assist with suturing the incision or by providing hemostasis (stoppage of bleeding). The *circulating nurse* (circulator) is an RN who works outside the sterile field. Duties include general management of the operating suite, including monitoring temperature, cleanliness, humidity, lighting, and fire safety. This nurse continually assists anesthesia personnel in monitoring the client and observes for breaks in technique by all personnel in the area, including ancillary personnel, such as laboratory or x-ray staff. The circulator also assists by opening sterile packs, delivering sterile supplies and instruments to the sterile team, delivering medications to the scrub person, weighing and labeling specimens, and keeping records during the surgical procedure.

IN PRACTICE
IMPORTANT MEDICATIONS 56-1 — Examples of Important Preoperative and Intraoperative Medications

Sedatives Used as Premedication Before Anesthesia
- Promethazine HCl (Phenergan)—used pre- or postoperatively, and in obstetrics
- Midazolam HCl—benzodiazepine, central nervous system (CNS) depressant, anxiolytic; causes some amnesia, can be used alone for IV moderate sedation (conscious sedation)

Sedatives Used to Assist Clients to Sleep
- Chlorpromazine (used in Canada)—especially to relieve preoperative apprehension, also antiemetic
- Secobarbital Na$^+$ (Seconal Na$^+$)—also can be premedication
- Temazepam (Restoril)—used pre- or postoperatively
- Trazodone HCl—antidepressant, with drowsiness side effects
- Propofol (Diprivan)

Antibiotics and Cephalosporins
- Amoxicillin trihydrate (Amoxicillin)
- Ampicillin—used in some high-risk clients undergoing cesarean section
- Cefotaxime Na$^+$ (Claforan)
- Ceftriaxone Na$^+$ (Rocephin)—used especially in coronary surgery and in potentially contaminated procedures
- Cefoxitin sodium (Mefoxin)
- Cefuroxime axetil (Ceftin)
- Ertapenem (Invanz)—used in adults to prevent infection after colorectal surgery
- Erythromycin—used in clients allergic to penicillin, with valvular heart disease
- Penicillin (various forms)
- Vancomycin HCl (Vancocin)—used in clients allergic to penicillin

Narcotics (Used for Pain)
- Fentanyl (Sublimaze)
- Hydromorphone (Dilaudid)
- Meperidine HCl (Demerol HCl)
- Morphine SO$_4$ (Morphine)

Drying Agent
- Atropine sulfate (anticholinergic)—prevents or reduces respiratory tract secretions

Nursing Considerations

When Sedatives and Narcotics are Given
- Observe for respiratory distress or bradypnea (very slow respirations). These medications often are contraindicated in clients with severe respiratory disorders.
- Observe for inability to arouse client, extreme lethargy, drowsiness, and/or fatigue.
- Observe for other CNS symptoms, such as dizziness, blurred vision, severe nightmares, and ataxia (difficulty in coordination).
- Keep in mind that the medications may potentiate (abnormally enhance) the action of oral anticoagulants and antihypertensive drugs.
- Watch for paradoxical excitement in older adults or children (a reaction opposite the desired reaction).
- Observe for constipation and/or bowel obstruction; routine medications, such as senna or colace, are often prescribed.

When Antibiotics are Given
- Instruct the client to inform the caregiver of any untoward effects, such as a rash, stomach upset, or diarrhea.
- Instruct the client to drink plenty of water and other fluids.
- Some antibiotics are to be taken on an empty stomach and some with food. Check the specific instructions.
- Instruct the client to take all of the medication for the prescribed length of time.
- If the client is taking an oral contraceptive, advise her to use another means of fertility control while taking antibiotics.
- Avoid alcohol.

When Atropine is Given
- Atropine is given to reduce the production of saliva, mucus, or other secretions in the airway during a surgery.
- Know that atropine is given cautiously to clients with glaucoma and certain other eye disorders and may be contraindicated. Atropine is also contraindicated in clients with certain GI conditions, such as achalasia, peptic ulcer, or pyloric obstruction, and with asthma, chronic obstructive pulmonary disease (COPD), heart conditions, symptomatic prostatic enlargement, Down syndrome, brain damage, and liver or kidney dysfunction.
- Inform the client about the experience of a dry mouth; relieve with moistened cloth, ice chips, sips of water, and hard candy, as tolerated and allowed. Report if dry mouth does not gradually resolve postoperatively.
- Observe for side effects such as dizziness, agitation, confusion, diarrhea, constipation, urinary retention, blurred vision, and sensitivity to light.
- Be alert for other more serious side effects, including skin rash, eye pain, difficulty breathing, irregular heartbeat, hallucinations, and difficulty swallowing. Report any of these immediately.

NURSING PROCESS

ASSESSMENT AND DATA GATHERING PRIORITIES
- Client's understanding of the proposed surgical procedure (clarify any misperceptions)
- Past experiences with surgery
- Fears (e.g., fear of the unknown, of pain or death, or of changes in body image/self-concept)
- Factors that increase surgical risk or the potential for postoperative complications:
  - *Past and present illnesses:* Cardiovascular/pulmonary disorders, alterations in renal/liver function, metabolic disorders (especially diabetes), seizure disorders
  - *Medications:* Such as anticoagulants, diuretics, tranquilizers, adrenal steroids, antibiotics
  - *Lifestyle factors:* Nutrition (history of eating disorders, malnutrition, or obesity); use of alcohol or recreational drugs (can cause unexpected withdrawal); activity level; use of herbal supplements (many are mild anticoagulants or can adversely interact with medications); smoking history
- Adequacy of coping patterns and support systems
- Pertinent sociocultural factors (e.g., health beliefs and practices, economic concerns, cultural considerations, such as language barriers or ethnic beliefs related to surgery and healing)
- Vital signs the morning of surgery (report any significant deviation from normal)
- Accurate height and weight (medications may be calculated on the basis of these data, especially for children)
- General systems review, noting in particular any new cardiopulmonary developments that place the client at high risk
- Results of all preoperative diagnostic tests; any abnormalities are reported to the surgeon
- Presence of an escort or driver (for same-day surgery)

POSSIBLE NURSING DIAGNOSES
- Anxiety
- Ineffective coping
- Decisional conflict
- Fear
- Anticipatory grieving
- Deficient knowledge
- Powerlessness

PLANNING
Assist in the development of a plan of care with the client and family to achieve the following general client goals. Before surgery, the client
- Demonstrates physical preparedness for surgery (absence of significant deviations from normal vital signs; no signs of infection)
- Verbalizes any concerns or fears related to the surgery
- Provides *informed consent* for the surgery
- Correctly demonstrates how to turn, deep breathe, use equipment (e.g., incentive spirometer), and perform splinting of incision, when appropriate
- Correctly demonstrates how to use any special equipment that will be in place following surgery
- Verbalizes understanding of postoperative pain management program
- Verbalizes understanding of postoperative activity plan
- Demonstrates the presence of adequate caregivers at home after discharge

IMPLEMENTATION
- Establish a supportive and trusting nurse–client relationship.
- Develop and implement a teaching plan that
  - Familiarizes the client and family with what to expect on the day of surgery
  - Prepares the client to participate in the pain management program
  - Enables the client to state the purpose of deep breathing and to demonstrate it, as well as procedures such as incentive spirometry, leg exercises, and turning in bed
- Counsel the client and family about helpful coping strategies and available resources. At the client's request, invite a spiritual counselor to see the client.
- Maintain nutrition and hydration; if the client is to be NPO (nothing by mouth) for a specified time before surgery, ensure that the client understands the reason for this restriction, and remove all food and fluids from the bedside. If the client is in the facility, place an NPO sign on the door of the room. If the client performs preparation at home, make sure that they remained NPO.
- Evaluate the client's bowel status and determine the need for an order for bowel elimination.
- If an indwelling catheter is ordered before surgery, explain its use before insertion.
- Carry out preoperative skin and hygiene orders.
- Facilitate sleep and rest in the immediate preoperative period. A sleeping aid may be ordered.
- Remember that many clients are not admitted until the morning of surgery. The nurse must determine what teaching has been done previously and perform the remainder of the preoperative teaching at that time.

EVALUATION
Determine the effectiveness of the plan of care by evaluating the client's achievement of the preceding identified preoperative goals. If the client is unable to meet key goals, modify the plan. Key evaluative criteria are as follows:
- Client's physical preparedness for surgery
- Client's mental preparedness for surgery
- Client's understanding of and ability to participate in care postoperatively
- An uneventful course of recovery

The client's family is included in all preparation, as needed.

POSTOPERATIVE NURSING CARE

The Postanesthesia Care Unit

Nearly all hospitals have an area designated for the care of clients immediately after surgery. Various names are used to identify this area, including PACU and PAR room. (The LVN/LPN requires additional education in order to work in the OR or PACU.) The client is carefully monitored in the PACU until they have recovered from anesthesia and are medically cleared to leave the unit. Specific monitoring includes the basic ABCs of life: airway, breathing, and circulation (Chapter 43). A complete systems assessment of the client is performed immediately on arrival in the PACU; measures are taken to prevent postoperative complications. It is important to identify clients who are particularly at risk. Because the PACU is located next to the OR, surgeons and nurses, as well as specialized equipment, are readily available in case of emergency (Fig. 56-6). Concentrating postoperative clients in a limited area makes it possible for nurses to observe immediate postoperative clients closely. Articles that may be needed for care are located near the client's unit in the PACU:

- Breathing aids: Oxygen, suction equipment, nasal and oral airways, pulse oximeter, mechanical breathing bag or other resuscitation equipment, and emergency equipment, such as a laryngoscope, tracheostomy set, or endotracheal tube
- Specialized equipment, such as an otoscope or ophthalmoscope
- Circulatory aids and related medications: BP and pulse monitor, stethoscope, IV solution and pumps, tourniquets, syringes and needles, cardiac monitor, cardiac arrest equipment, cardiac drugs, medications to counteract narcotic overdose, respiratory stimulants, the defibrillator, and a backboard for CPR
- Drugs: Narcotics, sedatives, and drugs for emergency situations
- Other supplies: Surgical dressings, sandbags, warmed blankets or a forced-air warming blanket (Fig. 54-1), extra pillows, and various other items. A crash cart is also available. Special equipment for a particular client, such as a traction setup or back brace, is also present.

Each client unit has a recovery bed/cart equipped with side rails, poles for IV medications, wheel brakes, and a computer. The cart can be moved easily and adjusted to elevate or lower the head or feet or the entire cart. The bedside stand holds supplies and equipment, such as a bedpan and/or urinal, tissues, an emesis basin, tongue blades, a face cloth, and a towel. Each unit has outlets for piped-in oxygen, suction, hooks for IV bags, and BP and other monitoring equipment. Warmed bath blankets or warming blankets are available to assist the client with the normal body chilling that usually follows anesthesia.

> **Key Concept**
>
> In the case of ambulatory day surgery, clients may recover in a special reclining lounge chair (Fig. 56-7). They still require careful nursing observation, and client and family teaching are a vital part of care before discharge.

Moving the Client to the PACU

When a client is moved from the OR to the PACU, every effort is made to avoid unnecessary strain or injury to the client and to accomplish the transfer as quickly as possible, with the least exposure. Enough people must be available for the safe transfer of the semiconscious client from

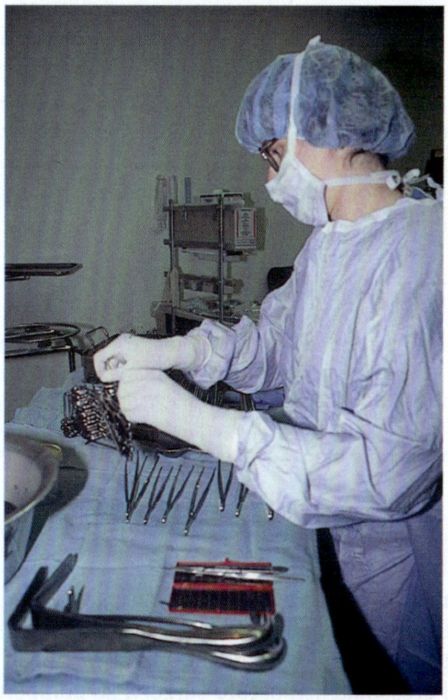

Figure 56-5 The scrub nurse or surgical technician prepares sterile instruments for the surgeon's use.

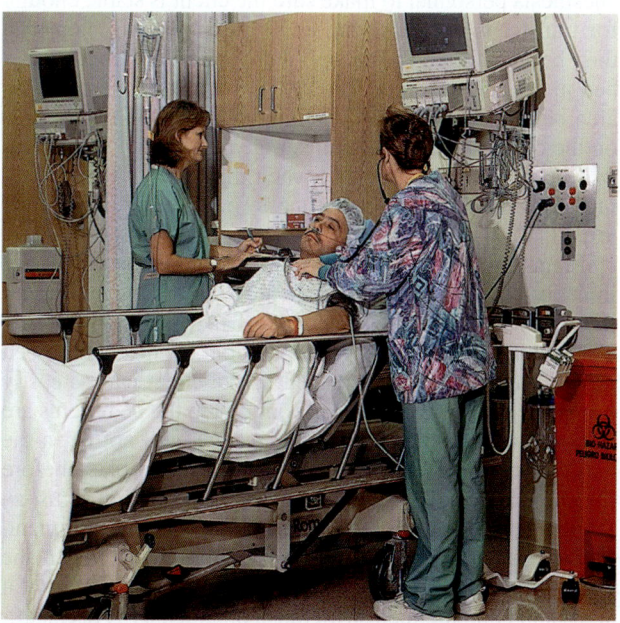

Figure 56-6 The PACU contains special equipment, to deal with any postoperative emergency. (Photo by B. Proud.)

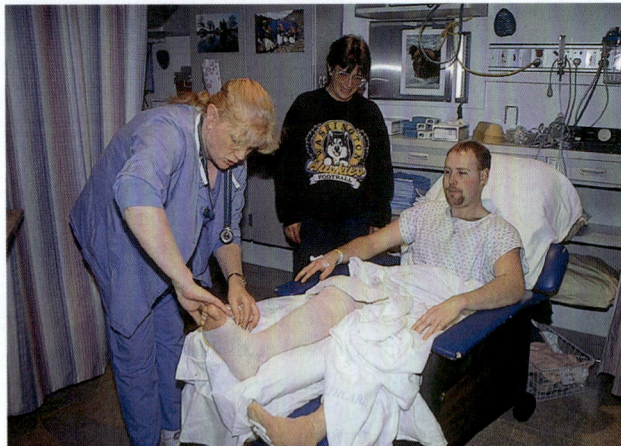

Figure 56-7 In ambulatory surgery, the client may be placed in a lounge chair for recovery from anesthesia.

the OR table to the PACU cart. The anesthesia person and circulating nurse accompany the client to the PACU, to make certain the client's condition is stable. Having been responsible for monitoring the client's condition throughout the surgical procedure, the anesthesia person reports the client's condition to the PACU nurse and leaves the surgeon's postoperative orders and any required special instructions. The care of the client then transfers to the PACU nurse. The client remains in the PACU until they are stabilized.

> **Key Concept**
>
> All preoperative orders are null and void when the client enters the OR. New orders (postoperative orders) must be written.

Receiving the Client in the Nursing Unit

When the client is nearly awake, the PACU staff confers with anesthesia personnel to make sure the client is stable enough for transfer to the receiving unit. The stabilized client can then be transferred to the ambulatory recovery area or to a bed in the acute facility. The PACU staff calls the receiving area before the client's discharge from the PACU to report on the client's condition, indicating what special equipment will be needed for the client when they arrive. The receiving nursing staff must have time to prepare for the client's arrival.

Preparation of a hospital room for a postsurgical client includes all clean linens and opening the bed by pulling all the top linens to the foot or side of the bed (Fig. 49-1C). The bed is placed in its highest position; the head of the bed is flat. The furniture is arranged so the client can be easily transferred from the recovery room cart to the bed. Items are removed from the bedside stand, so they will not be in the way. All necessary equipment must also be in place before the client arrives. This includes equipment for vital signs, an IV pole, emesis basin, bed protector pad, suction equipment, oxygen, and other items specific to that client. When the client arrives from the PACU, immediately check their vital signs and compare them with those obtained by PACU staff. Remember to include pain as the fifth vital sign (Chapter 55) and be sure to check to see if any PRNs have been given for pain in the PACU. Any significant variation in vital signs must be reported immediately. The client's airway must remain patent (open) with effective breathing to provide adequate oxygen saturation levels. The client's neurologic status is also monitored. If the client has had local, spinal, or regional anesthesia, the sensory and motor functions must be monitored as well.

> **Key Concept**
>
> The client's blood pressure and respiratory effort are often lowered initially as a result of anesthesia. Pulse is often elevated, due to administration of anticholinergic medications, such as atropine. Vital signs should stabilize before the client leaves the PACU. Remember that the client's VS may have been elevated before surgery, as a result of apprehension. It is important to know the baseline VS for each client.

> **Nursing Alert** Leave no client alone until they have fully regained consciousness. Check the healthcare provider's orders and carry them out immediately.

The PACU nurse will provide an additional report to the unit staff. In Practice: Nursing Procedure 56-1 reviews information needed for receiving the client from the PACU. When the client is settled in bed, and after initial vital signs have been taken and all immediate orders have been carried out, notify the client's family that the client is back in the room. The family can reassure the client by their presence, although they should allow the client to rest.

Immediate Postoperative Complications

It is the nurse's responsibility to measure frequent vital signs, including pain, after surgery. Observe the client postoperatively for immediate complications, including hemorrhage, shock, hypotension (low blood pressure), hypertension (high blood pressure), *tachycardia* (rapid pulse), *bradycardia* (slowed pulse), *hypoxia* (inadequate oxygen), *hypothermia* (below normal body temperature), *hyperthermia* (above normal temperature), and neurologic complications.

> **NCLEX Alert**
>
> NCLEX examination scenarios may test your knowledge of the signs of surgical complications, both those that can develop shortly after surgery and later complications. Your selection of nursing actions during the examination will demonstrate that you know *your* priority steps to take as a member of the healthcare team.

Hemorrhage

Hemorrhage (excessive bleeding) during or after surgery can lead to shock, requiring blood transfusions or other fluid replacement. Usually, the client's blood has been routinely typed and crossmatched before surgery, so compatible blood is available. Prompt action is necessary in the event of hemorrhage because this condition could be fatal. *Secondary* *hemorrhage* sometimes occurs postoperatively; consequently, inspect the client's wound dressings frequently. If bleeding is noted, report it. Be sure to look *under the client* because blood may pool there. However, concealed (*occult*) bleeding or *internal bleeding* is revealed mainly through signs of shock.

> **Key Concept**
> If hemorrhage is internal, the client may need to return to the OR for repair of blood vessels. This is a very dangerous situation.

Hypotension and Shock

The blood pressure may be dangerously low (hypotension) following surgery. This may be caused by blood loss but may also be caused by withholding of food, fluids, and medications before surgery. Anesthetics and pain killers used may also cause hypotension. Many times, hypotension can be alleviated by the anesthesia personnel before the client is released from the PACU. Hypotension should be reported immediately, as it can indicate shock. The most dangerous type of postoperative shock is known as *circulatory* or **hypovolemic** *(low blood volume) shock*, caused by severe hemorrhage (Chapter 43). Severe blood loss is life threatening; cells cannot live without the oxygen carried by the blood. Be on constant alert for signs of shock, many of which are listed in Box 56-4.

Nursing Alert If shock occurs, take these steps:

- Call for help first.
- Control hemorrhage, using direct pressure, if needed.
- Position the client in a supine position with the legs elevated approximately 20°. **Rationale:** *The Trendelenburg position is no longer recommended because it causes the abdominal organs to press against the diaphragm, limiting respirations.*
- Administer oxygen, as ordered by the practitioner. Administer blood, plasma, or other parenteral (IV) fluids, as ordered. Electrolytes will probably be added to the IV line. **Rationale:** *These actions help prevent hypoxia and help restore the client's blood volume and fluid balance.*
- Anticipate that vasopressor or other medications may be ordered. **Rationale:** *Vasopressors increase BP. Other medications may be ordered to support circulation.*
- Observe the client very closely. **Rationale:** *This can be a life-threatening situation.*

Postoperative Hypertension and Abnormal Pulse Rates

The client may also exhibit high blood pressure after surgery. This may be a result of withholding regular antihypertensive medications before surgery or may be caused by the trauma of surgery. Other causes include anxiety, pain, bladder or bowel distention, extreme chilling, hypoglycemia (low blood sugar), and some medications, particularly anticholinergics (e.g., atropine). One of the greatest dangers of hypertension is the risk of stroke. A diastolic reading of 100 mmHg or above is a *serious danger sign* and immediate action must be taken. This is a particularly dangerous situation if the client also complains of blurred vision, dizziness, headache, or a decrease in level of consciousness.

> **Box 56-4 Signs of Shock**
>
> - Hypotension (low blood pressure)
> - Narrowed pulse pressure (the narrowing of the range of the systolic and diastolic readings)
> - Tachycardia; rapid, thready pulse
> - Restlessness and anxiety
> - Difficulty breathing (dyspnea)
> - Cyanosis or dusky skin color
> - Extreme thirst
> - Cold, clammy skin
> - Hypothermia (low body temperature)
> - Low oxygen saturation (measured by pulse oximeter)
> - Slowed capillary refill

Treatment is symptomatic, if the cause of hypertension can be determined. In very high blood pressure, a medication which may be used is clonidine (Catapres), which must be administered very cautiously, to prevent the blood pressure from falling too low. The client's pulse rate may also be excessively rapid (tachycardia) or slow (bradycardia). In cases of extreme deviations from normal, the situation should be reported. Symptomatic treatment is provided and may involve specific medications.

Hypoxia and Hypoxemia

Anesthetics and preoperative medications sometimes depress respirations (*hypoventilation*) and interfere with blood oxygenation (**hypoxemia**). This can lead to a lack of oxygen in the tissues, a condition known as **hypoxia** (Chapters 86 and 87). Mucus blocking the trachea or bronchial passages may also reduce the amount of oxygen entering the lungs, thereby reducing oxygen available for transport to the tissues. Oxygen and suction equipment should always be readily available for emergency use. Symptoms of hypoxia include dyspnea, rapid pulse, dizziness, and cyanosis, as well as initial elevated BP, followed by lowered BP. Some symptoms of shock, as listed in Box 56-4, are also related to hypoxia. Untreated hypoxia may lead to cardiac dysrhythmias (abnormal heart rhythms). The most dangerous are the ventricular dysrhythmias, which can reduce the amount of circulating blood and thus the amount of oxygen available to the tissues. Treatment for hypoxia depends on its cause. The client's oxygen saturation is monitored with a *pulse oximeter*, a device that can be attached to the client's nail bed (finger or toe) or earlobe. Usually, if the client's oxygen saturation falls below 92%–95% on room air, the client receives oxygen by nasal cannula or mask. Respiratory exercises can also help raise the oxygen saturation. Steps for using a pulse oximeter are described and pictured in Chapter 46. Oxygen therapy is described in Chapter 87.

Hypothermia

Clients often complain of feeling cold after surgery. This is commonly associated with anesthesia. However, severe chilling can cause hypoxemia, hypoxia, and cardiac stress. The following are significant signs and symptoms of postoperative *hypothermia*:

- Temperature below 36.4 °C (97.5 °F). Taking a rectal measurement is the most reliable way to obtain a

noninvasive temperature value. However, it is often recommended that it be obtained with the infrared tympanic temperature monitor.
- Chills, shivering, and "goose flesh," unrelieved by warmed blankets.
- Client complains of being extremely cold.
- Confusion, disorientation, difficulty with speech. (*Note:* Because the client is recovering from anesthesia, it is difficult to determine if these symptoms are related to the anesthesia or to hypothermia.)

The nurse can apply warmed blankets without an order. If the client is found to be hypothermic, follow the instructions of the surgeon or other primary caregiver. Treatment in the PACU often involves the use of an overbed warmer (which is usually available only in the PACU). A forced-air warming blanket may also be used (Fig. 54-1). In an extreme case, other treatments, such as warmed IV solution, may be given to raise the client's core temperature.

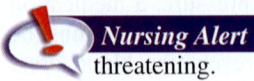 ***Nursing Alert*** Severe hypothermia can be life threatening.

Hyperthermia

In some cases, the client's body temperature will be excessively elevated. This can also be a dangerous situation and measures are taken to restore normothermia. A hypothermia (cooling) blanket is the most common measure used in this case (Chapter 54). A condition known as *malignant hyperthermia* (significantly elevated body temperature) is not common, but may occur. It usually begins in the OR and is the result of overcontraction of skeletal muscles. It has a genetic base, but may be triggered by anesthetics. Specific recognition and treatment are beyond the scope of this book, but if the client's temperature is elevated, report it immediately.

Neurologic Complications

Neurologic complications include *delayed awakening* (not regaining consciousness within 60–90 min), which may be caused by hypoxia, hypothermia, or electrolyte imbalances. *Abrupt awakening* may also occur. The client awakens in a confused and disorganized state of *emergence excitement* or delirium, which may be related to preoperative anxiety or to the type of surgery and age of the client. This may also be caused by certain intraoperative medications or by postoperative hypoxia, hypothermia, hypoglycemia, or dehydration. *Prolonged paralysis* may occur. Another complication is *compartmental syndrome*, ischemia in a confined space, such as the muscle compartments of the leg (Chapter 77). This is caused by prolonged tissue pressure, due to fluid and blood accumulation within the stationary fascia surrounding muscles. Treatment measures are instituted immediately, to prevent injury and/or permanent damage.

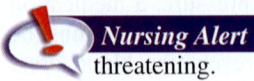 ***Nursing Alert*** In all postoperative complications, preoperative substance abuse must be considered. Many clients will not report drug or alcohol abuse, and sudden withdrawal of the abused substance may lead to unexpected and dangerous postoperative complications. Withdrawal from alcohol is particularly dangerous.

NCLEX Alert

The concepts relating to physical and psychological changes of aging are commonly incorporated in an NCLEX scenario. You should be aware of aging factors that impact a client's surgical risks and how you will approach the client/family's pre- and postoperative needs for educational interventions. Other situations may reflect your ability to respond to pre- and postoperative difficulties.

Postoperative Discomforts

By the time the client returns from the PACU to the ambulatory receiving area or nursing unit, they are usually awake and aware of a number of discomforts. One measure used to relieve these discomforts is the administration of medications (In Practice: Important Medications 56-2).

Pain

Pain, the fifth vital sign, is usually the first postoperative discomfort the client notices. Pain is usually most severe immediately after the client's recovery from anesthesia. If the client receives medication early and subsequent doses are spaced properly, they usually will be relatively comfortable. Make sure the client is conscious and that their vital signs are stable before giving pain medications. *Rationale: Analgesics are associated with respiratory depression, placing the client at high risk.* Common pain medications are narcotics similar to those given preoperatively, in addition to analgesics, such as ibuprofen (Advil) (Chapter 55).

Thirst

Thirst is almost always present postoperatively, usually because of NPO status preoperatively, fluid loss during surgery, anesthetic recovery, and dryness caused by drying agents (e.g., atropine). Most clients receive IV fluids during surgery and immediately postoperatively. These fluids help prevent thirst, as does rinsing the mouth. In some cases, the client may be allowed to suck on a wet cloth, sip water, or suck ice chips in small amounts soon after surgery. Hard candy or chewing gum may also be permitted.

Abdominal Distention

Temporary halting of intestinal peristalsis allows gas to accumulate in the client's intestine, causing abdominal *distention* (bloating). Handling of the intestines, anesthesia, drugs, lack of solid food, and restricted body movements also disturb normal peristalsis during surgery. Accumulated gas (*flatus*) may cause sharp pains that often are more distressing than incisional pain. Moving from side to side, sitting up in bed, or ambulating soon after surgery helps the client to expel flatus (gas). *Do not offer fluids or solid food until bowel sounds have returned.*

Key Concept

If a client complains of distention or "gas pains," do not give ice or allow the client to take fluid through a drinking straw. *Rationale: These tend to add air to the bowel and increase gas.*

IN PRACTICE
IMPORTANT MEDICATIONS 56-2 | Examples of Important Postoperative Medications

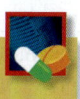

Postoperative Nausea (Antiemetics)
NOTE: Most of the antiemetic medications are also used to treat nausea associated with chemotherapy and/or radiation treatments.

- Aprepitant (Emend)—may be given preoperatively or during surgery, to prevent postoperative vomiting.
- Dolasetron mesylate (Anzemet)—if client is unable to swallow tablets, injectable form may be diluted in juice and taken orally or may be given IV.
- Granisetron HCl (Kytril, Sancuso)—available as injection, oral solution or tablets, or as a transdermal patch
- Hydroxyzine HCl (Vistaril, Atarax)—helps control nausea and allows reduction in use of opioids. Is also given for anxiety or pruritus (itching). Available in oral tablets, syrup, or injectable forms.
- Metoclopramide HCl (Reglan)—used for postoperative nausea when nasogastric suction is undesirable. Available in oral tablets or syrup, intramuscular (IM), and IV forms. May be given at the end of surgery as a preventive measure.
- Ondansetron HCl (Zofran)—used to prevent further vomiting or when vomiting must be avoided (oral); prophylactic use (parenteral). Available in tablets, orally disintegrating tablets or solution and as injection.
- Palonosetron HCl (Aloxi)—can be used for up to 24 hr postoperatively, given IV.
- Prochlorperazine (Compro)—given for preoperative nausea and for severe postoperative nausea. Available in injectable, rectal suppository, and sustained-release tablet forms.
- Promethazine HCl (Promethegan)—Be aware that the drug could lead to severe or fatal breathing problems. It is used for preoperative, postoperative, and obstetric sedation and as an antiemetic.

Nursing Considerations
- Allergy to any drug may cause anaphylaxis.
- Side effects of most antiemetics include drowsiness, dizziness, lethargy, dry mouth and respiratory passages, orthostatic hypotension, and constipation.
- If the client has glaucoma, this condition may be aggravated (increased intraocular pressure) by drugs. Certain other physical conditions preclude the use of specific medications. Many medications are carried across the placenta or in breast milk and must be used cautiously in pregnant or nursing women. The provider considers these factors when ordering medications.

Postoperative Constipation
Stool Softener
- Docusate sodium (Colace, Diocto-C)

Laxatives
- Bisacodyl (Dulcolax)
- Docusate, casanthranol (Peri-Colace)
- Lactulose (Cephulac)
- Magnesium oxide (Mag-Ox, milk of magnesia [MOM])
- Senna (Senokot)

Bulk-Forming Agents
- Polycarbophil (FiberCon)
- Psyllium (Metamucil, Genfiber): chewable pieces, effervescent powder, granules, powder, wafers

Nursing Considerations
- Make sure bowel sounds are present before administration.
- May stimulate excessive GI motility. Avoid administering to clients with GI bleeding, obstruction, or perforation.
- May endanger abdominal suture line.
- Be alert for diarrhea.
- Monitor older clients for extrapyramidal side effects, due to a possible *paradoxical* (opposite) *reaction* (Chapters 92 and 94).

Postoperative Flatus
- Famotidine (Pepcid)
- Ranitidine (Zantac)
- Simethicone (Gas-X, Mylicon)

Nursing Considerations
- Make sure bowel sounds are present before administration.
- Be alert for adverse side effects, including constipation, headache, diarrhea, nausea, and skin lesions.

Other
Bacitracin is an antibiotic, often used topically to prevent or treat incisional infections.

If the client's discomfort increases and nursing measures bring no relief, insertion of a rectal tube may be ordered (Chapter 51). Medications to relieve pain and intestinal gas also may be ordered to be given rectally or IM (In Practice: Important Medications 56-2). These medications reduce stomach acid, slow peristaltic movements, and lessen heartburn and gastric distress. When the client is no longer NPO, these medications may be given orally. Simethicone (Mylicon) is also given orally, to reduce gas. During each shift, assess the client for the presence of bowel sounds (Chapter 51). If bowel sounds have not returned within 2–3 hr following surgery, report this. If *intestinal paralysis* persists, a serious complication, **paralytic ileus**, may develop, in which the bowel has no peristaltic activity. Any ingested food, fluids, and digestive juices may accumulate and cause considerable discomfort. This may be life threatening because a *bowel obstruction* may occur and the bowel may perforate or rupture. A nasogastric tube is inserted to decompress or empty the stomach of its contents and may provide relief, but does not resolve the problem. Emergency surgery is often required to eliminate a bowel obstruction.

> *Key Concept*
>
> Symptoms of a *bowel obstruction* are lack of bowel movement, with the presence of bowel sounds. Symptoms of a *paralytic ileus* are absence of bowel motility and absence of bowel sounds. In addition, the client complains of bloating, gas pains, nausea, and vomiting. The client should not take anything by mouth until either of these situations is resolved.

Nausea

If the client complains of nausea, give ordered medications, in an effort to prevent emesis. Often such medications are given IM or rectally. Some also may be given IV (In Practice: Important Medications 56-2). It is important to prevent vomiting, if at all possible, because this can cause added complications. In reports, postoperative nausea and vomiting may be abbreviated to **PONV**.

Urinary Retention

Many clients leave the OR with a urinary catheter in place. After its removal, the client may have difficulty voiding because of anesthesia's effects. To aid urination, help the client sit upright, pour warm water over the vulva or penis, place the client's hands in warm water, and run water so the client can hear it. If the client has not voided within 8 hr after surgery, catheterization may be ordered (Chapter 57). This client is usually on intake and output (I&O). Monitor the amount of fluid taken through IV infusion and by mouth to judge the amount of urine likely to be accumulating in the bladder. I&O should be approximately equal (Chapter 52). The postoperative client may be permitted to take a sitz bath, a warm shower, or a warm tub bath (Chapter 54). This often facilitates voiding and/or defecation.

Constipation

Disruption of the normal diet and daily elimination schedule, drying medications (e.g., atropine), pain medications (particularly morphine and its derivatives), inactivity, and slowed peristalsis following anesthesia may cause constipation (decreased frequency of stools, difficult passage, or hard, dry stools). As soon as the client can eat or drink, encourage fluid intake, specifically fruit juices (especially prune juice). Help the client to the commode or bathroom. Encourage ambulation, to stimulate peristalsis. Some healthcare providers routinely prescribe a stool softener (e.g., Colace), both pre- and postoperatively. A laxative may be given as well to prevent constipation (In Practice: Important Medications 56-2).

Restlessness and Sleeplessness

The client may be restless and have difficulty sleeping postoperatively. Provide comfort measures and PRN medications, as ordered.

Prevention of Later Postoperative Complications

Dangers of prolonged bed rest following surgery include respiratory and circulatory complications, including hypostatic pneumonia, blood clots (thrombophlebitis or deep vein thrombosis [**DVT**]), pulmonary embolism, pressure wounds, generalized edema, contractures and muscle atrophy, difficulty in weight bearing and balance, formation of renal calculi (stones), scrotal edema, constipation, urinary retention, loss of appetite, and general depression and disorientation. Consequently, the sooner the client can move about after surgery, the better it is for the client.

> *Key Concept*
>
> Postoperative skin assessment is particularly important, as the client may have remained in the same position for an extended period of time in the OR and PACU.

Postoperative Activity

Follow the instructions of the provider. The client may dangle the legs over the edge of the bed, then sit in a chair, and finally walk (Chapter 48). The nurse helps clients to ambulate as soon as possible, per orders. Early ambulation, preferably on the day of surgery, assists circulation, improves respiration, prevents lung congestion, and aids in voiding and bowel activity. The client who is out of bed and walking will eat better and sleep more soundly. They can become more self-sufficient, promoting a rapid recovery. Many subsequent disorders are prevented by early ambulation.

Respiratory Complications

A high percentage of complications following surgery are respiratory in nature. Preventing these complications requires vigilant nursing care. Respiratory insufficiency (hypoventilation) leads to hypoxemia and may cause respiratory arrest. Other respiratory complications include hypostatic or aspiration **pneumonia** (inflammation of the lung or accumulation of fluid in the lung) and atelectasis. *Hypostatic pneumonia* is caused by immobility, particularly lying on the back. This condition does not involve invasion by microorganisms. *Aspiration pneumonia* can result when fluid (e.g., emesis) or mucus is aspirated or sucked into the lungs. Inhibition of normal clearance mechanisms (e.g., coughing) caused by anesthesia can be a contributing factor. (Postoperative pneumonia caused by infectious microorganisms is less common.)

Atelectasis is the collapse of air sacs in the lungs, usually caused by mucous plugs or blood clots that close the bronchi; it may involve all or part of a lung. The postoperative client often is reluctant to cough or breathe deeply because of incisional pain: this can also lead to atelectasis. This client may become somewhat cyanotic, as respirations and pulse become very rapid and breathing becomes difficult. Listen to lung sounds at least once per shift for evidence of fluid accumulation, dyspnea, atelectasis, or other respiratory symptoms (Chapter 47). Other important signs are fever and cyanosis.

Prevention of Respiratory Complications

In addition to exercise, respiratory exercises or treatments (e.g., turning, coughing, and deep breathing [**TCDB**]), chest percussion, and using the incentive spirometer can reduce or eliminate respiratory complications (In Practice: Nursing Care Guidelines 56-3). **Splinting** the incision helps relieve some pain and discomfort when coughing. Be sure to provide ample analgesia about one half hour prior to coughing and deep breathing exercises. *Rationale: To maximize pain relief and allow greater client participation.*

The **incentive spirometer**, which forces the client to concentrate on inspirations while providing immediate

---

IN PRACTICE
NURSING CARE GUIDELINES 56-3 — Assisting the Client With Postoperative Exercises

General Guidelines
- Remember that the postoperative client will be better able to perform these exercises if they learn them during the preoperative period.
- *Wear gloves for these procedures if the client has any open drainage.*
- Explain procedures to the client before you assist with them.
- Document all procedures, client reactions, and results.

Splinting an Incision
- Splinting relieves pressure on the abdominal suture line and thus relieves pain.
- Use a pillow, folded bath blanket, or large towel as a splint to distribute pressure evenly across an incision. Assist the client to hold the splint for the first few postoperative days; the client will be able to hold it in place after that.
- Grasp the pillow or bath blanket at the edges and stretch it across the client's incision. Apply pressure firmly by pushing down on the splint for the client who is lying in bed or by pulling the splint toward you from behind when the client is sitting. Do this as the client coughs.

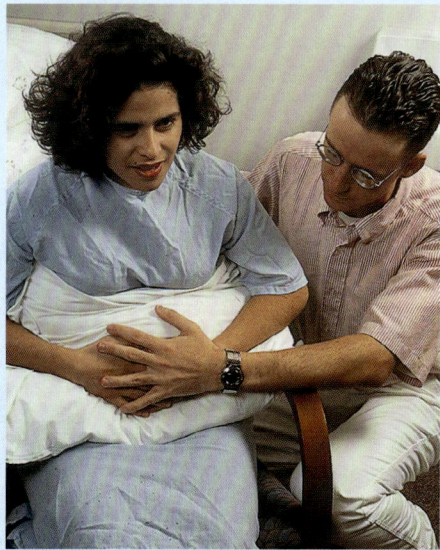

Holding a pillow or a folded bath blanket and pulling it tightly against the incision splints the incisional area.

This helps make coughing or deep breathing more comfortable and promotes better oxygenation.

- Anticipate the timing and strength of each client's cough. Count aloud and feel the movement of the client's breathing as they prepare to cough.
- **Turning, coughing, and deep breathing (TCDB)**
- Instruct the client to take a deep breath and hold it for 2–5 s. (The incision may require splinting during TCDB.) *Rationale: Holding a deep breath allows air to reach the lung's most severely deflated areas.*
- Instruct the client to do a strong double-cough with the mouth open. *Rationale: The double-cough maneuver helps the client to mobilize and remove secretions.*

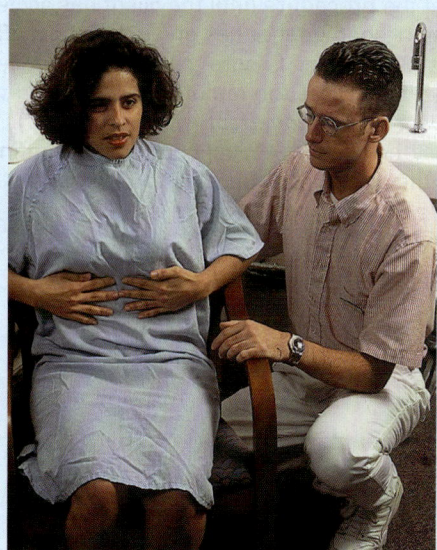

Instruct the client to take a deep breath, hold it for 2–5 s, and then do a strong double-cough (or "hack out" three short coughs) with the mouth open.

- Repeat this process several times each hour, especially for the first few days after surgery and while the client remains bedridden.

Huffing
- Teach the client to take a deep abdominal breath and then force air out in several short, quick breaths. The client should then take a second, deeper breath and force it out in short, panting movements. The

NURSING CARE GUIDELINES 56-3: Assisting the Client With Postoperative Exercises (Continued)

client should then take an even deeper third breath and exhale it quickly in a strong huff. *Rationale: This series helps loosen more secretions than just coughing.*
- Instruct the client to repeat this series of breaths as many times or for as long as is ordered.

Using the Incentive Spirometer
- Wear gloves if the client has any infectious drainage. Position the client as upright as possible without causing discomfort. *Rationale: An upright position allows the client to maximize the use of the diaphragm.*
- Explain the operation of the spirometer to the client (Fig. 56-4). Set a goal, number of seconds, or specific volume to be attained. Agree on the number of times and how often the procedure is to be done, within healthcare provider's orders.
- Instruct the client to cough to remove as much mucus as possible before the treatment. *Rationale: This enables the client to achieve maximum inhalation.*
- Teach the client to take slow, deep breaths and hold each breath at the end of inspiration for 2–5 s. *Rationale: This enables air to reach the lung's most severely deflated areas.*
- Repeat the procedure until the client has achieved the established goal or has given their best effort at least 8–10 times. Ensure that the client does not repeat the process too rapidly. *Rationale: Prevent the client from inadvertently hyperventilating.*
- Instruct the client to repeat coughing or huffing after using the spirometer. *Rationale: The client must clear the lungs as much as possible.*

Using the volume-activated spirometer. The client can observe her progress by watching the diaphragm rise in the tube. This exercise should be repeated 5–10 times every hour.

- Dispose of gloves, if used, and wash hands thoroughly at the end of the procedure. *Rationale: These procedures reduce the risk of infection transmission.*

Leg Exercises
- Position the client in a semi-Fowler position.
- Have the client wiggle the toes. *Rationale: This is the first action that the client can do immediately after surgery. This helps promote circulatory function.*
- Bend the client's knee and raise their foot. Hold this position for a few seconds.
- Extend the client's leg and lower it to the bed.
- Do this five times for each leg. *Rationale: Repetition helps maintain muscle tone and decrease venous stasis.*
- Have the client trace circles with the feet by bending them down, in toward each other, up, and then out. Repeat this procedure five times with each foot. *Rationale: This motion promotes circulation and contributes to optimal respiratory exchange.*
- Position the client in a side-lying position.
- Flex and extend the client's hip joint by using a bicycling motion. Repeat this five times on each side. *Rationale: This motion promotes contraction of the muscle, which is strengthened with repetition.*
- Encourage the client to exercise their legs as much as possible when in bed. Remind the client that they will get out of bed as soon as possible. *Rationale: These actions promote circulatory function and prevent contractures, foot drop, and complications of immobility.*

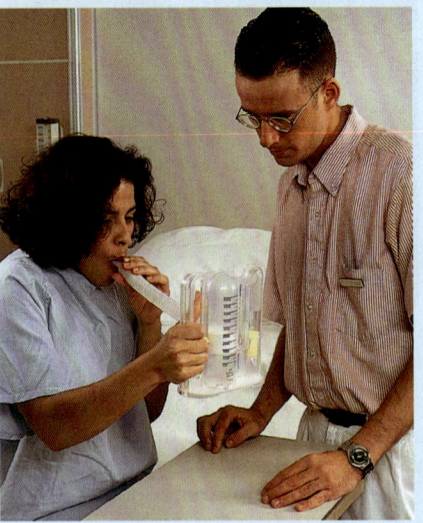

feedback, aids deep breathing (Fig. 56-4). Incentive spirometers are *flow activated* (flow generated) or *volume activated* (volume generated). The flow-activated incentive spirometer usually consists of one or more balls in a vertical tube. Because deep breaths (volume) are the objective, the length of time the client suspends the ball at the top of the tube determines the depth of the breath. Volume-activated devices come in many shapes, but because they measure volume directly, they make it easier for the client to understand when they have accomplished a deep breath. (Other devices can be used in pediatrics, such as the blow-out toy noisemaker.)

> **Key Concept**
> Breathing exercises will be more effective if the client learns and practices them preoperatively. The client takes the incentive spirometer home at discharge, so these exercises can be continued.

Circulatory Complications
Serious circulatory complications can develop postoperatively.

Thrombophlebitis and Deep Vein Thrombosis
A dangerous circulatory complication is **thrombophlebitis**, inflammation of a vein, associated with formation of a blood clot, a *thrombus*. This condition, **DVT**, is caused by factors such as *venous stasis* (slowing/stopping of venous circulation) due to increased clotting, lack of activity, or increased intravascular pressure. DVT most often develops in the calves of the legs. Clients at highest risk for DVT are those older than 40 years with prior thromboembolism and who are undergoing major surgery on the lower extremities. This particularly includes those who are having hip or knee replacements. Other risk factors include obesity, smoking, and a sedentary lifestyle. These clients are often given preoperative prophylactic medications. In addition, the use of graduated compression stockings and the intermittent (sequential) pneumatic compression device (Fig. 53-2) can help prevent DVT.

Symptoms of DVT and thrombophlebitis include swelling, warmth, redness, and tenderness in the area. If thrombophlebitis occurs, the following supportive measures may be ordered by the primary provider:

- Elevate the affected body part on a soft pillow when in bed.
- Administer thrombolytic and/or anticoagulant medications, as directed (see below).
- Avoid rubbing the body part (may dislodge clot).
- Apply warmth, as directed (Chapter 54).
- Maintain the client on bed rest, in rare cases.

Embolism
An **embolus** (plural: emboli) is a piece of a clot or thrombus that breaks off and enters the person's circulatory system, usually obstructing the blood flow in a smaller vessel (an *embolism*). Symptoms of embolism depend on its location, but include severe pain and shock, and may include nausea and vomiting, as well as other symptoms. Probably the most life-threatening embolism is a blood clot that lodges in the small vessels of the lung, a *pulmonary embolism*. Signs of pulmonary embolism include difficult breathing, sharp chest pain, cough, cyanosis, rapid respirations and heart rate, and severe anxiety. A pulmonary embolism rapidly can be fatal. If an embolism is in an arm or leg, distal circulation is often cut off, causing related symptoms, such as numbness, pain, and the absence of pulse. An embolism often can be treated with immediate administration of special medications that dissolve or split up existing blood clots (**thrombolytic** *agents*), such as alteplase (t-PA, Activase), a thrombolytic enzyme. Thrombolytic agents must be used with caution after surgery, because they may interfere with clot formation in the surgical incision, while dissolving the thrombi that caused the embolism. These medications are also used cautiously in clients with liver disorders because they may be difficult to eliminate. One means of avoiding circulatory disorders is to apply elastic stockings, elastic roller bandages, or antiembolism (TED) stockings, as ordered. Other nursing measures used to prevent circulatory disorders include performing leg exercises every 2 hr, complete range of motion exercises every shift, and ambulation as soon as possible after surgery. As stated previously, sometimes, a pneumatic/sequential compression device is used to help keep blood circulating, by alternating external pressure on the legs (Fig. 53-2).

Other Complications
Infection
A temperature elevation occurring 2 or 3 days after surgery, severe pain, redness or swelling around an incision, excessive drainage, or an elevated white blood count (WBC) are usually signs of infection. The nurse should observe for, and teach the client signs of, infection, to prevent complications. Observe the condition of the client's incision at least every 4 hr and document findings. Compare the condition of the incision with previous observations and document carefully. Sterile technique and careful handwashing are important when changing dressings. Wear gloves and carefully dispose of all waste materials, according to agency protocol. These activities help prevent infections and spreading of existing infections to others.

> **Key Concept**
> All used dressings are considered grossly contaminated, if there is any drainage. They must be disposed of in a red biohazard bag, according to agency protocol.

Treatment of infection includes administration of antibiotics, increased fluids, rest, and an adequate diet, to build up resistance. If necessary, the wound is drained. In some cases, the wound is cleaned or flushed with a solution (*wound irrigation*) (Chapter 58). A serious situation is the development of an infection caused by an antibiotic-resistant organism. One such organism is the methicillin-resistant *Staphylococcus aureus* (**MRSA**), which is very difficult to treat, because it does not respond to penicillin and related drugs (Chapter 40). A number of other organisms are developing resistance to antibiotics, making it necessary to continue to develop newer, stronger, and more broad-spectrum antibiotics.

> **Key Concept**
> Because most postoperative clients return home soon after surgery, it is vital to instruct the client and family about signs and symptoms of infection. They should be instructed to report any problems immediately.

Dehiscence and Evisceration
Dehiscence is the splitting open or separation of the surgical incision. If the incision opens enough so abdominal organs (viscera) protrude, this is known as **evisceration** (Fig. 56-8). Clients at risk for dehiscence and evisceration include those

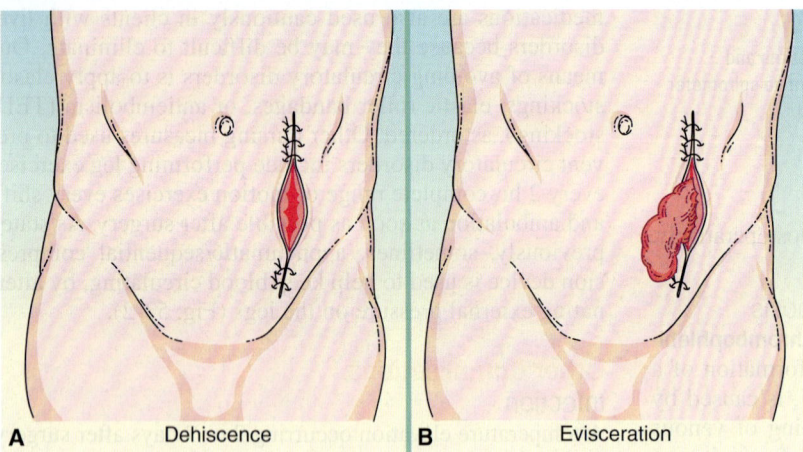

Figure 56-8 Serious postoperative complications. **A.** *Dehiscence* is the splitting open or separation of the surgical incision. **B.** *Evisceration* is dehiscence with protrusion of viscera. Both are emergency situations.

with poor wound healing (e.g., diabetic clients), older adults with *friable* (fragile) skin, morbidly obese individuals, and persons with invasive abdominal cancer or a postoperative infection. Violent coughing, vomiting, or excess movement also can cause dehiscence or evisceration. Usually, the client describes this sensation by saying "something gave." The condition is uncommon, but the nurse should be prepared to deal with it. This is an urgent situation. Wear gloves (sterile, if possible). Cover protruding structures with sterile large abdominal (ABD) pads that have been moistened with sterile normal saline. Report the incident immediately. The greatest dangers of dehiscence and evisceration are infection, intestinal strangulation, and hemorrhage.

Additional Supportive Measures

Providing Adequate Nutrition

To rebuild tissue after the trauma of surgery, the client requires nutrients in excess of normal body needs. Protein is particularly necessary, to rebuild wounded or diseased tissue (Chapter 32). The client should return to oral intake of adequate food and fluids as soon as bowel sounds return. Most people who have had uncomplicated surgery can function on IV therapy for a short time but should resume oral intake as quickly as possible. Usually, the client starts with a *progressive diet*, to avoid abdominal distention that may occur if peristalsis is sluggish. As ordered, offer the client a clear liquid diet first. Progress to a full liquid diet and finally a soft or general diet (Chapter 32). Usually, the sooner the client tolerates food, the sooner they recover overall. This progression is often ordered as **DAT** (diet as tolerated).

Certain clients require more extensive diet therapy and should be evaluated by a dietitian, in cooperation with the healthcare provider. Special attention is needed for clients with

- mental illness or who have an intellectual disability
- dementia or who are confused
- advanced age or who may be debilitated
- obesity or who are underweight
- eating disorders
- diabetes
- malabsorption and/or digestion disorders
- dietary restrictions, such as those who adhere to a vegan or strict vegetarian diet (particularly if no eggs or dairy products are used)
- allergies to foods
- a high fever (for any length of time)
- a client who has experienced severe trauma and/or amputation
- infection, especially a systemic infection
- burns covering a large portion of the body
- severe diarrhea or constipation

Special attention is also needed for the following clients:

- Clients who have experienced severe trauma and/or amputation
- Clients who have experienced vomiting for an extended period
- Clients who are unable to resume oral intake within 8–10 days after surgery
- Clients experiencing extensive drainage from any body orifice or wound

> **Key Concept**
> In many cases, a nutritional drink, such as Boost or Ensure, is given with meals after surgery, to supplement solid foods. Many clients find they are able to drink, even if it is difficult to take solids.

Wound Irrigation

Many clients have wounds that must be irrigated. The healthcare provider will order the type of solution to use and may suggest a particular irrigation method. Otherwise, check the facility's policies and procedures to determine the method of wound irrigation. In some cases, irrigation follows sterile technique; in others, the procedure is clean (Chapter 58).

Dressing Changes

A *dressing reinforcement* is the application of additional dressing materials to an already existing dressing. A *dressing change* is removing the dressing entirely and replacing it with a fresh one. Depending on the institution's policy and the surgeon's orders, nurses can reinforce a dressing without a specific order. A healthcare provider's order usually is needed to *change* a dressing. Use sterile technique and always follow Standard Precautions when changing dressings (Chapter 57).

> **Key Concept**
> The surgeon usually does the first postoperative dressing change, so the wound can be carefully inspected. After that, there may be an order for nurses to change dressings.

Suture and Staple Removal

Sometimes, there is an order for the nurse to remove **sutures** (stitches) or staples. This is more common in the healthcare provider's clinic than in the hospital. In many cases, the nurse will assist with this procedure. In assisting with or performing suture removal, a disposable suture removal kit is used and sterile technique is followed (Fig. 58-13A). Staples are also used frequently to close surgical incisions because they are inert, do not cause infection, and are quickly inserted and removed (Fig. 58-1A). A special staple remover is required to remove staples (Fig. 58-13B). Sterile adhesive skin closures (Steri-Strips) are often applied after sutures or staples are removed, to reinforce wound healing. A dressing may be applied after suture or staple removal, but often, the wound heals faster if exposed to the air. The procedures for suture and staple removal are contained in Chapter 58.

IV Therapy

Most clients leave the OR with an IV infusion running. Several solutions are commonly used, including dextrose 5% and water (D_5W) and dextrose 5% and normal saline (D_5NS). Normal saline is 0.9% sodium chloride, NaCl, and is *isotonic*—of the same concentration as the fluids surrounding normal body cells. Another commonly used solution is dextrose 5% in half-normal saline ($D_5\frac{1}{2}NS$—0.45% NaCl). Often, antibiotics and other medications and/or several electrolytes are added to the IV. In most cases, the IV will be regulated by an electronic pump or controller. It is important for the nurse to know the techniques necessary when giving daily care, ambulating the client, and positioning the client who has an IV in place. It is important to recognize when the IV catheter has *infiltrated* (moved out of the vein) and to know how to discontinue it safely. Observe and monitor the infusion site at least once per hour to make sure the infusion is running. Chapter 64 contains more information and illustrations regarding management of IVs. The IV fluid infused with medications is recorded as part of the client's total I&O.

Venous Access Lock

Almost all clients will have an IV in place during surgery. Some clients will return to the nursing unit with an *intermittent infusion device* (saline lock, **venous access lock**—Fig. 64-14) in place. In this case, fluids and medications can be given via the lock. They may be given with a needle and syringe, a needleless system, or by using an IV bag and tubing. In this case, the tubing is disconnected after the medication is given and the lock remains in place so it is available to be used again without restarting the IV. The access lock is often used postoperatively to administer antibiotics. A time period between 8–24 hr is suggested, to maintain patency. The flush solution most often used is sterile normal saline, although heparin is occasionally ordered. Removal or discontinuance of the venous access lock is the same as for an IV and is ordered by the provider (Chapter 64).

STUDENT SYNTHESIS

KEY POINTS

- The client who is having surgery needs both physical preparation and empathetic emotional support. The nurse is in a unique position to provide that support.
- The client's family caregivers are vital members of the healthcare team because they will be assisting the client when they go home. They need careful instruction and support, since the client will be doing most of the recuperation at home.
- Preoperative teaching is the first line of defense against postoperative complications. Teaching also helps clients to feel more at ease during this stressful time.
- Surgery may need to be canceled if the client has a cold or other illness or if the client is extremely apprehensive.
- Before giving any pre- or postoperative medication, always check the client for drug and/or latex allergies.
- All permits must be signed before any preoperative medications are given.
- Use of narcotics and sedatives can cause serious side effects. Watch carefully for these side effects, especially respiratory depression.
- Early postoperative complications include hemorrhage, hypotension and shock, hypoxia and hypoxemia, hypertension, pulse disorders, hypothermia and hyperthermia, and neurologic complications. Be alert for early indications of these complications and report and respond to them quickly.
- Postoperative discomforts may include pain, thirst, abdominal distention, nausea, urinary retention, constipation, restlessness, and sleeplessness. Anticipate client needs and take appropriate steps to prevent or alleviate these discomforts.
- Other later postoperative complications include circulatory complications, such as thrombophlebitis, DVT, infection, and dehiscence or evisceration. The nurse must report signs of any of these complications immediately.
- Pulmonary hygiene is extremely important in the prevention of later postoperative respiratory complications.
- Early postoperative mobility helps decrease the possibility of respiratory or circulatory complications.

CRITICAL THINKING EXERCISES

1. Discuss the levels of urgency of various types of surgery. Where might each type be performed?

2. Develop a teaching plan for clients who will use the incentive spirometer postoperatively. Practice coaching a classmate in its use.

3. Discuss the importance of pre- and postoperative teaching to the surgical client and their family.

NCLEX-STYLE REVIEW QUESTIONS

1. The nurse is caring for a client in the postoperative phase after an appendectomy. The client feels hungry and wants to eat but no bowel sounds are auscultated. What is the best response by the nurse?
   a. "I can give you some water but no solid foods."
   b. "You can't be hungry if you don't have bowel sounds."
   c. "You will have to wait until your bowel sounds return or you may vomit."
   d. "I will be able to give you something to eat once you are ambulating."

2. When providing instructions to a client preparing to have a surgical procedure with general anesthesia, what should the nurse be sure to include?
   a. Discontinue antihypertensive medications 3 days prior to the procedure.
   b. Do not have anything to eat or drink 24 hr before the procedure.
   c. Continue to take herbal supplements that are presently being used.
   d. Discontinue the daily dose of aspirin for 7 days before surgery.

3. The nurse is administering fentanyl to an older adult client. What should the nurse observe specific to this client?
   a. Paradoxical excitement
   b. Increased thirst
   c. Tachypnea
   d. Irregular heart rate

4. The nurse is preparing a client with severe asthma for a surgical procedure. What order would the nurse seek clarification, prior to implementing?
   a. Promethazine for nausea
   b. Ceftriaxone to prevent infection
   c. Fentanyl for pain
   d. Atropine to inhibit secretions

5. The nurse is caring for an older adult client who has undergone abdominal surgery. Which prescribed interventions would the nurse provide to reduce the risk for pneumonia? Select all that apply.
   a. Instruct the client how to turn, cough, and deep breathe.
   b. Force fluids before the surgery.
   c. Provide chest percussion.
   d. Instruct the client how to use the incentive spirometer.
   e. Suction the client every 2 hr.

CHAPTER RESOURCES

Enhance your learning with additional resources on **thePoint***!*

Student Resources related to this chapter can be found at **thePoint.lww.com/Rosdahl12e**.

CHAPTER 56   Preoperative and Postoperative Care   839

Welcome Steps

Look at healthcare provider's orders.

Protocol for procedure.

Necessary equipment/supplies.

Wash hands using proper hand hygiene; put on gloves.

Explain the procedure and reassure the client.

Locate two identifiers to confirm correct client.

Comfortable and efficient position for nurse and client.

Obtain privacy.

Make sure to follow correct steps and body mechanics with good technique.

Ensure safety and observe deviations from normal.

End Steps

Ensure comfort and safety.

Note questions or concerns from client or nurse; note significant data.

Dispose of materials properly.

Disinfect the area and your hands.

Document and report the procedure and your findings.

IN PRACTICE

NURSING PROCEDURE 56-1   Receiving the Client From the Postanesthesia Care Unit (PACU)

Supplies and Equipment
Blood pressure (BP) apparatus and other monitoring equipment
Emesis basin/bag
Frequent vital signs sheet or computer database
IV stand
Oxygen equipment and pulse oximeter
Stethoscope
Suction apparatus
Gloves
Temperature measuring equipment
Tissues
Pillow
Protective bed pads under pillow and on bed
Any other supplies or equipment needed for this client
Location of the nearest crash cart

Steps
Follow LPN WELCOME Steps and Then

1. Carefully identify the client. Check the name band with another nurse. Check the health record with the name band before the PACU nurse gives report. *Rationale: Because the client is not fully conscious, identification depends on the name band.*

2. Always wear gloves. *Rationale: This client has nonintact skin. Wear gloves to protect yourself against exposure to body substances.*

3. Attach any drainage apparatus such as wound drainage, a urinary catheter, or chest tubes, as ordered. Attach gastric or other tubes to the appropriate suction device. Plug in the IV pump and make sure the IV is patent and flowing at the correct rate. Make sure to have additional IV fluids available. Attach any monitors. Make sure to know how to operate all equipment and that it is working properly before the PACU nurse leaves. *Rationale: All equipment must be in proper working order. For example, the chest tube suction must operate properly, to maintain life.*

4. Maintain a *patent* airway. Feel for the client's exhaled breath by holding a hand in front of the client's nose. *Just because the client's chest or abdomen moves does not necessarily mean the client is breathing adequately.* Watch for any signs of respiratory distress (rapid breathing, cyanosis, panic) or for evidence of reduced oxygen saturation, as measured by the oximeter. *Rationale: Anesthesia and sedatives can depress respirations.*

5. Keep the client flat, often in Sims or modified Sims position, until they fully awaken, unless specifically ordered otherwise. Keep side rails up. *Rationale: The semi-anesthetized client could fall.*

6. Perform any orders for drug or oxygen administration. *Rationale: Immediately ordered interventions help stabilize and make the client comfortable as soon as possible.*

7. Monitor level of consciousness. If the client received spinal anesthesia, evaluate sensation in, and ability to move, the extremities. Record the advancing level of sensation and movement. Reassure the client that the anesthesia will wear off and movement and sensation will return. *Rationale: This is part of ongoing nursing care and documentation.*

8. Take vital signs (VS) as ordered (Chapter 46). Measure VS at least every 15 min for the first hour and gradually less often, as ordered, if VS are stable. Remember to ask about pain each time vital signs are measured. Record VS on the frequent vital signs sheet or in the computer. Continuously watch for signs of shock (Box 56-4). Check the client's temperature every 2–4 hr. *Rationale: Complications, such as hemorrhage, are most likely to occur in the immediate postoperative period. Changing BP values and pulse rate often are the first indicators of hypovolemic shock, a consequence of blood loss. It is important to evaluate pain, so medication can be given early. This helps prevent severe pain, which is much more difficult to treat.*

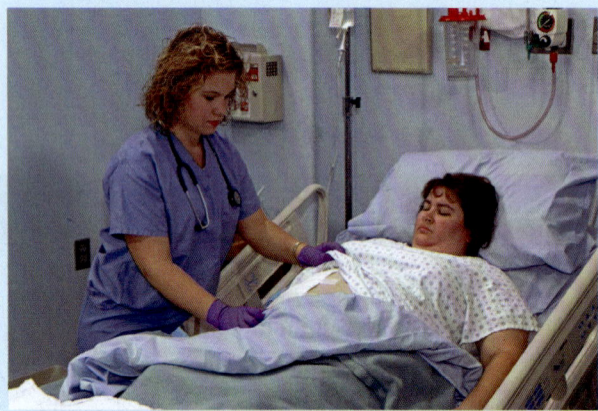

Inspect dressings for drainage in addition to measuring vital signs and asking about pain.

1. Inspect dressings; note signs of hemorrhage and any unusual amount of drainage. If necessary, reinforce but *do not change* dressings. Report any untoward signs. *Rationale: The surgeon may wish to see the drainage's character; the dressing may be weighed to determine exact blood loss. Removing the dressing might upset the suture line. The surgeon makes the first dressing change after the procedure.*

2. If the client is nauseated or if vomiting occurs, turn the client's head to the side, unless contraindicated. Place a protective pad under the client's head. Use the emesis basin/bag to catch the emesis. Check to see if antiemetics can be given. *Rationale: Turning the head helps empty the mouth, preventing aspiration, which is life threatening. The airway must remain patent; emesis could obscure the airway. The emesis basin is specially shaped to fit around the client's neck. Antiemetics help prevent excessive vomiting and are given rectally or by injection. The protective pad eliminates the need to change the entire bed, if soiling occurs.*

3. If the client vomits excessively or violently, check to make sure dressings and incisions are intact and that suction equipment operates properly. *Rationale: The quick and violent movements of vomiting can interfere with the suture line. Stitches or staples can rip out. If vomiting occurs, it may mean the suction is operating improperly. This may be an emergency situation.*

4. Measure emesis, noting the time, amount, and character (TAC) of emesis on the client's health record. Report your findings. Save the emesis if it appears unusual. *Rationale: This information is important for monitoring I&O and fluid and electrolyte balance; unusual appearance of vomitus may suggest a problem, requiring notification of the surgeon. A specimen may be required.*

5. If the client is receiving IV fluids or blood, check the rate of flow and the time for the next bag (Chapter 64). Make sure the IV catheter is not infiltrated. Check the IV site for swelling, warmth, pain, blanching, or redness. Report any problems immediately. Be sure to have a new IV bag ready. *Rationale: Maintaining a patent (open) IV is necessary for adequate hydration and in case emergency medications must be given. The signs listed above may indicate IV infiltration. It is important to have fluids on hand so the IV is not interrupted*.

Follow ENDDD Steps

Special Reminder
- Documentation includes input and output (I&O). Include any oral and IV fluids, as well as drainage, voiding, and emesis. Also document level of consciousness, if the client had general anesthesia, and document the progress of returning sensation in the extremities, if the client had spinal or regional anesthesia. *Rationale: I&O is monitored to identify normal output and other fluid or blood loss. The elimination of the anesthetic is important information.*

57 Surgical Asepsis

Learning Objectives

1. List examples of areas of the body considered sterile and nonsterile.
2. Differentiate between medical and surgical asepsis.
3. Differentiate between disinfection and sterilization.
4. List guidelines to follow when using sterile technique.
5. Demonstrate the proper technique for opening a sterile tray and a sterile package.
6. Demonstrate the correct method for handling sterile supplies or pouring solutions when working with a sterile field.
7. Describe the procedures for female and male catheterization, demonstrating each on a laboratory model. Identify what information must be documented following catheter insertion.
8. Explain the procedure for removal of a retention catheter.

Important Terminology

autoclave
clean
contaminated
dirty
disinfection
medical asepsis
sterile
sterile technique
sterilization
surgical asepsis

Acronym

IC/ISC

Keeping the client and the environment *clean* is necessary to maintain comfort and well-being, as well as to reduce the risk of infection transmission. In addition, in specific circumstances, keeping aspects of the environment *sterile* is critical, to ensure that the client does not develop an infection. This chapter explains the differences between *medical asepsis* (clean technique) and *surgical asepsis* (sterile technique). This chapter also discusses how to perform selected procedures in which surgical asepsis (sterile technique) is necessary.

ASEPSIS

To limit the transfer of microorganisms effectively, the nurse must understand the differences between commonly used terms, *as they apply to medical asepsis*. **Dirty** is a term for any object that has not been cleaned or sterilized to remove microorganisms. A **contaminated** object is any object that is not sterile. This includes items that are dirty, as well as those that are considered to be only clean. An object that is *grossly contaminated* contains visible body fluids, discharges, or dirt. (Most body fluids are considered to be contaminated.) The term, **clean**, implies that *many* of the most harmful microorganisms have been removed. Mechanical cleaning of inanimate objects, such as tops of medication vials, counters, or blood-drawing chairs, is done with a special soap or an antiseptic cleanser. Careful handwashing, including careful cleaning of fingernails, is also part of this process (see Chapter 41). Both mechanical cleansing of inanimate objects and handwashing are sufficient to provide *medical asepsis*; the skin or countertop is now considered to be clean. **Sterile** means that the item or area is free of *all microorganisms and spores*. (A *spore* is the resting stage of some microorganisms and is resistant to environmental changes [see Chapter 40].)

> **Key Concept**
> If a sterile item touches a nonsterile item, the sterile item *is always considered contaminated.*

Many body parts are clean but not sterile. Examples include the skin, mouth, gastrointestinal tract, and upper respiratory tract. These areas are open to the outside and are inhabited by microorganisms at all times. Other body parts are considered to be sterile. Either they do not normally open to the outside (e.g., the abdominal cavity or the ovary) or they do not normally contain microorganisms. Some areas (e.g., the urinary bladder) are susceptible to infection. (The bladder is normally considered to be sterile, even though it is open to the outside.)

DISINFECTION AND STERILIZATION

Disinfection

Disinfection is a process that results in the destruction of most pathogens but not necessarily their spores. Common methods of disinfection include the use of alcohol wipes or chlorhexidine gluconate (Hibiclens) soap scrub, or a povidone-iodine (Betadine) scrub, to kill microorganisms on the skin. A surgical hand scrub takes longer than regular handwashing and is considered to be a disinfection process. The skin is considered to be disinfected, rather than just clean. Stronger disinfectants include phenol and chlorine bleach, which are generally too strong to be used on living tissue. They are used on surfaces, such as floors and countertops. Boiling also can be used to *disinfect* inanimate objects; however, it does not destroy all organisms and does not destroy spores. *Boiling does not make objects sterile.*

> **Key Concept**
>
> It is possible to *disinfect* the skin; it is not possible to sterilize the skin.

Sterilization

Sterilization is the process of exposing articles to steam heat under pressure or to chemical disinfectants long enough to kill *all microorganisms and spores.* After a client leaves a healthcare facility, the equipment they used is either sterilized or discarded. For example, the Aqua-K pad is discarded; the pump that runs it is sterilized. At discharge a client may take items such as washbasins, water pitchers, mouth care utensils, and incentive spirometers; if they do not take them, they are discarded. Occasionally, large or very expensive medical equipment is sterilized for reuse. This includes machines such as the dialysis or heart–lung machine and certain nondisposable surgical equipment.

As stated, *sterilization destroys all organisms and spores.* Exposure to steam in a sterilizer, the **autoclave** (18 lb pressure, at a temperature of 125 °C [257 °F], for 15 min) will kill even the toughest organisms and spores. Some chemicals also can be used to sterilize an object. However, *chemical disinfectants* powerful enough to destroy spores and all pathogens or the extreme temperatures of the autoclave cannot be used on certain articles, such as plastic or knife blades. Thus, these items are disposable. In addition, moist heat such as that found in an autoclave dulls the sharp cutting edges of some instruments; therefore, if special items are not disposable, dry heat or chemicals are used to sterilize them. (Sharps, such as scalpels and suture removal scissors, are disposable.) Needles used for injections or acupuncture and all materials used for IVs are always discarded after one use. Other methods of sterilization include *radiation* and *gas sterilization* (with ethylene oxide).

MEDICAL AND SURGICAL ASEPSIS

Medical asepsis is *clean* technique. Surgical asepsis is a *sterile* technique.

> **NCLEX Alert**
>
> It will be important to know and understand the definitions of and differences between surgical asepsis and medical asepsis, and disinfection and sterilization, as they relate to the prevention of infection and complications.

Medical Asepsis or Clean Technique

The purpose of maintaining **medical asepsis** is to prevent the spread of disease from one person to another, whether it is from client to nurse, client to client, nurse to client, or from a person to the environment. Chapter 41 discusses techniques of medical asepsis, also called *clean technique.* Remember, *handwashing* is the most important medical asepsis technique; skin cannot be sterilized, but it can be cleaned. Chapter 41 also introduces the concept of *standard precautions* to be used in the *delivery of all healthcare.* This is medical asepsis in action.

Surgical Asepsis or Sterile Technique

To maintain sterility, **surgical asepsis** or **sterile technique** is used. Surgical asepsis uses sterile technique for all procedures. Use of effective sterile technique means that *no organisms are carried to the client.* All microorganisms and spores are destroyed before they can enter the body. The remainder of this chapter explains sterile technique and selected applications.

In some cases, sterile and clean techniques are combined. For example, for many dressing changes or for procedures such as tracheostomy care or emptying a catheter drainage bag, sterile materials are used, but clean gloves are worn. This means that clean technique (medical asepsis) is performed, using sterile supplies. In other cases, sterile technique is used throughout the entire procedure. Sterile technique (surgical asepsis) is used when administering injectable medications and performing surgical and other procedures, such as urinary catheterization. With surgical asepsis, first, the articles are sterilized and then their contact with any nonsterile articles is prevented. When a sterile article touches a nonsterile article, the sterile article *always* becomes contaminated—it *is no longer sterile.*

STERILE TECHNIQUE (SURGICAL ASEPSIS)

Reasons for Sterile Technique

To prevent the spread of infection, the supplies used for surgical and other sterile procedures must be free of all microorganisms. Anything that either touches an open wound or skin break, enters a sterile body cavity, or punctures the skin must be sterile, to prevent introducing microorganisms (see Chapters 58 and 64). Many healthcare facilities prepare sterile supplies in a central supply room (CSR), also called central sterile supply (CSS), or purchase them in a sterile package and dispose of them after use. Some items, such as surgical towels or drapes, are packaged, secured with special masking tape, labeled, and sterilized by autoclave (Fig. 57-1). Items such as syringes and needles are packaged individually by the manufacturer, sterilized before distribution, and discarded after one use.

> **Key Concept**
>
> **Disinfection** is the destruction of most pathogens but not spores.
> **Sterilization** is the destruction of all microorganisms and spores.
> Always think before you touch anything. If a sterile article touches an unsterile article, it becomes contaminated. Sterile to sterile remains sterile. Sterile to clean, dirty, or contaminated becomes contaminated. Discard any article if you are not sure whether or not it is contaminated.

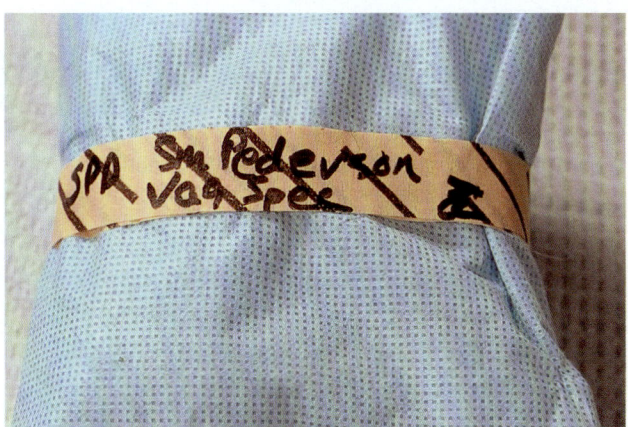

Figure 57-1 Some items, such as surgical towels, nondisposable instruments, and surgical linens, are packaged, secured with special masking tape, labeled, and sterilized. The tape changes color or shows black stripes when the items are sterilized. The facility specifies the length of time the item will still be considered sterile. When that period of time has elapsed, the item must be resterilized.

Every step in an aseptic procedure is a link in a chain. If one link is broken by contaminating anything, the entire chain has been broken, and infection can occur (see Chapter 40). Learning to perform correct sterile technique requires understanding the meanings of *dirty, contaminated, clean,* and *sterile.* The skill of maintaining sterile technique requires a great deal of practice. In Practice: Nursing Care Guidelines 57-1 provides general tips for using sterile technique. In Practice: Nursing Procedure 57-1 describes the steps associated with opening a sterile package; these techniques are basic to many sterile procedures. Also refer to Figure 58-7, which illustrates the method for a clean nurse to hand sterile supplies to a nurse wearing sterile gloves and performing a sterile procedure.

Healthcare providers entering sterile environments, such as an operating room (OR), must wear protective clothing, to prevent contaminating the area from the skin, hair, and clothing. Because many clients today are sent home with catheters, intravenous (IV) lines, and other tubes in place, it is vital to teach the client and family how to lessen the possibility of infection at home. Typically, the client and family are taught to manage specific equipment at home; this equipment is kept sterile, if possible. However, because the client will be exposed only to microorganisms within their own home, clean technique may be used for some procedures that would require sterile technique in the healthcare facility. In these cases, the equipment is considered contaminated specifically to that person. In Practice: Educating the Client 57-1 highlights some examples and tips for teaching family caregivers how to prevent spreading infection.

Hair Covering

In sterile environments (especially the OR) workers must completely cover the hair. If the hair is long, a hood is worn; if the hair is short, a surgical cap is used. The nurse with a moustache or beard wears a full-face surgical hood, to cover the entire face, except the eyes.

IN PRACTICE
NURSING CARE GUIDELINES 57-1 — Sterile Technique

- After sterile gloves (and/or gown) have been put on, the nurse cannot touch anything that is not sterile. Keep hands between nipple and waist level, whether or not a gown is worn.
- Reaching over a sterile field contaminates the sterile area, unless sterile clothing and gloves are being worn.
- If a sterile wrapper becomes wet, the wrapper *and its contents* are no longer sterile.
- If a mask becomes wet, it no longer screens out microorganisms; the mask must be changed for a new mask.
- When wearing sterile gloves to perform a sterile procedure, keep them in front, between the nipple line and waist. If gloves move above or below these areas, they are considered contaminated.
- A person's back is not sterile, even if a sterile gown is being worn.
- Objects are considered contaminated if there is any uncertainty whether contamination has occurred. *When in doubt, consider the objects in question to be contaminated.*
- Skin cannot be rendered sterile; it can only be made clean.
- Parts of the body that are not normally exposed to the outside are considered sterile. These parts include the abdominal cavity, the urinary bladder, and usually the uterus.

Surgical Mask and Eye Protection

Chapter 41 illustrates how to put on a *surgical mask* (see Nursing Procedure 41-3). Masks are used in the OR, in protective isolation, and in certain other types of client isolation (see Chapter 42). The mask covers the mouth and nose. Its purpose is to provide a barrier against pathogens. In the OR or during sterile procedures, the mask prevents harmful microorganisms in your respiratory tract from spreading to the client. When the client has an infection, the mask protects you from the client's pathogens.

Key Concept
Remember: The mask is contaminated because it touches the nurse's face. Do not touch the mask with sterile gloves. If the mask becomes wet, it must be changed, because it is no longer effective.

Eye protection is often worn in the OR or in other areas, such as the dental office, Emergency Department, or acute psychiatric services. The nurse's eyes must be protected from splashing or spitting of body fluids. If a sterile gown is to be worn, the mask/eye protection and hair protection are donned *first.*

Sterile Gown

In-service education is required before wearing a sterile gown. A *sterile gown* is commonly worn by scrub personnel

IN PRACTICE
EDUCATING THE CLIENT 57-1 — Preventing the Spread of Infection at Home

Examples of Client and Family Teaching
- Emptying the catheter drainage bag.
- Safely changing catheter tubing (usually, not the catheter itself).
- Hanging a new IV bag.
- Giving an injection.

Additional Tips for Teaching
- Demonstrate the skill to be performed.
- Ask the client and family to repeat the demonstration.

- Explain how to recognize problems or complications, such as postoperative infections.
- Describe when to seek medical care immediately.
- Give the client/family printed instructions, to reinforce teaching.
- State where to obtain needed supplies.
- If indicated, make a referral for home care nursing follow-up.

---

in the OR, in protective isolation, and sometimes in the delivery room. When putting on the sterile gown, the hands touch only the parts of the gown that will touch the body after it is in place (only the inside). Another person must tie the strings. The back of the gown and any part of the gown below waist level or above nipple level is considered contaminated, even though it was sterile when put on. When wearing a sterile gown, be careful not to touch anything that is not sterile.

Sterile Gloves

When a sterile gown is worn, *sterile gloves* are also required. (Sterile gloves are sometimes worn alone.) Practice is required in order to put on sterile gloves without contaminating the gloves or anything else in the sterile area. Remember that once gloves are put on, touching anything nonsterile contaminates them. Therefore, make all preparations before putting on sterile gloves. In Practice: Nursing Procedure 57-2 describes a method of gloving called *open gloving*.

A procedure called *closed gloving* is often performed when a sterile gown is used. You will learn that procedure if you work in an OR, short-stay surgery, or assist with minor surgery in a healthcare provider's clinic.

> **Key Concept**
> Whenever the cover on a sterile tray, or a gown, mask, dressing, drape, or other sterile cloth or paper item becomes wet, it is contaminated.

Removal of Sterile or Nonsterile Gloves

To remove gloves, whether they are sterile or clean, pull one glove down over the other. Place the gloved fingers of your first hand only under the *outside cuff* of the glove being pulled off (Fig. 57-2A). *Rationale: This keeps your hand and arm away from contamination that might be on the glove.* The glove that was pulled off is held in the gloved hand. Then, slide the ungloved fingers of the other hand inside the second glove, pulling it off and over the first glove. This time, put your fingers *inside the glove* and avoid touching the outside of the gloves with your ungloved fingers. Keep the outsides

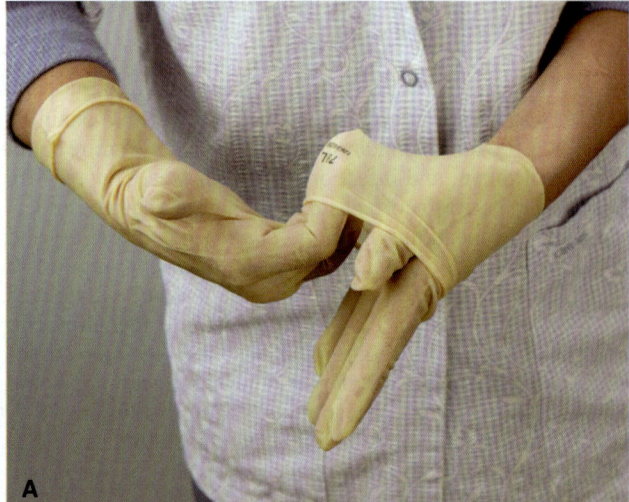
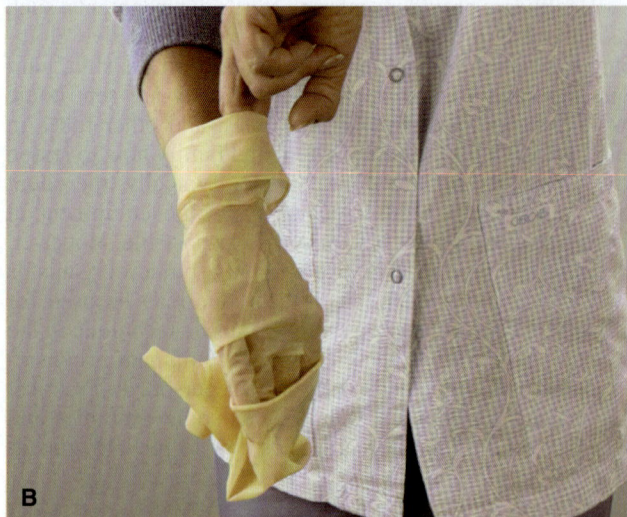

Figure 57-2 Safe removal of gloves. A, Touch only the outside of the contaminated glove (inside a folded-down cuff) with gloved fingers. B, Touch the skin only with bare fingers. Roll gloves together, with contaminated areas inside the roll and discard appropriately. Wash hands carefully. (Evans-Smith, 2005.)

of the gloves inside the rolled-up gloves (Fig. 57-2B). ***Rationale:*** *By following this procedure, if the gloves are contaminated most of the contamination will be contained within the gloves. Discard gloves per protocol and carefully wash your hands. Remember: Handwashing is your most important defense against the spread of microorganisms.*

PROCEDURES REQUIRING STERILE TECHNIQUE

A number of procedures require the use of sterile equipment and/or sterile technique. Several of these are described elsewhere in this book. They include:

- Care of the indwelling catheter—Chapter 51 (see Nursing Care Guidelines 51-3)
- Surgical intervention and invasive procedures—Chapter 56
- Sterile dressing change—Chapter 58 (see Nursing Procedures 58-1 and 58-2)
- Suture and staple removal—Chapter 58 (see Fig. 58-13)
- Administration of parenteral medications—Chapter 64
- Venipuncture and Management of IVs—Chapter 64

Urinary Catheterization

The bladder is the reservoir for urine. Normally, when about 250 to 300 mL of urine collects in the bladder, the urge to void (urinate) occurs. If the bladder cannot empty normally, it becomes distended (enlarged or stretched out) as urine collects. Urine may dribble from the urethral opening, and chronic kidney disorders can result. *Urinary catheterization* is the procedure of inserting a tube (*catheter*) through the urethra into the bladder, to remove urine. Although urinary catheterization is related to elimination of urine, it is in this chapter because it is an important sterile procedure, helping to prevent the introduction of pathogens into the bladder. Only disposable sterile equipment is used. (Other procedures related to elimination of body wastes do not require sterile technique [see Chapter 51].)

A *straight catheter* (*intermittent catheter*, e.g., the Robinson) is used only for one sample, removed, and discarded. A *retention catheter* or *indwelling catheter* (e.g., *Foley catheter*) remains in the bladder. Other types of indwelling catheters include the *mushroom, Malecot,* and *Pezzer*. A special type of catheter, the *coudé-tip* catheter, has a curved tip and is often used in male catheterization because it is easier to pass through the prostatic curvature. It may be used in the female if there is abnormal placement of the urinary meatus. A special *hematuria catheter* may be used following removal of the prostate, to control bleeding (see Chapter 89). (A *condom catheter* [Texas catheter, external catheter] is a device that is placed over the tip of the penis. Because it fits around the penis and is not inserted, it carries less possibility of infection. For initial application, a sterile condom catheter is used.)

Most providers order *midstream* or *clean-catch* specimens to obtain an uncontaminated urine specimen (see Chapter 52). Catheterization may be required to determine the amount of urine residual (remaining) after voiding or to instill dye or contrast media for certain urinary system studies. The need for catheterization after surgery has diminished because early ambulation is the norm (which helps all body systems to return more rapidly to normal).

Generally, no more than 750 to 1,000 mL of urine can be safely removed from the bladder at any one time, particularly if the client has had urine retention or abdominal distention for some time. If urine flow seems undiminished after withdrawal of this quantity, clamp or remove the catheter and report the findings to the provider. (If there is any possibility of excess urine, a Foley-type catheter should be used.) The procedure for removal of the retention/indwelling catheter is explained later in this chapter.

Intermittent Self-Catheterization

Some clients are taught to catheterize themselves (intermittent catheterization [**IC**], *intermittent self-catheterization* [**ISC**]) on a regular basis (four to six times daily), usually with a straight catheter. This may be done by the paraplegic client or the client with chronic neurologic bladder atony (lack of muscle tone). In this case, the procedure may continue at home, using clean, rather than sterile, technique, because the catheter is contaminated only to that client. (In the healthcare facility, sterile technique is always used.)

> **Nursing Alert** Before performing any catheterization, make sure the client is not allergic to latex (rubber). Although catheters today usually are not latex, the client with a latex allergy could also have a severe reaction to another type of catheter, even though a special nonallergenic catheter (e.g., polyurethane, Teflon, silicone) is used. If the client's allergy is severe, specific allergy testing must precede catheterization.

Catheterizing the Female Client

Placement of a retention catheter may be necessary when a woman has had pelvic surgery or bladder tumors. In Practice: Nursing Procedure 57-3 summarizes steps for catheterizing the female client. (In some cases, a suprapubic catheter is inserted during surgery [see Chapter 51].)

The Side-Lying Position

If a female client is unable to lie on their back for catheterization, or cannot relax their legs because of contractures, use the side-lying position (Fig. 57-3). Many clients are more comfortable in this position than on the back and some nurses prefer to always use this position for this procedure. This position facilitates accurate sterile technique because the nurse needs to hold only one side of the labia in position. Contamination of the catheter is less likely because this position is easier for the client to maintain, and the nurse does not need to reach over the client's leg. The client lies on their side with knees drawn up to the chest. If the nurse is right-handed, the client lies on their left side and vice versa. Raise the level of the bed to a comfortable height. Position the client's buttocks near your side of the bed, and the client's shoulders near the far side. Stand behind the client, near her buttocks. Sterile technique and general steps are the same as for the supine client.

Catheterizing the Male Client

Catheterization of the male client offers challenges because the male urethra is longer and more curved and the man

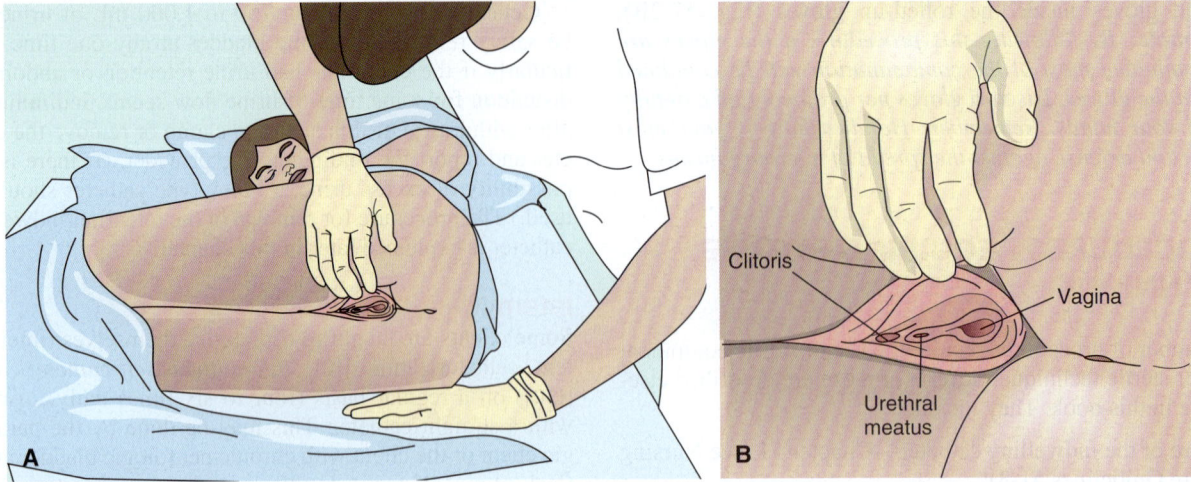

Figure 57-3 The side-lying position for female catheterization. Shown here is the position for the *left-handed nurse*. **A**, The client is positioned on her side. *After the client is positioned,* the nurse must put on sterile gloves (because these gloves were contaminated during positioning). **B**, The urinary (urethral) meatus is exposed and the catheter inserted. (Taylor, Lillis, & LeMone, 2005.)

may have an enlarged prostate constricting or obstructing the urethra. Previous urethral infection can also cause strictures. In Practice: Nursing Procedure 57-4 describes male catheterization.

Caring for the Client After Catheterization

After catheterization, reposition the client to ensure that they are comfortable and the signal cord is within reach. Be sure that the balloon of an indwelling catheter is inflated and the catheter tubing is secured externally, to avoid pulling and discomfort. Use hypoallergenic tape or use the stabilization device that comes with the kit to hold the catheter to the man's abdomen or thigh or to the woman's thigh. Explain to the client that they may feel the urge to void, because of the catheter's presence in the urethra, particularly within the first 30 min of insertion. This feeling should diminish and usually goes away within an hour.

> **Nursing Alert** If the client continues to feel a very strong urge to void or severe discomfort after catheter insertion, report this to the provider.

The drainage tubing extends straight down from the bed level to the bag (*straight drainage*) with extra tubing placed on the bed with the client, so movement is possible. *Rationale: Loops hanging down can promote urinary stasis and infection.* If a retention catheter is left in place, attach the drainage apparatus to the bed frame (not the side rails), maintaining its sterility (see Chapter 51). When the client is out of bed, a leg bag may be used during the day and a "down drain" bag at night. If the client is to wear a bag permanently, a "belly bag" may be fastened around the waist and inside the clothing, where it does not show.

> **Key Concept**
> The drainage bag must be lower than the client's bladder for the urine to drain properly and to help prevent infection.

Removing the Retention Catheter

Removing a retention catheter is a simple procedure. The balloon is deflated and the catheter gently pulled out, preventing urethral trauma. In Practice: Nursing Procedure 57-5 describes retention catheter removal. In Practice: Educating the Client 57-2 lists important self-care points for the client.

> **Nursing Alert** A catheter is *never cut* for removal. This could cause the catheter to be pulled back into the urethra or bladder. In that case, surgical removal would probably be necessary. This would also be a prime source for introducing pathogenic organisms into the urinary bladder.

IN PRACTICE
EDUCATING THE CLIENT 57-2 — After Catheter Removal

Client education encourages cooperation and lessens anxiety. Teach the client to
- Drink plenty of fluids (to facilitate voiding).
- Report the urge to void for the first time after catheter removal.
- Understand that some discomfort may be felt with the first voiding.
- Report any severe pain or blood in the urine.

STUDENT SYNTHESIS

KEY POINTS

- *Clean* applies to medical asepsis. It denotes removal of gross contamination and many microorganisms.
- *Sterile* identifies an item that is free of all microorganisms and spores.
- When a sterile item touches anything unsterile, the sterile item becomes contaminated.
- If a sterile item becomes contaminated or if there is uncertainty whether or not it is contaminated, it is considered contaminated and must be discarded.
- Catheterization is the procedure of inserting a flexible tube through the urethra into the bladder to remove urine. This procedure requires sterile equipment and technique.
- The balloon is deflated when removing a retention catheter. The catheter is never cut for removal.
- Client and family teaching is vitally important, especially if the client or family will need to perform sterile procedures, such as IV therapy or catheter care, after discharge.

CRITICAL THINKING EXERCISES

1. A 48-year-old female client has been unable to void since having abdominal surgery approximately 6 hr ago. Her bladder is distended (swollen) and she complains of discomfort. The provider has ordered straight catheterization to relieve her bladder discomfort. How will you explain the procedure to her? Include its purpose, how it will be done, and what she will be expected to do.
2. Describe how you would explain to a client of the opposite sex that you are about to perform a catheterization.

NCLEX-STYLE REVIEW QUESTIONS

1. The nurse is assisting with a surgical procedure and hands the surgeon an instrument free of microorganisms and spores to prevent surgical site infection. The nurse is ensuring that this is which category of instrument?
   a. Clean
   b. Sterile
   c. Contaminated
   d. Disinfected

2. The nurse accidentally touches a sterile instrument with a nonsterile object. What is the best action for the nurse to take next?
   a. Discard the instrument in the trash.
   b. Wash the instrument with soap and water and reuse.
   c. Obtain another sterile instrument to use.
   d. Use the instrument since it has limited exposure to the unsterile object.

3. The nurse is disinfecting a client's skin prior to a surgical procedure. What method would be most effective? Select all that apply.
   a. Chlorhexidine gluconate scrub
   b. Povidone-iodine scrub
   c. Soap and water scrub
   d. Hydrogen peroxide scrub

4. A client is being discharged from the acute care facility after successful treatment for pneumonia. An incentive spirometer is left behind. What would the nurse do with the incentive spirometer that was left behind?
   a. Soak the incentive spirometer in a chemical disinfecting solution for reuse.
   b. Have the incentive spirometer sterilized for reuse.
   c. Discard the incentive spirometer.
   d. Clean the incentive spirometer with alcohol wipes and reuse.

5. The nurse is setting up a sterile field for a client's surgical procedure and spills sterile water on the sterile wrapper covering an instrument tray. What would the nurse do next?
   a. Obtain another surgical instrument tray because it is contaminated.
   b. Cut the wet area away with sterile scissors.
   c. Use the tray because the saline was sterile.
   d. Remove the wrapping and use the tray.

CHAPTER RESOURCES

Enhance your learning with additional resources on thePoint!

Student Resources related to this chapter can be found at thePoint.lww.com/Rosdahl12e.

Welcome Steps

Look at healthcare provider's orders.

Protocol for procedure.

Necessary equipments/supplies.

Wash hands using proper hand hygiene; put on gloves.

Explain the procedure and reassure the client.

Locate two identifiers to confirm correct client.

Comfortable and efficient position for nurse and client.

Obtain privacy.

Make sure to follow correct steps and body mechanics with good technique.

Ensure safety and observe deviations from normal.

End Steps

Ensure comfort and safety.

Note questions or concerns from client or nurse; note significant data.

Dispose of materials properly.

Disinfect the area and your hands.

Document and report the procedure and your findings.

IN PRACTICE

NURSING PROCEDURE 57-1 — Opening a Sterile Package

Supplies and Equipment
Sterile supplies (as needed for procedure).
Waist-high table.

Steps
Follow LPN WELCOME steps and then

1. Check the expiration date on sterile supplies. Prepare a waist-high working area. *Rationale: Sterile objects must be kept above waist level to maintain their sterility. Outdated packages are considered contaminated.*

2. Place the sterile package on the working area. Remove the outer covering or plastic wrap if present. *Rationale: The outer covering protects the sterile contents.*

3. Grasp the edge of the outermost flap of the inner wrapper and open the package away from you, toward the back of the table. *Rationale: Opening the top flap away from you prevents reaching over a sterile field and contaminating it.*

4. Using your left hand, fold the flap on the left side down toward the table. Using your right hand, repeat with the right side flap. Then, after opening both side flaps, push up on the underside of the wrapper, to bend it up in the middle and pull the near flap out flat, grasping only its tip. Do not touch any part of the sterile field. Pull the flaps taut and flat onto the table. *Rationale: Folding each side outward allows access to the remaining flap(s); pushing the wrapper up in the middle and pulling the flaps out taut keeps the wrapping from curling back into its original position (which would contaminate the area). When the flaps are unfolded, the inside is sterile.*

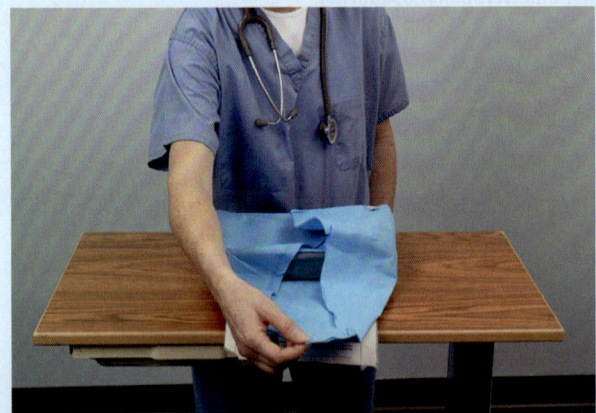

Opening outermost top flap away from the body without reaching over the sterile field. (Evans-Smith, 2005.)

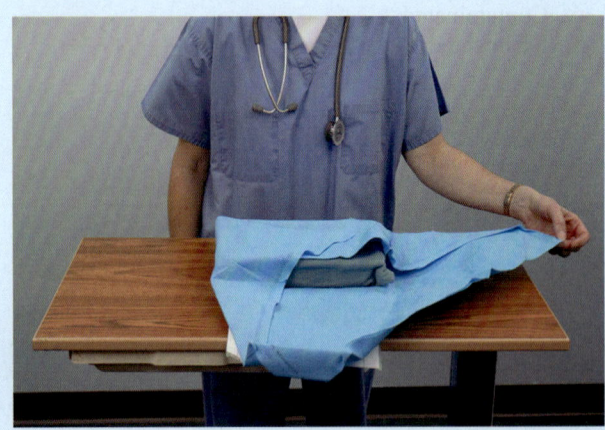

Opening left side flap away from the center. (Evans-Smith, 2005.)

CHAPTER 57 Surgical Asepsis **849**

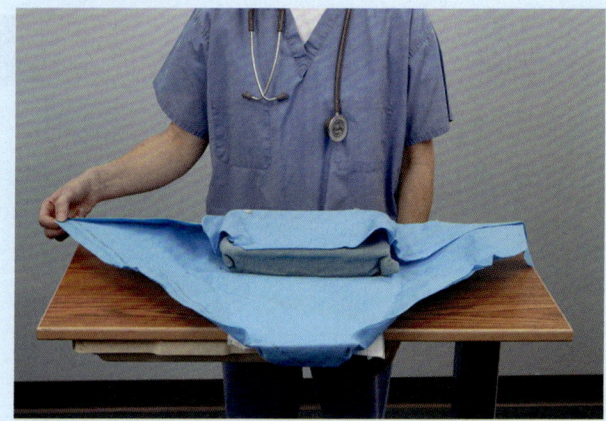

Opening right side flap. *(Evans-Smith, 2005.)*

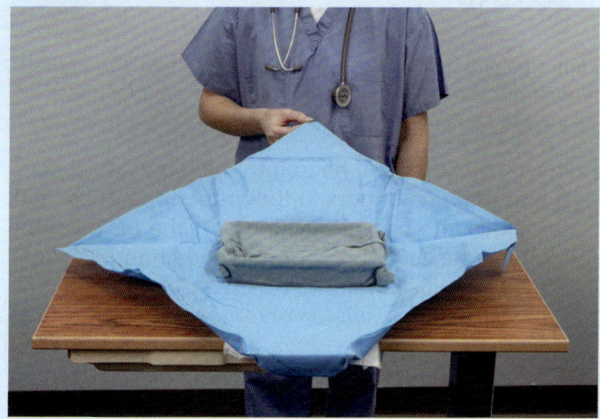

Dropping sterile contents on the sterile field, keeping at least 2 in. from the edge of the sterile drape. *(Evans-Smith, 2005.)*

5. Open any additional sterile packages without touching the contents. Drop these items onto the sterile field, staying at least 2 in. from the edges. Do not allow the wrappings from these packages to touch the sterile field; dispose of the wrappers appropriately. Do not reach over the sterile field more than absolutely necessary. Do not touch the sterile drape with your body or clothing. *Rationale:* Sterile touching sterile maintains surgical asepsis. The outer 2 in. of any sterile field is considered contaminated. All packages touched by unsterile gloves, hands, or packages are contaminated.

6. Pour any sterile solutions into basins or cups, as instructed. Hold the bottle with the label upward. Do not touch the inside of the bottle, its cap, or the basin into which the solution is poured. Place the cap, with inside up, on a nonsterile area. If the bottle has been previously opened, "lip" it by pouring a small amount off first, into a sink or lined trash receptacle, before pouring onto the sterile field. Pour solution slowly into the basin or cup, to prevent splashing solution. Do not touch the sterile drape with your body or clothing. *Rationale:* Pouring off a small amount of solution ensures that the solution will be sterile and will not be contaminated from the bottleneck or cover. The cap is placed with the inside up, to keep it sterile. Touching any part of the inside of the bottle, the cap, or the basin would cause contamination. Protect the label from becoming wet, which might make it illegible. If the drape becomes wet, it is contaminated. The entire procedure would then need to start again.

Follow ENDDD steps

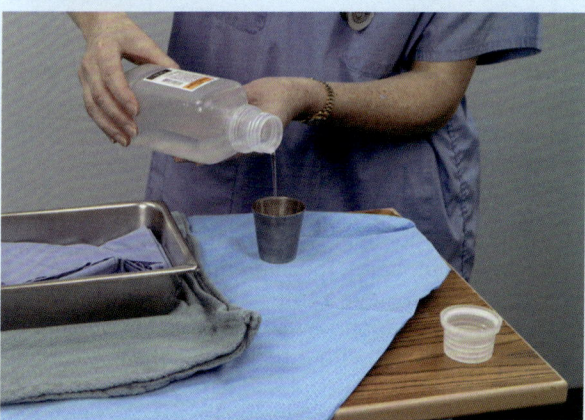

Pouring sterile solution into sterile cup without touching the sterile field and without splashing. *(Evans-Smith, 2005.)*

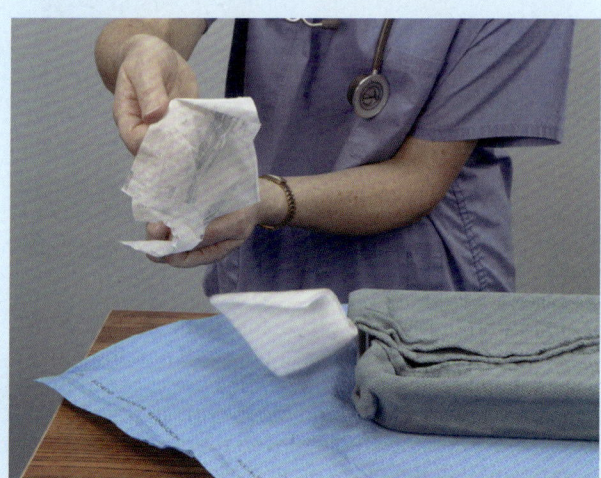

Opening bottom flap toward the nurse's body and folding it backward to prevent it from reentering the sterile field. *(Evans-Smith, 2005.)*

IN PRACTICE
NURSING PROCEDURE 57-2 — Putting on Sterile Gloves (Open Gloving)

Supplies and Equipment
Wrapped sterile gloves of the appropriate size.

Steps
Follow LPN WELCOME steps and then

1. Open the outer glove package, following In Practice: Nursing Procedure 57-1, on a clean, dry, flat surface at waist level or higher. *Rationale: Properly opening the sterile package of gloves protects them from becoming contaminated.*

2. If there is an inner package, open it in the same way, keeping the sterile gloves on the inside surface with cuffs toward you. *Rationale: This ensures that the gloves remain sterile and ready to apply.*

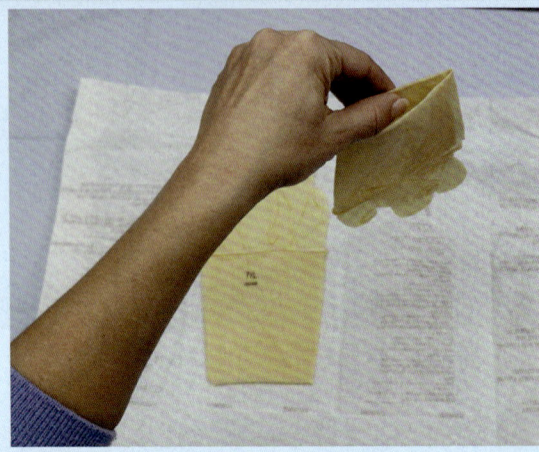

Lifting the glove up and away from the package. The right-handed nurse uses the left hand to pick up the first glove. (Evans-Smith, 2005.)

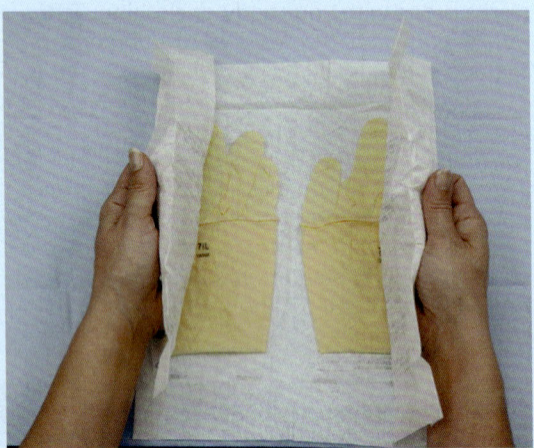

Opening the inner glove package. Both gloves are cuffed at the wrist to allow the nurse to pick them up without contaminating the outside sterile surface of the glove. (Evans-Smith, 2005.)

3. Use the nondominant hand to grasp the glove for the dominant hand, touching only the *inside* upper surface of the glove's cuff. Lift the glove up and clear of the wrapper. Avoid touching the outside of this glove with either hand. *Rationale: Touching only the cuffed inner surface of the glove with your clean hand allows the outer surface to remain sterile. The outside of the glove will later come in contact with sterile items. The inside is now considered to be only clean because it is touching your clean (not sterile), ungloved fingers. Lifting the glove clear of the wrapper prevents the glove from touching the wrapper, which is considered contaminated in the area from which the glove has been removed.*

4. Insert the dominant hand into the glove, placing the thumb and fingers in the proper openings. Pull the glove into place, touching *only* the *inside* of the glove at the cuff with your ungloved hand. Leave the cuff in place. *Rationale: Attempts to unfold the glove cuff may result in contamination. Touching only the inside of the glove with the ungloved hand preserves the sterility of the outside of the glove.*

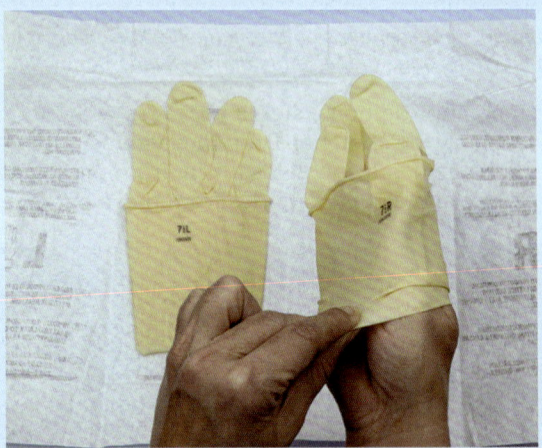

Inserting the dominant hand into the first glove. (Evans-Smith, 2005.)

5. To put on the second glove, insert the fingers of the sterile gloved hand between the cuff and the glove (on the outside of the glove). Be sure to touch only the *outside* of the second glove with sterile gloved fingers. Keep the sterile gloved thumb pointed outward. Lift the glove up and clear of the wrapper.

Rationale: The sterile fingers of the first gloved hand will be protected by the cuff as the second glove is pulled on. Touching only the outside of the second sterile glove with the sterile gloved fingers maintains the sterility of the outsides of both gloves. Holding the thumb outward keeps it out of the way and prevents it from touching the sterile area.

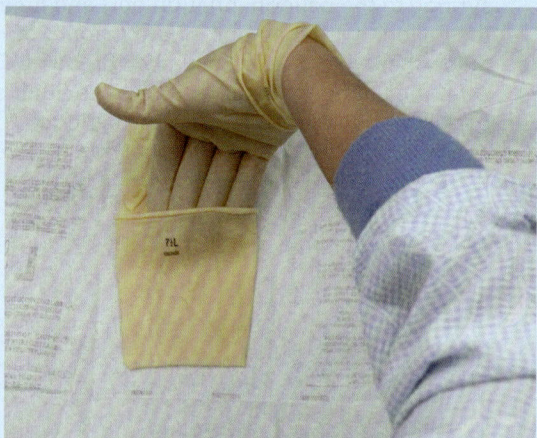

Slipping sterile gloved fingers under the sterile cuff of the second glove, keeping the thumb up and out of the way. (Evans-Smith, 2005.)

a. Insert the ungloved hand into the glove.
b. Pull the second glove on, touching *only* the *outside* of the sterile glove with the other sterile gloved hand and keeping the fingers of the first hand between the cuff and the sterile glove.
c. Adjust gloves and snap cuffs into place. Avoid touching the inside glove and wrist areas with the sterile gloves. *Rationale:* Gloves remain sterile when touching other sterile areas.

6. Keep the sterile gloved hands between waist and nipple level. Make sure not to touch the clothes or anything that is unsterile. Keep hands folded when not performing the procedure. *Rationale:* Holding the hands above waist level keeps them within sight. Raising them too high could possibly cause them to touch the face, hair, or other unsterile objects. Keeping the sterile gloved hands folded when not performing a procedure helps maintain control. It is important to prevent accidental contamination of the gloves.

Follow ENDDD steps

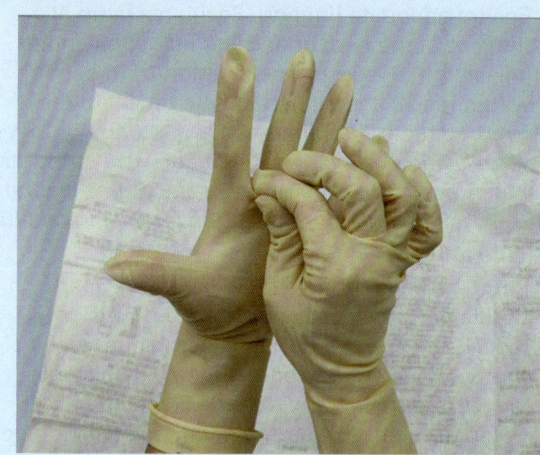

Inserting the nondominant hand into the second glove and pulling the fingers of both gloves into place from the outside. (Evans-Smith, 2005.)

IN PRACTICE
NURSING PROCEDURE 57-3 Catheterizing the Female Client

Supplies and Equipment
Sterile catheterization tray.

Note: Depending on the manufacturer, kits may contain different items. It is important to read the label to determine if any additional supplies must be added. Most kits contain the following:

Basin
Cotton balls
Antiseptic solution (usually Betadine) and cup
Straight or indwelling catheter (size appropriate for client). Catheters are sized by the "French scale" and range from 10 F (3.3 mm) to 28 F (9.3 mm)
Lubricant (unless the catheter is prelubricated)
Forceps
Drapes: Plain; fenestrated drape (containing an opening or window)
Syringe prefilled with water or saline (no needle)
Specimen container

Additional items needed:

Sterile gloves
Urine collection bag (usually attached to catheter)
Examination lamp
Plastic biohazard bag for trash
Waterproof pad
Velcro leg strap or nonallergenic tape
Bath blanket
Clean gloves, soap, and water
Washcloth and towel
A stabilization device

Note: Not all of these items are needed for side-lying insertion. The basic steps remain the same.

Steps
Follow LPN WELCOME steps and then

1. Adjust the bed to a comfortable working height. If right-handed, stand on the client's right side (if left-handed, stand on the client's left side). *Rationale:* Proper positioning prevents back strain.
2. Determine if the client is allergic to any antiseptic, such as Betadine, or to latex. *Rationale:* If the client is allergic, the procedure could cause great discomfort or life-threatening anaphylaxis. Determining

allergies before starting the procedure allows the nurse to obtain alternate materials, allowing the procedure to proceed without interruption.

3. Assist the client into a supine position with feet spread apart and flat on the mattress and their knees flexed. Use a bath blanket to drape the client. *Rationale: This dorsal recumbent position allows visualization of the urinary meatus. A bath blanket provides warmth and privacy.*

4. Put on clean gloves. Wash the client's perineal area with soap and water, rinse, and dry. Remove gloves and wash your hands. *Rationale: Cleansing the perineal area ensures that the area is as free of microorganisms as possible.*

5. Ensure adequate lighting. Position a lamp at the foot of the bed, or another nurse may hold a flashlight. Place an opened biohazard bag within reach. It is often handy to tape it to the overbed table. *Rationale: Good lighting improves visualization of the urinary meatus. The biohazard bag is accessible, so contaminated items can be discarded without contaminating the sterile field or the nurse's sterile gloves.*

6. Raise the bedside table to waist height. Open the sterile catheterization tray on the bedside table using appropriate sterile technique (see In Practice: Nursing Procedure 57-1). Put on sterile gloves (see In Practice: Nursing Procedure 57-2). Grasp the sterile drape and gently allow the drape to unfold. Grasp the upper corners and fold the drape back over your hands (which are within the sterile gloves), making a cuff with the drape. Keep the hands inside this cuff. Ask the client to lift their buttocks. Place the drape between the thighs with the upper edge under their buttocks. If desired, place the fenestrated drape over the perineal area so only the labia are exposed. Do not touch the client's skin with the sterile gloved hands. *Rationale: Protecting the gloves with the drape maintains sterility during draping. The fenestrated drape offers the client additional privacy. (This drape is often used when catheterizing a male client.)*

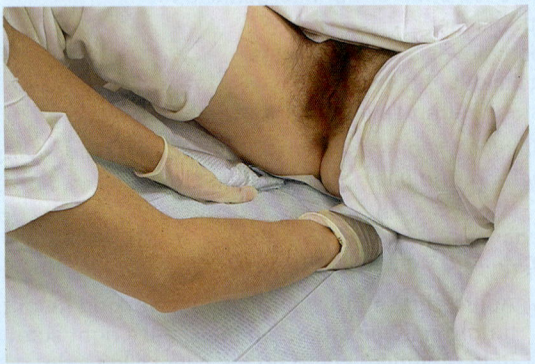

Placing the drape while protecting sterile gloved hands inside the cuff of drape.

7. Set up equipment on the open sterile tray:
   a. Place the cotton balls into the cup or into the receptacle of the molded tray. Open the package containing antiseptic (usually Betadine) and pour it over the cotton balls.
   b. Remove the plastic covering from the catheter. For an indwelling catheter, attach the prefilled syringe to the balloon inflation port and inflate the balloon with the appropriate amount of fluid to test the balloon (usually 5 or 30 mL). After the balloon inflates, aspirate the fluid back into the syringe, leaving the syringe connected to the port and the *balloon deflated.*

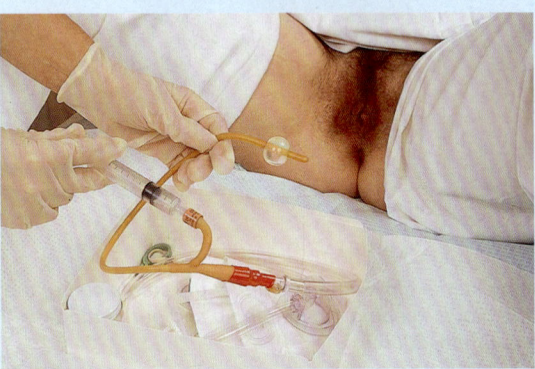

Testing the balloon on an indwelling catheter.

   c. Open the lubricant and lubricate the catheter's tip 1 to 2 in. (You may leave the catheter tip inside the sterile lubricant package until you need it.)
   d. Unscrew the cap from the specimen container if a specimen is ordered.
   e. If a straight catheter is being used, position the drainage end of the catheter in the basin to catch the urine. *Rationale: Correct preparation ensures that all equipment is present. Inflating the catheter balloon before use checks for leaks or a nonfunctioning balloon. Lubrication of the catheter increases comfort on insertion.*

8. Move the catheterization tray with the equipment onto the sterile drape between the client's thighs. If performing a straight catheterization, move the collection basin close to the perineum. *Rationale: All supplies are easily available, decreasing the likelihood of contaminating equipment. Having the collection basin close by provides ease in collection and helps prevent spills.*

9. Before proceeding, make sure you have all supplies and equipment and are ready to contaminate the nondominant hand. Using the nondominant hand, separate and gently spread the labia minora to expose the urinary meatus. Keep this hand in position; do not move it once you have touched the client. *Rationale: Spreading the labia allows for easier cleansing and visibility. Your nondominant hand is now considered contaminated. Moving your hand would spread contamination.*

10. With the dominant hand, use the forceps to pick up cotton balls that have been soaked with the antiseptic solution (Betadine). Use cotton balls to cleanse, as follows: labial fold on the side farthest from you; labial fold on the near side; and urinary meatus. Use a new cotton ball for each stroke, moving from top to bottom (front to back). Discard each used cotton ball in the biohazard bag. Never cross a sterile field with used cotton balls or any other contaminated item—move your hand around the sterile field. *Rationale: Moving from clean to dirty (front to back) lessens the chance of introducing microorganisms into the client's bladder. Using a new cotton ball each time helps keep the area as clean as possible. Moving around, rather than over a sterile field, ensures that no particles or debris can drip or fall onto the sterile field.*

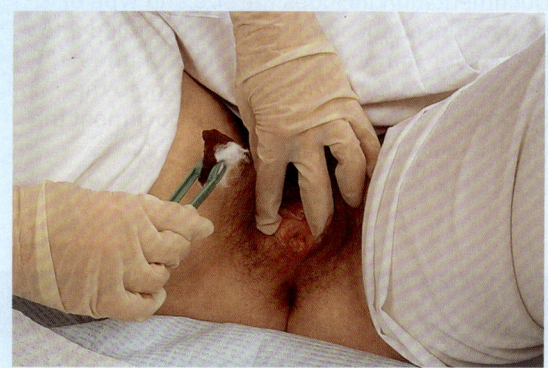

Spreading the labia with clean, gloved hand and cleansing from front to back, using a new cotton ball, held in forceps, for each stroke. The dominant hand remains sterile.

11. Pick up the catheter approximately 3 in. from the tip with the dominant hand. Make sure the drainage end of the straight catheter is in the basin to catch the urine flow. (If a specimen is ordered, place the drainage end into the specimen container.) If the catheter is indwelling, it is usually attached to the drainage tubing and collection bag. *Rationale: Think ahead and make sure urine is collected appropriately. Urine is considered to be sterile. It can safely be collected within the sterile field.*

12. Locate the urinary meatus on the perineum. Ask the client to breathe deeply and slowly through the mouth. Insert the catheter gently into the urinary meatus, advancing it 2 to 3 in. until urine begins to drain. If the catheter is indwelling, advance it another 1 to 2 in. *Never force insertion of the catheter if resistance is felt.* Do not let go of the catheter during this insertion and do not withdraw it. When the catheter is in place, move the nondominant hand to hold it in place between two fingers, bracing the rest of this hand against the client's perineum. Collect a urine specimen if one is ordered. *Rationale: Asking the client to focus on breathing relaxes the sphincter and ensures that the catheter meets with less resistance on entering the meatus. Forcing the catheter's advancement may injure the meatus or mucous membranes. If you let go of the catheter during this procedure, the pressure of urine in the bladder may force the catheter out of the meatus. If the catheter is withdrawn prematurely, it becomes contaminated. (If contamination should occur, an entire new sterile setup is required.)*

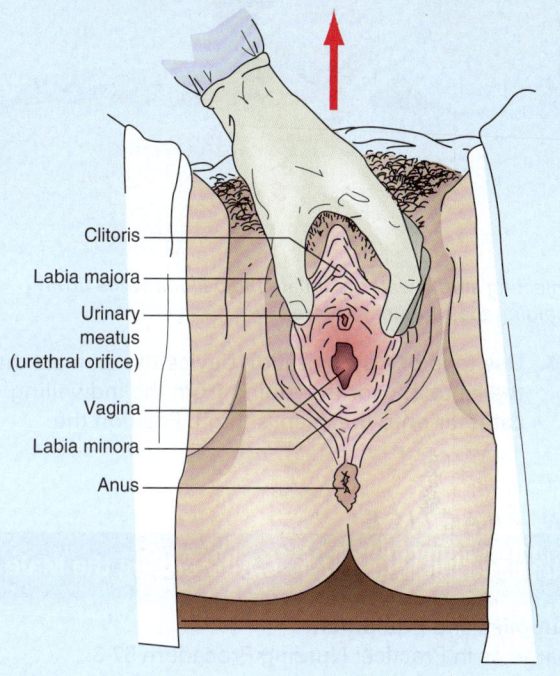

Accurately locate the urinary meatus between the clitoris and the anus. (Picture depicts nurse using the left [nondominant] hand). (Craven & Hirnle, 2007.)

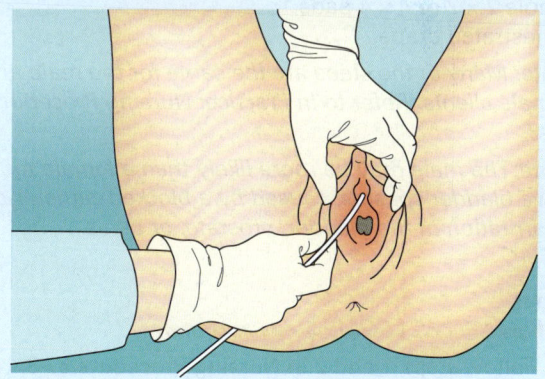

Inserting the catheter gently into the meatus with the sterile, gloved hand.

13. If the catheter is not to be indwelling, allow urine to drain into the basin. Remove the catheter after urine has drained. For an indwelling catheter, inject sterile water (or normal saline) to inflate the balloon. Pull very gently on the catheter to check that the balloon is inflated and the catheter is secure (Seating the balloon). Then, push back on the catheter a fraction of an inch. *Rationale: The balloon holds the catheter in place in the bladder. Pushing slightly back on the*

catheter helps relieve pressure on the mouth of the bladder. (Pressure on the sphincters can cause the urge to void and other discomfort.)

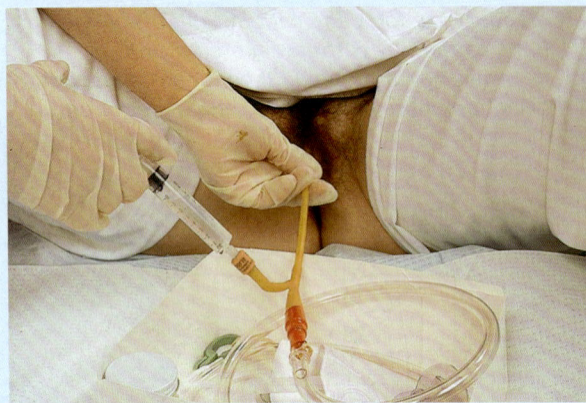

Injecting sterile water to inflate the balloon while firmly holding the catheter in place.

14. Use tape or a stabilization device that comes with the kit to anchor the tubing from the indwelling catheter onto the client's thigh. Position the drainage bag below bladder level. The catheter should pass *over the client's leg.* Allow some slack in the catheter tubing. *Rationale: Properly positioned tubing decreases tension on the catheter. The drainage bag positioned below bladder level uses gravity to promote urinary flow and decreases the risk of urinary stasis, prevents backflow of urine, and thus helps prevent infection. Some slack in the catheter tubing allows the client to turn in bed.*

15. Clean the Betadine off the client's perineum and dry the area. Measure the urine amount. See Chapter 51 for catheter care. *Rationale: These measures ensure comfort, safety, and accuracy.*

Follow ENDDD steps

Special Reminder

- Documentation includes the size and type of catheter inserted, amount of fluid instilled into the balloon, amount and character of urine obtained, and if a specimen was sent to the laboratory. It is also important to document the client's reactions, if significant.

IN PRACTICE
NURSING PROCEDURE 57-4 Catheterizing the Male Client

Supplies and Equipment
Same as In Practice: Nursing Procedure 57-3.

Additional Supplies
Coudé tip catheter, if available
Syringe lubricant, if available
Sterile 2 × 2 or 4 × 4 pads
Fenestrated drape

Note: Many of the steps are the same for the male and female clients. Refer to In Practice: Nursing Procedure 57-3.

Note: The male may be more likely than a female to have bladder spasms, caused by a blocked catheter or by irritation of the bladder, prostate, or penis.

Steps
Follow LPN WELCOME steps and then

1. Follow steps 1 and 2 in Nursing Procedure 57-3.
2. Assist the client to lie on their back with legs slightly apart. Bath blankets may be used to cover the client, except for the perineal area.
3. Follow steps 4 and 5 in Nursing Procedure 57-3.
4. Follow step 6 in Nursing Procedure 57-3; however, place the sterile drape over the client's thighs, with the fenestrated opening over the client's penis and the longer portion between the client's thighs, without contaminating the drape. *Rationale: Proper positioning and covering prevent chilling and protect the client's privacy. The setup and sterile procedures are the same for all clients.*
5. Follow step 7 in Nursing Procedure 57-3.
6. Move the catheterization tray onto the sterile drape between the client's legs, keeping your sterile gloved hands inside the wrapper of the tray. *Rationale: All supplies are easily available, decreasing the likelihood of contaminating equipment. Equipment and supplies are moved in such a way as to avoid contamination of the gloved hands.*
7. Pick up the catheter approximately 3 in. from the tip with your dominant hand. Place the drainage end in the basin. If the catheter is indwelling, it usually is attached to the drainage tubing and collection bag. If a lubricant syringe is not available, apply lubricant to the catheter on the tip and for about 5 to 7 in. of its length. *Rationale: This enables you to collect a urine specimen or to set up the indwelling catheter. Lubricant assists in catheter insertion. A longer portion of the catheter must be lubricated for a man because of the longer length of the urethra.*
8. Use your nondominant hand to grasp the penis. (This hand is now contaminated to the client.) If the penis feels slippery, use a sterile 2 × 2 or 4 × 4 pad to grasp it. Hold the penis upright. If the client is uncircumcised, retract the foreskin before cleansing. With the forceps in your dominant hand, pick up a cotton ball and cleanse from the meatus outward in a circular motion. Do not touch the penis with your dominant hand. Repeat three times, using each cotton ball only once. Remember: Your nondominant hand is now contaminated and must stay in the same position. *Rationale: Holding the penis upright helps to straighten the*

urethra and aids in insertion of the catheter. The foreskin needs to be out of the way for adequate visualization of the urethral meatus. Moving in a circular motion from the center outward (from clean to dirty) lessens the chance of introducing microorganisms into the bladder. Moving your contaminated hand would spread contamination.

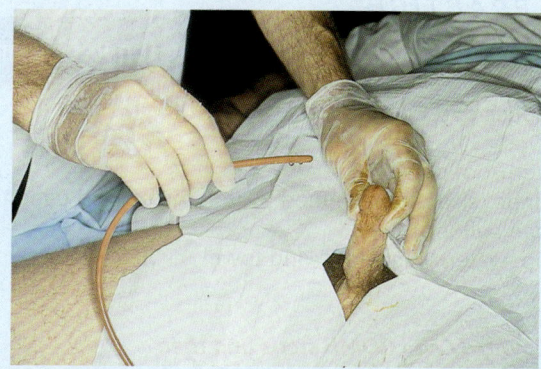

Holding penis upright and gently pressing sides, to insert catheter. (Pictured is a circumcised penis.)

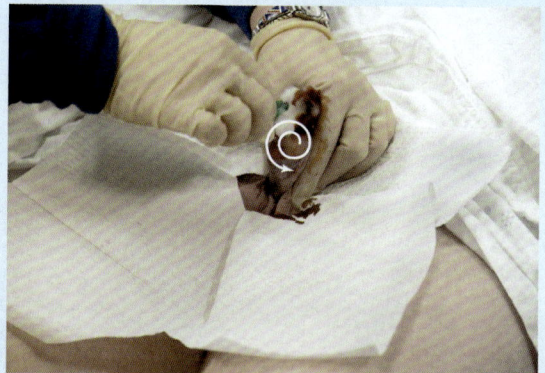

Lifting penis with gloved nondominant hand; this hand is now contaminated to the client. Holding cotton balls in forceps with sterile gloved hand and cleansing head of penis in circular motion, from meatus outward. (Evans-Smith, 2005.)

9. With the penis upright, gently insert the tip of the lubricant syringe (if available) into the urethra and instill the lubricant. Gently pressing the end of the penis from two sides may help to open the meatus. *Rationale: Holding the penis upright straightens the urethral canal. Instilling lubricant directly into the urethra helps distend the urethra and increases the ease and comfort of catheter insertion.*

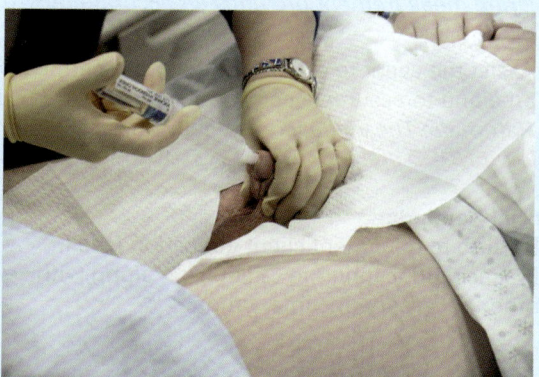

Instilling lubricant into urinary meatus. (Evans-Smith, 2005.)

10. Ask the client to bear down as if voiding and breathe deeply. Insert the catheter gently into the meatus, following the natural curvature, and advancing it 7 to 9 in. or until urine begins to drain. If you encounter resistance when passing the catheter, rotate it slightly or withdraw it, rather than forcing it. *Rationale: Rotating the catheter helps ease it past the client's prostate gland.*

11. For an indwelling catheter, advance it another inch. Collect a urine specimen if one is ordered. *Rationale: Additional catheter advancement ensures that the balloon inflates in the bladder rather than in the urethral canal.*

12. Follow steps 13 to 15 of In Practice: Nursing Procedure 57-3. Make the following exceptions for the male client:

   a. Tape or secure the catheter with a stabilization device that comes with the kit to the lower abdomen or upper thigh, allowing some slack in the tubing.

   b. Return the foreskin to its original position in the uncircumcised man. *Rationale: Securing the catheter to the lower abdomen or upper thigh may reduce urethral pressure at the angle of the penis and the scrotum. Some slack is allowed so the client can turn in bed. Returning the foreskin to its original position prevents impaired circulation in the penis and pressure on the urethra.*

Follow ENDDD steps

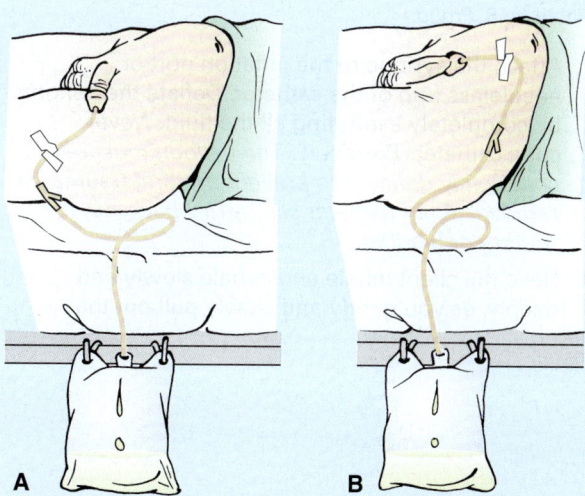

A, Securing catheter to upper thigh. B, Securing catheter to lower abdomen. Note that the drainage bag is secured below the level of the bladder.

IN PRACTICE

NURSING PROCEDURE 57-5: Removing the Retention Catheter

Supplies and Equipment
Gloves
Waterproof pad
Syringe (size is determined by volume of fluid used to inflate balloon)
Soap, water, washcloth, and towel

Steps
Follow LPN WELCOME steps and then

1. Adjust bed to a comfortable working height. Place a waterproof pad between the client's thighs and under the buttocks. Wash hands and put on gloves. *Rationale: Proper positioning prevents back strain. The waterproof pad prevents soiling of the bed linen. Hands are washed just before the procedure. Hands should be as clean as possible, to prevent transmission of microorganisms. Gloves are always worn when body fluids will be present.*

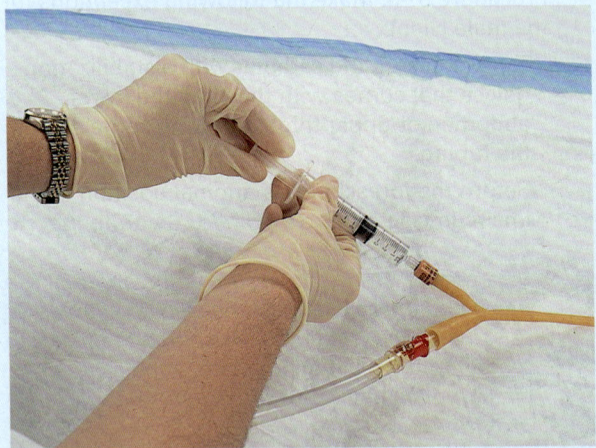

Deflating the balloon with a syringe using the inflation port. (Photo by B. Proud.)

2. Attach the syringe to the inflation port or needleless hub of the catheter. Deflate the balloon by completely aspirating all the fluid. *Never cut a catheter. Rationale: The balloon must be completely deflated to prevent urethral trauma on removal. A cut catheter can retract back into the urethra or bladder.*

3. Have the client inhale and exhale slowly and deeply, as you gently and slowly pull out the catheter. *Rationale: Taking deep breaths helps the client relax and makes removal more comfortable. Easing the catheter through the urethra minimizes the risk of trauma.*

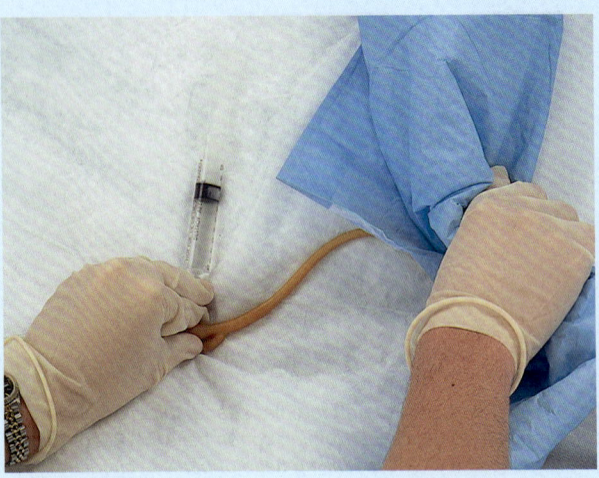

Pulling the catheter out gently and slowly and wrapping it in a waterproof pad. (Photo by B. Proud.)

4. Wrap the catheter in the waterproof pad. Remove the catheter, drainage bag, and equipment from the bedside. Dispose of apparatus, according to agency policy. Remember that the catheter and collection bag are considered to be grossly contaminated because they have been in contact with body fluids. Measure urine in the drainage bag and record in the designated location. *Rationale: Proper disposal helps prevent transmission of microorganisms. Urine measurement provides an accurate record of output.*

5. Assist the client to cleanse and dry the perineal area and to assume a comfortable position. *Rationale: These measures ensure comfort.*
Follow ENDDD steps

Special Reminder
- Be sure to document client education (see In Practice: Educating the Client 57-2) along with other necessary documentation.

58 Special Skin and Wound Care

Learning Objectives

1. Identify and describe the following types of wounds: abrasion, puncture, laceration, and surgical incision.
2. Describe the concept of skin breakdown, including the causes, most common locations, and staging of pressure injuries.
3. Describe the evaluation of risk factors for skin breakdown and how these data are used.
4. Describe nursing measures that help prevent skin breakdown.
5. Give examples of procedures and equipment used to care for a pressure injury or other open wounds.
6. Describe the three types of wound healing.
7. Explain three purposes of wound dressings.
8. Demonstrate how to change a dry, sterile dressing; how to apply a wet-to-dry dressing; and how to irrigate a wound.
9. Describe common types of wound drainage systems, including the VAC.
10. Describe how sutures and staples are removed.

Important Terminology

abrasion	eschar	pressure	surgical incision	wet-to-dry dressing
debridement	exudate	pressure injury	suture	wound
diabetic ulcer/ wound	friction	puncture	tunneling	
drain	granulation	shear	undermining	
drainage	laceration	sinus tract	venous stasis	
	packing	slough	ulcer	

Acronyms

ABD
IAD
NPUAP
NPWT
VAC
WOCN

The skin acts as the body's protective barrier against the potentially harmful external environment. When the skin's *integrity* (intactness) is broken, the body's internal environment is open to microorganisms that may be harmful.

Any abnormal opening or break in the skin is a **wound**. It is an important nursing responsibility to inspect the client's skin carefully on admission to a facility and frequently thereafter for *any signs of pressure or skin breakdown*. It is vital to prevent skin breakdown and, if it occurs, to report it immediately and treat it as ordered. (If skin breakdown occurs in the facility, that facility is responsible and will not be reimbursed for expenses.)

> **Key Concept**
> Skin breakdown is a particular problem in clients who are obese (bariatric clients).

WOUNDS

A wound is described as a physical injury causing a break in the skin or mucous membrane. The most common types of wounds are trauma (accidental or self-inflicted) wounds, surgical incisions, and several types of ulcers. (An external ulcer is a defect or break in the skin produced by sloughing away of dead inflammatory tissue. Ulcers may also occur in mucous membranes.) Other types of skin abnormalities include infections, rashes, lesions, and burns (see Chapters 47 and 75). A wound may be *accidental* or *unintentional*, such as an **abrasion** (rubbing off of the skin's surface [e.g., a skinned knee]); a **puncture** wound (stab wound); or a **laceration** (wound with torn, ragged edges [e.g., an accidental or self-inflicted cut]). A non–self-inflicted wound may be *intentional*, such as a **surgical incision** (a wound with clean edges). A wound that occurs accidentally or that is self-inflicted is assumed to be contaminated; intentional surgical incisions are made under sterile conditions and are kept as free from microorganisms as possible (Fig. 58-1).

Inspection and Description of Wounds

Skin inspection includes visual inspection as well as palpation, with special emphasis on body prominences, and careful and accurate documentation. Special inspection sites include the back of the head, ears, heels, coccyx, shoulder blades, and elbows, as well as sites of intravenous (IV) infusions, IM injections, and tracheostomies or other invasive procedures (see Fig. 58-2). Note whether the skin blanches when pressed or if it remains red or discolored. The first sign of skin irritation is often itching. Prediction of possible skin breakdown is discussed later in this chapter. (TED stockings, splints, and other devices are removed for skin inspection.) A group of procedures, called the *Skin Bundle*, are implemented to prevent skin breakdown in clients at risk.

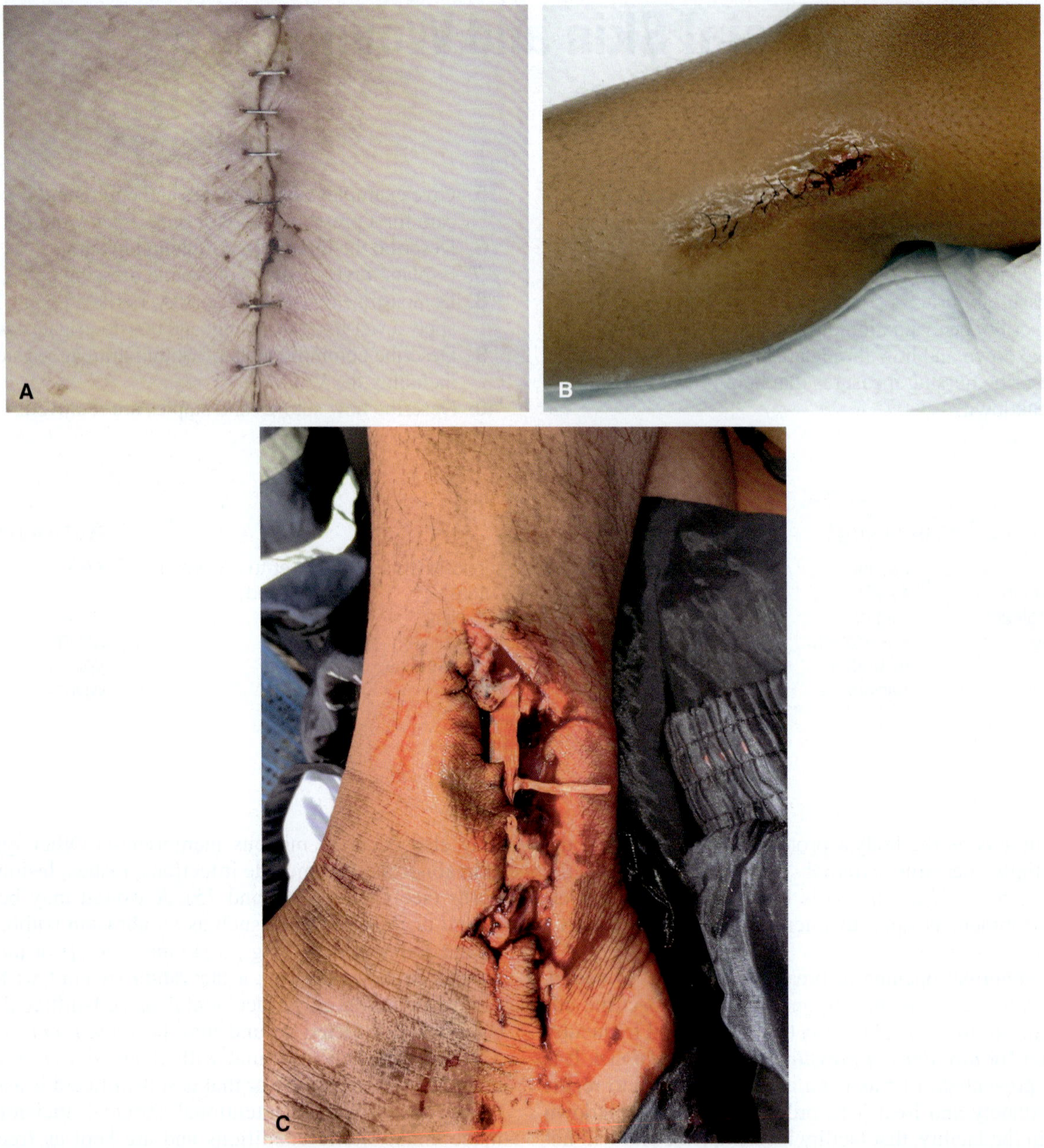

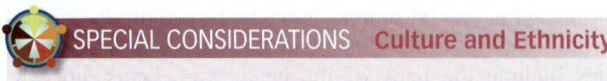

Figure 58-1 Types of wounds. **A.** A surgical incision is an *intentional* wound. Here, the edges are brought together and stapled (Craven & Hirnle, 2007). **B.** A surgical incision closed with sutures (stitches) (Lynn, 2008). **C.** An *unintentional* wound, shown here, results from trauma. Open unintentional wounds have a high risk of infection. (C: Dr P. Marazzi/Science Photo Library.)

SPECIAL CONSIDERATIONS — Culture and Ethnicity

Skin Observation: Color Changes Caused by Pressure Injuries

Darkly pigmented skin—damage may show as purplish, bluish, or gray and shiny.

Olive tone skin—not likely to have red tones—compare with surrounding skin or opposite side.

Lightly pigmented skin—defined area of persistent redness or purple appearance.

Wounds are diagnosed by the healthcare provider by several methods. Vascular (blood vessel) ulcers may be evaluated by using angiograms or the laser Doppler. Laboratory testing, including biopsy and wound culture, yields information about the cause and appropriate treatment of a wound. It is important for the nurse to observe, describe, and document all wounds carefully, including pressure injuries and surgical incisions. Report pertinent observations to the provider. In Practice: Data Gathering in Nursing 58-1 lists items that must be addressed for all wounds. Computer documentation contains a wound evaluation template, to ensure consistency between caregivers. See In Practice: Nursing Procedure 58-1 to review steps for inspecting, cleaning, and dressing a wound. (Chapter 47 contains key points for skin inspection.)

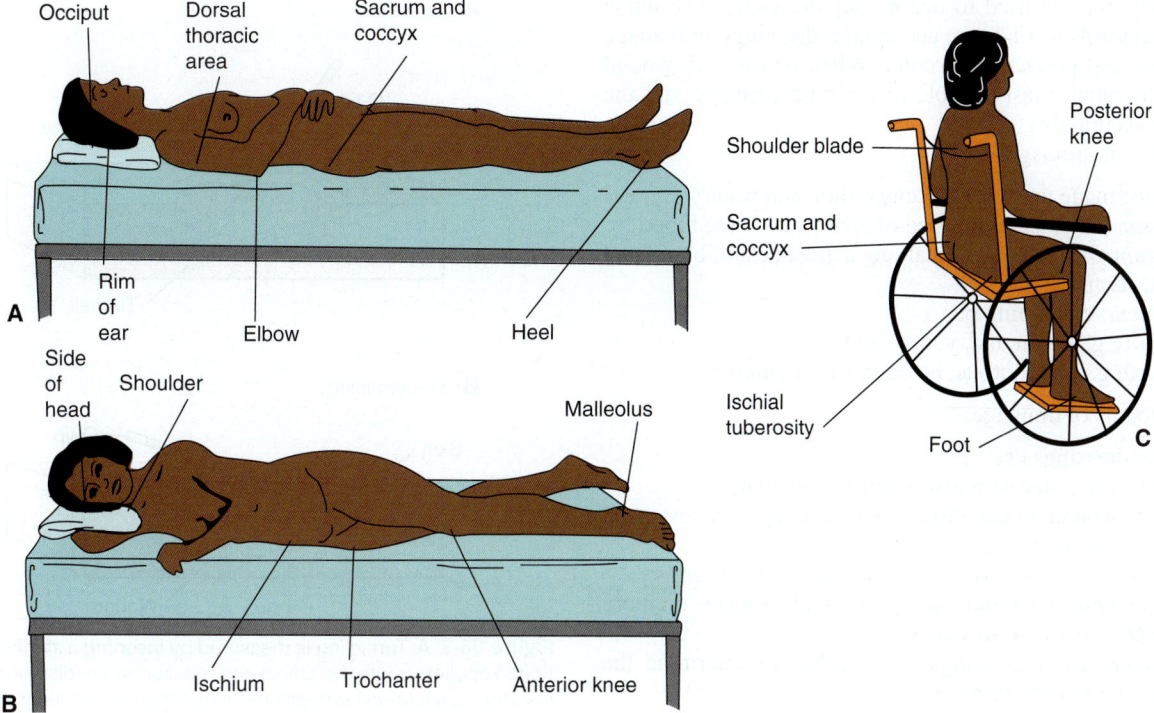

Figure 58-2 Common sites for pressure injuries **A.** Supine position. **B.** Side-lying position. **C.** Sitting. Included also are sites of tube insertion (e.g., IV, NG tube, catheter, drains).

> **Nursing Alert** Avoid inspecting wounds under fluorescent lights when observing wound/skin color. *Rationale:* Fluorescent lights may create an incorrectly diagnosed abnormal skin color or may mask variations in the client's skin tone.

Drainage

Discharge from a wound is called **drainage**. Wounds, particularly unintentional wounds, often have drainage. Drainage containing a great deal of protein and cellular debris, usually as a result of inflammation, is called **exudate** (although

---

IN PRACTICE
DATA GATHERING IN NURSING 58-1 | Describing a Client's Wound

Clearly describe a wound by including the following:
- Exact anatomic location (e.g., include distance in centimeters [cm] or millimeters [mm] from wrist, elbow, knee)
- Duration of wound (how long has it been there?)
- Exact dimensions: width, length, and depth (in mm/cm). Measure depth with a sterile cotton-tipped applicator
- Color and appearance of wound bed and of surrounding (*periwound*) tissue (closed or rolled, open, calloused, macerated, color)
- Presence of undermining or tunneling
- Specific appearance of areas of the wound, identified by using the hands of the clock as a reference
- Extent of tissue loss; percentage of each type of tissue (granulation, subcutaneous, muscle, eschar, leathery, slough)
- New tissue formation in margins; appearance of wound edges
- Presence or absence of exudate (drainage) and its description (odor, amount, color, general appearance)
- Warmth, coldness, hardness, softness, and other observations around wound
- Subjective complaints (and description) of pain, tightness, itching, or other symptoms
- Presence of any foreign bodies (sutures, staples, gauze, dressings, medications)
- Diagram of wound, if irregular in shape
- Other objective assessments (e.g., body temperature, blood tests)
- To determine changes in skin color and possible areas of damage, look at surrounding skin for comparison or compare one side of the client's body to the other
- Other signs of damage may include skin that is tender, indurated (swollen), boggy, or edematous to palpation.

this term may be used to denote any drainage). The nurse often performs wound care and applies dressings, to manage drainage and protect the wound. When performing wound care, the nurse must be able to describe drainage and the wound accurately.

Types of drainage:

- *Serous*: made up of serum; clear, thin, and watery
- *Serosanguineous*: composed of serum and some blood
- *Sanguineous*: bloody, containing a great deal of blood and some serum
- *Purulent*: containing pus
- *Color* (e.g., green, tan, yellow, red)
- *Odor* (e.g., malodorous, no odor, sweet-smelling)

Amounts of drainage:

- *None*: dressings dry
- *Scant*: wound tissue moist, no visible exudate
- *Small*: wound moist throughout, drainage on less than 25% of dressings
- *Moderate*: drainage on about 30%–60% of dressings
- *Large/copious*: wound tissues saturated; drainage on more than 60%–75% of dressings
- In some cases, dressings are weighed to determine the exact amount of drainage.

SPECIAL CONSIDERATIONS

All clients must have a complete skin inspection on admission to any nursing facility. This must be carefully documented. (In some facilities, Psychiatric and Obstetric clients are exempt, unless a wound is obvious.) Skin inspection must be performed on a regular basis thereafter, per facility protocol, and documented carefully (to monitor for any sign of skin breakdown). Any skin breakdown or apparent infection must be reported immediately.

> **NCLEX Alert**
>
> This chapter provides information on your role in inspecting clients' skin integrity and describing wounds. This information may be integrated into test scenarios and must be considered as you answer test questions.

Other Characteristics of Wounds

Tunneling
Tunneling refers to the one or more channels within or underlying an open wound. Each tunnel extends in only one direction. Tunneling depth is measured by inserting a sterile cotton-tipped applicator into the tunnel and then measuring the distance it was inserted (Fig. 58-3A).

Undermining
If tissue recedes beneath the skin, creating a shelf of skin or free edge with a space underneath, this is referred to as **undermining** (Fig. 58-3B). The distance the undermining extends behind the edge of the shelf is also measured with a sterile applicator and documented (see Fig. 58-4C).

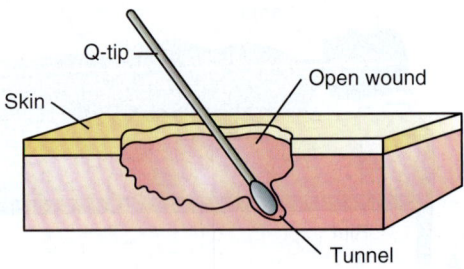

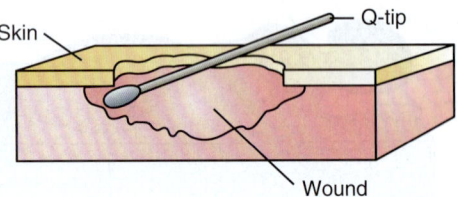

Figure 58-3 A. Tunneling is measured by inserting a sterile cotton-tipped applicator into the tunnel and measuring the distance of insertion. Each tunnel is measured and documented separately. **B.** Undermining is also measured using a sterile applicator. Usually, the undermining extends around the entire circumference of the wound, although the extent of the undermining may vary.

Wound Edges
The appearance of wound edges should be documented. For example, they may be *rolled under*—the top layer of epidermis is rolled down over the lower edge of the wound (closed), *macerated* (softened by moisture), or *calloused* (very hard, yellow to white). The wound edge may be *open*; the edge looks healthy, with evidence of tissue growth at the rim.

Periwound Area
Note the appearance of the area around the wound. Descriptive terms include intact, pink, erythema (redness), excoriated (scratch or abrasion), blistered, ecchymotic (hemorrhagic spot, blue or purple), denuded (skin stripped away), blistered, macerated, and many others. Include a descriptive comment, if necessary.

Wound Base
In some cases, the wound base cannot be visualized. Otherwise, describe the color, character, and appearance of the wound base. Does it contain **granulation** (soft and pinkish) tissue, slough, or eschar? Does it appear moist or dry? Is it beginning to resurface? Describe the color and percentage of different types of tissue.

Wound Measurement
There are a number of ways in which wounds may be measured. These include

- *Linear measurement*—a ruler is used to measure the width and length of a wound. This does not measure wound depth and is not well suited to an irregular wound.

CHAPTER 58 Special Skin and Wound Care

- *Planimetry*—graph paper is used to duplicate the shape of a wound. This can allow a large, irregular wound to be drawn to scale and is best used for a flat wound. Be sure to indicate the scale used (e.g., 1 cm = 1 in.).
- *Stereophotogrammetry*—a special video camera downloads to a computer. This method allows for color images and is noninvasive. It also gives some indication of wound depth.
- *Wound photography*—photos of the wound illustrate the color of the wound bed and its edges, as well as giving an indication of the condition of surrounding skin.
- *Wound tracing*—transparent paper may be laid over the wound and the edges lightly traced. This is effective for flat, irregular wounds.

Additional description of wounds is contained in the discussion of pressure injuries below.

Causes of Skin Breakdown

Disruption of skin integrity, nonintact skin, commonly called *skin breakdown*, is a potential complication for any client, but particularly those confined to a bed or wheelchair. This also includes the person with a body cast, traction, or the person who is paralyzed or otherwise cannot move without assistance. In other cases, skin breakdown can occur as a result of factors such as moisture, external pressure, infection, or rash, in any client. A common cause is *shearing force* (friction) caused by clothing, bed linens, or client safety devices.

Conditions contributing to skin breakdown are

- Immobility, low level of activity (lying/sitting in one position for extended periods of time, paralysis)
- Inadequate nutrition (very thin person; inadequate protein, insufficient calories)
- Hydration levels (inadequate fluid intake, excess fluid retention—edema)
- Presence of external moisture (including perspiration, urine, and feces); incontinence
- Impaired mental status, alertness, or cooperation; heavy sedation and/or anesthesia; mental illness, intellectual impairment
- Sensory loss; coma
- Fever; low blood pressure (particularly diastolic < 60 mm)
- Advancing age, friable skin
- Infancy
- Impaired immune system (AIDS, cancer chemotherapy)
- Presence of cancer or other neoplasms
- Circulatory disorders; anemia
- Diabetes

These factors are to be considered for all clients. Good nursing care can alter some of these factors, to prevent skin breakdown. The client with a past history of skin breakdown is particularly vulnerable.

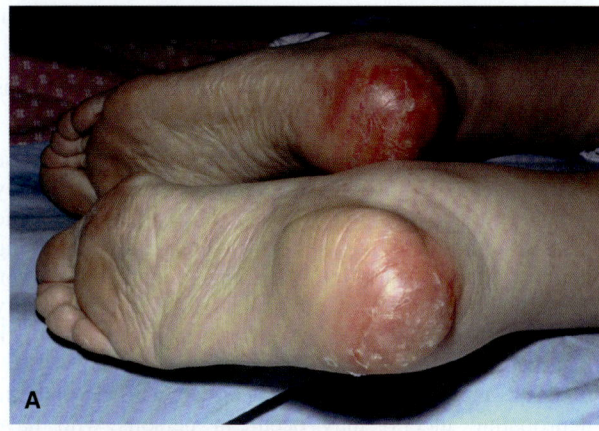
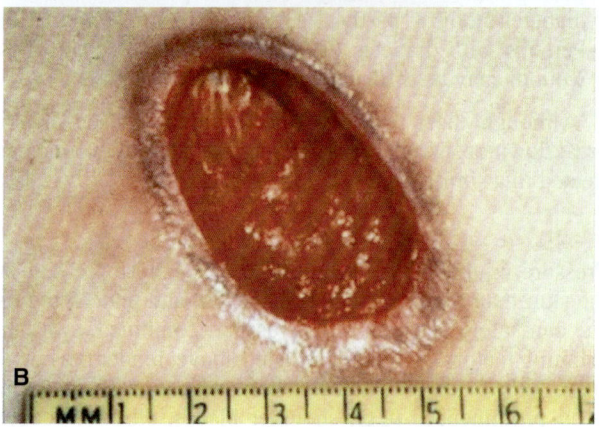
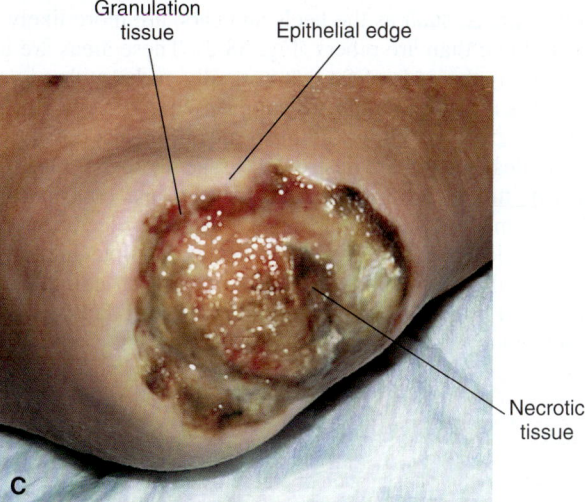

Figure 58-4 Stages of pressure injuries (see also Box 58-1). Stage I (reversible) includes pressure-related changes in intact skin, when compared with adjacent skin (not shown). Some pressure injuries are not stageable. The pressure injuries shown here are **(A)** Stage II: partial-thickness tissue loss. No sloughing; may appear as a blister. **B.** Stage III: full-thickness tissue loss, with subcutaneous damage and drainage. May show tunneling or undermining. (Note procedure for measuring the size of the wound.) **C.** Stage IV: full-thickness tissue loss, extensive destruction of muscle, bone, or other structures. Note undermining shown on the upper edge of the wound. (A: Mike Devlin/Science Photo Library; B: Lynn, 2018; C: Timby, 2013.)

NCLEX Alert

It will be important for you to understand the causes of skin breakdown and types of wounds/ulcers as they relate to client teaching and nursing actions to prevent skin and tissue damage. For example, you may be asked to select the appropriate nursing actions to prevent the development of pressure injuries during your NCLEX examination.

Types of Skin Breakdown

The discussion of unintentional wounds in this book is based, in large part, on prevention and treatment of skin breakdown and pressure injuries (formerly known as decubitus ulcers [plural: decubiti] or pressure injuries). Prevention of skin breakdown is a primary nursing responsibility. Types of skin breakdown include

- *Incontinence-associated dermatitis* (**IAD**). The client who is incontinent of urine or stool must have meticulous skin care, to prevent skin breakdown. Several means are available to help prevent IAD and new products are constantly being developed. Using an incontinence cleanser (e.g., Remedy Spray Cleanser, which does not dry skin) and a moisture barrier paste (e.g., Calazime, which protects skin) *before damage occurs* can be helpful. Special *barrier cream wipes* are available, for the client with chronic incontinence. Disposable paper washcloths should be used instead of cloth washcloths; dispose of them in the trash—do not flush. *Do not use* Bag Bath, shaving cream, or alcohol-based cleansers, which can irritate and dry out the skin. Hemorrhoidal ointment, as well as glycerin, lanolin, or mineral oil, can also be helpful. Be sure to keep the client as dry and clean as possible. Table 58-1 compares IAD with pressure injuries.
- Pressure injury: This wound is a localized injury to the skin and/or underlying tissue, usually over a bony prominence. Most often this is caused by **pressure** or pressure combined with **shear** and/or **friction**. Pressure causes a disruption in circulation, leading to tissue death (necrosis). Friction is the rubbing of one surface against another, and shear is the interaction of friction and gravity when tissue is moved across a material (such as a bedsheet). Some of the stages of a pressure injury (formerly called "bedsore" or pressure sore) are pictured in Figure 58-4. The stages and treatment of pressure injuries are discussed later in this chapter.

In addition to pressure injuries, two other skin ulcerations may occur:

- **Venous stasis ulcer** (venous insufficiency wound)—these wounds develop most often in the lower extremities. They are the result of local hypoxia (lack of oxygen) to specific tissues. A number of theories exist to their cause, including poor oxygen diffusion into the tissue, venous congestion caused by overly large white blood cells, and the inability of cells in the affected area to obtain appropriate growth factors.
- **Diabetic ulcers**—these wounds (also called diabetic neuropathic ulcers) may occur in persons who have diabetes mellitus, partly as a result of impaired circulation. Persons with diabetes often are slow to heal, and these wounds may be difficult to treat (see Chapter 79).

Although there are a number of other causes of skin breakdown or disruption of skin integrity, many wounds are treated in a similar manner.

Pressure Injuries

Pressure injuries are usually the result of more pressure on the skin than the particular client's skin and underlying tissue can safely tolerate. Skin pressure, combined with contributing factors such as those listed above, render the person susceptible to skin breakdown. Certain body areas, including bony prominences (e.g., shoulder blades, elbows, coccyx, hips, knees, sides of the ankles, and back of the head), as well as areas, such as the heels and ears, are more likely to break down than are others (Fig. 58-2). These areas are not covered by the pads of fat that normally cushion blood vessels. When blood vessels are compressed and blood flow is reduced, oxygen supply diminishes, skin breaks down, and the tissues beneath are destroyed (tissue necrosis). Insertion sites of tubes can also become irritated and contribute to skin or mucous membrane breakdown. An ulceration can also develop in an obese person, under pendulous breasts or abdominal folds. This type of wound is often complicated by a yeast infection. It is important to keep all these areas as clean and dry as possible.

> **NCLEX Alert**
>
> Be alert to the classification of pressure injuries, as well as the objectives and methods of wound care. You may be asked to demonstrate your knowledge in the NCLEX examination.

Prediction of Pressure Injury Risk

All clients must be evaluated for the risk of developing pressure injuries or skin breakdown on admission and regularly thereafter, according to facility protocol. Protocol usually requires more frequent skin examinations of clients in the intensive care unit (ICU) and pediatric unit. Several methods are used to predict the risk of pressure injury development. Two of these are the Braden Scale (Fig. 58-5) and the Norton Scale. If a client is found to be at high risk, special measures must be taken to prevent the development of pressure injuries before they occur.

TABLE 58-1 Differences Between Incontinence-Associated Dermatitis and Pressure Injury

	INCONTINENCE-ASSOCIATED DERMATITIS	PRESSURE INJURY
Cause	Moisture; irritants in feces and urine	Pressure or rubbing
Prevention	Meticulous skin care; keep client clean and dry; apply barrier creams	Prevent pressure areas, turn often, etc.
Location	May be located anywhere on the body	Usually on a bony prominence or area that rubs
Pattern of redness	Diffuse; extends to the perineum and upper thighs	Surrounding the pressure area only
Tissue loss	Usually limited to dermis and epidermis	May extend to muscle and bone

BRADEN SCALE FOR PREDICTING PRESSURE SORE RISK

Patient's Name _____ Evaluator's Name _____ Date of Assessment _____

	1	2	3	4				
SENSORY PERCEPTION Ability to respond meaningfully to pressure-related discomfort	**1. Completely Limited** Unresponsive (does not moan, flinch, or grasp) to painful stimuli, due to diminished level of consciousness or sedation. OR limited ability to feel pain over most of body.	**2. Very Limited** Responds only to painful stimuli. Cannot communicate discomfort except by moaning or restlessness OR has a sensory impairment which limits the ability to feel pain or discomfort over ½ of body.	**3. Slightly Limited** Responds to verbal commands, but cannot always communicate discomfort or the need to be turned OR has some sensory impairment which limits ability to feel pain or discomfort in one or two extremities.	**4. No Impairment** Responds to verbal commands. Has no sensory deficit which would limit ability to feel or voice pain or discomfort.				
MOISTURE Degree to which skin is exposed to moisture	**1. Constantly Moist** Skin is kept moist almost constantly by perspiration, urine, etc. Dampness is detected every time patient is moved or turned.	**2. Very Moist** Skin is often, but not always moist. Linen must be changed at least once a shift.	**3. Occasionally Moist** Skin is occasionally moist, requiring an extra linen change approximately once a day.	**4. Rarely Moist** Skin is usually dry, linen only requires changing at routine intervals.				
ACTIVITY Degree of physical activity	**1. Bedfast** Confined to bed.	**2. Chairfast** Ability to walk severely limited or non-existent. Cannot bear own weight and/or must be assisted into chair or wheelchair.	**3. Walks Occasionally** Walks occasionally during day, but for very short distances, with or without assistance. Spends majority of each shift in bed or chair.	**4. Walks Frequently** Walks outside room at least twice a day and inside room at least once every 2 hours during waking hours.				
MOBILITY Ability to change and control body position	**1. Completely Immobile** Does not make even slight changes in body or extremity position without assistance.	**2. Very Limited** Makes occasional slight changes in body or extremity position but unable to make frequent or significant changes independently.	**3. Slightly Limited** Makes frequent though slight changes in body or extremity position independently.	**4. No Limitation** Makes major and frequent changes in position without changes.				
NUTRITION Usual food intake pattern	**1. Very Poor** Never eats a complete meal. Rarely eats more than ⅓ of any food offered. Eats two servings or less of protein (meat or dairy products) per day. Takes fluids poorly. Does not take a liquid dietary supplement OR is NPO and/or maintained on clear liquids or IVs for more than 5 days.	**2. Probably Inadequate** Rarely eats a complete meal and generally eats only about ½ of any food offered. Protein intake includes only three servings of meat or dairy products per day. Occasionally will take a dietary supplement OR receives less than optimum amount of liquid diet or tube feeding.	**3. Adequate** Eats over half of most meals. Eats a total of four servings of protein (meat, dairy products) per day. Occasionally will refuse a meal, but will usually take a supplement when offered OR is on a tube feeding or TPN regimen which probably meets most of nutritional needs.	**4. Excellent** Eats most of every meal. Never refuses a meal. Usually eats a total of four or more servings of meat and dairy products. Occasionally eats between meals. Does not require supplementation.				
FRICTION & SHEAR	**1. Problem** Requires moderate to maximum assistance in moving. Complete lifting without sliding against sheets is impossible. Frequently slides down in bed or chair, requiring frequent repositioning with maximum assistance. Spasticity, contractures, or agitation leads to almost constant friction.	**2. Potential Problem** Moves feebly or requires minimum assistance. During a move skin probably slides to some extent against sheets, chair, restraints, or other devices. Maintains relatively good position in chair or bed most of the time but occasionally slides down.	**3. No Apparent Problem** Moves in bed and in chair independently and has sufficient muscle strength to lift up completely during move. Maintains good position in bed or chair.					
				Total Score				

Figure 58-5 Braden Assessment Scale for Predicting Pressure Injury Risk. Total possible points = 23. *The lower the score, the greater the risk.* The client is identified as at risk for pressure injury development if the score is less than 18. (Some facilities use scores from 15 to 18 as the risk prediction score.) A modified scale (Braden Q) is available for use with pediatric clients. The Braden Q also considers tissue perfusion and oxygenation; the risk cutoff score on the Braden Q for children is usually 23. (© 2021 Health Sense Ai. All rights reserved. All copyrights and trademarks are the property of Health Sense Ai or their respective owners or assigns.)

> **Nursing Alert** If a client is admitted to a facility with an existing wound or pressure area, this must be carefully documented as "present on admission." As stated before, if this is not documented, the facility will become liable for this and any additional skin breakdown. In addition, if a wound exists, plans can be made to begin immediate treatment.

A "facility-acquired" pressure area is considered to be a *sentinel event* and must be reported to the appropriate authorities. If stage III, IV, or nonstageable injuries develop within a facility, this usually must be reported to the Health Department and investigated. It is important to note that pressure injuries usually occur within 12–24 hr in the compromised client. The wound begins deep in the tissue and may not be observed on the skin surface for several days. Signs of an evolving pressure injury are nonblanching erythema (redness that does not lighten when pressed), pain, and induration (swelling).

> **Nursing Alert** Do not rub or massage any area if the above signs/symptoms are present. This added pressure may cause breakdown of small blood vessels, thereby worsening the skin's condition.

The Braden Scale

One of the evaluative scales used to predict a client's risk of developing pressure areas is the Braden Scale (see Fig. 58-5). This scale considers the primary factors related to pressure injury development—*intensity and duration* of pressure and *tissue tolerance* of pressure. The following factors are included in the rating scale: sensory perception, moisture level, activity, mobility, nutrition, and friction/shear. The use of such a scale allows healthcare personnel to take steps to prevent the development of skin breakdown in clients at high risk. (*The lower the score, the greater the risk.*) Table 58-2 identifies factors in management of clients at risk for skin/tissue breakdown. All clients should have a risk evaluation on admission and regularly during their stay in a facility.

TABLE 58-2 Preventive Measures for Common Causes of Wounds

CAUSES OF WOUNDS	LOCATION	PREVENTION[a]
Pressure		
External force sufficient to occlude blood in capillaries, resulting in tissue anoxia (lack of oxygen) and tissue death (necrosis)	Especially bony prominences	Establish a turning schedule at least every 2 hr. Use supportive measures to relieve pressure (see Box 58-3). Keep pressure off bony prominences and other vulnerable areas, by elevating them with pillows and by using padding and special beds. Have a minimum of linens under the client. Avoid donut devices. Assist the client to be out of bed and/or walking as soon as possible.
Shear		
Interaction of gravity and friction against the skin's surface (appears as a cut or tear)	Surfaces exposed to bed or chair, especially if skin turgor is poor; coccyx most common site	Use draw sheet and lifting/turning sheet or client lift. Use logroll turns. Avoid dragging client's body over sheets. Limit elevation of head of bed to 30°. Position feet against footboard before head elevation. Request assistance when necessary.
Friction		
Superficial abrasion, resulting from the skin rubbing another surface (results in scrape, abrasion, or blister)	Surfaces that rub on bed or chair surfaces or against each other. Sites of tube insertion, IV, NG tube, drains, etc.	Apply transparent dressings to areas of friction (to prevent rubbing and facilitate observation without dressing removal). Move client carefully. Use trapeze, client lift, etc. Use elbow protectors and elevate heels off bed. Keep skin adequately hydrated. Use lotion and special skin barrier products. Use friction-reducing sheets for turning and positioning. Use a bridge (transfer board) to move clients (be sure linens are between client's skin and the bridge). Use a client lift, when needed.
Stripping		
Unintentional removal of epidermis by mechanical means, such as with tape removal	Surfaces where applied	Use only porous tapes and apply without tension, if possible. Use saline, to help remove dressings that adhere to the skin. Remove tape by slowly pulling tape away with one hand, while supporting surrounding skin with the other. Use alternatives to tape, such as Montgomery straps or Kerlix to wrap a limb, or use a stockinette. Use tube-gauze dressing, rather than tape.

TABLE 58-2 Preventive Measures for Common Causes of Wounds (Continued)

CAUSES OF WOUNDS	LOCATION	PREVENTION[a]
Urine or Stool Urinary and fecal incontinence	Perianal skin	Use containment equipment (e.g., absorptive products, condom catheters, fecal pouches). Keep perianal skin cleansed, moisturized, and protected with barrier ointments or creams. Investigate cause (e.g., urinary infection, incontinence, need for toileting schedule, impaction, diarrhea, constipation, organisms in stool, tube-feeding intolerance, lactose intolerance, reactions to medications). Offer bedpan/urinal and fluids each time client is turned.
Perspiration	Areas where moisture can get trapped and air cannot circulate (e.g., skin folds, under breasts)	Keep areas of skin folds dry. Use barrier ointments, as prescribed. Use antifungal powder or other prescribed medication, if yeast infection is present. (Creams are often contraindicated.)
Arterial Insufficiency Arterial perfusion jeopardized	Feet, toes, and lower leg; edematous areas	Avoid compression. Protect from mechanical, chemical, or thermal injuries. Provide adequate remoisturizing. Take special care with diabetic clients, paralyzed persons, or persons with a bleeding disorder. Elevate edematous feet and legs.
Maceration		
Burns/Frostbite Improper use of heat or cold sources	Under pendulous breasts or folds of abdomen Any area	Wash thoroughly at least once per day. Expose to air, if possible. Apply powder or prescribed medicinal cream. Encourage female client to wear a bra when up, if possible. Cautious use of any external heat source, including a fireplace, or holding a laptop computer on the lap for an extended length of time. Very careful use of ice packs, etc.

IV, intravenous; NG, nasogastric.
[a]*Special note:* Some of these measures require a specific order by the primary provider. Check local protocols. A risk evaluation should be performed on each client and measures taken to prevent skin breakdown in all clients, particularly those most vulnerable.

Classification of Pressure Injuries

Pressure injuries are classified according to their stages of development (Box 58-1 and Fig. 58-4). In the fourth stage, a thick, leathery black crust of necrotic (dead) tissue, called **eschar**, often develops around the edges (see Figs. 47-17 and 58-4C). Eschar that separates from living tissue is called **slough** and is often tan or yellow. **Debridement** (de-breed-ment; removal of dead or infected tissues) allows healthy tissue to grow, progressing from internal tissue outward. Box 58-2 lists other types of wounds that are treated in a manner similar to that used for pressure injuries. Two national sources of information regarding wound prevention and pressure injury staging, prevention, and treatment are the National Pressure Injury Advisory Panel (**NPIAP**) and the Wound, Ostomy, and Continence Nurses Society (**WOCN**). Remember: If a client with a pressure injury or any other wound is to be sent to the operating room, x-ray, or any therapy, notify that department so appropriate measures can be taken to protect the wound and prevent the spread of infection.

Prevention of Pressure Injuries

Always remain alert for signs of pressure on the client's body (see Box 58-1). Be particularly observant when giving a bath or a back rub. The client may also report painful spots. Report any signs of pressure or *reddened/darkened* areas that do not return to normal hue (color) after pressure is removed. Follow the suggestions in the text for all clients at risk and those with obvious skin breakdown (see also discussion of Braden Scale). Turn and reposition immobile clients frequently, to prevent pressure on any one body area. Assist clients who cannot lift themselves. Do not pull the client across bed linens, which could cause a shearing-force injury (see Chapter 48).

Donut devices *are not used* to prevent pressure injury development. Their use is specifically contraindicated.

Assist clients to obtain adequate nutrition and hydration. Clients at risk should have a nutrition consult. To promote wound healing, a high-calorie, high-protein diet with supplemental vitamins (particularly vitamins A, C, and E) may be ordered. The client at risk often requires protein supplements between meals as well. The nurse is often ordered to encourage fluids (of varying types) for these clients, to promote adequate hydration. *Rationale: It is important to maintain skin hydration and elasticity. Dry, scaly skin is more subject to breakdown than is well-hydrated skin.*

| Box 58-1 | Stages of Pressure Injury Classification (see also Fig. 58-4) |

Stage 1 (I): Pressure-related alteration of intact skin, as compared with adjacent/opposite body area. May include changes in (one or more) *skin temperature* (warmth/coolness), *tissue consistency* (firm/boggy/mushy), *induration* (swelling), or *sensation* (pain/itching). Wound/ulcer appears as a defined area of persistent redness in lightly pigmented skin; in darker skin, may appear as persistent red, blue, or purple hue. (The color does not blanch/lighten when pressed.) Reversible, if pressure is relieved (by frequent turning, positioning, and pressure-relieving devices).

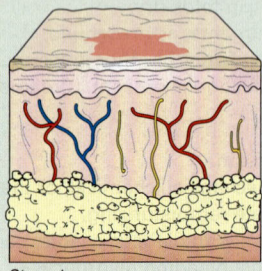
Stage 1

Stage 2 (II): Loss of epidermis with damage into dermis (partial-thickness tissue loss); appears as shallow crater/blister with red/pink wound bed, with no sloughing. May also appear as an intact or ruptured serum-filled blister or abrasion. Swollen and painful; several weeks needed to heal after pressure is relieved, often by maintenance of a moist environment (e.g., saline irrigation or special occlusive dressing).

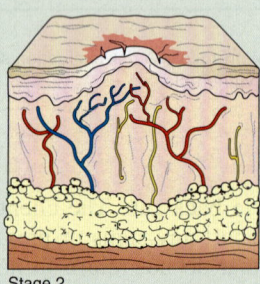
Stage 2

Stage 3 (III): Subcutaneous tissues involved (full-thickness tissue loss); subcutaneous fat may be visible (no bone, tendon, or muscle exposed). May show undermining or tunneling. Usually not painful; possible foul-smelling drainage; months may be needed to heal after pressure is relieved (e.g., by debriding with wet-to-dry dressings, surgery, or proteolytic enzymes).

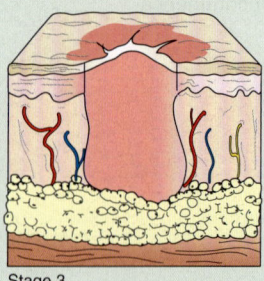
Stage 3

Stage 4 (IV): Extensive damage to underlying structures; full-thickness tissue loss, with exposed bones, tendons, or muscles. (Wound possibly appearing small on surface, but with extensive tunneling underneath.) Slough or eschar may be present. Usually foul-smelling discharge; months or years may be needed for healing (often requires skin grafting).

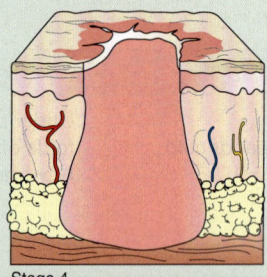
Stage 4

Nonstageable: The base of a full-thickness wound, covered by slough and/or eschar.

Deep-tissue injury: Purple or maroon intact skin, or blood-filled blister.

As a pressure wound heals, the stages do not reverse (e.g., a stage IV wound cannot become a stage III). This wound could be referred to as a "healing (or healed) stage IV pressure wound." Do not confuse a pressure wound with skin damage caused by incontinence or friction/shear.

Key Concept

A shallow wound on an area such as the nose, ear, occiput, or malleolus may be stage III or IV, even though it is not deep.

Keep the skin free of external moisture and body fluids, such as urine and feces. External moisture, particularly when combined with continuous pressure, predisposes the skin to breakdown. Pathogens from an infected wound or feces can be dangerous, particularly where a skin break exists. The incontinent client is particularly vulnerable to skin breakdown. Always wear gloves when caring for any wound. Wash hands thoroughly before and after any treatment. Table 58-2 and Box 58-3 list preventive measures used for the client at risk for skin breakdown. It is important to remember that as soon as a skin break occurs, the path to infection is open. In addition, the individual client's physical condition and probable extent and duration of illness or disability help determine the most effective prevention

| Box 58-2 | Other Wounds Treated in a Manner Similar to That Used for Pressure Injuries |

- Frostbite (often treated as a burn)
- Thermal burns
- Venous stasis ulcers/wounds
- Pressure injuries (difficult to treat because of high blood sugar, compromised circulation, poor kidney function, and other complications of diabetes)
- Large gunshot wounds or other large open wounds (may be left open to heal from the inside outward)
- Surgical incisions that have become seriously infected or that have opened (dehiscence, with or without evisceration)

> **Key Concept**
>
> Deep open wounds must granulate in (heal) from the inside outward. If the outside becomes sealed before the area underneath has healed, an abscess often forms. This abscess may be sterile or infected (containing pathogens). An abscess is painful and dangerous and must be treated. Reporting of granulation tissue is a part of pressure injury documentation.

Box 58-3 Prevention of Skin Breakdown

SKIN, MUCOUS MEMBRANE PROTECTION
- Careful and frequent skin cleansing
- Drying powder and dry lubricants
- Humidification
- Gauze or other protection between skin folds
- Heel protectors, if heel elevation not possible
- Hydrocolloids; skin barrier cream
- Incontinence pads
- Lip lubricant and careful oral hygiene
- Protective mittens (prevent scratching)
- Protective footwear for ambulatory clients
- Pouching devices (to catch drainage)
- Skin sealant/moisture barrier
- Topical antibiotics
- Transparent film, to cover wounds
- Minimum layers of linens under the client
- Use of products such as Oxi-Ears and InterDry Silver nitrate
- Special attention to the client with diabetes

PRESSURE-REDUCING TECHNIQUES
- Very frequent client examinations
- Turn/reposition client at least every 2 hr (with specific, documented, turning schedule)
- Use of logroll turns (prevent shear)
- Use of client lift (prevent shear and nurse injury)
- Elevate heels off bed (better than padding heels)
- Elevate head of bed no more than 30° (prevent shear)
- Nutritional consult, to determine best dietary plan
- Careful perianal care (use of protective creams, ointments, sitz baths, skin barriers)
- Careful personal hygiene (e.g., hair removal, nail care, oral hygiene)
- Careful use of standard precautions for all staff

PRESSURE-REDUCING DEVICES
- Chair cushion, gel pads, heel elevators
- Padding of chin and nose
- Elbow protectors
- Mechanical lifts
- Transfer board
- Trapeze over bed
- Use of turning sheet
- Positioning supports
- Specialty beds and mattresses (e.g., air mattress, rotating mattress)

efforts. Many immobile clients are placed on special beds or mattresses, to help reduce pressure and prevent skin breakdown (see Chapter 49). Encourage all clients to move themselves as much as possible. The major consideration with regard to pressure injuries is *prevention*. After a pressure injury has developed, it is usually very difficult to treat.

WOUND HEALING

Special Skin and Wound Care, Animation: Wound Healing

Wound healing differs according to how much tissue has been damaged. Wound healing occurs by first, second, and third intention (Fig. 58-6).

First-intention healing (healing by *primary intention*) occurs in wounds with minimal tissue loss, such as surgical incisions or wounds sutured (stitched) soon after injury. Edges are *approximated* (close to each other); thus, they

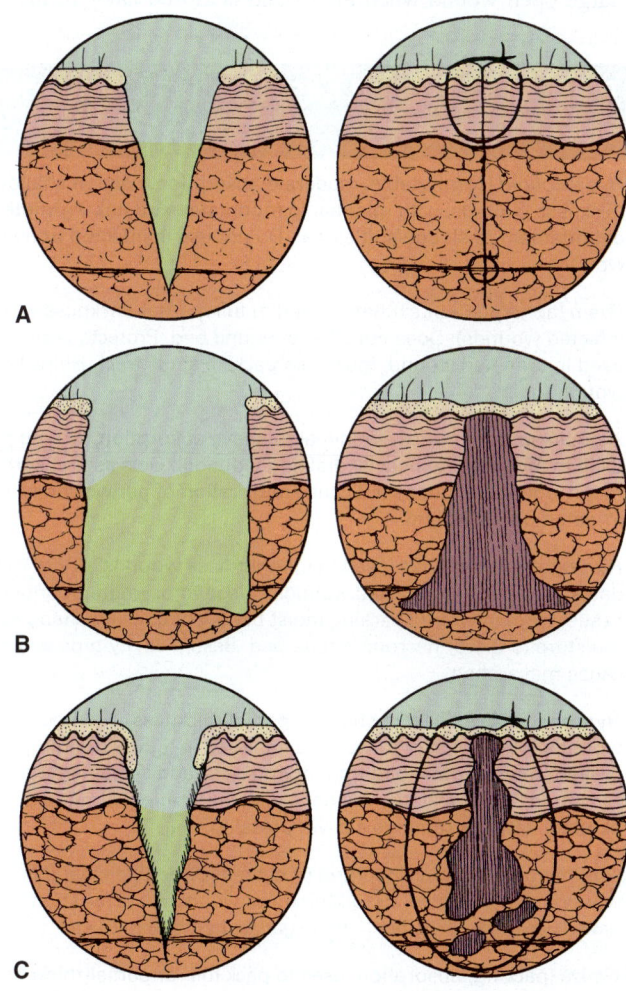

Figure 58-6 Wound healing. **A.** First (primary) intention (most surgical incisions). Clean incision, early suturing, hairline scar. **B.** Second (secondary) intention (tissue must granulate in). Irregular wound, granulation, skin grows over the scar. **C.** Third (tertiary) intention (wound edges brought together sometime after the wound occurs). Open wound, increased granulation, late suturing, wide scar. (Timby, 2013.)

seal together rapidly. Scarring and infection rates with first-intention healing are low.

Second-intention healing (healing by *secondary intention*) occurs with tissue loss; the wound edges are widely separated. Secondary intention healing occurs in injuries such as deep lacerations, burns, and pressure injuries. Because edges do not approximate, openings fill with *granulation tissue* that is soft and pinkish. This tissue grows slowly and must grow in from the inside outward, to prevent abscess. When the granulation tissue is in place, epithelial cells grow over the top. (Drainage or other wound debris slows the healing process.) Scarring often occurs, and the risk of infection is greater than that for first-intention healing. New technologies have been developed to treat such wounds more successfully; some of these are discussed later.

Third-intention healing (healing by *tertiary intention*) occurs when there is a delay in the time between the injury and the closure of the wound. For example, a wound may be left open temporarily to allow for drainage or removal of infectious materials. Tertiary-intention healing sometimes occurs after surgery when there is an infection, or in a large open wound when the wound is closed later. In the meantime, wound surfaces start to granulate in. Deep scarring almost always occurs.

Hundreds of products and procedures are in use today to assist in wound healing, including electrical stimulation, diathermy, and hyperbaric chamber treatment. These treatments are beyond the scope of this book.

Medications

Some available wound care products are external medications, such as antibiotics and antiseptics. Usually, the wound is cleaned and then patted dry with sterile gauze or other dressing. Follow the orders carefully; in addition, read the manufacturer's package insert. Apply medication to the wound itself, but not to the skin's edges, unless ordered otherwise. **Rationale:** *The medication may be damaging to surrounding tissues.* In many cases, an open wound will be filled in with a prescribed cream or ointment. In the case of a large wound, this is often performed with a tongue blade. For smaller wounds or sinus tracts, a cotton-tipped applicator is used. (Oral or IV antibiotics and other medications are often given as well, to speed the healing process.) Table 58-3

TABLE 58-3 Wound Care Product Categories

PRODUCT CATEGORY	EXAMPLES
Hydrocolloid (comfortable, moderate absorption, used in shallow, partial-thickness wounds, with minimal to moderate exudate). Promotes enzymatic debridement of slough/soft eschar. Do not use in infected or heavily draining wounds.	Tegasorb, DuoDERM, Comfeel, Tegaderm
Foam (absorption of exudates; used in full-/partial-thickness wounds and infected wounds). Does not stick to wound bed. Protects periwound skin. If used in tunneled wound, must also pack/fill sinus tract. Helps keep a shallow wound moist.	Optifoam, ALLEVYN, Biatain nonadhesive, and Mepilex—sacral-shaped silicone foam dressing (mark with "T," if used for wound treatment; mark with "P," if used for prevention; and date)
Alginate and Hydrofiber (minimal to heavy absorption, wound packing; used in moderate to heavily draining wounds). Gels as it absorbs; maintains moist wound bed; does not cause maceration of periwound skin; must be irrigated out of wound.	Maxorb, KALTOSTAT, SeaSorb calcium alginate, Algiderm
Hydrogel—amorphous (used in full-thickness wounds; dry to minimal exudates; necrotic and infected wounds). Used to promote debridement of dead tissue, to keep wound packing moist between dressing changes, and to add moisture to dry or necrotic wound bed. Best in cavity-type wound, but may cause maceration.	Woun'Dres hydrogel
Hydrogel—sheet (best in shallow [partial-thickness] and necrotic, dry wounds). Will not stick to wound bed. Used in lightly draining wounds or to prevent moist wound bed from drying out—adds small amount of moisture to wound; bacteriostatic; will not cause maceration. Limited ability to absorb exudate. Usually requires a cover dressing.	DermaGel sheet hydrogel
Antimicrobial products (control or decrease microbes; used in contaminated wounds and in partial- or full-thickness wounds). Preparations include alginate, Hydrofiber, hydrogel, foam, gauze, hydrocolloid, etc.	AMD packing gauze, SeaSorb Ag (contains silver)
Gauze (packing, absorption; used to pack full- or partial-thickness wounds, sinus tracts, cavities). Dries out unless used with another product, such as amorphous hydrogel or impregnated layer. May stick to wound bed; may shred or give off lint in wound bed.	Kerlix, Kerlix fluffs, packing gauze, Telfa nonadhesive dressings
Impregnated gauze (used to pack cavity or cover a dressing, to maintain moisture; used to dress full- or partial-thickness wounds; packing in cavities or sinus tracts). Easily conforms to shape of wound.	Oil emulsion dressing

TABLE 58-4 Objectives of Wound Care

OBJECTIVE	PRODUCTS USED	COMMENTS
Wound cleansing	Normal saline, Techni-Care	Techni-Care must be rinsed off.
Removal of dead tissue (not debrided unless there is adequate blood flow for healing)	(Thin layer or small amount of slough): sheet hydrogel (DermaGel), hydrocolloid (DuoDERM)	Hydrocolloid leaves a yellow, slimy layer; may have foul odor.
	(Dry eschar or thick, tenacious slough): hydrogel, gauze, and transparent dressing. Used for full-thickness wounds with cavities	Gauze moistened with hydrogel, covered with gauze, and covered with transparent dressing. Left in place 24–48 hr, to soften eschar.
Prevention/management of infection	Cover wound, to protect from additional microbes; cleanse wound with dressing change; apply antimicrobials. AMD packing gauze, SeaSorb Ag Alginate	Try not to use tape to hold dressing.
Elimination of empty spaces	Fill cavities, sinus tracts, tunnels, or undermining, to allow granulation. For heavily draining wounds: gauze, alginate	Do not pack tightly; completely fill spaces; use cotton-tipped applicator.
	For dry, cavities or tunneling wounds: hydrogel, strip packing gauze	Fluff packing; add saline, as ordered; fill wound bed loosely; pack deeply into wound.
Maintaining ordered moisture level	Foam dressing, hydrocolloid, sheet hydrogel, oil emulsion dressing	Added moisture usually not needed.
Reducing pain	Foam dressing, oil emulsion dressing, Vaseline gauze	Moisten dressings, if stuck to wound bed.
Protecting wound and periwound skin	Foam dressing, alginate	Heavily draining wounds require more absorbent dressing and frequent dressing changes.

presents wound care product categories, and Table 58-4 outlines the objectives of wound care and the products used. Do NOT use hydrogen peroxide or iodine, as these substances damage new skin cells developing in the wound.

Dressings

Many types of dressings are used to treat wounds. These include compression dressings and various types of manufactured dressing materials. *Dressings* serve to protect wounds from contamination, collect wound exudate (drainage, exuded material), assist in debridement, and protect against further damage during healing. The type of wound and its condition determine the type of dressing ordered and the frequency of dressing changes. The primary provider or wound care specialist orders the type and frequency for dressing changes. Always follow standard precautions for any wound care.

Key Concept
The technique used for most dressing changes is clean technique, using sterile dressings. Unless otherwise ordered, the surgeon performs the first dressing change after surgery or other procedure to close a wound. **Rationale:** *It is important for the surgeon to assess the wound and determine if healing is taking place or if there is a concern.*

Dry, Sterile Dressing

A *dry, sterile dressing* is often ordered for a wound to protect it from contamination (also known as a *dry-to-dry dressing*). This dressing is most often used for clean wounds healing by primary intention, such as surgical incisions. The materials used for this type of dressing include gauze (e.g., 2 × 2 or 4 × 4 gauze), Telfa pads, and larger abdominal (**ABD**) pads, also called Surgi-Pads (Fig. 58-7). These materials collect drainage and protect the wound. The used dressing is removed to evaluate healing, and a new, dry dressing is applied. In Practice: Nursing Procedure 58-1 outlines steps to follow when changing a dry, sterile dressing.

> **Nursing Alert** All used dressings are disposed of in red biohazard bags. This is particularly important if there is any drainage or blood on the dressing, or if it has been used as a packing.

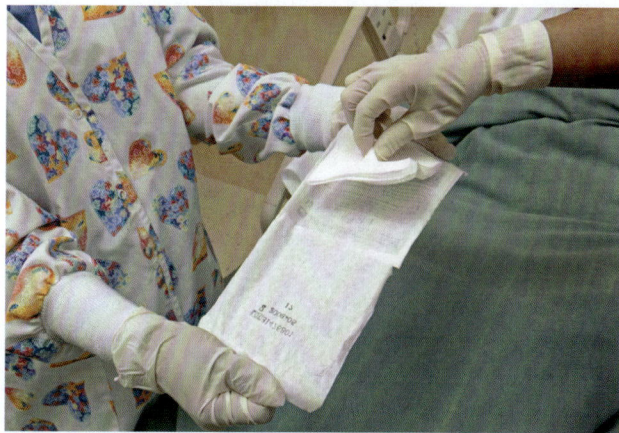

Figure 58-7 A large sterile ABD (abdominal) pad is used for a large wound. The "clean" nurse on the left holds the sterile package open so the "sterile" nurse on the right can remove the ABD without contaminating it (Carter, 2012).

> **Key Concept**
>
> The primary provider determines if debridement is appropriate or not. If any wound does not have adequate arterial blood flow to heal it, or if the wound contains stable, dry eschar and the circulation is questionable, current practice is to dry the wound and not debride. If a wound has adequate circulation to heal, it is usually kept moist and cleaned by debridement.

Wet-to-Dry Dressing

In some cases, mechanical debridement or cleansing of a wound can be accomplished by saturating a sterile dressing with normal saline or another sterile solution, placing the dressing on or packing it into the wound, and leaving it to dry. This is called a wet-to-dry dressing. **Wet-to-dry dressings** are not as commonly used as they were in the past, but still can be used for infected wounds healing by secondary intention. An infected wound has exudate composed of serum, tissue debris, and infectious material or pus. The wound will not heal unless these substances are removed. Debridement occurs as the dried dressing is removed; tissue debris and drainage that sticks to it also are removed. Follow the facility protocol to perform the wet-to-dry dressing change. *Remember:* Do not loosen a wet-to-dry dressing with normal saline or any other solution before removing the dried dressing material. **Rationale:** *This would defeat the purpose of the intended debridement.*

Packing

In some cases, **packing** is placed into a wound (Fig. 58-8). This may be performed by the healthcare provider at first and then by a specially trained nurse. Packing is done most often in the case of a puncture wound or a wound with a **sinus tract**, an abnormal tube-like channel or fistula, usually draining pus. The packing material may be dry or it may be impregnated with petrolatum (Vaseline) or another medication. A special sponge material or Gelfoam also may be used. When packing, the entire wound is packed with the material, no thicker than the wound bed. Some wounds are packed tightly, and some are packed loosely. Follow the provider's orders and the facility's protocols. Packing is inserted and removed with forceps, assisted by a cotton-tipped applicator.

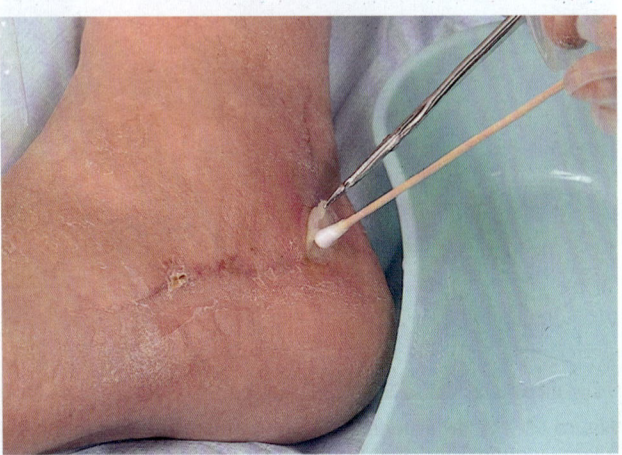

Figure 58-8 Packing material, such as Vaseline gauze, is held with forceps and pushed into the open wound with a cotton-tipped applicator (Lynn, 2015).

Wet-to-Wet Dressing

Wet-to-wet dressings are used on clean, open wounds or wounds that are granulating in. These dressings provide warmth and moisture, which aid the healing process and make the client more comfortable. Thick exudate also can be removed in this manner. Sterile saline or an antibiotic solution is used to saturate the dressing, and the dressing is not allowed to dry. These dressings are remoistened and/or replaced as ordered.

Commercially Prepared Special Dressings

A very large number of wound care products are available and can be supplied in sheets, ribbons, or pads, depending on the intended use. These include *alginates*, such as SeaSorb or Algiderm (calcium alginate), containing fibers derived from seaweed, and dressings containing silver. Many other debridement products are available, including hydrocolloids, hydrogels, and biologic, enzymatic, and mechanical products, as well as circumscribed maggot therapy, used in rare cases. It is important to note that wound care products are continually being improved. Follow the protocol of your facility.

Some wound care products interact with moisture on the skin to produce a gel; this provides a moist healing environment (see Table 58-4). These dressings are most often used in shallow to moderate-depth wounds and when drainage is minimal. They aid in healing, while also sealing the wound against air and water. An example of this type of dressing is DuoDERM, a *hydrocolloid dressing* (Fig. 58-9A). DuoDERM is self-adhesive and remains in place for 3–7 days. It absorbs drainage into its matrix while protecting the wound. Other dressings, such as polyurethane dressings, are not self-adhesive and must be taped in place. Sometimes, dressings are also covered with a transparent dressing (film), such as Tegaderm or OpSite (Fig. 58-9B). If using any special dressing, follow the manufacturer's instructions for correct application and use.

> **Key Concept**
>
> When applying any special dressing, make sure to adequately cover the wound. There should be at least a 1-in margin of the dressing on all sides of the wound.

Debridement

In addition to mechanical debridement by application of wet-to-dry and other chemical-containing dressings, mechanical debridement may be accomplished by hydrotherapy (whirlpool treatment), and by wound irrigation. *Sharp debridement* involves cutting away necrotic (dead) tissue with a scalpel or scissors, exposing living tissue; it is a very painful process. *Enzymatic debridement* is accomplished in an uninfected wound by use of chemical substances that break down wound debris, allowing this to be easily removed. *Autolytic debridement* is self-dissolution of necrotic tissue in a non-infected wound. If dressings are applied, it is important to observe for development of infection.

The Wound Drain

If a wound is deep or if there is a great deal of drainage, a **drain** may be used to facilitate drainage and help the wound heal

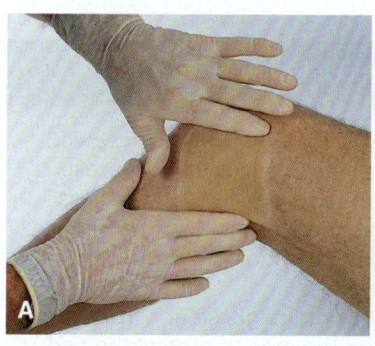
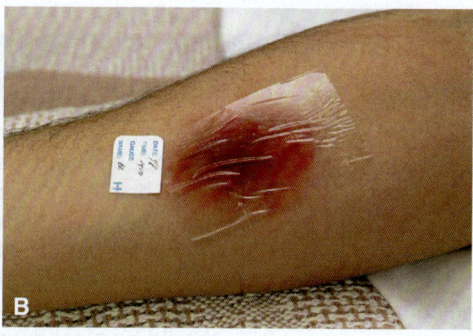

Figure 58-9 Commercially prepared dressings. **A.** Hydrocolloid dressing absorbs drainage into its matrix; aids healing by providing moist environment. **B.** Transparent dressing may be applied over another dressing or directly over a wound, providing visualization of the wound. (Carter, 2012.)

faster. Several types of drainage systems are commonly used. In Practice: Nursing Care Guidelines 58-1 lists some important nursing considerations when handling any drainage system.

> **Key Concept**
>
> If a drain is present, the provider often orders skin barrier protection to be applied around the drain. Dressings may also be used in conjunction with a drainage system, to further protect the skin.

The Penrose Drain

One type of drain, the Penrose drain (Fig. 58-10), is usually flat and is hollow. It wicks drainage out of a wound. A safety pin or other device is attached to the drain near its entrance to the skin, to prevent it from being pulled into the wound. A dressing or receptacle is placed over the open end of the drain, to catch drainage. The drain may be *advanced* (pulled out) a specified amount each day until it is completely removed. In this case, careful measurement of the drain length is necessary to make sure it is being advanced as ordered.

Closed Drainage Systems

Three common types of closed drainage systems are the Jackson–Pratt, the Hemovac, and the Davol. Using these devices, which provide gentle suction, can help deep or heavily draining wounds to heal faster. The *Jackson–Pratt* (Fig. 58-11A), also called the *grenade* drain, allows drainage to collect in a bulb about the size of a large lemon. A plug is removed to empty the contents. To reestablish suction, the bulb is squeezed until the inside walls of the bulb touch and then the plug is replaced. As the bulb expands, it creates gentle suction. The *Hemovac* (Fig. 58-11B) is used most often in a wound in which bloody drainage is expected after surgery. To establish suction, press on the top or both sides of the device, which is spring-loaded, and replace the plug. This creates suction as it slowly expands. The receptacle is emptied and the suction reactivated when it is full. The *Davol* is a drainage bottle with a rubber bulb on top. The bulb functions as a pump to inflate a balloon within the bottle. The balloon creates suction as it slowly deflates. The surgeon will usually place the specific type of suction device during surgery and order its postoperative management.

Other Equipment Used in Wound Care

A number of other devices are available to assist in wound care. These devices have promoted healing in otherwise difficult or previously untreatable wounds.

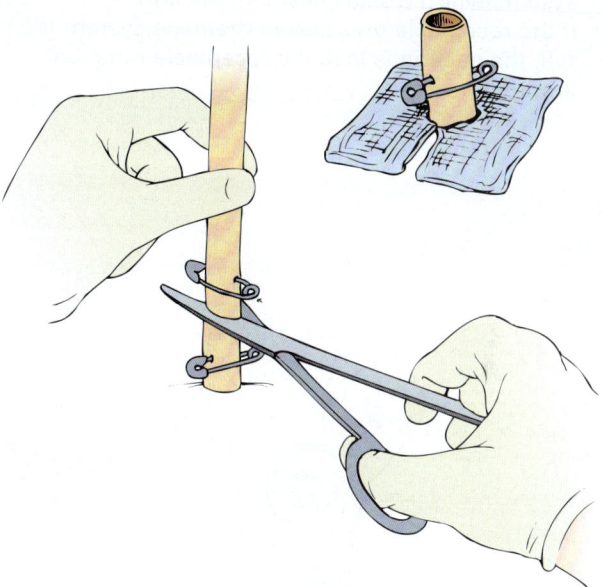

Figure 58-10 Open drainage apparatus. Penrose drain pulled from wound, excess portion cut, drain sponge replaced, and the wound covered with gauze. The safety pin prevents retraction of the drain back into the wound. (Timby, 2013.)

Vacuum-Assisted Closure—Negative Pressure Wound Therapy

The vacuum-assisted closure (**VAC**) machine, which resembles a suction machine, applies controlled localized negative pressure to a wound site (Fig. 58-11C). This speeds the growth of granulation tissue and decreases healing time. The VAC is particularly useful in the treatment of stage III and stage IV pressure injuries and other types of deep wounds (see Box 58-1). The system uses a special dressing that is applied within a wound or over a graft. The VAC is turned on, and the vacuum draws the wound edges toward the center. The direct pressure of the dressing on the wound also assists in removal of fluids, reducing swelling, stimulating growth of healthy cells, and increasing blood flow, thus promoting faster healing.

Wound Irrigation Systems

Wound irrigation helps remove debris from an open wound after injury or from an infected surgical incision. Wounds, even though they are draining or infected, are usually irrigated with sterile solution. **Rationale:** *This helps prevent introduction of additional pathogens.*

IN PRACTICE
NURSING CARE GUIDELINES 58-1 — Nursing Considerations in Handling Drainage Systems

- When working with any wound drainage, it is vital to wear gloves. If the drainage is excessive or obviously contains blood or pus, *double gloving* may be desired. Drainage is discarded according to agency protocol.
- Drains may or may not be sutured in place. Use extreme care when emptying drainage containers, so the drain is not dislodged.
- Be sure to check for leaks in a closed drainage system, which would negate the suction.
- If the receptacle on a closed drainage system is full, the suction is lost; the receptacle must be emptied.
- If there is a receptacle (e.g., the Hemovac or Davol), on an open drainage system, such as the Penrose drain, be sure it is emptied when needed. If this is not done, the drainage could retract back up into the wound and cause an infection, abscess, or great discomfort for the client.
- If there is a great deal of drainage, an absorbent pad should be placed under the area to protect the bed and keep the client's skin dry. A skin barrier cream may also be needed.
- The amount and character of drainage is carefully measured and recorded each time the receptacle is emptied.

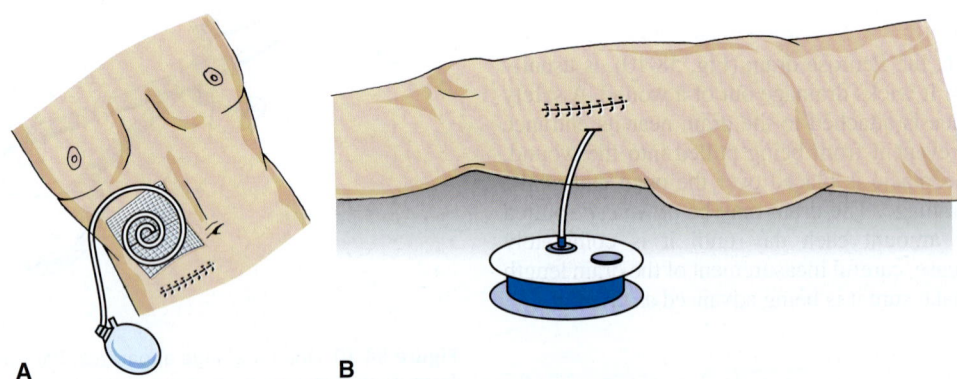

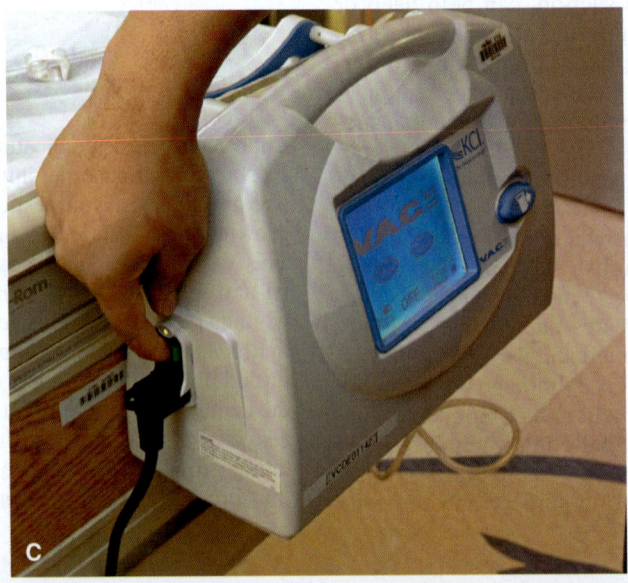

Figure 58-11 Closed drainage systems apply gentle suction to a wound. **A.** Jackson–Pratt. **B.** Hemovac (Smeltzer, Bare, Hinkle, & Cheever, 2008). **C.** The vacuum-assisted closure (VAC) device (negative pressure wound therapy [NPWT]) applies gentle suction directly to a wound site (Ellis & Bentz, 2007). In-service education is required before working with a VAC.

Several types of wound irrigation systems are available. They wash out debris and provide moisture to wounds, using saline, a biologic solution, or an antibiotic. One device, called the *Simpulse VariCare* System, is handheld and can provide irrigation under pressure (*pulsed lavage*), as well as suction. The tip is narrow so it can enter tunneling wounds, such as fistulas or deep decubiti. The tip is also marked to allow measurement of the depth of the wound. This system is used most often for heavily contaminated, infected, or deep wounds, and also in burns and cases involving several wounds. Another system, the *EnzySurge,* provides continuous irrigation and can also provide suction. This continuous streaming therapy involves a hand-held antiseptic wand, which can also be combined with an ultrasonic device. (The ultrasonic waves enlarge skin pores, enabling antiseptics to permeate the skin more easily.) This device is used most often to treat diabetic, venous, and pressure injuries. Other irrigation systems include *continuous wound irrigation* with an infusion-type setup and *intermittent irrigation,* alone or combined with gentle suction, such as the Hemovac.

Manual Wound Irrigation

Manual irrigation is performed with a hand-held syringe, usually sterile. Heat or medications also may be applied using this method. In Practice: Nursing Procedure 58-2 describes how to perform a manual wound irrigation, using sterile solution and dressings.

Sutures or Staples

After surgery, the wound may be closed with a tissue adhesive, such as DermaBond, or by a process called *laser soldering*. However, most incisions are closed with **sutures** (stitches) or staples (see Fig. 58-1). A common stitch pattern is called *interrupted sutures*; each stitch is inserted and knotted separately. Suture/staple removal is generally performed 7–10 days after surgery. Careful inspection of the wound must be made to determine if enough healing has occurred to remove the staples or sutures safely.

The nurse usually does not remove sutures or staples in the acute care facility, but may often do so in the clinic (following in-service training). A sterile "suture removal kit" is used. Sterile scissors are used to cut the suture *close to the skin*, while sterile tweezers firmly grip the knot. Then, the knot is pulled firmly, *straight-up* (Fig. 58-12A). Be sure to *pull on the knot. Rationale: Pulling on the knot prevents drawing the knot through the wound, which would interfere with the suture line and cause pain. Cutting the suture close to the skin avoids pulling contaminated suture material through the wound.*

Staples are used frequently to close surgical incisions, because they are inert, do not cause infection, and are quickly inserted. A special "staple remover" is required (Fig. 58-12B). Staples are removed following the manufacturer's recommendations and specific facility protocol. The staple remover is placed as shown in Figure 58-12B and the handles pressed together. When the prongs of the staple are straightened, the staple can easily be pulled straight out without injury to the client.

In some cases, *retention sutures* are interspersed with interrupted sutures. The retention sutures ensure that the incision remains closed after other sutures (or staples) are removed. Retention sutures are removed *only by the surgeon*. It is important for the nurse to recognize the difference between retention sutures and interrupted sutures.

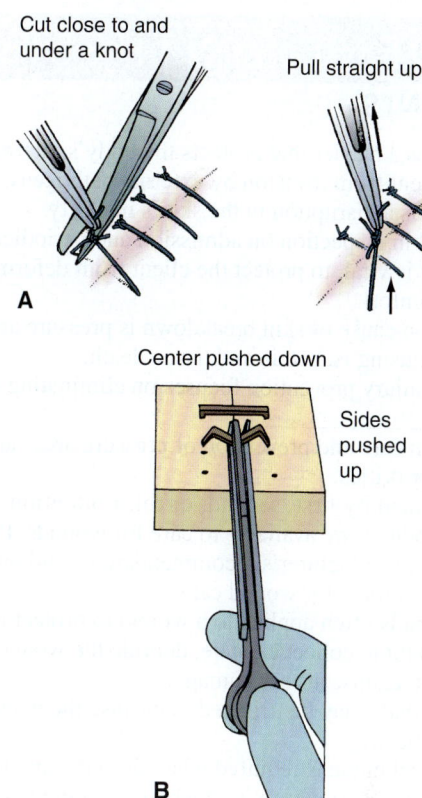

Figure 58-12 Removal of sutures and staples. Use a sterile suture or staple removal kit and wear gloves. **A.** Interrupted sutures. Place the scissors so as to cut beneath the knot, as close to the skin as possible, while applying the forceps firmly to the knot of the suture. Be sure to pull straight upward *on the knot*. **B.** Staples. The two lower side tips of the scissors-like instrument are placed *under* the staple and moved upward, while the upper center tip *presses down* on the center, when the handles are depressed. This bends the staple and causes the prongs to become vertical, so they can be easily pulled out. (Timby, 2009.)

> **Nursing Alert** When removing staples or interrupted sutures, first remove every other one and carefully inspect the wound edges after removal of each. In some cases, this is all that is done on the first day. **Rationale:** *Inspection will show if there is any evidence that the wound edges are pulling apart. If this happens, stop the procedure and report this immediately. The procedure may need to be postponed. If alternate stitches/staples are left in place, the wound has a chance to heal more, with the additional support.*

Often, narrow adhesive skin closures (Steri-Strips) are applied after staples/sutures have been removed. They may be applied after all staples or sutures have been removed or as each staple/suture is removed. An antiseptic, such as tincture of benzoin, may be applied to the skin around the incision where the Steri-Strips will be placed. The Steri-Strips are applied from one side of the incision to the other, with a slight pulling as the strip is placed. *Rationale: The antiseptic cleanses the wound and helps it dry, making the Steri-Strips stick better. The Steri-Strips help keep the wound edges together. Clients are instructed to shower, instead of taking a tub bath. Rationale: This allows the Steri-Strips to fall off on their own, rather than being soaked off.*

STUDENT SYNTHESIS

KEY POINTS

- The skin is a barrier that protects the body's internal environment from invasion by external pathogens.
- A wound is a disruption in the skin's integrity.
- Careful skin inspection on admission and periodically thereafter is vital, to protect the client from deformities and discomfort.
- A common cause of skin breakdown is pressure against tissues, causing ischemia and tissue death.
- Pressure injury prevention focuses on eliminating all causes.
- Good skin care and prevention of pressure areas are nursing priorities.
- Wounds heal by first, second, or third intention.
- Many products are available to care for wounds. Be sure to follow manufacturer's recommendations and primary provider's orders for wound care.
- A dressing is often applied to a wound to protect it from contamination, collect exudate, debride the wound, and/or protect against further damage.
- Open wounds may be irrigated to cleanse the wound and promote healing.
- Careful technique is required when dressing any wound.
- Standard precautions are used when changing any dressing, to help prevent the spread of infection to the nurse or others and to avoid contaminating the wound. Wear gloves and properly dispose of all used dressings.
- Removal of staples or sutures may be performed by the nurse after specific in-service education and practice.

CRITICAL THINKING EXERCISES

1. A client injured in an automobile accident is now paralyzed from the neck down. Identify this client's most vulnerable areas for skin breakdown. Explain how you will prevent pressure injury formation. What are the special nursing considerations for this client? Address physical and emotional aspects of care.
2. Visit a burn clinic or unit. Carefully describe in writing three wounds you see there. Include measurements and diagrams. Ask a burn nurse to critique your descriptions. Describe the types of dressings used in the burn unit and explain why each is used.

NCLEX-STYLE REVIEW QUESTIONS

1. Which client does the nurse determine is at greatest risk for impaired skin integrity?
   a. A client who is paralyzed on the right side after a stroke
   b. A client with pneumonia
   c. A client receiving a blood transfusion for anemia
   d. A client having a colonoscopy

2. The nurse is caring for a client at risk for skin breakdown. Which priority nursing actions may help prevent this development? Select all that apply.
   a. Apply moisture barrier cream to the skin.
   b. Determine the presence of dehydration and report findings.
   c. Immediately report any sign of skin redness.
   d. When skin redness is observed, massage vigorously.
   e. Turn an immobile client every 4 hr.

3. The nurse is obtaining data from a newly admitted client with a sacral pressure injury and observes a full-thickness wound with tissue loss, subcutaneous damage, and a purulent drainage. How will the nurse document the classification of this pressure injury?
   a. Stage I
   b. Stage II
   c. Stage III
   d. Stage IV

4. A client with a pressure injury has developed tunneling. When collecting data, how will the nurse measure the amount of tunneling?
   a. Insert a cotton-tipped application into the tunnel and measure the distance of insertion.
   b. Measure the width of the tunnel with a measuring tape.
   c. Estimate the depth according to the width.
   d. Pack the tunnel with a sterile 4 × 4 gauze pad and determine how much drainage is on the dressing.

5. The nurse is preparing a client for discharge and is reinforcing wound care instructions with the caregiver. Which findings would the nurse instruct the caregiver to report immediately? Select all that apply.
   a. Pink wound edges
   b. Redness around the wound
   c. Excess wound drainage
   d. Severe pain
   e. Hardness around the wound

CHAPTER RESOURCES

Enhance your learning with additional resources on **thePoint**!

Student Resources related to this chapter can be found at **thePoint.lww.com/Rosdahl12e**.

CHAPTER 58 Special Skin and Wound Care 875

Welcome Steps

Look at healthcare provider's orders.

Protocol for procedure.

Necessary equipment/supplies.

Wash hands using proper hand hygiene; put on gloves.

Explain the procedure and reassure the client.

Locate two identifiers to confirm correct client.

Comfortable and efficient position for nurse and client.

Obtain privacy.

Make sure to follow correct steps and body mechanics with good technique.

Ensure safety and observe deviations from normal.

End Steps

Ensure comfort and safety.

Note questions or concerns from client or nurse; note significant data.

Dispose of materials properly.

Disinfect the area and your hands.

Document and report the procedure and your findings.

IN PRACTICE

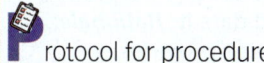

NURSING PROCEDURE 58-1 | **Changing a Dry, Sterile Dressing**

From Taylor's Interactive Nursing Skills: Cleaning a Wound and Applying Sterile Dressing

Supplies and Equipment
Clean gloves
Marked red biohazard bag
ABD (abdominal) pad or Surgi-Pads, if required
Sterile dressings, as ordered
Sterile saline or water, if required
Sterile cotton-tipped applicators or tongue blades
Medication, as ordered
Pen, paper, and measuring device
Waterproof marker, if ordered
Bath blanket
Sterile gloves, as ordered
Tape or Montgomery straps
Waterproof pads
Sterile forceps optional

Steps
Follow LPN WELCOME steps and then

1. Check the orders for type of dressing to apply. Check previous nursing notes to determine the presence or absence of drainage, its character and amount, and size and condition of the wound. Place a waterproof pad under the client, if necessary. *Rationale: The nurse needs a reference point for observation when the wound is exposed. This enables accurate documentation and reporting. If there is excessive drainage, the pad will protect the bed.*

2. Prepare a marked biohazard bag for soiled dressings. Fold back the cuff and place it within reach of your working area (often, it is handy to tape it to the end of the overbed table). If you are using tape on the new dressing, tear strips of the appropriate size and lightly tape the ends to the overbed table. *Rationale: The biohazard bag identifies materials that are soiled with body substances. This alerts others to the presence of microorganisms on the soiled dressings. Taping the bag to the table helps keep it open, facilitating safe disposal of biohazardous materials. Preparation of tape strips facilitates taping the new dressing in place while wearing gloves.*

3. Put on clean gloves. Untie the Montgomery straps or gently loosen the tape on the used dressing. Remove the used dressing, being careful not to tear the wound or dislodge any drains. Use sterile saline to moisten the dry dressing, if it is sticking to the wound. Lift the soiled side of the dressing away from the client's view. *Rationale: Gloves act as a barrier. Using caution while removing the dressing maintains the integrity of sutures and helps prevent discomfort. Sterile saline helps loosen the dressing, to minimize pain. (Do not use saline on a wet-to-dry dressing.) The sight of drainage or blood may upset the client.*

876 UNIT 8 Client Care

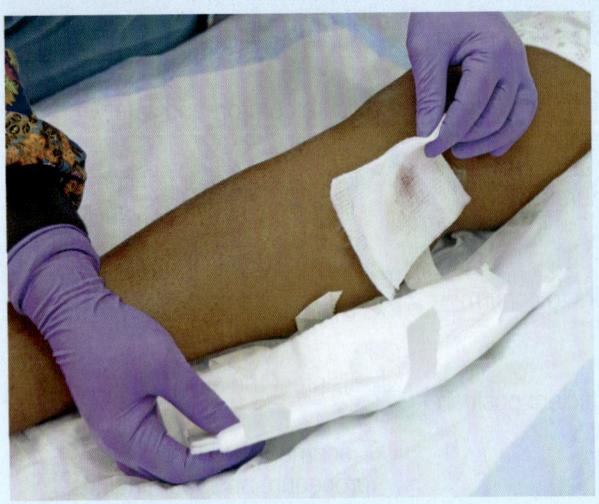

4. Determine the amount, color, odor, and consistency of any drainage. Observe the condition of the wound and surrounding tissues. Measure and describe the wound. Draw a picture of an irregular wound. If ordered, draw a line around the wound with a waterproof marker and date it. *Rationale: Data collection about the wound provides an indication of the wound's healing and presence or absence of infection. Careful description of the wound helps evaluate the healing process. A line will help to indicate later if the wound is becoming larger or smaller.*

Remove the used dressing, being careful not to tear the wound. Carefully dispose of the dressing (Evans-Smith, 2005).

A small device for measuring wounds. These paper strips are discarded after each use.

5. Remove gloves and place them in the biohazard bag. Wash hands. Prepare a sterile field on the bedside or overbed table and open sterile dressings onto it (see In Practice: Nursing Procedure 57-1). Uncap the sterile saline or other prescribed solution and pour it into a sterile receptacle. Place additional sterile dressings or swabs for cleansing onto the sterile field. *Rationale: The used gloves are contaminated with wound drainage. Dressing changes are carried out in as sterile a situation as possible. Organization ensures that needed sterile supplies are present and placed in the order of use.*

6. Put on sterile gloves (see In Practice: Nursing Procedure 57-2), as ordered. (Gloves are put on after all sterile materials are prepared and in place.) *Rationale: Using sterile gloves maintains surgical asepsis. Once sterile gloves are put on, you cannot touch anything unsterile without contaminating the gloves. (Some dressing changes may be carried out using clean gloves and sterile dressing materials.)*

7. Moisten sterile dressings or swabs and cleanse the wound, if ordered, moving from top to bottom or from the center of the wound outward (you may use sterile forceps). Use a new swab or gauze pad for each cleansing motion and discard the used materials in the biohazard bag. If necessary, clean the area around the wound as well. Do not use alcohol or soap. *Rationale: Cleansing from clean to dirty prevents introducing microorganisms into the wound. Alcohol and soap are drying and may cause further skin breakdown.*

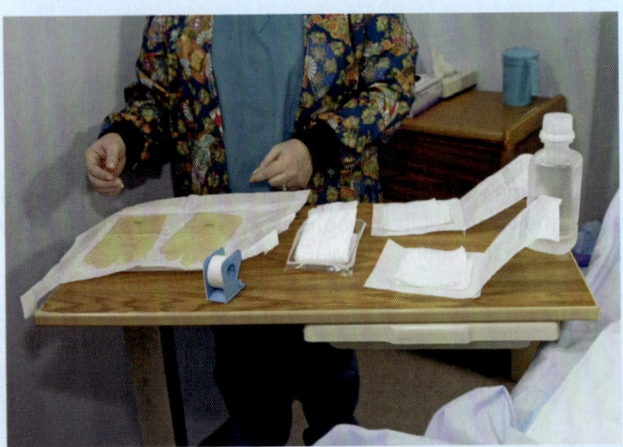

The sterile field and all supplies and equipment must be set up before putting on sterile gloves (Lynn, 2015).

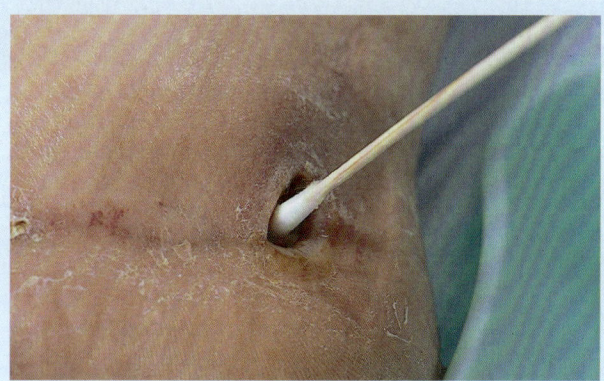

Cleansing the wound with a cotton-tipped applicator.

8. If necessary, use a gauze pad to dry the wound with the same motions as in step 7. Carefully inspect the wound. Be prepared to describe the wound accurately. *Rationale: Moisture provides a medium for microorganisms to grow and multiply. The wound should be kept as dry as possible. Visual inspection determines if the wound is healing and if there is any evidence of infection.*

9. Apply any ointments or medications to the wound, as ordered. Do not touch the wound with your hands. Apply a layer of dry sterile dressings over the incision and wound area, as ordered. Pad with additional dressings and cover with a sterile ABD pad if the wound is large or heavily draining. *Rationale: Medications assist in wound healing. The inner layer of dressings acts as a wick. Additional dressings and the outer pad absorb drainage and provide further protection for the wound. The dressings are kept as sterile as possible.*

10. If tape is to be used, use the previously torn strips. Apply at least one piece of tape immediately, to hold the dressing in place. In some situations, you may then remove your gloves and complete the taping of the dressing. An alternate method is to tie the dressing with Montgomery straps (see Fig. 53-2), to avoid frequent tape removal. *Rationale: Tape is difficult to tear and apply while wearing gloves. The previously prepared strips aid in this process. Taping or using Montgomery straps secures the dressing in place. Montgomery straps help to prevent skin irritation. Special note: It is not feasible to remove gloves before taping the dressing if the client is restless or if the dressing is in an awkward location. In this case, the dressing must be taped quickly, with gloves on.*

11. Remove gloves and wash hands. Reposition and cover the client, while preventing pressure on the wound. Handle only the outside of the biohazard bag, keeping hands inside (under) the cuff on the outside of the bag, and carefully closing it. Dispose of the bag according to agency policy. Wash hands again. *Rationale: Standard precautions and proper disposal help prevent transmission of microorganisms. The inside of the bag is grossly contaminated and must be handled as such. Keeping pressure off of the wound prevents further damage and minimizes pain.*

Follow ENDDD steps.

Special Reminder
- Completely describe the wound and any drainage in your documentation.

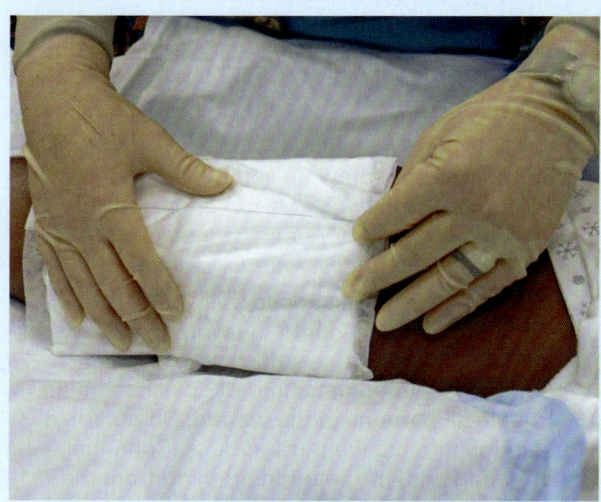

Applying a dry sterile dressing over the wound area with gloved hands (Lynn 2015).

NURSING PROCEDURE 58-2 Performing a Sterile Wound Irrigation

Special Skin and Wound Care, Video: Skin Integrity and Wound Care: Irrigating a Wound Using Sterile Technique

Supplies and Equipment
Disposable sterile irrigation pack
Sterile irrigation solution, as ordered
Marked biohazard bag
Clean gloves
Waterproof bed pad
Bath blanket
Eye shield or face guard
Sterile dressings, as ordered
Tape and other supplies needed to apply new dressing
Sterile gloves, if ordered
Clean basin or irrigating pouch

Steps
Follow LPN WELCOME steps and then

1. Put on clean gloves and an eye shield or face guard. *Rationale: Using appropriate barriers minimizes the risk of infection transmission. Gloves protect the hands. If there is any danger of splashing, eye shields or face guards are necessary.*

2. Position the client so the solution will run from the upper end of the wound downward. Place the waterproof bed pad and clean basin or irrigating pouch under the area to be irrigated. *Rationale: The bed pad protects the bed linens. The clean basin or pouch will catch the irrigating solution.*

3. Drape the client with a bath blanket to expose only the wound. *Rationale: Exposing only the area for treatment maintains the client's privacy and prevents chilling.*

4. Remove the used dressing and discard it as described in In Practice: Nursing Procedure 58-1. Discard gloves. Wash hands again. *Rationale: Handwashing and proper disposal of contaminated equipment help reduce the risk of infection transmission.*

5. Open the irrigation tray, using sterile technique. Open the irrigation solution; place the cover on the table, with the inside facing upward. Carefully pour the solution from the supply bottle into the irrigation bottle. (Pour solution with the bottle label facing your palm.) If the bottle has been opened previously, pour off a small amount of the solution into a trash receptacle. Leave the cover off the irrigation supply bottle, with the inside of the cover pointing upward. *Rationale: The inside of the bottle cover is protected from contamination by keeping the inside from touching the table, and the cover is left off so the irrigation syringe can be inserted. The outside of the bottle is no longer sterile. You must pour the solution before you put on sterile gloves. Spilled solution will cause contamination and make the label unreadable. Pouring off a small amount of solution washes potential microorganisms from the lip of the container so solution poured later will not be contaminated. You cannot touch the bottle once you have put on sterile gloves.*

6. Place the bottle close to the client on the overbed table. Date and initial the bottle after opening it. Include the client's name and facility ID number. *Rationale: You will use the solution for one client only. It must be clearly identified and kept handy. The date is needed to prevent using outdated solutions.*

7. Open the sterile dressing tray, if one is to be used, and put on sterile gloves. *Rationale: Maintaining sterile technique helps prevent the introduction of microorganisms.*

8. Prepare the inside of the irrigation and dressing trays. Place the irrigation syringe into the bottle. Open dressing packages and prepare other items. *Rationale: Proper setup of sterile equipment maintains sterility of the materials.*

9. Carefully assess the amount and character of drainage and the size and condition of the wound and surrounding tissue. *Rationale: Data collection about the wound determines the progress of the wound's healing. Be sure to report and document this information.*

10. While explaining the following steps to the client as you proceed, draw up solution into the syringe. *Rationale: Explanations foster cooperation and provide the client or family with teaching, should irrigation need to be continued at home.*

11. Hold the syringe just above the wound's top edge, and force fluid into the wound, slowly and continuously. Use sufficient force to flush out debris, but do not squirt or splash the fluid. Irrigate all portions of the wound. Do not force solution into the wound's pockets. Continue irrigating until the solution draining from the wound's bottom end is clear. *Rationale: Flushing the wound until drainage is clear ensures that as much debris and products of infection as possible are removed from the wound, without damaging the wound.*

CHAPTER 58   Special Skin and Wound Care   879

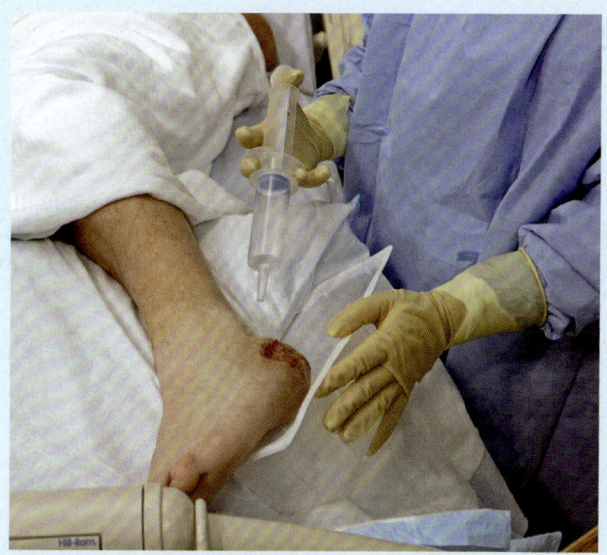

Flushing the wound with solution. The solution collects in the basin for disposal (Lynn, 2015).

12. Using sterile 4 × 4 pads, gently pat dry the wound's edges (if the wound is to have a wet-to-dry dressing, then dry only the surrounding skin). Work from the cleanest to the most contaminated area. *Rationale: This measure helps prevent further contamination by removing culture media for microorganisms. Moving from clean to contaminated helps prevent the spread of pathogens. If the wound is dry, the dressings will remain dry longer, and contamination will not spread.*

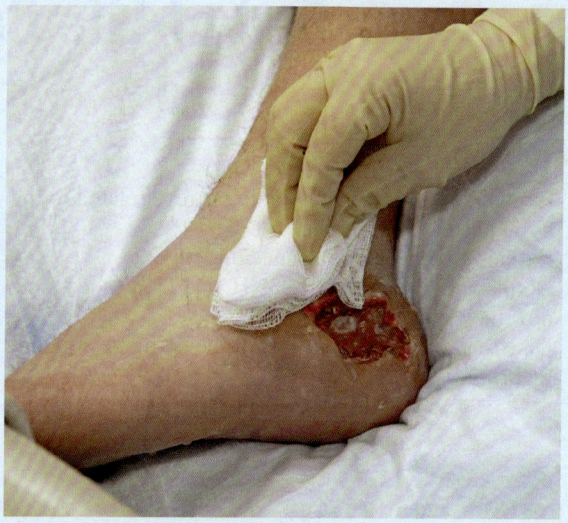

Patting dry the skin around the wound, without contaminating the wound (Lynn, 2015).

13. Apply sterile dressings as ordered. *Rationale: Applying sterile dressings protects the wound from contamination.*

Follow ENDDD steps.

Special Reminder

- Teach the client or caregiver to observe for excess drainage, severe pain, redness, or hardness around the wound. Include any other pertinent observations. *Rationale: The client's observations may alert staff to problems, resulting in quick action. Pertinent observations may assist the team in further care planning and treatment.*

59 End-of-Life Care

Learning Objectives

1. Explain how end-of-life nursing care is related to the basic needs of all people.
2. Explain two types of advance directives.
3. Define and discuss DNR, DNH, and DNI orders and how they relate to end-of-life care.
4. Discuss the emotional needs of the dying person and their family.
5. Briefly discuss pain management in the terminally ill client.
6. Identify nursing activities that may assist the family to cope with the death of their loved one.
7. Describe postmortem care of the body.
8. Discuss how members of the healthcare team can help each other when a client dies.

Important Terminology

antiemetic
autopsy
brain death
Cheyne–Stokes respiration
hospice
Kussmaul breathing
palliative care
postmortem examination
respite care

Acronyms

AD
DNH
DNI
DNR
PSDA
TPN

Working with clients at the end of their lives and with their families is a privilege and a challenge. Assisting clients with end-of-life care allows nurses to use many of the technical and life mental health skills learned throughout the nursing program. Assisting clients with end-of-care is a valuable learning experience, not only for the nurse, but also for the client and the family. You have an opportunity to provide physical and emotional support and care to the client and to involve the family deeply in that care. Nurses may encounter a person at the end of life in various settings, such as a hospital, long-term care facility, hospice care, or in the client's own home.

Western medicine has traditionally emphasized the preservation of life at all costs. This may be a challenge for the nurse when assisting a client through the death experience. It is important to remember that nursing care can provide needed physical care and comfort, as well as respect, empathy, and understanding; given without prejudice or bias. Nurses who dedicate their careers to end-of-life care must be compassionate and caring and must understand their own feelings regarding life and death. By drawing on spiritual and emotional reserves and by facing the crisis of death, the nurse can grow emotionally and spiritually. When caring for clients who are dying and their families, listen to them and offer unconditional support. It is often helpful to offer resources for spiritual counseling for the client and family (Fig. 59-1). A positive end-of-life experience is impeded when the client, the family, and the nurse do not have the same expectations and goals.

STAGES OF DYING

A number of years ago, Elisabeth Kübler-Ross, in landmark work, identified stages of dying. Kübler-Ross stated that most people pass through these stages at the end of their lives. Although there are other theories, Kübler-Ross' stages of dying are still generally accepted today. These stages are:

- Denial (*"This isn't* happening to me!")
- Anger (*"Why* is this happening to me?")
- Bargaining ("I promise I will be a better person *if only*…")
- Depression ("I *don't care* anymore.")
- Acceptance ("I'm *ready* for whatever happens.")

These stages, as well as other aspects of the dying experience, are discussed in more detail in Chapter 14. Hospice nursing is discussed in Chapter 100. This chapter focuses primarily on the physical nursing care required during end-of-life care.

Key Concept

The client's family often goes through the same stages of grief and loss related to the dying experience as does the client. In addition, not all people go through the grief experience in the exactly same sequence or the same way.

THE CLIENT'S WISHES

It is important that the client's wishes about their care be known to the healthcare staff and be carried out as requested by the client. This information must be carefully documented in the client's record.

NCLEX Alert

You should be alert during the examination to the meanings of acronyms found in this chapter: DNH, DNI, DNR, AD, and your nursing role in explaining these to clients and their families and ensuring that the client's wishes are carried out during their end-of-life experience.

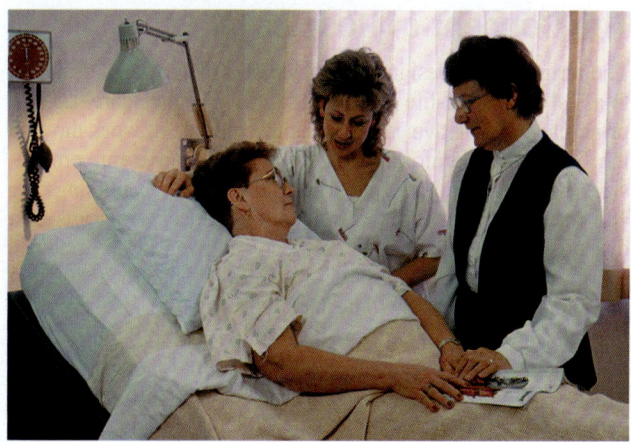

Figure 59-1 Offer to secure spiritual counseling or grief counseling for the client and/or family. (Photo by Mark Gibson.)

Advance Directives

An advance directive (**AD**) is an expression of the client's wishes about the kinds of treatment and care that they want to receive if terminally ill or unable to make decisions about healthcare. In 1990, the U.S. Congress passed the Patient Self-Determination Act (**PSDA**), a step toward increasing the autonomy of dying persons. Healthcare facilities that receive federal funds must ask every client on admission if they have an AD. The client's response must be entered into the client's health record. The client also must be given assistance if they wish to make a living will or other healthcare directive.

An AD can take several forms. The most common ADs are the living will and the durable power of attorney for healthcare. The *living will* is a document in which clients state the types of treatment they desire to receive or not to receive if a terminal situation arises or if they are unable to make decisions or express their wishes. A *durable power of attorney for healthcare* designates a person of the client's choice to make these healthcare decisions should the client become incompetent (unable to make or express decisions about care). Signed copies of advance directives may be carried by a client and presented to the healthcare facility on admission. An electronic form is also available in a device called the E-HealthKEY (see Chapters 4 and 43).

Codes

The AD informs healthcare personnel about procedures the client requests to be performed or not to be performed if they become terminally ill. Several healthcare "codes" are involved in these instructions. An individual may have a *do not resuscitate* (**DNR**), *do not intubate* (**DNI**), or both orders in their health record. Healthcare personnel are thus informed that if this person experiences cardiopulmonary arrest, a "code blue" (or the code name for arrest in that facility) should not be called. The person will be allowed to die naturally, without mechanical or chemical intervention. The use of tube feedings may also be specified as a treatment the client does or does not want. Clients who are DNR or DNI or who refuse tube feedings will be kept as comfortable as possible and given emotional support. It is important to carry out a client's wishes as a component of responsible healthcare delivery.

> **Nursing Alert** A written healthcare provider's order is needed for a client in a healthcare facility to be DNR/DNI. A copy of the signed advance directive must also be in the client's record.

In the nursing home or in the client's home, the nurse may see a *do not hospitalize* (**DNH**) order, in addition to a DNR or DNI order. Clients need to inform their families and significant others of their wishes regarding hospitalization and resuscitation. The client and family should know the policies of ambulance and emergency transport agencies in their area. Many such service personnel are trained to give cardiopulmonary resuscitation (CPR) to *anyone* under their care. When a client does not wish to be hospitalized or resuscitated, the family needs maximum support in the home if the person's condition becomes critical.

> **Nursing Alert** A copy of each person's living will should be readily available so it can be taken to the acute care facility in an emergency.

Some individuals with terminal illnesses are on *full code*, meaning that the CPR team is to be called in the event of cardiopulmonary arrest, even though natural death is imminent. When working in environments in which death occurs frequently, it is particularly important to know in advance which individuals are DNR and which are full code.

> **Key Concept**
> Healthcare personnel do not determine whether a code should be called. Clients, healthcare providers, or family members must have already decided in advance, and written instructions must be on file. If a client does not have a specific DNR order, a code is always called if the person should experience respiratory or cardiac arrest or another medical emergency, such as critical hypoglycemia.

The Ethics Committee

Healthcare facilities are required to have an *ethics committee*. This committee assists in making difficult client care decisions. This committee may discuss situations, including whether to discontinue a feeding tube or ventilator for a client when there is no living will, when there is an unclear advance directive, or when family members do not agree on what care should be given. The ethics committee may become involved in situations involving donation of organs or tissues for transplantation. The committee may also discuss types of medications to be used for symptom control. These are examples of the difficult decisions to be made by this committee; each case is different.

Organ and Tissue Donation

Advance directives or the client's driving license may indicate the wish to donate tissues (e.g., cornea, bone, skin) or organs (e.g., kidney, heart, lung). However, after death, in most states, the next-of-kin or legal guardian gains custody of the body and must give permission for donation.

Generally, a remaining spouse has the legal authority to consent to donation and must be included in all decision-making. If there is no living spouse, the next closest relative or the person with power of attorney has the legal authority for consent. Most states have a law (often called the Uniform Anatomical Gift Act) that requires healthcare facilities to approach each family regarding donation of their loved one's organs or tissues if a person dies or is expected to die very soon. In some cases, the client's entire body is donated for research or education. Special courses are available to assist nurses in approaching family members at this difficult time. In many cases, being able to help another person by organ or tissue donation assists the family in dealing with the death of their loved one. *Be sure your family knows about your wishes in relationship to organ and tissue donation!*

A nurse or other person specially trained in dealing with organ and tissue donation should be involved, if at all possible. The role of this person is to educate the family about all aspects of donation and answer any questions the family may have. Commonly asked questions regarding organ and tissue donation are:

- Can we still have an open casket? (Yes)
- Is there any cost to us? (No)
- Will we know who receives the organs or tissues? (Usually not)
- Can we donate some organs/tissues but not all? (Yes)

Key Concept

The nurse who approaches the family for organ and tissue donation should see the family through this time of decision making and not transfer the responsibility to another nurse or healthcare provider unless absolutely necessary.

It is important for nurses to be sensitive to the need of the family to have privacy to discuss the matter of donation. Provide a private place for them. Be sure all the family's questions are answered, and make sure they do not feel forced to donate. *Rationale: People are very vulnerable at this time; they should not feel pressured into consenting to donation.*

In some cases, special procedures (e.g., maintaining the client on a ventilator or heart/lung circulation until organs can be harvested) may be necessary to preserve the organs in sufficiently good condition to be transplanted successfully. This situation does not usually arise for tissues.

The Client Who Chooses to Die at Home

If the client's death has been anticipated and the client has chosen to die at home, a home care or hospice nurse will usually be assigned to the case. This nurse discusses plans for the client's care with the family beforehand. Usually, the nurse is not present at the actual time of death, so the family must be prepared ahead of time. The family is instructed to call the home care nurse if the client's condition significantly worsens or if the client dies. Most agencies have a nurse on call 24 hr a day to answer questions and to come to the home if necessary.

The Concept of Hospice

The term **hospice** designates a place or a plan of care designed to assist the end-of-life client and family. Hospice care uses the principles of **palliative care** to aid these people to work through the situation as comfortably as possible. Palliative care emphasizes comfort and pain control, so it encompasses nursing care and medical treatments that relieve or reduce symptoms of a disease or illness. Palliative care can be given at any point in a disease process and may be provided in a healthcare setting or in the client's home. The hospice principle also provides **respite care** (time away) for the family. (To be admitted to a hospice program, the client must be certified as eligible by a medical practitioner, and usually the client's life expectancy cannot exceed about 6 months [see Chapter 100].)

Key Concept

Palliative care is not aimed at curing disease or illness; its aim is to relieve symptoms.

Cultural Considerations

Death and dying are viewed differently in various cultures. Some cultures look at death as a natural progression toward a better future; others look at death as a finality (Box 59-1). Chapter 8 presents some aspects of transcultural healthcare in more detail. Chapter 14 identifies basic religious aspects related to end-of-life care. It is important for the nurse to respect the beliefs of each client and family. Allow them to grieve and minister to their loved one in their own way. Offer to call their spiritual advisor or the facility chaplain if they would like this type of support.

SPECIAL CONSIDERATIONS Culture and Ethnicity

Organ/Tissue Donation and Transplantation
Ethnic and religious groups may have differing beliefs and concerns about organ and tissue donation. Below are some common beliefs that may serve as an introduction to different cultures; however, it is *always* important to communicate with clients to ascertain their individual beliefs and concerns. Nurses should *never* assume a client's beliefs based on generalizations.
- African American—many oppose donation
- Hispanic—may oppose donation
- Islam/Muslim—generally not allowed
- Jewish—may agree to donation, with consent of rabbi
- Roman Catholic—generally allow donation
- Most Protestant faiths—generally allow donation
- Christian Scientist—usually do not allow donation
- Jehovah's Witness—personal decision, but donated material must be cleansed with nonblood product
- Church of Jesus Christ of Latter-day Saints (Mormon)—discuss with the church elder
- Seventh-Day Adventist—personal choice
- Hindu/Buddhist—no stated view, personal opinions vary

NCLEX Alert

As you study this chapter, you are referred back to concepts and skills studied previously: technical or client-care skills, such as positioning, bathing, supplemental oxygen, communication skills, providing emotional support to clients and families, and the relationship of Maslow hierarchy of needs to the death experience. These may be incorporated into the NCLEX test scenarios.

> **Box 59-1** Acceptable Death Versus Good Death
>
> One description of death, as related to different cultures,[a] involves "acceptable death" and "good death." An acceptable death is defined as "nondramatic, disciplined, and with very little emotion." The definition goes on to say that most deaths in Western society fall into this category, particularly those occurring in a structured setting, such as a hospital.
>
> A good death is defined as one that allows for "social adjustments and personal preparation by the dying person and the family." In this description, the dying person attempts to complete unfinished tasks, says farewells, and the family begins to prepare for life without the person. A goal of nursing care is to move toward the concept of the good death for all clients and their families.

[a]Kellahear, A. (1990). *Dying of cancer: The final year of life.* Harwood Academic Publishers.

BASIC NEEDS, AS RELATED TO THE DEATH EXPERIENCE

In Chapter 5, Maslow hierarchy of needs was presented. The dying client has the same basic needs as anyone else, although some needs may be approached in a slightly different way. In the case of the client who is dying, the nurse must often assist the client to meet even the most basic of needs. The goal is that the client and family will be able to work through the stages of dying successfully. In this way, they will be able to meet their *basic needs, so they can go on* to attain self-actualization and other *higher-level needs*. The needs of the dying person are addressed here in terms of the following:

- Oxygen and the airway
- Hydration and nutrition
- Elimination
- Hygiene
- Activity
- Pain control
- Higher-level needs

The major function of nursing is to be supportive and empathetic (Fig. 59-2). Assist clients to meet their needs, but allow them to maintain self-esteem and personal dignity; never do things for clients that they can do themselves. See the Nursing Process at the end of this section. The Rule of Threes applies to end-of-life care, as well as in survival situations (Box 59-2).

Oxygen and Maintenance of the Airway

As stated in Box 59-2, oxygen is the most basic of needs. Life cannot be sustained for more than a very few minutes without oxygen. One of the major priorities in assisting the dying person is the maintenance of a patent (open) airway. The client who can breathe will be more comfortable and less fearful. Nursing measures to assist in breathing include

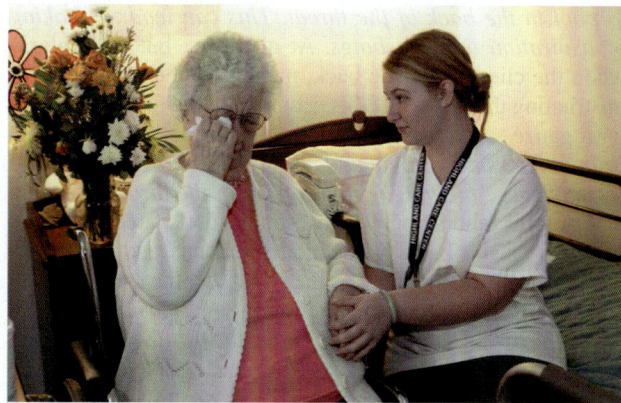

Figure 59-2 This nurse is practicing therapeutic use of touch to help the client work toward acceptance.(From Carter, P. [2019]. *Lippincott textbook for nursing assistants: A humanistic approach to caregiving* [5th ed.]. Wolters Kluwer.)

positioning of the client, keeping the nostrils clear, suctioning, and administering supplemental oxygen, as prescribed.

Various *breathing patterns* may be seen in the client who is dying. **Kussmaul breathing** often occurs if a person experiences acidosis. This type of breathing is fast (>20 breaths/minute), labored, and deep. It can rapidly become Cheyne–Stokes respiration, as heart failure occurs. **Cheyne–Stokes respirations** are characterized by alternating periods of *apnea* (absence of breathing) and *hyperpnea* (rapid breathing). As death approaches, the apneic periods gradually lengthen.

Positioning

Individuals who are dying may be unable to report that they are uncomfortable or that they would like to change position; therefore, expect to turn these clients frequently. Frequent position changes help prevent skin breakdown and usually assist clients to breathe more easily. For example, the client can be propped into a partially sitting position (low Fowler's) or sitting upright (orthopneic position; see Chapter 48). Pillows or other means are used to support the client and to prevent them from bending too far forward. *Rationale: If the client slumps down or bends over, it can put undue pressure on the chest and respiratory muscles and make it even more difficult to breathe.*

A lateral (side-lying) position is often comfortable and may make breathing easier. The lateral position also helps with drainage of excess oral and nasal secretions. Pillows and supports can be used to help the client maintain this position. The head may be kept flat, or it may be raised, to further assist with drainage. Often, the client prefers to lie on the back. Try to encourage alternate positions, as much as possible. *Rationale: Lying on the back may cause secretions*

> **Box 59-2** Rule of Threes
>
> **A person can live:**
> - 3 min without oxygen
> - 3 hr without warmth
> - 3 days without water
> - 3 weeks without food

to pool in the back of the throat. *This can lead to choking or aspiration into the lungs.* At all times, but particularly when the client is on the back, make sure the tongue is not obstructing the airway. If this occurs, pull the tongue forward with gauze, and assist the client into a side-lying position. *Rationale: As neurologic and muscular control is lost, gravity may cause the tongue to fall back in the throat.* Usually, it is helpful (and safer) to have the head elevated when the client is on the back. Collection of mucus and secretions may cause a "death rattle" as the client breathes, particularly when on the back. Gentle suctioning or a position change may relieve this sound. In rare cases, the healthcare provider may order a very small dose of atropine, to dry secretions.

> **Key Concept**
>
> Careful positioning is important to help the client to be more comfortable and to maintain a patent airway. The airway is of prime importance in caring for the dying client and helping to provide comfort.

Supplemental Oxygen and Suctioning

Oxygen may or may not be ordered for the client who is dying. Some clients request not to receive oxygen and, in some cases, oxygen makes the client more uncomfortable and anxious. Suctioning secretions from the nose and throat also may be ordered to assist in maintaining the airway. Sometimes, the suctioning is so uncomfortable and makes the client so panicky that it is not ordered. The nurse can keep the client's nostrils free of encrusted material by using a cotton-tipped applicator or swab moistened with normal saline. The nostrils can then be moistened and soothed by applying mineral oil.

Hydration and Nutrition

A person can survive longer without food than is possible without fluids (see Box 59-2). The dying person often does not want to eat or take fluids, but sometimes, with encouragement, will take small amounts. Clear, cold liquids, such as gelatin or juice, often are preferred to hot liquids or solids. Ice chips are often desirable. Milk is usually contraindicated in the final stages of life, because it may form a coating or membrane-like mucus in the throat and interfere with breathing. In some cases, the client refuses to eat because of nausea. If the client refuses to take anything by mouth, tube feeding or total parenteral nutrition (**TPN**) is possible. The healthcare provider, together with the client and family, determines what course of action to take, using the client's living will or durable power of attorney for healthcare as the guide (if available). In rare cases, the ethics committee becomes involved in this matter.

Nausea

Nausea and *vomiting* are quite common. The nurse can be helpful in providing supportive care. Teach the client to place a cool, damp cloth on the forehead; take slow, deep breaths; lie on the right side; and eat dry foods, such as soda crackers. The client's family should be taught these measures also, so they can assist. A number of **antiemetic** (antivomiting) medications are available (see Chapter 100).

Medications used to control nausea include metoclopramide (Reglan), trimethobenzamide hydrochloride (Tigan), ondansetron (Zofran), prochlorperazine (Compazine), an antipsychotic, and dronabinol (Marinol), a derivative of THC. (Marinol also stimulates appetite and is most often used for clients with acquired immunodeficiency syndrome [AIDS].) Antiemetics can be given orally or by injection; some are available as rectal suppositories. Sometimes, sustained-release tablets are available and may be scheduled on a regular basis to prevent nausea before it occurs (see Chapter 51).

Mouth Care

Swab the client's mouth with mouthwash as often as necessary. *Rationale: This helps to keep the mouth clean and to prevent a foul taste and bad breath.* If the client's tongue is dry, moisten it with saline swabs. In extreme cases, a very small amount of water-soluble lubricant may be applied. *Rationale: This helps prevent the tongue from sticking to the roof of the mouth.* Use mineral oil or water-soluble lubricant to keep the client's lips from cracking. Prepared mouth swabs are available to provide cleansing and a refreshing taste.

Elimination

Another basic need is that of elimination. Many very ill clients require assistance to meet this basic need, either to be able to void or to defecate, or to maintain cleanliness. These clients may also have a colostomy, ileostomy, ureterostomy, or indwelling catheter.

Incontinence

The client who is very ill may not be able to control bowel and/or bladder function. Urinary incontinence is more common than bowel incontinence. It is important to keep clients dry and clean (see Chapter 58). Use the prescribed skin cleanser and apply a moisture barrier substance. (Soap, shaving cream, cloth washcloths, and bag bath products are not used, because they can be irritating and dry the skin too much.) *Rationale: Careful skin care helps prevent skin breakdown and infection, minimize odors, and make the client more comfortable.*

Urinary Retention or Suppression

In some cases, the client is unable to void (urinate) or voids very little. Notify the provider if a client does not void for 8 hr or as specified in the care plan. Remember that in some cases, the client's body produces only a very small amount of urine. *Rationale: This can be due to causes, such as kidney failure and electrolyte imbalance, or may be the result of diaphoresis, emesis, or very limited fluid intake.* Urinary retention (inability to void) is also possible, as a result of poor innervation to the bladder and sphincter muscles, obstruction, or other disease processes. Notify the provider if the client's abdomen is hard and distended or if the client complains of unusual abdominal pain.

Constipation

In many cases, the very ill client may not have a bowel movement for several days. This can be a result of low food intake; bowel disorders; lack of stimulation to the bowel;

lack of exercise; and in rare cases, a bowel obstruction. Many very ill clients have constipation as an unwanted side effect of pain medications, particularly the opioids, such as codeine, meperidine (Demerol), and morphine and its derivatives. A mild laxative, such as magnesium hydroxide (Milk of Magnesia), may be given, but laxatives are given carefully. *Rationale: Overuse of laxatives may cause diarrhea and can lead to other disorders, particularly electrolyte imbalance and skin breakdown.* A stool softener, such as docusate sodium (Colace), or a mild bulk-producing laxative, such as psyllium (Metamucil), may be given routinely with the opioids, to prevent constipation. It is important to observe closely and report if a client complains of continued constipation or severe abdominal pain, to make sure a bowel obstruction is not present.

> **Nursing Alert** Remember: A client may be having diarrhea, even with a bowel obstruction. (In this case, the diarrhea stool is flowing around the obstruction.)

Diarrhea

Diarrhea is not uncommon in clients who are very ill. This can be a side effect of medications or can result from lack of solid food, a bowel obstruction, overuse of laxatives, or the disease process itself. It is very important to assist this client to keep the perineal area clean and dry if the client is unable to so. *Rationale: Diarrhea stool is very caustic and irritating to the skin.* The client with diarrhea is much more susceptible to bowel incontinence than the client who is constipated. This client may wish to wear an adult incontinence garment, such as Attends. An absorbent cloth bed pad (not paper, which can irritate the skin) should be in place as well.

Hygiene

The very ill client will usually be more comfortable if they are as clean as possible. The nurse may need to assist if the client is extremely ill. Even if a client is unconscious, it is important to keep the person clean and dry.

Bathing

If a client cannot bathe without assistance, the nurse needs to assist. In some cases, the client is too ill or too weak for a complete bed bath and can tolerate only a partial bath. The client can be assisted to brush the teeth or clean the dentures, or special mouth care is given by the nurse (see Chapter 50). The bedding is changed when necessary. This helps make the client more comfortable. A gentle backrub or hand or foot massage is often relaxing for the client.

Eye Care

Keep the client's eyes clean and moist by gently wiping them with gauze pads moistened in normal saline. Remember to wipe from the inner canthus outward and to use a separate gauze pad for each eye. *Rationale: This helps prevent spreading infection from one eye to the other.*

If the client's eyes are extremely dry, or if the client cannot blink, the care provider may instruct that the eyes be taped shut. In this case, paper tape is used and the tape is removed at least every 8 hr so the eyes can be cleansed and moistened with normal saline.

Hair Care

The very ill client will often have difficulty withstanding much attention to the hair. Usually if the client has long hair, a simple braid to the side will be sufficient. Use a shampoo cap or dry shampoo to cleanse the hair gently (see Chapter 50). *Rationale: Keep the braid out of the way, so the client will not lie on it. Do not subject the client to a bed shampoo with water; this would probably be too strenuous.* A satin pillowcase prevents stress on the hair. If the client has short hair, a surgical cap may be comfortable. The nurse can try to make the client feel as well-groomed as possible.

Odor Control

When a client is very ill, there may be unpleasant-smelling drainage or discharge from a wound or from the perineal area. Incontinence and emesis are common. The nurse can help control unwanted odors for the comfort of both client and family. Keep dressings clean and dry, and drainage bags empty. Use incontinence briefs and bed pads. *Rationale: This makes changing the client easier and more comfortable for the client.* Subtle deodorizers may be helpful. A small amount of oil of wintergreen on a gauze pad makes an effective deodorizer if nothing else is available.

Activity

As described in the preceding paragraphs, the nurse can perform many actions to make the client more comfortable. After addressing basic needs necessary to support life, such as oxygen, hydration, nutrition, and elimination, the nurse can work to meet the client's other needs, including activity. The client is assisted to be as active as possible. This may mean helping the client to dangle or to get up in the chair. The client may be assisted to walk to the bathroom or in the hall. Encourage the family to assist the client to move and walk. If the client cannot move, passive range of motion is performed by the nurse (see Chapter 48).

Pain Control

End-of-life care often involves the use of medications, including narcotics, to relieve and manage pain (see Chapter 100). In many cases, the provider will order regularly scheduled pain medications for very ill clients, to help manage distress and exhaustion, make them more comfortable, and overall make dying easier. Large doses of narcotics may be given; usually, there is no concern about drug abuse or dependency. Patient-controlled analgesia (PCA) may be used, so the client can self-administer opiates (see Chapter 55). Many clients find measures such as self-hypnosis and guided imagery to be helpful. In addition, therapies, such as acupuncture and acupressure, are often used. Other therapies, such as homeopathy, use of flower essences or essential oils, herbal remedies, or various traditional cultural remedies, have proved helpful for many clients. Just before death, pain may ease or disappear, often indicating impending death.

The Environment

The client's environment is kept as peaceful and comfortable as possible. Heating and air conditioning are controlled, so a comfortable temperature is maintained. The room should be kept well ventilated. Air is allowed to circulate, but should not be blowing directly on the client. The room should have some lighting, but not so much as to interfere with the client's ability to rest or sleep. At night, keeping a light on in the room is often helpful. *Rationale: Darkness is frightening to many people. Often, a dying client will turn toward a light. Clients may be more uncomfortable and afraid if left in the dark. Soft music is often soothing.*

Higher-Level Needs

If the client's basic needs have been met, the client will be able to work on achieving higher-level needs. This applies to the family as well.

Self-Esteem

People who are dying need to feel that they are worthwhile, that they have contributed to the world, and that they are an important member of the family. Many clients want to plan their funeral or write their will. Many clients choose to write a memoir or make a scrapbook of their life. The person can be encouraged to record memories, if they are not able to write a memoir. Fixing a client's hair or helping them to write a letter can provide comfort. Be sure to help clients perform any self-care they can manage. Clients may feel inadequate when they are no longer able to perform activities of daily living (ADLs) without assistance. Emphasize the things that the client *can do*. Encourage the client to focus on life achievements. Remember that having raised a family is a great contribution to the world.

Diversion

It is important for the client to have some diversion, if possible. A soft radio or CD playing can be soothing. Many clients enjoy watching television or reading a book or magazine. Helping the client to obtain and listen to audio books is a way to provide diversion, with minimal effort on the part of the client. Most clients enjoy outings, if they are able. Encourage friends and family to take the client on short outings and to come and visit. If outings and visits are too tiring for the client, encourage people to send cards, emails, and Facebook messages.

Emotional Support

Short visits from family and friends are encouraged, unless the client is in a great deal of pain. The client can visit with others and have an opportunity to let them know how they are feeling and to reassure them that everything will be OK. Often, the client or family members have questions that can be answered; this often makes everyone feel more comfortable. The nurse can be available to offer support and a "listening ear" for clients as they work toward acceptance of their situation. As clients move closer to death, many are more fearful if they are left alone, especially at night. Encourage the family to stay with the client if this is the case.

NURSING PROCESS

CARE OF THE DYING PERSON

Assessment and Data Gathering Priorities
- Understanding of medical condition/prognosis
- Attitudes toward death (personal, ethnic, religious)
- Psychological and spiritual needs of client and family
- Preferences: desire to be home, in hospital, enrolled in hospice program
- Decisions concerning resuscitation, aggressive treatment, advanced life support, organ and tissue donation
- Existence and documentation of advance directives, durable power of attorney
- DNR, DNI, DNH status
- Stage of grief and death reactions, coping behaviors
- Available resources
- Physiologic needs of the client

POSSIBLE NURSING DIAGNOSES
- Anxiety
- Risk for caregiver role strain
- Decisional conflict
- Ineffective coping
- Interrupted family processes
- Anticipatory grieving
- Hopelessness
- Pain
- Powerlessness
- Self-care deficit
- Social isolation
- Spiritual distress

Other diagnoses will depend on physiologic responses of client to the disease process.

PLANNING
Design a plan of care with the client and family to achieve the following general goals. The client and family will:
- Verbalize that they feel free to express needs, fears, and emotions.
- Identify preferences concerning death (these are documented).
- Demonstrate positive methods of coping.
  The client will:
- Report sufficient pain relief, in order to interact meaningfully with family and friends and attend to everyday matters.
- Participate in self-care to the extent possible.
  The long-term goal is death with dignity, which leaves the family unit intact.

IMPLEMENTATION
- Establish supportive, trusting relationship with client and family.
- Express warmth, care, and concern in interactions with client and family; do not be afraid to cry.
- Explain the client's condition/treatment to client and family.
- Maintain open communication with all concerned.
- Ensure that the client's basic physiologic needs are met.
- Provide appropriate pain relief.

- Talk with the client, even if they are comatose.
- Provide simple explanations of what is being done and what is expected.
- Support the client and family; avoid being judgmental.
- Encourage client and family to be actively involved in planning and providing care.
- Arrange spiritual counseling, if requested.
- Encourage family members to express needs and encourage respite time for them.
- Assist at the time of death, including caring for the body, placing identification tags, supporting the family and answering questions, and preparing necessary documentation.
- Offer the opportunity for organ and tissue donation.
- Offer support to other clients and staff.

EVALUATION

The plan of care is evaluated by determining if the above goals are met. Evaluative criteria include:
- Client's death with dignity
- Intact family, appropriately progressing through stages of grief

NURSING CARE OF THE DYING CLIENT'S FAMILY

The family of the dying client requires the empathetic support of nursing and medical staff. In many cases, the client's family members experience the stress of this period more keenly than does the client. They are dealing with a sense of loss, yet they often feel they must appear as though everything is normal. Family members should understand that crying and being sad in front of the client are acceptable behaviors and are actually recommended. Showing their feelings tells the client that they care deeply.

> **Key Concept**
>
> Encourage the family to express their emotions and to let the client see how they feel about the situation. Let them know that it is OK to cry. Some families hide their feelings and refuse to allow the client to talk about death. The danger here is that the client may feel that no one cares that they are dying.

If a client is in pain or is very apprehensive, explain to family members that they can make the death easier by taking turns staying with the client (Fig. 59-3). Some cultures require a family member to be present at all times when a client is dying. Show the family comfort measures they can take to ease the individual's pain (e.g., hand massage, offering fluids, or fluffing up the pillows). Encourage family members to continue to communicate with the person, even if they do not respond. *Rationale: The client may be too ill or too weak to respond, but usually can hear.* Family and friends can repeatedly tell the individual of their love. They may be reluctant to tell the client that they will be missed. However, this will strengthen the person's sense that they have made an impression on the world. Family members need to assure the dying person that they can manage after the death of the

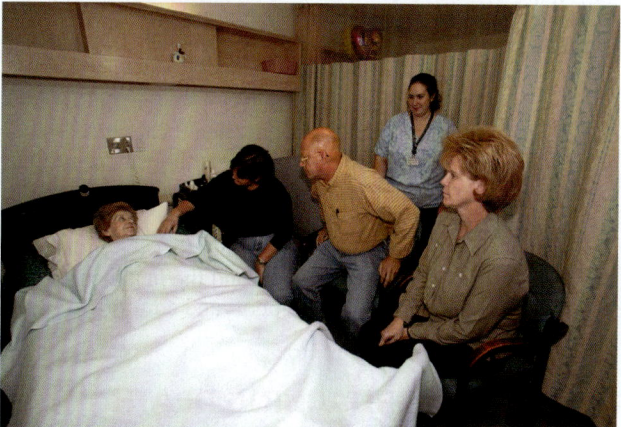

Figure 59-3 The family of the dying person can provide support and comfort just by being there. As a practical matter, the nurse makes sure they have enough chairs. (From Carter, P. [2019]. *Lippincott textbook for nursing assistants: A humanistic approach to caregiving* [5th ed.]. Wolters Kluwer.)

person. They can reassure their loved one that the love they share will support them in the future. Often, people struggling with death need their closest loved ones to give them permission to move on to the next stage of life's journey, that of death. Dying clients can offer comfort to the family by sharing feelings and thoughts. Encourage such communication. Support groups are available for assistance. If the client is well enough, they can attend the support group with the family. Otherwise, the family can attend and discuss their feelings. Families often need help in knowing what to do for their loved ones during the dying process. Explain to them the physical and emotional stages associated with dying.

Family Respite

It is important for family members to remember that they need personal rest and refreshment, as much as the client. This is called *respite care*. It is kind to offer a cup of tea or coffee or a snack when a visit with the client has been exhausting. Show them where facilities are located, including telephones and public computer terminals, bathrooms, or the cafeteria. Many facilities have a lounge or chapel for family members where they can be alone. Often, the lounge includes a place to nap. If a waiting period is likely to be long, encourage family members to go out for meals and rest, assuring them that they will be called immediately should any change occur. Suggest that they carry a cell phone for this purpose.

> **Key Concept**
>
> Clients who have been confused or unconscious may abruptly become lucid and alert when they are about to die. If possible, call family members at this time so everyone has a chance to say a final good-bye.

The Role of Hope

Dying individuals may cling to hope and not give up until the very end, when they finally reach acceptance or withdrawal. Families also may cling to the hope that an unexpected recovery may occur. Individuals and the family may resist entrance into a hospice program (see Chapter 100) because giving up seems impossible or wrong. Do not destroy this hope with logical arguments, but do not give false hope either. The role of the nurse and other healthcare professionals is to be honest with clients and to support them in their own way of coping. Clients and family members may ask, "Is there any hope at all?" An honest answer is that nobody truly knows when a person will die, but that the individual will receive the best care available, and the healthcare team will do all they can to provide support and comfort.

SIGNS OF APPROACHING DEATH

The dying process proceeds from the distal portions of the body inward. Therefore, the legs and then the arms lose sensation and the ability to move before internal organs cease to function. *Rationale: Blood flow is directed toward the brain and the vital organs in the center of the body.* Peripheral circulation diminishes first and then stops; the client often experiences *diaphoresis* (sweating) or elevated temperature, and then the body cools. The sense of touch is usually diminished, although the person can feel pressure. Box 59-3 lists some common signs of approaching death.

> **NCLEX Alert**
>
> It is important to know signs of approaching death as you read the examination scenarios and select your nursing actions for the test options.

Failing Circulation

As circulation begins to fail, the client's body temperature lowers, but the client may be perspiring. Heavy blankets may make the person restless. Provide light covering, and keep it loose over the client's feet, using a bed cradle if necessary (see Chapter 49). Warmed blankets are often comforting.

Failing Senses

Research has shown that hearing is the last sense that is lost. Most clients can hear until the final moment. Speak distinctly, and do not whisper or talk about the client; talk to the client, even if they are not able to answer. It is soothing for the client if someone holds their hand. Try not to leave the client alone. The dying client is likely to feel a sense of increasing darkness as vision begins to fail and may turn toward a window or other source of light.

> **Key Concept**
>
> Assist the family to be near the client as death approaches. Encourage them to talk to the client and hold the client's hand. This is helpful for the client and for the family, as they gain closure.
>
> Include the family in the care of the client, as the client and family desire. They can help bathe the client or help the person to walk, if they are comfortable in doing this.

> **Box 59-3 Signs of Approaching Death**
>
> The following signs may be noted in the client who is dying, as death approaches and eventually occurs. Keep in mind that there is no specific order to these changes and each of these changes *may or may not* occur.
>
> - Loss of control over bladder and bowel. Rationale: *Neurologic control may be lost.*
> - Intake of food and drink will diminish, and general nutritional requirements are less. Rationale: *The client is not moving and body processes are slowed, causing lowered requirements for food and fluids. The brain also may not be receiving neurologic stimuli for hunger and thirst.*
> - The extremities will feel colder to the touch. Rationale: *General circulation slows and blood flow is directed toward the body's core.*
> - The person experiences increased fatigue and difficulty waking. Rationale: *Circulation to the brain slows, as general circulation diminishes.*
> - Recognition of familiar people, places, or objects decreases, and visions of people or things that do not exist may occur. Rationale: *This is also a function of diminished circulation to the brain.*
> - Occasionally, restlessness increases. Rationale: *This is often caused by oxygen hunger.*
> - Dry mouth and accumulation of thick secretions in the back of the throat often occur. Rationale: *The client's swallow and gag reflexes are diminished.*
> - Noisy breathing is common. Rationale: *This is caused by secretions collected in the mouth, throat, or lungs.*
> - The pattern of breathing changes, such as rapid breathing followed by periods where breathing is slow or absent for as long as 15 s (Cheyne–Stokes respirations). Rationale: *As the breathing centers in the brain receive less oxygen, breathing patterns are affected.*
>
> At the point of death:
> - Breathing, heartbeat, and pulse stop entirely.
> - The person is entirely unresponsive to shaking or shouting.
> - The person does not respond to painful stimuli.
> - The eyelids may be open or closed, and the pupils are dilated and fixed in one direction.
> - Loss of bladder and bowel control occurs.
>
> *Note:* Not all of these changes occur in each death.

Stanford School of Medicine. (n.d.). *Signs of impending death.* https://palliative.stanford.edu/transition-to-death/signs-of-impending-death/ and Crossroads Hospice and Palliative Care. (n.d.). *A guide to understanding end-of-life signs and symptoms.* https://www.crossroadshospice.com/hospice-resources/end-of-life-signs/.

CARE FOLLOWING THE DEATH OF A CLIENT

At the actual time of death, a number of activities must be carried out, either by the nurse or by the family. The family can assist with the care of the body after death in the healthcare facility or their home, if they desire to do this. Some cultures require this care to be performed by the family.

Clinical Versus Biologic Death

Death is generally defined as the *cessation of all physical and chemical processes*. However, more specialized definitions of death apply in medical care.

Clinical death occurs when respiration and heartbeat both stop. (Clinical death may be reversible if resuscitation efforts are successful.) For the client who is DNR/DNI, note the exact time when respiration stops (usually first), and the exact time when the heart stops beating. Notify the healthcare provider or other primary care provider.

Biologic death is defined as the *irreversible* cessation of heart and lung functioning. Sometimes, a differentiation is made for the definition of **brain death** or *cerebral death*. Brain death is formally defined as the irreversible cessation of total brain function, including the brain stem, as determined by clinical examination. Mechanical or chemical means can maintain the client's vital functions (ventilation and circulation) even *after* brain death occurs. Therefore, the determination of brain death is made under carefully controlled conditions. In certain situations, a client's cardiovascular functions may continue to be maintained mechanically until some of their organs may be removed for transplant.

Determination of brain death varies slightly across different states and provinces, but generally, brain death means that the client's electroencephalogram (EEG) shows no brain wave activity ("flat line"). The EEG determination is often combined with other criteria to pronounce biologic death. Other criteria include:

- Total unresponsiveness to stimuli
- Cessation of all spontaneous movement, breathing, and heartbeat
- Complete absence of cephalic reflexes
- Fixed, dilated pupils

Cerebral circulation studies also may be done.

Two exceptions to the usual criteria for biologic death are a hypothermic condition (e.g., drowning) and central nervous system depression secondary to drug overdose. These situations require additional studies. The ethics committee may be involved in some determinations of brain death and procedures to be followed.

> **Key Concept**
>
> The determination of death while the client is being maintained on a ventilator and cardiac stimulants is difficult for the family. They need to understand fully and accept that even though the client appears to be breathing, it is the machine that is actually ventilating the client.

Pronouncement of Death

The formal pronouncement of death varies slightly among states and provinces. In most states, the healthcare provider must make the pronouncement of a death occurring within a healthcare facility. In the case of death in the client's home or the community, the pronouncement of death varies between situations and between states. If the client was previously accepted into a hospice program, often the professional hospice nurse can pronounce cardiovascular death. In the event of an accident, suicide, or homicide, death may be pronounced by the coroner. This person may or may not be a healthcare provider.

Caring for the Family

When a person dies, the family often does not know what to do next. Family members may need time just to sit with the body. Help them make the transition to bereavement. Care of the family now becomes the nurse's major focus. Allow them to talk and express their feelings. Answer questions. Offer them privacy and help them in locating local resources, such as calling the chaplain or social worker, or giving them a list of funeral homes in the area. The family may need to decide between cremation and full burial; funeral directors or hospice nurses can assist.

SPECIAL CONSIDERATIONS Lifespan

Family Coping After a Death

Many variables surrounding death influence how family members will cope. All these factors interact to influence how the family responds to the death. Individual family members most likely will respond in different ways. Variables include:

- Personalities of individual family members
- Personality and values of the client
- Relationships between client and other family members
- Family stability/unity
- Relationships among survivors
- Cultural, ethnic, and religious practices and customs
- Age of the client (infant, child, adult, older adult)
- Suddenness of death (time for preparation and resolution)
- Length and severity of illness
- Manner of death (natural, accidental, traumatic, homicide, suicide)

After the person has been pronounced dead, and if an **autopsy** (*"postmortem"* examination of the body after death) is not to be performed, remove nasogastric tubes, remove intravenous (IV) lines, and turn off monitors. Prepare the body so the family can see it. Try to make the client appear comfortable. Be sure the body is clean. Place a clean sheet over the client, but do not cover the face (Fig. 59-4). Allow family members to stay in the room as long as they wish, knowing that help or support is available if needed. Muted lighting is comforting. Offer to call their clergy, social services, friends, or other family members.

> **Key Concept**
>
> In the event of a sudden or accidental death, the client's family has had no time to prepare for the event. The nurse working in rescue or in areas such as the Emergency Department or the Coronary Care Unit needs to possess special communication and interpersonal skills. In many cases, special training is available for nurses and other healthcare providers who work in these areas.

Postmortem Care of the Body

In the healthcare facility, the primary provider pronounces that the client is dead and signs the death certificate. The body is then prepared for transport to the morgue or pickup by the funeral director. In Practice: Nursing Procedure 59-1 reviews caring for the body after death. In the healthcare facility, these procedures are usually performed by nursing staff. If the client plans to die at home, the home care nurse is responsible for adapting these procedures and teaching them to the family. In the home care

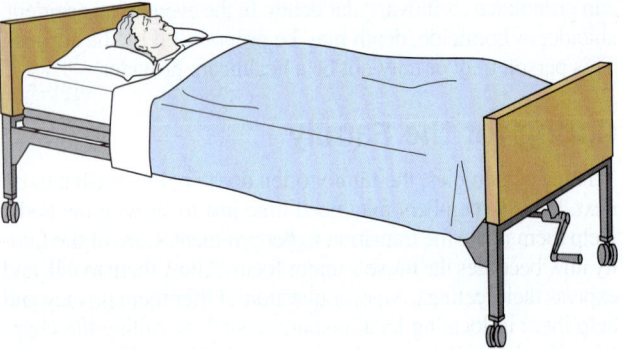

Figure 59-4 Prepare the client's body to be viewed by the family. (The shroud was previously placed under the client.) (From Carter, P. [2019]. *Lippincott textbook for nursing assistants: A humanistic approach to caregiving* [5th ed.]. Wolters Kluwer.)

situation and in some cultures, the family may have been taught and may be willing and able to carry out the preparation of the client's body. The funeral director or religious representative picks up the body directly from the home, unless an autopsy is to be done. In the event of an anticipated death of a hospice client at home, the healthcare provider usually does not need to travel to the home to pronounce death. (In the case of sudden or suspicious death, the coroner is called and pronounces the death and then determines who will manage the scene, which may now be considered a *crime scene*.)

The Postmortem Examination

In many cases, a **postmortem examination** (autopsy) is desirable or required by law. In the event of a sudden, unexpected death and certainly with any suspicion of foul play, a postmortem examination is required. This is known as a "coroner's case" and no consent is required. In other situations, such as if the client had been undergoing special therapy or experimental treatment, the healthcare team may feel that an autopsy would be helpful from a research standpoint. In some cases, an autopsy is requested by the provider or family to establish the exact cause of death, even though the person was known to be ill.

> **Key Concept**
> In some cases, the family may opt not to allow a postmortem examination for personal or religious reasons. Unless an autopsy is required by law, this is their right.

If an autopsy is to be done, the family may have questions about it. Answer their questions as completely and accurately as possible. In nearly all cases, the family may obtain a copy of the autopsy report at a later time.

When a loved one dies, a family may be required to make major decisions, involving:

- Performance of an autopsy
- Donation of organs or tissues
- Choice of funeral home or crematorium
- Cremation versus traditional burial
- Memorial service or other recognition of the client's life
- Posting of death notices in the newspaper or on-line
- Contacting special agencies, such as the VA, for a military funeral

Nurses often are involved in answering questions about these decisions. If you are not sure of the answers, obtain appropriate assistance. Be aware that in some cultures, burial must occur *within 24 hr* of death and in some cultures *cremation* is required or forbidden. Other specific *religious or cultural rituals* may also be required.

FEELINGS OF THE NURSE

The death of any client is traumatic for the nurse, even if the death was expected. The nurse has been concentrating on caring for the client and the family. Now, the nurse must remember to care for themselves.

Support for the Nurse on the Death of a Client

One of the greatest challenges facing the nurse is providing care for a dying person. Most nurses cannot just walk away from a situation where a person has died. Colleagues can be an informal help, by allowing time for grieving. Many healthcare facilities have meetings following the death of an individual who was receiving care. In such meetings, team members give each other mutual support. Discuss feelings with others who can provide support (e.g., supervisor, coworker, spouse, spiritual advisor). Formal support groups often exist in hospice units where nurses frequently encounter client death. Expressing sadness to coworkers and to the person's family is also appropriate. Chapter 100 discusses hospice nursing in further detail.

STUDENT SYNTHESIS

KEY POINTS

- Advance directives, codes, and organ and tissue donation are three types of client wishes that nurses must be familiar with when caring for dying individuals.
- The ethics committee may become involved in making determinations about care to be given to clients who cannot make decisions for themselves.
- Remember, when delivering end-of-life care, that this person has the same basic human needs as any other person.
- Changing the client's position frequently may promote comfort, prevent skin breakdown, and ease breathing.
- Maintaining a patent airway is a primary nursing responsibility for all clients.
- The dying client who is incontinent needs to be kept as clean and dry as possible.
- Tube feeding or total parenteral nutrition may be instituted if the dying client is unable to eat or drink. The client also may choose not to receive nourishment.

- Pain relief may provide comfort and help ease the dying process.
- Brain death occurs when no brain function can be identified by EEG or specific other means.
- The client's family needs nursing comfort in the form of understanding and support. They also need to have their questions answered.
- The family may choose to donate their loved one's tissues or organs after death.
- After death, the nurse often gives physical care to the client's body and offers emotional support to the family.
- When a family member chooses to die at home, the family assumes the role of caregiver and usually manages most of the postmortem care.
- Cultural and religious considerations must be taken into account when working with dying clients.
- Nurses must take care of themselves after the death of a client. Staff members can offer support to each other.

CRITICAL THINKING EXERCISES

1. Review Maslow hierarchy of needs (Chapter 5). Discuss how the needs of the dying person relate to Maslow basic needs. Make a chart showing the relationships.
2. You are aware of the need for more people to donate organs and tissues for transplant use. The wife of a terminally ill person on a ventilator has been asked to donate the organs for transplant. The wife is having difficulty deciding what the client would have wished and asks you to help think about the decision. How could you help? What resources are available?
3. A.M., a 35-year-old Muslim man, is brought to the hospital's emergency room in critical condition following a motor vehicle accident. He is not expected to live. "Donor" is printed on their driver's license. Describe your responsibilities in the nursing care of this client What issues might the medical and nursing staff discuss with this client's family? What support could you give to the family? What pertinent resources are available in your hospital and in your community? Discuss cultural aspects of this client's care as they relate to organ donation, family dynamics, and religious practices. What type of after-death activities would you expect if this man should die?
4. Discuss the differences in the dying experience in the following situations: the client who has had cancer for 1 year, a person involved in a fatal automobile accident, the older adult person who dies in their sleep, and the child who is dying of a fatal disease.

NCLEX-STYLE REVIEW QUESTIONS

1. The nurse is caring for a dying client. Which is the priority nursing action during the care of this client?
   a. Offer fluids every hour.
   b. Alleviate anxiety.
   c. Turn the client every 2 hr.
   d. Maintain a patent airway.
2. Which signs observed by the nurse indicate the client is approaching death? Select all that apply.
   a. Increased thirst and hunger
   b. Increased alertness and awareness
   c. Difficult to arouse
   d. Extremities feel colder to touch
   e. Loss of bowel/bladder control
3. The nurse is implementing a plan of care for a dying client. Which nursing action can assist the client in maintaining dignity?
   a. Apply restraints when the client becomes confused.
   b. Allow the client to do as much as possible.
   c. Give pain medication even when the client rejects it.
   d. Restrict visitors to immediate family only.
4. The nurse observes a family member of a dying client crying by the client's bedside. Which response by the nurse is appropriate?
   a. "Don't cry, you are going to upset the client."
   b. "The client can't hear you anyway."
   c. "Is there anything that I can do to help?"
   d. "You should expect this, the client has been ill for a long time."
5. A client has a terminal diagnosis and wants to be specific about what treatment and care is rendered when unable to make those decisions. What should the nurse encourage the client to obtain?
   a. A general will
   b. Advance directives (AD)
   c. Durable power of attorney (DPOA)
   d. Do not resuscitate (DNR) order

CHAPTER RESOURCES

Enhance your learning with additional resources on **the Point***!*

Student Resources related to this chapter can be found at **thePoint.lww.com/Rosdahl12e**.

WELCOME STEPS

Look at healthcare provider's orders.

Protocol for procedure.

Necessary equipment/supplies.

Wash hands using proper hand hygiene; put on gloves.

Explain the procedure and reassure the client.

Locate two identifiers to confirm correct client.

Comfortable and efficient position for nurse and client.

Obtain privacy.

Make sure to follow correct steps and body mechanics with good technique.

Ensure safety and observe deviations from normal.

END STEPS

Ensure comfort and safety.

Note questions or concerns from client or nurse; note significant data.

Dispose of materials properly.

Disinfect the area and your hands.

Document and report the procedure and your findings.

IN PRACTICE
NURSING PROCEDURE 59-1 | Postmortem Care of the Body

Supplies and Equipment
Disposable gloves (two pairs)
Protective gown
Chipped ice and extra gloves (if needed)
Postmortem kit or the following:
- Towel or chin strap
- Tape and safety pins
- Self-sealing property bag
- Fresh dressings
- Shroud or zippered bag
- Incontinence pad
- Gauze squares for padding and to cover wounds
- Ties for wrists and ankles
- Identification tags (at least two, usually three)

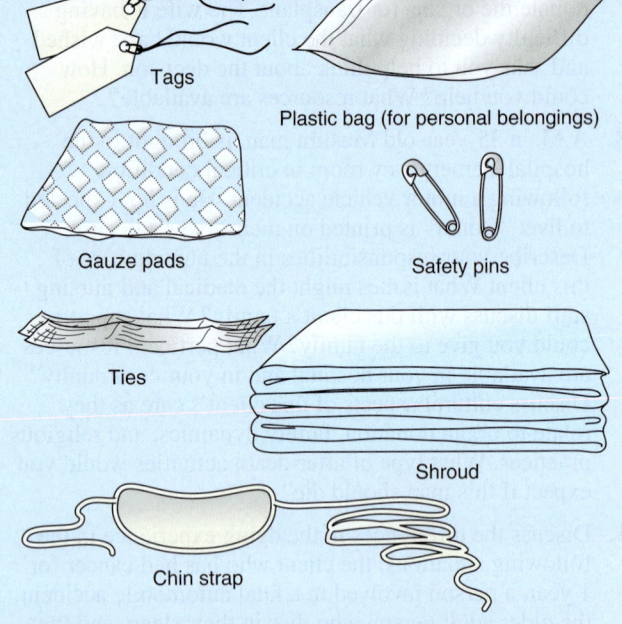

Most postmortem kits contain a shroud or special zippered body bag, as well as other materials for preparing the body for transport to the morgue. (From Carter, P. (2019). Lippincott textbook for nursing assistants: a humanistic approach to caregiving (5th ed.). Wolters Kluwer.)

Steps
Follow LPN WELCOME Steps and Then

1. Obtain a postmortem kit or assemble the needed supplies. You may wish to wear two pairs of gloves. Wear a protective gown. *Rationale: The contents of the postmortem kit may vary among institutions. Make sure you have what you need. The person has most likely been incontinent and may have had a communicable disease. You need to protect yourself against exposure to body fluids.*

2. Carefully identify the body. Straighten the body, and place a small pillow under the head. *Rationale: Checking the person's identity helps prevent errors. Proper positioning immediately after death prevents potential problems. The body will assume this position in a casket.*

3. If the person's eyes are to be donated, close them, and place a small ice pack on each eye. A glove with a few ice chips works well. *Rationale: Ice helps prevent swelling and discoloration and preserves the corneas.*

4. Remove any jewelry. If there is a specific order, tape a wedding ring in place. Carefully document this. List all client property and place it in the designated property bag. Give the client's property bag to the family and have them sign for it. Send all flowers and cards home with the family. Make sure to check the closet, dresser, and vault for property. *Removing jewelry and documenting its removal ensure that none of the client's property is lost. Some clients never take off their wedding rings. The family takes possession of the client's belongings and may wish to write thank you notes.*

5. Close the client's mouth by placing a chin strap or rolled towel under the chin. *Rationale: This closes the mouth and prevents the jaw from falling down.*

6. Remove all intravenous (IV) lines, monitors, and other equipment, unless ordered otherwise or this is a Coroner's case. Remove all extra equipment from the room. *Rationale: Equipment is no longer needed. It will stay in the facility to be sterilized for reuse or will be disposed of according to hazardous waste disposal policies.*

7. Remove all top bed linens, except the sheet that covers the client. Bathe any part of the body that has been soiled with discharges. Place a clean incontinence pad under the person. *Rationale: Bathing preserves the client's dignity. Additional urine or feces may escape from the body. The pad protects the bed.*

8. Remove soiled dressings, dispose of them properly, and replace with clean ones. Pad the wrists and ankles with gauze squares, and tie them loosely together. *Rationale: This procedure makes handling the body easier and prevents the arms and legs from falling down. Standard precautions are always followed.*

9. Give the client's dentures and glasses to the funeral director. Most funeral directors prefer to place dentures in the client's mouth themselves. The family may take the client's glasses to the funeral home. *Rationale: Dentures may be broken when being placed in the mouth. They will be placed in the mouth before the funeral, to preserve the shape of the client's face. Glasses are important so the person looks natural; the family can make sure they do not get lost en route.*

10. Attach two tags to the body: one tied to the foot (usually the right great toe) and the other to the hand or wrist. Another is usually attached to the covering sheet. (In some cases, a tag is placed in a slot on the morgue cart.) These tags are stamped with the client's name, facility identification number, facility name and address, client's diagnosis, attending healthcare provider, and the date and time of death. *Rationale: The client must be correctly identified.*

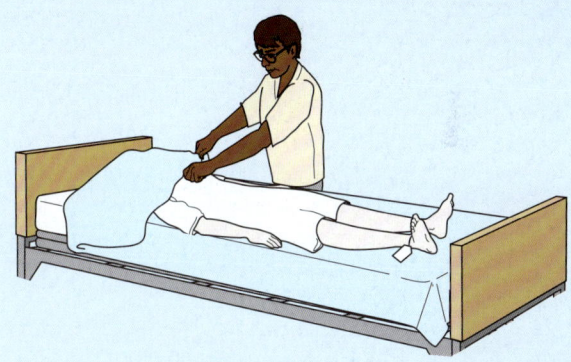

An identification tag is placed on the client's right foot or right great toe and on the wrist. If a shroud is used, the top of the shroud is folded over the person's head and the bottom over the client's feet. (From Carter, P. (2019). *Lippincott textbook for nursing assistants: a humanistic approach to caregiving* (5th ed.). Wolters Kluwer.)

11. Wrap the body before it is taken to the morgue according to facility protocol. Usually, a shroud or zippered bag is provided. A special morgue cart is used to transport the body. *Rationale: Properly wrapping the body covers the client, demonstrates respect, and maintains their dignity.*

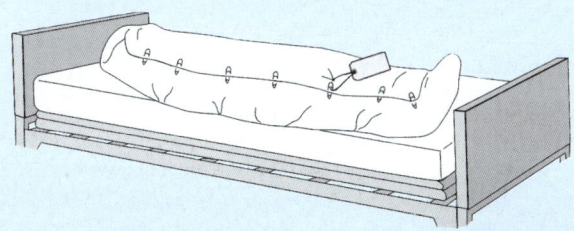

The sides of the shroud are brought up and fastened with pins or tape or zipped up, as per protocol. An additional identification tag is usually secured to the outside of the shroud. (From Carter, P. (2019). *Lippincott textbook for nursing assistants: a humanistic approach to caregiving* (5th ed.). Wolters Kluwer.)

UNIT 8 Client Care

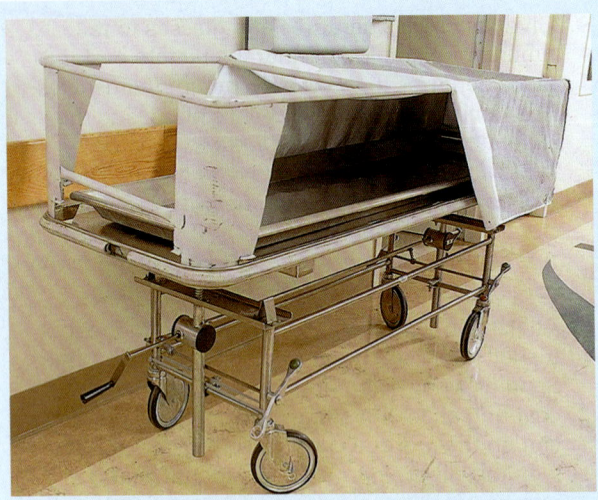

The client's body is transported to the morgue in a special covered morgue cart. A sheet is placed over the morgue cart for transport. (Photo by B. Proud.)

12. If the client had a known communicable disease, note this on the shroud or covering. *Rationale: Special precautions may need to be taken with the body.*

Follow ENDDD Steps

Special Reminders
- Standard precautions are used in caring for the body, as in any other procedure.
- *Do not remove any lines or appliances* if the death is a Medical Examiner or law enforcement case.

UNIT 9
Pharmacology and Administration of Medications

60 Review of Mathematics

Learning Objectives

1. Explain why an understanding of basic mathematics is essential when studying pharmacology.
2. Briefly state the historical uses of the household and apothecary systems of measurement. State one value in each system still used in healthcare.
3. Describe the most commonly used system of measurement in healthcare; state why this system is used.
4. State the basis of metric measurement.
5. Demonstrate the ability to convert among milligrams, grams, and kilograms.
6. Demonstrate the ability to convert between kilograms/grams and pounds; explain why this is necessary.
7. Give examples of formerly used drug-related abbreviations and symbols that are no longer acceptable; state the reasons for this.
8. Demonstrate the use of ratio and proportion to calculate medication dosages.
9. Demonstrate the ability to multiply and divide simple fractions.

Important Terminology

decimal fraction
denominator
fraction
gram
liter
meter
metric
numerator
percentage
pharmacology
proportion
ratio
units

This chapter discusses the basics of **pharmacology**, the study of chemical substances, and their effects on the body. Pharmacology is closely related to mathematics; basic mathematical principles are introduced here. The nurse needs a general understanding of mathematics to follow medication orders and safely administer medications, a primary nursing responsibility. This chapter emphasizes the metric system of measurement, the most common system used in pharmacology. Although in most cases, nurses are not required to calculate dosages, it is important to understand the basics. Thus, several methods of dosage calculation are introduced.

Nursing Alert Administering drugs is one of the most important nursing functions. Take this responsibility seriously. A medication error could cause a client's death.

SYSTEMS OF MEASUREMENT

Historically, three different systems of measurement were used in dispensing and administering medications: household, apothecary, and metric. In some cases, the measurements were not exact. In addition, the use of three systems was confusing, contributing to medication errors. Today, the metric system is used almost exclusively. Table 60-1 identifies some examples of the different systems and how they relate to each other.

One measurement system used in the past, the *household system*, used measurements used in the home. Common household units are familiar (e.g., drop, teaspoon, tablespoon, cup, pint, quart). These units are rarely used in healthcare, except in the case of a specified number of eye or ear drops.

The *apothecary system*, based on volume and weight, is the oldest system of measurement. (It is based on the "average weight" of one grain of wheat or the size of an "average" drop.) This system was used for many years in prescribing and dispensing medications but is the least accurate system. It is possible that a home care nurse could encounter an apothecary dosage (usually with outdated medications). The most common of these is "grains V," the dose of one regular size aspirin tablet (325 mg). You may also see an order for "one *fluid ounce*" of a medication, such as Milk of Magnesia, equivalent to 30 mL (milliliters). If you encounter household or apothecary measurements, or if you have questions, consult a pharmacist. Both of these older systems have been replaced by the metric system of measurement.

TABLE 60-1	Approximate Liquid Equivalents of Household, Apothecary, and Metric Measurement Systems	
HOUSEHOLD	APOTHECARY	METRIC
1 teaspoon (tsp)	—	5 milliliters (ml)
1 tablespoon (tbsp)	—	15 ml
2 tbsp	1 ounce (oz)	30 ml
1 cup	8 oz	240 ml
1 pint (pt)	16 oz	480 ml
1 quart (qt)	32 oz	960 ml (1 L = 1,000 ml)

TABLE 60-2	Symbols Used in Metric Measurement
UNIT	ABBREVIATION OR SYMBOL
Milligram	1 mg = 1/1,000 of a gram
Gram	G
Kilogram	1 kg = 1,000 g
Microgram	1 μg = 1/1,000 μg
Liter	1 L = 1,000 ml
Milliliter	1 ml = 1/1,000 L

Key Concept

Medications may also be ordered in **units** (a specific measurement used for certain drugs, such as insulin). The term "units," or International Units, is also used in nutrition to identify specific nutrients, including vitamins.

Be aware that a number of abbreviations and symbols have been identified as confusing and are no longer recommended for use (see Chapter 37; Table 37-5). If you have any question about an abbreviation or symbol, check with your instructor or team leader.

THE METRIC SYSTEM

The **metric** system is very simple to use and is the most widely used measurement system in the world today. It is used almost exclusively in drug dosages. The metric system is a **decimal** system based on the number 10. (The monetary system of the United States is based on the metric system.)

In healthcare, metric measurements are based on the meter, gram, and liter. The **meter** (M) is a measurement of length or distance; the **gram** (g) is a measurement of weight; and the **liter** (L) is a measurement of liquid volume. Greek and Latin prefixes are used to describe various increments of these basic units. For example:

  deci—divide by 10; 1/10
  centi—divide by 100; 1/100
  milli—divide by 1,000; 1/1,000
  micro—divide by 1,000,000; 1/1 millionth
  deca—multiply by 10; ×10
  hecto—multiply by 100; ×100
  kilo—multiply by 1,000; ×1,000

Refer to Table 60-2 for metric symbols or abbreviations most commonly used in computing dosages. In addition to medication administration, nurses use the metric system in other aspects of care. For example, amounts of oral fluid intake and urinary output are measured in milliliters (ml); newborns are weighed in grams (g) and measured in centimeters (cm). Clients are often weighed in kilograms (kg) to facilitate medication and anesthetic dosage calculations for surgery. When measuring the size of an incision or skin ulcer, healthcare personnel measure the area in centimeters (2.54 cm = 1 in.). Cervical dilation during delivery is stated in centimeters. (Ten centimeters—about 4 in.—is usually considered to be full dilation.) Reactions to purified protein derivative (PPD) tests and other skin tests are measured in millimeters (mm).

Key Concept

Adults are often weighed in kilograms. Infants are weighed in grams. These values may be converted to pounds and ounces for the client's information.

- 1 kg = 2.2 lb: multiply kilograms by 2.2 to determine pounds
- 1 oz = 28.35 g: divide grams by 28.35 to determine ounces; 16 oz = 1 lb: divide ounces by 16 to determine pounds and ounces

Conversion of Values Within the Metric System

Most healthcare facilities dispense each client's medications in unit-dose format; that is, each tablet or dose is packaged individually. In addition, many facilities utilize a computer with dosages already calculated. However, you may still occasionally need to compute the number of tablets or unit doses to be given. In home care, you are more likely to encounter medications dispensed in multiple-dose bottles. In this case, you will need to determine how many tablets of each medication to administer.

Sometimes, a prescription is stated in milligrams (mg), but a drug is available only in grams (g). This requires accurate completion of metric conversions to ensure administration of the proper dose. Because the metric system is a decimal (based on 10) system, conversion is easy by using multiplication or division. For instance, to convert grams (g) to milligrams (mg), multiply by 1,000. To convert milligrams to grams, divide by 1,000. Another quick and easy method to complete the conversion simply involves moving the decimal point (see "Decimal Fractions" section for rationale). To convert grams to milligrams, move the decimal point three places to the right; to convert milligrams to grams, move the decimal point three places to the left. Box 60-1 lists some common metric measurements and equivalents.

CHAPTER 60 Review of Mathematics

Box 60-1 Common Metric Measurements and Equivalents

Some metric equivalents are used more frequently than others. Memorize the following measures and equivalents:

DISTANCE
1 meter (M) = 100 centimeters (cm) = 1,000 millimeters (mm)
1 cm = 0.01 M
1 mm = 0.001 M
2.54 cm = 1 in.
(A meter is slightly longer than a yard—approximately 39.37 in.)

WEIGHT
1 kilogram (kg) = 1,000 grams (g) = 2.2 pounds (lb)
1 milligram (mg) = 0.001 g = 1,000 micrograms (μg)
1,000 mg = 1 g
1 μg = 0.001 mg = 0.000,001 g
(approximately) 454 g = 1 lb (1,000 g ÷ 2.2 = 454)

VOLUME
1,000 milliliters (ml) = 1 liter (L)
1 ml = 0.001 L
1 ml = approximately 1 cm^3 (cc)^a

^{a}A milliliter (ml) is approximately equal to a cubic centimeter (cc); the two were used interchangeably in the past. The preferred value today is milliliter.

Key Concept
To convert from large to small, move the decimal point to the right.
Example: *g to mg (large to small)*
- 1 g = 1,000 mg
- 1.5 g = 1,500 mg

To convert from small to large, move the decimal point to the left.
Example: *mg to g (small to large)*
- 1,000 mg = 1 g
- 1,500 mg = 1.5 g

NCLEX Alert
Safe medication administration is a primary nursing responsibility; it relates to the overall responsibility to provide safe and effective care to the client. During the NCLEX examination, you will need to demonstrate your general math skills. A general understanding of math is necessary to understanding basic pharmacology.

DOSAGE CALCULATION

Ratio and Proportion

Ratio and proportion are frequently used to calculate medication dosages. A **ratio** is the relationship of one quantity to another. A ratio may be written as a fraction or as numbers separated by a colon; for example, 2/3 or 2:3 or 2 is to 3.

When two ratios are set equal to each other, they are said to be *in proportion* to each other. A true **proportion** consists of two equal ratios separated by an equals sign (=) or a double colon (::). For example:

$$\frac{2}{3} = \frac{6}{9}$$

or
2:3 :: 6:9
or
2:3 = 6:9
or
2 is to 3 as 6 is to 9

This is a valuable relationship. When written with the double colon, the first and last numbers are referred to as the *extremes* and the second and third (middle) numbers are the *means*.

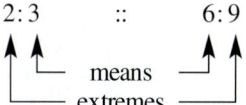

Rules

There are four rules that apply when using ratios and proportions:

1. The product of the means equals the product of the extremes. (The *product* is the answer you get when you multiply.) Therefore, 2 × 9 = 18 (product of the extremes) and 3 × 6 = 18 (product of the means).
2. The product of the means divided by one extreme yields the other extreme. Therefore, 3 × 6 = 18 and 18 ÷ 2 = 9.
3. The product of the extremes divided by one mean yields the other mean. Therefore, 2 × 9 = 18 and 18 ÷ 6 = 3. Therefore, when 3 of the 4 factors of a proportion are known, the missing factor can be found using simple mathematics.
4. **MAJOR RULE:** Whatever is done on one side of the "equals" sign must be done on the other side as well.

Dosage Calculations

The ratio and proportion method is probably the most commonly used method of calculating dosages. To use the ratio and proportion method, the numbers to be multiplied must be in the same units of measurement. Therefore, it is necessary to convert if this is not true.

1. EXAMPLE: The prescription is 1 mg haloperidol (Haldol) IM (intramuscularly), and the medication is available in an ampule with a strength of 5 mg/1 ml. How many milliliters (ml) should be given?

SOLUTION: Set up a ratio. Known factors:

- Medication available = 5 mg (strength): **Factor 1**
- Volume = 1 ml: **Factor 2**
- Prescribed dosage = 1 mg: **Factor 3**
- Volume (ml) needed to give = X ml: **Unknown factor**

One of the rules of ratio and proportion is that the product of the means, divided by one extreme, equals the other extreme. *Remember:* Units of measure must cancel properly during calculations (see equation below).

Set up units in the same position on each side of the double colon:

Set up ratio—1 ml : 1 mg = 5 mg : X ml

5 mg is to 1ml as 1 mg is to X ml

5 mg   1 ml   1 mg   X ml

$$\frac{1 \text{ ml} \times 1 \text{ mg}}{5 \text{ mg}} = X \text{ ml}$$

$(1 \text{ ml} \times 1 = \text{ml})$

$$\frac{1 \text{ ml}}{5} = X \text{ ml}$$

$(1/5 \text{ ml})$

$$\frac{1}{5} = \frac{2}{10} \text{ ml} = 0.2 \text{ ml}$$

Answer: Measure 0.2 (2/10) ml in the syringe. (Above, the fraction 1/5 is converted to tenths [2/10] and then to the decimal fraction 0.2 ml because syringe measurements are in decimal tenths of a milliliter.)

A nurse can also calculate tenths of a milliliter from a fraction by dividing the numerator (top number) by the denominator (bottom number) (see the section on fractions in this chapter):

$$\frac{1 \text{ (numerator)}}{5 \text{ (denominator)}} = 5\overline{)1.0}^{0.2} = \frac{2}{10} \text{ or } 0.2 \text{ ml}$$

The nurse would give 0.2 ml.

2. EXAMPLE: The prescription of benzathine (penicillin G) (oral tablets) is for 375 mg. Tablets are supplied in 250 mg *scored* (able to be divided in half) tablets. How many tablets should be given?

SOLUTION: Set up a ratio:

250 mg is to 1 tablet as 375 mg is to X tablets

250 mg : 1 tablet :: 375 mg : X tablets

Multiply means and extremes:

250 mg × X tablets = 375 mg × 1 tablet

Next, divide both sides by 250 mg, to isolate the X:

$$\frac{250 \text{ mg} \times X \text{ tablets}}{250 \text{ mg}} = \frac{375 \text{ mg} \times 1 \text{ tablet}}{250 \text{ mg}}$$

Then cancel equal values:

$$\frac{\cancel{250 \text{ mg}} \times X \text{ tablets}}{\cancel{250 \text{ mg}}} = \frac{375 \cancel{\text{ mg}} \times 1 \text{ tablet}}{250 \cancel{\text{ mg}}}$$

Therefore, you now have:

$$X \text{ tablets} = \frac{375 \times 1 \text{ tablet}}{250}$$

$(375 \times 1 = 375)$

Divide:

$$X \text{ tablets} = \frac{375}{250} = 1.5 \text{ tablets}$$

The nurse would give 1.5 tablets.

One of the scored tablets would need to be split in half. (Tablets can safely be divided only at the score mark.) See Nursing Care Guidelines 63-3. Occasionally, tablets are double-scored so they can be divided into halves, thirds, *or* fourths.

3. EXAMPLE: The prescription is 75 mg trazodone (Desyrel). The medication is provided in 150 mg scored tablets. How many tablet(s) are needed?

SOLUTION: Set up a ratio:

150 mg is to 1 tablet as 75 mg is to X tablets.

150 mg : 1 tablet :: 75 mg : X tablets.

You want to isolate the X, so divide both sides by 150 mg:

$$\frac{150 \text{ mg} \times X \text{ tablets}}{150 \text{ mg}} = \frac{1 \text{ tablet} \times 75 \text{ mg}}{150 \text{ mg}}$$

This is done by canceling out equal values:

$$\frac{\cancel{150 \text{ mg}} \times X \text{ tablets}}{\cancel{150 \text{ mg}}} = \frac{1 \text{ tablet} \times 75 \cancel{\text{ mg}}}{150 \cancel{\text{ mg}}}$$

Now we have:

$$X \text{ tablets} = 1 \text{ tablet} \times \frac{75}{150}$$

So, $X = \frac{75}{150} = 0.5$

The nurse would give 0.5 (½) tablet.

Note: If the dosage for tablets does not come out exactly, the prescribed dosage *cannot* be given.

4. EXAMPLE: A client is to receive a tube feeding at 75 mL/hr (hour). The bag contains 500 ml. How many hours will this feeding bag last?

SOLUTION: Set up a ratio:

75 ml : 1 hr :: 500 ml : X hours

Multiply means and extremes:

75 ml × X hours = 1 hr × 500 ml

Divide both sides by 75 ml to isolate X:

$$\frac{75 \text{ ml} \times X \text{ hours}}{75 \text{ ml}} = 1 \text{ hr} \times \frac{500 \text{ ml}}{75 \text{ ml}}$$

Cancel equal values:

$$\frac{75\,\text{ml} \times X \text{ hours}}{75\,\text{ml}} = 1\,\text{hr} \times \frac{500\,\text{ml}}{75\,\text{ml}}$$

Therefore:

$$X \text{ hours} = 1\,\text{hr} \times \frac{500}{75} \qquad 75\overline{)500.00}^{\,6.66}$$

$X = 6.66\,\text{hr} = 6^2/_3\,\text{hr} = 6\,\text{hr}\ 40\,\text{min}$
The bag will last 6 hr, 40 min.

Fractions

A **fraction** is a portion or a piece of a whole that indicates division of that whole into equal parts. Fractions can be either common fractions or decimal fractions.

Common Fractions

Common fractions, also called *simple fractions*, have a numerator (top number) and a denominator (bottom number). For example:

$$\frac{3}{4}\begin{pmatrix}\text{numerator}\\\text{denominator}\end{pmatrix}$$

$\frac{3}{4}$ can be pictured as

The **numerator** refers to a *part* of the whole and is the top number (in this example, 3). The **denominator** refers to the *total number of parts* and is the number on the bottom (in this example, 4). This example is interpreted as *three parts out of a total of four parts*. In order to multiply or divide, the numerator and denominator must be compatible.

Multiplying Fractions
To multiply fractions:

$$\frac{2}{3} \times \frac{3}{4}$$

a. Multiply the numerators to get the new numerator.

$$\frac{2}{3} \times \frac{3}{4}\,(2 \times 3 = 6)$$

b. Multiply the denominators to get the new denominator.

$$\frac{2}{3} \times \frac{3}{4}\,(3 \times 4 = 12)$$

c. The new value is 6/12.
d. Reduce the fraction to its lowest terms. (Here, divide both numbers by their largest common divisor, 6.)

$$\frac{6}{12} = \frac{1}{2}$$

Dividing Fractions
To divide fractions:

$$\frac{3}{4} \div \frac{2}{3}$$

a. Write the problem.

$$\frac{3}{4} \div \frac{2}{3}$$

b. Invert the divisor.

$$\frac{3}{4} \times \left(\frac{3}{2}\right)$$

c. Multiply the numerators and denominators.

$$\frac{3}{4} \times \frac{3}{2} = \frac{9}{8}$$

d. Reduce the fraction to its lowest terms. (In this example, divide 9 by 8. The result is 1, with 1 out of 8 leftover—the remainder.)

$$\frac{9}{8} = 1\frac{1}{8}$$

Decimal Fractions

Decimals are fractions in which 10 is always the denominator. The 10 is sometimes omitted when fractions are written, and a decimal point is inserted in the numerator as many places from the right as there are ciphers (zeros) of 10 in the denominator. Therefore, 1/10 = 0.1 and 1/100 = 0.01.

A fraction like 3/4 can also be written as a decimal by converting it to tenths, or in this case, hundredths: 4 goes into 100 25 times and 25 × 3 is 75. Therefore, 3/4 = 75/100ths or 0.75.

$$\frac{3}{4} = \frac{X}{100} \quad \overset{\text{cross-multiply}}{} \quad 4X = 300 \quad X = 4\overline{)300}^{\,75} \quad X = 75$$
$$X = \frac{300}{4} \qquad \underline{28}$$
$$\phantom{X = \frac{300}{4}\quad}20$$
$$\phantom{X = \frac{300}{4}\quad}\underline{20}$$

In fraction, X with 75 : $\frac{75}{100} = 0.75$

>  **Nursing Alert** When writing decimals in nursing, follow these rules:
> - Do not use a "trailing zero" after a decimal point (when dosage is expressed as a whole number). For example, if the dosage is 2 mg, do not insert the decimal point or the trailing zero. This is confusing and could be mistaken for "20" if the decimal point is not seen.
> - Do not leave a "naked" decimal point. For example, if the dosage is 2/10 of a milligram, it should be written as 0.2 mg. In other words, if a number begins with a decimal, it should be written with a zero and a decimal point in front of it. If it is not written that way, it could be mistaken for 2 instead of 2/10.
>
> (Institute for Safe Medical Practices, 2017.)

The Formula Method

When the prescribed or desired dosage is different from what is available, a dosage calculation is necessary to determine the quantity of drug to give. Use ratio and proportion to solve dosage calculations. Because the calculations are in fractions, follow the rules for working with fractions (see the section on fractions).

The formula method can be used only when calculating dosages in the *same system* and the *same units of measurement*. The following formula can be used to calculate the amount of medication needed:

$$\frac{\text{Desired amount or prescribed amount (D)}}{\text{Available dosage (what's on hand) (A)}} \times \text{Quantity} \begin{pmatrix} \text{e.g. 1 pill or} \\ \text{1 tablet or 5 ml} = X \end{pmatrix}$$

$$\frac{\text{Desired amount}}{\text{Available dosage}} \times \text{Quantity} = \text{Amount to give}$$

1. **EXAMPLE:** The prescribed dose is 1¼ mg clonazepam (Klonopin), and the medication is supplied as ½ mg tablets. Known factors:

- **D**esired amount: 1¼ mg (or 5/4)
- **A**vailable dosage: ½ mg
- In what **Q**uantity: 1 tablet

Set up the problem:

$$\frac{D}{A} \times Q = X \qquad \frac{1\frac{1}{4}}{\frac{1}{2}} \times 1 \text{ tablet} = X$$

Use the rules for calculating fractions:

1. Write the problem.

$$\frac{\frac{5}{4}}{\frac{1}{2}} \times 1 \text{ tablet} = X$$

2. Invert the divisor.

$$\frac{5}{4} \times \left(\frac{2}{1}\right) \times 1 \text{ tablet} = X$$

3. Multiply the numerators and denominators.

$$\frac{5}{4} \times \frac{2}{1} \times 1 \text{ tablet} = X$$

$$\frac{10}{4} \times 1 \text{ tablet} = X$$

$$\frac{10}{4} \times 1 = \frac{10}{4}$$

4. Reduce the fraction to its lowest terms.

$$\frac{10}{4} \text{ tablet} = 2\frac{2}{4} = 2\frac{1}{2} \text{ tablets} \quad 4\overline{)10.0}$$

(2.5 tablets)

The nurse would give 2.5 (2½) *tablets*. Because the tablets are scored, the nurse can give medications in ½ tablet increments. (Remember, some tablets cannot safely be split.)

2. **EXAMPLE:** Nitroglycerin (Nitrolingual) is ordered for a client. The prescribed dose is 6/10 mg. The medication is supplied as 3/10 mg sublingual tablets. (Remember, 6/10 means 6 parts out of 10 and 3/10 means 3 parts out of 10.)

Known factors:

- **D**esired amount: 6/10 mg
- **A**vailable dosage: 3/10 mg
- In what **Q**uantity: 1 tablet

Set up the problem.

$$\frac{D}{A} \times Q = X$$

$$\frac{\frac{6}{10} \text{ mg}}{\frac{3}{10} \text{ mg}} \times 1 \text{ tablet} = X$$

Use the rules for calculating fractions:

1. Write the problem.

$$\frac{6}{10} \div \frac{3}{10} \times 1 \text{ tablet} = X$$

2. Invert the divisor.

$$\frac{6}{10} \times \left(\frac{10}{3}\right) \times 1 \text{ tablet} = X$$

3. Multiply the numerators and the denominators.

$$\frac{6}{10} \times \frac{10}{3} \times 1 \text{ tablet} = X$$

$$\frac{60}{30} \times 1 \text{ tablet} = X$$

$$\frac{60}{30} \times 1 = \frac{60}{30}$$

4. Reduce the fraction to its lowest terms.

$$\frac{60}{10} \text{ tablets} = \frac{6}{3} \text{ tablets} = \frac{2}{1} \text{ tablets} = 2 \text{ tablets}$$

The nurse would give two tablets.

> **Key Concept**
> In a fraction, a larger denominator denotes that the item is divided into more pieces. Therefore, 1/10 is half as much as 1/5.

Significant Figures

The term *significant figure* refers to numbers that have practical meaning or dosages that can be measured. For example, a dosage prescribed is 1.325 ml. When measured with a syringe that has markings of 1.3, 1.4, and 1.5 ml, the last two numbers (the "25") cannot be measured. Therefore, the amount given is 1.3 ml because this amount is closer to the prescribed dosage than it is to 1.4 ml. (The dosage that can be measured, 1.3 ml, is the *significant figure*.) When rounding, the dosage is rounded to the closest amount. Therefore, using the example, values ranging from 1.301 to 1.349 are rounded down to 1.3, and values from 1.350 to 1.399 are rounded up to 1.4.

> **Key Concept**
>
> In some cases, a liquid medication is ordered in a dose that is too small to be measured accurately in a medication cup. In this situation, a syringe can be used to draw up the correct amount of medication, and then the medication can be transferred to a medication cup for administration.

Percentages

The term **percentage** refers to the number per hundred. Therefore, 20% equals 20 per hundred. Percent has no specific units of measure. It is actually a ratio. To convert from percentage to a fraction, the percent number becomes the numerator, and 100 is always the denominator.

Example: 20% = 20/100.

Fraction to Percent

To convert a fraction to a percent, multiply both the numerator and the denominator by the number required for the denominator to equal 100. The numerator becomes the percentage.

1. EXAMPLE:

$4/10 \times 10/10 = 40/100 = 40\%$ (multiply both sides by 10)

2. EXAMPLE:

$\dfrac{9}{20} = \dfrac{X}{100}$ cross-multiply $20X = 900$ $X = \dfrac{900}{20}$

$X = 20\overline{)900}$ subtract 80, then 100, 100, 0

$100\overline{)45.0}$ subtract 40.0, then 500, 500, 0 giving 0.45

Replace X with 45: $\dfrac{9}{20} = \dfrac{45}{100} = 45\%$.

Alternatively, looking at the original equation, 20 goes into 100 five times.

$9 \times 5 = 45$

Another way to look at it is: $9/20 = 4.5/10$

$4.5/10 \times 10/10 = 45/100$ or 0.45 or 45%.

Percent to Fraction

You can also determine the percentage designated by any fraction by dividing the numerator by the denominator.

$\dfrac{9}{20}$ $20\overline{)9.00}$ giving 0.45 (subtract 80, then 100, 100) $0.45 = \dfrac{45}{100} = 45\%$

> **Key Concept**
>
> Use references for any questions about dosage conversions. It is advisable to have another nurse double-check all calculations of medication dosages.

STUDENT SYNTHESIS

KEY POINTS

- The metric system is the most commonly used measurement system in the world; it is used for most measurements and dosages in medicine.
- The nurse must understand how to convert between systems of measurement. Occasionally, a drug order is stated in a different unit of measurement than what is available.
- Many symbols and abbreviations are used in medication orders.
- Some abbreviations and symbols are too similar to be used safely (and are not recommended).
- The nurse must be proficient in the use of ratios, proportions, and fractions.
- It is vital to ask if any questions arise about a medication or a dosage. A pharmacist is an excellent resource.
- Weights may be converted to pounds and ounces for the client's benefit but are usually recorded in grams and kilograms in the medical record.

CRITICAL THINKING EXERCISES (SHOW YOUR WORK)

1. A label on a cephalexin (Keflex) bottle states: "cephalexin (Keflex) 250 mg capsules." The healthcare provider's order reads "administer 500 mg." How many capsules would be given?

2. A label reads "docusate sodium (Colace): 150 mg/15 ml." The provider's order reads "100 mg." How many milliliters would the nurse administer?

3. A client weighs 95.45 kg on the hospital scale. He wants you to calculate his weight in pounds. A newborn weighs 3,061.8 g at birth. His parents want to know his weight in pounds and ounces.

4. Haloperidol (Haldol) is available in 50 mg/ml as a long-acting injection. The prescribed dose is 75 mg. How much should the nurse give?

NCLEX-STYLE REVIEW QUESTIONS

1. The nurse is preparing to administer warfarin (Coumadin) 5 mg po to a client for treatment of deep vein thrombosis. The dose on hand is 2.5 mg tablets. How many tablets will the nurse administer?

2. The nurse is to administer cephalexin (Keflex) 250 mg suspension to a client. There is cephalexin (Keflex) 125 mg/5 ml suspension on hand. How many milliliters of cephalexin will the nurse administer?

3. The nurse is to administer heparin 2,500 units subcutaneously to a client with a pulmonary embolism. The nurse has on hand a vial with 5,000 U/ml. How much heparin will the nurse administer?

4. The nurse is preparing to administer a liquid medication but the dose is 1.24 ml. Which action should the nurse take?
    a. Estimate the amount that should be given.
    b. Administer the dose in a syringe.
    c. Withdraw the correct amount in a syringe and put in medicine cup to administer.
    d. Inform the primary care provider the order is too small for the medicine cup.

5. The nurse has an order to administer promethazine (Phenergen) 25 mg IM to a client with reports of nausea. The medication comes in a vial of 50 mg/ml. The nurse will administer _____ ml.

CHAPTER RESOURCES

Enhance your learning with additional resources on thePoint!

Student Resources related to this chapter can be found at thePoint.lww.com/Rosdahl12e.

61 Introduction to Pharmacology

Learning Objectives

1. Explain how the Controlled Substances Act regulates the storage of, and accountability for, specific medications. Describe the proper procedure for monitoring these *schedule* drugs in the healthcare facility.
2. Describe specific client rights, related to prescribed medications.
3. List sources of drug information for nurses.
4. Define the terms chemical, generic, official, and trade/brand names of medications. State which medication names are most commonly used.
5. Describe dosage formats for oral medications.
6. List and describe routes of medication administration.
7. Discuss factors influencing medication dosage.
8. Differentiate between prescribed and over-the-counter medications.
9. List required components of a prescription.

Important Terminology

agonists, antagonist, brand name, caplet, capsule, chemical name, dosage, enteric-coated, generic name, inhalant, injectable, interaction, medication, official name, oral, over-the-counter, paradoxical, pharmacokinetics, pharmacology, potentiation, prescription, sublingual, synergistic, tablet, topical, trade name, transdermal, translingual, transmucosal, troche

Acronyms

DEA, DR, ER, FDA, IR, MDI, ODT, OTC, PDR, Pharm D, RPh, SR, TD, TORB, USP-NF, VORB, XR

A **medication** is an agent that modifies body functions. A medicine or drug is any substance(s) used to prevent disease or pregnancy, aid in diagnosis and treatment of disease, and restore or maintain bodily functions. **Pharmacology** is the science that deals with the origin, nature, chemistry, effects, and uses of medications.

A Doctor of Pharmacy (**Pharm D**) or Registered Pharmacist (**RPh**) is a healthcare professional licensed to prepare and dispense medications on the order of a licensed medical provider. Medication orders can legally be written by a healthcare provider (Doctor of Medicine [MD] or Doctor of Osteopathy [DO]), dentist (Doctor of Dental Surgery [DDS] or Doctor of Medical Dentistry [DMD]), or veterinarian (Doctor of Veterinary Medicine [DVM]), and in many states by a physician's assistant (PA). In many states, prescriptive authority extends to advanced practice nurses/nurse practitioners (CNP/NP), certified registered nurse anesthetists (CRNA), or the certified nurse midwife (CNM). This chapter provides an introduction to the basics of pharmacology and general information concerning medications, all very important throughout a nurse's career.

The primary nursing obligation is to "do no harm," including when administering medications. Thus, a general knowledge of pharmacology is essential. Because in the current healthcare delivery system, clients must take more responsibility for their own healthcare, nurses often bear most of the responsibility for medication teaching. Teaching should include the desired effects, methods of administration, actions, and possible adverse reactions or side effects of medications.

Key Concept

Important in nursing practice is teaching clients about the desired effect and possible side effects of their medications. It is vital to document this teaching and the client's response. Ask the client to "teach back," to help verify their understanding.

NCLEX Alert

It will be important for you to understand the nurse's responsibility for teaching clients about their medications. This information may be integrated into NCLEX examination questions.

LEGAL ASPECTS

Federal Drug Standards

The U.S. Food and Drug Administration (**FDA**) operates under the enforcement of the U.S. Department of Health and Human Services. Its Canadian counterpart is Health Canada (Santé Canada), which is a part of the Health Products and Food Branch (HPFB) of the government. These agencies ensure that medications and therapeutic agents are safe and effective for public use before they are available. Standards of strength and purity help protect the public. For example, several medications have been removed from the market in recent years. These include terfenadine (Seldane), a histamine antagonist; troglitazone (Rezulin), an oral antihyperglycemic agent; and rofecoxib (Vioxx), a medication used to treat osteoarthritis pain. Although these medications seemed to be effective, their side effects were so serious that they were deemed unsafe for use. (In some cases, a drug not available in the United States is still marketed in other parts of the world.) The FDA and Health Canada are constantly doing research to ensure the efficacy and safety of medications. There are a number of publications that define standards for medication approval. These publications are used primarily by pharmacists and primary care providers.

Nursing Alert It may be dangerous to obtain medications from other countries because not all countries have the stringent safety precautions of the United States and Canada.

Controlled Substances

A federal law, the Comprehensive Drug Abuse Prevention and Control Act of 1970, commonly referred to as the "Controlled Substances Act," is enforced by the Drug Enforcement Agency (**DEA**). It regulates the manufacture, prescription, and distribution of psychoactive medications, including narcotics, depressants, stimulants, and hallucinogens. There are five classifications, or "schedules," of controlled substances. The degree of control depends on the medication's actions, which range from Schedule I (high potential for abuse) to Schedule V (relatively low potential for abuse) (Box 61-1). A similar schedule has been established in Canada by the National Drug Scheduling Advisory Committee.

Protection of Controlled Substances

Controlled substances must be managed carefully, and an accurate inventory and dispensing record must be kept. In a healthcare facility or pharmacy, controlled substances must be kept in a *double-locked* area. This may be a locked medication room or cart with a separate locked "narcotics cabinet." The keys must be in a licensed nurse's possession at all times or access must be controlled electronically. Only licensed nurses are allowed to access schedule drugs. Each healthcare facility incorporates specialized forms or computer documentation for the management of controlled substances. The client's name, medication name, dose, time of administration, and signature or personal identification number (PIN) of the licensed nurse who administered it must be recorded. In some cases, the name of the prescribing person is also listed. Schedule drugs must be documented in the client's record within 5 min of administration.

Most acute care facilities use some sort of computerized dispensing unit (Fig. 61-1). This unit dispenses and keeps records of controlled substances and other medications. Medications are accessible only with the entry of a PIN assigned to each individual nurse or by fingerprint identification. In this way, a computerized record is maintained for each medication removed from the machine, as well as the

Box 61-1 Schedule of Controlled Substances

Controlled substances (schedule drugs) are classified on the following basis:
- *Schedule I (C-I):* High potential for abuse; no accepted medical use (e.g., heroin, LSD; not kept in healthcare facilities or pharmacies)
- *Schedule II (C-II):* High potential for abuse; severe dependence liability (e.g., narcotics, amphetamines, and some barbiturates)
- *Schedule III (C-III):* Lower potential for abuse than Schedule II drugs; moderate dependence liability (e.g., anabolic steroids, nonbarbiturate sedatives, nonamphetamine stimulants, limited amounts of certain narcotics)
- *Schedule IV (C-IV):* Lower potential for abuse than Schedule III drugs; limited dependence liability (e.g., some sedatives, antianxiety agents, nonnarcotic analgesics)
- *Schedule V (C-V):* Limited potential for abuse; primarily small amounts of narcotics (e.g., codeine) used as antitussives and antidiarrheals

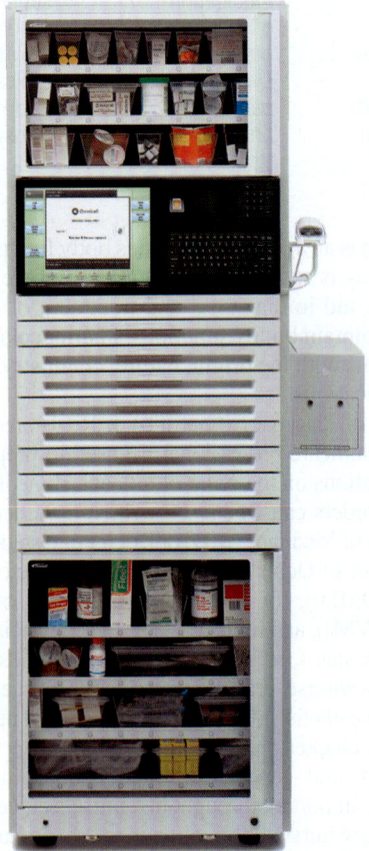

Figure 61-1 Omnicell XT Automated Dispensing Cabinet provides a comprehensive, end-to-end solution to track medication inventory and usage pattern to support regulatory compliance and safe medication administration workflows at the point of care. Medication access is controlled by the system to ensure medication security. (Courtesy of Omnicell, Inc.)

client for whom it was signed out, the nurse, the time and date, and the amount of medication remaining.

Controlled Drug Count Verification

To ensure that schedule drugs are properly controlled, all counts must correspond with documentation. If there is a locked narcotics cabinet, two licensed nurses, one going off duty and the other coming on duty, review the documentation and count the number of remaining controlled medications. (*The oncoming nurse counts; the outgoing nurse records.* This assures the oncoming nurse that all drugs are there.) The documentation must match the number of remaining medications in the controlled substances cabinet. If the count does not agree, no one is allowed to leave the unit until a search is undertaken or the discrepancy resolved. If narcotics are dispensed by a computerized system, the count is maintained by the machine, but a visual count may be required once a day. This may be done by pharmacy staff and is done during the night or when they refill the machine. Documentation regarding schedule drugs and other drugs in the machine downloads to the pharmacy at least every 24 hr. In addition, pharmacy computers can access the inventories in the machines at any time.

In many cases, even though there is a dispensing machine, a separate narcotics cabinet is in place for unusual medications. In this case, the keys to the narcotics cabinet are locked in the machine and can only be accessed by authorized personnel, using a PIN number. Medications kept in the separate cabinet are counted each shift.

If there is no medication dispensing machine, the narcotic keys should be in possession of the nurse to whom they have been assigned. The keys are not to leave the unit at any time. In the event a nurse forgets to give the keys to the oncoming nurse and takes them out of the healthcare facility, they must return the keys immediately when realizing the error. In addition, the locks to the narcotic cabinet containing controlled medications may need to be changed and new keys assigned.

> **Key Concept**
> Nursing students usually do not give schedule medications without direct supervision by the licensed instructor.

When additional controlled drugs are brought to the nursing unit, only a licensed nurse or pharmacy representative is allowed to add them to the inventory, whether using a narcotics cabinet or machine. In some facilities, two nurses must perform this procedure. A record is signed by the nurse and verified by the pharmacist to ensure that all the medications were, in fact, added to the unit inventory. If schedule medications are sent to the nursing unit by pneumatic tube, they must be sent in "secure" mode and can be accessed only using special codes.

> **NCLEX Alert**
> To administer medications safely, you need to be alert to concepts presented in this unit—uses of medications, rationales for medication standards, factors affecting client reactions to a medication, and the rights of clients related to medications. During the examination, you may need to demonstrate knowledge and understanding of these concepts.

Client Rights

Clients have the right to know the *name, action,* and possible *side effects* of their medications. They also have the right to *refuse* medications, unless a court order is in place. (If clients are endangering themselves or others or are considered a "medical emergency," medications may be given against their will.) Clients also have the right to request the *generic form* of prescribed medications, if available. Generic forms of medications are often less expensive than their brand name counterparts.

Drug References

Many references regarding medications are available. These references are valuable tools for learning about the classification, use, abuse, desired actions, recommended dosage, and adverse actions of medications. The *Physicians' Desk Reference* (**PDR**) is published annually in the United States, with free updates. A free PC and mobile app download is also available. This recognized source contains extensive information concerning therapeutic dosages, expected therapeutic effects, possible side effects, contraindications, drug interactions, and FDA pregnancy categories (levels of danger to a fetus). The PDR contains a number of sections, including a product identification section and product information section. This reference also contains a list of national poison control centers and a guide to managing overdose. A companion handbook for nurses is available, as is an online version. A list of drugs removed from the *PDR Nurse's Drug Handbook* is archived on the Internet yearly.

> **Nursing Alert** The emergency telephone number for poison control centers in the United States and U.S. Territories is 1-800-222-1222. The numbers vary by province in Canada. Note: These telephone numbers are to be used *for emergencies only.*

Facts & Comparisons is another drug reference in hard copy and online. It lists medications under the following classifications: nutritional products, blood modifiers, hormones, diuretics, cardiovascular drugs, autonomic drugs, central nervous system drugs, gastrointestinal drugs, anti-infectives, and biologicals. This resource, used by many pharmacies, is updated monthly and provides the most current medication information available. The *United States Pharmacopeia/National Formulary* (**USP-NF**) is a book containing national standards for drugs, chemicals, and dietary supplements marketed in the United States. The USP-NF is recognized in over 37 countries. This reference is continually updated and is published annually.

Many other publications, such as *Lippincott's Nursing Drug Guide,* and the *Nursing Drug Reference* and *Handbook of Drugs for Nursing Practice,* are published annually. These sources are designed to meet the needs of nursing students and practicing licensed nurses. They incorporate nursing considerations, in addition to mechanisms of action, uses, contraindications, precautions, dosages, preparations, interactions, **pharmacokinetics** (actions of drugs), side effects, and treatment of overdose. They also emphasize client and family teaching. In addition to the above sources, much information about medications is available at various Internet Websites (see Web Resources on Pharmacology).

Nursing Considerations

When a client is admitted to a healthcare facility, initial assessment must include a detailed medication history. Information must be obtained from the client and family, as well as from the client's pharmacy and/or personal healthcare provider. In addition, any medications brought in by the client must be cataloged and kept in a safe location. Each facility has a specific protocol for this.

It is vital to identify and indicate in the client record any client drug allergies and what adverse reaction is caused by each medication, as well as the date of the reaction. This information will enable the primary provider to decide which medications are safe and would be effective for this client. All clients wear an allergy wristband, verifying that an allergy assessment has been done. This wristband either identifies allergies or notes that the client has no known allergies.

> **Nursing Alert** Some adverse reactions to medications (such as a rash) are usually not considered true allergies. True allergies are differentiated from other adverse reactions by the primary healthcare provider. A pharmacist is a good source of information if there are any questions about drug interactions or allergic responses. A client usually does not experience an adverse or allergic reaction on first exposure to a medication. Therefore, stay alert for adverse reactions, even if the client has received the medication previously.

Before administering any medication, the nurse must know about the medication (Fig. 61-2). Before administering any medication, be sure to confirm the client has not had a previous adverse or allergic reaction to it. Failure to do so may jeopardize the client's well-being and may be life-threatening.

> **Key Concept**
> Nurses are obligated to know the generic and common trade name, classification, use, recommended dosage, desired effects, possible adverse or untoward effects, and route of administration of any medication administered. Should a client experience an adverse reaction that the nurse does not recognize and appropriately respond to, a medication error has been committed, just as if the wrong medication had been given.

MEDICATION PREPARATIONS AND ACTIONS

Medications are used for many different purposes and may be administered in various ways. The *route of administration* refers to the method by which a medication is given

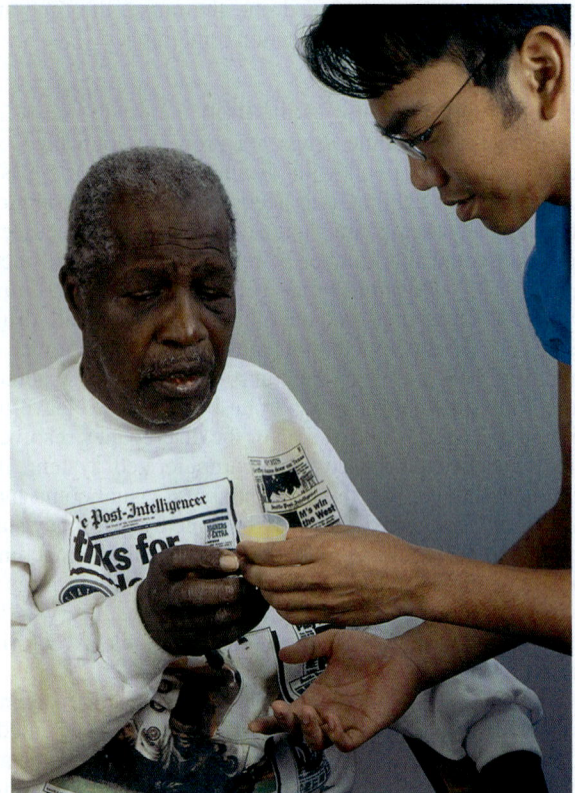

Figure 61-2 A nursing student or licensed nurse is responsible for knowing vital information about medications the client is receiving.

(Chapter 63). Examples of medication preparations include **oral** (administered by mouth), **topical** (applied to the skin or mucous membranes), **inhalant** (inhaled or breathed in), **injectable** (given via a needle), and **transdermal** (applied to and absorbed through the skin).

Medication Names

The number of medications available, as well as the variety of names often given to the same medication, can be confusing. Medications are named in four categories: chemical, generic, official, and trade or brand name. The **chemical name** describes the medication's chemical composition. The **generic name** is often similar to the chemical name and is assigned by the medication's first manufacturer. The generic name may be simpler than the chemical name and may be used in any country by any manufacturer. The **official name** is the name identified in the *USP-NF* or in *Health Canada's publications*. The **trade name** or **brand name** is the copyrighted name assigned by the company manufacturing the medication and is usually followed by the symbol ®. If more than one company makes the same medication, it will have the same generic name, but different trade names. For this reason, many healthcare providers order medications using only the generic name. Box 61-2 gives examples of various names for one medication.

Many medication labels and inserts contain both the generic and trade names. Should the healthcare provider use

CHAPTER 61 Introduction to Pharmacology

> **Box 61-2 Medication Names**
>
> The following is an example of the different names used for one medication:
> - *Chemical formula:* $C_9H_8O_4$
>
> [chemical structure of acetylsalicylic acid]
>
> - *Chemical name:* 2-acetoxybenzenecarboxylic acid
> - *Generic name:* acetylsalicylic acid (ASA)
> - *Official name:* acetylsalicylic acid
> - *Selected brand names:* Aspirin, Aspergum, Bayer, Ecotrin, Heartline, St. Joseph (also many combination products)

> **Box 61-3 Example of Side Effects/Adverse Reactions**
>
> Medication: diphenhydramine (Benadryl)
> - *Desired effect:* Antihistamine; relief of itching and allergy symptoms
> - *Negative, but usually not life-threatening, side effects:* Dry mouth, hypotension
> - *Positive, helpful side effects:* Cough suppression, relief of motion sickness
> - *Mixed side effects:* Sedation that could lead to problems with driving or operating machinery; also helpful as a sleep aid or sedative
> - *Life-threatening adverse effects:* Anaphylaxis

> **Key Concept**
>
> Be aware that in drug reference books all secondary or side effects, whether negative or positive, are listed as "adverse effects."

one form of the name and the label states another, verify the names in a designated reference to make sure that the correct medication will be given. Make sure that this medication is correct before administering it to the client. These references commonly list generic and one or more trade names for most medications.

Medication Actions

A medication that produces a desired response is called an **agonist**; one that has an opposing effect, or acts against another medication, is called an **antagonist**. A medication that enhances the effects of another medication has a **synergistic** or **potentiating** effect. The actions of synergistic medications taken together are greater than the combined action of the two medications taken separately; the effects are multiplied. Smaller doses of each medication should be used because their combined effects are greater than normal. There may also be **interactions** between drugs, some of which are dangerous.

Side Effects and Adverse Responses to Medications

Be aware not only of the desired actions of medications but also of undesired or secondary reactions. It is important for nurses to be alert constantly for adverse reactions and unwanted side effects of drugs, so appropriate actions can be taken.

Side effects are *secondary effects* that are other than the initial desired goal of the medication. Some side effects are considered to be *adverse or negative reactions* and can even be life threatening. However, side effects sometimes can be positive or helpful (Box 61-3).

Interactions of Prescription Medications With Herbal Supplements and Homeopathic Remedies

It is important to ask clients if they take dietary supplements, herbs, or homeopathic remedies. Record in the clinical record the type and amount of herb or remedy taken and call it to the attention of the primary care provider. Some of these substances have potential interactions with prescribed medications or with each other. The supplement may increase or decrease the desired effect of a prescribed medication. Combinations of herbal supplements or of supplements and prescribed medications may produce life-threatening adverse effects (Chapters 56 and 62).

Medication Forms

A medication's form, properties, and desired effects determine its dosage and route of administration. Medications are available in several forms. These include liquids, solids, semisolids, metered-dose inhalants, and transdermal medications. Many medications are available in more than one form for different administration routes. For example, promethazine (Phenergan), an antiemetic, is available in rectal suppository, liquid (syrup), and injectable forms. The medication nitroglycerin, used to relax vascular smooth muscle (primarily to relieve or prevent angina in the heart), is available in many forms, including intravenous (IV) injection, sublingual tablets, sustained-release oral tablets, topical paste, transdermal patches, translingual spray, and transmucosal tablets (Chapter 63).

Liquids

Liquids are administered orally, *parenterally* (by some means other than the gastrointestinal [GI] tract), or topically.

Oral Administration of Liquids

Oral administration of liquid medications is used most often for pediatric, psychiatric, and geriatric clients. Oral liquid medications, usually in syrup form, are given to ensure medication compliance, as well as to assist a client who has difficulty swallowing a tablet. Some liquid medications are mixed with juice or another substance to mask the taste. A *syrup* is a liquid that contains a sweetener, usually sugar. A *tincture* is a form of liquid medication containing alcohol.

Some liquids are designed to be held under the tongue and absorbed through oral mucosa. Atropine, the liquid medication used to treat enuresis (involuntary nighttime voiding), is administered sublingually and homeopathic remedies are often given by this method as well. Other liquids are designed to be gargled for their therapeutic effect, such as a warm saline (salt water) gargle for a sore throat. Some are swished in the mouth and then expectorated ("swish and spit" mouthwash; e.g., viscous lidocaine). Another type of medicated mouthwash is designed to be gargled or held in the mouth as long as possible and then swallowed ("swish and swallow" mouthwash, e.g., nystatin). Medications such as nystatin can also be prepared in other forms, such as frozen flavored ice pops, to assist in compliance. Another form of many medications, including nystatin, is the oral **troche**, which is a medicated tablet that dissolves in the mouth.

Topical Administration of Liquids
Liquids for topical use include *instillations* (as into the eye or ear) and *irrigations* (as in flushing out a wound).

Solids
Solid medications are those given by mouth. In addition to liquid oral medications, medications given by mouth may be in the form of pills, tablets, capsules, caplets, liqui-gel capsules, gel, or chewing gum (Fig. 61-3). Capsules or tablets may contain medications that are absorbed slowly or rapidly (discussed below). Typically, most tablets can be either chewed or swallowed. (Exceptions include those that are enteric coated, which should be swallowed whole.) Some solid or semisolid medications are designed to be placed *under the tongue* (**sublingual**) or *on the tongue* (**translingual**). An example of translingual administration is the orally disintegrating tablet (ODT), discussed in the next section. Another route for medication administration is **transmucosal**. In this case, a tablet or gel is placed *between the cheek and gum* and absorbed through the oral mucosa. An example is glucose in gel form, administered to the client with a dangerously low blood sugar level. When medications are absorbed via the oral mucosa or skin, they bypass the GI tract. Technically, a *pill* is absolutely round. However, tablets, capsules, and caplets are commonly referred to as "pills," even though they are of different compositions and shapes. A **tablet** is a compressed, spherical form of a medication; tablets may be **enteric-coated** (the coating does not dissolve until the tablet reaches the intestine because the medication can irritate the stomach mucosa), or they may be plain. A **capsule** is a medication in powdered or pellet form enclosed in soluble, cylindrical, gelatin-like material. The capsule may be used to delay the medication's absorption over time or because the medication has a disagreeable taste. The capsule's smooth covering also makes swallowing easier than a tablet, which may dissolve in the client's mouth if they do not swallow it quickly. A **caplet** is a tablet in the shape of a capsule. This shape makes it easier for the client to swallow. A liqui-gel is a liquid-filled capsule that can provide faster absorption than a tablet. Medications in the forms of tablets, capsules, or caplets may be made to release over time (*slow release* [**SR**], *delayed release* [**DR**], or *extended release* [**ER, XR**]) or may be *immediate release* [**IR**], designed to release all at one time.

Orally Disintegrating Tablets
ODT is solid, but dissolves very quickly when exposed to saliva in the client's mouth. These tablets are designed to improve medication compliance, particularly in psychiatric clients or very small children. The ODT form of a drug often has its own trade name. For example, the ODT form of olanzapine (Zyprexa) is Zyprexa Zydis; of clozapine (Clozaril) is FazaClo; of risperidone (Risperdal) is Risperdal M-TAB; and of loratadine is Claritin ODT. Special techniques are used to administer these tablets (Chapters 63 and 94).

Powders
A *powder* is another type of solid. Powders are most often mixed with liquids or soft foods for oral administration. They may also be applied topically, inhaled, or combined with a sterile diluent for injection.

Chewing Gum
Chewing gum is used as a medium for delivery of nicotine (Nicorette gum), to assist in smoking cessation.

> **Nursing Alert** Many tablets and pills can be crushed for easier swallowing or to make sure the client takes them. However, not all medications can be crushed safely. Capsules, time-released medications, ODTs, and enteric-coated tablets should not be crushed or split. Many facilities require a provider's order to crush any medication.

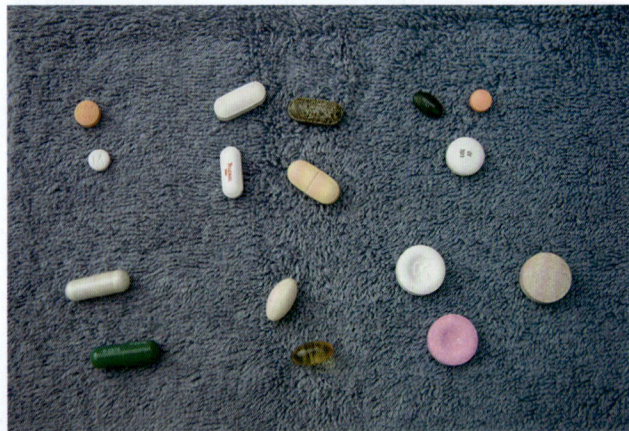

Figure 61-3 Solid oral medications come in many forms. (**Left to right, top**) Tablets, caplets, and enteric-coated tablets. (**Bottom**) Capsules, gelcaps, chewable tablets, and troche. (Photo by Caroline Bunker Rosdahl.)

Semisolids

Semisolid medications are usually given by rectal, vaginal, or urethral routes. Systemic medication may also be administered by topical paste applied to the skin or a gel given orally. (Other semisolid creams are intended for topical application and are not absorbed systemically.)

Semisolid medications (e.g., a suppository), used for systemic purposes, are designed to melt at body temperature and are absorbed through mucosa or skin (often rectal or vaginal). Suppositories usually are kept refrigerated, to maintain their shape. Other semisolid drugs include ointments and pastes. An example of a systemic medication administered by topical paste is nitroglycerin (Nitro-Bid). The dosage of Nitro-Bid is written in measurements of length, such as "1 in." (Fig. 61-4).

Inhaled Medications and Nasal Sprays

Oral or nasal *inhalers and nebulizers* deliver medications topically to the area of desired effect (e.g., lung or nasal mucosa). Inhalers are either an aerosol (metered-dose inhaler [**MDI**]) or a nonaerosol powder inhaler (e.g., Flexhaler, Diskus). They deliver a measured amount of medication with each inhalation. A nebulizer is a device that delivers liquid medication to the airways in the form of a mist as the client inhales. Each dose typically can take as long as 5 min to nebulize. The advantage of this delivery is that the inhaled drug provides a topical administration to the lung tissue and reduces the systemic side effects on the body, such as rapid heart rate. These considerations are especially important when using steroids or sympathomimetics.

Other inhaled medications are intended to cause systemic effects. An example is nicotine for inhalation (Nicotrol Inhaler), used to assist in smoking cessation. A medication D.H.E. is a form of ergotamine and is available as a nasal spray to treat migraine headaches. DDAVP, a form of desmopressin in a nasal spray, is used to treat enuresis.

Transdermal Medications

Transdermal (**TD**) *medications* are designed to be absorbed through the skin ("trans" = through; "dermal" = skin) into the body. Transdermal medication is incorporated into a resin and prepared in the form of a patch or paste. The patch or paste is placed on the body, and the skin absorbs the medication in controlled amounts over time. Medications that the GI system would destroy can be given effectively via the transdermal route. In addition, the patches are convenient to use. In most cases, transdermal medications require smaller doses than oral medications to achieve the same desired effects. Examples of medications supplied in transdermal patch include fentanyl (Duragesic, Sublimaze), nicotine patches (Nicoderm), nitroglycerin patches, and estrogen patches (Vivelle-Dot). As mentioned, Nitro-Bid is a paste applied to the skin and absorbed transdermally.

Injectable Medications

Injectable medications are given by needle into tissues or a blood vessel or by a catheter into a blood vessel. Injectable medications may be given within the layers of the skin (*intradermal*), under the skin into the subcutaneous tissue layer (*subcutaneous*), into the muscle tissue (*intramuscular* [IM]), into the blood vessels (*intravenous* [IV] or *intra-arterial* [IA]), or into the area surrounding the spinal cord (*intrathecal*). The latter is a highly invasive method and is used only when absolutely necessary and only by specially trained personnel (Chapter 64).

PRESCRIBED MEDICATIONS

A *dose* is a single amount of a medication administered to achieve a therapeutic effect (e.g., 250 mg penicillin). A **dosage** contains the dose *and* scheduled times (e.g., penicillin, 250 mg, three times a day, in equal intervals). A *therapeutic dose* is the amount of medication required to obtain a desired effect in most clients. A blood sample may be obtained to determine the client's *blood level* of a drug. This helps establish the therapeutic dose for that client. The *minimal dose* is the smallest amount of drug necessary to achieve a therapeutic effect. A *loading dose* (larger than the usual continuing dose) may be given as the first dose of a newly prescribed medication, to establish a minimum blood level. A *maximal dose* is the largest amount that can be given safely without causing an adverse reaction or toxic effect. A *toxic dose* is the amount of medication that causes symptoms of poisoning or toxicity. A *lethal dose* is the amount that will cause death. These doses may vary between individuals and often depend on the client's weight.

Factors Affecting Medication Prescription

When healthcare professionals prescribe medications, numerous factors must be considered.

Age

Children cannot tolerate the same amount of medication as adults because of their smaller size and different metabolism. Older adults also may be unable to tolerate normal adult dosages of medications because of the effects of the aging process on liver and kidney function, which may lead to incomplete metabolism of some medications. This can cause the drug to accumulate in the body or to be excreted without being absorbed. Either situation can result in serious adverse reactions. In addition, older adults, as well as children, may exhibit **paradoxical** responses to medications—the opposite of the desired response.

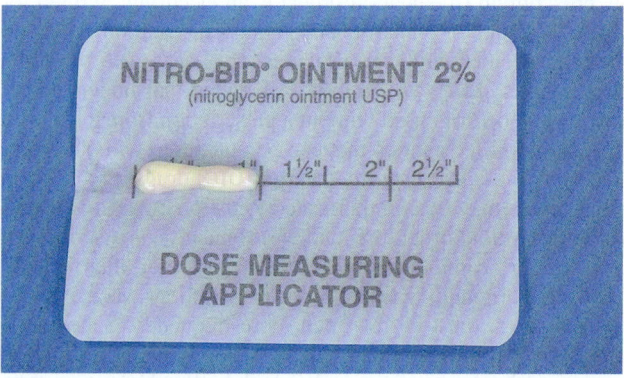

Figure 61-4 Nitro-Bid is available in a paste and is ordered in inches. (Photo by B. Proud.)

Gender
Some medications are more soluble in fat; others are more soluble in water. Because women usually have more body fat and tend to be smaller, and men have more body fluid, effects of medications differ across genders. Women usually require smaller doses than men. In addition, many medications and herbal supplements cross the placental barrier and can harm the fetus in a pregnant woman. Breast milk absorbs some medications in lactating women, which could harm breast-feeding babies. Therefore, pregnant or lactating women should consult their maternal–child healthcare provider before taking any medications, including over-the-counter medications, dietary supplements, and herbal preparations.

Weight
Dosage is often prescribed in relation to a client's weight. This is especially true for children. Heavier clients may require larger dosages than thinner clients to reach therapeutic levels. Body weight is usually expressed in grams or kilograms for dosage calculations.

Client's Condition
A disease's nature and severity may influence the prescribed dosage of a medication. For example, the person in severe pain will often will require a higher level of pain-relieving medication than does the person experiencing less pain. The client's condition may also affect their activity level, which can influence medication absorption.

Disposition and Psychological State
The client's personality and culture may affect the amount of medication needed. For example, a client with a relatively high pain threshold will require less pain medication than the client with a very low pain threshold. A highly agitated individual may require a larger dose of a sedative than the person experiencing less anxiety. A client's cultural values and ethnic background may also affect the client's reactions to pain and willingness to take medications (Chapter 8).

Method of Administration
Administration route affects the amount of time for the medication to enter the general circulation and become effective. IV and IM injections act more rapidly than do oral medications. Rectally administered and transdermally applied medications often are absorbed more slowly than are those administered by injection. Sublingual medications are usually absorbed quickly.

Distribution
The body distributes some medications evenly to reach all cells; other medications reach only certain body fluids or tissues. For example, nitroglycerin targets vascular smooth muscles; acetaminophen (Tylenol) reduces fever by acting on the heat-regulating center in the hypothalamus; acyclovir (Zovirax) inhibits the DNA replication of viruses and is used to help manage human immunodeficiency virus (HIV) infections; and simvastatin (Zocor) inhibits a specific enzyme involved in cholesterol synthesis. However, penicillin kills bacteria throughout the body.

Environmental Factors
Temperature may influence a medication's speed of absorption. For example, heat causes vasodilation and therefore faster absorption, whereas cold causes vasoconstriction and decreases absorption. This might be a factor in administering IM medications and in treating the client with a high fever.

Some medications are damaged by exposure to light and must be stored in dark bottles or opaque containers (e.g., nitroglycerin). Some medications require refrigeration to maintain their effectiveness. Certain liquid medications, when mixed in a syringe or cup, must be given immediately to prevent deterioration related to exposure to room air or to prevent becoming so thick they are not possible to drink (e.g., psyllium). Some liquid medications cannot ever be mixed because they destroy or interact with each other. Other medications may also interact with each other and may need to be separated in administration times to ensure proper absorption. An example is the combination of calcium and fluoroquinolones (a family of antibiotics; for example, ciprofloxacin [Cipro XR]).

Time of Administration
Time is an important factor. For example, the body will absorb a medication taken with meals more slowly than one taken on an empty stomach, although some medications must be taken with food, to avoid stomach upset. A diuretic is best taken in the morning, so frequent voiding does not disrupt the client's sleep. Antidepressants and vitamins are usually given in the morning, to prevent interfering with sleep. Medications with sedative effects or side effects are usually given in the evening or late afternoon. Certain insulins must be given before meals, whereas others are administered with meals. The goal is to provide insulin close to the same time carbohydrates enter the bloodstream. For example, insulin glargine (Lantus) is usually given in the evening and is used to provide a basal level of insulin throughout the entire 24-hr day.

Elimination
The body eliminates medications through urine, feces, breath, and perspiration. Some medications leave the body in their original forms; others are made inactive by chemical changes. If these processes are slowed, a medication's effects may be prolonged. Medication that leaves the body too quickly may be excreted before it has a therapeutic effect. If the body cannot eliminate a medication because of kidney or liver dysfunction, toxic levels may accumulate in the blood. Chemical changes may also form substances that are harmful to the body if it is unable to dispose of them rapidly enough. Excess fluid intake can flush medications out of the body before they can take effect.

Prescriptions
A **prescription** (medication order) is an electronic, written, or verbal formula for preparing and giving a medication. As stated before, specific healthcare providers are licensed to prescribe medications. A *legend drug* is a medicine that under federal law cannot be dispensed without a prescription from a licensed practitioner. Medications that can be purchased without a prescription are called **over-the-counter** (**OTC**) drugs. Prescription drug orders may be communicated to the pharmacist via written order, verbal order, fax, and electronically via e-scribe. All prescriptions cannot be refilled more than 1 year after the date they were originally written. Some prescriptions, such as those for narcotics, must be rewritten more frequently. Schedule II drugs are not refillable and require a new written prescription each time the drug is dispensed. Schedule III to V drugs may be phoned in or written, but are limited to five refills in a 6-month period (from the date originally written). Each state or province

TABLE 61-1 Parts of a Prescription

PART	PURPOSE
Client's full name	Avoids confusion with another client with the same surname; in some facilities, or if two clients have the same name, the client's room number, medical record number, and/or birth date may also be included.
Date and time of day	Tells when order is to be started; may tell when order is to be discontinued; prescription must be rewritten if medication is to be continued after discharge date.
Name of drug	States the exact name (generic name preferred to trade name; sometimes both are used).
Dosage/amount of drug	States measurement system used by healthcare facility; may also be expressed as number of capsules or tablets or as fluid volume.
Time/frequency of dose	Aids in determining the schedule for administration; nursing service usually determines medication routine schedules, such as the hours for medications ordered four times per day or those ordered every 6 hr; the prescribing healthcare provider may give less-definite directions. (However, the nurse needs to know that certain medications must be given before meals, whereas others must be given with or after meals for maximum effect, e.g., it is important to differentiate between a medication to be given every 6 hr and one that is to be given four times a day.)
Method/route	Determines the route by which the medication is to be given (e.g., oral [PO], intramuscularly [IM]). In most situations, giving a medication via the wrong route could be dangerous, possibly fatal, e.g., administration of an IM medication given intravenously (IV) could increase the dose received or speed of absorption.
Primary healthcare provider's signature (written or electronic)	Identifies the prescribing individual; essential for legal reasons or if some question exists about the order. An unsigned order may mean that the person has not finished writing it or that it was not written by an authorized person.

may have specific regulations relating to prescription drug orders. It is important to be aware of the laws of the area in which you are practicing. Nurses may give medications only on direct orders from a recognized healthcare provider.

A licensed *pharmacist* prepares medications following the practitioner's orders in the prescription. In the healthcare facility, the prescription is entered by the provider and sent to the hospital pharmacy for preparation. The orders contain a start time and date. The medication is to be given for the specific length of time stated in the order or until the order changes or is discontinued. Table 61-1 lists the parts of a prescription. Nurses need to be aware of medical terminology, symbols, and abbreviations used in prescriptions (Chapter 37 and Appendix B).

> **Nursing Alert** Be aware that some abbreviations and symbols used in the past are not used today because of the danger of misinterpretation and errors (Chapter 37).

Verbal Orders

In emergencies, healthcare providers may give verbal medication orders, either directly or by telephone. Most acute care facilities allow only registered nurses to accept verbal orders; however, practical/vocational nurses in extended-care facilities and healthcare provider's clinics may be allowed to take them as well.

If, as a licensed nurse, you are permitted by your facility to take verbal orders, be sure to read the order back to the healthcare provider and to document it in the prescribed location. It is important to document that the order was taken by a nurse and that it was read back to the provider. *Rationale: Reading back the order helps assure that the order as written is the order that was intended. Documentation states who gave the order and who took the order and verifies that it was read back. This provides a permanent record of events for reference and protection of clients and healthcare personnel.*

A verbal order must be verified and is documented as **VORB**, "verbal order, read back," or **TORB**, "telephone order, read back." Make sure the order is cosigned by the prescribing person as soon as possible, at least within 24 hr.

> **Key Concept**
> A verbal or telephone order is not legal unless the nurse reads it back to the primary provider. Only licensed nurses are permitted to take verbal or telephone orders. Nursing students or other unlicensed personnel cannot legally take verbal or telephone orders at any time.

Clarification of Orders

Nurses are responsible for carrying out orders as given and cannot make any changes to them. If there is any reason to question an order, if handwriting is not legible or if the order is confusing, clarify it with the provider. If an order is clarified by telephone, it is written as a "clarification" under the order in question, dated, and signed by the nurse as a TORB. The primary care provider who was consulted is also identified. This clarification is treated as a telephone order and must be cosigned by the ordering healthcare provider within 24 hr.

> **Key Concept**
> All medication and other orders must be clear, understandable, and open to only one interpretation before the nurse takes any action. If you cannot read or understand an order, it must be clarified. The safe administration of medications is one of the nurse's most important responsibilities. If you have any question, you must clarify the order.

STUDENT SYNTHESIS

KEY POINTS

- Medications are substances that modify body functions. They are used to prevent disease or pregnancy, to aid in diagnosis and treatment of disease, or to restore and maintain bodily functions.
- Many laws, rules, and regulations concern the prescription, storage, and administration of medications.
- Clients have the right to know what medications they are receiving and to request available generic forms of medications. They may refuse to take medications, unless it is an emergency or a court order exists to the contrary.
- Medication administration is a nursing task that must be taken very seriously, to prevent harm to clients.
- Nurses are required to know how and where to obtain information concerning medications.
- Drugs are available in many forms: liquids, solids, semisolids, and transdermal patches.
- Factors that affect medication dosages include the client's age, gender, weight, condition, and psychological state.
- Many medications are considered unsafe for use without a healthcare provider's supervision and, thus, require a specific prescription. OTC medications can be purchased by the consumer without a prescription.
- Medication orders must be carried out exactly as written. If any questions arise, the prescribing healthcare provider must be consulted for clarification. No medication can be given legally without a valid and clear order.

CRITICAL THINKING EXERCISES

1. You are working as a licensed nurse in a long-term care facility. On the way home from work, you realize you have forgotten to turn over the keys to the medication cabinet. What do you do next? What steps could you take to make sure that you always remember to submit the keys at the end of your shift?
2. An older adult is experiencing what appear to be toxic effects of a medication. Discuss factors that could be contributing to this finding.
3. Describe how drug allergies are determined and documented in your facility.

NCLEX-STYLE REVIEW QUESTIONS

1. The nurse is administering a new medication to a client in the hospital. Which nursing action should be performed to ensure the client's rights are adhered to? Select all that apply.
   a. Inform the client of the chemical content of the drug.
   b. Inform the client of the cost of the drug.
   c. Inform the client about the name of the drug.
   d. Discuss what the possible side effects may be.
   e. Discuss how the medication will work.

2. Which instruction should the nurse include to the client who has been prescribed a diuretic once daily?
   a. Take the medication in the morning.
   b. Take the medication prior to going to bed.
   c. Take the medication with food.
   d. If you miss a dose, double the next dose.

3. A nurse in the long-term care facility accepts a verbal telephone order from a healthcare provider. Which priority action should the nurse take after receiving the order?
   a. Have another nurse review the order.
   b. Carry out the healthcare provider's order.
   c. Read the order back to the healthcare provider.
   d. Refuse to carry out the order.

4. A healthcare provider writes an order for a client and leaves the facility. The nurse is unable to read the order due to the illegible handwriting. Which action by the nurse is appropriate?
   a. Notify the charge nurse.
   b. Do not transcribe the order until the healthcare provider comes back to sign it.
   c. Have another person read it and then carry out the order.
   d. Call the healthcare provider to clarify the order.

5. A client states, "I feel nauseous and do not want to take my medications now." Which response by the nurse is best?
   a. Inform the client to put on the call light when ready to take the medicines.
   b. Inform the client that if the medicine is not taken now, the client will not be able to take it.
   c. Inform the client that if the medicine is taken, the client will feel better.
   d. Inform the client that the medicine can be taken with some food.

CHAPTER RESOURCES

Enhance your learning with additional resources on **thePoint**!

Student Resources related to this chapter can be found at **thePoint.lww.com/Rosdahl12e**.

62 Classification of Medications

Learning Objectives

1. Describe the following classifications of medications, including actions, possible side effects, adverse reactions, nursing considerations, and examples of each: antibiotics, analgesics and narcotics, hypnotics and sedatives, anticonvulsants, steroids, antihypertensives, diuretics, and cardiotonics.
2. Discuss implications associated with drug-resistant bacteria.
3. Discuss major side effects of prolonged steroid therapy.
4. Describe the most common side effects of narcotics, hypnotics, and sedatives.
5. Demonstrate ability to research information about medications accurately.

Important Terminology

analgesic	bronchodilator	narrow-spectrum antibiotic	transdermal	ASA	MOM
antiarrhythmic	catecholamine	nephrotoxicity	vasoconstrictor	CR	NSAID
antibiotic	cathartic	opiate	vasodilator	DDAVP	NTG
anticonvulsant	cross-sensitivity	ototoxicity	wide-spectrum antibiotic	DR	ODT
antihypertensive	depressant	photosensitivity		ER	PCN
antineoplastic	diuretic	sedative	**Acronyms**	HCTZ	PPF
antitussive	emetic	septicemia	ACE	HRT	PT
bactericidal	expectorant	steroid	APAP	HTN	PTT
bacteriostatic	hypnotic	stimulant	ARB	INR	SA
broad-spectrum antibiotic	insulin	topical		IR	SR
				LMWH	TCN

With thousands of medications available today, remembering the action and particulars of every available medication would be impossible. Without a system of *classification,* a drug reference would need to be constantly consulted. Quite simply, classification of medications is similar to a filing system, in which medications are filed according to their actions and body systems affected. Medications that specifically affect each body system are available—those medications with similar actions on a body system can be grouped together. For example, bronchodilators affect the bronchioles, which are part of the respiratory system. Antihypertensive medications lower blood pressure by several different mechanisms. Likewise, medications that share common actions may also share common adverse effects (**cross-sensitivity**) (Chapter 61). Becoming familiar with medication classifications helps the student to recognize possible adverse client effects, providing a basis for implementing appropriate nursing actions, should undesirable effects occur.

> **Nursing Alert** Severe, total-body life-threatening adverse reactions are *anaphylactic* reactions and may result from administration of any drug. Although these reactions are rare, death can result if proper treatment is not instituted immediately.

Classification of medications is also helpful for implementing appropriate nursing actions *before* administering medication to a client. Proper data gathering and follow-up can prevent possible overdose or other adverse reactions that could be life threatening. For example, if an antihypertensive agent is being administered, the nurse should know that it is important to check the client's blood pressure before giving the medication. Another example would be to check the potassium level of a client who is receiving potassium replacement therapy.

Most drugs are considered to be dangerous to a developing fetus if taken during pregnancy. Drug reference books typically identify a pregnancy category for each medication (Box 62-1).

> **Key Concept**
> A person can be allergic to any medication at any time. Always watch for signs of allergic reaction, including anaphylactic, life-threatening reactions. Also, determine if the client is taking any over-the-counter (OTC) medications or herbal supplements. Many of these, in combination with prescribed drugs, can cause serious undesired effects (Box 62-2).

INTERACTIONS BETWEEN FOOD AND MEDICATIONS

Some medications interact negatively with certain foods (e.g., *monoamine oxidase inhibitors* [MAOI]) (Chapter 94). Certain medications, if taken with grapefruit juice, can cause toxicity (Box 62-3). Some medications should always be taken with food, whereas others should be taken on an empty stomach.

> **Box 62-1 FDA Pregnancy Categories**
>
> The U.S. Federal Drug Administration (FDA) has established categories of risk potential during pregnancy, as related to benefits.
> - Category A: A risk has not been documented during pregnancy.
> - Category B: Animal studies have not shown a risk, but there is inadequate documentation in humans, OR animal studies have shown adverse effects, but this has not been demonstrated in humans.
> - Category C: Animal studies have shown adverse effects, but there are no adequate studies in humans, OR the benefits to the pregnant woman may outweigh potential risks, OR there are no adequate studies in humans or animals.
> - Category D: There is evidence of human fetal risk, but the benefits may outweigh potential risks.
> - Category X: Abnormalities have been documented. The risk of use in pregnant women precludes the use of the medication.
> - Category N: FDA has not yet classified the drug.
>
> It is important to remember that no drugs should be administered to pregnant women unless absolutely necessary.

INTERACTIONS BETWEEN DRUGS (DRUG–DRUG INTERACTIONS)

Medications are very complex and care must be taken when using two or more drugs for a client. This includes the use of prescription drugs, OTC drugs, vitamins, and herbal supplements. The possible interactions vary from decreased drug effectiveness to overdose. If you are not familiar with your client's medications, always consult a reliable reference to ensure maximum benefit to your client.

INTRODUCTION TO DRUG CLASSIFICATIONS

This chapter provides an introduction to major drug classifications and their actions. Addressing every medication that affects the body systems is impossible in a text of this length; however, some commonly prescribed medications, their classifications, actions, forms available, routes of administration, and special nursing considerations are presented. More common Canadian trade names are identified as (Can). Tables in this chapter are available for quick reference and convenience. Common dosages are listed here, but always refer to a drug reference if you have questions. Some drug reference sources contain photo guides to assist in recognition of pills and capsules (Fig. 62-1).

Major drug classifications introduced in this chapter include anti-infective agents and medications that affect the integumentary, nervous, endocrine, sensory, cardiovascular, respiratory, gastrointestinal (GI), and urinary systems. Many drugs are available in more than one form and act at differing rates of speed. In addition, some drug preparations are absorbed over a longer period of time (Box 62-4).

ANTIBIOTICS AND OTHER ANTI-INFECTIVE AGENTS

An anti-infective agent is used to treat an infection. An **antibiotic**, one type of anti-infective, is a chemical compound used specifically to treat bacterial infections. It is

> **Box 62-2 Contraindications for Herbal/Dietary Supplements and Complementary Therapies**
>
> Remember that many herbal and dietary supplements and alternative/complementary therapies are very useful and aid in treating various conditions. Many clients believe they are harmless because they are "food." However, some of these can interact negatively with prescribed medications or exacerbate selected medical conditions. A primary care practitioner should be consulted regarding complementary therapies in any of the following situations.
>
> | Herbal/Dietary Supplement | Contraindication |
> |---|---|
> | Angelica and Chinese angelica (dong quai), cat's claw, chamomile, chondroitin, feverfew, garlic, ginger, ginkgo, ginseng, goldenseal, grape seed extract, green tea leaf, horse chestnut seed, ledum tincture, turmeric | May contribute to bleeding tendencies, particularly if combined with oral anticoagulants (Chapter 56) |
> | Bee pollen, celery, coriander, dandelion root, fenugreek, garlic, ginseng, juniper berries, ma huang, Momordica charantia (Karela), xuan shen | May cause problems in persons with diabetes |
> | Ashwagandha, barberry, black cohosh root, burdock, cat's claw, chamomile, dandelion root, false unicorn root, ginger, ginseng, licorice, nettle, octacosanol, schisandra, went rice | May cause problems in pregnancy and/or lactation |
> | Black cohosh root, chaste tree berry, Chinese angelica (dong quai), ginseng, licorice, saw palmetto, St. John wort | May have adverse reaction if taken with hormone replacements or hormonal contraceptives |
> | Chamomile, evening primrose, fish oil, ginkgo, ginseng, kava, ma huang, passionflower vine, psyllium (may block lithium), St. John wort, thyme, valerian, yohimbe | May interact or cause overdose with antidepressants or other psychiatric medications |
> | Allspice, evening primrose | May exacerbate seizure disorders |

> **Box 62-3** Examples of Medications That Should Not Be Taken With Grapefruit Juice

A number of medications should not be given with grapefruit juice. Chemicals in the grapefruit juice inhibit the metabolism of these medications, which can lead to increased blood levels and medication toxicity.

Do not take the following medications with grapefruit juice:

- albendazole (Albenza)
- alfentanil (Alfenta)
- amiodarone (Cordarone)
- amlodipine (Norvasc)
- alprazolam (Xanax)
- atorvastatin (Lipitor)
- 17beta-estradiol
- budesonide (Pulmicort)
- buspirone (BuSpar)
- caffeine
- carbamazepine (Tegretol)
- carvedilol (Coreg)
- cilostazol (Pletal)
- clarithromycin (Biaxin)
- clomipramine (Clomid)
- cortisol
- cyclophosphamide (Cytoxan)
- cyclosporine A (Gengraf)
- dextromethorphan (Delsym, Robitussin)
- diltiazem (Cardizem)
- erythromycin (Erythrocin)
- estrogens (e.g., Premarin)
- etoposide (Toposar)
- felodipine (Plendil)
- fentanyl (Duragesic, Sublimaze)
- fexofenadine (Allegra)
- fluoxetine (Prozac)
- fluvastatin (Lescol)
- fluvoxamine (Luvox)
- indinavir (Crixivan)
- itraconazole (Sporanox)
- losartan (Cozaar)
- lovastatin (Mevacor)
- methadone (Dolophine)
- methylprednisolone (Medrol)
- midazolam (Versed)
- nelfinavir (Viracept)
- nicardipine (Cardene)
- nifedipine (Procardia)
- nimodipine (Nymalize)
- nisoldipine (Sular)
- progesterone
- quinidine
- ritonavir (Norvir)
- saquinavir (Invirase)
- sertraline (Zoloft)
- sildenafil (Viagra)
- simvastatin (Zocor)
- sirolimus (Rapamune)
- sufentanil (Sufenta)
- tacrolimus (Prograf)
- tadalafil (Cialis)
- tamoxifen (Nolvadex)
- temsirolimus (Torisel)
- testosterone
- theophylline
- triazolam (Halcion)
- troleandomycin
- vardenafil (Levitra)
- verapamil (Calan)
- vinblastine (Velban)
- vincristine (Oncovin)
- warfarin (Coumadin)

a product of living cells formed naturally by other living cells (e.g., bacteria, yeasts, or molds) or is produced semi-synthetically in a laboratory. Although living cells produce antibiotics, the term *antibiotic* may also be used to mean any medication that acts as an antimicrobial agent. Antibiotics are classified as **broad spectrum** if they are effective against many organisms and **narrow spectrum** or *specific* if they are effective against only a few microorganisms. Antibiotics that retard the growth of bacteria are called **bacteriostatic** agents; those that kill bacteria are referred to as **bactericidal** agents. Table 62-1 lists common anti-infective medications.

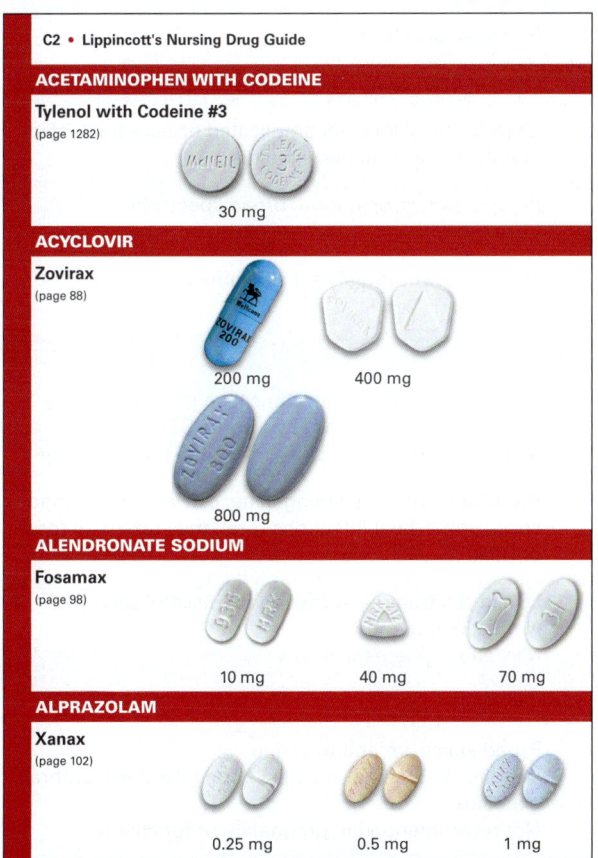

Figure 62-1 Photo guides are available to assist in recognition of pills and capsules. This portion of a photo guide is found in a reference book. The drugs are labeled with their generic and trade names, as well as strength. (Karch, 2003.)

> **Box 62-4** Speed of Action of Medications

Several terms refer to the length of time a medication will be effective. Some are used interchangeably.

Controlled release (**CR**): Drug slowly released over a period of time

Delayed release (**DR**): Medication will begin to take effect after a period of time

Extended release (**ER**): Drug released over a longer period of time

Immediate release (**IR**): Drug released immediately after being taken

Sustained release (**SR**): Drug released over a period of time

Depot, decanoate injections: Drug released for 2 to 3 weeks

Transdermal patches: Drug released for 12 hr to 30 days

TABLE 62-1 Selected Anti-Infective Medications[a]

NAME OF MEDICATION[b]	DOSAGE FORM	NOTES
Penicillins		
amoxicillin (Amoxil)	Capsules: 250-500 mg	Extended spectrum
amoxicillin/clavulanate (Augmentin)	Tablet: 250/125-1,000/625 mg Oral suspension	Otitis media, sinusitis Take with food; commonly causes diarrhea in children
dicloxacillin (Dycill)	Capsules: 500 mg	Best absorbed of the oral antistaphylococcus drugs Oral form used for mild to moderate infections with penicillin-sensitive organisms
penicillin G, aqueous (Benzathine)	Injectable: IM, IV	Parenteral route used for severe infections
penicillin G procaine, aqueous (Bicillin)	Injectable: IM	Long-acting: moderate to severe infections
penicillin V (VK)	Tablets: 250-500 mg	Mild to moderate bacterial infections; prophylaxis, particularly for streptococcus
ticarcillin/clavulanate (Timentin)	IV	Effective against gram-negative, gram-positive, and anaerobic bacteria
Cephalosporins		
cefadroxil (Duricef, Novo-Cefadroxil [Can])	Capsules: 500 mg	Used for skin infections and tonsillitis caused by β-hemolytic streptococcus (can cause renal impairment)
cefdinir (Omnicef)	Capsules: 500 mg Liquid: 125-250 mg/5 mL	To treat specific diseases caused by *Haemophilus influenzae* and some staphylococcus organisms; otitis media
cefepime (Maxipime)	Injectable: IM; IV	Possibly nephrotoxic; may potentiate anticoagulants
cefotaxime (Claforan)	Injectable: IM; IV	Extended spectrum
cefoxitin (Mefoxin)	Injectable: IM; IV	Used against gram-negative and anaerobic organisms
cefuroxime axetil (Ceftin)	Tablets: 250-500 mg	Used for tonsillitis, uncomplicated urinary tract infection (UTI), otitis media, sinusitis
cefuroxime sodium (Kefurox, Zinacef)	Suspension: 250 mg/5 mL Injectable: IM; IV	Preoperative preparation; broad spectrum
cephalexin (Biocef, Keflex)	Capsules: 250-500 mg Suspension: 125-250 mg/5 mL	Used most commonly for skin infections
Tetracyclines		
doxycycline (Apo-Doxy [Can])	Tablets: 20-150 mg Capsules: 50-150 mg IV	Long duration of action; can cause photosensitivity Used to treat infections (e.g., some STIs, traveler diarrhea) and as malaria prophylaxis, Lyme disease
minocycline (Minocin)	Capsules: 50-100 mg IV	Broad spectrum, including acne; carriers of meningococci; gonorrheal infections (oral: may take with food or milk)
tetracycline (Sumycin, Panmycin, Actisite)	Capsules: 250-500 mg	Use in children may cause tooth discoloration Not used in pregnancy May cause photosensitivity
Fluoroquinolones		
ciprofloxacin (Cipro, Ciloxan)	Tablets: 250-750 mg Oral suspension 250-500 mg/5 mL IV Ophthalmic; otic	Broad-spectrum anti-infective Used for UTI, acute sinusitis, bone infections, anthrax exposure Not recommended in pregnancy or for children
levofloxacin (Levaquin)	Tablets: 250-750 mg IV	Used for community-acquired pneumonia, UTI IV form infused over 60-90 min; not for IM use

TABLE 62-1 Selected Anti-Infective Medications[a] (Continued)

NAME OF MEDICATION[b]	DOSAGE FORM	NOTES
Aminoglycosides		
amikacin (Amikin)	IM; IV	Treatment of gram-negative infections, including pseudomonas and bacterial septicemia (nephrotoxic, ototoxic)[c]
gentamicin (Garamycin, Alcomicin [Can], Cidomycin [Can])	Ophthalmic Topical IM; IV	Nephrotoxic and ototoxic[c]; reserved for serious gram-negative infections
neomycin (Neo-Fradin, Mycifradin, Neo-Tab)	Tablet: 500 mg	Toxicity with continued systemic use May be used as bowel preparation
tobramycin (Nebcin, Tobrasol, Tobrex)	IM; IV Ophthalmic	Similar to gentamicin in all aspects
Macrolides		
azithromycin (Zithromax)	Tablets: 250-500 mg Suspension: 100-200 mg/5 mL IV Ophthalmic	10% cross-sensitivity to erythromycin allergies Long acting; client takes for 5 days, but medication effect lasts for 10 days Indicated uses: otitis media, strep infections, community-acquired pneumonia, and sexually transmitted infections
clarithromycin (Biaxin)	Tablets: 500 mg Suspension: 125-250 mg/5 mL	Used for chronic bronchitis, sinusitis, pneumonia; larger doses for duodenal ulcer Used with omeprazole and tetracycline to treat *Helicobacter pylori*
erythromycin (Erythrocin, E-Mycin)	Tablets: 250-500 mg Oral suspension: 200-400 mg/5 mL IV Ophthalmic; topical	Gastrointestinal (GI) distress with oral forms
Sulfonamides and Urinary Antiseptics		
co-trimoxazole (trimethoprim and sulfamethoxazole) (Septra, Bactrim)	Tablets: 400/80 mg-800/160 mg Suspension: 200/40 mg/5 mL IV	A combination of two sulfa drugs for UTI and otitis media in children; other infections in adults
nitrofurantoin (Macrodantin, Furadantin)	Capsules: 25-100 mg Oral suspension: 25 mg/5 mL	Must be taken with food or milk; urinary antiseptic; urine becomes rust colored
sulfasalazine (Azulfidine, Salazopyrin [Can], S.A.S. [Can])	Tablets: 500 mg	Ulcerative colitis; can cause *oligospermia* (lack of sperm cells) and infertility in men (withdrawal of drug reverses adverse effect)
Antifungals		
amphotericin B (Fungizone)	IV	This product is reserved for use in clients with severe life-threatening fungal infections
fluconazole (Diflucan)	Tablets: 100-200 mg Oral suspension: 10-40 mg/mL IV	Broad-spectrum antifungal; 150 mg oral one-time dose for vaginal yeast infections
itraconazole (Sporanox)	Capsules: 100 mg	Histoplasmosis Pulse dosing used for nail infections Used with caution, due to numerous drug interactions
ketoconazole (Nizoral)	Tablets: 200 mg Topical	Antifungal Also available as shampoo (OTC)
miconazole (Monistat)	IV Vaginal; topical	Severe systemic fungal infections For vaginal yeast infection Intrathecal[d] for fungal meningitis

(Continued)

TABLE 62-1 Selected Anti-Infective Medications[a] (Continued)

NAME OF MEDICATION[b]	DOSAGE FORM	NOTES
nystatin (Mycostatin)	Capsule: 0.5 million units Tablets: 0.5 million units Oral suspension: 100,000 units/mL Topical Vaginal	Antifungal agent Swish and swallow for thrush; also component in Magic Mouthwash (swish and spit)
Antivirals		
acyclovir (Zovirax, Alti-Acyclovir [Can], Avirax [Can])	Tablets: 200-800 mg IV Topical	Used for herpes simplex virus types I and II and shingles
amantadine (Symmetrel, Endantadine [Can])	Capsules: 100 mg	Antiviral: influenza type A virus, respiratory tract infections
valacyclovir (Valtrex)	Tablets: 500-1,000 mg	Shingles (herpes zoster); most effective if started within 48 hr of onset; also for genital herpes
zidovudine (AZT, Retrovir) (many other antivirals exist and are used in HIV infections)	Tablet: 100-300 mg Capsules: 100-300 mg Syrup: 50 mg/5 mL IV	Treatment of HIV infections, AIDS, advanced ARC: adjust dose PRN for hematologic changes
Other Antibiotics and Anti-Infectives		
chloramphenicol (Chloromycetin Sodium Succinate, Chloromycetin, Chloracol)	IV	Very broad spectrum; can be toxic to bone marrow
chloroquine phosphate (Aralen)	Tablets: 500 mg, IM	Antimalarial; amebicide; antirheumatoid
clindamycin (Cleocin, C [Can], ClindaMax)	Capsule: 150-300 mg Oral suspension: 75 mg/5 mL IV; IM Vaginal; topical	Available in topical, oral, and injectable forms; effective against gram-positive infections Therapy with this drug can cause severe and possibly fatal colitis
isoniazid (INH; Isotamine [Can], Nydrazid)	Tablets: 100-300 mg Syrup: 50 mg/5 mL IM	Treatment of tuberculosis (take with food)
metronidazole (Flagyl, MetroCream [Can], NeoTric [Can], NidaGel [Can], Noritate, Novonidazol [Can], Trikacide [Can])	Tablets: 250-500 mg IV Vaginal; topical	Treatment of anaerobes; treatment of trichomoniasis; Severe interaction with alcohol
polymyxin B sulfate	IV; IM; intrathecal Ophthalmic	Acute eye infections, when less toxic, drugs are ineffective (IM, IV, and intrathecal[d] forms are very toxic)
rifampin (Rifadin, Rofact [Can])	Capsules: 300 mg IV	Treatment of tuberculosis (discolors urine); for prophylactic use after *H. influenzae* meningitis exposure
vancomycin (Vancocin)	Capsules: 125-250 mg IV	Used for resistant staphylococcal infections in penicillin-allergic clients; used to treat *Clostridium difficile*–associated diarrhea

AIDS, acquired immunodeficiency syndrome; ARC, AIDS-related complex; HIV, human immunodeficiency virus; IM, intramuscular; IV, intravenous; mcg, microgram (one-millionth of a gram); mg, milligram (one-thousandth of a gram); OTC, over-the-counter; PRN, as needed; STI, sexually transmitted infection; UTI, urinary tract infection.
[a]Always consult a current drug reference to confirm the recommended dose before administering any drug.
[b]A trade name in parentheses following the generic name of the medication [Can] indicates the Canadian trade name.
[c]*Nephrotoxic:* damaging to kidney cells; *ototoxic:* damaging to eighth cranial nerve, causing hearing and balance disorders.
[d]*Intrathecal:* injection through the sheath (theca) of the spinal cord into the subarachnoid space.

> **Key Concept**
> Many antibiotics function by reducing the virulence (strength) of a pathogenic organism (bacteriostatic). The body's natural defenses must then take over to actually kill the pathogen.

Effectiveness

Several factors influence the effectiveness of an antibiotic. It must be water soluble and must diffuse readily into body tissue. It should not cause adverse reactions, nor should it affect the normal *flora* (normal and useful bacteria) that usually reside in the human body. Furthermore, if given orally, it should be well absorbed by the GI tract and it should not be antagonistic to other antibiotics.

Antibiotic-Resistant Organisms

If an antibiotic is used indiscriminately, particularly for minor ailments, or is administered improperly, certain pathogens may mutate or build a tolerance to it. Eventually, the antibiotic's action is rendered ineffective against that particular microorganism and the microorganism is termed *resistant* to the antibiotic. For example, a common pathogenic bacterium that may become penicillin resistant is *Staphylococcus aureus*. A dangerous organism known as methicillin-resistant *S. aureus* (*MRSA*) can cause life-threatening illness because it does not respond to antibiotics. This has become a serious problem, particularly in healthcare facilities (Chapter 40).

> **Key Concept**
> Some clients, who are subject to frequent "strep" infections or who have a history of rheumatic fever, take a small daily prophylactic (preventive) dose of oral penicillin, sometimes for years. This dosage schedule generally does not build up resistant strains of streptococcus and generally does not have side effects. In these individuals, antibiotics can be used in increased dosages to treat occasional infections and they are usually effective.

Selection of the Appropriate Antibiotic

Healthcare providers often order a *culture and sensitivity* (C&S) test to determine the specific microorganism causing an infection (culture) and the medication most effective against that organism (sensitivity). Cultures may be obtained from blood, stool, sputum, pus, wound drainage (exudate), urine, or drainage from mucous membranes (Chapter 52). A culture is grown in the laboratory and the cultured bacteria are tested for sensitivity against several antibiotics, to determine which antibiotic most successfully inhibits the bacterial growth.

> **Key Concept**
> To ensure accurate C&S results, antibiotic therapy should not start until after the specimen is obtained and forwarded to the laboratory.
> *Rationale:* If antibiotic therapy begins before the specimen is secured, the numbers and types of bacteria present in the specimen could be reduced, which may result in inappropriate, and perhaps ineffective, antibiotic selection.

Presently, the most effective and widely used antibiotics include penicillins, cephalosporins, tetracyclines, aminoglycosides, macrolides, and sulfonamides. In some infections, any one of the several antibiotics will be effective. In others, only one specific antibiotic will be of value. Sometimes, a combination of antibiotics is required to control an infection. Antibiotics may also be used in conjunction with other medications, to improve their effectiveness.

Penicillins

Penicillin (**PCN**), derived from a specific mold, inhibits the growth of susceptible bacteria. It is also *bactericidal* (kills bacteria) in sufficiently high concentrations or blood levels. It is most effective against gram-positive organisms, such as streptococci, staphylococci, and pneumococci. It is also active against some gram-negative organisms, such as gonococci and meningococci, and against the organism that causes syphilis. PCN has also proven effective in treating early Lyme disease in some cases. It is excreted rapidly in the urine and is remarkably free of toxic effects. PCN is ineffective against the tubercle bacillus, all viruses, and the organisms causing typhoid fever. Therefore, is a fairly narrow-spectrum antibiotic.

Penicillin is available in liquid, tablet, and parenteral forms. The dosage is usually expressed in milligrams and will vary with individual needs and with the type used. It can be given by several routes (Chapters 63 and 64). The oral route is the easiest and safest way to administer PCN and is usually effective for all but the most severe infections. Gastric secretions destroy some PCN, so the oral dose is often larger than that ordered parenterally. The intramuscular (IM) route is most often used with slower acting PCNs. The intravenous (IV) route is used for severe infections when a high blood level is desired as quickly as possible. PCN is a pregnancy category B drug.

Penicillin has few side effects, even in large doses, except for the person who is sensitive or allergic to it. Penicillin sensitivity occurs in about 5% of North Americans. In some cases, PCN causes a comparatively mild allergic reaction, such as nausea, sore mouth, or diarrhea. More serious adverse effects, such as hives, a skin rash, fever, dyspnea, or unusual bleeding, should be reported. In milder PCN reactions, symptoms may be delayed and may occur 5 to 14 days after administration.

> **Nursing Alert** Penicillins share *cross-sensitivity* or the potential for causing allergic reactions. However, some individuals who are allergic to benzathine (penicillin G) may not be allergic to one of the other forms of penicillin. Nevertheless, if a client is allergic to one type of penicillin, use extreme caution when administering another. Penicillins also share cross-sensitivity to cephalosporins, which are similar in molecular structure.

If the client experiences an anaphylactic reaction (Chapter 43), treatment includes immediate oxygen administration, epinephrine 1:1,000, and IV aminophylline (Norphyl) or theophylline (Theo-Dur) for respiratory distress. Steroidal anti-inflammatory agents are usually administered after the client's condition stabilizes. A mild allergic reaction is usually treated with an antihistamine, such as diphenhydramine (Benadryl). Clients with a history of previous reaction to a drug should not receive therapy with that drug or related drugs without first being tested for sensitivity.

Cephalosporins

Cephalosporins, like PCN, were originally derived from a mold. Because cephalosporins are structurally similar to PCN, clients receiving cephalosporin therapy should be asked about previous sensitivity to PCN. Monitor these clients very carefully for adverse or allergic reactions. Approximately 10% of clients with a history of allergy to PCN are also allergic to cephalosporins.

The cephalosporins are divided into three groups: first, second, and third generations. These divisions are based on the range of the medication's specificity, with third-generation agents being more broad spectrum or **wide spectrum** (effective against more pathogens). Most cephalosporins are bactericidal. They are produced semisynthetically and are active against gram-positive cocci, including PCN-resistant staphylococci and gram-negative bacteria, including *Escherichia coli*, *Proteus mirabilis*, and *Klebsiella* species. The cephalosporins are used frequently for mixed infections (those caused by more than one pathogen).

Cephalosporins are available in oral and injectable forms and have become the most widely used antibiotics in the hospital setting. Adverse effects are usually minimal but may include GI symptoms such as flatulence (excessive intestinal gas) and diarrhea. Some cephalosporins can cause more serious adverse effects, such as bone-marrow depression. As with any drug, allergic reactions are possible. Cephalosporins are pregnancy category B agents.

> **Nursing Alert** If the client drinks alcohol while taking a cephalosporin, severe nausea and vomiting are likely.

Tetracyclines

Tetracyclines (**TCN**) are broad-spectrum antibiotics effective against a wide variety of organisms, including *Rickettsia*, *Chlamydia*, and *Mycoplasma*. They are sometimes used in clients who are allergic to penicillin. TCNs are well absorbed orally and are also available for IM or IV use. The presence of food and some dairy products (especially milk) in the stomach decreases oral absorption. To promote GI absorption, clients should receive tetracyclines on an empty stomach at least 1 hr before or 2 to 3 hr after eating.

> **Key Concept**
>
> The presence of iron, calcium, magnesium, or aluminum in the stomach influences tetracycline absorption. Therefore, clients taking tetracyclines should not take antacids such as aluminum hydroxide (Gelusil, Mylanta), calcium carbonate (Tums, Maalox), or magnesium hydroxide (milk of magnesia). Oral calcium supplements will also inhibit absorption and should be taken at least 1 hr before or 3 hr after taking tetracyclines.

Tetracyclines have relatively few side effects. Side effects usually involve the GI system—nausea, vomiting, or diarrhea. Intestinal infections or digestive difficulties are possible because tetracyclines may kill the normal digestive flora. **Photosensitivity** (sensitivity to light) may develop. Adverse reactions include skin rash, burning eyes, and vaginal or anal itching. Tetracyclines, pregnancy category D, cause a brownish discoloration of the enamel in developing teeth and are contraindicated for pregnant women and for children who do not yet have their permanent teeth. Allergic reactions are also possible.

> **Key Concept**
>
> The nurse should instruct the client to take the full prescribed dose of any antibiotic, even though symptoms subside. *Rationale: Taking less than the prescribed dose can contribute to development of antibiotic-resistant strains of pathogens.*

Aminoglycosides

Aminoglycosides are potent bactericidal antibiotics. They are active against many aerobic gram-negative organisms, particularly those causing urinary tract infections (*UTIs*), meningitis, and life-threatening **septicemias** (generalized sepsis or infection throughout the body). Aminoglycosides are considered the medication of choice for hospital-acquired (*nosocomial*) gram-negative infections. They are also used preoperatively in some clients who are scheduled for surgery of the GI tract because the action of these medications reduces the number of normal bacterial flora found there. Aminoglycosides are most often administered parenterally.

Aminoglycosides can have toxic effects, namely, ototoxicity and nephrotoxicity. **Ototoxicity**, caused by damage to the eighth cranial nerve, is manifested by dizziness, tinnitus, and gradual hearing loss that can occur even several days after the medication has been discontinued. **Nephrotoxicity** (kidney damage) is manifested by blood and protein in the urine. Monitor clients receiving aminoglycosides carefully for any signs and symptoms of toxicity. Aminoglycosides are pregnancy category C agents.

Macrolide Antibiotics

Macrolide antibiotics are narrow-spectrum bacteriostatic agents. Macrolides include azithromycin (Zithromax, "Z-Pack"), clarithromycin (Biaxin), dirithromycin (Dynabac), and erythromycin (Erythrocin). They are effective against most microorganisms that are sensitive to PCN and are used to treat respiratory tract infections in clients who are allergic to PCN. Macrolides are usually administered orally; erythromycin also may be administered parenterally. Adverse reactions include skin rashes, abdominal pain, nausea, and cramping. Macrolides are pregnancy category B agents.

> **Key Concept**
>
> Azithromycin oral suspension and erythromycin should be given 1 hr before or 2 to 3 hr after a meal. Clarithromycin (Biaxin) and dirithromycin (Dynabac) should be taken with food.

Sulfonamides and Other Urinary Antiseptics

Sulfonamides (commonly called *sulfa drugs*) are used as antimicrobial agents, chiefly because of their low cost and effectiveness in treating common bacterial infections. They are bacteriostatic agents, requiring normal body processes to eradicate infection. Although sulfa drugs are effective, they are not used as frequently today, particularly due to increasing bacterial resistance to them. The use of specific sulfonamides may be indicated in chancroid, trachoma, toxoplasmosis, uncomplicated UTIs, specific cases of malaria, meningococcal meningitis, *Haemophilus influenzae* infections of the middle ear, and as an alternative to PCN for PCN-sensitive clients with rheumatic fever. Sulfonamides may be used with PCN or erythromycin in conditions such as otitis media.

Encourage clients taking sulfonamides to drink large amounts of fluids, to dilute the urine. **Rationale:** *Sulfa drugs are excreted via the kidneys and tend to form crystals in the urine, which causes kidney irritation and possible kidney stone formation.* The intake of large amounts of fluid will minimize the possibility of crystal formation.

Observe this client for signs and symptoms of adverse reactions including nausea, vomiting, diarrhea, electrolyte imbalance, cyanosis, or jaundice. Kidney damage or failure is possible and is a serious adverse effect. Sulfonamides are considered pregnancy category C drugs during pregnancy and category D drugs at term.

Sulfamethoxazole/trimethoprim (Bactrim, Bactrim DS) is a combination drug often considered the medication of choice for UTIs. As with all other medications of this type, Bactrim should not be given to infants younger than 2 months. (Bactrim is *not* recommended for streptococcal or upper respiratory infections.)

Other Anti-Infectives

The previously discussed antibiotics are the most effective and widely used anti-infective agents. Other antibiotics and anti-infectives are available and may be used when the causative organism has shown resistance to the more popular antibiotics or when the client is allergic to other medications. Some are used to treat nonbacterial infections, such as fungal and viral infections.

The medications in Table 62-2 are not all derived from living organisms, such as mold or algae. Thus, some of those listed are *technically not antibiotics*. They do have antimicrobial actions and thus are commonly referred to collectively as *antibiotics*.

> **Nursing Alert** Symptoms of a serious reaction to clindamycin (Cleocin) include diarrhea with liquid feces and shreds of intestinal lining. Although rare, this reaction can be fatal, especially in children or older adults. Therefore, a client receiving clindamycin must report any diarrhea *at once*.

MEDICATIONS THAT AFFECT THE INTEGUMENTARY SYSTEM

The condition of sweat glands and pores that penetrate the epidermis from subcutaneous (SC) tissue and the adequacy of blood supply to the area affect absorption of medication through the skin. Absorption increases if the skin is *macerated* (softened), either by water or perspiration. Chapter 75 describes skin disorders and specific methods of administering dermatologic medications. Table 62-2 lists common medications affecting the integumentary system.

Medications applied to the skin or into external body structures, such as the ear or eye, are called **topical** agents. Topical *dermatologic agents* are medications applied to the skin to treat localized skin conditions. Examples include soothing agents, antiseptics, anesthetics, corticosteroids, antifungals, and pediculicides (to kill lice). Sterilizing the skin is impossible, but sufficient cleansing will remove most bacteria. Strong antiseptics can cause skin irritation that may interfere with the skin's protective function as a natural barrier against bacterial invasion. **Transdermal** *medications* are topical agents *designed to be absorbed through the skin* for systemic effects (Chapter 63).

> **NCLEX Alert**
>
> The classifications of medications into major groups, such as analgesics, sedatives, and antibiotics, contain important NCLEX concerns. As you will be responsible for monitoring clients for expected and unexpected reactions to any medications a client receives, it will be important for you to know the typical, normal effects and side effects of each classification. Side effects of medications must be known for the NCLEX.

MEDICATIONS THAT AFFECT THE NERVOUS SYSTEM

The central nervous system (CNS) regulates the body's vital control centers, in addition to many other body processes (Chapter 19). When CNS functions are disturbed, medications may be used to increase or decrease the activity of vital brain and nerve structures. **Stimulants** speed mental and physical processes; **depressants** slow them. (Psychiatric medications are described in Chapter 94; drug abuse and dependency are described in Chapter 95.) Table 62-3 lists common medications affecting the CNS.

Many medications stimulate the CNS, but only a few are medically valuable for this purpose. The most valuable are those that stimulate the brain's respiratory centers, usually to counteract toxic effects of depressants, such as barbiturates. Other than for this purpose, stimulants are rarely prescribed today because they have a high potential for abuse and many adverse side effects.

Medications that depress the CNS include analgesics; hypnotics and sedatives that bring rest and sleep; and general anesthetics that cause loss of consciousness. In addition, some medications are *selective depressants* and are used for symptomatic treatment. Table 62-3 describes commonly used medications affecting the CNS.

Analgesics

Analgesics are medications that relieve pain. They are divided into two groups: narcotics and nonnarcotics. An example of a narcotic analgesic is morphine. Examples of nonnarcotic analgesics are aspirin (acetylsalicylic acid [**ASA**]) and acetaminophen (**APAP**, known as Tylenol). Analgesics interfere with a person's perception of pain but do not cause unconsciousness. Because they relieve pain, they promote comfort and relaxation and allow the client to sleep.

TABLE 62-2 Selected Dermatologic Agents

TYPE	EXAMPLES[a]
Soothing Agents	
Emollient preparations	*dexpanthenol* (Panthoderm): Relieves itching, aids in healing mild skin irritations
	glycerin: In pure form, tendency to dry skin; if mixed with rosewater, has moisturizing effect
	lanolin: Used as ointment base; purified fat of sheep's wool with water
	urea (Aquacare, Carmol 10 or 20, Nutraplus): 2%-40%, promotes hydration and removal of excess keratin in dry skin
	vitamin A & D ointment: Relieves minor burns, chafing, irritation
	zinc oxide ointment: 15% zinc oxide in simple ointment base; relieves burns, abrasions, diaper rash
Pain Relief	
Lotions and solutions	*capsaicin (Capsin):* Apply maximum 3-4 times per day for temporary arthritis relief
	Burow solution: Aluminum acetate used for its *astringent* (drying) properties; used for poison ivy, insect bites
	Calamine lotion: Used for *dermatitis* (itching, inflamed skin) caused by poison ivy, insect bites, prickly heat
Anesthetics	
Benzocaine, lidocaine	Sprays, lotions, or creams used for *pruritus* (itching) and pain due to wounds, minor burns, prickly heat, chickenpox, insect bites, sunburn
Antiseptics	*benzalkonium chloride (Zephiran):* Detergent-type agent; germicidal for many pathogens; activity reduced by soap solutions; most effective in 1:750 solution
	chlorhexidine gluconate (Hibiclens): Antimicrobial activity against wide range of microorganisms; used as surgical scrub and cleanser for preoperative bathing and wound cleansing
	iodine: Generally in alcohol solution (*tincture of iodine*), in concentration to 7%
	povidone-iodine (Betadine): Stable compound slowly releases iodine; relatively nonirritating; contains 1% available iodine
Antifungals	*butenafine hydrochloride (Mentax):* Used for athlete's foot, ringworm
	tioconazole (Vagistat-1): One-dose treatment for vaginal fungal infections; mild increase of burning or itching may occur
	clotrimazole (Lotrimin): Antifungal used topically for athlete's foot and diaper rash; used vaginally for yeast infection; both forms available OTC
	ciclopirox (Loprox, Penlac): Treatment of *onychomycosis* (fungal infection of the nails) in immunocompromised individuals
	Gentian violet: Antifungal; external application of solution of 1% of the dye; do not apply to active lesions; stains clothing
	nystatin (Mycostatin): Antibiotic; used for fungal infections of skin and mucous membranes; used in mouthwashes for thrush
	terbinafine HCl (Lamisil): Antifungal cream; used for athlete's foot, ringworm; available OTC
	tolnaftate (Tinactin): 1% in cream or solution to treat infections caused by *Trichophyton,* the organism of athlete's foot and other dermatologic infections
Corticosteroids	*betamethasone dipropionate (Diprosone):* Available in varying strengths and emollient bases; used for anti-inflammatory, antipruritic, and antiproliferative actions; avoid contact with eyes; apply sparingly
	desoximetasone (Topicort): Available as cream, gel, or ointment (use cautiously in viral diseases; may macerate skin if covered with occlusive dressing)
	hydrocortisone: Available as aerosol, cream, gel, lotion, ointment, topical solution, rectal foam; used for dermatitis; may be used on face, groin, axillae, and under breasts; clean area before application; avoid eyes; use as directed

TABLE 62-2 Selected Dermatologic Agents (Continued)

TYPE	EXAMPLES[a]
Pediculicides (kill lice)	*crotamiton (Eurax):* Thorough massaging into skin needed; bed linens and clothing should be changed the next day *lindane (Kwell):* Available as lotion or shampoo. Avoid eyes and mouth; potential for CNS toxicity in infants and children; by prescription only *malathion (Ovide):* Lotion; applied to dry hair and left on for 8-12 hr; repeated in 7-9 days; prescription only *Permethrin (Nix):* Shampoo (combing of nits [lice eggs] not required); will prevent reinfection to 2 weeks; available OTC; no CNS toxicity if used as directed
Miscellaneous	
Chigarid	*Camphor 2.8%, phenol 1.5%, menthol 0.1%, collodion, oil of eucalyptus:* Applied externally to relieve pain and itching of insect bites; OTC

CNS, central nervous system; OTC, over-the-counter.
[a] A trade name appears in parentheses following the generic name of a medication.

TABLE 62-3 Selected Central Nervous System Medications[a]

NAME OF MEDICATION[b]	DOSAGE FORM	NOTES
Narcotic Agonist Analgesics (given for pain)		
codeine	Tablets: 15-60 mg IM; SQ	Oral form is combined with acetaminophen (as Tylenol #3) for moderate to severe pain
fentanyl (Innovar, Oralet, Sublimaze, Duragesic)	IV; buccal; intranasal Topical patch	Dosage depends on use (induction of anesthesia, maintenance of anesthesia, versus pain management)
hydromorphone (Dilaudid)	Tablets: 2-8 mg Syrup IM	Shorter duration of action than morphine
levorphanol (Levo-Dromoran)	Tablets: 2 mg IM	For relief of moderate to severe pain
methadone (Dolophine)	Tablets: 5-10 mg Soluble tablet: 40 mg Oral solution Oral concentrate IM	Longer duration of activity; used as narcotic replacement to facilitate withdrawal; also to manage severe pain
Morphine	Tablets: 15-30 mg ER tablets/capsules: 10-200 mg Oral solution Oral concentrate IV; IM	Used to treat severe pain (e.g., MI, cancer); ER formulations used for chronic pain; oral concentrate used commonly in hospice clients
oxycodone (Endocodone, M-Oxy, OxyContin, OxyFAST, Supeudol [Can], Roxicodone, Intensol)	Tablets: 5-30 mg ER tablets: 15-80 mg Oral solution Oral concentrate	Often combined with aspirin (as Percodan) or acetaminophen (as Percocet); oral concentrate commonly used for hospice clients; OxyContin has history of abuse
Narcotic Antagonist (antidote)		
naloxone (Narcan)	IV preferred; IM; SQ; oral	Used as antidote in narcotic overdose; prevents or reverses effects of opioids
Nonsteroidal Anti-Inflammatory Drugs (NSAIDs)[c] and Antirheumatics (given for pain)		
acetaminophen (Aceta, Atasol [Can], Tylenol)	Tablets: 325-500 mg ER tablet: 650 mg Chewable tablet: 80-160 mg Oral drops, liquid and suspension Rectal suppository	Analgesic and fever reducer (antipyretic); used in aspirin-allergic clients and children; does not contribute to bleeding or impair clotting

(Continued)

TABLE 62-3 Selected Central Nervous System Medications[a] (Continued)

NAME OF MEDICATION[b]	DOSAGE FORM	NOTES
acetylsalicylic acid, ASA, aspirin	Tablets: 81-650 mg Rectal suppository	Antipyretic, nonopioid analgesic, anti-inflammatory, may cause GI distress in high doses; mild anticoagulant; low dose (81 mg) used daily to prevent stroke and/or MI
celecoxib (Celebrex)	Capsule: 100-200 mg	Selective COX-2 inhibitor; treatment of osteoarthritis, rheumatoid arthritis; contraindicated for those allergic to sulfonamide or NSAIDs; can be given with warfarin
diclofenac (Nu-Diclo [Can], Voltaren, Rapide [Can]), Flector Patch, Voltaren Gel	Tablets: 25-100 mg ER tablet: 100 mg Ophthalmic Transdermal	Used in arthritis and ankylosing spondylitis; transdermal forms treat without unwanted GI side effects
ibuprofen (Motrin, Advil)	Tablets: 200-800 mg oral drops, solution, and suspension	Antipyretic; used for arthritis; give with meals or milk if GI distress occurs; available OTC in 200-mg tablets, and in liquid for children
indomethacin (Indocin, Indotec [Can], Indocid P.D.A. [Can])	Capsules: 25-50 mg ER Capsule: 75 mg IV Suppository	Commonly used in arthritis and acute gout; gastric distress common
naproxen (Naprosyn, Aleve)	Tablets: 220-500 mg	Long-acting drug (BID dosing); used for arthritis; OTC version is Aleve 220 mg
Nonnarcotic Analgesic		
tramadol (Ultram)	Tablet: 50 mg ER tablets: 100-300 mg	No respiratory depressant effects; used for moderate to severe pain; ER form used for chronic pain
Hypnotic, Sedative, and Antianxiety Medications		
barbiturates amobarbital (Amytal)	IM; IV	Hypnotic; intermediate duration of action
pentobarbital (Nembutal)	IM; IV	Short-acting hypnotic; may be used as preanesthetic
phenobarbital (Barbilixir [Can], Barbita [Can], Belatol)	Tablets: 15-100 mg Oral elixir IV IM	Long-acting sedative; used principally as anticonvulsant
secobarbital (Seconal)	Capsules: 100 mg	Short-acting hypnotic and preanesthesia sedative; used occasionally in pregnancy
Benzodiazepines		
alprazolam (Xanax)	Tablets: 0.25-2 mg ER tablets: 0.5-3 mg ODT: 0.25-2 mg Oral concentrate	Intermediate acting; indicated for anxiety disorders; 2-mg dose used to treat panic attacks
diazepam (Valium)	Tablets: 2-10 mg IV; IM Rectal	Used to treat acute seizures, muscle spasm, anxiety, tetanus; IV form for status epilepticus; used in alcohol detoxification to control BP and prevent DTs
flurazepam (Somnol [Can])	Capsules: 15-30 mg	Hypnotic only; use dose of 15 mg in elderly
lorazepam (Ativan)	Tablets: 0.5-2 mg Oral concentrate IV; IM	Intermediate acting; sublingual administration or Intensol (solution) absorbed faster than oral; oral concentrate used for hospice
midazolam (Versed)	Injection Syrup	IV or IM sedation, anxiolytic, preanesthetic; or used alone in procedures, such as colonoscopy; provides amnesia

TABLE 62-3 Selected Central Nervous System Medications[a] (Continued)

NAME OF MEDICATION[b]	DOSAGE FORM	NOTES
temazepam (Restoril)	Capsules: 7.5-30 mg	Intermediate acting; prescribed for insomnia
Anticonvulsants and Antiepileptic Agents		
carbamazepine (Tegretol)	Tablets: 100-200 mg ER tablets: 100-400 mg Oral suspension	Used in mixed seizures, generalized tonic–clonic seizures, and treatment of pain associated with trigeminal neuralgia
clonazepam (Klonopin, Apo-Clonazepam [Can], Clonapam [Can], Rivotril [Can])	Tablets: 0.5-2 mg ODT: 0.125-2 mg	Used in specific seizures not responsive to other drugs; also used for panic attacks and generalized anxiety; ODT formulation provides easy administration for unresponsive/uncooperative clients
magnesium sulfate	IV	Used for prevention and control of seizures in toxemia of pregnancy
phenytoin (Dilantin)	Capsules: 30-300 mg Tablets: 50 mg Oral suspension IV; IM	Anticonvulsant for generalized tonic–clonic and psychomotor seizures (gingival hyperplasia is frequent side effect)
Other CNS Medications		
buspirone (BuSpar)	Tablets: 5-30 mg	Management of anxiety disorders, antidepressant; not related chemically to benzodiazepines, barbiturates, or other sedative hypnotics; fewer sedative effects than benzodiazepines
carbidopa/levodopa (Sinemet)	Tablets: 10/100-25/250 mg ER tablets: 25/100-50/200 mg ODT: 10/100-25/250 mg	Antiparkinsonism agent; may cause hemolytic anemia, cardiac arrhythmias; contraindicated in glaucoma, melanoma; may interact with antihypertensive agents
cyclobenzaprine (Flexeril, Amrix)	Tablets: 5-10 mg ER Capsules: 15-30 mg	Centrally acting muscle relaxant; structurally related to tricyclics (may cause drowsiness, dry mouth)
dantrolene sodium (Dantrium)	Capsule: 25-100 mg IV	Skeletal muscle relaxant used for cerebral palsy, multiple sclerosis; also used for malignant hyperthermia
dextroamphetamine (Dexedrine)	Tablets: 5-10 mg ER capsules: 5-15 mg Oral solution	Used in adults for narcolepsy (sleep disorder); in children for ADHD
DHE (Migranal)	Injection Nasal spray	Ergot derivative; used in acute migraine or cluster headache; possible coronary artery vasodilation
eszopiclone (Lunesta)	Tablet: 1-3 mg	Sleep aid; take immediately before bedtime; potential for depression; may cause withdrawal if stopped abruptly; do not use with alcohol
methocarbamol (Robaxin)	Tablet: 500-750 mg IV; IM	Centrally acting muscle relaxant (may cause drowsiness); used to treat tetanus
methylphenidate (Ritalin, Concerta, Metadate, Daytrana patch)	Tablets: 5-60 mg ER: 10-60 mg Chewable tablets: 2.5-10 mg Oral solution Transdermal patch	Adults: Narcolepsy Children: ADHD; various forms available to ease administration and increase compliance
ramelteon (Rozerem)	Tablet: 8 mg	Melatonin receptor agonist; to treat insomnia, in difficulty falling asleep; minimal side effects
sumatriptan (Imitrex)	Tablet: 25-100 mg SQ Nasal spray	Treatment of severe migraine headaches; available by prescription (prefilled syringes) for home administration; oral form also available

(Continued)

TABLE 62-3 Selected Central Nervous System Medications[a] (Continued)

NAME OF MEDICATION[b]	DOSAGE FORM	NOTES
zolpidem (Ambien)	Tablet: 5-10 mg	Sleep aid
	ER tablet: 6.25-12.5 mg	Minimal next-day residual effects; dosage decreased in elderly or clients with hepatic insufficiency
Antidepressants and Antipsychotics		
See Chapter 94		

ADHD, attention-deficit hyperactive disorder; BID, twice daily; BP, blood pressure; DTs, delirium tremens; ER, extended release; GI, gastrointestinal; IM, intramuscular; IV, intravenous; mcg, microgram (one-millionth of a gram); mg, milligram (one-thousandth of a gram); MI, myocardial infarction; ODT, orally disintegrating tablet; SQ, subcutaneous.
[a]Always consult a current drug reference to confirm the recommended dose before administering any drug.
[b]A trade name appears in parentheses following the generic name of the medication. [Can] indicates Canadian trade name.
[c]NSAIDs are contraindicated when clients are taking any medication that may cause kidney damage, such as lithium.

Narcotic Agonist Analgesics

Narcotic agonist analgesics, the **opiates**, are opium derivatives or have opium-like actions. They can occur naturally or be produced synthetically. The most common opiates are morphine and codeine, which are very potent and mainly affect the CNS. These drugs generally are considered pregnancy category C agents. Opiates are highly addictive and subject to narcotic regulation, as described in Chapter 61 (Boxes 61-1 and 62-5). Opiates depress the brain's cerebral cortex, altering the client's awareness of pain, and some are more potent than others.

> **Nursing Alert** The first sign of narcotic overdose is usually respiratory depression. Therefore, monitoring the client's vital signs, particularly respirations, is extremely important when administering narcotics.

Morphine Sulfate

Morphine sulfate (MS) is a very potent narcotic analgesic used to relieve severe pain such as that produced by myocardial infarction (MI, "heart attack"), passage of renal calculi (kidney stones), or terminal conditions (e.g., advanced cancer). Morphine is most effective when given before the client's pain becomes severe. Morphine's analgesic effect allows the client to rest more comfortably and also produces a feeling of well-being, reducing fear and anxiety. Thus, it may be used preoperatively and is usually administered in conjunction with atropine, a drying agent used to reduce secretions of the respiratory tract.

Nausea and vomiting are common morphine side effects that can be relieved by antiemetics (antinausea drugs). However, these preparations *potentiate* (increase) the actions of narcotics. Therefore, carefully monitor the client's vital signs, especially if the client is also receiving an antiemetic. Morphine and other opiates delay stomach emptying and

Box 62-5 Management of Controlled Substances

Stringent legal requirements apply to anyone handling controlled substances (Box 61-1). The medication must be tracked from the time it is manufactured until it is administered to the client and documented (or wasted and witnessed).

- All controlled substances must be ordered by an approved healthcare provider.
- An override is permitted only in an emergency. The override must be immediately backed up by an appropriate order.
- The nurse who obtains the medication from the supply should be the person who administers and documents it.
- All controlled substances must be accounted for, either by the count in the machine or by a manual count. Manual counts must be witnessed and signed off by two licensed nurses at least every 8 hr.
- Controlled substances must be given immediately after their removal from the supply. They cannot legally be saved for later administration.
- These medications must be documented as given, immediately after administration.
- If a controlled substance is not given, this must be recorded. If the package is opened, the medication is disposed of in the appropriate container. If the package is unopened, it may be returned to the pharmacy. In either case, two nurses must witness the disposal or returning of the medication.
- If there is a discrepancy in the controlled substances count, it must be resolved immediately.
- Controlled substances brought from home by clients or sent home on discharge must be accounted for, according to agency policy.
- Any healthcare professional who suspects inappropriate diversion, use, or handling of controlled substances is legally and ethically bound to report this.

slow peristalsis. They can be used to treat severe diarrhea or for surgical interventions involving the intestines. However, this slowed peristalsis can also cause constipation (a very common side effect) and abdominal pain and distention. Allergic reactions are fairly common. Morphine is not recommended for pain that can be relieved by administration of a less-potent analgesic. Clients receiving morphine may develop a tolerance to it and, thus, may require increasingly larger doses.

Morphine poisoning is often the result of attempted suicide. Significant early symptoms of poisoning include decreased respirations (<12/min), deep sleep, and constricted pupils. Emergency treatment involves the use of narcotic antagonists, such as naloxone (Narcan), that counteract the action of morphine. If respirations are severely depressed, the medical goal is to maintain the person's airway and to initiate emergency respiratory care measures. The nurse must be prepared to assist with rescue breathing, oxygen administration, emergency endotracheal intubation, or tracheostomy.

Fentanyl
Fentanyl (Sublimaze), a pregnancy category C agent, is a potent synthetically produced opioid analgesic. It has a rapid onset of action, coupled with a short duration of action, which makes it ideal for use before, during, and after surgery. A fentanyl dose of 100 mcg is equivalent to 10 mg of morphine and usually causes less nausea and vomiting than morphine. Fentanyl slows the respiratory rate; the respiratory effect is dose related. Postoperative clients' vital signs must be monitored routinely, and adequate facilities to treat all degrees of respiratory depression must be available. Possible side effects include depression, nausea, vomiting, constipation, and headache. A toxic dose may cause circulatory collapse, seizures, cardiac arrest, and pulmonary edema and may be fatal. The patch form of fentanyl (Duragesic) is used only in clients who are opioid dependent.

Hydromorphone Hydrochloride (Dilaudid)
This medication is prepared from morphine and has about five times its analgesic effect. Although the effect of hydromorphone hydrochloride (Dilaudid) is shorter than morphine, it can be prolonged *if given by suppository.* The medication causes very little drowsiness, nausea, or vomiting but does depress respiration. Nursing considerations are similar to those for morphine.

Codeine
Codeine is a derivative of morphine, but its action is milder. A pregnancy category C agent during pregnancy and a category D agent during labor, this drug is recommended for relief of mild to moderate pain. Codeine has a depressant effect on the cough reflex and, therefore, is especially effective in relieving cough and is a common ingredient in cough mixtures. Codeine depresses the CNS to a lesser degree and is less addictive than morphine. However, it may be as constipating as morphine.

Other Narcotic Analgesics
Other narcotic analgesics, such as *meperidine hydrochloride* (Demerol), are effective pain relievers and have fewer adverse reactions than morphine. However, Demerol is rarely used today since other drugs are as effective and cause fewer side effects.

> **NCLEX Alert**
>
> Side effects of medications can include life-threatening anaphylaxis, changes to various physical functions (e.g., loss of electrolytes, hypotension), or unexpected reactions (idiosyncratic responses). Each pharmaceutical intervention must be considered as only one piece of a bigger clinical picture. NCLEX situations and options will require that you understand not only the medication but also your choice of nursing interventions.

Methadone hydrochloride (Dolophine), a pregnancy category C agent, is much like morphine in that it is an effective pain reliever and has similarly lasting effects. However, it does not cause euphoria, so it is used to manage heroin addiction. Methadone is slightly more effective than morphine in relieving chronic pain and is effective in depressing the cough reflex. It may cause nausea and vomiting, itching, constipation, and respiratory depression (Chapter 95).

Oxycodone, typically combined with aspirin (Percodan) or acetaminophen (Percocet), is effective for the treatment of moderate pain. Side effects are similar to those found with other narcotics. Onset of action is approximately 15 min, and the duration of action is 4 to 5 hr. *OxyContin* is the extended-release (ER) version of oxycodone. ER tablets are designed to release a controlled amount of oxycodone over a 12-hr period. The tablet should be taken whole; do not break, crush, or chew. ER tablets are intended to be used in clients with moderate to severe pain when around-the-clock pain control is necessary; OxyContin can be used for an extended period of time, but carries a high risk of abuse.

> **Nursing Alert** All opiates and opiate-like medications can be addictive; their administration must be monitored closely. Evaluate the type and intensity of the client's pain. More potent opiate medications, such as morphine, should be used only when the client's pain level is severe. Expect to institute appropriate tapering doses or substitute less-potent narcotic analgesics, as ordered, as the client's pain level decreases. Be particularly cautious in administering opiates to any person who is otherwise chemically dependent, including alcohol dependent. These clients may become dependent on opiates very quickly.

Nonnarcotic Analgesics and Nonsteroidal Anti-Inflammatory Drugs
Nonnarcotic analgesics are less potent than narcotic analgesics and are available over the counter (OTC). Aspirin, ibuprofen (Advil, Motrin), and acetaminophen (Tylenol) are the most commonly used examples. *Antipyretic analgesics* are medications that reduce both pain and fever.

Salicylates
The *salicylates* derive from salicylic acid (**SA**). *Acetylsalicylic acid* (ASA, aspirin) is available in tablets and rectal suppositories. Flavored chewable tablets are available in dosages

appropriate for administration to children; however, *aspirin is not recommended for children* because it is believed to contribute to the development of Reye syndrome. Acetylsalicylic acid (Aspirin) is commonly used in adults and is highly effective for the treatment of mild to moderate pain.

Acetylsalicylic acid (Aspirin) and other salicylates have three separate actions: analgesic (pain relief—headache, arthritis), antipyretic (fever reduction), and anti-inflammatory (arthritis, neuralgia [nerve pain]), in addition to mild anticoagulation (by reducing platelet aggregation, preventing blood clots). Daily low dose acetylsalicylic acid (aspirin) (81 mg) is often recommended to reduce the incidence or severity of stroke and MI. The salicylates have remarkably few side effects, the most common of which is gastric irritation, which can be eliminated by the use of enteric-coated tablets. ASA is not recommended for clients with active gastric ulcers or bleeding disorders, for those taking warfarin (Coumadin) or other agents that affect blood coagulation, or for use immediately before and after surgery or obstetric delivery. It is a pregnancy category D agent. Overdose or toxicity can occur; the most common symptoms are dizziness, tinnitus (ringing in the ears), and visual disturbances. Severe anaphylactic reactions may also occur.

> **Key Concept**
>
> The use of acetylsalicylic acid (aspirin) and other anticoagulants is contraindicated for 7 to 10 days before any surgery, dental work, or invasive procedures, such as biopsy or colonoscopy. In addition, some herbal supplements can contribute to operative and postoperative bleeding (Chapter 56). The client should consult the surgeon or dentist for specific instructions.

Nonsalicylate Analgesics

Acetaminophen (Tylenol, Atasol [Can]), a nonnarcotic analgesic, has the same analgesic and antipyretic properties as aspirin, but fewer side effects. Acetaminophen (Tylenol), a pregnancy category B agent, is often prescribed for people allergic to salicylates and is usually used for infants and children. It also has few GI side effects. Acetaminophen (Tylenol) is not an anti-inflammatory agent and, therefore, is less useful than aspirin for treating arthritis and other inflammatory conditions. The maximum daily dose of acetaminophen (Tylenol) is 4,000 mg (4 g) from all sources, including combination medications.

Tramadol (Ultram) is a centrally acting semisynthetic analgesic. It does not contain salicylate and is unrelated to the narcotics. Clients who cannot tolerate salicylates or nonsteroidal agents often use it. Tramadol (Ultram), a pregnancy category C agent, does not cause respiratory depression. Side effects include dizziness, constipation, and nausea. Because it may contribute to increased risk of seizures, the drug is contraindicated in clients with a seizure disorder. Tramadol (Ultram) was classified as a schedule IV drug in 2014 because of its high abuse potential.

D.H.E. (dihydroergotamine mesylate) is used to treat pain, particularly migraine and cluster headaches. DHE (Migranal) is an ergot derivative available as an injection or nasal spray. Its specific action is unknown, but it constricts cranial blood vessels and decreases pulsation in these arteries, thus relieving pain. This drug is a pregnancy category X medication and thus should not be used in pregnancy or lactation.

Nonsteroidal Anti-Inflammatory Drugs

The nonsteroidal anti-inflammatory drugs (**NSAIDs**) are used primarily to treat inflammation, but also have analgesic and antipyretic actions. This large class of medications is used to treat mild to moderate pain. Most NSAIDs can cause gastric upset and should be taken with food. They *should not be given* with salicylates or anticoagulants or with certain psychiatric medications (especially lithium) because they reduce renal (kidney) clearance, and toxicity or kidney damage may occur. NSAIDs also reduce the effectiveness of some diuretics and antihypertensive agents. Clients receiving cyclosporine (to prevent organ transplant rejection) should not receive NSAIDs. NSAIDs should not be combined with other OTC agents because of the possibility of duplication. These drugs are generally considered pregnancy category B agents, although some variation exists.

Ibuprofen (Motrin, Advil, Midol Liqui-gel, Genpril) is a potent NSAID used to relieve mild to moderate pain. Ibuprofen is available OTC and is indicated for minor aches and pains, fever reduction, and dysmenorrhea (painful menstruation). It also is available in children's drops, suspension, and chewable tablets to control pain and fever in children. Monitoring liver and kidney function is necessary for the client receiving ibuprofen.

Indomethacin (Indocin) belongs to the NSAID group, but is chemically unrelated to other medications in this class. It is a pregnancy category B agent during the first two trimesters and a category D agent during the third trimester. Indomethacin (Indocin) is effective in treating arthritis, bursitis, and other joint diseases. Clients should always take it with meals or milk because it may cause severe gastric distress.

Celecoxib (Celebrex) is a newer type of NSAID. It inhibits (blocks) the cyclo-oxygenase-2 (COX-2) enzyme, which is activated in inflammation. However, the drug does not inhibit cyclo-oxygenase-1 (COX-1), an enzyme that protects the lining of the GI tract and plays a role in blood clotting and kidney function. COX-2 inhibitors have excellent anti-inflammatory and analgesic properties, with fewer GI side effects. Celecoxib (Celebrex), a pregnancy category C agent, is often the drug of choice for clients with arthritis or peptic ulcer disease. It should not be given to clients who are allergic to sulfonamides, NSAIDs, or aspirin. Side effects include headache, dyspepsia, and diarrhea. This medication is the only anti-inflammatory drug that can be safely taken by clients who are taking warfarin (Coumadin) for anticoagulation.

Hypnotics and Sedatives

A **hypnotic** is a medication that produces sleep. It is usually taken at bedtime. A **sedative** is a medication that has a calming or quieting effect. Depending on the dose, medications in this class can have either a hypnotic or sedative effect. To achieve a calming or relaxing effect, small doses of sedatives may be administered throughout the day. If given in a large dose at bedtime, a sedative's calming effect may induce sleep. The ideal hypnotic acts quickly, brings a natural sleep without "hangover," is nonaddictive, and has few or no harmful, adverse effects. The search for this medication has resulted in the manufacture of hundreds of barbiturates, only a few of which approximate these requirements.

Barbiturates

Barbiturates are derived from barbituric acid and, in the past, have been referred to as "sleeping pills." However, the use of barbiturates to produce sleep has greatly decreased since the advent of benzodiazepines. Nonetheless, some barbiturates are still prescribed. Their action is classified as long acting (10-16 hr), intermediate acting (6-8 hr), or short acting (3-4 hr). Long-acting barbiturates, such as phenobarbital, are used to control and prevent seizure activity. Intermediate-acting barbiturates are used primarily as daytime or day-surgery sedatives and for their sedative effects during labor or before anesthesia. Short-acting barbiturates, such as secobarbital (Seconal), are used primarily at bedtime, or as a preanesthetic, because there are fewer hangover reactions (because of their short-acting effect). Barbiturates are easily absorbed and can be given orally or parenterally. They are pregnancy category D agents and schedule II drugs (Chapter 61). When barbiturates are used as hypnotics, they interfere with normal sleep patterns. Commonly experienced side effects of barbiturates include morning hangovers, drowsiness, lethargy, mood change, and depression. Clients should be warned not to operate machinery or drive when taking barbiturates. Alcohol potentiates the action of barbiturates, and clients using barbiturates for extended periods may develop a physical dependency on them. Withdrawal from barbiturates may cause very uncomfortable symptoms, which vary with the length of time they have been used, as well as the dosage. Observe for alterations in vital signs and for hallucinations, delirium, or seizures. Barbiturate therapy must not be discontinued abruptly, but rather doses are tapered down slowly.

> **Key Concept**
> Habituation, addiction to, many drugs, especially narcotics and barbiturates, is common. Be alert to this possibility when working with any client (Chapter 95).

Benzodiazepines

In addition to barbiturates, many other medications, including *benzodiazepines* ("benzos"), are used as hypnotics and sedatives. The benzodiazepines, available since the 1960s, are safer than barbiturates, with a wide margin of safety between therapeutic and toxic dosages. In addition to their sedative and hypnotic effects, some benzos are used as anticonvulsant agents or to manage anxiety. Most of these drugs are pregnancy category D agents and are primarily schedule IV drugs.

Common side effects are similar to those of the barbiturates, including morning hangover, drowsiness, lethargy, and sleep disturbances. Due to the risk for addiction, the administration of benzos is monitored closely. If clients discontinue these medications rapidly, severe withdrawal symptoms, similar to those that accompany the abrupt withdrawal of barbiturates, may occur. Withdrawal symptoms may be delayed, possibly appearing several days after discontinuation. For this reason, the dosages of these medications are tapered down gradually during a period of 2 to 3 weeks.

Flurazepam (Dalmane), a long-acting benzodiazepine, is useful in the treatment of insomnia. Smokers may metabolize it more quickly; women taking oral contraceptives may metabolize it more slowly. *Temazepam* (Restoril) is an intermediate-acting hypnotic used to treat insomnia. *Diazepam* (Valium), also a benzodiazepine, is not prescribed often today because of its high potential for abuse. However, it is used in managing withdrawal from alcohol (Chapter 95). *Lorazepam* (Ativan), an antianxiety agent, is also classified as a sedative but is not recommended for routine treatment of insomnia. It is most often used to control anxiety, acting-out behavior, and for preoperative sedation. *Alprazolam* (Xanax) is indicated for clients with panic disorders and is available in a short- or long-acting (XR) formula. *Midazolam* (Versed), a short-acting benzodiazepine, is used mainly as a relaxant and amnesiac before surgery and during induction of anesthesia. The onset of action with IV administration is 3 to 5 min; afterward, the person usually does not remember the procedure.

Miscellaneous Hypnotics and Sedatives

Although *diphenhydramine* (Benadryl) is primarily an antihistamine, it also has sedative effects. It is available in a number of forms, such as capsules, chewable tablets, liquid, and injectable solution. Many OTC sleep aids contain diphenhydramine (Benadryl), which also helps prevent side effects from other medications. This medication is safe and effective for many clients.

Some previously used sedatives have been discontinued or are rarely used. One of the oldest such medications is *chloral hydrate,* which is used in Canada. It is available in capsules, syrup, and rectal suppositories. It is a pregnancy category C medication and is also a controlled substance. It may be used for older clients because it is relatively safe.

Newer medications to treat insomnia include *eszopiclone* (Lunesta), a pregnancy category C drug available in oral tablets. Dosages are reduced in older clients and clients with liver impairment. The most common side effect of this drug is an unpleasant taste. Another frequently used nonbarbiturate sedative is *zolpidem tartrate* (Ambien, Ambien CR), a pregnancy category C medication. The CR formula is unique in that it releases some medication immediately to induce sleep and then slowly releases medication to keep the client sleeping for 6 to 8 hr. Ambien is available in oral tablets and is associated with fewer side effects than many of the barbiturates. Long-term use is not recommended, and withdrawal must be gradual to avoid dangerous withdrawal symptoms. Ramelteon (Rozerem) is a melatonin receptor agonist that is useful for people who have difficulty in falling asleep. It is unrelated to other drugs in this class. It has relatively few side effects but can cause withdrawal reactions if stopped abruptly. It may also be difficult for the client to sleep for a few days after stopping many of the sleep aids.

Anticonvulsants

Seizures, involuntary and abnormal nervous system activity, are indicative of disorders associated with changes in the brain's electrical activity. The most serious seizure disorders are classified as *epilepsy*. Seizures include tonic–clonic, petit mal, Jacksonian, and complex partial-type seizures (Chapter 78). There are many **anticonvulsant** medications, CNS depressants that help prevent or control various types of seizure activity. The dosage of anticonvulsants is usually adjusted for the individual client, with gradually increasing dosages administered until the desired blood level is achieved or until seizure activity is controlled. Many anticonvulsants require periodic dosage adjustment with prolonged use. Most are pregnancy category D agents. Some anticonvulsants are used in psychiatry as adjunct drugs, combined with antipsychotics (Chapter 94). Most commonly used anticonvulsants are discussed here.

One of the most commonly used anticonvulsants is *phenytoin* (Dilantin). It depresses the brain's sensory areas located in the motor cortex. It is available in tablet, capsule, suspension, and injectable forms. Its most common side effects include muscular incoordination, dizziness, gastric irritation, weight loss, and skin rash.

Clonazepam (Klonopin), a benzodiazepine, is most commonly used for the treatment of petit mal and absence seizures. It is also used as an anxiolytic (antianxiety) in psychiatry. Common side effects include alterations in behavior, incoordination, and drowsiness, and clients may build up resistance or tolerance to it.

Carbamazepine (Tegretol) is primarily used to control seizures. However, it has many serious side effects, including heart failure, liver dysfunction, and urinary retention. This medication is not recommended if other, less-toxic, medications are effective.

Diazepam (Valium), a benzodiazepine, has been used parenterally for control of acute seizure activity, such as *status epilepticus*. A serious adverse reaction that may occur with IV administration is respiratory arrest. The client's vital signs must be carefully monitored, and resuscitation equipment must be readily available. Diazepam (Valium) can be used in conjunction with other medications for the treatment of seizures. However, used singularly, it is not the medication of choice. Diazepam (Valium) is used to manage alcohol withdrawal and anxiety.

Valproic acid (Depakote) is used to treat many types of seizures and is also used to treat the manic phase of bipolar disorder (as a mood stabilizer). It is available in a number of forms, including capsules, sprinkle, and syrup (Depakene), and as an IV infusion. The delayed-release form is called *divalproex sodium* (Depakote ER or DR). Depakote is a pregnancy category D medication and should be given with food.

Levetiracetam (Keppra) is used to treat partial, myoclonic, and tonic–clonic seizures in clients from 1 month old to adult. Serious dermatologic adverse reactions have occurred; clients should report any sign of a rash to their healthcare provider immediately. Other side effects include dizziness, somnolence, and behavior changes, such as aggression, anger, or agitation.

Magnesium sulfate is usually used only in an emergency to prevent or treat seizure activity associated with pregnancy-induced hypertension (PIH). It is a pregnancy category A agent, making it relatively safe for use in pregnancy. When administered IV, it has an immediate onset of action; however, its duration is only about 30 min. Magnesium sulfate is not generally used to treat seizure activity associated with epilepsy. A number of side effects can occur.

Adrenergic Medications

An adrenergic is epinephrine or a substance that acts like epinephrine. Adrenergics mimic the actions of the sympathetic division of the autonomic nervous system (ANS) and, thus, are referred to as *sympathomimetics*. The major classifications of adrenergics are catecholamines and noncatecholamines.

Catecholamines

Catecholamines are neurotransmitters that play an important part in the body's response to stress. Their release at sympathetic nerve endings increases cardiac output by increasing the strength of cardiac muscle contractions, constriction of peripheral blood vessels, rising blood pressure, and bronchodilation. Epinephrine (adrenaline) and norepinephrine are catecholamines.

Epinephrine's major sympathomimetic action is to constrict peripheral blood vessels. The medication may be applied locally or administered parenterally. Local application constricts blood vessels and controls capillary bleeding; however, it does not control hemorrhage from larger vessels. Given parenterally, it increases heart rate, raises blood pressure, constricts surface blood vessels, and relaxes smooth muscles in the respiratory tract, causing bronchial dilation. It is the medication of choice for the treatment of *anaphylactic* (severe allergic) and hypersensitivity reactions. Epinephrine's bronchodilating effect is also helpful in treating airway obstruction caused by acute asthma attacks, bronchitis, and emphysema. It may also be used to reverse cardiac arrest.

Epinephrine is extremely potent, and very small doses are needed to be effective. It is available for SQ and IV injection. Its onset of action is almost immediate; however, its duration of action is short, lasting only about 30 min. It is important to monitor the client's vital signs. Major side effects include restlessness, nervousness, tachycardia, heart palpitations, dizziness, pallor, tremors, nausea, vomiting, and severe headache. These reactions are temporary, common side effects. Clients with existing heart disease, hypertension, hyperthyroidism, or diabetes may be more sensitive to epinephrine's adverse effects. Epinephrine crosses the placental barrier and is also secreted in breast milk. A pregnancy category C agent, it is contraindicated during pregnancy and in the breastfeeding woman. However, it may be used in an emergency. EpiPen and EpiPen Junior autoinjectors are available as a prescription for the treatment of severe allergic reactions. The pens are preloaded to give the precise dose in case of an emergency, such as a bee sting or exposure to peanuts in a severely allergic person.

Norepinephrine (levarterenol, Levophed), a pregnancy category D agent, is a potent sympathetic neurotransmitter. Its primary action is to increase blood pressure as a result of vasoconstriction of peripheral blood vessels. Increased blood pressure slows the heart rate. Norepinephrine may be used to treat heart failure. This medication is available in parenteral form. Side effects include bradycardia (slow pulse) and hypotension (low blood pressure). Overdose can lead to seizures and severe hypertension. If not administered properly or if IV infiltration occurs, norepinephrine can cause sloughing of tissue. This medication should not be used in the presence of hemorrhage.

Noncatecholamines

Dopamine hydrochloride (Dopamine), also a sympathomimetic agent, is not a catecholamine. It is an adrenergic agonist that affects the contractility of heart muscle and increases blood pressure. It is used to treat severe shock and hypotension. Dopamine hydrochloride (Dopamine) is available for IV administration. Side effects include restlessness, nervousness, headache, tachycardia (rapid pulse), palpitations, and anginal-type chest pain. The client receiving dopamine requires close monitoring.

A number of other sympathomimetic amines are available. They often are used to relieve bronchospasm or symptoms of asthma. These agents are discussed elsewhere in this chapter.

> **Nursing Alert** It is important to remember that great care must be taken when giving medications. Some medications are more likely to cause adverse effects than others. In addition, some medication names are very similar. Box 62-6 lists selected "high-alert" medications.

MEDICATIONS THAT AFFECT THE ENDOCRINE SYSTEM

The endocrine glands secrete hormones carried by the bloodstream to various target organs, where they have specific regulating effects. Hormone replacement therapy (**HRT**) is given to reduce symptoms caused by various hormonal deficiencies. Endocrine disorders and examples of hormonal agents are discussed in Chapter 79.

Thyroid Replacement Hormones

Thyroid preparations are used to treat primary hypothyroidism and for clients who have had a thyroidectomy. Thyroid replacement hormones consist of one or both thyroid hormones: thyroxine (T_4) and triiodothyronine (T_3).

Steroids

Steroids include the adrenocortical hormones produced by the adrenal glands. The most common adrenocortical hormone is *cortisone,* a very effective anti-inflammatory agent. In addition, steroids have immunosuppressive and salt-retaining effects. Prolonged cortisone therapy has many serious side effects, including changes in physical appearance. (See In Practice: Educating the Client 62-1.) Cortisones may cause GI upset to occur; administer steroids with food, to prevent or reduce gastric upset. In addition, the client may take antacids, to prevent GI upset or gastric ulcer formation. The client and family also must be able to recognize signs and symptoms of more serious side effects, such as thrombophlebitis. Reassure the client that most side effects will disappear on discontinuation of steroid therapy. Prolonged steroid therapy should be reduced gradually. If cortisone is administered artificially, the adrenal glands are not stimulated to produce it; if cortisone therapy is discontinued abruptly, the adrenal glands are unable to immediately produce sufficient amounts of naturally occurring cortisone. This client could suffer adrenal crisis, a life-threatening condition requiring immediate intervention.

Prednisone, hydrocortisone (Cortef), and *prednisolone* (Hydrocortone) are examples of other steroidal anti-inflammatory medications. They should be used with caution in individuals with peptic ulcers because of the increased risk for worsening the ulcer. They are contraindicated for individuals with serious infections, such as tuberculosis or spinal meningitis, because these agents interfere with the immune response.

> **Nursing Alert** The anabolic steroids (e.g., nandrolone decanoate—Deca-Durabolin; oxandrolone—Oxandrin; and oxymetholone—Anadrol-50) carry a high risk of abuse and are on schedule III of the controlled substance list. These drugs may be abused by athletes and other people who wish to build muscle bulk and strength. Abuse of anabolic steroids is very dangerous; people abusing them may become assaultive, and sudden withdrawal can be life-threatening (Chapter 95).

Insulin

One of the best known replacement hormones is **insulin**. Insulin, produced by the beta cells of the islets of Langerhans in the pancreas, is essential for carbohydrate metabolism. Several types of insulin preparations exist, and new types are being developed constantly. Newer products are more

---

Box 62-6 High-Alert Medications

Some medications look alike or their names sound alike. Be particularly careful when administering these medications. Examples include the following:
- OxyCONTIN and oxyCODONE
- hydrALAZINE and hydrOXYzine
- ePINEPHrine and ePHEDrine
- hydroMORPHONE (Dilaudid) and MORPHINE
- loRAZEPAM (Ativan) and ALPRAZolam (Xanax)
- METROnidazole and METformin
- CeleBREX (celecoxib), CeLEXA (citalopram), and CereBYX (fosphenytoin)
- cloNIDine (Catapres) and KlonoPIN (clonazePAM)
- vinBLASTine and vinCRISTine

Other medications carry high potential for life-threatening effects, if used incorrectly. These include the following:
- chemotherapy agents
- any intravenous (IV) narcotics
- heparin
- any insulin preparation
- digoxin and derivatives
- blood products

Often, agency protocol requires nurses to double-check any high-alert medications before administration.

IN PRACTICE

EDUCATING THE CLIENT 62-1 — Side Effects of Long-Term Steroid Therapy

- Feelings of euphoria, general well-being
- Increased appetite and subsequent weight gain
- Tendency to bruise easily
- *Hirsutism* (increased facial and body hair)
- Aggravation of adolescent acne
- Generalized weakness
- Hypertension
- Elevated blood glucose levels
- Increased susceptibility to infection
- Cataract formation
- Thrombophlebitis or embolism (or both)
- *Moon facies* (puffy, round face)
- Buffalo hump
- Osteoporosis

---

effective and have fewer allergic properties than do older insulins. Various insulins have different lengths of onset and duration of action. Injectable insulin must be administered SQ, or via insulin pump (hydrochloric acid in the stomach destroys its action), with the exception of regular insulin, which can be administered IV. Injectable insulins are supplied in the U-100 dosage (100 units of insulin per 1 mL). A new dosage is now available as 500 units insulin per 1 mL.

Clients with type 2 diabetes may also control the symptoms of the disorder by using oral hypoglycemic agents. Some clients manage their diabetes by using a combination of oral and injectable agents. Oral hypoglycemics are not insulin derivatives. They have a number of actions, one of which is the lowering of blood glucose levels by stimulating the pancreas to release available insulin (Chapter 79).

MEDICATIONS THAT AFFECT THE SENSORY SYSTEM

Medications Affecting the Eye

Ophthalmic medications include agents that dilate or constrict the pupil, antibiotics, and agents that reduce intraocular pressure. Some ophthalmic medications produce their effects by causing the ANS to relax and to contract smooth muscle. Others act directly on eye tissues.

> **Nursing Alert** Only those medications clearly marked "for ophthalmic use" may safely be used in the eyes.

Mydriatics and Miotics

Mydriatics are ophthalmic preparations used to dilate pupils. They are used primarily during physical examination of the eye. Examples include cyclopentolate (Cyclogyl) and homatropine. Atropine eye drops are sometimes used orally for clients with excessive secretions caused by drug-induced side effects or end-of-life symptoms. *Miotics* are ophthalmic preparations used to constrict pupils. Examples include dapiprazole (Rev-Eyes) and carbachol (Carbostat). A direct-acting miotic agent that can be used to counteract drug-induced mydriasis is pilocarpine (Pilocar, Piloptic).

Ophthalmic Antibiotics

Eye infections may be treated with antibiotics or sulfonamides specific to the causative organism and prepared for ophthalmic use in the form of solutions or ointments. Examples include bacitracin (AK-Tracin), tobramycin (Tobrex), ofloxacin (Ocuflox), and moxifloxacin (Vigamox).

Agents That Reduce Intraocular Pressure

Elevations in *intraocular* (within the eyeball) pressure can occur, leading to glaucoma or ocular hypertension. The term *glaucoma* refers to a group of disorders characterized by an increase in intraocular pressure. The most common type of adult primary glaucoma is open-angle glaucoma. Another type is angle-closure glaucoma, which can be acute or chronic. *Ocular hypertension* is a situation in which intraocular pressure is elevated without any other signs of glaucoma. A number of medications can be used to treat ocular hypertension and the various types of glaucoma. These include brimonidine tartrate (Alphagan), brinzolamide (Azopt), dorzolamide (Trusopt), latanoprost (Xalatan), levobetaxolol (Betaxon), levobunolol (AKBeta, Betagan), and metipranolol (OptiPranolol). Epinephrine (Adrenaline) also may be used to decrease production of aqueous humor.

Other Ophthalmic Medications

Nepafenac (Nevanac) and Ketorolac (Acular) are anti-inflammatory agents used in incisional refractive surgery (LASIK) and other laser surgeries to offset pain and photophobia. Azelastine (Optivar), emedastine (Emadine), levocabastine (Livostin), and olopatadine (Patanol) are used to treat allergic conjunctivitis.

Medications Affecting the Ear

Most medications that affect the ears are applied directly into the ears to treat localized conditions. Commonly used medications include anti-infectives (to treat ear infections), analgesics (to treat the pain of otitis media, especially for children), and *cerumenolytics* (to loosen and remove impacted earwax).

Chapter 80 describes disorders of the sensory system and their treatment.

MEDICATIONS THAT AFFECT THE CARDIOVASCULAR SYSTEM

Some cardiovascular medications are used for their effects on the heart's action; others affect blood vessels. Medications that stimulate or strengthen the heart's pumping actions are called *cardiotonics*. Medications that regulate heart rhythm are called *antiarrhythmics*. Those that primarily act on blood vessels are *vasoconstrictors* (constrict or narrow the blood vessels) and *vasodilators* (dilate or widen blood vessels). Often, vasodilators are used to lower and control blood pressure. In addition, a number of other medications are used to control blood pressure. Table 62-4 lists common medications related to the cardiovascular system. Cardiovascular disorders and their treatment are discussed in Chapter 81.

Cardiotonics

Cardiotonics are heart stimulants. Commonly used cardiotonics include digoxin (Lanoxin, Novo-Digoxin [Can], Digitek), a derivative of the digitalis leaf. The main action of cardiotonics is to strengthen the force of ventricular contractions and, in doing so, to increase cardiac output. Increased cardiac output results in a slower heart rate and less heart workload. Digoxin is available in oral and parenteral forms. Dosages vary by individual. The initial dose, the *digitalizing dose*, is prescribed to reduce the heart rate to the desired rate

TABLE 62-4 Selected Cardiovascular System Medications[a]

NAME OF MEDICATION[b]	DOSAGE FORM	NOTES
Cardiotonic		
digoxin (Lanoxin)	Tablets: 0.125-0.25 mg Oral solution IV; IM	Toxicity increased with low potassium levels; IM administration extremely painful
Antiarrhythmics		
disopyramide (Norpace)	Capsules: 100-150 mg ER capsules: 100-150 mg	Depressed contractility of heart, reserved for life-threatening ventricular arrhythmias
lidocaine (Xylocaine)	IV	Action primarily on ventricles; increased toxicity with reduced hepatic function
procainamide (Pronestyl, Procanbid, Procan SR, Pronestyl-SR)	IV; IM	Half-life of 4 hr; adverse effects include arthritis-like symptoms
propranolol (Inderal)	Tablets: 10-80 mg ER capsules: 60-160 mg Oral solution IV	Decreased conduction, contractility, and automaticity of heart; hypertension, prophylaxis of migraine
quinidine sulfate	Tablet: 200-400 mg ER tablet: 300 mg IV	Similar in action to procainamide; ventricular arrhythmias; gastrointestinal (GI) distress common
verapamil HCl (Calan, Isoptin)	Tablet: 40-120 mg ER tablet: 120-240 mg ER capsule: 100-360 mg IV	Calcium channel blocker; depresses phase 4 of depolarization of heart
Vasoconstrictors and Sympathomimetics[c]		
dobutamine (Dobutrex)	IV	Less increase in heart rate and cardiac arrhythmias than with other drugs
dopamine (Revamine [Can])	IV	Results in increased cardiac output and renal blood flow
epinephrine (Adrenalin HCl, EpiPen, Primatene Mist)	IV; IM Nasal spray	Used in *anaphylaxis* (severe allergic reaction) and as *hemostat* (to stop bleeding)
isoproterenol (Isuprel)	IV; IM	Cardiac contractility stimulated; increased heart rate and cardiac output
norepinephrine (Levophed)	IV	Restores blood pressure in acute hypotensive states
Vasodilators and Antianginal Agents		
amyl nitrate	Inhalation	Relief of acute angina; excessive side effects limit use; may be abused
isosorbide mononitrate (Imdur, Monoket)	Tablet: 10-20 mg ER tablet: 20-120 mg	Antianginal agent; administer immediate release tablets twice a day 7 hr apart

(Continued)

TABLE 62-4 Selected Cardiovascular System Medications[a] (Continued)

NAME OF MEDICATION[b]	DOSAGE FORM	NOTES
nitroglycerin (Nitrostat, Nitrolingual, NitroMist Nitro-Bid, Nitro-Dur)	Sublingual tablets: 0.3-0.6 mg Oral spray: 0.4 mg/spray ER capsules: 2.5-9 mg IV Topical: ointment; patches	Sublingual tablets or spray are drug of choice in angina; rapid action, short duration; prophylactic use (patch or ER forms); excess dose may cause headache; patch applied daily; alternate application sites; use location with minimal hair
verapamil (Calan)	Tablets: 40-120 mg ER tablets: 120-240 mg ER capsules: 100-360 mg IV	Used for vasospastic and unstable angina at rest; arrhythmias; hypertension; prevention of migraine
Antihypertensives		
atenolol (Tenormin)	Tablets: 25-100 mg	Used alone or with diuretics; acts mostly on the heart
candesartan cilexetil (Atacand)	Tablets: 4-32 mg	Angiotensin II receptor blocker, used to treat HTN
captopril (Apo-Capto [Can], Gen-Captopril [Can], Novo-Captopril [Can])	Tablets: 12.5-100 mg	ACE inhibitor; sometimes combined with thiazide diuretics to lower blood pressure; also used for heart failure
eprosartan mesylate (Teveten)	Tablets: 400-600 mg	Angiotensin II receptor blocker, used alone or with other medications, especially diuretics and calcium channel blockers
irbesartan (Avapro)	Tablets: 75-300 mg	Angiotensin II receptor blocker, used to treat HTN and diabetic neuropathy in type II diabetes
labetalol (Trandate, Normodyne)	Tablets; 100-300 mg IV	Beta blocker; lowered peripheral resistance with direct action on the heart
lisinopril (Prinivil, Zestril)	Tablets: 2.5-40 mg	ACE inhibitor; used in hypertension; as adjunct in congestive heart failure (CHF); used in diabetic clients for kidney protection
losartan (Cozaar)	Tablet: 25-100 mg	Angiotensin II receptor blocker (ARB), used to treat HTN, diabetic neuropathy, and for reduction of stroke risk
Methyldopa (Aldomet)	Tablets: 250-500 mg IV	Drowsiness possible during first days of therapy; with prolonged use, clients can develop positive Coombs test (indicative of blood disorder); off-label use for HTN in pregnancy
metoprolol (Lopressor, Toprol XL, Betaloc [Can], Novometoprol [Can], Nu-Metop [Can])	Tablets: 25-100 mg ER tablets: 25-100 mg IV	Action mostly on the heart; beta blocker without side effects of bronchospasm; indicated for treating HTN, heart failure, angina
nitroprusside sodium (Nitropress)	IV	Used in HTN crisis—for immediate lowering of blood pressure—and in cyanide toxicity with overdose
propranolol (Inderal)	Tablets: 10-80 mg ER tablets: 60-160 mg IV	Beta blocker Used to treat arrhythmia, angina, migraine, and stage fright; not indicated for asthmatic clients (can cause bronchospasm)
verapamil (Calan)	Tablets: 40-120 mg ER tablets: 120-240 mg ER capsules: 100-360 mg IV	Calcium channel blocker (effects observed in first week)
valsartan (Diovan)	Tablets: 40-320 mg	Angiotensin II receptor blocker (ARB); used to treat HTN and heart failure in clients who cannot take ACE inhibitors

ACE, angiotensin-converting enzyme; ER, extended relief; HTN, hypertension; IM, intramuscular; IV, intravenous; mcg, microgram (one-millionth of a gram); mg, milligram (one-thousandth of a gram).
[a]Always consult a current drug reference to confirm the recommended dose before administering any drug.
[b]A trade name appears in parentheses following the generic name of the medication. [Can] denotes Canadian trade name.
[c]These medications mimic the action of the sympathetic nervous system; they are used to raise blood pressure.

of 60 to 80 beats/min. When a stabilizing dose maintains desired heart rate, the client is placed on a *maintenance dose*, administered daily. Most clients taking digoxin continue the medication for life.

Because heart rate slows in response to digoxin, the *apical pulse* rate is counted for *1 full minute before administration*. If the client's heart rate is below 60 beats/min or if irregularities in heart rhythm are present, withhold the medication and report the information. **Rationale:** *The primary healthcare provider may wish to change or omit the dose for that day.* When a client is receiving digoxin, observe closely for toxicity. Overdose of digoxin can dangerously lower heart rate or cause cardiac arrest. Signs and symptoms of toxicity or overdose include nausea, vomiting, headache, premature ventricular contractions, diarrhea, confusion, drowsiness, blurred vision, or visual disturbances in which lights appear much brighter than they really are or appear to have halos around them.

> **Nursing Alert** Digoxin (Lanoxin, Novo-Digoxin [Can], Digitek) doses are very small (approximately 0.125-0.425 mg/day). Because these doses are so small, they are usually ordered as micrograms (mcg). (Thus, the doses above would be ordered as 125-425 mcg/day.) Because these dosages are so minute, even a small overdose could be fatal. Providers routinely check the client's digoxin level, to ensure that the dose is still correct.

The nurse must be aware that digoxin toxicity occurs very quickly if the client's potassium (K^+) level is low. Many clients with cardiovascular disorders are on potassium-wasting diuretics, and low potassium levels are common. (Potassium is necessary for proper functioning of muscles, including cardiac muscles.)

Antiarrhythmics

Antiarrhythmics act on the heart's electrical conduction system to regulate and slow heart rate. *Quinidine sulfate* (Quinidine) is an antiarrhythmic used to treat atrial arrhythmias. Quinidine sulfate's (Quinidine) action regulates the number of times the atria contract in a given period. It may be administered orally or IM. Side effects include dizziness, headache, ventricular tachycardia, angina, bradycardia, and nausea.

Procainamide hydrochloride (Pronestyl) is used to treat atrial fibrillation; however, it is more commonly used for ventricular arrhythmias, such as ventricular tachycardia or premature ventricular contractions. It can be administered orally, IM, or IV. Side effects include anorexia, nausea, vomiting, skin rash, urticaria (hives), and arthralgia (joint pain).

Verapamil hydrochloride (Calan, Isoptin) is a calcium channel blocker used to treat cardiac arrhythmias. It also has antianginal and antihypertensive effects. Verapamil hydrochloride (Calan, Isoptin) slows the electrical conduction rate of the atrioventricular (AV) node, resulting in a slower heart rate and decreased cardiac workload. Side effects include bradycardia, heart block, and constipation.

Propranolol hydrochloride (Inderal), a beta blocker, reduces myocardial irritability, thus decreasing heart rate and the force of ventricular contraction. It results in increased cardiac output and lowered blood pressure. Increased cardiac output improves coronary circulation, which helps to decrease vasoconstriction, spasm, and pain associated with angina pectoris. By decreasing myocardial irritability, propranolol (Inderal) is also effective in treating and preventing atrial arrhythmias, such as atrial flutter and atrial fibrillation. Propranolol (Inderal) may be administered orally or IV. Side effects include dizziness, fainting, drowsiness, insomnia, weakness, confusion, depression, vivid dreams, and loss of libido. It is also used to prevent migraine headaches, treat essential tremor, and help prevent subsequent MIs.

Lidocaine hydrochloride (Xylocaine) is used to treat life-threatening ventricular arrhythmias following MI. It is available for this use only in IV or IM forms and should be used only in intensive care settings.

Other antiarrhythmics include acebutolol HCl (Sectral), adenosine (Adenocard), amiodarone (Cordarone), carvedilol (Coreg), flecainide acetate (Tambocor), ibutilide fumarate (Corvert), and tocainide HCl (Tonocard). The antiarrhythmics are generally pregnancy category C agents.

Medications That Affect the Blood Vessels

Many abnormal conditions can affect the body's arteries and veins. Medications that constrict blood vessels are *vasoconstrictors*; those that dilate the blood vessels are *vasodilators*.

Vasoconstrictors

Vasoconstrictors (vasopressors) are used to control superficial hemorrhage, increase the heart's pumping action, raise blood pressure, and relieve nasal congestion.

Norepinephrine bitartrate (Levophed, Levarterenol) is a potent medication used to raise and sustain blood pressure in acute states of hypotension, such as those caused by hemorrhage or shock. It is also used in cardiac arrest. Given IV in solution, this medication should be administered only in intensive care units.

Metaraminol bitartrate (Aramine), a pregnancy category D agent, indirectly affects the release of norepinephrine, to raise blood pressure. It is used to prevent hypotension or to raise or maintain blood pressure in cases of hemorrhage, hypotension related to spinal anesthesia, trauma, and surgical complications. It may be given IV in a solution of normal saline or it may be given SQ or IM.

Phenylephrine hydrochloride (Neo-Synephrine), a pregnancy category C agent, relieves congestion in mucous membranes. It is also used to treat some types of shock and to raise and stabilize blood pressure. It is available in ophthalmic solution, as chewable tablets, as a decongestant nasal spray, and for injection.

Vasodilators

Medications that dilate blood vessels are used to treat peripheral blood vessel disease, coronary artery disease, and hypertension (**HTN**). **Vasodilators** increase the lumen size of blood vessels and thereby increase blood flow.

Nitrates

Nitrates have been used for many years to treat and prevent acute episodes of angina pectoris (heart pain). The nitrates dilate blood vessels, particularly in the coronary arteries, by inducing relaxation of peripheral vascular smooth muscle fibers located in blood vessel walls, increasing blood flow to myocardial tissue. This decreases the constriction and spasm of coronary blood vessels and reduces or relieves anginal pain.

Nitroglycerin (**NTG**), a pregnancy category C agent, is a potent vasodilator that has long been the treatment of choice for acute angina pectoris. Nitroglycerin is available in several forms, including tablets for *sublingual* (under the tongue) administration (Nitrostat, NitroQuick) and a spray for *translingual* (sprayed onto the tongue) administration (Nitrolingual). The tablet form can also be placed in the buccal pouch (cheek) or between the lip and gum above the incisors. The mucous membranes quickly absorb the medication and provide immediate symptom relief, usually within 1 to 2 min. The duration of action is approximately 30 min. The date should be noted when initially opening the bottle because the shelf life of NTG tablets is only approximately 6 months.

Nitroglycerin is also available in long-acting capsules (Nitro-Time), as an ointment for topical administration (Nitro-Bid), as transdermal patches (Nitro-Dur), or in IV solution. Nitroglycerin should be protected from exposure to light; it is provided in brown bottles and should be kept in a dark, dry place.

> **Nursing Alert** Nitroglycerin tablets should not be crushed, chewed, or swallowed. Translingual spray should *not be inhaled or swallowed.* Sustained-release forms should be given with water.

Clients who have recently had an MI or who have severe asthma, angle-closure glaucoma, severe anemia, increased intracranial pressure, or hypotension should not use nitroglycerin.

Amyl nitrate, a pregnancy category C agent, is an antianginal drug used to treat acute angina. It relaxes the smooth muscles of blood vessel walls, causing vasodilation and increased blood supply to affected myocardial tissue. It is administered by inhalation. It is supplied in liquid form contained in a hard capsule and wrapped in a protective cloth covering. When administering amyl nitrate, crush the capsule between thumb and forefinger and pass it back and forth under the client's nose. Amyl nitrate has a very strong, disagreeable odor. Its vasodilating effect is immediate and lasts approximately 3 to 5 min. Side effects include nausea, vomiting, headache, dizziness, and flushing. The drug should be protected from light and kept in a cool place. The client should be advised not to drink alcohol after amyl nitrate is used.

Other Vasodilators

Hydralazine (Apresoline), a pregnancy category C agent, relaxes arterial smooth muscle, causing vasodilation. As a result, blood pressure is lowered. It is available for oral or parenteral administration. Side effects include headache, palpitation, fluid retention, nausea, and vomiting.

Prazosin HCl (Minipress) acts by reducing peripheral vascular resistance, allowing arteries and veins to dilate, thus lowering blood pressure. It is used to treat chronic HTN. Unlike other agents, such as phentolamine (Regitine), prazosin (Minipress) does not cause reflex tachycardia. It is available in oral capsules. Side effects include shortness of breath, *orthostatic hypotension* (sudden drop in blood pressure on standing), pounding heartbeat, fluid retention, dizziness, headache, and drowsiness. Because prazosin (Minipress) tends to cause fluid retention, it is often prescribed with a diuretic.

Antihypertensives

Medications specifically used to reduce blood pressure on an ongoing basis are called **antihypertensives**. Some antihypertensive agents have been discussed previously. Other medications used to treat chronic HTN, or in conjunction with other antihypertensives, include diuretics, beta blockers, calcium channel blockers, and angiotensin-converting enzyme (**ACE**) inhibitors.

Diuretics

Diuretics increase the amount of urine excreted by the kidneys. Thus, they decrease the body's circulating fluid volume, thereby lowering blood pressure. Indications for use include edema, HTN, heart failure, and PIH. One side effect of some diuretics is excessive excretion of potassium (K^+), *potassium-wasting diuretics.* Hydrochlorothiazide (**HCTZ**; HydroDIURIL) and *furosemide* (Lasix) are examples of potassium-wasting diuretics. This client will usually require supplemental potassium. The potassium levels of clients taking diuretics are closely monitored. Diuretics also increase sodium excretion, thereby reducing edema. Most diuretics are pregnancy category C agents.

Some diuretics, such as *amiloride HCl* (Midamor), *spironolactone* (Aldactone), and *triamterene* (Dyrenium), and the combination *triamterene/hydrochlorothiazide* (Dyazide) are *potassium-sparing diuretics.* Their action on kidney tubules promotes potassium reabsorption. Nonetheless, potassium levels are monitored.

Beta (β) Blockers

Blood vessels contain adrenergic-blocking receptors, called alpha (α) and beta (β) receptors. Stimulation of alpha receptors causes vasoconstriction and rising blood pressure.

There are two types of beta receptors. The beta-1 receptors are primarily located in the myocardium of the heart. The beta-2 receptors are located in the bronchial tree and in the smooth muscles of blood vessels. Stimulation of beta receptors causes vasodilation of arterioles supplying these muscles. Because the heart has mainly beta-1 receptors, specific β-adrenergic *blockers,* pregnancy category C agents, are commonly used as first-line therapy for HTN. They act directly to decrease heart rate and blood pressure by depressing AV node conduction and decreasing the strength of myocardial contraction.

Other beta blockers are type 2 blockers, which act primarily on the bronchial tree to relieve asthma and conditions such as chronic obstructive pulmonary disease (COPD). Because nonspecific beta blockers can cause bronchospasm, clients with asthma are given a cardioselective beta blocker, which acts only upon the heart.

Examples of nonselective beta blockers are *propranolol* (Inderal) used to treat angina, HTN, arrhythmias, and migraine; nadolol (Corgard) used to treat angina and arrhythmias; and timolol ophthalmic drops (Timoptic) used to treat glaucoma. Cardioselective beta blockers include *atenolol* (Tenormin) and *metoprolol* (Lopressor).

> **Nursing Alert** It is important to remember that most cardiac medications, particularly the beta blockers, cannot be discontinued abruptly. This creates a high risk of rebound angina.

Calcium Channel Blockers

Calcium channel blockers, pregnancy category C agents, inhibit or block movement of calcium ions across cell membranes, reducing peripheral vascular resistance and resulting in lowered blood pressure. *Diltiazem* (Cardizem, Cardizem CD, Apo-Diltiaz [Can], Dilacor XR) is used to treat chronic HTN. It is available for oral and IV administration. Side effects include headache, fatigue, bradycardia, dizziness, and weakness. *Nifedipine* (Procardia) and *verapamil* (Calan) are used to treat HTN and angina. Verapamil (Calan, Isoptin) is also used to treat arrhythmias. Other calcium channel blockers include amlodipine (Norvasc), felodipine (Plendil), and nisoldipine (Sular).

Angiotensin-Converting Enzyme Inhibitors

ACE inhibitors reduce peripheral vascular resistance in the hypertensive client by blocking the activation of angiotensin, a powerful vasoconstrictor. ACE inhibitors are often used alone or in combination with thiazide diuretics. They are the most widely prescribed antihypertensive agents. Examples include *captopril, enalapril,* and *lisinopril* (Prinivil, Zestril). Diabetic clients are often prescribed an ACE inhibitor to prevent kidney damage and diabetic neuropathy, regardless of their blood pressure. ACE inhibitors are typically pregnancy category C or category D agents.

> **Nursing Alert** An unrelenting cough is an undesirable side effect of ACE inhibitors and may require discontinuation of the medication.

Angiotensin II Receptor Blockers

The angiotensin II receptor blockers (**ARBs**) selectively block the binding of angiotensin II to specific receptors in the smooth muscle of blood vessels and in the adrenal gland. This blocks the vasoconstriction effect of the renin-angiotensin system. These medications are used in the treatment of HTN, alone or in combination with other drugs. They are also used to treat heart failure and help reduce the risk of stroke. Drugs in this category include candesartan cilexetil (Atacand), eprosartan mesylate (Teveten), irbesartan (Avapro), losartan potassium (Cozaar), and valsartan (Diovan).

Miscellaneous Agents

Guanethidine monosulfate (Ismelin) is a potent antihypertensive used to treat chronic and renal HTN. Side effects include orthostatic hypotension, dizziness, fainting, and bradycardia. Instruct clients to monitor blood pressure regularly and caution them to rise slowly from sitting. *Methyldopa* reduces blood pressure by lowering peripheral vascular resistance. This drug is pregnancy category B (oral) and category C (IV).

An antihypertensive that may be used on a continuing basis or in a hypertensive emergency is *clonidine HCl* (Apo-Clonidine [Can], Dixarit [Can], Catapres). The medication's onset varies according to the route of administration. It is available in oral, transdermal, and epidural (applied to the dura mater of the brain or spinal cord) forms, with the epidural form having the fastest onset. Clonidine has numerous off-label uses, such as smoking cessation, alcohol withdrawal, opiate withdrawal, Tourette syndrome, migraine headaches, attention-deficit hyperactivity disorder (ADHD), and hot flashes.

MEDICATIONS THAT AFFECT THE BLOOD

Blood is composed of plasma, as well as blood cells, including erythrocytes (red blood cells [RBCs]), leukocytes (white blood cells [WBCs]), and platelets. RBCs contain *hemoglobin*, the main component of which is iron. When hemoglobin combines with oxygen, *oxyhemoglobin* forms. The circulatory system transports oxyhemoglobin to body cells, providing them with oxygen. Normally, a balanced diet provides essential iron and other nutrients necessary for blood formation. Blood and lymph disorders are discussed in Chapter 82.

Other medications and products also affect the blood, assisting in blood clotting or preventing clots from forming and serving to replace blood volume or components lost by events such as hemorrhage. *Epoetin alfa* (erythropoietin), a glycoprotein that stimulates RBC production, is indicated in the treatment of anemia in clients receiving chemotherapy and those with chronic renal failure. It is an injectable drug used both on an inpatient basis (IV and SQ) and outpatient basis (SQ only).

Iron Replacement Preparations

The adult male needs only small amounts (15 mg) of daily iron intake. Premenopausal and pregnant women need up to four times as much iron as men. An inadequate intake of iron-rich foods can contribute to iron-deficiency anemia. However, many women need iron supplements, even with a healthy diet.

Prolonged bleeding, such as seen with bleeding ulcers, excessive menstrual bleeding, or injury resulting in hemorrhage, also can lead to iron-deficiency anemia. Many women experience iron-deficiency anemia during pregnancy because of increased demands of the fetus. Iron supplements are commonly given as a routine prophylactic supplement during pregnancy.

Ferrous sulfate (Feosol) is the most commonly used form of iron replacement therapy and is available in tablets and liquid. *Ferrous fumarate* (Femiron, Hemocyte) is also available in chewable tablets. The liquid form is administered through a straw. **Rationale:** *This helps to prevent staining the teeth.*

Remind clients who take the nonchewable tablet form to swallow the tablet whole to avoid the unpleasant taste and prevent tooth staining. Oral iron preparations can irritate gastric mucosa; they should be taken with food. Some oral iron preparations are designed for slow absorption and cause less gastric irritation. The addition of vitamin C aids in the absorption of iron; teach clients to drink a glass of orange juice or take a vitamin C tablet, to maintain iron levels.

> **Key Concept**
> Iron preparations turn the stool black; alert the client to this normal side effect.

Iron preparations also can be administered parenterally as *iron dextran* (DexFerrum), a pregnancy category B agent. Because injectable iron is irritating to the tissues, it should be administered using the Z-track method, deep into the muscle (Chapter 64). Iron can also discolor the skin if administered superficially. Iron administration over a prolonged period may cause appetite loss, nausea, vomiting, headache, stomach pain, diarrhea, or constipation. Large doses can cause poisoning, especially in children. Symptoms of iron overdose include headache, fever, and *urticaria* (hives).

Vitamins

Folic acid (folacin, folate, Folvite) is indicated for clients with megaloblastic anemia, a condition characterized by abnormal RBCs. Folic acid stimulates the production of RBCs and WBCs and is necessary for normal maturation of RBCs. Folic acid is commonly prescribed in combination with vitamins and minerals before conception and during early pregnancy to reduce the incidence of birth defects in infants. Folic acid therapy has proved particularly effective in preventing neural tube (spinal cord) defects. It also is routinely given to clients who abuse alcohol (Chapter 95), as well as to clients receiving methotrexate (Otrexup, Xatmep, Trexall) (for rheumatoid arthritis).

Vitamin B_{12} (cyanocobalamin) is necessary for the manufacture of erythrocytes and healthy nervous system functioning. It is absorbed in the small intestine and cannot be absorbed without the presence of intrinsic factor, which the stomach secretes. Clients who lack intrinsic factor develop pernicious anemia. Injections of vitamin B_{12} (given deep IM) can help control pernicious anemia. Vitamin B_{12} administration is not usually associated with undesirable side effects.

Coagulants

Medications that promote blood coagulation are *coagulants*. *Vitamin K,* a fat-soluble vitamin, is necessary for the formation of prothrombin, essential for normal blood clotting. Vitamin K deficiency results in a tendency to hemorrhage. Several preparations of vitamin K are available. *Phytonadione* (Mephyton) is an emulsion of vitamin K available in tablet form, used to control active hemorrhage. *Phytonadione injection* (AquaMEPHYTON) is a colloidal solution of vitamin K that may be administered parenterally, by the SQ, IM, or IV route. *Absorbable gelatin sponge* (Gelfoam) is used as a packing to stop capillary bleeding. It can be left in a surgical wound, where it will be completely absorbed. *Oxidized cellulose* (Oxycel) comes in the form of a treated cotton or gauze pack that is absorbable and can be applied to check hemorrhage.

Anticoagulants

Anticoagulants increase the time it takes blood to coagulate. They are used to treat *thrombophlebitis* (blood clots), to prevent thrombus formation after surgery, and to treat blood disorders in which blood viscosity is abnormally high. Observe any client receiving anticoagulant therapy for evidence of bleeding, including bleeding gums or unexplained bruising. Check the stool for *occult* (hidden) blood.

Heparin, a pregnancy category C agent, prevents platelets from attaching to blood vessel walls, the first step in thrombus formation. Heparin is useful in preventing postoperative thrombosis and embolism. Heparin is administered SQ, most often in the abdominal area, or IV. Apply an ice pack to the area of administration 10 to 15 min before injection. This causes vasoconstriction and decreases the possibility of bleeding.

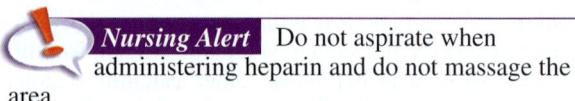

> **Nursing Alert** Do not aspirate when administering heparin and do not massage the area.

Laboratory tests, specifically prothrombin time (**PT**), partial thromboplastin time (**PTT**), and/or international normalized ratio (**INR**), are obtained before beginning therapy and then used to monitor effectiveness of anticoagulant therapy. These tests measure the length of time it takes for the blood to clot. The specific test needed will be determined by the primary provider, depending on the medications being prescribed.

For the client receiving heparin or any other "blood thinner," check for use of alternative therapies or herbal supplements. A number of these substances can interfere with blood clotting, contribute to bleeding, or interfere with heparin (Box 62-2). This is also true if the client regularly takes aspirin and, to a lesser degree, NSAIDs (e.g., ibuprofen). Conversely, psyllium can block the absorption of anticoagulants, such as warfarin, and of other medications, such as digoxin and lithium.

Warfarin sodium (Coumadin, Warfilone [Can]), a pregnancy category D agent, is an anticoagulant used to treat venous thrombosis and pulmonary embolism. It prevents thrombophlebitis by inhibiting synthesis of all types of prothrombin. It is available in tablets for oral administration and also in parenteral form for dilution in sterile water. IV administration is used only when oral administration is not possible. Side effects include skin rash and potential for hemorrhage. Client and family teaching is important because clients are often sent home on warfarin therapy. PT and/or PTT values are closely monitored. Low-molecular-weight heparins (**LMWHs**), pregnancy category B agents, are injectable anticoagulants. LMWHs are indicated for prevention and treatment of deep vein thrombosis (DVT) and pulmonary embolism. They specifically target certain clotting mechanisms and, thus, are effective in preventing blood clots, with a lesser risk of hemorrhage than is associated with heparin and warfarin. LMWHs are the drugs of choice for postoperative prophylaxis after knee and hip replacement surgery until the client is able to switch to oral warfarin. They are administered once or twice a day by SQ injection into the abdomen. Local side effects following SQ injection include mild irritation, pain, hematoma, and erythema. Clients are often discharged from the hospital on this therapy and must be taught to administer the SQ injection. Examples of LMWHs are enoxaparin (Lovenox) and dalteparin (Fragmin).

> **Nursing Alert** Clients receiving any anticoagulant therapy should have regular PT or PTT evaluations to ensure the blood is not becoming "over anticoagulated." If the blood takes too long to clot, the anticoagulant dose is decreased. An order for the daily anticoagulant dose is written, based on the outcome of daily blood tests. This may be written as a "sliding scale" dosage by the healthcare provider for several days or may be ordered daily.

Blood Products

Whole Blood

Whole blood is indicated primarily when there is a rapid loss of both RBCs and plasma, such as in massive hemorrhage. A transfusion of whole blood quickly increases the number of erythrocytes, restoring blood volume and, thus, raising blood pressure. It may save a client's life when survival depends on quick action. The blood given must be compatible with the client's blood group. For most transfusions, packed red cells are preferred because they provide only the blood component needed, without extra fluid. Administration of packed RBCs helps prevent circulatory overload. Chapter 82 describes the administration of blood and blood products.

> **Key Concept**
> Careful blood banking and testing techniques ensure a safe, disease-free blood supply.

Blood Components

Blood components include plasma, plasma proteins, and fractions, such as albumin, plasma protein fraction (**PPF**), immune globulin, and antihemophilic factor preparations. Because of the risk of blood incompatibilities, nonplasma solutions are preferred for rapid fluid replacement. *Fibrinogen,* a component of blood plasma, can be applied locally to stimulate blood clotting. *Antihemophilic factor* is used as a temporary aid to the person with hemophilia.

Platelets

Platelets also can be removed from a fresh unit of blood. They are administered to clients who have inadequate platelet production, are undergoing intensive cancer chemotherapy, or are receiving large amounts of stored bank blood. Platelets may also be administered to clients with aplastic anemia and leukemia.

ANTINEOPLASTIC MEDICATIONS

Chemotherapy is the administration of **antineoplastic** medications (Chapter 83). In some cases, *antineoplastic* ("against cancer") medications are used as a palliative measure for tumors that are no longer curable by surgery or for cancers such as leukemia that spread throughout the body. Antineoplastic medications can be divided into several large groups based on their probable mode of action. These include the following:

- Alkylating agents (e.g., cisplatin—interferes with DNA synthesis)
- Antineoplastic antibiotics (e.g., doxorubicin [Adriamycin]—inhibits DNA synthesis)
- Antimetabolites (e.g., 5-fluorouracil [Adrucil]—inhibits vital metabolic functions for DNA growth)
- Antimitotics (e.g., vincristine [Oncovin]—interferes with cell mitosis)
- Hormonal agents (e.g., tamoxifen [Soltamox, Nolvadex]—antiestrogenic effects; produces temporary regression of metastasis)
- Corticosteroids (e.g., prednisone [Deltasone]—anti-inflammatory and immunosuppressive actions)
- Antiangiogenics (e.g., endostatin—interferes with formation of tumor-feeding blood vessels)
- Biologicals

MEDICATIONS THAT AFFECT THE IMMUNE SYSTEM

Medications Used to Treat Allergies

Antihistamines are most effective in relieving the uncomfortable symptoms of allergic rhinitis and chronic urticaria (itchy rash). These medications are not curative, but do bring temporary relief. Their benefits are short lived, and they are merely adjuncts to more specific treatment (Chapter 84). The most common side effects of antihistamines are drowsiness, decreased mental alertness, dry mouth, dizziness, confusion, and constipation. Advise clients to maintain adequate fluid intake because the action of antihistamines is drying. Clients with asthma should not take antihistamines because of their drying effects on the respiratory tract.

Diphenhydramine (Benadryl) is an antihistamine available in oral and injectable forms. It is more sedating than other antihistamines and is sometimes prescribed as a sleep enhancer. *Chlorpheniramine* (Chlor-Trimeton) is slower acting, but has fewer side effects than diphenhydramine. Loratadine (Claritin), Cetirizine (Zyrtec), and fexofenadine (Allegra) are long acting (24 hr) and have the advantage of once-daily dosing. They cause the least drowsiness of drugs in this class. Combinations of antihistamines and decongestants (Claritin-D, Zyrtec-D, Allegra-D, Dimetapp) are useful in treating sinusitis, rhinitis, nasal congestion, and postnasal drip.

Corticosteroid nasal spray is used when antihistamines are ineffective in controlling the symptoms of allergic rhinitis. They are very effective and the newer forms have few, if any, side effects. They are available OTC (Nasacort) and by prescription (Nasonex). If the inhaled form of corticosteroid is not effective, oral corticosteroids may be needed to bring the situation under control. Oral agents may be used only for a maximum of 10 days. If a person needs to take oral corticosteroids more frequently, *immunotherapy* (allergy shots) should be considered.

> **Nursing Alert** The discontinuance of steroids must be carefully tapered down because abrupt removal can cause severe discomfort, including abdominal and back pain, anorexia, dizziness, fever, headache, and syncope (sudden loss of consciousness, heart arrhythmias).

Immune Sera and Vaccines

A number of products have been developed to protect children and adults from diseases. The concept of immunity is presented in Chapter 24. Chapter 71 discusses childhood immunizations.

MEDICATIONS THAT AFFECT THE RESPIRATORY SYSTEM

The respiratory system delivers oxygen to the lungs, which in turn helps deliver oxygen and remove wastes to and from the body's cells (Chapter 25). For this to occur, clear airways and a properly functioning respiratory center in the brain's medulla must exist. Chapter 86 describes adult respiratory disorders, and Chapter 87 describes the delivery of supplemental oxygen. Medications that affect the respiratory system include bronchodilators, corticosteroids and antiasthmatic medications, respiratory stimulants, antitussives, expectorants, antihistamines, and decongestants (Table 62-5). Most medications related to the respiratory system are administered by inhalation, to reduce systemic effects. If such a medication is given orally, it must reach sufficient blood levels to induce the desired response. Blood samples may be drawn at intervals to measure and determine the appropriateness and effectiveness of the therapy.

Bronchodilators

Bronchodilators act to relax smooth muscles of the tracheobronchial tree, thereby dilating (increasing) the size of the lumen. Certain diseases, such as asthma and bronchitis, constrict or narrow the size of the lumen, resulting in obstruction of airflow. Bronchodilators remove the obstruction by opening the airways, thus relieving symptoms.

Epinephrine (adrenaline) is a potent bronchodilator available in several preparations, including injection, aerosolized mist (Primatene Mist), and solutions for nebulization. It also is available as a nasal spray and an ophthalmic solution. Other bronchodilators include albuterol (Proventil, Ventolin), ipratropium (Atrovent HFA), levalbuterol (Xopenex), salmeterol (Serevent), theophylline, and tiotropium (Spiriva). These medications generally are pregnancy category B or D. Adverse effects of bronchodilators include tremors, nervousness, tachycardia, palpitations, and dizziness. Side effects are dose related and tend to be less severe with inhaled preparations than with those taken orally.

Antiasthmatic Medications

A number of bronchodilators and other medications, including steroids, function specifically to relieve asthma symptoms. Steroids are helpful in treating *status asthmaticus,* a situation in which an asthma attack does not respond to routine treatment and, if continued, is life threatening. Inhaled corticosteroids, such as fluticasone (Flovent) and budesonide (Pulmicort), are very effective for long-term management of asthma, without the serious side effects of their oral counterparts. Other medications used daily by clients to help prevent asthmatic symptoms include montelukast (Singulair), roflumilast (Daliresp), and zafirlukast (Accolate). Most of these medications are pregnancy category C agents.

Respiratory Stimulants

Medications that stimulate deeper respirations and an increased rate of respiration act directly on the brain's respiratory center in the medulla. Respiratory depression caused by drug overdose or following general anesthesia is the most common indication for the use of these chemical agents.

IV *Naloxone hydrochloride* (Narcan), a specific antidote to opiates, is most often used to reverse respiratory depression resulting from opiate overdose. *Doxapram HCl* (Dopram) is a CNS stimulant often used to reverse respiratory depression immediately after surgery or to treat acute respiratory failure in COPD.

Antitussives

Coughing is a protective reflex to clear the respiratory tract of foreign bodies or secretions. A cough is *productive* when it brings up and removes secretions, such as sputum and mucus, as well as exudates from a lung infection. A cough is *nonproductive* when it is dry and irritating and no secretions are produced. Treatment of cough is secondary to treatment of the underlying disorder. Medications used to relieve cough include narcotic and nonnarcotic **antitussives**.

Narcotic Antitussives

Narcotics, such as morphine, codeine (most common), and hydrocodone bitartrate (Hycodan), are effective antitussives (cough suppressants). The use of narcotic cough medications is limited to a short time because of their undesirable side effects, particularly constipation, and the potential for habituation (Chapter 95).

Nonnarcotic Antitussives

Nonnarcotic antitussives are widely used, but are less effective than narcotics. One is *dextromethorphan* (DM), contained in many OTC cough and cold preparations, such as Delsym, Mucinex DM, and Robitussin DM. Benzonatate (Tessalon Perles) is a prescription antitussive.

Expectorants

Expectorants liquefy secretions in the bronchi, thus making it easier to cough up and expel mucus. Clients should take expectorants with ample amounts of liquid to help reduce the viscosity of bronchial secretions. The most common expectorant is guaifenesin (Mucinex, Robitussin), a pregnancy category C agent.

TABLE 62-5 Selected Respiratory System Medications[a]

NAME OF MEDICATION[b]	DOSAGE FORM	NOTES
Bronchodilators		
albuterol (Proventil, Ventolin)	Tablets: 2-4 mg ER tablets: 4-8 mg Inhalation: MDI or nebulizer	Most selective bronchodilator available; most commonly administered by MDI or nebulizer
epinephrine (Adrenalin)	SQ	Short duration; side effects include CNS stimulation and heart palpitations
epinephrine bitartrate (Primatene, Medihaler-Epi)	Oral inhalation	For temporary use only; available OTC
levalbuterol (Xopenex)	Oral inhalation	Used for treatment or prevention of bronchospasm; vials require protection from light; few cardiac side effects
salmeterol (Serevent)	Oral inhalation	Used for long-term maintenance in clients with asthma and prevention of bronchospasm; not for acute attacks; long-acting drug (12 hr per dose)
Antitussives (Control Cough)		
benzonatate (Tessalon)	Capsules: 100-200 mg	Anesthetizes receptors in respiratory tract, to reduce cough reflex
codeine	Tablets: 15-60 mg IM; SQ Syrup	A narcotic, generally combined with other products in cough syrup; causes constipation
Dextromethorphan (Delsym, DM Cough)	Capsules: 15 mg Syrup	Available in many OTC syrups; said to be as effective as codeine for cough
diphenhydramine (Benadryl)	Tablet: 25 mg Capsule: 25 mg ODT Chewable tablet Oral solution; IV, IM	Antihistamine with antitussive properties; causes drowsiness, short-acting (4-6 hr)
Expectorants		
guaifenesin (Robitussin, Mucinex)	Tablets: 200-600 mg Syrup	Widely used, but some doubt as to clinical efficacy; thins mucus
Antihistamines		
cetirizine (Zyrtec)	Tablet: 5-10 mg Chewable tablet: 5-10 mg Capsule: 10 mg Syrup	Indicated for allergies and hay fever; used for hives; OTC; combination with pseudoephedrine is Zyrtec-D
chlorpheniramine (Chlor-Trimeton)	Tablets: 4-8 mg ER tablet: 12 mg Oral suspension and solution	Short-acting agent (4-6 hr); available OTC
diphenhydramine (Benadryl)	Tablet: 25 mg Capsule: 25 mg ODT Chewable tablet Oral solution IV; IM	Sedative effects pronounced; also indicated for motion sickness and as sleep aid
fexofenadine (Allegra)	Tablets: 30-60 mg ER tablet: 180 mg	Used for seasonal allergies Less drowsiness than diphenhydramine; Allegra-D contains pseudoephedrine with fexofenadine
loratadine (Claritin)	Tablet: 10 mg Chewable tablet: 5 mg ODT: 5-10 mg Syrup	Used for allergic rhinitis and urticaria; ODT tablets available (used without water); take on empty stomach; available OTC; minimal drowsiness

(Continued)

TABLE 62-5 Selected Respiratory System Medications[a] (Continued)

NAME OF MEDICATION[b]	DOSAGE FORM	NOTES
promethazine (Phenergan)	Tablets: 12.5-50 mg Syrup IM Rectal suppository	Marked sedative action; also used for postoperative nausea and vomiting; may lower seizure threshold
Corticosteroids and Antiasthmatic Medications		
budesonide (Pulmicort)	Oral inhalation	Used for maintenance treatment of asthma and as prophylactic therapy; respules administered via nebulizer
fluticasone (Flonase, Flovent, Flovent Diskus)	Nasal inhalation Oral inhalation: BID	Fewer side effects than systemic steroids; nasal: for treatment of seasonal or perennial rhinitis; oral: use 5 min after bronchodilator. Not for acute asthmatic attacks; for preventive use only
mometasone (Nasonex)	Nasal inhalation	Long-acting steroid for once-daily dosing used for seasonal rhinitis
Respiratory Stimulants		
naloxone (Narcan)	IV; IM (after initial crisis only)	Complete/partial reversal of opioid depression; reversal of alcoholic coma; may be used postoperatively
doxapram (Dopram)	IV	Drug-induced respiratory depression/apnea (postoperatively; overdose); also used in obstructive sleep apnea and COPD
Decongestants		
oxymetazoline (Afrin)	Nasal inhalation	Long duration of action (12 hr)
phenylephrine HCl (Sudafed PE; Neo-Synephrine, Rhinall, Dionephrine [Can], Vicks Sinex)	Tablets: 15 mg Syrup Nasal inhalation	Oral form is contained in many OTC cold preparations
pseudoephedrine (Sudafed, Sudafed 12 Hr, Nexafed)	Tablets: 30-60 mg ER tablets: 120-240 mg Syrup	Avoid use in clients with HTN; available OTC (requires signature at time of purchase)
Miscellaneous Products		
cromolyn sodium	Oral inhalation; nasal inhalation	Antiasthmatic, antiallergic, and mast cell stabilizer; used for prophylactic management of bronchial asthma (not for acute attacks)
montelukast (Singulair)	Tablet: 10 mg Chewable tablets: 4-5 mg	Used as prophylaxis for chronic asthma and allergies in persons aged 2 years and older; not for acute attacks
zafirlukast (Accolate)	Tablet: 10-20 mg	Used to decrease daytime asthma symptoms; not for treatment of acute attacks

CNS, central nervous system; COPD, chronic obstructive pulmonary disease; ER, extended release; IM, intramuscular; IV, intravenous; mcg, microgram (one-millionth of a gram); MDI, metered-dose inhaler; mg, milligram (one-thousandth of a gram); ODT, orally disintegrating tablet; OTC, over-the-counter; SQ, subcutaneous.
[a]Always consult a current drug reference to confirm the recommended dose before administering any unfamiliar drug.
[b]The trade name appears in parentheses following the generic name of the medication. [Can] denotes Canadian trade name.

Antihistamines

Antihistamines arrest the action of histamine, a body chemical believed to cause allergy symptoms. Antihistamines have been used for the treatment of various types of allergic reactions (see previous discussion). Their vasoconstrictive effects have the greatest impact on nasal mucous membranes. They are particularly helpful in controlling the symptoms of allergic rhinitis ("runny nose"). Antihistamines relieve symptoms, but do not provide a cure. They should be regarded as accessory agents to more specific treatment. Antihistamines are contraindicated in clients with diabetes mellitus or glaucoma. Commonly used antihistamines include cetirizine (Zyrtec), chlorpheniramine maleate (Chlor-Trimeton), clemastine fumarate (Tavist), diphenhydramine (Benadryl), fexofenadine (Allegra), loratadine (Claritin), and promethazine (Phenergan). Many of these agents are used to treat systemic allergic reactions, such as pruritus or sequelae of bee stings, not just those limited to the respiratory system. Diphenhydramine, in particular, is used to treat or prevent undesirable side effects of other medications, such as antipsychotics. These medications generally are pregnancy category C agents.

Decongestants

Decongestants act by reducing swelling of nasal membranes and opening nasal passages. They may be administered orally as tablets or liquids or topically as nasal sprays or nose drops. Nasal decongestants should not be used for longer than 3 days; after this time, they cause rebound congestion (the client becomes congested again). Oral decongestants, such as *pseudoephedrine HCl* (Sudafed) are contraindicated in clients who have HTN because they can increase blood pressure. Pseudoephedrine is classified as a sympathomimetic amine and does not cause drowsiness. This drug is currently regulated by the federal government, which limits where the drug can be purchased and the quantity allowed for purchase (because it is a component of methamphetamine). This drug is OTC but is only available behind the pharmacy counter. The purchaser must provide a photo ID and signature. Loratadine (Claritin-D), cetirizine hydrochloride (Zyrtec-D), and pseudoephedrine HCl (Sudafed) contain pseudoephedrine as well. Phenylephrine (Suphedrine PE) is available OTC and does not require a signature. This is the decongestant in many OTC products, such as Sudafed PE, Tylenol Cold, DayQuil, and NyQuil.

MEDICATIONS THAT AFFECT THE GASTROINTESTINAL SYSTEM

Medications affect the GI tract in numerous ways (Table 62-6). They cleanse the mouth, stimulate or control peristalsis, and produce or relieve vomiting. Chapter 88 describes GI disorders and treatment.

Medications That Affect the Mouth and Teeth

Oral hygiene, including flossing, is the most effective form of mouth care in prevention of disorders that affect the mucous membranes of the mouth. Mouthwashes are not very potent microorganism killers because they cannot be used in strong enough concentrations without harming the mouth's mucous membrane lining. However, they are useful in removing mucus from the mouth and throat. They are also helpful in managing *halitosis* (bad breath). A 1% sodium bicarbonate (baking soda) solution (1/2 teaspoon soda in a glass of water) also is effective for removing mucus, or NaCl (table salt), mixed with water, can be used. A solution of warm salt water (saline solution) is also helpful as a gargle for a sore throat. Zinc lozenges also help relieve sore throat pain.

"Swish and swallow" and "swish and spit" mouthwashes, described previously, are used to treat various mouth disorders. A special mouthwash, called "Magic Mouthwash" in some parts of the country, is made up of a number of medications. It is used to treat oral yeast infections (e.g., *thrush*, most often caused by a candida organism) and other mouth infections, particularly in clients with human immunodeficiency virus (HIV) and other immunosuppressive disorders. Viscous lidocaine may also be used to treat the open sores of thrush.

Stannous fluoride is recognized as having beneficial effects in preventing tooth decay. It is found in many dentifrices (tooth pastes). The American Dental Association has recommended the fluoridation of drinking water as a method for reducing dental caries (decay). A 2% solution of sodium fluoride applied to children's teeth has also been found to be effective in preventing dental caries. In some cases, fluoride treatments are recommended for adults as well. Sodium fluoride tablets, drops, solution, and lozenges are available for those who do not have access to fluoridated water or fluoride treatments. A dentist should be consulted about the specific dose.

In certain conditions, and in clients taking particular medications, such as *clozapine* (Clozaril), the client may have a tendency to drool. In this case, *sublingual* atropine ophthalmic drops may be helpful.

Medications That Affect the Stomach

Certain medications are used to control excess production of hydrochloric acid in the stomach and to relieve distention from gas.

Antacids

Antacids are used to treat common "upset stomach." They are also used to reduce and control stomach acidity, giving peptic ulcers a chance to heal. Some of the most commonly used antacids include *magnesium-aluminum hydroxide* (Mintox) and calcium carbonate (Tums, Maalox). Liquid forms are generally more effective than tablet forms.

Histamine Antagonists

Histamine (H_2) antagonists inhibit gastric secretions that are mediated by histamine. They are used in the treatment of ulcers, gastric reflux, and hypersecretory conditions. Results are usually immediate, but complete healing can take as long as 6 weeks or more. Cimetidine (Tagamet), famotidine (Pepcid), and ranitidine (Zantac) are examples of H_2 antagonists. Most of these medications are pregnancy category B agents and are available OTC.

Proton Pump Inhibitors

Proton pump inhibitors inhibit gastric acid secretion in its final stage. They are used in the treatment of ulcers and in gastroesophageal reflux disease (GERD). Omeprazole (Prilosec), esomeprazole (Nexium), rabeprazole (Aciphex), pantoprazole (Protonix), and lansoprazole (Prevacid) are proton pump inhibitors. They are also used in combination with antibiotics for the treatment of *Helicobacter pylori* infections. Omeprazole (Prilosec), esomeprazole (Nexium), and lansoprazole (Prevacid) are available OTC.

> **Key Concept**
> Antacids alter the absorption of many other medications. Therefore, antacids should be taken at least 1 hr before or 2 to 3 hr after other medications.

Antiflatulents

Antiflatulents are used to treat symptoms associated with excess *flatus* (gas) in the digestive tract. Simethicone (Mylicon, Gas-X) is the most common antiflatulent. It is safe to use in infants with colic. It is dosed after meals and at bedtime.

TABLE 62-6 Selected Gastrointestinal System Medications[a]

NAME OF MEDICATION[b]	USUAL ADULT DOSE	NOTES
Antacids		
aluminum hydroxide	Oral suspension	May have constipating effect; may impair absorption of certain drugs; OTC
aluminum–magnesium hydroxide-simethicone (Mintox)	Chewable tablets Oral suspension	Combination products tend to be less constipating, with equal acid-reducing ability; OTC (simethicone is added as antiflatulent)
calcium carbonate (Titralac, Tums)	Chewable tablet Oral suspension	High dose may cause hypercalcemia; may reduce absorption of tetracycline antibiotics; OTC; often used as calcium supplement
magnesium hydroxide–calcium carbonate (Rolaids)	Chewable tablet	Some forms have been recalled
Antiemetics		
dimenhydrinate (Dramamine, Gravol [Can], Traveltabs [Can], Triptone)	Tablet: 50 mg Chewable tablet Syrup IV; IM	An antihistamine; for nausea, vertigo, and motion sickness; OTC
meclizine (Bonine)	Tablets: 12.5-50 mg Chewable tablets	Prevention and treatment of nausea and vomiting of motion sickness; treatment of Ménière disease; OTC
metoclopramide (Reglan, Apo-Metoclop [Can], Maxeran [Can], Maxolon, Reclomide)	Tablet: 5-10 mg Oral solution IV; IM	GI stimulant with antiemetic properties; may be used in chemotherapy; may cause extrapyramidal side effects similar to tardive dyskinesia—closely monitor client
ondansetron (Zofran)	Tablet: 4-8 mg ODT Oral solution IV	Used to prevent nausea and vomiting associated with cancer chemotherapy and radiation therapy; off-label use for nausea in pregnancy
prochlorperazine (Compazine, Stemetil [Can], Nu-Prochlor [Can])	Tablet: 5-10 mg IM Rectal suppository	For postoperative nausea and vomiting; also used after cancer chemotherapy or radiation therapy
scopolamine hydrobromide (Transderm-Scop, Scopace)	Tablet: 0.4 mg IV; IM; SQ Transdermal patch Ophthalmic	Topical patch provides sustained release over 72 hr; used in hospice and preoperatively to control secretions; used for motion sickness and to relieve spasticity; ophthalmic solution used to produce mydriasis (pupil dilation) and cycloplegia (paralysis of specific eye muscles)
Antispasmodics		
dicyclomine (Bentyl)	Tablet: 20 mg Capsule: 10 mg Oral solution IM	Slowing of hypermotility of bowel; do not give IV
glycopyrrolate (Robinul)	Tablet: 1-2 mg IV; IM	Used in peptic ulcer therapy and to reduce secretions during anesthesia
propantheline (Pro-Banthine)	Tablet: 15 mg	Used in peptic ulcer therapy; has antisecretory and antispasmodic capabilities
Cathartics (Laxatives)		
bisacodyl (Dulcolax)	Tablet: 5 mg Rectal suppository	Must be swallowed whole, not chewed; action occurring in 6-10 hr; not to be taken within 1 hr of antacids; bowel stimulant; possible urine discoloration
castor oil	Oral liquid	Stimulant laxative; action occurring in 2-6 hr; possible severe abdominal cramping

TABLE 62-6 Selected Gastrointestinal System Medications[a] (Continued)

NAME OF MEDICATION[b]	USUAL ADULT DOSE	NOTES
docusate and senna (Senokot-S, Peri-Colace)	Tablet: 50/8.6 mg	Laxative, combined with stool softener
glycerin suppository (Fleet Babylax, Colace)	Rectal suppository	Hyperosmolar agent (adds fluid to feces); insert high into rectum, retain for 15 min; action occurring in 15-30 min
lactulose (Kristalose)	Oral syrup	Hyperosmolar agent; mix with juice or milk to mask taste; action occurring in 24-48 hr
magnesium hydroxide (milk of magnesia, MOM)	Oral suspension	Saline laxative with onset of action in 0.5–3 hr; flavored varieties available; also acts as mild antacid; shake well before giving
calcium polycarbophil (FiberCon, Konsyl Fiber)	Tablet: 625 mg	Bulk-forming laxative; action occurring in 12-24 hr; follow tablet with 8 ounces of liquid
polyethylene glycol electrolyte solution (Colyte, GoLYTELY) powder (Miralax)	Powder for oral solution	Solution used for bowel cleansing prior to GI surgery or examination; action occurring within 1 hr; not to be used with bowel obstruction; powder used daily for laxative
psyllium (Metamucil, Hydrocil, Konsyl, Genfiber)	Capsule: 520 mg Powder for oral solution Wafer	Bulk-forming laxative; considered to be safest laxative; onset about 12-24 hr; mix with full glass of juice, to mask taste and texture; mix well and instruct client to drink immediately because it will thicken
senna (Fletcher Castoria, Senokot, Ex-lax)	Tablet: 8.6 mg Syrup Suppository	Stimulant laxative; possible cramps; action occurring in 6-10 hr; do not use in bowel obstruction
Stool Softeners		
mineral oil	Oral solution	Emollient that lubricates intestinal mucosa, softens stool; action in 6-8 hr
docusate (Colace, Surfak, Doxinate)	Capsule: 50-240 mg Oral solution Oral syrup	Fecal softener; take with full glass of water; higher doses required for initial therapy; gentle action, occurring in 24-72 hr
Antidiarrheals		
bismuth subsalicylate (Pepto-Bismol)	Tablet: 262 mg Chewable tablet Oral suspension	Used for traveler diarrhea, indigestion, nausea, gas; may cause black, tarry stools. Caution for children: risk of Reye syndrome
diphenoxylate with atropine (Lomotil)	Tablet: 2.5/0.025 mg Oral syrup	Related to meperidine (subject to drug abuse); used for traveler diarrhea; can be harsh
kaolin-pectin mixture	Oral suspension	For symptomatic treatment of diarrhea; absorbs excess fluid and reduces intestinal inflammation
loperamide (Imodium)	Tablets: 2 mg Capsules: 2 mg Oral solution	Clinical improvement noted within 48 hr; gentle action; possible constipation; OTC for traveler diarrhea. Also used in other combination drugs
Miscellaneous GI Drugs		
chenodiol (Chenodal)	Tablet: 250 mg	Used to dissolve gallstones; indicated only in clients of poor surgical risk; possible hepatotoxicity
esomeprazole magnesium (Nexium)	Capsule: OTC 20 mg; prescription 40 mg	Inhibits gastric secretion; used to treat gastric reflux, esophagitis; may be used with antacids
lansoprazole (Prevacid)	Capsule: OTC 15 mg; prescription 30 mg ODT: 15-30 mg	Suppresses gastric acid secretion; used to treat duodenal ulcer, gastric reflux

(Continued)

TABLE 62-6 Selected Gastrointestinal System Medications[a] (Continued)

NAME OF MEDICATION[b]	USUAL ADULT DOSE	NOTES
omeprazole (Prilosec)	Tablet: OTC 20 mg; prescription 40 mg Capsule: 20-40 mg	Proton pump inhibitor, OTC; used to treat gastric ulcer, reflux
ranitidine (Zantac)	Tablet: 75-300 mg Oral solution IV; IM	Histamine-2 antagonist; similar in almost all respects to cimetidine; longer acting, so is given only twice/d, some strengths are OTC
simethicone (Mylicon, Mylanta Gas)	Tablets 60-95 mg Chewable tablets: 40-150 mg Capsules: 125 mg Oral drops	Defoaming agent, relieves excess gas in GI tract; may be combined with antacids: drops used for infants with colic
sucralfate (Carafate)	Tablet: 1 g Oral suspension	Used in treatment of ulcers; forms a protective barrier at ulcer site to protect against acid; take 0.5 hr prior to food

Bid, twice daily; CNS, central nervous system; ER, extended release; GI, gastrointestinal; IM, intramuscular; IV, intravenous; ODT, orally disintegrating tablet; OTC, over-the-counter; SQ, subcutaneous.
[a]Always consult a current drug reference to confirm the recommended dose before administering any drug.
[b]A trade name appears in parentheses following the generic name of the medication. [Can] denotes Canadian trade name.

Antispasmodics

The ideal *antispasmodic* agent reduces gastric secretions and slows GI motility. Although there are a number of these medications, they are associated with adverse effects, including blurred vision, dry mouth, and rapid heart rate. Antispasmodics include dicyclomine HCl (Bentyl) and glycopyrrolate (Robinul).

Medications That Produce or Stop Vomiting

Emetics

Emetics are agents given to induce vomiting. Emetics were formerly used as a first-aid measure for prompt stomach evacuation. However, rescue experts now recommend the use of activated charcoal (to neutralize irritants) or stomach lavage (to empty the stomach) in an emergency department. Vomiting may cause additional damage, subjecting the throat to the poison for a second time.

> **Nursing Alert** In any case of poisoning, contact the local Poison Control Center (1-800-222-1222 in the United States). They will advise as to the best action to be taken. Usually, the client is within range of an emergency department (Chapter 43).

Antiemetics

Antiemetics produce symptomatic relief from nausea and vomiting. Effective long-term treatment usually depends on removal of the cause. Causes of nausea and vomiting include emotional stress, motion sickness, pregnancy, side effects of medications or treatments, chronic illness, or diseases such as influenza.

Dimenhydrinate (Dramamine) inhibits nausea, vomiting, and vertigo, but has a strong sedative effect. It is frequently used to control motion sickness.

Prochlorperazine HCl (Compazine) is an antipsychotic drug that is also used to control nausea and intractable hiccoughs.

Ondansetron (Zofran) is used for the prevention and treatment of nausea and vomiting associated with chemotherapy, radiotherapy, and that following surgery. It is available for administration IV or orally in tablets, oral solution, and orally disintegrating tablets.

Another drug used to prevent nausea in chemotherapy is *metoclopramide* (Reglan), which is often given 15 to 30 min before chemotherapy is administered. Reglan functions as an antiemetic because it increases gastric motility, thus increasing gastric emptying time, which can lead to a decrease in nausea. Metoclopramide has the possibility of adverse side effects, including Parkinson-like dyskinesias and akathisia.

Medications That Affect the Intestine

Cathartics

Cathartics (*laxatives*) are used to relieve constipation. A healthy person who eats a normal diet, pays attention to the impulse to defecate, drinks adequate fluids, and exercises sufficiently generally does not need laxatives. *Constipation* usually results from a low-residue diet, dehydration, lack of exercise, or stress. Physical activity stimulates peristalsis; thus, clients on bed rest are at risk for constipation. Certain medications, such as opiates and some antipsychotics, also can cause constipation. Nursing care includes providing natural means of relieving constipation before administering laxatives. Prolonged use of cathartics can result in dependency. Do not administer laxatives to clients experiencing abdominal pain, particularly if it could be caused by appendicitis. Increased gut motility could result in serious problems. Many older clients believe they need to move their bowels daily and need reassurance. Cathartics are classified according to their mode of action: bulk-producing agents, irritants, lubricants, saline cathartics, and osmotic agents.

Bulk-Producing Agents
Bulk-producing agents stimulate peristalsis by increasing the bulk of feces, thereby modifying stool consistency. Their mechanism of action is based on a normal stimulus; therefore, these laxatives are among the least harmful to the body. However, bulk-producing substances can cause fecal obstruction and impaction. They must be given with adequate fluids; observe the client for any untoward symptoms. An example of a bulk laxative is psyllium hydrophilic mucilloid (Metamucil, Konsyl).

Irritant Cathartics
As the name implies, *irritant cathartics* irritate the large intestine, causing increased peristalsis, which promotes evacuation. Examples of irritant cathartics are senna, cascara sagrada, and castor oil.

Lubricant Cathartics
Liquid petrolatum or mineral oil is a *lubricant* used to soften feces. It is given to prevent straining on bowel movements after rectal surgery or for chronic constipation in less-active persons. Mineral oil taken orally interferes with absorption of fat-soluble vitamins (A, D, E, and K). Therefore, give it between meals or at bedtime, to avoid interfering with food absorption.

Saline Cathartics
Saline cathartics are soluble salts that cause water retention by osmosis (Chapter 17). Given with large amounts of water, they increase intestinal bulk and cause distention. The distended colon stimulates smooth muscle contraction, followed by a thorough, quite rapid emptying of the bowel. Examples are milk of magnesia (**MOM**), magnesium citrate, and magnesium sulfate. These medications are usually given once a day at bedtime, as needed, or as a bowel preparation before general surgery or GI examinations.

Osmotic Agents
In some situations, such as preparation for bowel surgery or GI examination (e.g., colonoscopy), total bowel emptying is required. One common agent for this process is *polyethylene glycol electrolyte solution* (Colyte, GoLYTELY). *Osmotic agents* are not absorbed and, thus, do not result in electrolyte imbalance. The client must drink the total amount of solution over 3 hr. Because the total prescribed amount is contained in 4 L of solution, monitor intake and encourage the client to drink the total amount.

Polyethylene glycol 3350, NF powder (Miralax), is an OTC laxative. It is an osmotic product that draws water into the stool, softening the stool and increasing the frequency of bowel movements. The dose is 17 g of powder, mixed in 8 oz of water. It may take 2 to 4 days to produce a bowel movement. It should not be taken for more than 2 weeks without a specific provider's order. This medication may also be used to prepare clients for bowel surgery or GI examinations, usually mixed with Gatorade.

Fecal Softeners
Fecal softening agents act like a detergent by helping permit water and fatty material to mix with fecal contents. They cause stools to become moist and bulky, thus stimulating the bowel and softening the stool so it can be expelled more easily. These agents have a wide safety margin and few undesirable side effects. Examples of fecal softening agents include dioctyl sodium sulfosuccinate—docusate sodium (DSS, Colace)—and dioctyl calcium sulfosuccinate—docusate calcium (Surfak). Gel caps are available. Mix liquid forms with fruit juice to mask the taste.

Antidiarrheals
An *antidiarrheal agent* is a medication given to slow GI peristalsis and stop diarrhea, while allowing normal bowel movements. Examples are diphenoxylate hydrochloride in combination with atropine (Lomotil) and loperamide (Imodium).

Atropine (Lomotil) is a schedule V controlled substance. It reduces intestinal motility and increases intestinal tone. It must not be given to children younger than 2 years. Side effects include paralytic ileus, toxic megacolon, bloating, constipation, stomach pain, nausea, vomiting, confusion, dizziness, and drowsiness. Encourage clients taking Lomotil to drink at least 2 L of fluid daily. Loperamide (Imodium), available without prescription, is as effective as Lomotil, with fewer side effects. Imodium Multi-Symptom Relief contains loperamide and simethicone, to relieve symptoms of diarrhea and bloating.

MEDICATIONS THAT AFFECT THE URINARY TRACT

Table 62-7 provides information on common urinary system medications. Chapter 89 discusses urinary disorders and their treatment.

Diuretics
When urine flow is inadequate, water and salts accumulate in the tissues, causing edema. *Diuretics* rid the body of excess fluids by increasing urine formation. The use of certain diuretics (e.g., *furosemide* [Lasix] and *hydrochlorothiazide* [HydroDIURIL, HCTZ]) can result in the loss of potassium and sodium. Because these are non–potassium-sparing diuretics (also called potassium-wasting diuretics), clients using them usually require a potassium supplement or must increase sources of potassium in their diet (e.g., bananas and orange juice). Diuretics are often prescribed in conjunction with antihypertensive agents to control HTN.

Thiazide Diuretics
The *thiazide diuretics* are synthetic medications, chemically related to sulfonamides. Their development marked a major breakthrough in the search for a potent oral diuretic. All thiazides are equally effective, although dosage and duration of action vary. The thiazides have many advantages over other diuretics—ease of administration (oral), low cost, effectiveness over long periods, low toxicity, and few side effects. *Hydrochlorothiazide* (HydroDIURIL, HCTZ) is the most common drug in this class. A thiazide-like diuretic is *indapamide* (Lozide [Can]), which is often used to treat edema associated with congestive heart failure (CHF) and to treat HTN.

TABLE 62-7 Selected Diuretics and Bladder Stimulants[a]

NAME OF MEDICATION[b]	DOSAGE FORM	NOTES
bethanechol (Myotonachol, PMS-Bethanechol [Can])	Tablets: 5-50 mg	Used to stimulate bladder contraction
bumetanide (Bumex, Burinex [Can])	Tablets: 0.5-2 mg IV; IM	Action similar to furosemide; much smaller doses needed
furosemide (Lasix, Furoside [Can], Myrosemide [Can])	Tablets: 20-80 mg IV	*Concomitant* administration (at same time) with gentamicin may increase ototoxicity[c]; potassium wasting
hydrochlorothiazide (HCTZ, Apo-Hydro [Can], Ezide, Urozide [Can])	Tablets: 12.5-50 mg Capsules: 12.5 mg	Usual initial drug for HTN treatment: potassium wasting
indapamide (Lozol)	Tablets: 1.25-2.5 mg	Used in CHF, diabetes insipidus, HTN; relatively few side effects; may be dangerous in kidney/liver disease, systemic lupus erythematosus, or diabetes mellitus
mannitol (Osmitrol, Resectisol)	IV	Osmotic diuretic; rapidly excreted
spironolactone (Aldactone, Novospiroton [Can])	Tablets: 25-100 mg	Often combined with HCTZ; potassium sparing; used in HTN; off-label use for acne
triamterene (Dyrenium)	Capsules: 50-100 mg	Often combined with HCTZ (as Dyazide, Maxzide)

CHF, congestive heart failure; HCTZ, hydrochlorothiazide; HTN, hypertension; IM, intramuscular; IV, intravenous.
[a]Always consult a current drug reference to confirm the recommended dose before administering any drug.
[b]A trade name appears in parentheses following the generic name of the medication. [Can] denotes Canadian trade name.
[c]Ototoxic: Damaging to eighth cranial nerve, causing hearing and balance disorders.

Loop Diuretics

Furosemide (Lasix) and *bumetanide* (Bumex) are effective, potent, rapidly acting diuretics. Because of their potency, clients taking them require close supervision of fluid and electrolyte balance. Supplemental potassium is usually required. These medications are called *loop diuretics* because they inhibit reabsorption of sodium and chloride in the loop of Henle in the kidney.

Other Diuretics

Spironolactone (Aldactone) promotes diuresis and helps counteract potassium loss. It is effective in promoting diuresis in clients resistant to more common diuretics. *Triamterene* (Dyrenium) is a mild, potassium-sparing diuretic. Its onset of action is slow; thus, it should be used in combination with other diuretics when rapid diuresis is required. Dyazide is a combination of *triamterene* and HCTZ and is a mild, potassium-sparing diuretic, with a slow onset of action.

Medications That Affect the Muscle Tone of the Urinary Bladder

Bladder dysfunction can result in urinary retention or urinary frequency. In either case, the problem is one of poor muscle tone in the bladder. *Neostigmine methylsulfate* (Prostigmin) and *bethanechol chloride* (Urecholine) improve the bladder's muscle tone. *Oxybutynin* (Ditropan) is an antispasmodic used to treat clients who have bladder dysfunction with urinary frequency. *Desmopressin acetate* (**DDAVP**) is a hormone administered as a nasal spray or orally. DDAVP is administered at bedtime to treat *enuresis* (bed wetting). This condition is often a side effect of certain medications, including psychotropics. Desmopressin acetate (DDAVP) is also used to treat the excessive voiding of diabetes insipidus.

Urinary Antiseptics and Antispasmodics

Urinary antiseptics are effective in the treatment of urinary tract bacterial infections. A sulfonamide commonly used to treat UTIs is co-trimoxazole (Bactrim). The tetracyclines, erythromycin, fosfomycin (Monurol), ciprofloxacin (Cipro), and urinary tract anti-infectives, such as cinoxacin (Cinobac), and nitrofurantoin (Furadantin) are also used to treat UTIs.

Phenazopyridine (Pyridium) is a urinary antiseptic commonly prescribed for its prompt analgesic effects. The client usually experiences relief of symptoms of urgency and frequency, as well as burning when voiding, within 30 min of the initial dose. This drug is available OTC (AZO Standard) and by prescription phenazophyridine (Pyridium). Urine cultures are not compromised by the use of phenazopyridine (Pyridium) before specimen collection.

> **Key Concept**
> Advise the client that phenazopyridine (Pyridium) will turn the urine reddish orange.

MEDICATIONS THAT AFFECT THE REPRODUCTIVE SYSTEMS

Male Sex Hormones (Androgens)

Androgens are essential for the development and maintenance of male sex characteristics. Both sexes produce male and female hormones, but their effects are antagonistic to each other. Androgen replacement therapy may be administered to men whose circulating hormone levels are insufficient to maintain male sex characteristics. Androgens may also be administered to female clients in an effort to retard the growth of estrogen-dependent cancers. Disorders of the male and female reproductive systems are discussed in Chapters 90 and 91.

Ovarian Hormones

The ovaries secrete two important hormones: *estrogen* and *progesterone* (progestins).

Estrogen
The Women's Health Initiative (*WHI*) revealed that estrogen alone for the treatment of postmenopausal women increased the risk of developing stroke, deep vein thrombosis (DVT), and dementia. The current goal of treatment is to use the lowest possible dose to control the client's symptoms. Topical patches and vaginal creams are the most common dosage forms because fewer drugs are needed to obtain the desired effect.

Progesterone
The corpus luteum secretes progesterone, which influences uterine and ovarian conditions during pregnancy. Progesterone prepares the lining of the uterus for implantation of the ovum. It suppresses ovulation during pregnancy and reduces the irritability of uterine muscle, to prevent premature labor or spontaneous abortion. *Medroxyprogesterone acetate* (Provera) may be used in dysmenorrhea, menorrhagia, metrorrhagia, or threatened spontaneous abortion.

Sometimes, estrogen and progesterone are given in various combinations, such as in Prempro, Premphase, and oral contraceptives.

Medications That Affect the Uterus

The uterus is a highly muscular organ capable of great distention and elasticity. Medications that act on the uterus are used either to increase or to decrease contraction of uterine muscle (Chapters 65 and 66).

Medications Used in Family Planning

Oral contraceptives are hormonal preparations containing estrogen and progesterone; they are used to prevent pregnancy. Estrogen suppresses ovulation by affecting the release of follicle-stimulating hormone (FSH). Side effects of oral contraceptives include nausea, vomiting, breast tenderness, headache, nervousness, emotional lability, and *venous thrombosis* (blood clots). Estrogen can promote the growth of existing cancers of the breasts and uterus. Hormonal preparations are also used to enhance fertility in women who have difficulty conceiving (Chapter 70).

Medications Used in Treating Sexually Transmitted Infections

Antibiotics are used to treat many sexually transmitted infections (STIs), including syphilis and gonorrhea. Viral STIs, such as herpes, are resistant to antibiotic therapy and must be treated with antiviral agents, such as acyclovir sodium (Zovirax) or zidovudine (Retrovir). Acyclovir (Zovirax) and zidovudine (Retrovir) are also used to treat HIV and acquired immunodeficiency syndrome (AIDS). Immune disorders and related medications are highlighted in Chapters 84 and 85. Medications used to treat STIs are discussed further in Chapter 70.

Medications Used to Treat Erectile Dysfunction

A number of medications have been released in the past few years to treat erectile dysfunction in men. The most commonly used medications of this type are *sildenafil* (Viagra), *vardenafil* (Levitra), and *tadalafil* (Cialis), as well as a number of herbal supplements. Some of these medications are taken about an hour before sexual activity; others are taken on a daily basis. If an erection lasts more than 3 to 4 hr (*priapism*), the client should call the primary care provider. Disorders of the male reproductive system and their treatment are discussed in Chapter 90.

STUDENT SYNTHESIS

KEY POINTS

- A wide variety of medications are available to treat or prevent illness or other body dysfunctions. The major groups include antibiotics, analgesics, sedatives, anticonvulsants, and medications specific to disorders affecting each of the body systems.
- Because of the large number of medications available, the nurse must be knowledgeable in the use of drug references. The nurse is legally obligated to know basic information about any medication that he or she administers.
- Drugs are classified according to their risk to a developing fetus. However, the pregnant woman should not take any medications without medical supervision.
- In some cases, medications are prescribed even though they have undesirable side effects. Their benefits are judged to outweigh the risks and disadvantages.
- It is important to document if a client is taking any herbal supplements or using any homeopathic remedies because these can counteract or potentiate the effects of prescribed medications.
- Medications are often prescribed using their generic name, to avoid confusion.
- Special procedures and regulations apply to the administration of schedule drugs. The nurse must follow these procedures exactly.
- A number of medications are susceptible to errors. The nurse must be particularly careful when administering these high-risk medications.

CRITICAL THINKING EXERCISES

1. The healthcare provider writes a medication order that does not seem correct to you. Describe what actions you would take.

2. Choose three commonly used medications from different classifications. Using available drug references, write the following information for each: generic name, trade name(s), pregnancy category, general and specific drug classes, therapeutic (desired) actions, reasons for use (indications), contraindications and precautions, forms in which the medication is available, average adult dose, average pediatric dose, and how the dose is calculated; pharmacokinetics, including how the drug is distributed to the body or target areas and how it is excreted; adverse effects, identifying those that are and are not life threatening; special nursing considerations; and client teaching points.

NCLEX-STYLE REVIEW QUESTIONS

1. A client is scheduled for a surgical procedure in 2 weeks. Which information should the nurse include in the preparation information?
   a. "Do not take your daily acetylsalicylic acid (aspirin) for 10 days before the procedure."
   b. "You may continue to take your herbal supplements since they are natural."
   c. "If you have a headache, it is okay to take acetylsalicylic acid (aspirin) before your surgery."
   d. "You won't be able to take acetylsalicylic acid (aspirin) but you can take your clopidogrel (Plavix)."

2. The nurse is caring for a client with a seizure disorder. Which medication order would the nurse question for this client?
   a. Acetaminophen (Tylenol) PO PRN for a headache
   b. Phenytoin (Dilantin) TID for seizures
   c. Diazepam (Valium) PRN for seizures
   d. Tramadol (Ultram) for back pain

3. A client develops a severe allergic reaction while receiving an IV antibiotic. Which medication should be immediately administered by the nurse with a healthcare provider's order?
   a. Prednisone (Deltasone)
   b. Norepinephrine (Levophed)
   c. Tylenol (Acetaminophen)
   d. Epinephrine

4. A client taking digoxin (Lanoxin) has a heart rate of 50 bpm, vomiting, diarrhea, and confusion and reports seeing a halo around the visual field. Which action by the nurse is appropriate?
   a. Administer the antiemetic prescribed by the healthcare provider.
   b. Administer the next dose of digoxin and monitor the client.
   c. Administer epinephrine since the client is having an allergic reaction.
   d. Withhold further doses and report findings to the healthcare provider immediately.

5. A client is prescribed lisinopril (Prinivil) for the treatment of hypertension. Which undesirable side effect does the nurse inform the client may be experienced that requires discontinuation of the medication?
   a. Nausea
   b. Dry cough
   c. Increase in urination
   d. Constipation

CHAPTER RESOURCES

Enhance your learning with additional resources on thePoint*!*

Student Resources related to this chapter can be found at **thePoint.lww.com/Rosdahl12e.**

63 Administration of Noninjectable Medications

Learning Objectives

1. Review and describe how medications are stored and supplied in healthcare facilities.
2. Discuss the importance of accurate documenting of medication administration.
3. Differentiate between STAT, PRN, and bedtime medications.
4. Discuss the importance of the "Five Rights, Plus Two" of medication administration, including steps to observe before administering medications.
5. State the approved means of identifying a client before giving medications.
6. Differentiate between desired and undesired effects, and local and systemic medication effects.
7. Differentiate between enteral and parenteral administration.
8. Describe and demonstrate methods of enteral medication administration: oral administration (including translingual, sublingual, buccal), and administration via NG tube and rectally.
9. Describe procedures for administration of transdermal, vaginal, eye/ear, and aerosolized medications.

Important Terminology

adverse effect, anaphylaxis, buccal, enteral, local effect, ophthalmic, otic, paradoxical, parenteral, potentiation, sublingual, suppository, systemic effect, topical, toxicity, transdermal

Acronyms

G-tube/NG tube, H_2H, MAR, MDI, PO, PR, SL, STAT, TD

Administering medications is one of the most important functions in nursing. It also is one that has an extremely high risk of danger for the client. Administering medications involves much more than just "giving pills." It is important to faithfully follow the rules of safe medication administration. To ensure each client's safety, every nurse must be familiar with recommended administration routes, dosages, desired actions, possible side effects, and nursing considerations for prescribed medications. This chapter considers the administration of *enteral* medications, that is, those given via the digestive system. In addition, selected noninjectable methods, such as vaginal, transdermal, ophthalmic, otic, and inhalation will be considered. In Chapter 64, the discussion will center on *parenteral* medications, including injections and intravenous administration.

PREPARATION FOR ADMINISTRATION

Before administering medications, it is important to interpret the medication order accurately. It is also vital to correctly follow administration instructions. The nurse must be familiar with commonly used abbreviations, acronyms, and terminology, some of which are listed at the beginning of this chapter. Many of these are also defined in the Glossary and Appendix B. It is also important to be familiar with abbreviations no longer recommended for use, because they can be misinterpreted (see Table 37-5). All nurses must know the procedures used in their facility for supplying and dispensing medications and how administration is documented.

A number of medications have been identified as having a high potential for confusion/error or as being very potent. These include "look-alike/sound-alike" medications and those most likely to cause injury or death when used incorrectly (see Box 62-6). Become familiar with these medications; use appropriate safeguards when administering them. Some facilities require two nurses to double-check certain medications.

Storage

Healthcare facilities must have a secure medication storage area. This may be a locked mobile cart, allowing medication set-up close to the clients' rooms. In this case, medications are in individual locked client drawers. The cart is kept locked except when a licensed nurse is using it. Some medications require refrigeration to preserve their potency; these are kept in a designated refrigerator, which cannot be used for anything else. The temperature of this refrigerator must be monitored and documented at least daily. If the temperature is not within safe limits, the medications must be moved.

Many acute care facilities use a computerized dispensing machine (see Fig. 61-1). In the long-term care facility, a locked medication cabinet may be within the client's room or close by, or medications may be in a locked "med cart." All medications must be properly labeled, with the client's name, medication name, dosage, and expiration date. *If a label is illegible, return the container to the pharmacy for replacement.* A nurse NEVER relabels a medication.

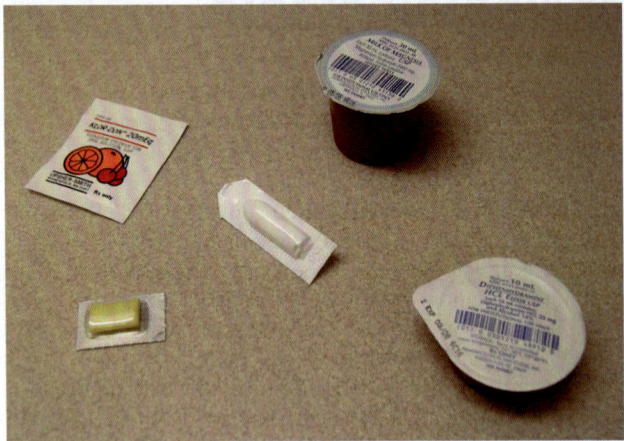

Figure 63-1 Unit-dose medications, clockwise from left: powder to mix with liquid, rectal suppository, two liquid medications for oral use (not to be diluted), and nicotine gum. (Photo Copyright © Caroline Bunker Rosdahl.)

All narcotics and other controlled substances (schedule medications) are kept double-locked, as described in Chapter 61. Follow the protocol of your facility for storage and inventory of drugs.

Dispensing and Supply Systems

Stock Supply
In the client's home or assisted living facility, you may encounter stock supply medications, such as acetaminophen (Tylenol) or acetylsalicylic acid (Aspirin), comfort medications (e.g., throat lozenges), stomach preparations (e.g., aluminum hydroxide [Maalox]), or bowel preparations (e.g., magnesium hydroxide [milk of magnesia]). Usually, only OTC medications are supplied in this manner. Even then, in a healthcare facility, these medications are kept locked until they are needed. Acute care facilities rarely have stock medication supplies.

Unit-Dose Systems
Acute care facilities and most skilled long-term nursing facilities use unit-dose medications (packaged in single-dose units) because they provide greater safety. They are supplied by pharmaceutical companies or the facility's pharmacy in individual prepackaged containers and include tablets, liquid, and injectable medications (Fig. 63-1). These packages identify the medication's generic name, the dose contained, and the expiration date. Moreover, in acute care facilities, usually only an 8-, 16-, or 24-hr supply of medication is supplied for each client, preventing duplication. In long-term care facilities, a week's supply may be supplied at one time.

In many facilities, the pharmacy labels unit doses with each client's name and client number before sending them to nursing units. The nurse should take unopened unit-dose packages to the client's bedside. This provides an additional safety check for nurse and client and also prevents waste, if the medication is not given. Some unit-dose packages are difficult to open. Box 63-1 describes opening of these packages.

> **Box 63-1 Opening Unit-Dose Packages**
>
> Unit-dose packages open in one of several ways:
> - The top layer will separate at one end and peel off.
> - One corner can be loosened and then the top layer will peel off. (Sometimes, you must first bend the corner at a designated spot.)
> - There is a tiny slit or cut in one corner or near the top of a foil-type package. Fold over the corner in the middle of the slit. The package will then tear down from there.
> - There may be a notch, which will facilitate tearing the package.
> - Some packages have a top layer that must be peeled off, exposing a thin foil layer underneath. The medication can then be pushed out through this foil layer.
> - Some packages cannot be opened unless they are cut. Usually, they have lines to indicate where they should be cut. Be careful not to cut the contents.
>
> Special considerations in opening unit-dose packages:
> - Do not push a tablet, capsule, or other medication through the wrapper unless it is specifically designed to be used in this way. (The medication could be broken or crushed.)
> - Be careful that the tablet or capsule does not fall out of the package when it is opened.
> - Be careful in opening liquids. They are susceptible to splashing when the top is peeled off.

Automated Systems
Many facilities use a computerized system to dispense medications. The pharmacy often sends medications via conveyor, pneumatic tube, or courier or may program the medication dispensing unit so medications can be removed by nurses. Providers' orders are electronically transmitted to the pharmacy.

Self-Administered Medications
In some facilities, a responsible client is allowed to keep certain medications at the bedside and manage the administration. Examples include creams and ointments, nicotine gum or inhaler cartridges, throat lozenges, and emergency inhalers. In addition, some clients manage their own pain, using patient-controlled analgesia (PCA) pumps (see Chapter 55). Some clients with diabetes also dispense their own insulin via an insulin pump or insulin pen. Clients at home or in an assisted living facility may manage their own medication administration. Often these are set up weekly by staff or the visiting nurse.

Medication Records
Healthcare facilities use various systems to document medication administration. In the skilled nursing facility, the *medication administration record* (**MAR**) may be a computer-generated sheet, generated daily or weekly, with updates if a client's medication orders change. Paper MARs may be kept on a med cart, in the med room, or next to each client's medication cabinet or drawer. In the acute

care facility, most often the MAR is in the computer and administration of medications is entered directly into the computer.

Whatever system a facility uses, all MARs include the client's name, medication's generic name, dosage, administration route, and scheduled times. As-needed (PRN) medications are also included. The nurse is responsible for checking the accuracy of the MAR by comparing it with the original provider's order. The nurse cosigns or acknowledges each new order. (In the case of handwritten orders, the orders should be double-checked every 24 hr, usually during the night shift.) Each nurse is responsible for checking frequently for any new orders and for double-checking the MAR at the end of each shift, to make sure all medications have been given and documented. *Rationale: Even though a computerized scanner is used, errors or omissions in recording may occur.*

Setting Up Medications

Although each facility's routine for administering medications varies, it is important to conscientiously observe universal rules for safe administration. *Remember:* Safety rules protect nurses, as well as clients. In Practice: Nursing Care Guidelines 63-1 highlights important actions in setting up medications.

> **Nursing Alert** In addition to determining a client's history of drug allergies, inquire as to possible food allergies and allergies to OTC products, tape, or latex. (Regular gloves, catheters, and tourniquets often contain latex.) In most facilities, latex-free products are used when possible. Always double-check for allergies *before* giving medications or performing any procedures.

IN PRACTICE
NURSING CARE GUIDELINES 63-1 | Setting Up Medications

Before Beginning
- Check the order with the MAR. They must be identical. Resolve any inconsistencies by checking the original order. *Rationale: This is necessary to prevent an error.*
- Check for client allergies. Do not give any medications to which the client is allergic. *Rationale: An error could cause serious illness or death.*
- Make sure all medications being given are compatible. If you have any questions, ask. *Rationale: Drug interactions could render the drug useless or dangerous. Interactions and incompatibilities can be double-checked online.*
- Wash/sanitize your hands. *Rationale: Standard Precautions are followed in all nursing procedures.*
- Sanitize your work area by wiping with a disinfectant solution. *Rationale: This helps prevent the spread of microorganisms.*
- Wear gloves, if necessary. (If in doubt, wear gloves.) *Rationale: Some medications, such as chemotherapy agents and hazardous to handle (H_2H) drugs, are toxic. Gloves should also be worn when administering eye/ear drops, ODT medications, transdermal patches, and any other medication that could come in contact with your skin.*
- Locate all appropriate medications and needed equipment.
- Keep medications with you or keep the medication cart or drawer locked whenever it is not in use. Never set up a medication and leave it unattended or unlocked. *Rationale: It might be taken by the wrong client or used inappropriately. Safety must be maintained.*

Setting Up Medications
- Work from the top to the bottom of the MAR when setting up medications. If using a paper MAR, check off medications as they are set up. *Rationale: This helps prevent omitting any medications.*
- If using an electronic medication scanner, set up all medications and then scan the bar codes one at a time. *Rationale: The electronic scanner verifies the client's name, the medication, the dose, and time to be given. It will alert you if any medications are incorrect or missing. This system interfaces with the client's electronic medical record, and if the medications are all correct, they are electronically documented in the client's MAR. (The bar code system can also be used for IV medications.)*
- Set up medications for one client at a time. Administer medications as soon as possible after setting them up. *Rationale: This helps prevent errors.*
- Compare each medication label with the MAR. They must be identical. If there is any question, double-check. *Rationale: This helps prevent errors and gives you a background if the client has questions.*

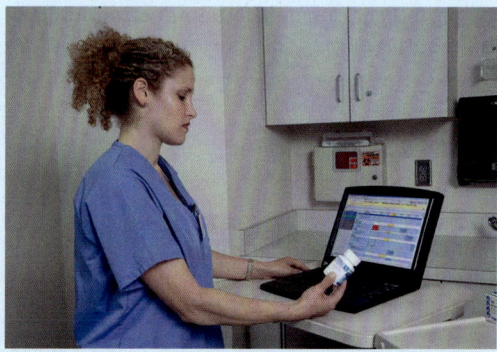
Comparing medication label with the MAR.

- Always pay close attention when setting up medications. Do not talk to coworkers in the medication area. *Rationale: A medication error could cause serious injury or death. It is important not to be distracted.*
- Read the medication label at least three times: (1) when taking the medication from the client's drawer or the computerized machine; (2) before

NURSING CARE GUIDELINES 63-1 Continued

- putting the sealed package into a cup or envelope; and (3) before opening the package and giving the medication. Check each time against the MAR or scanner. *Rationale: Checking the label at least three times helps ensure safe administration.*
- Remove unit-dose packages and set aside for that client. Liquid medications are sealed in individual cups. Place unit-dose packages into a cup or envelope to keep them together. Do not take medications out of the packages or open liquid cups until you get to the bedside. *Rationale: This helps prevent mix-ups. The packages keep the medications clean and safe and facilitate their identification.*
- Have scissors available, in case certain packages are difficult to open. *Rationale: This facilitates opening of the packages.*
- *Never* give a medication if you are unable to read the label. *Rationale: Doing so increases the risk of a medication error.*
- Be familiar with abbreviations and generic and trade names. Use extreme caution with medications that have similar names. *Rationale: Every effort is necessary to ensure that an error does not occur.*
- Check each medication, to make sure it is not spoiled or outdated. *Rationale: Medications may lose their effectiveness or become toxic. Nearly all medications have an outdate; they must not be used after that date. Return these to the pharmacy.*
- Do not open unit-dose packages until ready to give the medication. *Rationale: If the client refuses a medication it will not be wasted. Clients can also be sure they are receiving the correct medication. You will be able to identify medications if there are any questions.*
- Pour tablets into clear cups. *Rationale: If the client tries to "cheek" a medication, you will be able to see it in the cup.*
- Shake liquid medications before administration. *Rationale: In some cases, portions of the medication may settle out.*
- If you must set up medications for more than one client in advance, be sure that each client's medications are carefully labeled and in a separate container or envelope. Do not remove schedule drugs from the locked machine or cupboard until ready to administer them. *Rationale: It is important to give medications to the correct client. Schedule drugs must be under lock and key at all times. They must be tracked from manufacture to administration.*
- Wash/sanitize your hands again after drawing up parenteral medications. *Rationale: Excess medication may have gotten on your hands and you could absorb the medication through your skin.*
- When all medications have been set up, recheck each one with the MAR or scanner. *Rationale: This gives you a final check, to ensure accuracy.*

Using Stock Supply Medications
In some facilities or in the client's home, you may encounter medications that are not in unit-dose packages. In this case:
- Measure the dose with appropriate equipment. When measuring liquids, hold the measure at eye level, with the thumbnail on the line of the desired amount, using the meniscus (lower part of the curve at the surface of the liquid) to indicate the level. Pour liquid medications from the unlabeled side of the bottle. *Rationale: Pouring from the unlabeled side helps to avoid soiling the label. A soiled label may be unreadable.*
- Use a syringe to measure small amounts of liquid. *Rationale: This enables you to get an accurate measurement.*
- Shake the required number of tablets or capsules into the cap of a multidose container. Small plastic cups are usually available for passing medications. Never handle medications with the fingers. *Rationale: If too many tablets are shaken out, they can be returned to the container if they have not been touched. If tablets are handled, they are contaminated. In this case, they must be discarded.*

SAFETY

Safe administration of medications is an absolute priority. The Joint Commission published a list of National Patient Safety Goals for Hospitals, several of which directly apply to medication administration (Box 63-2).

The "Five Rights, Plus Two"

To ensure accuracy, nurses follow the "Five Rights, Plus Two" of medication administration:
- Right client
- Right medication
- Right dose
- Right time
- Right route
- Right documentation
- Right programming (of medication pumps)

A sixth "right," *right documentation,* has been added to this list (Fig. 63-2). In addition, when using pump administration, a seventh "right," *right programming,* is also included.

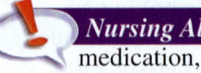 **Nursing Alert** Before administering any medication, always follow:
- Standard Precautions
- The "Five Rights, Plus Two" of medication administration
- Steps listed in Nursing Care Guidelines 63-1

In Practice: Nursing Care Guidelines 63-2 provides tips for safe administration of medications. It also provides documentation guidelines to follow if clients refuse medications.

CHAPTER 63 Administration of Noninjectable Medications

Box 63-2 Safety Goals for Administration of Medications

- *Improve the accuracy of client identification.*
- Use at least two client identifiers (neither to be the client's room number nor bed tag) or a scanner whenever administering medications or providing any other treatments or procedures.
- *Improve the effectiveness of communication among caregivers.*
- For verbal or telephone orders, verify the complete order by having the person receiving the order read back the complete order.
- Standardize a list of abbreviations, acronyms, and symbols that can safely be used throughout the organization.
- *Improve the safety of using medications.*
- Take action to prevent errors involving the interchange of look-alike/sound-alike drugs.
- Label all medications (e.g., syringes, medicine cups) in procedural settings.
- Implement a process for obtaining and documenting a complete list of the client's current medications when the client is admitted to the facility. This is part of the *Medication Reconciliation* process.
- Communicate a complete list of the client's medications to the next provider of service when a client is transferred to another setting. This is the other component of the *Medication Reconciliation* process.

© Joint Commission Resources. Adapted from The Joint Commission (2020). *National patient safety goals effective July 2020 for the hospital program.* Oakbrook Terrace, IL: Joint Commission on Accreditation of Healthcare Organizations. Reprinted with permission. Available at https://www.jointcommission.org/-/media/tjc/documents/standards/national-patient-safety-goals/2020/npsg_chapter_hap_jul2020.pdf

NCLEX Alert

Administration of medications is one of the most important nursing functions, of which ensuring client safety is a major component. This chapter provides you with procedures for meeting client safety goals: accuracy of client identification, timely documentation of medication administration or client refusal, and communicating a complete list of the client's medications to the next provider of service. You may be asked to select safe nursing actions related to medication monitoring or administration in the examination.

The Right Client

Take special precautions to ensure that the *correct medication* is given to the *correct client*. Direct total attention to giving medications.

"Check Two for Safety." Always check at least two forms of identification before giving any medications:

- Scan the bar code on the client's wrist band. *Rationale: This verifies that this is the correct client.*

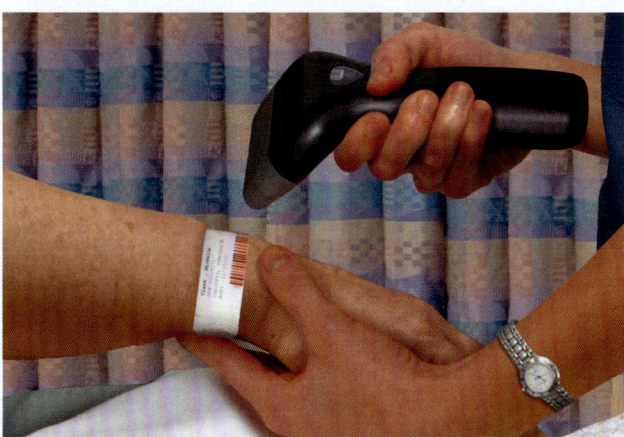

Scanning the bar code on the client's identification bracelet.

- Compare the MAR with the client's identification band. Check the medical record number on the identification (ID) band, as well as the client's name.
- Compare the client's name and medical record number on the medication package with the client's name band.
- Ask the client their name.
- Ask the client to state their birth date.
- Obtain corroboration from another nurse or responsible family member *as a last resort.*

The Identification Band

The best way to identify a client is to check the wrist band. It is important to check the client's medical record number, as well as their name. *Rationale: Many clients have common names or similar names.* Do not administer medications if the client does not have a wrist band. (A name tag taped to a bed or door does not necessarily mean that this is the correct client.) This is particularly true in long-term or psychiatric facilities, where clients freely move about. Some clients in these facilities may be confused or may deliberately mislead the nurse. In some situations, such as in psychiatry or rehabilitation, clients may refuse to wear ID bands because they may be embarrassed when going on outings or passes. Sometimes, such clients are allowed to carry ID bands in their pockets. In this case, the client's identity must be positively determined by other means of identification. Some clients in special areas are allowed to wear the ID band on the ankle, where it is less conspicuous.

> **Be sure you have the:**
>
> 1. Right client
> 2. Right medication
> 3. Right dose
> 4. Right time
> 5. Right route
> 6. Right documentation
> 7. Right programming (with pump)

Figure 63-2 The "Five Rights, Plus Two" of medication administration.

IN PRACTICE
NURSING CARE GUIDELINES 63-2: Administering Medications Safely

- "Check two for safety." Make sure to use at least two objective means of identifying the client (not including bed or room tag) before administering any medications. *Rationale: Client identification is vital, to prevent errors.*
- Scan or visually check the client's wrist band and ask their name and birth date. *Rationale: The wrist band is an objective form of ID. The client is not likely to give the wrong birth date. If you simply ask the client if he is Mr. Jones, the reply may be "yes," because the client did not hear you, did not speak English, or simply wanted to mislead you. The scanner will indicate if this is the wrong client.*
- Make sure you have the correct medications, correct dosages, and correct forms of medications. Double-check the time the medications are due. *Rationale: Medications should have been checked at least twice before being carried to the client, to prevent errors. If you have any questions, check before giving any medications. Medications must be given within a specified time limit, to prevent error.*
- Check *very carefully* for medication allergies. Ask the client if they are allergic to anything (including foods, latex) before giving any medication. Note any allergies in the client's record and make sure the client is wearing an allergy band, whether they are allergic or not. *Rationale: Checking for allergies is essential to prevent client injury. It is important to know the allergy status of each client.*
- Take the electronic scanner or paper MAR with you when giving medications. Follow the "Five Rights, Plus Two" of medication administration. *Rationale: This provides a final check before giving medications. It is vital to administer medications to the correct person by the correct route. Having the scanner or MAR with you allows documentation of the administration before leaving the client. This prevents forgetting to document or documenting incorrectly.*
- Administer medication for each client as it is prepared. *Rationale: This helps avoid medication errors. This will avoid mixing up medications for various clients.*
- Keep all unit-dose medications in individual packages until you are with the client. Open the packages in front of the client and pour the medications into a clear medication cup or the client's hand, if the client requests this and is reliable. *Rationale: This will provide a last check before giving the medication. If the client refuses a medication, it will not be wasted and you and the client can identify which medication is being refused. If the client questions which medication is which, you can respond. Using a clear cup allows you to see if the client takes all of the medications. If the client is not reliable, they can keep a medication in the hand and not take it ("cheeking").*
- Do not leave a medicine tray, package, or cup within client's reach unless there is a specific provider's order that the client can have it at the bedside. If you must leave the room, take the medication with you. Lock the medication cart each time you leave it. *Rationale: The wrong person may take medications or the client may not take them. You must observe the client actually taking medications.*
- Follow the facility's policy for established medication administration times. *Rationale: If medications are not given within the established time limits, a medication error has occurred.*
- If using a scanner, indicate "given" or "accept." Document medication administration on the paper MAR as soon as medications are given. *Never* chart a medication before it is given. Record the time, medication, and dose. *Rationale: The scanner will record the administration in the computer. The MAR is a legal document and must be accurate.*
- Initial each entry or accept it in the computer. If using a paper MAR, initial and sign and print your full name and status (e.g., LVN/LPN, RN, student) at the bottom. *Rationale: Doing so ensures that other members of the healthcare team will know who gave the medication. The MAR is a legal document and may be used in court. The computer will automatically record this information when you acknowledge giving the medication on the scanner.*
- Record and *report immediately* any unusual client reaction, an unfavorable change in the client's condition, a client's refusal to take medicine, their inability to take all of it, or any attempts to cheek medication. *Rationale: The client may need immediate medical attention. If the client cheeks medication, they are not obtaining the therapeutic effect and a different route of administration may be required.*
- If a client questions a medication, says it is the wrong medication, or says they have an allergy, stop and double-check. *Do not give the medication until you are sure it is correct.* Report and document what occurred. *Rationale: Most clients are knowledgeable about their medications, providing an extra safety factor. Double-checking and explaining help clients to understand if medications are correctly prescribed for them. If it was an incorrect medication, an error has just been prevented.*
- Be aware that sometimes the same medication from a different manufacturer can look different. Explain this to the client. *Rationale: After double-checking, even though the client has not seen this format before, it may be the correct medication.*
- If a medication has been forgotten, report this promptly. *Rationale: This is a medication error.*
- Discard any open medication dose. An unopened unit-dose package may be returned to the client's drawer or the pharmacy. *Rationale: An open dose is considered contaminated and no longer properly*

NURSING CARE GUIDELINES 63-2 Continued

identified. An unopened package may be reused because it is sealed and labeled.
- Dispose of medications according to facility policies. Have a witness cosign if a controlled substance is being discarded or returned. Medications to be disposed of, as well as all medication packages, are usually required to be placed in the hazardous waste receptacle, not in the general trash or the sink. *Rationale:* The nurse is legally required to maintain an accurate record of all controlled substances. Medications are considered hazardous medical waste and must be disposed of in special ways to protect the environment and the sanitation workers. Toxic medications are handled only with special nitrile gloves and are discarded in a special "hazardous to handle" container.
- Client refusal can be documented on the scanner. If using a paper MAR, document as usual and then circle the time and write "ref" next to it. Follow the same procedure for any other reason a scheduled medication is not given on time—circle the time, and indicate a reason (e.g., "refused," "emesis," "on pass"). *Rationale:* Proper and accurate documentation helps prevent medication errors. In addition, it provides a means of communication with other healthcare personnel. In many cases, if a medication has been missed for a logical reason, it may safely be given later.
- Do not give medications that someone else has prepared without double-checking the medication packages against the MAR. Make sure another nurse has not already given the medication. *Rationale:* Each nurse is personally responsible for all medications they give.
- Wash your hands after administering medications. *Rationale:* You may have a minute amount of medication residue on your skin, which could be absorbed into your body. This also helps prevent cross-contamination.
- If you must set up medications for several clients at one time, keep the setups separate and do not set up controlled substances until you are ready to give them. *Rationale:* It is important to prevent errors. Controlled substances must be locked or with a licensed nurse at all times.

Note: If your facility uses stock medication supplies, follow the local protocol. Remember: Stock supply medications carry a greater risk of error than do unit-dose systems.

Asking the Client's Name
After checking the client's identification band, if the client is conscious and oriented, ask the client to state their name. Do so in a polite, friendly manner. Do not ask the client "Are you Mr. Brown?" *Rationale: Phrasing a question this way does not help in determining who the client is. Some clients with hearing or psychological disorders or who do not speak English well will answer "yes" to any question they are asked.*

Asking the Client's Birth Date
Most clients are able to tell you their birth date. This is very good identification, but not foolproof. For example, in some countries, everyone is considered to have been born on January 1. In this case, the birth date is only limited to the year they were born and is not definitive. In other cases, clients may not know their actual birth date.

Verification by Another Responsible Person
This method is a last resort for identifying a client. It may be used if there is no other way to identify the client positively.

The Right Medication
Compare and confirm the *medication's name* and dosage with the client's MAR at least three times before administering it.
1. The first check: when removing the medication from storage.
2. The second check: when scanning it and placing it in the medication cup or envelope.
3. The third check: when opening the unit-dose package at the client's bedside.

> **Nursing Alert** Following the three simple checks will drastically reduce the possibility of a medication error.

Remember to check both the generic and trade name of a medication. If the medication is ordered by trade name and only the generic name is on the package, you must look it up. *Rationale: It is important to make sure you are giving the correct medication.*

As a general rule, do not administer a medication that someone else has prepared or to a client assigned to another nurse. However, in an emergency, if a labeled unit-dose medication has been set out by another nurse, you can compare the packages to the MAR to make sure they have been prepared correctly and have not been given. In this case, it would be as though you had set up the medication. This practice is not without risks, however.

> **Nursing Alert** If you give a medication to a client who is not assigned to you, it is vital to document the administration and report this to the assigned nurse. *Rationale: This helps prevent duplication of doses.*

The Right Dose
To ensure the *right dose,* double-check that the amount of medication supplied matches the amount needed for the ordered dose. Make sure to calculate the dose if the supplied medication is not exactly the same amount as the ordered dose (see Chapter 60). In addition, verify that the dose ordered is appropriate for the client. Moreover, always listen

to the client. If they question the medication's color, number of tablets being given, or administration route, recheck the MAR, order, and medication label *before* giving the medication.

The Right Time

Administer all medications at the *time* for which they are ordered. Most facilities allow 30 min on each side of the scheduled time for administering medications. For example, a medication ordered for 0900 usually may be administered anytime between 0830 and 0930 and still be considered "on time." Administering medications as ordered is important, to maintain the medication's therapeutic effects. Deviation from the "time window" is considered a medication error.

> **Nursing Alert** Some medications must be administered at the correct time. For example, some insulins must be given within 15 min of a meal. Other medications must be given before meals or with food, or cannot be given with food or milk. Antibiotics may be ordered for administration at equal intervals around the clock. Sometimes, pain medications or sedatives are given a specified length of time before a special treatment or rehabilitation exercise. *Rationale: If these medications are not given at the correct time, they will not have the desired effect and may actually be detrimental.*

Devising a method to ensure delivery of medications at the specified time is advisable. Nurses have devised many different systems of "reminders." You can make a chart containing each client's name and location, with separate boxes for each hour. You then can indicate medications and treatments to be given at specified times. This helps the nurse to plan a schedule and administer medications on time. An area for "Notes" is helpful when you are documenting. Allow time for lunch or for performing special treatments. Be consistent with your organizational plan.

STAT Doses

An **STAT** order means that a medication must be administered *immediately*. First, check the order against the original provider's order. Then, make sure the order appears on the MAR. Prepare and administer the medication as soon as possible. If the medication is not readily available, inform the team leader and notify the pharmacy. As with all medications, *scan and document STAT medications as soon as they are given.* This helps to prevent duplication of an STAT order. Write or enter "given," the date, time, and your initials next to the original order, if the order is handwritten. If a paper MAR is used, the medication is marked as "given." This procedure informs the provider that the order was carried out and when.

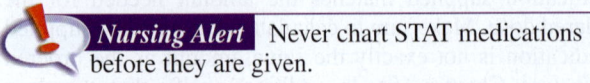

> **Nursing Alert** Never chart STAT medications before they are given.

PRN Doses

Evaluating a client's need for PRN (*as needed* or *on request*) medication is an important nursing responsibility that is learned with experience. If a client requests a PRN medication, first gather information about the client's symptoms. For example, if the client is complaining of pain, determine the pain's location and the client's discomfort level, based on the designated rating scale in your facility. One such scale rates pain as 0 (no pain) to 10 (extreme pain) (see Chapter 55). Next, consult the MAR to determine when the client last received the PRN or a regularly scheduled pain medication. If the appropriate time has elapsed, administer the medication as soon as possible. If it is too soon to give the medication, inform the client when the next dose is due. If the pain is extreme, consult the provider to determine if an additional dose or another medication can be given. Sometimes, pain medications are given on a regular basis, to prevent pain before it begins. The nurse and client together determine the need for this procedure. PRN medications are usually available for sleep and situations such as diarrhea, constipation, and gastric distress, as well as for pain.

Hour of Sleep (HS, Bedtime) Doses

Providers often order sedatives and hypnotics, "sleeping pills," on a PRN basis. Technically, the client should request these but may be unaware that these are ordered. Thus, it is appropriate to offer HS medications to the client and to inform the client to ask for this medication in the future, if needed. Bedtime sleep medications should be given as close to the time the client will be retiring as possible.

The Right Route

Check the provider's orders and the MAR to verify the *route* by which medication is to be given. Remember the three checks. Administering a medication by the wrong route, even though it is the correct medication, could be fatal. *Rationale: Medications are absorbed at different rates, depending on the route of administration. Dosages also may be different when using different routes. For example, an oral medication may require a larger dose than if it were to be given IV. Giving an oral dose by the IV route could cause the client's immediate death.*

The Right Documentation

Documentation is vital in medication administration. *Actions not documented are considered not to have been done.* Proper documentation communicates to other members of the healthcare team which medications were administered and when. If a medication is PRN or a first-time administration, documentation *must* include the medication's effects. Chapter 37 describes documentation. Drug orders and documentation of administration may be on the same treatment record or computer record.

In many healthcare facilities, all recording is done using *military time* (the 24-hr clock). For instance, 0000 denotes midnight, 0800 is 8 AM, 1200 is noon, and 2000 is 8 PM (see Table 37-3). This method eliminates errors in interpreting whether the entry designates AM or PM. Some facilities require nurses to wear a sign saying, "Please do not disturb during medication administration."

> **Nursing Alert** Be sure to check the MAR before giving any PRN medications and to document all PRN medications immediately on giving them. *Rationale: This will help prevent duplication, should the client ask another nurse for the same medication.*

The Right Programming

When medications are given by programmable pump, the programming must be done as carefully as if portions of medication were to be given by the nurse. It is vital to program in the correct dosage, times of administration, and alarm parameters. An error in programming would cause the client to receive an inaccurate dose of medication and would be considered a medication error. Two nurses should check for accuracy whenever a medication pump is programmed. If the client is to manage self-administration of medications via pump, it is vital to program in the upper limits of medication allowed, to prevent accidental or intentional overdose.

Other Considerations in Giving Medications

Medication Errors

Although every nurse hopes never to commit a medication error, chances are that this will happen sometime during their career. Students and new graduates, because they are learning, must be particularly careful. Report any medication error to the clinical instructor or charge nurse as soon as it is discovered. In some cases, immediate emergency action is necessary to prevent undesirable or potentially fatal effects. Medication errors include administering to the wrong client, administering the wrong medication or dose, administering at the wrong time, or administering by the wrong route. Failure to document a medication or to document it incorrectly is also considered a medication error in many facilities.

For any doubts about a medication, consult a drug reference and ask the team leader before giving it. If the possibility of a medication error exists, do not hesitate to report it. *The greatest error is to avoid reporting.* The client's well-being is the major concern.

> **Nursing Alert** The nurse who discovers an error and does not report it is endangering the client and may be subject to disciplinary action.

Medication Compliance

After determining that the client is the right client, stay with the client until they have taken the medication. Make sure the client has swallowed the medication. Do not leave medications at the bedside, except in special circumstances, as stated earlier. *Rationale: Some clients may deliberately dispose of the medication, or the wrong client may take it.*

In some instances, checking the client's mouth to make sure the medication has been swallowed may be necessary. Some clients, particularly in long-term care or psychiatry, are required to remain out of their room for a period of time after taking medications, to make sure they have swallowed the medication and are not disposing of it or causing themselves to vomit. Other methods used to ensure medication compliance include the use of liquid or crushed medications, orally disintegrating tablets (ODTs), or long-lasting (depot or decanoate) injections.

Client Refusal

The nurse is obligated to encourage the client to take all medication; however, a client has the right to refuse a medication unless there is a court order to the contrary or a medical emergency has been declared. If a medication package is unopened, it may be returned to the pharmacy. In the case of a controlled substance, two nurses must witness its return. In some facilities, all returned medications require a witness. Usually, there is a special receptacle on the machine for the return of unused medications (see Fig. 61-1).

> **Nursing Alert** If a medication package has been opened, the medication must be disposed of, using specific procedures. Most medications are discarded in the designated hazardous waste receptacle. A controlled substance requires signature by two nurses, one of whom is the designated witness. Never sign that you witnessed the disposal of a controlled substance if you did not see the actual disposal.

Documenting Client Refusal or Held Medications

If a medication is not given, the nurse must indicate this, according to facility protocol. The reason the medication is not given is also indicated. There are several reasons for not giving a medication, including client refusal, medication not available, medication held for a procedure, or client not in the room. There is usually a space for comments as well. If a comment is made, it is not necessary to enter this information in the nurse's notes. If a previously refused or held medication is given later, it is documented, indicating the actual time of administration.

Hazardous to Handle Medications

Some medications are considered "hazardous to handle" (H_2H). Drugs that might be toxic to staff, such as chemotherapy agents, or might be dangerous to the pregnant nurse, such as divalproex and other psychotherapeutic agents, require special handling. The nurse is required to wear nitrile gloves and packages should be disposed of in the special H_2H container. (This is different from the "hazardous waste" container.)

Proper Disposal of Medication Packages

In most facilities, medications are not disposed of in the sewer system; they are placed in a hazardous waste container for environmentally safe disposal. Medication packages are often disposed of in the same container. *Rationale: They may contain minute traces of medication.* See In Practice: Nursing Care Guidelines 63-2.

Discontinued or Changed Medications

Each healthcare facility has a method for indicating when medications (or treatments) have been discontinued or changed. This also applies when other factors, such as dosage, time, or route of administration, have been changed. The nurse acknowledges the change in orders in the computer or on the MAR. The pharmacy is electronically notified, or otherwise informed, so the correct dose or medication will be dispensed. *Rationale: This helps ensure that the order has been recorded correctly and the client will be receiving medications as ordered.*

Client Teaching

Client teaching is an important safety consideration for medication administration. Teach clients the following information concerning their medications:

- Which medications they are given (generic and trade name)
- Why they are taking them
- Dosage and frequency
- How to administer or take them at home
- Medications from different manufacturers may look different
- Expected effects
- Possible undesirable side effects
- How long they will need the medications
- What to do if they miss a dose
- Signs and symptoms clients should report to healthcare provider

Clients should be able to verbalize this information ("teach back"), to indicate their understanding. They should be able to demonstrate specific related procedures (e.g., the injection technique for administering insulin). All teaching *must* be documented, because it is an important component of the nursing care plan and is required by the Joint Commission. If teaching is not documented, it is considered not to have been done. Clients and families should also be provided with written information, in addition to verbal instruction, to reinforce their knowledge and understanding.

> **NCLEX Alert**
>
> As you administer medications and monitor clients for their effects, it will be important to consider your responsibility to teach clients/family members about their medications. The importance of documentation is emphasized: note what was taught and the client's verbalized or demonstrated understanding of your teaching. On reading test scenarios, you may be asked to select answers demonstrating your understanding of this nursing role.

GENERAL PRINCIPLES OF MEDICATION ADMINISTRATION

Desired and Undesired Effects

Medications have many effects on the body, both desired and undesired. These include:

- *Therapeutic effect.* The medications desired effect; the medication produces the result for which it was given.
- **Adverse effect**. A response that is not intended or desired. Some adverse effects are minor (*side effects*) and, although bothersome, can be ignored or treated easily. Constipation is an example of a side effect.
- *Serious adverse effect.* Some side effects, such as respiratory depression or neurologic damage, are disabling or potentially fatal.
- *Anaphylaxis.* The medication causes the client to experience a severe, immediately life threatening, allergic reaction (**anaphylaxis**) manifested by vasodilation, low blood pressure, and shock. Anaphylaxis is a medical emergency; it must be recognized and treated immediately.

Medication **toxicity**. A harmful, undesired effect resulting from an increased blood level of medication beyond its therapeutic level. Administering a medication in too large a dose or via the wrong route can lead to drug toxicity. In some cases, the client can also build up toxicity as a result of a disorder, such as inadequately functioning kidneys. *Remember:* clients, particularly those with dementia or depression, may also accidently or intentionally take extra medications, resulting in a harmful or life-threatening response.

- **Paradoxical** *effect.* This client's response is *opposite* to that which is desired. For example, a client may become extremely agitated and restless in response to a sedative given for sleep. Paradoxical responses are most common in very young and elderly clients.
- **Potentiation**. Two drugs may potentiate each other. The effects of the two medications together are greater than would be the two individually. Potentiation *multiplies* or enhances the effects of the drugs. This can become a very dangerous situation.

Local and Systemic Effects

A medication's effects may be local or systemic. **Topical** application (applied directly to the skin or mucous membranes) can cause a **local effect**. Anti-inflammatory creams and lotions and medications to relieve itching are examples. These may be applied to mucous membranes of the eye, mouth, nose, throat, or vagina by instillation, irrigation, swabbing, or spraying. Rectal suppositories most often supply laxatives (a systemic effect); vaginal suppositories are used most often to treat localized vaginal infections. The effects of local medications are limited to the area of application, thus reducing the possibility of undesired systemic reactions.

Medications can be administered in a number of ways to achieve systemic effects (to be absorbed into the general circulation, blood and lymphatic fluids) and transported to a specific area or to the entire body. To achieve **systemic effects**, medications often are administered by transdermal application, mouth, or injection, although other methods, such as nasal inhalation, can also produce systemic effects (see Table 63-1).

Medication Administration to Children

Children, because of their smaller size, can tolerate only a fraction of adult dosages. To ensure that correct dosages of medications are administered to children, body weight is often considered (see Chapter 71). The primary provider is responsible for determining these dosages. Carefully check the healthcare facility's protocol, a drug reference, and the dosage before administering any medications to children.

TABLE 63-1 Common Routes for Medication Administration

ROUTE	PROCESS OF ADMINISTRATION	TERM USED TO DESCRIBE ROUTE
Enteral Methods		
By mouth	Client swallows medication (e.g., tablet, capsule, liquid) Medication placed on tongue and dissolves instantly (orally disintegrating tablets [ODTs]), then swallowed	Oral (PO) administration A form of oral administration
Applied to oral mucous membranes	Medication placed under tongue Medication placed between the cheek and gum (buccal pouch), e.g., chewing gum (aspirin, nicotine replacement)	Sublingual (SL) administration Buccal administration
By feeding tube	Medication instilled through feeding tube into stomach or intestine	Types of tubes: Nasogastric (NG) Gastrostomy (GT) Jejunostomy (JT)
Given by suppository or enema	Medication inserted into rectum	Rectal administration (R, PR)
Parenteral Methods		
Suppository or applicator	Medication inserted into vagina	Vaginal administration (V)
Applied to mucous membranes via dropper or tube	Medication instilled into eye (cream, ointment, liquid) Medication instilled into ear (ear drops)	Eye (ophthalmic) administration Ear (otic) administration
Given via respiratory tract	Client inhales the medication Client uses nasal spray Client receives nasal drops	Nasal inhalation Aerosolized administration Nasal gtts (drops)
Absorbed through the skin	Medication patch or ointment placed on the skin	Transdermal (TD) administration
Given by injection (see Chapter 64)	Medication injected into: Corium (under epidermis) Subcutaneous tissue Muscle tissue Vein Large vein (e.g., subclavian) Artery Heart tissue Peritoneal cavity Spinal canal Bone Subarachnoid space of spinal column Bone marrow cavity	Intradermal (ID) injection Subcutaneous (SubQ) injection Intramuscular (IM) injection Intravenous (IV) injection Total parenteral nutrition (TPN) Intra-arterial (IA) injection Intracardiac injection Intraperitoneal injection Intraspinal injection Intraosseous injection Intrathecal injection Intramedullary injection

Enteral Versus Parenteral Administration

Enteral indicates medication administration by way of the digestive (GI) tract. This route includes administration orally, **buccally** (inside the cheek), and via gastrointestinal tubes (**G tubes/NG tubes**). Other forms of oral administration include **sublingual** (under the tongue) and *translingual* (through the tongue). Medications may be dissolved in the mouth (ODTs) or may be sprayed onto the tongue (see Chapter 61). Technically, rectal (**PR**) administration also is a form of enteral administration. However, some healthcare personnel consider this route to be *parenteral* because it is not "by mouth."

Parenteral administration means medication administration into any part of the body other than the GI tract. This route includes medications administered via the vagina, eye, ear, nose and respiratory tract, skin, and by injection. (In common usage, the term has come to refer to medications administered by injection.) Chapter 64 describes methods of administering medications by injection, including IV administration. Table 63-1 lists various routes of medication administration.

Rate of Absorption and Onset of Action

A medication's rate of absorption depends on its route of administration. Clients usually prefer oral administration, which is used most frequently. A disadvantage of drugs administered orally is the slower absorption rate, which results in a slowed onset of action. Absorption and onset of action with injected medications are more rapid than with orally administered drugs. Of the commonly used injection methods, IV medications are absorbed most rapidly. Medications absorbed through oral mucosa are also absorbed rapidly.

Key Concept

Many medications are available in different forms, suitable for various routes of administration (see also Chapter 62). Examples include

- prochlorperazine (Compazine)—available in oral form (tablets, spansules, syrup), injectable form, or in rectal suppositories
- gentamicin (Alcomicin [CAN], Garamycin)—available for injection, as an ophthalmic solution or ointment, implantable beads, and as a topical ointment or cream
- nitroglycerin—available for IV injection, as sublingual tablets, translingual spray, transmucosal tablets (extended-release [ER] buccal tablets), oral tablets (sustained release [SR]), transdermal patch, and topical ointment
- acetaminophen (Tylenol)—available as suppositories; chewable tablets; oral tablets (immediate release [IR], ER), orally disintegrating tablets (ODTs), caplets, gel-caps, and capsules; oral elixir, liquid, solution, and drops; and in sprinkle capsules
- risperidone (Risperdal)—available as tablets, ODTs (M-Tab), oral solution, fast-acting injection, and long-lasting injection (Consta—given every 2-3 weeks).

Other medications are available in only one form. Examples

- procaine penicillin, naloxone (Narcan), and heparin—only injectable
- tolterodine (Detrol) and celecoxib (Celebrex)—only oral tablets/capsules

Nursing Alert Some medications cannot be crushed safely (e.g., enteric-coated tablets, time-release tablets, orally disintegrating tablets, or capsules). Some medications in capsules would not be effective if the capsule were opened (e.g., extended-release medications or those designed not to dissolve until reaching the small intestine). Always consult a pharmacist or reliable reference before crushing any medication or opening a capsule.

liquid medication has an unpleasant taste, a client may dull the taste buds by sucking on ice chips before taking it. Some liquid medications are best taken through a straw. *Rationale: This helps minimize contact with the taste buds in the mouth.* Nearly all liquid medications come in premeasured unit-dose containers or oral syringes.

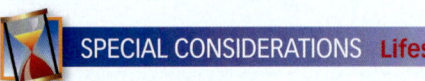

SPECIAL CONSIDERATIONS Lifespan

Liquids and Children

Administer oral liquid medications to small children directly from a syringe or calibrated pediatric dropper.

ENTERAL ADMINISTRATION METHODS

Oral Administration

The oral route of medication administration is used most frequently (see In Practice: Nursing Procedure 63-1). Medications administered orally (by mouth) are referred to as **PO** (Latin: "per os"). A PO medication can be in many forms, including tablets, capsules, caplets, sprinkles, or in liquid or gel form to be swallowed or sprayed on the tongue or applied to the mucous membranes of the mouth. Most oral medications are swallowed, but some are designed to be absorbed in the mouth.

Although the oral method is convenient, economical, and preferred by most clients, it has disadvantages. Some medications have an unpleasant taste or odor; others are harmful to the teeth or oral mucous membranes. Clients experiencing nausea and vomiting often cannot retain PO medications. Some clients have difficulty swallowing and, therefore, risk choking on PO medications; others have just had mouth or throat surgery; and some clients are noncompliant, refusing to swallow medications.

If a client is unable or unwilling to swallow tablets, in some cases, tablets can be crushed and dissolved in water or juice or mixed with applesauce or other food (gelatin, ice cream). Some capsules may also be opened and the contents used in the same manner as crushed medications. Make sure there is an order to crush medications or open capsules. Split tablets, if required, to obtain the correct dose. In Practice: Nursing Care Guidelines 63-3 describes the procedure for crushing or splitting tablets.

Some liquid medications are given full strength. Other liquid medications are diluted with water, juice, or milk. If a

Sublingual Administration

Sublingual (**SL**) medications (e.g., nitroglycerin) are placed under the tongue, where they are dissolved and absorbed. Clients should not chew or swallow SL medications. *Rationale: Chewing and/or swallowing speeds absorption too much.* Tell clients to keep SL medications under the tongue until the medication dissolves.

Translingual Administration

Translingual (TL) medications are placed on the tongue, where they are absorbed or dissolve. These medications may be in the form of a spray or may be a troche, which dissolves slowly. The medication is absorbed through the tongue or is swallowed with saliva.

Orally Disintegrating Tablets

The ODT is an excellent choice for noncompliant clients and small children. This tablet is placed on the client's tongue and dissolves instantly, thus ensuring medication compliance (see In Practice: Nursing Care Guidelines 63-4). The client should be instructed not to chew or break up the ODT, because this interferes with the timing of the drug's release.

Buccal Administration

Buccal administration involves placing medication between the client's cheek and gum. Clients should not chew or swallow buccal medications but should leave them between the cheek and gum until they dissolve or are discarded, as in the case of Nicorette gum. *Rationale: These medications are designed to be absorbed via the mucous membranes of the cheek.* Buccal administration may be in

CHAPTER 63 Administration of Noninjectable Medications

IN PRACTICE
NURSING CARE GUIDELINES 63-3 Crushing or Splitting Tablets

To Crush a Tablet
- Place the tablet within a paper soufflé cup and place this into a mortar. Cover the tablet with another paper soufflé cup (placed inside the first one with the tablet between the two layers). Crush the tablet with the pestle until it is in powder form. If using a pill-crusher, place the tablet within the special plastic bag and lower the handle, or otherwise follow the manufacturer's instructions. Unit-dose medications may also be crushed within their package. Remember that only certain types of tablets can safely be crushed. *Rationale: This prevents medication from being left in the mortar or pill crusher. The medication must be in powder form to be mixed with food and swallowed. Crushing some types of tablets will deliver an inappropriate dose of medication.*
- Dissolve crushed tablets in water or juice or mix with applesauce or other food, such as gelatin or ice cream, or administer via nasogastric (NG) tube. *Rationale: Dissolving helps mask the taste and allows the powder to be swallowed.*
- Clean the mortar, pestle, and/or pill crusher after use. *Rationale: This prevents medication from being mixed with another client's medications.*

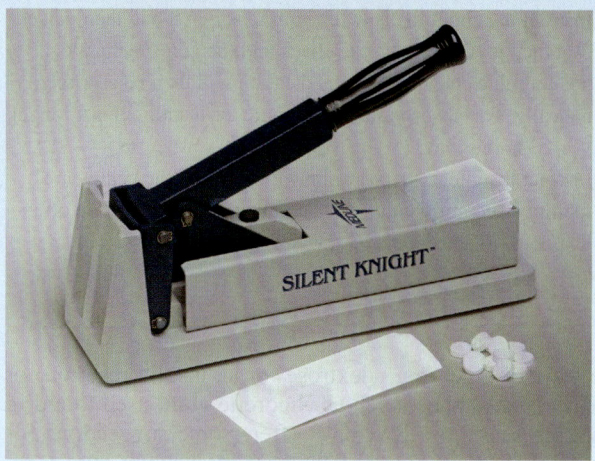

Instead of the traditional mortar and pestle, a "pill crusher," such as that shown here, may be used. The tablet is placed into the supplied plastic bag and fitted into the device. When the handle is pulled down, the tablet is crushed evenly. (Photo: Medline Industries.)

To Split a Tablet
- Cut tablets at the score mark only. Place the tablet into the pill cutter, with the score mark exactly lined up with the blade. Lower the blade carefully. Make sure the two halves or thirds are the same size. *The blade is very sharp; prevent injury.* Remember that certain types of medications cannot be safely split. *Rationale: Using the score mark ensures accurate dosing. You cannot safely split an unscored tablet or split a tablet if the dose does not come out exactly. It is important to obtain the correct dose.*

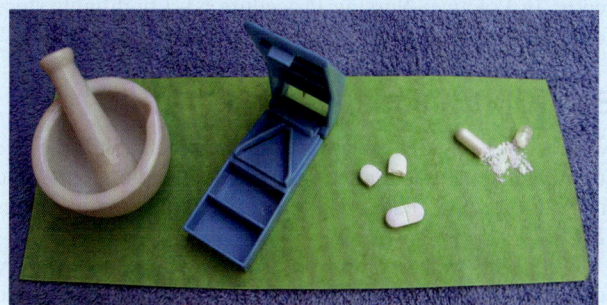

Materials needed to crush or split tablets. Mortar and pestle, pill splitter, scored tablet, and opened capsule. (Photo Copyright © Caroline Bunker Rosdahl.)

IN PRACTICE
NURSING CARE GUIDELINES 63-4 Administering Orally Disintegrating Tablets

- Follow the steps in Nursing Care Guidelines 63-1 and 63-2 before administering any medication.
- Wear gloves. Scan the medication package. Do not touch the ODT with bare fingers. *Rationale: This prevents the nurse from absorbing any of the medication.*
- Be sure to leave the tablet in its sealed bubble package until it is ready to be administered.
- Peel back the foil on top of the package, to expose the tablet.
- Do not push the tablet through the foil or the package. *Rationale: This could crush the tablet and make it impossible to administer safely.*
- Explain that the ODT will dissolve immediately. Ask the client to touch their tongue to the medication while it is still in the package. The tablet will then be on the tongue and will not have been touched by the fingers. If the client refuses to do this, make sure their fingers are dry. *Rationale: Moisture of any sort can begin to melt the tablet, making it very difficult to remove from the package and altering the dose.*
- Instruct the client to keep the entire tablet in the mouth and not to chew it. *Rationale: Chewing is not necessary, because the tablet will dissolve instantly. In some cases, breaking up or chewing the ODT alters the medication's effectiveness.*

Note: ODTs cannot safely be split or crushed.

Box 63-3 Administering Nicotine Replacement in Chewing Gum Form

- Wear gloves.
- Instruct the client to chew the gum to soften it and then place it in the mouth between the cheek and the gums/teeth. Do not continue chewing. The medication will then be absorbed buccally. The absorption will be more even and will last longer if used in this way.
- Instruct the client not to swallow the gum. In the healthcare facility, used gum, wrappers, and nicotine cartridges are often disposed of in special containers.
- Nicorette gum is commonly available in 2- or 4-mg strengths. For smoking cessation, reduce the strength and lengthen the time between pieces of gum as much and as quickly as possible.
- The client should not smoke or use another type of nicotine replacement while using the gum.
- Do not touch the gum yourself. You would then be receiving nicotine through your skin and also would be contaminating the gum.

---

the form of a gel (e.g., dextrose for an insulin reaction) or may be a substance, such as Nicorette gum, used to aid in smoking cessation. Box 63-3 offers some suggestions for administering nicotine replacement in chewing gum form (see also Fig. 63-1).

Administration Through a Gastric Tube

Clients with nasogastric (NG) tubes or other types of GI tubes generally receive their medications through the tube. Medications administered by this route should be in liquid form, although they can be quite thick (see In Practice: Nursing Procedure 63-2). If medications are unavailable in liquid form, obtain an order from the primary provider before crushing any medication and mixing it with liquid for administration (see In Practice: Nursing Care Guidelines 63-3). In some cases, capsules may be opened and the contents mixed with liquid and instilled into an NG tube; this also requires a specific order. *Do not crush enteric-coated or time-release medications.* Only medications specified as *enteral* may be given via GI tube. Medications to be given by GI tube are set up separately; they are not mixed together. *Rationale: Crushed medications tend to clog GI tubes. Crushing an enteric-coated or time-release medication may interfere with its desired action.*

Nursing Alert To avoid undesired medication effects, consult a drug reference, pharmacist, or team leader with any doubts about restrictions or incompatibilities of medications.

Rectal Administration

Typically, medications given rectally are in the form of a **suppository**, a bullet-shaped semisolid medication designed to melt at body temperature (see Fig. 63-1). Suppositories are usually stored in the refrigerator until needed. Suppositories are usually prelubricated. If this is not the case, lubricate the pointed tip of the suppository with water-soluble lubricant (e.g., K-Y) before insertion. In Practice: Nursing Procedure 63-3 outlines steps for rectal suppository administration. Additionally, fluid or medication can be instilled into the rectum as an enema (see Chapter 51).

PARENTERAL ADMINISTRATION METHODS

Parenteral administration includes noninjection methods and injection methods. Noninjection methods are discussed here. Injection methods are discussed in Chapter 64.

Vaginal Administration

Vaginal medications are supplied in the form of suppositories, foams, creams, and tablets that usually involve the use of an applicator, to ensure that the medication is placed correctly. In Practice: Nursing Procedure 63-4 highlights steps for vaginal suppository administration.

Eye (Ophthalmic) Administration

Medications instilled or administered directly into the eye (**ophthalmic** medications) include liquids, ointments, and medication-impregnated disks that resemble contact lenses (Fig. 63-3).

If applying ointment or drops to both eyes, take great care to avoid spreading infection from one eye to the other. Do not allow the applicator tip to touch either eye during administration. In some cases, a separate tube or blister pack is used for each eye. Many times, eye ointments are given at bedtime. *Rationale: Ointments may cause blurred vision.* See In Practice: Nursing Procedure 63-5.

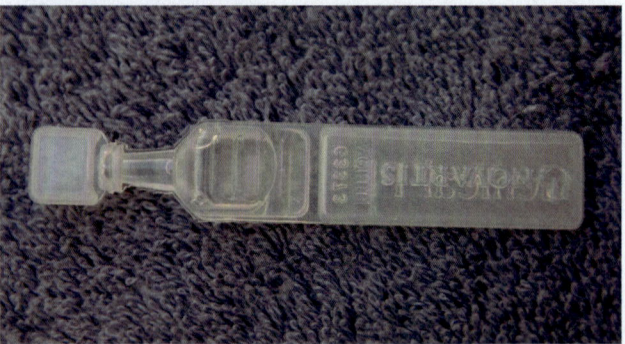

Figure 63-3 Some types of eye drops are supplied in unit-dose modules (blister packs), as shown here. (Solutions for nebulization are often packaged the same way.) (Photo Copyright © Caroline Bunker Rosdahl.)

> **Key Concept**
>
> Eye drops and ointments are instilled for various reasons—to contract or dilate the pupils, treat an infection, provide lubrication, or produce a local effect (e.g., anesthesia). Nurses are often responsible for carrying out the procedure and for instructing clients and their families in the procedure.

Ear (Otic) Administration

Ear (**otic**) medications may be given by instillation from a squeeze bottle or dropper. Occasionally, ear suppositories are used. To better visualize the ear canal and help ensure proper medication delivery, position the auditory canal correctly (see In Practice: Nursing Procedure 63-6). Position the squeeze bottle tip or dropper slightly above the ear canal while instilling the drops. Never insert the dropper or applicator tip into the ear canal.

Nasal or Respiratory Administration

Drugs may be given by drops, inhalation, or through nebulizer delivery systems for disorders of the respiratory tract. Some nasal medications have systemic effects as well.

Inhalants and Nebulizer Systems

Inhaled medications have a very rapid rate of absorption and onset of action. They may be delivered by inhaler or nebulizer delivery system.

> **Key Concept**
>
> An inhaler or nebulizer setup is used for one client only. It is kept in a sealed bag in the client's medication drawer or other designated place.
> *Rationale: This helps prevent cross-contamination.*

> **Nursing Alert** Never leave a client alone during nebulizer treatments, because of the effects of the medication. Encourage the client to breathe deeply, but not rapidly. *Rationale: Should the client breathe too rapidly, they may experience dizziness or possibly tetany (muscle spasms). This is the result of hyperventilation, caused by excess oxygen in the system.*

Handheld inhalers are devices that deliver a specific dose of topical medication to the mucous membranes of the respiratory system with each inhalation (Fig. 63-4). These inhalers are often called *metered-dose inhalers* (**MDIs**). Some inhalers deliver aerosolized medication; Diskus inhalers deliver nonaerosol powdered medication.

Medications delivered by handheld inhalers include

- Aerosol examples: albuterol (Proventil, Ventolin) and metaproterenol (Alupent).
- Nonaerosol inhalation powder examples: salmeterol (Serevent Diskus) and Advair Diskus (a combination of fluticasone and salmeterol).

Nebulizer treatments are based on the use of compressed air or oxygen, which forces a mist of medication through tubing to a mouthpiece or mask (Fig. 63-5). The client then inhales the medication. Nebulizer therapy is often administered by Respiratory Therapy personnel in the acute care facility. The treatment takes about 5 min. Many of the same medications available in the MDI form are available in nebulizer solutions. The advantage of the nebulizer over the MDI is that the medication mist is absorbed in the lungs better and the client will receive faster results. After initial setup in acute care facilities, nurses in long-term facilities or the client's home often regularly administer nebulizer treatments. Medications used for nebulizer treatments include albuterol, budesonide (Pulmicort), ipratropium (Atrovent), and levalbuterol tartrate (Xopenex).

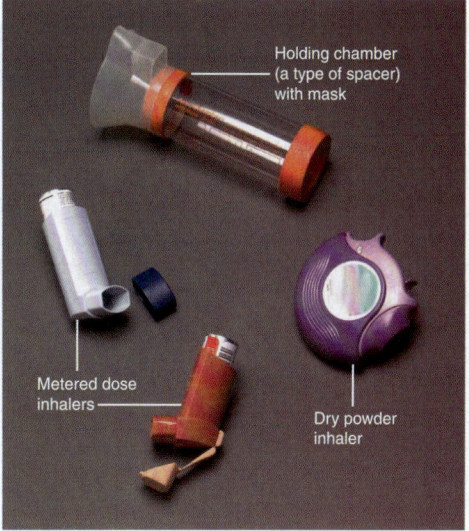

Figure 63-4 Handheld metered-dose inhaler (MDI), spacer, and dry powder inhaler (Taylor C, Lynn P, Bartlett J. *Fundamentals of Nursing, 9th edition*. Philadelphia, PA: Wolters Kluwer Health, 2018.).

> **Key Concept**
>
> As a nurse, you will often be required to teach clients or their families to perform nebulizer treatments. This is most common in pediatric nursing.
>
> In Practice: Nursing Care Guidelines 63-5 provides more information about administering inhaler and nebulizer medications.

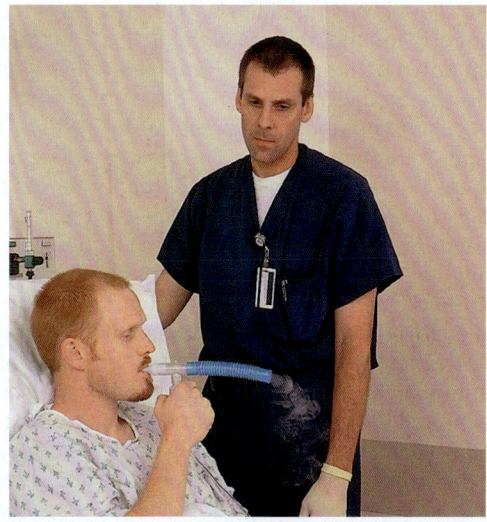

Figure 63-5 Administering a nebulizer treatment, using a flexible tube-type spacer. (Photo by B. Proud.)

IN PRACTICE
NURSING CARE GUIDELINES 63-5 — Administering Aerosolized and Powdered Respiratory Medications

General Information
- Follow the steps in Nursing Care Guidelines 63-1 and 63-2 before administering any medication.
- Wear gloves. Teach the client how to use their particular device and to check the device to see if there is remaining medication or is empty. The metered dose inhaler (MDI) can be shaken to see if medication remains. The Diskus shows a number indicating the number of remaining doses; if the number is zero, the device is empty.
- Avoid treatments immediately before and after meals. *Rationale: Avoiding these times helps decrease the chance of vomiting or appetite suppression, especially with medications that cause the client to cough or expectorate or those that are taken in conjunction with percussion/bronchial drainage.*
- If the client is to continue treatments at home, be sure they completely understand the medication and have demonstrated the ability to perform the treatment. *Rationale: At home, the client may not have access to teaching, which could result in incorrect dosing or inability to use or maintain the equipment.*
- Be sure to document all teaching and the client's ability to return your demonstrations.

For an Inhaler
- Shake the inhaler well immediately before use. *Rationale: Shaking aerosolizes the fine particles.*
- Instruct the client to take a deep breath and then to exhale completely through the nose. *Rationale: This empties the respiratory passages as much as possible so the medication will have the greatest effect.*
- Have the client position the inhaler just in front of their mouth, push down on the canister, and inhale as slowly and deeply as possible through the mouth. If the client is having difficulty with this, have the client grip the mouthpiece with the lips and then push down on the canister. *Rationale: These steps allow the medication to come into contact with mucous membranes of the respiratory system for the maximum amount of time. The inhaler will deliver a fine mist of medication into the oropharyngeal area, which the client will inhale into the lungs.*
- *Extenders,* also called *spacers* or *chambers,* are available to increase the volume of medication delivered (see Fig. 63-5). They deliver the medication into a closed chamber and increase the inhalation's effectiveness. In addition, this helps ensure that the client receives the complete dosage. When using a spacer, tell the client to close their lips around the mouthpiece and then depress the canister, releasing the medication. *Rationale: Closing the lips around the mouthpiece helps prevent unwanted escape of medication.*
- With either the inhaler alone, or when using a spacer, instruct the client to take and hold a deep breath or to take two to three short breaths. Each depression of the MDI directly into the client's mouth or into a spacer is considered to be one "puff." The healthcare provider usually orders one or two inhalations (puffs) several times a day. *Rationale: Deep breaths are required to move the medication as far into the respiratory tree as possible.*

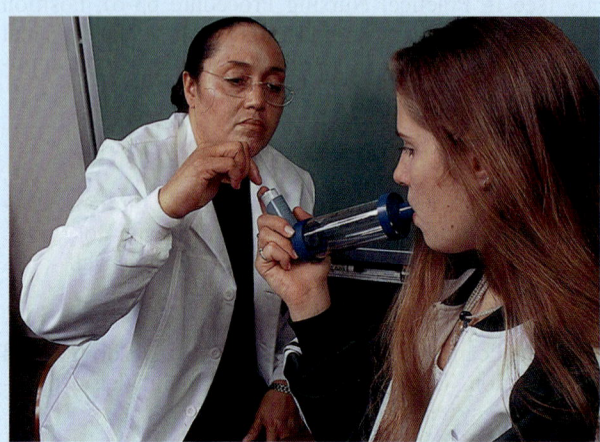

A chamber-type spacer may be used with a hand-held inhaler, to increase the effectiveness of the inhalation.

- Instruct the client to hold their breath for about 10 s and then slowly exhale with pursed lips. *Rationale: This helps the medication to be absorbed.*
- Repeat the above steps for each ordered "puff," waiting 5 to 10 min or as prescribed between puffs. *Rationale: This method achieves maximum benefits.*

For a Nebulizer
- Always inspect the nebulizer tubing for moisture. If moisture is present, replace the tubing. *Never wash nebulizer tubing. Rationale: Excess moisture could cause aspiration.*
- Fill the nebulizer cup with the ordered amount of medication. In the healthcare facility, these medications are often supplied in a blister pack (see Fig. 63-3). In the home, a multiuse bottle is often provided, which requires measuring. *Rationale: Use of a blister pack or measuring ensures that the required medication amount is given.*
- Turn on the oxygen or air at the prescribed liter flow. *The oxygen or air must be on before giving the mouthpiece to the client. Rationale: This aerosolizes the medication and forces it into the lungs.*
- Instruct the client to close the lips around the mouthpiece and breathe through the mouth (see Fig. 63-5). If the client is using a mask, they should breathe normally, with the mouth closed. *Rationale: Breathing through the mouth or normally with a mask helps the medication travel to the lungs.*

NURSING CARE GUIDELINES 63-5 Continued

- Instruct the client to continue the treatment until the mist can no longer be seen on exhalation (from the opposite end of the mouthpiece) or vent holes (in the mask). **Rationale:** Lack of mist indicates the client has inhaled the entire dose.
- Cleanse the nebulizer cup and mouthpiece with warm, soapy water. Rinse and dry it after each use. Follow facility protocols for the frequency of changing the tubing and cup for each client. Wash or sanitize your hands. **Rationale:** Proper cleaning and following guidelines decreases the possibility of pathogens entering the client's respiratory tract.

IN PRACTICE
NURSING CARE GUIDELINES 63-6 Administering Nasal Sprays or Drops

- Follow the steps in Nursing Care Guidelines 63-1 and 63-2 before administering any medication.
- Wear gloves. Scan the bar code on the medication bottle. Assist the client to a high Fowler or sitting position with the head tilted back.
- Place the tip of the bottle just inside the nares, aimed toward the nose's midline. Activate the nebulization or squeeze the bottle while the client inhales. **Rationale:** This position allows the medication to come into contact with nasal mucous membranes for maximal therapeutic effect.
- Offer the client a tissue. Instruct the client to maintain the position for approximately 1 to 2 min. **Rationale:** This position will inhibit drainage of the medication from the nares due to gravity flow.
- When administration is completed, always perform handwashing and document the procedure.

SPECIAL CONSIDERATIONS Lifespan

Aerosol and Inhalation Therapy

To ensure that a young child receives an accurate dose, hold the mouthpiece closely to the nose and mouth or use a mask.

Nasal Sprays or Drops

Nasal sprays or drops may be ordered for conditions such as nasal congestion or after nasal surgery (see In Practice: Nursing Care Guidelines 63-6).

Key Concept

Nose drops or sprays are used for one client only. They are labeled and kept in a plastic bag in the client's medication drawer or other designated area.

SPECIAL CONSIDERATIONS Lifespan

Administering Nasal Sprays or Drops

A child who must receive nasal medications may be more receptive if a family caregiver administers them. The child may be the most comfortable if held on a caregiver's lap during the procedure. If a family caregiver is unavailable, hold the child with the head tilted back while gently restraining the arms and legs. Make every effort to administer nasal medications with care. Be gentle and reassuring, especially for a small child.

Transdermal Administration

Many medications are now available in **transdermal** (**TD**) patches (Fig. 63-6). There are several types of TD patches. These include

- The reservoir membrane-modulated system
- The microreservoir system
- The drug-in-adhesive layer system
- The matrix system

As a general rule, it can be very dangerous to cut a TD patch. For example, if a reservoir membrane-modulated system patch is cut, the entire dose of medication is available immediately. This could cause a life-threatening overdose. If a microreservoir patch is cut, there is no accurate way to measure the dose available to the client. In some cases, the manufacturer describes a safe way to cut a patch, but *this is not a nursing decision*.

Many clients use nitroglycerin and hormone replacement patches (e.g., estrogen). Nicotine patches are commonly

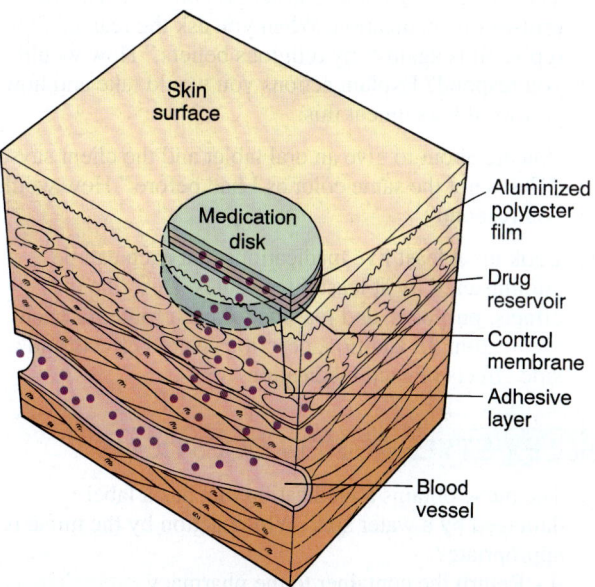

Figure 63-6 Structure and mechanism of action of a transdermal (TD) disk medication. Be sure not to tear or cut a TD patch (Timby, 2005).

used for smoking cessation. Another common transdermal patch is the fentanyl patch, used to manage pain. The skin absorbs these medications systemically (see Fig. 63-6). In Practice: Nursing Procedure 63-7 describes steps in administering a transdermal patch.

> **Nursing Alert** Some clients may tell you that their patch "fell off." It is important to make sure they do not have the old patch somewhere. *Rationale: Some clients are seeking double doses of medications, particularly nicotine or pain medications.*

STUDENT SYNTHESIS

KEY POINTS

- Because administration of medications is perhaps the single most important and potentially dangerous nursing function, follow the rules of safe administration precisely.
- The "Five Rights, Plus Two" of administration are the right client, right medication, right dosage, right time, right route, and right documentation, as well as right programming of medication pumps.
- Document all medications immediately *after* administering them.
- Local effects of a medication are restricted to the area in which they are administered. Topical medications often have local effects. Systemic effects spread throughout the body.
- STAT medications are to be given immediately; PRN medications are given as needed; bedtime (HS) medications are given in the evening to help clients sleep.
- Enteral administration means through the gastrointestinal (GI) system (most commonly, this is PO or via NG tube). Parenteral administration is administration by any other method; it most commonly refers to administration by injection.
- Enteral medication administration methods include oral, sublingual, translingual, buccal, and through a gastric tube. Rectal administration is technically considered enteral administration as well.

CRITICAL THINKING EXERCISES

1. You are ready to administer a medication to a client. The client is conscious and seems coherent. The client refuses the medication. When you ask the reason, they reply, "It is against my religious beliefs." How would you respond? Explain actions you would take and how you would document this.
2. You are about to give an oral tablet and the client says, "That's not the same color as I had before." How would you respond?
3. Look up at least five medications that each can be administered by at least three routes. Describe the effects, purposes, and reasons for each route for each medication. In addition, describe desired effects and side effects of each medication.

NCLEX-STYLE REVIEW QUESTIONS

1. The nurse obtains a medication that has a label damaged by a water spill. Which action by the nurse is appropriate?
   a. Return the container to the pharmacy.
   b. Change the label.
   c. Use the medication.
   d. Discard the medication in the trash.

2. The nurse is preparing to administer medications to a client but observes there is no identification bracelet. Which is the best action by the nurse?
   a. Take the client's word that he is who he says he is.
   b. Have another nurse identify the client.
   c. Do not administer the medication until the ID band has been replaced.
   d. Only administer the most important medication and then get the ID bracelet.

3. The nurse is administering medication to a client. The client states, "I don't take this medication." Which is the best response by the nurse?
   a. "You need to take your medication so that you can get well."
   b. "I will go and double check the order."
   c. "It probably doesn't look like the one you take at home, but I'm sure it's the same."
   d. "I will just document that you refuse the medicine."

4. The nurse is working on a busy acute care unit. At 1,300, a client states to the nurse, "I was supposed to take my medication with my meal at 9 o'clock." Which action by the nurse is appropriate?
   a. Inform the client that it is too late to take the medication now.
   b. Omit the dose for the day.
   c. Report the error to the charge nurse.
   d. Double the dose at 0900 the next morning with breakfast.

5. A client is scheduled to take a narcotic for pain, but when the nurse offers it, the client states it is not needed. How should the nurse dispose of the medication?
   a. Have another nurse witness and cosign the waste.
   b. Throw it in the trash in the client's room.
   c. Return the medication to the pharmacy.
   d. Pour the medication down the sink.

CHAPTER RESOURCES

Enhance your learning with additional resources on **the Point**!

Student Resources related to this chapter can be found at thePoint.lww.com/Rosdahl12e.

CHAPTER 63 Administration of Noninjectable Medications

Welcome Steps

Look at healthcare provider's orders.

Protocol for procedure.

Necessary equipment/supplies.

Wash hands using proper hand hygiene; put on gloves.

Explain the procedure and reassure the client.

Locate two identifiers to confirm correct client.

Comfortable and efficient position for nurse and client.

Obtain privacy.

Make sure to follow correct steps and body mechanics with good technique.

Ensure safety and observe deviations from normal.

End Steps

Ensure comfort and safety.

Note questions or concerns from client or nurse; note significant data.

Dispose of materials properly.

Disinfect the area and your hands.

Document and report the procedure and your findings.

IN PRACTICE

NURSING PROCEDURE 63-1 Administering Oral Medications

Supplies and Equipment
Medication scanner or MAR
Disposable medication cups (clear cups preferred)
Water or juice and drinking cup
Medication cart or unit-dose medications (per facility protocol)
Straws, if needed
Scissors, if needed
Spoon and juice or applesauce, if needed
Gloves, if needed
Hazardous waste container

Note: Follow steps in Nursing Care Guidelines 63-1 and 63-2 before proceeding.

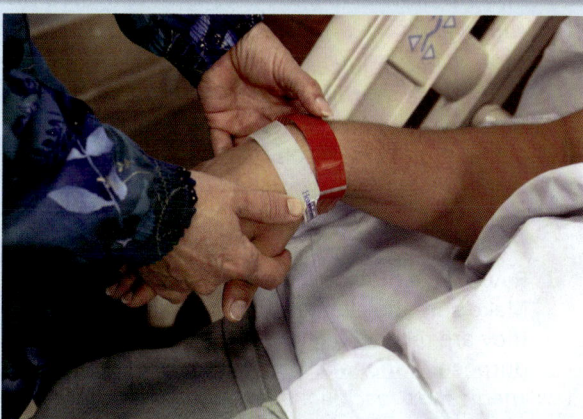

Checking the client's identification bracelet (Evans-Smith, 2005).

Steps

Follow LPN WELCOME steps and then

1. Take medication to the client. Give medication as close to the ordered time as possible. Carefully identify the client. *Rationale:* Agency policy usually considers 30 min before or after the ordered time as acceptable. Make sure you have the right client. "Check two for safety."

2. Complete necessary assessments before giving medications. *Rationale:* Checking helps reduce the risk of problems after drugs are administered. Ask the client about allergies, and assess blood pressure, apical pulse rate, or respiratory rate, depending on the medication's action.

3. Scan each medication package or double-check each. *Rationale: Make sure you have the correct medications. Scanning medications begins the process of electronic charting in the client's medical record and will alert you to any errors.*

4. Assist the client into sitting position. Scan the client's wrist band. *Rationale: Sitting as upright as possible makes swallowing medication easier and less likely to cause aspiration. Do not allow a client to swallow medication lying down unless absolutely necessary. In any case, the client must be very carefully monitored. The wrist band is the final check of client identity.*

5. Administer the medication:
   a. Ask the client how they prefer the medication (e.g., one at a time, all at once, from the cup or hand). *Rationale: Including the client's preferences involves the client in the process.*
   b. Open unit-dose medication packages. Often, it is easiest to transfer tablets from the package into a medication cup. Allow the client to see the packages. Cut open any packages that cannot be ripped. *Rationale: If the client can see the packages, they are less likely to question the medications. Some packages cannot be opened without scissors. If the client is paranoid, they may be allowed to open packages, with careful supervision.*
   c. Offer water or juice. Be aware of fluid or dietary restrictions. *Rationale: Fluids make swallowing solid medications easier. Be aware that clients from some cultures prefer room temperature water, rather than ice water. Bring a large cup of water if several pills are to be given. Usually, juice is not offered to clients with diabetes.*
   d. Review the medication's name and purpose. Make sure the client knows what medications they are receiving and can tell you their purpose. *Rationale: Use this opportunity for medication teaching. It is important that the client know about their medications.*
   e. Assist the client to put tablets in their mouth or take crushed medications in food with a spoon, if necessary.
   f. Mix powder medications with fluids at the bedside. Stir thoroughly. The client may want to use a straw, if permitted. *Rationale: Powdered forms of drugs may thicken when mixed with fluid; give them immediately.*
   g. Discard any medication that falls on the floor. *Rationale: This medication is contaminated.*

6. Observe the client swallowing the medication. Check the client's mouth, if necessary. *Rationale: This ensures that the client has taken the medication and does not choke. Some clients hide medication between the gum and cheek (called "cheeking"). Leaving medication at the bedside is unsafe and illegal.*

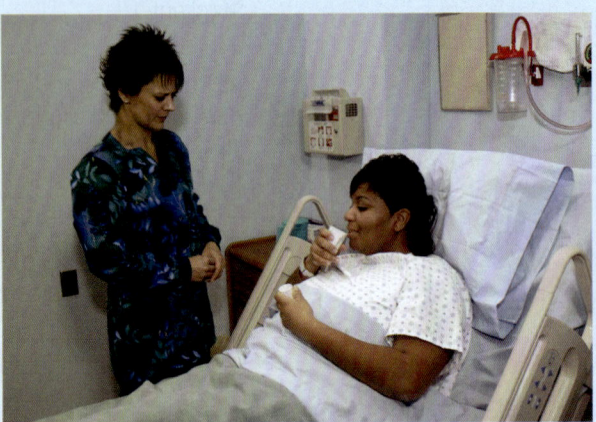

Observing the client swallowing the medication (Evans-Smith, 2005).

7. Indicate "accept" on the scanner or chart the administration on the MAR. *Rationale: This records the medication in the client's record.*

8. Record fluid intake if the client is on intake and output (I&O). *Rationale: This maintains accurate documentation.*

Follow ENDDD steps

Special Reminders
- Documentation includes specific assessments, such as blood pressure or pulse, depending on the medication given.
- Check the client within 30 min after giving medication. This is particularly important following pain medication or any PRN (as needed) medication. *Rationale: Follow-up after administration verifies the client's response, particularly pain relief, after administration of an analgesic.*
- Double-check the chart, to make sure the scanner has functioned properly or you have recorded properly.

IN PRACTICE
NURSING PROCEDURE 63-2 Administering Medications Through a Gastrointestinal Tube

Supplies and Equipment
Medication scanner or MAR
Gloves
Medication
Large syringe
Fluids, as needed

Stethoscope
Mortar and pestle or pill crusher, if there is an order to crush medications
Hazardous waste container

Note: Follow steps in Nursing Care Guidelines 63-1 and 63-2 before proceeding.

Steps
Follow LPN WELCOME steps and then

1. If there is an order to crush or otherwise prepare medications, do this before beginning the procedure. (Scan the packages first.) Do not crush time-release, enteric-coated, or orally disintegrating tablets (ODTs). *Rationale: It is important to complete the procedure as quickly as possible, to maintain client comfort. Crushing special tablets may alter the dosing or effectiveness of the medication.*

2. Place the client in a high Fowler position and verify placement of the tube.
   a. Wear gloves. Using a syringe, aspirate the nasogastric (NG) tube gently. Stomach contents should return. Do not aspirate button-type gastrostomy (G-tube) or jejunal tube (J-tube). *Rationale: Aspiration could damage the antireflux valve of the G-tube or J-tube.*
   b. Check placement of the NG tube again or check placement of G-tube or J-tube by placing the stethoscope over upper aspect of the stomach. Quickly insert several milliliters of air. You should be able to hear the air enter the stomach. *Rationale: Correct placement of the tube ensures that medication will be delivered into the stomach and not the lungs.*

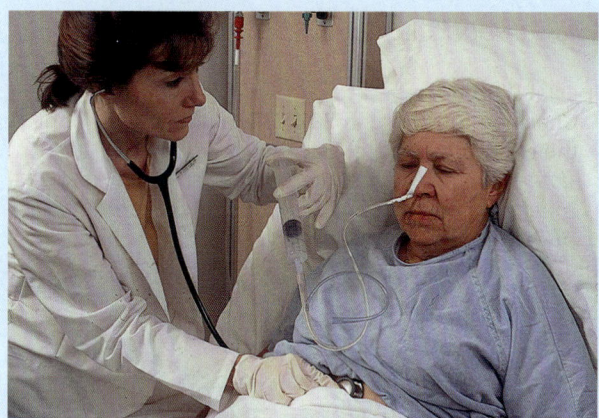

Checking placement of the NG tube with a stethoscope.

   c. If the tube is not in the stomach, *do not instill the medication.* Stop the procedure and check with the provider. *Rationale: If the tube has migrated to a lung, instilling air will not cause harm; instilling medication would cause aspiration into the lung and could be life threatening.*

3. After checking the tubing's placement, clamp the tubing and remove the syringe. *Rationale: Clamping the tube prevents gastric contents from escaping through the tubing and ensures that no air enters the stomach, causing client discomfort.*

4. Remove the plunger from the syringe first and then reconnect the syringe to the tube. *Rationale: The syringe will deliver the medication into the tube. If you remove the plunger while it is still in the tube, it will aspirate stomach contents.*

5. Pour 15 to 30 mL plain water into the open syringe and release the clamp. Let the water flow in by gravity. It should flow freely. *Note:* If water does not flow freely down the tube, insert the plunger of the syringe and *gently* apply a *slight* pressure to start the flow. *Rationale: Instilling water flushes the tube and reduces the surface tension within the lumen of the tube. If the tube is slightly plugged, sometimes a small amount of pressure will start the flow.*

6. If flow does not start, the tube may be plugged. If you have questions, report the situation and consult the provider or team leader. Do not force medication into the tube! *Rationale: Forcing medication into a plugged tube could cause serious intestinal damage.*

7. Pour medication into the open syringe. *Note:* NG medication is usually diluted. Follow the facility protocol. Instill each medication separately and flush the tubing with 5 to 10 mL of water between each instillation. Do not let the syringe become empty before or between instillations. It may be necessary to reinsert the plunger into the syringe. *Rationale: Flushing the tube ensures that all medication is administered and that the medications do not interact with each other or plug the tube. If the syringe becomes empty, air will enter the stomach, causing discomfort. The medication may be thick and the plunger may be needed, to facilitate the flow of liquid medications.*

8. After administering all medication, flush the tube with approximately 30 mL of water. *Rationale: Flushing clears the tube and decreases the chance of tube blockage. It also ensures that all medication was given.*

9. Clamp the tubing and remove the syringe. If the tubing will be reconnected to suction, replace the plug on the tubing. The tube should remain clamped for *at least 30 min.* If a continuous NG feeding is to be given, the tubing can be reconnected to the tube feeding immediately. *Rationale: Clamping the tubing and then removing the syringe prevents excessive air from entering the tubing. If suction will be reconnected, it is necessary to clamp the tubing, to allow absorption of the medications. Otherwise, the medication would be suctioned out immediately and would not be absorbed. If a feeding will be given, the medications will not be suctioned out. Reconnecting the feeding reestablishes the client's nutrition.*

10. Keep the head of the bed elevated for at least 30 min after administering medications. *Rationale: This helps prevent aspiration into the lungs.*

Follow ENDDD steps

Note: Check back with the client after about 20 min, to determine effectiveness of the medication and check for discomfort.

IN PRACTICE

NURSING PROCEDURE 63-3 Administering a Rectal Suppository

Supplies and Equipment
Medication scanner or MAR
Gloves
Medication (suppository)
Lubricant, if needed
Applicator, if needed
Scissors
Hazardous waste container

Note: Follow steps in Nursing Care Guidelines 63-1 and 63-2 before proceeding.

Steps
Follow LPN WELCOME steps and then

1. Assist the client to the Sims position and cover the client as much as possible. Generally, the left-side lying position is preferable. Wear gloves. *Rationale: This position provides easy visualization of, and access to, the rectum.*

2. Leave the suppository in the refrigerator as long as possible before the procedure, unless it is a nonrefrigerated type. Cut the wrapper off the suppository. *Rationale: The suppository will retain its shape better if it is cold. By the time it is inserted, it will not be uncomfortably cold. Cutting the wrapper or foil helps preserve the shape of the suppository. (Squeezing the suppository out of the wrapper melts it and distorts the shape.)*

3. Lubricate the suppository, if necessary. Wearing gloves, insert the suppository into the client's anal canal, pointed end first. It is inserted at least 4 in. for an adult and 2 in. for a child. You should be able to feel the suppository pass through the anal sphincter as you insert the suppository. *Rationale: Inserting it this far ensures placement of the suppository above the client's internal sphincter and helps the client to retain it, maximizing medication absorption.*

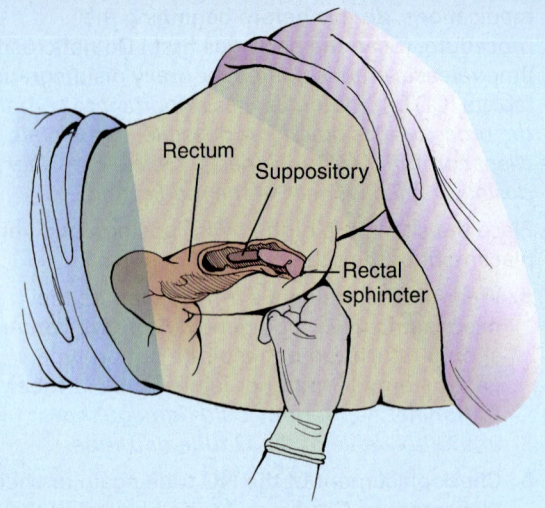

Inserting the rectal suppository past the internal anal sphincter against the rectal wall, with gloved finger (Timby, 2005).

4. Ask the client to maintain the Sims position for 15 to 20 min and not to expel the suppository. *Rationale: Maintaining the position allows time for the suppository to melt and release the medication.*

Follow ENDDD steps

Special Reminder
- Check on the client in 20 to 30 min and document the client's response. *Rationale: Follow-up determines if the medication was effective and maintains communication with other members of the healthcare team.*

IN PRACTICE

NURSING PROCEDURE 63-4 Administering a Vaginal Suppository

Supplies and Equipment
Medication scanner or MAR
Gloves
Medication
Lubricant, if needed
Applicator, if needed
Scissors
Hazardous waste container

Note: Follow steps in Nursing Care Guidelines 63-1 and 63-2 before proceeding.

Steps
Follow LPN WELCOME steps and then

1. Position the client in the modified lithotomy position (on her back). *Rationale: This position enables visualization of the vaginal area and easy access for insertion of the suppository.*

2. Prepare the medication and/or applicator. Scan the medication package.
   a. Cut the foil wrapper off the suppository. If the suppository is to be placed with an applicator,

place it on the end of the applicator. ***Rationale:*** *Cutting the wrapper or foil helps preserve the suppository's shape. Squeezing it out of the foil melts it and distorts the shape. The applicator helps with insertion of the suppository.*

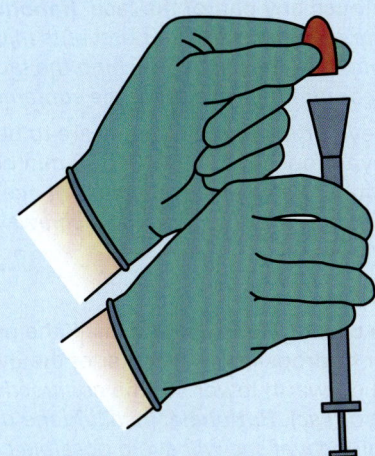

Positioning the vaginal suppository in the applicator (Timby, 2005).

    b. If vaginal cream is to be used with an applicator, draw the cream up into the applicator. Pull out the plunger to the "fill" line.

3. Insert the medication.

    a. Wear gloves. If using an applicator, insert it into the vagina, just past the sphincter (about 2-3 in.). Push in the plunger to instill the cream or the suppository.

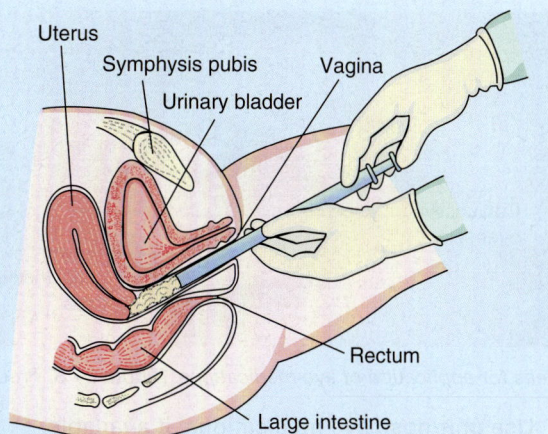

Inserting vaginal cream, using an applicator (Evans-Smith, 2005).

    b. If inserting a suppository without an applicator, insert the suppository approximately 2 to 3 in. into the vagina, using your gloved finger. ***Rationale:*** *Proper placement will ensure absorption.*

4. Instruct the client to remain on her back for 15 to 20 min. ***Rationale:*** *This position will maximize retention and absorption of the suppository.*

5. Offer the client a sanitary pad. ***Rationale:*** *It will absorb excess drainage and protect the client and bed.*

Follow ENDDD steps

Note: Check back with the client after about 20 min, to determine the effectiveness of the medication or check for discomfort.

IN PRACTICE
NURSING PROCEDURE 63-5   Administering Eye Medications

Supplies and Equipment
Medication scanner or MAR
Goggles or face shield, if needed
Medication (with dropper), if needed
Clean cotton balls
Gloves
Disposable tissues
Separate droppers for each eye (if droppers are used)
Hazardous waste container

Note: Follow steps in Nursing Care Guidelines 63-1 and 63-2 before proceeding.

Steps
Follow LPN WELCOME steps and then

1. Ask the client to lie down or sit with the head tilted backward. Medications will be instilled into the lower conjunctival sac. ***Rationale:*** *This position will help facilitate instillation and dispersion of medication.*

2. Provide the client with two tissues, if both eyes are to be treated. ***Rationale:*** *There may be an overflow of medication or tears. A separate tissue should be used for each eye.*

3. Wear gloves. If administering medication to both eyes, use a separate clean cotton ball, moistened with water, to clean each eyelid and the lashes, if they contain debris. Wipe gently from the inner canthus to the outer canthus. Wash your hands before and after treating each eye. Wear goggles if there is any possibility of splashing of fluids. ***Rationale:*** *These actions clean the eyelids. Using a separate cotton ball for each eye helps prevent the spread of infection from one eye to the other. Wiping from inner to outer canthus moves debris away from the nasolacrimal ducts. Goggles protect the nurse.*

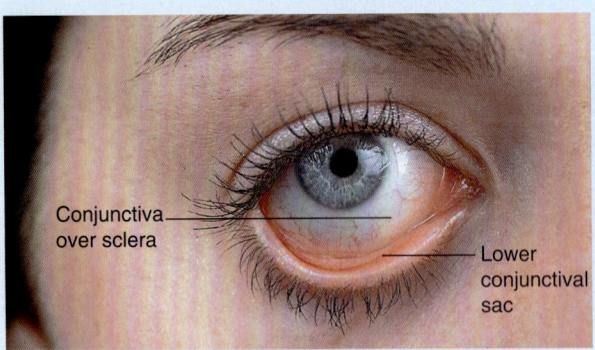

Areas for application of eye medications. (Photo by B. Proud.)

4. Use unit-dose eye medications, if available. However, many eye medications come in multiuse tubes or bottles. In this case, they are used more than once for a *single client*. The medication must be labeled specifically for the client and kept in a plastic bag with the client's other medications. ***Rationale:*** *Stock supply eye medications are to be used for only one client to prevent cross-contamination between clients. In some cases, a separate bottle is labeled for each eye.*

5. Check the bottle's label; do not instill any medication in the eye unless it is labeled *ophthalmic.* Make sure the label is readable. ***Rationale:*** *The only type of medication that can be safely used in the eye is that labeled specifically as ophthalmic. Other medications could endanger the client's vision. Fluid might have damaged the label.*

6. Warm eye drops or ointments, by holding them in your hand, if they have not been stored at room temperature. ***Rationale:*** *Cold eye medications are very uncomfortable for the client.*

7. Instruct the client to look toward the ceiling. Move the container from below the client's line of vision or from the side. ***Rationale:*** *These actions help prevent the client from blinking as the medication is instilled.*

8. Gently retract the lower eyelid with the first two fingers of your nondominant hand. You can also gently pinch the lower eyelid together to form a sac. Do not press on the eyeball. Apply gentle pressure on the cheek bone. ***Rationale:*** *Pulling on or pinching together the lower eyelid exposes the lower conjunctival sac, allowing for proper medication administration. Pressure on the cheek bone anchors the fingers holding the eyelid.*

9. Brace your dominant hand on the bone over the eyebrow while instilling drops or ointment. Do not touch the eye with any part of the container. Do not touch any part of the face. ***Rationale:*** *This helps steady your hand and prevents injury and/or discomfort for the client. Touching the face or eye would contaminate the tip of the container.*

10. If both eye drops and ointments are to be given, instill eye drops first. Allow 5 to 10 min between instillations. ***Rationale:*** *Instillation of eye drops after ointments would tend to wash away ointment.*

For eye drops

11. Ask the client to look up, and instill the prescribed number of drops into the center of the *everted* (turned outward) lower lid (the *conjunctival surface or sac*). ***Rationale:*** *Instilling the drops into the conjunctival sac will avoid possible corneal injury.*

12. Instruct the client to close the eyelids and place gentle pressure on the inner canthus (near the bridge of the nose) after instilling eye drops. Maintain this pressure for 1 to 2 min. ***Rationale:*** *Applying gentle pressure helps prevent the solution from draining into the lacrimal duct. It also minimizes the risk of systemic effects or bacteria being washed into the lacrimal duct. Closing the eyelid while applying gentle pressure facilitates better distribution of medication.*

13. Gently pat off excess medication with a clean cotton ball or tissue. ***Rationale:*** *It is important to prevent irritating the eye or spreading infection.*

14. If ordered, repeat the procedure for the other eye. Use separate tissues or cotton balls for each eye. Use separate droppers, if ordered. ***Rationale:*** *It is important to prevent spreading infection from eye to eye.*

For eye ointments

15. Before administration, wipe the tube with a clean cotton ball and discard a small amount of ointment. ***Rationale:*** *Discarding the first portion of ointment maintains the ointment's sterility.*

16. Apply the ointment inside the lower lid, in a thin line, from inner to outer canthus. Ask the client to blink a few times. ***Rationale:*** *The medication is placed into the lower conjunctival sac. Blinking aids in medication distribution.*

CHAPTER 63 Administration of Noninjectable Medications

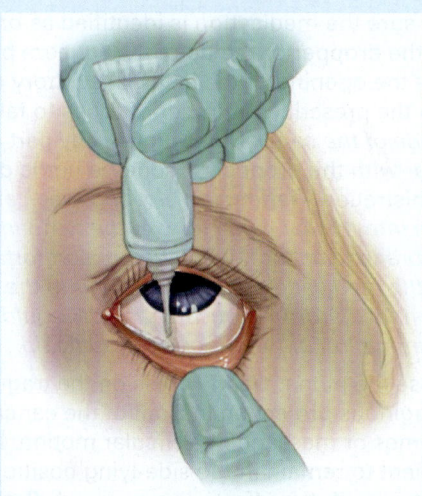

Applying a narrow ribbon of eye ointment within the lower conjunctival sac (Kyle, T., Carman, S. (2012). Essentials of pediatric nursing (2nd ed.). Wolters Kluwer Health.).

17. Use a clean cotton ball or tissue to wipe away any excess medication. Repeat for the other eye, if ordered. **Rationale:** *Removing excess ointment provides client comfort.*

Follow ENDDD steps

Note: Check back with the client after about 20 min, to determine the effectiveness of the medication or check for discomfort.

IN PRACTICE
NURSING PROCEDURE 63-6 Administering Ear Medications

Supplies and Equipment
Medication scanner or MAR
Disposable tissues
Medication
Cotton balls
Gloves
Hazardous waste container

Note: Follow steps in Nursing Care Guidelines 63-1 and 63-2 before proceeding.

Steps
Follow LPN WELCOME steps and then

1. Ask the client to lie on the side of the unaffected ear. Wear gloves. **Rationale:** *This position facilitates instillation of medication into the affected ear.*
2. Remove excess drainage with a dry wipe or cotton ball. If the drainage has dried, use a damp, warm washcloth to clean the area. **Rationale:** *Dried drainage or crusting may limit the medication's effectiveness. Removal of debris aids in client comfort.*
3. Expose the external ear canal by properly adjusting the client's ear lobe. For adults, pull the lobe up, back, and outward. For children older than 3 years, pull the lobe straight back. For children younger than 3 years, pull the lobe down and back. **Rationale:** *Proper positioning of the ear facilitates delivery of medication into the external auditory canal.*

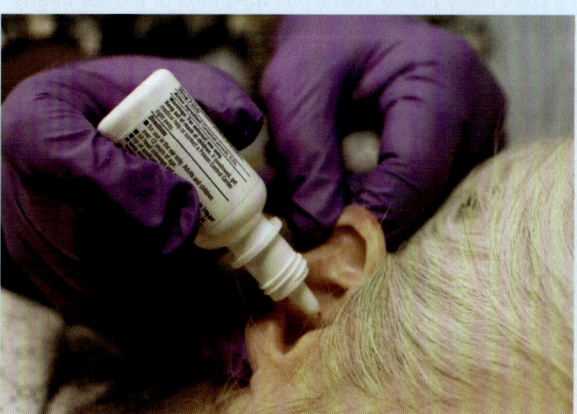

Position for administering ear drops. Wear gloves. In an adult, pull the pinna of the ear up and back to straighten the ear canal. Hold the tip of the bottle above the auditory canal opening (Evans-Smith, 2005).

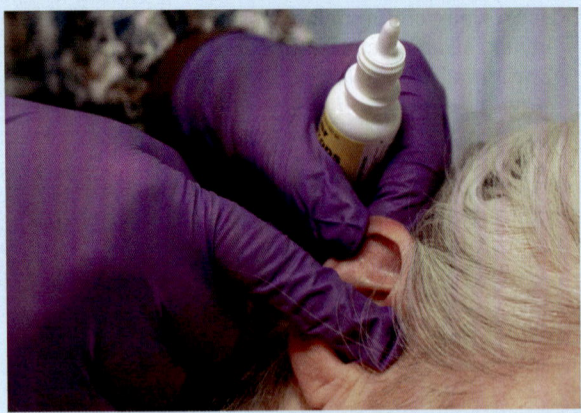

Gently press or massage the tragus and ask the client to remain on the side for a short time (Evans-Smith, 2005).

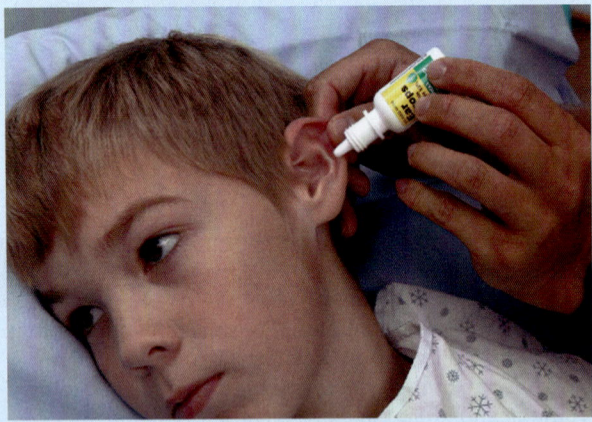

In a child older than 3 years, pull the pinna of the ear nearly straight back to straighten the ear canal (Evans-Smith, 2005).

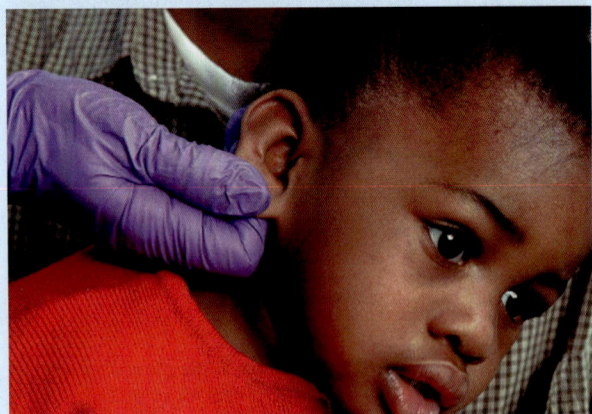

In a child younger than 3 years, pull the pinna down and back (Evans-Smith, 2005).

4. Make sure the medication is identified as *otic*. Hold the dropper or the tip of the squeeze bottle above the opening of the external auditory canal. Allow the prescribed number of drops to fall *on the side of the canal.* Do not touch any part of the ear with the dropper or squeeze bottle during administration. **Rationale:** *Allowing medication to run into the ear canal toward the tympanic membrane (eardrum) will be more comfortable than the medication falling directly into the canal and on the eardrum. Touching the ear could cause contamination of the dropper or bottle tip.*

5. Release the pinna. *Gently* press on the tragus (the cartilaginous projection in front of the ear canal) a few times or massage in a circular motion. Instruct the client to remain in the side-lying position for 5 to 10 min with the affected ear upward. **Rationale:** *Pressure on the tragus causes medication to move toward the eardrum. The side-lying position also helps the medication to run into the ear canal, for maximum effectiveness.*

6. If ordered, place a cotton ball into the external ear. **Rationale:** *This will help to keep the medication from running out of the ear.*

7. If the procedure is ordered for both ears, allow 5 to 10 min between instillations. Repeat the above steps for the other ear. **Rationale:** *Waiting allows medication to come into adequate contact with the first ear (and not to run out) before the second ear is treated.*

Perform ENDDD steps

Note: Check back with the client after about 20 min, to determine the effectiveness of the medication or check for discomfort.

IN PRACTICE

NURSING PROCEDURE 63-7: Administering a Transdermal Patch

Supplies and Equipment
Medication patch
Scissors
Gloves
Medication scanner or MAR
Permanent marking pen
Hazardous waste container

Note: Follow steps in Nursing Care Guidelines 63-1 and 63-2 before proceeding.

Steps
Follow LPN WELCOME steps and then

1. Wear gloves during the entire procedure, including preparation of the patch. *Rationale: Because the patch contains medication that can be absorbed through the skin, you need to protect yourself from absorbing any medication.*

2. Check with the team leader if the provider does not indicate the area of patch placement. The order will include the dosage and frequency of patch replacement (e.g., every 12 hr, daily, weekly, monthly). *Rationale: Patches such as nicotine patches are often replaced daily. Other patches, such as those for fertility control, are replaced monthly. Some patches used for pain control, such as lidocaine (Lidoderm), are on for 12 hr and then off for 12 hr. (In this case, be sure to document "on" and "off" times.) Be aware that some patches are given in reducing (tapering-down) dosages, as well.*

3. Note carefully the location of the current patch before removing it. Be sure to cleanse the skin carefully after removal. *Rationale: It is important to rotate sites for patch placement. Patches may irritate the skin.*

4. Remove the old patch before placing the new patch. *Rationale: Leaving the previous patch in place may result in an increased and undesired dosage of medication.*

5. Using a clean scissors, cut open the package, following the "cut" mark indicated. Be very careful not to cut into the patch itself. *Rationale: These packages are designed so they will not rip. Ripping, tearing, or cutting into the patch can distort the patch and release medication inappropriately. The scissors must be used to cut the package before cutting anything else, to maintain cleanliness.*

6. It may be necessary to trim excess hair from the intended site. Cut hair after cutting the patch package. *Rationale: Patch removal is painful if excess hair is present. Hair may also interfere with medication absorption. The patch must remain uncontaminated.*

7. Take the patch from the package and remove its backing. *Rationale: The back of the patch contains adhesive. This must be exposed so the patch will stick to the skin.*

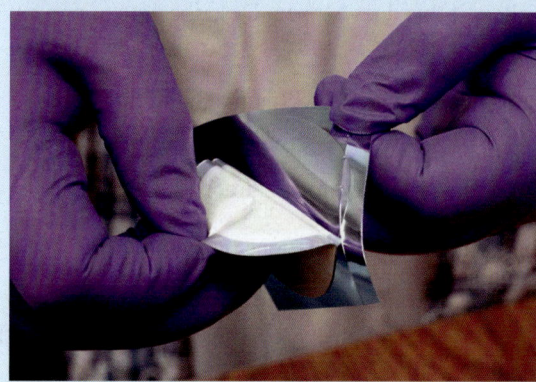

Removing backing from transdermal patch (Evans-Smith, 2005).

8. Place the patch on a clean, dry, hairless area. *Rationale: Moisture and hair interfere with patch adherence and comfort.*

9. Press firmly on all parts of the new patch, to position it firmly in place. *Rationale: The body area where the patch is applied may affect its absorption rate. It is important to press firmly, so the patch will adhere.*

10. Use a permanent marking pen to indicate the date and time the patch was applied and your initials. Document the patch placement. *Rationale: It is important to monitor patch placement. Your initials allow others to know who applied the patch and when.*

11. The proper way to dispose of a transdermal patch is to fold it over on itself and dispose of it in the designated hazardous waste container. *Rationale: This prevents any medication from being transferred to another worker or into the environment.*

Follow ENDDD steps

Note: Check back with the client after about 20 min, to determine the effectiveness of the medication or check for discomfort.

> **Nursing Alert** Cutting a transdermal patch does NOT reduce the dose. It may actually increase the dose, because the medication is able to escape faster than intended. Do not cut TD patches!

64 Administration of Injectable Medications

Learning Objectives

1. Describe different types of syringes and parts of a syringe. State the intended use of each type of syringe.
2. State the hazards of needlestick injury and procedures to follow if this does happen. Describe how to prevent needlestick accidents with safety syringes and with nonsafety syringes.
3. Demonstrate the proper technique for administering intradermal, subcutaneous, and intramuscular injections.
4. Identify the procedure for a Z-track injection; state when it is used.
5. Identify nursing considerations related to total parenteral nutrition.
6. Describe how to flush a saline lock, as well as how to administer medications, discontinue a lock, and cap off an existing IV into a lock.
7. Describe medication administration via IV piggyback, volume-controlled infusion, and existing IV infusion.
8. Describe accurate programming of the IV pump or electronic IV controller used in your facility.
9. Describe the role of the nurse in assisting with venipuncture; describe the process of venipuncture.
10. State the most common signs of IV infiltration and what actions to take.
11. Describe the role of the nurse in management of IVs, within the legal scope of practice.
12. Describe the process of setting up an intravenous infusion.

Important Terminology

ampule
bolus
butterfly needle
central line
diluents
induration
infiltration
infusion
intradermal
intramuscular
intravenous
needleless system
phlebitis
phlebotomy
piggyback infusion
prefilled syringe
saline lock
subcutaneous
tourniquet
transfusion
vacutainer
venipuncture
vial
Z-track (zig-zag)

Acronyms

$D_5 1/2NS$
$D_5 NS$
$D_5 W$
G
ID
IM
IV
IVF
IVPB
KVO
NaCl
NS
PCA
PICC
SubQTKO
TPN
VAD

The administration of medications via injection or **intravenous** (IV) infusion is more invasive than administration by mouth, rectum, or transdermally. This chapter introduces concepts of medication administration by injection. Be aware that regulations vary among states and provinces related to procedures legally performed by a licensed practical nurse or licensed vocational nurse (LVN/LPN). Injection is a method of introducing liquid medications within body tissues. Common methods of injection include intradermal, subcutaneous (**SubQ**), intramuscular (**IM**), and intravenous (**IV**). Other methods include *intracardiac* (within the heart), *intramedullary* (within the spinal cord), *intrathecal* (into the subarachnoid space around the spinal cord), *intraosseous* (within bone), and *intraperitoneal* (within the peritoneal cavity) (see Table 63-1). Only certain licensed primary providers can legally use the latter routes; therefore, they are not addressed in this text.

Although the nurse may give injections by various routes, general principles apply for every method. Because any injection is an invasive procedure, new sterile equipment is always used to avoid introducing pathogens into the client's body and disposed of after use. In addition, the nurse must be protected against exposure to the client's body fluids.

A medication may be administered by injection for several reasons:

- The medication is most effective by injection.
- The medication is unavailable in any other form.
- The client needs the desired action quickly.
- Dosage accuracy is critical; the client must obtain the entire dose.
- The client is nauseated or vomiting and cannot retain oral medications.
- The client's mental or physical condition renders them unable or unwilling to swallow oral medications.
- The digestive system cannot absorb the drug.

In most cases, the body absorbs injected medications more quickly than it absorbs oral medications. Generally, IV injection achieves the fastest method of systemic absorption.

The nurse must know appropriate administration sites and specific actions of medications being injected. For example, accidental injection into a nerve could result in damage and/or paralysis. Injection directly into a blood vessel could cause the medication to be absorbed too rapidly, with an adverse, possibly fatal, reaction. Failure to inject certain medications, such as injectable steroids, into deep muscle

CHAPTER 64 Administration of Injectable Medications

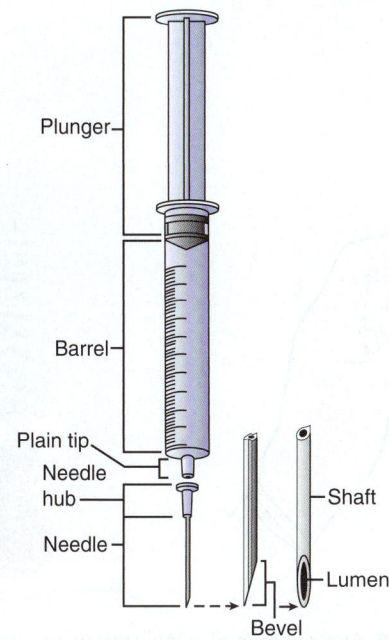

Figure 64-1 Parts of a syringe (*plain tip*) and needle.

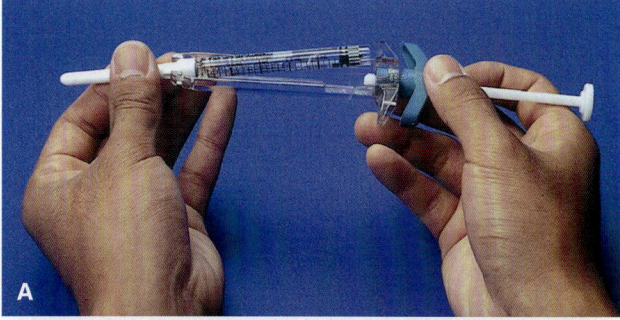

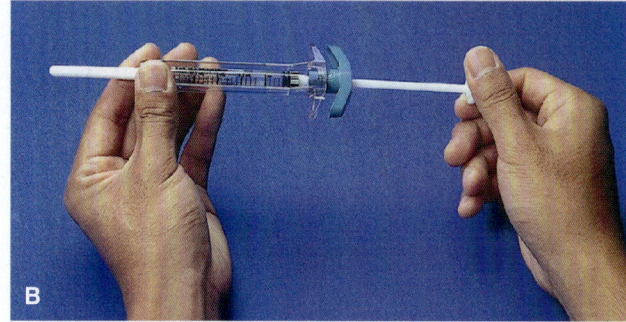

Figure 64-2 Using prefilled syringes. **A.** The prefilled cartridge is inserted into the holder/injection device. **B.** The plunger section is positioned over the cartridge and screwed on to tighten it, to hold the cartridge in place. The cartridge may need to be pushed firmly into place (to break its seal) before injection. The injection is then given as with any syringe. Shown is not a safety syringe; the needle must be protected after use (see Fig. 64-4B).

tissue may cause tissue atrophy, with resultant pitting or deformity. Neglecting to rotate insulin injection sites often causes tissue atrophy and indentation (*lipodystrophy*).

SYRINGES AND NEEDLES

Syringes

Disposable syringes are available in various sizes, ranging from 0.5- to 100-mL capacity. They consist of three parts: tip, barrel, and plunger (Fig. 64-1). The *tip* is the portion of the syringe attached to the needle or needleless adaptor. A syringe may have either a Luer–Lok or plain tip (shown in the figure). The *barrel* is clearly marked with a calibrated measurement scale. When preparing an injection, the medication is drawn into the barrel section. The *plunger* is the inner portion that fits inside the barrel. The plunger is pulled out to create a vacuum and withdraw medication; it is pushed in to inject medication. Milliliters are subdivided into tenths on the barrel of the syringe. The volume of medication drawn into the syringe is read at the point where the rubber flange of the plunger is even or parallel with the marked measurement scale on the barrel.

Some syringes contain a needle; others do not and the needle must be attached separately. Other syringes, called *cartridges* or prefilled syringes, contain premeasured amounts of medication. One type of prefilled syringe is shown in Figure 64-2. This cartridge-type unit is inserted into a reusable holder containing a plunger.

Needles

Needles are also disposable and consist of three parts: hub, shaft, and beveled tip (see Fig. 64-1). The *hub* or *hilt* attaches to the tip of the syringe. The *shaft* is the elongated portion. The *bevel* (area containing the hole or bore) can vary from regular bevel (long, allowing for easy entry through the skin) to intradermal bevel (blunt, used exclusively for intradermal injections). Needles usually are made of stainless steel and come in various sizes. The needle's gauge and length are both important when choosing the correct type for injection. The gauge (**G**) is the needle's inner diameter (bore), through which medication is administered. The gauge is stated using numbers. *The larger the number, the smaller the bore.* A 25-G needle has a very small opening and would be used for SubQ or intradermal (**ID**) injections; a 23-G needle, which has a larger bore, may be used for IM injections of more viscous (thicker) liquids; an 18-G needle has a very large bore and may be used for IV injection of large amounts of medication. Insulin syringes are marked differently (regularly 100 U/mL) and are not used for anything but insulin (see Fig. 64-3 and Chapter 79). Needles commonly used range in length from 3/8 to 2 in. The SubQ injection is given with a short needle (usually 3/8 in. in length); an IM injection requires a longer needle, with a larger bore, to ensure delivery into muscle tissue. Although the provider's order identifies the type of injection, needle size depends on the medication's volume (amount) and viscosity. Additionally, some medications, such as steroids, need to be injected deep into muscles and, therefore, will need longer needles for accurate delivery.

Needles and syringes are packaged in sterile wrappers. Be sure to maintain their sterility (see Chapter 57). Check to ensure wrappers are intact. Also, check expiration dates. If in doubt, obtain a different syringe and/or needle.

980 UNIT 9 Pharmacology and Administration of Medications

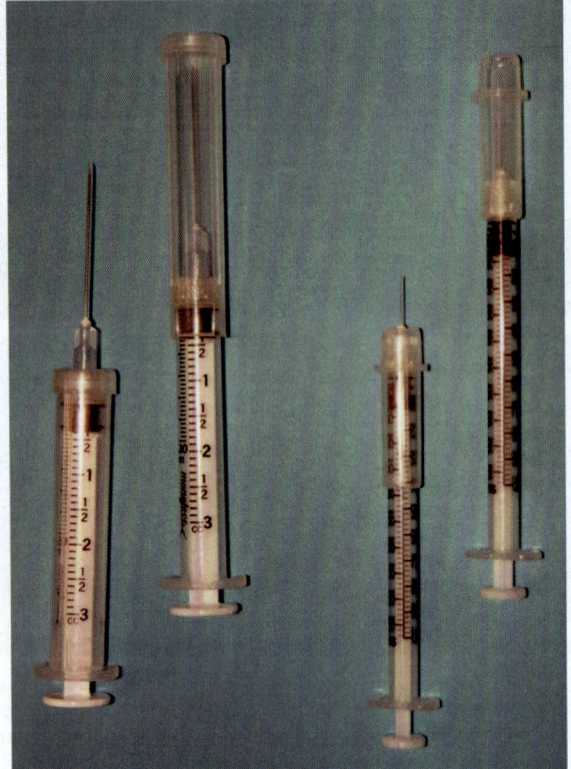

Figure 64-3 One type of safety syringe. After drawing up the solution to be injected or drawing blood, the sheath is pulled straight out, clicked into place, but not locked. This covers the needle while it is transported. The sheath is retracted straight back to administer the injection and is again pulled out and *twisted* to lock it in place, when the injection is completed. Needles are not recapped. Shown are a 3-mL syringe with a 22-G, 1.5-in. needle (for IM injections), and a 1-mL insulin syringe with a 29-G, 0.5-in. needle. Each is shown with the sheath retracted and with the sheath in place. (Photo Copyright © Caroline Bunker Rosdahl.)

> **Nursing Alert** *Always dispose of all syringes and needles in the sharps container provided (even if the injection was not given).* This helps prevent needlestick injuries to nurses and environmental personnel. A needlestick injury can cause serious infections and/or other disabilities.

The Safety Syringe

Most syringe-and-needle combinations are a type of *safety syringe*. One type has a plastic sheath that is pulled down to protect the needle after drawing up medication and again after administering the medication (Fig. 64-3). The circular sheath will click into place, but will not lock if pulled straight out. When ready to give the injection, the sheath is pushed straight back until it clicks. After giving the injection, the sheath is pulled out and *twisted until it clicks*. This will lock it into place; now it cannot be retracted.

The articulated sheath is often found on prefilled syringes or prepackaged needles. In this case, the needle is protected by a sterile needle cover, which is removed when the injection is given. After the injection is given, the index finger pushes the sheath over the needle (Fig. 64-4A). The sheath

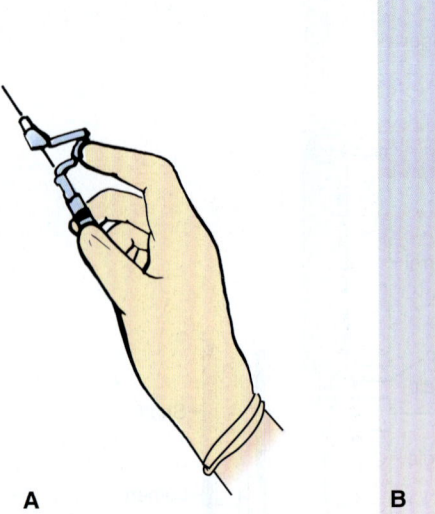 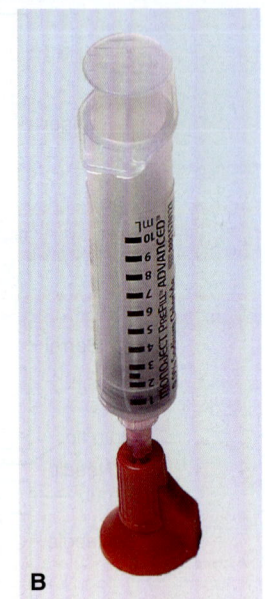

Figure 64-4 A. Another type of safety syringe has an articulated, levered shield that is pushed over the needle after use. Because it is pushed from above, the fingers do not come in contact with the needle. (Timby, 2005.) **B.** If a safety needle system is not available, the needle must be protected after use. This method shows the needle pushed into a protective cap (Point–Loc device) that locks into place, making needle removal impossible. (Photo Copyright © Keith Bunker Rosdahl.)

clicks into place, protecting the needle. Safety syringes help prevent accidental needle sticks.

If a safety syringe is not available, the needle can be injected into a special cap, the Point–Loc device, which locks the tip of the needle in place, to prevent needlestick injuries (Fig. 64-4B). Recapping of needles, even with the "scoop method," in which the fingers do not touch the needle, is no longer recommended, because of the danger of an accidental needlestick.

> **Key Concept**
> If a nurse or environmental worker sustains a needlestick, this must be reported immediately to the employee health service and an incident report filed. The staff member and involved client require blood tests. If the client has an infection, such as human immunodeficiency virus (HIV) or methicillin-resistant *Staphylococcus aureus* (MRSA), the healthcare worker may require immediate treatment. Blood tests should be repeated in 6 months, to determine any subsequent infection. Some states require reporting of needlestick injuries as well. Because serious health consequences can result from a needlestick injury, it is important to take steps to prevent them.
>
> All needles, syringes, ampules, and glass vials are disposed of in the sharps container. *Rationale: Other containers do not protect against needle sticks or injury from broken glass. The sharps container is managed using special procedures.*

Needleless Systems

Another injection system that prevents needle sticks allows medication to be drawn up into a syringe and injections made into IV tubing without an exposed needle. There are several types of **needleless systems**. They are more commonly used

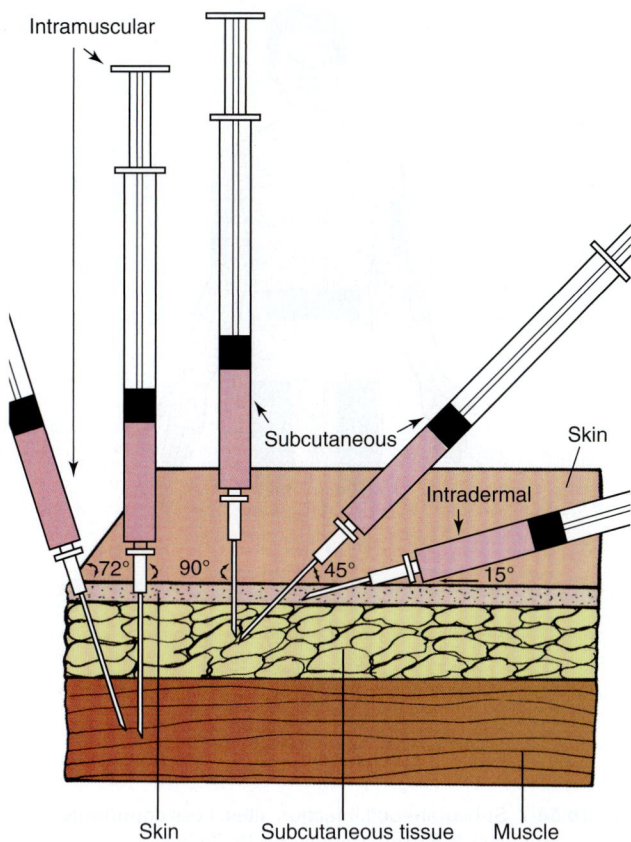

Figure 64-5 Comparison of the angles of insertion for intramuscular (IM), subcutaneous, and intradermal injections. An IM injection is given at a 72° to 90° angle. A subcutaneous injection is usually given at a 45° angle but may be given at up to a 90° angle, if a short needle is used or if the person is heavy. The intradermal injection is given holding the syringe nearly parallel to the skin (10°-15° angle).

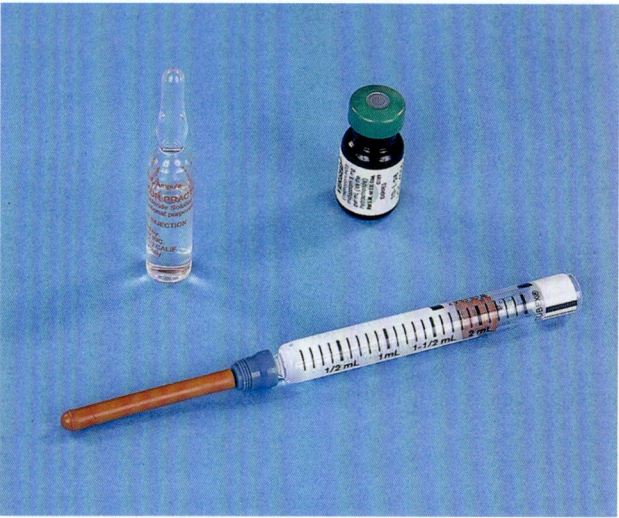

Figure 64-6 Examples of an ampule, vial, and prefilled medication cartridge. (Photo by B. Proud.)

in the hospital than in other settings. The most commonly used type consists of a rubber-type sheath covering a short needle. When the needle is injected into a firm rubber stopper, the sheath retracts. When the needle is withdrawn, the sheath moves back into place to recover the needle. Because it must be pushed into an object with resistance on all sides to push the sheath out of the way, the sheath will not retract when pushed against a finger.

Systems for Various Injection Methods

Subcutaneous injections usually are given using 1- or 2-mL syringes with 5/8- to 1-in. needles. When injecting more than 1 to 1.5 mL subcutaneously, the dose usually is divided into two syringes and administered in two injections.

Depending on the type and amount of medication, *IM injections* usually require 2- to 3-mL syringes with 1- to 1.5-in. needles. The angle of injection is also different (72°-90°), depending on the type of injection given (Fig. 64-5). For an IM injection, 2 to 3 mL is the maximum volume that can safely be injected into one site. (In some cases, less than that would be considered the maximum.) If a greater volume is to be given, two separate injections into different sites must be used.

Intradermal injections often test for exposure to TB and are given using 1-mL tuberculin syringes. Needles should be 25- to 26-G with a 3/8-in. intradermal bevel (see Nursing Procedure 64-2). The intradermal bevel is blunter than a regular bevel and allows easier access to the epidermis. *Rationale: Regular-bevel needles are much more difficult to use for intradermal injections because their added length makes it almost impossible not to enter the dermis. Because the dermis contains blood vessels, the medication would be absorbed too quickly, causing an unwanted systemic reaction and defeating the purpose of the test.*

PREPARATIONS

Injectable medications are packaged in many ways. Some are supplied as powders that must be reconstituted with a **diluent** (liquid). When mixed with liquid, these medications are often unstable and may deteriorate rapidly. They must be used within the time specified by the manufacturer. Common diluents include sterile water and sterile normal saline. The manufacturer's instructions will specify the diluent and amount to be used. In some cases, the diluent, the powder, and the syringe are supplied by the manufacturer. Follow the specific instructions for mixing any of these solutions.

Many parenteral medications are premixed by the manufacturer. Medications for injection may be supplied in a single-dose ampule, single- or multidose vial, or prefilled syringe (Fig. 64-6). An **ampule** is a glass container holding a premeasured, single dose of medication.

> **Key Concept**
> Discard any unused portion of an ampule's contents, because it is not possible to prevent contamination of an open ampule.

A **vial** is a glass container topped with a self-sealing rubber stopper. It may contain a single premeasured medication dose or maybe a multidose vial. When drawing up any injection, use strict aseptic technique, to prevent contamination. Label all multidose vials with the time, date, and your initials, detailing first use. (Some medications require refrigeration before and/or after being opened.) In Practice: Nursing Procedure 64-1 describes drawing up medication from an ampule and from a vial.

A **prefilled syringe**, such as Tubex or Carpuject, provides a single-medication dose prepared by a manufacturer or pharmacy. If the entire amount of medication is not needed, discard the excess amount into the designated receptacle before administration. This is done by pushing the plunger until the correct quantity remains. *Remember,* if the medication is a controlled substance, another licensed nurse must witness this procedure and document it in the designated manner. Sometimes, prefilled syringes do not have safety needle covers. Therefore, other measures must be taken to prevent accidental needle sticks (see Fig. 64-4B).

> **Key Concept**
> Remember: Medications and their packaging are usually not disposed of in the community sewer system but are placed in the hazardous waste container. All vials, ampules, needles, syringes, and prefilled syringes must be disposed of in the sharps container.

INTRADERMAL INJECTIONS

Intradermal injections, often used for diagnostic testing (skin tests), are shallow injections given just beneath the epidermis. The inner aspect of the forearm is the common injection site. If a number of substances are to be tested, the back may be used. Tuberculin syringes, which identify hundredths of a milliliter and can hold a total of 1 mL, are commonly used. Because the *tuberculin syringe* has a very small diameter, it can be graduated in hundredths and tenths of a milliliter for accurate measurement of very small amounts of medication (In Practice: Nursing Procedure 64-2 and Fig. 84-1).

> **Key Concept**
> If administering an intradermal injection, instruct the client not to scratch or pinch the site. *Rationale: This could irritate the area and alter the results of the test. This could also cause the injected material to be absorbed systemically.*

SUBCUTANEOUS (SUBQ) INJECTIONS

Subcutaneous injections may be injected into various body sites. They are administered into *subcutaneous* or *adipose* (fatty) tissues located below the dermis (Fig. 64-7; see also Fig. 64-5). This method is used for small amounts of medication that require slow, systemic absorption. Generally, the duration of SubQ medications is longer than that of other parenteral medications. Many medications cannot be given by the subcutaneous route. If the volume of medication is greater than 1 mL, the subcutaneous route is usually not recommended or two sites must be used.

SubQ medications must be soluble and of sufficient strength to be effective, yet safe for surrounding tissues. Common SubQ medications are insulin and heparin, as well as allergy injections and some pain medications. SubQ injections are given in areas where bones and blood vessels are not near the skin's surface. One common site is the outer

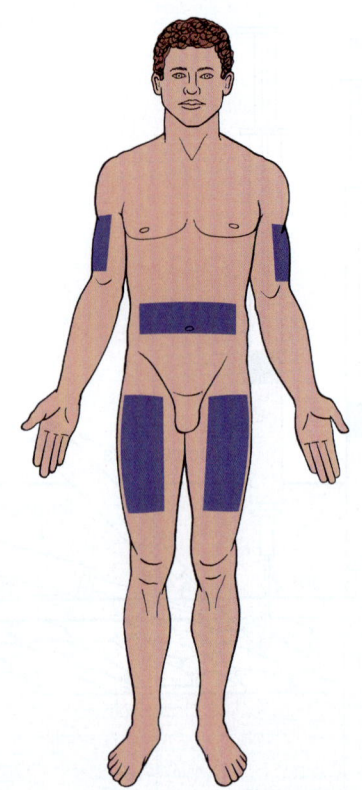

Figure 64-7 Subcutaneous injection sites. Less commonly, sites on the back are used. (Evans-Smith, 2005.)

aspect of the upper arm, above the halfway mark between the elbow and the shoulder.

There are a number of commonalities between the administration of SubQ and IM injections. The major difference is the choice of the site, the needle used, and the angle at which the needle is inserted. In Practice: Nursing Procedure 64-3 explains general considerations in administering a SubQ or IM injection. Nursing Procedure 64-4 describes specific steps for SubQ injections.

> **Key Concept**
> Always rotate injection sites for clients who receive injections on a regular basis.

Intramuscular (IM) Injections

Intramuscular injections are given in muscles situated below the dermal and subcutaneous skin layers (see Fig. 64-5). IM medications must be injected deep into muscles. The body absorbs IM injections much more rapidly than SubQ injections because of the greater amount of blood supply to muscle tissue. It is important for the nurse to be thoroughly familiar with IM injection sites and the technique for administering these injections. The most common areas for IM administration are the following (Fig. 64-8):

- Dorsogluteal (back of hip) *Use this site with caution due to close proximity to sciatic nerve
- Ventrogluteal (side of hip)
- Deltoid (upper arm)

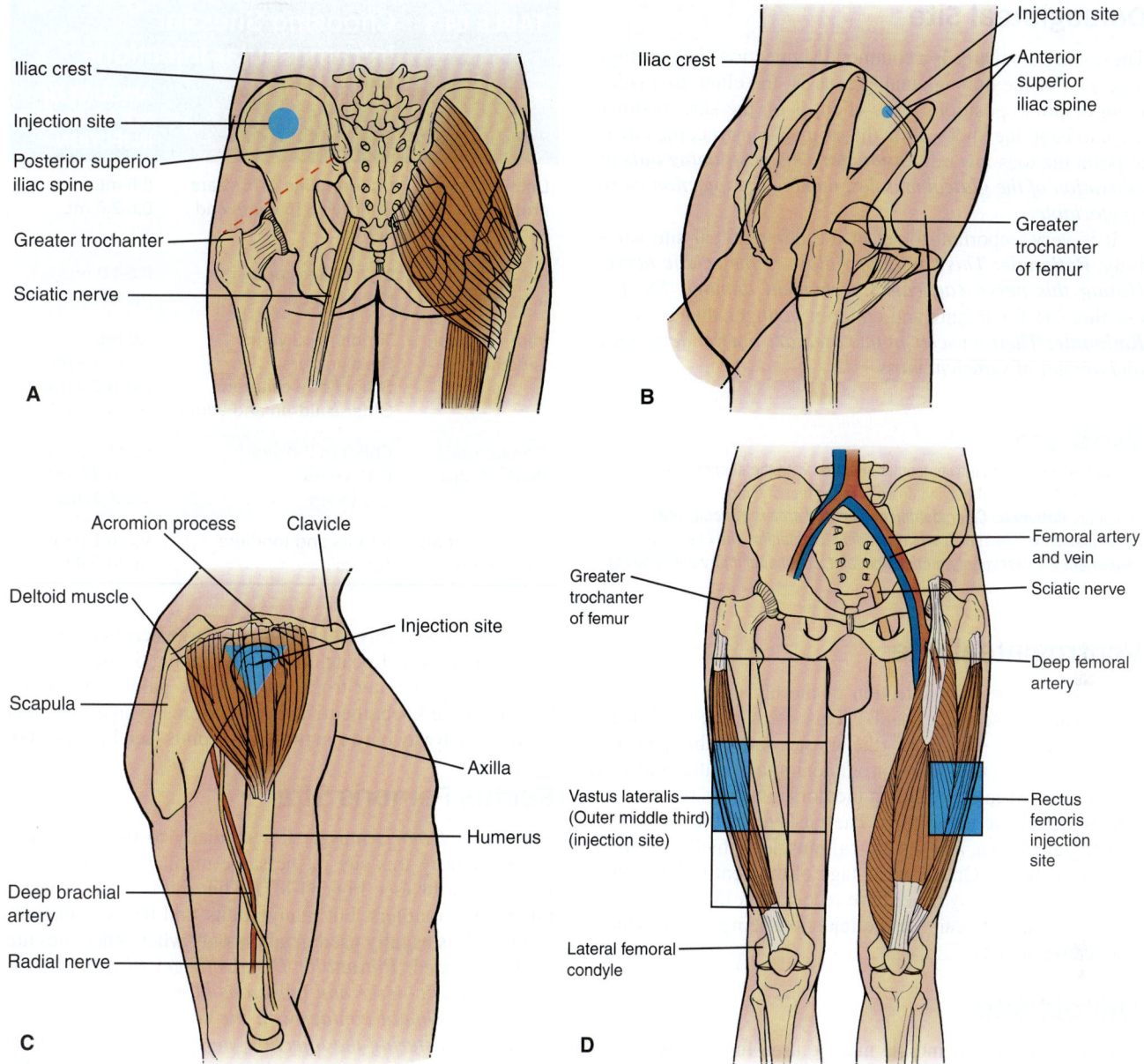

Figure 64-8 Intramuscular injection sites. **A.** Dorsogluteal (posterior view): lateral, slightly superior to midpoint of line drawn from trochanter to posterior superior iliac spine. **B.** Ventrogluteal (side view): palm placed on greater trochanter and index finger toward anterior superior iliac spine; middle finger spread posteriorly away from index finger as far as possible; injection site is in middle of the triangle. **C.** Deltoid (side view): lower edge of acromion process palpated; at midpoint, in-line with axilla on lateral aspect of upper arm, a triangle is formed. (Deltoid site not used for children younger than 4 years.) **D.** Vastus lateralis: divide thigh into thirds, horizontally and vertically. Give injection in outer middle third. (Vastus lateralis site used in infants and toddlers, as well as adults.) The rectus femoris site is on the anterior aspect of the thigh, approximately one-third of the way between knee and hip. This site is uncomfortable and not commonly used.

- Vastus lateralis (side of thigh)
- Rectus femoris (anterior thigh), used only when other sites are not available

IM injection is preferred when medications given less deeply irritate the client's tissues or when large amounts of medication are necessary. IM injections are given in much the same way as SubQ injections. However, a longer needle with a larger bore is used, most often a 1.5- to 2-in., 20- to 22-G needle, depending on the type of medication. Use an angle of 90° for the injection (see Fig. 64-5; see also In Practice: Nursing Procedures 64-3 and 64-5). In addition to requiring a longer and larger gauge needle, IM injections are more difficult and dangerous than SubQ injections. The needle must be injected deeper into the client's body, penetrating the epidermal, dermal, subcutaneous, and muscle tissues. If the medication is thick, injecting into the muscle may be more difficult (see In Practice: Nursing Procedure 64-5).

Nursing Alert When administering IM and SubQ injections, insert and remove the needle *quickly* (unlike the intradermal injection).

Dorsogluteal Site

The dorsogluteal area is a common IM injection site (see Fig. 64-8A). For the dorsogluteal site, assist the client to a side-lying or prone position. If the client is on the side, instruct them to bend the knees. If on the stomach, instruct the client to point the toes inward. *Rationale: This positioning aids in relaxation of the gluteal muscles, making the injection more comfortable.*

It is very important to select the dorsogluteal site carefully. *Rationale: This site is very close to the sciatic nerve. Hitting this nerve can cause permanent damage.* Do not use this site for infants and children younger than 3 years. *Rationale: Their muscles in this area are not yet developed and are not of sufficient mass.*

> **Key Concept**
> Do not administer an intramuscular injection with the client standing. Explain to the client that lying down is the safest and most comfortable position. *Rationale: Clear identification of the area is difficult, and the muscles will be tenser while standing. In addition, the client may experience a vasovagal reaction and faint, sustaining injury when falling.*

Ventrogluteal Site

The preferred site for injection in the hip area is the ventrogluteal site (see Fig. 64-8B). This site can be used if the client is in the side-lying (the most comfortable), prone, or supine position. The ventrogluteal site is safer and less painful for IM injections than the dorsogluteal site, through which the sciatic nerve runs. The fat layer is thinner in the ventrogluteal area, and the gluteal muscle is thicker, even in very thin clients. One disadvantage of the ventrogluteal site is that the client may never have received an IM injection in this area and also, can see the injection being given, which may cause anxiety.

Deltoid Site

Although the *deltoid* muscle may be used for IM injections, it is large enough only for small amounts of medication, and there is a risk of brachial artery or radial nerve damage. In most cases, 1 mL is the maximum amount of medication that can safely be given in this site. Use this route in children *only* if they are older than 4 years, if the medication is not irritating to the tissues, the volume is very small, and the medication will be absorbed quickly. This site is *not used* for infants and toddlers.

The deltoid muscle is located on the lateral aspect of the upper arm, 1 to 2 in. below the acromion process (see Fig. 64-8C). Identify the injection site by placing the index and middle fingers over the acromion process. The injection site is 1.5 to 2 in. below the middle finger. Hepatitis B vaccine and tetanus toxoid are examples of medications often given in the deltoid muscle.

Vastus Lateralis Site

The *vastus lateralis* is a thick muscle located on the anterior, lateral area of the thigh. This muscle may be used for IM injections in infants and children younger than 3 because it is the largest muscle mass in this age group. Little risk of injury exists with this site because no large nerves or arteries surround the area. Locate this site by placing the palm of one hand over the greater trochanter and the palm of the other hand over the knee; identify the injection site anteriorly and laterally, halfway between these two points (see Fig. 64-8D).

Rectus Femoris Site

The *rectus femoris* muscle lies medially to the vastus lateralis. Identify this site in the same manner as that for the vastus lateralis (see Fig. 64-8D). This site is often used for infants and toddlers, but many adults find this site uncomfortable. It is usually used in adults only when other sites are contraindicated. *Rationale: Disadvantages of this site are that the sciatic nerve and numerous blood vessels run very close to it. Should contact with the sciatic nerve be made while administering the injection, nerve damage—resulting in permanent damage or paralysis—may occur.* Table 64-1 presents further guidelines for site selection.

> **Nursing Alert** IM injections must be given into *healthy* muscle tissue for proper absorption to occur. If a client requires frequent IM injections, rotate the sites and note on the client's MAR or a "site rotation map," which site was used.
>
> Rotating insulin injection sites is particularly important because insulin can atrophy tissue (*lipodystrophy*) with repeated injection in the same site.

Z-Track or Zig-Zag Method

Certain medications, such as iron preparations and steroids, irritate the skin's dermal and subcutaneous layers. These medications must be injected deeply into muscle tissue. The **Z-track** method ("**zig-zag**" method) is recommended for administering these or any other medications that irritate skin and other body tissues (Fig. 64-9).

TABLE 64-1 Choosing Sites for Intramuscular Injections

SITE	AGE GROUP	AMOUNT OF SOLUTION PER INJECTION
Deltoid (upper arm)	Children age 4-15 years Children >15 years and adults	0.5 mL 0.5-2.0 mL
Rectus femoris (anterior thigh)	Infants and toddlers Preschoolers	0.5-1.0 mL up to 1.5 mL
Ventrogluteal (side hip)	Toddlers >3 years Preschoolers School-age children Older children and adults	1.0 mL up to 1.5 mL up to 2.0 mL up to 2.5 mL
Dorsogluteal (back of hip)	Children 3-6 years 6-15 years ≥15 years	up to 1.5 mL up to 2.0 mL 2.0-2.5 mL
Vastus lateralis (side thigh)	Infants and toddlers Adults	up to 2.0 mL up to 3.0 mL

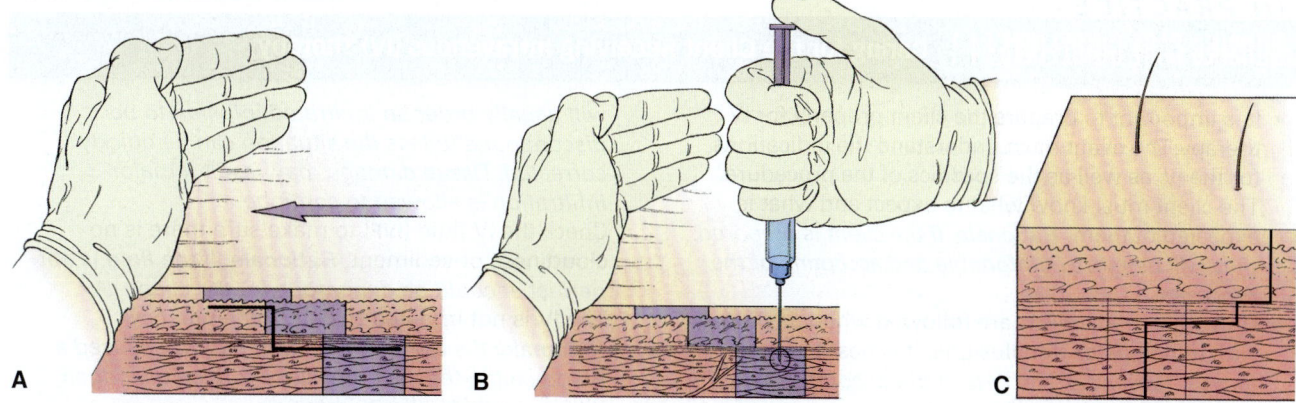

Figure 64-9 Z-track (zig-zag) injection. **A.** The tissue is tensed laterally at the injection site. This pulls the skin, subcutaneous tissue, and fat planes into a "Z"-formation. **B.** The needle is inserted. **C.** After the injection, the tissues are slowly released while the needle is withdrawn. As each tissue plane slides by the other, the track is sealed. (Timby, 2005.)

The Z-track method helps prevent medication from leaking back onto the skin and is used only in the gluteal muscles. To administer medication by Z-track, pull the skin of the injection site to one side. Insert the needle, aspirate, and inject the medication. Keep the skin taut and pulled to one side; wait a few seconds before withdrawing the needle. Allow the skin to return to its original position slowly while removing the needle. As the tissues slide past each other, they close the needle track. *Do not massage the injection site* when using the Z-track administration method.

INTRAVENOUS ADMINISTRATION

Fluids are administered via the circulatory system to correct or prevent fluid and electrolyte imbalance. For example, the client who is given nothing by mouth (NPO) for surgery often receives IV fluids pre- and postoperatively. IV access is also used to administer medications (see Nursing Care Guidelines 64-1). In nearly all cases, IV solutions are supplied in plastic bags. Glass bottles are almost never used; special instructions are required in this case. Peripherally placed catheters are used for short-term administration of fluids and nutrients. **Central lines** are used for longer term administration and for certain products that cannot be administered through a peripheral line.

In some states and provinces, an LVN/LPN does not work with intravenous lines. However, it is becoming more common for these nurses to monitor IVs and, in some cases, to administer medications via IV. This is particularly true if the home care client is receiving IV therapy. In this case, family caregivers are taught to manage the IV and the nurse assists them. Nursing assistants usually do not work with IVs, except to report problems.

The IV infusion may be run as a *primary* infusion, with one IV line running continuously. IVs may also be run in *tandem*, that is, a primary infusion plus a smaller bag. The smaller bag is connected at the same level as the primary bag. In this case, both the primary and the tandem bag infuse in at the same time. The IV infusion may also be run as a **piggyback infusion**, which will be discussed later in this chapter.

> **Nursing Alert** If a tandem bag is not clamped off immediately when the medication is infused, the fluid from the primary infusion will back up into the tandem line.

Intravenous injections and infusions allow the introduction of fluid solutions of electrolytes, nutrients, vitamins, and medications directly into the bloodstream. Medications are absorbed more rapidly via the IV route than any other commonly used route. Large quantities of a solution may be given IV by way of an infusion. A solution flows at a constant, continuous rate into the client's vein with the aid of gravity or an infusion pump or controller. IV infusions are commonly given for fluid replacement caused by dehydration or excessive blood loss, electrolyte replacement, antibiotic therapy, chemotherapy, or nutrition. If blood or blood products are administered IV, the procedure is referred to as a **transfusion**. (Transfusion is discussed in Chapter 82, in relation to blood and lymph disorders.)

Infusions

Healthcare facilities, as well as home care agencies and clinics, commonly use IV infusions. Although the LVN/LPN may or may not be responsible for initiating the infusion, they are often responsible for monitoring it. Careful monitoring of IV infusions is a must. Monitor the IV site for *patency* (openness), inflammation, infection, or **infiltration** (the flowing of fluid into tissues instead of the vein). In Practice: Nursing Care Guidelines 64-1 presents information regarding monitoring an IV. It is important to note the rate of administration and type of fluid being administered. Nurses document at

> **NCLEX Alert**
> The NCLEX can use situations that include equipment for administering medications. You will need to know concepts of administration by injection or IV, such as needle gauge, syringe size, type of IV pump, and the best injection site. You may also need to consider the client setting, such as acute care, hospice, or home.

IN PRACTICE
NURSING CARE GUIDELINES 64-1: Caring for the Client Receiving Intravenous (IV) Therapy

- It is important to prepare the client properly for IV therapy. The client must understand the indications for the IV, as well as the specifics of the procedure. The client must know what to expect and what is expected of them. *Rationale: If the client is prepared, they will be more comfortable and accepting of the process.*
- Universal precautions are followed when dealing with infusions or transfusions. It is best to wear gloves. *Rationale: The IV is in direct contact with the client's blood.*
- Monitor the IV site for swelling, coolness, fluid leaking, or pain. Lower the bag below the level of the insertion site, to determine if blood returns. Visually inspect the insertion site. *Rationale: Swelling, coolness, and leaking fluid are signs of infiltration. If blood returns when the bag is lowered, the infusion is most likely in the vein, but may still be leaking into the tissues.*

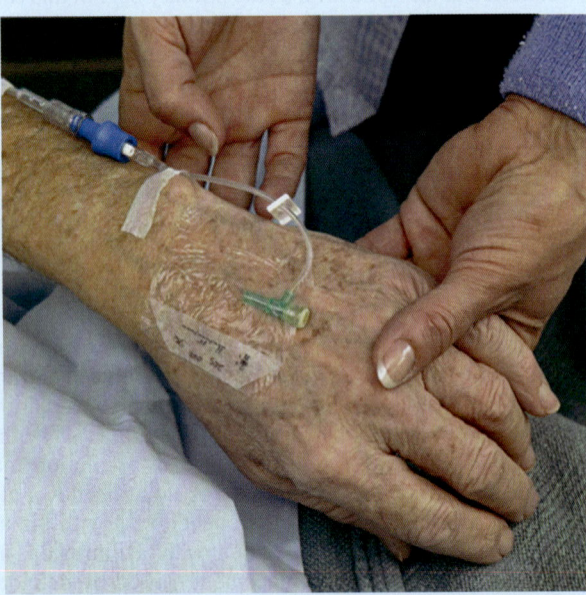

Inspecting the IV site. Note that it is covered with a transparent dressing, for easy viewing. The date of application is written on the dressing. Make sure the slide clamp (white) is open when the IV is running. Gloves are worn if the IV is to be discontinued or tubing or dressing changed. (Lynn, 2018.)

- It is helpful if the client (or family) also knows what to watch for. *Rationale: If they know how the infusion should operate, they can report signs of infiltration, an emptying bag, pump alarm, or other concerns. Thus, problems can be dealt with immediately. It is important for the client and family to realize that these situations are not life-threatening and can usually be easily rectified.*
- If signs of infiltration exist, stop the infusion and report the situation immediately. The provider will determine if the *infusion should continue or be discontinued. Rationale: The primary provider will usually order an infiltrated infusion to be discontinued unless the situation can be quickly corrected. Tissue damage may result if major infiltration is allowed to continue.*
- Check the IV fluid (**IVF**) to make sure there is no cloudiness or sediment. *Rationale: If the fluid is not perfect, it could be dangerous for the client.*
- The IV is not irrigated to determine patency. *Rationale: If a clogged or stopped IV has caused a blood clot in the vein, the clot could be dislodged, which would be life-threatening.*
- Monitor the infusion site for redness or hardness that follows the vein. *Rationale: This is a sign of phlebitis, which can also be life-threatening.*
- The rate of flow and amount and type of solution present are carefully monitored. The pump or controller is frequently checked. Most IV tubing today is continuous, so loose connections between parts of the tubing are usually not a concern. However, it is important to make sure the bag spike and connection to the venous access device are firmly in place. Remember that correct programming of the pump is one of the "7 Rights" of medication administration. *Rationale: It is important to ensure that all settings are correct and that the fluid is flowing properly.*
- A pump alarm must be investigated immediately. *Rationale: This is reassuring to the client and any difficulty can be quickly corrected.*
- Do not write on an IV bag with a felt tip marker or pen. To label a bag, use a preprinted sticker or piece of tape. *Rationale: The ink may penetrate the plastic bag and contaminate the IV fluid. The tip of a pen could also pierce the bag.*
- It is important for the designated nurse to replace IV bags before they become totally empty. *Rationale: It is hazardous for the client if air has collected in the tubing. In addition to removing the air from the tubing, the pump controller also must be reset if the bag has been allowed to empty completely. The venous blood may also clot if the bag runs dry; this can be very dangerous.*
- The infusion site is carefully protected. It is important for nurses to be aware of the tubing and pump during transfers, ambulation, or other activities. Remember, the IV controller works on the principle of gravity. *Rationale: If the tubing gets in the way, the client could trip and fall or dislodge the tubing from the bag or the insertion site. If the bag of solution is too low, blood will flow up the tubing and may cause complications.*
- All clamps and connections are double-checked when changing tubing, adding medications, or removing IV tubing from a pump or controller. *Rationale: If the flow rate is not regulated properly, the client could receive a bolus of medication, causing overdose. In addition, the client may not receive the required amount of fluids or fluid may be lost if tubing is not properly clamped.*

IN PRACTICE
NURSING CARE GUIDELINES 64-1 Continued

- Prevent the IV site from getting wet or soiled. *Rationale:* This helps reduce the possibility of infection and loosening of tape. Moisture is a route of transmission for pathogens.
- If the client will be away from the nursing unit for tests or procedures, nursing staff must make sure there is adequate solution to be infused while they are gone. A pump or controller usually has a backup battery so the client can be transported from place to place. It is important to make sure the battery is charged. *Rationale:* This allows the client to receive the infusion without interruption. The backup battery also is important in the event of a power failure.
- Plug the unit back in if the client will be waiting for any period of time. *Rationale:* This recharges the battery.
- IV dressings are changed according to facility policy. For example, dressings over Hickman catheters often are changed every 72 hr. In addition, the dressing is changed if it becomes wet or contaminated. It is standard practice to use clear dressings over the IV site. *Rationale:* Each time the dressing is changed, there is a chance of contamination or dislodging the catheter. However, dressings must be changed at appropriate intervals, to allow staff to inspect the site and to prevent infection. Clear dressings provide an opportunity to observe the site without removal of the dressing.
- IV tubing is changed, per agency protocol. (Most facilities require specific in-service education or test-out for any nurses changing IV tubing.) A preprinted sticker is attached, dated, and initialed when tubing is changed. It may be necessary to change IV tubing before the scheduled time (see Nursing Procedure 64-6). *Rationale:* The label allows other staff to know when tubing was last changed. New tubing is required if the tubing seems to be in danger of becoming clogged, if it becomes severely kinked, and in other circumstances.
- Gloves are worn at all times when starting or discontinuing an IV, and often when adding medications. *Rationale:* An IV site presents direct exposure to the client's body fluids, particularly blood. Gloves also help protect the client from risk of infection.
- The less the nurse handles dressings and connections to the bag or IV catheter, the lower the client's risk of infection.
- If the client is receiving total parenteral nutrition (TPN), it is run through a filter (see Nursing Care Guidelines 64-2). Other instances in which a filter is used include the administration of blood or blood products (see Chapter 82), during pediatric IV administration (in most cases), and sometimes if the client is at high risk for infection. Lipids (fats) are not to be run through a filter.

 Nursing Alert Remember to watch for the following complications when working with IVs:
- Infiltration
- Phlebitis
- Embolism (thrombus)
- Infection (sepsis)

---

least hourly regarding site condition, infusion rate, and specific medications or fluids being given.

Over-the-needle or inside-the-needle catheters are nearly always used to initiate IV infusions (see Fig. 64-19). The initial IV is often started in the hand. If this IV infiltrates, the IV may be restarted in the outer aspect of the forearm. The wrist and inner aspect of the forearm may also be used, but they are more painful when started (Fig. 64-10A). Veins located over bony prominences or joints are poor insertion choices, because the vein can easily become occluded, interfering with the infusion's delivery (Box 64-1). After the needle has been inserted into the vein and the catheter placed, the needle is withdrawn, leaving only a flexible plastic catheter in the vein. A length of IV tubing is attached to the catheter hub, which is in turn attached to the plastic bag that contains the prescribed solution. If a pump or controller is not used, a roller clamp on the tubing regulates the flow rate. If the clamp is completely closed, the flow is occluded and stops completely (Fig. 64-11).

Initiating the Intravenous Infusion

In some areas of the country, an LVN/LPN is allowed to initiate IV infusions. In this case, supervised practice and a procedural test out are often required. The nurse must carefully follow the provider's orders regarding the type of venous access device to use, the amount and type of IV solution, and the rate at which the infusion is to be administered.

IV Solutions

The most commonly used IV solutions include normal saline (0.9% **NS**/0.9% **NaCl**), 5% dextrose in normal saline (**D₅NS**), 5% dextrose in sterile water (**D₅W**), and 5% dextrose in 0.45% normal saline (*half-normal saline;* **D₅1/2NS**). Follow the same safety precautions when administering IV solutions as for administering any medication. Always observe the "7 Rights" of administration (including accurate programming of pumps) and sterile technique very carefully. If you are permitted to initiate IVs, Nursing Procedure 64-14 outlines the basic procedure.

UNIT 9 Pharmacology and Administration of Medications

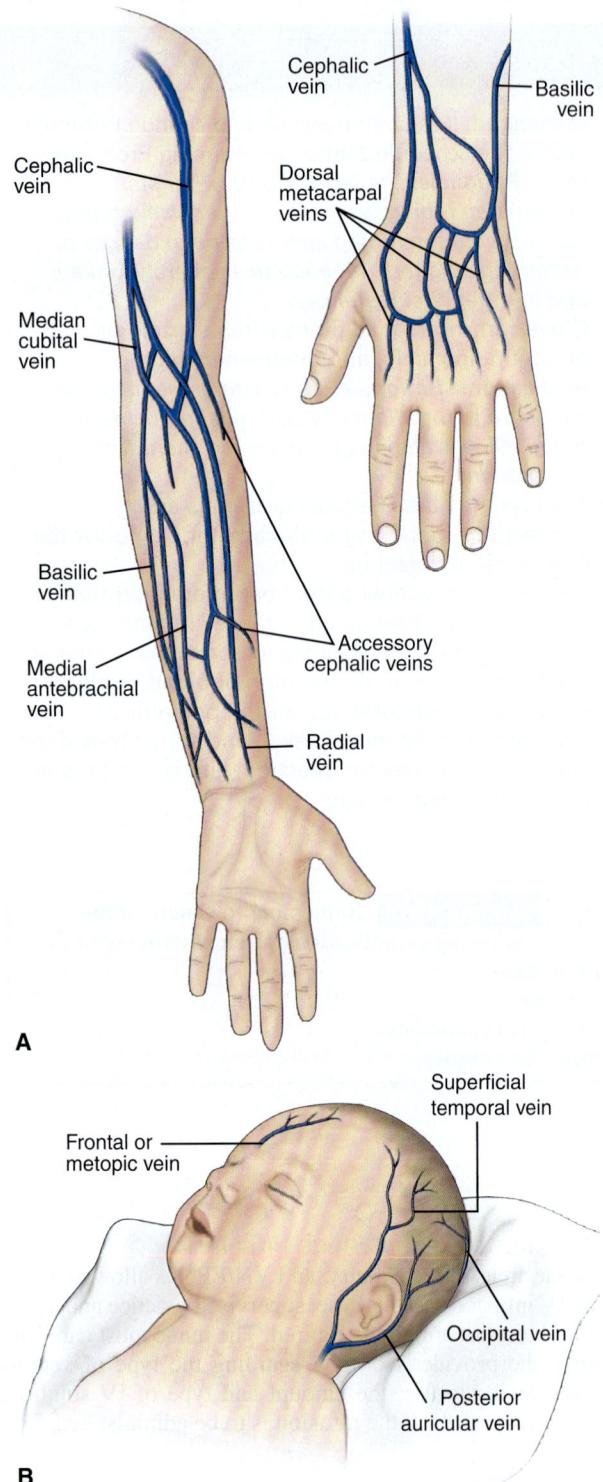

BOX 64-1 Considerations in Determining Venous Access Sites

- Peripheral veins vary in size. Choose a vein by considering its size for the purpose, length of time the vein will be accessed, mobility requirements, and comfort for the client.
- If the client is dehydrated, the peripheral veins may be partially collapsed; it may be difficult to locate a vein.
- It may be difficult to locate a vein in an obese client. A longer needle may be needed.
- Small children and infants have smaller veins. Different venipuncture sites and different needles and tubing are often used. Special techniques may be required.
- Older adults may be dehydrated, maybe debilitated, and often have friable skin. Access may be difficult.
- A client who is very ill may have poor circulation. Access may be difficult.
- If there is any doubt, seek assistance.

Key Concept

Signs of infiltration include:
- Swelling or puffiness
- Coolness
- Pain at the insertion site (sometimes)
- Surrounding tissues appear white or red
- Feeling of hardness in the area and possible leaking of fluid evident around the catheter

Rationale: The area feels cool because IV solutions are typically at room temperature, which is cooler than body temperature. The symptoms listed indicate the IV fluid is flowing not into the vein but into the surrounding tissues. The fluid may be leaking around the site, even though the catheter is in the vein; this can indicate that the flow of fluid is too fast.

Figure 64-10 Commonly used infusion sites. **A.** Ventral and dorsal aspects of arm and hand. **B.** Scalp veins (usually only used for infants. [Lynn, 2018].)

Infiltration of the IV

If the IV fluid is not flowing into the client's vein, but into surrounding tissues, this is known as *infiltration*. This can be a dangerous and painful situation and must be corrected as soon as possible.

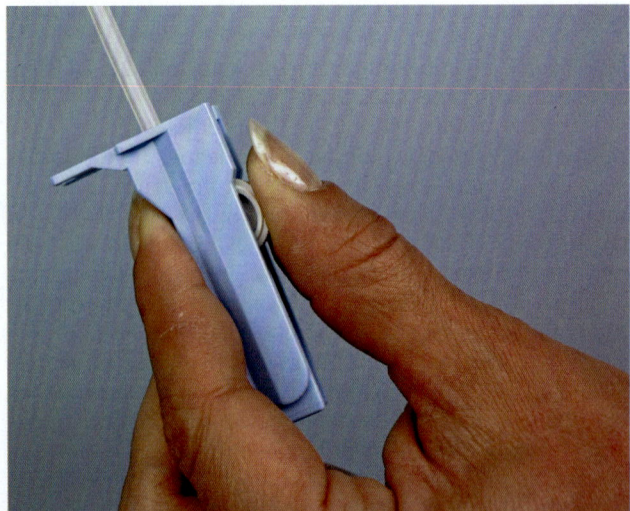

Figure 64-11 The roller clamp is used to control or stop the flow of intravenous (IV) fluid. When the roller is moved down to the narrower part of the clamp, the flow is stopped. When it is moved up to the larger part, the fluid is allowed to flow. (Lynn, 2018.)

Phlebitis

Another complication is **phlebitis**, inflammation of a vein. In this case, there may be redness and a cordlike mass, which follows the route of the vein. Other symptoms of phlebitis include pain and tenderness, swelling, and warmth in the area. This can be life-threatening if a blood clot forms.

Pumps and Controllers

Infusion pumps use positive pressure to deliver a preset fluid volume (see In Practice: Nursing Procedure 64-14). The disadvantage of pumps is that, in some cases, they continue to pump fluids even though the catheter may have been displaced from the vein. It is important that the nurse watch for adverse reactions. All IV sites should be checked at least hourly.

Electronic infusion controllers are most often used in the nonacute setting. They use gravity to maintain the flow of IV fluids at a preset rate. The height of the IV bag must be sufficient to take advantage of the force of gravity. Controllers sense the number of drops infusing and control the rate and amount of IV fluid. It is important to inspect the infusion site frequently, to make sure it is not infiltrated.

Both the IV pump and controller sound an alarm if air is in the tubing, the bag is empty, or the flow is obstructed.

Programming an infusion pump or electronic controller varies with the manufacturer; however, both can be programmed to deliver a preset fluid amount at a preset infusion rate. In addition, both units are equipped with memory systems that continuously total the volume of fluids infused. The nurse must have access to the instruction manual or receive specific in-service education in the local facility before programming pumps or controllers and otherwise working with IVs. Safety features are built into each machine to avoid erroneous programming. When a client at home is receiving fluids using an infusion pump or controller, instruction is vital. The client and family must understand the pump and its safety features, especially the sounding of an alarm if the tubing becomes obstructed or the IV bag becomes empty. Tell the client and family not to shut off the alarm until the situation has been corrected.

> **Nursing Alert** Because IVs are considered medications, it is important to remember that correct programming of controllers and pumps is the "7th right" in the guidelines for administration of medications. Many facilities require that two nurses double-check pump programming.

Patient-Controlled Analgesia and Portable Pumps

Sometimes, the client with chronic or intractable pain has a patient-controlled analgesia (**PCA**) pump. Medications commonly administered in this manner include morphine, fentanyl, and hydromorphone, as well as a combination of drugs called *BAD* (Benadryl, Ativan, and Decadron), often used in oncology. The pump, such as the CADD-Solis Intravenous Pump, is preprogrammed to deliver a set dose of medication. The medication may be delivered by continuous infusion or in the PCA mode (the client activates the pump when needed). Limits are preset, as well as time intervals between PCA doses (PCA lockout). A number of regulations apply to the use of PCA pumps

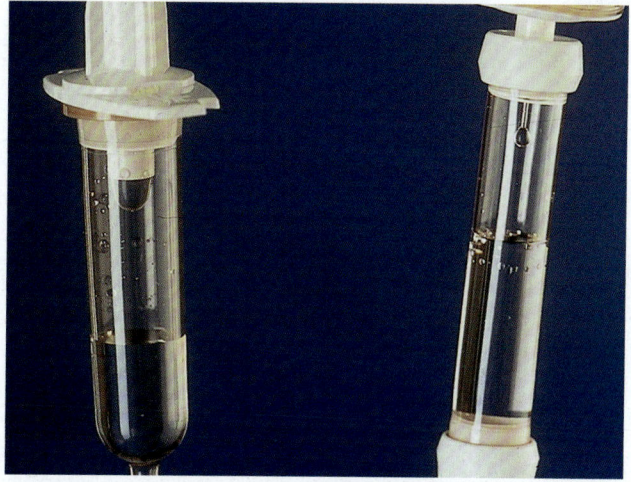

Figure 64-12 A macrodrip intravenous (IV) drip chamber (left). This device delivers approximately 10 to 15 drops per milliliter of fluid. The microdrip setup delivers approximately 60 drops per milliliter (right). (Ellis & Bentz, 2007.)

and many of the safety procedures are the same as those for administering any controlled substance (see Chapter 61).

In other situations, clients are also allowed to manage their own medication pumps. This includes the insulin pump for diabetics and a pump containing an antiemetic, such as metoclopramide (Reglan) or ondansetron (Zofran), for the client undergoing cancer chemotherapy or who has hyperemesis of pregnancy.

Microdrip Setup

A nurse may encounter an IV in a long-term care setting or in the client's home that is not controlled by a device. This client often uses the microdrip setup, which allows IV solution to be administered in very small "mini" drops that allow better regulation of fluid flow (Fig. 64-12). The microdrip usually delivers approximately 60 drops per milliliter of fluid. (The more commonly used system, the macrodrip, delivers 10-15 drops per milliliter, depending on the tubing's manufacturer.) The microdrip system is often used without a pump or controller but has many advantages over the conventional macrodrip setup, using only gravity. Because the microdrip delivers fluid in very small drops, it can be used in situations in which careful flow rate regulation is necessary to prevent overload when a pump or controller is not feasible or available (e.g., in children and confused adults, or for clients in long-term care settings or at home).

Regulating the Infusion Rate

An infusion pump or controller may not always be used, even though it is the safest choice. When a pump or controller is not used, the size of the catheter, the height of the solution bag or bottle, and the position of the insertion site influence the infusion rate. A catheter with a larger inner diameter (bore) allows solution to flow faster. The higher the IV bag, the faster the infusion will flow. Calculation of drip rates is usually the function of the registered nurse (RN) or pharmacist. The new nurse will require assistance in setting up the infusion and determining the rate of flow (Box 64-2). If no pump is used, tape is applied to the bag, indicating the times the fluid should reach each level. *Do not write directly on the bag.* It is important to monitor the infusion, to make sure the ordered amount of fluid is being infused.

Box 64-2 Calculating the Rate of Infusion

In most cases, LVs/LPNs are not expected to calculate the rate of an intravenous (IV) infusion. However, in the long-term care facility or home care, when a pump is not used, this may be necessary. Follow the policies of the agency. General guidelines are:
- Check the tubing wrapper to determine the drip rate factor of the tubing being used.
- For example, if the microdrip tubing set delivers 60 drops per milliliter (mL) of fluid, an example of calculations would be as follows:

$$\text{Drops per minute} = \frac{\text{volume (in mL)} \times \text{drip factor (drops per mL)}}{\text{time (in min)}}$$

So, if the order is to give 1,000 mL in 10 hr, the formula would be written thus:

$$\text{Drops per minute} = \frac{1{,}000 \text{ mL} \times 60 \text{ (drops per mL)}}{600 \text{ minutes } (10 \text{ hours} \times 60 \text{ minutes})}$$

Therefore,

$$\text{Drops per minute} = \frac{60{,}000}{600}$$

The answer would be 100 drops per minute.
Another method is to find milliliters per hour by dividing 1,000 mL by 10 hours. This would be 100 mL per hour. Therefore,

$$\text{Drops per minute} = \frac{100 \text{ mL} \times 60 \text{ (drip rate factor)}}{60 \text{ (minutes)}}$$

The formula would set up as:

$$\text{Drops per minute} = \frac{6{,}000}{60 \text{ (minutes)}}$$

The answer would be 100 drops per minute.
If a macrodrip setup is used, the drip rate factor would be much different but would still yield 100 mL per hour. However, to attain 100 mL per hour, it would require many fewer drops per minute.

If the insertion site allows a great deal of movement (e.g., the arm) and the IV is inserted into the antecubital area (inner aspect of the elbow), the solution can flow freely if the client extends the arm. However, should the client bend the arm at the elbow, the IV fluid flow will be obstructed. In some instances, immobilization of the insertion site is desirable, to allow a regulated flow. An arm board can be attached to the arm that will keep the insertion site stable but will not restrict arm movement completely.

A slower rate of infusion is usually necessary for older adults, small children, clients with kidney or heart disease, or clients with a head injury. A rapid infusion rate may cause circulatory overload or increased intracranial pressure in these clients (see Chapter 78). However, a faster infusion rate is often desirable for persons who have lost large amounts of body fluids and are severely dehydrated.

Nursing Considerations

In Practice: Nursing Care Guidelines 64-1 highlights major considerations in caring for any client receiving IV therapy. Be sure to closely monitor this client, to determine adverse infusion reactions. In addition, monitor the rate of flow and the appearance of the administration site, checking for signs of problems. Document all findings on an IV flow sheet or on the computer. Report any untoward findings immediately.

Changing the IV Bag
When the IV bag is nearing empty, the bag must be discontinued and a new bag added. It is important to prevent the bag from becoming completely empty because this can introduce air into the line and/or cause blood clotting. The nurse may also be requested to change the IV tubing or the dressings over the IV site. These procedures are outlined in In Practice: Nursing Procedure 64-6.

Long-Term Infusions, Central Lines, and Infusion Ports

There are several types of IVs called *central lines, central venous access devices (CVAD),* or *central venous catheters (CVC),* because they deliver fluid into a large central vein or directly into the heart. The first brand of tunneled central venous catheters was the Hickman. The term *Hickman* generally refers to all standard tunneled central catheters (Fig. 64-13D). The Hickman may have one, two, or three lumens. It is large enough to draw blood, as well as to infuse fluids. Another brand, the Broviac, is smaller and can only be used for intravenous infusions. Another type, the double-lumen catheter, may be used to deliver nutrients, such as TPN, through a smaller lumen. A larger lumen allows blood to be drawn and medications to be administered. There are many other brand names and types of central venous catheters.

The type of catheter used depends on the fluids to be delivered, the client's condition, and the length of time the CVC will be in place. A short percutaneous (through the skin) CVC may be surgically threaded from its entrance site (usually the subclavian vein) into a large central vein, such as the vena cava. This CVC may consist of one, two, or three lumens (tubes) and is used for several purposes. For example, if incompatible fluids are being infused, they may be delivered into different areas. The short CVC is sutured to the skin at the insertion site. A long CVC, the peripherally inserted central catheter (PICC) has a single lumen and is threaded through veins from an entrance site, often in the antecubital area of the arm, into the superior vena cava or the right atrium of the heart. The short CVC is most suitable for short-term use. The PICC can be left in place for a longer time and can be used to administer blood transfusions or medications and to measure central venous pressure. The PICC line is frequently used in home care. Central lines lower the risk of IV infiltration and infection because of their deep placement.

An LVN/LPN often is not allowed to work with central lines in the acute-care facility, but should be aware of the basics. In any case, special in-service education is required before working with these lines. Check with the state or province for guidelines. In nearly all cases, the LVN/LPN's

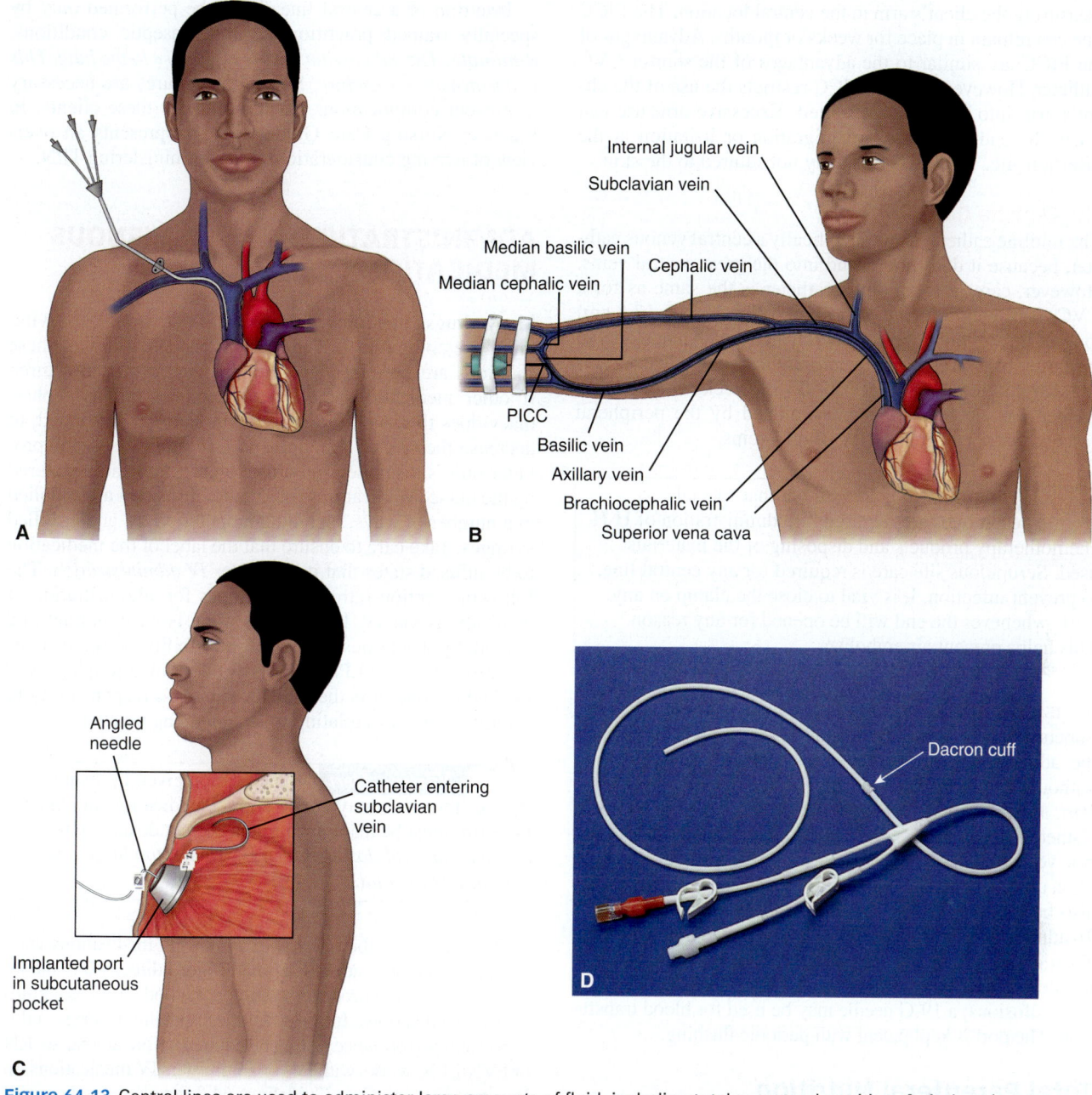

Figure 64-13 Central lines are used to administer large amounts of fluid, including total parenteral nutrition. **A.** A short (nontunneled) triple-lumen percutaneous (through the skin) central venous catheter, inserted into the subclavian vein and threaded up into the superior vena cava. (Lynn, 2018.) **B.** The peripherally inserted central catheter (PICC) line is inserted into the antecubital space and is sufficiently long to be threaded up into the superior vena cava. (Lynn, 2018.) **C.** The implanted port allows long-term, intermittent access to the central vein, without the need for a catheter protruding from the skin. Shown here with the 90° noncoring needle inserted, to administer medications or transfuse blood products. (Lynn, 2018.) **D.** A double-lumen Hickman catheter showing snap clamps and two types of ports. Dacron cuff helps hold it in place. (Ellis & Bentz, 2007.)

role is to assist the RN. LVs/LPNs may observe the insertion site and make sure the fluid is infusing properly and, in some cases, are allowed to change site dressings. An *LVN/LPN does not change the infusion rate.*

The Short Central Venous Catheter

The short CVC is used for the client who requires large amounts of supplementary fluids or total parenteral nutrition (**TPN**) for a limited length of time (Fig. 64-13A). This CVC can also be tunneled under the subcutaneous skin into the subclavian vein for longer term use. Tunneling allows the skin exit site to be a distance from the catheter's placement in the vein. (TPN is discussed in the next section.) TPN can be administered only by way of a large central venous catheter because it is very concentrated. A peripheral blood vessel would not have sufficient blood flow to dilute the TPN solution.

The PICC Line

One type of long central catheter is the **PICC**. The PICC is inserted into a peripheral vein, at the antecubital space or another site, and threaded up through the vein to a large central vein (Fig. 64-13B). This catheter is not tunneled. The catheter's length (12-16 in. or more) is determined by measuring the client's arm to the central location. The PICC line can remain in place for weeks or months. Advantages of the PICC are similar to the advantages of the shorter CVC catheter. However, use of a PICC restricts the use of the client's arm into which it is inserted. Excessive arm use can cause the catheter's outward migration or irritation at the insertion site. The PICC is usually not sutured to the skin.

The Midline Catheter

The midline catheter is not specifically a central venous catheter, because it does not extend into the great central veins. However, care of the midline catheter is the same as for a CVC. It is a shorter catheter (about 4-8 in. or 8.8-17.6 cm) long. It is inserted in the antecubital area and extends only to the larger blood vessels in the proximal area of the arm. This catheter can remain in place for 2 to 4 weeks and supplies greater volume than can be assimilated by the peripheral vessels, but not as great as the central veins.

> **Nursing Alert** Remember that special techniques are required for administration of H_2H chemotherapy products and disposing of the materials used. Scrupulous site care is required for any central line, to prevent infection. It is vital to close the clamp on any CVC whenever the end will be opened for any reason. This helps prevent air embolism.

Infusion Ports

Subcutaneously implanted (under the skin) CVC devices have the advantage of long-term access for frequent infusions, without any part of the catheter outside the skin. *Infuse-a-Port, Mediport,* and *Port-a-Cath* are examples (Fig. 64-13C). Catheters used in these systems are often placed in the superior vena cava via the subclavian vein. Implanted ports are often used for cancer chemotherapy (see Chapter 83) and may also be used to administer blood products (see Chapter 82). To administer medications, the port is palpated under the skin. Then a special angled needle (e.g., a Huber 90° *noncoring* needle) is inserted into the port. A 20-G needle is used for most infusions; a 19-G needle may be used for blood transfusion. The port is kept patent with periodic flushing.

Total Parenteral Nutrition

TPN, formerly known as *hyperalimentation,* is also called *central parenteral nutrition (CPN).* In addition to fluids, *nutrients* are also administered in this way. The volume administered is approximately equal to that of a routine maintenance IV, but additional components can be added, making it much thicker than IV solution. TPN solution often contains amino acids, dextrose (10%-70%), and electrolytes, and sometimes vitamins and trace elements (e.g., zinc, copper, manganese, or chromium). Lipids (fats) can also be given by a special method. TPN can help maintain adequate levels of nutrients for clients who are unable to receive adequate nourishment by mouth. Infusion of TPN requires insertion of an IV line in a large blood vessel, such as the subclavian vein, the internal jugular vein in the neck (*IJ line*), or the superior vena cava (*SVC line*). *Rationale: The nutritive solution is concentrated and could cause irritation, clots, or swelling if administered into a smaller vessel. The larger vessel provides sufficient blood to adequately dilute the TPN solution.*

Insertion of a central line should be performed only by specially trained practitioners, under aseptic conditions. *Rationale: The subclavian vein is very close to the lung. This is an invasive procedure.* Special procedures are necessary to prevent complications when caring for these clients. In Practice: Nursing Care Guidelines 64-2 presents an overview of nursing considerations when administering TPN.

ADMINISTRATION OF INTRAVENOUS MEDICATIONS

Many drugs, including antibiotics, electrolytes, and vitamins, are commonly added to IV infusions. Many of these solutions are premixed and supplied by the manufacturer. If other medications must be added, the facility's pharmacy does this, working in a special laminar flow hood, to decrease the risk of contamination. In other cases, the provider orders a smaller amount of a drug to be administered by the nurse. Medications for IV administration are supplied in a number of ways, including ampules, vials, and prefilled syringes. Take care to ensure that the label of the medication to be infused states that it is *safe for IV administration.* The following section introduces methods for administration of medications via IV. IV administration is an important and potentially dangerous nursing responsibility; in some states and provinces, the LPN/LVN is not permitted to administer IV medications. It is the individual nurse's responsibility to determine the laws relating to local nursing practice.

> **Nursing Alert** A medication given IV, even though it may be the correct medication and in an IV form, must be also given in the correct dosage. *For example, an oral dosage given IV is often too large and can rapidly be fatal.*

In some cases, the order is to administer medications via a continuous IV or to administer medications directly into the IV line. This section introduces common methods used to administer IV medications. In most facilities, specific in-service education and performance testing is required before any nurse, RN or LVN/LPN, works with IVs or administers IV medications. In Practice: Nursing Care Guidelines 64-3 details special considerations for administration of IV medications.

> **Nursing Alert** Never administer IV medications into tubing that is infusing blood, blood products, or TPN solutions.

Converting the Continuous IV Infusion to a Saline Lock

In some cases, the client no longer needs a continuous IV infusion but will need intermittent IV administration of medications or fluids. The IV line can be capped, leaving venous access (saline lock) available. Facilities use a number of procedures and devices for this; it is important to determine the policies in your facility. In Practice: Nursing Procedure 64-7 presents an overview of one procedure used to cap an IV line and convert it into a saline lock.

IN PRACTICE
NURSING CARE GUIDELINES 64-2 Managing Parenteral Nutrition

- Specific in-service education is required before working with central lines. Most facilities require two nurses to check before any total parenteral nutrition (TPN) bag is hung. Be sure to check every element of the provider's order—dextrose, electrolytes, protein, vitamins—with the pharmacy label. The bag should be at room temperature for at least 30 to 60 min before being hung. *Rationale: Double-checking helps prevent errors, which could be fatal. Administration of cold fluid is uncomfortable and could cause shock.*
- Be sure the appropriate inline filter is being used. Filters of different sizes are used for specific purposes. TPN solutions usually require a 1.2-micron filter. If a new filter is added or the tubing is changed, be sure to saturate the filter with IV fluid and remove all air bubbles. *Rationale: The filter prevents the passage of particles too large to be safely infused, as well as undesirable materials, such as bacteria or fungi. The introduction of air bubbles into the IV could be life-threatening for the client.*

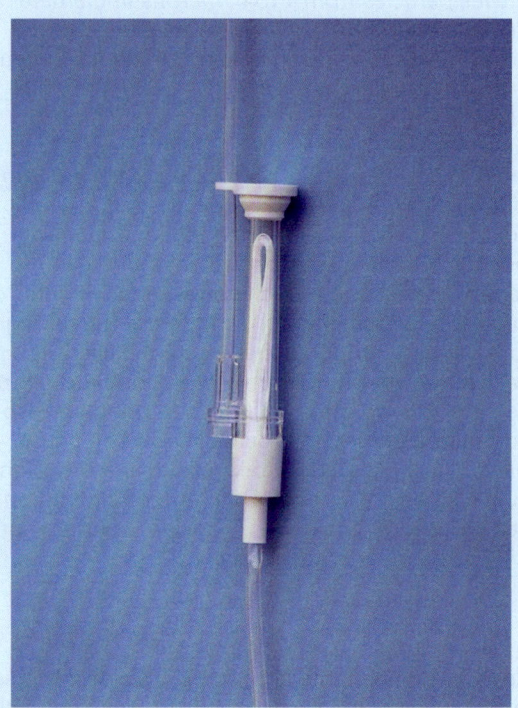

One type of inline IV filter, used with TPN and some other infusions, is shown here. The filter tube may be color-coded to denote the size of particles to be filtered. A special filter is also used for transfusion of blood and blood products and in some other situations. (Timby, 2005.)

- TPN solution should be checked for discoloration or precipitates. *Rationale: Any deviation may cause problems and should be discarded.*
- After a central line is inserted, a sterile dressing is applied to the site, which must be monitored carefully. Some central catheters are sutured in place. Make sure the sutures are intact. *Rationale: It is important to monitor for signs of infection and for the tubing's patency. The short catheter will advance or come out if sutures are not in place.*
- Specially trained nurses perform sterile dressing changes with central lines. Sterile technique is also very important when changing bags, tubing, or filters. Dressings at the insertion site are kept clean. Infection is always a concern. *Rationale: The high concentration of dextrose (D-glucose, a simple sugar) contained in TPN provides an excellent medium for bacterial growth. Bacteremia (bacteria in the blood) can be rapidly fatal. Because the catheter is in a major blood vessel, any infection would spread rapidly throughout the body.*
- The client's vital signs are monitored carefully, at least every 4 hr. *Rationale: It is important to discover any developing infection as soon as possible.*
- Many of the same precautions are used for TPN as when managing any other IV (see In Practice: Nursing Care Guidelines 64-1).
- The TPN line is usually continuous, without any connections between the bag and the insertion site. The insertion site is covered with a transparent dressing, which is changed every 4 to 7 days or as needed. Follow the facility's protocol. *Rationale: The continuous line prevents loose connections. A transparent dressing allows visualization of the site without removal of the dressing. Tubing changes are necessary, to prevent fluid build-up and infection.*
- The facility often uses "click-lock" or special Luer–Lok connections at the insertion site (see Nursing Procedure 64-10). *Rationale: This ensures that the connections are secure and air cannot enter the system. An air embolus in the general circulation is life-threatening.*
- The client's blood glucose level is monitored, usually several times daily. Higher concentrations of dextrose are used when the client's fluids must be restricted; lower concentrations help prevent hyperglycemia. This client is on intake and output (I&O) and daily weights. *Rationale: Metabolic and fluid balance changes can occur quickly. It is important not to raise the blood sugar to a dangerous level, to make sure the client is not retaining too much fluid and is voiding in appropriate amounts. In addition, these clients are often in very poor physical condition.*
- The rate of infusion for TPN must be constant. An infusion pump is used. *Rationale: This helps prevent episodes of hypoglycemia or hyperglycemia.*
- Lipids (fats) can be administered through a separate peripheral line, through a central line via a Y-connector, or as an admixture in the TPN solution. This provides supplemental kilocalories, and prevents fatty acid deficiencies and thus, deficiencies of fat-soluble vitamins (A, D, E, and K). When lipids are added, this is called a 3:1, three-in-one, or total nutrition admixture (*TNA*). The addition of lipids can cause complications, which are beyond the scope of this book. *Rationale: The addition of lipids to TPN allows the lipids to be infused slowly, decreasing carbon dioxide (CO_2) production and accumulation of fats in the liver.*

IN PRACTICE
NURSING CARE GUIDELINES 64-3: Administering Intravenous (IV) Medications

General Considerations:
- Prepare IV medications for only one client at a time. *Rationale: It is vital to ensure that IV medications are prepared and given accurately. Confusion must be avoided.*
- Extra care is required when administering IV medications. *Rationale: Because IV medications are entering the general circulation immediately, it is nearly impossible to reverse their effect after being administered. An error can be rapidly fatal.*
- Absolute sterile technique is required. *Rationale: Introduction of any microorganisms will immediately enter the client's bloodstream.*
- The nurse must protect themselves. *Rationale: Because the IV exposes the nurse to the client's blood, it is particularly important to observe universal precautions.*
- Several methods are used to administer IV fluids and medications. They include:
  - Continuous infusion: IV fluids are administered without stopping, until ordered otherwise. Sometimes, this is *to keep open* (**TKO**) or *keep vein open* (**KVO**) and is run very slowly.
  - Intermittent infusion: A medication dose or specific volume of fluid is infused over a designated period of time, usually between 15 min and 2 to 3 hr, stopped and repeated at specified intervals.
  - IV push: Injection of a single small dose of medication through a venous access device.
  - Bolus infusion: A special solution, such as a colloid, is rapidly infused for volume replacement. The specified quantity is run in as fast as possible, unless ordered otherwise.
  - Piggyback (superimposed) infusion: A secondary bag of fluid is infused as an intermittent infusion, usually while the primary infusion is stopped.
  - Volume-controlled infusion: Use of a device such as the Buretrol allows medication to be added to a specific volume of fluid. Usually, this is infused as a piggyback.
- An infusion pump is required in certain situations, such as infusion of TPN and lipids, any use of a central catheter, when it is vital to control the exact amount of fluid infused, and when administering drugs that have been identified as particularly dangerous (e.g., KCl). *Rationale: The infusion pump helps prevent errors in speed of administration.*
- Usually, drugs that have been identified as high risk require double-checking by two nurses; some facilities require double-checking for all IV medications. *Rationale: It is vital to prevent errors.*
- Some medications require special tubing or use of a filter. *Rationale: These facilitate safe administration of medication (or blood) and help prevent difficulties.*
- Even if an *inline filter is present, a filter needle is recommended for drawing up IV medications, particularly if the medication is drawn up from a glass ampule. Rationale: Minute particles of glass or other contaminants may be present. The filter needle catches particles from 1 to 5 microns in diameter and prevents them from being introduced into the IV.*
- Be sure that tubing used is appropriate for the pump or controller used. *Rationale: Use of the wrong tubing could be dangerous. The correct tubing facilitates the safety features of the pump used. These include free-flow prevention, accurate rate control, and the antisiphon device.*
- Most facilities require an *independent double-check* by another nurse before any IV infusion is started. The second nurse verifies the "7 Rights" of medication administration, and traces the tubing from the bag through the pump to the client to make sure everything is correct. A double-check of the pump's programming (the "7th right") is also required (see Nursing Procedure 64-5). In some cases, the client's laboratory results and/or weight must also be considered. Both nurses sign off on the medical record. *Rationale: These procedures provide additional safety for the client.*

The Saline Lock

A **saline lock** (formerly called a "heparin lock") is sometimes referred to as a *hep lock, intravenous infusion port (IIP), peripheral saline lock, intermittent infusion device,* or simply as a *lock*. This is an IV catheter inserted in a vein and left in place, either for intermittent administration of medication or to provide an open line in case of an emergency (Fig. 64-14). The saline lock provides continuous peripheral IV access without continuous infusion. A seal or cap is attached to the hub (end) of the IV catheter, "locking" it. To reduce the possibility of clotting, the lock may be flushed with 2 to 3 mL of saline every 8 hr or as ordered. A needleless system is usually used to flush the lock (Fig. 64-15). *Rationale: Frequent needle insertion could cause the lock to leak.* Some locks are not flushed. (In the past, heparin was used to flush locks; however, today, saline is the solution of choice, but you may still hear this device referred to as a "heparin lock.") On the other hand, central lines, such as PICC lines, are often flushed with heparin.

The main advantage of the lock is freedom for the client because they are no longer "attached" to an IV line and pump. Many times, clients are sent home with a lock in place. A provider's order prescribes which type of lock to use; an order is required to convert a continuous IV to a lock or to discontinue a lock. Some facilities have "lock kits" that contain syringes prefilled with normal saline. In Practice: Nursing Procedure 64-8 describes how to flush the lock and how to give medications via the lock. (See also Nursing Care Guidelines 64-3.)

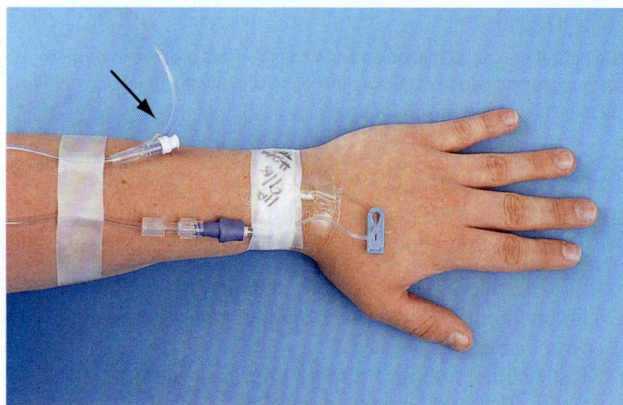

Figure 64-14 An intermittent infusion device (saline lock, intravenous [IV] port). This lock allows an IV to be restarted or small amounts of medication to be given with a syringe, without an additional venipuncture. The *arrow* points to the IV port on the extension tubing. This port is used to connect an IV tubing for continuous administration or to administer medications with a syringe. Note the blue slide clamp positioned above the client's hand; it is used to shutoff flow in the lock. The notations on the tape indicate the date the lock was placed and the initials of the nurse. (Photo by B. Proud.)

Discontinuation of an Infusion or Saline Lock

When the nurse receives an order to discontinue an infusion or a saline lock, the tubing will be clamped and the catheter removed from the vein. In Practice: Nursing Procedure 64-9 describes the process of discontinuing an IV or lock.

Administration of Medications Via Piggyback

Frequently, IV medications are given at scheduled intervals (e.g., twice daily) using a separate premixed IV bag and additional IV tubing to be connected to an existing IV infusion (Fig. 64-16). This method of administration is referred to as "IV piggyback" (**IVPB**) or a *superimposed infusion*. (It may also be called a *small-volume parenteral delivery system,* a

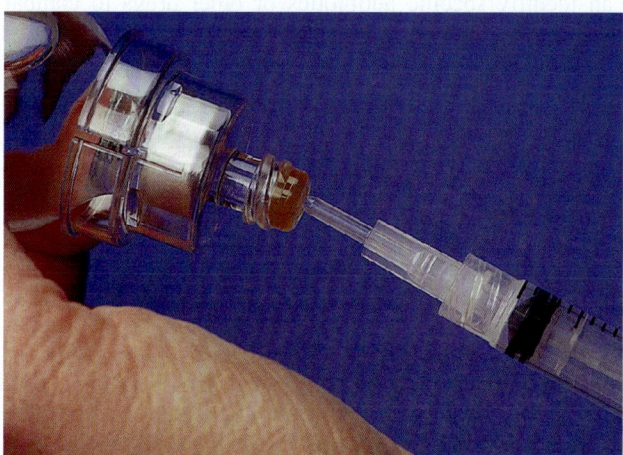

Figure 64-15 Some type of needleless system is usually used to prevent needlestick injuries when administering intravenous (IV) medications, flushing saline locks, or drawing blood. Some needleless systems require the use of a vial adapter, shown here, to draw up medications or saline from a vial.

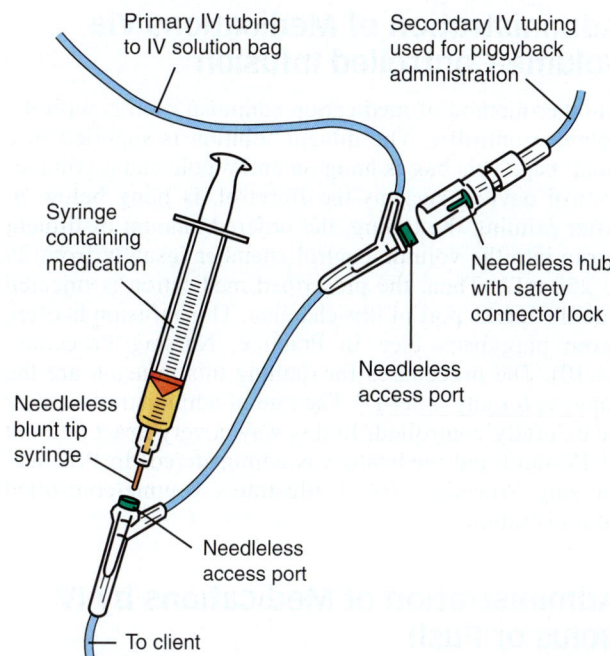

Figure 64-16 A basic intravenous (IV) setup includes tubing to deliver basic IV fluids via the client's venous access. Also shown are the access port on the tubing, used for injection of small amounts of medication by syringe (below) and the access port used for piggyback administration of larger amounts of medication (above). These needleless ports prevent needlestick injuries to staff. (Blood and total parenteral nutrition [TPN] are administered through a different type of IV tubing [Timby, 2005].)

partial fill, or a *mini bottle*.) The client receiving an IVPB also has a "primary" IV, which is usually one of the more commonly ordered IV solutions (e.g., normal saline—0.9% NaCl). A small bottle medication may also be delivered into a lock.

Following the provider's order and using a second infusion bag, the pharmacist adds medication to a predetermined volume (usually, 50 or 100 mL) of a compatible IV solution. The smaller infusion, containing medication, commonly an antibiotic, is referred to as the *secondary* infusion, *superimposed* infusion, or IVPB. The IVPB is connected to the primary infusion by way of secondary tubing and a needle or needleless setup. The IVPB is administered over a period of up to 1 hr (e.g., for mycins), or as ordered by the healthcare provider.

A controller or pump can be programmed to deliver the contents of the secondary bag. When the total contents of the secondary bag have been administered, the controller or pump automatically switches back to the primary infusion bag. The secondary bag must be hung higher than the primary bag to allow for a greater force of gravity. In Practice: Nursing Procedure 64-10 describes the process of IVPB medication administration.

Nursing Alert If a pump or controller is not used, the drip rate must be calculated (see Box 64-2). Request assistance if you have questions.

Administration of Medications Via Volume-Controlled Infusion

Another method of medication administration is with the volume controller. The diluent solution is supplied in a small bag. This bag is hung on an IV pole and a volume-control device, such as the Buretrol, is hung below it. After priming the tubing, the ordered amount of diluent is run into the volume-control chamber (usually from 25 to 250 mL). Then, the prescribed medication is injected into the intake port of this chamber. This infusion is often given piggyback (see In Practice: Nursing Procedure 64-10). The procedures for running this infusion are the same as for any other IV. The rate of administration must be carefully controlled. In this way, a very exact amount of IV fluid and medication is administered. In Practice: Nursing Procedure 64-11 illustrates volume-controlled administration.

Administration of Medications by IV Bolus or Push

Medications may be given by IV "push," also called a **bolus**, given in a short period of time (not intermittent). The IV push or bolus uses only a small amount of fluid. Thus, it is often recommended for a client at risk for fluid overload. Many facilities have firm policies regarding which medications may be given by IV push, because this method introduces a concentrated dose of medication directly into the circulation. This procedure is introduced in In Practice: Nursing Procedure 64-12, although the nurse must receive specific in-service education before performing the procedure. In some cases, a "smart pump" is used. This pump can identify dosing limits and other factors, to aid in safe administration (Fig. 64-17).

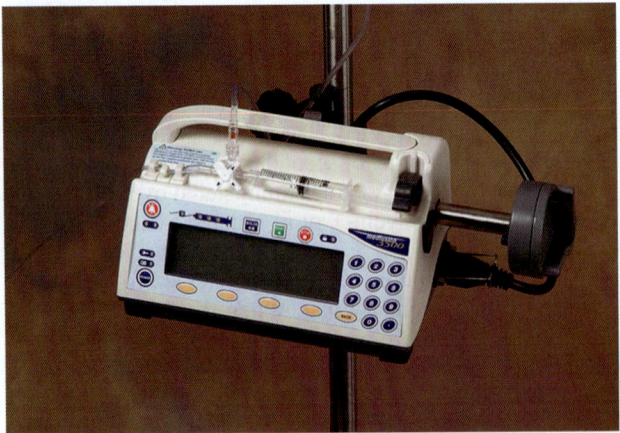

Figure 64-17 A computerized syringe-infusion pump or mini-infusion pump (smart pump) holds a syringe containing medication in a small amount of solution; it is connected to a primary infusion. The pump applies mechanical pressure to the plunger of the syringe, to deliver the medication; it can be programmed to repeat the same infusion at regular intervals (e.g., every 4 hr) around the clock. This pump is able to identify dosing limits and has other safeguards to protect the client. (Lynn, 2018.)

> **Key Concept**
> Do not refer to a medication as an "IV push" if it is ordered to be given over a specific period of time. In this case, identify the procedure as "an IV to be given over 5 min," for example.

The IV push has associated dangers. In many areas, an LVN/LPN is not allowed to perform this procedure.

Special nursing considerations include:

- It is vital to calculate the dosage exactly.
- This method of administration does not allow any time to correct an error.
- Most facilities require double-checking by two nurses for any IV push medication.
- The IV push may irritate the lining of the blood vessel.
- It is vital to confirm that the IV catheter is in the vein and the fluid is flowing freely.
- If the IV appears to be infiltrated, DO NOT give the push. If IV push medication is injected into surrounding tissue, rather than the vein, serious problems can occur, including abscess or tissue sloughing.
- If an IV push is given too fast, it can cause very serious complications, including death.

If in doubt, do not give medication by IV push!

VENIPUNCTURE

Venipuncture (**phlebotomy**) is the process of puncturing a vein to obtain a blood specimen (drawing blood) or to establish an intravenous access site. Blood tests are very commonly used diagnostic tools. A blood specimen can yield valuable information regarding the client's nutritional, metabolic, hematologic, immune, or biochemical status. Blood tests can reveal many disorders, as well as response to treatment. Blood levels of various drugs, illegal and prescribed, can be determined. A blood pregnancy test confirms or denies pregnancy. DNA testing is used for many purposes. A blood culture identifies microorganisms that might be causing disease; when combined with a sensitivity test, this can identify specific antibiotics or other drugs to combat offending pathogens.

For a simple blood draw, a butterfly needle is often used (Fig. 64-18); if an IV site is to be established, several devices are available (Fig. 64-19).

The **Vacutainer** system, shown in Figure 64-18, is often used for venipuncture. It consists of a disposable plastic sleeve into which a double-ended needle setup or butterfly needle is inserted. This device has a needleless connector on one end and a venipuncture needle or butterfly needle on the other end. The needleless end is screwed into the plastic sleeve, with the needle or butterfly outward and the needleless access device inside the sleeve. The needle often contains an articulated shield, which is pushed over the needle after the venipuncture (see Fig. 64-4A). If this is not present, a Point–Loc device must be used (see Fig. 64-4B). One disadvantage of the Vacutainer needle with the articulated shield is that this system contains a large needle, which might not be appropriate for some venipunctures. If a smaller needle is desired, a **butterfly needle** is used. Butterfly needles are available with adaptors to be used with Vacutainer sleeves

CHAPTER 64 Administration of Injectable Medications

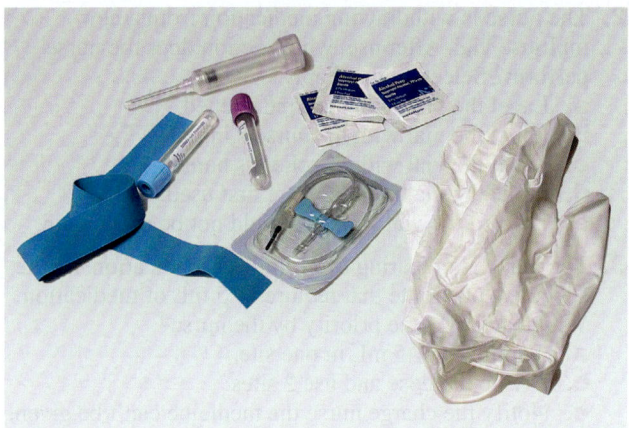

Figure 64-18 The nurse will often be expected to gather materials and equipment for venipuncture (phlebotomy). Some of the items needed to obtain a blood specimen are shown here (clockwise, from bottom left): **tourniquet**, Vacutainer (vacuum) blood tubes, safety syringe with needle, alcohol sponges, and gloves. Shown also is a butterfly needle pack with a needleless Vacutainer adaptor, used to puncture a Vacutainer blood tube. Also needed are 2 × 2 gauze squares and tape or a Band-Aid, identification stickers, and a red biohazard bag. A Vacutainer sleeve and/or needle system may also be used. (If the butterfly needle is used, the syringe and needle are not required.) Additional items are needed to initiate an IV infusion. (Photo Copyright © Keith Bunker Rosdahl.)

(Fig. 64-18) or for initiating IVs. After the vein is accessed, the needleless connector is pushed into a Vacutainer (vacuum) tube, which draws the blood into the tube.

A blood specimen can also be obtained by a skin puncture (capillary puncture), as in blood sugar testing for persons with diabetes. In addition, an arterial puncture can be performed to obtain values, such as blood gas analysis. In some cases, a blood sample can be taken from an existing IV infusion.

The procedure for venipuncture is contained in In Practice: Nursing Procedure 64-13. Arterial puncture is beyond the scope of this book. In the case of blood cultures, the facility will identify specific procedures to follow.

Key Concept

Venipuncture is not without some discomfort. In addition, the sight of a needle is frightening to many people, particularly children. A small butterfly needle is used when possible. It is up to the nurse to reassure the client and make them as comfortable as possible.

The sequence of blood collection is important. Blood cultures should be collected first, followed by other blood samples. Tube colors are used as dictated by the healthcare facility.

In addition, some tubes must be inverted several times immediately after collection. Some must be sent to the laboratory on ice. Follow the facility's protocol.

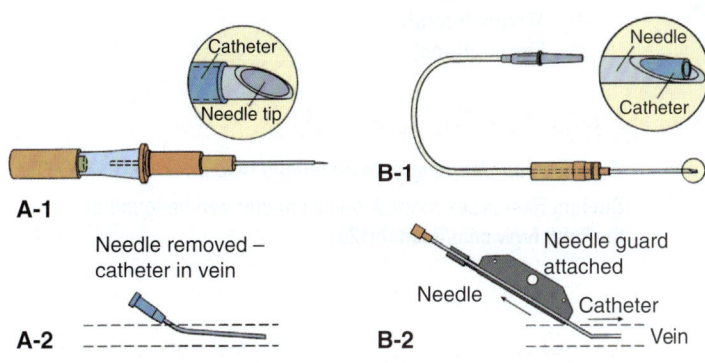

Figure 64-19 Venous access devices (VAD). In addition to the butterfly needle, two types of intracatheters are commonly used, allowing fluid to flow through a flexible catheter into the vein. (**A-1**) An over-the-needle catheter is inserted into the vein and, (**A-2**) the needle is removed, leaving the catheter in the vein. (**B-1**) A through-the-needle catheter is passed through the needle after the needle is inserted into the vein. (**B-2**) The needle is pulled out, leaving the catheter in the vein. Both devices have a locking guard mechanism that locks the needle guard in place, to prevent needle sticks when the catheter is in place and when it is removed. (Timby, 2005.)

STUDENT SYNTHESIS

KEY POINTS

- Parenteral administration of medications carries more risk than does oral administration.
- The nurse must be particularly careful in preparing medications for injection.
- It is important to take precautions to prevent needlestick injuries.
- Proper technique and site preparation for intradermal, subcutaneous, intramuscular, and intravenous injections are essential to prevent errors, infections, and/or injury to the client.
- Monitoring of IV infusion solutions, rates, and sites is very important. Prevention of infiltration, phlebitis, and/or infection is necessary.
- Administration of medications via the intravenous route requires accuracy, because errors can be immediately life-threatening.
- The nurse needs great skill to administer IV medications by any method. Special in-service education is usually required before any nurse is permitted to administer IV medications, perform venipuncture, and/or start IVs.
- It is important to know what materials to assemble in order to assist with, or to perform, venipuncture, including starting an IV infusion. The equipment must all be ready before beginning.
- It is important to seek assistance if there are any questions about IV administration.

- Each pump is programmed differently (the "7th right"). Follow the manufacturer's instructions, which are usually kept attached to the pump.

CRITICAL THINKING EXERCISES

1. You receive a medication order for a 2-year-old child. The order states that you should give an IM injection in the dorsogluteal area. Which steps would you take next?

2. You are giving an IM injection. When you draw back on the plunger, a small amount of blood returns in the syringe. What is the significance of this? Which action should you take?

3. Describe materials needed to assist with venipuncture. Demonstrate where these are located in your facility. Describe the procedure of venipuncture.

4. State why the "7th right" of medication administration (programming of pumps) is so vital. Demonstrate how an infusion pump is programmed in your facility.

5. A client tells you that he does not want another injection in his left hip. How would you respond? Which actions would you take? Why?

6. The IM injectable medication ordered for Mrs. Shapiro totals 4 mL. Describe how you would administer it.

7. State the role of the LVN/LPN in working with IVs in your facility and in your state/province.

8. Describe key points in observing the client who has a continuous infusion running. State what would be documented and which situations must be reported immediately.

NCLEX-STYLE REVIEW QUESTIONS

1. The nurse is preparing to administer an intradermal tuberculin skin test. Which type of needle should the nurse place on the syringe?
   a. 22-G with a 5/8 in. bevel
   b. 20-G with a 3/4 in. bevel
   c. 18-G with a 1/4 in. bevel
   d. 25-G with a 3/8 in. bevel

2. The nurse is withdrawing medication from a new multiuse vial. After use, which action does the nurse perform? Select all that apply.
   a. Label the vial with the time opened.
   b. Label the vial with the nurse's initials.
   c. Label the vial with the client's name.
   d. Label the vial with the date first used.
   e. Discard the vial since it should not be used again.

3. The nurse is preparing to administer medication via the subcutaneous route that requires 1.5 mL of medication. Which action is the priority by the nurse?
   a. Administer 1.5 mL in one site.
   b. Divide the dose and use 2 sites.
   c. Notify the charge nurse the medicine can't be given.
   d. Obtain a larger syringe.

4. When preparing to administer an intramuscular injection into the dorsogluteal area, what instructions should the nurse give to the client?
   a. Stand and bend over the stretcher.
   b. Sit in the chair and expose the upper arm area.
   c. Lie on your back and bend the knees.
   d. Lie on your side and bend the knees.

5. The nurse is administering an immunization to an 18-month-old child. Which site does the nurse use to administer this injection?
   a. Deltoid
   b. Ventrogluteal
   c. Vastus lateralis
   d. Dorsogluteal

CHAPTER RESOURCES

Enhance your learning with additional resources on thePoint!

Student Resources related to this chapter can be found at **thePoint.lww.com/Rosdahl12e**.

CHAPTER 64 Administration of Injectable Medications

Welcome Steps

Look at healthcare provider's orders.

Protocol for procedure.

Necessary equipment/supplies.

Wash hands using proper hand hygiene; put on gloves.

Explain the procedure and reassure the client.

Locate two identifiers to confirm correct client.

Comfortable and efficient position for nurse and client.

Obtain privacy.

Make sure to follow correct steps and body mechanics with good technique.

Ensure safety and observe deviations from normal.

End Steps

Ensure comfort and safety.

Note questions or concerns from client or nurse; note significant data.

Dispose of materials properly.

Disinfect the area and your hands.

Document and report the procedure and your findings.

IN PRACTICE

NURSING PROCEDURE 64-1 Drawing Medication From an Ampule or Vial

Supplies and Equipment
Syringe and needle (or needleless adapter)
Ampule or vial of medication
Filter needle for use with ampule
Alcohol swabs
2 × 2 gauze squares, if opening an ampule
Gloves

- Wear gloves for most medications. *Rationale: You need to protect your hands. In some cases, it is vital to prevent any contact with your skin, to prevent absorption.*
- Check the medication's expiration date. Discard any outdated medications. *Rationale: Outdated medication may be ineffective or dangerous.*

For an Ampule

Steps

Follow LPN WELCOME steps and then

1. *Sanitize hands, put on gloves, and then:* Hold the ampule upright. Use the finger to tap on the ampule's stem, or hold the ampule by the stem and rotate the hand in a circular motion. *Rationale: All medication in the ampule should be in the lower part before the stem is removed.*

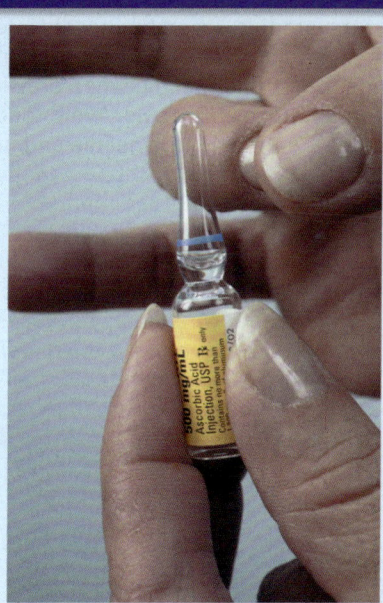

Tapping the stem of an ampule. (Evans-Smith, 2005.)

2. Cleanse the ampule's neck with an alcohol swab. Let it dry. Grasp the ampule with a 2 × 2 gauze and snap off the ampule's top at the line, *away* from your hands and face. *Rationale: Alcohol disinfects as it dries. The gauze square protects the fingers from glass particles when the stem is snapped. Snapping away from the body protects the nurse's face from small glass particles or medication.*

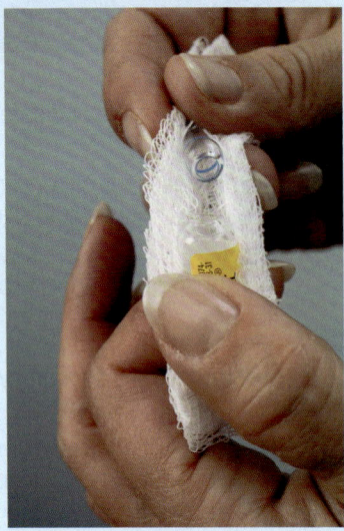

Snapping off the top of an ampule away from the nurse's face, while protecting the fingers with a gauze square. Gloves may be worn for additional safety. (Evans-Smith, 2005.)

3. Uncap a filter needle and insert into the ampule, using one of the following methods.
   a. Keeping the ampule upright on a flat surface, insert the needle into the solution and aspirate medication into the syringe.
   b. Invert the ampule, insert the needle into the solution, and aspirate the medication into the syringe. Use a filter needle when drawing medication from an ampule. Avoid touching the ampule's rim with the needle and injecting any air into it. *Rationale: Keeping the needle in the solution prevents aspiration of air. Touching the sterile needle against the ampule rim contaminates the needle. Injecting air into the ampule is not needed because its contents are not under pressure. Because of its shape, an ampule can be inverted without losing its contents. The filter needle ensures that no minute fragments of glass are in the solution.*

4. Remove the needle from the ampule. Remove the filter needle from the syringe and replace with an appropriate injection needle. Hold the needle upright and eject any air that was drawn into the syringe. Discard any excess medication into the designated receptacle and the used ampule in the sharps container. *Rationale: Checking the amount of medication withdrawn from the ampule ensures that the correct dose is administered. Proper disposal prevents accidental injury.*

5. Pull the safety sheath over the needle. Do not twist it. *Rationale: The cap maintains the needle's sterility. Twisting the sheath would lock it.*

Follow ENDDD steps

For a Vial

Steps
Follow LPN WELCOME steps and then

1. Sanitize hands and then:
   Remove the metal or plastic cover from the vial and cleanse the rubber port with an alcohol swab. Let the alcohol dry. *Rationale: This decreases the possibility of introducing contaminants into the vial. Alcohol disinfects as it dries.*

2. Remove the needle cap and draw an amount of air into the syringe equal to the amount of medication that will be withdrawn from the vial. (In some cases, a filter needle will be used.)
   Insert the needle through the center of the rubber stopper and inject air into the vial, keeping the needle above the solution.
   Rationale: Injecting an equal amount of air into the vial prevents buildup of negative or positive pressure. By injecting air into the air space, formation of bubbles is prevented. This facilitates withdrawing an accurate dose.

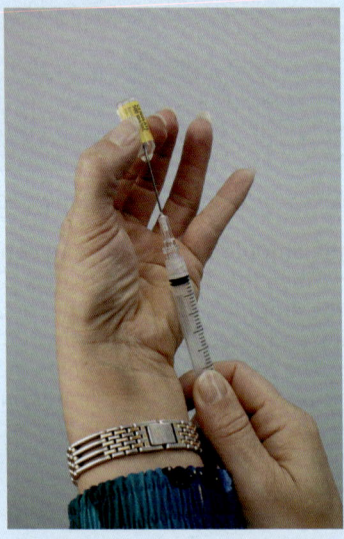

Withdrawing medication from an inverted ampule. (Evans-Smith, 2005.)

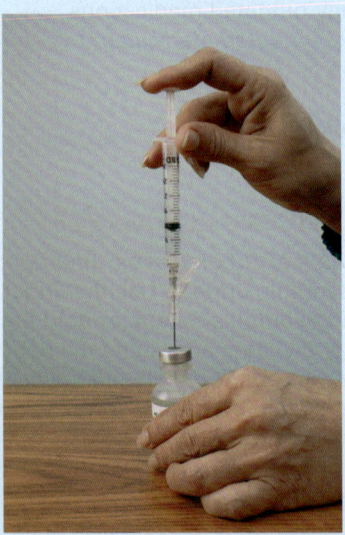

Adding air to the vial with the needle in the air space above the medication. This syringe has an articulated needle shield. (Evans-Smith, 2005.)

3. Invert the vial. Steady the vial and syringe in the nondominant hand at eye level. Brace the little finger against the barrel. Firmly hold the plunger in the dominant hand. *Rationale: Holding the vial and syringe securely prevents contamination of the medication. Hold the plunger, in case negative pressure already exists in the vial, which could force out the plunger.*

4. Move the needle into the solution without allowing the plunger to come out. *Rationale: Doing so allows medication, rather than air, to be aspirated into the syringe.*

5. Use the dominant hand to pull back on the syringe's plunger. Withdraw an accurate dose into the syringe. Remove the needle from the vial. *Rationale: Positive pressure in the vial promotes easy aspiration of fluid into the syringe.*

6. Hold the needle upright and recheck the syringe's contents for the presence of air. Tap the barrel of the syringe to move air bubbles upward; then expel them. Reinsert the needle into the solution, if any additional medication is needed. *Rationale: Removing air bubbles ensures an accurate dose of medication.*

7. Change the needle, if necessary, or pull the safety sheath over it. Do not lock the shield. *Rationale: Capping maintains the needle's sterility.*

8. Discard the used single-dose vial in the sharps container or date, initial, and store the multidose vial according to agency policy. *Rationale: Proper disposal prevents infection transmission; proper storage provides for future use without wasting the medication.*

Follow ENDDD steps

IN PRACTICE

NURSING PROCEDURE 64-2 Administering Intradermal Injections

Supplies and Equipment
Medication scanner or MAR
Medication (often the syringe will be prefilled)
Alcohol swab
Gloves
Sterile tuberculin syringe and 25- to 26-G needle with intradermal bevel (see Fig. 64-3)
Permanent marking pen
Note: Follow steps in Nursing Procedure 64-1 before proceeding. Use of a prefilled syringe is illustrated in Figure 64-2; safety syringes and needle guards are shown in Figures 64-3 and 64-4.

Steps
Follow LPN WELCOME steps and then

1. Choose an injection site on the inner aspect of the forearm that is not heavily pigmented or covered with hair. For a single purified protein derivative (PPD) test, the left forearm is usually used. For allergy tests, both arms or the back may be used. Cleanse with alcohol and make sure the alcohol thoroughly dries. *Rationale: Hair or discoloration may interfere with assessment of the site after injection. Any alcohol will alter the results of the test if it is wet.*

2. Use the nondominant hand to pull the skin taut over the injection site, pulling from the side opposite the injection. *Rationale: Firm skin makes injection into the epidermis easier.*

   a. Hold the syringe across the palm of your hand. Turn your hand slightly so the syringe and needle are at a sharp angle to the arm's surface (see Fig. 64-5).

   b. Place the needle, bevel down, near the skin surface at approximately a 10° to 15° angle.

   c. Rotate the syringe between the index finger and the thumb 180°, while exerting slight forward pressure so that the bevel is up when it is inserted. Insert the bevel just under the epidermis. *Rationale: The rotating action makes insertion into the epidermis much easier and less traumatic to the tissue. Be sure the bevel is up for proper injection.*

3. Transfer the thumb to the end of the plunger and slowly inject the medication (usually 0.3 mL). *Do not aspirate.* Watch for the formation of a *wheal* (small elevation similar in appearance to a hive). *Rationale: A wheal indicates correct delivery of the medication into the epidermis.*

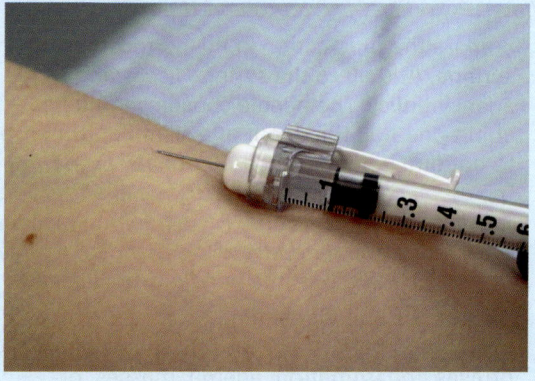

Inserting the needle at a 10° to 15° angle. (Evans-Smith, 2005.)

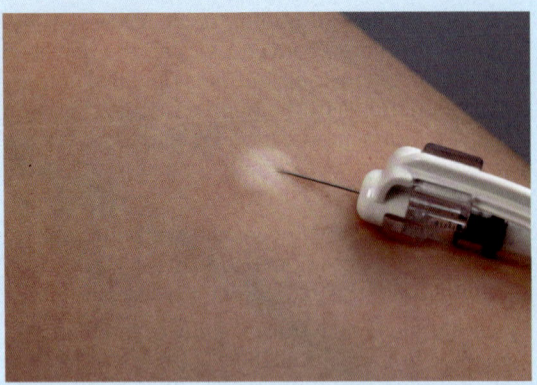
Injecting the solution to form a wheal. (Evans-Smith, 2005.)

4. Withdraw the needle at the same angle at which it was inserted. *Rationale: Doing so minimizes skin damage.*
5. Do not massage the site. Instruct the client not to scratch it. *Rationale: Massaging or scratching increases absorption and can irritate the skin and interfere with the results of the test.*
6. Draw a circle around the site with the permanent marking pen. Some facilities request that the date be added also. (Reading of the test is done by feeling for a swelling or bump [induration] at the end of the test period [2-3 days]. The size of the induration is measured and recorded. Erythema [redness] does not indicate a positive reading.) *Rationale: Marking ensures that the person reading the test will be examined in the correct location. Measuring the induration gives an accurate evaluation of the amount of reaction to the test.*

Follow ENDDD steps

Special Reminders
- The needle is inserted and withdrawn more slowly than for intramuscular (IM) or subcutaneous (SQ) injections.
- Usually, a special form or card is filled out when a PPD test is administered. In some cases, the manufacturer and lot number of the serum must be recorded, depending on agency protocol.
- A notation is made in the client's record, to make sure the test is read in 48 and/or 72 hr.
- In some cases, a negative PPD (or appropriate management of tuberculosis [TB]) is required before the client can be transferred from a hospital to a long-term care facility or group home.

IN PRACTICE
NURSING PROCEDURE 64-3 — Administering Subcutaneous or Intramuscular Injections

Supplies and Equipment
Medication scanner or MAR
Medication
Appropriate syringe and needle (see Fig. 64-3)
Gloves
Alcohol swabs
Note: Follow steps in Nursing Procedure 64-1 before proceeding.

Steps
Follow LPN WELCOME steps and then

1. Prepare the medication in the correct type of syringe. Add air to the syringe according to agency policy. The needle chosen should be about one-half the depth of a skinfold, from top to bottom, when pinched. *Rationale: Preparing the medication before entering the client's room facilitates administration. For a heparin injection, 0.1 mL of air is generally recommended, to clear the medication from the needle when injected.*
2. Choose the site, depending on the type of injection to be given. Choose a site with no bruises, inflammation, edema, masses, or tenderness. Heparin is usually given in the abdomen. Wear gloves for all injections. *Rationale: Site selection is very important for client comfort and safety and for the medication to be effective. Gloves are particularly important because this poses a risk for contact with the client's blood.*
3. Open at least two alcohol swab packages. Cleanse the injection site with an alcohol pad in a circular motion, from the center outward. Allow to dry. *Rationale: Cleansing in this manner removes skin microorganisms and prevents contaminating a clean surface with a dirty one. Alcohol disinfects as it dries. Also, wet alcohol might mix with the medication, causing damage and/or discomfort.*
4. Remove the needle cap, if a prefilled syringe, or retract the safety sheath. *Rationale: This readies the needle for injection.*
5. For a subcutaneous injection, use the nondominant hand to pull the skin taut or bunch the skin over the injection site, depending on the situation (see Nursing Procedures 64-4 and 64-5). For an average-size client, the skin may be spread tightly over the injection site or bunched together. For an obese client, the skin is usually bunched. *Rationale: The client's size determines the choice of site preparation. Skin that is spread taut facilitates needle entry. Bunching the area, if the client has excess tissue or loose skin, may be necessary to ensure that the needle is placed in*

subcutaneous tissue. Firm skin makes injection easier and more comfortable.

6. For an intramuscular injection, the skin is often held taut. ***Rationale:*** *This usually allows the medication to be given into muscle tissue.*

7. Hold the syringe in the dominant hand as though it were a pencil or a dart. Keep the first finger on the side of the plunger during insertion. ***Rationale:*** *This position prevents accidental medication loss while inserting the needle.*

8. Insert the needle quickly at the correct angle. ***Rationale:*** *Quick needle entry is less painful for the client. The correct angle delivers medication into the proper tissue.*

9. Release the skin. Adjust the nondominant hand to hold the syringe near the skin. ***Rationale:*** *You will use your dominant hand to manipulate the plunger and inject the medication.*

10. Aspirate for a blood return by pulling back on the plunger with the dominant hand. If blood enters the syringe, remove the needle and prepare a new injection. Aspiration is usually contraindicated for heparin and certain other injections. ***Rationale:*** *Blood return indicates needle placement in a blood vessel. The injection would then be intravenous (IV), which could be life-threatening. Blood contaminates the medication, which must be redrawn. Aspiration is not done with heparin because of its anticoagulant activity.*

11. If no blood appears, transfer the thumb of the dominant hand to the plunger of the syringe. Inject the medication at a slow and steady rate. ***Rationale:*** *Rapid injection may be painful for the client.*

12. Remove the needle quickly at the same angle at which it was inserted. ***Rationale:*** *Slow needle withdrawal may be uncomfortable for the client. Removing it at the same angle minimizes discomfort.*

13. Apply pressure on the site gently with a new alcohol swab, unless contraindicated for specific medication. ***Rationale:*** *It is recommended that gentle pressure be applied over a heparin injection for 30 to 60 s.*

14. Pull the sheath over the safety syringe and twist until it locks, cover the needle with the attached sheath, or insert the needle into a protective cap (see Figs. 64-3 and 64-4). Do not recap the needle. Place the needle and syringe in the sharps container. ***Rationale:*** *Most accidental needle sticks occur during recapping of needles. Proper disposal prevents injury to nurses and environmental workers.*

Follow ENDDD Steps

IN PRACTICE
NURSING PROCEDURE 64-4 Giving a Subcutaneous (SubQ) Injection

Note: Assemble supplies and equipment as in Nursing Procedure 64-1 and review the preparation steps in Nursing Procedures 64-1 and 64-3 before proceeding.

Steps
Follow LPN WELCOME steps and then

1. The most common method of giving a subcutaneous (SubQ) injection is to bunch the skin at the subcutaneous site. ***Rationale:*** *Usually, bunching the skin will ensure that the injection is made into the subcutaneous tissue and not the muscle beneath. Spreading the skin would not allow sufficient subcutaneous tissue to prevent intramuscular injection.*

2. Assess the client for body mass of subcutaneous tissue and choose the appropriate needle and angle of injection. The angle of injection varies with the amount of available tissue (Fig. 64-7). Most subcutaneous injections are given at a 90° angle. However, a thin client may need to be injected at an angle of a lesser degree (as small as 45°). ***Rationale:*** *It is important to choose an injection angle that will ensure the medication is delivered into the subcutaneous tissue and not muscle.*

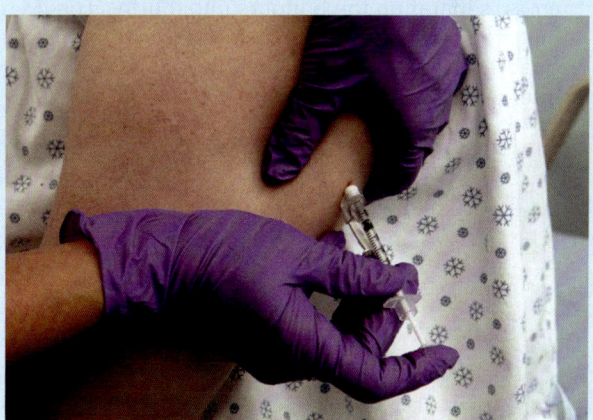

Injecting the medication. (Evans-Smith, 2005.)

3. The amount of the client's adipose tissue also determines the length of needle to use (generally between 5/8 and 1 in.). ***Rationale:*** *It is important to*

have a needle that is short enough to just reach the subcutaneous tissue and not extend into muscle.

4. Take care not to inject the medication too closely to the skin's surface. **Rationale:** *Shallow injection will allow for faster absorption and onset of action of the medication and may cause local irritation. (This might actually be an intradermal injection if it is very shallow.)*

5. Injection at the correct angle is important. **Rationale:** *The usual rule is 45° for a 5/8-in. needle or 90° for a 0.5-in. needle. Check your agency's policy.*

6. Indicate that the medication was administered subcutaneously. If the client is to receive repeated injections, identify the exact site used. **Rationale:** *Documentation provides coordination of care. Site rotation prevents injury to subcutaneous tissue.*

7. Check the client's response to the medication within an appropriate period. **Rationale:** *Drugs administered parenterally have a rapid onset.*

8. Dispose of syringe and needle in the sharps container.
Follow ENDDD steps

IN PRACTICE
NURSING PROCEDURE 64-5 Giving an Intramuscular (IM) Injection

Note: Assemble supplies and equipment as in Nursing Procedure 64-1, and review the preparation steps in Nursing Procedures 64-1 and 64-3 before proceeding.

Steps
Follow LPN WELCOME steps and then

For dorsogluteal administration

1. Drape the client, to maintain privacy, while exposing the buttock to determine the proper administration site.

2. Position the client on the side or prone. Draw an imaginary line from the posterior superior iliac spine to the greater trochanter of the femur (see Fig. 64-8A). Another method of identifying the correct site is to draw two imaginary lines that cross, separating the buttocks into fourths. The IM injection can be given safely in the upper, outer quadrant, approximately 1 to 2 in. above the intersection of the imaginary lines.

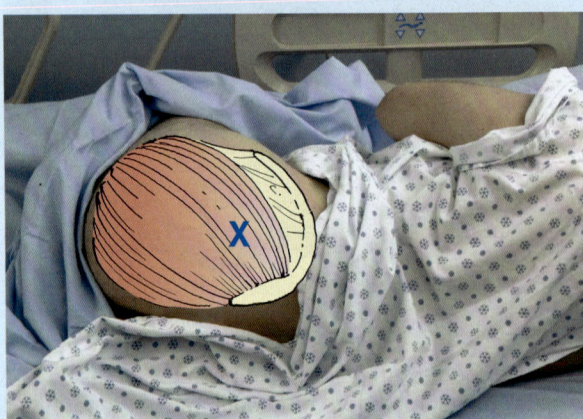

Side-lying position for dorsogluteal intramuscular (IM) injection (client on the right side). (Evans-Smith, 2005.)

3. Take care not to touch the client's buttocks while drawing this imaginary line. **Rationale:** *This is invasive and might cause unnecessary anxiety and embarrassment.*

4. Before administering the injection, encourage the client to relax the gluteal muscles by pointing the toes inward. **Rationale:** *This will ease discomfort caused by the medication being injected into muscle tissue.*

5. The skin at the injection site can be bunched or spread, depending on the client's size and the nurse's preference. **Rationale:** *It is important that the medication be injected only into muscle tissue.*

6. Safely give the injection anywhere along the imaginary line below the curve of the iliac crest.
Follow ENDDD steps

For ventrogluteal administration

1. Move the client into a side-lying position. To locate the ventrogluteal site, place the palm on the lateral aspect of the greater trochanter of the femur.

2. Move the index, or first, finger to position on the anterior superior iliac spine. Extend the middle finger to the iliac crest. With the fingers and palm in this position, a "V" is formed between the index and middle fingers (see Fig. 64-8B). **Rationale:** *The injection site is in the center of the "V".*

3. Ask the client to turn his or her toes inward to relax the muscle used for the injection. **Rationale:** *This position will relieve the discomfort of the medication being injected into the muscle tissue.*

CHAPTER 64 Administration of Injectable Medications

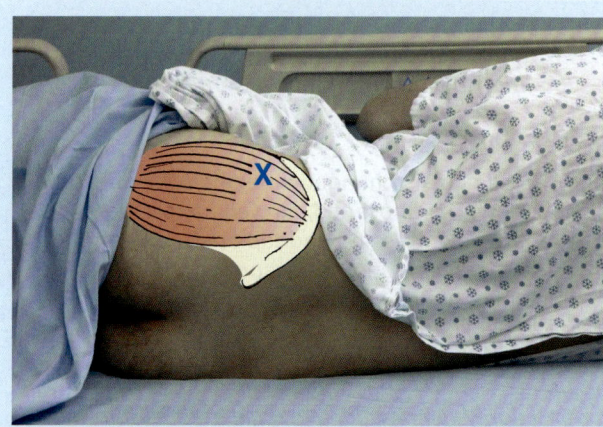

Side-lying position for ventrogluteal intramuscular (IM) injection (client on the right side). (Evans-Smith, 2005.)

Follow ENDDD steps

Special Considerations
- Intramuscular medication can also be given in the deltoid site or the vastus lateralis site. In rare cases, the rectus femoris site is used.

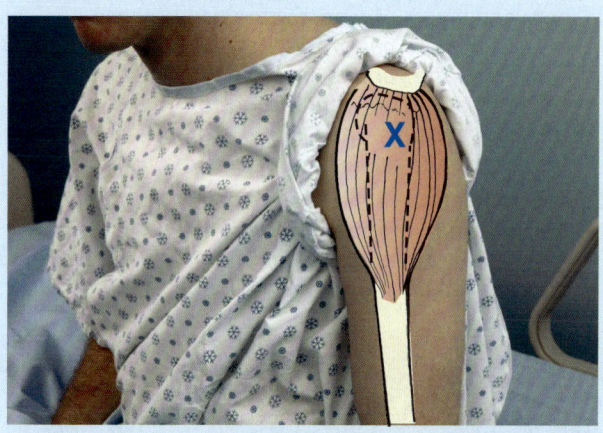

The deltoid site. (Evans-Smith, 2005.)

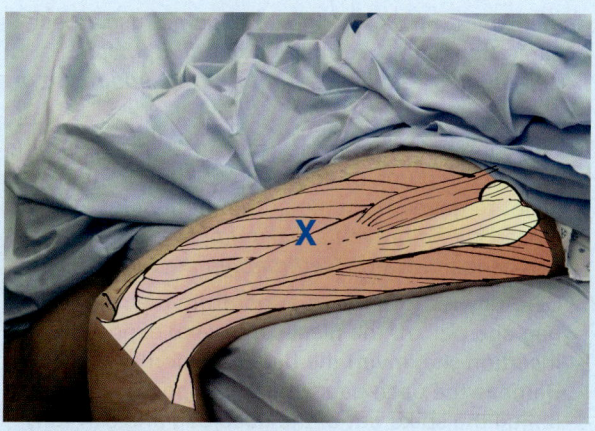

The vastus lateralis site. (Evans-Smith, 2005.)

- Indicate that the medication was administered intramuscularly. If the client is to receive repeated injections, identify the site used. ***Rationale:*** *Documentation provides coordination of care. Site rotation prevents injury to subcutaneous tissue.*
- Check the client's response to the medication within an appropriate period. ***Rationale:*** *Drugs administered parenterally have a rapid onset. Dispose of syringe and needle in the sharps container.*

Follow ENDDD Steps

IN PRACTICE
NURSING PROCEDURE 64-6 Changing the Intravenous (IV) Bag, Dressing, and/or Tubing

Note: Review the steps in Nursing Care Guidelines 64-1 and 64-3 before proceeding.

Follow LPN WELCOME steps and then
1. Always follow universal precautions when changing an IV bag or tubing.
2. To change an IV bag, gloves, an antimicrobial swab, and a disposal site for used materials are needed, in addition to the correct IV fluid. If also changing the dressing and tubing, it will be necessary to add dressings, tape, and the correct tubing. In addition, tape remover and skin protectant are required, if ordered. Make sure to have a good light source.

To change an IV bag,
1. If an IV bag is running low, it is necessary to replace it with a new bag. Make sure you have the ordered solution, as specified by the provider. ***Rationale:*** *A life-threatening air embolus or blood clot can form if the IV fluid is not flowing into the vein. In addition, an empty bag may require that the IV be restarted in a new location, causing unnecessary discomfort and the possibility of infection for the client. The infusion of incorrect IV fluid could be life-threatening.*
2. Examine the new bag carefully for sediment, cloudiness, particles, leakage, or any cracks or holes; do not use it if any of these exist. Check

the expiration date of the fluid; do not use if past expiration date. **Rationale:** *Using fluid that is not perfect or is past its expiration date could result in harm to the client.*

3. Close the roller clamp (see Fig. 64-11) on the tubing and set the pump or controller to "hold." The tubing is not removed from the pump. **Rationale:** *The closed clamp prevents leaking of fluid. The pump can be reset without rethreading the tubing.*

4. Carefully remove the wrapper from the new IV bag and pull off the plastic sleeve to expose the insertion site. Invert the bag (insertion site up). Remove the used bag from the IV pole and invert it. Pull the spike out of the used bag and carefully insert it into the new bag, without contaminating the spike or the insertion site. Some facilities require that the insertion site be wiped first with an alcohol swab. **Rationale:** *All these procedures must be performed carefully, to prevent contamination of the IV fluid. The bags are inverted to prevent fluid leakage.*

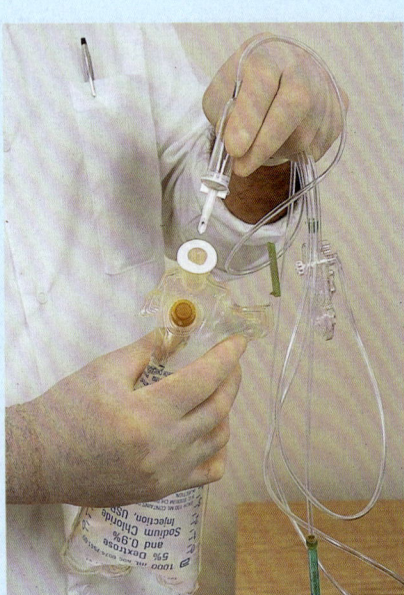

"Spiking" the new intravenous (IV) bag, with bag inverted. The fluid shown here is D_5NS (5% dextrose in 0.9% sodium chloride). (Lynn, 2018.)

5. Hang the new bag on the IV pole, making sure the drip chamber is half full (squeeze to fill; do not overfill) and the tubing is filled, "priming the tubing" (see Nursing Procedure 64-6). Turn "on" the pump. Check to make sure the preprogrammed rate of flow is correct; if not, reprogram the pump and have another nurse double-check. Label the IV bag, as per agency protocol; do not write directly on the IV bag. Document the amount of fluid infused from the old bag. **Rationale:** *Remove all air from the tubing, to prevent air embolism. If the drip chamber is completely full, you are not able to see the drops as they infuse. Follow the "7 Rights" of medication administration. Labeling is important for continuity of care. Writing on the bag may cause ink to leach through the plastic and contaminate the fluid. Documentation is essential.*

To change IV dressing

1. IV dressings are changed whenever they become soiled, wet, or loosened, as well as routinely. Prepare new dressing and tape before beginning. Stick necessary lengths of tape loosely by their ends on a handy surface; open the dressing package, keeping it sterile. **Rationale:** *The tape and dressings must be readily available because both hands will be needed to stabilize the access device and apply the new tape. It is also difficult to tear tape wearing gloves.*

2. Put on gloves and remove the transparent semipermeable dressing from over the venous access by pulling it sidewise from both sides, toward the middle, while holding the catheter hub. Remove tape from the old dressing, one layer at a time, pulling toward the insertion site. Leave the innermost layer of tape (holding the catheter hub) in place. Be careful if the tubing is entangled between layers of tape. **Rationale:** *All these procedures are performed very carefully, to prevent disturbing the venous access and/or pulling out the catheter, and to prevent discomfort to the client as much as possible. The last piece of tape stabilizes the access site until everything is ready.*

3. Carefully observe the IV site, making sure there is no infiltration or irritation. **Rationale:** *If irritation or infiltration exists, report it immediately. Discontinue the infusion, if so ordered.*

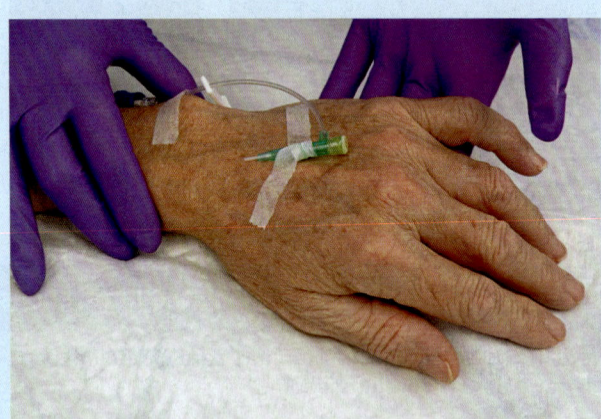

Carefully examine the insertion site. Note here how the last piece of tape was applied, sticky side up, under the catheter hub, with the ends crossing over. (Lynn, 2018.)

4. While stabilizing the venous access device (**VAD**) gently remove the last strip of tape securing the VAD. Pull each end toward the center. Roll or fold the tape. **Rationale:** *Pulling the tape toward the middle helps keep the VAD in place. Folding the tape keeps it from sticking to other things and getting in the way. Be sure to stabilize the VAD carefully, because it is no longer taped in place.*

CHAPTER 64 Administration of Injectable Medications 1007

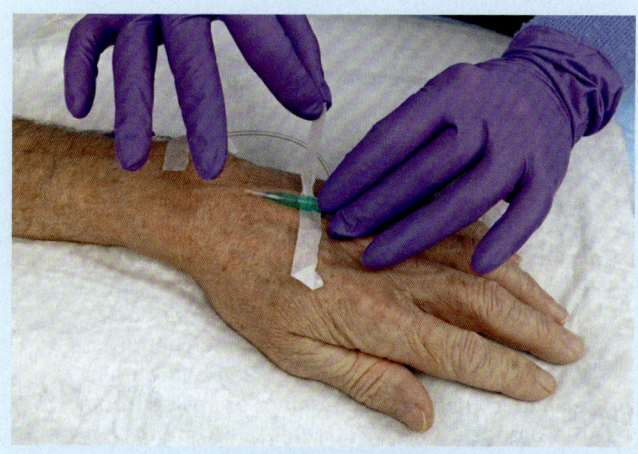

While stabilizing the insertion site, carefully remove the last piece of tape. The ends are pulled toward the venous access device (VAD) and folded over or rolled. After the site is cleansed, new tape is applied. (Lynn, 2018.)

5. Still stabilizing the VAD, remove excess tape residue with adhesive remover. Then, cleanse the insertion site with alcohol or other antimicrobial swabs, moving horizontally, then vertically, and lastly, in a circular fashion. Change swabs between each motion. Cleanse from the site outward. Allow the antiseptic to dry thoroughly. The protocol may be to apply skin protectant, such as Skin Prep or No Sting Barrier Film, before redressing the site. Allow this to dry also. *Rationale: It is vital to keep the insertion site as free of microorganisms as possible. This site is the most common source of infection for IVs. Antimicrobials continue to work as they dry. Skin barriers help prevent skin breakdown and itching.*

6. Reapply tape and/or dressings, per facility policy. Make sure the IV insertion site is protected and the VAD is firmly in place. The first piece of tape is applied as follows: Pass the tape under the catheter hub, sticky side up. Cross the ends over the hub, one at a time (in a chevron pattern), making sure the VAD is securely in place. The tape should pass over both the connecting hub on the VAD and the tubing. It should look like the earlier photo in this procedure when completed. Then, the remainder of tape strips and the transparent dressing are applied. *Rationale: By attaching the first strip of tape directly to the VAD and then taping it to the skin, the device will be more secure. Other tape and dressings are added, as needed. A transparent dressing is placed over the insertion site and connections to facilitate inspection and stabilize the site further.*

To change IV tubing

1. If tubing is to be changed, the bag should also be changed. *Rationale: This helps preserve the sterility of the system. Tubing is changed periodically, to prevent clogging and/or infection.*

2. Unwrap the new tubing, maintaining sterility of the bag spike. Be sure you have chosen the correct tubing (vented or nonvented spike; with or without filter [see Nursing Care Guidelines 64-2 for inline filter]). Do not uncover the distal catheter connection yet. Spike the new IV bag (which is inverted), as described above. Turn the bag over and hang on the IV pole. Control the flow of fluid with the roller clamp (see Fig. 64-11). Prime the tubing and fill the drip chamber about half full. Close the clamp or regulator to stop the flow of fluid temporarily. *Rationale: Uncover only the portion of tubing you will be using immediately, maintaining the sterility of the catheter connector. The tubing must be primed, to prevent air from entering the client's vein.*

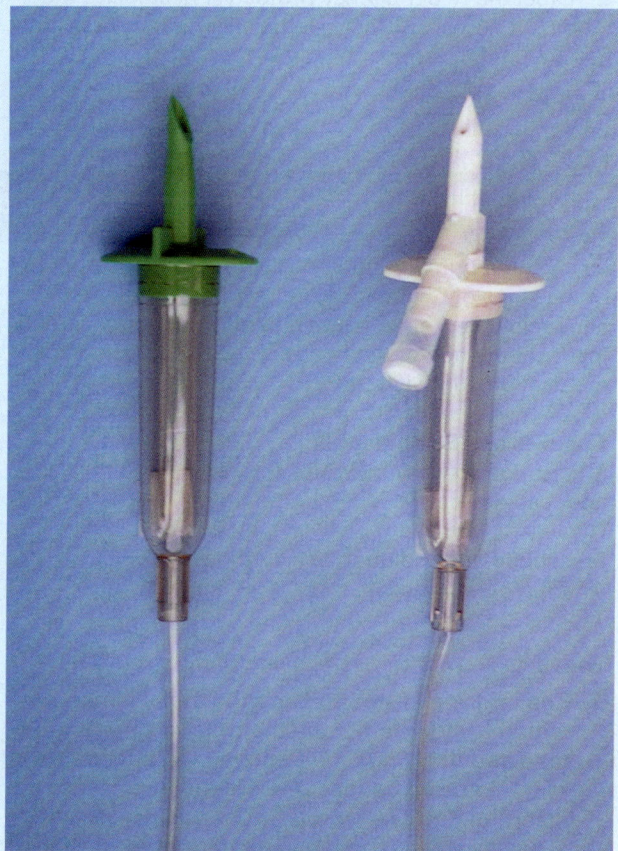

Intravenous (IV) tubing spikes. A nonvented IV spike (left) is used in most cases. In unusual cases, a glass IV bottle is used; in this case, a vented IV spike (right) is necessary to allow the fluid to flow. The vented spike often contains a filter as well, to prevent impurities in the air from entering the bottle. (Timby, 2015.)

3. Insert the tubing into the pump, according to the manufacturer's specifications (see Nursing Procedure 64-5). *Rationale: The procedures for setting up the pump must be followed exactly in order to maintain the safety features of the pump.*

4. Maintain sterility of the system. Remove dressings, as needed, to expose the insertion port in the client's

vein. Do not untape the VAD. Disconnect the old tubing. Uncover the new catheter connector and connect the end of the new IV tubing, which has been primed, to the hub of the insertion port. Make sure the connection is solid. Reapply tape and dressings, as needed. Open the clamp on the tubing and observe carefully to make sure fluid is flowing into the vein. Reprogram the pump. Most facilities require this to be double-checked by two nurses. *Rationale: It is important to have a solid connection between the bag and the spike and between the tubing and the catheter, to prevent leakage, disconnection, and/ or backflow. The tubing must be primed, to prevent introduction of air into the system. It is vital to program the pump correctly to make sure the client gets the ordered amount of fluid.*

5. Label the IV per agency protocols. Restabilize the site, if necessary. Instruct the client if there are any moving restrictions. *Rationale: It is important that all personnel know when the tubing was changed. An arm board or other stabilizing mechanism is used in some cases (see* Nursing Procedure 64-5). *It is important to prevent the IV from being dislodged.*

Follow ENDDD steps

Special Considerations

- Documentation involves date/time, type and amount of solution infused, assessment of IV site, and whether or not a tubing change was done. In many facilities, used IV tubing is placed in the sharps container or sealed into a red biohazard bag. *Rationale: Documentation provides communication with other healthcare workers. It is important to protect nurses and environmental workers from the client's body fluids.*

IN PRACTICE
NURSING PROCEDURE 64-7 — Converting a Continuous Intravenous (IV) Infusion to an Intermittent Line (Saline Lock)

To cap off a primary infusion line to a saline lock, many of the steps of IV initiation are reversed. The locks shown in this chapter contain extension tubing extending from the hub of the IV access device, to allow for medication administration.

Supplies and Equipment
Medication scanner or MAR
Lock cap device
Gloves
Prescribed flush solution in a syringe
Antimicrobial wipes
Tape

Follow LPN WELCOME steps and then

1. The infusion is stopped and the tube clamped with the slide clamp *and* the roller clamp. Enough tape and dressings are removed to allow removal of the infusion connector from the hub of the insertion device. *Rationale: Clamping prevents air from entering the line and blood from escaping.*
2. Remove the primary IV tubing from the extension device. Cleanse the device with an antimicrobial wipe. *Rationale: Cleansing helps deter the spread of microbes.*
3. Insert the tip of the syringe into the extension tube. Unclamp the extension tube and flush with the prescribed solution, usually normal saline, over 1 min (see Nursing Procedure 64-8). Reclamp the extension tube and remove the syringe. *Rationale: The tubing must be clamped when not being used for injection of medications; this prevents bleeding. The clamp is opened to allow the flush solution to be injected. Flushing helps keep the lock clear and open.*
4. Insert the lock cap device firmly into the extension tubing. Tape firmly in place. *Rationale: It is important to secure the lock firmly, to keep the access sterile and to prevent it from migrating or leaking.*

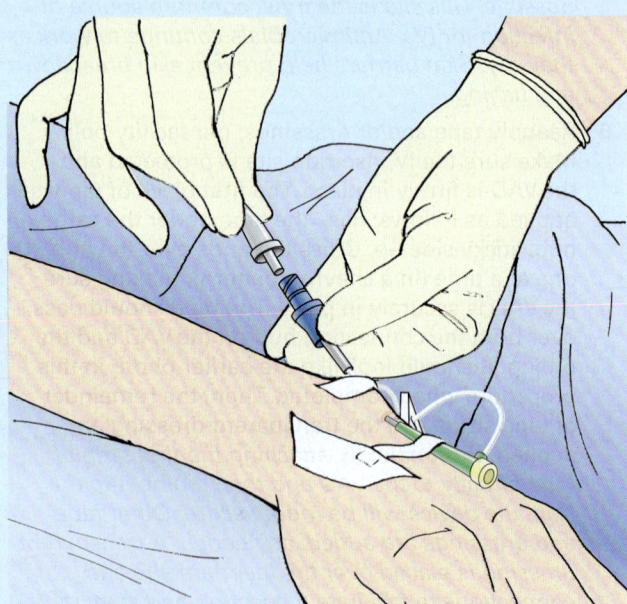

Insert the cap device firmly into the extension catheter, making this a saline lock. The lock is kept clamped until needed for flushing, or for a medication injection or IV infusion. (Lynn, 2018.)

5. Document the procedure and the amount of fluid that has been infused. *Rationale: Documentation is vital.*

Follow ENDDD steps

CHAPTER 64 Administration of Injectable Medications

IN PRACTICE
NURSING PROCEDURE 64-8 Flushing the Saline Lock; Administration of Medications Via Saline Lock

Supplies and Equipment
Medication scanner or MAR
Prescribed medication
Flush solution
Alcohol or other antimicrobial swabs
Gloves
Watch with a second hand
Needleless access syringe and hub

For Flush, Add:
Saline vial and syringe and needles or
Prefilled syringes (2-3) with needleless tip/hub

For Bolus or Push Injection, Add:
Syringes with needleless hub, containing medication

For Intermittent Infusion, Add:
IV bag or bottle with 50- to 100-mL premixed solution
IV tubing and tape
Syringe with needleless access hub
Needle lock device (see Nursing Procedure 64-10)
IV pole and pump

Note: Review Nursing Care Guidelines 64-1 and 64-3 and follow the steps in Nursing Procedure 64-1 before proceeding.

Steps
Follow LPN WELCOME steps and then

For Bolus Injection or Saline Flush

1. (See also Nursing Procedure 64-12.) Draw up the solution to be injected into a syringe, using the needleless system (see Fig. 64-15). Label the syringe carefully with the client's name and ID number, as well as the medication and dosage. Locate the "bull's eye" (needleless) port of the lock. *Rationale: The needleless system is safer for both client and nurse. The bull's eye is the area into which the medication or saline will be injected.*

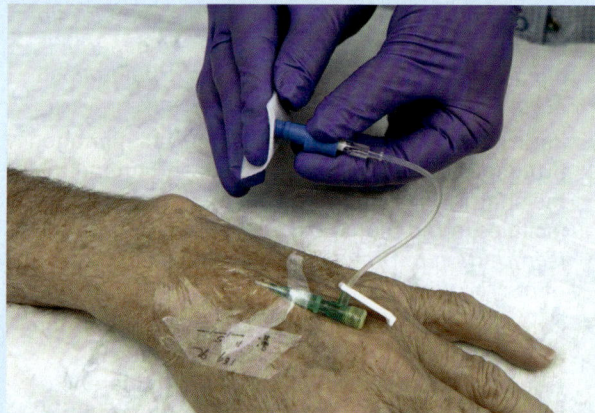

After the "bull's eye" port is cleansed with alcohol, it is prevented from touching anything else, to deter the spread of microorganisms. (Lynn, 2018.)

2. Steady the port with the nondominant hand. After cleansing the port with alcohol or the prescribed antimicrobial swab, insert the needleless hub of a syringe containing 1 mL of saline into the center of the port. Release the slide clamp on the extension tubing of the port. Aspirate *gently* for blood return (in this case, blood should usually return). *Rationale: It is important to steady the device, because it could be pushed further into the vein, which would contaminate the area. In addition, it will not be possible to insert the needleless hub into the port unless it is held firmly. The syringe should be in the port before releasing the clamp, to prevent external bleeding. Blood usually should return into the tubing when aspirating because the lock is in a vein, although blood return does not always occur.*

3. To flush, gently inject the saline after the clamp is released. *Do not force the solution.* Clean the port again with a new antimicrobial swab. *Rationale: The saline clears the lock and ensures that it is patent (open). A new antimicrobial swab should be used each time, to deter the spread of microorganisms. If the lock has clotted off, forcing the solution could cause an embolism.*

4. If injecting medication, inject according to the prescribed rate, using a watch with a second hand. A needle may have been required to draw up the medication. If so, change to a needleless hub before bringing it to the client. Be sure the syringe is labeled until you reach the client. *Rationale: Many medications would be too stressful to the system if injected too quickly (speed shock). It is important to follow the* "Rights of Medication Administration."

5. Remove the medication syringe and insert a new syringe of saline into the lock. Inject approximately 5 to 10 mL of saline after injecting the medication. *Rationale: The saline fills the lock and pushes the medication out, so the client receives the full dose of medication.*

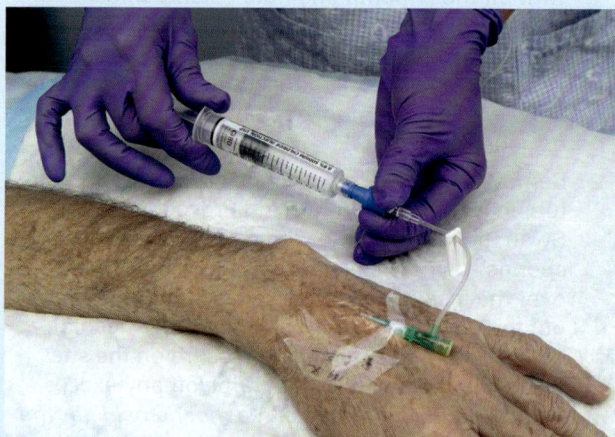

After cleansing the port, the syringe with the needleless device is inserted. Stabilize the hub with the nondominant hand. The slide clamp (shown here as white) is released. After aspirating for blood return, the medication or saline is injected slowly. The clamp is reapplied, to prevent bleeding and/or leakage of medication, and the syringe removed. An IV bag is attached in the same manner. (Lynn, 2018.)

6. Before removing the needleless hub, close off the saline lock, using the slide or snap clamp. *Rationale: It is important to clamp off the device, to prevent bleeding and/or loss of solution.*

For Intermittent Infusion Via Saline Lock

1. Use premixed IV solution. Pull the cover off the tubing spike and spike the bag. Add the needleless component to the distal end. Prime the tubing, making sure all air is out. Fill the drip chamber about half full. Hang the bag and insert the tubing into the pump, as prescribed. *Rationale: Preparing the medication before entering the client's room facilitates administration. Air injected into the client's vein could be dangerous.*
2. Follow steps 2 and 3 above, if the tube is to be flushed. Insert the needle or needleless component attached to the IV into the access port. Lock it in place or tape securely. (Locks are illustrated in Nursing Procedure 64-10.) Regulate the flow rate. *Rationale: The connections must be secure. The flow rate must be regulated carefully; injection of medication too rapidly can lead to shock.*
3. Clamp the tubing and withdraw the needle from the lock when all solution has been infused. Follow agency policies regarding equipment disposal (usually in the sharps container). *Rationale: Proper disposal maintains safety.*
4. Flush the lock again after the medication has infused. *Rationale: This action ensures that all of the medication has been administered.*

Follow ENDDD steps

Special Reminder

- Check the client's allergy band, to make sure they are not allergic to medication being administered. Make sure the medication is compatible with the IV solution. *Rationale: It is important to prevent errors or unwanted side effects.*
- Remember to record the fluid volume in the bag (often 50 mL) on the client's intake and output (I&O) record. Check the client's response to the medication within the appropriate time frame. *Rationale: Drugs administered parenterally have a rapid onset of action.*
- In special cases, the lock is flushed with heparin. Follow the facility's protocol.

IN PRACTICE
NURSING PROCEDURE 64-9 — Discontinuing an Intravenous (IV) Infusion or Saline Lock

Supplies and Equipment
Medication scanner or MAR
Gloves
Alcohol sponges
2 × 2 sponges
Tape or Band-Aid

Follow LPN WELCOME steps and then

1. Turn off the IV pump and note volume infused for documentation. Clamp the tubing, using the roller clamp, the slide clamp, or both (see Figs. 64-11 and 64-14 and Nursing Procedure 64-6). *Rationale: This prevents overflow of fluid after the IV is discontinued.*
2. Remove all tape and dressings on and around the tubing (see figures in Nursing Procedure 64-6). Swab the insertion site with an antimicrobial sponge. Using an alcohol sponge, press gently over the insertion site. Gently and smoothly pull out the VAD (intracatheter, tubing, or IV needle), without stopping. Maintain pressure on the site while withdrawing the VAD. Wipe off any excess blood and fluid. *Rationale: Alcohol helps deter the spread of microorganisms. Pressure helps prevent a bruise (hematoma) at the insertion site. Steady removal is more comfortable for the client.*
3. Continue to apply pressure over the venipuncture site for about 5 min. Sometimes, it is helpful to elevate the limb. Apply a Band-Aid or folded 2 × 2 sponge and tape tightly over the puncture site. Some facilities specify the application of antibiotic ointment as well. *Rationale: Continued pressure also helps prevent hematoma formation. The antibiotic helps prevent infection.*
4. Check the catheter tip carefully, to make sure it is intact. *Rationale: Although such an occurrence is uncommon, a small portion of the catheter tip could break off the catheter, enter the general circulation, and form an embolism. Should this occur, it must be reported immediately.*
5. Return the pump to the designated site, per agency protocol. Discard all used IV bags and tubing in the sharps container or designated area. In some facilities, a red biohazard bag is used. *Rationale: It is important to prevent needle sticks and the spread of microorganisms.*
6. Carefully document the procedure. It is important to document if the catheter's tip was intact, where the IV was located, the site's appearance at discontinuation, and the total amount of fluid infused. *Rationale: Accurate documentation is important, for continuity of care.*

Follow ENDDD steps

CHAPTER 64 Administration of Injectable Medications

IN PRACTICE

NURSING PROCEDURE 64-10: Administration of IV Medications Via Piggyback Setup (Small Volume Delivery System)

Supplies and Equipment
Medication scanner or MAR
Gloves
Antimicrobial swabs
IV piggyback solution, containing medication
Needleless connector
Piggyback tubing
IV pole with hooks on two levels or separate extension hook
Labels to identify client, solution, date, and other pertinent information

Steps
Follow LPN WELCOME steps and then

1. Make sure you have the correct intravenous (IV) solution and medication; scan the client's name tag. The IV piggyback medication (IVPB) is often contained in 25 to 100 mL of fluid (often normal saline), although it may be as much as 250 mL. The IVPB medication must be given within 30 min of the scheduled time. *Rationale: Most piggyback medications are antibiotics or chemotherapy agents and must be timed correctly for maximum effectiveness.*

2. Check to make sure the IV solution in the IVPB is compatible with the primary infusion. *Rationale: Incompatible solutions could cause clotting or other untoward effects.*

3. The IVPB will usually be timed. Make sure to follow the orders. If using a pump or controller, this can be programmed into the unit. If using a drip setup, the number of drops per minute must be calculated (see Box 64-2). *Rationale: Administration over the correct period of time is essential. If it is run too fast, shock could occur.*

4. Open the IVPB solution package and the tubing, maintaining sterility. (Sometimes, the IVPB solution comes with attached tubing.) Make sure the clamp on the tubing is closed. Spike the new IVPB solution bag, open the clamp, prime the tube, and half fill the drip chamber. Close the clamp. Attach a needleless connector or safety needle connector to the distal end of the tubing and keep it sterile. *Rationale: Make sure everything is ready before proceeding.*

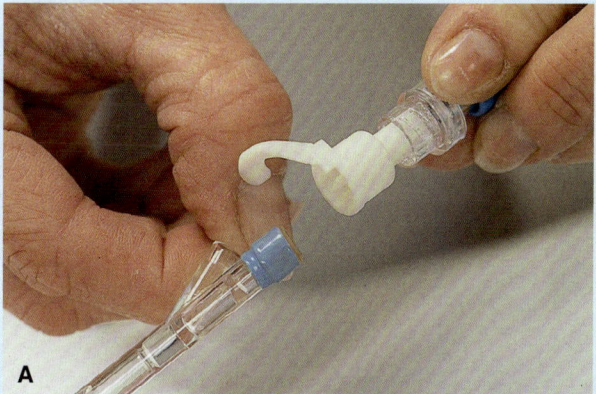
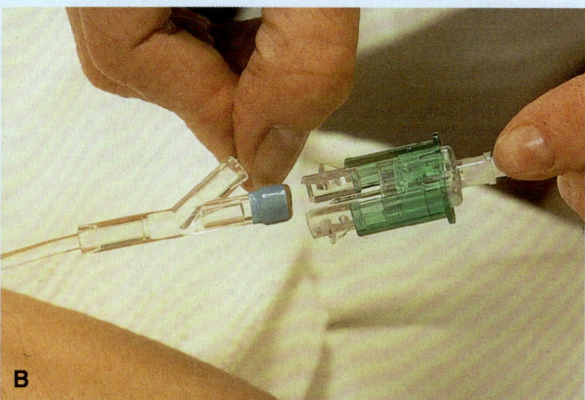

An illustration of two types of safety connectors that can be used for piggyback administration. This photo is for demonstration purposes only. If connecting a working IV, gloves should be worn. **A.** The needleless system often includes an IV locking clamp. The needleless cannula is pushed into the injection port and the hook locks it into place. **B.** If a needle must be used, it should be a safety needle. This needle is surrounded by a clear plastic guard, which slides over the injection port, guides the needle into the port, and anchors the needle in place. (Ellis & Bentz, 2007.)

5. Hang the IVPB on the IV pole. Move the primary IV to a lower position on the pole or add an extension hook. Make sure the primary IV is infusing properly. *Rationale: It is important to make sure that lowering the primary infusion did not stop the flow. The primary infusion must be lower than the piggyback, so atmospheric pressure will allow the piggyback to run, stopping the primary infusion (via a back-check valve). Whichever infusion bag is higher on the pole will run first.*

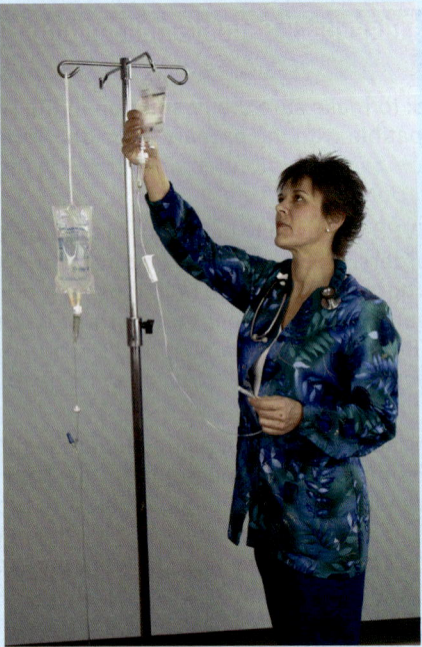

Hanging the piggyback solution at a higher level than the primary IV bag (right). The primary bag (left) is lowered by a hook supplied by the manufacturer of the piggyback solution. (Lynn, 2018.)

6. Swab the infusion port of the primary tubing with the antiseptic solution. Insert the needleless connector or needle, with a safety connection, into this port. *Rationale: The antimicrobial solution deters microorganism spread. The needleless connector prevents needlestick injuries. The lock feature prevents the IVPB from being dislodged.*

7. Open the clamp on the IVPB, to allow fluid to infuse. When the IVPB is completed, close the clamp and raise the primary infusion to the higher position. Disconnect the IVPB and discard appropriately.

8. Document the amount of fluid infused. *Rationale: Documentation is vital for continuity of care.*
Follow ENDDD steps

Special Considerations
- In some facilities, a stopcock port is used. This will be turned to the "open" position to run IVPB fluids and closed when the piggyback infusion is completed.
- In some cases, two IVs are run in tandem. That is, the primary IV and piggyback are hung at the same level and run at the same time. This setup must be monitored closely and clamped off immediately when the piggyback solution has infused. *Rationale: If the piggyback is not clamped off, the primary solution will flow back up into the tandem line.*
- If incompatible IV solutions are being infused, the primary IV is clamped off and the tubing flushed with normal saline. Then, the secondary bag is run, the line flushed again, and clamped off. Then, the primary infusion is unclamped and run.

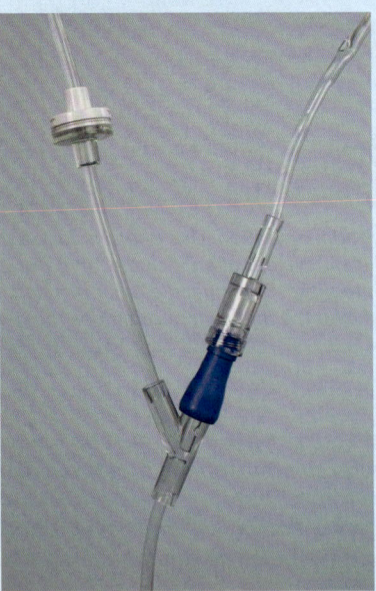

After cleansing the access port, the piggyback tubing is connected to the port using a system similar to the one shown above. (The primary IV is shown on the left; the piggyback is on the right [Lynn, 2018].)

IN PRACTICE

NURSING PROCEDURE 64-11: Administration of Medications Via Volume-Controlled Infusion

Supplies and Equipment
Medication scanner or MAR
Prescribed medication
Ordered diluent solution
Large syringe with needleless adaptor
Antimicrobial sponges
Gloves
Volume-control setup
Appropriate tubing
IV pole
Note: Review Nursing Care Guidelines 64-1 before proceeding.

Steps
Follow LPN WELCOME steps and then

1. The volume-controlled infusion is usually used as a piggyback with an existing intravenous (IV) infusion (see Nursing Procedure 64-10). It is also possible to use with a saline lock, and in this case, the facility may require that the lock be flushed before and after administration of the medication. *Rationale: It is important that the client get all the medication, as ordered. The volume-control setup is a convenient method of determining that all medication is given.*

2. Close the roller clamp on the diluent solution and attach the bag to the tubing in the same manner as any IV bag. Hang the diluent bag on the IV pole. If being given piggyback, this bag is above the primary infusion. The volume-control chamber is attached below the diluent bag. Often, the entire setup comes packaged as a unit. *Rationale: The solution will flow by gravity and must be high enough so it will flow freely. This is true, whether flowing by gravity or controlled by a pump. Aseptic technique is used in working with any IV.*

3. Open the roller clamp to prime the tubing and half fill the drip chamber. Then, run the prescribed amount of solution from the diluent bag into the volume-control chamber. This amount must be measured exactly. Then, securely close the roller clamp between the diluent bag and the control chamber (above the control chamber). *Rationale: The diluent solution is run into the chamber before medication is added. This method ensures that the medication is diluted with an exact amount of IV solution. This method is effective for small amounts of medication and diluent solution.*

4. Cleanse the intake port on the volume-control chamber. Using the needleless adaptor, inject the prescribed amount of medication into the chamber. *Rationale: Cleansing the port helps deter the spread of microorganisms. By using the syringe, the amount of medication can be measured exactly. The needleless adaptor prevents needlestick injuries.*

5. Run this IV in the same manner as any other. Be sure to regulate the rate of flow—calculate the flow rate or use a pump or controller. Usually, a specific length of time for this infusion is part of the provider's order. When all the medication has been infused, clamp off the volume-control tubing. Disconnect this tubing from the primary IV or from the saline lock and discard appropriately. *Rationale: The volume-control infusion is completed and is discarded. This helps prevent the spread of microorganisms and is less cumbersome for the client.*

The volume-controlled infusion setup. The bag on top contains diluent solution. The roller clamp above allows fluid to flow into the volume-control chamber and is closed after the tubing is primed and the prescribed amount of fluid is in the chamber. The slide clamp below is kept closed until the infusion is ready to administer. (Lynn, 2018.)

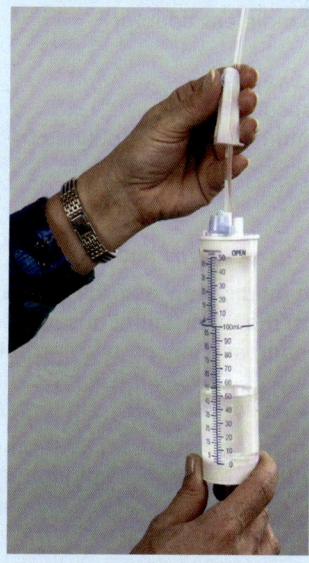

Opening the roller clamp to fill the volume-control chamber with the prescribed amount of IV fluid. (Shown here, the amount is 50 mL, a commonly used volume for this procedure [Lynn, 2018].)

1014 UNIT 9 Pharmacology and Administration of Medications

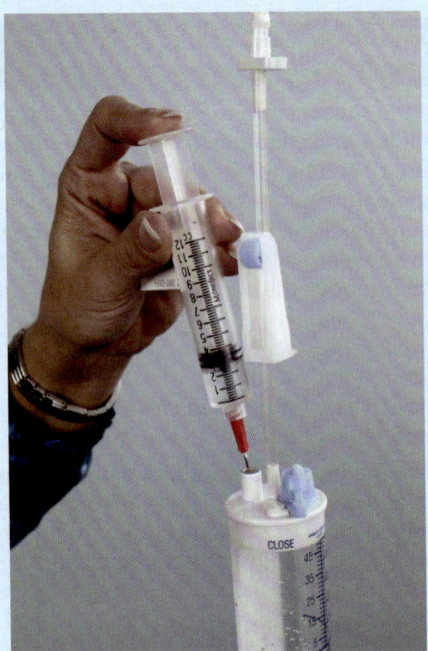

After cleansing the port with an antimicrobial swab, injecting the prescribed medication into the needleless port of the volume-control chamber with a large syringe. (Lynn, 2018.)

6. If this medication is run as a piggyback, the primary IV should restart automatically. Make sure the pump is set correctly. If the client has a saline lock, many facilities require the lock to be flushed again after the administration of medications. In some cases, a primary IV is also flushed. *Rationale: Flushing the lock or IV tubing ensures that all the medication has been given.*

7. Document the amount of fluid infused. *Rationale: Documentation provides continuity of care.*
Follow ENDDD steps

Special Considerations
This method of administration infuses medication in a fairly concentrated form. Be sure to observe the client carefully during the infusion and for a period of time after the infusion is completed.

IN PRACTICE
NURSING PROCEDURE 64-12 Administration of Medications Into a Continuous Infusion (IV Push)

Supplies and Equipment
Medication scanner or MAR
Prescribed medication
Syringe with needleless adaptor
Gloves
Antimicrobial swabs
Watch with a second hand
Note: Review Nursing Care Guidelines 64-1 before proceeding.

Steps
Follow LPN Welcome steps and then

1. Prepare the medication, as ordered. Label the syringe with the medication, dosage, client's name, record number, and any other information required by the facility. *Rationale: It is important that this medication be correct and be accurately identified.*

2. Swab the injection port on the IV tubing closest to the client with antimicrobial solution. Allow to dry. *Rationale: The antimicrobial solution continues to kill microorganisms as it dries.*

3. Many facilities require two nurses to double-check any IV push medication. In addition, many facilities do not allow LVs/LPNs to administer medications by this method. *Rationale: This is a very dangerous method of medication administration.*

4. After swabbing the injection port, insert the needleless hub of the syringe into the center of the port. Stop the flow of the primary infusion by pinching the tubing just above the injection site. Pull back gently on the plunger of the syringe, to aspirate for blood return. *Rationale: Pinching the tubing during the injection allows blood to return when aspirated.*

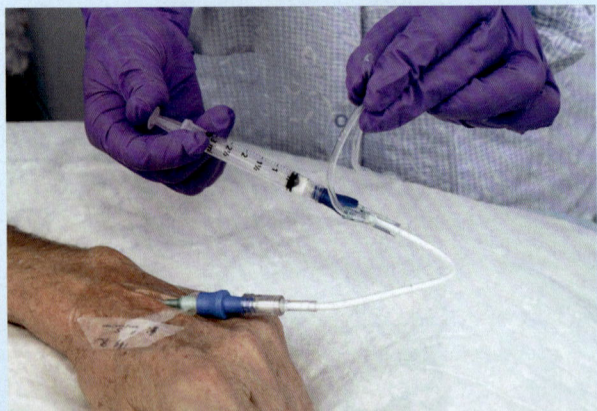

Pinching the IV tubing above the injection port, to interrupt the flow of fluid from the primary IV. Injecting the medication into the port. (Lynn, 2018.)

CHAPTER 64 Administration of Injectable Medications

5. Smoothly inject the medication into the port. If the injection is given in less than 1 min, it is referred to as a push or bolus. Release the tubing. *Rationale: Remember this is a very dangerous procedure.*

6. In some cases, the injection is timed with a watch, as per orders. In this case, the medication is referred to as "medication given over _X_ minutes." Some facility policies recommend pinching the tubing while injecting and releasing between pushes. In any event, be sure the primary IV solution is infusing when not pushing the medication. *Rationale: It is important to follow the primary provider's instructions, in order to help prevent complications. The flow of IV fluid helps to dilute the medication.*

7. After injecting the medication, withdraw the syringe and recheck the infusion rate. *Rationale: Make sure the solution is infusing properly.*

8. Recheck the client frequently after the administration of this medication. *Rationale: It is important to make sure the client is not having any complications.*

Special Considerations

- In some cases, medication must be diluted before administration. If the volume of medication is less than 1 mL, the medication should be diluted in 5 to 10 mL of normal saline or sterile water before injection. Document the amount of fluid infused. *Rationale: This prevents the medication from being lost in the injection port or the IV cap. Documentation is vital.*
- In some cases, particularly when using a very small needle, blood may not return when aspirated. This does not necessarily mean that the IV is not patent. If there are no signs of infiltration and the IV is running freely, the IV push may be given. If you have any questions, be sure to request assistance.

Follow ENDDD steps

IN PRACTICE
NURSING PROCEDURE 64-13 | Venipuncture (Phlebotomy)/Obtaining a Blood Specimen

Supplies and Equipment
Gloves
Alcohol or chlorhexidine swabs
Vacuum-type blood tubes
Tourniquet
2 butterfly needles (with vacutainer connection or adaptor), syringes and needles, or
Vacutainer sleeve and needles
2 × 2 gauze squares (and/or Band-Aid)
Tape
Tube labels and pen or preprinted stickers
Laboratory request forms (or request programmed into computer)
Biohazard bag and sharps container
Eye protection (optional)
Light source

Steps
Note: Review Nursing Care Guidelines 64-1 before proceeding.

Follow LPN WELCOME steps and then
Venipuncture (phlebotomy), using the butterfly needle.

1. Assemble materials needed (see Fig. 64-19). Be sure you have the correct tubes for the specimens ordered and to sequence the tubes as per facility protocol. Have name stickers or labeling materials available. Use the smallest needle possible. *Rationale: Specific tests require different types of tubes. Specimens should be collected in the prescribed order. A specimen collected in the wrong tube or not handled properly will not yield an accurate test and must be redrawn. All specimens must be clearly identified. The smaller the needle, the less discomfort for the client.*

2. Open the butterfly needle package, keeping the contents sterile. Screw the needle assembly into the vacutainer sleeve with the needleless access device inside the sleeve. Hold the first vacuum tube loosely in the sleeve; do NOT plug it into the tube. If the butterfly does not have a vacutainer connection, an adaptor will be required. Wear eye protection, if there is any chance of blood splash. *Rationale: It is important to have everything ready before accessing the vein. Protect yourself from the client's body fluids.*

3. Check for presence of a radial pulse. Locate a peripheral vein. The ideal vein is straight and prominent, without hematoma or swelling. The antecubital fossa is often the site used; the hand may also be used. Apply the tourniquet about 4 to 6 in. (10-15 cm) above the proposed insertion site. Do not apply too tightly. If the client's skin is friable, the sleeve of the client's gown may be under the tourniquet. A blood pressure cuff may also be used. Inflate to just below the client's normal diastolic pressure—about 50 mm Hg. *Rationale: The client must have a radial pulse for an appropriate vein to be accessed. Protect the client from skin breakdown.*

4. Ask the client to alternately open and close the fist, ending with a closed fist. If a vein is difficult to locate, lower the arm below the level of the heart and/or tap or stroke the area, while gently moving away from the heart. As a last resort, a warm pack may be applied for about 10 min before the venipuncture. *Rationale: Various methods are used to make the vein accessible. Having the tourniquet in place for a few seconds helps the vein to fill and stand out.*

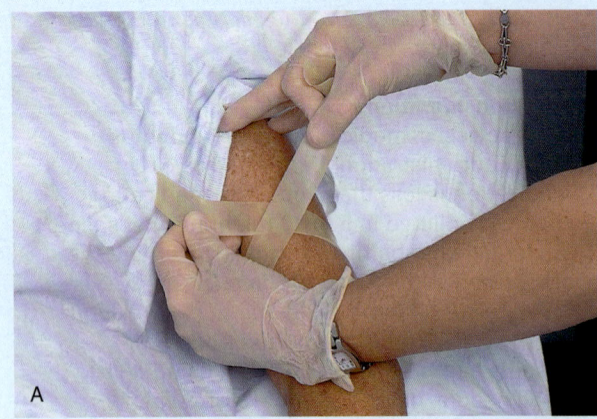
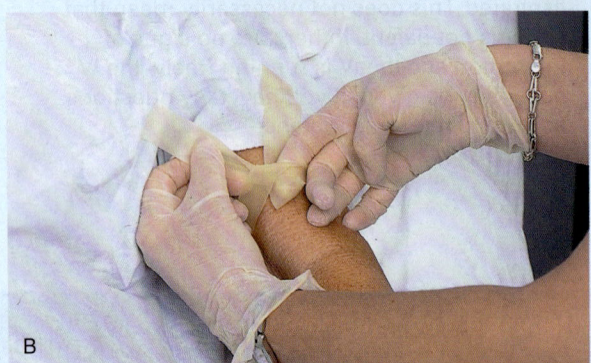
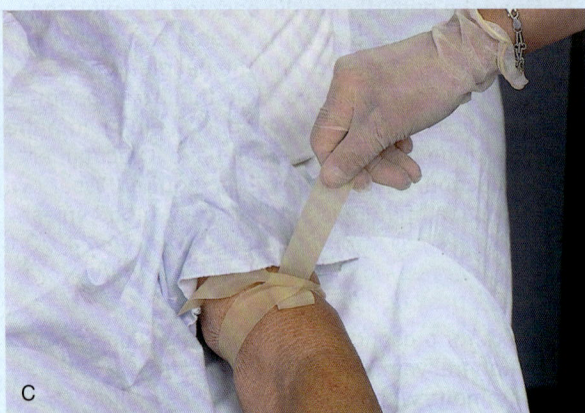

To apply a tourniquet: **A.** Cross the two ends over each other and pull them tightly in opposite directions. **B.** Tuck one end under the other side. **C.** To release the tourniquet, pull one of the free ends. Dispose of the tourniquet per agency policy. (Copyright © B. Proud.)

5. Ask the client to hold the arm straight, from shoulder to wrist. A small pad may be applied under the elbow, to keep the arm straight.
   Rationale: The more clearly the vein can be felt, the more likely it is that the venipuncture will be successful. The arm needs to be straight to allow the best access.

6. Locate the vein by *feeling* it (palpation). It should feel firm, but not hard, and slightly rebound when palpated. Do not use a vein that feels rigid or rolls when palpated. *Rationale:* Palpation is much more accurate than visualization. In this way, the nurse can determine the location and quality of the vein. It is important to use the best possible vein.

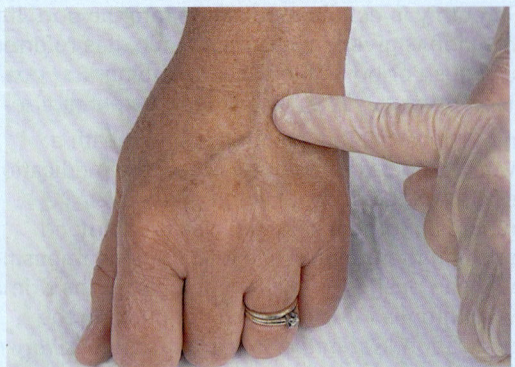

Palpating the vein, to determine the best access site. (Timby, 2005.)

7. Release the tourniquet. Make sure the vein decompresses. Clean the area with prescribed antiseptic. If using alcohol, move in a circular motion from the site outward. If using chlorhexidine, move horizontally over the site. Allow to dry. Do not touch the area after it has been cleaned. *Rationale: The vein should decompress when the tourniquet is released. Clean from the site outward, making the actual site as clean as possible. The antiseptic kills microorganisms as it dries. This also prevents burning when inserting the needle. Touching the site would contaminate it.*

8. Reapply the tourniquet. Grasp the wings on the butterfly needle, so the needle's bevel is up (see Figs. 64-18 [butterfly] and 64-19 [other devices]. Bevel up is shown in the current procedure). This will render the butterfly unit flat on the bottom, with the bumpy sides of the wings outward, toward your fingers. Remove the protective cover from the needle (nearest the wings). Without contaminating the site, pull the skin downward until it is taut. Alternatively, the skin may be held taut on each side of the insertion site. *Rationale: Grasping the wings of the butterfly firmly allows best control of the needle. The needle will be easier to insert if the setup is flat against the skin, which will position the needle with the bevel up. The rough sides of the butterfly wings make them easier to grip. Pulling on the skin will move it slightly away from the needle. The vein must be stabilized or it will move away when the needle touches it.*

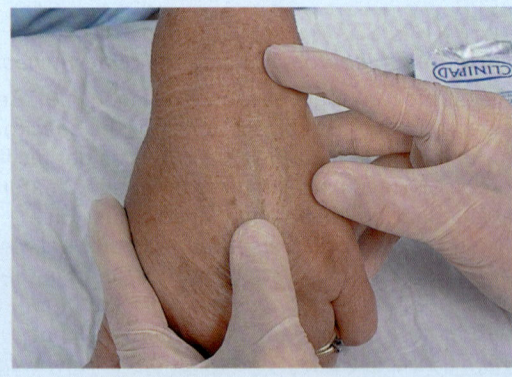

Stabilizing the vein by pulling the skin downward until it is taut. (Timby, 2005.)

9. Insert the needle into the vein at an angle of 15° to 30° with the *bevel up.* You may puncture the vein from the top or the side. You will feel a "give" (change in resistance) when the needle enters the vein. When blood returns, the specimen can be obtained. Shown in the accompanying figure is the vacutainer system for venipuncture. The basic procedure is the same as for the butterfly needle. *Rationale: The butterfly needle is small, making the procedure as comfortable as possible. The vein must be stabilized or it will move when the needle touches it. The butterfly needle may be used for a continuous infusion, although other devices are also commonly used* (see Figs. 64-18 and 64-19).

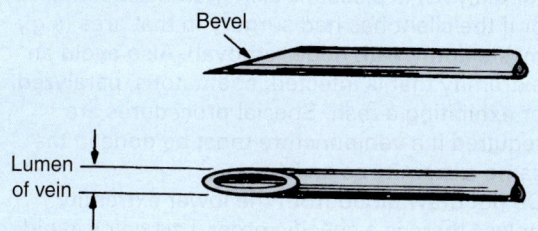

After applying the tourniquet, locating the vein, and cleaning the site, the needle is injected with the bevel of the needle upward. Follow the lumen of the vein when inserting the needle. (Timby, 2005.)

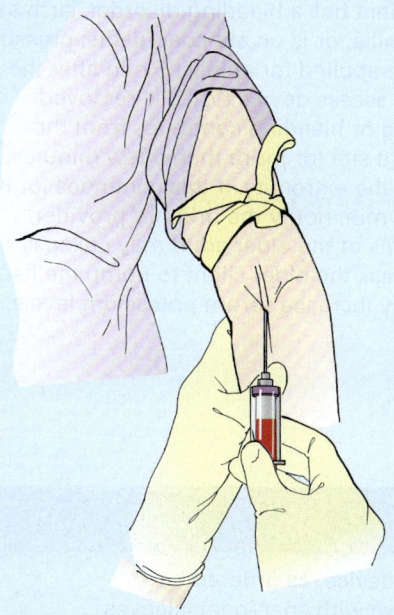

Shown here is the vacutainer method of blood collection. Visualize blood return before puncturing the stopper of the vacutainer tube. (Lynn, 2018.)

10. If blood does not return, the needle may be rotated or advanced slightly. It also may be withdrawn slightly. The needle may NOT be advanced after being withdrawn. Lower the hub of the butterfly close to the skin. *Rationale: These procedures are important to prevent contamination. Lowering the hub causes blood to displace the air in the tubing and facilitates the flow of blood.*

11. Stabilize the vacutainer sleeve and push the needleless device into the required blood tube, puncturing the rubber stopper of the blood tube. Each tube has a vacuum to draw blood into it. Allow the vacuum in the tube to draw the desired amount of blood into the tube. Pull the blood tube off the needle and apply additional tubes, as needed. Gently rotate each tube as it is removed from the access device. *Rationale: It is important to have blood return before inserting the butterfly into the collection tube. The vacuum provides gentle suction to draw the desired amount of blood into the tube. Rotating the tubes ensures that the blood will be mixed with any special media in the tube.*

12. Follow the sequence of tubes to be collected, as specified by the facility. *Rationale: If the tubes are filled in the wrong sequence, the tests may not be accurate.*

13. The tourniquet may be removed after the first tube is filled if the blood flow is adequate. Always remove it before removing the needle. After sufficient blood is obtained, ask the client to relax the fist. *Rationale: If the tourniquet is not released, a hematoma will form and bleeding may occur.*

14. Gently withdraw the needle and engage the needle guard or use a Point-Loc device. Apply firm pressure over the site for several minutes with an antiseptic swab. Fold a 2 × 2 gauze in half or fourths and apply firmly over the site. Tape securely. Tell the client that this dressing can be removed in about 30 min. *Rationale: Protect from needle sticks. Hematoma formation can usually be prevented by the above procedures.*

15. Carefully label all specimens with the client's name, record number, and other pertinent data. The label must be applied before you leave the client. In most facilities, stickers are available for this purpose. Place the sticker on the tube and not the top. Make sure to angle the sticker on the tube so it does not overlap. In some facilities, each sticker is for a specific test. If this is the case, make sure stickers are applied to the correct tubes. *Rationale: It is vital to make sure the labels are for the correct client. Any tubes that are not labeled or are labeled incorrectly will not be tested by the laboratory and must be redrawn.*

16. Place blood tubes in a biohazard bag and send to the laboratory immediately, accompanied by the appropriate requests. If requests are programmed into the computer, double-check them. Indicate that specimens were drawn. If using a pneumatic tube system, make sure the foam rubber inserts are in the tube. *Rationale: The biohazard bag identifies body fluids. The tube should be padded, to prevent breaking the tubes.*

17. Dispose of all materials, per agency policy. Be sure needles are placed in the sharps container. Used tourniquets and vacutainer sleeves are disposed of as well, according to agency policy. *Rationale: It is important to prevent injuries and contamination.*

Follow ENDDD steps

For Vacutainer Blood Draw

1. Screw the needleless (black) end of the double-ended needle unit into the vacutainer sleeve with the needle outside. Place the first blood tube loosely into the vacutainer sleeve; do not puncture the rubber stopper. Uncover the access needle and insert it into the vein, holding the vacutainer at a 20° to 40° angle with the bevel of the needle up. Push the needleless connecter inside the sleeve into the blood tube after the vein is accessed. This will allow the vacuum to draw the blood into the tube.

2. After blood is drawn, remove and protect the sharp needle with the articulated shield or a Point-Loc device before placing it in the sharps container. The plastic vacutainer sleeve and tourniquet are also discarded. *Rationale: The basic procedures are the same, no matter how the blood is obtained for a specimen. The same blood tubes are used as in the procedure above.*

For Syringe Draw

1. A syringe and needle may also be used to obtain a blood specimen. The procedure is the same as above.

2. After the blood is drawn into the syringe, the tops of the blood tubes are cleansed, and the needle is inserted into the blood tubes, allowing the vacuum to fill the tubes to the desired level.

Follow ENDDD steps

Special considerations

- Some types of testing require special handling. For example, in some cases, the tubes must be pre-warmed (cryoglobulin) or must be placed on ice for transport to the laboratory (ammonia, ionized calcium). When testing for lactic acid level, a tourniquet is not used (to prevent artificially raising the levels). For vitamin levels, the tube must be protected from exposure to light (to avoid destroying the vitamins).
- Tubes for transfusion testing are never drawn by LVs/LPNs.
- After the tourniquet is applied, a brachial pulse should still be able to be palpated. If the tourniquet is too tight, arterial blood flow will be impeded.
- Unless absolutely necessary, do not draw blood from the same extremity in which an IV is running, an arteriovenous shunt (access device for dialysis) is placed, a skin graft has been done, or if the client has had surgery in that area (e.g., mastectomy with node removal). Also avoid an extremity that is infected, edematous, paralyzed, or exhibiting a rash. Special procedures are required if a venipuncture must be done in the same extremity as an IV site.
- Do not draw blood from the lower extremity, unless there is a specific order. This helps avoid thrombophlebitis.
- If the client has large, distended veins, the venipuncture may be performed without a tourniquet. This helps prevent hematoma formation.
- If the client has a bleeding disorder, such as hemophilia, or is on anticoagulants, pressure must be applied for at least 5 min after the venous access device (VAD) is removed.
- If oozing or bleeding continues from the puncture site for more than a few minutes, elevate the extremity. If this continues for more than 10 min, notify the primary provider.
- The veins of the older adult may collapse easily. Do not ask the older client to pump the fist, as this may increase serum potassium levels.

IN PRACTICE
NURSING PROCEDURE 64-14 — Initiating Intravenous Infusions

Note: Review Nursing Care Guidelines 64-1 and Nursing Procedure 64-13 before proceeding.

Supplies and Equipment
Medication scanner or MAR
Gloves
Chlorhexidine, povidone-iodine, or alcohol swabs
Ordered IV solution
Tourniquet
IV pole
Dressings and tape, including transparent dressing
Waterproof pad
Appropriate IV tubing
IV access device, as ordered
Client gown with snap-open sleeves
Light source
Electronic controller or pump, or microdrip setup
Printed label or marker
Anesthetic (numbing) cream, such as Numby Stuff (optional)
Lidocaine 1% and syringe (optional)
Syringe with saline flush (optional)
Arm board (optional)
Razor (optional)
Scissors (optional)

Steps

Follow LPN WELCOME steps and then

1. Assist the client to don a gown with snap-open sleeves. Open IV tubing set, using sterile technique (see below, Chapter 57, and also Figs. 64-18 and 64-19). Open intracatheter (or butterfly) to be used. *Rationale: The snap-open sleeves facilitate changing the gown, without needing to thread the equipment through closed sleeves. Sterile technique is necessary, to deter the spread of microorganisms. This is particularly important since the IV is in direct contact with the client's bloodstream.*

2. Have client in a low-Fowler position. Raise the entire bed to a comfortable height for you. Place a waterproof pad under the client's arm. If necessary and permitted in the facility, shave a small area of the client's arm. Otherwise, excess hair may be clipped with scissors. Apply numbing cream or inject lidocaine, if ordered. It may be necessary to remove the client's watch or move his or her ID band. *Rationale: This is the most convenient position for the nurse and is comfortable for the client. The pad will keep the bed from becoming soiled. Some facilities do not permit shaving the site, because of the danger of nicking the skin and providing a possible site for infection. If the area is hairy, shaving or clipping hair will enable the nurse to visualize the site better and will make tape removal more comfortable later. In addition, hair can harbor microorganisms. Numbing the area makes insertion of the catheter more comfortable. Applying these medications now gives them time to take effect while you are preparing the infusion materials. A watch or ID band may be in the way or may impede the flow of IV fluids.*

3. Inspect the IV solution, to make sure there are no impurities, and unwrap it. Invert the bag and spike it with the IV tubing (see Nursing Procedure 64-7). Turn it upright and hang on the IV pole. Loosen the protective cover on the hub of the tubing that will attach to the venous access device. Keep it sterile. Prime the tubing (fill with IV fluid) and squeeze the drip chamber until it is one-half full of fluid. Thread the tubing through the pump or controller. Make sure all bubbles are out of the tubing.

4. Program the pump, following the manufacturer's guidelines. Another nurse is usually required to double-check the programming. *Rationale: Remember the "7 Rights" of medication administration.* Set the pump on "hold." *Rationale: These procedures help you to have everything ready, so when the vein is accessed, there will be no delay in attaching the infusion. Two nurses are required to set the initial IV flow rate, to avoid errors. Each machine has a different method of setup.*

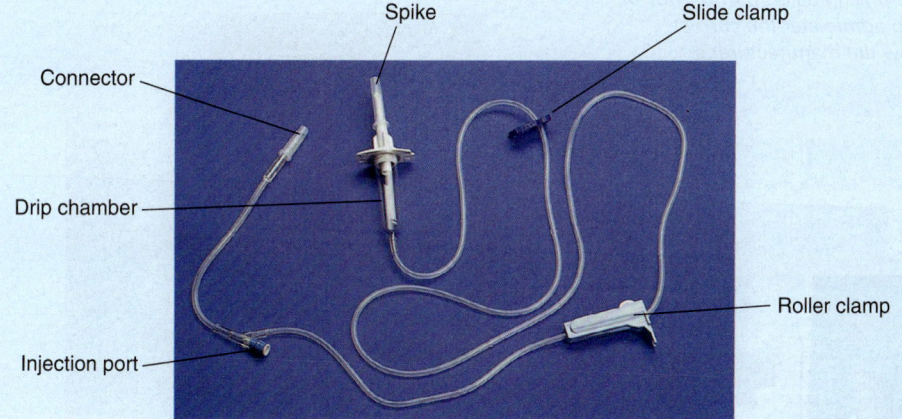

A basic tubing set for IV therapy. Note the injection port for administration of medications and the two clamps for controlling the flow of fluid. The connector and bag spike are both kept sterile until used.

UNIT 9 Pharmacology and Administration of Medications

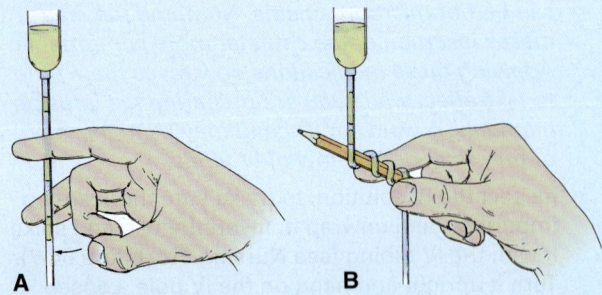

Removing air bubbles from the IV tubing. **A.** Tapping the tubing firmly usually will cause bubbles to rise to the top and be discharged into the drip chamber. **B.** If this is not effective, the tubing may be wrapped around a pencil, while the tubing is crimped below. This will force the bubbles upward. (Timby, 2005.)

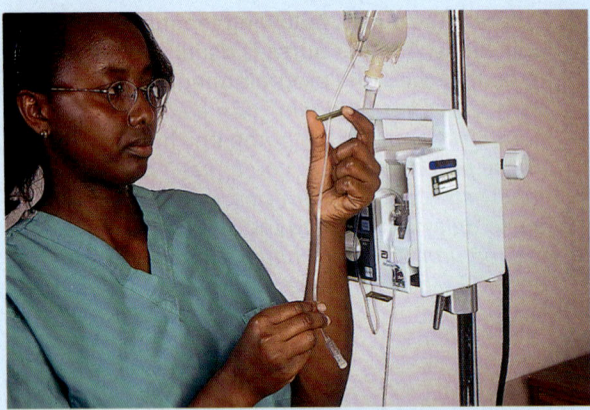

This nurse is setting up an IV infusion. A special tubing and cassette are required for this electronic infusion pump. The pump will then be programmed to administer the correct volume of fluid to the client. Follow the manufacturer's instructions.

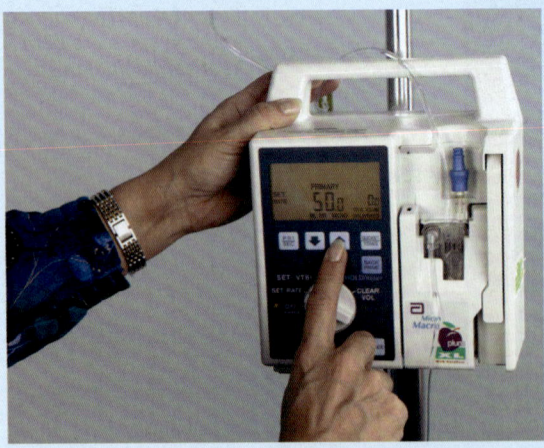

The IV infusion pump or controller is carefully programmed to administer the correct amount of fluid to the client. This is the "7th right" of medication administration. (Lynn, 2018.)

5. Tear several tape strips, about 4 in. (8.8 cm) long and place them in a convenient place. Open the transparent dressing package, keeping it sterile. Carefully inspect the venous access device and catheter. *Rationale: Tear tape ahead of time, to make sure everything is ready. Make sure there are no defects in the venous access device (VAD).*

6. Check for an appropriate site. Use the client's nondominant hand or arm. Look for a vein that is straight and palpable. Choose an access site that is as distal as possible. Use the hand instead of the antecubital space, for example. Wipe numbing cream, if used, off insertion site. Follow the pertinent steps in Nursing Procedure 64-14 to access the vein. *Rationale: The steps for venipuncture are the same, whether drawing a blood specimen or initiating an IV infusion.*

7. Apply the tourniquet and ask the client to make a fist. (Application of a tourniquet is illustrated in Nursing Procedure 64-14.) Feel for an appropriate vein. Gently insert the venous access device into the top or side of the vein by holding the device by the hub, and keeping the bevel side of the needle up. When blood enters the device, advance the needle to almost its full length. Then, thread the cannula/intracatheter into the vein, following the manufacturer's instructions. Most intracatheters are about 1 to 2 in. (2.2-4.4 cm) long. Gently follow the course of the vein to thread it in. As the catheter is being threaded in, the needle is withdrawn. When the needle is totally out of the vein, pull it into the needle guard and pull or twist, to snap it into place (see Fig. 64-19). Release the tourniquet. *Rationale: The catheter is advanced into the vein up to the hub of the device.*

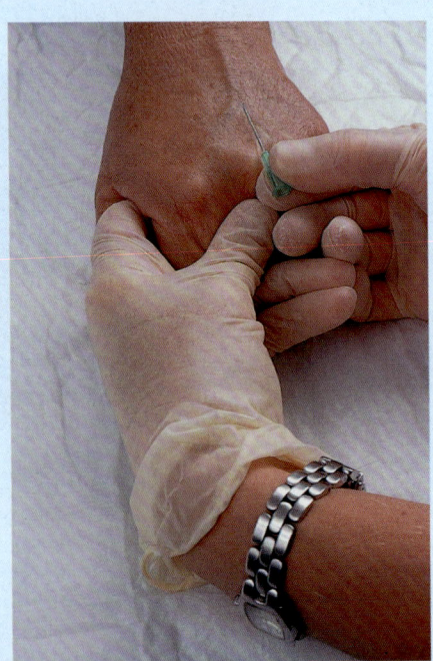

After entering the vein, the intracatheter or needle is advanced into the vein. (Timby, 2005.)

8. Attach the IV tubing of the primary infusion to the insertion hub immediately. Start the flow of fluid slowly. *Rationale: The hub must be*

attached immediately, to avoid loss of fluid and/or bleeding.

9. Secure the cannula hub with tape. The first piece of tape should be placed under the hub with the sticky side up. It is then crossed over the hub and taped securely on both sides in a chevron pattern. Another piece of tape is placed horizontally over the top of the hub and tape strips. *Rationale: It is vital to secure the device firmly.*

10. If a winged (butterfly) access device is used, place a strip of tape under the hub, sticky side up. Then pass one end of the tape back over each wing, parallel to the cannula. A second piece of tape is applied across the hub, the wings, and the first piece of tape, perpendicular to the cannula. *Rationale: This method secures the butterfly device firmly.*

11. Add other tape, as required. A transparent (moisture-vapor-permeable) dressing, such as OpSite or Tegaderm, is applied over the top after the VAD is secured. Seal this dressing around the cannula hub and make sure all the edges are secure. A 2 × 2 gauze may be gently inserted under the VAD hub, if necessary. *Rationale: Transparent dressings allow visualization of the site without removal of the dressing. If the insertion site is oozing or if the client is diaphoretic, the gauze will absorb the moisture and prevent the tape from loosening.*

12. Make a loop of tubing near the access site and tape it in place. Add other tape as needed. Start the pump and make sure it is operating properly. *Rationale: This will keep the weight of the tubing from pulling on and possibly dislodging the cannula. It is important that the fluid is infusing accurately.*

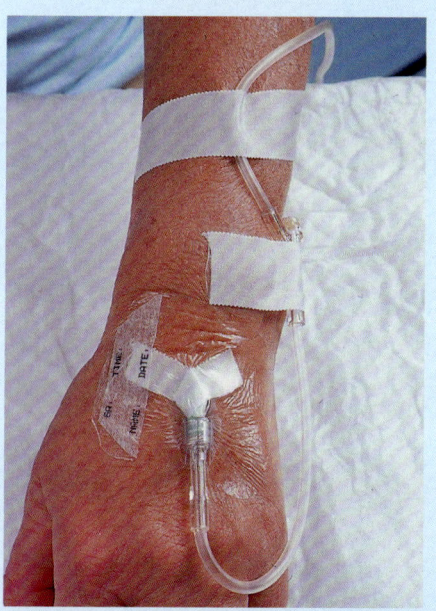

The hub of the VAD is taped securely, using the chevron pattern. Then the proximal lengths of the tubing are secured to the client's arm, to prevent dislodging the access. The date of insertion, initials of the nurse, and other pertinent information are added to the dressing.

13. Label the site with date, time, and type and size of catheter used; add your initials. A sticker is often supplied for this purpose. *Rationale: It is important to communicate with other members of the staff.*

14. Apply arm board, if needed. Check for pump operation and infiltration before leaving the client and check back in a few minutes. *Rationale: The venous access must be secured firmly in place. An arm board is needed if the site is near a joint or otherwise in danger of being compromised. Make sure the infusion is operating properly.*

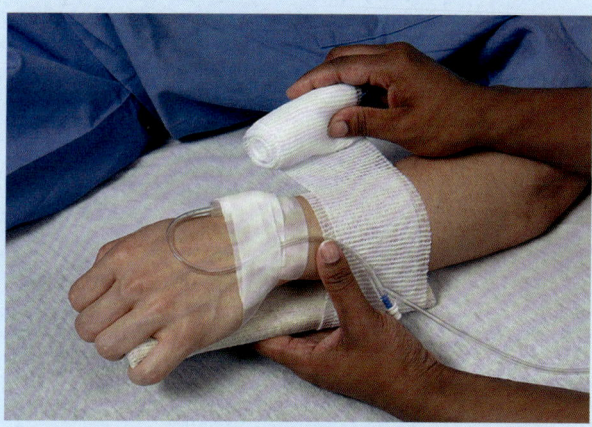

An arm board is used if there is any danger that the VAD will be dislodged by the client's movements. (Ellis & Bentz, 2007.)

15. Documentation includes the site, size, and type of venous access device used, rate of infusion, date, time, and the client's response. *Rationale: Documentation ensures continuity of care. It is important to identify when the access was placed.*

Follow ENDDD steps

Note: Many facilities supply an "IV Start Kit." Common contents of such a kit include tape, gauze, transparent dressing, antiseptic skin prep, alcohol swabs, sterile or clean gloves, skin protector, and tourniquet. Other items may be included, depending on the facility. Also needed will be the items listed above that are not in the kit. Be sure to check to see if any additional materials are needed.

Special Considerations
- Selecting the shortest and smallest IV cannula that will accomplish the IV administration is important for the client's safety and comfort.
- Some facilities require the application of antimicrobial ointment to the venous access site after insertion of an IV.
- Be sure to have adequate lighting when performing any venipuncture or initiating an IV.
- Sometimes, the client will be more comfortable if jewelry is removed on the side of the IV.
- If the rate of infusion must be calculated, two nurses should double-check the calculations for the number of drops per minute (see Box 64-2).

Maternal and Newborn Nursing | UNIT 10

65 Normal Pregnancy

Learning Objectives

1. Identify the components of preconceptional care and state the nursing considerations related to preconceptional care.
2. Describe the processes of conception, implantation, and placental development.
3. Differentiate the major events of the development of the embryo and the growth of the fetus.
4. Describe the structure and function of the placenta, umbilical cord, fetal membranes, and amniotic fluid.
5. Outline the pathway of fetal blood circulation.
6. Contrast the presumptive, probable, and positive signs of pregnancy. State the significant nursing considerations for each.
7. Describe the changes in a client's anatomy and physiology that occur during each trimester of pregnancy.
8. Discuss anticipatory guidance for pregnant clients related to changes in the body's structure and function.
9. Identify the major teaching concepts related to prenatal care.
10. Prepare a nursing care plan teaching healthy lifestyle behaviors for pregnant clients.
11. Identify recommended nutritional guidelines during pregnancy.
12. Describe the major and minor discomforts of pregnancy, how they might be alleviated, and how a client can differentiate them from more serious problems.
13. Summarize the major nursing considerations and nursing interventions for the pregnant client.
14. Explore ways to support preparing for parenthood and expanding the family.

Important Terminology

amnion
amniotic fluid
antepartum
ballottement
blastocyst
cephalocaudal
certified
   nurse-midwife
Chadwick sign
chorion
colostrum
conception
congenital
decidua
Doppler
ductus arteriosus
ductus venosus
embryo
fetoscope
fetus
foramen ovale
fundal height
gestation
Goodell sign
grand multipara
gravida
Hegar sign
hyperemesis
   gravidarum
implant
lactation
linea nigra
lordosis
melasma
morula
multifetal
multigravida
Nägele rule
obstetrician
obstetrics
para
pica
placenta
preconception
prenatal
primigravida
ptyalism
quickening
trimester
ultrasound
umbilicus
viable
Wharton jelly
zygote

Acronyms

BBT
BMI
CNM
EDC
EDD
HCG
HPL
LMP
LNMP
MSAFP
PIH
PMP
PPD
PPROM
PROM
PTL
RH Immune
   Globulin
   (R$_H$oGAM)
STI
TST

During the female client's reproductive years, the body is designed for conceiving and bearing children. Every month, it experiences a complex system of hormonal and physical changes for the sole purpose of producing an egg and supporting the earliest days of pregnancy. When pregnancy does not occur, the client has a menstrual period. When the egg that is produced meets with a sperm and conception occurs, they become pregnant. This initiates a sequence of events that, if all goes well, will result in the birth of a healthy infant.

Key Concept

Pregnancy is a normal physiologic process, not a disease.

In this chapter, you will learn about normal healthy pregnancy, the amazing changes that occur in the client's body during pregnancy, and the process of human development. You will learn how to help the client experience the healthiest pregnancy possible and prepare them for the changes in their life and family that are soon to come.

DEFINING PREGNANCY AS A NORMAL PROCESS

Gestation is the period of time that occurs from the moment the sperm fertilizes the egg until the birth of the newborn. Fertilization usually occurs 2 weeks after a client's last normal menstrual period (LMP or LNMP); most textbooks consider these 2 weeks as part of the gestational period. The total length of gestation, including these 2 weeks, is 40 weeks (10 lunar months or 9 calendar months). Based on the common use of the calendar year, pregnancy is divided into three 3-month periods (trimesters). If we break these trimesters into weeks, the first trimester begins on the first day of the client's last period and ends on the last day of week 13. The second trimester includes weeks 14 through 27, and the third trimester begins at week 28 and extends until the pregnancy is expected to end at 40 weeks (Table 65-1).

During the 40 weeks of pregnancy, the client may be referred to as a gravida, the Latin term for a pregnant client. If it is the client's first pregnancy, they are a primigravida; if they have had other pregnancies they are a multigravida. The word para refers to the parting of the client and baby or the birth itself. A client who has given birth many times (specifically, at least five times) is called a grand multipara. See Table 65-1 which shows the terminology and classifications of a pregnancy history.

Pregnancy is also called the antepartum period; therefore, prenatal care (care before the birth) may also be called *antepartum care*. Prenatal care can be provided in a private practice, at a clinic, or at home. Good prenatal care is one of the most important factors in the health of clients and babies. Even with the best prenatal care, it is possible for problems to occur; however, without adequate prenatal care, the risk for problems is much higher for both the client and the baby.

Obstetrics is the branch of medicine concerned with pregnancy and birth. An obstetrician is a medical doctor (MD or healthcare provider) who has had specialized training in the areas of obstetrics and gynecology. Healthcare providers, such as the *obstetrician* or other specialists, can obtain voluntary Board Certification showing advanced training via passing rigid, certifying examinations as designed by the American Board of Obstetrics and Gynecology, a subset of the American Board of Specialties. A nursing specialty in obstetrics means that a registered nurse has received specialized training in the management of pregnancy, labor, and birth. To be called a *certified* nurse-midwife (CNM), the RN must successfully complete advanced theory and clinical nursing education and have passed the comprehensive nursing certification requirements (Chapter 2 has further discussion of advanced nursing credentials.) CNMs work with healthy clients during their pregnancies. They help them to maintain wellness and attend at vaginal births. A CNM will refer a client who has known for suspected serious health risks to an appropriate healthcare provider (e.g., cardiologist) or to an obstetrician specializing in high-risk pregnancies. A healthy pregnancy and uncomplicated birth is a goal of all healthcare professionals.

TABLE 65-1 Abbreviations and Terminology Used in Obstetrics

G	Gravida	The number of pregnancies regardless of outcome
P	Parity	The number of deliveries
T	Term	A pregnancy greater than 37 weeks or less than 42 weeks or greater than 2,500 g
GTPAL	Gestations, Term pregnancies, Preterm pregnancies, Abortions, Living children	
TPAL	Term births (37 weeks' gestation), Premature births, Abortions, Living children	
Gestation	Also known as gestational age or the number of weeks from a client's last menstrual cycle to the current date. Normal ranges 38–42 weeks.	
Live births	The total number of children who survived birth but may have died any time later. Often confused with reference to "Living children."	
Living children	The number of children living as of today (does not include live births who died previously). Can be confused with reference to "Live birth."	
Preterm*	*A pregnancy of about 20–37 weeks, or more than 500 g or less than 2,500 g	
Postterm	An infant who is older than 42 weeks of gestational age	
Abortion	The delivery of an embryo or fetus by spontaneous or therapeutic means	
Puerperium	The time period between birth and 42 days after delivery	
Trimesters	First trimester = Week 1–12 Second trimester = Week 13–28 Third trimester = Week 29 (to delivery)	

NOTE TO STUDENT: The number of weeks of viability and of notation of preterm infants is not standardized and varies from 20 to 24 weeks. The delineation of viability and preterm infant can lead to misinterpretation of the actual gestational age of the infant.

Preconceptional Care

Preconceptional care is the care of the client *before* they are pregnant; it is an important healthcare priority. The health of a client before pregnancy influences the physical changes during pregnancy as well as the overall general health of the client and the fetus after the start of a pregnancy. The goal of preconceptional care is to have the best possible pregnancy outcome for every client and baby. This goal can be accomplished by performing a complete health assessment that includes a review of high-risk situations such as known hereditary conditions, environmental issues such as exposure to alcohol, or overall poor nutrition due to dieting or weight loss. The role of the nurse is to familiarize the family with existing or potential health conditions and to recommend any lifestyle, dietary, or environmental changes that will make the pregnancy safer for both client and baby. Preconceptional care is important because the health of the client affects the earliest weeks of pregnancy for both the embryo and the mother. Some clients often do not realize that they are pregnant until several weeks after conception. *These weeks are the most critical in human development.* Another good reason to start care before pregnancy is that some of the most important changes are difficult to accomplish and take a lot of effort by the client (e.g., better nutrition and the elimination of alcohol). Seven areas need to be addressed in preconceptional care:

1. Eating a healthy diet, including 400 mg (microgram, also seen as µg) of folic acid a day.
2. Stopping harmful or addictive behaviors, such as smoking, drinking alcohol, or using drugs.
3. Stopping the use of prescription drugs that are known to be harmful to a developing infant. Obtaining prescriptions for alternate drugs that are safer for use during pregnancy.
4. For the client with diabetes: Changing to insulin instead of an oral diabetic agent and making sure their blood sugar is under excellent control.
5. Referring a couple at risk of having a baby with a genetic defect for genetic testing and counseling before the pregnancy.
6. Testing the expectant client for infectious diseases, and either providing immunizations (e.g., rubella vaccine) or treating any infections that are found, including human immunodeficiency virus (HIV) and other sexually transmitted infections (**STIs**).
7. Reducing psychosocial risk factors. For example, helping a client who is being battered to find services and help or linking these clients with community resources.

For additional precautions, see In Practice: Educating the Client 65-1.

There are two types of preconceptional visits: (1) visits by a client or couple planning a pregnancy, and (2) visits by a client who is not planning to become pregnant soon but who may become pregnant. In the ideal world, every client or couple would seek healthcare when they are in the planning stages before a pregnancy occurs.

IN PRACTICE
EDUCATING THE CLIENT 65-1 — Pregnancy Precautions

The following is a summary of essential precautions to discuss with each client who is pregnant or who may become pregnant.

- Do not take any medication or drug, unless it was prescribed by a practitioner who knows that the client is trying to conceive or is already pregnant.
- Avoid x-rays whenever possible. If an emergency x-ray is indicated following an injury or due to a disease, it should not be refused because of pregnancy. An abdominal/pelvic shield should be used whenever possible. The pregnant client should inform both the healthcare provider and the x-ray technologist of their pregnancy. Elective x-ray examinations should be deferred until after delivery.
- Avoid substance use, including limiting caffeine intake; avoiding tobacco in any form, including passive smoke exposure; and abstaining from alcohol and recreational drugs.
- Avoid or limit exposure to known environmental toxins.
- Avoid exposure to infections, including rubella, influenza, tuberculosis, and sexually transmitted infections.
- Avoid hyperthermia-producing situations, such as hot tubs, excessive exercise, or prolonged sitting in hot water (>100 °F).

Stages of Human Development

Conception and Sex Determination

Human life begins with the union of two cells: the *ovum* and the *sperm* (Fig. 65-1). This union, known as *fertilization* or **conception**, usually occurs when the ovum is in the outer third of the fallopian tube (oviduct). At the time of conception, the sperm determines the sex. An ovum carries only one type of chromosome to determine sex: the X chromosome. A sperm cell may carry either an X or Y sex chromosome. If a sperm cell carrying a Y chromosome fertilizes the ovum, a boy (XY) will result; if the sperm cell carries an X chromosome, the result will be a girl (XX).

Period of the Zygote and Implantation

The fertilized ovum, or **zygote**, is the beginning of potential individual human development. During this time, the zygote divides rapidly until it forms a ball of about 16 identical cells, which is then called a **morula**. At this stage, the first differences among cells develop.

The morula is then swept down the fallopian tube and into the uterus, a process that takes approximately 7–9 days. The lining of the uterus, or *endometrium,* has become rich in nutrients in preparation for the pregnancy.

Just before the morula reaches the uterus, the cells begin to form layers; first one, then two layers surround a fluid-filled space, called a **blastocyst** (Fig. 65-2). A blastocyst is a thin-walled hollow structure of early embryonic growth and development. The

1026 UNIT 10 Maternal and Newborn Nursing

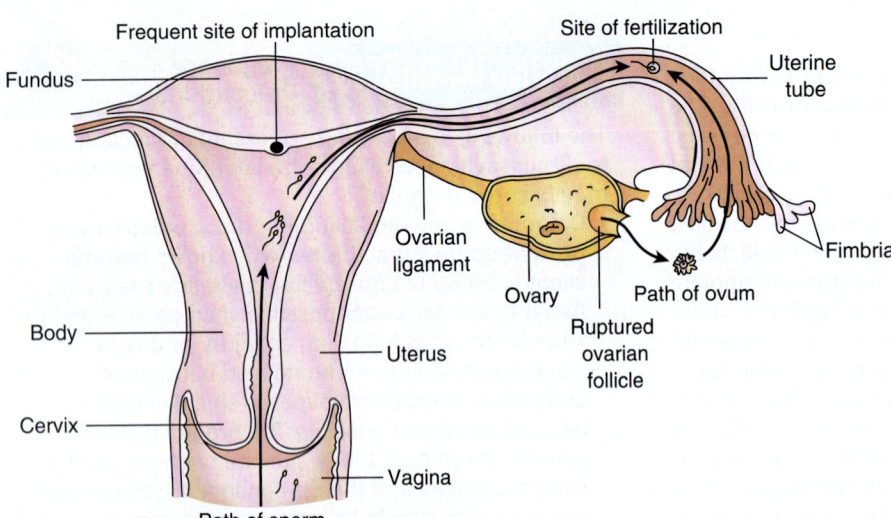

Figure 65-1 Fertilization: the union of ovum and sperm.

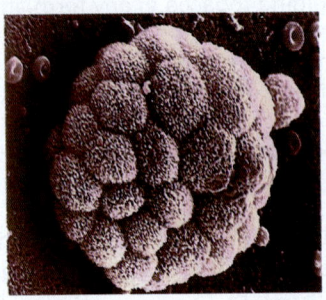

Figure 65-2 Blastocyst 7–8 days after fertilization. (Klossner & Hatfield, 2006.)

inner cell mass will form the body tissues and will develop into an **embryo**. The outer layer evolves into the placenta and other supporting tissues needed for fetal development. As the blastocyst enters the uterus, the outer cell layers secrete an enzyme that permits it to burrow (**implant**) into the endometrium (or, as it is known during pregnancy, the **decidua**). (see Fig. 65-3 for a diagram depicting early human development and implantation.)

Period of the Embryo

The period of the embryo lasts from the time that the developing blastocyst becomes fully implanted in the

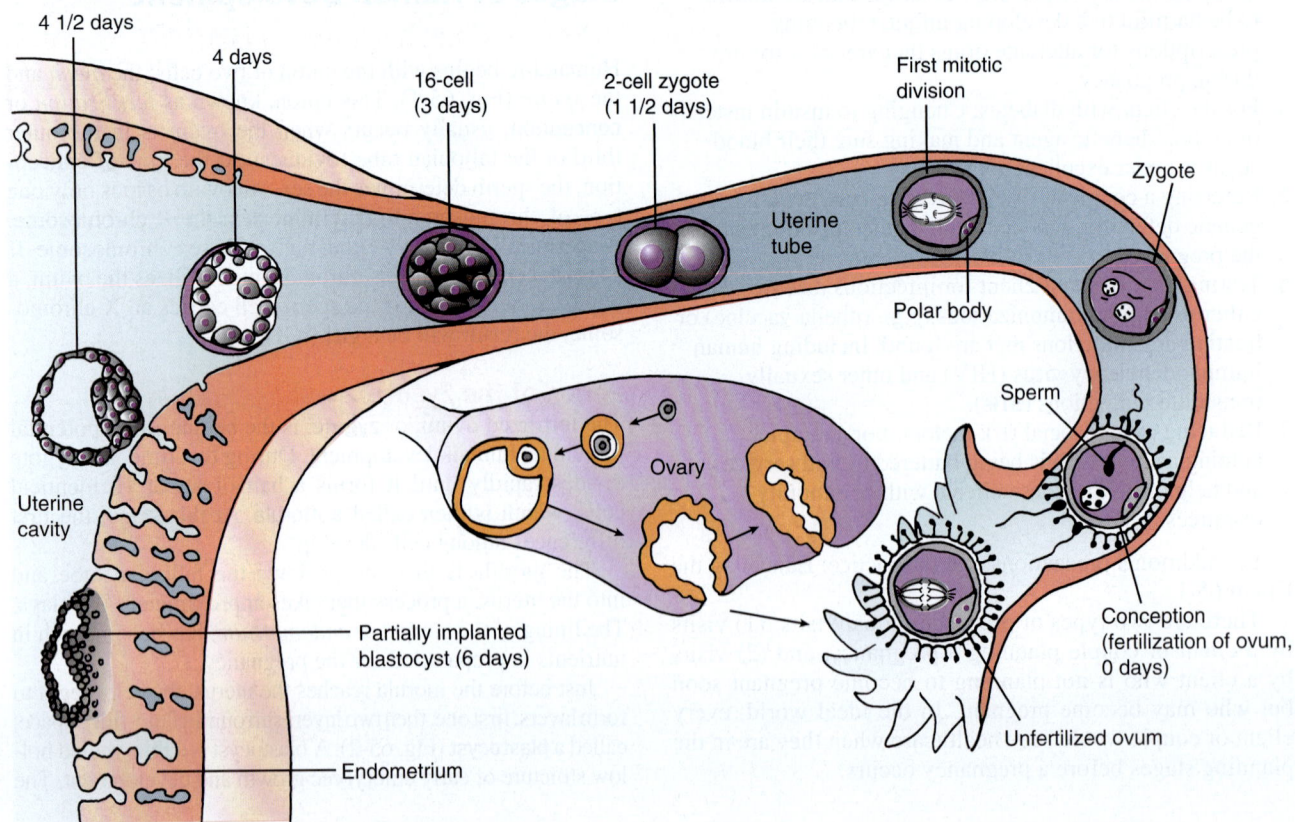

Figure 65-3 Early human development and implantation.

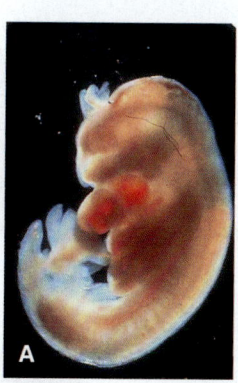 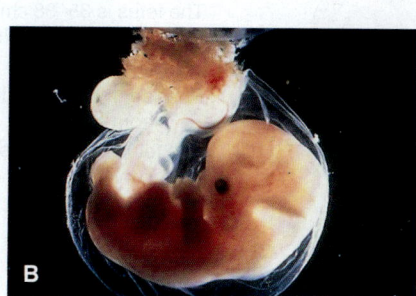 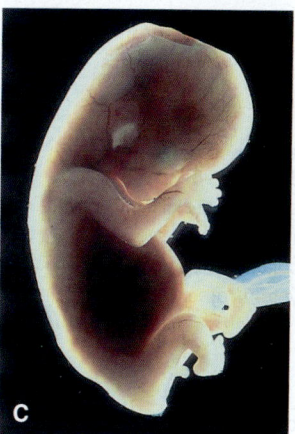

Figure 65-4 **A.** A 4-week embryo. **B.** A 5-week embryo. **C.** A 6-week embryo. (Klossner & Hatfield, 2006.)

uterus until the eighth week after conception (Fig. 65-4). During these weeks, all the organs and structures of the human are formed and are most susceptible to damage (Fig. 65-5). The embryo is in what is called the *critical phase of human development.* The outermost cell layer that surrounds the embryo and fluid cavity is called the **chorion**. Some of these outer cells send out projections (*chorionic villi*), which are the "roots" through which the developing embryo receives its oxygen and nourishment from the mother.

The embryo, and to a lesser degree the fetus, is vulnerable to a number of potentially harmful influences that could result in **congenital** (literally, "born with") defects. Genes determine the basic embryonic structure; therefore, a defective gene may be responsible for certain congenital defects. Environmental factors, such as direct or indirect exposure to tobacco smoke or the consumption of alcohol, can cause *congenital anomalies,* also known as *birth defects* (see Chapter 74).

> **Key Concept**
>
> The first 8 weeks of pregnancy are the critical period of human development; during this time, all major systems of the embryo develop.

> **NCLEX Alert**
>
> The terminology associated with pregnancy is related to specific nursing knowledge and, therefore, certain applicable nursing interventions. It is important that the student learn to associate specific levels of the pregnant uterus with the responsibilities of observance, teaching, and documentation.

Critical Phase of Human Development

4 weeks

The embryo is 0.75–1 cm in length.
Trophoblasts embed in decidua.
Chorionic villi form.
Foundations for nervous system, genitourinary system, skin, bones, and lungs are formed.
Buds of arms and legs begin to form.
Rudiments of eyes, ears, and nose appear.

8 weeks

The embryo is 2.5 cm in length and weighs 4 g.
Embryo is markedly bent.
Head is disproportionately large, owing to brain development.
Sex differentiation begins.
Centers of bone begin to ossify.
Heart pulsates.

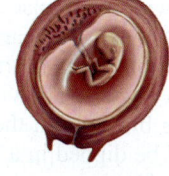

Figure 65-5 Critical period of development.

Period of the Fetus

The period of the **fetus** lasts from the beginning of the 9th week after fertilization through birth, which is usually at about the end of the 40th week of pregnancy. This is a period of increasing growth, differentiation, and functional development of the tissues that appeared during the embryonic period (Fig. 65-6). Healthcare technology may be able to sustain life for a very premature infant, but a **viable** fetus of less than 24 weeks is unusual and will need significant healthcare resources for maintenance of life.

Normal fetal growth and development follow a definite and predictable pattern (Fig. 65-7). Growth and development,

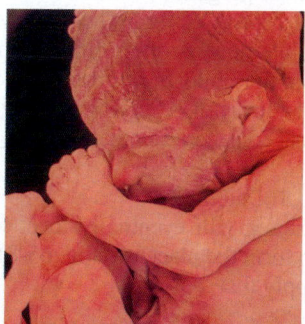

Figure 65-6 A 12- to 15-week fetus. (Klossner & Hatfield, 2006.)

Normal Fetal Growth

12 weeks

The fetus is 7–9 cm in length and weighs 28 g.
Fingers and toes are distinct.
Placenta is complete.
Fetal circulation is complete.
Organ systems are complete.

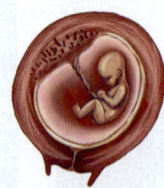

28 weeks

The fetus is 35–38 cm in length and weighs 1,200 g.
Skin is red.
Pupillary membrane disappears from eyes.
The fetus has an excellent chance of survival.
Eyes open and close.

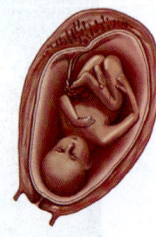

16 weeks

The fetus is 10–17 cm in length and weighs 55–120 g.
Sex is differentiated.
Rudimentary kidneys secrete urine.
Heartbeat is present.
Nasal septum and palate close.

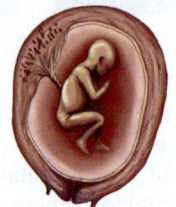

32 weeks

The fetus is 38–43 cm in length and weighs 1,500–2,500 g.
Fetus is viable.
Eyelids open.
Fingerprints are set.
Vigorous fetal movement occurs.

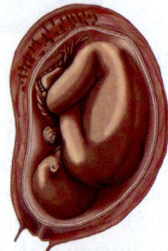

20 weeks

The fetus is 25 cm in length and weighs 223 g.
Lanugo covers entire body.
Fetal movements are felt by mother.
Heart sounds are perceptible by auscultation.

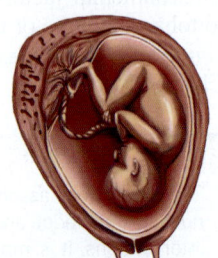

36 weeks

The fetus is 42–49 cm in length and weighs 1,900–2,700 g.
Face and body have a loose wrinkled appearance because of subcutaneous fat deposit.
Lanugo disappears.
Amniotic fluid decreases.

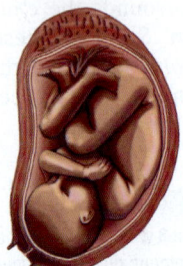

24 weeks

The fetus is 28–36 cm in length and weighs 680 g.
Skin appears wrinkled.
Vernix caseosa appears.
Eyebrows and fingernails develop.

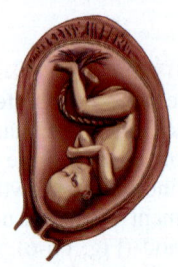

40 weeks

The fetus is 48–52 cm in length and weighs 3,000 g.
Skin is smooth.
Eyes are uniformly slate colored.
Bones of skull are ossified and nearly together at sutures.

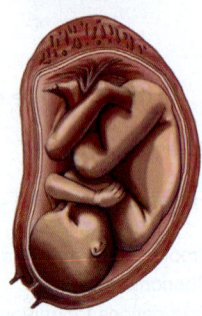

Figure 65-7 Different stages of fetal development.

before and after birth, follows the **cephalocaudal** (head to toe) principle.

Heredity and the pregnant client's nutritional status have influence on the growth of the fetus. A newborn weighing 10 lb (4,540 g) or more is often difficult to deliver; however, the smaller the child is at birth, the less likely their chances are for survival. A newborn weighing less than 2.2 lb (1,000 g) is considered immature.

Placenta and Umbilical Cord

The fetus' chorionic villi eventually meet with an area of uterine tissue to form the **placenta** (Fig. 65-8), an organ with a rich blood supply that

- Supplies the developing organism with food and oxygen
- Carries waste away for excretion by the pregnant client
- Slows the pregnant client's immune response so that the client's body does not reject the fetal tissue
- Produces hormones that help maintain the pregnancy

The fetal blood is entirely within blood vessels. Blood vessels may be found within the fetus's chorionic villi. These villi within the placenta are bathed in a pool of maternal blood, making this area the only place in the body (with the exception of the heart) where blood is not contained within blood vessels. The villi are suspended in this pool of nourishing blood from the client, much like a cluster of grapes could be dipped in a bowl of water that is continuously circulated by being pumped into the bowl and then drained.

Using its chorionic villi within the placenta, the fetus secures its oxygen and food directly from the client's blood, instead of using its own lungs and digestive system. The

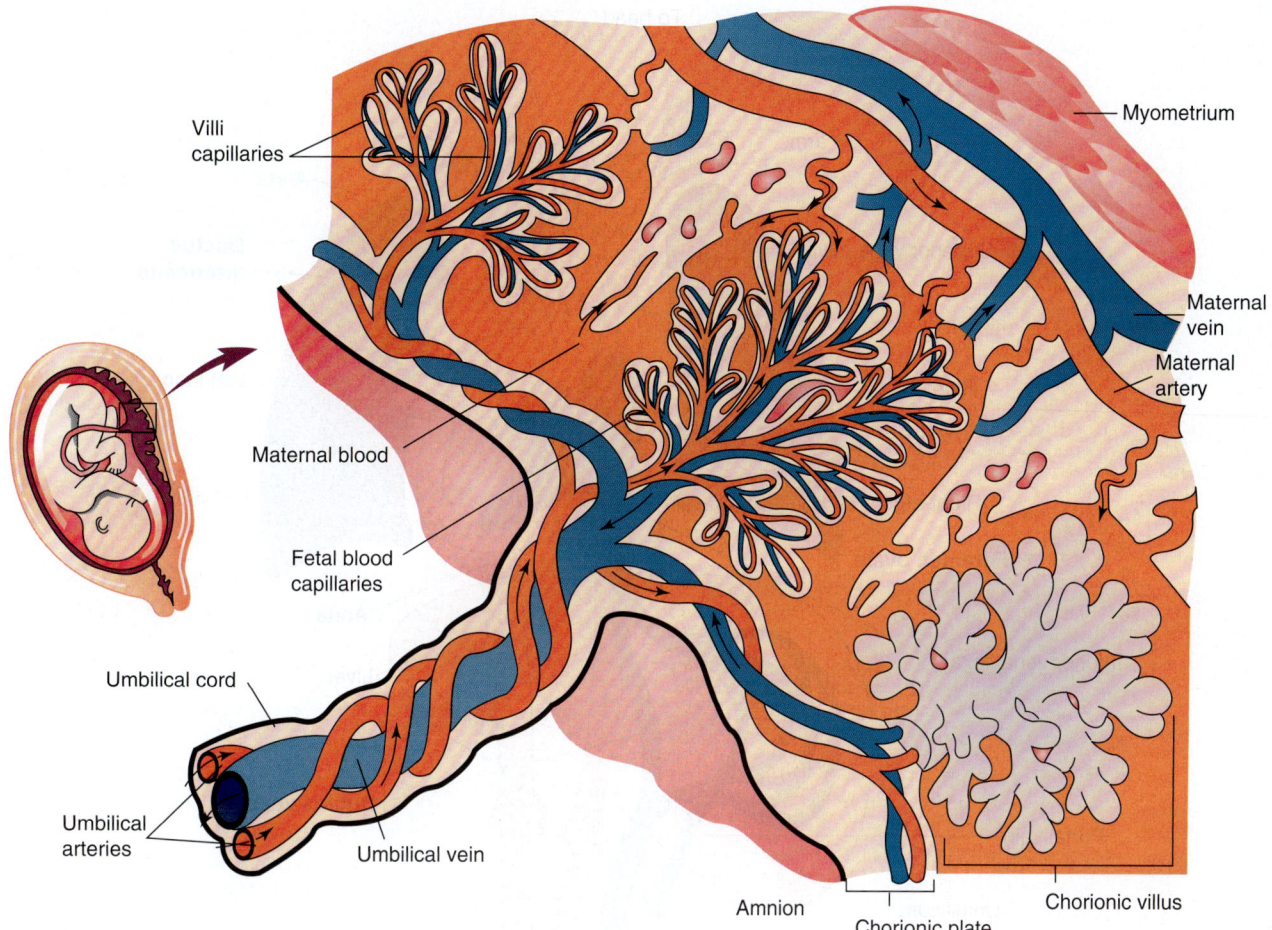

Figure 65-8 Placenta.

absorption of nutrients, excretion of wastes, and exchange of gases occur across the walls of the placental villi and the fetal blood vessels they contain. The fetal and the maternal blood are separate.

By term, the placenta is approximately 15–20 cm in diameter, 2–3 cm thick, and weighs between 500 and 600 g. The weight of the placenta is about one-sixth the weight of the infant if both are healthy.

The *umbilical cord* connects the fetal blood vessels contained in the villi of the placenta with those found within the fetal body. The umbilical cord consists of two arteries and one large vein twisted around each other. The umbilical cord is approximately 20 in. (51 cm) long. A soft, jelly-like substance called **Wharton jelly** protects the cord, which enters the fetus' body approximately in the middle of the abdomen at the **umbilicus**, or *navel*.

Fetal Blood Circulation

Fetal circulation differs from newborn and adult circulation (Fig. 65-9). The client's blood supplies food to—and carries wastes away from—the fetus. The uterus expels the placenta, which is also called the *afterbirth*, following the newborn's delivery. While the fetus is in utero, the placenta returns *deoxygenated* (low in oxygen) blood from the fetus to the mother through the two *umbilical arteries*. The placenta returns *oxygenated* (oxygen-rich) blood to the fetus via a single vessel, the *umbilical vein*. This process is an exception to the usual pattern, in which all arteries carry oxygenated (bright-red) blood, and all veins carry deoxygenated (dark-red) blood. Some oxygenated blood from the umbilical vein passes through the fetal liver, but most of it enters the fetus' inferior vena cava through the **ductus venosus**. This short duct is found only in the fetus and atrophies after birth. From the inferior vena cava, the blood flows into the fetus' right atrium.

Because the fetal lungs are not yet functioning, most of the blood is shunted to the heart's left atrium. This shunt occurs through another fetal structure, the **foramen ovale**, which is an opening between the right and left atria. This structure permits most of the blood to bypass the right ventricle. A small amount of blood passes from the right atrium to the right ventricle and makes its way into the pulmonary artery. This blood is then shunted through the **ductus arteriosus**, a connection between the pulmonary artery and the aorta that allows shunting of blood around the fetal lungs.

Normally, with the newborn's first few respirations, the lungs expand as soon as the pressure within the chest alters. The foramen ovale closes, and the ductus arteriosus and ductus venosus shrivel and become fibrous ligaments. Congenital heart defects in a child occur when these events do not take place after birth.

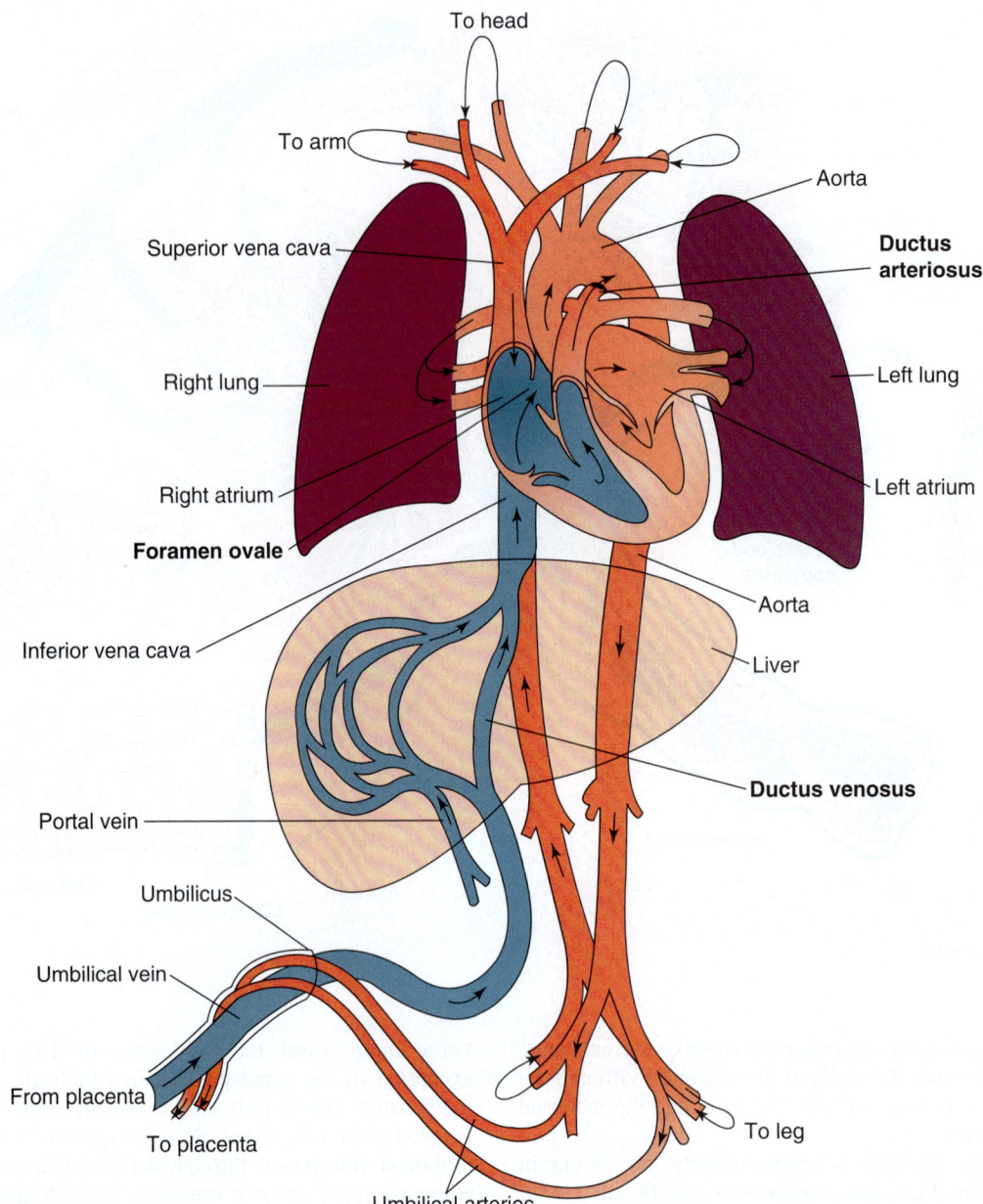

Figure 65-9 Fetal circulation. Notice the two arteries, the one vein, the ductus venosus, the ductus arteriosus, and the foramen ovale, which are unique to fetal circulation.

> **NCLEX Alert**
>
> Transference from fetal circulation to adult-type circulation is a common cause of post-birth problems. The nurse, who is generally caring for the newborn in the client's room, must be aware of a wide variety of post-birth anatomical complications and their nursing interventions.

Membranes and Amniotic Fluid

In the earliest human developmental stage, the chorionic plate that gives rise to the villi resembles a fuzzy ball. As the embryo grows, most areas of the villi atrophy, leaving only a disc of villi that develops into the placenta. The rest of the chorion becomes a smooth *outer membrane* for the embryo. Inside it, other cells eventually form a fluid-filled sac, the *amnion*, in which the fetus floats. The **amnion** is the inner membrane surrounding the fetus. These two membranes form a tough, protective bubble for the developing embryo and fetus, protecting it from organisms that might infect the pregnant client's cervix. In addition, the membranes are important to hormone production and also play a role in the onset of labor. The **amniotic fluid**, kept inside the amnion, performs the following functions:

- It cushions the fetus against injury.
- It regulates temperature.
- It allows the fetus to move freely inside it, which allows normal musculoskeletal development of the fetus.

In late pregnancy, the amniotic fluid is made up primarily of fetal urine and fetal lung fluid. Near term, the fetus swallows almost 400 ml of amniotic fluid each day and then excretes it in the urine; therefore, a defect in either the ability of the fetus to swallow or in its kidney function can dramatically change the quantity of amniotic fluid. The quantity of amniotic fluid increases to about 1,000 ml by 37 weeks of gestation; decreases slowly until 40 weeks; and then decreases much more quickly if the baby is not born by the end of the 40th week. Because of this predictable pattern in the quantity of fluid, one measurement of postterm fetal well-being is the volume of amniotic fluid.

Changes in a Client's Body During Pregnancy

Many of the changes in a client's body during pregnancy can be seen externally. However, there are also many changes in their internal structure and function. Some of these changes are caused by the growing size of the fetus, but even more changes result from the unique hormonal environment caused by pregnancy. These changes begin to occur soon after fertilization, when the production of hormones changes from that of a normal menstrual cycle.

Signs of Pregnancy

The signs of pregnancy are grouped into three categories (Box 65-1).

- *Presumptive signs* generally appear early and are subjective; that is, they may be noted only by the client. When a client experiences these symptoms, they may assume that they are pregnant. However, these symptoms could indicate a condition other than pregnancy.
- *Probable signs* also appear early in pregnancy, but they are more objective. Often, both healthcare personnel and the client themselves can observe probable signs. Although probable signs are more definite, they still are not absolute. Presumptive and probable signs are primarily caused by the hormonal changes that occur during pregnancy.
- *Positive signs* of pregnancy provide proof that there is a developing fetus.

> **Key Concept**
> Pregnancy is not confirmed until the existence of a fetus can be proved.

Presumptive Signs of Pregnancy
Amenorrhea
Amenorrhea, the absence of menstruation, is often one of the first indications of pregnancy. A missed menstrual period,

> **Box 65-1 Signs of Pregnancy**
> - **Presumptive:** *Possible signs,* appear in first trimester, often only noted subjectively by the client (e.g., breast changes, amenorrhea, morning sickness)
> - **Probable:** *Likely signs,* appear in first and early second trimesters, seen via objective criteria but can also be indicators of other conditions (e.g., hydatidiform mole)
> - **Positive:** *Proof exists* that there is a developing fetus in any trimester; objective criteria seen by a trained observer and/or diagnostic studies (e.g., ultrasound)

however, does not always signify conception. Pregnancy is dated from the first day of the client's LNMP. To be considered normal, the period should have come on time, lasted as long as is usual for the client, and have been the normal flow for them. If any of these three items are not true of that period, ask the client to recall the first day of their previous menstrual period (**PMP**).

Nausea
Nausea may begin soon after the first missed menstrual period and usually disappears after the third month of pregnancy. Approximately half of all pregnant clients experience some nausea or vomiting, usually owing to hormonal changes. Although it is sometimes called "morning sickness," the nausea or vomiting of pregnancy may happen at any time during the day. If this condition lasts beyond the fourth month, results in a weight loss of 8 lb or more, or affects the client's general health, it is considered a complication of pregnancy, **hyperemesis gravidarum**. Chapter 68 further discusses this condition.

Frequent Urination
The enlarging uterus presses against the urinary bladder. This action may cause the client to feel the need to urinate more frequently than usual. As the uterus grows upward into the abdominal cavity, the pressure eases. Late in the pregnancy, the client again feels the need to empty their bladder frequently. Once again, this is caused by pressure, as the fetal head moves downward before birth.

Fatigue
During the early months of pregnancy, the client may feel drowsy and may tire easily. They may find that they require more rest and sleep than usual and that even if they get the extra rest, they still feel tired. Although the exact causes of this fatigue are unknown, tiredness is probably caused by the body's increased use of energy because it works harder than normal during this time.

Quickening
The first fetal movements that the pregnant client feels are called **quickening**. The client usually experiences quickening between 18 and 20 weeks of gestation, but it may occur a week or two earlier in a multigravida. Women describe quickening as a light, "fluttery" sensation. This "feeling of life" is not considered a positive sign of pregnancy because it cannot be confirmed objectively by anyone other than the client themselves. The movement of gas within the colon can also simulate this feeling.

Breast Changes
The earliest breast changes that occur in pregnancy are similar to those a client may experience before their menstrual period. However, the sensations during pregnancy are more intense than premenstrual changes. The sensations include enlargement, heaviness, tingling, throbbing, or tenderness. The breasts may be so tender that the discomfort awakens a client who rolls over onto their stomach during sleep. As the pregnancy progresses, the areolae and the nipples enlarge and darken. By the 14th week, the client's breasts begin to

produce **colostrum**. This clear or slightly milky fluid will be produced in very small amounts throughout the rest of their pregnancy and in a greater quantity during the first day or two after birth. After that, their true milk will come in.

Pigment Changes

Pregnancy causes some skin changes. A suntanned, bronzed masking may appear across the face of dark-haired women. This is known as **melasma** (or *chloasma gravidarum*), or the "mask of pregnancy." A line of darker pigmentation, known as the **linea nigra**, often appears on the lower abdomen and extends from the umbilicus to the pubic bone. Hormone level changes cause these pigment changes.

Probable Signs of Pregnancy

Probable signs of pregnancy are more objective than the presumptive signs. An obstetrician or CNM may observe them during examination. They are more reliable indicators of pregnancy than the presumptive signs but still are not proof that a pregnancy exists.

Basal Body Temperature Elevation

The body temperature at rest, or basal body temperature (**BBT**), rises slightly (usually less than 1°) as one of the earliest signs of pregnancy. For accuracy, however, comparisons require that the temperature also must have been taken and recorded before pregnancy occurred.

Positive Urine Pregnancy Tests

Pregnancy tests check for the presence of the hormone called human chorionic gonadotropin (**HCG**, HCg, or hCG). This hormone is produced by the cells that will become the placenta. It can be found in small amounts in a client's urine or blood by about the 7th to 10th day of pregnancy.

Home pregnancy testing allows the client to know they are pregnant at a very early stage and lets them process the possibility of pregnancy in privacy. They can then make their own decisions about both the pregnancy and their lifestyle. The manufacturers of home pregnancy tests recommend confirmation of the results through professional examination and clinical testing. This advice should be followed because home tests may not have the same accuracy as clinical tests. Errors may occur in as many as 20%–30% of the home tests performed. The most common error (a false-negative) results from urine testing that is performed too early to obtain an accurate finding. The user must be able to read, follow directions, and perform the test correctly for the results to be accurate.

Cervical Changes

At about the eighth week of gestation, the cervix softens. This is known as **Goodell sign**. Before pregnancy, the cervix feels firm (like the tip of a nose); during pregnancy, it feels softer (more like the earlobe). The cervix also looks blue or purple when examined; this is **Chadwick sign** and may occur as early as the sixth week of pregnancy.

Vulvar and Vaginal Changes

The blueness due to increased blood supply (Chadwick sign) also occurs on the vulva and vagina.

Uterine Changes

At about 6 weeks, the lower uterine segment (the portion between the body of the uterus and the cervix) softens. This softening is called **Hegar sign**. A softening of the uterine *fundus*, where the embryo has implanted, also occurs by about the seventh week. The fundus enlarges by the eighth week. The uterus as a whole enlarges steadily throughout the pregnancy. The uterus rises above the symphysis pubis by about the 12th week and reaches the umbilicus between the 20th and 24th weeks.

Ballottement

After about 16–18 weeks of pregnancy, gently tapping one side of the pregnant client's abdomen will cause the fetus to "bounce" in the amniotic fluid—because the fetus is small compared with the amount of fluid. Examiners can feel this rebound tap, known as **ballottement**, against their hand.

Enlargement of the Abdomen

As the uterus increases in size, the abdomen is forced outward.

Positive Signs of Pregnancy

The *positive signs* of pregnancy, described below, can only occur in pregnancy.

Visualization of the Fetus

A fetus can be seen either on an ultrasound or, less commonly, on an x-ray examination. **Ultrasound** is the most common method used to evaluate fetal size, development, and due date. Using ultrasound, it is possible to diagnose pregnancy as early as the fourth week of gestation. The ultrasound examination is safe, painless, and relatively inexpensive.

Fetal Heartbeat

An examiner can detect the fetal heartbeat (fetal heart tones [FHTs]) by using either a *Doppler* or a special manual stethoscope called a **fetoscope** (Fig. 65-10). The **Doppler** (an electronic stethoscope) converts ultrasonic frequencies (high-frequency sound waves) into audible frequencies or onto a video monitor. An examiner can hear FHTs with the Doppler as early as the 10th week. They can be heard with the fetoscope at about the 18th to 20th week. A normal fetal heart rate ranges from 120 to 160 beats per minute (BPM). When assessing fetal heart rate, the examiner must be aware of two other sounds to avoid confusion. The *funic souffle* is a swishing sound produced by the pulsation of blood as it is propelled through the umbilical cord. Its rate is the same as the fetal heart rate. The *uterine* (or *placental*) *souffle* is a swishing sound produced by the pregnant client's blood as it flows through the large vessels of the uterus. Its rate is the same as the client's heart rate. The examiner should feel the client's radial pulse at the same time they are checking the fetal heart rate, to avoid confusing the two. Listening to *FHTs* is an important part of caring for a pregnant client. FHTs should be evaluated at every prenatal visit and at very frequent intervals during labor (see Chapter 66). In Practice: Nursing Procedure 65-1 provides information on obtaining FHTs.

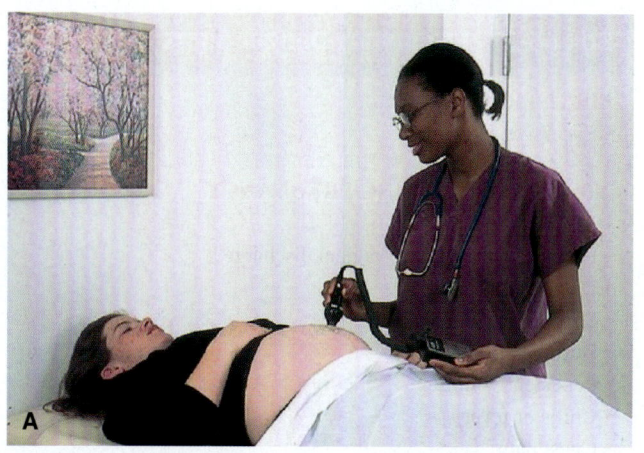
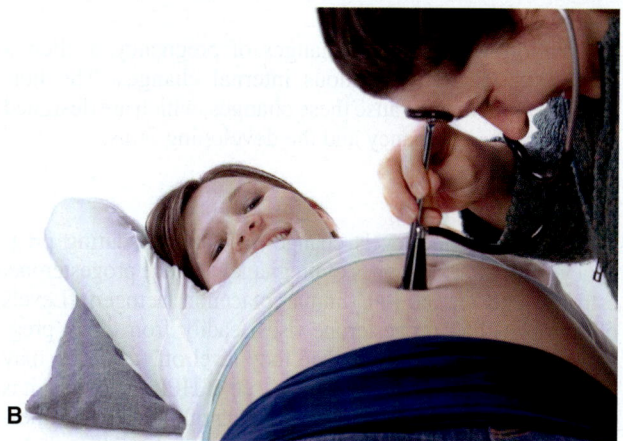

Figure 65-10 **A.** Checking fetal heart tones (FHTs) using a Doppler. (Photo by B. Proud.) **B.** Checking FHTs via auscultation, using a fetoscope. (Photo by Beth VanTrees/Shutterstock.)

Nursing Alert If you are unable to hear fetal heart tones, you must notify the healthcare provider, certified nurse-midwife, or nurse practitioner immediately.

Fetal Movement Felt by an Examiner
An examiner may be able to feel fetal movement after about week 20. At first, the movements are faint; however, as the fetus grows and muscle strength increases, the movements become stronger. These fetal movements must be differentiated from other movements within the client's body (e.g., peristalsis).

Important Changes in Maternal Anatomy and Physiology
As you learned at the beginning of this chapter, many of the changes that occur in a client's body are due to the increasing size of the fetus. Other changes result from the altered hormonal environment. The placenta produces so many hormones, and in such great quantity, that some people think of it as a "hormone factory." These hormones are needed to help the client sustain the pregnancy, to nourish the rapidly developing fetus, to prepare for breastfeeding (**lactation**), and for the client to still have enough energy to support themselves. Refer to In Practice Educating the Client 65-2 for several anatomical changes and concerns that occur in pregnancy.

> **Key Concept**
> Hormones and the size of the growing fetus both result in changes in the client's body.

External Changes
After the first trimester of pregnancy, most clients look pregnant. Their abdomen changes in contour, becoming increasingly more round as the pregnancy progresses. As the abdomen enlarges and their center of gravity shifts forward, the client's posture and gait alter as well. They develop an inward curve of the lower back, known as **lordosis**. During late pregnancy, their rib cage flares outward, making more room for the fetus.

IN PRACTICE
EDUCATING THE CLIENT 65-2 — Common Concerns in Pregnancy

- A client should not have bleeding during pregnancy, and they should tell their provider promptly if they do bleed. Note that some women have a spot or two of bleeding when implantation occurs, just about the time they expect a period. However, you should inform the healthcare provider, certified nurse-midwife, or nurse practitioner about *any* bleeding that a pregnant client reports.
- A pregnant client may wake up feeling very hungry. You might advise them that it could help to eat a starchy food, such as a baked potato, just before bedtime. If they eat sweets, they will probably have a rapid rise in blood sugar, followed by a sharp drop. Either of these changes can cause uncomfortable symptoms. Advise them to try to avoid consuming concentrated sweets to prevent this from occurring.
- As their blood volume rises, the pregnant client's heart has to work harder (pump more strongly) to deal with the increased workload. They may feel palpitations or a rapid and pounding heartbeat. This is normal unless they also feel dizzy or light-headed.
- The extra blood vessels that form in the gastrointestinal system, along with the slowing of peristalsis, may combine to cause constipation and hemorrhoids. The pregnant client should consume plenty of fiber and water to prevent this.
- As the ligaments relax and the pregnant client's center of gravity changes, their balance may be "off." They should avoid wearing high heels, especially during late pregnancy.
- Breast enlargement is normal. The pregnant client may need to buy a larger-sized bra. Some women need a bra that is larger in both chest and cup sizes.

Internal Changes

In addition to the visible changes of pregnancy, a client's body experiences tremendous internal changes. The hormones of pregnancy cause these changes, which are designed to support the pregnancy and the developing fetus.

Hormone Levels

A client's hormone levels change dramatically during pregnancy. Important hormones of pregnancy include progesterone, estrogens, HCG, and **HPL** (human placental lactogen). Levels of estrogens and progesterone rise steadily from early pregnancy until close to term, when they level off (and then may slowly decline). A similar pattern is true of HPL except that it is not produced until close to the beginning of the second trimester. It then rises rapidly until about 34 weeks, when it decreases. On the other hand, HCG is the primary hormone of early pregnancy; its level drops significantly during the second trimester.

Together, these hormones create an environment that supports the pregnancy. Some of the most important hormonal effects include

- Maintaining the endometrium so that the embryo can implant
- Causing changes in the pregnant client's metabolism so that nutrients will be available for their own needs as well as the needs of the growing fetus
- Causing an increase in the client's blood volume and red blood cell mass to provide the extra oxygen needed for both the fetus and their own increased demands
- Increasing the blood supply to the gastrointestinal tract and slowing the peristaltic waves, changes that result in increased absorption of nutrients
- Relaxing the ligaments that connect the pelvic bones, allowing them to spread slightly to increase the space available for the fetus to pass through
- Preparing the breasts for lactation, while keeping the milk from coming in until after the baby is born

Signs of Possible Problems During Pregnancy

Each stage, or trimester, of pregnancy carries its own risks. Any time a client reports one or more of the following symptoms, they should be advised to visit their healthcare provider or an emergency department promptly.

Danger Signs During the First Trimester

The primary danger of the first trimester is *spontaneous abortion (miscarriage)* (Box 65-2). Signs of threatened abortion include the following:

- *Vaginal bleeding or spotting:* Bleeding does not mean that the client will miscarry, but it does indicate that they might do so. Bleeding due to a threatened abortion reflects a partial separation of the placenta from the decidua. Blood may appear either bright red, darker red, or brown. The amount of blood loss does not predict the outcome unless it becomes very heavy (enough to saturate more than one pad per hour).
- *Pelvic/abdominal cramping:* Cramping that increases over time, especially if accompanied by vaginal bleeding, indicates threatened abortion.

Box 65-2 | **Pregnancy Danger Signs**

FIRST TRIMESTER
- Excessive vomiting

AT ANY TIME DURING PREGNANCY
- Vaginal bleeding
- Excessive or irritating vaginal discharge
- Dizziness or fainting
- Decrease in urine output
- Burning with urination
- Persistent vomiting
- Chills or fever
- Chest pain

LATE IN PREGNANCY
- Leaking or gushing of amniotic fluid
- Swelling in the client's extremities or face
- Dyspnea
- Blurred vision or spots before the eyes
- Severe headaches
- Abdominal, epigastric, or severe back pain
- Decreased fetal movement
- Lower abdominal pressure

- *No longer feeling pregnant:* If the embryo or fetus has died and the placenta has ceased to function, the hormonal environment changes rapidly. The most common statement about this change is, "I just don't feel pregnant anymore." Specific symptoms of pregnancy that quickly subside with missed abortions are nausea, breast tenderness, and headaches.

Danger Signs During the Second and Third Trimesters

The complications for which early signs may develop during later pregnancy include incompetent cervix, placenta previa, placental abruption, preterm labor (**PTL**) and/or preterm premature rupture of the membranes (**PPROM** or **PROM**), decreased fetal movement, and pregnancy-induced hypertension (**PIH**) (see Chapter 68). Danger signs during the second and third trimesters include the following:

- *Vaginal bleeding, with or without cramping, pressure, or pain:* Painless vaginal bleeding may be a sign of *placenta previa,* a condition in which the placenta lies partly over the cervical opening. The first episode of bleeding often occurs at about 26–28 weeks. It may follow sexual activity or occur spontaneously. The bleeding is generally bright red, and the flow is fairly heavy—at least as heavy as a normal menses.
- *Bleeding with severe abdominal pain:* This symptom is a sign of *placental abruption* or premature separation of the placenta. The fetus can die if not delivered quickly, usually by cesarean section.
- *Vaginal or lower abdominal pressure:* This may occur when the cervix is *incompetent* or not strong enough to hold the fetus inside the uterus. This symptom is

especially worrisome if the client also has increased vaginal discharge.
- *Preterm labor:* Early signs of PTL include backache, pelvic/abdominal cramping, rhythmic pelvic pressure, diarrhea, change in vaginal discharge, vaginal spotting, leaking fluid, and malaise.
- *Premature labor/Premature rupture of the membranes: PPROM/PROM* is a condition identified by either a gush of fluid or a continuous steady trickle of fluid. The gush is usually easily recognized, but the client may not realize that a slow, steady leak is a problem.
- *Decreased fetal movement:* Regular fetal movement is a sign of fetal well-being. Each fetus has its own pattern of activity; a marked drop-off in a fetus' activity is a cause for concern about the health of the fetus.
- *PIH* is suspected when the following symptoms are noted:
  - *Severe headache,* which does not respond to over-the-counter remedies.
  - *Visual changes:* double vision, suddenly blurred vision, seeing spots or flashing lights.
  - *Sudden edema or swelling,* especially of the face, eyes, and hands.
  - *Epigastric pain* or pain in the upper abdomen.

HEALTHCARE DURING PREGNANCY

The prenatal period refers to the period between conception and the onset of labor. The goals of good prenatal care are to

- Promote physical and mental wellness of the mother during the pregnancy and afterward
- Help the client give birth safely and without complications
- Ensure a healthy baby

Many clients seek prenatal care as soon as they suspect pregnancy. In recent years, the healthcare industry has emphasized health promotion measures, such as preconceptional examination, to encourage positive maternal and child health for the future. Ideally, the client's health at the end of pregnancy will be as good as or better than it was at the beginning. Regular prenatal care is associated with lower infant mortality and better client and infant outcomes.

Pregnancy involves all members of the family. Having a baby has a powerful influence on the family system. Each member of the family reacts to pregnancy from their own point of view and as related to individual needs, beliefs, and experiences.

Choosing a Healthcare Provider

Preconceptional and prenatal care, at its best, is a partnership between the client and the healthcare provider. The client should choose a provider who will help them make decisions about the best healthcare for themselves and their family. Above all else, the provider should be someone who genuinely listens to the client and their concerns.

A client may choose an obstetrician, other healthcare provider, a certified nurse-midwife, or a nurse practitioner for their prenatal care. They may go to a public health clinic, a private office, or a community-based organization. Each of these sites and providers has strengths and limitations. Some examples of questions a client might ask as they select a prenatal care provider include

- *Which gender would I prefer when choosing a provider?*
- *Should my provider speak the same native language that I do?*
- *When I have a question or concern about my pregnancy, will my provider talk with me about it?*
- *Is the location convenient? How will I get to the provider's office? Will I walk, drive, or take the bus?*
- *Is the staff courteous, friendly, and respectful toward me?*
- *Do I have a choice of the hospital at which I'll give birth?*
- *Are there other services (e.g., dietitian or social worker) available to me through my provider?*
- *Can my partner come with me for my prenatal visits?*

After a client has chosen a provider, they will have an initial preconceptional or prenatal visit. When possible, the client's partner should be encouraged to accompany them on the first visit to the practitioner. If the partner is the child's father, they can provide the practitioner with important information about their medical history and any genetic concerns they may have. Any partner who is present to learn important facts about pregnancy will also be in a better position to support and encourage the client who is expecting. A partner's presence is helpful at subsequent visits, also, to allow the couple to hear and discuss information together.

Components of Prenatal Care

There are three basic components of adequate prenatal care:

1. Early and regular prenatal care
2. Maintenance of maternal health; promotion of good health habits
3. Recognition and treatment of physical, mental, and social/economic problems

Risk Assessments

The goal of risk assessment is to identify clients and fetuses who have a chance of having a complication development during pregnancy, labor, birth, or the neonatal period. After a risk is identified, the healthcare team can provide the appropriate type and level of care, which results in better outcomes. There is no perfect risk-assessment system.

The best health for pregnant client and baby results when the client has their first visit before the end of the first trimester (before the end of week 13) and then has regular visits until after they have delivered the baby. The usual timing for visits is about once every 4 weeks for the first 28 weeks, then every 2 weeks until 36 weeks, and then weekly until the birth. The postpartum visit is usually scheduled at 4 or 6 weeks after birth, although many providers also like to see the client at 2 weeks postpartum.

The Initial Prenatal Visit

The following are key components of the initial prenatal visit.

- *Health history:* The provider takes a complete health history of the client and their partner, if possible, to learn about past illnesses and any pattern of certain inherited diseases that might affect this pregnancy (e.g., Tay-Sachs, diabetes, or sickle-cell anemia). The provider is also interested in learning whether a **multifetal** pregnancy (twins or more) has occurred in either family. The healthcare provider, certified nurse-midwife, or nurse practitioner needs to know if the client has had any difficulties during previous pregnancies or births, or if they have had any serious infections, including STIs or HIV. It is also important to assess the client's lifestyle, including risk due to infections, substance use, or domestic violence. A thorough health history provides an accurate record of the client's past and present health and gives the provider important data.

- *Physical examination:* A complete physical examination, including a pelvic examination, is part of the initial prenatal visit. This head-to-toe assessment includes examination of the gums, teeth, thyroid gland, heart, lungs, breasts, and all body systems. Also, the client's height and weight should be measured and recorded at the first prenatal visit. During the pelvic examination, the provider checks the reproductive organs for signs of pregnancy, the bony pelvis for approximate size and shape, and looks for indications of any health problems. Pelvic measurements help in determining whether the bony passageway is large enough for delivery of a normal-sized newborn, an especially important consideration in a primigravida. A Pap test and test for STIs (gonorrhea and chlamydia) are also routinely performed as part of the pelvic examination.
- *Laboratory tests:* The client's blood type and Rh factor are determined. If the client is Rh-negative, they should receive Rho(D) immune globulin (**RhoGAM**, Gamulin Rh) at the 28th week of gestation and following any episode of bleeding or any invasive procedure (e.g., amniocentesis). The purpose of giving RH Immune Globulin (RhoGAM) is to prevent Rh isoimmunization (see Chapters 68 and 69).
- *Other blood tests* that are routinely obtained include a syphilis test (RPR or VDRL), complete blood count (CBC), antibody screen, and rubella titer. A rubella titer is done to determine if the client is immune to rubella, or German measles. If they are not immune, they are *not vaccinated during pregnancy.* The client should wait until after giving birth and avoid getting pregnant for 4 weeks after vaccination with the MMR vaccination because the rubella could have a harmful effect on a fetus.
- *HIV testing* should be offered to every pregnant client, according to the Institute of Medicine and the American College of Obstetricians and Gynecologists. If a client tests positive for the virus and begins treatment for HIV during the pregnancy, the risk of transmitting the virus to the fetus drops significantly.
- *Urine testing* looks for albumin (protein), glucose, and the presence of harmful bacteria. A urine pregnancy test may be needed to confirm the pregnancy. Each time a urine sample is collected from a pregnant client, the nurse needs to provide client with materials for a clean-catch urine specimen. A clean-catch specimen is used to enhance detection of bacteria in the urine. If the UA does show the presence of bacteria, a urine culture may be ordered.
- *Tuberculosis testing:* The pregnant client should be given a Mantoux tuberculin skin test (**TST**), which is the standard test for tuberculosis. The TST determines if an individual is infected with *Mycobacterium tuberculosis.* Refer to the latest information TB, pregnancy, and testing procedures provided on the Centers for Disease Control and Prevention (CDC) Website.

> **Nursing Alert** The TST contains 0.1 tuberculin purified protein derivative (**PPD**) given intradermally into the inner surface of the forearm. A specific tuberculin syringe must be used with the needle bevel facing upward. Correct procedures of administration and reading are necessary. The TST must be read between 48 and 72 hr later. In reading the test, only the raised area, not the reddened area, should be measured. A normal response may produce a pale elevation or wheal of 6–10 mm in diameter; erythema (redness) is not measured.

- *Genetic background* information is obtained about both baby's biologic parents. Genetic background information may reveal sickle cell anemia, Tay–Sachs, or a variety of other genetically transmitted disorders. A referral for counseling and testing should be given to the couple if needed.
- *Determining the baby's due date:* A client who thinks they are pregnant is wise to consult a healthcare provider after they have missed one menstrual period. A full-term pregnancy is approximately 280 days from the first day of the last menstrual period or 266 days after fertilization. The 280 days equal 40 weeks. Many clients do not keep an accurate record of their menstrual periods or may not have regular periods for many different reasons. In these cases, the practitioner determines the estimated date of delivery (**EDD**), also called the estimated date of confinement (**EDC**), based on the size of the uterus during the physical examination and/or by an ultrasound estimate of fetal age. See In Practice: Data Gathering in Nursing 65-1 for more information on determining the anticipated birth date. The actual duration of pregnancy varies greatly, and the EDD is an approximate due date. Only about 4% of women actually deliver on their EDD.

Return Prenatal Visits

At each return appointment, also called a *revisit,* the following measures should be performed and charted by a member of the healthcare team:

- *Weight:* This reading is then compared with their prepregnancy weight and their previous weight measurements.
- *Blood pressure.*
- *Urine:* A "dipstick" analysis is performed for protein, glucose, and sometimes nitrites and leukocytes (indicators of bladder infections).
- *Uterus:* Measurement of the size of the uterus, called **fundal height**, and an evaluation of its growth since the last visit are performed.
- *FHTs.*
- *Edema:* Check the face, hands, legs, and feet for edema.
- *Continuing risk assessments:* At each prenatal visit, the risk profile should be updated. If new information indicates a change in the client's risk status, the provider will develop a new plan of care with them to address their needs.

The client should be asked about any problems or complications that they have experienced since their last visit; how

IN PRACTICE
DATA GATHERING IN NURSING 65-1: Nägele Rule: Determining the Anticipated Date of Birth or Due Date

Pregnancy is dated from the first day of the client's *last normal menstrual period (LNMP)*. To be considered normal, the period should have
- Come on time
- Lasted as long as is usual for them
- Have been the normal flow for them

If any of these three items is not true of that period, ask them to recall the first day of their previous menstrual period (PMP).

When you have an accurate date for their last period, the due date for the baby is determined either by using a gestational wheel or by applying Nägele rule. The due date is usually called the *estimated date of confinement* (EDC) or the *estimated date of delivery* (EDD).

Nägele Rule
- Determine the date of the first day of the client's LNMP.
- Add 7 days.
- Subtract 3 months.
- The resulting date is the EDD.
- *Initial risk assessment:* The provider determines the degree of risk to the client and fetus based on information from the history, physical examination, laboratory results, and due date. Commonly used terms for risk status are *low risk* and *high risk*. Although there is certainly such a thing as moderate risk, it is very hard to define. Based on their risk assessment, an individualized plan of counseling, classes, referrals, and prenatal care appointments is developed with the pregnant client.

---

they are feeling; whether they have any concerns or worries; and how often the fetus is moving (after quickening has occurred).

Additional Tests Performed During Pregnancy
Many clients have an ultrasound examination done between 16 and 20 weeks of pregnancy. This is a very accurate time at which to determine gestational age and also to examine the fetus for normal development. If there is a problem or a concern at a different point during the pregnancy, the ultrasound examination may be repeated.

Between weeks 15 and 19, a blood test called the *maternal serum alpha-fetoprotein* (**MSAFP**) is done. The primary purpose of this test is to screen for fetal neural tube defects. It may be combined with two other tests (HCG and estriol), which increases the number of neural tube defects that may be identified and also screens for Down syndrome. This test is called a *triple marker screen.*

Between 24 and 28 weeks, all pregnant clients should be screened for diabetes. The test used during pregnancy is a 1-hr random glucose tolerance test. The client eats normally until their prenatal or laboratory appointment, then drinks a 50-g glucose beverage. Their blood is drawn 1 hr later to be tested for glucose. Elevated glucose levels may indicate gestational diabetes.

The Rh antibody test is repeated at 26–27 weeks, and RH Immune Globulin (RhoGAM) is given at 28 weeks if the antibody test remains negative (In Practice: Important Medications 65-1).

Many providers repeat STI testing at 36 weeks and may also do a vaginal culture for group B streptococcus.

Health Promotion
Health promotion through education of the pregnant client is recognized as an important aspect of prenatal care. Education before and during pregnancy is related to the increase in scientifically acquired knowledge and the client's perception of self-care and empowerment. The nurse's responsibilities

IN PRACTICE
IMPORTANT MEDICATIONS 65-1: RH Immune Globulin (RhoGAM)

Microdose: 50 µg (used after spontaneous or elective abortion at <13 weeks' gestation).
Full dose: 300 µg at 28 weeks' gestation.
Expected effect: In an Rh-negative client, RH Immune Globulin (RhoGAM) prevents antibodies to Rh-positive fetal blood cells from forming. The 28-week dose provides protection for about 12 weeks; another dose should be given after delivery.
Adverse side effects: Pain, soreness at injection site.

Nursing Considerations
- RH Immune Globulin (RhoGAM) should also be given if an Rh-negative client has any bleeding during the prenatal period or if they have invasive testing performed, such as chorionic villus sampling or an amniocentesis.
- RH Immune Globulin (RhoGAM) is a blood product, but unlike whole blood or red blood cells, it is a processed immunoglobulin. It is safe for pregnant clients to use. The method of its preparation includes viral inactivation. Human immunodeficiency virus (HIV) is not a concern with this blood product.
- Because RH Immune Globulin (RhoGAM) is a blood product, clients who do not take blood products for religious reasons may refuse to take it.

---

include providing and promoting knowledge related to the day-to-day care and concerns of pregnancy.

Elimination and Hygiene
A daily bowel movement is preferable for the pregnant client, although not all clients normally have one. A client who

has a tendency toward constipation may face increased difficulties during pregnancy due to decreased peristalsis. Plenty of water, fruits, vegetables, moderate exercise, and adequate fiber intake encourage regular elimination.

The body's oil and sweat glands are more active than usual during pregnancy, so a daily warm (not hot) bath or shower is important. Of course, the client must be careful not to slip or fall in the tub or shower. During the last few weeks of pregnancy, the client should not take a tub bath if they are home alone because they may have difficulty getting out of the tub and may require assistance. The client's hair may be oilier than usual and may need frequent shampooing.

Oral Hygiene

The pregnant client should practice good oral hygiene. The client should eat a balanced diet and see their dentist regularly. Dental and gum issues are not uncommon during pregnancy. Necessary dental work should be performed and sources of infection treated. Some dentists do not want to perform oral surgery (e.g., root canal) on pregnant clients unless it is an emergency. **Ptyalism** is an increase in salivation during pregnancy. Although annoying to the client, ptyalism does not cause tooth decay or gum irritation.

Vaginal Infections

If there is an infection with an odor or itching, the client should be checked for a vaginal infection. Douching can actually increase their risk of vaginal infection and sometimes can cause an existing infection to be pushed up into the cervix and uterus. Pregnant clients should be advised not to douche.

Breast Care

Except for the use of a supportive bra, elaborate breast care is unnecessary before breastfeeding. Clients who plan to breastfeed should bathe as usual and use little or no soap on the nipples. They should gently pat their nipples dry. The nipple secretes its own natural moisturizer, which should not be removed with soap or other chemicals. Clients should also avoid applying alcohol, tincture of benzoin, and lanolin ointments. These substances may damage the areola and nipple and have not been shown to be effective in preventing sore and cracked nipples. Lanolin is also a common allergen and may contain insecticide residuals and DDT.

Wearing a nursing bra with the flaps down and exposing the nipples to air and sunshine may help to condition them. Harsh treatment may cause sore and cracked nipples and should be avoided. Nipple exercises and stimulation should not be done, especially in the third trimester, when they can cause uterine contractions and premature labor. Flat nipples should be treated with breast shields that are worn during the last trimester and after delivery between feedings. Inverted nipples are rare and can be treated with a nipple shield.

Rest

The pregnant client tires more easily and should have enough rest to avoid fatigue. Preventing fatigue is better than having to recover from it. The client should know how much rest they ordinarily require and plan to get more if needed. Going to bed earlier, getting up later, or taking an afternoon nap may help. Short daytime rest periods are beneficial if the client really relaxes. Pregnant clients are able to carry on normal household activities without harm if they avoid heavy work and get additional rest.

Sleep

As pregnancy advances, the client may have a hard time finding a comfortable sleeping posture. Simple measures, such as additional pillows at the back, or a pillow supporting the weight of the abdomen or the top arm while the client lies on their side, will usually relieve these common problems.

During the pregnancy's last months, advise the pregnant client not to sleep or lie on their back to avoid *supine hypotension syndrome (aortocaval compression)* (Fig. 65-11). The weight of the uterus can interfere with the circulation in the aorta and the vena cava, thus depriving the client and the fetus of oxygen (Fig. 65-11B). The side-lying position relieves fetal pressure on the renal veins, helps the kidneys excrete fluid, and increases flow of oxygenated blood to the fetus. If the client must remain on their back, place a small pillow or towel roll under one hip. The goal is to keep the client's circulation unimpeded by displacing the weight of the uterus to the side rather than on the major blood vessels.

Exercise and Posture

Exercise improves circulation, appetite, and digestion; it also aids in elimination and helps the client to sleep better. Unless contraindicated by the healthcare provider, the client, generally, may safely continue customary exercises.

Swimming in a pool can be beneficial; however, swimming in lake water in later stages of pregnancy is not advised because of the danger of infection. Specific prenatal exercises are a part of childbirth education. Walking in fresh air is excellent exercise. Whatever the exercise, it should not be fatiguing. Exercise should be daily rather than sporadic (see In Practice: Educating the Client 65-3 and 65-4).

Activity

Weight gain, stability, and activity involve the balance between energy sources (diet and stored fuel) and energy expenditure. Energy use in this energy equation is the combination of basal metabolic rate, body heat production, and physical activity. The average total additional energy (calorie) requirement is about 2,500–3,500 calories per day. Changes in daily physical activity are individual, leading either to an increase or a decrease in energy used throughout the pregnancy.

Sexual Relations

Some individuals may consider the sight of a pregnant client beautiful, sensual, and erotic. Other individuals, including the client themselves, may view the pregnant body as misshapen, awkward, and not particularly sexual.

During pregnancy, a client continues to have sexual needs. If the pregnant client has a partner, the partner also continues to have sexual needs. Both partners have needs for intimacy and closeness, which may differ from their sexual

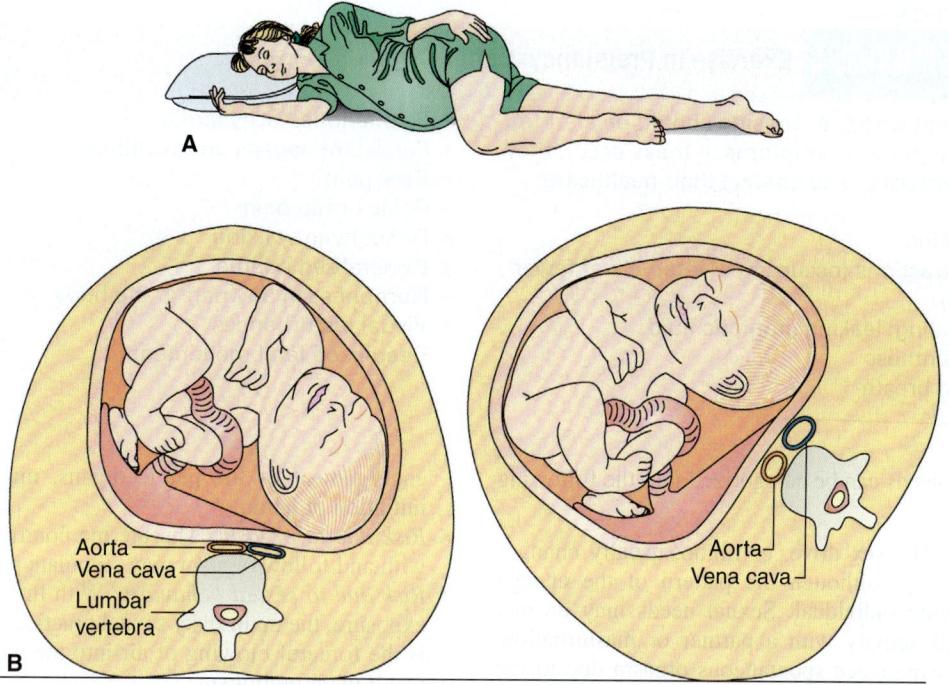

Figure 65-11 A. Rest position during pregnancy. The knees and elbows should be slightly bent, the muscles limp, and the breathing slow and regular. Notice that the weight of the fetus is resting on the bed. **B.** Supine hypotension syndrome can occur if a pregnant client lies on their back, trapping blood in the lower extremities. If a client turns on their side, pressure is lifted off of the vena cava.

IN PRACTICE
EDUCATING THE CLIENT 65-3 Exercise Guidelines During Pregnancy

The goal of prenatal exercise is physical fitness within the limitations of pregnancy. If a client does not have contraindications, as designated by their healthcare provider, to exercising during pregnancy, these general guidelines should be followed:

- Clients with uncomplicated pregnancies can continue a moderate exercising program, with these modifications:
  - Reduce the intensity of the exercise by about 25%.
  - Maximum maternal heart rate should not exceed 140 bpm.
  - Periods of strenuous activities should be limited to 15–20 min, interspersed with low-intensity exercise and rest periods.
- Extremely active clients, athletes, and clients who perform vigorous aerobic exercise should reduce the level of exertion.
- Sedentary clients should begin to exercise very gradually.
- The types of exercise that provide the best cardiovascular and psychological benefits throughout pregnancy are walking, cycling, and swimming.
- Relaxation and stretching exercises (yoga) may be continued throughout pregnancy. Muscle-strengthening exercises, such as Kegel exercises to strengthen the pelvic floor and pelvic tilts or pelvic rocks to strengthen the lower back and relieve back pain, may be done by all pregnant clients. These provide no cardiovascular benefits.
- Jogging and weight-bearing aerobic programs should be moderated to avoid injury caused by ligament relaxation and increased joint mobility during pregnancy.
- Clients who lift weights may continue to lift light weights during pregnancy, with the following modifications:
  - Avoid heavy resistance on machines.
  - Avoid use of heavy free weights.
  - Breathe properly to avoid the Valsalva maneuver.
- Sports that pose a potential risk to the mother or fetus include
  - Contact sports—football, soccer.
  - Sports involving potential joint or ligament damage—basketball, volleyball, gymnastics, downhill skiing, skating.
  - Horseback riding.
- Sports that are safe to continue during pregnancy include
  - Racquet sports—tennis, racquetball, squash (avoid heat stress; decrease intensity as pregnancy progresses).
  - Golf (may need to modify golf swing).
  - Slow-pitch softball (avoid sliding into bases, blocking bases).
  - Cross-country skiing.
- Avoid any strenuous exercise or sport in adverse conditions—extreme heat, high humidity, air pollution, high altitudes.

IN PRACTICE
EDUCATING THE CLIENT 65-4   Exercise in Pregnancy: Danger Signs

A pregnant client who is exercising should be alert to the following signs and symptoms. If these occur, they should stop exercising and contact their healthcare provider:
- Pain of any kind
- Uterine contractions (occurring at intervals of fewer than 15 min)
- Vaginal bleeding; leaking amniotic fluid
- Dizziness; faintness
- Shortness of breath
- Palpitations; tachycardia
- Persistent nausea and vomiting
- Back pain
- Pubic or hip pain
- Difficulty in walking
- Generalized edema
- Numbness in any part of the body
- Visual disturbances
- Decreased fetal movement

---

needs. Intimacy needs can be categorized into the following three groups:

- *Sexual needs:* The sex drive, or libido, usually changes during pregnancy—although the pattern of the change in libido is quite individual. Sexual needs may be met through sexual activity with a partner or masturbation. Some clients experience spontaneous orgasm due to the increased pelvic blood supply during pregnancy. Pregnancy diminishes sexual desire in some clients and increases it in others. Communication between the pregnant client and their sexual partner helps to eliminate conflicts.
- *Touch needs:* Pregnancy is a time of a heightened need for touch. Part of this need can be met via sexual interactions, but sensual needs of protection, loving, or caring are also important. Nonsexual touch needs include massage, caressing, or holding.
- *Comfort and reassurance needs:* The need of the pregnant client for comfort and reassurance stems both from their changing body image and from the developmental processes of pregnancy. These factors bring fears and concerns for the pregnant client about safety for themselves and the fetus, their desirability, and their need for continued love and support.

Sexual Safety During Pregnancy

In general, expressions of sexuality during pregnancy are quite safe. Sexual intercourse is often physically difficult and awkward late in the pregnancy, and couples may wish to experiment with a variety of positions and sexual practices. Sexual intercourse during pregnancy is not harmful as long as it is not unduly uncomfortable and no high-risk factors are present (e.g., placenta previa, preterm labor, or ruptured membranes). There are a few exceptions to these safety rules, and these risks can be categorized by the causative factor. Categories of risk include the following:

- *Risk due to penetration:* Clients who experience bleeding during pregnancy should avoid vaginal penetration until the problem is diagnosed.
- *Risk due to possible infection:* There are two primary areas where infection is a risk with sexual activity: sex with a partner who has an STI; and sex after the rupture of membranes, which normally protect the fetus and placenta from infection.
- *Risk due to arousal:* For a client at risk for preterm labor, sexual arousal, and the accompanying increased engorgement of the pelvic organs, might stimulate the initiation of labor.
- *Risk due to orgasm:* The uterine contractions that occur with and follow orgasm may stimulate preterm labor.
- *Risk due to sexual behaviors:* With the exception of STI exposure, the main risky sexual practice during pregnancy is the forceful blowing of air into the vagina, which may result in air embolism.

Clothing

By about the third month, the pregnant client will discover that their clothing is becoming tight, and they need to wear looser clothing. Some clients wear special maternity clothing; others opt for bigger and looser versions of normal, everyday clothing (e.g., oversized sweaters, elasticized pants and skirts). Garters, constrictive knee socks, and knee-high pantyhose should not be used because they restrict blood flow. Clients should wear comfortable shoes; flat heels are less awkward and provide a better base of support. The pregnant client will probably have difficulty tying shoelaces or fastening buckles late in the pregnancy.

The pregnant client should wear a wide-strapped bra that supports the breasts without causing nipple pressure. An underwire bra is usually more comfortable for the client with heavy breasts. A good nursing bra is essential after delivery if the client plans to nurse. They should purchase two or three bras of their normal chest size but with a larger cup size.

Travel and Employment

Most clients continue driving during pregnancy, at least until the last months, when it may become uncomfortable (the fetus, client, and steering wheel cannot occupy the same space at the same time). The client must be sure to buckle their seatbelt under their enlarging abdomen. They should use the shoulder strap, placing it to the side of their abdomen (Fig. 65-12). Seatbelts are particularly important during pregnancy to protect the client and the fetus. Airbags provide added protection.

Long trips are exhausting for anyone, but because today's families are often on the move, the pregnant client may find regular travel necessary. If the client is to travel by car, they should plan to stop at least every 2 hr to go to the bathroom, stretch, relax, and walk around for at least 10 min. This movement helps to prevent blood from pooling in the lower

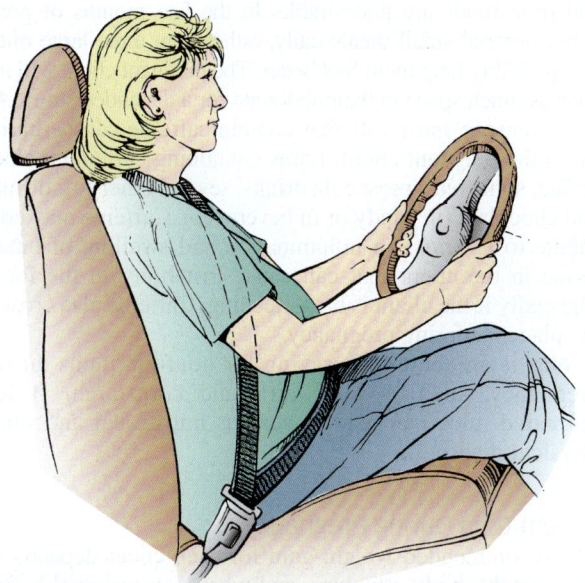

Figure 65-12 Pregnant clients should wear a seatbelt with the shoulder strap above the uterus and below the neck and a lap belt low and under the abdomen.

extremities. The pregnant client should never fly in a small plane that is not pressurized because the lower atmospheric pressure decreases the supply of oxygen to the fetus. The expectant client should consult with their healthcare provider about travel plans because special conditions and times during pregnancy may rule out traveling. The possibility of starting labor while on a long trip away from home needs to be part of the considerations when considering travel.

Many clients continue to work outside the home during pregnancy. The law states that in most situations, a maternity leave of absence, without loss of seniority, must be granted to a client who requests one. Jobs that involve heavy lifting, operating dangerous machines, continuous standing, or working with toxic substances are contraindicated during pregnancy. Radiation should also be avoided.

Teratogenic Factors

Some fumes, chemicals, substances, and infections are known to cause fetal defects. These environmental, damaging agents are called *teratogens*. Most teratogenic effects occur in the first trimester of pregnancy, during the critical period of development of the embryo. The client may not even know yet that they are pregnant.

Teratogenic events occur after fertilization and are not genetic (inherited), although they are congenital (present at birth). Maternal dietary deficiencies and food, air, and water pollutants may play a role. Radiation is particularly dangerous.

The following are some examples of teratogens:

- *Diseases:* Rubella (German measles), herpes, toxoplasmosis, and syphilis are some of the problematic infectious disorders in pregnancy. Rubella outbreaks in the United States are not uncommon due to avoidance of vaccines for immunization and the migration of nonimmunized populations into the United States (CDC, 2017). If exposed, rubella is difficult to prevent and is hazardous to the fetus. To avoid the infection of toxoplasmosis, the pregnant client should not handle cat litter and should cook meat well, especially poultry. They should wash their hands carefully after handling raw meat and wash all raw fruits and vegetables thoroughly before eating them. They should wear gloves while gardening or cleaning.
- *Prescribed medications:* Phenytoin (Dilantin), lithium (Lithobid), valproic acid (Depakene), isotretinoin (Zenatane), and warfarin (Coumadin) have each been associated with teratogenesis.
- *Substances of abuse:* The provider should obtain a complete substance use history at the first preconceptional or antepartum visit. If the client uses tobacco, alcohol, or recreational drugs, they are strongly advised to stop. Street or recreational drugs, such as amphetamines and stimulants, can cause fetal difficulties. The danger seems to be greatest early in pregnancy. Alcohol is the most widely used substance and also the most damaging to the fetus. Heroin can cause congenital addiction. Cocaine may be associated with long-term behavioral and attention problems in the child born to a mother who used it during pregnancy. Other recreational drugs are either known or suspected teratogens. Chapter 95 discusses substance abuse and chemical dependency further. Chapters 68 and 69 present some harmful effects of drugs and alcohol on pregnancy and the fetus in more detail.
- *Ionizing radiation:* This is the type of radiation exposure that is used in treating cancers or that occurs with a nuclear plant accident.

> **Nursing Alert** Caution the pregnant client not to take any herbs, drugs, or medications without asking the healthcare provider. Laxatives, diuretics, stimulants, and depressants are particularly dangerous. Many herbs also are not proven safe for the fetus.

> **Nursing Alert** If you suspect any type of drug abuse in a pregnant client, notify the healthcare provider.

Nutrition During Pregnancy

One of the earliest and most important purposes of prenatal care has been to counsel clients and ensure that they receive adequate nutrition to support themselves and their growing fetus during pregnancy. Studies show that a newborn's chances for good health are greater with a reasonably high birthweight. The nutritional requirements of a pregnant client differ from those of a nonpregnant client. The client's caloric needs increase during pregnancy because they need to meet energy requirements for fetal, placental, and maternal tissue development. The quality of the diet, not the quantity, matters most, and the pattern of weight gain is more important than the total amount.

To obtain the necessary distribution of nutrients, foods for the pregnant client should be selected from all food groups. Exclusion of any group may lead to a deficiency of one or more nutrients. The guidelines for pregnant women are basically the same as the general guidelines for healthy eating. It is suggested that the pregnant client increase their intake of milk and milk products. The pregnant client should make the following dietary adjustments:

- Increase caloric intake by approximately 300 calories daily.
- Increase calcium intake before the last half of the pregnancy. Increase milk intake to 3–4 cups daily. Supplemental calcium is sometimes prescribed. (*Rationale: Calcium is essential to the development of the fetus' bones and teeth and for blood clotting.*)
- Maintain iron intake. Most providers order an iron supplement during pregnancy because of its dietary importance. (*Rationale: Iron is essential in the production of hemoglobin. Because breast milk contains little iron, the developing fetus stores iron for use after birth.*)
- Maintain folic acid intake. Taking 400 µg daily of folic acid (folate) in a supplement is recommended for all women of childbearing age when not pregnant, in addition to food sources of folate. During pregnancy, the recommendation increases to 600 µg from a supplement, plus food sources. Most prenatal vitamins contain 1 mg of folic acid. (*Rationale: Folic acid, a B vitamin, helps to prevent congenital neural tube defects, most notably spina bifida.*)
- Increase intake of most vitamins. Many healthcare providers prescribe supplemental vitamins during pregnancy.
- Increase protein intake. (*Rationale: Protein is essential to the building and repair of all body tissues and aids in the production of milk for the nursing mother.*)
- Avoid empty calories, including alcohol, sugared soda drinks, other sweets, and salty foods.
- Use iodized salt. (*Rationale: It promotes proper functioning of the thyroid gland.*)
- Eat a wide variety of foods. (*Rationale: A variety of foods will encourage proper nutrition, especially during the first few months of pregnancy if the client is experiencing nausea.*)
- Avoid laxatives and enemas unless the healthcare provider specifically orders them. Stool softeners, such as docusate sodium (Colace), are ordered more often than laxatives. Fiber is also essential to prevent and to treat constipation.
- Increase fluid intake to 10 glasses daily to assist in kidney and bowel function. Water is the preferred fluid.

When providing prenatal nursing care, keep in mind a client's general health, age, cultural and religious background; and their likes and dislikes, food allergies or sensitizations, and socioeconomic status. These factors will affect their diet and pattern of weight gain. Dietary counseling should begin at the first visit and continue throughout all follow-up visits. Instructing the client to make a sample diet for review is useful in determining needed dietary changes.

Appetite

Changes in the client's body during the early part of pregnancy may interfere with their appetite, so attention must be given to supplying them with proteins, vitamins, and iron throughout pregnancy.

Many pregnant clients find that they are extremely hungry after the first few weeks. They should monitor what they eat and be careful not to fill up on empty calories. Rich, highly spiced, and fried foods are undesirable. In the late months of pregnancy, several small meals daily, rather than three large ones, will probably help them feel better. The pregnant client will not have as much space in their abdomen for a distended stomach.

Beverages and foods that contain caffeine can be harmful to the pregnant client. Items containing caffeine include coffee, some teas, most cola drinks, several other soft drinks, and chocolate (in candy or in beverages). Caffeine may contribute to *mastitis,* an inflammation and swelling of breast tissue in the client that can cause irritability in the fetus, especially if the client is breastfeeding. Caffeine also crosses the placenta during pregnancy.

Pica is an abnormal craving for nonfood items during pregnancy, such as clay, dirt, and cornstarch. If left untreated, pica can lead to serious nutritional and other physical disorders.

Weight Gain During Pregnancy

The recommended weight gain for each client depends on their height, body structure, and what they weighed before they got pregnant. This comparison, known as the body mass index (**BMI**), provides a starting place to determine how much weight is ideal to gain during this pregnancy. At the initial prenatal visit, the client's height and weight will be measured. They will be asked what they weighed prior to pregnancy. Finally, a BMI chart will be used to determine whether they are underweight, of average weight, overweight, or obese.

The pregnant client's weight should increase gradually from the sixth week after conception until the end of the full term.

The variables of weight gain include body size and condition of being underweight, of normal weight, overweight, or obese. Not only do clients prepregnant body size and weight gain in pregnancy affect birthweight, but they also have an impact on perinatal mortality. Although weight gain itself is critical, the quality of the calorie is important; empty sugars provide calories but not nutrition. If not stated by the obstetrician or healthcare provider, the pregnant client should ask their provider for guidance for their particular situation. Most normal-weight clients will gain about 10 lb by the 10th gestational week. Weight loss, especially during the first trimester, needs to be evaluated by the healthcare professionals. Nutritional and caloric advice is easily attainable using qualified Websites such as the CDC.gov or FDA.gov.

> **Key Concept**
> All pregnant clients should gain weight.

Common Discomforts of Pregnancy

Even in normal pregnancy, it is common for the client to have some unusual, and sometimes uncomfortable, sensations. These are the "common discomforts of pregnancy." They are considered minor, not in the sense that they do not cause true discomfort, but because they are not serious and do not threaten the life of the fetus or the client. However, sometimes it is difficult to tell what is truly a common discomfort or when a symptom may be a warning sign of a more serious problem. Table 65-2 describes the possible

TABLE 65-2 Common Discomforts of Pregnancy

SYMPTOM	PROBABLE CAUSE OR CONTRIBUTING FACTORS	RELIEF MEASURES[a]	DANGER SIGNS
Integument Itching of skin	Stretching of skin over breasts and abdomen	Bathe with baking soda, cornstarch, or colloidal oatmeal in bathwater. Use little, if any, soap. Watch for sensitivity to soaps and detergents. Use moisturizers.	None
Stretch marks (*striae gravidarum*)	Hormonal changes of pregnancy Heredity	Use soothing oils: coconut, olive, vitamin E *Recipe:* ½ cup virgin olive oil ¼ cup aloe vera gel 6 capsules vitamin E (cut) 6 capsules vitamin A (cut) Mix; refrigerate. Apply twice daily See above if stretch marks itch	None
Melasma	Increased pigmentation	Avoid sun exposure Wear hats; use sunblock Adequate folic acid intake (1.0 mg/day) Advise client that it may or may not resolve after the birth	None
Sleeplessness	Over-exhaustion Dreams Stress Excitement Hard to find a comfortable position	Use pillows to help find a comfortable position Use herbal teas: chamomile, lemon, marjoram; or hot milk with honey No heavy meals before bedtime If cannot sleep, get out of bed and read or take a warm bath or shower	Depression
Moodiness	"Superwoman" syndrome Hormonal changes Adaptation to life changes	Emotional self-care Spoil yourself! Nurturing from family and friends	Depression Suicidal thoughts Extremely moody
Musculoskeletal Low-back pain or backache	Relaxation of joints and ligaments Weight of enlarging uterus Increased lordosis	Practice good posture Wear flat shoes with good support Pelvic rocking Walking Good body mechanics Apply small amount of salve to back, such as Tiger Balm (camphor, menthol, peppermint, clove, and cajuput)	Kidney infection (one-sided pain) Fever, chills
Braxton Hicks contractions	Uterus readying itself for labor May occur with breast stimulation or orgasm	Reassurance Take warm baths or showers Use herbal teas: red raspberry, sarsaparilla.	Preterm labor
Round ligament pain	Enlarging uterus stretches ligaments May be felt on sides of the abdomen, in the groin, and outside the vagina	Heat, massage, rest Avoid sudden movements Bend slowly toward pain to allow relaxation	Preterm labor Abdominal problem Infection
Reproductive Vaginal discharge	Estrogen stimulation of glands of cervix and vagina	Avoid soaps to the vulva Wash with clear water as needed Do not douche Avoid "anti-itch" creams containing steroids	Severe itching, odor, lesions, pain with intercourse; bleeding after intercourse; pain Partner with complaints of discharge from penis or lesions

(Continued)

TABLE 65-2 Common Discomforts of Pregnancy (Continued)

SYMPTOM	PROBABLE CAUSE OR CONTRIBUTING FACTORS	RELIEF MEASURES[a]	DANGER SIGNS
Breasts Breast enlargement and tenderness	Hormonal changes Preparation for lactation	Wear a supportive bra Practice good posture Breast care: Wash with water only to keep the oily secretions from Montgomery follicles on the nipple and areolae	Breast masses
Nose Nasal stuffiness or bleeding	Allergies Common cold Increased number of capillaries	Use normal saline nose drops Use cold compresses Use cool-mist humidifier Decrease dairy products in diet	Severe nosebleed may indicate high blood pressure
Mouth Sore or bleeding gums	Increased blood supply Poor oral hygiene Gingivitis	Vigorously brush teeth and gums with soft toothbrush Floss regularly Massage gums Consume adequate vitamin C	Overgrowth of gums onto teeth (this may require oral surgery)
Excess saliva production (ptyalism)	Cause unknown Ask about pica	Consume small, balanced, frequent meals Chew gum Suck on oral lozenges or hard candies Increase fluid intake to compensate	None
Gastrointestinal Food cravings	May be social custom May indicate lack of certain nutrients in diet	Reassurance Complete diet review Avoid unhealthy foods Limit consumption of nonfoods (pica)	Pica may replace nutritious foods Excessive weight gain due to consuming "junk" foods or excessive sweets
Heartburn	Slow stomach emptying Acid reflux into the esophagus	Consume small, frequent meals Avoid caffeine Sip on water, milk, soda water Eat a tablespoon of yogurt Sit up (if happens when lying down) Try to avoid antacids Try herbs: Papaya (has digestive enzymes); anise or fennel-seed tea after meals; slippery elm powder (1 teaspoon with honey, or in a tea)	Ulcer Gastrointestinal bleeding
Constipation	Slowed gastrointestinal (GI) motility Pressure of uterus on intestines Iron therapy Limited water intake Trying to avoid having a bowel movement when it is painful due to hemorrhoids or fissures	Increase fluid intake Increase fiber: bran, fruits, dark breads, vegetables, prunes, raisins If laxative needed, use only bulk laxative, such as Metamucil Increase activity level	Fecal impaction
Nausea and vomiting of pregnancy	Decreased stomach motility Increased hCG level Hereditary, dietary, socioeconomic factors	Eat small, frequent meals Eat snacks high in complex carbohydrates at onset of nausea Avoid heavy meals, excessive fats, excessive spices Try peppermint tea, soda water, ginger tea Eat sour, salty foods (potato chips and lemonade)	Weight loss >8 lb Starvation Loss of appetite Eating disorders GI disease (ulcers, gallstones, liver disease)

TABLE 65-2 Common Discomforts of Pregnancy (Continued)

SYMPTOM	PROBABLE CAUSE OR CONTRIBUTING FACTORS	RELIEF MEASURES[a]	DANGER SIGNS
Hemorrhoids	Varicose veins or hemorrhoidal veins Increased pressure from constipation	Avoid constipation Use cold witch-hazel compresses Try topical anesthetics Take sitz baths Rest on the left side with feet slightly raised	Excessive pain Excessive bleeding
Neurologic Headaches	Cause usually unknown Possible causes: sinus infection, eye strain	Rest Darkness Take acetaminophen as needed	One-sided headache Associated sudden visual change Not relieved by acetaminophen
Dizziness Syncope	Pressure of uterus on inferior vena cava when lying down Decreased cardiac return Decreased cardiac output Low blood pressure	Avoid lying on the back (supine) after 24–26 weeks' gestation Left lateral position increases blood flow Get up slowly from lying down	Fainting
Urinary Frequency, urgency nocturia	Pressure of enlarging uterus on the bladder	Maintain good fluid intake Void frequently Decrease evening fluid intake	Pain or burning with urination Sweet smell to urine
Cardiovascular Varicose veins	Heredity Weight of enlarging uterus Relaxation of smooth muscle in vein walls due to progesterone	Avoid prolonged standing or sitting Rest several times daily with legs elevated Use elastic stockings If varicosities on vulva, apply pressure with a thick sanitary pad inside underwear	Signs of blood clots: heat, swelling, pain Pain with walking
Swollen feet	Increased estrogen and progesterone Decreased venous return to heart	Elevate legs when sitting Elevate legs above heart when lying down or rest on the left side Perform leg exercises while standing and sitting Ensure adequate calcium and potassium intake	Preeclampsia (high blood pressure, swelling, protein in the urine)

[a]Advice or recommendations must first be approved by the client's healthcare provider.

causes of many discomforts, suggestions that may decrease discomfort, and warning signs of more serious problems.

> **Key Concept**
> It is important to differentiate a common discomfort of pregnancy from a warning sign of a complication.

Medical Interventions

The pregnant client should not take any medications, herbs, or nutritional supplements unless they are absolutely necessary and ordered by their healthcare provider. Prescribed medications should be taken in the smallest effective dose and discontinued as soon as possible. The safety of any drug in pregnancy is unpredictable; even commonly used medications can cause fetal problems. For example, a client's use of acetylsalicylic acid (Aspirin) late in the pregnancy can cause a clotting problem in the fetus. Medications such as nose drops, diet pills, diuretics, and cold remedies can also cause serious difficulties.

Some medications taken during pregnancy cause defects that appear many years later in the child. Diethylstilbestrol (DES), previously taken in pregnancy to prevent miscarriage, has been linked to later cervical cancer in girls and infertility in boys born to women who took DES. Antineoplastic drugs (used to treat cancer) are particularly teratogenic.

The U.S. Food and Drug Administration (FDA) has established five categories of drugs based on their potential for teratogenic effects in humans. Box 65-3 lists these categories of drug safety in pregnancy as rated by the FDA.

PREPARING TO BE A PARENT

When approaching pregnancy in a holistic manner, there is an obligation to see the client not just as a container for the fetus but also as an individual in the context of their family and community. It is important to determine how we can best help them and their family members make the necessary transitions. This section examines several aspects of becoming a parent, whether it is for the first or the sixth time.

> **Box 65-3 Categories of Drug Safety in Pregnancy**
>
> The FDA has rated drugs according to their relative safety during pregnancy as follows:
> - *Category A:* Controlled studies in women do not demonstrate a risk; possibility of fetal harm appears remote.
> - *Category B:* Animal studies fail to demonstrate fetal risks, and there are no controlled studies in women; *or* animal studies show an adverse effect, but the same effect was not confirmed in studies in women.
> - *Category C:* Animal studies have demonstrated fetal risks, but no controlled human studies are available; *or* studies in women and animals are not available. Drugs in this category should be given only if the potential benefit to the mother outweighs the possible risk to the fetus.
> - *Category D:* Human fetal risks exist, but the benefits of use in pregnant women may be acceptable despite the risk—such as when a life-threatening situation exists, or for a serious disease for which safer drugs cannot be used or are not effective.
> - *Category X:* Proven fetal risks exist; drug is contraindicated in women who are or may become pregnant.
>
>   **NOTE:** Most drug handbooks identify the pregnancy risk for each drug.
>
>   **NOTE:** Drugs are particularly dangerous to the fetus in the first and third trimesters. In the first trimester, the fetus is being formed and is particularly sensitive to teratogens. Drugs administered in the third trimester are dangerous to the fetus because when the fetus is born, the client's circulatory system is no longer available to help metabolize or excrete drugs, and the newborn's immature circulatory and excretory systems must take over.

Adapting to Pregnancy

Pregnancy can be seen as a developmental crisis, a time of both challenge and opportunity. In the earliest stages of pregnancy, it is very common for a client to feel shock, disbelief, and sometimes denial. To adapt to the pregnancy, there are several stages through which a client must progress.

Pregnancy Validation: First Trimester (Weeks 1–13)

The task of this period of the pregnancy is to accept the pregnancy and all that it means as a reality. Common responses include ambivalence, shock, disbelief, self-focus, and fear (particularly if this client had a prior negative pregnancy experience).

Fetal Embodiment: Second Trimester (Weeks 14–27)

During this phase, the task of the pregnant client is to incorporate the fetus into their body image and to begin to see themselves as a parent. Often, the client becomes more able to identify with their own parent. They may relive and reevaluate all aspects of this relationship.

Common responses during the second trimester include increased dependency, excitement when quickening (first sensation of fetal movement) occurs, calmness, increased libido, and buying maternity clothes.

Fetal Distinction: Third Trimester (Week 28 to Term)

At this stage, the pregnant client must learn to see the fetus as separate from herself in preparation for the birth. This is often called a period of "watchful waiting." The client may exhibit "parent-like" behavior, such as reading to the fetus, stroking their abdomen, preparing clothes, choosing a name, and reading books about childbirth and parenting. They also may experience fear related to the birth, their survival, and the survival of the infant. Often these fears lead to dreams of danger. Many women experience a slight depression late in the third trimester.

Separation From the Fetus: Labor and Birth

With the onset of labor, the inevitability of separation becomes clear. Although in many ways this separation is desired, there is usually some ambivalence about the loss of being the center of attention, the physical separation from the baby, and the fear about the process of labor and birth.

Common manifestations of this fear include frequent visits to the hospital or birth center to assess the onset of labor and needing constant reassurance that they and the baby are doing well and can complete this step.

Transition to Parenthood: Postpartum

Parent–infant bonding is a process that begins during the pregnancy and accelerates immediately after the birth. Strong bonding increases the client's commitment to the infant and also their ability to be an effective parent. Bonding of the client and child is helped by immediate client–infant touch, visual contact, suckling, and vocalizations by both the client and the infant. Behaviors that indicate positive attachment include fondling, kissing, cuddling, and gazing.

Preparing for Labor and Birth

As the client enters the final phase of pregnancy, they become more focused on labor and birth, and typically is eager to plan for these events. Planning may include choosing a site for the birth and a birth attendant (if this has not already done) and developing a plan that reflects their desires regarding the conduct of labor and birth, including analgesia and anesthesia alternatives. Safety for themselves and the fetus is the overriding concern in planning for labor.

Safety, however, means different things to different people. For some clients, safety means immediate access to, and probably use of, the highest level of technology available. For others, the hospital environment may seem inherently unsafe. For these clients, safety may lie in attendance by a trusted certified nurse-midwife or healthcare provider, maintaining control over any interventions considered, and having family and/or friends with whom they choose to have stay with them during the labor and birth. For most clients, safety lies somewhere in between these two choices.

Only the pregnant client themselves can decide what safety means to them and how to have the need for safety met during labor and birth. During the prenatal period, they may wish to explore all the alternatives open to them and evaluate them in light of their own values, beliefs, and goals. As a nurse, your task is to support them in the choices they make.

Approaches to Childbirth Preparation
Common Methods of Childbirth Preparation
Natural childbirth consists of progressive relaxation and abdominal breathing techniques that are taught to the expectant mother and their partner. *Hypnosis,* when used in childbirth, is a combination of relaxation and conditioned reflexes. It uses a normal breathing pattern. A healthcare provider trained in hypnosis and childbirth works with the mother and their significant other.

The Lamaze Method of Childbirth
The most well-known model for childbirth preparation is the Lamaze method. The two components of this method are education and training, using the theory of conditioned reflex. Expectant women are trained in toning and relaxation exercises and breathing techniques, which use three levels of chest breathing for different stages of labor.

Current Childbirth Preparation Trends
Currently, the childbirth preparation movement is steering away from specific breathing techniques and toward assisting the client to find their natural ways of coping with stress and pain. Many clients find the following methods helpful: vocalization, massage, water therapy, visualization, relaxing music, and subdued lighting.

Regardless of the approach to childbirth preparation, it is essential to communicate to the family that the goal of childbirth is to have a healthy mother and baby. Health is more than the physical event of labor and birth; it includes family interactions, bonding with the infant, and the successful transition to a new phase of life. Preparation for childbirth will require knowledge and understanding of the anatomical processes and the emotional tendencies of pregnancy. Refer to In Practice 65-5 Educating the Client for several topics that provide information and understanding relating to childbirth.

Responses to Parenthood: The Partner
In many pregnancies, the partner is the one person whose changing role and developmental tasks do not receive serious consideration. The pregnant client receives attention, the children in the home receive attention, but the partners needs are often unrecognized and unmet. Partner responses to pregnancy include the following:

- *First trimester:* Fears losing the pregnant client and the child and has self-doubt as to their capability as a future parent
- *Second trimester:* Has increased respect and awe as quickening occurs; sees the fetus as a new person; begins to consider names for the fetus
- *Third trimester:* Fears harming the fetus during sexual intercourse (yet finds sexual abstinence is difficult); has envy or pride at their partners creativity; worries over the birth; and is keenly aware of male and female differences

---

IN PRACTICE
EDUCATING THE CLIENT 65-5 Childbirth Education

There are many excellent topics about childbirth that will help clients and their partners or support persons develop understanding of the processes. Childbirth education topics should include the following:
- Information about the process of birth.
- Exploration of individual fears about birth.
- Mechanisms for alleviating the pain and working through the fears of childbirth.
- Discussion of options in labor and birth and how to promote having a normal labor. This may include choosing the site and attendant, discussing positions for labor and activity, hydration during labor, nutrition during labor, analgesia/anesthesia, options surrounding the birth itself (presence of family/friends/siblings, positions for birth, use of labor/delivery/recovery rooms), episiotomy, immediate contact with the neonate, and immediate breastfeeding.
- Discussion of possible complications and potential interventions (this should not be the primary focus of the course).
- Postpartum options, such as the amount of contact with and care of their baby; establishing breastfeeding, or breast care if bottle feeding; time of discharge; danger signs; basics of infant care; and postpartum contraception.

- *Throughout the pregnancy:* Has increased romanticism, increased nurturing, increased participation in family life, anxiety about costs, and concern about their lack of skills in infant care

Preparing for the Expanding Family
Family Dynamics
The family unit will evolve with the new changes. Major changes in the family occur because of the economic cost of pregnancy and a new family member. Healthcare costs escalate during a pregnancy. The pregnant client may need additional emotional support, as well as additional physical care if a complication develops during the pregnancy. The client who is at risk of preterm labor, or who is simply 39 weeks pregnant and ungainly, may not be able to perform their usual household and familial chores.

Siblings often react to a pregnancy by regression in behavior and attitude because they fear that they will be replaced or unloved. If older children originated in another biologic family (i.e., if they are stepchildren, adopted, or living in a blended family), such fears and behaviors may be magnified. It is common for a child to regress in developmental stage, but it is often difficult for the parents to cope with this occurrence.

The changing hormones of pregnancy can keep the client slightly out of touch with their usual methods of coping. Although they may normally interact and communicate in quite mature ways, during a pregnancy they may become depressed, anxious, withdrawn, or angry as they accomplish their own developmental tasks. Such behavioral changes can be hard for a child or partner to tolerate, just as the behavioral changes of children are hard for parents to accept.

Preparing for the Newborn

The family's emotional and physical environment will change significantly with the addition of a newborn. Preparations for the newborn, such as prenatal classes or the creation of a sleeping space for the infant, will directly concern the mother and indirectly involve other members of the family. Preparations for the newborn maybe even more important for that family who has had a previous negative experience such as an unsuccessful attempt to breastfeed or giving birth to a child with physical deformities.

Client Education: Infant Care

Client education regarding general infant care should include the following:

- The range of normal physical characteristics of newborns
- Neonatal and infant response: adjusting to the needs expressed by the infant (attunement), sleep–wake patterns, vision, hearing, startle reflex, and so forth
- Holding the infant
- Skin care and bathing
- Care of the umbilicus
- Diapering options
- Infant stool patterns
- Newborn and infant safety, including the importance of using a car seat

Client Education: Infant Feedings

Widespread agreement is that breast milk is the best milk for a baby. The only exceptions are clients who might transmit a disease (e.g., HIV) or a medication (e.g., lithium [Lithobid]) through the breast milk.

Little preparation is involved in breastfeeding. In the past, sources recommended a variety of activities to be performed, including nipple toughening, nipple rolling, and nipple pulling. None of these methods has been proven to be of any benefit to lactation, either in establishing suckling or in preventing nipple soreness and cracking, and they are no longer recommended. Some guidelines for lactation teaching are found at In Practice: Educating the Client 65-6.

However, deciding between breastfeeding and formula-feeding a baby is a complicated decision for many women. They may be shy, modest, or have concerns about the reactions of other people if they breastfeed. Throughout the pregnancy, healthcare staff should make the information known that "breast is best," but respect each client's decision as the best for them.

Summary

For the client and their family, pregnancy is a time of hope, dreams, anxiety, and fears. Often it can be the nurse who makes the difference for a pregnant client in adjusting to their pregnancy, preparing for the baby, and maintaining a healthy state for themselves and their child. By listening, teaching, and caring, you can be the one to make that difference.

IN PRACTICE
EDUCATING THE CLIENT 65-6 | Lactation

Generally, new parents need information regarding the following topics:
- Nutrition and hydration during lactation
- Supply-and-demand concept
- Nipple care
- Let-down reflex
- Appearance of breast milk
- Positions for breastfeeding
- Expressing/pumping and storing milk

After a client has decided which method they will use to feed their infant, the preparation for that method should be focused on their specific learning needs.

The client who opts to formula-feed the infant may have educational needs about formula preparation and storage (e.g., the frequency and amount of feedings). Each client should be treated individually, so that education can focus on their particular needs.

For the client and their family, pregnancy is a time of hope, dreams, anxiety, and fears. Often it is a nurse who makes the difference for a pregnant client in adjusting to the pregnancy, preparing for their baby, and maintaining a healthy state for themselves and their child. By listening, teaching, and caring, you can be the one to make that difference. Many resources are available for the mother who chooses to breastfeed; e.g., The Leche League's Guide to Breastfeeding is located on the Internet.

THE NURSING PROCESS FOR AN OBSTETRIC CLIENT

DATA COLLECTION/ASSESSMENT

The nursing process for an obstetric client retains the same format as for a medical or surgical client. The data collection/assessment phase is often documented and recorded using standardized formats with spaces provided for an individual's information. Table 65-3 provides the overall content that is typically collected for the initial visit, which is used as a baseline for follow-up return visits. Some information is collected at all visits to the healthcare provider. When collecting the data, the nurse must remember that each client is unique and may have problems or disorders that are not related to a pregnancy. This information is also collected and used as part of the care plan.

PLANNING AND GOALS

The nursing process and its nursing care plan will distinguish the individual client via the plans and goals related to this specific client. Short-term goals and long-term goals may relate to any specific problem, prenatal concern, or to another physiologic issue such as diabetes or an infection.

Short-term goals are often designed to be completed within the time-frame of "by the next office visit," for example:
- Changes in behaviors that could be problematic for the mother or fetus, such as avoidance of alcohol, tobacco, and secondhand smoke
- Evaluation of nutrition requirements for mother and for fetal growth and development
- Psychosocial evaluation, often based on statements by the client, family, or partner, which affirm the client's capability to cope with the physical and emotional changes accompanying pregnancy
- Use of appropriate strategies for dealing with any of the discomforts of pregnancy

Long-term goals tend to relate to the entire pregnancy and the outcome of the pregnancy:
- Demonstration by actions or words that the client can adapt to changes and to the developments related to the psychological aspects of being a parent
- Comprehension of anticipated needs related to the care of a newborn

IMPLEMENTATION

The implementation of the nursing process for an obstetric client includes a variety of factors. Actions or interventions are determined by the information gained in the data collection/assessment phase of the nursing process. The nursing goals provide the overall direction of these actions. For example, implementation of the plan or the actions needed to complete a goal varies according to the client's previous experience with pregnancy, their age and life experiences, their support system, and the available resources they may need. Past medical history, surgeries, or other healthcare concerns must be considered when the nurse implements obstetric nursing care. Examples of implementation include
- Development and implementation of a teaching plan that corrects any knowledge deficits about conception, fetal growth and development, general health practices for the client, and the labor and delivery experience
- Providing educational resources and instructing the client the available methods or strategies for dealing with any of the discomforts of pregnancy that present, such as morning sickness or leg cramps
- Referral to prenatal classes for the client and their significant others

EVALUATION

The evaluation must look at the overall picture, that is, the actual, factual results of the planning and implementation phases. It is idealistic and not realistic to believe that all plans and actions will be effective. To improve outcomes, it will be necessary to evaluate the success of the plan of care. Guidelines are provided within standardized core measures and developed through reviewing the client's and their family's achievement of the above goals. Changing goals may involve incorporating different nursing actions, educating the client, or accepting that a less lofty goal might be more practical for the client. The following are some examples that might be included within an evaluation:
- Modification of the plan, goal, or outcomes if stated goals cannot be met

- Determination of actual versus idealized changes in the physical and mental health of the client throughout pregnancy
- Delivery of a healthy newborn
- Uncomplicated delivery and a healthy mother

TABLE 65-3 Overview of Data Collection for Initial Visit, Return Visits, and All Visits

PHYSICAL EXAMINATION: *INITIAL VISIT*	PHYSICAL EXAMINATION: *RETURN VISIT*
General info - Height - Prepregnant weight - Blood pressure	**General info** - Weight, weight comparison - Blood pressure - Urine dipstick tests for sugar, albumin (protein), nitrites, and leukocytes
Physical examination including a pelvic examination	**Presence of edema**
Obstetric history - Last menstrual period - First day of period - Was it normal?	**Abdominal examination** - Fundal height - Fetal heart tones
Pertinent lifestyle factors - Risk factors (medical, surgical, or lifestyle) - Nutrition - Balance between activity and rest - Sexual activity - Exposure to teratogenic factors, including secondhand smoke - Cultural or ethnic considerations - Use of prescription or OTC medications - Use of drugs of abuse, e.g., alcohol, nicotine, caffeine, cocaine, heroin	**Laboratory and diagnostic tests** - Blood test as requested - Urine culture if requested - Ultrasound if indicated
Presence of common discomforts of pregnancy - Morning sickness - Shortness of breath - Leg cramps - Constipation - Hemorrhoids - Vaginal discharge - Gingivitis - Edema - Varicose veins - Stretch marks	
Psychosocial concerns - Recognition of danger signs in pregnancy and ability to state appropriate action - Preparedness for labor and delivery experience - Preparedness for parenting - Effect of pregnancy on self-concept - Adequacy of coping skills and resources - Concerns, superstitions, and fears	

STUDENT SYNTHESIS

KEY POINTS

- Gravida refers to the number of pregnancies a client has had; para refers to the outcomes of those pregnancies.
- Preconceptional care includes addressing client's habits, nutrition, and psychosocial needs, as well as risks due to medications, diseases, and genetic defects.
- The fertilized ovum, or zygote, will eventually develop into the fetus and all the supporting structures: placenta, membranes, and umbilical cord.
- The period of the embryo is the critical period of human development when the organs and systems are formed; the period of the fetus is a period of further growth and development.
- The placenta provides a place for exchange of gases, nutrients, and fluid between the client and the fetus.
- In fetal circulation, oxygenated blood travels from the placenta through the umbilical vein, whereas deoxygenated blood is carried back from the fetus to the placenta through the two umbilical arteries.
- Of the presumptive, probable, or positive signs of pregnancy, only the positive signs demonstrate proof of a fetus.
- A client's body changes in both structure and function owing to the size of the growing fetus and the hormones produced during pregnancy.
- Anticipatory guidance about the changes that are coming with pregnancy gives a client or a couple time to prepare for those changes.
- A healthy lifestyle for a pregnant client includes maintaining adequate nutrition, avoiding harmful substances, and exercising.
- Good nutrition during pregnancy depends on the client taking in sufficient calories to provide energy and sufficient protein to support themselves and the rapidly growing fetus, as well as consuming the recommended amount of vitamins and minerals every day.
- All pregnant clients should gain weight; the amount that is ideal for each client is based on their height and weight before the pregnancy.
- The common discomforts of pregnancy do not threaten the health of the mother or the fetus but may be similar to warning signs of more serious problems. It is important to know how to distinguish common discomforts and warning signs and to report them as necessary.
- The psychological changes of pregnancy are just as tremendous as the physical changes; every client and family deserves support in dealing with these changes.

CRITICAL THINKING EXERCISES

1. Discuss ways that you would need to individualize a nursing plan of care to address a pregnant client's cultural beliefs.
2. Plan interventions that you would use to provide supportive care during pregnancy to a client when the partner is present and involved. How would you adapt the plan to meet the needs of a client whose partner is not interested or involved?

NCLEX-STYLE REVIEW QUESTIONS

1. A client arrives at the clinic stating to the nurse, "I have a positive urine home pregnancy test and a set of twins at home that were born at 32 weeks gestation." Using the G-P system, how will the nurse document these findings?
   a. G2 P2
   b. G1 P1
   c. G2 P1
   d. G3 P2

2. A client is demonstrating presumptive signs of pregnancy. Which symptoms described by the client should the nurse document as presumptive? Select all that apply.
   a. Nausea
   b. Frequent urination
   c. Breast fullness and tenderness
   d. Positive urine home pregnancy test
   e. Basal body temperature elevation

3. The nurse is providing instruction to the client with a recently confirmed pregnancy at 5 weeks gestation. Which information would the nurse be sure to include in the instructions to prevent congenital anomalies in the embryo?
   a. Avoid exercise during the pregnancy.
   b. Maintain a diet of only fruits, vegetables, and grains.
   c. Avoid the consumption of alcohol.
   d. Over-the-counter medications are allowed but avoid all prescription medications.

4. A pregnant client states to the nurse, "I have a darkening of the skin on my face since I got pregnant and don't know what it is." Which response by the nurse is best?
   a. "I am sure that you had this before pregnancy and just didn't notice it."
   b. "There are medication and creams that you can take to remove this."
   c. "This is an abnormal response to the pregnancy, and we will notify the doctor."
   d. "This is melasma and is caused by hormonal changes during pregnancy."

5. A client reports their last menstrual period was on July 1, 2020. When calculating the estimated date of confinement using Naegele rule, what will the nurse document?
   a. April 1, 2021
   b. June 18, 2021
   c. April 8, 2021
   d. May 8, 2021

CHAPTER RESOURCES

Enhance your learning with additional resources on **thePoint**!

Student Resources related to this chapter can be found at thePoint.lww.com/Rosdahl12e.

CHAPTER 65 Normal Pregnancy 1051

Welcome Steps

Look at healthcare provider's orders.

Protocol for procedure.

Necessary equipment/supplies.

Wash hands using proper hand hygiene; put on gloves.

Explain the procedure and reassure the client.

Locate two identifiers to confirm correct client.

Comfortable and efficient position for nurse and client.

Obtain privacy.

Make sure to follow correct steps and body mechanics with good technique.

Ensure safety and observe deviations from normal.

End Steps

Ensure comfort and safety.

Note questions or concerns from client or nurse; note significant data.

Dispose of materials properly.

Disinfect the area and your hands.

Document and report the procedure and your findings.

IN PRACTICE

NURSING PROCEDURE 65-1 | Listening to Fetal Heart Tones (FHTs)

Purpose
To determine the well-being of the fetus.

Supplies and Equipment
Fetoscope with tubing <10 in. long or Doppler and water-soluble ultrasound gel.

Steps
Follow LPN WELCOME Steps and Then

1. Be sure that the room is quiet and that the client has recently emptied their bladder.
2. Ask the client to lie down on their back (supine position). If they are >28 weeks pregnant, place a small rolled towel under one hip, to tilt them slightly to one side.
3. If you are using a Doppler, apply a small amount of gel to the end of the instrument.
4. If you are using a fetoscope, place the padded cone on the client's abdomen, just above the pubic bone, and the headpiece solidly against your forehead.
5. Exert a little pressure as you place the instrument immediately above the pubic bone.
6. Slowly rotate it 360° until you hear the fetal heartbeat.
7. If you hear nothing, move the instrument 1 cm at a time up toward the umbilicus until you are halfway between the pubic bone and the umbilicus. If you have not yet heard the heartbeat, move 1 cm to one side of the midline and proceed back down toward the pubic bone. If the FHTs are still not heard, do the same on the opposite side.
8. Be sure to rotate the instrument at each new position, as it must be directed at the fetal heart.
9. Count the FHTs for 15 s and multiply by 4 to get the rate per minute. Chart the FHT rate.
10. In late pregnancy, also chart the location on the client's abdomen at which you heard the FHTs. This is done by placing an X, or the rate, in a simple diagram of the abdomen:

    In this diagram, the *curved lines* represent the sides of the abdomen, the *vertical line* is the midline, and the *horizontal line* is an imaginary line drawn through the umbilicus of the client. The FHTs were heard in the *right lower quadrant* of the abdomen.

    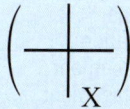

11. If no FHTs are heard with a Doppler by 13 weeks or a fetoscope by 20 weeks, request a sonogram.
    Rationale: Listening to fetal heart tones (FHTs) is an important part of caring for a pregnant client. FHTs should be evaluated at every prenatal visit and at very frequent intervals during labor.

Follow ENDDD Steps

Adapted from Hatfield & Kincheloe (2018); Johns Hopkins Medicine (2020); Stanford Children's Health (2020).

66 Normal Labor, Delivery, and Postpartum Care

Learning Objectives

1. Identify several choices or options for locations for birth. Discuss the advantages and disadvantages for each option. Identify the nursing considerations for each choice.
2. Define the differences between true labor and false labor. State the nursing considerations related to each type of labor.
3. Explain the significance of lightening, Braxton Hicks contractions, effacement, dilation, "show," SROM and AROM, engagement, nulliparous, and parous.
4. Differentiate among the following terms related to contractions: increment, acme, decrement, rest interval, frequency, duration, intensity, and length of relaxation time.
5. Define and discuss the nursing considerations for each of the following terms: lie, presentation, station, and position.
6. Discuss the events that indicate the onset of the first stage of labor. Differentiate among the three phases of the first stage of labor. Identify the nursing considerations for the latent phase, the active phase, and the transitional phase.
7. Identify the events of the second stage of labor and the significance of bearing down and crowning. Identify the nursing considerations related to this stage.
8. Identify the events of the third stage of labor and explain the significance of the expelled placenta. Identify the nursing considerations related to this stage.
9. Identify the events of the fourth stage of labor and explain the significance of involution. Identify the nursing considerations related to this stage.
10. Compare the advantages and disadvantages of comfort measures related to contractions. State the nursing considerations related to epidural and general anesthesia.
11. Discuss the nursing considerations related to external fetal monitoring.
12. Differentiate among the following terms: acceleration, deceleration, early deceleration, late deceleration, and decreased variability.
13. Identify the nursing responsibilities to the newborn and the postpartum client immediately after birth.
14. Define and differentiate among the following terms: lochia rubra, lochia serosa, and lochia alba. State the nursing considerations for each.
15. In the nursing skills laboratory, demonstrate the techniques of postpartum care, including fundal massage, episiotomy and perineal observation, peripad changes, Homans sign, and bladder assessment.
16. In the nursing skills laboratory, present a client-teaching session on the advantages of breastfeeding. Include the following concepts: colostrum, lactation, the "let-down reflex," engorgement, and expression of milk.
17. Discuss the chances of becoming pregnant when a client is breastfeeding. Differentiate between the return of menstruation and ovulation.

Important Terminology

acme	cardinal	engorgement	labor	postnatal	CNM
after-pains	movements	epidural	labor contractions	postpartum	CRNA
amnihook	cervical os	episiotomy	lactation	presentation	FHR
amniotomy	colostrum	false labor	lie	show	LDRP
birth assistant	contractions	fetal monitor	lightening	stages of labor	MD
birth attendant	crowning	frequency	lochia	station	NP
birth center	decrement	fundus	lochia alba	tocodynamometer	OB
birth plan	dilation	increment	lochia rubra	true labor	OB/GYN
birthing room	doula	intensity	lochia serosa		PA
Braxton Hicks	duration	interval	nuchal cord	**Acronyms**	4 P's
contractions	effacement	intrapartum	obstetric		SROM
	engagement	involution	perinatal	AROM	SVE

LABOR AND BIRTH AS NORMAL PROCESSES

In Chapter 65, you learned about normal pregnancy and how to provide nursing care for the expectant family. In this chapter, you will learn about the process of normal labor and delivery, as well as how to provide nursing care during the **perinatal** period (the weeks before the time of birth), the **postnatal** period, and **postpartum** period (4-6 weeks after birth).

A client's body is designed for conceiving, carrying, and bearing children. The process of labor is normal, but it is a process that most women experience only a few times in their lives. It is an intense process that requires enormous amounts of physical and emotional energy.

CHAPTER 66 Normal Labor, Delivery, and Postpartum Care

In this chapter, you will learn how to promote the normal progression of labor and how to recognize signs of possible complications. You will also learn to care for the emotional needs of the laboring client and their family. Although most families have looked forward to delivery for many months, the individuals involved will have unique concerns. As a nurse, you will be expected to provide encouragement, support, and education to assist family members during this intense event. Through the nursing process, you can provide comprehensive care to the growing family.

Careful observations of both the postpartum client and newborn are necessary after delivery. You will perform tasks that prevent the development of complications and promote rapid healing of tissue. You will also function as a teacher to provide knowledge the family needs for maternal and newborn care. For many women, the most important role of the nurse during the postpartum period is the role of educator. Whether this baby is the client's first child or their fifth, each baby brings changes and challenges to the new parents.

The Four Stages of Labor

Labor is a series of events during which a client's uterus contracts and expels a fetus and completes the birthing process. There are four **stages of labor**, which will be discussed in more detail later in this chapter:

- *Stage I, Dilation*: **uterine contractions** (also called **labor contractions**) cause the **cervical os** (mouth) of the cervix to open (dilate) and move the fetus downward into the birth canal. Stage I has **three phases of labor**, which include *latent, active,* and *transitional*.
- *Stage II, Birth or Expulsion*: uterine contractions continue and increase in intensity until the baby is delivered through the vaginal opening.
- *Stage III, Delivery of Placenta*: uterine contractions expel the placenta after the delivery of the newborn.
- *Stage IV, Recovery*: uterine contractions continue and close off open blood vessels to prevent excessive blood loss.

Although there are many theories, no one is certain what causes labor to begin. Approximately 38 weeks after fertilization (the 40th week after the last menstrual period), the fetus is ready to be born. **Intrapartum** is the time period during which labor and delivery take place; it is followed by the **postpartum** period, which lasts until the end of the sixth week after the birth.

Choices in Labor and Birth

Because each birth is an important life event, many clients and their families have a clear sense of what they would like to occur during the process. There are choices in many areas of intrapartum care. The following are some of the options that should be considered.

Choices for a Birth Attendant

One of the choices available to an expectant client and their significant other is the choice of the **birth attendant**. Many choose healthcare providers, who may be a medical doctor (**MD**) specializing in either family practice or obstetrics or obstetrics-gynecology (**OB/GYN**). Others may choose to receive pregnancy and birth care from a certified nurse midwife (**CNM**). Women who have received prenatal care from a nurse practitioner (**NP**) or physician assistant (**PA**) will have a different care provider for the birth; the role of these professionals does not typically include attending at births.

This choice may depend on the availability of **obstetric** (**OB**) healthcare professionals, socioeconomic factors, and geographic location. Isolated areas may use the terminology *birth attendant* to mean an individual who "attends" the expectant client by providing basic and emergency healthcare during the prenatal months, the childbirth process, and the postpartum period. Educational requirements, clinical training, and licensure examination requirements vary for different types of birth attendants. A birth attendant may be a single person, usually a lay midwife or nurse-midwife, who works with available professional members of the pre- and postnatal healthcare team. In isolated communities with limited resources, a **doula** or **birth assistant** may work in tandem with more formally educated healthcare members. The World Health Organization recognizes the importance of the birth attendant and the birth assistant (doula) in the prevention of maternal–infant mortality and morbidity.

SPECIAL CONSIDERATIONS Culture and Ethnicity

A *doula* or *birth assistant* is traditionally a respected individual in a community who provides emotional support, basic advice, and healthcare during pregnancy. This individual assists the birth attendant or midwife. Sometimes referred to as a birth worker, labor support person, or childbirth educator, the doula works with the expectant family providing education of the obstetrical needs and childbirth processes.

Obstetrics Healthcare Team

In a society with available resources, the OB healthcare team typically consists of trained and well-educated professionals, and may include the RN, the LVN/LPN, and a general medical physician (MD, medical doctor) for care of the client's overall health. Resources may be restricted in isolated areas and may combine a lay midwife with the highly trained nurse and other obstetric healthcare providers. OB healthcare professionals assist with prenatal visits, perinatal issues, and postnatal care. A specific OB healthcare professional may also be part of the team. Specialists in the various forms of family practice, obstetrics, neonatology, or OB/GYN may be needed for some higher-risk pregnancies. Other clients choose to receive pregnancy and birth care from a certified nurse midwife (*CNM*). Clients may receive prenatal care from an *NP* or *PA* or an MD. The role of these professionals does not always include attending at births.

Birth Setting

Another choice families can make when preparing for birth is the location of the event. Options available for OB prenatal, perinatal, and postnatal care include an acute care hospital, a birthing center, or delivery at home. Most clients choose to deliver in a hospital setting. In a few acute care hospitals, the laboring client may be assigned to a traditional labor and delivery unit, in which the client labors in one room, but is taken to a delivery room for the birth. More commonly available is a hospital **birthing room**, in which labor and the delivery take place in the same room. In some hospitals, these rooms are called **LDRP** rooms, or labor/delivery/recovery/postpartum rooms. A client might be moved to the obstetric operating room if a cesarean section delivery or delivery complication develops.

A free-standing (not in a hospital) **birth center** is another option for giving birth. Free-standing birth centers promote the concept of safe, satisfying, and cost-effective childbirth. Birth centers often become accredited. Rigorous and specific standards of quality must be met before a birth center can advertise an accreditation status. More than one type of accreditation is possible and different types of accreditation are available for the various healthcare facilities. The American Association of Birth Centers has developed standards and criteria for care and safety in childbirth centers.

Finally, clients may choose to give birth at home. Home births may be attended by either a CNM or, less frequently, a physician or other healthcare provider. One reason some choose this option is that the home is their territory, which is not the case in either a birth center or a hospital.

Only clients in good general health whose pregnancies have progressed normally should be candidates for any type of out-of-hospital birth (birth center or home). At the first signs of complications for the client or fetus, a transfer to a hospital is indicated to ensure the safety of both.

Birth Plan

A **birth plan** is a written document in which the expectant client expresses their desires for labor and birth. Some are brief, whereas others are long and very detailed. Some items that may be included are:

- The client's choice of a partner for support during labor
- The type of pain-relief measures the client desires
- The client's feelings about having an intravenous (IV), electronic fetal monitoring, or an episiotomy

It is the nurse's role to inform the client or couple preparing a birth plan of the policies of the birth setting and birth attendant, and of the need for flexibility if complications develop. The family should discuss the birth plan with their healthcare provider before the onset of labor.

> **NCLEX Alert**
> The nursing graduate should be especially alert to terminology used on an NCLEX-PN. OB examples include *lie, presentation, station*, and *position* of the in utero fetus, and the *four stages of labor*, and the *three phases of stage I*. What do these words mean in relationship to nursing care of the client and fetus? What does the nurse need to consider when these words are used in a NCLEX scenario?

The Process of Labor

Lie, Presentation, Station, and Position

To understand the process of labor and birth, it is helpful to understand the relationship of the fetal body to the maternal body. Several terms are used to describe how the fetus is lying within the expectant client.

Lie

Lie is a term used to compare the position of the fetal spinal cord (the "long part") to that of the client. The normal lie of the fetus is *longitudinal* (up and down), which means that the fetal spine is parallel to the client's. In a *transverse lie*, the fetus is lying crosswise in the uterus and cannot be delivered until the lie is altered.

Presentation

Presentation refers to the body part of the fetus that lies closest to the pelvic inlet, thus will enter the birth canal first.

Cephalic Presentation The most common position in childbirth is when the fetus is in a longitudinal lie and the occipital bone of the head enters the pelvis first, the *cephalic presentation*. The occipital portion of the fetal head is deepest into the pelvis as the fetus becomes engaged into the pelvic inlet. (*Engagement* is described below.) Cephalic presentations, within the pregnant uterus, show flexion of the fetus's body so that the chin is in contact with the thorax.

Cephalic can be subdivided by the locations of the head and what structures of the head face the pelvis (the presenting part). Presentations include *vertex* (occiput), *sinciput* (forehead), *brow* (eyebrows), or *chin* (face) presentation. Vertex presentations are further described according to the position of the occiput such as right, left, transverse, anterior or posterior (Fig. 66-1A). Figure 66-4 shows the cardinal movements and the vertex presentation. See Figure 66-1A for views of types of cephalic or vertex presentations and compare this with Figure 66-1B which shows a *face presentation* and *brow presentation*.

Breech Presentation When the buttocks, foot, or knee is the presenting (lowest) part, it is called a *breech presentation* (Fig. 66-1C). Complicated labor often occurs when body parts other than the fetal head present (see Chapter 68).

Shoulder Presentation Rarely, the shoulder may be the presenting part, if the fetus is lying in a transverse (horizontal) position. If the fetus cannot be turned from this shoulder presentation to a cephalic presentation, the baby must be delivered by cesarean birth.

Station

Station refers to the descent level of the fetal presenting part into the birth canal. Station is measured as the relationship of the fetal presenting part's lowest bony portion to the level of the ischial spines of the client's pelvic bones (Fig. 66-2).

During pregnancy, the fetus is floating in the amniotic fluid above the level of the symphysis pubis. Near term, the fetal presenting part dips into the pelvis, but can still be dislodged upward. **Engagement** is the term used when the fetal head has moved downward in the birth canal until it can no longer be pushed up and out of the pelvis. In *nulliparous* (first time delivery) women, engagement often occurs before the onset of labor. In *parous* (having a history of more than one birth) women, engagement usually occurs during labor. Box 66-1 contains some terms related to pregnancy and birth that are important for you to know.

The station at which the fetus is said to be *fully engaged* is called station 0; that is, the widest part of the presenting part of the fetus has lodged in the pelvic inlet, and the lowest part

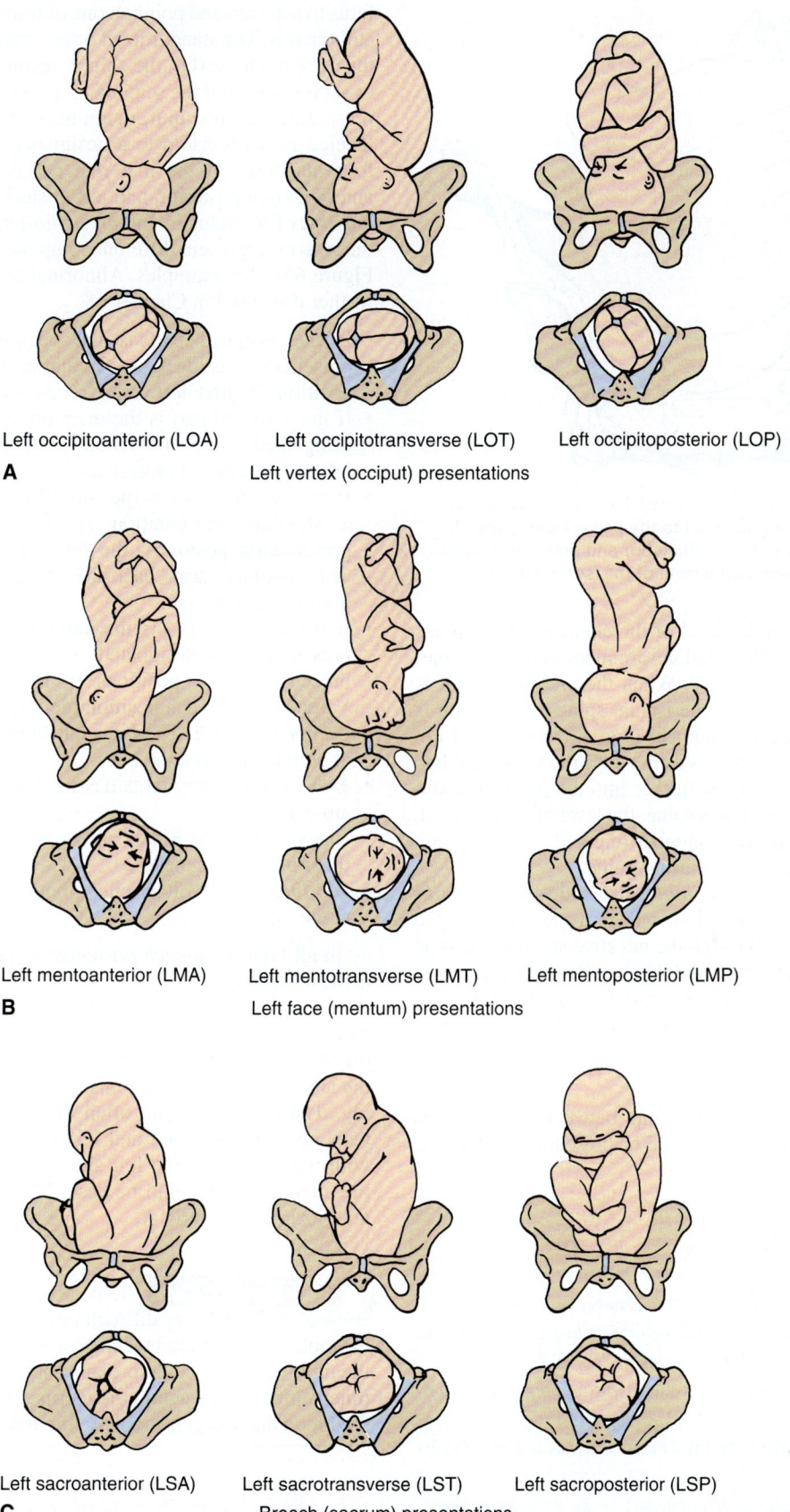

Figure 66-1 Left fetal presentations. A, Vertex presentations. B, Face presentations. C, Breech presentations. Each position can be left or right, and anterior, posterior, or transverse. Each presentation has a possibility of six positions: LOA, left occiput anterior; LOP, left occiput posterior; LOT, left occiput transverse; ROA, right occiput anterior; ROP, right occiput Posterior; ROT, right occiput transverse.

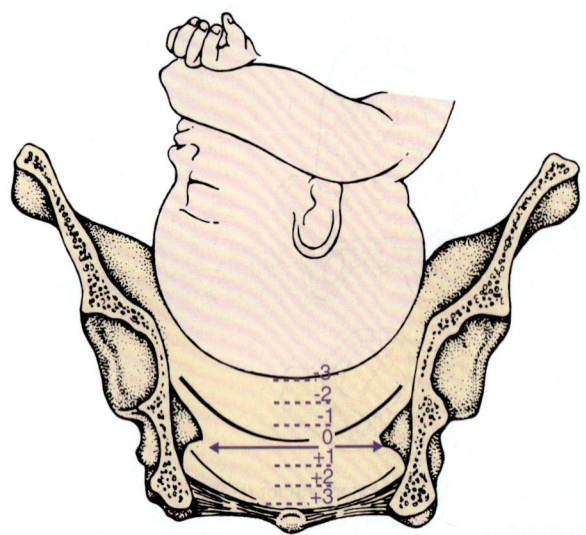

Figure 66-2 Stations of the fetal head. This diagram shows the relationship of the fetal head to the pelvic bones, specifically the ischial spines, during the labor and delivery process. Station zero (0) represents the level of the ischial spines.

of the fetal skull is at the level of the client's ischial spines (see Fig. 66-2). The other stations are measured in centimeters above or below station 0. When the presenting part is higher (above) the level of the ischial spines, the station is expressed with a negative number (e.g., −1 station is 1 cm above the spines; −2 station is 2 cm above the spines). When the presenting part descends further into the pelvis, the station is at or below the client's spine, the level of engagement, it is expressed as a positive number (e.g., +1 station), again using centimeters as the measuring guide.

During the *mechanisms of labor*, also known as the *cardinal movements*, the contractions will move a fully engaged skull so that it passes through the negative stations, become engaged in the pelvic inlet, and then are described as a positive number. (The *mechanisms* or *movements* are discussed in more detail later, in the section on the stages of labor.)

Position

Position refers to the relationship between standardized points on the lowermost structure or presenting part of the fetus to a designated point on one of four quadrants of the client's pelvis. The standardized or assigned points can include the occipital bone (O), the chin or mentum (M), the buttocks or sacrum (S), and the scapula or acromion process (A). The presenting part (occiput, mentum, sacrum, or acromion) is labeled in relationship to a designated point of one of the four quadrants of the maternal pelvis: right anterior, left anterior, right posterior, and left posterior. There are several *positions* for a fetus in any *presentation*. While interrelated, these terms represent different components of labor. Refer to Figure 66-1 for examples. Abnormal fetal presentations are further discussed in Chapter 68.

- If the assigned part is the occipital bone, a vertex presentation is designated. Figure 66-1A shows three positions in three left vertex (occiput) presentations.
- If the assigned part is the mentum, a face presentation is designated. Figure 66-1B shows three positions in three left face (mentum) presentations.
- If the assigned part is the shoulder or acromion process, a shoulder presentation is designated. In shoulder presentation positions, the fetus is on a *transverse lie*. The shoulder, arm, backside, or abdomen may be the presenting part.
- If the assigned part is the buttocks or sacrum, a breech presentation is designated. Figure 66-1C shows three breech (sacrum) positions in three left presentations. Variations of breech position include:
- *Complete breech:* The fetus has both legs drawn up, bent at both the hip and the knee.
- *Frank breech:* The fetus has the hips bent, but the knees are extended.
- *Kneeling breech:* Either one or both legs are extended at the hip, flexed at the knee.
- *Footling breech:* Either one or both legs are extended both at the hip and knee.

In all types of *breech presentation* positions, the sacrum is the assigned point.

After you learn which body part is presenting, you can then accurately describe the position of any fetus. For example, the occiput may be on the client's right or left side and in the anterior, posterior, or transverse area of the pelvic opening. These positions are often designated by the obstetric personnel and recorded and initialed in the charts. A fetus with the occiput in the left side of the anterior portion of the client's pelvis could be described as LOA (left occiput anterior) (see Fig. 66-1A).

> **Nursing Alert** Some positions of the fetus make delivery difficult or dangerous. For example, in a footling breech position, there is a chance the umbilical cord could prolapse because there is so much empty space within the uterus. This could cut off the blood and oxygen supply to the fetus before it is born.

Signs That Labor Is Approaching

The common variables of labor, known as the **4 P's** of labor, are passage, passenger, powers, and psyche. The *passage* includes the diameter of the body pelvis and its soft tissues. The *passenger* includes the fetus, umbilical cord, and

---

Box 66-1 Terminology Relating to Pregnancy and Birth

Nulligravida refers to a client who has never been pregnant.

Nullipara (adjective: nulliparous) refers to a client who has never delivered a live child; also seen as "para 0."

Primigravida relates to the client who is pregnant for the first time.

Multigravida is the term for a client who has had more than one pregnancy.

Primipara (adjective: primiparous) is the term for a client who has given birth to one child.

Multipara (adjective: multiparous) is a client who has given birth to more than one viable infant.

placenta. The *powers* are the uterine contractions. The *psyche* includes the process of birthing, the attitude and behaviors of the parents, and the evaluation process of the stages of labor.

Lightening
Lightening is the settling of the fetus into the pelvis. Lay people often say, "the baby has dropped." Lightening usually occurs 2 to 3 weeks before the onset of labor in primigravidas (clients having their first child). If the client is a multigravida (has had more than one pregnancy), lightening may not occur until labor begins. Although lightening allows the pregnant client to breathe more easily, they will notice an increase in pelvic pressure and urinary frequency and may also have leg cramps and increased leg edema.

Braxton Hicks Contractions
During pregnancy's late stages, the uterine muscles prepare for labor and delivery by tightening and relaxing at intervals. These contractions, called **Braxton Hicks contractions**, are usually painless, short, and irregular. They are also known as *false labor*. As labor approaches, these contractions may become stronger and somewhat regular. The client may sometimes mistake these false labor contractions for true labor. They may experience false labor anytime in the last trimester, but more often during the final 2 or 3 weeks of pregnancy. A change in activity, such as walking, may provide the client some relief.

Show
A mucous plug seals the cervix during pregnancy. Just before labor, the cervix opens slightly and this plug dislodges. At the same time, some capillaries of the cervix rupture, staining the sticky mucus a pinkish color. This process is called the **show**, or *bloody show*, and indicates that labor is about to begin.

False Versus True Labor
A pregnant client may find that distinguishing between true and false labor contractions is difficult. **False labor** (prodromal labor) is the term for Braxton Hicks contractions occurring toward the end of the pregnancy. They are generally felt low in the abdomen. Overall, they occur in an irregular pattern, and their intensity does not grow substantially with time. Although false labor may be annoying, the contractions come and go, and a change of position or activity can relieve the discomfort. In false labor, no change is found in the cervix on internal examination, and there is no bloody show. A pelvic examination may dislodge the mucous plug and cause some spotting that resembles show. Walking for an hour or more can decrease or eliminate the Braxton Hicks contractions, however, no cervical changes are noted.

In **true labor**, the involuntary uterine contractions are rhythmic, grow stronger over time, and begin the true work of labor. These contractions occur at fairly regular intervals, starting at about 20 to 30 min apart and increasing until they are about 2 to 3 min apart. True labor contractions usually last about 30 s initially and increase in duration as labor progresses. The **interval** (**frequency**), or time from the start of one contraction until the start of the next one, in true labor gradually decreases (gets shorter), whereas the **intensity** (strength) and **duration** (length) of each contraction increase. The bloody show usually appears during this time. Usually, the true labor contraction feels like lower-back pain that moves gradually around to the abdomen. These contractions help create *effacement* (thinning) and *dilation* (opening) of the softened cervix. The most important difference between true and false labor is whether or not the cervix changes. During labor, the cervix will become 100% effaced, meaning almost paper-thin, and 10 cm dilated, which will permit the fetus to pass through it (Table 66-1). In Practice: Educating the Client 66-1 provides information about when the client should notify their practitioner.

TABLE 66-1 False Versus True Labor

	FALSE LABOR	TRUE LABOR
Contractions		
Timing	Irregularly spaced	Regular, rhythmic
Duration	Variable	Increases over time
Frequency	Variable	Becomes closer over time
Intensity	Variable	Becomes stronger over time
Effect of position or activity change	Contractions lessen	Becomes stronger with ambulation or activity
Location where felt	Primarily in low abdomen	Starts in back, radiate to abdomen
Cervical Change	None	Progressive effacement and dilation
Presence of "Show"	None	Usually present

IN PRACTICE
EDUCATING THE CLIENT 66-1 — Notifying the Practitioner

A client should notify their practitioner when they are having regular, rhythmic contractions that are getting closer together, lasting longer, and becoming stronger. They should also notify their practitioner immediately if the membranes ("bag of waters") break or leak—whether or not they are having any uterine contractions. The practitioner will need to know if the client is having contractions before, during, or after the membranes rupture.

The time between contractions is called the *relaxation time* or *rest interval* and is equally as important as the contractions themselves. If the relaxation time is short or absent, the fetus may suffer from lack of oxygen, and the client may become extremely tired.

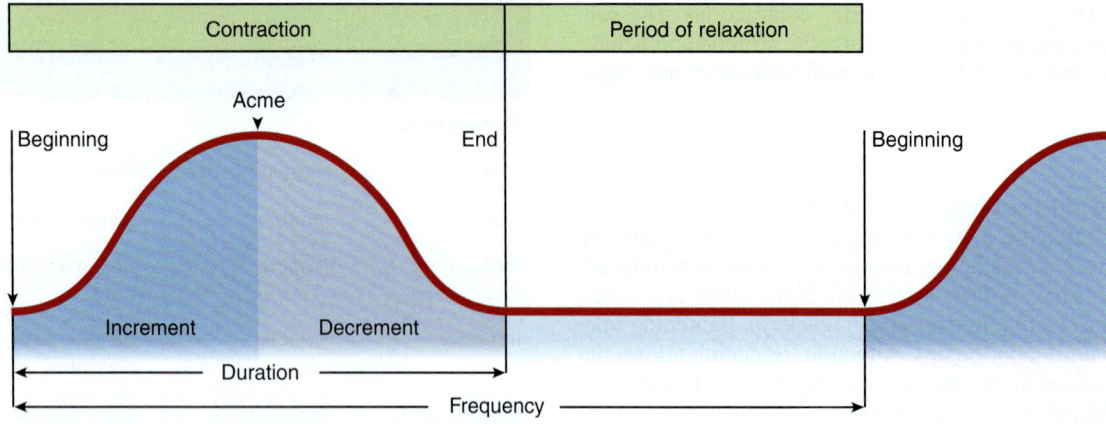

Figure 66-3 The basic three phases that occur during the *duration* of a single uterine contraction. The *increment* is an increasing muscle tone or intensity. The *acme* is the peak or greatest intensity. The *decrement* is lessening of muscle tone or decreasing intensity. Note the *rest period* that follows between contractions. Rest periods become shorter as delivery of the infant becomes imminent (Hatfield, 3e, Fig. 8-10).

> **NCLEX Alert**
>
> Important concepts to consider for examinations relate to differentiation between true and false labor, nursing considerations/interventions, and client teaching.

Uterine Contractions

Contractions of the uterine muscles bring about the birth of the fetus. The uterine muscle is a smooth muscle, and the contractions are involuntary; therefore, the client cannot hurry, slow, lengthen, or shorten them.

During each contraction, the muscle fibers of the uterus tighten. When the contraction ends and the uterus is at rest, the muscles remain slightly shorter than when it started. This is called *retraction* of the muscles. As this process continues over the hours of labor, the shorter muscles pull against the point of least resistance, or the cervix, and cause effacement, and later dilation (Fig. 66-3). The pressure from the taut bag of waters or the presenting part of the fetus helps maintain the dilation of the cervix. Each labor contraction has three phases:

1. **Increment:** This phase, during which the contraction builds from the resting phase to full strength, is longer than the other two combined.
2. **Acme:** This is the time during which the contraction is at full intensity. This phase becomes longer as labor progresses.
3. **Decrement:** During this phase, the uterine contraction eases, until the resting state is achieved.

> **Nursing Alert** Report immediately if contractions come more often than every 2 min or if each contraction lasts 90 s or longer. *Rationale: There is not enough relaxation time for the fetus to be well oxygenated. This event is rare during normal labor but must be carefully watched for when oxytocin is used for labor augmentation or induction.*

Some people refer to contractions as "labor pains." When giving nursing care, the term *contraction* is preferred to avoid reinforcing the idea of pain. You may inform the client that they may feel some discomfort and prepare them for the experience. However, if they insist that they are in pain, do not ignore or correct them. Instead, work with them on ways to relieve the pain. Such methods may include relaxation techniques, breathing techniques, vocalizations, and the use of pain medication.

Rupture of the Membranes

The fetus lies in a two-layered sac filled with amniotic fluid commonly called the "bag of waters." By the pregnancy's 40th week, the amniotic fluid volume has reached approximately 1,000 mL (about 1 quart). Before the birth of the fetus, the membranes break, and the fluid is released. If left to nature, this usually happens just before delivery and provides additional protection for the fetal head during labor, by serving as a dilating wedge against the opening cervix.

When the membranes break, either a sudden gush or a gentle trickle of fluid results. The breaking of the bag of waters without medical intervention is termed *spontaneous rupture of membranes* (**SROM**) and occurs in approximately 25% of all births.

In the remaining 75% of births, the birth attendant may perform artificial rupture of the membranes (**AROM**), a procedure called **amniotomy**. This procedure is performed using a special hook (**amniohook**) under sterile conditions. This procedure may stimulate true labor to begin or may speed the active labor process.

> **Nursing Alert** Report any yellow, green, or cloudy amniotic fluid. *Rationale: Normal amniotic fluid is clear and colorless, and has a slightly salty odor. Yellow or green fluid may indicate the fetus has passed meconium (stool) while still in utero. White or cloudy fluid may indicate the presence of pus in response to an infection.*

A simple test, known as the Nitrazine test, will determine if the amniotic sac has ruptured. A strip of Nitrazine paper is placed against the client's vaginal wall and is compared with a color standard. The normal pH of the vagina is 5.0 (acidic); the pH of the amniotic fluid is 7.0 to 7.5 (neutral to slightly alkaline). If the paper turns blue, it is probably stained with amniotic fluid, indicating the amniotic sac has ruptured. If the test or urine strip remains yellow, it is probably in contact with vaginal secretions only. Blood or urine may also turn the paper blue, so it is important to avoid touching these body fluids with the paper.

When providing nursing care to a client whose membranes have ruptured, record the time, method of rupture (SROM or AROM), color of fluid, and fetal heart rate (FHR).

When the membranes are ruptured, microorganisms from the vagina can travel through the cervix and enter the uterus, which poses a risk of infection to both the client and infant. For this reason, the nurse should obtain a baseline maternal temperature at the time the bag of waters ruptures and continue to assess the client's temperature every 2 hr until delivery. If the client's temperature begins to increase, the practitioner will usually initiate measures to prevent infection of the fetus. These measures may include giving intravenous antibiotics to the client and planning the immediate delivery of the infant.

The practitioner will also assess the FHR for the possibility of a *prolapsed cord* (cord presenting before the fetal head) if the presenting part is not engaged at the time of membrane rupture. If there is any question about whether the presenting part is engaged, a client who was ambulatory should be placed on bed rest. Providers differ in their practices regarding ambulation for a client with ruptured membranes when the fetus is of normal size, in cephalic presentation, and engaged. In this instance, there is little risk of cord prolapse, and ambulation may be permitted or encouraged. The healthcare facility policies and the client's practitioner provide individual guidelines regarding activity.

Stages of Labor

The entire labor process lasts on average between 8 and 18 hr for the primigravida and between 1 and 14 hr for the multigravida. As stated previously, there are four stages of labor: stage I (dilation), stage II (birth or expulsion), stage III (placental), and stage IV (recovery).

Stage I (Dilation)

Stage I begins with the onset of true labor contractions and ends with complete cervical effacement and dilation. Stage I is divided into three *phases: latent, active, and transitional* (see Tables 66-2 and 66-3). Stage I can begin with the spontaneous rupture of the membranes ("breaking of the bag of waters"). Uterine muscles contract with increasing strength and frequency to supply the pressure needed for cervical stretching and dilating.

Two distinct cervical changes occur during stage I: effacement and dilation. **Effacement** refers to the thinning of the cervix. The cervix, normally long and thick (approximately 1-2 cm in length), shortens or thins as a result of contractions. This thinning is measured in percentages. The higher the percentage, the thinner or shorter the cervix. Complete effacement is known as "100% effaced," which describes a cervix that has become almost paper-thin. In **dilation**, the cervical os (opening), normally held closed in a tight circle, begins to open. Dilation is measured in centimeters from 1 to 10. Complete dilation (10 cm or about 3.9 in.) is necessary to allow the uterus to expel the fetus. Cervical dilation is the result of uterine contractions.

Medical personnel are able to estimate the amount of dilation and effacement by feeling the cervix during a rectal or sterile vaginal examination. In a primigravida, effacement usually occurs first, then dilation. In a multigravida, effacement and dilation occur simultaneously.

TABLE 66-2 Average Time Frames of Labor

STAGE	NULLIPARA		MULTIPARA	
	AVERAGE (HR)	UPPER NORMAL (HR)	AVERAGE (HR)	UPPER NORMAL (HR)
Stage I, *latent phase*	9	20	5	14
Stage I, *active phase*	6	12	2.5	6
Stage I, *transitional phase*	1	2	15 min	1
Stage II	1	2	15 min	1

> **Key Concept**
> Effacement of the cervix is expressed in percentages. Full effacement is 100%. Dilation is expressed in centimeters, according to the diameter of the cervical opening. Complete dilation is 10 cm.

Stage II (Birth or Expulsion)

Stage II begins with complete cervical effacement and dilation and ends with the expulsion of the fetus. Required for fetal descent through the birth canal, the fetal body must undergo a series of adjustments in position. These very important position changes are referred to as **cardinal movements** (Fig. 66-4) and provide the capability or *mechanisms of delivery*. The onset of these cardinal movements occurs when the fetus has engaged or dropped down into the client's pelvic inlet. The cephalic presentation is the most common and associated with the fewest delivery complications is the vertex presentation (head first). The sequences for a spontaneous vaginal birth are *engagement, descent, flexion, internal rotation, extension, external rotation* or restitution, and *expulsion*. Cardinal movements involve changes in the position of the fetus's head during its passage in labor as described in relation to a vertex presentation. Normal birth involves the birth of the head, with the face downward. The head then immediately rotates to one side. The shoulders are born, one at a time, and the rest of the newborn follows quickly.

The overall timeframe for stage II is about 1 to 2 hr for a primigravida and usually about 25 min for a multigravida, but can take as long as 1 hr (about 10-15 contractions). The cardinal movements may overlap or occur simultaneously. An expulsive grunt from the client as they exhale is a classic sign of stage II.

During this stage, the client's abdominal muscles and diaphragm join the uterine muscles to push the newborn out

TABLE 66-3 Phases of Stage I

PHASE	FREQUENCY OF CONTRACTIONS (MIN)	DURATION OF CONTRACTIONS (S)	CHARACTER AND INTENSITY OF CONTRACTIONS	CERVICAL DILATION (CM)	CLIENT'S BEHAVIOR
Latent	5-20	30-50	Irregular, mild	0-4	Follows directions, excited, talkative
Active	2-4	45-60	Regular, moderate to strong	4-8	Serious, apprehensive
Transitional	2-3	60-90	Regular, very strong	8-10	Difficulty following directions Frustrated, irritable

of the client's body. The client may say they feel "pushing pains" or a "bearing down" feeling. The rectum dilates, the perineum bulges, and the top of the fetal head appears. This is known as **crowning**. The birth of the infant ends the second stage of labor. The cord is clamped in two places and cut between the clamps.

Stage III (Delivery of Placenta)

Stage III extends from the time the newborn is delivered until the placenta and membranes are expelled. The placenta is attached to the uterine wall; after the newborn is delivered, the uterine muscles contract. With this contraction, the uterus becomes much smaller in size, and the

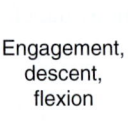
Engagement, descent, flexion
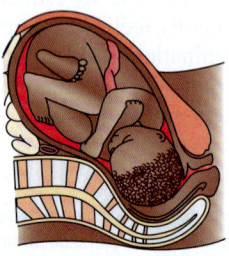
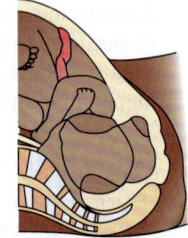
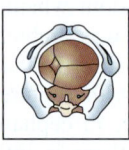

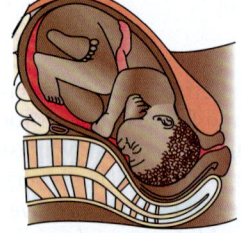
Internal rotation
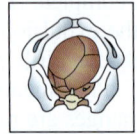
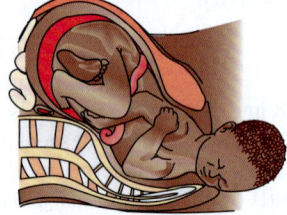
External rotation (restitution)
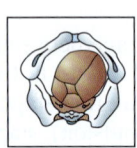

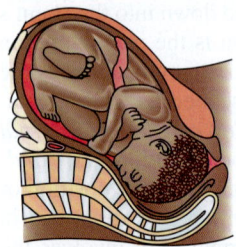
Extension beginning (rotation complete)
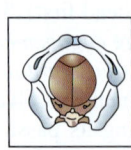
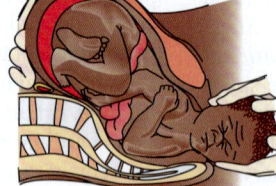
External rotation (shoulder rotation)
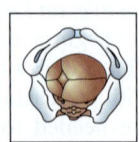

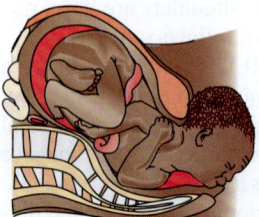
Extension complete
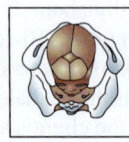
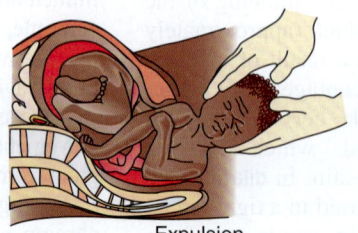
Expulsion

Figure 66-4 The cardinal movements of labor. (**Row 1**) **Engagement** occurs when the fetal presenting part descends to its widest diameter at the level of the ischial spine within the pelvis. **Descent** is complete when the biparietal diameter of the fetal head reaches the pelvic inlet. During **flexion**, the fetal head reaches the pelvic floor and bends forward onto the chest, which results in the presentation of the smallest anteroposterior diameter. (**Row 2**) As the fetus enters the maternal pelvic inlet, an **internal rotation** occurs. Further fetal adjustments through the bony pelvic inlet allow the infant to move through this confined space. Extension occurs when internal rotation is complete. The fetal head flexes and passes beneath the synthesis pubis. (**Row 3**) The fetus is nearly ready to leave the client's body. As the fetus begins to exit, detailed movements occur which include fetal **extension**. In order for the shoulders to exit, an **external rotation** occurs. Internally, the shoulder rotates, followed by an external rotation of the body. (**Row 4**) After passage of the shoulders under the symphysis pubis, **extension** is complete and the newborn is born, that is, **expulsion** (Nettina, 9e).

placenta is sheared away from the wall and then expelled. Stage III can last as long as 30 min for a primigravida, but usually takes only 5 to 15 min for either the primigravida or multigravida.

The placenta is delivered after the uterus contracts. With the contraction, the uterus rises into the abdomen and becomes round, or globular. As the placenta moves into the vagina, the umbilical cord lengthens, and there may be a sudden trickle or gush of blood. The birth attendant (or the nurse) keeps a hand firmly over the empty uterus until it feels firm and hard, indicating that the muscles and the blood vessels are contracted, and minimal danger of hemorrhage exists. If the placenta is expelled with the shiny (membranous) side out, it is called a Schultze presentation (it helps to remember this as "shiny Schultze"); this is the fetal side of the placenta. Schultze presentation occurs in approximately 80% of births. If the placenta is expelled with the dull side out, it is called a Duncan presentation ("dirty Duncan"). This is the maternal side, which is rough and irregular. Excessive bleeding is more likely with this type of placental presentation.

The birth attendant examines the expelled placenta and membranes to determine if the placenta is intact. Retained placental fragments are a major cause of hemorrhage following delivery. The birth attendant also examines the cervix, vagina, and perineum and then sutures the episiotomy, if performed, or any lacerations. Blood loss during a normal delivery is usually estimated to be 300 to 350 mL.

Stage IV (Recovery)

Stage IV includes the first 1 to 4 hr following the expulsion of the placenta. During this time, the client's body begins the process of *involution*, as their reproductive organs begin to return to their normal prepregnant size. Total involution takes about 6 weeks. During stage IV, the nurse must closely observe for signs of hemorrhage, urinary retention, hypotension, and undesirable side effects from anesthesia.

The other critical event of this stage is *bonding* (attachment) between the parents and infant. The more time the client, baby, and other family members spend together during this time, the better the chance of good parental–infant attachment. Bonding is important to the development of a solid relationship between the parents and infant (Fig. 66-5).

> **NCLEX Alert**
>
> Common questions on nursing examinations relate to the nursing care and interventions necessary for each stage of labor.

NURSING CARE DURING LABOR

Nursing Care During Stage I

Maternal Comfort and Care

Stage I nursing care focuses on frequent monitoring of the client's vital signs, contractions, and cervical change, as well as the fetus' well-being to ensure the safety of both. These findings help the birth attendant to determine the fetus' condition and the client's progress. Of equal importance is the role of the nurse in the physical and emotional support of the client.

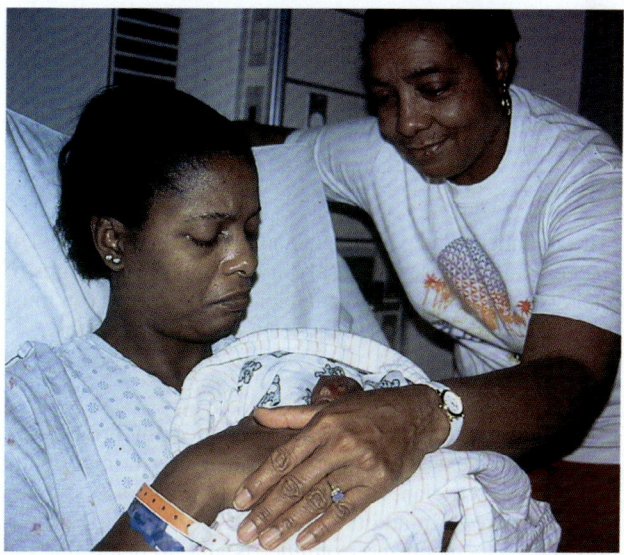

Figure 66-5 Bonding during stage IV.

Admission

Admission procedures for clients in labor vary among healthcare facilities. However, the important elements of an admission history are standard in all institutions. The admitting nurse asks about the estimated date of delivery and confirms this by comparing the information obtained with the prenatal record, which may already be on file at the hospital or may be brought by the client. If the newborn is preterm, special precautions are taken, and special equipment is readied. The nurse also obtains the following information:

- When labor began
- How close are the contractions
- How long each contraction lasts
- Whether the client has noticed any bleeding
- Whether the bag of waters has ruptured

The anesthesiologist or certified registered nurse anesthetist (**CRNA**) will also want to know when the client last ate.

> **Nursing Alert** Report any bright-red bleeding at once. *Rationale:* A client who is bleeding should never be examined vaginally until ultrasound rules out placenta previa.

Other routine procedures include checking temperature, pulse, respirations, and blood pressure; urine dipstick testing for sugar and albumin; and blood tests for hemoglobin, hematocrit, and confirmation of the client's blood type. The fetal heart tones should first be checked at the time of admission. The birth attendant may examine the client's heart, lungs, and abdomen and will also listen to the fetal heartbeat. In most facilities, an external fetal monitor is applied to the client's abdomen to obtain a baseline FHR tracing. A sterile vaginal examination often determines how far labor has progressed.

> **Nursing Alert** Be sure to ask the client upon admission about allergies to povidone-iodine (Betadine), lidocaine (Xylocaine), any other drugs, and latex. ***Rationale:*** *Allergic reactions can range from uncomfortable to fatal.*

Remember to keep the client and their partner informed of progress and to observe closely at all times for any signs of fetal distress. Box 66-2 lists danger signs in labor. You must report any of these signs to the team leader immediately.

Observation and Data Gathering

Uterine contractions are one means of checking progress. A sterile vaginal examination (**SVE**), usually performed by the midwife, obstetrician, or registered nurse, also assesses the labor's progress. In addition to the degree of cervical dilation and effacement, the examiner is able to determine the presenting part, station, size of the pelvic outlet, and status of the membranes.

Nursing students may assist by ensuring that the client is draped properly and that the examiner has the needed supplies (sterile gloves, lubricant, and, if necessary, an amniohook). Students should not be asked to perform SVEs. If, as a graduate, you are asked to perform an SVE, you must receive in-service instruction in the procedure from the healthcare facility first.

Emotional and Physical Support

Nursing support during stage I is directed toward making the client as comfortable as possible and encouraging them to do the things (e.g., breathing) that promote the normal progression of labor. Labor is exactly what it implies, hard work. In the past, clients were encouraged to be passive during labor, to lie down and rest. More current thinking is that the client should be an active participant in the labor process. By laboring in different positions or walking in the room or around the unit, the healthy client is more likely to have a normal progression of labor.

Carefully observe the client's physical state during labor and delivery. Measure and record their vital signs at least every 4 hr and the fetal heart tones at regular intervals. Follow healthcare facility routines carefully.

Stay with the client and do everything possible to help them work with the contractions and relax and rest between them. Encourage the support person to be as involved as the couple wishes. Remind the client to breathe slowly and deeply and to use any techniques learned in childbirth preparation classes to relax their muscles and allow the contractions to do the work. Sponge the client's face and hands occasionally, rub their back, offer them a sip of water or ice chips from time to time, change their gown or bedding if they become damp or soiled, and see that the air in the room is fresh.

Ensure that the client's bladder is empty. A full bladder prevents the fetal head from descending into the client's pelvis and thereby slows labor's progress. A full bladder during labor may also result in trauma, urinary incontinence during delivery, or urinary retention in the immediate postpartum period, in which case catheterization may become necessary.

Early labor is best spent out of the bed. The healthy client may choose to walk, sit in a rocking chair, shower, and engage in diversionary activities such as card games or conversation. As the labor becomes more intense, they will concentrate more and more on the contractions and may have little tolerance for suggestions that they earlier would have welcomed.

For those times when the client is in bed, they might prefer to have the head of the bed elevated. If they do lie flat, however, they should lie on their left side, rather than on their back, to prevent hypotension, which results from compression of the aorta and vena cava by the weight of the uterus falling backward against the spine (see Fig. 65-11).

Some hospitals allow the client to be ambulatory only as long as the bag of waters is intact; other hospitals allow a client whose membranes have ruptured to be up and about if the fetal presenting part is well applied to the cervix. Be sure to know and follow the policies of your institution and the client's birth attendant.

Water and clear fluids are usually allowed during the very early stages of labor. Some believe that solid foods may cause the client to vomit, particularly if they are to have a general anesthetic; others would prefer that the gastric acid be diluted by oral intake, even if a general anesthetic becomes necessary. It has become common practice in many hospitals to give IV solutions to maintain caloric and fluid intake and to lessen exhaustion and dehydration. However, be aware that a full liter bag of 5% dextrose contains only about 125 calories and, if given at a slow infusion rate, will not be sufficient to prevent maternal exhaustion.

Relief of Discomfort

If the client desires, after labor is well established, they may be given medication to make them more comfortable and relaxed. The type of drug may vary with the locale, the provider, and the client's condition. Analgesics reduce the discomforts of labor, sedatives promote rest, and tranquilizers

---

Box 66-2 Danger Signs in Labor

- Sharp, unremitting pain
- Prolonged contractions or failure of the uterus to relax (rigid uterus after a contraction)
- Change in character of the fetal heartbeat; abnormal deceleration pattern on fetal monitor
- Maternal bleeding
- Extreme maternal exhaustion
- Cessation of labor after it has begun
- Hypotension or increased pulse rate of the client
- Prolapse of the umbilical cord
- Irregular fetal heartbeat
- Passage of meconium-stained amniotic fluid when fetus is in vertex position
- Exaggerated movement of the fetus
- A pH value below 7.2 of fetal blood drawn from scalp veins (indicating fetal acidosis)

relax the client. Sometimes a combination of two drugs is administered. Anti-emetics may also be given for women who experience nausea or vomiting during labor.

> **Nursing Alert** After consulting with their provider, a client often makes a decision about when to use medication during labor. **Rationale:** *Medications may slow labor if given too early or may cause the newborn to be lethargic if given too late.*

Many clients receive some form of anesthesia during labor and delivery. One of the most common methods of anesthesia is **epidural** anesthesia, also called the *lumbar epidural block*. A small catheter is inserted into the epidural space within the spinal column. The catheter is taped into place, and a test dose of the anesthetic drug is given. If no undesired side effects arise, the drug can be carefully administered through the catheter during labor and delivery—either intermittently or continuously—using a pump. Most women receive pain relief within 20 min. An anesthesiologist should monitor the administration of this type of anesthesia because serious side effects (e.g., maternal hypotension) can occur.

The client receiving epidural anesthesia during labor should be positioned on their side, with their head slightly raised. If they lie on their back, a small firm pillow should be placed under their right hip so that the uterus tilts to the left. This measure will help prevent the compression of the client's aorta and vena cava. Monitor the client's blood pressure frequently (at least every 15 minu). The FHR should be monitored either continuously with an electronic monitor, or frequently with a fetoscope. Disadvantages of delivery using epidural anesthesia include the blocking of the urge to push in stage II and an increased chance of forceps delivery.

Other anesthetics can be injected into the spinal canal (*saddle block*), the caudal space (*caudal block*), or the pudendal nerve (*pudendal block*). Sometimes the local anesthetic is injected around the cervix (*cervical block*). Although the client is awake during delivery, they lose sensation in the anesthetized site. The following anesthetic agents are frequently used:

- Tetracaine hydrochloride (Pontocaine)
- Dibucaine hydrochloride (Nupercainal)
- Lidocaine hydrochloride (Dilocaine, Xylocaine)

General anesthesia is rarely used because the client receiving this type of anesthesia is asleep when the newborn arrives. Babies born this way may not breathe spontaneously and may be difficult to awaken. General anesthesia is used in emergencies only (e.g., emergency cesarean delivery) because of the possibility of newborn central nervous system depression. In most cesarean deliveries, general anesthesia is not given until after the baby is delivered, with either spinal or epidural anesthesia used before that.

Each type of anesthesia has distinct advantages and disadvantages. The client's needs and wishes and the availability of medications dictate the form used. Many women view labor as a natural function and desire to deliver with little or no medication.

For the client receiving anesthesia, report the following findings *immediately:*

Inability to move the legs

- Numbness in the legs
- Ringing in the ears
- Dizziness
- Metallic taste
- Hypotension or seizures

Rationale: *These serious side effects of anesthesia can be fatal to the client and/or the fetus.*

Assessing Fetal Well-Being

The well-being of the fetus is of utmost concern during the course of labor. The best indicator of fetal health is the **FHR**. The normal FHR is 120 to 160 beats per minute (bpm).

The frequency with which the FHR is evaluated should depend on the absence or presence of risk factors. FHR evaluation may be done using a fetoscope to perform intermittent auscultation; an electronic monitor may be used for continuous monitoring or periodic test strips. Electronic monitors can be used externally or internally. To permit internal electronic monitoring, the membranes must be ruptured.

Intermittent Auscultation

When there are no risk factors with the laboring client or the fetus, the standard practice is to evaluate and record the FHR at least every 30 min during stage I, and at least every 15 min during stage II. When risk factors are present, the FHR should be evaluated at least every 15 min during stage I, and every 5 min during stage II.

> **Key Concept**
> The most important factor in fetal monitoring is the relationship between the fetal heart rate and the contractions of the uterus.

Electronic Fetal Monitoring

Continuous electronic monitoring of the FHR during labor is routine in many facilities. The purpose of the **fetal monitor** is to record the rate and quality of the fetal heartbeat during contraction and relaxation. It can give an early warning of fetal distress so that corrective measures can be started immediately. The nurse will periodically print out (run off) strips of the monitor's graphic record and place them into the client's chart as part of the documentation of labor. Documentation of periods of distress is particularly important and needs to be placed in the permanent record (see In Practice: Nursing Procedure 66-1). An electronic fetal monitor is usually used in the following situations:

- If the fetus seems to be in distress
- If the delivery is being induced
- If the client has a chronic health problem
- If a complication of pregnancy exists

External monitoring of the FHT is most commonly used. This approach is based on the Doppler effect, in which high-frequency ultrasound waves directed to the fetal heart bounce back to a transducer strapped onto the client's abdomen. The receiver amplifies the fetal heart sounds. The signal is converted to sound and is printed on electrocardiograph paper. In addition, a pressure-sensitive device, called a **tocodynamometer**, is used to monitor the frequency of contractions. When placed directly over the client's **fundus** (upper curve of the uterus), the device transfers an electrical impulse to the monitor, creating a readout. The tocodynamometer does not give information about the strength of uterine contractions. The relationship between the fetal heartbeat and uterine contractions can be studied because the information is printed simultaneously.

Advantages of external monitoring are that it is noninvasive, has no contraindications, and is easy to apply. Disadvantages include the need for frequent adjustments and its sensitivity to fetal and maternal movements.

If the external monitor's printout signals a fetal or maternal problem, an internal or direct monitor is used because it is more accurate. An electrode, such as the *scalp clip* or *spiral*, is passed through the client's dilated cervix and carefully attached directly to the presenting part of the fetus. The internal monitor can provide precise information, including a fetal electrocardiogram. The external sensor may still be used to measure the frequency and length of uterine contractions, or a catheter (*intrauterine pressure catheter*) may be inserted into the uterus so that the intensity of contractions may also be measured.

The advantages of internal monitoring include a high-quality tracing and fewer *artifacts* (interference from other sources) than external monitoring. The disadvantages are that membranes must be ruptured, the cervix must be dilated, and the presenting part must be accessible.

Evaluation of Fetal Monitor Information

As a nursing student or licensed practical/vocational nurse, you most likely will not be responsible for the interpretation of electronic fetal monitoring. However, you should understand basic theory and terminology. Notify the team leader immediately if any signs of fetal distress appear on the fetal monitor, such as:

- *Accelerations:* Accelerations are brief increases of the FHR of 15 bpm or more. It is a sign of a healthy fetus for the FHR to accelerate after movement or stimulation. Any acceleration of 60 bpm or more is considered a complication, and the fetus may be in danger.
- *Decelerations:* Decelerations (slowing) of the FHR are categorized according to when they occur in relation to a contraction. Some decelerations are expected; others are warning signs of possible problems. An *early deceleration* begins early in the contraction, hits its low point at the peak of the contraction, and returns to baseline at the end of the contraction; it mirrors the contraction pattern. Early decelerations are caused by vagal nerve stimulation, resulting from pressure on the fetal head, and are considered a normal response of the fetus to labor. A *late deceleration* begins as the contraction eases, and lasts longer than the contraction—into the resting phase of the uterus. This is a sign of a possible problem and should be reported to your team leader.
- *Decreased variability:* Little to no fluctuation in the FHR on an internal electronic monitor tracing is a danger sign and may indicate an abnormality in the fetal nervous system. It might also indicate that the client has taken or been given central nervous system depressants. Report this observation to the team leader for further evaluation.

> **Nursing Alert** *Variable decelerations* in fetal heart rate occur anytime during or after contractions. They usually indicate umbilical cord compression and can usually be altered by changing the client's position or by giving them oxygen. *Late decelerations* begin late in the contraction, and the fetal heart rate recovery occurs after the contraction is over. Decelerations are related to placental insufficiency and indicate fetal distress. The fetal heart rate should not fall below 100 bpm.

Nursing Care During Stage II

Maternal Care

Either a licensed practical nurse or licensed vocational nurse (LVN/LPN) or RN will assist in delivery. If you are assigned to assist during the birth, you most likely will help with the transfer to the delivery room (in a traditional labor and delivery suite) and then stand at the client's side, instructing them on how to breathe and when to push, and informing them of what is occurring. If you are assisting the birth attendant, you may be responsible for handing their necessary equipment, medications, and other items. If you are caring for the newborn, you will need to make sure that the infant is breathing and kept warm (see Chapter 67).

Aseptic conditions must be maintained during delivery. You and any of the client's support people will wear a clean scrub suit, a cap to cover your hair, and a mask.

If the client is going to deliver in a hospital delivery room, they are transferred on the bed and moved over to the delivery table, with the assistance of the circulating nurse. The table, which is split across the middle, is opened (broken), and the client's buttocks are positioned at the break in the table. Their feet are placed in stirrups simultaneously to prevent strain on the pelvic ligaments. Perineal preparation is done to cleanse the skin and to remove secretions from the genitalia. (Shaving is rarely done today.) In some cases, a *birthing chair* or *squat bar* is used.

Coaching the Client

In stage II, the client actively helps the birth process. As each contraction begins, they take a deep breath, hold it, and then push with each contraction. Clients often make grunting noises during pushing. If the client relaxes between contractions, they can work better when the next contraction comes. Encourage the client to push only with contractions and to rest between them.

If a client tells you the baby is coming, you should trust their judgment. Get assistance immediately, and check for crowning. If a delivery occurs suddenly, without advance warning and aseptic preparation, it is called a *precipitous delivery* (this is different from a *precipitous labor*, in which fewer than 3 hr elapse from the onset of labor to birth). A client may "precipitate" in the labor room bed if

CHAPTER 66 Normal Labor, Delivery, and Postpartum Care

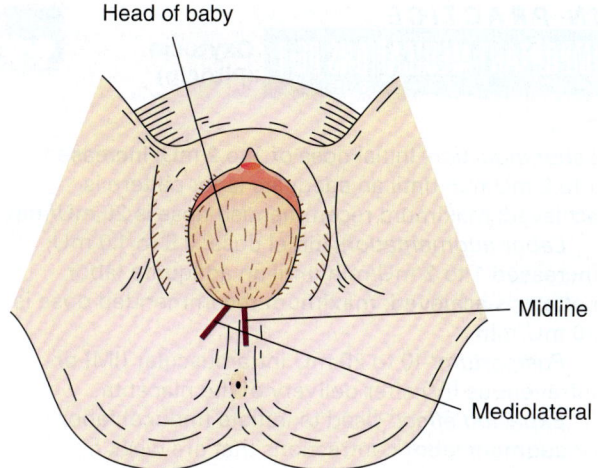

Figure 66-6 Position of episiotomy incision in a client during stage II. The baby's head is presenting to the vaginal outlet (*crowning*).

their claim that birth is imminent is ignored. Encourage the laboring client to pant or blow forcefully when told not to push. Remember that only one person should give the client instructions: during this challenging experience, too many different voices and directions can be overwhelming.

Episiotomy

Often the birth attendant makes an incision in the perineum, called an **episiotomy**, which enlarges the vaginal opening and allows an easier delivery of the fetus. Some birth attendants believe that episiotomy helps to preserve the structure and strength of the perineal muscles and prevents a jagged laceration or a tear extending to the anus. Other birth attendants believe that a laceration, should one occur, will be less extensive than the episiotomy. Extensive lacerations are difficult to repair and could leave permanent damage.

Note the type of episiotomy (midline, or right or left mediolateral), as well as any lacerations that occurred, on the client's chart (Fig. 66-6).

Neonatal Care

After the baby's head is delivered, the birth attendant will check for any loops of cord that have become wrapped around the infant's neck (**nuchal cord**) and remove them. Next, they will suction the nose and mouth of the newborn with a bulb syringe. The anterior shoulder is delivered, then the posterior shoulder and the remainder of the body. The newborn cries out, and the lungs expand. The time of delivery of the baby should be noted for legal records. This entire portion of the delivery often takes only a few seconds.

The baby may be handed to the client immediately, before the umbilical cord is clamped. Assist the client in placing the baby on the bare skin of their chest. Dry the baby, remove any damp towels or sheets, and cover the baby with a clean, dry cloth. Most babies calm quickly after experiencing the warmth of the client and the security of their embracing arms. You should observe for the infant's breathing pattern and suction the mouth if needed.

When the umbilical cord stops pulsating, two Kelly clamps are applied to it, and the birth attendant or support person cuts the cord between them. An umbilical clamp is later applied near the baby's abdomen. Make certain it is attached securely but does not pinch any skin folds. Some hospitals and birth attendants prefer that the infant be stabilized first in a radiant warmer. After the newborn is stable, the parents may hold the infant. However, healthcare personnel are responsible for the newborn's care. Newborns must be kept warm, yet parents should have time to hold and to bond with them. Overhead warmers allow you to observe the newborn. Observations of the newborn include assessment of the Apgar score at 1 and 5 min of life (see Chapter 67).

For each delivery, a staff person skilled in neonatal resuscitation should be available to provide resuscitation if needed. If the infant is depressed or not fully responsive to stimulation, the neonatal resuscitation expert should be called immediately. Every minute is critical; never delay summoning help in the hopes that the baby's condition will improve.

Nursing Care During Stage III

Stage III is relatively short, but may be a dangerous period for the client because of the possibility of hemorrhage. The nurse should record the following information about the delivery of the placenta:

- The exact time the placenta was delivered.
- Whether the placenta was delivered spontaneously or removed manually.
- Which side of the placenta presented.

After the placenta is delivered, an oxytocic medication may be administered to assist the uterus to contract and to minimize the risk of bleeding. You may be instructed to administer these oxytocics or to massage the fundus gently to minimize blood loss.

After the birth attendant has examined the cervix and vagina and sutured the episiotomy or lacerations, the vulva and perineum should be cleansed. If stirrups were used, remove the client's legs from them.

> **Key Concept**
> Bring the client's legs down from the stirrups slowly and together.
> **Rationale:** Doing so helps to avoid further trauma and discomfort.

Change the client's gown, apply perineal pads, and cover them with a warm blanket. Some healthcare facilities transfer clients to a recovery room; in others, clients recover in the room where they deliver.

Before the client leaves the delivery or birthing room, complete the necessary documentation. Box 66-3 lists information required for the health record.

Nursing Care During Stage IV

Following delivery, the client might feel chilled and shake uncontrollably, possibly in response to a cool room, sudden hormonal shifts, or the sudden change in intra-abdominal pressure after the fetus and placenta are expelled. Be sure they have several warm blankets available if needed.

Box 66-3 Necessary Documentation for Delivery

- Complete information about the type of delivery and procedures used; who was present
- Sex and condition of the baby (include Apgar score)
- Time of birth
- Time at which the placenta was expelled and presentation; indicate manual removal or spontaneous delivery
- Condition of the fundus
- Any medication administered
- If an episiotomy was done, and its type
- Condition and vital signs of the client
- Measured maternal blood loss
- Any other events (e.g., maternal incontinence, infant resuscitation, perineal tears)

Many healthcare facilities have a recovery room where the client and newborn are taken after delivery and where the parents can bond with and care for their newborn during the first hours. In some facilities, the newborn is first taken to the nursery for an initial admission examination and then returned to the recovery room. Others admit the newborn when the parent arrives in the postpartum area.

Immediately following delivery, the client may experience extreme fatigue, close to exhaustion, just as they would after any extremely vigorous physical activity or hard work. At the same time, they are usually relieved and excited. They are usually interested in seeing and holding the newborn and having a visit with their partner. The bonding between parents and newborn should be encouraged immediately. Allow time for the family to be together as soon as possible. If both the postpartum client and infant are stable, you should provide the family with privacy during this time. Observe the client closely for several hours after delivery for signs of complications. In addition, document any maternal complaints.

Observations and Data Gathering

Check the postpartum client's blood pressure and pulse at least every 15 min for the first 1 or 2 hr or until it is stable and then every half hour for 1 hr or longer. Usually after the first 12 hr, you will check vital signs every 4 hr for 12 hr and then every 8 hr if no difficulties arise.

When taking vital signs, also check the fundus of the uterus and the perineum. The reason for keeping a close check on the fundus is to ensure that it remains firm and contracted. If it becomes soft and boggy, hemorrhage could

IN PRACTICE
IMPORTANT MEDICATIONS 66-1 Oxytocin (Pitocin)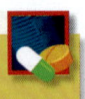

Dose
Labor induction: Initial dose of 1 to 2 mU; increased 1 to 2 mU/min until an adequate labor pattern is achieved; maximum recommended dose is 20 mU/min
  Labor augmentation: Initial dose: 0.5 to 1.0 mU; increased 1 to 2 mU/min until an adequate labor pattern is achieved; maximum recommended dose is 20 mU/min
  Postpartum: 10 to 20 mU intramuscular (IM) or intravenous (IV) after delivery of the placenta
  Expected effect: Used to initiate (induce) labor or augment labor contractions that are weak or ineffective; also used after the delivery of the placenta to contract the uterus

Adverse Side Effects
Client: Unpredictable individual response; hypertonic uterine contractions; tetanic uterine contractions; cervical and vaginal lacerations; amniotic fluid embolism; water intoxication
  Fetus: Fetal distress, birth injury

Nursing Considerations
- *Contraindications to use:* Any obstruction that would interfere with the descent of the fetus; hypertonic or uncoordinated uterine contractions; fetal distress; any contraindication for vaginal birth.
- Amount and rate of administration must be carefully controlled; this can be done effectively only by use of the IV route, using an infusion pump.
- Type of solution, amount of oxytocin added, and rate of infusion vary according to agency protocols or healthcare provider preference.
- Evaluate fetal heart rate every 15 min when given during labor.
- To prevent water intoxication, give in electrolyte solution, avoid infusing high volumes of fluid, and avoid using high doses of oxytocin for prolonged periods.

occur. Teach the client to assess their own uterine fundus. If nursing measures are not effective, the healthcare provider may order administration of an IV or intramuscular (IM) oxytocic drug. Common oxytocic drugs are oxytocin (In Practice: Important Medications 66-1) and methylergonovine maleate (In Practice: Important Medications 66-2).

IN PRACTICE
IMPORTANT MEDICATIONS 66-2 Methylergonovine Maleate (Methergine)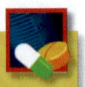

Dose: 0.2 mg intravenous (IV), intramuscular (IM), or oral (PO) (IV only for emergencies)
  Expected effect: Strong, persistent uterine contractions that last for hours
  Adverse side effects: Hypertension is primary side effect; may also cause headache, some chest pain, palpitations, and dyspnea

Nursing Considerations
- Methylergonovine should never be given until the fetus and placenta have been delivered.
- Check the client's blood pressure before giving the medication; if elevated, do not administer this drug.

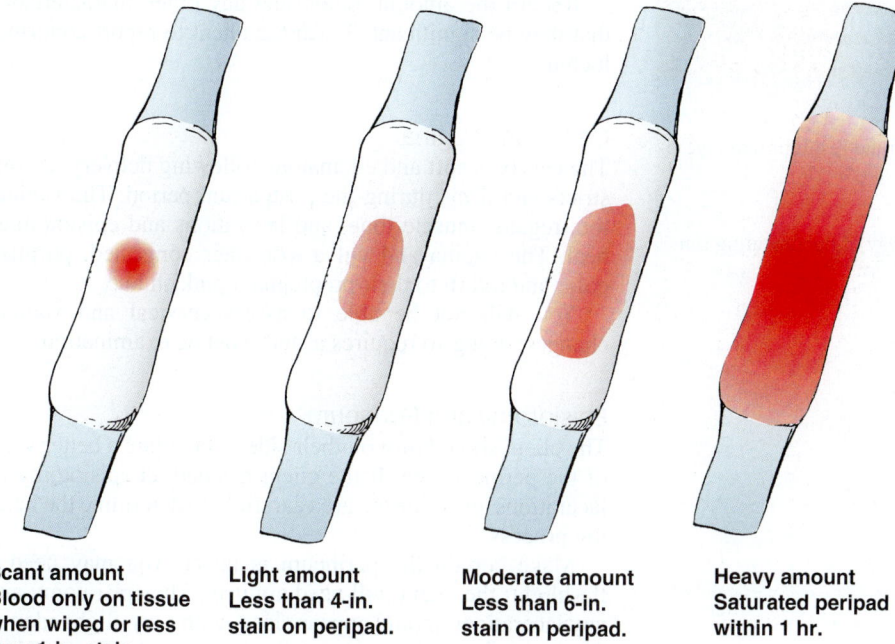

| Scant amount
Blood only on tissue when wiped or less than 1-in. stain on peripad. | Light amount
Less than 4-in. stain on peripad. | Moderate amount
Less than 6-in. stain on peripad. | Heavy amount
Saturated peripad within 1 hr. |

Figure 66-7 Determine the volume of lochia by peripad saturation.

A rising fundus may indicate uterine hemorrhage. If the fundus does not become firm with massage, report this finding immediately. A fundus located to the right of the midline often indicates a full bladder. Voiding will usually return the fundus to its earlier location. If this does not occur, notify the team leader. Check the perineum to make sure the stitches are intact. Be sure no excessive bleeding, edema, or bruising is found.

Lochia is the vaginal discharge that occurs following delivery. It consists of blood and the tissues of the uterine lining as it breaks down. Immediately following delivery, lochia is bloody and should be moderate in amount. While wearing gloves, check lochia during the immediate postpartum period. Observe the amount, character, and color. The amount is described as scant, light, moderate, or heavy; it should have a fleshy or metallic, never foul, odor (Fig. 66-7).

Observe and record the client's first voiding after delivery. Failure to void may indicate swelling or injury to the urinary system. Report if the client feels the urge to void but is unable to do so or if the fundus shifts to one side. If they are unable to void within 6 to 8 hr after delivery, catheterization may be necessary.

Maternal and Newborn Feeding

The new parent may be thirsty and hungry after delivery. Encourage them to drink fluids to replace those lost during labor and delivery; they can have solid foods as tolerated.

If the client plans to breastfeed, encourage them to put the newborn to their breast in the delivery or recovery room. The newborn usually is alert at this time, and the stimulation of the breast encourages the secretion of natural oxytocin to contract the uterus.

Transitioning After Birth

The postpartum client remains in the recovery room or is closely observed in the birthing room long enough to ensure that their condition is satisfactory (usually 1-2 hr). When their condition is stable, they are transferred to a postpartum room if they delivered elsewhere.

Record complete information about the delivery and other procedures on the client's health record before they are moved. Check the charting from the delivery room and the recovery room to make sure the record is complete. Transfer this documentation with the client (see Boxes 66-3 and 66-4).

Postpartum Care

Postpartum refers to the first 6 weeks following delivery, the time during which the client's reproductive organs return to their normal, nonpregnant state. The general care of the postpartum client is similar to that of other clients. Observe the client's overall state, appetite, activity, patterns of sleep and rest, and interactions with their newborn. Note the client's vital signs. Postpartum women are usually discharged from the hospital within a day or two. Client teaching on all aspects of postpartum care and documentation of this teaching are vital. The client must know what to expect as their body undergoes the rapid changes of the postpartum period and when to call the practitioner for assistance.

Important Changes in Maternal Anatomy and Physiology

The process by which the reproductive organs return to their nonpregnant state is called **involution**. To provide competent and safe nursing care to the postpartum client, you must understand the physiologic changes that occur following childbirth.

Uterus

Immediately after delivery, the uterus weighs approximately 2 lb (900 g) and is about the size of a grapefruit. It can be felt at the level of, or slightly below, the umbilicus. After delivery, it

> **Box 66-4** **Necessary Documentation Regarding the Postpartum Client**
>
> Assessment of the fundus:
> - Firmness (*consistency*)—firm, boggy (and result of massage)
> - At center or deviated (*location*)
> - Height (*position*)
>
>   Height of the fundus. One possible way of documenting fundal position is shown below:
>
>   2/U = 2 finger widths over umbilicus
>   1/U = 1 finger width over umbilicus
>   UU = fundus at level of umbilicus
>   U/1 = 1 finger width below umbilicus
>   U/2 = 2 finger widths below umbilicus
>
>   Lochia:
> - Rubra, serosa, alba (*character*)
> - Excessive, moderate, scant (*amount*)
> - Odor

begins to return to its normal position and smaller size. When this process is complete, the uterus will weigh about 2 oz (50 g) and will be low, at or near the center of the pelvic cavity.

During the postpartum period, the uterus should be positioned midline and feel firm to the touch. The height of the fundus indicates the progress of involution. By palpating the abdomen, the fundus can be located; measure its height in finger widths above or below the umbilicus. Normal involution is occurring when the fundus descends one finger width each day. Record the fundal height as indicated in Box 66-4.

Abnormal findings include the following:

- If the uterus is deviated to the side, suspect a distended bladder. Increased bladder size will prevent the uterus from contracting and will contribute to excessive bleeding. The uterus should contract after the client voids.
- A soft or boggy uterus indicates relaxation of the uterine muscles and is also a danger sign.

Lochia

Normally the flow of lochia continues for 3 to 4 weeks, with the following gradual changes:

Lochia rubra is seen for the first 2 days. It is mostly red and bloody. It should smell like blood (slightly metallic); a foul odor indicates infection.

Lochia serosa starts after the bleeding diminishes. The color of the lochia changes to pink or brown-tinged for approximately the next 7 days. Lochia serosa has a slightly earthy odor.

Lochia alba, which is yellow or white, starts on about day 10. At this point, the lochia has decreased greatly in amount. Lochia alba also has an earthy smell.

The amount of lochia after delivery should be about the same as the blood flow during normal menstruation. Abnormal findings include:

- Large clots
- Foul odor
- Lochia that does not change color and characteristics as described

Record the amount, color, and any other characteristics that may be significant. Teach the client to report abnormal lochia.

Cervix and Vagina

The cervix is soft and edematous following delivery. It constricts and firms during the postpartum period. The vagina, too, regains muscle tone, and lacerations and episiotomies heal. The vagina and vulva lose their congested, purplish color and return to their prepregnant pinkish hue.

You will not be able to assess cervical and vaginal changes; doing so requires a sterile pelvic examination.

Episiotomy and Perineum

The client should turn on their side to facilitate a better view of the perineal area. If the client has had an episiotomy or lacerations, examine the area carefully to determine the healing process.

Make certain the perineum is intact. You may need a flashlight; the client will need a mirror. The episiotomy and any lacerations should appear clean, with very slight edema. The sutures should not be pulling against the tissue. Note any hemorrhoids to initiate measures to alleviate them.

Abnormal findings include:

- Inflammation, redness, and discharge from the episiotomy or lacerations
- Hematomas, ecchymosis, and edema

If the client is unable to ambulate, administer perineal care. Apply a fresh perineal pad, usually to the panties, and pull the panties straight up. If using tabbed pads, attach the front first.

Abdominal Wall and Weight Loss

The client's abdominal wall often remains soft and flabby for several weeks following childbirth, because of the extensive stretching of the tissue and loss of muscle tone. By approximately 6 weeks after delivery, the client should regain muscle tone. The client can begin an exercise program gradually as the birth attendant recommends. The length of time it takes for a client to regain their figure depends on the amount of weight they gained during the pregnancy, the amount of weight they lost during the delivery, the amount of exercise they have after delivery, their diet and eating patterns, and whether or not they are breastfeeding. Body weight decreases by approximately 12 to 15 lb (5,440-6,800 g) at delivery and by about 5 lb (2,270 g) during the next few days due to loss of excess body fluid.

Breasts

Changes in the breasts following childbirth prepare for the newborn's nourishment. During the last half of pregnancy and the first few days postpartum, the breasts produce **colostrum**, a thin yellowish secretion that provides vitamins and immune substances that protect the newborn against infection. On about the second or third day postpartum, the breasts begin to secrete milk.

Each time a newborn is put to a breast, milk is secreted. **Lactation**, the production of milk, occurs because of the release of two hormones: prolactin and oxytocin. As the newborn sucks the nipple, a reflex reaction occurs whereby

IN PRACTICE
EDUCATING THE CLIENT 66-2 Engorgement

The following measures help to relieve the nursing client's engorgement:
- Wearing a supportive bra
- Frequent breastfeeding
- Applying warm packs to the breast for 15 min before nursing or standing in the shower with warm water spraying on the breast for 15 min before nursing

The following measures can help to relieve the nonnursing client's engorgement:
- Wearing a supportive bra
- Avoiding excessive fluid intake
- Placing cold packs on their breasts three to four times per day
- Avoiding stimulation (e.g., hot shower spray)
- Avoiding manual expression or pumping their breasts
- Using medications (usually acetaminophen) as prescribed for discomfort

---

the posterior pituitary gland releases oxytocin, which stimulates cells to produce milk and to move it to the milk ducts. The oxytocic hormone also results in uterine contractions, and the client may often experience abdominal cramping while breastfeeding. This entire process is commonly known as the "let-down reflex"; the milk is said to "let down" or "come in." Because the risks outweigh the benefits, medications to suppress lactation are rarely given to nonbreastfeeding clients.

For the first few days, the breasts should be soft. The nipples should be intact, without drying, cracking, or fissures. When the milk comes in, the breasts will feel full and firm to touch. **Engorgement** is the response of the breasts to the presence of an increased volume of milk and a sudden change in hormones. It usually occurs on the third to fifth postpartum day. The breasts become tender, swollen, hot, and hard. The swelling may extend into the axilla. The breasts may look shiny and red. The client may experience a headache, breast discomfort, and a slight temperature elevation at this time (see In Practice: Educating the Client 66-2).

Bladder
Pregnancy and labor place added strains on a client's urinary system. The abdominal muscles may be weakened. In addition, bruising and swelling of the urethra and general loss of muscle tone are common. The involution process places an increased demand on the kidneys and bladder, as the client's fluid balance is restored. Because of these factors, new parents may have stress incontinence or difficulty voiding.

Palpate the bladder for a rounded bulge in the suprapubic region, which indicates distention. By questioning the client regarding voiding, you can gain information related to urinary symptoms.

Abnormal urinary system findings include:
- Voiding in small amounts
- Residual urine
- Dysuria
- Bladder infection
- Urinary retention

Gastrointestinal System
The client may be constipated for 1 to 2 weeks following delivery because the abdominal muscles have been stretched, and the intestines have been inactive.

Whether or not the individual had hemorrhoids during pregnancy, they may have problems with them after the birth.

Extremities
To check for thrombophlebitis, the client's legs should be exposed. Ask the client to straighten their legs on the surface of the bed and to flex their feet toward their face. Abnormal findings in the legs include the following:

- Redness, pain, and swelling along the path of a vein may indicate a superficial thrombophlebitis.
- Pain behind the knee on flexion of the feet indicates a positive Homans sign and suggests thrombophlebitis.

Observation and Data Gathering
To prepare the client for the postpartum assessment, ask them to empty their bladder and then lie flat in bed. Always follow Standard Precautions when contact with body secretions is possible. Teach the client to check themselves frequently.

Measure and record the client's vital signs (see In Practice: Nursing Care Guidelines 66-1). Ask them about any problems they may be having with their breasts, bleeding (lochia), sutures, cramping, constipation, or hemorrhoids.

Begin the postpartum observation with the fundus. Palpate the fundus. If it is boggy, perform fundal massage to encourage muscle contraction of the uterus and reduce blood loss (see In Practice: Nursing Procedure 66-2). If the boggy uterus does not become firm with massage or if large clots are expressed with fundal massage, notify the team leader.

> **Nursing Alert** Never massage a contracted fundus. *Rationale: Massage of an already contracted uterus may cause it to invert, which can present an emergency situation.* Observe the amount, color, and odor of the lochia.

For the first few days after delivery, the client may have painful cramps as the uterine muscles contract. These cramps are called **after-pains** and are more likely to occur in multigravidas. Breastfeeding stimulates uterine contractions and therefore often brings on the cramping. An analgesic may be ordered as needed for these pains. Heat application is sometimes helpful.

Observe the episiotomy or lacerations for healing. Provide perineal care; change the sanitary pad. While tucking it in at the back, ask the client to roll onto their left side. Lift the right buttock and examine the anus for hemorrhoids. Ice packs, witch-hazel pads (Tucks), suppositories, creams, ointments, or sitz baths may be necessary for hemorrhoids.

Wash your hands, and then examine the breasts. Observe the breasts for tightness and redness, and palpate for fullness

IN PRACTICE
NURSING CARE GUIDELINES 66-1 | Postpartum Period

Immediate Postpartum Care
- Check blood pressure (BP) and pulse every 15 min × 1 to 2 hr or until stable; then every 30 min × 1 hr; then every 4 hr × 12 hr or as ordered.
- Check uterine fundus, lochia, and episiotomy at the same time as BP and pulse.
- Check for any signs of hemorrhage (check the perineal pad, and be alert to the possible pooling of blood under the client).
- Monitor for urinary distention and document first voiding for quantity of urine. Ask the client if they had any difficulty voiding because urinary retention is not uncommon. Swelling of the urethra and around the perineal area can inhibit the patency of the urinary meatus. If voiding has not occurred in 6 to 8 hr, or if they void in small, frequent amounts (<100 mL), notify the healthcare provider.
- Monitor interactions with infant. If signs of bonding are not present, determine cause (e.g., pain, complications, exhaustion) and address these issues. Psychological and emotional issues that interfere with normal bonding need to be addressed as soon as possible.

General Postpartum Care
- After the first 12 hr, check vital signs every 4 hr × 12 hr and then every 8 hr.
- Check breasts, fundus, lochia, stitches (if present), and legs (for signs of thrombosis) at least once every shift. (Memory aid: BUBBLLEEE—breast, uterus, bladder, bowels, legs, lochia, episiotomy, emotions, education.)

In the Breastfeeding Client
- Observe that the breasts begin to produce milk by the third or fourth day.
- Monitor that the breasts are not engorged.

In the Nonnursing Client
- Observe that breast engorgement does not last more than 2 or 3 days.
- Check that the fundus remains firm and contracted and moves downward. If the fundus is soft and spongy, cup a hand around the fundus, and massage it gently until it becomes firm and contracted.
- Monitor elimination patterns (urinary and bowel) until they return to the normal, prepregnant state. Check that client demonstrates correct perineal care.
- Evaluate for thrombophlebitis in the legs. Check for presence of a positive Homans sign.
- Observe that lochia progresses on schedule from lochia rubra to lochia alba.
- Monitor incision (episiotomy or cesarean incision, if present) for healing.
- Evaluate quality of maternal/newborn bonding and family dynamics.
- Educate client, family, and significant others so they know what to expect after discharge.

IN PRACTICE
IMPORTANT MEDICATIONS 66-3 | Docusate Sodium (Colace)

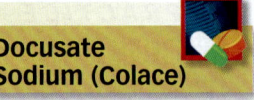

Dose: 100 mg oral (PO) three times daily (t.i.d.) as needed (PRN)
Expected effect: Stool softener
Adverse side effects: None

Nursing Considerations
- Colace is not a laxative but simply makes the stool softer to pass.

---

and temperature. Observe the nipples for drying, cracking, or fissures. Teach the client to examine the nipples to determine that they are in good condition and to observe them for cracking, caking, dryness, or bleeding. If the client is breastfeeding, observe whether their nipples protrude sufficiently for adequate nursing. They can palpate the breasts gently to determine if they are soft, firm, or engorged.

Engorgement in the nursing individual generally subsides within 48 hr if the client feeds the infant from both breasts every 2 to 3 hr, alternating the breast that they use first on each feeding. Engorgement in the nonnursing individual is treated with breast binders and ice packs (see Chapter 67).

Constipation is a common problem for some clients. Diet, adequate fluids, and activity help to regulate this condition. Many birth attendants routinely order stool softeners, such as docusate sodium (Colace) (In Practice: Important Medications 66-3), or mild laxatives until good bowel function is reestablished. The client may need a suppository or small enema if a laxative is ineffective.

> **Nursing Alert** Postpartum clients should never take an enema without a specific order from the healthcare provider. An enema could cause the rupture of episiotomy sutures and could be the source of incisional infection.

Client Teaching

Client teaching begins early (at the time of admission) because clients are often discharged a short time after delivering. The individual receives instruction in these aspects of self-care:

- Breast care and nursing
- Perineal care and care of the stitches
- Fundus observation
- Fluid intake
- Voiding
- Ambulation
- Engorgement
- Involution

Teach the client how to massage their uterine fundus and document this teaching. The client should use a mirror to check the stitches. Teaching the client the normal sequence of lochia changes is important, as they will probably go home the first or second postpartum day. They must know danger signs so they can spot a problem early and report it to their birth attendant. See In Practice: Educating the Client 66-3 for client information on changing the perineal pad.

IN PRACTICE
EDUCATING THE CLIENT 66-3 — Changing the Perineal PAD

When removing a soiled pad, the client should pull their underwear straight down. If using a sanitary belt, they should unhook the pad from the front first. Advise the client always to start removal of the perineal pad by first removing the pad from "clean" areas in the front and then removing the pad from the "dirty" area near the rectum. When applying a clean pad, they should hook it onto the front first, which helps prevent infection.

Breastfeeding

Reinforce the benefits of breastfeeding for the client and newborn. Nursing the newborn is beneficial for many reasons:

- Breast milk is readily available and convenient.
- Breast milk is always the correct temperature.
- Breast milk contains antibodies.
- Nursing helps in the bonding process.
- Nursing speeds involution.
- Breast milk is less likely to cause allergic reactions and other difficulties.
- Breast milk is cheaper than formula.

Most clients can nurse their babies unless complications, such as severely retracted nipples, infections, or breast malformations, arise. The first requirement for breastfeeding is a good supply of milk; the client's emotional status, diet, fluid intake, and amount of rest all influence milk production. Generally, the client who is happy, wants to nurse their newborn, and is not worried or overly tired has an excellent chance to have a good milk supply. An adequate diet based on the MyPlate Framework (see Chapter 30) and ample fluids are essential. Intake of dairy products and fluids may be increased. Supplemental vitamins are often prescribed for breastfeeding women.

"Expression of milk" means artificial emptying of the breasts. It may be used when a preterm newborn must be fed in the newborn intensive care unit or for the convenience of a working client. An electric breast pump offers the best method for expressing milk because the suction is steady and controlled. Milk also can be expressed by hand. Milk that is to be used later should be collected in a sterile bottle and refrigerated. Refrigerated milk should be used within 48 hr. Breast milk can be kept in a home freezer for 1 month or in a frozen food locker for 6 months.

Bottle Feeding

Although breast milk is the preferred milk for most infants, there are times when it is not the best milk for a particular baby. For instance, some blood-borne infections, such as HIV, may be transmitted through breast milk. The client who has chosen to bottle-feed should receive equal support from nursing staff.

The client who does not choose to nurse their newborn should wear a bra that gives firm support. They may have fluids as desired for the first 24 hr after delivery, but after this time, fluids are often restricted. Ice packs and a breast binder can be applied to reduce discomfort.

Perineal Care

Perineal care provides comfort and cleanliness and prevents odor and infection. Encourage the client to use a peri-bottle (a flexible plastic bottle containing clear, warm water), a sitz bath, or surgigator (a handheld sprayer device) after toileting, whether or not they had an episiotomy. In addition to promote healing, these methods help keep the perineum clean and decrease the risk of infection. You may give initial perineal care with the client in bed on a bedpan. When the client is ambulatory, they may attend to it themself. Methods vary, but the purpose is the same: to avoid contamination from fecal material.

Perineal care is necessary after the client voids or has a bowel movement. Teach the client to wash their hands and to change the perineal pad every 2 to 3 hr during the day. Help remove the pad they are wearing carefully, moving from front to back, and place it in a paper bag for later disposal.

After voiding or a bowel movement, teach the client to spray tepid water onto the perineum from the peri-bottle, sitz bath, or surgigator. Use fresh toilet tissues to pat dry from front to back, on each side, and then in the middle. Discard the tissues in the toilet. Do not use undue pressure, which can cause discomfort. Without touching the inner surface of the perineal pad, the client should fasten the tab of the sanitary belt, or attach the adhesive side of the pad to their panties, from front to back so that it will not slip forward.

A soothing analgesic ointment or spray may be applied as ordered. Witch hazel (Tucks) pads may be used. Frequent sitz baths (four times a day) will increase the client's comfort and promote healing of the episiotomy. Oral analgesics and warm or cold compresses may be ordered to relieve discomfort. Squeezing the buttocks together before sitting down helps provide a cushion.

Bathing

When the client is ambulating and stable, they are permitted to take a shower. You will need to assist them the first time, assembling supplies and instructing them on the procedure. Instruct the nursing client to avoid using soap on the nipples (soap will cause the nipples to dry and crack). The client usually receives a bed bath on the first day after a cesarean delivery.

Activity, Rest, and Diet

The client needs a combination of rest and activity. In most cases, they are up within 4 hr after a normal delivery, which helps to prevent respiratory and circulatory complications. Encourage the client to nap during the day. In some cases, visitors may need to be restricted. Analgesics may facilitate their ability to rest.

Assist the client in their initial ambulation. Encourage them first to sit on the edge of the bed and to take deep breaths. If they feel dizzy, they should not get up further until that sensation passes. When they get up, they should move slowly. Remain with them the first few times until they feel totally stable.

Sometimes the client experiences an increase in lochia while ambulating, which may cause them alarm. Monitor the flow and assure the client that the increase is likely due to gravity when arising. Explain that the increased lochia helps the uterus to drain and to return to its normal position and size.

The client should have a nutritious, balanced diet. If they are nursing, extra quantities of milk and other liquids may be added.

Discharge

Examination by the Birth Attendant

The birth attendant checks the client before discharging them from the healthcare facility. They are told to return for a follow-up examination at the end of 6 weeks, and they are usually advised not to have sexual intercourse or use vaginal douches until then.

Discharge Procedures and Teaching

Routine discharge procedures are followed when the client and their newborn leave the facility, and specific obstetric procedures also are performed. The client should be informed that menstruation will resume in 6 to 8 weeks if they do not nurse their newborn. If they do nurse, menstruation is usually delayed for 4 to 5 months or until they stop nursing.

Although ovulation does not usually occur during the nursing period, prolonging nursing is no guarantee that pregnancy will not occur. To a great extent, the degree of protection from pregnancy depends on whether the infant has all its sucking needs met at the breast. A baby who uses a pacifier or sucks on its fists will not provide as much stimulation to the nipple, and therefore provides less contraceptive benefit. Many nursing clients do become pregnant. The client should be made aware that pregnancy is a possibility before the first normal menstrual period because as a rule, ovulation occurs before menstruation.

Discharge teaching should also include normal maternal responses to sex and sexuality, contraception, and when to resume intercourse.

At the time of discharge, rubella vaccine and Rho(D) immune globulin (RhoGAM, Gamulin Rh) may be administered to the Rh-negative client as indicated. The newborn may be given the first hepatitis vaccine. All these medications require informed consent. If the client receives rubella vaccine, they must be cautioned to avoid pregnancy for 3 months to avoid harm to the next fetus.

The practitioner examines the client and newborn approximately 6 weeks after delivery. The purpose of this examination includes making sure the client's uterus has returned to normal size, the episiotomy has healed, and no infection is present. The examiner will advise the client at that time regarding resumption of regular activities.

STUDENT SYNTHESIS

KEY POINTS

- The role of the labor and delivery nurse is to ensure maternal and fetal well-being.
- The onset of true labor may be difficult to recognize, even for the multigravida.
- Rhythmic uterine contractions causing cervical dilation and effacement, and the descent of the fetal presenting part characterize true labor.
- Normal labor has four distinct stages. In stage I, cervical dilation and effacement occur, along with fetal descent; in stage II, the neonate is born; in stage III, the placenta is delivered. Family bonding, maternal recovery, and infant stabilization occur in stage IV.
- An important nursing responsibility during labor is performing frequent assessments of the client's progress and any deviations from normal for the client or fetus.
- FHR can be heard and assessed using a fetoscope, Doppler ultrasound device, or electronic fetal monitor.
- Various patterns of fetal response to uterine activity can be identified with electronic fetal monitors, and appropriate interventions can be started early.
- Stage IV is a critical time for the client and their newborn. The major concerns during this time are preventing maternal hemorrhage, maintaining the newborn's respiratory and cardiac function, and initiating family bonding.
- In the postpartum client, major changes (involution) occur in most body systems, restoring them to their normal prepregnant state.
- The uterus decreases in size, the placental site and episiotomy heal, and lochia progresses from rubra to serosa, then to alba, during the 6 weeks following delivery.
- Breasts will begin producing milk within 2 to 4 days after delivery.
- Lactation may be suppressed by mechanical means, such as ice packs and compression binders, and by avoiding breast stimulation. Medications usually are not used because the risks outweigh the benefits.
- Client teaching regarding fundal height and consistency, lochia, perineal care, nursing and breast changes, uterine cramping, backache, and fatigue ensures that these important self-care concepts are learned by the client.

CRITICAL THINKING EXERCISES

1. Discuss expectations of labor with at least three other students or friends. Explore what is common and what is different in your expectations.

2. Find a source to learn about the labor and birth practices of a different culture. Discuss with colleagues how these practices might be accommodated in our country.

NCLEX-STYLE REVIEW QUESTIONS

1. A client delivered a 3.80 kg infant 1 hr ago and is experiencing a large amount of rubra lochia with clots. Which is the first action by the nurse?
   a. Call the primary healthcare provider.
   b. Have the client turn to the left side.
   c. Reinforce the maternity pads.
   d. Palpate the fundus and massage.

2. A pregnant client in the third trimester experienced "lightening." Which instructions would the nurse provide the client regarding this sensation? Select all that apply.
   a. They may observe vaginal bleeding.
   b. There will be an increase in urinary frequency.
   c. They may experience an increase in indigestion.
   d. They may notice increase in leg edema.
   e. Leg cramps may be experienced.

3. A client who is 36 weeks' gestation calls the clinic and states, "I'm not sure if I'm really in labor or if it is false labor." Which is the best response by the nurse?
   a. "It is too early for the baby to be born, go to bed and put your feet up."
   b. "Change your activity and walk around the house. If it is false labor, you will feel relief."
   c. "I am sure that it is true labor because it is so close to the due date so it is advisable that you come in to the birthing center."
   d. "True labor contractions are usually painless, short, and irregular."

4. A client in labor is 100% effaced and fully dilated at 10 cm. Which stage of labor does the nurse document the client is experiencing?
   a. First stage
   b. Second stage
   c. Third stage
   d. Fourth stage

5. A client receives epidural anesthesia during labor at 6 cm dilation for pain control. Which nursing action is appropriate after initiation of the epidural?
   a. Have the client begin pushing.
   b. Allow the client to sit up in the chair.
   c. Position the client on the side with the head of bed slightly elevated.
   d. Position the client supine with the head of bed flat.

CHAPTER RESOURCES

Enhance your learning with additional resources on **the**Point*!*
Student Resources related to this chapter can be found at thePoint.lww.com/Rosdahl12e.

Welcome Steps

Look at healthcare provider's orders.

Protocol for procedure.

Necessary equipment/supplies.

Wash hands using proper hand hygiene; put on gloves.

Explain the procedure and reassure the client.

Locate two identifiers to confirm correct client.

Comfortable and efficient position for nurse and client.

Obtain privacy.

Make sure to follow correct steps and body mechanics with good technique.

Ensure safety and observe deviations from normal.

End Steps

Ensure comfort and safety.

Note questions or concerns from client or nurse; note significant data.

Dispose of materials properly.

Disinfect the area and your hands.

Document and report the procedure and your findings.

IN PRACTICE

NURSING PROCEDURE 66-1 — Application of External Monitor

Supplies and Equipment
Fetal monitor and paper
Doppler (ultrasound [US] transducer)
Electronic fetal monitor (tocodynamometer)
Two straps
Conductive jelly

Steps

Follow LPN WELCOME Steps and Then

1. Elevate the head of the bed 15° to 30° or place client in lateral position. *Rationale: Elevation and uterine displacement decrease aorta and vena caval compression.*
2. The obstetrical RN will perform Leopold maneuvers (a series of four steps used to palpate the abdomen to determine fetal presentation, position, and lie). When the fetal placement within the uterus is estimated, place two straps under the client. *Rationale: This locates fetal position and best placement of the Doppler so the heart rate can be clearly heard.*
3. Apply conductive jelly to Doppler and place on the client's abdomen until strong fetal heart rate (FHR) is heard and consistent signal is obtained. *Rationale: The jelly helps locate the area of maximum FHR signal.*
4. Attach straps to Doppler and secure. *Rationale: Straps should be snug but not tight.*
5. Push recorder button if not already on. *Rationale: Machine will not record data if machine is off.*
6. Place the tocodynamometer on the abdomen between umbilicus and top of fundus. *Rationale: Fundus is the contractile portion of the uterus; take care to avoid placing too high on fundus; respirations will record on monitor.*
7. Attach straps to tocodynamometer and secure. *Rationale: Straps should be snug but not tight; if too tight, pressure-sensitive button will not record data.*
8. Adjust sound and equipment as needed, particularly when a procedure is performed or client's position is changed. *Rationale: The monitor is sensitive to change or disturbance to equipment.*

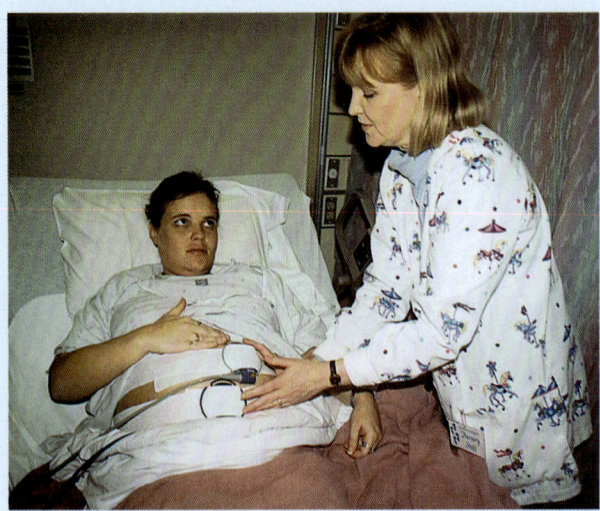

Client being monitored with external transducers secured to their abdomen.

9. Review FHR and US data with client and family. Use thorough descriptions of data. *Rationale: This review promotes understanding of what the client and family will be observing on the monitor.*

Follow ENDDD Steps

Adapted from University of Rochester Medical Center (2020).

IN PRACTICE
NURSING PROCEDURE 66-2 Fundal Massage

Supplies and Equipment
Gloves
Perineal wipes or washcloths
Perineal pad

Steps
Follow LPN WELCOME Steps and Then

1. Cup your hand around the uterine fundus (at about the level of the umbilicus). *Rationale:* This is the best position to start to palpate the fundus.

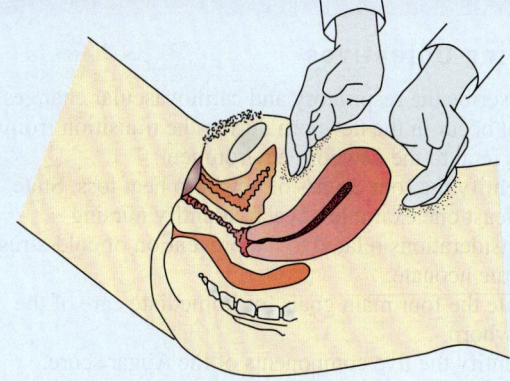

The fundal massage as viewed from the side.

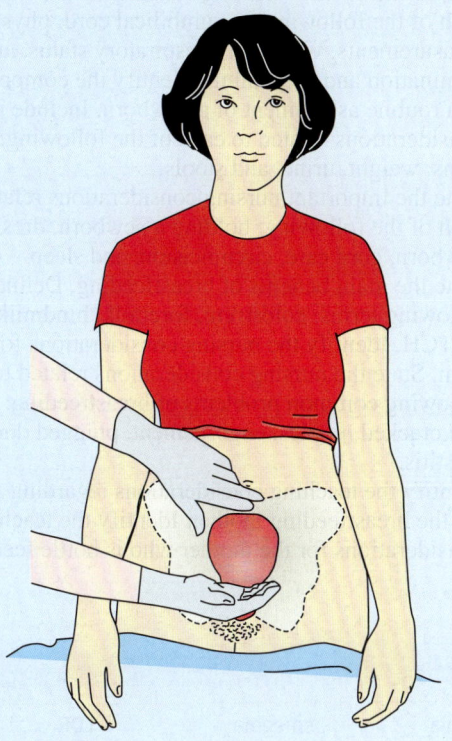

The upper hand is around the uterine fundus at about the level of the umbilicus. The other hand stabilizes the uterus at the level of the symphysis pubis.

2. Place your other hand over the symphysis pubis to stabilize the uterus. *Rationale:* Two-hand technique stabilizes the fundus in the abdomen.

3. Rotate your fundal hand gently. *Rationale:* Your touch must be firm but still gentle so that the fundus can be massaged but has a minimal amount of pain for the client.

4. Continue this massage until you feel the uterus become a firm globe. *Rationale:* The uterine muscle responds to stimulation by contracting. When contracted, the figure-eight muscles of the uterus clamp off the blood vessels, reducing bleeding.

5. Observe for passage of large, numerous, or frequent clot(s). Notify healthcare provider of changes or worsening status. *Rationale:* Numerous, frequent, and/or large clots indicate a soft and spongy, noncontracted (boggy) uterus and/or active hemorrhage.

6. Clean the client's vulva and perineum. *Rationale:* Blood is an excellent growth medium for bacteria. Good hygiene in this area helps to prevent urinary tract and postpartum infections.

7. Apply a clean perineal pad. *Rationale:* A clean pad provides accurate, baseline observations during the periodic inspections of postpartum bleeding. Clean pads decrease the chances of bacterial growth. Also, the client feels clean and refreshed.

Follow ENDDD Steps

67 Care of the Normal Newborn

Learning Objectives

1. Describe the respiratory and cardiovascular changes that occur in the newborn during the transition from the fetal to the newborn environment.
2. Identify the four causes of newborn heat loss. State at least one example of each. Identify nursing considerations related to the prevention of cold-stress of the neonate.
3. State the four main goals for immediate care of the newborn.
4. Identify the five components of the Apgar score. Identify nursing considerations related to each component.
5. Discuss the procedure for proper identification of a newborn. State nursing considerations related to safety precautions, prevention of nosocomial infections, and completion of birth documentation.
6. State nursing considerations related to Standard Precautions, eye prophylaxis, vitamin K administration, and parental bonding.
7. Discuss the normal ranges of weight and length of the neonate. State nursing considerations related to molding, caput succedaneum, cephalohematoma, anterior fontanel, and posterior fontanel.
8. Define and discuss the nursing considerations related to the following terms: pseudomenstruation, phimosis, acrocyanosis, milia, Epstein pearls, erythema toxicum, petechiae, Mongolian spots, lanugo, and vernix caseosa.
9. Define the following reflexes of the newborn: rooting, palmar grasp, Moro, tonic neck, Babinski, stepping, and sucking.
10. Identify the important elements of information regarding the process of labor and birth that must be reported to the newborn nursery nurse.
11. Identify the components of the initial assessment of a newborn. Include nursing considerations related to each of the following: the umbilical cord, physical measurements, vital signs, respiratory status, and elimination and meconium. Identify the components of a routine assessment of a newborn. Include nursing considerations related to each of the following: vital signs, weight, urine, and stools.
12. State the important nursing considerations related to each of the following: holding a newborn, dressing a newborn, cord care, circumcision, and sleep.
13. State the main benefits of breastfeeding. Define the following terms: colostrum, foremilk, hindmilk, and LATCH. Identify the nursing considerations for each term. State the nursing considerations related to the following common problems of breastfeeding: sore and cracked nipples, engorgement, plugged ducts, and mastitis.
14. Identify the teaching considerations regarding nutrition for the breastfeeding mother. Identify the teaching considerations for the mother who is bottle feeding.

Important Terminology

acrocyanosis
alveoli
Apgar
bonding
brown fat
caput succedaneum
cephalohematoma
circumcision
desquamate
en face position
epispadias
Epstein pearls
erythema toxicum
fontanels
foremilk
galactosemia
hindmilk
hypospadias
hypothyroidism
inner canthus
lanugo
mastitis
meconium
milia
molding
Mongolian spots
neonate
ophthalmia neonatorum
outer canthus
petechiae
phimosis
port-wine stain
prepuce
pseudomen-struation
smegma
stork bite
surfactant
vernix caseosa

Acronyms

G_6PD
LATCH
LDR
LDRP
PKU
SIDS

The care babies receive and the bond they form with their parents during the first several weeks of life have many effects. These factors influence the growth and development of healthy infants and the closeness of the entire family. As a nurse, you play a special role as a teacher and advocate for family caregivers and their newborns.

A normal baby is born with the reflexes and body systems needed to live outside the woman's body. By no means, however, is the baby ready to live on its own. The infant cannot meet its own basic needs without help. You will learn to assist neonates, which is the term used for the infant in the first 28 days of life. For both the parents and the neonate, a nurse is a great resource and a major support system. In this chapter, you will be introduced to the concepts related to immediate care for healthy newborns, their physical and behavioral characteristics, and the typical care of the infant from the time of birth until the time of discharge.

IMPORTANT CONCEPTS IN NEWBORN CARE

At the time of birth, the neonate must quickly make four dramatic changes to adapt to the world outside the shelter of the womb. These changes are temperature regulation, circulation, respiration, and source of nourishment.

The neonate must also complete these transitions quickly; the first 24 hr of life are critical for the newborn. In providing initial care, the focus is on monitoring and assessing the newborn's vital systems and keeping the infant warm. The baby's well-being depends on having a clear airway and effective respiration. Assessing the respiratory and circulatory systems, checking vital signs, and administering cord care are important skills that you will need to master.

Respiration

The changes in respiration are the greatest challenge for the newborn. The baby must begin breathing immediately after birth. Before birth, all of the fetus' oxygen had been provided through the placenta, where gases and nutrients from the maternal blood diffused into the fetal blood. As soon as the cord is clamped, however, the infant's lungs become the organs of gas exchange.

Excess secretions in the airway can block breathing and, if inhaled, can cause aspiration pneumonia. Immediately after delivery of the baby's head, the birth attendant removes secretions first from the mouth, then the nose with either gloved fingers or with a small, soft-bulb syringe (In Practice: Nursing Procedure 67-1).

The change from being enclosed by the muscular walls of the uterus and the bag of amniotic fluid to an air-filled room with light, noises, and stimulation must be quite a shock. The healthy infant responds to the changes in pressure, temperature, gravity, and stimulation by taking the first breath. When the newborn takes the first breath, they usually make the first sounds.

Although the fetus had some breathing movements in utero, the lungs were filled with fluid, and no gas exchange occurred across the lung sacs (**alveoli**). The first breath expands the air passages and the alveoli. The healthy newborn has enough **surfactant**—a chemical that stabilizes the walls of the alveoli—to allow the sacs to remain open rather than collapsing after each breath. This means that the next breath will not require as much effort.

The first few breaths set into process events that (1) assist with the conversion from fetal to adult-type circulation, (2) empty the lungs of liquid, and (3) establish neonatal lung volume and function in the newborn. The baby's respirations may not stabilize for about 2 hr after birth. During that time, some breaths may sound noisy and wet. However, it is abnormal for the respiratory rate to be greater than 60 breaths per minute at 2 hr of life.

If the mother has been medicated or has had a long-lasting anesthetic, the newborn may not breathe at once and must be stimulated.

> **Nursing Alert** By 2 hr of life, the baby's respiratory rate should be less than 60 breaths per minute. Apgar numbers are significant and might also be related to NCLEX questions.

Circulation

Review the information about fetal circulation in Chapter 65 to help you understand the dramatic changes that occur in the circulatory pathway during the first few hours and days of life. The circulatory pathway changes abruptly when the umbilical cord is clamped and then cut. At birth, the fetal circulatory structures (the foramen ovale, ductus arteriosus, and ductus venosus) must close to allow blood to flow to the heart, lungs, and liver. If these circulatory changes do not occur spontaneously, the newborn will have inadequate oxygenation because of persistent fetal circulation. Surgical intervention is required to correct this problem.

> **Nursing Alert** It is important to remember that the changes in the circulatory system happen at the same time as the changes in respiration; the transitions to support life after birth by these two systems are completely interrelated.

Body Temperature

When the fetus was inside the mother's uterus, the temperature was very stable. The fetus had no need to expend energy to maintain its own temperature. After being born, however, the baby must work to keep warm. The baby loses heat by four mechanisms: conduction, convection, evaporation, and radiation (Fig. 67-1).

To counteract the heat loss, the baby has three ways to maintain its temperature: shivering, which is not very efficient; muscle movements, which have only a little benefit; and the production of heat caused by using a stored fat known as **brown fat**. Only infants born at term have much brown fat, and after it is used, the baby cannot create more. This is one reason that it is so important for the nurse to take steps to keep the baby warm. If the baby needs to work hard to keep their temperature elevated, the baby may become cold-stressed. A chain of events then occurs that can be harmful to the baby's blood sugar, oxygenation, and acid–base balance.

A newborn's skin has a bluish or dusky tinge at first. As soon as oxygen enters the circulating blood in quantity, the white newborn's skin turns lighter and assumes a pink tone. Newborns of other races remain slightly darker.

> **NCLEX Alert**
> The concepts of conduction, convection, evaporation, and radiation are very important thermoregulation issues that may be found in an NCLEX scenario. The adverse effects of cold-stress are safety concerns that can lead to respiratory and circulatory distress. See Figure 67-1 for a more detailed description.

CARE OF THE NEWBORN IMMEDIATELY AFTER BIRTH

It is important to set goals for the immediate care of the newborn. Without goals, actions become merely routines; but if the goals are clear, then it is possible to make a plan to meet them. The importance of each goal and the way that it is

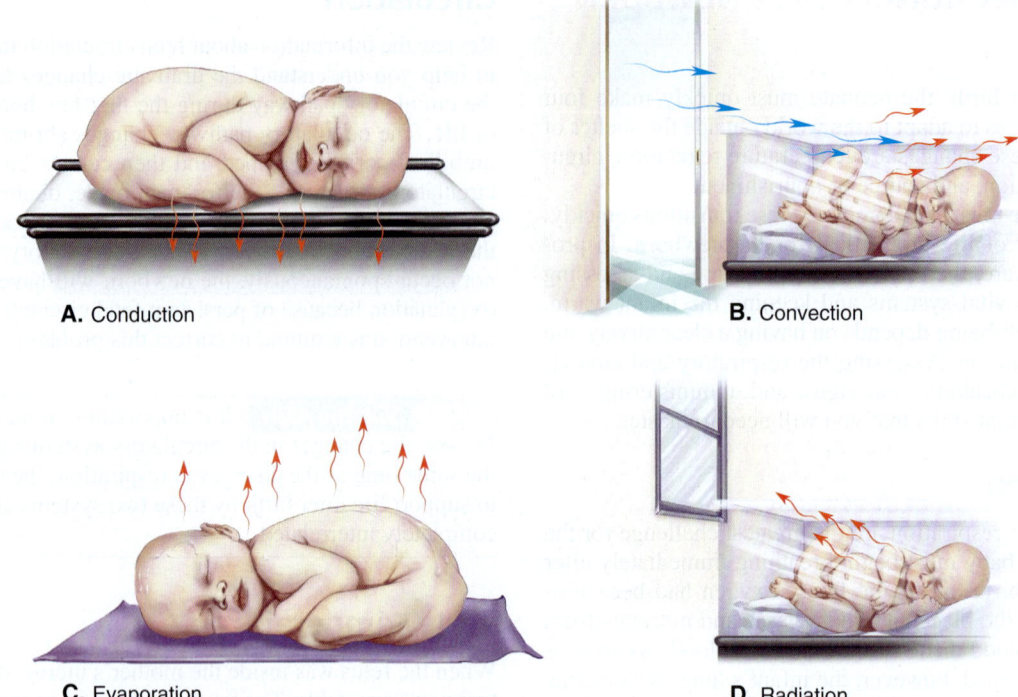

Figure 67-1 Heat loss in the newborn can be caused by anyone, or a combination, of the following factors: **(A)** *Conduction:* heat loss due to direct contact with a colder surface. **B.** *Convection:* heat loss due to air movement. **C.** *Evaporation:* heat loss due to the cooling effect of water loss on the skin. **D.** *Radiation:* heat loss via infrared heat rays due to body metabolism. (Adapted from Ricci, 2007.)

addressed will vary from one place to another. Four goals for immediate management of the newborn are to

1. Establish and maintain an airway and respirations.
2. Provide warmth and prevent hypothermia.
3. Provide a safe environment and routine preventive measures.
4. Promote maternal–infant attachment.

NCLEX Alert

Clinical situations may ask you to differentiate between the normal newborn and a newborn who needs nursing interventions. Respirations, body temperature, or reflexes may be described in the scenario. Be sure to know how to use the Apgar scores.

Initial Assessment: Apgar Score

The **Apgar** score was named for the healthcare provider who developed it, Dr. Virginia Apgar. A mnemonic for the five criteria of the Apgar score is **a**ppearance, **p**ulse, **g**rimace, **a**ctivity, **r**espiratory effort. It provides a quick and accurate means to assess the newborn's physical condition at the time of birth. The score is used to determine whether the baby needs immediate assistance or resuscitation. It should be determined at 1 min and again at 5 min after birth. The 1-min score is most accurate in predicting immediate survival, whereas the 5-min score may be better in predicting long-term survival and any neurologic damage. If the Apgar score is less than 7 points at the 5-min measurement, a third Apgar reading may be obtained at 10 min after birth.

Five criteria are assessed each time (Table 67-1). To obtain an Apgar score, give a number from 0 to 2 on each area of the Apgar scoring chart to the infant. Then total all the numbers. Record both the 1- and 5-min Apgar scores on the newborn's chart. The following list describes the meanings of the Apgar scores:

- If the total score is 10, the newborn is in the best possible condition.
- If the score is 7 to 9, the newborn usually does not need resuscitation.
- If the score is 4 to 6, the newborn is in danger.
- If the score is 0 to 3, the newborn needs emergency resuscitation.

TABLE 67-1 The Apgar Score

	SCORE		
	0	1	2
Heart rate	Absent	<100	>100
Respiratory effort	Absent	Slow, irregular	Good, crying
Muscle tone	Flaccid	Some flexion of extremities	Active motion
Reflexes, irritability	No response	Weak cry or grimace	Vigorous cry
Color	Blue, pale	Body pink, extremities blue	Completely pink

Nursing Alert If the Apgar score is 7 or less, a person who is skilled in neonatal resuscitation should evaluate the infant and provide immediate assistance.

Neonatal Resuscitation

If breathing does not begin either spontaneously or following tactile stimulation, the newborn's respiratory center is probably depressed. You must take emergency action. The newborn must be resuscitated immediately; permanent brain damage can occur if the newborn is without oxygen for more than approximately 4 min.

The purpose of resuscitation is to establish an airway, provide oxygen to the lungs, and stimulate the newborn to breathe. When respiratory difficulties develop in the delivery room, the birth attendant or anesthesiologist assists the newborn. When a baby develops complications in the newborn nursery, however, you may be the person to begin the resuscitation efforts (see In Practice: Nursing Procedure 67-1).

Maintaining Body Temperature

Even with the birthing room temperature set at 75 °F (23.9 °C), the air is a cold shock to the baby emerging from the warm mother's body, still wet with amniotic fluid. Lifting the newborn onto the mother's bare stomach or chest, perhaps even before the cord is clamped or cut, lets the heat of the mother's body transfer to the newborn. The baby should also be quickly dried, and all wet towels and blankets should be promptly removed and replaced with dry ones. Warm towels or receiving blankets should be placed over mother and newborn. The infant will lose a great deal of heat from its head, so many hospitals and birth centers place a cap on the baby's head to conserve warmth. When it is time for the infant assessment, using a radiant warmer, a prewarmed mattress, and warm instruments provides a heat-gaining, rather than a heat-losing, environment (Box 67-1). The goal of thermoregulation is to balance heat loss and heat production and create a neutral thermal environment.

Clamping and Cutting the Cord

The birth attendant will decide when to place two Kelly clamps on the umbilical cord. Delaying this procedure allows the infant to receive additional blood from the placenta. Whether or not this is best for the baby depends on the gestational age of the baby, the health of the mother and baby, and other factors. After the cord is clamped, the infant must obtain oxygen through its own respiratory effort. The cord is cut between the two clamps; usually a cord blood sample is obtained from the portion of the cord still attached to the placenta.

After the baby is dried, they are handed either to a nurse or to the mother for skin-to-skin contact. This can be done before the Kelly clamp is replaced with a plastic umbilical cord clamp. When replacing the Kelly clamp with a plastic umbilical cord clamp, be careful to place the clamp 1 to 2 cm above the umbilicus, taking particular care not to clamp any of the baby's skin along with the cord. The Kelly clamp is removed only after the plastic clamp is applied.

BOX 67-1 Conserving Heat for a Newborn

There are several things you can do to help a newborn maintain its temperature.

IN THE DELIVERY OR BIRTH ROOM
- Prewarm any blankets, towels, hats, or clothing before the birth.
- Dry the baby immediately.
- Replace wet blankets or towels after drying the baby.
- Prewarm the infant resuscitation area.
- Set birth room temperature at 75 °F (23.9 °C).
- Do not lay the baby on wet sheets while being suctioned.

IN THE NURSERY
- Transport the newborn in an isolette with the portholes closed.
- Place newborn care areas away from windows, outside walls, doorways, and drafts.
- Keep the newborn's head covered and the body well wrapped for the first 48 hr.
- Postpone the newborn bath until the baby's temperature has been stable for 2 hr at about 97.6 °F to 98.6 °F (36.5 °C-37 °C).
- Bathe the newborn under a radiant heater.
- Do not wash off all vernix (protective material on skin) initially.
- Cover work table and scales so they are not cold.
- Organize work so that the newborn is uncovered only briefly.
- Heat any oxygen or humidified air given.

Nursing Alert Leave the Kelly clamp on the cord stump until after the plastic umbilical cord clamp has been applied. Otherwise, the infant will lose blood through the cord stump.

Identification

Identification Bands

While the infant is still in the delivery or birth room, it is the nurse's responsibility to prepare and initiate some form of identification. Each hospital differs in what is required; most use flexible plastic bands that come in sets of three or four with identical numbers on them. The nurse writes the mother's name and admission number; the birth attendant's name; the date and time of birth; and the baby's sex on each band. One band is placed around the mother's wrist, two on the infant (wrist and ankle), and the fourth on the significant other. The printed number on the band should be recorded in the baby's and mother's records.

Properly identifying each newborn following birth is extremely important. Protective measures include identification bands, electronic bracelets, footprinting, and the completion of necessary records.

Electronic Bracelets
Another mechanism of ensuring infant safety is an electronic bracelet that creates an alarm if the baby is taken off the obstetrical unit without the bracelet having been deactivated by hospital personnel.

Footprinting
Some hospitals also use newborn footprints and maternal fingerprints as means of identification. These prints are taken before either the mother or the newborn leaves the delivery room, and they become part of the permanent health record.

Completing Birth Information in the Health Record
The client record must include information about the newborn's sex, hour of birth, condition, and type of delivery. Document any identifying marks, care of the eyes, vitamin K administration, and the mother's Rh status. You must complete the chart before the newborn leaves the delivery room. Be especially careful if someone in the family has a common name. In all cases, the mother's full name and the date and time of the newborn's birth are of critical importance and should be carefully documented.

The birth attendant who delivered the newborn should complete and sign a certificate of birth as soon as possible. The birth certificate is filed with the State Department of Vital Statistics. To best prevent later confusion, advise parents to choose a name for the newborn before the birth certificate is filed.

Protection Against Disease

Standard Precautions
Infection control is not only very important for the mother and the new infant but is also important for members of the healthcare team. Many body fluids and substances are involved in the birth process, including amniotic fluid, blood, and sometimes stool. It is essential that all members of the healthcare team practice Standard Precautions, including thorough handwashing and gloving, before handling the baby or providing care to the mother.

Eye Prophylaxis
If the mother has gonorrhea or chlamydia infecting her reproductive organs, the birth process could result in the infant being exposed to those organisms. Even babies born by cesarean section may have been exposed. Each of these organisms can cause blindness, or **ophthalmia neonatorum**, if left untreated. Therefore, specific protection against them is required in most states.

Erythromycin ointment, which is effective against both gonorrhea and chlamydia, is the drug of choice (see In Practice: Important Medications 67-1). Treatment may safely be delayed for 2 to 3 hr while the baby and parents are getting to know each other (see In Practice: Nursing Procedure 67-2).

Vitamin K Administration
Newborns are at risk for bleeding problems during the first week of life because their gastrointestinal tract is sterile. The lack of intestinal bacterial flora means that the newborn is unable to produce an adequate amount of vitamin K, which is important for production of certain clotting factors by the liver. Therefore, an intramuscular injection of 0.5 to 1.0 mg of vitamin K is usually administered during the first hour after birth (see In Practice: Important Medications 67-2). The nurse should document and report this injection.

Vaccinations
All newborns receive the first vaccination against hepatitis B shortly after birth (In Practice: Important Medications 67-3). It is important to educate parents about the need for the remaining doses to be given according to the guidelines of the Centers for Disease Control and Prevention (CDC). It is safe for the mother to breastfeed, even if the mother is a hepatitis carrier, if the baby has been immunized.

Promoting Parental–Infant Bonding
The best relationship between a parent and infant occurs when they are able to have early and extended contact. The nurse assists in the attachment, or **bonding**, process by encouraging parents to see, touch, and hold their newborn baby. With a healthy baby, practices to promote attachment rarely interfere with its transition to extrauterine life.

Immediately after birth, one of the most important events that occur is the formation of family relationships. The healthy, nonmedicated baby is in a state of "taking in" his or her environment. The mother is in a period called the "maternal sensitive period," which fosters the process of bonding.

Forming a bond with the baby begins during pregnancy. During the first hour after birth, the infant and parents take the next step in bonding, setting the stage for a loving relationship. It may seem obvious, but for bonding to happen,

---

IN PRACTICE
IMPORTANT MEDICATIONS 67-1 — Erythromycin 0.5% Ophthalmic Ointment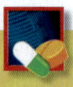

Dosage
Apply a thin line, 1 to 2 cm long, of ointment along the conjunctival sac.
Move from the inner to the outer canthus (see In Practice: Nursing Procedure 67-2).
Expected Effects: Prevention of gonorrheal or chlamydial ophthalmia neonatorum.

Adverse Side Effects: May cause temporary blurred vision in the neonate.

Nursing Considerations
- Be careful not to touch the newborn's eyelid or eyeball with the tip of the tube.
- Delay administration until after the initial bonding period with the mother and/or father.

IN PRACTICE
IMPORTANT MEDICATIONS 67-2 Vitamin K (Phytonadione, Aquamephyton)

Dosage
Apply 0.5 to 1.0 mg IM one time within the first hour of life.

Expected Effects
Vitamin K is used to prevent and treat blood clotting problems in the newborn. It is a necessary component for the production of certain clotting factors by the body. The infant cannot produce vitamin K until the gastrointestinal tract is populated with microorganisms after several days of feedings.

Adverse Side Effects
Local irritation, such as pain and swelling were injected.

Nursing Considerations
- Administer the injection into a large muscle, such as the anterolateral muscle of the newborn's thigh.

IN PRACTICE
IMPORTANT MEDICATIONS 67-3 Vaccination for Hepatitis B

Hepatitis B vaccination for infants should be administered according to the following guidelines:
- **Mother is HBsAg-negative:**
  - Infant weighs >2,000 g: one dose within 24 hr of birth for **all** medically stable infants ≥2,000 g.
  - Infant weighs <2,000 g: administer one dose at chronological age 1 month or hospital discharge.
- **Mother is HBsAg-positive:**
  - Administer **HepB vaccine** and **hepatitis B immune globulin (HBIG)** (in separate limbs) within 12 hr of birth, regardless of birth weight.
  - For infants <2,000 g: administer three additional doses of vaccine (total of 4 doses) beginning at age 1 month.
- **Mother's HBsAg status is unknown:**
  - Administer **HepB vaccine** within 12 hr of birth, regardless of birth weight.
  - For infants <2,000 g, administer **HBIG** in addition to HepB vaccine (in separate limbs) within 12 hr of birth. Administer three additional doses of vaccine (total of 4 doses) beginning at age 1 month.
  - Determine mother's HBsAg status as soon as possible. If mother is HBsAg-positive, administer **HBIG** to infants ≥2,000 g as soon as possible but no later than 7 days of age.

Three Doses Required
- First dose within 12 hr after birth
- Second dose at age 1 to 2 months
- Third dose at 6 months of age

  Expected effects: The infant will develop antibodies to hepatitis B, which will protect the child from infection with the virus.
  Adverse side effects: Pain with injection.

Adapted from information provided by the Centers for Disease Control. (2020). *2020 Recommended Child and Adolescent Immunization Schedule for ages 18 years or younger, United States, 2020.* Retrieved on January 11, 2021 from https://www.cdc.gov/vaccines/schedules/downloads/child/0-18yrs-child-combined-schedule.pdf

---

the parents and the baby must be together. Behaviors that indicate this beginning attachment include the following:

- The mother moves from touching with her fingertips only to stroking and massaging her baby.
- The mother and baby assume the **en face position**, in which their heads align as they look at each other.
- The parents speak to the infant in high-pitched voices.

The nurse can facilitate bonding by keeping the baby and mother together; placing the naked baby between the mother's breasts (skin-to-skin contact); delaying eye prophylaxis until after this critical time period; and joining in the parents' happy exploration of the miracle of their newborn.

CHARACTERISTICS OF THE NORMAL NEWBORN

Each newborn is different, but some characteristics are common to all newborns.

Weight and Length

At birth, the weight of a healthy newborn ranges from 5.5 to 9.5 lb (2,500-4,250 g). The average full-term infant weighs 7.5 lb (3,500 g). Girls usually weigh less than boys (see Fig. 67-2A and In Practice: Nursing Procedure 67-3).

> **Nursing Alert** Be sure to assemble all needed supplies and equipment before starting to weigh the baby. Never leave the baby unattended for even a moment.

> **Key Concept**
> Weigh the baby each day to note the baby's condition and progress. Expect a weight loss of 5% to 10% from the birthweight before the baby begins to gain weight from feedings.

Normal newborn length ranges from 18 to 22 in. (46-56 cm), with boys usually being approximately one-half inch longer than girls. The easiest way to measure an infant's length is to make a mark on the crib sheet at the top of the baby's head, then stretch the legs downward to their full length. Make another mark on the sheet, and measure between the two marks (Fig. 67-2B).

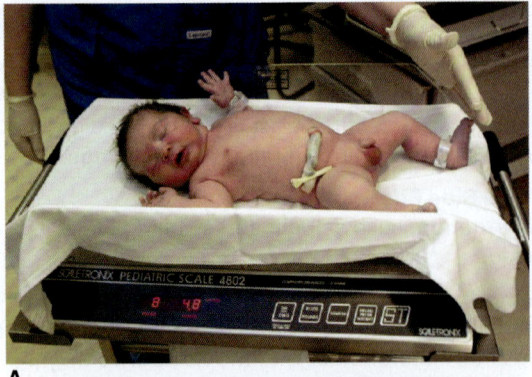

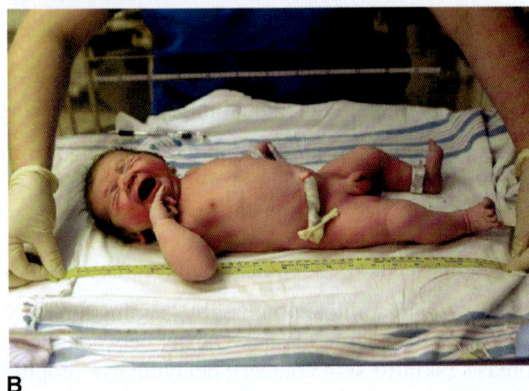

Figure 67-2 **A.** Weighing a newborn. Notice the protective handheld over the infant. **B.** Length should be measured soon after birth, to serve as a baseline from which to judge future growth. (Hatfield, 2014.)

Head and Body

The newborn has a large head, averaging 13 to 14 in. (33-35.5 cm) in circumference. A short neck supports it. The chest is somewhat smaller than the head, 10 to 12 in. (25.5-30.5 cm) in circumference. The head usually measures 1 to 2 in. (2.5-5 cm) more than the chest (Fig. 67-3 and In Practice: Nursing Procedure 67-4).

Head

The newborn's head may have an irregular shape due to the events of labor and birth. If the newborn was born by cesarean delivery without the mother laboring, the head is usually round. If the newborn was delivered vaginally, the head may show temporary **molding** (elongation) because of the overlap of skull bones during the birth process (Fig. 67-4).

Caput succedaneum results from an accumulation of fluid within the newborn's scalp (Fig. 67-5A). This swelling is caused by pressure to the head during delivery. The fluid causes the scalp to be puffy and edematous, and the edema crosses the midline of the baby's scalp. The condition disappears within a few days. **Cephalohematoma** is an accumulation of blood between the bones of the skull and the periosteum, the membrane that covers the skull (Fig. 67-5B). This swelling stops at the midline. The newborn's appearance may upset the parents. It is important to reassure them that the fluids will eventually be absorbed.

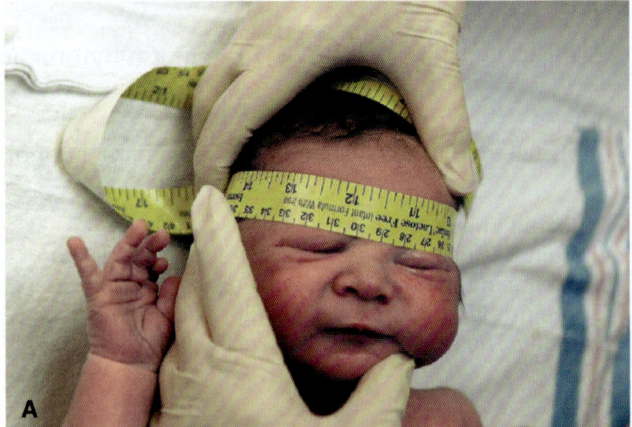

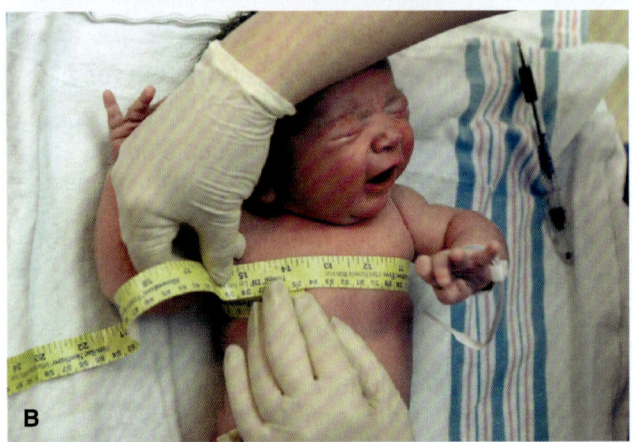

Figure 67-3 **A.** The circumference of the head is measured by placing a nonstretchable tape measure just above the eyebrows and over the most prominent part of the occiput. **B.** Measuring the chest circumference. (Hatfield, 2014.)

Fontanels

The **fontanels** are the "soft spots" in the newborn's skull, formed at the junction of the individual skull bones. These bones do not fuse completely before birth so that the head can mold to fit through the mother's birth canal. Two major fontanels can be felt. The *anterior fontanel* is found just above the forehead; it is diamond shaped. The anterior fontanel closes between the ages of 12 and 18 months. The *posterior fontanel,* located on the crown of the head (near the

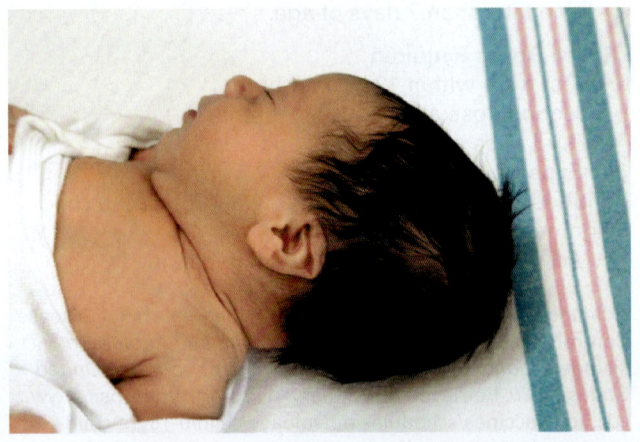

Figure 67-4 Molding in the newborn's head. (Hatfield, 2014.)

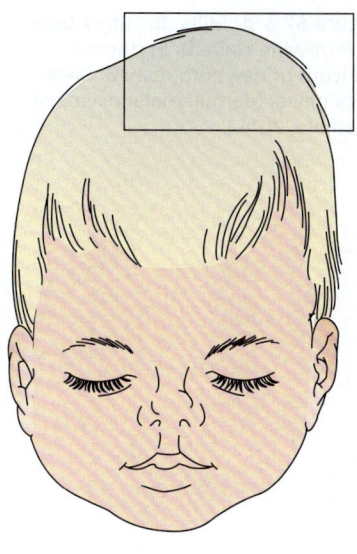 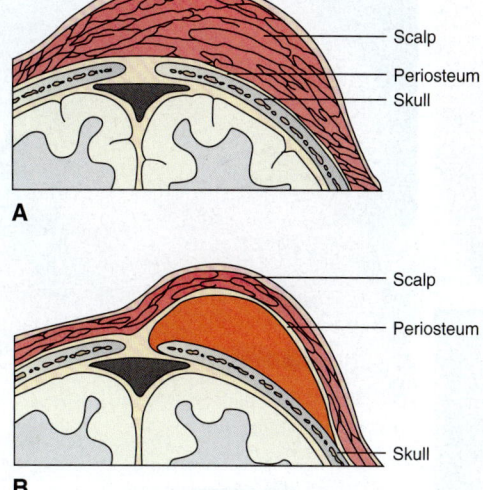

Figure 67-5 **A.** Caput succedaneum: From the pressure of the birth canal, an edematous area is present beneath the scalp. Note how it crosses the midline of the skull. **B.** Cephalhematoma: A small capillary beneath the periosteum of the skull bone has ruptured and blood has collected under the periosteum of the bone. Note how the swelling now stops at the midline. Because the blood is contained under the periosteum, it is necessarily stopped by a suture line.

back of the head or *occiput*), is smaller and more triangular. It closes by the third month of life.

Face

Newborns typically have small faces, flattened noses and ears, and receding chins. The newborn's eyes appear blue or gray at birth. He or she may look cross-eyed because the eyes are unable to focus. The newborn usually has eyelashes and eyebrows at birth. They keep the eyes closed most of the time because they are still sensitive to bright lights. During the first several weeks, the newborn is unable to produce tears because the lacrimal (tear) glands are not yet functioning.

The top of the ear should be at or above an imaginary line drawn from the **inner canthus** of the eye to the **outer canthus**. The ears are functional at birth, but hearing improves over the first 2 or 3 days, as the fluid in the eustachian tube is replaced with air.

Body

The normal newborn has a round chest and a slightly protruding abdomen. Engorgement of the breasts is common for the first 2 or 3 weeks of life in all newborns. This is one result of no longer being under the influence of the hormones of pregnancy from the mother's body. Another effect is that the baby's breasts may produce a small amount of fluid, known by the unusual term *witch's milk*. The nurse should assure the parents that this is common and that trying to express the milk may result in the complication of infection.

The genitals may be swollen, particularly in girls, as well as in any baby who was born in a breech position. The genitals of the female infant may be enlarged and have a mucoid, white, or blood-stained discharge. This is called **pseudomenstruation**. The swelling and discharge will disappear spontaneously within about a week.

In male newborns, the scrotum usually appears relatively large and may have darker pigmentation than the parents expect. This is because of the mother's hormones and will fade within a few weeks.

At term, the boy's testes usually can be either felt inside the scrotum or easily stroked down from the inguinal canal. The foreskin, or **prepuce**, covers the glans of the penis and is often adherent at birth. If the opening of the foreskin is so small that it cannot be pulled back at all, the condition is called **phimosis**. The penis should be inspected to determine the location of the urinary meatus, which should be at the very tip of the penis. If it is located on the underside of the penis (near the scrotum), it is termed **hypospadias**. A less common location is on the upper side of the penis; this is called **epispadias** (see Chapter 69).

Skin

Skin Color and Texture

A white newborn's skin is pink or red in the first few days after birth. The skin of nonwhite babies may appear pink or tan, with some pigment changes occurring within hours or days of delivery. The newborn's skin should become smooth and of a color typical of its ethnic background within 2 weeks.

Because of slowed peripheral circulation, the newborn's arms and legs may appear cyanotic; this condition is called **acrocyanosis**. It is common in the first 24 hr of life and is more prominent when the newborn is exposed to cold. It is not a serious condition.

Nursing Alert Report generalized cyanosis or pallor (paleness), which may indicate a heart defect or respiratory disorder. Report at once any jaundice that appears, especially within the first 24 hr.

The newborn's skin may be dry and peeling for a few days, and the skin may even show dry cracks in the folds of the wrists and ankles. The skin also may **desquamate** (peel) in large or small flakes.

Bumps, Rashes, and Other Marks

The nose and cheeks may have pinhead-sized white spots, caused by unopened oil and sweat glands. These spots are called **milia** (Fig. 67-6A). Sometimes white or gray bumps known as **Epstein pearls** are found on the mouth's hard and soft palate.

You may see various types of marks on the skin. Some disappear early in life; others are permanent birthmarks. If forceps or a vacuum extractor has been used for delivery, small bruises or swollen areas may appear on the face or head.

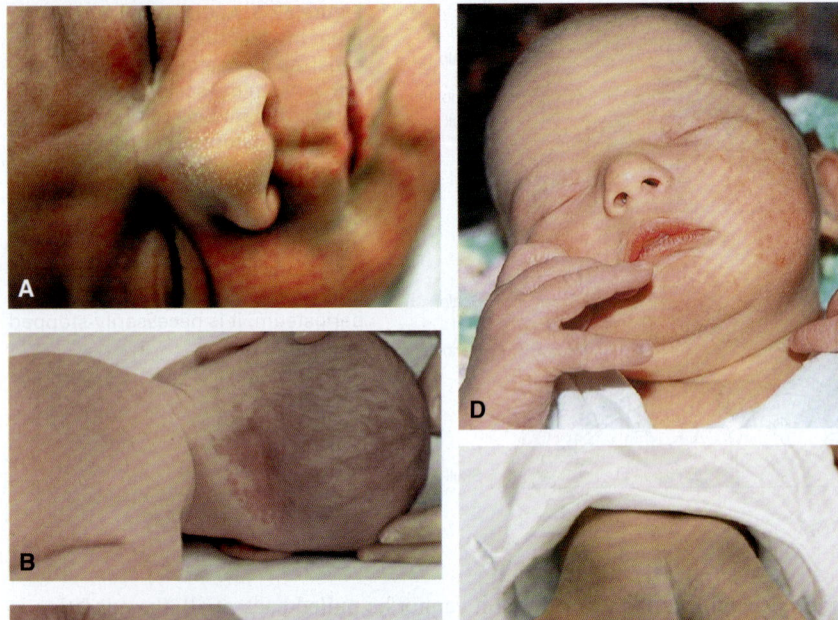

Figure 67-6 **A.** Milia. **B.** "Stork bites." **C.** Port-wine stain. **D.** Erythema toxicum or newborn rash. **E.** Slate gray nevus (dermal melanocytosis). (Hatfield, 2014.)

A mark that often appears on the newborn's eyelid or forehead is called a **stork bite** (Fig. 67-6B). This type of mark generally fades during infancy, although it sometimes persists into adulthood. A **port-wine stain** is a flat, purple-red area with sharp borders; this is a permanent birthmark (Fig. 67-6C). The skin of some newborns is sensitive; many newborns develop a red, raised rash known as **erythema toxicum** (Fig. 67-6D).

Petechiae, small purplish dots on the skin, are due to pressure caused by labor and will fade. Veins may be visible over the entire body. Dark blue areas of discoloration called **Mongolian spots** often appear on the buttocks, lower back, or upper legs of nonwhite babies (Fig. 67-6E). These spots usually disappear by early childhood. It is important to know that they have no relationship to Down syndrome.

Hair and Vernix

Fine, downy hair, called **lanugo**, may be seen on the face, shoulders, and back. A white, thick, cheesy material may also cover the skin. Called the **vernix caseosa**, it is composed of epithelial cells and the secretion of glands (Fig. 67-7). It protects the skin from the drying effects of amniotic fluid in utero and is especially noticeable in the hair and skin creases. Both the quantity of lanugo and the amount of vernix decrease with gestational age; a term infant will usually have less than a preterm infant.

> **NCLEX Alert**
>
> Be alert to questions discussing the physical appearance and typical behaviors of a neonate. The clinical scenario may reflect the need for teaching any of the multiple aspects of care of the infant. Safety issues might be the focus of an NCLEX question.

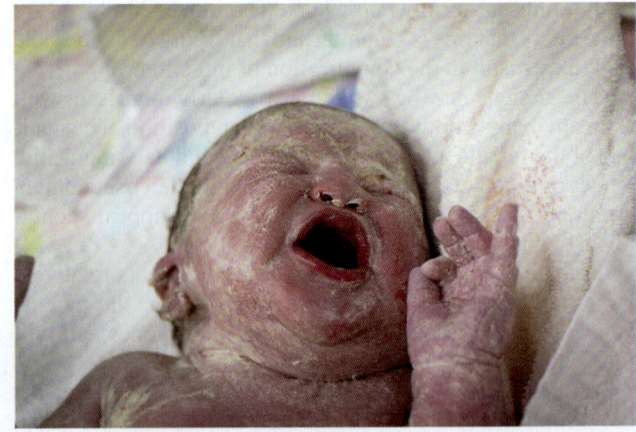

Figure 67-7 Newborn with vernix-coating skin (Hatfield, 2014).

Movement and Activities

Maturity
Generally, each facility will have a gestational age maturity guide in the form of a table. The birth attendant observes the infant's posture, tests flexibility and reflexes, and identifies specific physical characteristics to determine the newborn's physical maturity. The form will allocate scores and identify criteria related to maturity. If the scores are too low, the newborn is treated as premature.

Behavior
Typical newborns sleep approximately 17 hr a day. They awaken easily and cry when hungry or uncomfortable. Their arms and legs move freely and symmetrically. They often flex their extremities. They are unable to support the weight of the head.

Reflexes
Certain reflexes are present at birth, although the newborn's nervous system is immature. These reflexes indicate adequate neurologic functioning; their absence indicates abnormalities.

- *Rooting reflex:* When stroked on the lip or cheek, the newborn reacts by turning the head toward the direction of the stimulus (Fig. 67-8A).
- *Palmar grasp reflex:* The newborn tightly grasps a finger or other object placed into his or her hand. This reflex disappears as the newborn grows older (Fig. 67-8B).
- *Moro* or *startle reflex:* Sudden noises or jarring movements cause the newborn to throw out the arms and to draw up the legs (Fig. 67-8C).
- *Tonic neck reflex:* When the newborn is lying on the back and turns the head to one side, the leg and arm of that side extend, and those of the opposite side flex (Fig. 67-8D).
- *Babinski reflex:* Hold the newborn's foot and stroke up the lateral edge and across the ball of the foot. The big toe fans out and hyperextends in a positive response (Fig. 67-8E).
- *Stepping reflex:* The newborn steps with one foot, and then the other, when held upright with the feet touching a surface (Fig. 67-8F).
- *Sucking reflex:* As the newborn grasps the nipple with the lips, sucking should be automatic.

Other reflexes include gagging, crawling, blinking, sneezing, and coughing.

Senses
Newborns can see shades of light and darkness following birth. They blink in response to bright lights; however, they are unable to focus their eyes for more than a few seconds at a time. They respond to faces by staring.

Babies can hear at the time of birth. Caregivers should talk to them in soothing tones. It is typical for adults to speak in high-pitched voices to a baby; this is a sign of attachment.

Touch is well developed in newborns. They respond to discomfort, such as pain and wetness. Less is known about the senses of smell and taste. Newborns are known to increase sucking when offered glucose water. Research has shown that newborns at 1 week of age are able to distinguish their mother's milk by smelling their mother's breast pads.

CARE OF THE NEWBORN AFTER DELIVERY

In a labor-delivery-recovery room (**LDR**) or a labor-delivery-recovery-postpartum (**LDRP**) setting where the birth has just taken place or if the baby is transferred from the delivery room to a separate newborn nursery, healthcare personnel who take responsibility for the care of the infant must receive certain information as follows:

- Length of first and second stages of labor
- Length of time the membranes were ruptured
- Type of delivery and any difficulties; use of forceps or vacuum extraction
- Analgesics and anesthetics that were used in delivery
- Newborn's condition at delivery
- Newborn's Apgar scores
- Whether resuscitation was needed
- Newborn's vital signs
- Whether vitamin K was given
- Whether eye prophylaxis was performed
- Whether or not the baby voided or passed the meconium plug or stool

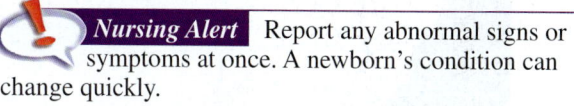
Nursing Alert Report any abnormal signs or symptoms at once. A newborn's condition can change quickly.

Data Gathering

Initial Observations
The first hours after birth are a time of continuing transition for the infant as they adapt to life outside the uterus. If you work in the newborn nursery, you will observe the newborn on admission. Note physical characteristics, including the newborn's appearance, behavior, and reflexes.

Umbilical Cord
Observe the cord and make certain that the clamp is securely attached. Count the number of vessels in the umbilical cord. Normally, you will find three vessels: two arteries and one vein. If you observe only two vessels, you must report this because it indicates a strong possibility of congenital defects in the newborn.

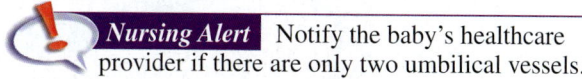
Nursing Alert Notify the baby's healthcare provider if there are only two umbilical vessels.

Measurements
Weigh the newborn immediately after their arrival in the newborn nursery. Record the weight on the health record in grams and convert it to pounds for the mother's benefit. Measure the length of the baby along with the head and chest circumference. These measurements are often recorded in centimeters (see In Practice: Nursing Procedures 67-3 and 67-4).

Vital Signs
Take respiration, pulse, and temperature, and record them every hour or two immediately after birth and then every

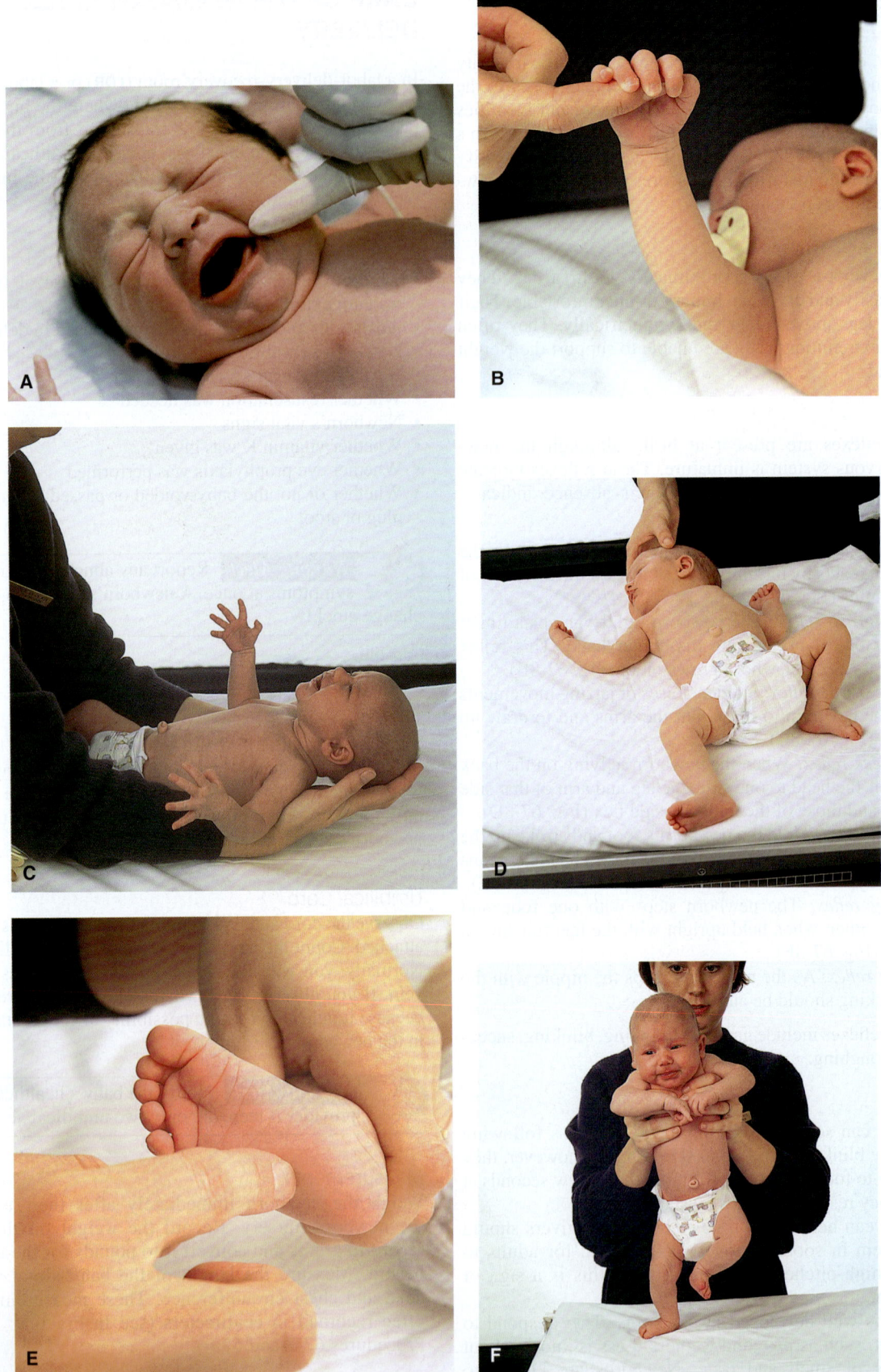

Figure 67-8 **A.** Rooting reflex. **B.** Palmar grasp reflex. **C.** Moro reflex (startle reflex). **D.** Tonic neck reflex. **E.** Babinski reflex. **F.** Stepping reflex. (Ricci, 2007.)

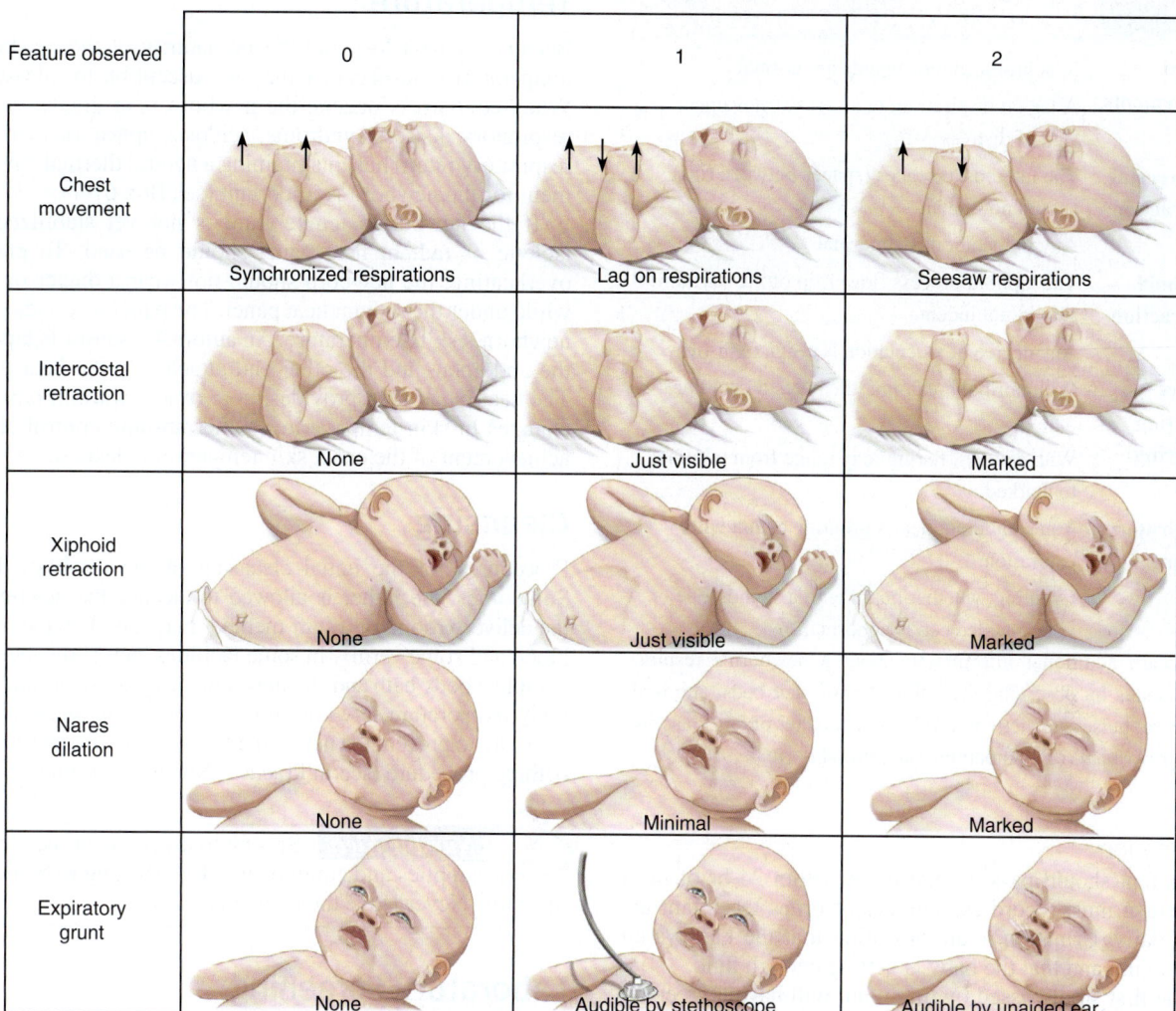

Figure 67-9 Grading of neonatal respiratory distress based on the Silverman–Andersen index. (Reproduced with permission from Silverman, W. A., & Andersen, D. H. (1956). A controlled clinical trial of effects of water mist on obstructive respiratory signs, death rate and necropsy findings among premature infants. *Pediatrics*, 17(1), 1–10. Copyright © 1956 by the AAP.)

4 hr for the first 24 hr. In the past, the initial temperature was taken rectally to establish the patency of the rectum. Currently, the passage of the *meconium* (stool) is accepted as validation that the anus is patent. Tympanic and axillary temperatures are considered safe and accurate.

Ongoing Observations
Respiratory Status
For several hours after birth, continue to observe the newborn's respiratory status. Respiratory status is normal if the movements of the newborn's diaphragm and abdominal muscles are synchronized. The newborn's chest should expand as a whole, and the muscles of the chest wall should not show great effort with breathing. The nares should not flare out with the breath, and the baby should not make grunting noises when breathing.

Observe the baby's general condition and evaluate respiratory status by skin color, rate of respiration, and general activity (Fig. 67-9). Newborns are obligatory nose breathers, with a respiratory rate of 30 to 60 breaths per minute. The reflex response of opening the mouth to breathe when the nasal passage is blocked is absent in most newborns until they are 3 weeks old. Box 67-2 explains the signs of newborn respiratory distress.

Nursing Alert Immediately report any signs of respiratory distress; an infant in distress can worsen very quickly.

Crying
The newborn cries and tightens the muscles in response to sudden loud sounds, changes in position, the feel of something cold touching the skin, or any interference with movements. Crying is the only way a baby can ask for help. They cry when hungry, wet, disturbed, uncomfortable, or sick. The cry of the healthy newborn is lusty. The baby who gets more care usually cries less. Hunger cries are healthy, demanding cries, and the newborn may put fingers in the mouth as an additional sign of hunger. After being fed, the baby is quiet unless they have swallowed air from the bottle and need to bubble (be burped). The baby relaxes when held, rocked, and patted lightly.

Box 67-2	Signs of Newborn Respiratory Distress
Chest Movements	Synchronized movements are normal.
	A lag on inspiration, or a seesaw movement, is a sign of distress.
Intercostal Retractions	The intercostal spaces (spaces between ribs) should not indent.
	Any indentation is abnormal.
Xiphoid Retraction	The xiphoid process (lower tip of the sternum) should not indent.
	Any degree of indentation is a sign of distress.
Nares Dilating (Flaring)	With normal breathing, the nares do not flare out.
	With distress, flaring may range from minimal to marked.
Expiratory Grunt	You should not hear a grunting sound with expiration.
	Grunting, whether heard with a stethoscope or your unaided ear, is abnormal.

Learn additional information about a newborn's respiratory status by observing the color of skin, nail beds, and oral mucosa; pulse rate; activity level; and character of cry. Gasping and *tachypnea* (rapid breathing) are also abnormal.

Elimination

The infant should pass its first urine within 24 hr of birth. The nurse must record the number of times the infant urinates daily. Urination is an indication that the kidneys are functioning and that the baby is getting enough fluid.

The first stool passed by the infant will have a greenish-black, tarry appearance. This stool, called **meconium**, was formed during fetal life and is composed of shed skin cells and **lanugo** hair that the fetus has swallowed. The greenish-black color is due to bile pigments. The first stool is usually passed within 12 hr after birth and should be recorded in the infant's hospital record. If no stool has passed by 24 hr of life, the nurse should report this; it could be due to an anatomic defect of the baby.

Examination by the Healthcare Provider

In addition to the Apgar scoring, the baby's healthcare provider or the birth attendant examines the newborn to determine obvious physical defects. This thorough examination should occur within 24 hr of birth. The healthcare provider reviews the chart, including the prenatal records as well as the labor and delivery records. The physical examination will include the newborn's circulatory, respiratory, digestive, and neurologic systems. Patency of the nose and esophagus can be determined by passing a French suction catheter (number 5-8) through the newborn's nares (nose) and into the esophagus. The healthcare provider also carefully observes the reproductive, urinary, musculoskeletal, and endocrine systems. The nurse's observations and charting during the first few hours are important to this detailed examination.

Maintaining the Infant's Body Temperature

Because of heat loss and the immaturity of the newborn's temperature control center, they are susceptible to cold-stress. When cold-stress occurs, the newborn is at greater risk of respiratory distress syndrome, acidosis, apnea, or increased respiratory rate. Thus, maintaining a neutral thermal environment for the newborn is important (see Box 67-1).

If the newborn's temperature is not yet stabilized, an isolette or radiant heat panel should be used. To prevent overheating, the newborn should not wear a diaper or shirt while under the radiant heat panel. The panel responds to the newborn's skin temperature. An automatic sensor is taped to the abdomen, and the other end attaches to the heat panel. The heat panel then provides more or less warmth based on changes in skin temperature. A thermostatic control allows achievement of the exact skin temperature desired.

Cleansing

Procedures for the initial cleansing of the newborn differ. Sometimes, the father is allowed to cleanse the newborn in the delivery room, or a staff member may merely wipe off the blood and some vernix. In some facilities, newborns receive a complete body bath and shampoo after they are stable and their body temperature is within normal limits. The nurse should take care to prevent the newborn from being chilled during any bathing procedure (see In Practice: Nursing Procedure 67-5).

> **Nursing Alert** Be sure to assemble all needed supplies and equipment before starting to bathe the baby. Never leave the baby unattended.

Laboratory Screening

When the newborn is a few hours old, hemoglobin and hematocrit tests are often ordered. Because a newborn has increased blood volume for size, the hemoglobin is normally 15 to 18 g/100 mL blood. The normal hematocrit for the newborn is 45% to 60%. Hemoglobin and hematocrit results lower than these normal ranges may indicate anemia.

The healthcare provider may also order a test to monitor the newborn's blood glucose level. A small sample of blood is obtained with a heel stick and tested with a blood glucose monitor. If a Dextrostix heel stick reading is less than 40 to 45 mg/100 mL of blood, it suggests hypoglycemia (see In Practice: Nursing Procedure 67-6).

Most states in the United States require testing for specific diseases. Tests are done to rule out phenylketonuria (**PKU**), an inherited disorder caused by the body's inability to digest protein normally. Tests are also made for **galactosemia**, a hereditary disease in which the newborn cannot digest galactose, a certain type of sugar. Tests of thyroid function can rule out **hypothyroidism**. Individuals with many of these disorders have a much better prognosis if they are treated before the age of 3 months. Blood tests can also determine the sickle cell trait and maple syrup urine disease. A test for glucose-6-phosphodehydrogenase (**G_6PD**) deficiency may be done, especially in babies of African, Asian, or Mediterranean origin.

The newborn's urine may be tested for drugs, such as cocaine or heroin. The presence of these substances indicates maternal substance abuse (see Chapter 69).

> **Key Concept**
> The heel stick is the preferred method for obtaining routine blood samples from a newborn. The sample may be used for glucose, PKU, or other necessary blood tests.

Protecting the Newborn

Identification
When starting to care for the infant, double-check the identification bands. Nurses must be diligent in this practice. Cross-check the infant's identification with that of the mother to ensure that the correct mother and child are together.

Security
Nurses must also be alert to the possibility of infant kidnapping or abduction (Box 67-3). Hospitals should have a written critical incident response plan in case an abduction occurs or a person is observed acting suspiciously.

Sleeping Position
An important measure to teach new parents is that the best sleeping position for newborns is on the back. An alternate position is on the side. This reduces the risk of sudden infant death syndrome (**SIDS**) in infants under 1 year old.

Protection From Nosocomial (Hospital-Acquired) Infection
A newborn nursery can be a dangerous place if an infection is present. Epidemics of skin infections, such as impetigo, and staphylococcus may occur. A fatal type of newborn diarrhea is a particular danger.

Nursery personnel must use techniques that isolate all newborns from direct contact with other babies. Everyone in the nursery, hospital workers and visitors alike, must follow a specific handwashing and scrub technique. Nursery personnel usually wear scrub suits, and visitors wear gowns over their clothes. People with infectious diseases are not allowed in the obstetric area. Each newborn has his or her own equipment and supplies.

> **Key Concept**
> Equipment and supplies are never shared between babies.

When working in the nursery, place each newborn in a separate crib or radiant heat warmer equipped with a firm, waterproof mattress. The crib has clear sides to facilitate constant observation of the newborn.

The nursery is well lighted and heated to approximately 75 °F (23.9 °C). The nursery is never left unattended, and newborns are within sight at all times.

DAILY NEWBORN CARE

Routine care of the newborn requires careful observation for signs of abnormalities or problems. It also requires meeting the basic needs of food, cleanliness, comfort, and safety. Teaching for the mother and other caregivers is vital. They must know what is normal and when to consult the primary caregiver should possible problems occur.

> **Key Concept**
> As part of the routine care, the nurse should document the following on the newborn's chart:
> - Rate of respirations (note if crying or sleeping)
> - Type of respirations (note abnormal symptoms, such as retraction, dilation of nares, expiratory grunts, and unusual crying sounds)
> - Pulse
> - Temperature
> - Weight (daily)
>
> The nurse should make these observations (with the exception of weight) several times a day for the first day of life and then on a daily basis. If complications are suspected, assessments should be performed more often.

In Practice: Nursing Care Guidelines 67-1 summarizes important responsibilities of the nurse when caring for a newborn.

Data Gathering

Respirations
Count the respirations first, then the pulse. Chart whether the newborn was sleeping, awake, or crying when respiration and pulse were taken. (Respiration rate and pulse increase when the newborn is disturbed. Values are inaccurate if the newborn is moving or crying.)

Count respirations for 60 s. The newborn breathes through the nose. Observe the abdomen's rise and fall with

---

Box 67-3 The "Typical" Abductor of a Baby

For more information visit The National Center for Missing and Exploited Children at: www.missingkids.com/

1. Female, 12 to 55 years old, often overweight
2. Uses manipulation, lying, and deception to gain access
3. Frequently has lost a baby or is incapable of having one
4. Often married or cohabiting; her companion's desire for a child may be the motivation for the abduction
5. Considers the newborn her own after the abduction occurs
6. Usually lives in the community where the abduction takes place
7. In many cases, visits more than one nursery unit before the abduction; asks detailed questions about hospital procedures and the maternity floor layout
8. Plans the abduction but does not necessarily target a specific newborn; when an opportunity presents itself, the abduction is simply a matter of "snatch and run"
9. Frequently impersonates a nurse or other hospital personnel
10. Frequently uses a fire exit stairwell for escape
11. Abductions may occur from a home setting
12. Often acquainted with hospital personnel, staff work routines, and the victim's parents

Adapted from the National Center for Missing and Exploited Children. (n.d.). https://www.missingkids.org/theissues/infantabductions

IN PRACTICE
NURSING CARE GUIDELINES 67-1: Care of the Normal Newborn

Immediately After Birth
- Obtain Apgar score (see Table 67-1).
- Place identification bands on the newborn and the mother.
- Take the newborn's footprints and the mother's thumbprint if indicated by facility protocol.
- Complete the delivery information on the chart before the newborn leaves the delivery room.
- Obtain newborn's weight and length.
- Complete physical examination by healthcare provider on admission to the newborn nursery.
- Follow the facility's procedures for the initial cleansing and daily bathing of the newborn.

Continuing Care
- Obtain vital signs.
- Monitor rate and type of respirations (note if the newborn is crying or sleeping while the rate is taken), apical pulse, blood pressure, and temperature.
- Monitor for signs of respiratory distress (see Box 67-2).
- Clear mouth and nares of mucus.
- Perform glucose (Dextrostix) checks according to agency parameters.
- Perform cord care as per agency protocol; monitor cord condition.
- Obtain daily weight.
- Document approximate amount of breast milk taken or measure amount of bottle feeding.
- Describe amount, color, and consistency of voiding and stools.
- Monitor skin color for signs of jaundice or cyanosis.
- Observe and report condition of circumcision or perineum.
- Be observant for any signs of difficulty or abnormalities.
- Observe sleep–activity patterns, behavior patterns.
- Be alert to character of cry (e.g., whining, sharp, or high pitched).
- Facilitate the mother's breastfeeding or bottle feeding.
- Role model healthy parenting behaviors for the parent(s) if indicated.
- Observe bonding process and adequacy of parenting behaviors.

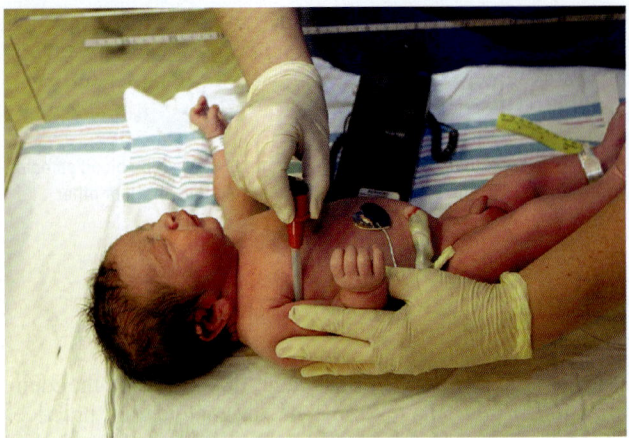

Figure 67-10 Measuring the newborn's axillary temperature. (Hatfield, 2014.)

Temperature
Many newborn nurseries use the tympanic (ear) method to measure the newborn's temperature. The tympanic temperature probe may be set to convert to the rectal temperature equivalent. Insert the tympanic probe into the newborn's ear, while holding his or her head steady. The probe will record temperature within a few seconds.

If the tympanic method is not used, axillary temperatures may be ordered (Fig. 67-10). The normal newborn's axillary temperature is between 97.6 °F and 98.6 °F (36.5 °C and 37 °C). In some cases, a rectal temperature may be ordered. To measure rectal temperature, gently insert the temperature probe no more than 0.5 in. (1.3 cm). Place infant on their side while taking a rectal temperature. Place a dry diaper over the newborn's genitals so you will not get wet if he or she voids. Keep the probe in place until the instrument beeps. Hold the probe at all times. Many healthcare facilities no longer perform rectal temperatures because of the potential for injury.

Blood Pressure
The newborn's blood pressure usually is low compared to adult readings, ranging from 50 to 80 mm Hg systolic and 30 to 50 mm Hg diastolic. Follow protocols for the location to use; the leg is the most commonly used site. Use an appropriately sized cuff.

Weight
Weigh the newborn once a day without clothing or diaper for the most accurate measurement. Bath time is an excellent time for weighing.

Urine
Continue to record the number of voidings per day in the hospital record.

Stools
The stools gradually change in character as the baby begins to eat. These next several stools are called *transitional* stools, and the appearance depends on whether the baby is breastfed or bottle-fed.

By the fifth day of life, the daily number of stools ranges from four to six. As the baby grows, the number usually drops to one or two per day. During the infant's hospital

each breath. Respirations should be quiet and may be somewhat irregular. The normal respiratory rate ranges from 30 to 60 breaths per minute when the newborn is at rest. Review Box 67-2 for signs of respiratory distress in the newborn that you must report immediately.

Pulse
Take the pulse by listening with a stethoscope over the baby's heart (apical pulse) for 60 s. The pulse is rapid and may be slightly irregular; the normal range is 120 to 160 beats per minute (bpm). Warm the stethoscope in your hand before taking the pulse, to avoid chilling the baby.

stay, the number, color, and consistency of stools should be recorded in the hospital record.

Basic Needs

The newborn has the basic human needs for safety, security, and love. Nursing care is designed to provide the newborn with warmth, hygiene, nutrition, rest, and affection, making sure that he or she is protected and thriving. You will also teach essential skills to the family to ensure that they will be able to continue to meet the newborn's needs after nursing care ends.

Handling the Newborn

There is no one right way to hold a baby, but movements should be smooth and firm to help the baby feel secure. Keep in mind that:

- The head, neck, and buttocks need support.
- Newborns wiggle! Be sure you have a firm hold on the baby.
- It is easier to pick up a newborn when he or she is lying on the back (supine) rather than on the stomach (prone). If the infant is on the stomach, turn him or her over before picking up, to make the process more secure.
- Hold the baby close to your body to provide security. The "football" hold is a convenient method because it provides a free hand with which to perform additional tasks.

Dressing and Wrapping the Newborn

Handle the baby gently but firmly when dressing them. Stretch the neck opening of a shirt or gown before bringing it over the head. Reach into the sleeves and pull the baby's hand through, to avoid catching a small finger in the cloth. Fold the diaper beneath the cord stump. Wrap the baby securely in a blanket. This process is known as *swaddling* and helps many babies feel more secure.

Cord Care

Because the umbilical cord maintained fetal circulation, the newborn faces the danger of rapid hemorrhage through it. Therefore, the clamps or ties must be secure until they can be safely removed. When caring for the newborn, assess the cord for bleeding at frequent intervals during the first few hours of life. The stump of the cord begins to shrivel and darken soon after birth. The clamp is usually removed after 24 h, as long as no bleeding is evident. (Removal of the clamp prevents tension on the drying stump.)

Triple Dye may be applied to the cut cord and around the umbilicus to prevent infection. One application of Triple Dye is usually sufficient, although some healthcare providers order daily application. The stump is usually swabbed with alcohol with each diaper change. The diaper should not be placed over the stump of the cord but rather folded beneath it so that the cord is exposed to the drying effects of room air.

When bathing, do not submerge the baby in tub water until the cord falls off (see In Practice: Educating the Client 67-1).

Care of the Genitals

To prevent irritation of the infant's sensitive skin, thoroughly clean their buttocks following each voiding and bowel movement. Report any rash or irritation. (Broken skin can be an entry for infection.)

IN PRACTICE
EDUCATING THE CLIENT 67-1 — Cord Care

- The cord will dry and fall off naturally. This should happen at about 10 to 14 days after birth.
- Clean the cord stump with isopropyl (rubbing) alcohol at each diaper change. Allow to air dry.
- Fold the diaper below the cord stump.
- Do not give the baby a tub bath until after the cord falls off.
- Call your baby's doctor if the cord shows any of these signs of infection:
  - Red streaks around the cord
  - Foul odor
  - Pus

In male babies, the foreskin (prepuce) covers the glans penis or extends beyond it. The opening may be very small, a condition known as *phimosis*. **Smegma** (excess secretions and dead skin cells) may collect beneath the foreskin, and drops of urine also may remain, causing irritation.

Some male newborns may be circumcised (part or all of the foreskin is removed). **Circumcision** is most often done for cultural reasons. Ritual circumcision is performed on Jewish male babies, usually on the eighth day of life. If the baby has been circumcised, they must be kept clean and assessed for bleeding, swelling, and voiding. A sterile dressing may be applied after each voiding for 24 to 48 hr, to keep the diaper from sticking. Circumcision is usually performed shortly before the newborn leaves the healthcare facility or after discharge. For this reason, instruct the parents in the care required and document teaching. Never place the infant on their stomach following circumcision. Observe circumcision every 15 min for the first 4 hr. Report any excessive bleeding immediately.

If circumcision is not performed, the healthcare provider may order that the foreskin be gently stretched and retracted over the glans penis for cleaning once every day. In some babies, the foreskin will not easily stretch over the glans. Do not force it. Cleaning must be gentle and careful. Replace the foreskin immediately; a tight foreskin causes edema and pain.

In female babies, gently clean between all the folds of the labia, wiping from front to back. You may notice mucus or a blood-tinged discharge from the vagina. This is normal and is caused by the sudden absence of the mother's hormones; it will last only a few days.

Sleep

Except when being fed, the newborn sleeps most of the time, although not deeply. The baby will awaken and cry when hungry or uncomfortable. The baby should be placed on his or her back or side to sleep. Pillows should not be used because of the danger of suffocation.

NUTRITION

Breastfeeding is the best source of nutrition for infants. Differences have been found in the breast milk of mothers of preterm infants and term infants; each mother produces breast milk that is ideally suited for her own baby. However, not all mothers will choose to breastfeed. It is important that the nurse supports each woman in her own choice and provides client teaching tailored to the needs of each new mother.

Birth attendants differ in their preferences for the first feeding of newborns. It is ideal if mothers who breastfeed are encouraged to do so in the delivery room. A few birth attendants prefer that the newborn remain NPO (nothing by mouth) for 3 to 4 hr after birth. When the first feeding is not from the breast, it usually consists of sterile water and is sometimes given by a nurse. If all is normal, the mother gives the newborn as many other feedings as desired.

If the baby eats too much or too fast or is improperly burped (bubbled), they may regurgitate. (Regurgitation is simply an overflow; do not think of it as vomiting.) Food remaining in the esophagus may cause hiccups. Giving the infant sips of water can usually stop the hiccups. However, because of the difference in the method for sucking from a bottle versus the breast, many breastfeeding mothers do not wish the baby to have anything from a bottle.

Feeding Schedule and Bringing the Baby to the Mother for Feedings

All babies should be fed when they are hungry. Babies are all different, and their nursing patterns will vary. Newborns are usually fed "on demand" or approximately every 2 to 4 hr.

If the baby and mother are not "rooming-in," an important nursing skill to learn is bringing the newborn to the mother for feeding. The following are recommended guidelines:

- Wash your hands.
- Dress the newborn warmly.
- Some hospitals have a policy that requires that you weigh the breast-fed baby before feeding and again after feeding. Other authorities believe this is unnecessary and feel that adequate breastfeeding can be determined by the baby's contentment and number of voids and stools daily.
- Carry the baby carefully; use the football hold.
- Instruct the mother to wash her hands to prevent infection.
- Compare the wristband of the mother with that of the baby to ensure the right baby is with the right mother.
- Provide privacy.
- Assist the mother into a comfortable position because she will be in the same position for about 20 min.
- Show the mother how to hold and bubble the newborn. Have her do a return demonstration.
- When the feeding is finished, check with the mother about how the baby fed or determine the amount of formula missing from the bottle if the baby was bottle-fed. Check if the baby was bubbled.
- Make sure the baby is clean and dry before placing them in the crib. Place the baby on the back or side because sleeping on the back decreases the risk of SIDS.
- Wash your hands and document the feeding on the baby's chart, including how well the baby breast-fed or how much formula was taken and any other pertinent observations.

Breastfeeding

In summary, breastfeeding provides the following:

- Better nutrition
- Lower risk of the baby developing allergies
- Reduced risk of infections in the newborn because maternal antibodies pass through the breast milk
- Enhanced maternal–newborn bonding
- Involution of the uterus promoted by breastfeeding
- Delayed ovulation for women who breastfeed only (no supplements or pacifiers). Breastfeeding provides a measure of contraceptive protection for 6 months or until the woman's first period after the birth (whichever comes first)
- Correct temperature of breast milk
- Availability and convenience of breast milk
- Economical aspects

It is important for the nurse to educate the parent about the advantages of breastfeeding to enable them to make a decision based on this information and lifestyle needs.

Assisting a Nursing Client

During the first few days, the client's breasts produce *colostrum,* which is rich in disease-fighting immunities and nutrients. Although the client's true milk is not in yet, the newborn should nurse often to receive the health benefits of colostrum, to condition the client's nipples for nursing, and to stimulate milk production. Frequent nursing also prevents engorgement and related complications. The newborn's sucking stimulates milk production (see In Practice: Educating the Client 67-2).

Help the breastfeeding client the first few times so that they learn the best positioning. Proper positioning helps the newborn to receive milk easily. It minimizes nipple soreness, plugged ducts, and mastitis. It also provides comfort for both the client and the newborn during feedings. The client can use the cradle or football hold, or they can lie on their side.

Teach the client the following steps:

- Use the arm to support the newborn. If using the cradle hold, place the back of the newborn's head in the crook of your arm, with your hand holding the newborn's bottom or thigh.

IN PRACTICE
EDUCATING THE CLIENT 67-2 Assisting a Nursing Parent

The parent will often nurse their newborn immediately after birth and again within 4 hr. If the parent does not ask to nurse, the birth attendant may suggest it. You may do so as well. The delivery room staff should cooperate if the parent agrees. Use thermal heat or a radiant warmer to heat the nursing couple if the room is cool or if the parent is shivering from strenuous labor or medication. Breast-fed newborns usually do not receive supplementary water or bottles in the nursery to avoid nipple confusion and to encourage nursing at the breast.

- Support the nursing breast with your opposite hand. Place the hand below the breast on your rib cage. Use as many fingers as necessary to support the breast without covering any of the nipple. Place your thumb above the nipple. This grasp is called the *C-hold* or *palmar grasp*.
- Turn the newborn's body toward yours so that you are stomach-to-stomach.
- Tickle the newborn's bottom lip or corner of the mouth to trigger the rooting reflex. You will coax the newborn to open their mouth. Wait until the newborn's mouth is open wide. *Rationale: If the mouth is not wide open, the newborn will grasp the tip of the nipple, causing soreness.*
- Pull the newborn close. As soon as their mouth is wide open, move the baby quickly to the breast so that the nipple passes the gums well into the mouth. The newborn should have the whole areola in the mouth, not just the nipple. Use your arm to support the newborn. The newborn's chin should touch the breast. If the newborn's nose is covered, press the breast away from the nose so that the baby can breathe easily.
- To stop nursing, place a finger between the baby's mouth and your areola to break suction.
- If you feel pain while nursing, break suction and begin again. *Rationale: Pain is not a normal part of breastfeeding.*
- Offer both breasts at each feeding, first offering the breast used last at the previous feeding. *Rationale: Each breast needs to be emptied regularly.*

Many breastfeeding clients feel a slight tingling sensation when they begin to nurse, called the *let-down reflex*. The newborn's sucking action triggers hormones that cause the client's brain to release milk from the alveolus. Many "let downs" occur during a single nursing session. The let-down reflex can be impaired when the client is stressed, cold, or in pain. Alcohol use can also inhibit milk flow.

It is common for newborns to be too sleepy to nurse. Sleepy babies can often be roused by a diaper or clothing change or a sponge bath. Falling asleep while nursing is also normal for newborns.

When the client's true milk "comes in" by the second, third, or fourth day, a breastfeeding baby typically nurses 8 to 12 times per day. The client should first offer the breast from which the baby nursed last because it may not have been emptied completely. Deciding which breast to offer first is often easy because one feels fuller than the other. The baby should nurse at least 10 min on one breast before being offered the other breast. Letting the baby signal when they want to switch is best for the newborn to get the right balance of calories. When the baby first begins nursing, they will get **foremilk**, which is relatively low in fat. **Hindmilk** appears at the end of the feeding and is higher in fat and calories.

Many women seem concerned about their milk supply after a few weeks because their breasts feel softer and less full. This is normal and due to the body's adjustment to the newborn's needs. Often, a baby who has settled into a nice feeding pattern begins to nurse more often for a day or two. This baby is probably experiencing a growth spurt. Although the client may not have enough milk the first day, their body will quickly adapt, and their milk supply will increase. Then the baby will once more be satisfied and will again reduce the frequency of wanting to nurse. During the early days and months, many babies suck for pleasure, which is called *nonnutritive sucking*. When a baby is actually nursing, the client will hear a "suck-suck-swallow" pattern. No swallow occurs during nonnutritive sucking.

Signs that the breast-fed newborn is receiving adequate nutrition are at least six to eight wet diapers and at least two stools per day. Once the neonate has finished passing the meconium (within 24-48 hr), the breast-fed baby's stool will be loose and unformed, and range in color from pea soup to yellow to tan. The stool may appear seedy and will have little odor. By 6 weeks, most breast-fed babies have only one to two daily soft bowel movements because breast milk is so well absorbed.

One approach to documenting a client's progress and success with breastfeeding is the **LATCH** (latch, audible swallowing, type of nipple, comfort, hold) breastfeeding charting system (Table 67-2).

TABLE 67-2 LATCH Breastfeeding Charting System

	0	1	2
L Latch	Too sleepy or reluctant. No latch achieved.	Repeated attempts. Hold nipple in mouth. Stimulate to suck.	Grasps breast. Tongue down. Lips flanged. Rhythmic sucking.
A Audible swallowing	None.	A few with stimulation.	Spontaneous and intermittent under 24 hr old. Spontaneous and frequent over 24 hr old.
T Type of nipple	Inverted.	Flat.	Everted (after stimulation).
C Comfort (breast/nipple)	Engorged. Cracked, bleeding, large blisters or bruises. Severe discomfort.	Filling. Reddened/small blisters or bruises. Mild/moderate discomfort.	Soft, nontender.
H Hold (positioning)	Full assist (staff holds infant at breast).	Minimal assist (i.e., place pillows for support, elevate head of bed). Teach one side; mother does other. Staff holds and then mother takes over.	No assist from staff. Mother able to position and hold baby by self.

Jensen, Wallace, and Kelsey (1994).

Common Problems of Breastfeeding

Breast care for the client who is nursing their newborn varies. The goal is to simplify procedures while avoiding infection. In some facilities, the client rinses their nipples before each feeding. In other facilities, however, this practice is not followed because it is believed that breast milk contains lactic acid, which acts as a natural cleanser for the nipples. Previous practices of "toughening" the nipples, washing them vigorously, and applying creams are not currently recommended. Nursing clients are at risk for the following common problems.

Sore and Cracked Nipples

Improper positioning is most often the cause of sore nipples. Prevention of sore nipples is very important. The suction of the baby at the breast is strongest in the first minutes of feeding, so a longer feeding period may actually reduce the chance of nipple soreness rather than make it worse. Also, changing the position in which the mother holds the baby at the breast for each feeding session helps to change the area of greatest suction.

In the early days of nursing, a baby with a vigorous suck may cause discomfort. Nipple soreness caused by an enthusiastic baby should ease as the client's nipples become conditioned. Treatment of sore nipples includes swabbing the affected nipple with breast milk and allowing it to air dry; wearing a nursing bra and leaving the flaps down for a few minutes after feeding to air dry the nipples; changing breast pads when wet; and assisting the infant to "latch on" to the nipple and areola properly.

Other remedies may also be helpful. The tannic acid in brewed tea is believed to help speed healing. The client can apply it by blotting a steeped, cool tea bag on the sore nipple or areola after feeding. Vitamin E oil may be used sparingly, but it must be rinsed off with clear water before the next feeding to prevent the buildup of a toxic level of vitamin E being ingested from the nipple.

Soap should not be used on the breasts because it is drying, and it promotes nipple cracking. Flexible nipple shields are available but may actually contribute to sore nipples by rubbing against the nipple as the baby sucks. In addition, the baby may be unable to grasp the breast effectively for complete emptying at feeding time.

A well-fitting nonwaterproof cotton bra is essential. Waterproof bras hold in moisture, which can cause irritation or maceration of the nipples. The breasts should be firmly supported.

Engorgement

Engorgement is extreme fullness of the areola and/or breast. Some degree of engorgement is normal. Two or 3 days after giving birth, a breastfeeding client may feel the tingling and fullness that indicates their milk is "coming in." It is a good idea to provide anticipatory guidance about this event and to suggest that the client nurse the baby as soon as this sensation is felt. Doing so may help prevent engorgement of the breasts. Frequent nursing also helps in the prevention of engorgement.

If engorgement is already present, have the mother shower or use warm, moist heat before it is time to nurse, and then manually express some milk to soften the breast. This measure allows the newborn to get a proper grasp on the nipple and prevents further pain for the mother. Massaging from the outer breast toward the nipple also helps to soften the engorged breast, to allow for easier hand expression or nursing. The most important treatment is to nurse frequently.

Plugged Ducts

Incomplete emptying of the breasts may cause plugged ducts or tender lumps in the breasts of an otherwise healthy lactating woman. The treatment is to continue nursing. Massaging the area and applying heat before nursing helps ensure complete emptying. Nursing on the opposite breast first will allow the affected breast to "let down," easing the affected side. Proper positioning also may help. The mother's bra should be checked for proper fit.

Mastitis

Mastitis is almost always caused by bacteria from the baby's mouth that enter the mother's breast through a crack in the nipple. Preventive measures include reducing those steps that decrease the chances of soreness and cracking of the nipple: changing positions, nursing more frequently, and nursing at least 10 min on each breast.

Signs of mastitis include a sore, red area that feels warm to the touch. Because the bacteria came from the baby's mouth, continued nursing is not harmful to the baby and is helpful to the client. The best advice for this client is to continue nursing during treatment for mastitis. Treatment includes heat, antibiotic therapy, rest, and plenty of fluids. Many antibiotics are safe for nursing clients to take; the client's healthcare provider will select the one that is best.

> **Nursing Alert** Complications of the postpartum period may also include hematoma, hemorrhage, uterine atony, thrombophlebitis, puerperal infections, cystitis, and depression. These subjects are discussed in Chapter 68.

Nutrition for a Breastfeeding Mother

A well-nourished client ensures an adequate and nutritious milk supply for their newborn and protects their own health. On the other hand, a poorly nourished client who is breastfeeding or one who is restricting their calories may not produce enough breast milk. Nursing clients should receive about 500 calories a day above their nonnursing caloric intake. Adequate fluids are also important for milk production. Usually, following the nutritional guidelines for pregnancy provides the nursing mother with adequate food intake. If the client exclusively nurses the infant beyond 4 months of age, their dietary needs will increase as the infant's nutritional needs increase. The nursing client need not restrict their intake of favorite foods just because they are nursing, although a few foods and beverages cause concern.

Alcohol does appear in breast milk, and large quantities in the maternal diet have been shown to inhibit the let-down reflex. Babies of heavy alcohol drinkers nurse less often and for shorter periods. Alcohol does relax the breastfeeding client, but there is not sufficient information about a safe level of alcohol intake to assure a client that drinking any alcohol while nursing is absolutely safe for their baby.

Caffeine also transfers to breast milk. A moderate intake (1-2 cups of coffee daily) is fine; however, if the baby appears wakeful, restless, or irritable, the client should cut down on or eliminate their caffeine intake.

The use of cow's milk by the client has possibly been linked to colic in newborns. If the baby is colicky, the client may want to eliminate milk from their diet for 2 weeks to see if it makes a difference. Colic usually worsens if a breast-fed baby is switched to a formula. Strongly flavored foods may cause temporary colic in some babies. This colic usually lasts approximately 24 hr. Common offenders are onions, garlic, beans, and rhubarb.

Use of Medications While Breastfeeding

Breast milk passes many medications from nursing client to infant. The nursing client should consult the baby's pediatrician before taking any drugs (Box 67-4).

> **Nursing Alert** A nursing client should not take any medication or drug without asking their healthcare provider.

Box 67-4 Medications and Breastfeeding

Many drugs pass into breast milk from the nursing parent. Many factors determine whether a medication is safe for a nursing parent to take. Not all drugs pass in the same concentration or remain in breast milk at a stable concentration. The concentration in the breast milk depends on fat solubility, water-solubility, the rate at which the parent's body metabolizes the drug, the time between taking doses of the medication, and other factors. The effect on the nursing baby depends on the drug concentration, as well as on the age and the maturity of the baby.

GUIDELINES FOR DRUG SAFETY IN BREASTFEEDING

Drugs taken by the breastfeeding client that are *particularly dangerous* to the nursing newborn are as follows:
- Anticancer drugs (chemotherapy)
- Radioactive substances (e.g., those used for diagnostic tests or treatment of cancers)
- Lithium (used to treat psychiatric disorders)
- All drugs of abuse, including
  - Amphetamines
  - Cocaine
  - Heroin
  - LSD
  - PCP

   Excessive nicotine and alcohol

These drugs are *generally considered compatible* with breastfeeding:
- Acetaminophen (Tylenol)
- Many antibiotics (penicillins, cephalosporins, erythromycin)
- Codeine
- Phenytoin (Dilantin)
- Pseudoephedrine (Sudafed)

Bottle Feeding

Although it is widely accepted that "breast is best," formulas have been developed that are satisfactory breast milk replacements. Breastfeeding may be undesirable when the client has a chronic disease (e.g., HIV infection), if the nipples are severely inverted, or if the baby has certain abnormalities.

In the event of a premature delivery and in some other situations, the client may express their breast milk, which may be bottle-fed to the baby. Some clients choose to bottle feed for social or personal reasons.

Many formulas are available; each product has its own advantages. The baby's healthcare provider orders the specific formula appropriate for the newborn's needs.

During the first week of feeding, most babies take from 1 to 3 oz per feeding, with a total intake of 12 to 15 oz every 24 hr. This amount increases to approximately 20 oz in 24 hr by the end of the second week. Intake increases rapidly thereafter. By the third week, many babies drop an evening or a night feeding and sleep longer without hunger.

The person feeding the baby must wash their hands before receiving the newborn. Use care in keeping the nipple of the bottle clean. Check the rate of flow from the nipple to make certain that it has a constant drip. Nipple openings are made either with a "cross-cut" or with holes. If the opening is not large enough, the hole can be enlarged by putting a red-hot needle through it. If the opening is too large, the baby may tend to choke.

While the baby is eating, the person who is feeding the newborn should tilt the bottle, so that milk is in the neck of the bottle at all times or so the plastic liner folds in on itself, to keep the baby from swallowing air. The baby should be bubbled at intervals during the feeding.

Feeding does not just provide nutrition, it also gives the baby a sense of security and of being loved. The baby should not be left alone with a propped bottle either in the nursery at the hospital or at home. The parents or other caregivers should always hold the baby and cuddle them during the feeding.

If you are using a bottle to feed a baby, hold the baby exactly as you would the breast-fed baby and teach family caregivers to do the same. To prevent aspiration of milk and to promote bonding, do not prop the bottle. A propped bottle may also contribute to ear infections because the milk can flow from the throat into the baby's eustachian tube.

Because bacteria thrive in milk, the parents should be taught to exercise care when preparing the newborn's formula. Many families use either a premixed formula or a formula that is simply mixed with water. If the formula is purchased in small, disposable bottles, the bottles are already sterilized. When using disposable bottles, caregivers must be sure that the plastic bag is securely fastened into the holder and that the baby cannot pull the end of the bag through the side of the holder while feeding. Bottles usually do not need to be disinfected if they are cleaned in an automatic dishwasher.

Formula is usually given at room temperature. A bottle should not be warmed in a microwave; this creates "hot spots" in the formula that may burn the baby's mouth and throat unexpectedly. The person feeding the baby should also check the temperature of the formula. Room or body temperature is appropriate.

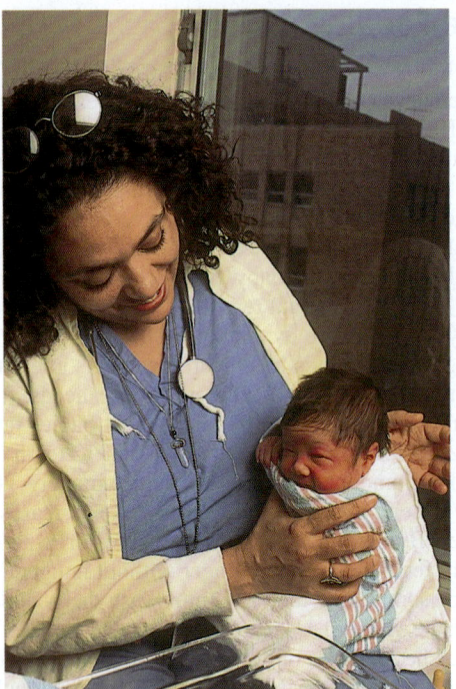

Figure 67-11 The nurse demonstrates a sitting position for burping a newborn. The infant's head is supported by the nurse's hand.

Bubbling (Burping) the Baby

> **Key Concept**
> Bubbling must be done whether the baby is breast-fed or bottle-fed.

Newborns must be properly bubbled (burped) during and after each feeding to prevent regurgitation of food and possible aspiration of food into the lungs. The breast-fed baby should be bubbled when switching from one breast to the other; the bottle-fed baby should be bubbled after every 1/2 to 1 oz of fluid for the first day or so. All babies should be bubbled after a feeding. The time between bubblings gradually increases, but caregivers must be sure that the baby is not retaining any gas in the stomach at the end of the feeding.

Several methods for holding the baby during bubbling are recommended. Hold the baby so that they expel gas in the stomach without regurgitating. You can hold the newborn upright on your knee or against your shoulder. Gently pat or rub the baby's back (Fig. 67-11). Alternatively, you may place the baby prone over your knees, gently rubbing their back.

Supplements

The healthcare provider may suggest that vitamin concentrates be added to feedings when the newborn is 2 to 3 weeks old. Breast milk or formula contains the other essential nutrients for the first 6 months of life, although iron is often given as a supplement to prevent iron deficiency anemia.

Breast milk or formula alone is the only source of nutrition that the baby needs for the first 4 to 6 months of life. Parents should be taught that adding other foods, such as cereals, too early can lead to digestive problems and allergies.

DISCHARGE

Before the newborn is discharged, the birth attendant examines him or her thoroughly. All birth and newborn records are completed. The family is instructed regarding the care of the newborn, including how to bathe him or her (see In Practice: Educating the Client 67-3).

The family is also notified when to return the newborn to the healthcare provider's office for an examination. Sometimes there is a need for a Public Health Department or home care referral. If so, a visiting nurse will contact the caregivers after they arrive home with the baby. The home visit is quite common and is particularly valuable when the mother and baby have been discharged very soon after the birth.

Ensuring Safety

Identification
At discharge, the nurse should remove one of the newborn's identification bands and place it on the chart, which the mother then signs.

Use of Infant Car Seat
All babies should be sent home securely restrained in an infant car seat, which is installed as recommended in the back seat of the car. The car seat for the newborn should be rear-facing.

IN PRACTICE

EDUCATING THE CLIENT 67-3 — Giving the Newborn a Tub Bath

Teach parents and other family caregivers the following steps when bathing their newborn.
- Do not give a tub bath until the baby's cord falls off.
- Be sure that the room is warm enough and that the newborn is protected from drafts.
- Never talk on the telephone or leave the baby unattended—even for a moment!—during the bath, to prevent accidents, such as falling or drowning.
- Have all equipment ready and conveniently placed: baby bathtub, bath thermometer, two washcloths, towels, baby soap, clean clothes and diaper, and lotion. You cannot leave the baby after you start the bath.
- Wash your hands to prevent spreading infection.
- Check the water temperature carefully; it should be warm, not hot (98.6 °F or 37 °C is the usual maximum temperature).
- Carefully support the newborn's head and body with a moderately firm grip when you put them in the tub.
- Use a soft washcloth, towel, and only a small amount of soap.
- Rinse off all soap.
- Dry the baby, paying particular attention to drying the skinfolds well.
- Look for skin irritation or abnormalities.

STUDENT SYNTHESIS

KEY POINTS

- The Apgar score is used for immediate assessment of the newborn based on heart rate, respiratory effort, muscle tone, reflex irritability, and color. The maximum score is 10. The evaluation is done at 1 min after birth and again at 5 min. An Apgar score of 7 or less indicates a need for neonatal resuscitation.
- Newborns can lose heat by convection, conduction, radiation, and evaporation.
- To prevent cold-stress, the nurse should keep the baby dry, provide a hat or cap to prevent heat loss from the head, provide a heat source for the baby until their temperature stabilizes (skin-to-skin contact with a parent, isolette, or radiant warmer), and maintain the room's temperature at about 75 °F (23.9 °C).
- At the time of delivery, neonatal assessments include the Apgar score, further evaluation of need for resuscitation, temperature regulation, and neonatal adaptation to life outside the uterus.
- When an infant is admitted to the nursery, ongoing assessments include evaluation of respiratory status, temperature regulation, umbilical cord, body measurements, and elimination.
- Daily newborn assessments include weight, respiration, elimination, and feeding. Each of these items should be reviewed at the time of discharge.
- Newborn identification is essential to ensure that the mother goes home with her own baby.
- Identification measures used in many hospitals include using matching identification bands, taking footprints, using electronic bracelets, and keeping an accurate and complete hospital record. The identification should be confirmed each time the mother and baby are brought together and again at hospital discharge.
- The normal newborn has a respiratory rate of less than 60 breaths per minute, a heart rate of 110 to 150 bpm, and a normal body temperature. The infant may have a variety of temporary or permanent skin markings. Effects of maternal hormones on the baby's breasts and genitals may last for a few weeks.
- When weighing the infant, take care to avoid cold-stress; the baby must never be left alone. In measuring the infant, use the crib sheet to mark where the crown of the head is, then stretch the legs, make another mark, and measure between the marks.
- Daily care of the neonate includes cord care, skin care, assessment of possible problems, and attention to the baby's needs for security, safety, and bonding with the parents.
- A circumcised infant needs frequent changes of a sterile dressing over the wound and assessment for complications; the infant should not be placed on their stomach.
- Normal newborn stools progress from meconium to transitional stools as feeding begins. Breast-fed babies have loose, yellow stools; babies drinking formula have firmer stools that may be darker in color.
- The nursing client needs information regarding helping the baby latch on; taking care of the nipples; alternating breasts; using different positions; and recognizing complications.
- Bottle-fed babies should be held during feedings just as breast-fed babies. The bottle should not be propped, and the infant should not be left unattended.
- All babies should be bubbled during and after feeding. This can be accomplished by sitting the baby on your lap, holding the baby on your shoulder, or laying the baby across your knees and gently patting his or her back until bubbling occurs. Some spitting up is normal.

CRITICAL THINKING EXERCISES

1. Review the list of newborn reflexes. Why do you think that each of these might exist? Find a book or article that discusses at least one reflex and write down an explanation that you could give to a new parent as you demonstrate the baby's reflex.

2. Heat loss is a critical factor for newborns. Develop a plan to protect a newborn from the major sources of heat loss in an acute care facility. Compare and contrast that plan with an infant delivered at home.

NCLEX-STYLE REVIEW QUESTIONS

1. The nurse is assisting with the care of a newborn after delivery. The newborn has an Apgar score of 10 at 1 min and 5 min. What action does the nurse prepare for?
   a. The newborn is in danger and should be closely monitored.
   b. No action is required since the baby is in the best possible condition.
   c. The newborn requires immediate resuscitation measures.
   d. The newborn requires tactile stimulation.

2. Immediately after the delivery of a newborn, what initial action by the nurse can assist with avoiding heat loss by evaporation?
   a. Lay the infant on the mother's bare chest or stomach.
   b. Wipe the infant's head.
   c. Place the infant in the radiant warmer.
   d. Give the infant a warm bath.

3. The nurse is preparing to administer erythromycin 0.5% ophthalmic ointment to the newborn's eyes. What condition is the nurse preventing the newborn from contracting?
   a. Herpes simplex
   b. Human immunodeficiency virus (HIV)
   c. Ophthalmia neonatorum
   d. Syphilis

4. A newborn received a hepatitis B vaccine after birth. What instructions should be given to the parents by the nurse prior to discharge of the newborn?
   a. This immunization will last throughout the newborn's life.
   b. The newborn should be monitored for signs of hepatitis B.
   c. The newborn will need to be tested for immunity in 1 month.
   d. Be sure remaining doses are given according to CDC guidelines.

5. A parent calls the clinic and states to the nurse, "I changed my newborn daughter's wet diaper and saw a spot of blood on it." What is the best response by the nurse?
   a. "This is known as a pseudomenstruation and should disappear within a week."
   b. "The baby needs to be checked for hormonal disturbance."
   c. "This finding may indicate a serious female reproductive problem."
   d. "You must be mistaken, that isn't possible in a newborn."

CHAPTER RESOURCES

Enhance your learning with additional resources on thePoint!

Student Resources related to this chapter can be found at **thePoint.lww.com/Rosdahl12e**.

CHAPTER 67 Care of the Normal Newborn

Welcome Steps

Look at healthcare provider's orders.

Protocol for procedure.

Necessary equipment/supplies.

Wash hands using proper hand hygiene; put on gloves.

Explain the procedure and reassure the client.

Locate two identifiers to confirm correct client.

Comfortable and efficient position for nurse and client.

Obtain privacy.

Make sure to follow correct steps and body mechanics with good technique.

Ensure safety and observe deviations from normal.

End Steps

Ensure comfort and safety.

Note questions or concerns from client or nurse; note significant data.

Dispose of materials properly.

Disinfect the area and your hands.

Document and report the procedure and your findings.

IN PRACTICE
NURSING PROCEDURE 67-1 — Assisting a Newborn With Breathing

Supplies and Equipment
Gloves
Bulb syringe
Oxygen mask, oxygen tubing
Bag valve mask device (e.g., AMBU bag)
Endotracheal tube and intubation supplies (as found on a crash cart)

Steps
Follow LPN WELCOME Steps and Then

1. Place the newborn in the supine (back-lying) position, with head slightly lower than the body. *Rationale: This position facilitates drainage and counteracts shock.*

2. Maintain the neck in a neutral or "sniffing" position. *Rationale: Hyperextension can cut off the airway. The purpose of resuscitation is to establish an open airway, provide oxygen to the lungs, and stimulate the newborn to breathe.*

3. Provide gentle suction. If using a bulb syringe, compress the bulb before insertion. Suction the mouth before the nose. *Rationale: Suctioning the nose first may trigger a reflex gasping motion, which can lead to aspiration of meconium or mucus in the mouth. In most cases, newborns respond by crying, which clears their respiratory tract of mucus. If suctioning is ineffective, more aggressive techniques will be done.*

4. Physical stimulation, such as rubbing the newborn's chest and feet, may help breathing. However, if the baby does not respond to stimulation, do not keep trying it. *Rationale: Stimulation may not be successful in an infant with moderate to severe respiratory distress, and time should not be taken for stimulation when more aggressive resuscitation efforts are necessary. Physiologic complications, especially during the transitions immediately after birth, may be the reasons for poor respiratory effort.*

5. Provide oxygen by mask or AMBU bag. The mask must be of the proper size to seal over the newborn's mouth and nose. *Rationale: Oxygen deficit may lead to further respiratory compromise, an increase in distress, and eventually death of the newborn.*

6. Occasionally a newborn needs to be intubated, a procedure that can safely be performed only by specially trained personnel. *Rationale: Intubation is performed by individuals who have had training and practice in neonatal resuscitation.*

7. Medication may be necessary to stimulate the newborn to breathe on his or her own. *Rationale: Medications are used according to protocols and criteria established for neonatal resuscitation.*

8. The newborn usually takes nothing by mouth (NPO) until respiration is stabilized. *Rationale: This prevents aspiration.*

9. Administration of antibiotics may be necessary if extensive resuscitation has been done. *Rationale: Because the newborn has been exposed to potentially threatening microorganisms, antibiotics reduce the risk of infection.*

Follow ENDDD Steps

1100 UNIT 10 Maternal and Newborn Nursing

IN PRACTICE

NURSING PROCEDURE 67-2 Prophylaxis for the Eyes of the Neonate

Supplies and Equipment
Gloves
Sterile cotton balls
Sterile water

- Erythromycin (0.5%) ophthalmic ointment or drops (most commonly used)
- Tetracycline (1%) ophthalmic ointment or drops
- Silver nitrate (1%) solution (rarely used)

Steps
Follow LPN WELCOME Steps and Then

1. Clean over the baby's closed eyelids and surrounding area with sterile cotton balls moistened with sterile water. Dry area with soft, sterile gauze. *Rationale: This action removes blood and body fluids left on the skin following birth and reduces the risk of transmitting hepatitis B or HIV through the mucous membrane of the eye.*

2. Stabilize the baby's head, shade the eyes from overhead lighting, and gently separate the lids of one eye by pressing on the lower and upper lids. *Rationale: This allows the medication to reach the conjunctival sac, to prevent blindness caused by eye infection with gonorrhea or chlamydia.*

3. If using ophthalmic drops:
   a. Instill two drops in the conjunctival sac and allow to run across the whole sac. *Rationale: Instillation into the conjunctival sac avoids direct contact with the sensitive cornea.*
   b. Repeat in the other eye. Note: If using silver nitrate, use one ampule for each eye. *Rationale: This provides the proper amount of medication.*
   If using ophthalmic ointment:
   c. Place a thin 1- to 2-cm line of ointment along the conjunctival sac, moving from the inner canthus (angle of eye nearest the nose) to the outer canthus. Be careful not to touch the eyelid or eyeball with the tip of the tube. *Rationale: The tip of the tube could cause injury to the newborn's eye or eyelid or carry infection from one eye to the other.*
   d. Repeat in the other eye. Note: When using eye drops or ointments, use one container (tube, dropper) for each newborn. Some facilities may require that the container be discarded after use in one eye and a new container be used for the other eye. *Rationale: Using a new tube prevents cross-contamination from one baby to another or from one eye to another.*

4. Close the eye and count to 5. Carefully manipulate the eyelids. *Rationale: This technique ensures that the medication is spread thoroughly underneath the eyelid.*

5. After 1 min, gently wipe excess solution or ointment from eyelids and surrounding skin with sterile water. *Rationale: Wiping helps avoid irritation of skin.*

6. Do not irrigate eyes. *Rationale: Irrigation may decrease the effectiveness of the prophylaxis.*

Follow ENDDD Steps

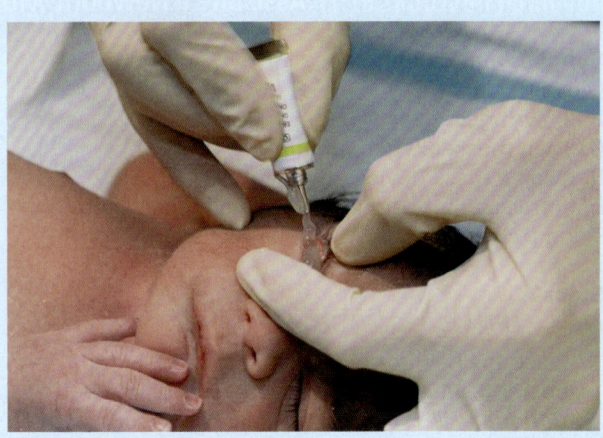

Applying ophthalmic ointment. (Ricci, 2007.)

IN PRACTICE

NURSING PROCEDURE 67-3 Weighing a Neonate

Supplies and Equipment
Towel
Clean diaper
Infant scale

Steps
Follow LPN WELCOME Steps and Then

1. Pad the scale with a towel. Deduct the towel's weight to ensure accuracy. *Rationale: Providing a pad prevents excess heat loss and startling the baby.*

2. Remove all the newborn's clothes and weigh the newborn as quickly as possible. *Rationale: Weighing the baby quickly minimizes the newborn's exposure and discomfort.*

3. Keep your hand close above the newborn at all times. Never leave the newborn unattended (see Fig. 67-2A). *Rationale: This protects the newborn from falling.*

CHAPTER 67 Care of the Normal Newborn   1101

4. Dress the newborn. Use a clean diaper. Place the newborn back in the crib. Discard the towel. Make sure the baby is safe before cleaning up the area. *Rationale: It is important to keep the infant warm. The area needs to be cleaned before being used by another infant to prevent the spread of infection.*

5. Record the weight in grams on the chart for consistency and accuracy. Convert to pounds for the mother's information. *Rationale: Weight must be carefully monitored and documented. Appropriate weight gain is an important aspect of normal infant growth and development. Most medical facilities use the metric system, so converting grams to pounds makes weight more easily understood by a person who is not familiar with the metric system.*

Follow ENDDD Steps

IN PRACTICE
NURSING PROCEDURE 67-4   Measuring Head Circumference

Supplies and Equipment
Disposable paper tape

Steps
Follow LPN WELCOME Steps and Then

1. Explain the procedure to parents and newborn. *Rationale: To lessen anxiety, family members need to be aware of what you are going to do. Infants may respond to a soothing voice.*

2. Place the tape measure over the most prominent part of the occiput and around the forehead, just above the supraorbital ridges (eyebrows) (see Fig. 67-3). *Rationale: The measurement is done in the same place each time so that a consistent point of reference is used and accuracy is maintained.*

3. Hold the child's head in a stable position. *Rationale: The child is stabilized for safety reasons and because movement may cause inaccurate readings.*

4. Tighten the tape so that the reading is accurate. *Rationale: Accuracy and consistency are important because these measurements are compared with previous readings.*

5. Read the measurement over the forehead. Discard the tape. *Rationale: The tape is used for only one infant to prevent possible cross-contamination of microorganisms.*

6. Compare readings with previous measurements or a growth chart and report and document any significant deviations. *Rationale: Interventions may be indicated if measurements are not within normal limits.*

IN PRACTICE
NURSING PROCEDURE 67-5   Bathing a Neonate

Supplies and Equipment
Stethoscope
Pan of warm (98.6 °F or 37 °C) water
Baby wipes, soft cloth, or other material used in your hospital
Baby soap
Cotton balls
Alcohol or antiseptic for cord stump
Cleanser for buttocks
Clean clothes and diaper
Clean crib linens
Trash bag
Fine comb or brush
Watch or clock with second hand
Temperature probe

Steps

1. Check the baby's respiration, pulse, and temperature first, if ordered. Then undress and weigh the newborn before giving the bath (see In Practice: Nursing Procedure 67-3).

2. Wipe each eye with a cotton ball dampened with clear water only. Stroke from the inner to the outer corner of each eye, using a clean cotton ball for each eye. Wipe the rest of the face, including the ears, with a soft cloth; do not use soap. *Rationale: Always go from "clean" to "dirty" areas. Soap is not necessary and is irritating if it gets into the eyes, and it can cause excess skin dryness.*

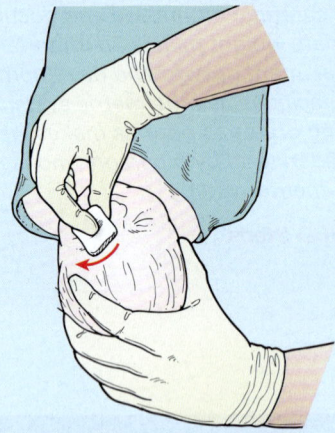

Stroke from the inner to outer corner of each eye.

3. Moisten and wash the hair with a baby shampoo. **Rationale:** *Hair can contain dried blood.*

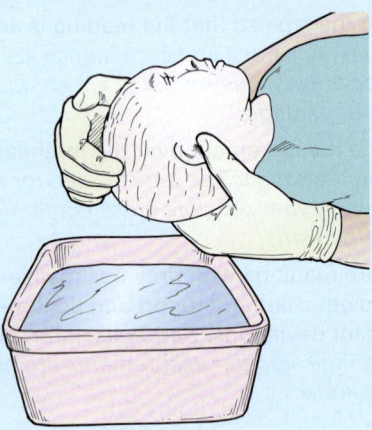

Wash the hair with a baby shampoo.

4. Cleanse the genital area last, checking for signs of rash or irritation. Use cotton balls or baby wipes to cleanse the vulva and perineum from front to back for girls, separating the folds of skin and removing all smegma or discharge. For boys, use the soft cloth to clean the penis, scrotum, and perianal area. **Rationale:** *To prevent contamination of clean areas, always take care to wash from the cleaner areas toward the less-clean areas (clean to dirty).*

5. If a baby boy has been circumcised, provide care as prescribed at your hospital. Check for any unusual swelling or bleeding. Cleanse the penis carefully; report foreskin adhesions immediately. **Rationale:** *Early intervention may prevent more severe problems.*

6. Keep unhealed cord dry. The healthcare provider may order alcohol or Triple Dye cleansing or application of an antibiotic ointment to the cord stump. Be sure to carefully clean the base of the umbilical cord. **Rationale:** *A cord stump that gets wet is more likely to get infected. These substances help speed healing and prevent infection.*

7. Dry the baby's body and hair. Gently comb or brush the hair. Dress the newborn, folding the diaper below the cord stump, and wrap the baby in a blanket. Hold the newborn in a football hold with one arm while changing the crib's linen. **Rationale:** *It is important to prevent the infant from getting cold caused by having a wet body or being on wet linens.*

8. Place the baby on his or her back to sleep. **Rationale:** *Sleeping in a supine position is considered the safest position and is used as one form of protection against sudden infant death syndrome.*

Follow ENDDD Steps

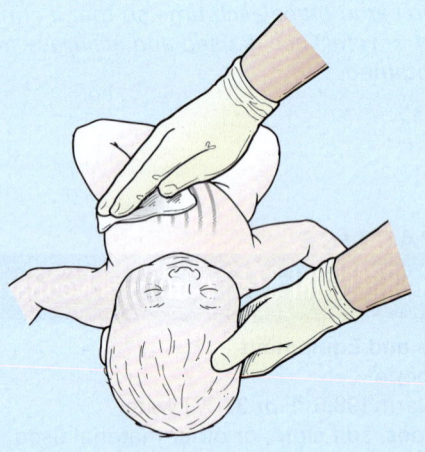

Work from the head down.

IN PRACTICE
NURSING PROCEDURE 67-6 Performing a Heel Stick Procedure on a Newborn

Supplies and Equipment
Nonsterile latex gloves
Warm, moist compress
Alcohol wipe
Sterile gauze
Disposable lancet
Test strip(s) or capillary tube(s)
Small sterile bandage

Steps

Follow LPN WELCOME Steps and Then

1. Warm the newborn's foot. Hold it in the palm of your hand or wrap it in a warm (not hot) moist compress for 3 to 5 min. Do not squeeze the foot too vigorously when obtaining the sample. *Rationale: This may dilute the blood with tissue fluid or cause hemolysis or tissue damage.*

2. Position the newborn with the foot lower than the body to increase blood flow to the foot. Hold the foot dorsiflexed (against the shin), with your thumb and forefinger encircling and exposing the heel and the other fingers stabilizing the ankle. *Rationale: This will reduce the chance of the infant reflexively withdrawing the foot and jerking it away from the stimulus, resulting in either a laceration or an ineffective puncture.*

3. Clean the heel with alcohol; allow to air-dry or completely dry with a sterile gauze square. *Rationale: Alcohol should not enter the puncture wound or dilute the sample.*

4. Use a disposable lancet to make a quick, clean stab in the outer (lateral) surface of the heel. Do not make the puncture wound near the center of the heel or on the sole of the foot. *Rationale: Correct placement minimizes tissue trauma.*

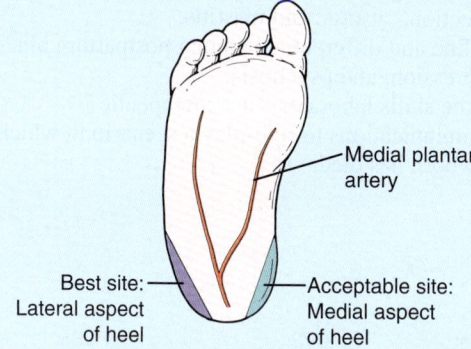

Approximate sites for the heel stick procedure.

5. Wipe off the first drop of blood with a sterile gauze square. *Rationale: Remove blood that could be mixed with skin cells.*

6. When a second large drop forms, without excessive squeezing allow it to fall onto the test strip to cover the sensitive area completely or lightly touch a capillary tube to the drop of blood. *Rationale: Squeezing may dilute blood with tissue fluid. Inadequate sampling may give false results.*

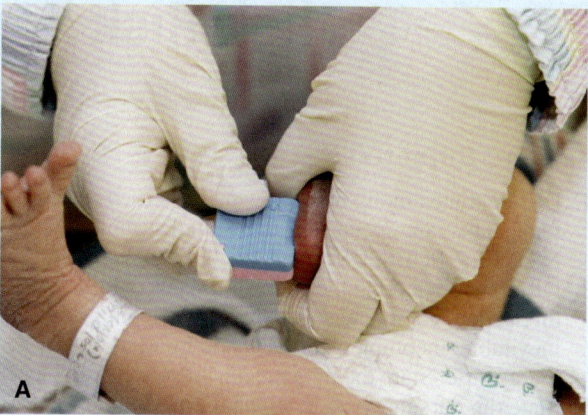

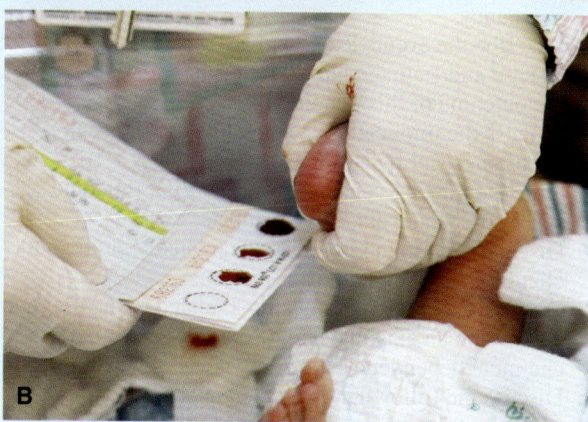

A. Performing a heel stick. **B.** After discarding the first drop of blood, the nurse collects the next drops onto a test strip or a capillary blood tube. (Ricci, 2007.)

7. If the blood flow slows or stops before the sample is complete, wipe the area with a sterile, dry gauze square. This may increase the blood flow. *Rationale: Do not use any liquid on the gauze that would dilute the blood sample.*

8. Follow the manufacturer's directions for the particular test that has been ordered. *Rationale: Each test has specific timing and sample requirements. Not observing these can result in needing to repeat the test.*

9. Apply a small, sterile bandage to the heel; apply gentle continuous pressure over the wound until bleeding stops. *Rationale: Applying pressure controls the bleeding.*

Follow ENDDD Steps

68 High-Risk Pregnancy and Childbirth

Learning Objectives

1. Differentiate among the following tests used to assess fetal status: amniocentesis, ultrasound scanning, OCT, NST, FBP, PUBS, CVS, and MSAFP.
2. Differentiate among the following types of abortions: threatened, complete, septic, recurrent spontaneous, inevitable, incomplete, missed, and induced or therapeutic. State the nursing considerations for each.
3. State the nursing considerations for an ectopic pregnancy.
4. Describe the events leading to gestational trophoblastic disease and state the nursing considerations related to the outcome of this condition.
5. Discuss the implications to client and fetus when hyperemesis gravidarum exists.
6. State the nursing considerations for PIH, mild and severe preeclampsia, and eclampsia.
7. Discuss the nursing implications related to a pregnant client with existing diabetes mellitus.
8. Discuss the nursing implications related to the pregnant client with an existing cardiac disorder or who has a chemical dependency.
9. Discuss the following disorders and state nursing concerns for each condition: maternal infection, Rh sensitization, erythroblastosis fetalis, ABO incompatibility, and polyhydramnios.
10. Differentiate among placenta previa, abruptio placentae, and placenta accreta and discuss the nursing considerations for each condition.
11. Discuss the nursing implications related to each of the following: prolonged pregnancy, multiple pregnancy, adolescent pregnancy, and pregnancy in the client older than 35 years.
12. Develop a nursing plan of care for a client with the following complications: maternal hemorrhage, PROM, preterm labor, precipitate labor and delivery, uterine rupture, uterine inertia and fetal dystocia, CPD, and abnormal fetal presentation.
13. Differentiate the aspects of nursing care related to a prolapsed cord and a nuchal cord.
14. Discuss the nursing considerations related to the induction of labor with drugs and amniotomy.
15. Discuss the nursing considerations related to version, forceps delivery, and vacuum extraction.
16. Discuss the nursing considerations related to preoperative and postoperative care following a cesarean delivery. Identify the special considerations related to care of the newborn.
17. Discuss common complications of the postpartum period, including postpartum hematoma, postpartum hemorrhage, uterine atony, thrombophlebitis, puerperal infection, cystitis, and mastitis.
18. Define and differentiate among postpartum blues, depression, and psychosis.
19. In the skills laboratory, use therapeutic communications to role-play a scenario in which a newborn has died.

Important Terminology

ABO incompatibility
abruptio placentae
amniocentesis
amniotomy
atony
breech
cerclage
cesarean delivery
choriocarcinoma
cystitis
delivery forceps
dystocia
eclampsia
ectopic pregnancy
erythroblastosis fetalis
gestational diabetes
high-risk pregnancy
hydatidiform mole
hyperemesis gravidarum
induction
macrosomia
mastitis
nuchal cord
perinatologist
placenta accreta
placenta previa
polyhydramnios
postpartum hematoma
postpartum hemorrhage
preeclampsia
premature cervical dilation
products of conception
prolapsed cord
puerperal
station
stress test
thrombophlebitis
transverse lie
uterine inertia
vacuum extraction
version
vertex

Acronyms

AB
BOA
BOW
CPD
CVS
D&C
DIC
FBP
FHT
IUGR
LOP
LS
MSAFP
NST
OCT
OP
PIH
PROM
PUBS
ROP
SGA
STI
SVE

Although pregnancy, labor, and delivery are normal physiologic processes, complications can arise at any time, with serious consequences for the client and fetus. The term **high-risk pregnancy** (or *at-risk pregnancy*) is used when physiologic or psychological factors could significantly increase the chances of mortality or morbidity of the client or fetus. Early antepartal care helps to identify these problems so that interventions can begin quickly.

Complications related to childbirth have a physical and an emotional impact. The client faces many hazards to their own well-being, and they have concerns about their baby. For example, prolonged and difficult labor is physically and emotionally draining; this fatigue can interfere with the initial bonding between client and newborn.

TESTS TO ASSESS FETAL STATUS

Various tests are used to assess fetal status and fetal maturity. The most commonly used tests include amniocentesis, ultrasonic scanning, the oxytocin challenge test, and the nonstress test.

Amniocentesis

Amniocentesis is the insertion of a needle through the maternal abdominal wall into the amniotic sac to withdraw amniotic fluid. This invasive test can be performed in the examiner's office or on an outpatient basis. *An ultrasound scan should always precede amniocentesis* to determine the location of the placenta and the fetal parts. The examiner confirms the fetal position by palpation, cleanses the area, and anesthetizes the skin site. They insert a long, sterile needle through the client's abdominal and uterine walls into the amniotic sac. They then withdraw approximately 20 mL of fluid, remove the needle, and cover the insertion site with a bandage. Amniocentesis involves some risk. Placental and fetal damage, premature labor, or abortion may result, although the use of ultrasound minimizes these risks.

Information Provided
Testing of amniotic fluid can reveal a number of abnormalities. It can diagnose some disorders causing fetal intellectual impairment, such as *Down syndrome* or the genetic condition known as *Tay–Sachs* disease. Other conditions can be diagnosed, including the congenital conditions of *muscular dystrophy* and *cystic fibrosis,* as well as some fetal abnormalities, such as *spina bifida.* Amniotic fluid analysis will also reveal a test for fetal lung maturity, called the *LS ratio* (see Chapter 69). Amniocentesis is frequently used to determine the status of an Rh-positive fetus in an Rh-negative client.

The birth attendant may order an amniocentesis when they suspect intrauterine growth restriction (**IUGR**), which generally results in an infant who is small for gestational age (**SGA**) (see Chapter 69). IUGR can begin at any time during pregnancy and is linked to inadequate amounts of oxygen and nutrients necessary for fetal growth. Causes related to maternal conditions include diabetes (gestational or long-standing), placental growth or functioning, intrauterine infection, or pregnancy-induced hypertension (PIH).

Nursing Considerations
Instruct the client to empty their bladder before the test (to prevent bladder rupture). Monitor the client's vital signs during the test and for at least 1 hr afterward. Monitor fetal heart tones (**FHTS**) to ensure that the fetus is not in distress; the external fetal monitor is most often used. Instruct the client to notify the birth attendant if they have any difficulties after returning home, including any bleeding or cramping.

Ultrasonic Scanning

An *ultrasound scan* uses high-frequency sound waves to visualize intrauterine activity and structures. The graphic recording of this picture is called a *sonogram.* From this image, the examiner can learn much about the developing fetus.

A *transducer,* placed on the skin of the abdomen, passes sound waves into the fetus. Because of various densities of body tissues (e.g., bone and muscle), the waves are echoed back to the transducer at different rates. A computer transforms the echo into an image on the monitor.

Information Provided
An ultrasound scan can determine gestational age, fetal head size, location of the placenta, and some fetal abnormalities. It can identify multiple pregnancies, and in some cases, it can also determine the sex of the fetus. Ultrasound is commonly used in conjunction with tests such as amniocentesis. The client is often allowed to watch the fetus move and listen to the heartbeat. They are usually given a print or DVD of the ultrasound to take home.

Nursing Considerations
Explain to the client that a full bladder is necessary for the test so that the fetal parts will move up into the abdomen, allowing for better visualization of the fetus. Ask the client to drink large amounts of liquids. Tell them they will not be allowed to empty their bladder. This test takes 20 min with no known harmful effects. The test is noninvasive.

Oxytocin (Pitocin) Challenge Test

The oxytocin (Pitocin) challenge test (**OCT**), also known as the contraction **stress test**, is a way to evaluate the response of the fetal heart to contractions. Nipple stimulation can initiate uterine contractions, but most often intravenous (IV) oxytocin (Pitocin) is used. An IV administration of oxytocin (Pitocin) by infusion pump is begun. Its rate of administration increases until three contractions occur within 10 min. The reaction of the fetal heart is determined using the fetal monitor. If, toward the end of a contraction, the fetal heart rate decreases (*late deceleration*), uteroplacental insufficiency is indicated, which may lead to fetal death.

Information Provided
The OCT provides information on how well the placenta is supplying oxygen to the fetus. Therefore, it is particularly useful in detecting fetuses that are beginning to experience difficulty because of inadequate placental circulation. An OCT is classified as *positive* when there are persistent late decelerations with more than 50% of the contractions. A decision is made about continuing the pregnancy or performing a cesarean delivery.

Nursing Considerations
Although the OCT is not dangerous in itself, it may stimulate labor. Therefore, it is generally performed in the labor and delivery area of the healthcare facility—rather than in the clinic setting—after the fetus is viable (able to survive outside the uterus: 20–24 weeks' gestation).

Nonstress Test

The nonstress test (**NST**) provides information on the fetal heart rate in response to fetal activity and gives the healthcare provider an indirect measurement of uteroplacental function. The healthy fetus is active in utero, and the fetal heart rate normally increases as the fetus moves in the uterus. To perform the NST, an external fetal monitor is strapped to the client's abdomen, and they are asked to press a button each time they feel the fetus move. This monitoring process is carried out for approximately 40 min. The procedure is usually performed after 28 weeks' gestation. As with the OCT, the NST is generally performed in a location that is close to a place where the client can deliver the baby if necessary.

Information Provided

An NST is classified as *reactive* when at least two episodes of fetal heart rate accelerations of 15 beats per minute (bpm) last at least 15 s within a continuous 10-min period. A reactive test shows that the fetal heart rate increases with every fetal movement and that the fetus is doing well.

A *nonreactive* test shows that the fetal heart rate did not increase with activity, so the fetus may be experiencing lack of oxygen. The fetus may not be active during the course of the test. The fetus is then stimulated by other methods, which include palpating or shaking the uterus, making loud noises, or stimulating the client's nipples.

Nursing Considerations

Explain the steps of the testing and assisting the client physically and emotionally during the procedure. The client needs an empty bladder and should be positioned in a semi-Fowler position. The nurse maintains documentation of the procedure. After the testing period, the nurse assists the client off the table and allows them to void. Fluids may be encouraged at this time. If serial NSTs are scheduled, discuss the date and time of the next test with the client. The healthcare provider will generally discuss the results of the testing.

Fetal Biophysical Profile

The fetal biophysical profile (**FBP**) combines an NST with ultrasonic fetal assessment to check for fetal well-being. Using ultrasound, the examiner evaluates fetal breathing, fetal movement, fetal tone, amniotic fluid volume, and placental grade. These components, including the NST, are scored between 0 (abnormal) and 12 (normal). With a score of 8–12, the fetus is considered to be doing well.

Other Tests

Newer tests providing information from direct access to the fetus are percutaneous umbilical blood sampling (**PUBS**) and chorionic villus sampling (**CVS**). These tests diagnose fetal defects early in pregnancy. They are invasive procedures and carry serious risks for both the client and fetus. Usually, these tests are done if the client is considering an abortion because of a serious genetic defect. PUBS has also become the preferred method of intrauterine blood transfusion for Rh-sensitized fetuses because it can be done early in the pregnancy.

Maternal serum α-fetoprotein (**MSAFP**) levels are increasingly used as a screening tool to detect the presence of fetal neural tube defects and open abdominal wall defects early in pregnancy.

INTERRUPTED PREGNANCY

Pregnancy may be interrupted due to abortion, premature cervical dilation, ectopic pregnancy, or hydatidiform mole. The loss or termination of a pregnancy has physical, psychological, and emotional consequences for the client. Nursing care focuses on meeting the client's immediate needs and providing support.

Abortion

Abortion (**AB**) describes the natural or artificial (through medical intervention) termination of a pregnancy. Abortions occur commonly in nature. Medically induced abortion remains a controversial issue. Certain groups oppose most medically initiated abortions for various reasons. Roman Catholic hospitals, for example, may not perform abortions unless specific criteria are met, such as a life-threatening situation for the client. A healthcare professional may refuse to participate in an induced abortion based on religious or moral grounds.

If the client undergoing abortion is Rh negative, a specific anti-D immune globulin, such as Rh immune globulin (RhoGAM), should be given as a precautionary measure against Rh sensitization.

The two major categories of abortion are (1) *spontaneous* (by natural cause or without medical intervention; often called a *miscarriage* or *pregnancy loss* by laypeople) and (2) *induced* or *therapeutic* (with medical intervention by way of mechanical assistance or medical agents).

Spontaneous Abortion

It is estimated that approximately 10%–20% of all pregnancies end in *spontaneous abortion*. Fetal abnormalities or defects are the most frequent causes of spontaneous abortion. Maternal alcohol use and cigarette smoking may contribute. Other causes include maternal disorders, trauma (e.g., a motor vehicle accident), dietary factors, and abnormalities of pregnancy.

Threatened Abortion

This condition exists any time bleeding or cramping occurs in the first 20 weeks of pregnancy without major cervical dilation. Many birth attendants will not take extreme measures to save such a pregnancy because a spontaneous abortion is often nature's way of dispelling a fetus with malformations or anomalies that may not be compatible with life. If bleeding is slight, however, hormones or muscle relaxants may be given. The client is put to bed with their feet elevated for 48–72 hr. If bleeding stops, they may resume limited activities. If true uterine contractions occur, the prognosis is more guarded.

Complete Abortion

This occurs when the client spontaneously expels all the **products of conception** (i.e., the placenta and fetus). The uterus then contracts toward normal size, and the cervix closes. The same care that routinely follows a normal delivery is given to the client. Observe the client closely for signs of hemorrhage. Check their blood pressure to see that it remains stable. Note and report any changes in skin color, especially pallor or cyanosis. Check their pulse (a weak, rapid pulse is a sign of shock). The birth attendant checks to make sure the uterus is contracted. Document the number of perineal pads the client uses and the amount of bleeding.

Septic Abortion
This is the term given when the contents of the uterus become infected before or during an abortion or when the uterus becomes infected later. *Septic (endotoxic) shock* may occur and may cause maternal death.

Recurrent Spontaneous Abortion
Referred to in the past as *habitual abortion,* this term means that a client has spontaneously lost three or more successive pregnancies. Recurrent spontaneous abortion is often caused by an incompetent cervix that dilates prematurely. In such a case, the birth attendant usually makes every possible effort to save the pregnancy. Attempts are made to determine the cause of the recurrent abortions and to correct the situation if possible. Sometimes, surgery may correct a problem causing the loss.

Some habitual and spontaneous abortions are the result of **premature cervical dilation** during the second or early third trimester of pregnancy. This situation is also called *incompetent cervix.* Premature cervical dilation simply means that the cervix is unable to support a pregnancy. The weight of the fetus is sufficient to force the cervix to dilate, causing a spontaneous abortion. Causes of this condition include cervical infections (e.g., chlamydia), cervical or vaginal cancer, previous cervical biopsies or conizations, and prior multiple dilation and curettage procedures. The cervical weakness may be congenital; one such cause is maternal exposure to diethylstilbestrol in utero.

Minor surgical procedures are often used for the pregnant client with an incompetent cervix. A nonabsorbable suture called a cervical **cerclage** or cervical ring is placed around the cervix. This suture holds the cervix closed during the remainder of the pregnancy; when the client begins labor, the suture or ring is removed. If the cerclage is permanent, the client requires a cesarean delivery.

Inevitable Abortion
An abortion in which the loss of the products of conception cannot be prevented is known as an *inevitable abortion.* Increased cramping and blood loss, with progressive cervical dilation, characterize this type of abortion.

Incomplete Abortion
This type of abortion occurs when the uterus expels some products of conception but retains others. Extensive bleeding may occur. In this case, the healthcare provider may perform a dilation and curettage (**D&C**), which may also be called a dilation and evacuation, of the uterus. In a D&C, the surgeon dilates the cervix and then inserts instruments into the uterus. The uterine walls are scraped to remove any products of conception.

Missed Abortion
A *missed abortion* occurs when the fetus has died but remains in the uterus. If the fetus is not expelled spontaneously within 1 month, the pregnancy will be terminated, and a D&C performed.

For inevitable, incomplete, and missed abortions occurring between 16 and 20 weeks of pregnancy, a drug called dinoprostone (Prostin E2) may be administered to the client. The drug causes the uterus to expel the fetus.

Induced Abortion
Therapeutic Abortion
A *therapeutic abortion* is the legal termination of pregnancy under a healthcare provider's direction. Induced abortion before the 16th–20th week of gestation is legal in the United States and in many other countries, although an abortion may be difficult to obtain in some areas. It may be done for medical or personal reasons.

A therapeutic abortion may be recommended for a client whose life is in jeopardy due to the stress of pregnancy. Medical reasons for therapeutic abortion include severe maternal cardiac disease, severe renal or hypertensive disorder, or a fetus with a high probability of congenital anomaly. In some situations, abortion is performed as an elective procedure.

Certain congenital disorders, which amniocentesis can determine at about the 14th week of gestation, are an indication for abortion to avoid the birth of a severely impaired child. If the client has rubella (German measles) during pregnancy, especially during the first trimester, the likelihood of fetal defects is strong, and an abortion may be performed (see Chapter 74).

Criminal or Illegal Abortion
An intervention in pregnancy performed without medical or legal justification is a *criminal* or *illegal abortion.* When appropriate professionals or facilities are not available, a client may reach out to alternate nonmedical or unprofessional individuals to obtain an abortion. Facilities, the equipment, and the procedure may not be sterile, and the risks to the pregnant client are great. Major risks include hemorrhage, infection leading to sepsis, and a high mortality rate.

Complications of Abortion
When the placenta separates from the uterus, large blood vessels are exposed, which can lead to severe infection or hemorrhage. During the time when most abortions were performed illegally and, generally, under unsanitary conditions, sepsis was a common concern.

Untreated, postabortion sepsis can be fatal. *Sterility* (the inability to conceive) is another common result. Therefore, maintaining *surgical asepsis* (sterile conditions) and removing all the products of conception from the uterus are vitally important.

Therapeutic abortions involve complex and difficult decisions. Regardless of the decision, depression, guilt, and anger are not uncommon psychological concerns.

> **Nursing Alert** A client's blood pressure that spontaneously and rapidly drops may indicate maternal hemorrhage.

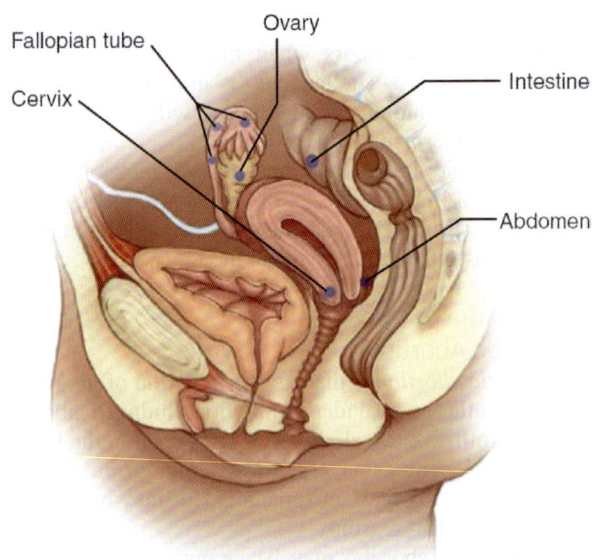

Figure 68-1 Possible sites of ectopic pregnancy. (Klossner & Hatfield, 2010.)

> **Box 68-1 High-Risk Pregnancies**
>
> - Maternal age older than 35 years
> - Preconception health issues
>   - Addiction
>   - Smoking
>   - Poor eating habits
> - Preexisting medical conditions
> - Medical conditions that develop during pregnancy
>   - Premature labor
>   - Multiple births
>   - Placenta previa
>   - Fetal problems
> - Preeclampsia and eclampsia

Ectopic Pregnancy

The word **ectopic** means *outside;* therefore, an ectopic pregnancy is one that implants outside the uterus (Fig. 68-1). The most common ectopic pregnancy is a *tubal pregnancy*. In rare cases, *abdominal* and *ovarian pregnancies* are seen.

Factors predisposing to ectopic pregnancy are tubal occlusion, an intrauterine contraceptive device, tumors, pelvic infections, endocrine imbalances, and abnormal tubal development. The symptoms of an ectopic pregnancy begin with spotting or bleeding 2–3 weeks after a missed menstrual period. Often pain accompanies the bleeding, which may be quite severe. A tubal pregnancy requires surgical removal of part or all of the affected tube to prevent rupture, a dangerous complication. An untreated ectopic pregnancy can be rapidly fatal due to shock from blood loss after tubal rupture.

> **NCLEX Alert**
>
> Common questions may include situations that need immediate nursing actions, such as with ectopic pregnancy.

Gestational Trophoblastic Disease (Hydatidiform Mole)

In *gestational trophoblastic disease,* also known as **hydatidiform mole**, trophoblasts, the cells that normally develop into the placenta, grow at an abnormal rate forming grape-like clusters (Mayo Clinic, 2017). At first, the pregnancy appears normal; however, over time the uterus enlarges more rapidly than usual. The client has episodes of spotting and bleeding, with brownish-red discharge of "tapioca-like" vesicles. The mole can become very large. Typically there is no fetus formed in a gestational trophoblastic disease pregnancy. However, in the case a fetal tissue forms, the fetus does not survive and is miscarried during the pregnancy (Johns Hopkins, 2020).

The signs and symptoms of hydatidiform mole include vaginal bleeding, a uterus that is larger than expected for the weeks of pregnancy, anemia, excessive nausea and vomiting, and signs of PIH occurring before 24 weeks of pregnancy. No fetal heart rate, fetal movement, or palpable fetal parts are detectable. After diagnosis is certain, a healthcare provider usually performs a careful D&C.

Documentation following a client's D&C should include the amount and character of the expelled tissue, which should be saved and sent for pathologic examination. Aseptic techniques should be used to avoid infection. Because the experience is frightening, the client needs a great deal of emotional support.

Follow-up after delivery of a hydatidiform mole is essential. A *human chorionic gonadotropin (hCG) titer* must be done; the titer ratio should fall after delivery. Titer that remains high or rises often indicates a situation known as **choriocarcinoma**, which can be fatal and is treated with chemotherapy. The client should be counseled to avoid pregnancy for at least 1 year until a series of negative hCG levels are found and chemotherapy treatment is finished. Any contraceptive method, other than an intrauterine device, is acceptable. If the client is Rh-negative, administration of an anti-D gamma globulin (e.g., RhoGAM) is required to prevent Rh sensitization.

MATERNAL COMPLICATIONS DURING PREGNANCY

In addition to the complications related to an incomplete or interrupted pregnancy, many types of complications can occur during a pregnancy that becomes known as a high-risk pregnancy. An obstetrician called a **perinatologist**, specializing in maternal–fetal medicine, may be part of the OB team. The loss of the fetus or long-term damage to the client's health is not necessarily directly related to a complication. Many disorders that affect the client, fetus, placenta, or amniotic fluid require early treatment and careful monitoring. Clients with existing medical conditions who become pregnant often have special requirements and need special attention. Box 68-1 lists some of the most common causes of high-risk pregnancy.

PRAMS, the Pregnancy Risk Assessment Monitoring System, is a surveillance project of the CDC and state health departments, with the goal of collecting information about state-specific maternal attitudes and experiences before, during, and shortly after pregnancy. The data are used to identify groups of clients and infants at high risk for health problems, to monitor changes in health status, and to measure progress toward goals for improving the health of clients and infants. The goals include the collection and use of reproductive health and advocate programs that reduce health problems among clients and infants.

> **Key Concept**
> Any bleeding in pregnancy or labor is a serious sign and must be reported immediately to the healthcare provider.

The most common disorders related to pregnancy that affect the client are hyperemesis gravidarum and PIH.

Hyperemesis Gravidarum

Hyperemesis gravidarum, or *pernicious vomiting*, is more severe than normal morning sickness. Its cause is unknown; however, various theories include toxins in the client's bloodstream, possible hormonal imbalances, and emotional conditions related to digestive disturbances. For example, clients whose established reaction to stress involves gastrointestinal disturbances often react the same way to pregnancy.

Morning sickness usually begins between the second and fourth week of gestation and ends at approximately the 12th week, although it may continue throughout the pregnancy. Persistent vomiting to the point of excessive weight loss, dehydration, severe loss of appetite, and acetone in the urine are signs of hyperemesis gravidarum. The client also may have excessive salivation (*ptyalism*), epigastric and rib discomfort, constipation or diarrhea, nutritional anemia, and electrolyte imbalances. Few drugs can be used without potential harm to the fetus. The client may receive IV glucose and water with electrolytes, antiemetics, and sedatives. In the more advanced stages, severe headache, mental aberrations, delirium, coma, jaundice, and cyanosis may occur. In severe cases, an abortion may be necessary to save the client's life.

Pregnancy-Induced Hypertension

Hypertension, edema, and proteinuria are conditions that characterize **PIH**. Not all of these parameters must be present for the diagnosis of PIH. *Edema* is more indicative of advancing disease and multiorgan involvement. PIH may occur antepartally, intrapartally, or postpartally. It is a major contributor to maternal and fetal morbidity and mortality.

The symptoms of PIH result from vasoconstriction and vasospasm of blood vessels throughout the body. The central nervous system, kidneys, and liver may be affected. Decreased blood flow to the placenta and uterus may endanger the fetus.

Prompt treatment of PIH includes controlling symptoms as much as possible and allowing labor to start normally or initiating it when the safety of the client and fetus best permits.

Following delivery, the client with PIH must continue to be monitored. If the elevated blood pressure continues for more than 42 days after delivery, they are diagnosed with *chronic hypertension*. A 6-week checkup should include extensive evaluation of the client's blood pressure, complete blood count, blood urea nitrogen, urinalysis, and creatinine level. Magnesium sulfate, the drug of choice for PIH, is often continued for 24 hr after delivery.

PIH is divided into preeclampsia and eclampsia, depending on the symptoms (Table 68-1).

TABLE 68-1　Signs and Symptoms of Preeclampsia and Eclampsia

MILD PREECLAMPSIA	SEVERE PREECLAMPSIA	ECLAMPSIA
Weight gain: 1 lb/week during second and third trimesters; 4.5 lb in a week anytime during pregnancy	Weight gain, as in mild preeclampsia	Symptoms of severe preeclampsia plus below
1+ or 2+ proteinuria (0.3 g/L in 24-hr urine)	3+ or 4+ proteinuria (≥5 g in 24-hr urine) in two random urine specimens collected at least 6 hr apart	
Urine output ≥30 mL/hr; output = intake	Abnormally small amount of urine secretion (*oliguria*) in relation to fluid intake with fluid retention and edema. Urine output: ≤30 mL/hr or 120 mL/4 hr	Maximum urine albumin level with scanty urine output
BP ≥140/90 mm Hg or elevated by ≥30 mm Hg systolic or ≥15 mm Hg diastolic on two occasions 4–6 hr apart	BP ≥160 mm Hg systolic or ≥110 mm Hg diastolic or elevation of ≥30 mm Hg diastolic recorded on two occasions, 6 hr apart while the client is on bed rest	Very high blood pressure (>170/110 mm Hg; systolic can be above 200 mm Hg)
Hyperreflexia—no clonus	Hyperreflexia—with clonus	
Edema—fingers, face, legs, feet	Severe, unremitting frontal or occipital headache Nausea and persistent vomiting Abdominal pain, epigastric pain Visual disturbances Localized arterial spasms of retina	Fever Seizures, coma

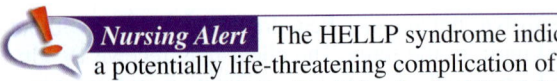

Nursing Alert The HELLP syndrome indicates a potentially life-threatening complication of PIH:
- **H**emolysis (destruction of red blood cells [RBCs])
- **E**levated **L**iver enzymes
- **L**ow **P**latelet count

Preeclampsia

The client who previously was experiencing normal progression of pregnancy but who develops PIH with edema, proteinuria, or both (usually after the 20th week of gestation) has **preeclampsia**. Preeclampsia develops in approximately 5% of pregnancies, most often in primigravidas and in clients with a history of high blood pressure or vascular disorders. Although the symptoms most often allow the obstetrician to intercept preeclampsia and treat it early, it can occur explosively, perhaps the day after an examination. An expectant client should report symptoms to the birth attendant immediately.

Predicting preeclampsia is also possible with a test in which the client's blood pressure is measured while they lay on their back and again while they lay on their left side. This test is referred to as the "roll-over test." It is performed most often in the examiner's office. If the client's diastolic blood pressure is 20 mm Hg higher (or greater) when they are lying on their back, preeclampsia is likely. They should be advised to rest on their left side as much as possible. The birth attendant usually sees this client every 2 days during the entire pregnancy.

Mild Preeclampsia

This condition may be treated at home with sedation or tranquilizers and a regular diet (with salted foods omitted in some cases). Resting in a lateral position (particularly on the left side) aids in placental circulation. The client is encouraged to rest most of the time and avoid climbing stairs.

Severe Preeclampsia

The symptoms of severe preeclampsia are identified in Table 68-1. These clients must be admitted to a healthcare facility because the eclampsia that may follow is one of the leading causes of maternal death in North America.

When treating the client with preeclampsia, check intake and output and body weight daily. Output must be at least 30 mL/hr. The client may have an indwelling catheter. Take vital signs at least every 2 hr; use the fetal monitor to assess fetal status. A low-fat, high-protein diet may be necessary, or the client may be NPO (nothing by mouth) and have an IV, such as Ringer solution. Check the urine for albumin at least twice daily. Reduce external stimuli as much as possible. In Practice: Nursing Care Plan 68-1 discusses an adolescent with PIH.

Ensure that the client and their family understand the following precautions:

- Visiting is restricted.
- The room is kept quiet and fairly dark.
- Sedatives are given.
- The client is on bed rest.

IN PRACTICE
NURSING CARE PLAN 68-1 The Adolescent Client With Severe Preeclampsia

Medical History: D. L., a 15-year-old, single, primipara client at 30 weeks of pregnancy, comes to the emergency department complaining of a persistent headache for the past 3 days and blurred vision. Blood pressure is 190/110 mm Hg with hyperactive deep-tendon reflexes and mild clonus. Urine sample is obtained and reveals 3+ for protein. Marked edema is noted in the face and lower extremities. Client states, "I've been to the clinic once since I became pregnant." Client's medical history is negative, except for being underweight for height. Prepregnancy weight of 102 lb; height of 5 ft 6 in. The client is admitted to the hospital for evaluation and treatment.

Medical Diagnosis: Pregnancy-induced hypertension (PIH), severe preeclampsia

I. DATA COLLECTION/NURSING OBSERVATION

Client is an adolescent with marked edema of face, ankles, and feet. Edema is +1 pitting. They stated, "I noticed that my feet looked a bit puffy and that my shoes felt tight. And I gained almost 3 lb since the day before yesterday." On admission to the unit, client's weight is 124 lb and vital signs are as follows: Temperature, 98.2 °F (36.8 °C); pulse, 98 bpm and regular; respirations, 22 breaths per minute. Blood pressure is 190/102 mm Hg. Fetal heart rate at 154 bpm. Fundal height is 30 cm. Client reports that they have felt the baby move earlier today. Urine sample obtained reveals 3+ for protein. Client states, "I haven't been going to the bathroom as much over the last couple of days even though I've been drinking a lot of fluids." Dietary history reveals intake of large amounts of carbohydrates and minimal protein. Hyperactive patellar (knee-jerk) reflex is noted, with mild ankle clonus.

II. NURSING DIAGNOSIS

(Although several nursing diagnoses may be appropriate, a priority nursing diagnosis is addressed below.) Injury risk (maternal and fetal) related to physiologic effects of severe preeclampsia as evidenced by hypertension, proteinuria, edema, headache, and blurred vision.

CHAPTER 68 High-Risk Pregnancy and Childbirth   1111

3. PLANNING (Outcomes/Goals)	4. IMPLEMENTATION (Nursing Actions)	5. EVALUATION
Short-term goals		
A. Prevent onset of seizures.	• Obtain baseline VS and physical data. *Rationale: Baseline information will be the foundation of medical and nursing treatment. As VS crisis and seizures are a possibility, it is essential that data gathering and physical assessments are completed ASAP.* • Set up client's unit for possible emergency intervention. *Rationale: Preparation ahead of a crisis will save valuable time if seizures occur.*	Day 1—1,800 hr. Hypertension, weight gain, protein in urine, and hyperactive reflexes noted. **Goal A complete.** Observations continue.
B. Educate client and caregivers/family of potential, urgent, and emergency changes of maternal–fetal situation.	• Explain condition and necessity for treatment to the client, including measures to help them participate in care. *Rationale: Understanding of events and treatments fosters compliance and helps to alleviate anxiety and stress. Participating in care helps client to regain some control over the situation.*	Day 1—1,815 hr. Client and caregivers/family notified of seriousness of client's condition. Confusion stated as to how condition began but client and caregivers state understanding of current status. **Goal B met.**
C. Promote sedate environment that caregivers/significant others (family, friends) and client will observe during hospitalization.	• Place the client in a private room. • Dim any lighting and keep the room as quiet as possible. • Restrict visitors to only the client's immediate family. *Rationale: With PIH and preeclampsia, the client's central nervous system is irritable. Decreasing external stimuli (e.g., light, sound, and noise) and stress help to reduce the risk of seizures.*	Day 1—2,000 hr. Client maintaining bed rest reporting that headache is lessening. **Goals A, B, and C met.**
D. Reduce maternal blood pressure and heart rate gradually to within acceptable parameters, with diastolic controlled between 90 and 100 mm Hg.	• Monitor VS and status every 15 min for 1–2 hr (or more often). *Rationale: During preeclampsia, effects of BP medications can be variable with sudden onset of hypotension or hypertension possible.* • Administer an antihypertensive agent such as hydralazine (Apresoline). *Rationale: An antihypertensive such as hydralazine (Apresoline) medication is needed. BP med reduces the client's BP while protecting the fetal circulation.* • Continue to monitor every ½ hr gradually decreasing VS monitoring to 1–2 hr. • If possible, alternate arms when taking BPs. *Rationale: Increases in BP can be a warning of imminent problems needing emergency measures. However, obtaining VS can be painful especially if taken frequently. Pain can increase blood pressure which can lead to further hypertensive complications.*	Day 2—0,300 hr. VS demonstrated significant decrease. Stabilized for 4 hr. BP maintained less than 130/85 mm Hg. **Goal D in progress.** Observations continue.

3. PLANNING (Outcomes/Goals)	4. IMPLEMENTATION (Nursing Actions)	5. EVALUATION
E. Follow hospital protocol for administration of antihypertensive medications for prevention of seizures r/t PIH and preeclampsia.	• Assist with the monitoring of antiseizure medications such as IV infusions of magnesium sulfate. *Rationale: Magnesium sulfate acts to reduce edema and depress central nervous system irritability.* • Frequently check level of consciousness (LOC), deep-tendon reflexes, and respirations. *Rationale: Decreases in LOC, respirations, and reflex activity can occur indicating toxicity.* • Have calcium gluconate readily available at the bedside. *Rationale: Calcium gluconate (Kalcinate) is the antidote for magnesium toxicity.* • Assist with obtaining laboratory specimens, including serum magnesium levels, as ordered. *Rationale: Laboratory specimens provide valuable information about the client's condition.*	Day 1—2000 hr. IV rate and infusion site monitored by RN and LPN. IV without infiltration or infusion complications. Deep-tendon reflexes are within normal range. No signs and symptoms of magnesium toxicity or seizures. Client's LOC demonstrates sleepiness, but they do awaken with light skin touch. **Goal E met.** Observations continue.
F. Follow hospital protocol for administration of sedatives, hypnotics, and anti-anxiety medications for PIH and preeclampsia.	• Monitor blood pressure every 5–30 min until stabilized. • Continue monitoring of hydralazine (Apresoline) or nifedipine (Procardia). *Rationale: Clients status can change rapidly. An increase in BP can lead to eclampsia (seizures and deterioration of client). An antihypertensive agent is needed to reduce BP while maintaining fetal circulation.* • When VS stable, monitor BP and LOC every 1–2 hr, as indicated by client's vital signs and needs for increased sedation. *Rationale: Continued monitoring necessary as preeclampsia may worsen without major physical changes. Antiseizure, sedatives, or hypnotic meds,* e.g., *phenytoin (Dilantin), phenobarbital (Luminal), or diazepam (Valium) may be needed to lessen anxiety and to decrease impulses to CNS.* • Have emergency supplies readily available at the client's bedside. *Rationale: Having emergency resuscitation equipment and medications near to client which saves time—an important consideration in a crisis.*	Day 1—2000 hr. Blood pressure decreasing gradually from initial readings to 140/94 mm Hg. Respirations at 20 breaths per minute; client alert and oriented. Emergency equipment with additional meds positioned just outside of client's room. **Goals E and F partially met.** Observations continue.
G. Urinary output at least 30–50 mL/hr.	• Assess intake and output frequently. If ordered, insert a retention catheter to monitor urine output hourly. *Rationale: Oliguria is a sign of preeclampsia and also magnesium toxicity. Urine output needs to be at least 30 mL/hr to indicate adequate renal function.* • Check urine for protein. *Rationale: Checking urine for protein helps to determine the severity of the preeclampsia.*	Day 2—0300 hr. Urine output at 50 mL/hr for 3 hr. Urine 1+ for protein. **Goal G partially met.** Observations continue.

3. PLANNING (Outcomes/Goals)	4. IMPLEMENTATION (Nursing Actions)	5. EVALUATION
H. Fetal circulation retains adequate placental and cord blood flow.	• Monitor fetal status at least hourly or more often if conditions indicate increased risk to fetus. *Rationale: The client's hypertension can decrease placental perfusion and subsequently the nutrient and oxygen supply to the fetus.* • Encourage client to lie on their side as much as possible. *Rationale: The left side-lying position, compared to the supine position, enhances blood flow to the uterus, the placenta, and the fetus.*	Day 1—2000 hr. Fetal heart rate ranging from 144–156 bpm; client maintaining left lateral (left side-lying) position; client reports no signs and symptoms of labor. Membranes intact. **Goal H met.** Observations continue.
Long-Term Goals		
I. Client is able to maintain pregnancy to term.	• Monitor client for signs of impending labor. *Rationale: Adolescents have an increased risk for preterm labor. Preeclampsia clients at high risk for early labor.* • Monitor VS, weight gain/loss, and urine output at least daily. • Encourage a moderate-to-high protein, moderate-sodium diet. *Rationale: Large amounts of protein are being lost in the client's urine and must be replaced. Moderate amounts of sodium are necessary to maintain electrolyte balance. The client's weight is a valuable indicator of fluid balance.*	Day 2—0900 hr. Weight decreased to 122 lb (2 lb loss since admission). Blood pressure maintained about 128/85 mm Hg for 8 hr. Edema of face, hands, and lower extremities decreased to moderate; no pitting noted. **Goal I met.** Observations continue.
J. Healthy neonate delivered as close as possible to 40 weeks' gestation.	• Observation and documentation of maternal and fetal status to continue at regular intervals, e.g., q (every) 4 hr. *Rationale: As maternal condition stabilizes, fetal environment also stabilizes. Client will need continued monitoring until delivery of infant.*	Day 2—0900 hr. FHR averages 142 bpm. Maternal BP stable. No sign of seizure activity. Fetal heart rate and maternal vital signs within acceptable parameters. **Goal J met.** Observations continue.

- The client should lie on their left side as much as possible. (*Rationale: This helps to facilitate renal circulation in the client and placental circulation for the fetus.*)
- All intake and output are measured.
- Vital signs are taken often; weight is taken daily.
- Level of consciousness and reflexes are checked often.
- Blood is drawn periodically for testing.
- The fetus is monitored.
- Hospital protocol initiated regarding the use of (padded) side rails which may be required to prevent injury or falls from bed during a seizure.

The drug of choice in the treatment of severe preeclampsia (and prevention of eclampsia) is magnesium sulfate given via IV or intramuscularly (IM). This potent anticonvulsant drug slows neuromuscular conduction and depresses central nervous system irritability, thus reducing muscle excitability and hyperreflexia. Although the vasodilating effects of magnesium sulfate will lower the blood pressure slightly, this action is only transient. The main reason for administering magnesium sulfate is to prevent seizures, not to lower blood pressure.

Because of the drug's effects on the central nervous system, assess the client's respirations and deep-tendon reflexes frequently. Observe and report any changes. Also, monitor urinary output because oliguria can result from excessively high levels of magnesium sulfate in the blood. Calcium gluconate (Kalcinate) is the specific antidote for magnesium sulfate. It is kept at the bedside at all times while the client receives magnesium sulfate and is used if toxicity occurs.

If magnesium sulfate does not control seizures, diazepam (Valium) may be used. Furosemide (Lasix) may be needed to stimulate urine output. Potassium (K^+) often is given with furosemide (Lasix).

An IV is usually kept running to administer fluids and to keep the vein open in case emergency drugs must be given. Electrolytes are replaced via the IV, as blood tests determine needs. If blood pressure remains dangerously elevated, additional medications may be ordered. Hydralazine HCl (Apresoline) is the antihypertensive agent of choice, although labetalol HCl (Normodyne), methyldopa (Aldomet, Dopamet [Canada]), and nifedipine (Adalat, Procardia) are sometimes used. However, the client's blood pressure should not be reduced too much or too quickly to avoid causing fetal anoxia. Maintain blood pressure in the range of 90–100 mm Hg diastolic.

> **NCLEX Alert**
>
> Medications, indications, and contraindications for specific obstetric or neonatal situations may be found on examinations. Be sure to know nursing actions for these medications.

When the client at or near term is stabilized, the fetus will usually be delivered. *Induction,* stimulating labor by using a medication such as oxytocin (Pitocin), will be done if the cervix is ripe. If it is not ripe, cesarean (surgical) delivery is performed. If the fetus is not mature enough to survive, the pregnancy may be sustained for a short time. If the client's condition worsens, the fetus will usually be sacrificed to save the client's life.

Eclampsia

Because of the availability of successful medical therapies, few clients progress to the serious stage called **eclampsia**, which is likely to occur if preeclampsia is left untreated. Eclampsia is one of the most severe complications of pregnancy. Generalized tonic–clonic seizures, very rapid pulse, and very high blood pressure (see Table 68-1) characterize eclampsia, which develops in 1 of every 200 clients with preeclampsia.

After a seizure, the client may regain consciousness within a few minutes, or they may remain in a coma for several hours or days. Seizures may recur in either instance. Even when a client awakens after seizures, they may be confused. The treatment for eclampsia is basically the same as that for severe preeclampsia, with delivery performed as soon as possible.

If seizures continue, the coma deepens. The "slushy" respirations characteristic of lung edema are audible, and the client's prognosis is now poor. The primary causes of maternal death caused by hypertension are circulatory collapse, cerebral hemorrhage, and renal failure. A major complication is abruptio placentae with maternal hemorrhage.

EXISTING DISORDERS COMPLICATING PREGNANCY

Some pregnant clients have existing conditions that may complicate pregnancy and that require special attention. Such conditions include diabetes mellitus and cardiac disorders. Chemical dependency is another existing condition that requires special considerations to protect both the client and the fetus (see Chapter 69).

Diabetes Mellitus

Diabetes mellitus is an endocrine disorder in which the pancreas fails to produce sufficient insulin for proper use of glucose (see Chapter 79). A diabetic client needs special care and monitoring during pregnancy because insulin requirements fluctuate. Even when diabetes is monitored carefully, the pregnant client and the developing fetus are at risk. Clients with diabetes ideally should receive optimal care and client education before conception to prevent interrupted pregnancy and congenital malformations in their babies. Tight metabolic control can be achieved with intensive self-management and preparation for pregnancy.

Potential problems during pregnancy include fetal death, **macrosomia** (oversized fetus), a fetus with a respiratory disorder, difficult labor, preeclampsia or eclampsia, polyhydramnios, and congenital malformations.

Diabetes is usually more difficult to control during pregnancy. The client may become *hyperglycemic,* with resulting acidosis or diabetic coma. They also may become *hypoglycemic,* with resulting fetal hypoxia. The pregnant client with insulin-dependent diabetes will need to learn to administer their own insulin injections during the pregnancy. Depending on the condition of the client and fetus, clients with diabetes may deliver early (36–38 weeks) by induction or cesarean delivery.

> **Nursing Alert** A reaction to too little or too much insulin is a danger to the client, especially during labor and immediately after delivery. The client's body reacts to the trauma of birth, and their glucose level is easily upset.

Blood glucose testing, dietary adjustments, and danger signs that must be reported are necessary teaching for the diabetic client and their family. Family teaching is important because the client may be unable to recognize these signs in time to be able to take action (In Practice: Educating the Client 68-1).

Clients with diabetes should be under the care of an internist and an obstetrician during pregnancy. Frequent antepartal visits are essential. Careful fetal monitoring is necessary during labor, and the newborn must be assessed carefully. Generally, these newborns are treated as premature babies.

IN PRACTICE
EDUCATING THE CLIENT 68-1 — The Pregnant Client With Diabetes

Client and family teaching for the pregnant client with diabetes includes the following:
- Method for self-testing blood for glucose several times per day
- Insulin and diet adjustments based on glucose level
- Method for insulin injections if the client has not used insulin previously
- Signs of hyperglycemia and hypoglycemia
- Actions to take if hyperglycemia or hypoglycemia occurs
- Signs and symptoms of beginning preeclampsia

An increasing number of pregnant clients develop diabetes for the first time during pregnancy, a condition called **gestational diabetes**. Although management of gestational diabetes through diet alone works for some clients, others will require insulin. Most clients will return to prepregnancy glucose levels following delivery. Clients with gestational diabetes mellitus and clients who have delivered a baby weighing more than 9 lb are known to develop type 1 or 2 diabetes in later years. These clients should be advised that they are at higher risk than others.

Cardiac Disorders

Pregnancy places additional strain on the heart. Because of the increased blood volume, the greatest dangers are during the last trimester, labor, and delivery. During labor, clients with a history of cardiac problems should be assessed for dyspnea, chest pain, and pulmonary edema.

During pregnancy, the client with a cardiac condition should get plenty of rest and avoid activities that result in shortness of breath. They should maintain a diet that will prevent excessive weight gain and water retention. Usually, sodium (salt) is restricted. The client's prognosis depends on their age and the severity and type of heart disease.

Clients with cardiac disorders often successfully deliver their babies. Current belief is that a vaginal delivery is safer for the client than a cesarean delivery because of the added strain of surgery. However, induced labor and early delivery may prevent a difficult labor.

Chemical Dependency

The pregnant client with an addiction may be malnourished. Their addiction may result in a failure to seek antepartal care. Drug use may account for stillbirth, spontaneous abortion, abruptio placentae, and numerous congenital defects. The pregnant client who is chemically dependent may lack parenting skills. Child protection authorities should be involved early in the pregnancy of a client who is chemically dependent.

DISORDERS AFFECTING THE FETUS

Some disorders present special concerns for fetal health and well-being. Infections, including *sexually transmitted infections* (STIs), not only require careful maternal treatment but also can compromise fetal health (see Chapter 70). *Hemolytic conditions,* such as Rh sensitization and ABO incompatibility, also warrant careful evaluation.

Infection

Maternal infections can harm the fetus. For instance, a severe respiratory disease, such as *viral pneumonia*, can cause fetal anoxia. If the client contracts *rubella* early in pregnancy, fetal malformation is a strong possibility. A client whose rubella titer is low (<1:10) does not have the antibodies to fight rubella. If this client is exposed to rubella, gamma globulin may be given. An abortion may be an option. After the pregnancy, the mother is immunized for rubella. They should be cautioned not to become pregnant for at least 3 months after this immunization to avoid harm to the next fetus.

Maternal STIs are often transmitted to the fetus. Maternal/fetal circulation transmits syphilis, gonorrhea, herpesvirus 2, and human immunodeficiency virus or acquired immunodeficiency syndrome (HIV/AIDS; see Chapters 70 and 85).

Rh Sensitization

Rh sensitization is preventable in most cases. In Rh sensitization, the pregnant client is Rh negative, but Rh-positive red blood cells from the fetus cross the placental barrier and enter the maternal circulation. Because the Rh-positive cells become antigens in the Rh-negative client, they stimulate the formation of antibodies within the client's circulatory system. These antibodies return to the fetus, destroying the fetal erythrocytes. An Rh-negative client who has produced these antibodies is said to be *sensitized*. The newborn in this situation is born with a condition known as **erythroblastosis fetalis**.

The sensitization of the client in erythroblastosis fetalis usually occurs at or near the delivery, so the antibodies do not always affect the fetus being carried at that time. However, in subsequent pregnancies with Rh-positive fetuses, the already sensitized client usually produces large numbers of antibodies. Some newborns are only mildly affected, whereas others are severely affected. Efforts to save the fetus may include *intrauterine transfusion* (exchange of fetal blood in utero) if the pregnancy is less than 32 weeks' duration or early delivery at 34–38 weeks.

Administering *anti-D gamma globulin,* also known as *Rho (D) immune globulin* (RhoGAM, Gamulin Rh), to the Rh-negative client can prevent erythroblastosis fetalis. This drug should be administered at 28 weeks' gestation and again after 72 hr: or after the birth of an Rh-positive baby, any abortion, or any invasive procedure, such as an amniocentesis. *Rho (D) immune globulin* (RhoGAM) prevents the client's body from building up anti–Rh-positive antibodies. Erythroblastosis fetalis is thus prevented, even in Rh-positive fetuses. *Rho (D) immune globulin* (RhoGAM's) availability has made this disorder rare in the United States.

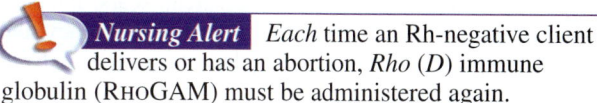 **Nursing Alert** Each time an Rh-negative client delivers or has an abortion, *Rho (D) immune globulin* (RhoGAM) must be administered again.

ABO Incompatibility

ABO incompatibility, a type of hemolytic disease of the newborn, can arise if the client's blood type is A and the fetus's is B or AB; if the mother is B and the fetus is A or AB; and if the mother is O and the fetus is A, B, or AB (see Chapter 69).

ABO incompatibility is not detectable before birth. It can occur in a first pregnancy and does not increase in severity with subsequent pregnancies. It is usually clinically milder than Rh sensitization. The problem is indicated by jaundice in the newborn within the first 24–36 hr. Phototherapy is often initiated to treat jaundice (see Chapter 69).

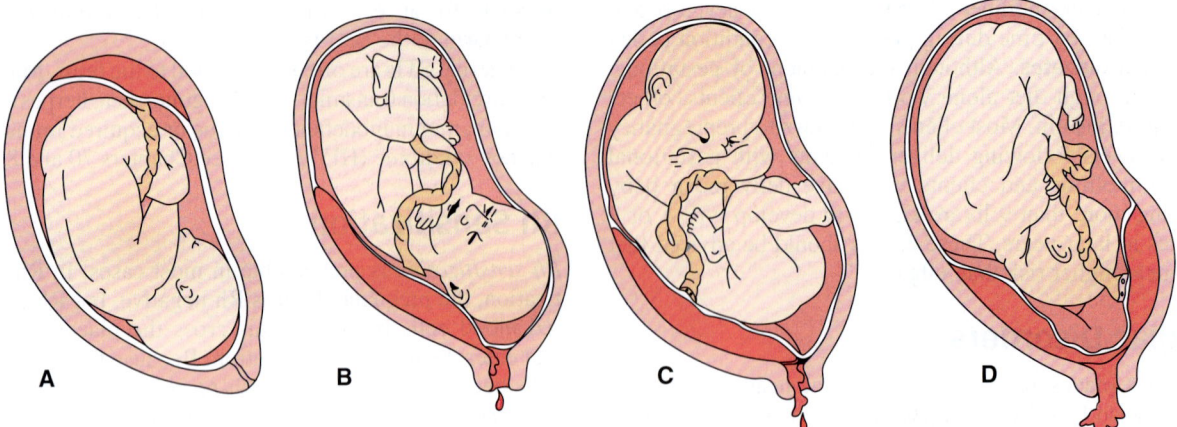

Figure 68-2 Placenta previa. **A.** Normal placenta. **B.** Low implantation. **C.** Partial placenta previa. **D.** Total placenta previa. (B, C, & D from Pillitteri, 2007.)

PLACENTAL AND AMNIOTIC DISORDERS

Placental disorders include placenta previa and abruptio placentae. *Placenta previa* means that the placenta implants in the wrong place within the client's uterus. *Abruptio placentae* is a condition in which the placenta tears abruptly and prematurely from the uterus. Both conditions can be life-threatening to the client and fetus. *Polyhydramnios,* or excessive amniotic fluid, presents serious dangers to the fetus.

Placenta Previa

Placenta previa is a serious condition that occurs when the placenta implants in the lower segment of the uterus, rather than in the upper wall (Fig. 68-2). *Low implantation* is placental attachment at the opening or border of the cervical os but not covering it. If the placenta partially obliterates the cervical os, it is a *partial placenta previa.* Placenta that totally covers the cervical os is called *total placenta previa.*

Predisposing factors for placenta previa are numerous and include closely spaced pregnancies, abnormalities in uterine structure, late fertilization, and old cesarean scars. Painless vaginal bleeding during the later months of pregnancy, the primary symptom, is caused by the placenta separating from the uterine wall.

If undetected before labor begins, placenta previa will result in hemorrhage because the cervical dilation causes increased tearing of the placental tissue. The severity of hemorrhage in relation to the progress of labor determines the method of delivery to be used. In total placenta previa, cesarean delivery is performed. In partial placenta previa, the amount of cervical involvement dictates the method of delivery, although cesarean delivery is usually performed if the placenta previa covers more than 30% of the cervical os when the cervix is fully dilated. A client may be hospitalized several times before hemorrhaging becomes severe enough to warrant cesarean birth.

Other potential complications of placenta previa are loss of uterine muscle tone (*atony*), uterine rupture, retention of placental tissue, and *air embolism,* a serious complication caused by exposure of uterine sinuses and blood vessels to the air. The fetus is at considerable risk, and fetal shock and maternal or fetal death are possible.

Diagnosis and Management

If vaginal bleeding occurs, the client should be hospitalized *immediately* and placed on bed rest. The need for fetal monitoring, IV and blood administration, possible cesarean delivery, vaginal packing, and emergency infant resuscitation should be anticipated.

Diagnosis is most often obtained by ultrasonography (Doppler ultrasound), which can usually identify the exact placental location. In some situations, x-rays may be used (including *placentography*) to visualize the placenta.

If the fetus is diagnosed as viable, a sterile vaginal examination (**SVE**) may be done (by the healthcare provider only) in the operating room. The operating room should be prepared with a double setup to allow for an emergency cesarean delivery if necessary.

Vaginal birth is not usually considered unless the previa is minimal. If the fetus is under 36 weeks' gestation, the pregnant client is put on strict bed rest either in the healthcare facility or at home. If no bleeding occurs, ultrasound scanning may be done every 2–3 weeks along with nonstress testing and biophysical profile. If bleeding is found, a cesarean delivery is anticipated.

Although placenta previa is still considered serious, modern surgical methods and the use of blood transfusions have greatly reduced maternal mortality. The prognosis for the fetus depends on the effect of maternal hemorrhage on fetal circulation and oxygenation.

Nursing Considerations

Observe the client carefully for hemorrhage following a placenta previa delivery. If bleeding continues to be severe and attempts at control are unsuccessful, an emergency hysterectomy may be performed.

Abruptio Placentae

Abruptio placentae, the abrupt premature separation of the normally implanted placenta from the uterine wall, is a

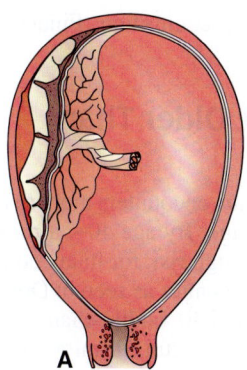
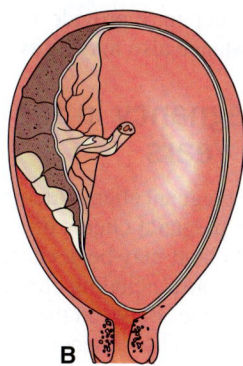
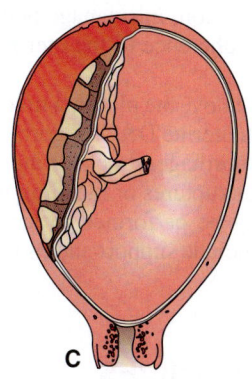

A
Partial separation
(Concealed hemorrhage)

B
Partial separation
(Apparent hemorrhage)

C
Complete separation
(Concealed hemorrhage)

Figure 68-3 Premature separation and abruptio placentae. **A.** Separation is low and incomplete; vaginal hemorrhage is evident. **B.** Separation is high, causing fundus of uterus to rise. Fetus is in grave danger. External hemorrhage is not present, but amniotic fluid is port-wine color. **C.** Complete abruption, with fetus in grave danger. External hemorrhage is prevented because fetus's head is in cervical os. (Pillitteri, 2007.)

grave complication of late pregnancy (Fig. 68-3). It usually develops after the 20th week of gestation, and it often occurs without labor.

> **Nursing Alert** Abruptio placentae is an emergency that may require immediate cesarean delivery. Report vaginal bleeding, signs of shock, or a rising uterus (which becomes very hard without contractions) immediately. *Rationale: Blood may be trapped inside the uterus.*

Some predisposing factors are hypertension, preeclampsia, poor placental circulation, substance abuse, grand multiparity, and numerous abortions or stillbirths. Physical trauma, such as a motor vehicle accident, also can cause immediate placental separation. The extent of the separation determines the amount of danger to the fetus. Abruptio placentae is a common cause of *stillbirth.*

Diagnosis and Management
Abruptio placentae can occur any time in pregnancy before the birth, giving rise to fetal distress. The bleeding that results from the separation may be apparent or hidden. If bleeding is externally visible, it is often dark. The uterus becomes tender and rigid, and symptoms of maternal shock may occur. Fetal movement may increase or decrease. If the client experiences extreme pain or the uterine fundus rises, it may indicate bleeding and pooling behind the placenta (*retroplacental hemorrhage*).

Other possible maternal complications include bleeding into the uterine muscle, *precipitous labor* (fast and uncontrolled), loss of uterine tone (*atony*), and oliguria leading to acute renal failure. Disseminated intravascular coagulation (**DIC**) and maternal death may occur (see Chapter 82). Dangers to the fetus include anemia, anoxia, and death.

Nursing Considerations
The diagnosis of abruptio placentae is based on the client's history, physical examination, and laboratory studies. Sonograms are used to rule out placenta previa, but they are not diagnostic for placental abruption. The amount of vaginal bleeding seen can be misleading because blood may be trapped behind the placenta. The nurse must be aware of changes in vital signs and indicators, such as sudden extreme pain or aberrations in uterine shape.

Treatment depends on the severity of maternal blood loss, determined by laboratory findings, fetal maturity, and the biophysical condition of both the client and the fetus. Continuously monitor the fetus if a fetal heart rate is present. Identify the upper limit of the fundus and mark it on the client's abdomen with a felt-tip pen. Observe the fundus for changes in shape or movement upward. Measure abdominal *girth* (the distance around) with a flexible tape measure. If the abdomen increases in girth or moves upward, blood may be collecting within the uterus; this dangerous situation usually calls for immediate cesarean delivery.

Before a cesarean birth, lost maternal blood must be replaced and circulating blood volume restored. During this time, constantly monitor maternal vital signs and fetal heart rate (if present). In a few cases, a hysterectomy may need to be performed to control the bleeding.

With modern treatment, abruptio placentae is rarely fatal to the client. However, the outlook for the newborn's survival depends on the severity of the separation and the degree to which their oxygen supply has been affected.

Polyhydramnios

Polyhydramnios (sometimes called **hydramnios**) means an excessive amount of amniotic fluid (>2 L or 2000 mL). Seen in approximately 10% of pregnant clients with diabetes, polyhydramnios also accompanies neural tube defects, such as spina bifida and anencephaly. The client's abdomen is excessively large, producing dyspnea and difficulty with movement. The skin is stretched tightly, and excessive stretch marks (*striae gravidarum*) may be present. Uterine muscles also have been stretched, which may lead to ineffective contractions (*dystocia*) and failure of the uterus to contract following childbirth.

Placenta Accreta

A placenta that fails to separate, fails to be expelled within 20–30 min after delivery, or leaves remnants in the uterus is a danger to the client. This condition is called **placenta accreta** or *retained placenta*. The tissue must be removed soon after delivery so that infection or hemorrhage does not develop. Retained placenta may result from partial separation of a normally attached placenta, entrapment of the separated placenta by uterine constriction, mismanagement of labor's third stage, or abnormal adherence to the uterine wall.

The birth attendant may need to remove the placenta manually and may perform a postpartum uterine D&C. Vigorous attempts at removal may lead to hemorrhage, shock, or uterine rupture or inversion. If the uterus ruptures or bleeding is uncontrollable, a hysterectomy may be performed to save the client's life. Nursing measures include support and monitoring vital signs.

OTHER HIGH-RISK PREGNANCIES

Prolonged Pregnancy

A pregnancy continuing beyond 42 weeks is known as a *prolonged* (*postdate* or *postterm*) pregnancy. In this case, the obstetrician may induce labor or perform a cesarean delivery. The condition of the fetus is a determining factor. If any indication of fetal distress exists, a cesarean delivery is the most likely option. Risks to be considered include *placental insufficiency,* a condition in which the placenta deteriorates and uteroplacental circulation is compromised.

Multiple Pregnancy

A multiple pregnancy is one in which more than one fetus is developing in the uterus at the same time. If a multiple pregnancy is suspected, ultrasound is diagnostic. Labor is not ordinarily more difficult than in a normal pregnancy, although preterm and *precipitate* (sudden, progressing faster than normal) deliveries are relatively common.

Adolescent Pregnancy

More than 1.2 million adolescent clients in the United States become pregnant each year, representing nearly 20% of births. Pregnancy in a client younger than 16 years places a particular strain on their body; this adolescent is undergoing not only the normal changes of adolescence but also those needed to sustain a pregnancy. Iron requirements are high for both adolescence and pregnancy, and anemia may result. The young client who is pregnant may need special dietary instructions or vitamin supplements.

Complications of adolescent pregnancy often involve preeclampsia, eclampsia, and spontaneous abortion. Babies are often preterm and small for their gestational age. Perinatal mortality is increased, and newborns often develop slowly. Pregnant adolescents are at high risk for infections and STIs.

Childbirth preparation classes are offered through local public health departments or healthcare facilities. Pregnant clients, particularly adolescents, should attend these classes to understand their nutritional needs and the process of pregnancy.

The adolescent client who is pregnant should also receive information about continuing their education. By law, public school education must be made available to pregnant teenagers. Counseling services should be offered because the client may be afraid to go to their parents for help. Local church groups or clergy members, Planned Parenthood of America, local social service agencies, and the family healthcare provider may provide resources and counseling. Financial assistance also may be available.

Pregnancy in the Client Older Than 35 Years

The pregnant client older than 35 years encounters more risks than pregnant clients of a younger age. By age 40+, a pregnant client may be at exceptionally high risk for many complications, including chromosomal changes as seen in Down syndrome. Between the ages of 35 and 40, bodily changes in preparation for menopause may have begun. Primigravidas of this age have an increased incidence of complications in pregnancy (e.g., ectopic pregnancy, gestational diabetes, and hypertensive disorders) in addition to problems during labor and delivery, such as *hypertonic* or *hypotonic dystocia* (contractions too weak or too strong, respectively) and hemorrhage. They also face greater than normal chances of having cognitively impaired or malformed children. The older grand multipara may be more likely to have a precipitate delivery, placenta previa, hydramnios, hypotonic dystocia, or hemorrhage because of an *atonic uterus* (one that does not contract following delivery).

COMPLICATIONS OF LABOR AND DELIVERY

Approximately 85% of all deliveries are considered *normal;* 15% are considered *complicated.* One nursing duty in the labor and delivery area is to assess for possible complications.

Maternal Hemorrhage

Intrapartum and *postpartum maternal hemorrhage* are life-threatening events that may occur without warning and are often not recognized until the client experiences profound symptoms. Carefully observe the client immediately after delivery for signs of hemorrhage or shock. Maternal hemorrhage requires aggressive measures to locate the cause. Begin localized and systemic therapy to avoid maternal mortality. Monitor fundal firmness because *uterine atony* is the number one cause of postpartum hemorrhage.

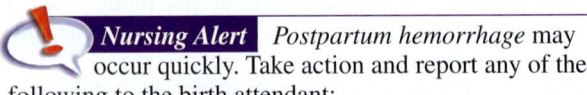

Nursing Alert *Postpartum hemorrhage* may occur quickly. Take action and report any of the following to the birth attendant:
- Copious vaginal bleeding
- Boggy uterus (*massage first* and then report)
- Uterus high in the abdomen
- Signs of maternal shock

Premature Rupture of Membranes

Normally, the amniotic sac ruptures with a large gush slightly after the onset of labor. However, in 2%–18% of all pregnancies, the amniotic sac, also referred to as the bag of waters (**BOW**) by the layperson, may have a small leak. In this scenario, the client may not go into labor for several days because the rupture is generally a small leak that they may not detect. When the amniotic sac loses fluids before the onset of labor, the condition is called premature rupture of membranes (**PROM**). Several complications may arise with PROM:

- Premature labor
- Intrauterine infection (the fetus is particularly susceptible to infections)
- Malpresentation and prolapsed cord

Nitrazine tests may be used to detect amniotic fluid in the vagina.

The client should be admitted to the healthcare facility when PROM occurs. The client and fetus are then assessed. Ultrasound and amniocentesis will determine fetal maturity, and labor is induced if the fetus is sufficiently mature.

Preterm Labor

Labor that occurs before the end of the 37th week of gestation is *preterm*, but it often still produces a viable fetus. Because prematurity is a leading cause of infant mortality, the birth attendant often attempts to postpone delivery until the baby is more mature.

The client is placed on bed rest. *Tocolytic agents* (uterine relaxants) may be given to stop the contractions if there is no fetal distress, the membranes are intact, and the cervix is dilated fewer than 4 cm (see In Practice: Important Medications 68-1). Medications are usually administered IV until contractions cease, after which they may be administered orally. The client and fetus must be followed up closely for the remainder of the pregnancy.

Precipitate Labor and Delivery

A precipitate labor is one that is brief (<3 hr) and in which contractions are unusually severe. It most often occurs in induced labor or multiparity. A precipitate delivery may be so rapid that the client cannot be taken to the delivery room or prepared for delivery; the obstetrician or midwife is not always present.

IN PRACTICE
IMPORTANT MEDICATIONS 68-1 — To Stop Labor (Tocolytic Agents)

Ritodrine HCl (Yutopar)
    Terbutaline sulfate (Brethine, Bricanyl)
    Magnesium sulfate
    Indomethacin (Indocin)
    Nifedipine (Procardia)

Nursing Considerations
- Side effects of these drugs include dizziness, headache, tremor, and gastrointestinal symptoms.
- Side effects of ritodrine HCl (Yutopar) include maternal hypotension, maternal pulmonary edema, and maternal or fetal tachycardia.
- Dexamethasone (Decadron) may be given to speed maturation of fetal lungs.
- Indomethacin (Indocin) also may be given to the premature infant after birth to close a patent ductus arteriosus.

When providing nursing care for a client experiencing precipitate labor, stay with them, put the signal light on for help, remain composed, and assist the client as much as possible until help arrives. Apply the principles of asepsis as the situation allows. Never prevent delivery in any way. Simply assist with the birth and make sure that the newborn is breathing adequately.

Because of the force and speed of labor, possible trauma can occur to the client and newborn. Dangers to the client include perineal laceration, hemorrhage, infection, and uterine rupture. Anoxia, subdural hematoma, and fractures may occur in the newborn. Hospitals usually have protocols on determining under what circumstances an infant born out of asepsis (**BOA**) (i.e., in an unsterile environment) needs isolation to prevent spread of infection to other infants.

Uterine Rupture

A *ruptured uterus* is one of the most serious complications of labor; fortunately, it is rare. Predisposing factors include a previous cesarean delivery or any uterine scar. Severe tonic contractions with no period of relaxation, dystocia (difficult labor), cephalopelvic disproportion, or injudicious use of drugs, such as oxytocin to stimulate uterine contractions, also may predispose to rupture.

When uterine rupture threatens, the client complains of continuous and intense pain. A *Bandl ring* may be noticeable as a thickened upper segment and a thin distended lower segment of the uterus. The client appears apprehensive and restless. Contractions are tonic, pulse is rapid, and urination is frequent. If the threat of rupture occurs before delivery, the fetus is usually in great distress, as shown by irregular or absent FHTs.

Constant fetal monitoring is vital. The client at high risk of, or with, a uterine rupture may need an emergency cesarean delivery to save their life and the life of the fetus. A hysterectomy may be needed to save the client's life.

Symptoms of rupture are a sharp, tearing pain followed by its sudden cessation. The client is anxious and shows signs of shock and hypotension; their pulse is rapid and weak. (They are hemorrhaging internally.) Use emergency measures to treat them for shock and hemorrhage. Prepare them at once for an emergency cesarean delivery and possible hysterectomy.

Maternal Dystocia

Dystocia is prolonged, painful labor that does not result in effective cervical dilation or effacement. Labor is long but does not progress. Dystocia may be related to fetal factors, uterine or passageway abnormalities, or faulty contractions. Dystocia not only exhausts the client but also predisposes them and the fetus to possible danger and even death.

Uterine Inertia

Uterine inertia refers to insufficient, uncoordinated contractions that do not produce effective dilation. It is also called *hypotonic dystocia*. Causes include emotional stress, a thick and rigid cervix, and excessive or premature use of analgesic medications. Uterine inertia occurs most often in primigravidas. However, it also is identified in some grand multiparas who have weak uterine muscle tone. Other clients may suffer from uterine inertia if they have an overdistended uterus because of an extremely large fetus, multiple pregnancy, or hydramnios.

Nursing care includes early recognition, prompt notification of the obstetrician, assessment of cervical dilation (if any), accurate evaluation of pain, assessment of the fetal heart rate related to the pattern of contractions by monitor, and positive emotional support and reassurance. Anticipate and be prepared to assist with treatments, such as IV fluids or efforts to stop the ineffective labor with medications such as morphine. Sleep and rest often enable the client's uterus to achieve a normal pattern when labor resumes. Other treatments may include IV oxytocin infusion or cesarean delivery.

Dystocia Caused by the Fetus

Sometimes the size of the fetus as compared with the size of the client's pelvis or the position or presentation of the fetus causes dystocia.

Cephalopelvic Disproportion

Cephalopelvic disproportion (**CPD**) means that the presenting part, usually the fetal head, is too large to pass through the client's pelvis. It may be related to maternal diabetes (which often results in large babies), heredity, or maternal nutrition. Cesarean delivery should be anticipated; however, some birth attendants use cesarean birth as a last resort. An ultrasound or x-ray pelvimetry is performed to determine CPD. Often the client has dilated and effaced, but the presenting part fails to descend.

Fetal Positions and Presentations

The normal fetal presentation is the **vertex** (head-first) position. If the fetus assumes an abnormal position within the uterus, labor is difficult, and vaginal delivery may be impossible. Depending on the head's position, difficulties may occur. For example, if the face is the presenting part, vaginal delivery is often impossible because this angle causes a CPD. An abnormal position also may cause a hand or foot or the buttocks to present. Ultrasonography can identify fetal position, as can the location of FHTs. A cesarean delivery may be done for an abnormal position or presentation.

Abnormal Fetal Presentations
Posterior Positions

Normal fetal presentations and positions are discussed in Chapter 66. The most common abnormal fetal presentation is *occiput posterior,* where the occiput, or back of the fetal head, is toward the client's back. Posterior positions are designated right occiput posterior (**ROP**), left occiput posterior (**LOP**), or direct occiput posterior (**OP**). Delivery can be difficult or impossible because the fetal neck is overflexed, the face is uppermost, and the head diameter may be too large to pass through the birth canal. This presentation can occur if the maternal pelvic floor is relaxed. The client typically complains of a continuous low backache, and FHTs are heard on the client's *flank* (side).

Medical management may include manual rotation of the fetus (**version**) before engagement, forceps-assisted delivery, or cesarean delivery, which are discussed later in this chapter. Help the client do pelvic rocking exercises. Pelvic rocking is done while the client lies flat in bed. They rock the abdomen from top to bottom, alternating back and forth. First, they press their backbone against the bed and rocks the hips away from the bed, while tightening the vaginal muscles. They then press their buttocks into the mattress, while lifting the small of the back. Give emotional support, and massage the client's lower back.

Transverse Position

The **transverse lie** usually results in a *shoulder presentation.* The fetus lies across the client's abdomen in the uterus, so a risk of prolapsed cord or descent of a fetal arm exists if the membranes rupture. Management may include version, but a cesarean delivery will most likely be performed.

Face-Brow Presentation

Face-brow presentation (occipitomental) occurs when the fetal head is unfavorably positioned for delivery. Predisposing factors include multiparity, polyhydramnios, and a low-lying placenta. The client may deliver spontaneously if flexion of the fetal neck occurs. Reassure the client, and anticipate treatment to include an attempted version or cesarean delivery if fetal position cannot be altered.

Breech Presentations

Breech presentation occurs in 3% of all deliveries. In a *complete breech,* the buttocks present, with the knees bent and the feet next to the buttocks. A *footling breech* is one in which one or both feet present (*single footling* or *double footling*). In a *frank breech,* the buttocks present, with the legs extended straight up (the legs and feet are entwined around the face). Predisposing factors include placenta previa, CPD, multiple pregnancy, small fetus, tumors, and polyhydramnios. If the mother has had a previous breech birth, a subsequent one is more likely (see Breech Presentations, Chapter 66).

Fetal mortality is higher in breech deliveries than in any other kind of delivery. The risks to the client include laceration and hemorrhage; to the fetus, the risks include birth injuries and fetal anoxia, which may be caused by early rupture of the bag of waters and by cord prolapse. Because the head is delivered last, asphyxia can occur; the fetal head cannot undergo normal molding and may become caught in the birth canal.

Treatment may include diagnostic ultrasound and fetal maturity studies, the use of forceps for the head, or cesarean delivery. Nursing care is the same as for any client in labor. Anticipate that FHTs will be located at or above the umbilicus, and meconium-stained amniotic fluid may be present. Prepare for newborn resuscitation if a spontaneous delivery occurs.

UMBILICAL CORD COMPLICATIONS

The umbilical cord can be a potential problem during delivery. Possible complications include prolapsed and nuchal cord.

Prolapsed Cord

In a **prolapsed cord**, the umbilical cord precedes the baby. The cord may protrude from the cervix or may drop as low as the vulva. An *occult* (hidden) prolapse is difficult to determine because the cord is compressed between the fetus and the uterine wall. A prolapsed cord is a serious complication because as the fetus's head descends, it may press the cord against the hard structures in the client's pelvis, cutting off fetal circulation. This condition usually requires an emergency cesarean delivery.

A prolapsed cord can result from any factor that interferes with the engagement or adaptation of the presenting part to the pelvis, such as multiple pregnancy, a transverse lie, an abnormal presentation (e.g., a footling), hydramnios, or a high presenting part when the membranes suddenly rupture.

Sometimes electronic fetal monitoring detects this condition early. The birth attendant or nurse must insert a sterile gloved hand into the vagina to hold the fetal presenting part away from the cord. This measure ensures that fetal circulation is not cut off while the client is prepared for an emergency cesarean delivery. If the cord has prolapsed outside the vagina, it is covered with sterile towels and moistened with warm, sterile normal saline. This measure prevents drying and caking of the cord and fetal blood. Place the client in the Trendelenburg or knee-chest position as ordered. Fetal monitoring is essential. Notify the healthcare provider at once and prepare for resuscitation of the newborn. A postoperative complication may be maternal puerperal infection.

Nuchal Cord

As the fetus moves within the uterus, the umbilical cord may become wrapped around the neck. This condition is known as **nuchal cord**. If this condition is discovered before labor, cesarean delivery may be done. If it is not discovered until the client is in labor, the cord may have become so tightly wrapped around the neck that the fetus is unable to receive oxygen. In this case, the birth attendant may use forceps to speed delivery, and the cord is cut immediately. If the nuchal cord is loose, the birth attendant may be able to slip it over the fetus's head.

CONSIDERATIONS RELATED TO DELIVERY

Induction of Labor

The start of labor by medical interventions is called **induction**. Induction of labor may be initiated by a birth attendant for various reasons before labor begins naturally.

Labor is induced only in certain instances because it is not without risk. Reasons for induction include the possibility of fetal death without labor, worsening signs of PIH, a large or postterm fetus, and maternal diabetes mellitus.

The birth attendant must determine if the client's birth canal is large enough before inducing labor. If a CPD exists, induction should not be attempted. Fetal maturity also must be evaluated to make sure that the fetus is viable. Amniocentesis can determine maturity by assessing the **LS ratio**.

Nursing Considerations

Nursing assessment is important during induction. Carefully monitor the fetus for signs of distress. Take the client's blood pressure and pulse every 10–15 min during an IV or

---

IN PRACTICE
IMPORTANT MEDICATIONS 68-2 For Induction of Labor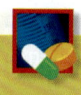

Oxytocin (Pitocin, Syntocinon)

Nursing Considerations
- Oxytocin (Pitocin) is given intravenous (IV), using a piggyback setup with a solution of normal saline or D$_5$W (5% dextrose in water) to keep the vein open.
- Adjust the drip rate for optimum flow rate, character of contractions, and optimum relaxation time between contractions.
- Use the infusion pump to ensure accurate measurement and delivery of the drug.
- Use a fetal monitor to make sure the fetus is not in danger.

---

suppository induction and at least every half-hour following the rupture of the bag of waters. Any sign of maternal or fetal distress is *an emergency that you must report immediately*. Be sure to provide physical and emotional support to the client and family during induction.

Induction With Drugs

Drugs may be administered parenterally, orally, or vaginally to induce labor (In Practice: Important Medications 68-2). Oxytocin (Pitocin) is the drug most commonly used to induce labor. Prostaglandin vaginal suppositories or gel may also be administered before oxytocin to ripen the cervix.

Amniotomy

Labor also can be induced by **amniotomy**, which means rupturing the amniotic membranes with a special hook. A healthcare provider performs this procedure under sterile conditions, at times with nursing assistance. Labor usually follows quickly. Chart the time of the amniotomy, the color and approximate amount of fluid, and the effects on the client. If labor does not begin spontaneously after amniotomy, induction with medications will usually follow. Watch the client for signs of uterine infection if delivery does not occur within 24 hr.

Emergency Delivery

Sometimes, not enough time is available for the client to get to the healthcare facility for delivery. In this case, police officers, rescue personnel, or nurses may be asked to assist with emergency childbirth. A BOA pack of necessary delivery supplies and equipment is generally kept available at all times in emergency departments and ambulances and on obstetrical units.

Nursing Considerations

Never delay delivery. Preventing delivery can cause great damage to the client and fetus. Remain calm and deliver the baby as safely as possible, following the best possible aseptic technique (In Practice: Nursing Care Guidelines 68-1).

Usually, few complications arise in a precipitous delivery. Important interventions in the care of the newborn include ensuring respirations and proper body temperature. Cutting the cord is inadvisable unless the services of the birth

UNIT 10 Maternal and Newborn Nursing

IN PRACTICE
NURSING CARE GUIDELINES 68-1: Assisting in an Emergency Delivery

- Provide as much privacy as possible for the client.
- Wear gloves.
- Do not attempt to prevent delivery.
- Follow aseptic technique as closely as possible.
- Make sure the membranes have ruptured.
- Make sure the newborn's airway is clear before they take the first breath.
- Initiate respiration in the newborn.
- Keep the newborn warm.
- Tie off the umbilical cord in two places.
- Do not cut the umbilical cord.
- Have the client hold the newborn and put it to their breast.
- Get medical assistance as soon as possible.
- Make sure the client's uterus contracts after delivery of the newborn and placenta.
- Write down the time of birth of the newborn and delivery of the placenta. Write down the client's name and address.
- Keep the client warm.
- Reassure the client.

attendant are unavailable. However, *tie the cord in two places* when the newborn is breathing or the placenta is delivered. Keep the newborn and placenta together if you anticipate a birth attendant's or hospital's services. Putting the newborn to the mother's breast immediately helps the uterus to contract and prevents maternal hemorrhage. The mother will be examined for retained placental tissue, lacerations, and other complications when they receive medical assistance.

Lacerations

During a precipitous or emergency delivery, a laceration or tear into the perineal tissue and anus may occur. All lacerations are repaired while the client is still on the delivery table or in the emergency department. Cervical tears are also repaired to prevent hemorrhage.

Lacerations are classified into several categories:

- *First degree* involves the perineal skin and vaginal mucous membranes.
- *Second degree* involves muscles of the perineal body.
- *Third degree* involves the anal sphincter.
- *Fourth degree* extends to the anal canal.

Operative Obstetrics

Sometimes assisting the client with the delivery of the baby through operative obstetrics becomes necessary. This section discusses version, forceps delivery, vacuum extraction, and cesarean birth. The student needs to be familiar with the concepts of normal labor, delivery, and postpartum care (see Chapter 66).

Version

Version is used to turn the fetus to a more desirable presentation. In *external version,* the client lies on their back with their knees flexed, and the birth attendant maneuvers the fetus with the hands outside the abdominal wall to a more favorable presentation. In *internal version,* the fetus is turned with the birth attendant's sterile gloved hand inside the uterus. Because the cervix must be dilated to perform the internal version, the fetus is generally delivered at the same time. You must have long, sterile version gloves available for the birth attendant.

Forceps Delivery

Sometimes the birth is assisted with **delivery forceps**, which are double-bladed, curved instruments that fit around the fetal head. Their purpose is to increase traction and to assist in rotating the fetus during delivery.

Maternal indications for forceps delivery include the following:

- Exhaustion
- Heart disease
- Prolonged labor

Fetal indications for forceps delivery include the following:

- Fetal distress
- Decreased heart rate of <100 bpm
- Late deceleration pattern on the fetal monitor
- Prolapsed umbilical cord

Forceps deliveries are classified according to the **station** of the presenting part, that is, the position of the fetal head in relation to the ischial spines (see Fig. 66-2). *Midforceps* delivery is used when the head is at the ischial spines (*engaged*), and the station is 0. The most commonly used forceps procedure is the *low forceps,* in which the fetal head is on the perineal floor (+3 station).

Before the practitioner applies forceps, the FHTs are checked (preferably with the fetal monitor), an SVE is done to determine whether cervical dilation and effacement are complete, and the membranes are ruptured. The client is usually catheterized before the SVE if forceps delivery is anticipated.

You will be responsible for documenting the time of delivery and the use of forceps and for observing the newborn. If any marks or injuries result from the forceps, document them on the newborn's chart. Document the mother's physical status, vital signs, and emotional reactions.

Vacuum Extraction

An alternative to forceps delivery is **vacuum extraction**, whereby a round, soft plastic cup is placed on the fetal head. Suction is created by a special pump to secure the cup to the presenting part (the fetal head), and traction is exerted to ease the fetus gently out of the birth canal. The client's cervix must be fully dilated before the vacuum extractor can be used. Document the procedure and observe the newborn and the mother.

Cesarean Delivery

A **cesarean delivery** is a surgical procedure used to deliver the baby through an incision in the abdomen and the uterus. Any complication of labor may be an indication for performing cesarean delivery. In some instances, the client may have an elective cesarean birth. If the client has had previous cesarean births, the healthcare provider may prefer to do another to avoid the risk of a ruptured uterus. The high number of cesarean births in the United States is a matter of controversy.

Preoperative Care
Cesarean delivery may be scheduled in advance or may be an emergency procedure. A cesarean delivery is not usually done if the fetus is dead.

As a nurse, you will prepare the family for the procedure. Family members are likely to be concerned about the safety of the client and fetus, as well as the client's recovery, not only from childbirth but also from major surgery. A complete explanation of the procedure is given to the partner or coach. Many healthcare facilities allow significant others in the operating room during cesarean delivery because they can support the client during this procedure, just as they can during vaginal delivery.

Chapter 56 discusses preoperative care in abdominal surgery. One difference in cesarean delivery is that the client does not receive narcotics or strong sedatives because fetal respiration could easily become depressed. Check for symptoms of fetal distress or any unusual discomfort the client might experience.

> **NCLEX Alert**
> Pre- and postoperative care in obstetrics has additional concerns to those of the typical surgical client such as fundal massage and breast care. Be sure to learn these differences, especially sources and types of hemorrhage.

Prepare the operating room for abdominal surgery and for care of a newborn. An *isolette* or *radiant heat panel* and resuscitation and suction equipment are required. Surgical nurses and a special nurse to care for the newborn are present at the delivery.

Anesthesia
As with vaginal births, the typical obstetrical anesthesia during labor is the *epidural* form of anesthesia. Medication is injected into the epidural space in the sacral area of the spine. Depending on the dose administered, epidurals can be used for either analgesia or anesthesia. Epidural analgesia is usually not started until the client has dilated greater than 5 cm. Epidural analgesia is often supplemented with an opioid such as fentanyl or morphine. The client may have a continuous infusion drip to assist with pain management.

Spinal anesthesia is injected a little below the epidural space into the subarachnoid space. A technique known as *combined spinal-epidural* (CSE) analgesia gives rapid relief from pain while maintaining the client's ability to ambulate. Whatever procedure is used, the nurse must be vigilant and observe for maternal hypotension, fetal distress, and respiratory depression. Generally, the mother is awake for at least part of a cesarean delivery.

Postoperative Care
The client should be given routine postoperative care. Check vital signs, observe *lochia* (vaginal discharge) and the incision, and check the fundus. Although fundal assessment may be difficult because of the abdominal dressing, it is important to prevent hemorrhage. Record intake and output for 24–48 hr. IV fluids are usually continued for 24 hr after surgery. Advance the diet as tolerated. Administer perineal care and oxytocic drugs as ordered. Early ambulation and breathing exercises are important. The client usually goes home on the third or fourth postoperative day.

Care of the Newborn
Carefully check the newborn's respiratory status for the first few days of life because they are more likely to experience respiratory distress than a newborn delivered vaginally. During a vaginal delivery, approximately 40% of the fluid in the fetal lungs is squeezed out when the fetal chest compresses while passing through the birth canal. A newborn delivered by cesarean birth does not experience this compression and may suffer respiratory distress due to retained fluids. This newborn also has not had the stimulation of the birth experience. (See Chapter 69 for a discussion of *transient tachypnea of the newborn* and *respiratory distress syndrome*.)

COMPLICATIONS OF THE POSTPARTUM PERIOD

If undetected and untreated, a postpartal or **puerperal** (occurring following the birth of a baby) complication can become so severe that the mother may require rehospitalization within days of discharge. Therefore, the postpartum assessment provides valuable information in detecting problems. Postpartum complications include circulatory disturbances, infectious processes, and emotional disorders.

Postpartum Hematoma
Bleeding into the subcutaneous tissue in the perineal area is called a **postpartum hematoma**. A precipitous delivery, prolonged pressure during labor and delivery, large varicosities in the pelvic area, or a vein that has been cut or pricked during an episiotomy or its repair may cause hematoma. The client experiences severe pain in the perineal area, especially after a bowel movement or if the bladder becomes overly distended.

Observe the perineal area for discoloration and swelling. You may give the client cold compresses or a medicated pad, such as Tucks (containing witch hazel); sometimes, you will use compresses soaked in a magnesium sulfate solution. Sitz baths may be soothing. You may give analgesics to relieve discomfort. The client may be returned to the delivery room for incision and ligation of a blood vessel. Small hematomas will be absorbed without treatment.

Postpartum Hemorrhage
Average blood loss during a normal delivery is approximately 300 mL. Depending on agency guidelines, **postpartum hemorrhage** is defined as any blood loss from the uterus between 500 and 1,000 mL within 24 hr. A postpartal hemorrhage is classified as *early* if it occurs within 24 hr

after delivery. A *late* hemorrhage may occur from 2 days to 6 weeks following delivery.

Symptoms of hemorrhage include steady or gushing external vaginal bleeding. The uterus is usually located high in the abdomen and feels boggy. The client's pulse is often rapid, and the blood pressure drops in relation to the severity of the hemorrhage.

The hemorrhaging client's life depends on prompt nursing care. Grasp the abdominal area over the uterus, cupping it with both hands. While supporting the lower part of the uterus with one hand, use the other hand to massage gently but firmly. If you cannot locate the uterus because it is boggy, massage the lower abdomen until the uterus contracts. Place the client into the Trendelenburg position, and monitor her vital signs. Notify the healthcare provider, and anticipate IV oxytocin (Pitocin) infusion.

If the cause of the bleeding appears to be a laceration or retained placental tissue, the nurse will likely need to prepare the client for an SVE and treatment, including D&C. If the blood loss is extensive, the client will probably require a blood transfusion.

Uterine Atony and Other Causes

Uterine **atony**, or lack of uterine muscle tone, prevents the uterine muscles from contracting and closing the venous sinuses, which usually causes postpartum hemorrhage. Other causes of hemorrhage are retention of *placental fragments* (which prevents the blood vessels from contracting) and *tears* in the reproductive tract as a result of delivery.

Thrombophlebitis

Thrombophlebitis involves a clot in a blood vessel with resultant inflammation. In a new mother, thrombophlebitis typically occurs in the femoral vessels in the leg. Early ambulation greatly lessens the occurrence of thrombophlebitis in new mothers.

Symptoms include swelling, slight temperature elevation, pain, and redness or whiteness in the affected area. A positive *Homans sign* occurs (calf pain on passive dorsiflexion of the foot). The symptoms most often develop in the second postpartal week and may persist for months.

Treatment consists of bed rest with elevation of the affected part, local application of heat, analgesics, antiembolism stockings, and anticoagulants. After the acute stage has passed, the client may need to wear a support stocking for some time. Assess lochia, which might become heavier due to anticoagulants.

> **Nursing Alert** Carefully observe the client with thrombophlebitis. ***Rationale:*** *If the clot breaks away, it can enter the circulation as an embolism and cause death.*

Puerperal Infections

Puerperal infection is an infection in any part of the reproductive tract following childbirth. Before the practice of asepsis, it was the major cause of maternal death. Predisposing conditions include the presence of injured tissues or retained pieces of placenta and lowered maternal resistance. Infection may be mild or severe, local or general; however, as with any infection, it is preventable and treatable.

Staphylococcus and *Streptococcus* are common organisms causing puerperal infection. Because healthcare facility personnel can carry these organisms, those who work in the labor room wear caps, clean or sterile suits or gowns, and gloves. In the delivery room, aseptic technique is practiced, and masks are worn. The partner or coach also wears hospital garb in the delivery or birthing room. Handwashing before and after all examinations is absolutely necessary. Practice asepsis when handling the client's articles, such as perineal pads, and teach the client proper perineal care. Personnel with upper respiratory or gastrointestinal symptoms should not be in contact with the client.

Signs and Symptoms

Fever with a possible chill is the outstanding symptom of puerperal infection. Suspect infection if the client's temperature elevates to 100.4 °F (38 °C) orally on any 2 successive days during the first 10 postpartum days. A tender, enlarged uterus, headache, general malaise, and dark-colored, foul-smelling lochia are other symptoms of infection. The episiotomy may appear red, swollen, and tender. The suture line may not be intact. There may be *purulent* (pus-filled) drainage. Assess the characteristics of the lochia, the height of the fundus, and the appearance of the perineum.

The infected mother may be isolated or moved to another floor. The newborn may be isolated and may not be brought to the mother for feeding. Administer antibiotics and encourage fluids. Place the bed in Fowler position to promote drainage of lochia.

Cystitis

Cystitis, an inflammation of the bladder, is caused by a microorganism. It occurs frequently following childbirth because of urinary retention, residual urine, and trauma to the bladder and urethra during delivery. When urine remains in the bladder, it becomes a breeding place for bacteria.

Signs and Symptoms

The symptoms of cystitis include urination frequency, urgency, pain, burning; hematuria; low abdominal pain; fever; and malaise. After obtaining a urine specimen, administer antibiotics as ordered, and encourage fluids.

Mastitis

Mastitis is a breast infection most commonly caused by *Staphylococcus aureus* (which comes from the baby's mouth), *Escherichia coli*, and rarely *Streptococcus*. These organisms usually enter the body through cracked or injured nipples. The highest incidence occurs in the second or third postpartum week.

Predisposing conditions to mastitis are plugged milk ducts, poor breast drainage, the presence of a pathogenic organism, stress and fatigue, and tight-fitting clothing. Treatment of mastitis includes local massage, moist heat, antibiotic therapy, rest, and frequent nursing (see In Practice: Educating the Client 68-2).

> **IN PRACTICE**
> **EDUCATING THE CLIENT 68-2** — **Prevention of Mastitis Complications**
>
> Teach the client and family the following measures to prevent mastitis complications:
> - Continue to nurse the newborn on both breasts, beginning with the unaffected breast to ease the let-down reflex on the other side.
> - Bed rest is mandatory.
> - Follow antibiotic therapy regimen as directed by the healthcare provider.
> - Use hot packs on the breast for comfort.
> - Drink plenty of fluids.
> - Use mild analgesics (for example, acetaminophen (Tylenol), ibuprofen (Motrin)) for pain relief.
> - Wear a well-fitting support bra.

Signs and Symptoms

The signs and symptoms of mastitis include localized tenderness, redness, heat, fever, malaise, and sometimes nausea and vomiting. Mastitis should be treated immediately to avoid abscess and chronic mastitis, which may last for up to 4 months and require extensive antibiotic therapy.

Postpartum Blues, Depression, and Psychosis

Clients are at risk for "the blues," depression, and psychosis in the months following childbirth. These *mood disorders* are often undiagnosed and therefore may not be treated. The etiology of the psychological aspect of the postpartum period is most likely caused by gonadal hormone imbalances (imbalances in the levels of reproductive hormones). Family and genetic tendencies are also implicated in the development of postpartum mood swings.

Postpartum Blues

Approximately 25%–85% of all clients experience a mild depression, called *postpartum blues,* 3–10 days after delivery. Symptoms generally start about 1 week after delivery. The symptoms tend to peak about 5 days after onset and generally resolve spontaneously in about 2 weeks.

Typical maternal behaviors may include crying, anxiety, poor appetite, irritability, and insomnia. Many consider these symptoms a normal adjustment phase of the postpartum period. However, these behaviors may also be a warning and indicator of a more serious depression. Treatment generally consists of understanding, reassurance, and support. Members of the family should be made aware of the possible development of "the blues," as well as be told of the importance of follow-up treatment if the symptoms get worse or do not resolve.

Postpartum Depression

Postpartum depression occurs in about 10%–20% of postpartum clients. Depression is more serious than "the blues." Depression begins about 4 weeks after delivery, and clients are at increased risk for major depression for several months. The depression may last 6 months or more. A risk factor assessment for depression may be helpful in the early detection of this condition. Risk factors for depression include

- *Psychological risk factors:* Family history of blues or depression, personal psychiatric history, premenstrual mood swings
- *Social risk factors:* Limited or nonexistent emotional support (from partner, parents, or friends), relationship conflict and concerns, stressful living conditions, nominal recreational activities
- *Physical risk factors:* Fatigue, poor general health, thyroid dysfunction, sleep disturbances, use of intramuscular progesterone contraceptive
- *Infant risk factors:* Child health problems, feeding or sleep problems, consensus that the child is a "difficult child"
- *Employment risk factors:* Parental leave of less than 6 weeks, long work hours with few work rewards

Treatment for depression generally consists of medications such as fluoxetine (Prozac) and/or psychotherapy. The nurse assists by supporting the need for postpartum and well-baby visits. The client's family and other members of their support system should be advised to notify the healthcare provider of significant, persistent mood changes between visits.

Postpartum Psychosis

A *postpartum psychosis* can be suspected if the client exhibits manic-depressive behaviors, generally starting within the first 4 weeks after delivery. Postpartum psychosis occurs in less than 1% of the postpartum population. Initially, the symptoms may include irritability, restlessness, sleeplessness, agitation, and avoidance of the infant. The condition may progress to include incoherence, with delusions or hallucinations relating to the child or childbirth. Postpartum psychosis is considered a *medical emergency;* suicide or infanticide is not uncommon.

Treatment consists of hospitalization with suicide precautions and medications such as lithium, antipsychotics, or antidepressants. Child protective services may be necessary. Prognosis, with appropriate medications, is usually good, but the condition may recur following subsequent deliveries. Generally, 95% of these clients improve within 3 months after starting therapy. This condition rarely occurs in clients with no previous psychiatric history.

WHEN A NEWBORN DIES

Occasionally, despite excellent antepartal care, a fetus or newborn dies. Such an event is very difficult for family members. Provide them with as much support as possible and give them a chance to express their feelings. They may or may not appreciate a visit from a chaplain or counselor; ask if the family wishes to have someone special called.

Depending on the client's wishes and the healthcare facility's policies, the client may be moved from the obstetric unit. However, moving the client from the OB unit may intensify emotions and add further trauma to the experience.

Some facilities prepare a small package of mementos from the baby, such as the tee shirt worn in the nursery, a lock of hair, some photos, an identification bracelet, and the birth certificate. Such articles are given to the client for them to open or to keep sealed as they choose. In this way, the baby's existence is acknowledged, along with the loss. Be familiar with policy, and respect the family's wishes. Allow the client to hold the child and take photos if they wish. The family also may choose to donate fetal tissues.

The family should be given the opportunity to have a funeral or cremation. Referral to an appropriate support organization is often helpful.

STUDENT SYNTHESIS

KEY POINTS

- A high-risk pregnancy is one in which complications of the pregnancy or preexisting health conditions endanger the life or well-being of the client or fetus.
- Diagnostic techniques for assessing fetal status include amniocentesis, ultrasound, nonstress testing, oxytocin challenge testing, and biophysical profile.
- Some spontaneous abortions occur for unknown reasons; however, fetal maldevelopment and certain maternal factors account for many cases. The type of spontaneous abortion dictates medical and nursing management.
- Ectopic pregnancy is a significant cause of maternal morbidity and mortality.
- Discharge of a client with hyperemesis gravidarum occurs when they regain fluid and electrolyte balance and begin to gain weight.
- Careful management of the client with pregnancy-induced hypertension is crucial.
- Existing medical disorders—such as diabetes mellitus, cardiac disorders, and chemical dependency—will complicate pregnancy and require special care.
- Maternal insulin requirements in the client with insulin-dependent diabetes increase as the pregnancy advances. Control of maternal blood glucose is essential to prevent hydramnios, dystocia, and other complications.
- Placenta previa and premature separation of the placenta are differentiated by the type of bleeding, uterine tone, and the presence or absence of pain.
- Complications of labor and delivery are related to the status of the membranes, the pace of labor, the effectiveness of contractions, the passageway, and the passenger.
- Dystocia is active labor that does not result in effective cervical dilation or effacement.
- Operative obstetrics concerns procedures that involve manipulating the fetus to facilitate birth. Version, forceps, vacuum extraction, and cesarean birth are examples.
- Hemorrhagic (hypovolemic) shock is an emergency in which sufficient blood does not reach vital organs in the client or newborn; death may ensue.
- The primary purpose of a cesarean delivery is to preserve the life and health of the client and the fetus.
- Infection control measures are essential to protect the client and newborn from transmission of infectious organisms.

CRITICAL THINKING EXERCISES

1. Identify risk factors for noncompliance with the treatment regimen for a client who is pregnant and has diabetes.

2. You are caring for a client who is 32 years of age. Three previous pregnancies have been full-term without complications. One previous pregnancy ended in a stillbirth. During this pregnancy, the client developed preeclampsia during the third trimester. They are now at 38 weeks' gestation and have been admitted with a large amount of painless vaginal bleeding. List nursing interventions according to priority.

3. Compare the effect of amniotomy for induction of labor with various other methods. Consider risks and benefits for the client and newborn.

4. Place yourself in the position of a client who has just been told they must have an emergency cesarean birth because of complications. Describe your feelings. Discuss which information you will need and the nursing care you would like to receive.

NCLEX-STYLE REVIEW QUESTIONS

1. A pregnant client at 6 weeks' gestation just expelled all products of conception. Which is the priority action by the nurse after this occurrence?
   a. Force oral fluids.
   b. Dispose of the products of conception.
   c. Observe for hemorrhage.
   d. Insert an indwelling catheter.

2. The nurse is gathering data from a client who suspects they are pregnant. Which data obtained by the nurse is of most concern regarding the presence of an ectopic pregnancy?
   a. The client has one living child.
   b. The client has early morning nausea.
   c. The client has a history of a lengthy labor with the first child.
   d. The client has a history of several pelvic infections.

3. A 36-week pregnant client is diagnosed with pregnancy-induced hypertension (PIH). Which laboratory studies reviewed by the nurse may be an indication that the client is developing HELLP syndrome? Select all that apply.
   a. Elevated liver enzymes
   b. A decreased platelet count
   c. An elevated white blood cell count
   d. An elevated glucose level
   e. Low red blood cell count

4. A pregnant client with eclampsia is being treated with intravenous magnesium sulfate. Which medication would the nurse keep at the bedside in the event toxicity occurs?
   a. Calcium gluconate (Kalcinate)
   b. Potassium chloride (KCl)
   c. Protamine sulfate (Prosulf)
   d. Phytonadione (vitamin K)

5. The nurse is planning the discharge of a client at 32 weeks' gestation with placenta previa. Which information is important for the nurse to discuss with the client before discharge?
   a. The client will have to return every 2 weeks to have a vaginal examination.
   b. The client must remain on strict bed rest at all times.
   c. The client will have to have a blood transfusion every week.
   d. The client may not be able to have any more children after this.

CHAPTER RESOURCES

Enhance your learning with additional resources on thePoint!

Student Resources related to this chapter can be found at thePoint.lww.com/Rosdahl12e.

69 The High-Risk Newborn

Learning Objectives

1. Discuss the healthcare influence and technologic significance relating to high-risk newborns, infant morbidity, and infant mortality.
2. Name the two main classifications of high-risk newborns.
3. Differentiate the morbidity and mortality healthcare consequences of the following terms: appropriate for gestational age, low birth weight, very low birth weight, and extremely low birth weight.
4. Compare and contrast the following terms: gestational age, small for gestational age, large for gestational age, macrosomia, intrauterine growth restriction (asymmetric and symmetric), preterm infant, and postterm infant.
5. State the major nursing observations necessary and discuss the nursing considerations needed for the care of the high-risk newborn.
6. Relate the physiologic causes to the nursing care necessary for the following complications in the high-risk newborn: diabetes, respiratory distress disorders, hyperbilirubinemia, neurologic consequences, retinopathy of prematurity, necrotizing enterocolitis, meconium aspiration syndrome, and sudden infant death syndrome.
7. Differentiate the causes of hemolytic disease of the newborn including erythroblastosis fetalis and ABO incompatibility; state the nursing interventions required.
8. State nursing interventions for the following congenital musculoskeletal disorders: talipes, congenital dislocated hip, polydactylism, and syndactylism.
9. Describe the following congenital neural tube defects: hydrocephalus, spina bifida, anencephaly, and microcephaly, and state the nursing interventions for each disorder.
10. State nursing interventions for the following cardiovascular disorders: patent ductus arteriosus, ASD, VSD, tetralogy of Fallot, and coarctation of the aorta.
11. List nursing interventions for the following gastrointestinal and genitourinary disorders: cleft lip, cleft palate, esophageal atresia, tracheoesophageal fistula, pyloric stenosis, imperforate anus, PKU, galactosemia, exstrophy of the bladder, hypospadias, and epispadias.
12. Relate physiologic causes to the nursing care necessary for the following congenital or acquired intrauterine disorders: fetal alcohol syndrome, Down syndrome, and thrush.
13. Relate physiologic causes and the nursing care necessary for each of the infections associated with a TORCH infection.
14. Identify the consequences to the fetus if the pregnant client has a history of substance abuse; identify the nursing considerations related to neonatal abstinence syndrome.

Important Terminology

ABO incompatibility, acquired disorders, anencephaly, Ballard Score, Ballard Maturational Assessment, choanal atresia, cleft lip, cleft palate, cluster care, congenital, endotracheal tube, epispadias, erythroblastosis fetalis, esophageal atresia, exstrophy, galactosemia, high-risk newborn, hydrocephalus, hyperbilirubinemia, hypospadias, iatrogenic, imperforate anus, infant mortality, jaundice, kangaroo care, kernicterus, LS ratio, macrosomia, microcephaly, phototherapy, pyloric stenosis, Rh sensitization, spina bifida, thermoregulation, toxoplasmosis, tracheoesophageal fistula

Acronyms

AGA, ASD, CMV, CPAP, CSF, ECMO, ELBW, ET tube, FASD, FAS, GA, HDN, IUGR, IVH, LBW, LGA, MAS, NEC, NICU, NTD, PKU, RDS, ROP, SGA, SIDS, TORCH, TTN, VLBW, VSD

At birth, the newborn assumes the functions of breathing, eating, digesting, eliminating, and stabilizing their own body temperature. If problems related to any of these vital functions develop, the newborn is likely to have difficulty surviving. The newborn with a complication is considered a compromised or **high-risk newborn**. Due to advanced technology and improved healthcare measures, high-risk newborns have ever-increasing chances for survival. However, lifelong complications are potential complications of major technical interventions.

Infant mortality, the death of infants before their first birthday, averages about 5.7 deaths per 1,000 live births (Ely and Driscoll, 2020). In spite of improvements in maternal–fetal healthcare, these numbers have been relatively unchanged for at least a decade. Healthcare professionals need to be aware that the five leading causes of infant mortality remain:

- Serious birth defects
- Born too small or too premature
- Sudden infant death syndrome (SIDS)
- Maternal complications of pregnancy
- Victims of injuries

Infant health is considered to be a reflection of the well-being of a nation and its entire population. Information gathered by the CDC and other health agencies are used to promote research into causative factors of mortality, projects that promote improved healthcare, and education for both healthcare workers and parents.

Families often are shocked when learning their newborn has a problem. Remember when caring for newborns, nurses also care for the whole family. Family members need to express their fears, hopes, and disappointments. Sometimes, they require more knowledge so that they can make decisions related to treatment. Lifelong physical and mental challenges develop in some of these children. Most of all, families appreciate a caring nurse—someone who listens with compassion and understanding.

The morbidity and mortality of high-risk pregnancies and newborns have improved greatly in the past few decades. The successful outcomes are generally possible only with the intervention of obstetric technology. The lives of many high-risk neonates may be saved. However, many of these infants are often born with or develop serious, lifelong problems. Hospitalization and posthospital care will most likely be required for these high-risk neonates. Teams of medical professionals, including individuals who specialize in medical ethics, are often used to discuss medical options and to educate the family of the short-term risks and lifelong consequences of the survival of the high-risk infant. Hospitalizations for high-risk situations may involve weeks to months of intensive care, which increase the risks for iatrogenic problems. Iatrogenic refers to an inadvertently acquired problem that results from medical or surgical treatments. Mechanical or highly evolved technical environments can be responsible for eyesight problems, neurologic damage, infections, and developmental difficulties. Examples of long-term consequences related to the care of a high-risk infant include intellectual disabilities, brain hemorrhage, blindness, cerebral palsy, and necrotizing enterocolitis (NEC; a bacterial infection resulting in bowl necrosis).

Healthcare professionals and society in general have become more aware of the positive and negative possibilities of high-tech interventions. Additional questions to be discussed and debated by neonatal healthcare teams include the societal issues and financial commitments involved with long-term care.

> **Key Concept**
> Good preconception self-care (care before getting pregnant) has a significant effect on the health outcome of a pregnancy. A safe, healthy lifestyle and the stabilization of health-related conditions, such as diabetes, have an especially positive effect on the maternal and fetal outcome.

The client who has just given birth, their family, and the high-risk newborn are highly vulnerable. Basic priorities for any newborn include adequate oxygenation, hemostasis of fluids and electrolytes, sufficient nutritional (caloric) intake, thermoregulation (an appropriately warm environment), and protection against infections. The high-risk newborn's basic needs are essentially the same but more complex. These infants need constant observation. The baby's survival and well-being depend on the collaborative efforts of the healthcare team. Through accurate data collection and assessments, the healthcare team can often detect abnormalities early and report them promptly. Nurses are typically among the first to receive the newborn after delivery and, as such, have a primary responsibility to recognize and report any potential issues that could be related to the well-being and survival of a high-risk newborn. Difficulties can often be alleviated or corrected when treatment begins quickly.

CATEGORIES OF HIGH-RISK NEWBORNS

High-risk newborns can be categorized according to birth weight and gestational age. Other concerns are often related to these two major categories. Many high-risk neonates have a combination of problems. Variations in gestational age, such as preterm or postterm births, plus low birth weight (LBW) are the most prevalent issues. For example, preterm birth typically results in LBW, inadequate formation of body systems, and a decreased incidence of ability to thrive. Risk factors for high-risk newborns are often related to maternal conditions affecting pregnancy. Examples include pregnancy-induced hypertension, preeclampsia, and preexisting maternal disorders such as cardiac issues. Box 69-1 summarizes many of the most common high-risk categories. See Box 68-1 for a more complete list of maternal issues.

Newborn Birth Weight

Appropriate-for-Gestational-Age Newborn

Appropriate for gestational age (**AGA**) is the term used for newborns whose weight and size are appropriate for their estimated gestational age (**GA**). GA is discussed further in the next section. Comparisons of normal of weight, height, head size, and developmental level are obtained. Children of the same gestational age and sex should weigh within the standard normal ranges for a term delivery, or about 2,500 to 4,200 g (about 5 lb 8 oz to 9 lb 6 oz). AGA babies tend to have a lower risk for mortality and morbidity than babies who are born small or large for their GA.

Low–Birth-Weight Newborn

LBW babies, who typically weigh less than 2,500 g (about 5 lb 8 oz), can be born as full-term or *preterm* infants. LBW is one of the most common characteristics of high-risk infants.

Very Low–Birth-Weight Newborn

Very low–birth-weight (**VLBW**) babies weigh about 1,500 g (about 3.3 lb), are at a higher risk than LBW newborns, and are generally born before their expected birth date. LBW babies are more likely to be born to adolescent clients.

Extremely Low–Birth-Weight Newborn

Extremely low–birth-weight (**ELBW**) newborns, or "micropremies," are infants born with a birth weight of less than 1,000 g (about 2 lb 3 oz). They are also the youngest of the

Box 69-1 High-Risk Newborns

The following conditions may contribute to high-risk newborns:
- **Low birth weight**—The less the infant weights, the greater risk the infant has for complications.
- **Gestational age: (preterm or postmature)**—An infant of less than 30 weeks or more than 42 weeks is at greater risk than an infant born close to 37 weeks.
- **Apgar score <4 to 5**—An infant with two low Apgar scores 5 min apart has a greater risk than an infant with a low rate at 1 min and a 7 or above at the 5-min postbirth interval.
- **Birth defects**—Some of these conditions include congenital heart defects, acquired defects, or genetic birth defects.
- **Birth infections**—Examples include maternal sepsis, infant HIV exposure, TORCH, or an aseptic birth environment.
- **Infants of clients with diabetes**—Diabetes increases the risk of hypoglycemia and birth injuries.
- **Respiratory distress syndrome**—Increased risk of respiratory disorders is often corelated with the problems associated with high-risk newborns, for example, small for gestational age.
- **Meconium aspiration syndrome**—Meconium aspiration can be a significant factor in the survival of a newborn.
- **Infants of clients who misuse substances**—Infants have significant neurologic problems as well as neonatal abstinence syndrome (withdrawal).
- **Preconceptive disorders or problems**—Pregnant clients who have fertility problems, cardiovascular disorders, or diabetes often give birth to high-risk newborns.
- **Previous familial history of high-risk pregnancies or newborns**—High-risk newborns may result from a variety of conditions that have been seen in previous pregnancies, for example, Down syndrome.

Adapted from Hatfield (2018); https://www.cdc.gov/reproductivehealth/maternalinfanthealth/index.html

premature neonates, typically born at 27 weeks' gestational age or younger. ELBW survival rates have improved due to the availability of life-saving drugs such as respiratory surfactant agents, given to the at-risk neonate. Prebirth steroids given to the pregnant client support lung maturity in the fetus. The advancements in neonatal technologies have shown that a minimum age of viability can be seen in infants of 23 weeks' gestation, with an occasional successful outcome for infants of 21 to 22 weeks' estimated gestation. Although mortality rates for ELBW infants have decreased, morbidity (i.e., life-long complications) often accompanies survival. Examples include chronic lung disease, cognitive delays, cerebral palsy, deafness, and blindness (Medscape, 2020).

Gestational Age

Gestational age (**GA**) refers to the weeks of fetal growth and development between conception and birth, which typically results in an infant of appropriate gestational age (discussed in the previous section). The time period from the first day of a client's last menstrual cycle to the current date determines the GA, which by the time of birth normally ranges from 38 to 42 weeks. Within a few hours after birth, a gestational age assessment is completed, usually by an RN. One of the most common methods of ascertaining basic age is the **Ballard Score or Ballard Maturational Assessment**, which looks at neuromuscular diagrams and descriptions of various ages of known physical maturity. Each diagram and description is given a numerical rating or score. The New Ballard Score can assess premature maturation starting at age 20 weeks. The total score indicates the GA listed for the newborn. A more detailed GA will be assessed by the appropriate healthcare provider (e.g., pediatrician, neonatologist), who will do the more detailed physical examination of the infant. If the initial Ballard Score is not within normal ranges, the nurse must notify the healthcare provider as soon as possible.

Small-for-Gestational-Age Newborn

Small for gestational age (**SGA**) is a condition in which an infant may not grow normally in utero, for a variety of reasons. SGA includes infants born at 10% or less of expected weight. High-risk protocols are generally initiated for any SGA infant. Examples of SGA risk factors include genetic abnormalities, cytomegalovirus (CMV) infection, or fetal alcohol syndrome (FAS). Some infants who can be classified as SGA may be small for reasons related to family characteristics (genetics) and may have actually met their in utero growth potential.

Characteristics of the SGA newborn include poor skin turgor, loose and dry skin, sparse or absent hair, wide skull sutures caused by inadequate bone growth, and diminished muscle and fatty tissue. Weight, length, and head circumference are below normal expectations as defined on growth charts. These infants are at high risk during normal labor or cesarean deliveries. Common problems associated with the SGA newborn immediately after birth include respiratory distress, hypoglycemia, and problems with regulation of body temperature (*thermoregulation*).

Other problems faced by the SGA newborn include prolonged infantile apnea, delayed neurologic development, and **SIDS**. If hypoxia occurred during early fetal development, the infant has an increased risk for abnormal development of the nervous system, with resulting developmental delays after birth.

Large-for-Gestational-Age Newborn

The *large-for-gestational-age* (**LGA**) newborn is a fetus or newborn who is larger than expected as compared with infants of that same age and sex. They exceed the 90th percentile of newborns of the same gestational age. LGA term birth weights are over 4,000 g (about 8 lb 13 oz). LGA neonates are born most often to clients with diabetes or who have a prolonged pregnancy (>40 weeks). Genetics and family characteristics may also influence the size of an infant. Clients who are obese or who have previously had an LGA infant are more likely to have another LGA birth. LGA neonates, from clients with existing diabetes or obesity, are more likely to be obese in childhood and to develop type 2 diabetes in adulthood.

Macrosomia

Macrosomia refers to excessive intrauterine growth regardless of gestational age. Due to inability to accurately predict prenatal fetal weight, macrosomia can only be confirmed after delivery and affects less than 10% of all pregnancies.

If full-term, an infant with macrosomia has a birth weight greater than 4,000 or 4,500 g (about 8 lb 13 oz to 9 lb 15 oz) or greater than 90% for gestational age after correcting for neonatal sex and ethnicity. As with LGA infants, the condition of macrosomia increases morbidity. Factors associated with fetal macrosomia are similar to those of LGA infants and include genetics, duration of gestation, presence of gestational diabetes, and sex. Male newborns generally weigh more than female newborns. Some racial and ethnic backgrounds have a genetic influence on birth weight and size.

Although LGA newborns and those who have macrosomia are large and appear fat, they are not necessarily healthy. Elevated blood glucose levels in the pregnant client increase the glucose available to the fetus, which stimulates additional insulin production by the fetal pancreas. When the baby is delivered, often by cesarean section, the supply of excess glucose is suddenly terminated. This newborn quickly uses all available carbohydrates and may develop hypoglycemia. Poor glucose control in the fetus increases the risk of intrauterine death and hypoglycemia in the newborn can occur suddenly. Further discussion regarding hypoglycemia follows in the section on newborns of clients with diabetes.

Other problems facing the large newborn include birth injury. Examples include fractured clavicle, skull fracture, and brachial nerve palsy, respiratory disorders, and brain injuries. Long-term consequences may result in delayed mental and physical development.

Intrauterine Growth Restriction

Intrauterine growth restriction (**IUGR**) or *fetal growth restriction* describes a condition of insufficient *fetal* growth. The fetus does not reach its genetic growth potential. The etiology of IUGR includes fetal, placental, and maternal causes or a combination of causes. Many cases involve instances of poor maternal nutrition and interference with oxygen supply via the placenta. The specific etiology is not always known. Mortality and morbidity rates are high when compared with the AGA infant. IUGR is the most common causative factor leading to SGA or LBW. The term *SGA associated with IUGR* is used when the baby has not reached its expected growth or weight. The terms IUGR and SGA are not synonymous, however; common usage may see the acronyms used interchangeably.

There are two typical growth patterns associated with IUGR: *asymmetric* and *symmetric*.

- *Asymmetric IUGR* develops in the third trimester and is the most common type of IUGR. Typically, asymmetric IUGR results because of a redistribution of maternal–fetal blood flow. Poor blood flow means that some fetal organs get inadequate circulation and do not develop fully. Fetal weight, length, and/or abdominal circumference are affected. However, in asymmetrical cases, the head circumference is spared (not affected). Maternal factors affecting the fetus in later pregnancy include preeclampsia, chronic hypertension, and uterine anomalies.
- *Symmetric IUGR* usually occurs in early pregnancy with uniform abnormalities noted. Genetic abnormalities, maternal alcohol consumption, and TORCH syndrome can be causative factors for early gestational growth restriction. As discussed later in this chapter, TORCH is an acronym for a group of serious infections that can occur during pregnancy. Most of these affected children have permanent neurologic problems.

The IUGR neonate typically appears wasted (too thin) and pale. The face looks shrunken; the ear cartilage and female genitalia appear less mature than those of an AGA infant. Meconium staining and meconium aspiration are common findings. (See Meconium Aspiration Syndrome later in this chapter.) Neurologic abnormalities including a shrill cry, hyperalertism, and irritability may be observed.

> **NCLEX Alert**
>
> Examination considerations for the high-risk newborn and client would typically involve accurate identification of problems and selection of required nursing interventions. When responding to the clinical situation described, be sure to respond to the *actual problem presented*. It is possible that an NCLEX question may present several facts within the scenario but you will need to provide the correct response only to the *pertinent facts*.

Preterm Newborn

Newborns classified as preterm are those born before the end of the 37th week of gestation. A category called *late preterm* occurs between weeks 34 and 37. The preterm infant appears thin, with minimal subcutaneous fat. *Lanugo* (fine hair) may appear on the face, back, arms, and legs. Skin is transparent and breast tissue is barely palpable. In male newborns, the testes may be undescended. Breathing is irregular and weak. Body temperature is frequently subnormal, and the baby's cry is weak. Neurologic assessments reflect an immature central nervous system, as demonstrated by diminished or absent reflexes. Mortality and morbidity improve as the infant's gestational age comes closer to term; therefore, accurate determination of GA is essential.

Postterm Newborn

The fetus who remains in the uterus beyond 42 weeks is called *postterm*. Such newborns are not necessarily in better condition than full-term newborns. Postterm newborns often have respiratory or nutritional problems because the placenta is unable to provide adequately for them after the normal gestation period. As a result, they may be SGA. They often have long fingernails and hair, dry parched skin, and no vernix caseosa. These babies look wrinkled and old at birth. They may have swallowed meconium or aspirated it into their lungs, which can result in serious problems with oxygenation and may result in the demise of a newborn.

NURSING CONSIDERATIONS FOR THE HIGH-RISK NEWBORN

Nursing Observations

In addition to the care of the normal newborn described in Chapter 67, the high-risk newborn needs specific and careful observations, generally accomplished by an experienced nurse in a *neonatal intensive care unit* or **NICU**. Norms for gestational age need to be considered. Respiratory symptoms are a common early sign of pending complications and further problems. Apnea, cardiac, and pulse oximetry monitors are commonly used. Heat-controlled environments, such as the radiant warmer, are used. Neurologic assessments are performed on all newborns to determine their maturity. Maternal history (e.g., diabetes, existence and quality of prenatal care, maternal infection), which is available with the client's medical records, is an important source of information about potential risk factors. Oxygen is supplied if necessary (see Fig. 69-1 and In Practice: Nursing Care Plan 69-1). Document all findings. Report any abnormal symptoms immediately because newborn conditions change rapidly. Specific newborn disorders are discussed later in this chapter. Consider the following when making observations:

- *General appearance:* active or sleeping, sleep patterns, symmetrical movements of all extremities
- *Respirations:* normal versus abnormal rate, thoracic retractions, nasal flaring, expiratory grunt, stridor, crackles with auscultation
- *Pulse:* rate, rhythm, strength, equality

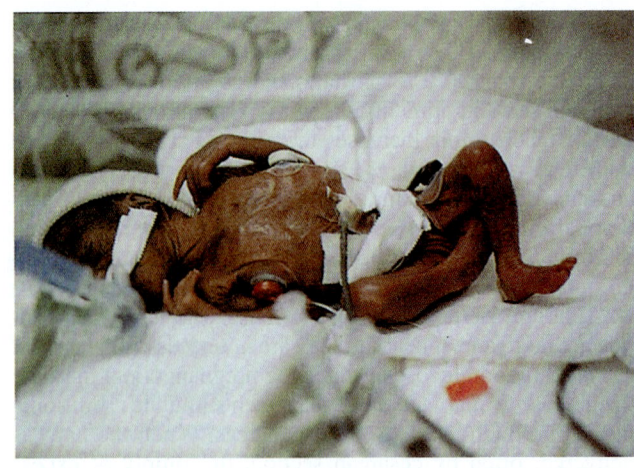

Figure 69-1 A newborn in the intensive care unit. Note the electrodes for constant monitoring and the cap on the head to maintain body heat.

IN PRACTICE
NURSING CARE PLAN 69-1 — The Preterm Neonate Experiencing Difficulty Regulating Body Temperature

Medical History: Baby boy Darrell, born vaginally at 30 weeks' gestation, has an Apgar score of 4 and 6 (at birth and at 5 min, respectively) and weighs 2,250 g. Mother had received betamethasone at 24 and 12 hr prior to birth to enhance lung maturity.

Medical Diagnosis: Prematurity.

I. DATA COLLECTION/NURSING OBSERVATION

Neonate born at 30 weeks. Temperature (axillary) fluctuates, ranging between 96.8 °F (36 °C) and 99.0 °F (37.2 °C). Client, although preterm, is appropriate for gestational age. Skin appears ruddy with vernix caseosa seen on the face, chest/abdomen, and back. Minimal subcutaneous fat noted. Acrocyanosis is evident. Respirations are slightly irregular at 66 breaths per minute; no bradycardia is noted.

II. NURSING DIAGNOSIS

(Although several nursing diagnoses may be appropriate, a priority nursing diagnosis is addressed below.)

Ineffective thermoregulation, related to immaturity and large body surface area with minimal fat stores, as evidenced by fluctuating axillary temperature readings.

3. PLANNING (OUTCOMES/GOALS)

Short-Term Goals

A. Client will exhibit no signs of cold-stress or hypothermia during the first 8 hr post delivery.

4. IMPLEMENTATION (NURSING ACTIONS)

- Cover the neonate's head.
  Rationale: Covering the neonate's head, a large body surface area for heat loss, minimizes the amount of heat loss.
- Dry neonate thoroughly and place in isolette or under a radiant warmer.
- If using an isolette, minimize the number of times the portholes are opened.
  Rationale: Drying helps to prevent heat loss by evaporation; an isolette or radiant warmer provides a neutral thermal environment. Opening the portholes provides a means for heat to escape from the isolette.
- Cover any surfaces that the neonate is to lie on and position the neonate away from doors, windows, or other areas that may cause drafts.
  Rationale: Lying on a cold surface increases the loss of body heat via conduction. Keeping the neonate away from areas that may cause drafts minimizes the amount of heat lost via convection and radiation.

5. EVALUATION

Day 1—05:45 hr
Neonate's temperature ranging between 97.6 °F and 98.6 °F (36.5 °C-37 °C) for past 4 hr.
Goal A complete.
Observations continue.

3. PLANNING (OUTCOMES/GOALS)	4. IMPLEMENTATION (NURSING ACTIONS)	5. EVALUATION
B. Client will demonstrate gradual stabilization of body temperature within acceptable range for weight.	• Keep the handling of the neonate to a minimum. • Refrain from bathing the neonate until the temperature is maintained between 97.6 °F and 98.6 °F (36.5 °C-37 °C) or wait 24 hr post birth. • Consolidate procedures and treatments to avoid tiring the neonate. *Rationale: Minimizing handling helps the neonate to conserve energy and have energy available for stabilization of temperature.* • Continue to monitor neonate's heart rate and respirations for changes indicating possible cold-stress. • Begin to increase time out of isolette from 10 to 30 min for each session with mother. • Monitor temperature closely for changes. *Rationale: Cold-stress increases the neonate's consumption of oxygen, increasing the workload of the heart.* • Weigh the neonate daily • Report any significant decreases. *Rationale: Cold-stress can increase the consumption of energies (calories) and, thus, decrease the rate of weight gain in the neonate.*	Day 1—10:00 hr Neonate warm, color pale pink; head covered; axillary temperature at 97.6 °F (36.5 °C); being maintained in isolette. No evidence of cold-stress at end of first 8 hr post delivery. **Goal A complete.** Observations continue. Day 1—21:30 hr Neonate's temperature, respirations, and heart rate within normal limits. Tolerates being out of isolette for at least 3 hr duration. **Goal B partially met.** Observations continue. Day 2—09:00 hr Neonate in mother's room and tolerated being out of isolette for 8 hr without significant change in VS. **Goal B met.**
Long-Term Goal C. At time of discharge, mother will state understanding of infant's energy (caloric) needs.	• Instruct client and neonate measures for continued conservation of energy techniques • Arrange for nursing follow-up after discharge. • Written discharge instructions given. *Rationale: Knowledge about necessary therapy and follow-up aid in decreasing the risk for recurrence.*	Day 2—09:45 hr Neonate's temperature ranging between 97.6 °F and 98.6 °F (36.5 °C-37 °C); heart rate (120-130 beats/min) and respirations (56-60 breaths/min) within age-acceptable parameters. **Goal C met.**

- *Color:* pink, acrocyanosis, overall cyanosis, jaundiced
- *Stools and voiding:* occur within a few hours after delivery, meconium in amniotic fluid, urine clear or dark, urine quantity
- *Weight:* gain or loss, appropriate for gestational age
- *Temperature:* normal, hypothermic, or febrile (state specific method/equipment used to take temperature), use of crib, isolette, incubator, or radiant warmer. **Kangaroo care** (skin-to-skin contact between a parent and infant) can also be used to keep an infant warm.
- *Nutrition:* breast or bottle, supplemental feedings, intravenous (IV) infusions
- Medications: routine postdelivery medications, antibiotics, vaccine

> **Nursing Alert** General observations made in the first 30 to 60 s of infant contact are valuable indicators. Remember the ABCs = Airway, Breathing, and Circulation. With newborns, also observe symmetrical movements, body temperature, and vocalization (a lusty cry is normal). Follow-up on any concern.

Nursing Care Considerations

Immediate postbirth care includes interventions that sustain and promote the well-being of the high-risk newborn. Nursing care needs to include teaching plans that address the long-term issues that accompany the infant after discharge from the hospital. Nursing care will include actions that deal with the following actual or potential problems.

Respiratory Difficulties

If the newborn does not establish initial breathing, they turn blue or dusky, a condition known as *cyanosis*. Cyanosis may be the first sign of respiratory difficulties. Many factors can be responsible for cyanosis, including lack of newborn respiratory surfactant, a prolapsed cord during delivery, a congenital heart defect, faulty respiratory apparatus, birth injury to the brain, a congenital defect in the brain stem, or medications including the analgesic or anesthetic given to the client during labor.

Prompt initiation of treatment for newborns who do not breathe as soon as they are delivered is crucial. First, it is necessary to determine whether the air passages are clear of obstructive substances, such as amniotic fluid and mucus. Soft catheters, bulb syringes, and mechanical suction are used to remove this material. The newborn's head is lowered, to facilitate postural drainage. The back is rubbed to stimulate respiration. If the baby fails to respond, additional resuscitation measures, for example, mechanical ventilation, are begun. Further discussion of serious respiratory complications is found later in this chapter.

Thermoregulation

Immediate postbirth care includes controlling the infant's temperature, or *thermoregulation*. Special considerations should be taken to keep these babies warm. Factors that alter the infant's physical environment, for example, turning, touching, repositioning, or opening an enclosed, thermodynamic space, will cause an increase in oxygen and caloric consumption while interfering with weight gain, fluid levels, and electrolyte stability. Air temperature, ambient humidity, and clothing help to decrease evaporative heat loss, convection, and radiant heat loss, as well as insensible water loss, in an unstable newborn.

Typically, the infant is not bathed immediately. Wetness promotes cold-stress so the infant must be dried and kept warm. Use a *stockinette cap* to prevent heat loss from the head. Frequent or continual temperature monitoring may be required. Heat loss via convection, conduction, evaporation, and radiation is discussed in more detail in Chapter 67. Refresh your knowledge of these important concepts and review Figure 67-1.

Hypoglycemia

All babies have the potential for *hypoglycemia* (decreased blood sugar) soon after birth. Infants of clients with gestational diabetes are at high risk for the first few days post birth. Any condition that results in physiologic stress on the fetus can increase the risks for and result in newborn hypoglycemia (Box 69-2). High-risk categories and newborns of clients with diabetes will need additional observations.

> **Key Concept**
> A newborn can be hypoglycemic and have no observable symptoms or history of risk factors. Most facilities include a routine heel stick after delivery to determine a newborn's blood sugar level.

Box 69-2 Risk Factors for Newborn Hypoglycemia

- Maternal diabetes
- Macrosomia (large for gestational age [LGA])
- Intrauterine growth restriction (IUGR)
- Small for gestational age (SGA)
- Prematurity
- Postmaturity
- Fetal distress during labor
- Prolonged labor
- Low Apgar score with respiratory or cardiovascular depression
- Erythroblastosis fetalis
- Congenital heart disease
- Galactosemia
- Maternal gestational hypertension
- Maternal infection
- Clients who have received ritodrine or terbutaline to stop preterm labor

Box 69-3 Typical Signs of Hypoglycemia

- Jitteriness and exaggerated Moro reflex (main signs)
- Tremors or irritability
- Seizures
- Apnea
- Tachycardia
- Cyanosis or paleness
- High-pitched or weak cry
- Eye rolling
- Listlessness
- Eating poorly

A capillary blood sugar test via heel stick is usually done within 2 hr after birth (see In Practice: Nursing Procedure 67-6). Although somewhat controversial, a typical normal newborn's blood sugar level ranges from 40 to 60 mg/dL in the first 24 hr after birth. Transient blood glucose levels can be as low as 30 mg/dL and still be considered adequate for the healthy infant. Glucose levels should stabilize within the first 3 to 4 hr post delivery. If the capillary sugar (heel stick) is low, a venous blood sample may be ordered. In either instance, the infant may be breast-fed, bottle-fed, or given glucose via IV line.

It is important to check the baby carefully for changes in status, monitor blood sugar levels, and decrease supplemental sugar as the infant becomes more physiologically stable. Box 69-3 lists typical signs of hypoglycemia in a newborn. However, it is important to remember that *there may be no signs of hypoglycemia*. The importance of the consequences of hypoglycemia episodes and maintenance of stable blood glucose levels cannot be understated. Untreated, severe hypoglycemia can result in brain damage.

Cluster Care

To conserve the energy of small newborns, handle them as little as possible. Care provided in an organized manner is known as **cluster care**, which helps conserve the infant's energy, avoid exhaustion, and prevent excessive heat loss. Minimal handling promotes the internal homeostasis of the infant and external stability of the environment. The results of planning care are better thermoregulation, continual humidity and oxygen levels, and less caloric stress (energy use). Contact with the infant is essential for survival, so do not ignore or avoid the basic, therapeutic needs of gentle touch or a back massage. Neonates often prefer to be placed in a flexed position. Nonnutritive sucking, for example, a pacifier, helps develop the motor skills needed for feedings.

Environment

The atmosphere and environment of the NICU is typically an active place with nurses, parents, healthcare providers, laboratory technicians, and incidental hospital staff often in and out of the unit. The nurses are responsible for the traffic flow of individuals as part of their concerns for infant safety. The NICU environment contains protective devices, including the *radiant warmer* and the *isolette* (Fig. 69-2), which are artificial intrauterine substitutes designed for protective isolation and thermoregulation of the neonate. The environment needs to be quiet, calm, and stress-free. Disturbances to the physical environment can interfere with the infant's ability

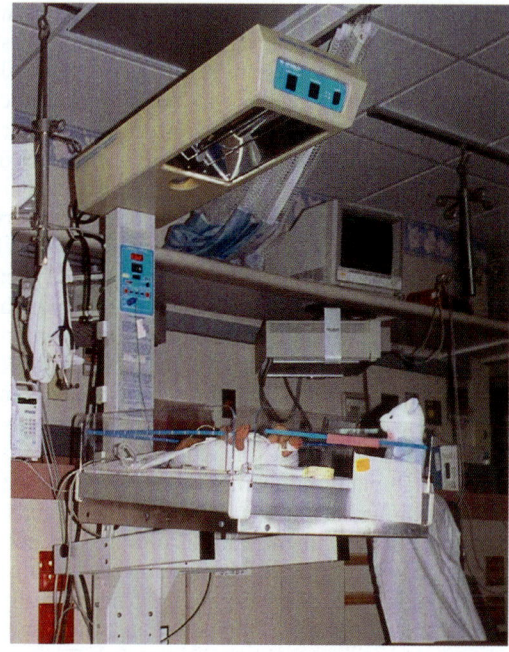 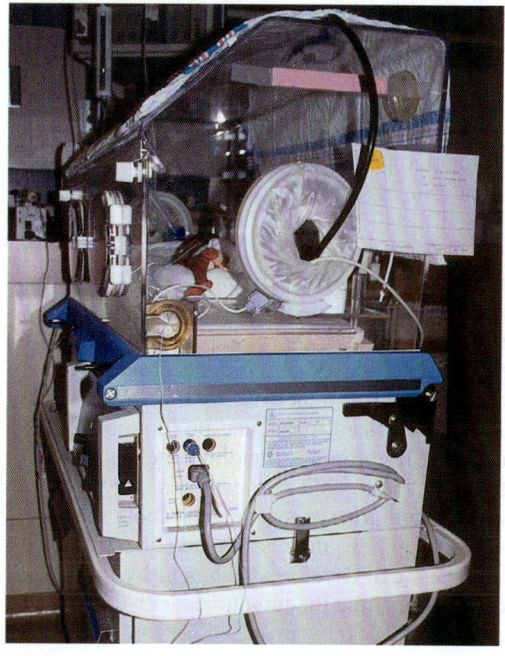

Figure 69-2 Thermoregulation devices, such as (A) the open radiant warmer and (B) the enclosed isolette, are designed to sustain body temperature and to maximize homeostasis of the newborn (Hatfield, 2014).

to maintain homeostasis. The radiant warmer is an open unit with an overhead heat source that allows for frequent access to the infant. The isolette is a closed, transparent microenvironment where specific temperatures, oxygen, and humidity are maintained. Access to the isolette is by portholes at the side of the unit or a hood that covers it. Most nursing care is given through portholes. Generally, these newborns are not dressed, so that nurses can observe their breathing, skin color and condition, and neurologic symptoms.

Fluid and Electrolytes

The greatest concern with newborn vomiting or diarrhea is dehydration, which may lead to electrolyte imbalance if unchecked. Dehydration develops quickly because the baby has so little reserve fluid. Start treatment immediately, or the newborn may die. Give IV fluids as ordered, along with humidified oxygen. Lost electrolytes must be replaced.

Newborn *vomiting* may be a symptom of a congenital defect, for example, esophageal atresia, birth injury, intracranial hemorrhage, or infection. A distinct difference exists between vomiting and normal spitting-up in the newborn.

Bacteria most commonly cause *diarrhea,* although an incompatible formula or an allergy may also be the culprit. In newborn diarrhea, the stool is formless, greenish-yellow, and foul-smelling. Evidence of diarrhea requires isolation of the baby to prevent possible infection of other newborns. Obtain stool cultures.

Nutrition

The feeding of small newborns varies. Caloric intake and nutritional needs are the main concerns of postbirth feedings. In some instances, small newborns receive no food for 36 hr because digestion is an additional burden on their bodies. In other instances, they receive formula or expressed breast milk using a nipple or a nasogastric tube, called *gavage feeding.* Formula is prescribed in very small amounts on a 2- to 3-hr schedule, to avoid distending their small stomachs or adding to respiratory distress. Caloric intake needs to be monitored. Daily weightings and constant monitoring of intake and output are crucial.

Elimination

Because their kidneys are not fully developed, small newborns may have difficulty eliminating wastes. The nurse should determine accurate output by weighing the diaper before and after the infant urinates. The diaper's weight difference in grams is approximately equal to the amount of milliliters voided.

Infection

Handwashing is the primary method of infection control. Very small newborns are very susceptible to infection. Bacteria are spread via touching the infant or the infant's supplies, which include items such as the isolette, IV tubing, respiratory equipment, suction, or infant's articles. Signs of infection in a newborn may be subtle and develop into major infections quickly, as newborns have minimal ability to fight infections. Contact with people is limited as much as possible. Personnel from other departments, for example, laboratory technicians, put on a cover gown and gloves when working with an infant. Family members must be taught how to put on protective gloves and gowns. NICUs typically have their own trained staff and may use cover gowns when leaving the unit.

The following list may indicate the presence of problems, including developing infections.

- Temperature instability: up or down, also seen with cold-stress

- Glucose instability: hyperglycemia, hypoglycemia
- Lack of weight gain: poor feeding, sucking, or nutritional intake
- Vomiting or diarrhea: electrolyte disturbances, lethargy
- Respiratory distress: cyanosis, apnea
- Hyperbilirubinemia: jaundice
- Changes in neurologic status: seizures, lethargy

Parental Concerns

Normal emotional attachment or *bonding* may be physically and psychologically difficult or impossible during the first hour post birth. Infants and/or their mothers may be physically removed from the delivery environment and placed in separate units or moved to another facility that has a NICU. Nursing considerations need to include promotion of family–infant bonding. To promote bonding, the parents are encouraged to touch and to hold the newborns, if conditions permit. Allow the parent to express concerns about the crisis and to grieve. Guilt, anxiety, depression, and anger are normal feelings. Parents can develop attachment by providing care and holding or touching the infant.

POTENTIAL COMPLICATIONS IN THE HIGH-RISK NEWBORN

Many of the possible complications in the high-risk newborn are related to maternal complications. High-risk newborn categories include metabolic disorders, infections, respiratory surfactant issues, cardiac abnormalities, and problems relating to substance misuse by the pregnant client. Box 69-4 reviews causative factors for high-risk newborns. General nursing considerations that are necessary for these high-risk newborns are discussed in the previous section.

The Newborn of a Client with Diabetes

Due to the epidemic of obesity, inadequate healthy lifestyles, and/or genetic influences, diabetes has become a major metabolic disease of the 21st century. A client with diabetes who becomes pregnant, or one who develops gestational diabetes as a result of pregnancy, will have a high-risk pregnancy. The newborn is at high risk for complications such as macrosomia, preterm birth, respiratory distress syndrome (RDS; with or without prematurity), and hypoglycemia. Preexisting conditions of type 1 and type 2 diabetes are discussed in Chapter 79.

Gestational diabetes typically develops during the last 3 months of a pregnancy. Therefore the client's blood sugar levels will rise during these later months. The extra glucose in the client's blood crosses the placenta, which raises fetal blood sugar levels, and, in turn, triggers the infant's pancreas to make additional insulin. At birth, the placenta no longer connects the client and infant; thus the excess maternal glucose is no longer available to the child. Shortly after birth, the newborn is at risk for hypoglycemia because the infant is still habitually producing higher levels of insulin than is needed. It may take several days for the infant's blood sugar (pancreatic adjustment) to return to normal neonatal levels. The problem during this timeframe is the high possibility of hypoglycemia. Sudden onset of newborn hypoglycemia can result in seizures. Immediate nursing intervention with intravenous or oral glucose is needed. Treatment includes frequent measurement of blood glucose levels (heel stick or venous) and replacement of either glucose or insulin, depending upon the current glucose level. Intravenous therapy, respiratory surfactant, and monitoring of calcium and magnesium levels are also part of postbirth therapies.

The characteristic appearance of the infant of a client who has diabetes at birth is due to increased subcutaneous fat. The placenta and umbilical cord are notably large. Typically, the infant is LGA, covered with vernix caseosa, is plump, and has a full face and a bulky shoulder appearance. Diabetic newborns often have *macrosomia*, a term confused with LGA, as discussed in the section above regarding newborn birth weight. Other problems commonly seen in the diabetic infant include traumatic birth injuries, hypoglycemia and glucose instability post birth, respiratory distress, electrolyte disturbances, congenital problems, and polycythemia with jaundice.

Nursing considerations for the pregnant client who has existing diabetes or develops gestational diabetes begin at the first prenatal appointment. Education for the client and caregivers must include the importance of stabilizing maternal blood sugar levels. Consultation with the diabetic specialist and dietician is scheduled. During the pregnancy, blood sugar levels are closely monitored. High-risk obstetricians or diabetic specialists may require frequent prenatal checks. Nursing monitoring and care of hypoglycemia is discussed in an earlier section of this chapter.

> **Nursing Alert** It is critical to differentiate between "jitteriness" caused by hypoglycemia and what might be mistaken as "shivering." If the newborn startles easily or has shaky movements, think hypoglycemia and obtain a blood glucose level.

Respiratory Disorders

Transient Tachypnea of the Newborn

Transient tachypnea of the newborn (**TTN**) is a generally mild and transitory form of respiratory distress. Typically, it develops within the first few hours after birth, with the

---

Box 69-4 Causative Factors Associated with High-Risk Newborns

- Maternal history of chronic problems before and during pregnancy, such as cardiac disorders, kidney disease, or hypertension
- Maternal conditions related to pregnancy, such as pregnancy-induced hypertension and preeclampsia
- Poor maternal nutrition before and during pregnancy
- Intrauterine infections
- Maternal substance abuse, including alcohol
- Maternal cigarette smoking and exposure to secondhand smoke
- Multiple gestations (e.g., twins, triplets)
- Placental abnormalities (placenta previa or placental abruption)
- Congenital defects
- Chromosomal abnormalities
- Other—An infant may be at risk even without reaching an acceptable maturation age (after 37 weeks' gestation).

greatest respiratory distress occurring at about 36 hr after birth. TTN generally disappears about the third day after birth. The cause of TTN is a delayed absorption of fetal lung fluid after delivery. The most vulnerable infants are those of clients who deliver by cesarean section. These infants do not have the benefits of compression of the thoracic cavity, which helps eliminate the fetal fluid from the newborn lungs. Infants who are delivered via the vaginal birth canal have most of the fetal lung fluid eliminated as part of the birthing process. Other infants at risk include preterm or SGA infants or those whose mothers have asthma, have smoked during pregnancy, or had diabetes during pregnancy.

Diagnosis is made when the infant demonstrates mild respiratory distress and a sustained respiratory rate of greater than 60 breaths per minute. Mild retractions, respiratory grunting, nasal flaring, and cyanosis may occur. Feeding can be difficult because the infant may be unable to suck while maintaining the high respiratory rate associated with TTN. Diagnostic tests include arterial blood gases, which may show low oxygen levels and high carbon dioxide levels, and a chest x-ray, which may indicate fluid in the central portion of the lungs.

Nursing Considerations

The nurse monitors oxygen saturation levels via routine pulse oximetry. Supplemental oxygen is given, if indicated, according to the healthcare provider's order. Frequent vital signs are taken. The nurse observes nutritional intake and hydration levels. Feeding by gavage and IV fluids may be necessary if the infant cannot feed adequately by breast or bottle. The infant may fatigue easily and thus must be observed closely, because respiratory arrest is a possibility. More serious disorders, such as RDS and group B streptococcal pneumonia, which have similar initial findings, may be detected by early nursing observations and data collection. If other risk factors, such as gestational age, infection, and extent of respiratory distress, are affecting overall status, more in-depth treatment may be necessary, such as IV antibiotics and respiratory assistance by mask or intubation with mechanical ventilation.

Respiratory Distress Syndrome

Respiratory distress syndrome (**RDS**) is a serious breathing disorder caused by a lack of alveolar surfactant. Gestational age and the level of surfactant are directly linked with postbirth survival of the newborn with RDS. Thus birth is delayed, if possible, by the use of medications so the fetal lungs can become more mature, increasing the infant's chances of survival. When possible, betamethasone, a glucocorticosteroid, is given to the pregnant client 12 to 24 hr before the preterm birth to help reduce the severity of RDS.

The typical infant with RDS has respiratory symptoms soon after birth that worsen within a few hours. Similar disorders that may initially imitate RDS include TTN and various types of pneumonias.

Diagnosis of RDS is made based on a chest x-ray and the clinical symptoms of increasing respiratory distress (see Fig. 67-9), crackles, generalized cyanosis, and heart rates exceeding 150 beats per minute. Assisting with the lung profile analysis, a specimen may be taken from amniotic fluid or from a newborn's trachea to obtain a lecithin-to-sphingomyelin ratio or **LS ratio**. This biochemical marker can be used as an indicator of the probable severity of RDS.

Nursing Considerations

Without treatment, RDS will worsen. The infant typically is transferred to the NICU for complex, multidisciplinary therapies, including IV antibiotics, total parenteral nutrition, and administration of high concentrations of oxygen. The infant with RDS typically improves when artificial surfactant is administered by the intratracheal route until respiratory status and lung maturity allow natural alveolar surfactant to be produced in sufficient quantities. Oxygenation using hood, cannula, or mechanical ventilation via **endotracheal tube** (**ET tube**) is used according to the severity of symptoms. Continuous positive airway pressure (**CPAP**) treatments and exogenous surfactant by ET tube may also be included. In some instances, *extracorporeal membrane oxygenation* (**ECMO**) might be used. ECMO requires the use of a pump to circulate oxygenated (oxygen-rich) blood to the infant's bloodstream by the use of an artificial device or heart–lung bypass support system.

Hyperbilirubinemia

Bilirubin is a yellow-colored pigment that is released when red blood cells (RBCs) are broken open or destroyed, which is known as *hemolysis*. During fetal growth, the placenta removes bilirubin. RBC products like bile and bilirubin go through a variety of chemical processes as they travel in the bloodstream, through the liver, and back out into the bloodstream to the colon. Before reaching the liver, bilirubin is fat-soluble and is called *unconjugated* or uncombined. Within the liver, bilirubin becomes water-soluble and is called *conjugated* or combined. Conjugated bilirubin exits the liver, goes into the colon, and is converted back into the unconjugated form as it is excreted from the body.

Hyperbilirubinemia, a condition of too much bilirubin in the blood, often occurs with the birth of a newborn. The immature liver may not be able to manage the production and release of RBCs. *Hemolysis* results, in which RBCs break down into their component parts and enter the bloodstream. Newborns have a problem with elevated levels of unconjugated (fat-soluble) bilirubin, causing release of bilirubin's yellow-pigment into cells that can be seen as yellowing of the skin known as **jaundice**. The development of **jaundice**, if untreated, can lead to brain damage, or **kernicterus** (*bilirubin encephalopathy*). Bilirubin levels change daily after birth. Normal bilirubin levels range from 2 to 10 mg/dL during the period of 3 to 5 days after birth. Typical laboratory testing for hyperbilirubinemia includes detection of total, direct, and indirect bilirubin. Total bilirubin is the sum of direct (conjugated) and indirect (unconjugated) bilirubin. Kernicterus tends to occur around levels of 20 mg/dL. In the newborn, two types of hyperbilirubinemia may be seen: physiologic and pathologic. Diagnosis consists of a heel stick blood test to determine the degree of hyperbilirubinemia (see In Practice: Nursing Procedure 67-6).

Physiologic Jaundice

Physiologic jaundice is fairly common, especially with an infant who has a difficult or traumatic delivery, which could lead to RBC damage. When RBCs are damaged, their cellular components, which include bilirubin, are released into the bloodstream. In a newborn, the by-products of RBC damage can result in the accumulation of bilirubin in the skin, making the skin appear yellow. Physiologic jaundice manifests in about 48 to 72 hr after birth.

Pathologic Jaundice
Pathologic jaundice is a hemolytic disorder. It usually presents within the first 24 hr of life and has a rapid rise in bilirubin levels usually related to a serious illness.

Nursing Considerations
Treatment for hyperbilirubinemia varies according to the results of laboratory bilirubin tests (direct, indirect, and total) to determine the most effective course of treatment. Depending on the level that is normal for that time frame, **phototherapy** may be indicated if the bilirubin level is sufficiently high. For phototherapy, the infant is placed in an isolette equipped with special fluorescent overhead lights. The infant is nude, but some healthcare providers allow a diaper to be used during treatment. The eyes are shielded from the overhead phototherapy ultraviolet light. An additional source of phototherapy ultraviolet light is the fiberoptic blanket, which can be placed under the infant in the isolette or over the infant when outside of the isolette. Photo therapy may be continued at home, thus decreasing the time for hospitalization.

The nurse should monitor the amount of exposure the infant receives from the light source. Manufacturer's instructions regarding distance from lights to infant must be followed or the infant can be injured. Provide additional fluids because infants who are receiving phototherapy need more fluids to prevent dehydration. Monitor serum bilirubin levels to ensure that they are decreasing. Parents and family members need to be aware that dehydration, skin rashes, loose greenish stools, priapism (sustained abnormal erection of the penis), and hyperthermia are common but treatable side effects of phototherapy.

> **Nursing Alert** Physiologic jaundice usually appears at about the third day of life. Report jaundice that appears immediately after birth. *Rationale: An immediate case of jaundice (pathologic jaundice) is likely to indicate hemolytic disease of the newborn.*

Neurologic Complications

Intraventricular Hemorrhage
Intraventricular hemorrhage (**IVH**) occurs because the fragile capillaries and the pressure within the brain (cerebral pressure) cause spontaneous bleeding into the ventricles of the brain. IVH can also be caused by the necessary mechanical devices used for life support of the compromised infant. It is a dangerous birth injury that is primarily a problem for preterm newborns of less than 32 gestational weeks. Additional causes include respiratory distress at birth, hypotension, LBW, difficult delivery, *precipitate* (sudden, progressing faster than normal) labor and delivery, or prolonged labor. Symptoms may be subtle such as generalized pallor (poor blood perfusion to the skin), bradycardia, or twitching. Convulsions, stupor, bulging fontanelles, cyanosis, and hypotonia (muscle weakness) may develop. Seizures, respiratory distress, apnea, a shrill cry, and increased head circumference indicate critical changes. Diagnosis is made via ultrasounds, CT scans, MRIs, and clinical observations. Prognosis varies with the extent of the intracranial injury and the course of treatment.

Nursing Considerations
Preventative care is vital. Increased intracranial pressure and IVH can be assisted by gravity flow; position the newborn with the head of the bed slightly elevated. Avoid stimulation, abrupt setting changes related to use of mechanical devices, such as suctioning or ET ventilation, and sudden movements that jar the head. Monitor the NICU environment for potential causative factors. Supportive care includes maintenance of acid–base balance. Administer oxygen, vitamin K, antibiotics, anticonvulsive medications, and sedatives as ordered. Feeding is by *gavage tube.* Complications that may result include cerebral hemorrhage (cerebrovascular accident, brain damage), cerebral palsy, hydrocephaly, and intellectual disabilities.

Brachial Plexus Injury
Injury to the *brachial plexus* results from trauma during a difficult delivery, for example, shoulder dystocia. One example of brachial plexus injury is *Erb–Duchenne paralysis,* which results from trauma to the fifth and sixth cranial nerves. The baby is unable to elevate the affected arm, which lies limply at the side. Grasp reflex is present. *Lower plexus injury* results in symptoms in the hand and forearm, with the grasp reflex absent. Nursing care includes range-of-motion exercises and possible splinting. Prognosis depends on the degree of nerve damage.

Facial Paralysis
Also known as *Bell palsy,* facial paralysis occurs when the newborn's facial nerves are injured, usually as a result of forceps delivery. If nerve tissue is damaged, paralysis may be permanent. Usually only one side of the face is affected, and the eyelid and mouth may droop on that side. The baby's sucking mechanism may be impaired, requiring special feeding. The newborn also may need saline irrigation or patching of the eye to retain moisture. Plastic surgery is sometimes effective in improving appearance. Fortunately, most cases of facial and brachial paralysis are temporary. Nursing care focuses on nutritional needs of the infant.

Retinopathy of Prematurity
Retinopathy of prematurity (**ROP**) is a serious complication of the retina of the eyes that can occur when oxygen is given long term or in a concentration that is too high for the neonate. It is most common in a preterm infant of less than 28 weeks. Varying degrees of visual damage including blindness can occur. This degenerative disease of the retina is caused by abnormal growth, scarring, and/or detachment of immature retinal blood vessels. Nursing care includes careful monitoring of blood oxygen (PO_2) levels to keep oxygen levels as close to acceptable for that newborn as possible. Treatments for infants at risk include consultation with an ophthalmologist or a neonatal specialist. If too much oxygen is given, ROP may occur; if too little oxygen is given, irreversible brain damage can result. Laser surgery has proved effective in the treatment and preservation of many infants with ROP.

> **Nursing Alert** Oxygen supplied to a newborn can cause permanent blindness. Oxygen levels to the newborn must be closely monitored and used with extreme caution.

Necrotizing Enterocolitis

Necrotizing enterocolitis (**NEC**) is a serious, often fatal, disorder of preterm infants. Surviving infants typically have chronic health conditions and disabilities. The specific etiology is unknown. NEC develops when bacteria invades the bowel, which becomes ischemic (poor blood flow), eventually leading to an acute inflammatory disease and necrosis (death) of varying amounts of the intestine. Bottle-fed babies are more susceptible. Symptoms include lethargy, abdominal distention, vomiting of bile, hypothermia, apnea, and irritability. Diagnosis is by x-ray and ultrasound. Nursing considerations are consistent with many high-risk disorders. Using a nasogastric tube and suction allows the bowel to rest. Supportive care includes parenteral fluids and total parenteral nutrition, antibiotics, infection control, and surgical resection as needed.

Meconium Aspiration Syndrome

Meconium aspiration syndrome (**MAS**) is a serious condition in which either the fetus or the newborn inhales meconium mixed with amniotic fluid, resulting in respiratory distress. Meconium is the thick, dark greenish-black pasty substance that forms in the fetus's bowel. During labor, either before birth or with the first breaths of birth, the infant's anal sphincter relaxes, allowing meconium to pass into the amniotic fluid. If the first breath is taken before suctioning, the newborn may aspirate meconium and amniotic fluid into the lungs. As a consequence, the airways become partially or completely blocked, which leads to a *hypoxic* fetus (one who is lacking oxygen) and a cyanotic newborn. Any aspirated fluid can lead to atelectasis, pneumonia, and other pulmonary problems. Risk factors for MAS include fetal distress, maternal history of diabetes or hypertension, difficult delivery, postterm birth, or IUGR. An x-ray confirms diagnosis but meconium-stained amniotic fluid is typically noted first. Additional symptoms may be corelated to other high-risk complications that typically include a low Apgar score, cyanosis, apnea or tachypnea, retractions, hypothermia, and hypoglycemia.

Nursing Considerations

Nursing considerations include having and using the aspiration bulb syringe (a personal suction device) or wall suction to clear the mouth and upper respiratory passages. Give oxygen, encourage fluids, and regulate temperature. Provide antibiotics as ordered. If breathing does not begin shortly after birth, the healthcare provider intubates the infant, which will permit suctioning below the trachea and vocal cords and into the bronchial tubes. ECMO may be considered.

Sudden Infant Death Syndrome

Sudden infant death syndrome (SIDS), or what formerly was called "crib death," is the sudden, unexpected death of an apparently healthy infant, less than 1 year of age, in whom the postmortem examination fails to reveal an adequate cause. SIDS is a not diagnosis but a description of the syndrome. No single cause has been identified. The incidence of SIDS has dropped significantly in the 21st century, possibly because of the initiation of the supine position as the infant's only recommended sleeping position. The American Academy of Pediatrics recommends avoiding the prone position for sleep until the age of 12 months. High-risk factors include LBW, preterm birth, maternal age of less than 20 years, and smoking during pregnancy. Symptoms are vague or nonexistent. If high-risk situations are suspected, the caregivers are taught emergency measures, for example, CPR.

Nursing considerations focus on the traumatic psychological effects to the caregivers. Grief and guilt evoke high emotions. Disbelief, hostility, and anger toward the spouse or other caregivers often respond to counseling. Resources for the family of a SIDS infant or for families who have concerns are available locally and online. The nurse may make the initial call to a community SIDS support group.

HEMOLYTIC DISEASE OF THE NEWBORN

ABO Incompatibility

Hemolytic disease of the newborn (**HDN**) is a hemolytic condition causing destruction to the RBCs. HDN often results from an *Rh factor* or *ABO blood incompatibility*. The Rh factor involves the D antigen only (one of the many proteins on RBCs), which is either positive (present) or negative (absent) on an RBC. The major blood groups are A, B, AB, and O and are referred to as ABO blood groups. With **ABO incompatibility**, the neonate's RBCs are positive for A or B antigens (or both) and the client's RBCs are usually negative for both of these antigens. ABO incompatibility is more common than Rh problems. In both conditions, the pregnant client builds up antibodies against antigens from their own fetus.

Erythroblastosis Fetalis

An HDN, **erythroblastosis fetalis**, can occur when an Rh-negative client is pregnant with an Rh-positive fetus, resulting in **Rh sensitization** (*Rh incompatibility*). The disease does not occur in the first pregnancy, but occurs with increasing severity in future pregnancies. The condition causes the client's antibodies to destroy fetal RBCs (see Chapter 68).

This condition is uncommon today because it is preventable. The Rh-negative client receives *anti-D gamma globulin* or RhoGAM prophylactically at 28 weeks' gestation, following any invasive procedure, for example, amniocentesis, or any abortion. When discussing RhoGAM, consider using the lay term *miscarriage* instead of the medically appropriate word *abortion*, which has emotional associations. It is also important to give RhoGAM within 72 hr following delivery of an Rh-positive baby. Some cases of erythroblastosis fetalis still occur in women who did not have antepartal care or who did not receive RhoGAM following a previous abortion.

Nursing Considerations

Nursing considerations for HDN relate to the most common symptoms resulting from anemia, such as fatigue, cyanosis, and hyperbilirubinemia (e.g., jaundice). Pathologic jaundice may develop in less than 24 hr after birth. Phototherapy is used to treat milder cases after birth. Refer to the previous section on hyperbilirubinemia for more details and information about treatments.

> **NCLEX Alert**
>
> Rh sensitization and ABO incompatibilities are not uncommon concerns in any clinical practice and are likely to be seen as an NCLEX question.

INTRAUTERINE DISORDERS: CONGENITAL AND ACQUIRED INFECTIONS

Intrauterine disorders often result from *congenital* factors or *acquired* intrauterine problems. A **congenital** disorder is any abnormality that exists at birth regardless of cause. **Acquired disorders** are often due to *teratogenic* interference with fetal growth. Teratogenic problems are a result of something that happens inside the pregnant uterus. Sources may be acquired from the placenta prenatally, from a maternal vaginal infection during labor and delivery, or from contaminated amniotic fluid via aspiration of amniotic fluid. Teratogenic disorders can be the result of maternal illness or infections; use of drugs, alcohol, or tobacco; or exposure to external toxins. For example, a pregnant woman's exposure to rubella can result in cataracts, brain damage, and deafness of her newborn. Congenital heart defects are reviewed below and discussed in more detail in Chapter 72. Associated with intrauterine disorders, Chapters 70 and 74 discuss sexually transmitted disease (STD)-related infections and children with special needs.

Iatrogenic issues result from problems that are inadvertently caused by a healthcare professional. For example, iatrogenic issues include cross contamination of an infection from one newborn to another or a clavicular fracture that occurs during delivery. Iatrogenic infections and associated problems can be the result of teratogens that are known to cause fetal and newborn disabilities.

Fetal Alcohol Spectrum Disorder

Fetal alcohol spectrum disorders (**FASDs**), also referred to as *fetal alcohol syndrome* (**FAS**), are a group of conditions that occur in an individual whose mother drank alcohol during pregnancy (see Fig. 74-1), contributing to fetal physical defects, behavioral problems, and learning difficulties. Effects of FASD include growth deficiency, microcephaly, facial abnormalities, cardiac anomalies, and intellectual disabilities. The degree of defect relates to the client's level of alcohol intake while pregnant; safe levels of intake are currently unknown. Chapter 74 discusses FASD in more detail.

> **Nursing Alert** Advise pregnant women to avoid alcohol completely. *Rationale: Safe levels of alcohol intake during pregnancy have not been established.*

Down Syndrome

Down syndrome, also called *trisomy 21,* is a genetic disorder often associated with clients who give birth after age 40. It is commonly identified in the newborn nursery by typical physical features, although only chromosomal analysis can make a final diagnosis. Physical and mental manifestations may range from mild to severe. One deep crease runs horizontally across the hands. Eyes are slanted, and the tongue is large and protruding. The infant is flaccid. Usually, accompanying intellectual disabilities and heart defects exist, and cataracts and gastrointestinal disorders may be present. See also Chapter 74.

TORCH Syndrome

TORCH syndrome is an acronym of the most common and serious high-risk infections during pregnancy. Both the client and the fetus are affected. Examples of such infections include STDs, rubella, toxoplasmosis, thrush, and CMV.

The acronym **TORCH** is used as a reminder of the most serious infections:

T = **T**oxoplasmosis
O = **O**ther (other infections: thrush, staphylococcus, streptococcus, hepes zoster)
R = **R**ubella
C = **C**ytomegalovirus
H = **H**erpes simplex virus

Toxoplasmosis

The protozoa responsible for **toxoplasmosis** are found in cat feces and in rare or raw meat. Although the pregnant client may have no symptoms, possible fetal effects include stillbirth, premature delivery, microcephaly, hydrocephaly, seizures, and intellectual disabilities.

> **Nursing Alert** Infections can be transmitted to nursing personnel. Therefore, follow Standard Precautions in the care of all clients and newborns.

Rubella

The virus of *rubella (German measles, 3-day measles)* can be dangerous in pregnancy, but has no permanent ill effects on the woman. It does, however, cause fetal defects, known as *congenital rubella syndrome.* Common defects are cataracts, deafness, congenital heart defects, cardiac disease, and intellectual disabilities. The concerns regarding congenital rubella syndrome have increased because of a generalized population decrease in MMR (measles, mumps, rubella) immunizations.

Cytomegalovirus

An asymptomatic client can transmit **CMV**, which belongs to the herpesvirus group, to their fetus through the placenta, or through contact during delivery. Possible effects on the newborn include SGA, microcephaly, hydrocephaly, and intellectual disability.

Herpes Simplex Virus

Herpes simplex virus (HSV type 1 and type 2) or *genital herpes* can complicate a pregnancy and can be harmful to a newborn. Neonatal herpes is potentially fatal for the newborn. HSV can be difficult to diagnose, especially if the blisters are not present. It is not possible to differentiate between HSV-1 and HSV-2 without laboratory tests. If the virus becomes active before the 20th week of gestation, a spontaneous abortion ("miscarriage") may occur. HSV-2 infection acquired late in pregnancy is very dangerous to the fetus. HSV may cause premature labor or local infection of the eyes, skin, or mucous membranes.

A client who is known to be infected with herpes and is near term will usually undergo a cesarean delivery, unless the amniotic fluid is considered contaminated. In this case, the fetus probably is already infected. After delivery, the newborn is isolated to prevent transmission of the virus to others in the nursery.

Gonorrhea

If the organism causing *gonorrhea* gets into the newborn's eyes during delivery, it causes a bilateral *conjunctivitis* (eyelid inflammation). If untreated, this condition can lead to blindness (*ophthalmia neonatorum*). The prophylactic installation of antibiotic ointment into the eyes soon after birth prevents this condition (see Fig. 69-3 and In Practice: Nursing Procedure 67-2). Law requires this treatment in all states. If a newborn should contract conjunctivitis, they receive large doses of antibiotics and are kept in isolation to prevent spreading the infection to others.

Syphilis

In most states, law requires testing of pregnant clients for *syphilis*. If the test is positive, prompt treatment with penicillin early in pregnancy will prevent harmful effects on the newborn. Untreated syphilis can lead to premature labor and delivery. Complications for the infant include congenital infection, anomalies (defects), and *stillbirth* (born dead).

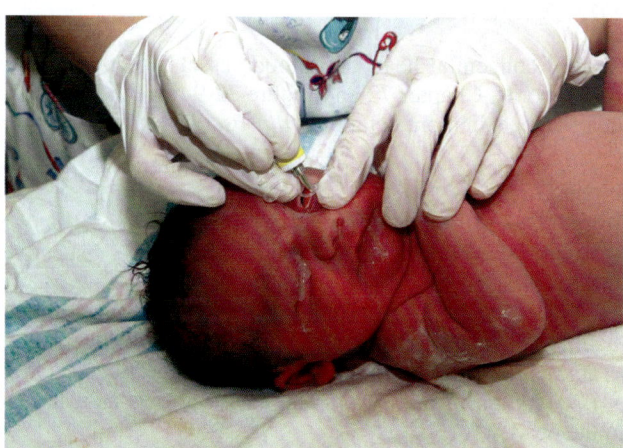

Figure 69-3 Ointment is applied to the eyes of a neonate within the first hour after birth. The most common treatment to prevent eye infections related to birth is the use of erythromycin ophthalmic ointment. Erythromycin ointment is effective against the organisms of both gonorrhea and chlamydia (Klossner & Hatfield, 2006).

Signs of syphilis in the newborn are general skin eruptions of *rose spots, blebs* (blisters) on the soles and palms, *snuffles* (a catarrhal discharge from the nasal mucous membrane), hoarse cry, cracks and ulcerations around the anus and mouth, and a positive blood test. Isolate the affected newborn and treat him or her with antibiotics as ordered.

HIV and AIDS

HIV can be transmitted during pregnancy via the placenta, during delivery, or through breastfeeding. Treatment with HIV/AIDS antiretroviral medications is the most effective approach. When HIV is detected early and treatment is provided before, during, and after birth, HIV maternal–fetal transmission is greatly reduced in infected pregnant client.

Although not all pregnant client who are HIV positive will transmit the virus to their babies, continual monitoring and treatment are essential. Both clients and babies benefit from preventive measures, early diagnosis, and consistent treatment, which can lead to longer and healthier lives. Nursing care for the HIV-infected client is focused on educating them about consistent and appropriate medication use. The pregnant client and their sexual partners also need to be aware that several other STDs are associated with HIV infections. Therefore, the client may need treatment for more than one type of infection. Refer also to Chapter 70.

Thrush (also known as a *monilial infection*) is a yeast infection, in which milk-like spots form in the newborn's mouth. Thrush is transmitted to the newborn during delivery if the client has it. Infected healthcare personnel, or family members who fail to use proper aseptic technique, can also spread thrush. The infected newborn is isolated and treated with nystatin (Mycostatin, Nilstat) by mouth or, less frequently, with a 1% to 2% aqueous solution of gentian violet.

Nursing Considerations

Clean equipment and good handwashing technique are essential to prevent reinfection. Wiping the newborn's mouth with a gauze sponge after each feeding is important because lactose (milk sugar) promotes the growth of *Candida albicans*, the causative organism.

CONGENITAL MUSCULOSKELETAL DISORDERS

Various injuries may occur during the birth process and are considered congenital disorders. Some are serious but most can be corrected. Several of these conditions are also discussed in Chapter 72.

Fractures

Fractures, which occur at birth, are rarely complicated and usually heal without difficulties. One common birth injury that infants may have is a *fractured clavicle*. Signs and symptoms of a fractured clavicle include asymmetric *Moro reflex* and crying when the affected arm is moved.

Talipes

Talipes is also known as *clubfoot*. In clubfoot, one or both feet turn out of the normal position. The condition occurs more often in boys. Early diagnosis and treatment usually yield an excellent prognosis. Exercise, corrective shoes, braces, casts, and surgery also may be helpful.

Developmental Dysplasia of the Hip

Developmental dysplasia of the hip is also called a *congenital dislocated hip,* which is an instability of the hip joint in a newborn. Faulty embryonic development of the hip joint is the likely cause. The head of the femur fails to sit securely in the acetabulum. Early treatment is necessary to prevent permanent damage. Any infant can be born with an unstable hip joint but it is more common in girls and with first-time pregnancies. All infants are routinely checked for the condition.

The first sign of this condition may be a limitation of abduction on the affected side when the thigh is flexed (*Ortolani sign*). The affected femur is shorter than the unaffected femur; the skinfolds of the thigh and buttocks are asymmetric, and a slight click may be heard with hip abduction. X-ray studies usually confirm diagnosis.

Treatment usually consists of stabilizing the head of the femur into the acetabulum and holding it there for a certain length of time. A "triple" diaper, providing bulk in the groin region to force the leg into abduction, may resolve the problem, as may thick foam pads or splints. In extreme cases, the baby may need a cast.

Polydactylism and Syndactylism

Polydactylism is an often congenital, but not always genetic, condition of having more than five digits (fingers or toes) per hand or five toes per foot. *Syndactylism* is the webbing or fusing together of two or more digits. The extra digits may be poorly developed or may be well-formed and completely functional. The little finger may have a small stalk attached to a poorly developed finger. Treatment of polydactyly may be surgical or simple occlusion of the finger so it does not grow.

NEURAL TUBE DEFECTS

Some central nervous system disorders of the newborn involve *neural tube defects* (**NTDs**) which are congenital disorders related to genetic abnormalities, teratogenic drugs, or environmental toxins that affect fetal development of the neural tube or neurons in the fetal brain. Normally the neural tube develops into the spinal cord and fetal neurons develop into the brain. Location, size, and severity of the abnormalities are related to the specific sections involved. Many factors are involved with NTDs (Box 69-5).

The use of folic acid supplementation, antenatal diagnostic testing, and the selective termination of some affected fetuses have decreased the incidences of NTDs. Chapter 72 has more information regarding the following congenital disorders.

Hydrocephalus

Hydrocephalus is an excess of cerebrospinal fluid (**CSF**) in the ventricles and subarachnoid spaces of the brain. Untreated, it results in an enlarged head, brain damage, and death. The newborn may also exhibit bulging fontanels and nervous irritability. Hydrocephalus is treated by surgically inserting shunts that drain the ventricles.

> **Box 69-5 Causative Factors of Neural Tube Defects**
>
> - Genetics
> - Fetal exposures
>   - Environmental toxins
>   - Teratogenic drugs
> - Nutritional deficiencies
>   - Folic acid deficiency
>   - Vitamin and zinc deficiencies suspected
>   - Maternal obesity
> - Maternal age
> - Birth order—first-born children at highest risk, next pregnancies may receive genetic counseling.
> - Socioeconomic status—lower socioeconomic status may be corelated with other conditions such as lack of prenatal healthcare, vitamin deficiencies, or generalized poor nutrition.

Spina Bifida

Spina bifida is a congenital NTD in which the vertebral spaces fail to close, allowing a *herniation* (*bulging*) of the spinal contents into a sac. When the meninges covering the spinal cord herniates through the vertebral space, it is called a *meningocele.* When spinal cord nerve fibers and meninges herniate, it is referred to as a *myelomeningocele.* Surgery may correct these problems; prognosis depends on the deformity's extent.

Anencephaly and Microcephaly

In children with **anencephaly**, part or all of the brain is missing. The skull is flat, and these newborns live for only a short time, if at all. Children with **microcephaly** have abnormally small heads. They may live or die, depending on the extent of the deformity. Because the brain does not develop as normal, these newborns almost always have intellectual disabilities.

CONGENITAL CARDIOVASCULAR DISORDERS

Several congenital heart and blood vessel defects are seen in newborns. Chapter 72 and Figure 72-9 review congenital heart defects in more detail. *Cardiovascular defects* include:

- *Patent ductus arteriosus:* The ductus arteriosus fails to close at birth.
- *Atrial septal defect* (**ASD**) and *ventricular septal defect* (**VSD**): Abnormal openings exist between the respective heart chambers.
- *Tetralogy of Fallot:* Four major heart defects occur simultaneously: pulmonary stenosis, VSD, overriding aorta, and hypertrophy of the right ventricle.
- *Coarctation of the aorta:* The aorta narrows as it leaves the heart.

Nursing Considerations

One characteristic feature of many congenital of the more severe heart disorders is cyanosis, which becomes more pronounced when the newborn cries. The birth attendant and nurse must assess carefully for heart murmurs. Other signs may be respiratory difficulty, easy tiring, and abnormal vital signs. The newborn will be treated symptomatically. Medications, such as cardiotonics, may be ordered; surgical repair may be necessary.

CONGENITAL GASTROINTESTINAL DISORDERS

Cleft Lip and Palate

Cleft lip, which occurs in approximately 1 in 1,000 births, is a vertical opening in the upper lip. It may appear as a notch in the lip or extend upward into the nose (see Fig. 72-7). When the palate is split, the condition is known as **cleft palate**; this condition occurs less frequently than cleft lip. Cleft palate can be one-sided (*unilateral*) or two-sided (*bilateral*). Clefts also are classified as *complete* or *incomplete*.

Cleft lip and palate cause feeding difficulties if the newborn is unable to suck effectively. In addition, milk that goes into the mouth may be expelled through the nose. Special nipple and feeding devices assist in feedings. The treatment is surgical repair, usually between 6 and 12 weeks of age. Nursing care is discussed in Chapter 72.

Gastrointestinal Obstructions

- **Choanal atresia** occurs when the newborn's nostrils are closed at the entrance to the throat, so that air cannot pass through to the lungs. Because newborns are obligatory nose breathers, atresia must be quickly corrected through surgery to open the nostrils.
- **Esophageal atresia** occurs when the upper end of the newborn's esophagus ends in a blind pouch, making it impossible for the baby to obtain food. Surgery must be performed quickly. The baby sometimes is maintained on total parenteral nutrition until after surgery.
- **Tracheoesophageal fistula** occurs when an esophageal atresia is accompanied by a tracheal fistula; it is referred to as a *tracheoesophageal fistula*. The situation is life-threatening because the esophagus channels food and mucus directly into the lungs. This condition must be corrected immediately or the child will suffocate. Emergency surgery is performed immediately, with no feedings before surgery.
- **Pyloric stenosis** is a congenital anomaly in which an increase in size of the musculature at the junction of the stomach and small intestine occurs, causing the pyloric opening to constrict. Food cannot pass through. The newborn initially vomits a milky substance. Later, the vomiting becomes projectile. The baby is fussy and hungry, loses weight, and becomes dehydrated. Surgical correction is necessary.
- **Imperforate anus** occurs when the baby's rectum ends in a blind pouch, causing an obstruction to the normal passage of feces that must be corrected immediately. Imperforate anus is suspected if the newborn does not pass a stool within 24 hr of delivery.

Phenylketonuria

Phenylketonuria (**PKU**) is a genetic defect that renders the newborn incapable of metabolizing certain amino acids, which spill into the blood and tissues in the form of phenylalanine. No cure exists for this disease, but it can be controlled with a special diet. Treatment is initiated as soon as possible after birth. Untreated, PKU results in mental impairment, behavioral problems, intellectual disabilities, and other abnormalities. All newborns are tested for PKU before discharge from the healthcare facility and at the 6-week checkup (see Chapter 67).

Galactosemia

Galactosemia is a genetic disorder in which the newborn is incapable of metabolizing galactose, which is a sugar found in all foods that contain milk. Galactose is made up of lactose and glucose. If galactose cannot be broken down into its two components, it builds up in the body, causing vomiting, diarrhea, jaundice, seizures, liver damage, brain impairment, and death. Symptoms typically start a few days after birth. Failure to thrive (lack of weight gain and growth) may be noted. The infant feeds poorly, has vomiting and diarrhea, and is often irritable. Hypoglycemia and abnormal sleeping patterns are common. Early diagnosis and dietary management, usually continued throughout life, are required in order for the child to survive and thrive.

CONGENITAL GENITOURINARY DISORDERS

Exstrophy of the Bladder

Bladder **exstrophy** results from abnormal development of the bladder, abdominal wall, and symphysis pubis, causing exposure of the bladder, urethra, and ureteral openings to the abdominal wall. Infection is a common problem, and surgery is necessary. Surgical reconstruction is done in steps; it is usually completed by the time the child is of school age.

Hypospadias and Epispadias

The male newborn has **hypospadias** when his urethra opens on the bottom side of the penis. This condition causes problems later during toilet training because the child is unable to direct his urinary stream. Surgical repair involves the use of the foreskin, so circumcision should not be performed on this newborn. Less common is **epispadias**, in which the meatus is located on the upper side of the penis.

SUBSTANCE MISUSE AND THE NEWBORN

Substance misuse is the excessive use of a drug without therapeutic medical justification. It is seen as a pattern of continued and inappropriate use of substances that cause substantial emotional, psychological, and physiological effects. Substance misuse may include stimulants, opiates, inhalants, marijuana, hallucinogens, tranquilizers, and sedatives. All drugs, including alcohol and nicotine, can adversely affect a fetus. Polydrug use (more than one drug) is common. The newborn of a client who uses any chemical is likely to have symptoms because drugs reach the fetus through the placenta. As a result, this newborn is at high risk for a vast variety of complications. Many of these infants experience withdrawal symptoms, known as *neonatal abstinence syndrome*, after birth. This section provides an overview of the effects on the neonate related to the use of stimulants and opioids that are pharmacologically different but may cause similar symptoms. Both typically produce abstinence syndrome. The effects of marijuana are also discussed.

Lifestyle risk factors need to be considered when working with these clients and infants. High-risk newborns of clients who drink, smoke, or use drugs are more likely to be preterm, of LBW, and to have intellectual impairments. Spontaneous abortions, abruptio placentae, and stillbirths also are more common in these women.

Stimulants: Cocaine and Methamphetamine

Stimulants cause major vasoconstriction throughout the body, which also affects the fetus and placenta. Many medications are potential *teratogens*, but certain drugs, such as cocaine and methamphetamine, are known to be teratogenic which means they cause abnormal development of an embryo or fetus. Some drugs may cause spontaneous abortions (miscarriages). Hypoxia is a leading cause of teratogenic defects which include severe brain damage, genitourinary malformations, arm and leg abnormalities, and cardiac defects. Preterm pregnancy is very common.

Opioids: Medical Narcotics and Heroin

Opioids, also referred to as narcotics, are CNS depressants and are physiologically different from stimulants. Opioids act on the CNS and induce feelings of relaxation. Included in this grouping are codeine, heroine, methadone, morphine, and heroin. Many of these substances are available by prescription or by illicit drug dealers. They are addictive and readily cross the placenta. Stimulants are often used in addition to opioids. Opioids such as heroin that are present in the client will also be present in the newborn for at least 2 to 6 days. The symptoms appear shortly after birth and progress in severity and frequency.

The following are examples of opioid narcotics:

- codeine (only available in generic form)
- fentanyl transdermal patch (Duragesic, Fentora)
- hydrocodone (Lorcet, Lortab, Norco, Vicodin)
- hydromorphone (Dilaudid)
- meperidine (Demerol)
- methadone (Dolophine)
- morphine (MS Contin, Ora-Morph SR)
- oxycodone (OxyContin, Oxyfast, Percocet, Roxicodone)

Newborns experiencing neonatal abstinence syndrome typically demonstrate many of the following signs and symptoms:

- Irritability, jitteriness, tremors
  - Hyperactivity
  - Hypersensitivity to environmental stimuli
  - Shrill, high-pitched persistent cry
  - Frequent sneezing or yawning
  - Increased tendon reflexes
  - Increased muscle tone
  - Decreased *Moro reflex*
- Irregular sleep patterns
- Feeding problems
- Diarrhea
- Weight loss or lack of adequate weight gain

Key Concept

The addicted newborn is hypersensitive. Suggestions for handling an addicted newborn include providing eye contact, touching the newborn gently, and rocking up-and-down (not side-to-side).

Marijuana

Marijuana (also known as pot, weed, or cannabis) is one of the most commonly used drugs in the United States. In some states the purchase and use of marijuana is legal. However, marijuana use is not well studied during pregnancy, so its effects on the fetus are not completely accepted or understood. As do many other drugs, it crosses the placenta. Smoking of any drug is known to disrupt the fetus's supply of oxygen and nutrients, which can result in high-risk newborns. If used during pregnancy, marijuana is associated with preterm births and LBW. The National Institute on Drug Abuse states that exposure to the chemicals in marijuana has negative effects on short- or long-term brain development (National Institute on Drug Abuse, 2019). Long-term consequences seen in children of clients who used this drug include problems with memory, behavior, skill-solving, and attention deficit. Neonatal abstinence syndrome can occur when the baby gets addicted to a drug before birth and goes through withdrawal after birth. Use of stimulants or opioids, in conjunction with marijuana, is common and can increase risks for the pregnant client and their fetus. More research is needed for long-term follow-up studies of these newborns.

Nursing Considerations

Most babies born to clients who use chemicals experience symptoms of neonatal abstinence syndrome serious enough to require treatment. The nurse includes a maternal history of the presence or absence of prenatal care. If approached in a nonjudgmental manner, pregnant clients may provide information regarding the use of drugs. Most symptoms of opioid use are gone in 3 days but may continue for 4 to 6 weeks or longer, depending on the drug. Cocaine-dependent newborns often experience a significant withdrawal syndrome, which can last 2 to 3 weeks. The cocaine-exposed neonate may not show specific withdrawal behaviors but may only demonstrate irritability several weeks after birth. Specific symptoms include increased muscle tone, tremors, and persistence of primitive reflexes that are slow to progress in maturity.

Care of these newborns is based on the type and extent of withdrawal symptoms, and focuses on ensuring adequate respiration, nutrition, and temperature. The stimulants of the environment such as light, sound, or noise must be minimized; sedation may be necessary. Pre- and postbirth legal issues typically need to be considered. Depending on maternal history, for example, prenatal care, hospital protocols may require maternal blood testing, social services, and home care monitoring. Infant urine samples may be sent for toxicology (drug testing). Home care may be initiated because babies who have been exposed to drugs, alcohol, or inhaled toxins are at higher risk for SIDS.

STUDENT SYNTHESIS

KEY POINTS

- High-risk newborns have a greater risk of morbidity and mortality with physical and emotional issues that persist for a lifetime.
- Newborn birth weight is an important indicator of a newborn's survival and lifelong well-being.
- Gestational age and birth weight are strong indicators of potential problems for the newborn.
- Low birth weight, very low birth weight, and extremely low birth weight respectively, result in an increased possibility of severe to very severe physical problems.
- Large-for-gestational-age infants have special problems, including hypoglycemia, respiratory disorders, and injuries such as fractures of the clavicle and skull.
- Intrauterine growth restriction is possible when the fetus does not receive adequate nutrients, the placenta oxygen supply is blocked, or the client's physical status is poor.
- Preterm and postterm neonates both have problems that interfere with appropriate growth, size, and weight.
- The nurse's observations of an infant's status, combined with accurate documentation and prompt reporting of abnormalities, promote the newborn's welfare.
- Nursing observations and subsequent nursing care include monitoring respiratory status and changes, thermoregulation, hypoglycemia, nutrition, and prevention of iatrogenic infections.
- Parental concerns and questions need to be part of the nurse's teaching plan.
- Immediately after birth, the source of fetal glucose decreases and the infant will commonly become hypoglycemic.
- Hyperbilirubinemia may result in a mild physiologic or more severe pathologic jaundice.
- Intraventricular hemorrhage in the newborn can be the result of prematurity or environmental stressors and cause lifelong problems.
- Severe complications after birth include retinopathy of prematurity, necrotizing enterocolitis, and meconium aspiration syndrome.
- Neural tube defects are problems of growth of the fetal spinal cord and brain.
- Numerous congenital or acquired intrauterine disorders can be the result of genetics, teratogenic medications, or various infections, such as those associated with TORCH syndrome.
- Substance abuse by the pregnant client may be responsible for neonatal abstinence syndrome in the newborn.

CRITICAL THINKING EXERCISES

1. A 2-day-old SGA newborn in your care has developed diarrhea. Describe your actions. Explain why diarrhea is dangerous to this newborn and to other newborns in the NICU.
2. Imagine caring for a newborn with bilateral cleft lip and palate. Describe your reaction to the baby's physical appearance. Explain how you would prepare the family members for caring for their child.
3. A newborn of a client who is addicted to cocaine has just arrived in the NICU. Describe what you expect to see in the newborn, and how you will handle each of these problems.

NCLEX-STYLE REVIEW QUESTIONS

1. What is the priority for the nurse when caring for a macrosomic newborn who was born by a cesarean section to a client with diabetes?
   a. Vomiting
   b. An inability to immediately pass a meconium stool
   c. The presence of hyperthermia
   d. The presence of hypoglycemia
2. What observations by the nurse would indicate that a newborn may be "late premature"? Select all that apply.
   a. Increased amount of subcutaneous fat
   b. Lack of vernix caseosa
   c. Presence of lanugo on face, back, arms, and legs
   d. Diminished reflexes
   e. Respirations irregular and weak
3. A preterm newborn is receiving gavage feeding every 2 hr. What action by the nurse is a priority while these feedings are being administered? Select all that apply.
   a. Monitor caloric intake.
   b. Refrigerate the formula.
   c. Obtain daily weights.
   d. Monitor intake and output.
   e. Increase the amount if the newborn is still hungry.
4. A newborn in the nursery begins to have greenish-yellow foul-smelling diarrhea. What is a priority action by the nurse?
   a. Supplement the next feeding with formula.
   b. Insert a gavage feeding tube.
   c. Take a rectal temperature.
   d. Isolate the newborn.
5. An Rh-negative client who did not receive antenatal care gives birth to an Rh-positive newborn. When should the nurse administer the RhoGAM to the client?
   a. It is not necessary to administer the RhoGAM because the delivery was normal.
   b. Within 72 hr after delivery.
   c. When the client returns for their first postpartum appointment in 2 weeks.
   d. After becoming pregnant with their next child within 12 weeks.

CHAPTER RESOURCES

Enhance your learning with additional resources on **thePoint**!
Student Resources related to this chapter can be found at thePoint.lww.com/Rosdahl12e.

70 Sexuality, Fertility, and Sexually Transmitted Infections

Learning Objectives

1. Define and discuss the evolving terminology and concepts of sex, sexuality, sexual orientation, sexual identity, and gender.
2. Discuss the interconnecting aspects of sexual violence, intimate partner violence, sexual abuse, child abuse, elder abuse, and community violence.
3. Identify the primary causes of sexual dysfunction. Describe the medical and surgical interventions for each of these disorders.
4. Define the terms and discuss the treatment differences between artificial insemination and assisted reproductive technology.
5. Define and discuss the following contraceptive methods: abstinence, withdrawal, fertility awareness methods, breastfeeding, hormonal-based contraception, emergency contraception, hormonal patches, hormonal ring, hormonal implants, intrauterine device, chemical and mechanical barriers.
6. Differentiate between infertility and sexual dysfunction. Relate the risk factors of impotence, dyspareunia, and vaginismus to the causes of sexual dysfunction. Describe medical and surgical interventions for each of these disorders.
7. Present a client teaching demonstration that reviews the most common side effects of birth control. Include discussion regarding the most significant side effects of hormonal birth control methods.
8. Identify which forms of birth control are most effective against the spread of sexually transmitted infections. Discuss the reasons why some birth control methods do protect while others do not protect against the spread of sexually transmitted infections.
9. Discuss aspects of client teaching related to sterilization by tubal ligation, vasectomy, and hysterectomy.
10. Differentiate the signs and symptoms of viral sexually transmitted infections including herpes simplex, human papillomavirus, and cytomegalovirus.
11. Differentiate and discuss aspects of client teaching related to the following types of STIs: HIV/AIDS, chlamydia, gonorrhea, syphilis, candidiasis, trichomoniasis, and bacterial vaginosis.
12. Discuss the benefits of prophylaxis against human papillomavirus and cancer using HPV vaccinations.

Important Terminology

adhesions
artificial insemination
assisted reproductive technology
bacterial vaginosis
candidiasis
chancre
chancroid
chlamydia
coitus interruptus
congenital syphilis
contraception
dyspareunia
external condom
genital herpes
gestational carrier, gestational surrogacy
gonorrhea
impotence
infertility
inflammatory process
internal condom
intimate partner violence
neurosyphilis
orgasm
outercourse
priapism
rape
sex
sexual dysfunction
sexual health
sexual orientation
sexual rights
sexual violence
sexuality
spermicide
sterility
surrogate
transitioning
trichomoniasis
tubal ligation
vaginismus
vasectomy

Acronyms

AI
ART
BC
BCP
BV
CMV
EC
ED
eSET
FAM
GC
GIFT
HPV
HSV-1
HSV-2
ICSI
IPV
IUD
IVF
KOH
LGBT, LGBTQ
LH
PCOS
PID
POI
PTSD
RPR
SANE
STD, STI
SV
TET
TSS
VDRL
VVC
ZIFT

Sexuality, fertility, and the potential for sexually transmitted infections (**STIs**) are topics that involve some of the most basic needs, desires, and fears that rule the individual. STIs have affected humankind since the beginning of human relationships. Before proceeding in this chapter, you may want to review anatomy in Chapters 28 and 29, respectively, as well as Chapters 90 and 91, which discuss reproductive disorders.

> **NCLEX Alert**
>
> NCLEX situations may relate to communicating and teaching information that pertains to the various aspects of a client's sexual concerns. Correct responses on an NCLEX examination will typically include responses to questions that are informative, sensitive, and accurate.

HUMAN SEXUALITY

Sexuality is the way in which individuals physically, emotionally, and socially experience and express themselves as sexual beings. The vocabulary of human sexuality is in the process of changing. The World Health Organization (WHO) states that "sexuality is influenced by the interaction of biological, psychological, social, economic, political, cultural, legal, historical, religious, and spiritual factors" (WHO, 2006). As an important aspect of being human, sexuality is associated with intimate sexual contact, the ability to reproduce, and the concepts associated with *sexual health*. The term **sexual health** encompasses the way in which we see ourselves and how we physically and emotionally relate to other human beings.

The WHO defines *sexual health* as a state of physical, emotional, mental, and social well-being in relation to sexuality; it is not merely the absence of disease, dysfunction, or infirmity. *Sexual health* requires a positive and respectful approach to sexuality and sexual relationships, as well as the possibility of having pleasurable and safe sexual experiences, free of coercion, discrimination, and violence (WHO, 2006).

Many components of nursing include discussions related to the multifaceted aspects of sexual health. For example, discussing a client's postoperative physical limitations may include queries from the client regarding resuming sexual activities after surgery. In the nursing world, you are expected to be sensitive to the spectrum of human feelings and be able to deliver nursing care in a nonjudgmental manner.

Sex, Gender, and Sexual Orientation

The word **sex** has more than one definition. Sex can be defined as the physical union of genitalia, accompanied by the rhythmic movements of *coitus*, also known as *sexual intercourse* or sexual activity. The category of sex refers to the biological characteristics, anatomical organs, and sexual functions a person may possess, including male, female, and intersex.

Gender or *gender identity* is not the same as sex but rather refers to the socially constructed characteristics that pertain to how a person is recognized in the world. Categories like gender are socially constructed and change over time and geography. Some cultures have more than two genders. In the United States, the pervasive categories known as the gender binary consist of man and woman. Relevant terminology related to gender and gender identity in the contemporary United States are as follows (GLADD, 2016; American Psychological Association [APA], 2020; Planned Parenthood, 2020):

- *Cisgender:* A term for individuals whose gender identity or self-expression of gender matches the expectations for the biological sex assigned at birth
- *Nonbinary:* A term for individuals who define their gender as falling somewhere in between man and woman, or they may define it as wholly unrelated to the gender binary
- *Transgender:* A general term for individuals whose gender identity or self-expression of gender is different from the expectations for the biological sex assigned at birth

Individuals may not identify as male or female (nonbinary); they may also feel that their gender does not match the sex to which they were assigned at birth. *Transgender* is an umbrella term for individuals whose gender identity or self-expression of gender is different from their sex assigned at birth (e.g., a client assigned as a boy at birth based on visual inspection of male genitalia may identify as a woman). Transgender individuals may live overtly as one gender but psychologically and internally know that their gender identity is something else. **Transitioning** is a process that some transgender people pursue in order to be recognized as the gender identity they feel that they are. *Gender transition* is a process consisting of personal, medical, and legal steps. Medical aspects of transition may include hormone therapy, sexual reassignment surgery (also known as *gender confirmation surgery)*, or other medical procedures.

Sexual orientation refers to a person's physical, romantic, and/or emotional attraction to other people. Research suggests that genetic, hormonal, social, and environmental influences are factors relating to sexual orientation. An individual's orientation may involve the use of the following terms (GLADD, 2016; American Psychological Association [APA], 2020; Planned Parenthood, 2020):

- *Asexual:* Refers to individuals who are not particularly attracted to any gender
- *Bisexual:* Refers to individuals who are attracted to people of the same gender or another gender, recognizing the masculine and feminine
- *Gay:* Describes men who are sexually attracted to other men
- *Heterosexual:* Refers to individuals who are attracted to persons of the other sex
- *Homosexual:* Refers to individuals who are attracted to persons of the same sex
- *Lesbian:* Describes women who are sexually attracted to other women
- *Pansexual*: Refers to individuals who have the capacity to be attracted to people of any gender, recognizing fluidity and nonbinary people

To summarize the terms of gender identity, the acronym **LGBTQ+** was developed. It stands for **l**esbian, **g**ay, **b**isexual, and **t**ransgender, **q**ueer or **q**uestioning, and more (Griffith et al., 2017; APA, 2020; Planned Parenthood, 2020). Beginning in the 1990s, more terms were initiated by the gay community to reflect the evolving diversity of gender identity within contemporary culture. The word *queer* has developed new meanings (Planned Parenthood, 2020) and, if acceptable to the individual, might be used in a nonpejorative way to express gender identity. The alternative word *questioning* reflects the questioning process that some individuals use as they explore their identity. The plus sign represents the fragility of categories and boxes and includes pansexuality and gender fluidity.

> *Key Concept*
> Teach all people, no matter what their sexual orientation, methods of safer sex, for example, sex within a committed relationship or the use of condoms and spermicides.

Violence

Violence is the intentional use of force or power (physical or psychological), threatened or actual, against oneself or a person, group, or community. The results of violence include the likelihood of injury, death, acute psychological harm, or deprivation plus lifetime psychological damage. Research has identified that categories of violence such as child abuse, sexual violence, intimate partner violence, and elder abuse share the same root causes as does violence in a local or world community. The most likely victims and perpetrators of violent behavior are adolescents and young adults aged 15–24 (UNICEF, 2017).

> **Key Concept**
> Women who are in relationships that have a history of violence have four times the risk for contracting STIs, including HIV, than in women in relationships without violence. Sources: https://www.cdc.gov/violenceprevention/index.html; https://www.cdc.gov/hiv/basics/index.html

Violence can be classified according to how the actions are inflicted: physical, sexual, psychological, and deprivation or neglect. Socioeconomic factors, age, alcohol and drug use, prior history of violence, dysfunctional relationships, and desire for dominance, power, or control are among the common predictive factors of abuse. Violence is a learned behavior. The most effective method of treatment for all types of violence is prevention. Prevention should focus on teaching conflict resolution with training in social skills such as self-control, communication, resisting peer pressure, and being assertive rather than aggressive. You might want to review the introductory concepts of violence and the risk factors involved for the individual, a relationship, or a community found in Chapter 6.

Sexual violence (SV) is an identified, significant problem in the United States. SV refers to sexual activity that is not obtained by freely given consent. Anyone can be the victim of sexual violence, but statistics show that most victims are female. The person most commonly responsible for an assault is a male known to the female victim. Other individuals involved in SV include a friend, coworker, neighbor, or family member. **Intimate partner violence (IPV)** describes threats or acts of physical violence, sexual violence, coercive tactics, stalking, or physical aggression by a current or former partner or spouse. IPV occurs among heterosexual or same-sex couples and does not require sexual intimacy. **Rape** is a violent crime committed against an individual, without their consent, that involves penetration via objects or body parts. *Lack of consent*, a key factor of the definition of rape, suggests the use of force, the incapacity to make an informed judgment, and the inability to provide appropriate consent, as occurs with children, the mentally disadvantaged, or individuals who are under the influence of alcohol and/or drugs.

Crisis intervention centers, women's shelters, and special telephone services are available to provide emergency advice and counseling. In some centers, group therapy sessions are held that aim to help victims regain their emotional health. Chapter 72 addresses the sexual abuse of children.

Victims of rape, childhood sexual abuse, or other sexual assault may feel that they want to put the experience behind them as quickly as possible, which cause them not to seek out initial physical or mental care. They may refuse to seek help or leave treatment early. Many may later experience flashbacks and other symptoms of *posttraumatic stress disorder* **(PTSD)**. PTSD can occur in the weeks, months, or years following trauma. Early psychological treatment after traumatic events is an effective measure that lessens the negative effects of trauma.

Nursing considerations related to care of a client after violence often involve treatment of both physical and psychological traumatic injuries. Initially, a complete and thorough medical history is obtained from the victim. Observable physical injuries are documented and often photographed. In addition to having damage to internal sexual tissues, the client may have numerous exterior physical injuries that may involve genital and rectal areas. Helping to collect evidence is a key nursing intervention. It is important to follow hospital and police policies regarding any evidence obtained during the examination. Careful and factual documentation is essential in the client's health record. The nurse should follow protocols regarding the handling of the victim's clothes and other pieces of evidence. Doing so ensures that the victim's rights are protected and that the appropriate information is available for legal purposes. The health record is often used in court as evidence. Additional interventions for the client include prophylaxis for STIs and unintended pregnancy. Emergency contraceptive measures may be indicated. STIs and contraception are discussed later in this chapter.

Victims of sexual assault are often seen initially in a healthcare facility, generally in an emergency department. A prepared package, with a name such as "rape kit," "sexual assault evidence collection kit," "physical evidence recovery kit," or "sexual assault forensic evidence kit" will contain specimen collection containers to be used later for legal purposes. The kit will contain instructions for obtaining specimens as well as for collection and packaging of specimens so that they are not contaminated by extraneous substances, which could make specimens useless. The evidence collected is maintained under the local jurisdiction's chain of evidence and given to the appropriate police official. If you know or suspect an assault, encourage the victim to seek physical and psychological treatment immediately. Many healthcare agencies allow only trained personnel or the sexual assault nurse examiner **(SANE)** to assist in sexual and intimate partner violence situations. A person who has been raped should not shower, bathe, or douche before examination. The nurse will assist the healthcare provider with the pelvic examination and provide emotional support to the rape victim. Sensitivity for the client during these examinations should include having the healthcare providers be of the same gender as the victim. For example, a female client/victim may feel less intimidated when being examined by female healthcare providers.

> **SPECIAL CONSIDERATIONS   Culture and Ethnicity**
>
> **Sexual rights** involve the growing consensus that sexual health cannot be achieved and maintained without respect for, and protection of, certain human rights. The fulfillment of sexual health is tied to the extent to which human rights are respected, protected, and fulfilled. Sexual rights embrace certain human rights that are already recognized in international and regional human rights documents and other consensus documents and in national laws (WHO, n.d.).

Sexual Dysfunction

Sexual dysfunction is the inability to enjoy or to engage in sexual activity. The person may be reluctant to seek help because of difficulty in speaking about a personal problem with a stranger. Sexual dysfunctions involve the inability to become physically aroused during sexual activities, the inability to achieve or to sustain an erection (impotence), the inability to achieve or the absence of **orgasm** or orgasms, and the presence of **dyspareunia** (pain during sex, generally affecting women). A variety of physical and psychological factors can cause sexual dysfunction. Sexual dysfunction can lead to relationship problems, infertility, low self-esteem, anxiety, stress, and unsatisfactory sex life.

> **NCLEX Alert**
>
> The NCLEX may provide situations (clinical scenarios) relating to communication, documentation, and education. Subjects can include communication problems related to coping mechanisms for couples diagnosed with infertility, complications of birth control, or how to approach sensitive topics such as STIs. Options (responses) for the NCLEX situations might present various nursing techniques, such as teaching the client self-care or demonstrating the use of a birth control device, but only one response will be the *best response* for the given situation.

Male Sexual Dysfunction

The most common sexual dysfunction in males is **impotence** or *erectile dysfunction* (**ED**). ED is the inability to achieve or to sustain an erection. An occasional episode of impotence is fairly common and should not alarm the client. The continued inability to perform sexually merits careful investigation.

Medical causes of ED include risk factors that decrease or occlude (prevent) blood flow to the penis necessary for sexual intercourse. Multiple diseases and disorders can result in damage to the arteries of the penis. Risk factors include STIs, heart disease, vascular disease, atherosclerosis, hypertension, prostate disorders, metabolic or hormonal disorders (especially diabetes mellitus), age, obesity, mumps, exposure to radiation, and reproductive anatomical dysfunctions. Abuse of substances such as tobacco, alcohol, or cocaine is a modifiable risk factor. Some medications or chemicals, some types of neurologic damage, and certain degenerative disorders, such as Peyronie disease (scar tissue in the penis), Parkinson disease, or multiple sclerosis, may also be risk factors for ED.

Psychological factors are often important concerns in ED. Examples include anxiety, depression, fatigue, or stress. If no physical cause can be found, psychological counseling of both partners is recommended. Extreme tension, feelings of guilt or inadequacy, obesity, and exhaustion can be contributing factors.

Treatment

In addition to physical examinations and counseling, several treatment options are available. The specialist in reproductive systems will ascertain the medical necessity for the treatment of ED prior to initiating any treatment. Existing medications or a combination of medications, including over-the-counter (OTC) supplements, must be analyzed to ascertain if they are a causative factor in sexual dysfunction. To improve sexual function, it is sometimes possible change the client's medical regimen, for example, by reducing dosages, eliminating some drugs, or changing to alternate medications. Lifestyle changes related to nutrition, obesity, smoking, alcohol and drugs, and physical activity (e.g., taking up bicycling) can be effective treatments for many sexual disorders. Risk Factors for ED are reviewed in Box 90-1.

Endocrine abnormalities, such as diabetes mellitus and prostate or thyroid disorders, need to be treated. Chronic disorders, such as cardiac and vascular issues, need to be addressed. Several prescription medications are available to treat ED. These *oral medications* include sildenafil (Viagra), tadalafil (Cialis), and vardenafil (Levitra). The goal is to induce erection directly by chemically stimulating an increase in blood flow in the penis, which causes an erection. *Intracavernous injection* is another method; it involves the injection of alprostadil directly into the base or side of the penis. Alprostadil intraurethral therapy involves insertion of a suppository inside the penis via a special applicator. In Practice: Important Medications 90-1 reviews the most common medications. Occasionally, *intramuscular injection* of a long-acting testosterone treatment can normalize hormone levels; in some cases, men may use oral testosterone. Side effects of these medications may be significant and serious. Hypotension and cardiac complications may result. Another possible complication is **priapism**, continued erection accompanied by pain. Chapter 90 has more information on reproductive disorders in men.

> **Nursing Alert** Medications, such as nitrates, anticoagulants, alpha blockers, and some antihypertensive drugs, can interact with medications used to treat ED. Significant, even fatal, side effects can occur.

If medications are unsuccessful, other options are available for treating impotence. Two options include a *penile pump* and a *penile implant*. A penile pump, also known as a vacuum constriction device, creates negative pressure and promotes blood flow for an erection. The pump is removed when erection has occurred and intercourse can be attempted. A penile implant, also known as a penile prosthesis, is either bendable or inflatable. With the bendable prosthesis, a pair of rods is implanted within the erection chambers of the penis, forming a permanent semirigid penis. To penetrate, the male lifts or adjusts the penis to the erect position. The inflatable option, considered more natural, allows the client to inflate the device when an erection is desired. A more extensive surgical option is *penile revascularization*, which is a surgery done to bypass an occlusion of an artery in the penis. Various types of prosthetic devices are available that assist in the ability to make and sustain an erection. Each device has its own advantages and disadvantages. Surgical implants may need to be replaced and can be sources of infection, pain, and mechanical failure.

Female Sexual Dysfunction

Female sexual dysfunction refers to difficulty during any phase of the female sexual response that prevents the individual from experiencing satisfaction from sexual activity. As with male dysfunctions, many physical and medical issues interfere with blood flow to female sexual tissues and can be causative factors. The main problematic conditions include diabetes and other endocrine disorders (e.g., thyroid), hormonal imbalances such as occur in menopause, and acute and chronic diseases of the cardiovascular, urinary, or hepatic organs. Lifestyle factors such as drug use, alcohol consumption, and exposure to or use of tobacco products are also known to inhibit blood flow. Prescription medications, for example, antidepressant drugs, can interfere with sexual satisfaction. Psychological factors may be direct or indirect causative agents of sexual dysfunction. All individuals experience stress, anxiety, relationship problems, and everyone occasionally has some experience with depression. Feelings of guilt and memories of past sexual trauma are also known to be psychological risk factors.

Women experiencing sexual dysfunction should be referred for medical and psychological counseling. Medical causes for female sexual dysfunction include the following:

- *Dyspareunia:* Painful intercourse as seen in endometriosis, ovarian cysts, or vaginitis
- **Vaginismus**: Painful, involuntary spasms of vaginal outlet muscles, which prevent penetration
- *Hormonal imbalances*, especially loss of estrogen, as seen with menopause, hysterectomy, or some chronic illnesses (e.g., diabetes)
- *Poor vaginal lubrication and decreased genital sensations* as seen with changes in estrogen and testosterone levels

Treatment

In 2015 the drug flibanserin (Addyi) was the first medication approved by the FDA to treat female sexual dysfunction. Flibanserin (Addyi) may be prescribed for premenopausal women with diagnosed hypoactive sexual desire disorder. As with all new medications available to the public, overall health must be monitored, and the client and healthcare provider must maintain vigilance for potential harmful side effects.

INFERTILITY

Infertility refers to the inability to conceive and to produce live babies after adequate sexual exposure. Infertility is generally defined as inability to conceive after 1 year of trying or 6 months if a female client is 35 years of age or older. Individuals who are able to get pregnant but are not able to stay pregnant may also be diagnosed with infertility. Infertility is fairly common, affecting approximately 10%–15% of all couples. Finding causes and treating infertility is typically a long and emotional process. Approximately one-third of infertility is due to male-related factors. Another third is related to female-related factors. The remaining third of infertility cases results from a combination of male, female, and other factors. Many factors inhibit the blood flow to the reproductive tissues or cause blockages in the male or female reproductive passageways. Lifestyle risk factors, such as tobacco smoke, have been shown to negatively affect reproductive functioning in a female and to destroy sperm cells in a male. The causes of some cases of infertility are unknown. The vast majority (up to 90%) of infertility cases are treated with medications, for example, antibiotics, hormone replacement, or surgical repair of the reproductive organs or passageways (Centers for Disease Control and Prevention [CDC], 2019).

Sterility is the absolute inability to procreate. In other words, the client is unable to produce eggs or does not produce adequate amounts of sperm. Without eggs or sperm in adequate amounts, conception will not be possible.

Male Infertility

Anatomical, environmental, and psychological factors must work together, or the ability to reproduce is limited or prevented. Normally, the volume of semen ejaculated needs to be about 2–5 mL, with a density of sperm at about 20 million/ml. In addition to the number of sperm, the *motility* (movement), *viability*, and *morphology* (shape) of the sperm must be within normal limits.

> **Key Concept**
>
> Although the client may be considered infertile, they may or may not be impotent. Infertility relates to the ability to conceive, and impotence refers to the ability to ejaculate.

The number of normal, active spermatozoa or the *sperm concentration* or *sperm count* within ejaculate is the important consideration in a client's ability to be fertile. Semen contains anywhere from 15 to 150 million sperm cells per milliliter, but this value varies depending on the laboratory, the actual fluid being examined, and the details needed for the diagnosis of infertility. The volume of semen ranges from 1.5 to 5 mL per ejaculation; thus, the amount of sperm available after each orgasm will influence the man's potential fertility. Often, combinations of risk factors exist that increase the client's chances of being infertile (Box 70-1).

Treatment

Generally, infertility is treated with medications or surgery. The types of treatments are commonly used in combination. Treatment begins with the healthcare provider doing an infertility checkup, which will include a physical examination, sexual histories of the partners, and evaluation of the sperm. Several tests exist to validate the function of sperm, such as cervical mucus penetration tests. Sperm antibody testing and numerical counts of sperm ("sperm counts") may also be required to determine the cause of infertility. Several factors are reviewed, including test results, the age of the partners, the health of the partners, and personal preferences for treatments. Medication may be given to treat an infection or hormone disturbance. Male hormonal levels are typically checked. Surgery may be required when the cause (e.g., an obstruction or a congenital anomaly) is not treatable by medical therapies.

Artificial insemination (AI) is a procedure that involves direct insertion of semen into the uterus or oviduct. AI may be considered when the sperm count is low but otherwise healthy. AI is discussed below in detail. Infertility may also be treated by assistive reproductive technologies, which are presented in the next section.

CHAPTER 70 Sexuality, Fertility, and Sexually Transmitted Infections

Box 70-1 Risk Factors Affecting Male Infertility

Heredity, Congenital, or Anatomical—Deformed structures or the impossibility to create sufficient sperm Azoospermia or oligospermia (no or few sperm cells produced)
- Cryptorchidism (undescended testicles)
- Cystic fibrosis
- Kidney disease
- Age

Lifestyle, Injury, or Infection—Causing acute or chronic changes to vascular system
- Hormonal disturbances (e.g., diabetes mellitus or the use of hormonal-based drugs used to treat prostate or breast cancer such as *goserelin* [Zoladex] or *leuprorelin* [Lupron])
- Injury or adhesions to reproductive tissues (e.g., sports injuries that block passage of sperm)
- Infections, such as orchitis (e.g., inflammation of the testes after mumps or testicular injury)
- Smoking or secondhand smoke (e.g., damage to blood vessels and cardiopulmonary system)
- Alcohol consumption (e.g., chronic liver problems combined with poor nutrition and existence of high-risk lifestyle factors)
- Some types of prescription drugs (e.g., antihypertensives, antidepressants)
- Some over-the-counter drugs (e.g., decongestants, antihistamines)
- Sexually transmitted infections (e.g., resultant scarring or adhesions of reproductive and genital tissues)
- Obesity (e.g., difficulty maintaining adequate physiologic support of reproductive organs)
- Psychological stress (e.g., causes physiologic problems leading to difficulty maintaining adequate support of reproductive organs)

Environmental Exposure—Causing damage or death to reproductive sperm
- External environmental temperature, which can change the number or size of sperm
- Irradiation of the testes (e.g., exposure to x-rays)
- Chemotherapy and radiation treatments
- Exposure to mercury or lead
- Exposure to pesticides

Female Infertility

In order for pregnancy to occur, a client must be able to release an egg (ova) during their ovulation cycle. To become an embryo, the egg must then become fertilized by a sperm. The fertilized embryo, generally inside a fallopian tube, travels and implants inside the uterus. This process can take up to 6 days. All of the ova that a client will ever produce are present in their ovaries at birth. Damage to the ovaries at any time may cause a permanent inability to produce viable ova. The causes of these situations may be hormonal, anatomical, situational, or environmental.

For example, when long-term starvation occurs, such as in anorexia nervosa, the body may not be able to sustain required hormonal reproductive functions. During this time, the body maintains its focus on its own life, not on the ability to reproduce. Lifestyle risk factors, which can be identified and often modified by the client, include obesity, diabetes, age, smoking, alcohol, stress, poor diet, and extensive athletic activities. Protection during sexual intercourse, such as condom use, can prevent infections from STIs and their harmful consequences on the reproductive organs (e.g., adhesions). Box 70-2 reviews the many reasons that exist for female infertility. The following conditions are some of the causes of infertility:

- *Polycystic ovarian syndrome* (**PCOS**) is the most common cause of infertility due to hormone imbalances that interfere with normal ovulation, that is, eggs maturing or being released properly.
- *Primary ovarian insufficiency* (**POI**) is a disorder that occurs before the age of 40 that causes a client's ovaries to stop normal functioning. POI is not the same as early menopause.
- *Uterine fibroids* are benign tumors or clumps of tissue on uterine walls that inhibit the fertilized egg from implanting in the uterus.
- *Pelvic inflammatory disease* (**PID**) is a serious complication of infections of the reproductive tract caused by invading organisms, such as chlamydia, gonorrhea, herpes, or genital warts. Chronic infections produce scar tissue and blockages within the reproductive tract. Refer to the STI section in this chapter and Chapter 91.
- Endometriosis, ectopic pregnancy and surgery, displaced uterus, obstructed oviducts, cancer, and vaginal infections may form blockages related to scar tissue and inhibit movement or transplantation of an ova.

Diagnosing Causes of Infertility

If desired conception does not occur after 1 year of regular, unprotected intercourse, the concerned parties should consult a healthcare provider. Clients in their 30s may wish to consult a specialist earlier if they suspect a problem because conception decreases considerably after the age of 30. A healthcare provider will check the general health of both clients. Routine laboratory tests will be done, such as a complete blood count, thyroid levels, and an analysis of the reproductive gonadotropic hormonal levels. Tests of semen and vaginal and cervical secretions are often done as well. Checking the client's ability and consistency to ovulate may be the initial step. Home ovulation test kits are available OTC, or the healthcare provider may order blood tests to check ovulation. Ultrasound of the ovaries may be the next step. If these initial tests do not demonstrate a cause of infertility, more extensive testing can be ordered.

- *Rubin test* is a procedure in which oviducts are inflated with carbon dioxide to determine *patency* (openness) of the fallopian tubes.
- *Hysterosalpingogram* is an x-ray study that looks for problems within the fallopian tubes and uterus.
- *Laparoscopy*, generally an outpatient surgery, uses a small flexible tube with a light on the distal end (the part inserted into the body) to examine the ovaries, fallopian tubes, and uterus for disease, scar tissues, and structural deformities.

Box 70-2 Risk Factors Affecting Female Infertility

Heredity, Congenital, or Anatomical—Deformed structures, tissue scarring, or ovulation problems
- Displaced uterus
- Vaginal or cervical infection (e.g., syphilis, herpes)
- Endometriosis
- Painful, irregular, or no menstrual periods
- Ovarian cysts or tumors
- History of spontaneous abortions (miscarriages)

Lifestyle, Injury, or Infection—Complications of the inflammation → infection process that leads to adhesions (scar tissue that does not function as normal tissue) of fallopian tubes
- Pelvic inflammatory disease or sexually transmitted infections—often related to scarring or adhesions
- Vaginal infection (e.g., chlamydia, herpes, or genital warts, often related to scarring or adhesions)
- Overweight or underweight—often relating to poor physiologic support of the body's conditions needed for reproduction
- Nutritional inadequacies—often relating to poor physiologic support of the body's conditions needed for reproduction
- Hormonal disturbances—conditions in which the body cannot support a pregnancy (e.g., diabetes mellitus, thyroid disorders, ovarian disorders)
- Age, with increasing problems after 30–40 years of age—reproductive problems increase with age, often related to ovulation dysfunction or ova problems
- Smoking or secondhand smoke (e.g., damage to blood vessels and cardiopulmonary system)
- Excess alcohol consumption (e.g., chronic liver problems combined with poor nutrition and existence of high-risk lifestyle factors; refer also to fetal alcohol syndrome)
- Some types of prescription drug (e.g., antihypertensives, antidepressants)
- Some over-the-counter drugs (e.g., decongestants, antihistamines)
- Athletic-level training (e.g., sports injuries can cause menstrual dysfunctions or inflammations, infections with resulting damaged, scarred tissues)
- Psychological stress (e.g., physiologic problems leading to difficulty maintaining adequate support of reproductive organs or hormonal needs for ovulation and pregnancy)

Environmental—Causing damage or death to ova and damage to hormone-producing glands (e.g., thyroid)
- Chemotherapy
- Radiation treatments

- A laparoscopy can also identify scarring and excessive tissue growth due to endometriosis.
- *Curettage*, generally an outpatient surgery, is a scraping of the inside lining of the uterus performed to determine whether the uterine lining is undergoing the normal changes necessary to receive a fertilized ovum.

Treatment

Clients are fertile for only a few days per month, generally within 48 hr of ovulation (release of an egg from an ovary). Ovulation testing is used to determine the time during the menstrual cycle when a client is most fertile. Fertility, and therefore, pregnancy, is most likely to occur around the time of ovulation. *Luteinizing hormone* (**LH**) rises 24–36 hr prior to ovulation. A client can determine when they ovulate by using commercial OTC ovulation kits, which have small, chemically infused test sticks that monitor LH levels. Symptoms of ovulation also include a slightly elevated temperature and changes in appearance and consistency of cervical mucus. The client who wants or does not want to become pregnant uses ovulation kits.

AI and *assisted reproductive technologies* are also treatments for infertility. These treatments involve procedures that are invasive, expensive, and not always successful. They are not attempted unless other methods to induce pregnancy are nonproductive or have been shown to indicate anatomical problems that are known to prevent pregnancy. These are discussed in the next sections.

Artificial Insemination

AI involves the insertion of semen artificially into a female reproductive tract. There are several methods of AI (e.g., intracervical, intratubal, or intrauterine tuboperitoneal). AI is not a form of assisted reproductive technology because it does not involve a transfer of eggs; AI involves only the distribution of sperm. With AI, the female generally receives fertility drugs to enhance the production of more eggs (ova). Sperm are introduced into the female's body after ovulation. More than one egg may be fertilized, resulting in multiple embryos (fertilized eggs). AI may be used if the male's sperm count is too low or if the female's body interferes with sperm motility.

Assisted Reproductive Technology

Assisted reproductive technology (ART), also known as in vitro *fertilization* (**IVF**), uses both eggs and sperm. In general, ART procedures involve removal of eggs from a client, which are surgically taken from the ovaries, and combined with sperm in a laboratory for fertilization. The eggs may be newly retrieved (fresh) or previously frozen and then thawed. The fertilized egg is then returned to the uterus of the egg *donor* or to the uterus of another client (nondonor). ART is considered after other medical or surgical options have been attempted to counteract infertility.

Sometimes a couple uses a donor who is a substitute for either or both of the individuals who want a baby. That is to say, a person supplies eggs or sperm for another individual. Donors are used when a client cannot produce their own eggs or adequate sperm or when either individual has infertility. On occasion, a donor is used when a couple wants to avoid passing on a genetic condition. Couples may use a donated embryo (fertilized egg from a nongenetically related couple), which is inserted into the uterus of the client who desires a baby; this child will not be genetically related to either parent.

Traditional *surrogacy* involves an individual who acts as a **surrogate** (substitute) and agrees to carry and give birth to a child resulting from AI or the implantation of a fertilized egg (IVF). The fertilized egg may originate from a couple, but that cannot or should not give birth, or from an egg donor. Sometimes the surrogate is the egg donor who is, therefore, genetically related to the child. In these cases, the sperm may be from the intended parent or from a sperm donor. The surrogate becomes pregnant, has the child, and, after birth, relinquishes the child to the couple. Surrogacy involves issues of trust as well as financial and legal issues. **Gestational surrogacy** may utilize a variety of egg and sperm combinations. It can occur when intended parents give their embryo, fertilized from their own egg and sperm, to the gestational surrogate, who acts as the **gestational carrier** (surrogate) during the intrauterine growth (gestation) of the child. In this case, the infant will be genetically related to the couple who donated the egg and the sperm. Other variations include donated eggs and/or sperm or donated embryos. In any case, the gestational surrogate carries a pregnancy to delivery.

ART has varying success rates, with resulting medical, financial, and psychological considerations. Success rates should be considered by the hopeful couple because the process is emotional, time-consuming, and expensive. Factors that affect success rates include the age of the couple, reason(s) for infertility, the type of ART chosen, the use of fresh or frozen eggs or embryos, and the clinic chosen for the procedures.

Research suggests that babies conceived through use of ART are more likely to have cleft lip or cleft palate and some heart and gastrointestinal disorders (U.S. Department of Health and Human Services [USDHHS], 2019). However, these birth defects although still under study, do not seem to be due to ART technologies but rather to risk factors such as the age of the parents. The most common complication of ART is *multiple pregnancies* (the production of two, three, four, or more fetuses). Mortality and morbidity are significant concerns of multifetal pregnancies; major complications and a variety of health issues are involved for both the fetuses and the mother. Although multiple pregnancies can often be prevented or minimized, decisions regarding resultant fetuses may involve personal, spiritual, and societal considerations.

The types of ART include the following:

- IVF is the most effective type of ART. It involves fertilization of the egg by selected sperm outside of the body in a prepared laboratory Petri dish (in vitro means "in glass"). A female is initially given medications that cause the ovaries to produce multiple eggs. Once the eggs are mature, some are removed from the client's ovaries and put into the prepared growth medium with the sperm. Fertilization of the eggs with the provided sperm is anticipated. The embryos are left in the dish for 3–5 days and then implanted into the client's uterus.
- *Zygote intrafallopian transfer* (**ZIFT**) or *tubal embryo transfer* (**TET**) also uses fertilized eggs (zygotes), which are transferred via laparoscope into the client's fallopian tubes in lieu of the uterus. The difference between ZIFT and TET is the date of implantation after fertilization.
- *Gamete intrafallopian transfer* (**GIFT**) transfers the unfertilized eggs and sperm directly into the fallopian tubes via an abdominal laparoscopic procedure; thus,

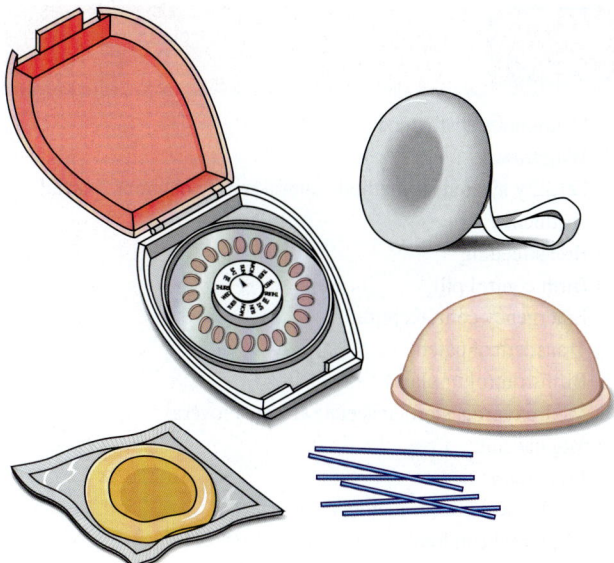

Figure 70-1 Birth control methods: Condom, birth control pills, birth control sponge, diaphragm, and birth control implants.

fertilization takes place within the client's body. Only a few clinics perform GIFT.
- *Intracytoplasmic sperm injection* (**ICSI**) may be used for couples who have significant difficulties with sperm or with an older couple. With ICSI, a single sperm is injected into a mature egg. After fertilization, the embryo is transferred to the uterus or a fallopian tube.
- *Elective single-embryo transfer* (**eSET**) is a procedure that uses one selected embryo taken from the embryos after successful IVF. The single embryo is placed in the uterus or fallopian tube. The eSET procedure avoids multifetal pregnancy, thus avoiding the risks associated with multiple fetuses.

CONTRACEPTION

Contraception, commonly called *birth control* (**BC**), is the artificial prevention of pregnancy. Several methods or devices of BC are available. Some methods inhibit ovulation, and other methods are designed to avoid implantation of an embryo in the uterine wall. Unintended pregnancies can be prevented by the use of various hormones, devices, sexual practices, or surgical procedures. Any contraceptive method used should be safe, effective, and affordable. It should also have minimal side effects and be easy for individuals to obtain and to use (Fig. 70-1).

This chapter provides an overview of many forms of BC but is not intended as the personal, educational foundation for individuals seeking comprehensive information. Individuals need to consult with their healthcare providers, the local public health department, or specific agencies that have comprehensive knowledge and experience in this field. A vast amount of reliable information is available on the Internet including sites such as www.cdc.gov, www.plannedparenthood.org, or www.nlm.nih.gov. Discussions regarding contraception require diplomatic and knowledgeable communication between the healthcare provider, the nurse, the

UNIT 10 | Maternal and Newborn Nursing

Box 70-3 | Most Commonly Used Types of Birth Control

- Continuous abstinence
- Withdrawal
- Fertility awareness method, natural family planning, partial abstinence
- Breastfeeding
- Birth control pill
- Emergency contraception
- Transdermal patch
- Birth control implant
- Medroxyprogesterone acetate (Depo-Provera)
- Vaginal ring
- Intrauterine device
- Mechanical barrier methods
  - External condom
  - Internal condom, cervical cap, diaphragm
- Chemical barrier methods for males and spermicide for females
- Sterilization
  - Nonsurgical—hysteroscopic tube insertion
  - Surgical—tubal ligation, hysterectomy, vasectomy

client, and the sexual partner(s) to ensure the best method for the individual or the couple. No single ideal method exists for everyone. The individual using a particular method of contraception must be comfortable with it and committed to *using it correctly and consistently* to attain optimum effectiveness (Box 70-3 and In Practice: Nursing Care Plan 70-1). Box 70-4 lists important points to consider when working with clients to choose a method that is right for them.

Contraception or Abortion

Treatments to prevent unintended pregnancies include the therapies of contraception, emergency contraception, or BC, which differ from treatments used to stop a pregnancy by either an induced abortion or taking an "abortion pill." A drug used to induce an abortion is called an *abortifacient*. The two-drug abortifacient regimen in the United States uses mifepristone (Mifeprex, RU-486) to block the hormone progesterone needed for pregnancy to continue, and, 2 days later, the drug misoprostol (Cytotec), which induces uterine contractions. Specially qualified healthcare providers monitor the administration of the drugs, ensure that drug protocols are maintained, and monitor the health of clients who are taking the medications. Some legal regulations may apply if the client is younger than 18 years. Some states require notification of one or both parents prior to an abortion. In some situations, a judge can make the decision in lieu of a parent.

Prior to using the mifepristone/misoprostol regimen, the client participates in a counseling session. Side effects are noted by nearly all clients after taking the combination of drugs, who state that they experience cramping, vaginal bleeding, or spotting for about 2 weeks. Mifepristone (Mifeprex), the initial drug, is given up to 7 weeks (49 days) after the first day of the client's last menstrual period (LMP) but may be effective up to 9 weeks (63 days) after that date. Misoprostol (Cytotec), the second drug, is given 2 days after mifepristone. Some states limit use of this technique to within 49 days after the LMP. After taking the drugs, an observation period is indicated to monitor the client for potential complications, such as excessive bleeding or incomplete termination of the pregnancy. Contraindications for the use of this technique include the presence of an IUD, ectopic pregnancy, hemorrhagic disorders, and specific adrenal disorders.

IN PRACTICE
NURSING CARE PLAN 70-1 | The Client Requesting Information About Birth Control

Medical History: L. C. is a 21-year-old, Southeast Asian client who delivered a healthy baby at term 2 days ago. L.C. is requesting information regarding BC. Past medical history includes having previously smoked one pack per day before becoming pregnant. "I quit as soon as I found out I was pregnant." Otherwise, own medical history is negative for major health problems, including sexually transmitted infections. Client's pregnancy progressed without problems or complications. Menarche occurred at age 12 with menstrual cycles averaging approximately every 29–30 days with moderate flow lasting approximately 5–6 days. Client does report occasional cramping with menses. Family history is positive for kidney stones and heart disease. Client's father died at age 55 of heart attack.

1. DATA COLLECTION/NURSING OBSERVATION

Client states, "We really didn't plan on having this baby like we did. We've only been married for a little over a year. I'm not sure we can handle more than one child for a while, at least not until we both get ourselves settled. My partner and I talked, and we don't know much about the different methods of contraception and which would be best for us." Client lives with partner, who is enrolled part-time in school. Client is currently on family leave of absence from work as a pharmaceutical sales manager for 6 weeks.

2. NURSING DIAGNOSIS

(Although several nursing diagnoses may be appropriate, a priority nursing diagnosis is addressed below.)

Knowledge deficiency related to appropriate contraception methods as evidenced by client's questions and statements.

CHAPTER 70 Sexuality, Fertility, and Sexually Transmitted Infections

3. PLANNING (Outcomes/Goals)	4. IMPLEMENTATION (Nursing Actions)	5. EVALUATION
Short-Term Goals		
A. Client and partner identify BC options.		Office Visit 1—1,830 hr. Client and partner enroll in clinic's teaching session titled "New Parents and Birth Control." Teaching Session 1 Couple voices numerous questions about condoms, oral contraceptives, and diaphragms. **Goal A complete.**
B. Client and partner choose an appropriate method of contraception.	• Provide general overview of the various methods of contraception available. • Compare and contrast effectiveness, preparation and use, risks, and possible side effects of BC methods. *Rationale: An overview provides the couple with necessary summary information from which to make an informed decision on a specific choice. Discussions of the varieties are proactive steps of preventative healthcare, e.g., first signs or symptoms of a blood clot.* • Listen to couples' concerns. • Discern existence of any physical, religious, or economic situations that may affect choice. *Rationale: Listening to concerns and reviewing background information helps to enhance client's learning and strengthen understanding. Long-term compliance and successful BC are more likely if couples understand personal and healthcare issues involved with choices.* • [a]Provide brochures, diagrams, charts, and pictures for couple to read at home. • [a]Encourage individual research on the Internet and bring questions to the next appointment. *Rationale: Individuals learn differently. Providing material in different forms enhances learning. Allowing the couple time to look over and process the information reinforces their ability to ask specific, individually based questions.* • Using anatomical models, demonstrate and have couple return-demonstrate insertion technique of diaphragm and condom. *Rationale: Return demonstration and discussions provide a means for evaluating the couple's understanding. The method is only effective if it is used consistently and correctly.*	Teaching Session 2—1,745 hr. After initial discussions, couple focusing discussion on two major methods: oral contraceptives (BCPs) and diaphragm. Couple states that they need more time before finalizing decision. **Goal B partially met.**

3. PLANNING (Outcomes/ Goals)	4. IMPLEMENTATION (Nursing Actions)	5. EVALUATION
Long-Term Goals		
C. Client and partner state decision to start a BC method.	• Support couple's decision. • Emphasize specific instructions regarding use of BCPs such as consistent and regular use of BCPs. *Rationale: The client's choice, not the nurse's choice, will be the most effective choice.*	Teaching Session 3—1,730 hr. Couple states that they are considering BCPs. Office visit appointment made with healthcare provider for prescription and further discussions. Client is able to verbalize major complications associated with BCPs. **Goal C met.**
D. Client and partner verbalize satisfaction with method chosen.	• Review with the couple the specific instructions about early danger signs and possible complications. *Rationale: Knowledge of potential complications, danger signs, and necessary follow-up helps to minimize the risks associated with the method chosen.* • Schedule necessary follow-up appointments, e.g., yearly pelvic examinations, and routine screening. *Rationale: Assisting with follow-up promotes compliance and helps to determine the couple's satisfaction with the method chosen.*	Office Visit 2—1,730 hr. Follow-up appointment with healthcare provider scheduled for 3 and 6 months. Couple verbalizes danger signs and symptoms independently. Couple stating they are satisfied with their choice. **Goal D met.**

[a]Note to Students: Suggestions for Internet research.
Sources for Healthcare Providers: www.cdc.gov/reproductivehealth/UnintendedPregnancy/Contraception_Guidance.htm
Sources for Research on Topic: https://www.cdc.gov/reproductivehealth/contraception/contraception_guidance.htm; Free Materials | Birth Defects | NCBDDD | CDC; https://www.cdc.gov/ncbddd/birthdefectscount/freematerials.html

> **Key Concept**
> There is no "totally safe sex." Use of a condom provides safer sex.

> **Box 70-4 Factors to Consider When Choosing Birth Control**
>
> • Lifestyle
> • Age and sexual activity
> • Number of partners
> • Need or desire for spontaneity
> • Level of maturity
> • Understanding of personal health
> • Comfort with touching own body
> • Religious and cultural beliefs
> • Effectiveness
> • Reaction to unplanned pregnancy
> • Plans for future pregnancy
> • Ability to take or to use contraceptives as prescribed
> • Client's or partner(s)' health history
> • History of sexually transmitted infections

Continual Abstinence

Continual abstinence is the only 100% effective method of BC and protection against STIs. The individual does not have intimate physical contact or intercourse with any partner. The advantages of continual abstinence include the knowledge that no STIs can be transmitted and no pregnancies will result. However, it may be difficult to abstain from sex for long periods of time.

Outercourse is a term used occasionally when discussing abstinence. Some individuals define *outercourse* as having intimate activity without having penetrative intercourse. Others use the term meaning sexual activity without penile penetration of the vagina, oral cavity, or anal area. Outercourse includes kissing, masturbation, manual stimulation, and body-to-body rubbing. Sexual activity without penile penetration of the vagina is a safe and effective method of BC. It greatly reduces the chances of HIV/AIDS or other STIs unless other body fluids are exchanged through oral or anal intercourse.

Withdrawal

Withdrawal, technically known as **coitus interruptus**, is an ancient form of BC. The male must be aware of the approach of their climax (*ejaculation*) and withdraw from the vagina prior to it. This method involves a need for tremendous awareness and disciplined control. It is controversial and risky because most males release small amounts of pre-ejaculatory fluid, which could contain spermatozoa. Unplanned pregnancies are not uncommon with this method. When the best techniques are used, this method has about an 80%–90% protection against pregnancy, which is increased to nearly 100% when a condom is used.

Fertility Awareness Method

Fertility awareness methods (**FAMs**) can also be called the *rhythm method* or *periodic abstinence*. Sometimes this technique is called *natural family planning*. FAMs involve determining when an egg is released from the ovary (ovulation) when a client is most likely to be fertile. *Periodic abstinence* may be useful for the couple who can avoid vaginal intercourse but may allow other types of sexual activity. Fertility awareness methods are reliable only for female individuals who ovulate regularly. OTC ovulation kits are available in many retail stores. They contain instructions and equipment that assist a female client in determining the specific time of their ovulation. A female client is generally considered fertile during the 2 days before and the 2 days after ovulation. To avoid pregnancy, they should avoid intercourse during these days. Another option is to supplement FAM by using a separate form of BC during the time of fertility.

The rhythm method is only about 75%–99% effective. It does require training and awareness of the days of ovulation. Illness, lack of sleep, and vaginal or other infections may affect temperature patterns. FAMs offer no protection against STIs. FAMs are not expensive and offer alternatives to people who find hormonal or barrier methods of BC unacceptable.

Breastfeeding

Breastfeeding can be a fairly reliable method of BC for the first 6 months after birth. Breastfeeding prevents ovulation. As a BC method, it is healthy, free, and does not require a prescription or supplemental BC device. To ensure effectiveness, the breastfeeding parent does not feed the infant anything besides breast milk, feeds the infant on a regular daily schedule, for example, every 4 hr during the day and every 6 hr at night, and has not had a period since giving birth. After 6 months, the client should start using another form of BCP. Breastfeeding does not provide any protection against HIV/AIDS or STIs for the client but does provide antibodies and excellent nutrition for the infant.

Hormonal Methods

Hormonal methods of BC alter a client's normal hormone level to prevent ovulation and thus the chances for conception. Hormonal contraception inhibits ovulation, fertilization, or implantation.

> **Key Concept**
> During educational sessions with a client, it is important to emphasize the fact that many forms of contraception do not protect against STIs.

Oral Contraceptives

Oral contraceptives, also called birth control pills (**BCPs**), or "the pill" are widely used in the United States and Canada. They are prescription drugs containing hormones. Single hormone BCPs contain progestin, sometimes referred to as the mini-pill. Other forms of BCPs contain estrogen and progestin. The pill works by preventing ovulation, which is needed for egg–sperm contact, and by making cervical mucus thicker, which inhibits sperm from reaching eggs. The effectiveness rate for BCPs is between 95% and 99%. A client must take BCPs correctly and consistently to ensure effectiveness. Progestin-only BCPs must be taken at the same time every day because it helps to maintain the needed hormonal level.

Hormonal BCPs are dispensed in a package of 21 or 28 pills. A client can choose the option of taking a pill for 21 days and no pills for 7 days. The 28-day option contains 21 pills that contain hormones and 7 days of placebo (no active ingredients) pills. The 28-day method is often used because it is simpler not to have to start and stop taking BCPs every 3 weeks as with the 21-day method. A brand of BCPs called levonorgestrel/ethinyl estradiol (Seasonale) or levonorgestrel/ethinyl estradiol (LoSeasonique) has an extended cycle of pills with the goal of reducing the total number of menstrual periods per year. The number of menstrual cycles per year will depend on which extended-cycle BCP is taken.

BCPs have side effects that can be problematic but generally not serious. These side effects include nausea, weight gain, swollen and tender breasts, spotting between menstrual cycles, lighter periods, and mood changes. Rare but serious health problems can occur with BCPs. Clients may complain of chest or abdominal pain, severe headaches, and blurred vision. Swelling or aching in the legs and thighs can be an indicator of a *thrombus* (blood clot) in the legs. A thrombus can break from its site of origin and become an *embolus* (a traveling clot). Emboli can cause serious or fatal consequences related to blockage of blood vessels in the lungs (pulmonary emboli), heart (myocardial infarctions), or brain (strokes). Female clients older than 35 years who smoke are among those at highest risk for these serious conditions. Some BCPs contain drospirenone, a synthetic progestin that is different from other progestins found in many BCPs. These pills are linked to migraine headaches, uncontrollable uterine bleeding, a higher risk of blood clots, hyperkalemia (high blood potassium levels), and heart and kidney problems. Examples include drospirenone/ethinyl estradiol (YAZGianvi, YASMIN, and Ocella) Some women should not take BCPs. Typical contraindications for the use of BCPs include the following:

- High blood pressure
- Heart defects
- Blood or clotting disorders
- Women older than 35 years
- Smoking
- Obesity
- Diabetes

Certain medications and supplements are known to or are suspected of interfering with the effectiveness of BCPs. Research regarding the degree to which drugs may or may not decrease effectiveness is not conclusive. Therefore, if a client is taking medications, in addition to BCPs, they should consult with their healthcare provider and consider a secondary method of BC. Common at-risk concerns relate to the following:

- Rifampin (Rifadin)—An antibiotic used for treatment of TB or other serious infections; it decreases BCP effectiveness
- Ampicillin (Omnipen)—An antibiotic that may cause menstrual irregularities in female clients taking BCPs; it may affect BCP effectiveness
- Tetracyclines—A class of antibiotics used to treat many bacterial infections; it is suspected of initiating irregularities in a menstrual cycle that may decrease BCP effectiveness
- Griseofulvin (Grifulvin V)—An antifungal thought to decrease BCP effectiveness
- HIV/AIDS medications—Some of the antiviral medications used to treat HIV/AIDS decrease effectiveness of BCPs
- Phenytoin (Dilantin)—An antiseizure medication that may decrease BCP effectiveness
- Barbiturates—A class of sedatives that may decrease BCP effectiveness
- St. John wort—An OTC supplement often used to treat mild depression or forms of anxiety

Health benefits from oral contraceptives include decreased rates of ectopic pregnancy, PID, cancers of the ovary and endometrium, recurrent ovarian cysts, benign breast cysts, and fibroadenomas, and discomfort from menstrual cramps. Some protection may be available for bone thinning, iron deficiency anemia, premenstrual symptoms (e.g., headache and depression), severe abdominal cramping, and heavy and/or irregular periods.

> **Key Concept**
> Breastfeeding mothers should be aware that breast milk will contain traces of the hormones from BCPs. It is unlikely that these hormones will affect the baby.

Emergency Contraception

Emergency contraception (**EC**) consists of two safe and effective methods of BC. Emergency contraception does not imply use of an *abortifacient*, a pill that initiates abortion. Most commonly, EC consists of the hormones levonorgestrel (Plan B One-Step) or ulipristal acetate (brand name Ella). Another type of EC is the insertion of the copper-based ParaGard IUD. EC can be used to prevent pregnancy after unprotected sex when the male's condom falls off or breaks, the male does not exit the vagina before ejaculation (withdrawal), or after forced unprotected sex. EC is also referred to as the "morning-after pill." Emergency BC can be used up to 120 hr (5 days) after unprotected intercourse but is less effective 72 hr (3 days) after sex.

Information provided to clients about EC includes the following subjects: EC offers no protection against STIs. Plan B One-Step is available OTC to anyone; no age or ID is required to purchase the product. Obesity decreases the effectiveness of Plan B One-Step. The ParaGard IUD or the brand Ella is recommended for clients who are significantly overweight. Nausea, vomiting, and cramping are the most common side effects. The ParaGard IUD needs to be inserted by a healthcare provider within 5 days of unprotected sex.

Additional Hormonal Contraceptives

Transdermal Patches

Transdermal patches with time-released hormones are convenient for a client to use. It may not be available in all communities as it is not being produced by some manufacturers. The patch is worn like an adhesive bandage and is changed once a week for 3 weeks, followed by 1 week in which no patch is worn. It is not effective against STIs.

Birth Control Implant

Similar to other hormonal methods, the BC implant releases progestin. Lack of progestin prohibits ovulation and increases cervical mucus. Known by the brand names of *Implanon* and *Nexplanon*, the implant is a cardboard matchstick-sized, thin, flexible plastic rod. It is inserted by a healthcare provider subcutaneously into the upper arm. It is effective for up to 3 years. Side effects mimic other hormonal BC methods. The client needs to monitor the insertion site for infection. It is not effective against STIs.

Depo-Provera

Medroxyprogesterone acetate (*Depo-Provera*) is a hormone similar to progesterone. It is administered by a healthcare provider every 3 months by injection and is about 99% effective in preventing pregnancy. Medroxyprogesterone acetate (Depo-Provera) works by preventing ovulation. When the drug is discontinued, the return of fertility can take anywhere from 3 to 18 months. Medroxyprogesterone acetate (Depo-Provera) is not effective against STIs.

If a pregnancy does occur, it is more likely to be in a fallopian tube (*ectopic pregnancy* or *tubal pregnancy*). Medroxyprogesterone acetate (Depo-Provera) may aggravate diabetes mellitus, kidney disease, seizure disorders, cardiac disorders, and mental illness. Additional possible side effects of Medroxyprogesterone acetate (Depo-Provera) include the following:

- Weight gain
- Depression
- Headaches
- Abdominal pain
- Irregular or loss of menstrual cycle
- Nervousness
- Increased or decreased libido
- Breast tenderness or excessive enlargement
- Pulmonary embolism

Contraindications of medroxyprogesterone acetate (Depo-Provera) include the following:

- Pregnancy
- Cancer of the breast or reproductive organs
- History of strokes
- History of liver disease
- History of blood clots in legs
- History of bone fractures
- Currently taking the medication aminoglutethimide (Elipten), a treatment for Cushing syndrome

> **Nursing Alert** Any client using hormones is at risk for heart disease, hypertension, stroke, deep vein thrombosis, emboli, breast cancer, and impaired liver function. Clients must be warned of these possibilities. Clients who take hormones have an even higher risk of complications if they also smoke.

Vaginal Ring

A vaginal ring, known by its brand name, *NuvaRing*, is a hormonal vaginal contraceptive ring. It slowly releases progestin and estrogen. Considered a safe and simple contraceptive device, the client inserts the ring once every 3 weeks; then, it is removed for 1 week when menses will occur. The ring is 98%–99% effective in preventing pregnancy. Common side effects, which are relatively mild when compared with other hormonal BC methods, include lighter periods, bleeding between periods, breast tenderness, and nausea and vomiting. Longer lasting side effects can include increased vaginal discharge, vaginal irritation, or infection.

Intrauterine Devices

An *intrauterine device* (**IUD**) is a small, T-shaped, flexible, plastic insert that a healthcare provider inserts into a client's uterus. IUDs inhibit the sperm's ability to reach the egg or prevent ovulation (hormonal IUDs). The IUD can prevent the fertilized ovum from implanting in the uterus. One benefit of the IUD is that it offers continuous protection without the need for a client to have to remember to insert it prior to sex. It is 97%–99% effective. IUDs give no protection against STIs and may cause an increased, albeit uncommon, incidence of PID, tubal pregnancies, and infertility. The greatest danger is uterine or cervical perforation, although these situations occur rarely.

In the United States, there are two types of IUDs. One is copper (ParaGard), and the other type contains hormones (Mirena or Skyla). The hormonal IUD continually releases small amounts of progestin. Mirena needs to be replaced every 5 years, and Skyla is effective for 3 years. The copper IUD, ParaGard, needs replacement after a maximum of 12 years. This copper device should not be used if the client is allergic to copper. During the time an IUD is in place, a very small string will exit the cervical opening (cervical os) and be felt in the vagina. The string indicates the presence, but not always the correct placement, of the IUD. The client should not pull on the string because the IUD can be pulled out of position. The presence of the string should be monitored at least every month.

After insertion, it is common for the client to have mild to moderate pain, cramping, or a backache for the first few days. During the next 3–6 months, the client may notice irregular periods (hormonal IUDs) or heavier, more intense menstrual cramps (copper IUD).

Most symptoms are mild or moderate and decrease over time. However, severe, sharp abdominal pain that radiates to the shoulder, neck, or rectum may indicate an ectopic pregnancy and is a medical emergency. In Practice: Educating the Client 70-1 provides information that you can share with clients about the IUD.

> **NCLEX Alert**
>
> NCLEX clinical situations may discuss a client's choice of a hormonal or a barrier type of contraception. Clinical options require knowledge about methods, complications, and the client's specific needs for information regarding their personal BC options.

An IUD may be contraindicated when any of the following situations exist:

- STI, pelvic inflammatory disease, or pelvic tuberculosis. The IUD may become a site for infection, which can cause scarring and later infertility.
- Pregnancy, known or suspected, can result in a spontaneous abortion if an IUD is inserted.
- Unexplained bleeding from the vagina or copious vaginal discharge can indicate a uterine perforation with hemorrhage or infection.
- Severe menstrual cramps, abnormally heavy menstrual flow, or spotting between periods can indicate possible perforation of the uterus or a misplaced IUD.
- Anemia, hypotension, dizziness, or syncope (fainting spells) can indicate hemorrhage.
- Severely displaced or flexed uterus or another gynecologic problem can indicate a misplaced IUD.
- Cancer of the cervix or uterus, diabetes, circulatory problems, or atherosclerosis may interfere with effectiveness or create problems such as infection.

IN PRACTICE
EDUCATING THE CLIENT 70-1   Considerations Related to an Intrauterine Device (IUD)

- The client may feel a sharp pain when the IUD is inserted.
- The client may have cramps for a few days, but these should not continue.
- Menstrual flow may be heavier, or last longer than normal, after IUD insertion.
- The device may be expelled within the first few months. (If the client does not expel it within 2–3 months, it probably will remain in place.)
- The client should check monthly to make sure the IUD is in place. (Slender threads attached to the device can be felt protruding from the cervix.)
- The client should have a yearly Pap test and pelvic examination to assure there is no irritation from the IUD.

> **Nursing Alert** If a client becomes pregnant with an IUD in place, the device is usually removed immediately to avoid spontaneous abortion, ectopic pregnancy, septic abortion, or premature labor.

Barrier Methods

Barrier methods interfere with conception by physically preventing sperm from fertilizing ova. Barriers work through mechanical and chemical means. Mechanical devices are more effective when used in combination with chemical barriers. For barrier methods to be effective, those who use them must be consistent and follow appropriate instructions. When discussing BC with a client, keep in mind their need for follow-up instructions, such as how to insert a condom or how to care for a cervical cap. Much information is available, often in an online video or step-by-step instruction. Healthcare professionals should routinely suggest that their clients read and review these materials before sexual intercourse.

Mechanical Barriers

There are a variety of mechanical barrier methods that may be used depending on client health, preference, and anatomy. These consist of various types of internal and external condoms, cervical caps, and diaphragms. **External condoms** are thin latex or plastic sheaths designed in the shape of a penis. An external condom is packaged as a flat disk that can be placed or rolled over the erect penis before sexual intercourse. There are many brands of packaged external condoms, for example, dry, lubricated, colored, scented, spermicidal, which are designed for ease of use, sexual stimulation, or personal preference. When used correctly, they are effective methods of BC. Advantages of external condoms include their ability to protect against STIs when the penis is covered during vaginal, anal, or oral sex. Condoms are relatively inexpensive OTC or are free at some clinics.

The *cervical cap*, *diaphragm*, and *internal condom* are both a mechanical and a chemical barrier because they require a spermicide to be effective. A healthcare provider is needed to examine the client who may become pregnant and prescribe the appropriate size for either the cervical cap or the diaphragm; the prescription may be filled at a local drugstore or clinic. Barrier methods must be inserted into the vagina each time before intercourse.

The *cervical cap*, brand name FemCap, is a thimble-shaped silicone cup that is inserted into the vagina to cover the cervical opening. To protect against pregnancy, these devices are left in place for 6–8 hr after having sex. The cap should not be left in for longer than 48 hr, and the diaphragm should not be left in for more than 24 hr.

The *diaphragm* is a silicone, dome-shaped shallow cup that covers the cervix. Urinary tract infections, vaginal irritation, or unusual discharge from the vagina may be related to the placement and use of a diaphragm. Some preexisting conditions may make the use of a diaphragm unwise. Examples of potential problems include a sensitivity to silicone or spermicide, recently giving birth, certain anatomical issues, and a history of infections such as toxic shock syndrome or urinary tract infections.

An *internal condom* is worn inside the client's vagina. It is a pouch made of thin latex attached to two flexible rings; one ring is inserted internally, and the other is left to open externally. The internal ring is inserted into the vagina, and the ring at the open end stays outside the vagina during intercourse. It can also be inserted into the anus. The condom protrudes from the vagina or anus, providing protection for the external genitalia. As with an external condom, the internal condom is for one-time use, but the internal condom can be inserted up to 8 hr before sexual intercourse.

The *vaginal sponge* is a combination method of BC using a barrier, made of polyurethane foam and a spermicide, nonoxynol-9 (see next section). In the United States, the vaginal sponge is available as the Today Sponge. It is effective for as long as 24 hr. It is an OTC product, so it is important to advise the client to read and follow all instructions carefully before beginning sexual intimacy. It needs to remain in place for at least 6 hr after intercourse but be removed within 30 hr of insertion. A risk of toxic shock syndrome (**TSS**) exists if it is left in for more than 30 hr. TSS is a serious acute systemic disease caused by infection with strains of *Staphylococcus aureus*. (Refer to Chapter 91 for more information on TSS.) The sponge does not protect against STIs or HIV/AIDS, and the client can become sensitive to the spermicide, which can cause mucosal irritation.

> **Nursing Alert** Hormonal forms of BC and most barrier methods of BC have little or *no protection* against STIs, including HIV/AIDS and, in some cases, may actually increase the risk for STIs.

Chemical Barriers

Chemical barriers involve the use of a **spermicide**. *Spermicides* are chemicals that immobilize or kill sperm and block the cervix to inhibit sperm from traveling to an egg. They are available in a variety of forms, including spermicidal creams, vaginal foams, film, gels, and suppositories. They are available in most drugstores or retail markets. The most common side effect is skin irritation to the vagina or the penis; changing brands of spermicide may be a simple alternative if irritation results. Spermicides are not very effective if used as the only contraceptive method. They offer added contraceptive protection when used with barrier methods such as a male or female condom or with the withdrawal method. Spermicides do not prevent the risk of STIs, but when used with a condom the STI risk is decreased. A spermicide is used in combination with a diaphragm or a cervical cap. The spermicidal foams are most effective in preventing pregnancy when used with a diaphragm or condom. The spermicide must be inserted each time vaginal intercourse occurs and, to be most effective, the client needs to wait 10 min prior to having intercourse. After intercourse, spermicides remain effective for only about an hour.

> **Nursing Alert** The most commonly used spermicide is nonoxynol-9 (N-9). It is considered an effective spermicide, but many clients may develop sensitivities to the drug, leading to irritation and breakdown of protective mucosa. The irritation may result in an increase in susceptibility to STIs and HIV or acquired immunodeficiency syndrome (AIDS).

Sterilization

Sterilization is permanent BC. There are options for sterilization available to all sexes. Methods of sterilization for a client include chemical scarring, or by making cuts inside the fallopian tubes that produce scar tissue, which inhibits fertilization. Surgical methods include a tubal ligation for the client (removal of some or all of the female reproductive organs) or a vasectomy for clients with male reproductive organs. Surgical procedures are more invasive than nonsurgical BC methods. Complications can occur, including hemorrhage, infection, or reaction to anesthesia. Chapter 91 discusses female reproductive issues. The benefits of sterilization include the knowledge that sexual intercourse need no longer be associated with fear of an unintended pregnancy. Disadvantages of permanent BC include the possibility of future life changes and the prospective desire to have children. It is often helpful to discuss the pros and cons of sterilization with a partner; however, individuals do not need their partner's permission for sterilization to be performed. Client education will include emphasis on the remaining need for protection against STIs.

Nonsurgical Methods
Chemical
Chemical methods of tubal sterilization are commonly used for permanent BC. Specific chemicals can be introduced into the tubes to induce scarring of the inside of the fallopian tubes.

Hysteroscopic Tube Insertion
Another nonsurgical method is the hysteroscopic insertion of a thin tube through the vagina and uterus and into each fallopian tube. As scar tissue forms, a natural mechanical barrier is created that prevents the egg from contact with sperm (i.e., prevents conception).

Surgical Methods
Tubal Ligation
Tubal ligation is the most common and effective procedure for permanent sterilization in clients with female reproductive organs. The fallopian tubes are cut and tied (ligated), sealed by electric current, or closed with clips, clamps, or rings. The fallopian tubes transport the ova to the uterus. If the ova cannot travel through the fallopian tubes, the client will not become pregnant.

Tubal ligation is usually done in a same-day surgery center under epidural, spinal, or general anesthesia via endoscope (*laparoscopic* tubal ligation). Each tube is usually ligated in two places, cut, and a portion removed. The client can expect to leave the healthcare facility as soon as they have recovered from the anesthesia. Someone should be available to drive them home after surgery. They may experience a slight vaginal discharge or spotting for a few days after the procedure. Normal menstrual periods and libido should resume after tubal ligation.

Often a client may have a tubal ligation performed after a vaginal delivery. It is easier to perform following childbirth because the fallopian tubes are easily accessible. Tubal ligation may be performed at the time of other abdominal surgery through an abdominal incision; all or part of the tube may be removed. It also may be done vaginally.

Mild postoperative cramping may result from manipulation of the ovaries, or referred pain to the shoulder may occur after abdominal distention with carbon dioxide, which is used for better visualization of the tubes.

Abortion
An *induced* or *therapeutic abortion* may be performed to interrupt a pregnancy. Chapter 68 discusses abortion. Abortion is a controversial means of family planning and is discouraged by healthcare providers as a primary means of controlling pregnancy.

Hysterectomy
A *hysterectomy* is the removal of the uterus. It is a significant surgery used to correct a variety of medical conditions and not usually done for BC. After a hysterectomy, the client ceases to have a menstrual period, but the individual will still have their ova and fallopian tubes. Other serious conditions may require the removal of all female reproductive organs, including both ova and each fallopian tube. Recovery after surgery will take several weeks; sexual intercourse should not resume until the surgeon states that healing of the tissues is adequate. Chapter 91 discusses female reproductive issues.

Vasectomy
A **vasectomy** is the most common surgical method for sterilization in clients with male reproductive organs. This procedure involves the ligation (tying off) and sometimes the removal of a small part of the vas deferens (ductus deferens). The vas deferens is part of the long tube that transports viable sperm in the testes to the outside of the client's body. When it is cut, the sperm cannot reach the ova during intercourse, and pregnancy is prevented.

The client who chooses to have a vasectomy should anticipate that they will remain sterile but will not be impotent (will be able to have an erection). Reversal (reattaching the vas deferens) of a vasectomy is not uncommon, but this revision procedure often is unsuccessful.

The vasectomy is relatively easy and has few complications. It may be performed in the healthcare provider's office under local anesthesia. Only two small scrotal incisions are made, and the postoperative course is usually uneventful. A vasectomy reversal may need to be done in an outpatient setting.

Postoperative complications of vasectomy may be scrotal tenderness, swelling, and impotence for 1–2 days. Infection may occur, but usually it is mild. Sitz baths, ice packs, and analgesics are usually all that are needed to relieve postoperative discomforts.

To ensure the success of a vasectomy, regular sperm counts following the procedure are important. The client must be told that it may take up to 6 weeks after a vasectomy for the semen to be totally free of sperm because the body stores semen. A sperm count is usually taken 6 weeks–2 months after the procedure. If the sperm count is zero, the vasectomy was most likely successful.

Client teaching includes reminding the client to use BC measures until their sperm count remains at zero for

6 weeks. However, a sperm count should be taken again after 6 months and then yearly to assess the continuing effectiveness of the surgery. In rare cases, sperm find an alternate pathway, and the client is then no longer sterile.

The client should feel confident in their decision to have a vasectomy. Emotional aspects of vasectomy can be stressful, even more so than physical concerns. Talking with others who have had a vasectomy may reassure a client that they will not lose their sexual potency or drive.

SEXUALLY TRANSMITTED INFECTIONS

STIs are infections obtained by having sexually intimate contact with an individual who has an STI. The WHO uses the term *sexually transmitted infections (STIs)* because not all infections are diseases with specific, unpleasant symptoms. Individuals may think of an infection as something treatable and be encouraged to seek help. At least 25 types of STIs exist. Etiologies of STIs include bacteria, parasites, and viruses.

STIs are a significant health challenge for the United States. State and national Public Health Departments have requirements for healthcare providers for the reporting of STIs. Many cases are undiagnosed, and many are unreported (e.g., human papillomavirus, herpes simplex virus [HSV], and trichomoniasis).

> **Key Concept**
> Women are 10–20 times more likely than men to get STIs. Those most vulnerable to STIs are teens and young girls and pregnant individuals. The increased STI susceptibility is related to the anatomic structural differences between women and men.

Individuals between the ages of 15 and 24 account for about one-half of the cases of STIs, especially chlamydia and gonorrhea. Since these cases occur in the younger, sexually active population, acute and chronic (i.e., lifetime) problems develop for the individual. Younger populations tend to have more sexual partners as well as more instances of unprotected sex, which increases proliferation of new cases of STIs. In addition to problems related specifically to each STI, infertility, ectopic pregnancy, and mortality and morbidly of newborns are known outcomes of many untreated STIs. **Adhesions** initiate as scar tissue, which leads to the development of chronic infections that have frequent acute episodic outbreaks. (Refer to In Practice: Educating the Client 70-2: The Inflammatory Process below.) This type of scar tissue is often seen in individuals, especially individuals who have had acute or chronic pelvic inflammation such as PID or abdominal surgery.

Younger people are often reluctant to seek treatment and counseling related to STI. Confidentiality, embarrassment, lack of finances or insurance, and lack of transportation also factor into the high rates of adolescent infections. Box 70-5 reviews important concerns related to STIs.

> **Nursing Alert** STIs and BC must be considered as *connected but separate issues*. Certain BC methods—such as withdrawal, IUDs, and oral or implanted contraceptives—factor into the *spread of STIs*. These BC methods have no mechanism to prevent the spread of bacteria, viruses, or other microorganisms.

Contraception is discussed in the previous section. Several BC methods provide some protection against both STIs and pregnancy (e.g., barrier methods). *Safer sex*, but not *safe sex*, is possible with the use of condoms. Additional precautions, for example, spermicides and barrier methods of BC, provide better protection against STIs. Continual sexual abstinence is the only guarantee of protection against STIs.

IN PRACTICE
EDUCATING THE CLIENT 70-2: The Inflammatory Process

Inflammation is a critical first-response of healing. If tissues become damaged for any reason (cut, bruise, infection, surgery), the **inflammatory process** will commence. Increased blood flow to the damaged area causes the classic signs of inflammation: redness, warmth, tissue swelling, and pain. Pain develops because of increased pressure from swollen tissues as well as the release of prostaglandin chemicals on localized nerves. An irony of healing is that the inflammatory process can become excessive and be the actual cause of many autoimmune and other problems. The inflammatory process has an acute and chronic nature that may be deleterious in many situations such as with PID or STIs. *Adhesions* can develop and are particularly problematic in the abdomen. *Adhesions* are bands of scar-like, damaged tissues that form on the internal surfaces of the mucous membranes that line body cavities. Scar tissue does not function as normal tissue; its design is basically for use as connective tissue. The scar tissue of adhesions adheres to linings and internal organs, which inhibits the normal flexible activity and movement of tissues. Normal mucous membrane linings are designed to move or shift but are not supposed to adhere to each other. Chronic abdominal tissue damage results in an increasing amount of scar tissue and abdominal adhesions. In addition to scarring of the internal structures, pain can become extreme and severely interfere with an individual's capability to function.

When discussing STIs with a client, it is important to emphasize the effects of inflammation, infection, and the likely development of abdominal adhesions in a female client. The client may be less hesitant to seek early treatment of an infection if they understand that the long-term consequences can be severe pain, sterility, and lifestyle changes.

> **Box 70-5 Lifetime Considerations Related to STIs**
>
> Sexually transmitted infections may
> - Increase your chances of infection with human immunodeficiency virus (HIV).
> - Increase your chances of infection with other STIs (coinfections).
> - Have significant side effects for the individual including minor symptoms that range from irritation, discharge, or pain to significant permanent consequences such as PID, inability to reproduce, and death.
> - Have few, inconsistent, confusing, or no symptoms.
> - Cause significant side effects and/or death in newborns.
> - Cause infections that lead to pelvic inflammatory disease (PID) and/or infertility.
> - Cause infections of the mouth, throat, respiratory tract, urethra, and reproductive organs in any individual.
> - Cause infections that reoccur when reexposed by a partner who has not been diagnosed or who had incomplete treatment.
> - Can occur at any age but are most common in sexually active young adults.
> - Are less common in individuals who are tested for STIs and are in monogamous relationships.

Treatment of STIs is often difficult. Individuals themselves may become more resistant to antibiotics. They may have received antibiotic therapy for STI exposure, but individuals can be reexposed and infected several times during a lifetime of sexual activity. Because STIs are now so prevalent, antibiotic resistance is problematic. No specific antibiotic, antiviral, or other treatment has been found that will prevent or cure HIV/AIDS or herpes simplex virus type 1 or 2. *Individuals infected with viral STIs are infected for life.* A person also may have more than one STI simultaneously, which complicates treatment.

HIV and AIDS

A link connecting HIV and other STIs has been established. A person who has an STI and is exposed to HIV is two to five times more likely to acquire HIV than is a person who does not have an STI. HIV/AIDS is discussed in more detail in Chapter 85.

Women are more easily infected by unprotected sex because the delicate tissues of the female reproductive tract can become scratched or irritated. These little fissures offer direct routes of invasion for the HIV virus. Individuals can transfer the virus to their unborn children during pregnancy, birth, or through breastfeeding. Clients with HIV can often prevent the transfer of HIV to their unborn children with proper prenatal care.

Signs and Symptoms

HIV infection can mimic many other illnesses. Diagnosis by laboratory testing is the only accurate HIV detection method. A person who has had any STI should consider getting tested for HIV. Warning signs of possible HIV infection include rapid weight loss, fever, night sweats, enlarged lymph nodes, severe diarrhea, purplish blotches on or under the skin, and a change in neurologic behaviors. Refer to Chapter 85 for more information regarding HIV/AIDS.

Symptoms that HIV-positive women have frequently differ from those in men. HIV treatment is delayed because the initial symptoms often appear as common problems, such as frequent yeast infections or pelvic pain. This may lead clients to self-treat symptoms at home. However, frequent problems, such as yeast infections, abnormal Pap smears, or pelvic pain, can be early symptoms of HIV infection.

Nursing Considerations

In keeping with *Standard Precautions*, nurses wear gloves when coming in contact with any body fluids to protect themselves against the possibility that their clients might be positive for a communicable disease. The best defense against contacting an infectious disease, such as an STI, in a healthcare work environment is the fastidious implementation of Standard Precautions.

> **Key Concept**
>
> *Standard Precautions* are the minimum infection prevention practices that apply to all client care in any setting where healthcare is delivered, regardless of suspected or confirmed infection status of the client. These practices are designed to both protect healthcare professionals and prevent healthcare personnel from spreading infections among clients (CDC, 2016).

Chlamydia

Chlamydia trachomatis is the bacterial species that is the leading cause of preventable infertility in women and the most common STI in the United States. **Chlamydia** is transmitted during vaginal, anal, or oral sex, leading to infections in the associated tissues of these areas.

Signs and Symptoms

Approximately 50% of affected individuals are asymptomatic. Chlamydia may be called a "silent STI." Symptoms may be mild, absent, or misdiagnosed. Three of four women have no symptoms, and half of men have no symptoms. If symptoms occur, they typically occur 1–3 weeks after exposure. Often the infection is not diagnosed until complications or damage occurs. Box 70-6 presents the many signs and symptoms of chlamydia.

For men, the symptoms of chlamydial infection include painful urination, a watery penile discharge, and pain and swelling in the testicles. Untreated chlamydia infection generally causes urethral infections, epididymitis, and potential infertility.

Women initially may have *dysuria* (burning, painful, or difficult urination), vulvar itching and burning, grayish-white or abnormal vaginal discharge, or spotting between menstrual periods. Although symptoms may begin in the urethra and cervix, which ascend to the fallopian tubes, recognizable problems may start with abdominal pain, low back pain, fever, and dyspareunia (painful sex). PID occurs in women who may or may not receive treatment for chlamydia. PID

> **Box 70-6** **Signs and Symptoms of Chlamydia**
>
> - Absent, mild, or nonexistent symptoms
> - Burning or itching with urination in all individuals
> - Urinary discharge in all individuals
> - Vaginal discharge
> - Low back pain
> - Nausea
> - Fever
> - Dyspareunia
> - Abnormal menstrual cycles
> - Pelvic inflammatory disease
> - Infertility
> - Epididymitis
> - Rectal pain, discharge, or bleeding in all individuals
> - Genital papules
> - Rectal ulcers
> - Swollen lymph glands in infected areas

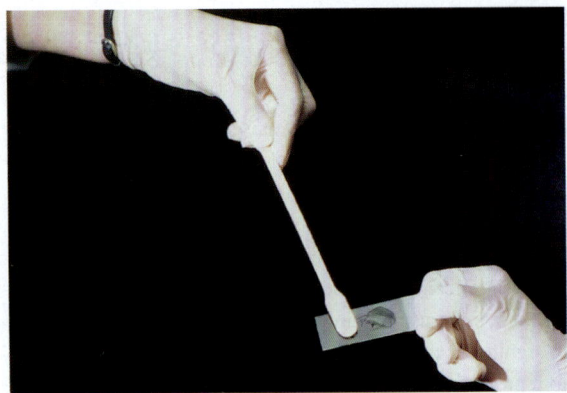

Figure 70-2 The nurse is assisting the practitioner during a pelvic examination. Notice that the nurse holds the microscope slide on the frosted portion so that the practitioner can smear the clear portion with vaginal secretions.

often results in chronic pelvic pain, permanent damage to the female reproductive organs, ectopic pregnancies, and infertility. Chlamydia can be the cause of preterm births, newborn pneumonia, and *conjunctivitis* ("pink eye").

Diagnosis and Treatment

Diagnosis is made with a stained smear test that includes urine or specimen collection from the penis or cervix. Because of the reinfection frequency, retesting when changing partners is highly recommended (Fig. 70-2).

Treatment includes the medications azithromycin (Zithromax) and tetracycline (doxycycline). For clients who are pregnant or allergic to tetracycline (doxycycline), erythromycin (Erythrocin) is used. Because 40%–60% of clients with gonorrhea also are infected with chlamydia, treatment with ceftriaxone (Rocephin) may also be indicated. People with chlamydia must use condoms when engaging in sexual activity, and all sexual partners must be treated simultaneously to avoid reinfection, which is common.

> **Nursing Alert** Tetracyclines (doxycycline) are contraindicated in pregnancy or in infants because they permanently stain teeth. Alternative antibiotics such as erythromycin (Erythrocin) or azithromycin (Zithromax) are used when necessary.

Gonorrhea

Gonorrhea is caused by invasion of the bacteria *Neisseria gonorrhoeae*, also known as gonococcus (**GC**). It is spread through vaginal, oral, or anal sexual contact between partners. It can infect the cervix, urethra, rectum, anus, and throat. Gonorrhea can be spread from one part of the body to another, such as by touching infected genitals and then the eyes.

During delivery, an individual can infect their infant with gonorrhea. Untreated infection in a newborn can lead to blindness, joint infection, or sepsis. Healthcare facilities have standard criteria, such as administration of antibiotic eye drops to newborns, to prevent gonorrheal eye infections. Prenatal care and STI screening are important teaching considerations for the nurse.

Signs and Symptoms

Typical symptoms appear within the first 2 weeks after exposure, but it is possible not to have any symptoms; this is especially true for women. When initially infected, the client may have a burning sensation during urination and a yellowish-white discharge from the penis. Painful or swollen testicles are common. Prostatitis, infection of the seminal vesicles, and sterility may develop. Without treatment, the infection progresses to the epididymis. Gonorrhea can spread to bones, joints, or the bloodstream, resulting in arthritis, heart disease, liver damage, or central nervous system damage.

Many women with gonorrhea are asymptomatic. Clinical findings in women include cervical tenderness, dyspareunia, purulent anal discharge, dysuria, a yellow-green purulent discharge, or a change in vaginal discharge. PID with abdominal adhesions is common, and sterility may result. Douching, sexual intercourse, and menstruation may spread the infection to the ovaries and cause abscess. Individuals infected with gonorrhea are more likely to contract HIV than are noninfected people.

> **Nursing Alert** After treatment of an STI, such as gonorrhea, immunity does not occur. The person is susceptible to *reinfection* (a "ping-pong effect"). Reinfection by a carrier or by an object (e.g., a diaphragm or other device used during intercourse) is common. To avoid reinfection, it is important to trace and treat all of the person's sexual contacts.

Diagnosis and Treatment

A smear of the discharge is cultured and examined microscopically, obtaining a Gram stain of the gonorrhea bacterium, often referred to as a GC Gram stain (Fig. 70-3A). Some healthcare providers advocate obtaining urethral, vaginal, anal, and throat cultures. One treatment for gonorrhea is intramuscular injection of ceftriaxone (Rocephin) or

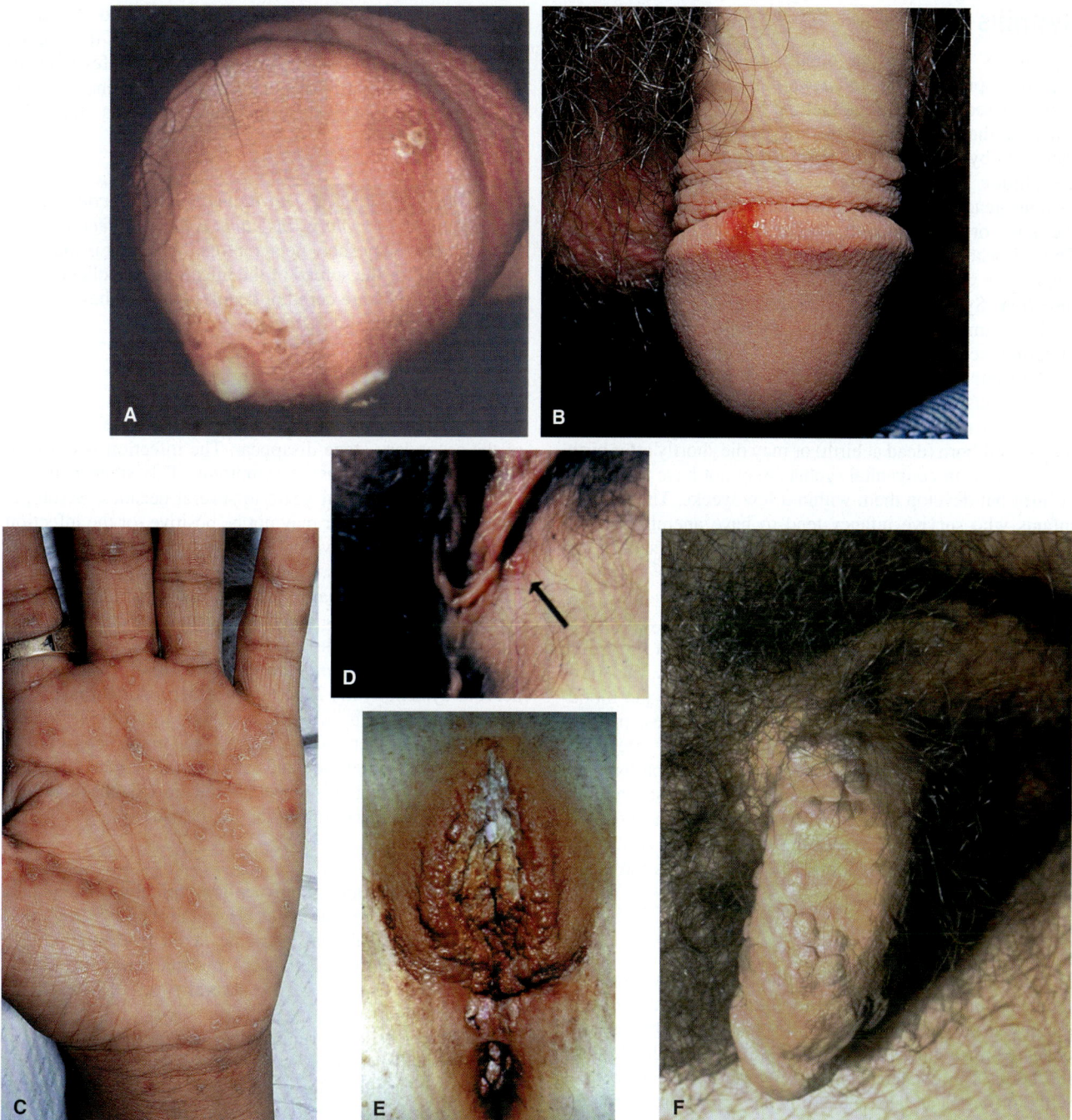

Figure 70-3 **A.** Gonococcal urethritis is the most common symptom of gonorrhea seen in men. Note the purulent penile discharge from the meatus and the gonorrheal lesions on the foreskin. **B.** The painless chancre of primary syphilis seen on a penis. **C.** The rash of secondary syphilis is often seen on the palms of the hands or the soles of the feet. **D.** Herpes simplex virus is seen as shiny, small blisters in the vulva area (arrow). **E.** Genital human papillomavirus, also known as *condyloma acuminatum* (pl. *condylomata acuminata*), causes genital warts, as seen here in the vulva region. **F.** Genital human papillomavirus of the penis. Note the raised, round lesions on the shaft of the penis. (A and B from Strayer, D. S., Saffiz, J. E., & Rubin, E. (2019). *Rubin's pathology* (8th ed.). Wolters Kluwer Health.)

cefixime (Suprax). Drug-resistant strains are problematic in many areas. Coinfection with chlamydia is very common. Treatment consists of antibiotics that treat both infections. Individuals with gonorrhea should also be tested for other STIs, including HIV.

All sexual partners also must be treated simultaneously to prevent reinfection. When the infection is active, teach the client about the use of Standard Precautions; that is, to wear gloves when coming into contact with their own body secretions. Frequent and careful handwashing is critical. Eyes are particularly susceptible to gonorrheal infection.

With an advanced infection, the client needs bed rest and may require Sitz baths and massive doses of intravenous antibiotics. The individual is not considered infection-free until cultures have been negative for at least 7 days without antibiotics.

Syphilis

Syphilis is caused by a highly contagious, destructive bacterial spirochete (*Treponema pallidum*) that can have grave consequences throughout the body. The CDC (2018) reported that between 2014 and 2018 cases of syphilis increased by 74%. Syphilis is spread by direct contact with a syphilitic lesion (chancre) via vaginal, anal, or oral sex. Lesions generally occur on the external genitals, the vagina, the anus, or in the rectum, on the lips, and in the mouth. The spirochetes can enter through cuts or breaks in the skin. Healthcare workers must use Standard Precautions to avoid infection. Syphilis cannot be spread by toilet seats, doorknobs, swimming pools, hot tubs, bathtubs, shared clothing, or eating utensils.

Pregnant individuals can pass syphilis to a fetus. Spontaneous abortions (*miscarriages*) are not uncommon in cases of maternal syphilis. An infant born with syphilis may be stillborn (dead at birth) or may die shortly after birth. Newborns with **congenital syphilis** may not have symptoms at birth but develop them within a few weeks. The infected infants who survive infancy tend to have anemia, skeletal deformities, neurologic problems, liver disease, speech and motor delays, or seizures.

Signs and Symptoms

The spirochetes thrive in moisture and live for a short time outside the human body. After entering the body, the spirochetes immediately multiply and gain access to the bloodstream. Syphilis progresses through three stages: primary and secondary, in which the individual is highly infectious, and, if left untreated, will progress to tertiary syphilis in the latent stage. Within 10 days–3 months, the first syphilitic lesion (**chancre** or *primary lesion*) appears. The presence of a chancre greatly increases the likelihood of HIV exposure and contamination. Table 70-1 summarizes the stages of syphilis.

Primary Stage

Within 10–90 days of infection, the chancre may appear on the penis, on the anus, inside the vagina, on the nipple, or in a crack at the side of the mouth (Fig. 70-3B). One or more chancres may appear at the spot where syphilis has entered the body. The chancre lasts 3–6 weeks and heals with or without treatment. The chancre is deep, painless, hard, and oval-shaped, with serous drainage. It contains millions of spirochetes. Sometimes, enlarged lymph nodes also appear. Blood tests are usually positive during the primary stage. Without treatment, the infection progresses to the secondary stage.

> **Nursing Alert** A syphilitic chancre is *not* to be confused with the "blisters" of herpes simplex virus type 1 or 2.

Secondary Stage

Approximately 2–4 weeks after the initial infection, the *secondary stage* begins; it may last 2–6 weeks. A macular copper-colored rash can appear on the abdomen, the soles of the feet, or the palms (Fig. 70-3C). Wart-like spots may develop on the mucous membranes or around the anus. These spots are extremely infectious. Patches of the client's hair may come out, and he or they may have a fever, headache, or sore throat. The person may have none of these symptoms and may feel normal and well. This stage also ends spontaneously.

> **Nursing Alert** *During the first and second stages of syphilis*, the client is highly infectious, although they may show no symptoms. This fact is the main reason for the spread of the infection. The client believes that they are cured or decides that they have never had syphilis.

Latent Stage and Tertiary Syphilis

Latent (hidden) *stage* syphilis occurs when the symptoms of the secondary stage disappear. The infection is dormant (inactive) without causing symptoms. This stage may last anywhere from several years to several decades. Serologic laboratory tests may or may not be positive for the infection (Table 70-2). The individual may not be infectious to others during the later stages. *Tertiary syphilis* is the end stage of the infection. Dementia, lack of muscle coordination, paralysis, gradual blindness, and death occur.

The lack of muscle coordination with syphilis, called *tabes dorsalis (locomotor ataxia)*, involves invasion of the nervous system by the *T. pallidum* bacterium (**neurosyphilis**). It is accompanied by a sharp, burning pain in the legs; legs feel numb, and then cold or warm. The person seems not to know where their legs are and cannot walk without watching them closely. The gait is jerky, and the individual cannot find their way in the dark. Joint function is lost.

Diagnosis and Treatment

Tests for syphilis and gonorrhea are typically done as part of antepartal care. Some states also require premarital blood tests for these disorders. A smear taken from a syphilitic lesion can provide diagnostic information. More commonly, diagnosis comes from several types of blood tests (see Table 70-2).

Treatment will be related to the length of time that the individual has had syphilis. If contaminated for less than a year, a single, large dose of long-acting injectable penicillin may be sufficient. Tetracycline, doxycycline, or other antibiotics are alternatives. Individuals who have had repeated treatments, incomplete courses of antibiotics, and/or are in a later stage of the infection will need additional antibiotics. Treatment can destroy the syphilis organisms at any stage of the infection; however, drugs cannot reverse any damage already present. Syphilitic damage is irreversible.

> **Key Concept**
> Do not confuse the words *chancre* with the word *chancroid*. A chancre is a painless, hard lesion, often the first indicator of syphilis. A **chancroid** is a painful genital ulcer caused by *Haemophilus ducreyi*, previously a common STI generally occurring in warm, humid climates. Sporadic outbreaks of chancroid lesions are now seen, but incidences have decreased worldwide.

TABLE 70-1	Stages of Syphilis		
STAGE	TIMEFRAME	SYMPTOMS	IMPORTANT TOPICS
EXPOSURE to *Treponema pallidum*	1–9 days	No symptoms	• Transmission of syphilis occurs during vaginal, anal, or oral sex. • Pregnant clients with the infection can transmit it to unborn.
PRIMARY syphilis	10–90 days	Chancre appears	• Appearance of a single sore or multiple sores at the location(s) where the bacteria entered the body. • Chancre (sore) is usually firm, round, and painless and can easily go unnoticed. • Chancre lasts 3–6 weeks and heals regardless of treatment. • Without treatment, syphilis continues to the next stage.
SECONDARY syphilis	6 weeks–6 months	Skin eruptions	• Rash, called mucous membrane lesions, on one or more areas of the body. • Can appear from the time when the primary sore is healing to several weeks after the sore has healed. • Rash usually does not itch and is unusual in that it can occur on palms of hands and soles of feet. • Symptoms from this stage will go away whether or not treatment is received. • Without the appropriate care, the infection moves to the latent and possibly late stages of syphilis.
LATENT syphilis	Begins when primary and secondary symptoms disappear		• Latent syphilis is defined as having serologic proof of infection without symptoms of infection. • *Late* latent syphilis is asymptomatic and not as contagious as early latent syphilis. • *Early* latent syphilis may have a relapse of symptoms which makes the individual very contagious. • Early latent syphilis is latent syphilis where exposure occurred within the past 12 months. • Late latent syphilis is latent syphilis that occurred more than 12 months ago.
LATE or TERTIARY syphilis • Neurosyphilis • Gummatous syphilis • Cardiovascular syphilis	10–30 years		• Tertiary syphilis may occur approximately 3–15 years after the initial infection and may be divided into three different forms. • *Neurosyphilis* may be early and asymptomatic. or • *Neurosyphilis* may occur later involving degenerative changes to the central nervous system which include poor balance, lightning pains in the lower extremities, numbness, paralysis, gradual blindness, dementia, damage to internal organs, cardiovascular lesions, and death. • Neurosyphilis typically occurs 4–25 years after initial exposure. • *Gummatous syphilis* occurs about 1–46 years after exposure; average 15 years. • Gummas form. They are soft, tumor-like balls of inflammation of variable sizes affect the skin, bone, liver, and other areas. • *Cardiovascular syphilis* occurs 10–30 years after exposure, which may result in the formation of an aneurysm. • Without treatment, the individual can have syphilis for years without any signs or symptoms and about a third of the infected will die. • Individuals with tertiary syphilis are not infectious to others.

Note: The content of this table refers to untreated syphilis.
Note: First-time infection provides no immunity; reinfection can occur if exposed a second time.
Adapted from https://www.cdc.gov/std/syphilis/stdfact-syphilis.htm; https://www.mayoclinic.org/diseases-conditions/syphilis/symptoms-causes/syc-20351756; https://www.healthline.com/health/std/syphilis#symptoms-by-stage

TABLE 70-2 Laboratory Tests for the Various Stages of Syphilis

Antibody Tests for Syphilis	Exposure to *Treponema pallidum*	Primary Syphilis Chancre appearance	Secondary Syphilis Skin eruptions	Tertiary Syphilis Neurologic disease
Nontreponemal Used to • screen for or • confirm a positive treponemal antibody test Also used as a guide for treatment.	• VDRL • **RPR**	Highly sensitive; positive screening results must be confirmed with treponemal antibody test, as it may be positive in other conditions. Nontreponemal antibodies typically disappear in an adequately treated person after about 3 years.	Same as primary stage	VDRL is primarily performed on CSF and used to detect neurosyphilis.
Treponemal Antibody Tests Used to • screen or • Confirm a positive nontreponemal antibody test.	• FTA-ABS • TP-PA and • Various automated immune-assays	Highly specific; positive screening results must be followed by nontreponemal antibody test to differentiate between active and past infection. These antibodies remain positive for life even after treatment.	Same as primary stage	The CSF FTA-ABS is less specific than VDRL, but the test is highly sensitive; can be used to exclude neurosyphilis.
Direct Detection Tests (much less common than antibody testing)				
• Microscopic examination • Darkfield examination Sample from chancre is placed on a slide and examined with a special microscope.		If the bacteria are seen, a definitive diagnosis of syphilis is made.	N/A	N/A
• Polymerase chain reaction (PCR)		Detects genetic material of bacteria in sample from chancre	Detects genetic material of bacteria in the blood	Detects genetic material of bacteria in the blood and/or CSF sample

Adapted from https://labtestsonline.org/tests/syphilis-tests and https://www.cdc.gov/std/syphilis/stdfact-syphilis.htm

Herpes Simplex Virus (Genital Herpes)

Herpes simplex virus type 1 (**HSV-1**) and the more common STI, *herpes simplex virus type 2* (**HSV-2**), are the causes of **genital herpes**, sexually transmitted viral infections. It is difficult to differentiate between HSV-1 and HSV-2. Direct contact with the saliva of an infected person, such as by kissing, can transmit the infection from one person to another. Viruses embed themselves in the body's nerve fibers. HSV-1 appears as fever blisters or cold sores on the lips but can infect genital regions through oral–genital or genital–genital contact (common canker sore; see Fig. 70-3D). HSV-2 typically causes painful watery skin blisters around the genital or anus. Many contaminated individuals have no symptoms. Outbreaks happen spontaneously or during times of stress or illness. New blisters form which are infectious to others during intimate contact. The first infection can take 2–4 weeks to disappear, and, commonly, other outbreaks will appear within weeks or months. After the initial outbreak, the following outbreaks tend to be less severe and heal more rapidly. The virus is small enough to penetrate a condom.

Genital herpes infection makes individuals more susceptible to HIV infection. Persons with existing HIV infection are more likely to become infected with HSV, as well as other STIs (Box 70-7).

Pregnant individuals can shed the virus at the time of delivery, causing potentially fatal infections in the newborn. Cesarean delivery is commonly scheduled if a client has active or a history of genital herpes.

Risk factors for genital herpes infections include the following:

- Multiple sexual partners
- Age ranging from 14 to 50 years
- Low socioeconomic status
- Ethnic minority
- Female
- Same-sex sexual activity
- HIV infection

Signs and Symptoms

Symptoms of HSV range from none, mild, or severe. The initial lesions will disappear without treatment, although the condition usually recurs. Two-thirds of people who have an initial outbreak will have a recurrence. Systemic flu-like symptoms, such as headache, general malaise, fever, and node tenderness, often exist concurrently. Precipitating

CHAPTER 70 Sexuality, Fertility, and Sexually Transmitted Infections

> **Box 70-7** **Considerations Related to Herpes Simplex Virus (HSV)**
>
> **PREDISPOSING AND PRECIPITATING FACTORS TO HSV-1 AND HSV-2 INFECTION**
> - Existing oral, anal, or vaginal lesions (blisters)
> - Multiple sexual partners
> - Anxiety or fatigue
> - Vaginal or labial irritation
> - Sunburn
> - Tight clothes, especially synthetics or wet bathing suits
> - Fever
> - Certain time of menstrual cycle
> - Birth control pills
> - Hormonal imbalance
>
> **OTHER CONSIDERATIONS**
> - HSV-2 closely associated with cervical cancer
> - HSV-2 closely associated with prostatic cancer
> - HSV-2 closely associated with Hodgkin disease and lymphosarcoma
> - Great danger to the newborn if mother has active HSV
> - Disease is very contagious at certain times
> - The virus can penetrate a condom

Screening for HSV should be done at the same time as screening for syphilis and gonorrhea. Cultures should be taken for any suspicious lesion. HSV testing can include HSV-2 blood tests, which will generally be considered diagnostic for a genital herpes infection. Only viral cultures can differentiate HSV-1 from HSV-2. The virus may bury itself, perhaps in the central nervous system, between outbreaks and become nonobservable.

> *Key Concept*
>
> If herpes is present, a condom offers minimal, if any, protection against the spread of the infection.

Genital herpes is closely associated with cervical and prostate cancer. Because HSV is not curable, the client needs routine examinations and emotional support. Treatment is mostly symptomatic and directed at reducing discomfort and preventing secondary infection. Oral analgesics, such as aspirin, acetaminophen (Tylenol), or other nonsteroidal anti-inflammatory drugs (NSAIDs), may reduce systemic discomfort. Cleanliness and dryness are essential to promote healing. Cotton underwear is useful. Individuals with herpes should avoid unprotected sexual contact, especially when lesions or any symptoms are present.

Client teaching includes instruction on use of standard precautions and restricting others from using items that come in contact with the lesions, such as a toothbrush. During active outbreaks, an infected person should not share food or engage in kissing. Meticulous handwashing is necessary to prevent the spread of the lesions to another part of the body.

factors include anxiety, fatigue, excessive sexual activity, excessive vaginal or labial irritation, sunburn, tight clothes (especially synthetics), and fever. The lesions may be extremely painful. However, a significant number of all people infected are unaware of being infected.

In women, the lesions begin on the external genital labia approximately 6 days after exposure. From there, they spread and usually become painful. However, they may be painless if they spread into the vagina. The lesions often look like pimples surrounded by a reddened area; they then progress to papules, vesicles, and finally crusts. This sequence lasts 1–3 weeks. Recurrence also seems to be related to hormonal imbalance; the recurrence of herpes often coincides with the menstrual cycle or during times of stress. BCPs increase the possibility of infection. Other symptoms of primary infection in women include dysuria, vaginal discharge, perineal discomfort, and dyspareunia.

In men, the major symptom is a painful lesion, usually on the penis, which may be mistaken for the chancre of syphilis. The uncircumcised clients may carry the HSV in the *smegma*, a secretion that collects under the foreskin.

Diagnosis and Treatment

Treatment is generally palliative. Four or five outbreaks per year are common. No cure for genital herpes exists. Antiviral medications can shorten and prevent outbreaks when the client is taking the drugs. *Episodic* or *suppressive treatment* exists using antiviral medications. Episodic treatment (i.e., antiviral medication taken only during outbreaks) helps to speed healing and shorten the length of the outbreaks. *Suppressive therapy* is used if outbreaks are frequent or severe; antiviral medications are taken every day.

Cytomegalovirus

Cytomegalovirus (**CMV**) is a viral infection related to the large family of HSVs that includes chickenpox (varicella) and mononucleosis (Epstein–Barr virus or EBV). As with other herpes viruses, CMV has periods of dormancy. CMV is transmitted by exposure to body fluids, including blood, urine, saliva, tears, and breast milk, and by intimate sexual contact (e.g., intercourse, kissing, or exposure to genital body fluids). Testing has shown that by age 40 at least 50% of the adult population has been infected with CMV; however, CMV of the newborn can be asymptomatic or result in serious infections affecting the liver, spleen, and central nervous system. CMV in adults rarely causes obvious illnesses. Exceptions do occur, and some adults acquire a CMV infection similar to infectious mononucleosis. Immunocompromised individuals, for example, organ transplant recipients, HIV/AIDS clients, or individuals with chronic severe illnesses, are at a high risk of the more severe complications of CMV. Mild symptoms include general malaise, upper respiratory symptoms, generalized pain, fever, and, the most common symptom, retinitis. More serious symptoms include severe eye infections, gastrointestinal problems, and encephalitis.

Treatment includes symptomatic relief, for example, through bed rest or acetaminophen; no specific treatment or vaccine for CMV currently exists. Immunocompromised individuals (e.g., persons with HIV/AIDS or those who are undergoing cancer chemotherapy) may be given immunotherapy and an antiviral agent to control symptoms. Pregnant individuals should avoid contact with CMV.

Genital Human Papillomavirus

There are about 100 varieties of *human papillomavirus* (HPV) that can cause warts on sundry parts of the body. They are one of the most commonly reported STIs in the United States, and the vast majority of individuals do not know that they have HPV and that they can spread HPV to others. Four main areas of HPV infections exist. One variety of warts can affect the genital areas and are known as *genital warts* or *venereal warts* (*condylomata acuminata*); they resemble flat lesions, small cauliflower-like bumps, or tiny stem-like protrusions. Other HPV warts affect hands, fingers, and elbows (known as common warts), the feet (known as plantar warts), and the face and neck of the younger population (known as flat warts) (Fig. 70-3E,F).

About 40 variations of HPV are associated with genital warts, which infect the vulva, labia, anus, mouth, and throat. The types of HPV that cause genital warts are not the same types of HPV that cause HPV-related cancers. Cancerous HPV is caused by specific viruses, and there is no way to differentiate between these varieties; individuals can have both types. In men, warts appear on the penis, scrotum, or around the anus. In women, some of the warts appear around the vulva, cervix, vagina, or anus. Oropharyngeal cancer can occur as growths in the throat, at the base of the tongue, and on the tonsils. Any sexually active person is at risk for genital HPV. Predisposing factors for genital warts include the following:

- Oral contraceptive use
- Frequent sexual intercourse
- Multiple sexual partners
- Cigarette smoking
- Presence of other STIs
- Sex without condom use
- Being immunocompromised
- Damaged or scratched skin

Signs and Symptoms

HPV infections are very common but have very few signs or symptoms. Most of the time, warts appear and seem to disappear without any treatment. Genital warts appear as small bumps or group of bumps in the genital areas, which may be single or multiple soft, moist, pinkish growths. Sometimes the genital warts form a cauliflower-like shape appearing on and around the genital structures and the anus. Lesions may not appear for several weeks or 2–3 months after exposure. Additional clinical signs include *pruritus* (itching), dyspareunia, and chronic vaginal discharge. Self-inspection and healthcare follow-up are particularly important steps for individuals because warts, which may cause itching, rarely cause discomfort or pain.

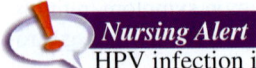 **Nursing Alert** The greatest danger with an HPV infection is the *predisposition to cervical cancer.*

Diagnosis and Treatment

Cancer of the cervix is the most often diagnosed problem associated with genital HPV. The best treatments for cancer of the cervix are preventative HPV vaccinations and pelvic examinations to obtain a Pap smear, which typically detects precancerous, abnormal cervical cell changes. Cervical cancers are often discovered when a Pap smear shows abnormal cell changes that may or may not be HPV; that is to say, not all cervical cancers are caused by HPV. Follow-up is necessary as soon as possible if the Pap test is positive, and particularly if the virus is discovered. Cancer of the anus and penis are also possible with HPV.

The best form of treatment for HPV is *prevention* via HPV immunizations (Box 70-8). Standard treatment should begin with self-inspection and observation of vaginal discharge or unusual pain. Routine examination by healthcare professionals is important because many individuals are asymptomatic and, thus, not aware that they are infected. Healthcare testing, for example, Pap smears or HPV DNA testing, can be done to check for genital cancers. With early detection, cervical cancer has a high cure rate.

Symptomatic treatment is done by removal of visible genital warts and/or use of topical medications. Lesions must be actively treated to reduce the possibility of cancer. There are several topical medications or local treatments that diminish or destroy a lesion. Several applications of the topical medications are generally necessary before symptoms are affected. Examples of medications and treatments include the following:

- *Salicylic acid.* OTC topical solution used on common warts. Causes skin irritation and is not used on the face.
- *Imiquimod* (Aldara, Zyclara). A prescription cream used topically against HPV. Common side effects include redness and swelling at the application site.

Box 70-8 Vaccination for Prevention of HPV-Related Cancers

The cancers caused by HPV can develop years after infection with HPV. Immunization against HPV is possible and is most effective if given before the individual becomes sexually active. The vaccine needs adequate time to become effective. Giving the vaccine to both males and females by age 11–12 is the most effective method of protecting individuals against genital warts and HPV-related cancers. There are three types of HPV vaccines. *Gardasil* and *Gardasil* 9 protect against the strains of HPV that cause genital warts and HPV-related cancers for both females and males. Another vaccine, *Cervarix*, protects against cervical cancer but not against genital warts. Vaccines are administered in three doses over 6 months. The CDC recommends HPV vaccination using the following guidelines:

- Vaccinate all boys and girls ages 11 or 12 years.
- Vaccinate males through age 21 and females through age 26 if these individuals were not vaccinated when younger.
- Vaccinate any man who has sex with a man through age 26.
- Vaccinate individuals with compromised immune systems (e.g., HIV/AIDS) through age 26 if they were not fully vaccinated at a younger age.

Adapted from materials at https://www.cdc.gov/vaccines/vpd/hpv/hcp/recommendations.html and https://www.mayoclinic.org/diseases-conditions/hpv-infection/symptoms-causes/syc-20351596

IN PRACTICE
EDUCATING THE CLIENT 70-3 — Prevention of STIs

Personal responsibility is an important component in the prevention of STIs. Educating your client about prevention of STIs should include the following topics:
- Vaccinate for HPV prior to becoming sexually active.
- Avoid or abstain from oral, anal, or vaginal sex.
- Maintain a mutually monogamous sexual relationship.
- Limit sexual activity to individuals whose STI status is known.
- Use latex or polyurethane condoms every time sex occurs.
- Apply latex condoms appropriately.
- Use a barrier method (e.g., condom), which can prevent some, but not all, STI and HIV infections.
- Know the limits of the effectiveness of condoms.
- Be in a relationship with someone who has tested negative for STIs, including HIV.
- Have open and honest conversations with a sexual partner to ascertain if an untreated or partially treated STI exists; avoid sexual activity if concerns develop.
- Medicate or treat *both partners* simultaneously, and avoid sex if one partner has an STI.
- Suggest mutual partner testing for STIs and HIV and wait for test results prior to having sex.
- Be alert for signs of STIs prior to having sex (e.g., a foul, fish-odor discharge, or unusual growths).

https://www.cdc.gov/std/prevention/default.htm

- *Podofilox* (Condylox). A prescription topical solution used to destroy genital wart tissue. May cause local pain and itching when applied.
- *Trichloroacetic acid.* A chemical burn treatment used to burn off genital warts. Causes temporary, local irritation.
- *Cryotherapy.* Freezing the wart with liquid nitrogen, which causes local tissue death.
- *Electrocautery.* Burning with a small device that delivers an electrical current.
- *Surgical removal.* Small incisions or cutting out infected areas.
- *Laser surgery.* Use of a laser light to destroy infected areas.

In Practice: Educating the Client 70-3 discussions actions that clients may take to prevent STIs.

Other STIs

Other common infections can be spread by sexual contact. As with all STIs, both sexual partners should be treated simultaneously (*concomitant* treatment) to prevent reinfection. The three most common causes of microorganism-produced vaginitis are vulvovaginal candidiasis, trichomoniasis, and bacterial vaginosis.

Candidiasis or Vulvovaginal Candidiasis

Candidiasis or vulvovaginal candidiasis (**VVC**) is a fungal infection caused by yeasts that belong to the genus *Candida*. More than 20 species of the yeast *Candida* exist. They are found on the skin, in the gastrointestinal tract, and the vagina, usually without causing problems. An overgrowth of *Candida albicans* is the most problematic. *C. albicans* is also known as moniliasis, thrush, fungal infection, or yeast infection. It is one of the most common causes of vaginitis (Fig. 70-4A). Oropharyngeal candida (mouth or throat) is also possible. Normally, there is a homeostatic balance among this organism and others in the body. Under certain conditions, overgrowth of the normal fungal population has been linked to antibiotics, high sugar intake, hormone disturbances, BCPs, corticosteroid therapy, malnutrition, too-frequent douching, immunosuppression, and diabetes.

Symptoms include pruritus (intense itching), pain, swelling, and redness of the vulva, burning after urination, and a white, cottage cheese-like (curdy) vaginal discharge. A pelvic examination is done and samples of the vaginal discharge are obtained. Diagnosis is made by putting a sample of the discharge on a microscopic slide. The healthcare provider typically requests a slide for a Gram stain and a "wet prep," that is, a slide prepared with potassium hydroxide (**KOH**). A culture and sensitivity may be ordered also but, since *Candida* is known to normally be found in the vagina, a positive result may not be a helpful diagnostic indicator for this STI.

Treatment is available with prescription and nonprescription medications. OTC intravaginal creams include butoconazole 2% (Femstat 3) or miconazole 2% (Monistat). Prescription medications include nystatin 100,000-unit vaginal tablet or terconazole 0.4% (Terazol) creams. Creams are available in disposable applicators and are used for 1–7 days depending on product. Fluconazole (Diflucan), a single-dose pill, can also be used, especially in cases of reinfection.

Clients tend to self-treat this problem due to the availability of OTC medications. Some clients report relief from symptoms by swallowing acidophilus capsules, eating yogurt, or instilling yogurt directly into the vagina. Unnecessary or inappropriate use of OTC medications or self-care remedies can result in serious complications that do not respond well to short-term therapies. Client teaching should include the awareness that a healthcare provider should be seen for persistent problems. Recurrent problems, bad-smelling greenish discharge, and severe pain are not associated with *Candida*.

Trichomoniasis

Trichomoniasis, also known as trichomonas or "trich," is caused by the parasitic protozoan *Trichomonas vaginalis*. The parasite is common in young, sexually active female clients and, less frequently, in male clients. Transmission is by vaginal, anal, or oral sex with an infected individual and via any device (sex toy or douche tip) that has been exposed to the protozoa. Condoms help prevent cross-transmission. In female clients, signs and symptoms include itching and burning of the vulva accompanied by a copious, foul-smelling, greenish-yellow or gray, frothy or bubbly discharge (Fig. 70-4B). Red ulcerations may be seen on the vaginal wall or cervix. Both sexes may have frequent, painful, burning urination. Pain may be present

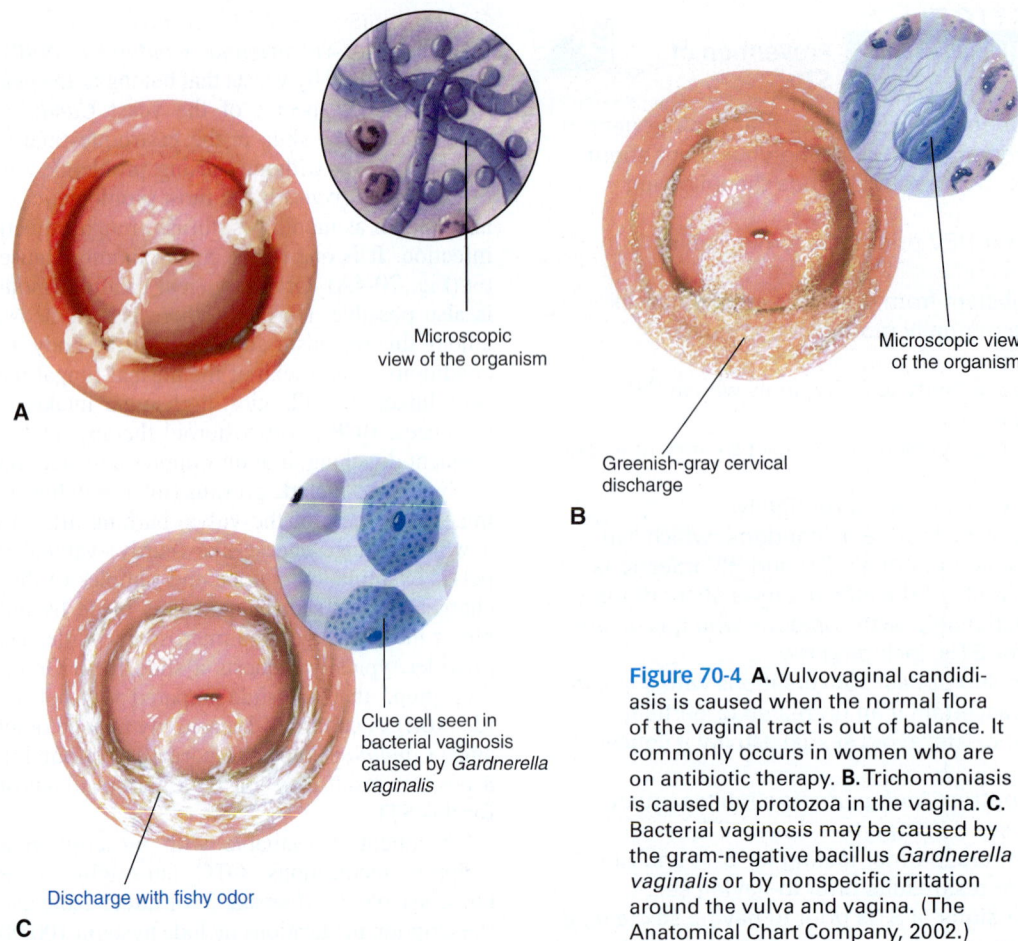

Figure 70-4 A. Vulvovaginal candidiasis is caused when the normal flora of the vaginal tract is out of balance. It commonly occurs in women who are on antibiotic therapy. **B.** Trichomoniasis is caused by protozoa in the vagina. **C.** Bacterial vaginosis may be caused by the gram-negative bacillus *Gardnerella vaginalis* or by nonspecific irritation around the vulva and vagina. (The Anatomical Chart Company, 2002.)

in both sexes during sexual activity or when urinating, leading to urinary tract infections. Individuals may not have any symptoms, and, if untreated and nonsymptomatic, individuals can still infect or reinfect partners.

Factors that trigger growth of trichomoniasis include the following:

- Pregnancy
- Sexual activity
- Irritation of vaginal walls
- Trauma to the vaginal walls
- Systemic illness
- Menstruation
- Emotional upsets

Key Concept

In sexually active women with STIs, HIV infection is more likely than in non–STI-infected individuals. The rationale seems related to the presence of irritated vaginal tissues, which makes access for HIV transmission more probable. Treatment of STIs will reduce the capability of the HIV virus to gain entry to a non–HIV-infected individual.

Diagnosis is confirmed by physical examination and laboratory testing. Treatment consists of metronidazole (Flagyl), which is a highly effective antiprotozoal and antibacterial drug.

Bacterial Vaginosis

Bacterial vaginosis (**BV**) or *vaginitis* is a nonspecific term that implies inflammation and possible bacterial infection of the vagina. The gram-negative bacillus *Gardnerella vaginalis* is a common bacterial etiology of BV. It is commonly found in sexually active women but can occur in women who have never had sex. The condition also may be called *nonspecific vaginitis*. Many things cause *vaginitis* (inflammation of the vagina), including personal hygiene products such as soap, laundry detergent, bath oil, frequent douching, spermicides, tampons, diaphragms, condoms, or sexual activity. Infections occur when normally healthy bacteria found in the vagina or alkaline semen from the male disturb the balance normally found within vaginal acidic tissues. The client may have no symptoms or may complain of an odorous discharge. BV causes a "stale fish" vaginal odor with a vaginal discharge. The discharge is a thin, gray-white leukorrhea that may be mild or profuse (Fig. 70-4C). Without treatment, BV can result in PID and sterility. With many cases of BV, no itching or burning exists as is associated with candida or trichomonas infection.

A pelvic examination is done by the healthcare provider. Diagnosis is obtained by looking at a small smear of the vaginal secretion on a microscopic slide (at least two slides needed); a pH of the vaginal smear is also done. A Gram stain determines the relative quantity and type of bacteria that are present. The potassium hydroxide (KOH) test is done to ascertain a fishy odor associated with the vaginal samples of BV. Treatment is generally successful with topical creams, metronidazole (Flagyl), or clindamycin (Cleocin T).

STUDENT SYNTHESIS

KEY POINTS

- Human sexuality involves the whole body, mind, and spirit.
- Violence is a learned behavior. Prevention is the most successful mode of treatment.
- Sexual dysfunction is a person's inability to enjoy or engage in sexual activity for any reason.
- Infertility can be caused by multiple factors. Common factors include decreased sperm production, ovulation disorders, tubal obstruction, pelvic inflammatory disease, and endometriosis. Untreated, many STIs cause infertility.
- Infertility carries deep physiologic and psychological effects but can often be treated by artificial insemination or assistive reproductive technology.
- Contraception is an important consideration for individuals during their fertile years. Counseling in this area must be nonjudgmental and geared to meet the needs and preferences of the individual.
- STIs are often asymptomatic but, left untreated, have the potential to cause serious health problems, sterility, and death.

CRITICAL THINKING EXERCISES

1. Consider the concepts of sex, gender, and sexual orientation. How can knowledge of these concepts improve client care?
2. You are working with a couple in their early 30s. They have been trying unsuccessfully for about 6 months to conceive. They are eager to begin fertility testing and have mentioned an interest in discussing fertility drugs and other options with their healthcare provider. What is your initial reaction? How would you approach this couple? What advice would you give them?
3. J.P. is 15 years of age. They come into the clinic with symptoms indicative of chlamydial infection. Tests confirm this diagnosis. J.P. currently has two sexual partners. Which type of information would you discuss with J.P.? Explain treatment and other measures for them to avoid reinfection and to prevent infecting others.

NCLEX-STYLE REVIEW QUESTIONS

1. A 28-year-old client informs the nurse that they are unable to become pregnant and have been trying for about 3 months. Which response by the nurse is best?
    a. "That is a long time to try without having any results."
    b. "What do you think might be wrong with you?"
    c. "Maybe your partner should be tested because it probably isn't you."
    d. "You should consult a fertility specialist after 1 year of regular unprotected intercourse."

2. A client who is a victim of intimate partner violence (IPV) comes to the clinic for treatment of various bruises and lacerations. Which nursing action is the priority in the care of the client?
    a. Document observable physical injuries with photographs.
    b. Inform the client that they will have to be tested for a sexually transmitted infection.
    c. Ask the client if this partner has had similar behaviors in other relationships.
    d. Inquire as to why the client continues to remain in an abuse situation.

3. A client informs the nurse that he is unable to achieve or maintain an erection. Which medications would the nurse anticipate teaching the client about? Select all that apply.
    a. Sildenafil (Viagra)
    b. Tadalafil (Cialis)
    c. Doxycycline (Monodox)
    d. Vardenafil (Levitra)
    e. Flibanserin (Addyi)

4. A client has been given the abortifacient drug, mifepristone (Mifeprex). Which information would the nurse provide the client?
    a. There are no contraindications to taking the medication.
    b. You can only take this medication once because it will not work again.
    c. You may experience cramping and vaginal bleeding for 2 weeks.
    d. There may be severe vomiting and diarrhea, which are normal side effects.

5. The nurse is caring for a group of clients in the health clinic. Which client requesting birth control pills (BCPs) is at greatest risk for complications?
    a. A 38-year-old client who smokes cigarettes
    b. A 22-year-old client with a bladder infection
    c. A 30-year-old client who has had an IUD removed 2 months previously
    d. A 27-year-old client who was previously on BCP a year ago

CHAPTER RESOURCES

Enhance your learning with additional resources on thePoint!

Student Resources related to this chapter can be found at thePoint.lww.com/Rosdahl12e.

Pediatric Nursing | UNIT 11

71 Fundamentals of Pediatric Nursing

Learning Objectives

1. Explain the concepts of prevention and health maintenance as they pertain to children.
2. State the rationale for providing immunizations to children. Identify three nursing considerations related to immunizations.
3. Discuss five specific nursing observations needed for the care of an infant, toddler, preschooler, school-age child, and adolescent.
4. Provide three topics of therapeutic communications with a toddler, preschool-age child, and school-age child.
5. Define and differentiate among the stages of separation anxiety. Differentiate between separation anxiety and loss of control.
6. State the normal limits of pulse, respiration, temperature, blood pressure, height, and weight for infants and children of different ages.
7. Identify five concerns related to pediatric safety during a hospital admission.
8. List four types of pediatric restraints. State three nursing concerns regarding pediatric restraints.
9. In the skills laboratory, demonstrate the application of a urine collection device on an infant. State three nursing concerns for this procedure.
10. Identify three nursing concerns for bathing an infant.
11. Define and differentiate among the following: oxygen mask, mist tent, and hood. State two nursing concerns for each.
12. Identify nursing considerations for each of the following: venipuncture, heel stick, and lumbar puncture. State three nursing concerns for each procedure.
13. Differentiate and discuss the treatments for fever lower than 102 °F (38.8 °C) and higher than 102 °F (38.8 °C). State three nursing concerns for each.
14. State three nursing concerns when administering PO and IM medications to an infant, a toddler, a preschool-age child, and a school-age child.
15. State eight nursing considerations for a child before and following a surgical procedure.
16. Identify five concepts that need to be discussed with the caregivers of a child who is scheduled to undergo a surgical procedure.

Important Terminology

circumoral
  cyanosis
health
  maintenance
health supervision
immunization
pediatrician
pediatrics
well-child visit

Acronyms

APRN
DDST
HELP
IPPB
NPO
OFC
PICC
TPN
URI
VIS

Pediatrics is the area of care that deals with children and adolescents. Nursing care of children is called *pediatric nursing*. Generally, the healthcare provider in this field is a **pediatrician**, although family practitioners, nurse practitioners (NP) or advanced practice nurses (**APRN**), and physician assistants (PA) also provide pediatric care. Changes in healthcare delivery have greatly decreased the number of children cared for in a standard acute care hospital. The primary emphasis in current pediatric healthcare is on prevention of diseases and accidents, maintenance of good health, safety awareness, and positive lifestyle promotion. The healthcare role of the APRN has increased in conjunction with the preventative care needs of the younger population.

As a nurse, you will encounter children in various healthcare settings. You may care for well, ill, physically challenged, and mentally challenged children. Family or other primary care providers will be a part of situations involving children. Possible settings for healthcare delivery include the home, school, community healthcare facility, day-surgery center, healthcare provider's office, summer camp, residential setting, or hospital. The fundamentals of pediatric nursing discussed in this chapter apply regardless of where you provide care. Note that the nursing procedures in this chapter can be used or adapted for children of all ages. Many skills in Unit 8 also are applicable to and adaptable for pediatric nursing.

> **NCLEX Alert**
>
> Always consider a child's age and developmental stage when responding to the query in the NCLEX clinical scenario (situation). The responses may all be true but only one response will be the most accurate for the given pediatric scenario.

HEALTH MAINTENANCE

Prevention of disease, disorders, and disability is the goal of pediatric nursing. The concept of well-baby and well-child visits for **health maintenance** or **health supervision** has proved to be the most effective method of promoting the growth and development of healthy children. Caregivers must be aware of the importance of routine, scheduled trips to a primary provider or community health facility. Preventive healthcare monitors growth rates and achievement of developmental milestones and provides opportunities for early detection of health problems.

Well-child visits allow for immunization appointments, school and athletic physicals, and screening for eye and ear problems. The child also may visit one of these settings for specific complaints of distress or injury. Well-child visits are also excellent opportunities for the nurse to provide teaching about health, safety, and nutrition issues. Health facilities offer excellent spaces to display educational brochures, pamphlets, or booklets that are often free from Websites such as the American Academy of Pediatrics, the Centers for Disease Control and Prevention (CDC), and many other reliable healthcare sources. The nurse has an opportunity to observe family interactions and can notify the healthcare provider of behaviors that suggest family dysfunction.

Counseling of family caregivers can be provided before crises develop (In Practice: Educating the Client 71-1).

Remember that some children are cared for in families headed by persons other than their biologic parents. Gather data that include information about the relationships within a child's immediate family when you initiate care. Also consider the child's cultural and religious background.

You may find that a review of Chapters 6 and 7 will be beneficial at this time. As you are now in the more advanced and specific units of this textbook, you will better understand the importance of the topics in the preliminary chapters, and how these fundamental issues do affect the daily life of clients and healthcare personnel, as well as nursing considerations.

> **Key Concept**
>
> Basic principles of safety and child care apply for both well and ill children.

During each visit, the nurse should obtain specific information related to the child's age. **Well-child visit** information includes vital signs, height and weight, and occipital–frontal circumference (**OFC**) of the head (to 2 years of age). Plot the child's height and weight on a growth chart that allows comparison with other children of the same age. At each visit, the child's growth should be compared with what is considered "normal limits" and compared to their previous growth trends. Early detection of abnormal trends can lead to preventive treatments. You can view comprehensive facts about child development on the Centers for Disease Control and Prevention Website.

Tools for a more detailed preliminary assessment of child development are available. The Denver II Developmental Screening Test (**DDST**) is a tool used to identify developmental delays in infants, toddlers, and preschoolers. The Hawaii Early Learning Profile (**HELP**) charts are designed to

---

IN PRACTICE

EDUCATING THE CLIENT 71-1 — Family Caregiver Instruction for Children of Different Ages

Infant
- Proper diet and feeding techniques
- Teething
- Feeding routine, colic, and spitting up
- Need to suck; pacifiers
- Positioning and sleep habits
- Diaper rash
- Bathing and bathing safety
- Urinary and bowel habits
- Crib safety
- Use of a car restraint or safety device
- Accident prevention: suffocation, drowning, poisoning, and falling
- Beginning dental care: wipe the infant's gums with a damp cloth to remove excess food

Toddler
- Dental care: dental visits
- Weaning from the bottle
- Diet and solid food
- Behavior patterns: separation anxiety, negativism, and temper tantrums
- Discipline and limit setting
- Poison prevention
- Toilet training

Preschooler
- Eating habits: dawdling over food, "picky" eating
- Night waking, bedtime fears, and nightmares
- Development of a positive self-concept and body image
- Aggressive behavior and sibling rivalry
- Preparation for school
- Thumb-sucking; dental care
- Care for common childhood illnesses

help determine a child's developmental level. The charts are available in sets that cover six primary domains, including cognitive, language, gross motor, fine motor, social–emotional, and self-help. They provide "normal limits" of development and also compare a child's developmental growth to general trends. If a delay is identified or suspected, a more detailed evaluation of the child may be performed.

Physical Examination

The primary caregiver will complete a physical examination that will become a reference point for evaluating future illnesses. Many examiners use a head-to-toe checklist. Some protocols use a body system approach (e.g., cardiovascular, neurologic, pulmonary). In this way, patterns are established, and nothing is overlooked. When an exception to the established normal trend is noted, it is described in detail on the child's chart.

Immunization

Immunization provides people with temporary or permanent protection against certain diseases. The immunization program begins shortly after the child's birth and should be continued on a regular schedule. Family caregivers must present records of immunizations to the child's school; failure to do so may result in the child's exclusion from the school. Most immunizations can be given even when the child has a mild illness. (Immunizations are discussed in more detail in Chapter 72.) Immunizations are very important healthcare actions designed to help not only the individual child but also society in general. It is, therefore, very important that individuals receiving immunizations have the most current and verified information available regarding both the productive expected effects and the nonbeneficial effects of each immunization, as well as the effects related to combinations of immunizations given throughout an individual's lifetime. The CDC provides Vaccine Information Statements (**VIS**) that explain both the benefits and possible risks of a vaccine to parents or vaccine recipients. In addition, yearly recommended immunizations are easily viewed on printable summary tables available on the CDC immunization web pages. See the *Recommended Child and Adolescent Immunization Schedule for ages 18 years or younger* on the CDC Website (http://www.cdc.gov/vaccines). Federal laws require that healthcare workers provide a VIS to a client, parent, or legal representative before each dose of certain vaccines (for additional information, go to https://www.cdc.gov/vaccines/hcp/vis/index.html). Individual states may also have pertinent regulations regarding the immunization of school children.

Some individuals have objections to vaccination protocols. Extensive research is available to the public regarding these concerns (Box 71-1). The CDC and numerous professional healthcare agencies strongly support immunization. Taking time to listen and educate families is important to correct misinformation.

Specific Care for Age Groups

Infant Care

Infant health supervision includes documentation of milestones of development and growth, as well as documentation of immunizations and family teaching, which center around discussion with family caregivers and anticipatory teaching.

> **Box 71-1 Resources and Information About Vaccines**
>
> The following sources have more specific discussions and concerns regarding vaccination, which will be useful for client teaching:
> - IAC's Talking About Vaccines (Immunization Action Coalition)
>   www.immunize.org/concerns
> - CDC Vaccine Information Statements (VISs)
>   https://www.cdc.gov/vaccines/hcp/vis/index.html
> - National Foundation for Infectious Diseases
>   https://www.nfid.org/immunization/
> - National Network for Immunization Information
>   http://www.immunizationinfo.org/professionals/
> - CDC's Vaccines, Healthcare Providers/Professionals
>   https://www.cdc.gov/vaccines/hcp/

General observations include the following:

- How family caregivers hold the infant
- If the infant "cuddles" with family caregivers
- General cleanliness of the infant
- The infant's response to painful procedures
- The infant's appearance of health or illness; weight compared with length

Specific observations include the following:

- Equal, active movement of all extremities
- General activity level
- Alertness
- Skin color, warmth, and texture
- Tone and pitch of the infant's cry
- General respiratory status
- Fontanels, reflexes
- Achievement of developmental milestones

Toddler Care

As a toddler's growth progresses, independence and autonomy become important. Documentation for a well-child checkup will include the following:

- Age of weaning from breast or bottle to cup (usually achieved by age 12 months)
- Ages at which toilet training was started and completed
- Language development
- Play patterns and activities
- Sleep patterns

Discuss with family caregivers their child's behavior patterns and the type of discipline they use at home. Encourage caregivers to begin dental checkups for toddlers as early as 12 months of age.

Teaching requires a strong focus on safety. Toddlers are very mobile, but lack the judgment to protect themselves. Observe caregiver–toddler interaction.

Preschooler Care

The physical examination for preschool children focuses on readiness for school. Use a systems checklist to evaluate each child's physical condition. Focus attention also on sleep patterns, safety, and relationships with peers, siblings, and family caregivers.

Evaluation of speech, hearing, and vision is critical in the preschool years. Each must be within normal limits to facilitate learning. Determine if a child's developmental age is commensurate with their chronologic age. An adequate attention span is essential. Your observational skills are important, and you will need to document each child's ability to pay attention, follow directions, and focus on a task. Evaluate gross and fine motor control. These characteristics are evaluated earlier, but they become a special focus in the preschool examination.

School-Age Child Care

Continue to plot the school-age child's height and weight on the growth grid to establish a comparison with other children of the same age. Emphasize successful completion of schoolwork and relationships with peers, siblings, and family caregivers. Evaluate nutrition, elimination, and sleep patterns. Immunization status needs to be reviewed, using the most current immunization recommendations. Some healthcare providers may have specific guidelines they prefer.

Adolescent Care

Health supervision issues for adolescents focus on puberty and a smooth transition to young adulthood. Adolescents require an update of the diphtheria–tetanus–pertussis and meningococcal immunization, and they are old enough to begin the human papilloma vaccine series.

> **Key Concept**
> Adolescents may be too embarrassed to ask questions, particularly about their health. A bulletin board or brochure rack well stocked with informational pamphlets about common concerns can aid communication.

Adolescents are capable of expressing individual concerns; therefore, you will benefit from talking separately with caregivers and with adolescents. A tactful approach to care includes detailed explanations of procedures you are to perform. The transition from childhood to adolescence can be difficult. The adolescent may present with such problems as acne vulgaris, menstrual dysfunction, inadequate nutrition, sexually transmitted diseases, suicidal ideation, or chemical abuse. Adolescents may benefit from professional counseling.

Adolescents need certain accommodations to preserve their self-respect and identity. They do not belong either with young children or only with adults. Adolescents feel more comfortable and are able to relate better with healthcare personnel in a setting customized for them. The healthcare staff should be chosen to work specifically with adolescents. If a specialized setting is unavailable, the adolescent should be placed with others close to their age. In any situation, clear rules should be posted so that all adolescents know the setting's guidelines.

Illness or injury can seriously threaten self-image. Many young people worry about damage to their bodies or about death, whether the threat is real or not. In addition, they are often acutely aware of their emerging sexuality; therefore, their modesty should be respected. Include adolescents in planning and performing care as much as possible to encourage their emerging independence.

Adolescents need nonbiased and accurate information regarding their rapidly changing bodies and the issues they may encounter during this transition to young adulthood. Health education should include information concerning sexually transmitted diseases and prevention, including HIV/AIDS, sexual identity, pregnancy, and birth control. Teenagers also need clear and nonjudgmental information about substance use and abuse, depression, and suicide.

> **NCLEX Alert**
> Clinical scenarios involving infants and children often relate to appropriate levels of care for a specific age group. When reviewing question options, be sure to keep in mind the age of the pediatric client and the expected behaviors for that age group.

THE HOSPITAL EXPERIENCE

Short- or long-term hospitalization can be traumatic and disturbing for children and families. Small children usually do not understand what is happening or why they are being taken away from home. Illness threatens body image at any age. You will see nurses in the pediatric department dressed in colorful scrubs. The units are decorated with pictures of animals or cartoon characters to make the children feel more comfortable.

> **Key Concept**
> Pediatric nurses provide care not just for the sick child but for the entire family.

Age-Related Concerns

Infants, Toddlers, and Preschoolers

Even before children are 1 year of age, they become frightened of strangers and are aware of their family's absence. From ages 1 to 5 years, children often exhibit anxiety when separated from home and family. Stranger and separation anxiety are also discussed in Chapter 10.

Very young children have concrete thought processes and often misinterpret what they hear. The following statements are examples of what to avoid saying when caring for children. (The statements in parentheses give an example of what the child might be thinking.)

- "I am going to take your blood pressure." (Where are you taking it?) Instead you might say: "I am going to find out how strong your heart is beating right now."
- "I am going to give you a shot." (Are you going to shoot me with a gun?) Instead, you might say: "I am going to give you some medicine."
- "This will only feel like a little bee sting." (Oh, no, I'm afraid of bees!) Instead you might say: "This may hurt a little. Hold your teddy bear tightly to help you."

Keep sentences short, and phrase statements so the child knows what to do, not what to avoid (e.g., instead of saying, "Don't cross the street alone," say to the child, "Always cross the street with an adult"). Tell children who are to remain in the hospital overnight that nurses work at night also, in case

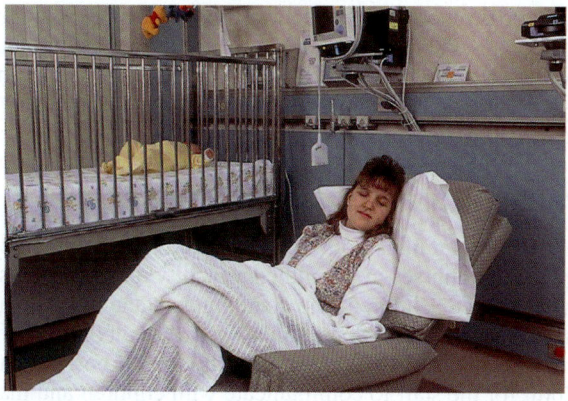

Figure 71-1 Rooming-in helps alleviate anxiety for both the child and the caregiver.

they are worried that they will be alone (In Practice: Nursing Care Guidelines 71-1).

School-Age Children and Adolescents

As a rule, older children are able to understand the need for hospitalization, although they often hide many fears. Younger school-aged children may experience fear of separation when they are ill. Peer relationships are important to children, especially adolescents. Most healthcare facilities allow friends to visit, but activities should be regulated to prevent sick teens from becoming overtired. A telephone should be available for the child client; however, rules for its use should be clearly established.

> **Key Concept**
> A smile is a universal language.

Family-Centered Care

Most healthcare facilities make every effort to meet a child's need to be part of a family unit. Family-centered care may include rooming-in (Fig. 71-1). Healthcare personnel encourage family caregivers to remain with children during their hospital experience. Participation in care by family members promotes a less-stressed child and parent.

If family members are unable to remain with their children, caregivers should assure the children that they will return. All caregivers need to state the time of their return in terms that children will understand (e.g., "before lunch," "after your nap"). They can also give children a possession to hold until their return. Nurturing measures, such as providing a doll, a toy, or a teddy bear, can help to relieve anxiety; the object becomes a physical reminder that the family caregiver will return.

Family caregivers react in various ways to hospitalization. Reactions often depend on the following factors:

- The seriousness of the child's illness
- The immediate threat to the child's life
- Family situation
- Ego resources of the family caregivers
- The family's former experiences with illness and hospitalization
- The family's style of coping with stress
- The caregivers' beliefs and values

Preparation

Hospitalization often causes apprehension and fear in families. Helping children successfully adjust is an important nursing goal. One way to ease this adjustment is to prepare children for the experience at their own level of comprehension. Tell children what to expect and help them avoid feeling abandoned or punished. If possible, a tour of the healthcare facility before admission provides a foundation for preparing the child. Encourage family caregivers to include the child in packing for the trip to the facility. Remind them to be sure to bring along special items.

Separation Anxiety and Loss of Control

As discussed in Chapter 10, *separation anxiety* is a developmental milestone for children under normal circumstances. A frequent initiating factor of anxiety is a child's separation from a familiar person and environment (e.g., parent and home) and the initiation of an unfamiliar, and therefore stressful, new lifestyle (e.g., hospital caregivers and facility environments). When separated from the primary caregiver and surroundings, children typically experience anxiety, a fear associated with the separation and changes in routine. They feel threatened and unsafe. Separation anxiety is often, initially, a panic reaction, with behaviors that include crying, resisting attention or treatment, and screaming. *Loss of control* often accompanies separation anxiety and affects most children in a hospital setting. Loss of control refers to the child's inability to maintain newly learned concepts associated with autonomy, such as walking, being potty trained, or feeding oneself.

There are three phases of separation anxiety: *protest*, *despair*, and *denial*. Each phase extends into the next. The phases of separation anxiety manifest themselves as behavioral changes (Box 71-2). Protest takes the form of crying and rejection of new caregivers. The child in the phase of despair appears sad or apathetic. Denial has the appearance of resolved stranger anxiety because the child may seem to identify and

---

Box 71-2 Stages of Separation Anxiety

Separation anxiety—a normal developmental milestone for children that can become more acute or problematic when experienced by a child being hospitalized. Stages of separation anxiety include the following:

- *Protest:* In the protest phase, the child's need for family caregivers is conscious and sorrowful. The child cries and reacts aggressively, rejecting healthcare personnel. Fear of the unknown and anxiety cause the child to demand their own caregivers. Such a reaction is normal and denotes a healthy attachment to the caregivers.
- *Despair:* In the despair stage, the child becomes inactive and sad. Usual comfort measures, such as thumb-sucking and clutching a blanket, become prominent. He or she watches constantly for family caregivers, is quiet and withdrawn, and is uninterested in food or play.
- *Denial:* The denial phase (detachment) may be interpreted as a sign that the child is protecting himself or herself from anxiety by rejecting family caregivers. In truth, the child's need for caregivers is more intense than ever.

accept the new environment and staff while seeming to deny and avoid parental attention. Infants and preschool-age children have only minimal abilities to comprehend abstract concepts such as time, consequences, or illness. Older children have a better understanding of these concepts; therefore, for the older child, separation is not perceived as a threat.

Prior to a hospitalization, children benefit from pre-exposure to a new environment. Many hospitals offer hospital tours designed for the pediatric client and the family. The nurse needs to assure the child that a parent is waiting and let the child know where the parent will be during any procedure. If possible, some medical professionals encourage a parent to be with the child at all times, for example, during treatment in an emergency room. Because of the concerns related to separation anxiety and loss of control, nursing considerations must include an understanding of age-appropriate growth and developmental milestones. For example, at the toddler stage, it is important to help the child maintain as much independence as possible, by encouraging self-feeding and dressing, and age-appropriate communication between child and caretaker. Nursing Care Guidelines 71-1 provide techniques that can minimize the intensity of stressful experiences.

Transcultural Considerations

Children and families from a culture that differs from most of the clients or nurses in a healthcare facility may be confused and frightened. Children who do not understand the language may be especially frightened and have a difficult time. Family caregivers should translate for their children, if possible. It is helpful for the staff to communicate with children and make them feel comfortable and relaxed. Allowing them to be with other children as much as possible is also beneficial. Keeping pictures of common items available can help children to communicate their needs, thereby making them feel less isolated.

IN PRACTICE
NURSING CARE GUIDELINES 71-1 — Reducing Anxiety and Calming Children for Procedures

General Guidelines
- Explain the procedure in terms that the child can understand.
- Explain the procedure to family caregivers.
- Never tell the child something will not hurt if it might.
- Avoid performing painful or frightening procedures in the child's bed or the playroom. Use the examination or treatment room. The bed or playroom should be a "safe place."
- Never make a promise to a child that you cannot or will not keep.
- Give an analgesic before a painful procedure, if possible.
- Crying is a normal response to pain and fear. Never tell a child not to cry because it may shame or embarrass them.
- After the procedure, explain to the child and family caregivers any undesired effects that they should note and what to do if they occur.
- Report test results to family caregivers and the child, if possible.
- Check the child's condition frequently and reassure the child that you are close by if needed.
- Document any unusual reactions. Also note on the nursing care plan any tips to help make a repeated procedure less disagreeable the next time.

Infant
- Change the infant's diaper before the treatment.
- Feed the infant before the treatment, unless a danger of vomiting exists.
- Offer the baby a pacifier.
- Talk and play with the infant before performing the procedure.
- Position the infant in their accustomed sleeping position, if possible.
- Release the thumb for sucking if the infant does not use a pacifier.
- Sing repetitious songs softly to encourage sleep. If singing does not work, try whistling.
- Rub the infant's arms and back soothingly.
- Hold the infant in your arms.

Toddler
- Let the child play with and explore the equipment before the procedure.
- Explain the procedure to the toddler using simple words and short sentences.
- Encourage family caregivers to participate by supporting and comforting the child when possible.
- Allow the child to hold a security object (e.g., doll, stuffed animal, blanket) during the procedure.
- Distract, rather than restrain, whenever possible.
- Praise the child for being "helpful."
- Allow the child to cry without feeling ashamed.
- Allow the child to hold equipment or help whenever possible.
- Allow the child to play with equipment after the procedure.

Preschooler
- Use simple words to prepare the preschooler for sensations he or she will experience.
- Use dolls or puppets to explain procedures.
- Allow the preschooler to play with the teaching aids.
- Ensure privacy for the preschooler.
- Encourage the preschooler to talk about the procedure; clarify any misunderstandings or questions.
- Encourage the preschooler to help in a reasonable way with the procedure that might help him or her achieve a sense of control.
- Verbally praise the preschooler and reward him or her in some way (e.g., stickers, stars).

CHAPTER 71 Fundamentals of Pediatric Nursing

TABLE 71-1 Average Range of Vital Signs for Children

AGE	AVERAGE PULSE (BEATS/MIN)	AVERAGE RESPIRATION (BREATHS/MIN)	SYSTOLIC BLOOD PRESSURE (MM HG)	DIASTOLIC BLOOD PRESSURE (MM HG)
Infant	80–180	20–40	74–100	50–70
Toddler	80–140	20–30	80–112	50–80
Preschooler	70–115	20–25	82–110	50–78
School-age	65–110	17–22	84–120	54–80
Adolescent	60–90	15–20	94–120	62–80

Adapted from Flynn J. T., Kaelber D. C., Baker-Smith C. M., Blowey D., Carroll A. E., Daniels S. R., de Ferranti S. D., Dionne J. M., Falkner B., Flinn S. K., Gidding S. S., Goodwin C., Leu M. G., Powers M. E., Rea C., Samuels J., Simasek M., Thaker V. V., Urbina E. M., & Subcommittee On Screening And Management Of High Blood Pressure In Children. (2017). Clinical practice guideline for screening and management of high blood pressure in children and adolescents. *Pediatrics*, 140(3), e20171904. https://doi.org/10.1542/peds.2017-1904

BASIC PEDIATRIC CARE AND PROCEDURES

Admitting Children to the Healthcare Facility

Although the process of admitting children to a healthcare facility is similar to that for admitting adults, a special effort should be made to be alert to the needs of both the family caregivers and the child. Make family members as comfortable and secure as possible; it is important to earn their confidence and cooperation. Often, if children see that their family caregivers accept and trust you, they become more willing to accept you as well.

Ask family caregivers about their child's special needs, likes and dislikes, allergies, and special vocabulary, especially for items such as the "potty." You can include children in gathering this information by directing the questions to them. You should also introduce them to roommates. The playroom is a nonthreatening environment in which the family and nursing staff can get to know each other, thereby helping to put children at ease.

> **Key Concept**
> You can collect most of the admission data for a small child while they sit on the caregiver's lap.

Assisting With the Physical Examination

The equipment for the physical examination of a child is the same as that for an adult, except that some pieces are smaller. The child's cooperation is of utmost importance. A little extra time helping children become comfortable often works wonders. Show the child the equipment and let them handle it to promote a sense of control. If the child is too young, ill, or frightened to understand how to cooperate, you may need to restrain them for parts of the examination. Use restraint only as a last resort because it makes children feel more threatened and frightened.

Data Collection on Admission

Observe the child carefully for any signs of rash, abrasion, discharge, or alteration in consciousness level. Note complaints of pain or other symptoms, as you would for an adult. Carefully document all observations. If you have reason to think a child has been battered or abused in any way, report your beliefs to your supervisor—this is a legal responsibility (Chapter 72).

Vital Signs
Obtain and document vital signs on admission (Table 71-1).

Respiration
Take respirations before taking other vital signs because you will be unable to obtain an accurate respiratory rate if a child is crying. Count the respiratory rate for 1 minute. If you cannot obtain a respiratory rate because of crying, observe for signs of respiratory distress by checking skin color, pallor, and the presence of breath sounds. Sites of respiratory distress are shown in Figure 71-2. Signs of respiratory distress include xiphoid retraction, nares

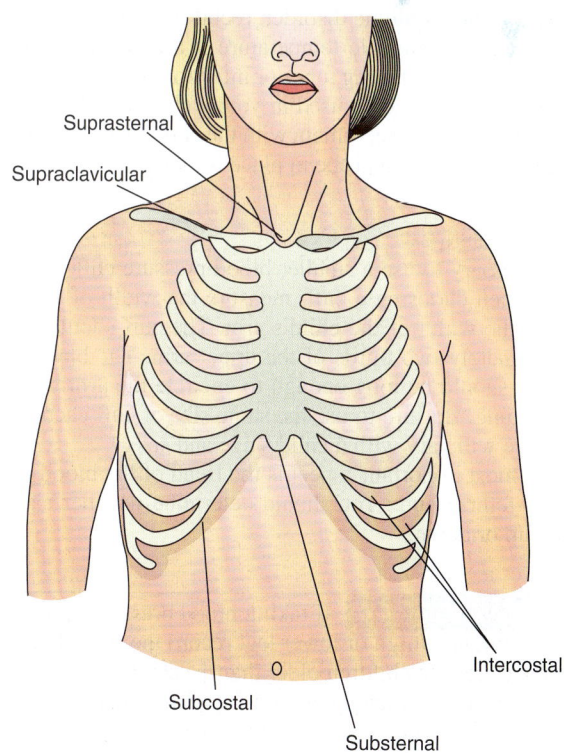

Figure 71-2 Sites of respiratory retractions.

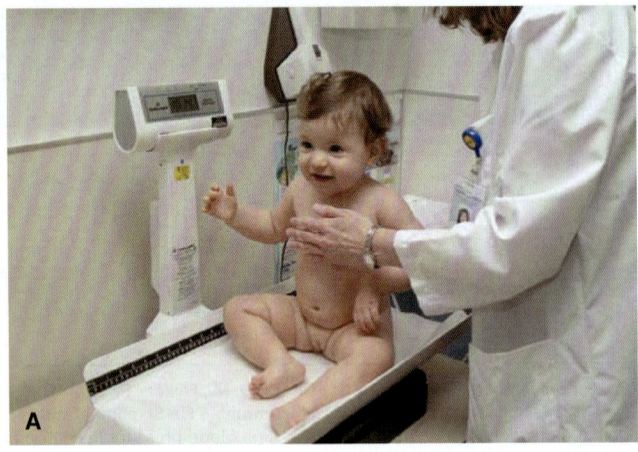 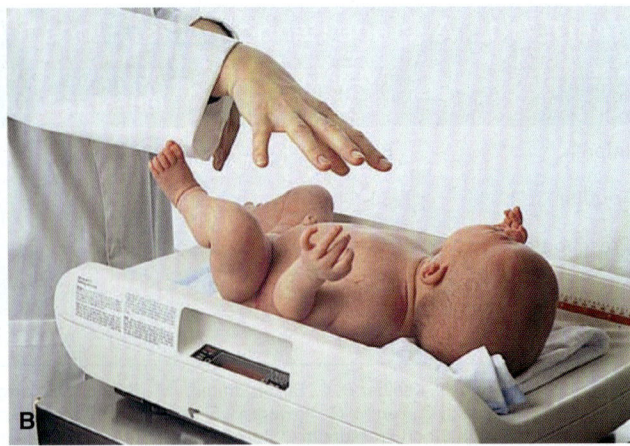

Figure 71-3 **A.** Children who can sit may be weighed in a sitting position if this is less frightening for them. **B.** Infants are weighed lying down. (Pillitteri, 2009.)

dilation, and expiratory grunt (Box 67-2). Appropriately document your findings.

Pulse
For children older than 2 years, you may take the radial pulse; for those younger than 2 years, take the pulse apically. Count the pulse for a full minute. The sizes of the bell and diaphragm of the stethoscope are smaller for children than for adults.

Temperature
Take an oral or tympanic temperature for children older than 6 years. Take a tympanic, axillary, or rectal temperature for children who are younger than 6 years or those who are disoriented, unconscious, or in severe respiratory distress. Rectal temperatures are not routinely used due to risk of tears.

Do not take a rectal temperature if a child has had any immune or hematologic disorder, rectal surgery, or diarrhea. Do not take a tympanic temperature if a child has had ear surgery or has ventilating tubes or infection. Axillary method can be safely and easily used in young children. Regardless of the method you use, remain with the child to ensure safety. Hold the temperature probe in place for the required time.

Blood Pressure
It is necessary to use a smaller blood pressure cuff for children. When choosing a cuff, measure the width of the cuff against the width of the child's arm. The cuff should cover approximately two thirds of the upper arm. The bladder of the cuff should be long enough to encircle the arm without overlapping. Be sure to use the same size of cuff each time. Cuff size will vary with a child's age and size.

The most important aspect is the trend of the blood pressure or temperature: You should determine whether each is going up or down.

> **Nursing Alert** If taking blood pressure at an infant's thigh or lower leg, record the limb that you measured. In children older than 1 year, thigh pressure is approximately 20 mm Hg *higher* than arm pressure. If you must use the radial artery (wrist), radial blood pressure is 10 mm Hg *lower* than that of the brachial artery. Note use of the radial artery on the record.

Weight and Height
All children should be weighed on admission. Weigh small children on an infant or child scale, always keeping a hand near them for safety (Fig. 71-3). Older children are weighed standing up if they are able (Fig. 71-4). Measure the weight in kilograms. Often, you will need to convert this weight to pounds for the benefit of family caregivers (2.2 lb = 1 kg). Documenting weight in kilograms allows accurate dosage calculation for medication administration and intravenous (IV) fluids.

To maintain medical asepsis, place a clean paper on the infant scale before weighing a child and disinfect the scale after the procedure. After weighing is finished, discard the paper and document the weight. Wash your hands before and after weighing. Use Standard Precautions throughout the procedure. You should report any deviations in weight immediately. Observe and document any signs of edema, dehydration, and the child's nutritional state.

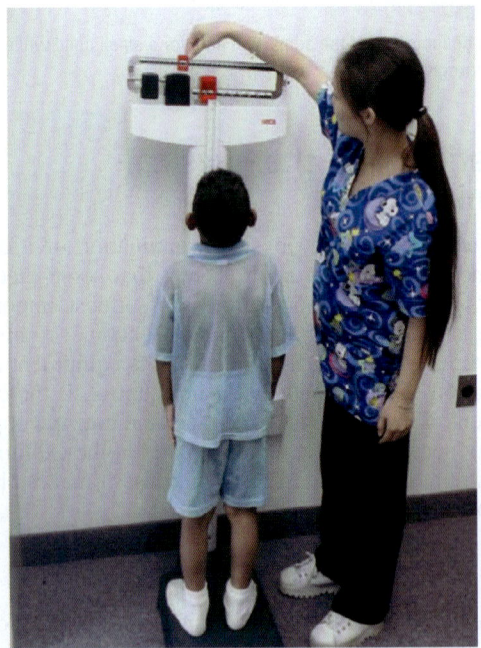

Figure 71-4 Weighing an older child. (Pillitteri, 2009.)

Use the following guidelines when weighing an infant:

- Weigh the infant at the same time each day, before feeding.
- Balance the scale carefully before obtaining the infant's weight.
- Weigh the infant without clothes or diaper.
- Note additional equipment being weighed (e.g., IV, arm board, brace, cast).

One way to measure a child's length is to mark the child's length from head to toe on the bed and then measure between the marks, rather than trying to measure a moving child.

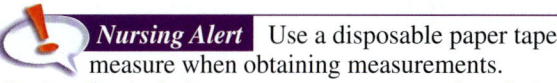 **Nursing Alert** Use a disposable paper tape measure when obtaining measurements. ***Rationale:*** *A cloth tape measure may stretch and alter measurement findings. Disposable tape measures also prevent cross-contamination.*

Head Circumference
Measure the OFC of the head for children to 2 years of age and for any child with a head size that is in question (Chapter 67). Plot measurements on a growth chart and compare them against normal sizes for the child's age group to determine any abnormalities.

> **Key Concept**
> The OFC reflects intracranial volume pressure, which is a significant finding. Factors that affect head circumference include brain development, intracranial pressure, hydrocephalus, brain tumor, and some congenital defects, such as microcephaly and hydrocephalus.

Chest Circumference
Measure and compare the child's chest circumference with the OFC. Normally, the newborn's head is larger than the chest. Chest and head measurements are approximately equal for children aged 1–2 years, after which the chest begins to become larger than the head. By age 5, a child's chest is about 2–3 in. (5–7.6 cm) larger than the head. Measure the chest at the child's nipple line, using a paper tape.

Other Measurements
Other important measurements may include abdominal circumference, extremity length, and extremity circumference. Be sure to note where on the extremity you took a circumference measurement. Measure the abdomen at the child's umbilicus.

Daily Collection and Documentation
Observe and document all information about the child, including normal behavior and reactions, abnormal symptoms, and unfavorable signs. Check the child's nonverbal signals. A child who is pulling at the ears, for example, may have an ear infection.

Because children often cannot tell how they feel, whether they have voided or had a bowel movement, or how much they have eaten, in a hospital setting, the nurse is responsible for recording this information.

Diet
Observe how much a child eats and drinks throughout the day. Intake and output (I&O) for children does not mean just fluid I&O; it also means food intake and all types of output. Accuracy is important because it is easy for small children to become dehydrated. Note if an infant spits up formula or if a young child does not want to eat. Many healthcare facilities have special menus that cater to children's appetites. Common menu items include pizza, macaroni, soup, corn dogs, hamburgers, and ice cream. Observe and document the number, color, and consistency of stools and any emesis (vomiting), voiding, or other drainage. Weigh diapers to obtain an accurate assessment of urine output.

Nursing Alert Illness and separation from family and home can greatly change a child's appetite. Be alert for candy and other snacks visitors bring. Eating empty-calorie snack foods can decrease a child's appetite for regular meals. Be sure to include such snacks when documenting intake.

General Appearance
Note the child's activity level, skin color and warmth, comfort level, cry (lusty or weak), response to environment, and general respiratory status.

Family Caregivers' Comments
Note statements that family caregivers make about their child's condition. Family caregivers are more familiar with the child's normal activity and appearance and often notice signs that others miss.

Physical Signs
Be alert for changes in vital signs, cough, congestion, wheezing, nasal discharge, rash, or any other abnormality, such as a fever, seizure, or the lack of achievement of physical milestones.

Visitors
Note whether family caregivers are at the bedside or if they visit frequently. Lack of visits may indicate a family problem. Also observe and report interaction between family caregivers and children.

Discharging Children
Children are discharged from the healthcare facility in much the same way as adults, except that they are taken home by their family caregivers who are responsible for follow-up care. Be sure children have been properly discharged by the provider and have appointment slips, prescriptions, and provider's orders. Teach family caregivers follow-up care and document this teaching. Family members should carry children to a car or use a wheelchair or wagon to do so. Healthcare personnel must accompany children and family caregivers to the facility's exit. All states require placement of children in a car seat or restraining safety device. Some facilities make car seats available to families who are unable to afford one by the time of discharge. If a car seat or restraining device is not present, one should be made available.

INTERMEDIATE PEDIATRIC CARE AND PROCEDURES

Providing for Pediatric Safety

Nurses are legally responsible for the safety of children in their care (In Practice: Nursing Care Guidelines 71-2).

Safety Devices

Special measures are necessary to prevent accidents or injuries from falls. Children may also need restraints to remind them not to pull on tubes or pick at suture lines. Sometimes, enforcing bed rest by applying a child safety device called a *restraint* is necessary. Small children also should be restrained whenever they are in a high chair, wheelchair, or other device. Restraints typically have procedural guidelines. Use restraints only in combination with the regulations for that device. Common sense safety practices and good observations are important nursing considerations. Also, be aware that a restraint can be the cause of damage, or even death, of a child if used inappropriately or without checking the device regularly.

A healthcare provider's order is usually required for application of any restraint device. Release and reapply restraints every 1–2 hr. Check the child's skin and circulation each hour. Document these safety measures (In Practice: Nursing Care Guidelines 71-3).

IN PRACTICE
NURSING CARE GUIDELINES 71-2 — Providing Pediatric Safety

- Wash your hands before and after giving care. Follow Standard and Transmission-Based Precautions, as necessary. **Rationale:** *Pediatric nursing often involves contact with body fluids. Following these guidelines will protect against contamination or exposure to biohazardous substances.*
- Make sure side rails on beds and cribs are up at all times. Beds should always be in the lowest position unless you are performing specific procedures. **Rationale:** *Prevent injuries from falls.*
- Adequately support children when you carry or transfer them. Always support their heads and necks, and watch the position of their extremities carefully. **Rationale:** *Correct positioning decreases the possibility of injury and gives children a sense of security.*
- Supervise ambulatory children.
- Be aware of facility procedures for fire, severe weather, external alerts, and so forth. **Rationale:** *Children will need more attention and assistance than adults in emergencies.*
- Keep children away from electrical equipment, cords, and outlets. Keep them away from heat sources (e.g., radiators, lamps, heat vents). If using heat therapy, check the child's temperature and closely monitor the child's skin. **Rationale:** *A child's skin is more sensitive to heat and burns more easily than does adult skin.*
- Never leave a child younger than 10 years of age alone in any amount of water. Frequently check on older children. **Rationale:** *Prevent drowning, which can occur in a very small amount of water for a young child.*
- Use safety restraints when transporting a child. Never leave the child unattended. Always use the provided safety devices when a child is in a high chair.
- Use disposable diapers unless the child is sensitive to them. **Rationale:** *Disposable diapers do not require pins and therefore are safer to use.*
- If you must use safety pins, keep them closed whenever you remove them. Do not leave pins exposed because children can swallow them easily. Put your fingers between the child's skin and the pin when applying a pin. **Rationale:** *Prevent choking or injuries to yourself or the child.*
- Check all toys for small, removable, or broken pieces. **Rationale:** *The child can swallow them and choke.*
- Supervise children who are using pens, pencils, or scissors. **Rationale:** *Sharp objects can cut children.*
- Use only toys that can be disinfected. Remind family caregivers that toys that cannot be disinfected may need to be thrown away. Disinfect toys regularly (always between use by different children or if dirty or contaminated). **Rationale:** *Disinfection decreases the possibility of contamination.*
- Do not allow children to use latex balloons; Mylar is acceptable. **Rationale:** *Latex balloons can pop, and the child can aspirate the pieces. Mylar balloons will not pop.*
- Be alert for any broken equipment, furniture, or glass items. **Rationale:** *Prevent accidents.*
- When taking a child's temperature, consider their ability to cooperate. **Rationale:** *If the child is uncooperative, the thermometer could break, or the reading could be inaccurate.* Check the graphic sheet to see which route to use for temperature taking. Sometimes, the provider orders a specific route. Always stay with a child when you take their temperature. Hold the thermometer in place.
- Supervise children when they are out of their room. They should never be in the medication, diet, kitchen, or utility room. **Rationale:** *Decrease the risk of injury.*
- Never prop bottles. **Rationale:** *Prevent choking, aspiration, and ear infections.*
- Never leave a young child unattended during eating. Cut food into small bites. Avoid giving foods that are slippery or hard to chew.
- Teach family caregivers good safety practices, and make sure they understand the reasons behind them. **Rationale:** *Family caregivers will be more receptive to safety practices if they understand the reasons for their use. Teaching helps prevent home accidents.*

CHAPTER 71 Fundamentals of Pediatric Nursing

IN PRACTICE
NURSING CARE GUIDELINES 71-3 — Using Pediatric Restraints

General Guidelines
Explain to family caregivers and the child what you are doing and why. Be sure the child does not view the restraint as punishment. *Rationale: Teaching helps to decrease fears and prepares family caregivers to see the child in a restraint.*

Commonly Used Restraints
Bubble top—Made of clear plastic and attached to the top of the crib.
- Be sure it is firmly attached to the crib. *Rationale: You need to prevent the child from being able to climb out around it or from getting their head stuck.*
- Use for any child who may be able to climb or jump over the sides of the crib.

Jacket—A smaller version of that used for adults; can be used in cribs, highchairs, beds, or wheelchairs (Fig. A).
- Apply over clothing or gowns. *Rationale: This decreases skin irritation.*
- The straps come out on each side and usually cross in front and tie in back.
- Tie the straps to the back of the chair or to the frame of the bed or crib. Tie to a movable part of the bed. Do not tie straps to side rails. *Rationale: Preserve the ability to raise or lower side rails without needing to tighten or loosen restraints. A restraint tied in the wrong place can interfere with the use of equipment or could strangle the child.*
- Check the child's circulation every 1–2 hr; allow the child to exercise. *Rationale: These activities prevent skin breakdown, promote circulation, maintain muscle function, and decrease the possibility of respiratory complications.*
- Document and report any evidence of skin irritation.

Clove hitch or commercial wrist device—A Kerlix bandage or stockinette applied in a figure-eight knot, or a manufactured device, can be used to restrain one or more extremities (Fig. B).

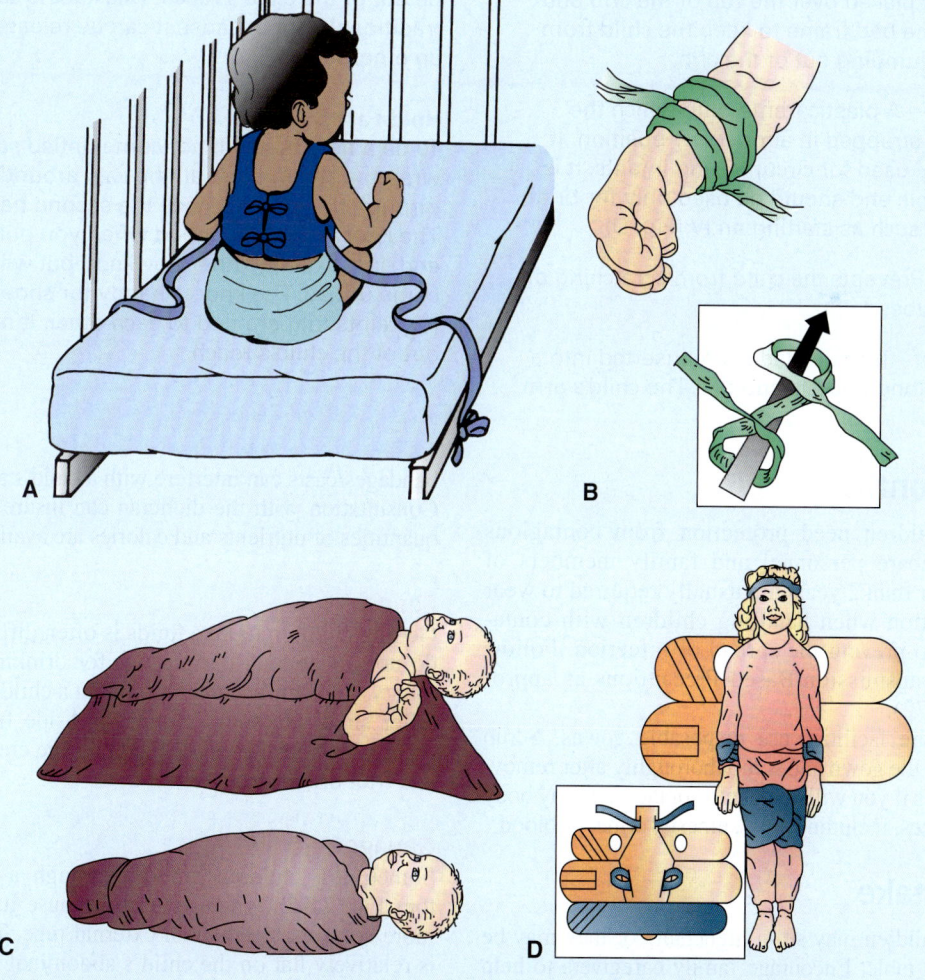

Types of pediatric restraints. **A.** Jacket device. **B.** Clove hitch restraint. **C.** Mummy device. **D.** Papoose board.

NURSING CARE GUIDELINES 71-3 — Using Pediatric Restraints (Continued)

- Apply padding under the restraint.
- Tie a knot so the device cannot become too tight.
- Check the extremity every hour for circulation and signs of skin breakdown.
- Remove restraints every 2 hr, and allow the child to exercise the extremity.

Arm boards—Used to protect intravenous (IV) sites.

- Pad the board with a washcloth or small towel and fasten with tape. **Rationale:** *The cloth will absorb perspiration and provide comfort. Also, the nurse can change and wash it if it becomes soiled.*
- Secure the arm board to the client's extremity after the IV is in place and secure. **Rationale:** *Ensure the security of the IV even if the board needs removal.*
- Check the child's circulation to the arm each hour.
- Loosen or reapply tape, as needed.
- Document your findings.

Less Commonly Used Restraints

Mummy restraint—Used to restrain the entire body with a small blanket. Only the head is exposed (Fig. C).

Crib net—A net placed over the top of the crib and secured to the bed frame to keep the child from climbing or jumping out of the crib.

Papoose board—A plastic frame onto which the child can be strapped in almost any position. It is commonly used for circumcising infants. It is uncomfortable and should be used only for brief procedures, such as starting an IV (Fig. D).

Mitt or *glove*—Prevents the child from scratching or pulling on tubes.

Sleeve restraint—Tongue blades are inserted into a sleeve with long pockets and ties. The child's arm is slid into the sleeve, and straps are tied under the opposite arm. This device is used to keep a child from bending their arm, pulling on tubes or other devices, or disrupting a facial suture line.

Documentation

You may use a checklist to document the use of such devices. This list allows you to state the child's specific reactions and the number of times you applied and removed safety devices.

Knots Used for Restraints

- Make sure straps are not too long or too tight. **Rationale:** *The child might become caught or might strangle. The child's circulation should not be affected by the restraint.*

Quick-Release Knot

Figure 48-21A demonstrates how to make a quick-release knot. If the child pulls on the strap from their end, the knot will tighten. However, when you pull on the free end, it will release easily. The free end must be out of the child's reach. This knot is safer than a traditional knot because it can be released quickly in an emergency.

Hold-Fast Bow

To tie a bow that will not come untied spontaneously, wrap the second end all the way around before pulling through the loop to make the second half of the bow. The knot will come untied when you pull on the free end, just like any other bowknot, but will not easily come untied. The knot is handy for shoelaces and for restraints that are tied to each other. It must be kept out of the child's reach.

Infection Control

Hospitalized children need protection from contagious diseases. Healthcare personnel and family members of children younger than 2 years are usually required to wear isolation protection when handling children with contagious diseases to prevent the spread of infection. Follow Standard and Transmission-Based Precautions as appropriate (Chapter 72).

Most healthcare facilities use disposable gowns. Scrub before putting on the gown and scrub thoroughly after removing it. Wear gloves if you will come into contact with any body fluids or substances, including stool, emesis, urine, or blood.

Nutrient Intake

At mealtimes, children may sit in highchairs or they may be seated at a small table. Encourage family caregivers to help feed their child because most children eat better for family members. Always supervise children who are eating. Record all food and fluid the child consumes. Caloric intake and fluid intake vary according to age. Illness, IV placement, or bandages/casts can interfere with a child's ability to self-feed. Consultation with the dietician can insure that the adequate quantities of nutrients and calories are available to the child.

Fluids

Getting children to take fluids is often difficult because they do not understand the reasons for drinking if they are not thirsty. Ask family caregivers about a child's favorite liquids. Offer small amounts frequently. Aside from actual fluids, acceptable substitutes are ice pops, ice cream, gelatin, soda, and fruit drinks.

Gavage Feeding

Sometimes, children are fed through a gastrostomy button (Fig. 71-5), which is used because it is less bulky and more comfortable than an external tube. The gavage button is relatively flat on the child's abdominal wall and connects to a tube that leads into the child's stomach. A syringe or tube-feeding bag is attached to an adapter and is primed with the tube feeding. The adapter is then attached to the button, and the tube feeding is administered. A bolus tube feeding the IV site is monitored closely to ensure that the catheter is within the vein. Because an infusion pump literally pumps fluid into a person, it is possible that fluid can be pumped into the wrong spaces, causing tissue damage.

> **Nursing Alert** Do not assume that the alarm on an infusion pump will provide warning of IV infiltration, especially for children. Fluids intended for the infusion into a vein (e.g., IV) can be unintentionally routed and forced into the tissue spaces, causing edema. If there are additives to the fluids, such as aminophylline, tissue damage to the child's arm can be a consequence.

You may need to restrain the child to prevent them from pulling on the tube. The IV may be administered into the scalp or neck veins in infants and toddlers and the arm or neck veins in older children. Protective devices for IV sites are shown in Figure 71-6.

Children who are receiving long-term cancer chemotherapy or other IV medications may have a central venous line. Examples of these lines include Hickman, Broviac, jugular, and peripherally inserted central catheter (**PICC**) lines. These devices allow for prompt access to blood specimens, the infusion of IV chemotherapy or antibiotics, and total parenteral nutrition (**TPN**) therapy (In Practice: Nursing Care Guidelines 71-4).

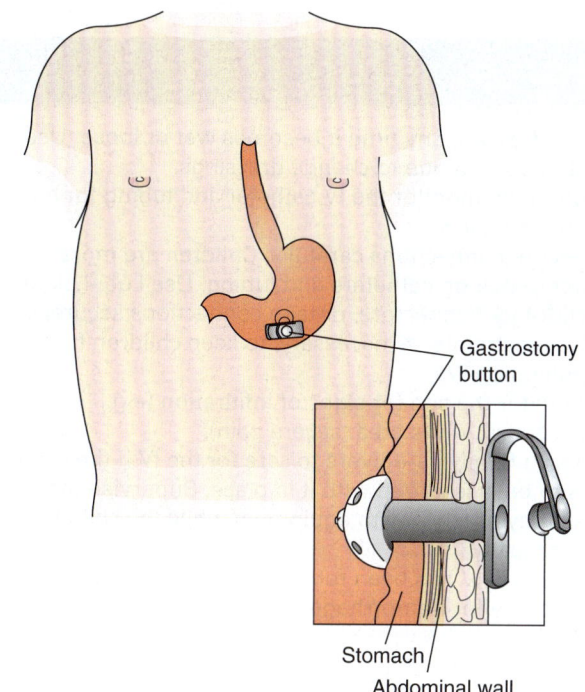

Figure 71-5 Placement of gastrostomy button.

is usually administered over 30 min, using only gravity. In some cases, an infusion feeding pump, such as the Kangaroo, is used to give continual feedings.

Parenteral Fluid Administration

Because between 65% and 80% of children's weight is water, they become dehydrated more easily than adults. Children who have diarrhea, a high fever, or difficulty excreting wastes may have a fluid or electrolyte imbalance. Parenteral administration of fluids and electrolytes may be necessary to maintain homeostasis.

Too much fluid is dangerous for children. Equipment that controls the rates and amounts of fluids is used to minimize the danger of fluid overload. An infusion pump may be used to control the exact amount a child can receive. This device delivers fluids at a precise, preselected rate. It is critical that

Elimination

For children who are not yet toilet trained, use disposable diapers to promote cleanliness, unless they are allergic to them or have a bad diaper rash. In such cases, use cloth diapers.

Collecting a Urine Specimen

Use the pediatric urine bag to collect a urine specimen. The bag is sterile, disposable, and has an adhesive neck applied to the infant's skin (In Practice: Nursing Procedure 71-1). Verify with facility that this sample can be submitted for a urine culture requisition.

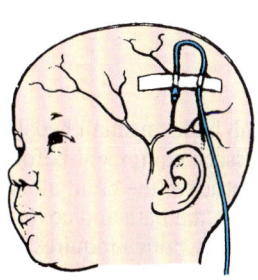
Venipuncture of scalp vein

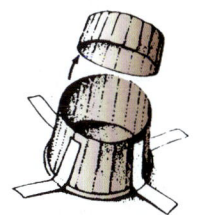
Paper cup taped over venipuncture site for protection. A clear plastic cup may also be used.

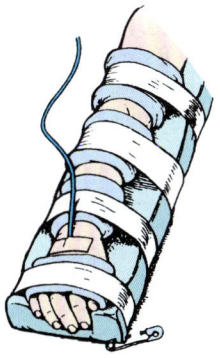
Restraint of arm when hand is site of infusion

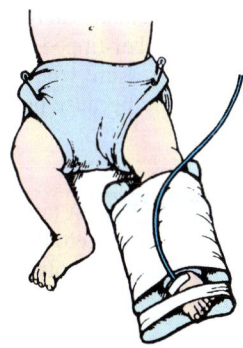
Infant's leg taped to sandbag for immobilization (IV site should be visible)

Figure 71-6 Intravenous (IV) fluid therapy protective devices.

IN PRACTICE
NURSING CARE GUIDELINES 71-4: The Child and IV Therapy

- The most common sites for IV therapy in infants are scalp veins, a foot, a hand, and a forearm. From about the toddler stage to adult, the most popular IV sites are the nondominant hand or arm. The foot may also be used in a young child.
- Infiltration and infection are the most common complications of IV therapy, especially if the therapy uses a long-term IV line or central line. Monitor for the following signs and symptoms of infection at the site: redness, pain, elevated white blood cell count, and temperature. Document observable signs and symptoms making note of laboratory findings that may indicate infection.
- If your nurse practice act allows the LVN/LPN to change central line dressings, change dressings every 24 hr, if using gauze, and every 72 hr, if using a transparent dressing (e.g., Tegaderm). Change the dressing any time it becomes wet or loose. Use sterile technique to change dressings.
- Carefully monitor the IV catheter and tubing for any tears or leaks.
- Secure connections carefully. Children are more apt to pull on catheters and tubing. Use Luer-Lok or click-lock connectors, or tape connections securely.
- Use restraints, as necessary, to keep children from pulling on IVs.
- Monitor the site for signs of infiltration (e.g., hardness, white area, severe pain).
- Teach family caregivers to care for the IV if the child is to be discharged with it in place. Supervise them as they practice with equipment while the child is in the facility.
- After the IV has been removed, monitor the site carefully for hemorrhage.

Catheterizing the Child

Children are not catheterized unless it is absolutely necessary because the procedure can cause distress and damage delicate structures. Catheterization also can introduce bacteria into the bladder, causing urinary tract infections.

If catheterization is necessary, you will need to restrain small children during the procedure. The most common means of restraint is the papoose board. Restrain children in this manner for the absolute minimum length of time only. Assistance from another nurse is helpful.

Administering Enemas

For infants and young children, oral laxatives are usually preferred. If absolutely necessary, an enema is given. Give enemas to children in the same way as you would for adults, but use a smaller quantity of solution. Disposable enemas are most often used; disposable pediatric enemas are available in measured amounts. If another type of enema is to be given, follow the protocol of your healthcare facility. Isotonic solutions are necessary.

Give disposable enemas at room temperature. For infants, you may use a rubber-tipped bulb syringe. Be careful not to use too much pressure when instilling the fluid; squeeze the container gently because pressure from fluids can cause tissue damage.

> **Nursing Alert** A tap-water enema is particularly dangerous for small children because it can cause fluid and electrolyte imbalances and dehydration.

Often, children are unable to retain the solution on their own. Place a child on the bedpan before administering an enema. You may need to restrain a small child or ask for assistance. Remember, this experience is frightening for young children. Praise and reassure them.

Using Suppositories

Drugs commonly administered through suppositories include Tylenol (acetaminophen) and anticonvulsive or antinausea drugs. Suppositories may also be used to promote bowel elimination. Explain the procedure to the child. Tell the child if the suppository is to be retained or expelled. Use a clean glove when inserting the suppository. Lubricate the suppository with water-soluble lubricant before insertion, if needed. Insert the suppository and hold it in place by gently pressing on the child's anal sphincter from the outside until the child no longer feels the urge to expel it.

Treating Diarrhea

When young children have diarrhea, the main dangers are dehydration and spread of disease. Small children become dehydrated very quickly as a result of diarrhea; therefore, you must take quick preventive measures. Carefully follow Standard and Transmission-Based Precautions when children have diarrhea. Close observation for signs of dehydration and for skin *excoriation* (breakdown) is essential so that nursing interventions are established before damage is done to the skin.

Daily Cleanliness

Infant Bath
Infants are usually given tub baths in small bedside tubs. Be sure to gather all the necessary equipment before you start the bath because you cannot leave the child alone once you begin. Weigh the child before the bath and cover him or her with a bath blanket or as facility policy requires (In Practice: Nursing Care Guidelines 71-5 and Chapter 67).

Oral Hygiene
Provide oral hygiene for the infant by wiping the baby's gums with a damp washcloth or gauze pad after each feeding. Pediatric dentists encourage early oral hygiene for all infants. As soon as the child's teeth erupt, begin to use a brush to clean them.

IN PRACTICE
NURSING CARE GUIDELINES 71-5 — Giving an Infant a Bath

- Generally, the infant does not need to be bathed every day. In place of giving a tub bath, wash the face, hands, and diaper area daily.
- Some children need a shampoo daily to prevent seborrhea, a scaly scalp condition known as cradle cap.
- Place a young infant into a plastic tub. Use this time to talk to the child and make the bath a pleasant experience. Depending on facility guidelines, you may use a mild soap or give the bath with clear water only. Give perineal and genital care. *Never leave an infant in a bath unsupervised.*
- Cleanse the eyes first with clear water from the inner to outer canthus using a separate cotton ball for each eye, and then wash the rest of the baby's face. Do not probe the outer ear canals.
- The application of a diaper ointment such as Desitin or A&D is good prophylaxis and should be used on irritated areas. Do not use oil because it may lead to clogged pores and possible infection.
- After the bath, dress the infant, and comb and dry the hair. Clean the child's fingernails and toenails. Many healthcare facilities do not allow nails to be trimmed without a specific healthcare provider's order.

By age 3 years, children should be able to brush their teeth with adult supervision. By age 8 years, children should be brushing and flossing independently, with occasional adult supervision. Teach children these procedures, if necessary.

Assist children with brushing their teeth. Encourage all children to rinse often with water. If children are mature enough to rinse the mouth and spit out the solution, they may use a well-diluted mouthwash. Do not allow children to swallow toothpaste.

Oxygen

The primary cause of cardiopulmonary arrest in children is respiratory in origin. Small children have respiratory tracts that differ anatomically from adults. These structural differences, in addition to immature immune systems, place infants and young children at high risk for respiratory problems. Babies and small children are unable to tell you that they are having difficulty breathing. A child's status can change quickly, and early signs can be difficult to see.

If you work as a pediatric nurse, you must be skilled at counting respirations in young children.

Nursing Alert A change in the respiratory rate of an acutely ill child is significant. An infant with a rapid respiratory rate expends a great deal of energy. When the respiratory rate becomes too slow, it may indicate that the infant is becoming too tired. This infant is at high risk for respiratory arrest (Chapter 67 and Box 67-2, Signs of Newborn Respiratory Distress).

Be alert for the following signs of pediatric respiratory distress:

- Restlessness, apprehension, panic
- Tachycardia
- Tachypnea
- Nasal flaring
- Wheezing
- Stridor
- Change in color (e.g., pallor, **circumoral cyanosis**—a darkening of skin color, particularly around the nose, eyes, and mouth that is a significant sign of poor oxygenation)
- Expiratory grunt—a significant indicator of impending respiratory arrest
- Retractions: substernal, subcostal, intercostal, suprasternal, supraclavicular (Figs. 71-2 and Box 67-2)
- Gasping and shallow, labored breaths
- Head bobbing

Nursing Alert Do not use an infant seat for a child with respiratory distress. Because of the lack of head control, the infant's head tends to fall forward, thereby closing off the airway. In addition, the infant tends to "scrunch" down in an infant seat. In this position, the abdominal organs push up on the diaphragm, preventing full lung expansion (*excursion*). The head of the crib is elevated instead.

Administering oxygen (O_2) to the small child by nasal catheter or face mask is difficult because of the child's limited ability to understand and cooperate. If only humidity is needed, you may use an oxygen mask. Place the mask *near* the child's face, which allows humidity to reach the child without the use of a restricting mask on the face. The child's oxygen saturation should be monitored and recorded at regular intervals during oxygen administration. In Practice: Nursing Care Guidelines 71-6 lists general considerations for oxygen administration, and Table 71-2 compares some methods of oxygen administration to the pediatric client.

Key Concept
Too much O_2 can be toxic. Too little O_2 will not be effective. Monitor the child and the equipment closely.

Nursing Alert Check toys to determine if they are safe and appropriate for the moist, oxygenated atmosphere. Stuffed toys become waterlogged very easily. Electrical or mechanical toys can cause sparks, creating a fire hazard. Toys that are easily wiped clean and do not absorb moisture are best.

Mist Tent
You may place a child with a respiratory condition in a mist tent, which provides oxygen and/or humidity to liquefy secretions and aid breathing. This device may be used to administer humidity, oxygen, or medications.

IN PRACTICE
NURSING CARE GUIDELINES 71-6 — General Considerations for Oxygen (O_2) Administration

1. For newborns and young infants, O_2 must be warmed to prevent loss of heat by the body, leading to further respiratory distress.
2. Oxygen must be humidified because it can dry mucous membranes, leading to thickened secretions and worsening breathing difficulties. Equipment must be changed according to facility protocol to prevent growth of microorganisms.
3. Monitor O_2 concentration carefully. Too little O_2 will result in a delivery system that is not therapeutic. Causes of too little O_2 include leakage via a cannula or mask that is not in the correct position or leakage from a hood or tent caused by frequent opening of the equipment. Too much O_2 can be toxic and lead to lung damage, such as thickening of the alveoli with loss of elasticity; higher concentrations of 70%–80% can be the source of these problems. In addition, in newborns and infants, high concentrations can lead to retinopathy of prematurity. Use of high concentrations for extended periods will require serial arterial blood gases. Use facility protocols for all therapies and make sure that all equipment is working properly.
4. Anxiety about O_2 therapy is common. Reassurance and education about therapy often helps relieve anxiety and support compliance.
5. Oxygen supports combustion. Keep O_2 away from sources of flame and sparks.
6. Children in respiratory distress may be inclined to vomit, which could lead to aspiration. Keep suctioning equipment available (e.g., a bulb syringe or suction catheter).
7. Plan nursing care efficiently so that interruptions to O_2 therapy are minimized.

TABLE 71-2 Methods of Oxygen Administration

METHOD OF O_2 ADMINISTRATION	APPROXIMATE AGES FOR USE	NURSING CONSIDERATIONS	COMMENTS
Isolette or incubator	Newborn or infant	O_2 not humidified, therefore can cause dryness.	Used in delivery room or nursery or LDRP (labor, delivery, recovery, postpartum)
Hood	Newborn or infant Fits over head and neck of infant	Monitor placement so gas does not blow directly onto face. Do not let hood rub against neck, chin, or shoulders.	Can keep O_2 saturation at 100%
Nasal cannula	Infant (recommend humidifying to help with small airways and tolerance) Child Adolescent Adult	Make sure nares are clear of mucus. Make sure prongs are correctly placed into nares. Monitor for pressure areas because pressure can cause necrosis on nasal mucosa and nasal septum.	May be uncomfortable in younger child; at 4 L, can provide 50% O_2 saturation
Mask	All ages Many sizes available Fits over nose and mouth	Choose appropriate size. Plan treatment so that mask is off only for short periods. With healthcare provider's orders, sometimes a nasal cannula can be substituted for a mask when the client is eating.	May not be tolerated well by children because it can be uncomfortable and obstruct the child's view, ability to eat, and to talk Can supply 100% O_2 saturation Frequently used in an emergency
Tent	Young children to adult	Allows child to move unrestricted inside tent. May be difficult for child to see out or for others to see child in tent. Because of constant moisture in air, frequent linen and clothing changes needed.	Child may feel that they are being punished Difficult to maintain a specific O_2 concentration within tent when tent opened/closed frequently, such as for meals, changing, and medications

Adapted from Hatfield, N. T. & Kincheloe, C. (2018). *Introductory maternity & pediatric nursing* (4th ed.). Wolters Kluwer.

Place a bath blanket on top of bed linens to absorb moisture so the child stays warm and dry. Flush the tent with oxygen or air before placing the child in it. Tuck the plastic tent securely around the mattress and seal it with a folded bath blanket if the bottom edge does not reach the foot of the bed. Fill the reservoir with distilled water. Document the procedure, its effects, and any signs of dyspnea, cyanosis, or other difficulties. Change linens often (Table 71-2).

Hood
The hood, sometimes called an oxyhood, is a clear plastic box that fits over the small child's head (Fig. 71-7). In the hood, an oxygen–air blender that can administer oxygen in any concentration is contained. The blender controls the amount of oxygen that mixes with room air and then enters the hood. The oxygen must be humidified to prevent damage to respiratory mucosa. The flow rate must be sufficiently high so that carbon dioxide flushes out of the hood. The advantage of the hood is that it maintains a constant oxygen concentration because the child is in a high-flow atmosphere (Table 71-2).

Intermittent Positive Pressure Breathing
Another method of administering oxygen in combination with medication is intermittent positive pressure breathing (**IPPB**). IPPB is used almost exclusively for children with cystic fibrosis (Chapter 72).

Resuscitation
Resuscitation of children poses a special challenge for all healthcare personnel. The pediatric nurse must be skilled in emergency medication administration. Pediatric emergency drugs are calculated according to a child's body weight, so it is important to have an accurate weight. Pediatric units have a specialized emergency cart, known as a "crash cart" or "code blue cart," which is stocked with medication and equipment of various sizes. On the crash cart you may find a Broselow tape, which is a color-coded system that facilitates the use of correct pediatric drug calculations based on the length of the child in an emergency if a weight is not known. Those caring for children in emergencies must be familiar with the sizes and use of this equipment.

Nurses caring for children should receive training each year in pediatric basic life support. Ventilation and chest compressions must be done with the utmost care to prevent further complications.

Diversion and Recreation
Play is an important aspect of growth and development. Play is the work of children. Providing diversional activities in the healthcare facility helps the child physically, socially, and psychologically. Play activities are more than just ways to entertain children or to pass the time; they are also therapeutic tools that can aid recovery. Children can express their fears, frustrations, and anxieties through role-playing with dolls and teddy bears.

Many play activities are suitable for use in the hospital setting. All activities should be selected for their age and developmental appropriateness. Computers and computer games are appealing to preschool children, school-aged children, and adolescents. Children of all ages enjoy reading. Children also need to be included in conversations and have a great need for someone to listen to them. Therefore, avoid using the television as a "babysitter" for the ill child. Activities that strengthen the child's muscles and improve coordination should also be planned.

Play is important in a child's social development and can be an emotional outlet for the ill child who is experiencing the stress of strange surroundings and painful procedures. Play helps children to learn more about the world. Play can also be used to teach children and to prepare them for certain clinical procedures. For example, you may playact deep breathing or taking medications. Use dolls or teddy bears to describe planned procedures and to help the child understand what is going to happen.

Many children regress to previous developmental stages when they are frightened, ill, or injured. By observing children at play, you can learn a great deal about their physical, mental, and social states. Healthcare facilities with large pediatric departments have child life specialists who are specifically trained to address diversional and therapeutic play.

ADVANCED PEDIATRIC CARE AND PROCEDURES

Nurses perform or assist healthcare providers with many procedures. They also assist in comforting children during painful and frightening procedures.

Diagnostic Procedures
Several procedures are used to assist the healthcare provider with diagnosis. The role of the nurse is to reassure the child, provide the appropriate equipment, and assist the healthcare provider with care. The child's caregivers may be allowed to stay during the procedure, depending on hospital policy (In Practice: Nursing Care Guidelines 71-7).

Therapeutic Procedures
Managing a Fever
Fever in a child does not always indicate serious illness; teething or a recent immunization can be the cause. Fever is one way the body fights pathogens so letting a low-grade fever run its

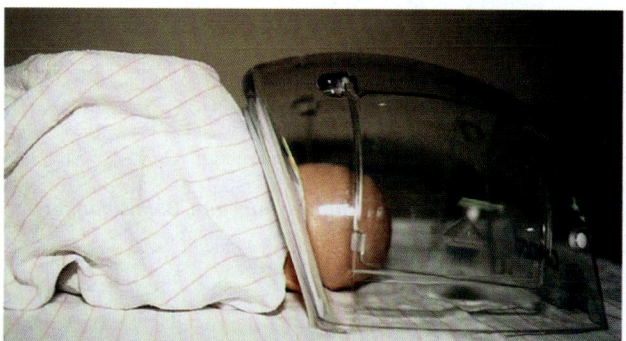

Figure 71-7 Oxygen hood for an infant. (Pillitteri, 2009.)

IN PRACTICE
NURSING CARE GUIDELINES 71-7 — Diagnostic Procedures

Venipuncture
- One site for venipuncture in infants is the femoral (thigh) area, which may be used for an ABG. When this site is used, stand at the child's head and hold the child on the back with legs spread apart ("frog-leg" position). Hold the child securely while the healthcare provider does the procedure. You can easily talk to the child when he or she is in this position. Cover the perineum with a washcloth; apply firm pressure to the puncture site for 5 min and check the site every 15 min for 1 hr (Fig. A).
- There may be access devices in place to easily collect a blood sample from a very young child. However, if a blood sample from a very young child is to be taken from the *jugular vein*, assist the healthcare provider by holding the child. Restrain the child with the head extended over the edge of the table, and pad the table edge. Hold the child perfectly still. After the procedure, note any signs of swelling or bleeding around the puncture site. Apply firm pressure to the site for the child who is sitting upright (Fig. B).

Heel Stick Blood Samples
- Blood may be obtained from an infant by heel stick. Apply a disposable heel warmer first to increase blood supply to the area.
- Use a sterile lancet to obtain the sample after cleansing the area with an alcohol sponge (In Practice: Nursing Procedure 67-6).

Lumbar Puncture
- When lumbar puncture is being performed, hold the infant (Fig. A) or child (Fig. B) with the back curved while restraining the legs with a sheet.

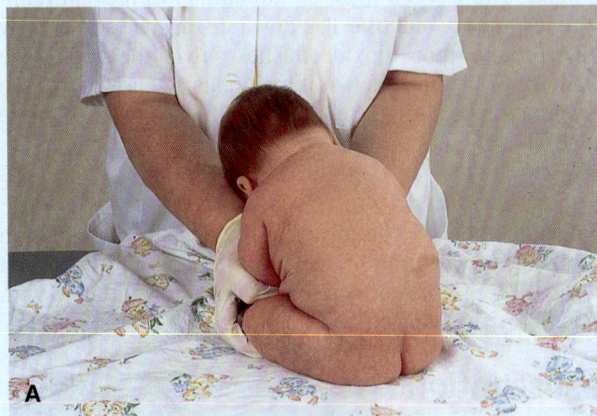

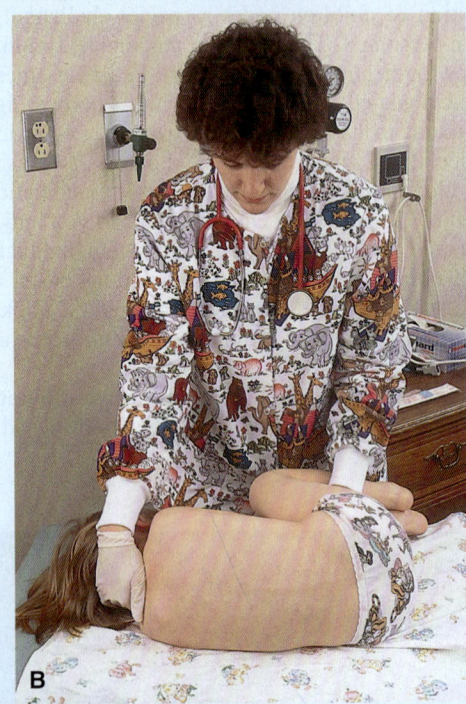

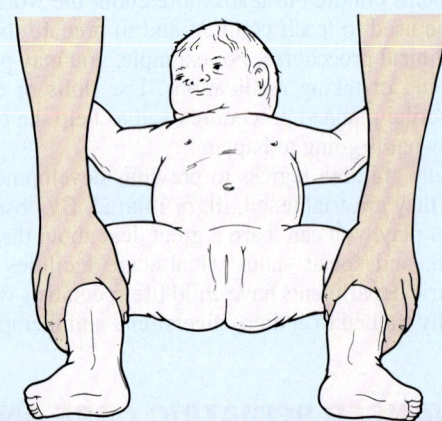

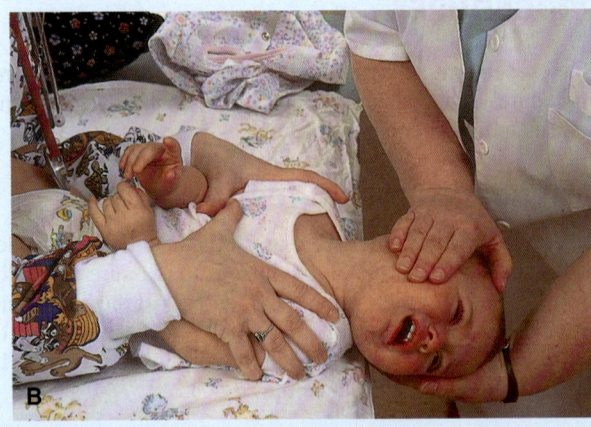

A. Position of infant or young child for femoral venipuncture. **B.** Position for jugular venipuncture. The infant's head is held sideways over the edge of the table by one nurse, while his body is restrained by a second nurse.

A. Positioning an infant for lumbar puncture. **B.** Positioning a young child for lumbar puncture.

course may be better than giving antipyretic (fever-reducing) medications (In Practice: Nursing Care Guidelines 71-8).

> **Nursing Alert** Fevers above 104 °F (40 °C) must be immediately brought under control in children who have neurologic problems, history of febrile illness, or cardiac or respiratory problems (e.g., hypoxia).

Medication Administration

More opportunities for errors occur when administering medication to children than to adults. The dosage and routes may differ. There may be specific techniques that need to be adapted to children. Usually, the novice must successfully complete a course in medication administration before giving medications to anyone, particularly children. Therefore, nursing students or new graduates sometimes are not allowed to administer medications to young children in a healthcare facility (In Practice: Nursing Care Guidelines 71-9).

> **Nursing Alert** Know the side effects of each drug being administered so that your observations of the child will be complete.

IN PRACTICE
NURSING CARE GUIDELINES 71-8 — Managing a Fever

Managing a Fever Lower Than 102 °F (38.8 °C)
- Keep the child quiet and comfortable. Prevent crying.
- Do not overdress the child; use minimum clothes for comfort.
- Encourage fluids.
- Generally do not use antipyretics unless ordered by the healthcare provider or if the child is very uncomfortable.

Managing a Fever Higher Than 102 °F (38.8 °C)
If the oral temperature is between 102 °F and 104 °F (38.8 °C and 40 °C), use the preceding measures and add the following:
- Call the healthcare provider; antipyretics may be ordered.
- Put the child to bed.

If the oral temperature is >104 °F (40 °C), use all the preceding measures and add the following:
- Give nonaspirin fever-reducing medication. *Do not give aspirin* because of the danger of Reye syndrome (Chapter 72). Check the child's temperature every 30 min.
- Sponge the child with lukewarm water until you receive further instructions from the healthcare provider.
- Check the child's temperature every 10–15 min during sponging.

Children who do not respond to routine fever treatment may respond to a tepid sponge bath. **Do not use alcohol or ice.** *Rationale: They lead to hypothermia. Alcohol fumes are irritating and may be inhaled or absorbed through the skin.* If the child shows signs of chilling (e.g., shivering), discontinue the sponge bath temporarily and wrap the child in a blanket until shivering stops. Generally, the water's temperature should be 85 °F–95 °F (29.4 °C–35 °C). This procedure is very appropriate for home use. It may be used infrequently in the acute care facility because a cooling blanket is more efficient. Follow the procedure for giving an adult a tepid sponge bath as described in Chapter 54, keeping in mind the previous points.

IN PRACTICE
NURSING CARE GUIDELINES 71-9 — Administering Medications to Children

- Always check the child's identification band before giving a medication. *This cardinal rule in giving medications applies to people of all ages.*
- Always approach a child in a positive, kind, and firm manner. Never give the child a choice of whether or not to take medicine. Do not say, "Are you ready for your pill now?" Give choices that allow the child some control over the situation, such as the injection site or the number or placement of bandages, such as Band-Aid.
- Be sure young children understand that medicine is not a punishment for being "bad" or refusing to cooperate. Use simple terms to explain why they are receiving medication.
- Do not surprise or sneak up on a child or give an injection while the child is sleeping. Doing so will destroy the child's feeling of security, causing psychological trauma.
- After administering an injection, use the term "brave." Do not tell the child he or she has been "good."
- Reassure the child that crying is okay.
- Keep explanations brief and simple. Use words the child will understand.
- Never refer to medicine as candy. *Rationale: This could lead to accidental overdose or poisoning.*
- Never lie to the child. Do not tell the child an injection will not hurt.
- If the child is to receive an intravenous (IV) medication, be sure to explain that after the initial insertion, the child will not get another "poke" with each dose.
- Avoid prolonging a procedure. Keep the time of administration to a minimum.
- Most medication doses are calculated based on the child's weight in grams or kilograms. Always have

NURSING CARE GUIDELINES 71-9: Administering Medications to Children (Continued)

- another person double-check any calculations before administration.
- Accuracy in administration is vital. Liquids are usually the best method of measurement because you can measure small doses and because you can be sure the child swallows it.
- Oral catheter tip syringes are usually used for administering liquids to infants. Use the smallest syringe possible to ensure accuracy. You may give infants liquid medications through a nipple.
- You can crush pills or empty capsules and place their contents in small amounts of applesauce or pudding or dissolve them in ice cream, juice, or formula. Because some medications cannot be mixed with certain types of foods, check a drug reference before using this technique. If adding a medication to any of these foods, use only a small amount of the food. For instance, do not add a medication to an entire bottle of formula or cup of juice. *The child may not finish it and thus may not receive the prescribed medication dose.*
- The anterior thigh (the vastus lateralis muscle) is the preferred site for intramuscular (IM) injections in children younger than 3 years of age. **Rationale:** *Their other muscles are not well enough developed.* You may use the deltoid site if no alternative is available and if there is sufficient muscle mass.
- Children are smaller and have a higher metabolic rate than adults; therefore, they absorb and excrete medications quickly. Watch closely for side effects.
- Determine pain through verbal and nonverbal communication. Use developmentally appropriate pain scales (e.g., smiling and frowning faces) to document the child's pain level.
- Be sure to monitor the child's respirations when giving narcotics. **Rationale:** *Prevent respiratory depression.*
- Children may be more likely than adults to experience a paradoxical reaction to medication (a reaction *opposite* of what is expected).

THE CHILD HAVING SURGERY

Many pediatric procedures are now completed in a same-day surgery setting. Examples of such procedures include circumcision, insertion of polyethylene tubes, detailed dental work, hernia repairs, and cystoscopy.

Most preparation for surgery is done at home before admission. Teaching is of primary importance because children are discharged from same-day surgery to the home. Thoroughly instruct family caregivers in the care of the child at home, making certain that the caregivers understand the teaching and instructions. Documentation of teaching and instructions given to the family is essential.

Although many preoperative and postoperative procedures are similar for adults and children, certain differences exist:

- Children often cannot verbalize the discomfort or symptoms they are experiencing. The nurse is responsible for noting any untoward signs and using appropriate pain scales in their assessments. Make every effort to help children understand what is happening.
- The normal ranges of vital signs differ with age. Children's lungs and hearts are smaller, their respirations and heart rates are more rapid, and their urine volumes and their body blood levels are less. Therefore, small deviations from normal are more significant for children than they are for adults.
- Children need analgesia appropriate for their body size after surgery to control pain and should receive medicine, as needed, for comfort.
- A characteristically rapid rate of metabolism and growth in children increases the healing ability of their tissues.
- Children can become dehydrated very quickly.
- Electrolytes are not as stable in children as they are in adults.
- The high metabolic rate in infants and small children dictates a high caloric intake.

Consider family caregivers and their emotional needs. If you include family members in preoperative and postoperative care, everyone will be more comfortable and cooperative. The teaching of care measures is vital.

Family caregivers are usually permitted to be with the child until the child is taken into an operating room (OR). Tell the child exactly where he or she will be and what will happen when he or she awakens. Permit family caregivers to be with the child as soon as possible.

A visit from a nurse or anesthesiologist before surgery helps to acquaint the child with those whom he or she will see in surgery and may help to relieve some anxiety. The child's waiting period should be as short as possible after arriving in the OR.

Preoperative Care

Before elective surgery, children should have an opportunity to tour the facility and touch equipment, as well as to meet the nurses. If the child is to go directly to the OR on the morning of surgery, try to alleviate fear of the unknown by giving calm explanations (In Practice: Nursing Care Guidelines 71-10).

Postoperative Care

Prepare the room to receive the child. The room should have available an IV stand, emesis basin, tissues, blood pressure apparatus, drainage equipment, and any other necessary supplies. If the child is being cared for in a same-day surgery unit, they will return to the unit in the same bed on which they left. However, if the child is returning to a pediatric unit, arrange the room so that the gurney from the recovery room can be easily moved in.

A child usually recovers from anesthesia much more quickly than an adult. However, considerate care and close observation are essential (In Practice: Nursing Care Guidelines 71-11).

IN PRACTICE
NURSING CARE GUIDELINES 71-10: Preoperative Care for Children

Many of the same principles prevail for care of children who undergo surgery as for adults. Review general preoperative and postoperative care (Chapter 56).

Preparation
- Involve family caregivers as much as possible. Most preoperative preparation is done at home by family caregivers, who need careful instructions.
- Send an admission questionnaire home with the family caregivers. They are to complete and return this form to the facility on the child's admission. Provide assistance if the caregivers are unable to read the questionnaire. Handle such a situation nonjudgmentally to avoid embarrassment.
- Review the admission questionnaire with family caregivers to ensure it is accurate and understandable.
- The healthcare provider, APRN, or physician's assistant obtains the medical history and performs a physical examination. The licensed practical nurse or nursing student may do part of the nursing history. The family caregivers may come to the facility with the child and stay during the history and physical examination. Be sure to include the family caregivers when obtaining the nursing history.
- General laboratory work is completed. Much laboratory testing may be done in a preadmission appointment. The child may go to the facility a day or so before surgery for preadmission blood work and x-ray examinations. Blood type and crossmatch are done, if necessary. Blood is not given unless absolutely necessary.
- The child returns home and is admitted the morning of surgery to the pediatric or same-day surgery unit.
- The child will probably need to have nothing by mouth (**NPO**) after midnight the day before the surgery.
- The family caregivers will have performed preoperative procedures as instructed.
- The family caregiver signs the operative permit because the child is not of legal age. (The nursing student may not be a witness on the operative permit.)

Nursing Observations
- When the child arrives on the morning of surgery, observe and document any signs of upper respiratory infection (**URI**), such as fever, cough, or runny nose. URI makes respiratory complications more likely and will probably cause surgery to be delayed until the infection clears.
- A child is more likely than an adult to have a URI.
- Be sure to chart the presence of any open wounds, rashes, or other unusual conditions.

Immediate Measures Before Surgery
- Ask the child to void if developmentally appropriate.
- Measure and record vital signs. Weight (in grams/kilograms) *must* be recorded.
- Remove any hairpins, barrettes, or jewelry.
- The child should wear an appropriate gown and must wear an identification band.
- Perform ordered surgical preparation and check to see that all laboratory reports are on the chart and that blood work is complete.
- Take everything, including toys, out of the bed (some facilities permit children to take a special toy or headphones into the surgical suite).
- If the child will be taken to the operating room in a crib, change the sheets.
- Keep the child NPO (nothing by mouth).
- Preoperative medication is often omitted in children, confirm with the healthcare provider. If you do give medications, an important safety factor is to remind the child and family caregivers to limit activity.
- The child may rest in bed or may be held by a family caregiver, but if the child has to go to the bathroom, you must provide help if the child has been sedated.
- When everything is ready, sign the chart. Give emotional support to family caregivers and the child. Family members may wish to consult a chaplain or clergy person; facilitate this discussion.
- Tell family members where they can wait during surgery so that the healthcare provider will know where to find them. Usually, the family caregivers can accompany the child to the door of the operating room.
- Make sure the appropriate parent or guardian has signed the operative permit. Reports of all blood work and preoperative x-ray studies must be on the chart.
- Explain the operative procedure to the family caregiver and child as simply and frankly as possible; explain the general procedures of the postanesthesia care unit (PACU), such as what it will be like to wake up after surgery and the likelihood of an IV.
- Explain the need for early ambulation, turning and deep breathing, and encouraging fluids.
- Explain the need for any special equipment, such as nasogastric suction, chest tubes, or catheters.
- Teach family caregivers how to perform any care they will provide when they take the child home.
- Carefully document all preoperative procedures and teaching.

IN PRACTICE
NURSING CARE GUIDELINES 71-11: Postoperative Care for Children

- Reorient the child to the room—explain the intravenous (IV), oxygen, suction and drainage tubes, and dressings to the child and family.
- Notify the family caregivers when the child returns to the unit.
- Observe the child carefully. Measure vital signs, according to the facility's policies and the healthcare provider's orders. Children's vital signs may change quickly. Most facilities provide a postoperative checklist on which the nurse documents vital signs.
- Inspect the operative site for discharge or bleeding; note equipment in use, such as a retention catheter, suction drainage, bottles, casts, or traction. Be sure everything is connected and operating properly.
- Check color, motion, and sensitivity of toes or fingers if a cast is in place. If ordered, reattach weights to traction.
- Monitor flow of IV, or program the controller or infusion pump; monitor fluid intake and output (I&O).
- Check the child's positioning; the side or abdominal position is best (to prevent aspiration).
- Turning, coughing, and deep breathing exercises are important, especially for an older child.
- Younger children do not seem to have as much difficulty with postoperative respiratory complications. (Be sure to support an abdominal incisional site with a bath blanket or pillow while encouraging the child to deep breathe.)
- Encourage the older child to move their toes, ankles, and legs (if permitted) to prevent thrombophlebitis.
- Check for voiding; take a positive approach, and follow the healthcare provider's orders. Many times a child is up and around the afternoon following surgery. (Remember, the child's oral intake may be diminished, but the child has probably had 500–1,000 mL of IV fluids.) Say that you will "help the child to the bathroom" rather than forcing or coercing the child to void.
- Check for return of peristalsis (e.g., flatus, bowel sounds/movement). If bowel sounds are absent, consult your supervisor before you give fluids or ice, to prevent gas pains.
- Give fluids according to healthcare provider's orders. Usually about 1 hr after the child returns from the PACU, you can give sips of water or ice chips.
- Refresh the child, when permitted; wash the face and hands, and change the gown and bed linens.
- Evaluate pain or discomfort. Use medications, as needed. Remember, children experience pain and may have difficulty describing it. Also, children may try to hide pain, so watch them as they move about, to ascertain their discomfort. Use pain scales (Fig. 55-4) to help the child express their level of discomfort; a simple pain scale for children shows a smiling face on one end and a crying face on the other, with gradations in between. Early ambulation prevents complications.
- Document thoroughly and report accurately.
- Children often recover from surgery quickly. Many children are discharged the afternoon of surgery or the next day. Teach family caregivers specific postoperative procedures and observations for the child's safety and the family's feelings of security. Carefully document all teaching.

STUDENT SYNTHESIS

KEY POINTS

- Basic care in pediatrics is similar to care for adults, but some procedures need modifications.
- Pediatrics requires knowledge of developmental milestones to help determine developmental delays.
- Children may need assistance to meet basic needs simply because of their age and development.
- Educating the family caregivers is a vital component of caring for a child. After discharge, pediatric care is given at home and the family caregivers must be able to understand any new procedures (e.g., administering medications and changing dressings) or following a new diet (e.g., for diabetes).
- Very young children are especially susceptible to communicable diseases.
- Protecting children from hazards includes monitoring IV infusions, preventing falls, and using safety devices, such as restraints.
- Vital signs vary according to a child's size and age.
- Children's respiratory tracts are small and susceptible to infection.
- Play is children's work and their means of communication.
- Administration of medications to children involves precise calculation; it is usually based on body weight in kilograms.
- Special teaching considerations are made for the preoperative and postoperative care of children.

CRITICAL THINKING EXERCISES

1. A 4-year-old girl, J.L., is admitted to the acute care facility for abdominal surgery. Using your knowledge of growth and development and client teaching, design a preoperative and postoperative teaching plan for J.L. and her family.

2. An 18-month-old male, K.O., is in the emergency room with pneumonia. His parent states that the he clings to his teddy bear "all the time." When it is time for K.O. to be admitted, he is to be placed in a humidified oxygen tent environment. Discuss the possible consequences

related to this situation. What toys would be appropriate for his age and situation?

3. A 24-month-old child is being admitted to the pediatric unit for a 2-week treatment of intravenous medication. Separation anxiety is a concern. The child clings to their parents, cries loudly if left alone, and becomes angry if a stranger approaches them. Discuss the fears and anxieties that are normal for a child of this age. What diversional activities would be appropriate? In your discussion, include the phases of separation anxiety, that is, protest, despair, and denial. Develop an educational plan that will assist the child and his parents that can be implemented during this toddler's stay in the hospital.

NCLEX-STYLE REVIEW QUESTIONS

1. The nurse is discussing typical behavior patterns with the parents of a toddler. Which issues should the nurse include in the discussion? Select all that apply.
   a. Aggressive behavior
   b. Separation anxiety
   c. Sibling rivalry
   d. Negativism
   e. Temper tantrums

2. The nurse is obtaining data from a child who will be having a surgical procedure this morning. The nurse observes that the child has a cough, runny nose, and temperature of 100 °F. What is the priority action by the nurse?
   a. Notify the surgeon of the findings.
   b. Continue gathering data so the surgery will not be delayed.
   c. Administer acetaminophen.
   d. Give the child some water for the cough.

3. A preschool child requires hospitalization and states, "I want my mom and dad to stay with me!" What is the best response by the nurse?
   a. "You will be okay by yourself. We will take care of you."
   b. "Be good and let us do what we need to do so you can go home with your parents."
   c. "You can have your parents stay with you if they are able to."
   d. "Your parents can stay until bedtime."

4. The nurse is caring for a hospitalized child and observes the child's behavior as apathetic and sad. The child is most likely experiencing which of the following phases of separation anxiety?
   a. Protest
   b. Despair
   c. Denial
   d. Anger

5. The nurse is obtaining vital signs on an 18-month-old child. What data should the nurse obtain first?
   a. Respiratory rate
   b. Heart rate
   c. Blood pressure
   d. Temperature

CHAPTER RESOURCES

Enhance your learning with additional resources on thePoint!

Student Resources related to this chapter can be found at **thePoint.lww.com/Rosdahl12e**.

Welcome Steps

Look at healthcare provider's orders.

Protocol for procedure.

Necessary equipment/supplies.

Wash hands using proper hand hygiene; put on gloves.

Explain the procedure and reassure the client.

Locate two identifiers to confirm correct client.

Comfortable and efficient position for nurse and client.

Obtain privacy.

Make sure to follow correct steps and body mechanics with good technique.

Ensure safety and observe deviations from normal.

End Steps

Ensure comfort and safety.

Note questions or concerns from client or nurse; note significant data.

Dispose of materials properly.

Disinfect the area and your hands.

Document and report the procedure and your findings.

IN PRACTICE

NURSING PROCEDURE 71-1 — Collecting a Pediatric Urine Specimen

Supplies and Equipment
Urine collector of appropriate size and type
Washcloth
Gloves
Water for cleansing
Towel for drying
Note: Offer the child fluids half an hour before applying the collector bag.

Steps
Follow LPN WELCOME Steps and Then

1. Position the child on their back with the legs apart and knees bent ("frog-leg" position). You may need another adult's assistance to position the child properly so you can accurately apply the collector. *Rationale:* This is the best position to secure the collection bag so the bag does not leak and cause loss of the urine specimen.

2. Gently cleanse and dry the child's perineal area. You may use plain water and a washcloth to cleanse the labia or penis. Remove any powder or lotion. *Rationale:* Clean, dry skin is necessary for the adhesive to stick.

3. Peel off the backing of the adhesive surface and apply the bag to the child's perineum. For girls, sealing from the bottom up to the pubis is easiest; do the opposite with boys. Be sure to smooth the skin during application by gently pulling on it, as needed. *Rationale:* The surface must be attached securely to prevent leakage.

4. For boys, place the penis in the bag and apply the bag to the pubis and scrotum. In an uncircumcised boy, be sure the foreskin is in its normal position before you apply the bag. *Rationale:* Keep the skin smooth to form a tighter seal and to prevent the specimen from leaking.

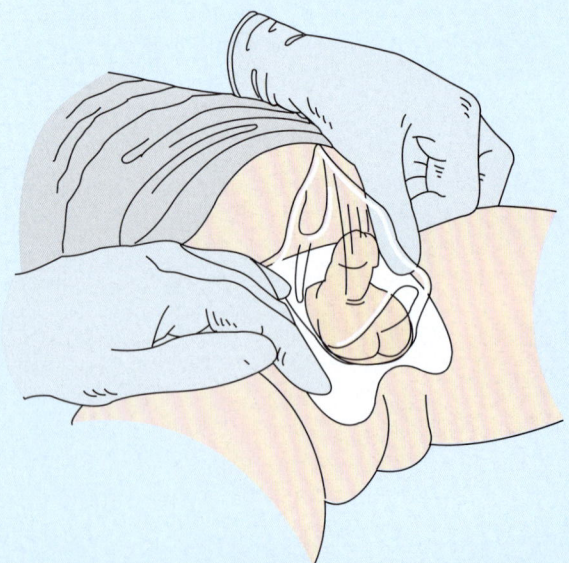

The trick to making the collection bag adhere is to make sure that the child's skin is dry.

5. Cover the bag with a loose-fitting diaper or underpants. *Rationale: This action discourages the child from pulling on the bag. Tight-fitting diapers or pants may dislodge the bag or cause the seal to burst after the child voids.*
6. Offer fluids after you apply the bag. *Rationale: Fluids encourage voiding.*
7. Check the bag every 15–30 min to see if the child has voided. *Rationale: You will want to collect the specimen and send it to the laboratory as soon as possible after voiding before urine has had time to become contaminated with skin surface bacteria. The bag may become too full and leak. The sealant may cause skin irritation if left on for an extended period.*
8. After the child has voided, gently remove the bag as soon as possible. *Rationale: This prevents loss of the specimen and makes the child more comfortable.*
9. Cleanse the child's perineum. *Rationale: Urine on the skin is likely to cause skin irritation (excoriation).*
10. Apply a clean diaper or underpants. *Rationale: A clean diaper makes the child feel more comfortable.*
11. Place the urine in a specimen cup, through the emptying port provided on the outside of the bag. Be sure that the specimen gets to the laboratory in 30 min or less or is placed in a refrigerator that is designated for specimens only. *Rationale: If the specimen is left at room temperature, it is likely to grow microorganisms, thus leading to results that are inaccurate.*

Follow ENDDD Steps

72 Care of the Infant, Toddler, or Preschooler

Learning Objectives

1. Compare and contrast the symptoms, treatment, and immunizations for the following preventable communicable diseases: hepatitis B, rotavirus, diphtheria, tetanus, pertussis, *Haemophilus influenzae*, pneumococcal infection, inactivated poliovirus, influenza, measles, mumps, rubella, varicella, hepatitis A, and meningococcal infection. State three nursing considerations for each disease.
2. Compare and contrast the symptoms of streptococcal infections and roseola. Identify three nursing considerations for each of the following: scarlet fever, "strep throat," and rheumatic fever.
3. Compare and contrast the treatment and control of common parasitic infections in children, including scabies, lice, pinworms, giardiasis, and roundworms. Identify three family teaching concerns for each.
4. Discuss nursing considerations for each of the following common injuries: fractures, lacerations, cuts and puncture wounds, foreign objects, and animal bites.
5. Identify methods of prevention and treatment for each of the following: burns, poisoning, suffocation, and drowning.
6. In the skills laboratory, practice a therapeutic communication with the parents of a child who has died of SIDS.
7. Identify potential clues to each of the following: neglect, physical abuse, and sexual abuse. Discuss the nurse's role and responsibility related to these conditions.
8. Describe the physical and/or psychological causes of FTT. State nursing considerations related to FTT.
9. Define and discuss nursing implications of each of the following skin disorders: nevi, rash, and eczema.
10. Define and discuss the nursing implications of each of the following musculoskeletal disorders: dysplasia, talipes, and torticollis.
11. Define and discuss the nursing implications of each of the following neurologic disorders: Reye syndrome, meningitis, spina bifida, hydrocephalus, febrile seizures, and breath-holding spells.
12. Define and discuss the nursing considerations for each of the following metabolic and nutritional disorders: marasmus, biliary atresia, celiac disease, and PKU.
13. Define and discuss the nursing considerations for each of the following eye disorders: strabismus, amblyopia, and cataracts in children.
14. Define and discuss the nursing considerations for each of the following ear disorders: otitis media, epistaxis, tonsillitis, cleft lip and cleft palate, and baby bottle syndrome.
15. Differentiate and state the nursing considerations for each of the following cardiovascular disorders: ASD/VSD, PDA, TGV, TOF, COA, stenosis, and tricuspid atresia.
16. Differentiate and state the nursing considerations for each of the following blood and lymph disorders: Kawasaki disease, iron deficiency anemia, sickle cell anemia, ITP, and hemophilia.
17. Define and differentiate between ALL and AML. State the nursing considerations for each type of leukemia.
18. Differentiate and state the nursing considerations for each of the following respiratory disorders: URIs, pneumonia, croup, epiglottitis, asthma, bronchiolitis, and cystic fibrosis.
19. Define and state the nursing considerations for each of the following gastrointestinal disorders: pyloric stenosis, Meckel diverticulum, intussusception, and megacolon.
20. Identify the types of hernias commonly seen in children. State three pre- and postoperative nursing considerations for hernias.
21. Discuss the nursing considerations for possible electrolyte disturbances and dehydration related to diarrhea in children.
22. Discuss the physical and psychological factors related to encopresis and lactose intolerance.
23. Define and state the nursing considerations for each of the following urinary system disorders: enuresis, HUS, urinary obstruction, UTI, pyelonephritis, glomerulonephritis, nephrotic syndrome, Wilms tumor, hypospadias, and epispadias.
24. Define and state the nursing considerations for each of the following reproductive disorders: ambiguous genitalia, cryptorchidism, and hydrocele.
25. Demonstrate a parent–child teaching session related to the nutritional concerns of childhood.

Important Terminology

amblyopia	cleft palate	encephalitis	glomerulonephritis	hydrocele	leukemia
apnea monitor	colic	encephalocele	hemangioma	hydrocephalus	lymphangiomas
asthma	collagen diseases	encopresis	hemophilia	hypospadias	mandatory reporter
biliary atresia	cryptorchidism	enuresis	hernia	intussusception	marasmus
bronchiolitis	cystic fibrosis	epiglottitis	herpes zoster	Kawasaki disease	Meckel diverticulum
celiac disease	diphtheria	epispadias	Hirschsprung disease	Koplik spots	megacolon
child abuse	dysplasia	epistaxis		kwashiorkor	meningitis
cleft lip	eczema	giardiasis	Hodgkin lymphoma	lactose intolerance	meningocele

meningomyelocele	rheumatic carditis	streptococcal ("strep") throat	ASD	HBV	PE
Mongolian spots	rheumatic fever		ASO	HepA	PIA
mumps	rickets	talipes	BMT	HepB	PKU
nephrotic syndrome	roseola	tetanus	CLL	Hib	RSV
nevus	rubella	tonsillitis	CML	HPV	RV
otitis media	rubeola	torticollis	COA	HUS	SGA
pediculosis	scabies	toxoplasmosis	CPT	IPV	SIDS
pertussis	scarlet fever	Transmission-Based Precautions	CRP	ITP	SUID
pinworms	scurvy		CRS	LTB	T&A
plumbism	shingles	varicella	DT	MDI	Td
pneumonia	sickle cell crises	Wilms tumor	DTaP (formerly DTP)	MMR	Tdap
poliomyelitis	sickle cell disease		EEG	O&P	TGA, formerly TGV
ptosis	spina bifida	**Acronyms**	ESR	OPV	TOF
pyelonephritis	spina bifida occulta		FTT	ORS	URI
pyloric stenosis	status asthmaticus	ALL	GABHS	PCV	UTI
Reye syndrome	strabismus	AML	HAV	PDA	VSD

Chapter 71 introduced general pediatric nursing care. This chapter discusses many conditions that are first seen in infants, toddlers, and preschoolers, but may also be seen in adolescents or adults. Infections, natural curiosity, lack of experience, accidents, and traumatic injuries are common for young children. In addition, congenital defects are responsible for a number of health-related disorders requiring nursing support. Many diagnostic, x-ray, and laboratory procedures are similar for children and adults.

> **NCLEX Alert**
>
> Immunizations help prevent many contagious diseases. On the NCLEX, a clinical scenario may pertain to these types of diseases and their side effects. NCLEX scenarios may also suggest instructional plans designed to teach family members about immunizations. Your option would be to choose the best teaching plan for that family situation.

COMMUNICABLE DISEASES

Communicable diseases are infections or they are diseases transmitted from one person to another. Many communicable diseases are preventable. However, preventing exposure to contagious diseases can be problematic. One reason for this is that these conditions are often most infectious before symptoms appear. The period between exposure and the development of symptoms is the *incubation period.* Children who contract communicable diseases are hospitalized only if they require acute treatment. When treating individuals who have highly contagious conditions, use **Transmission-Based Precautions**. Chapters 41 and 42 also discuss medical asepsis and Standard and Transmission-Based Precautions.

Transmission-Based Precautions

Transmission-Based Precautions supplement Standard Precautions when suspecting or caring for individuals with specific infectious diseases. They are based on the awareness of the mode(s) that a causative microorganism uses to spread an infection. Transmission-Based Precautions include isolation procedures, which require the use of personal protective equipment such as N95 quality oropharyngeal filtering masks, gowns, or eye protection. Infectious diseases can be spread by one or more of three primary methods. The names of the type of isolation precaution(s) reflect the method(s) of transmission:

- For direct contact with the infectious agent, use *Contact Precautions.*
- For moisture droplets that connect with humans through close respiratory or mucous membrane contact, use *Droplet Precautions.*
- For respiratory routes that transmit infectious microorganisms through longer distances suspended in the air (infectious aerosolization), use *Airborne Precautions.*

Transmission-Based Precautions may be initiated singly or in combination by a nurse or healthcare provider as part of hospital or facility protocols. These types of isolation procedures can also be initiated in the home, when appropriate. Conditions that create the unnecessary spread of preventable diseases include lack of immunization, not completing the series of immunization, or the waning of the original strength of an immunization. Additional conditions include global human migrations that have led to exposure of formerly rare infectious diseases to new populations. Immunizations protect children and adults from many preventable communicable diseases, but many of the immunizations are not being effectively used. The mixture of partially immunized and nonimmunized populations heightens the needs of public health awareness and protocols for prevention.

> **SPECIAL CONSIDERATIONS** **Culture and Ethnicity**
>
> **Preventive Healthcare**
> Children of low-income, migrant, or transient families may often lack preventive healthcare, especially in receiving immunizations or preventing parasitic infestations. Medical records are often absent or incomplete. Healthcare is usually received only for severe, acute illnesses. These populations are at risk for communicable disease epidemics that could be prevented with immunizations.

Diseases Preventable Through Immunization

The long-term, ultimate goal of immunization is to eradicate a communicable disease. This goal has been achieved with smallpox and, perhaps very soon, polio. The short-term purpose of the administration of vaccines via immunizations is to prevent an individual from contracting the disease from one person and then passing on the infection to another person. Prevention of the disease is important because of the many serious complications that occur when a communicable disease is acquired. Problems such as pneumonia, meningitis, sepsis, and liver cancer are among the most common complications. Your major responsibility, as a nurse, is to stress to families with children the importance of up-to-date immunizations. Numerous clinical studies have demonstrated that immunizations are safe, even for newborns, and may be administered as recommended. Refer to Chapter 71, which also provides information regarding VIS data sheets and immunizations.

It is important for healthcare professionals to be aware that "preventable" diseases may still occur in susceptible individuals, both children and adults, for example, pertussis (whooping cough). Concerns pertaining to the use of immunizations include the additives and ingredients, such as the antiseptic and antifungal preservative thimerosal, which, except for some flu vaccines, has not been used in routinely recommended childhood vaccines since 2001. Some suggest that a child receives too many vaccines and/or too many vaccines at a time, but this issue has not been proven to be problematic for a child who has a normal immune system. The persistent myth that autism is associated with immunizations has been disproven by numerous scientific studies. This textbook defers to the extensive scientific data available through the NIH, American Academy of Pediatrics, American Academy of Family Physicians, and the CDC Websites, which provide recommendations and guidance for immunization usage, in-depth discussions regarding vaccinations, and issues related to possible complications. Figure 72-1, a downloadable and printable CDC table available on the CDC Website, includes an extensive amount of information regarding vaccine-preventable diseases and the vaccines that prevent them. Transmission-Based Precautions for these diseases can be determined from Figure 72-1, column 3: *disease spread by*. This table also lists the yearly recommended immunizations for children from birth through age 6 years.

Hepatitis B

Hepatitis B (**HepB**) is one of a large group of disorders that involves some form of inflammation of the liver. HepB is a serious disease and is typically the first immunization received by a newborn prior to leaving the hospital after birth. It is spread by contact with the hepatitis B virus (**HBV**) found in infectious blood, semen, sexually related body fluids, contaminated needles, and transmission from infected mother to a newborn. It can be an acute mild case, but commonly results in serious chronic illness, liver disease, and liver cancer. Treatment is symptomatic. Prevention via vaccination is recommended for all infants and unvaccinated children, adolescents, and adults. Healthcare workers are commonly provided with HepB immunization as a part of employment protocols if they were not previously vaccinated.

> **Key Concept**
> Education of parents and other caregivers is a necessary nursing intervention. Box 72-1 lists the treatment of symptoms.

Rotavirus

Rotavirus (**RV**) is a virus that causes a severe form of gastroenteritis in infants and young children. Epidemics are not uncommon during the winter seasons, generally November to April. Adults can be infected, but their symptoms are less severe than those in children. It is spread via the fecal–oral route, contaminated food or water, contact with contaminated surfaces or, occasionally, via respiratory tract secretions. The incubation period is about 2 days. Symptoms include vomiting, watery diarrhea, fever, and abdominal pain for 3–8 days. Diagnosis may be made via rapid antigen detection of RV in stool specimens. Generally a self-limiting infection, RV treatment is symptomatic, with emphasis on rehydration of the client. Hospitalization may be required to treat dehydration via intravenous (IV) fluids.

Diphtheria

Diphtheria, which is transmitted through droplets, begins with a sore throat, fever, and often generalized aching and malaise. Typically the disease presents with throat inflammation, but also may appear in the nose, larynx, or trachea, and is followed by the formation of a whitish-gray membrane that is closely adherent and cannot be removed without causing bleeding. The causative bacillus produces a poison that can weaken the child's cardiac muscle. The child is very ill and requires close observation. People who show no symptoms of diphtheria may be carriers and are treated prophylactically with antibiotics.

Tetanus

Tetanus, also known as *lockjaw*, is a highly fatal disease caused by the *Clostridium tetani* bacteria. Tetanus is not passed from one person to another; rather, anaerobic bacteria enter through breaks in the skin, especially deep puncture wounds. Early symptoms include the inability to open or close the jaw, difficulty in swallowing, and stiffness in the neck and abdomen. Later symptoms manifest with the characteristic convulsive contractions of all voluntary muscles, seizure-like activity, and severe nervous system problems. Tetanus is preventable through the administration of a scheduled series of immunizations using tetanus toxoid, which is often combined with diphtheria or acellular pertussis as **DtaP**, **Tdap**, **DT**, or **Td** vaccines. Booster immunizations are necessary in adults because immunization against tetanus is known to wane over time.

Pertussis

Pertussis, or "whooping cough," is a highly contagious bacterial respiratory disease occurring most commonly in young children who have not been immunized. In the last decades, it has become epidemic in some areas and is seen more commonly in adults and young adults than in previous years. The causative agent, *Bordetella pertussis*, is a gram-negative coccobacillus. It is transmitted through direct contact and through droplets. Pertussis can be prevented in younger children through the diphtheria, tetanus, acellular pertussis (DTaP) immunization. Booster immunizations for adolescents or adults are given via the **Tdap** combination vaccine.

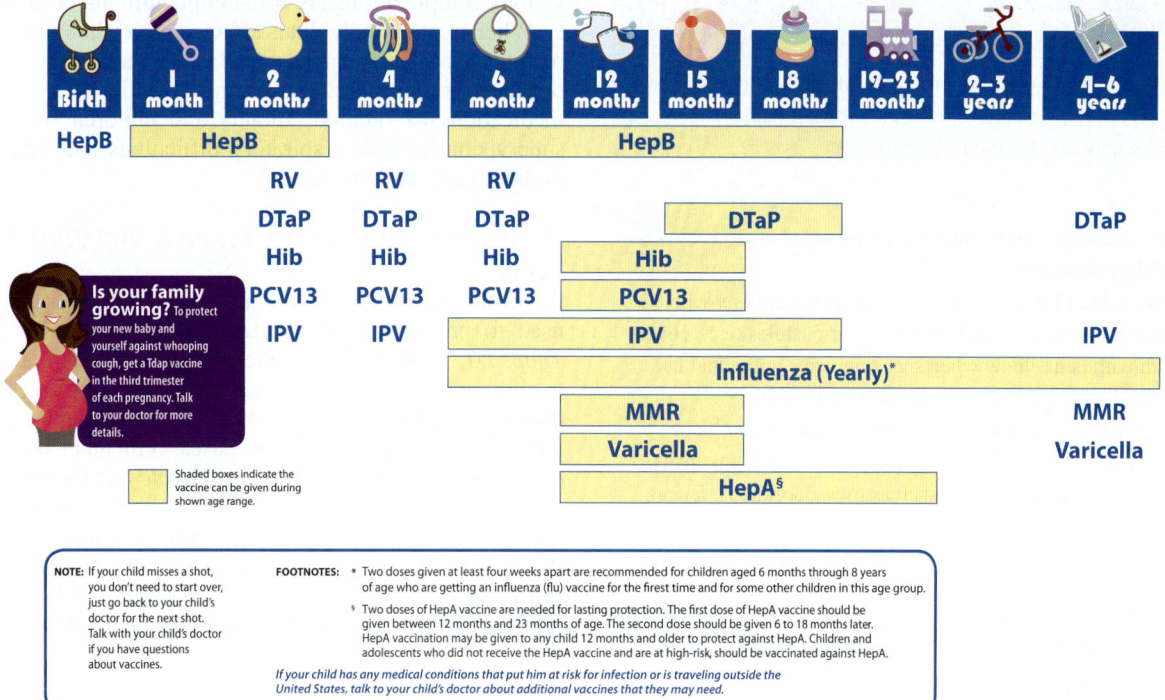

Figure 72-1 2020 recommended immunizations for children from birth through 6 years old.

Box 72-1 Nursing Considerations: Symptom Relief

Treatment or relief of common symptoms such as *general body malaise, mild headache, sneezing, stuffy or runny nose, or coughing* may include the following:

GENERAL
- Rest—decrease activity and encourage naps.
- Wash hands frequently.
- Protect self and family members from *direct contact* with secretions, rashes, papules (pimples), or pustules (e.g., cover mouth with bent elbow when sneezing, have individual use own wash cloth, and clean secretions from face).
- Protect self and family members from *indirect contact* of potentially infected items (e.g., do not share eating utensils; disinfect common surfaces, such as toys, doorknobs, faucet handles).
- Maintain adult supervision when using any type of medication.

AIRWAY MAINTENANCE
- Elevate head of bed—use pillows, if appropriate for age of child (do not use with infants).
- Use humidifier or cool mist vaporizer (maintain clean air filter in machine).
- Avoid environmental pollutants, such as any type of smoke, airborne chemicals, and irritants (e.g., cleaning products).
- Use saline nasal spray for relief of nasal symptoms or rubber suction bulb for infants.

MONITOR FLUID STATUS
- Offer small amounts (25–50 mL) of fluids every 1–2 hr.
- Increase fluid intake as tolerated (e.g., clear fluids or soup).
- Alternate types of fluids (e.g., ice chips, popsicles, noncarbonated drinks).

PAIN AND/OR FEVER TREATMENTS
- Ear pain—try warm moist cloth over painful ear.
- Throat pain—use ice chips, throat sprays.
- Medicate with *age-appropriate* over-the-counter medications *per label directions* using ibuprofen, acetaminophen, or naproxen.
- Remember, antibiotics have limited uses and must be taken for the full dosage if prescribed.

NOTIFY HEALTHCARE PROVIDER IF
- Temperature is >100.4 °F (38 °C).
- Symptoms persist or get worse.

The incubation period is 5–21 days. Symptoms begin with bronchitis and a slight temperature elevation. The cough steadily worsens, leading to paroxysms (spasms) of coughing, characterized by a "whooping" sound. The person may cough so hard that they vomit or become *dyspneic* (labored breathing). The first stage lasts about 1 week. The severe coughing stage lasts 2–3 weeks. It usually takes another 2–3 weeks for the cough to disappear, but whooping cough can last for several months. The most serious complications are bronchopneumonia or death.

When treating individuals affected with whooping cough, maintain droplet Transmission-Based Precautions throughout the whooping period. Administer antibiotics and other medications as ordered. Infants and children need close supervision because respiratory difficulties and nutritional problems are likely to occur.

Summary of Diphtheria, Tetanus, and Pertussis Vaccines

According to the CDC, there are four combination vaccines used to prevent diphtheria, tetanus, and pertussis: *DTaP, Tdap, DT, and Td*. Two of these (DTaP and DT) are given to children younger than 7 years, and two (Tdap and Td) are given to older children and adults. To understand the rationale of using upper and lower cases, remember that *upper case letters* in these abbreviations *denote full-strength doses* of diphtheria (D) and tetanus (T) toxoids and pertussis (P) vaccine. *Lower-case* letters "d" and "p" *denote reduced doses* of diphtheria and pertussis used in the adolescent/adult formulations. In addition, the "a" in DTaP and Tdap stands for "acellular," meaning that the pertussis component contains only a part of the pertussis organism.

SPECIAL CONSIDERATIONS Lifespan

Age-appropriate vaccines for diphtheria (D, d), pertussis (aP, ap), and tetanus (T)
  DTaP—a series of immunizations used for children younger than 7 years
  DTP—replaced by DtaP, no longer in use in the United States
  Tdap—single-dose booster recommended for ages 11 years and older and may be repeated every 10 years as needed
  Td—Td or Tdap are recommended every 10 years for older children and adults as protection against tetanus and diphtheria

---

Adapted from U.S. Department of Health and Human Services: CDC Website www.cdc.gov, Vaccine Information Statement, Diphtheria, Tetanus and Pertussis.

Haemophilus influenzae Type b

H. influenzae serotype b (**Hib**) is a serious, bacterial infection that may affect many organ systems, causing pneumonia, meningitis, epiglottitis, endocarditis, osteomyelitis, cellulitis, otitis media, and septic arthritis. Consequences of infection with Hib can be death or morbidity, with problems such as permanent hearing loss, brain damage, or other long-term sequelae. Direct contact with respiratory droplets causes spread of the infection and indicates the need for in-home or in-facility respiratory droplet isolation. Initial symptoms may be "flu-like," including fever, malaise, and respiratory tract problems and secretions. Symptoms can quickly become severe, with febrile seizures occurring. Treatment is symptomatic, including the use of antipyretics for fever, monitoring nutrition, and observing respiratory function.

Pneumococcal Infection

Pneumococcal bacterial infection is caused by *Streptococcus pneumoniae* (pneumococcus). There are numerous causes of pneumonia, but pneumococcal disease may be preventable when the client is injected with one of the available forms of pneumococcal vaccine (**PCV**). Initially, the pneumonia may present with a fever, cough, dyspnea, otitis media, and chest pain. Later symptoms of pneumococcal disease include pneumococcal pneumonia, meningitis, or bacteremia. All of these later symptoms are serious, with long-term or fatal outcomes. Brain damage, hearing loss, or loss of a limb is a known complication. The causative bacteria are often found in an individual's oropharyngeal passages and spread through contact with respiratory secretions directly or indirectly by droplets from coughing or sneezing. Individuals may carry the bacteria without having the serious pneumonia; the reason for the development of the specific pneumonia is not known.

Poliomyelitis

Poliomyelitis (polio) used to be a feared pandemic, contagious, viral disease. Still existing in pockets of the world, polio causes serious damage by attacking the central nervous system (CNS). Some of the symptoms that occur in sufferers are temporary or permanent paresthesia (the feeling of pins and needles in the legs), paralysis (inability to move body parts), and meningitis (infection of the spinal meninges), leading to temporary or permanent loss of the ability to move, significant muscle weakness, and severe head pain. Two types of vaccine exist. Inactivated poliovirus vaccine (**IPV**) is the only vaccine in use in the United States since 2000. Oral poliovirus vaccine (**OPV**) is still used in many parts of the globe. The administration of IVP, the inactivated form, has replaced OPV in many parts of the world, including the United States. Treatment of polio is symptomatic, with an emphasis on maintenance of respiratory function and long-term physical therapy rehabilitation. Adults who have had polio in their youth may develop *postpolio syndrome* 15–40 years after having had polio symptoms, which is characterized by muscle pain, worsening weakness of muscles, or paralysis. Postpolio syndrome is not contagious, and victims do not spread the poliovirus.

Influenza

Influenza or "the flu" is a general term for a variety of seasonal viruses or a specific endemic virus. Typically in the fall, a virus develops and spreads through vulnerable populations, such as infants, the immunocompromised, or older adults. Symptoms vary from mild to severe, usually involving respiratory difficulties, fatigue, and malaise. Influenza is different from what is often referred to as a cold or the common cold (Chapter 73). Symptoms may be similar but are more severe, and, generally, it takes longer for the client to recuperate. Treatment for influenza is symptomatic for fever and vomiting. Antiviral or antibiotic medications are used for some individuals (Box 72-1). Vaccines for immunization against specific influenza strains are typically developed annually as needed, generally requiring several months to develop. No vaccines are yet available against what is considered the "common cold." Immunizations against influenza are available through healthcare providers as per the recommendations of the CDC and other professional organizations.

> **Key Concept**
>
> **M**easles, **M**umps, and **R**ubella (**MMR**) are among the most easily avoided communicable diseases. Most frequently, they are abbreviated as MMR, which stands for the *rubeola* **m**easles, the **m**umps, and the **r**ubella measles. Rubeola measles generally attacks young children. Rubella measles is extremely hazardous to the unborn infant and commonly associated with serious fetal malformations. To avoid confusion, the word "measles" is identified with rubeola. The word rubella is identified as a disease that affects the unborn child. Refer to the CDC immunization chart in Figure 72-1.

Rubeola (Measles)

Rubeola, also known as the *red measles, 10-day measles, or measles*, is caused by the measles virus found in the nose, mouth, throat, eyes, and their discharges. It is transmitted through direct contact with an affected individual and through airborne droplets. Measles is highly communicable and difficult to recognize in its early stage because the symptoms resemble those of the common cold, roseola infantum, and rubella (*German measles, 3-day measles*). The incubation period is 10–20 days. The disease begins with a slight temperature elevation, a runny nose, and watery eyes. By day 2 or 3, diagnostic bluish-white pinpoint spots with a red rim, called **Koplik spots**, appear in the person's mouth. Small, dark-red areas appear on the face and spread downward throughout the body. These red areas grow large and group together, giving the skin a blotchy appearance. Respiratory symptoms increase and pneumonias are possible. The child sneezes frequently, the eyes are sore, and the discharge becomes purulent; light hurts the eyes (*photophobia*). The child also develops a sore throat and a hacking cough. The rash, which may last for up to 10 days, is greatest at about the fourth day. During the second week, the skin begins to flake off in tiny powderlike flakes (*desquamation*) for 5–10 days. The child itches all over and soothing, antipruritic nursing measures are important to manage itching.

Measles is most hazardous to the very young child. The infection may spread to the middle ear, causing **otitis media**, pneumonia, and encephalitis. **Encephalitis** is an inflammation of brain tissue and occasionally accompanies meningitis, an infection of the meninges. Permanent brain damage, learning disabilities, or death can result from measles encephalitis.

All children should be immunized against measles because of the seriousness of the complications. Measles outbreaks occur periodically in populations in which a large group of individuals have not received necessary immunizations.

Mumps

Mumps, also called *epidemic parotitis*, is a viral disease that affects the salivary glands, especially the parotids. It is transmitted through direct and indirect contact and through salivary secretions. Children younger than 2 years and adults seldom contract mumps. However, adults who contract mumps may suffer serious after effects, including sterility in men.

Close contact is required for mumps to be transmitted. The incubation period is 2–3 weeks. The first sign is usually a swelling of the parotid gland, on one side or both. Sometimes, the individual has a low-grade fever, headache, and general malaise before the swelling appears. The swollen gland is painful, and opening the mouth and eating are uncomfortable. The swelling begins to disappear by the second or third day and is usually gone by day 10. The disease is considered communicable until the swelling disappears. Treatment of the symptoms is the typical nursing measure.

Rubella

Rubella (*German measles, 3-day measles*) is a viral infection that is mild and lasts only a short time. However, *rubella can cause serious fetal malformations if a pregnant woman contracts the disease.* Congenital rubella syndrome (**CRS**) occurs in about 90% of infants exposed to rubella (World Health Organization, 2020). The baby, if it survives birth, commonly has congenital (born with) brain damage, blindness, and heart disorders. Rubella is transmitted through direct contact or airborne transmission. All children should be immunized, not only for their own protection but also for the protection of pregnant women with whom they may come in contact.

The symptoms of rubella are similar to those of other disorders that develop a rash. Unlike measles (rubeola), spots do not appear on the oral mucous membrane. Sometimes, the facial rash is the first noticeable sign of infection. Swelling of the lymph nodes in the occipital region is another frequent symptom. The rash spreads quickly and disappears just as rapidly. Although complications are uncommon, they can be serious. Treatment is symptomatic.

> **Key Concept**
>
> A rash may be the first symptom of a contagious disease. Most emergency departments, outpatient clinics, and healthcare offices require that rashes be evaluated before the child is allowed into a waiting room. It is important to protect others from exposure to an infectious disease.

Varicella

Varicella (chickenpox) originates with the varicella zoster virus, which is the same virus that causes **herpes zoster** (**shingles**), found in adults who had chickenpox in earlier years. Following or concurrent with a rash, a fever develops. The itchy rash develops first into papules then vesicles and finally pustules that turn into crustlike lesions that fall off in 1–3 weeks. A highly infectious disease, the varicella virus is found in the nose, throat, blisters, and crusts. The blisters generally concentrate on the face, scalp, and trunk. Severe complications, including bacterial dermatitis, encephalitis, and pneumonia, are more common in adolescents and adults than in infants and children. Immunized persons may get milder forms of the disease than nonimmunized individuals. Transmission is by highly infectious droplets from coughing and sneezing or by direct contact. Treatment includes droplet and contact precautions as well as symptomatic treatment for the fever and rash. The most common complication is infection caused by scratching the blisters, which can leave scars or "pock marks." Caregivers should keep the child's fingernails short to prevent scratching. Antihistamines (diphenhydramine [Benadryl]) and antiitching measures, such as antipruritic medications in a bath, may relieve intense itching. The administration of antiviral medications, such as acyclovir (Zovirax), may be helpful in reducing symptoms.

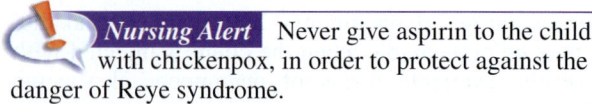 **Nursing Alert** Never give aspirin to the child with chickenpox, in order to protect against the danger of Reye syndrome.

Hepatitis A

Hepatitis A (**HepA**) belongs to the list of disorders causing inflammation of the liver. Hepatitis A is caused by the hepatitis A virus (**HAV**). Unlike some other forms of viral hepatitis, it does not lead to long-term infection. Transmission is by ingestion of microscopic amounts of fecal matter, close person-to-person contact, or ingestion of contaminated food or drinks. Before HepA immunization, HAV was commonly found in preschools and day-care centers where young children may not have been practicing consistently good bathroom hygiene.

 SPECIAL CONSIDERATIONS Lifespan

Many individuals, including adolescents, adults, and older adults, should consider visiting their local Public Health Department for an immunization evaluation. Global populations include vast numbers of travelers and migrating populations, many of whom are not or are only partially immunized. There may be new vaccines or recommended booster shots needed for vacationers, business travelers, adolescents, seniors, and migrating populations. Immunization recommendations, which change periodically, are available on the CDC Website. The publication of the CDC Health Information for International Travel 2020 (the Yellow Book) has detailed information about global destination sites and recommendations for pretravel health considerations.

Meningococcal Infection

Meningitis is a general term describing inflammation of the membranes that cover the brain and spinal cord. Bacteria and viruses can directly or indirectly cause this serious infection that can leave the individual with brain damage, hearing loss, and learning disabilities. Bacterial meningitis, for example, was a common side effect of *H. influenzae* type b before the initiation of Hib vaccine. The viruses that cause measles, mumps, and chickenpox may also result in the complication of meningitis. Bacterial meningitis is currently more common in adolescents and young adults than in children because of the effectiveness of childhood vaccinations.

Meningococcal immunizations are designed to protect individuals directly against specific forms of meningitis. *Neisseria meningitides* and *S. pneumoniae* are bacterial forms of meningitis for which there is a specific vaccine.

> **Key Concept**
>
> Teach family caregivers the importance of immunizations.

Contagious Diseases

Recommended vaccinations for contagious diseases are continuously under review and updated as technology and research advances. Additional immunizations for communicable diseases, such as that for types of genital human papillomavirus (**HPV**), which is known to cause certain cancers, are available (Chapter 73). Other infectious diseases that do not currently have vaccines include those listed below. As with other infectious diseases that used to occur primarily in the young, trends show that adolescents, young adults, and older adults may have these disorders.

Respiratory Syncytial Virus

Respiratory syncytial virus (**RSV**) is a very common seasonal virus that infects the upper respiratory tract, the lungs, and the bronchioles of nearly all infants by their second birthday. It is believed to cause more than half the cases of bronchiolitis and pneumonia of vulnerable infants, children, and older adults. RSV is easily transmissible by direct or indirect contact with tears, nasal, or oral secretions; thus, it is important to protect against cross-contamination from secretions from the eyes, nose, and mouth. Sneezing spreads airborne viruses. Contamination by kissing or touching environmental surfaces, such as doorknobs, cribs, or toys, spreads the virus. The peak RSV season typically begins in the fall and ends in the spring. Strict handwashing and the use of Transmission-Based Precautions are very important interventions to avoid the spread of this highly contagious disease.

Most symptoms occur within 4–6 days of infection and may affect infants (especially premature infants), children, and older adults. Typically, the child presents with symptoms similar to the common cold, such as a runny nose, low-grade fever, sore throat, mild headache, sneezing, loss of appetite, and dry cough. Cases of RSV are generally mild but may be life threatening in at-risk populations, such as those who are very young, those who are older, and those who have chronic health disorders. Severe cough, wheezing, lethargy, irritability, and breathing difficulties with cyanosis may also occur or be the only symptoms, especially in the young infant. Pneumonia or bronchiolitis is possible in severe cases. Recovery generally occurs in 1–2 weeks, but the virus can remain active (infectious) for up to 3 weeks. Hospitalization is sometimes required, but most clients with RSV are treated at home. Diagnosis of RSV is based on symptoms and a positive respiratory secretion.

Treatment is based on symptoms, typically using antipyretics, fluids, and rest. For children at high risk, treatment may include suctioning of secretions, supplemental oxygen, and medications. For the hospitalized infant, respiratory symptoms are treated by the use of an antiviral agent, ribavirin, which is administered by mist tent or face mask.

> **Nursing Alert** *Ribavirin* is often teratogenic to the fetus and is therefore listed in Pregnancy Category X. Pregnant or lactating clients and partners of pregnant clients should avoid contact with children who are receiving ribavirin.

Streptococcal Infections

Group A beta-hemolytic streptococcal infections (**GABHS**) are fairly common among children older than 2 years. GABHS are disease-causing strains of the genus *Streptococcus*, which are gram-positive bacteria normally found in the respiratory, alimentary, and female genital tracts. GABHS are spread by direct contact and large droplets.

Streptococcal Pharyngitis

Streptococcal pharyngitis ("**strep throat**") is common in young children older than 2 years. It is treated with antibiotics, most often penicillin. To prevent complications, treatment should be started as soon as possible after receiving a positive culture for strep. A rapid diagnostic test ("rapid strep screen") or culture can differentiate strep throat from other types of throat problems. White patches on the tonsils can be caused by streptococcal pharyngitis. An elevated temperature that does not fall after giving an antipyretic (acetaminophen, ibuprofen) may also point to strep. Children may complain of a "lump" in the throat or their neck hurting rather than a sore throat since they describe things differently.

The most serious complications of "strep throat" are rheumatic fever, rheumatic heart disease, and nephritis. The prognosis is good if treated promptly. Make certain that family caregivers understand that children with this illness must finish their prescribed antibiotic to ensure complete eradication of the bacteria, even if symptoms improve before the medication regimen is completed.

Scarlet Fever

Scarlet fever, sometimes referred to as scarlatina, is also GABHS but more often considered another type of strep infection. Symptoms develop after an incubation period of 1–7 days; they include the appearance of a generalized flush or redness caused by a sandpaper-like rash of pinpoint-like red spots crowded together (macular rash). Desquamation follows. The tongue becomes coated with a white substance that later disappears, leaving prominent papillae ("strawberry tongue"). The most common complications are ear infections, nephritis, arthritis, cardiac problems, and pneumonia. Prognosis is favorable when scarlet fever is treated promptly.

Rheumatic Fever

Rheumatic fever, an autoimmune reaction to GABHS, belongs to a group of diseases called **collagen diseases** (diseases of connective tissues). It is believed to result from continued streptococcal infections (e.g., scarlet fever, streptococcal sore throat), in which the child becomes sensitive to streptococci or develops an autoimmune response. Prompt and complete treatment of streptococcal infections greatly reduces the child's risk of contracting rheumatic fever. *Rheumatic heart disease* is the most common complication of rheumatic fever. The incidences of rheumatic fever and rheumatic heart disease have decreased in countries with access to healthcare resources, although they continue to be a problem in many countries where healthcare is limited.

Signs and Symptoms. Symptoms of rheumatic fever vary in degree from mild to severe. Loss of weight and appetite, fatigue, irritability, aches, joint pain, and tenderness in the extremities may be signs. Fever may begin suddenly, especially after a cold or sore throat, and becomes highest in the evening. The most significant symptom of rheumatic fever is *polyarthritis*, in which the child's shoulders, elbows, wrists, or knees swell and become excruciatingly painful. Pain travels or migrates from one joint to another and may affect several joints at the same time. It usually lasts for a few days to a week in each joint and then subsides gradually. Fortunately, the polyarthritis does not cause joint deformities, and the joints usually return to normal after the attack.

Diagnostic tests with the following results may indicate rheumatic fever (not all findings need be present):

- Elevated white blood cell (WBC) count
- Elevated erythrocyte sedimentation rate (**ESR**), commonly known as "sed rate"
- Positive C-reactive protein (**CRP**)
- Elevated antistreptolysin-O (**ASO**) titer

Signs to watch for include jerky, uncontrolled movements of the face, neck, arm, and leg muscles, which are known as *Sydenham chorea;* small nodules under the skin over the elbows, ankles, legs, knuckles, and at the back of the head; and frequent nosebleeds.

A common and serious complication of rheumatic fever is **rheumatic carditis** or *rheumatic heart disease*, in which valvular lesions impair mitral valve efficiency. The consequence of valvular inefficiency can eventually lead to severe cardiac failure.

Medical Treatment. Most children recover from rheumatic fever and lead normal lives. When severe instances of carditis or heart failure (HF) occur, hospitalization is necessary; however, most cases of rheumatic fever are treated in the home. The disease's course depends primarily on the degree of heart damage. The degree of carditis directly affects recovery time. Recovery may be complete, but carditis can also be fatal.

Rheumatic fever's active phase usually lasts 1–4 months, but other outbreaks are likely to follow. The key to treating rheumatic fever is to prevent permanent heart damage. Complete bed rest is maintained until the child is afebrile. Keeping the child inactive is fairly easy during the acute phase because they are very sick; however, aggressive family teaching is important during convalescence, when regulating the child's activity may be difficult.

Drugs, such as acetaminophen, are given for pain relief and fever reduction. Aspirin may be used for its anti-inflammatory properties (as opposed to aspirin's effects as an antipyretic). Cortisone reduces inflammation, but is prescribed only if absolutely necessary because of associated adverse reactions. Antibiotics are administered. Because recurrence is probable, prophylactic antibiotic medication may be prescribed for up to 5 years. For example, if the child needs dental work, has an infection, or is having an invasive procedure, antibiotics are typically given as prophylactic treatment. Some children continue on prophylactic antibiotics for many years. Surgical replacement of a cardiac valve, particularly the mitral valve, may be necessary.

If any sign of a strep throat exists, family caregivers should consult a healthcare provider immediately.

Roseola

Roseola is a benign disease of infancy. A very high fever lasting a few days is followed by a rash appearing first on the trunk and then spreading to the neck, face, and extremities when the child's temperature falls. Theorists believe roseola is caused by a virus, which is not as communicable as with many other diseases. The affected child may experience febrile seizures, but other complications are rare. One attack seems to confer lifelong immunity.

PARASITIC INFESTATIONS

Parasites live in or on the body of another living organism. Skin parasites spread easily from one person to another (Chapter 75). Common parasites that invade a human's gastrointestinal (GI) tract include bacteria, protozoa, fungi, insects, and worms. A hookworm infection is a parasitic infection caused by bloodsucking roundworms, which are found in the ground in unhygienic areas. These worms survive in the small intestine of a human, dog, cat, or bird and can cause mild to severe gastrointestinal problems. *Giardia* (causing **giardiasis**) or *cryptosporidium* (causing cryptosporidiosis) can affect all ages, including infants, children, and adults. These microscopic parasites are a common cause of diarrhea spread through infected feces or drinking contaminated water. Breeding sites for giardiasis as well as cryptosporidiosis ("crypto") include swimming pools or other recreational waters. **Toxoplasmosis**, infection from the *Toxoplasma gondii* parasite, is caused by infected cat or dog feces from cat litter or ground soil.

You may collect a stool specimen for ova and parasites (**O&P**) to determine their presence. When handling stool specimens, always wear gloves, and take care to avoid self-contamination. Refer to Nursing Care Guidelines 72-1 and Box 72-2.

Pediculosis, scabies, and pinworms are discussed in more detail below.

IN PRACTICE
NURSING CARE GUIDELINES 72-1 — Obtaining a Stool Specimen for Pinworms

- The primary caregiver may assist or may be asked to perform this minor procedure at home. *Rationale: The early morning hours before the child awakens are most favorable for finding ova.*
- Obtain assistance and provide privacy. *Rationale: The procedure may be considered invasive of the child's personal space.*
- Obtain a piece of clear cellophane tape and a tongue blade. *Rationale: To obtain and identify pinworms.*
- Wind the tape around the end of a tongue blade with the sticky side out. *Rationale: The sticky side of tape will touch the skin where ova may be located.*
- Spread the child's buttocks and press the tape against the child's anus. *Rationale: The anal area is where the worms are most likely to be seen, and where to obtain a specimen.*
- Transfer the tape to a clear microscope slide and send it to the laboratory for examination for eggs. *Rationale: Infestation is confirmed when the pinworm eggs are seen visually or under the microscope.*

> **Box 72-2 Nursing Considerations for Parasitic Care**
>
> - Teach the child and family caregivers good personal hygiene and careful handwashing.
> - Treat all family members simultaneously.
> - Teach client or caretaker to avoid food preparation during treatment.
> - Discuss careful washing and cleaning of all household items and clothing when teaching about treating for lice.
> - Observe carefully the person with a seizure disorder, kidney malfunction, severe malnutrition, or anemia. They may be unable to use these medications.
> - Observe for side effects of dizziness, drowsiness, headache, seizures, diarrhea, nausea, and vomiting.
> - Avoid applying parasitic lotions to open lesions, a rash, the face, eyes, mucous membranes, or urethral meatus.
> - Use of antipruritic medication (oral or topical) may help if itching continues for a few days after treatment.
> - Observe those receiving piperazine treatment for roundworms; monitor for the side effect of hemolytic anemia.
> - Observe those receiving treatment for lice for the common side effect of skin irritation.
> - Repeat the treatment, as needed, especially for lice.

Pediculosis

Pediculus pubis (lice, pubic lice, "crabs") are tiny parasites that attach themselves to pubic hair follicles and cause intense itching. The condition of having lice in the pubic area is known as *pediculosis pubis*. Pediculosis can spread through sexual contact, infested bed linens and clothing, or close physical contact. The most common lice infestation (**pediculosis**) in children occurs on the head (*pediculosis capitis*).

As discussed in Chapter 75, body lice are different forms of pediculosis, but they all have the same three stages: the egg (nit), the nymph (young adult), and the adult. Nits lay their yellow or white oval eggs near the waistlines or seams of clothing and under armpits, or they are attached to body hair. Nits take 1–2 weeks to hatch into nymphs, a smaller-sized louse, which in 9–12 days grows into an adult louse. Adult lice are tan to grayish-white and about the size of a sesame seed with six legs. Nymph and adult lice feed on blood.

Bedding and clothing generally become infested when used by infected people. Direct physical contact with the infested person, clothing, bed, bed linens, or towels can spread the parasite. Regular bathing and clean clothes are necessary to prevent infestations. Children are most vulnerable, as are the homeless and transient individuals.

Diagnosis is based on viewing the lice or their eggs (nits) attached to the hair follicles. Treatment consists of applying over-the-counter pediculicides, such as pyrethrins (Nix, RID), to the affected area and thoroughly cleaning all clothing and personal articles. Generally, scalps or bodies need at least two separate treatments to ensure the death of any nits that hatch after the first treatment. The lice die within 24 hr after being separated from the body, but the nits can live for approximately 2 weeks. A repeat treatment is needed at that time. Sexual partners and household members must be treated simultaneously. If an infestation occurs, the entire family needs to be treated. Teach the family household control measures.

> *Key Concept*
>
> Contact Precautions are necessary to prevent the spread of lice and scabies. Healthcare providers are best protected when using Standard Precautions and Transmission-Based Precautions.

Scabies

Scabies is a microscopic mite that is easily transmitted among children and adults of all socioeconomic classes. The mite burrows into the epidermis where it lives and lays its eggs. Intense itching and pimple-like red rashes are the most common symptoms. Direct, skin-to-skin contact spreads the mite from one person to another. High-risk places for infection include childcare centers, long-term care facilities, and prisons. It is not uncommon to have seasonal outbreaks of scabies or to find the mite on healthcare providers who are infested by caring for others who have scabies.

> *Key Concept*
>
> Family caregivers are often embarrassed when they find out that their child has a parasitic infestation. The entire family needs to be treated when infestation occurs.

Pinworms

Pinworm infections (enterobiasis) are one of the most common infestations in children because they typically do not yet have good hygiene habits and often put their dirty fingers into their mouths. Children ingest the eggs, which mature in the cecum. The hatched worms lay ova in anal and perineal folds, causing local itching. Signs that a child may have pinworms include scratching, especially around the anus; teeth grinding during sleep; fatigue; anorexia; and irritability. Worms may appear in the anal region or on stool. Treatment consists of the administration of *anthelmintics* (antiworm medications), which are given to all family members as well. See In Practice: Nursing Care Guidelines 72-1—Obtaining a Stool Specimen for Pinworms.

TRAUMA

Children are susceptible to injury from accidents, including falling, choking, drowning, poisoning, and burns. Because young children do not have the judgment or experience to protect themselves and are constantly on the move, watching them every moment is difficult. Accidents are the number one cause of death in children older than 1 year through young adulthood. Family caregivers and others who care for children must constantly be alert to prevent trauma. See In Practice: Educating the Client 72-1 to learn more about choking prevention.

IN PRACTICE
EDUCATING THE CLIENT 72-1 — Choking Prevention

- Cut children's food into small pieces.
- Teach children to eat slowly.
- Teach children not to laugh and talk when they have food in their mouth.
- Serve foods appropriate to a child's age. Avoid serving nuts, popcorn, chewing gum, hard candy, raisins, carrot sticks, and hot dogs to children younger than 4 years.
- Keep small objects, such as coins, marbles, beads, and small toy pieces, away from children younger than 4 years.
- Store small household items, such as pins, buttons, toothpicks, nails, screws, and thumbtacks, away from children's reach. Monitor children when they are in an area where such items are being used.

SPECIAL CONSIDERATIONS — Lifespan

Unintentional injuries are the leading cause of morbidity and mortality between the ages 0 and 19 years in the United States. Traumatic injuries include drowning, falls, burns, and injuries involved during transport. Accidents involving transport include occupants of motor vehicles, pedestrians, and individuals on or around pedal cyclists. Prevention is the major objective that will improve these current statistics (CDC, n.d.).

Fractures

Although children's bones are not as brittle as those of adults, children receive more accidental blows and injuries and, consequently, suffer many fractures. Falls are frequent among children with nervous system disorders because of their impaired balance and coordination. Some fractures result from abuse. Fractures most commonly seen in children are those involving the radius, ulna, clavicle, tibia, and femur. Treatment of fractures includes casts and traction. When a child is in a cast or traction, check circulation by observing skin color, sensitivity, temperature, motion, and pulse distal to the injury (Chapter 77).

NCLEX Alert

Safety concerns are commonly integrated into NCLEX clinical scenarios. Correct clinical responses may integrate age, development, disease, physical immobility, or any instance of the need for supervision.

Lacerations, Cuts, and Puncture Wounds

Many children come to an emergency department (ED) with cuts and punctures from knives, forks, pencils, or other sharp objects found in the home. The preventive measure is for family caregivers to keep such objects out of children's reach.

Children also may sustain crushing injuries from being caught in car doors or under heavy pieces of furniture, or from being hit by moving vehicles or bicycles. Serious injuries can also occur with electric car windows or garage doors. Bruises and abrasions can result from falls from tricycles, wagons, or playground equipment.

When caring for such injuries, the healthcare provider will suture lacerations, apply antiseptics and dressings, and send children for x-ray examinations if necessary to determine the presence of fractures. A tetanus booster may be given, depending on the injury and immunization status. Remind caregivers that a tetanus immunization does not protect against any other form of infection and that wounds need to be kept clean and dry. Educate the caregivers to monitor the wound for signs of infection, such as increasing redness, odors, and drainage.

Foreign Objects

Children learn about the world by exploring. Part of this exploration may include picking up small objects and trying to put them into any convenient body opening, including the mouth, ears, nose, rectum, or vagina. Young children need close observation from family caregivers to avoid injuries resulting from this kind of exploring.

Animal Bites and Scratches

Animal bites can be very serious. Children should be warned never to go near a dog that is eating (even a family dog) or to pet any unfamiliar dog. Sometimes, a dog will bite a child's face, necessitating plastic or reconstructive surgery. When a dog bites a child, determine if the dog has received a rabies immunization. If not, the dog must be isolated and watched for signs of rabies or distemper. If the dog becomes ill or cannot be found, the child must receive prophylactic rabies injections; a tetanus booster also may be necessary. Very few documented cases exist of the survival of humans who were infected with rabies.

A cat scratch that becomes infected is referred to as *cat scratch disease* or *cat scratch fever.* It is caused by the bacteria *Bartonella henselae,* which is present in the saliva of about 40% of cats. Because cats lick their paws frequently, a cat scratch is treated as a bite and requires wound cleaning and antibiotics.

Cleanse scratches carefully and apply an antibiotic ointment. Prophylactic antibiotics may be prescribed. If a scratch becomes infected, the child should see a healthcare provider immediately. The child may have a low-grade fever and malaise. Lymphadenopathy may last 2–3 months. As with dogs that bite, cats that scratch must be watched for signs of rabies.

Wild animals also bite people, particularly when trapped or frightened. They are often carriers of rabies or other diseases. Report such bites, and treat and monitor the victim to avoid serious complications.

Burns

Chapters 43 and 75 discuss burns in more detail. Most information found in these chapters applies to children as well as adults. (In Practice: Educating the Client 75-2 lists methods of burn prevention.)

The chief nursing concerns in treating burns are combating shock, alleviating pain, and restoring fluid and electrolyte balance. Secondary interventions include the prevention of infection and contractures, and the reconstruction or repair of damage. Children who have been severely burned are best cared for in a specialized burn unit.

Treatment for burns is long term. Frequently, pressure garments are used to prevent contractures and scarring. Children may need to wear pressure garments continuously for 12–18 months; these garments require replacement to accommodate growth. Family members need understanding and support during a child's rehabilitation period. Children younger than 5 years have difficulty recovering from burns because their thin skin receives deep burns, they have incomplete immune systems, and they dehydrate easily.

SPECIAL CONSIDERATIONS Lifespan

Burns

Even a superficial burn is critical if it covers two thirds or more of an infant's body.

The extent of burns is determined on a percentage basis. Burns may be classified as *partial thickness* or *full thickness*, relating to the type of grafting that may be needed. Because a child's body surface differs in proportion from that of an adult, the following method should be used to determine the extent of a burn. Remember that an infant's head is large in proportion to the body.

- *The newborn:* The head is 17% of the entire body surface; each arm, 8%; each leg, 13%; the front or back, 20%; and genitals, 1%.
- *The 3-year-old:* The head is 15%; each arm, 8%; each leg, 14%; the front or back, 20%; and genitals, 1%.
- *The 6-year-old:* The head is 11%; each arm, 8%; each leg, 16%; front or back, 20%; and genitals, 1%.
- *Older than 12 years:* The "rule of nines" applies (Chapter 75): the head is 9%; each arm, 9%; each leg, 18%; front or back, 18%; and genitals, 1%.

Poisoning

More than 80% of poisonings occur in the home. Inquisitive toddlers, who put anything and everything into the mouth, can easily ingest one or more of these substances. See In Practice: Educating the Client 72-2 for poisoning prevention measures.

Cleaning compounds are a major problem because they are usually kept under the sink or on the floor of the bathroom closet and, therefore, are easily accessible. There has been a notable decrease in accidental poisonings since drug companies began installing safety caps on bottles. However, many older adults with arthritic hands ask their pharmacists to dispense prescriptions with a regular cap rather than a safety cap. Consequently, medications continue to contribute to accidental poisonings. Another factor that contributes to the problem of accidental poisoning is the appearance of medications manufactured for children. Often these drugs are packaged attractively, taste good, and are in "fun" shapes. As a result, many small children mistake these medications for candy. Children can also be poisoned by consuming an overdose of a medication that had been prescribed for them.

Poisonous house plants and cigarette butts, which are poisonous if eaten, should be kept out of children's reach. **Plumbism** (lead poisoning) results from inhaling or eating leaded substances, such as flakes of lead paint.

Poison Treatment

In the event of poisoning, family caregivers should call their local poison control center or the *American Association of Poison Control Centers at 1-800-222-1222* immediately. Special personnel can determine the best treatment for the particular poison. The person calling the center should take the container of the substance to the telephone in order to give information as quickly as possible. The poison control center's number should be placed on all telephones used by family members. In most areas of the United States and

---

IN PRACTICE
EDUCATING THE CLIENT 72-2 Poison Prevention

- Post the local poison control center number (1-800-222-1222) on all telephones in the house.
- Label all poisonous chemicals with warning labels and store them in locked cabinets.
- Keep medications and poisonous materials in their original containers. Never put any poisonous substance in a soda or drink container.
- Use childproof caps whenever possible. Always close them properly.
- Teach children the dangers of poisonous materials and medications. Keep medications in a locked cabinet.
- Keep edibles in separate cabinets from inedibles.
- Never leave children alone when poisonous materials are nearby.
- Never treat medicines and vitamins as though they are candy. Do not purchase medicines resembling candy, animals, people, or cartoon characters.
- Read product labels carefully and follow precautions. Never give medications in the dark.
- Dispose of poisonous materials and medications carefully. Follow current guidelines for disposing of medications, which currently involve taking them to a designated drop-off. Do not throw them in the trash or flush them down the toilet.
- Never smoke around children. Keep all fresh or used smoking materials, including ashtrays and butts, away from children.
- Watch children when visiting relatives and friends. A new setting is frequently an invitation for children to explore.
- Remain calm in an emergency. Dial the emergency number, give all information, and follow directions.
- Take the container of the medicine or poison to the emergency department with you. If you are uncertain what was ingested, list all possible substances.

Canada, dialing 911 provides immediate access to emergency assistance.

When a poisoned child arrives in the ED, specific procedures are performed. Sometimes, the stomach is washed out (*gastric lavage*), usually with normal saline, in an effort to remove as much poison as possible. This procedure must be done quickly to prevent as much absorption of the harmful substance into the bloodstream as possible.

Nursing Considerations

The nurse may be asked to assist with gastric lavage. In most EDs, the needed equipment is packaged as a "gavage set." You should assist with procedures, document all pertinent information, and support the child and family. If several hours have passed since the child ingested the toxin, stomach lavage is usually not performed because the child has probably already absorbed most of the substance. In this case, the symptoms are treated. Be ready to assist with suctioning (to prevent aspiration), oxygen administration, resuscitation, catheterization, blood sampling, x-ray studies, and electrocardiograms (ECGs). After lavage, the child generally remains in the ED for 1–2 hr before discharge, unless their bloodstream has absorbed much of the poison. In this case, the child is admitted to the facility for observation. When the child is released from the healthcare facility, instruct family caregivers to watch for unfavorable symptoms that are specific to the type of poison ingested. Advise them to return the child to the ED if such symptoms develop.

Nursing care involves observing the child for any change in level of consciousness (LOC), dizziness, nausea, vomiting, unusual behavior, extreme drowsiness, or excitement. Sometimes irreversible physical or mental changes occur.

Surgery must be performed occasionally to correct physical damage caused by ingested caustic substances. In severe poisonings, the child may have renal failure and may require *dialysis*, a process whereby wastes are removed from the body when the kidneys are not functioning. In the worst case, the child could die.

> **Key Concept**
> Poisonings and accidents sometimes occur during periods of change for the family because adult members are distracted. Typical changes include a move to a new home, the death of a family member, the birth of a new baby, or divorce or separation.

Suffocation

The many causes of suffocation in infants and children include the aspiration of a foreign object or smothering with a pillow or plastic bag. Infants or children should not use pillows until they are able to turn themselves over freely. Mattresses should never be covered with any type of plastic bag.

Infants are obligatory nose breathers who have not yet learned mouth breathing. Suffocation can result if an infant with an upper respiratory infection (**URI**) cannot clear mucus plugging the bronchi. Humidity and normal saline nose spray usually helps to loosen secretions. A bulb syringe should be available to assist in keeping the infant's nasal airway clear of mucus accumulation.

Children can suffocate if they become trapped in discarded refrigerators or other enclosed spaces. Children seeking treats in large freezers have been known to fall into the freezers and be unable to rescue themselves. Trunks and toy chests can also be fatal traps. State laws generally call for the removal of doors from all discarded refrigerators and upright freezers or for them to be turned tightly against a wall.

Drowning

Danger areas for drowning are age related. Infants are subject to drowning in bathtubs, toilets, or containers of standing water (e.g., a dog dish or a pail). Residential swimming pools are danger zones for children. The resuscitation of drowning victims depends on the amount of time that the victim was without oxygen and the temperature of the water.

> **Key Concept**
> Drownings can occur in any body of water. Keep small buckets of any fluid away from young children. Never allow children to swim alone. Constant vigilance is the key component to safety.

Sudden Unexpected Infant Death and Sudden Infant Death Syndrome

Sudden unexpected infant death (**SUID**) is the term used when an infant dies suddenly and unexpectedly. The causative agents for SUIDS are not immediately known before investigation. Causes of SUIDS may include metabolic disorders, poisonings, hypothermia, hyperthermia, neglect, abuse, and accidental suffocation or can remain unknown.

Sudden infant death syndrome (**SIDS**) is the sudden, unexplained death of a seemingly healthy infant. Half of all defined SUIDS cases are owing to SIDS. SIDS occurs while the infant is asleep and is the primary cause of death in infants 1 month to 1 year of age. This diagnosis can be made only following a thorough autopsy, forensic evaluation of the scene of death, and a review of the child's clinical history.

Although the etiology of SIDS is unknown, one theory suggests that an abnormality in brain stem functioning results in faulty respirations. Sleeping in a prone position has a strong connection to SIDS. Additional causes may include incomplete bubbling after feeding, secondhand smoke, and the use of a pillow. Small-for-gestational-age (**SGA**) infants are at a greater risk.

Prolonged infantile apnea (**PIA**) is defined as cessation of breathing for at least 20 s or for a shorter time with accompanying bradycardia, cyanosis (bluish skin), and/or pallor. When this condition is discovered (via a "near miss"), an **apnea monitor** can be used to prevent SIDS. Some infants at high risk are placed on an apnea monitor until about 1 year of age. The apnea monitor functions through electrodes placed on the infant that are attached to a small bedside monitor. The machine sounds an alarm when there is a breach of preset respiratory parameters (e.g., no respirations for more than 15 s).

> **SPECIAL CONSIDERATIONS   Culture and Ethnicity**
> **Cyanosis**
> Cyanosis is more difficult to determine in dark-skinned children; however, a definite duskiness is present in the skin, lips, and nail beds regardless of the child's skin tone.

In addition to experiencing profound shock and grief, families of children who die suddenly often feel overwhelming guilt. When this tragedy occurs, be particularly sensitive and offer support and compassion. Provide families with information regarding support groups that are available locally.

CHILD ABUSE

Child abuse is a widespread social problem and, as a consequence, has serious healthcare implications. Definitions of **child abuse** and neglect vary according to state or federal legislation, but generally include the following: actions that are seen as threats (e.g., words), situations with a potential for harm (e.g., unsafe environments), exploitation (e.g., having a child earn money, leaving a child to care for younger siblings, or having a child cook for the family), injury, or death. The definition of "child" varies but technically includes an individual younger than 18 years who is not an emancipated minor. Most abuse by either commission or omission is caused by a caregiver, for example, a parent, relative, or teacher. Neglect is more often considered an act of omission, that is, the failure to provide for a child's basic needs. Abuse and neglect can have profound short- and long-term consequences. If the situation of abuse or neglect is reversed or corrected, thriving is possible. Many children die or are temporarily or permanently injured each year as a result of abuse.

Child abuse takes several forms, including physical neglect, emotional neglect, physical abuse, emotional abuse, and sexual abuse. As a nurse, you are considered a **mandatory reporter**. If you suspect child abuse or neglect, you are obligated by law to report it to your supervisor, a healthcare provider, or the police authorities. Being aware of the signs and symptoms of child abuse begins by knowing the normal growth and developmental milestones. Children who have had difficulties thriving may not achieve these milestones within expected normal ranges.

Signs and symptoms of child abuse or neglect may not always be clearly recognizable. Children who have been mistreated may be afraid to tell others of their situation. Physical and emotional signs or symptoms may be confused with the activities of normal growth and development. The different forms of child abuse (e.g., physical, emotional, sexual) may bring about variable behaviors in the child. To assist with accurate detection, many facilities offer healthcare specialists who have had additional training and experience in child abuse pediatrics. When available, the *child abuse pediatrician* or other healthcare specialist in child abuse should be among the first personnel called to interact with and to observe the child. Advanced training helps such specialists to visualize any causative factors and to provide effective interventions for the welfare of the child. Individuals who do not have this training or experience may not be effective caregivers for the child and family. The specialist may also be able to explain the overall situation to other caregivers nonjudgmentally. See In Practice: Data Gathering in Nursing 72-1 for significant considerations in suspected child abuse.

> **Key Concept**
> A sudden change of behavior in a child of any age is a clue that something in that child's life may be causing a problem. Abuse may be recognized by anger, silence, acting out, depression, or other changes in behavior.

Anger is likely to be your first response to any kind of child abuse. If you observe a suspicious situation that could be child abuse or neglect, take the time to remain objective. Be aware of possible personal problems of the suspected abuser, such as low self-esteem, rejection, and isolation. Include objective explanations and be consistent in your approach. Suspected abusers are often in an environment that is out of control.

> **Key Concept**
> If you suspect child abuse, you must, by law, report it immediately. Nurses who do not do so are committing a crime. Those reporting suspected abusers are legally protected against recourse.

Support groups throughout the country assist abusers in breaking the cycle of abuse. The goal of support groups is to provide ongoing help via counseling programs and to promote day-to-day assistance in pursuing nonabusive lifestyles.

Your role as a mandated reporter of suspected child abuse is important. Following are guidelines for reporting abuse:

- *Reporting abuse is mandated.* Follow your facility protocol or call your local child protection agency if you have any concerns about a child or about appropriate procedure.
- *Believe the child.* If a child confides in you, assume that they are telling the truth.
- *Observe the child's reactions.* Look not only for marks and bruises but also for reactions. An abused child may draw away when touched or avoid contact or interaction with others. The child may attempt to protect the abuser by making excuses for "accidents."
- *Document your observations.* Carefully observe the signs of abuse. Be objective. Identify and document every observation to the last detail. Measure bruises, abrasions, and other signs of injury. Take photographs.
- *Teach the child.* The child needs to learn what activities are inappropriate, what to do if someone tries to exploit them, and that mistreatment is not something they "deserve."

For more information, see In Practice: Nursing Care Plan 72-1.

Neglect

Neglect involves the failure to meet emotional and physical needs or offer the basic protections from harm or potential harm related to childcare. Child maltreatment can also include the lack of attention to educational or medical needs. It is the duty of caregivers to ensure that every child receives an education and medical preventative care (e.g., immunizations or medical treatments) if the need arises. An *emotionally neglected* child is deprived of love, affection, and attention from family caregivers, or is continually berated, called derogatory names, and told that they are stupid. A *physically neglected* child does not receive adequate food, water, clothing, or medical care (In Practice: Data Gathering in Nursing 72-1). Child abuse specialists and trained social workers may be needed to help discern the often vague differences between normal incidents or accidents and neglect or abuse. In any situation of concern, remember that the priorities are related to protecting the child and providing guidance to a family

IN PRACTICE
DATA GATHERING IN NURSING 72-1 | Detecting Child Abuse

Adults and Risk Factors
Adults who have risk factors for committing child abuse include the following:

- Adults who have suffered abuse, neglect, or rejection in their past
- Adults with a history of dependency on others
- Adults with a history of depression or mental health problems
- Adults who feel isolated and alone (e.g., parents whose spouse is away on a military tour)
- Adults with one or more of the following personality traits: hostility, tendency to blame others, punitiveness, low self-esteem, or impulsiveness
- Adults who are caring for unwanted or foster children
- Young and immature family caregivers
- Individuals in troubled relationships who have unmet needs or who are subject to excessive demands, rejection, or abuse from their partners
- Individuals who live in poverty or in low-income environments
- Those who use drugs excessively
- Adults with high expectations of their children, or those who are overcritical and who do not view the child positively
- Adults who use extreme discipline measures
- Family caregivers who have exhibited a loss of control in disciplining, such as slapping, shaking, and hitting the child
- Adults who are overwhelmed by their children's emotional and physical needs and demands
- Individuals who are unable to cope with daily activities, which can lead to irritability and frustration
- Family caregivers who seldom touch or look at their child, react with impatience, or ignore their child's crying

School-Age Children
Suspect abuse when you encounter school-age children who exhibit the following behaviors:

- Lying about an injury
- Behavior problems
- Expectation of abusive behavior
- Lawbreaking
- Use and abuse of drugs, especially at an early age
- Truancy
- Self-injurious behavior; suicidal thoughts or attempts
- Promiscuous behavior

Young children
Suspect abuse when you encounter infants, toddlers, and preschoolers who exhibit the following:

- Injuries at various stages of healing (could not have happened at the same time)
- Inappropriate sexual knowledge
- Agreement with family caregivers on illogical causes of injury
- Burns, lacerations, or serious bruises without the appearance of accidents; unexplained fractures; missing chunks of hair
- Attempts to stay away from home
- Attempts to hide scars with clothing
- Frequent injuries
- Extreme fear of adults; fear of being touched
- An appearance of neglect: dirty, unkempt, extremely thin, lethargic
- Stomach problems, colitis, rectal/vaginal bleeding, frequent headaches

Neglect
Suspect child neglect in the following instances:

- Abandonment of child by caregiver
- Inadequate medical or dental care, hygiene, clothing, supply or quality of food, sleep
- Unmet needs relating to physical or mental problems
- Isolation of family from usual social contacts
- Excessive demands placed on the child (expected to do all the housework or accept total care of younger siblings)
- Child left without custodial care or supervision

---

or caregiver. In many early contacts with healthcare providers, the caregivers/parents may seem incapable of working with a child in distress, be excessively emotional or lacking in emotion, and be seemingly unaware of the seriousness of the child's urgent physical or emotional needs.

Physical Abuse

Physical abuse generally refers to a situation in which a child has been physically harmed and injury has occurred; standardized definitions of abuse are not yet available. The injury is inflicted intentionally and can vary from minor bruising to death. *Shaken baby syndrome* is an example of physical abuse. In these cases, an adult violently shakes the baby. It usually occurs when the adult becomes frustrated after attempts to quiet the crying infant. The immature development of the infant's neck muscles (leading to lack of head control), along with the violent shaking, results in cerebral trauma or hemorrhage. Visual impairment, including blindness, motor impairment, serious intellectual impairment, and death, can result.

Evidence of physical abuse can take a variety of forms. Unexplained bruises in various stages of healing, cigarette burns, scars, and numerous unexplained fractures that have healed are common indicators.

IN PRACTICE
NURSING CARE PLAN 72-1: The Child Who May Be a Victim of Abuse

Medical history: F.M. is a 4-year-old boy admitted to the pediatric unit from the emergency department following treatment for an asthmatic attack secondary to pneumonia. Client is receiving continuous intravenous (IV) therapy along with nebulized bronchodilators administered every 2 hr. He is receiving oxygen via mask at 4 L/min. This is his fifth admission for asthma; his first admission was when he was 30 months old. His appearance is apathetic, and he does not interact with nurses or physical therapy staff. His face and clothes are unclean with the appearance of not being washed for several days. Parents state that they ran out of his asthma medicine last week. Past medical history (from previous admission records) reveals visits to the emergency department for spiral fracture of the left forearm and a mild concussion.

Medical diagnosis: Asthma, pneumonia; rule out suspected physical abuse

DATA COLLECTION/NURSING OBSERVATION	NURSING DIAGNOSIS
A 4-year-old male client sleeping off and on. Client unable to provide any history. On examination, bruises are noted on the back and torso in several stages of healing. Small circular burnlike area approximately 1/4 in. in diameter is noted on buttocks (appears to be a cigarette burn). When questioned about the bruises, his family caregivers state, "He's so clumsy and he falls a lot." When questioned about the client's asthma regimen, the caregivers state, "We tried giving them for a while but he never got better so we stopped." Child withdraws but does not cry when touched. Child neglect and possible abuse are suspected.	(Although other nursing diagnoses pertaining to asthma or respiratory distress may be appropriate, this NCP presents the priority nursing diagnosis as addressed below.) • Impaired parenting related to unmet social/emotional/maturational needs of the family caregivers and lack of knowledge about child's needs, as evidenced by the bruising and frequent visits to the emergency department and hospitalizations relating to inadequate home management of asthma.

PLANNING (Outcomes/Goals)	IMPLEMENTATION (Nursing Actions)	EVALUATION
Short-Term Goals A. Child will be placed in a safe environment pending observations of respiratory status and interactions with others, plus observations of discussions and activities between caregivers and parents. (*Note to Student: See *In Practice Data Gathering in Nursing 72-1: Detecting Child Abuse*)	• Reassure child that he is in a safe place with people who will protect him from harm. • Report the case to child protective services. • Maintain protective status of child until child protective service assumes control. • Monitor respiratory status. • Continue nebulized, short-acting bronchodialators. *Rationale: All states have mandatory laws for reporting child maltreatment; reassuring the child helps to foster the development of trust. Maintaining the child's safety is the priority. Respirations need to be monitored but, at this time, do not seem to be the priority problem. Maintaining a safe environment may help assist the child's asthma.* • Observe child's behaviors and document present physical condition with notations and photos made of bruises, and skin conditions (e.g., burns, lesions). • Document presence of old vs new injuries. • Obtain x-rays as ordered by healthcare providers or social service healthcare advisor. • Research past history of sibling abuse. *Rationale: Not all children receive the same type of parental attention. Some children are more likely to be abused than other children.*	Pediatric unit Day 1—15:00 hr Child observed playing quietly in bed with play therapist at bedside. When family caregivers visiting, nurse present at all times. Respiratory status with good aeration. No wheezing at this time. Nebulized, short-acting bronchodilators improving asthma symptoms. **Goal A complete.** Observations continue.

PLANNING (Outcomes/ Goals)	IMPLEMENTATION (Nursing Actions)	EVALUATION
Short-Term Goals		
	• Interview or have pediatric medical or social services interview caregivers. • Consider any history of abuse of caregivers as a child. • Obtain baseline of parenting skills and expectations of children. • Consider factors that may lead to lack of knowledge of parenting skills such as feelings of isolation or lack of resources to deal with multiple life stresses. *Rationale: Determining the caregivers' potential for abuse provides a baseline for further investigation and inquiry. Abusive caregivers were often abused as children. Determine the family's ability to cope with issues such as isolation from support (as may occur in military families) or lack of resources (healthcare, basic finances).*	
B. Family caregivers will identify the need for help and to adapt to positive child-rearing behaviors.	• Provide consistent behaviors that promote positive parenting/caretaking. • Promote feelings of acceptance of, and affection for, the child. • Implement a program of attention based on play, group interaction with other children, and quiet time with the child. • Ensure that someone is in the child's room at all times when parental caregivers are present. *Rationale: Parental acceptance is critical to the child's welfare. Meeting the child's anxiety needs is fundamental to care and safety. Having someone present when family caregivers are present reduces the risk of trauma to the child.* • Attempt to establish a supportive relationship with caregivers. • Acknowledge the difficulties of parenthood and child-rearing. • Promote opportunities to act as a role model for positive interactions with the child and to teach parenting skills. *Rationale: Establishing a supportive relationship is essential to building trust with the caregivers and to accept the problem of inadequate parental skills. Role modeling provides an opportunity for teaching.*	Day 2—1830 hr Caregivers deny any problem on admission. Communications between nursing staff, child protective services, and parents occur throughout the day. Caregivers continue to deny abuse of child and refer to bruises as being the child's fault or that child was punished for bad behavior. Caregivers mentioned their own family experiences during childhood. Many experiences involved having frequent episodes of verbal and physical assaults by their own parents. At suggestion of nursing staff, caregivers request a conversation with counselor. After speaking to counselor, an appointment is made for parents and child protection services to discuss parent's current child-rearing behaviors. **Goal B partially met.** Observations and interventions continue.

PLANNING (Outcomes/Goals)	IMPLEMENTATION (Nursing Actions)	EVALUATION
Long-Term Goals		
C. Family caregivers actively participate in group counseling for parenting.	• After trust and a supportive relationship are established, assist the caregivers in acknowledging the problem and recommend that the caregivers voluntarily seek professional counseling. *Rationale: Abusing caregivers have rarely learned to trust others and may feel defensive about their deficiencies. A caregiver needs to acknowledge the problem before being able to seek help.* • Observe and document behaviors, effect, and comments made by child. • Encourage caregivers to continue to meet with counselor and to practice positive role model parenting behaviors. • Observe caregivers for imitation of these behaviors. *Rationale: Emotionally neglected children may demonstrate self-destructive behaviors or be passive and withdrawn. They may have difficulty sleeping, experience nightmares, and show signs of depression. Physically neglected children may appear disheveled, unclean, and malnourished. They may show evidence of untreated dental problems.*	Day 3—1500 hr Caregivers currently state that they will be attending weekly counseling sessions. Caregivers demonstrating beginning awareness of ability to differentiate child abuse from productive parenting. **Goal A met.** Progress to meeting Goals B and C.
D. Family caregivers begin to demonstrate effective parenting skills.	• Observe caregivers for signs of readiness for discharge. • Arrange continuation of parenting education of asthma therapies for after discharge. *Rationale: Continuing to meet with a counselor aids in working through the problems. Caregivers demonstrating behaviors indicates learning.*	Day 4—discharge plans Social service workers inform nursing staff that in-home visits are scheduled. Asthma controlled by oral and inhaled medications. **Goals B, C, and D met.** Observations and interventions continue.

*Note to Student: Knowledge and experience are necessary in the detection and treatment of any form of child abuse. Refer to In Practice Data Gathering in Nursing 72-1: Detecting Child Abuse.

> **Key Concept**
> Accidental brain injury can occur when a child is thrown into the air and caught. Caution caregivers about the dangers of this type of play.

Emotional Abuse

Emotional neglect, which may include social or emotional isolation, may be defined as the intentional omission of positive words or behaviors that would encourage the development of self-esteem and self-respect. *Emotional abuse* is often difficult to document with certainty. An observer may notice frequent verbal comments that result in loss or destruction of a child's self-esteem. Rejecting and threatening the child may also be observed or reported. Lack of supportive emotional concern may be combined with overactive criticism, especially of relatively minor events. Emotional abuse is often combined with varying degrees of physical neglect or abuse.

Sexual Abuse

Sexual abuse of children ranges from exposure and fondling to anal, vaginal, or oral intercourse. The typical pattern is one of secrecy. The abuser may be a stranger, someone the child knows well, or a family member (incest). They can be an adult, adolescent, or an older child. The abused child may be as young as 1 year of age or younger.

As the abused child grows older, the abuser tells them to keep the abuse a secret and may threaten the child. By the time an abused individual is old enough to realize that what is happening is wrong, they are too ashamed and afraid to reveal the truth. Their reaction is typically guilt and fear. In many cases, the child represses the abuse, only for it to surface in flashbacks, nightmares, and self-injurious or self-defeating behavior years later. Sexual abuse of children includes child pornography.

Sexual abuse is difficult to identify and harder to prove. Following are signs of sexual abuse:

- Sudden behavioral changes
- Abdominal pain, gastric distress, or headaches
- Emotional disturbances
- Avoidance of touching or physical contact
- Vaginal or rectal bleeding or lesions

Many schools now have programs that teach young children about sexual abuse and incest. These programs demonstrate "good touch and bad touch" and help children learn to say "no" and to seek help. Children learn to avoid strangers and to report any uncomfortable incidents to persons in authority. These programs encourage a strong feeling of self-worth.

Failure to Thrive

Inadequate physical growth is termed *failure to thrive* (**FTT**). FTT may involve only weight or it may involve weight and height. Characteristic developmental symptoms include retarded motor development, inadequate social response, and delayed language development. FTT children are withdrawn and apathetic, do not relate to their environment, and do not cry. Psychologically, these children show a *flat affect*, which means that the child has little or no emotional expression in response to external stimulation.

A physiologic problem, such as cystic fibrosis, celiac disease, gastroenteritis, parasites, or congenital heart disease, may cause FTT. More commonly, FTT has a psychosocial rather than a congenital physical cause. If the cause is related to a difficult social or home situation, commonly owing to a disturbance in the parent–child relationship, the FTT child may appear malnourished and may have spindly arms and legs, a potbelly, and an unnaturally old appearance (Fig. 72-2).

Infants diagnosed or suspected of having FTT may be passive and withdrawn and may have developmental delays. Family caregivers of FTT children may not be able to afford food, may have inadequate nutritional knowledge, or have health beliefs (dietary restrictions) that prevent the child from receiving adequate nutrition. Avoid judgment or blame of family caregivers. Recommend family counseling and education. New or alternative parenting skills can be reinforced. Nutritional needs of children of different ages can be another area of focus.

Take a developmental history of FTT children. If the family caregivers are the biologic parents, examine their feelings about pregnancy and having to care for children. See In Practice: Data Gathering in Nursing 72-2 for additional considerations. Healthcare providers trained in child abuse and neglect may be able to help differentiate between actual abuse and lack of parenting skills.

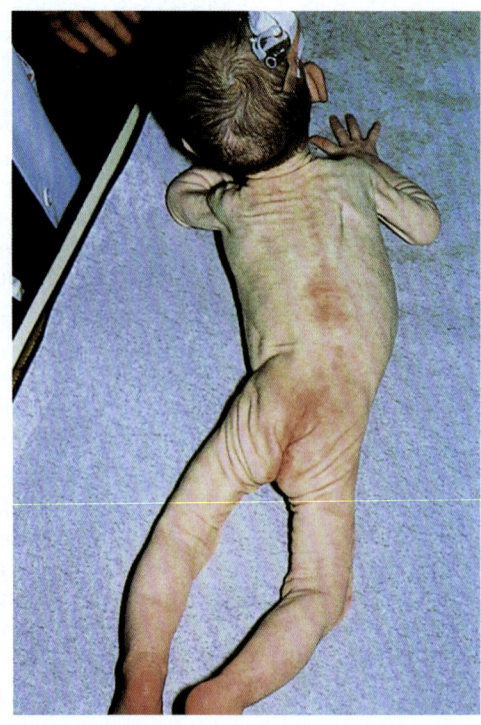

Figure 72-2 Failure to thrive (FTT). The child with failure to thrive experiences a loss of subcutaneous fat, muscle wasting, and skin breakdown.

IN PRACTICE
DATA GATHERING IN NURSING 72-2 — Failure to Thrive Danger Signals

Familial Causes
- Early separation of mother from infant, which leads to inadequate bonding
- Major depression or mental illness of a prominent caregiver early in the child's life
- Major family crisis that disrupts normal family interaction
- Serious illness of the infant, which leads to an inability to form strong familial bonding
- Family caregivers who isolate themselves or who have marital problems
- Very young caregivers or caregivers with minimal parenting skills
- Serious illness or death of caregiver or sibling

Infant-Related Causes
- Prematurity, illness, congenital malformation, malabsorption disorders
- Reduced responsiveness and interaction with others in the environment
- Dislike of cuddling, slow social development (e.g., does not smile), difficulty in feeding
- Disorders, such as severe autism or mental retardation

The FTT infant is often hospitalized from 10–14 days. The child is fed on demand, at least every 2–3 hr. If the resulting weight gain is appropriate, FTT is a definite diagnosis. If the child does not gain weight, physiologic reasons must be sought. A physical examination is essential, including a complete blood workup.

Family caregivers should be with their infants to provide care and to spend as much time as possible. Tender loving care and stimulation are essential. Hold such children and rock and cuddle them. Educate caregivers to look for positive signs (smiles, responsiveness).

Accurate recordings of intake and output (I&O) are essential. Be sure to follow the feeding schedule. In older children, record accurate food and fluid intake.

SKIN DISORDERS

Nevi

A **nevus** (plural: nevi) is an abnormal skin mark that can be either hereditary or acquired as a result of *teratogens* (substances that damage the development of a fetus). A nevus may be pigmented or vascular. Some types are called "birthmarks." Pigmented nevi (birthmarks or moles) are either simple brown spots or dark hairy spots composed of cells containing melanin. Although normally harmless, nevi require close observation because they can develop into malignant melanomas. Pigmented nevi are removed if any chance exists that they are malignant. They are sometimes removed for cosmetic reasons.

A vascular nevus (*angioma*) may be of two types. **Lymphangiomas** are overgrowths of lymph vessels. **Hemangiomas** are overgrowths of blood vessels. A *capillary hemangioma* ("port-wine stain," *nevus flammeus*) is a red or purple lesion that usually does not fade. Port-wine stains, especially on the face, can be treated with a series of pulse laser treatments under anesthesia. An immature hemangioma ("strawberry mark," *nevus vasculosus*) usually regresses and disappears, making treatment unnecessary. A *cavernous hemangioma* is a raised, red lesion that does not regress.

Mongolian spots are irregular dark, blue–green areas generally found on the lower back. The shapes have regular edges and are NOT a sign of abuse. They are almost always present in Asian infants and are frequently found in Mediterranean and African infants. They usually disappear by about the age of 2–3 years and should be documented for reference.

Rash

Many small babies experience rashes of unknown cause. Infant and toddler skin is very delicate and easily irritated. Some rashes are symptomatic of infectious diseases. If no cause can be determined, treat the rash symptomatically. Exposure to air, topical ointments, or lotions may relieve the rash. Symptoms, such as itching, may be treated with medicated baths or antipruritic medications.

Eczema

Eczema, a severe atopic dermatitis, is characterized by remissions and exacerbations accompanied by vesicle formation, oozing, crusting, excoriations, and itching. Usually beginning on the cheeks, it may move to other parts of the body and usually decreases as the child ages. It appears to worsen in cold weather and tends to run in families. Eczema may occur owing to an allergy, although often the cause is unknown.

The baby with severe eczema is miserable; they cry and want to scratch constantly. Scratching can lead to severe excoriation, streptococcal or staphylococcal infection, scarring, or a dangerous complication called *eczema herpeticum* (eczema complicated by herpes virus). Spending a lot of time with this baby is a good idea because when the baby is alone they will probably need to be restrained to prevent scratching. An effective restraint is the elbow restraint. A child can be restrained in a rocking chair so that they can move but cannot scratch.

Dermatitis packs or therapeutic colloidal baths often relieve itching. Sometimes antibiotic or cortisone ointments are applied (Chapter 75).

Adjust the child's diet to eliminate identified allergy-producing substances. Dietary adjustments often include trial of various types of formulas. Gradually, foods are added to the diet at the rate of one new food per week (known as an elimination diet). Instruct family caregivers to use nonallergenic coverings on crib mattresses. Pets may need to find new homes.

Cradle cap is seborrheic dermatitis of the scalp. It often occurs when a caregiver is apprehensive about hurting the infant's soft spot. Teach the family caregiver that regular shampooing and brushing of the baby's head is important.

MUSCULOSKELETAL AND ORTHOPEDIC DISORDERS

Chapter 77 discusses orthopedic nursing. Before caring for a child in a cast or in traction, be sure to examine specific related procedures in that chapter.

Developmental Dysplasia

One or both hips may be improperly located in the ball and socket joints; the head of the femur may be displaced, or the acetabulum may develop improperly. These conditions are known as **dysplasia**, causing hip dislocation. If the disorder is unilateral (on one side only), the buttock on the affected side has an additional crease, and the child's two knees are not level when they lay on the back with the hips and knees flexed and the soles flat on the bed (*Allis sign*). The child's knee on the affected side is lower.

Radiographic studies are diagnostic. In addition, the child shows limited abduction on the affected side when the knees are flexed while in the supine position. This condition occurs more frequently in girls; it is uncommon among African Americans; and it occurs most often on one side only. It is common in breech intrauterine position, especially frank breech, and in multiple births.

If untreated, the dislocation causes deformity in later life, characterized by a shorter leg and limited abduction on the affected side; the person limps and has *lordosis* (concave curvature of the lumbar spine) and a protruding abdomen.

Medical Treatment

Early diagnosis and treatment are essential. If dysplasia is diagnosed before complete dislocation occurs, the condition

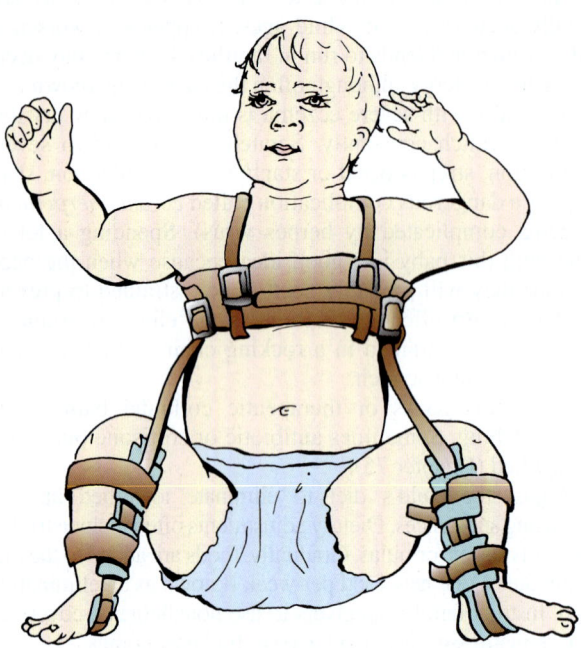

Figure 72-3 An infant in a Pavlik harness. The harness consists of shoulder straps, stirrups, and a chest strap. It is placed on both legs even if only one hip is dislocated. (Nettina, 2006.)

can be treated medically. Most affected infants have dysplasia without dislocation. This disorder is usually discovered when the child is in the newborn nursery or at the 6-week checkup.

To treat dysplasia, the infant is placed in a splint brace or Pavlik harness for 3–6 months to maintain the hips in an abducted position (Fig. 72-3). The problem may be corrected in the small infant with the use of multiple diapers, which keep the hips abducted. These measures keep the head of the femur within the acetabulum, promoting bone development.

If the hip has been dislocated, it must be repositioned and maintained in that position. If ligaments or muscles have been torn, the child may wear a spica (body) cast for between 6 weeks and 9 months. Traction may be necessary before casting.

When the child has been walking for several years before diagnosis, skeletal traction may be used to try to abduct the hips gradually. If this measure is unsuccessful, surgical repair is necessary. If closed reduction under general anesthesia and casting are unsuccessful, an open reduction (through an incision) is performed. A *tenotomy* (transection of a tendon) may also be necessary. If the child has not been treated and is older than 6 years, the prognosis for prolonged maintenance of the repair is poor.

Nursing Considerations

Handle the child carefully, but pick them up to encourage normal social development. Protect the pillow splint or cast from soiling and wetting. Cover the perineal area with moisture-proof protection. Normal rules for cast care apply (Chapter 77). Watch for any signs of irritation or pressure. Turn the child often. Help the child to exercise, if possible, and take them to the play room and to meals. Monitor the child's toys because small toys can be placed inside a cast, causing skin irritation or skin ulcers.

Instruct family caregivers in the child's care. It is helpful to obtain a hospital bed with a special overhead frame to suspend splints and/or an overhead trapeze or to hang weights and pulleys. The child can change positions more easily without disruption of orthopedic therapies.

> **Nursing Alert** Skin care is especially important for the infant or child in a corrective device. Avoid using powders and lotions because "caking" or "pilling" can occur, causing added skin irritation and breakdown.

Talipes

The term *clubfoot* or **talipes** describes a foot that is twisted or bent out of shape as a result of hereditary factors or an abnormal fetal position (Fig. 72-4A). It may be flexible (owing to intrauterine positioning) or rigid and fixed. The condition occurs more commonly in boys and more often in multiple than in single births. Unilateral clubfoot is slightly more common than bilateral clubfoot.

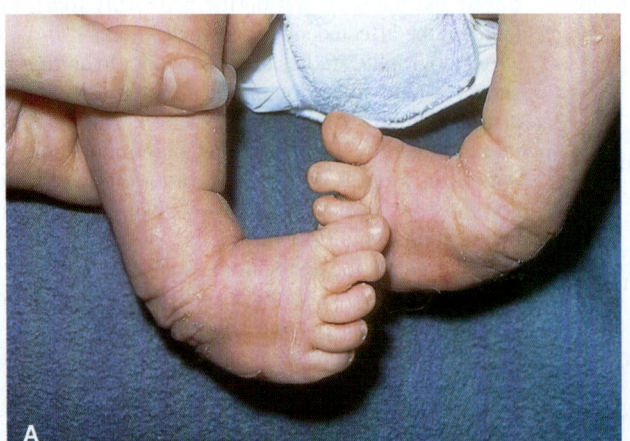
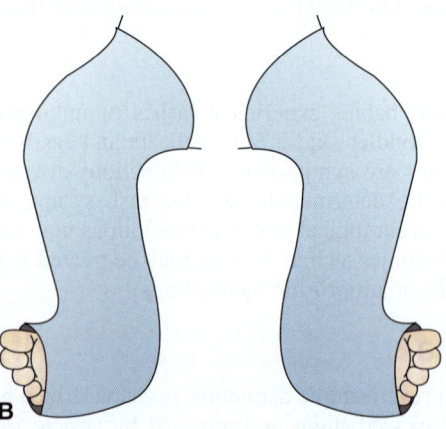

Figure 72-4 **A.** Talipes equinovarus. **B.** Casts are applied to treat bilateral clubfoot.

Medical Treatment

Treatment includes casting or splinting to correct the deformity (Fig. 72-4B); sequential casting at 1- to 2-week intervals is usual. Surgery may be necessary for older children or for those with severe defects. The type of surgery depends on the specific defect. In young children, usually only the soft tissues need to be repositioned because bones are not yet calcified. In older children, the bones may require repositioning and casting.

Nursing Considerations

Follow the usual procedures and precautions for observing and caring for children in casts. Teach family caregivers what symptoms and complications to look for. Remind them that they need a great deal of patience because a child may be in a splint or cast for several years.

Torticollis

Torticollis, also called "wryneck," may be congenital or acquired by damage to the nerves or muscles. The congenital type is caused by failure of the sternocleidomastoid muscle to lengthen as the child grows. It must be corrected, or curvature of the upper spine and abnormal elevation of the shoulders will result.

Treatment includes passive or active exercises, surgical correction, or casting. The child must be examined periodically until after puberty to prevent recurrence.

NEUROLOGIC DISORDERS

Reye Syndrome

Reye syndrome is an acute and potentially fatal childhood disease that causes swelling in the liver and brain. The condition is rare and its etiology is unknown but may be associated with inherited metabolic disorders in which the body is unable to break down fatty acids due to deficient or absent enzymes. It may also be an underlying metabolic condition that is unmasked with exposure to certain toxins such as insecticides, herbicides, or paint thinners. Generally, it affects children and teenagers. The signs and symptoms of Reye syndrome appear 3–5 days after the onset of a viral illness, such as a URI (a cold), influenza (the flu), or varicella (chickenpox).

Initial signs and symptoms for the very young may include diarrhea and tachypnea (rapid breathing). For older children and teenagers, signs and symptoms may include continuous vomiting and lethargy. As the disease worsens, symptoms become more aggressive and may require emergency treatment. Such developments include a change in mentation (mental status) such as becoming irritable, aggressive, confused, and irrational. New symptoms that include weakness or paralysis in the arms and legs, seizures, and, potentially, a decreased level of consciousness develop. Defining characteristics of Reye syndrome will show cerebral edema, impaired liver function, and severely impaired LOC. Elevated blood ammonia levels are also present.

Treatment is supportive. There are no specific diagnostic tests for the syndrome; rather, the individual has blood and urine testing that looks for metabolic oxidation or other metabolic disorders. Elevated blood ammonia levels indicate the potential for serious outcomes. Additional diagnostic procedures may include a spinal tap (lumbar puncture), liver biopsy, CT, MRI, and skin biopsy to test for fatty acid oxidation disorders. Glucose and electrolyte IV solutions are given to maintain homeostasis. Diuretics to decrease intracranial pressure known as osmotic diuretics will decrease fluid pressure within the brain. Vitamin K, plasma, and platelets are given to prevent hemorrhagic complications. Seizures may require the use of sedatives and barbiturates. Nursing considerations require the close monitoring of the child's respiratory rate as well as potential changes in breathing patterns, the onset of seizures, or the deepening of coma.

Public education regarding the dangers of aspirin use for sick children has been credited for the drastic reduction in incidences of this disease. Early diagnosis and aggressive medical intervention have greatly improved the prognosis for children who contract it.

Meningitis

Meningitis is an acute inflammation of the meninges of the brain. It may be caused by bacteria or viruses. In neonates, meningitis is most commonly caused by group B streptococci and *Escherichia coli* organisms. Immunizations, as indicated in the above section, can prevent many causes of meningitis, such as *S. pneumoniae* and *Neisseria meningitidis (meningococcal meningitis)*. In children older than 2 months, the common organism formerly was *H. influenzae*, also referred to as "H flu." This type of influenza has decreased as a cause of meningitis by 90% since the Hib immunization became common.

Symptoms of meningitis include fever and *nuchal rigidity* (neck stiffness). A lumbar puncture determines the presence of organisms in the spinal fluid. Viral meningitis is treated symptomatically. In bacterial meningitis, intravenous fluids and antibiotics are administered. Isolation is necessary until the child has been on antibiotics for 24 hr. Decreased environmental stimulation and neurologic checks are essential. Elevate the head of the bed to lessen the increased intracranial pressure that is caused by edema. Monitor I&O.

Serious complications may result from meningitis, such as hydrocephalus, learning disabilities, seizure disorders, and deafness. Chemoprophylaxis with antibiotics or antivirals may be necessary for healthcare workers, family members, and daycare workers who come in close contact with meningitis. Provide support to the family and keep them informed of the child's progress. Encourage them to express their feelings of blame and guilt.

Encephalocele

If the bones in the fetal skull do not close correctly, a portion of the brain may *herniate* (protrude) through the opening. This condition is known as **encephalocele**. The degree of damage to the child's functioning depends on the encephalocele's size and location, and on the presence or absence of strangulation or rupture in the brain. The chief danger in this condition is possible rupture of the meningeal sac, leading almost inevitably to meningitis or encephalitis. The defect can be surgically corrected; surgery is sometimes delayed until the child is 1 year old.

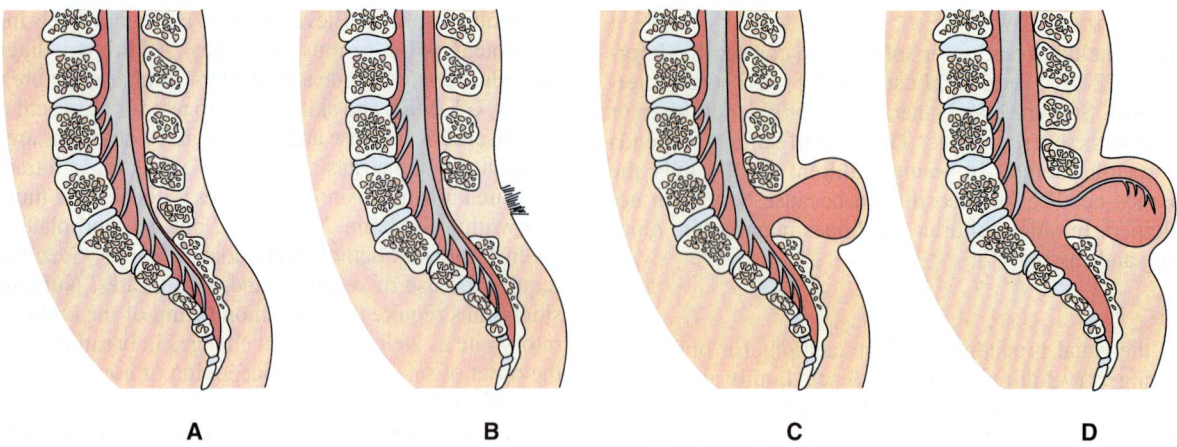

Figure 72-5 Spina bifida. **A.** Normal spine. **B.** Spina bifida occulta. **C.** Spina bifida with meningocele. **D.** Spina bifida with myelomeningocele.

Spina Bifida

Spina bifida is a malformation in which a part of the vertebral or spinal column (usually the lower spine) is open or missing (Fig. 72-5). The condition may be asymptomatic or may cause severe paralysis, depending on how large the opening is and whether the meninges or spinal cord herniate through the opening. Amniocentesis or ultrasound can detect this disorder in a fetus. The examiner checks the amniotic fluid for α-fetoprotein, which, if present, indicates an abnormality. The pregnant woman may have an elective abortion. Genetic counseling may be indicated.

Folic acid (folate) taken during pregnancy helps to prevent spina bifida (and other neural tube defects). The three forms of this disorder are spina bifida occulta, meningocele, and meningomyelocele:

- **Spina bifida occulta** is an opening in the child's vertebral column with no apparent symptoms (Fig. 72-5B). It is discovered only if an x-ray examination of the child's spine is done for an unrelated reason, or if an investigation is done because a dimple is present over the backbone. A small tuft of hair or a port-wine stain sometimes appears in the vertebral area. Although this condition may cause the child problems during the pubescent growth spurt, it generally does not cause any difficulty. It may be corrected by surgery if necessary.
- **Meningocele** occurs when one layer of the meninges (the spinal cord covering) herniates through an opening in the vertebral column (Fig. 72-5C). The child with a meningocele will have a visible sac on the back, but may show no disability; conversely, they may experience muscle weakness, difficulty with bowel and bladder control, and (rarely) paralysis. Corrective surgery is needed. **Meningomyelocele** or *myelomeningocele* (Fig. 72-5D) is the most serious form of spina bifida. The meninges and part of the spinal cord protrude through an opening. The child has a visible sac on the back. They are usually paralyzed and may have bladder and bowel control problems. Serious possible complications include meningitis (inflammation of the meninges covering the spinal cord), encephalitis, and hydrocephalus. You must handle the defect with great care to avoid injury to the sac or damage to the spinal cord. Surgery is necessary to prevent infection and to preserve as much nerve function as possible. It is often done soon after birth.

Nursing Considerations

A nursing goal in treating children with spina bifida is to prevent further damage. The most common problem is loss of leg sensation, so be sure to protect the child against possible leg injury. Careful examination is necessary to eliminate pressure areas and tight clothing, which can be irritating and cause skin breakdown or lack of sufficient circulation. Give good skin care, and change diapers immediately and with great care after the child voids or defecates.

Assist in preoperative and postoperative surgical management. Take precautions to protect the child from infection in the defect area. Another common site for infection is the bladder because the child is often catheterized. The child can be predisposed to infection if the catheter is improperly managed. Teach caregivers to clean the catheter every few hours. If kidney damage or other urinary system damage occurs, a urinary tract diversion may be required.

Pay special attention to the child's positioning because preventing musculoskeletal deformities is important. Also assist the child with range of motion exercises (passive or active). A physical therapist usually sees the child regularly. Frequently, orthopedic surgery must be performed to correct accompanying deformities, such as hip dysplasia or clubfoot. Children with spina bifida may need support services involving many specialists throughout their life. Urinary incontinence is one of the most difficult complications that threatens social acceptance. Your role as a nurse is to provide psychological support to family caregivers and the child.

> **Nursing Alert** For some reason, many children with spina bifida tend to be extremely sensitive to latex. Make sure such children do not come in contact with items such as tourniquets, catheters, rubber bands, gloves, balloons, or various tubes made of latex.

Hydrocephalus

Spinal fluid, which circulates constantly, encloses the CNS. If this circulation is disrupted, spinal fluid collects, causing head swelling and brain damage. This condition is called **hydrocephalus**. It often results from improper development of the brain or spinal cord or from a spinal cord defect (e.g., spina bifida). It can also occur as a complication of meningitis, head injury, or cranial hemorrhage.

Symptoms and Treatment

The symptoms of hydrocephalus include a progressive increase in the head's circumference. The sutures between the cranial bones open because of increased fluid accumulation. Brain tissue *atrophies* (shrinks) progressively as cranial cavity pressure increases. Be alert to the possibility of seizures. The severely affected or untreated child cannot control voluntary muscle movements and may die from respiratory complications, malnutrition, or infection. Diagnosis of hydrocephalus is made on the basis of lumbar puncture, computed tomography (CT) scan, positron emission tomography (PET) scan, or magnetic resonance imaging (MRI) studies. An electroencephalogram (**EEG**) may also be done.

Treatment for hydrocephalus is to insert a *shunt* (bypass) surgically, allowing the fluid to circulate around the defect or blockage (Fig. 72-6). Shunts are *ventriculoperitoneal* or *ventriculoatrial* (from the ventricles of the brain to the peritoneal cavity or into the heart). The ventriculoperitoneal shunt is the preferred route. The shunt should be inserted as soon as possible after birth because brain damage is irreversible.

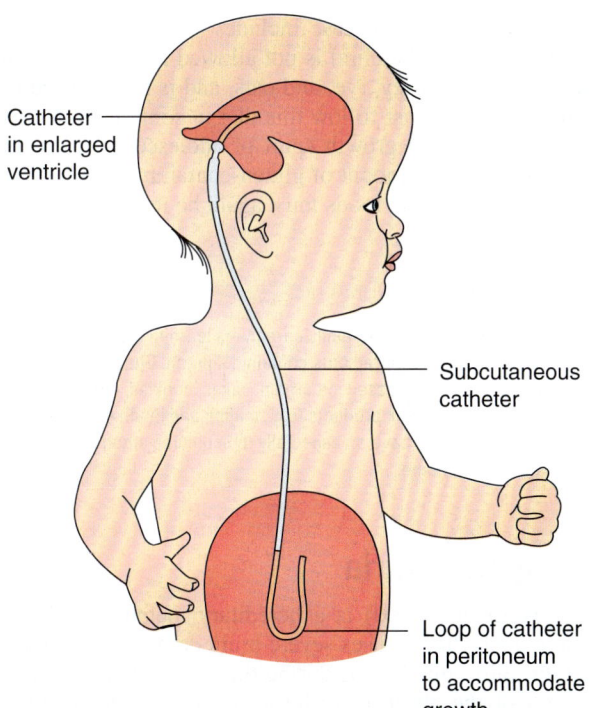

Figure 72-6 A ventriculoperitoneal shunt removes excessive cerebrospinal fluid from the ventricles and shunts it to the peritoneum. A one-way valve is present in the tubing behind the ear.

Nursing Considerations

Preoperatively, give skin care to prevent skin breakdown and take precautions to prevent infection. Turn the child frequently from side to side to prevent aspiration and pressure sores. Especially prevent pressure areas on the enlarged, fragile head and the ears. Place the child's head, neck, and shoulders on a soft pillow, evenly distributing the pressure that would otherwise be exerted on the infant's head. Keep the head clean and dry. Observe the child's head carefully. Monitor the fontanels for tension or fullness; measure and record the occipital–frontal circumference (OFC) daily (Chapter 67).

Postoperatively, observe for signs of shock or hemorrhage and check the incisional area for spinal fluid leakage. Take vital signs according to your facility's routines or as directed by the healthcare provider. Position the child away from the operative side to prevent pressure and damage to the shunt valve and the suture line. Restraints may be needed. Record I&O accurately to determine if the child is retaining fluids.

You may need to give gavage feedings or total parenteral nutrition (TPN) to prevent malnutrition in a child with hydrocephalus because this child often has difficulty eating. Feed the child carefully and slowly.

Because shunts are not always effective, observe carefully for any signs of increasing intracranial pressure, such as increasing irritability, bulging fontanels, and changes in eye signs or LOC. Another frequent complication is infection; report any sign of it immediately. If the shunt is performed before brain damage occurs and is successful, the child can lead a normal life.

Family caregivers need to know major developmental milestones to identify any problems their child has after discharge. Encourage them to prepare goals for their child that are appropriate to their ability and potential. Focusing on the child's strengths is important. Referral to special education programs may be necessary.

> **Key Concept**
> Head measurements (OFC and other measurements, as ordered) are an important aspect of nursing care in hydrocephalus. An increase in head size indicates increasing fluid in the brain. For this reason, measure the head's circumference at the same site every time. Mark the head with ink or indicate on a drawing exactly where you are taking measurements so that each nurse will measure in the same location, allowing for accurate comparison. Use a disposable paper tape. Document your measurements carefully, usually in centimeters (cm).

Febrile Seizures

Febrile seizures are generalized convulsions of unknown etiology, which occur in children between the ages of 6 months and 3 years and are more common in males. Febrile seizures are often related to acute illnesses in which a child's body temperature rapidly rises above 101.8 °F (38.8 °C). Risk factors include a family or personal history of febrile seizures and neurologic disorders.

Treatment of febrile seizures is aimed at controlling fever with antipyretics (acetaminophen, ibuprofen), tepid sponge baths, or other measures. Medications also may include lorazepam (Ativan) or phenobarbital. Febrile seizures are usually benign and related to the high fever only; thus, long-term antiepileptic drugs are not usually prescribed for prophylactic care.

Reassure the parents of the benign nature of the seizure and of the fact that most children do not develop a seizure disorder. Teach early management of fever and seizures at home.

Breath-Holding Spells

A *breath-holding spell* is an episode during which a child holds their breath and becomes unconscious (usually following a period of intense crying). Most authorities counsel parents to ignore these benign episodes because the child will usually outgrow them by 5 years of age.

One type of breath-holding episode may occur following a fall in which the child hits their head. The child begins to cry violently and holds their breath, resulting in a period of unconsciousness, with some myoclonic (muscle-jerking)-type movements. This activity mimics a seizure and can be frightening for family caregivers. If the child does not begin to breathe spontaneously and quickly recover, but must be stimulated to begin breathing, advise the parents to have the child seen as soon as possible in a local urgent care or emergency department. Other injuries and tantrums may result in breath-holding episodes.

METABOLIC AND NUTRITIONAL DISORDERS

Marasmus

Marasmus describes a general FTT condition. It seems to be related to such conditions as **kwashiorkor** (protein deficiency), **rickets** (vitamin D deficiency), and **scurvy** (vitamin C deficiency). Marasmus is a unique condition often caused by a general systemic disease, an absorption problem, neglect, or abuse.

Symptoms of marasmus include wasting and atrophy of body tissues. In contrast to kwashiorkor, no edema is present. The child's eyes are sunken, head size is small, and body temperature is low. The child is generally weak and listless. Physical growth lags behind that of other children of the same age. Mental development may or may not be slowed, but severe malnutrition in infancy contributes to slow brain growth and threatens future mental ability. These children are truly starving and will suck on anything available (e.g., clothing or fingers).

Nursing care involves restoration of hydration and nutrition, maintenance of body temperature, and general tender loving care. The child usually responds well to treatment.

Many caregivers are not knowledgeable about diets and parenting. An important part of nursing care in such cases is to teach caregivers nutrition and general aspects of childcare. Include the importance of hygiene, affection, and play. Teach caregivers feeding routines (e.g., giving solids), holding the baby, keeping air out of the neck of the bottle, and bubbling.

Biliary Atresia

One cause of malnutrition may be **biliary atresia**, a defect in the bile ducts that prevents bile from escaping from the liver. The lack of bile causes defective digestion and elimination.

In most cases, surgery must be performed to relieve the obstruction. Liver transplantation may also be considered.

Celiac Disease

The most common malabsorption syndrome in children of European descent is **celiac disease**, a chronic intestinal disorder. It involves small bowel inflammation and nutrient malabsorption. Celiac disease is thought to be congenital, although its effects may not appear for several months or years after birth. Usually, however, the condition manifests itself within 6 months after birth.

Children with celiac disease have an intolerance of the protein *gluten* found in wheat, oats, barley, and rye. When children with celiac disease eat foods containing glutens, the small intestine gradually becomes less able to absorb food through the intestinal villi into the bloodstream. These children are specifically unable to absorb fats. Remission usually occurs when family caregivers omit gluten-containing foods from the child's diet. Breastfeeding seems to postpone the appearance of symptoms because breast milk lacks glutens.

Celiac disease is characterized by large, floating, fatty stools; anorexia; undernutrition and FTT; distended abdomen and wasted buttocks; excessive flatus; and arrested growth. A jejunal biopsy and the child's clinical improvement when placed on a gluten-free diet verify the diagnosis. Before treatment, the child may also have a lactose intolerance, which improves with treatment. More than one child in a family may have the disorder, indicating a familial tendency. The disorder varies in degree from mild to severe. The severe form of the disorder is discussed here.

Medical Treatment

Treatment of celiac disease includes strict adherence to a gluten-free diet. The child is not allowed any cereal grains, such as wheat, barley, rye, and oats, and is not allowed any malt. The child must follow this diet in some form for life. However, after the growth spurt of adolescence, they may introduce a small amount of gluten-containing foods. If any difficulty occurs, the foods must again be removed from the diet.

> *Key Concept*
>
> Celiac disease requires that family caregivers learn to read labels very carefully to avoid ingredients containing gluten. Gluten is found in prepared soups, processed ice cream, cakes, cookies, other baked goods, pastas, some milk products (e.g., malts), and lunch meat. The school-age child may have an especially difficult time when planning meals away from home.

Phenylketonuria

Phenylketonuria (**PKU**) is a hereditary metabolic disorder. If untreated, PKU causes severe brain damage and intellectual disability that begins during the first months of life. As a result of the absence of the liver enzyme *phenylalanine hydroxylase*, phenylalanine is not converted to tyrosine and phenylketones build up in the blood and tissues, causing permanent brain damage. In addition, melanin is not formed; therefore, children with PKU are most often blue eyed and blond with sensitive skin. A blood test obtained by a heel stick after the newborn has consumed formula or breast milk for at least 2 days detects PKU. The blood test is inaccurate until the newborn has had several feedings of formula or breast milk. Because the baby is usually discharged from the birthing facility soon after delivery, the test needs to be repeated when the baby is 2 weeks old. If the baby is born at home, caregivers will need to take the baby to a healthcare facility for testing no later than 2 weeks after birth. The test is required by law in most states.

Existing damage is irreversible, but treatment, which must begin as soon as possible, prevents further damage. The only treatment is a diet very low in phenylalanine, an essential amino acid necessary for growth and repair of body cells. Family caregivers should use a low-phenylalanine formula in place of the usual milk in the diet. The child should avoid phenylalanine-containing foods, including most breads, eggs, meat, milk, cheese, legumes, nuts, and some artificial sweeteners. The child can eat low-protein natural foods, such as fruits, vegetables, and certain cereals. A dietitian will prescribe a diet that provides a safe amount of phenylalanine, yet will maintain the serum amounts below the toxic level. Reading product labels will be a very important part of any caregiver's responsibilities.

These dietary restrictions usually continue until late childhood or adolescence, when the person has achieved most brain growth. The time to discontinue the diet is controversial, with some experts recommending indefinite adherence to the restrictions.

DISORDERS OF THE EYES

Strabismus

Strabismus, commonly known as "squint" or "crossed eyes," is an inability to appropriately move the eyes. Although strabismus is usually congenital, it may result from a childhood disease. The normal newborn appears cross-eyed because they have not yet developed control of the eye muscles (*pseudostrabismus*). However, strabismus found in a child older than 6 weeks of age requires evaluation.

The two chief classifications of strabismus are *paralytic strabismus* (the muscles of one eye are underactive) and *concomitant strabismus* (both eyes move, but the deviation of the affected eye is always the same). Other terms associated with strabismus are *convergent* (both eyes looking toward the center), *divergent* (both eyes looking outward), and *vertical* (the affected eye [or eyes] moves only on a vertical plane).

Concomitant strabismus may involve the same eye (*monocular*), both eyes alternately (*alternating*), or both eyes (*binocular*). The child uses the unaffected eye at any particular time. If the child uses one eye all the time, the other eye does not participate in vision, and the resulting double vision (*diplopia*) causes the unused eye to weaken.

In *alternate strabismus*, each eye is dominant at different times and monocular weakness is less likely. In *latent strabismus*, great effort is needed to overcome the muscle imbalance, so the child complains of eye strain, headache, and diplopia.

Medical Treatment

The unaffected eye is patched to stimulate the unused eye; corrective eyeglasses, which can be prescribed as early as 1 year of age, are ordered. Eye exercises and miotic drugs are prescribed to contract the pupils of the eyes. Treatment begins early to prevent further damage and to improve the child's appearance.

Surgical intervention may be done to the affected muscles to match the unaffected muscles.

Nursing Considerations

Prepare the child preoperatively if they are to be on bed rest or have the eyes covered following surgery. Surgery is done in a same-day or outpatient surgery setting. Often elbow restraints are necessary after surgery to prevent the child from touching the eyes. Speak to the child whose eyes are covered before touching, to avoid frightening them.

The child is usually up and moving about soon after surgery. Many children with strabismus have photophobia; sunglasses may help. Teach the child and family caregivers preoperative and postoperative care.

Other Eye Disorders

Infants may have *congenital glaucoma*, an increase in intraocular pressure with symptoms of an enlarged, edematous, and hazy cornea and increased tearing, pain, and photophobia. Surgery may be necessary.

Cataracts may be present at birth or can occur because of eye trauma or disease. The pupil appears to be white and the red reflex cannot be elicited. Surgical removal, with insertion of internal contacts, is necessary.

Amblyopia ("lazy eye") is subnormal vision in one eye, which may fail to develop due to lack of visual stimulation because the child always uses the good eye for vision. Blindness may develop in the "lazy eye." Strabismus or refractive errors may contribute to amblyopia. Treatment consists of patching the good eye to force the child to use the underdeveloped eye. Correction of strabismus and refractive errors is also essential.

A small child's eye muscles are not sufficiently developed to permit normal pupil accommodation. However, because other factors also may be involved, the child should be examined regularly after 3 years of age (or earlier if symptoms appear). Red, puffy, and watering eyes, or frequent rubbing of the eyes, may indicate difficulty in seeing. The child also may complain of dizziness, headache, or double vision. Determine whether visual difficulties arise from an error of refraction, which can usually be corrected by eyeglasses, or from another problem, such as a brain tumor.

Ptosis, or drooping eyelids, is usually congenital. In most cases, it is corrected by surgery.

DISORDERS OF THE EARS, NOSE, THROAT, AND MOUTH

Otitis Media

Otitis media, an acute infection of the middle ear, is the most common bacterial infection of early childhood, most often caused by nasopharyngeal reflux or eustachian tube dysfunction. Most children have at least one episode of otitis media. Bacterial organisms can travel through the eustachian tube in an infant or young child much more readily than in an adult. This is because the eustachian tube is wider and more horizontal in children, allowing bacteria from the nasopharynx to readily enter the middle ear.

Otitis media is defined as *acute* if its onset is rapid and short, *subacute* if fluid involvement lasts between 3 weeks and 3 months, and *chronic* if it lasts longer than 3 months. Complications include hearing loss, a scarred or ruptured tympanic membrane (eardrum), inner ear infection, mastoiditis (inflammation of the mastoid process), or meningitis.

Infants and young children who live in homes with smokers have a higher incidence of otitis media due to passive smoke inhalation. Bacterial infections, viral nasopharyngitis, enlargement of nasopharyngeal lymphoid tissue, tumors, foreign bodies, allergies, and other physiologic factors may cause eustachian tube dysfunction. Breastfed babies have a lower incidence of otitis media perhaps because they receive immunoglobulin A, which protects against respiratory viruses and allergies. Breastfed infants are also held in a more upright position than are bottle-fed babies. Propping a baby's bottle may allow fluid to flow through the eustachian tube, causing otitis media.

Pain may be present with otitis media. The infant may express the pain by pulling on or scratching the ear and being irritable. Older children will complain of pain. Signs of infection, a temperature as high as 104°F (40°C), swollen glands, and loss of appetite (sometimes with vomiting) are other symptoms. Occasionally, family caregivers are surprised when a healthcare provider points out a child's red, swollen eardrum because the child had not indicated any type of ear discomfort.

Definite diagnosis is made when a bulging tympanic membrane is seen on otoscopic examination. Landmarks of the bony prominences are obscured. If the tympanic membrane ruptures, bleeding or purulent drainage may occur.

The most serious complication of otitis media is hearing loss, which may be permanent. Hearing loss occurs from scarring as a result of repeated infections. In many children, hearing loss may go undetected until they enter school. Other complications include mastoiditis and, occasionally, encephalitis or meningitis. These conditions are rare with the administration of antibiotic therapy.

Medical Treatment

Antihistamines and decongestants may be administered for otitis media. Warm, moist packs may provide comfort. Some children experience more comfort with an ice pack because it tends to reduce edema. Acetaminophen for fever and pain may be prescribed. Antibiotics are also prescribed. After 10 days, the healthcare provider inspects the child's ears. If the tympanic membrane remains red or if other symptoms persist, another course of antibiotic therapy may be indicated.

Surgical Treatment

If repeated medical therapies with antibiotics are unsuccessful, surgical options may be considered. Treatment of otitis media involves restoring the normal eustachian tube function and maintaining or improving hearing.

An ear, nose, and throat healthcare provider specialist called an *otolaryngologist* may perform an outpatient procedure called a *myringotomy*. This procedure involves making a surgical opening into the eardrum and inserting a polyethylene (**PE**) ventilating tube as a temporary or permanent accessory eustachian tube. The PE tube allows drainage of the accumulated fluid from the middle ear and equalization of pressure on each side of the eardrum (Fig. 72-7). Hearing is usually restored after placement of the PE tube.

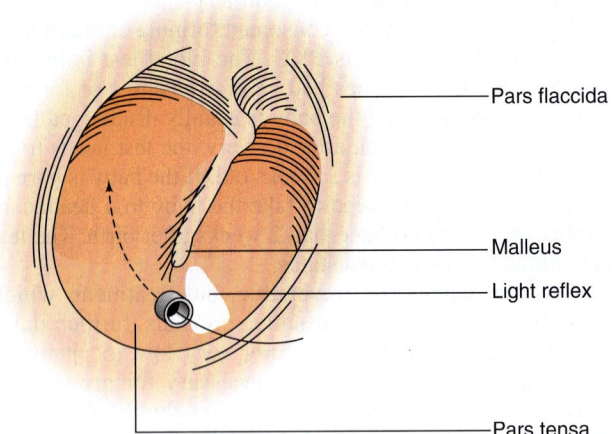

Figure 72-7 A myringotomy tube provides air to the middle ear to prevent serous otitis media.

The child with a PE tube must avoid getting water into the ears when swimming, taking a shower, or shampooing the hair. Special ear plugs may be prescribed.

Other surgical procedures in otitis media are *tympanoplasty*, which involves reconstruction of the middle ear, either with the placement of a homograft transplant of the structure or with a prosthesis, and myringoplasty. A *myringoplasty* is reconstruction of the eardrum, usually with a graft of temporalis fascia.

Epistaxis

Epistaxis (nosebleed) is common in children and usually originates in the anterior portion of the nares. Common causes of epistaxis include foreign objects pushed into the nose, systemic disorders, trauma, allergy, and dry mucous membranes. Dry mucous membranes lead to cracking, crusts, and nose picking. Treatment consists of applying pressure or cold compresses across the bridge of the nose for 5–10 min. Usually the bleeding will stop. Have the child sit up and tilt the head forward, to minimize pressure on the nasal blood vessels and to prevent blood from running down the posterior pharynx.

For serious or stubborn nosebleeds, a healthcare provider may need to pack the child's nose to stop hemorrhage. A child's blood volume is lower than an adult's, so epistaxis is potentially dangerous. Also, the child may swallow blood. Report any symptoms, such as vomiting "coffee-ground" material. Cautery, or application of a substance such as silver nitrate, is used to control epistaxis if it occurs frequently.

> **Nursing Alert** If a child with a nosebleed also has a head injury, do not stop the bleeding without specific healthcare provider's orders. *Rationale: Holding blood inside the nasal cavity can increase intracranial pressure.*

Tonsillitis

Tonsillitis, an inflammation of the tonsils, is caused by a virus or bacteria. Symptoms include a sore, reddened throat with swelling and sometimes exudate on the tonsils. Swallowing is difficult, and the child's WBC count and temperature may be elevated. A throat culture can determine the offending organism, and drug sensitivity tests will signify the treatment of choice. Viral infections are treated symptomatically. Refer to the discussion of sore throats in Chapter 73.

> **Key Concept**
>
> Because the tonsils are so close to the eustachian tubes, tonsillitis can easily spread to the middle ear and cause otitis media. Infants and toddlers are most often affected because their eustachian tubes are shorter and straighter than those of adults.

Medical and Surgical Treatment

The child is kept in a high-humidity environment and antibiotics are administered if the cause is bacterial. If the child has difficulty swallowing, a soft diet may be offered. Fluids are encouraged, and antipyretics (naproxen, acetaminophen, ibuprofen) are given to lower temperature and relieve discomfort.

If the child has had numerous streptococcal infections in a short time, removal of the tonsils (*tonsillectomy*) may be indicated, although this procedure is controversial. Tonsillectomy also may be done in the case of a recurring *peritonsillar* (around the tonsil) abscess. Tonsillectomy is rarely done following a single episode of tonsillitis. Removal of the tonsils and adenoids is called a tonsillectomy and adenoidectomy (**T&A**).

Nursing Considerations

Most T&A surgery is performed in same-day surgery centers. Before surgery, the child must be free of URIs. Accurate documentation of observations is necessary on admission.

Instruct family caregivers in preoperative measures to perform at home. Routine preparation includes giving the child nothing by mouth (NPO) after midnight. When the child arrives at the facility, check to determine if they have a URI. Report and document the presence of loose teeth. Preoperative medication may be given to young children.

Direct postoperative nursing care for preventing hemorrhage, the most common complication. Observe the child for spitting up of a great deal of bloody sputum or vomiting of "coffee-ground" material. The child may swallow blood, so some vomiting of dark blood is not unusual. Observe and document the presence of bloody sputum or vomiting. Position the child on the side or abdomen or with the head of the bed elevated to prevent aspiration.

Encourage fluids after the child is awake and fully responding. Clear, bland fluids are best; milk tends to form a film in the throat. Children usually accept popsicles, non-acidic fruit drinks, gelatins, and sherbet very well.

> **Nursing Alert** Avoid giving red juices and red frozen pops to the child after T&A surgery. Emesis of red juice may be difficult to differentiate from bloody emesis.

Many healthcare providers write "diet as tolerated" as the order for meals meaning that the client is allowed foods that are preferred and that will be eaten without difficulty. Allow children to help choose the foods and liquids that are most appealing within these limits. Do not permit the child to drink fluids through a straw. Sucking can dislodge clots or stitches and lead to hemorrhage. Normal drinking, chewing, and swallowing promote healing. Supervise gum chewing carefully; chewing gum promotes the flow of saliva, which is soothing and facilitates healing.

Use pain medications as needed so that the child can drink more comfortably and rest more easily. Be alert for an elevated temperature postoperatively, which may indicate dehydration and the need to force fluids. Temperature elevation also may point to infection, although infection is uncommon.

The child is usually discharged the day of or the day after surgery. Sometimes an antibiotic prescription may be given as prevention against infection. Give home care instruction to family caregivers, including signs of hemorrhage and respiratory distress. The child should continue with high fluid intake and soft foods. They should play quietly and rest in bed for approximately 1–2 weeks before returning to school and other normal activities.

Cleft Lip and Cleft Palate

Cleft lip and **cleft palate** are deformities that commonly occur together at birth. They result from failure of the upper lip and palate to close completely during the second and third gestational months (Fig. 72-8). Each of these defects may also occur separately. Cleft lip is more common in boys; cleft palate is more common in girls. Evidence also indicates a slight tendency for familial occurrence. Developmental delays and intellectual disability are not related to cleft lip or cleft palate.

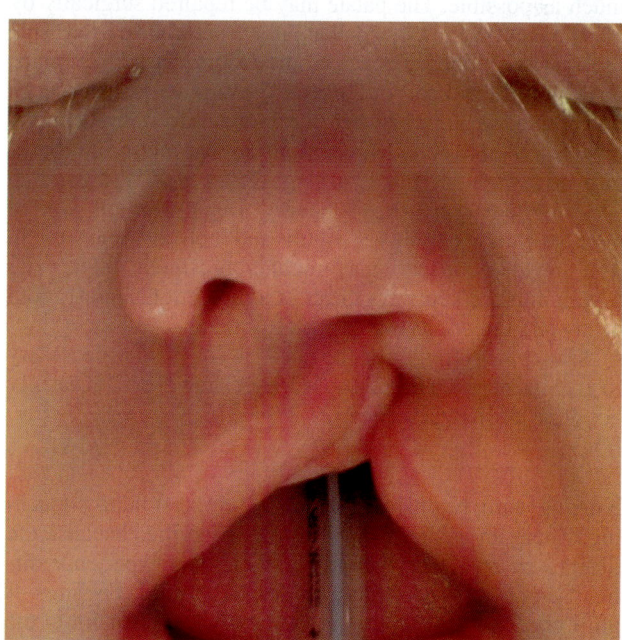

Figure 72-8 Unilateral cleft lip. (From Thorne, C. H., Chung, K. C., Gosain, A. K., Gurtner, G. C., Mehrara, B. J., Rubin, J. P. & Spear, S. L. (2013). *Grabb and Smith's plastic surgery* (7th ed.). Wolters Kluwer Health/Lippincott Williams & Wilkins.)

Cleft lip may be no more than a notch in the upper lip, or it may extend up into the nostril on one or both sides. The cleft may be *complete* or *incomplete* and may be complicated by other factors, such as a lip muscle separated by the cleft, skin that is thinner than normal, missing hair follicles and sweat glands, a flattened nostril on the affected side, and a missing part of the jaw and teeth.

Surgical Treatment

Surgical repair of cleft lip is called a *cheiloplasty*. The cleft is sutured, generally when the child is quite young, to facilitate sucking. Very little preoperative preparation is needed for an infant. The goal of surgery is to restore lip function and to improve the child's appearance.

A skin graft or revision of the scar is often necessary at a later date. The scar is quite prominent immediately after the operation, but usually becomes unnoticeable as the child grows older. A young client may grow a moustache to cover the scar.

Immediate postoperative care is directed toward maintaining the airway, preventing shock or hemorrhage, using proper feeding techniques, and preventing injury to the suture line. Sometimes a Logan bow (curved metal bar) is placed over a repaired cleft lip to decrease tension on the suture line. Often these children need to have PE ventilating tubes inserted in their tympanic membranes to reduce the incidence of ear infections. An elbow restraint may be used to keep children from rubbing the suture lines.

Cleft palate appears as an opening in the roof of the mouth that leads into the nose. The cleft lip is repaired at a very early age. The cleft palate, however, is repaired later.

Surgical repair of cleft palate is called a *palatoplasty*. It is done when the child is 2–6 years of age. Repairing the palate before the child develops poor speech habits is desirable. The goals of this surgery are to restore normal speech, to avoid damage to the lip's suture line, and to close the palate as much as possible. The palate may be repaired surgically by placement of a graft, or a dental prosthesis may be used. This prosthesis is either attached to the teeth or used to replace missing teeth and part of the jaw. The prosthesis aids speech by closing the hole between the mouth and nose. Surgical repair of the palate is usually done in one procedure, but it may be carried out in several stages if the cleft is severe.

Consistent dental care is needed. Dental surgery is often necessary to rebuild missing gums and replace missing teeth. The prosthetic palate may include prosthetic teeth. The mouth must be kept very clean as a protection against tooth decay and infection.

Rhinoplasty (repair of the nose) is sometimes necessary to give the nose a balanced appearance; however, it is usually not done until adolescence.

Nursing Considerations

Nursing care begins at birth and involves family teaching. These anomalies may upset their families because the defects are so visual. Family members may experience difficult emotions when they first see their child. Feelings of guilt may play a great part in the family's adjustment to the child. Be sensitive to the family's feelings. Also be careful not to reveal any personal negative feelings about the infant's appearance.

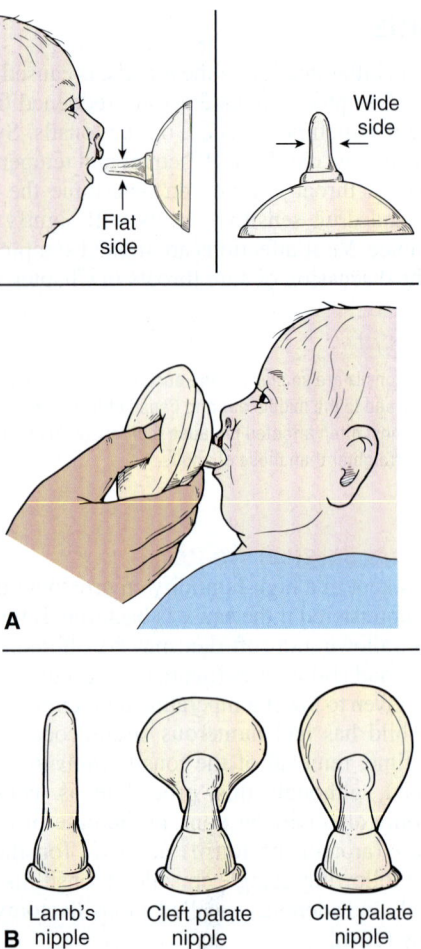

Figure 72-9 Nipples used for feeding newborns with cleft lip and palate. **A.** Beniflex nurser. **B.** Other types of nipples. (Courtesy of Mead Johnson, Evansville, IN.)

Feeding

Part of the child's soft palate is missing in cleft palate, and the uvula is almost always absent, as is a part of the hard palate. As a result, the child's mouth and throat are not separated from the nose. Therefore, if the baby is fed by usual methods, they regurgitate milk through the nose. If they also have a cleft lip, sucking is difficult.

You can feed some of these babies by using a soft nipple with large holes. Hold the baby upright so that they do not draw milk into the nose. Occasionally, you may use a special flattened nipple ("duckbill" nipple) or a cleft palate nipple with a flap to cover the hole in the palate. In other cases, you will use a special feeder (Fig. 72-9).

Following are recommendations for feeding infants with cleft lip and/or palate:

- Feed slowly in small amounts, and bubble frequently.
- Hold the infant upright, but cuddle and talk to the infant while feeding.
- Clean the mouth and cleft carefully after each feeding.
- Dilute solids and spoon-feed them.
- Prevent aspiration.
- In extreme cases, gavage feeding may be necessary until part of the palate is covered.

Providing Oral Care

Oral hygiene is essential. Encourage the older child to use mouthwash and to brush their teeth often.

Preventing Infection

Because the pathway is open between the mouth and nose, swallowing does not equalize pressure in the eustachian tubes. Infections develop easily and may cause partial hearing loss. Instruct caregivers in ways to prevent ear infections. They should protect these children against colds and URIs.

Addressing Emotional Aspects

How a child adjusts to a cleft lip or palate depends largely on how family caregivers and others react to the deformity. Group discussion with other family caregivers who have faced the same problem provides support. Caregivers can learn to help their child deal with teasing.

Providing Postoperative Care

Aim nursing care at preventing strain on the suture line and preventing deformities or complications. Do not allow sucking or insert anything into the mouth.

Baby Bottle Syndrome

If bottle feeding continues after a child has teeth, or if a child uses a bottle as a pacifier, a deformity called *baby bottle syndrome* (nursing bottle mouth) can occur. Baby bottle syndrome is caused by the bottle's contents continually coming into contact with the baby's teeth for prolonged periods, resulting in numerous dental caries. This condition most frequently occurs in children between 18 and 36 months of age. Instruct caregivers how to prevent this condition (In Practice: Educating the Client 72-3).

IN PRACTICE

EDUCATING THE CLIENT 72-3 — Baby Bottle Syndrome Prevention

- Never prop a bottle.
- Do not give the infant a bottle in bed to fall asleep with.
- Clean the child's mouth and brush their teeth after feeding.
- Wean the infant to a cup by 1 year of age.
- Do not allow the child to walk or run around with a bottle.
- Begin regular dental checkups after tooth eruption.
- Do not give juice.
- Keep pacifiers clean.

CARDIOVASCULAR DISORDERS

Disorders of the cardiovascular system can result from defects, diseases, hemorrhage, fluid and electrolyte imbalance, neurologic disorders, or poison ingestion. Some children are born with a structural abnormality of the heart, called a *congenital cardiac anomaly* or *defect*. These disorders can quickly result in respiratory distress, shock, and death in the infant or small child. Some cardiac disorders are associated with other conditions, such as Down syndrome, congenital rubella syndrome, or fetal alcohol syndrome (Chapter 74).

Various types of congenital cardiac anomalies may occur. Major cardiac abnormalities can be divided into cyanotic and acyanotic defects (Table 72-1). *Cyanotic defects* may cause a right-to-left shunt, in which venous (deoxygenated) blood is mixed with arterial (oxygenated) blood within the heart and then circulated to the body. The total amount of blood sent to the tissues has a decreased amount of oxygen because the blood that is sent is only partially saturated with oxygen. *Acyanotic defects* have a left-to-right shunt, which sends oxygenated blood into the venous system.

An infant with a significant heart defect may eventually show evidence of HF and poor peripheral oxygen tissue perfusion. *Perfusion* refers to the body's ability to send and receive oxygen to the cells. Without adequate oxygen and perfusion of the oxygen, the skin appears *cyanotic* (bluish).

The infant with a heart defect may show signs of cyanosis, depending on the origin of the condition. Other symptoms include *dyspnea* (difficulty breathing), coughing or choking, persistent tachycardia (>200 beats/min), heart murmurs, failure to gain weight, difficulty in feeding, listlessness, and a general sickly appearance. Observe the child for symptoms of respiratory distress and changes in pulse rate and rhythm.

The severity of CHF may depend on the severity of the heart defect and the amount of the abnormal mixture of arterial and venous blood within the chambers of the heart. The result of this abnormal mixture is an increase in the work of the cardiac muscle, which *hypertrophies* (enlarges). An enlarged heart is the body's attempt to provide oxygen to tissues throughout the body. This enlarged heart eventually becomes ineffective (Chapter 81).

The older, untreated child often has poor physical development, low tolerance for physical activity, and clubbing of fingers and toes owing to chronic hypoxia; cyanosis, in certain cases; elevated blood pressure and pulse rate; and, possibly, an enlarged heart. Frequently, the child may need to squat or sit to facilitate breathing, especially on exertion. With pulse oximetry, providers can measure the child's level of peripheral oxygenation.

TABLE 72-1 Major Cyanotic and Acyanotic Heart Defects

CYANOTIC DEFECTS	RIGHT-TO-LEFT SHUNT	ACYANOTIC DEFECTS	LEFT-TO-RIGHT SHUNT
Tetralogy of Fallot (**TOF**) Transposition of the great arteries (vessels) (**TGA, TGV**)	Deoxygenated (venous) blood on the right side of the heart mixes with oxygenated (arterial) blood on the left side of the heart. The left ventricle sends this blood to the body. The cells of the body do not receive enough oxygenated blood. Signs and symptoms include cyanosis, shortness of breath, and fatigue.	Atrial septal defect (**ASD**) Ventricular septal defect (**VSD**) Coarctation of the aorta (**COA**) Patent ductus arteriosus (**PDA**)	Oxygenated blood on the left side of the heart mixes with deoxygenated blood on the right side of the heart. The heart sends this blood to the lungs, where more oxygen is picked up. Signs and symptoms may not be obvious. Untreated, heart failure (HF) may develop.

Definite diagnosis of congenital heart disease is made by auscultation (listening for heart sounds), x-ray studies, echocardiogram, ECG, careful physical examination, complete blood gases, and a complete history. At times, cardiac catheterization and angiocardiography may be done. However, because these procedures carry some risk, they are done only when necessary.

Children with a congenital heart disease (repaired or unrepaired) need prophylactic antibiotics at times of invasive procedures to prevent subacute bacterial endocarditis.

Septal Defects

Ventricular septal defect (**VSD**) is the most frequent congenital anomaly of the circulatory system (Fig. 72-10A). An abnormal opening is found between the left and right ventricles. This defect is usually acyanotic because the greater pressure in the left ventricle causes a shunt from left to right, so the blood pumped to the body is oxygenated. If pulmonary hypertension exists, the shunt may go the other way, and the child will be cyanotic. Open-heart surgery can usually correct such defects; the surgeon places a patch made of surgical elastic into the opening. If the opening is small and no pulmonary hypertension exists, the child may be asymptomatic and the septum may grow to cover the opening. Surgery may be unnecessary or postponed until the child is older. In some cases, an "umbrella" occluder is placed via catheter, thereby postponing or preventing surgery.

Atrial septal defect (**ASD**) is an abnormal opening between the right and left atria. Most of these defects occur in the area of the foramen ovale (Fig. 72-10B). Defects found lower in the septum are more likely to involve the mitral and tricuspid valves and the AV node. Usually, the shunt is from left to right, so the child is acyanotic. Surgery or an occluder can usually close this defect unless severe pulmonary hypertension exists. If the valves are involved, the operation is much more complicated and may include valve replacement.

Patent Ductus Arteriosus

In the fetus, the *ductus arteriosus* is a blood vessel between the aorta and the pulmonary artery that allows the fetal circulation to bypass the lungs. It normally closes before birth or very soon after. If the ductus remains open (*patent*) after birth, the defect is called *patent ductus arteriosus* (**PDA**) (Fig. 72-10C).

In a child with this defect, when the left ventricle pumps blood that should go to the body into the aorta, some oxygenated blood returns to the pulmonary circulation via the patent ductus because of the higher pressure in the aorta. Lung pressure thereby increases, as does the volume of oxygenated blood, which may cause pulmonary hypertension. The heart must work harder, and the child's body cells lack oxygen.

Infants may be given indomethacin (Indocin), a prostaglandin inhibitor, to promote closure of a PDA. In some heart anomalies (those with decreased blood flow to the lungs), the patency of the ductus is beneficial to increase blood flow to the lungs for oxygenation. Administration of prostaglandin E keeps the ductus arteriosus open in conditions where increased blood flow to the lungs is needed (e.g., transposition of the great arteries). A foam plug or an umbrella occluder placed via cardiac catheterization may close the ductus. If these measures do not work, surgical ligation and severing of the ductus is performed. This closed-heart procedure was one of the first surgeries performed. It is usually done even if a child shows no symptoms because of the danger of lung damage from pulmonary hypertension.

Transposition of the Great Arteries

In *transposition of the great arteries* (**TGA**), also known as transposition of the great vessels (TGV), the aorta and the pulmonary artery are reversed, so that each connects to the wrong side of the heart. If no shunts or septal defects exist, the child dies early owing to lack of sufficient oxygenation to the body cells because only unoxygenated blood circulates systemically (Fig. 72-10D).

Immediate intervention includes maintaining patency of the ductus arteriosus to increase pulmonary blood flow and removal of the atrial septum to facilitate mixing of oxygenated blood into unoxygenated blood. Medication (prostaglandin E) may be given to maintain patency of the ductus arteriosus. Surgical correction involves an arterial switch procedure or construction of an intracardiac baffle to divert the blood to the appropriate vessel.

Tetralogy of Fallot

Tetralogy of Fallot (**TOF**) is a combination of four major defects (Fig. 72-10E):

- *Pulmonary stenosis:* Narrowing of the pulmonary artery
- *VSD:* A hole in the septum separating the ventricles
- *Overriding aorta (dextroposition of the aorta):* The aorta shifts to the right over the septal defect and receives both venous and oxygenated blood
- *Right ventricular hypertrophy:* An enlarged right ventricle due to the heart pumping harder in an attempt to increase blood flow to the lungs for oxygenation

The infant with a severe defect in any of these areas is cyanotic. The repair is done in the first year of life if the infant can withstand surgery. If complete repair is impossible, a temporary repair is performed to increase pulmonary blood flow, usually through a subclavian shunt to the pulmonary vessels.

The infant with this condition may first be seen as an FTT infant. Such infants may go on to have periods of cyanosis and hypoxia, called "blue spells" or "tet spells." If the diagnosis is not made early and the child does not at least have palliative surgery, they often have increasing pulmonary stenosis. As this child gets older, clubbed fingers and squatting to breathe may become evident.

Improved diagnosis and surgery have greatly decreased the death rate in TOF. Reconstructive surgery is highly successful.

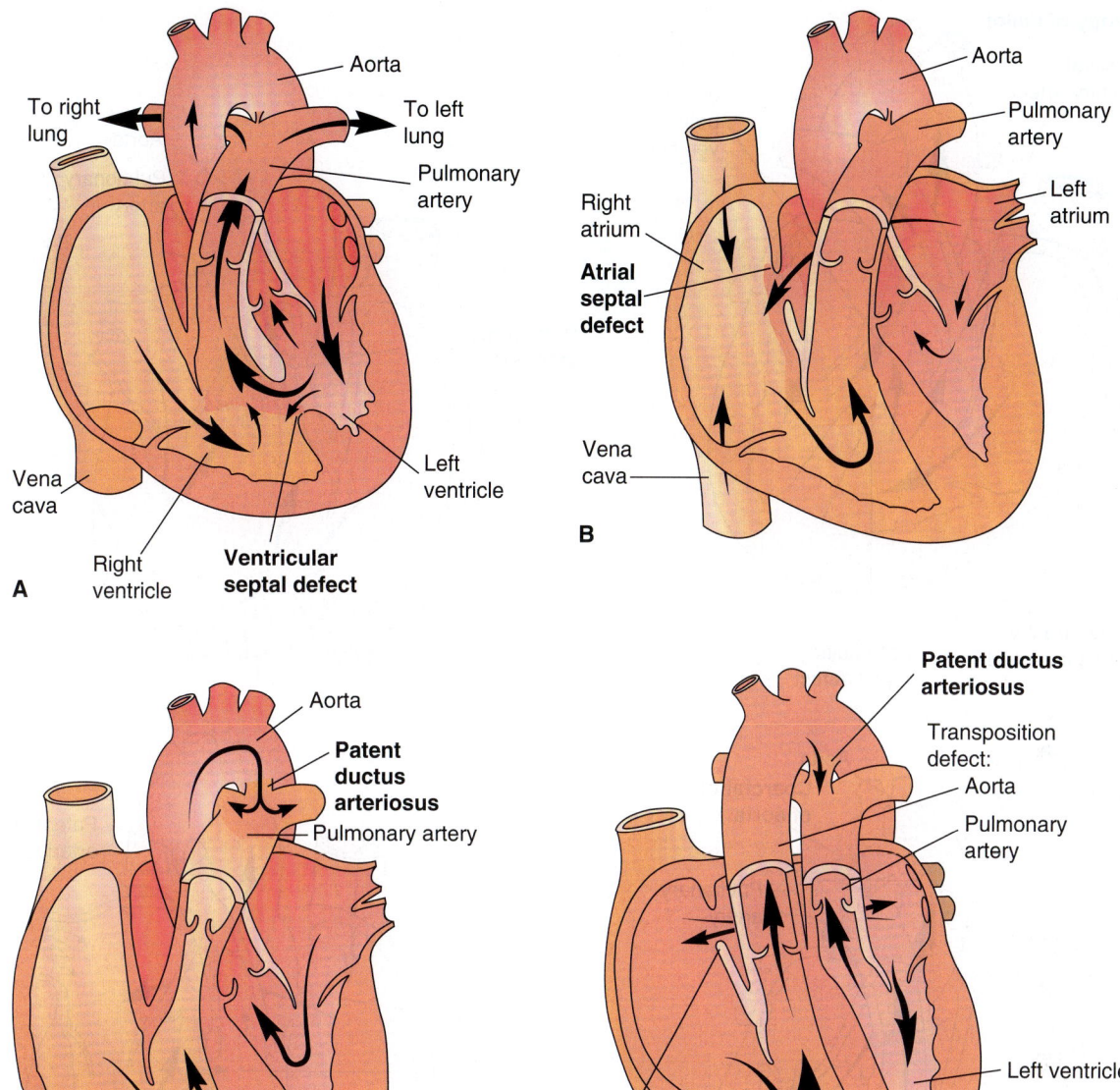

Figure 72-10 **A.** In a *ventricular septal defect*, a hole is in the wall of the septum that separates the left and right ventricles. Normally, deoxygenated blood flows through the superior vena cava and inferior vena cava into the right atrium, right ventricle, and pulmonary artery. In a ventricular septal defect, some oxygen-rich blood from the left ventricle flows through the defect and recirculates through the lungs. **B.** In an *atrial septal defect*, an abnormal communication exists between the atria, allowing blood to be shunted from the left atrium to the right atrium through the atrial septum. This hole is usually the area of the foramen ovale, which normally closes at birth. **C.** A fetal vascular connection called the *ductus arteriosus* directs blood from the pulmonary artery to the aorta. Functional closure of the ductus normally occurs soon after birth. In *patent ductus arteriosus*, the ductus remains patent, and the direction of blood flow in the ductus is reversed owing to the higher aortic pressure. **D.** *Transposition of the great arteries.* The aorta exits the right ventricle; the pulmonary artery exits the left ventricle. The fetal foramen ovale, now an atrial septal defect, allows blood to mix and provides some oxygenation of the blood.

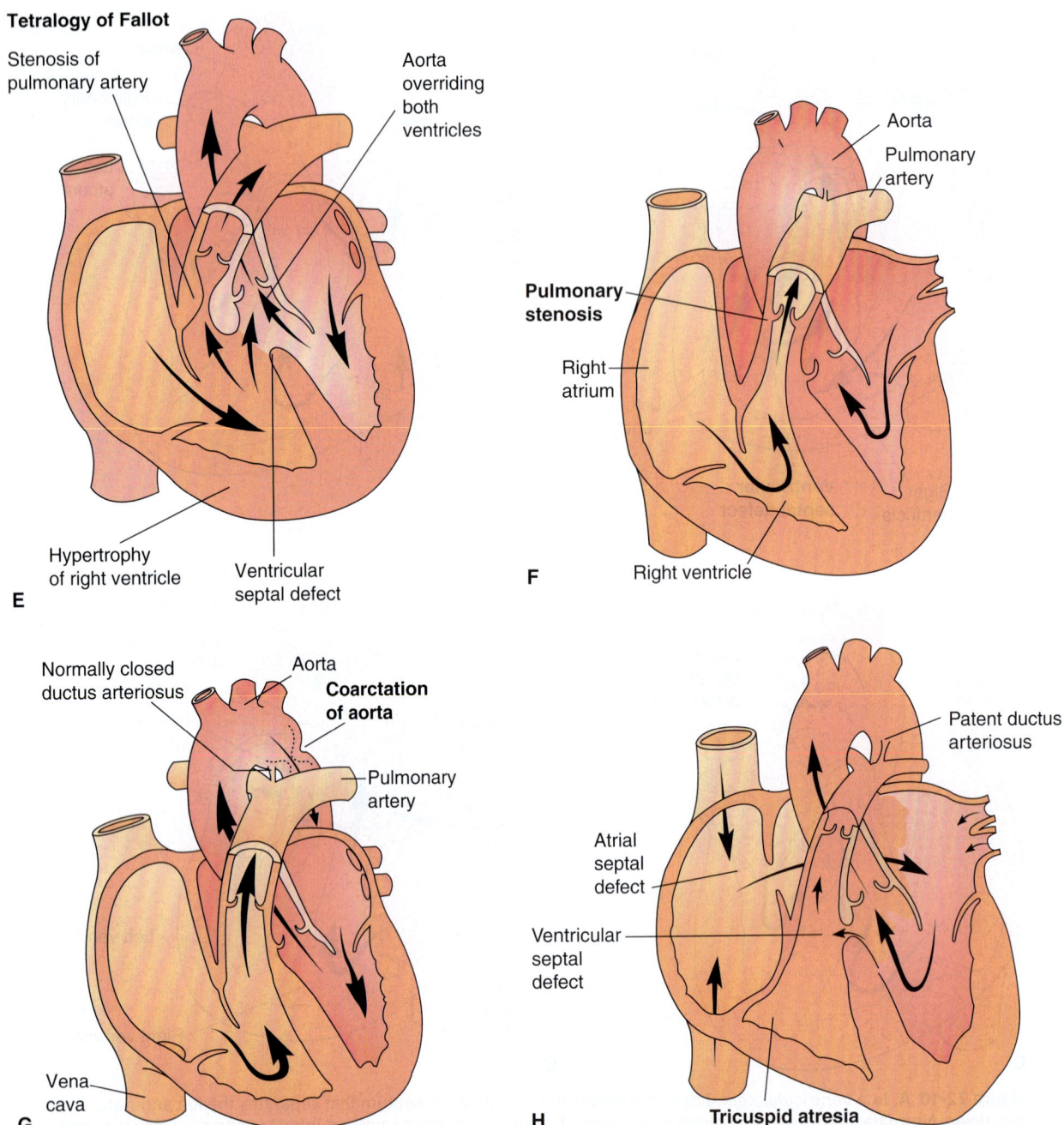

Figure 72-10 **E.** *Tetralogy of Fallot* is characterized by the combination of four defects: (1) pulmonary stenosis, (2) ventricular septal defect, (3) overriding aorta, and (4) hypertrophy of the right ventricle. It is the most common defect causing cyanosis in children who survive beyond 2 years of age. Symptom severity depends on the degree of pulmonary stenosis, the size of the ventricular septal defect, and the degree to which the aorta overrides the septal defect. **F.** In *pulmonary stenosis*, the right ventricular outflow tract narrows, causing decreased blood flow to the lungs and, therefore, decreased oxygenation of the blood. **G.** In *coarctation of the aorta*, abnormal narrowing of the aorta causes an obstruction of the blood flow from the left side of the heart. Because of this narrowing, pressure in the aorta and left ventricle increases. To help carry blood through the narrowing, blood vessels around it and the left ventricle enlarge. **H.** *Tricuspid atresia*. The absence of a tricuspid valve prevents blood from entering the right ventricle, causing decreased blood flow to the lungs for oxygenation.

Stenosis

Pulmonary stenosis is the narrowing of the right ventricular outflow tract, including the valve (Fig. 72-10F), which decreases blood flow into the lungs. On rare occasions, pulmonary stenosis also involves a narrowing of the pulmonary artery. If symptoms are present, the valve is surgically corrected (*commissurotomy*). Closed- or open-heart surgery may be indicated, and an artificial valve may replace the defective valve. If a pulmonary artery is greatly stenosed (*narrowed*), a vessel graft may be done.

In *aortic stenosis*, an aortic valve malfunction causes the heart to work harder to pump blood to the body. The treatment is similar to that for pulmonary stenosis. The aorta itself may also be stenosed.

Coarctation of the Aorta

In *coarctation (constriction) of the aorta* (**COA**), the aorta narrows, obstructing blood flow (Fig. 72-10G). The condition appears similar to aortic stenosis, except that the coarctation is usually further from the heart and, therefore, causes circulation problems in the arms, head, and lower extremities. Blood pressure is higher in the upper extremities than in the lower extremities. Upper body pulses are usually stronger; lower extremity pulses are weak. In children, conservative medical treatment may be attempted because surgery is difficult. Surgical correction consists of either excising the coarctation and suturing the two ends of the vessel together, or using a blood vessel graft.

Tricuspid Atresia

Tricuspid atresia is the absence of an opening between the right atrium and the right ventricle, allowing no blood to flow from the right atrium to the right ventricle, greatly decreasing pulmonary blood flow (Fig. 72-10H). The only routes by which the blood can get to the lungs are through an atrial or ventricular septal defect or a patent ductus arteriosus. The child dies soon after birth, unless corrective surgery is performed. Because oxygenated blood mixes with unoxygenated blood, the child is cyanotic.

Generally, the older a child is when surgery is performed, the better their prognosis will be. However, surgery must be performed earlier for a child who exhibits symptoms of heart failure, pulmonary hypertension, or severe cyanosis.

Sometimes, palliative surgery is performed early, and corrective surgery is attempted when the child is older. In some cases, activity is reduced to lessen strain on the heart, and medications are administered to strengthen the heart's activity and to decrease fluid accumulation, the heart's workload, and the chance of infection.

Medications may include digoxin, diuretics, and antibiotics. Some children regularly receive oxygen. The child should be in the best possible physical and mental condition before surgery.

Open-Heart Surgery

In *open-heart surgery*, bypassing the heart circulation by means of a heart–lung pump (pump oxygenator) is necessary. The heart's action is temporarily stopped. Closed-heart surgery is much safer, although any open-chest surgery is serious. A heart transplant is also possible.

Surgery may be done under hypothermic conditions, which reduces body temperature, thereby slowing all body processes, or performed under hyperbaric conditions, in which the atmospheric pressure is increased to force the blood to carry more oxygen.

BLOOD AND LYMPH DISORDERS

Kawasaki Disease

Kawasaki disease (mucocutaneous lymph node syndrome) is a febrile, multisystem disorder resulting in inflammation of the blood vessels (*vasculitis*). The platelets in the blood tend to be caught in the vessels. It occurs in children younger than 5 years. If untreated, as many as 25% of children with Kawasaki disease develop severe cardiac problems. Its cause is unknown.

Symptoms of Kawasaki disease include the following:

- Prolonged fever of 5 days or more
- Red and infected eyes
- "Strawberry tongue" and cracked, dry lips and oral mucous membranes
- Edema of hands and feet; reddened and peeling soles and palms
- Rash (particularly in the perineal area)
- Swollen lymph nodes
- Pain

Diagnosis of Kawasaki disease is based on the healthcare provider's assessment of these symptoms. Blood work may reveal increased ESR and anemia; urinalysis may be abnormal.

SPECIAL CONSIDERATIONS — Culture and Ethnicity

Kawasaki Disease

Kawasaki disease was first identified in Japan. The incidence is highest in clients of Asian descent.

Medical treatment includes administration of gamma globulin and medications with antipyretic, anti-inflammatory properties (acetaminophen, ibuprofen). Later, an antiplatelet dose is given until the child's platelet count comes down to normal. Nursing care is supportive and should include frequent oral care, skin care, and cardiac monitoring.

Anemia

Anemia results from an abnormally low number of red blood cells (RBCs), low hemoglobin content, or defects in RBC functioning. Some children develop anemia when bottle feeding continues for too long, and they do not eat iron-rich foods. Anemia can also result from hemorrhage, hemolytic disease, malabsorption of vitamin B_{12}, and hereditary factors (Box 82-1).

Iron Deficiency Anemia

The most common childhood type of anemia is iron deficiency anemia. Infants should be kept on breast milk, which contains some highly absorbable iron, or an iron-fortified commercial formula until 1 year of age to prevent this condition. Maternal iron stores are exhausted in a term infant by 4–6 months of age, and the healthcare provider may encourage iron supplements. Iron-fortified cereal should be the first solid food introduced. Some forms of anemia respond to vitamins and iron. Emphasize to family caregivers the need for the child to follow a nutritious diet, especially with complete proteins, vegetables, and fruits. Caregivers should include foods high in iron, such as egg yolk, green vegetables (peas, green beans, lettuce, spinach), dried beans, dried peas, peanut butter, organ meats, poultry, fish, and fruits.

> **Key Concept**
>
> Liquid iron preparations can be administered through a straw or placed on the back of the tongue with a dropper, to prevent staining of the teeth and to mask the taste. Rinsing of the mouth after ingestion also reduces staining. Iron preparations (Feosol) are best absorbed if taken on an empty stomach. If gastric distress occurs, the medication can be taken with, or immediately after, meals. Orange juice enhances the body's iron absorption if taken at the time of medication administration.

Sickle Cell Disease

Sickle cell disease is a genetic disorder that is primarily seen in descendants of people from Africa, Saudi Arabia, India, and the Mediterranean area. *Sickle cell disease* includes any of the diseases having the presence of hemoglobin S and sickle cells. *Sickle cell trait* occurs in the person with one defective gene and one normal gene. *Sickle cell anemia* occurs in the child when both parents carry the recessive gene. The carrier does not show symptoms of the disease. Testing of newborns (*hemoglobin electrophoresis*) can be done to diagnose sickle cell disease or sickle cell trait.

Sickling, or the formation of an abnormal, curved, sickle-shaped RBC, is key to this disorder. These misshapen RBCs are ineffective as oxygen carriers and therefore cause anemia. The sickle shape allows the RBCs to clump together, thereby blocking capillaries. Because blood cannot circulate properly and carry oxygen to the body cells, anemia and circulatory occlusion result.

Clinical symptoms of the disease usually do not appear until the child is about 6 months old because sufficient fetal hemoglobin is still present to prevent sickling. Eventually, the child develops chronic anemia and splenomegaly. Episodes of lethargy, weakness, and fever are sporadic or daily. *Thrombosis* (formation of blood clots) is not uncommon.

Sickle cell crises are severe, painful episodes of sickle cell anemia, which are caused by clumping and occlusion of blood vessels. With blood vessel occlusions and without proper oxygenation, tissues become ischemic and can eventually die (*infarction*).

Common sites of pain include the abdomen and the hands and feet; any joint pain may migrate to other joints or be constant. Organs can be damaged, causing a stroke, headaches, convulsions, hearing or visual disturbances, paralysis, pulmonary emboli, and hematuria.

Treatment of sickle cell crisis includes analgesics, transfusions of RBCs, oxygen therapy, and hydration. Constant monitoring of the child during a crisis is necessary because of the possibilities of stroke, shock, or hypoxic episodes. Individuals with a severe active form of the disease usually do not live past middle adulthood.

Nursing considerations include the administration of pain medications, oxygen, and rest. The application of warmth may help diminish pain and promote circulation. Cold therapy is contraindicated because it can worsen clumping. Client and family teaching should include suggestions to avoid cold environments and high altitudes and, when traveling by air, to fly only in a pressurized cabin. (For more information about sickle cell disease, see Chapter 82.)

Idiopathic Thrombocytopenic Purpura

Idiopathic thrombocytopenic purpura (**ITP**) is the most common acquired bleeding disorder of childhood. The acute form is seen most often in children between the ages of 3 and 7 years. Symptoms include easy bruising, often without an obvious cause; *petechiae* (tiny internal hemorrhages) on the mucous membranes; frequent epistaxis; and bleeding into the bladder or GI tract. Symptoms appear suddenly, and the child may look as though they have been beaten.

The disease is seldom fatal in children. In most cases, symptoms run an acute course and then clear, with recovery within 6 weeks. The greatest risk is intracranial hemorrhage. Sometimes, the cause of the disease cannot be identified, although an affected mother can transmit it to her fetus.

Nursing care involves close observation for hemorrhage, avoidance of injury, and bed rest. Keep the side rails of the bed raised and pad them to prevent accidental bruising. Use a soft toothbrush for oral care to avoid gum injury. Do not give the child intramuscular (IM) injections because of the danger of hematoma formation. Rectal temperatures or enemas are not recommended because of the possibility of trauma to the mucous membranes. Avoid urinary catheterization because of the danger of hemorrhage and infection. Avoid invasive procedures, such as venipuncture, for the same reason. If venipuncture must be done, exert pressure on the puncture site for at least 20 min after inserting the needle to prevent hemorrhage. Transfusions of platelets are of limited benefit. The child may receive steroids. In extreme cases, a *splenectomy* (surgical removal of the spleen) is performed.

Hemophilia

Hemophilia is a sex-linked, hereditary bleeding disorder in which a deficiency exists in one or more of the factors necessary for blood clotting. Generally, the missing factor is factor VIII or factor IX. Males become symptomatic with hemophilia. Females are carriers of the gene, but are very rarely symptomatic.

Internal and external hemorrhage can occur with even a minor injury. Bleeding into soft tissues, the GI tract, and joints (most commonly the hip, knee, ankle, and elbow) results in severe pain. Bleeding into joints may first be noticed when the child begins to walk. Joint contractures can result from scarring and fibrosis of damaged joint synovial membranes. Death can occur as a result of hemorrhage.

Nursing considerations include the prevention of injury. Gently touch or move the child. Use measures to try to stop hemorrhage. Take tympanic temperatures to reduce the risk of hemorrhage. Periodic transfusions of blood products may be required. Factor VIII has been genetically produced, which allows for safe replacement of the missing clotting factor.

Teach the family to recognize the symptoms of bleeding, to get medical assistance immediately when needed, and to protect the child from injury without being overprotective.

Leukemia

Leukemia is a group of associated disorders characterized by malignancies in the bone marrow and lymphatic system. The highest rates occur in children younger than 4 years. A child's survival may depend on the risk factors involved. Factors relating to prognosis include the type of cell involved, age at onset (the child aged 2–8 years has a better prognosis), initial WBC count (a low WBC count has a better prognosis), and the child's sex (girls have a better prognosis). Rapid remission usually means a better prognosis.

Types of Leukemias

Leukemia is classified into four major types:

- Acute lymphoid leukemia (**ALL**)
- Acute myeloid leukemia (**AML**)
- Chronic lymphoid leukemia (**CLL**)
- Chronic myeloid leukemia (**CML**)

Leukemia may be inherited, especially CLL. Genetic abnormalities, such as those associated with Down syndrome, also carry higher risks for specific forms of leukemia. Risk factors to leukemia include exposure to ionizing radiation and benzene, a chemical found in unleaded gasoline. ALL has a better prognosis.

Diagnosis

Diagnosis is made on the basis of medical history, which often indicates sudden illness with general malaise, high fever, joint pains, bleeding from body orifices, and enlargement of the liver, spleen, and lymph nodes. The WBC count is usually elevated, with characteristic abnormal cells. The child is anemic, with a hemoglobin count as low as 4–8 g/dL (grams per deciliter [100 mL]); normal is about 13–14 g/dL. Bone marrow and lymph node biopsy can produce a positive diagnosis. Further testing may include genetic studies.

Symptoms

Symptoms of leukemia include fatigue, aches in bones and joints, headaches, fever, swollen lymph nodes, unexplained weight loss, bleeding of gums or nose, frequent bruising, and slow healing. The individual is pale and lethargic and bruises easily. Sometimes, the client becomes ill gradually, with increasing weakness and pallor.

Acute Leukemias

In *acute leukemias*, normal bone marrow is relatively rapidly replaced by large numbers of immature lymphoid or myeloid cells. These primitive cells do not mature normally and, therefore, are incapable of functioning as effective WBCs. Over time, the abnormal cells crowd out normal blood cells. Anemia can develop as the primitive cells interfere with the production and maturation of RBCs. In addition, the cancerous cells can collect in lymph nodes and cause swelling. Organ function can be disrupted when these cancerous cells spread.

Acute Lymphoid Leukemia

Acute lymphoid leukemia is sometimes called *lymphocytic, lymphatic, lymphoblastic, stem cell,* or *blast cell leukemia*. ALL is the most common kind of cancer in children younger than 15 years.

Acute Myeloid Leukemia

Acute myeloid leukemia is also called *granulocytic, myelocytic, monocytic, myelogenous, monoblastic,* or *monomyeloblastic leukemia*. AML is the most prevalent form of leukemia in adults and usually presents in young people, from teenagers to people in their 20s, but rarely presents in young children.

Chronic Leukemia

With *chronic leukemias*, the characteristic excessive production of cells occurs in abnormal but apparently mature cells. Chronic leukemia does not attack as swiftly as acute leukemia and progresses more slowly. As with acute leukemia cells, the cells of chronic leukemia do not fight infection well. They invade bone marrow and lymph nodes. Children with CLL and CML have wide ranges of lifespans after disease onset. Factors that affect survival rates include early diagnosis, the age of the child, and the individual success of therapies. Chronic leukemia is discussed in Chapter 82 because it is a disease that affects adults more than children.

Medical and Surgical Treatment

Aggressive treatment of leukemia is necessary to inhibit the production of leukemic cells. Treatment includes chemotherapy and radiation and also may include stem cell transplant or platelet transfusions.

Treatment occurs in phases. A phase is determined by factors such as the client's overall condition and whether the disease is newly diagnosed, in *remission* (controlled but not cured), or in relapse after a remission. Chemotherapy may be given initially, with the goal of putting the disease in remission. Various chemotherapies may be combined with radiation as prophylaxis to prevent metastasis. When the child has achieved remission, maintenance of treatment consists of scheduled visits to the health provider, who monitors the child's overall condition and reviews laboratory tests. *Recurrent leukemia* happens when a child has a relapse or recurrence of the disease. When a relapse occurs, the child is given additional chemotherapies to maintain a remission.

Chemotherapy

Chemotherapy consists of potent antineoplastic (*anticancer*) drugs. These drugs must be carefully administered. Many drugs are given intravenously through a central line in a large vein. Oral drugs are sometimes used, alone or in combination with IV therapy. Medications and protocols vary.

Side effects and adverse reactions of chemotherapy include *alopecia* (hair loss), bleeding, *oliguria* (low urine volume), fluid retention, edema, anorexia, nausea and vomiting, rashes, skin lesions, severe headache, fluctuations in body temperature, and tissue necrosis around the injection site.

Inflammation and ulceration of the GI tract may occur, with ulcerated sores in the mouth often appearing as the first symptom, followed by anal ulcerations. Check the child's mouth each day with a flashlight to make sure no ulcerations, reddened areas, or white patches are present. Report any unusual symptoms immediately (In Practice: Important Medications 72-1).

Platelet Therapy

Platelet apheresis is a process through which only the platelets are removed from a donor's blood. The amount of platelets removed is equivalent to that collected from 6 to 10 U of whole blood. The platelets are then transfused into the leukemic child. Platelet therapy is performed in the hope of forestalling death by hemorrhage until a chemotherapeutic cure is found. This therapy is used primarily in children with AML.

Radiation Therapy

Radiation therapy may be a part of the regimen; however, it can cause vomiting, diarrhea, severe electrolyte imbalance, and rapid dehydration. Appropriate nursing considerations are necessary when caring for children receiving radiation therapy.

Combination Chemotherapy and Radiation

In some cases, chemotherapeutic agents and radiation are combined for maximum effectiveness. This therapy may be hard on the client and may reduce antibody levels to the point at which infections occur. The individual may be kept in protective isolation during treatment.

IN PRACTICE
IMPORTANT MEDICATIONS 72-1 For Leukemia Treatment

Acute Lymphoid Leukemia
- prednisone (Meticorten, Orasone)
- vincristine (Oncovin)
- asparaginase (Elspar)
- doxorubicin HCl (ADR, Adriamycin)
- cytarabine (Cytosar-U)
- methotrexate (MTX, Amethopterin)
- mercaptopurine (6-MP, Purinethol)

Acute Myeloid Leukemia
- doxorubicin (ADR, Adriamycin)
- daunorubicin citrate (DNR, DaunoXome)
- cytarabine (cytosine arabinoside, Ara-C, Cytosar-U)

Chronic Lymphoid Leukemia
- chlorambucil (Leukeran)
- Combination therapy of Cytoxan, Oncovin, and prednisone (COP)

Chronic Myeloid Leukemia
- busulfan (Myleran)
- hydroxyurea (Hydrea)
- Combination therapy of daunorubicin, Ara-C, thioguanine (DAT)

Nursing Considerations
- Chapter 62 discusses side effects for corticosteroid use.

Hematopoietic Stem Cell Transplantation

Previously referred to solely as bone marrow transplantation (**BMT**), hematopoietic stem cell transplantation (HSCT) uses a variety of sources for stem cells, including those derived from the bone marrow, umbilical cord blood, or placenta hematopoietic stem cells. If a client does not improve with other treatments, HSCT may be done. HSCT, donors, and grafting treatments are discussed in Chapter 82.

Stem cells are transplanted through an IV infusion, similar to a blood transfusion. The transplanted marrow naturally grafts itself within the recipient's bones, replacing diseased marrow and making new blood cells.

Nursing Considerations

The child with leukemia can be severely anemic and *thrombocytopenic* (low platelets), which leads to easy bruising and bleeding. Death from hemorrhage is a possibility because of insufficient platelets. Because WBCs are defective, the child is highly susceptible to infection.

The greatest threat to the child during treatment is *bone marrow suppression* (decreased WBCs, RBCs, and platelets), which may lead to life-threatening infection, anemia, or hemorrhage.

Treat symptoms, and make the child as comfortable as possible. Encourage the child to be as active as the disease permits. Prevent infections and injuries. Do not take rectal temperatures because of the danger of injury. Report a cough or any other symptom of a URI immediately; any infection can result in generalized septicemia and can cause death.

The client and family need skilled emotional support. Help caregivers accept the course of the disease; always offer hope of remission. The sick child is a part of a family unit; they should be involved in family life and friendships as much as possible.

 Nursing Alert The individual undergoing treatment for leukemia usually has very low immunity to disease; the greatest danger is infection. Excellent nursing technique is essential for the client's protection.

Other Cancers

Malignant lymphomas, such as **Hodgkin lymphoma** (Chapter 82), lymphosarcoma, and other sarcomas (e.g., osteogenic sarcoma) are not uncommon in children. Children with such conditions may have a poor prognosis because malignancies in children often progress quickly and are not detected early. The most common cancers in children are those of the brain, kidney, adrenal glands, bones, and structures of the CNS.

Any brain tumor is serious; the increase in size puts undue pressure on the brain and can cause brain damage. Very young children are less likely to have malignant tumors than are older people. In children, the most common brain tumors are gliomas of the cerebellum, the brain stem, the optic nerve, tumors of the pituitary, and congenital brain tumors. They are most likely to be fast growing and may be inoperable. Whenever possible, immediate surgery and follow-up radiation or chemotherapy is required to prevent further complications.

Dealing with the emotional impact of childhood cancer may require the most nursing assistance. Chapters 82 and 83 also discuss the need to provide emotional support to the child and the family dealing with cancer.

RESPIRATORY TRACT DISORDERS

Upper Respiratory Infection

URIs are common in children and adults; they may be caused by a virus or a bacterium. Symptoms of URI may include a fever; varying degrees of dyspnea with thick, tenacious sputum and mucus; and throat edema. If no cough is present, the child may have difficulty getting rid of secretions. Children are usually cared for at home unless complications develop.

General treatment includes fluids humidity and rest. Oxygen may be necessary. The child may be put in a mist tent, or a bedside cool-air humidifier may be used. If hospitalized, the child with a contagious disease is kept in their room, and only adults may visit. At home, caregivers should try to keep ill children separate from well children and encourage the use of separate glasses and utensils. Frequent handwashing is a must.

Pneumonia

Pneumonia, an inflammation of the lungs, usually with consolidation and drainage, is common in children and adults. It may initially be an infectious disease (see pneumococcal pneumonia immunization earlier in this chapter), or a disease that is secondary to another disease, or it may result from aspiration. The healthcare provider differentiates pneumonia from other URIs by means of a chest x-ray examination. Pneumonia is usually treated with antibiotics, rest, and fluids.

When caregivers administer antibiotics for any reason, they should understand that the child must take the medication for the prescribed number of days. If the prescribed regimen is not followed, resistant strains of pathogens can develop.

Laryngotracheobronchitis

Laryngotracheobronchitis (**LTB**), a viral infection of the upper airways, usually follows several days of URI. It is also known as *croup*. Croup is a syndrome that results in a harsh, "barky" cough, *inspiratory stridor* (shrill sound on inhalation), hoarseness, and other signs of respiratory distress.

Croup syndromes that affect the larynx, the trachea, and bronchi are serious in children because of the smaller diameter of their airways. Acute spasmodic croup is an inflammation of the subglottic area characterized by the barking cough and varying degrees of respiratory distress occurring primarily at night. Copious, tenacious secretions and edema of the airway make breathing difficult. Cyanosis may be present. The child usually has a low fever, rapid pulse, cold and clammy skin, and flushed face. Treatment consists of cool, humidified air and keeping the child calm.

The child is placed in a mist-tent humidifying device. Oxygen may be given to assist respirations. A pulse oximeter may be used to detect hypoxia. A chest x-ray examination

may be ordered. Expectorants are often given to loosen secretions and to assist the child in coughing up mucus. A semi-Fowler position may ease respiratory efforts. Antipyretics (acetaminophen, ibuprofen) are used to reduce temperature. Oral fluids are encouraged. If the child cannot take fluids orally, IV fluids are given. Frequently offer clear liquids, ice pops, gelatin, and other fluids.

Epiglottitis

Acute **epiglottitis** is an acute, rapidly progressive, life-threatening inflammation of the epiglottis usually caused by a bacterium. Severe respiratory distress, high fever, absence of cough, and drooling of saliva (with refusal to swallow owing to an extremely sore throat) are the cardinal symptoms. Intravenous antibiotics result in a rapid recovery. Endotracheal intubation for 1–3 days may be necessary to ensure a patent airway.

> **Nursing Alert** If epiglottitis is suspected, do not attempt to examine the throat, obtain a throat culture, or do anything that might upset the child because this might cause respiratory obstruction.

Asthma

Asthma is a chronic inflammatory disorder of the airways affecting millions of adults and children. Asthma is caused by edematous airways and excessive mucus production, which cause airway obstruction. The incidence of asthma has been steadily increasing globally as a result of multiple environmental factors. Other triggers may include strenuous physical exercise, high humidity or cold temperatures, some foods and food additives, and some medications. Emotions may play a part in asthma because the stress of the disorder complicates the person's ability to maximize the use of their personal defense mechanisms. Asthma has become a common chronic illness of childhood and is a primary reason for school absences. Most clients with asthma have their first symptoms by the age of 4 years.

Symptoms

The disorder is chronic, but acute asthma attacks generally occur when triggers or irritants affect the lungs. Attacks may occur abruptly or may gradually build over several days. Wheezing is not always present, but is a common symptom. Wheezing occurs when expired air is pushed through obstructed bronchioles. Other common symptoms include difficulty breathing, chest tightness, and coughing, particularly at nighttime or in the early morning. During an attack, the lungs become inflamed and edematous. The small bronchiole muscles constrict airways so that less air goes in and out of the lungs. Mucus forms and can clog the small airways.

Treatment

Prevention is the most important aspect of treatment. Children and their families must learn to recognize the symptoms that lead to an attack and begin treatment as soon as possible. Family caregivers should work toward eliminating any possible allergens in the home. Their children need protection against smoke inhalation. In addition, family caregivers must alert teachers, school nurses, babysitters, and others involved with the child of their asthma so that they can provide support as needed.

The drug of choice is bronchodilators during an asthma attack, including albuterol. Additionally, steroids may be administered orally or through metered-dose inhalers (**MDI**). Prophylactic medications that may be used daily also include leukotriene antagonists, such as montelukast (Singulair) or zafirlukast (Accolate). Long-term management of asthma includes bronchodilators albuterol (Ventolin). Mast cell stabilizers, such as cromolyn sodium (Intal) or nedocromil (Tilade), may also be used as daily therapy to prevent asthma attacks. Treatment for asthma varies with the duration and intensity of the illness. In an acute attack, epinephrine may be used. Corticosteroids, either orally or, preferred, by inhalation, may be used for the short-term management of acute or chronic inflammation of the respiratory tract.

The child learns to use the nebulizer or MDI to administer medications. Use of a spacing unit makes the MDI easier to use and aids in delivering the correct dosage of the medication to the lung tissue (Fig. 72-11).

Chest physical therapy (**CPT**) is also a useful addition to treatment; it includes breathing exercises, physical training, postural drainage, and inhalation therapy.

> **Nursing Alert** Acute severe asthma, often called status asthmaticus, is a condition that can be fatal. It exists when medications do not relieve an acute episode of asthma. Treatment includes administration of IV fluids, bronchodilators (e.g., aminophylline), antibiotics, and anti-inflammatory agents.

Bronchiolitis

Bronchiolitis is a viral respiratory infection resulting in inflammation of the bronchioles. It is seen most often in children younger than 2 years and tends to be a seasonal illness, occurring in winter and early spring.

The illness begins with symptoms of a cold, which gradually worsen. Chest x-ray studies reveal air trapping in the lungs. The illness usually resolves within 10 days. A severe case of bronchiolitis may require hospitalization and treatment with IV fluids and oxygen administered by mist tent. RSV, discussed earlier in this chapter, is believed to cause more than half the cases of bronchiolitis.

Cystic Fibrosis

Cystic fibrosis, a multisystem chronic and lifelong condition, is a major dysfunction of the exocrine glands. It is the most common genetic disease among European American individuals, inherited as an autosomal recessive condition. It is rare in African American and Asian American individuals. It affects the respiratory system, GI system (pancreas, liver), and, in adult men, reproductive organs. In cystic fibrosis, mucus-producing glands secrete abnormal quantities of thick mucus. These secretions collect in the child's lungs, pancreas, and liver, disrupting the normal functions of these organs. Many children with cystic fibrosis eventually die of cardiopulmonary complications; however, with active treatment, children often live past adolescence.

Symptoms and Diagnosis

Symptoms may occur at any age. Some children show symptoms in infancy, including *meconium ileus* (causing bowel obstruction), bile-stained emesis, a distended abdomen, and no stool. The skin of these infants may have a salty taste because of the high sodium chloride content in their sweat. FTT, despite a good appetite, is common. In some children, a hard, nonproductive cough may be the first indication. Frequent respiratory infections follow. A barrel chest, finger clubbing, and signs of malnutrition may be evident.

Diagnosis is based on family history, elevated sodium chloride levels in the sweat (as determined by a sweat test), analysis of duodenal secretions for trypsin content (obtained via a nasogastric tube), and a history of frequent respiratory infections and FTT. If the sweat test is positive for high levels of sodium, only one other criterion must be met for a positive diagnosis.

Medical Treatment

During an acute infection, the client is treated with antibiotics to prevent infection. Drugs, such as pancreatin and pancrelipase, seem to be useful in counteracting pancreatic insufficiency. These pancreatic enzymes are given with meals or snacks to aid in digesting fats and proteins. Pancreatic enzymes have an enteric coating that protects stomach acid from destroying them and delivers them safely to the duodenum. They should be administered at the beginning of the meal with cold—not hot—food because heat decreases the activity of the enzyme.

The high-calorie, high-protein, moderate-fat diet should include supplementary water-soluble forms of fat-soluble vitamins A, D, E, and K, which are necessary because of poor fat digestion. Weight should be frequently monitored. Salt should not be restricted, especially in hot weather. Fluids should be encouraged to prevent dehydration, which causes the mucus to become thicker.

Treatment for maintaining optimum pulmonary function includes chest physical therapy, inhalation therapy, antibacterial drugs for the prophylaxis or treatment of infection, as indicated, and immunization against childhood communicable diseases. All immunizations should be maintained and

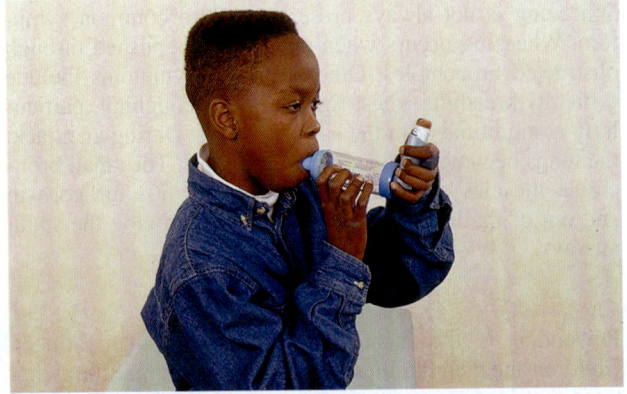

Figure 72-11 Child using a metered-dose inhaler with spacer. (Klossner & Hatfield, 2006.)

given at appropriate intervals. Encourage physical activity because it improves mucus secretion as well as a positive self-image. Encourage the child to participate in any aerobic activity they enjoy. Limit activity, along with physical therapy, only according to the child's endurance.

Inhalation therapy is prescribed as a preventive or therapeutic measure. A bronchodilator drug (albuterol) is usually administered by a hand-held nebulizer. Agents that break down DNA molecules in sputum result in a breakup of the thick mucus in the airways. The addition of a mucolytic agent, such as acetylcysteine (Mucomyst), may be prescribed during periods of acute infection. A humidifier can provide a beneficial moist atmosphere. During the summer, a room air conditioner can help provide the child with comfort and controlled humidity.

Chest physical therapy is performed regularly. CPT is a combination of postural drainage and chest *percussion* (clapping and vibrating of the affected areas). Chest percussion that is performed correctly helps to loosen and move secretions out of the lungs. A nurse, physical therapist, or respiratory therapist can teach family caregivers to perform this routine as an essential part of home care.

The family needs much teaching and support. Because cystic fibrosis is a genetic disease, more than one child in a family can be affected. Caregivers should avoid overprotecting the child or children. Caregivers will need to learn CPT, postural drainage, administration of IV antibiotics, and enzyme regulation, according to the child's needs. In summer, the active child may need extra salt. Caring for the child places enormous stress on the family's financial resources. The Cystic Fibrosis Foundation, a national organization, provides education and services for these children and their families. In addition, assistance may be available through local sources. The caregivers must also learn to take time to care for themselves.

GASTROINTESTINAL DISORDERS

Review the information on general surgery in Chapter 56 and pediatric surgery in Chapter 71 before caring for children who are undergoing surgery for GI disorders.

Pyloric Stenosis

In **pyloric stenosis**, also called congenital hypertrophic pyloric stenosis, the child's pyloric sphincter thickens, narrowing the canal through which food passes from the stomach to the intestine. This condition is more common in boys than in girls. An infant usually does not show signs of pyloric stenosis until they are about 2 months old. The stenosis may be so extensive that the obstruction is complete; the pylorus then closes, and food cannot pass into the intestine. As a result, the child regurgitates food into the esophagus, causing severe projectile vomiting. Vomiting is the most common symptom of pyloric stenosis. Other symptoms include loss of weight, hunger, irritability, and dehydration. Often, constipation and oliguria are associated with it. Diagnosis is made on the basis of an upper GI ultrasound examination.

Medical and Surgical Treatment

The treatment of choice for pyloric stenosis is surgery (*pyloromyotomy*). However, if the child is a poor surgical risk and if the stenosis is not life-threatening, medical means of treatment may be used, including sedation, antispasmodic drugs, and thickened feedings.

Nursing Considerations

Before surgery, IV fluids should be given to correct fluid and electrolyte imbalance caused by vomiting. Electrolyte laboratory studies identify the type of solution to administer. An accurate record of I&O and the amount and type of vomitus is essential.

After surgery, precautions should be taken to prevent aspiration. Position the child on the right side, with their head slightly elevated. Schedule care so that you give the child a bath *before* feeding. Glucose water feedings are started 2–3 hr after surgery; bubble the child frequently. Increase the amount of feedings when the infant is able to retain more. Progress the diet from glucose water, to half-strength formula, to full-strength formula. Recovery is usually complete, and the child experiences no further problems.

Meckel Diverticulum

Meckel diverticulum is a congenital disorder in which a small portion of the child's ileum ends in a blind pouch just before its junction with the colon. Symptoms include the passage of bloody or tarry stools. The child experiences no pain unless the diverticulum is inflamed; the condition may exist without ever causing symptoms. When symptoms do occur, surgical removal of the pouch is necessary. Complications are rare. Preoperative and postoperative care is routine.

Hernia

A **hernia** is the protrusion of part of an organ through an abnormal opening. In children, a congenital defect is most often the cause of hernia. Hernias take various forms:

- *Diaphragmatic hernia*, which occurs rarely, is a condition in which a portion of the intestine protrudes through the diaphragm. It is usually diagnosed at birth and repaired through immediate surgery.
- In *umbilical hernia*, a portion of the intestine protrudes through a weak umbilical ring, producing a bulge beneath the child's navel. Because this condition commonly disappears by the time the child is 3–4 years old, surgery is usually unnecessary. Strangulation of the protruding part is rare, with surgery necessary only if the protruding part is large or if other congenital defects are present.
- In *indirect inguinal hernia*, which is most frequent in boys, the intestine protrudes through the round ligament into the inguinal area and may descend into the scrotal sac. Surgery is required if strangulation develops. In girls, an inguinal hernia may involve the ovary or the uterus, and immediate surgery is needed to prevent damage to these structures.
- A *direct inguinal hernia* protrudes through the weakest part of the abdominal wall. Because the peritoneum overlying the protruding abdominal contents is transparent, all or part of the abdominal contents may be seen. Should the hernia rupture, severe hemorrhage, peritonitis, a generalized septicemia, or strangulation of the hernia could occur. Surgery is usually performed early in life.

Treatment

The treatment of choice for most hernias is surgery. The specific procedure varies with the condition. Preoperative and postoperative care is routine. Often hernia repair is completed in the same-day surgery suite and may be done by laparoscopy.

Diarrhea

Diarrhea is a sudden increase in frequency of loose and watery stools. It is most often caused by pathogens in the GI tract. Stress, prolonged temperature elevation, and spoiled food are other causes. Certain antibiotics can alter the bacteria normally present in the intestine, resulting in an increased number of stools.

Diarrhea can be very dangerous for young children. Smaller and younger children are at increased risk for fluid and electrolyte imbalance and dehydration. Severe diarrhea can be rapidly fatal in an infant.

Medical Treatment

Mild forms of diarrhea are treated at home. Family caregivers should administer an oral rehydration solution (**ORS**), such as Pedialyte, to children with diarrhea. ORSs are available in different flavors. Clear liquids with sugar and/or caffeine should be avoided. An age-appropriate diet should be offered within 24 hr. Family caregivers should avoid giving salty broth to children with diarrhea because the salt content may further disturb their electrolyte balance.

In severe diarrhea, stools are frequent and forceful and are green or yellow liquid. The child is lethargic and irritable. Skin turgor is poor, mucous membranes are dry, the eyes and anterior fontanels are sunken, urination is decreased, and the pulse is weak and rapid, indicating dehydration. Usually IV fluids, based on electrolyte studies, are necessary to replace water loss and to restore fluid and electrolyte balance. A chest x-ray examination determines any complicating respiratory condition, and a stool culture identifies the causative organism.

Nursing Considerations

Transmission-Based Precautions should be followed when caring for the child with diarrhea. IV therapy is necessary to replace body fluids. Be sure to comfort the child, and to release restraints periodically so that the child can change position at will.

Maintain accurate I&O records and carefully describe the amount and character of all stools. Continue food and fluids, except in cases of severe vomiting. Teach caregivers to use ORSs and observe the child for any signs of dehydration. Clear fluids and juices are inadequate because they are high in carbohydrates but low in electrolytes. Encourage the early reintroduction of regular nutrients.

Good skin care is essential because the child's buttocks can become sore and irritated. Thorough, gentle cleansing from the front of the perineal area to the back is necessary each time the child defecates. Expose the child's buttocks to air as much as possible. Sitz baths in clear, tepid water and protective ointments help ease discomfort.

Encopresis

Encopresis is incontinence of feces without physical cause. It occurs in previously toilet-trained children. Usually, symptoms begin with stool withholding late in infancy.

Treatment should be geared toward improving family relationships and understanding personality patterns. Nursing support and a nonjudgmental, nonpunishing approach from family caregivers is fundamental to the therapeutic plan. The child with prolonged encopresis and the caregivers may need counseling. Increased dietary fiber and fluids is recommended. Additional medications, such as polyethylene glycol, are usually initiated after disimpaction.

Lactose Intolerance

If a child has frequent attacks of diarrhea, the problem may be **lactose intolerance**, an inherited disorder characterized by an inability to metabolize lactose in milk and milk products. It is more common in Asian American individuals and African American individuals than in other ethnic groups.

The child who is lactose intolerant cannot drink milk or eat dairy products. Not only does the lactose-intolerant person's body improperly absorb and metabolize dairy products, but the presence of such substances also interferes with the absorption of other foods. If the problem is not recognized and treated in a child, they could die from malnutrition.

Symptoms of lactose intolerance include diarrhea, abdominal pain, vomiting, listlessness, and FTT. These symptoms may appear 1–2 weeks after birth. The baby is switched to a lactose-free formula. Yogurt, which has inactive lactase that is activated by the temperature and pH of the duodenum, is an excellent source of calcium. Teach family caregivers to observe for hidden sources of lactose that the child must avoid.

Intussusception

Intussusception is the telescoping of one bowel part into another. It is usually caused by hyperactive peristalsis in one bowel part and hypoactivity in another. Cardinal symptoms include abdominal pain and passage of a currant jelly stool (clear mucus with blood). One danger of this condition is that the bowel's blood supply may be blocked, causing gangrene and possible bowel rupture.

Intussusception is most common in infants; yet affected babies usually appear to be thriving. A definite diagnosis is based on the findings of a barium enema. The x-ray examination itself may reduce the intussusception; if not, surgery is necessary to prevent complications. Preoperative and postoperative care is routine, and the healthy child seldom has complications.

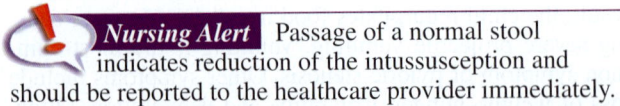

Nursing Alert Passage of a normal stool indicates reduction of the intussusception and should be reported to the healthcare provider immediately.

Colic

Colic is paroxysmal abdominal pain, most commonly occurring in the first 3 months of an infant's life. The baby almost always outgrows the condition by the time they are 3–4 months old. Although colic is not serious, it can be extremely frustrating for family caregivers. Affected babies have frequent crying episodes. These children double up as though they are in great pain. Symptoms seem to worsen in the evenings.

Treatment consists of feeding the baby slowly and reducing the amount of air that the infant swallows. A pacifier may help by promoting nonnutritive sucking. Soothing the infant through touching, rocking, and gently speaking is also recommended. Family caregivers need a break from the baby's constant crying; encourage them to develop a support system of relatives, friends, and babysitters.

Megacolon

In **megacolon**, also known as **Hirschsprung disease** or *aganglionic megacolon*, the child's colon lacks parasympathetic nerve supply. Because of a lack of peristalsis, the abdomen becomes abnormally enlarged with stool and flatus. If a large colon segment is affected, palliative treatment may be the only alternative. Surgical treatment may be effective if the damaged or malfunctioning portion can be removed.

Symptoms and Diagnosis

Feces accumulation in the child's bowel causes symptoms that include diarrhea, constipation, nausea, and vomiting. The abdomen becomes distended, and bowel movements are abnormal, resulting in malnutrition. Usually, the effects of megacolon appear shortly after birth when the newborn fails to pass meconium within 24–48 hr.

Signs of obstruction, such as bile-stained or fecal vomiting, abdominal distention, irritability, feeding problems, FTT, or dehydration, may occur. The older child exhibits intractable constipation that usually requires laxatives and saline enemas. Surgery is usually required.

Diagnosis is made on the basis of medical history, x-ray studies, barium enema, and palpation of the distended abdomen. A proctoscopy usually reveals an empty rectum and lower colon, and biopsy of the rectal wall usually indicates an absence of nerve fibers.

Medical and Surgical Treatment

If possible, corrective surgery is delayed until the child is about 1 year old and better able to withstand the procedure. During the waiting period, preventing constipation is important. Small saline enemas, stool softeners, and digital removal of fecal impactions are used. Sometimes colonic irrigations are done. These are similar to enemas, except that they require a larger tube to be passed into the descending colon.

Drugs that act on the parasympathetic and sympathetic nervous systems may be given to improve peristalsis. Surgery often involves a temporary *colostomy* (opening of the large intestine onto the abdominal wall).

> **Key Concept**
> Watch for abdominal distention, temperature spikes, and irritability after surgery for megacolon. These are signs of possible anastomotic leaks (leakage where the two ends of the bowel are sewn together).

Nursing Considerations

Preoperative preparation may include saline enemas for colon evacuation. Keep accurate records of the quantity of solution administered. The return solution should be clear of fecal particles. Administer ordered antibiotics as a bowel preparation.

Keep the surgical wound clean and dry after surgery. Do not take rectal temperatures. The child's first liquid bowel movement will be approximately 3–4 days after surgery. Observe for the presence of blood in the child's urine because bladder trauma can result from extensive surgical manipulation.

Clear oral feedings usually begin after active bowel sounds are audible. The diet progresses according to the child's tolerance. Instruct family caregivers to watch closely for foods that increase the child's number of stools and to avoid including them in the child's diet at home. Assure caregivers that the child will eventually achieve sphincter control and be able to eat a normal diet. Complete continence may take several years for the child to attain. Encourage caregivers to participate in the child's care as much as possible, to gain confidence in caring for the child at home.

URINARY SYSTEM DISORDERS

Enuresis

Enuresis is the involuntary passage of urine. When it occurs at night, it is classified as nocturnal enuresis in a child older than 5 years. More commonly, this condition is known as "bed wetting." Enuresis is more common in boys than in girls. A complete urologic workup is necessary to discover any physical cause, including severe infection, bladder trauma, diabetes mellitus, small bladder capacity, meatal stenosis (narrowing of the urinary opening), or bladder spasm. Any such physical cause is treated directly. Other possible physical factors may be that the child does not empty the bladder completely on voiding, or that they are an exceptionally sound sleeper.

If no physical cause is found, providers will investigate a possible underlying emotional problem. Family stress or school problems are associated with enuresis. Family caregivers should not shame or criticize the child for bed wetting. If the condition persists, desmopressin may be used since it has a quick onset of action without long-term effects. For difficult cases, low dosages of an antidepressant, such as imipramine hydrochloride (Tofranil), have been used to promote continence. Oxybutynin chloride (Ditropan) may be used in children older than 5 years. Counseling can sometimes assist the child and family.

Hemolytic Uremic Syndrome

Hemolytic uremic syndrome (**HUS**) is an acute condition occurring in children usually between the ages of 1 and 10 years and primarily between the ages of 6 months and 4 years. Three conditions occur in this illness: renal failure, hemolytic anemia, and thrombocytopenia. HUS is the leading cause of acute kidney failure in children.

Cases of HUS are associated with infection by a toxic strain of *E. coli* (0157:H7). This strain (*E. coli* 0157:H7) causes HUS due to contamination of numerous food sources, such as contaminated meat, raw milk, raw vegetables, and water. Thorough cooking of meat products is critical in preventing this illness. *E. coli* can also be transmitted person to person because it can be transmitted in diarrheal stools. Proper handwashing is essential.

HUS usually presents as a flu-like illness and gastroenteritis. Nausea, vomiting, abdominal pain, fever, and bloody diarrhea may be present. Pallor, lethargy, and oliguria typically follow the onset of the milder symptoms. The affected child appears pale, bruised, and hypertensive, with diminished or absent urine output. As the disease progresses, acute renal failure, hemolytic anemia, thrombocytopenia, and microemboli lead to multisystem organ failure. Seizures, disorientation, decreased LOC, and death may follow.

Treatment includes management of hypertension, dialysis, blood transfusions, and nutritional support.

Urinary Obstruction

Urinary obstruction can result from a *neoplasm* (cancer), *calculi* (stones), or severe infection. Relieving the obstruction is necessary to prevent complications such as hydronephrosis. Catheterization or antibiotics can be effective; otherwise, surgery is performed.

Urinary Tract Infection

Infection of the urinary tract (**UTI**) is most commonly caused by perianal microorganisms, most commonly *E. coli*, and is accompanied by frequency, urgency, and dysuria. The short urethra in the female anatomy contributes to a higher incidence of UTIs in females. Anatomic anomalies may also contribute to the cause of the infection. The occurrence of a UTI in a male warrants urologic evaluation.

Diagnostic evaluation consists of a urine specimen for urinalysis and culture and sensitivity (C&S). Treatment consists of antibiotics, encouraging frequent voiding, and copious fluids. Prevention is the most important goal (In Practice: Educating the Client 72-4). Children who have chronic UTIs may be maintained on low-dose antibiotics.

Pyelonephritis

Pyelonephritis (*pyelitis*) is a potentially dangerous infection of the upper urinary tract and kidneys (Chapter 89). The causative bacterial infection can migrate to the kidneys by way of the bloodstream or ascend from the bladder because the urinary tract has a mucous membrane.

Symptoms of pyelonephritis include *dysuria* (painful voiding), urinary frequency and urgency, fever, chills, lower back pain, and headache. There may be nausea, abdominal tenderness, and pain. C&S tests are done to determine the causative organism so that appropriate antibiotics can be prescribed. Pyelonephritis is curable in most cases if treated promptly.

Glomerulonephritis

Acute **glomerulonephritis**, also called *acute poststreptococcal glomerulonephritis*, is the most common form of nephritis found in young children between the ages of 5 and 10 years. It results from an immunologic reaction to infection (most often, streptococcal) elsewhere in the body. Damage to the glomeruli may cause urinary output to decrease or cease.

The initial and main symptom is smoky urine or hematuria. The child's eyes may be puffy and the blood pressure elevated. A throat culture may reveal GABHS. Kidney enlargement may also be present. Blood tests show mildly to moderately elevated blood urea nitrogen (BUN) and creatinine. The urine shows the presence of RBCs (*microscopic* or *gross hematuria*) and elevated WBCs. The urine values, including abnormal protein, indicate impaired renal function. There may be an elevated ASO titer.

The child is kept on bed rest; activity is allowed when the hematuria clears and blood pressure returns to normal. Keep people with URIs away from the child. Provide a diet high in calories and low in sodium, protein, and potassium. Fluids may be restricted. Take daily weights to determine if the child is accumulating fluid in the tissues. Take vital signs regularly and compare new findings with previous readings. Antibiotics and corticosteroids may be prescribed, although the use of steroids is controversial.

In most cases, recovery is complete. In a few cases, chronic nephritis may develop, and the client may need to be maintained on dialysis.

Chronic glomerulonephritis may be a complication of acute glomerulonephritis or may occur without preceding illness. Symptoms are unpredictable, and kidney damage usually is progressive. Chronic glomerulonephritis can lead to hypertension, proteinuria, hematuria, and uremia.

The disease tends to progress in three stages. The first stage is the *latent stage*, in which the child shows few outward symptoms. Albumin appears in the urine, and the child may be anemic. No special treatment is needed at this time. In the second stage, called the *edema stage*, the child retains fluid. Treatment includes a high-protein, low-salt diet. Corticosteroid use is controversial; these drugs are sometimes prescribed, but are not as widely used as they once were. In the third stage, the stage of *uremia*, the child's kidneys begin to fail. No medical treatment is available for this stage. The child may be maintained on dialysis until a suitable donor for a kidney transplant is located. These children are often excellent candidates for kidney transplantation.

IN PRACTICE
EDUCATING THE CLIENT 72-4 — Prevention of Urinary Tract Infections in Females

- Wipe the perineal area from front to back.
- Wear white cotton underwear because they are not irritating and allow good air circulation.
- Do not use bubble bath because it is irritating.
- Drink plenty of fluids.
- Thoroughly rinse soap off the perineum.
- Use white, unscented toilet paper.

The components of nursing care for clients with chronic glomerulonephritis include the following:

- Accurate taking and documentation of vital signs, I&O, and daily weight
- Monitoring daily laboratory studies of renal function
- Observing for signs of fluid, electrolyte, and acid–base imbalance
- Encouraging a low-sodium, high-calorie diet with adequate protein
- Providing good skin care (because of itching and edema)
- Providing good oral hygiene (take care not to damage fragile gums)
- Family teaching: the child needs to take medications as ordered and diuretics in the morning so as not to disrupt sleep; report symptoms of UTIs; avoid having the child come into contact with people with URIs
- Explaining to the child and caregivers about side effects of corticosteroids if they are to be given

Nephrotic Syndrome

In **nephrotic syndrome**, changes in the basement membrane of the glomeruli cause the kidneys to excrete massive amounts of protein. It occurs most often in children between 18 months and 5 years of age and is characterized by generalized edema, proteinuria, and hematuria. Urine output is scanty, and blood pressure is elevated. The abdomen is distended, and the child is uncomfortable. They do not eat because fluid in the abdomen and chest causes discomfort. The child is susceptible to other infections.

Palliative measures are symptomatic. Edema is reduced by administering corticosteroids and by limiting fluid and salt intake. Diuretics may be used to reduce edema. Encourage the child to eat. Protect the child against infection. Provide careful skin care and assist the child to move about in bed. If the child is having difficulty breathing, they may be more comfortable sitting up.

The child is very ill and needs expert nursing care and emotional support. Corticosteroids may induce a remission, and the prognosis for eventual recovery is good in most cases. Children who respond to steroid therapy have fewer relapses as time progresses. If the disease is diagnosed and treated early, the child can expect to regain normal (or near-normal) renal functioning. Nursing care is similar to that in chronic glomerulonephritis. Check the child's weight at the same time each day, on the same scale, with the child wearing the same amount of clothing. Monitor vital signs and I&O regularly. During periods of edema, decrease the child's sodium intake by not adding salt to the diet. A high-protein diet is unnecessary. Do not restrict fluids. Offering frequent small meals (six per day) may help the child's nutritional intake during periods of *exacerbation* (flare-up of symptoms). Protect the child from contact with others who have URIs.

Wilms Tumor

Wilms tumor, also called *nephroblastoma*, is a malignant adenosarcoma of the kidney. It is most common in children aged 3–4 years. One of the most common neoplasms of childhood, it usually affects only one kidney.

In most cases, the child shows no symptoms until the tumor is far advanced. Microscopic hematuria may be present, but usually not until late in the disease's course. Diagnosis is based on palpation of the abdominal mass, x-ray studies, and biopsy during a *laparotomy* (surgical exploration of the abdomen).

Treatment for Wilms tumor depends on the extent of disease spread. Surgical removal, when done, is followed by irradiation of the tumor site and both sides of the spine. Chemotherapy is often used.

Whenever a child is to have surgery, prepare the family caregivers and child. If the child is old enough to understand, you may use dolls, puppets, and drawings to explain placement of tubes and to play out fears. After surgery, prepare the child and family for the child's hair loss resulting from chemotherapy.

Nursing Alert When treating a child with Wilms tumor, never unnecessarily palpate the abdomen preoperatively. The tumor could rupture and disseminate. Use extreme caution when handling this child at all times. Post a clear warning sign at the child's bedside.

Hypospadias and Epispadias

In **hypospadias**, the male child's urinary meatus is located on the bottom of the penis; in **epispadias**, the meatus is located on top of the penis. These conditions can usually be surgically corrected and are not life threatening. In severe instances of hypospadias, the newborn's sex may be in doubt because the position of the meatus may appear to be the female urethra, especially when undescended testes are part of the presentation (Chapter 69).

Minor hypospadias is common and usually requires no correction. If surgery is required, it is sometimes done in two stages. Circumcision is contraindicated before surgical correction of this displacement of the urinary meatus because the foreskin may be used for the procedure. Prepare the caregivers intellectually and emotionally for surgery, which is scheduled between 6 and 18 months of age, before the child develops a strong body image.

REPRODUCTIVE SYSTEM DISORDERS

Intersex

Intersex is a term used to describe the newborn who exhibits undifferentiated sexual anatomy or differences between external and internal sexual anatomy. For instance, in some cases of hypospadias, the newborn's sex is unclear. In other cases, a child may have both testes and ovaries. If any doubt exists about a baby's sex, studies are performed immediately. Examiners study the buccal mucosa or skin structure microscopically for a female or male chromosomal pattern. Hormonal and anatomic studies also may be done. Surgery may be necessary to revise or to remove structures. Appropriate hormone administration may also be required. This may cause confusion and emotional strain for the newborn's family. Explaining the role of accurate biologic sexual identification, surgery, and hormonal treatment are of foremost importance in helping the family.

Cryptochidism

Cryptochidism is an undescended testicle. It is common at birth, but usually corrects itself spontaneously. If not, surgical treatment (*orchiopexy*) is performed in early childhood to prevent sterility. Because undescended testes are often associated with hernia and hydrocele, surgical repairs are usually completed together. If an undescended testicle is found in an older child, surgery must not be postponed. A delay could result in sterility because sperm cannot tolerate the heat inside the body.

Surgery is usually performed on an outpatient basis. Postoperatively, the child is sent home after bowel sounds return and the child takes and retains fluids, voids, and ambulates properly. The child may return from surgery with an abdominal dressing as a result of accompanying hernia repair. Observe the dressing often for drainage. Teach caregivers what to look for if the child goes home soon after surgery.

Hydrocele

A **hydrocele** is an accumulation of serous fluid within the scrotal sac, causing the scrotum to become large and painful. If the fluid is not reabsorbed spontaneously, excision and drainage may be necessary. A hydrocele is often associated with a hernia.

NUTRITIONAL CONSIDERATIONS IN YOUNG CHILDREN

Normal growth implies a state of health and absence of a major chronic disease. Growth parameters of height, weight, head circumference (up to 36 months), and body mass index (BMI) should be monitored at each well-child visit and graphed on the appropriate chart. (BMI is the ratio of weight in kilograms divided by the height in meters squared.)

The explosive growth during infancy demands adequate nutrition to facilitate proper growth and development. Protein and fat are especially important for CNS development. Infants require 110–120 cal/kg of body weight per day for the first 6 months, and 95–100 cal/kg of body weight per day for the remainder of the first year. Commercial formulas supply 20 cal/oz and are fortified with vitamins and minerals (especially iron). Formula should be fed at room temperature.

The introduction of solid foods may begin at 4–6 months of age when the GI tract has matured and is less sensitive to potentially allergenic foods.

The signs of readiness for the introduction of solid foods include the following:

- The ingestion of 32 oz of milk daily without hunger satisfaction
- The disappearance of the extrusion reflex (at about 4 months)
- The doubling of birth weight
- The ability to sit unsupported and lean forward with an open mouth to receive food or to lean back and turn the head away, thereby indicating fullness

The order of solid food introduction is not crucial, but rice cereal is usually introduced first, followed by vegetables and fruit. Highly allergenic foods should be avoided. Parents should introduce one new food at a time in small amounts for a period of 5–7 days to determine the infant's response to the food. Solid food should be fed with a spoon and not placed in bottles with formula. As the quantity of solid food increases, the quantity of milk should be decreased to prevent overfeeding. Milk should be introduced in a cup at 6–7 months of age, with the goal of weaning completely from the bottle to a cup by 1 year of age to prevent dental caries. Soft, mashed table foods may be introduced gradually.

The toddler's growth slows, requiring decreased energy and caloric requirements (100 kcal/kg/day). Appetite decreases dramatically (*physiologic anorexia*), and the desire for self-feeding increases. Introducing finger foods and allowing food choices facilitate independence. Avoid foods that may induce choking, such as round foods (wieners cut into slices), hard foods (e.g., raw carrots), or smooth, sticky foods (e.g., peanut butter). The toddler's diet should consist of a wide range of nutritious foods from all food groups in small-sized servings and should include nutritious snacks.

The preschool period is not a time of rapid growth and requires only 90 kcal/kg/day. Food fads and strong taste preferences are common. Engaging the child in food preparation and offering food in small portions in an attractive manner promote food acceptance. All snacks should be nutritious and not empty calories. The general consumption of food at this age is about one half of an adult's portion. Children should never be forced to eat. Preschool children tend to be deficient in zinc, calcium, and iron.

> **NCLEX Alert**
>
> Questions on a nursing examination that relate to children often include factors relating to nutrition. Keep in mind that both breast milk and cow's milk are deficient in iron.

CHAPTER 72 Care of the Infant, Toddler, or Preschooler

STUDENT SYNTHESIS

KEY POINTS

- Many childhood communicable diseases can be prevented through immunization.
- Streptococcal infections can lead to serious cardiac complications.
- Parasitic infections generally involve the entire family and home environment.
- The most common cause of injury to a child is trauma.
- SUIDS, including SIDS, is the sudden, unexplained death of an apparently healthy child.
- Abuse must be reported.
- Common skin disorders include nevi, rashes, and eczema.
- Neurologic disorders include Reye syndrome and meningitis.
- Meningomyelocele, the most serious form of spina bifida, may cause paralysis or other disorders.
- Hydrocephalus can be detected by OFC measurements.
- Otitis media may require medical or surgical therapies.
- Children with celiac disease must avoid dietary intake of food containing gluten.
- Structural defects of the heart may result in abnormal shunting of oxygenated and deoxygenated blood.
- Leukemias may be acute or chronic.
- Cystic fibrosis is an autosomal recessive disease of the exocrine glands resulting in serious damage to the lungs, pancreas, and liver.
- Serious respiratory tract illnesses include RSV, LTB, epiglottitis, and asthma.
- Illness of the GI tract places the young child at high risk for fluid and electrolyte imbalance or dehydration.
- Urinary tract problems may be structural, autoimmune, cancerous, or infections.
- Intersexality and cryptorchidism are the most common reproductive disorders.
- Solid foods are generally introduced at 4–6 months of age.

CRITICAL THINKING EXERCISES

1. P.D., a 16-month-old child, has a congenital hip location. Describe activities that are appropriate for stimulating growth and development after surgery if the child is confined in a hip spica cast. What measures can be taught to the caregivers to prevent urinary tract infections and maintain good perineal care?

2. J.J., a 4-year-old boy with nephrotic syndrome, is eating poorly. Although edema gives him a plump appearance, he is actually becoming undernourished. Identify suggestions you will give his caregiver to improve his nutritional intake.

3. You are caring for T.M., an 8-month-old infant who is recovering from the surgery for a bilateral cleft lip. What information will you give the family to help them understand the child's care and how they can assist with protecting T.M. from postsurgical infection and injury?

NCLEX-STYLE REVIEW QUESTIONS

1. The nurse is preparing to administer immunizations to an infant. The parent states, "Won't those vaccinations give my child autism?" What is the best response by the nurse?
   a. "There is always a possibility but it would be worse to get the diseases."
   b. "That only occurs with children who have weak immune systems."
   c. "Recent research shows no connection between vaccines and autism."
   d. "You can refuse them but your child won't be able to go to school."

2. A child is found to be asymptomatic but tests positive as a carrier for diphtheria. What action does the nurse anticipate providing?
   a. Informing the parents about the importance of adhering to prophylactic antibiotics
   b. Informing the parents that the child will need to be quarantined
   c. Informing the parents that the child will eventually get the disease
   d. Informing the parents that the child will have to take antiviral medications for at least 6 months

3. A parent of a newborn asks the nurse, "When should I start introducing solid foods into my child's diet?" What is the best response by the nurse?
   a. "Whenever you feel like your child is still hungry after eating."
   b. "When your child is about 4–6 months old."
   c. "You can start in a couple of weeks with rice cereal in the bottle."
   d. "After the child drinks 6 oz of milk without hunger satisfaction."

4. A child is diagnosed with varicella (chickenpox). What medication should the nurse inform the parents to avoid when treating the fever?
   a. Diphenhydramine
   b. Acetaminophen
   c. Ibuprofen
   d. Aspirin

5. The nurse is caring for a child preoperatively with Wilms tumor. When following the plan of care for this child, what intervention is essential?
   a. Palpate the tumor to be sure it has not grown.
   b. Place a clear warning sign over the bed to not palpate the abdomen.
   c. Limit visitors.
   d. Place the child in isolation.

CHAPTER RESOURCES

Enhance your learning with additional resources on **thePoint**!

Student Resources related to this chapter can be found at thePoint.lww.com/Rosdahl12e.

73 Care of the School-Age Child or Adolescent

Learning Objectives

1. Compare the symptoms and treatment of conjunctivitis, mononucleosis, and Lyme disease and differentiate the use of the term *sore throat* as a general term and a specific symptom.
2. Define and discuss the nursing implications of each of the following skin disorders: acne vulgaris, impetigo contagiosa, and tinea pedis.
3. Define and discuss the nursing implications of each of the following musculoskeletal disorders: lordosis, kyphosis, scoliosis, juvenile rheumatoid arthritis, Legg–Calvé–Perthes disease, dental malocclusion, and malignant bone tumors.
4. Compare and contrast the nursing implications for diabetes mellitus type 1 and diabetes mellitus type 2.
5. Define and discuss the nursing implications of retinitis pigmentosa and juvenile glaucoma.
6. Define and discuss the nursing implications of IBD and appendicitis.
7. Define and discuss the nursing implications of mittelschmerz and dysmenorrhea.
8. Present a therapeutic teaching session for a family with an adolescent who has concerns about sexual development.
9. Present a therapeutic teaching session for an adolescent with a known or suspected STI.
10. Define and discuss the nursing implications of narcolepsy, nightmares, somnambulism, night terrors, somniloquism, and insomnia.
11. Identify and differentiate between anorexia nervosa and bulimia nervosa. State the nursing considerations for each condition.
12. Present a therapeutic teaching session to the parents of a child who is obese.
13. Define and discuss the nursing implications for enuresis and encopresis.
14. Identify the nutritional concerns for a school-age child and state the nursing considerations for each concern.

Important Terminology

acne vulgaris
amenorrhea
anorexia nervosa
biologic agents
biologic response modifiers
biologics
bowel obstruction
bulimia nervosa
conjunctivitis
dermabrasion
dysmenorrhea
endometriosis
exacerbation
fibrostenosis
fistula
fomite
giant papillary conjunctivitis (GPC)
impetigo contagiosa
insomnia
kyphosis
lordosis
Lyme disease
malocclusion
mittelschmerz
mononucleosis
narcolepsy
orthodontia
polydipsia
polyphagia
polyuria
refractive errors
remission
sarcomas
scoliosis
sleep apnea
somnambulism
somniloquy
tenesmus
vector

Acronyms

BMI
DMARD
EBV
GPC
HAI
IBD
IBS
IDDM
JCA
JIA
JRA
LCPD
NIDDM
NSAIDs
PMDD
PMS
PTLDS
REM
RP
UC
VCE

Pediatric nursing continues with the study of common conditions found in school-age children and adolescents. Older school-age children and adolescents often feel uncomfortable in healthcare settings in which most clients are young children. Healthcare personnel must be sensitive to these feelings and make every effort to provide a comfortable atmosphere for them.

COMMUNICABLE DISEASES

Communicable diseases are a group of diseases that are spread from one person to another, and in many circumstances, from an animal to a person. They are also known as infectious or contagious diseases. Communicable diseases are spread in various ways, for example, via airborne routes, blood and body fluids, or direct contact. Many situations involve a **vector** or living agent, such as a flea, tick, or mosquito, which indirectly transmits an infection. Some infections involve a **fomite** or nonliving object such as a doorknob, restaurant menu, toy, or pen, which directly transmits a pathogen to a person. *Hospital-acquired infections (HAIS)* often involve direct contamination by way of a fomite such as a bathroom faucet, bedding, or stethoscopes. Standard precautions and transmission-based protocols are designed to limit the sources of contact and thus to prevent the spread of most infectious diseases in healthcare facilities.

The younger population is greatly affected by the variety of ways communicable diseases are transmitted. Problems with cross-contamination from mother to baby begin at conception. Sexually transmitted infections (STIs) often cause mortality or morbidity in a fetus (e.g., syphilis and rubella). Prevention of communicable diseases begins in the home. Children benefit from immunizations via vaccinations. Effective handwashing and proper cooking habits can greatly minimize

Box 73-1 Teaching Individuals and Family Members: Reducing the Spread of Infectious Diseases

1. Wash your hands frequently using soap and water or an alcohol-based hand sanitizer. *Rationale: Pathogens and nonpathogens survive on surfaces for different lengths of time, ranging from a few minutes to several months. Frequent handwashing is the best, most effective method of preventing cross-contamination. Consider the number of objects that you touch in a day: cell phone, computer keyboards, refrigerator handle, microwave buttons, door knobs, light-switch, handbag/wallet, countertops, desktops, ATM machines, restaurant menus. Wash hands after touching animals.*
2. Get the vaccinations that are recommended for childhood, adolescents, older adults, or travelers. *Rationale: The immunizations induce your immune system to develop memory cells and encourage resistance against communicable diseases. Your body develops its own defenses and the disease does not develop. Without immunizations, the body cannot enhance its own defenses against communicable infections. The nonvaccinated, exposed individual typically develops the disease. An infectious disease involves many serious complications (e.g., fever, rash, pain, respiratory and neurologic problems).*
3. Use arm, sleeve, or crook of elbow to stop the spread of transmissions by coughing or sneezing. *Rationale: Coughing or sneezing can spread pathogens via microscopic droplets transmitted through the air. The current recommendation is to cover your mouth with your arm, sleeve, or crook of the elbow, but handwashing remains the most effective method of pathogen destruction.*
4. Practice safe sex using barrier birth control methods or abstinence. *Rationale: Barrier birth control methods (e.g., use of condoms) can be helpful in the prevention of the spread of STIs. Safer sexual practices are a personal responsibility. STIs affect the personal and societal cost of healthcare and the health of the fetus, the child, and the adult, and are on the list of most preventable infectious diseases.*
5. Use safe cooking practices to control the microorganisms (both pathogens and nonpathogens) that thrive on foods. Wash hands between food groups, keep countertops clean, and wash all fruits and vegetables well prior to eating. Use separate cutting boards for raw meats and vegetables. Heat foods to properly designated temperatures. Refrigerate foods within 2 hr of cooking. *Rationale: Illness is often related to improperly prepared food, such as not cooking thoroughly or permitting food to develop more microorganisms when left at room temperature.*
6. Be a smart traveler to avoid contracting infectious diseases. Prepare for travel by checking to see if any immunizations are recommended for you or any member of your travel group. If water or food sources may be contaminated, provide your own safe water sources (e.g., bottled water) and use it for eating, drinking, and brushing teeth. Eat foods that have been adequately cooked; avoid raw vegetables and fruits. *Rationale: Some communities or countries have limited resources, and the same quality of safe water and food sources are not available. Citizens from one area may become ill when exposed to conditions in new areas.*
7. Avoid cross-contamination with zoonotic diseases (diseases that are passed from an animal to a human via vector transmission). Toxoplasmosis is a common parasitic infection that is transferred from animals to humans, often by cat feces or saliva; it is very serious to the pregnant woman. Bird flu, rabies, fleas, and ticks (that spread Lyme disease) are common causes of human illnesses. Monitor the health of your home pets by getting the vaccinations that are available for pets. Some areas need special enclosed trash containers to prevent infestation of rats, raccoons, coyotes, bears, or other local animal inhabitants and any pathogens that these animals may carry (e.g., rabies). *Rationale: Animal parasites can lead to serious human illnesses, but there are many measures available to prevent problems.*
8. Watch local and global news reports, which are often a first notification of pending problems. Local news may report the public notification of a local flu epidemic or an outbreak of *Salmonella* in lettuce. Bird flu may be seen to be epidemic in another country. *Rationale: Business travelers, vacationers, and migrating populations cause constant movement of pathogens with distribution of infectious diseases. Travel plans should include a review of information provided by WHO and CDC Websites.*

www.cdc.gov/Features/Rhinoviruses/index.html, https://www.verywellhealth.com/tips-to-prevent-infections-1958877.

the transmission of disease from one family member to another. Improper handling and undercooking beef, pork, chicken, or lamb can be sources of pathogens (c.g., *Escherichia coli* [*E. coli*], *Giardia*, *Salmonella*). Family pets can be a source of illnesses in children (e.g., toxoplasmosis). *Zoonotic diseases* are caused by viruses, bacteria, parasites, and fungi and are passed from animals to humans (e.g., malaria). Children and caregivers can learn behaviors that produce good hygiene and lessen transmission of disease. Box 73-1 presents several areas of focus for teaching clients methods of preventing cross-contamination.

Outbreaks of communicable diseases can have serious regional health implications. Country-wide and global disease epidemics are referred to as *pandemics*. All U.S. local, state, and county health departments have specific written and often online protocols for containment of communicable diseases. Many diseases are on a *mandatory report list* or *Reportable Communicable Disease List,* which requires healthcare personnel to notify specific regional, state, or federal agencies of the suspicion or confirmation of a disease within a specific timeframe of hours to days. Some diseases must be immediately reported to the appropriate healthcare agency by telephone; others can be reported by email or fax.

Key Concept

Handwashing: The CDC recommends washing thoroughly and vigorously with soap and water for at least 20 s, followed by hand-drying with a paper towel. In the absence of running water, an *alcohol-based* hand gel or wipe will suffice.

The Common Cold

The common cold is a viral infection that includes more than 200 known viruses. The *rhinovirus* is known to cause colds and sinus and ear infections, as well as to trigger asthma attacks. Typically, a cold starts with *rhinorrhea* (a runny nose) with clear mucus. As the infection is attacked by the body's own immune system, the clear rhinorrhea can start to look white, yellow, or greenish. Other symptoms of a cold include sneezing, sore throat, mild fever, coughing, malaise (body aches), mild headache, and watery eyes. The typical common cold lasts about up to 14 days. It is not uncommon for adults and children to have two to three colds per year while children tend to have more minor upper respiratory infections a year than adults.

Diagnosing a cold generally involves differentiating between its symptoms and those of other similar physical presentations. A fever is a helpful immune response; however, notify the healthcare provider if the fever persists or exceeds 100.4 °F (38 °C) for more than 3 days. The common cold differs from influenza by the intensity of symptoms and the severity of illness. (See Influenza in Chapter 72 as well as Box 72-1 for Nursing Considerations: Symptom Relief.) Treatment consists of rest, fluids, and over-the-counter (OTC) symptomatic medications such as acetaminophen or ibuprofen for aches and fever. Antibiotics are not recommended for viral infections. The healthcare provider needs to be called if symptoms worsen or persist longer than 10–14 days. High-risk individuals are more likely to develop complications such as pneumonia.

Nursing considerations involve teaching the client the ways that viruses are transmitted, handwashing techniques, and discussion regarding measures for symptomatic relief. Another important related subject for client teaching is the relationship between smoking and infections (Box 73-2).

Sore Throat

A *sore throat* is a common condition identified by pain, inflammation, or infection in the throat, generally caused by a bacteria or virus. The typical sore throat makes swallowing painful and dry, and the throat feels "scratchy." Many sore throats are accompanied by a low-grade fever. The term *sore throat* may indicate a localized problem, for example, strep throat (a streptococcal infection) or a sign of more serious problems, such as laryngeal tracheal bronchitis (an infection of the larynx also known as LTB or croup), or other respiratory tract infections.

Signs and Symptoms

When a sore throat occurs, monitor the individual for fever, dry mouth, drooling, difficulty breathing, poor skin turgor, lethargy, decreased intake and output, headache, and few or no tears when crying. A healthcare provider needs to be contacted if breathing or swallowing difficulty develops, pus forms on the back of the throat, a body rash develops,

---

Box 73-2 | Smoking and Contagious Illness

Smoke is transmitted by respiratory routes from person to person and, in this sense, can be considered a contagious substance. The tissues of both the smoker and the victims of secondhand smoke are harmed. Smoke is so damaging to young lungs that healthcare providers need to teach children, as well as their caregivers, about the effects of both smoking and inhaling secondhand smoke.

A child is exposed to thousands of toxic chemicals in tobacco smoke. Smoke is known to trigger asthma attacks, which can result in respiratory arrest and death. Toxic fumes lead to a weakened immune system; thus, the smoke-exposed child who gets a common cold virus becomes ill more frequently, has more intense symptoms, and often has an illness that stays longer than the nonsmoke-exposed child. This child becomes very vulnerable to other illnesses throughout adolescence and adulthood. Smoke-exposed individuals do not grow to normal potential; their growth is stunted. Toxic damage to DNA increases instances of cancer almost everywhere in the body, not just the lungs. Smoke is linked to development of many chronic conditions seen in adulthood. Bronchitis, emphysema, and dementia are among the serious conditions associated with exposure to tobacco smoke in youth that are seen in older and senior adults.

Smoking is the leading cause of preventable death in the United States. No vaccine is necessary to prevent the cross-contamination of smoke from the smoker to the nonsmoker. Individuals can prevent the toxic, infectious properties of smoke from occurring by not smoking.

Centers for Disease Control and Prevention (n.d). *Smoking and Tobacco Use*. U.S. Department of Health and Human Services, National Institutes of Health. https://www.cdc.gov/tobacco/index.htm

---

or blood-tinged secretions occur. Excessive drooling may indicate a swollen esophagus or blocked trachea caused by inflammation. *Drooling or difficulties swallowing* or *breathing* can indicate an occluded (blocked) trachea or esophagus. *These symptoms may indicate an emergency.*

Treatment

Diagnosis of the etiology of a sore throat will determine its treatment. Recurring sore throats can indicate minor problems such as allergies, dry air, and exposure to smoke or other forms of pollution. However, sore throats that happen several times per year can be more serious problems, including non- or partially treated bacterial throat infections, such as strep throat, which need medical interventions. Most sore throats can be treated at home by taking throat lozenges, ibuprofen, or acetaminophen; drinking plenty of warm fluids such as tea, soup, or water; gargling with warm salt water; and avoiding environmental allergens that act as irritants such as smoke, ragweed, or household cleaning products, especially aerosols.

Conjunctivitis

Conjunctivitis is a very common eye condition in all age groups. The conjunctiva is the thin, transparent membrane that lines the sclera (white part of the eye) and the tissue inside of the eyelid. There are three basic categories of conjunctivitis: bacterial, viral, and allergic. Bacterial and viral conjunctivitis are highly contagious and easily pass from one eye to the other, as well as to someone else who is infected by contact with infectious conjunctivitis' secretions. Allergic conjunctivitis usually occurs simultaneously in both eyes; it is not passed from person to person.

Signs and Symptoms
The eye becomes inflamed and swollen, making the white part of the eye appear pink or red, thus the nickname "pink eye." Eye symptoms also include tearing, itching, redness, eye irritation, a "gritty feeling," and, sometimes, photophobia (sensitivity to light). While sleeping, a crust forms around the eyelids, and the client complains of difficulty opening the eyes.

Diagnosis and Treatment
Diagnosis and treatment depend on the etiology of the problem. The three basic types of conjunctivitis include the following:

- *Bacterial conjunctivitis* infections are treated with topical antibiotics (e.g., eyedrops or gel ointments). STIs, like chlamydia and gonorrhea, are common causes of *ophthalmia neonatorum* conjunctivitis in newborns, which is why prophylactic measures (prevention) occur at birth. This serious condition could lead to permanent eye damage unless it is treated immediately.
- *Viral conjunctivitis* infections can be caused by a member of the adenovirus family, which is associated with the common cold, and members of the herpesvirus family such as herpes simplex, varicella-zoster, and Epstein–Barr virus. Rubeola and rubella viruses cause redness and eye irritation, with secretions that expose these viruses to others.
- *Allergic conjunctivitis* occurs seasonally or year-round, especially with individuals who have a history of allergies related to hay fever, eczema, or sensitivity to dust mites and animal dander. Often causative factors are environmental, such as dust particles, chlorine in swimming pools, cosmetics, or hair-care products. With allergic conjunctivitis, both eyes are typically affected simultaneously. Treatment for allergic conjunctivitis is generally the use of OTC eye drops designed for allergies. OTC medications are generally designed to treat one or more symptoms such as irritated eyes or rhinorrhea. Teaching the client will include teaching the definitions and differences of the OTC medications and which would be best for specific symptoms. Examples include antihistamines, mast-cell stabilizers, steroids, and/or anti-inflammatory eye drops.

Nursing Considerations
The nursing considerations for conjunctivitis include teaching clients to avoid touching or rubbing the area around the eyes. Urgent care is needed if symptoms such as eye pain, light sensitivity, or if blurred vision occur. An ophthalmologist or optometrist should be seen by the client. If contacts are worn, discharge instructions by the healthcare provider for individuals with conjunctivitis typically include

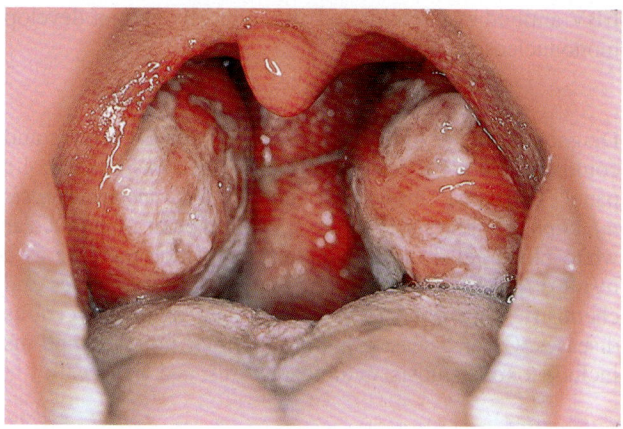

Figure 73-1 Appearance of tonsils in a child with infectious mononucleosis. Note the degree of erythema, enlargement, and purulent covering.

instructions to remove and discard any contact lenses, storage solutions, or storage containers. Regular glasses need to be worn during the entire time of the infection. There is a high probability of recurrent conjunctivitis due to cross-contamination if lenses or storage supplies are not replaced. *Never* use mouth saliva on a lens. Conjunctivitis in contact lens wearers can be an early symptom of more severe and permanent eye damage. **Giant papillary conjunctivitis** (**GPC**), a type of severe allergic conjunctivitis, is the result of chronic use of contact lenses. In GPC, the papillae (glands) of the upper eyelid greatly enlarge. Itching and mucus discharge are early symptoms. Most clients with GPC recover in weeks to months by discontinuing the wearing of contact lens and wearing prescription eyeglasses.

Acute Infectious Mononucleosis

Mononucleosis or *mono* is an infection of the Epstein–Barr virus (**EBV**). EBV is a member of the herpesvirus family. Saliva is the most common mode of transmission. The salivary glands are infected by EBV, and the virus is transmitted by droplets in saliva, coughs, and sneezes and by direct contact with mucous membranes of the mouth. Mono is often referred to as the "kissing disease" because of the mouth-to-mouth saliva contact.

Signs and Symptoms
Symptoms develop within 4–8 weeks after contact with the EBV. Clients complain of a headache, low-grade fever, anorexia, cervical lymphadenopathy, and a sore throat (Fig. 73-1). Fatigue can range from mild to severe and tends to be a long-lasting symptom. EBV infections may cause hepatitis and enlargement of the spleen. Upper airway obstruction, severe dysphagia, and dehydration can occur during the first weeks of the acute phase. The illness typically is self-limiting, but the recovery period can last several months. Acute symptoms generally improve over 3–4 months, but therapy may be needed for 6 months or more.

EBV can be an acute or a chronic infectious disease. It is possible that an individual can have EBV and not be infectious. Some adults may carry EBV throughout their lifetime and never develop mononucleosis but can pass it on to others who might develop the illness. Many individuals develop

EBV antibodies in childhood and, typically, do not develop mononucleosis.

Diagnosis
Diagnosis is done by a "mono spot" test or EBV titers and could include a CBC with differential and basic metabolic panel. The name "mono spot" and the term *mononucleosis infection* are references to the specific type of mononuclear white blood cells, the B lymphocytes, which increase as a result of the EBV spleen infection. Laboratory studies and chemistries are done to rule out other serious infectious diseases. Other diseases that have similar initial symptoms include toxoplasmosis, cytomegalovirus, and HIV.

Treatment
Treatment for mononucleosis is symptomatic. Rest, fluids, and analgesics are essential in the treatment plan. Acetaminophen (Tylenol) can be given for fever, headaches, sore throat, or body aches, also referred to as general malaise. Fatigue and weakness may persist for several weeks. Antibiotics, such as penicillin or erythromycin (E-Mycin, Ilosone), may be given if strep throat is also diagnosed. Antiviral drugs are not recommended and may lengthen recovery time. Both caregivers and client need to be informed of the need for the client to avoid physical activity such as contact sports, a necessary precaution because severe hemorrhage and death are possible if the enlarged spleen ruptures. The greatest risk of rupture of the spleen occurs during the first 2–4 weeks of the illness.

Nursing Considerations
It is essential to teach both caregivers and clients the importance of absolute rest. Rest does not need to be total bed rest. A sedentary lifestyle and frequent naps are necessary therapies for mononucleosis. Reassure them that the acute phase (severe sore throat) is worse in the first 1–2 weeks and the painful lymph nodes subside by the third week. However, the major recovery period tends to persist for weeks, gradually lessening until symptoms disappear over the next 6–12 months.

Lyme Disease

Lyme disease is a zoonotic bacterial spirochete infection (*Borrelia burgdorferi*) in humans that is transmitted by way of infected pinhead-sized ticks. This disease and a few other tickborne diseases are most likely to infect individuals who spend time outdoors or near wooded areas populated with deer and certain other animals. Lyme disease is endemic in many areas of the continental United States. Diagnosis is based on symptoms, physical assessment, and a history of exposure or possible exposure to infected ticks.

Signs and Symptoms
Symptoms may appear 3–31 days after the bite. An early characteristic skin rash called *erythema migrans,* which is a type of *annular rash* (a circular or oval lesion with a clear center). Erythema migrans appears commonly around the original tick bite site as a distinctive ring-shaped red rash surrounding a clear ring inner space. As the ring fades, a central clearing with red edges develops. This rash may develop in other locations such as the thighs, groin, trunk, armpits, and on the face, especially in children. The rash does not appear in all cases, and the lack of this common symptom may lead to a delay in treatment, which can result in long-lasting complications.

Flu-like symptoms such as fever, headache, fatigue, and regional lymphadenopathy (glandular swelling) commonly appear. In a few individuals, fatigue, pain, joint and muscle aches continue for 6 months or longer. The long-term illness may be referred to as *chronic Lyme disease* or, more properly as, *posttreatment Lyme disease syndrome* (**PTLDS**). The etiology of PTLDS is unknown, but healthcare provider awareness of this complication is important since future autoimmune problems are possible. If left untreated, the infection can cause serious problems. Arthritis develops as a result of inflamed joints. Damage to the heart can result in conduction abnormalities. Bell palsy is an example of difficulties related to the nervous system.

Diagnosis
The symptomatic rash and the flu-like symptoms are typical of this disease. Laboratory testing can be done. Treatment consists of 2–4 weeks of antibiotics (doxycycline, amoxicillin, erythromycin). Early treatment usually prevents the development of more serious illnesses and long-lasting systemic illness.

Nursing Considerations
People who cannot avoid potentially infested areas must take preventive measures (see In Practice: Educating the Client 73-1). Individuals should develop self-protective behaviors that include using insect repellent, checking for the presence of ticks on oneself and on children, and washing outdoor clothing. Pesticides can be used in the environment that harbors ticks, and minimizing overgrowth and brush will reduce tick habitats.

SKIN DISORDERS

Acne Vulgaris

Acne vulgaris or **acne** is a very common chronic skin disease of the hair follicles seen on the face, chest, and back. It affects nearly all teens and young adults during puberty. Sebum (skin oil) is a natural substance produced in the sebaceous glands that lubricates and protects the skin. However, during puberty, the androgen hormones in the adrenal glands (e.g., testosterone) become active in males and females. Overactive sebaceous glands become inflamed and plugged. Acne typically appears as *comedones* (occluded pores) or blackheads (oxidized oils), whiteheads (closed pores under the skin surface), tender red bumps (pimples, zits), pustules (bumps filled with fluid or pus), and cysts. Cysts or cystic lesions are large, deep pimples (Fig. 73-2), which can become painful and cause skin scarring.

Causes of acne include genetics, age, pressure on the skin (e.g., helmet straps), cosmetics, severe stress, and a few medications (e.g., prednisone and lithium). Cigarette smoking increases the frequency and severity of acne. The steroids that bodybuilders may take are known to cause acne. It is generally accepted that food does not cause acne, with the possible exception of milk and chocolate. Foods that

IN PRACTICE
EDUCATING THE CLIENT 73-1 — Prevention of Lyme Disease

When in a known, unknown, or potentially infested outdoor area, prevention of Lyme disease should include the following:
- Wear long sleeves and long pants tucked into the socks or boots (and tape them). Wear closed shoes or sneakers (no sandals).
- Wear light-colored clothing so ticks can be seen more easily.
- Check skin and clothing frequently.
- Brush clothing off before going indoors.
- Insect repellants, such as DEET, may be used but use with caution on infants and children because of toxicity dangers. Permethrin can be sprayed on clothing to prevent tick attachment.
- Apply spray repellants outdoors.
- Walk on paved areas or cleaned paths rather than through brush, if possible.
- Check the entire body after leaving an infected area. Have someone else assist with the inspection.
- Wash clothes after being outdoors.
- To remove a tick, use tweezers; grasp the tick at its head and slowly pull it straight out without crushing its body. Crushing the body may force some of the infected fluid into the wound.
- Wash the wound with soap and water and apply an antiseptic.
- Use tick and flea collars on pets that are outside in possible infected areas. Inspect them regularly. Common pet ticks do not carry the offending spirochete, but pets can pick up the tick if they are in infested areas outdoors.
- Keep areas where children play free from tall grass, weeds, scrubby areas, and leaf litter.

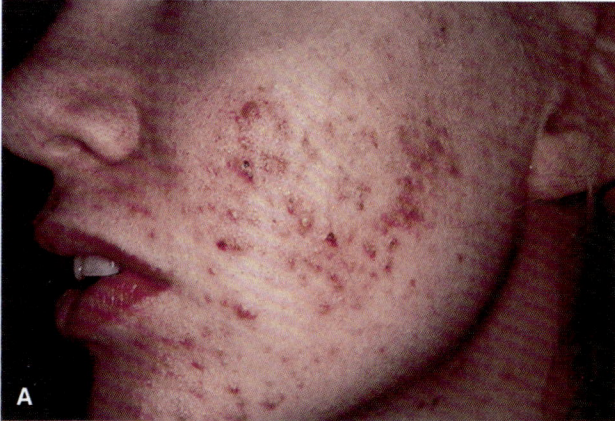
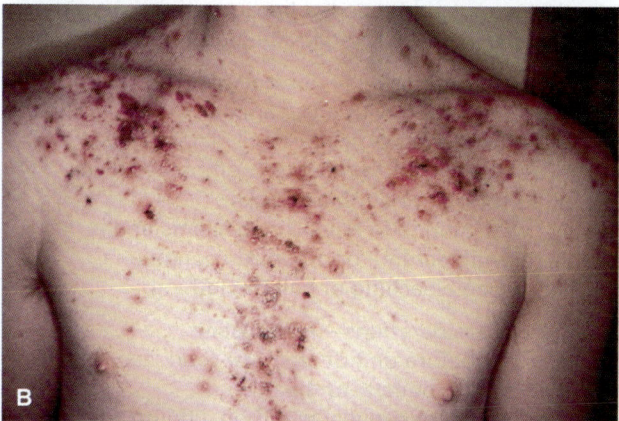

Figure 73-2 **A.** Acne of the face. **B.** Acne of the chest.

increase an individual's blood glucose level (glycemic load) are associated with worsening acne, for example, sugars, candy, carbohydrates.

Treatment
Treatment for acne includes keeping the skin clean, avoiding irritating the skin by using strong soaps or cleansers. Individuals who are prone to acne should check the labels of cosmetics to ensure that they are noncomedogenic. Treatment includes topical and systemic medications. In Practice: Important Medications 73-1 contains a list of key medications for acne. A well-balanced, nutritional diet is essential for good overall health. Mild cleansers, exfoliating (skin peeling) cleansers and masks, and retinol (a nonprescription derivative of vitamin A) are helpful topical agents to minimize acne and promote exfoliation.

Nursing Considerations
Emotional support is an important aspect of the care for adolescents with acne. Accept and acknowledge that physical appearance is important to the adolescent. The emotional stress, social withdrawal, and anxiety that accompany acne can greatly affect a young person's development. Education needs to include a review of personal hygiene, good general health, and diet. Be sure to educate the client about the side effects of different acne medications. Skin care is discussed further in In Practice: Educating the Client 73-2.

Impetigo

Impetigo contagiosa is an infection caused by *Streptococcus pyogenes, Staphylococcus aureus,* or mixed bacteria. Methicillin-resistant *Staphylococcus aureus* (MRSA) and gentamicin-resistant *Staphylococcus aureus* strains have also been reported to cause impetigo. There are two types of impetigo: nonbullous impetigo (impetigo contagiosa) and bullous impetigo. Impetigo contagiosa is the most common bacterial infection of children 2–5 years of age. Generally, it begins in the superficial layers of the epidermis as a red inflamed vesicle near the nose, mouth, face, neck, hands, or, if a child wears diapers, on the diaper region. Rarely occurring in adults, impetigo may follow another skin condition or infection. The vesicle breaks, leaking pus or fluid, which forms a honey-colored scab. The last stage is a red mark, which heals without leaving a scar. The sores may be itchy but not painful (Fig. 73-3). Impetigo is highly contagious. Touching or scratching the sores easily spreads the infection. Scratching the skin can result in scarring. Transmission-based precautions are necessary to prevent the spread of infection.

Diagnosis is usually made through observation by a healthcare provider. A culture may be done in specific cases. Healing takes place within 2 weeks with proper antibiotics

IN PRACTICE
IMPORTANT MEDICATIONS 73-1 — For Acne Vulgaris

Topical Agents

Salicylic acid—available in many over-the-counter topical agents

Benzoyl peroxide—available in many over-the-counter topical agents

Retinoic acid, tretinoin (Retin-A)

Tetracycline cream

Erythromycin cream

Systemic Agents

Tetracycline (e.g., Panmycin, Achromycin)

Isotretinoin (Accutane)—*careful monitoring* by healthcare provider needed because of serious side effects; use only when other agents not effective.

Nursing Considerations—Topical Agents

- When combined with other agents, they may cause excessive drying of skin.
- Avoid application to mucous membranes, eyes, inflamed skin, or sunburned skin.
- Use with caution in fair-skinned clients and in clients with eczema or other skin conditions.
- May cause bleaching of hair or clothing.

Nursing Considerations—Tetracycline

- Take 1 hr before or 2 hr after any food, especially milk, dairy products, or meat.
- May interact negatively with iron, lithium, and oral contraceptives.
- Do not use with renal (kidney) or hepatic (liver) dysfunction.
- Drink plenty of water.
- Contraindicated in pregnancy and lactation; may cause permanent staining of teeth of infants.

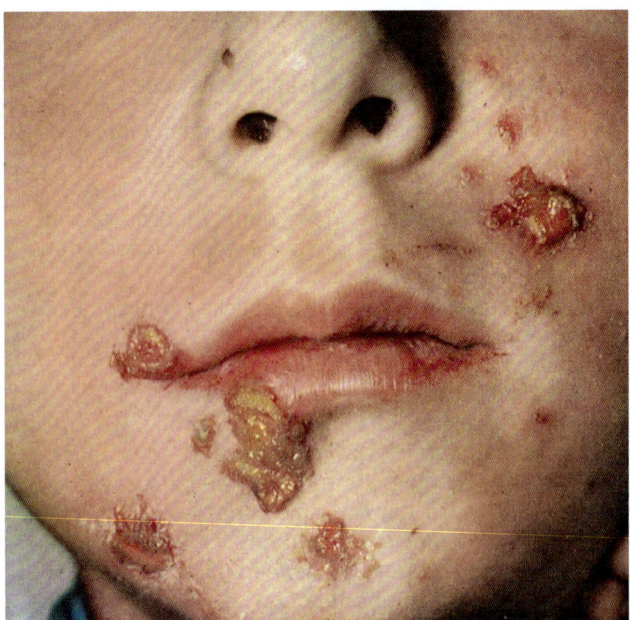

Figure 73-3 Impetigo of the face. (Reprinted from Abner Kurten. *Folia Dermatologia.* No. 2. Geigy Pharmaceuticals. Copyright © Novartis AG.)

if the infection does not contaminate other parts of the skin. Complications may occur if *S. aureus* invades other parts of the body, for example, the heart (rheumatic fever) or kidneys (glomerulonephritis).

Treatment consists of topical, oral, or intravenous antibacterial antibiotics, such as mupirocin, fusidic acid, or antistaphylococcal penicillins. Remove crusts with soap and water. Nursing considerations are aimed at preventing the spread of infection. Thorough and frequent handwashing is essential. Clip fingernails, which harbor the bacteria. Keep the infected person's washcloths, towels, and linens away from others. Discourage the child from scratching or touching infected sites; wearing cotton gloves can be helpful. A cotton mask over the nose and mouth may help limit scratching and might make the child feel more like a pirate than a client.

Tinea Pedis

Tinea pedis, also known as "athlete's foot," or "ringworm of the foot," is a common fungal infection that attacks the skin between the toes or on the heels. A photograph of tinea pedis is in Figure 47-12G. Tinea pedis is the most common of the tinea fungal infections. It is easily spread from a surface to the skin and recontamination is common. The fungus thrives in warm, moist areas, such as athletic shoes, or in areas that are wet for long periods of time, such as around a swimming pool or in a locker room. The infection is spread by contact with contaminated shoes, socks, or wet surfaces. Symptoms include cracked, flaking, and peeling skin between the toes or the side of the foot. The fungus forms watery blisters in moist, weepy spots that burn, itch, or sting. Blisters form that ooze or get dry and crusty. Infection can spread to fingernails, which can become thick, flaky, and discolored.

Diagnosis is made by visual examination. Sometimes a KOH (potassium hydroxide) examination or a skin culture may be done. For the KOH examination, skin cells are

IN PRACTICE
EDUCATING THE CLIENT 73-2 — Acne Care

- Follow skin care instructions carefully and patiently. Acne takes a long time to clear up.
- Use gentle cleansing to avoid further skin damage. Avoid scrubbing the face.
- Review side effects and instructions for use of any prescribed medications (especially Accutane).
- Inspect the skin for any adverse reactions following any treatment.
- Avoid pinching or picking at pimples. This results in inflammation and possible scarring, as well as an increased risk of infection.
- Use a clean washcloth and towel with each washing. Shampoo frequently.
- Maintain good health practices, including regular exercise and balanced nutrition.
- Maintain careful skin care, even after acne lesions have cleared.

IN PRACTICE
EDUCATING THE CLIENT 73-3 — Tinea Pedis (Athlete's Foot)

- Expose the feet to dry air when possible.
- Wear sandals, cotton socks, and shoes that let foot moisture evaporate.
- Wash the feet daily. Dry thoroughly, particularly between the toes.
- Use a separate towel for each foot; use a clean towel with each bath.
- Apply antifungal medication after each bath; continue medication for 1–2 weeks after topical results are noticed.
- Wear flip-flops in public areas, such as swimming pools and locker rooms.
- Discard contaminated footwear, if possible, as the fungus may survive for long periods of time.
- Keep shoes ventilated; expose to sunlight and fresh air.
- Alternate wearing at least two pairs of shoes.

obtained by lightly scraping the infected area; the sample is placed on a microscope slide with KOH and gently heated. The technician then looks for fungus cells under the microscope. The KOH procedure takes only a few minutes; a skin culture requires 24–48 hr on a growth medium before cell growth is obtained.

Treatment consists of OTC antifungal medications such as powders or creams that contain medications such as miconazole, clotrimazole, terbinafine, or tolnaftate. To prevent reinfection, treat or discard contaminated shoes or socks and apply medications topically for 1–2 weeks after the infection has cleared. Persistent tinea pedis may need oral antifungal medications and, possibly, antibiotics to treat open skin lesions. Client teaching should include the topics in In Practice: Educating the Client 73-3.

MUSCULOSKELETAL DISORDERS

Trauma

Because school-age children and adolescents are usually active, they are subject to many kinds of muscle and bone injuries. Chapter 77 discusses musculoskeletal disorders, such as fractures, traction, complications of orthopedic disorders, and their treatments.

Postural Defects

Other than trauma, postural defects involving the spine are the most common musculoskeletal problems affecting school-age children and adolescents. The spine is made of the stacked vertebrae separated by discs. When viewed from the side, the normal spine has mild curves or, if viewed from the back, the spine should run up and down in the middle of the back. These curves absorb stress that results from body motion. Abnormalities of the spine involve the natural curves, which become exaggerated and misaligned in some areas. Common defects of the spine include lordosis, kyphosis, and scoliosis.

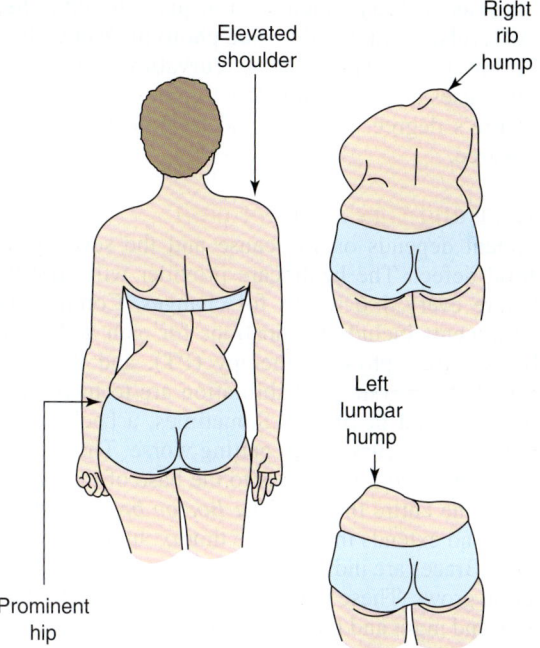

Figure 73-4 Scoliosis. Abnormalities to be determined at the initial screening examination. (Gore, Passhel, Sepic, & Dalton, 1981.)

Lordosis, or swayback, is an exaggerated inward curvature of the lumbar spine in which the pelvis tips forward. It may result from a disease process such as osteoporosis. Osteoporosis is a common condition in which the vertebrae become fragile because of a loss of bone mineral density and bone mass, which can be a precursor to compression fractures. Lordosis may be *idiopathic* (of unknown cause). It may be associated with obesity, in which excess abdominal weight distorts the person's center of gravity. It is also associated with hip dislocations or contractures and is accompanied by pain.

Kyphosis is an abnormal curvature of the thoracic spine that results in a "hunchback" appearance. It can result from disease (e.g., tuberculosis), compression fractures, or osteoarthritis. Kyphosis can be congenital related to abnormal vertebrae development in utero, such as spina bifida. Postural kyphosis is related to poor posture or slouching. Spine tumors and infections can cause kyphosis.

Scoliosis is a lateral (sideways) curvature, resulting in an S-shaped or C-shaped spinal appearance. It tends to be familial and is seen more frequently in girls than in boys. Scoliosis can also result from injury, infection, or a birth defect. The two types of scoliosis are functional and structural.

Diagnosis

Diagnosis is made by observation and radiography. Postural defects, especially scoliosis, are often discovered by the child's pediatrician (Fig. 73-4). The examination is simple and takes relatively little time. The child faces the screener and stands straight with the feet 2–3 in apart. The examiner looks at the symmetry of the upper torso. The healthcare provider then instructs the child to place the chin on the chest and the hands together and bend over, allowing the hands to hang freely. The screener looks for any asymmetry, such as unequal shoulder height, elbow levels, or hip height. (See photo in Data Collection in Children in Chapter 47.) If curvature is present, the screener uses a *scoliometer* (leveling device) to detect the curvature's degree. Referral and treatment are based on this degree.

Medical and Surgical Treatment
Treatment depends on the cause and the severity of the postural defect. The healthcare provider will observe the curvature every 4–6 weeks for changes. Common medical treatments include medications for pain and swelling, daily exercises, physical therapy (PT), and weight loss. The goals for physical rehabilitation are to increase muscle strength and flexibility. Sometimes, a back brace can help prevent the curve from getting worse. The *Milwaukee brace* extends from the pelvis to the base of the skull (i.e., it covers the entire thorax). The *Boston brace* starts under the arm and extends through the thorax, lumbar, and sacral regions. Braces are individualized and regularly adjusted as the child grows. These braces are typically worn for most of the day and night and may be worn for many years. Surgery may be needed to correct severe, worsening, or congenital curvatures. Surgical intervention may be necessary to correct a postural defect. Untreated postural defects are generally permanent and can cause respiratory compromise, pneumonias, and death. To secure unstable or damaged vertebrae, a spinal fusion or artificial disc replacement may be done. Specific devices, for example, hook, rod, wire, are attached to the spine to help realign the bones and keep them secure. A kyphoplasty is a procedure in which a balloon is inserted inside the spine. The goals of all surgeries are to straighten and stabilize curvatures and to relieve pain. One well-known spinal device is the *Harrington rod*, which is actually secured to the vertebral bones following spinal fusion. The child's growth is arrested following rod implantation. After surgery, the child may require a cast or brace for immobilization. Surgery is done only after more conservative treatment of the defect is unsuccessful. Physical therapy exercises may help in some cases of scoliosis and are typically used as a part of postoperative surgical intervention.

Nursing Considerations
Postural defects are often lifelong problems. They may cause pain and disfigurement. The child or adolescent may not be able to play with peers or participate in activities that are common for the adolescent. Loneliness and isolation are common. The nurse must emphasize the importance of weight loss, if needed, and appropriate physical exercises. It may be possible to prevent worsening of the abnormal curves. Support for the parental caregivers is as important as is an understanding of the needs of the client. The use of braces can seem overwhelming. Postoperative care needs individualized attention.

> **Key Concept**
> Scoliosis most often affects preadolescent girls. Screening and early treatment of structural scoliosis prevent long-term, permanent, and disabling disorders.

Juvenile Rheumatoid Arthritis
Juvenile rheumatoid arthritis (**JRA**), *juvenile idiopathic arthritis* (**JIA**), or *juvenile chronic arthritis* (**JCA**) are arthritic diseases of the musculoskeletal system in persons younger than 17 years old. In the United States, JRA is the most commonly identified condition. Classification of these diseases is ongoing, and each type seems to be unique; etiology focuses on both heredity and environment. A viral infection may affect the musculoskeletal system, which then initiates an autoimmune disease, that is, an abnormal immune response. Swollen lymph nodes, rashes, and fever are causes of the pain, swelling, and stiffness that are associated with juvenile arthritis. Some individuals have symptoms for a few months, and for others, it is a lifetime problem. Many children experience a spontaneous remission with no recurrence.

Symptoms
Symptoms can be persistent or intermittent. Painful joints, pain with movement, swelling, and stiffness are likely the primary symptoms that lead caregivers to seek medical care. In lieu of the child complaining of pain, the caregiver may notice limping, especially after getting up in the morning. Swelling typically appears first in the larger joints, such as the knee joints. Stiffness makes the child appear clumsier than usual, unable to manage fine motor skills. Eye inflammation may be an indicator of serious eye problems such as uveitis, which can lead to cataracts, glaucoma, and blindness. The child's growth may be arrested; malformation may result from uneven maturation of bones or joints.

Treatment
The focus of treatment is pain relief and alleviation of symptoms. If the adolescent has less pain, movement is more likely to improve, which is important in the prevention of swelling and stiffness. The primary group of drugs used for treatment includes the nonsteroidal anti-inflammatory drugs (**NSAIDs**) and, on occasion, corticosteroids, which help to relieve swelling, fever, pain, and inflammation. Newer classifications, for example, DMARDs and biologics (discussed below), may be used in combination with steroids and NSAIDs.

Disease-modifying antirheumatic drugs (**DMARDs**) suppress the entire immune system. Examples of DMARDs include methotrexate (Trexall), tofacitinib (Xeljanz), or leflunomide (Arava), which may slow the progress of JRA. DMARDs help prevent joint damage and deformity, which is a significant advance from earlier types of treatments that could only affect symptoms, such as pain and swelling. They are usually administered in pill form and target the entire immune system. It may take several months before noting any beneficial effects. Side effects of methotrexate, one of the most common DMARDs, include liver damage, bone marrow suppression, and spontaneous abortion or birth defects. Each DMARD is known to have its own set of side effects.

Biologic agents (**biologics**) or **biologic response modifiers** are genetically engineered proteins derived from human genes. Technically, they are a type of DMARD but differ from other DMARDs because they inhibit only specific parts of the inflammatory process. Examples of biologics include abatacept (Orencia), rituximab (Rituxin), anakinra (Kineret), and tocilizumab (Actemra). Biologics show results typically within 4–6 weeks and are more expensive than DMARDs. Biologics are given subcutaneously or by intravenous solution. The frequency of administration depends upon the specific drug and can range from daily to monthly. Pneumonia is a common risk factor of biologics. Side effects of biologics include skin reactions at the site of injection; increased changes of skin cancer are known to occur.

Nursing considerations during the acute phase include pain relief, exercising the limbs, helping the child with daily activities, and sometimes, applying heat in the form of hot baths, packs, or whirlpool treatments. Cold packs may also be helpful. It is important to educate the client and the family caregivers regarding handwashing and avoidance of infectious diseases because both DMARDs and biologics have the potential to increase the risk for infections by affecting the functioning of the immune system. NSAIDs and corticosteroids may mask the effects of infections since they are effective in the treatment of fevers and pain. Adequate nutrition needs to emphasize adequate calcium intake because JRA children are at risk for the development of osteoporosis. Weak bones may be the result of the disease, use of corticosteroids, decreased weight-bearing exercises, and minimal physical activity.

Legg–Calvé–Perthes Disease

Legg–Calvé–Perthes disease (**LCPD**) is a disease of one or both hips, affecting boys five times more commonly than girls, occurring in children aged 4–10 years. The condition results from a lack of blood supply to the hip joint, a ball-and-socket joint, causing avascular necrosis or death of the joint. Poor blood supply to bones results in fractures and poor bone healing. The cause of this spontaneous, yet temporary, reduction of blood flow to the femoral head is unknown. It may be caused by an injury or another disease process and tends to run in families. Signs and symptoms of Legg–Calvé–Perthes disease include painless limping, pain with walking, and difficulty or stiffness in the hip, groin, upper leg, and knee. The child has a limited range of motion in the affected hip joint. Both hips can be affected but typically at different times. The disease progresses through identifiable stages. Regeneration and bone growth occur gradually, up to 3 years.

Diagnosis

X-ray, MRI, or bone scan studies will be ordered to assist in diagnosing the condition. Changes on an x-ray may be difficult to see initially; the x-ray could read as normal. It may take up to 2 months after the onset of problems before bone damage can be identified by an x-ray with symptoms associated with the LCPD. An MRI can identify bone and soft tissue damage more clearly than an x-ray. A bone scan uses a small amount of radioactive material, which is attracted to areas where bone destruction is active.

Treatment

Treatment is geared toward prevention of permanent hip deformities, such as loss of the round shape of the femoral head, which occur when the weakened hip bones fracture. The condition typically clears spontaneously. Although the parental caregivers may be fearful and desire more aggressive therapies, common medical treatment is observation, symptomatic treatment for pain, mild to moderate physical exercise (e.g., stretching, limited playing). Hot or cold packs help relieve pain and can loosen tight muscles before PT exercises. Crutches, traction, and casts are occasionally used to protect the joint, prevent weight-bearing on the joint, or to keep the femoral head within the acetabulum.

Reconstructive orthopedic surgery may be necessary in a child older than 6–7 years who may have more significant and fixed hip deformity. These children need treatments that will fix contractures, remove excess bone or cartilage growths, reform the shape of the acetabulum, or replace all or part of the hip joint.

Nursing Considerations

Nursing interventions vary with the stage of LCPD. It is important to remember that, along with bone destruction, muscles and ligaments are affected. Soft tissue (i.e., muscles, ligaments) damage leads to the development of contractures and deformities, which can be permanent if not treated very early in the disease process. Stretching exercises help flexibility and encourage the muscles and ligaments to support the hip within its socket. Stretching can also prevent contractures. Nursing considerations must include emphasis on the importance of appropriate physical therapy.

Dental Malocclusion

Malocclusion of the teeth refers to any degree of irregular contact of the teeth of the upper jaw with the teeth of the lower jaw. Most malocclusions are minor, and no treatment is necessary. Significant faulty tooth positioning, such as overbite and underbite, jaw joint disorder, or poorly aligned jaw position, results in improper contact of the jaws and teeth. Malocclusion commonly causes problems with chewing, gum tissue, speech development, and cosmetic appearance. There are several causes of malocclusion, including genetics and environmental factors. Children who suck their thumbs or fingers after the age of 5 years are more prone to the development of faulty tooth positioning. Problems may occur in the phase between the loss of primary teeth (baby teeth) and the eruption of permanent teeth.

Diagnosis of malocclusion may be initially made by a dentist, who may refer the client to an *orthodontist* who will determine the need for correction. *Orthodontists* are dentists who are trained in the specialty of **orthodontia**, the correction of tooth positioning, and jaw deformities. Orthodontists learn to correct some facial abnormalities and disorders of the jaw but are most often associated with correction of irregularities of the teeth, bite, and jaw. Orthodontic screening should begin after the child's permanent teeth erupt, no later than age 7, after the first 6-year permanent molars erupt. Screenings may begin as early as age 2 years to watch for early dental or malocclusion problems.

Treatment

Treatment may begin as soon as possible after a thorough dental evaluation, or it may be delayed until the child is older, depending on the problem's severity. The initial evaluation by a dentist or orthodontist will include a history, oral examination, x-rays, and imprints (impressions) of the mouth in dental plaster. Oral health in general and factors such as age, general health, medical history, and cosmetic expectations and preferences are considered. Adolescents commonly have dental caries (cavities) that need regular attention to prevent further tooth, gum, and bone damage. Signs of STDs, diabetes, pregnancy, tobacco use, and lesions that indicate systemic problems may be discovered. Treatment may take several years and, typically, is done in phases, depending on the individual's growth. Some teeth may be extracted, such as third molars (wisdom teeth), which appear between the ages of 15 and 25. Appliances such as retainers may be inserted and removed by the child. Braces, a type of fixed appliance, are made of plastic, metal, or elastic bands. *Orthognathic surgery* (jaw surgery) may sometimes be indicated and may be done by a surgeon specializing in facial repairs (a maxillofacial surgeon).

Nursing Considerations

Nursing considerations focus on good mouth care, which includes toothbrushing twice a day, flossing, and regular dental visits. Soft bristle toothbrushes, toothpaste with fluoride, and fluoridated drinking water are recommended. It is important to maintain good preventative care of retainers, braces, or other appliances. Precautionary measures include avoidance of chewy foods like popcorn, gummy candy, nuts, and caramels. Professional cleaning is recommended about every 6 months. Long-term effects of poor oral health can be addressed by encouraging the adolescent to consider oral care as an important part of physical health.

> **SPECIAL CONSIDERATIONS** — **Culture and Ethnicity**
>
> Children of European descent are more likely to develop Legg–Calvé–Perthes disease than are children of African descent. Ewing sarcoma is more common in young children among those of European descent.

Malignant Bone Tumors

Malignant bone tumors or **sarcomas** are primary bone cancers. A primary sarcoma originates in the bone, that is to say, malignant cells are first found in bone tissues and later can metastasize (spread) to other areas, commonly the lungs. Secondary bone cancers are cancers that have been metastasized from another site (e.g., pancreas or cervix) and spread to the bone. Sarcomas are fairly rare and are more likely to be diagnosed in children than adults. A bone cancer specialist, either a pediatric oncologist or an orthopedic oncologist, will typically be the primary healthcare provider. Treatment for sarcomas may result in *late effects,* which are health problems that occur months or years after treatments have ended. Clients who have had chemotherapy, radiation, surgery, or stem cell transplants are at risk for late effects. Chapter 83 discusses cancer in more detail.

Osteosarcoma, also known as *osteogenic sarcoma,* is a type of cancerous bone tumor which is more commonly seen in young men between the ages of 10 and 30 years. The osteoblasts of the ends of the long bone are frequently involved, and other bones may be involved as well. The cancer metastasizes by way of the circulatory system, often to the lungs first. Symptoms vary but often include limping, sharp or dull pain, swelling, and redness at the site of the tumor. Range of motion on the affected side is decreased.

Diagnostic x-rays would show suspicious bone lesions, which would need further evaluation. Additional studies include bone scans, MRI, CT scan, and bone biopsy. Laboratory tests include a standard CBC and blood chemistries.

Treatment typically may involve surgical biopsy, surgical resection, amputation, chemotherapy, and/or radiation of the affected extremity. Postoperative treatment includes fitting of a prosthetic with training and rehabilitation if needed. Aggressive treatment can reduce the risk of death.

Nursing considerations involve care of the physical and psychological needs of the child and parental caregivers. Adolescents need to adapt to pain, frequent rehabilitation, and significant changes of body image. Client teaching and support are required as the amputation site heals, and adjustments are made to accommodate living with a prosthesis. Infection control and pain relief are important. Continuous follow-up care includes long-term responses to treatment, detection of recurrent cancers, and management of the side effects of radiation and chemotherapy.

Ewing sarcoma is a primary bone malignancy that arises from the bone marrow, affecting the long and flat bones and occasionally muscles and tissues. It is one of the cancers belonging to the *Ewing sarcoma family of tumors* (ESFT or EFT). Ewing sarcoma develops after birth and is not a genetically inherited disease, but it is a disorder of chromosomes. It can be seen typically in children and young adults between the ages of 10 and 30 years and has no identifiable etiology. Ewing sarcoma can be cured in many cases, especially if discovered in its early stages.

Symptoms resemble many other conditions (e.g., infections, accidental injuries); therefore, early, accurate diagnosis is important. The most common signs and symptoms are pain or swelling that gets progressively worse occurring in the arm, leg, chest, back, or pelvis. Affected bones may have spontaneous fractures (breaks for unknown reasons). Swelling without pain, redness, or localized heat may be an indicator. Limited range of motion is noted.

Diagnosis uses imaging tests such as x-ray, MRI, CT scan, PET scan, and bone scan. Physical examinations and blood testing will be done to identify other issues (e.g., infection). A tissue biopsy with testing for DNA changes confirms the diagnosis. The oncologist will also determine the extent of the cancer. Chapter 83 discusses cancer grading and staging.

Treatment begins with chemotherapy; it is intense and can continue for several months. Surgery and/or radiation are done to remove or destroy as much of the tumor as possible. Chemotherapy is resumed for several more weeks or months. Long-term monitoring is necessary to look for late side effects of chemotherapy such as impaired hearing or vision, growth and development difficulties, or development of problems with the heart or respiratory system.

Nursing considerations will involve supporting the client and parental caregivers throughout the months of treatments.

> **SPECIAL CONSIDERATIONS** — **Educating the Client**
>
> The American Cancer Society recommends that caregivers maintain copies of medical records associated with treatments for cancer. This information will be helpful to future healthcare providers. Included should be copies of biopsy reports, the list of drugs used for chemotherapy, a summary of the types and doses of radiation, and copies of hospital discharge summaries.

ENDOCRINE DISORDERS

Of all endocrine disorders that can affect school-age children and adolescents, diabetes mellitus is the most prevalent. Diabetes is discussed in more detail in Chapter 79. Other, relatively uncommon, endocrine conditions include diabetes insipidus and pituitary disorders that result in changes in growth.

Diabetes Mellitus

Diabetes mellitus type 1 or *insulin-dependent diabetes* (**IDDM**) and *diabetes mellitus type 2* or *non–insulin-dependent diabetes mellitus* (**NIDDM**) are significant and growing healthcare concerns for children and adolescents in the United States. The incidence of both types of diabetes has increased, largely due to issues related to obesity in children.

Type 1 diabetes results from lack of the body's ability to produce insulin. Etiologic factors in IDDM include genetics, autoimmune factors, progressive, uncontrolled type 2 diabetes, and environmental factors, such as viruses and infant nutrition (see Chapter 79).

Type 2 diabetes is most likely to occur in overweight female clients. Female children and adolescents have increased risk factors such as a family history of being overweight or having diabetes, gestational diabetes, or having insulin resistance. American Indian, African American, Asian, or Hispanic/Latino ancestry is also considered a risk factor. Unhealthy eating and lack of physical activity contribute to the risk factors.

At first, symptoms of diabetes, such as dry mouth, itchy skin, or fatigue, may be difficult to distinguish because they can be associated with many issues. Classic symptoms of diabetes include **polyuria** (dramatic increase in urinary output, probably with enuresis), **polydipsia** (abnormal thirst), and **polyphagia** (increased hunger). These symptoms are usually accompanied by weight loss or failure to gain weight and lack of energy. General malaise, irritability, blurred vision, and yeast infections accompany the symptoms because blood sugar is out of control. Failure to note symptoms and to refer children for diagnosis may result in the rapid progress of the disorder to diabetic ketoacidosis and eventually to diabetic coma.

Diagnosis is made by a physical examination, review of family history, and assorted laboratory studies. A random blood sugar test can be done several times a day, and A1C levels are measured every 3 months. (Refer to Chapter 79 for more discussion of diabetes and blood sugar testing.)

Nursing Considerations

Treatment of diabetes in children can be overwhelming due to the significant number of changes needed in daily activities. Treatment starts with stabilization of blood sugar levels by way of insulin therapy. Exercise, weight loss, nutritional changes, and psychological support are also important in managing the disease. Involve the whole family in the diabetic child's care and treatment. The child will need close supervision by the healthcare team until he or she adjusts to the insulin dosage and the condition stabilizes. Typically, a family may need a year after initial diagnosis to begin to feel comfortable with their new adaptations. Infections must

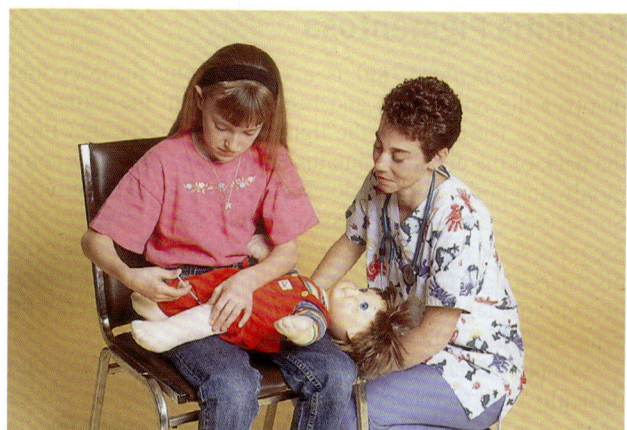

Figure 73-5 A school-age child is taught insulin administration using a teaching doll for practice.

receive immediate medical care because they can lead to ketoacidosis. Encourage insulin-dependent diabetic youngsters as early as possible to test their own blood glucose level, self-administer their injections, and lead a normal, independent life (Fig. 73-5). Encourage family caregivers to inform other appropriate adults, as needed, about the child's condition, such as teachers, school nurse, camp nurse, scout leader, or athletic coach. All adults caring for a diabetic child must learn the signs and symptoms of hypoglycemia and hyperglycemia and how to respond to each. Adolescents often go through an adjustment period in which they rebel against treatment. They need patience, understanding, and support. The adolescent will need close regulation of dietary intake and insulin administration. A third major component of diabetes management is physical activity, which affects both dietary intake and insulin needs. The amount of glucose may be increased in an appropriate diet while the insulin needs may be decreased. More glucose is consumed when the adolescent is active. Hypoglycemia is of special concern during times of activity and growth, that is, metabolism changes.

> *Key Concept*
>
> Encourage parental caregivers to seek independent information regarding the care of diabetes. Many agencies have Websites with valuable and useful information for the child, adolescent, and parent, including the American Diabetes Association and the Centers for Disease Control and Prevention.

VISION DISORDERS

Early detection of learning-related vision problems is a fundamental but often overlooked healthcare step for parental caregivers and healthcare providers. Correction of visual disorders in the child and adolescent can prevent many difficulties that would interfere with an individual's potentials and goals. Common visual disorders, known as **refractive errors**, including *myopia* (nearsightedness), *hyperopia* (farsightedness), and *astigmatism* (unequal eye curvatures), are discussed in Chapter 80 and summarized in Table 80-1. Prescription eyeglasses and/or contact lenses help the majority of individuals with these problems.

Retinitis Pigmentosa

Retinitis pigmentosa (**RP**) is a rare, genetic disorder that involves the breakdown and loss of cells in the retinas of both eyes. The *retina* is the light-sensitive tissue that lines the back of the eye that contains photoreceptors. RP is commonly diagnosed during adolescence but can occur at birth. Some types are nonprogressive, while other cases of RP progress slowly. RP can be associated with specific hearing disorders (e.g., *Usher syndrome*) in which RP and neural hearing loss are seen. Usher syndrome is the most common cause of deaf-blindness in the United States.

Symptoms include progressively poor night vision and difficulty with peripheral vision (difficulty seeing the side or edges of a visual field). The client loses increasing amounts of peripheral visual acuity as vision seems to concentrates to the center. To the client, it appears as if one is inside a tunnel looking out, that is, *tunnel vision*. Tunnel vision can be present for years or decades but vision eventually deteriorates to blindness. The timeframe for this process can range from childhood or adolescence to the 40s.

Diagnosis is obtained using family medical history and physical eye examination. Initial complaints of poor night vision and retinal changes unique to RP are seen by the ophthalmologist when a fundoscopic examination is done. A *fundoscopic examination* uses an ophthalmoscope to see through the pupil to the retina at the back of the eye. The ophthalmologist will also perform visual field testing, which will help assess the severity of tunnel vision. Electrophysiologic testing can be done, but the eye equipment may only be available in specialized eye care facilities.

Treatment is palliative as there is no cure. Some research studies suggest the use of certain fat-soluble vitamins, as prescribed by the ophthalmologist, in conjunction with stem cell therapy. An early diagnosis may help the family and the client prepare for gradual vision loss. Low-vision services are helpful, such as visual field-expanding glasses, adaptive eye equipment, and in-home lifestyle consultations.

Nursing considerations will be based on the current and future needs of the client and the client's caregivers. Coping with the diagnosis of blindness requires psychological adjustments as well as physical adjustments to the environment, for example, loss of ability to drive, placement of furniture, and development of new skills and habits.

Glaucoma

Glaucoma refers to abnormally high *intraocular* (within the eyeball) pressure due to the inability of the fluid of the eye, the aqueous humor, to drain properly. Fluid pressure increases and damages the optic nerve, resulting in eventual blindness. Refer to Chapter 80 for more information on glaucoma. There are two types of glaucoma in children: congenital and juvenile.

Congenital glaucoma, also called *infantile glaucoma*, is found in babies born with glaucoma and is typically diagnosed in the first year of life. Infantile glaucoma is the diagnosis given typically if glaucoma develops during childhood, commonly after ages 4 or 5. Parental observations and intervention are critical. The parental caregivers may notice excessive tearing, cloudy corneas, large eyes, and avoidance of bright lights (e.g., shutting eyes tightly). Successful preservation of vision will depend upon early diagnosis and interventions. Treatments include medications and, sometimes, surgery. Long-term follow-up with the ophthalmologist will be necessary because visual changes will continue to occur. Visual results for most children will be good.

Juvenile glaucoma is a type of open-angle glaucoma often associated with myopia (nearsightedness). It may be caused by trauma, hemorrhage into the eye, tumor, inflammatory eye disease, or developmental abnormalities during infancy and early childhood. Noticeable symptoms include frequent tearing, *photophobia* (sensitivity to light), problem adjusting to the dark, excessive blinking, chronic red eyes, and cloudiness of the cornea. The adolescent may complain of head or eye pain. Vision loss may not be noticed at first and considerable damage may have occurred before the client seeks treatment. Surgery is performed as early as possible to prevent further damage to vision. Medications to control intraocular pressure are also used.

Retinoblastoma

Retinoblastoma is a cancer of the retina of the eye that occurs in young children and rarely in adults. It may occur in one or both eyes. Etiology is genetic mutation that may be inherited, but the reason for mutation is not understood. The cancerous retinal cells can invade the eye, brain, and spine. Retinoblastoma may return in or around an eye that had been treated. Years after treatment, recurrent retinoblastoma or cancers in other parts of the body tend to occur. Symptoms include eye redness, eye swelling, and eyes that appear to be looking in different directions. Also noticeable is a white color in the pupil (center dark circle of the eye) when light is shone in the eye, such as when taking a flash photo.

Diagnosis is made after completion of a thorough review of family medical history, eye examination, and imaging tests, for example, CT scan, MRI, or ultrasound. The healthcare provider will also be looking for metastasis to other structures.

Treatment depends upon the size and spread of the tumor. The goal will be to preserve vision if possible. Consultations with pediatricians who specialize in oncology, surgery, or eye disorders are recommended. Laser photocoagulation may be done to destroy blood cells that supply the cancerous cell growth. Cryotherapy (extreme cold therapy) (e.g., liquid nitrogen) or thermotherapy (extreme heat therapy, e.g., microwaves or lasers) may be used to destroy malignant cells. Therapies include various protocols of chemotherapy, radiation, and surgery. Enucleation (removal) of the eyeball may be necessary to prevent spread of the cancer. Immediately after the eyeball is removed, the surgeon places an eye implant into the eye socket. The eye muscles are attached to the implant so that the eye will move naturally. Several weeks after surgery, the implant is replaced with a personalized artificial eye that will appear to move as does the normal eye. The child will adapt to the use of one eye but must be aware that some peripheral vision will be lost due to the enucleation.

Nursing considerations depend upon the stage of therapy and disease. Children and caregivers need emotional support. Enucleation may be difficult to consider as a therapy. If an artificial eye is used, the child and caregivers may need assistance learning to insert the eye behind the eyelids. Long-term goals will be to reinforce the need for follow-up visits to check for reoccurrences of cancer. A genetic counselor may be suggested so that the family will be aware of any existing or future children's chances of development of cancer, as well as those children's chances of passing on the cancer to their offspring.

GASTROINTESTINAL DISORDERS

Gastrointestinal disorders in the child and adolescent include a variety of common conditions that are often seen with the symptoms of abdominal pain, nausea, vomiting, diarrhea, and constipation. GI problems may be mild and resolve without intervention, or they can be severe and significantly interfere with daily activities and be the cause of frequent school absences. Due to the relative position and location of the organs, urinary tract infections and disorders of the reproductive organs need to be differentiated from disorders of the GI tract.

Irritable bowel syndrome (**IBS**) refers to a pattern of symptoms affecting the large intestine (colon) that includes abdominal pain, abdominal cramping, bloating, gas, and constipation or diarrhea. In the past, IBS had a variety of names, including colitis, spastic colon, nervous colon, and spastic bowel. It does not have an identifiable cause and occurs more often in females than males. It is considered a *functional disorder,* meaning that the GI tract behaves abnormally but the colon's tissues are not damaged. Triggers have been identified that seem to irritate the bowel and instigate symptoms. Triggers include gas-producing foods (e.g., broccoli or beans) or food sensitivities (e.g., milk, cheese), as well as situations in which physical or psychological stress are present. It is thought that females have IBS more often than males due to female reproductive hormones; IBS may be more prevalent during menses.

Diagnosis

Diagnosis is made by physical examination, medical history, standard laboratory studies, and, possibly, a colonoscopy. A culture and sensitivity of stool may be indicated if diarrhea is present. The symptoms of IBS are similar to other GI disorders that might include more serious problems such as GI bleeding, unexplained weight loss, or worsening abdominal pain. A blood test to rule out celiac disease may be ordered. Medications may be prescribed for specific symptoms. Box 88-4 and Table 88-3 list GI drugs, classifications, and their indications for use.

Treatment

Treatment is palliative. Initially, a food diary (record of what is eaten) is helpful in identifying triggers to be avoided. Educate the client and other caregivers about ways to avoid common triggers, such as caffeine, fatty foods, dairy products, and alcohol, and the use of OTC and prescription medications for symptomatic relief. Dietary fiber is beneficial but can result in either diarrhea or constipation for the client with IBS; therefore, fiber content should be considered individually. Also, consider omitting gas-producing foods such as beans, cabbage, broccoli, and cauliflower. For some patients, additional medicines may be used.

Nursing Considerations

Individuals are able to successfully control most signs and symptoms of IBS through dietary choices, lifestyle adjustments, and palliative medications. However, most clients would prefer a cure rather than palliative treatments, and frustration is common. Provide positive feedback to adolescents and parental caregivers when changes are successful. During acute episodes of IBS, it is important that the client receive adequate fluids and electrolytes.

Inflammatory Bowel Disease

Inflammatory bowel disease (**IBD**) is a term that describes major inflammatory reactions of the intestines. Autoimmune reactions are considered to be the most likely cause. The two most common types of IBD are *Crohn disease* and *ulcerative colitis* (see also Chapter 88). Both of these conditions have cyclic periods called **exacerbations**, which are flare-ups of acute disease, with intermittent periods of **remission** or absence of symptoms. The symptoms of both conditions range from mild to severe. Signs and symptoms for both Crohn disease and ulcerative colitis include the following: diarrhea several times a day, fever, fatigue, general malaise, abdominal pain, abdominal cramping with pain, bright red or occult blood in the stool, poor appetite with occasional nausea and vomiting, and unintended weight loss. Clients may become malnourished because of decreased caloric and nutrient intake and the inability of the food to properly digest due to damage inside the intestinal walls where nutrients are absorbed.

Crohn Disease

Crohn disease is an IBD that may affect any part of the gastrointestinal tract, from the mouth to the anus. In addition to the autoimmune disorder etiology of Crohn disease, it is known that cigarette smoking is also a risk factor for its development. Crohn disease attacks different areas of the large and/or small intestinal wall, leaving normal intestine between damaged areas. The most commonly affected areas are the ileum (last section of the small intestine) and the colon. It affects the entire depth, or "full thickness," of the intestinal wall. *Fibrostenosis, fistulas,* and *bowel obstructions* occur. **Fibrostenosis** is a narrowing of the intestinal lumen due to scaring and inflammation of the tissue. A **fistula** is an abnormal, unintended open section between two areas of bowel wall. **Bowel obstructions**, causing potentially fatal intestinal necrosis and infarction, occur because the narrowing of the intestinal lumen blocks passage of stool. These three problems can instigate serious complications, bowel infarction, and death. Symptoms are challenging and include abdominal pain, diarrhea or bloody diarrhea, and weight loss. In children and adolescents, the disease can delay puberty, weaken bones, and stunt growth. Symptoms may include **tenesmus**, which is the unyielding feeling or need to pass stool, accompanied by straining, pain, and cramping, even if the bowels are already empty.

Diagnosis

Diagnosis is made by a history and physical examination, standard and specific blood tests, and by ruling out other possible causes of symptoms. Blood tests will look for anemia, inflammation, or infections. A stool sample may show *occult blood,* which is blood in the stool that is not obvious to the naked eye. Imaging studies are done, such as an abdominal x-ray and a barium swallow (a procedure to visualize the small bowel after the client swallows liquid barium). The diagnostic workup may also include a CT scan, MRI, colonoscopy, sigmoidoscopy, and, perhaps, more specific types of endoscopy, such as a *video capsule endoscopy* (**VCE**). The client swallows a capsule that has a camera inside it; these pictures are transmitted to a computer. The capsule is passed through the intestinal tract and exits painlessly from the body.

Treatment

Treatment for Crohn disease is largely palliative, involving exercise, lifestyle changes (e.g., smoking cessation), and a diet that does not exacerbate symptoms. OTC anti-inflammatory and antidiarrheal medications are helpful, as are nutritional supplements such as vitamin B, iron, calcium, and vitamin D. Surgery may be done to remove a portion of the GI tract that has fistulas, abscesses, or strictures. Many medications are available to treat autoimmune disorders. Refer to Box 88-4 and Table 88-3 for more information.

Nursing Considerations

Crohn disease is a long-term acute and chronic condition that greatly affects one's lifestyle. Nursing considerations depend upon the client's current condition. The client may need the nurse to be a good listener. At other times, the client or the caregivers may need to have information about a new issue or to be referred to resource Websites and materials.

Ulcerative Colitis

Ulcerative colitis (**UC**) is a relatively common disorder in adolescents and young adults between the ages of 13 and 30 years. It results in inflammation and ulcers of the lining of the colon and rectum but does not affect the entire thickness of the wall of either the large or small intestine. One of the most pronounced symptoms of UC is severe diarrhea, which may contain blood or pus, and which may be accompanied by weight loss, anorexia, and growth delays. Unlike Crohn disease, obstructions, stenosis, and fistulas are not associated with ulcerative colitis. UC can greatly affect one's lifestyle and, during exacerbations, can be debilitating or life-threatening. Weight loss, fever, and fatigue are noted. A delay in the appearance of secondary sex characteristics also may be evident if the disease occurs before puberty. The distal colon or rectum can show evidence of ulceration, inflammation, and bleeding. Symptoms may include tenesmus, in which the client may have the urgency to defecate but not be able to pass any stool. Complications of UC include *toxic megacolon* (a rapidly swelling colon), thrombosis and emboli, perforated colon, osteoporosis, hemorrhage, and aphthous ulcers of the mouth. Additional problems include liver disease, inflammation of the skin, joints, and eyes, and an increase in the risk for cancer.

Diagnostic tests include standard blood studies (i.e., CBC, UA, electrolytes, liver enzymes, and renal function) plus a review of studies that indicate inflammation, such as an erythrocyte sedimentation rate (ESR) or C-reactive protein (CRP). Testing is focused on differentiation between the two major types of IBD, that is, Crohn disease and ulcerative colitis. UC affects only the colon and rectum; therefore, imaging and endoscopic examinations, such as a VCE, can confirm the UC disorder.

Treatment is based upon the severity and extent of involvement of the tissues of the colon and rectum. There is no cure, but long-term remission is possible. Medications include analgesics and anti-inflammatory medications. Systemic corticosteroids are used with caution in acute exacerbations. Immunomodulators (e.g., azathioprine/6-MP, methotrexate, and cyclosporine) and biologic agents (e.g., infliximab [Remicade]) have been effective in many cases. As stated earlier, refer to Box 88-4 and Table 88-3 for more information regarding gastrointestinal medications. A *colectomy,* which removes the diseased portion of the colon, or a total *proctocolectomy* (removal of the entirety of the large bowel and rectum) results in the alleviation of symptoms. Surgical intervention is considered if medical interventions are ineffective.

Nursing considerations are similar to those of Crohn disease or any chronic inflammatory bowel disease. Clients benefit from an explanation of diagnostic procedures and from support for dietary and lifestyle changes. Assist with the understanding of medications and their side effects.

REPRODUCTIVE SYSTEM DISORDERS

Reproductive system disorders typically begin in puberty, generally between the ages of 11 and 14 years. During the years of early adolescence, a client may experiment with different types of behaviors, some of which are high risk and can have long-term consequences. Sexual intercourse, one of the common high-risk adolescent behaviors, can lead to serious outcomes such as unintended pregnancy and STIs. Refer to Chapter 70 for an in-depth discussion of STIs.

Menstruation and Menstrual Difficulties

Menstruation or *period* is the normal shedding of blood and tissue from the endometrium of the uterus, which occurs over a 3- to 5-day timeframe (range 2–7 days). A period occurs about every 28 days (range 21–45 days). Additional signs and symptoms that accompany a period include abdominal pain, pelvic cramping, lower-back pain, bloating, sore breasts, food cravings, irritability, mood swings, headache, and fatigue. Menstrual cycles are often irregular for up to 6 years after onset. If a client does not start their menses by the age of 15–16, a healthcare provider should be consulted.

Menstrual difficulties include pain, delayed onset, discomfort, and altered patterns. **Mittelschmerz** is a word that refers to the one-sided, lower abdominal pain occurring around the time of ovulation.

Dysmenorrhea is painful menstruation, a common problem for young clients whose bodies are establishing regular cycles. Occasionally, dysmenorrhea is due to a disorder within the pelvis such as **endometriosis**. Endometriosis may not be diagnosed until the mid-20s, but it is not uncommon for a young client to have excessive bleeding and to complain of abdominal or pelvic pain that differs from, or is worse than, the standard period-based dysmenorrhea. Chapter 91 discusses endometriosis in more detail. Delayed onset of more than 3 months or an absence of a period, **amenorrhea**, is a reason to consult with a medical professional.

Premenstrual syndrome (**PMS**) is a group of symptoms that start before the onset of a period and can continue throughout menses. PMS symptoms range from mild to significant and involve a variety of emotional and physical factors. Fluctuations in hormones are considered to be the standard etiology of PMS. The client may have mild to moderate symptoms of depression and anxiety. They may have mood swings and be irritable or have crying spells. Physical symptoms include appetite changes and food cravings, weight gain, abdominal bloating, breast tenderness, headaches, and acne flare-ups.

Premenstrual dysphoric disorder (**PMDD**) is similar to PMS, but the monthly symptoms are often disabling. The lifestyle and daily activities of clients with PMDD are affected. They have depression and feel overwhelmed. They may not be able to concentrate. The anger, irritability, and tension that they feel can become a spontaneous outburst with exaggerated inappropriate behaviors. Counseling and medical intervention to address the symptoms are typically necessary.

Treatment

Treatment of menstrual difficulties is symptomatic. Administration of NSAIDs 1–2 days before the beginning of menses prevents the formation of prostaglandins and helps reduce discomfort and inflammation. Warm baths and relaxation techniques also help reduce pain. In severe cases, oral contraceptives may be used to regulate menstrual cycles. Treatment of PMDD includes counseling, emotional support, and antianxiety or antidepressant medications.

Nursing considerations for menstrual disorders involve consideration of phases appropriate to the client's age. The onset of menses is a time of emotional and physical change for the client. Their self-concept and body image depend on their concept of "what is normal" as they transition from child to adult. Nursing educators can provide resources that will facilitate understanding of normal physical and emotional changes. Parental caregivers often expect and accept physical changes but are unprepared for the fluctuating emotions (e.g., mood swings or irritability) that develop.

SLEEP DEPRIVATION AND DISORDERS

Sleep Deprivation

Sleep deprivation is a chronic or acute state of not having adequate sleep. Sleep deprivation in school-age children and teenagers has been associated with a variety of emotional and behavioral problems, as well as with negative effects on academic progress, which can be a result of chronic fatigue. Lack of sleep results in slower reaction time, which can be a risk factor for accidents and injuries. Accidents are the third leading cause of death in the United States (Xu et al., 2020). Sleep deprivation may be seen in children who are inattentive, hyperactive, or restless, which are also symptoms associated with various nervous system disorders such as ADHD. A child could be misdiagnosed with ADHD, which could result in stereotyping and expectations for self-control that are not appropriate for a child. To differentiate between sleep deprivation and various nervous system disorders, consider the totality of existing symptoms.

The amount of time that a child should sleep depends upon the child's age. A 1-month-old infant may sleep for a total of 15–16 hr out of 24 hr. Children of ages 12–18 years sleep about 9 hr a night. Adults need about 7–8 hr of sleep per night.

Sleep disorders or *parasomnias* are conditions that disturb or prevent sleep. They are fairly common in the school-age child and the adolescent. Symptoms of a sleep disorder include restless sleep, excessive snoring, frequent awakening at night, difficulty getting to or maintaining sleep, gasping for air, grinding of teeth, and a sudden inability to move. Consider sleep disorders if bedwetting occurs in children older than 6 years. Other behaviors that may indicate sleep deprivation include a decline in school performance, hyperactivity or unusual movements during sleep, sleepwalking, and falling asleep during the daytime.

Sleep Hygiene

Sleep hygiene refers to the behaviors and environmental factors that precede the time set aside for sleep. Poor sleep hygiene may interfere with sleep. Specific symptoms of poor sleep hygiene include daytime sleepiness, trouble getting to sleep, and difficulty staying asleep. Physical and emotional problems are often accompanied by poor sleep hygiene. Parental caregivers need to plan behaviors and habits around bedtime that establish good sleep hygiene. Habitual routines around bedtime are essential for the child and continue into adolescence. Rituals that immediately precede sleep are important routines, such as washing and brushing teeth followed by reading a book to help establish a low-key sleep-ready atmosphere. The sleeping room should be between 60 °F and 67 °F or 15.5 °C and 19.4 °C or slightly cooler than during waking hours. Eliminate distracting lights and noises, such as any type of media monitor, phone, or game.

Types of Sleep Disorders

The following is a list of common sleep disorders in the child and adolescent, many of which are also found in the adult.

Insomnia is difficulty falling asleep. It may be caused by *hyperkinesis* (hyperactivity) or may be a symptom of an emotional problem.

Sleep-onset anxiety is a problem falling asleep because of overwhelming fear or anxiety. Stressful events that occur during the day may dominate the individual's thoughts before bedtime. While anxieties are common in adults, a school-age child also worries, for example, feels the stress of competition in the classroom or becomes fearful of the words and actions of others (bully-type behaviors). Parental caregivers should not dismiss a child's worries as being insignificant. Good sleep hygiene, which promotes nighttime relaxation, is helpful. Successful strategies would include active listening, providing safety and reassurance, and children to develop coping methods to address their concerns.

Sleep apnea occurs when a person stops breathing for short periods of time during regular sleeping hours. Physical defects may be the causative factor, and this condition is not uncommon in individuals who are obese. Typical results of sleep apnea include difficulty staying alert and awake and difficulty with concentration during the regular waking hours.

Night terrors are sudden, partial awakenings accompanied by significant emotional outbursts, such as screaming, panic, fear, and increased motor activity. Family members cannot console the child, who may be incoherent. When awake, the child typically does not remember the event.

Night terrors most often occur between the ages of 4 and 8 years, during periods when the child is not dreaming (*non-REM sleep*). Rapid eye movement (REM) sleep occurs when the individual is dreaming. Parental caregivers are advised not to waken the child but to ensure safety and comfort. In extreme situations, night terrors may require counseling and medications. If night terrors occur often or they worsen, a sleep study (*polysomnogram*) may be helpful.

Somniloquy (talking during sleep) is common in young people. It may or may not be associated with sleepwalking. The person can often carry on a logical conversation but will not remember it the next morning.

Somnambulism (sleepwalking) usually occurs during the later stages of non-REM sleep, most commonly in children 8–12 years old. The child sits up in bed with eyes open but does not see and may walk through the house. Sleepwalking episodes can last from several minutes to half an hour or longer. Children usually do not recall sleepwalking episodes the next morning. Sleepwalking is more common in boys than in girls, is more likely to occur when children are fatigued or under stress, and is usually outgrown by adolescence. The major concern with sleepwalking is physical protection. Do not threaten or abruptly awaken a sleepwalker, but observe safety measures to avoid injuries.

Narcolepsy is a brief attack of irresistible sleep. It is a rare and potentially dangerous condition that generally first appears in adolescence and may be seen in adults. Narcolepsy can include sleep-onset paralysis or sleep-onset hallucinations. A sleep specialist is needed to assist with this disorder. Treatment may include medications, scheduled naps, and ensuring a 12-hr nighttime sleep schedule.

EATING DISORDERS

An eating disorder is a type of psychological disorder characterized by abnormal eating behavior, which can range from eating extremely small amounts of food to eating excessive quantities followed by vomiting. Most commonly seen in adolescent female clients, eating disorders can also occur during young adulthood. Possible causes of these disorders include family factors (e.g., genetics and environmental behaviors); psychological factors (e.g., low self-esteem, depression, perfectionism, or impulsive behaviors); and sociologic factors (e.g., peer pressure, media representations of body images, or poor relationships). Diagnosis is based on criteria for various eating disorders as identified by the American Psychiatric Association. Treatment consists of psychological and medical interventions. Examples include anorexia nervosa, bulimia, and binge eating.

Anorexia Nervosa

Anorexia nervosa or anorexia is a condition of severe, obsessive, self-imposed undernourishment, sometimes to the

---

Box 73-3　Signs and Symptoms of Anorexia Nervosa

- Extremely low body weight
- Extreme weight loss
- Intense fear of weight gain
- Denial of the seriousness of malnutrition and low body weight
- Severe self-imposed food restrictions—making excuses not to eat, eating meals different than others in family, severe restriction to diets or dieting
- Consumption of high-fat foods or sweet foods
- Eating in secret
- Use of dietary supplements or laxatives
- Menstrual irregularities, unexplained amenorrhea
- Infertility
- Self-induced vomiting—callouses may be noted on knuckles from induced vomiting
- Loss of tooth enamel—a side effect of repeated vomiting
- Leaving meals to use the toilet (to vomit)
- Weakness
- Fatigue
- Lightheadedness
- Constipation
- Low blood pressure
- Low body temperature
- Dry skin
- Bradycardia (slow pulse)
- Electrolyte imbalance, e.g., hypokalemia (potassium deficiency)
- Thinning hair
- Distorted body image—frequently looks in mirror, describes flaws
- Self-esteem that focuses on body weight and shape
- Withdrawal from friends or social activities
- Excessive exercising
- Acid reflux disorder

Adapted from materials at https://www.nimh.nih.gov/health/topics/eating-disorders/index.shtml, https://www.mayoclinic.org/diseases-conditions/eating-disorders/symptoms-causes/syc-20353603.

---

point of starvation and death, which interferes with health and growth. Before the start of anorexia, the client's concept of weight loss begins with "dieting" but spirals out of control to an extreme point where food, even in small amounts, becomes an enemy. Individuals use extreme efforts to control their weight and shape. It is a potentially life-threatening eating disorder that occurs mostly in adolescent females. Symptoms include an abnormally low body weight, intense fear of weight gain, and a distorted perception of weight gain (Box 73-3).

Bulimia Nervosa

Bulimia nervosa, or bulimia, is an eating disorder characterized by loss of control during overeating, followed by purging. It most commonly occurs in the older adolescent and young adult female, but males have also been affected. The individual has habitual episodes of eating large amounts of food followed by forced vomiting, excessive use of laxatives or diuretics, and extreme exercise, or a combination of these behaviors. The cycle fluctuates between binge eating and purging, which can happen several times a day to several times a week. Unlike anorexia, clients are not usually underweight. They may have a healthy or normal weight or be slightly overweight. Clients feel guilt and depression, fear weight gain, and often complain about their body size and shape. Purging is often done secretly. Recurrent vomiting (as with anorexia) can cause dental caries, erosion of enamel from the front teeth, and throat irritation from stomach hydrochloric acid. Electrolyte imbalances and even death are possible.

Binge-Eating Disorder

Binge-eating disorder occurs when a client regularly eats too much food. A lack of control is the main concern. Unlike with anorexia or bulimia, the client does not follow eating with purging or exercise. The client may be of normal weight, overweight, or obese. Eating quickly or excessive amounts, even if the client is uncomfortably full, can lead to social embarrassment. Eventually, eating alone is preferred. Extreme obesity will occur if the condition is not controlled.

NUTRITIONAL CONSIDERATIONS

During the school-age period, children are spending more time away from home and assume more control over their daily intake of foods. School-age children need a nutritious breakfast to prevent hypoglycemia and discomfort due to hunger, which may cause poor concentration and a shorter attention span. The rapid growth of adolescents is accompanied by increased nutritional requirements and a ravenous appetite. There is an increased need for protein as body mass increases and a need for calcium to promote bone density and prevent future osteoporosis. Iron intake is important, especially for girls beginning menses, to prevent iron deficiency anemia. Middle childhood and adolescence provide parental opportunities to demonstrate food preparation and cooking methods. The use of nutritional guidelines should have beneficial preventative effects against diabetes, obesity, atherosclerosis, and osteoporosis (see Websites www.ChooseMyPlate.gov or https://health.gov/our-work/food-nutrition). Advise parents and guardians to teach children how to make good food choices and to avoid nonnutritive, high-calorie snacks. Encourage parents to provide a calm, relaxed atmosphere free of conflict at mealtime.

Obesity

Obesity is the condition of having too much body fat. The terms obesity and overweight are often used interchangeably, but technically, they are not the same. Being *overweight* means weighing too much, but the excess weight might be due to body water, muscle, bone, or fat. However, both terms imply that an individual's weight is greater than what is considered to be healthy for that person's age, height, and gender.

Childhood obesity occurs when the child's weight greatly exceeds the normal or healthy weight for age and height. As with obesity in adults, obesity in children is a complex issue involving a combination of factors. Genetics is one factor, which can involve many inherited disorders, some of which affect body weight (e.g., Cushing syndrome). Environment and family lifestyle issues are another factor, influencing eating habits, amount of physical exercise, food preparation, and the ability to make informed judgments about food. Family rituals can promote a lifetime of good eating habits or can be the basis for multiple food-related disorders in adults, such as atherosclerosis, hypertension, and obesity.

Diagnosis of a child with obesity is based on body mass index (**BMI**). The internet has BMI calculators that can be helpful. In children and adolescents, BMI is then charted on the CDC's BMI percentile chart based on height, weight, and gender which then gives a category of healthy weight, overweight, or obese. The number of children with obesity and the number of children with diabetes, both type 1 and type 2, have increased significantly in this century. The effects of the pattern of *obesity → diabetes → health problems* have extremely significant overall public health consequences on current and future costs for unhealthy children who become unhealthy adults.

Treatment of obesity is achieved through reduction of body fat by gradual but persistent weight loss in adults. Weight loss in children and adolescents should be discussed and under the care of a healthcare provider as children are still growing. Fad diets typically deprive individuals of essential nutrients while creating cravings for foods, creating a yo-yo effect, that is, weight loss followed by weight gain, which usually results in an overall weight gain. Weight loss can be accomplished by control of nutritional intake, exercise to increase caloric consumption, and education about nutritional concepts. Education should focus on ways good nutrition can promote improved health.

STUDENT SYNTHESIS

KEY POINTS

- The common cold, sore throat, conjunctivitis, and mononucleosis are common in young adults; typically, they are treated with fluids, rest, and analgesics.
- Lyme disease can be misdiagnosed because it imitates other disorders. Unless treated, it can cause serious health problems.
- Acne vulgaris is treatable with topical and systemic medications.
- Impetigo is highly contagious.
- The most important aspect of treatment of Legg–Calvé–Perthes disease is maintaining the affected extremity as non–weight-bearing.
- Scoliosis is more common in girls and must be treated to prevent serious defects related to curvature of the spine.

- Anorexia nervosa and bulimia, although related to nutrition, are psychological disorders requiring long-term treatment.
- Juvenile rheumatoid arthritis can lead to deformities, contractures, and impaired movement.
- Children with IDDM and NIDDM need to monitor medications, diet, and exercise closely.
- Retinitis pigmentosa is characterized by progressive, bilateral retinal degeneration that causes blindness.
- Irritable bowel disease in adolescents is seen as Crohn disease and CUC.
- Dysmenorrhea is the most common menstrual complaint of adolescents who menstruate.

CRITICAL THINKING EXERCISES

1. Explain the developmental characteristics of a 15-year-old male adolescent that may create adjustment problems for him as a client with diabetes. Compare and contrast the male adolescent issues with the concerns of a 15-year-old female adolescent who has recently been diagnosed with diabetes.

2. While you are providing care for 13-year-old A.Y., she confides in you that she is worried about her sexual development. What help and guidance will you give her?

3. D.E., age 13 years, has recently begun wearing a Milwaukee brace for scoliosis. Previously, she was active in softball, cheerleading, band, and other school activities. Now you find that she has abandoned most of those activities. She claims that she needs more time to study now that she is in the eighth grade. What is your response to her?

NCLEX-STYLE REVIEW QUESTIONS

1. An adolescent arrives in the clinic reporting a rash and feeling "flu-like" after finding a tick embedded in the leg 2 weeks ago on a camping trip. What does the nurse anticipate discussing with the teen?
   a. The laboratory results that will give a definitive diagnosis
   b. The use of physical therapy to prevent contractures from arthritis
   c. The use of an antibiotic for 2–4 weeks
   d. Handwashing to prevent disease transmission

2. An adolescent client is diagnosed with irritable bowel syndrome, and the nurse is providing nutritional information to assist with control of symptoms. Which of the following substances is most likely to act as an irritant food trigger and should be avoided by the adolescent? Select all that apply.
   a. Fatty foods
   b. Dairy products
   c. Chicken and fish
   d. Caffeine
   e. Bread and pasta

3. A school-age child is diagnosed with the common cold. The child's guardian is concerned that the child did not receive an antibiotic and wants to know how the child can get rid of the cold without it. What is the best response by the nurse?
   a. A virus causes a cold, and antibiotics are used for bacterial infections.
   b. The primary care provider must have forgotten to write the prescription.
   c. An antibiotic will worsen the cold symptoms.
   d. If the cold is not better in 3 days, an antibiotic will be prescribed.

4. A parent brings a school-age child to the clinic with a sore throat due to a *Streptococcus* infection. Which of the following actions is a priority concern for the parents?
   a. Seek immediate medical attention.
   b. Gargle with warm saline solution.
   c. Use ibuprofen to decrease the swelling.
   d. Increase the dose of the antibiotic.

5. An adolescent is treated for bacterial conjunctivitis. Which of the following actions would be the most appropriate subject for a discharge teaching session?
   a. Save the eye drops not used in case the infection comes back.
   b. Avoid touching or rubbing the area around the affected eye.
   c. Contact lenses may continue to be worn during treatment.
   d. Use a little bit of saliva on the contact lenses to clean them.

CHAPTER RESOURCES

Enhance your learning with additional resources on **thePoint**!

Student Resources related to this chapter can be found at **thePoint.lww.com/Rosdahl12e**.

74 The Child or Adolescent With Special Needs

Learning Objectives

1. Define and differentiate between the following terms: special needs, intellectual disability, developmental disability, and special learning disabilities.
2. Discuss the alterations in lifestyle, ADLs, and behaviors if an individual has special learning disabilities such as impairments in vision, hearing, and speech.
3. Compare the needs of a 5-year-old, 10-year-old, or 15-year-old when preparing a teaching plan for the individual with disabilities.
4. Define and differentiate between a genetic disorder, a congenital disorder, and an acquired disorder.
5. Discuss the circumstances that occur if a genetic disorder is also a congenital disorder.
6. Under what circumstances would the nurse suggest genetic counseling to a family, a parent, or an individual?
7. Discuss the signs and symptoms, types of treatments, and the nursing interventions for the following disorders: color blindness, hemochromatosis, neurofibromatosis, polycystic kidney disease, Tay–Sachs disease, and Prader–Willi syndrome.
8. Discuss the signs and symptoms, types of treatments, and the nursing interventions for the following disorders: fetal alcohol spectrum disorder, neonatal abstinence syndrome, Down syndrome, Fragile X syndrome, attention deficit hyperactivity disorder, plumbism, cerebral palsy, and muscular dystrophy.
9. State and discuss the lifelong challenges for an individual with intellectual and developmental disorders.
10. Identify any preventable intellectual and developmental disorders listed in this chapter.
11. Differentiate between mental health and mental illness.
12. Discuss the etiology, types of treatments, and the nursing interventions for the following disorders: depression, suicide, and schizophrenia.

Important Terminology

ataxia
athetosis
autism spectrum disorder
cerebral palsy
chelation
chorionic villus sampling
color blindness
contracture
coprolalia
developmental disability
diparesis
diplegia
Down syndrome
Duchenne muscular dystrophy
dysarthria
dysfluency
dyskinesia
dyslexia
dysphagia
echolalia
fragile X syndrome
genetic
Gowers sign
hemiparesis
hemiplegia
hemochromatosis
neurofibromatosis
nystagmus
plumbism
Prader–Willi syndrome
quadriparesis
quadriplegia
rigidity
shaken baby syndrome
simian line
spasticity
special learning disabilities
special needs
suicidal ideation
Tay–Sachs disease
tic
tremors
trisomy 21

Acronyms

ADD
ADHD
ALT
ARBD
ARND
ASD
BAL in Oil
BLL
BMD
CK
CP
CVS
DABS
DD
DMD
DSM-5
FAS
FASD
IADL
IQ
MD
MMD
NAS
OCD
PKD
SLD
TS

Special needs is an expression or global term used to describe the circumstances of some individuals who may need assistance due to intellectual, medical, and psychological disorders. Most persons with special needs have a combination of disorders that involve disabilities that range in severity from mild to severe and, occasionally, fatal. In healthcare, nurses are often asked to explain the problems, to discuss treatments, and to provide care for individuals with special needs. (See In Practice: Nursing Care Guidelines 74-1: Working with an Individual with Special Needs.)

To diagnose disabilities, healthcare professionals depend upon specific terminology and descriptions of signs and symptoms found in the most current edition of the standard diagnostic reference book, the *Diagnostic and Statistical Manual of Mental Disorders*, 5th Edition, or **DSM-5**. The DSM-5 is able to delineate specific disorders but is not able to differentiate the special needs associated with each of these disorders. Each individual and disorder will have unique properties and manifestations that differ according to age, gender, current level of disability, and environmental support systems. An individual, especially a young person, will need clinical and functional diagnosis of any disorders in order to obtain the most appropriate medical treatments, financial resources, and community support.

> **Key Concept**
>
> Family caregivers of a physically or mentally challenged child may go through a grieving process. Grieving may occur intermittently, as the child reaches or fails to reach major developmental milestones. Such grieving does not mean that caregivers do not love the child. Your support and understanding can help caregivers cope.

IN PRACTICE

NURSING CARE GUIDELINES 74-1: Working With an Individual With Special Needs

- Use behavioral modification techniques
  - Focus on actions that the individual can do successfully.
  - Break down each desired behavior into small steps.
    Example: The steps for brushing teeth would be as follows: holding the toothbrush; putting toothpaste on the brush; holding toothbrush against teeth; moving toothbrush up and down; spitting out excess toothpaste; rinsing the mouth; rinsing toothbrush; storing toothbrush
  - Make instructions simple and specific for each step.
  - Use positive words and emotions after each step.
  - After each instruction, allow the person to attempt the action.
  - Acknowledge the individual's attempts—even if an attempt failed.
  - Praise and reward successful accomplishments as soon as possible after completion.
- **Increase complexity of behavior**
  - Do not act impatient or in a hurried manner.
  - Realize that individuals with learning disabilities have difficulty processing directions.
  - Provide one level of direction at a time.
    Example: Avoid generalizations such as "get ready for bed." Start with a learned behavior (e.g., brush your teeth) and then proceed to the next level (e.g., wash face and hands, put on night clothes, get into bed).
- **Build self-esteem**
  - Encourage self-care.
  - Help with activities but do not take over control of individual's attempts.
  - Reinforce self-esteem and the ability to do ADLs by repeating instructions and watching (not doing) the behavior.
- **Act as a role model**
  - Let the individual watch the mentor (parent, teacher, or peer).
  - Encourage the individual to attempt similar actions (e.g., playing ball, picking up the bedroom).
  - Encourage participation in support groups where the person is among others with similar problems.
- **Be consistent with discipline**
  - Ensure that others interacting with the person will follow the same or similar discipline methods.
- **Establish and follow routines**
  - Have consistency in activities such as getting up in the morning, getting ready for school, completing homework, or playing after school.
- **Establish normalcy**
  - Have standards of acceptable behaviors for each member of the family that will be considered "normal" for this family or situation.
  - Provide equality of discipline for individuals at home or at school.
  - Involve all family members—other siblings may feel neglected and resentful that one individual gets most of the attention.
  - Support social interaction, such as sports, support groups, or school activities.
- **Watch and listen**
  - Family members might see changes in behavior instead of verbalized emotions or concerns.
  - Allow for self-expression, behavioral changes (acting out, withdrawal, or aggressive statements).
  - Offer and accept emotional support from others.
  - Expect failures as a normal part of the growth process.
  - Anticipate successes but expect success to be less common than hoped for.
- **Be observant for signs of depression**

Adapted from www.cdc.gov/mentalhealth, https://www.mayoclinic.org/healthy-lifestyle/childrens-health/in-depth/mental-illness-in-children/art-20046577, and http://www.webmd.com/anxiety-panic/mental-health-illness-in-children

DISABILITIES AND DISORDERS

In this chapter, we will look at a variety of *disabilities*, many of which involve complex *disorders*. Some of these conditions have genetic origins, and others are acquired. Several disorders have both genetic and acquired etiologies (see later discussion). Disorders can be noticeable at birth or during early infancy. Some disorders do not appear until adolescence or adulthood. The underlying causes and risk factors of a disorder, as well as its symptoms, produce effects that will determine the definition of each individual's special needs. Special needs and disabilities are usually interrelated and include the ability to succeed in the following areas:

- To learn new things (i.e., intellectual capability or lack of ability)
- To succeed at a specific pace (i.e., developmental milestones)
- To communicate with others and socialize in a group (i.e., behavior and mental health capabilities)
- To have a continuum of health (i.e., medical issues)

Intellectual Disability

Intellectual disability refers to a problem for an individual who has cognitive impairment, demonstrated by below-average ability to learn and to use knowledge. Intellectual abilities are given numerical designations based on a standardized test. The overall designation of intellectual capability is known as an intelligence quotient (**IQ**). A numerical IQ score is derived from the test results. Average baseline normal score is about 100. An individual with an

IQ between 70 and 85 has limited intellectual functioning and may require assistance performing activities of daily living (ADLs) or other areas identified as special needs.

IQ tests are widely used but are known to have limitations. IQ tests are good predictors of academic achievement but are highly criticized for not being able to indicate other types of intelligence. Many indicators of success in life and the working world include factors such as persistence, self-confidence, motivation, interpersonal skills, creativity, intuition, and verbal and nonverbal skills. Intellectual functioning, or intelligence, refers to a general mental capacity such as learning, reasoning, or problem-solving.

Adaptive behaviors are responses to everyday needs, which include social needs, such as making friends and keeping a job; practical day-to-day activities, such as self-care, hygiene, and dressing; and personal responsibility, such as safety and the ability to use money. The Diagnostic Adaptive Behavior Scale (**DABS**) provides comprehensive, standardized observations of adaptive behaviors for individuals from 4 to 21 years old. The identification of significant limitations in adaptive behaviors can be used to determine an individual's potential to function in a community. Intellectual disability encompasses a combination of intellectual functioning and adaptive behaviors.

Intellectual impairment reflects deficits in cognitive (learning) capacity. Impairment can be related to genetic inheritance. Sometimes genes mutate after conception and the child is born with a deficit. Many times impairment is related to maternal complications during pregnancy, such as infections, for example, rubella (German measles), varicella, syphilis, or toxoplasmosis. Impairment can occur because of brain injury during fetal development, such as exposure to lead or radiation. Impairment perinatally can be due to birth trauma related to hypoxia or anoxia, multiple fetuses, low birth weight, and breech birth. After birth, intelligence can be impaired by kernicterus and jaundice of hyperbilirubinemia. Infants are more susceptible to brain damage if they develop bacterial meningitis or viral encephalitis, or have a head injury due to a fall or child abuse. Many substances that may be safe for the mother are unsafe to the unborn child. *Teratogens* are substances that cause congenital malformations during pregnancy. A fetus exposed to a teratogen will be born with some type of disorder. For example, rubella (German measles) is a teratogenic virus that will cause congenital problems in the newborn if the mother was exposed to the virus during the first trimester of pregnancy. Other teratogens include alcohol, drugs, or exposure to radiation. The U.S. Food and Drug Administration (FDA) has designated pregnancy categories for drugs, an important reference for the nurse (see Box 62-1).

> *Nursing Alert* Abusive head trauma (**shaken baby syndrome**) is a type of physical abuse. It is a leading cause of intellectual, speech, and learning disabilities, other permanent disorders such as blindness, paralysis, seizures, and hearing loss, or even death in children younger than 5 years (CDC, n.d.). Whiplash motions occur if the child is held by the arms, legs, chest, or shoulders, and vigorously shaken. Damage will occur to an infant's fragile blood vessels and delicate brain.

Developmental Disability

Developmental disability (**DD**) is a term that not only includes intellectual disability but also involves physical disabilities. In general, the term is associated with an individual's failure to meet developmental milestones, often related to damage to the brain that resulted in chronic physical problems (e.g., deformed extremities, poor muscle control, or muscle spasms). The terms related to disabilities, including developmental, intellectual, language, and movement, often coexist and are interrelated.

SPECIAL LEARNING DISABILITIES

Special learning disabilities (**SLDs**) are disorders in which one or more parts of the central nervous system do not function normally. Abnormalities of the brain result in difficulty perceiving, understanding, remembering, reasoning, and communicating. The individual has difficulty reading, writing, developing or using social skills, and maintaining an emotional balance. The child or adult with SLDs typically (but not always) has a lower than average IQ, has visual or hearing impairment, and processes thoughts and ideas differently than do others without SLDs. Communication is difficult, whether through vocal or nonvocal behaviors (body language) or language (written speech). Individuals with SLDs may have a different learning style and require education tailored to their unique needs. When caring for a child with an SLD, learn about the specific disabilities from parental caregivers and set achievable goals. Consider individual needs and limitations, and set goals. Plan ADLs carefully according to the individual's physical and emotional needs as well as the requirements of any medical treatment plan. Consider age, sex, developmental level, family environment, medical problems, and prognosis. Individuals must have a sense of security; therefore, meeting basic needs is a priority. Some disorders may require special feeding techniques or other assistance in meeting the basic survival needs of the child. (See In Practice: Nursing Care Guidelines 74-2: Feeding the Intellectually Impaired Child.)

Visual Impairment

The most frequent causes of *visual impairment* include genetic or congenitally acquired cataracts (often caused by exposure to rubella during fetal development), optic nerve atrophy, and retrolental fibroplasia resulting from oxygen toxicity. Other causes are amblyopia, retinitis pigmentosa, refractory errors, strabismus, and trauma (see Chapters 72 and 80). **Dyslexia** is one of the most common disorders in which the person has difficulty with reading, spelling, or writing words. Often the dyslexic child reverses letters or numbers.

Nursing Considerations

Clocks with large numbers, calendars with large letters, and books with large print may decrease frustration for children who have partial sight. Encourage nonsighted children to participate in activities with their peers, such as music, guided skiing, swimming, and so forth. Family caregivers should encourage nonsighted infants and toddlers to explore

NURSING CARE GUIDELINES 74-2: Feeding the Intellectually Impaired Child

- Ensure correct positioning, preferably in a sitting position. For the infant or child, flex the head slightly. **Rationale:** This position helps to close the larynx against the epiglottis.
- Teach the individual to suck by massaging the cheeks or by using a special nipple. A nipple or bottle is appropriate for the infant and young toddler; as the individual becomes older, use a cup or glass. A straw may be helpful. Encourage blowing, too. **Rationale:** These actions build up muscles used in speech.
- Assist the person to learn to drink from a cup by using sucking movements. **Rationale:** Drinking from a cup uses different muscles than sucking liquid from a bottle. Teaching sucking movements will help the individual to transition from a bottle to a cup.
- Teach or remind the individual to chew. If necessary, manipulate the jaw up and down; demonstrate using a mirror. **Rationale:** The impaired individual may not be able to coordinate muscle movements or may lose the ability over a period of time (e.g., muscular dystrophy), needing tactile sensations and visual clues.
- Remind the individual to swallow. **Rationale:** The person may have difficulty following many directions and loses focus easily. Prevents aspiration.
- Place food on the side of the mouth, not in the center. Do not rush. **Rationale:** Prevent choking.
- Encourage the individual to use the lips to remove the food from the spoon, to bite off pieces of food, and to move food around in the mouth with the tongue. **Rationale:** These exercises also prepare the muscles for speech. Occupational and speech therapy are helpful.
- Allow the person to do as much self-feeding as possible. Keep the table neat and clean. **Rationale:** The impaired individual needs to succeed to support personal self-esteem and independence. A tidy area has fewer distractions which is helpful to the person who has difficulty focusing.

their environment, while at the same time ensuring their safety. Community resources and support groups are beneficial to the family unit as well as to the individual with the disability.

Hearing Impairment

Hearing impairment can result from fetal exposure to cytomegalovirus, herpes, rubella, or syphilis. Meningitis, chronic ear infections, Down syndrome (DS), exposure to loud noises, and certain medications also can cause hearing damage. Manifestations of hearing impairment in a child include avoiding social interaction, playing alone, acting timid, not learning to talk, and displaying poor socialization skills. Children with impaired hearing face the coexisting problem of poor speech development. Communication and safety are major issues for families with hearing-impaired children.

Nursing Considerations

Speech therapy and sign language are important tools for learning and communication. School environments can be challenging. Classmates need to understand that a child with special needs is not always intellectually impaired.

Speech Development

Be patient and encourage children with speech difficulties to say each word slowly and clearly. Do not use baby talk. Encourage children to listen. Even if they cannot answer, be sure to talk to them. Explain to children what you are doing, and try to anticipate their questions. Read to children, and encourage them to look at pictures. Children with speech difficulties may be able to communicate by using specially designed computers.

Speech Impairment

Impairment of speech can result from a hearing deficit, muscular disorders, or cleft lip or palate. Environmental and emotional factors can also influence speech. Disorders in articulation are related to the ability to produce the correct sound. An example of speech impairment is the child who speaks with a lisp (pronounces "th" instead of "s"). A **dysfluency** is an interruption in the natural flow of speaking. An example is the child who stutters. Stuttering is normal for preschool children because, at this age, the ability to understand is more developed than vocabulary and command of the language. Stuttering in school-age children requires evaluation.

Nursing Considerations

Most children benefit from speech therapy. Some require surgical intervention or orthodontics. Evaluation by an otolaryngologist or neurologist also may be appropriate, depending on the specific circumstances. Specialists will test hearing. They will also make necessary referrals to psychologists or counselors for children with emotionally related speech disorders. Computers and tablets are especially valuable for these children to aid in the ability communicate.

> **Key Concept**
>
> Hearing disorders are common causes of speech disorders in children. A professional audiologist should test the hearing of a child who is having speech problems. Learning to talk is difficult for one who has never heard anyone speak. If a person loses their hearing later, they can often maintain speech.

Activities of Daily Living

Some children with physical, learning, or intellectual impairments have great difficulty achieving success in performing basic ADLs. There are specific techniques for teaching dressing skills, feeding skills, toilet training, and other ADLs. Patience is the most important factor in training the intellectually impaired child. Teaching should occur in a quiet place with few distractions. The site for learning should be neat and kept in the same order at all times. If an individual progresses with ADLs, additional levels of functioning may be considered, including *instrumental activities of daily living* (IADLs), such as cleaning, purchasing food or clothes, or preparing meals. In Practice: Nursing Care Guidelines 74-1 reviews working with an individual with special needs. In Practice: Nursing Care Guidelines 74-2 outlines teaching techniques for feeding the intellectually impaired child.

Behavior Modification

Behavior modification is a technique that uses positive reinforcement to encourage an individual to repeat desired behaviors, rather than relying on verbal criticism or punishment of undesired behavior. Behavior modification is commonly used to develop skills related to ADLs and speech development. The desired behavior may need to be repeated many times before it becomes habitual.

Nursing Considerations

A child with intellectual and developmental deficits will commonly have special learning disabilities. Having a child with these needs will require the cooperation of the total family unit plus a variety of community services. Use a team approach for medical and social needs. Most intellectual and developmental disorders will require more than one specialized type of medical care, physical rehabilitation, and occupational care. A team will include many of the following:

- Parents, siblings, and relatives who provide support and understanding
- Primary healthcare pediatrician
- Healthcare providers who specialize in pediatric or developmental disabilities in the areas of cardiology, endocrinology, gastroenterology, neurology, ophthalmology, audiology, and otorhinolaryngology (ear, nose, and throat)
- Therapy providers who specialize in pediatric or developmental disabilities, to provide physical rehabilitation, speech and language therapy, and occupational therapy for activities of daily living
- Community support system, including social workers who can help locate financial support and community resources such as public health and immunizations, in-home nursing services, hospice care, and respite care. In addition, other sources of support may be found in spiritual or individualized support groups (e.g., a cerebral palsy support group)
- Educational services for the disabled individual, home-schooling, or specialized classrooms

> **Key Concept**
>
> Encourage the young person with a disability to participate in educational, social, and recreational activities.
>
> Keep the lines of communication open by developing active listening skills. Observe verbal and nonverbal cues for potential problems.
>
> Working with people with long-term disorders and their families offers you the opportunity to use all your technical skills and interpersonal nursing skills.

ETIOLOGY OF DISABILITIES AND DISORDERS

Genetic Disorders

Genetic disorders are those conditions that are passed from one generation to the next, that is, they are hereditary, resulting from defective chromosomes or genes (e.g., DS). The defective gene can be *familial,* which means that one or both of the biologic parents has the defective gene and passes it on to the offspring. In contrast, a defective gene can occur for no apparent reason. A genetic disorder is inborn and present at birth, but it may not be immediately apparent. Some conditions can be either genetic or acquired, for example, color blindness and hemochromatosis, which are discussed later in this chapter.

Genetic Counseling

Genetic counseling is the process of helping people understand and adapt to the medical, psychological, and familial implications of genetic contributions to disease. This process integrates family and medical histories, education about genetic inheritance, testing, management, prevention, resources, and research, and counseling to promote informed choices about risks and adaptation to the condition.

Counseling is available for people who are seeking information about the possibility of genetic disorders in their families. Based on this information, the counselor designs a family tree or genetic profile. Counseling includes education regarding genetics, how disorders are inherited, and individual risks of genetic disorders. The role of the genetic counselor is one of providing information, support, and options, from which the individual or couple can make decisions about family planning.

Congenital and Acquired Disorders

Congenital means "present at birth"; therefore, a congenital disorder is one that exists at birth. A congenital condition can be caused by a defective gene. The defective gene, in some cases, can be hereditary, that is passed on from its parents from either the sperm or ova. If the congenital condition results from a mutation of the fertilized or embryonic cells (not the sperm or ova cells), the condition is a genetic congenital disorder but not an inherited genetic disorder. If that child passes on the defective gene, the next generation will have a congenital, genetic, and hereditary disorder. Some disorders that had previously been thought to begin in childhood may develop later in life, that is to say, have a late onset (e.g., some types of muscular dystrophy).

Other disorders commonly seen in adults can be identified in children, in which case they are said to have an early onset (e.g., schizophrenia). These changes in diagnosis may be due to better understanding of complete or partial changes in genetic inheritance, such as a total or partial lack of fundamental chromosomal proteins, and a better ability to identify acquired pathologies such as exposure to radiation or environmental hazards (e.g., lead poisoning).

Acquired disorders occur throughout a person's lifetime, including the months in utero. Acquired disorders, before birth, occur as a result of maternal factors or conditions that happened during pregnancy. A condition can be acquired during the trauma of birth, shortly after birth, or later in life. Due to various and specific circumstances, some genetic disorders can have acquired equivalents. It is possible that pathologic anatomic changes can occur during an individual's lifetime from injury, medications, or environmental conditions combined with the effects of age, which cause acquired, not inherited, conditions. For example, there is a common, genetic form of color blindness, but over time and under certain conditions, the cones in the retina can become damaged, resulting in an acquired disorder of poor color vision.

COMMON DISORDERS

Color Blindness

Color blindness, also known as color vision deficiency, is a decreased or lack of ability to see certain colors. Typically, it is an inherited problem, but it can become an acquired color vision problem due to aging, side effects of some medications, injury to the eye, and visual disorders such as glaucoma, cataracts, macular degeneration, or diabetic retinopathy. The cells that see color are the cone cells in the macula, the portion of the retina with the highest concentration of cone cells. Normally, the individual can differentiate between the colors red, green, or blue. With color blindness, the cone cells are either damaged or absent, meaning that the individual perceives colors differently, that is, sees a different shade, or does not see the color at all. Color blindness does not imply a vision loss or total blindness.

Symptoms of color vision deficiency will vary, and some individuals may not be aware of any color vision problems. Typically, an individual will be able to see some colors but not others. The most common example is the inability to see reds and greens. Blue-yellow color blindness is less common. Some individuals may be able to see a few shades of color but not the hundreds of different hues available for each color. A few individuals see only black, white, and gray, a condition known as monochromacy. Reduced visual acuity, myopic vision, and **nystagmus** (uncontrollable eye movements) are noted with some forms of color blindness.

Diagnosis is made during eye examinations, often using Ishihara color blind test charts or the Cambridge color test. These tests are visual evaluations of specialized charts designed to differentiate and diagnose color blindness.

There is no treatment for this disorder. The individual with red-green color blindness may have success seeing colors if special lenses are worn. If the color blindness is acquired, locating and eliminating the causative factor (e.g., a medication) may restore color vision.

Nursing Considerations

Color blindness may be undetected unless eye examinations are done. For children, especially boys, a physical should include an eye examination. Difficulties may be miscategorized as learning disabilities; for example, a green chalkboard may disguise writing if yellow chalk is used. Many educational materials are color-coded. The child may be labeled as having a reading disorder. If examined by the eye care providers, a diagnosis can specify the problem and treat the issue appropriately. The child with color vision deficiencies should be encouraged to ask for assistance if a task requires color recognition. Daily activities may be disrupted if an individual cannot distinguish colors. For example, the red-orange-green stop signal may be difficult to differentiate. Parental caregivers need to learn the importance of color differentiation, for example, picking out a ripe fruit or knowing when food is cooked. Color blindness is not a typical learning disability and adapting to this disorder generally occurs with time.

Hemochromatosis

Hemochromatosis is either a hereditary or an acquired condition in which the body absorbs iron from foods and stores excess iron in body tissues and organs. Common locations for excess stored iron include the liver, heart, pancreas, reproductive organs, and skin. There are several types of hemochromatosis: *juvenile, neonatal,* and *secondary*. Hemochromatosis typically develops in men aged 50–60 years but can also develop in women after menopause. Juvenile hemochromatosis is similar but becomes symptomatic during the teenage years up to the age of about 30 years. Neonatal hemochromatosis occurs when iron accumulates rapidly in the developing fetus and may be an autoimmune disease. Secondary hemochromatosis is an acquired form of the disease due to iron deposit accumulation secondary to anemia, chronic liver disease, or an infection. Uncontrolled iron deposits can cause side effects such as cirrhosis, liver cancer, diabetes, heart failure, erectile dysfunction, joint pain, and skin color changes. Early signs and symptoms are nonspecific and can mimic other disorders, which can make diagnosis difficult. Later, organ damage may be the first indicator of excess iron overload and be the etiology of diabetes, loss of libido, cardiac dysrhythmias, or heart failure. Lifespan for individuals with hemochromatosis is similar to other individuals of the same age except when complications of cirrhosis or diabetes have developed. Diagnosis is based on symptoms, specific blood tests, and a review of family genetics.

Treatment

Treatment is to reduce the amount of iron in the body. The most common method of iron reduction is removal of blood from the body at regularly scheduled phlebotomy sessions. About 1 unit of blood (about 1 pint or 470 mL) is removed during each session depending upon overall health, age, and severity of iron overload. The maintenance schedule depends on how rapidly iron accumulates in the body as determined by testing iron levels. Phlebotomy can slow the progression of the disease but will not reverse cirrhosis or improve joint pain. Periodic screening for cirrhosis and liver cancer involves laboratory studies and an abdominal ultrasound. Some individuals cannot tolerate scheduled phlebotomy due to medical history of anemia or cardiac complications, and chelation may be advised. **Chelation** is a process in which a chemical is injected into the bloodstream to remove heavy metals or minerals from the body. Heavy metals include iron, lead, mercury, copper, arsenic, and aluminum. The mineral calcium may be chelated. A chemical called EDTA (ethylenediaminetetraacetic acid) is injected and binds to the metal. The EDTA causes the body to expel the substance through stool or urine. The process is controversial in some instances.

Nursing Considerations

Nursing implications for the treatment of hemochromatosis include teaching the client methods that will help prevent complications. Avoid iron supplements, multivitamins containing iron, and vitamin C. Vitamin C, especially if taken with food such as orange juice, will increase the absorption of iron. Avoid eating raw shellfish because individuals with hereditary hemochromatosis are more susceptible to infections caused by bacteria in raw shellfish. Avoid alcohol, which has the risk of increasing liver damage. Drink tannin-rich teas that may slow the storage of iron.

Neurofibromatosis

Neurofibromatosis refers to genetically inherited conditions in which benign painful tumors develop as growths on nerve tissue (neurofibromas). In some cases, a benign tumor will become malignant. There are three types of neurofibroma, type 1 (NF1) and type 2 (NF2), and schwannomas. Neurofibromas from NF2 grow on the eighth cranial nerve (vestibulocochlear nerve). Schwannomas grow on cranial, spinal, and peripheral nerves. Men and women are affected equally, but each individual will have a different severity of the disorder. Symptoms are typically related to the type of neurofibromatosis and the growth and pressure of these tumors upon nerves. The individual may have extensive café au lait spots on the skin of the facial area and large neurofibromas on the legs. A café au lait spot is a harmless, light brown spot on the skin and can be a strong indicator of NF1 if there are more than six spots that are greater than 0.5 cm in children prior to puberty. They are present at birth or may appear during the first 5 years. Possible effects on the skeletal system include bones that form abnormally (e.g., scoliosis), bowing of the legs, osteoporosis, and fractures that do not heal. Commonly, an individual will have some degree of hearing deficit or loss, vision deficit or loss, learning and cognitive impairment, cardiovascular complications such as hypertension or blood vessel abnormalities, and severe pain. Severe, debilitating pain, associated with schwannomas, can require surgical intervention and pain management by a pain specialist. Meningiomas (multiple benign brain tumors) or spinal tumors may require surgeries to remove the growths.

Diagnosis is usually confirmed in childhood or early adulthood by a medical review of symptoms and a genetic family history. The healthcare provider will look for the café au lait spots and differentiate symptoms according to the known types. General and specialized eye and ear examinations help specify the diagnosis. Genetic counseling and testing can be done for the individual or prenatally.

Treatment is palliative. Pain relief, surgical removal of some problematic lesions, and physical therapy are the most common types of palliative treatments. Scoliosis may benefit from braces, which help to reconfigure the direction of growth of the bones.

Polycystic Kidney Disease

Polycystic kidney disease (**PKD**) is an inherited disorder in which clusters of cysts develop, primarily within the kidneys, but the liver and other areas can also be affected. Cysts are noncancerous, round sacs filled with fluid. The cysts can increase in size as they accumulate fluid. Complications develop as the cysts put pressure on the functional areas of the organs (parenchymal tissue). Hypertension and headaches are common with PKD and may be precursors to kidney failure. Other signs and symptoms include chronic back or side pain, abdominal distension, urinary frequency, hematuria, kidney stones, and urinary tract or kidney infections. Serious cardiovascular complications include the development of an aneurysm (balloon-like bulge in a blood vessel) in the brain and the development of mitral valve prolapse.

Diagnosis is made using the physical examination, family medical history including inherited disorders, blood testing, urinalysis, and blood chemistries. A CT scan, ultrasound, or MRI will assess kidney structure and look for cysts.

Treatment looks first at controlling hypertension, which is an essential method for protecting kidney function. Antihypertensive drugs, such as ACE inhibitors, are often used, but it may be necessary to take more than one type of antihypertensive to maintain control of blood pressure.

Nursing interventions will include discussion of a low-salt diet, fluid intake, and dietary intake of fruit, vegetables, and whole grains. It is important to maintain a healthy weight and to take any medications, especially antihypertensive medications, as ordered. Monitor BP at home. Avoid smoke and exercise about 30 min five to six times per week or as directed by a healthcare provider. Surgical intervention may involve removal of problematic cysts, that is, cysts that cause pressure or pain or interfere with parenchymal tissues.

Tay–Sachs Disease

Tay–Sachs disease (**TSD**) is a fatal inherited metabolic disorder. It occurs most commonly in young children, who have the most severe symptoms, but can become obvious at an older age. Certain lipids accumulate in the body due to the absence of a fundamental enzyme, resulting in progressive destruction of the neurons (nerve cells) within the nervous system. As the fatty lipid proteins accumulate, damage occurs to the neurons of the brain, in turn causing damage to the eyes, ears, movement, and mental development. Destruction of neurons can occur in the fetus during pregnancy, but signs and symptoms may not become obvious until 3–6 months of age, when development slows. By about 2 years of age, the child has had recurrent seizures and shows a diminished capacity to function mentally and physically. Motor abilities gradually regress until the child can no longer crawl, turn over, or sit.

Diagnosis is typically made after the family notices that the child is not progressing in growth and development. The healthcare provider will do a physical examination and test for milestones of growth and development. A characteristic of TSD is an eye abnormality called a cherry-red spot, which develops at the back of the child's eyes. Between the ages of 3 and 4 years, the child becomes severely cognitively disabled, blind, paralyzed, and unresponsive. By the age of 5 years, the child dies because the nervous system can no longer function. Rare forms of TSD with milder symptoms include juvenile TSD, where symptoms develop in early childhood and death occurs in the midteens. Late-onset TSD affects adults, causing neurologic and intellectual impairment. There is no cure for TSD.

Treatment involves support for the parents and palliative management of the child's symptoms. Genetic counseling is strongly suggested for individuals who may carry the TSD trait. Individuals with origins in eastern and central Europe, such as those of Ashkenazic Jewish heritage, are at risk for this genetic abnormality. TSD is also seen in populations living in certain French–Canadian communities of Quebec, the Old Order Amish community in Pennsylvania, and the Cajun population of Louisiana. Prenatal testing via **chorionic villus sampling** (**CVS**) between the 10th and 12th weeks of pregnancy is available to screen for condition. An amniocentesis can be done between the 15th and 18th weeks of pregnancy.

Prader–Willi Syndrome

Prader–Willi syndrome (**PWS**) is a complex genetic disorder that occurs equally among genders and all races. Most cases of PWS are not inherited but occur as random events during the formation of the eggs and sperm or in early embryonic development. There is no family history of this disorder. Considered a *multiphase syndrome,* signs and symptoms develop in stages. Initially noted are hypotonia (poor muscle tone) and feeding difficulties. Later, *hyperphagia* (chronic feelings of hunger), and weight gain are noted. The individual's metabolism is slow; calories are not used efficiently for energy. The combined effects of insatiable hunger and slow metabolism will lead to excessive eating, weight gain, life-threatening obesity, and diabetes type 2. Intellectual impairment, learning disabilities, and behavioral problems range from mild to moderate in severity. As the child ages, a short stature is noted and growth hormone may be prescribed; small hands and feet are common. Typically the individual has incomplete sexual development. A variety of unique and complex medical issues may be accompanied by social and behavioral problems in childhood. The child may have outbursts of temper, compulsiveness (e.g., picking at the skin) and stubbornness but may also be loving and friendly at times. Distinctive facial features are common, such as a narrow forehead, almond-shaped eyes, and triangular mouth. Unusually fair skin and light-colored hair are typical. Underdeveloped genitals and delayed or incomplete puberty may also occur. Most individuals are infertile (unable to conceive children).

> **NCLEX Alert**
>
> Clinical scenarios on an NCLEX examination may include nursing considerations related to disorders where education and counseling for caregivers are the primary nursing interventions. Genetic counseling is particularly indicated for adults who have known genetic disorders.

Fetal Alcohol Spectrum Disorders and Fetal Alcohol Syndrome

Fetal alcohol spectrum disorders (**FASDs**) is the general term that describes the wide range of physical, mental, behavioral, and learning disabilities known to be directly related to maternal alcohol consumption during pregnancy. *Fetal alcohol syndrome* (**FAS**) is the most severe form of the FASD categories. FAS may also be known as *fetal alcohol abuse syndrome.* As with other syndromes, FAS consists of a group of signs and symptoms that appear together and indicate a specific problem. Mental and physical birth defects are the most well-known problems related to a person's use of alcohol while pregnant. In addition to FAS or FASD, other conditions associated with alcohol consumption and pregnancy include *alcohol-related neurodevelopmental disorder* (**ARND**) and *alcohol-related birth defects* (**ARBDs**). Infants with ARND may not have all of the typical diagnostic features of FAS, but they do have some degree of functional or mental health problems referred to as *fetal alcohol effects* (*FASs*). Children with ARBD have birth defects that involve the heart, kidneys, bones, and/or hearing. The etiology of these problems is due to the fact that alcohol readily crosses the placenta.

> **Key Concept**
>
> Any drink containing alcohol can damage a fetus. The alcohol content is about the same in a 4-oz glass of wine, a standard 12-oz glass of beer, and a 1-oz shot of straight liquor. Wine coolers, malt beverages, and mixed drinks generally contain more alcohol.

Alcohol and the Fetus

The detrimental effects of alcohol (i.e., wine, beer, or liquor) on a fetus are permanent. All cases of FASDs are preventable if a pregnant client does not consume alcohol. FAS is the leading known preventable source of cognitive impairment and birth defects. Birth defects caused by alcohol consumption can occur at any time throughout pregnancy. People may not be aware that they are pregnant during the early weeks of pregnancy, so any person in their childbearing years needs to be concerned about alcohol consumption and the possibility of becoming pregnant. When a pregnant person stops drinking, the health of the fetus improves, but the fetus does not recover from the damage that has been done. It is not known why some people who drink heavily during pregnancy do not have children with FAS. Abstinence is the only known way to prevent FAS and other alcohol-related disorders.

> **Nursing Alert** The effects of alcohol on a fetus are permanent. The effects of alcohol are also 100% preventable when the fetus is not exposed to alcohol.

> **Key Concept**
>
> Special educational programs, rehabilitative mental and physical therapies, and an extensive use of social services may be needed by children with disabilities to achieve their maximal developmental and educational potentials.

Signs and Symptoms

Most infants with FAS experience facial abnormalities (Fig. 74-1), slowed growth, developmental delays, below-normal mental functioning, and dysfunctions of the central nervous system. The effects can be mild to severe. The diagnosis

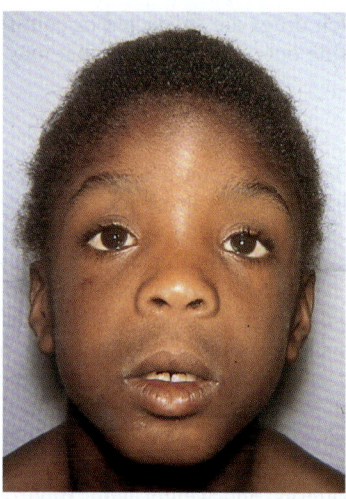

Figure 74-1 A child with fetal alcohol syndrome. Babies born to pregnant clients who chronically consume alcohol are at increased risk for growth deficiency, microcephaly, and mental impairment. Facial characteristics shown here include short palpebral fissures, a wide and flattened philtrum (the vertical groove in the midline of the upper lip), and thin lips.

of FASD or FAS occurs when a child has some of the following characteristics and/or exhibits some of the following behaviors.

Typical abnormal facial features (e.g., small, wide-set narrow eyes with drooping upper lids; short upturned nose; flattened cheeks; small jaw):

- Small for gestational age
- Failure to thrive
- Microcephaly
- Sleep and sucking abnormalities in infancy
- Extreme irritability
- Epilepsy, seizures
- Eye and ear defects
- Heart defects (e.g., septal defects, tetralogy of Fallot)
- Delayed gross motor skill development: difficulty rolling over, sitting, crawling
- Delayed fine motor skill development: cannot grasp using thumb and index finger
- Impaired language skills development; does not learn new words adequately
- Impairment of fine motor abilities and poor coordination
- Poor organ and bone development
- Learning disabilities; memory deficits, shortened attention span
- Hyperactive behavior, distractibility, impulsiveness
- Poor socialization skills
- Belligerence or stubbornness
- Problems adjusting to daily living
- Poor judgment and reasoning skills
- Inability to live independently
- Difficulty understanding or following rules, regulations, and laws
- Worsening social, behavioral, and comprehension difficulties when approaching adulthood

Diagnosis

Diagnosis is made by obtaining a thorough maternal history and observing characteristic signs and symptoms of the child. There is no single diagnostic test for alcohol-related disorders. Children with fetal alcohol effects, who typically have milder FAS symptoms, may not be diagnosed. Many conditions may coexist with alcohol-related disorders. For example, growth and developmental delays, hyperactivity, and specific learning disorders may also be diagnosed.

Treatment

Treatment consists of early recognition and referral to support services. Medical management of conditions, such as seizures, may be indicated, and counseling and emotional support should be offered to the individual and the family. Repair of physical defects may involve several surgeries.

Nursing Considerations

Every pregnant client should be encouraged to stop drinking any form of alcohol during the entire prenatal period, including the preconceptual period. Early identification and intervention are necessary to maximize the potential of the children with FASD or FAS. Support needs to be encouraged among peers, family or significant others. The key to prevention of alcohol-related disorders is public education regarding the dangers of consuming any alcohol during pregnancy. Client education should discuss the lifetime consequences of mental retardation, learning disabilities, and serious behavioral problems. Chronic lifelong health disorders are major concerns to the individual, the family, and society in general. Children with FASDs are at risk for psychiatric problems, abnormal social behaviors, unemployment, incomplete education, and dysfunctional familial lifestyles.

Neonatal Abstinence Syndrome

Neonatal abstinence syndrome (**NAS**) is a group of medical problems that occur in a newborn who was exposed to addictive opiate or narcotic drugs as a fetus (Box 74-1). These drugs include prescription or illegal narcotics such as heroin, codeine, oxycodone (Oxycontin), methadone (Methadose), or buprenorphine (BuTrans). The infant becomes addicted (i.e., physically dependent) to narcotics because the mother consumed the drug during pregnancy. After birth, the source of the drug is gone, and the abrupt discontinuation of the drug causes withdrawal in the newborn. Withdrawal symptoms include anxiety, insomnia, diaphoresis, vomiting, muscle pain, and goose bumps. Depending upon the severity of exposure during fetal development, the syndrome can last from a week to about 6 months. A second type of NAS can occur if opiates (e.g., fentanyl or morphine) are used as long-term analgesics for an infant in severe pain, for example, a victim of burns. Other drugs, either legal or illegal, may be addictive or problematic to the infant such as nicotine, amphetamines, barbiturates, cocaine, and marijuana. Alcohol abuse, STDs, and drug abuse often coexist in a pregnant woman.

Withdrawal symptoms in NAS may range from mild to severe depending on the type and quantity of the drug used by the mother, the length of time the drug was being used, and how long the drug takes to metabolize in the infant. Conditions change if the baby is premature or full-term. The premature infant going through withdrawal is at greater risk for infection, neonatal respiratory problems, and death.

Box 74-1 Neonatal Abstinence Syndrome: Opiates and Narcotics

An *opiate* is a synthetic drug, originally derived from the opium poppy, which mimics opium's effects as a sedative, hypnotic, or analgesic. Opiates include heroin or morphine. A *narcotic* is any one of a number of substances, including opiates plus other addictive substances such as alcohol and belladonna that are known to affect the senses and produce euphoria, stupor, or coma. Opiates and narcotics affect mood, behavior, and sensation to pain and can cause habituation and addiction. Legally, they are used as analgesics, sedatives, or hypnotics. The terms *opiate* and *narcotic* are often used interchangeably.

Drugs frequently associated with neonatal problems include the following:

Opiates and Narcotics
- Codeine
- Fentanyl
- Heroin
- Methadone
- Meperidine (Demerol)
- Oxycodone
- Morphine
- Hydromorphone (Dilaudid)
- Butorphanol (Stadol)
- Pentazocine
- Chlordiazepoxide
- Buprenorphine

Other Addictive-Type Drugs
- Barbiturates
- Caffeine
- Cocaine
- Selective serotonin reuptake inhibitors (SSRIs)
- Antihistamines (diphenhydramine, hydroxyzine)
- Ethanol
- Marijuana
- Nicotine
- Phencyclidine
- Meprobamate
- Glutethimide
- Ethchlorvynol
- Diazepam and lorazepam

Other complications may develop that are related to an unhealthy pregnancy, such as birth defects, failure to thrive, sudden infant death syndrome, and long-term developmental and behavioral problems.

Signs and Symptoms
Signs and symptoms include tremors, hyperactive reflexes, high-pitched crying, irritability, seizures, and excessive crying. The skin mottles (turns shades of reddish-blue). The infant may have diarrhea, vomiting, fever, and diaphoresis. Despite excessive sucking, the infant does not feed well, has tachypnea (rapid breathing), has difficulty sleeping, and shows a failure to thrive. Symptoms may start in the first 3 days or may take up to a week, depending upon when drugs were last ingested by the mother.

Diagnosis
Diagnosis is based on observation of the infant's behaviors and toxicology tests. A drug test may be done by urine. Meconium (the first bowel movement) may be tested for drugs. A maternal drug history may be helpful; however, the mother may deny use of any drugs for fear of legal repercussions. Facilities may require notification of child protective services if illicit drugs are suspected or confirmed. It is also important to rule out other disorders that may mimic symptoms of NAS.

Treatment
Treatment will depend upon the severity of the symptoms, the type of drug or drugs involved, and the overall health of the infant. Symptoms need to be prioritized according to which symptom is most life-threatening. In severe cases, the neonate may be hospitalized in an NICU and receive pharmacotherapy, that is, decreasing small doses of an opiate until symptoms abate. But in-hospital treatments may interfere with maternal–child bonding and increase time spent in the hospital. Phenobarbital may be useful if the child has opioid withdrawal seizures. Nonpharmacologic treatment is preferred. The nurse will monitor vital signs, sleeping habits, feeding patterns, and weight gain. Environmental stimuli such as lights, noise, and handling must be minimized to prevent neurologic stress. Nonnutritive sucking (e.g., a pacifier) and swaddling are generally comforting to the infant. If the child has difficulty feeding or does not gain weight, frequent high-calorie formula or nasogastric tube feedings are initiated.

Nursing Considerations
Nursing interventions will include postnatal checkups in the home. Nutritional support and education will promote growth and healthier lifestyles. Some of the difficulties of addicted newborns may also result from a dysfunctional home environment, in which the mother continues her drug use. Women who use drugs regularly are often malnourished and frequently exposed to infections during pregnancy.

> **Nursing Alert** Substance abuse is one of the most common causes of cognitive impairment and physical disabilities in children. Behavioral and psychosocial problems may result.

> **Key Concept** Some genetic and congenital disorders are not identified until the child fails to achieve certain developmental milestones. Typically, early treatment promotes maximal progress.

Down Syndrome

Down syndrome (DS) is a genetic disorder caused from abnormal cell division of chromosome 21, resulting in extra genetic material. A chromosome is a structure that contains small packages of genes. Normally, the mother and father each contribute 23 chromosomes to form a fertilized cell of 46 chromosomes (or 23 pairs). An infant with DS has extra amounts of chromosome 21. Although degrees of the disorder vary in severity, children with DS have lifelong intellectual disabilities and developmental delays, that is, decreased mental acuity and decreased physical development. Additionally, numerous and significant health disorders coexist, such as heart defects, leukemia, and early-onset dementia. There are three variations in cell division that cause the three types of this disorder: *trisomy 21, mosaic DS,* and *translocation DS.* **Trisomy 21** is the most common form, occurring when either the sperm cell or the egg cell has abnormal division before fertilization; generally, the egg cell is the problem. Mosaic DS is rare and caused by abnormal cell division after fertilization (i.e., in the embryo). In translocation DS, the only form of the disorder is considered to be inherited, the mother or father has genetic material that is different or rearranged. In this situation, the mother or father is said to be a *balanced carrier* of DS, that is, exhibiting no signs or symptoms of the disorder but able to pass on the translocation (rearranged chromosomes) to a child.

There are several risk factors accounting for appearance of DS, including the possibility of inheriting the translocation form. Advancing maternal age increases the chances of giving birth to a baby with DS because the mother's eggs are older and at a greater risk of improper chromosomal division. A woman aged 25 years has a 1 in 1,250 risk; by the age of 30 years the risk is 1 in 1,000. Increasing significantly at the age of 35 years, the risk is about 1 in 350, and by the age of 40 years, the risk is about 1 in 100. At the age of 45 years, the risk is about 1 in 30. If a mother has already given birth to a DS child, she has a 1 in 100 chance of having another impaired child (Mai et al., 2013). Both men and women can be carriers of the genetic translocation form of the syndrome; therefore, one or both parents may have a high risk of passing on the abnormal chromosome.

Signs and Symptoms

Typical physical characteristics of DS include multiple characteristic facial features listed below (Fig. 74-2). At birth or shortly thereafter, healthcare providers may notice that the hands of newborns with DS have an abnormal crease straight across the palms called a **simian line**. The presence of the simian line and other facial features is likely to lead to further examinations and diagnostic testing. Symptoms may be mild to severe:

- Small flattened nose
- Small head and neck
- Tongue that protrudes
- Eyes that slant upward (not typical of child's ethnic group)
- Brushfield spots (tiny white spots on the iris)
- Ears that are unusually shaped or small
- Short stature
- Slow growth; remains smaller than peers
- Delayed developmental milestones
- Tendency toward overweight and obesity
- Hypotonia (poor muscle tone, appears flabby)
- Extreme flexibility (joints can be hyperextended without causing pain)
- Broad, short hands with a single crease in the palm (called a simian line)
- Small hands and feet with fingers that are shorter than normal
- Wide space between the big toe and the rest of the toes
- Transverse crease across the soles of the feet

External signs and symptoms may be obvious, but a DS baby typically has additional health problems. Obesity is common. Heart defects may require surgery. Leukemia and a variety of blood disorders are common. Abnormalities in

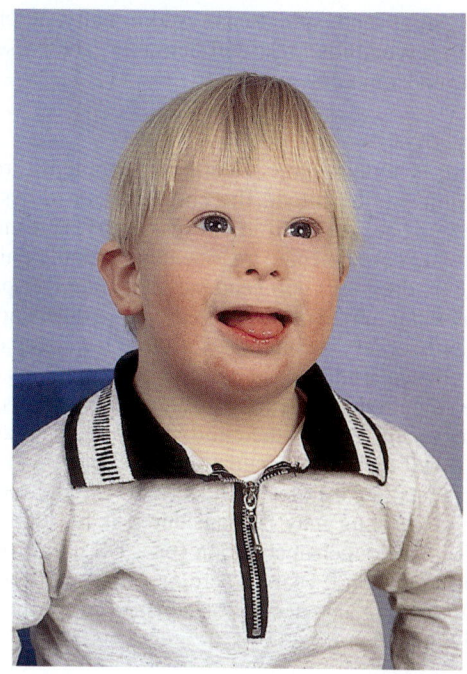

Figure 74-2 A child with Down syndrome. (Marks, 1998.)

their immune system increase risks of infectious diseases, such as pneumonia. Sleep apnea is due to the soft tissue and skeletal abnormalities causing an obstructed airway. Dementia, Alzheimer disease, and seizures may begin around the age of 50 years. Additional problems occur throughout life, such as poor vision, ear infections, hearing loss, gastrointestinal blockages, thyroid problems, psoriasis or other skin problems, skeletal deformities, and early-onset menopause.

Diagnosis

Diagnosis is based upon physical examination with follow-up genetic studies. If there are risk factors, testing may be done during pregnancy. Screening tests are initial tests used to help identify the chances of carrying a DS baby but are not sufficient for diagnostic confirmation. Genetic counseling is beneficial in these situations. Parents need to balance decisions (e.g., therapeutic abortion) and consider potential lifelong issues relating to the infant, as well as consequences to the family unit.

Screening tests during the first trimester would include pregnancy-associated plasma protein-A (PAPP-A) and the hormone human chorionic gonadotropin (HCG). An ultrasound may show abnormalities of increased fluid buildup (nuchal translucency). After 10 weeks of gestation, specific DNA tests of maternal blood may indicate high risk for the presence of DS. Second trimester testing measures four pregnancy-associated substances: alpha fetoprotein, estriol, HCG, and inhibin A. *CVS* is done in the first trimester after 10 weeks of gestation to analyze fetal cells from the placenta. An *amniocentesis* might be ordered in the second semester after week 15 to analyze fetal chromosomes. *Cordocentesis* or *percutaneous umbilical blood sampling (PUBS)* uses blood from a vein in the umbilical cord between 18 and 22 weeks to check for chromosomal defects. After birth, the initial diagnosis is based upon physical signs and symptoms. Additionally, a chromosomal karyotype blood test will determine the presence of extra chromosome 21.

Treatment

Treatment is symptomatic. Healthcare problems are acute and chronic. As an infant, the child may need assistance with feeding because of difficulty suckling. Gastrointestinal problems are common, and treatment is generally palliative. ADLs (e.g., dressing) will need parental caregiver patience and understanding. Surgical repair of cardiac anomalies and other disorders is common. Children may need chemotherapy for leukemia and antibiotics for infections. Vision may be impaired and require prescription glasses. Team members for the care of the child may include an audiologist, physical therapist, occupational therapist, and pediatric specialists in cardiology, endocrinology, and oncology. Genetic counseling may be considered if not done previously. It is no longer uncommon for a DS child to have a life expectancy of 60 years. Therefore, the conditions associated with aging also need to be considered for the care of the individual.

Nursing Considerations

After birth of the affected child, grief counseling is generally necessary. Nursing interventions focus on prevention of complications. Treat disorders, such as ear infections, leukemia, or cardiac problems, as they occur. Education and support for the family are important. Respite care is often recommended for caregivers. Social, healthcare, and financial resources are needed to provide the care for these children. Special education may also be required, but many DS children attend regular schools.

Fragile X Syndrome

Fragile X syndrome (FXS) is an inherited intellectual disability carried on the X chromosome, which means that either parent may be a carrier. The condition occurs because a specific protein is absent or, in milder fragile X-associated disorders, is deficient. About half of the children with FXS are also diagnosed with autism. Many of the children have some variation of an attention deficit disorder (ADD) or attention deficit hyperactivity disorder (ADHD) (discussed in more detail later in this chapter). Intellectual disabilities range from mild to severe. Boys are more severely affected than girls, who may have normal or borderline learning difficulties.

Signs and Symptoms

Signs and symptoms of FXS fall into five categories: intelligence and learning deficits, physical characteristics, social and emotional problems, speech and language difficulties, and sensory problems. The first developmental delays noticed typically are related to the child's difficulty with balance, which makes sitting, moving, or walking difficult. The child may stutter and have disorganized speech. Physical characteristics include an elongated face, protruding ears, large testes, and a heart murmur. Behavioral characteristics include stereotypic movements such as hand flapping, or shyness and social anxiety.

Diagnosis and Treatment

Diagnosis is made by chromosomal studies. Treatment is symptomatic. No cure exists for FXS.

Nursing Considerations

Early interventions are essential to maximize the child's potential and should involve the entire family and a team of professional healthcare providers. Educating family members about reasons for behavioral problems or intellectual deficits help them understand the acute and chronic nature of this lifelong condition. Many of the nursing interventions for children with DS are appropriate for those with FXS. The child will benefit from speech and occupational therapy. Table 74-1 compares the characteristics of DS and FXS.

TABLE 74-1 Characteristics of Down Syndrome and Fragile X Syndrome

FEATURE	DOWN SYNDROME	FRAGILE X SYNDROME
Head	Round, small, short	Abnormally large
Face	Flattened profile	Long, large, protruding jaw
Ears	Small, low set	Large, protruding
Eyes	Upward, outward slant; epicanthal folds; Brushfield spots	Wide set; epicanthal folds
Nose	Small; depressed nasal bridge	Flattened nasal bridge
Hands	Short, square; simian creases	Simian creases
Mouth	High-arched palate; protruding tongue; mouth curved downward	High-arched palate
Behavioral	Low-normal intelligence to severe intellectual impairment; language delay	Mild to profound intellectual impairment; short attention span, hyperactivity; temper tantrums; autistic-like behaviors; speech delays

> **Key Concept**
>
> A child who does not appear to follow directions can cause frustration. Such behavior may indicate a behavioral problem or a learning disorder. Patience and sensitivity are necessary, along with praise and positive reinforcement.

> **NCLEX Alert**
>
> Nursing considerations are always important aspects of clinical scenarios. Remember that teaching, also known as educating the client, is an important aspect of nursing care.

Attention Deficit Hyperactivity Disorder

ADHD, also known as ADD, is a condition associated with three categories of symptoms: inattentiveness, impulsivity, and hyperactivity. ADHD always begins in childhood and may continue through adolescence and adulthood. There are three predominant types of ADHD: *inattentive, hyperactive-impulsive,* and *combined* inattentive with hyperactive-impulsive behaviors. Inattentive ADHD was formerly called ADD. All normal children occasionally have the three main symptoms, but to be diagnosed with ADHD, the symptoms must be severe, occur for at least 6 months, and significantly affect the child's developmental milestones.

Signs and Symptoms

Examples of the three main symptoms include:

- Inattentiveness
  - Easily distracted and cannot focus on one single task
  - Seems forgetful; cannot remember where items were placed
  - Daydreams and becomes easily confused
  - Becomes bored with an activity shortly after starting it
  - Cannot seem to follow directions or understand something new
  - Has difficulty organizing a task or completing homework
- Hyperactivity
  - Talks nonstop
  - Wants to be constantly moving
  - Cannot sit still; fidgets or squirms during meals or at school
  - Touches everything within sight
- Impulsivity
  - Interrupts other's conversations
  - Is emotionally inappropriate; shows no emotional restraint
  - Acts out with inappropriate comments
  - Shows impatience; cannot wait to be given attention

Diagnosis

The diagnostic criteria for ADHD indicate that the behaviors must persist for at least 6 months and to such a degree that they are maladaptive and interfere with developmental milestones. There is no single diagnostic test. Diagnosis is made by an examination of behaviors and the ruling out of other disorders with similar problems (e.g., depression or anxiety).

Treatment

Treatment involves a multifaceted approach that will include the parental caregivers and the child. Early intervention with psychological counseling and medication therapy are considered beneficial. Vision and auditory testing should be done to ensure that behaviors are not due to the possibility that the child cannot see well enough to read or cannot hear language or sounds. A scan called the Neuropsychiatric EEG-Based Assessment Aid (NEBA) measures theta and beta brain waves. The ratio (difference between the resulting scores) of these two types of brain waves is greater in children with ADHD. Categories of medications will include stimulants, such as amphetamines (Dexedrine) or methylphenidate (Ritalin), nonstimulants, such as atomoxetine (Strattera), plus other classifications such as antidepressants (Wellbutrin) and antihypertensives (Catapres). Stimulants, while somewhat controversial, are helpful in decreasing hyperactivity and improving concentration. These medications and the client's overall mental and physical health must be monitored for untoward side effects. For example, the drug atomoxetine (Strattera) is associated with suicidal ideation in children and adolescents, and the drug classification of amphetamines is known to be used for illicit, nonmedical reasons.

Nursing Considerations

As with all chronic disorders, long-term therapies are emotionally draining. Support groups are helpful. Teach family caregivers to minimize environmental stimuli, use consistent discipline, set limits, and focus on positive behaviors. Encourage caregivers to give directions one step at a time, such as "brush your teeth" or "wash your face and hands." Avoid generalizations such as "get ready for school," so that the child is not overloaded with details to remember and organize. Words of praise such as "good job" are more effective than criticisms. Routines in daily activities are important (see In Practice: Nursing Care Guidelines 74-1).

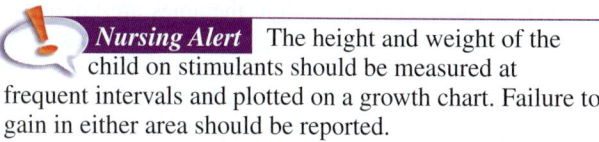

> **Nursing Alert** The height and weight of the child on stimulants should be measured at frequent intervals and plotted on a growth chart. Failure to gain in either area should be reported.

Tourette Syndrome

Tourette syndrome (TS) is an inherited, neurologic disorder of unknown cause characterized by repetitive, multiple involuntary movements and uncontrollable vocalizations called tics. Current research suggests a possible genetic relationship of TS with some forms of ADHD or obsessive-compulsive behaviors (OCD) (National Institutes of Health, 2014). Genetic counseling may be necessary to review a family's medical history and be able to identify potentially inherited traits. According to the rules of genetic inheritance of TS (autosomal dominant), at-risk males are more likely to have tics and at-risk females risk are more likely to have obsessive-compulsive symptoms.

Signs and Symptoms

TS is a chronic condition with lifelong symptoms that vary in frequency, severity, and location. Signs and symptoms of

TS are usually first noticed in childhood, in the head and neck areas, generally between the ages of 3 and 9 years. The worst tic symptoms tend to appear in the early teens and diminish in severity in the late teens into adulthood. Some individuals will have progressive or disabling tics for the duration of their lifetime.

Tics can be simple or complex and consist of two types: motor and vocal. Both types range in severity from barely noticeable to embarrassing, affecting social and career interactions. Motor tics include arm and head jerking, blinking, making a face, mouth twitching, and shoulder shrugging. Vocal tics include barking, yelping, grunting, coughing, and clearing of the throat. Simple tics involve a limited number of muscle groups, such as blinking or making a face. Complex tics are specific, coordinated patterns involving several muscle groups plus the use of words or phrases; for example, jumping and swearing. Many situations can affect the intensity of tics, such as stress, illness, fatigue, or emotions. Some tics result in self-harm, such as head banging or punching oneself. **Coprolalia** and **echolalia** are conditions that occur in a small percentage of individuals with TS. During episodes of coprolalia, the individual uses socially inappropriate words. Echolalia involves meaningless repetition of the words or phrases of others.

Diagnosis is made after the healthcare provider verifies the presence of both motor and vocal tics for at least 1 year. Other neurologic and psychiatric conditions need to be eliminated as a source of the problem. Standard blood testing and imaging studies may be done to rule out infections, tumors, or trauma, but no definitive test for TS is available. Many individuals are undiagnosed because their symptoms (e.g., eye blinking or sniffling) may mimic other problems, such as seasonal allergies.

Treatment is not always necessary. Tics are involuntary actions and often difficult or impossible to suppress. Some individuals may need neuroleptic drugs, such as haloperidol (Haldol), to suppress severe or significant tics that interfere with ADLs. Long-term medication therapies are known to cause significant side effects (e.g., tardive dyskinesia), a motor disorder not related to TS. Certain physical or emotional experiences can trigger tics. Individuals often adapt to or change behaviors that act as triggers. Tics tend to be minimized during calm, focused activities. During sleep, tics are diminished but not absent.

Nursing considerations will focus on educating the client and family. For children or teenagers, social adjustment may be challenging. Psychiatric counseling does not decrease tics, but may be effective in helping the child and family cope. Educational settings should be tailored to the individual's needs and may involve tutoring, home schooling, or special classrooms. Compassion, tolerance, and patience are needed, both by the affected individual as well as by others (e.g., colleagues, schoolmates). Reinforce positive facts about the disorder. For example, TS is not a degenerative condition, and it does not impair intelligence. Many adults become less symptomatic or symptom free.

Autism Spectrum Disorder

Autism spectrum disorder (**ASD**) is a lifelong, complex developmental disorder characterized by intellectual, social, and communication deficits. It is an umbrella term that covers a spectrum of neurodevelopmental disorders that impair a child's ability to communicate and interact with others. ASD can greatly diminish the individual's ability to function and perform social, occupational, and behavioral interactions. Terms still in use, but not diagnostically used include *autism* and *Asperger syndrome*. Autism is not actually a disease, but a syndrome of behaviors that vary widely. *Asperger syndrome* is a term formerly used to indicate autism that is at the mild end of the autism spectrum. ASD can show signs in early infancy. Some children develop normally for many months or years but suddenly become withdrawn, aggressive, or lose language skills that they have acquired. Each pattern of symptomatic behaviors is unique and abilities range from low to high functioning.

The cause or causes of ASD are not well understood but are possibly both genetic and environmental. Risk factors for ASD do include gender; boys are more likely to develop problems than girls. A family who has one child with ASD is more likely to have another child with the disorder. Also, if one child is diagnosed with ASD, another child may have noticeable problems related to behavioral, communication, and social interactions. Some children may have other medical disorders that have behaviors similar to those of ASD, for example, FXS or TS. Risk factors also include extremely preterm infants (i.e., infants of 26 weeks or less gestation). A variety of scientific studies have provided strong clinical evidence that there is no link between ASD and childhood vaccinations, such as that for measles, mumps, and rubella (MMR).

Signs and Symptoms

Signs and symptoms of ASD may develop suddenly, without warning. Some children succeed in reaching their developmental milestones for many months or years, but for an unexplained reason, these abilities are lost. The child initially becomes withdrawn, aggressive, and may lose previously acquired language skills. Autistic children typically demonstrate a profound lack of social interaction and communication. They do not respond to verbal stimuli and do not like to cuddle or be touched. They may show bizarre attachments to mechanical objects. These children are believed to be preoccupied with themselves, perhaps having fixed delusions and hallucinations. They sometimes become very upset or aggressive when interrupted.

The "spectrum" or range of disorders is highly unique and variable. A child might be said to have *low-support needs,* meaning that abilities are adequate or near normal for the age. Or, the child may have severe problems and have *higher support needs*. As the child matures, they may develop a higher level of social interaction and more age-appropriate behaviors. However, the teen years can often be very problematic and challenging. The following list provides examples of ASD-related social interactions and behavioral patterns:

Examples of social interactions

- Passive, aggressive, or disruptive when with other people
- Appears to avoid others, does not respond when called or when talked to
- Lacks expressive facial expression
- Avoids eye contact
- Uses "sing-song," rhythmic vocalizations when speaking
- Does not speak and can lose previous ability to use words or sentences

- Prefers solitary play, avoids conversations
- Shows a flat affect (lack of emotion) and does not seem to understand another's feelings
- Does not appear to understand directions or have ability to respond to questions

Examples of behavioral patterns

- Performs repetitive movements, for example, rocking, spinning, hand-flapping, head-banging
- Moves constantly
- Makes exaggerated, unusual body movements; is clumsy and uncoordinated
- Develops specific routines or rituals and becomes very upset if any detail is changed
- Resists any change in daily routine
- Is fascinated by a detail, for example, spinning wheels of a toy car, but does not understand the purpose of the car
- Has an exaggerated response to sensations, for example, light, sound, touch, but does not seem to feel pain
- Eating habits are atypical; eats only certain foods or foods with a specific texture

About 10% of individuals with ASD possess an exceptional ability in some area, such as memory, music, art, calendar calculation, or mathematics; such individuals are referred to as *autistic savants*. In the nonautistic population, the chance of having "savant" ability is less than 1%. "Savant" ability may also appear in an individual with some form of central nervous system injury or disease.

Diagnosis
There is no specific diagnostic test for ASD. An official medical diagnosis is made only when the professionally defined diagnostic criteria in the DSM-5 have been met. Parental caregivers and healthcare providers may agree that the child has difficulties with social interactions and behaviors, but a diagnosis of ASD may be delayed so that other intellectual, genetic, or behavioral disorders can be eliminated as the source of problems. Because there is no specific test or procedure to diagnose autism, recognition at the earliest possible age of obvious delays in social interaction and language skills is crucial. Intervention should begin immediately, even during the weeks or months of clinical observation and testing before diagnosis. Early intervention is shown to improve social skills and language development. Delayed intervention is detrimental to the child and the family's success in dealing with this chronic disorder.

Treatment
No known cure exists for autism. Treatment is individually structured using a child's existing abilities and maximizing each individual's potentials. Intensive, early treatment helps the child reach potentials in functioning. Family education is a preliminary area of focus. The family learns about the disorder and how it affects their child. The goal is to teach daily living skills, identify problematic behavioral patterns, and assist with communication and social interactions. Outside the home, highly structured educational environments are beneficial. A team of professionals who are knowledgeable in the complexities of ASD is needed. Medications are given if behaviors need symptomatic control (e.g., for hyperactivity). Antianxiety, antidepressant, and some antipsychotic drugs are considered on a case-by-case basis.

Nursing Considerations
Emphasize the positive and focus on the child's skills. Teach family caregivers to give the child immediate feedback and to continue interaction with the child using short sentences and simple commands. Remind caregivers to be concerned with the child's safety and to maintain normal daily routines. Family respite services may be helpful.

Plumbism

Plumbism is *lead poisoning*. Lead is a metal that can naturally be present in water, dirt, food, or air. Lead is toxic to both adults and children, but lead is especially dangerous to children. Unlike most poisonings that result in emergency therapies, lead poisoning usually occurs slowly over a period of weeks or months. At high levels, lead poisoning can be fatal.

Individuals who work with batteries or are in the mining industry are at risk for the presence of lead. Water pipes can be sources of lead at home or work. Living in a home that contains lead paint is a well-known risk factor. Lead was removed from paint in 1978. Hobbies such as making pottery or stained glass use lead. Lead in paint on toys can cause serious health problems.

Signs and Symptoms
Some individuals do not have obvious signs of plumbism. Signs and symptoms may not appear until large quantities have accumulated in the body's organs and tissues. Children develop anemia, severe stomach aches, hearing loss, muscle weakness, and mental and physical damage. Brain damage is permanent. Adults with plumbism have hypertension, are often infertile, have muscle and joint pains, and have nerve disorders. Other symptoms include pain, headache, irritability, memory loss, decline in mental functioning, and mood swings. Adult symptoms may mimic other disorders or conditions that are seen with aging and, therefore, go undiagnosed. A fetus can acquire plumbism prenatally, which will result in a newborn with delayed physical and developmental capabilities.

The signs and symptoms of plumbism include the following:

- Blue or blue-black line on the gums near the teeth
- Hyperirritability
- Anorexia, nausea, and vomiting
- Intermittent vomiting (lead colic)
- Abdominal pain
- Joint pain
- Headache
- Fatigue and decreased play
- Anemia, pallor, and decreased RBCs
- Constipation
- Behavior changes (sudden changes may indicate acute lead poisoning)
- *Ataxia* (unsteady gait), weakness, or clumsiness
- Decrease in intellectual and mental abilities (e.g., memory loss and poor school performance)
- Impaired level of consciousness
- Seizures
- Coma
- *Encephalopathy* (brain degeneration)

Diagnosis

Blood lead level (**BLL**) should be obtained from children who are at high risk or who demonstrate symptoms. Other disorders need to be eliminated as causes of symptoms. Healthcare providers should consider this problem if risk factors are present. Some, but not all, communities have regulations for lead testing at the ages of 1, 2, and 6 years.

> **Key Concept**
> Eating nonfood items is termed *pica*.

> **Nursing Alert** Lead is contained in items other than paint, such as leaded pottery or dishes, home remedies, shoes, old toys, old eating utensils, old pipes and plumbing, soil containing lead from old chipped paint, sand and dirt on playgrounds, air pollution from unleaded gasoline, and family members who bring lead dust home on their clothes. A child who inhales the dust from scraped, leaded paint can suffer the same deleterious effects as the child who eats paint. The buildup of lead typically occurs gradually.

Treatment

The individual first must be removed from the lead source. High-risk children should be screened for elevated BLL. If the case is mild, the child is treated symptomatically. Anemia is treated with diet and iron supplements; seizures are treated with antiseizure medications. If lead levels are high, *chelation* is considered (see the earlier section on hemochromatosis). The drugs of choice for chelation are edetate acid (EDTA) given intravenously (IV) and the heavy metal antagonist dimercaprol (**BAL in Oil**) given via deep intramuscular injection. Of special consideration: BAL in oil ampules are manufactured with *peanut oil*; thus, the oil may be a cause of *significant allergic reactions* in tree nut–sensitive individuals.

Nursing Considerations

Plumbism may easily be missed as a possible cause of childhood disorders. During well-baby and well-child checkups, the nurse should consider plumbism if the child is at risk or demonstrates symptoms. Changes in play activities, new aches and pains, and altered intellectual abilities may be seen by parents but not reported to healthcare providers. The source of lead must be eliminated. Educate the parents about media alerts that concern lead in children's toys. Practical teaching should also include the importance of the following: avoiding areas where lead might have contaminated the soil (e.g., around mining sites or construction zones); washing hands before eating; and avoiding tap water when making formula or cooking if old lead-lined pipes or lead-based solder are a concern.

> **Key Concept**
> Public education and prevention are the most effective approaches for eliminating the problem of lead poisoning.

Cerebral Palsy

Cerebral palsy (**CP**) is a general term used to describe movement and coordination disorders, or "palsies," in children that are the result of damage to the parts of the developing brain that affect muscle movement. Lack of voluntary muscle coordination (**ataxia**), uncontrollable movements (**dyskinesia**), and stiff muscles with exaggerated reflexes (**spasticity**) are commonly seen with CP. It may be accompanied by intellectual and learning deficits, epilepsy, blindness, or deafness. Impaired movements of CP include floppiness or rigidity of the limbs or trunk, abnormal posture, or unsteady gait. The individual may have *dysphagia* (difficulty swallowing). Some children are able to walk, some walk with difficulty, and others are unable to walk. Unlike other movement disorders, CP is not progressive, which means that the symptoms may improve or worsen, but the initial brain damage does not worsen. Symptoms may appear at any time before the age of 2–3 years.

Cerebral palsy appears to have many etiologies. Brain injury during the fetal development, which is present at birth, is the most common cause and may not be detected at birth. Congenital CP may be the result of infections during pregnancy (e.g., rubella [German measles], syphilis, varicella, cytomegalovirus, or toxoplasmosis). Multiple births, premature births, low birth weight, and breech births are associated with CP. Genetic conditions often have an impact on motor, intellectual, and developmental abilities. Rh incompatibility between the mother and the fetus can cause problems. Brain injury during the birthing process can occur; however, cerebral *anoxia* (absence of oxygen) or severe *hypoxia* (serious deficiency of oxygen) is diagnosed in only a small percentage of CP cases. CP can also result from exposure to toxins, such as lead or mercury, in utero or during infancy. After birth, CP can be acquired as a result of kernicterus, excessive bilirubin and jaundice in the newborn, bacterial meningitis, viral encephalitis, head injury secondary to a fall, child abuse, or a motor vehicle accident.

For a few months or a few years, the child may appear normal until infant developmental and intellectual milestones do not appear or appear late. Milestones related to movement are often absent or delayed, such as rolling over, sitting, standing, or walking. Early CP may be initially diagnosed as a variety of other disabilities.

Signs and Symptoms

Characteristics of CP generally include the following to varying degrees:

- Spasticity—stiff muscles and exaggerated reflexes
- **Rigidity**—stiff muscles with normal reflexes
- Ataxia—lack of muscle coordination
- **Athetosis**—slow, writhing movements
- **Tremors**—involuntary muscle movements
- **Contractures**—muscles and tendons become inflexible leading to deformity, rigidity, and disuse of extremity
- Rapid variations of muscle contractions and relaxations—too stiff or too floppy
- Abnormal gait—difficulty walking: walking on toes, scissors-like gait with knees crossing or a wide gait
- Increased stretch reflexes
- Muscle weakness
- Limited range of motion
- Bilateral favoritism, using only one side of body to reach or move
- Lack of muscle tone of affected extremities

- Delayed motor development: unable to sit, crawl, or walk per milestone schedules
- Poor fine motor abilities
- **Dysarthria**—speech abnormalities
- **Dysphagia**—problems with swallowing and eating, excessive drooling
- Abnormal sense perception: touch or pain
- Difficulty with vision or hearing
- Urinary incontinence
- Seizures
- Oral disorders
- Psychiatric disorders

Classifications

There are four major classifications of CP and several subclassifications for the most common type.

1. Spastic cerebral palsy is the most common type of CP. Spastic refers to a condition of having sudden, involuntary contractions of muscle groups. Muscle tone is increased significantly (i.e., muscles are stiff). Awkward movements are noted with walking. Spastic CP is subclassified according to what parts of the body are affected.
   - *Spastic diplegia/diparesis* is mainly in the legs with arms partially or not at all affected. **Diplegia** is symmetrical paralysis of corresponding parts on both sides of the body, for example, both legs or both arms. **Diparesis** refers to the weakness affecting the symmetrical parts. Walking is difficult due to *scissoring,* which occurs when hip and leg muscles cause legs to adduct (turn inward toward midline of the body) and cross at the knees.
   - *Spastic hemiplegia/hemiparesis* refers to CP that affects only one side of the body, generally an arm and occasionally a leg. **Hemiplegia** is paralysis on one vertical half of the body. **Hemiparesis** is weakness of the entire left or right side.
   - *Spastic quadriplegia/quadriparesis,* the most severe form of spastic CP, involves both legs and both arms. The trunk and the face are included with the paralysis (**quadriplegia**) or weakness (**quadriparesis**). Individuals with spastic quadriplegia or quadriparesis are typically unable to walk and have significant intellectual disabilities, including seizures and problems with vision, hearing, and speech.
2. *Dyskinetic* (or *athetoid*) **cerebral palsy** is characterized by slow, writhing involuntary movements or rapid and jerky movements. The condition of *dyskinesia* refers to involuntary muscle movements. *Athetoid* refers to uncontrolled rhythmic writhing or weaving motions often of the fingers, hands, head, and tongue. The muscle tone can vary in intensity from extremely tight to flabby and loose, over a timespan of hours. These movements disappear during sleep and increase with stress or excitement. The child may have difficulty swallowing, sucking, sitting, and walking because of the involuntary movements. Speech and language disorders (dysarthria) are common with athetoid CP children.
3. *Ataxic cerebral palsy* causes problems with balance and coordination. Gait is unsteady and walking is difficult. Tremors cause these clients to have difficulty controlling their hands and arms when they reach for an object. *Nystagmus* (rapid, repeated movements of the eyeball) may be seen.
4. *Mixed cerebral palsy:* Some individuals have symptoms of more than one type of CP, most commonly a mixture of spasticity and dyskinetic/athetoid movements.

Diagnosis

Cerebral palsy is primarily considered as a possibility due to signs and symptoms the child demonstrates during infancy. The child will fall behind in developmental milestones. Laboratory and genetic studies will be needed to rule out other causes, such as infection, various hereditary conditions, metabolic disorders, or other brain and nervous system conditions. Imaging studies may be done to pinpoint brain abnormalities, as well as hearing and visual screening to determine sensory disabilities.

Treatment

Treatment is multidisciplinary, using a team that includes physical, occupational, and speech and language specialists (Fig. 74-3). Their goals are to prevent complications, such as injuries from falls or contractures, and to maximize the child's potential for walking, self-care, and communication. There is no cure for CP. Disabilities associated with CP are permanent. Medications are supportive and used symptomatically. Muscle relaxants can reduce tremors and spasticity. Seizures can be controlled with anticonvulsants. Isolated muscle spasticity may benefit from onabotulinumtoxinA (Botox) injections directly into the muscle and/or nerve about every 3 months. Medications to reduce drooling include Botox, scopolamine (Scopace), or glycopyrrolate (Robinul). Generalized spasticity may benefit from oral muscle relaxants such as diazepam (Valium), dantrolene (Dantrium), and baclofen (Gablofen). Braces, splints, crutches, and walkers help with movement and ambulation. Surgical interventions may be necessary to realign bones, correct deformities, and minimize muscle and tendon shortening that cause contractures.

Nursing Considerations

Cerebral palsy does not necessarily affect the length of life, but it does profoundly affect the quality of life. Nursing considerations begin at the time of diagnosis, often just after birth, and continue throughout the lifetime. Client and

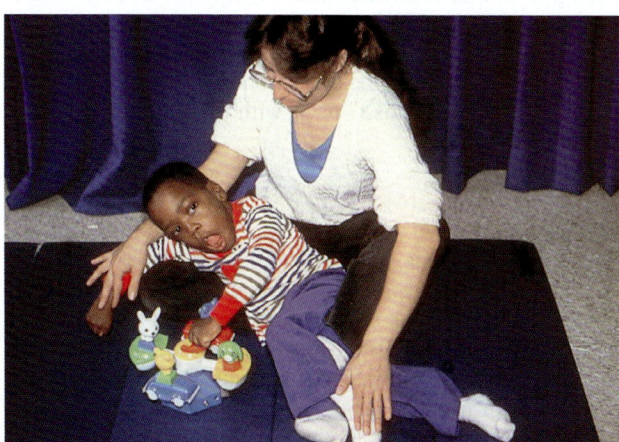

Figure 74-3 A physical therapist works with a child with cerebral palsy to maximize mobility.

family teaching are very important. Teams of professionals are often necessary to cover all the needs of the child, family, and family unit. Social workers design community and financial resource plans for the family. Behavioral therapists help with learning deficits and day-to-day emotional needs. The child will have individualized plans for physical needs such as occupational, speech, and physical therapy. Eating difficulties will need consultations with a dietician. Adaptive care devices, such as hearing aids, glasses, vision-enhancing equipment, braces, and walkers help with mobility and ADLs. Education must be adapted to the needs and capacities of the child. Surgical interventions require individualized preoperative and postoperative care. The family and the child will need much respite care and emotional support, which can be found in support groups or through individual counseling.

Muscular Dystrophy

Muscular dystrophy (**MD**) is a group of about 30 genetic diseases characterized by gradual, progressive weakness and loss of muscle mass with degeneration of the skeletal muscles. Genetic mutations cause a deficit or a total lack of the protein dystrophin in the muscles, resulting in progressive muscle wasting (atrophy) with gradual loss of strength and increasing muscle deformities. The forms of MD are related to the location and extent of muscle weakness, age that symptoms appear, and rate of progression of symptoms. Some types of MD affect cardiac muscle. Muscular dystrophy can be inherited or it can occur in a family with no previous medical history of progressive muscle degradation and weakness. Some forms of MD appear in both sexes, some occurring in infancy or childhood in boys, while other forms do not appear until middle age or later.

<u>Duchenne muscular dystrophy</u> (**DMD**) is the most common form of MD, characterized by progressive atrophy of symmetrical groups of skeletal muscles in boys between the ages of 2 and 6 years. DMD progresses rapidly. By the age of 12 years, most boys are unable to walk. At some point, the teenager may not be able to breathe without mechanical assistance. The mutated gene of DMD is inherited in about 50% of female children, and they are able to pass on the genetic defect to their children.

Becker muscular dystrophy (**BMD**) is another form of MD; it is similar to DMD, but the symptoms are less severe. *Myotonic MD* (**MMD**) is the most common adult form of the disorder. It causes sustained muscle spasms, endocrine problems, cataracts, and cardiac abnormalities. Adults with MMD have a "swan-like" neck with a long, thin face, and drooping eyelids.

Signs and Symptoms

Symptoms of DMD begin to appear around the age of 3 years. Before this time, the child may have noticeable developmental delays. The child may not be able to walk upstairs, run, or get up off the floor. The child's gait appears as a waddle and a positive **Gowers sign** occurs, in which the child uses the upper extremity muscles to compensate for weak hip muscles (Fig. 74-4). The child may walk on the toes, fall frequently, and have difficulty hopping or running. These children often develop lordosis, scoliosis, and contracture deformities, especially of the hips and knees.

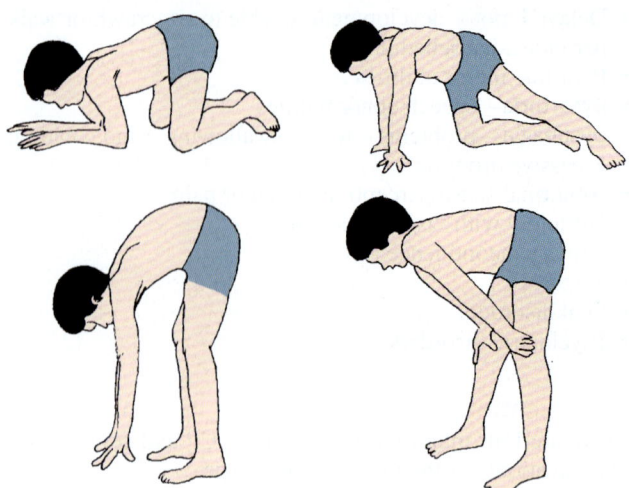

Figure 74-4 Positive Gowers sign. The child gets up by pushing to an upright position, using the hands to climb up the legs to a standing position: The child starts at the ankles, alternating hands; he then gradually pushes to an upright position, using the legs as the climbing pole.

Delayed intellectual development and borderline IQ may be present. Gradual muscle atrophy occurs, and by the age of 11 or 12 years, the child is unable to walk and becomes wheelchair bound.

Health issues related to immobility are problematic, such as pneumonia and skin problems.

Due to the inability to perform fine motor movements, the child will lose the ability to feed themself. Muscles involved in swallowing are also affected, and tube feeding may be necessary. The child has difficulty breathing and begins to have cardiac failure. In some cases, assisted respiratory ventilation can extend life.

Diagnosis

Muscular dystrophy is diagnosed by the presence of symptoms, electromyogram, muscle biopsy, and elevated enzyme levels, such as aspartate aminotransferase (**ALT**) and creatine kinase (**CK**). Genetic testing may be recommended. As the disease progresses, cardiac and lung function tests will be ordered to monitor cardiopulmonary function.

Treatment

There is no cure for any of the forms of muscular dystrophy. Treatment is supportive. Medications will include the use of corticosteroids, anticonvulsants, immunosuppressants, and antibiotics, depending on the individual's current level of health. Wheelchairs are needed as the child loses the ability to walk. A pacemaker may be inserted. Feeding tubes may be necessary if the child can no longer swallow. As the disease progresses, supportive respiratory therapies, such as ventilators, may be set up in the home or in a long-term care facility.

Nursing Considerations

Muscular dystrophy is a chronic and long-term disorder with episodes of acute illnesses and complications. The goal is to maintain physical function for as long as possible. Prevention of complications such as pneumonia, urinary tract infections, dehydration, or injury from falls is an ongoing process. This disease is devastating, and emotional support must be provided for the child and family. Genetic counseling may be helpful for families who have known or suspected histories of muscular dystrophy. Grief counseling should also be considered.

> **NCLEX Alert**
>
> When taking an examination, be alert for descriptive terms in the clinical scenario, such as *ataxia, dysphagia, atrophy, nystagmus,* or the expressions *intellectual* or *developmental disability.* Each of these clues could influence the choice of the correct response.

Mental Health and Illness

The CDC states that *mental health* in childhood means reaching developmental and emotional milestones, learning healthy social skills, and using coping skills when problems occur (CDC, n.d.). *Mental illnesses* are alterations in thinking, mood, behavior, communication, or a combination of these. Mental health disorders in children and adolescents are similar to conditions that develop in adulthood. However, children have fewer life experiences and are less able to apply knowledge and experiences to new circumstances. Mental health issues need to be assessed while balancing the total capabilities and disabilities of each individual. A child with special needs, that is, intellectual, physical, and developmental disabilities, has fewer coping skills than the unimpaired child. Disabilities also include a variety of chronic medical conditions, such as heart and lung pathologies, diabetes, movement difficulties, or difficulty communicating. Mental illness is often a consequence of inadequately treated physical disorders resulting in poorly developed coping mechanisms. Successful treatment of the physical aspects of disabilities will increase the incidences of improved mental health.

Mental illnesses in the younger person are often diagnosed with one or more of the following issues:

- *Depression or affective (mood)* disorders are seen in individuals who have persistent feelings of sadness, sometimes with rapidly fluctuating moods.
- *Schizophrenia* is a serious psychological condition involving distorted ideas of reality and thoughts.
- *Anxiety* disorders are very common. Situations become overwhelming and change is difficult. Fear, dread, nervousness, tachycardia, and diaphoresis are noted.
- *Eating disorders* may be displays of psychological issues. Anorexia nervosa, bulimia, and binge eating are discussed in Chapter 73.
- *Intellectual and developmental disabilities* can be linked to a variety of disruptive behavioral disorders. Examples include ADHD and ASD.

Depression

Depression is a mental illness defined by periods of sadness, hopelessness, mood swings, and negative thoughts about one's self. An individual may become withdrawn and have difficulty expressing feelings and emotions. The cause of depression is generally considered to be a combination of genetic, biologic, environmental, and psychological factors. Depression often develops over a period of time (weeks, months, or years) but can also develop in response to unexpected situations involving grief and loss. Depression is discussed in more detail in Chapter 94.

Serious depression interferes with daily life and eventually has a destructive effect on others in a family unit. A child or teenager who is depressed may feign illness in order not to go to school or may become negative, moody, and angry, often acting out aggressive behaviors. The symptoms may go unnoticed or unaddressed if they are perceived as a passing phase, temporary crisis, or a personal weakness that will resolve or disappear. Or, parental caregivers and school educators may be aware of these symptoms but believe them to be typical of a developmental stage that will pass with time and patience.

> **Nursing Alert** Depression is the risk factor most often identified with suicide. An individual who talks about committing suicide should be taken very seriously. Most communities have a local suicide hotline and support groups for depression. Additional help may be available from the *National Suicide Prevention Lifeline* **1-800-SUICIDE (1-800-784-2433)**, or at **1-800-273-TALK (1-800-273-8255)**, or visit the Website which has additional information for young adults and veterans www.suicidepreventionlifeline.org.

Signs and Symptoms

Symptoms of depression are often subtle and not all symptoms occur in an individual. The severity, frequency, and duration of symptoms will vary depending upon the individual's circumstances and the source or causes for the depression. Generally, symptoms are noticeable if a caregiver can perceive the overall circumstances and view details as risk factors. Details, such as missing school, giving excuses for not doing homework, complaining of vague physical symptoms, plus significant changes in behavior are worth investigating. The following list provides a review of some of the most common signs and symptoms of depression.

- Change(s) in behavior: for example, loss of interest in a favorite activity, poor school performance, change of appearance, drinking alcohol, taking drugs, changes in language (more aggressive or passive)
- Not eating or excessive eating; not sleeping or excessive sleeping
- Continually appears to be sad and lonely
- States feelings of helplessness, hopelessness, worthlessness, or guilt
- Increased sensitivity to rejection, low self-esteem, low self-worth
- Extreme low energy or bursts of activity
- Withdrawal from friends, family, or social contacts (e.g., sports)
- Inability to concentrate
- Vague physical complaints, for example, stomachaches or headaches that do not get better with treatment
- Risk-taking behaviors, for example, sexual promiscuity, racing cars, extreme sports
- Vocal outbursts, crying, emotional sensitivity to comments from others

- Talking about another person's suicide, for example, a media celebrity or friend
- Focusing on morbid, negative themes
- Giving away possessions
- Talking about committing suicide

Treatment

The first step in treating depression is identifying the symptoms. Although recognizing depression in children may be difficult, it is important to understand that all behavior is meaningful. Psychotherapy and counseling are necessary and may be provided on an outpatient basis. More serious cases of depression may require hospitalization. Family counseling is always helpful. Antidepressants are often effective medication therapies. Unintentional side effects of antidepressants may occur with some individuals, especially adolescents and young adults, including suicide attempts or suicide.

Contemporary antidepressants are fairly effective in the treatment of depression. Classifications include selective serotonin reuptake inhibitors (SSRIs) such as fluoxetine (Prozac), sertraline (Zoloft), escitalopram (Lexapro), paroxetine (Paxil), and citalopram (Celexa). Fluoxetine has been noted to be effective for children and teenagers with depression from the ages of 8–18 years. Bupropion (Wellbutrin) is another commonly used drug, which is similar to SSRIs but acts on a different neurotransmitter. Another classification of antidepressants is called serotonin and norepinephrine reuptake inhibitors (SNRIs), which include venlafaxine (Effexor) and duloxetine (Cymbalta). Older medications, which may be of assistance in some cases of depression, include tricyclics imipramine (Tofranil), nortriptyline (Aventyl), and amitriptyline (Elavil). The oldest category is the monoamine oxidase inhibitors (MAOIs), which have significant side effects. Individuals must avoid foods and beverages that contain tyramine, such as cheese and red wine. MAOIs cannot be taken with SSRIs, some birth control pills, prescription pain relievers, cold and allergy medications, and some herbal supplements. Severe hypertension, confusion, hallucinations, seizures, and other life-threatening conditions may result when taking MAOIs.

Nursing Considerations

The care of individuals with depression, especially of the adolescent or young adult, typically involves cooperation of parental caregivers. Caregivers may not be able to accept that noted signs or symptoms are abnormal and need healthcare intervention. Denial is part of a generalized social stigma pertaining to mental illnesses. It is not unusual for caregivers and healthcare providers to consciously or unconsciously ignore the symptoms accompanying depression in a child, teenager, or adult. All children have adjustment difficulties associated with growth and development, but it is not normal for these problems to persist for weeks or months and increase in frequency and severity.

Client teaching must be done patiently and in phases; learning new concepts can become overwhelming to the stressed mind. Education will help the family recognize the symptoms of depression in adolescents and young adults and understand that depression is often a long-term disorder with acute exacerbations over a lifetime. Nursing interventions should also include discussion of the necessity of taking medications daily and monitoring for side effects (including signs of *suicidal ideation,* see below). Maintaining physical health, for example, through exercise, eating right, and avoiding substance abuse, will be as important as the routines necessary to deal with depression. The feelings of loss of self-control associated with depression can be a frustrating and frightening experience; avoid giving advice or placating the client by saying, "it will get better" or "just get over it." Develop and utilize active listening skills, which typically take practice.

Suicide

Suicide is taking one's own life. It is often a response to a stressful situation or an accumulation of stressful situations. Risk factors associated with suicide include depression, prior suicide attempts, family history of a mental disorder or suicide, family history of substance abuse, domestic violence, child abuse, incarceration (being in prison or jail), or exposure to the suicide of another family member, such as a mother or sibling. Adolescents, who are experiencing the physical and emotional changes typical of their age group, have less developed coping skills, which are often needed in relationships and stressful situations. Women attempt suicide more impulsively, often by poisons or drugs, than do men. Men are usually more successful in suicide because they use more lethal methods, such as guns or hanging. Risk factors for suicide are reviewed in Box 74-2. Individuals with long-term, permanent

---

Box 74-2 Risk Factors for Suicide

- Depression
- Previous suicide attempt(s)
- Suicidal ideation (thoughts)
- History of mental disorders, particularly depression
- Family member or friend's history of suicide
- Family history of domestic violence or child abuse
- Family history of child maltreatment and child abuse
- Feelings of hopelessness
- Impulsive or aggressive tendencies
- Barriers to accessing mental health treatment
- Grief and loss of friends or family, unemployment, financial concerns
- History of alcohol and substance abuse
- Medical illnesses with chronic issues that interfere with the quality of life, e.g., chronic pain, traumatic brain injury, end-stage renal disease, diabetes, systemic lupus erythematosus, HIV/AIDS
- Easy access to lethal methods
- Unwillingness to seek help because of a perceived stigma attached to mental health
- Cultural and religious beliefs; for instance, the belief that suicide is a noble resolution of a personal dilemma
- Media attention to a celebrity who has committed suicide
- Isolation, a feeling of being cut off from other people

Adapted from Centers for Disease Control and Prevention, Program Performance and Evaluation Office. www.cdc.gov/mentalhealth and The National Institute of Mental Health: http://www.nimh.nih.gov/health/publications/suicide-faq/index.shtml

medical health issues, associated with chronic, unrelenting physical problems, have increased incidences of suicide attempts. Examples of these conditions include chronic pain, traumatic brain injury, cancer, end-stage renal disease, HIV/AIDS, and systemic lupus erythematosus.

Causes
Causes for suicide vary greatly. Untreated or unrelenting depression is the most common basic risk factor for suicide; it is common, however, for suicide to have more than one causative factor. Most individuals who attempt suicide have a history of a mental disorder. An accumulation of negative life events or risk factors may also trigger suicidal thoughts or attempts (see Box 74-2). Some individuals may have a genetic basis for their depression, and in such cases, symptoms may not have been noted before the suicide.

Signs and Symptoms
Suicidal ideation is the term given to thoughts or ideas of suicide. Suicidal ideation usually precedes a suicide attempt. A *suicide gesture* is an attempt at inflicting personal injury; the injury is not intended to cause death. Suicidal ideation and gestures are symbolic cries for help. Ignoring these symptoms of despair can result in an individual's death. Both are key warning signs that must not be ignored. See Box 74-3: Warning Signs or Symptoms of Mental Illness.

Diagnosis
There is no specific test to determine the state of depression or inclination toward suicide. Key warning signals include depression, morbid discussion of, and preoccupation with, death, giving away personal belongings, and a sudden cheerfulness following a somber, withdrawn, depressed period. This sudden cheerfulness may indicate that the individual has decided to commit suicide and is relieved about the decision. This warning sign can be easily missed.

Treatment
Warn the family to take suicidal ideation, gestures, and attempts seriously. Have the individual see a professional therapist immediately. Suicidal ideation and gestures will need follow-up psychological counseling, often accompanied by medications. Intensive and long-term psychological therapies are essential. If one type of therapy is not successful, do not allow the client to be discouraged. It is common for an individual to try several types of therapy and search for the therapist who seems to be the best "fit" for the circumstances. Adolescents with severe depression and suicidal thoughts may require hospitalization and close monitoring until suicide is no longer an immediate threat.

Nursing Considerations
Be aware of early signs of depression. Listening is more effective than talking to individuals about sadness, unhappiness, or depression. Keep in mind that all individuals need to feel wanted and to have feelings of self-worth. Consider using a no-suicide contract, wherein the person agrees not to attempt suicide for a specified period and will contact help immediately if he or she feels suicidal. The younger person is usually more conscientious about wanting to keep their word, and a no-suicide contract can be effective in some situations.

Box 74-3 Warning Signs or Symptoms of Mental Illness

- **Actual suicide threats:** a suicide note, overuse of drugs; constant talk of death, willingness to die, or being ready for death; stating a sense of being worthless or no good; stating that death is a release from pressure and pain
- **Any suicidal gesture:** drug overdose, carrying a weapon, talking about suicide as a possibility
- **Mood changes:** withdrawal from friends and family; sadness, anxiety, tension, or mood swings
- **Behavioral changes:** drastic, out-of-control behaviors, impulsivity, frequent fighting, use of weapons, expressing desire to hurt others
- **Personality changes:** the individual does not seem to be the same person; extremes in emotion (e.g., sad or excessively cheerful, or happy without a reason)
- **Learning deficits:** inability to concentrate, sit still, or focus on a topic; interrupts others; sudden changes in school academic or social activities
- **Physical changes:** complains of physical pain, stomachaches, headaches; begins a rigorous exercise routine; loses too much weight, and may take substances that encourage muscle growth
- **School and social changes:** lack of involvement in school, lack of any social interaction with friends or acquaintances; loneliness and isolation
- **Home environmental changes:** problems in family relationships, refusal to talk to parents or siblings
- **Depression:** deep, lingering anxiety and sadness, with a loss of energy and desire
- **Self-harm:** deliberately harming one's self, e.g., cutting arms or inflicting cigarette burns; lack of self-esteem, self-respect, and self-worth
- **Intense feelings:** anxiety (fear for no apparent reason) that interferes with daily activities
- **Dangerous lifestyle:** playing "Russian roulette" with a loaded gun, or driving at excessive speeds
- **Substance abuse:** experimentation with a variety of drugs

Adapted from the following sources: www.cdc.gov/mentalhealth and https://www.mayoclinic.org/healthy-lifestyle/childrens-health/in-depth/mental-illness-in-children/art-20046577, and http://www.webmd.com/anxiety-panic/mental-health-illness-in-children

---

Schizophrenia
Schizophrenia is a psychotic disorder, a loss of connection with reality that includes a range of problems with thinking, behavior, and emotions. The usual onset of schizophrenia is in the late teens to the early 20s. A genetic predisposition or early central nervous system damage may account for an earlier onset of the disorder. *Childhood schizophrenia* is considered to be a virulent childhood version of the same adolescent or adult psychosis. Early-onset schizophrenia may start around 12 years of age or younger. In schizophrenia, the individual has difficulty interpreting reality. Hallucinations, delusions, and disordered thinking occur. It is a devastating disorder. The effect of this psychosis on a child's behavior, learning, information processing, and

understanding has a great influence on the child's development, as well as on the dynamics of the family unit. Childhood schizophrenia may interfere with the child's ability to go to school, or cause difficulties in coping with the emotional changes of puberty and communicating with others. It is a lifelong disorder but may be managed with a team approach to therapy.

The causes of schizophrenia are not totally clear but appear to include both genetic and environmental etiologies. Familial inheritance has been identified. Possible environmental risk factors include exposure to viruses, fetal malnutrition, perinatal difficulties, and perhaps unknown psychosocial factors. Individuals who develop this disorder before adolescence have less success overall in life. They have few, if any friends, are more likely to be unemployed as adults, and are more often not capable of living independently. They may not benefit from psychotherapy and have minimal beneficial effects from pharmacotherapy. Individuals with schizophrenia have a high risk for suicide; about one third will attempt suicide. Overall, suicide occurs in about 10% (1 in 10) of the individuals with this psychosis).

Signs and Symptoms

Schizophrenia symptoms involve an impaired ability to function. Abnormalities in thinking (cognitive function), behavior, and emotions are among the most common symptoms, such as the following:

- Paranoia—an unreasonable fear; can be a source of violence
- Aggression—behavior that is inappropriate, negative, or physically abusive
- Delusions—firm, false beliefs that are not based on facts
- Hallucinations—seeing or hearing things that do not exist
- Auditory hallucinations—hearing voices that no one else can hear (most common type of hallucination)
- Abnormal, disorganized behaviors—useless or excessive motions, inappropriate or bizarre posture, unpredictable agitation
- Negativity—lacks ability to function normally; apathetic, unable to organize or complete a task; social withdrawal
- Word salad—language that may be a jumble of incomprehensible or meaningless words or phrases
- Flat or inappropriate affect—shows no emotions or laughs at a sad event
- Out of touch with reality—distorted sense of what is real
- Confused—may not know location, date, or time
- Impaired relationships—not able to make friends or have appropriate social manners

The younger person with this psychosis is less likely to have delusions but more likely to have visual hallucinations. Symptoms are difficult to differentiate from typical behaviors of the adolescent years. The more common symptoms include the following:

- Withdrawal from friends and family
- Changes in school performance and activities
- Mood changes, irritability, depression, sadness
- Trouble sleeping

Diagnosis

Initially, standard blood tests are completed in order to rule out infections, hormone imbalances, or substance abuse. Other tests may include an MRI or CT scan to screen for abnormalities or tumors and psychological evaluations performed by a specialist in mental health disorders. The diagnosis is made by considering the criteria listed in the DSM-5. Other types of mental health disorders, substance abuse, or a variety of medical conditions can mimic schizophrenia. The DSM-5 diagnosis states that the individual must have at least two significant symptoms occurring most of the time for at least 6 months. Significant symptoms include extremely disorganized behavior, thinking, or speech and language patterns; catatonic behavior; hallucinations; delusions; and an extremely reduced ability to function normally.

Treatment

Treatment requires a team of specialists knowledgeable in this disorder. In-home treatment is typical, but hospitalization in a mental health facility may be required. At times of great stress, the individual may not be able to function and may require hospitalization to stabilize an acute crisis or to establish a medication regimen. Adolescents are especially vulnerable and may need in-hospital therapy that will continue for weeks or months. The potential for violence or suicide should be considered.

When symptoms are stable, the individual will need to develop ADLs, IADLs, and coping skills. Social interactions and vocational skills will be part of a lifelong therapy plan. Antipsychotic medications, plus behavioral modification and psychotherapy, are the most effective treatments. Family therapy is highly recommended.

Some medications used to treat schizophrenia, particularly first-generation antipsychotics such as chlorpromazine (Thorazine), are known to cause significant side effects. Many schizophrenic clients do not follow their medication regimen, sometimes due to uncomfortable side effects and sometimes due to the paranoia or hallucinations that accompany the disorder. Newer types of antipsychotics have fewer serious side effects than do earlier classifications. Examples of these include aripiprazole (Abilify), risperidone (Risperdal), clozapine (Clozaril), and quetiapine (Seroquel).

Nursing Considerations

Educating the client and any caregivers will be an essential component of nursing care. The disabilities that accompany schizophrenia are complex, and it takes experience to understand the priorities of care. Long-term therapy is required. Family and caregivers will need supportive counseling. A program of home care with respite care, medical assistance, and social service assistance is preferred to hospitalization. The nurse may be a case manager who coordinates medical, psychological, and other necessary therapies. The case manager can assist by helping to locate social and financial services as well as Internet and local support groups. Improvement in symptoms will take time; several weeks of medication may be necessary before results are evident. It is essential that the child and the caregivers maintain the regimen of medications. When symptoms diminish or disappear, it means that the medications are effective. It is important to differentiate the concept of medical management from the false hope that the disorder has gone away and the medications are no longer necessary.

STUDENT SYNTHESIS

KEY POINTS

1. Individuals with special needs may require assistance due to vision, hearing, speech, or behavioral problems.
2. Visual and hearing impairment may be the result of genetic or acquired problems, for example, color blindness.
3. Intellectual and developmental disabilities are unique to the person. Symptoms may be mild or severe and may vary in intensity and frequency.
4. A genetic disorder results from an abnormality in genes passed from one generation to another. A congenital disorder is one that is present at birth. An acquired disorder may occur any time after birth and be the result of newborn exposure to teratogens, infections, or trauma.
5. Maternal use of alcohol or drugs and other teratogens during pregnancy can result in physical or mental abnormalities in a newborn.
6. Fetal alcohol spectrum disorder is preventable if the pregnant parent abstains from drinking alcohol during pregnancy.
7. Individuals with neuromuscular disabilities often have motor, sensory, and developmental delays, and feeding problems.
8. A multidisciplinary, team approach is essential to achieve the best possible outcomes for the individual with an intellectual or developmental disability.
9. Down syndrome and fragile X syndrome are chromosomal abnormalities with resulting physical and intellectual impairment.
10. Individuals with ADHD have difficulty with attention span, impulsivity, and hyperactivity.
11. Individuals with Tourette syndrome have involuntary movements called tics and uncontrolled vocalizations.
12. Autism spectrum disorder is complex and often characterized by intellectual, social, and communication deficits that vary in severity.
13. Plumbism can be acute, chronic, or fatal. Lead sources in the home and environment are the major causes.
14. Cerebral palsy may be a result of prenatal infections, fetal hypoxia, birth trauma, meningitis, or head trauma.
15. Duchenne muscular dystrophy is an inherited degenerative disorder, which eventually is fatal.
16. The risk factors for suicide include depression, poor self-esteem, and schizophrenia.

CRITICAL THINKING EXERCISES

1. C. J. is a 6-year-old boy who has been diagnosed with ADHD. Using your understanding of ADHD, build a teaching plan that will help to organize his daily health habits.
2. K. K. is a 32-year-old woman with schizophrenia who lives at home with her parents, who are in their late 50s. Consider the issues and possible concerns for the aging parental caregivers. Compare and contrast the issues of adults with intellectual and developmental disorders with the issues of a newly diagnosed special needs child.

NCLEX-STYLE REVIEW QUESTIONS

1. A client with Ashkenazi Jewish ancestry is suspected to be pregnant. The client is concerned about the child having Tay–Sachs disease. For what testing option should the nurse prepare the client?
    a. A complete blood count (CBC) at 16–18 weeks
    b. An MRI upon confirmation of pregnancy
    c. Chorionic villus sampling between 10 and 12 weeks
    d. An amniocentesis between 4 and 5 weeks
2. A client is diagnosed with hemochromatosis. What should the nurse be sure to include when reinforcing education? Select all that apply.
    a. Avoid vitamin C supplements
    b. Avoid iron supplements
    c. Avoid vegetables
    d. Avoid eating raw shellfish
    e. Avoid alcohol intake
3. A newborn is observed to have tremors, hyperactive reflexes, a high-pitched cry, and irritability. What action does the nurse anticipate performing first?
    a. Obtain urine and meconium for drug screen.
    b. Report the mother to child protective service.
    c. Increase stimulation of the newborn.
    d. Withhold all feedings.
4. Which pregnant client is at greatest risk for having a child with Down syndrome?
    a. A 25-year-old client who smokes
    b. A 35-year-old client with four children
    c. A 16-year-old client without prenatal care
    d. A 45-year-old client with a previous child with Down syndrome
5. A child with attention deficit hyperactivity disorder is taking methylphenidate (Ritalin). What information should the nurse give the parents?
    a. Healthcare providers will regularly measure height, weight, and plot on growth chart.
    b. Give several directions at one time so the child can learn to prioritize.
    c. Alter routines to prevent boredom.
    d. Point out negative behaviors.

CHAPTER RESOURCES

Enhance your learning with additional resources on thePoint!
Student Resources related to this chapter can be found at
thePoint.lww.com/Rosdahl12e.

Adult Care Nursing | UNIT 12

75 Skin Disorders

Learning Objectives

1. Differentiate among the following diagnostic tests: Wood light examination, Tzanck smear, tissue biopsy, and scabies scraping.
2. Discuss the two major types of skin grafts, including nursing considerations for the care of skin grafts.
3. Identify types of skin lesions, providing an example of each type.
4. State possible nursing diagnoses for a client with a chronic skin disorder.
5. Relate three nursing interventions for the care of a client with pruritus.
6. Discuss the following conditions, including nursing considerations for each condition: acute and chronic skin conditions (urticaria, vitiligo, dermatitis, eczema, and psoriasis); infections (warts, impetigo, and folliculitis); parasitic infestations (scabies, lice, and bedbugs); and sebaceous gland disorders (sebaceous cysts, seborrhea, seborrheic dermatitis, and dandruff).
7. Identify the four mechanisms that cause burns, and explain how burns are classified according to depth and size.
8. Describe the three phases of recovery in burn therapy, including evaluation protocols and treatment of fluid and electrolyte imbalances, respiratory dysfunction, renal changes, infection, and pain.
9. Describe four types of dressings, four types of topical medications, and the processes of débridement and skin grafting that may be used when treating burns.
10. Identify the complications that can occur during burn recovery, and discuss nursing considerations during the rehabilitative stage of burn healing.
11. Identify three common nonmalignant and malignant skin lesions, and discuss interventions that can be used to prevent skin cancer.

Important Terminology

allograft	débridement	furuncle	neoplasm	warts	
angioedema	dermatitis	graft	pruritus	Wood light	
angioma	dermatology	heterograft	psoriasis	xenograft	
autograft	eczema	homograft	scabies scraping		
biopsy	electrodesiccation	impetigo	Tzanck smear		
carbuncle	eschar	isograft	urticaria		
cryosurgery	folliculitis	keloid	vitiligo		

Acronyms

CEA
NPWT
UV
UVA
UVB

The *integumentary system* is composed of the skin (the epidermis and dermis) and its accessory organs, including epithelial and connective tissue, nerves, and sweat and oil glands (Chapter 16).

Dermatology is the study of skin diseases; a *dermatologist* is a healthcare provider who specializes in this field. Nurses specializing in the care of people with skin disorders are called *dermatologic nurses*. Nurses commonly see skin problems in their clients. For instance, infants sometimes have rashes, and older people may have problems with itching. Common terminology for skin disorders is found in Box 75-1. Some systemic disorders include skin manifestations. These conditions are discussed throughout this unit along with the body system that is primarily involved in the condition.

One of the most common skin conditions that affects the client and nursing care is the development of skin breakdown. Dermatology has several names for skin breakdown. The term *pressure injury* is also known as decubitus ulcer, dermal ulcer, pressure wound, pressure sore, or skin ulcer. The National Pressure Injury Advisory Panel (NPIAP) defines a pressure injury as an area of unrelieved pressure over a defined area, usually over a bony prominence, resulting in ischemia, cell death, and tissue necrosis. Pressure injuries are discussed in Chapter 58.

Box. 75-1	Commonly Used Terminology in Skin Disorders
Abrasion	Scraping of the skin surface
Dermatitis	Skin inflammation
Desquamation	Flaking or shedding of outer layers
Escar	Dead skin tissue, often crusty, scabbed, or leathery black in appearance
Excoriation	Abrasion of the epidermis; scraped area
Laceration	Jagged cut through the skin or tissue
Pruritus	Itching
Purpura	Discoloration of skin due to blood in the tissue outside a blood vessel (e.g., ecchymosis, petechiae, or hematoma)

DIAGNOSTIC TESTS

Direct observation is often the diagnostic tool used first to determine disorders of the integumentary system. However, many skin conditions are manifestations of disorders involving other body systems. If a systemic disorder has skin manifestations, the systemic disorder is first diagnosed, and then the symptoms appearing in the skin are treated. Some diagnostic tests used to determine the origin of a skin disorder include allergy skin testing, laboratory tests for blood dyscrasias (e.g., leukemia or systemic lupus erythematous), and blood glucose tests for diabetes mellitus. Other diagnostic tests may include the following:

- *Wood light* examination: Use of a special high-pressure mercury lamp that produces long-wave ultraviolet (**UV**) rays to diagnose pigmentary abnormalities and to detect superficial fungal and bacterial skin infections.
- *Tzanck smear:* Examination of cells and fluids from *vesicles* (blisters), such as those found in herpes zoster and varicella. Tissue is scraped from the base of the vesicle and applied to a glass slide, and then a specific stain is applied. Under a microscope, multinucleated giant cells are diagnostic for herpesvirus or varicella.
- *Biopsy:* The procedure of removing a skin tissue specimen with scalpel excision, punch instrument, or shaving technique for microscopic examination to rule out malignancy or diagnose a skin disorder.
- *Scabies scraping:* Diagnoses scabies (a parasite that burrows under the skin): Obtained by shaving the top of a suspected lesion, placing the specimen on a microscope slide that has been covered with immersion oil, and examining the slide under a microscope.

COMMON MEDICAL TREATMENTS

Clients with skin disorders often are uncomfortable. Therefore, treatment is aimed at providing comfort and treating systemic problems. The healthcare provider may order moist dressings, packs, or therapeutic baths.

Assisting the Client Who Has Pruritus

Pruritus (itching) is often a symptom of a skin disease, but may also arise from other systemic disorders, such as kidney or liver disease, iron deficiency, cancer, diabetes mellitus, and thyroid disturbances. Dry skin may cause pruritus, particularly for older adults. The main problem with pruritus is that the client is almost irresistibly compelled to scratch. Scratching can lead to skin breaks, which can become infected and cause scarring.

Telling a client not to scratch probably will be futile. Try to divert their attention with other activities. Antianxiety drugs, antihistamines, or topical corticosteroids are sometimes ordered. Educate clients about the proper use of such medications. In Practice: Important Medications 75-1 summarizes the most common medications used to control pruritus.

Be sure to document the client's reactions, noting which measures are effective. Most clients appreciate advice on how to cope with itching (In Practice: Educating the Client 75-1).

IN PRACTICE
IMPORTANT MEDICATIONS 75-1 For Pruritus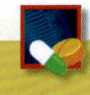

Antihistamines
- Chlorpheniramine (Chlor-Trimeton)
- Diphenhydramine HCl (Benadryl)
- Fexofenadine (Allegra)
- Loratadine (Claritin, Alavert)

Antianxiety Drugs/Antihistamines
- Hydroxyzine HCl (Atarax, Vistaril)

Nursing Considerations
- These medications often cause drowsiness. Warn the client not to drive or work around machinery.
- Alcohol and other sedating drugs potentiate these medications. Urge the client to avoid these.
- Dry mouth is a common side effect. Encourage the client to drink juices and other fluids, not just water. Sucking on hard candy or ice chips, popsicles, or chewing sugarless gum is helpful.
- Other side effects may include stomach distress, diarrhea, constipation (administer medication with milk or food), and urinary frequency or retention.
- Before any allergy skin testing, antihistamines should be discontinued for 4 days before the testing to preserve test accuracy.
- Sunscreen use is recommended to avoid photosensitivity reactions.
- Older adults should use these medications with caution because the risk for sedative effects is greater in this population.

CHAPTER 75 Skin Disorders

IN PRACTICE
EDUCATING THE CLIENT 75-1 — Pruritus Prevention and Treatment

- Perform skin testing to determine allergens. Eliminate allergens if possible.
- Wash new clothes before wearing them.
- Rinse clothes in clear water. Avoid using fabric softeners, starch, and antistatic chemicals.
- Wear cotton clothing. Keep irritating materials away from the body. Avoid wool or lanolin.
- Shower immediately after swimming.
- Use nonallergenic makeup.
- Take only cool or lukewarm baths.
- Use soothing baths (colloidal oatmeal, starch) or localized skin preparations as ordered.
- Use lotion on dry skin if healthcare provider allows.
- Take medications as prescribed.
- Avoid activities that cause the body to become overheated.
- Keep fingernails short. Wear cotton gloves or cotton socks at night.
- Lightly slap, rather than scratch, the itching area. Slapping will provide the same stimulation as scratching but without continued irritation.
- If unable to exercise, sit in a rocking chair to provide some exercise without further skin irritation.
- Use relaxation audiotapes to assist in falling asleep.

Nursing Alert Follow Standard Precautions and appropriate Transmission-Based Precautions when caring for clients with skin problems. Such clients often have open, draining, or weeping wounds. Remember to wear gloves whenever there is possible contact with any body fluids or drainage; wear eye goggles and a gown if any possibility of splashing exists.

IN PRACTICE
NURSING CARE GUIDELINES 75-1 — Giving a Therapeutic Bath

- Follow Standard Precautions. Disinfect the tub or tank before and after use according to facility policies and procedures. *Rationale: Colloids and oils used in these baths are often difficult to remove.*
- Give a therapeutic bath in a bathtub or whirlpool tank. *Rationale: The fluid environment of water reaches irritated or burned areas readily. The whirlpool is therapeutic because it increases circulation, helps remove dead skin cells, and promotes healing.*
- Use tepid water (not hotter than 100 °F/30 °C). *Rationale: A very hot bath aggravates pruritus.*
- Protect the client from falling. *Rationale: The tub will be very slippery, particularly if oil is used.*
- Follow the provider's orders regarding the substance to use, the length of time the client is to be in the bath, and other treatments to perform at the same time. *Rationale: Agents added to bath water often contain oatmeal or other cereals, starch, tars, and baking soda. Detergents and antipruritic preparations may be ordered. These agents help in the treatment of pruritus. Additional therapies, such as range of motion or removal of eschar, may be performed at the same time as the bath.*
- Use medicated bath oil instead of soap. *Rationale: Soap has drying effects, which can aggravate pruritus.*
- Pat the client's skin dry after the therapeutic bath. *Rationale: Rubbing increases irritation or pruritus.*
- Use nonirritating linens, which are typically kept separately from standard facility linen supplies. *Rationale: Nonirritating linens protect the client's skin from coming in contact with abrasive or allergenic chemicals typically found in standard facility linens.*
- Place soiled linens in a labeled laundry bag and send it to the laundry according to facility protocols. *Rationale: Facilities have special laundering procedures or purchase special commercial linen packages that are used for burn clients or clients with special skin care needs.*

Giving Therapeutic Baths

A therapeutic bath is used not only to cleanse the body but also to soothe the skin and relax the client. It promotes wound healing, relieves itching, and helps remove **eschar**, the dry crust that results after trauma (e.g., pressure injuries), infection (e.g., skin infections), or injury (e.g., burns). One type of therapeutic bath, often to a specific body part, is the whirlpool bath typically found in physical therapy. Therapeutic baths offer a way of applying medication to the entire body at one time. The therapeutic bath also provides warmth so that the client can perform physical therapy and range of motion (ROM) exercises more comfortably (In Practice: Nursing Care Guidelines 75-1).

Applying Moist Dressings

Moist packs are applied to reduce swelling and weeping in acute **dermatitis** (skin inflammation), to soften and remove exudate and crusts, and to relieve pruritus and discomfort. These dressings may be clean or sterile, depending on whether the client's skin is intact. The moist dressing may be closed or open. A *closed dressing* is covered with plastic or a firm material. An *open dressing* is not covered because the lack of oxygen may cause tissue necrosis. In an open dressing, fluid evaporates rapidly, and the dressing requires frequent changing or resoaking. Chapter 58 has additional information regarding wounds and wound care. In Practice: Nursing Care Guidelines 75-2 provides information about the application of dressings.

Débriding a Wound

Débridement of a wound is the removal of dead, devitalized, contaminated tissue, foreign materials, or eschar. Foreign materials in a wound can include necrotic tissue, bone fascia, and nonviable tissue such as muscle or ligaments.

IN PRACTICE
NURSING CARE GUIDELINES 75-2: Application of Moist Dressings

- Explain the procedure to the client. Medicate with analgesics and anxiolytics (antianxiety) 30–60 min before the procedure. *Rationale: These medications provide pain relief and relaxation. The client's cooperation is necessary when applying dressings. Premedicating to minimize pain during the procedure facilitates cooperation and promotes healing.*
- Follow Standard Procedures. Wear goggles and sterile gloves when changing dressings. Wear gown and mask if splashing is likely. *Rationale: Assume that the wound is contaminated and be proactive in preventing the spread of microorganisms.*
- Use aseptic technique throughout the procedure. *Rationale: Infection is commonly the cause of morbidity and mortality of clients with large wounds or burns. Sterile technique protects the client and the nurse.*
- Premoisten existing dressings with warmed, sterile, normal saline if ordered. *Rationale: When the dressing is being removed, the use of premoistened dressings is less traumatic to the wound because the moisture helps to prevent damage to new, fragile healing areas.*
- Use the correct type of solution and the specific type of dressing as directed by the primary healthcare provider. *Rationale: Many solutions, such as aluminum acetate (Burow solution), silver nitrate, and potassium permanganate, can be used on moist dressings. Generally, a pharmacy will provide the prepared solution. Dressings are available in many varieties and may have specific properties or uses for healing. Use of the wrong type of dressing can be harmful to the client.*
- Apply dressing according to specific protocol. Use provided commercial directions and/or follow facility policies and procedures. *Rationale: Sometimes it is necessary to soak the pack in the solution and apply it, lightly dripping, to the affected area. With other types of dressings, it is necessary to apply a layer of ointment over the burned area.*
- Change the dressing as indicated by healthcare provider or policy. *Rationale: Directions for the different types of dressings will be available in the facility's policy and procedure manual and/or in the commercial product directions. Sometimes it will be necessary to keep the pack wet and to change or resaturate the moist pack at least every 2 hr. Some types of dressings are changed completely three or four times per day.*
- Protect the bed, the rest of the client's body, and the nurse's body from contact with the medication or solution. *Rationale: The medications or solutions may be caustic or cause staining of skin or clothing or linens.*
- Use a bed cradle when applying packs to the client's legs or torso. Place blankets over the cradle. *Rationale: Keeping the linens off the client's legs or torso prevents wicking of the solutions into the linens. Wet areas can cause a loss in body temperature and skin cooling due to the effects of evaporation, convection, and conduction. Extra blankets over a bed cradle can keep in warm air, minimize heat loss, and protect the client from chilling.*
- Be sure to document the procedure and your observations when removing packs. *Rationale: Documentation is a legal requirement and promotes communication between healthcare providers.*
- Documentation should include general skin condition: extra dry indicates dehydration; wet, soupy texture and strong odor indicate infection; redness and swelling at the edge of the wound indicate cellulitis; and clean, pink, shiny appearance indicates healthy healing. *Rationale: Documentation of progress or lack of progress is essential. Changes in the nursing care plan must be made according to need, that is, changes in type of dressings applied.*
- Additionally, document improvement or lack of improvement noted since last dressing change, skin color, signs of infection, presence of eschar, presence or absence of pain, and how well the client tolerated the procedure. *Rationale: Overall improvement or lack of improvement in the client's condition will affect the healing process. Implementation of changes to nursing care plans depends upon accurate observational and documentation skills.*
- Used dressings are considered contaminated; dispose of them correctly. *Rationale: Standard Precautions and facility policies will dictate the correct disposal procedure for dressings that have been removed.*

The presence of nonviable tissue and foreign bodies increases the chances for active infection, reduces the client's ability to fight any local infection, and increases the possibility of a systemic infection or sepsis. The rationale for débridement is to reduce a source of infection, such as bacteria, that inhibits the healing process. It is a sterile procedure that is often performed when changing moist packs. The nurse may assist with débridement. Receive full instruction how to carry out the procedure because each client requires different treatment.

Several methods can be ordered by the healthcare provider for wound débridement. The débridement method will depend upon many factors, including age of wound, age of client, size, position, original cause of wound, and factors that are inhibiting healing, such as infection. Some types of wound care are more expensive than other types of treatments. Additional factors of débridement include pain management during dressing changes and pain control for the client's overall condition. The amount of exudate, the risk of infection, or the presence of infection is also considered.

Autolysis (autolytic) is a method that uses the body's own enzymes and moisture to rehydrate the wound and dissolve wound slough. With this method, an occlusive or semiocclusive dressing is used to cover the wound; frequency of dressing changes is determined by the healthcare provider.

Enzymatic débridement involves the use of commercially prepared chemical enzymes applied to the necrotic tissue of the wound. Considered a highly selective method of wound débridement, it uses naturally occurring proteolytic enzymes that are manufactured by the pharmaceutical and healthcare industry specifically for wound débridement. These exogenous enzymes work in collaboration with natural endogenous enzymes. There are several types: collagenase-based, papain-based (papain/urea), fibrinolysin/DNAse, trypsin, a streptokinase–streptodornase combination, and subtilisin. The most commonly used are the collagenase-based and papain-based enzymes. *Collagenase-based débridement* is often used because it has the advantage of being painless, causing minimal amounts of blood loss, and is selective in removing dead tissue. It is appropriate for both long-term and home care. *Papain-based débridement* is useful for clients who have decreased sensations of pain (e.g., spinal cord injury) because this therapy causes more localized pain.

Mechanical débridement utilizes wet-to-moist or wet-to-dry dressings. As the dressing dries and is then removed, some of the necrotic tissue that adheres to the dressing is removed with the dressing change.

Surgical débridement (sharp débridement) is normally done by the healthcare provider. Either a scalpel or scissors is used to remove slough and eschar. This can be done at the bedside or in the operating room.

Biosurgical débridement (myiasis) is a technique that uses sterile maggots, which are known to débride and heal wounds without damaging surrounding healthy tissue.

COMMON SURGICAL TREATMENTS

Plastic Surgery

Although skin disorders make clients physically uncomfortable, disfigurement is one of the most damaging psychological effects. Plastic surgery is one way to improve or correct disfigurement. It may be performed for cosmetic effects, to repair congenital defects, or to repair the results of trauma. Plastic surgery is also called *reconstructive surgery*.

Skin and Tissue Grafts

Skin grafts are used to cover areas of skin lost through wounds, burns, or infections. A **graft** is a transplant of skin taken from the client (autograft) or a donor (allograft) that is placed on clean, viable tissue. Grafting is a painstaking procedure that may be done in stages. Grafting may take many months, depending on the size and number of areas to be covered and the success of each step.

There are several types of grafts. One type is called a *free graft*, which means that skin has been completely removed from its original site and grafted onto the recipient site. The other type is *pedicle-flap graft*. In this type of graft, one end of the graft remains attached to the donor site so that it can continue to receive nourishment until new circulation is established. The other end is attached to the recipient site on the same client's body. In some situations, the client must assume an unnatural position until the graft begins to grow in the new site, at which time the graft can be separated from the donor site. A pedicle-*free* graft is used when a large area of skin is to be replaced, such as on an ear, part of a hand or foot, or a large part of the face.

Other types of grafts are named in relation to the donor and are described in more detail in the section of this chapter on burns.

Nursing Considerations

Before reconstructive or graft surgery, prepare the client by explaining what they can expect. Postoperatively, the surgical site may be swollen and bruised. Pay scrupulous attention to aseptic technique, protect the grafts, keep new grafts immobilized, and prevent infection at donor sites.

Emotional support is an important part of nursing care in reconstructive surgery. The client is often self-conscious about his or her appearance and may avoid others. Encourage family and friends to visit. Provide the client with emotional support and reassurance.

NURSING PROCESS

DATA COLLECTION

Carefully observe and document the skin condition of all clients. Establish a baseline for future comparison and report any changes that occur. Compare skin color with the client's usual color, texture, and turgor. Note whether the skin is intact; examine for any lesions or pressure injuries. Carefully document the size, color, texture, location, pattern of disruption, or any other distinctive characteristics of the lesion. Figure 75-1 highlights several types of common skin lesions. Always use correct terminology to describe variations from normal skin appearance (Box 75-1). In addition, ask the client about subjective symptoms, such as itching (pruritus).

NCLEX Alert

As a major component of nursing care, observation of the skin is a normal clinical task. Therefore, on an NCLEX examination, expect to answer questions relating to your observations and the priority for interventions needed for these observations.

SPECIAL CONSIDERATIONS — Culture and Ethnicity

Variations in Skin Appearance
All color types of skin can become sunburned. Be aware of normal biocultural variations in the skin's appearance. If possible, ask the client or family to describe any variations from normal skin appearance.

Primary lesions (originating from previously normal skin)

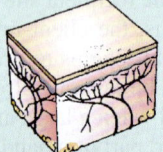

Type: Macule
Description: Flat, discolored spot on skin with sharp borders
Example: Freckle

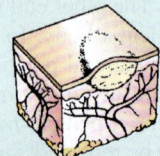

Type: Papule
Description: Solid elevations without fluid with sharp borders
Example: Mole

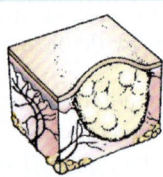

Type: Nodule, tumor
Description: Palpable, solid, elevated mass Nodules with distinct borders Tumors extending deep into the dermis
Example: Wart (nodule) Large lipoma (tumor)

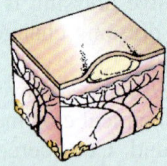

Type: Vesicle
Description: Small distinct elevation with fluid
Example: Blister caused by herpes simplex

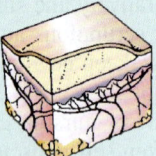

Type: Bulla
Description: Large distinct elevation with fluid
Example: Large friction or burn blister

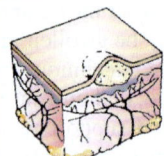

Type: Pustule
Description: Vesicle or bulla filled with purulent fluid
Example: Acne, carbuncles

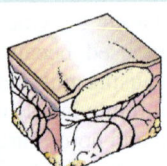

Type: Wheal
Description: Localized area of edema, often irregular and of variable size and color
Example: Hive, insect bite

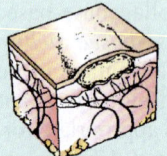

Type: Plaque
Description: Larger, flat, elevated, solid surface
Example: Psoriasis

Secondary lesions (originating from a primary lesion)

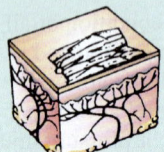

Type: Scale
Description: Thin or thick flake of skin varying in color; usually secondary to desquamated, dead epithelium
Example: Dandruff

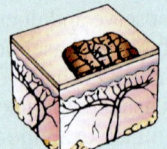

Type: Crust
Description: Dried residue of exudates
Example: Residue of impetigo

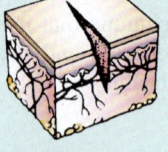

Type: Fissure
Description: Linear crack in the skin
Example: Athlete's foot

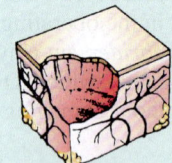

Type: Ulcer
Description: Opening in the skin caused by sloughing of necrotic tissue, extending past the epidermis
Example: Pressure ulcer, stasis ulcer

Figure 75-1 Common skin lesions.

Fluid and Electrolyte Balance

Data collection should include an understanding of the client's fluid and electrolyte status. A client's fluid and electrolyte balance and general nutrition may be difficult to maintain because of developing exudates or serum loss stemming from inflammation or burns. Encourage the client to drink and eat. Provide a high-calorie, high-protein diet. Carefully document the client's intake and output (I&O). Initiate a calorie count for clients who are at risk for poor nutrition. Individuals who have large surface area grafts or deep burn injuries usually require electrolyte replacement.

Allergies

As part of data collection, ask the client if they have known food or drug allergies. Food allergies may cause or aggravate skin disorders. Clients may also be sensitive to products such as tape, iodine, latex, or fragrances. Clients may know their allergies, or skin tests may determine them. Use more than one approach with the client when discussing allergies. For example, the client may deny being allergic to all antibiotics. Instead, ask the client specific questions such as, "Have you ever had an unexpected reaction to penicillin, shellfish, peanuts, or other foods or medicines?" Protect the client from exposure to known allergens.

Emotional Support for Clients With Skin Disorders

During data collection, determine your client's support system and coping mechanisms. A relationship may exist between emotional difficulties and skin problems—an underlying psychological problem may manifest itself in some type of skin eruption. Furthermore, the itching that accompanies many skin disorders gives rise to emotional distress; pruritus is often more irritating and difficult to control than pain.

Observe the client's emotional response to the skin disorder or disease by answering the following questions. Is the client so disabled by pain or itching that they need assistance or encouragement to meet daily needs? Is the disorder so disfiguring that it affects social activities or self-esteem? Is the client anxious or fearful of the outcome? Is the situation life threatening?

PLANNING AND IMPLEMENTATION

Involve the client when planning effective care (based on the nursing diagnoses) to meet their needs. Provide preoperative and postoperative care for the client undergoing plastic surgery or skin grafting. For the client with severe burns, assist in débridement of dead tissue or in life-sustaining treatments. The client with a skin disorder may also require assistance in meeting daily self-care needs, dealing with itching or pain, or working through the emotional aspects of a disfiguring or chronic disorder. Teach the client about the disorder and its necessary treatments. Develop a nursing care plan to meet each individual's needs.

Planning and implementing care includes relieving pruritus, providing therapeutic baths, and applying dressings. Basic nursing care, such as turning the client, assisting with hygiene, and observing and preventing pressure injuries, is also essential.

Chronic skin problems can present emotional challenges. Often, the same disorder flares up at intervals throughout the client's life. The client may require assistance to cope. Group therapy may be helpful.

As a result of the skin disorder, the client may feel that their outward appearance is unattractive. Foster an atmosphere of acceptance and support. Allow the client to express their feelings and provide companionship.

The use of touch can be therapeutic. The nurse may touch the client who has a skin condition with clean, ungloved hands, unless the client is contagious or has open or draining lesions. Touch can be equally effective with gloved hands.

EVALUATION

Routinely evaluate outcomes of care. Include the client, family, and all members of the healthcare team. Have you met short-term goals? Are long-term goals still realistic? What rehabilitation, home care, or other community services (if any) does the client need, especially if the skin disorder is chronic or requires continued treatment? In planning for further care, consider the client's prognosis, complications, and responses.

ACUTE AND CHRONIC SKIN CONDITIONS

Urticaria

Urticaria, commonly called *hives*, is characterized by the sudden appearance of edematous, raised pink areas called *wheals* that itch and burn. Hives may disappear quickly or they may remain for several days. In most instances, acute urticaria is a manifestation of an allergic reaction to medications, foods, spores, or pollens.

Contact allergens, such as face powder, can cause contact dermatitis. The most common contact allergens are soaps, nickel-based jewelry, perfumes, dyes, plants (e.g., poison ivy), chemicals, rubber, and insecticides. Stress and anxiety are thought to be important aggravating factors.

Urticaria that lasts more than 6 weeks is called *chronic urticaria*. Its exact cause remains unknown in the vast majority of people. Examine the client with an unexplained rash for the possibility of Lyme disease.

Edema associated with urticaria is only a temporary annoyance, unless it involves extensive vital areas. However, **angioedema** (swelling) can be a life-threatening condition that is similar to urticaria, but involves deeper dermal and subcutaneous tissues. Angioedema commonly affects the lips, eyelids, skin, gastrointestinal tract, hands, feet, genitalia, tongue, and larynx. If the larynx becomes edematous, the client may develop severe respiratory distress due to airway obstruction.

The best treatment for urticaria is identification and removal of its cause. Treat mild reactions with cold compresses or tepid colloidal oatmeal or baking soda baths. Antipruritic lotions, such as calamine, may help. Nonsedating antihistamines, such as fexofenadine HCl (Allegra), are often used for chronic urticaria. In severe cases, epinephrine may be administered. Chapter 84 discusses specific nursing care of the client who has an allergy.

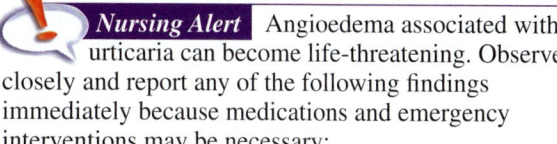

Nursing Alert Angioedema associated with urticaria can become life-threatening. Observe closely and report any of the following findings immediately because medications and emergency interventions may be necessary:
- Extreme swelling of the lips
- Swelling around the eyes
- Dyspnea (difficult breathing)

Vitiligo

Vitiligo occurs when areas of the skin are completely lacking in pigmentation. Pigment cells (*melanocytes*) cannot be detected in the depigmented areas, resulting in patches or areas of very pale, white-looking skin. The cause of vitiligo is unknown. No effective remedy is known. Surgical treatments include minigrafting and melanocyte transplantation. The treatment is prolonged and time consuming and must take place under a healthcare provider's supervision. Cosmetics designed to cover birthmarks may be used to mask vitiligo. Areas of skin that are not pigmented are more susceptible to sunburn and skin cancers; thus, it is important for clients with vitiligo to use a sunscreen with a high sun protection factor (SPF) and to monitor closely for any skin changes that appear cancerous.

> **SPECIAL CONSIDERATIONS** **Culture and Ethnicity**
>
> **Detecting Pigment Changes**
> Vitiligo is more obvious in darker-skinned individuals.

Eczema

Eczema, also known as *atopic dermatitis*, is a form of dermatitis (Fig. 75-2). This condition causes small vesicles to appear, as well as reddened and pruritic skin. Sometimes, the vesicles burst and ooze, forming crusts. Persistent irritation and scratching make the skin appear leathery and thick. Affected individuals may develop viral, bacterial, or fungal skin infections. Eczema may spread to other areas, but it is commonly found in the folds of the elbows, the backs of the knees, and on the face, neck, wrists, hands, and feet. It may disappear completely for months or sometimes years but can recur at any time.

Although the exact cause is unknown, eczema is known to be associated with heredity, allergy, and emotional stress. There may also be an autoimmune component. Sometimes, a family history indicates an allergy, such as hay fever or asthma. Children who have eczema often develop these conditions later. As a client grows older, emotional factors can aggravate eczema.

The goal of treatment is to prevent skin dryness, cracking, and itching. Treatment consists of applying moisturizing creams, corticosteroid ointments, tar solutions, or wet dressings to inflamed skin or using starch baths. Antihistamines may relieve the itching, and antianxiety drugs may relieve the tension or anxiety that contributes to the condition. Instruct the client to use soaps that are less alkaline and contain no lanolin. Recommend the use of lanolin-free lotions. Teach clients to avoid contact with wool.

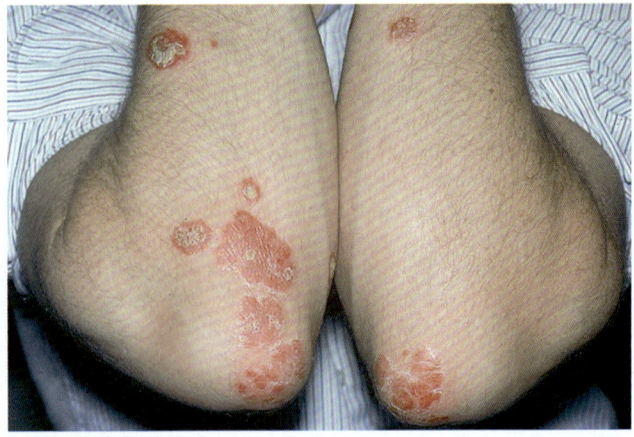

Figure 75-3 Characteristic primary lesions of psoriasis.

> **NCLEX Alert**
>
> On NCLEX examination questions, skin conditions or disorders can contain concerns related to priority observations and interventions. For example, does the clinical scenario provide an example of an emergency case of urticaria as with anaphylaxis? For other conditions, such as psoriasis, be observant for self-esteem concerns.

Psoriasis

Psoriasis is a chronic, noncontagious, proliferative skin disorder that most commonly affects young adults and people of early middle age (Fig. 75-3). Epidermal cells rapidly proliferate and form small, scaly patches of skin. The primary cause is unknown, although hereditary, environmental, metabolic, or immune factors contribute to an outbreak of psoriasis. The course of the disorder is unpredictable. In most clients, the disease remains localized.

In some individuals, however, the severity is incompatible with a productive life. Spontaneous clearing is rare, but unexplained exacerbations (flare-ups) and improvement are common. Stress and anxiety frequently precede the disease's exacerbations.

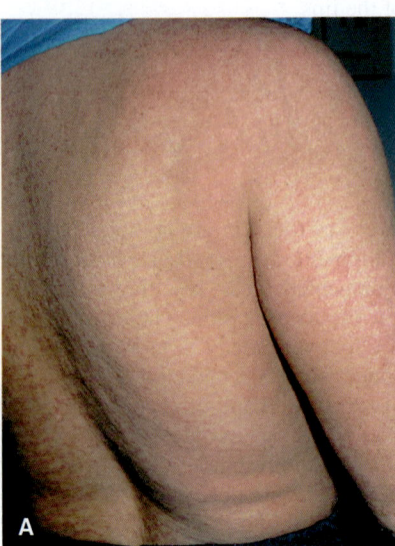
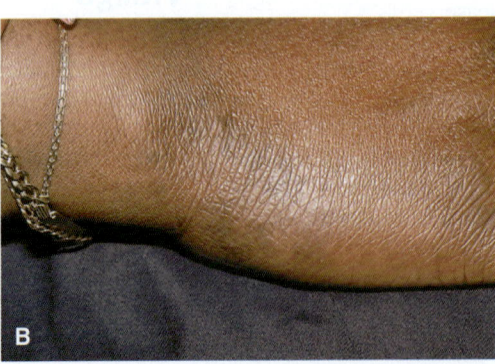

Figure 75-2 Examples of atopic dermatitis (eczema). Atopic dermatitis with reddened and pruritic skin is present on the **(A)** upper torso and **(B)** arm of a patient.

Signs and Symptoms

The hallmark of psoriasis is red papules covered with silvery, yellow–white scales that the client constantly sheds. These patches appear mainly on the extensor surfaces of the elbows and knees, on the scalp, and on the lower back. The nails may begin to loosen at the beginning of the fingertips (*onycholysis*).

Medical Treatment

Generally, treatment of psoriasis is never completely successful. The main objective is to reduce scaling and itching. Therapeutic baths, wet dressings, or lubricating ointments may be helpful, followed by application of emollient creams to soften the scaling. Specialized shampoos are used to treat scalp psoriasis. Corticosteroids may be injected into psoriatic lesions. UV light treatment or sun exposure may be useful but requires careful supervision. Methotrexate, cyclosporine (Gengraf), and oral retinoids (synthetic derivatives of vitamin A) are useful in clients with severe, extensive psoriasis. However, methotrexate may cause hepatic or renal damage, bone marrow suppression, nausea, and fatigue. Biologic agents may be helpful, such as etanercept (Enbrel), alefacept (Amevive), efalizumab, and infliximab (Remicade). Photochemotherapy, which combines a photosensitizing agent (psoralen) with UV light, may also be used.

INFECTIONS

Warts

Warts (verrucae) are small, flesh-colored, brown or yellow papules caused by the human papillomavirus (HPV). Most warts are not painful, with the exception of the plantar wart that occurs on the sole of the foot and grows inward due to the pressure of body weight.

Common warts are found most often on the hands, especially of children, or on other sites often subjected to trauma. They may grow anywhere on the skin. *Filiform warts* are slender, soft, thin, fingerlike growths seen primarily on the face and neck. *Plantar* or *palmar warts* are firm, elevated, or flat lesions occurring on the soles or palms.

Common, plantar, and palmar warts are most often treated with salicylic acid or liquid nitrogen (cryosurgery). Flat warts are most often treated with cryotherapy or topical applications of 5-fluorouracil, imiquimod (Aldara), or tretinoin (Renova). Filiform warts are most often treated with snip or shave excision or contact freezing of the wart. Some warts resolve without treatment.

Bacterial Skin Infections

Impetigo and folliculitis are the primary bacterial infections of the skin.

Impetigo, most commonly caused by streptococcal or staphylococcal bacteria, is contagious among infants and young children (Chapter 73). Adults are also susceptible to impetigo, but generally have better handwashing techniques than do young children, so adult outbreaks are usually not as severe. The characteristic vesicles ooze a clear exudate, which develops a golden yellow crust that causes local discomfort and pruritus. When the crust is removed, a smooth, red, moist surface remains.

Medications for topical treatment of impetigo are mupirocin (Bactroban) and retapamulin (Altabax). Impetigo caused by *Staphylococcus aureus* and streptococcal infections can be treated with systemic antibiotics (e.g., dicloxacillin [Dycill] and cephalexin [Keflex]). Daily bathing with an antibacterial soap helps remove the crusts. Because the bacteria transfer from the infected client to another person through touch, teach clients to avoid touching the exudates and crusts to prevent the spread of infection. Wear gloves when bathing the client or treating the lesions.

Folliculitis is a staphylococcal infection starting around the hair follicle. Prolonged moisture, trauma, and poor hygiene often contribute to this problem. Lesions consist of white pustules or follicular nodules that are superficial or deep. The face is a common site for *deep folliculitis*. *Superficial folliculitis* may respond to aggressive topical hygiene with antibacterial soaps and the use of topical antibiotics. Folliculitis of the beard can be difficult to treat and may require the use of systemic antibiotics. Clients with curly facial hair often have more difficulty because their hairs easily become ingrown. Teach clients to change their razor blade daily and to avoid shaving too closely.

Folliculitis may lead to the production of a **furuncle**, also called a *boil*. A furuncle starts as a firm, red, tender nodule. After a few days, the furuncle may drain pus and finally extrude the core. The core is dead tissue that can drain spontaneously or be reabsorbed into the skin. A boil can also be surgically removed by incision and drainage (I&D). Furuncles are found most frequently in areas of hair-bearing skin that are subject to friction, irritation, and moisture, especially the face, scalp, buttocks, and axillae.

Furunculosis, the term for recurrent boils, develops in individuals who are unable to get rid of the *Staphylococcus* organism. No evidence has shown that these individuals harbor a particular strain of *Staphylococcus* or have any deficiency in their host defense mechanisms. A **carbuncle** is composed of several interconnecting boils in a cluster. A carbuncle usually drains at multiple sites; carbuncles are commonly found on the back of the neck, the back, and the thighs.

Wearing clean gloves, apply warm, wet dressings or soaks to localize boil and carbuncle infections to one spot. A healthcare provider may carefully incise and drain large boils after they come to a point. After boils are drained, the client will need only topical antibiotics. Furuncles or carbuncles associated with surrounding cellulitis or fever, or that are located on the upper lip, nose, cheek, or forehead, may be treated with oral antibiotics that are active against *Staphylococcus* organisms. A sensitivity test is obtained before starting treatment to determine the most effective antibiotic.

> **Nursing Alert** Picking or squeezing a boil is dangerous. Doing so may spread infection to surrounding tissues and possibly to the bloodstream. Advise clients to take special precautions with boils on the face because the skin area drains directly into the cranial venous sinuses. Microorganisms in that area can cause encephalitis or meningitis.

PARASITIC INFESTATIONS

Parasites live on another organism and take nutrition from it, often damaging the host organism. Scabies, lice, and bedbugs are common parasites found in humans. (See Chapter 72 for additional information regarding scabies or lice in children.)

Scabies

Scabies is caused by mites (*Sarcoptes scabiei*) that burrow under the outer layer of the host's skin. One month or more after the mites enter the body, the host's skin develops intense itching, especially when heavily covered. Red spots appear, with a row of blackish dots that are one-eighth to one-half inch long with tiny vesicles and depressions. Scabies is found especially between the fingers. Other possible sites include the wrist, front of the elbow, elbow points, axillary folds, nipples, umbilicus, lower abdomen, genitalia, and gluteal cleft (between the buttocks). Adults rarely have scabies above the neck; however, the mites may affect children on any body surface. Mites can live for months or years in persons who are untreated or who have poor hygiene.

Typically, people acquire scabies primarily through close personal contact. However, the infection can be transmitted through clothing, linens, or towels. Because the parasites can live a long time without a host, and usually get into bed clothing and personal garments, use special precautions to keep scabies from spreading. If possible, examine and treat all family members for scabies simultaneously. Begin treatment by having the affected individual bathe and towel dry to remove crusts and open infected spots. Application of the prescribed medication (e.g., permethrin [Nix] and diphenhydramine [Benadryl]) to the entire body from the neck down is the treatment of choice for children older than 2 months and nonpregnant adults. Systemic or topical antibiotics may be needed for secondary infections. Instruct the client to cover all body surfaces, including around the nail beds, between the fingers and toes, the genital area, and the cleft between the buttocks. Inform the client to leave the medication on for 8–24 hr, depending on the product used, and then to bathe thoroughly. The client will be instructed to repeat the treatment in 1 week.

Lice

Humans can be infested by three types of lice, called *pediculosis* (head lice; *Pediculus humanus capitis*), body lice (*Pediculus humanus corporis*), and *pubic lice* (*Pthirus pubis, Pediculosis pubis*), which inhabit the genital region. Lice may inhabit the hair of the axillae, beard, eyebrows, and eyelashes. Lice survive by sucking blood. They are difficult to eradicate because their eggs, called *nits*, can live for a long time on clothes, bedding, or upholstered furniture. Signs and symptoms include the presence of nits and extreme pruritus (itching). The disease is most common in children. Outbreaks are fairly common in schools and daycare centers.

> **Nursing Alert** Be alert for the presence of parasites, such as lice or scabies, when caring for a person who has lived on the streets or in shelters. Treat the infected person immediately to prevent transmission to others.

Medical Treatment

Head and pubic lice can be treated by over-the-counter preparations, but prescription medications may be needed. Instruct the client to follow product directions meticulously. It may be necessary to remove nits (lice eggs) by combing the hair with a fine-toothed comb. Warn the client not to apply pediculicidal agents near the eyes. Rather, apply petroleum jelly to the eyelashes and eyebrows and remove the nits by hand. For body lice, preparations containing lindane (Kwell) are highly effective. These preparations are applied directly to the affected area, allowed to remain for 8 hr, and then completely removed with soap and water. Lindane (Kwell) is also available as a shampoo. The treatment usually is repeated in 1 week. The first treatment should kill most live lice. The second treatment kills lice that hatch after the first treatment. After each treatment, inspect the client; treated nits are expected to remain. Look for live bugs. All lice must be killed and nits destroyed to prevent reinfestation. Refer also to Box 72-2, which describes nursing considerations for parasitic care.

Nursing Considerations

Treat everyone in the family and close contacts at the same time. Instruct the client to wear clean clothing. The client should use clean bed linens and should wash and dry clothing, bed linens, and towels using hot laundry water. The client should have unwashable items dry-cleaned and stored in a plastic bag for 30 days.

Bedbugs

The *bedbug (Cimex lectularius)* measures 4 to 5 mm and can survive up to 1 year without food. Bedbugs live in clothing or bedding and are difficult to eradicate. Bedbug bites appear as red macules that develop into nodules. The bites often appear in groups of three. Bedbugs usually bite the legs and feet, causing itching and burning. Lotions containing menthol, phenol, or 0.5% hydrocortisone are applied to the bitten areas. Spraying all crevices in furniture, mattresses, walls, and floors with an insecticide usually eliminates the insect.

SEBACEOUS GLAND DISORDERS

Sebaceous Cysts

Sebaceous glands secrete oils. When such glands become plugged, small hard nodules form, called *cysts*. *Sebaceous cysts* are not treated unless they become large and annoying, in the case of which they are drained or excised surgically.

Seborrhea, Seborrheic Dermatitis, and Dandruff

An excessive sebaceous discharge that forms large scales or cheeselike plugs on the body is known as *seborrhea*. *Seborrheic dermatitis* is a condition that causes scaling, primarily of the scalp, that is often associated with itching. This inflammatory condition erupts on body areas that have a large concentration of sebaceous glands (e.g., scalp, eyebrows, eyelids, ears, axillae, groin, and skin under the ears and the breasts). The dry form of seborrheic dermatitis (also known as *dandruff*) is characterized by scales ranging from small and dry, to thick and powdery, with little to no redness. The oily form of seborrheic dermatitis is characterized by greasy or oily scales and crusts on a red base.

Frequent shampooing is the mainstay of treatment, as advised by a provider. Some shampoos contain selenium sulfide suspension (e.g., Selsun Blue); others contain coal tar, salicylic acid and sulfur, or zinc pyrithione. Instruct the client to leave the shampoo on for 5–10 min. In some cases, lotions or solutions containing corticosteroids are prescribed. The client should use such products sparingly—once or twice daily—according to the provider's directions.

If the seborrheic dermatitis exists in a location other than the scalp, corticosteroid creams or ointments are prescribed. Although no known cure is available, a low-fat diet, exercise, sunlight, stress reduction, and rest can be helpful in management (In Practice: Educating the Client 75-1).

BURNS

Burns are traumatic injuries that result in tissue loss or damage. A burn destroys cells by increasing capillary permeability and damaging cellular proteins. Prevention is key. In Practice: Educating the Client 75-2 covers essential burn

---

IN PRACTICE
EDUCATING THE CLIENT 75-2 — Protection From Fires and Burns

Around the Home
- Do not leave an iron on unattended.
- Place portable heaters where no danger of falling over or brushing against them exists.
- Do not leave portable heaters on when sleeping.
- Place portable heaters and lamps away from curtains, bedspreads, or furniture that can easily catch fire from the heat or flames. Use the type of heater that will shut off automatically if the heater tips over.
- Do not use candles for heat or light. Burn candles only when someone is in the room.
- Place electrical appliances where no one will trip over them.
- Never use equipment that has a frayed cord.
- Do not use multiple outlet plugs.
- Do not run a cord under a rug.
- Use special care around a plugged-in appliance (e.g., never use a fork to remove toast from a toaster).
- Wear safety goggles when working with chemicals such as household cleaners.
- Avoid inhaling chemical fumes in enclosed places.
- Never mix bleach with other cleansers.
- Keep the hot water heater's thermostat below 120 °F.
- Develop an escape plan: practice weekly until the entire household is familiar with the procedure and then practice monthly.
- Identify a central meeting place in case of fire or mass casualty event.
- Do not depend on availability of landline phones or cell phones.
- Place smoke alarms throughout the house; check batteries regularly (one good rule of thumb is to check them in the spring when setting the clocks forward and in the fall when setting the clocks back).
- Hire a qualified electrician to do work in the home.

- Teach children not to touch hot stoves, ovens, and radiators. Turn handles of pans on the stove inward. Keep the oven door closed.
- Place matches and cigarette lighters in a safe place, out of children's reach.
- Place hot liquids out of the reach of infants and toddlers.
- Carefully follow the manufacturer's instructions for heating pads and other equipment.
- Never go back into burning building once you have exited the site.

Outside the Home
- Use a sunscreen that blocks both UVA and UVB rays.
- Consider wearing clothing that contains sunscreen properties.
- Be aware of loose clothing or flowing sleeves that could catch fire when cooking.
- Never add lighter fluid to a fire. Gasoline and kerosene fumes are extremely flammable.
- Do not bury coals in the sand. This will create an oven.
- Be aware of overhead wires in the yard or neighborhood. Do not touch wires with metal ladders.
- Prevent children from climbing poles or flying kites near wires.
- Have an expert check any wires found disconnected or on the ground, particularly after a storm.
- Use care when operating electrical appliances around water.
- Use special lights and equipment for swimming pool areas and for outdoor decorating.
- Insist that schools and places of employment have routine fire drills.

Adapted from the Centers for Disease Control and Prevention fact sheets www.cdc.gov/safechild (including www.cdc.gov/safechild/burns/index.html) and U.S. Fire Administration education materials (https://www.usfa.fema.gov/prevention/outreach/#materials).

> **Box 75-2 First Aid for Minor Burns**
>
> - *Cool the area for 10 or more minutes or until the pain diminishes—Do NOT use ice*
>   - Use cool, not cold, running water *or*
>   - Immerse burned area in cool water *or*
>   - Cover area with moist, cool compresses
> - *Cover the burn with sterile gauze*
>   - Do wrap bandage loosely because the area will swell, which can lead to pressure on skin
>   - Do NOT use fluffy materials, which leaves behind lint and promotes infection
>   - Do NOT break blisters, which can lead to infection and promote scaring
> - *Relieve pain*
>   - Do use over-the-counter nonsteroidal anti-inflammatory drugs (NSAIDs; ibuprofen, naproxen), aspirin, or acetaminophen *or*
>   - Do use prescription medications as ordered
>   - Do NOT use butter or other ointments, which can lead to infections.
> - *Monitor*
>   - For respiratory distress that can happen up to 24 hr after inhalation of smoke
>   - For infection: redness, swelling, fever, suppuration (pus formation), fluids oozing
>   - For tetanus immunization status
>   - Against additional trauma for at least a year and use sunscreen to prevent extensive increase in pigmentation of area

Adapted from the Centers for Disease Control and Prevention (www.cdc.gov) and the Mayo Clinic (https://www.mayoclinic.org/first-aid/first-aid-burns/basics/art-20056649) fact sheets.

prevention information. Warn children and adults about the danger of burns, how to prevent them, and what to do if they occur (Box 75-2).

> **Nursing Alert** The very young and very old are more likely to have accidents that might cause burns. Consider special preventive measures for these individuals.

Burn Classification

Burns are classified according to the mechanism of injury and according to burn depth and size.

> **Key Concept**
>
> Most victims of fires die from smoke or toxic gasses. Airway and respiratory compromise, via nose, mouth, trachea, or lungs, may not be obvious but should be considered.

Mechanism of Injury

- *Thermal burns*, the most common type of burn, are caused by steam, hot water scalds, flames, and direct contact with heat sources.
- *Electrical burns* are potentially life-threatening burns caused by electric shocks due to exposure to the AC or DC current of electricity or lightning.
- *Chemical burns* are caused by exposure to strong acids, alkalis, or other substances such as detergents or solvents. The skin and eyes are commonly affected by these substances.
- *Radiation burns* result from exposure to radioactive sources, such as the ionizing radiation used in industry, or therapeutic radiation. Sunburns are another type of radiation burn.

> **Key Concept**
>
> Exposure to both ultraviolet A (**UVA**) and ultraviolet B (**UVB**) rays of the sun is the leading cause of skin cancer; such cancer is linked with excessive and/or multiple sunburns throughout a person's lifetime. UVA and UVB rays from the sun are strongest during the summer months between the hours of 10 AM and 3 PM, so exposure during those times should be avoided. Tanning beds and salons use UVA-type bulbs, which are linked with cumulative skin damage, premature skin aging, and skin cancer.

Burn Depth and Size

Burns are classified as superficial, superficial partial-thickness, deep partial-thickness, and full-thickness injuries. Table 75-1 summarizes the characteristics of first-, second-, and third-degree burns.

> **Nursing Alert** The severity of injury is related to the burn's depth, extent, and location and the length of exposure to the burn agent, as well as the victim's age and health status at the time of injury.

The extent of burn damage depends on the depth of the burn as well as the extent, location, and size of the injury. Burns can be treated initially at the scene of the injury, a healthcare provider's office, or in an urgent care clinic or emergency department. There are situations in which the victim of a burn may be transferred or sent directly to a specialty care center's Burn Unit. All factors must be considered when estimating burn damage and overall recovery time. For example, an individual with a 5% full-thickness burn on the outer forearm can have a quicker recovery than an individual with 3% partial-thickness burns on the hands or face.

The differentiation between partial-thickness and full-thickness burns is often left to the professional judgment of the initial healthcare provider and/or the specialists of the Burn Unit. The thickness (or depth), as well as the degree, of the burn will frequently increase or "mature" and, thus, be redefined, from the time of injury to about 24–48 hr after injury.

> **Nursing Alert** Severe burn injuries are often obvious and distressing. Be observant for other concomitant injuries, such as spinal cord injury and fractures.

Most institutions use some modification of the "rule of nines" for estimating percentage of body burned. This method divides the body into multiples of 9%. For instance, one arm equals 9%;

CHAPTER 75 Skin Disorders

TABLE 75-1 Characteristics of Burns of Various Depths

DEPTH	TISSUE INVOLVED	USUAL CAUSE	CHARACTERISTICS	EXTENT OF PAIN
Superficial, partial-thickness	Minimal epithelial damage; part of epidermis involved	Sun, steam	Dry, mild swelling Blisters after 24 hr Pinkish-red color Blanching with pressure Peeling of dried skin for about a week No scar	Painful
Superficial, partial-thickness	Epidermis; superficial layers of the dermis involvement	Flash burn Hot liquids	Moist Pinkish or mottled-red color Blisters Some blanching New epidermal growth in 1–3 weeks Loss of skin barrier protection	Pain Hyperesthetic (very sensitive)
Deep partial-thickness	Entire epidermis into the deep layers of the dermis, damage to hair follicles and glandular tissue	As above, plus hot solids, flame, and intense radiant injury	Dry, pale, waxy No blanching Thick-walled blisters Grafting may be needed	Painful when blisters break
Full-thickness	Every body system and organ; extends into subcutaneous tissue layer; muscle bone; and interstitial tissue damage	Sustained flame, electrical, chemical, and steam	Leathery, cracked, avascular, white, cherry red, or black Wound sepsis	Painless because of extensive nerve damage

Adapted from The Centers for Disease Control and Prevention (www.cdc.gov), the National Institutes of Health (https://www.nigms.nih.gov/education/fact-sheets/Pages/burns.aspx) definitions, and http://www.medscape.com/viewarticle/579832_3

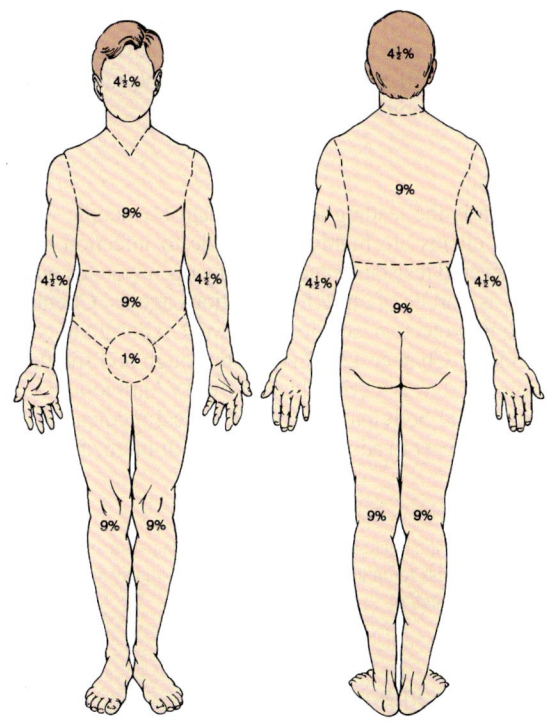

Figure 75-4 Rule of nines in an adult.

the entire back equals 18% (Fig. 75-4). Actual percentages to body areas may vary with individual burn institutions.

Phases of Burn Injury Management

The immediate or emergency response to a burn is to stop the burning process and to apply cold packs or cold water to the affected area. As in other emergencies, the care priorities are maintaining the airway, breathing, and circulation (Box 75-2). When the client is transported to the nearest emergency department, the three phases of burn injury management begin:

- *Resuscitative:* Initial hours after burn, stabilization of immediate health concerns
- *Acute:* Occurs several hours to days after burn, process of acute burn healing
- *Rehabilitative:* Begins at time of initial treatment of burn, maximization of physical repair of tissue, and psychological restoration of individual

Nursing Alert Any burn of the hands, face, feet, groin, buttocks, or joints needs to be evaluated by a healthcare professional.

Resuscitative Phase

Usually, the burn client is admitted to a specialized unit called the Burn Center or Burn Care Unit. If a burn unit is unavailable, the client is admitted to an intensive care unit. A client with significant burns may be stabilized in an emergency room and transferred via qualified personnel to a regional burn center. During the *resuscitative phase*, the client's physiologic condition is unstable; the goal of this phase is to achieve physiologic stability.

When working with a client who has been burned, wash hands thoroughly and frequently, wear sterile gloves, and use aseptic technique when preparing the room and handling supplies. When the client arrives at the healthcare facility, carefully remove his or her clothes, taking care not to further damage burn sites. Place the client on sterile sheets if the burn is severe. Show concern and give encouragement: the client is probably fearful, in pain, and experiencing a sense of loss. The primary provider performs a comprehensive physical examination immediately.

Vital Signs
Record vital signs, and obtain height and weight measurements. Because the client is subject to shock, monitor vital signs frequently. Place a cardiac monitor on the client. Note any changes in vital signs, such as tachycardia (which may indicate a worsening condition) or a rise in temperature (which may indicate dehydration or infection).

> **Nursing Alert** Initially, never apply ointments or salves to an extensive burn; removing them causes further discomfort, and their presence makes determining the extent of the burn difficult. Salves may also introduce pathogens into wounds.

> **Nursing Alert** Avoid using silver sulfadiazine on the face to prevent permanent facial discoloration.

Respiratory Status
Suspect inhalation injuries if the burn victim was in a closed area with the fire and smoke. Singed nasal hairs, facial burns, and soot-stained sputum are clear indications of smoke inhalation. Unless the client is suctioned, however, soot-stained sputum may not be apparent. The individual may also be hoarse or have a cough. Inhalation injuries may also be present in chemical exposure.

Smoke inhalation is often the cause of death for clients who do not have noticeable external burns. Carefully monitor the client's respiratory status, including the rate and depth of respirations. The client probably inhaled smoke and may have sustained lung burns. Carefully observe individuals who have head and neck area burns because such individuals are more likely to have respiratory damage.

Initiate Oxygen Therapy
Because of possible respiratory complications, keep an endotracheal tube or tracheostomy set, or both, at the bedside. Begin immediate measures to prevent hypostatic pneumonia. Measure pulse oximetry, blood gases, and pH frequently to determine respiratory status and general body status. Monitor serum carbon monoxide level if an inhalation injury is suspected. Administer respiratory therapy as prescribed.

> **Nursing Alert** Report the presence of a cough immediately. Note the amount and character of any sputum. Black or gray sputum indicates smoke inhalation.

Fluid and Electrolyte Balance
The client who has experienced burns loses body fluids from capillary leaks and open wounds. Thus, the client requires large amounts of intravenous (IV) fluids. To maintain survival, give such individuals large quantities of sodium-containing fluids. Fluid replacement maintains circulating volume and prevents circulatory collapse, which contributes to serious or fatal shock. Burn care management has specific IV fluid replacement formulas and criteria for administration of these fluids.

The client usually has a retention catheter inserted and a nasogastric tube attached to suction.

Record I&O Accurately
The goal is for a urinary output of 0.5–1 mL/kg/hr, heart rate less than 120 beats/min, and systolic blood pressure greater than 100 mm Hg.

Carefully monitor and record the client's electrolyte status. Hyperkalemia, hypokalemia, and hyponatremia may occur after a burn injury (Chapter 76). Monitor serum electrolytes and gastric secretions to determine electrolyte levels. A drug such as cimetidine (Tagamet) may reduce gastric secretions.

Renal Function
Monitor urine output closely because renal function commonly slows or stops after the body undergoes severe shock. Measure urinary output at least hourly for the first few days. A very high or a very low urine output is significant. Also monitor the specific gravity of the urine. Note a very high urine specific gravity (very concentrated urine). If the output is too low (<30 mL/hr), dialysis may be needed. Acidosis also is a common complication.

Infection
Infection is the leading cause of death for people with burns. Burned clients are highly susceptible to infection because of their lowered resistance and the many open wounds on the body acting as portals of entry for infectious agents. Clients may be placed in protective isolation to prevent exposure to pathogenic organisms (Chapter 42). Practice thorough and frequent handwashing and wear sterile gloves. Give IV antibiotics as ordered. Antibacterial body packs or other topical medications may be applied. Expect to administer a tetanus immunization.

> **Key Concept**
> Burns disrupt the integumentary system and place the individual at increased risk for infection. Note early signs and symptoms of a developing infection.

Pain Management
Depth of injury, anxiety level, previous experiences with pain, cultural beliefs, and the type of invasive monitoring and wound care procedures needed affect the client's pain level. Individuals with superficial burns experience a great

deal of pain. Those with full-thickness burns are not in as much pain because their nerve endings have been destroyed. Narcotic administration via a patient-controlled analgesia (PCA) device is the standard for pain relief. Morphine is often given to relieve pain; be alert for symptoms of respiratory depression. Imagery, hypnosis, distraction, and music therapy may help the client learn to tolerate the pain (In Practice: Nursing Care Plan 75-1).

IN PRACTICE
NURSING CARE PLAN 75-1: A Client With Burns

Medical History: L. D., a 66-year-old man, was admitted to the Regional Burn Center with superficial partial-thickness burns extending over 10% of the right side of his body, involving his upper thigh and lower abdomen. Client reports, "I was making tea and I accidentally spilled a pot of boiling water on myself. Oh, it hurts so much!" Initial intravenous (IV) bolus of morphine sulfate administered with patient-controlled analgesic (PCA) with morphine to be initiated.

Medical Diagnosis: Thermal burns.

DATA COLLECTION/NURSING OBSERVATION

Client is well-nourished older adult male who is alert and oriented. History reveals no major health problems. Burned areas on upper thigh and lower abdomen appear moist, mottled red, with some blisters and blanching noted. Client moving about in bed and grimacing; rates pain as 9 on a numerical scale of 1–10. Vital signs are as follows: temperature, 98.6 °F (40.0 °C); pulse, 92 beats/min and regular; respirations, 26 breaths/min; and blood pressure, 146/90 mm Hg. Client reports that pulse rate and blood pressure are elevated from his usual readings.

NURSING DIAGNOSIS

(Although other nursing diagnoses may be appropriate, a priority nursing diagnosis is addressed below.)

Pain related to thermal burn injury as evidenced by client's rating of 9, grimacing, and elevation in vital signs.

Planning (Outcomes/Goals)	Implementation (Nursing Actions)	Evaluation
Short-Term Goals		
A. Obtain baseline data for pain relief.	• Have client rate pain using a numerical pain rating scale. • Observe the client for nonverbal indicators of pain. • Give initial bolus of 5 mg morphine sulfate as ordered. *Rationale: Effective and therapeutic pain relief promotes psychological and physiologic healing. Using the numerical pain rating scale allows for a consistent method of evaluating the client's pain. Nonverbal indicators provide additional evidence for determining effectiveness of pain relief.* • Place the client in a position of comfort, using pillows for support as necessary. *Rationale: Nonpharmacologic measures, including proper positioning, can enhance the effects of analgesia.*	• Client reports pain at 7 following bolus injection of morphine. • Respiratory rate 20 breaths/min and regular; pulse rate, 88 beats/min; blood pressure, 138/88 mm Hg. • Client is lying in bed quietly; minimal grimacing is noted. **Goal A met.**
B. Provide continuous IV pain relief.	• Initial IV PCA pump as per order. • Follow protocol per pain pump. *Rationale: Depending on size, location, and depth, burns will remain painful. Must be monitored to ensure good pain relief.*	• Client states that pain has decreased to 5 or less on 1–10 scale within 12 hr of initial burn. **Goal B met.**
Long-Term Goals		
C. Client reports that pain is at acceptable level.	• Question client about level of pain as part of routine assessment, e.g., with vital signs. • Question client about other nonpharmacologic measures used in the past for pain control. • Assist with implementing these measures. *Rationale: Clients need to be reassured that pain management is considered a routine part of therapy. Psychological stress inhibits the healing needed for the process of burn healing.*	• Within 18 hr after initial burn injury, client reports continuous relief of pain stated as 4 on numerical rating scale. Vital signs are as follows: pulse, 80 beats/min; respirations, 18 breaths/min and regular; blood pressure, 130/82 mm Hg. • Client lying in bed quietly on his side, listening to music. • PCA in use. **Goal C met.**

SPECIAL CONSIDERATIONS — Culture and Ethnicity

Pain Management
Culture influences responses to pain. Recognize cultural differences and avoid stereotyping others. Some cultures commonly practice nonpharmacologic pain relief measures, such as biofeedback, yoga breathing techniques, acupuncture, meditation, and hypnosis.

Acute Phase

During the *acute phase*, the client remains very ill and requires continuing vigilant observations and interventions. After the client's physiologic condition is stabilized, the focus is on managing the burn wound.

Dressing

Several types of solutions and substances are used as dressings, including gauze impregnated with an antibiotic or drug, and moist packs soaked in a substance such as silver nitrate. Synthetic dressings, such as DuoDERM, OpSite, Vigilon, and Biobrane, promote wound healing or temporarily cover the wound (Fig. 75-5).

Continue to use aseptic technique and sterile dressings (In Practice: Nursing Care Guidelines 75-2). Open dressings are continuously applied as wet dressings. Because wounds heal better if kept moist, closed dressings are not often used. Often the client wears a tight occlusive dressing, face mask, or pressure dressing. The pressure may be applied to a specific burn area, such as an arm, or the client may wear a full-body pressure suit. These devices help to prevent the development of **keloid** (scar) tissue.

Topical Agents

The application of topical agents to the burned area is currently the most widely used therapy. Agents used may include the following:

- *Mafenide acetate (Sulfamylon):* An effective bacteriostatic cream used against many gram-negative and gram-positive bacteria; applied in a thick layer to the entire burned area with a sterile, gloved hand; area usually allowed to remain open to the air. This agent is associated with complaints of burning after application and development of metabolic acidosis.
- *Silver sulfadiazine (Silvadene, Thermazene):* Bacteriocidal cream used against many gram-negative and gram-positive bacteria; applied in a thin layer to the burned area with a sterile, gloved hand; covered with petroleum jelly (Vaseline)–coated Adaptic or sterile dressings, commonly held in place with Kling or Kerlix. This agent is associated with leukopenia; monitor the client's complete blood count. (Some gram-negative bacilli are resistant to the effects of Silvadene. If this condition develops, Silvadene is used in conjunction with other antimicrobial agents.)
- *Bacitracin ointment:* Used for superficial and facial burns applied as a thin layer two or three times per day as ordered.
- *Silver nitrate:* Rarely used today; applied as a 0.5% solution to gauze dressings placed on the burn areas, with dressings kept moist with bulb syringe used to apply the solution.

Nursing Alert Silver nitrate will blacken anything with which it comes into contact, permanently staining it. Therefore, take measures to prevent staining of clothes, linen, walls, and floors.

Débridement

Eschar is usually thick, dry, and black or dark brown dead tissue. It must be débrided to expose viable (living) tissue. In this way, grafting can be successfully performed.

Although packs and externally applied medications assist in loosening and softening eschar, the whirlpool is more commonly used for débridement because it is the most comfortable method. Débridement may also be performed in the operating room. Healthcare providers now use laser scalpels for excision (removal) of eschar. This method causes minimal blood loss and less pain than previously used methods. Enzymatic débridement involves the application of proteolytic substances that digest necrotic tissue.

Nursing Alert Offer the client an as needed (PRN) pain or anxiolytic (antianxiety) medication approximately one-half hour before any painful procedure, such as débridement.

Skin Grafting

Full-thickness burns destroy all skin tissue; therefore, skin grafting is performed to replace tissue that cannot heal by itself. Grafting is also done for cosmetic reasons to limit the amount of scarring. Skin grafts can be either partial thickness where a thin layer is peeled away from the body or full thickness, which involves cutting away thicker donor sections. If the client has sufficient intact, undamaged skin, an **autograft** (or *autologous graft*)—a graft using the client's own skin—is performed. When healing begins and the eschar is completely removed, the plastic surgeon, often using a *dermatome*, peels or cuts specific thicknesses of skin from an unaffected part of the client's body and places these grafts on the affected area.

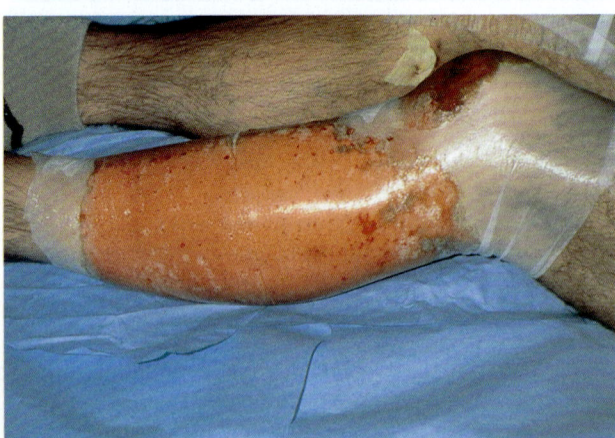

Figure 75-5 Biobrane, a type of synthetic membrane burn dressing, protects the wound from fluid loss and bacterial invasion.

If the client's own skin cannot be used, cadaver skin or skin from another person—a **homograft** (*homogeneic*) or **allograft** (*allogeneic*)—may be used. Immunosuppressive medications may be given to prevent rejection of the foreign skin. In many cases, the foreign skin is allowed to be rejected, but it is left in place long enough to allow new tissue growth underneath. If the donor and recipient are genetically identical an **isograft** (*isogeneic*) can be done.

In some severe burns, especially in areas such as the hands, which are susceptible to contractures, pigskin—a **heterograft** or **xenograft** (*xenogeneic*)—is grafted into place. The client's body will reject the pigskin in approximately 1 week, but before this occurs, the pigskin will aid in body fluid retention, protect the open wound from infection, and promote healing.

Clients who are severely burned do not have sufficient unharmed skin to graft onto injured areas. It is possible to perform a biopsy on unburned skin and grow new skin. These *cultured epithelial autografts* (**CEA**) are useful in covering extensive burns. *Prosthetic* grafts using synthetic materials, such as plastic, ceramic, or metal pieces, may be implanted.

Skin grafting sites need special attention. A pre- and postoperative wound management technique involves the use of *negative pressure wound therapy* (**NPWT**). This system consists of a vacuum unit, foam wound coverage, and negative pressure, which combine to seal the edges of the wound. It promotes healing by minimizing excessive blood and fluids, promotes the development of new blood vessels, and increases the chances that the wound graft will be successful.

Skin grafts are delicate; take care not to disturb them so that they can attach to the live tissue underneath and grow. Observe the graft and report if it seems to be detaching. Follow the protocols of the healthcare facility for care of both the graft and the donor sites.

> **Key Concept**
> Wound management in burns is critical. The key to increased survival is early wound closure.

Other Care Management Priorities

Electrolyte imbalances, which are related to wound leakage and impaired kidney function, may occur. Monitor gastric pH, electrolytes, and renal function test results. Administer electrolyte replacement as ordered.

Balanced nutrition with some supplemental nutrients to rebuild injured tissues is vital. The burned client may need as many as 6,000 calories daily. The diet should be high in calories, nitrogen, and protein. Vitamin supplements, extra between-meal protein supplements, tube feedings, or total parenteral nutrition (TPN) may be used. If the client is allowed oral intake, urge the client to eat. (Medications ordered earlier to prevent excess acid formation in the stomach may be continued.)

Accurate recording of food intake is often ordered; record exactly what the client eats and any significant observations (e.g., refusal to eat, choking, difficulty in swallowing, or vomiting). Also monitor daily weights.

Often, stool softeners such as docusate sodium (Colace) are given to avoid straining. Record all bowel movements (time, amount, consistency, and other characteristics).

> **Nursing Alert** Circumferential burns of the extremities or chest may compromise circulation or breathing. Monitor perfusion of distal extremities and respiratory status. Notify the healthcare supervisors and document all events in the client's written records. An escharotomy may be needed to restore tissue perfusion or ease breathing.

Rehabilitative Phase

During the *rehabilitative phase*, which can last for months or years, clients require extensive recuperation and healing. During this phase, the emphasis is on recovery of strength and function.

Services

The client often goes to the Physical Therapy Department for whirlpool treatment and exercises. The whirlpool serves several purposes: it helps clean the body and assists in removing eschar; it can be used to apply external medication; it provides warmth, so that the client can exercise with less pain; and it helps to stimulate viable tissue growth and wound healing. When the client completes whirlpool treatment, the physical therapist exercises the client's extremities.

The seriously burned client is usually in the healthcare facility for a considerable length of time and needs diversional activity. The client may also need counseling or job retraining after discharge, as well as help in learning how to manage household activities. The occupational therapist provides these services or referrals to vocational counseling.

Because of the long-term nature of the healing of a severe burn, assistance in arranging for care of the client's family during hospitalization and the rehabilitation period may be necessary. Financial assistance may be needed as well. Inform the client and family about available support groups.

Complications

Various complications can occur following a burn, including infection, general gastrointestinal disturbances, hypostatic pneumonia, kidney failure, anemia, skin ulcers, and contractures.

Impaired circulation or difficulty in moving or breathing may occur, as eschar begins to tighten and constrict vital areas. An *escharotomy* (incision into eschar) may be needed to relieve difficulties.

Multiple stomach and duodenal ulcers, called *Curling ulcers*, may develop approximately 1 week after the injury, causing significant gastrointestinal bleeding. Curling ulcers occur when the gastric mucosa becomes ischemic, when there are excess hydrogen ions, or when there is inadequate mucosal cell proliferation. Prevent Curling ulcers by monitoring gastric pH, providing enteral (tube) feedings, and administering medications such as cimetidine (Tagamet), ranitidine (Zantac), famotidine (Pepcid), sucralfate (Carafate), or antacids. The first symptom of Curling ulcers often is bleeding, as evidenced by bloody sputum or emesis or by tarry stools.

Contractures, caused by abnormal shortening of muscles, tendons, or scar tissue, result in deformity and limited joint movement. Contractures are the most serious long-term complication of burns but are now usually preventable with passive and active ROM exercises. The client may be reluctant to move because of pain or fear of pain. Therefore, encourage exercise and explain its importance. Splinting the extremities in antideformity positions is essential in preventing contractures. If the burn is near a joint, contractures are more likely to form and may need to be released surgically. Give PRN medications before exercises to reduce pain.

> **NCLEX Alert**
>
> A clinical situation regarding any aspect of burn care could be a component of the correct answer on an NCLEX question. Be sure that you are aware of the needs of the client during the different aspects of burn care, the medications used for a client with burns, and the psychosocial needs of the burned client.

Emotional Aspects

Many emotional aspects accompany burns. The client may become demanding, expecting much attention in later stages of care because they received so much attention immediately after the injury. Allow the client to express their feelings. At the same time, be honest, understanding, and firm. Encourage the client and family members to participate in developing a realistic nursing care plan. If the client requires infection control precautions, an added element is loneliness. The client may be realistically concerned about their appearance. Help by listening and by encouraging the client to become involved in a support group.

Discharge Planning

Inpatient hospital stays for burn injuries are becoming increasingly shorter. Prepare families for discharge and home care. Teach about wound care, medication use, and signs and symptoms of infection. Make referrals for outpatient care as indicated.

Prognosis

Although the course of treatment is long and arduous, current techniques help the client return to optimum functioning. Most people are able to live productive lives.

SPECIAL CONSIDERATIONS *Lifespan*

Burns and the Older Adult

- Older adult and diabetic clients may not realize they are being burned; they may be unable to feel the burn because of poor circulation, paralysis, or confusion.
- Older adult clients and all diabetic clients may have more difficulty recovering from burns. The cardiovascular and immunologic systems may be compromised.
- Older adults are at high risk for hypostatic pneumonia.
- Cardiovascular disease increases the risk factors for infection, which could mean that the elderly are unable to withstand the additional trauma (i.e., physiologic stress) of a burn.

NEOPLASMS

A **neoplasm** is a new growth, often called a *tumor*, which may be *malignant* (invasive) or *benign* (not invasive). Cancer is a malignant neoplasm.

Nonmalignant Tumors

Nonmalignant tumors of the skin include warts, cysts, **angiomas** (birthmarks), keloids, and nevi. A *wart* is a tumor that can be caused by an infection (e.g., human papillomavirus [HPV]) or by other nonmalignant neoplasms.

Moles

Moles, or *pigmented nevi*, are usually benign. However, they may become malignant, especially if they are very dark, hairy, and elevated. A biopsy procedure should be performed if a mole has these characteristics.

Angiomas

Angiomas, or *birthmarks*, are vascular skin tumors, involving underlying tissues and blood vessels. Some angiomas, such as the *port-wine angioma*, are difficult to remove. If they are very large, they are inoperable. Other *strawberry angiomas* tend to involute (regress or disappear) spontaneously. Most angiomas are neither very noticeable nor very dangerous.

Keloids

Keloids are painless, benign overgrowths that develop at the site of a scar or trauma. Keloids occur more often in darker-skinned individuals. Plastic surgery, for cosmetic reasons, may be performed to hide these scars.

Skin Cancer

Skin cancer is the most common and most curable form of cancer. Because the lesion is visible, the client usually seeks treatment early. There are three main types of skin cancer: basal cell carcinoma, squamous cell carcinoma, and malignant melanoma (Fig. 75-6).

Exposure to the sun is the leading cause of skin cancer. Light-haired, fair-skinned, light-eyed people are at highest risk for skin cancer. Also at high risk are individuals who are susceptible to sunburn or who do not tan. People older than 40 years are more susceptible than younger people. A client who, as a child, had a severe sunburn has an increased chance of developing skin cancer at that site later in life. Smoking also seems to increase susceptibility.

Observation and early investigation of changes in a mole and of new growths is vital; a deeply pigmented mole should be checked. The American Cancer Society has developed a helpful ABCDE rule for evaluating a mole (American Cancer Society, 2019):

Asymmetry: One half of the mole does not match the other half.
Border: Edges are irregular, ragged, notched, or blurred.

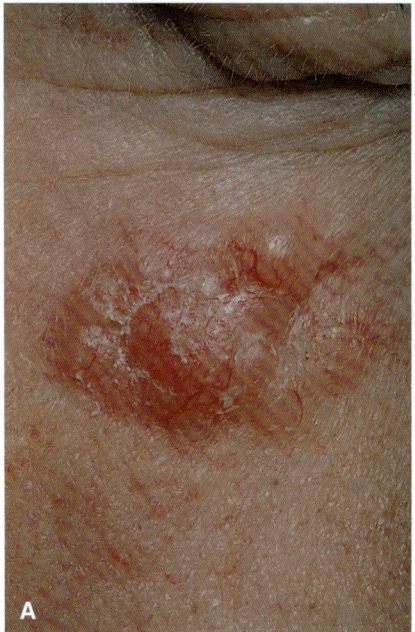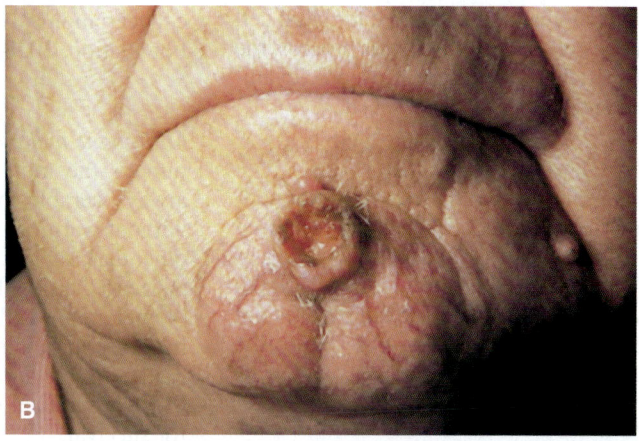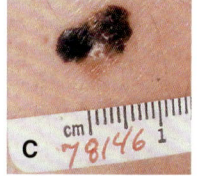

Figure 75-6 Skin cancers. **A.** Basal cell carcinoma. **B.** Squamous cell carcinoma. **C.** Malignant melanoma.

Color: Color is not uniform, but it appears as differing shades of tan, brown, or black, sometimes with patches of red, white, or blue.
Diameter: Spot is larger than 6 mm (about the size of a pencil eraser [about 1/4 in.]).
Evolving: The mole or spot is changing in size, shape, or color over time.

Teach clients to consult a healthcare provider when any changes occur in a wart or mole, including such factors as size, shape, color, flaking, bleeding, sudden elevation, hair growth, or sudden itching or burning.

Preventive teaching is of utmost importance in controlling skin cancer (In Practice: Educating the Client 75-3).

IN PRACTICE
EDUCATING THE CLIENT 75-3 Skin Cancer Prevention

- Avoid bright sunlight, especially midday or tropical sun, primarily during the hours of 10:00 AM–3:00 PM.
  - The middle of the day is when the sun's rays are most harmful.
  - Use sunscreen with a sun-protection factor (SPF) of *at least* 15 that is waterproof or water resistant. Higher SPF coverage is often recommended. Protect your body from the sun.
- Sunscreens absorb UVA and UVB rays. Products are labeled with a sun protection factor (SPF). SPF of 15 or higher is called a sunblock.
  - Products with an SPF of 20–30 provide better protection against sunburn and prevent tanning.
  - Apply the lotion 30 min before going out into the sun and reapply it several times during the day.
  - Include skin areas, such as the rims of the ears, back of the neck, tops of the feet, and the lips.
- Wear UV-blocking sunglasses, a wide-brimmed hat, and clothing with a tight weave and long sleeves.
  - Skin cancer is associated with cumulative exposure to the sun and, currently, the majority of total lifetime skin exposure occurs before the age of 20 years.
- Keep babies younger than 6 months out of direct sunlight.
- Except for minimal amounts over small areas, such as the face and hands, do not use sunscreen on children younger than 6 months.
- Use adequate clothing and shade whenever possible, instead of sunscreen, for infants.
- Avoid the use of sunlamps and tanning beds.
  - Premature aging of the skin and subsequent skin cancer is associated with UVA rays of the sun and the bulbs in tanning salons.
- Observe the skin for changes in pigmentation; changes in warts or moles; abnormal growths; hair growing in or on a mole; or sudden itching, burning, flaking, or elevation of any skin lesion.
  - Observe your children's or partner's skin, including the back.
- Have warts or moles removed if they are irritated or exposed to friction from clothing.
  - Consult a healthcare provider if any of the above features occur.

Most forms of skin cancer are treated by curettage (scraping), **electrodesiccation** (removal with intermittent electric sparks), **cryosurgery** (tissue destruction by freezing), or wide excision (surgery). A pathologist examines the tissue to ensure complete removal. Radiation therapy may supplement surgical removal or may be used for older adults or for those in whom excision is impractical or impossible. Mohs micrographic surgery is the treatment of choice for basal cell carcinoma and squamous cell carcinoma. In this process, the tumor is removed layer by layer, until a microscopic examination reveals that the entire tumor was removed.

Basal Cell Carcinoma

Basal cell carcinoma appears as a small, fleshy bump or nodule. It usually is found in areas that are repeatedly exposed to the sun or other UV light. It is the most common form of skin cancer in Caucasians. This cancer occurs mostly on the head and neck; it is very slow growing and usually does not metastasize. However, it may extend below the skin to the bone and cause considerable local damage.

SPECIAL CONSIDERATIONS   Lifespan

Skin Cancer

The older adult population has the greatest incidence of precancerous and cancerous skin lesions.

Squamous Cell Carcinoma

Squamous cell carcinoma may appear as a nodule or as a red, scaly patch. Squamous cell carcinoma is the second most common type of skin cancer found in Caucasians. It is typically found on the rim of the ear, face, lips, or mouth. This cancer increases in size and develops into a large mass; the cancer may metastasize. The cure rate for squamous cell carcinoma is 95% with early treatment (Skin Cancer Foundation, 2020).

Malignant Melanoma

Malignant melanoma is a darkly pigmented mole or skin tumor—the most virulent of all skin cancers, but almost always curable in its early stages. Melanoma may appear without warning, but it may also begin in or near a mole or other dark spot on the skin. It has a strong tendency to metastasize to the skin, bone, liver, brain, and lung. When colonies of melanoma cells reach vital internal organs, the disease becomes more difficult to treat. The treatment of choice for malignant melanoma is wide excision of the primary lesion. Elective regional node dissection also improves the chances for survival.

STUDENT SYNTHESIS

KEY POINTS

- Dermatology is the study of skin diseases.
- Common diagnostic tests used to determine skin disorders are Wood light examination, Tzanck smear, tissue biopsy, and scabies scraping.
- A variety of pharmacologic and nonpharmacologic measures are used to treat pruritus.
- Various allergies may cause urticaria and contact dermatitis.
- Chronic skin disorders include vitiligo, dermatitis, and psoriasis.
- Folliculitis and carbuncles are common bacterial skin infections.
- Parasitic skin infestations include scabies, lice, and bedbugs.
- The four types of burns are thermal, electrical, chemical, and radiation.
- The three major phases of client recovery after a burn are resuscitative, acute, and rehabilitative.
- Extent of burns is determined by a variety of means. Burn depth and percentage of body surface area burned are significant.
- The major types of skin grafts include autografts, allografts, heterografts, and cultured epithelial autografts.
- Moles, angiomas, and keloids are nonmalignant skin tumors.
- Basal cell carcinoma, squamous cell carcinoma, and malignant melanoma are types of skin cancer. Basal cell carcinoma is the most common type of skin cancer and usually does not metastasize.

CRITICAL THINKING EXERCISES

1. A homeless shelter recently experienced an outbreak of lice. Identify the factors that place shelters at risk for lice. How will you instruct the staff at the shelter to manage the problem?

2. You are caring for a client with severe facial burns. The client's partner desires to visit; however, the partner is afraid of the client's appearance. Discuss how you can support this couple.

3. Your client, who has a circumferential burn to the right forearm, informs you that their fingers are cold and painful. Discuss the possible causes and treatments for this finding.

4. You are participating in a health fair at a shopping mall. An adolescent individual asks you if they could develop skin cancer. What would you consider to be the individual's risk factors for skin cancer? Discuss specific recommendations for how the individual could reduce their risk for skin cancer.

NCLEX-STYLE REVIEW QUESTIONS

1. The nurse is preparing to apply a moist dressing to a sacral pressure injury. Which is a priority action by the nurse?
   a. Medicate with analgesics one-half hour prior to the procedure.
   b. Have the client sign a consent form to perform the procedure.
   c. Document the procedure so that it will not be forgotten.
   d. Remove the necrotic tissue with forceps.

2. A client is prescribed hydroxyzine HCl (Atarax) for the treatment of pruritus. Which information should the nurse provide to the client? Select all that apply.
   a. The medication may cause drowsiness.
   b. Drink water, juice, and other fluids.
   c. Use sunscreen when exposed to the sun.
   d. Administer medication on an empty stomach.
   e. Discontinue medications 1 week before skin testing.

3. A client developed angioedema after taking prinivil (Lisinopril). Which priority nursing action is essential when caring for this client?
   a. Start an IV.
   b. Insert an indwelling catheter.
   c. Apply antipruritic lotion.
   d. Maintain a patent airway.

4. A child has been treated for head lice but has remaining nits attached to the hair shaft. Which instruction would the nurse provide to the parent?
   a. Apply petroleum jelly.
   b. Apply a hair cap to smother them.
   c. Soak the hair in water.
   d. Comb the hair with a fine tooth comb.

5. The nurse observes a client with facial burns and suspects smoke inhalation. Which observations lead the nurse to suspect this condition? Select all that apply.
   a. The facial burns
   b. Singed nasal hairs
   c. Soot around nares
   d. Soot-stained sputum
   e. Report of pain at the burn site

CHAPTER RESOURCES

Enhance your learning with additional resources on thePoint*!*

Student Resources related to this chapter can be found at **thePoint.lww.com/Rosdahl12e**.

76 Disorders in Fluid and Electrolyte Balance

Learning Objectives

1. Discuss the major nursing responsibilities associated with laboratory tests ordered by a clinician.
2. In the clinical laboratory, demonstrate a client and family teaching session, emphasizing the importance of fluid and electrolyte balance and the types of care that may be needed for the client.
3. Identify the possible causes of the two major types of fluid imbalances (fluid volume excess and fluid volume deficit), including the nursing considerations for each cause.
4. State the nursing considerations for each of the following: dependent edema, sacral edema, pitting and nonpitting edema, and pulmonary edema.
5. State the normal serum levels for the following electrolytes: sodium, potassium, calcium, magnesium, chloride, and phosphorus.
6. Identify the causes of each type of electrolyte imbalance. Discuss the major symptoms associated with each type of electrolyte imbalance, stating the nursing considerations related to each condition.
7. Differentiate among the four major types of acid–base imbalances: respiratory acidosis, respiratory alkalosis, metabolic acidosis, and metabolic alkalosis.
8. Identify the nursing considerations related to the data collection, assessment, monitoring, and care of a client with acidosis and a client with alkalosis.

Important Terminology

acidosis, alkalosis, anasarca, fluid volume deficit, fluid volume excess, homeostasis, metabolic acidosis, metabolic alkalosis, nonpitting edema, overhydration, pitting edema, respiratory acidosis, respiratory alkalosis, turgor (skin turgor)

Acronyms

ABG, ADH, ATP, BMP, Ca++, Cl−, CMP, H+, HCO$_3$−, H$_2$CO$_3$, K+, KCl, LFT, mEq, mEq/L, Mg++, mg/dL, Na+, P, pH, PO$_4$−, SI

A normal balance between the body's fluids and electrolytes, and acids and bases, must exist for a person to be healthy. **Homeostasis**, the dynamic process by which the body constantly adjusts to internal and external stimuli, is disrupted by abnormalities of fluid levels and electrolyte content.

The body constantly uses feedback mechanisms to maintain fluid and electrolyte balance. The nervous and endocrine systems are most intimately involved in feedback. The integumentary, respiratory, digestive, and urinary systems also respond to feedback mechanisms.

Any disorder, disease, or injury can disrupt homeostasis. The risk of serious disturbances in fluid–electrolyte or acid–base balance increases in clients at the extremes of the age spectrum, in those with burn injuries, and in those with preexisting conditions or chronic illnesses. Nurses play a major role in monitoring clients for actual or potential threats to homeostasis, with nursing care being directed toward monitoring and maintaining this balance.

Chapter 17 introduced the concepts of body fluids, fluid compartments, and electrolyte balance. This chapter continues the discussion of fluids and the major electrolytes. Emphasis is given to data collection and nursing concerns related to excesses or deficiencies of fluids and electrolytes.

DIAGNOSTIC TESTS

Many laboratory tests are aimed at evaluating the body's fluid and electrolyte or acid/base balance. Chemical studies of electrolytes are probably among the most commonly ordered laboratory studies. The healthcare provider may order the determination of levels of a single electrolyte or a combination of electrolytes. In general, a *basic* metabolic panel (**BMP**) or a comprehensive metabolic panel (**CMP**) consists of laboratory testing of specific numbers of certain important chemicals found in blood plasma. Most clinical facilities have standard panels identified with terms such as *BMP 6*, *BMP 8*, or *CMP 24*. Each facility defines the components of these chemistry panels. The fundamental chemistry panel consists of the basic electrolytes (sodium, potassium, and chloride) plus glucose.

Other commonly ordered tests include hematologic tests of the complete blood count (CBC), clotting factors, and liver function tests (**LFTs**). In addition, arterial blood gas (**ABG**) evaluations may be performed to determine the **pH** (potential of hydrogen in concentration) of blood, a valuable indicator of acidosis or alkalosis. The basic components and values of an ABG are listed in Table 17-5.

Urine and other body fluids also are studied for composition and abnormal components. In some cases, urine is collected for 24 hr so that an entire day's chemical and fluid output can be analyzed.

Key Concept
Fluid and electrolyte disturbances are possible in anyone, but they are particularly common in an ill and hospitalized client, including those undergoing surgical and diagnostic procedures, and in young children and older adults.

NCLEX Alert
A clinical situation on an NCLEX may provide chemistry or hematologic levels for an individual. It is imperative that the student know normal and abnormal levels for common laboratory tests.

COMMON MEDICAL TREATMENTS

When an excess of body water exists in the extracellular fluid (ECF), which is found in the interstitial and intravascular spaces, or electrolyte excess is detected, medications may be given to facilitate removal of the excessive substance from the body. Oral or rectal medication may be given to draw electrolytes out of the body through the gastrointestinal system. Oral or intravenous (IV) medications may draw fluids or certain electrolytes from the body for elimination through the urinary system.

When a deficit of body water exists in the ECF or electrolyte deficit is determined, fluids, electrolytes, and other substances can be administered to the client to help restore homeostasis. Some substances, such as potassium, can be administered orally. In certain clients, either the body cannot absorb electrolytes taken orally or the body will not absorb them quickly enough to prevent serious problems. In such cases, IV administration of electrolytes is usually the treatment of choice.

Specific electrolytes may be added to a large-volume infusion (e.g., 1,000 mL of $D_5$1/2NS with 20 milliequivalents [**mEq**] of potassium chloride [**KCl**]), or given in a smaller volume via intermittent infusion (e.g., 100 mL of NS with 20 mEq KCl via IV piggyback). The person's blood electrolyte levels are monitored, and the dosage is adjusted accordingly. After critical deficits are corrected and any oral restrictions are removed, oral fluid or electrolyte replacements may be initiated. Chapter 64 discusses administration of IV fluids.

NURSING PROCESS

DATA COLLECTION
Carefully observe and monitor all clients for potential disorders in fluid or electrolyte balance. Obtain ordered laboratory studies and report results to the clinician. Chapter 47 describes nursing data collection. A baseline is important for future comparison and to determine the presence of suspected abnormalities. *Report any abnormalities or changes in the baseline level.*

> **Nursing Alert** In the normal flow of information in clinical facilities, the nurse is often the first care provider to see the laboratory results. Although laboratory personnel may have highlighted or noted critical values, generally the nurse is responsible for notifying the primary healthcare provider of significant changes in laboratory values or of critical laboratory values. *Critical values* are those laboratory levels that are considered serious or life threatening. The nurse documents that the laboratory values have been reported (e.g., "0815 Dr. B. Smith notified by phone of K⁺ result of 3.0 mEq/L. Stat order for K supplement given. 0830 Client received ordered medication").

When collecting and documenting data about a client's fluid and electrolyte balance, observe factors such as the skin's appearance and **turgor** (elasticity or tonus), urine's volume and specific gravity, the relative balance between intake and output (I&O), and comparisons of daily weights (In Practice: Data Gathering in Nursing 76-1).

PLANNING AND IMPLEMENTATION
The healthcare team plans together with the client and family for effective care. The client with a fluid or electrolyte imbalance may require assistance in meeting daily needs, maintaining a balance between I&O, and understanding more about the disorder, its prognosis, and its treatment. The client needs to follow the prescribed regimen to resolve the imbalance. A nursing plan of care is developed to meet these needs. To meet desired outcomes, the nurse may also need to map a care plan for the client's use.

Teaching the Client and Family
Teach the client and family about fluid and electrolyte problems, especially if the person will be cared for in the home. Include the client and family as much as possible in planning the diet, monitoring dietary restrictions, and following the schedule and amounts of food and fluids to be consumed. If the client understands the rationale for special diets or limitations, they are more likely to comply. This understanding is also important for the individuals who will do the shopping and food preparation in the home.

Treating Edema
Handle edematous areas carefully. Edematous skin is friable and susceptible to skin breakdown, sloughing, and ulceration. Change the person's position frequently for maximum comfort. Elevating an edematous body part, usually the feet and ankles, to a position higher than the heart's level helps alleviate the edema.

IN PRACTICE
DATA GATHERING IN NURSING 76-1 — Possible Indicators of Fluid and Electrolyte Imbalances

- Presence or absence of edema
- Poor skin turgor
- Changes in skin color
- Sudden weight gain or loss
- Hypertension or hypotension
- Increased heart rate
- Change in respiratory pattern
- Significant difference between intake and output
- Dyspnea, orthopnea, or crackles (fluid in the lungs) on auscultation
- Abnormal electrolyte levels (on laboratory report)
- Elevated temperature
- Decreased or increased urine specific gravity
- Psychological or sensorium abnormalities
- Changes in urine volume
- Thirst

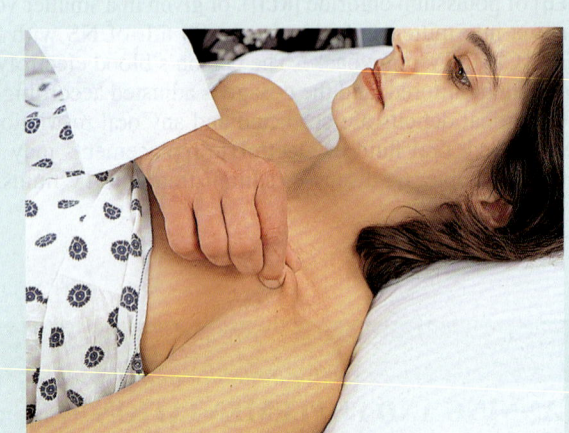

Figure 76-1 Testing for skin turgor. The nurse is pinching the skin over the clavicle. Other testing sites include the skin over the sternum and over the forehead. With normal skin turgor, when the skin is released, the skin will return to its normal position immediately. If turgor is diminished, the pinched skin will remain in position briefly. *Tenting* is the term used to describe a finding of poor skin turgor. (Photo by B. Proud.)

Monitoring Daily Fluid Balance
Keep accurate I&O records. Normally, fluid I&O amounts are roughly equal. If the amounts differ greatly, evaluate the client's hydration level. Check the urine specific gravity. Evaluate the client's skin turgor by lifting a fold of skin between your thumb and forefinger (Fig. 76-1). Check the extremities or any dependent areas for edema. To detect a serious complication of pulmonary edema, auscultate anterior and posterior lung fields for crackles or rhonchi. Document and report abnormal lung sounds. Monitor IV fluid administration to prevent circulatory overload. Closely watch and document any drainage. Note any watery stools and significant *diaphoresis* (sweating). Weigh the client daily to detect rapid, unexplained weight loss or gain.

Administering Medications
Administer medications as ordered; observe their results and side effects. Correcting an acid–base imbalance may be necessary to correct a fluid–electrolyte imbalance. Give diuretic drugs, to increase urinary output, and electrolytes, as ordered. The client's urinary output should increase soon after diuretic therapy is started. Monitor for signs of potassium deficit, dehydration, or acid–base imbalance that may occur with the extended use of diuretics.

Assisting With Mouth and Skin Care
The skin and mucous membranes of the client with a fluid imbalance are susceptible to breakdown, cracking, and infections. Give the client good mouth and skin care (Chapter 50). Perform these actions at least every 2 hr.

EVALUATION
Periodically, the healthcare team evaluates the outcomes of care. Have short-term goals been met? Are long-term goals still realistic? Planning for further nursing care considers the client's prognosis, any complications, and the client's responses to treatment.

MAINTENANCE OF FLUID BALANCE

A person needs to maintain a homeostatic balance of the amount of water in all body fluid compartments. Fluid is constantly moving among compartments. For example, blood contains *plasma fluids,* which circulate to all body areas. *Tissue fluids* and *lymph fluids* also travel from one fluid compartment to another. *Intracellular fluids* (ICF) are relatively stable. However, if disturbances occur in the ICF balance, the client is critically compromised. If the balance among compartments is upset, several problems can occur, including fluid volume excess and fluid volume deficit (Chapter 17).

Fluid Volume Excess

Fluid volume excess (FVE) is excessive retention of water and sodium in the ECF. **Overhydration** refers specifically to excess water in the extracellular spaces. The following are possible causes of FVE:

- Increased fluid intake, as in too-rapid administration of IV fluids containing sodium, or too-rapid administration of enteral tube feedings (e.g., nasogastric tube feedings)
- Decreased urine output, as in kidney or liver disorders
- Physical disorders (e.g., heart failure [HF] or cardiac insufficiency) that result in a decreased ability of the heart to pump effectively

- Excess ingestion of sodium (e.g., from substances that contain large amounts of sodium chloride; overuse of table salt; or medications that contain large amounts of sodium)
- Stress from surgery or other physical trauma that causes aldosterone and antidiuretic hormone (**ADH**) production, resulting in sodium and water retention

Nursing care includes daily observations, collection of data, and documentation. Administration and observation of the effects of diuretics may be indicated. Often a sodium-restricted diet is ordered.

Edema

The excessive accumulation of interstitial fluid is known as *edema*. Edema can be a local or generalized clinical manifestation of many disorders involving FVE, such as the following:

- *Heart failure, thrombophlebitis, and liver cirrhosis,* all of which increase venous pressure and cause faulty reabsorption of fluids and electrolytes
- *Low protein levels* owing to conditions such as malnutrition or liver disease, which cause fluid to be drawn out of blood vessels and into tissue spaces
- *Poor lymphatic drainage,* which reduces osmotic pressure, causing more fluid to be retained
- *Sodium retention* owing to conditions such as kidney or endocrine disorders, which cause sodium to be reabsorbed rather than excreted; increased sodium levels cause water to be drawn out of the circulation and into the tissues
- *Inflammation,* which dilates the arteries and increases the permeability of the capillary walls
- *Physical stress,* such as surgery, which may cause increased amounts of interstitial fluids (third-spacing) owing to tissue trauma and responses by the endocrine system

Dependent edema occurs in an area that hangs down, that is, in a *dependent* position. In an ambulatory person or one who remains in a sitting position, dependent edema is common in the feet and ankles.

Sacral edema, as the name implies, is dependent edema in the sacral area. Typically, sacral edema is noted in the client who remains in bed, and no limb edema is noted.

Pitting edema is the descriptive term used to describe serious observable edema that dents under slight finger pressure. The healthcare provider can indicate the extent of pitting edema by using a finger to press against the area of swelling. Generally, a scale of +1 to +4 is used to describe the intensity of the edema. For example, the nurse presses against the lower extremity and a slight dent remains after the finger is removed. The dent remains for only a second or so. This example could be described as plus one (+1) pitting edema. When a dent remains for 2, 3, or 4 or more seconds, the observation is charted as +2, +3, or +4 pitting edema, respectively. If the dent in the skin remains for some time in edematous tissue, as in a +4 pitting edema, **anasarca** (generalized body edema) may also be noted (Fig. 76-2).

Nonpitting edema, which can also be severe, refers to swelling that does not indent when slight pressure is applied.

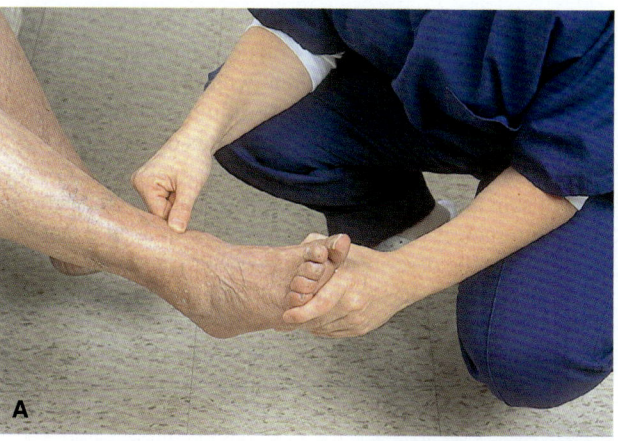
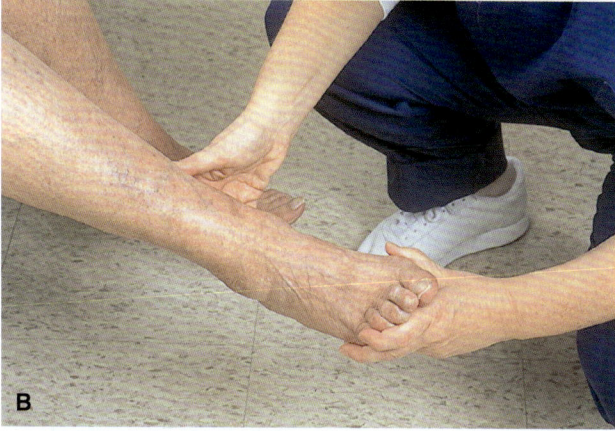

Figure 76-2 Testing for pitting edema. **A,** The nurse is pressing her thumb into the skin on the ankle of the client. **B,** The impression left by the thumb is called pitting edema and indicates significant fluid retention.

Be sure to chart that the edema is either pitting or nonpitting on the +1 to +4 scale. Also include the location, and be sure to notify the primary healthcare provider.

Pulmonary edema is an accumulation of interstitial fluid in the lungs. It is a symptom of various heart and blood vessel disorders, nephrosis, cirrhosis of the liver, and IV therapy that is administered too fast.

Fluid Volume Deficit

Fluid volume deficit (FVD) is a deficiency of fluid and electrolytes in the ECF. *Dehydration* refers to a decreased volume of water, but it does not occur without electrolyte changes. The following are possible causes of FVD:

- Inadequate fluid intake and starvation
- Loss of body fluids (e.g., from excessive sweating, diarrhea, vomiting, excessive urine output, excessive drainage, such as from wounds or burns, or GI suctioning)
- Prolonged fever
- Inability of the body to conserve and reuse water by concentrating the urine. This occurs with renal failure or some endocrine disorders.

The cause of FVD needs to be identified and treated. Younger and older clients are at the highest risk for dehydration because of inadequate oral fluid intake. Encourage oral fluid intake unless the person is nauseated or in danger of aspiration. Oral fluids are the easiest and safest way to restore proper hydration. In Practice: Nursing Care Plan 76-1 highlights the care of a client with FVD.

The person with FVD may need fluid replacement therapy or total parenteral nutrition (Chapters 64 and 88).

Monitor results from increased fluid intake via observations of skin turgor (Fig. 76-1) and urine output. When checking skin turgor, if the skin remains elevated, as in a tent, the condition can be described as *tenting*. Skin tenting is an indication of dehydration. A scale of +1 to +4 is commonly used to describe tenting. For example, if the skin does not return to normal position in 4 or so seconds, the nurse would chart, "*Poor skin turgor as seen by +4 tenting over sternum.*"

Key Concept

FVD can occur as a result of many disorders. Monitor the client's level of hydration and observe for FVD in all clients.

MAINTENANCE OF ELECTROLYTE BALANCE

For the body to function properly in all aspects, electrolytes must be properly balanced. Electrolyte imbalances (Table 76-1) can have serious consequences on the body.

Units of measure for electrolytes include milliequivalents per liter (mEq/L), which is a calculated concentration

---

IN PRACTICE

NURSING CARE PLAN 76-1 — The Client With Fluid Loss

Medical History: J.J., a 68-year-old woman, comes to the emergency department complaining of vomiting for the past 2 days. She states, "I can't keep anything down. I've tried to drink because I'm thirsty, but it's no use. Everybody in my bridge club has been sick with a GI virus." Complete blood count (CBC) and serum electrolyte levels are obtained. Results are consistent for viral infection. Urinalysis shows dark, concentrated amber urine with a specific gravity of 1.027. Intravenous (IV) fluid therapy is initiated at 125 mL/hr; client is placed on nothing by mouth (NPO) status.

Medical Diagnosis: Gastroenteritis with dehydration.

DATA COLLECTION/NURSING OBSERVATION

Client is alert and oriented. Skin and mucous membranes are pale pink and slightly dry. Skin tenting test reveals a 1+ to 2+ slow return when pinched. Vital signs are as follows: temperature, 99°F (37.2°C); pulse, 92 beats/minute and regular; respirations, 22 breaths/minute; and blood pressure, 110/62 mm Hg. Client scale weight at 132 lb (59.8 kg) in ER. She states, "I've lost a little over 2 lb since I've been sick." Client states she has gone to the bathroom "once or twice today" (within the last 12 hr). UA specimen is noted to be concentrated, dark amber in color. She states she is very thirsty but gets nauseous when "even thinking of drinking anything."

NURSING DIAGNOSIS

(Although other nursing diagnoses may be appropriate, a priority nursing diagnosis is addressed below.)

Fluid volume deficit related to persistent vomiting from probable gastroenteritis as evidenced by the client's report of vomiting for the past 2 days, minimal to no oral intake, and coworkers being similarly ill.

Planning (Outcomes/Goals)	Implementation (Nursing Actions)	Evaluation
Short-Term Goals		
A. Client will report that she has not had any episodes of nausea, vomiting, and complaints of thirst for 3 hr.	• Monitor electrolytes per laboratory studies. • Administer antinausea medications as per order. • Maintain status of NPO order for 4 hr as per order. • If no nausea reported, begin to offer ice chips and sips of clear fluid, approximately 30 mL/hr, as ordered. • Gradually increase amount according to client's tolerance. *Rationale: Offering ice chips and small amounts of clear fluids gradually helps to reestablish oral intake without overstressing the GI tract.*	Day 1—1,730 hr. • Client demonstrates ability to tolerate ice chips and sips of clear liquids. **Goal A met.**

Planning (Outcomes/Goals)	Implementation (Nursing Actions)	Evaluation
B. Observations of client's skin turgor, I&O, and vital signs demonstrate improvement in fluid volume deficits from baseline data.	• Maintain IV fluid therapy as ordered. • Maintain NPO status as ordered. **Rationale:** IV fluid replacement therapy is needed to prevent further fluid imbalance that could have an impact on renal function. Maintaining NPO status aids in resting the gastrointestinal (GI) tract. • Continue to monitor I&O, vital signs, mucous membranes, skin turgor, and urine specific gravity at least every 2 hr. **Rationale:** Continued monitoring is necessary to provide a means for evaluating improvement or deterioration in the client's status.	Day 1—2,300 hr. • Client reports ability to tolerate approximately 2-3 oz of oral fluid over the past hour with decreased complaints of thirst. • No episodes of vomiting since during the last 3 hr. • Client has voided 450 mL since admission. • Urine color appears less concentrated. **Goal B met.**
Long-Term Goals		
C. Client will demonstrate ability to tolerate progressive diet intake.	• Continue to advance oral intake and diet, as ordered, offering small amounts of full liquids and then diet as tolerated. • Monitor IV fluid therapy, decreasing rate as ordered. **Rationale:** Advancing oral intake aids in promoting the resumption of pre-illness diet. As oral intake increases, the need for IV fluid replacement decreases.	• Day 2—0800 hr. • Weight 133 lb (60.3 kg). • Urine is clear yellow, with a specific gravity of 1.020. • Output is approximately 350 mL in 8 hr. • No further episodes of vomiting. • Clear liquid diet tolerated. • IV DC'd at 1,330 hr. **Goal C met.**
D. Client will demonstrate signs and symptoms of adequate fluid balance.	• Obtain weight and compare with baseline. • Continue to monitor I&O and laboratory test results. • Check mucous membranes and skin turgor. **Rationale:** Parameters, such as weight, I&O, mucous membranes, skin turgor, and laboratory test results, are reliable indicators of fluid balance.	• Client able to tolerate full liquid to bland diet. • IV fluid therapy discontinued. • No weight loss since admission. • Vital signs, CBC, and electrolyte levels are within acceptable parameters. • Mucous membranes pink and moist. • Skin returns quickly when pinched. **Goal D met.**

of electrolytes in a specific volume of solution. Some laboratories report levels using the International System of Units ("Système International," or **SI** units), such as milligrams per deciliter (**mg/dL**). A deciliter is equal to 0.1 L or 100 mL.

Sodium

Sodium (**Na⁺**), as the main extracellular ion, induces water movement between ICF and ECF to help achieve homeostasis of water within those compartments. The severity of symptoms seen with imbalances of sodium concentration is most greatly affected by the cause of the problem, the speed at which the change takes place, and the degree of change in the sodium level.

Hypernatremia, a serum sodium level of 145 mEq/L or greater, is most commonly caused by water loss and an excess of sodium. Hypernatremia occurs in endocrine disorders (e.g., diabetes insipidus) or in situations involving an increased insensible loss of water (e.g., hyperventilation or serious burn injuries). Less commonly, it results from

TABLE 76-1	Electrolyte Functions and Imbalances		
ELECTROLYTE	MAJOR FUNCTIONS	EXCESS	DEFICIENCY
Potassium (K)	Major electrolyte in intracellular fluid (ICF) Controls cellular osmotic pressure Activates enzymes Regulates acid–base balance Maintains nerve and muscle function Influences kidney function Influences sugar uptake	*Hyperkalemia:* Vague muscle weakness (usually the large muscles of the lower extremities) initially, with skeletal muscle weakness possibly progressing to paralysis, paresthesias, and dysrhythmias	*Hypokalemia:* Vague fatigue and general malaise initially; muscle weakness, paresthesias, diminished deep tendon reflexes, hypotension, and cardiac dysrhythmias
Sodium (Na)	Major electrolyte in extracellular fluid (ECF) Influences distribution of water Maintains acid–base balance Maintains nerve function	*Hypernatremia:* Thirst, dry mucous membranes, flushed dry skin, and hypotension (if accompanied by fluid volume deficit [FVD]); neurologic findings (due to dehydration of the brain cells) such as weakness, lethargy, irritability, twitching, spasticity, and seizures; in extreme cases, coma and death	*Hyponatremia:* Anorexia, nausea, and abdominal muscle cramps; neurologic dysfunction, including headache, lethargy, and seizures (due to hyposmolarity and cellular swelling), possibly resulting in coma, respiratory arrest, and death; optic disc possibly swollen (papilledema); sternal edema with severe hyponatremia
Calcium (Ca)	Major component of bones and teeth Affects permeability of cell membranes Plays a role in blood coagulation and maintenance of heartbeat Affects nerve function	*Hypercalcemia:* Dysrhythmia, hypertension, muscular weakness, depressed reflexes, and altered states of consciousness progressing to coma	*Hypocalcemia:* Dysrhythmia, hypotension, tetany (muscle spasms), paresthesias, altered mood, and confusion; seizures are possibly the primary observed symptoms
Magnesium (Mg)	Thought to be needed in activation of enzymes Aids in some neuromuscular functions	*Hypermagnesemia:* Weakness, diminished deep tendon reflexes, and muscle weakness; hypotension with peripheral vasodilation	*Hypomagnesemia:* Hyperexcitability with muscle weakness, tremors, and generalized seizures; apathy, confusion, delirium, vertigo, ataxia (defective muscle coordination), and coma; and dysrhythmias. These symptoms are most commonly seen when levels are less than 1 mEq/L and are possibly difficult to identify because of hypokalemia and hypocalcemia occurring simultaneously
Chloride (Cl)	Plays a key role in acid–base balance Helps to maintain water balance	*Hyperchloremia* (usually associated with hypernatremia and metabolic acidosis)	*Hypochloremia* (usually associated with deficit of sodium and potassium, and metabolic alkalosis)
Phosphorus (P) and phosphate (PO_4)	Component of bone Involved in most metabolic processes	*Hyperphosphatemia:* Few symptoms caused by hyperphosphatemia alone; symptoms of hypocalcemia; deposits of calcium phosphate salts around joints and in soft body tissues, causing pain on movement with long-term hyperphosphatemia	*Hypophosphatemia* (common with levels less than 1 mg/dL): Anemia, infections, and bleeding (because of impaired function and survival time of red blood cells [RBCs], white blood cells [WBCs], and platelets); muscle weakness (including the respiratory and cardiac muscles), irritability, and paresthesias progressing to coma; renal symptoms; symptoms related to loss of magnesium and bicarbonate; hypercalciuria (excess Ca^{++} excretion in urine) resulting in osteomalacia (bone softening in adults) and rickets as possible secondary effects

sodium gain that cannot be dissolved in the body's water, such as through excess IV or oral intake.

SPECIAL CONSIDERATIONS Lifespan

The Thirst Sensation

In some individuals, especially the elderly, the thirst sensation may be diminished or depressed. Individuals with impaired sensations, altered mental status, or communication difficulties may be unable to perceive, communicate, or respond to thirst. Thirst is also a major symptom of hypernatremia.

Hyponatremia, a serum sodium level of less than 135 mEq/L, usually results from excessive water retention. Water retention in excess of salt retention may be caused by an excess production of **ADH**, owing to pulmonary disorders such as pneumonia, asthma, oat cell carcinoma, or acute respiratory failure or to malignancies, such as lymphomas, leukemia, or Hodgkin disease.

Monitor closely the neurologic status of the client because lethargy and/or confusion can be caused by both hypernatremia and hyponatremia. Client safety is always a concern when there is noted confusion. Sodium loss may occur because of diuretic therapy, renal disease, adrenal insufficiency, or loss of gastrointestinal (GI) fluids owing to vomiting or GI suction. Sodium deficiencies because of inappropriate intake may be seen with a low-sodium diet or inappropriate oral or IV fluid (10% dextrose in water [$D_{10}W$]) intake of water.

SPECIAL CONSIDERATIONS Lifespan

Factors Predisposing Older Adults to Fluid and Electrolyte Imbalances

- Older adults have decreased renal and respiratory functioning.
- The thirst mechanisms of older adults are depressed, so encouraging fluids is vital.
- Many medications taken regularly by older adults (e.g., blood pressure medications) affect renal and cardiac function and fluid balance.
- Routine procedures, such as administering laxatives before colon x-ray examinations, may induce serious fluid volume deficits in older adults.
- Signs and symptoms of fluid and electrolyte disturbances, such as confusion, may be subtle or atypical.
- Skin turgor is a *less valid observation of dehydration in older adults* because of the decreased elasticity of their skin. Check mucous membranes for dryness and cracking.
- Older adults may deliberately limit fluid intake to avoid the embarrassment of incontinence. Intervention may be necessary to prevent imbalances.
- Self-medication with enemas, laxatives, or remedies, such as baking soda, can cause severe electrolyte imbalance.

Potassium

Even though potassium (K^+) is the major electrolyte in the ICF, the portion of potassium located in the ECF is important for neuromuscular function, especially cardiac function. Excretion of potassium is done primarily by the kidneys (80%). Potassium is also lost through the bowel (15%) and sweat (5%). Potassium cannot be stored and must be taken in daily. Many different types of drug therapy are associated with potassium imbalances.

Hyperkalemia, a serum potassium level of 5.5 mEq/L or greater, can result from inadequate excretion (e.g., renal failure). However, sustained hyperkalemia is not likely for the individual with normal renal function. Shifts of potassium out of body cells that result from *acidosis* (increased hydrogen ion concentration in the blood), tissue damage, or burns can lead to hyperkalemia. Rapid IV infusion of potassium solutions, excessive intake of salt substitutes, or decreased production of aldosterone are also common causes of hyperkalemia. Because stored blood cells gradually release potassium, transfusion of aged blood can also result in hyperkalemia.

Hypokalemia, a serum potassium level of less than 3.5 mEq/L, can result from decreased potassium intake, possibly associated with starvation and alcoholism. Excessive excretion of potassium can occur in renal disease, vomiting, diarrhea, gastric suctioning, excess sweating, diuretic use, or endocrine disorders. Alkalosis can lead to intracellular shifts of potassium, leading to serum potassium deficits. Hypokalemia also contributes to hyperglycemia because of potassium's effect on both insulin release and organ sensitivity to insulin.

When there is an imbalance of potassium, either hypokalemia or hyperkalemia, the client is at risk for cardiac dysrhythmias. Monitor the cardiac status of the client closely. Check for irregular pulse rhythms and report these to the healthcare provider. Carry out orders for electrocardiograms (ECGs) and/or telemetry as ordered.

Calcium

Calcium (Ca^{++}), by exerting a relaxing effect on nerve cells, plays a major role in nerve impulse transmission and muscle contraction. Calcium is also involved in hormone secretion and blood clotting. Hormonal control of the calcium level is achieved by parathormone (from the parathyroid gland) and calcitonin (from the thyroid gland). Calcitriol, the active form of vitamin D, is a regulator of calcium metabolism.

Hypercalcemia is based on a classification of mild, moderate, or severe levels of total serum calcium and ionized calcium levels. Mild hypercalcemia ranges from total Ca 10.5 to 11.9 mg/dL (2.5-3 mmol/L) or ionized Ca 5.6 to 8 mg/dL (1.4-2 mmol/L). Severe or hypercalcemic crisis levels of hypercalcemia range from a total Ca 14 to 16 mg/dL (3.5-4 mmol/L) or ionized Ca 10 to 12 mg/dL (2.5-3 mmol/L). Hypercalcemia most commonly results from cancer or primary hyperparathyroidism. However, immobilization, which promotes bone resorption (*decalcification*), other endocrine disorders, medications, and abnormal vitamin D metabolism could cause hypercalcemia.

Although rare, *hypocalcemia*, a total serum calcium level of less than 9 mg/dL (4.5 mEq/L) or ionized calcium less than 4.6 mg/dL, is most commonly caused by a parathyroid hormone deficit, owing either to surgical or primary hypoparathyroidism or abnormal vitamin D metabolism. In many instances, alkalosis causes a decrease in ionized serum calcium. Other conditions—such as hypoalbuminemia, hyperphosphatemia, hypomagnesemia, cancer, acute pancreatitis, malabsorption, chronic alcoholism, and some drugs—cause hypocalcemia.

Magnesium

The balance of magnesium (Mg^{++}) depends on normal intake, absorption, and renal excretion. Intracellular and extracellular magnesium concentrations are significant for many important cellular processes, including enzyme reactions, neuromuscular transmission, and cardiovascular tone. Mg^{++} is closely related to calcium, phosphorus, and potassium.

Hypermagnesemia, a serum magnesium level of greater than 2.5 mEq/L (3.0 mg/dL), is seen in clients with decreased renal excretion owing to diminished renal function. Clients with normal renal function but who have been aggressively treated with over-the-counter medications (antacids and laxatives) or prescribed doses of magnesium may develop hypermagnesemia. Calcium gluconate is the specific antidote for magnesium intoxication.

Hypomagnesemia, a total serum magnesium level of less than 1.5 mEq/L (1.8 mg/dL), is most commonly caused by chronic alcoholism and severe HF that is being aggressively treated with diuretic therapy. Decreased magnesium intake, malabsorption, and GI losses, including suctioning, vomiting, diarrhea, and fistulas, result in hypomagnesemia. Renal or endocrine diseases, drugs, burns, or shifts of magnesium into cells or bone may also result in hypomagnesemia.

Chloride

Chloride (Cl^-) plays a key role in acid–base balance. An excess is called *hyperchloremia*; a deficit is called *hypochloremia*. Both of these conditions are associated with acid–base imbalance.

Phosphorus/Phosphate

Phosphorus (P) is a critical component of all tissues. In the human body, phosphorus is often found in the form of phosphate (PO_4^-). More than 70% of phosphorus is found in combination with calcium in bones and teeth. To absorb and metabolize phosphorus, vitamin D is needed.

Phosphorus, an important intracellular messenger, is critical for energy production in the form of adenosine triphosphate (ATP). Glycogen needs phosphorus to convert glycogen to glucose. An efficient intestinal tract and normal renal conservation mechanisms are crucial to the normal level of phosphate.

Hyperphosphatemia, an elevation of serum phosphate above 4.5 mg/dL, is commonly caused by decreased renal excretion; redistribution from the ICF to the ECF; or increased intake or intestinal absorption of phosphate. Clients with metabolic acidosis, such as those with renal failure, will often have more ionized calcium present and may exhibit no symptoms of hypocalcemia.

Hypophosphatemia, a serum phosphate of less than 2.5 mg/dL, is unusual but often occurs with respiratory alkalosis owing to prolonged hyperventilation and extensive burn injury. Decreased oral intake or absorption from the GI tract, a shift of phosphate from ECF to ICF, or a loss of phosphate owing to hyperparathyroidism or renal tubule disorder are other causes. Because only 1% of phosphate is in the ECF, decreased serum levels do not necessarily reflect low total body phosphate.

MAINTENANCE OF ACID–BASE BALANCE

The body must maintain acid–base balance to carry out its functions adequately. The body's cellular activity requires a slightly alkaline medium. ECF is normally maintained at a pH of approximately 7.4 or between 7.35 and 7.45. ICF has a slightly lower pH. Alterations of even a few tenths can be incompatible with cellular activity. An overview of the causes and symptoms of acidosis and alkalosis is presented in Table 76-2.

TABLE 76-2 Causes and Symptoms of Acidosis and Alkalosis

ACID–BASE IMBALANCE	POSSIBLE CAUSES	SIGNS AND SYMPTOMS
Metabolic acidosis	Uncontrolled diabetes mellitus, fasting and starvation (anorexia and bulimia), lactic acidosis, salicylate poisoning (aspirin overdose), alcoholic ketoacidosis, kidney dysfunction and failure, and loss of intestinal secretions (diarrhea, intestinal suctioning, fistulas)	Decreased pH, decreased HCO_3^-, diarrhea, nausea and vomiting, anorexia, weakness, lethargy, malaise, altered mental status, coma, peripheral vasodilation, shock, bradycardia, cardiac dysrhythmias, and warm and flushed skin
Respiratory acidosis	Respiratory center depression (sedative overdose, head trauma); lung disorders, such as pneumonia, emphysema, asthma, and pulmonary edema; respiratory distress syndrome; and airway obstruction owing to airway or injury to the thorax, extreme obesity, respiratory muscle paralysis, and kyphoscoliosis	Decreased pH, increased PCO_2, hypoventilation, and shallow respirations; headache, weakness, altered mental and behavioral changes (disorientation, confusion, depression, paranoia, hallucinations), tremors, paralysis, stupor, and coma; warm, dry skin; drowsiness; nausea and vomiting; diarrhea; fruity-smelling breath; acidic blood; and acidic urine
Metabolic alkalosis	Excess ingestion or administration of sodium bicarbonate, total parenteral nutrition (TPN) solutions containing acetate, parenteral solutions containing lactate, or blood transfusions containing citrate; gastrointestinal (GI) loss of hydrogen ions via vomiting, gastric suction, bulimia, diuretic therapy, and loss of chloride and body fluids	Increased pH, increased HCO_3^-, confusion, hyperactive reflexes, tetany, convulsions, hypotension, and dysrhythmias
Respiratory alkalosis	Hysteria, hyperventilation, high fever, salicylate (aspirin) poisoning, elevated blood ammonia levels, encephalitis, and mechanical ventilation	Increased pH, decreased PCO_2, accompanied by deep respirations with rapid breathing; irritability, panic, light-headedness, dizziness, paresthesia, positive Chvostek and Trousseau signs, seizures; nausea, vomiting, and diarrhea; muscle twitching, tetany, and tremors; alkaline urine; and electrocardiogram (ECG) changes

Chapter 76 Disorders in Fluid and Electrolyte Balance

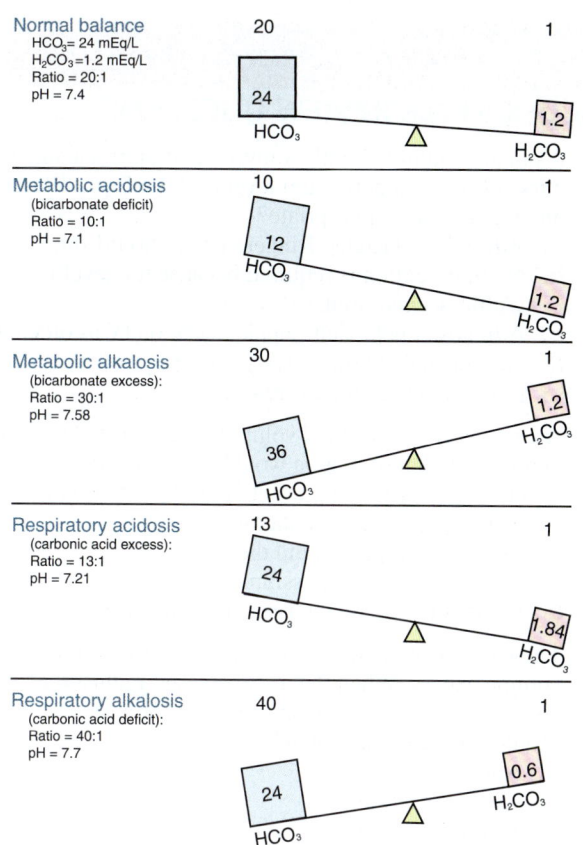

Figure 76-3 The pH of fluid is balanced using bicarbonate ion (HCO_3^-), carbonic acid (H_2CO_3), and hydrogen ions (H^+). This figure illustrates pH changes and the balance between HCO_3 and H_2CO_3.

Acidosis

When the blood is more acidic than normal, a state of **acidosis** exists. A deficit in bicarbonate ions (HCO_3^+) or an excess in hydrogen ions (H^+) causes a condition called **metabolic acidosis**. Excess loss of bicarbonate or excessive retention of hydrogen ions owing to renal disease is a common cause. Figure 76-3 illustrates normal and abnormal pH balance (hydrogen ion or H^+) using bicarbonate ion (HCO_3) and carbonic acid (H_2CO_3).

An increase in carbon dioxide in the blood characterizes a condition called **respiratory acidosis**. It may occur in pneumonia, emphysema, and asthma, and after administration of large doses of certain drugs (barbiturates, narcotic analgesics), all of which cause hypoventilation.

> **Key Concept**
>
> ABGs are common diagnostic tests frequently drawn by the respiratory therapist or an RN. Table 76-3 provides a general view of the major aspects of respiratory or metabolic acidosis or alkalosis using the main components of pH, CO_2, and bicarbonate (HCO_3^-).

The treatment of choice is correction of the underlying condition. Administer IV infusions, as ordered. The clinician may order bicarbonate for severe metabolic acidosis; however, it should not be given for respiratory acidosis. Lactated Ringer solution may be ordered.

The character of respirations and the respiratory rate can indicate changes. Notify the healthcare provider of respiratory changes. The person can be compensating for the condition, or the situation may be worsening. The client may need stimulants or narcotic antagonists to reverse respiratory depression caused by medications. Nursing interventions include placing the client in a position that promotes breathing, such as elevating the head of the bed, or placing the client in the orthopneic position, and administering ordered oxygen. The client may need a mechanical ventilator for severe respiratory acidosis.

Carefully document changes in vital signs. The acidosis may worsen or the client may become alkalotic as an overreaction to the treatment. Monitor laboratory values carefully. Observe the person's level of consciousness because any change may be significant. The client can lose consciousness if acidosis worsens. The pH of urine can be an indicator of serum acidosis or alkalosis. Acidosis can cause electrolytes to shift, leading to electrolyte imbalances. For example, potassium ions may shift out of the cells in response to metabolic acidosis, resulting in hyperkalemia.

Alkalosis

When the blood is more basic than normal, because of a loss of body acids or excessive retention of alkaline substances, a state called **alkalosis** exists. **Metabolic alkalosis** is caused by an excess of bicarbonate, often owing to excess bicarbonate antacid administration or a loss of acids, such as through vomiting or excessive gastric suctioning.

A condition called **respiratory alkalosis** is a deficit of plasma CO_2 (carbonic acid [H_2Co_3]). This situation is usually caused by hyperventilation. Symptoms are similar to those of metabolic alkalosis. Direct treatment includes reducing the cause of the hyperventilation. Interventions may involve the client using a rebreathing mask or breathing into a paper bag so that they will rebreathe their own CO_2, thus replacing the CO_2 needed by the body.

Alkalosis can result in shifts in electrolytes and subsequent electrolyte imbalances. Potassium ions may shift into cells as hydrogen ions shift out of cells in response to metabolic alkalosis. Calcium ions are deionized in states of alkalosis, resulting in symptoms of hypocalcemia. In cases of respiratory alkalosis, serum phosphate may move into the cells, resulting in hypophosphatemia.

Attention to detail is vital. Monitor laboratory values carefully. Administer IV solutions, as ordered, to treat any electrolyte imbalances. Treatment of choice for GI causes is often sodium chloride or potassium chloride because these electrolytes are usually lost with hydrochloric acid in vomiting. Make sure the alkalosis does not worsen or result in the opposite imbalance. *Paresthesia* (tingling in the fingers and toes) and muscle twitching are ominous signs of electrolyte loss—particularly the loss of ionized calcium.

TABLE 76-3 Clues to Respiratory or Metabolic Acid–Base Balance

	ACIDOSIS	ALKALOSIS
	↓ pH < ±7.35[a]	↑ pH > ±7.45[a]
Respiratory	↑ CO_2 >45	↓ CO_2 <35
Metabolic	↓ HCO_3^- (bicarbonate) > ±22 mEq/L	↑ HCO_3^- (bicarbonate) > ±26 mEq/L

[a]Note: Read symbols in the table as *approximately or about 7.35* because there is a great deal of variability in actual levels.

STUDENT SYNTHESIS

KEY POINTS

- Fluid and electrolyte disturbances can occur in anyone, but they are commonly seen in ill and hospitalized clients, including those undergoing surgical and diagnostic procedures. The risk of serious disturbances increases in clients who are at the extremes of the age spectrum.
- Measurement of I&O and daily weight is an important component in the determination of fluid balance.
- Edema is a symptom of many disorders, but most commonly indicates fluid overload. Edematous skin is very friable and susceptible to breakdown. Good skin care is imperative, as is client positioning.
- Electrolyte imbalances commonly involve either an excess or a deficit of the electrolyte. In certain cases, more than one electrolyte imbalance may be occurring.
- The body's cellular activity requires a slightly alkaline medium. ECF is normally maintained at a pH of approximately 7.4 or between 7.35 and 7.45. ICF has a slightly lower pH. Alterations of even a few tenths can be incompatible with cellular activity.
- Respiratory acidosis, if not corrected, could lead to the need for mechanical ventilation.
- A simple treatment for respiratory alkalosis, usually caused by hyperventilation, is for the client to breathe into a paper bag, thereby retaining needed CO_2 in the body.

CRITICAL THINKING EXERCISES

1. You have just admitted an older adult from a nursing home. The client has poor skin turgor, a dry mouth, and cracked, bleeding lips. They are awake and oriented, but refuse oral fluids. Which further actions would you take? Which strategies might be effective in restoring fluid balance?
2. Your client has been diagnosed with respiratory alkalosis caused by hyperventilation secondary to head injury. Which primary symptoms would you monitor? Which symptoms might be attributed to acid–base imbalance and which might be caused by electrolyte imbalance? What might be symptoms of head injury? What major treatments would you expect to administer to this client?

NCLEX-STYLE REVIEW QUESTIONS

1. A client is admitted with vomiting and diarrhea and the nurse observes a potassium level of 2.9 mEq/L. Which nursing action is appropriate?
   a. Administer lactated Ringers IV at 150 mL/hr.
   b. No intervention is required because the level is within normal limits.
   c. Administer potassium supplementation IV as ordered.
   d. Administer sodium polystyrene (Kayexalate) to promote potassium excretion.

2. A client is at risk for fluid volume excess related to heart failure. Which information would the nurse provide to the client to assist with prevention of this occurrence?
   a. Comply with diuretic therapy
   b. Maintain a high-sodium diet
   c. Increase level of potassium in the diet
   d. Drink 8 to 10, 8-oz glasses of fluid per day.

3. The nurse is obtaining data from a client with fluid volume excess. When the nurse presses against the lower left leg, a slight indent remains for a second. How should this be documented?
   a. Anasarca
   b. +1 pitting edema
   c. +3 pitting edema
   d. +4 pitting edema

4. A client is hyperventilating and has a pH of 7.52 and a PCO_2 of 68 mm Hg. Which intervention by the nurse will assist in correcting this acid–base imbalance?
   a. Have the client use a rebreather mask.
   b. Administer oxygen.
   c. Administer lactated Ringers IV.
   d. Elevate the head of the bed.

5. The nurse is observing a client with a calcium level of 4.2 mEq/L. Which clinical manifestations may correlate with this level? Select all that apply.
   a. Paresthesia
   b. Hypotension
   c. Muscular weakness
   d. Depressed reflexes

CHAPTER RESOURCES

Enhance your learning with additional resources on **thePoint**!

Student Resources related to this chapter can be found at **thePoint.lww.com/Rosdahl12e**.

77 Musculoskeletal Disorders

Learning Objectives

1. In relationship to a client with a musculoskeletal disorder, discuss the diagnostic benefits of the following tests: laboratory tests including ESR, CBC, RF, uric acid, CK, calcium, and phosphorus levels; x-ray; arthrogram; myelogram; CT scan; MRI; bone scan; ultrasound; arthrocentesis; arthroscopy; bone biopsy; and EMG.
2. Describe the components of data collection for a client with a musculoskeletal disorder.
3. Identify the major components of nursing care necessary to protect the client from the hazards of immobilization.
4. Discuss the important areas of nursing care for the client who has had an amputation and now has a new limb prosthesis.
5. Explain the aspects of nursing care needed for a client who has been surgically treated for IVD or HNP.
6. State the nursing considerations for clients with TMJ, muscular dystrophy, and osteoporosis.
7. Differentiate among the following conditions: inflammatory disorders (RA, OA, ankylosing spondylitis, bursitis, and tenosynovitis); repetitive strain injuries (carpal tunnel syndrome and lateral epicondylitis); and systemic disorders with musculoskeletal manifestations (gout, SLE, scleroderma, and rickets or osteomalacia), stating the nursing considerations for each disorder.
8. Compare and contrast the following: strain, sprain, and fracture. Identify the four categories and five types of common fractures.
9. Describe the nursing implications for the care of a client in a cast.
10. Differentiate between skin traction and skeletal traction, including indications and nursing considerations for each type of traction.
11. Discuss the nursing measures for care of clients with the following treatments: external fixation, open reduction/internal fixation (ORIF), and arthroplasty.
12. Identify the complications of fractures or bone surgery.
13. Explain the difference between primary and metastatic bone tumors.

Important Terminology

acrosclerosis	fasciotomy	osteomalacia	
amputation	fracture	osteomyelitis	
ankylosis	gangrene	prosthesis	
arthritis	gout	replantation	
arthrocentesis	halo device	rickets	
arthrogram	kyphosis	sclerodactyly	
arthroplasty	laminectomy	scleroderma	
arthroscopy	lordosis	scoliosis	
bursitis	myelogram	sequestration	
cast	neurovascular	skeletal traction	
dislocation	checks	skin traction	
electromyogram	orthopedics	spinal stenosis	

Acronyms

sprain	AEA	IVD
strain	AKA	IVDD
synovectomy	BEA	OA
tenosynovitis	BKA	ORIF
	CK	RA
	CMS	RF
	CPM	SLE
	DJD	THA
	ECG	TLSO
	EEG	TMJ
	ESR	
	HNP	

The medical specialty that examines and treats diseases and injuries of the musculoskeletal system is called **orthopedics** (*orth/o* = straight). Surgeons who specialize in this area of medicine are *orthopedists*. Orthopedic nursing involves preventing further complications for clients with musculoskeletal conditions (Chapter 18 for a review of musculoskeletal anatomy and physiology).

DIAGNOSTIC TESTS

Nursing care for clients with musculoskeletal disorders is likely to involve preparation for physical examinations, radiographic tests, and other diagnostic procedures. Be sure to explain the actual procedures to reduce tension or anxiety that clients may experience. Teach post-procedure activities that ease discomfort and promote wellness. Carry out physical preparation and document all aspects of care.

Laboratory Tests

Several laboratory tests are available to monitor the condition of bones and muscles. Complete blood cell count (CBC), uric acid levels, and blood levels of calcium and phosphorus help indicate the overall condition of the musculoskeletal system. Erythrocyte sedimentation rate (**ESR**), rheumatoid factor (**RF**), and creatine kinase (**CK**) tests may show inflammation related to an infection or inflammatory condition.

Radiography (X-Ray)

Radiography is the most common method of assessing the general state of bones. An x-ray study visualizes bones and other internal structures noninvasively so that the healthcare provider can diagnose abnormalities and monitor the effectiveness of treatments. Some types of radiographic examinations require the use of dye to visualize cavities within bony parts. Before giving a radiopaque dye, ask clients if they have any sensitivity to foods, especially any shellfish or medications containing iodine, as well as any sensitivities to latex or medications. Before a female client undergoes any x-ray procedure, determine if they are pregnant. Special precautions must be taken to protect the reproductive organs of all clients from potentially harmful radioactivity.

> **Key Concept**
>
> Rather than asking your client, *"Are you allergic to anything?"* ask your client, *"What sensitivities do you have to food, iodine, latex, medications, or other substances?"* If your client has sensitivities, your next question should be, *"What happens when you are exposed to this substance?"*

Arthrogram
An **arthrogram** is an x-ray study of a joint (e.g., knee or shoulder). A radiopaque or radiolucent substance is injected, and then a sequence of x-rays films is taken to determine the joint's condition.

Myelogram
The **myelogram** (*myello* = spinal cord; bone marrow) is an x-ray examination of the spinal cord and vertebral canal after injection of a contrast medium or air into the spinal subarachnoid space. This diagnostic procedure is particularly valuable for evaluating spinal cord abnormalities caused by tumors, herniated intervertebral disks, or other lesions.

Computed Tomography
Computed tomography (CT) scanning provides a three-dimensional radiographic view of a body part. CT scanning is painless and can be performed with or without the use of contrast agents. The amount of radiation the client receives is the same as what they would receive during a conventional chest x-ray. The scanner takes a series of cross-sectional pictures of the body part in minute slices across the *coronal plane* (vertically, from front to back). A CT scan is useful in diagnosing bone, ligament, and tendon injuries, soft-tissue disorders, and tumors.

Other Diagnostic Tests

Magnetic Resonance Imaging
In *magnetic resonance imaging* (MRI), a powerful magnetic field enables a scanning machine to produce detailed images of internal organs without the use of potentially dangerous ionizing radiation or x-rays. The use of a magnetic field and radio frequencies produces measurable signals, which a computer translates into three-dimensional visual images. MRI is safer and less expensive than invasive procedures such as biopsy, surgery, or the use of radioactive isotopes or dyes. For these reasons, many examiners prefer to use MRI whenever possible. MRI units are expensive, however, and not all institutions have MRI capabilities. Portable MRI units are often available for rural facilities.

> **Nursing Alert** Clients who have metallic implants, such as orthopedic screws, may not be eligible for MRI scanning. Severe damage and death can result if metallic implants are exposed to the intense magnetic fields of an MRI.

Bone Scan
A *bone scan* is used to detect primary bone tumors, metastatic bone disease, osteomyelitis, osteoporosis, inflammation, bone or joint infections, and stress fractures. It requires the intravenous (IV) injection of a radioisotope, such as technetium-99m, which then enhances the visualization of abnormal tissue areas. The client must lie quietly during the entire scan. After the test, instruct the client to drink extra fluids, to increase excretion of the isotope.

Ultrasound
Ultrasound technology, which uses sound waves and their echoes to display images, helps to evaluate soft-tissue masses, osteomyelitis, infection, congenital and acquired pediatric disorders, bone mineral density, sports injuries, and fracture healing. This method is noninvasive, inexpensive, readily available, and safe because it does not involve ionizing radiation.

Arthrocentesis
An **arthrocentesis** is aspiration of synovial fluid, blood, or pus from a joint cavity. By examining these fluids, a healthcare provider can diagnose infections, inflammatory conditions, and bleeding. After the test, a compression dressing is applied and the joint is rested for 1 day.

Arthroscopy
Arthroscopy is a minimally invasive procedure used in viewing joints for diagnostic and treatment purposes. It uses a special endoscope, called an *arthroscope,* which has a lens and a light source at its end that transmits a picture to a video monitor in the operating room (OR). Because the flexible scope can bend inside the joint, the surgeon views and operates on the joint's interior, using only a very tiny incision referred to as a "stab wound." The procedure is known as a *closed procedure* because the joint does not need to be laid open.

The procedure is performed in the OR or same-day surgery facility, often under local anesthesia. Surgeons use arthroscopy to diagnose and treat joint disorders. For example, foreign or loose objects (e.g., a piece of cartilage, a bone spur) can be removed. A rough and worn joint can be made smoother and more comfortable. Tissue samples can be obtained via biopsy, and a torn meniscus or ligament can be diagnosed and possibly repaired. Arthroscopic surgery is much safer, more comfortable, and more cost effective than open surgery, and for these reasons, it is used whenever possible.

Following the procedure, elevate the client's joint and apply ice to control edema and pain. Teach the client how to monitor the site for evidence of infection.

Biopsy

A *biopsy* of bone, tissue, or muscle may be performed using local anesthesia to diagnose tumors, infections, muscle inflammation or atrophy, and various other problems. After the procedure, monitor the biopsy site for bleeding, swelling, infection, or hematoma.

Electromyogram

The **electromyogram** (EMG) is a test of electrical conductivity, similar to the electrocardiogram (**ECG**) or the electroencephalogram (**EEG**). The provider places fine needles into the client's muscles (*my/o* = muscle) and measures the electrical impulses within the muscles, both at rest and during activity. The provider can then determine whether the client's muscles respond appropriately to stimuli.

> **Nursing Alert** Do not confuse the term *myogram* with the term *myelogram*. The combining form my/o refers to muscle, whereas the combining form mye/lo refers to the spinal column.

COMMON MEDICAL TREATMENTS

Joint, bone, and muscle disorders often cause pain and limit movement. Common treatments for these disorders include application of heat or cold through hot baths or soaks, hot or cold compresses or packs, or paraffin baths. Heat causes vasodilation, thereby drawing oxygen, leukocytes, and nutrients to an injured or diseased area to promote healing and prevent infection.

Physical therapy is another common medical treatment for joint, bone, and muscle disorders. The simplest therapies for joints are passive range of motion (PROM) and active exercises (AROM). *Massage,* if joints are not damaged or inflamed, often helps to soothe aching joints.

Muscle, bone, or joint fractures or diseases accompanied by damage to surrounding soft tissues are treated by external immobilization devices to alleviate pain and discomfort, prevent further injury, and promote healing. External immobilization is achieved through the use of braces, corsets, splints, casts, and traction.

COMMON SURGICAL TREATMENTS

Common surgical treatments for muscle, bone, and joint disorders are performed to remove or repair damaged or diseased parts. Disorders that may require surgery include fractures, ligament ruptures, arthritic joints, or accidental limb amputation.

Surgery is necessary if a fractured joint or bone cannot heal with external immobilization alone. A bone fracture that results in multiple fragments usually cannot be realigned without surgically opening the body part and reattaching the fragments using surgical hardware such as pins, screws, or plates. *Joint replacement surgery,* or *arthroplasty,* is a common treatment for the client with either arthritis or severe fractures that may not heal. Various surgical procedures are performed to immobilize or repair the spinal column if trauma or disruption of the spinal space and cord occurs. *Amputation* is the surgical choice if a limb is damaged by injury or disease beyond repair.

NURSING PROCESS

DATA COLLECTION

Carefully observe and document the status of a client with a musculoskeletal disorder. Establish a baseline for future comparison. Report any changes from the baseline findings.

Observe for any skeletal deformity. Observe posture, coordination, and body build, noting any asymmetry or deformity. Palpate soft tissues, joints, and muscles. Measure muscle mass. Palpate the skin temperature for warmth and document any swelling, crepitation, tenderness, skin discoloration, or other abnormality.

To determine the client's musculoskeletal function, perform range of motion (ROM) exercises. Check for bilateral muscle strength, as well as for balance and gait. A healthcare provider may refer the client to a specialist if limited mobility is suspected. Also evaluate the client's ability to use mobility aids, such as a wheelchair, walker, cane, or crutches safely (Chapter 48).

Observe the client's emotional response to the disorder or disease. Do they need assistance to meet daily needs? Does the disorder affect social activities or self-esteem? Is the client anxious or fearful of the outcome?

Immobilization Devices

The nurse must carefully monitor clients who have immobilization devices in place because it is extremely important to prevent and promptly treat any complications (In Practice: Data Gathering in Nursing 77-1). Areas of concern include pressure, infection of the wound or bone, and hemorrhage.

A primary concern while observing such clients is to watch for signs of pressure. Undue pressure of any kind can cause serious neurovascular compromise or damage to nerves and blood vessels. Pressure, and its accompanying lack of blood or nerve supply, can cause tissue *necrosis* (death) and other complications.

> **Nursing Alert** Follow Standard Precautions when providing care for clients with compound fractures, wound infections, or the possibility of hemorrhage.

PLANNING AND IMPLEMENTATION

When planning care, include clients and their families. For clients undergoing surgical procedures (e.g., lumbar decompression, joint replacement, insertion of a fixation device or prosthesis), provide preoperative and postoperative care.

Clients with musculoskeletal disorders may also require assistance with mobility, pain control, cast care, nutritional needs, and emotional problems. They need to understand their disorder, prognosis, and treatment. Develop nursing care plans that meet the client's individual needs.

IN PRACTICE
DATA GATHERING IN NURSING 77-1 | Key Findings With an Immobilization Device in Place

Complications of Pressure
- *Edema:* Swelling under the device, at the edges of the device, or of the entire extremity
- *Skin color:* Blanched, mottled, or cyanotic; inspect the client's fingers and toes frequently and separately for signs of circulatory impairment
- *Numbness, tingling, or the inability to move:* Inability to move the fingers or toes and to identify specifically which digit is touched; inability to flex the foot (dorsiflexion and plantar flexion) if the ankle and foot are not casted
- *Cool temperature of digits:* Sensation of being colder on affected side if pressure exists
- *Severe pain:* Most likely caused by swelling if medication fails to relieve severe pain
- *Lack of distal pulse:* Indicative of inadequate blood flow
- *Slow capillary refill:* Lack of color return in 2 to 4 s after nail bed is compressed

Wound Infection
- Elevated temperature, pulse, and respirations; the client may develop hypotension if infection is developing
- Odor of decaying tissue
- Elevated leukocyte count
- Drainage of blood or serous fluid from the fracture area (may be seen at pin insertion sites or in cast window or may soak through cast)
- Redness and swelling in surrounding tissues
- Pain
- Swelling

Infection of the Bone (Osteomyelitis)
- Fever
- Pain
- Redness and heat
- Elevated leukocyte count
- Nausea, with or without vomiting
- Headache
- Swelling and pressure

Hemorrhage
- Diminished color, motion, and sensitivity of distal limb
- Tachycardia
- Hypotension
- Rapid respirations
- Anxiety, panic, or confusion
- Diaphoresis
- Oliguria (decreased urine output) or anuria (no urine output)

Preventing Disorders of Immobility
Prolonged bed rest is dangerous for clients with musculoskeletal disorders because of the increased risk for complications such as skin breakdown, contractures, constipation, and thromboembolism (also referred to as deep vein thrombosis [DVT]). Provide teaching to prevent such complications. Work closely with physical therapists to help clients regain mobility.

Providing Comfortable Positioning and Proper Alignment
Some clients must remain in bed. Maintaining proper body alignment is essential. Turn clients frequently to prevent skin breakdown. Pillows, sandbags, splints, and trochanter rolls help prevent footdrop and contractures. PROM and AROM exercises promote and maintain joint mobility and muscle strength. Encourage clients to move independently as much as possible.

Providing Skin Care
Maintain skin integrity and protect against irritation. When bathing clients, minimize the use of soap. Use lotion for cleansing and for soothing dry skin. Reduce friction and shear forces through proper positioning. Keep sheets smooth and clear of crumbs after meals. If necessary, use special beds, air mattresses, foam pads, and flotation pads to help reduce pressure; however, their use is not a substitute for frequent skin care. Nursing observations with documentation of the client's circulation, motion, and sensation (**CMS**) distal to the injury are important aspects of monitoring musculoskeletal problems. CMS checks are also known as **neurovascular checks** because they monitor the function and status of nerves and blood vessels, as well as the movement of muscles that could be damaged. Preventative skin care is important because many musculoskeletal problems involve difficulty with movement and prolonged immobility. If a client has an incision or pins in place, give special care to these skin breaks. Use the protocol prescribed by the healthcare facility. Use Standard Precautions and wear sterile gloves, if necessary, for pin site care.

Providing Adequate Nutrition
To promote healing, the client with a musculoskeletal disorder should receive a high-protein diet. Increased fiber and fluids help to maintain normal elimination. Record intake and output. Observe for signs of urinary infection or constipation. Give IV fluids, as ordered. Many clients receive nutritional supplements, such as Ensure.

Providing Activity and Exercise
Determine how much activity clients are allowed. Too little or too much exercise can be harmful. Place a trapeze on the bed frame of clients who are confined to bed so they can help lift their bodies for nursing care. Clients can also use a trapeze for exercise. Encourage clients to exercise unaffected body parts as much as possible.

Remind clients in casts or splints to flex and extend unaffected joints and muscles frequently. Usually, casted extremities are most comfortable when they are elevated. Remind clients to wiggle the fingers or toes of the affected extremities. Instruct clients to do *isometric* (muscle-setting) exercises of immobilized parts as often as possible. A continuous passive motion (**CPM**) machine is sometimes used to exercise extremities. Assist clients to be out of bed as much as possible. Help them use crutches, walkers, or other assistive devices.

EVALUATION
Periodically evaluate outcomes of care with clients, families, and members of the healthcare team. Have short-term goals been met? Are long-term goals still realistic? In planning for further nursing care, such as the need for follow-up care at home or continued physical therapy, consider prognosis, the presence of any complications, and responses to care.

> **NCLEX Alert**
>
> Nursing interventions for conditions such as hemorrhage, infection, and pain are very common clinical situations. Be sure that you are aware of these interventions and can decide which intervention has priority (e.g., *generally* hemorrhage before infection because excessive bleeding can be life threatening), but read the situation carefully.

COMMON MUSCULOSKELETAL DISORDERS

Amputation

Amputation is the absence or removal of all or part of a limb or body organ. An amputation may be congenital, or it may result from an injury or surgery. Reasons for surgical amputation include malignancy, trauma, gangrene, infections, and neurovascular compromise related to diabetes mellitus or cardiovascular disease.

A *surgical amputation* is the treatment of choice only when other means cannot control or arrest a disease process. In such cases, amputation is often a life-saving measure. In malignant disease, surgery may offer improved comfort, increased function, and greater potential longevity. Amputation does not always cure malignancies.

Level of Amputation
The disease process for which the procedure is necessary determines the level of amputation. Amputation of any extremity is performed at the most distal point possible. When a surgeon is able to preserve joints and maximize limb length, prosthetic fitting is easier and clients retain more functional ability.

Amputations are classified according to the affected limb and the level of the amputation. An amputation of the hand is called a below-the-elbow amputation (**BEA**); an amputation of the forearm and any part of the upper arm is called an above-the-elbow amputation (**AEA**). Amputation of the leg may be below-the-knee amputation (**BKA**) or above-the-knee amputation (**AKA**). Sometimes, only a finger or toe is amputated. An example of this description is "amputation of first finger, right hand, below second knuckle."

Residual Limb Pain
Residual limb pain, a frequent after effect of amputation, refers to the sensation of pain, pressure, or itching that occurs in the area of the amputation and the feeling that the absent body part is still present. If possible, discuss this concept with the client before surgery because they may be too embarrassed to mention residual limb pain when it occurs. Encourage clients who seem to be disturbed and uneasy following amputation to discuss their feelings. If residual limb pain or discomfort is causing the distress, explain that the sensation is common and results from damage to the nerves in the residual limb. Reassure clients that residual limb pain generally disappears in time. For pain relief, tell clients to "move" the missing limb. By activating the damaged nerves leading to the amputated limb, clients usually feel great relief. Other interventions include use of analgesics, transcutaneous electrical nerve stimulation (TENS), ultrasound, and visual imaging. Persistent pain can interfere with prosthesis fitting.

Prosthesis
A **prosthesis** is an artificial device that replaces part or all of a missing extremity. Over the years, the design of prostheses has improved, and they have become more lightweight and reliable. The use of computer technology has resulted in better-fitting prosthetic devices that are more functional and natural looking.

Clients are fitted with prostheses as soon as possible after surgery; sometimes surgeons attach temporary prostheses while clients are still anesthetized. Leg prostheses are most successful. Skirts and trousers can conceal leg prostheses, which can be equipped with shoes that match. Therapists and specially trained nurses assist the person in learning to walk with the new prostheses (Fig. 97-6).

Typically, arm prostheses are more complicated because the hand is an exquisite motor and sensory organ. Functional artificial hands usually do not look real. Above-the-elbow amputees can use either functional or cosmetic prostheses. A practical prosthetic hand is fashioned with a mechanical hook, consisting of metal prongs placed opposite each other to replace the fingers and thumb. The opposition placement is necessary to allow the amputee to hold articles in a normal manner. Clients can activate their prostheses by body movements or an external electrical power source.

Nursing Considerations
After amputation surgery, a *rigid* or *compression dressing* is applied to the residual limb to protect the limb, permit healing, control edema, and minimize pain and trauma. Two sets of compression bandages are needed so that bandages can be changed at least twice per day, or more often if a client perspires freely. Teach clients and their family members how to apply bandages. Correct residual limb wrapping reduces edema and is important to later use of a prosthesis. Wrap the residual limb so that it forms a cone shape. Obtain instructions for the recommended wrapping of each client's residual limb.

Preventing Complications
Potential complications following amputation include hemorrhage, infection, failure of the residual limb incisions to

heal, and deformity of proximal structures. Use the following nursing actions to prevent complications:

- Keep a tourniquet within reach at all times to be applied if severe, life-threatening bleeding occurs.
- Observe the dressing for bleeding.
- Change the dressing using aseptic technique.
- If the surgeon has inserted drains, monitor and document the amount, color, consistency, and odor of drainage.
- Avoid dislodging drains when turning the client.
- When changing dressings, check the incision closely for signs of healing. Report any signs of dark-red to black tissue, opened areas along the incision line, unusual drainage, or lack of healing. Dark-red or black tissue is a sign of **gangrene**, which is necrosis of tissue caused by insufficient or lack of blood supply.
- Encourage the client who has had a leg amputated to lie in a prone position, rather than on the back. To prevent hip contractures, do not place pillows under the residual limb when the client is on the back. Reduce residual limb edema by elevating the foot of the bed.
- If ordered, apply skin traction to the residual limb as soon as the client returns from surgery. A cast of lightweight material is sometimes applied to the residual limb to maintain its shape.
- If no cast is in place, cleanse, dry, and carefully inspect the residual limb according to the institution's protocols. Report any redness or irritation because any irritation or skin breakdown will interfere with the use of a prosthesis and may lead to infection.

Client Teaching

Teach and encourage prosthesis self-care as soon as possible. Show clients how to wash, rinse, and dry the residual limb. Teach clients how to inspect the residual limb for signs of complications and how to use prostheses. Teach clients who are wearing limb socks to avoid skin problems by keeping the socks free of wrinkles. Instruct clients how to maintain the actual prostheses.

Providing Emotional Support

Clients who have amputations naturally react with grief because of their limb loss and change in body image. They may exhibit irritability, anger, depression, and other emotions. Allow time for clients to express such feelings. Listen to their concerns and provide support. Refer clients to support or recreation groups. Help family members adjust to the change and provide support for them as well through listening, understanding, and encouragement.

Assisting With Exercise

When clients undergo foot or leg amputations, they are prepared for walking by increasing the strength of upper extremities. Exercises to increase arm strength for crutch walking may start preoperatively. Encourage ROM exercises. Physical therapists may show clients how to maintain muscle tone. Direct your efforts to help clients prevent contractures. Usually, by the first or second postoperative day, most clients can sit up at the edge of the bed and soon progress to a wheelchair. Periodic bed rest is advisable because prolonged sitting may cause contractures and edema. Crutch walking should begin as soon as possible. Amputation changes a person's sense of balance; thus, clients who have experienced amputation require close supervision as they resume movement and ambulation.

Replantation of Severed Limbs

Replantation is the reattachment of a completely severed body part. With the advent of microvascular surgery, some clients who suffer traumatic amputations may have their limbs successfully replanted, although this procedure is sometimes impossible. Factors affecting the success of this type of surgery include the availability of a specialist and equipment for the procedure, the client's general condition, and the condition of the severed extremity. Usually, reattachment of lower extremities is less successful than reattachments of upper extremities because of the large and complex sciatic nerve system that innervates the legs.

Postoperative management includes anticoagulation therapy, a caffeine-free diet to prevent vasospasm, wound care, administration of antibiotics, and continuous inspection of the replanted part. Perform frequent neurovascular checks of the replanted limb. Monitor for complications, such as bleeding, arterial or venous compromise, infection, or decreased ROM.

Chronic Back Pain

Back pain, particularly lower back pain, is a malady that affects nearly 80% of all individuals. It has many causes, but perhaps the most common contributing factor is that the human body stands and walks upright, with most of its weight centering on the lumbar region of the pelvis. The stresses of upright mobility may cause lumbosacral ligament strain and aching muscles. As the body grows older, the combination of prolonged muscular and ligament strain, pressure on the lumbosacral vertebrae, and the aging process itself results in problems such as osteoarthritis, **spinal stenosis** (narrowing of the intervertebral space), and intervertebral disk problems. All of these conditions cause pain because of pressure on the nerves or inflammation of the lower back muscles.

Back pain may be caused by abnormal or exaggerated curvatures of the vertebral column. **Lordosis** ("swayback") is an abnormal curvature of lumbar vertebrae. **Kyphosis** ("humpback" or "hunchback") is an abnormal curvature of the thoracic spine. **Scoliosis** is a lateral (side-to-side) angulation of the spinal column. Abnormal spinal column curvatures may be caused by poor posture, congenital disease, malignancy, compression fractures, osteoarthritis, rheumatoid arthritis, rickets, or aging. Treatment for these conditions will include combinations of therapies, including exercise and electrical muscle stimulation. In more severe cases, braces, casts, or traction may be used. Scoliosis is more common in adolescence and may require insertion of spine-strengthening braces (Milwaukee brace) and support rods (Harrington rod; Chapter 73).

> **NCLEX Alert**
>
> Clinical situations on an NCLEX may contain terminology that will affect the correct response. Be sure that you are aware of the nursing interventions, side effects, client teaching, and other issues associated with the terminology.

Herniated Intervertebral Disc Disease

The *intervertebral disc* (**IVD**) is a small pad or disc of rubberylike cartilage (*nucleus pulposus*) located between two vertebrae. The spelling of *disc* is often used interchangeably with *disk*. With age or trauma, the disc can push some of its softer interior jellylike substances through a crack in the exterior of the disc. The result is pressure against the spinal nerves and pain that radiates out from the spinal cord. Typically, disc problems occur in the cervical or lumbar areas. The phenomenon is referred to as *herniated IVD disease, intervertebral disc disease* (**IVDD**), or *herniated nucleus pulposus* (**HNP**). Commonly, the condition is referred to as a "slipped disc." The problem of pain with this dislocation is known as *sciatica* because the sciatic nerve is commonly a site of damage and resulting pain.

IVDD's signs and symptoms include limited ability to bend forward, gait difficulty; back, shoulder, or neck pain; and *paresthesia* (numbness) and muscle spasm. Risk factors include advancing age, obesity, stress, congenitally small lumbar spinal canal, degenerative joint disease, and progressive bone disorders, such as osteoporosis. Persons whose occupations require exposure to vibrating equipment, repetitive work movements, or frequent bending, twisting, heavy lifting, pushing, or pulling are at risk for IVDD.

Diagnostic Tests

Diagnosis can be made with a CT scan or MRI, performed in conjunction with the presentation of a positive history and physical examination. The CT scan and MRI can identify spinal stenosis, soft-tissue abnormalities, and spinal cord compression. X-rays of the spine can show degenerative changes and can evaluate the disk's internal structure.

Medical and Surgical Treatment

Clients are rarely immobilized. Instead, physical therapists recommend a treatment plan that includes regular walking or aquatic exercise. Lumbosacral corsets or braces may be used to improve muscular support of the lower back; however, they do not significantly decrease long-term pain. Clients wear them only for a short time because prolonged use weakens the supporting abdominal muscles. Antispasmodic and analgesic medications may be helpful. The therapist may also prescribe ultrasound, heat or ice application, intermittent traction, or TENS therapies.

If such methods are unsuccessful in relieving symptoms, clients may choose surgery. Spinal disorders caused by pressure on a spinal nerve can often be treated surgically by removing the causes of pressure, if possible.

In an operation called a *lumbar decompression,* the surgeon removes a portion of the vertebra to expose the spinal cord and takes out the bone fragment, herniated disk, tumor, or clot pressing on neural elements. A **laminectomy** is a type of lumbar decompression that exposes the spinal canal and allows for relief of compression of the spinal cord and spinal nerve roots. A *diskectomy* removes the herniated disk, which can relieve pressure on the nerves. This procedure can usually be performed on an outpatient basis using an endoscope, resulting in only a very small incision.

Microdiskectomy may also be used to remove a herniation. The surgeon makes a small incision and uses a microscope to help visualize the disk. Because microdiskectomy is quicker and less traumatic than more invasive surgeries, the client experiences a shorter hospital stay and recovers more rapidly. Sometimes, the weakened vertebra can be strengthened by the attachment of a steel rod or by grafting a piece of bone from the tibia or iliac crest, or from donated bone, onto several vertebrae or between a vertebra and the sacrum in a process called *spinal fusion*. When the graft heals, the spine in that area will be stiff.

Another surgical procedure is the *interbody fusion*. In this procedure, bone grafts or substitutes are placed between the vertebrae after the disk space is cleaned out. The bone graft is supplemented with a metal fusion cage or other instrument. The surgeon determines the specific type of fusion to be done after careful testing to determine the cause of spinal instability.

Nursing Considerations

For the client undergoing surgery, provide routine postoperative care and assist with pain management. Give meticulous wound care to prevent contamination because infection could lead to meningitis. Watch closely for signs of bleeding and other drainage, leakage of cerebrospinal fluid, or shock caused by trauma. Evaluate the client's neurologic function at frequent intervals. Carefully follow the healthcare provider's orders for the client regarding turning, positioning, and getting out of bed.

When a lumbar decompression has been performed, carefully observe the client's level of sensation and mobility in the legs. Observe for further complications, such as spinal nerve damage or spinal cord damage, which may have occurred during surgery. Immediately report any complaints of tingling, numbness, or difficulty in moving the legs.

Be alert for the edema that may be an inflammatory response to the trauma of surgery. Edema around the tissues of the surgical site may cause pressure on the spinal cord and may also lead to fluid collection in the legs. In Practice: Data Gathering in Nursing 77-2 provides information on factors to consider following lumbar decompression.

In addition, if a cervical laminectomy or decompression was performed, monitor the client's upper extremities for evidence of nerve damage or impaired respiratory function.

Although adequate rest is required, encourage clients to move to prevent respiratory complications. Assist the client in participating with the turning procedures prescribed by the healthcare provider. For example, the client can hold the body straight and keep the arms crossed over the chest while being rolled as a single entity (*logroll turn*). Use a turning sheet if necessary.

Manage postoperative pain. Pain medication is often given via a patient-controlled analgesia (PCA) pump or epidural catheter. Offer analgesics before moving, turning, or ambulating the client. Encourage the use of pain medications so that the client is reasonably comfortable both at rest and with activity.

> **Key Concept**
> Clients with acute or chronic pain need consistent, reliable pain relief.

The client is usually allowed out of bed on the day of surgery. Assist the client to their side, and then gradually and

IN PRACTICE
DATA GATHERING IN NURSING 77-2 — Postlumbar Decompression Concerns

- *Nerve damage:* Change in sensation or mobility of legs; tingling, numbness of legs, urinary retention
- *Edema:* Collection of fluid in legs; severe pain, which could indicate edema within spinal column
- *Change in level of consciousness:* Possibly indicative of encephalitis or meningitis
- *Muscle spasms:* Leg pain; possibly prevented by exercises
- *Thrombophlebitis:* Leg pain; can be prevented by surgical stockings, exercises, and ambulation
- *Additional injury:* Prevented by avoiding heavy lifting for a period
- *Infection:* Fever, wound drainage, erythema

Following *cervical* decompression, also observe for nerve damage suggested by the following:

- Difficulty or change in sensation of arms
- Difficulty in moving arms
- Difficulty in breathing

---

smoothly move the legs over the side of the bed as the client pushes up with the arms to a sitting position. Finally, help the client rise to a standing position, while maintaining spinal support and alignment at all times.

Most clients wear a thoracic–lumbar–sacral orthosis (**TLSO**) brace or a corset to support the back and to maintain the effects of surgery. Before applying a brace, put a thin cotton shirt on the client to protect the skin. Be sure to smooth all wrinkles to avoid unnecessary pressure against the skin. Follow the institution's policy and manufacturer's instructions for applying the device. When placing a bedpan, never lift the client, but rather roll the client onto the pan. Always use a fracture bedpan. *Rationale: It is smaller and the client does not arch the back when using it.* Teach the client never to reach or stretch for articles.

During the first few postoperative days, the client may develop muscle spasms, especially in the legs. The healthcare provider may order exercises to relieve these spasms. Teach the client isometric exercises for the quadriceps because they can perform these exercises without moving in bed. Apply antiembolism stockings and intermittent pneumatic compression devices (also known as sequential compression devices). These items help prevent thrombus formation related to immobility.

After lumbar decompression surgery, the client is gradually allowed to do light work but must always avoid heavy lifting. Instruct the client to take caution when lifting anything for at least 1 year after surgery. Reinforce proper body mechanics and appropriate lifting techniques. Emphasize that disregarding precautions—even once during convalescence—may result in injury.

If a spinal fusion has been performed, the client may encounter more limitations. They usually must wear a brace or corset whenever leaving bed. Occasionally, the healthcare provider orders the client to wear the brace at all times. Sometimes, the healthcare provider applies a body cast. Tell the client to avoid prolonged sitting because it places extra strain on the back. The client is never moved unless the healthcare provider has ordered it and healthcare personnel have learned the correct procedure. The client who is paralyzed also needs care appropriate to the degree of paralysis.

After a cervical diskectomy, the client usually wears a cervical collar to limit neck extension, rotation, and flexion. Teach the client to keep their neck in a neutral and aligned position. Instruct the client to wear the collar as directed by the healthcare provider. Show the client how to open the cervical collar and wash and dry the neck. Assist the client with sitting by supporting the client's neck and shoulders.

Temporomandibular Joint Disorders

Temporomandibular joint (**TMJ**) disorders are painful, aching disorders involving the facial bones and muscles around the joint between the mandible and the temporal bones. TMJ may affect one side or both sides of the face. Chewing may make the condition worse. The joints may have limited movement, and the client may note clicking sounds during chewing. In more severe cases, tinnitus and deafness may be present. Stress, *malocclusion* (malpositioning) of the upper and lower jaw, poorly fitting dentures, rheumatoid arthritis, and neoplasms are the most common causes of TMJ. Successful treatment involves identifying the cause, physical therapy, anti-inflammatory agents, and braces or surgery, if indicated.

Degenerative Disorders

Muscular Dystrophies

Muscular dystrophies are chronic, degenerative diseases of skeletal muscles that are often inherited. These disorders are characterized by various degrees of progressive weakening and wasting of the muscles.

Although causes of muscular dystrophies are unknown, some researchers believe that they are related to a disruption in enzyme production. Treatment focuses on support. Encourage clients to continue all activities as normally as possible. Exercise programs and splints may help prevent deformities. Often, clients can use special braces to permit ambulation. Inform clients of the need to prevent upper respiratory infections, to maintain ideal weight, and to strive for general good health (Chapter 74).

SPECIAL CONSIDERATIONS — Lifespan

Muscles of the Older Adult

With advanced age, a person experiences a decrease in muscle strength. Joints become stiff and slightly more flexed with age.

Repetitive Strain Injuries

Repetitive strain injuries commonly occur in the workplace because of the necessity of performing certain motions, such as keyboarding, repeatedly in some occupations. These injuries may also be identified as *overuse disorders*.

Carpal Tunnel Syndrome

Carpal tunnel syndrome is a compression neuropathy of the median nerve in the wrist. Often, its cause is repetitive movements, such as knitting or keyboarding. Other causes include arthritis, trauma, myxedema, gout, or tumors.

Signs and symptoms include forearm and wrist pain, numbness, and tingling. Symptoms often increase at night. The client's grip is weak. When the provider taps the median nerve, the client experiences paresthesia and pain in the thumb and first three fingers (Tinel sign).

Treatment includes wrist splinting, rest, nonsteroidal anti-inflammatory drugs (NSAIDs), and corticosteroid injections. If these therapies are unsuccessful, surgery may be done to decompress the carpal tunnel.

SPECIAL CONSIDERATIONS   Lifespan

Pregnancy
Pregnant clients may experience carpal tunnel syndrome related to fluid retention in that area.

Lateral Epicondylitis

Repeated forceful wrist and finger movements that stress the origins of muscles cause *lateral epicondylitis*. Lateral epicondylitis is often related to activities such as tennis, bowling, pitching, and golf and thus may be called "tennis elbow."

Clients with lateral epicondylitis often complain of pain along the outer aspect of the elbow, radiating to the forearm. Pain increases on stretching and on resisted wrist and hand flexion. Common treatments include splinting, analgesics, rest, and corticosteroid injections. Surgery is generally not needed but is usually successful if performed.

Rotator Cuff Injury

Injury to the rotator muscles in the shoulders may be caused by repetitive injury or sudden trauma. The injury can vary in severity. Pain, weakness, and loss of shoulder movement generally result. Less severe injuries may be treated with extended physical therapy to increase ROM and muscle strength. With more severe injuries, surgical intervention often is necessary because these injuries tend not to heal by medical intervention alone.

Inflammatory Disorders

Bursitis

The *bursa* is a sac filled with synovial fluid that pads bony prominences in the joints. **Bursitis** is inflammation of a bursa related to mechanical irritation, bacterial infection, trauma, or gout. In response to inflammation, fluid increases, causing distention. With chronic inflammation, calcification may result. Pain and tenderness in the joint limit movement.

Usual treatment includes heating and resting the affected part. Anti-inflammatory medications may be indicated. The healthcare provider may inject the bursal sac with corticosteroids or aspirate fluid from it to provide relief. A surgical drainage is performed for infectious bursitis. If these treatments are ineffective, the bursa is excised surgically.

Tenosynovitis

Tenosynovitis, an inflammation of the tendon sheath that may result from irritation or an infection, typically affects the wrist or ankle. The infected tendon swells and is painful and disabling. Noninfectious tenosynovitis is caused by strains, blows, or prolonged use of a particular set of tendons (e.g., playing the piano over a long period). Symptoms include pain and tenderness, especially on movement. Treatment involves the following:

- Resting the affected body part; application of a splint
- Application of ice for 1 to 2 days to decrease swelling
- Physical therapy
- Use of NSAIDs, when indicated
- Surgery, if needed
- Antibiotics
- Elimination of activities that exacerbate symptoms during the inflammatory phase

Arthritis

Arthritis means joint inflammation. More than 100 arthritic disorders are known. The most common types include the following:

- Rheumatoid arthritis (**RA**)
- Osteoarthritis (**OA**), degenerative joint disease (**DJD**), hypertrophic arthritis
- Ankylosing spondylitis, rheumatoid spondylitis, RA of the spine
- Gouty arthritis
- Systemic lupus erythematosus (**SLE**), lupus
- Scleroderma, progressive systemic sclerosis

Arthritis affects many people in the United States. *Monoarticular arthritis* affects one joint; *polyarticular arthritis* affects many joints. Most types of arthritis, except for ankylosing spondylitis and gouty arthritis, are more common in women than in men. Several factors may be associated with the cause of arthritis:

- Infection of a joint by a virus or microorganism (*infectious arthritis*)
- Direct injury to a joint (*traumatic arthritis*)
- Degeneration or deterioration of a joint (*degenerative arthritis*)
- Metabolic disorder, such as gout (*metabolic arthritis*)

Many researchers believe that some types of arthritis have an autoimmune component and/or familial tendencies. In most cases, the cause of the arthritis and its cure are unknown. However, control of the disorder or correction of its crippling effects may be possible. Arthritis occurs in both *acute* and *chronic* forms. Acute exacerbations may also occur with chronic forms of the disease.

> **Key Concept**
>
> Arthritis can interfere with an individual's ability to perform both basic (hygienic) and instrumental (functioning) activities of daily living. For example, because of pain and physical joint deformations, arthritis interferes with using one's hands (buttons, laces, handling coins) or lifting objects (shopping, gardening, cleaning). The individual can have difficulty maintaining social activities owing to the interrelationship of pain, fatigue, and frustration.

Monocyclic arthritis, which accounts for approximately 35% of cases, has a sudden onset, usually responds well to medications, and may never return. *Polycyclic arthritis,* accounting for approximately 50% of cases, is marked by exacerbations and remissions. *Progressive arthritis,* accounting for approximately 15% of cases, continues to worsen, not stopping without treatment.

The clinical features of arthritis include the following:

- Persistent pain and stiffness on arising lasting for 6 weeks or more
- Stiffness aggravated by damp weather or strenuous activity
- Pain or tenderness in the joints, often symmetrical
- Swelling in the joints
- Recurrence of symptoms, particularly when more than one joint is involved
- Obvious redness and warmth in a joint
- Unexplained weight loss, fever, or weakness, combined with joint pain
- *Bouchard nodes* (enlargement of proximal interphalangeal joints) or *Heberden nodes* (growths on the terminal phalangeal joints) with DJD

Box 77-1 describes goals and pain management in the treatment of arthritis.

Rheumatoid Arthritis

Rheumatoid arthritis is probably the most painful and crippling form of arthritis. It occurs worldwide and, until age 65 years, is three times more common in women than in men. Theories suggest that a triggering mechanism, possibly a virus, causes the immune system to become overactive. A genetic predisposition to the disorder seems to exist; several members of one family may be affected (Table 77-1).

Signs and Symptoms

Chronic inflammatory changes thicken the synovial membrane. The joint capsule swells, the synovial membrane becomes inflamed, and the cartilage is eaten away. An overgrowth of synovial lining occurs. When the cartilage and bone erode, the joint becomes painful because bone rubs against bone. If the *joint* becomes calcified, movement is impossible. The condition of an immovable joint is called **ankylosis**; however, it does not occur in all persons with RA. If the opening in the *spinal column* becomes calcified, its diameter becomes smaller, a condition called *spinal stenosis*. Spinal stenosis can place pressure on the spinal cord.

Rheumatoid arthritis often begins with systemic symptoms such as fatigue, weakness, weight loss, and general body aches. Joints become painful, tender, stiff, swollen, and warm. As tendons and ligaments become shortened and less flexible, joint deformities, such as *hyperextension, contractures,* and *subluxation* (dislocation), can occur (Fig. 77-1).

Box 77-1 Management of Arthritis

GOALS
- Relieve inflammation (medication)
- Relieve pain (medications, local treatments)
- Maintain optimal functioning (exercise, adaptive devices)
- Educate the client (prevention, treatment)

PAIN MANAGEMENT
- Splinting/casting/night splinting/traction
- Positioning
- Heat (paraffin baths, diathermy) and cold (ice packs)
- Physical therapy
- Massage (if joint is not acutely inflamed)
- Medications (most commonly salicylates and nonsteroidal anti-inflammatory drugs [NSAIDs])
- Low-impact exercise; isometric exercises (improves muscle strength without overexerting joints)
- Rest (physical and emotional); avoidance of fatigue and overexertion (10 or more hours of rest daily)
- Sleeping on a firm bed
- Placement of bed and chair at same level, to facilitate transfer; chair that helps client to stand is possibly necessary
- Chair 3 to 4 in. higher than regular chair to avoid bending too much at hips. (Do not use pillow in chair; promotes slouching, which is tiring.)
- Emotional support
- Adaptive devices to make activities of daily living easier to perform

---

Medical Treatment

The goal of treatment is to help the client maintain function and reduce inflammation before joints are permanently damaged. Treatment is multidisciplinary and includes drug therapy (In Practice: Important Medications 77-1), client education (In Practice: Educating the Client 77-1), physical therapy, occupational therapy, and psychosocial therapy. Physical therapists design exercise programs that help clients prevent contractures, strengthen muscles, and improve function. Occupational therapists teach clients how to protect their joints and how to use adaptive devices. Measures to increase body resistance to disease, such as rest and a well-balanced diet, are also helpful.

> **Nursing Alert** Many drugs used to treat arthritis have serious side effects, such as gastrointestinal bleeding. Be sure to check drug reference sources before administering any drugs. Be alert to possible side effects and report any difficulties immediately.

TABLE 77-1 Rheumatoid Arthritis Versus Osteoarthritis

RHEUMATOID ARTHRITIS	OSTEOARTHRITIS (DEGENERATIVE JOINT DISEASE)
Systemic (fatigue, weight loss, anemia)	Not systemic (results from wear and tear)
Fever	No fever
Systemic inflammation	Local inflammation (joint only)
Probably autoimmune origin	Most common type of arthritis
3:1 in women	2:1 in women
Affects young adults (ages 20-30 years)	Affects middle and older adults (>45 years) Common in women after menopause More common in obese people
Affects small and large joints (symmetrical); most common in fingers, knees, elbows, ankles	Affects primarily large weight-bearing joints and knuckles (knees, hips, knuckles, spine)
May remain the same for life	May progress
Causes inflammatory process in other body parts (lungs, kidneys, eyes)	Sets up local inflammation Can be hereditary
Surgery does not help (condition returns)	May surgically replace or fuse joints (last choice for treatment)
May have lumps (nodules) on joints, which are painful	Often have lumps, but they do not restrict activity and are not painful
Fingers may swell; joints feel cold and moist; bluish color to skin; muscles may become weakened	Joints usually do not swell; muscles remain firm
Joints are distorted and dislocated	Not as likely to be disabling; may remain localized in body
Joints may ankylose (fuse)	Joints usually do not ankylose
Abnormal laboratory values (rheumatoid factor, sedimentation rate high; hemoglobin low)	

Adapted from https://www.uwhealth.org/health/topic/special/comparing-rheumatoid-arthritis-and-osteoarthritis/aa19377.html; https://www.arthritis.com/about-arthritis/rheumatoid-arthritis-vs-osteoarthritis

Osteoarthritis or Degenerative Joint Disease

Osteoarthritis, believed to have a genetic cause or predisposition, is caused by wear and tear on a joint. The cartilage wears away and exposes the bone (Fig. 77-2). Next, bony *hypertrophy* (overgrowth) occurs, with the creation of bone spurs. Particles of cartilage break off and float in the joint, making movement painful. **Synovectomy,** excision of the synovial membrane, helps to prevent further inflammation in some cases. Arthroscopic surgery may be done to remove loose bodies and bone spurs. Total arthroplasty (joint replacement) is the last resort and, in many cases, is effective. In other cases, the joint must be fused to prevent pain (Table 77-1).

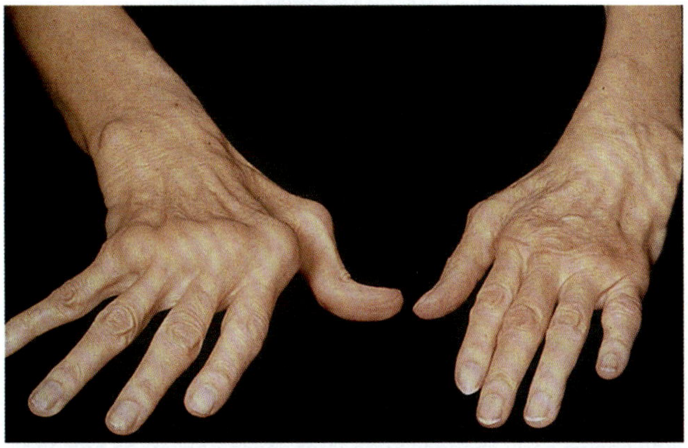

Ankylosing Spondylitis

Ankylosing spondylitis, also called *rheumatoid arthritis of the spine,* primarily affects the facet joints and the stabilizing ligaments of the spinal column. It mainly affects men and often begins in adolescence or young adulthood. The most common early symptoms are hip and lower back pain and stiffness. Other symptoms include pain and limited chest expansion, anorexia, weight loss, mild fatigue, fever, and iritis. Hip contractures and flexion of the neck and back may occur. Breathing may be impaired because chest expansion is impeded. The osteoporotic spine increases the risk of spinal fractures. In severe cases, spinal stiffening also occurs, with resultant humpback and chest curvature. Neck stiffness may make turning the head impossible.

Treatment is similar to that for other types of arthritis. NSAIDs, sulfasalazine, and tumor necrosis factor alpha antagonists such as etanercept (Enbrel) are given. Teach the

Figure 77-1 A severe dislocation called *subluxation of the fingers* in rheumatoid arthritis.

IN PRACTICE
IMPORTANT MEDICATIONS 77-1 — For Arthritis

Nonsteroidal Anti-Inflammatory Drugs
Ibuprofen (Motrin, Advil, Nuprin)
Indomethacin (Indocin)
Piroxicam (Feldene)
Sulindac (Clinoril)
Naproxen (Naprosyn, Aleve)
Ketoprofen (Frotek)
Ketorolac tromethamine (Toradol)
Nabumetone (Relafen)

Gold Salts
Auranofin (Ridaura)
Antimalarials
Hydroxychloroquine sulfate (Plaquenil sulfate)
Chloroquine (Aralen)

Corticosteroids
Cortisone (Cortone)
Hydrocortisone (Cortef)
Prednisone (Deltasone)

Immunosuppressives
Methotrexate (Abitrexate)
Azathioprine (Imuran)
Cyclophosphamide (Cytoxan)
Cyclosporine (Gengraf)
Sulfasalazine (Azulfidine)
Leflunomide (Arava)
Hydroxychloroquine sulfate (Plaquenil)
D-penicillamine
Azathioprine (Azasan)

Biologic Agents
Rituximab (Rituxan)
Infliximab (Remicade)
Adalimumab (Humira)
Golimumab (Simponi)
Etanercept (Enbrel)

IN PRACTICE
EDUCATING THE CLIENT 77-1 — Exercising With Arthritis

- Keep your body in the best possible physical condition. Control weight, rest, and exercise.
- Exercise daily even if you have pain. Do specific exercises and not just daily work.
- Apply heat before exercise to lessen pain. Do not overdo exercise because of lessened pain.
- Prepare for exercise with gentle stretching.
- When possible, do active exercise. If not possible, do isometrics or have someone perform passive exercise. You may use a continuous passive motion machine. Stretching and exercise are better when they are done actively (self-movement) rather than passively (by a nurse or therapist).
- Engage in low-impact exercises such as swimming, slow walking, or bicycling.
- Stop exercising if pain becomes too severe.
- Use an adaptive brace or corrective corset or brace as needed.
- Prevent contractures: turn doorknobs to radial (thumb) side when possible. Flatten hand as much as possible.

client to refrain from lying on the side, to prevent excess sideways spinal curvature. Light exercise may be more comfortable than prolonged bed rest. The client may wear a back brace.

SYSTEMIC DISORDERS WITH MUSCULOSKELETAL MANIFESTATIONS

Gout

The body produces substances called *purines* during metabolism. If the body is unable to metabolize these substances, uric acid accumulates in the bloodstream and forms crystal deposits in the joints. This arthritic condition, called **gout** or hyperuricemia, usually affects the big toe, instep, ankle, or knee, but it may appear in any joint. Gouty arthritis is more common in men. Alcohol, allergies, surgery, injury, infection, nitrogenous or fatty foods, a fasting diet, emotional stress, or a change in the person's environment can trigger a gout attack. Secondary gout may be associated with drugs such as thiazide diuretics and cyclosporine (Sandimmune) or associated with other diseases such as diabetes mellitus, hypertension, or hypothyroidism.

Signs and Symptoms

Periodic gout attacks are characterized by joint swelling, redness, and severe pain. The slightest touch or weight on the affected area is unbearable during an attack. The person may have fever, *tachycardia* (rapid heartbeat), and anorexia. An attack lasts from 3 to 14 days, after which it disappears

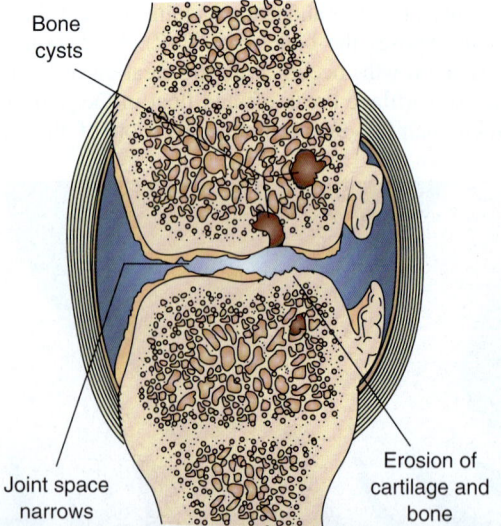

Figure 77-2 Joint changes in osteoarthritis. Notice that the left side shows early changes, with joint space narrowing and cartilage breakdown. The right side shows severe progression, with lost cartilage.

suddenly. It may return at any time. However, at other times, the joint is normal. Eventually, repeated attacks permanently damage the joint and limit its ROM. Renal damage and vascular damage (especially atherosclerosis) can follow.

Medical Treatment

Gout cannot be cured, but attacks can be prevented and controlled by adhering to prescribed routines and making regular visits to healthcare providers. Some healthcare providers instruct clients to avoid high-purine foods (e.g., liver, anchovies, mussels, trout, veal, salmon, turkey, and sardines); other healthcare providers prescribe no dietary changes. Gradual weight loss and avoidance of excessive alcohol intake are encouraged.

Colchicine (Colcrys) is usually effective in relieving gout symptoms. This medication must be administered within 24 hr of the onset of acute gout symptoms for it to be effective. Side effects include gastrointestinal disturbances (nausea, vomiting, abdominal pain, and diarrhea). The healthcare provider also may order corticosteroids or NSAIDs. Probenecid (Probalan) is used in long-term management because it prevents the kidney's reabsorption of uric acid. Allopurinol (Zyloprim) or febuxostat (Uloric) inhibits uric acid formation. Instruct clients taking any of these medications to drink at least 3 L of a variety of fluids each day to promote excretion of a large urine volume. When taking these medications, clients should not take acetylsalicylic acid (Aspirin) or any other salicylate because they counteract the effects of gout-relieving drugs.

Nursing Considerations

The affected joint needs protection. If the client is in bed, use a bed cradle to protect the joint. If necessary, hang a warning sign in a prominent place to prevent jarring or bumping of the bed. Gentle application of warm or cold compresses is sometimes ordered. Elevate the affected joint for comfort. To prevent the joint from stiffening, start ROM exercises as soon as the pain and the redness clear.

Lupus Erythematosus

The two types of *lupus erythematosus* are discoid and systemic. *Discoid lupus erythematosus* is a chronic disease with skin manifestations of disc-like patches with raised, reddish edges and depressed centers. *SLE* ("lupus") is an autoimmune systemic disorder that affects many body systems.

People with SLE produce autoantibodies that ultimately contribute to immune complex formation and tissue damage. SLE primarily affects women. It can be acute or chronic, marked by remissions and exacerbations. It causes widespread damage to the collagen system, affecting any organ system, including the kidneys, heart, and lungs. The characteristic sign of SLE is a butterfly rash on the face. However, a rash may appear over other body parts as well. Arthritic symptoms include joint pain and muscle aches. Other symptoms include anorexia, nausea, vomiting, swollen glands, and general malaise. In severe cases, the inflammatory process may involve the lining of the lungs and heart, with damage to the kidneys, central nervous system, or brain.

Medical Treatment

Although SLE has no known cure, early intervention can often prevent serious joint damage. Treatment, which is focused on preventing complications, minimizing disability, and preventing organ dysfunction, is based on manifestations of symptoms.

Commonly used medications include NSAIDs, corticosteroids, and immunosuppressive drugs. Teach clients to avoid sunlight because it can intensify skin manifestations. If clients cannot avoid the sun, instruct them to apply sunscreen lotion with a sun protection factor (SPF) of at least 22. Adequate rest and prevention of exhaustion are essential. Treatment of the musculoskeletal symptoms of SLE is similar to the treatment of other types of arthritis: medication, exercise, and physical therapy.

Scleroderma

The term **scleroderma** means "hard skin." Scleroderma is considered a collagen disorder that involves chronic hardening and shrinking of connective tissues. Most often, this condition affects women, usually beginning in middle age. Its most severe forms commonly affect men, African Americans, and older people. Scleroderma may have an autoimmune component. The disorder may be localized or generalized.

Localized scleroderma primarily involves the skin, muscles, and bones and is a less severe form. *Generalized scleroderma* involves the skin, muscles, joints, and internal organs, such as the heart, digestive tract, lungs, and kidneys. **Sclerodactyly** is scleroderma of the fingers and toes; **acrosclerosis** is scleroderma of the distal extremities and face.

The disorder begins on the face and hands, where the skin becomes hard and unwrinkled and cannot be raised from the underlying structures. The condition slowly spreads. The person often has joint pain and difficulty moving. *Raynaud phenomenon,* evidenced by hands or fingers that are cold, numb, tingling, or blanched, is usually an early symptom. Over time, the face appears tight, shiny, and rigid. The fingers may become flexed and atrophied. Death may result from respiratory or renal failure or cardiac dysrhythmias.

Treatment is symptomatic. Joint manifestations are treated in the same manner as in other arthritic conditions. Drug therapy has been ineffective in treating scleroderma.

Nursing Considerations

Because of the client's hardened skin, take measures to prevent skin breakdown. Also consider the condition of the client's hardened skin when giving injections. Teach clients to avoid smoking and exposure to cold. Emotional support is vital.

Rickets and Osteomalacia

Rickets is a disease that results from a deficiency of vitamin D during childhood. The adult form of vitamin D deficiency, which results in softening of the bones, is called **osteomalacia**. The deficiency causes faulty absorption of calcium and phosphorus, both of which the body needs for normal bone hardening.

In rickets, bones remain soft and become distorted as the child grows. When the bones finally do harden, they remain in this deformed state. Severely bowed legs are an example of an effect of rickets. Children with rickets are slow to walk and cut teeth; they are pale, irritable, and inactive. Exposure to sunshine and vitamin D from an early age prevents rickets, making it rare in developed countries. Milk with vitamin D and exposure to sunshine are preventive measures.

TRAUMATIC INJURIES

Sprains

A **sprain** is a traumatic injury to the tissues around a joint. The tissues, such as tendons, muscles, and ligaments, can stretch and tear. Bone fractures may result, as the tearing forces of the tendons and ligaments pull against the bone.

Sprains cause swelling, pain, and interference with movement. At first, a sprain may seem mild with minimal swelling. Rupture of the nearby blood vessels often leaves bruises (*ecchymosis*). Tissue damage can be mild or quite severe. If the sprain is left untreated and the client continues to use the extremity, the tissue damage can become worse. X-ray examinations may be indicated to rule out fractures.

Treat a sprain by elevating the injured part and using an elastic bandage or splint to immobilize and support the affected area. Relieve pain and swelling by applying ice for 24 to 48 hr. After the first 24 to 48 hr, use warm, moist packs to provide pain relief and prevent muscle spasms. Occasionally, the healthcare provider will apply a cast to keep the area immobile and to facilitate healing. Ligament rupture may require surgical repair.

Strains

A **strain** generally involves damage to the muscle and sometimes to the attached tendon. A strain is a less severe injury than a sprain. Signs and symptoms include pain, swelling, ecchymosis, loss of function, and muscle spasm. Treatment includes application of ice packs for 24 to 48 hr, elevation of the affected part, and rest. Surgical repair may be needed.

Dislocations

When a ligament gives way so completely that a bone displaces from its socket, the resulting injury is called a **dislocation**. Dislocations cause severe pain, abnormal bone position, and inability to manipulate the joint. Following an x-ray examination, the healthcare provider is usually able to put the bone back into position by stretching the ligaments and manipulating the joint. The client may receive sedation or anesthesia for this procedure. Occasionally, the dislocation cannot be reduced. In this case, the area must be surgically opened and realigned. A splint, a brace, or an elastic bandage is applied to immobilize the parts until they heal.

Apply ice to reduce swelling. Perform neurovascular checks above and below the affected area. The joint capsule and surrounding ligaments may take several weeks to return to their normal position.

Fractures

Any break or crack in a bone is called a **fracture** (Fx). Fractures occur when stress placed on a bone is greater than the bone can withstand. *Pathologic fractures* are bones that break spontaneously or with nominal trauma, in diseases such as osteomalacia, osteoporosis, bone cancer, and osteomyelitis. An older adult client may experience a pathologic fracture to an ankle, hip, or wrist by the ordinary act of getting up out of a chair.

> **Key Concept**
>
> Fractures involving any part of the vertebral column are very serious. *Cervical fractures, especially C1 to C4, can be immediately life threatening.* Cervical fractures can result in long-term respiratory dependency. All vertebral fractures can result in various levels of paralysis, with motor and nerve impairment. If you suspect any vertebral injury, immobilize the client and call for help immediately.

Most fractures, however, result from significant trauma. Usually surrounding structures, such as muscles, blood vessels, ligaments, and tendons, are injured as well. Traumatic events that cause fractures include striking a hard surface, a hard fall, or being subject to an indirect force that exerts a strong pulling force on the bone, such as getting a foot caught between rocks and the body falling away from the rocks.

SPECIAL CONSIDERATIONS Lifespan

Child Abuse

Child abuse is a common cause of fractures in children. Suspect abuse in a child who presents with fractures if the child's medical history is inconsistent, the child is younger than 1 year, the fracture is inappropriate for the child's developmental level, fractures have occurred at different times, a sibling is blamed for the injury, other evidence of abuse exists, or family caregivers delay seeking treatment.

Until age 45 years, more men than women have fractures; however, after this time, more women are affected because menopausal changes may cause decalcification of bones (osteoporosis). Many women take oral calcium in an effort to prevent osteoporosis. Some healthcare providers advise women to take the hormones estrogen and progesterone. A bisphosphonate, alendronate (Fosamax), increases bone density and reduces the risk of fractures and deformities.

SPECIAL CONSIDERATIONS Lifespan

Slippery floors and bathtubs, loose rugs, and dark stairways or corners are hazardous, especially for older adults.

Types and Patterns

The following are basic categories of fractures:

- *Complete:* An entire cross section of the bone is involved; the bone is usually displaced, which means that the bone fragments are out of alignment.
- *Incomplete:* A portion of the cross section of the bone is involved.
- *Closed:* The overlying skin is intact (this is sometimes called *simple fracture*).
- *Open:* The overlying skin is broken (this is sometimes called *compound fracture*), with various grades of tissue involvement.

CHAPTER 77 Musculoskeletal Disorders 1335

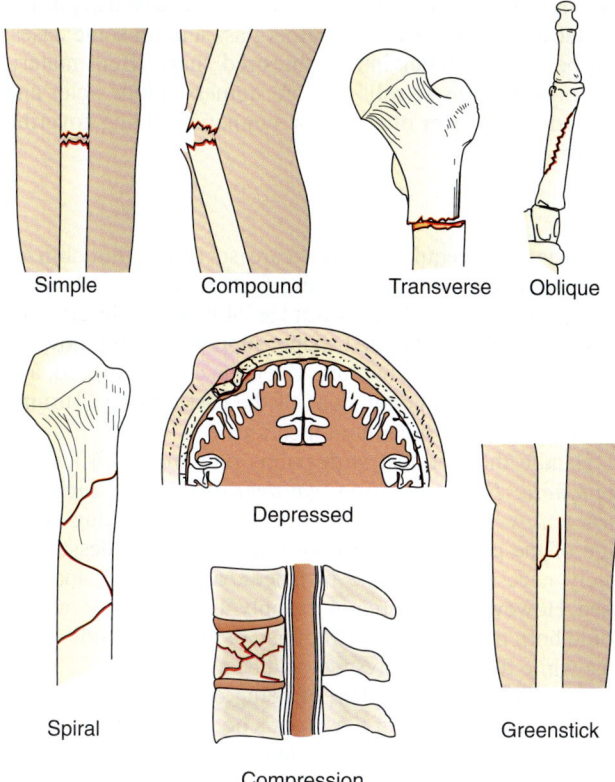

Figure 77-3 Fracture types and patterns. Fractures are classified according to type (complete, incomplete, closed [simple], or open [compound]) and the direction of fracture line (transverse, oblique, spiral, depressed or compression, and greenstick).

The pattern of the break defines some fractures. For instance, there are *transverse, oblique,* and *spiral fractures,* which are defined according to the direction of the fracture in the bone. A fracture may be *depressed,* in which bone splinters are driven into underlying tissue. In a *compression fracture,* the bone collapses in itself. In a *greenstick fracture,* one side of the bone breaks, while the other side bends (Fig. 77-3).

Signs and Symptoms

The most pronounced symptom of a fracture is pain that becomes more severe with movement of the part or when pressure is placed over the affected area. Loss of function and *deformity* (an unnatural position of the part) may accompany pain. Other symptoms include swelling over the part and discoloration caused by bleeding within the tissues.

> **Nursing Alert** A complicated fracture may result in the loss of the pulse distal to the fracture. Perform frequent neurovascular checks of the affected extremity. Compare skin color, pulse strength and symmetry, and movement proximally and distally to the injured areas.

TRAUMA CARE AND MANAGEMENT

With any traumatic musculoskeletal injury, x-ray films of the injured area are taken to determine the injury and its extent, such as a fracture and the resulting positions of bone fragments. A portable high-quality video machine is available to make the first determination of fracture. Such machines help in sports injuries because they can be carried onto the playing field before the injured person is moved.

The treatment objective is to restore the bone to natural alignment to ensure proper healing. The method chosen depends on the location and extent of the break and the client's condition and age. The fragments must be brought back into place (*reduction*) and held in that position (*immobilization*) until the broken parts heal. The two types of reduction are closed and open. In *closed reduction,* external manipulation realigns the bone ends; in *open reduction,* surgery accomplishes the realignment.

Different types of immobilization devices may be used, including casts, internal and external fixation, splints, and traction. The use of computers helps determine the exact type of prosthesis or reconstruction needed in some cases.

Many healthcare facilities have a special cast-and-splint room. In large facilities, specialized technicians work in this area. If the nurse is asked to assist, the healthcare provider will specify the desired cast or splint material to be used and will direct its application.

Often, clients receive analgesics or anesthetics before cast application; medications are given less frequently for splint application. If a general anesthetic is used, the immobilizing device is applied in an operating room or day-surgery center. Give routine preoperative and postoperative care.

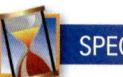 **SPECIAL CONSIDERATIONS** Lifespan

Casts
Sometimes, older clients with casts do not move sufficiently to counteract the dangers of hypostatic pneumonia. Encourage deep breathing exercises and the use of an incentive spirometer as a good preventive measure. Older persons may have difficulty learning to use crutches or other mobility aids safely.

Splints

Immediately after an injury, a temporary splint is necessary to immobilize the affected body part before treatment begins or until swelling subsides. Splints are also used for therapeutic purposes.

A common splint is the *half-cast,* in which a full cast is applied, then sawed in half lengthwise (*bivalved*). The bottom half of the cast may be used alone, or both halves may remain in place. Half-casts are held in place with an elastic roller bandage, which may also be used alone after healing begins, to give support. The half-cast may be taken off at intervals and reapplied, or it may remain in place for the full period of immobilization.

Another type of splint is the *inflatable splint,* consisting of a plastic bag that is inflated inside a second plastic bag with a zipper on one side. Although they are most often used in emergency first aid, acute care facilities also use inflatable splints. These splints are available in different sizes to fit various body parts, including the leg, ankle, and arm.

If an inflatable splint is to remain in place for some time, loosely apply a light stockinette to the affected extremity.

Apply the splint, zip it, and inflate it just enough to immobilize the part. This splint is comfortable because it is lightweight. It is also convenient for healthcare personnel to use because it is transparent and does not need to be removed when x-ray films are taken. Be careful not to puncture an inflatable splint.

Other splints include *Thomas* or *ring splints* (which may be used in combination with traction), molded aluminum splints, and other metal splints. Nursing care of a client in a splint is similar to that of a client in a cast.

> **Nursing Alert** Never ignore a complaint of pain or pressure from a person wearing a cast or splint. *Check the extremity's circulation, motion, and sensation (CMS), elevate the extremity, and report the situation immediately.*

Casts

A **cast** is a solid mold that is used to immobilize a fracture, relieve pain through rest, and stabilize an unstable fracture. The cast remains on the affected area until the bones have rejoined, a process called *fusion*. A cast may be applied in a client's room, emergency department, operating room, healthcare provider's office, or clinic. Nurses may be asked to assist with cast application. Specific in-service training is usually required (In Practice: Nursing Care Guidelines 77-1).

Types of Casts

Casts are typically made of plaster or a synthetic material such as fiberglass. Although fiberglass is lighter in weight, longer wearing, and allows better air circulation than plaster, plaster is less expensive than fiberglass and, in some cases, can be molded better into the desired shape. Both materials come in strips or rolls that are immersed into water and applied over a layer of cotton or synthetic padding covering the injured area.

Plaster Cast

A plaster cast requires proper care so that it immobilizes the injured part without causing further damage or injury. A large plaster cast remains wet for 24 to 48 hr. Because the cast must dry in its applied shape, support it with pillows to preserve the original contours. Keep the cast uncovered, and turn the client so that all sides of the cast will dry. Turning also helps prevent other complications.

Handle the wet cast with palms only, not with fingers. *Rationale: Finger pressure can dent a cast, creating pressure points.* Move the client's extremity by grasping either side of the casted area. Do not grasp the cast unless absolutely necessary. In some instances, a cast dryer may be used. However, take care not to apply intense heat because it could burn the client, crack the cast, or dry the outside of the cast while the inside stays wet and becomes moldy.

The client may complain of being cold while the cast is drying. Cover the rest of the client's body with a blanket and prevent drafts. If the weather is hot, the client may complain of being too warm. Cool liquids and a cool cloth applied to the forehead may help. If necessary, lower the room temperature slightly. Ice packs can be applied around the cast to offset the heat the drying plaster emits.

If a cast's edges are rough, cover them with tape, a procedure called *petaling*. If a stockinette is placed inside the cast, cover the rough edges by pulling the edge of the stockinette out, folding it over the cast's edge, and taping it in place. Doing so can help prevent irritation to the extremity caused by plaster crumbs and rough cast edges.

Protect a cast applied near the client's genital area against moisture. Even after a plaster cast dries, it must not become wet or the plaster will dissolve.

Synthetic Cast

Light synthetic casting materials, such as fiberglass, are often more convenient to use than are plaster casts. Most casts applied to the extremities are fiberglass. They are sometimes more durable and take less time to dry, drying in approximately 15 min. Synthetic casts are lighter and stronger than plaster casts. Some synthetic casts can be exposed to some water. X-ray films can be taken through this material. However, the synthetic cast is firm and has little, if any, flexibility, which some clients cannot tolerate.

> **Key Concept**
> If a cast or splint becomes dented, softened, or broken, it will not serve its purpose: immobilization of a body part.

Caring for Clients in Casts

In Practice: Nursing Care Guidelines 77-2 and In Practice: Educating the Client 77-2 provide fundamental information for the nurse, the client, and the family about cast care.

IN PRACTICE
NURSING CARE GUIDELINES 77-1 — Preparing for Casting

- Gather all materials beforehand, including a stockinette and padding materials. Be sure a source of water is available.
- Follow the manufacturer's instructions regarding preparation.
- Wear gloves if the fracture involves blood and to protect your hands from the casting materials.
- Prepare the injured area. In many cases, wash the area (without soap), carefully dry it, and shave it. Apply an astringent or alcohol if ordered.
- Lubricate the area, as ordered.
- Have sterile dressings available for an open (broken-skin) compound fracture.
- Position the client as directed.
- Assist or restrain the client, as needed.
- Reassure the client during the procedure.
- Be aware that a follow-up x-ray examination is necessary after the cast is applied. Ensure that the client is comfortable.
- Clean up immediately after the procedure, before the cast or splint material hardens and becomes difficult to remove. A special sink with a plaster trap is usually available. *Do not* put plaster or cast material in a regular sink.

IN PRACTICE
NURSING CARE GUIDELINES 77-2 Performing Cast Care

Synthetic Cast
- Check for rough edges. Petal as necessary. Pull sock or nylon stocking over the cast to prevent it from snagging on clothing. *Rationale: It is important to protect the skin from any form of irritation.*
- Do not immerse the cast totally in water. However, it is not necessary to prevent all contact with water. *Rationale: Although the cast is not likely to dissolve, when the cast or padding is soaked, the padding may begin to rot. Also, the underlying skin can itch or necrose.*
- Keep in mind that the fiberglass cast is solid and does not give, as does a plaster cast. The fiberglass cast, as a result, may be too tight for comfort. *Rationale: The tissues under casts can swell for as long as 3 days after injury. Any type of cast can become too tight, leading to damage to the nerves and blood vessels.*
- Carefully wash, dry, and gently massage the skin around the cast daily. *Rationale: A nursing priority is to monitor skin condition.*
- Caution the person against being too active. *Rationale: The cast can break, injuring the extremity further.*
- Perform neurovascular checks frequently. *Rationale: Checks to monitor circulation, motion, and sensation are needed to identify problems early and to remedy the problem with the goal of preventing long-term complications.*

Spica (Body) Cast
- Turn the client frequently. *Rationale: Frequent turning prevents development of pressure points, venostasis, and circulatory complications.*
- Reassure the client when turning them. *Rationale: Turning may cause apprehension and fear of falling.*
- Be sure no crumbs or other foreign substances get inside the cast. *Rationale: Foreign material inside the cast can lead to itching and skin breakdown.*
- Provide air conditioning, if possible. Hot weather is particularly uncomfortable for the client in a cast. *Rationale: Perspiration under a cast causes itching and promotes skin breakdown.*
- Give special attention to bladder and bowel elimination and to the area near the buttocks. *Rationale: Cast breakdown because of moisture from urine or stool can result in skin breakdown and infections.*
- Use a fracture bedpan for elimination. Remove these bedpans slowly. *Rationale: They overflow easily.*
- Apply powder or lotion to the bedpan before placing it under the client. *Rationale: This helps to slip the pan into place. Protect the bed with a waterproof pad.*
- Report symptoms such as abdominal pain and a bloated feeling. The area of the cast over the stomach should be cut out. *Rationale: Cutting out the area over the stomach helps to prevent superior mesenteric syndrome, also known as body cast syndrome. If the stomach area is not cut out, the stomach has no place for expansion after eating or if the person has gas. This could lead to partial or complete strangulation of the bowel.*
- Encourage the client to exercise as much as possible. Isometric exercises should be done inside the cast. *Rationale: Exercises encourage circulation and help prevent complications.*
- Move the client out of the room on a stretcher or in a standing wheelchair. *Rationale: The cast could break, resulting in loss of immobility and further damage to the client.*
- Encourage diversional activities. *Rationale: Boredom and restlessness are common problems.*
- Use several people or a hydraulic lift or chair to move the client. *Rationale: Assistance is needed when moving the client to prevent injury to staff and the client.*
- Encourage the client to do as much self-care as possible. *Rationale: Participating in self-care helps to improve self-image and provides meaningful exercise.*

Cast Removal

Casts are removed with a cast saw, which oscillates back and forth, although it appears to rotate. The blade moves only a fraction of an inch and will not cut the client. Because cast removal can be frightening, explain the procedure and show the client the cast saw before removal begins. A client who realizes that cast removal is safe will be better able to tolerate the noise and dust. Wear gloves, protective eyewear, and a mask to avoid irritation and inhalation of small dust particles.

Before a cast is removed, explain to the client that the skin under the cast may be covered with scales or crusts of dead skin. Also inform the client that muscles may appear atrophied and that the limb may be weak or stiff. After cast removal, the client may wear a brace for a week or two to provide additional stability to the injured area. All healthcare team members (e.g., healthcare provider, nurse, physical therapist) will instruct the client about therapeutic exercises for the affected body part.

Traction

Another means of immobilization is *traction*, which may be used with other types of immobilization, such as surgical internal fixation. Traction exerts a continuous pulling force on broken bones to keep them in the natural position for proper healing. In traction, continuous pulling force is controlled through the use of weights; a healthcare provider

IN PRACTICE
EDUCATING THE CLIENT 77-2 — Wearing a Cast

- Follow the healthcare provider's instructions regarding physical activity and limitations.
- Exercise the muscles. Move the fingers or toes frequently to reduce swelling, prevent joint stiffness, and maintain muscle strength. Do muscle-setting exercises (contracting and relaxing without movement) inside the cast to maintain muscle mass, tone, and strength.
- With a foot or leg cast, wear a cast walking shoe at all times, except when sleeping or showering.
- Elevate the cast extremity to prevent swelling.
- Avoid bumping the cast.
- Never stick anything inside the cast. It could result in itching, infection, or decreased circulation. (This consideration is especially important for children.)
- Never trim or cut back the cast.
- Keep a plaster cast dry. If a synthetic cast becomes wet, pat it dry with a towel and dry it with a hair dryer, using the low setting.
- When resting the cast on furniture, protect the furniture with a pad.
- Contact your healthcare provider if any of the following problems develop: unrelenting itching; foul odor from cast; drainage present through or around cast; pain unrelieved by medication; cast that feels very tight or too loose; cast that breaks, cracks, or becomes dented; painful rubbing or pressure inside the cast, especially in one particular place; limb that constantly feels cold; fingers or toes that are numb or tingling; fingers or toes that are white, blue, or the color of which does not return when pressed.

---

determines how much weight to apply by using principles of physics. The strength of the *traction forces* (weights) on the bones must be sufficient to counteract the overall pull of the body's muscles. The location and number of pulleys help determine the direction and degree of the pull. *Countertraction forces* pull against traction forces and may be produced with weights, bed position, or the client's body weight. An overhead frame attached to the bed holds the traction pulleys and equipment in place. A trapeze may also be attached to the bed so the client can pull their head and shoulders off the bed. With any type of traction, never remove or change the weights on *any* traction device without a healthcare provider's order.

Skin Traction

In **skin traction**, the pull is applied to the client's skin, which transmits the pull to the musculoskeletal structures. Skin traction, such as Bryant or Buck extension traction, is typically left on for shorter periods than skeletal traction, often for 3 weeks or less. A belt, head halter, foam rubber wrapped with an elastic bandage, or a foam boot is applied to the client's skin before the appendage is attached to traction. A disadvantage of skin traction is that it can provide only 8 to 10 lb of pull.

Irritation and breakdown of the skin are complications. Skin traction may be supplemented or replaced entirely by physical therapy and medications for muscle spasms. It is often used for children, minor fractures in adults, muscle strains or spasms, and temporary traction for adults with a hip fracture. If skin traction is being used to immobilize a fracture, the traction is left on. However, if skin traction is used to minimize muscle spasms, the healthcare provider may allow for periods without traction. Types of skin traction are described in Box 77-2. Figure 77-4 illustrates some types of skin traction.

Skeletal Traction

In **skeletal traction**, a healthcare provider surgically inserts metal pins or wires into the client's bones so that traction is applied directly to them. Skeletal traction can use up to 30 lb of weight and can be applied for continuous periods as long as 4 months. Adults with serious fractures typically use skeletal traction, although it can also be used for children. There are two main types of skeletal tractions: balanced suspension traction and skull tongs traction.

Clients with skeletal traction are allowed to move slightly in bed while maintaining the correct position. Skeletal traction can be successful and cost effective in the home setting. To prevent infection, pin insertion sites require the same care as any incision. Immediately report any signs of infection, and teach clients and family caregivers about these signs. Infection in the incision site can spread to the bone, causing the serious complication of *osteomyelitis*, a bone infection discussed later in this chapter. Other complications of skeletal traction include skin damage owing to the shearing forces of skin against bed linens, skin breakdown, and the numerous hazards of immobility. As with skin traction, CMS checks are part of routine nursing care.

Balanced Suspension Traction

Balanced suspension traction is a type of skeletal traction that is used to stabilize fractures of the femur (Fig. 77-5). A wire (e.g., Kirschner wire) and a pin (e.g., Steinmann pin) are inserted through the femur. The femur is then supported or balanced on a Thomas splint with a Pearson attachment. The Thomas splint is a ring that supports the thigh. The Pearson attachment is a canvas sling that supports the calf portion of the affected leg. Traction is applied via parallel rods using ropes, pulleys, and weights. Padding the areas touching the skin, prevention of skin breakdown, and pin care are of special importance.

Skull Tongs Traction

Skull tongs are also used for cervical injuries or fractures. Gardner-Wells tongs are commonly used today because they are considered less likely to pull out of place than are Crutchfield tongs. Holes are drilled into the sides of the skull, and the tongs are inserted into these holes (Fig. 77-6A).

Box 77-2 Types of Skin Traction

BUCK TRACTION
One or both legs are wrapped with an elastic roller bandage or tape. Traction is applied with a weight attached to a spreader bar below the foot. A foam boot may also be used. The traction pull is toward the pulley at the bottom of the bed. Buck traction may be used temporarily to manage a hip, lower spine, or simple fracture, often before surgical repair (Fig. 77-4A).

BRYANT TRACTION
Bryant traction is a variation of Buck traction often used for a child aged 2 years and younger with unstable hip or femur fractures (Fig. 77-4B).

CERVICAL HALTER TRACTION
Cervical halter traction is used for neck pain, neck strain, and whiplash. The pull of cervical skin traction should be felt as an upward pull on the back of the neck. A slight change in the level of the head of the bed is often the key to correct application of this type of traction. Because this is a form of skin traction, it cannot be used for prolonged periods. This type of traction is often used by the client at home with the client sitting in a chair (Fig. 77-4C).

DUNLOP (SIDE-ARM) TRACTION
Generally used as temporary skin traction for stabilization of fracture before surgery, Dunlop skin traction is used for fractures of the upper arm and for shoulder dislocations. The client is supine with the arm positioned with weights at an angle of 90°. Skin breakdown, especially over the elbow, and problems with neurovascular functions are common. Circulation, motion, and sensation (CMS) checks of the fingers and forearm are very important.

RUSSELL TRACTION (BALANCED TRACTION)
Downward pull, as in Buck traction, may be applied to the leg, but an additional overhead pulley system is incorporated into the traction apparatus, with the leg supported by a sling. The pull is up (toward the ceiling) and toward the foot of the bed. It is commonly used to reduce or realign femur fractures or to treat knee injuries. Because of the need for a greater weight and pull system, the use of Russell traction in adults is usually skeletal, not skin, traction. The nurse must be aware of possible damage behind the knee in the popliteal space due to the sling, which can cause pressure, swelling, and damage to nerves and blood vessels. CMS checks must be done as long as the client is in traction.

PELVIC TRACTION AND PELVIC SLING TRACTION
Used in pelvic fractures to support separated bones, this traction may be applied by either a belt or a sling. The pelvic belt causes downward pull on the pelvis, whereas the pelvic sling supports the pelvis off the bed. With a pelvic belt, the upper rim of the belt should rest at the top of the iliac crest and not around the abdomen. This type of traction is used in treating a herniated intervertebral disk or a muscle spasm of the back. It is usually applied intermittently (on 2 hr, off 2 hr) while the client is awake. Weights on the traction are increased gradually. As the name implies, a client in *pelvic sling traction* has the pelvic area elevated off the bed in a sling attached to weights. It may be used for an individual who has a fracture of the pelvis that has separated the pelvic bones.

Lynn (2018); Russell & Jarrett (2020).

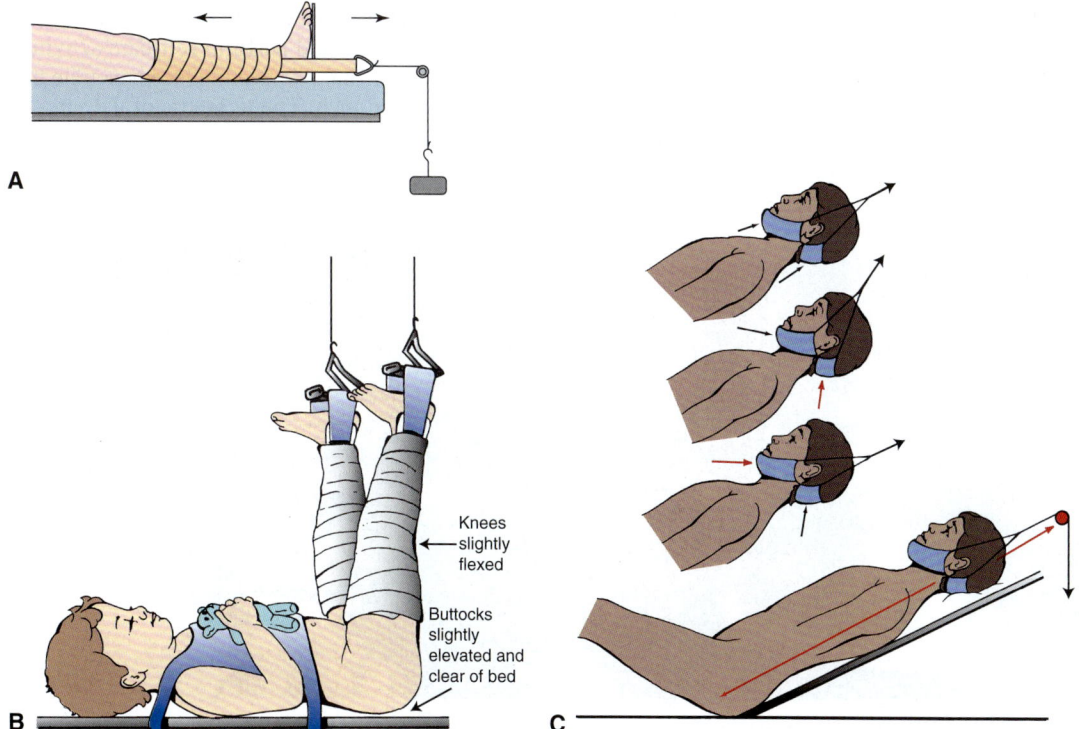

Figure 77-4 **A.** Buck traction. **B.** Bryant traction. **C.** Cervical halter traction. (Ellis & Bentz, 2007.)

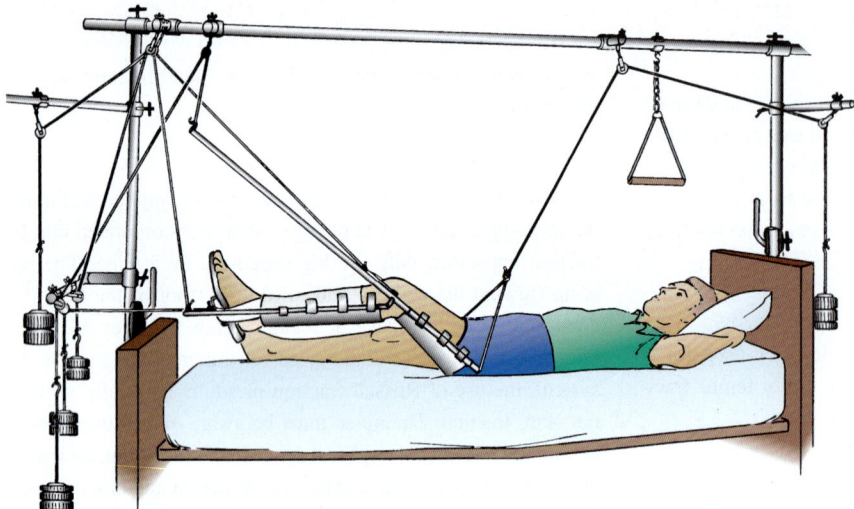

Figure 77-5 The client in a balanced suspension traction with a Thomas leg splint. The client uses the trapeze to help move vertically. It is important that the line of pull on the traction is maintained. Note that the weights hang freely at the head and foot of the bed.

Traction is applied to the tongs to stabilize the cervical spinal cord. The client stays in bed and must remain immobile until the injury heals, surgery is performed, or a halo device is applied. For the client with skull tongs, keep in mind the following:

- Provide client and family teaching and support. *Rationale: If the client has sustained a sudden injury, they will be frightened and, in addition, may be newly paralyzed. Thus, remain with the client during the entire procedure.*
- Explain the procedure to the client. After the client receives local anesthesia, the healthcare provider drills shallow holes into the sides of the client's skull. Be aware that the healthcare provider will either shave the area around the tong insertion sites or instruct the nurse to shave a specific area. Warn the client that they may experience some pain during the drilling, although most clients feel pressure rather than severe pain. The noise from drilling is loud and may be frightening to the client.
- Once the healthcare provider inserts the tongs, pay attention to the insertion sites. Check the institution's policies for routine care. Immediately report any signs of infection. *Rationale: The tongs are in close proximity to the brain, and any infection could be fatal. Headache is a serious sign that could indicate encephalitis or osteomyelitis. Report a client's headache immediately.*
- If possible, place the client in an antidecubitus bed.
- Routinely check the client's level of consciousness (LOC) and pupils (eye signs).
- Restlessness and boredom are common problems.
- Insertion site care, skin care, ROM exercises, and good nutrition are priority nursing considerations.

Halo Device

The **halo device** (Fig. 77-6B) is a form of external fixation device. A halo device consists of skeletal traction used for cervical fractures that is applied to the skull and allows the client to ambulate and perform self-care activities. The four pins holding the halo device in place penetrate the skull only a fraction of an inch. The tightness of the screws influences the amount of traction.

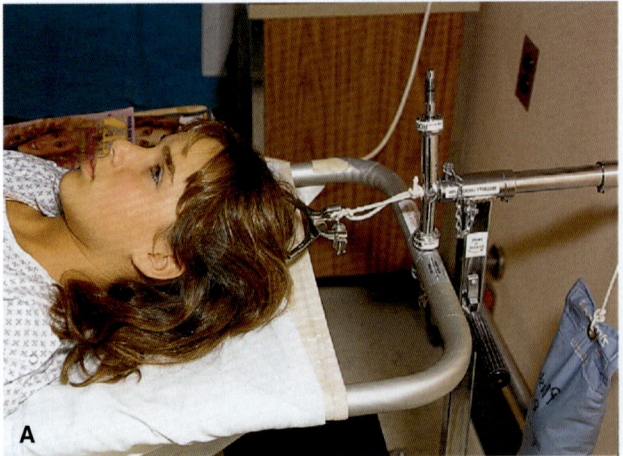 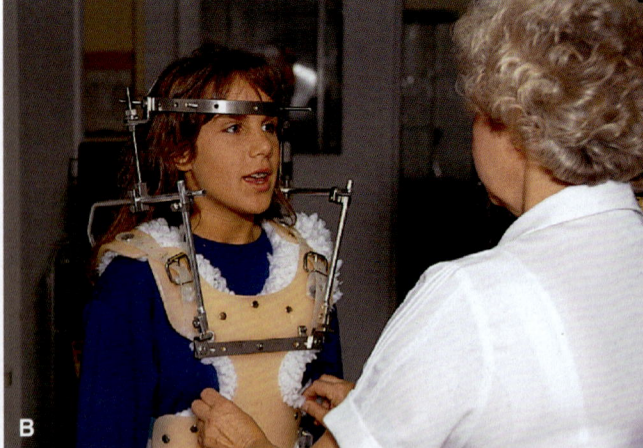

Figure 77-6 Methods of cervical skeletal traction. **A.** Crutchfield tongs. **B.** Halo.

> **Nursing Alert** The halo device comes with a wrench. Always tape the wrench to the halo device so that the device can be quickly removed in an emergency.

Nurses may assist healthcare providers with applying halo devices. Explain to clients what will be done. Provide the healthcare provider with the halo, vest, special wrench and positioning plate, regular wrench, and Xylocaine. Follow Standard Precautions as well as sterile technique when indicated.

- Be prepared to place a client in a special bed or chair before the application of the halo device. Use caution not to change the alignment of the head or neck. Support the client's head and neck on movement and during application. After the device is applied, help the client to sit up slowly. *Rationale: The client may become dizzy or faint.* Support the client in a sitting position while the healthcare provider adjusts the halo's vertical bars.
- Give good skin care around the device and at the pin sites. Using a sterile cotton-tipped applicator, apply sterile hydrogen peroxide to the pins; rinse with sterile normal saline. Even though the insertion sites are small, watch for evidence of infection. Wear gloves.
- Administer analgesics, as ordered. Typically, the client may experience some mild discomfort. Immediately report pain that is not relieved by medications.
- Monitor the client for possible complaints of difficulty in swallowing, inability to open the mouth all the way, or persistent neck pain; report such findings immediately because they are signs that the vertical connecting bar is too long.
- Note if the client complains of not being able to see straight ahead, a sign that the apparatus is not straight. If any complications occur, a healthcare provider must readjust the apparatus.
- Provide emotional support. Always encourage clients to be as independent as possible. Inform them about community resources and support groups.

> **Nursing Alert** Severe headache is a specific danger sign for the client wearing a halo device.

Clients will wear the halo device for about 10 to 12 weeks, during which time they or their families will become responsible for care. Teaching is vital (In Practice: Educating the Client 77-3). Carefully document all teaching.

Caring for Clients in Traction
In Practice: Nursing Care Guidelines 77-3 highlights the basic principles for care of clients in traction.

External Fixation
The *external fixator* is a device used to manage complex fractures that are associated either with soft-tissue damage

IN PRACTICE
EDUCATING THE CLIENT 77-3 — Wearing a Halo Device

- Report the following danger signs immediately: severe headache, difficulty swallowing, inability to open mouth completely, and persistent neck pain.
- If the halo device loosens, do not try to tighten it. Report the situation to your healthcare provider.
- Wash the skin under and around the vest. Conduct pin care as directed.
- Report the following signs of infection: fever, drainage, redness, and warmth.
- Report any complaints from the client of not being able to see straight ahead.
- Never use the halo frame for lifting or turning.

or open wounds in the fracture area. *Rationale: Wounds associated with the injury can be observed closely for signs of infection because casting material is not covering them.* A healthcare provider inserts multiple pins that protrude through the client's skin into the bone fragments. The *external fixation device* is a metal frame on the outside of the body that holds the pins in place and maintains immobilization (Fig. 77-7). The healthcare provider adjusts the frame to maintain traction and to keep the fracture in proper alignment. This alignment must continue until the bone heals. Another advantage of external fixation devices is that they allow the client to be more mobile than if confined to a bed in traction, thus minimizing some hazards of immobility.

Nursing care is consistent with traditional care of a fracture and also includes care of the pin sites. The healthcare provider will order the type and frequency of pin care required. In general, use a sterile cotton-tipped applicator to apply sterile hydrogen peroxide. Rinse with sterile normal saline. If dressings are present, be sure to change them using sterile technique. Avoid the formation of scar tissue around the pin sites; thus, whenever giving pin care, put traction on the skin by slightly and gently pulling the skin away from the pin site. Wear sterile gloves.

Be alert for possible rejection—an adverse reaction to the nails, screws, or plates used. It can occur even though such materials are made of a special metal alloy that, in most cases, is nonirritating. The device itself needs to be cleaned with soap and water. Do not allow water to seep into the pin insertion sites.

> **Nursing Alert** Never move a limb by grasping the frame of the external fixation device because you could disrupt the positioning of the healing fracture site.

Open Reduction and Internal Fixation
Surgery, called an open reduction and internal fixation (**ORIF**), is usually necessary if a client has a compound (open) fracture or if multiple bone fragments are present.

IN PRACTICE
NURSING CARE GUIDELINES 77-3 | Caring for Clients in Traction

- Follow the healthcare provider's order for the exact amount of weight to use. *Rationale: The ordered specific weight is designed as a main component of the traction and countertraction.*
- Be sure the weights hang free; they must never rest on the bed or the floor. Take care not to bump into the weights. *Rationale: Releasing the pull defeats the purpose of traction.*
- When adding weights or attaching traction, release the weights gradually onto the rope. *Rationale: Suddenly adding weights causes an uncomfortable jerk and may disrupt alignment of the fracture.*
- Never remove weights without an order. *Rationale: Traction usually is ordered to be continuous.*
- If the footpiece is touching the pulleys at the bottom of the bed, report it at once. The client should be moved up in bed when this happens. *Rationale: The footpiece touching the pulleys would negate the effects of traction.*
- Inspect pulleys and ropes regularly. *Rationale: The ropes can slip out of their grooves or become untied.*
- Be certain to understand the healthcare provider's orders completely regarding the client's body positioning, that is, the degree to which the head of the bed may be elevated and to which side the client with a fracture may turn. *Rationale: Prevent complications and maximize effects of the treatment.*
- Do not use a pillow under an extremity in traction, unless specifically ordered by the healthcare provider. *Rationale: Placement of the pillow might counteract the effects of the traction.*
- Encourage the client to exercise the feet periodically and to keep the ankles in neutral position. *Rationale: Make every effort to prevent footdrop, a deformity caused by nerve damage because the foot has been allowed to remain in an abnormal position.*
- Maintain the client's body alignment. Be sure to obtain specific guidelines from the healthcare provider before allowing the client to change position. *Rationale: The ends of the bones must remain in good alignment to heal properly.*

- Reposition frequently as needed. *Rationale: The weight of the traction may tend to pull the client out of alignment.*
- Guide the weights if the client is allowed to use a trapeze to slide up in bed. *Rationale: This ensures that the weights hang freely and are not impeded when the client moves.*
- Follow the healthcare provider's orders for range of motion (ROM) exercises. If ROM is not ordered for the client, find out what kind of exercise or positioning is needed. *Rationale: ROM exercises can minimize loss of muscle tissue caused by immobility, but the healthcare provider may not want certain muscle groups to have exercise until the bones are stabilized.*
- Provide diversional activities. *Rationale: Boredom and restlessness are common problems.*
- Use the fracture bedpan. *Rationale: This type of bedpan is easier to slip under the client's hips than the large conventional pan.*
- Maintain skin integrity. Be sure that the rubber strips, elastic roller bandage, or tape does not irritate the client's skin. Clean, dry thoroughly, and gently massage the skin daily. *Rationale: The hazards of immobility related to being in traction can lead to skin breakdown in otherwise healthy areas. Traction and external fixation devices can become sources of skin irritants because of perspiration, shearing forces, or pressure.*
- Apply lotion to the client's elbows. Frequent skin care is required. *Rationale: These measures prevent skin breakdown. If the elbows become irritated, apply elbow protectors.*
- If the client has skeletal traction, give pin site care, as ordered. Wear gloves when caring for the client with skeletal traction. *Rationale: Osteomyelitis, a serious bone infection, is very difficult to treat successfully once it has occurred and often results in severe, chronic pain. Prevention of bone infection is a nursing priority.*

With an *open reduction*, the surgeon makes an incision so that the injured or damaged area can be seen. After the wound is *débrided* (dead and damaged tissue removed) and irrigated with antibiotics, peroxide, normal saline, or other solutions, the surgeon looks at the bone fragments and determines exactly how to rejoin them. The fractured ends of the bone are placed in alignment (i.e., the fracture is "reduced"), which promotes bone healing. With *internal fixation*, the surgeon places a pin, wire, screw, plate, nail, or rod into or onto the bone to keep it reduced (properly aligned), immobilized, or both.

The ORIF is the treatment of choice for certain fractures in which casting is generally impossible (e.g., hip fracture) or if multiple fragments are impossible to realign. Internal fixation eliminates the need for traction. In addition, the client's recovery is usually quicker (Fig. 77-8).

Internal fixation can be performed using various devices. It is used most frequently for fractures of the leg's long bones, in which case the spike is called an *intramedullary nail*. Usually internal fixation is done if the client has more than one transverse fracture or if the client's history includes fractures that do not align or heal easily with casting.

The surgeon may apply a metal plate with screws to the outside of the bone; such a device often must remain in place permanently. This procedure is usually performed when a bone is fractured in several places. Screws are sometimes inserted to hold the bone fragments in place without using a plate. Wires may be used to hold fragments of bone together.

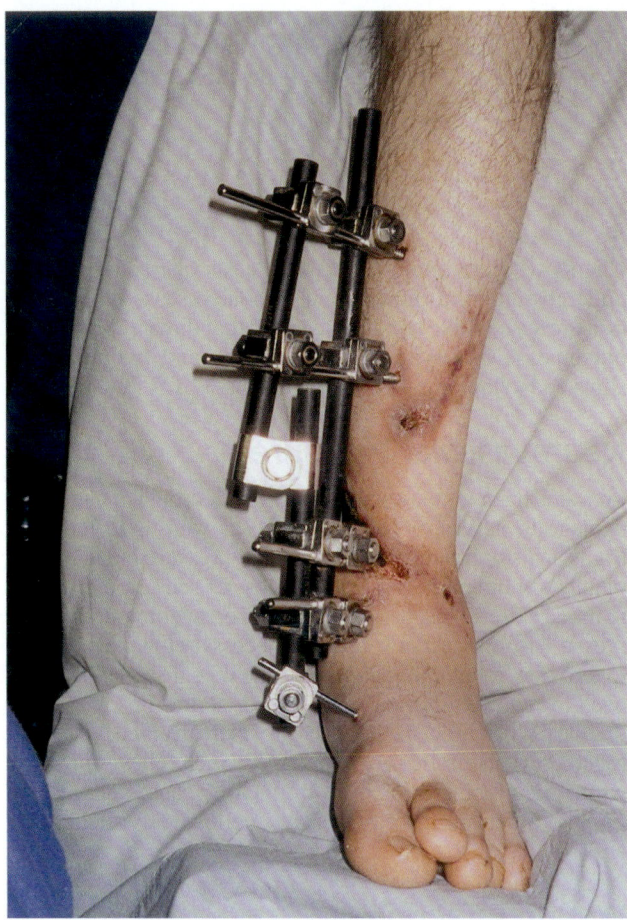

Figure 77-7 Pins are inserted directly into the bones in this external fixation device used to realign broken bony parts.

Although the client with internal fixation may have no visible form of immobilization, a fracture that requires careful handling still exists. Sometimes, internal fixation is combined with another form of immobilization, such as splinting or casting.

Nursing Alert Clients who have internal fixation devices must avoid future MRI studies because of the implanted metal.

Arthroplasty

Repair or replacement of a joint is called **arthroplasty**. For example, in some cases of fractured hip, the femoral head is replaced; in other cases, the hip socket is also replaced with a studded cup, which may be cemented into a deepened hip socket. This procedure is called *total hip replacement* or *total hip arthroplasty* (**THA**). Other joints that can be totally or partially replaced include the ankle, knee, shoulder, elbow, and wrist.

Total joint replacement is done in clients with severe injuries or severe degenerative arthritic disorders, when joints become injured, fused, or too malformed to be functional. Postoperative care is similar to that described for open reduction of the hip or other joint.

Shoulder joint replacement has been less successful than hip joint replacement. Because of minimal bone contact, the

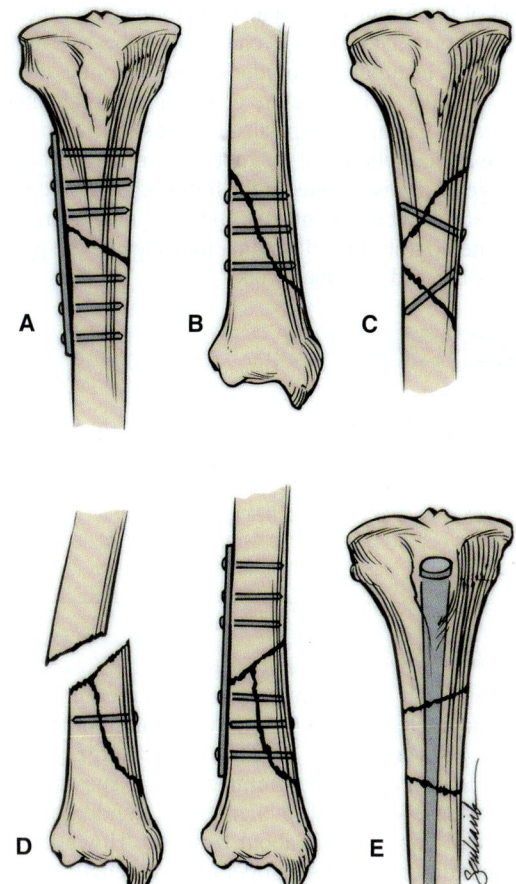

Figure 77-8 Types of internal fixation. **A.** Plate and screws secure a transverse fracture. **B.** Screws secure a long oblique fracture. **C.** Screws secure a long butterfly fragment of bone. **D.** Plates and screws secure a short butterfly fragment. **E.** A medullary nail secures a segmental fracture of the femur.

shoulder joint is less supported, less stable, and more subject to trauma and disease. For clients with minimal shoulder damage, a *hemiarthroplasty* may be done; in this procedure, only the head of the humerus is replaced.

Hip Fractures

Hip fractures include fractures of the head and neck of the femur or of the trochanter. These fractures often heal poorly because the healing process in such large bones disrupts nutrition to the bone matrix. In addition, hip fractures are more common in older adults (particularly older women), whose bones heal slowly and who are more likely to have osteoporosis. Risk factors for hip fractures include decreased bone mass, advancing age, female gender, difficulty with ambulation, and poor arterial perfusion.

Signs and Symptoms

Whenever an older person falls or complains of pain in the hip, groin, or knee, suspect a hip fracture. Although the exact location of the fracture causes symptoms to vary, many hip fractures involve shortening of the leg on the affected side and external foot rotation.

In most cases, if the neck of the femur is fractured, the client complains of severe pain that worsens with movement. If the head of the femur is compacted onto the neck, the client may have less pain and may even be able to bear weight. For this reason, a healthcare provider should examine any older person who falls. If the fracture occurs at the trochanter, the client usually has muscle spasms, obvious shortening of the leg, and external rotation of the foot. They report severe pain, and a large bruise is visible on the hip. Radiographic studies can indicate a specific diagnosis. Bleeding may decrease the person's hemoglobin level; trauma may elevate the person's blood glucose and enzyme levels.

SPECIAL CONSIDERATIONS Lifespan

Osteoporosis

Osteoporosis, a condition in which bone mass decreases, occurs in men and women of all races. Risk factors include white females, advanced age, family history, early menopause, low intake of dietary calcium, excessive alcohol or caffeine intake, sedentary lifestyle, and smoking. Osteoporosis can cause pathologic bone fractures, difficulty in weight bearing, loss of height, and the spinal curvature *kyphosis*.

Medical and Surgical Treatment

The fracture will first be immobilized by traction, typically Buck skin traction. Buck traction is a temporary device applied for several hours or days before surgery because the skin traction can help minimize muscle spasms and the pain from these spasms. If a client cannot undergo surgery, traction will continue for about 6 weeks. However, if the client's condition permits an operation, an ORIF of the hip is done as soon as possible. This procedure allows mobility soon after the injury, thus preventing severe complications of immobility, which can be particularly dangerous for older adults.

Sometimes called a "hip pinning," the ORIF involves lining up the bone fragments (reduction) and attaching the bones together (internal fixation) by using pins, nails, screws, metal plates, or an intramedullary nail. If these devices fail to provide stabilization, the surgeon removes the head of the femur and replaces it with a prosthesis. Some surgeons implant a hip prosthesis in all cases of fractured hip. Hip prostheses provide stabilization and also prevent complications, such as nonunion of bones and the death of joints, which can result from poor blood supply to joints or bones. Surgeons often perform THA or replacement, which provides even more comfort and quicker mobility than ORIF.

Nursing Considerations

In addition to routine pre- and postoperative care, special teaching is required to prevent hip dislocation after hip replacement surgery. Three major teaching and nursing considerations are necessary for postoperative care of the hip replacement client to maintain alignment of the affected hip:

- Never allow the affected leg to cross the center of the body (e.g., do not cross legs when sitting in a chair).
- Never allow the body to bend more than 90° (e.g., avoid bending forward to put on shoes).
- Never allow the affected leg to turn inward (e.g., avoid bending or flexing the hip when putting on slacks or stockings; In Practice: Nursing Care Plan 77-1).

Additional limitations or restrictions concern weight bearing on the affected side. In Practice: Nursing Care Guidelines 77-4 details care for clients with new hip replacements.

COMPLICATIONS OF FRACTURES OR BONE SURGERY

Clients who are immobilized with casts or traction or who undergo surgery to repair joint or bone disease or dysfunction are susceptible to complications that threaten successful outcomes. Observe the client carefully and frequently for signs and symptoms of these problems.

Neurovascular Pressure

Pressure from an external immobilization device can cause damage to nerves or blood vessels, as well as to the skin. Signs and symptoms of neurovascular pressure include complaints of numbness and tingling, loss of sensation, inability to move extremities, pallor, cool skin, or swelling. If you find pressure from a cast or splint, it is necessary to take measures to provide relief *immediately*. A healthcare provider may need to remove all or part of a cast or splint. In some cases, the cast will be cut in half lengthwise (bivalved) and held together by an elastic roller bandage, which relieves pressure while maintaining immobilization. Other causes of pressure may be a dent in the cast, tissue swelling, or crutches that are too long.

Wound Infection

Any compound (open) fracture or open reduction involves a skin break, making infection a possibility. Always use sterile gloves when caring for clients with any wound. Carefully observe for signs of infection.

Osteomyelitis

Osteomyelitis is a serious bone infection that is curable if it is detected early and treated appropriately. Modern antibiotics have greatly improved the chances for recovery from this infection.

Acute Osteomyelitis

Acute osteomyelitis may result from a compound fracture that exposes bone to infection. Because blood supply to the bone is compromised, the bone becomes necrotic. Pus drains through the primary wound. *Acute hematogenous osteomyelitis* is most common in children and occurs when the bloodstream carries organisms, such as staphylococci or streptococci, to the bone from infection elsewhere. Pus forms in the bone's shaft and under its covering (*periosteum*), thereby separating the periosteum from the bone.

Signs and symptoms of osteomyelitis include pain, fever, flushed appearance, elevated white blood cell (WBC) count and ESR, and positive blood cultures. The skin over the affected area may be warm, red, and swollen. Early detection is imperative to prevent bone necrosis. When osteomyelitis is suspected, blood cultures are obtained and vigorous antibiotic therapy is started. After the offending organism is

IN PRACTICE
NURSING CARE PLAN 77-1: The Older Adult Client With a Fractured Hip

Medical history: I.M., a 65-year-old widowed woman with a history of osteoporosis, was hospitalized after falling at home and fracturing the neck of their left femur. They underwent an open reduction and internal fixation of the left hip 24 hr ago.

Medical diagnosis: Fracture of the left hip with open reduction and internal fixation.

DATA COLLECTION/NURSING OBSERVATION

Client is alert and oriented 1 day following open reduction with internal fixation. They report pain is adequately controlled with analgesic therapy. Surgical site dressing is clean, dry, and intact. Vital signs are within acceptable parameters. Client demonstrates coughing, deep breathing, and incentive spirometry every 2 hr. Client states, "How will I ever be able to walk again? I'm even afraid to move. The doctor said that I have to watch how I move my leg." Before the client's fall, they were living independently in their own home, frequently babysitting their grandchildren.

NURSING DIAGNOSIS

Decreased physical mobility is related to repair of fractured left hip as evidenced by client's statement about walking and prescribed postoperative restrictions.

(Although other nursing diagnoses may be appropriate, a priority nursing diagnosis is addressed below.)

PLANNING (Outcomes/Goals)	IMPLEMENTATION (Nursing Actions)	EVALUATION
Short-Term Goals		
A. Client participates in proper alignment while in bed.	• Check the healthcare provider's instructions about position and activity. • Discuss weight-bearing goals with client for the first time getting out of bed. • Coordinate client's mobility with physical therapy's post–hip surgery protocol; PT to be with client when getting out of bed. • Reinforce preoperative instructions regarding rules of postoperative hip alignment. • Maintain hip in neutral position, using abductor pillow when in supine position. *Rationale: Specific instructions for activity and positioning are determined by the orthopedic surgeon. Maintaining the hip in a neutral position prevents stress on the operative site. An abduction pillow and sometimes a trochanter roll reduce the risk of external rotation, which could cause the femoral head to dislocate. Often, PT has initial responsibility, with coordination from nursing staff, of getting client to a sitting position and getting client out of bed.* • Enlist the aid of sufficient, qualified healthcare personnel to turn the client. • When turning the client, use an abductor pillow. *Rationale: An abductor pillow prevents adduction of the hip joint, which could cause the femoral head to dislocate. Using additional personnel ensures that the client's body is maintained in proper alignment during turning.*	Day 1—postoperative ORIF left hip 1,330 hr. • Client is maintaining abduction of left lower extremity with use of abduction pillow. • Client stated, "I really want to be independent again." • Abduction pillow used when client is lying in supine position. • Abductor pillow is in place when turning. • Client stated that the abductor pillow is "a little uncomfortable" but uses pillow to keep legs abducted. ***Goal A complete.***

1346 UNIT 12 Adult Care Nursing

PLANNING (Outcomes/Goals)	IMPLEMENTATION (Nursing Actions)	EVALUATION
B. Client demonstrates appropriate exercise techniques.	• Client using trapeze bar to help when moving up in bed. • Teach exercises the client can do in bed, including isometric, quadriceps-setting, and gluteal-setting exercises. • Have client return-demonstrate these exercises. • Encourage exercises every 1–2 hours. • Offer support and encouragement. *Rationale: These exercises help to strengthen the muscles needed for ambulation and aid in venous return.* • As ordered, assist PT, PRN, with client transfer from bed to chair, while maintaining proper positioning of the client's extremity and prescribed amount of weight-bearing allowed. *Rationale: Getting the client out of bed is important to prevent postoperative complications of immobility and to promote a sense of increasing independence.*	Day 1—postoperative ORIF left hip 2,130 hr. • Client demonstrates isometric in-bed exercises; observed performing exercises every 2 hr. • Client able to bear weight on both legs and get out of bed using appropriate precautions. **Goal B complete.**
Long-Term Goals		
C. Client demonstrates ability to transfer from bed to chair independently.	• PT and nursing staff monitor client's progress getting out of bed. • Client able to transfer without bending more than 90°. • Client able to transfer without twisting leg inward. • Client able to sit in chair without crossing legs. *Rationale: Explanations help to alleviate anxiety and promote client participation in care. Trapeze bar allows the client to participate in moving and repositioning and helps to strengthen upper extremity muscles.*	Day 2—postoperative ORIF left hip 0800 hr. • Client observed getting out of bed and ambulating to bathroom using walker. • Client seen using proper techniques for ORIF left hip. • Client transferred out of bed to chair without physical assistance but being monitored during procedure by PT. **Goal C complete.**
D. Client participates in physical therapy program for progressive ambulation in a home situation.	• Contact PT department to arrange for progressive ambulation program. • Work with PT and client to promote ambulation. *Rationale: Physical therapy is indicated to assist the client to achieve the maximum level of independent mobility that is possible. Working with the physical therapist and client is important to foster achievement. Transfer to a rehabilitation center or unit for PT before being discharged to home is a safety mechanism for protection of surgical incision as well as keeping hip securely in joint space.* • Reinforce the ambulation skills the client is learning in physical therapy and use them when assisting the client in transferring, getting out of bed to go to the bathroom, or for walks. • Take proper safety precautions with each interaction. • Praise the client's progress. *Rationale: Ambulation will increase muscle mass, tone, and strength and facilitate mastery.*	Day 3—postoperative ORIF left hip 1,030 hr. • Client demonstrates transfer from bed to chair with nurse watching at bedside. • Client reports ambulating with walker. • Client and family members state comprehension of transfer to unit that provides continued PT instruction. **Goal D complete.**

IN PRACTICE
NURSING CARE GUIDELINES 77-4 Caring for Clients With New Hip Replacements

- Provide routine postoperative care: deep breathing, high-protein diet, intravenous (IV) and oral fluid administration.
- Perform neurovascular checks every 15 min for 1 hr, every 30 min for 1 hr, every hour for 24 hr, every 4 hr for 24 hr, and every 8 hr thereafter.
- Initiate anticoagulation therapy, as ordered. Place antiembolism stockings or pneumatic compression devices, as ordered.
- Turn clients every 1 to 2 hr (from unaffected side to back). Always check the surgeon's orders before turning a client whose hip fracture was surgically stabilized. Place a special pillow called an *abduction pillow* between the client's legs when turning. *Rationale:* The pillow prevents adduction of the legs, which could result in dislocation of the prosthesis.
- Have another nurse or technician help turn the client to the *unaffected side* with a pillow between their knees to provide good alignment. Position the client comfortably and support them with pillows or sandbags and trochanter rolls so that the body is in correct alignment and contractures do not develop. The client usually remains in this position for 2 hr.
- Turn the client onto the back again. The client usually remains in this position for an hour. Elevate the head of the bed at least 30° when the client is on their back, to prevent aspiration.
- Turn the client to the *unaffected* side again. (*Note:* The client with a hip fracture is usually not placed on the affected side, although some surgeons allow this.)
- Prevent common complications: infection and dislocation of prostheses or pins.
- Frequently evaluate incisions for erythema, intactness, and drainage. If a drainage device is in place, empty it frequently and measure the drainage.
- Change dressings, as needed, maintaining sterile technique.
- Provide frequent skin care. Keep skin dry. Relieve pressure areas to prevent skin breakdown.
- Give back care every 2 hr while the client is on bed rest.
- Following insertion of a hip prosthesis (and sometimes following open reduction), maintain the client's leg in an abducted position and in neutral or slight external rotation. Carefully follow the surgeon's orders for positioning and movement.
- Provide active and passive ROM exercises, as ordered.
- Place a trapeze on the overhead frame. *Rationale:* The trapeze will help the client move and use the bedpan.
- Encourage early mobility, particularly for older adults. Complications of immobility cause more deaths than surgery itself.
- Assist clients into a chair two to three times per day. Check with the surgeon for any flexion restrictions before helping a client into a chair.
- Begin progressive ambulation as soon as ordered. The healthcare provider will determine how much weight a client is allowed to bear on the operative side. Do not ambulate clients before checking this information. Clients often use walkers.
- Instruct clients in routine postoperative procedures and precautions.

---

isolated, specific antibiotics are given IV or directly into the wound. A surgeon may drain the pus and may place a catheter into the wound for irrigation and drainage. Fragments of dead bone loosen (**sequestration**) and require surgical removal (*sequestrectomy*). Careful attention to rest, nutrition, fluid intake, elimination, and skin care is vital. Instruct clients to move about as ordered to prevent problems associated with prolonged bed rest; however, they must maintain complete immobilization of the affected part. If healing becomes impaired, remaining dead bone tissue (*sequestrum*) must be removed surgically.

Osteomyelitis is so painful that the affected part is sensitive to the slightest touch or motion. Do not move the affected part any more than is absolutely necessary. When the part must be moved, support and splint it with a pillow, and lift and move it with the rest of the body. Sandbags, a cast, or a brace help immobilize the limb. Take extreme care to avoid jarring the bed.

Promote healing through a diet that is high in proteins, calcium, carbohydrates, and fats. Encourage the client to drink fluids.

Report any swelling, redness, and pain in any other body part because these may be signs of spreading infection. Pathologic fractures are possible, but they may not be recognized because the pain is overshadowed by the greater pain of osteomyelitis. Growth of new bone may lengthen the infected bone, or bone destruction may shorten it. A break in aseptic technique when changing dressings could introduce pathogens into the wound.

Chronic Osteomyelitis

If antibiotics are ineffective in killing the offending microorganism, the microorganism may be resistant to the antibiotic and the bone infection persists. In these cases, *chronic osteomyelitis* occurs. Because of the possibility that a microorganism is drug resistant, a culture and sensitivity test should be done before a course of antibiotic therapy is initiated. Acute osteomyelitis may become chronic in immunosuppressed individuals (e.g., those receiving chemotherapy or those with human immunodeficiency virus or acquired immunodeficiency syndrome [HIV/AIDS]).

Signs and symptoms of chronic osteomyelitis include purulent drainage from a sinus tract over the affected bone, pain, swelling, and weakened bone. Changes in the bone's structure are visible on x-ray examination.

The treatment of choice for chronic osteomyelitis is surgical débridement of dead and infected tissue. The healthcare provider orders antibiotics and rest of the affected area.

Another type of chronic osteomyelitis is caused by the tubercle bacillus, which settles in the bone or joint (*tuberculosis osteomyelitis*). Signs and symptoms include pain, swelling, localized redness, and warmth. Tuberculosis of the spine, known as *Pott disease,* is characterized by kyphosis, abscess formation, and possible paralysis. Because skeletal tuberculosis is not spread via the air, it is less contagious than pulmonary tuberculosis. Treatment includes antimicrobial drugs, such as isoniazid, ethambutol, pyrazinamide, and rifampin.

Hypostatic Pneumonia and Atelectasis

Hypostatic pneumonia and *atelectasis* (collapse of all or part of a lung) are preventable complications that result from prolonged immobility. Signs of these conditions include elevated temperature, tachycardia, cough, *dyspnea* (difficulty breathing), decreased oxygen saturation by pulse oximetry, pleural pain, and anxiety. Encourage clients to turn and ambulate as much as possible and to cough and take deep breaths. Show clients how to perform incentive spirometry. Provide respiratory therapies, such as suctioning, postural draining, and chest percussion (Chapter 56).

Embolism

An *embolism* is the sudden blockage of one or more arteries by a piece of foreign material. The foreign material (*embolus*) can be a blood clot, bacteria clump, air bubble, piece of tissue, fat globules, or piece of an IV catheter. Embolism formation is another possible consequence of immobility, although other factors may be the cause.

The goal is to prevent embolism. Immobilize fractures, minimize fracture manipulation, and support fractured bones when moving clients. If an embolism occurs, be prepared to administer oxygen, steroids, and IV fluids, as ordered.

Fat Embolism

The most common embolism associated with fractures involves a bolus of fat. *Fat embolism* is most common in young people with multiple injuries, particularly fractures of the long bones (e.g., femur and humerus), pelvis, and ribs. This type of embolism travels through the circulatory system and causes an obstruction in the brain, the heart, or most commonly, the lungs.

Signs and symptoms of a fat embolism include dyspnea, tachycardia, fever, petechial rash, *hypoxemia* (low blood oxygen), chest pain, and pulmonary edema. Often, *crackles* (abnormal sounds) are heard on lung auscultation. Fat may be present in the blood, urine, or sputum. A change in the client's neurologic status is common. Fat embolism can lead to coma, pneumonia, heart failure, and acute respiratory distress syndrome.

Pulmonary Embolism

An embolism in the lungs is called a *pulmonary embolism* (PE). Risk factors include immobility, history of prior deep vein thrombophlebitis, or PE, trauma, and orthopedic surgery of the lower extremities or pelvis. Signs and symptoms include dyspnea, *tachypnea* (rapid respiration), hypoxemia, chest pain, tachycardia, cough, and *hemoptysis* (bloody sputum). PE may cause life-threatening cardiac dysrhythmias.

Prevent PE by encouraging clients to ambulate and to perform active exercises. Administer prophylactic anticoagulant therapy, as ordered. Pneumatic compression devices may be used on the legs. Antiembolism stockings or hose, such as TEDS, must be removed at least every 8 hr and reapplied.

PE is an emergency that requires immediate reporting and corrective action. Administer oxygen to relieve hypoxemia and dyspnea. Obtain blood gases, as ordered. Other common treatments include anticoagulation therapy and thrombolytic therapy. Emergency surgery to remove the embolus may or may not be life saving. Give clients emotional support and calmly explain what is being done.

Deep Vein Thrombosis

DVT is a primary complication of prolonged bed rest. *Venostasis* (pooling blood flow) occurs when clients are immobile for long periods, predisposing individuals to clot formation (*thrombosis*). *Venous thrombosis* occurs most often in the legs and pelvis and can be fatal if the clot moves and obstructs a vital blood vessel (causing an *embolism*). Doppler studies of the lower extremities are used to diagnose DVT.

Signs and symptoms include unequal leg circumference and pain, swelling, and redness of the affected leg.

Prevent DVT by applying support stockings or pneumatic compression devices to the legs. The healthcare provider may order prophylactic aspirin or low-dose subcutaneous heparin. Teach client's family passive exercises and encourage ambulation as soon as possible.

Hemorrhage

In many fractures, bone fragments damage blood vessels. Be alert for signs of internal hemorrhage, such as hypotension, tachycardia, change in mental status, anxiety, increased pain in the affected extremity, and decreased urine output.

Compartment Syndrome

Compartment syndrome and *Volkmann contracture* (also called *Volkmann paralysis*) result from inadequate or obstructed blood flow to muscles, nerves, and tissue. These disorders may also result from compression of the muscle compartment or from an increase in muscle compartment contents related to edema, hemorrhage, fracture, or soft-tissue injury. A tight cast, pneumatic compression stocking, or tissue swelling can cause pressure as well.

Compartment syndrome is a medical emergency. If left uncorrected, permanent muscle and nerve damage will result in 4 to 6 hr. Ischemia leads to muscle necrosis. Contractures develop because fibrous tissue replaces muscle tissue.

The cardinal symptom of compartment syndrome is pain that is unrelieved by medications and aggravated by passive stretching of the ischemic muscle. Other signs and symptoms include swelling, tightness, and *paresthesia* (numbness and tingling) of the affected extremity.

The first treatment for compartment syndrome is to remove the constricting dressing or cast and to elevate the extremity. A **fasciotomy** (excision of the fascia) may be needed to relieve internal pressure.

When caring for any client with a cast, severe sprain, or condition that causes swelling in an extremity, elevate the extremity and apply ice. Be alert for symptoms of nerve compression. Perform routine neurovascular checks according to the institution's policies. Immediately report any suspicions of compartment syndrome. Teach clients and their families how to monitor for compartment syndrome at home.

Other Complications

Numerous other complications can occur following fractures or musculoskeletal surgery. Confusion is not uncommon, especially in older adults. It often occurs at night, when clients tend to be more confused and restless. Constipation can occur because of age, inactivity, poor eating habits, and insufficient fluids. Kidney stones may form because of poor nutrition, inactivity, changes in mineral composition that may occur during the healing process, or overmedication with salicylates. Skin breakdown can result from poor circulation, immobility, infrequent turning, or poor skin care.

Nonunion (failure of the fracture site to fuse and heal), *malunion* (healing in improper alignment), and *delayed union* (slow healing) are complications of fractures. These complications may result from malnutrition, inadequate mobilization, infection, poor circulation, or older age. Poor positioning or lack of exercise may cause contractures, footdrop, and external rotation.

NEOPLASMS

Common *neoplasms* of the musculoskeletal system are *bone tumors*. Bone tumors are of two types: primary and metastatic. *Primary bone tumors* originate in the bone. They may be benign or malignant. Primary benign bone tumors are usually well circumscribed and slow growing and seldom spread. They include osteomas, chondromas, giant cell tumors, cysts, and osteoid osteomas. *Primary malignant bone tumors* are rare. They include osteogenic sarcoma, chondrosarcoma, and multiple myelomas (Chapter 83). These extremely malignant tumors metastasize early, often to the lungs.

Metastatic bone tumors travel to the bone from some other part of the body. They are relatively common. Metastatic bone tumors result from primary lesions in the lung, breast, prostate, kidney, ovary, or thyroid. Metastases occur most commonly in the vertebral bodies, ribs, pelvis, femur, and humerus bones. Carcinomas tend to metastasize to bone more commonly than do sarcomas. The client with metastatic bone disease has a poor prognosis.

Symptoms

Symptoms of bone tumor include pain, swelling, restricted motion, and aching. One of the most significant signs of a malignant bone tumor is pathologic fracture. The bone fractures because it is weakened, even though no external trauma has occurred.

Diagnosis

Diagnosis of bone tumor is made by x-ray, biopsy, frozen section, and laboratory evaluation. Whenever a care provider suspects malignant tumors, chest films are routinely taken to look for *pulmonary metastases* (spread to the lungs). A skeletal radiologic survey (*bone scintigraphy*), MRI, or CT scan is done to locate additional bone lesions.

Treatment

Treatment may consist of surgical removal of a primary tumor, chemotherapy, or radiation therapy. A bone excision or amputation may be necessary to save the person's life. Metastatic bone lesions are usually treated with palliative measures (as opposed to curative). Nursing care focuses on providing comfort, controlling pain, preventing pathologic fractures, and giving emotional support.

STUDENT SYNTHESIS

KEY POINTS

- Tests that are used to diagnose musculoskeletal disorders include blood tests, x-ray, MRI, CT scan, arthrogram, bone scan, ultrasound, arthrocentesis, arthroscopy, biopsy, and electromyogram.
- Be alert for signs and symptoms of damage to bone, muscle, tissue, nerves, and blood vessels, which may be noted during CMS checks.
- Be aware of, and try to prevent, the hazards of immobility and the subsequent complications caused by the client's decreased mobility.
- Early treatment of orthopedic complications is necessary to prevent further injury to the area involved.
- Treatment of musculoskeletal disorders and diseases, including the various forms of arthritis, can include drug therapy, exercise, surgery, amputation, physical therapy, diet, or resting the affected part.
- Traumatic musculoskeletal injuries, such as sprains, strains, dislocations, and fractures, require different forms of treatment.
- The many different methods of treating orthopedic injuries include casts, splints, internal fixation, external fixation, traction, and surgeries, such as arthroscopy, total joint replacement, and lumbar decompression.
- A cast stabilizes and immobilizes fractures. When clients are wearing casts, carefully observe and document their neurovascular status, provide pain relief, and protect the casts.
- In skin traction, the pull is applied to the skin; in skeletal traction, the traction is applied directly to the bones.
- Potential orthopedic complications include compartment syndrome, wound infection, osteomyelitis, hypostatic pneumonia, embolism, deep vein thrombosis, and hemorrhage.
- Primary benign bone tumors grow slowly and rarely spread. Metastatic bone tumors originate elsewhere in the body; the client has a poor prognosis.

CRITICAL THINKING EXERCISES

1. Your client with arthritis complains that they are having increased difficulty caring for themselves. What adjustments could they make? Explain how they can best live with the arthritis and the needed adjustments. Identify other medical professionals or community resources that could assist.

2. You work in an orthopedic unit of a large hospital. An 80-year-old client has a closed leg fracture. Formulate a teaching plan for them. How would your teaching differ if the affected individual is an 8-year-old with the same type of fracture?

3. You work in an elementary school. A first-grade child with an arm cast comes to see you. Their cast is wet and dented. They report increased pain; their fingers are cool and white. Discuss possible causes of these findings and how you would intervene.

NCLEX-STYLE REVIEW QUESTIONS

1. A client is experiencing residual limb pain following a surgical amputation to the right lower extremity below the knee. Which action by the nurse would help alleviate the pain?
   a. Instruct the client to "move" the missing limb.
   b. Apply ice packs to the residual limb.
   c. Encourage the client to discuss feelings of loss.
   d. Present reality and do not support the delusion of sensation.

2. The nurse is caring for a client who has had a lower extremity amputation. Which intervention by the nurse will best help prevent hip contractures?
   a. Change drains using aseptic technique.
   b. Elevate the foot of the bed.
   c. Inspect the limb for signs of infection.
   d. Do not place a pillow under the residual limb.

3. The nurse is caring for a client postoperatively who has had cervical decompression. Which symptom(s) reported by the client would the nurse immediately report to the primary care provider? Select all that apply.
   a. Reports of discomfort when moving
   b. Reports of change in sensation of arms
   c. Difficulty breathing
   d. Difficulty moving arms
   e. No bowel movement for 2 days

4. A client is diagnosed with arthritis and wants to maintain an active lifestyle. Which exercises would the nurse recommend to the client? Select all that apply.
   a. Swimming
   b. Jumping rope
   c. Bicycling
   d. Running
   e. Slow walking

5. The nurse is preparing to administer allopurinol (Zyloprim) for a client with gout. Which information would the nurse include in the instructions?
   a. Use acetylsalicylic acid (Aspirin) to additionally relieve pain.
   b. Eat foods high in purine.
   c. Drink at least 3 L of fluids each day.
   d. Alcohol may be used while taking this drug.

CHAPTER RESOURCES

Enhance your learning with additional resources on **thePoint**!

Student Resources related to this chapter can be found at **thePoint.lww.com/Rosdahl12e**.

78 Nervous System Disorders

Learning Objectives

1. Differentiate among the following diagnostic tests: CT, PET, MRI, cerebral angiography, cerebral arteriography, myelography, brain scan, electroencephalography, and video telemetry.
2. Discuss the nursing care involved for a client before and after an LP.
3. Compare and contrast migraine and cluster headaches, including nursing considerations for each condition.
4. Identify the main characteristics of partial (focal) seizures and general seizures. Identify the key components of nursing care for a client with a seizure disorder or status epilepticus.
5. Discuss the causes, signs and symptoms, and nursing implications for the following disorders involving nerves: trigeminal neuralgia, Bell palsy, and herpes zoster.
6. Compare paraplegia with tetraplegia, including a discussion of differences in nursing care for each condition.
7. Describe the signs and symptoms of autonomic dysreflexia.
8. Discuss the causes, signs and symptoms, therapies, and nursing considerations for each of the following degenerative disorders: multiple sclerosis, Parkinson disease, myasthenia gravis, Huntington disease, and amyotrophic lateral sclerosis.
9. Discuss the causes, signs and symptoms, therapies, and nursing considerations for each of the following inflammatory disorders: brain abscess, meningitis, encephalitis, Guillain–Barré syndrome, postpolio syndrome, and acute transverse myelitis.
10. Explain causes of increased intracranial pressure. Identify pre- and postoperative nursing considerations for a client undergoing craniotomy.
11. Explain the nursing care required for clients with concussion, brain laceration and contusion, skull fractures, and hematoma.
12. State nursing considerations related to care of a client with a brain tumor.

Important Terminology

ataxia	concussion	intracranial pressure	parkinsonism	tetraplegia	EEG
aura	contusion		photophobia	tonic phase	GCS
autonomic dysreflexia	craniotomy	laceration	ptosis	transection	HD
	diplopia	neuralgia	rhinorrhea	vertigo	ICP
bradykinesia	dysphagia	neurology	seizure	**Acronyms**	↑ICP
cephalgia	dysphasia	nuchal rigidity	seizure disorder		LOC
chorea	flaccidity	opisthotonos	shingles	ALS	LP
clonic phase	focal point	otorrhea	status epilepticus	CNS	MG
	halo sign	paraplegia	subdural hematoma	CSF	MS

The medical specialty related to the nervous system is neurology. Healthcare providers trained in this specialty are called *neurologists;* surgeons are called *neurosurgeons.* Nurses specializing in the care of people with nervous system disorders are called *neuroscience* nurses. Review the normal anatomy in Chapter 19 before learning about the disorders of the nervous system. You will better understand why this system is a highly specialized major center for communication and control.

Key Concept
To understand the rationale of nursing interventions, it is very important to understand both the normal functioning and the pathology of the body's anatomical systems.

DIAGNOSTIC TESTS

Many diagnostic tests are used to determine the integrity or functioning of the nervous system.

Visualization Procedures

Numerous tests can be used to visualize nervous system structures. Two commonly used tests are *computed tomography* (CT) scan, a test that incorporates x-rays and computer technology to produce an image of a transverse body plane; and *magnetic resonance imaging* (MRI), a test that uses a powerful magnetic field to align hydrogen nuclei, which emit signals that are converted into precise images. An MRI can distinguish between normal and abnormal tissues in all parts of the body, even identifying chemical changes within cells. MRI is helpful in identifying strokes and cancerous lesions before clinical signs and symptoms appear. It is particularly sensitive in identifying multiple sclerosis plaques and other abnormal changes in demyelinating diseases (see Chapter 47). Other visualization procedures may include positron emission tomography, cerebral angiography and arteriography, myelography, and brain scan.

SPECIAL CONSIDERATIONS Lifespan
CT and MRI Scans and Children

A child may be permitted to take a favorite toy or blanket along for the test. For an MRI, make sure the toy contains no metal. Because sedation is often required, the child's safety must be maintained.

Positron Emission Tomography

Positron emission tomography (PET) is a type of tomography used to study changes within the brain. Glucose containing a radioisotope is injected into the brain. After the scan, the client remains flat in bed for a few hours and is observed for signs of irritation, such as a stiff neck or pain when bending the head forward. The client is also observed for signs of *anaphylaxis* (severe allergic response).

Cerebral Angiography and Arteriography

In some instances, angiography or arteriography may be performed. An *angiogram* is an x-ray study of any blood vessel, and an *arteriogram* is an x-ray study of an artery. The procedure involves injecting a radiopaque substance into the femoral, brachial, or radial artery. X-ray films are then taken of the brain's blood vessels to detect any abnormalities. Be alert for any signs of allergy to the drug injected for the test. If severe anaphylaxis occurs in a client, it usually occurs immediately.

Before the procedure, obtain a baseline neurologic assessment. A possibility exists that a thrombus can become dislodged, causing an embolus. An embolus could travel to the heart, lung, or brain. During the procedure, also observe for symptoms of muscular weakness, twitching in the face or extremities, and respiratory difficulties. If any of these occur, notify the healthcare provider immediately.

After the procedure, a sandbag or a specialized pressure device is applied to the insertion site to reduce edema and to prevent bleeding and hematoma formation. Check the area for bleeding every 15–30 min for several hours. Observe the leg's color, temperature, and pedal pulse if the femoral artery was used as the injection site. Because of the radiopaque dye used, encourage intake of fluids unless contraindicated.

Nursing Alert If you cannot find a pulse distal to the injection site or if active bleeding occurs, notify the healthcare provider immediately.

SPECIAL CONSIDERATIONS Lifespan
Dye Procedures and the Older Adult

Monitor the older adult client's blood urea nitrogen (BUN) and creatinine before and after any procedure that uses dye. The aging population is at increased risk for kidney damage; promptly report any elevations in BUN and creatinine.

Myelography

In some cases, a *myelogram* is performed to visualize the spinal cord. However, this test is less commonly used if CT or MRI scanning is available. A lumbar puncture is done, and a radiopaque substance is injected into the spinal canal. The client, in the prone position, is tilted so that dye flows around the spinal cord; then x-ray films are taken to detect tumors or a ruptured intervertebral disk. The radiopaque substances used today are water-soluble and reabsorbed into the body with little, if any, side effects.

SPECIAL CONSIDERATIONS Lifespan
Lumbar Puncture in Children

Expect the need to hold young children in the proper position for LP because often they are extremely frightened by someone who is doing something to their back who cannot be seen. They may try to turn over to see what is happening. Sometimes, family caregivers are willing to hold the child, which may be less frightening to the child. Because needles are smaller, insertion may be easier in children.

Brain Scan

A *brain scan* involves the injection of a radioactive substance (*radioisotope*), which is then detected by a scanner that generates images as the substance circulates within the brain vasculature. This test is used to evaluate vascular lesions, neoplasms, abscesses, and areas of cerebrovascular ischemia. The rationale for this procedure is that the radioisotope will accumulate in a greater amount at a site of pathology than in normal brain tissue.

Other Diagnostic Tests

Lumbar Puncture

The *lumbar puncture* (LP, *spinal tap*) involves the insertion of a hollow needle with a *stylet* (guide) into the subarachnoid space of the lumbar region of the spinal canal (Fig. 78-1). A healthcare provider performs the LP under strict sterile conditions. Nurses play a role in assisting with the procedure (see In Practice: Nursing Procedure 78-1).

An LP may be performed to:

- Measure pressure of cerebrospinal fluid (CSF)
- Obtain a sample of CSF for culture and sensitivity, blood, pus, or other substance levels (e.g., protein, glucose, red blood cells, white blood cells)
- Inject an anesthetic or other drug
- Inject air for special tests

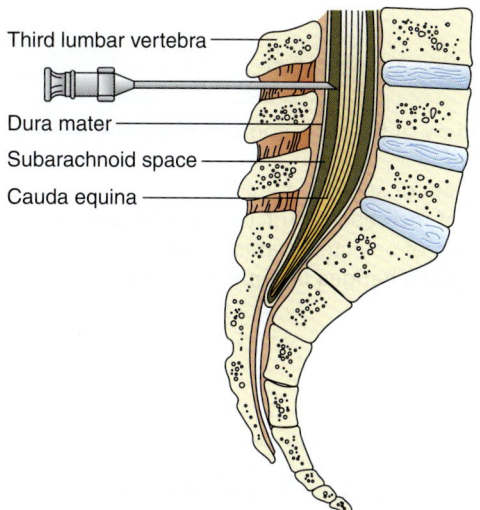

Figure 78-1 Lumbar puncture. Note that the spinal needle is inserted into the subarachnoid space.

After LP, complications may occur, including the following:

- Severe pounding headache, unrelieved by mild analgesics
- Malaise
- Nausea, with or without vomiting
- Irritation/hematoma at injection site
- Temporary leg or buttock pain
- Central nervous system (CNS) infection
- Brain herniation (most severe complication, but extremely rare)
- Bleeding into the spinal canal
- Leakage of CSF
- Paralysis (spinal cord injury, which is very rare)

> **Nursing Alert** Document the client's ability to move all extremities before and after the procedure. If the spinal catheter goes in too far, it can damage the spinal cord.

> **Nursing Alert** During the procedure, observe the client closely for signs of an adverse reaction, for example, elevated pulse rate, pallor, or clammy skin.

Electroencephalography

Electroencephalography (EEG) records the brain's electrical impulses as a graph. This test is used frequently in the diagnosis of seizure disorders, brain tumors, intracranial lesions (in Parkinson disease, Alzheimer's disease, and narcolepsy), blood clots, infections (meningitis, encephalitis), and sleep disorders. Another important use of the EEG is to confirm brain death (*electrocerebral silence*).

Electrodes are placed on the client's forehead and scalp by means of a special glue called *collodion;* these electrodes are connected to the machine. In some cases, a cap containing the electrodes is placed on the head; a few clinics use tiny needles. The procedure is painless, has no after effects, and requires 1–2 hr to conduct.

In preparation for an EEG, the client may be asked not to sleep the night before the test (for a *sleeping EEG*), or they may receive sedation (for a *resting EEG*). It may be necessary to wash and dry the client's hair before the procedure.

Explain to the client that no electric shock will be given and that the EEG procedure cannot determine thoughts or mental ability. Tell the person that they will be asked to open and close the eyes and sometimes to perform other movements on command. In some cases, lights will be flashed, the client will be asked to watch a repeating pattern on a television monitor, or a small electrical stimulus will be given. The brain's responses to these stimuli are recorded. These responses are called *evoked responses* or *evoked potentials*.

Stimulants, such as caffeinated beverages, chocolate, and tobacco, should be avoided for 8 hr before the test. Anticonvulsants, tranquilizers, barbiturates, and other sedatives may interfere with the test results. If needles are used, there is a slight possibility of infection. After the procedure, the client may need a shampoo to remove collodion.

Video Telemetry Monitoring

Healthcare facilities specializing in neurology and seizure disorders use a diagnostic tool called *video telemetry monitoring*. It involves video, audio, and EEG monitoring of a person 24 hr a day or all night. When the client experiences a seizure, it can be seen and heard on videotape as well as recorded electrically by EEG.

Seizure precautions are initiated to protect the client from injury. The client should wear a pajama bottom with a gown for protection of modesty. To allow for observation of extremities, which may be indicators of the types of seizures, make sure that the client is uncovered so that these areas can be seen. Make sure the client is within camera range, so the event will be filmed.

CRANIOCEREBRAL DISORDERS

> **NCLEX Alert**
> Neurovascular disorders typically need abundant and specific nursing interventions. An NCLEX clinical scenario might ask you to prioritize a given list of nursing interventions. For example, list in order of priority the concerns for a client who is having a seizure.

Headaches

Headaches can range in intensity from minor discomfort to extreme pain. Some people suffer from chronic headaches. The most common types are discussed here.

Symptomatic Headache

Cephalgia (headache) is one of the most common symptoms of a neurologic disorder. It is also associated with many other diseases and disorders. Headache is not a disease in itself, but rather it is a symptom of an underlying disorder. Do not confuse the occasional headache that disappears after taking an analgesic with persistent headaches that require further evaluation.

Headaches often appear with conditions such as eye strain, sinusitis, muscle strain, ligament strain, cervical degenerative changes, emotional tension, and stress. They are also associated with brain tumors, hypertension, and *increased intracranial pressure* (↑*ICP*). Persistent or recurring headaches are frequently associated with true neurologic diseases or disorders, such as brain tumors and aneurysms.

IN PRACTICE
DATA GATHERING IN NURSING 78-1 — Key Components of a Neurologic Assessment

- Neurologic nursing history, including history given by family
- Speech patterns
- Level of consciousness (LOC), particularly changes in LOC
- Neurologic status, using the Glasgow coma scale
- Gross evaluation of muscle tone/strength
- Overview of balance, coordination, and protective reflexes
- Overview of sensory function
- Signs of increased intracranial pressure (↑ICP)
- Function of selected cranial nerves
- Eye signs (changes in pupillary size and response)

NURSING PROCESS

DATA COLLECTION

Chapter 47 describes a head-to-toe assessment, including that of the nervous system. This assessment establishes a baseline for future comparison. Report any changes in the baseline level. Change in behaviors, mentation, level of consciousness (LOC), alertness, and orientation could be subtle but significant. For example, perhaps a client has been alert and cooperative with caregivers. Later, however, the nurse notices that this client is irritable and less cooperative. This change of action and behavior could be relevant. The nurse needs to gather further data to determine if the change could be a result of a physical dysfunction, such as an embolus in the brain; metabolic causes, such as low blood sugar; or effects of prescribed medications.

Observe and document the client's general appearance and mobility level, as well the major components listed in In Practice: Data Gathering in Nursing 78-1. Additionally, observe the client's emotional response to the situation. Does the disorder affect social activities, self-care, and self-esteem? Does the client seem anxious or fearful of the outcome?

PLANNING AND IMPLEMENTATION

The healthcare team plans together with the client and family for effective care to meet the client's needs. The client with a neurologic disorder may need help with activities of daily living (ADL), exercises, body alignment and position, elimination, nutrition, and sensory and emotional problems. They will need to learn more about the disorder, its prognosis, and its treatment. An individualized nursing care plan is developed to meet these needs.

Assisting With ADL

The client may need assistance with ADL: skin care, special eye care, mouth care, nail and hair care (see Chapter 50), and management of bowel or bladder elimination (see Chapter 51). Be sure to help the client maintain adequate nutritional status to rebuild strength and to prevent further deterioration (see Chapter 5).

Providing Exercise

The client with impaired mobility needs as much active and passive exercise as possible to prevent contractures, muscle atrophy, and other disuse deformities. Clients who are paralyzed or otherwise physically challenged can use many assistive devices, including lifts, wheelchairs, braces, and splints (see Chapters 48 and 97).

Providing Comfort With Special Devices

Clients with neurologic disorders who are immobilized may need to use a bed with specialized features designed to minimize some of the hazards of immobility. The most important goals of these specialized beds are to prevent skin breakdown and alleviate pain. Follow the manufacturer's specifications when using any of these special beds.

Special "neuro chairs" also help to transfer clients in and out of bed and serve as a comfortable place for the client to rest when out of bed. These chairs adjust to various positions and can be placed in high Fowler or Trendelenburg positions when necessary. Various commercial reclining chairs are also available. When assisting a client to move from the bed to the neuro chair and back, use good body mechanics and place the bed and chair in the flat position and raise both to high position. Maintain the client's safety by locking the wheels of the chair and bed, obtaining additional help to move the client, using safety devices as necessary, and placing the call light within the client's reach.

EVALUATION

Periodically, the nurse, client, and family evaluate outcomes of care. Have short-term goals been met? For example, is the client able to participate in self-care? Are long-term goals still realistic, especially if the client has a progressive neurologic disorder? Planning for further nursing care must consider prognosis, complications, and the client's response.

SPECIAL CONSIDERATIONS — Lifespan

Skin Care and Special Devices

Often the skin of older adults is very fragile (*friable*), which can increase the client's risk for skin breakdown. Specialized beds or mattresses may be routinely ordered for older clients with fragile skin and neurologic conditions.

Diagnosis of headaches is made by medical history, family history, and evaluation of the individual patterns of the headaches. Any history of trauma is relevant. Knowledge of changes in behaviors or LOC is particularly important. X-ray examinations of the head and sinuses; food elimination diets (particularly, dairy and cheese products); and diagnostic scans, such as CT, MRI, or PET, can also help to determine the cause of the pain.

Nonjudgmental acknowledgment of the individual's pain is essential because pain thresholds differ among clients. The nurse may assist by educating the client and family in the various treatment alternatives presented by the healthcare provider. Offer analgesics as needed (PRN) and encourage compliance with the medication regimen. If the headache is triggered by foods, major changes in eating habits may be necessary.

Migraine Headache

The specific cause of a *migraine headache* is not known, but it appears to result from a vascular disturbance in which the brain's blood vessels dilate abnormally. Migraine headaches are also called *vascular headaches*.

The person may have sensory warnings or premonitions (aura) that a headache will occur. Various auras include mood changes, anorexia, numbness of a body part, or visual symptoms, such as flashing lights or floating spots. Later, the person will experience unilateral throbbing or steady pain, sometimes accompanied by nausea and vomiting.

Migraine headaches run in families; they occur more frequently in people who have asthma, hay fever, and food allergies. Stress may bring on migraine headaches. Other triggers include caffeine (or its sudden withdrawal), nicotine, cheese, alcohol, and certain food preservatives (e.g., monosodium glutamate). Fasting and missing meals may serve as triggers, as may premenstrual fluid retention. Certain drugs, including oral contraceptives and reserpine, an antihypertensive agent, also may be triggers.

There are three categories of medical interventions for migraine headaches. *Abortive* therapy includes drugs designed to interfere with the cause of the headache, that is, to stop the headache. *Symptomatic* relief is used to treat headache's pain or nausea. *Preventative* therapy uses medications to prevent the headaches. These methods may be most effective when used in addition to dietary and lifestyle changes. Preventative therapies are used as adjuncts to relaxation exercises, biofeedback, acupuncture, or the application of cold to the back of the neck or the base of the skull (see In Practice: Important Medications 78-1). Each category of migraine medication has specific side effects, and each needs to be taken as part of supervised medical interventions.

Cluster Headache

Cluster headaches receive their name because they tend to occur in groups or clusters, often at night. As with migraines, they seem to result from vascular disturbances. These headaches can be severely disabling. They are more common in men than in women.

A cluster headache occurs suddenly and severely, often affecting only one side and involving the eye, neck, and face on that side. The eyes may appear to bulge, and other symptoms of vasodilation are seen, such as edema, *lacrimation* (tear formation), rhinorrhea (runny nose), *diaphoresis*

IN PRACTICE
IMPORTANT MEDICATIONS 78-1 — For Migraine Headaches

Category: Abortive—used when symptoms first begin or to halt process causing headache.

Triptans
- Naratriptan HCL (Amerge)
- Rizatriptan (Maxalt)
- Sumatriptan succinate (Imitrex)
- Zolmitriptan (Zomig)
- Almotriptan malate (Axert)
- Frovatriptan succinate (Frova)
- Eletriptan hydrobromide (Relpax)

Category: Preventive—used to lessen frequency and intensity of frequent migraine attacks.

Antihypertensive
- Beta-blockers: propranolol (Inderal), atenolol (Tenormin), nadolol (Corgard), and metoprolol tartrate (Lopressor)
- Calcium channel blockers: verapamil (Calan), diltiazem (Cardizem)

Antidepressants
- Amitriptyline (Elavil)
- Fluoxetine (Prozac)

Antiseizure
- Gabapentin (Neurontin)
- Topiramate (Topamax)
- Valproic acid (Depakote)

Category: Symptomatic
- Combination of nonsteroidal anti-inflammatory drugs (NSAIDs): acetylsalicylic acid (Aspirin), acetaminophen (Tylenol), and caffeine (Excedrin Migraine)
- NSAIDs: ibuprofen (Advil), naproxen (Aleve)
- Antiemetics: metoclopramide (Reglan), prochlorperazine (Compro), and promethazine (Phenergan)
- Ergot: Dihydroergotamine (DHE-45)

(sweating), and flushing of the affected side. The pupil constricts, and the face and head are sensitive to external touch. The condition may disappear as suddenly as it occurs, or it may continue for several days. Although no specific cure is known, some drugs have been effective in selected cases. These drugs include vasoconstrictor drugs, corticosteroids, and indomethacin (Indocin).

Seizure Disorders

A seizure, also known as a *convulsion,* is an episode of abnormal motor, sensory, cognitive, and psychic activity caused by erratic and abnormal electrical discharges of brain cells. Repeated episodes of seizures are called *seizure disorders.* Most seizures are self-limiting and benign, lasting a few seconds to a few minutes. Some known causes of seizures include birth trauma, genetic predisposition, head injuries, some types of brain infections and abscesses, toxicity, fever, metabolic and nutritional disorders, tumors, or brain malformations.

The duration of the seizure is called the *ictal phase*. The period following the seizure is called the *postictal phase*. During the postictal phase, the person may be confused or fall into a deep sleep lasting minutes or hours.

Seizure disorder may be associated with birth trauma, meningitis, traumatic injury, and a variety of metabolic or developmental disorders. An individual who has had a seizure does not necessarily have epilepsy. For example, a child who has had a febrile seizure or a pregnant client who has had eclampsia is not typically diagnosed with epilepsy.

Status epilepticus refers to the occurrences of a single, unremitting seizure that lasts longer than 5 min or frequent clinical seizures without an interictal return to baseline. The most common types of seizures are discussed below.

> **Nursing Alert** Status epilepticus is a *medical emergency* because 20% of adults who experience a first episode may die during the episode.

Classification

There are two major classifications of seizures: *partial* or *focal* seizure and *generalized* seizure. A partial or focal seizure may be subclassified as simple or complex. Each category may have several types. A *partial or focal seizure* initially involves smaller, localized sections of the brain and might spread within seconds or minutes to involve widespread areas of the brain. A *primary generalized seizure* begins with involvement of both sides of the brain. Box 78-1 reviews the common names and categories of seizures. With *unclassified seizures*, the origin of the abnormal electrical activity is not known.

A *tonic–clonic* or *grand mal seizure* is the most commonly known type of generalized seizure. At the onset of the seizure, the individual may cry out and experience an aura, knowing that a seizure is imminent. The seizure may commence with the person falling down because of brief loss of muscle tone (flaccidity). Rigid contraction of body muscles (tonic phase), which alternates with rhythmic jerking movements (clonic phase), follows. The tonic–clonic or grand mal seizure is perhaps the most life-threatening type of seizure.

Diagnostic Tests

Diagnosis of seizure disorders is made based on the client's history, physical examination, laboratory tests, and EEG findings. An accurate description of the seizure itself is essential to identify the type of seizure and appropriate treatment.

The EEG is a useful diagnostic tool because different seizure types produce specific electrical wave patterns. Just because the EEG looks normal does not necessarily mean that the person is not experiencing seizures. Video telemetry monitoring is helpful to the healthcare provider in diagnosing the specific seizure type.

> **Key Concept**
> The EEG of a person with a seizure disorder may look normal, especially if no seizure occurs at the time of the EEG.

Box 78-1 | Classification of Seizures

PARTIAL OR FOCAL SEIZURES

Partial or focal seizures occur in one part (focus) of the brain
- **Partial simple**—Localized shaking movements, usually does not result in a loss of consciousness
- **Complex partial (psychomotor)**—Consciousness is impaired but not totally lost; maybe associated with an aura (unpleasant sensation of impending seizure)
- **Jacksonian**—Rhythmic jerking movements start in one muscle group and spread
- **Adversive**—Person may become combative
- **Sensory**—Person has unpleasant hallucinations, talks unintelligibly, or experiences vertigo

PRIMARY GENERAL SEIZURES

Primary general seizures involves both hemispheres of the brain
- **Tonic–clonic (grand mal)**—stiffening of the body, repeated jerking, and loss of consciousness
- **Absence (petit mal)**—no convulsions; may see twitching facial muscles, fluttering eyelids, rapid blinking, or a few seconds staring into space
- **Tonic**—severe stiffening of muscles, especially of the back, legs, and arms
- **Clonic**—repeated bilateral jerking movements
- **Atonic**—brief periods, usually in children, complete loss of muscle tone and consciousness
- **Myoclonic**—quick jerking movements of one or more limbs or trunk; may be brief, but repetitive; no loss of consciousness
- **Status epilepticus**—a medical emergency; convulsions with intense muscle contractions and dyspnea lasting 15 min or more

UNCLASSIFIED EPILEPTIC SEIZURES

Unclassified seizures include all seizures that cannot be classified. These seizures may be caused by high fevers, genetic abnormality, or metabolic disorders, such as hyperglycemia, hypercalcemia, hypermagnesemia, or hypernatremia or structural damage caused by trauma, a stroke or a tumor. About half of the causes of seizures are unknown (idiopathic).

https://www.epilepsysociety.org.uk/about-epilepsy/epileptic-seizures.

Other diagnostic procedures may include the following:
- CT scan and MRI to identify a tumor, bleeding, or a brain lesion
- Cerebral angiogram to differentiate between brain tumor and blood vessel malformation
- Blood work to indicate electrolyte imbalance, drug toxicity, or underlying disorders

Medical and Surgical Treatment

The primary treatment of seizures is pharmacologic therapy with a group of medications referred to as *anticonvulsant drugs*. These drugs work by raising the individual's seizure threshold. Choice of drugs is based on the type of seizure the person experiences. Sometimes, several drugs are combined to control the seizures. Routine blood levels of the drug are monitored to ensure a therapeutic dose. If

IN PRACTICE
IMPORTANT MEDICATIONS 78-2 — For Seizures

- Anticonvulsants, such as oxcarbazepine (Trileptal), levetiracetam (Keppra), phenobarbital (Solfoton), phenytoin (Dilantin), carbamazepine (Tegretol), ezogabine (Potiga), zonisamide (Zonegran), and valproic acid (Depakene), according to the type of seizure
- Ethosuximide (Zarontin) for absence seizures

For Status Epilepticus
- Diazepam (Valium)
- Lorazepam (Ativan)
- Midazolam (Versed)
- Phenobarbital (Solfoton)
- Phenytoin (Dilantin)
- Valproic acid (Depakene)
- Propofol (Diprivan)

Nursing Considerations
- Keep in mind that when these drugs are given intravenously (IV) for status epilepticus, there is danger of overdose.
- Be alert for central nervous system (CNS) signs (e.g., drowsiness and lethargy), respiratory depression, and cerebrovascular signs, which may range from hypotension to cardiovascular collapse.
- Monitor kidney function. Some of these drugs may also cause kidney damage.

---

the person is experiencing status epilepticus, anticonvulsant drugs are typically given intravenously (IV) (see In Practice: Important Medications 78-2).

Surgery may be performed in certain circumstances in which the seizure's focal point can be clearly identified in the brain. Electrodes are placed directly on the brain to obtain more specific information as to where the seizure originates. Brain tissue that is thought to initiate the seizure is removed. The neurosurgeon must take great care to protect healthy brain tissue from damage during surgery. A procedure called *brain mapping* is done before surgery to identify the important brain structures to avoid.

Nursing Considerations

When a client with a history of seizures or of taking certain medications is admitted to a healthcare facility, they are placed on *seizure precautions*, an expression implying that staff must take special steps to ensure that injury does not result from a seizure (Fig. 78-2). Necessary equipment should include the following:

- Oral airway. **Rationale:** *It assists in maintaining a patent airway. Note: Do not insert if seizure activity has already begun.*
- Suction setup. **Rationale:** *This is useful if the client has difficulty in handling secretions.*
- Setup of piggyback port on an open IV. **Rationale:** *This provides a ready access if the client needs emergency drugs.*
- Rectal or tympanic temperature probe. **Rationale:** *Oral thermometers are unsafe to use. The staff must tailor precautions to the type of seizure the client experiences.*

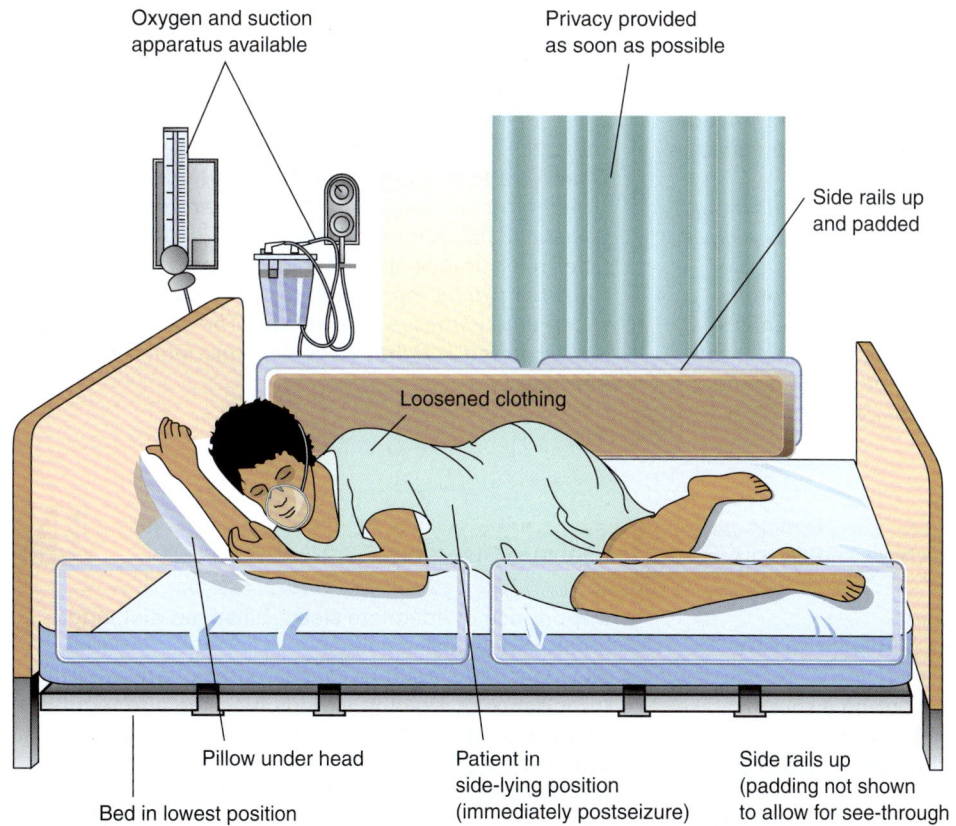

Figure 78-2 This client unit is set up for seizure precautions. After a seizure, the client is placed in a protective position. Hospital protocol may require documentation for the use of side rails because side rails can be considered a restraint.

- Blankets on the bedside rails, headboard, and footboard fastened with adhesive tape. *Rationale: It is important to protect the client's limbs, head, and feet from injury during a seizure while in bed.*
- Bed in low position. *Rationale: To minimize injuries that may occur if the client climbs over the rails.*

In Practice: Nursing Care Guidelines 78-1 highlights important measures to ensure the client's safety.

Careful documentation of the seizure helps in identifying its origin and developing a treatment plan. Some facilities have an event form on which to document all seizures. Documentation must include what the person was doing at the seizure's onset, where the seizure began, if and how the person fell, time of day, triggering events, seizure progression and symmetry, eye response, responsiveness, results of commands and memory tests, duration, direction of eye gaze and eye movements, confusion, incontinence, drooling, and diaphoresis. Document what the client says about the seizure and how they behave; check eye signs and LOC. Describe clusters of seizures.

> **Nursing Alert** The nurse's role during a seizure is to protect and observe. During a seizure, observe the client for respiratory depression and have emergency airway equipment readily available.

Client and family teaching for seizure disorders is essential. In Practice: Educating the Client 78-1 lists the important topics to address when teaching about seizures. The client

---

IN PRACTICE
NURSING CARE GUIDELINES 78-1 Maintaining the Client's Safety During a Seizure

- Protect the client from nearby hazards. Move the overbed tray table and other dangerous items away from the client. *Rationale: The client will be unable to control muscle movements or reactions during the seizure.*
- Loosen restrictive clothing, such as a client's tie or shirt collar. *Rationale: Loosening clothing helps to maintain an unobstructed airway.*
- Do not place anything in the person's mouth after a seizure has begun. *Rationale: Doing so could cause the client's teeth to break by forcing an object into the mouth.*
- Do not attempt to restrain the client. *Rationale: Injury may result from forcible restraint against the contraction of the muscles.*
- Place a small, soft padding beneath the client's head, such as a folded jacket. *Rationale: Padding the area helps to protect the head from injury.*
- Turn the client's head to the side. *Rationale: Turning the client's head to the side helps to maintain a clear airway and prevent aspiration.*
- Monitor the seizure activity and location carefully. Note the exact time the seizure begins and ends. Test the extremity strength and tone. *Rationale: This information is important to aid in determining the type of seizure that the client experienced.*
- Call the client's name. Give a simple command, such as asking them to grab your hand and to let go. *Rationale: Responses to these evaluative techniques assist in evaluating the type and severity of the seizure.*
- Give the client a "memory test" by asking them to remember two unrelated words. *Rationale: Whether or not the client is able to remember the words helps provide additional information about the type of seizure.*
- After the seizure, ask the client if there was an aura (warning). *Rationale: The client may learn to take protective measures before a seizure occurs.*
- Check the tongue and oral cavity for any bite injuries. *Rationale: The client may have injured themselves during the seizure; evidence of injury indicates a need for treatment.*
- Observe and document carefully. *Rationale: Documentation helps to provide communication and assists healthcare personnel in treating the client.*
- Offer reassurance and emotional support. *Rationale: Seizures can be frightening to the client and to those who witnessed the seizure. The client is often embarrassed and may have been incontinent or confused.*

IN PRACTICE
EDUCATING THE CLIENT 78-1 Teaching Topics to Address for Seizure Disorders

- Explanation of seizure disorder
- Specific information about the particular seizure type the client experienced
- Safety and prevention of injury during a seizure
- Care of the client during and after a seizure
- Importance of taking medications as prescribed
- Medication side effects
- Importance of family observation of seizure, so they can fully describe it to the neurologist
- Importance of adequate sleep, balanced diet, and suitable physical activities
- Avoidance of situations that can precipitate a seizure
- Importance of wearing a MedicAlert tag and regular follow-up with healthcare provider
- Importance of having blood drawn to determine blood levels of antiepileptic medications

needs to know how to adapt their lifestyle to the disorder, living as normally as possible. Most people with seizure disorders have seizures that are controlled with medication. Individuals and family members must understand the importance of regular medication administration and periodic medical evaluations.

Stroke

A sudden or gradual interruption of blood supply to a vital center in the brain is a *stroke*, also known as a *cerebral (brain) infarct*, and formerly referred to as a cerebrovascular accident. A stroke may cause complete or partial paralysis or death. The underlying cause of this disorder often involves atherosclerosis of the cerebral blood vessels (see Chapter 81). In Practice: Nursing Care Plan 78-1 addresses the client experiencing hemiplegia resulting from a stroke.

NERVE DISORDERS

Neuralgia

The term *neuralgia* literally means "pain in a nerve." Neuralgia often applies to fleeting pain in the shoulder and upper arm or pain caused by a herniated intervertebral disk. If application of external heat and administration of analgesics, such as acetylsalicylic acid (Aspirin), do not relieve the pain, medical evaluation is needed.

Trigeminal Neuralgia

In *trigeminal neuralgia (tic douloureux)*, the root of the trigeminal (fifth cranial) nerve becomes painful. The cause is unknown, and it generally occurs in the older population. The pain is excruciating and comes in spasms that can last for seconds to hours, occurring in the jaw and parts of the face.

The pain may be triggered by the slightest touch to various parts of the face, or even by a breeze, a change in temperature, or a mouthful of food, depending on the trigger zone's location. Treatment consists of medications or surgery. Some drugs may help temporarily, but surgery is the treatment with the most satisfactory results. Partial removal of the nerve roots eliminates the pain permanently, although it may leave burning, tickling sensations for several weeks or months.

After surgery, various symptoms may occur, depending on which nerve branches were sectioned. In addition to adjusting to a certain amount of numbness, the client may have some eye irritation or difficulty eating. The client learns to avoid situations that previously triggered pain.

Bell Palsy

Bell palsy is a temporary, partial, one-sided facial paralysis and weakness caused by ischemia or inflammation of the seventh cranial nerve. A Bell palsy-type syndrome may result from a brain lesion.

The paralysis may result in a lopsided facial appearance. The eye on the affected side will not close. The client cannot control the mouth on the affected side, which often leads to drooling. In addition, the mouth does not turn up when the client smiles. These symptoms can be emotionally upsetting for the client. Special eye care may be necessary. Heat and massage may be helpful. In the early stages, prednisone (Deltasone) may be used. Usually, symptoms subside gradually, but they may take months to do so.

Shingles (Herpes Zoster)

Shingles, *or herpes zoster*, is an acute viral inflammation of a nerve caused by the varicella-zoster virus (the same virus that causes chickenpox). The disease results from reactivation of latent virus cells residing in dorsal root or cranial nerve ganglion cells.

Signs and Symptoms

Mild to moderate pruritus (itching), tenderness, or pain frequently precedes the appearance of vesicles. The interval between pain and eruption of vesicles averages 3–5 days. Lesions erupt for several days and usually disappear within 3–4 weeks. Vesicles follow the distribution of sensory nerves, causing excruciating pain. Sites of vesicle distribution include the forehead, face, and buttocks. Normally, only one site is affected, and it is usually limited to either the left or right side. However, the eruption may encircle the trunk. This is common in clients with HIV/AIDS. Some scarring may occur. Pain can be quite severe even if vesicles are not visible on the skin. The pain can last for several weeks or months. Some clients also experience gastrointestinal upset and general malaise.

Generally, the disorder is self-limiting and localized. Herpes usually heals without complications. The eruption of herpes zoster vesicles is sometimes associated with other diseases, particularly in clients with suppressed immune systems, such as those with tuberculosis, HIV/AIDS, and lymphoma. Sometimes, an injury or an injection of a drug may trigger the inflammation.

In rare cases, the infection may invade the eyes and cause conjunctivitis. If it is not checked, blindness may result in the affected eye (*ophthalmic zoster*). In clients with serious underlying conditions that suppress the immune system, serious complications may develop.

Postherpetic neuralgia (pain along the nerves after a herpes infection) may cause pain and discomfort for 8 weeks or more. Postherpetic neuralgia is most common in clients older than 60 years.

Treatment

Shingles vaccination is recommended for adults age 60 and older. A single dose of the vaccination (Zostavax) can prevent shingles or decrease its symptoms. Pediatric immunization against chickenpox is recommended (see Chapter 72). Treatment of shingles is symptomatic, focusing on relief of pain and pruritus. Narcotics and/or anti-inflammatory agents may be helpful in obtaining pain and pruritus relief. Wet dressings with Burow solution may be useful during the vesicular stage of the infection. Calamine lotion and antihistamines may treat pruritus. IV acyclovir (Zovirax) has improved the rate of healing of skin lesions and shortened the period of pain. Oral corticosteroids have been used in clients aged 50–60 years and older to decrease postherpetic neuralgia.

IN PRACTICE

NURSING CARE PLAN 78-1 — The Client With a Stroke and Hemiplegia

Medical History: I. K., a 55-year-old African-American female with a history of hypertension, was admitted to the hospital 3 days ago with a left-sided stroke resulting from cerebral thrombosis. Client has right-sided hemiplegia.

Medical diagnosis: Left-sided stroke with right-sided hemiplegia.

DATA COLLECTION/NURSING OBSERVATION

Client is alert and oriented to person, place, time, and situation. Vital signs within acceptable parameters. Slight residual slurring of speech is noted. Gag reflex is intact. Client demonstrates ability to swallow without problems. Client is able to tolerate small amounts of liquids by mouth, approximately 30–45 mL at one time. Intravenous (IV) is infusing at a rate of 125 mL/hr. Right side flaccid and weak. Client is right-handed and uses the left side to move extremities on the right. Currently, they require moderate assistance with self-care. Skin inspection reveals 8-mm circumference reddened area on the right heel. No skin breakdown. Urine output is approximately 350 mL over the past 8 hr. Urine is clear and yellow. Client moved bowels 2 days ago. Scattered crackles auscultated at both bases that clear with coughing. Client lives with a 60-year-old husband in a two-story home in the country. Their family lives approximately 20 min away by car.

NURSING DIAGNOSIS

(Although other nursing diagnoses may be appropriate, a priority nursing diagnosis is addressed below.)

Altered tissue integrity risk related to hemiplegia as evidenced by right-sided flaccidity and weakness and reddened areas on heel and elbow.

(Although other nursing diagnoses may be appropriate, a priority nursing diagnosis is addressed below.)

Planning (Outcomes/Goals)	Implementation (Nursing Actions)	Evaluation
Short-Term Goals A. Anticipate problems that enhance development of skin breakdown. B. Initiate nursing measures that help prevent skin breakdown and other hazards of immobility.	• Change the client's position every 2 hr. • Provide passive and active range of motion. • Eliminate pressure area on the right heel. • Encourage the use of a trapeze bar with left arm and hand. *Rationale: Frequent position changes help to prevent disorders caused by immobility–disuse disorders. Splints or high-top sneakers aid in maintaining normal anatomical alignment of the joints. Use of trapeze bar allows the client to assist with position changes and to reduce the shearing forces that can lead to skin breakdown.* • Protect bony areas from pressure, especially those areas on the right side. • Provide orthopedic shoes designed to eliminate pressure on heels and eliminate foot drop. • Use a standing wheelchair, tilt table, or rehabilitation chair as soon as possible to get client out of bed. • Use measures to prevent foot drop, such as splints or high-top sneakers. • Auscultate lung fields to detect rales. *Rationale: Pressure on bony prominences increases the client's risk for skin breakdown. The client's right-sided hemiplegia contributes to this risk. Mobility will prevent respiratory complications. Movement will help the client to maintain self-esteem and promote independence.* • Overview nursing care measures by others, e.g., nurses' aides, to ensure that the sheets are smooth, without wrinkles, and the bed is clean, without potential hazards to skin. *Rationale: The skin of the client with hemiplegia is subject to pressure areas and skin breakdown.*	Day 1—1,030 hr. • Pressure-relieving shoe in place on both feet. • Bilateral heels checked every 2 hr. • Decrease in size right heel redness from 8 to 4 mm since admission assessment. • Area appears less red with improved skin color. • No new reddened areas are noted on left heel or coccyx. • Lung fields are clear to auscultation. Goals A and B met. Observations ongoing.

Planning (Outcomes/Goals)	Implementation (Nursing Actions)	Evaluation
C. Client will verbalize measures to reduce or prevent hazards of immobility.	• Teach client about measures to reduce the risk for problems related to immobility. • Encourage client to turn, cough, and deep breathe every hour. • Encourage client to drink about 1 L fluids per shift. • Encourage client to use overhead trapeze when moving self in bed. *Rationale: Client participation in the plan of care helps to promote a sense of control over the situation, thereby helping to promote self-esteem.*	Day 2—1,700 hr. • Client is able to state measures to reduce risk of skin breakdown. • Asks for assistance with sitting up in bed. • Actively uses trapeze bar to change positions. • Client is observed using incentive spirometer every 2–3 hr. • Lungs clear to auscultation. *Goals A–C met.* *Observations ongoing.*
D. Client actively participates in measures to reduce or prevent complications related to hazards of immobility.	• Provide respiratory care instructions using bedside incentive spirometers. • Encourage coughing and deep breathing and use of incentive spirometer at least every 2 hr. • Provide written instruction materials for family and caregivers regarding importance of movement, fluids, and respiratory interventions (hazards of immobility). • Provide opportunities for family/caregivers to demonstrate interventions when client is at home. *Rationale: Respiratory care measures are necessary to prevent pulmonary complications. Pneumonia is a particularly dangerous complication. Family/caregiver participation encourages compliance with regimen and fosters improved at-home care.* • Encourage fluid intake to approximately 2–3 L/day. • Observe urinary output for color and amount. • Monitor intake and output at least every 4–8 hr. • Teach the client and family the signs and symptoms of urinary tract infection and kidney stones, e.g., flank pain. *Rationale: Adequate fluid intake helps to prevent kidney stones and bladder infections. Changes in the color or clarity of the urine may suggest a potential problem. Adequate client understanding of signs and symptoms of potential problems helps to ensure prompt detection and early intervention should any problems occur.*	Day 3—1,600 hr. Predischarge to rehabilitation center • Client is able to state and actively demonstrate measures to prevent problems of immobility. • Client is scheduled to attend physical therapy this afternoon and occupational therapy in the morning. • Lungs are clear to auscultation. • Client drank 2.5 L yesterday; voiding clear yellow urine in adequate amounts. • No complaints of flank pain. • Right heel's skin coloring without signs of redness or breakdown. • No signs of breakdown in coccyx or either heel. *Goal D completed.* *Observations ongoing.* Family/caregivers encouraged to continue interventions after discharge.
E. Client remains free of hazards of immobility.	• Maintain nutritional status, gradually increasing the client's diet as ordered, including high-fiber foods. *Rationale: Adequate nutrition is necessary to promote healing and to maintain health. The intake of fiber helps to reduce the risk of constipation.* • Encourage client to perform active range-of-motion exercises to left side and passive range-of-motion exercises to right side. • Contact physical therapy to assist with muscle strengthening, endurance, and mobility. • Contact occupational therapy to assist with self-care activities at home. *Rationale: Continued exercise helps to maintain function of the extremities; contacting physical therapy and occupational therapy professionals promotes development of a beginning rehabilitation plan for the client.*	• No further evidence of skin breakdown is noted. • Lungs are clear to auscultation. • Client states, "I'm looking forward to PT and OT." *Goals A–E met.* Encouraged family/caregivers to monitor skin for pressure wounds and other hazards of immobility while in rehabilitation center as well as at home when client returns to home.

Nursing Considerations

All causes of neuralgia need adequate evaluation of pain and pain control measures. Environmental conditions may need to be adjusted so that the client can have a quiet environment with minimal stimulus.

With herpes zoster, infection control measures are necessary to prevent cross-contamination. It is possible for individuals who have never had chickenpox to develop chickenpox from contact with someone with shingles. Transmission-based precautions are necessary. All healthcare providers should avoid touching the lesions directly. Be sure to wear gloves whenever there is a possibility of exposure to drainage and secretions.

Instructions on how to avoid pain triggers and measures for appropriate pain management are key areas to stress in client and family education. Emotional support also is important because the client may have a disturbed body image related to paralysis, muscle twitching, or outbreaks of vesicles.

SPINAL CORD DISORDERS

An understanding of several basic concepts is necessary when caring for persons with spinal cord disorders. Application of these concepts will help healthcare providers to understand these disabilities better and initiate appropriate care:

- The *spinal cord* is the communication system between the brain and the periphery of the body. It is composed of a tight cluster of nerve cell bodies (*gray matter*), surrounded by the ascending (*sensory*) and descending (*motor*) tracts (*white matter*). If the spinal cord is severed or compressed, communication between the brain and the rest of the body is literally cut off.
- The spinal cord lies in an enclosed and confined space called the *vertebral column.* Any invasion into this space can cause devastating effects.
- The spinal cord is responsible for the *reflex arc* (see Chapter 19), which is a built-in protective mechanism. For example, it allows a person to jerk the hand quickly away from a hot stove, thus bypassing the brain and preventing further injury.

Categories of Spinal Cord Disorders

Spinal cord problems can be divided into three main categories: congenital defects, tumors, and trauma. *Congenital defects of the spinal cord* are malformations that occur in the developing fetus. They most often affect the CNS by disrupting the flow of CSF (see Chapter 72).

A *spinal cord tumor* is located within the vertebral column, taking up space and causing compression of the cord. It interferes with blood supply and CSF circulation. Tumors may be surgically removed. Resulting neurologic deficits will vary, depending on the type of tumor and the length of time compression has occurred. If a tumor involves the cord itself, damage is usually most severe and is often permanent.

Trauma to the spinal cord can be caused by blunt or penetrating forces. Examples of penetrating objects include displaced vertebrae or foreign objects such as bullets. Transection (severing) of the cord can be incomplete (partial) or complete. If the transection is *complete,* all sensation and voluntary movements below the site of injury are lost. A *partial* or *incomplete transection* has the best prognosis. In this case, the resulting deficits will depend on whether ascending (sensory) or descending (motor) nerve tracts were severed. Trauma to the spinal cord also includes bruising, in which case the person may regain total function.

Level of Injury

The level of the spinal cord injury determines which body functions are affected. Paraplegia means paralysis of the legs and lower body; it usually results from injury to the cord below the first thoracic vertebra. Clients with paraplegia have damage to the thoracic, lumbar, or sacral nerve segments. The trunk, pelvic organs, and lower extremities are affected. Generally, the arms are not affected.

Tetraplegia (also referred to as quadriplegia) means paralysis to the cervical segments of nerves from C1 to C8, resulting from impaired function of the upper extremities, trunk (including respiratory involvement), pelvic organs, and lower extremities.

The extent of all spinal cord injuries depends on the injury's location and severity. Injuries occurring at the second and third cervical vertebrae are usually fatal. Clients who experience any damage at the level of C4 and above require respiratory assistance because innervation to the respiratory muscles is damaged, and the client cannot breathe independently. Figure 78-3 identifies the structures that are affected by spinal cord injury at various locations.

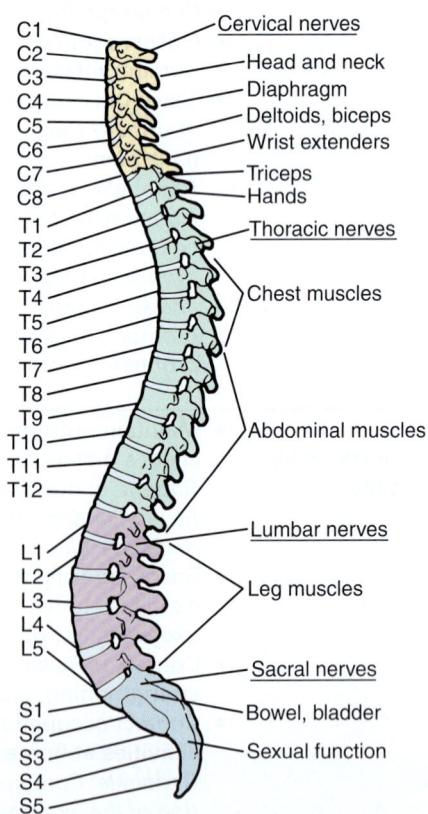

Figure 78-3 Structures affected by spinal nerves.

Sometimes, the final outcome of a spinal cord injury is uncertain for a long period. This time can be highly stressful for the person's family and loved ones. When a diagnosis of paralysis is made, the emotional shock to the person and family is usually devastating.

Adjustments, ranging from minor modifications to total alterations in lifestyle, need to be made. Changes may include adaptations in a home's physical setup, installation of an elevator and ramps, and changes in employment. Assistance with ADL is generally necessary. Adaptations can be made to accommodate the client's needs for transportation, including driving a car. Rehabilitation and occupational therapy can be very helpful.

Effects of Injury

Immediately after a spinal injury, the client is at risk for spinal shock and respiratory arrest. Long-term damage to the spinal cord can have various effects. Sensory deficits can range from numbness and tingling in the extremities to total loss of body sensation. Movement disabilities can also range from muscle weakness to partial or complete paralysis.

> **Key Concept**
> Many persons with varying degrees of paralysis have an active sex life. Adaptations and understanding on the partner's part may be necessary. Paralyzed individuals can conceive and bear children.

Complications of spinal cord injury include impaired circulation, bowel and bladder incontinence, bone demineralization, skin breakdown, anemia, muscle spasms, contractures, increased body temperature, gastric distention, atelectasis, pneumonia, autonomic dysreflexia, neurogenic shock, and respiratory complications. Blood clots may develop in the legs. The lower the location of the cord transection, the fewer the complications.

The client may experience severe, shooting pain that results from nerve damage. Many stimuli may trigger the pain—injections, kidney stones, or fecal impactions can aggravate pain. A person may feel *phantom pain* in a paralyzed area of the body because of nerve damage, or it may occur in a ringlike fashion at the level of injury.

Autonomic Dysreflexia

Autonomic dysreflexia (also known as *autonomic hyperreflexia*), an exaggerated response to stimuli below the level of the lesion in clients with lesions at or above T6, *is a medical emergency that requires prompt treatment*. Physical events or occurrences may trigger or be the precursor to autonomic dysreflexia. Triggers include a distended bowel or bladder; fecal impaction; urinary tract infection; constrictive clothing, shoes, or device; or noxious stimuli such as pain, pressure, or strong smells. Signs and symptoms of autonomic dysreflexia include the following:

- Sudden, significant increase in blood pressure (systolic and diastolic) of 20–40 mm Hg above baseline
- Sudden onset of a pounding headache
- Bradycardia, arrhythmias
- Profuse sweating (diaphoresis), goosebumps (piloerection), and flushing above the level of injury
- Blurred vision, or spots in the visual field
- Nasal congestion
- Apprehension, anxiety

Immediate treatment is required if a client displays these signs and symptoms. Elevate the client's head or have the client sit up, if possible, and notify the healthcare provider. Loosen any constrictive clothing or devices. Quickly check the client for possible causes of pressure, such as a blocked urinary catheter. Monitor the client's blood pressure every 2–5 min.

Nurses need to be ever vigilant in monitoring the client for possible triggers. Treatment involves elimination of the triggering stimulus. In cases of severe hypertension, antihypertensive medications are used. Teach the client and family preventive measures, such as preventing constipation and visually inspecting catheters to ensure that they remain patent.

Paralysis in Female Clients

For female clients with paralysis from a spinal cord injury:

- Menses usually resume within 3 months following the injury. *Rationale: It takes time for the body to adjust to the injury.*
- The use of tampons is dangerous. *Rationale: The client may forget that a tampon is in place because they have no sensation.*
- The use of birth control pills is not recommended. *Rationale: They can lead to thrombus formation, particularly if the client is not exercising or is immobile. Effectiveness often decreases because of interactions with other medications.*
- The use of intrauterine devices (IUDs) is not recommended. *Rationale: They can promote thrombus formation or infections. This client would not be able to tell if the device had fallen out. They also would not be able to feel the pain associated with a perforated uterus.*
- Labor and childbirth may be dangerous. *Rationale: The individual may not be aware of the onset of labor. The likelihood of a cesarean birth is increased because the client may not be able to assist with the delivery, and the uterus may not have adequate muscle tone. In addition, labor and delivery may serve as a trigger for autonomic dysreflexia.*

Emergency Treatment and Diagnostic Tests

After any trauma, extreme care is necessary to prevent further damage when injury to the spine and cord is suspected or known. The head, neck, and spine must be stabilized with the person lying flat on a firm surface. Never lift the person with a known or suspected spinal cord injury by the head, shoulder, or feet. A victim of trauma should never be moved without proper precautions unless the circumstances are such that the individual's safety is compromised and remaining in place would jeopardize the client's life. Treatment for shock and hemorrhage may also be necessary (see Chapter 43). An x-ray examination to determine the extent of injury is a medical priority.

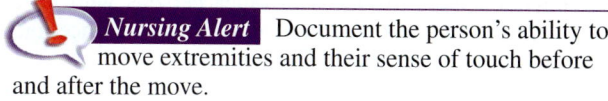

Nursing Alert Document the person's ability to move extremities and their sense of touch before and after the move.

Medical and Surgical Treatment

If the cause of paralysis is trauma, skeletal traction may be applied to immobilize the damaged cervical vertebrae. Several different devices can be used (see Chapter 77). Surgery may be necessary to remove a portion of vertebral bone pressing on the spinal cord or to stabilize the vertebrae to prevent further damage. If the spinal column is unstable, spinal fusion is done to prevent further damage to the spinal cord and to enable more mobility later.

Rehabilitation must begin immediately on hospitalization to maintain the client's cardiac and pulmonary reserves. The client must be rehabilitated in all spheres—body, mind, and spirit. It is best for the person with a spinal cord injury to enter a rehabilitation center as soon as possible. Usually, most acute-care facilities are not equipped to handle all the lifestyle adjustments that must occur.

Nursing Considerations

The nurse plays a vital part in the care and progress of the client with a spinal cord injury. Observe the client closely when providing care. Check for minute changes in the client's condition that are not yet evident to others.

Rehabilitation focuses on preventing disabilities from becoming worse and on strengthening function. Begin measures immediately to prevent disuse disorders, such as skin breakdown and plantar flexion (*foot drop*). Initiate passive and active exercises to develop the client's muscle strength and movement. The degree of success depends on the nature and the extent of nerve damage, as well as the client's own perseverance. Despite paralysis, many clients are able to move about and perform ADL. In Practice: Nursing Care Guidelines 78-2 highlights care for the client with paralysis.

Encourage the client to make every effort to maximize abilities and perform self-care. Remind the client that, at first, even accomplishing the simplest tasks may be overwhelming. The client may become discouraged and angry. Allow the client to express frustration and discouragement and acknowledge these feelings. Provide realistic feedback and encouragement, pointing out the positive gains that the client has made, regardless of how small they may be.

DEGENERATIVE DISORDERS

Degenerative disorders of the nervous system affect people of all ages, with loss of neurologic function at various rates. In addition to all the physical problems the person with degenerative disorder experiences, they will often show major emotional and psychological problems. Such problems may include profound mood swings and outbursts of frustration or anger. The person may exhibit inappropriate sexual behavior, signs of regression, and even infantile behavior. Help by allowing clients and their families to express their feelings and anxieties.

Support groups are available for most degenerative disorders. Numerous resources are available. Assist clients and their families to find appropriate support groups. Encourage all family members to talk with other persons who have faced similar situations. Talking can offer reassurance and helpful suggestions for management.

Multiple Sclerosis

Multiple sclerosis (MS) is one of the most common nerve disorders in the United States, typically affecting young adults and people living in northern temperate climates. It is slightly more common in females. In MS, the myelin sheath covering the nerves is destroyed. Myelin maintains electrical impulse strength. Loss of myelin (*demyelination*) results in weak electrical impulses and weak muscle contractions.

The cause of MS is unknown. A current theory proposes that MS is an autoimmune disease. Some experts believe MS is viral in origin; the Epstein–Barr virus, the cause of infectious mononucleosis, is under consideration. Table 78-1 summarizes the four courses of clinical progression of MS. Each course may have mild, moderate, or severe symptoms.

Signs and Symptoms

Initially, MS may be manifested as difficulty in walking, tremors, lack of coordination, "pins and needles" numbness, and visual changes, including loss of vision. Symptoms are few at first but can increase in number and seriousness over time. Symptoms may disappear in the early stages, and the person may appear normal and well for years. Each time symptoms reappear, they are more severe and of longer duration. Thus, the disease can be marked by remissions and exacerbations. A person may live 20 years or more after the disease is diagnosed, but disabilities develop over time.

Individuals who have few attacks or who have long intervals between attacks are less likely to develop more severe symptoms. However, clients with early symptoms of difficulty walking, tremors, frequent attacks, and incomplete recoveries have a more rapid progression of the disease.

With recurrent episodes, increasingly severe symptoms, such as paralysis, dysphagia (difficulty in swallowing), and bladder and bowel dysfunctions develop. Cognitive dysfunction, depression, and emotional upsets are common. The client may complain of fatigue, headaches, and pain. Seizures, tremors, and spasticity, as well as hearing and visual losses, are common. The client experiences dizziness, nausea, or vomiting or has spastic paraplegia (exaggerated reflexes and muscle tone) and muscle tremors. The individual may have increasing difficulty thinking, reasoning, and remembering and may have sudden emotional upsets, becoming either depressed or exuberant and euphoric.

Diagnosis

Diagnosis of MS is difficult until certain symptoms appear together and create widespread disturbances. An MRI best detects changes in the myelin sheath. About 95% of clients with MS show plaque changes correlating with the person's symptoms. MRI is said to be conclusive for MS if it identifies two areas of plaque changes.

Other causes of symptoms, such as Lyme disease or collagen–vascular diseases, such as lupus erythematosus, need to be ruled out. Other causes of neurologic lesions may present with similar symptoms but have different etiologies. There are no specific diagnostic blood tests for MS.

Medical Treatment

No cure is known for MS. The client needs to maintain general health with periods of rest, adequate sleep, and a

IN PRACTICE
NURSING CARE GUIDELINES 78-2 Caring for the Client With Paralysis

- Use measures to prevent foot drop, such as shoes that control foot positioning or orthopedic shoe splints. *Rationale: Splints aid in maintaining normal anatomical alignment of the joints.*
- Change the client's position frequently and provide passive and active range of motion. *Rationale: Prevent disorders caused by immobility–disuse disorders.*
- Give respiratory care, as needed. *Rationale: This is necessary to prevent respiratory complications. Pneumonia is a particularly dangerous complication.*
- Encourage the client to sit up as much as possible with adequate support. Use a standing wheelchair, tilt table, or "neuro" chair as soon as possible. *Rationale: Mobility will prevent respiratory complications and will help the client to maintain self-esteem.*
- Use special devices (beds, chairs, and other mechanical devices) in the early phases of treatment. Trochanter rolls and sandbags may also be used. *Rationale: These devices help to maintain proper body alignment and positioning, thus helping to prevent orthopedic deformities.*
- Give special skin care. Make sure the sheets are smooth, and the bed is clean. *Rationale: The skin of the client with paralysis is subject to pressure areas and skin breakdown.*
- If cervical traction, tongs, or a halo device is in place, visually inspect the pin site. Give site care as ordered by the healthcare provider. Give incisional care postoperatively. *Rationale: Infection must be prevented because it can be particularly dangerous to a paralyzed person whose physical condition is already compromised.*
- Teach the client and family the warning signs of genitourinary infection. *Rationale: Genitourinary infection is a common complication of immobility.*
- Encourage fluid intake. *Rationale: Adequate fluid intake helps to prevent kidney stones and bladder infections.*
- Institute bladder retraining and rehabilitation early, if possible. *Rationale: Bladder retraining and rehabilitation help restore the client's independence and self-esteem.*
- If urinary retention is present, use a urinary appliance, retention catheter, or self-catheterization. *Rationale: The client may not be able to tell when the bladder is filled. Retention of urine can lead to autonomic dysreflexia, infection, or hydronephrosis.*
- If a catheter is used, make sure it is draining properly and is handled in as clean a manner as possible. Teach the client and family to care for the indwelling catheter or urinary appliance as early as possible if bladder retraining is not an option. *Rationale: Proper drainage and care are needed to avoid bladder and urinary tract infections.*
- If disposable pads or incontinence products are used, give special attention to keeping the skin clean and dry. *Rationale: Keeping the skin dry and clean helps to prevent skin irritation, pressure areas, and infection.*
- Teach the client to do manual disimpaction for a fecal impaction. *Rationale: Damage to the bowel can trigger autonomic dysreflexia. Some clients do a manual disimpaction daily as their bowel maintenance program.*
- Give injections above the level of injury, if possible. *Rationale: Circulation is impaired below the level of injury, and the action of the drug is delayed. The skin is more subject to breakdown below the level of injury.*
- Avoid applying external heat to areas of decreased sensation, particularly to the penis or testes. Take care to avoid pressure on the client, and keep sharp objects from touching the client. *Rationale: The client may experience decreased sensation and be unable to detect changes that could result in injury.*
- Monitor temperature of bathwater. *Rationale: Burns occur easily because of lack of circulation and sensation: The client would not feel the injury, and skin stimulation can cause autonomic dysreflexia.*
- Maintain nutritional status. *Rationale: Nutrition is necessary to promote healing and to maintain health.*
- Establish some sort of communication system if the client cannot speak. It can involve blinking the eyes, moving a finger, or using a computer. *Rationale: The person's mind is usually active; there must be some way for the person to make needs, wants, and thoughts known to others.*

balanced diet. Stress reduction is important. Stressful situations include physical triggers, such as exposure to infection, and emotional triggers, such as employment stress, excitement, and depression.

Preventive interventions may help reduce exacerbation of the symptoms. Physical therapy helps prevent deformities and maintain muscle strength. Occupational therapy may be necessary to provide rehabilitation for lost abilities.

During significant exacerbations, clients may receive IV corticotropin (ACTH) on an out-client or in-client basis. ACTH is given for 6–7 days and then decreased, with weekly injections for another month.

Nonsteroidal immunosuppressive drugs are effective in treating MS, targeting the disease itself rather than just the symptoms. Interferon drugs, such as beta-1b (Betaseron) and beta-1a (Avonex), are used to reduce the number and severity of acute exacerbations. Newer drugs, such as fingolimod (Gilenya), teriflunomide (Aubagio), and dimethyl fumarate (Tecfidera), might be able to reduce relapses and delay disability in some clients.

TABLE 78-1 The Clinical Progression of Multiple Sclerosis

COURSE OF MS	CHARACTERIZED BY	COMMENTS	MS POPULATION (%)
Relapsing-remitting (RRMS)	Partial recovery after attacks (exacerbations with relapses)	Most common form of MS	75%–85% of clients start with RRMS
Secondary-progressive (SPMS), aka "galloping MS"	RRMS course becoming steadily progressive	SPMS develops within 10 years of RRMS	50% of people with RRMS progressed to SPMS approximately 10 years after their first diagnosis
Primary-progressive (PPMS)	Continually progressive disabilities	No periods of remitting (lessening) of symptoms	This type of MS is not very common, occurring in about 10% of people with MS. PPMS is characterized by slowly worsening symptoms from the beginning, with no relapses or remissions
Progressive-relapsing (PRMS)	Continually progressive, with noticeable periods of acute attacks	Rare	5% of MS population have neurologic steady decline

https://www.nationalmssociety.org/; https://www.multiplesclerosis.com/global/treatment.php.

Nursing Considerations

Nursing care focuses on encouraging the client to schedule periods of rest and adequate sleep. In addition, encourage a well-balanced diet and good skin care. As the individual's body manifests more symptoms of muscle wasting and paralysis, the client is less able to prevent the hazards of immobility, such as the complications of contractures, pneumonia, and social isolation.

Elimination problems usually occur. Monitor diet and fluid intake and output. The client may experience urinary incontinence or retention. If the client requires an indwelling urinary catheter, take steps to prevent infection and teach the client and family how to prevent infection. Because constipation often occurs, a bowel training program may be initiated (see Chapter 51).

The client and caregivers need to encourage body repositioning and deep breathing to prevent pneumonia. Give attention to maintaining proper body alignment because paralysis and weakness can lead to deformities.

Unless physically necessary, do not confine the client to bed. Instead, encourage the person to lead as normal a life as possible. The person with MS can live at home as long as they can perform independent physical care or family members are able to assist. Sometimes, the client can work at home until the disease's progression makes this impossible.

Provide support to the client with MS and the family. The client and family members may need to alter aspects of their lifestyles and to readjust goals in accordance with the client's condition. Also, alert the client and family that stress, temperature changes, fatigue, and illness exacerbate or worsen MS. Frequent rest periods during the day are important.

Parkinson Disease

Parkinson disease, also called parkinsonism, is second only to Alzheimer's disease as the most common neurologic disease in older adults. It is a chronic, progressive disease affecting the dopamine-producing cells of the brain. *Dopamine* is a neurotransmitter (chemical messenger) that sends signals within the brain. Without dopamine, neurons fire out of control, and individuals cannot control muscle movements.

Parkinson disease affects slightly more men than women. Although the disorder usually appears in people in their 60s, it can occur in much younger individuals. It is not considered an inherited disorder. Side effects of some medications, such as tricyclic antidepressants, may present with Parkinson-like symptoms.

Signs and Symptoms

Early signs and symptoms often go unnoticed because they occur gradually. This progressive brain disease is characterized by bradykinesia (slowness of movement) and fine, rhythmic tremors of the hands, arms, legs, jaw, and face. The limbs and trunk become rigid and stiff. The person has difficulty maintaining balance and coordination (ataxia). A shuffling and unsteady gait is common. Postural instability occurs. The effects of the disorder may lead to a state of immobility.

Clients have progressive difficulty with walking, talking, eating, and completing ADL because the disease affects automatic movements. Movement of small muscles that control facial expressions is affected. The person may be unable to blink or smile. As muscles become rigid, the face presents as masklike. The person with Parkinson disease often drools. Typical features are seen in Figure 78-4.

In the early years, tremors are regular but typically mild so that they are scarcely noticeable. They may affect only one side, then spread to the other side, which may occur immediately or after a period as long as 15 years. Tremors may start in the fingers, extend to the arms, and finally spread to the entire body. Severe tremors are constant—two to five shakes in a second with the thumb beating against the fingers in a sort of pill-rolling movement. Tremors worsen if the person gets excited but may cease if they move voluntarily. Tremors disappear during sleep, except in the disease's final stages. All muscles become rigid, with slightly flexed limbs and slowed movements.

Because the disease can affect the neck muscles, the person sits or stands in a stooped position. The arms no longer swing when the person walks, and they are unable to shift position quickly to keep balance. The walking gait is characterized as *shuffling,* a motion that helps to keep the client

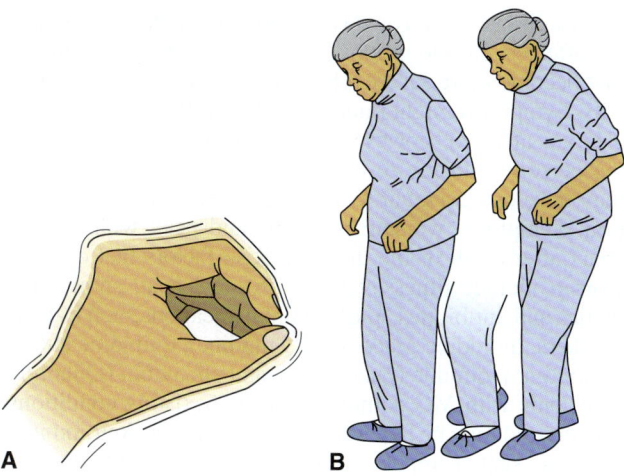

Figure 78-4 Parkinson disease signs. **A.** "Pill-rolling" tremor. **B.** Forward stoop and shuffling gait.

from falling. If pushed a little, the person loses balance, going faster in the direction of the push.

Although mental changes may accompany this disease, their intensity varies. Common changes include emotional lability (*fluctuations*) and a slowed thinking process. Many people with Parkinson disease become clinically depressed.

Medical and Surgical Treatment

Currently, there is no test to predict Parkinson disease. No preventive treatment is known. Although many medications are used, the most effective antiparkinsonism drug found to date is carbidopa-levodopa (Sinemet) (see In Practice: Important Medications 78-3).

Surgery, such as deep brain stimulation, may be performed in carefully selected cases. An electrode is implanted deep in part of the brain that controls movement. Control of the stimulation is via a pulse generator (a pacemaker-like device) placed subcutaneously that attaches wires to the electrodes. Surgery may help clients with advanced Parkinson disease or poor responses to medication. It is not effective for all individuals.

Nursing Considerations

Physical therapy promotes activity and enables self-feeding, dressing, and transferring from bed to chair. The person can learn range-of-motion (ROM) exercises for the legs and fingers and ways to maintain balance and to prevent neck muscles from contracting. Exercising does not eliminate tremors but does help prevent rigidity.

Because handling food, chewing, and swallowing are difficult, the person may not eat enough nutritious food. Specific vitamins (except vitamin B) and a high-calorie, high-protein diet are prescribed. Provide teaching for the client and family (see In Practice: Educating the Client 78-2).

While the client is in the healthcare facility, check the consistency of food and teach the client and family about food preparation. They should prepare food that is easy to chew and swallow. Meat should be ground and potatoes mashed; a straw should be provided for liquids. Stress the need to prevent injury, especially burns. The client may be embarrassed by eating difficulties, so encourage them to eat. Help the client to make agreeable and safe menu selections.

CHAPTER 78 Nervous System Disorders

IN PRACTICE
IMPORTANT MEDICATIONS 78-3 — For Parkinson Disease

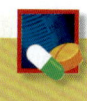

- **Levodopa** (L-dopa, Dopar, Levodopa)
- **Carbidopa-levodopa** (Sinemet)—The initial drug of choice replenishes missing dopamine, a neurotransmitter found in the brain; helps reduce tremors and rigidity of Parkinson syndrome, and because it is combined with carbidopa, it prevents nausea.
- **Dopamine agonists:** bromocriptine mesylate (Parlodel), pramipexole (Mirapex), ropinirole (Requip)—Mimic effects of dopamine; used to promote consistency of levodopa's effects.
- **MAO B inhibitors:** selegiline (Emsam), rasagiline (Azilect)—Help to prevent breakdown of dopamine.
- **Anticholinergics:** trihexyphenidyl and benztropine (Cogentin)—Assists in reduction of the tremors of Parkinson syndrome.
- **N-methyl-D aspartic acid inhibitors:** amantadine (Symmetrel)—Used alone, may help in early stages of syndrome; used in later stages to reduce dyskinesia.

Nursing Considerations
- Levodopa may cause hemolytic anemia and dyskinesia (involuntary muscle movements).
- The beneficial effects of levodopa tend to diminish or become less consistent as the disease progresses.
- All classifications of Parkinson syndrome drugs have significant side effects.

Constipation may develop because of lack of physical activity, absence of adequate roughage in the diet, or the effects of various medications. Usually, a stool softener, such as docusate sodium (Colace), is given. Encourage fluid intake (at least four to six glasses of water and juice each day).

Help the client learn how to use adaptive techniques and devices (see Chapters 48 and 97). Help the family make adaptations to the home and in homemaking. Families

IN PRACTICE
EDUCATING THE CLIENT 78-2 — Parkinson Disease

- Be as independent as possible.
- Protect against unnecessary stress and fatigue.
- Use adaptive techniques and devices.
- Protect against injuries.
- Take medications on time. Avoid foods and vitamins that negatively interact with medications.
- Be sure to eat a well-balanced diet with plenty of fluids for optimum functioning.
- Have regular eye examinations to check intraocular pressure.
- Follow pertinent exercises, as prescribed or recommended.
- Use adaptive feeding utensils, as necessary.

should do a house safety check and eliminate hazards such as throw rugs and highly waxed floors. *Rationale: The client has poor balance and can easily fall.* Arrangements for bathroom facilities and a bedroom on the first floor may be necessary. *Rationale: The client should avoid stair climbing, which can be dangerous and maybe impossible.* Handrails may need to be installed in bathrooms, stairs, and hallways. Night-lights are also helpful. *Rationale: These measures can help the client to be more self-sufficient.*

Myasthenia Gravis

Myasthenia gravis (MG) is a progressive disorder of weakness of the voluntary muscles. Generally considered an acquired autoimmune disorder, it also can involve genetic factors. Two forms affect children. Some children are born with *neonatal myasthenia gravis;* if treated promptly, these children generally recover within 2 months after birth. The other type affecting children is called *congenital myasthenic syndrome,* a rare hereditary form of myasthenia. For adults, there is no cure for the progression of MG, but treatment and rest can help the symptoms. MG can affect individuals of any age or race but is more common in women younger than 40 years and in men older than 60 years.

The cause of MG is a breakdown in the normal communication between nerves and muscles, which leads to episodes of weakness in the striated (skeletal) muscles, most commonly the extraocular, pharyngeal, facial, and respiratory muscles. One type of MG involves the *neurotransmitter* (chemical messenger) *acetylcholine,* which inhibits transmission of messages because *antibodies* block, alter, or destroy acetylcholine's receptor sites at the neuromuscular junction. Another version of this disorder is referred to as *antibody-negative myasthenia gravis* because it is not caused by antibodies blocking neuroreceptors. The thymus gland is abnormal in individuals with MG. The thymus may trigger or maintain production of the antibodies that block neuroreceptors such as acetylcholine. In adults with MG, the thymus is abnormally large, with abnormal clusters of lymphoid tissues, which can include tumors of the thymus gland (*thymomas*). Generally, these tumors are benign, but malignancies can occur.

Signs and Symptoms

Myasthenia gravis can affect any voluntary muscle groups, but some groups are more prone to problems than are others. Initially, symptoms involve the eye muscles. Double vision (diplopia) and drooping of one or both eyelids (ptosis) are noted. Diplopia may be horizontal or vertical and improves or resolves when one eye is closed. The client may appear sleepy, expressionless, and be unable to smile. A percentage of affected individuals have facial and throat muscles involved first. These muscles will affect speech, making the voice seem soft or nasal sounding. Consequences of weakened facial and throat muscles include difficulty breathing, dysphagia (difficulty in swallowing), dysphasia (difficulty in speaking), choking, difficulty chewing, and inability to control facial expressions. Neck and limb muscles will eventually become affected. The individual tends to have greater weakness in the arms than in the legs. Weakened leg muscles result in a waddle-like gait. The individual has difficulty holding the head upright.

The disease usually evolves gradually. In the early stages, the affected muscle groups will have intermittent problems that become more severe when the muscles are used repeatedly. Symptoms might improve with rest. If respiratory muscles are affected, however, breathing becomes difficult. If the person is unable to expectorate secretions, pneumonia may develop. Eventually, the person tires with slight exertion. Symptoms worsen over time and peak within a few years after onset of the disorder. Risk factors that cause to worsen include illness, fatigue, extreme heat, some anesthetics and antibiotics, and certain medications such as beta-blockers, quinidine gluconate (Quinidine), quinidine sulfate (Quinidine), quinine (Qualaquin), and phenytoin (Dilantin).

Clients with MG commonly have coexisting conditions. The thyroid may be hyperactive or hypoactive. Autoimmune disorders such as lupus erythematosus or rheumatoid arthritis are commonly seen in conjunction with MG.

Myasthenic crisis, a life-threatening condition, can occasionally occur. The crisis has a sudden onset as respiratory muscles become too weak to function. The client needs immediate mechanical ventilation. Dysphagia, dysphasia, ptosis, diplopia, and respiratory distress are the usual manifestations. Maintaining an open (*patent*) airway can be lifesaving. Pulmonary function studies can be used as predictors of respiratory abilities and indicators of potential myasthenic crisis. Treatment involves respiratory assistance, medications, and plasmapheresis, a blood-filtering therapy that helps remove the antibodies that block the receptor sites.

Diagnostic Tests

Because the onset of signs and symptoms is slow, diagnosis is often delayed. In addition, similar signs and symptoms are seen in other disorders. Neurologic testing of reflexes, strength, muscle tone, coordination, and balance will be examined. Sight and touch will be assessed. Positive results will demonstrate muscle weakness that improves with rest. Additional testing includes injection of the medication edrophonium chloride (Tensilon), which blocks an enzyme that breaks down the necessary neurotransmitter acetylcholine. After the injection, the client will have temporary improvement in muscle strength. An ice pack test is a noninvasive method of testing for MG. If the client has diplopia, an ice pack over the eyelid for 2 min will result in improvement of eye symptoms. Standard and specific laboratory testing will be completed. One test will look for the presence of abnormal antibodies that disrupt the neuroreceptor sites.

Other tests include nerve conduction studies (repetitive nerve stimulation) and electromyography (EMG), which help determine electrical activity and muscle fiber sensitivity. CT and MRI scans can be used to identify thymus or thyroid tumors. Pulmonary function tests are done to evaluate the client's respiratory status.

Medical Treatment

Myasthenia gravis can be controlled with several available therapies used to reduce weakness and improve muscle strength. Muscle strength can be increased by promoting neuromuscular transmission. Anticholinesterase agents, also referred to as cholinesterase inhibitors, such as neostigmine and pyridostigmine (Mestinon), are commonly used to improve muscle contraction and muscle

IN PRACTICE
IMPORTANT MEDICATIONS 78-4 — For Myasthenia Gravis

- Neostigmine methylsulfate (Bloxiverz)
- Pyridostigmine bromide (Mestinon, Regonol)
- Immunosuppressant drugs: prednisone, azathioprine (Imuran), cyclosporine (Neoral), tacrolimus (Prograf), cyclophosphamide (Cytoxan), mycophenolate mofetil (CellCept)
- Diagnostic drugs: edrophonium chloride (Enlon, Tensilon)

Nursing Considerations
- These medications play a vital role in the client's ability to swallow and to handle respiratory secretions.
- Medications must be given on time and can be given with food (to minimize side effects).
- Side effects must be reported immediately.

IN PRACTICE
EDUCATING THE CLIENT 78-3 — Myasthenia Gravis

- Wear a MedicAlert tag at all times.
- Use a self-dialing telephone or voice-activated phone. *Rationale: These phones are useful in emergencies. A voice-activated phone is necessary if the client cannot dial or hold the receiver.*
- Take medications on time. Use an alarm clock as a reminder. *Rationale: Medications need to be taken on time to maintain a constant blood level.*
- Maintain a regular exercise schedule and conserve energy for essential activities.
- Avoid exposures to temperature extremes. *Rationale: They may trigger myasthenic crisis.*
- Follow a well-balanced diet to maintain optimum health and strength.
- Avoid exposure to infections.
- Be alert for signs of myasthenic crisis—respiratory distress, muscular weakness, dysphagia, fever, and general malaise. Keep a suction device available for emergencies; maintaining an open airway is a priority should crisis occur.

strength. Potent immunosuppressive drugs, such as the corticosteroid prednisone, or other agents, such as cyclosporine and azathioprine, can suppress the production of the antibody (see In Practice: Important Medications 78-4). Immunosuppressive medications have significant side effects such as increased incidences of infections, as well as liver and kidney damage.

Nursing Alert For the client with MG, avoid the use of sedatives, tranquilizing drugs, and morphine because these drugs may cause respiratory or cardiac depression.

Plasmapheresis, a procedure in which antibodies are removed from the blood, can be beneficial for a few weeks. Additionally, high doses of IV immune globulin may be given to provide the client with a temporary dose of normal antibodies. These procedures may be performed during periods of severe weakness.

Surgical Treatment
In many clients with MG, signs and symptoms are abated with a *thymectomy* (surgical removal of the thymus gland). A stable, long-term remission is the goal of a thymectomy. Some individuals may be cured by the surgery.

Nursing Considerations
Assure clients that current medications and therapies can greatly improve their muscle strength. Generally, individuals can lead normal or nearly normal lives. The client should also be aware that emotional upsets and infections can intensify the disease and precipitate a crisis. Teaching is an important aspect of care (see In Practice: Educating the Client 78-3).

During acute episodes, tube feedings or total parenteral nutrition (TPN) may be necessary. Suctioning may be needed to remove secretions. Keep an oral suction machine at the client's bedside; it may be lifesaving in a case of choking or threatened aspiration.

Warn the client of the signs of myasthenic crisis, and instruct them to take precautions regarding medical assistance before the crisis develops. Be prepared to assist with intermittent positive pressure breathing (IPPB) treatments, which are often indicated. In the case of severe respiratory involvement, a tracheostomy may be performed.

Huntington Disease

Huntington disease (HD), also known as *Huntington chorea,* is a chronic, progressive, hereditary condition in which brain cells in the basal ganglia prematurely die. The disorder involves a combination of physical, intellectual, and emotional symptoms.

A child with a parent who has the HD gene has a 50-50 chance of inheriting the gene. Only children who inherit the gene will develop the disease. Only children who inherit the gene can pass the gene to the next generation. All children who inherit the gene eventually will develop HD. The age of onset varies, although symptoms generally do not appear until the person is about 30–40 years of age. If symptoms develop before age 20, the disorder is referred to as *juvenile Huntington disease,* which presents with different symptoms and faster disease progression than does the adult version.

Signs and Symptoms
The disease progresses at different rates. HD usually starts with abnormal involuntary movements, called chorea, such as fidgeting, jerking, and spasms. Personality changes include irritability, mood swings, depression, loss of judgment, and carelessness. Early intellectual symptoms include difficulty making decisions and learning new things. These symptoms progress to constant writhing and uncontrollable movement, changes in speech and ability to swallow, great weakness, severe personality disorders, and psychosis.

Eventually, the person loses bowel and bladder control and all purposeful movement and is confined to bed rest.

Death usually results from pneumonia or another disorder-related complication associated with immobility.

Diagnostic Tests

A thorough medical and family history is important. A genetic test to confirm the presence of the HD gene is available, but a positive genetic result cannot estimate an age of onset of the disorder or what symptoms are likely to appear. Neurologic tests and laboratory tests can be used to differentiate HD from other nervous system disorders. PET scan (positron emission tomography) may confirm the diagnosis, showing reduced glucose utilization and lowered dopamine receptor binding. MRI may show characteristic butterfly dilation of the brain's lateral ventricles. CT scans may show brain atrophy and possibly enlarged lateral ventricles.

Treatment

There is no cure for HD. Symptoms cannot be reversed. Treatment is aimed at symptomatic relief of physical symptoms, such as fatigue, restlessness, or hyperexcitability. Medications can be given for agitation and depression.

Nursing Considerations

This disorder is disabling and disturbing to the individual as well as to the family. Genetic counseling is strongly suggested. Initially, the client may be able to remain at home until ADL cannot be managed. Home care adaptations can provide a better quality of life. The person with HD can use lamps with a touch base and handrails at the proper height that are strong enough to support full body weight. The person can use an electric razor and toothbrush. To steady the hands and arms, they can sit down and rest the elbows on a table when shaving or brushing the teeth.

If the person can swallow thin liquids, they can use two straws cut to just above the rim of the glass. Sometimes, a thickening agent such as Thick-It is used to make swallowing easier. Cutting a spot out of a Styrofoam cup for the person's nose can make drinking easier and safer. *Rationale: The person does not have to tip the head back to drink; this measure prevents choking.*

Amyotrophic Lateral Sclerosis

Amyotrophic lateral sclerosis (ALS), also known as *Lou Gehrig disease,* is a rapidly progressive, fatal neurologic disorder resulting in destruction of motor neurons of the cortex, brain stem, and spinal cord. Voluntary muscle movement gradually degenerates. ALS usually strikes between ages 50 and 70 years and affects more men than women.

Signs and Symptoms

The loss of motor neurons causes muscles to atrophy. Initially, the individual may fall frequently and lose motor control of the hands and arms. The individual experiences weakness, fatigue, and spasticity of the arms. As the disease advances, muscles atrophy, with flaccid quadriplegia. Eventually, the respiratory muscles are involved. The course of the disease is consistent, with no remissions. ALS always progresses to respiratory dysfunction and death, generally within 5 years after onset, although the course of the disease may vary.

Treatment

There is no cure or therapy that will lessen the progress of or reverse the disorder. The first drug shown to prolong survival of ALS clients is riluzole (Rilutek). Additional treatments are palliative only, focusing on support and symptom management.

Nursing Considerations

As with many other neurologic disorders, the nurse can provide physical, emotional, and spiritual support to the client and family. The nurse may provide direction and compassion to the family when discussing subjects such as disease progression and death and dying.

> **Key Concept**
> The individual with ALS retains intellectual and sensory function throughout the course of the disease.

INFLAMMATORY DISORDERS

Brain Abscess

A *brain abscess* is a collection of pus that may result from an infection of the ears, mastoid, sinus, or skull. It can also directly result from brain surgery. If left untreated, the encapsulated pus pocket eventually ruptures and spreads, causing further abscesses and *meningitis,* infection of the meninges.

Findings associated with a brain abscess mimic those of a brain tumor. The person may also experience a fever if the primary infection site is still infected. Those with brain abscesses are at risk for ↑ICP and seizures, as well as spread of the infection. Surgical treatment is necessary to drain the abscess. Massive doses of IV antibiotics are given preoperatively and postoperatively. The person may be left with some brain damage or may be completely cured.

Meningitis

Meningitis is an inflammation of the meninges, the membranes that cover the brain and the spinal cord. Bacteria, viruses, fungi, or other microorganisms can cause meningitis. Brain damage, hearing loss, disabilities, and death are known to occur more often with bacterial meningitis than with viral meningitis. Meningitis can be a secondary infection caused by microorganisms which have traveled to the meninges from nearby structures, such as the sinuses or the middle ear. The bloodstream also may carry the infection as sepsis. The causative organism is often related to age, and children are particularly susceptible. Prevention of many causes of meningitis is available via immunizations against preventative infections. (Chapter 72 discusses both immunizations and meningitis.)

Meningitis can be a contagious infection. Direct contact with respiratory secretions can transmit the organism from one person to another. People living in close proximity to others, children and caregivers in daycare centers, and individuals who have contact with another person's secretions (as in kissing) are most at risk for meningitis. Specific high-risk groups include refugees, military personnel, college students living in dormitories, and infants and young children. People who are exposed to active or passive tobacco smoke are also at risk.

> **Nursing Alert** The best protection for healthcare providers against meningitis is thorough and frequent handwashing.

Vaccines are available for *Streptococcus pneumoniae, Neisseria meningitides,* and *Haemophilus influenzae* meningitis type b, which cause most of the cases of bacterial-related meningitis. *S. pneumoniae* is commonly called *Pneumonococcal meningitis. N. meningitides* is also known as *meningococcal meningitis* and is particularly contagious. *N. meningitides* has an incubation period of 2–10 days, which is pertinent because the causative organisms are present in the throat as well as in the CSF.

Viral meningitis, also known as *aseptic meningitis,* may resolve without specific treatment. Many types of viruses can be causative agents of meningitis, such as the enterovirus, herpesvirus, and the mumps virus. The illness lasts 7–10 days, and the person generally recovers without disability. The client needs bed rest, good hydration, and adequate nutrition. Analgesics for headache and fever may provide symptomatic relief. Antiviral medications may be useful.

Signs and Symptoms
Signs and symptoms of meningitis usually appear abruptly. Symptoms of viral and bacterial meningitis are often the same. Many symptoms are due to ↑ICP.

Signs and symptoms include fever, chills, severe headache, nausea and vomiting, nuchal rigidity (stiff neck), and irritability. A change in LOC is present. Two neurologic signs are present: positive Kernig sign and positive Brudzinski sign (Fig. 78-5). Photophobia (intolerance to light) and pain when the eyes move from side to side occur. The affected person may have seizures. A petechial purpuric rash is also possible. Opisthotonos, an acute spasm in which the body is bowed forward, with the head and heels bent backward, is often present. Children have tense or bulging fontanels and a high-pitched cry.

Diagnostic Tests
Meningitis is diagnosed based on a general neurologic examination that includes two special neurologic signs:

- *Kernig sign:* The client lies on the back and brings one leg up so that the hip and knee are both flexed at 90°. They then straighten the knee (the sole of the foot toward the ceiling). Pain or resistance indicates meningeal and spinal root inflammation. Kernig sign is considered a positive indicator of meningitis (Fig. 78-5A).
- *Brudzinski sign:* The client lies on the back and brings the head forward toward the chest. Pain or resistance indicates meningeal irritation, arthritis, or a neck injury. If the person responds by flexing the hips and knees, meningeal inflammation is indicated. Brudzinski sign is also considered a positive indicator of meningitis (Fig. 78-5B).

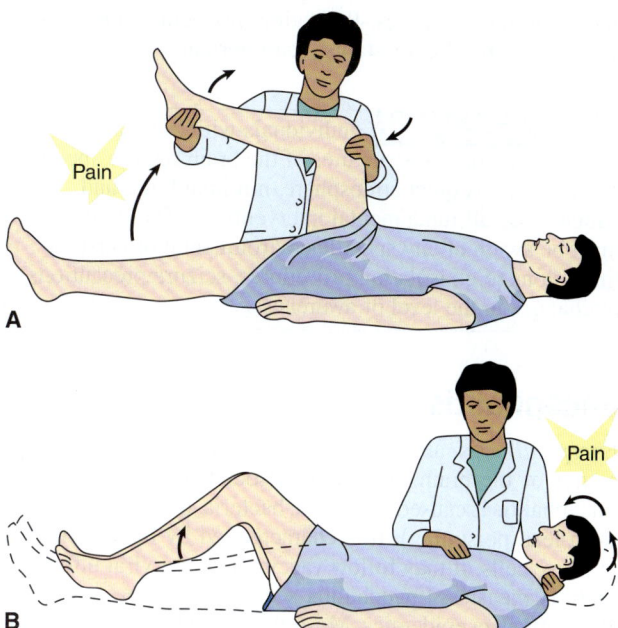

Figure 78-5 Signs of meningeal irritation. **A.** Kernig sign. **B.** Brudzinski sign.

Medical Treatment
When a diagnosis of meningitis is suspected, an LP is done. A culture and sensitivity test of CSF may be ordered to determine the causative organism. The client is given antibiotics.

If it is possible to identify the causative organism, the healthcare provider prescribes large doses of antibiotics that have been identified as effective in treating the specific organism. Antibiotics are highly effective in treating bacterial meningitis. If the infection is exceedingly virulent, drugs may prove useless, and the person may die. Sometimes, nerves of sight and hearing are damaged.

Nursing Considerations
Provide nursing care with the awareness that the person is critically ill. Transmission-based Precautions are likely, especially in the early days of meningitis. The person is generally placed on seizure precautions. Side rails should be raised and padded for the client's protection. Elevate the head of the bed to at least 30°, unless otherwise ordered. Monitor the client's LOC. Keep the environment subdued, both in visual and auditory sensations (e.g., do not turn on bright over-the-bed lighting and do speak quietly in the room). Minimize traffic in and out of the room.

Carefully monitor the person's respiratory status; endotracheal intubation may be necessary if the client's respiratory status deteriorates. A hypothermia blanket and antipyretic medications may be ordered for high fever. Analgesics may be given for pain. Give IV fluids and nourishing liquids, as ordered. Tube feedings or TPN may be necessary.

Caution caregivers and the client not to flex the individual's neck because doing so can obstruct venous flow and increase ICP. The client should also avoid acute hip flexion because it can cause increased intra-abdominal and intrathoracic pressures. These increased pressures interfere with cerebral blood vessel drainage and cause ↑ICP. Caregivers need to be aware that the individual may become confused and disoriented at times. Repeating instructions and closely monitoring the client's status are important.

> **Nursing Alert** Individuals with trauma or infection of structures of the brain require specific nursing care. A quiet atmosphere, minimal light, and patience are all fundamental interventions. The family must be aware of any specific environmental or personal limitations (e.g., isolation procedures, seizure precautions) or changes in the level of awareness.

Encephalitis

Encephalitis is an inflammation of the white and gray matter of the brain. It may be associated with meningitis. Encephalitis is caused by a virus, bacteria, or chemicals (such as in lead poisoning). It is characterized by the destruction of nerve cells. It may follow vaccination or a viral infection, such as measles. Encephalitis seems to be more prevalent after influenza epidemics. Mosquitoes and ticks are common vectors.

Some types of viral encephalitis are more lethal than others. The death rate varies from 5% to 70%, depending on the infection's cause. Many people who recover from encephalitis are left with mental changes, seizure disorders, or parkinsonian symptoms, all of which become increasingly disabling.

Signs and Symptoms
Encephalitis can attack suddenly, causing violent headache, fever, nausea, vomiting, and drowsiness. The person may show muscular weakness, tremors, or visual disturbances.

Medical Treatment
No drug for the specific treatment of encephalitis has been found. Treatment is similar to the care of a client with meningitis.

Nursing Considerations
Nursing care focuses on reducing fever and maintaining a quiet environment. Warm, moist packs may be ordered to relieve muscle spasms. Tube feedings or TPN is necessary for clients who are unresponsive. If acute respiratory distress occurs, endotracheal intubation and mechanical ventilation may be required.

The client with encephalitis is subject to seizures. Side rails should be in place. Hospital policy may require a signed release when side rails are used. The family needs instructions for safety to prevent injury. The family also needs to be aware that the client may exhibit mental changes such as irritability and confusion.

Guillain–Barré Syndrome

Guillain–Barré syndrome is an autoimmune disorder of the peripheral nervous system. In Guillain–Barré syndrome, antibodies start to destroy the myelin sheath of peripheral nerves. When the sheath is damaged, it cannot transmit nerve signals to the muscles. The muscles atrophy, leading to weakness, numbness, and eventually paralysis. *Paresthesia* (tingling sensation) develops; the nerves cannot transmit sensory messages such as pain, heat, or texture. There are several forms of this disorder, but all forms have some form of muscle weakness. *Acute inflammatory demyelinating polyradiculoneuropathy* (AIDP) is the most common form in the United States. AIDP is presented as muscle weakness that starts in the lower part of the body and spreads upward over the next few weeks. Guillain–Barré syndrome is considered rare, and the exact cause is unknown. However, it typically is preceded by bacterial or viral infectious illnesses such as a respiratory tract infection or gastroenteritis.

Signs and Symptoms
After a nonspecific febrile illness, onset is often sudden, although sometimes 3–4 weeks may pass before signs and symptoms develop. Symmetrical pain and weakness follow. The AIDP form usually begins in the lower extremities, ascends, and may progress to total paralysis. Disability ranges from muscle weakness to total body paralysis. Vital functions, such as breathing, heart rate, and blood pressure, can be compromised. Eventually, the progression of the disease stops and stabilizes. The client generally then begins a gradual recovery. Partial or complete recovery is possible.

Diagnosis
Diagnosis is made after obtaining a careful history and review of systems. No differential diagnostic procedure or laboratory test exists. An LP may be done, possibly revealing increased protein levels in CSF. An EMG and nerve conduction study will determine activity and speed of nerve signals in the muscles.

Treatment
Some success has resulted from two types of treatments: plasmapheresis and injection of high-dose immunoglobulins. However, the effects of both are temporary. *Plasmapheresis* may be helpful because it removes the antibodies that are destroying the myelin sheaths. *Immunoglobulin therapy* may be effective because it provides normal support to an immune system that is under abnormal attack.

Steroid therapy is controversial because, although it may reduce symptoms, steroids have significant nonbeneficial side effects that can affect the client's overall health.

Nursing Considerations
The nurse must keep in mind that the client with Guillain–Barré syndrome has an excellent chance of total or nearly total recovery. Therefore, excellent nursing care is necessary to prevent permanent damage. Emergency interventions, such as endotracheal intubation and mechanical ventilation, may be necessary when the respiratory muscles fail.

Maintenance of muscle function is required to prevent atrophy and skeletal deformities. Nursing interventions, such as providing passive ROM exercises and working with physical therapy, are very important from the very beginning of the diagnosis. Adequate nutrition may necessitate tube feedings or TPN. Family and other caregivers will need instruction in ROM exercises, skin care, positioning, and ADL.

Recovery is usually slow, lasting weeks, months, or years, depending on the severity of symptoms. Emotional support is essential. This condition is frightening for the client and family. If the acute phase of the disease is correctly managed, however, recovery is often complete.

Acute Transverse Myelitis

Acute transverse myelitis is an inflammatory condition affecting the spinal cord. It results from inflammation or destruction of the myelin of the spinal cord neurons. The person experiences impaired bowel and bladder function, generalized weakness of the extremities, and loss of sensation.

Acute transverse myelitis has several causes. If the disease is diagnosed as *postinfectious,* it usually begins 5–20 days after a viral infection. The cause may also be related to collagen–vascular disease, syphilis, or HIV/AIDS. Prognosis varies; some individuals recover fully, and others do not.

Nursing Considerations

Nursing care for the client with acute transverse myelitis involves supportive and preventive measures. Be alert for urinary retention, constipation, skin breakdown, thrombus formation, and other complications of immobility.

HEAD TRAUMA

Trauma to the brain is a common cause of motor and sensory symptoms, including brain damage, coma, and paralysis. Normally, the skull's thick bones, as well as the tough outer membrane of the meninges (the dura), protect the brain. In addition, CSF acts as a shock absorber. However, violent blows to the head can cause several kinds of injury to the brain and skull. A major complication of head trauma is increased pressure within the brain. Numerous factors can cause swelling including hemorrhage, or an inflammatory process. Head injuries may be the cause of seizures and epilepsy later in life.

> **Nursing Alert** Serious symptoms can appear up to several days after a head injury. Observe the client carefully.

Increased Intracranial Pressure

Intracranial pressure (ICP) is the pressure that the brain, blood, and CSF exert inside the cerebrospinal cavity. Normally, ICP is 4–13 mm Hg. If one of the normal components of the cranial or spinal cavity (e.g., brain tissue, blood, or CSF) increases in size, volume, or shape, pressure increases. This increase in pressure can cause the delicate structures to be moved, damaged, or destroyed.

The increase in pressure is caused by the limited space within a rigid bony skull, leaving little or no room for expansion because of brain edema, hemorrhage, or increased amounts of CSF. Examples of conditions that may lead to ↑ICP include head injury, brain tumor, CNS infection, brain surgery, stroke, and hydrocephalus. Normal body functions, such as straining at stool (the *Valsalva maneuver*) and coughing, may increase ICP.

Sustained ICP over 15–20 mm Hg is called *increased intracranial pressure* (↑ICP). It is an abnormal and dangerous condition. The first consequence of ↑ICP is venous compression, resulting in a decrease in blood flow to the brain. This results in cerebral hypoxia or cellular hypoxia. Brain cells are extremely sensitive to levels of oxygen. Neuron tissue death will begin within 4–6 min if oxygen is not supplied.

An elevation in ICP can occur suddenly and progress rapidly. Usually, ↑ICP begins on one side of the brain, although both sides quickly become involved. Early detection and treatment are vital before complications occur (see In Practice: Data Gathering in Nursing 78-2). The earliest and most important sign of ↑ICP is any change in LOC.

ICP Monitoring

In special circumstances of ↑ICP, devices that are surgically inserted into the brain can monitor the levels of ICP. The most common monitor is the intraventricular catheter. Other monitors include the subarachnoid (subdural) bolt (or screw), intraparenchymal bolt (fiberoptic), and epidural sensor (least invasive). The neurosurgeon places the devices under strict sterile technique, using the information that these devices relay via computer to determine the plan of care (Fig. 78-6). The clients are generally in an intensive care unit (ICU), and trained ICU nurses monitor the ICP pressures as part of nursing care. Medications and possibly surgical interventions are

---

IN PRACTICE
DATA GATHERING IN NURSING 78-2 — Signs of Increased Intracranial Pressure (ICP)

- Any change in level of consciousness (loss of consciousness, lethargy, confusion, seizures)
- Any change in sensory–motor function (slowed reflexes, slowed response time, restlessness, ataxia, aphasia, slowed speech)
- Headache, which becomes progressively worse or is aggravated by movement
- Change in eye signs or vision (change in pupil size, unequal pupils, slowed or no response to light, inability to follow examiner's finger, difficulty seeing)
- Change in vital signs (pulse <60 or >100, increased blood pressure, widening of pulse pressure, increased or lowered body temperature)
- Change in respirations or evidence of respiratory distress (occurs late—caused by pressure on brain stem)
- ↑ICP recorded on a monitoring device
- Nausea and vomiting (especially projectile vomiting)
- Urinary incontinence
- Bulging fontanels (in infant); elevation of bone segments
- Sudden changes in condition
- Leakage of cerebrospinal fluid (CSF) (clear yellow or pinkish) from nose or ear

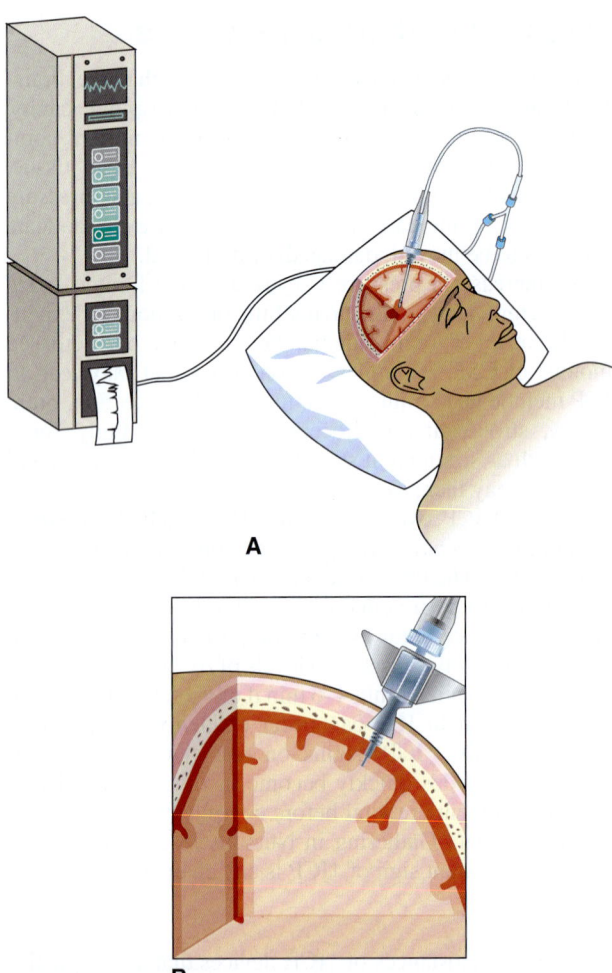

Figure 78-6 Monitoring intracranial pressure. **A.** Fiberoptic, transducer-tipped pressure and temperature ventricular monitoring catheter. **B.** Ventricular bolt that is connected to a pressure transducer and display system.

calculated based on the results of ICP monitoring. Mannitol (Osmitrol) is an osmotic diuretic specifically ordered by the healthcare provider to lower ICP caused by swelling.

> **Nursing Alert** Report any break in an ICP monitoring system to the healthcare provider immediately. The system must remain sterile. Never move the client's head up or down without specific orders from the healthcare provider.

The intraventricular catheter *(ventriculostomy)* may also be used to drain CSF to relieve pressure. The drained CSF can then be sent for laboratory analysis.

Herniation of the Brain

When ↑ICP exerts enough pressure to displace a portion of the brain, *herniation* (an upward, downward, or lateral pushing of a portion of the brain through an opening) can occur. This opening can be a natural intracranial opening, such as the foramen magnum. The brain herniates (pushes) through the large foramen (opening) in the occipital bone, which lies between the cranial and spinal cavities.

Herniation can also occur through a previous *craniotomy* site or through an opening caused by trauma. Herniation causes severe injury to the brain because of prolonged hypoxia to parts of the brain that control the vital functions of the body—breathing and blood circulation. The result is brain death and death of the individual.

When ICP is elevated, an LP is contraindicated because the withdrawal of even a small amount of CSF can cause the brain to shift or herniate. Therefore, a safer method of determining ICP is ICP monitoring.

Concussion

A concussion is the result of any blow to the head. The concussion may not damage any brain structures, but temporary unconsciousness is possible. The length of time a person remains unconscious varies. Some clients recover from concussions with no apparent ill effects apart from the inability to remember the event; others have blurred vision or severe headaches. A client who has had anything other than a very minor concussion should see a healthcare provider immediately for a thorough neurologic examination.

In *acceleration–deceleration* injuries, damage occurs in two places. Acceleration occurs when a blow to the head suddenly causes the brain to move from a stationary position to another position. The cranium (skull) hits the brain on the acceleration side of the blow or injury. Deceleration occurs when the moving cranium is abruptly stopped, but the brain continues to move forward and impacts at the site where the cranium has stopped. Serious injuries may also occur to the brain stem because of the acceleration–deceleration action. The brain stem is attached and floats in CSF within the cranium. With direct and rebound trauma, blood vessels, nerve tracts, brain tissue, and other structures are bruised and torn. After the original injury, a postconcussion syndrome may persist for several weeks to months. Symptoms include headache, anxiety, fatigue, or vertigo (a sensation of rotation of self or one's surroundings; not true dizziness).

Laceration and Contusion

A laceration is tearing of the brain tissue caused by direct impact or penetrating injury. Lacerations are commonly associated with depressed skull fractures, which are discussed below. In contusion, the brain tissue is bruised.

Skull Fractures

A *skull fracture* may be open, closed, simple, depressed, or *comminuted* (fragmented), depending on whether the skull and scalp are intact. Many skull fractures are minor, being no more than cracks in the bone. Usually, they heal without difficulty. Any scalp lacerations must be thoroughly examined to determine if the cranium has been opened.

Open skull fractures potentially expose the brain to external microorganisms, which could lead to meningitis or encephalitis. However, open skull fractures are less likely to produce rapid elevations in ICP. The fracture allows for some brain swelling.

A *depressed skull fracture* is caused by a severe blow to the head. The fracture breaks the bone and forces the broken edges to press against the brain, resulting in a significant risk for ↑ICP and meningitis. Effects vary with the injury's severity and location. If, for example, the bone fragment presses on the brain's speech center, the client's speech may be impaired until the pressure is relieved.

IN PRACTICE
NURSING CARE GUIDELINES 78-3: Determining Cerebrospinal Fluid (CSF) in Drainage

- Wet a chemical reagent strip, such as a Dextrostix, with drainage from the nose or ear.
- Observe the color change and whether it indicates the presence of glucose. The presence of glucose in the fluid suggests that the fluid is CSF; the test is positive.

If the test is positive and there also is blood (which also contains glucose) in the drainage:

- Collect droplets of drainage on a white absorbent pad.
- Inspect the wet area after a few minutes for a halo sign: If a yellow ring encircles a central ring that is red, the red ring indicates blood, and the yellow ring suggests CSF.

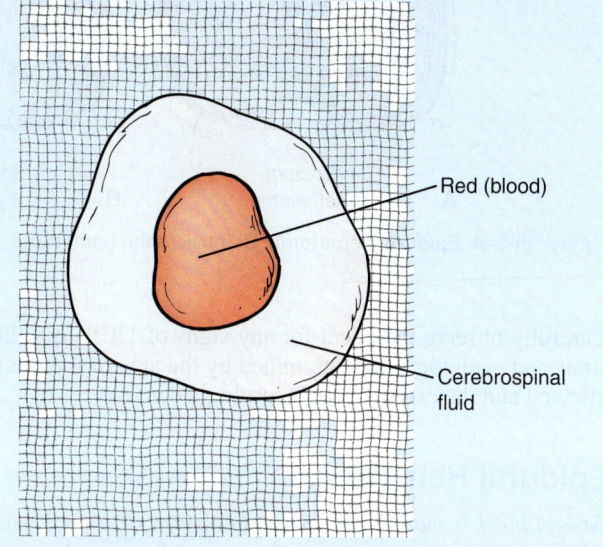

Halo sign. Clear drainage that separates from bloody drainage suggests the presence of CSF.

A *basilar skull fracture* is a fracture at the base of the skull. It may injure the nerves entering the spinal cord or interfere with CSF circulation. Basilar skull fractures can tear the dura.

In a basilar skull fracture, rhinorrhea, leakage of CSF from the nose (otorrhea), or leakage of CSF from the ear may occur. The nurse may be asked to test this fluid for the presence of CSF. A positive test for CSF is known as a *halo sign* (see In Practice: Nursing Care Guidelines 78-3).

Figure 78-7 illustrates the effects of a basilar fracture with *periorbital ecchymosis* (raccoon's eyes) and *periauricular ecchymosis* (Battle's sign). A basilar skull fracture is especially dangerous because of potential damage to the vital centers that control blood pressure and respiration.

Hematoma

A *hematoma* refers to a blood clot within the skull. Hypertension and trauma are the most common causes. With any type of cranial hematoma, ICP may dangerously elevate. The swelling or mass of blood compresses brain tissue, creating further damage. Herniation of brain tissue is possible.

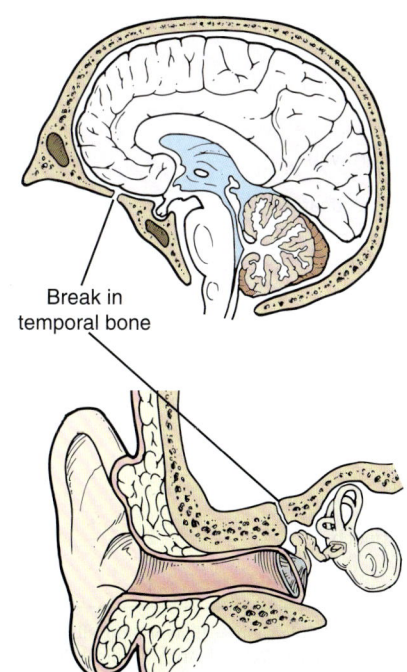
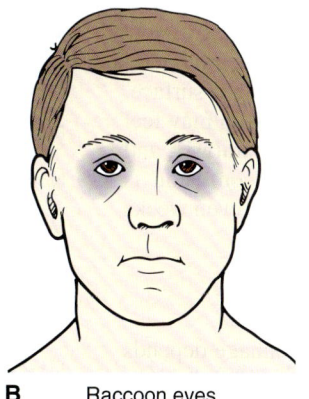
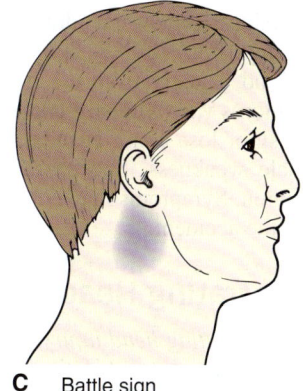

B Raccoon eyes   C Battle sign

Figure 78-7 **A.** Basilar skull fracture in the temporal bone can cause cerebrospinal fluid (CSF) to leak from the nose or ear. **B.** Periorbital ecchymosis, called *raccoon eyes*. **C.** *Battle sign* over the mastoid process.

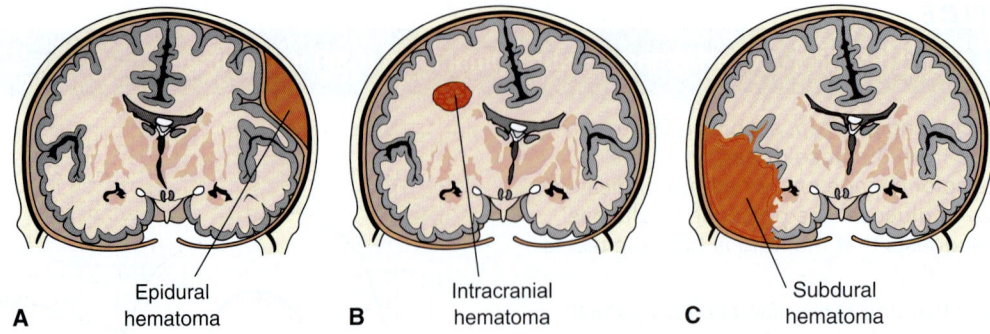

Figure 78-8 **A.** Epidural hematoma. **B.** Intracranial hematoma. **C.** Subdural hematoma.

Carefully observe the client for any signs of ↑ICP. Specific signs and symptoms are determined by the area of the brain affected and the extent of any neurologic damage.

Epidural Hematoma

An *epidural hematoma* is an accumulation of blood, usually from the temporal artery, between the dura and the skull (Fig. 78-8A). The pressure of an epidural hematoma can quickly cause seizures, paralysis, and death. One or both of the person's pupils may be dilated. Usually, the person is unconscious immediately after the injury, lucid for a brief period, then unconscious again as blood accumulates in the epidural space and causes pressure. Epidural hematomas are most common in children. The mechanism of injury is typically a blow to the side of the head.

Intracranial Hematoma

An *intracranial (intracerebral) hematoma* is caused by hemorrhage and edema that results from bleeding within the skull (Fig. 78-8B). The cause may be rupture of delicate blood vessels owing to hypertension or a cerebral aneurysm. Ruptured blood vessels within the brain are one cause of strokes.

Subdural Hematoma

A subdural (below the dura) hematoma is typically slow forming (Fig. 78-8C). It is caused by an accumulation of blood, usually from a torn vein on the brain's surface. Symptoms vary with size and location. The person may feel drowsy or lose consciousness, with seizures, paralysis, and muscle weakness. Speech may be affected; confusion is common. Symptoms may not appear for days or even weeks after the accident.

Penetrating Head Injuries

In a *penetrating head injury*, the degree of damage depends on the penetrating object's velocity and location. A high-velocity object, such as a bullet, typically causes more damage than a low-velocity object, such as a stab wound.

Medical and Surgical Treatment

Immediately after any potential or actual injury to the brain, a neurologic evaluation should be done. The Glasgow coma scale (GCS) is commonly used as a broad indicator of the severity of brain injury (Table 78-2). Three areas are given numerical values: eye-opening, best verbal response, and best motor response. Each area is evaluated according to standard criteria, and the numbers are totaled. The highest possible number of 15 indicates that the individual has no impairment; the lowest possible number of 3 indicates brain death. The range of 6–8 is associated with a coma state.

TABLE 78-2 The Glasgow Coma Scale

TEST	SCORE
Eye Opening (E)	
Spontaneous	4
To voice	3
To pain	2
None	1
Motor Response (M)	
Obeys commands	6
Localizes pain	5
Normal flexion (withdrawal)	4
Abnormal flexion (decorticate)	3
Extension (decerebrate)	2
None (flaccid)	1
Verbal Response (V)	
Oriented	5
Confused conversation	4
Inappropriate words	3
Incomprehensible speech	2
None	1

GSC score = E + M + V. Best possible score = 15; worst possible score = 3. Adapted from Glasgow Coma Scale, Womack Army Medical Center, Fort Bragg, NC, and https://www.cdc.gov/masstrauma/resources/gcs.pdf; https://www.brainline.org/article/what-glasgow-coma-scale.

Medical treatment consists of methods to limit swelling and damage caused by ↑ICP. Osmotic diuretics may be given. Immediate neurosurgery may be necessary to prevent death. Surgery involves tying off the bleeding vessel and cleaning the area of debris and any accumulated blood or blood clot. Burr holes may be made in the skull, or an intraventricular catheter may be inserted to relieve ↑ICP by draining CSF or blood.

Nursing Considerations

Head injury requires sensitive nursing care related to the specific needs resulting from the trauma. Loss of consciousness does not always follow a severe head injury. Every client who suffers a blow to the head, no matter how minor it appears, needs careful observation until it is certain the injury has not damaged the brain. Care providers need to be aware that symptoms of brain damage do not always appear immediately.

The conscious client should remain absolutely quiet, with complete bed rest. Observe for the following signs of ↑ICP: headache, dizziness, visual impairment, hearing loss, nausea, or clear or bloody drainage from the ears, nose, or mouth. *Projectile* (forceful) vomiting is indicative of brain injury. Also, observe the client for changes in blood pressure and pupils. If the client is hospitalized, monitor LOC frequently and note any personality or behavior changes.

Advise a client who is preparing for release after receiving first aid treatment following a head injury to see a healthcare provider immediately if they have any recurring symptoms. In addition, teach the family these symptoms because the client may be unable to detect deterioration of functioning (see In Practice: Educating the Client 78-4).

> **NCLEX Alert**
>
> NCLEX clinical scenarios may present client's symptoms that the nurse must be able to translate into nursing actions. For example, trauma or infection of the brain may result in a headache. As a symptom of this clinical example, a headache could indicate nursing care that includes close monitoring of LOC, elevating the head of the bed, and notifying the healthcare provider of projectile vomiting or pupil changes.

NEOPLASMS

Brain tumors occur in all age groups. Only a small percentage of brain tumors are malignant, and they may result from metastasis from another part of the body. Even a benign brain tumor can be fatal, however, because of the pressure that it exerts on the brain. Benign tumors may also later become malignant. Regular follow-up is essential after treatment for any brain tumor.

Signs and Symptoms

The signs and symptoms of brain tumor include headache, sudden projectile vomiting, and visual abnormalities, all caused by ↑ICP. Additional signs and symptoms may develop, depending on the area of the brain that is affected. For example, if the motor area is affected, numbness or twitching in the arm may occur; a tumor on the brain's frontal lobe may cause personality changes and may affect memory or reasoning abilities.

Often, a seizure is the first symptom of a brain tumor. If ↑ICP near the brain stem is unrelieved, severe respiratory difficulties and possibly death owing to respiratory failure may occur. As brain tumors grow, signs and symptoms progressively worsen.

Diagnostic Tests

Neurologic assessment and history are necessary to make a diagnosis. By questioning the client and family, the healthcare provider can determine the progress of any neurologic deficits. Diagnostic tests, such as the CT scan and EEG, are performed to determine the tumor's location, size, and neurologic effects.

Treatment

Treatment options include surgery, chemotherapy, and radiation therapy, or all three. The specific treatment is determined

---

IN PRACTICE
EDUCATING THE CLIENT 78-4 After a Head Injury

- Know that the client may not be sufficiently coherent to recognize dangerous symptoms.
- Be alert that some symptoms may not appear until several days, weeks, or even months following a head injury.
- Have the client rest quietly for 24 hr. Every 2 hr for the first 24 hr, check the client's ability to state orientation to place (e.g., at home, in bed), time (e.g., middle of the night), and situation (e.g., I hit my head when I fell). Family caregivers need to understand that the orientation checks must continue throughout the night. Suggest that the caregivers set an alarm for every 2 hr and plan to stay within the client's room for these first 24 hr.
- Immediately report the following to the healthcare provider:
  - Unusual or increased drowsiness
  - Weakness of arms or legs; muscle twitching
  - Nausea and vomiting (*especially forceful or projectile vomiting*)
  - Headaches—localized or generalized, unrelieved by mild analgesic
  - Dizziness
  - Visual or hearing disturbances, abnormal eye movements
  - Difficulty arousing from sleep, particularly during the first 24 hr
  - Personality changes, such as forgetfulness, irritability, speech difficulties
  - Bleeding or clear drainage from the mouth, nose, or ears
  - Seizures
  - Blood pressure changes

according to the tumor's type and location. One type of surgery is a *craniotomy*.

Craniotomy

Surgical entry into the skull (cranium) is called a craniotomy. This invasive procedure is performed for many reasons, one of the most common being a brain tumor. Any tumor near the brain is removed when possible because its growth would put pressure on the brain. A *craniectomy* is a procedure that removes a portion of skull bone.

Surgical success for a brain tumor depends on the tumor's location and whether it can be removed without causing brain damage. Some tumors are *inoperable* (impossible to remove without causing severe brain damage or death). Even successful brain surgery can result in neurologic deficits.

Nursing Considerations

Providing Preoperative Care

Before a craniotomy, follow routine preoperative preparation. In addition, the client's head or a portion of it may need to be shaved. If this is the case, inform the client before doing so. Often, hair is not shaved until the client is in the operating room. The client (or legal guardian, if the client is a child) must sign an informed consent before hair can be removed or surgery is done. (Shaved hair is put into a paper bag and labeled. This hair can be used later for a wig or hairpiece, if the client desires.)

The surgeon will inform the client if it is necessary to remain awake during the craniotomy. Mild sedatives may be given to relax the client, but the client must still be able to respond to questions or other stimuli. Inform the client beforehand if the surgeon will ask questions or ask for specific movements during surgery. Midazolam may be given, so the client does not recall the procedure.

The client and family are almost certain to be apprehensive before such surgery. Provide concerned, competent preoperative care. Reassure the client that little pain is involved in brain surgery because the skin is locally anesthetized. Although the procedure can be noisy because the surgeon will drill out a part of the skull bone, the client will feel no pain because the skull and brain have no sensory nerves. However, warn the client about the possibility of a headache after surgery. Surgery may take 2–6 hr.

Providing Postoperative Care

During the immediate postoperative period, the client requires expert observation and nursing care, usually provided in the ICU. Monitoring by ICU nurses is done continuously, with comparisons performed between the client's present condition and the initial neurologic examination (the baseline assessment). Any changes, such as signs of ↑ICP, are noted.

Nursing care focuses on the following activities:

- Monitoring the client's vital signs and respiratory status regularly.
- Elevating the head of the bed.
- Performing nasogastric suction to help prevent aspiration.
- Positioning the client according to healthcare provider's orders.
- Checking dressings for blood and CSF, especially at the back and on the side where drainage accumulates by gravity.
- Monitoring the client's LOC, orientation to time and place, and ability to speak clearly.
- Checking the client's ability to grasp equally in both hands and to move each foot in any position on command.

These activities are continued even after the client is discharged from the ICU to the nursing unit.

When the client is allowed out of bed, check their ability to stand with the eyes closed (*Romberg test*). The client should be able to stand on each foot without holding on to anything. Immediately report any deviation from normal. If in doubt, notify the surgeon. The client's neurologic status can change very rapidly.

During convalescence, the client needs encouragement and understanding. For example, the client may find that it takes time to regain control of bodily movements or that they are spilling food, dropping things, and feeling dizzy when walking. Reassure the client and give assistance as needed.

STUDENT SYNTHESIS

KEY POINTS

- Because the nervous system controls the body's movements, disorders in this system may cause unwanted movement or immobility.
- Seizure disorders have different manifestations, ranging from generalized tonic–clonic movements to uncontrolled movements without loss of consciousness.
- Spinal cord injuries can result in a range of physical and mental deficits, including paralysis.
- Degenerative disorders of the nervous system can cause difficulties in movement, sensory deficits, or varying degrees of alteration in mental status.
- Inflammatory disorders of the nervous system can quickly become life-threatening.
- Increased ICP has many causes. It is a significant sign of a brain disorder. One of the first and most important signs of ↑ICP (and other disorders of the brain) is a change in LOC.
- Most brain tumors are nonmalignant. Benign tumors, however, cause pressure on the brain and can be fatal.

CRITICAL THINKING EXERCISES

1. Discuss how your nursing care would differ for a client paralyzed from the waist down and a client paralyzed from the neck down. Give explanations for your answers.

2. Female client H. C., age 40 years, has recently been diagnosed with MS. They are married with two children, ages 9 and 12 years. Their partner is very

concerned about H.C.'s condition. When you ask H.C. how they feel about their diagnosis, they respond, "I don't understand what all the fuss is about. I don't think it's that serious since I'm feeling fine now." How would you respond to the couple? Which types of changes should the family prepare for?

3. You are working with a 70-year-old individual who has Parkinson disease and their family. The client's condition has made it impossible for them to continue to live on their own, and they are planning to move in with their family. Which types of home care adaptations can be made for the client? Which suggestions would you make for the family to adapt to this situation successfully?

NCLEX-STYLE REVIEW QUESTIONS

1. The nurse witnesses a client having a tonic–clonic seizure in the bed. Which is the priority action by the nurse?
    a. Insert a tongue blade between the client's teeth.
    b. Place the client in the prone position.
    c. Turn the head to the side.
    d. Insert an indwelling catheter.

2. The nurse is caring for a client with herpes zoster. Which priority measures to avoid cross-contamination would the nurse provide?
    a. Use transmission-based precautions.
    b. Administer antiviral medications as ordered.
    c. Apply antihistamine cream to the lesions.
    d. Instruct the client to wear gloves.

3. A client with a T6 injury reports a pounding headache, blurred vision, and nasal congestion. The nurse observes profuse sweating above the level of injury. Which is the priority action by the nurse?
    a. Irrigate the client's indwelling catheter.
    b. Elevate the client's head.
    c. Place the client in Trendelenburg position.
    d. Obtain the client's temperature.

4. The nurse is reinforcing education for a female client paralyzed from a spinal cord injury (SCI). Which statement made by the client demonstrates understanding of the education?
    a. "I may begin to menstruate within 3 months following my injury."
    b. "I should use birth control pills as a means of contraception."
    c. "It is just as safe for me to become pregnant without an SCI."
    d. "I should use a tampon instead of a feminine pad when I am menstruating."

5. The nurse is requested to place an ice pack on the eyelid for 2 min for a client suspected of having myasthenia gravis (MG) with diplopia. Which outcome does the nurse anticipate if the diagnosis is confirmed?
    a. The client will experience an improvement in respiratory status.
    b. The client will experience blindness.
    c. The client will have a grave prognosis.
    d. The client will have a temporary improvement in eye symptoms.

CHAPTER RESOURCES

Enhance your learning with additional resources on thePoint!

Student Resources related to this chapter can be found at thePoint.lww.com/Rosdahl12e.

UNIT 12 Adult Care Nursing

Welcome Steps

Look at healthcare provider's orders.

Protocol for procedure.

Necessary equipment/supplies.

Wash hands using proper hand hygiene; put on gloves.

Explain the procedure and reassure the client.

Locate two identifiers to confirm correct client.

Comfortable and efficient position for nurse and client.

Obtain privacy.

Make sure to follow correct steps and body mechanics with good technique.

Ensure safety and observe deviations from normal.

End Steps

Ensure comfort and safety.

Note questions or concerns from client or nurse; note significant data.

Dispose of materials properly.

Disinfect the area and your hands.

Document and report the procedure and your findings.

IN PRACTICE
NURSING PROCEDURE 78-1 Assisting With a Lumbar Puncture

Supplies and Equipment
Sterile gloves
Dressing materials
Local anesthetic solution (sterile), usually lidocaine (Xylocaine)
Bath blanket
Prepackaged sterile, disposable lumbar puncture (LP) kit
Clean gloves
Antiseptic solution
Specimen labels
External light source (maybe needed)
Note: Before beginning, be sure the procedure has been thoroughly explained to the client and that the client has signed the consent form. (Nursing students do not witness these permits.)

Steps
Follow LPN WELCOME Steps and Then

1. Identify the client and ask the client to empty the bladder. *Rationale: Proper identification of the client is essential to ensure that the procedure is completed for the correct person. Emptying the bladder helps the client avoid the discomfort of a full bladder.*

2. Take and record the client's vital signs before the procedure. *Rationale: Obtaining vital signs before the procedure provides a baseline assessment for later comparison.*

3. Assist the client with removing any clothing and putting on a gown that opens in the back. Drape the client with a bath blanket or sheet. *Rationale: The gown provides easy access to the proper site. Draping provides privacy and warmth, if needed.*

4. Place equipment within the healthcare provider's reach. Open packs and make sure extra sterile gloves are available. Provide extra lighting, as necessary. *Rationale: Organizing supplies and equipment enhances efficiency.*

5. Position the client on their side with the lower part of the back at the edge of the bed. Help the client to draw their knees up toward the chin and to bend their head forward. *Rationale: This position increases the space between the lower vertebrae, making needle insertion easier.*

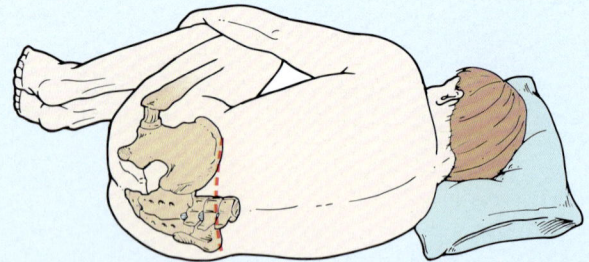

The intervertebral spaces between the spines of L3 and L4 are just below a line drawn between the anterosuperior iliac spines of the pelvis.

6. When the procedure begins, move the drape to uncover the client's back. Tell the person to lie very still, holding the client in place, if necessary. *Rationale: Any sudden movement is dangerous and could cause spinal cord damage.*

7. Talk to the client during the procedure, offering reassurance, as necessary. *Rationale: This*

procedure can be frightening. The client needs to relax and remain still.

8. Assist, as requested, such as with removing caps on bottles, labeling specimens, or assisting with dressing placement over the LP site. *Rationale: The procedure must be done using strict aseptic technique. Assistance helps to minimize the possibility of contamination.*

9. Note the beginning cerebrospinal fluid (CSF) pressure, as measured by the healthcare provider. Also, look at the color and clarity of the CSF, which should be pale and clear. *Rationale: This information is important in determining the client's disorder.*

10. Monitor the client for any difficulties or problems. *Rationale: Untoward side effects are rare, but they can occur.*

11. After the procedure, return the client to a comfortable position in bed. Keep the client's head flat (supine) for at least 6 hr or as otherwise ordered. *Rationale: Proper positioning promotes comfort while also decreasing the possibility of CSF leakage and postpuncture headache.*

Follow ENDDD Steps

Special Reminders
- Monitor and document the client's vital signs and neurologic signs, comparing them with baseline data. Determine the client's level of consciousness. Report any unusual findings to the healthcare provider.
- Encourage fluids (unless contraindicated) and record intake and output (I&O). Encourage the client to lie flat to minimize headache.
- Monitor the insertion site for leakage of CSF, hematoma formation, or edema.
- Determine the severity of any headache that occurs. Report severe headache unrelieved by mild analgesics or lasting more than 24 hr.

79 Endocrine Disorders

Learning Objectives

1. Name the common laboratory tests and radiology procedures performed to evaluate functioning of the pituitary, thyroid, parathyroid and adrenal glands, and pancreas.
2. Differentiate the four major tests used to test blood glucose levels.
3. Describe the difference between gigantism and acromegaly, and SIADH and diabetes insipidus.
4. Compare and contrast Graves disease, congenital hypothyroidism, and myxedema, including nursing considerations for each.
5. Identify preoperative and postoperative nursing considerations for a client who needs a thyroidectomy.
6. Explain the differences between hyperparathyroidism and hypoparathyroidism.
7. Describe the three major adrenal gland disorders: Cushing syndrome, primary aldosteronism, and Addison disease.
8. Differentiate among the following: type 1 and type 2 diabetes mellitus, gestational diabetes, and impaired glucose homeostasis.
9. List the three common types of insulins, stating their onset, peak, and duration of action; and the common groups of antidiabetic agents, identifying examples of each group.
10. Compare and contrast hypoglycemia, hyperglycemia, DKA, and nonketotic hyperosmolar state, including causes, signs and symptoms, treatment, and nursing considerations.
11. Identify two examples of macrovascular and microvascular complications of diabetes.
12. Prepare a teaching plan for a client with diabetes that addresses 10 topics for discussion.
13. Demonstrate the use of a blood glucose monitor in the skills laboratory.

Important Terminology

acromegaly
Addison disease
congenital hypothyroidism
Cushing syndrome
diabetes insipidus
diabetes mellitus
endocrinologist
exophthalmos
gigantism
glycemic index
goiter
Graves disease
Hashimoto thyroiditis
hyperglycemia
hyperparathyroidism
hyperthyroidism
hypoglycemia
hypoparathyroidism
hypothyroidism
insulin resistance
ketoacidosis
metabolic syndrome
myxedema
negative feedback system
nephropathy
neuropathy
pheochromocytoma
polydipsia
polyphagia
polyuria
prediabetes
retinopathy
Somogyi phenomenon
thyroidectomy

Acronyms

2-hr PG
A1c, HA1c, HbA1c
ACE
ACTH
ADH
BGM
BIDS
DKA
DM
eAG
FPG
FSH
GDM
GH
GI
IDDM
IFG
IGH
IGT
IVP
LH
NIDDM
NPH
OGTT
PH
PTH
PTU
RAI
RAIU
SIADH
SMBG
STH
T_3
T_4
TFT
TSH
VMA

The *endocrine system,* a highly integrated system, is intricately involved in regulating nearly all body processes. The *endocrine glands (ductless glands)* are groups of cells that produce chemical substances called *hormones.* The major sources of the hormones work in concert with other hormones to perform many functions, including the following:

- Helping to control water and electrolyte balance
- Assisting with the regulation of digestion
- Regulating carbohydrate metabolism
- Working as neurotransmitters
- Maintaining stress and inflammation
- Regulating reproductive functions

Endocrine glands and hormones often have more than one name or similar names (see Chapter 20). A healthcare provider trained in this specialty is called an **endocrinologist**. Other specialists also treat endocrine disorders.

Most endocrine disorders are caused by overproduction or underproduction of specific hormones (Table 79-1).

DIAGNOSTIC TESTS

Many blood and urine tests can diagnose endocrine disorders. Other tests, such as computed tomography (CT) and x-ray studies, also may be done. Table 47-3 summarizes Selected Diagnostic Tests. In addition, indirect and direct observations aid in diagnosing endocrine problems because some endocrine disorders lead to defects in growth or appearance.

TABLE 79-1 The Major Endocrine Glands and Their Hormones

GLAND	HORMONE	PRINCIPAL FUNCTIONS
Anterior pituitary	GH (growth hormone) TSH (thyroid-stimulating hormone) ACTH (adrenocorticotropic hormone) PRL (prolactin) FSH (follicle-stimulating hormone) LH (luteinizing hormone); ICSH (interstitial cell–stimulating hormone) in males	Promotes growth of all body tissues Stimulates thyroid gland to produce thyroid hormones Stimulates adrenal cortex to produce cortical hormones; aids in protecting body in stress situations (injury, pain) Stimulates secretion of milk by mammary glands Stimulates growth and hormone activity of ovarian follicles; stimulates growth of testes; promotes development of sperm cells Causes development of corpus luteum at site of ruptured ovarian follicle in female; stimulates secretion of testosterone in male
Posterior pituitary	ADH (antidiuretic hormone; vasopressin) Oxytocin	Promotes reabsorption of water in kidney tubules; stimulates smooth muscle tissue of blood vessels to constrict Causes muscle contraction of uterus; causes ejection of milk from mammary glands
Thyroid	Thyroid hormone (thyroxine and triiodothyronine) Calcitonin	Increases metabolic rate, influencing both physical and mental activities; required for normal growth Decreases calcium level in blood
Parathyroid glands	Parathyroid hormone (parathormone)	Regulates exchange of calcium between blood and bones; increases calcium level in blood
Adrenal medulla	Epinephrine and norepinephrine	Increases blood pressure and heart rate; activates cells influenced by sympathetic nervous system plus many not affected by sympathetic nerves
Adrenal cortex	Cortisol (95% of glucocorticoids) Aldosterone (95% of mineralocorticoids) Sex hormones	Aids in metabolism of carbohydrates, proteins, and fats; active during stress Aids in regulating electrolytes and water balance May influence secondary sexual characteristics in male
Pancreatic islets	Insulin Glucagon	Aids transport of glucose into cells; required for cellular metabolism of foods, especially glucose; decreases blood glucose levels Stimulates liver to release glucose, thereby increasing blood glucose levels
Testes	Testosterone	Stimulates growth and development of male sexual organs (e.g., testes, penis) plus development of secondary sexual characteristics, such as hair growth on body and face and deepening of voice; stimulates maturation of sperm cells
Ovaries	Estrogens (e.g., estradiol) Progesterone	Stimulate growth of primary female sexual organs (e.g., uterus, fallopian tubes) plus development of secondary sexual organs, such as breasts; changes pelvis to ovoid, broader shape Stimulates development of secretory parts of mammary glands; prepares uterine lining for implantation of fertilized ovum; aids in maintaining pregnancy

Pituitary Function Tests

Various tests are used to diagnose disorders of the pituitary gland. Most are specific to the client's suspected condition. Tests include x-ray examinations, CT scans, blood tests, urine tests, and others.

Thyroid Function Tests

Laboratory Tests
The thyroid gland secretes several hormones. Therefore, to monitor thyroid function, usually a combination of blood tests is done because no single test gives a complete picture. Multiple tests help determine the cause of the problem, which could be the thyroid gland itself, the pituitary gland that controls it, or both. Table 79-2 presents common thyroid function tests (**TFTs**).

Radiographic Evaluations
Thyroid Scan (Radioscan or Scintiscan)
For this test, the client ingests radioactive iodine or receives it intravenously (IV) (see Box 47-2 Precautions When Tests are Performed Using Dye). Then a scanogram (x-ray study) is obtained to indicate the amount of radioactivity in the entire body. If the thyroid absorbs a great deal of the

TABLE 79-2 Tests of Thyroid Function

TEST	PURPOSE
FT$_4$I (free thyroxine index)	Measures levels of T$_4$ and T$_3$U
T$_4$ (serum thyroxine)	Measures circulating levels of T$_4$
T$_3$ (serum triiodothyronine)	Measures circulating levels of T$_3$
T$_3$U (T$_3$ resin uptake)	Determines amount of radioactive resin bound to T$_3$
TSH (thyroid-stimulating hormone)	Measures levels of TSH produced by the pituitary gland
Provocative (Response-Inducing) Tests of Thyroid Function	
TRH (thyrotropin-releasing hormone) stimulation test	Measures TSH levels repeatedly after thyroid-releasing hormone (normally produced by the hypothalamus to stimulate TSH) is given IV
TSH stimulation test	Measures body's response to TSH by following levels of radioactive iodine uptake and protein-bound iodine uptake
Thyroid suppression test	Measures levels of radioactive iodine uptake and serum T$_4$ after 7–10 days of receiving thyroid hormone

radioactive iodine, the thyroid is hyperactive, suggesting possible hyperthyroidism. If a decreased amount of iodine appears in the thyroid, the gland is hypoactive, suggesting hypothyroidism or a malignancy. This test may also indicate locations of thyroid malignancy metastases to other parts of the body.

Radioactive Iodine Uptake

The *radioactive iodine uptake* (**RAIU**) test measures thyroid gland activity. After a period of fasting, a client drinks a small amount of radioactive iodine dissolved in distilled water or swallows a capsule of the radioactive substance. At various intervals for up to 24 hr, a scan of the thyroid gland is performed. As the radioactive material is metabolized and removed from the bloodstream, the amount that the thyroid absorbs can be measured. A normally active thyroid will remove from 15% to 45% within that period; in hyperthyroidism, it may remove as much as 90%. Certain drugs can influence the accuracy of an RAIU test, including oral contraceptives, anticoagulants, salicylates, and propylthiouracil (**PTU**) derivatives. Check to make sure that the client is not allergic to iodine or shellfish. Pregnant or lactating women should not take this test.

Before the test, knowing how much iodine the client usually consumes (ocean shellfish, iodized salt, saturated solution of potassium iodide, Lugol solution) is important. Testers should be aware if clients use iodine-containing antiseptics or if they have had recent x-ray studies using iodine-based contrast media or other recent studies involving radioactive substances. Question clients about the use of any of the medications mentioned above, plus thyroid-stimulating hormone (**TSH**), estrogen, aspirin, phenothiazines, or barbiturates. Clients must not use any of these substances for a week before the test. In addition, assure clients that the dose of radiation associated with the radioactive iodine is not dangerous. After the substance is given, make sure that the client knows exactly when to return to the laboratory.

Other Tests

Thyroid Ultrasound (Thyroid Echogram)
The *thyroid ultrasound* test determines the thyroid gland's size, shape, and position. Abnormal findings may indicate a cyst or a solid nodule, which is often cancerous. The test may also be done periodically during treatment to determine the effectiveness of therapy or to evaluate the thyroid during pregnancy (because RAIU examination is dangerous to the fetus).

The ultrasound examination will not hurt, nor will it disturb breathing or swallowing. The test takes approximately 15 min. The client will lie on the table, while a liberal amount of water-soluble gel is applied to the neck to ensure transmission of sound waves. The photos and computer printouts will then be evaluated by the healthcare provider. After the test, the client may need assistance to remove the gel from the skin.

Parathyroid Function Tests

Laboratory Tests

Blood tests to evaluate parathyroid function include serum parathormone (also known as parathyroid hormone; **PH, PTH**) levels, serum phosphate and calcium levels, urinary calcium, and serum alkaline phosphatase. Tests of other systems will also be ordered because normal calcium and phosphorus balance involves multiple body systems, including the musculoskeletal, gastrointestinal, and urinary systems.

Other Tests

Ultrasound, magnetic resonance imaging (MRI), thallium scan, and fine-needle biopsy can evaluate the function of the parathyroid glands and localize parathyroid cysts, tumors, and *hyperplasia* (abnormal increase in size).

Adrenal Function Tests

Laboratory Tests

Blood Tests
Common blood tests to determine adrenal function include the adrenocorticotropic hormone (**ACTH**) stimulation test, serum ACTH test, and plasma cortisol test. Plasma cortisol and ACTH follow a *diurnal* (daytime) pattern. They can be measured at 8 AM and 4 PM to establish whether the normal diurnal pattern is present.

Urine Tests
Urine tests can also be used to evaluate adrenal function. Measurement of metabolites of catecholamines in the urine is useful in diagnosis. Urinary metanephrine is the most diagnostic urine test of adrenal medulla function. A 24-hr urine specimen may be collected for determining vanillylmandelic acid (**VMA**), a metabolite of catecholamines.

A clonidine suppression test can help determine pheochromocytoma, a catecholamine-secreting adrenal tumor. In this condition, serum and urinary catecholamines are elevated and are not suppressed by clonidine. (Normally, clonidine suppresses catecholamines.) Side effects of the test include hypotension, bradycardia, and *somnolence* (extreme sleepiness).

In addition, a somewhat risky test involves histamine administration, which produces a hypertensive crisis when the client has pheochromocytoma. Similarly, phentolamine (Regitine) can be given to provoke a hypotensive situation. The drop in blood pressure is diagnostic of pheochromocytoma.

A 24-hr urine specimen may be collected for determining metabolites such as 17-hydroxycorticosteroids, 17-ketosteroids, and 17-ketogenic steroids. These 24-hr urine collections require special preservatives. Know the institution's requirements and make sure the appropriate container is available. Proper client education is necessary to ensure the collection of all urine.

Radiographic Evaluations

Radiographic evaluations of adrenal function include the adrenal angiogram and venogram, CT scan of the adrenals, MRI, ultrasonography, and retroperitoneal air sufflation, as well as an x-ray study of the sella turcica. These examinations detect benign and malignant tumors of the adrenal glands, as well as *hyperplasia* (excess multiplication of normal cells).

Adrenal Angiogram or Venogram

These tests involve insertion of a catheter and injection of a contrast medium (dye) so that x-ray contrast studies can be done. The client is usually *NPO* (nothing by mouth) before the test. The major complication is an allergic reaction to the dye. Therefore, be sure to determine the client's allergy to dye before the test, and observe other precautions (see Chapter 47). To prevent this complication, propranolol (Inderal), diphenhydramine (Benadryl), or other medications may be administered for several days before and after the test. The test may also cause hemorrhage or dislodging of an atherosclerotic plaque from the wall of the blood vessel used for dye injection. This may cause an infarction. If hemorrhage occurs within the adrenal glands, **Addison disease** (chronic adrenocortical insufficiency resulting from adrenal gland destruction) may result. If surgery is needed later, it is more difficult when any of these events have occurred.

Angiograms and venograms are also contraindicated in clients who are pregnant, unstable, or uncooperative and in those with hemophilia, a bleeding disorder, or measurable atherosclerosis.

General Pancreatic Function Tests

The pancreas secretes two enzymes: *amylase*, necessary for carbohydrate metabolism; and *lipase,* necessary for fat digestion. Serum levels of both of these enzymes can be obtained. Elevations suggest pancreatitis. Urinary amylase levels also may be obtained. The amylase level in urine remains elevated for a longer time than it does in serum.

Tests for Diabetes Mellitus

Blood Tests

A number of blood tests indicate the functioning of the endocrine portion of the pancreas. Some of these tests specifically relate to the detection and evaluation of diabetes mellitus (DM).

Random Blood Glucose

A *random blood glucose* is a blood test that looks at the amount of circulating blood sugar at the time of the blood draw. The client does not fast prior to the test. This test is often done to look at the circulating amounts of glucose at random times. The random test may indicate hypoglycemia or hyperglycemia, which need to be followed up with more specific testing procedures. Normal results range from 70 to 110 mg/dL.

Fasting Plasma Glucose

The *fasting plasma glucose* (**FPG**) test, formerly called *fasting blood glucose* (also referred to as *blood sugar*), is used for diabetes screening. In most cases, an elevated *fasting* (without eating) or nonfasting blood glucose level is an indication of *diabetes mellitus* (metabolic condition involving elevated levels of glucose in the blood). The FPG level is defined as the amount of glucose (sugar) present in the blood when the client has been fasting for the prescribed length of time (6–8 hr). The normal for FPG ranges about 65–115 mg/dL. An FPG greater than or equal to 126 mg/dL and obtained on two or more occasions confirms a diagnosis of DM.

Oral Glucose Tolerance Test

The *oral glucose tolerance test* (**OGTT**) is a timed test used to confirm the diagnosis of DM when the client's FPG is equal to or greater than 126 mg/dL, or when the client's FPG is above normal, but below the diagnostic level for diabetes. It is also used in screening for gestational diabetes in both the 1- and 3-hr formats. OGTT also can diagnose functional *hypoglycemia* (abnormally low blood glucose).

- The client should ingest at least 150 g of carbohydrate daily for 3 days before the test (most individuals following a good general diet easily meet this criterion).
- Tests of both blood and urine are done during the fasting state.
- The client drinks 75–100 g of glucose. They must consume this glucose completely and as quickly as possible. *Rationale: The starting point of this timed test must be as precise as possible.*
- Blood and urine specimens are again taken at prescribed intervals: 1/2, 1, 2, and 3 hr. Specimen collection is timed from the point of ingestion of glucose.
- The test begins with an empty bladder, although the pretest urine specimen is also saved as one of the fasting specimens to be examined.
- The laboratory technician takes the blood and urine specimens, labels them, and indicates the time when each was collected.
- The client may have water to drink during the test to provide comfort and to make voiding easier. Juice, other fluids, and food are not permitted.
- The client is not allowed to smoke or chew gum.

Normally, plasma glucose levels peak at 160–180 mg/dL within 1 hr after the client receives an oral glucose test dose; they return to fasting levels or lower within 3 hr. Urine glucose tests should remain negative throughout. Values greater than 200 mg/dL or above at 2 hr (2-hr postload glucose [**2-hr PG**]) indicate diabetes. (Actual blood glucose tolerance levels may differ per laboratory.) Some factors that may affect the test include thiazide diuretics, oral contraceptives, lithium, caffeine, and nicotinic acid. These substances elevate glucose levels.

Hemoglobin A1c

Hemoglobin A1c is also known as *glycosylated hemoglobin, glycohemoglobin, or glycated hemoglobin,* with various acronyms such as **HA1c**, **HbA1c**, or **A1c**. This is a measurement that reflects the client's average blood glucose level over the previous 2–3 months. It is measured by determining the amount of glucose attached to a certain portion of hemoglobin in red blood cells. This test is invaluable in monitoring blood glucose control and allows the client and healthcare team to set measurable goals. Although normal ranges vary depending on the laboratory, most healthcare providers want their clients to be in the range of 5% to 7%, depending on which exact subfactors they are measuring.

Estimated Average Glucose

Estimated average glucose (**eAG**) reports HA1c levels using the same units as standard handheld glucose monitors. For example, if the HA1c is 8%, the eAG will be about 180 mg/dL.

Glycemic Index

The **glycemic index** (**GI**) is a measurement of how foods containing carbohydrates (starchy foods such as potatoes, bread, or cereals) raise blood glucose levels. Carbohydrates are compared with a standard known carbohydrate, such as glucose or white bread. Some foods are known to raise the blood glucose levels significantly and are considered to have a high GI. Carbohydrate-containing foods can be rated as a high GI, medium GI, or low GI. The use of the GI can assist with stabilization of meal planning and blood glucose levels.

Urine Tests

Normal urine is free from sugar (*glucose*), acetone, and protein, but any of these may be present in the urine of a client with diabetes. Excess glucose in the blood spills over into the urine; acetone appears as a by-product of faulty metabolism. With the availability of a variety of sophisticated (but easy-to-use) blood glucose monitors, urine testing is now done infrequently, both in the healthcare facility and at home. The most common need for urine testing is the test for ketones if a client's blood glucose level is consistently high. Because only clients with type 1 diabetes are susceptible to diabetic ketoacidosis, these clients learn to test their urine for ketones if their blood glucose readings exceed 240 mg/dL.

> **! Nursing Alert** The test for urine ketones (acetone) is especially important if the client is vomiting, has a fever, or has a high concentration of glucose in the blood (>240 mg/dL).

Keto-Diastix Test

Acetone is a ketone body that is present when the body cells are starving because of faulty metabolism. Buildup of acetone leads to ketosis, which in turn leads to acidosis. Vomiting or excessive perspiration can alter electrolyte balance. The Keto-Diastix test, which detects both elevated glucose and ketone levels in urine, is typically done in the laboratory but can be done by healthcare providers using standardized urine dip sticks.

> **NCLEX Alert**
>
> Laboratory test results are commonly seen in nursing situations. NCLEX clinical scenarios might require knowledge of normal levels of many tests, including blood glucose, thyroid functioning, or hormone levels. Nursing reactions to abnormal levels (e.g., low or high blood glucose) are significant concerns.

COMMON MEDICAL AND SURGICAL TREATMENTS

The most common surgical treatment for some pituitary or thyroid disorders is removal of the affected gland. The pituitary gland also may be removed in some cases to slow or stop the spread of certain types of malignancies that are nourished by an endocrine hormone.

DM cannot be treated with surgery, although pancreatic or cellular transplants have had some success in reversing the symptoms.

NURSING PROCESS

DATA COLLECTION
Using the skills of physical examination and nursing assessment and data gathering, observe and document client status for possible endocrine disorders. This establishes a baseline for future comparison and helps determine the presence of suspected endocrine-related complications. Report any changes in baseline levels.

Much knowledge of endocrine function is based on laboratory examination of blood. Other testing (e.g., x-rays or ultrasound) is also done. Check reports of these evaluations, and report any abnormal results immediately. Nurses may perform blood testing for glucose and occasionally urine testing for ketones.

While caring for clients, note any signs and symptoms of endocrine disorders and report them. In addition, observe the client's emotional response to the disorder or disease. Does the client need assistance to meet daily needs? Is the client anxious or fearful of the outcome? Is the client having difficulty accepting a disorder's long-term nature?

PLANNING AND IMPLEMENTATION
Plan together with the healthcare team for effective care to meet the client's needs, based on the nursing diagnoses. Properly prepare clients for diagnostic tests. Provide preoperative and postoperative care for clients undergoing surgery.

Because disorders of the endocrine system can affect most body functions, listing all the nursing implications is difficult. An endocrine disorder can be a simple imbalance that is successfully rectified by administration of hormones or other medications. However, in some cases, such as end-stage renal disease caused by diabetes mellitus, a client may require total nursing care and assistance to meet all needs, including those related to death and dying.

Clients may have difficulty accepting an endocrine disorder's chronic nature and the fact that treatments, such as insulin injections or thyroid medications, must continue for life. Most clients need to learn about their disorder, its prognosis, and its treatment.

EVALUATION
Periodically, the healthcare team evaluates the outcomes of the client's care. Have short-term goals been met? For example, is the client's blood glucose level being maintained within an acceptable range? Are long-term goals still realistic? Planning for further nursing care considers the client's prognosis, any complications, and the client's response to care given. Client and family teaching is an important component of nursing care. Do the client and family understand the treatment required and the underlying reasons? For example, do they demonstrate an understanding of the need for lifelong thyroid hormonal replacement? Is teaching adequate and documented?

PITUITARY GLAND DISORDERS

Disorders of the Anterior Lobe
The anterior pituitary exerts control by a **negative feedback system**—after it has stimulated a target gland to produce a hormone and the hormone level rises sufficiently high, the anterior pituitary stops stimulating the target gland and stops the hormone release. The anterior lobe alone produces or releases the following hormones: growth hormone (**GH**; somatotropin [**STH**]), ACTH, TSH, prolactin, follicle-stimulating hormone (**FSH**), and luteinizing hormone (**LH**). These hormones are of vital importance in growth, maturation, and reproduction.

Gigantism and Acromegaly
Disturbances of the anterior lobe may cause overproduction of the growth hormone STH. If overproduction occurs in childhood, it causes excessive growth of bones, or **gigantism**. In adults, an excess of STH causes overgrowth of tissues, called **acromegaly**. The features of the person with acromegaly coarsen. They develop a massive lower jaw, thick lips, a bulbous nose, a bulging forehead, and hands and feet that seem enormous. In women, facial hair also appears (*hirsutism*) and the voice deepens. Headaches are common and partial vision loss may develop. The spleen, heart, and liver enlarge; muscles weaken; and joint pain and stiffness appear. Men may be impotent. Women may not menstruate (*amenorrhea*).

Acromegaly is treated by irradiation of the pituitary gland using proton-beam therapy or surgical intervention. Recently, certain drugs, such as bromocriptine mesylate (Parlodel) and somatostatin analogues, have shown promise in lowering the levels of STH. Treatment can stop the disease's progression, but therapy cannot alter abnormal growth that has already occurred.

Disorders of the Posterior Lobe
The posterior lobe of the pituitary secretes and releases hormones that affect blood pressure and control water balance in the kidney tubules. It releases *antidiuretic hormone* (**ADH** or *vasopressin*), which regulates the passage of water through the kidneys. It also releases oxytocin in women, which stimulates uterine contractions during labor and milk release during breastfeeding.

Syndrome of Inappropriate Antidiuretic Hormone
The *syndrome of inappropriate antidiuretic hormone* (**SIADH**) involves the excessive secretion of ADH. Clients with SIADH cannot excrete dilute urine. Fluid retention and ultimately water intoxication occur, along with sodium deficiency. SIADH can result from central nervous system (CNS) disorders, chemotherapy, ADH production by some cancers, and overuse of vasopressin therapy.

Urinary output decreases. The severity of the condition depends on how low the client's serum sodium levels fall (*hyponatremia*) and how much water they retain. The client may complain of a headache or experience confusion, lethargy, seizures, and possibly coma if sodium deficiency is severe. Hyponatremia may cause diarrhea. Weight gain also occurs with fluid retention.

Close monitoring of fluid intake and output (I&O), daily weights, and mental status is necessary. Institute safety measures to reduce the risk of possible injury. Fluids usually are restricted to 500–1,000 mL daily. To correct fluid retention and hyponatremia, medications such as hypertonic saline infusions and diuretics may be ordered. Also, medications such as demeclocycline and lithium carbonate, which interfere with the antidiuretic action of ADH, may be ordered. Treatment is aimed at correcting the underlying problem.

Diabetes Insipidus
Diabetes insipidus is a disease that results from underproduction of ADH. *Primary nephrogenic insipidus* is rare and is caused by kidney dysfunction due to a deficiency in ADH or to a lesion in the midbrain. *Secondary central diabetes insipidus* results from a tumor in the gland itself or pressure in the pituitary area from head trauma, infection, or other tumors. It may also occur after pituitary surgery that removes all or a portion of the gland.

In diabetes insipidus, the client voids copious amounts of urine, as much as 15–20 L in 24 hr. The urine is dilute, with a specific gravity less than 1.006, and contains no sugar or acetone. The client is constantly thirsty; restricting fluids may have some effect. Keep accurate I&O records to make sure the volume of output is being replaced; closely monitor electrolyte levels. Record daily weights in the early morning before breakfast. Despite an abnormally large appetite, the client is weak and may need assistance with self-care. Treatment consists of giving intranasal or oral desmopressin acetate (DDAVP) or subcutaneous vasopressin (ADH) to control urinary output.

Nursing Alert Monitor Pitressin administration closely because it can cause coronary artery constriction.

Pituitary Neoplasms

Neoplasms of the pituitary gland can affect various aspects of body function. An overgrowth of eosinophilic cells in the pituitary can result in gigantism. A basophilic tumor in the pituitary can upset production of the hormone that regulates the adrenal glands, leading to hyperadrenalism (*Cushing syndrome*). A chromophobic tumor can destroy the pituitary and result in hypopituitarism. A client with this disorder has fine, scanty hair; lowered basal metabolic rate; lowered body temperature; and a tendency toward obesity and slow movements.

Hypophysectomy

Hypophysectomy, surgical removal of the pituitary gland, may be done for a variety of reasons, including malignancy or to decrease diabetic retinopathy. Occasionally, the pituitary is removed to control pain associated with metastatic carcinoma of the breast or prostate. The client usually is admitted to the intensive care unit after surgery.

THYROID GLAND DISORDERS

The *thyroid gland* secretes the hormones thyroxine (T_4) and triiodothyronine (T_3), which regulate metabolism by stimulating *catabolism* (the breakdown of cells and foods, with release of energy). Too much of these hormones makes tissues burn oxygen rapidly; too little causes the reverse. The thyroid gland requires iodine to produce these hormones. Thyroid-stimulating hormone from the anterior pituitary gland influences the secretion of T_3 and T_4. In addition, the thyroid gland produces *calcitonin,* which helps to maintain calcium balance in the plasma (see Table 79-1).

Hyperthyroidism

Hyperthyroidism involves the overproduction of T_4, which leads to an increase in metabolic rate. **Graves disease** or *toxic diffuse* **goiter** (enlargement of the thyroid gland) is the most common type of hyperthyroidism (Fig. 79-1). The exact cause of this overactivity is unknown, but it may result from infection, physical or emotional strain, or changes related to puberty or pregnancy. Current theories point to an autoimmune origin, in which the person forms antibodies against thyroid cells, specifically the TSH receptor cells. Hyperthyroidism occurs most frequently in women and in the third and fourth decades of life.

Signs and Symptoms

The client is highly excitable and overactive and may have tremors that make eating impossible without help. The pulse is rapid; the person may have heart palpitations and an increased incidence of arrhythmias, which will cause damage if left untreated. The systolic blood pressure is elevated. The person feels hot, and eats voraciously—yet loses weight—because they burn calories so rapidly. The skin becomes thickened and takes on a characteristic salmon color. In women, menstruation may cease.

Another common symptom is bulging eyes (**exophthalmos**). The cause of this symptom is not fully understood. It can lead to blindness caused by stretching of the optic nerve or corneal ulceration. The neck is swollen, and pressure from the thyroid gland may cause hoarseness or difficulty swallowing.

If untreated, this disorder may cause intense nervousness, delirium, and finally death as a result of persistent cardiac overload.

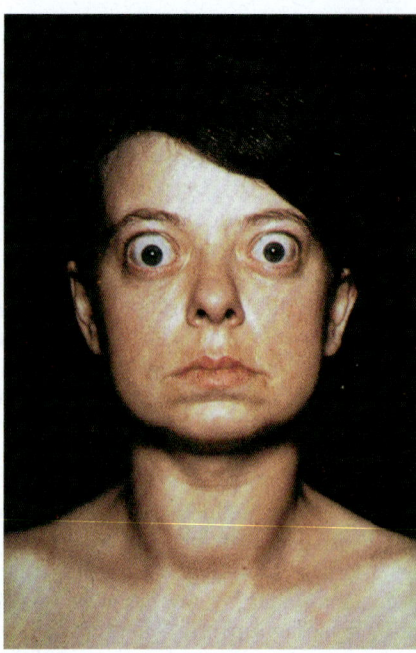

Figure 79-1 A woman with Graves disease. Note the exophthalmos and enlarged thyroid gland.

Treatment

Treatment for hyperthyroidism may be medical or surgical. Medical treatment consists of prescribing antithyroid agents, such as propylthiouracil or methimazole (Tapazole), which block secretion of the thyroid hormone. They may also be given as preparation for surgery. If prescribed as medical therapy, these drugs are given daily, generally over a long time. They may have toxic effects—fever, skin rash, and enlarged lymph nodes, with an increase in white blood cells. Therapeutic doses of radioactive iodine (**RAI**) may also be prescribed. RAI is administered as an oral solution absorbed through the gastrointestinal tract. The radioactive iodine is transported to the thyroid gland, where it destroys the gland's ability to make T_4 and T_3.

Thyroidectomy, removal of the thyroid gland, is no longer the treatment of choice and is done only after antithyroid drugs and radioactive iodine have proved unsuccessful, or when the goiter is so large that it constricts structures in the neck region.

Nursing Considerations

Nursing care focuses on minimizing overactivity, improving nutritional status, maintaining a normal body temperature, and improving self-esteem. Assist in providing a calm environment and minimizing the client's expenditure of energy by helping with activities and encouraging alternating periods of rest and activity. Provide increased calories and nutritional support to help improve the client's nutritional status. Diet therapy usually consists of increased caloric and protein needs, vitamins (especially B complex and D), minerals (especially calcium), and fluids. If exophthalmos is present, the client can use eye protection, such as patches, drops, or artificial tears. If body temperature is elevated, give acetaminophen (Tylenol) as ordered and use cooling blankets to reduce body temperature. Because the client is experiencing changes in appearance, appetite, and weight along with overactivity, convey understanding, concern, and willingness to help.

Hypothyroidism

Hypothyroidism occurs when a deficiency of T_4 slows down metabolic processes. It may be due to removal of the thyroid gland or to a decrease in its activity. It is more likely to affect women than men. The congenital form of this deficiency causes a condition called **congenital hypothyroidism**. Advanced hypothyroidism in the adult is called **myxedema**.

Signs and Symptoms

Untreated congenital hypothyroidism results in arrested physical and mental development and dystrophy of bones and soft tissues (Fig. 79-2). The person is dwarfed and has a large head, short arms and legs, puffy eyes, and a protruding tongue. The person also has dry skin and movements that are uncoordinated; sterility occurs in almost all cases. Intellectual impairment ranges from moderate to severe (see Chapter 74). If discovered early, this condition can often be successfully treated with administration of T_4 replacement, which must continue for life.

In adults, myxedema is evidenced by a slowing of physical and mental activity, accompanied by forgetfulness and chronic headache. The client's expression becomes masklike. The skin is dry; the voice is hoarse and low; hair is coarse and tends to fall out; and the client gains weight. The client may become chronically constipated and anemic, and heart rate may be affected. The RAIU uptake rate will almost always be normal; *menorrhagia* (excessive menstrual flow) may occur.

Treatment

Synthetic hormone levothyroxine sodium (T4, L-thyroxine sodium, and Synthroid) plus synthetic liothyronine sodium (Cytomel) are given to supply the hormone deficiency. The results are dramatic. The client becomes more alert, and the appearance becomes normal. Replacement therapy must be done gradually because a rapid change can be dangerous; for example, the heart rate may increase too rapidly and show signs of strain from increased activity.

Nursing Considerations

Nursing care focuses on the client's improvements in activity tolerance and independence, resuming normal bowel function, improving mental activity, and adhering to the medical regimen. Anyone with a thyroid deficiency is susceptible to respiratory depression from sedatives or hypnotics. Some people must take thyroid replacement preparations all their lives, but with regulated treatment, they remain well and healthy. Follow-up visits with healthcare providers for periodic examinations are essential.

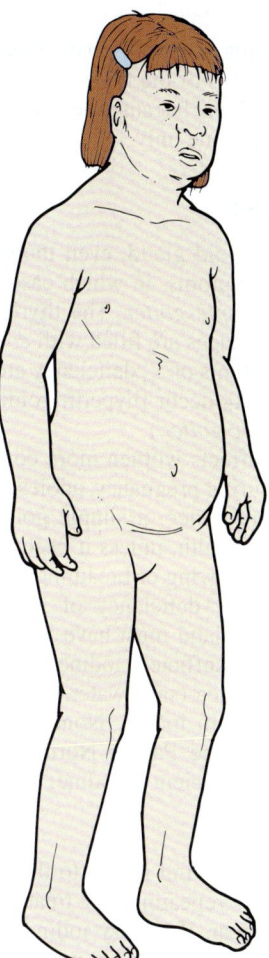

Figure 79-2 A client with congenital hypothyroidism.

> **Nursing Alert** Do not give sedatives, narcotics, and hypnotic drugs to the person with hypothyroidism or give them in very small doses.
> *Rationale: The client's respiratory and heart rates are already slow; additional depressants could cause respiratory or cardiac arrest.*
> Be alert for signs of myocardial infarction (MI).
> *Rationale: MI could result from the long period of slowed circulation to heart muscle.*
> Immediately report any complaints of anginal pain, which can occur when thyroid hormone therapy begins. Teach the client signs and symptoms of angina.
> *Rationale: This pain can be the first sign of an MI. A clot may block a portion of the coronary circulation.*

Long-term untreated hypothyroidism can result in *myxedema coma*, a medical emergency necessitating immediate but careful administration of thyroid hormone. Treatment of any depressed respiratory function that occurs and close monitoring of cardiac function are essential.

Hashimoto Thyroiditis

Hashimoto thyroiditis is hypothyroidism believed to be autoimmune in origin. It is of the type of autoimmune disorders known as *organ specific* because the body builds up antibodies against thyroid tissue only.

Simple Goiter

Sometimes, the thyroid gland, even though enlarged, does not cause toxic symptoms, in which case it is called a *colloid goiter* or a *simple goiter*. The thyroid gland enlarges and the distended spaces are filled with *colloid,* a gelatinous material. No symptoms of T_4 deficiency are noted. (If symptoms of too much T_4 occur [hyperthyroidism], the goiter is referred to as a *toxic goiter.*)

Simple goiter affects women more commonly than men and may appear during pregnancy, adolescence, or infection. Except for its appearance, a simple goiter usually has no harmful effects on health, unless it becomes so large that it interferes with swallowing or breathing.

Usually, a dietary deficiency of iodine causes simple goiter. The thyroid gland must have iodine to produce thyroid hormones. If a sufficient iodine supply is unavailable, the gland enlarges. Sea (salt) water, some soils, and inland drinking water contain iodine. Noncoastal areas—such as mountainous areas, the Pacific Northwest, and the Great Lakes region—are deficient in iodine.

Treatment

Goiter is treated by giving iodine to the client for a period of 2–3 weeks and repeating the treatment three or four times during the year, if dietary iodine intake is deficient. Administration of iodine does not cure simple goiter; it prevents it or stops its progression.

The most economical, suitable, and reliable goiter prevention program is the use of iodized table salt. Reinforcing the body's supply of iodine is simple because the thyroid needs a very small amount. Surgery may be necessary if a goiter causes excessive pressure.

Thyroid Neoplasms

A liquid or semisolid cyst sometimes forms in the thyroid. It can be located by ultrasound. A *simple cyst* can be aspirated. A *semisolid cyst* is most often malignant and must be surgically removed. A malignant tumor can occur any time from childhood to late adulthood. If a thyroid tumor is cancerous, it must be removed surgically or treated by irradiation with radioactive isotopes. A biopsy study will tell whether such a growth is malignant. Most common thyroid cancers are slow growing, although a fast-growing adenocarcinoma may metastasize and not respond to radiation therapy.

Thyroidectomy

Thyroidectomy is surgical removal of the thyroid gland. Surgery to remove tissue from the thyroid was once the primary method of treating hyperthyroidism. Today, however, surgery is reserved for special circumstances, such as for pregnant women, those who are allergic to antithyroid medications, and clients with large goiters. Generally, only part of the gland is removed (*subtotal thyroidectomy*) so that some thyroid hormone production continues postoperatively. Before surgery, antithyroid agents may be administered until signs of hyperthyroidism are minimized. In addition, β-adrenergic blocking agents (usually propranolol [Inderal]) may be used to reduce the heart rate. However, if these measures fail to achieve a normal thyroid state, iodine (Lugol solution or potassium iodide) may be given. Thyroid hormone levels and metabolic rate must be normalized before surgery to reduce the risk of thyroid storm (see discussion below).

A subtotal thyroidectomy usually prevents the recurrence of hyperthyroidism because only enough of the gland is left to maintain normal function. If a *total thyroidectomy* is done (because of injury or malignancy), the client requires thyroid hormone (thyroxine; T_4) for life.

Postoperative Complications

Postoperatively, the client is at risk for complications, including hemorrhage, hematoma formation, edema of the glottis, and injury to the recurrent laryngeal nerve. Keep airway equipment near the client's bedside postoperatively in case edema of the laryngeal area causes respiratory distress.

> **Nursing Alert** Internal hemorrhage and edema following thyroidectomy are postoperative threats. Inspect dressings for excessive bleeding. Check for edema in the neck or bleeding at the back of the neck. Keep an endotracheal tube available in the client's room, both preoperatively and postoperatively, because swelling may obstruct the airway, causing respiratory distress. In this event, an endotracheal tube is inserted, and the client is taken to the operating room for a tracheostomy.

Another potential and dangerous complication is *tetany,* a generalized continuous muscle spasm of the entire body. It is most often caused by accidental removal of the parathyroid glands during thyroidectomy. The *Chvostek sign* (abnormal spasm of the facial muscles in response to light taps on the facial nerve) and *Trousseau sign* (an abnormal carpopedal spasm induced by inflating a sphygmomanometer cuff on the upper arm to a pressure exceeding systolic blood pressure for 3 min) may be positive (Fig. 79-3). (The Trousseau sign also may be seen in clients with hypocalcemia and

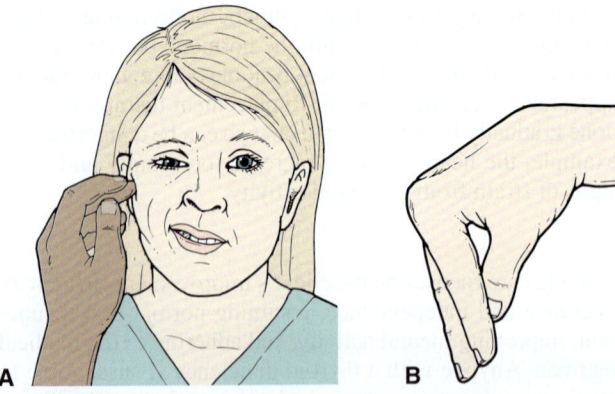

Figure 79-3 A. Chvostek sign. **B.** Trousseau sign.

hypomagnesemia.) Serum calcium levels also may be low. This condition may be fatal, resulting in seizures and cardiac arrhythmias. Emergency treatment of tetany is the IV administration of calcium gluconate, which must be kept available postoperatively. PTH may be administered, along with calcium gluconate, to treat the condition. If the parathyroid glands have been totally removed, administration of PTH must continue for life.

Thyroid crisis (*thyrotoxicosis* or *thyroid storm*) is another possible complication that can occur in the hospital or possibly after discharge. It is a dangerous condition caused by a sudden increase in T_4. Before and after surgery, be alert for symptoms such as tachycardia, anxiety, and an abrupt increase in vital signs. This extreme form of thyrotoxicosis can cause heart failure. Treatment focuses on maintaining oxygen and glucose levels in the body cells, while reducing fever. Sedatives, tranquilizers, and cardiotonics may be prescribed. Thyroid storm is less prevalent postoperatively with the use of antithyroid drugs and iodine preparations. In some cases, corticosteroids are given.

Nursing Considerations

Nursing considerations include encouraging the client to rest and avoid excessive physical activity and to increase nutritional intake to ensure adequate calories, vitamin D, and calcium. Teach the client the importance of continued medication therapy and the signs and symptoms of hypofunction and hyperfunction. Reinforce the need for close follow-up after surgery. Periodically, the client will need to have thyroid function tests done as part of the follow-up.

PARATHYROID GLAND DISORDERS

The *parathyroid glands* secrete PTH. Aided by vitamin D, PTH regulates the amount of calcium and phosphorus in the blood and, thus, regulates bone formation.

Hyperparathyroidism

Hyperparathyroidism stems from an excess of PTH that causes blood calcium levels to rise, resulting in calcium depletion in bones (*osteomalacia*). Bones become soft and weak, leading to skeletal tenderness. They tend to break easily, even in the absence of pressure or injury (*pathologic fractures*). The skull may enlarge. Muscles weaken, and the client complains of fatigue, nausea, and constipation. Kidney stones, urinary tract infections, and uremia may develop. The person may become disoriented and paranoid and may lose consciousness. This condition may be secondary to chronic nephritis.

Hyperparathyroidism is detected by a consistently high blood level of parathormone and by x-ray indications of skeletal changes or pathologic fractures.

A diuretic agent, such as furosemide (Lasix), and large amounts of fluids are often given to prevent renal disorders such as stones, which develop because of the high blood calcium levels. Phosphates may be given cautiously to reduce the serum calcium level. A thyroid lobectomy to remove part of the thyroid gland containing the parathyroid may be done.

Preoperatively, encourage exercise to help prevent the bones from releasing some calcium. Calcium in the diet is limited in some cases. If tetany occurs postoperatively, calcium gluconate is given to restore the blood's calcium–phosphorus balance.

Keep a tracheostomy tray and IV calcium at the bedside for emergency use. The postoperative diet is high in calcium, fat, and carbohydrate. The client needs special care to avoid injury until bones are recalcified.

Hypoparathyroidism

Hypoparathyroidism, the deficiency of PTH, results from lowered production of the hormone, with a consequent reduction in the amount of calcium available to the body and an accumulation of phosphorus in the blood. Accidental removal of the parathyroid glands during a thyroidectomy may cause hypoparathyroidism.

Lack of calcium causes tremors and tetany, the characteristic sign. Cardiac output decreases. A positive Trousseau sign (carpopedal spasm caused by blocking the blood flow to the arm for 3 min using a blood pressure cuff) or a positive Chvostek sign (twitching of the mouth, nose, and eye after tapping the area over the facial nerve just in front of the parotid gland and anterior to the ear) suggests latent tetany (see Fig. 79-3). This extreme muscular irritability may be so pronounced that laryngospasm or seizures occur. Other symptoms include hair loss, skin coarsening, brittle nails, arrhythmias, and possible heart failure.

Treatment is to increase the client's serum calcium level. Calcium salts (calcium gluconate) must be given, usually intravenously (IV). (Never give calcium preparations intramuscularly [IM]; they injure tissues.) Large doses of vitamin D are also given because vitamin D helps regulate body calcium levels. Administration of sedatives or anticonvulsants may also be necessary in the acute phase of hypoparathyroidism (to prevent seizures). Client teaching about medications and the need for follow-up is important.

ADRENAL GLAND DISORDERS

The *adrenal glands* contain two parts: the cortex and the medulla. The *cortex* (outer covering) secretes various types of steroid hormones that control many vital functions. These hormones regulate metabolism to supply quick energy, help maintain fluid and electrolyte balance, and regulate the development of secondary sex characteristics. The *medulla* is stimulated by the sympathetic nervous system; it secretes the hormones epinephrine (adrenaline) and norepinephrine (see Chapters 19 and 78).

Cushing Syndrome

Cushing syndrome (*hyperadrenalism*) results from overproduction of hormones secreted by the adrenal cortex. It can also result from overuse of corticosteroids or tumors of the adrenal glands or the pituitary.

Fat distribution is abnormal. The face is rounded ("moon face"), the abdomen is heavy and hangs down, and the arms and legs are thin. There is a noted fat pad in the neck and supraclavicular area sometimes referred to as a "buffalo hump." As the disease progresses, the client becomes weaker, the bones soften, and the client may have a backache. Edema develops and urinary output decreases. *Hypokalemia* (low blood potassium levels) is usually present. *Hypernatremia* (high blood sodium levels) and **hyperglycemia** (abnormally high blood glucose) follow. The client is hypertensive. Wounds do not heal, and the client bruises easily. Mood swings are common; the client may be irritable or euphoric. Striae may develop because of an enlarged abdominal girth.

If hyperadrenalism occurs in childhood, puberty starts early for boys. Girls develop masculine traits (e.g., hirsutism), owing to increased secretion of male sex hormones by the adrenal glands.

> **Nursing Alert** Many young people, especially athletes, use large doses of steroids to enhance muscle development. This dangerous practice often leads to long-term disability and can be fatal. In addition to sexual dysfunction and heart dysrhythmias, the person is at risk for severe behavior problems. In some cases, the person becomes aggressive, loses touch with reality, or shows manic symptoms.

Treatment
Treatment depends on the cause. Surgical removal of the adrenal gland may be indicated. Adrenocortical hormones are given as indicated. After surgery, the client is treated as for Addison disease. If the cause is pituitary in origin, various controversial methods of treatment are possible.

Nursing Considerations
Nursing care primarily is symptomatic. Institute measures to protect the client from injury and infection, such as monitoring and protecting skin integrity, promoting good hygiene, and removing or minimizing environmental hazards. Monitor the client's weight daily and take vital signs frequently. Check electrolyte and glucose levels for changes.

Primary Aldosteronism

A rare condition of the adrenal cortex, primary aldosteronism is characterized by excessive secretion of aldosterone. Symptoms include hypertension and muscle weakness owing to low potassium levels. If tumors or excessive growth of the adrenal glands exist, surgery to remove the glands is the treatment of choice.

Addison Disease

Destruction or degeneration of the adrenal cortex causes a condition called **Addison disease**, a relatively rare disorder. Tuberculosis, cancer, or a massive infection can be the underlying cause, but in most cases, the gland *atrophies* (wastes away) for unknown reasons. It may be a secondary response to pituitary malfunction. In this case, the pituitary gland fails to produce ACTH in sufficient amounts; thus, adrenal function diminishes.

Signs and Symptoms
With Addison disease, the production of adrenal hormones decreases, resulting in fluid and electrolyte imbalances and hypoglycemia. In addition, thyroid function is abnormally low, with hyponatremia and hyperkalemia.

The first symptom is usually a darkening of the skin and oral mucous membranes so that the skin looks bronzed. Dehydration, anemia, and weight loss are seen. Blood pressure drops. The hair thins. Strain or stress of any kind may cause adrenal shock, with abnormally low blood pressure, nausea and vomiting, diarrhea, headache, and restlessness. Tremors and disorientation may arise, progressing to loss of consciousness and seizures.

Addisonian crisis occurs when adrenal function falls to a critically low point. This condition is marked by nausea, vomiting, weight loss, and extreme hypotension, leading to vascular shock, which can be fatal. A stressful situation is usually the precipitating factor.

Intravenous administration of hydrocortisone is the treatment of choice. In some cases, vasopressors, such as dopamine hydrochloride, are given to raise blood pressure. Salts (sodium and potassium ions) lost by vomiting are replaced in an IV solution of saline with added electrolytes. The exact solution and electrolyte content, to be given several times daily, are determined by the laboratory test results.

Treatment
Treatment consists of supplying needed hormones (fludrocortisone acetate [Florinef]) to restore normal fluid and electrolyte balance. Typically, the prescribed diet is high in protein and sodium and low in potassium.

Nursing Considerations
Because this client is dehydrated, fluid replacement is key. Because sodium loss results from previous hormone imbalance, sodium also must be replaced in the diet. Although water intake is restricted, increased sodium will aid in fluid retention without excess fluid intake. *Rationale: Excess water overloads the system.*

Five or six small meals per day may be prescribed, or the client may receive between-meal snacks of milk and crackers. *Rationale: The person may be too weak to eat a large meal at one time. The diet is planned to combat dehydration.*

Watch the person for dizziness or lowered blood pressure and protect them from falling. Accurately record all food and fluid intake, including the type and amount. Also document the volume and specific gravity of each voiding. Daily weights are important. *Rationale: All these measurements help determine the body's fluid and electrolyte balance. Therapy continues until these values are normal.*

Client teaching is vital. Enlist the client's cooperation and urge the client to maintain regular follow-up visits with their primary healthcare provider and avoid strain or stress, such as overwork, infection, or exposure to cold. By protecting their health, the client with Addison disease can do very well.

> **Key Concept**
> The client should wear an identification tag with instructions for hormone dosage in case the prescribing healthcare provider cannot be contacted.

Adrenal Neoplasms

Pheochromocytoma is a tumor, usually benign, that originates in the adrenal medulla. A tumor of the adrenal medulla increases secretion of the hormones epinephrine and norepinephrine, which in turn causes extreme hypertension, tremor, headache, nausea and vomiting, dizziness, and increased urination. Treatment is surgical removal of the tumor—a dangerous operation because it may cause sudden and extreme changes in blood pressure. Before surgery, a 24-hr urine test (VMA test) will be ordered to confirm the diagnosis. In addition, a CT scan of the adrenal glands, along with IV pyelogram (**IVP**), may be used to locate the tumor. After surgery, a repeat 24-hr urine for VMA and catecholamines will be done to evaluate return-to-normal levels. If the client has a bilateral adrenalectomy, they must be treated for Addison disease postoperatively; adrenal hormones must be supplied artificially for life.

PANCREATIC ENDOCRINE DISORDERS

Hormonal disorders of the pancreas include hypoinsulinism and hyperinsulinism. *Hyperinsulinism* is not common, but it may be a precursor to *hypoinsulinism*. Lowered amounts, lack of, or ineffective use of insulin leads to the disorders of *diabetes mellitus*. DM has various forms, including type 1 diabetes, type 2 diabetes, gestational diabetes, and impaired glucose tolerance or homeostasis. Understanding the various types, treatments, and implications of DM is critical for any healthcare provider.

Diabetes Mellitus

Specialized cells of the pancreas produce a hormone called *insulin* to regulate metabolism. Without this hormone, glucose cannot enter body cells and blood glucose levels rise. As a result, the individual may begin to experience symptoms of hyperglycemia. Simply stated, this process is the development of **DM**.

Individuals who are significantly overweight or obese have steadily increased in the percentage of the population starting in the late 20th and early 21st centuries. *Overweight* is the term related to having excess body weight for the individual specifics of height, fat, muscle, bone, water, or a combination of these factors. *Obesity* is the term associated with excess body fat. Being overweight or obese greatly increases risk factors for the development of diabetes type 1 or type 2. As a consequence of the trend of oversized individuals, the number of people with diabetes is expected to double as more the populace lives to middle and old age.

Diabetes in children and adolescents is occurring at a rate higher in the 21st century than in previous decades. (Refer to Chapter 73.) Significant healthcare research demonstrates that diabetes in childhood or adolescents is no longer the singular effect of autoimmune damage to the pancreas. Rather, diabetes in the young is commonly associated with the inadequacy of the pancreas to deal with the chronic high sugar content and resultant burden on the pancreas. The incidence of increased diabetes is related to the epidemic of childhood obesity which has doubled for children and quadrupled in adolescents in the past 30 years (CDC, 2014k). Overweight or obese children have a greater tendency for caloric imbalance and increased stress and an inadequately functioning pancreas. Non-Hispanic white children and adolescents had the highest rate of new cases of both diabetes type 1 and type 2.

Classification
- *Type 1* (formerly known as *type I; insulin-dependent diabetes mellitus* [**IDDM**]; or *juvenile diabetes*)
- *Type 2* (formerly known as *type II; non–insulin-dependent diabetes mellitus* [**NIDDM**]; or *adult-onset diabetes*)
- *Gestational diabetes mellitus* (**GDM**): Occurring during pregnancy and disappearing on delivery; these women are susceptible to the development of DM later in life.
- **Prediabetes** is a term that refers to the condition of *impaired glucose homeostasis* (**IGH**) that occurs when blood glucose levels are higher than normal but not high enough for the definitive diagnosis of diabetes mellitus. This condition may also be referred to as *impaired fasting glucose* (**IFG**) or impaired glucose tolerance (**IGT**). Prediabetes is considered a risk factor for future diabetes. It is often possible for individuals with prediabetes to delay or prevent the onset of type 2 diabetes with diet and lifestyle changes.

Diagnosis of prediabetes can be made by either the fasting plasma glucose test (FPG) or the oral glucose tolerance test (OGTT). These tests consist of the client fasting overnight with follow-up blood glucose monitoring (**BGM**) testing in the morning. The FPG consists of documenting the blood glucose level in the morning before eating. The OGTT consists of checking blood glucose levels in the morning with a follow-up test 2 hr after drinking a high glucose drink. Prediabetes is determined if the BGM falls between 100 and 125 mg/dL. The diagnosis of diabetes is considered if the level is above 126 mg/dL or higher on two separate occasions.

Signs and Symptoms
Diabetes can present a wide variety of signs and symptoms. Often clients have no symptoms; but, when present, they may include the "classic symptoms" of the three "polys": **polyuria** (excessive urination), **polydipsia** (excessive thirst), and **polyphagia** (excessive hunger). **Metabolic syndrome** is a combination of at least three conditions that are commonly found in a prediabetic or diagnosed diabetic state. These symptoms include abdominal obesity, hypertension, high blood glucose, insulin resistance and/or *dyslipidemia*. Dyslipidemia (abnormal amounts of fat in the blood) may include low high-density lipoprotein (HDL), elevated cholesterol, and elevated triglyceride levels. Metabolic syndrome is associated with the complications of both type 1 and type 2 diabetes.

The classic symptoms of polyuria, polydipsia, and polyphagia are found more often in type 1 diabetes and come on rapidly.

Other signs and symptoms may include the following:
- Fatigue
- Blurred vision
- Mood changes
- Numbness and tingling in extremities
- Dry skin
- Infections (urinary tract, vaginal yeast infections)
- Weight loss (most often in type 1)

Type 1 Diabetes Mellitus

Type 1 diabetes results from destruction of the pancreatic beta cells because the beta cells of the pancreas have been damaged or destroyed by an autoimmune process. Research has shown an inherited tendency for developing the disease. Environmental factors, lifestyles, or unknown factors may contribute to triggering the disease.

When type 1 diabetes is diagnosed, the goal is to achieve metabolic stabilization, restore body weight, and relieve symptoms of hyperglycemia. Ongoing goals focus on achieving and maintaining normal metabolic functions and minimizing the negative impact of diabetes on the person's life (see In Practice: Nursing Care Plan 79-1).

Type 2 diabetes can occur at any age. It is not uncommon for type 2 diabetes to occur in overweight adults older than 40 years or in the youth younger than 20 years. Prediabetes can be the precursor to fully symptomatic diabetes type 2. The pancreas is often still functional at diagnosis, which means it still produces insulin. Levels may be normal, low, or elevated. The person may show decreased tissue sensitivity to insulin, called *insulin resistance*. The individual is unable to make adequate amounts of insulin to overcome this resistance. In lieu of going into the cells, blood glucose gathers in the blood stream, causing hyperglycemia. The etiology for type 2 diabetes is not clearly understood. Genetics, family lifestyle, and nutritional habits are some of the risk factors. Commonly—but not always—diabetes type 2 individuals are overweight or obese. Revision of lifestyle and weight loss are very beneficial to clients with prediabetes or type 2 diabetes. Initially, these clients do not depend on insulin injections to maintain blood sugar levels. They may require oral antidiabetic agents that will promote the production of insulin. It is not uncommon for an individual with type 2 diabetes to eventually need supplements of subcutaneous insulin for adequate glucose control.

Risk factors for developing diabetes include being overweight or obese, age, stress, and lack of exercise. Many of these factors combine to form a lifestyle characterized by inadequate eating habits and minimal physical exercise, which often reflects family habits that are passed on to new generations, leading to future problems. In addition to these controllable risk factors, the individual with type 2 diabetes may have an inherited tendency to develop diabetes type 1. Race is a risk factor for diabetes, as it occurs more often in clients who are African American, Hispanic, American Indian, and Asian American. Gestational diabetes and prediabetes are also known factors that preview the onset of diabetes. Other disorders are known to occur more often in the diabetic population. These conditions include high blood pressure, high triglycerides and abnormal cholesterol levels, metabolic syndrome, and, in women, polycystic ovary syndrome. The specific etiology of type 2 diabetes is yet unknown; however, autoimmune destruction of pancreatic beta cells does *not* occur. Combinations of factors are stronger indications for the development of diabetes than any single factor.

Most clients with this form of diabetes are significantly overweight or obese, which can cause some degree of insulin resistance. The muscle cells of obese people are less responsive to insulin than are the muscle cells of thinner people, and most glucose breakdown occurs in the muscle cells. Without the normal response to insulin in the muscle cells, the cells cannot take up glucose, leading to increased glucose concentration in the bloodstream (hyperglycemia).

Clients who are not obese may have an increased percentage of body fat in their abdominal regions. Ketoacidosis (see "Hyperglycemia" section) seldom occurs but may arise in the presence of another illness. Type 2 diabetes can remain undiagnosed for many years. Because hyperglycemia develops gradually, clients may not notice any classic diabetes symptoms. However, they are at increased risk for development of *macrovascular* (large blood vessels) and *microvascular* (small blood vessels) complications, discussed later in this chapter.

Diagnosis of diabetes is based on the results of a variety of factors. The individual with a body mass index of 25 who has coexisting conditions such as hypertension, a history of heart disease, high cholesterol levels, and a sedentary lifestyle needs evaluation of blood glucose levels. Other preconditions or risk factors include giving birth to an infant weighing more than 9 lb (4 kg), having a history of gestational diabetes, and having a close relative with diabetes. Anyone older than 45 years should receive basic blood screening (e.g., HA1c at least every 3 years) if a normal level below 5.7 results. HA1c levels of 6.5 or higher on two occasions indicate diabetes. HA1c levels are between 5.7 and 6.4 are considered prediabetes. Other blood glucose tests include the random blood sugar test, fasting blood sugar, and the oral glucose tolerance test.

The major goals of treatment are to achieve metabolic control and to prevent vascular complications. Recommended treatment includes meal planning, an exercise program, weight loss, and medication, if needed. Weight management is a primary concern because losing as little as 5–10 lb can significantly improve blood glucose control.

> **Key Concept**
>
> In type 1 diabetes, insulin deficiency is absolute; insulin injections are necessary for survival. In type 2 diabetes, insulin deficiency ranges from insulin resistance with relative insulin deficiency to a predominantly secretory defect with insulin resistance.

Treatment

Continuous research of diabetes has resulted in significant and changing information about diabetes. To simplify this vast amount of information, the nurse and the client should focus on the three main areas that support stabilized normal blood glucose levels:

1. Carefully plan a therapeutic diet that promotes good nutrition.
2. Maintain an individualized exercise plan.
3. Monitor medication effects and side effects.

The client's understanding of and adherence to a personalized treatment program greatly improves its effectiveness. Priority concerns involve regular BGM. BGM is achieved by standardized, personal handheld meters that are used in home or in healthcare facilities for frequent monitoring. Blood glucose levels are also periodically obtained by the laboratory tests called *glycosylated hemoglobin* (HA1c), which is written as a percentage, or an eAG, which is written as units in milligrams/deciliter (mg/dL). The HA1c is an average of blood glucose levels over the previous 2–3 months.

CHAPTER 79 Endocrine Disorders

IN PRACTICE
NURSING CARE PLAN 79-1: The Client With Type 1 Diabetes

Medical History: D. W., a 24-year-old male client, diagnosed with diabetes mellitus type 1 approximately 6 months ago, comes to the clinic for a follow-up visit. Fasting blood glucose this morning was 210 mg/dL. Vital signs are within acceptable parameters. Currently, they are prescribed insulin twice daily, in the morning and before dinner, with self-monitoring of blood glucose (SMBG) level before meals and at bedtime. Client states, "I forgot to check my blood and take my shot last night before dinner."

Medical Diagnosis: Diabetes mellitus, type 1, poorly controlled.

DATA COLLECTION/NURSING OBSERVATION

Client is an active 24-year-old sales executive. The client reports skipping meals several times a week. "When I'm on the road, I stop to get some fast food, like french fries and a milkshake." The client reports that they have not been keeping a log of their blood glucose results. They stated, "I'm too busy and I don't always have my monitor with me. So I forget." History reveals that client performs SMBG levels on the average of once a day. They state that they have been taking their insulin as prescribed but does admit to forgetting insulin on the average of one to two times per week. "I can give myself the injection without a problem. I just can't remember to do all these things."

NURSING DIAGNOSIS

(Although other nursing diagnoses may be appropriate, a priority nursing diagnosis is addressed below.)

Ineffective diabetes management related to lack of knowledge about control of blood glucose and difficulty integrating diabetes into daily routine as evidenced by client's statements of skipping meals, irregular insulin administration, and poor coordination of diabetic health needs into daily activities.

PLANNING (OUTCOMES/GOALS)	IMPLEMENTATION (NURSING ACTIONS)	EVALUATION
Short-Term Goals		
A. Client will verbalize the importance of adhering to prescribed regimen.	• Question client about usual activities for the day, including time spent in car on the road, at the office, and at home. • Work with the client to develop a plan for their daily schedule that includes the important aspects of the diabetic regimen. • Demonstrate the documentation of blood sugar and insulin administration in log. **Rationale:** *Determining the client's usual activities helps to develop an individualized plan for this client. Working with the client provides the client an opportunity to participate in the plan, providing them with some feelings of control over the situation.* • Review underlying physiologic components of the disorder and rationale for specific monitoring activities. **Rationale:** *Review of information reinforces the necessity and the reasons for adhering to the regimen.*	Clinic Visit—Day 1, 1,100 hr. • States, "I didn't realize that this disorder could be so long lasting and harmful. I thought a few shots would fix it." • Demonstrates techniques for blood glucose monitoring and insulin injection without difficulty. • Documents clinic glucometer's values and insulin into log book. • Reports understanding of the necessity and use of documentation. **Goal A not met.** Observations continue.
B. Coordinate dietary needs with dietician and spouse, who typically cooks meals at home.	• Consult dietitian to help with food choices. • Offer suggestions for appropriate food choices when client is on the road. • Coordinate team meetings with nurse, dietician, and spouse. **Rationale:** *Offering suggestions in conjunction with help from a dietitian provides the client with some alternatives and choices, enhancing their feelings of control over the situation. Family involvement with diet, exercise, and medication is a strong, valuable source of positive feedback. Family involvement encourages an overall nutritional improvement and dietary adjustment. Future meetings will need to be scheduled to reinforce past learning as well as to introduce new concepts of dietary maintenance, e.g., meals when traveling.*	Clinic Visit—Day 1, 1,100 hr. • Spouse states they understand the need for changes of some of the food habits. • Family willing to review Internet resources and dietary references provided by dietician. • Discussion planned for meals when client traveling on business. **Goal B met.**

PLANNING (OUTCOMES/ GOALS)	IMPLEMENTATION (NURSING ACTIONS)	EVALUATION
C. Client will demonstrate understanding of diet as part of diabetes management.	• Suggest individualized approach to buying food for the need of the client with diabetes; compare these choices with the existing habits of family purchases. • Suggest and document a 1-week meal plan for client when he is out of town. • Provide feedback and direction to food choices. • Anticipate blood sugar levels range from 110 to 145 mg/dL. *Rationale: Having the client propose methods for self-control promotes participation in their care. Incorporating family and spouse, who does majority of meal preparation, provides a sense of control over the situation. Chances for success and adherence to new habits improved with assistance of family environment.* • Discuss the correlation among diet, activity, and insulin. • Reinforce the need for a well-balanced diet with periodic snacks. *Rationale: Discussing the interconnection among diet, activity, and insulin helps to stress the need for adherence to the regimen.*	Clinic Visit—Day 7, 1,300 hr. • Family met as a group to develop a revised grocery list for the newly diagnosed diabetic. • Client and spouse went grocery shopping together with new, revised grocery list. • Client talking about ways to make sure they eat when out on the road. Stated, "I really need to take better care of myself. It's more work than I thought it would be. My spouse is worried about me." • After use of dietary changes, client stated that the last 3 days of blood glucose levels each morning ranged from 95 to 128 mL/dL. • Stated that the written log helps them to understand the connection between food, blood sugar, and insulin. **Goals B and C met.** Progress to meeting Goal A.
Long-Term Goals		

D. Client will demonstrate ability to integrate diabetes into their lifestyle.	• Arrange for follow-up visit for client with phone call follow-up for review of log and activities in
	  • 2 days
	  • 3 days
	  • 2 weeks
	  • 3 weeks
	  • 1 month
	
	Rationale: Follow-up provides a means for determining adherence to instructions and plan. Positive reinforcement and understanding of complexity of changes will help client maintain new lifestyle and medication regimen.
		Postdischarge phone calls
		Day 2—Stated that client will take fresh fruit with them to work and have some snacks available when on the road.
		Day 3—Verbalized appropriate food choices and times for insulin administration and blood glucose monitoring.
		Week 2–Reported blood glucose levels range from 92 to 130 mL/dL over the last week.
		1 month—Reported food choices seem to make blood sugar more stable. Stated, "I am ordering fresh foods and baked meats when traveling."
		Goal C met.
		Goal D partially met; blood sugar levels improving. Observations ongoing.

The numbers of an eAG resemble the readings of a standard handheld blood glucose monitor. The goals of treatment for diabetes include the following:

- Relief of symptoms
- Maintenance of normal weight
- Achievement of normal activity
- Maintenance of average daily blood glucose levels between 70 and 140 mg/dL (or as stated by a specific healthcare provider)
- Achievement of acceptable levels on HA1c or eAG laboratory tests
- Prevention of long-term and short-term complications
- Prevention of hypoglycemic and hyperglycemic reactions

Diet and Nutrition Therapy

Diet and nutrition therapy in diabetes is based on an individualized care plan of needs. The dietitian generally is responsible for establishing baseline parameters for the client's diet. The nurse reinforces the needs of nutrition and promotes the special needs of the client with diabetes, encourages diet maintenance, and provides client and family support.

To develop the most individualized dietary plan for the client, the following factors must be considered:

- Degree of diabetes control
- Presence of complications such as infection, decreased cardiovascular stamina, or neuropathies
- Presence of difficulties such as visual problems, the inability to prepare meals, or financial concerns
- Adequacy of current nutrient intake; usual eating habits, including snacks
- Intake of saturated and unsaturated fats
- Ability to read and understand food labels
- Treatment goals
- Personal schedule and lifestyle
- Measurement of the levels of carbohydrates or the glycemic index (GI)
- Client's medication regimen

In the early phases of nutritional therapy, clients are often encouraged to obtain blood glucose levels before and after meals. Individuals will vary in their responses to carbohydrates; thus, the glycemic index will vary from person to person. The results of BGM provide the client, the healthcare provider, and the dietitian with a more individualized picture of the client and their response to the diet. Thus, the healthcare team has a better understanding of how specific foods affect the individual's glucose level and can adjust foods or medications accordingly.

There are several ways to manage nutrition and diet therapy but all should begin with consultation with a diabetic specialist and/or a registered dietitian. Guidelines for the client with diabetes focuses on three main concepts. First, eat a variety of healthful foods. Second, eat smaller amounts of protein foods and fewer high-fat foods. Third, balance the carbohydrates eaten with insulin and exercise. *Carbohydrate counting* is one basic method of helping the individual with diabetes maintain blood glucose levels. The individual needs to understand that calories, that is, glucose, come from three sources of food: carbohydrates, proteins, and fat. Carbohydrates are the main nutrient that affects blood glucose levels. Within 2–3 hr after eating a carbohydrate, most of it has been changed to glucose (blood sugar). Proteins and fats have less effect on the blood glucose but are necessary to maintain a stable blood glucose level. The total amount of carbohydrate is more important than the source. Counting carbohydrates can be simpler and less structured than some meal-planning approaches because the client focuses on one nutrient rather than on several nutrients, such as proteins and fats.

Another way to introduce clients to basic nutritional guidelines is through the USDA's Dietary Guidelines for Americans, 2015–2020. Not often used, but still available, is the Diabetic Exchange List Diet. Exchange lists group foods together because they are similar, that is, they have about the same amount of carbohydrates, meat or proteins, fats, and calories per serving. Clients can interchange selections from several lists, such as fruit, starch, and milk. The dietitian or the nurse can demonstrate a typical meal pattern to the client. A simplified example could include dividing the plate into quarters, which should encourage smaller portions. Two quarters of the plate are starchy and nonstarchy (carbohydrate) foods, such as vegetables. Proteins make up one quarter and fats, drinks, or fruits make up the remainder. With any meal planning program, initial and follow-up appointments with a dietitian are important.

Resources on the Internet are numerous. Information regarding nutrition and diet therapy, medications, current research, and support groups can be found on Websites, such as those for the American Dietetic Association, American Association of Diabetes Educators, and the American Diabetes Association. Students should note that these professional sites often have basic information designed for the client with diabetes as well as more in-depth information designed for healthcare providers. Many professional Websites include access to free educational booklets, interactive pages, and informative videos.

Exercise

Although exercise is an important aspect of health promotion for all persons, it is a therapeutic tool for clients with or at risk for diabetes. Exercise increases circulation, helps control weight, decreases blood pressure, and reduces stress. It also helps regulate blood glucose levels. Effects will depend on the individual client and the type of diabetes. Clients must learn which effects may occur, as well as how to reduce the risk of hyperglycemia or hypoglycemia. This understanding is important because their bodies cannot compensate for changes in the same manner as can individuals who do not have diabetes.

Before beginning an exercise program, individuals with diabetes will undergo a detailed medical evaluation with appropriate diagnostic studies. Medical history and physical examination will focus on signs and symptoms that affect the heart and blood vessels, eyes, kidneys, and nervous system. Clients learn to properly warm up before and cool down after exercise. Precautions involving the feet are essential for people with diabetes. Proper hydration is also important because dehydration can adversely affect blood glucose levels and heart function. Clients must take precautions when exercising in extremely hot or cold environments.

Clients who use medications to control their blood glucose levels must understand the relationship of exercise to food intake and medication use and learn how and when to exercise. For those with type 1 diabetes, all levels of exercise, including leisure activities, recreational sports, and competitive professional performance, may be appropriate if they have effective glucose control. Exercise does not control this type of diabetes; thus, the purpose of exercise is for its multiple health benefits. These clients must learn to monitor blood glucose level before and after exercise, to ingest added carbohydrates if glucose levels are under 100 mg/dL, and to maintain adequate hydration. Making appropriate insulin adjustments based on blood glucose readings is essential.

The possible benefits of exercise for clients with type 2 diabetes are substantial. Long-term studies have shown that regular exercise helps improve carbohydrate metabolism, insulin sensitivity, and blood glucose control. Other possible benefits include weight loss and reduction of hyperlipidemia. The benefits of exercise in the prevention and management of type 2 diabetes are probably greatest when clients start early in the disease's progression.

Insulin

The goal of insulin therapy is to mimic the body's natural levels of this endogenous hormone. Normally, insulin levels fluctuate and adjust to the daily variations of blood glucose level. Proper insulin management is essential to ensure the longevity of the client with diabetes. If insulin were to be taken orally, digestive enzymes would destroy the effectiveness of the hormone; therefore, all insulin products are given by parenteral routes, such as subcutaneous injection, IV drip, IV, or injection (IVP; intravenous push). *All liquid insulins can be given subcutaneously, but only regular insulin can be given both subcutaneously and intravenously.*

Insulin concentrations are based on a standard 100 U/mL in the United States. Insulin syringes are designed to hold 100 or 50 U/0.5 mL. Insulins in the United States are synthetic human insulin derived from genetically engineered bacteria. The older animal-based (pork or beef) insulins may be available in other countries.

> **Nursing Alert** In some parts of Europe and Latin America, insulin may be found in the U-40 system (40 U/mL). The U-40 and U-100 systems are NOT compatible. Each system's dose must use the matching system's syringe. If traveling, the client must be sure to have the correct and matching measurement system of insulin/mL and syringes. U-40 insulin syringes have a red cap and red markings. U-100 syringes have an orange cap and black markings.

Onset, Peak, and Duration

The four main categories of insulin are separated according to the concepts of onset, peak, and duration (Table 79-3). *Onset* refers to the time that the insulin begins to become effective (starts to lower blood glucose). *Peak* occurs when the insulin has reached its maximum ability to lower blood glucose. *Duration* is the length of time that the insulin remains active (continues to lower blood glucose). Onset and duration time intervals typically do not have the same therapeutic strength as do insulins at their peak. Dosages of insulin are based on the individual insulin's therapeutic effects, which are designed to provide insulin through a specific length of time. The nurse and the client must be aware of these concepts because hyper- or hypoglycemic episodes may occur during the day based on the three factors of onset, peak, and duration.

Types of Insulin

The four main types or categories of insulin include the following:

1. **Ultrarapid, short-acting regular insulin**
   - Insulin analogues: lispro (Humalog), aspart (NovoLog), glulisine (Apidra)
   - Clear solutions
   - May be mixed in same syringe with intermediate-acting insulin
   - Typically given 10–15 min before a meal
   - Duration can be up to 5 hr, but typical duration is approximately 3 hr
2. **Rapid, short-acting, regular human insulin**
   - Biosynthetic recombinant DNA technology: Humulin R, Novolin R
   - Clear solutions
   - May be mixed in same syringe with intermediate-acting insulin
   - Typically given 30–60 min before a meal
   - May be given intravenously or subcutaneously
   - Duration is typically about 5 hr, but ranges from 3 to 10 hr
3. **Neutral protamine Hagedorn (NPH) insulin**
   - Biosynthetic DNA technology (Humulin N, Novolin N) and analogue mixtures
   - Cloudy solutions because NPH insulin contains regular insulin plus insulin bound in suspension to protamine or to zinc
   - Insulin released gradually from the protamine or zinc, producing a prolonged onset, peak, and duration
   - Goal is to provide one insulin injection that has both a rapid onset and a long duration (from 12 to 24 hr)
   - Examples of mixtures of biosynthetic NPH and regular insulin: Humulin 50/50 (50% NPH insulin and 50% regular insulin); Humulin 70/30 (70% NPH insulin and 30% regular insulin); Novolin 70/30 (70% NPH insulin and 30% regular insulin)
   - Examples of mixtures of analogue insulins include the use of ultrarapid insulin (lispro, aspart) and protamine analogue mixtures: Humalog 75/25 (75% lispro protamine suspension and 25% lispro solution); NovoLog 70/30 (70% aspart protamine suspension and 30% aspart solution)
4. **Long-acting insulin**
   - Synthetic insulins—analogues: glargine (Lantus), detemir (Levemir)
   - Absorbed in fairly uniform time frame without large fluctuations in insulin levels; thus, no typical "peak" is achieved and the client has a reduced chance of hypoglycemic episodes
   - Should not be mixed with any other insulins
   - Regular insulin in zinc suspension for extended release (Ultralente)
   - May last 24 hr or more

> **Nursing Alert** The "R" after an insulin means that the insulin is "regular" or short-acting insulin. The "N" stands for NPH or intermediate-acting insulin. The "L" indicates a long-acting insulin. DO NOT confuse or substitute one insulin for another type of insulin!

TABLE 79-3 Examples of Types of Insulins[a]

TYPE OF INSULIN	ONSET OF ACTION	PEAK EFFECT	DURATION OF EFFECT	CHARACTERISTICS
Regular, Short-Acting				
Ultrarapid regular • lispro (Humalog) • aspart (NovoLog) • glulisine (Apidra)	15–30 min	30 min–1½ hr	3–4, up to 5 hr	Clear Give just before a meal May be mixed with intermediate-acting insulins
Regular human • Humulin-R • Novolin R	½–1 hr	2–3, up to 5 hr	3–5, up to 10 hr	Clear May be given IV or SQ May be mixed with intermediate-acting insulins
Intermediate-Acting				
Isophane (protamine) suspension (NPH) • Humulin N • Novolin N	1–4 hr	6–10 hr	10–16, up to 24 hr	Cloudy Do not mix with other insulins
Zinc suspension • Humulin L • Novolin L	1–4 hr	6–12, up to 15 hr	12–20, up to 28 hr	Cloudy Do not mix with other insulins
Mixtures, NPH and regular • Humulin 50/50 • Humulin 70/30 • Novolin 70/30	30 min–1 hr	4–8 hr 4–12 hr 2–12 hr	10–16, up to 24 hr	Cloudy Do not mix with other insulins
Long-Acting				
Synthetic analogues • glargine (Lantus) • detemir (Levemir)	1–2, up to 5 hr	None	24 hr	Do not mix with other insulins
Zinc extended suspension • Ultralente	4–8, up to 10 hr	8–12, up to 16 hr	18–20, up to 36 hr	Cloudy Do not mix with other insulins

[a]Note to student: Onset, peak, and duration times vary with each client and with each type of insulin. The time frames given are estimated averages with ranges based on data collected from several sources.
IV, intravenous; SQ, subcutaneously.

Inhaled Insulin

A separate category included an insulin inhalation powder, Afrezza, which is a human insulin introduced to the public in 2014. Exubera, an earlier inhaled insulin, is no longer available. The inhalation method seemed to be an effective method of decreasing the number of daily injections and new research may result in inhaled insulins in the future.

Other Diabetic Injectable Medication

Normal body chemistry uses amylin, insulin, and glucagon to regulate blood glucose levels. A synthetic drug pramlintide (Symlin) is based on the hormone amylin, which is produced by the beta cells in the pancreas as is the hormone insulin. Pramlintide, which is injected at meal times, helps to improve average blood glucose levels (HA1c or eAG). It cannot be combined with insulin and, therefore, must be injected separately.

Use, Care, and Storage

Insulin deteriorates when it is exposed to excessive heat, cold, light, or agitation. Constant refrigeration is unnecessary as long as the client uses the vial within 30 days. Instruct clients to refrigerate extra bottles until they are needed.

Insulin preparations may be mixed to meet an individual's needs. Clients using regular insulin alone at breakfast may have elevated glucose levels by noon. To correct this condition, they may also take a prescribed amount of intermediate-acting insulin. These mixtures can be administered in the same syringe. Syringes may be prepared up to 3 weeks in advance and refrigerated. If 70/30 is the right proportion, Novolin 70/30 or Humulin 70/30 can be used. If lispro is prescribed, clients administer single doses before each meal, and administer intermediate- or long-acting insulin only once or twice a day as prescribed. Sometimes, clients use both regular and lispro insulin before meals. Many combinations can help individuals maintain good glucose control.

When administering insulin in a prefilled syringe to a client, roll and invert the syringe before administration to mix the solution well. Roll and invert insulin between the hands. Do not shake a vial. Shaking causes air bubbles to form, which would alter the dosage.

Vials or prefilled syringes should be crystal clear (regular insulin or lispro) or milky white, depending on the type of insulin. Discard if the liquid is discolored. Also discard vials that do not easily resuspend when you roll them. Other signs of unusable insulin are frosting or coating on the bottle (especially with NPH) and any settling or clumping. Note the expiration date printed on the side of the vial and do not use contents after that date. Make sure insulin is not decomposed. If in doubt, throw it out! Double-checking insulin dosages helps to prevent errors in the healthcare facility; adapt these guidelines for client and family teaching.

> **Key Concept**
>
> If regular and NPH insulin are to be mixed, the regular insulin must be drawn up first, after injecting air into both vials. Remember: "Clear to partly cloudy."

Insulin Coverage

Many people who have diabetes experience difficulty regulating insulin when they become ill, particularly from infections. For this reason, clients with diabetes who are hospitalized, regardless of the reason for hospitalization, almost always undergo routine blood testing for glucose and often have insulin coverage to control elevated blood glucose levels. The healthcare provider determines a sliding scale of regular insulin, based on the blood glucose levels. Clients receive this coverage three to six times per day, in addition to their usual intermediate-acting dose. Many clients whose conditions are usually well controlled with oral diabetes medications may require insulin during the course of an operation, pregnancy, or systemic disease. A client's insulin requirements are likely to increase during disease and other stressful events.

> **Nursing Alert** Many facilities require another nurse to double-check insulin before it is administered. Even if the facility does not have such a policy, it is a good idea. A tiny error in insulin dosage can cause serious adverse reactions.

Insulin Pumps

Insulin pumps are mechanical devices that inject insulin automatically (Fig. 79-4). They attempt to mimic pancreatic function by releasing insulin continuously to maintain an acceptable blood glucose level. Clients also may inject a bolus before eating.

Development continues with small implantable devices that automatically monitor blood glucose levels and deliver the appropriate insulin directly into the bloodstream. A type of insulin called *buffered regular* is often used in the pump. This insulin is not used in any other way.

Antidiabetic Medications

Insulin itself is ineffective orally, but several groups of medications given orally can lower the blood glucose levels of some clients with type 2 diabetes. These agents are not oral forms of insulin and are not to be regarded as insulin substitutes. Oral agents act within 2–6 hr, with effects lasting between 8 and 60 hr. Some oral hypoglycemic agents are

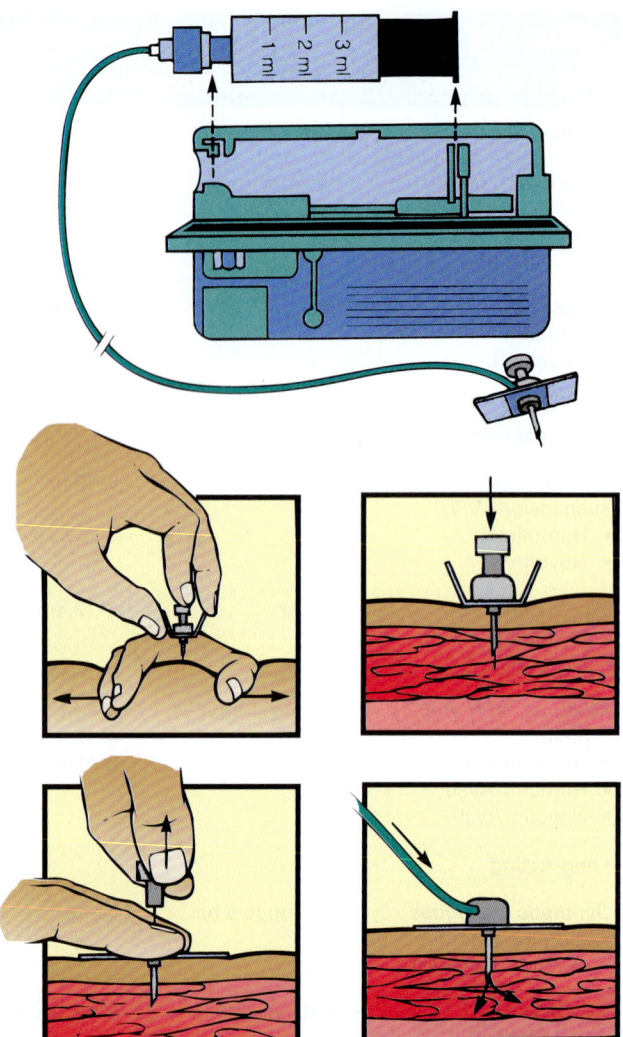

Figure 79-4 The insulin pump. Usually attached to the client's clothing, this external insulin pump has an insulin-filled syringe that is attached to a subcutaneous needle via tubing.

given two to three times per day. They can cause hypoglycemia. Four major mechanisms cause blood glucose levels to elevate in clients with type 2 diabetes. These are as follows:

- Impaired insulin secretion
- Altered carbohydrate absorption
- Increased basal hepatic glucose production
- Decreased insulin-stimulated glucose uptake

Several major categories of oral antidiabetic agents act to interfere with one or more of these mechanisms (Fig. 79-5). These categories include sulfonylureas, biguanides, alpha-glucosidase inhibitors, and thiazolidinediones. Another category is the insulin secretagogues or nonsulfonylurea hypoglycemic agents (meglitinides), which help the pancreas to make more insulin. An injectable medication called exenatide (Byetta), in a class of drugs known as incretin mimetics, is available; it is designed to lower blood glucose levels primarily by increasing insulin secretion.

Agents used to control blood glucose may be used in combinations (e.g., a sulfonylurea and metformin or a metformin and insulin). Box 79-1 and Table 79-4 review the major medications used for diabetes.

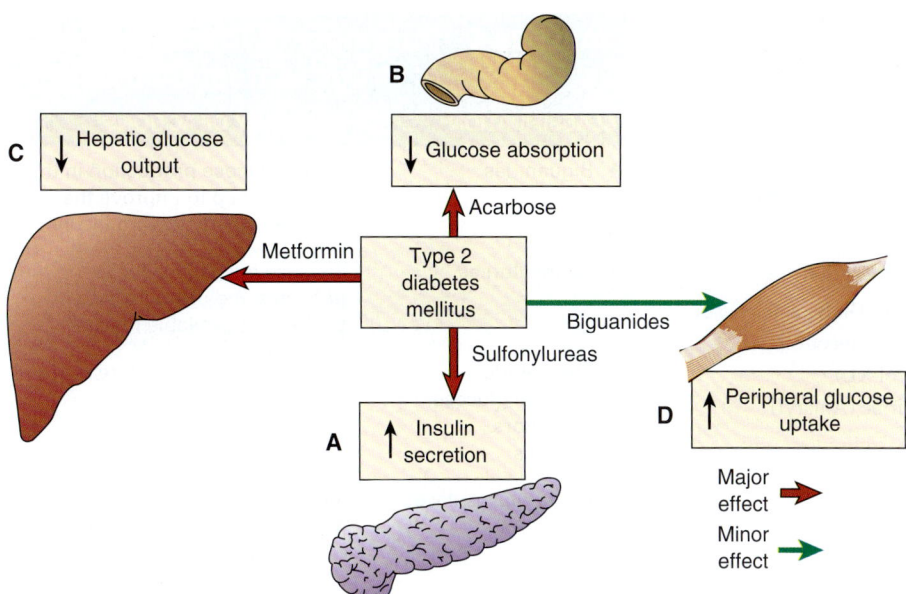

Figure 79-5 Oral hypoglycemic drugs use various mechanisms to lower blood glucose levels. There are several categories of oral hypoglycemic agents: sulfonylureas, biguanides (metformin), alpha-glucosidase inhibitors (acarbose), and thiazolidinediones. These drugs have various effects on the body to lower blood glucose levels. Note how the different categories of drugs have one or more of the following effects: (A) increases insulin secretion from the pancreas; (B) increases glucose absorption by the cells; (C) decreases production of glucose from the liver; and (D) increases the use of glucose by peripheral tissues.

The actions of the sulfonylureas (Diabinese, Glucotrol, DiaBeta, Micronase) are not fully understood. These medications are thought to stimulate the pancreas to produce more insulin, to improve the use of insulin at the cell's receptor sites, or to increase the effectiveness of endogenous insulin. Because they stimulate the pancreas to produce more insulin, they are useful only for people with type 2 diabetes who still produce their own (*endogenous*) insulin.

> **Nursing Alert** Advise clients receiving oral hypoglycemic agents or insulin about the use of alcohol; alcohol can exaggerate the hypoglycemic effect of these drugs. Alert clients that if they drink alcohol, they should do so in moderation and consume it with food (e.g., wine at mealtime).

Metformin (Glucophage), a biguanide, works by preventing the liver from overproducing glucose. Metformin does not increase insulin secretion and, thus, does not cause hypoglycemia. This drug is useful for clients who experience early morning fasting hypoglycemia. It is sometimes given to clients who are also taking sulfonylureas. Future types of metformin may be in the form of delayed-release capsules. Acarbose (Precose) and miglitol (Glyset) are alpha-glucosidase inhibitors that block enzymes that break down dietary starches so that starches can be absorbed more slowly in the small intestine. It helps clients who experience rapid increases in blood glucose after meals.

Clients can use oral antidiabetic medications alone or in combination with each other or with insulin. *Bedtime insulin and daytime sulfonylureas* (**BIDS**) is one such combination.

Glucophage and Precose do not cause hypoglycemia. However, when they are combined with drugs that do, dramatic lowering of blood glucose levels can occur. The client's participation through **SMBG** level is important in determining which pills or combinations to use and how effectively the medication regimen controls blood glucose levels.

Sulfonylureas are a class of antidiabetic agents for type 2 diabetes that typically end in "ide." Their purpose is to increase available stores and the effectiveness of insulin. They are also known as *secretagogues,* because they help the pancreas to *secrete* insulin. Examples include glyburide (*DiaBeta, Glynase*), glipizide (*Glucotrol, Glucotrol XL*), and *glimepiride* (*Amaryl*). Weight gain and hypoglycemia are fairly common side effects with this class of drugs.

For many years, a goal of diabetic management was to prevent an overflow of sugar from the blood into the kidneys and into the urine. However, a new category of antidiabetic agents work by inhibiting this mechanism so that sugar can be eliminated via the urinary system. These oral drugs are known as sodium-glucose transporter-2 inhibitors or *SGLT2 inhibitors*. Examples of SGLT2-inhibitors include canagliflozin (Invokamet, Invokana), dapagliflozin (Farxiga, Xigduo), and empagliflozin (Jardiance).

Another goal for diabetic medications involves drugs that are longer lasting. It is known that the intestines release the hormone GLP-1, which notifies the pancreas to increase insulin production. Medications called *GLP-1 receptor agonists* last several hours so that once-a-day injections can be given. Examples include liraglutide (Victoza). Drugs lasting 7 days are in process of production and include albiglutide (Tanzeum), dulaglutide (Trulicity), and the extended-release exenatide (Bydureon).

Pancreas Transplantation

Experimentation with pancreas transplantation in clients with diabetes has been under way for many years. Success has been limited because of the high rate of transplant rejection, but with new antirejection medications, results are improving. Research has also shown some success in implanting only the beta cells from the islets of Langerhans.

Complications of Diabetes Mellitus

Hypoglycemic Reaction

Doses of insulin (or oral diabetes medications) are calculated to control blood glucose levels. Too much insulin in relation to the amount of glucose reduces this level

Box 79-1 Categories and Examples of Major Antidiabetic Agents

Biguanides
- metformin (Glucophage)
- metformin extended release (Fortamet, Glucophage XR)

Sulfonylureas (Secretagogues)

First generation	Second generation
tolbutamide (Tol-Tab)	glyburide (DiaBeta, Glynase)
tolazamide (Tolinase)	glipizide (Glucotrol, Glucotrol XL)
acetohexamide (Dymelor)	
chlorpropamide (Diabinese)	glimepiride (Amaryl)

Meglitinides/prandial glucose regulators/glinides (short-acting secretagogues)
- repaglinide (Prandin)
- nateglinide (Starlix)

Alpha-glucosidase inhibitors
- acarbose (Precose)
- miglitol (Glyset)

Thiazolidinediones (TZDs)
- pioglitazone (Actos)

DPP-4 inhibitors/gliptins
- sitagliptin (Januvia)
- vildagliptin (Galvus)
- saxagliptin (Onglyza)
- linagliptin (Tradjenta)

Incretin mimetics/GLP-1 analogues (subcutaneous injection)
- exenatide (Byetta, Bydureon)
- liraglutide (Victoza)

Amylin analogues (subcutaneous injection)
- pramlintide (Symlin)

Bile acid sequestrants
- colesevelam (WelChol)

Combination pills: Use to maximize effectiveness of individual drug's actions
- pioglitazone and metformin (Actoplus Met)
- glyburide and metformin (Glucovance)
- glipizide and metformin (Metaglip)
- sitagliptin and metformin (Janumet)
- saxagliptin and metformin (Kombiglyze)
- repaglinide and metformin (PrandiMet)
- pioglitazone and glimepiride (Duetact)

Adapted from https://www.webmd.com/diabetes/default.htm and www.diabetes.co.uk/Diabetes-drugs.html.

TABLE 79-4 Summary of Classifications of Drugs to Treat Diabetes

CLASSIFICATION	SUMMARY OF ACTIONS
Biguanides	Inhibit glucose production in the liver and help to improve the cells' sensitivity toward insulin
Sulfonylureas	Increase insulin production in the pancreas and promote the effectiveness of available insulin
Meglitinides Prandial glucose regulators Glinides	Similar to the sulfonylureas but act for a shorter time
Alpha-glucosidase inhibitors	Inhibit the digestion of carbohydrates in the small intestine and reduce postprandial blood glucose spikes
Thiazolidinediones (TZDs) Glitazones	Stimulate the production of insulin; improve sensitivity to insulin for type 2 diabetics; and reduce the production of glucagon
DPP-4 inhibitors Gliptins	Decrease release of glucagon
Incretin mimetics GLP-1 analogues	Similar to DPP4 inhibitors that decrease the release of glucagon. Mimic production of insulin. Injectable treatment for type 2 diabetes
Amylin analogue	A hormone produced in small amounts by the pancreas that helps to suppress glucagon release and limit postprandial blood glucose levels. Injectable for type 2 diabetes
Bile acid sequestrants	Used with other antidiabetic agents to lower blood glucose.
Insulin	A natural or synthetically produced hormone which regulates blood glucose

Adapted from https://www.webmd.com/diabetes/default.htm and www.diabetes.co.uk/Diabetes-drugs.html.

Signs and Symptoms

In hypoglycemia, the client experiences symptoms of excess adrenaline, which the body releases in response to a low blood glucose level. Suddenly, the person feels weak, cold, and exhausted. This is followed by feelings of hunger and nervousness. The client trembles and perspires and may also experience headache, drowsiness, nausea, and vomiting. Without treatment, other symptoms develop, such as dizziness, confusion, combative behaviors, and speech loss. The person is unable to control body movements. Vision is double or blurry; if the condition is still untreated, seizures, loss of consciousness, and permanent brain damage may develop, sometimes causing death.

below normal. It causes a reaction called **hypoglycemia** (once called *insulin shock*). Hypoglycemia usually means that the person with diabetes has a blood glucose level of under 70 mg/dL. Table 79-5 compares hypoglycemia with hyperglycemia.

TABLE 79-5 Hypoglycemia Versus Hyperglycemia

	HYPOGLYCEMIC REACTION[a] (INSULIN REACTION)	HYPERGLYCEMIA (ACIDOSIS, DIABETIC KETOACIDOSIS, "DIABETIC COMA")
Reason	Too much insulin (blood glucose too low); also caused by too little food or too much exercise	Too little insulin (a frequent occurrence during a systemic infection); ketosis results from upset in acid–base balance
Onset	Sudden (may occur in clients who use insulin or who are taking oral hypoglycemics)	Slow—several hours to days (more rapid in active child)
Causes	Skipped meals, overdose of insulin, overexertion, vomiting, excessive dieting	Omitted dose of insulin, spoiled insulin, error in dosage, improperly mixed insulin, increased need for insulin due to stress of illness, exposure, surgery, or improper diet; also, undiagnosed diabetes or not following diet plan (especially in active child or adolescent)
Symptoms[b]		
• Skin	Pale, moist, cool and clammy, sweating	Flushed, dry, hot, no sweating
• Behavior	Shaky, nervous, irritable, trembling, confused, disoriented, strange actions, difficulty in problem-solving; later, unconsciousness (rarely, seizures); may first be evidenced by a personality change or drowsiness	Drowsy, lethargic, dizzy, weak; later, delirium and loss of consciousness; anorexia
• Breath	Normal odor	Fruity odor (acetone)
• Respiration	Normal, rapid, and shallow	Air hunger (Kussmaul breathing), labored, slow
• Blood pressure	Increased	Decreased
• Pulse	Increased	Increased
• Hunger	Great hunger, often sudden in onset	Anorexia, nausea—may have time of excessive hunger
• Thirst	None	Great thirst
• Vomiting	Absent	Present, with abdominal pain
• Sugar in urine	Absent in second voiding (in unusual circumstances, sugar may be spilled, depending on type and time of insulin administration and kidney function)	Present in high concentrations
• Acetone in urine	Absent	Usually present
• Urination	Small amount	Frequent, copious, diluted
• Blood glucose level	Low, <60	High, >140
• Chemistry	Electrolytes usually within normal limits	Blood electrolytes and BUN elevated
• Other	Blurred or double vision, dizziness, headache, sleepiness	Ringing in ears
Response to Treatment	Rapid	Slow
Treatment	Glucose—stop exercising; take simple sugar (regular soft drinks upset the stomach less than orange juice); glucagon for injection is available; 50% glucose; glucose tablets	Force fluids (usually IV), give antiemetics, keep client warm; administer regular insulin in low dosage

(Continued)

TABLE 79-5	Hypoglycemia Versus Hyperglycemia (Continued)	
	HYPOGLYCEMIC REACTION[a] (INSULIN REACTION)	**HYPERGLYCEMIA (ACIDOSIS, DIABETIC KETOACIDOSIS, "DIABETIC COMA")**
Nursing Considerations	Prepare to assist with blood samples, urine collection, IV administration of glucose; remain with client until they are fully conscious and watch for symptoms of recurrence; client is often nauseated after a reaction; nursing measures should prevent complications of emesis; institute seizure precautions	Prepare to insert catheter, assist with IV, gastric lavage, ECG; prepare to deal with circulatory or respiratory complications and, later, with nausea; remain with client and observe

[a]The symptoms of the hypoglycemic reaction are those of adrenaline overdose because the body secretes adrenaline when the blood glucose level gets too low in an attempt to raise blood glucose.
[b]A slow drop in blood glucose is most likely to result in confusion, sleepiness, and headache. A rapid drop in blood glucose (e.g., caused by exercise) is more likely to result in shakiness, pallor, rapid heart rate, and sweating.
BUN, blood urea nitrogen; ECG, electrocardiogram; IV, intravenous.

> **Key Concept**
> All persons with diabetes who use insulin or oral hypoglycemic medications should wear a MedicAlert tag at all times.

Treatment and Nursing Considerations

Hypoglycemia can develop so rapidly that a client may be having seizures or may become unconscious before anyone knows what is wrong. Be quick to recognize the early symptoms of hypoglycemia.

Carbohydrates are needed to counteract the insulin reaction in hypoglycemia. If the client is conscious, give sugar in some form (4 oz orange juice, 4 oz regular soft drink, 6–8 Life Savers, honey, or Karo syrup). Individually packaged glucose tablets are available in pharmacies; give such glucose to individuals who use Precose. *Rationale: The enzymatic action of Precose blocks the absorption of sucrose, which is found in table sugar and fruit juice.* Sugar in liquid form is easiest and safest. If the person is unconscious, 50% dextrose IV solution (D50%) is the initial treatment.

Glucagon administration is another treatment for hypoglycemia. *Glucagon* is not glucose; it is a hormone that causes the liver to release glucose into the bloodstream. It is available as glucagon for injection in IV and IM preparations. If the client shows no response within 5–10 min after the injection, administer 50 mL of 50% glucose IV.

> **Nursing Alert** Avoid chocolate bars and whole milk as treatment for a hypoglycemic reaction because the high fat content prevents quick release of glucose.

Hypoglycemia requires emergency treatment, followed by adjustment of the client's carbohydrate intake and insulin dosage to regulate the disturbed metabolism. Adjusting these factors is difficult in the first 24 hr after the reaction; the client requires close observation for symptom recurrence. Check the client's blood glucose levels frequently.

If medical assistance is unavailable, the client may use a substance called instant glucose, which contains 25 g of pure glucose and is packaged in a tube for squeezing into the client's mouth. If a client is unconscious, place the glucose between the lower lip and front teeth to prevent aspiration. The body will absorb glucose through the oral mucous membranes. Absorption in this manner is much slower than when glucose is given IV.

The **Somogyi phenomenon** occurs when hypoglycemia is followed by a compensatory period of rebound hyperglycemia as the body attempts to correct the initial problem by increasing glucose production. It most commonly develops late at night or early in the morning when the client is asleep. During this time, the body continues to absorb insulin from the injection site, although insufficient glucose is available for the insulin to act on. As a result, the body secretes glucagon, norepinephrine, and corticosteroids to correct the hypoglycemia but exceeds the necessary amounts. Treatment involves reducing insulin dosages until the optimum level is reached.

Hyperglycemia

Diabetic ketoacidosis (**DKA**) results from a lack of effective insulin, causing hyperglycemia. Glucose no longer enters the muscle cells. To make up for the loss of sugar as a source of energy, the body uses more fats and proteins, which it breaks down into ketones and sends to the muscles. If too many ketones accumulate (*ketosis*), body fluids become imbalanced, and a condition called **ketoacidosis** follows. In ketoacidosis, the body produces a volatile substance called *acetone*, which has a characteristic sweetish odor (like nail polish remover) that can be detected on the client's breath in late stages of ketoacidosis. Any condition that interferes with storage of glycogen in the liver and increases the body's need to burn fat and energy (e.g., lack of insulin, vomiting, surgery, or anesthesia) may increase production of ketone bodies.

Signs and Symptoms

Ketoacidosis develops over time. The client experiences weakness, drowsiness, vomiting, thirst, abdominal pain, and dehydration. They have flushed cheeks and dry skin and mouth. The breath may have the sweetish odor mentioned earlier; breathing and pulse may become rapid and deep, and blood pressure may become low. Unconsciousness may follow. Sometimes, the unresponsive client who is admitted to the healthcare facility is unaware that they have diabetes. Or, a person may have a diabetic condition that is hard to control, even when they follow the regimen faithfully.

Treatment and Nursing Considerations

Intervention must include IV fluids and electrolytes as well as insulin replacement. While laboratory examination of blood and urine specimens is being completed, apply blankets to the unresponsive client to support warmth and combat shock. Check vital signs frequently.

Continuous IV infusion of low-dose regular insulin, with a controlled-flow mechanism, is used. By lowering the body's production of ketones, insulin makes more carbohydrate available to the tissues and builds up the liver's glycogen supply. Regular insulin acts quickly.

Following the initial emergency, test blood specimens for sugar hourly and keep a record of fluid I&O. Monitor blood levels of potassium, chlorides, and bicarbonates hourly and sodium levels every 8 hr. Also check urine or blood ketones every 4–8 hr. All these tests are necessary to evaluate the client's progress and to assist the healthcare provider in determining how much insulin to prescribe and which electrolytes to replace. When the client's metabolism is in balance again, the healthcare provider prescribes a regimen specifically designed for that client.

> **Nursing Alert** If you are outside the healthcare facility and do not know whether a person is having a hypoglycemic or hyperglycemic reaction, give sugar. *Rationale: If you give sugar, and it is incorrect, an already high blood glucose level will only increase slightly. However, if you give insulin and the blood glucose is already too low, the reaction is faster, more severe, and more long lasting. Death is much more likely when insulin, not sugar, is incorrectly given.*

Nonketotic Hyperosmolar State

In this condition, the client has a blood glucose level in the vicinity of 1,000 mg/dL, without typical symptoms of ketosis. It occurs most often in older adults with no history of diabetes or with a history of type 2 diabetes. The mortality rate is 65%. Underlying causes include advanced age, severe stress, diuretics, undiagnosed diabetes, or response to anticonvulsant or hypnotic sedative drugs.

The client experiences hyperglycemia, hyperosmolarity, severe dehydration, and coma. The body produces some, but not enough, insulin. Hyperglycemia results in severe loss of fluids and electrolytes, resulting in dehydration.

Treatment is a continuous low-dose infusion of insulin and aggressive fluid and electrolyte replacement.

Nursing care focuses on measures to restore the fluid volume and correct the hyperosmolar state. Administer IV fluids and electrolyte replacements as ordered. Monitor fluid and electrolyte balance, I&O, and daily weights. Evaluate blood and urine glucose levels frequently.

Infections

Infections aggravate diabetes. When increased glucose concentration damages blood vessels, clients are more susceptible to infections. Clients with diabetes are particularly susceptible to yeast and fungal infections, carbuncles, and furuncles, as well as common colds and influenza. Because of sugar in the blood and reduced circulation, fighting infection is difficult. Effective diabetes management minimizes blood vessel damage and reduces infections. Injury prevention is important because people with diabetes heal slowly.

Surgical Complications

Persons with diabetes are considered greater surgical risks because of associated circulatory problems and difficulty in regulating insulin balance postoperatively. They are also more susceptible to infections in any wound, including a surgical incision, and heal less readily because of impaired circulation.

Postoperative nursing care includes frequent BGM, watching for possible complications, encouraging fluids, and following measures to prevent respiratory, circulatory, and wound complications. These individuals are susceptible to skin breakdowns. Practice meticulous skin care. Clients with type 2 diabetes who do not usually take insulin may require insulin during the perioperative period to control blood glucose elevations.

Macrovascular Complications

High blood glucose levels may increase *arteriosclerosis* (a condition that affects the peripheral blood vessels), especially in the lower extremities and the vessels of the kidneys and heart. These changes are the *macrovascular* (large blood vessels) complications associated with diabetes. When arteriosclerosis narrows the lumen of blood vessels, decreased blood flow causes oxygen deprivation in tissues. Diabetic ulcers can result (Fig. 79-6).

Other consequences of arteriosclerosis include hypertension, coronary artery disease, peripheral vascular disease, myocardial infarction, and stroke. Persons with diabetes are two to six times more likely to have a stroke and twice as likely to have a heart attack as the general population. Skin breakdown and a greatly slowed healing process also result from poor circulation and lack of oxygen. Theorists also believe that elevated glycosylated

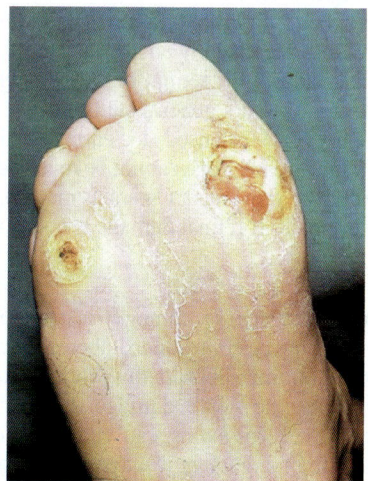

Figure 79-6 Diabetic ulcers. Ulcerations, particularly on the legs or feet, are serious for the client with diabetes. In many cases, an ulceration heals very slowly or may not heal at all. Gangrene is a serious threat and usually necessitates amputation.

hemoglobin is stickier than normal hemoglobin, so it is more likely to clump, clot, and occlude small blood vessels in the brain, heart, and kidneys.

> **Nursing Alert** Uncontrolled diabetes mellitus predisposes a person to long-term complications, such as hypertension, stroke, heart and kidney disorders, blindness, and amputation secondary to gangrene. Control of blood glucose levels greatly reduces the possibility of these complications.

Microvascular Complications

Diabetes causes unique microvascular changes in the capillary walls, resulting in diminished blood flow and poor oxygenation of tissues that are highly vascular. The retina of the eye and the kidneys are the primary organs that can be severely damaged by diabetes.

Nephropathy

Kidney disease (**nephropathy**) caused by microvascular changes can result in death from kidney failure. Kidney infections or albumin or blood in the urine, often the first indications, must be dealt with immediately. Three general approaches to slowing the progress of nephropathy include blood pressure control, blood glucose control, and diet.

Angiotensin-converting enzyme (**ACE**) inhibitors are used to treat high blood pressure and kidney disease in clients with diabetes. Research has shown that people with diabetes who have proteinuria respond better to ACE inhibitors than to other medications used to treat hypertension.

Retinopathy

One of the leading causes of blindness in this country is diabetic **retinopathy**, which is loss of the functional retinal tissue in the eye owing to microvascular damage. Many healthcare providers recommend yearly eye examinations for people with diabetes. Circulatory problems may appear first in the retinal arteries (in the retina of the eye) in the form of hemorrhage or inflammation. Disorders in the retinal blood vessels are usually visible through an ophthalmoscope. The condition of retinal blood vessels reflects the entire circulatory system's general status.

Laser therapy can be used to curtail pathologic eye changes. Damage already done cannot be reversed, but further damage can often be prevented. Cataracts may appear and can be removed surgically if retinal damage is not too great.

Neuropathy

Diabetic **neuropathy** (nerve damage) is another long-term complication of poorly controlled diabetes. It can occur as peripheral or autonomic neuropathy. Various theories exist about what causes the nerve damage. It may result from swelling of nerve cells or axons, caused by the accumulation of sorbitol (a type of sugar), or it may result from accumulation of end products of glucose metabolism.

Peripheral neuropathy usually starts as numbness or tingling in the toes and progresses gradually (over years) to the ankle and then the leg. Symptoms vary from unawareness to extreme pain or numbness. Painful neuropathy can be treated with gabapentin (Neurontin), amitriptyline, carbamazepine (Tegretol), or phenytoin (Dilantin). Lack of sensation in the feet can be dangerous because it can mask injury; ulcers may form that can ultimately lead to amputation.

Autonomic neuropathy can have various effects, including impotence, intestinal involvement (diarrhea with periods of constipation), urinary retention, stomach involvement (*gastroparesis*), *orthostasis* (dizziness on arising), and sweating abnormalities. These neuropathies are treated symptomatically because no cure for autonomic neuropathy exists.

Because neuropathy causes lack of sensation in peripheral tissues of the body, clients are more likely to develop skin infections or injury without being aware of the problem.

Long-Term Management of Diabetes Mellitus

Client Teaching

Because clients are ultimately responsible for self-care, the most important aspect of long-term management is educating clients and families to understand diabetes and its management. Much of this teaching is the responsibility of nursing staff and diabetes educators (In Practice: Educating the Client 79-1).

IN PRACTICE
EDUCATING THE CLIENT: 79-1 — Diabetes Mellitus Teaching Plan

- Ascertain the client's and family's knowledge about diabetes. Start by stating, "Tell me what you understand about diabetes." Focus on general and work toward specific concepts. Build on what the person already knows.
- Divide lessons into specific, small portions for short time periods (15–30 min).
- Ask which topic of the following survival skills needs to be discussed *at this time:*
  Basic meal planning
  Self-monitoring of blood glucose
  Recognition of hypoglycemia or hyperglycemia
  Insulin preparation and administration (if appropriate)
  Oral medication administration (if appropriate)
- Explain everything in terms the client can understand.
- Give ample opportunity for the client to ask questions. Be willing to repeat information given.
- Ask for return demonstrations. Make sure the person is not "agreeing" just to be cooperative.
- Use booklets, pictures, and Internet resources. Give materials to the client to keep.
- Recognize that people learn in different ways and at different rates of speed. Structure information to meet these needs.
- Promote independence to increase self-esteem and safety. Use positive reinforcement.
- Stress that seemingly trivial problems can be serious. Define when the client must notify the healthcare provider immediately.

Clients will understand the disease best if it is explained in simple terms. Review this sample explanation when working with clients with diabetes:

> When you have diabetes, your body can't use the sugar in your blood. That's why your blood glucose level is so high. The sugar stays in your blood instead of going into your body's cells where it can be used for fuel. That's why you have not felt well and have been lacking energy. You will learn the tools to use to control your blood glucose level: they consist of healthy food choices, medication, and exercise. There is a lot to learn about diabetes, but there is also a lot of support available to you. We can help you take it one step at a time. Eventually, you will gain the confidence you will need to self-manage your diabetes. What is it about all of this that you find most difficult?

Clients must understand that diabetes is never cured. It is considered *controlled* or *managed* when the following conditions exist:

- The person feels well.
- The person maintains normal weight on a balanced diet.
- The person's blood glucose level stays within 70–140 mg/dL (normal).

Clients must learn that they can reduce long-term complications by controlling their blood glucose levels. Injury prevention is crucial. Special care and regular examinations are necessary for the feet, hands, teeth, and eyes. Illness can quickly upset glucose control.

Clients will be responsible for managing food selection, blood testing, appropriate exercise, and medication administration. Observe performance of these procedures to ascertain the client's understanding and ability to perform certain tasks. Praise clients when they perform procedures correctly and assist with areas that need reinforcement.

> **Key Concept**
>
> Persons with diabetes are able to lead normal lives and live longer than in the past. They should maintain tight blood glucose control (70–140 mg/dL) to prevent complications of diabetes.

Healthcare Provider Contact

The healthcare provider will help the client determine the most appropriate schedule for medication dosage, as well as a diet and exercise regimen. Although some clients are able to adjust insulin dosage on their own, clients may need to contact their healthcare provider for changes in their blood glucose levels. In addition, clients need to report symptoms, such as loss of appetite, hunger, or any gastrointestinal upset persisting for more than 24 hr that is severe enough to prevent eating or to cause diarrhea or vomiting.

Glucose Monitoring

Many nurses in various healthcare facilities monitor blood glucose levels (see In Practice: Nursing Procedure 79-1).

Adapt these steps to teach clients how to self-monitor blood glucose levels. If they have type 1 diabetes, clients will also learn when and how to test their urine for ketones. These clients must notify their healthcare provider if their blood glucose level is consistently above 240 mg/dL for 3 days. Teach clients to perform these tests and document the results in a log or diary. Clients should take these records with them to follow-up appointments.

SMBG level is an important tool in the daily routine for any individual with diabetes. It allows clients to evaluate their diabetes management, aids in problem-solving and insulin adjustments, and provides invaluable information to the diabetes team. Keeping a blood glucose level diary helps everyone involved to understand when blood glucose levels fluctuate and why.

Numerous blood glucose meters are available. With recent advances in technology, these meters have become easy to use. Some models are made specifically for the visually impaired. Although they help clients to obtain quick and highly accurate results, these monitoring programs are expensive. However, because monitoring is so useful in preventing chronic hyperglycemia (and long-term complications), the cost is justified and usually covered by third-party payors.

Every meter is different; a healthcare provider who is familiar with the particular technology should teach the client how to select and use a meter. Clients must understand and be able to interpret the data the meter generates. Blood glucose levels in the normal range can assure clients that self-management techniques are working. Abnormal readings provide opportunities to identify what is not working and can assist clients to make any necessary changes.

Blood glucose testing can be done visually, in which a test strip is compared with a colored chart, or by using a meter in which a test strip is inserted into an electronic device that reads it. Visual testing is rarely used today because blood glucose meters have become easier and quicker to use. Meters are available for clients with visual, hearing, or other problems. SMBG is recommended for all clients who have diabetes.

Meal Planning

Meal plans for people with diabetes are individualized with help from a registered dietitian. These clients can achieve optimal blood glucose control by making realistic food choices that not only mimic their typical eating patterns but also reflect healthy eating approaches as well. They must be introduced to the concept of carbohydrate awareness. Explain meal plans in terms that clients can easily understand and follow. Foods containing sugar are not forbidden, but clients must count them as part of their total carbohydrate intake. Consider the client's cultural background when planning meals. Clients must understand the relationships among diet, medication, and exercise. Alcohol may be allowed, in moderation, provided it is accompanied by food to prevent hypoglycemia.

Lifestyle Factors

Often, clients have many questions about the effect of diabetes on their lifestyles. Assure them that they can participate in activities, as long as they allow for changes in exercise levels and control their blood glucose level. They should avoid fatigue. Genetic counseling may be advisable before deciding whether to have children.

Smoking

Smoking is definitely contraindicated because the vasoconstrictor effect of nicotine increases the likelihood of circulatory disorders. Strongly urge people with diabetes to stop smoking and provide assistance to do so by giving information about smoking cessation programs.

Insulin Injection

When insulin is prescribed, teach clients about the type of insulin and syringe, along with dosages and self-injection. Usually, clients fear the injection itself. Draw up the insulin the first time and immediately let the client inject it to get over the initial fear. After fear and anxiety are relieved, the client is better able to focus on the technique for drawing up the correct amount, site selection, and so forth. Use the type of syringe that the client will use at home. Encourage those clients who feel well enough in the healthcare facility to give all their own insulin injections. Doing so will allow you to observe the technique and provide reinforcement or correction as appropriate. Children older than 7 or 8 years are usually able to give their own insulin.

Rotating insulin injection sites will keep skin and tissue healthy and prevent lipodystrophy. Teach clients that standard injection sites include the outside or front of the thighs, the upper outer part of the buttocks, the outside of the upper arm, and the abdomen. Insulin absorption is fastest from the abdomen. Inform clients to use care when selecting sites. The body will rapidly absorb insulin from sites that are exercised shortly after administration (e.g., running after injecting into the thigh can cause too rapid insulin absorption, resulting in hypoglycemia).

Alternative Forms of Insulin Administration

In addition to the administration of insulin by injection, subcutaneous infusion set (also referred to as insulin infusers), or external insulin pump, manufacturers are actively pursuing alternative routes for insulin administration.

Hypoglycemia and Hyperglycemia

Clients must understand the symptoms of hypoglycemia and hyperglycemia (see Table 79-5). Because these reactions can be dangerous, clients, their families, and their caregivers must know how to identify and manage them. Encourage frequent monitoring of blood glucose levels. Clients who experience frequent reactions should have a sugar supply readily available at all times. Encourage the client to carry a simple carbohydrate snack, such as peanut butter crackers or five to six pieces of hard candy. A glucagon/glucose emergency kit is recommended for clients receiving insulin; family members and significant others should also learn how to use it.

Also encourage the client to wear a medical alert identification bracelet or tag (e.g., MedicAlert). This is very helpful in emergency situations, when the client might not be able to respond. In the home, a list of health conditions and medications should be kept (and updated periodically). Family or emergency personnel will need this information. This list needs to be placed in a central location, such as the outside of a refrigerator.

Sexuality

Many men with diabetes experience erectile dysfunction. Approximately 50% of men with diabetes are unable to achieve a satisfactory erection; the cause is believed to be neurogenic. Encourage male clients to bring this problem to a healthcare provider's attention. Some men with diabetes use penile implants or prostheses, as well as oral medications such as sildenafil (Viagra).

The literature provides very little discussion about sexual dysfunction in women with diabetes, although it occurs. Sexual dysfunction is not uncommon in women with type 2 diabetes, most likely because many of these clients are postmenopausal with diminished estrogen secretion. Treatments exist for sexual problems in female clients as well.

Exposure to Cold

Clients should be aware that exposure to extreme cold slows blood circulation, especially in the extremities, owing to vasoconstriction. Frostbite or hypothermia is a danger, especially because individuals with diabetes do not heal well.

Vision Impairment

Clients with diabetes must understand the importance of annual eye examinations with pupil dilation, which can detect early visual problems. Many assistive devices are available for use by visually impaired clients. Furniture can also be placed where clients are less likely to bump into it, as bumps can cause breaks in the skin.

Dental Examination

Persons with diabetes need regular dental examinations. Dental *caries* (decay) can lead to infection, which can upset glucose control. In addition, rough edges can irritate the mouth, exposing the mouth to infections.

Foot Care

Warn people with diabetes against foot injuries. Explain that poor circulation and diminished sensation can result in a wound that is not detected by the client and does not heal because of poor circulation. Left untreated, a wound can become infected and ultimately result in amputation. Teach preventive foot care to all people with diabetes (see In Practice: Educating the Client 79-2).

Traveling

Persons with diabetes who plan to travel great distances (across several time zones) should consult their healthcare provider before such trips. Often, they will need to adjust their daily insulin doses during travel days, until they achieve a regular morning schedule again. Clients must consider diet and exercise in their travel plans. People taking insulin and testing blood glucose levels must keep medications and equipment with them in carry-on luggage and give a spare supply to a companion, in case luggage gets lost. Some countries use a different type of insulin syringe (U40), so sufficient U100 syringes need to be taken when traveling. These clients must also carry a fast-acting carbohydrate and some food with them when traveling. They will probably be asked for a prescription if they try to buy syringes.

Identification

Every person with diabetes should wear a tag, such as a MedicAlert tag, that gives immediate and positive identification of the problem. Many times, a card in the wallet

IN PRACTICE
EDUCATING THE CLIENT: 79-1 — Foot Care and Diabetes Mellitus

- Inspect feet daily. If necessary, use a mirror to check the undersides of the feet or areas that are difficult to see. **Rationale:** *Daily inspection allows for prompt intervention should a problem arise.*
- Wash feet daily. Do not soak. **Rationale:** *Soaking softens the skin too much, making it more easily damaged.*
- Dry feet thoroughly yet gently, especially between the toes. **Rationale:** *Proper drying prevents cracking and breaks, which could lead to infections.*
- Massage gently with a good quality lotion. Do not use lotion between toes. **Rationale:** *Lotion keeps the skin soft. Lotion between the toes promotes moisture accumulation, which could lead to skin maceration and breakdown.*
- Cut nails only with a healthcare provider's permission. Cut nails straight across with a blunt-tipped scissors. See a podiatrist for treatment of corns, calluses, or ingrown toenails. Self-treatment in any form is dangerous and absolutely forbidden. **Rationale:** *Proper foot care prevents complications.*
- Never pick at sores or rough spots on the skin.
- Do not walk barefooted. **Rationale:** *Walking barefoot increases the risk of injury and possible infection.*
- Put lamb's wool between overlapping toes. **Rationale:** *Lamb's wool prevents rubbing and irritation.*
- Exercise daily. Walking is the best exercise. If you are unable to walk, sit on the edge of the bed and point toes upward, then downward. Do this 10 times. Make a circle with each foot 10 times. **Rationale:** *Exercise improves circulation.*
- Make sure that shoes fit well, are of high quality, and give good support. Inspect the inside of shoes for any rough areas. **Rationale:** *Properly fitting shoes prevent the development of any ulcerations or breaks in the skin of the feet. The circulation of the feet may be poor, and any ulceration is often difficult to heal.*
- Wear new shoes only for a short period each day for a few days. **Rationale:** *Minimizing the time in new shoes helps to avoid irritation.*
- Never wear constrictive stockings or socks. Avoid sitting with knees crossed. **Rationale:** *These actions restrict circulation.*
- Do not use adhesive tape on the skin. **Rationale:** *Adhesive tape abrades the skin when it is removed.*
- For cold toes, use warm socks and extra blankets at night. Select stockings that allow toe motion.
- Avoid using heating pads and hot water bags because they can be dangerous. **Rationale:** *Because circulation is poor and neuropathy may be present, the person can be burned more easily.*
- See a healthcare provider for a cut or burn, no matter how small it is. If first aid treatment is necessary, cleanse the area gently with soap and water. Do not use harsh antiseptics. Apply a dry, sterile dressing. It is essential to see a healthcare provider as soon as possible. **Rationale:** *Immediate therapy is necessary to prevent complications. Because of impaired circulation, gangrene is a possibility, which would necessitate amputation.*

is not easily found. Most paramedics and emergency room personnel are actually forbidden from looking through wallets and purses, presumably to protect against accusations of stealing and for privacy reasons. A tag worn on the body gives immediate and visible information to healthcare personnel.

> **NCLEX Alert**
>
> Diabetes is one of the most commonly seen clinical situations. Therefore, it is very important that your nursing knowledge include a thorough understanding of the types of diabetes, the types of medications and their side effects, and the nursing implications for care of the clients with diabetes.

STUDENT SYNTHESIS

KEY POINTS

- Endocrine glands secrete hormones that influence metabolism, growth, and development.
- Laboratory diagnostic tests for the endocrine system include serum hormone levels, various glucose tests, several urinalysis tests, radiology procedures, and occasionally iodine uptake tests. Many endocrine disorders affect growth, development, and appearance.
- Most endocrine disorders result from overproduction or underproduction of specific hormones.
- Nursing procedures in the care of a postoperative thyroidectomy client include careful monitoring and preparation for emergency care.
- Diabetes mellitus occurs when the pancreas does not make enough insulin or the body becomes resistant to insulin.
- Diabetes mellitus is classified as the following: type 1 diabetes, type 2 diabetes, gestational diabetes, and impaired glucose homeostasis (impaired fasting glucose or impaired glucose tolerance). Clients with type 1 diabetes must use insulin as part of their treatment

regimen. Clients with type 2 diabetes may use oral antidiabetic agents that affect insulin secretion and/or metabolism. Some clients with type 2 diabetes also use insulin.
- Meal planning, exercise, and medications, as needed, are essential components of diabetes management.
- Complications of diabetes affect all aspects of life. Members of the diabetes team work to provide accurate and thorough client teaching and to avoid related complications of the disease.

CRITICAL THINKING EXERCISES

1. A client comes to your healthcare facility. They have a rapid pulse and elevated systolic blood pressure. They say that, although they have been eating a lot more than usual, they have been losing weight. Their skin is a salmon color, and they have bulging eyes and a swollen neck. Based on these symptoms, which disorder might this client be experiencing? Which additional data would you want to collect? Which diagnostic test could help confirm the client's condition?

2. Your client is a child with diabetes mellitus. Their parents ask you to explain the differences among the various kinds of diabetes mellitus, particularly the differences between children and adults with the disease. Describe what you will tell them.

3. While riding a public bus in your community, you notice a man who is confused, appears sleepy, and is staggering down the aisle. As he bumps next to you, you notice that he is wearing a MedicAlert tag that identifies him as diabetic. What do you think may be happening to this man? How will you decide? What can you do to help?

NCLEX-STYLE REVIEW QUESTIONS

1. A client has a random blood glucose level drawn with results of 80 mg/dL. Which conclusion can the nurse draw from this result?
   a. The client is hyperglycemic and will require insulin.
   b. The client is hypoglycemic and needs dextrose 50%.
   c. The client requires further testing for confirmation.
   d. There is no further action required.

2. A client with type 1 diabetes has a consistent glucose reading of 200–320 mg/dL. For which test should the nurse prepare the client?
   a. Urine for detection of ketones
   b. Ice pack test
   c. Bladder ultrasound
   d. 24-hr urine collection for VMA

3. A client is suspected of developing diabetes insipidus after sustaining a head injury. Which observation made by the nurse should be documented that supports the diagnosis of diabetes insipidus? Select all that apply.
   a. Voiding 20 L in 24 hr
   b. Reports of severe thirst
   c. Concentrated urine, dark in color
   d. Urine specific gravity of 1.000
   e. Diarrhea

4. The nurse is caring for a client after undergoing a total thyroidectomy. Which action should the nurse take to prevent complications? Select all that apply.
   a. Massage legs to prevent clot formation.
   b. Inspect dressings for excessive bleeding.
   c. Check for edema in the neck.
   d. Keep an endotracheal tube at the bedside.
   e. Suction the client every 2 hr.

5. The nurse is caring for a client who has had a thyroidectomy with removal of the parathyroid glands. After observing positive Trousseau and Chvostek signs, which medication should the nurse prepare to administer?
   a. Morphine sulfate
   b. Calcium gluconate
   c. Levothyroxine
   d. Iodine

CHAPTER RESOURCES

Enhance your learning with additional resources on thePoint!

Student Resources related to this chapter can be found at thePoint.lww.com/Rosdahl12e.

CHAPTER 79 Endocrine Disorders 1411

Welcome Steps

Look at healthcare provider's orders.

Protocol for procedure.

Necessary equipment/supplies.

Wash hands using proper hand hygiene; put on gloves.

Explain the procedure and reassure the client.

Locate two identifiers to confirm correct client.

Comfortable and efficient position for nurse and client.

Obtain privacy.

Make sure to follow correct steps and body mechanics with good technique.

Ensure safety and observe deviations from normal.

End Steps

Ensure comfort and safety.

Note questions or concerns from client or nurse; note significant data.

Dispose of materials properly.

Disinfect the area and your hands.

Document and report the procedure and your findings.

IN PRACTICE
NURSING PROCEDURE: 79-1 — Testing for Blood Glucose Level

Supplies and Equipment
Blood glucose testing strips
Glucose testing meter
Sterile lancet
Lancet activating device (optional)
Cotton balls
Alcohol swab
Gloves

Steps
Follow LPN WELCOME steps and then

1. Remove a test strip from the container. Turn on the glucose testing meter. Check that the code number on the strip matches the code number that appears initially on the monitor screen (or follow the manufacturer's instructions). *Rationale: Matching code numbers on the strip and the meter ensures that the machine is calibrated correctly.*

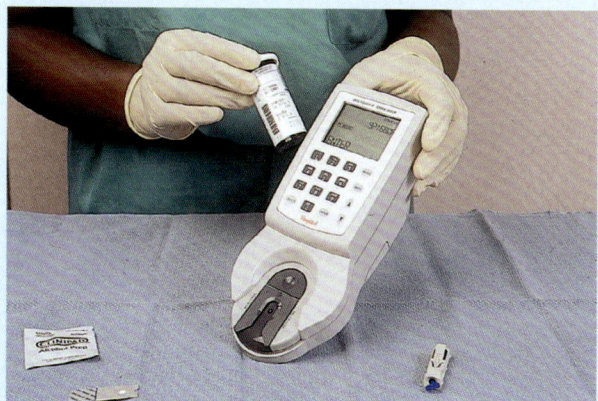

Match the code number on the glucose test strip with the code number on the monitor screen.

2. Prepare the lancet by twisting off the cap. Arm the automatic device by pushing back the plunger until it clicks. Attach the lancet. Remove the cap. Keep the tip sterile. *Rationale: Maintaining sterility of the lancet reduces the risk of transmission of microorganisms to the puncture site.*

3. Select the site on the client's finger for puncture, usually the fingertip in adults. *Rationale: Some devices allow for collection from alternative sites; consult the manufacturer's instructions.*

4. If necessary, dilate the capillaries by applying warm, moist compresses to the area for about 10 min. *Rationale: Warmth will cause the capillaries to dilate allowing more blood flow to the puncture area.*

5. If the client is able, have them wash the hands with soap and water and then dry them. *Rationale: Washing with soap and water will remove any sugar that may present on the skin from exposure to sugar-containing products.*

6. If the client cannot wash their hands, clean the site with alcohol and allow the area to dry thoroughly. (Clients may omit this step at home.) *Rationale: Alcohol can affect the blood sample and cause destruction of some red blood cells.*

7. Wearing gloves, prick the side of the client's finger with a lancet. Use a cotton ball to wipe away the first drop of blood, if recommended for the particular meter. *Rationale: Directions for some meters indicate that the first drop of blood should not be used because it may be diluted by serum and give a false reading.*

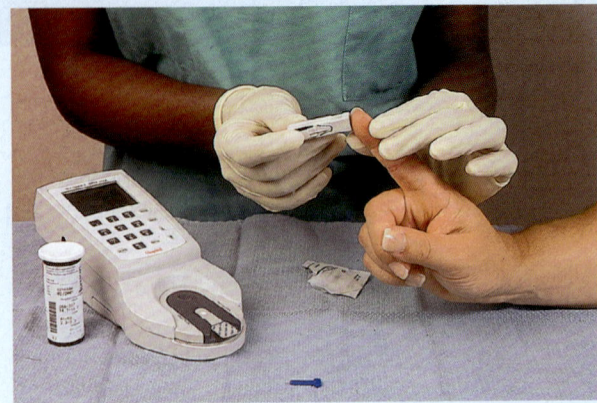

Wearing gloves, prick the side of the client's finger with the lancet.

8. Gently touch the drop of blood to the strip's target area, as instructed. Have the client hold a clean cotton ball to the puncture site for a few seconds.
Rationale: Blood must color the entire target area, but should not be smeared on the strip, or test results will be inaccurate. The person with diabetes often has slowed clotting.

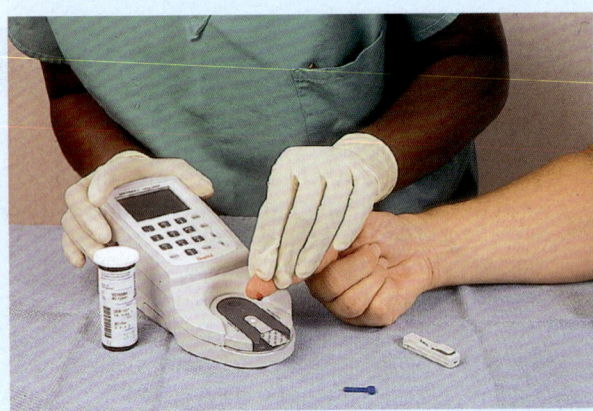

Note how the drop of blood is positioned over the sensing area of the test strip. Some test strips provide for the blood to flow directly onto the test strip.

9. Insert the strip as far as it will go into the meter, with the target area facing the red dot on the meter (or follow manufacturer's directions).
Rationale: Inserting the strip correctly enables the machine to determine the client's blood glucose level.

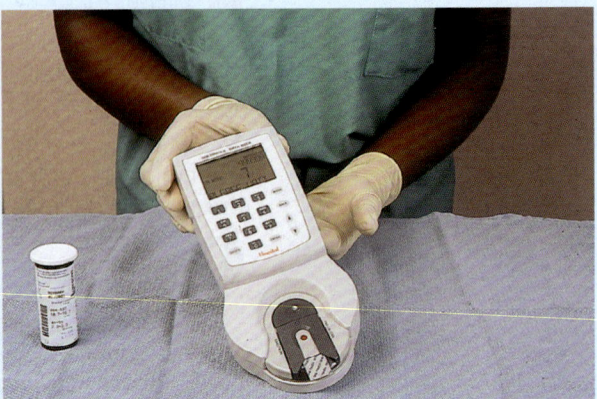

Wait 15–60 s, depending on manufacturer's instructions.

10. Read test results in 15–60 s on the meter face. Remove the strip and turn off the meter.
Rationale: Individual meters read test results within varying time frames.

Follow ENDDD steps

Special Reminder

- Record blood glucose reading on proper forms and check to see if the client is on insulin coverage. *Rationale:* Blood glucose reading may necessitate insulin coverage.

80 Sensory System Disorders

Learning Objectives

1. Identify nursing considerations for each of the following types of testing: refractive examinations, ophthalmoscope, otoscope, slit lamp, tonometry, ERG, audiometry, caloric test, and ENG.
2. In the skills laboratory, demonstrate use of a cotton-tipped applicator and an ear irrigation, differentiating between the techniques used for adults and children.
3. State nursing considerations for the care of the client with a visual deficit, including pre- and postoperative nursing considerations, and the client with a hearing deficit.
4. Define the following refractive errors: myopia, hyperopia, astigmatism, and presbyopia.
5. Identify the advantages and disadvantages of the following methods of visual correction: eyeglasses, hard contact lenses, soft contact lenses, and extended-wear lenses.
6. Define radial keratotomy, photorefractive keratectomy (PRK), and laser in situ keratomileusis (LASIK).
7. Describe the following: inflammatory and infectious eye disorders (conjunctivitis, blepharitis, hordeolum, chalazion, trachoma, and keratitis) and structural disorders (ectropion, entropion, and ptosis).
8. Differentiate chronic open-angle glaucoma, acute closed-angle glaucoma, and secondary glaucoma, identifying nursing considerations for each disorder.
9. Explain the causes and treatments for cataracts and macular degeneration.
10. Identify nursing considerations for each of the following types of eye traumas: hematoma, foreign bodies, hyphema, chemical burns, corneal abrasions, and detached retina.
11. Compare and contrast conductive hearing loss, sensorineural hearing loss, central hearing loss, and functional hearing loss.
12. Discuss the causes and nursing interventions for each of the following: disorders of the external ear (e.g., impacted earwax, furuncles, foreign objects, external otitis, fungal infections, punctured tympanic membrane) and disorders of the middle ear (e.g., otitis media, serous otitis media, acute purulent otitis media, chronic otitis media).
13. Describe the care for a client who is to undergo a tympanoplasty and myringotomy with insertion of PE tubes.
14. Discuss nursing considerations for a client with Ménière disease.
15. Identify two nursing considerations for clients with a tactile, gustatory, or olfactory disorder.

Important Terminology

age-related macular degeneration
astigmatism
cataract
cerumen
diplopia
drusen
ectropion
entropion
enucleation
glaucoma
gustation
hyperopia
hyphema
keratoplasty
labyrinthitis
Ménière disease
myopia
myringotomy
nystagmus
olfaction
otitis externa
otitis media
otosclerosis
ototoxic
phoropter
presbyopia
proprioception
ptosis
tactile sense
tinnitus
tonometer
tympanoplasty
vertigo

Acronyms

AMD
ENG
ERG
IOL
IOP
LASIK
PE
PRK
RGP
RK

The *sensory system* involves those organs and structures that give individuals information about the surrounding world through the senses of sight, hearing, touch, taste, and smell. The receptors for these senses are located in peripheral parts of the body. The nervous system (Chapter 19) transmits impulses sent from the sensory system to the brain for interpretation.

Any defect in a sensory organ or the brain itself or in the transmission of nerve impulses to the brain can cause a malfunction. Specific disorders of the nervous system and brain are discussed in Chapter 78. This chapter discusses disorders related to the senses of sight and hearing (Chapter 21) and briefly reviews conditions related to the other special senses.

DIAGNOSTIC TESTS

Eye and Vision Tests

Visual Acuity

The examination for *visual acuity* uses the standard Snellen chart to determine the person's ability to see at specified distances. This chart has a series of progressively smaller rows of letters. The person is usually positioned 20 ft from the chart and is asked to identify letters on a specific line.

The term *20/20 vision* means that the person can see an object at 20 ft that most people with normal vision can see at 20 ft. The person with 20/80 vision can see at a distance of

1413

20 ft what a person with 20/20 vision could see at 80 ft. The U.S. definition of blindness is visual acuity equal to or worse than 20/200, or a visual field of 20° or less, in the better eye.

Refractive Examination

The *refractive examination* is used to identify the degree of refractive error and determine the type of lens necessary to correct a visual defect. The pupils may or may not be *dilated* (opened) for examination. Drops such as cyclopentolate HCl (Cyclogyl), phenylephrine HCl (Mydfrin, Neo-Synephrine), scopolamine hydrobromide (Isopto Hyoscine), or tropicamide (Mydriacyl) are used to dilate the pupils.

Dilated pupils provide the examiner with a better view of the interior structures of the eyes and paralyze accommodation (ability to focus at various distances) in younger clients. This allows for more accurate testing for glasses. A **phoropter**, an instrument that simulates different corrective lenses, is placed in front of the client's eyes. Light from the examiner's retinoscope is streaked across the eye, while the lenses from the phoropter are adjusted until the light streak is neutralized. The final corrective lenses are selected by alternating similar lenses and having the client indicate which lens provides the clearest vision.

The Ophthalmoscopic Examination

The *ophthalmoscope* is an instrument used by the examiner to look through the pupil to see the retina and other interior structures (Fig. 80-1). The examination provides information about the blood vessels of the inner eye, especially those of the retina, as well as information about the presence of tumors and the condition of the optic nerve.

The blood vessels of the eyes suggest the general condition of blood vessels throughout the rest of the body. Atherosclerotic and hypertensive changes in the blood vessels of the eye are usually a sign that the same conditions exist elsewhere. Complications of diabetes mellitus can often first be seen in the eyes.

Slit Lamp Examination

The *slit lamp* is a special type of microscope that directs a beam of light onto or through the cornea to view the eye's anterior structures. The magnification of the images enables the examiner to identify abnormalities of the conjunctiva, cornea, anterior chamber, iris, lens, and anterior vitreous. The slit lamp also may be used in association with a type of magnifying lens to view the eye's posterior structures.

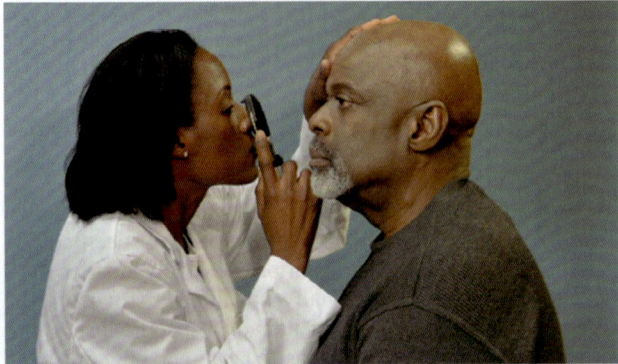

Figure 80-1 Technique for the proper use of the ophthalmoscope. The examiner uses the left eye to look into the client's left eye. They use the index finger to adjust the lens for proper focus.

Tonometry

An instrument called a **tonometer** can indirectly measure intraocular pressure (**IOP**), the pressure within the eye. Two devices, the *Schiøtz tonometer* and the more accurate *applanation tonometer*, are used to measure the pressure in the eye and detect glaucoma.

Other Tests

Other tests may be done to evaluate the function of the eyes and vision in specialized situations. The *retinal angiogram* is a visual depiction of the blood vessels in the retina, following the injection of radiopaque dye. *Ocular ultrasound* may also be used.

The *electroretinogram* (**ERG**) records the minute electrical impulses given off by the retina when it is struck by light, in much the same way as an electroencephalogram (EEG) is recorded. The ERG determines whether the retina is functioning. Local anesthesia is used for this test. A contact lens containing the *electrode* (measuring device) is placed on the eye. The client's head is under a "cone," and much of the test is done while the room is dark. The ERG can confirm a diagnosis of retinitis pigmentosa before the condition can be determined by other means.

Ear and Hearing Tests

The Otoscopic Examination

The *otoscope* is the fundamental piece of equipment used to examine the ear. Using the light and the magnifying lens of the otoscope, the healthcare provider can examine the external ear, the tympanic membrane, and anatomical points beyond the eardrum. Disposable plastic earpieces are used for each client. Several sizes for adults and children are available.

The nurse commonly assists the practitioner with eye and ear examinations by providing the appropriate equipment, checking to see that the light is working, and helping the client to remain still during the examination.

Audiometry

Audiometry is a test of hearing. Several types of audiometry may be used. *Pure tone audiometry* tests both conductive and sensorineural hearing deficits. *Bone conduction audiometry* tests only conduction loss.

Caloric Test or Caloric Study

The caloric test is designed to determine if an alteration exists in the vestibular origin of the acoustic nerve. Abnormal test results suggest a diseased labyrinth or a tumor of the acoustic nerve. This test can differentiate such disorders from disorders of the brain stem.

Procedure

The client is either seated or supine, and water is instilled into the external ear canal. Sometimes, warm and cold water are alternated. The affected side is tested first because less of a reaction is expected to occur there.

The normal response to this test is **nystagmus** (rapid, rhythmic eye movements), nausea, vomiting, *vertigo* (a feeling of spinning), and a feeling of falling. Decreased or absence of these responses within 3 min indicates an abnormality.

Contraindications

Water cannot be used for this test if the client's eardrum is punctured. Cold air may be substituted. The client who is having an attack of Ménière disease should not be tested until the symptoms of Ménière abate. Sedative and antivertigo agents may interfere with test results.

Nursing Considerations

Because nausea and vomiting are likely, keep the client NPO (nothing by mouth) or on clear liquids before the test and provide an emesis basin. The client is usually returned to the room by wheelchair or allowed to lie down until the nausea subsides, which is usually no more than an hour.

Electronystagmography

In *electronystagmography* (**ENG**), electrodes are placed near the client's eyes to assess for alterations in the vestibular system. In ENG, the caloric test is performed while eye movements are recorded on a graph. Other test components are the same as for the caloric test.

Other Tests

Magnetic resonance imaging (MRI) is used to detect tumors of the eighth cranial nerve. An EEG with evoked responses can be used to detect abnormalities of the nerve pathways between the eighth cranial nerve and the brain stem.

Another test of the function of the vestibular system and the semicircular canals involves seating the client in a chair that revolves in several planes and then evaluating the functioning of the client's sense of **proprioception** (location in space) and vestibular system.

COMMON MEDICAL TREATMENTS

Eye Patching

In some cases, a healthcare provider orders one or both of a client's eyes to be patched. Several types of patches are available. A *simple single patch* or *double patch* may be used to cover the eye for rest or protection. A *pressure patch* taped in place may be used to keep the eye closed. A metal shield over the patch is also commonly used to protect the eye.

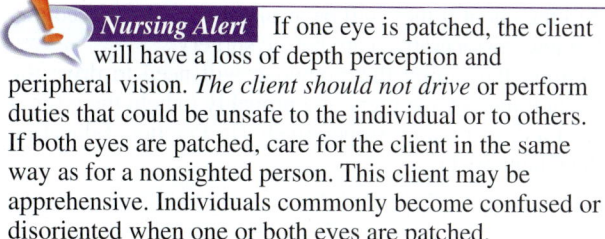

Nursing Alert If one eye is patched, the client will have a loss of depth perception and peripheral vision. *The client should not drive* or perform duties that could be unsafe to the individual or to others. If both eyes are patched, care for the client in the same way as for a nonsighted person. This client may be apprehensive. Individuals commonly become confused or disoriented when one or both eyes are patched.

Cotton-Tipped Applicator

A cotton-tipped applicator (or *dry wipe*) may be ordered to clean drainage out of the external auditory canal and the auricle (In Practice: Nursing Procedure 80-1).

Ear Irrigation

An *ear irrigation* may be performed to rinse drainage or medication from the ears and to remove wax or foreign bodies. It is done only with a healthcare provider's order. Do not irrigate the ear if the client's eardrum is punctured. Irrigating the ear or instilling medications requires different techniques for adults and children (Fig. 80-2). In Practice: Nursing Procedure 80-2 describes the procedure for ear irrigation.

COMMON SURGICAL TREATMENTS

Eye Surgeries

Most surgical procedures on the eye are performed as same-day surgery. In many cases, clients receive local anesthesia and are awake during such procedures. Eye surgeries involve precision. Often they are done with the aid of an operating microscope. The client's cooperation is essential; therefore, preoperative client and family teaching is important, including the following actions:

- Review activities permitted before surgery and restrictions following the procedure.
- Teach client and family how to administer eye drops or other medication prescribed to dilate the eye or treat infection.
- Review other procedures, such as eye patching.
- Outline the steps of the surgery: what will be done and what is expected of the client.

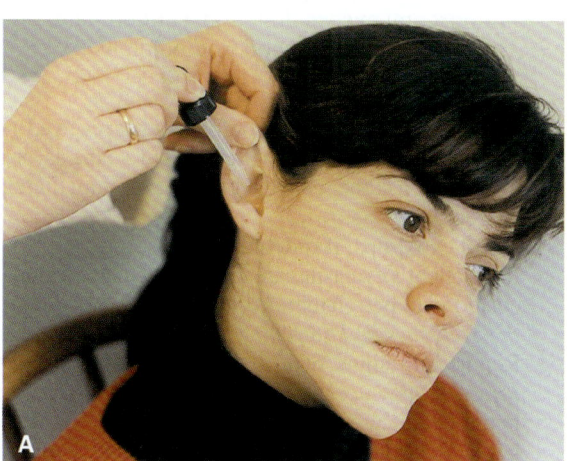
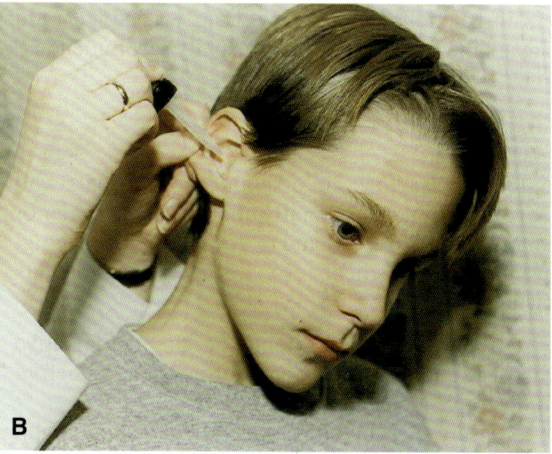

Figure 80-2 Technique for irrigation of the external auditory canal or instillation of ear drops. Note the difference in direction of pull on the pinna between **(A)** the adult (up and back) and **(B)** the child (down and back).

- Tell the client if they will be awake during the procedure.
- Review postoperative care before surgery.
- Remind the family that someone will need to drive the client home after surgery and probably to help them for at least a day or two postoperatively (In Practice: Educating the Client 80-1).

Enucleation

Enucleation is removal of the eyeball. This procedure may be done when disease or injury has destroyed the eye or if a malignant tumor develops. After the eye is removed, a metal or plastic implant is buried in the empty eye socket. The eye muscles attached to the capsule move the implant. After healing is complete, a glass or plastic prosthesis shaped like a shell is fitted over the buried implant, for cosmetic purposes. This shell is painted to match the other eye.

Care of the Prosthetic Eye

The client must learn how to insert and remove the prosthetic eye and how to care for it. Some types of prostheses are removed at night and placed in a solution. When practicing insertion and removal, the person leans over a soft or padded surface to prevent possible breakage of the prosthesis. The current versions of prostheses, which made of plastic, are not easily broken.

If the nurse is required to insert a prosthetic eye, do the following:

- Wear gloves.
- Wet the prosthesis. *Rationale: This action allows it to slip in easily.*
- Lift the upper eyelid. Slip the eye up under the top lid.
- Hold the prosthesis while pulling down gently on the lower lid.
- Slip the lower lid over the edge of the prosthesis.
- Ask the client to blink. Blinking should slip the lid over the prosthesis and seat it in place.

To remove the prosthesis:

- Pull down on the lower lid.
- Press inward on the bottom of the prosthesis, which should cause it to slip out.
- Be sure to work over a soft surface, to avoid breaking the prosthesis.

When caring for the eye socket, follow the healthcare provider's instructions. Rinsing with tap water or a mild solution available for this purpose is usually recommended.

Providing Care in Eye Surgery

Preoperative Care

Client and family teaching are essential for all clients who undergo eye surgery, and especially clients who are older or confused. Make sure to cover and to document all teaching.

When preparing the client for eye surgery, also include the following:

- Make sure to perform all items on the preoperative checklist. The client must sign an informed consent before any preoperative medications are given.
- Check to ensure that the client was NPO after midnight, if an early procedure is scheduled. Also note whether the client has taken a laxative or received an enema the night before surgery, if prescribed.

IN PRACTICE

EDUCATING THE CLIENT 80-1 | **After Eye Surgery**

- Do not remove your dressings; leave dressings in place.
- Do not use eye medications until you see the surgeon (usually on the first postoperative day). Bring your eye medications to that appointment.
- If a metal shield is prescribed, wear it while sleeping or napping, for up to 4 weeks to protect the eye from being accidentally bumped or touched.
- If both eyes are patched, be sure to ask your family for assistance; make sure they know how to help you.
- Do not sleep on the operative side for at least a week to prevent fluid and pressure from accumulating on the suture line.
- After the first postoperative day, clean the eye gently to remove mucus. Use cotton balls or tissues moistened with tap water.
- Follow these actions to avoid disrupting the suture line:
  - Avoid sudden movements.
  - Do not press on or rub the operative eye.
  - Avoid bending over with the head below the waist for about 2 weeks.
  - Avoid straining at stool.
  - Avoid vomiting; use antiemetics if prescribed.
  - Avoid activities such as coughing, sneezing, nose blowing, and vomiting.
  - Do not lift more than 10 to 20 lb for about a week.
  - Try not to bump or shake the head vigorously.
- Shampoo with the head back for at least a week.
- Avoid falls and jolts. Be careful walking on ice or up and down stairs. (Depth perception may be altered postoperatively.)
- Avoid getting soap in the operative eye. Bathing and showering are permitted.
- Read, watch TV, and ride in or drive a car, as vision permits.
- Follow the surgeon's instructions about your stitches, which may need to be removed or may be absorbable.
- Know that glasses will probably be fitted in about 6 weeks. They may need to be changed during the first year, as the eyes adjust.
- Report any excess drainage, sudden pain, or bleeding to the surgeon immediately.

- Assist the client if they are confused or has received a sedative.
- Wash the client's face with surgical soap, as ordered. If necessary, ask the male client to shave immediately before surgery.
- Instill eye drops, if ordered.
- If the client's eyelashes are to be clipped, use a blunt scissors coated with petrolatum. *Rationale: The petrolatum catches the eyelashes and prevents them from falling into the eye.*
- Report any signs of a respiratory infection. *Rationale: Infection may necessitate postponing the surgery.*
- If the healthcare provider has ordered the client's eyes to be patched preoperatively, find out what type of patch to use. Also check if a metal eye shield has also been ordered.
- Explain the reasons for patching to the client. *Rationale: Explanations reduce apprehension and confusion.*

- Have the client bring a hearing aid (if they wear one) to wear during the surgery. *Rationale: The client must be able to hear the surgeon's instructions. Be sure to document this on the preoperative checklist.*
- Perform and document all preoperative teaching. Answer any questions the client or family may have.

Postoperative Care

Because the client usually goes home soon after surgery, postoperative care centers around client and family teaching. The client is generally cautioned to avoid coughing, sneezing, lifting objects over 10 to 20 lb, and sudden head movements. These actions can cause sudden fluctuations in IOP that disrupt suture lines. Focus client teaching on preventing complications, such as hemorrhage, increased IOP, stress on the suture line, and infection (In Practice: Educating the Client 80-1).

Ear Surgeries

Because many ear surgeries are done on an outpatient basis, nursing care centers around client and family teaching. If the client is in an acute care facility, the same principles apply.

Nursing Alert Report any paralysis of the face or on the operative side or ptosis (drooping eyelid) immediately. *Rationale: These findings may indicate damage to the facial nerve or the presence of edema.*

Cochlear Implant

The *cochlear implant* is a surgically implanted device that emits an auditory signal, bypassing a damaged cochlear system and stimulating the remaining auditory nerve tissue. This procedure is for the profoundly deaf or severely hard of hearing person and allows sound perception.

There are several classifications of implants. Location and transmission of the auditory signals and the types of implanted electrodes and stimulation of nerve tissue determine the type and classification of implant. A cochlear implant has an internal coil with a stranded electrode lead that is surgically inserted into the cochlea. The external coil or transmitter aligns with the internal coil or receiver by a magnet. When the microphone receives sound, the stimulator wires receive the signal after it has been filtered. This filtering allows the sound to transmit comfortably for the client. Sound is then passed by the external transmitter to the inner coil receiver by magnetic conduction and is finally carried by the electrode to the cochlea.

The potential candidate for cochlear implant must be an otherwise healthy individual with no evidence of mental retardation or psychological disorder. The client must be unable to recognize words spoken away from the line of vision and be realistic and optimistic about the results.

Encourage clients to talk with others who have had the surgery to learn positive and negative aspects. Postoperatively, treat the client similarly to others who undergo middle ear surgery. Within a few weeks after the surgery, the controls on the implant are adjusted and the rehabilitation process begins. The client must learn to discriminate between sounds and voices. Listening will take patience and training.

Providing Care in Ear Surgery
Preoperative Care

Preoperative client and family instructions for ear surgery are similar to those for eye surgery. Prepare them for what will occur and what to expect before and after the surgery. The client is often awake for surgery and must be able to follow instructions. Be sure to let the client know this preoperatively. Ear drops may be instilled or the client's ear may require packing with cotton, as ordered.

Postoperative Care

If the client is to go home immediately after surgery, teach the client and family how to perform care (In Practice: Educating the Client 80-2). Usually the client is allowed out of bed as soon as they leave the recovery area. Someone must be available to drive the client home.

If the nurse is to change dressings or instill medications, be sure to follow strict aseptic technique and wear gloves. *Rationale: These actions help to prevent infection. Meningitis or encephalitis is possible because of the ear's close proximity to the brain. Instruct the client not to remove dressings.*

IN PRACTICE
EDUCATING THE CLIENT 80-2 — After Ear Surgery

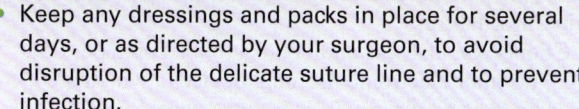

- Keep any dressings and packs in place for several days, or as directed by your surgeon, to avoid disruption of the delicate suture line and to prevent infection.
- Watch for signs of dizziness or prolonged nausea; these are symptoms of inner ear disturbance.
- Avoid vomiting because it can disrupt the delicate suture line. Take antiemetics, as ordered.
- Avoid abrupt changes in position. Do not sit up quickly. These actions may overstimulate or upset the semicircular canals of the inner ear.
- Avoid sudden movement, straining, lifting, or acts, such as sneezing or coughing. They may disrupt the suture line.
- Do not blow your nose. This can disrupt the suture line and possibly lead to infection.
- Watch for bleeding and any feelings of pressure or pain.
- Follow the surgeon's orders regarding positioning. Some recommend lying on the operative side to facilitate drainage. Some prefer the client to lie on the nonoperative side to prevent fluid and blood accumulation and stretching of the suture line after grafting.
- Watch for any fever, headache, vertigo, or ear pain or pressure over the implanted ear and notify your surgeon as soon as possible if you experience any of these effects.
- Although you can bathe, do not allow water to enter the operative ear.
- Resume your normal activities in about 2 weeks after being checked by the surgeon.

NURSING PROCESS

DATA COLLECTION
A sensory disorder may involve a disruption in vision, hearing, or one of the other senses. Carefully observe the client for signs and symptoms of a sensory disorder. Monitor and document the client's condition. Your observations and findings establish a baseline for future comparison and determine the presence of suspected complications (In Practice: Data Gathering in Nursing 80-1). Report any changes in baseline levels.

In addition, observe the client's emotional response to the disorder or disease. Is the client nonsighted? Is the client able to hear? What impact does the disorder have on the client? If vision or hearing has been lost, is the client able to communicate, and how do they communicate? Are they able to work? Can the client move from place to place? Do they need assistance to meet daily needs? Does the disorder affect social activities or self-esteem? Is the disorder correctable?

PLANNING AND IMPLEMENTATION
Nursing considerations for clients with sensory deficits include teaching and approaches to effective care for both client and caregivers or family. Whenever possible, make short-term and long-terms goals in conjunction with the client, caregivers, family members, and the healthcare team.

The client with a hearing disorder may require assistance with communication, maintaining balance, and meeting social and recreational needs.

A client with hearing or vision loss may need assistance in dealing with the disorder's emotional aspects. Help all clients to understand more about the disorder, the prognosis, and the treatment. Rehabilitation is designed to promote self-care.

Provide pre- and postoperative care for the client undergoing eye or ear surgery. The suture line is delicate in many of these operations. The client and caregivers at home will need to understand ways to protect these delicate suture lines because many eye and ear surgeries are done on an outpatient basis.

Nursing Considerations for the Visually Impaired Client
When caring for a client who is visually impaired and is hospitalized, include the following:
- Encourage clients to assume responsibility for their own care gradually.
- Identify yourself when you enter the room.
- Speak before touching clients to prevent frightening them.
- Speak in a normal tone.
- Keep the call light within reach and place the bed in the lowest position.
- Place food on the plate in the same "clock positions" for every meal. Tell the person what is being served and where it is located on the plate.
- When ambulating, walk slowly and allow the person to take your arm—do not push.
- Orient the client to the location of objects in the room, such as furniture, the door, grooming articles, and the water pitcher; keep these objects in the same place.
- Let the client know when you are leaving the room.

When a client is visually impaired, simple activities can become difficult or overwhelming. For example, medication administration ordered postoperatively can present problems. The side effects of some eye medications (e.g., timolol [Timoptic]) are bradycardia, dizziness, and syncope. Discharge teaching must include the common signs and symptoms of medication side effects. The nurse also can offer suggestions, such as the use of weekly pill reminder dispensers.

A home safety inspection should be performed. Scatter rugs, doors halfway open, and packages left in hallways are common hazards to the person with limited or no sight.

Individuals with a visual disruption often require rehabilitation to resume self-care. The visually impaired individual may need assistance moving around and learning to navigate in familiar surroundings. Meeting daily needs (e.g., preparing meals, shopping, hygiene, grooming) brings additional challenges. Moreover, the individual may need assistance in finding new modes of transportation and may experience possible changes in employment.

In addition, other options are available for the visually impaired or nonsighted client. These options include computer adaptations, Braille, guide dogs, and white canes.

Braille
The *Braille alphabet* is a system of raised dots on paper that correspond to the letters of the alphabet and punctuation marks. One of the hardest things that a person who has only recently become visually impaired must do is to become accustomed to the inability to read. Learning to read Braille can be of assistance to many individuals with permanent loss of sight.

The nonsighted person discerns these characters with the fingertips. Learning Braille takes patience. However, many books and other resources are available in Braille and will allow the person to continue to enjoy reading. Direct the person to local agencies for the nonsighted for more information.

Clients can also use audiobooks (books on tape, CD, MP3, or other electronic listening devices), which are recordings of books, articles, or magazines. Special Braille computer keyboards are also available. Some computer monitors, magazines, and newspapers are available in very large print for partially sighted people. Many are also available in Braille editions.

Guide Dogs
A *guide dog* (also called a *leader dog* or *seeing eye dog*) is used by many nonsighted individuals. These dogs are trained to recognize danger spots, such as curbs, obstacles, or holes. They learn to be careful of traffic. The dog wears

a harness fitted with a U-shaped handle that the nonsighted person can grasp; client and dog then communicate through the movements of the harness. A nonsighted person who wishes to use a guide dog must live at a training center for some time to learn how to use and take care of the dog.

The public accords these trained dogs certain privileges. They are allowed to enter restaurants, subways, hotels, and other public places that are usually off-limits to pets. If the client is not moving, the dog will lie quietly nearby. Airlines often reserve space for such dogs in the plane's cabin.

> **Nursing Alert** Never pet or play with a guide dog. Distracting a dog could place the visually impaired person in danger.

White Canes

A *white cane* is a signal that the person carrying it is nonsighted. Only a nonsighted person is allowed to use a white cane and that person has the right of way over all traffic. Some nonsighted persons, however, are reluctant to use a white cane unless absolutely necessary.

One type of collapsible white cane that a client can carry in a purse or pocket is longer than a normal walking cane and has a metal or plastic tip that transmits sound, thus providing the person with some guidance about their surroundings. As a part of the rehabilitation process, nonsighted people learn to use these canes to locate curbs and other obstructions.

Nursing Considerations for the Hearing-Impaired Client

A person with a marked hearing loss cannot hear sounds that warn of danger. This person loses the thread of a conversation and may ask questions or make comments that have no relation to the discussion. Sometimes, persons with hearing loss lapse into a silence that makes them seem uninterested or inattentive. People who are unable to hear their own voice may talk very loudly or in a monotone (In Practice: Nursing Care Plan 80-1).

Many people are generally less tolerant of hearing loss than they are of vision loss, thus they may become impatient when asked to repeat their words.

When caring for a client who is experiencing a hearing impairment, include the following:
- Get the client's attention before beginning to speak.
- Face the client on the same level.
- Place yourself in good light, so the client can see your mouth clearly.
- Do not chew, smoke, put objects in the mouth, or cover it while talking.
- Decrease background noises, such as television and radio.
- Speak slowly and clearly; repeat entire phrases rather than specific words.
- Restate the conversation with different words.
- Use contextual clues such as objects, persons, and hand motions to facilitate the conversation.
- Verify that the person understood the conversation.

Individuals with impaired hearing may stubbornly refuse to admit that they do not hear well. They may deny themselves the help of a hearing aid because of embarrassment. Hearing loss caused by advancing age (*presbyacusia*) cannot be restored, but there are ways of compensating.

Hearing Aids

Hearing aids operate either on the principle of bone conduction or air conduction, depending on the type of hearing loss. The device amplifies sounds. A tiny receiver is inserted in the ear, and an earpiece is molded to the wearer's ear. Many hearing aids today are so tiny they are barely noticeable.

The healthcare provider will determine whether a hearing aid will help and which type will be the most beneficial. Unfortunately, a hearing aid usually is less effective in improving hearing than glasses are in improving vision. Adjusting to a hearing aid takes time and patience.

Normally, an individual can adjust to, and focus attention on, specific sounds, such as human speech. Difficulties that clients encounter when wearing hearing aids include the resultant amplification of all sounds, including background sounds. These sounds can be distracting and annoying.

However, the client can overcome difficulties with perseverance and by wearing the aid at all times, not just occasionally. The earpiece should be washed every day with mild soap and water and dried well. A pipe cleaner will help to clean and dry the cannula. Batteries in hearing aids need to be checked regularly. Getting used to wearing a hearing aid and learning to adjust to it take time and patience.

Speech Reading

Individuals with a hearing loss may benefit from *lip reading (speech reading)* and facial expressions. To understand lip reading, the hearing-impaired person must directly face the speaking person.

Sign Language

Another means of communication is *sign language (signing)*. Sign language uses specific movements of the fingers and hands to form letters of the alphabet as well as concepts or words. Facial gesture, movements of the arms, and postures of the body combine with words to form a complete, complex language. In the United States, the most common form of sign language is *American Sign Language* (ASL). There are many varieties of sign language depending on the client's country of origin. No one sign language is universal. Different sign languages are used in different countries or regions. For example, in the United Kingdom the most common sign language is *British Sign Language* (BSL). ASL and BSL use different symbols and gestures; the person speaking one form may not be able to understand another form.

> **Nursing Alert** Lions International targets vision and hearing improvement as a major goal. If you come into contact with someone who needs eyeglasses, a guide dog, a hearing aid, or surgery, but cannot afford it, put the person in contact with their local Lions Club.

NCLEX Alert

Nursing care in healthcare facilities commonly include considerations for individuals who are visually or hearing impaired. Additionally, the aging process enhances alterations in most sensory abilities. When answering NCLEX questions, remember to consider nursing care options related to safety, nutritional needs, activities of daily living (ADLs), self-medicating, or any concept related to a sensory concern described in the NCLEX scenario.

Evaluation

Evaluate outcomes of care with the client, family, and other members of the healthcare team. Have short-term goals been met? For example, has the client's vision or hearing improved after surgery? Are long-term goals still realistic? For example, is the client adjusting to the use of a guide dog? Is the client able to perform self-care? Are family members available to assist? What type of rehabilitation, education, or assistive aids does the client need? Planning for further nursing care considers the client's prognosis, any complications, and the client's responses.

IN PRACTICE
DATA GATHERING IN NURSING 80-1 | Key Areas for Monitoring and Documenting the Sensory System

General Areas
- Nursing history, including information from family
- Presence of recent infections
- Medication use and recreational drug use
- General appearance of eyes and ears; examination with ophthalmoscope or otoscope
- Presence of foreign objects
- History of trauma to eyes and ears
- Documentation of cranial nerve function
- Neurologic status
- Signs of cardiovascular disorders (elevated cholesterol, hypertension)

Vision and Eye Documentation and Data Gathering
- Vision assessment with Snellen chart or similar tool (gross determination of visual acuity if person has poor vision)
- Screening for infection or injury
- Screening for color blindness
- Screening for visual field deficits
- Screening for extraocular muscle disorder
- Symptoms and history of vision loss
- Direct observation of disorders such as ptosis

Hearing and Ear Documentation and Data Gathering
- Prolonged noise exposure
- Presence of chronic respiratory or ear infections
- Screening with audiometer or similar instrument
- Complaints or symptoms and history of hearing loss

IN PRACTICE
NURSING CARE PLAN 80-1 | The Client With a Hearing Impairment

Medical History: S.S. is an 85-year-old client, widowed for 2 years, and a retired teacher. After being at an acute care facility for 3 days for pneumonia, they have been admitted to a long-term care facility. History upon admission to LTC reveals resolving pneumonia, hypertension, coronary artery disease, glaucoma, and severe degenerative joint disease. During their recent stay at the acute care facility, a hearing evaluation was completed and the client received a hearing aid for moderate hearing loss.

Medical diagnosis: Moderate hearing loss; history of hypertension, coronary artery disease, glaucoma, and degenerative joint disease.

DATA COLLECTION/NURSING OBSERVATION

Client is alert and oriented. Skin is pale pink, warm, and dry. S.S. has been living alone since the death of their partner 2 years ago. Over the past 2 years, the client's health has declined, necessitating increasing amounts of care. Client has one older sister who is in the same facility. Client reports joint stiffness and pain in the morning. "Once I get up and get started moving, they get a little better." Joints demonstrate limited range of motion. During the interview, client does not always respond to words spoken or responds inappropriately. When questioned about the use of the hearing aid and their ability to hear with and without it, the client states, "I usually leave it in my bag. Besides, what do I need this thing for? I can hear just fine." Further assessment reveals that client has a hearing deficit that is more severe on the left. When asked, client unable to demonstrate ability to insert, remove, or care for the hearing aid.

NURSING DIAGNOSIS

(Although other nursing diagnoses may be appropriate, a priority nursing diagnosis is addressed below.)

Altered sensory perception (auditory) related to diagnosed hearing loss as evidenced by resident's difficulty with responses when being spoken to and lack of use of prescribed hearing aid.

Planning (Outcomes/Goals)	Implementation (Nursing Actions)	Evaluation
Short-Term Goals		
Note to students: In a long-term care facility, individuals living there are generally referred to as "residents."		
A. Resident will acknowledge the need for using a hearing aid.	• Determine the resident's feelings and knowledge about hearing loss and using a hearing aid. • Clarify any misconceptions or misinformation. *Rationale: Determining the resident's feelings and knowledge about the hearing aid provides a baseline from which to plan further actions.* • Review the reasons for the use of the hearing aid. • Demonstrate insertion of device. *Rationale: Reviewing the reasons for the hearing aid helps to promote better understanding of the device. Demonstrating techniques associated with use and care of device aids in understanding of concepts.*	Day 2—0800 hr. • Resident states that they are embarrassed by the use of the hearing aid. • Nurse inserted hearing aid. Resident stated, "It does help a bit. Things don't sound so muddled." • Resident agreed to try wearing hearing aid for 2 hours per day. *Goal A partially met. Observations continue.*
B. Resident will respond appropriately to auditory stimuli with the use of the hearing aid.	• Get the resident's attention before beginning to speak. • Face the resident on the same level, making sure that lighting is appropriate to allow resident to see speaker's mouth. *Rationale: Getting the resident's attention and facing the resident when speaking help the resident to focus on the nurse and what is being said.* • Decrease background noises, such as television and radio. • Speak slowly and clearly, repeating, and restating information as necessary. *Rationale: Decreasing background noises helps to minimize distractions. Speaking clearly and slowly, repeating, and restating allow the resident to focus on what is being said, thereby fostering verbal communication.* • Use nonverbal behaviors to enhance verbal communication. *Rationale: Gestures and other nonverbal behaviors can help to clarify the message being communicated.*	Day 2—1,030 hr. • Hearing aid in place for 2 hr continuously. • Resident demonstrated appropriate responses to verbal communication. • Some difficulty with responses is noted after hearing aid removed. Resident stated, "I guess I'll try the hearing aid for a while longer." *Goals A and B met.*

Planning (Outcomes/Goals)	Implementation (Nursing Actions)	Evaluation
Long-Term Goals		
C. Resident demonstrates ability to insert, remove, and clean hearing aid without assistance. **REVISED GOAL** Resident cooperates with insertion and removal of hearing aid when done by nurse's aide or nurse.	• Have resident give return demonstration of insertion of the hearing aid. • Provide positive feedback and reinforcement when task is attempted by client. • Reinforce concept that procedures should become easier with practice. • While in long-term care facility, encourage resident to ask for aide's assistance to insert device when getting dressed in the morning. *Rationale: Feedback and positive reinforcement are necessary to aid in building self-confidence, thereby helping to foster compliance with the use of the hearing aid. Resident's physical disabilities, r/t osteoarthritis in hands and joints, may limit capabilities for self-care.* • Continue to assist and reinforce use of hearing aid. • Encourage resident to increase time spent using hearing aid. *Rationale: Continued assistance and reinforcement help to promote learning and to enhance self-confidence. Socialization improves when the resident is able to hear and talk with other residents in the LTC facility.*	Day 3—1,300 hr. • Resident unable to physically insert hearing aid. • Resident cooperated with assistant with inserting aid into ear, stating, "My fingers are so stiff that I can't always get the aid in my ear. I cannot do it by myself." • Resident unable to demonstrate proper technique for cleaning the device, stating their fingers "won't cooperate." • Responses are accurate and appropriate when hearing aid is in place. • Resident wears hearing aid from 8 AM until 12 noon every morning for the last 3 days. Goals A and B met. Goal C not met. Unable to physically insert or remove hearing aid due to physical limitations. New Goal C needed See REVISED GOAL C
D. Resident wears hearing aid during waking hours.	• Increase wearing time of hearing aid by 1 hr each day until resident can tolerate wearing the device for 8–10 hr or when awake during daytime hours. *Rationale: Hearing aids are better tolerated if wearing time is increased gradually. Wearing the device helps to maintain auditory function and promotes the individual's hearing capacity. Socialization with others in LTC facility improves with resident's ability to communicate with others.*	Day 4—1,530 hr. • Resident states that they can wear hearing aid for 3 or 4 hr without it "becoming annoying." • Stated that they enjoyed going to the dining room for meals so that they had someone to talk to. Goal D ongoing. Observations and assistance with hearing aid continue.

THE EYE AND VISION DISORDERS

Several specialists are involved in treatment of the eye.

- An *ophthalmologist* has received a Doctor of Medicine (MD) degree and has completed at least 3 years of postgraduate training in diseases and surgeries of the eye. This healthcare provider is licensed to diagnose and treat eye disorders, prescribe medications, perform surgery, and fit glasses or contact lenses.
- An *optometrist* has received a Doctor of Optometry (OD) degree following undergraduate and graduate studies. This individual is licensed to examine eyes, prescribe eyeglasses or contact lenses, and, in many states, treat some eye diseases with medications.
- An *optician* is responsible for grinding lenses and fitting spectacles as specified by either the ophthalmologist or optometrist.
- *Ophthalmic technicians* are certified by the Joint Commission to assist the ophthalmologist in performing tests on clients.

TABLE 80-1 Refractive Errors of the Eye

REFRACTIVE ERROR	CAUSE	RESULT
Myopia (nearsightedness)	Elongation of the eyeball	Light rays focus at a point in front of the retina; blurred distant vision
Hyperopia (farsightedness)	Shorter than normal eyeball	Light rays focus at a point behind the retina; blurred close vision
Astigmatism	Unequal curvature in shape of lens or cornea	Light rays focus on two different points on the retina; distorted vision
Presbyopia	Loss of elasticity of lens (poor accommodation)	Light rays focus at a point behind the retina; decreased close vision

Visual Changes

Changes in visual acuity are very common, affecting most people sometime during their lifetime. Visual changes may be corrected simply with lenses or surgery, or they may increase in severity until the person is unable to see light at all. The nurse is responsible for identifying early changes, teaching the client how to preserve vision or adapt to changes, and assisting the person when vision is impaired.

Refractive Errors

Vision occurs when light rays of an image pass through the lens and come to a focus point on the retina. From here, neurons send signals about the image to the brain for interpretation.

Refractive errors result when light rays focus in front of or behind the retina owing to variations in the shape of the lens. The person experiences blurred vision or other changes in acuity. Holding objects at a distance, squinting, and headaches are some signs of impaired acuity. Common refractive errors are **myopia** (nearsightedness), **hyperopia** (farsightedness), **astigmatism** (abnormal curvature of the cornea or lens), and **presbyopia** (loss of lens elasticity and accommodation owing to the aging process) (Table 80-1).

Correction of Refractive Errors

Refractive errors, which cause the most common changes in normal vision, are first identified by a Snellen test. The refractive examination pinpoints the degree of the error, which is necessary to determine the treatment. Corrective lenses (eyeglasses) or contact lenses are the most common treatment for refractive errors. The lenses are shaped as either concave or convex, thus *refracting* (bending) the light rays to focus on the retina.

Eyeglasses

Eyeglasses are prescribed to correct the refractive errors of myopia, hyperopia, astigmatism, and presbyopia and for some low-vision ("legally blind") individuals.

Bifocals, two lenses in one, may be prescribed to correct the problem of presbyopia. Each eyeglass lens has two parts: one part corrects the defect in near vision; the other corrects the defect in far vision. *Trifocals* are also available and provide an additional option for vision correction.

Contact Lenses

Contact lenses are designed to fit directly on the cornea, where they float on a layer of tears. Contact lenses may provide better vision than eyeglasses by eliminating minification or magnification of objects. Poorly maintained contact lens hygiene can cause significant problems, including corneal ulcerations.

Hard contact lenses are made of rigid gas-permeable plastic (**RGP**) and are paper thin. They are kept in place by capillary attraction and by the upper eyelid. Clients usually wear them daily. The lenses require special cleaning, rinsing, and storage solutions for care.

Soft contact lenses are made of hydrophilic plastic of a larger diameter and greater flexibility than RGP lenses. Soft contact lenses are more likely to be damaged by handling because they can easily tear.

Extended-wear soft contact lenses allow oxygen and carbon dioxide to pass freely through the lens. These lenses may be worn for up to 2 weeks before removal. However, extended-wear contact lenses have a greater risk of infection than daily-wear contact lenses. Some soft lenses are disposable and are discarded after an established period (e.g., daily, weekly) for a new set of lenses.

Many people take contact lenses for granted. Contact lens wearers must realize that prolonged wear or improper care can cause infections, particularly conjunctivitis, and injury to the sclera such as ulcerations. In some cases, blindness may result from *infectious keratitis* (inflammation of the cornea). Caution clients not to put contact lenses into the mouth to wet or clean them. Doing so can transfer unwanted pathogens to the eye. The greatest danger with the use of any type of contact lens is the possibility of injury to, or infection of, the cornea, which can permanently affect vision.

In the case of accident or unconsciousness, the wearer could become blind if hard contact lenses are not removed. When the eyes are closed, tears cannot circulate freely, and corneal ulcers can quickly develop. For this reason, clients should not wear contact lenses while sleeping unless they are designed for continuous use.

If the person wearing contact lenses is hit in the eye area, injury to the cornea may result. Contact lenses rarely break while they are in place because the eyeball will give with the blow and because the surrounding bony structure protects the eye. However, in the event of injury, severe swelling, or infection, a healthcare provider may need to remove the lenses.

Surgery

Surgical correction is done by *keratorefractive surgery* (surgical alteration of the corneal curvature), in which a laser or other microsurgical knife reshapes the cornea. Another procedure is *radial keratotomy* (**RK**), in which partial-thickness, radial incisions are made in the cornea to correct the refractive error. *Photorefractive keratotomy* (**PRK**) and *laser-assisted in site keratomileusis* (**LASIK**) are other procedures that correct refractive errors.

Inflammatory and Infectious Disorders

Conjunctivitis

Conjunctivitis, also called *pink eye,* is inflammation of the *conjunctiva,* the membrane lining the eyelids and covering the sclera (Fig. 80-3). A bacterial, viral, or an allergy may cause conjunctivitis. Infectious conjunctivitis is very

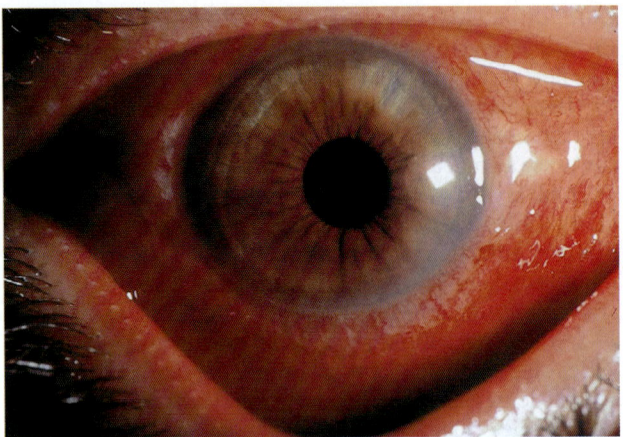

Figure 80-3 Conjunctivitis. Note the typical redness of the conjunctiva. (Smeltzer, Bare, Hinkle, & Cheever, 2008.)

contagious. It can develop in one eye and easily be transferred to the other eye when the eye or face is touched. Contact lens use is also a risk factor.

Conjunctivitis causes pain, redness, swelling, itching, and sometimes purulent discharge (*pus*). The discharge may be so thick and copious that the eyelids stick together. Antibiotic eye drops or ointments are prescribed for bacterial infections, and antiviral medications for viral infections. Proper handwashing, use of gloves, and proper cleaning of the client's linens are essential to prevent the spread of infection. Conjunctivitis can also be related to environmental allergies and not be considered an infection. Typically, allergic conjunctivitis is bilateral. Infectious conjunctivitis may be unilateral. Treatment of allergy-related conjunctivitis includes avoiding the offending allergen, taking antihistamines, and undergoing desensitization. Many over-the-counter antihistamine and prescription eye drops are helpful. Baby shampoo or saline solution irrigations or warm soaks may remove discharge, reduce swelling, and decrease pain and itching.

Giant papillary conjunctivitis (*GPC*), a type of severe conjunctivitis, can be the result of chronic, long-term use of contact lenses. (See conjunctivitis, Chapter 73.) GPC can be generally be successfully treated by discontinuing wearing of contact lenses for several weeks or months.

> **Key Concept**
> Teach the client not to rub the eyes, which can lead to corneal scaring. If eye drops are used, teach the client not to touch the eye with the dropper (which will contaminate the solution). Discard unused or partially used eye drops because the solution can become contaminated.

Trachoma
Trachoma is another form of conjunctivitis found in hot, dry climates. Its cause is the organism *Chlamydia trachomatis*, which may also cause the infection *inclusion conjunctivitis*. Trachoma is highly communicable and is one of the world's leading causes of preventable blindness.

Treatment includes topical and systemic antibiotics, which are very effective. Trachoma is rarely seen in the United States.

Blepharitis
Blepharitis, inflammation of the eyelid, is caused by excessive dryness of the eyes, excessive oiliness of the skin, or infection. This condition is usually characterized by red lid margins and purulent drainage. Treatment consists of applying warm packs to the eye to help loosen crusted drainage. Cleanse the eyelid gently with a mild soap and water once or twice a day. An antibiotic ophthalmic ointment may be prescribed to resolve infection and prevent recurrence.

Hordeolum
A *hordeolum* or *stye* is an acute inflammation of an oil or sweat gland of the eyelid. Styes are red, raised, swollen, and painful. They contain pus. After the area drains, pain is relieved and healing begins.

Treatment includes applying warm, moist compresses, and a topical antibiotic ointment to the area to help localize the infection. In severe cases, the abscess is incised and drained. Teach the client not to squeeze a stye, which could spread infection.

Chalazion
A *chalazion (meibomian cyst)* is an accumulation of *lipid* (fatty) material from a chronically obstructed *meibomian* (sebaceous) gland found on the eyelid. If the lesion is small and does not affect vision, treatment is unnecessary. However, if it becomes infected or interferes with vision or eyelid closure, incising and draining the area may be necessary.

Keratitis
Keratitis is an inflammation of the cornea caused by bacterial, viral, or fungal infections, often after trauma. *Herpes simplex keratitis* is the most common cause of unilateral visual loss from infectious keratitis in the United States.

Symptoms include pain, *photophobia* (sensitivity to light), blurred vision, purulent drainage, and redness of the sclera. Corneal ulceration is a common *sequela* (result). After culture studies are done, treatment consists of eye drops to dilate the pupil. Fortified antibiotic drops may be given hourly for bacterial disease. Antiviral or antifungal therapy, as necessary, may be given for viral or fungal causes.

Structural Disorders
Structural eye disorders may result from the aging process, injury, or a nervous disorder. They include the following:

- **Ectropion**, an outward turning of the eyelid, is caused by the aging process. The eye is no longer able to drain effectively and tearing occurs. Surgical intervention is necessary.
- **Entropion**, an inward turning of the lid margin, is common in older adults. The lower lashes turn inward and are often not visible, but they irritate the conjunctiva and cornea. Corrective surgery may also be necessary.
- **Ptosis** is drooping of the upper eyelid. Ptosis may result from muscular weakness, damage to the oculomotor nerve, or interference with the sympathetic nerves that maintain the lid's smooth muscle tone. Depending on the cause, corrective surgery and/or correction of the neurologic disorder may be necessary.

Glaucoma
Glaucoma is a condition of increased fluid (aqueous humor) pressure within the eye. It has an insidious onset, usually

occurring after age 40 years and having familial tendencies. Glaucoma is a leading cause of blindness in the United States. A disturbance in the normal balance between production and drainage of eye fluid causes glaucoma, leading to an increase in IOP. The increased pressure of glaucoma is also known as *ocular hypertension* or *high intraocular pressure.* Chronic elevated IOP permanently damages the retina and the optic nerve. If left untreated, visual changes and blindness can occur. Early diagnosis and treatment are of the utmost importance to prevent vision loss.

Angle-Closure Glaucoma

Angle-closure glaucoma is the most common type of glaucoma. In this condition, drainage of the aqueous humor through the *trabecular* (supporting) meshwork (located in the angle of the anterior chamber of the eye) is inadequate. The result is the accumulation of aqueous fluid in the anterior chamber, which causes an increase in IOP. Both eyes are commonly affected.

The onset of angle-closure glaucoma is slow, with gradual loss of peripheral vision. It is often diagnosed at a routine eye examination when increased IOP is discovered. Often symptoms are absent, mild, or intermittent. Therefore, a serious vision loss may occur before the condition is discovered.

When symptoms occur, they include eye discomfort, temporary blurring of vision, reduced peripheral vision, and headaches. Late signs are the appearance of halos around lights and central blindness.

Treatment

Angle-closure glaucoma may be treated with eye drops, to increase aqueous outflow, or oral medication, such as acetazolamide (Diamox), to decrease production of aqueous humor. Beta-adrenergic blockers, such as timolol maleate (Timoptic) and betaxolol hydrochloride (Betoptic), are used as well. Ophthalmic carbonic anhydrase inhibitors, such as brinzolamide–brimonidine tartrate (Simbrinza) and dorzolamide hydrochloride (Trusopt) reduce intraocular pressure by suppressing the rate of aqueous humor formation. They are effective ocular hypotensive agents but may have significant systemic side effects if used for long-term therapies. Ophthalmic prostaglandins, also known as prostaglandin analogs, such as travoprost (Travatan Z), latanoprost (Xalatan), or bimatoprost (Lumigan) reduce intraocular pressure by increasing the release of aqueous humor via the trabecular meshwork. Laser treatment is often used to facilitate the drainage of aqueous humor. In some cases, filtration surgery is required.

Primary Open-Angle Glaucoma

Primary open-angle glaucoma occurs when the aqueous humor is blocked by a bulge of the iris at the anterior chamber before it filters through the trabecular meshwork. The result is an accumulation of aqueous humor, with resultant increased IOP.

The cause is unknown; however, one theory identifies possible accumulation of mucopolysaccharides in the trabecular meshwork as the underlying mechanism. Risk factors include diabetes, cardiovascular disease, hypertension, and prolonged use of topical, periocular, inhaled, or systemic corticosteroids. Primary open-angle glaucoma occurs

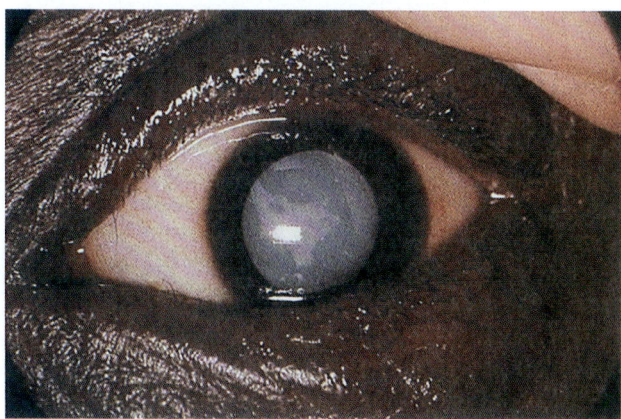

Figure 80-4 Cataract. The lens appears cloudy or opaque.

primarily in people older than age 40 years. It is three to four times more common in black clients than in white clients. The client may not be aware of any vision changes, but the IOP will fluctuate or increase and there will be visual field deficits and central field vision loss late in the disease.

Treatment

Treatment may include ocular hypotensive agents to decrease aqueous production, such as beta-adrenergic antagonists (timolol maleate [Timoptic], levobunolol hydrochloride [Betagan], carteolol hydrochloride [Ocupress], and betaxolol hydrochloride [Betoptic S]). Miotics, such as pilocarpine hydrochloride, oral (Salagen) or topical; carbonic anhydrase inhibitors, such as oral acetazolamide (Diamox), topical brinzolamide (Azopt)–brimonidine tartrate (Alphagan P); adrenergic agonists, such as brimonidine tartrate (Alphagan P), to suppress aqueous inflow; and prostaglandin analogues, such as latanoprost (Xalatan), bimatoprost (Latisse), or travoprost (Travatan Z), to increase aqueous outflow.

Early surgical intervention is indicated; it consists of an *iridectomy* (removal of a portion of the iris). This procedure involves making a hole in the iris so that the aqueous humor can flow uninhibited from the posterior chamber to the anterior chamber. Iridectomy is performed with a laser or by traditional surgery.

Cataracts

A **cataract** is an opacity or cloudiness of the lens (Fig. 80-4). Because light entering the eye must pass through the lens to reach the retina, vision is impaired when the lens loses its transparency. One of the earliest symptoms of cataract is seeing halos around lights. The person may also notice decreased visual acuity and double vision (**diplopia**).

Cataracts may be age-related, traumatic, complicated, or toxic. Age-related cataracts result from chemical changes in the protein of the lens in older adult clients. Traumatic cataracts result from a foreign object that causes the aqueous or vitreous humor to enter the lens capsule. Complicated cataracts result from systemic disease (such as atopic dermatitis), metabolic disease (such as diabetes or hypoparathyroidism), or secondary to an associated disease of the eye (such as retinitis pigmentosa or retinal detachment). Toxic cataracts have been associated with a drug or chemical toxicity, such as to corticosteroids or other drugs.

Treatment

The only remedy for cataracts is surgery to remove the lens. This procedure is one of the most frequently performed surgeries in the United States. Cataract surgery is usually done as an outpatient procedure using a local anesthetic.

In the person with cataracts, visual acuity that cannot be corrected to be better than 20/60 with eyeglasses is an indication for a cataract extraction. However, the main indication for surgery is when the client complains that vision loss interferes with ADLs.

Several types of surgical procedures are used to remove the lens. An *extracapsular cataract extraction* involves removal of the anterior capsule of the lens, followed by intact removal of the lens nucleus through a larger incision. Another alternative is ultrasonic fragmentation (*phacoemulsification*) of the lens nucleus through a smaller incision. An intraocular lens (**IOL**) implant is used with almost every procedure.

Age-Related Macular Degeneration

Age-related macular degeneration (**AMD**) can cause loss of central vision and partial or total blindness. The macula is the central portion of the retina that surrounds the optic disc, which is responsible for sharp, central vision. The macula is necessary for seeing fine detail or to see objects clearly, as is needed for reading or driving. Macular degeneration is a painless disorder that generally commences in the fifth decade and is the leading cause of vision loss in clients older than 60 years. Some forms of macular degenerations affect younger populations.

Risk factors for AMD include the formation of yellow cellular deposits or debris called **drusen**. Drusen accumulate between the retinal pigment and the choroid layer, which supplies nutrients to the macula. Drusen are often seen before vision changes and may be the first sign of AMD. The disorder can advance slowly or rapidly and may lead to blindness in both eyes. In the early stages, some individuals may not notice the visual changes or rationalize the changes by thinking, "I'm just getting older." Signs and symptoms include blurred vision, difficulty seeing faces or discerning colors, distorted vision, drastically decreased visual acuity, and the presence of drusen. Additional risk factors include tobacco smoking, aging, family history, hypertension, elevated cholesterol, obesity, and female gender. There are two forms of age-related macular degeneration: *nonexudative or dry macular degeneration* and *exudative or wet macular degeneration* (Fig. 80-5).

Nonexudative (dry) macular degeneration progresses slowly, and there is no cure for it; all forms of AMD begin with the dry form. Signs of the disease include needing more light to read, increased difficulty with reading, and noted blurred vision in the middle of the vision field. Treatment may include high doses of antioxidants, such as lutein. Exudative (wet) macular degeneration is a formation of fragile blood vessels behind the macula that can leak and cause vision problems. One of the first signs of the disease is wavy lines noted in the vision field as can be tested on an ocular testing grid. *Exudative macular degeneration progresses quickly and medical attention must be sought or blindness*

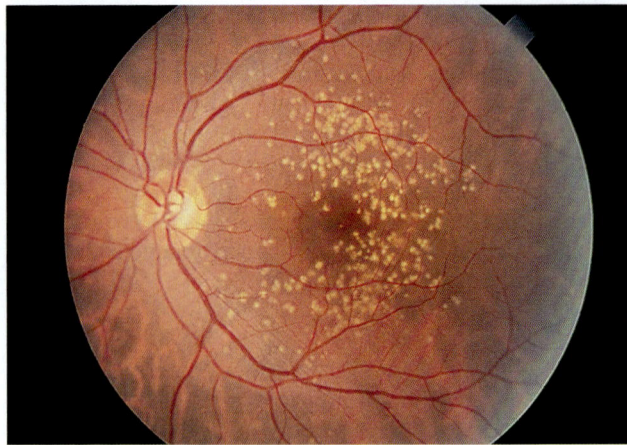

Figure 80-5 Age-related macular degeneration.

can occur. Testing for exudative AMD may include a fluorescein angiogram, which involves a peripheral injection of a specific dye and monitoring of the photos looking for blood vessels leaks in the eye. Treatment options include laser therapy, photodynamic therapy, eye injections, and vascular endothelial growth factor medications such as ranibizumab (Lucentis), bevacizumab (Avastin), or pegaptanib (Macugen) injected into the vitreous every 4 to 8 weeks. Multiple laser or photodynamic treatments may be required, as they are not a cure for the disorder. Advanced AMD does not respond to treatment, which means that early recognition and treatment are necessary to prevent or delay vision loss.

TRAUMA TO THE EYE

Contusion and Hematoma

A blunt injury to the eye may cause swelling and bleeding into the soft tissues surrounding the orbit, resulting in a *contusion* or *hematoma,* also known as a "black eye." Apply cold packs for the first 24 to 48 hr to decrease bleeding and edema. When the swelling has stopped, usually after 24 to 48 hr, use warm packs on the site to hasten the absorption of the blood from the tissues.

Foreign Bodies

Foreign bodies may be external or internal. External foreign bodies are found on the corneal or conjunctival surface. Internal foreign bodies may penetrate the cornea or sclera and enter the inside of the eye. The latter most often result from pounding metal on metal or trauma, such as a gunshot. To prevent damaging internal ocular structures, never attempt to remove a penetrating object from the eye. If an object is embedded in the cornea, a topical anesthetic may be ordered for severe ocular pain until the object can be removed. Ultrasound may be used to locate an embedded foreign body, and an electromagnet or surgery may be necessary for removal.

Hyphema

A **hyphema**, a hemorrhage into the anterior chamber of the eye, is usually caused by blunt trauma and can lead to glaucoma and vision loss. Clients should report signs of bleeding in the eye immediately. Treatment consists of mydriatic (dilating) or miotic (constricting) medications. Occasionally, an ophthalmologist may need to evacuate the accumulated blood.

Chemical Burns

Exposure to irritating acidic or alkaline chemicals can severely damage the eyes. Corneal abrasions and ulcerations with subsequent cataract formation may lead to permanent vision loss. The lens and the chambers of the eye can also be affected.

Treatment

If any accidental substance comes in contact with a person's eye, the eye should be irrigated with water for a minimum of 5 min. During irrigation of the eye, direct the flow of water so the solution does not come in contact with the other eye.

After this initial irrigation, the person should immediately report to an emergency department or an ophthalmologist's office for further treatment. There, the eye is *lavaged* (flushed out) for an extended period. This prolonged irrigation removes acids and alkalis that can continue to melt the eye, even after it seems that thorough irrigation has been performed.

After irrigation is complete, a topical antibiotic ointment is instilled. Continued follow-up with an ophthalmologist is necessary. *Keratoplasty* (corneal grafting), which is discussed in the next section, may be done.

> **Nursing Alert** Extreme caution is necessary when instilling any type of medication into the eye. Containers of eye medications are similar to bottles for other solutions. For example, some non–eye solutions come in small bottles with droppers (e.g., guaiac solutions used to test for occult blood). These solutions can be extremely caustic and can cause blindness.

Corneal Abrasions

Corneal abrasions, which involve the outer (epithelial) layer of the cornea, are often caused by tree branches, fingernails, paper, and contact lens injuries. Symptoms include severe pain, redness, and tearing (*lacrimation*). Corneal abrasions are easily diagnosed using fluorescein dye instillation. Following instillation, the area is viewed with a cobalt blue light. The abrasions appear green.

Treatment

Treatment of corneal injuries includes instillation of antibiotic drops or ointment and pressure patching. These measures should result in healing within 24 to 48 hr. If healing does not occur, prompt follow-up is required to prevent complications. A serious complication is *corneal destruction,* which often requires corneal transplantation.

If severe visual impairment results from irreversible changes in the cornea, vision might be restored by corneal transplantation (keratoplasty). **Keratoplasty** involves the replacement of damaged corneal tissue with human donor

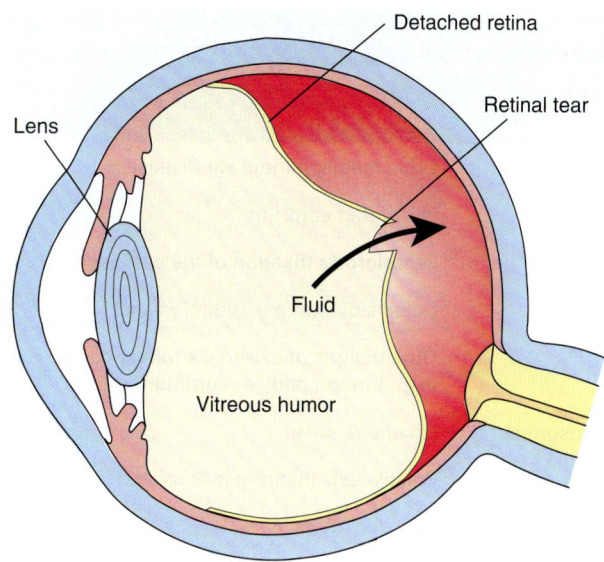

Figure 80-6 Retinal detachment.

tissue that is obtained within 6 hr after death. This tissue is rarely rejected because it has minimal blood supply.

Detached Retina

A *detached retina* (Fig. 80-6) is a separation of the retina from the choroid, thus depriving the image-receiving layer of its blood supply. Separation of these layers usually follows a hole or tear in the retina, which may result from a blow or injury, myopia, degenerative changes, surgery, tumor, diabetic retinopathy, or extreme hypertension. Because the sensory layer can no longer receive visual stimuli, vision in the affected area is lost.

Signs and Symptoms

Signs and symptoms may occur suddenly or gradually. If a large part of the central retina is affected, vision loss is greater than if the outer edges are destroyed. The person may see flashes of light (*flashers*) or moving spots (*floaters*). Vision may be blurry, or it may seem as though a shade has been pulled over part of the vision. Usually no pain occurs with a detached retina.

Treatment

One possible treatment for detached retina is a surgical procedure called *scleral buckling.* This operation shortens the sclera, thus allowing contact between the retina and the choroid. Procedures involving use of a laser beam (*photocoagulation*) and the application of extreme cold (*cryosurgery*) are also used to create an inflammatory reaction and promote healing.

THE EAR AND HEARING DISORDERS

The branch of medicine concerned with ear diseases and disorders is called *otology;* the healthcare provider in this specialty is known as an *otologist*. The otologist tests hearing, examines the ear for signs of disease, and determines the treatment. The *audiologist* tests hearing by various means.

TABLE 80-2 Types and Common Causes of Hearing Loss

TYPE	COMMON CAUSES
Conductive losses	Otitis media; middle ear disease
	Perforated eardrum
	Otosclerosis (fixation of the ossicles)
	Defects of external auditory canal
	Obstructions of external auditory canal (e.g., foreign body or cerumen)
Sensorineural losses	Excessive noise
	Presbycusis (hearing loss related to aging)
	Ototoxic drugs
	Tumors (e.g., acoustic neuroma)
	Ménière disease
	Congenital factors
	Trauma, skull fractures, brain damage (e.g., stroke)
	Viral infections (e.g., meningitis)

IN PRACTICE
EDUCATING THE CLIENT 80-3: Prevention of Hearing Problems

- Avoid excessive noise (e.g., loud music, televisions, work environment). Keep volume down and wear protective gear if working in a noisy area.
- Protect ears on cold and windy days. Be aware of dangers of riding in car with windows open, or in motor boats, or motorcycles.
- Wear ear plugs for swimming if ear problems are present.
- Dry ears thoroughly after bathing or swimming.
- Do not place foreign objects in ears.
- Do not clean ears excessively. Do not pick or pull ears excessively.
- Prevent and treat infection immediately. Ear infection is not to be treated personally; see a professional.
- Have ear piercing done by a healthcare provider or trained technician; follow instructions for follow-up care.
- At symptoms of hearing loss, see a healthcare provider immediately.

The *otorhinolaryngologist* or *otolaryngologist* treats disorders of the ear, nose, and throat (ENT). The acronym EENT refers to eye, ear, nose, and throat.

Types of Hearing Loss

Impaired hearing can occur at any age. Undetected hearing defects can be misinterpreted as lack of interest, attention deficit disorders, or mental retardation.

Injuries can affect hearing and cause deafness. Disease, exposure to excessive noise, or congenital factors may also impair hearing. Hearing loss may vary from slight to moderate or may be complete.

Total deafness usually cannot be corrected. A cochlear implant may be helpful to some deaf clients. Congenital deafness may result in the inability to speak or in speech that is very difficult to understand.

Conductive Hearing Loss

A *conductive hearing loss* is sometimes referred to as a *transmission hearing loss*, in which the conduction of sound waves to the organs of hearing is disrupted (Table 80-2). It may be caused by a disorder in the auditory canal, the eardrum, or the *ossicles* (tiny bones of the middle ear). Fluid in the middle ear is the most common cause. Conductive hearing losses are further classified as follows:

- *Air conduction loss* is caused by a defect in the external auditory canal.
- *Bone conduction loss* is caused by a defect in the bones of the middle ear.

Sensorineural or Perceptive Hearing Loss

Sensorineural or *perceptive hearing loss* involves a disturbance of the organs of the inner ear or of the transmitting nerve (Table 80-2). A sensorineural hearing loss involves the *organ of Corti* (cochlea) or the *auditory nerve* (eighth cranial nerve). Sensorineural hearing loss is further tested to differentiate between the following types:

- *Sensory* (cochlear): Factors such as trauma, viral infections, toxic drugs, or Ménière disease can result in cochlear hearing loss. These sensory conditions are usually not fatal.
- *Neural* (eighth cranial nerve defect): A tumor of the cranial nerve called an *acoustic neuroma* can cause a sensorineural hearing disorder. These tumors are potentially fatal.

Other causes of sensorineural hearing loss include excessive noise and congenital predisposition.

If the organs of hearing are impaired or deteriorating, the person has little chance of escaping deafness, unless the cause of the difficulty is discovered before damage occurs.

Central Hearing Loss

Central hearing loss refers to the brain's inability to interpret sounds after they have been transmitted. This sometimes occurs in atherosclerosis or after a stroke.

Functional Hearing Loss

In *functional hearing loss*, no organic cause is found and no damage to the auditory nerve is visible. Functional hearing loss is believed to stem from some underlying psychological problems. Professional counseling sometimes helps.

Prevention of Hearing Loss

All individuals should be aware of the dangers of infections and noise in regard to their hearing. The nurse can provide preventive teaching (In Practice: Educating the Client 80-3).

Prompt treatment of infectious diseases, such as upper respiratory infections that can spread to the ear, helps to prevent hearing loss. The use of antibiotics early in the course of an ear infection also helps to arrest the disease and to prevent later complications.

Noise pollution is of great concern, particularly for young people and workers in industry. Wearing protective ear devices can prevent many hearing disorders. The Occupational Safety and Health Administration (OSHA) has established standards for industries in general. The loud volume generated from audio equipment is often harmful to young people's hearing and can result in permanent hearing loss.

Disorders of the External Ear

Most external ear disorders are more annoying than they are serious. If proper treatment is given, the condition tends to heal without difficulty. Unfortunately, many people attempt to treat these disorders by themselves, and consequently complications develop.

Impacted Earwax

Impacted earwax (**cerumen**) in the auditory canal is one example of a minor condition that requires medical attention. Wax can be removed by irrigating the outer ear with a solution warmed to body temperature (98.6 °F or 37 °C).

Instruct the client not to attempt to remove wax or other objects from the ear. Pushing on a foreign object may damage the eardrum. If the client has a perforated eardrum, irrigation might force the wax and the solution into the middle ear and cause infection. Poking at the wax with a finger, a hairpin, or an applicator may injure the canal and cause infection. Additionally, the wax can be pushed in further.

Furuncles

Furuncles (boils) are infections of hair follicles, which drain purulent materials. A furuncle extends through the dermis into the subcutaneous tissue and can form small abscesses in the auditory canal. Ear furuncles commonly result from irritation due to scratching within the ear, such as using a cotton-tipped applicator to remove wax. Due to the location in the ear, these boils can be intensely painful. Symptoms may cause itching, irritation, and, occasionally, a temporary hearing loss, if infection is prevalent. If the furuncle bursts, discharge will drain from the ear and pain improves immediately. Heat may be applied, and antibiotics are sometimes given.

Foreign Objects

Children or persons who are emotionally or cognitively challenged may put objects into the ear. A healthcare provider must remove any objects. Pushing on the object may cause it to travel further into the canal or cause the eardrum to rupture. If the foreign object is a food substance such as a pea, bean, or piece of corn, moisture will cause swelling and extreme pain, often leading to damage of the eardrum.

Sometimes, insects enter the auditory canal. If they remain, they cause extreme distress by their fluttering and buzzing. If a flashlight is held to the ear, the light may draw the insect out. Sometimes, a few drops of mineral oil, alcohol, or anesthetic jelly will anesthetize or kill the insect, causing it to float out if the client's head is turned to the affected side. If none of these measures works, the client should see a healthcare provider at once. Trying to remove an insect with tweezers is dangerous. Removing an insect from the ear is a delicate process that requires great skill.

Otitis Externa

Otitis externa (external otitis), inflammation of the external ear, is most commonly caused by chronic external ear inflammation. Prolonged exposure to water often is the cause, and therefore it is sometimes called "swimmer's ear." The client receives antibiotics and is advised to avoid swimming until the infection clears. The client should then wear ear plugs when swimming.

Application of ear drops, composed of substances such as acetic acid (Domeboro Otic, VoSol Otic), boric acid (Ear-Dry, Swim-Ear), or chloramphenicol (Chloromycetin Otic), can be used for prevention.

Fungal Infections

Fungal infections in the auditory canal tend to occur in warm, damp climates, especially when the auditory canal has not been completely dried. Most of these fungi are opportunistic and feed on cerumen or dead skin cells. Ear drops containing antifungal medications, alcohol, and glycerin can treat such infections, which may resist treatment. Often treatment must continue for a number of weeks.

Punctured Tympanic Membrane

A punctured or perforated *tympanic membrane* (eardrum) is a serious threat to hearing later in life, as well as a possible source of middle ear infection. Although the perforation will often heal spontaneously, surgery is sometimes necessary. Occasionally, a **myringotomy** (surgical incision into the eardrum and drainage) is done for therapeutic reasons.

Piercing the Earlobes

Ear piercing is commonly done for cosmetic purposes. A healthcare provider or a trained technician using the correct sterile equipment and following sterile technique should perform this procedure. Client teaching is important. After the ears are pierced, the client is advised to keep the original earrings in place for at least 2 weeks, to turn them frequently, and to cleanse the earlobes often with an antiseptic solution, such as alcohol. The practice of piercing the external ears above the lobes is often more painful, but not as likely to cause infection, because the earlobes are thicker and not as quick to heal.

Disorders of the Middle Ear

Otitis Media

Otitis media is an inflammation of the middle ear. The ear is especially susceptible to upper respiratory infections, which can travel through the eustachian tube from the nose and throat. Children are especially vulnerable to these infections because their auditory tubes are straighter and shorter than those of an adult (Chapter 72).

The four different types of otitis media are acute, serous, chronic, suppurative, chronic serous, and chronic suppurative. *Serous otitis media* results from fluid that collects in the middle ear, causing an obstruction of the auditory tube. This condition may stem from infection, allergy, tumors, or sudden changes in altitude. Symptoms include crackling sensations and fullness in the ear, with some hearing loss.

If this condition is not treated promptly, fluid pressure may rupture the eardrum.

The treatment of choice remains controversial. It consists of antibiotic use or myringotomy. This is followed by analysis and treatment of the original cause of the difficulty, such as removal of a tumor in the nasopharynx.

Suppurative form is generally caused by an upper respiratory infection spreading through the auditory tube. Pus forms and collects in the middle ear to create pressure on the eardrum. Symptoms include fever, earache, and impaired hearing. The eardrum is inflamed and bulging and may rupture.

Initial treatment is often antibiotics. Myringotomy may also be indicated to prevent rupture of the eardrum. If spontaneous rupture of the eardrum occurs, scarring, which disrupts normal ossicle vibrations, can result. Often this permanently impairs hearing.

Chronic otitis media can develop if acute purulent otitis media is not treated promptly. In the past, mastoiditis, encephalitis, and meningitis were also complications. However, today these complications are rarely seen because of the use of antibiotics.

Other problems include nausea and vomiting, dizziness, injury to the facial nerve causing facial paralysis, or a brain abscess—all of which may start with a simple earache. Fortunately, these serious complications are less frequent owing to improved treatment for acute infections.

Chronic serous otitis media is usually associated with a punctured eardrum or may be a complication of acute otitis media, mastoiditis, or a severe upper respiratory infection. Symptoms include ringing in the ears, hearing loss, pain, and purulent drainage. Antibiotics are prescribed, and a mastoidectomy may be necessary in some instances. Steroids may be given to reduce inflammation.

Treatment

Myringotomy is the common procedure used to treat otitis media. It releases pressure and relieves pain. Healing proceeds rapidly. Discharge from the ear is bloody at first, then purulent. To avoid interfering with drainage, do not plug the ear with cotton. Place a small piece of cotton in the outer ear to absorb the drainage and change it frequently. Give ordered antibiotics. Rest, adequate diet, and prevention against chilling are recommended.

Polyethylene (**PE**) tubes are often inserted through the eardrum incision into the middle ear. This procedure is most commonly done in children with recurrent ear infections. PE tubes allow continuous drainage from the middle ear. In this case, the client must use caution to prevent water from entering the ear. Swimming and showering are contraindicated.

Tympanoplasty is the plastic reconstruction of the tiny ossicles of the middle ear. It is done when infection or tumor has destroyed or fused these bones together. The bones reconstructed involve the structures from the oval window to the tympanic membrane. Tympanoplasty is a delicate procedure, performed with the aid of an operating microscope. The goal of the surgery is to preserve and to maximize hearing.

Otosclerosis

Otosclerosis is a bony fixation of the stapes, one of the three ossicles in the middle ear that transmits sound to the inner ear. This condition slows or stops the vibration of the stapes and impairs or destroys hearing.

Otosclerosis usually develops slowly. It appears to have a hereditary basis because a familial tendency is found in its development. It is the most common cause of conductive deafness.

Signs and Symptoms

One of the first symptoms of otosclerosis is **tinnitus** (ringing in the ears), which is accentuated in quiet surroundings. It may occur for some time before the client notices a hearing loss. The client may not notice that they are losing the ability to hear, until ordinary conversation becomes difficult to hear—especially when others speak in low tones or there is background noise. Surgery or use of a hearing aid may help the client with this condition.

Treatment

Surgery to restore vibration of the stapes (*stapes mobilization*) may not be effective. Therefore, usually the client must make a decision about whether to have surgery. The operation is done under local anesthesia with an operating microscope and frees the stapes so it can vibrate. A more common procedure today is the removal of the stapes (*stapedectomy*) and replacement with a prosthesis.

Many clients are able to hear immediately after prosthesis placement. However, the return of hearing is not necessarily permanent; deafness may recur suddenly. Such deafness is owing to an infection or to formation of scar tissue. If stapedectomy is unsuccessful, *fenestration* (creation of a new oval window in the ear) may be done.

Disorders of the Inner Ear

Inflammation of the inner ear is called *otitis interna* or **labyrinthitis**. Almost every disorder of the inner ear is difficult to treat. Neither surgery nor hearing aids help inner ear deafness (*perceptive deafness*). Drugs used to treat conditions unrelated to the ear can harm the inner ear (**ototoxic**) and may cause an inner ear disorder. Streptomycin, for instance, may injure the auditory nerve. Some diseases or the aging process may also cause inner ear damage. Treatment often consists of preventing further injury and training in lip reading.

Ménière Disease

Ménière disease is a disturbance of the inner ear's semicircular canals, which are responsible for maintaining a sense of stability and balance due to fluid distention of the labyrinth leading to destruction of the cochlear hair cells. One theory suggests that the herpes simplex virus is a causative agent, but no specific cause is universally identified.

Signs and Symptoms

Symptoms are devastating and alarming. The affected individual has sudden attacks of severe and true **vertigo**, a sensation of spinning or rotating, either of oneself or of one's surroundings. (**Vertigo** is not the same as simple *dizziness*, although sometimes the terms are used interchangeably.)

Other findings include nausea, vomiting, and tinnitus. The person may be unable to walk. Migraine headaches may accompany the disorder. The person definitely should not drive. If the condition is untreated, hearing eventually deteriorates. Bed rest during an acute attack is sometimes necessary.

Sudden attacks of Ménière syndrome can be violent; they may last only a few minutes or several weeks, during which time the quantity of fluid in the space between the semicircular canals increases. During remission, the client's hearing and balance are often normal.

> **Key Concept**
> The person with Ménière disease is often frightened. Vertigo can occur at any time without warning.

Treatment

Medical treatment aims at relieving the symptoms. To decrease edema and pressure on the inner ear, which can cause vertigo and nausea, antihistamines, anticholinergics, corticosteroids, and mild diuretics may be used. Antiviral drugs, such as acyclovir, may help diminish the durations of the disease, but will not reverse existing damage. The person may receive sedatives or tranquilizers to subdue apprehension and accompanying anxiety. Vertigo may be treated by a device that provides transtympanic micropressure pulses (Meniett). Sometimes, when only one ear is affected, an operation to cut the auditory nerve is performed. This results in complete deafness in the affected ear. The client is advised to omit alcohol, coffee, tea, cola drinks, chocolate, and tobacco from the diet. A low-sodium diet may be suggested, although the benefits of this diet remain controversial.

Nursing Considerations

When caring for a client with Ménière disease, avoid jarring the bed, making sudden movements, turning on bright lights, or making loud noises. *Rationale: These actions may precipitate an attack.* Do everything slowly and explain actions to the client ahead of time. Protect the client from falls. *Rationale: If vertigo is severe, the client is in danger of falling.* Keep the bed in low position at all times to protect against dangerous falls.

Give fluids and foods in small amounts. *Rationale: The nauseated client is better able to tolerate small amounts.* Remember, the attacks are so devastating that the client is understandably apprehensive. Reassure the client that relief is possible.

DISORDERS OF OTHER SPECIAL SENSES

In addition to hearing and vision, the special senses include the senses of touch, taste, and smell.

Tactile Disorders

Tactile sense (sense of touch) includes the ability to feel softness, pressure, pain, heat, and cold. This sense also assists in proprioception and helps the inner ear to maintain balance. The body's muscles and tendons give information to the ear's labyrinth, which is involved in maintenance of balance.

A tactile sense disorder often results from a neurologic disorder. Persons with spinal cord injuries, nerve transmission deficits, or disorders in the brain's sensory area may be unable to feel or interpret pain. Diabetes mellitus causes peripheral neuropathy with subsequent loss of sensation, especially in the extremities.

Clients with tactile difficulties may be in danger because they cannot react appropriately to external injuries or internal disorders. They may be easily burned, for example, because they do not have the sensation that would warn them of the danger of heat.

In some cases of chronic pain, nerve transmission may be intentionally interrupted by surgery. In other cases, the person is unable to maintain balance and may easily fall or may be dizzy much of the time.

Gustatory Disorders

Gustatory sense or **gustation**, the sense of taste, involves the sensations of sweet, salty, sour, bitter, and others. Disorders in this sense are usually not life threatening. An absence or alteration in the sense of taste may reduce the person's interest in eating. The loss of the sense of taste is commonly associated with the loss of smell.

Olfactory Disorders

Olfactory sense or **olfaction** (sense of smell) greatly affects the sense of taste. Disorders in olfaction are usually not life threatening, but they may reduce pleasurable sensations in eating or in smelling flowers or perfumes. In certain cases, such as in gas leaks, lack of olfactory sense may be dangerous.

STUDENT SYNTHESIS

KEY POINTS

- The sensory system is important in enabling people to receive information from the surrounding environment.
- Most eye and ear surgeries are done during same-day surgery, using an operating microscope. Careful client and family teaching enables clients to resume daily activities.
- Clients with visual impairments may use eyeglasses, contact lenses, and large-print materials to enhance their sight.
- Visually impaired individuals can learn to read Braille, listen to books on tape, work with seeing eye dogs, and use white canes. Clients with total hearing loss can learn sign language and lip reading. Clients with partial hearing loss may use hearing aids to enhance remaining hearing.
- Refractive disorders result when light rays focus improperly on the retina.
- Most eye infections can be treated with the application of warm compresses and topical antibiotic ointments.
- Early recognition and treatment of glaucoma are essential to prevent visual changes and blindness.

- Surgery is the required treatment for cataracts.
- Hearing deficits may occur at any age. They are caused by diseases and congenital and environmental factors.
- Determination of the cause of a hearing deficit is important because it may point to a more serious problem.
- Ménière disease causes significant vertigo, nausea, vomiting, and tinnitus. The symptoms of the disorder typically are treatable with palliative medications.
- Disorders of touch, taste, and smell are considered to be hazards to safety.

CRITICAL THINKING EXERCISES

1. You are working in a school. One of your goals is to teach prevention of hearing loss to high school seniors. What would you include in your teaching plan? How will you communicate your teaching to the students?

2. Among the clients on your floor are a hearing-impaired person and a vision-impaired person. Identify ways in which your care would be the same for these two clients. Determine ways in which care would be different. Explain how the care would differ if one person were both hearing and visually impaired.

NCLEX-STYLE REVIEW QUESTIONS

1. The primary care provider orders ear irrigation for a client. Which situation requires the nurse to question this order?
   a. The client has a scratch on the external canal.
   b. The client has a foreign body in the ear.
   c. The ear canal has impacted cerumen.
   d. The eardrum may be punctured.

2. A client is being considered as a candidate for a cochlear implant. Which data gathered by the nurse would support the client's candidacy?
   a. The client has mild mental retardation.
   b. The client has a history of schizophrenia.
   c. The client is unable to recognize words spoken.
   d. The client expects hearing will resume normally after surgery.

3. The nurse is assisting a visually impaired client with meals. Which nursing interventions will assist the client with maintaining independence and dignity? Select all that apply.
   a. Place food in the same "clock position" on the plate.
   b. Tell the client what is being served.
   c. Feed the client so food will not spill.
   d. Tell the client where food is located.
   e. Prepare finger foods so the client will not have to use utensils.

4. The nurse is reinforcing education regarding the use of eye drops during treatment for a client who has been diagnosed with conjunctivitis. Which information will the nurse provide the client?
   a. Warm the solution briefly in the microwave prior to use.
   b. Save the unused solution for use if the infection returns.
   c. Ensure not to touch the eye with the dropper.
   d. Use the drops for the other member of the family who has conjunctivitis.

5. The nurse is caring for a client who was hit in the left eye with a softball. The eye is edematous and painful to touch. Which is the priority intervention by the nurse?
   a. Apply a cold pack.
   b. Apply a warm compress.
   c. Have the client lay flat for 12 hr to decrease swelling.
   d. Place drops in the eye to decrease pain.

CHAPTER RESOURCES

Enhance your learning with additional resources on thePoint!

Student Resources related to this chapter can be found at **thePoint.lww.com/Rosdahl12e**.

Welcome Steps

Look at healthcare provider's orders.

Protocol for procedure.

Necessary equipment/supplies.

Wash hands using proper hand hygiene; put on gloves.

Explain the procedure and reassure the client.

Locate two identifiers to confirm correct client.

Comfortable and efficient position for nurse and client.

Obtain privacy.

Make sure to follow correct steps and body mechanics with good technique.

Ensure safety and observe deviations from normal.

End Steps

Ensure comfort and safety.

Note questions or concerns from client or nurse; note significant data.

Dispose of materials properly.

Disinfect the area and your hands.

Document and report the procedure and your findings.

IN PRACTICE
NURSING PROCEDURE 80-1 — Using a Cotton-Tipped Applicator

Supplies and Equipment
Gloves
Cotton-tipped applicators

Steps
Follow LPN WELCOME Steps and Then

1. Straighten the ear canal, pulling up and back for an adult, or down and back for a child. *Rationale: Pulling on the pinna helps to straighten the ear canal and provide better visualization.*
2. Insert the sterile, cotton-tipped applicator only as far as can be seen. *Rationale: Going further than the line of sight could lead to puncturing of the eardrum.*
3. Use each applicator only once, drawing it out and rotation it. *Rationale: Applicators are not reused because they can spread infection.*

Follow ENDDD Steps

Special Reminder
Make sure that adequate light is available so you can see the ear canal.

IN PRACTICE
NURSING PROCEDURE 80-2 — Irrigating the Ear

Supplies and Equipment
Gloves
Plastic cover
Towel
Large emesis basin
Solution
Sterile, rubber-bulb syringe or sterile, large-volume medication syringe

Steps
Follow LPN WELCOME Steps and Then

1. Warm the solution to body temperature. *Rationale: Hot or cold solutions can stimulate the inner ear and cause nausea or dizziness.*
2. Help the client sit up and provide adequate back support. Have the client turn toward the affected side. *Rationale: Proper positioning helps to ensure that the client is comfortable. Turning to the affected side allows fluid to drain out.*
3. Drape the client with a plastic cover and towel. Have the client hold a large emesis basin under the ear to be irrigated. *Rationale: Draping and using an emesis basin help to prevent soiling the client's clothing.*
4. Straighten the ear canal (Fig. 80-2). *Rationale: This position provides better access to the ear canal.*

5. Expel air from the sterile syringe. Draw up the irrigating solution. *Rationale:* Air is purged from the syringe to avoid introducing air into the client's ear canal. A sterile syringe is used to prevent introducing pathogens into the ear.
6. Insert the syringe into the meatus as far as can be seen. Do not plug the canal with the syringe. *Rationale:* Inserting the syringe as far as can be seen prevents injuring the canal. Not plugging the canal allows the solution to flow out freely and prevents the buildup of too much pressure.
7. Irrigate gently with the prescribed solution. Note the client's reaction. Stop the procedure if the client finds it very uncomfortable. *Rationale:* This procedure can cause sudden and great discomfort. A person can become dizzy or nauseated. If this happens, let the client rest before continuing.
8. Allow the client to lie on the affected side. *Rationale:* Lying on the affected side allows the fluid to drain and helps to prevent any great pressure on the eardrum, which could cause it to rupture.
9. Dry the canal and ear. *Rationale:* Drying promotes client comfort.

Follow ENDDD Steps

81 Cardiovascular Disorders

Learning Objectives

1. Explain the rationales for the following laboratory tests: CK, LDH, AST, troponin, lipid levels, and BNP.
2. Differentiate an angiocardiogram from an arteriogram, including nursing considerations for each procedure.
3. Describe the role of the nurse during and after the following procedures: echocardiogram, ECG stress test, and an electrophysiology study.
4. Identify nursing considerations before and after a cardiac catheterization.
5. Identify the rationale for performing a PTCA.
6. Compare and contrast the following surgical procedures: closed-heart surgery, open-heart surgery, heart valve replacement, and heart transplantation, including postoperative nursing interventions for each.
7. Explain the role of each of the following conditions as they contribute to cardiovascular disease: arteriosclerosis, atherosclerosis, hypertension, and hypotension.
8. Differentiate the following cardiac rhythm abnormalities: sinus tachycardia, sinus bradycardia, PVC, heart block, and fibrillation.
9. Describe heart failure, including possible causes, signs and symptoms, diagnostic tests, treatment, and nursing care.
10. Define and differentiate the following terms: edema, ascites, anasarca, dependent edema, pitting edema, nonpitting edema, and pulmonary edema.
11. Define the following infectious and inflammatory heart disorders: **myocarditis**, **endocarditis**, and **pericarditis**.
12. Identify four major causes of coronary artery disease.
13. Describe three signs and symptoms for angina pectoris and myocardial infarction and nursing interventions for each condition.
14. Differentiate the following disorders: thrombophlebitis, deep venous thrombosis, phlebitis, and embolism.
15. Identify nursing considerations for each of the following conditions: intermittent claudication, Buerger disease, and Raynaud phenomenon.
16. Identify the main causes and common complications of strokes.
17. Identify nursing interventions that are important during the various phases of a stroke.

Important Terminology

anasarca
aneurysm
angina pectoris
angiocardiogram
angioplasty
aphasia
arrhythmia
arteriogram
arteriosclerosis
ascites
atherectomy
atherosclerosis
atrial ablation
cardiac catheterization
cardiogenic shock
cardiology
cardioversion
central venous pressure
claudication
dependent edema
dysrhythmia
echocardiography
embolus
endocarditis
fibrillation
heart block
hemianopsia
hemiplegia
hemodynamic monitoring
hypertrophy
ischemia
jugular venous distention
myocarditis
nonpitting edema
orthopnea
pancarditis
pericarditis
phlebitis
pitting edema
pulmonary artery occlusion (wedge) pressure
pulmonary edema
stenosis
stent
stress test
stroke
thrombolytic therapy
thrombophlebitis
transient ischemic attack

Acronyms

ACS
AED
AMI
AST
AV
BNP
CABG
CAD
CCU
CICU
CK, CPK
CPR
CVP
DVT
ECG
EPS
FAST
HF, CHF
HDL
HTN
ICD
JVD
LDH
LDL
MI
NT proBNP
PAOP, PAWP
PE
PROM
PT
PTCA
PTT
PVC
RIND
SBE
SGOT
SIE
TEE
TIA
TMLR
TNI
TNT
t-PA

Cardiovascular disorders include those conditions that interfere with the heart's ability to pump, those that disrupt blood flow within the coronary or cerebral vessels, and those peripheral vascular diseases that disrupt blood flow to a localized area (e.g., an extremity). The field of medicine that examines the cardiovascular system and its disorders is called **cardiology**; healthcare providers who specialize in this area are cardiologists. Nurses who work in this field are cardiac nurses.

The *Coronary Care Unit* (CCU) or *Coronary Intensive Care Unit* (CICU) is a specialized hospital unit designed for the care of people with heart disorders. The staff is specially trained in emergency measures and coronary care. Training in coronary care includes the following: normal anatomy and physiology of the heart; normal and abnormal electrocardiogram readings; laboratory tests and their significance; emergency drugs and resuscitation measures; use of special equipment (e.g., cardiac monitors and defibrillation equipment); hemodynamic monitoring (specialized devices to evaluate the pressure in the heart chambers); and the special emotional aspects of coronary care nursing. A detailed discussion of care in a CICU is beyond the scope of this text.

DIAGNOSTIC TESTS

Laboratory Tests

For clients with cardiovascular disorders, measuring the levels of serum enzymes is important. Nurses must know the laboratory levels of several cardiac enzymes. These enzymes include the following:

- Creatinine kinase (*CK*; formerly creatinine phosphokinase [*CPK*]) and isoenzyme CK_2 (or CK-MB)
- Lactic dehydrogenase (*LDH*)
- Aspartate aminotransferase (*AST*; formerly serum glutamic oxaloacetic transaminase [SGOT])
- Troponins: troponin I and troponin T (TnI or cTnI and TnT or cTnT)
- Myoglobin

These diagnostic markers are released into the bloodstream when muscle damage occurs, as in myocardial infarction (MI, heart attack, coronary occlusion). Levels of these enzymes rise and fall at specific times and, therefore, must be correlated with the client's medical history, as well as with other diagnostic tests. Currently, the enzymes relied on most heavily in conjunction with cardiac medical history are CK, CK-MB, myoglobin, and the troponins: troponin I and troponin T. Generally, two or three troponin laboratory tests are ordered over a 12- to 16-hour time frame. Troponin levels rise within 3 to 4 hr of the onset of chest pain. Troponin I and troponin T are specific cardiac markers for myocardial injury. Of the cardiac enzymes, troponin I returns to normal within 5–9 days, and troponin T returns to normal in 10–14 days.

Blood *lipid* (fat) studies may be ordered to determine *hyperlipidemia* (excess fat in the blood). Cholesterol is a blood lipid often associated with coronary artery disease (CAD). The BNP (brain-type natriuretic peptide) and the N-terminal (NT) pro-BNP laboratory tests help to confirm or exclude the diagnosis of heart failure (HF).

Other important tests measure the serum electrolytes, such as potassium, sodium, and magnesium. An increase or decrease in the level of these electrolytes may cause disturbances in the normal sequence of electrical cardiac impulses, also known as **arrhythmia** or **dysrhythmia**. Often used interchangeably, these terms refer to any irregular heartbeat such as tachycardia (heartbeats too fast), bradycardia (heartbeats too slow), or fibrillation (erratic heartbeat).

X-Ray Evaluations: Angiocardiogram and Arteriogram

An **angiocardiogram** (*angiogram*) is an x-ray study of the heart and major vessels performed after injection of a radiopaque dye into a vessel. The angiogram shows the movement of the dye from the heart to the lungs, back to the heart, then out through the aorta. An **arteriogram** is an x-ray study of an artery. Because these procedures are invasive, uncomfortable, and carry some risk, clients must sign an informed consent before these tests can be done. The procedures can provide information about structural abnormalities, atherosclerosis, and calcifications within the vascular system.

> **Nursing Alert** Ask clients if they are allergic to shellfish or iodine before performing any test using radiopaque dye. This dye could cause a severe anaphylactic reaction.

Nursing Considerations

Usually, the client does not eat breakfast before the procedure. They may receive a sedative 30 min to 1 hr before the test is scheduled. The groin area is often the site for insertion; the area may need to be prepared. Carry out other routine preoperative procedures. Ask the client to void just before the test.

Be alert for a possible allergic reaction to the dye during or after the procedure. Watch for signs of a delayed reaction after returning to the room, such as rapid pulse, diaphoresis, shakiness, skin rash, or a drop in blood pressure. The client may complain of a swollen throat or difficulty swallowing. The dye is irritating if it comes in contact with the skin, and sometimes the injection site becomes swollen and painful. Ice packs may be prescribed to relieve discomfort (see Box 47-3 for special precautions when dye is used).

Keep the client on bed rest until they are fully awake. Instruct the client not to bend the leg or flex the hip for up to 8 hr if the femoral site was used. Closely observe the insertion site for bleeding, and carefully monitor vital signs to check for internal hemorrhage. Check peripheral pulses distal to the site. Also, check the color and warmth of the affected extremity and assess motor and sensory function. Clots or other blockages in blood vessels are possible. If pulses are absent, take emergency measures.

> **Nursing Alert** After any study in which the femoral site is used, the client should lie flat for up to 8 hr. Lying flat helps prevent swelling, bruising, and bleeding at the puncture site. Follow healthcare provider orders for activity level.

Other Diagnostic Tests

Electrocardiogram

An *electrocardiogram* (ECG) is a graphic record or tracing that represents the heart's electrical action. It provides essential information about the heart, including rate, rhythm, and the presence of certain disorders.

The ECG may be done at the bedside or in a room set aside for this purpose. Tell the client that the test is painless and that they must lie very still. *Leads (electrodes)* are placed on the skin (the chest, wrists, and ankles) and connected to a machine called an *electrocardiograph* (Fig. 81-1).

The graph or tracing (ECG) is placed on the chart after the cardiologist has interpreted it and written a statement and summary of the findings. The client does not usually require any special treatment before or after the procedure. The person interpreting the ECG must be informed of any cardiac

CHAPTER 81 Cardiovascular Disorders 1437

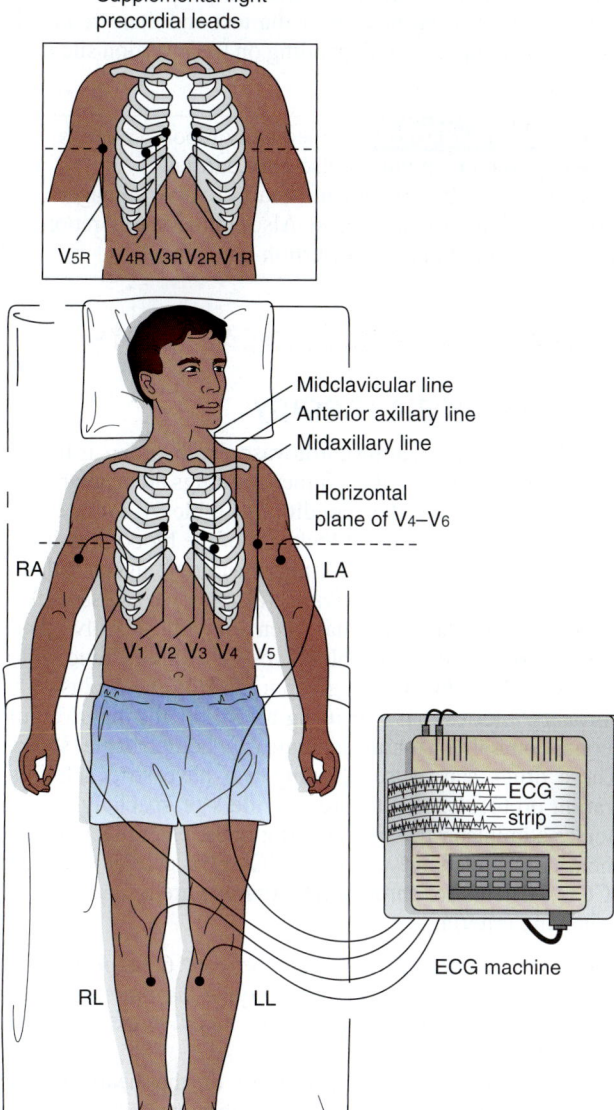

Figure 81-1 Twelve-lead electrocardiogram (ECG) electrode placement. aVF, augmented voltage left foot or leg; aVL, augmented voltage left arm; aVr, augmented voltage right arm; LA, left arm; LL, left leg; RA, right arm; RL, right leg; V_1–V_6, chest leads.

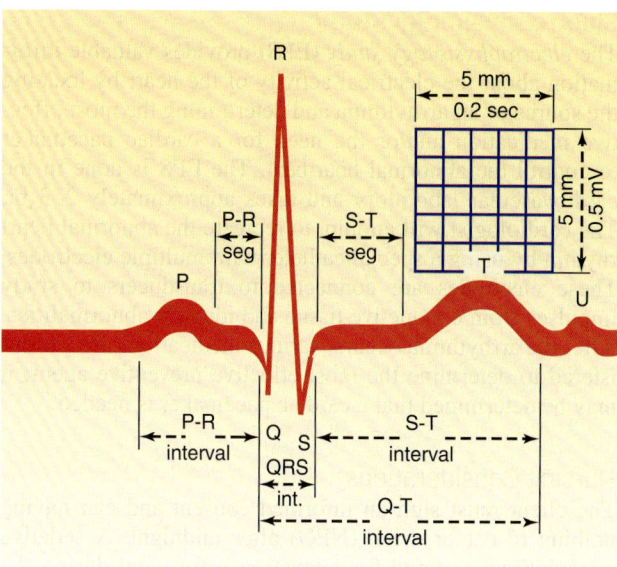

Figure 81-2 Diagram of the electrocardiogram (ECG) reading (lead II) and commonly measured components. Each small box on the horizontal axis represents 0.04 s; on the vertical axis, each small box represents 1 mm or 0.1 mV. The P wave represents atrial depolarization, the QRS complex ventricular depolarization, and the T-wave ventricular repolarization. Atrial repolarization, which occurs during ventricular depolarization, is hidden under the QRS complex.

medications the client is receiving. Data regarding the client's age, sex, blood pressure, height, weight, and symptoms must be available to the cardiologist. Figure 81-2 illustrates the basic ECG graphic recording, which is read as PQRST waveforms. Deviations from the normal PQRST waveforms indicate a variety of cardiac conditions.

Stress Test

A stress test is performed to assess the severity of symptomatic and *asymptomatic* (without symptoms) cardiac disease. The client pedals a stationary bicycle or walks on a treadmill while ECG and blood pressure measurements are taken. Various chemicals or medications (thallium, dipyridamole [Persantine], or dobutamine HCl) may also be injected before or during the test or used instead of exercise for older adults and those who cannot tolerate activity. The heart's response to physical activity or the medication is determined, and an appropriate exercise program or method of treatment is then prescribed for the individual.

Echocardiogram

Echocardiography uses sound waves to produce a three-dimensional view of the heart and its blood flow. An echocardiogram can assess heart size, detect the presence of excess fluid in the pericardial sac, assess valvular function, and it can show atrophy or distention of individual heart chambers. It is useful in the diagnosis and differentiation of heart murmurs, heart failure, and the amount of blood each ventricle ejects (pumps out) with every heartbeat. The percentage of blood ejected from a chamber is referred to as the *ejection fraction*. This percentage is a particularly important datum needed for diagnosing the amount of blood leaving a damaged left ventricle. Damage to the left ventricle inhibits the amount of oxygenated blood moving into the aorta and, thus, general circulation.

Transesophageal echocardiography (TEE) is another means of monitoring the heart. It is performed by inserting the ultrasound probe directly into the esophagus. This provides for a better visualization of the heart through the esophageal wall. TEE can be performed intraoperatively or in the healthcare provider's office.

Nuclear Scan

The *nuclear scan* is generally performed to detect *ischemic* patterns (lack of blood supply) and to assess for viable myocardium. During the scan, the client receives a weak radioactive chemical (thallium, technetium) intravenously to allow for a better view of the heart's chambers or myocardium.

Electrophysiology Study

The *electrophysiology study* (EPS) provides valuable information about the electrical activity of the heart by locating the source of an arrhythmia and determining the most effective medication and/or the need for a cardiac pacemaker to control the abnormal heartbeat. The EPS is done in the cardiovascular laboratory and takes approximately 2–3 hr. The cardiologist will attempt to recreate the abnormal heart rhythm by using a special catheter with multiple electrodes. These electrodes are connected to transducers to study impulses from conductive tissue and identify abnormalities. After the arrhythmia occurs, various medications are administered to determine the most effective preventive agent; it may be determined that a cardiac pacemaker is needed.

Nursing Considerations

The client must sign an informed consent and can having nothing to eat or drink (NPO) after midnight. A sedative is sometimes ordered for relaxation before and during the procedure.

After the procedure, the catheter insertion site is covered with a 4 × 4 bandage or Band-Aid. The client will be on bed rest for 1–2 hr after the procedure. Check the client's vital signs every 15 min initially and less frequently once they have stabilized. This procedure may be done on an outpatient basis.

Cardiac Catheterization

A **cardiac catheterization** is performed to obtain information about congenital or acquired heart defects, measure oxygen concentration, determine cardiac output, or assess the status of the heart's structures and chambers. It may be performed during an angiocardiogram to study the function of the heart or blood supply or to diagnose congenital anomalies or valvular disease. Therapeutic treatments may be done during the catheterization to repair the heart, open valves, or dilate arteries.

In this procedure, a long, flexible catheter is passed into the heart through a large blood vessel, usually the femoral or brachial artery. However, with the miniaturization of medical devices, an alternative approach is to use the radial artery (*transradial catheterization*). The pressure is measured as the catheter passes through each location, and blood specimens are taken in each area. A dye may also be injected. Notify the healthcare provider if the client has any allergies to shellfish, iodine, or contrast media. A team of healthcare providers, nurses, and technicians performs this procedure, which takes from 1–3 hr.

Nursing Considerations

Clients may be apprehensive about the procedure. Explain that it is not painful, although it may be slightly uncomfortable. A local anesthetic is given during the procedure. Warn the client that, during the procedure, they may feel a sensation of warmth as the dye is injected and a "fluttering" in the heart as the catheter passes through the blood vessels. A signed informed consent is required, and the client is NPO for at least 6 hr before the procedure. Exceptions to the NPO order are specific medications ordered by the healthcare provider.

Cardiac catheterization usually has no complications, but it is not entirely without danger. Assess the insertion site for bleeding or hematoma. Check the client's peripheral pulses every 15 min for an hour after the test and then frequently thereafter for up to 8 hr, depending on the insertion site used.

> **Nursing Alert** Immediately report a client's rapid or irregular pulse after cardiac catheterization. It may indicate heart or valve damage, clot formation, or hemorrhage. Also, immediately report any complaint of chest or insertion-site pain.

COMMON MEDICAL TREATMENTS

Pharmacologic Therapy

A major aspect of treating cardiovascular disorders is the use of pharmacologic therapy. Numerous drugs are available for the wide range of cardiac conditions (Table 81-1).

Clots cause *occlusion* (blockage) of the blood flow in situations such as acute MI. A pharmacologic agent called a *thrombolytic* alteplase (Activase) (also known as tissue plasminogen activator, t-PA), has been shown to dissolve these clots in arterial or venous blood vessels (Mayo Clinic, n.d.). For example, t-PA may be given to destroy the occlusion in coronary arteries that is causing an MI, or for massive pulmonary emboli, or for an ischemic (*not* hemorrhagic) stroke. These drugs can cause bleeding and have strict administration protocols. Healthcare providers or specially trained nurses administer the specific drug in the emergency department (ED), intensive care unit (ICU), or cardiac care unit (CCU). Clients for **thrombolytic therapy** are selected by the following criteria:

- History of chest pain within the past 6 hr. *Rationale: Studies have shown that the sooner the pharmacologic agent is administered, the less heart muscle damage results.*
- **Ischemia** (lack of blood supply) of the heart persists even after the administration of sublingual nitroglycerin. Ischemia is reflected on the ECG as ST-segment depression, T-wave inversion, or both.
- No recent history of surgery, organ biopsy, cardiopulmonary resuscitation, hemorrhagic stroke, bleeding abnormalities, intracranial neoplasm, recent head injury, pregnancy, or allergy to the thrombolytic.

General relief of chest pain occurs if the procedure is successful. Assess the client for complications, including arrhythmias, bleeding, allergic reactions, and fever. The client will be in the CCU for 1–2 days to facilitate close observation.

COMMON SURGICAL TREATMENTS

Percutaneous Transluminal Coronary Angioplasty

In *percutaneous transluminal coronary angioplasty* (PTCA), a surgeon inserts a balloon-tipped catheter into a client's narrowed coronary artery (Fig. 81-3). Injection of a radiopaque

TABLE 81-1 Common Classifications of Medications Used for Cardiovascular Disorders

CLASSIFICATION[a]	COMMON USES	GENERAL MECHANISM OF ACTION	EXAMPLES OF MEDICATIONS[b] (TRADE NAMES OF MEDICATIONS APPEAR IN PARENTHESES FOLLOWING GENERIC NAME.)
Inotropic agents Cardiac glycoside, Cardiotonic	• Heart failure • Often combined with other cardiac medications	Acts to slow and strengthen the heart; increases cardiac output; reduces workload and heart rate.	Digoxin (Lanoxin) NOTE—Antidote to digoxin is digoxin immune FAB (Digibind)
Antihypertensives *Diuretics* Thiazide Loop Potassium-sparing	• Hypertension • Heart failure	Increases excretion of water, which decreases total blood (water) volume and cardiac output, which lowers BP.	Thiazide diuretics: hydrochlorothiazide (Hydrodiuril) Loop diuretics: furosemide (Lasix) Potassium-sparing diuretics: spironolactone (Aldactone)
Angiotensin-converting enzyme (ACE) inhibitors	• Heart failure • Hypertension • Coronary artery disease • Postmyocardial infarction Often used with other cardiac medications	Decreases production of angiotensin II, resulting in vasodilation and lower BP.	Lisinopril (Prinivil) Captopril (Capoten)
Angiotensin receptor blockers (ARBs)	• Hypertension • Heart failure Often used with diuretic	Blocks angiotensin II receptors and lowers BP by decreasing systemic vascular resistance.	Irbesartan (Avapro) Losartan (Cozaar)
Beta-adrenergic blockers ("beta-blockers") *Note:* There are many types of beta-blocking agents that can vary in their effect on heart rate and blood pressure.	• Hypertension Some forms of tachycardia and angina	Inhibits simulation of specific beta-adrenergic sites, which result in lower heart rates and BP.	Atenolol (Tenormin) Metoprolol (Lopressor) Nadolol (Corgard) Propranolol (Inderal)
Calcium channel blockers *Note:* There are many types of calcium channel blockers that can vary in their effect on heart rate and blood pressure.	• Hypertension • Some tachyarrhythmias Angina	Slows cardiac conduction through AV node, which decreases heart rate, dilates peripheral arteries, and decreases peripheral vascular resistance.	Diltiazem (Cardizem) Nifedipine (Procardia) Verapamil HCl (Calan)
Centrally acting adrenergic inhibitors	• Hypertension Commonly given with a diuretic	Inhibits vasoconstriction and cardioacceleration, thus reducing peripheral resistance.	Clonidine (Catapres) Methyldopa (Aldomet)
Peripherally acting adrenergic inhibitors	• Hypertension Commonly given with a diuretic	Decreases vasoconstriction, thus increasing vasodilation.	Doxazosin (Cardura) Prazosin (Minipress) Reserpine (Serpasil)
Antianginals *Nitrates*	• Hypertension • Angina • Peripheral vascular disease • Heart failure	Causes vasodilation and lowers peripheral vascular resistance; reduces myocardial oxygen consumption.	Isosorbide dinitrate (Isordil) Nitroglycerin (Nitro-Bid)

(Continued)

TABLE 81-1 Common Classifications of Medications Used for Cardiovascular Disorders (Continued)

CLASSIFICATION[a]	COMMON USES	GENERAL MECHANISM OF ACTION	EXAMPLES OF MEDICATIONS[b] (TRADE NAMES OF MEDICATIONS APPEAR IN PARENTHESES FOLLOWING GENERIC NAME.)
Antiarrhythmics (also known as antidysrhythmics) *Classifications IA, IB, IC; miscellaneous Class I; Class II beta-adrenergic blockers; Class III potassium channel blockers; or Class IV calcium channel blockers*	Control arrhythmias, e.g., heart rates that are too fast or are life-threatening	Mechanisms depend on the specific drug; goal of therapy is to convert or reduce dysfunctional heart rhythms, such as ectopic heartbeats; slow conduction; prolong refraction; or increase heart rate.	Lidocaine (Xylocaine) Procainamide (Pronestyl) Quinidine Amiodarone See also beta-blockers and calcium channel blockers.
Antilipidemics *Bile acid sequestrants*	Hyperlipoproteinemia	Absorbs bile in GI tract, lowers LDL levels.	Cholestyramine (Questran)
HMG-CoA reductase inhibitors	• Hyperlipoproteinemia • Hypercholesterolemia • Hypertriglyceridemia	Inhibits cholesterol synthesis; decreases serum cholesterol and LDL.	Atorvastatin (Lipitor) Simvastatin (Zocor)
Blood coagulation agents *Anticoagulants Antiplatelets Thrombolytics (fibrinolytics)*	• Prevent clot formation • Treat thrombophlebitis • Dissolve clots	Heparin and warfarin inhibit clot formation, whereas alteplase and streptokinase will break up existing clots.	Enoxaparin (Lovenox) Warfarin (Coumadin) Alteplase (Activase) Streptokinase (Streptase)

Karch A., & Tucker R. (2021). *2020 Lippincott pocket drug guide for nurses.* Wolters Kluwer.
AV, atrioventricular; BP, blood pressure; GI, gastrointestinal; LDL, low-density lipoprotein.
[a]Many medications fall into more than one category and are used in different classifications.
[b]Medications are updated frequently, so it is important to seek references to the most current drug information available.

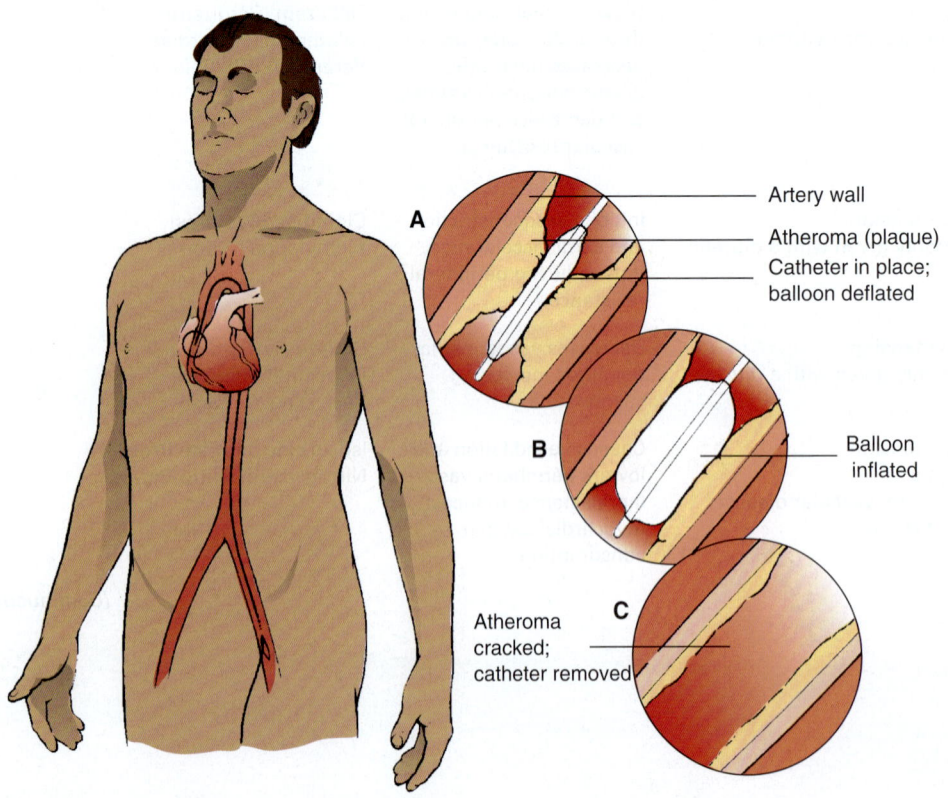

Figure 81-3 Percutaneous transluminal coronary angioplasty (PTCA) is a less invasive procedure than coronary artery bypass surgery in selected individuals. **A.** A balloon-tipped catheter is passed into the affected coronary artery and placed within the atherosclerotic lesion. **B.** The balloon is then rapidly inflated and deflated with controlled pressure. **C.** After the plaque is compressed, the catheter is removed, allowing improved blood flow in the vessel.

dye allows clear visibility of the coronary arteries by x-ray study so that the surgeon can see the vessels.

Sometimes, this procedure is simply called *angioplasty*. **Angioplasty** widens the artery's opening (*lumen*) and improves blood flow to the heart muscles. Another type of angioplasty, called **atherectomy**, involves use of a cutting device (*rotablator*) with a rotating shaver (*burr*) at the tip of the catheter. This is used to shave away plaque from the coronary artery. *Laser angioplasty* has also been used either alone or in conjunction with the balloon. The laser beam of light vaporizes the plaque in the coronary artery.

In some cases, angioplasty does not maintain arterial patency, and the artery closes. Some surgeons are finding long-term success through angioplasty with placement of a **stent**. The bare-metal stent (BMS) is commonly a wire coil similar to the coil of a ballpoint pen, although other types are used. Other stents called drug-eluting stents (DES) are coated with a medication that is slowly eluted (released) to prevent the growth of scar tissue in the vessel. This helps keep the artery open and smooth, allowing good blood flow. Both BMS and DES are left in the artery when removing the balloon catheter. Thus, the stent keeps the artery open. Researchers have found that DES have a lower rate of restenosis than do BMS (Mayo Clinic, 2019).

Cardiac Surgery

Heart surgery may help some people with heart disease. *Closed-heart surgery* refers to surgical procedures that are done without stopping the heart. *Open-heart surgery* involves opening or operating on the heart in such a way that the heart must be stopped and the circulated blood is oxygenated by a device, such as a *pump oxygenator* (*heart–lung pump*). Use of such a device is called *extracorporeal* (outside the body) *circulation*. As blood circulates through the machine, the machine removes carbon dioxide and adds oxygen through osmosis, filming, or bubbling. The machine also keeps the blood warmed to body temperature. A trained cardiopulmonary technician maintains the machine and determines if it is properly oxygenating the blood. A person can be maintained for several hours on the heart–lung pump. Various types of heart and blood vessel surgery may be done with the use of the pump oxygenator, or the pump oxygenator may be used as a support device in other types of surgery. In some cases, heart surgery is done after body temperature is lowered (*surgical hypothermia*) or under higher than normal atmospheric pressure with **hyperoxygenation** (in the hyperbaric chamber).

Coronary Artery Bypass Grafting

Coronary artery bypass grafting (CABG) is one example of heart surgery. Surgeons use healthy vessels, usually including the saphenous vein from a leg, and place it around the blockage in the coronary artery. One end of the vein is grafted to the aorta and the other end to the area of the heart that is not receiving blood from the blocked artery. The grafted vein supplies oxygenated blood from the aorta to the heart. This surgery is done when less invasive measures have failed or are not feasible. Usually, more than one blocked coronary artery requires bypass grafting during the surgery. Figure 81-4 illustrates common grafting sites that revascularize cardiac tissue by rerouting blood flow.

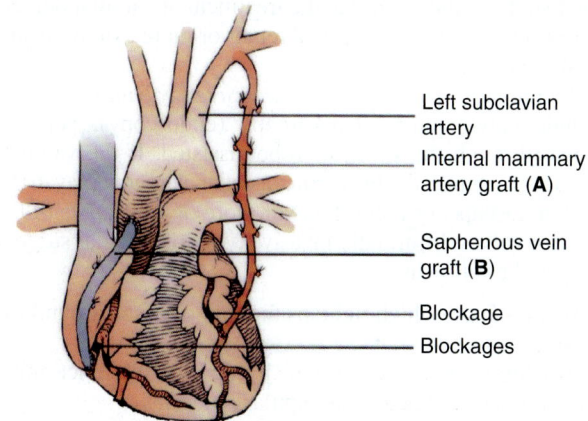

Figure 81-4 Coronary artery bypass grafting. **A.** Mammary artery bypass. The mammary artery is anastomosed to the anterior descending left coronary artery, bypassing the obstructing lesion. **B.** Saphenous vein bypass graft. The vein segment is sutured to the ascending aorta and the right coronary artery at a point distal to the occluding lesion.

A procedure called *transmyocardial laser revascularization* (TMLR) is used for the treatment of severe CAD in people who are unable to be treated with angioplasty or CABG surgery. This procedure uses a high-energy laser to create new channels through the heart muscle from the left ventricle. This allows blood to flow into the heart muscle even though the arteries are blocked. This laser surgery is performed on the beating heart; it does not require the use of a cardiopulmonary bypass machine (heart–lung oxygenator) and usually requires only a small left-chest incision. It is much less invasive than open-heart surgery.

Heart Valve Repair and Replacement

Cardiac valvular repair or replacement surgery is required when stenosis, regurgitation, calcification, congenital defects, rheumatic disease, or other disorders have significantly disrupted cardiac blood flow through the cardiac valves. Indications for heart valve surgery are listed in Box 81-1. Of the four heart valves (tricuspid, pulmonic, mitral, and aortic), most repairs are needed on the leaflets (flaps) of the ventricular valves (i.e., the mitral or aortic).

Box 81-1 Indications for Heart Valve Surgery

- Major cardiac symptoms: chest pain, angina, dyspnea, syncope, heart failure
- Mitral or aortic valvular insufficiency caused by *regurgitation* (The valves do not close completely, which allows blood flow to leak backward.)
- Mitral or aortic valvular insufficiency caused by *stenosis* (The valves are stiff and do not open completely.)
- Damage to valves caused by infection (endocarditis), trauma, blood clots, bleeding or deterioration of previously replaced valves
- Mitral valve prolapsed
- Pulmonary valve stenosis
- Tricuspid regurgitation

The two main approaches to the treatment of valvular defects involve either minimal surgical repair or more extensive surgical replacement.

Techniques of *minimally invasive valvular surgery* include valvuloplasty, laparoscopy (endoscopy), percutaneous (through the skin), or robot-assisted. If the valvular damage is minimal, the cardiovascular surgeon may trim, tighten, reshape, or rebuild one or more of the leaflets of the valve or valves. Minimally invasive types of valvular surgery include the following:

- *Annuloplasty*, which tightens the ring of tissue around the valve
- Structural support repair, which improves the functioning of chordae tendineae and papillary muscles
- Repair of a floppy or prolapsed valve leaflet

Heart valve replacement requires open-heart surgery. This technique involves removing the damaged valve and inserting a type of prosthetic (artificial) valve. There are two major categories of valves used for surgical replacement: one is a synthetic mechanical valve and the other is a biologic (tissue) valve.

Mechanical valves are made of cloth, stainless steel, titanium, or a type of ceramic. They are designed to be long-lasting and effective; however, they can create blood clots, leading to a thrombus or an embolus. The client who receives a mechanical valve will need to receive lifelong anticoagulant therapy, which in itself can cause bleeding or blood clotting problems. Anticoagulant therapies include warfarin (Coumadin) or aspirin. Postoperatively, mechanical valves may produce a clicking sound heard in the chest.

Biologic valves can be made from animal tissue, generally pork or bovine, and are known as *xenografts*. Valves or tissues from a donated heart can be used. This is known as an *allograft* or *homograft*. Occasionally, the client's own tissue, an *autograft*, can be used for the replacement. Biologic valves generally do not require anticoagulant therapy after replacement, but they may need to be replaced after 12–15 years.

Heart Transplantation

For clients with severe cardiac conditions, such as end-stage heart failure, severe cardiomyopathy, congenital heart defects, or significant CAD, surgical implantation of a donor heart may be considered. The heart recipient is considered a suitable candidate for heart transplantation if various medication regimens and/or cardiac surgeries have been tried without significant improvement, and the recipient has a significant chance of survival and improvement in their quality of life. Some cardiac replacement surgical centers consider factors such as smoking, alcohol intake, and recreational drug use as part of the criteria for future success as a replacement candidate. The donor heart is obtained from a recently deceased or brain-dead donor. Both preoperatively and postoperatively, the client undergoes a variety of stressful physical and emotional situations. It is standard for the recipient to undergo a variety of psychological and physical tests before surgery. After surgery, the client must take a variety of medications, including lifelong immunosuppressive therapy (cyclosporine [Sandimmune]) to inhibit rejection of the foreign cardiac donor tissue. Corticosteroid therapy may also be routine. Postoperative medications can have adverse reactions, such as nephrotoxic effects, bone loss, ulcers, atherosclerosis, and an increased risk for a variety of infections. Postoperative follow-up care includes routine monitoring of the new heart for rejection using cardiac biopsies, echocardiography, ECG, and laboratory studies. The client and their caregivers must recognize that a successful transplant will need to be followed by strict lifestyle routines.

Nursing Considerations and Cardiac Surgery

Sometimes, people who come into an acute care facility for surgery have been under intensive medical treatment for weeks or years. These clients have had time to prepare physically and emotionally for the experience, and many of them welcome heart surgery as an opportunity to improve their lifestyle, realizing that often no other treatment can help them. Other clients have little or no preparation when surgery must be initiated as an emergency measure (e.g., following a severe MI). In both cases, contemporary methods of treatment and surgical techniques allow many people who have cardiac surgery to live productive lives.

The following are important considerations before surgery:

- Preoperative teaching (e.g., deep breathing, expectations after surgery)
- Discharge planning, including plans for cardiac rehabilitation
- Client's nutrition and capacity for healing (e.g., need for supplemental protein)
- Supplemental oxygenation needs before and after surgery
- Vitamin and mineral therapy (e.g., supplemental B vitamins, iron)
- Routine tests and procedures (e.g., laboratory and radiologic testing, echocardiogram, heart catheterization, ECG, cardiac biopsies)

The main objective for this preparation is to promote the client's best possible physical condition before surgery.

Registered nurses are usually responsible for immediate postoperative nursing care; licensed practical/vocational nurses or nursing students may assist. The first 2 days after surgery are the most critical to survival. After surgery, nursing care focuses on the following:

- Maintaining airway and ventilation
- Providing adequate tissue oxygenation
- Monitoring and maintaining cardiac function
- Maintaining fluid and electrolyte balance
- Controlling chest drainage with suction
- Monitoring body temperature
- Identifying signs and symptoms of complications (e.g., infection, arrhythmias)
- Relieving pain

NCLEX Alert

Cardiovascular problems are among the most commonly seen conditions in hospitalized clients. Priority nursing concerns for NCLEX options include the ABC's (airway, breathing, circulation), nursing interventions, laboratory test results, medication uses and side effects, and teaching concepts for client and family.

NURSING PROCESS

DATA COLLECTION
Carefully observe the individual with a cardiac or blood vessel disorder. Establish a baseline for future comparison to determine the presence of suspected cardiovascular complications. Report any changes in baseline observations.

A complete cardiovascular assessment begins on admission. The nursing assessment includes a complete nursing history, as well as observations. When taking the health history, ask about any potential risk factors, such as family history of cardiovascular disease, smoking, lack of exercise, or poor nutrition. Also include any issues, such as shortness of breath or fatigue, which might interfere with the client's ability to perform activities of daily living (ADL).

Include observations of heart sounds, blood pressure, and pulse. Note any specific signs and symptoms, such as shortness of breath and edema in hands or feet, while taking the client's vital signs (see In Practice: Data Gathering in Nursing 81-1). Observe the client's emotional response to the disorder or disease and the person's understanding of ongoing treatment.

PLANNING AND IMPLEMENTATION
Together, the healthcare team, client, and family plan effective care to meet the client's individualized needs. For the client undergoing diagnostic tests, such as cardiac catheterization, and procedures, such as angioplasty, provide preoperative and postoperative care. The person with a heart or blood vessel disorder may require assistance in meeting daily needs. The person who has had a stroke may need total assistance and nursing care temporarily or on a long-term basis. The person with a chronic disability, such as hemiplegia or a damaged heart, may need assistance in dealing with psychosocial problems. Many clients need to understand more about their disorder, its prognosis, and its treatment. A nursing care plan is developed for each client to meet their individual needs.

Teaching About Prevention
To aid in the prevention of cardiovascular disorders, teach about predisposing factors (e.g., fat buildup in the arteries, hypertension, obesity, diabetes mellitus, or smoking). The goals of prevention and treatment with many cardiovascular disorders, including hypertension, include weight reduction, if necessary; reduction or elimination of dietary intake of cholesterol and salt; maintenance of a healthy pattern of sleep, rest, and relaxation; cessation of smoking; and learning ways to handle emotional upsets. If the client is taking antihypertensive drugs, teaching involves explaining the necessity of taking the prescribed medications even if they feel well. Antihypertensives help relieve cardiac stress, relax blood vessels, and reduce tissue fluid and blood volume. Describe possible side effects of these medications (see Chapter 62).

Suggest a consultation with a registered dietitian or a support group for weight loss and maintenance. Counseling about fat in the diet may be helpful.

Aerobic exercise (in moderation) is good for cardiovascular conditioning and helps in weight loss. Walking, especially at a good pace, is effective and inexpensive. The greatest exercise risk is avoiding it. Teach clients how to warm up before and cool down after exercise. Smoking cessation programs may be necessary for those who wish to stop smoking.

Clients can learn how to measure their blood pressure at home. Many authorities believe that when the person is involved in self-care more directly, they are more likely to comply with medications and required routines. In Practice: Educating the Client 81-1 lists teaching factors and actions individuals can take to reduce the risk of cardiovascular disease.

EVALUATION
Together, the healthcare team, client, and family evaluate outcomes of care. Have short-term goals been met? Is the client stabilized following any initial emergency? For example, have the client's vital signs and heart rate and rhythm stabilized? Are long-term goals realistic? For example, does the client accept the diagnosis of MI and the need for lifestyle changes, or are they denying the problem? Will the client need long-term nursing care or short-term rehabilitation placement? Does the client need home health aide/homemaker services or regular in-home medication administration? Has the client been referred to a "stop smoking" program? Do the client and family need a support group? When planning for further nursing care, consider the client's prognosis, as well as any complications, and the client's responses.

IN PRACTICE
DATA GATHERING IN NURSING 81-1: Signs and Symptoms of Cardiovascular Disorders

- Changes in the rate, quality, and rhythm of the pulse
- Rise or fall in blood pressure or central venous pressure (as can be noted by jugular venous distention)
- Edema, especially in the feet and ankles (faulty heart action causes the collection of fluids in the tissues)
- Weight gain due to excess fluid in the tissues
- Difficulty breathing and the presence of a cough, often caused by pulmonary edema
- Cyanosis, owing to a lack of oxygen in the blood or a circulatory disorder
- Clubbing of the fingers
- Needing to squat to breathe
- Pain (a significant symptom)
- Fatigue, for no apparent reason
- Intermittent **claudication**, which denotes a decrease in blood supply to the legs and feet

IN PRACTICE
EDUCATING THE CLIENT 81-1   Prevention of Cardiovascular Disorders

- Stop smoking and avoid smoking's harmful effects. *Rationale: Nicotine is a vasoconstrictor. It also increases heart rate and blood pressure.*
- Reduce sodium (salt) intake. *Rationale: Salt restriction minimizes fluid retention.*
- Maintain weight within standardized guidelines. *Rationale: Obesity increases the workload of the heart.*
- Avoid foods high in animal fats and cholesterol. *Rationale: Excess blood cholesterol can form plaque in blood vessels. Plan meals using* www.ChooseMyPlate.gov.
- Avoid foods that contain caffeine: coffee, cola drinks, tea, chocolate. *Rationale: Caffeine is a potent vasoconstrictor.*
- Exercise regularly and moderately (at least three times a week for 30 min). Walking is a healthful exercise. *Rationale: Exercise stimulates circulation and builds cardiac strength and endurance.*
- Avoid crossing the legs at the knees when sitting. *Rationale: Crossing the legs at the knees hampers circulation.*
- Have both feet comfortably touch the floor when sitting. *Rationale: This position avoids constriction of blood vessels in the groin area.*
- For a few minutes in the morning and evening, elevate the feet. *Rationale: This position encourages venous return.*
- Avoid constrictive garments, especially around the legs, arms, and waist. Tight-fitting garters or girdles should not be worn. *Rationale: These items restrict circulation.*
- Wear properly fitted shoes. *Rationale: They prevent irritation and skin breakdown. Ulcers on the foot or leg are difficult to heal if peripheral circulation is impaired.*
- Avoid and minimize environmental stress and anxiety-producing factors. Learn ways to handle stress effectively. *Rationale: Stress causes the release of substances called catecholamines, which constrict blood vessels and thus elevate blood pressure.*
- Follow medication regimens for prescribed medications. *Rationale: Routine administration of medications is necessary to maintain therapeutic drug levels.*
- Get plenty of rest and relaxation. Learn stress management and relaxation techniques, if necessary. *Rationale: Cardiac tissue is very sensitive to hypoxia, which occurs when the individual is emotionally or physically stressed. Under stressful situations, blood vessels will constrict, leading to increased blood pressure and a stroke.*

ABNORMAL CONDITIONS THAT MAY CAUSE CARDIOVASCULAR DISEASE

Some types of heart disease are curable; others are not, but they can be controlled with treatment. A client's attitude toward heart disease affects recovery. Some people are so frightened that they are afraid to move. Others deny the seriousness of their disease and disregard orders about diet, rest, and smoking. Several types of heart conditions are discussed here that, if left untreated, can lead to more serious cardiovascular conditions. Client teaching can help individuals understand the seriousness of these conditions and the value of diet, exercise, and medication.

Arteriosclerosis and Atherosclerosis

Arteriosclerosis applies to several pathologic conditions in which the walls of the arteries thicken, harden, and lose elasticity. It is also referred to as "hardening of the arteries." **Atherosclerosis**, the most common type of arteriosclerosis, is characterized by fatty deterioration of the arterial smooth muscle walls. Gradually, over several years, the walls absorb increasing amounts of circulating lipids, and the lumen of the arteries narrows (**stenosis**) or may close completely. This buildup of fat and mineral deposits is called *plaque*. Often the terms *arteriosclerosis* and *atherosclerosis* are used interchangeably. These diseases may affect the heart valves and may lead to hypertension or CAD.

A diet high in saturated fat is usually associated with an increased blood cholesterol level. Studies have shown that unsaturated fats (e.g., olive oil, corn oil) do not raise the blood cholesterol level as much as saturated fats (found in butter, eggs, and meats). Some people seem to metabolize cholesterol differently than others. In treating cardiovascular disorders, the healthcare provider periodically measures the client's blood cholesterol level and may attempt to control the amount of cholesterol through diet, medications, and exercise. The balance between high-density lipoprotein (HDL or "good" cholesterol) and low-density lipoprotein (LDL or "bad" cholesterol) is more important than is the actual total cholesterol value. However, as the total level rises above 150, a person's risk of CAD increases.

Hypertension

Hypertension (HTN) or *hypertensive heart disease* means *high blood pressure*. Hypertension is a leading cause of MI, cardiac damage, kidney damage, heart failure, and stroke. With advancing age, blood pressure tends to rise, although the exact reason is unclear. One thing is certain: the condition of the heart and blood vessels has the greatest effect on blood pressure. Although HTN cannot be cured, treatment can usually bring blood pressure to within the normal range.

 SPECIAL CONSIDERATIONS Culture and Ethnicity

Studies show that African American clients are more likely to have hypertension earlier in life, at higher levels, and more frequently than European American clients.

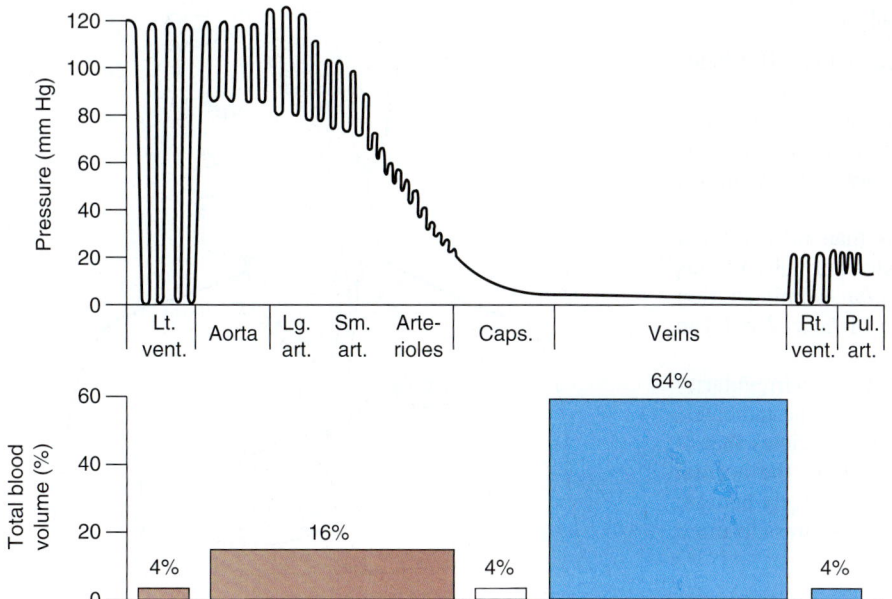

Figure 81-5 Pressure and volume distribution in the systemic circulation. The graphs show the inverse relationship between internal pressure and volume in different portions of the circulatory system. Notice that the arterioles and the capillaries have decreased pressure as compared with pressure in the aorta. Arteries and arterioles are damaged by high pressures and, in turn, damage the organs that they service.

High blood pressure is predominantly caused by a spasm of the small arterioles. Normal pressure gradients and normal volumes of blood are seen on the graph in Figure 81-5.

An increase in the pressure within the blood vessels can cause significant damage to small arterioles. The spasms increase blood pressure and thus contribute to arteriosclerosis (a vicious circle). Because the heart must pump harder to force blood through the arteries, the result is **hypertrophy** (enlargement) of the heart muscle.

Hypertension may exist owing to a known cause, such as kidney failure, malformations of blood vessels, certain tumors, and some specific endocrine disorders. However, the cause may be unknown (in most cases, a condition classified as *essential hypertension*). Symptoms other than elevated blood pressure may not occur for years, and no restrictions are imposed until other symptoms develop. Encourage clients with HTN to exercise, observe moderation in eating, and avoid tension and anxiety. Advise them to avoid smoking and to limit intake of alcoholic beverages, caffeine, and sodium. Symptoms of HTN may become severe, with headache, fatigue, dyspnea, edema, and nocturia.

Malignant hypertension (which is not cancer) refers to a sudden onset of severely elevated blood pressure that is controllable. It is most often seen in young people. The incidence is highest in African American clients, especially men younger than 40 years. Onset is sudden, and the disease progresses rapidly. In many cases, determining its cause is difficult. Malignant hypertension is known to cause rapid *necrosis* (death) of vital organs, such as the heart, brain, and kidney. Clients with malignant hypertension rarely survive more than a few years.

Hypotension

Hypotension is low blood pressure. Clinical manifestations differ depending on the underlying cause. Causes of hypotension can be classified under one of three mechanisms: a heart rate problem, a heart muscle or pump problem, or a volume problem. Treatment will depend on the underlying problem. Variations in blood pressure can also be caused by medications.

Rate problems include a heart rate that is too fast or too slow. *Pump problems* result from MI, *cardiomyopathy* (the heart cavity is enlarged and stretched), acute cardiac or aortic insufficiency, prosthetic valve dysfunction, *cardiac tamponade* (heart compression, caused by fluid buildup), pulmonary embolism, and medications that affect or alter the heart's function. Many other clinical problems can also affect how the heart muscle pumps. *Volume problems* include hemorrhage, gastrointestinal fluid loss, renal injury or disease, central nervous system injury, spinal injury, sepsis, medications or disease processes that affect vascular tone, and any other condition that causes large-volume fluid losses.

HEART DISORDERS

Conditions Affecting the Heart's Rhythm

The heart may be affected by normal physiologic factors (e.g., sleep, exercise) and medications (digoxin, calcium channel blockers, beta-blockers), which can cause a disturbance in the regularity of the heartbeat. In some cases, the irregularity can be the result of a disturbance in the heart's electrical conduction system.

Cardiac Arrhythmias

An arrhythmia (or dysrhythmia) is an irregularity in the heartbeat's rhythm. It is a complication of numerous disorders, such as an MI, electrolyte imbalances (especially potassium), and other heart and circulatory disorders. It may also result from severe trauma or electric shock. An arrhythmia is any change in the normal sequence of the electrical impulses in the heart. Arrhythmias are typically categorized according to their origination sites in the atria, septum, or ventricles. Abnormal electrical impulses occur in the SA node, AV node, bundle branches, or the Purkinje network.

Three common arrhythmias are as follows:

- *Sinus tachycardia:* Heartbeat is greater than 100 beats per minute. (This rate is normal in children.) It can be present postoperatively and in instances of high fever, decreased oxygenation, excessive fluid or blood loss, extreme emotion, overactive thyroid, or strenuous exercise.
- *Sinus bradycardia:* Heartbeat is less than 60 beats per minute. (This rate may occur in athletes normally.) Sinus bradycardia can occur with *digitalization* (administration of digoxin), or it can be a symptom of *heart block* (an abnormal situation discussed below).
- *Premature ventricular contraction* (PVC) is an irregularity in the heart's ventricular rhythm. As the name indicates, a PVC is a contraction initiated in the ventricles that is premature. In other words, it occurs before the normal SA node–conducted beat. PVCs can be relatively benign; indicators of early cardiac problems; or progress to more malignant ventricular arrhythmias.

Figure 81-6 depicts a few more common arrhythmias.

Atrioventricular Heart Block

Heart block is not a disease in itself but is associated with many types of heart disease, especially diseases of the coronary arteries and rheumatic heart disease. In atrioventricular (AV) heart block, heart contractions are weak and lack sufficient force to send blood from the atria into the ventricles. Pulse rate may be as low as 30 beats per minute.

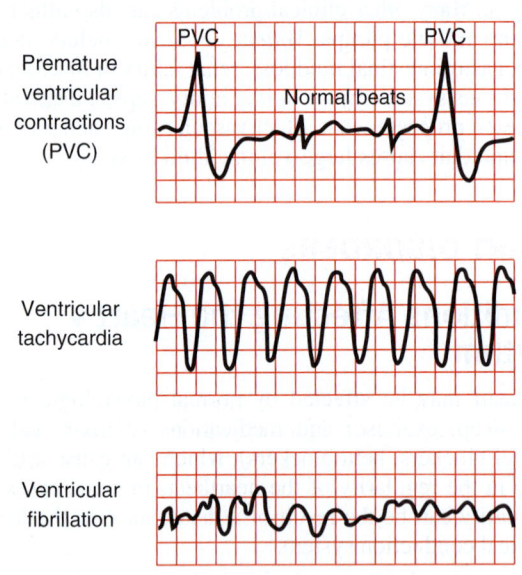

Figure 81-6 Electrocardiogram (ECG) tracings of ventricular arrhythmias. With premature ventricular contractions (PVCs) (*top tracing*), the QRS complex is distorted because the impulse is originating from an ectopic focus. Because the ventricle usually cannot repolarize sufficiently to respond to the next impulse that arises in the sinoatrial node, a PVC frequently is followed by a compensatory pause. With ventricular tachycardia (*middle tracing*), the ventricular rate is extremely rapid, ranging from 100 to 250 beats per minute; P waves also are not seen. In ventricular fibrillation (*bottom tracing*), there are no regular or effective ventricular contractions, and the ECG tracing is totally disorganized.

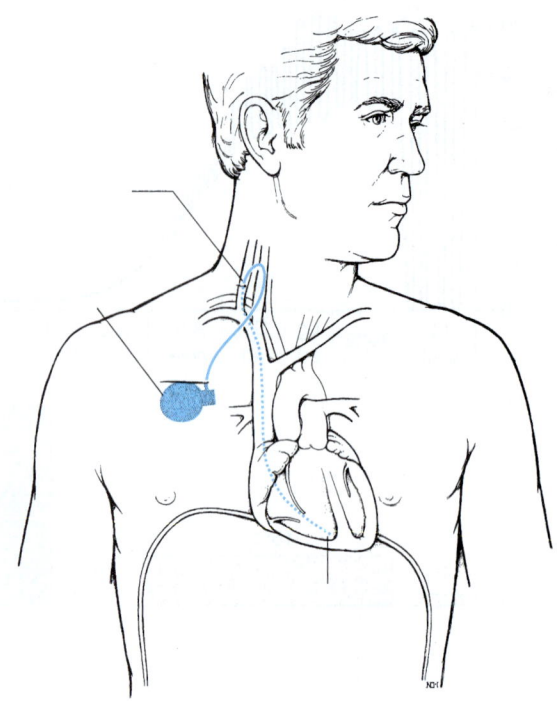

Figure 81-7 Pacemaker therapy. The pacemaker delivers an electrical impulse to the heart at specified intervals, causing the heart to beat.

An *electronic pacemaker* may be used to provide external stimulus to the heart. The electronic pacemaker stimulates heart contractions by means of wires connected to electrodes, which are inserted into the heart (Fig. 81-7). A pacemaker may be external, which is generally temporary, or internal, which is considered necessary for life-sustaining cardiac rhythms.

Clients who experience frequent difficulty with heart contractions may have a permanent pacemaker implanted. The problem with contractions may be result from a lack of initiation of electrical activity (e.g., heart block) or uncontrolled episodes of irregular or paroxysmal cardiac electrical conduction (e.g., assorted cardiac arrhythmias) in either the atria or ventricles. A portable pacemaker about the size of a cellular phone or an MP3 device is used in the clinical setting. If a permanent pacemaker is indicated, the surgeon implants the pacemaker pack underneath the client's skin, usually in the subclavian or lower abdominal area.

Some clients can discontinue use of a pacemaker gradually, depending on the heart's rhythm and etiology of the cardiac disruption. Other clients cannot live without it. For internal pacemakers, a battery replacement may be required every 5–10 years, which can often be done in an outpatient setting.

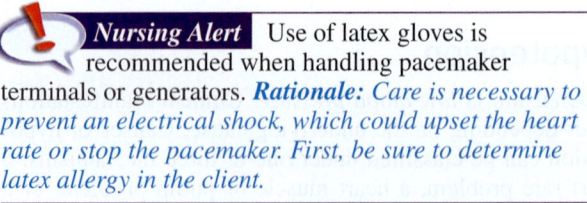

Nursing Alert Use of latex gloves is recommended when handling pacemaker terminals or generators. *Rationale: Care is necessary to prevent an electrical shock, which could upset the heart rate or stop the pacemaker. First, be sure to determine latex allergy in the client.*

The critical observation period is 3 days after the pacemaker's insertion. After a client has had a pacemaker implanted, do the following:

- Carry out routine postoperative care.
- Check all electrical equipment in the room for grounding.
- Carefully check the client's pulse, including cardiac rhythm and rate. The heart rate should correspond to the setting on the pacemaker. Report any deviation at once.
- Observe for neck vein distention or muffled heart sounds, which could indicate cardiac tamponade. These are serious signs that must be reported at once.
- Use sterile technique and keep the incision site clean to prevent infection.
- Provide active or passive range-of-motion exercises and incentive spirometer treatments to prevent complications.
- Reassure the client, who may find adjusting to dependence on the pacemaker difficult.

Nursing Alert If the client with a pacemaker notices any symptoms of dizziness or lightheadedness, instruct them to move at least 6 ft away from the source of any electrical interference.

A client with a pacemaker should wear a medical alert identification tag or bracelet (MedicAlert). Teach the client how to count the pulse and to report any deviation at once. Telecommunication or teletransmission of the ECG is used for clients with pacemakers. At a prescribed time and frequency, a client uses a special modem to transmit heart rate, rhythm, and battery life to a central location (usually, a hospital or healthcare provider's office), where heart rate and rhythm are transformed onto ECG paper for interpretation and follow-up.

Fibrillation

Fibrillation refers to the quivering of muscle fibers. A disorganized twitching of atrial muscles is known as *atrial fibrillation*. It is sometimes seen in clients with atherosclerosis and rheumatic heart disease. The pulse is irregular because coordination between the atria and ventricles is interrupted. Treatment depends on the cause, but unless the condition is life-threatening, the healthcare provider usually prescribes digoxin, beta-blockers, and calcium channel blockers to slow the transmission of electrical impulses from the atria to the ventricles. Anticoagulants may be given to prevent blood clots. Sometimes, it is necessary to perform **cardioversion** (changing of the cardiac arrhythmia, electrically or through medication administration). If all else fails to return the rhythm to normal, **atrial ablation** may be used. This procedure uses a catheter to determine the location of the abnormality; then, the diseased tissue is destroyed.

Ventricular fibrillation is a twitching of the ventricular muscles of the heart. The rhythm is totally disorganized, and blood does not circulate. It is the most dangerous type of fibrillation and is a medical emergency. It is fatal if untreated because it leads to cardiac arrest.

Defibrillation

Treatment for ventricular fibrillation is *electrical defibrillation*, which is done by a healthcare provider or a specialized critical care nurse. In defibrillation, a high-voltage electrical current is passed through the client's body in an attempt to shock the heart back into a regular beat. The electrical current necessary for cardioversion of atrial fibrillation is much less than that needed for ventricular fibrillation.

Nursing Alert During electrical defibrillation, everyone present must be careful not to touch the client or the bed; doing so will lead to shock and, possibly, injury.

If the client experiences cardiac arrest (asystole), external cardiac compression and cardiopulmonary resuscitation (CPR) are necessary. In an emergency inside a hospital, perform CPR until the code team arrives to perform electrical defibrillation. In many public places, as well as hospitals, it is common to find specific locations for an *automated external defibrillator* (AED), which is a user-friendly defibrillation device.

Implantable Cardioverter–Defibrillator

The *implantable cardioverter–defibrillator* (ICD) is an effective device in the management of lethal ventricular arrhythmias for clients whose condition cannot be managed by drug therapy.

The ICD is a lightweight (1/2 lb) lithium battery-powered pulse generator. It is surgically implanted under the skin, usually in the pectoral or abdominal region (similar to permanent pacemaker placement). Wires (called *leads*) placed in the heart sense the heart's rate and rhythm. Defibrillating heads attached to the heart deliver an electrical shock to the heart muscle when a ventricular arrhythmia is detected. If the first shock is unsuccessful, the ICD will deliver four to seven more shocks. The latest devices also provide backup pacing of the heart, as needed.

After placement of an ICD, the postoperative period allows for close observation of how the device responds to arrhythmias. Individuals receive continuous cardiac monitoring during this time. Assist the client with early ambulation, monitor the wound for signs of infection, and provide information and teaching about the device.

Teach the client to lie down when they feel a shock from the ICD. If the client is alone when this occurs, they should call 911 or the healthcare provider; if someone is with them, the client should lie down, and the other person should call the healthcare provider. When an electrical shock is delivered, it will cause a slight tingling to the individual and to anyone who touches them. If the person becomes unconscious, a family member or caregiver should call 911. All family members and caregivers will need to know how to perform CPR.

The battery on the ICD needs to be checked every 2 months. The batteries usually last at least 5 years. Be sure the client understands the need for wearing a tag that identifies the client as wearing an ICD. The client must notify airline personnel and healthcare workers who perform diagnostic tests (such as CT scans and MRIs) of the presence of the ICD, as possible disruption of the ICD by electrical or electronic devices can occur.

Conditions Affecting the Heart's Pumping Function

Tissue Perfusion
An important concept of cardiovascular homeostasis is the body's ability to send oxygenated blood to the body through the arterial system and return blood with metabolites (end products) back through the venous system to the right side of the heart. (Exception: The pulmonary artery sends deoxygenated blood to the lungs, and the pulmonary veins send oxygenated blood to the left atrium.) During the process of blood flow, the exchange of gases (e.g., O_2 and CO_2) and nutrients (e.g., glucose, minerals, enzymes, or hormones) occurs in the smallest capillary blood vessels, that is, the *microcirculation*. This exchange process is referred to as *tissue perfusion*. Poor tissue perfusion is an underlying cause of hypoxic signs and symptoms such as dyspnea, edema, or fatigue. Many disorders, such as heart failure, stroke, heart attack, or endocarditis, are affected by inadequate tissue perfusion. Tissue perfusion is also affected by hypertension and hypotension, as well as in instances of fluid volume excess or fluid volume deficits because blood pressures and fluids interfere with gas and nutrient exchange (Kalil & Bailey, 2020).

Heart Failure
Heart failure (HF), commonly known as congestive heart failure (CHF), may also be referred to as *cardiac decompensation, cardiac insufficiency,* or *cardiac incompetence*. Heart failure occurs when ventricular action and valves of the heart are inadequate and fail to maintain cardiac function, that is, the work of pumping blood efficiently throughout the body. The result is poor *cardiac output*, which is seen as a decreased volume of blood pumped by the heart. (Cardiac output is discussed in more detail in Chapter 22.) If the ventricles or valves become weak, ineffective, stiff, or enlarged, the heart cannot be an effective pump. Normally, as a functioning muscular pump, the heart will try to maintain tissue perfusion to the body's organs (Box 81-2). Generally, heart failure is a chronic, long-term progressive disorder; however, acute HF can happen without a previous onset of symptoms.

Causes of HF may include damaged or weakened cardiac muscle tissue. The major risk factors for HF include CAD, which involves arterial stenosis of the coronary arteries, hypertension, tobacco smoking, obesity, and diabetes. Most cases of HF are due to ventricles that have become dilated and incapable of acting with adequate force to pump blood, either to the lungs (right ventricle) or to the body's systems (left ventricle). Some HF is a result of the ventricles becoming stiff, which will result in insufficient filling with blood between beats. As the disorder worsens, the body becomes unable to meet basic life-sustaining oxygen demands of the body.

Left-sided heart failure occurs first in the majority of cases. The main culprits of left-sided heart failure are a weakened, dilated, or stenosed left ventricle—the main pumping chamber of the heart—and heart valves that are damaged.

The result of left-sided HF is poor tissue perfusion due to fluid buildup in the interstitial spaces of the lungs, which causes increased pressure in the pulmonary vessels. Pulmonary edema (PE), that is, fluid congestion in the lungs, develops. The term *heart failure* pertains to this increased amount and pressure of fluid in the interstitial spaces. If treatment, for example, with furosemide (Lasix), is not given, dyspnea will increase, and the client's condition will deteriorate.

Right-sided heart failure is the initial problem in some individuals, such as those with cystic fibrosis, because the right ventricle is affected first. Obstructive sleep apnea and emphysema may result from right-sided heart failure. The most common cause of right-sided heart failure is left-sided heart failure. Symptoms for right-sided heart failure will be **ascites** (fluid buildup in the abdomen) and edema in the extremities. If a client has failure of one side of the heart, eventually, failure will develop on the other side unless treatment is successfully initiated.

Signs and Symptoms
The first noticeable signs of a failing heart are excessive fatigue, arrhythmias, anorexia, nausea, dyspnea, and **orthopnea** (feeling short of breath while recumbent). These initial symptoms, often indicators of poor tissue perfusion, may develop gradually and not be considered medically important since the client can inaccurately rationalize that these problems are normal signs of aging. As the heart is unable to perfuse oxygenated blood to the brain, the client may develop altered levels of consciousness, such as difficulty concentrating or decreased alertness. Chest pain or angina may develop due to lack of oxygen perfusion to the cardiac muscles. Other symptoms include numbness or tingling in the fingers, *albuminuria* (albumin in the urine), cyanosis, edema, engorgement, and visible pulsation of neck veins, which is known as **jugular venous distention** (JVD). JVD is an indicator of heart failure that can be measured by obtaining a central venous pressure (CVP), which is discussed later in this chapter.

Diagnostic Tests
The usual tests for detecting heart disease, such as ECG, x-ray examination, echocardiography, and in some cases, cardiac catheterization, are performed. Heart failure may be diagnosed by evaluating the laboratory results of BNP and NT pro-BNP tests. Circulation time and arterial and venous blood pressure also are measured. Evaluation of urine reveals a diminished output (*oliguria*), elevated specific gravity, albuminuria, and the presence of blood (*hemoglobinuria*) and casts (tiny mineral deposits). Blood chemistry shows nitrogen retention by elevated blood urea nitrogen (BUN), uric acid, and creatinine concentrations.

Hemodynamic Monitoring
Hemodynamic monitoring looks at the cardiovascular status and tissue perfusion of a critically ill client. While a client is in an ICU or CCU, standard hemodynamic techniques involve continuous surveillance of the heart rate, blood pressure, temperature, cardiac rhythm, pulse oximetry, and arterial blood gases (ABGs). These methods provide basic knowledge of the client's cardiovascular status.

More invasive hemodynamic monitoring techniques include the **central venous pressure** (CVP) and a pulmonary artery occlusion (wedge) pressure (PAOP, PAWP). These methods are often used in determining and treating acute pulmonary edema, left ventricular failure, and mitral stenosis. A detailed discussion of these methods is beyond the scope of this textbook. A CVP reflects the amount of blood returning to the heart and the ability of the heart to pump blood into the arterial system. The PAOP reflects the degree of severity of many cardiovascular problems such as heart

Box 81-2 Edema and Heart Failure

Edema is the accumulation of fluid in the interstitial spaces. Normally, fluid remains balanced within the cells (intracellular) and in the tissue or *interstitial spaces* that surround cells. Edema develops for a variety of reasons, as summarized in Chapter 17, Box 17-1, Sample Causes of Edema. Several pathologies promote the increased interstitial fluids of edema. Inflammation of the capillaries and loss of plasma proteins (hypoproteinemia) in the capillary's blood promote fluid leakage into the surrounding tissues. Fluids within the body produce pressure (hydrostatic pressure), which leads to fluid movement and edema. Excessive sodium causes water retention and edema, which promote movement of fluids from one compartment to another, for example, from capillaries to interstitial spaces. Poor fluid drainage via the lymphatic system, which is designed to drain some fluids away from the cardiovascular system, causes more fluid back-up in the interstitial spaces.

Edema is associated with many disorders and has significant consequences when the heart muscles or heart valves are unable to be an efficient pump, as occurs in heart failure. Edema may be classified by location, such as pulmonary or cerebral edema. Edema's causes and consequences are important topics for nurses. Chapter 17 also discusses edema.

- Ascites is edema in the peritoneal cavity, generally associated with a damaged liver.
- **Anasarca** is widespread, significant edema of the body due to excess fluids in the interstitial spaces of the skin. This type of edema is found in heart failure, liver failure, and renal failure. Conditions that cause intravascular protein deficiency, such as severe malnutrition, cause the loss of intravascular proteins that promote fluid leakage from vessels into tissue spaces, leading to edema. Chemotherapy agents may cause anasarca because they cause the capillaries to leak fluids into surrounding extracellular spaces.
- **Pulmonary edema** is fluid in the interstitial spaces of the lungs, causing severe dyspnea (shortness of breath). It is associated with left-sided heart failure, which can progress to *acute pulmonary edema*, a medical emergency. Clients with pulmonary edema have a noticeable, persistent, and productive cough. Crackling or wheezing lung sounds are auscultated. Arrhythmias may develop due to lack of cardiac tissue perfusion or poor systemic tissue perfusion. Clients with pulmonary edema often have pink and frothy or blood-streaked sputum; they are treated with intravenous morphine sulfate, diuretics, supplemental oxygen, and a high Fowler position.
- **Dependent edema** is a type of swelling promoted by body positioning. It may occur with any type of HF. If the client is sitting up or walking, the feet, ankles, or legs swell. Edema in the lower legs lessens if the client is supine in bed; the edema may be noted in the posterior region (e.g., buttocks), which has now become the dependent location. However, the leg edema will again worsen as soon as the person is walking or sitting. Significant weight gain may occur, which is the rationale for weighing the client daily.
- **Pitting edema** and **nonpitting edema** are terms associated with the presence or absence of indentations in swollen areas of the body. They indicate poor tissue perfusion, poor cardiac output, and excessive fluid in the interstitial spaces. The difference between pitting and nonpitting edema is basically related to their causative factors. Pitting edema is generally related to a loss of cellular proteins and cardiovascular problems, whereas nonpitting edema is usually associated with a lymphatic problem. Nonpitting edema is typically seen in the upper arms or lower legs, for example, lymphedema. Pitting edema is noticeable when a finger pressed on a swollen area leaves a finger-sized indentation, usually on the lower legs. Pitting edema may also occur when any form of pressure (e.g., socks) has been exerted on the client's legs. In documentation, the edema may be quantified using the designations 1+, 2+, 3+, or 4+, which reflect the number of seconds an indentation remains before returning to normal. Nursing care is aimed at prevention of long-standing circular indentations around the calf since poor tissue perfusion to the skin can progress to inflammation, stasis ulcers, or thrombosis. A person with 1+ pitting edema of the leg has relatively mild edema that may disappear with diuretics and elevation of the extremity. In contrast, the individual with 4+ pitting edema has severe edema that may or may not disappear after a 4-second waiting period. This can occur with heart failure, cardiac myopathy, or mitral valve stenosis. No indentation is noticed with *nonpitting edema* after placing pressure on swollen areas. Nonpitting edema of the legs is difficult to manage because diuretics are not generally effective. Nonpitting edema responds best to elevation of the extremity and compression devices.

---

failure, pulmonary hypertension, pulmonary vascular resistance, and cardiovascular–pulmonary circulation.

To obtain a CVP, the healthcare provider inserts a catheter into the jugular vein and attaches it to a graduated cylindrical tube. The client is positioned and the CVP is obtained, usually by the RN who is trained in this technique. The more invasive PAOP uses a pulmonary artery catheter (PAC), also known as a Swan-Ganz catheter, to measure internal pulmonary pressures, which provide estimates of tissue perfusion. Placement of either catheter is an invasive procedure and is not without risk. The PAOP and its pulmonary arterial catheter are monitored by nurses who are specifically trained in this technique.

Medical Treatment

Treatment focuses on easing the workload of the heart. Rest, sedation, and proper diet are important. A *cardiac glycoside* (*digoxin*) is often used to slow the heart's rate, increase the force of systole (an *inotropic* effect), and decrease the heart's size. Digoxin is a cardiotonic glycoside that is given to slow and regulate the heart rate and to strengthen the heartbeat. Angiotensin-converting enzyme (ACE) inhibitors or other vasodilators should be added, as tolerated. These agents expand the blood vessels and decrease vascular resistance. Beta-blockers can be given because they improve left ventricular function. Diuretics help rid the body of excess fluid and salts. Salt (sodium) in the diet is restricted. Fluids also may be restricted, depending on the client's fluid balance status. If these measures are successful, systemic circulation will improve, increasing urinary output and reducing dyspnea and edema.

Nursing Considerations

Nursing observations and client teaching are important considerations when fatigue is identified. The person may have to rest after walking short distances or a few steps or may need two pillows at night to breathe comfortably. Pitting edema and nonpitting edema may be noticeable and should be documented. Lung sounds need to be auscultated. Key components of nursing care include measuring intake and output (I&O) and weighing the client daily to determine the client's fluid balance status and extent of edema. The healthcare provider needs to be informed of weight loss or gain; diuretics may need to be added to the dose adjusted.

Give oxygen if the blood is not receiving enough from the lungs. The high Fowler position usually aids breathing. Pressure-reducing devices often are used because the client with HF is at risk for skin breakdown. Dyspnea and fatigue can interfere with the client's ability to move. Plus, circulation is decreased in areas where edema is present. Another key aspect of nursing care is administering the prescribed medications and monitoring the client for the effectiveness of therapy. In Practice: Nursing Care Guidelines 81-1 highlights important areas for cardiotonic medication administration.

Nursing Alert Some medications have similar names. Look at the following list of commonly used drugs that are used to treat disorders of the circulatory system, such as hypertension, arrhythmias, or thrombophlebitis. Note the similarities of brand names. Using the wrong drug could be lethal. Always check your medication at least three times before giving it to your client.
- Carvedilol (Coreg), beta-adrenergic blocker
- Nadolol (Corgard), beta-adrenergic blocker
- Amiodarone (Cordarone), class III antiarrhythmic
- Captopril (Capoten), ACE inhibitor
- Doxazosin (Cardura), alpha-blocking agent
- Diltiazem (Cardizem), calcium channel blocker
- Verapamil (Calan), calcium channel blocker
- Warfarin (Coumadin), anticoagulant

Cardiomyopathy

Cardiomyopathy is a chronic, significant condition that occurs when the heart muscle is abnormal and prevents the heart from being an effective pump. Heart muscle can be damaged by acquired or congenital deformities. The result of the poorly functioning heart muscle is heart failure. Cardiomyopathy has three main types: *dilated* (enlarged) heart, *hypertropic* (thickened and stretched) heart walls, or *restrictive* (stiff and weakened) heart muscle.

Dilated or *congestive cardiomyopathy* is the most common form of this disorder. The heart cavity becomes enlarged or dilated, and usually, the condition progresses to HF. Dilation of the heart muscles affects the force of the muscle contraction, which results in poor cardiac output and diminished blood flow within the heart and to the pulmonary arteries. Arrhythmias and blood clots may also be problematic because blood flows more slowly through an enlarged heart. *Hypertropic cardiomyopathy*, another form of the disease, is hereditary in more than half of those diagnosed. The left ventricle hypertrophies, which may decrease the flow of blood from the left ventricle into the aorta. It may also cause mitral valve leakage. Symptoms include dyspnea, dizziness, and angina. Some people have arrhythmias. Often, a heart murmur can be heard. This form of cardiomyopathy is usually treated with a beta-blocker or calcium channel blocker, antiarrhythmics, as needed, or surgical treatment if medication treatment fails.

Restrictive cardiomyopathy is a less common form of the disease. The ventricles of the heart become rigid, making it difficult for blood to flow. This form of the disease causes fatigue, dyspnea on exertion, and peripheral edema. Another disease process usually causes this type of cardiomyopathy.

Treatment with anticoagulants and antiarrhythmics can help. Specific types of treatment relate to the symptoms of cardiomyopathy. Numerous medications are available to treat symptoms, for example, arrhythmias, poor cardiac output, and hypertension. Digoxin (Lanoxin) and diuretics, for example, furosemide (Lasix), improve cardiac blood flow and reduce pulmonary and dependent edema. Potassium chloride (KCl), a mineral replacement, typically accompanies furosemide (Lasix), as KCl is lost in the urine. Vasodilators may be given to relax the arteries, lower the blood pressure, and decrease the workload of the left ventricle. If the disease progresses despite medical treatment, surgically implanted devices may be beneficial. Sometimes, a heart transplant may be necessary.

Infectious and Inflammatory Heart Disorders

Rheumatic Heart Disease

Rheumatic heart disease is discussed in more detail in Chapter 73. As a consequence of this autoimmune disorder, several cardiac pathologies may be seen in the adult, including myocarditis, endocarditis, and pancarditis. *Myocarditis* refers to inflammation of the heart's muscular walls. *Endocarditis* refers to the inflammation of the heart's inner lining, usually involving the valves (as discussed below). *Pancarditis* refers to the inflammation of the entire heart. Symptoms typically include signs of poor tissue perfusion such as difficulty breathing, a cough, and sometimes cyanosis and *expectoration* (spitting) of blood. If the condition worsens, the client's feet and ankles swell, the liver enlarges, and the abdominal cavity fills with fluid (ascites). Systolic blood pressure may fall. Such signs indicate heart failure.

Mitral stenosis, a narrowing of the mitral valve, is the most common problem resulting from chronic rheumatic heart disease. As a result of stenosis, blood collects in the chambers of the left side of the heart, enlarging them and leading to a backup of blood in the pulmonary vessels, which causes pulmonary edema. The left side of the heart is affected first. The condition progresses to the right side.

IN PRACTICE
NURSING CARE GUIDELINES 81-1 — Administering the Cardiotonic Drug Digoxin (Lanoxin)

- Remember, the first administration of digoxin will be larger (*loading dose*) than later doses. The dosage will gradually be decreased until the amount needed to stabilize the heartbeat (*maintenance dose*) is found. If the dosage is too large, undesirable side effects will occur. When the medication slows the heart rate sufficiently, the client is said to be *digitalized*.
- Before administering digoxin, take the client's apical pulse for 1 full minute. Do not give the medication if the pulse is below 60 bpm (70 for a child), and report such a finding immediately. **Rationale:** Low pulse may indicate over digitalization.
- Be alert for possible side effects and adverse reactions of digitalization, including gastrointestinal symptoms, headache, and blurred vision. The client may say that everything has a yellow appearance. Bradycardia also occurs when digoxin slows the heart too much. For this reason, count the client's apical pulse before giving each dose. In some facilities, two nurses check digoxin dosages before giving such drugs to clients.
- If the client is discharged from the healthcare facility and prescribed digoxin, teach the client how to count the pulse rate, the symptoms of digoxin toxicity, and the significance of notifying the healthcare provider of any changes or symptoms. Document all teaching.

Heart failure is a common result unless treatment is successful. Surgical replacement of a valve may be indicated. The healthcare provider determines the particular valve design that best fits the client's needs.

Treatment

To best protect against chronic rheumatic heart disease, a person who has had rheumatic fever should avoid exposure to colds and streptococcal infections. General health goals include getting adequate sleep, eating a balanced diet, and not smoking. Complications may result from tooth extraction, oral surgery, or major surgery. Some clients take a daily maintenance dose of an antibiotic, such as penicillin G, as a prophylactic measure. Other clients may take a prophylactic dose of antibiotics prior to dental care. Preventing streptococcal infections is vital because each time a person has rheumatic fever, the possibility of cardiac complications increases.

Bacterial Endocarditis

Bacterial endocarditis is an infection of the surface membrane, the endocardium, which lines the heart. Endocarditis can be categorized as *acute* or *subacute*. Diseased or damaged heart valves usually exist before the development of endocarditis (Fig. 81-8). The source of the infection typically is the viridans streptococci bacteria but can also be fungi or other microorganisms. Initially, pathogens cross into the bloodstream and travel to the heart, where they attach to abnormal heart valves or damaged cardiac tissue. The bacteria present in the mouth, on teeth or gums, or in the throat, especially if these areas are unhealthy, are likely sources of the initial infection. Other sources of initial infection include sexually transmitted diseases, inflammatory bowel disease, invasive dental procedures, childbirth, upper respiratory infections, and contaminated syringes or intravenous catheters.

Subacute bacterial endocarditis (SBE) generally occurs on damaged valves and, if untreated, can become fatal within 6 weeks to a year. SBE is a relatively slow process of infection. The causative organism, usually streptococcus viridans, needs a previously damaged or diseased heart valve, which then becomes a site of colonization. However, in some cases, the bacteria that cause endocarditis can colonize a healthy heart valve. Risk factors include individuals who have damaged heart valves related to rheumatic fever, congenital heart defects, and artificial heart valves.

Signs and Symptoms

One of the first signs of bacterial endocarditis is a low-grade fever that gradually increases. The person perspires, has chills, aching joints, night sweats, anorexia, hematuria, and unexplained weight loss. Usually, the person is anemic and not enough oxygen is delivered to body tissues. Other cardiovascular symptoms include dyspnea, general pallor and paleness, persistent cough, and dependent edema. A heart sound that is new or changed, a murmur, may develop. The individual's face may have a brownish tinge, and tiny reddish-purple spots (*petechiae*) appear on the skin and mucous membranes. As the disease progresses, signs of heart failure appear. If untreated, endocarditis can lead to the development of *vegetations*, which are clumps of bacteria and cell fragments found at the site of the infection.

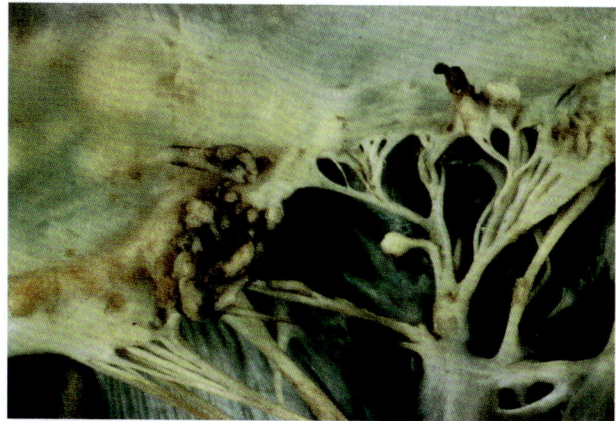

Figure 81-8 Bacterial endocarditis. The mitral valve shows destructive vegetations, which have eroded through the free margin of the valve leaflet.

Thrombosis and emboli can occur if all or part of a clump breaks loose, resulting in an occlusion in the brain, lungs, heart, kidneys, or extremities. Most cases of endocarditis, if treated promptly and effectively, can be cured without long-term side effects (e.g., heart failure or myocardial infarction).

Treatment
Blood culture and sensitivity can usually identify the specific causative organism. A complete blood count (CBC) will be able to guide treatment with knowledge about the number of RBCs, WBCs, platelets, Hgb, Hct, and various other standard blood values. Large doses of antibiotics are given to which the causative organism is sensitive. A transesophageal echocardiogram uses sound waves to look at cardiac structures, especially the heart valves. An ECG, CXR, CT, and MRI may be ordered. The healthcare provider will be searching for additional information regarding cardiac functioning and possible damage. Surgical intervention may be needed to remove an infected valve.

Nursing Considerations
Make the person as comfortable as possible and instruct them to conserve energy. Frequently, note the pulse rate and quality. Notify the healthcare provider of changes in vital signs, which can indicate complications. Provide all medications on time. Laboratory results of antibiotic cultures and sensitivities need to be given to the healthcare provider. Observe the client closely for fluctuation in body temperature; fever can indicate poor sensitivity to the prescribed antibiotic and, perhaps, development of sepsis. Symptoms of complications such as hematuria, pain, or impaired circulation can indicate an embolus (traveling blood clot), which results from diseased tissue of the valve. Client and family teaching concepts should include the notification of all healthcare providers, including dentists, of the possibility or existence of endocarditis. The American Heart Association can provide the client with an endocarditis wallet card.

Pericarditis
Pericarditis, an inflammation of the sac surrounding the heart, may be caused by infection, allergy, malignancy, trauma, or some other nonspecific problem. It is characterized by pain in the *precordial area* (over the heart and lower thorax), which is aggravated by breathing and twisting movements. A *friction rub*, a sign associated with pericarditis, is audible on auscultation. In most cases, pericardial infections are treated with antibiotics and anti-inflammatory agents.

Coronary Artery Disease

Coronary artery disease (CAD), also called *ischemic heart disease*, occurs when the coronary arteries become damaged or diseased. The main problems relate to cholesterol-containing deposits (plaque) that collect in the arteries and cause inflammation in a process called atherosclerosis. These plaques can break or rupture, causing further damage as platelets are drawn to the damage. The arteries become narrower, and the individual has decreasing amounts of blood flow to the heart. Dyspnea, angina, arrhythmias, heart failure, and myocardial infarction occur. CAD typically develops over decades and can be unnoticed until the individual has a myocardial infarction.

During the early middle years, more men than women are affected. However, after menopause, women's risk is increased. Although a familial tendency toward the disease seems to exist, anyone can be affected. A familial lifestyle that includes exercise, nutrition, and nonsmoking is known to positively affect the individual's risk for CAD. Therefore, all people should take precautions from an early age. In recent years, the healthcare community has given attention to preventing and discovering the disease early, before attacks occur and before atherosclerosis severely damages a person's heart and blood vessels. In addition, health promotion and disease prevention activities have focused on measures to reduce the risk factors for developing CAD, which include the following:

- Smoking tobacco
- Increased levels of cholesterol and lipids in the bloodstream
- Physical inactivity and obesity
- Diabetes

Angina Pectoris
Literally translated, **angina pectoris** (usually referred to as *angina*) means "pain in the chest." Angina occurs suddenly when extra exertion calls for the arteries to increase blood supply to the heart. Narrowed or obstructed arteries are unable to provide the necessary supply. Consequently, the heart muscle suffers.

In angina, the blood vessels of the heart are unable to supply the heart muscle with adequate amounts of oxygen. If this loss of oxygen supply continues, the result is *ischemia* (prolonged deficiency of oxygenated blood) and necrosis of heart tissue, or MI. For example, a major factor associated with the vessels' inability to supply adequate oxygen to the heart muscle is the development of plaques within the vessels, causing the vessels to narrow or become obstructed (Fig. 81-9).

When the underlying disease is coronary atherosclerosis, the prognosis may be more encouraging than when other factors are involved. The earlier the age of onset, the poorer the prognosis.

There are several types of angina pain. *Intractable angina* does not respond to therapy and often is so persistent that the person cannot work. *Unstable angina* is pain that increases and decreases in frequency, duration, and intensity. *Nocturnal angina* occurs at night. *Decubitus angina* occurs when the person is lying down and is relieved when the person sits up.

> **Nursing Alert** *Unstable angina pain is a medical emergency. This type of angina may last up to 30 min and not be relieved by antianginal medications. It could be a precursor to a heart attack. Often, it occurs at rest, feels different than one's usual angina, and feels more severe and lasts longer than stable angina.*

Signs and Symptoms
Pain is usually most severe over the chest, although it may spread to the shoulders, arms, neck, jaw, and back (Fig. 81-10). The person often describes the sensation as tightening, viselike, or choking. Indigestion is often the first complaint. The person is more likely to feel pain in the left arm because this is the direction of aortic branching. However, they may

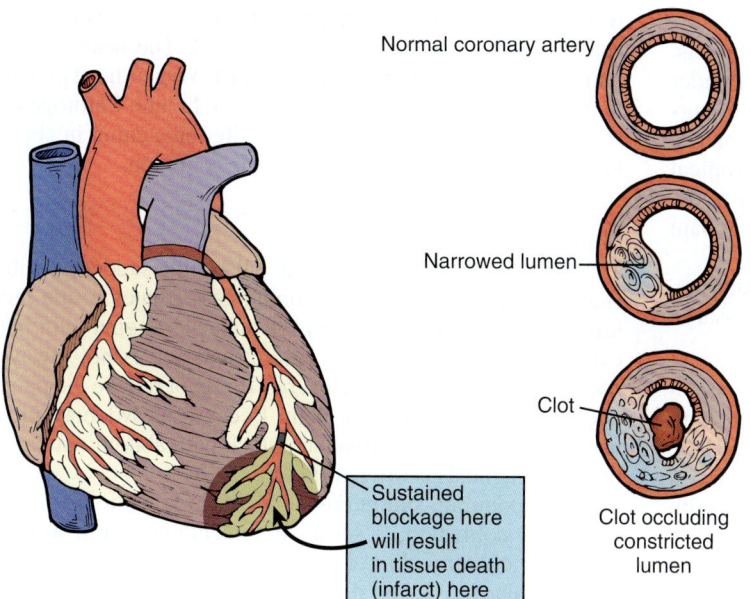

Figure 81-9 Progression of atherosclerotic plaque in the blood vessels. Over time, the buildup of fat, cholesterol, fibrin, cellular waste products, and calcium on an artery's endothelial lining may be complicated by hemorrhage, ulceration, calcification, or thrombosis. Infarction, stroke, or gangrene may also occur.

feel pain in either arm. The client may be pale, feel faint, or be dyspneic. Pain often stops in less than 5 min, but it is intense while it lasts. The pain is a warning signal that the heart is not getting enough blood and oxygen. People who ignore this warning are risking serious illness or sudden death if they do not immediately seek a healthcare provider's care. The client may have recurrent angina attacks, but treatment lessens the danger of a fatal attack.

Diagnostic Tests

Diagnosis is made on the basis of ECG, specific blood tests (especially cardiac isoenzymes), x-ray examinations, the client's medical history, and specific symptoms. If nitroglycerin relieves the attack, it is considered angina. Exercise, exertion, eating, emotions, and exposure often precipitate angina. A person who has diabetes may not feel angina pain because of peripheral neuropathy.

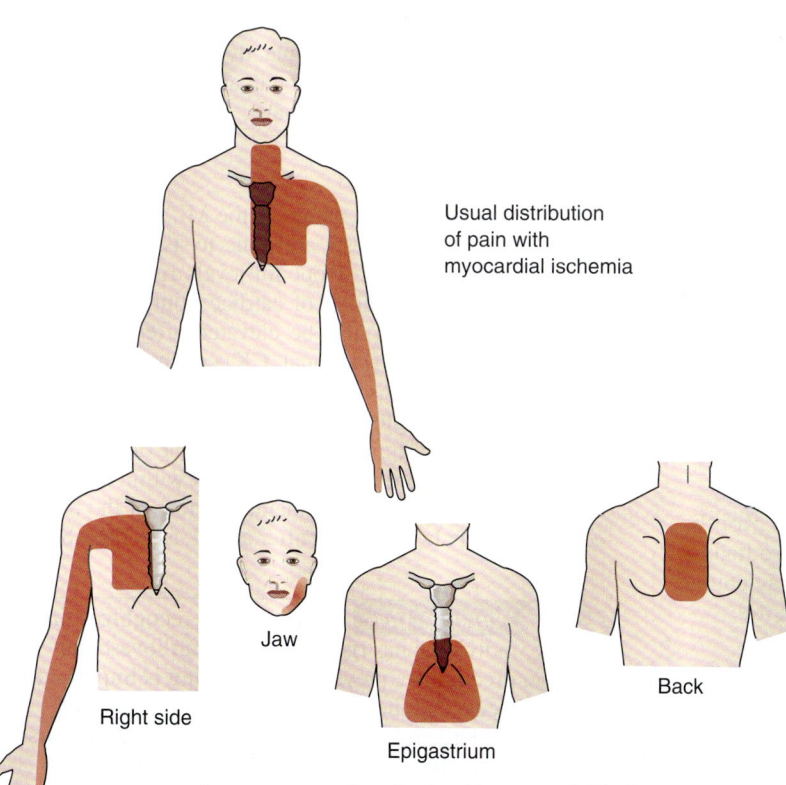

Figure 81-10 Pain patterns with myocardial ischemia. The usual distribution of pain is referral to all or part of the sternal region, the left side of the chest, the neck, and down the ulnar side of the left forearm and hand. With severe ischemic pain, the right side of the chest and right arm are often involved as well, although isolated involvement of these areas is rare. Other sites sometimes involved, either alone or together with pain in other sites, are the jaw, epigastrium, and back.

Medical and Surgical Treatment

Angina can usually be controlled with nitroglycerin tablets. As soon as an attack begins, the client places a tablet under the tongue, allowing it to dissolve. Nitroglycerin brings quick relief by dilating the coronary arteries; clients can use this drug safely for many years with no ill effects. Topical nitroglycerin ointment or nitroglycerin-impregnated transdermal pads are widely used to protect against anginal pain and promote its relief (see Table 81-1).

If medication fails to control the person's anginal attacks, PTCA or coronary artery bypass surgery may be necessary.

Nursing Considerations

Help the client by teaching about angina pectoris and how to prevent further attacks (In Practice: Educating the Client 81-2). Clients who know that certain stresses bring on angina can learn measures to avoid these stresses or better cope with them. Clients with angina need to quit smoking because nicotine constricts the coronary arteries and increases blood pressure and pulse rate.

Myocardial Infarction

A myocardial infarction (MI), also known as *heart attack, coronary thrombosis,* or *coronary occlusion,* is the sudden blockage of one or more coronary arteries. *Acute coronary syndrome* (ACS) includes conditions such as an acute myocardial infarction (AMI), diagnostic ST changes on an ECG, and unstable angina. If the blockage involves an extensive area, the person can die. If it involves a smaller area, necrosis of heart tissue and subsequent scarring will occur. After an MI, the heart can develop new cardiac blood vessels around the infarct (damaged) area. This rerouting of new blood vessels is referred to as *collateral circulation.*

Complications can occur at any time after an acute MI. Complications primarily result from damage to the myocardium and its conduction system that occurred because of diminished coronary blood flow. The major complications of MI are life-threatening arrhythmias and cardiac standstill. Abnormal heart rates and rhythms in the person with a recent MI often indicate that the left ventricle is pumping inadequately. As a result, HF may occur. **Cardiogenic shock** is a serious complication that sometimes occurs with an MI. The heart cannot pump effectively, and the body's unmet oxygen needs result in life-threatening hypotension and organ failure. Cardiogenic shock can be treated, but it remains life-threatening in about half of the individuals who develop the condition.

Signs and Symptoms

Typically, but not in all cases, an MI begins suddenly, with sharp, severe chest pain that sometimes radiates to the left arm, shoulder, and back. Pain is similar to angina pain but can last longer and is more severe; exertion is not always related to onset. Unlike angina, rest does not relieve the pain, and nitroglycerin does not help. Because an MI may imitate indigestion or a gallbladder attack with abdominal pain, definite diagnosis is often difficult.

Other common symptoms of MI include panic, restlessness, and confusion; a sense of impending death; ashen, cold, and clammy skin; dyspnea; cyanosis; rapid, thready, and irregular pulse; and drop in blood pressure and in body temperature. Nausea and vomiting may be present, and the person is often in shock. Silent attacks involving CAD, that is, MIs that show no overt symptoms, are common, especially among people with diabetes, and they may result in greater damage to the heart muscle. When chest pain or other symptoms of an MI occur, denial is often noted. The individual does not psychologically want to accept the potential seriousness of the symptoms. In this instance, family members may need to take responsibility for the client and to dial 911 for emergency medical services.

> **Nursing Alert** The location and severity of pain caused by an MI can vary greatly. Clients who are female, older adults, and who have diabetes can present with symptoms, such as back pain, jaw pain, right arm pain, indigestion, nausea, fatigue, dyspnea, and even no pain. The severity of pain is not an accurate indicator of the severity of myocardial damage.

Diagnostic Tests

Tests help determine the nature of the MI. An ECG and several diagnostic blood tests are done to assess the duration and severity of the MI. Troponin levels rise. Troponin I is an accurate cardiac marker of cardiac injury. Other cardiac isoenzyme levels will also be elevated after an MI. These isoenzymes include fractional CK enzymes (specifically, CK-MB, a cardiac muscle-specific enzyme), LDH, and myoglobin. Serum myoglobin is tested to estimate the amount of damage to the heart muscle. Within 1–2 hr of an MI, serum myoglobin starts to rise, reaching a peak within 6 hr after the onset of symptoms. The sedimentation rate of the red blood cells is almost always higher after an MI, as is the AST level.

> **Nursing Alert** When a nurse recognizes that an individual has risk factors for cardiovascular disease, preemptive, preventative teaching is important. Inform clients and their caregivers the importance of initiating emergency care before an MI or stroke occurs. Thrombolytic therapy, to be most effective, must be started as soon as possible after the client develops symptoms.

IN PRACTICE
EDUCATING THE CLIENT 81-2 — Treatment of Angina Pectoris

- Use medications properly. Take them at the same time every day. Do not stop or change dosages without a healthcare provider's approval.
- Do not expose nitroglycerin to sunlight or moisture. Keep nitroglycerin in its original container. Purchase a fresh supply every 3 months.
- Check with your healthcare provider before taking any nonprescription medications. They may cause harmful side effects when combined with the cardiac medications.
- Review your lifestyle. Make necessary lifestyle adjustments. Determine what risk factors can be adjusted and what may be inherited.
- Do not smoke. Avoid second-hand smoke.
- Exercise regularly and maintain an ideal weight.
- Keep cholesterol within the 150–200 mg/dL range.

Medical Treatment

Individuals complaining of chest pain should be evaluated promptly, with the goal of preventing further damage to the heart muscle. As previously discussed, thrombolytic therapy is an effective method of destroying the clot and preventing muscle damage, but it must be given in the very early phases of an MI. Pain indicates *anoxia* (lack of oxygen). Typically, morphine, administered IV, is the drug of choice for MI pain. Drugs also are given to dilate blood vessels, allowing more oxygen to reach heart muscle (see Table 81-1). Oxygen is administered by cannula or mask to assist with breathing and improve oxygenation, thereby relieving pain.

A low-cholesterol and restricted-sodium diet is usually ordered. Caffeine-containing beverages are usually not allowed. The client is informed of the hazards of smoking and is encouraged to quit as soon as possible.

Nursing Considerations

Immediately after diagnosis of an MI, continuous nursing care in the CCU is vital until the person's condition stabilizes. During this acute phase, nursing care typically includes the following elements:

- Frequent vital signs
- Electronic cardiac monitoring
- Hemodynamic monitoring
- I&O and daily weight
- Careful observation for restlessness, dyspnea, or chest pain
- Assessment for signs of HF, for example, dyspnea, frequent cough, crackles heard in the lung fields, and edema
- Assessment of skin color such as pallor or cyanosis
- Medications to promote pain relief and improve the heart's functioning
- Emotional support and stress reduction
- Observations and adjustments of diet, IV fluids, activity as condition improves or worsens

During recovery from an MI, rest is a priority. Bed rest may be ordered depending on the overall cardiac damage and the client's general status. The ischemic areas may form necrotic tissue, which can take from 3–6 weeks to form scar tissue. Tough scar tissue forms after about 8 weeks. The size of the area of scar tissue is important because scar tissue will inhibit normal myocardial electrical conduction, and it can inhibit normal contractions of the heart muscle. Cardiac arrhythmias are possible owing to these factors. In Practice: Nursing Care Plan 81-1 highlights the nursing care associated with a priority nursing diagnosis.

- Allow clients who are able to use a commode at the bedside for a bowel movement. A commode is preferable to a bedpan. *Rationale: Clients are more likely to strain on the bedpan, which could cause bradycardia owing to a vasovagal effect.* Stool softeners are usually prescribed. *Rationale: Stool softeners inhibit straining.*
- Assist the client with *isometric* (muscle-setting) exercises. *Rationale: They provide muscle exercise without causing exhaustion.* Incorporate a planned daily exercise program according to the cardiac rehabilitation program (Box 81-3).
- Use thromboembolic (antiembolism) stockings, as prescribed by the healthcare provider. *Rationale: Proper use of stockings prevents thrombophlebitis (inflammation of the vein wall; discussed below).*
- Place all necessary items within the client's reach. Be sure the call light is available. *Rationale: The client must not stretch or strain.*
- Perform physical care (e.g., baths, oral hygiene, skin care). *Rationale: Provide rest and comfort.*
- After giving the bath and before making the bed, allow the client to rest for a while. Positioning in a semi-Fowler position is often preferred. *Rationale: This position assists in breathing and relieves pain.*

Clients who are admitted with a diagnosis of "rule out MI," typically written as "R/O MI," are placed on bed rest until it is determined whether they have had a heart attack. Individualized care and activities are based on the client's overall condition as determined by the healthcare provider, usually the cardiologist. During this time, nursing care includes the reduction of stress and promotion of relaxation.

Clients who have had an MI can live a normal life and, generally, can return to previous employment, depending on the extent of myocardial damage. The goal is not to change a client's lifestyle completely but to have the client make necessary modifications to prevent recurrences. Before discharge, instruct clients and their families about patterns of healthy living and how to recognize emotional and physical stress. The client will more than likely be referred to a cardiac rehabilitation program to allow them a monitored and guided exercise program to resume their ADLs and activity level. If the client is taking antihypertensive drugs, emphasize the necessity of taking prescribed medications despite that they feel well. Discuss potential side effects when teaching. Also, include teaching about signs and symptoms that require immediate medical help (see In Practice: Educating the Client 81-3). Carefully and completely document this teaching.

BLOOD VESSEL DISORDERS

Inflammatory Disorders and Complications

Thrombophlebitis

Thrombophlebitis is inflammation of the wall of a vein, in which one or more clots form. *Deep vein thrombosis* (DVT) defines the condition wherein a *thrombus* (blood clot) has formed inside a deep blood vessel. The blood clot forms in response to the initial inflammation. **Phlebitis** is the inflammation of a blood vessel without clot formation.

In some situations, for example, following trauma, childbirth, heart attack, stroke, heart failure, or cancer surgery, excessive coagulability of the blood causes thrombophlebitis and thrombosis. Obesity is also a predisposing factor. Women who use birth control pills may have a higher than average risk of developing blood clots.

> **Nursing Alert** Never massage or rub a client's leg. *Rationale: Rubbing could dislodge a clot and cause embolism.*

IN PRACTICE

NURSING CARE PLAN 81-1: The Person With an Acute Myocardial Infarction

Medical History: C.F., a 37-year-old single white male accountant, presented in the emergency department with crushing chest pain. Cardiac enzyme levels and an ECG were obtained, revealing an anterior wall myocardial infarction of the left ventricle. He was admitted to the CCU approximately 18 hr ago. Oxygen at 4 L/min via nasal cannula and intravenous morphine were ordered. Cardiac medications, laboratory, and monitoring protocols initiated.

Medical Diagnosis: Acute MI of anterior wall of the left ventricle.

DATA COLLECTION/NURSING OBSERVATION

Client appears pale and diaphoretic. Skin is cool and clammy. States that chest pain is 5 on a 1–10 scale. Vital signs as follows: Temperature, 97.2 °F (37.2 °C); pulse, 120 bpm, irregular and thready; respirations, 26 breaths/min; blood pressure, 90/58 mm Hg. Intravenous morphine was given. Client stated that relief of pain occurred; pain currently rated as 2–3 on a scale of 1–10. Client is currently resting in bed with head of bed elevated 45°; oxygen being administered at 4 L/min per cannula. Oxygen saturation via pulse oximeter is at 96%. Continuous cardiac monitoring reveals frequent PVCs >5/min. Hemodynamic monitoring is in place. Urine output approximately 30 ml/hr.

NURSING DIAGNOSIS

(Although other nursing diagnoses may be appropriate, a priority nursing diagnosis is addressed below.)

Risk for impaired coronary tissue perfusion related to effects of coronary artery disease and cardiac tissue damage secondary to acute MI as evidenced by low blood pressure, frequent PVCs irregular, thready pulse, and cool pale skin.

PLANNING (Outcomes/Goals)	IMPLEMENTATION (Nursing Actions)	EVALUATION
Short-Term Goals		
A. Within 24 hr after admission, client will verbalize a decrease in complaints of chest pain.	• Assess for complaints of chest pain using a pain rating scale. • Assess peripheral pulses for signs of tissue perfusion and presence of pulse. • Medicate with morphine sulfate for pain and anxiety. *Rationale: Chest pain indicates myocardial ischemia and decreased cardiac tissue perfusion. Using a pain rating scale aids in quantifying the client's pain and provides a means for evaluating relief measures. Pulse in extremities can be an indicator of adequate tissue perfusion.*	Day 1—1,145 hr. • Client reports pain currently at 2 on a scale of 1–10 for the past 2 hr. • Pulse rate of 106 bpm with slight irregularity noted. • BP at 100/60 mm Hg; respirations 22 breaths/min and regular. • Occasional PVCs noted, approximately 1–2 per minute. **Goal A currently being met.**
B. Within 24 hr, client will exhibit pulse rate ranging between 60 and 100 bpm, BP within the range of 110–130 mm Hg/64–74 mm Hg, rare to absent PVCs, hourly urine output greater than 30 mL/hr; oxygen saturation of at least 97% with supplemental oxygen.	• Assess cardiopulmonary status for signs of cardiogenic shock. • Auscultate lung sounds and cardiac sounds. • Monitor vital signs, especially pulse rate and blood pressure, at least hourly or more frequently if indicated, until stable. • Monitor respiratory status and pulse oximetry closely after administration of morphine. *Rationale: Chest pain indicates cardiac ischemia. Frequent monitoring is essential to detect changes in the client's condition such as development of pulmonary edema or heart murmurs. Improvement can indicate improving cardiac output and tissue perfusion. Morphine is an effective analgesic for chest pain, but it is a central nervous system depressant that can cause respiratory depression.*	Day 2—1,315 hr. • Urine output last hour was 40 mL. • Skin color improved. Skin warm and dry, no sign of diaphoresis. • Oxygen saturation at 97% with 4 L of oxygen via nasal cannula. • Lungs clear to auscultation. • No cardiac murmurs noted. **Goal B in progress.** **Observations continue.**

PLANNING (Outcomes/Goals)	IMPLEMENTATION (Nursing Actions)	EVALUATION
Long-Term Goals		
C. Cardiac output remains stable as client's activity status increases.	• Increase level of activity as indicated by cardiologist's order. • Monitor for PVCs, dyspnea, and chest pain. • Administer morphine, as ordered, for complaints of pain. *Rationale: Client's ability to increase activity indicates stability of cardiac tissue perfusion and stability of cardiac output.*	Day 3—0800 hr. • Tolerated getting up to the chair for 30 min without development of chest pain or dyspnea. • Vital signs stable: pulse rate of 98 bpm and regular; BP 136/64 mm Hg; respirations at 22 breaths/min. • Oxygen saturation level at 98% with oxygen at 2 L/min via nasal cannula. • One to two PVCs noted in the last 30 min. **Goal C met.**
D. Initiate plans for discharge from CCU.	• Initiate pre-discharge protocol to cardiac telemetry unit and then home for outpatient rehabilitation. *Rationale: As client condition stabilizes, future plans for cardiac rehabilitation are needed.*	Day 3—2,330 hr. • Continuous relief of chest pain for 24 hr. • Pulse rate at 72 bpm and regular; BP 110/70 mm Hg. • Skin is pale pink and warm. • Continuous cardiac monitoring reveals no evidence of PVCs for 4 hr. • Urine output of 160 mL over the past 3 hr. • Oxygen saturation at 98% on room air. **Goal D met.**

Box 81-3 Postmyocardial Infarction Rehabilitation Plan

- In the healthcare facility, a gradual increase in the client's activity level, as ordered by the healthcare provider
- Exercise tolerance test and exercise progression
- Graded exercise program with monitoring of tolerance based on blood pressure and pulse
- Emotional support and counseling
- Stress management
- Sexual counseling
- Lifestyle changes, as needed
- Risk factor management
- Dietary changes (e.g., low-fat diet for hyperlipidemia or weight control)
- Smoking cessation
- Hypertension control
- Medication and compliance, as ordered

IN PRACTICE
EDUCATING THE CLIENT 81-3 Myocardial Infarction: When to Seek Medical Help

- Chest pain unrelieved with sublingual nitroglycerin
- Pain in left or right arm
- Pain in back or jaw
- Pain in gastrointestinal region or symptoms presenting as severe indigestion
- Severe shortness of breath
- Faintness or dizziness
- Unusual fatigue or weakness
- Palpitations or irregular or rapid heartbeat

Note: There are times when no symptoms may be present.

Pressure or prolonged inactivity may cause venous thrombosis. It may occur after surgery or any illness in which a person remains in one position for long periods or when sitting in a car or airplane for an extended length of time. The legs are most likely to be affected because venous blood does not return quickly enough, a condition known as *venous stasis* or *venous standstill*. Prevention of venous stasis is a major reason for early ambulation in illness. Clients with any condition that requires prolonged immobilization often receive low-dose prophylactic anticoagulants. (Some healthcare providers recommend that all adults take aspirin daily as a preventive measure.)

SPECIAL CONSIDERATIONS Lifespan

Thrombophlebitis

Older adults and those with heart disease or varicose veins are most susceptible to thrombophlebitis. Prolonged sitting may be a contributing factor. Inform older adults of the importance of frequent position changing. A rocking chair provides some exercise for people who find walking difficult. A large assortment of assistive walking devices with seats are available.

Most thrombi form in veins because venous blood moves more slowly than arterial blood. However, a thrombus may form in an artery (*arterial thrombosis*); this condition is usually related to arteriosclerosis, but it may result from infection, injury, or diabetes mellitus.

Signs and Symptoms
Signs and symptoms of thrombophlebitis include redness, swelling, and tenderness in the affected leg. There may be possible warmth in the affected leg or reddish-purple discoloration of the lower extremity. Positive Homans sign may not be a reliable indicator of thrombophlebitis.

Medical Treatment
Imaging studies are performed to differentiate between superficial thrombosis and DVT because each is treated differently. Clients with DVT only in the calf can be treated with outpatient therapy, receiving low–molecular-weight heparin. Those who must be admitted to the hospital require IV heparin bolus followed by continuous infusion for 3–5 days until adequate anticoagulation is achieved. Frequent blood tests to monitor clotting times are used to regulate the dosage of anticoagulants. The client may remain on oral anticoagulants for 3–6 months. In addition, clients are usually placed on bed rest for 1–5 days, gradually resuming their normal activities.

Nursing Considerations
All clients who are confined to bed should begin an exercise plan as soon as possible. The simplest exercises include periodic contraction and relaxation of the leg muscles and moving of the toes and feet. The bedcovers must be sufficiently loose to permit free movement. Most clients who must remain on bed rest wear antiembolism stockings and may have the foot of the bed elevated to help prevent venous stasis. Passive range-of-motion (PROM) exercises or the continuous passive motion (CPM) device may be used for clients who are unable to exercise actively. When caring for the client with thrombophlebitis, include the following:

- If exercise is ordered, encourage the client to wiggle the toes, bend the knees, and turn the ankle back and forth.
- In deep thrombophlebitis, immobilize the affected part.
- Prevent vigorous coughing or deep breathing (because of the danger of embolism; see next section). Try to keep the client from straining when defecating; administer stool softeners, as ordered.
- Use warm, moist packs (low temperature). *Rationale: Gently stimulate circulation and dissolution of the clot but avoid overdilation of blood vessels.*
- Enforce bed rest. *Rationale: Moving could cause embolism.* Elevate the affected leg on soft pillows. *Rationale: Promote comfort and enhance venous return from the leg.*

While the client is on anticoagulant therapy, follow the general nursing precautions and procedures to reduce the risks of injury and bleeding. The client usually receives IV heparin during the acute phase and warfarin (Coumadin) or another anticoagulant such as dalteparin sodium (Fragmin), tinzaparin sodium (Innohep), or fondaparinux sodium (Arixtra) as a prophylactic measure later. Routine prothrombin times (PT) for monitoring of Coumadin and partial thromboplastin time (PTT) clotting tests are done to monitor anticoagulant therapy. The dosage is based on daily blood tests. If clotting time is too high, the medication is temporarily discontinued. Provide education to the client and family about anticoagulants and when to contact the healthcare provider if problems occur (e.g., in cases of increased bruising, bleeding).

If the client is to wear an antiembolism stocking or an elastic bandage, apply it with even pressure from the toes to the thigh. *Rationale: Uneven pressure could cause another clot to form.* Remove elastic stockings or bandages at least once per shift for a short time. Gently cleanse the extremity and apply lotion, if necessary. Inspect the extremity carefully for any skin changes.

If the client is required to stay in bed for some time, help them to progress gradually from complete bed rest to ambulation, according to healthcare provider's orders. Constantly observe for any signs of embolism.

Embolism
Embolism is a severe complication of thrombophlebitis. An **embolus** is a blood clot that is carried through the circulation to some vital organ; it can lodge in a blood vessel and cause death. Urgent treatment is vital; refer to the earlier section on thrombolytic therapy.

Types
A *pulmonary embolism* is the result of a blood clot that travels to the lungs. If the obstruction occurs in a large pulmonary blood vessel (the most common site for the lodging of an embolus originating in the leg), it may cause sudden death. The obstruction of a small vessel may not be so damaging. A pulmonary embolism may cause sudden, sharp chest pain; breathing difficulty; violent cough; and bloody sputum. The client will become cyanotic, and symptoms of shock can develop rapidly. The immediate treatment is to administer oxygen and to provide for complete bed rest in a

high semi-Fowler position. Continuous IV anticoagulation therapy with heparin is a widely used treatment. Pain relief with the use of IV morphine is also indicated.

A *coronary embolus* is a blood clot that travels to a blood vessel in the heart. If the embolus lodges in a blood vessel within the heart, the heart tissue distal to the blockage will necrose. Depending on how large the vessel is, the necrosed area may cause instant death. Symptoms of a lesser blockage are sudden, severe chest pain and other characteristic symptoms of an MI, which were discussed earlier.

In *cerebral embolism*, the clot blocks one of the brain's blood vessels, causing a stroke. The amount of brain damage depends on the vessel's size and location. This situation is commonly known as an ischemic stroke.

Peripheral embolism and *thrombosis in a limb* involve an embolus that lodges in a blood vessel leading to an extremity. In this case, the first symptom is severe pain at the site of the blockage. The extremity becomes pale and cold to the touch; pulses distal to the blockage are lost. The limb becomes white and cold. Other symptoms of shock are seen if a large blood vessel is obstructed. Amputation below the level of the blockage may be necessary if a clot in a large vessel is not dissolved quickly or surgically removed. Without circulation, gangrene will occur.

Surgical Treatment

Certain surgical procedures may be performed to combat the danger of embolism. Emboli can be removed from pulmonary arteries, although this procedure is rare. If a thrombus is located in the femoral vein, the blood vessel can be *ligated* (tied off) at the blockage site in a procedure called *femoral ligation*. Sometimes, the vena cava is made smaller (*vena cava ligation*), or a filter is inserted in the vein to prevent clots from traveling to the heart.

Peripheral Vascular Disorders

Most peripheral vascular disorders are evidenced at one time or another by the following symptoms:

- *Intermittent claudication:* The person experiences no pain at rest; but exercise, particularly walking, causes excruciating pain in the limb, which disappears when the limb is again at rest. Smoking, vascular spasm, and atherosclerosis aggravate this condition. Intermittent claudication caused by venous stasis is called *venous claudication*.
- *Tingling and numbness:* The extremity or part of the extremity becomes numb, or the person feels a persistent tingling sensation, caused by poor circulation.
- *Coldness and difference in size:* The extremities may feel cold to the touch, or the person may sense that the hands and feet are cold. One leg may be markedly different in size, color, and temperature from the other.
- *Lack of new tissue growth:* The skin may become paper-thin, shiny, and easily subject to breakdown. Blood vessels are visible.

Simple changes to lifestyle can prevent or arrest peripheral vascular diseases. In Practice: Nursing Care Guidelines 81-2 lists general nursing measures for peripheral vascular disease.

Buerger Disease

Buerger disease, sometimes referred to as *thromboangiitis obliterans*, is inflammation of the arteries and veins of the extremities. It is one of a group of vasoplastic arterial diseases that cause obstruction of the arteries in the extremities, especially the legs. Initially, Buerger disease manifests in the hands and feet, and then progresses to the larger areas of the arms and legs. Due to the inflamed blood vessels, the vessels become edematous and may become blocked with thrombi. The disease typically strikes individuals between the ages of 20 and 45; the most typical age of onset is between 40 and 45. As the disorder progresses, the tissues become hypoxic; skin tissue is damaged and becomes infected. Without treatment, gangrene develops, and amputation of all or part of the extremity is necessary. The major risk factor is tobacco, which causes inflammation and spasms of the blood vessels that lead to the obstruction of blood vessels. Cigarette smoking or use of chewing tobacco is seen in nearly everyone with this disorder. Quitting all forms of tobacco may be the only way to avoid the disease. Other risk factors include cold; chilling aggravates the condition.

Usually, the first sign is cramps in the calf muscles, brought on by exercise, which disappear with rest. Other symptoms include tingling, burning, numbness, and edema, which may develop into pitting or *brawny* (hard) edema. Hardened, painful areas develop along the course of blood

---

IN PRACTICE
NURSING CARE GUIDELINES 81-2 | Caring for Clients With Peripheral Vascular Disease

- Protect the client's feet and legs from undue pressure of linens. **Rationale:** *Doing so prevents discomfort and skin breakdown.*
- Take great care in trimming the toenails. **Rationale:** *Cuts or abrasions on the feet are difficult to heal.*
- Be sure to dry carefully between the toes after washing them. **Rationale:** *Moisture promotes skin breakdown. Any break in the skin or subsequent infection heals much more slowly when circulation is poor.*
- Be very careful about application of heat. Use extra clothing rather than external heat to warm the extremities. **Rationale:** *This person is easily burned.*
- Report skin breakdown immediately. **Rationale:** *Ambitious therapy will be needed.*
- Use warm baths to help increase the circulation; be sure the water is not hot. **Rationale:** *Heat helps dilate blood vessels. This client is very susceptible to burns. Use a bath thermometer; the maximum temperature is 100 °F or 37.8 °C.*
- Do not attempt to treat corns or calluses. **Rationale:** *The client may be accidentally cut or injured, predisposing the client to infection.*

vessels. When the feet and legs hang down, they take on a mottled purplish-red hue; when raised, they become abnormally pale.

Medical and Surgical Treatment
Affected individuals must avoid anything that worsens this condition, especially chilling of hands and feet. Tobacco in any form is dangerous because nicotine constricts blood vessels. Advise clients to stop smoking, using electronic cigarettes, or using smokeless tobacco immediately.

Mild exercise is recommended if it is not painful. For this purpose, *Buerger–Allen exercises* are prescribed. They consist of alternately raising, lowering, and resting the legs. Sometimes, cramps occur with exercise (*intermittent claudication*). Clients may use an electrically operated rocking bed (*oscillating bed*) if they cannot exercise actively. Antibiotics, anti-inflammatory agents, and analgesics may be necessary to treat infection and pain. External heat is not used. Rather, clients are encouraged to wear extra clothing. Encourage fluid intake and advise clients to avoid constrictive clothing.

Sometimes, a *sympathectomy* is performed, whereby the sympathetic nerves, which innervate the smooth muscles, are cut to relieve vasospasms and increase blood flow to the lower extremities.

Raynaud Disease
Raynaud disease, also known as *Raynaud phenomenon* or *syndrome* is one of a group of vasoplastic arterial diseases in which the arteries have periodic narrowing or spasmodic constriction. It especially affects fingers and toes; often, it involves only the fingers. *Primary* or *idiopathic Raynaud disease* occurs without other illness. *Secondary* or *Raynaud syndrome* usually occurs in conjunction with another illness. It affects women more frequently than men, especially young women. Symptoms include narrowing and spasms of the distal arteries in the hands and feet. Hypoxia results in reducing the amount of blood flow causing pain, numbness, and discoloration. Extremity claudication (pain in legs related to exertion), headaches, hypertension, and blindness also occur. Chronic hypoxia will eventually lead to poor tissue perfusion to the skin or internal organs, which results in skin ulcers and organ failure. Cold and emotional stress can precipitate the condition.

Signs and Symptoms
Symptoms of Raynaud disease include blanched and cold extremities. They perspire and feel numb and prickly. Later they become blue—especially the fingernails—and are painful. As heat restores blood flow, the hands become red and warm. In the early stages, these symptoms disappear after an episode, and the hands seem normal again. But as the disease progresses, cyanosis persists between attacks, and ulcers, which are slow to heal, may develop on the fingertips. The skin looks tight and shiny, and the nails become deformed. The fingertips may develop gangrene.

Diagnosis
To rule out other disorders, the healthcare provider may order an antinuclear antibody test and an erythrocyte sedimentation rate. There is no specific blood test for diagnosis of Raynaud disease.

Treatment and Nursing Considerations
Clients must avoid chilling at all times. They must always wear warm clothing outdoors in winter (e.g., wool gloves and socks, and insulated boots). A goose down or other comforter at night provides steady warmth. Electric blankets may be dangerous because they may be too hot and could burn the client. Clients should avoid emotional upsets and tension of any kind. Smoking is contraindicated. Drugs to relieve spasm of arteries and dilate blood vessels provide considerable relief. A sympathectomy may be necessary.

Varicose Veins
Varicose veins result from weakening of the valves of the veins so that blood pools in the legs or another dependent area. Normal veins fill from below because of valvular action. With varicose veins, the veins fill abnormally. (Hemorrhoids and esophageal varices are also varicose veins.) Predisposing factors include heredity and weakening of the vein walls resulting from prolonged standing, poor posture, repeated pregnancies, round garters, obesity, tumors, HTN, and chronic diseases of the liver or kidneys. Varicose veins may also result from thrombophlebitis. Women are more commonly affected with varicosities of the legs than men, especially if they have had several pregnancies.

Signs and Symptoms
The main sign of varicose veins in the legs is the appearance of dark, tortuous superficial veins that become more prominent when the person stands and appear as dark protrusions. These superficial veins can sometimes rupture, causing a *varicose ulcer*. Internal or deep varicose veins cause symptoms such as pain, fatigue, a feeling of heaviness, and muscle cramps. Symptoms are much more severe in hot weather and at high altitudes. A diagnostic test involves putting the client into the Trendelenburg position to test blood drainage. Leg veins that do not fill normally on standing signify varicose veins.

Medical and Surgical Treatment
Treatment includes elevating the legs for a few minutes at 2- to 3-hour intervals throughout the day. It also includes avoiding constriction, standing for long periods, or restrictive clothing. The client should wear support hose. All measures aim at promoting venous return from the legs.

In severe cases, surgical ligation and stripping of varicose veins are done. The larger veins are surgically ligated, and smaller ones are stripped. Occasionally, sclerosing solutions are used for small varicosities: The solution is injected into the vessel that causes irritation and eventually fibrosis.

Nursing Considerations
The client needs teaching about measures that promote venous drainage to avoid the need for possible surgery. If surgery is necessary, apply antiembolism stockings to the leg postoperatively, and elevate the foot of the bed to encourage venous return. Analgesics may be ordered. Aspirin is often the drug of choice because of its anticoagulant action.

Early ambulation is important after surgical treatment. Often, the client must ambulate as soon as they recover from anesthesia. The client may be alarmed at the idea of walking so soon after the operation, while the legs are stiff and sore, and they will most likely need reassurance

CHAPTER 81 Cardiovascular Disorders   1461

IN PRACTICE
EDUCATING THE CLIENT 81-4 Discharge Teaching After Venous Stripping

- Elevate the legs while sitting.
- Be sure to walk and to avoid standing still in one place for any length of time.
- Avoid sitting for a lengthy time.
- Learn how to apply antiembolism stockings correctly.
- If possible, lose weight.
- Do not use tobacco.

and an explanation of the need for moving about. The order is often written for the client to walk 5–10 min each hour during the day and several times at night. Assist and encourage the client to follow this regimen. In Practice: Educating the Client 81-4 includes ideas for client teaching after venous stripping.

Instruct the client how to apply antiembolism stockings correctly and to avoid knee-high stockings and socks with elastic tops. If weight reduction is suggested, the clinical dietitian will give instructions.

Telangiectasia (Spider Veins)

Telangiectasia is a group of small dilated blood vessels. It is treated by *scleropathy*, the injection of a weak sodium chloride solution into nonfunctioning veins. Pressure is applied at specific points, and the veins stick together and are gradually absorbed. The lines almost disappear. The treatment is relatively painless.

Aneurysms

An **aneurysm** is an outpouching of a blood vessel. Although it may occur in any vessel, the most common site is the aorta. Figure 81-11 shows several types of aneurysms.

An aneurysm in the aorta or in a cerebral vessel represents an extreme emergency. If it ruptures, surgical intervention may be done if the aneurysm is in an operable site. However, if surgery is not done immediately, the vessel may hemorrhage, and the person may die. If the aneurysm is discovered before it ruptures, it is treated by surgical repairs, such as clamping or removal. Usually, a synthetic graft is substituted for the portion of the vessel affected.

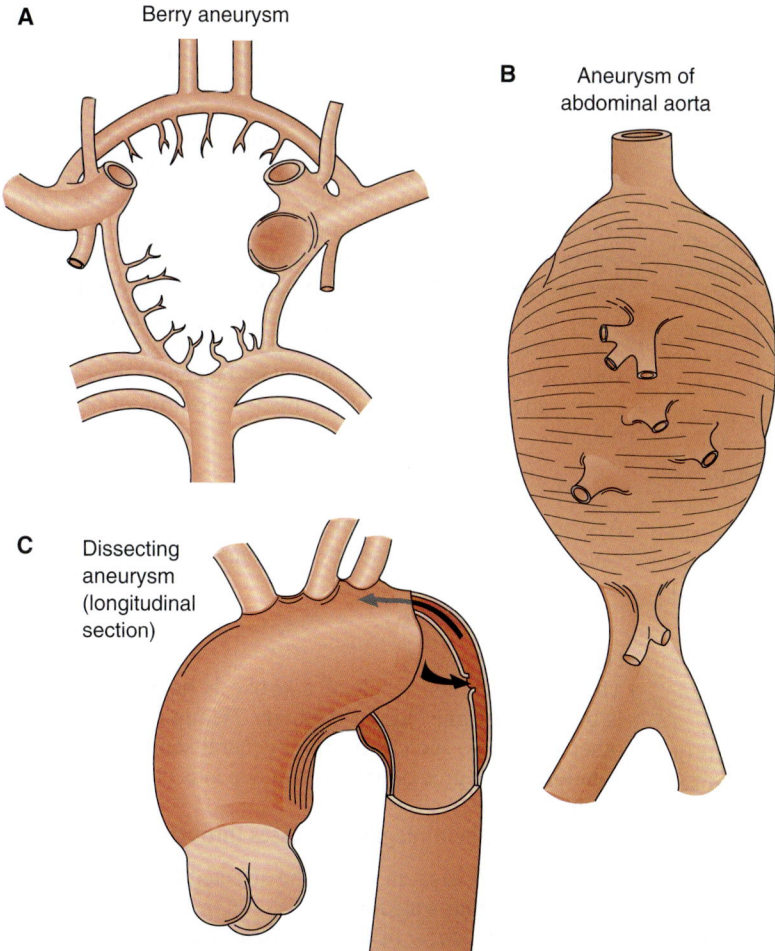

Figure 81-11 Three forms of aneurysms: **A.** Berry aneurysm in the circle of Willis, **B.** Fusiform-type aneurysm of the abdominal aorta, and **C.** A dissecting aortic aneurysm.

Aneurysms may be congenital, occur after trauma, or develop as a result of the increased pressure of arteriosclerosis. Unknown cerebral aneurysm rupture is often the cause of sudden death in healthy athletes.

Stroke

A **stroke**, also known as a *cerebrovascular accident* (CVA), is a sudden or gradual interruption of blood supply to a vital center in the brain. A stroke can cause complete or partial paralysis or death. Strokes are a major cause of death in America. Risk factors for strokes include hypertension, heart disease, and previous strokes or a history of transient ischemic attacks (TIA). If the client has diabetes mellitus, a family history of cerebrovascular disease, and cardiac arrhythmias, especially atrial fibrillation, the risk for a stroke increases. Smoking, obesity, and alcohol use are associated with this disorder. Women who use hormonal contraceptives, who also smoke, and have a history of hypertension are at higher risk of strokes. Individuals with certain blood disorders that have high RBC counts, which increase blood viscosity, are prone to strokes. Additionally, individuals with high serum triglyceride levels, elevated cholesterol levels, and triglycerides levels need to be monitored for signs and symptoms of a stroke.

Types of Strokes
- *Transient ischemic attack* (TIA), which may be called a mini-stroke, is a sudden, short-acting (not permanent) cerebral occlusion. The person recovers within 24 hr. TIA is often a warning that another, more serious, stroke will occur later. A *reversible ischemic neurologic deficit* (RIND) is similar to a TIA, except that the symptoms last for as long as a week. A brain scan may reveal that a brain infarction has occurred.
- *Ischemic strokes* are due to *cerebral thrombosis or cerebral embolism*. Plaques or fatty deposits within the arteries or a blood clot—usually a result of arteriosclerosis—block or narrow an artery, resulting in ischemia and infarction to a vital brain center. Cerebral thrombosis is local blockage of an artery. A cerebral embolus occurs when a blood clot breaks off from a thrombus elsewhere in the body and is carried to the brain. It lodges in a brain's blood vessel, which shuts off blood supply to part of the brain.
- *Hemorrhagic strokes* are due to *cerebral hemorrhage* or an *aneurysm*. An artery in the brain bursts because of arteriosclerosis, continuing weakening of the aneurysm wall, hypertension, or an acute, severe rise in blood pressure. The results are blood vessel rupture and hemorrhage.

Signs and Symptoms
Symptoms of stroke depend on its cause. In some cases of thrombosis and ischemia, the person has had dizzy spells or sudden memory loss for some time before the actual stroke. No pain accompanies these symptoms, so the client may ignore them. A cerebral hemorrhage may give warning. It causes dizziness and ringing in the ears (*tinnitus*), as well as a violent headache, often with nausea and vomiting. A hemorrhage may follow unusual exertion, such as shoveling snow, heavy eating, or vigorous exercise. Embolism usually occurs without warning, although the person often has a history of cardiovascular disease.

> **Nursing Alert** FAST—Identification of a stroke
> The American Stroke Association (2019) has developed a way to assist identification of the most common symptoms of a stroke by using the acronym *FAST*.
> - *Face:* Ask the person to smile and observe if one side of the **F**ace droops.
> - *Arms:* Ask the person to raise both **A**rms. If one drifts downward, a stroke is possible.
> - *Speak:* Ask the person to **S**peak a simple phrase and observe if their speech is slurred or strange.
> - *Time:* Since **T**ime is of the essence, it is imperative that someone who observes any of these signs and symptoms immediately call 9-1-1.

Nursing Considerations
Notice which side of the body is weak. If the client has the diagnosis of "left-sided stroke," then the paralysis will be on the opposite or right side of the body. After a stroke that occurs in the right side of the brain, the signs and symptoms will be evident on the left side of the body. However, a stroke that causes cranial nerve damage will result in signs and symptoms that are evident on the same side of the body as in the brain.

A sudden-onset stroke is usually the most severe. The victim loses consciousness; the face becomes red; breathing is noisy and strained. The pulse is slow but full and bounding. Blood pressure is elevated, and the person may be in a deep coma. *Stroke in evolution* (SIE) is a gradual worsening of symptoms of brain ischemia. The coma may deepen progressively until death occurs, or the person may gradually regain consciousness and eventually recover. The longer the time period that the person remains unresponsive, the less likely it is that the person will recover. The first few days after onset are critical. The responsive person may show signs of memory loss or inconsistent behavior; they may be easily fatigued, lose bowel and bladder control, or have poor balance.

Results of a Stroke
A stroke can result in numerous effects, depending on the cause and location of the stroke. Some of the major effects are discussed here.

Hemiplegia
The most common result of a stroke is **hemiplegia**, which is paralysis of one side of the body. Hemiplegia may affect other functions, such as hearing, general sensation, and circulation; the degree of impairment depends on the part of the brain affected.

Generally, hemiplegia progresses through three stages:
1. The *flaccid stage*, in which the affected side exhibits numbness and weakness
2. The *spastic stage*, in which muscles are contracted and tense and movement is difficult

3. The *recovery stage*, when therapy and rehabilitation methods are most successful

Aphasia and Dysphasia

Many people with stroke experience **aphasia**, a result of damage to the brain's speech center. Aphasia is a condition in which people are unable to speak. It can be frustrating and frightening because mental functioning usually is unimpaired. In Practice: Nursing Care Guidelines 81-3 highlights key measures for communicating with a client who has aphasia.

Another complication associated with a stroke is *dysphasia*, an inability to say what one wishes to say. Many clients regain some power of speech, but others never do. *Dysphagia* (swallowing difficulty) may also occur and can be life-threatening, as aspiration can occur. Therefore, all clients suspected of a stroke are to be kept NPO until a swallowing assessment can be performed by a trained individual.

Brain Damage

The extent of brain damage resulting from a CVA determines the client's chances for recovery. If the damage is slight, recovery will be more rapid and complete. Also, the chances of recovery are better for a younger person who suffers a CVA.

Hemianopsia (Hemianopia)

Hemianopsia is defined as blindness in half of the visual field of one or both eyes. It is a common occurrence with a stroke. Consider this condition in all aspects of care. For instance, always approach the client from the unaffected side. Teach the client to *scan* (move the head from side to side) to see things.

Pain

Usually, after a stroke, the client suffers very little pain. Problems such as infection, kidney or bladder *calculi* (stones), fecal impaction, or emotional disturbances may aggravate any existing pain.

Autonomic Disturbances

The person who has had a stroke may also have autonomic disturbances, such as perspiration or "goose flesh" above the level of the paralysis. They may have dilated pupils, high or low blood pressure, or headache. Disturbances of this kind may be treated with atropine-like drugs.

Personality Changes

Personality changes may be functional or organic. The *functional* type results from frustration at being unable to speak or walk or from the attitudes of other people. In either case, the individual may feel useless or helpless. *Organic changes* may result from blockage of blood supply to part of the brain. In this instance, the person may cry or become easily excited. These conditions cannot be consciously controlled.

Nursing Considerations

The person with a stroke may be admitted to the healthcare facility in the unresponsive state sometimes called a stroke in evolution (SIE). After careful examination and history, this individual may be eligible for thrombolytic therapy to resolve the clot. The quality of nursing care given during the acute phase often considerably affects how much rehabilitation is possible and how quickly it can be accomplished. The following are important nursing activities to implement during this time:

- Note changes in level of consciousness and any changes from the neurologic findings of the initial neurologic examination (see In Practice: Data Gathering In Nursing 78-1).
- Document every sign of improvement or lack of it.
- Position the unresponsive person on the unaffected side to keep the airway open and prevent aspiration. *Rationale:*

IN PRACTICE
NURSING CARE GUIDELINES 81-3 — Communicating With the Client With Aphasia

- If the client can read and write, supply a tablet and pencil or provide a board on which the person can write. Provide a pen or pencil that is easy to hold. Assistive devices for writing are available.
- If the client cannot write, provide a board or chart on which key words and phrases are printed. The client can point to these words and phrases to make any needs known.
- If the client is able to move a finger to indicate yes or no, check to see if the individual can let the staff know what is being said.
- If the client cannot move at all, ask the individual to blink. The client can blink once for "yes" and twice for "no."
- Talk to the client even if the person cannot answer. Chat while you perform daily nursing care.
- Do not talk to the client as if the client were mentally handicapped or has the understanding of a child.
- Never talk about the client to another person—including healthcare personnel—in the client's presence. Although the client might be unable to speak, the individual may be able to hear and understand everything being said.
- Keep in mind that some clients who are unable to speak can use computers. Assistive devices are available for those who cannot use conventional keyboards.
- Expect speech therapy to begin as soon as possible. After the speech therapist has decided what procedures to use, reinforce this with everyone involved in the client's care.

Proper positioning prevents contractures and undue pressure on any part.
- Avoid placing the unresponsive person on the back. ***Rationale:*** *The tongue may fall back and occlude the airway; secretions may accumulate in the back of the throat.*
- Provide adequate support for the affected limbs. Extremity splints are now routinely used. ***Rationale:*** *Positioning, support, and splints help prevent contractures.*
- Elevate the head of the bed. ***Rationale:*** *Reduce the chance of increased intracranial pressure.*
- Turn the person often, at least once every 2 hr, keeping the body in proper alignment.
- Provide suctioning, as necessary. A mechanical airway or tracheostomy may be required. Oxygen will most likely be administered.
- Monitor vital signs carefully. ***Rationale:*** *An elevated temperature and lowered pulse and respiration rates are signs of increased intracranial pressure—which you must report.*
- Keep the eyes lubricated with soothing eye drops, as ordered.
- Talk to the person and explain everything you do as if the individual were responsive. ***Rationale:*** *Although the person may not respond, they hear. Hearing is the last sense to be lost.*

When caring for the person who has regained consciousness, do the following:

- Continue to turn the client often, now from the unaffected side to a back-lying position.
- Encourage coughing and deep breathing.
- Encourage movement, if possible. ***Rationale:*** *Movement prevents hypostatic pneumonia, formation of kidney stones, fecal impaction, urinary retention, and other complications.*
- Provide PROM exercises as ordered.
- Encourage cooperation with the physical therapist.
- Administer ordered drugs (usually, heparin, dicumarol, or warfarin (Coumadin)) with care. Watch for side effects. ***Rationale:*** *These drugs prolong clotting time and prevent further clots from forming. However, danger of hemorrhage accompanies their use.* The client usually does not need analgesics for treatment of the stroke; however, other conditions, such as osteoarthritis, may need pain management.
- Begin bowel and bladder retraining as the client is ready for it.

Be aware of the various results of strokes. Treat clients with kindness and understanding. They need support, reassurance, and acceptance most of all (see In Practice: Nursing Care Plan 78-1).

> **Nursing Alert** Hearing and vision on the affected side are usually impaired as a result of a stroke. To avoid having to repeat what is said and perhaps embarrassing the person, approach from the unaffected side.

Rehabilitation

Immediately on admission, staff should begin planning for rehabilitation. If contractures are prevented, the client can learn to walk again much sooner. If the skin is kept intact, the client will not have to contend with ulcers and infections. If bowel and bladder training have begun, the client will be well on the way to independence. The goal of all rehabilitation is to return the client to the highest level of self-care in ADL. As soon as possible, teach adaptive ADL, such as transferring from bed to chair and to toilet; dressing; and feeding. Speech, physical, or occupational therapy also begins as soon as possible (see Chapter 97).

> **NCLEX Alert**
> Clients who have had a stroke need many nursing interventions. When taking NCLEX examinations, read the scenario carefully so that you are alerted to the priority nursing interventions. For example, initial, emergency nursing care of a client having a stroke differs from the interventions of a client who has existing hemiplegia, hemianopsia, dysphagia, or aphasia.

Members of the family play a vital role. They need to know what the client can do and how to encourage that person now and after discharge. They should also understand that because of brain damage, the person may behave differently after a stroke. Whatever the client's disability, members of the family should recognize their own, as well as the client's, emotional needs. They also need to learn how to perform various procedures that help the client, while allowing the person to do as much as possible. The family needs a lot of emotional support to deal with the client's limitations.

Many resources are available to assist in rehabilitation, including local social service agencies, the American Heart Association, and the state's division of vocational and occupational services. The local home health nursing services can help the family prepare for the client's homecoming and can assist the client in performing self-care at home.

STUDENT SYNTHESIS

KEY POINTS

- Cardiovascular disorders include conditions that interfere with the heart's rhythm and the heart's pumping ability and that disrupt the blood flow within the coronary, peripheral, or cerebral arteries.
- Hypertension can lead to such serious problems as myocardial infarction, kidney damage, heart failure, and stroke.
- Some types of heart disease can be cured, whereas others can be controlled by medical or surgical treatment.
- Heart failure means that the heart is failing, has lost its pumping ability, and is unable to do its work. It is a syndrome (group of symptoms) that affects individuals in different ways and to different degrees.
- Coronary artery disease develops over many years, so prevention of controllable risk factors should begin early in life.
- Angina pectoris is a temporary loss of oxygen to the heart muscle. If this loss of oxygen supply continues, the result is ischemia (prolonged deficiency of oxygenated blood), whereas death of heart tissue is called myocardial necrosis.
- Clients who complain of chest pains should be medicated promptly, as ordered by the healthcare provider, to prevent further damage to heart muscle due to anoxia.
- Hearing and vision are usually impaired on the person's affected side after a stroke; therefore, approach the client from the unaffected side.

CRITICAL THINKING EXERCISES

1. P. L., aged 25, comes to the healthcare provider's office because they have had chest pain off and on for a month. They are concerned because their family has a history of heart attacks. They ask you if they have had a heart attack. They want to know what they can do to prevent a heart attack. Formulate a plan you could use to teach P. L. preventive measures.

2. I. H., age 58, has recently suffered a stroke. He is dysphasic and has recently become very frustrated over their condition. Their family members are attentive and concerned; however, I. H. seems unhappy and angry when they are around. What measures could you take to assist I. H. with speech difficulties? How would you address their attitude toward their family members? How would you help their family cope with the condition?

NCLEX-STYLE REVIEW QUESTIONS

1. The nurse is reinforcing discharge instructions for a client who received a mechanical heart valve. Which statement made by the client indicates to the nurse that instructions are understood?
    a. "I will have to take lifelong anticoagulation therapy."
    b. "My valve will have to be replaced within 10 years."
    c. "I will not be able to exercise or participate in previous activities."
    d. "I will have to be on immunosuppressant therapy for the duration of my life."

2. A client is preparing to have an angiocardiogram in the morning. Which data would the nurse obtain in preparation for this test?
    a. Ask if the client has crutches or a cane to use after the test.
    b. Ask if the client has a family member that had this test.
    c. Ask if the client has received a yearly flu shot.
    d. Ask if the client is allergic to shellfish or iodine.

3. The nurse is reinforcing education for a client with hypertension. Which statement made by the client indicates that further education is required?
    a. "I will apply methods to reduce stress in my life."
    b. "I don't have to take my antihypertensives if I am feeling well."
    c. "I will reduce the cholesterol and salt intake in my diet."
    d. "I will measure my blood pressure routinely at home."

4. A client having an implantable cardioverter–defibrillator asks the nurse, "What should I do if I feel a shock and am alone?" Which is the best response by the nurse?
    a. "Lie down and call 911."
    b. "Continue previous activity."
    c. "Chew an aspirin tablet."
    d. "Take an extra dose of your antiarrhythmic medication."

5. A client is diagnosed with pulmonary edema and having pink, frothy sputum and crackles in both lungs. Which nursing intervention would be provided at this time? Select all that apply.
    a. Administer morphine sulfate as ordered.
    b. Administer furosemide (Lasix) as ordered.
    c. Place the legs in a dependent position.
    d. Administer oxygen as ordered.
    e. Place the client in high Fowler position.

CHAPTER RESOURCES

Enhance your learning with additional resources on thePoint!

Student Resources related to this chapter can be found at thePoint.lww.com/Rosdahl12e.

82 Blood and Lymph Disorders

Learning Objectives

1. State the main blood types, including the inherited antibodies and antigens for each blood type.
2. Describe the following diagnostic studies: indirect Coombs test, direct Coombs test, type and screen test, and type and crossmatch test.
3. State the functions of each of the following tests: RBC count, Hgb, Hct, WBC count, differential, platelet count, blood smear, PT, PTT, APTT, and bleed time.
4. Identify nursing considerations related to the following: ESR, blood culture, bone marrow biopsy, and lymph node biopsy.
5. Identify the advantages and the limitations for colloid solutions.
6. Identify the rationale for the administration of the following blood products: whole blood, packed RBCs, platelet concentrates, FFP, albumin, cryoprecipitates, plasmapheresis, IgG, and IgD.
7. Identify nursing considerations for autologous and allogeneic HSCT.
8. Discuss nursing considerations for each of the following RBC disorders: polycythemia, anemia, sickle cell disease, and thalassemia.
9. Compare and contrast the following types of anemia: iron deficiency, hemolytic, hemorrhagic, pernicious, and aplastic.
10. Define the causative factors for the following WBC disorders: neutropenia and leukemia. Identify nursing considerations related to each disorder.
11. Discuss nursing considerations for each of the following clotting disorders: thrombocythemia, ITP, DIC, hemophilia, and von Willebrand disease.
12. Identify the causative factors for the following lymphatic system disorders: Hodgkin lymphoma, non-Hodgkin lymphoma, and multiple myeloma.

Important Terminology

agranulocytosis, allogeneic, autologous, colloid solutions, hematology, hemophilia, Hodgkin lymphoma, leukemia, leukocytosis, leukopenia, neutropenia, oncologist, pancytopenia, phlebotomy, polycythemia vera, Rh factor, sickle cell disease, thrombocytopenia, thrombocytosis, von Willebrand disease

Acronyms

ALL, AML, APTT, BMT, CLL, CML, CSF, DIC, ESR, FFP, GVHD, HLA, HSCT, Ig, INR, ITP, NHL, PBSC, PT, PTT, SCD, vWD

The medical specialty concerned with the hematologic and lymphatic systems is called **hematology**. Healthcare providers educated in this specialty are *hematologists*. Blood and lymph are closely related to many other body systems and disorders (see Chapters 22 and 23). For example, cancer can originate in the blood or lymphatic systems. These transport systems can also be a route by which cancer cells travel and metastasize to other body areas. An **oncologist** (cancer specialist) often treats blood and lymph disorders (see Chapter 83).

Some blood and lymph disorders have systemic consequences and symptoms. Cardiovascular and blood and lymph disorders also affect children (see Chapter 72).

DIAGNOSTIC TESTS

Laboratory examination of blood can reveal the general condition of many body systems and can aid in the diagnosis of many disorders. Medical technologists, other laboratory personnel, and nurses perform many of these tests. This chapter discusses several indications for the use of many hematologic studies.

> **Key Concept**
> The nurse must be knowledgeable about the types of hematologic studies, the reasons for their use, and the implications of abnormal laboratory values. In many instances, it is the nurse's responsibility to notify the healthcare provider of routine and abnormal laboratory values.

ABO Blood Typing

There are four main types of blood—A, B, AB, and O—which comprise the ABO blood type (or blood group) system. Each of these four types has a unique combination of antigens and antibodies. Genetic heritage is responsible for the antigens on the surface of the red blood cells (RBCs). Antibodies develop within the first years of life and are found in the plasma. Following is a summary of the blood types:

- Type A has the A antigen and the anti-B antibody
- Type B has the B antigen and the anti-A antibody
- Type AB has both the A and B antigens and does not have either the anti-A or the anti-B antibody
- Type O has neither the A nor B antigen, but does have both the anti-A and the anti-B antibodies

> **Key Concept**
> ABO antigens may also be found in body fluids, such as saliva, tears, and urine. Referred to as the "secretor system," these antigens are used in forensic medicine to identify victims and criminals when blood samples are not available.

> **Nursing Alert** Transfusions of blood and blood products are common nursing actions. It is extremely important that the client receive blood that matches their own body's antigens and antibodies. If a client who is type A (with type A antigen and anti-B antibody) were to receive type B blood (with type B antigen and anti-A antibody) accidently, the client's immune system would identify the infused blood as foreign. The result would be agglutination (clumping) or hemolysis (destruction) of the infused RBCs.
> Type O blood is considered the *universal donor* blood type because it does not typically have the ABO antigens. Type AB blood is considered the *universal recipient* blood type because it has both A and B antigens but does not have the anti-A or anti-B antibodies. In reality, blood needs to be typed correctly and crossmatched before transfusion.

There are exceptions to the general guidelines of ABO transfusion compatibility. The most common additional factor is the aspect of the *D antigen* (D factor), which is more commonly known as the **Rh factor**. The D antigen is only one of at least five known inherited antigens for which blood is screened by the blood bank and the hospital laboratory. At birth, a person may have the Rh (or D) antigen on the RBC and is therefore Rh-positive (Rh+). If the individual does not have the D antigen, they are Rh negative (Rh–). When referring to blood type, the Rh status is stated along with the main ABO blood type, for example, O negative (O–), O positive (O+), B negative (B–), or B positive (B+). The D antigen is particularly pertinent in some hemolytic diseases, such as *erythroblastosis fetalis*, in the newborn. (Refer to Rh sensitization in Chapter 69 for discussion of this major newborn complication.)

Indirect Coombs Test

An *indirect Coombs test* screens for circulating Rh antibodies. It is ordered on an Rh-negative pregnant woman. If Rh antibodies are detected in the mother, the fetus is in jeopardy of developing erythroblastosis fetalis. RhoGAM is an anti-Rh antibody preparation that suppresses the mother's production of Rh antibodies.

Direct Coombs Test

A *direct Coombs test* will detect antibodies already attached to the RBC. This test may be ordered before blood transfusions and the administration of certain drugs. A positive or abnormal direct Coombs test may indicate transfusion reactions, erythroblastosis fetalis, hemolytic anemia, infectious mononucleosis, lymphomas, certain cancers and renal disorders, or autoimmune disorders, such as rheumatoid arthritis and systemic lupus erythematosus.

Type and Screen Test

A *type and screen test* of blood determines the ABO blood group, the Rh type, and an indirect Coombs test. A type and screen is often ordered for clients who have a low to moderate potential of needing a blood transfusion. It is a test that can be completed relatively quickly and reasonably inexpensively.

Type and Crossmatch Test

A *type and crossmatch test* is a more detailed test usually done for clients who have a greater potential of needing blood transfusions. The type and crossmatch includes testing for ABO groups and Rh factor. The ABO system is physiologically complex, and a laboratory examination may identify additional antibodies, so rarely is blood transfused that is not both typed and crossmatched. However, in some extreme emergency situations by specific healthcare provider order, blood that is typed, but not crossmatched, may be given. A type and crossmatch may take up to an hour to complete. Therefore, it is necessary to anticipate the need for blood transfusions in advance of their need.

Nursing Considerations

Nursing considerations related to blood typing include the awareness that blood of different types is often incompatible when mixed. The wrong type of blood could easily be fatal. Even with the safeguards of blood typing, screening, and crossmatching, be sure to observe the client very carefully while they receive a blood transfusion because dangerous reactions are still a possibility.

Complete Blood Count

The *complete blood count* (CBC) is the common analysis of blood that provides diagnostic information. A CBC usually includes a numerical estimate of the number of RBCs, white blood cells (WBCs), and platelets found in a blood sample. Deficiencies or excesses of any of the cells may indicate a specific problem. These numbers reflect the functioning of the person's bone marrow, the blood's ability to carry oxygen to the cells, and the client's infection-fighting status and clotting abilities. The components of a CBC include

- RBC count
- Hematocrit
- Hemoglobin
- RBC indices: mean corpuscular volume (MCV), mean corpuscular hemoglobin (MCH), and mean corpuscular hemoglobin concentration (MCHC)
- WBC count
- WBC differential count (granulocytes: neutrophils, basophils, eosinophils; agranulocytes: lymphocytes, monocytes)
- Blood smear

Red Blood Cell Count

The *RBC count* measures the number of circulating RBCs in a cubic millimeter of peripheral venous blood. Normal values vary according to age and sex.

The test for hemoglobin (Hgb, Hb) identifies the amount of hemoglobin in an RBC. The results of this test indicate the body's ability to carry oxygen to cells. The hematocrit (Hct) test identifies the percentage of RBCs in the blood.

Along with the RBC count, the Hgb and Hct tests can indicate different types of anemias or an overabundance of RBCs (*polycythemia*). With a client who has adequate overall hydration, the Hct result is about three times the Hgb.

The RBC indices are calculated measurements of the size of an RBC and the amounts of hemoglobin. Using the figures obtained for the MCH, MCHC, and the MCV, the diagnostician can differentiate among different types of anemias, including macrocytic, microcytic, thalassemic, aplastic, or pernicious anemia.

White Blood Cell Count and Differential

A *WBC count* is a valuable diagnostic aid. When an infection is present, the normal count of 5,000–10,000/mm^3 may increase to 25,000/mm^3 or higher. WBCs increase in number (**leukocytosis**) or decrease in number (**leukopenia**).

Under a microscope, the technician can estimate the numbers of each of the five types of leukocytes. In some diseases, the proportion of the kinds of WBCs varies. In bacterial infections, the number of neutrophils increases; in viral infections, the numbers of lymphocytes increase. Therefore, a differential count is made, in which the technician compares the number of granular leukocytes with the number of nongranular (agranular) leukocytes. The results are further diagnostic clues for the healthcare provider.

The *WBC differential* or "diff" may be ordered specifically to be done by mechanical estimates or to be visualized and counted by a trained laboratory technician.

Leukocytosis (increased total WBC count) is the body's normal response to injury or invading pathogens. Review the five major types of leukocytes in Chapter 23. The particular type of WBC involved may help to identify the cause of abnormal leukocytosis. For example, an increase in monocytes (*monocytosis*) would indicate mononucleosis. *Lymphocytosis* (increased numbers of lymphocytes), a useful indicator of leukemia, can be used to monitor the client's progress and response to treatment. Lymphocytes develop into B lymphocytes (B cells) or T lymphocytes (T cells), which are necessary for the development of antibodies (immunoglobulins).

Platelet Count

Platelets or *thrombocytes* are fragments of very large cells (megakaryocytes) formed in the bone marrow. They circulate until needed or are removed every 8–12 days, when they are destroyed by the spleen. The platelet count indicates the client's capacity of *hemostasis* (blood clotting).

Low platelet counts are associated with bruising, bleeding disorders, and hemorrhage. *Thrombocytopenia* (low numbers of platelets) can be seen in a number of conditions, including chemotherapy for cancer, radiation therapy, certain types of anemias, and leukemia. **Thrombocytosis** (increased platelets) can be an indication of certain types of anemias, leukemia, pregnancy, and polycythemia.

> **Nursing Alert** Possibly the most commonly seen laboratory test is the CBC. Therefore, an NCLEX question could require that the nurse know the components of the CBC, the normal levels, and the nursing actions required for abnormal laboratory test results.

Peripheral Blood Smear

The *peripheral blood smear* is an informative test performed by a qualified technologist. Under the microscope, the technician views a prepared smear slide for RBCs, WBCs, and platelets. The RBCs are examined for size, shape, color, and structure. A differential count of WBCs can be done. The number and appearance of platelets are also monitored.

Coagulation Studies

Prothrombin Time

The *prothrombin time* (**PT**, pro time, PT ratio/**INR**) is an actual amount of time that it takes for the blood to clot, generally given in seconds. This test can indicate the proper functioning of coagulation factors and the coagulation process. The *international normalized ratio* (**INR**) is often given along with the PT. The INR is a worldwide standard also used to monitor anticoagulation therapy. The PT will be longer when certain clotting factors are defective or not present in sufficient quantity. The factors that can affect the PT include fibrinogen I and prothrombins II, V, VII, and X. Normally, the PT is less than 12 s.

The PT/INR is commonly used to monitor the success of oral anticoagulation therapy using warfarin sodium (Coumadin). Adequate amounts of warfarin (Coumadin) will prolong clotting time—the desired effect of the therapy. However, too much of the drug can result in bleeding and hemorrhage. Intramuscular (IM) *vitamin K*, which reverses the effects of warfarin (Coumadin) in 12–24 hr, *is the antidote to warfarin (Coumadin)*. Therapeutic values for anticoagulation therapy of warfarin (Coumadin) are 1.5–2 times the normal ranges. If the client does not have adequate amounts of the anticoagulation drug, PT will be within normal limits, and *the healthcare provider will need to be notified*.

Measuring the PT daily is essential when the client begins anticoagulant drug therapy. When the therapeutic blood level of anticoagulant is stabilized, PT can be determined less often (approximately every 2 weeks). In Practice: Data Gathering in Nursing 82-1 highlights important findings for the client receiving anticoagulant therapy. When a client is receiving anticoagulant therapy, the following are important to reduce the risk of bleeding:

- Avoid IM injections and needlesticks, if possible
- Avoid taking temperatures rectally
- Avoid giving the daily dose of anticoagulant until after blood specimen for the PT is drawn
- Report results of PT or APTT test (see below) to healthcare provider (in case dosage needs to be adjusted)

> **IN PRACTICE**
> **DATA GATHERING IN NURSING 82-1** — The Client Receiving Anticoagulant Therapy
>
> **Adverse Signs and Symptoms**
> - Bleeding, no matter how slight
> - Headache
> - Unexplained abdominal pain
> - Changes in neurologic signs or level of consciousness

Partial Thromboplastin Time

Partial thromboplastin time (**PTT**) and activated partial thromboplastin time (**APTT**) are tests used to monitor the pathway of clot formation. The APTT differs from the PTT in that the APTT uses different chemicals in the testing process that accelerate or activate the clotting factors. Defective or deficient clotting factors that may affect the PTT or APTT include factors I, II, V, VIII, IX, X, XI, and XII. The tests can identify deficiencies of the clotting factors, prothrombin, and fibrinogen.

Control or normal values for the PTT range from 60 to 90 s. Control or normal values for the APTT range from 25 to 27 s.

The PTT and APTT may be used to monitor heparin anticoagulation therapy administered via an intravenous (IV) or subcutaneous route. Therapeutic ranges for both tests would be 1.5–2.5 times the normal ranges. Too much heparin may lead to bleeding and hemorrhage. *The antidote for heparin therapy is protamine sulfate.* One milligram of protamine sulfate will reverse the effects of 100 units of heparin.

> **Nursing Alert** When a client is on anticoagulation therapy, a "normal" laboratory value may indicate *too little* warfarin (Coumadin) or heparin. Successful anticoagulation therapies require a prolonged time for either the PT (Coumadin) or the PTT/APTT (heparin).

Bleeding Time

The *bleeding time* is a screening test used to detect platelet disorders, evaluate for capillary defects, and determine the client's ability to stop bleeding. It may also be referred to as an *aspirin tolerance test*, a *Duke bleeding time*, an *Ivy bleeding time*, or a *modified Ivy test*.

When a family history of bleeding is known or suspected, the bleeding time may be ordered before surgery as an indicator of hemostasis capability and during aspirin therapy when used for anticoagulation. Normal bleeding time is 3–8 min in adults.

Other Hematologic Studies

Erythrocyte Sedimentation Rate

The *erythrocyte sedimentation rate* (**ESR**) measures the speed (in millimeter per hour [mm/hr]) at which RBCs settle to the bottom of a tube of unclotted blood in 1 hr. Normal rate varies with age, sex, and testing method. Inflammation alters blood proteins, resulting in heavier than normal RBCs. The speed with which RBCs fall to the bottom of the tube corresponds to the degree of inflammation present.

Although ESR is a nonspecific test, it is useful in diagnosing infections, inflammatory processes, and autoimmune conditions. When performed in conjunction with a WBC count, the ESR can indicate infection. The ESR is also used to detect inflammatory processes, neoplasms, and necrotic processes. It can help to diagnose diseases and can be used to monitor treatment.

Blood Culture

A *blood culture* is done to discover the presence of bacteria in the blood or to determine the antibiotics that are most effective against a specific organism.

When obtaining a blood culture, it is important to follow the parameters established by the healthcare facility and the requesting healthcare provider for the proper timing. Because this test requires special collection procedures, laboratory technicians often draw the blood.

Hospital policy may indicate that routine blood cultures be taken at certain times of the day, using specific preparations before the venous stick. For example, a typical order may read, "Obtain blood cultures 2 times if temperature >101.5 °F [>38.6 °C]."

The culture should be obtained before any antibiotic therapy is started, to avoid interference with culture and sensitivity test results. A major nursing responsibility is to notify the laboratory when a client's temperature elevates so that the healthcare provider's order is followed promptly.

Bone Marrow Aspiration and Biopsy

A *bone marrow aspiration and biopsy* is done to evaluate the number, size, and shape of RBCs, WBCs, and *megakaryocytes* (platelet precursors). The aspirate provides a sample of cells that are examined under a microscope for a biopsy determination. This test can be helpful by assisting in the diagnosis and monitoring of many disorders, such as leukemias, hemorrhagic or hemolytic anemias, aplastic anemia, Hodgkin lymphoma, non-Hodgkin lymphoma, multiple myeloma, and infections (e.g., mononucleosis).

The procedure uses a large-bore needle with an attached syringe. The needle is used to aspirate marrow from the sternum, iliac crest, or anterior or posterior iliac spine (or the proximal tibia in children).

Although healthcare providers generally perform this procedure, nurses assist by ensuring that the client lies still and by providing support to the client. After the procedure, care includes applying pressure to the puncture site and observing carefully for bleeding.

Lymph Node Biopsy

A biopsy or excision of a lymph node is often performed to diagnose or stage a tumor or to diagnose immunodeficiency disorders. Staging a tumor helps identify its invasiveness. Staging is discussed in Chapter 83.

COMMON TREATMENTS

Transfusions of Colloid Solutions

Colloid solutions, often referred to as *plasma expanders*, are solutions, but not blood cells, used to replace circulating fluid volume. Depending on the components of an IV solution, plasma expanders may also be referred to as *hypertonic* solutions. The purpose of using hypertonic IV solutions is to promote movement of water between fluid compartments by initiating a change in fluid pressures. Colloid solutions have a higher osmolality than does normal plasma. Because of this change of fluid or osmotic pressure, water is pulled from interstitial areas to the intravascular (plasma) compartments. Therefore, the size of the intravascular compartments is "expanded." The result is an increase of intravascular fluid volume; that is, an increase in blood pressure.

Intravenous solutions such as 5% dextrose in 0.45% sodium chloride (D_5 1/2 NS) or 5% dextrose in 0.225% sodium chloride (D_5 1/4 NS) are examples of hypertonic solutions. Additionally, either a derivative of whole blood, such as plasma, or a synthetic product works by drawing interstitial (tissue) fluid into the intravascular (blood vessel) compartments. Synthetic plasma expanders include hetastarch (Hespan) and dextran (Macrodex, Rheomacrodex). Synthetic colloid products are economical and virus-free alternatives to blood.

Colloid solutions are given in critical or emergency situations when a hypotensive client is in jeopardy owing to excess loss of fluids (e.g., hemorrhage due to trauma, burns, or *anasarca* [total body edema]).

Synthetic colloid products are often used if blood products are not available, if the client refuses blood products, or if the client needs supplementation to the available blood products. Occasionally, a client needs more than fluid volume replacement. The client may need hemoglobin and oxygen-carrying capacity, which is not provided by the synthetic colloid products. Recombinant human erythropoietin (EPO, Epogen, Procrit) can be given to stimulate RBC production. At least 10 days before surgery, the client receives erythropoietin via IM injection. Additional doses are given on the day of surgery and 4 days after surgery.

Transfusions of Blood and Blood Products

The IV administration of blood and blood components is called a *blood transfusion*. When blood or blood products from donors are used, the procedure is called an **allogeneic** *transfusion*. A unit of blood can be transfused as whole blood. More commonly, the unit of blood is separated into individual components, which are given for specific purposes.

> **Key Concept**
> In some cultures and religions, clients are not allowed to receive blood products. Respect the client's beliefs.

Administering a blood transfusion involves practicing the essential principles of IV therapy as discussed in Chapter 64. See additional information in the clinical practice guidelines: In Practice: Nursing Care Guidelines 82-1, Precautions During Blood Transfusions, and In Practice: Data Gathering in Nursing 82-2, Blood Transfusion Reactions.

> **Nursing Alert** According to the policies of most healthcare facilities, two licensed personnel must identify both the client who is to receive a blood transfusion and the unit of blood. The client should be wearing an identification bracelet before the blood sample is drawn for type and crossmatch testing (no exceptions should be made). Misidentification of the client or use of the wrong test sample or blood unit can be fatal. Human error is responsible for most fatal transfusion reactions.

Blood Donation

Blood is obtained typically through blood donations. **Autologous** blood donations are self-donated; it is the safest blood for the client. Several types of autologous transfusion options are available, including preoperative autologous blood donation. Under certain criteria, blood can be collected ahead of time and used for surgery on that client. Autologous blood donations are generally limited to surgeries that typically require blood transfusions.

Perioperative blood infusions (intraoperative blood salvage and postoperative blood salvage) can use blood that is lost during and immediately after surgical procedures. Specialized training and equipment are necessary before attempting this procedure. *Acute normovolemic hemodilution* is the removal of blood and the simultaneous infusion of other solutions to maintain intravascular volume.

Directed blood donations (designated) are from donors the client selects, such as family members or friends. Directed donations are not as safe as the client's own blood. These blood donations are not equivalent to autologous donations but are considered as safe as any donation from a general community source.

> **Key Concept**
> Even though it is rare, a blood transfusion can transmit blood-borne diseases, such as hepatitis. Tests and procedures for screening blood and selecting blood donors have improved the safety of blood transfusions. When handling tested blood, always follow Standard Precautions.

Blood Products

Whole blood is rarely used for transfusions today, except to treat massive acute hemorrhage. The normal circulating blood volume in an adult is approximately 6 L (8–10 pints). Whole blood can be refrigerated for storage for up to 35 days.

Packed RBCs are produced by *centrifuging* (spinning) whole blood, which forces the RBCs to the bottom of the container. With the addition of a special preservative, packed cells can be refrigerated for storage for up to 42 days. Packed

IN PRACTICE
NURSING CARE GUIDELINES 82-1: Precautions During Blood Transfusions

For each unit to be given, follow all procedures for intravenous (IV) therapy PLUS the following:
- Obtain the unit to be infused just before the infusion.
- Double-check the label and the client ID with another nurse.
- Visually inspect the unit for any obvious abnormalities, such as gas bubbles, unusual color, or cloudiness (which may indicate contamination or hemolysis).
- Take and record the client's baseline vital signs:
  - Just before starting transfusion
  - After the first 15 min of the start of the transfusion
  - Hourly during the transfusion
  - At the end of transfusion
  - 1 hr after completion of the transfusion
  - More frequently during transfusion, if changes or concerns are noted or if required by the facility's policy
- Determine the client's understanding of the procedure.
- Obtain informed consent according to facility's policy.
- Instruct the client to report unusual symptoms immediately.
- Start the infusion slowly:
  - Remain with the client.
  - Observe closely for reactions during the first 15 min.
- After the first 15 min, if the client does not show any signs of a transfusion reaction:
  - Increase the infusion rate to the prescribed rate.
- Monitor the client for reactions throughout the entire transfusion.
- Provide emotional support to the client throughout the transfusion.
- Do not store blood components in the nursing unit or other unmonitored refrigerator.
- Do not keep blood out of a monitored refrigerator for more than 30 min before transfusion is started.
- Do not warm blood unless appropriate tubing and warming equipment is used.
- Do not allow any solution other than 0.9% normal saline to come in contact with the blood component or administration set.
- Never add IV medications to blood or components.
- Never infuse any other IV substance through the same tubing as blood components.
- Immediately stop the infusion and report signs of hemolytic reaction, including circulatory overload, sepsis, febrile reaction, allergic reaction, and acute hemolytic reaction.
- Document all procedures and nursing actions thoroughly, including the absence of untoward signs and symptoms.
- Return empty blood containers to the transfusion service, if this is facility policy. Many facilities discard blood containers according to a specific protocol.
- Never administer a blood component without the appropriate blood filter; change blood tubing and filter according to hospital policy.
- Do not transfuse a single unit of blood for more than 4 hr.

cells are given to clients with anemia who do not need increased circulating blood volume.

Platelet concentrates are used to prevent or to resolve bleeding caused by thrombocytopenia or for active bleeding disorders, such as disseminated intravascular coagulation (**DIC**).

Fresh frozen plasma (**FFP**) contains unconcentrated plasma with clotting factors. It can be used to produce various derivatives and may be used to supplement infusions of packed RBCs or for some bleeding disorders, such as DIC.

Serum albumin is a plasma protein that can be given in concentrated, small amounts to increase colloidal osmotic pressure by pulling interstitial fluids ("third-spaced fluids") into the intravascular compartment. Albumin is used to treat *hypovolemic shock* (low blood volume) or to replace albumin lost because of burns or kidney damage.

Cryoprecipitates are collected from fresh plasma that has been frozen and thawed. They contain factor VIII and other clotting factors that are used to treat hemophilia and other clotting disorders.

Plasmapheresis or *apheresis* is the separation and removal of specific components of blood. The remainder of the blood is returned to the client at the time of separation. Platelets are often collected by apheresis because a larger amount of the platelets from a single donor can be collected than by separating platelets from a unit of whole blood.

Immunoglobulins (**Ig**), a family of proteins that act as antibodies, include IgA, IgD, IgE, IgM, and IgG. IgG is the principal immunoglobulin in human serum. IgG is collected from multiple donors and may be given to a person who has been recently exposed to an infectious disease, such as hepatitis. IgD is the major component of RhoGAM, which is used to prevent erythroblastosis fetalis.

Immunoglobulins (antibodies) are a form of passive immunity because their effects are not permanent. Most immune globulins are given IM, except for one form, IV immune globulin.

Blood Administration

The first 10–15 min of a transfusion are the most critical, and the client must be monitored very carefully during this time. Note that if a major ABO incompatibility exists, the client will usually experience a severe reaction during the first 50 mm of transfusion. Therefore, take the client's baseline vital signs before the procedure, begin the transfusion very slowly, and observe the client carefully for the first 15 min. See In Practice: Data Gathering in Nursing 82-2 for major

IN PRACTICE
DATA GATHERING IN NURSING 82-2: Blood Transfusion Reactions

Possible signs and symptoms (changes from pretransfusion data):

General
- Fever (rise of 2 °F [1 °C])
- Chills
- Shaking muscle aches, flank pain
- Back pain, chest pain
- Headache
- Pain at site of infusion or along vein

Integumentary System
- Rashes, urticaria (hives), swelling, itching
- Diaphoresis (sweating)
- Oozing at surgical site

Nervous System
- Apprehension, impending sense of doom
- Tingling, numbness

Cardiovascular System
- Change in heart rate (slower or faster)
- Change in blood pressure (lower, raised, shock)
- Changes in peripheral circulation (cyanosis, facial flushing, cool/clammy, hot/flushed/dry, edema)
- Bleeding (generalized, oozing at surgical or transfusion site)

Respiratory System
- Increased or decreased respiratory rate
- Dyspnea (painful or difficulty breathing)
- Cough, wheezing, rales

Gastrointestinal System
- Nausea, vomiting
- Pain, abdominal cramping
- Diarrhea (may be bloody)

Urinary System
- Changes in urine volume (less, none)
- Changes in urine color (dark, concentrated, shades of red/brown/amber)

---

signs and symptoms of a transfusion reaction. If any of these occur, follow the guidelines of the healthcare facility (also see In Practice: Nursing Care Guidelines 82-2).

IN PRACTICE
NURSING CARE GUIDELINES 82-2: Managing a Transfusion Reaction

If a transfusion reaction occurs,
1. Stop the transfusion immediately.
2. Keep the IV open with 0.9% normal saline.
3. Report the reaction to both the transfusion service and the attending healthcare provider immediately.
4. Do clerical check at the client's bedside: identification band, blood bag, and accompanying materials.
5. Treat symptoms per healthcare provider's order and monitor vital signs.
6. Send blood bag with attached administration set and labels to the transfusion service.
7. Collect blood and urine samples and send to the laboratory.
8. Document all procedures and nursing actions thoroughly on transfusion reaction form and in the client's chart.

Nursing Alert Both mild and life-threatening reactions have similar symptoms. Therefore, consider every symptom as potentially serious. Discontinue the transfusion until the cause of the symptom can be determined.

HEMATOPOIETIC STEM CELL TRANSPLANTATION

Stem cell transplantation is a life-saving medical procedure that has been in use for many decades to treat diseases of the blood and bone marrow and certain cancers, such as leukemia or multiple myeloma. Formerly, only bone marrow was used for *bone marrow transplantation* (**BMT**). Only in selected cases is it still necessary to use bone marrow for stem cell collection. Currently, the goal is to use *pluripotential hemopoietic* stem cells, which provide the client with healthy *stem cells* (immature blood cells). Pluripotential hemopoietic stem cells are very young cells that have the potential to develop into a variety of different types of mature cells that can perform different actions. The process of using these cells for treatment is called *hematopoietic stem cell transplantation* (**HSCT**). HSCT is commonly used in leukemias and lymphomas (see Chapters 72 and 83).

Using specific growth factors, stem cells are derived and developed from bone marrow, umbilical cord blood, amniotic fluid, and peripheral blood stem cells (**PBSCs**). PBSCs are obtained by *apheresis* (removal through a large vein of blood that is then sent via tubing through special collection filters in a machine). Cancerous cells are treated or destroyed. The stem cells are harvested (collected), placed in frozen storage, and then reinfused into the client when needed.

Sources for bone marrow may be the client (*autologous*), a twin (*syngeneic*), or any other person (*allogeneic*). Donated bone marrow is matched to the tissues of the client's human leukocyte-associated (**HLA**) antigen on the surface of the client's WBCs. The stem cells that are in the bone marrow of an individual with cancer are commonly damaged by the types of therapies used to treat the abnormal cells, especially chemotherapy and radiation. The client receives the donated bone marrow after receiving chemotherapy and/or radiation. Preliminary results may be seen in 2–4 weeks. However, complete recovery with successful transplants may take 6 months to a year.

Stem cell recipients may experience complications associated with high-dose chemotherapy (called *ablative* or *myeloablative* treatment) that is administered before the actual transplant. Currently, some clients receive less chemotherapy and radiation before the transplant (called nonmyeloablative) or "mini" transplant. The goal of the pretransplant chemotherapy and radiation is to kill any cancer cells and to promote sites for new, noncancerous cells to grow. The most common complication of high-dose therapy is infection or sepsis. This is the result of the elimination of the body's neutrophils (WBCs that fight infection) along with the destruction of cancer cells. The client is generally placed on protective precautions for several weeks until the transplanted bone marrow is producing adequate amounts of WBCs.

The use of the client's own stem cells eliminates the complication of graft-versus-host disease (GVHD), which can occur in clients who receive bone marrow transplants from a donor. In GVHD, the donated bone marrow attacks tissues, such as the liver, skin, and the gastrointestinal (GI) tract. It can occur at any time, as long as years after a transplant. Drugs are given to suppress the risk of GVHD.

NURSING PROCESS

DATA COLLECTION
Carefully observe and monitor the client with a disorder of the blood or lymph. Examine the client's skin for petechiae, bruises, or other evidence of abnormal bleeding. Measure the client's blood pressure and pulse. Obtain a thorough nursing history that includes the client's nutritional status, dyspnea, elimination difficulties, difficulty in walking or moving, and pain. Does the person have frequent infections? Are injuries common? Signs and symptoms in these areas may indicate a blood or lymph disorder.

The data that are gathered establish a baseline for future comparison and determine the presence of suspected blood, lymph, or other disorders. Document and report any changes in this baseline level. Hematologic studies also are important indicators of disease status. Monitor and report abnormal laboratory values to the healthcare provider.

In addition, observe the client's emotional response to the disorder or the disease. Some blood or lymph disorders are chronic, and some are life threatening. What types of assistance does the client require? Do they need counseling? Will the client need assistance to meet daily needs? Will they need home care? Is the client anxious or fearful about the outcome? Do they understand the treatment regimen?

PLANNING AND IMPLEMENTATION
Together, plan with the client, family, and other healthcare team members for effective care that will meet the client's needs. Provide pretest, preoperative, posttest, and postoperative care for the client undergoing procedures such as bone marrow aspiration or HSCT. The client with a blood or lymph disorder may require nursing care that ranges from assistance with some daily activities to total nursing care.

In the case of a chronic, genetic, or fatal disorder, help the client and family to deal with the diagnosis, treatment course, and prognosis. Teach about the disorder, prescribed medications, precautions, and treatments to be conducted in the healthcare facility and at home. The nursing plan of care must meet these needs and include both the client and family.

EVALUATION
Periodically, the entire team evaluates the outcomes of care. Have short-term goals been met? For example, are the client's laboratory test results returning to within normal parameters? Are long-term goals still realistic? Is the client's prognosis the same, or has it changed? Is the client's disease in remission? Is a long-term cure anticipated? Will home care, social services, respite care, or rehabilitation services be necessary? Planning for further nursing care and community services considers the client's prognosis, as well as complications and the response to care given.

HEMATOLOGIC SYSTEM DISORDERS

Red Blood Cell Disorders

Polycythemia
Polycythemia means too many RBCs (erythrocytes) in proportion to blood volume. Hct levels of >55% can indicate polycythemia. There are several types of polycythemia. *Primary polycythemias* such as polycythemia vera and *polycythemia rubra* occur when excess blood cells are produced as a result of existing or acquired abnormalities of hematopoiesis. This process occurs when the bone marrow develops excess amounts of the formed elements, usually RBCs but sometimes WBCs and platelets (thrombocytes). Chapter 23 discusses blood, plasma, and formed elements. Figure 23-1 compares the different types of cells within bone marrow. The high numbers of RBCs, as well as WBCs and platelets, increase the *viscosity* (thickness) of the blood, which causes headaches, anginal (chest) pain, and difficulty breathing as a result of hypoxia and/or occlusions of blood vessels. The client is at risk for thrombosis, emboli, and hemorrhage. Other symptoms include hypertension, vertigo, and enlargement of the liver and/or spleen. Polycythemia can occur at any age, but it increases with age and is generally seen in individuals older than 60 years.

Secondary polycythemia is due to underlying medical problems that cause an overproduction of the enzyme erythropoietin, an important component in regulating RBC production. An overabundance of erythropoietin can lead to an overabundance of RBCs. The reason for the stimulus to increase RBC production is hypoxia. Secondary polycythemia can be related to hypoxic lung diseases such as COPD or the result of living in an elevated altitude. Chronic hypoxia, abnormal RBC structures, and malignant tumors can be the underlying disorders of secondary polycythemia.

Relative polycythemia is a condition in which the concentration or number of RBCs is highly "relative to" the fluid content of the blood. In this type of polycythemia, the client has lost intravascular water but has not lost RBCs in the blood's plasma. Thus, the RBCs numbers are higher in relation to the fluid in which the RBCs are found. This condition may occur with dehydration, which may be due to vomiting, diarrhea, profuse sweating, or, occasionally, with excess use of diuretics. Relative polycythemia is treated by increasing total fluid volume by oral or IV fluid intake.

Diagnosis
Polycythemia is inferred by noting a substantial increase in the number of RBCs or other bone marrow cells, for example, WBCs and platelets. Hct levels (the percentage of RBCs in the total blood volume) will be elevated. Hemoglobin (Hgb, Hb), the iron-rich protein that holds oxygen, is also elevated. Levels of erythropoietin may be abnormal. Bone marrow aspiration and a biopsy can indicate abnormal amounts of blood cells. Certain forms of polycythemia have genetic (but not always inherited) causes; bone marrow analysis may reveal a diagnostic cellular mutation.

Signs and Symptoms
The client may not recognize symptoms, and often the initial problem may be an Hct of greater than 55%. The client may also complain of headaches and vertigo, difficulty hearing, and an inability to concentrate. Physical examination can reveal hypertension and hepatosplenomegaly (enlarged liver and spleen). The client appears dusky red to cyanotic, especially the lips, fingernails, and mucous membranes. Night sweats, itching, and pain in the fingers or toes are common complaints. Hemorrhage, strokes, myocardial infarctions, and deep vein thrombosis can occur.

Treatment
The goal of treatment for primary and secondary polycythemia is to lower the numbers of RBCs. This is generally accomplished by **phlebotomy** (removal of blood through a vein). Oxygen therapy is generally initiated to relieve hypoxia. To reduce blood viscosity, the client may have regularly scheduled phlebotomy blood withdrawals on an outpatient basis. The therapeutic phlebotomy will reduce total RBCs and total blood volume. If the disorder is severe, chemotherapy may be given to suppress bone marrow function, thereby reducing the total numbers of RBCs, WBCs, and platelets. Low-dose acetylsalicylic acid (aspirin) reduces the risk of blood clot formation and may help burning pains that develop in the hands or feet. In addition or in place of phlebotomy, hydroxyurea (Droxia, Hydrea) can be given to suppress bone marrow function. Interferon alpha is sometimes used to stimulate the immune system's ability to decrease production of RBCs.

Nursing Considerations
Nursing considerations relate to the effects of hypoxia on the body's systems. Itching is a common annoying side effect and can be treated by antihistamines and ultraviolet light treatment. SSRIs, which are often used to treat depression, can be effective to reduce or relieve itching. Examples of SSRIs include paroxetine (Paxil) and fluoxetine (Prozac). Client and family teaching should include the awareness of complications of polycythemia, as well as the necessity for regular phlebotomy treatments for the disorder. Dehydration can result in thrombosis. Monitor skin turgor, encourage fluids, and be aware of the levels of RBCs and WBCs.

Anemias
Anemia, one of the most common hematologic problems affecting people of all ages, is defined as a condition of a lower than normal level of hemoglobin and fewer than normal RBCs within the circulation. Anemia is not considered a disease in itself. Rather, it reflects an abnormality in the number, structure, or function of RBCs. Anemia can be a manifestation of many abnormal conditions, such as the following:

- Dietary deficiencies of iron, vitamin B_{12}, and folic acid
- Bone marrow damage as a result of chemotherapy, radiation, or renal disease
- Malignancies
- Chronic infections
- Overactive spleen
- Bleeding from any organ or tract, or bleeding owing to cancer or trauma
- Hereditary disorders (e.g., sickle cell disease, thalassemia)

The incidence of anemia is more common in some underdeveloped countries because of poor nutrition and the presence of parasites that extract blood from the intestines. Studies suggest that older adults experience a higher incidence of anemia. However, the anemia in older adults is not caused by aging alone but by some other underlying cause.

The seriousness of anemia depends on factors, such as its speed of onset, whether it is chronic, and the client's overall health and nutritional status. The more rapidly anemia develops, the more likely it is to be serious.

Signs and Symptoms
Signs and symptoms of anemia relate to the loss of oxygen-carrying capacity, the severity of hypoxia, and the causative factors. In some types of anemia, the symptoms are insidious (develop slowly) (Box 82-1).

Diagnostic Tests
Diagnostic tests include the standard CBC, Hgb, and Hct. The simplest method of diagnosing anemia is by determining the blood's Hgb content. Mild anemia is generally diagnosed when the Hgb drops to 10–12 g per deciliter (g/dL). Severe anemia would be indicated by a drop of Hgb to less than 8 g/dL.

> **Nursing Alert** The common bedside aid known as a pulse oximeter reflects the ability of the RBC to carry hemoglobin, that is, its oxygen-carrying capacity. The pulse oximeter does not reflect the number of RBCs. Thus, in an individual with anemia, the client may have symptoms of hypoxia, such as dyspnea, but the pulse oximeter might read normal. You must take into consideration that the readings of a pulse oximeter may not truly coincide with the severity of dyspneic symptoms.

Box 82-1 Signs and Symptoms of Anemia

- Pallor and hypersensitivity to cold
- Fatigue and exercise intolerance
- Dizziness and weakness
- Symptoms of heart failure
- Gastrointestinal complaints (e.g., indigestion, loss of appetite)
- Jaundice
- Rapid pulse
- Hypotension
- Shortness of breath
- Irritability
- Difficulty sleeping
- Difficulty concentrating
- Menstrual problems; male impotence
- Decreased red blood cells (RBCs), hemoglobin, hematocrit
- Bone pain and sternal tenderness

Iron Deficiency Anemia

Iron deficiency anemia is the most prevalent anemia in all age groups in the world. It results from either an inadequate absorption or an excessive loss of iron. This condition occurs most often in women, young children, and older adults. Primary causes include trauma, excessive menses, bleeding from the GI tract, pregnancy, or a diet that lacks iron. Deficiency caused by faulty eating habits is especially prevalent in the adolescent and elderly populations.

Treatment for iron deficiency anemia includes treating the site of blood loss, increasing dietary iron intake, and introducing supplemental iron (see In Practice: Nursing Care Guidelines 82-3 and In Practice: Nursing Care Plan 82-1).

Hemolytic Anemia

Hemolytic anemia is caused by destruction of RBCs before their normal lifespan of about 120 days. The client will have an increase of immature RBCs (reticulocytes). Manifestations of hypoxemia symptoms relate to the impaired transport of oxygen and include dyspnea and limited exercise tolerance. The cause of hemolytic anemia is related to defects of the cell membrane of the RBC, inherited enzyme defects, certain drugs and toxins, antibodies, or physical trauma. Treatment of this type of anemia relates to diagnosis and to the causative factors. Corticosteroid hormones and splenectomy may also be of benefit.

Acute Hemorrhagic Anemia

Acute hemorrhagic anemia develops after a rapid and often sudden blood loss. Causes of such blood loss include trauma that leads to blood vessel rupture, aneurysm, or artery erosion caused by a cancerous lesion or ulcer.

Severity and prognosis depend on the total blood volume loss. A total blood volume loss of 20% is considered a marked insufficiency. A loss of 30% will cause failure in the circulatory system, coma, and shock. A loss that reaches 40% can be imminently fatal. In hypovolemic shock, the priority concern is related to the client's needs for fluids to sustain blood pressure. Immediate treatment is volume replacement,

IN PRACTICE
NURSING CARE GUIDELINES 82.3 — Administering Iron Supplements

Oral Administration of Iron

- Give liquid forms of iron with a straw. *Rationale: Liquid iron can stain the teeth. Using a straw may help prevent iron from getting on the teeth, avoids discoloring teeth, and minimizes unpleasant taste.*
- If the iron preparation must be given by a dropper, place the dropper on the back of the tongue. Follow this with water or juice. *Rationale: Liquid iron can have an unpleasant taste. The back part of the tongue has fewer taste buds.*
- Give oral iron preparations with meals. *Rationale: Iron is irritating to the gastrointestinal tract; it can have an unpleasant metallic taste and is easier to take if given with food.*
- Mix iron preparation with orange juice, fruit juice, tomato juice, or water. *Rationale: Vitamin C enhances absorption of iron.*
- If the teeth have iron stain, it may be possible to remove the stain by brushing with baking soda (sodium bicarbonate) or hydrogen peroxide 3%. *Rationale: Iron staining may be cosmetically problematic for the individual.*
- Explain to the client that iron will make stools black and might cause constipation. Stool softeners may be prescribed. *Rationale: The client may be alarmed by the black color of stool, as it can seem to be gastrointestinal bleeding. Iron preparations cause constipation, which is averted by stool softeners and mild laxatives.*

Intramuscular Administration of Iron

- After drawing up iron into a syringe, change the needle before administering the drug. *Rationale: Iron staining of the tissues will be minimized.*
- If oral administration is not feasible, administer iron dextran (INFeD) deep intramuscularly, using a 2- or 3-in., 19- or 20-gauge needle, into the upper outer quadrant of the buttock. Never administer IM into the arm or areas of minimal muscle density. *Rationale: Iron staining of the tissues will be minimized.*
- When administering IM, use the Z-track technique, i.e., displace skin laterally prior to injection. *Rationale: The Z-track technique will help avoid injection or leakage of iron into subcutaneous tissue, causing skin staining.*
- If in bed, have the client in a lateral position with the injection site uppermost. If the client is standing, have the individual bear weight on the leg opposite the injection site. *Rationale: Positioning relaxes the muscle prior to injection, which will lessen the chances of injection pain.*

Adapted from materials obtained on the following Websites:
http://www.drugs.com/ppa/iron-dextran.html
https://www.mayoclinic.org/drugs-supplements/iron-supplement-oral-route-parenteral-route/precautions/drg-20070148

IN PRACTICE
NURSING CARE PLAN 82-1: The Client With Iron Deficiency Anemia Who Is Receiving Iron Therapy

Medical History: S.H., a 32-year-old woman, comes to the clinic for a routine visit. During the visit, the client reports a history of heavy menstrual bleeding. CBC reveals a hemoglobin level of 10.1 g/dL and red blood cell (RBC) count of 3.7 million/mm^3. Client is scheduled for a dilation and curettage (D&C) in 2 days. Ferrous sulfate (300 mg) is ordered three times a day.

Medical Diagnosis: Iron deficiency anemia.

DATA COLLECTION/NURSING OBSERVATION

Client's skin is pale, warm, and dry. Mucous membranes and conjunctiva pale. Dietary history reveals adequate intake, although client states, "I'm not a big fan of fruits and vegetables." Client states, "I haven't had to take any medicines except for something for an occasional headache. What is this medication that the doctor has put me on and why?"

NURSING DIAGNOSIS

(Although other nursing diagnoses may be appropriate, a priority nursing diagnosis is addressed below.)

Knowledge deficit related to iron deficiency anemia and iron therapy as evidenced by client's questions.

Planning (Outcomes/Goals)	Implementation (Nursing Actions)	Evaluation
Short-Term Goals		
A. Client identifies reason for iron therapy.	• Monitor the client's current knowledge of iron deficiency anemia and possible causes. • Explore with client the possible factors contributing to development of iron deficiency anemia. *Rationale: Obtaining baseline knowledge provides a foundation for further teaching. Chronic blood loss, such as from excessive menses, and inadequate dietary intake of high-iron foods, such as green leafy vegetables, can contribute to iron deficiency anemia.*	Day 1–1,445 hr Clinic Appointment • Client reports, "I don't eat as many vegetables as I should, and I can see how the loss of blood with my periods would be a problem." • Client to make arrangements with dietician to review nutritional needs. **Goal A currently being met.** **Ongoing client teaching.**
B. Client verbalizes accurate information about iron therapy regimen.	• Review rationale for, and action of, ferrous sulfate. *Rationale: Ferrous sulfate improves red blood cell formation and replaces iron stores.* • Assist client with setting up a schedule for taking iron, based on usual activities. • Encourage client to take the iron 1 hr before or 2 hr after meals or with meals if stomach upset occurs. *Rationale: Assisting the client with scheduling medication aids in promoting compliance. Taking iron on an empty stomach enhances absorption. Taking the medication with food can help to reduce irritation to the gastrointestinal tract.* • Encourage the client to take iron with a citrus food or fluid. *Rationale: The acidity of the citrus food or fluid enhances absorption of the iron.* • Warn client that the iron can cause constipation, and stools may become black and tarry. • Recommend the intake of high-fiber foods to help with constipation. *Rationale: The client needs to be informed of these common side effects to prevent unnecessary anxiety and possible interruption in therapy. High-fiber foods promote peristalsis.*	Day 2–1,030 hr Phone call with office nurse • Client agrees to start oral iron supplements. • Client states, "I'll try before my meals first, but if my stomach gets upset, I'll take the medication with food." • Client able to verbalize appropriate choices for citrus foods and fruits. **Goals A and B met.**

Planning (Outcomes/Goals)	Implementation (Nursing Actions)	Evaluation
Long-Term Goals		
C. Following D&C, client's Hgb and Hct, nutritional changes, and medications maintain stability.	• Determine client's post D&C status. • Client to return in 2 weeks for follow-up testing and examination; has clinic phone number to call in case of problems. **Rationale:** Client will need to state status related to post-op bleeding, signs of fever, pain, or unexpected side effects after procedure. Reassurance and concern about client's condition is important. • Client to notify office if bleeding reoccurs. • Schedule laboratory work for 1 month. **Rationale:** Client will need to understand importance of additional bleeding and follow-up labs.	Day 3–1,015 hr 1 day post D&C—Phone call from office • Immediate post-op D&C laboratory studies for Hgb and Hct are low but improved since initial office visit. • Client states they have made an appointment with dietitian for a consultation. • Client denies significant problems related to taking iron supplements. • Client states they will get next laboratory work in 1 month. **Goal C partially met. Observations continue.**
D. Establish new nutritional needs and lifestyle changes.	• Assist the client with scheduling a return follow-up visit in 2 weeks. **Rationale:** A return visit helps to determine client's compliance with, and effectiveness of, therapy. • Discuss outcome of client's consultation with dietician. **Rationale:** Long-term dietary changes may be difficult to maintain. Reinforcement and encouragement are necessary.	Day 4–1,015 hr 2 weeks post D&C—Office visit • States, "I won't worry if my stool looks black. And I'll eat a salad every day for lunch now." **Goal D in progress.**

often with administration of IV plasma-expanding fluids, such as saline, albumin, or plasma, and transfusions with fresh whole blood. When fluid loss is controlled, the hypoxia resulting from the loss of RBCs must also be treated. Refer back to the earlier sections on "Transfusions of Colloid Solutions" and "Transfusions of Blood and Blood Products."

Chronic Hemorrhagic Anemia

Chronic hemorrhagic anemia is usually the result of conditions such as peptic ulcers, bleeding hemorrhoids, excessive emesis, or cancerous lesions in the GI tract. Chronic blood loss can eventually lead to iron deficiency anemia because available iron sources are depleted.

Treatment usually includes controlling the site of bleeding and replacing lost iron through diet and supplements.

Pernicious Anemia

Pernicious anemia is caused by a lack of a gastric substance called intrinsic factor, which is produced in the stomach. The body needs intrinsic factor to absorb vitamin B_{12} from food in the small intestine. Vitamin B_{12} is necessary for the body's proper absorption and use of iron and for the protection of nerve fibers.

Pernicious anemia generally affects middle-aged and older adults of northern European descent. Juvenile pernicious anemia, a rare congenital disorder in which the stomach secretes abnormal intrinsic factor, generally affects children younger than 10 years.

Pernicious anemia develops slowly; therefore, signs and symptoms are usually severe when a diagnosis is finally made. Early signs and symptoms include infection, mood swings, GI disorders, and cardiac and renal problems. Late classic signs and symptoms include weakness, fatigue, tingling, and numbness of the fingers and feet, sore tongue, difficulty walking, abdominal pain, and loss of appetite and weight.

Dietary modifications alone are ineffective. The client must take vitamin B_{12} (cyanocobalamin) for life, often by injection. Clients cannot take vitamin B_{12} (cyanocobalamin) orally because they lack the intrinsic factor necessary for absorption. Additionally, clients may receive iron supplements, folic acid, and digestants to enhance vitamin metabolism. Sometimes, blood transfusions are also necessary.

Aplastic Anemia

Aplastic anemia or bone marrow depression describes a condition in which the bone marrow is underdeveloped or has failed, resulting in a decrease in RBCs, WBCs, and platelets

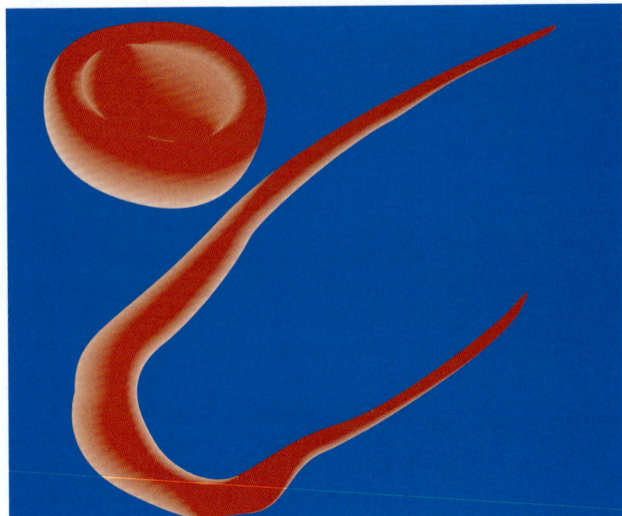

Figure 82-1 A sickled and a normal red blood cell.

(**pancytopenia**). This condition may occur at any age and develop very slowly or be rapid and very severe.

Causes may include excessive radiation, toxicity to various drugs (e.g., chloramphenicol and many anticancer drugs), tumors, insecticides, chemicals, and environmental toxins. It may develop as a complication of viral illnesses, such as hepatitis, human immunodeficiency virus or acquired immunodeficiency syndrome (HIV/AIDS), and mononucleosis. In many cases, the cause is unknown (idiopathic aplastic anemia). Some researchers believe that some cases of aplastic anemia may be autoimmune in origin.

Hematopoietic stem cell transplantation is the most successful therapy. Without transplantation, aplastic anemia has a poor prognosis and a high mortality rate. Prognosis improves dramatically when a stem cell transplant can be done. Antibiotics and transfusions may be given as palliative treatments.

The client with aplastic anemia is extremely susceptible to infection and bleeding. The following measures should be included in nursing care:

- Administer antibiotics per the provider's orders.
- Follow sterile technique in all invasive procedures.
- Handle the client carefully.
- Caution the client to avoid bruises and cuts. **Rationale: This client has a strong bleeding tendency**.
- Avoid taking rectal temperatures.
- Use protective isolation during exacerbations of the disease.

Sickle Cell Disease

Sickle cell disease (**SCD**), also known as *sickle cell anemia*, is a genetic disease in which the person's RBCs become crescent or sickle shaped because of a mutation in the hemoglobin gene. RBCs assume an abnormal, rigid, sickle shape that decreases the cell's ability to carry oxygen and promotes occlusive complications in blood vessels and organs (Fig. 82-1). If an individual has one sickle gene and one normal adult hemoglobin gene, the condition is referred to as *sickle cell trait*. Individuals with sickle cell trait are generally asymptomatic. Sickle cell disease is also discussed in Chapter 72.

Sickle cell anemia develops owing to hypoxemia and damaged RBCs. When sickled RBCs can enter the smaller blood vessels, they become caught, obstructing blood flow. Hypoxia ensues, which in turn causes more sickling. Strokes can occur in children and adults. Ischemia may cause aseptic bone necrosis, osteomyelitis, and renal failure. Severity of these symptoms relates directly to the percentage of abnormal cells (hemoglobin S [Hgb S]).

Sickle cell crisis occurs when the deformed RBCs collect (*aggregate*) in small blood vessels. These occlusions are painful owing to the hypoxic state of the affected tissues. Permanent damage to organs can develop.

Signs and Symptoms

Episodes of acute pain are the most common crisis of sickle cell disease. Main characteristics are severe pain in the abdominal and thoracic areas, muscles, and bones. Also seen are jaundice, dark urine, and a low-grade fever. Severe complications and death can occur (see Box 82-1).

Treatment

The goal of treatment is to prevent sickle cell crisis. Starting at the age of 2 months, children born with sickle cell disease may be required to take antibiotics to treat fever and infections with prophylactic penicillin therapy. Lifelong folic acid is necessary. When anemia or crisis does occur, packed RBC transfusions may be required. Oxygen may be administered to help decrease the pain of ischemia. Some clients may be treated with iron-chelating agents to remove excess iron from the blood and to counteract iron overload. Some *cytotoxic* agents (agents that destroy specific cells) are also used in sickle cell disease.

Nursing Considerations

Keep in mind that the client will have episodes of severe pain; thus, appropriate analgesia is important. Teach the client and family to monitor hydration, rest, and nutrition. Hospitalization may be necessary during a crisis.

Thalassemia

Thalassemia is an anemia characterized by deficient and damaged chains of hemoglobin. The thalassemias consist of two main groups of inherited hemolytic anemias caused by autosomal recessive genes. The two categories are alpha-thalassemia and beta-thalassemia. Depending on the number of genes affected, beta-thalassemia may be classified as either minor or major. As with sickle cell disease, these disorders are associated with geographic areas of ancient endemic malaria.

SPECIAL CONSIDERATIONS — **Culture and Ethnicity**

Thalassemias are found globally. Alpha-thalassemia is most common in people whose ancestry is of Western Africa. Beta-thalassemia has developed from people with Mediterranean, West Asian, and North African ancestry. South Asian people, including those from Cambodia, Thailand, India, Pakistan, and Iran, are also known to have thalassemia or similar pathologies of RBCs. Because of the healthcare, financial, and social aspects of these disorders, some countries require screening policies designed to reduce the incidence of thalassemias.

Signs and Symptoms

The signs and symptoms of anemia are related to the severity of the disease. *Thalassemia minor* does not affect a person's life expectancy. Mild anemias may be noted. The client generally has few changes of RBCs.

Thalassemia major, also known as *Cooley anemia*, is more serious and requires frequent transfusions. Without treatment, signs and symptoms start in infancy; they include fever, failure to thrive, and enlarged spleen. Rapid destruction of RBCs frees large amounts of iron, which can be deposited in the skin, heart, liver, and pancreas. With treatment, the individual's lifespan is two or three decades.

Growth and sexual development are usually impaired. The heart, liver, and pancreas become fibrotic and lose their capability to function. Heart failure may occur. Signs of thalassemia major also include those of other hemolytic anemias (see Box 82-1).

Treatment

Treatment consists of transfusion therapy with packed RBCs. Because these clients receive many transfusions, they are also at risk for iron overload, which is treated with iron chelation. Hematopoietic stem cell transplants offer some clients a cure.

> **Key Concept**
> Because of the seriousness of the diseases, genetic counseling should be considered for *clients who carry the genetic trait for sickle cell disease and thalassemia.*

White Blood Cell Disorders

Neutropenia and Agranulocytosis

Neutropenia, also known as *granulocytopenia*, is a decrease in neutrophils, one of the forms of leukocytes. Severe neutropenia is referred to as *agranulocytosis*, *granulocytopenia*, or *malignant neutropenia*. Agranulocytosis implies severe reductions of basophils and eosinophils, as well as neutrophils.

Neutropenia can be acquired or congenital. Most cases of neutropenia are the result of cytotoxic drugs used in cancer therapy, such as alkylating agents and antimetabolites, which are designed to suppress bone marrow function in clients with types of leukemias and lymphomas. Radiation therapies for cancer can also cause neutropenia.

Drugs other than the antineoplastic drugs can cause toxic idiosyncratic side effects that result in neutropenia. Examples of these drugs include barbiturates, phenothiazine tranquilizers, chloramphenicol, certain antipsychotic drugs, such as clozapine (Clozaril), and sulfonamides.

Idiopathic cases (of unknown cause) of neutropenia may be related to autoimmune disorders in which antibodies react against the normal human leukocyte antigens (HLA) on WBCs.

Agranulocytosis may also be seen in aplastic anemia. Agranulocytosis can develop during the course of another disease or from an overwhelming infection.

Signs and Symptoms

The most common signs and symptoms include respiratory infections. Typically seen are chills, fever, headache, malaise, extreme weakness, and fatigue. Bleeding may occur from ulcerations of the mucous membrane on any part of the GI tract, vaginal areas, or skin.

Treatment

Treatment begins by removing the causative agent. Colony-stimulating factor (**CSF**) may be given to stimulate the production, maturation, and differentiation of neutrophils.

Nursing Considerations

Because WBCs are depleted, the person is more susceptible to infection, especially respiratory infections. Extreme care is necessary to protect this person against exposure to pathogens. Protective isolation precautions may be initiated. Antibiotics may be ordered. If the cause is not a neoplastic disorder, bone marrow function may resume in 2–3 weeks after the cause is eliminated or resolved.

Leukemia

Leukemia is a malignant hematologic disorder of both children and adults that is characterized by an abundance of abnormal WBCs (see Chapter 72, which discusses leukemia with additional details). In leukemia, the factors that normally regulate the process by which cells differentiate and mature are lacking. Leukemias can be diagnosed as acute or chronic. In *acute* forms of leukemia, immature cells proliferate and accumulate in the person's bone marrow. In *chronic leukemia*, apparently mature cells become diseased. The type of leukemia depends on which cell line is affected: *lymphoid* or *myeloid*. With all types of leukemias, abnormal WBCs take over the normal marrow. RBCs and thrombocytes are also affected. The leukemic cells can proliferate and be released into the peripheral blood invading body organs causing metastasis.

In summary, the main types of leukemia are

- Acute lymphoid leukemia (**ALL**) or chronic lymphoid leukemia (**CLL**)
- Acute myeloid leukemia (**AML**) or chronic myeloid leukemia (**CML**)

Signs and Symptoms

Symptoms of leukemia result from anemia, neutropenia, and thrombocytopenia—damage to the RBCs, WBCs, and platelets. They can include fevers, malaise, anorexia, fatigue, bone pain, bruising, and bleeding. Clients also may present with anemia, enlarged lymph nodes, night sweats, shortness of breath, weight loss, tenderness over the sternum and spleen, and liver involvement.

Treatment

Treatments for all forms of leukemia are individual or combined therapies of antineoplastic drugs, radiation, and hematopoietic stem cell transplants.

Nursing Considerations

Symptom management relates to prevention and treatment of infections and anemia and bleeding precautions. Transfusion therapy is common, and thus, the nurse needs to monitor results, such as posttransfusion CBC, Hct, Hgb, and WBC with differential. During and after infusions, be mindful of any adverse side effects of the transfusion. Evaluation and precautions are key elements of preventative nursing care. Clients with leukemia require many treatments, procedures, tests, and frequent hospitalizations. Remember to include the client and family in the plan of care (see In Practice: Educating the Client 82-1). Emotional strain on the client and family is an effect of this disease. Provide therapeutic communication techniques to support the client and family. Refer the client and the family to spiritual leaders, social services, and support groups during the course of the disease and treatment.

> **IN PRACTICE**
> **EDUCATING THE CLIENT 82-1** | **Teaching Topic Areas for Leukemia**
>
> - Signs and symptoms of infection and bleeding
> - Precautions to avoid infections
> - Precautions to prevent tissue damage and bleeding
> - Good mouth care
> - Use of soft toothbrush only
> - Avoidance of constipation
> - Avoidance of aspirin-containing products
> - Good nutrition
> - Avoidance of smoking and alcohol
> - Possible side effects of chemotherapy and other treatment

Platelets and Clotting Disorders

Platelet disorders can include too many thrombocytes (*thrombocythemia*) and too few thrombocytes (*thrombocytopenia*).

Thrombocythemia

In many cases of *thrombocythemia*, also known as essential thrombocytosis, the disease is not diagnosed and may not be treated unless symptoms occur. The overproduction of platelets show laboratory platelet counts greater than 600,000/mm^3 and can be as large as 1 million/mm^3. Causative risk factors include smoking, peripheral vascular disease, atherosclerosis, and the previous formation of thrombi.

Signs and Symptoms
Because the platelets are dysfunctional, hemorrhage and *vaso-occlusion* (obstruction of blood vessels) are the primary concerns.

Treatment
Treatment may be low-dose aspirin therapy alone or in combination with more aggressive medications, such as hydroxyurea (Hydrea), an antineoplastic drug, or anagrelide (Agrylin), which inhibit the maturation of platelets.

Nursing Considerations
Nursing concerns relate to the risks of hemorrhage and the formation of thrombi. Teach the family and client to be aware of warning signs, such as purpura (bruising) and petechiae, bleeding from the nostrils or mouth, and menorrhagia (excessive menses). As with other platelet disorders, minor abrasions, lacerations, or trauma to internal organs can lead to hemorrhagic shock and death. Box 82-2 gives the signs of bleeding.

Thrombocytopenia

Thrombocytopenia, a stem cell disorder of the bone marrow, is diagnosed when a client's platelet count falls below 50,000/mm^3. It is the most common platelet complication of cancer and its treatments. The causes may be unknown (idiopathic) or related to the formation of antibodies against platelets (immune thrombocytopenic purpura). Several types of thrombocytopenia exist, and the names may be used interchangeably.

Idiopathic Thrombocytopenia Purpura
Idiopathic thrombocytopenic purpura (**ITP**) is one type of thrombocytopenia that can develop at any age but tends to occur more often in children and young women. The two forms of the disorder are acute and chronic. The acute form usually occurs in children. *Chronic ITP* is usually diagnosed in adults 20–50 years of age, with a higher incidence in women.

Acute ITP commonly occurs after a viral illness in children. Thus, it may be an autoimmune disorder in which the individual develops antibodies to his or her own platelets. The exact cause of many cases remains unknown. ITP may also accompany HIV infection, malignant disease, systemic lupus erythematosus, hepatitis C, or pregnancy.

Signs and Symptoms
Early signs may include bruises and low platelet counts. *Petechiae* (small hemorrhagic spots in the skin), headache, pain, and swelling, as well as any abnormal bleeding, such as from the nose, gums, and GI and urinary tracts, may be noted (see Box 82-2). The severity of ITP depends on the degree of the thrombocytopenia and the extent of the bleeding.

Treatment
Treatment for ITP is generally corticosteroids. If a drug is the suspected cause (e.g., quinine, heparin), the medication is discontinued. A splenectomy may be done. However, the effects of this surgery tend to be limited and transient.

Intravenous gamma globulin is commonly given for ITP. Some clients who are Rh-positive may receive anti-D antibodies against the D antigen. Platelet transfusions may actually result in a further drop in platelet count, but they may be beneficial to a client who is hemorrhaging.

Nursing Considerations
Nursing considerations are similar to those for all blood and bleeding disorders. Obtain a thorough medication history, including over-the-counter medications, aspirin, and sulfa-containing drugs. Because the client may be on corticosteroids, teaching about tapering down the medication may be indicated. Straining with the passage of stool (*Valsalva maneuver*) and constipation should be avoided. Electric razors and soft toothbrushes should be used. Client and

> **Box 82-2** **Signs of Bleeding**
>
> **SIGNS OF INTERNAL BLEEDING**
> - Restlessness
> - Rapid pulse and a drop in blood pressure
> - Unusual pallor
> - Headache
> - Signs of a stroke
> - Joint pain and swelling
> - Hematuria
> - Hematemesis
> - Blood in the stool
> - Shock
>
> **SIGNS OF EXTERNAL BLEEDING**
> - Purpura (bruising)—with or without known injury
> - Petechiae (small hemorrhagic spots)
> - Epistaxis (nosebleed)
> - Bleeding from the gums, mouth, or tooth extraction
> - Thrombocytopenia (low platelet counts)
> - Menorrhagia (excessive menses)
> - Death

family teaching should include information about determining the client's risk for injury. The client and family need to be aware of the appearance of petechiae, *ecchymosis* (purplish patches), or menorrhagia.

> **Nursing Alert** Because blood does not clot correctly in clients with bleeding disorders, even a slight injury can result in a serious hemorrhage. Watch for signs of internal bleeding, such as unusual pallor, rapid pulse, restlessness, and a drop in blood pressure. Protect these clients against injury.

Disseminated Intravascular Coagulation

Disseminated intravascular coagulation (DIC) is a complex and potentially fatal disorder in which clotting occurs in the microvascular system (small clots inside blood vessels) and, at the same time, hemorrhaging develops. The disorder usually has a rapid onset, further adding to its severity. It is not a disease, but a result of serious defects in clotting mechanisms related to underlying disorders.

Multiple conditions can cause DIC, including shock, acute bacterial and viral infections, septicemia, hemolytic transfusion reactions, tissue damage from trauma or burns, transplant rejections, various cancers, and complications of obstetrics. The mortality rate for DIC is high.

Signs and Symptoms

Symptoms of DIC may include petechiae, ecchymosis, or prolonged bleeding from a venipuncture site. Onset may also include severe and uncontrollable hemorrhage. Laboratory studies typically show very prolonged PT and APTT levels but reduced levels of fibrinogen. Severe thrombocytopenia may be seen.

Treatment

Treatment of DIC involves identifying the underlying cause. Symptomatic treatment involves administration of IV fluids, oxygen, and the administration of various clotting factors and platelets. Fresh frozen plasma, which contains coagulation factors and antithrombotic factors, may decrease bleeding but can adversely promote development of thrombi. Platelets, fibrinogen concentrates, or cryoprecipitate are also given. Anticoagulants, such as unfractionated heparin or low–molecular-weight heparin, may be given. Heparin is usually given to prolong bleeding times. For DIC, which causes hemorrhage, heparin may seem a contradictory treatment. However, as the pathology of DIC progresses, the development of emboli occurs. Heparin can often inhibit the development of microemboli. Emboli can cause massive organ damage, such as a myocardial infarction, stroke, or kidney damage. Successful heparin therapy is noted after an initial, but temporary, worsening of bleeding. Acting as a mechanism to inhibit microemboli, heparin will interfere with the clotting mechanisms of DIC and hemorrhage will decrease. Additional coagulation inhibitors, for example, recombinant activated protein C or antithrombin II, are given in addition to supplemental fluid replacement.

Nursing Considerations

Nursing considerations related to DIC include an awareness of the risk factors. The process of DIC may begin suddenly with little or no warning. Clients at risk will need to be closely monitored for signs and symptoms of bleeding, signs of shock, and the formation of thrombi (e.g., stroke). Nursing care of the client experiencing DIC will vary depending on severity.

Hemophilia

Hemophilia is a sex-linked genetic disorder in which the person's blood is slow to coagulate because of a lack of clotting factor VIII (*hemophilia A* or *classic hemophilia*) or factor IX (*hemophilia B* or *Christmas disease*) in the plasma. About one-third of new hemophilia cases occur without family history of the disease, which suggests new mutations to the gene.

Diagnosis

Almost all affected individuals are males, but females with certain genetic structures may have mild bleeding tendencies. Children with hemophilia are generally healthy but are always at risk for bleeding. Severity of bleeding relates to the level of deficiency of the clotting factor.

Signs and Symptoms

Unchecked bleeding may be severe. In clients with hemophilia, even a pinprick may cause prolonged oozing of blood. Early signs could be epistaxis (nose bleed) or continuous bleeding from a scrape or minor cut. Internal bleeding can manifest as blood in the urine, brain, or joints. The most minor surgical procedure is risky and is usually preceded by a transfusion of the appropriate blood factor (see Box 82-2).

Treatment

Treatment of hemophilia focuses primarily on either prophylaxis (ongoing) therapy or demand (as-needed) infusions. The goal is to increase the amount of clotting factors to prevent bleeding episodes. When a bleeding episode occurs, treatment involves the replacement of the deficient clotting factor. Clotting factors are obtained by isolating them from human blood, developing them using recombination techniques, or a combination of both methods. Clotting factors can be given in the home or at outpatient centers. Medication, such as the manufactured hormone desmopressin, is given by injection or nasal spray for mild to moderate hemophilia.

Nursing Considerations

Nursing considerations include awareness of the potential impact of any tiny cut or bruise. Dental work may require special bleeding precautions. Continuously monitor the family's needs, and include the family in the plan of care. Key areas of teaching include

- Maintenance of safety
- Injury prevention
- Lifestyle changes to meet the client's limitations
- Medication teaching
- Methods of administering factor VIII concentrate at home, if appropriate

> **NCLEX Alert**
>
> Bleeding disorders present challenges to nursing care. NCLEX questions may require that the nurse be aware of early signs of bleeding, including ecchymosis, petechiae, shortness of breath, abnormal hematologic laboratory levels, or increased pulse combined with lower blood pressure readings.

von Willebrand Disease

von Willebrand disease (vWD) is the most common hereditary bleeding abnormality in humans. There are four inherited types of the disease, and it is more common in women than men. This coagulation disorder can be also acquired as a complication of other medical conditions and may be autoimmune related. The disease is a result of a lack of sufficient or poor quality von Willebrand factor, which is required for platelet adhesion.

Diagnosis

Diagnosis is determined by searching for low levels of von Willebrand clotting factor and factor VIII. Clients with vWD typically have prolonged APTT and prolonged bleed time. PT and platelet counts tend to be normal.

Signs and Symptoms

As summarized in Box 82-2, the most common symptoms are various degrees of bleeding. Anemia may accompany the disease (see Box 82-1). Women may manifest menorrhagia (heavy periods) and have excessive blood loss during childbirth. Although internal bleeding and bleeding into the joints are not as common as with other bleeding disorders, they may occur.

Treatment

Generally, the client does not require routine treatment. Some women who routinely have menorrhagia may be prescribed a combined oral contraceptive pill, which may assist in the reduction or frequency of heavy periods. Prophylactic therapy, using factor VIII infusions, may be given before surgery to a client known to have the disease.

Nursing Considerations

Nursing considerations mimic those stated in the hemophilia section above. Any woman of childbearing years needs close monitoring because they may not be aware that they have inherited vWD until after the birth of a child.

Lymphatic System Disorders

Malignant lymphomas are a diverse group of diseases that arise from an uncontrolled proliferation of cellular components of the lymphatic system. The lymphomas are divided into two major groups: Hodgkin lymphoma and non-Hodgkin lymphoma. Clinical manifestations in both types are similar.

Hodgkin Lymphoma

Hodgkin lymphoma, also known as Hodgkin disease (HD), is a malignancy of the lymphatic system. There are four subtypes of Hodgkin lymphoma, but all types include the small vessels called lymphatics, the spleen, the thymus gland, and the bone marrow. Hodgkin lymphoma eventually involves the development of abnormal, cancerous B lymphocytes (or B cells) called Reed–Sternberg cells, which proliferate within the lymph system. B cells are extremely important types of specific lymph cells that fight against antigens (foreign invaders). B cells work with another type of lymph cell, the T cell; T cells are needed to fight infection. The Reed–Sternberg cells grow, eventually spreading beyond the lymphatic system, and thus compromise the body's ability to combat infection. Treated, Hodgkin lymphoma has a high cure rate.

Risk factors include ages between 15 and 34 and older than 55 years. It occurs in all races but is slightly more common in clients who are white. People with a family history and/or environmental exposures and male gender are at increased risk. A compromised immune system (HIV/AIDS, organ transplants) and past Epstein–Barr virus (EBV) infections are also risk factors.

> **Key Concept**
>
> Antigens are invading, foreign molecules that bind with antibodies. Antibodies (immunoglobulins) are specific proteins produced by the immune system. Antibodies combine with antigens by a lock and key mechanism to combat infections.

Diagnosis

Diagnosis is made by a biopsy study showing Reed–Sternberg cells in lymph node tissue. Hodgkin lymphoma studies suggest that it may be related to viral infections and suppressed immune systems. EBV, which causes infectious mononucleosis, also has Reed–Sternberg cells and may be one causative agent. Hodgkin lymphoma may be a result of an autoimmune disorder.

After Hodgkin lymphoma has been diagnosed, *staging*, or determining the extent of disease, must be ascertained.

Computed tomography (CT) scans, positron emission tomography (PET) scans, magnetic resonance imaging (MRI), x-ray examinations, and lymph biopsy assist in diagnosis. As with most cancers, staging will influence the client's treatment decisions. Hodgkin lymphoma spreads in an organized pattern, traveling from one node to another. The criteria for each stage are the numbers of lymph nodes involved, if the lymph nodes are involved on one or both sides of the diaphragm, and the extent of spread of the disease to the bone marrow or liver. Staging is discussed in Chapter 83.

Signs and Symptoms
Painless, enlarged lymph nodes are the most common finding. Progressive, painless lymph node enlargement continues unless the disease is diagnosed and treated. The client will demonstrate low-grade fever, fatigue, night sweats, itching, anemia, and unexplained weight loss. If the disease is allowed to advance, major organs, such as the lungs and liver, the GI tract, and the central nervous system, become involved. The individual becomes unable to fight infections.

Treatment
Treatment for Hodgkin lymphoma generally includes radiation, chemotherapy, or a combination of both. Hematopoietic stem cell transplantation may also be considered treatment, especially in those who have experienced recurrences. The prognosis for Hodgkin lymphoma depends on the disease's stage at diagnosis. Generally, 60%–70% of those who achieve complete remission after treatment will be cured.

Nursing Considerations
Nursing considerations are similar to those for other cancers and are often related to symptomatic relief of the side effects of treatment (e.g., nausea, vomiting, hair loss) (see Chapter 83).

Non-Hodgkin Lymphoma
Non-Hodgkin lymphomas (**NHLS**) are a group of lymphatic neoplasms that include any kind of lymphoma except Hodgkin lymphomas. NHLs are more common than Hodgkin lymphomas and do not have Reed–Sternberg cells (which are diagnostic of Hodgkin lymphoma).

The cause of NHL is unknown, but the disease occurs when abnormal lymphocytosis occurs. These abnormal WBCs grow, divide, and eventually overcome lymph nodes, which is the cause of lymph node swelling. Most NHLs arise from B cells; T cells are also involved, but to a lesser extent. If untreated, these cancerous lymphocytes will invade lymphatic vessels and lymphatic structures, such as the thymus, tonsils, adenoids, spleen, liver, and bone marrow.

Risk factors for NHL include immunosuppressive drug therapy, pesticide exposure, and age older than 60 years. The *Helicobacter pylori* bacteria associated with gastric ulcers and viruses, such as HIV, hepatitis C, and Epstein–Barr, are considered risk factors for NHL.

Diagnosis
Diagnosis for NHL is achieved with lymph node biopsy, bone marrow biopsy, and blood studies. CT scans and nuclear medicine studies may be added to determine the stage of the disease.

Signs and Symptoms
The most common findings in NHL are painless, enlarged lymph nodes in the neck, groin, or armpit. Other symptoms include abdominal discomfort, chest pain, back pain, and GI complaints, all of which result from node enlargement. The client with NHL may also experience night sweats, fever, fatigue, weight loss, coughing, and dyspnea.

Treatment
Chemotherapy, radiation, or a combination of both is the most common form of therapy. Hematopoietic stem cell transplantation may be used. Drugs that are designed to boost the body's immune system, such as the monoclonal antibody drug rituximab (Rituxan), can be beneficial. Other types of the monoclonal antibody drug ibritumomab (Zevalin) or tositumomab (Bexxar) are radioimmunotherapy drugs that allow the antibody to attach to cancer cells and deliver radiation directly to the cancerous cells.

Nursing Considerations
Infections are a primary concern because of the body's decreased immune system. Protective isolation may be necessary if the client is hospitalized. Teaching concerns for the client and family include promoting knowledge about the disease process, treatment options, and the side effects of therapy. As with any cancer, psychosocial issues and emotional support are important concerns.

SPECIAL CONSIDERATIONS Lifespan

Hodgkin Lymphoma and Non-Hodgkin Lymphoma
The older adult with either Hodgkin lymphoma or NHL may experience altered or impaired renal, cardiac, hepatic, or respiratory function caused by the aging process. Remember that many of the treatment options for Hodgkin lymphoma and NHL may also cause impairment of these organs. Monitor these clients carefully. Dose, schedule, or treatment changes and limitations may be indicated.

Multiple Myeloma
Multiple myeloma is a malignant cancer of bone marrow caused by malignant *plasma cells*. Plasma cells are the most mature form of B lymphocytes (B cells). Normally, plasma cells are activated to secrete antibodies (or immunoglobulins). With multiple myeloma, the plasma cells are abnormal and they develop and proliferate in bone marrow. Abnormal plasma cells also cause bone lesions as well as interfere with the development of RBCs, WBCs, and platelets. Without immunoglobulins, which plasma cells should provide, any infection can be life threatening.

Multiple myeloma occurs mostly in the middle-aged to older adult population, affecting males more than females; it is twice as common in the African American population when compared with the European American population. The etiology is unknown, and the onset may be *insidious* (slow). The individual may be without symptoms until the disease is advanced. The survival rate is 3–7 years after diagnosis, depending on the onset of treatment. Infection is the usual cause of death.

Diagnosis

The diagnosis of myeloma is made by the discovery of various classes of paraproteins (special immunoglobulins, such as IgG). Electrophoresis of the blood and urine will typically reveal the paraproteins. Bone marrow biopsy will yield the abnormal plasma cells. Tumors can occur in several sites. MRI, rather than standard x-ray or CT, shows bone lesions best. The mnemonic *CRAB* will reveal the four most common diagnostic symptoms: elevated *C*alcium levels, *R*enal failure, *A*nemia, and *B*one lesions.

Signs and Symptoms

Signs and symptoms can vary greatly, but typical multiple myeloma includes pathologic (or spontaneous) fractures and hypercalcemia with skeletal deformities. Bone pain of the back and ribs are commonly found with bone fractures. Infections include pneumonia and pyelonephritis. Fatigue, confusion, and weakness owing to anemia or hypercalcemia may occur. The hypercalcemia may also lead to excessive thirst, dehydration, constipation, osteoporosis, altered level of consciousness, and coma. Acute or chronic renal failure is possible. In late stages, paraplegia with incontinence of the bladder or bowel may occur.

Treatment

Treatment may include combinations of chemotherapy, corticosteroids, and radiation. Radiation is not effective alone in multiple myeloma because the plasma cells spread. The goal is to minimize proliferation and suppress growth of the abnormal plasma cells. Hematopoietic stem cell transplantation can be helpful in some clients. Palliative medications include erythropoietin to treat anemia and bone reabsorption inhibitors to treat osteoporosis.

Nursing Considerations

Nursing considerations focus on pain management, hydration, and prompt detection of fever or other signs of infection. Client and family teaching will include instructions on activity restrictions (e.g., lifting no more than 10 lb; proper body mechanics). Braces for support are occasionally used. The client generally can control the disease and live a relatively normal lifestyle for many years.

STUDENT SYNTHESIS

KEY POINTS

- The nurse must be aware of the normal and abnormal laboratory values for common tests of RBCs, WBCs, and platelets.
- Transfusions of blood products require careful identification of recipients, infusion techniques, and follow-up monitoring.
- Hematologic system disorders frequently manifest by fatigue, bleeding tendencies, infections, and cardiovascular complications.
- Anemias deprive a person of energy and oxygen to carry out the activities of daily living. Treatment of anemias is designed toward elimination of the causative factor and management of symptoms.
- Sickle cell disease and thalassemia are inherited disorders involving dysfunctional hemoglobin.
- White blood cell disorders affect a person's ability to fight infections.
- Neutropenia is a common side effect of antineoplastic drugs.
- All types of leukemia are generally treated by chemotherapy, radiation, hematopoietic stem cell transplant, or a combination of these.
- Blood disorders affecting clotting factors can cause serious and life-threatening bleeding problems. Bleeding disorders may result from damage to bone marrow by environmental toxins and autoimmune disorders, or as a side effect from chemotherapy.
- A major difference between Hodgkin lymphoma and non-Hodgkin lymphoma is that Hodgkin lymphoma develops Reed–Sternberg cells.
- An older client with the signs and symptoms of back pain with movement, hypercalcemia, and fractures should be tested for multiple myeloma.

CRITICAL THINKING EXERCISES

1. Signs and symptoms of disease relate directly to the pathophysiology and etiology of the disorder. Describe the effect of malfunctions of the five main types of white blood cells (neutrophils, basophils, eosinophils, lymphocytes, and monocytes). Discuss the relationship between low white blood cell counts and infection. Consider why a client with anemia is short of breath. Describe the relationship between osteoporosis and bone pain with hypercalcemia and spontaneous fractures. What are the presenting symptoms when a client does not have enough platelets or clotting factors?

2. A child with hemophilia has told you that their parent will not allow them to be involved in any extracurricular school activities. The child is angry and asks that you try to convince their parent otherwise. How would you handle this situation? What would you discuss with the mother and the child? Describe how you would include and support the mother in the plan of care.

NCLEX-STYLE REVIEW QUESTIONS

1. The nurse monitors a client's white blood cell count and observes an increase from 7,500/mm³ to 18,000/mm³. What does this increase indicate for the client?
   a. An infection
   b. Anemia
   c. Leukemia
   d. Bleeding disorder

2. A client taking warfarin sodium (Coumadin) for anticoagulation therapy has an increased INR with bleeding and hemorrhage. Which medication should the nurse anticipate administering?
   a. An antibiotic
   b. Protamine sulfate
   c. Heparin sodium
   d. IM vitamin K

3. The nurse is caring for a client with primary polycythemia. Which data obtained by the nurse should be immediately reported to the primary care provider?
   a. Dry cough
   b. Increase in urine output
   c. Report of no bowel movement for 2 days
   d. Pain in the calf

4. The nurse is reinforcing discharge instructions for parents of a child with hemophilia. Which statements made by the parents demonstrate understanding of the care? Select all that apply.
   a. "I will make sure he wears a helmet and protective gear when riding a bike."
   b. "I will sign my son up for the football team so that he can do what others do."
   c. "I will administer factor VIII at home if needed for bleeding."
   d. "I will make sure my child adheres strictly to a low-protein diet."
   e. "Swimming would be an appropriate activity for my child."

5. A client diagnosed with iron deficiency anemia is to begin iron supplementation. Which information would the nurse provide the client regarding therapy? Select all that apply.
   a. If the medication makes you constipated, discontinue and inform the primary care provider.
   b. If you forget a dose, double up when you remember to take it.
   c. Eat food with increased fiber content.
   d. Stools may be black and tarry.
   e. Take iron with citrus food or fluid.

CHAPTER RESOURCES

Enhance your learning with additional resources on the Point!

Student Resources related to this chapter can be found at **thePoint.lww.com/Rosdahl12e**.

83 Cancer

Learning Objectives

1. Describe the differences among carcinomas, sarcomas, leukemias, lymphomas, and myelomas.
2. List the most common sites of cancer in men and women in the United States.
3. State ways a client can assist with cancer prevention.
4. Define the following tumor markers: enzymes, cancer antigens, oncofetal proteins, hormones, genes, and miscellaneous markers.
5. Identify the noninvasive diagnostic procedures used to detect cancer and the four main modalities for cancer treatment.
6. Identify nursing considerations related to each of the following surgical techniques: incisional biopsy, excisional biopsy, cryosurgery, electrocauterization, fulguration, en bloc resection, exenteration, laser surgery and PDT, prophylactic and palliative surgery, and HSCT.
7. Compare and contrast the following biotherapy techniques: MOAB, IFN, CSF, IL, and retinoids. State the nursing considerations related to each technique.
8. Differentiate external radiation therapy from brachytherapy, and discuss the nursing considerations related to each procedure.
9. State the five main categories of chemotherapeutic agents. Identify concerns related to the safe administration of chemotherapeutic medications and safety considerations related to exposure to radiation.
10. Discuss the nursing considerations related to the following common side effects of cancer therapy: nausea and vomiting, stomatitis, fatigue, alopecia, secondary infections, pain, stress, and hormone therapy.

Important Terminology

adjuvant therapy
anaplastic cell
antineoplastic
apoptosis
benign
biopsy
biotherapy
blastoma
cachexia
cancer
carcinogen
carcinogenesis
carcinoma
chemotherapy
cryosurgery
cytology
differentiation
electrocauterization
fulguration
histology
immunotherapy
leukemia
lymphomas
malignant
melanomas
metastasis
myelomas
myelosuppression
neoplasm
oncogene
oncology
remission
replication
sarcoma
stomatitis
undifferentiated, poorly differentiated
xerostomia

Acronyms

AFP
BMT
BRM
CA
CEA
CSF
HCG
HGF
HSCT
IFN
IL
LITT
MOAB, MoAb
PCA
PDT
PIC
PICC
PSA
TNM

Oncology is the medical specialty concerned with cancer and its treatment. A nurse who works with clients with cancer is an *oncology nurse*. Treatment of cancer also can involve medical and surgical oncology specialists. Closely associated with these specialties is the *radiation oncologist*, who administers radiation therapy.

Clients may be seen and treated in many areas, including specialty care units of large hospitals or cancer specialty hospitals where nurses and healthcare providers focus on the prevention, management, and treatments of cancer. Clients may also be cared for in community hospitals, long-term care facilities, and at home. Hospice care for the terminally ill client may be done at home, in an acute care facility, or in special hospice care facilities.

CANCER DEVELOPMENT

Cancer is characterized by excessive growth (*proliferation*) of cells that lack the capabilities of normal cellular function (see Chapter 15). Unlike normal cells, cancerous cells have the abnormal ability to divide uncontrollably, to proliferate (spread), to infiltrate neighboring, normal cells, and to destroy existing cells and tissues. The development of cancer can occur in any tissue at any age. Although some cancers affect only the young, the adolescent, or the young adult, the overall incidence of cancer increases with age. Cancer ranks among the top three causes of death.

Signs and Symptoms

Cancer has many signs and symptoms that are similar (e.g., fatigue and pain). The most common signs and symptoms of cancer are found in Box 83-1. Carcinomas affect the parenchymal (functional) tissues of an organ; therefore, the most specific signs or symptoms typically include problems in the area where the cancer originates. For example, pancreatitis symptoms will appear as fever, pain, and weight loss, but will also cause the individual to have specific difficulties with food digestion. Some cancers, such as cancer of

> **Box 83-1 Signs and Symptoms of Cancer**
>
> Typical signs and symptoms of cancer include the following:
> - Fatigue
> - Unexplained weight loss
> - Fever
> - Pain
> - Sores that do not heal (e.g., mouth sore, genital lesions)
> - Leukoplakia (white patches inside mouth or white spots on the tongue)
> - Cough or hoarseness that does not go away
> - Dysphagia (difficulty swallowing) or indigestion
> - Changes in the skin (e.g., jaundice, erythema, pruritus, hyperpigmentation)
> - Changes in a wart, mole, or freckle (e.g., color, size, shape)
> - Changes in bladder function (e.g., frequency, hematuria)
> - Changes in bowel function (e.g., diarrhea, long-term constipation, size of stool)
> - Unusual bleeding in sputum, stool, urine, nipple, or vagina
> - Lump or thickening in breast, testicle, lymph nodes, or soft tissues

the ovaries and stomach, may have very few symptoms until they have metastasized, invading tissues that will produce symptoms.

Tumors

Tumors or **neoplasms** are growths that arise from normal tissues. (The terms *tumor* and *neoplasm* are interchangeable.) Not all cancers form tumors. Leukemia is an example of a cancer that does not form tumors. A tumor may be benign or malignant.

Benign tumors, although generally not life threatening, can cause serious problems. In cases where benign tumors push against normal tissues, they can threaten vital structures and functions. The following characterize benign neoplasms:

- Slow growth
- *Encapsulated* (contained within a fibrous cover)
- Composed of *differentiated* cells (resemble the cells of the tissue from which they develop)
- Lack **metastasis** (invasion of other tissues in the body)

Malignant tumors have different characteristics of growth; they also invade neighboring tissues. Malignant neoplasms are characterized by the following:

- Rapid growth with uncontrolled, progressive **replication** (reproduction).
- Nonencapsulated, infiltrating and invading other tissues.
- Composed of **anaplastic** (**undifferentiated**, **poorly differentiated**) cells (cells that do not have normal structure or function). The anaplastic cells of malignant tumors lack orderly growth and arrangement and do not function like the normal tissue cells from which they derive.
- Commonly metastasized, sending the abnormal cells to secondary sites via blood vessels or lymphatic vessels. Secondary sites will also eventually grow into malignant tumors.

Types of Cancer

There are over 100 types of cancer, which are categorized through the study of tissues or **histology**. Several general categories are discussed below. The most common types of cancers for males are cancers of the prostate, colon and rectum, and skin (i.e., melanoma). The most common forms of cancers in women include breast cancer, uterine corpus, also known as endometrial cancer, and colon and rectal cancer. The percentage of Americans with a history of cancer has increased, but this is due to the fact that individuals are living longer and the aging population is higher than in previous generations. Survival rates have improved as a result of the wider variety of drugs, improvements in surgical interventions, and the ability to radiate cancerous cells with precision. See Figure 83-1 for a summary of the top 10 types of cancer showing the 5-year survival rate for each type.

Carcinomas (**CA**) are the largest group of cancers. Nearly 80%–90% of all malignancies are carcinomas. These solid tumors develop from epithelial tissues that line skin, glands, gastrointestinal (GI), urinary, and reproductive organs. Examples of carcinomas include gastric adenocarcinoma, hepatomas, adenocarcinomas of the colon, and carcinomas of the glands, such as the thyroid, adrenals, breast, pancreas, and prostate. **Melanomas** are the most dangerous type of skin cancer, which originate in the pigment-producing melanocytes of the skin. Ultraviolet radiation from the sun or tanning beds causes genetic changes that promote the skin cells to multiply rapidly, forming tumors that can sometimes resemble moles.

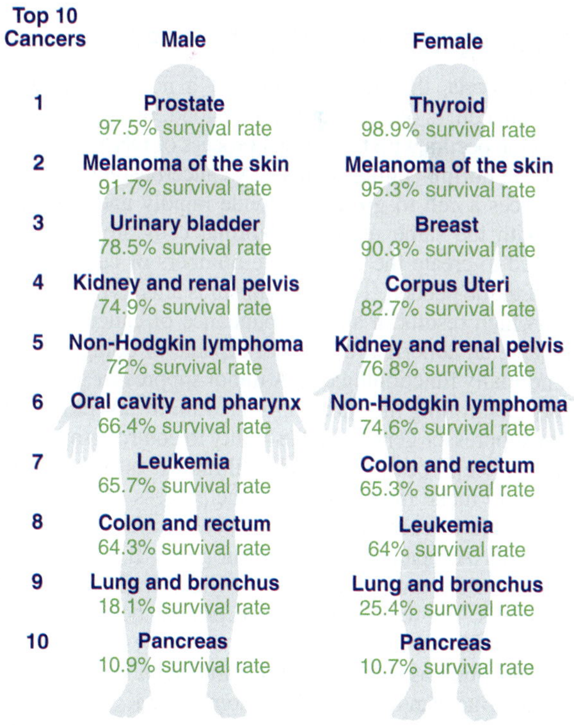

Top 10 Cancers	Male	Female
1	Prostate 97.5% survival rate	Thyroid 98.9% survival rate
2	Melanoma of the skin 91.7% survival rate	Melanoma of the skin 95.3% survival rate
3	Urinary bladder 78.5% survival rate	Breast 90.3% survival rate
4	Kidney and renal pelvis 74.9% survival rate	Corpus Uteri 82.7% survival rate
5	Non-Hodgkin lymphoma 72% survival rate	Kidney and renal pelvis 76.8% survival rate
6	Oral cavity and pharynx 66.4% survival rate	Non-Hodgkin lymphoma 74.6% survival rate
7	Leukemia 65.7% survival rate	Colon and rectum 65.3% survival rate
8	Colon and rectum 64.3% survival rate	Leukemia 64% survival rate
9	Lung and bronchus 18.1% survival rate	Lung and bronchus 25.4% survival rate
10	Pancreas 10.9% survival rate	Pancreas 10.7% survival rate

Figure 83-1 Top 10 cancers and 5-year relative survival rate in the United States, 2011-2017. (Howlader N, Noone AM, Krapcho M, Miller D, Brest A, Yu M, Ruhl J, Tatalovich Z, Mariotto A, Lewis DR, Chen HS, Feuer EJ, Cronin KA. (Eds). *SEER Cancer Statistics Review, 1975-2018, National Cancer Institute.* Bethesda, MD. https://seer.cancer.gov/csr/1975_2018/, based on November 2020 SEER data submission, posted to the SEER web site, April 2021.)

Sarcomas develop from connective or supportive tissues, such as cartilage, bone, adipose, muscle, bone marrow, lymph vessels, and blood vessels. Connective tissue tumors include the gliomas and neuroblastomas of the brain, as well as osteosarcoma, Ewing sarcoma, and leiomyosarcoma.

Leukemia is a cancer that originates in hematopoietic (blood-forming) tissue, such as bone marrow. Bone marrow is the main site of development of white blood cells (WBCs), red blood cells (RBCs), and platelets. Abnormal amounts and growth of the WBCs will enter blood and blood vessels. Leukemia has a variety of subtypes. In general, *acute* forms develop from proliferating young WBCs and *chronic* forms develop from diseased, mature WBCs. Leukemia is also categorized according to the specific differentiation of WBCs: *lymphoid* or *myeloid*. Further discussion of leukemia is found in Chapters 72 and 82.

Lymphomas and **myelomas**, which are cells that originate in the immune system, are the most common of the hematopoietic cancers. *Lymphomas* (from *lymphocyte,* one type of WBC) are a malignancy of either B cells or T cells. Burkitt lymphoma, Hodgkin lymphoma, and non-Hodgkin lymphoma are examples. *Myelomas* (from *myelo,* for bone marrow) are cancers of the plasma cells (mature forms of B cells). Multiple myeloma is an example.

Blastoma or *blastic tumors* are malignant tumors of immature or embryonic tissue. Many of these tumors are found in children. Blastomas derive from precursor cells, also known as blasts, meaning that the tumor has primitive, poorly differentiated cells. Examples include nephroblastomas, medulloblastomas, and retinoblastomas; that is, kidney, brain, or eye tumors.

Carcinogenesis and Carcinogens

Carcinogenesis, the transformation of a normal cell into a malignant cell, is only partially understood. It is known that a disruption occurs with the normal process of DNA replication occurring during cellular mitosis. A cancerous genetic mutation forces a cell to grow and divide rapidly and make new cells with the same mutation. Normal cells are genetically designed to create the appropriate numbers of cells for each type of tissue needed. This mechanism is altered in cancerous cells, which results in an overabundance of cancerous cells. Typically, an abnormal cell is not capable of doing the work of a normally functioning cell. A tumor suppressor gene is the genetic controlling mechanism for growth. In cancerous cells, tumor suppressor genes lose the ability to control growth. The cancerous cells proliferate and infiltrate. It is also possible for cells to make mistakes during the process of growth and development of each cell. Normally, cells have the capability to make DNA repairs via DNA repair genes. If a repair is not corrected, more errors can develop, which means more cancerous cells. The remaining normal cells can become overrun with the damaged cells. The functions that these normal cells would do, such as fight infection, carry nerve transmissions, or make urine, can no longer be accomplished.

Carcinogens are agents that cause damage to cellular DNA that leads to the development of cancer. At least 90% of cancers in the United States are caused by tobacco, viruses, alcohol, diet, obesity, lack of exercise, or environmental factors. Environmental pollutants include chemicals, radiation, and asbestos. Chronic irritation can predispose an individual to carcinogenesis.

Box 83-2 Types of Carcinogens

Chemical carcinogens are found in the environment.
- Hydrocarbons found in cigarettes, cigars, and pipe smoke
- Automobile exhaust, industrial chemicals, and asbestos
- Insecticides, dyes, and hormones

Radiation (a form of energy) can cause DNA damage and cellular mutations.
- Sunlight, x-rays, and radioactive materials
- Ultraviolet (UV) light radiation

Oncogenic viruses and retroviruses are the causative agents of cancer caused by DNA or RNA within viruses.
- Retrovirus of human immunodeficiency virus (HIV), which causes Kaposi sarcoma.
- Human T-cell leukemia virus (HTLV) is related to HIV and causes a form of adult leukemia.
- Human papillomavirus (HPV) can cause cervical cancer.
- Epstein–Barr virus, which is the cause of infectious mononucleosis, can also cause Burkitt lymphoma.

Key Concept

Viruses cause 15%–20% of all cancers. Viruses have the ability to cause cancer by integrating viral DNA into the host cell's DNA which will alter the capabilities of the host cell. Examples of viruses and cancer: Epstein–Barr virus and Burkitt lymphoma; hepatitis B and liver cancer; human papillomaviruses and cervical cancer.

In addition to carcinogens, oncogenetic and genetic causes are known. DNA can carry a cancer-causing gene called an **oncogene**, a piece of DNA that can cause normal cells to become abnormal malignant cells when they are activated by a mutation. Certain types of colon cancer and lymphomas are caused by genetically mutated oncogenes. RNA viruses are called *retroviruses* (see Box 83-2).

Heredity can cause the transfer of defective DNA through the sperm or egg cells. Through genetic screening, individuals can be tested for inherited cancer-causing genes. Inherited genes are implicated in the formation of some breast and ovarian cancers, *retinoblastoma* (retinal tumor), and Wilms tumor.

Cancer Grading and Staging

The place where cancer starts is called the *primary site*. *Cancer* in situ refers to tumor cells that have not invaded surrounding sites. Metastatic sites are called *secondary sites* or *secondary lesions*. Cancer may spread through the body by extending directly into nearby tissue or into a body cavity, such as the abdomen or chest. Secondary sites can also occur when cancerous cells travel through blood vessels or the lymphatic system from the primary site to other body parts, especially the lungs, bones, brain, and liver.

To assist in the diagnosis and treatment of cancer, classifications were developed to categorize the extent of cancer. The histologist looks for differentiation. A normal cell is well differentiated, containing the normal structures of typical, mature cells of a type of tissue.

Grading is a system of looking at abnormal cells under a microscope to determine the cells' degree of dedifferentiation

> **Box 83-3 General Classifications of Cancer Staging**
>
> STAGE I: The disease is limited to a single node or single extralymphatic site.
> STAGE II: The disease involves more than a single node but is confined to one side of the diaphragm.
> STAGE III: The disease is present both above and below the diaphragm.
> STAGE IV: The disease has extended to one or more extralymphatic organs or tissues.

or lack of maturity. Generally, a system of three to five grades is used. *Grade I* tumors closely resemble normal cells or well-differentiated cells. They retain much of their differentiation as specific tissue cells. *Grade II* or *III* tumors have intermediate phases of differentiation, ranging from slightly undifferentiated to extremely abnormal cells. *Grade IV* or *V* tumors are very anaplastic or poorly differentiated, often having little or no resemblance to the tissue cells from which they developed. Clients with a grade I tumor have a better *prognosis* (probable outcome) than do clients with higher grade tumors. Healthcare screening can be done as a detection and early prevention measure. Several types of tests are available for cervical testing, such as the Papanicolaou (Pap) test of uterine cervical cells. The Pap test has three general categories:

- Negative for intraepithelial lesion or malignancy
- Epithelial cell abnormalities
- Other malignant neoplasms

Staging is a method used to identify the spread of a tumor. Cancers are commonly segregated, or staged, based on the extent of disease spread away from the primary tumor site. The healthcare provider's prognosis or plan of treatment often depends on the progression of the tumor over time; that is, how extensive the spread of the tumor (metastasis) is (Box 83-3).

The tumor, node, and metastasis system is called the **TNM** system of staging. Subdivisions of the TNM system are used to designate the size and degree of involvement of each category, using a range from 0 to 4 or A to D. For example, a staging of $T_3N_4M_1$ would indicate a fairly large tumor with spread to distant nodes and distant metastasis. A tumor that is staged as $T_1N_0M_0$ is a small tumor without node involvement or metastasis.

Incidence and Risk Factors

Cancer, heart disease, and stroke are the top three major causes of adult deaths in the United States. Cancer can be diagnosed at any age, but occurrence increases as an individual ages. Therefore, most cancers affect adults of middle age or older. An individual can have genetic or acquired cancers. Inherited risk factors are a result of an individual's family medical history passed from one generation to the next. Acquired cancer can result from exposure to tobacco, secondhand smoke, alcohol, or unsafe sex. Chemicals can affect cellular mitosis and are a major cause of tobacco and secondhand smoke-related cancers. Exposure to asbestos and benzene are known risk factors for cancer. Radiation can involve exposure to the sun, that is, sunburns or occupational exposure to radioactive substances. Assorted health conditions raise the risks of cancer development, for example, ulcerative colitis or the human papillomavirus (HPV). Some cancers, such as HPV, have a vaccine which is effective in the prevention of many types of sexually transmitted cancers caused by HPV.

> **Key Concept**
>
> Many types of cancer are preventable since they are due to lifestyle choices such as smoking and tobacco use, poor diet, and physical inactivity. About 80% of the cases of lung cancer are due to smoking and tobacco.

Prevention and Early Detection

Lifestyle changes and early detection are of primary importance in the promotion of health and the prevention of deaths from cancer. Major emphasis on the reduction of cancer risks includes the following activities:

- Cessation of smoking and the use of smokeless tobacco (chewing tobacco) produces
- Changes in dietary habits
- Reduction in total dietary fats and calories
- Reduction of intake of red meat, salt-cured, or nitrate-containing foods
- Reduction of alcohol intake
- Increase in intake of fiber, fruits, and vegetables
- Reduction of exposure to sun
- Avoidance of artificial sources of ultraviolet light (tanning booths)
- Performance of self-examinations for breast and testicular cancer
- Healthcare screening and examinations for prostate and colorectal cancer (Box 83-4)
- Maintenance of an exercise regimen
- Improvement in educational strategies for cancer prevention

DIAGNOSTIC TESTS

Cytology

Cytology is the study of cells. A cytologic examination is done on sputum, bronchial washings, vaginal and cervical secretions, prostatic secretions, pleural secretions, and gastric washings. Cytology is less accurate than biopsy, but it has proven diagnostic value, particularly in cervical cancer. The test most frequently used to detect cancer of the cervix and uterus is the Pap test.

> **Key Concept**
>
> The Pap test is an important part of the physical examination of every woman who is older than 20 years or who is sexually active.

Laboratory Tests and Blood Studies

Many laboratory tests and blood studies help to diagnose cancer. Some malignancies can alter the blood's chemical composition, showing specific changes directly caused by the cancer. Healthcare providers may begin analysis for cancers by evaluating the results of routine tests, such as blood chemistries (e.g., enzymes, blood glucose, sodium,

Box 83-4 Cancer Screening Guidelines

BREAST CANCER
- Yearly mammograms starting at the age of 40–44 years (depending upon source of recommendation)
  - Women aged 40–54 years should receive an annual mammogram
  - Women aged 55 years and older may receive a mammogram every 2 years or continue to receive an annual mammogram
- Clinical breast examination (CBE) every 3 years for women in their 20s and 30s; every year for women of age 40+ years
- Breast self-examination (BSE) starting in the 20s
- Women at increased risk (e.g., family history, genetic tendency, past breast cancer) may start mammography screening earlier, have additional tests (e.g., breast ultrasound or magnetic resonance imaging [MRI]), or have more frequent examinations

American Cancer Society, 2020 Breast Cancer Screening Guidelines.

COLON AND RECTAL CANCER
Beginning at the age of 45 years, adults should follow one of these testing schedules:

Tests That Find Polyps and Cancer
- Flexible sigmoidoscopy every 5 years,[a] or
- Colonoscopy every 10 years, or
- Double-contrast barium enema every 5 years,[a] or
- Computed tomography (CT) colonography (virtual colonoscopy) every 5 years[a]

Tests That Primarily Find Cancer
- Yearly fecal occult bold test (gFOBT)[b], or
- Yearly fecal immunochemical test (FIT) every year[b], or
- Stool DNA test (sDNA), every 3 years

Risk Factors to Consider
- A personal history of colorectal cancer or adenomatous polyps
- A strong family history of colorectal cancer or polyps (cancer or polyps in a first-degree relative [parent, sibling, or child] younger than 60 years or in two first-degree relatives of any age)
- A personal history of chronic inflammatory bowel disease
- A family history of a hereditary colorectal cancer syndrome (familial adenomatous polyposis or hereditary nonpolyposis colon cancer)

American Cancer Society Screening Guidelines for Colorectal Cancer, 2020.

CERVICAL CANCER
- Beginning by the age of 21 years (women younger than 21 years should not be tested).
- Women between the ages of 21 and 29 years should have a Pap test performed every 3 years, and human papillomavirus (HPV) testing should not be used in this age group unless needed after an abnormal Pap result.
- It is preferred that women between the ages of 30 and 65 years should have a Pap test plus an HPV test (called "co-testing") done every 5 years. Also acceptable to have a Pap test alone every 3 years.
- Women older than 65 years who have had regular cervical cancer testing with normal results should not be tested for cervical cancer. Once testing is stopped, it should not be started again.
- Women with a history of a serious cervical precancer should continue to be tested for at least 20 years after that diagnosis, even if testing continues past the age of 65 years.
- Women who have had a total hysterectomy (removal of the uterus and cervix) may choose to stop having cervical cancer screening, unless the surgery was done as a treatment for cervical cancer or precancer.

American College of Obstetricians and Gynecologists Screening Guidelines for Cervical Cancer (2018).

ENDOMETRIAL (UTERINE) CANCER
- At the time of menopause, women should report any unexpected bleeding or spotting to their doctors. Consultation recommended: If there is a history of problems, some women may need to consider having a yearly endometrial biopsy.

American College of Obstetricians and Gynecology Endometrial Cancer (2019).

LUNG CANCER SCREENING
- Screening is not routinely recommended unless the client is at high risk due to cigarette smoking: if the client is 55–74 years of age, in fairly good health, and has at least a 30-pack-year smoking history AND is either still smoking or has quit smoking within the last 15 years. (A pack-year is the number of cigarettes smoked each day multiplied by the number of years a client has smoked).

American Cancer Society Lung Cancer Screening (2020).

PROSTATE CANCER SCREENING
- Informed decision: Consultation with healthcare provider to allow men about the age of 50 years to make an informed decision regarding testing for prostate cancer (e.g., prostate-specific antigen [PSA]). It is important that the individual know the potential benefits versus the risks of testing and treatment.
- Risk factors indicating possible need for PSA testing with or without rectal examination at the age of 45 years:
  - African American
  - Family history of prostate cancer before the age of 65 years (e.g., father, brother)

American Cancer Society Prostate Cancer Screening Recommendations (2019)

[a]If the test is positive, a colonoscopy should be done.
[b]The multiple stool, take-home test should be used. One test done by the doctor in the office is not adequate for testing. Follow-up with a colonoscopy if test is positive.

potassium, chlorine), a complete blood count with WBC differential (discussed in Chapter 82), and levels of hormones. Leukemia is a type of cancer that may be suspected as a result of a routine CBC because results show an unusually high amount or type of leukocytes (WBCs).

Tumor Markers

Tumor markers are specific enzymes, cancer antigens, oncofetal proteins, hormones, or genes that can indicate malignancies. Miscellaneous markers may be types of

TABLE 83-1	Tumor Markers
TYPE OF TUMOR MARKER	**EXAMPLES**
Enzymes	
Higher than normal enzyme levels can indicate specific tumors or can be nonspecific indicators of a problem	Prostate-specific antigen (**PSA**): Used as a detector for prostate cancer and an indicator of response to therapy Lactic dehydrogenase (LDH): Elevated in many types of cancer Neuron-specific enolase (NSE): Found in several neuroendocrine tumors and with neuroblastoma
Cancer antigens	
Type of protein that is associated with a few types of cancerous tumors	CA 125 tumor marker: Ovarian, colorectal, and gastric cancers CA 15-3 tumor marker: Metastatic or recurrent breast cancer CA 19-9 tumor marker: Helpful for diagnosis of gastrointestinal cancers and treatment of pancreatic cancers
Oncofetal proteins	
Normally found in high levels in the fetus, but not normal in the adult	Carcinoembryonic antigen (**CEA**): Breast, colorectal, and lung cancers Alpha-fetoprotein (**AFP**): Germ-cell tumors, liver cancer
Hormones	
Elevated levels of some hormones are possibly indicative of benign and malignant tumors	Beta–human chorionic gonadotropin (**HCG**): Testicular and certain types of ovarian cancers Thyrocalcitonin: Thyroid and other endocrine disorders and cancers
Genes	
Some genes are linked to specific types of cancer	WT1: Wilms tumor BRCA-1, BRCA-2: Breast and ovarian cancers
Miscellaneous markers	Philadelphia chromosome: Chronic myeloid leukemia Beta$_2$-microglobulin: Multiple myeloma and lymphomas Paraproteins: Multiple myeloma and lymphomas Serum ferritin: Hepatomas Thyroglobulin: Thyroid cancer and thyroid disorders

proteins or chemicals. Tumor markers can be found in the blood, and they are helpful in monitoring a tumor's response to treatment, evaluating the extent of tumor involvement, or detecting cancer recurrences (Table 83-1).

Some tumor markers can lack specificity. Therefore, they are used only as a general screening tool to detect cancer's initial presence. Additional testing is done to verify cancer, such as x-ray, computed tomography (CT), magnetic resonance imaging (MRI), and ultrasound studies.

Noninvasive Diagnostic Procedures

Imaging Studies

Imaging studies, often referred to as *radiologic (x-ray)* studies, allow visualization of the body's internal structures. The definitions of imaging studies and radiology studies are evolving, as diagnostic techniques are developed, but they may be used as synonyms. Imaging studies may include standard x-rays, CT, MRI, PET scans, ultrasounds, bone scans, or other diagnostic views of internal organs. They may be ordered to examine specific anatomical areas (e.g., chest x-ray examination), and various positions of the body (e.g., anterior, lateral, or posterior views). For example, a typical chest x-ray may be ordered as "*CXR, PA, and lateral.*" The healthcare provider is ordering two views of the chest. One is posterior to anterior, or back to front view, and the second is lateral or from the side. Imaging studies have the capability to visualize the function of an entire system, such as with a barium swallow or barium enema used to detect abnormalities of the GI system. Some procedures are given *with contrast,* which means to say that an iodine preparation is given IV during the procedure to enhance certain anatomic structures in order to show tumors, narrowing of spaces, or other problems.

Mammograms are specific x-ray studies used to detect abnormal cellular growth in the breasts. Generally, if an area of concern is detected, the woman will undergo further testing, such as a biopsy.

Computed Tomography

CT scanning can provide sectional views of various body structures. CT scanning is one of the most useful tools in the staging of malignancies. It is most useful for tumors of the chest, abdominal cavity, and brain.

Ultrasonography

Ultrasonography is a noninvasive technique that uses sound waves directed into specific tissues. It is most applicable in detecting tumors within the pelvis, retroperitoneum, and peritoneum. Ultrasound has many clinical diagnostic applications in the detection and diagnosis of disorders of all body systems.

Magnetic Resonance Imaging
MRI can provide detailed sectional images of the body without the use of ionizing radiation. With the use of magnetic fields, it can aid in detecting, localizing, and staging malignant disease in the central nervous system, musculoskeletal system, spine, head, and neck.

Invasive Diagnostic Techniques

Endoscopy
Sometimes, healthcare providers find an abnormality and need to evaluate findings more closely. Instruments, such as the *sigmoidoscope, colonoscope, gastroscope, bronchoscope,* and *laryngoscope,* may be used for visual observation of internal organs.

Exploratory Surgery and Biopsy Examination
In some cases, surgery must be done to visualize, examine, and take a sample of cells (biopsy specimen) from internal lesions or lymph nodes. **Biopsy** examination is the most definitive method of diagnosing cancer. The pathologist studies the sample of cells or tissue removed from the organ in question. In almost all cases, biopsy examination can determine whether a lesion is benign or malignant by determining if the cells look normal, meaning of normal size, shape, and organization. If the cells appear to be different from normal tissues, which is to say without organization, structure, or size, it is possible that the cells are malignant. The term *differentiation* refers to a process of cell maturation. Normally, an immature cell of a particular type of tissue (e.g., cardiac, blood, kidney) will become a mature cell with the specific functions and duties of its normal tissue, which means that it is *well differentiated.* A cancerous cell does not have the same growth and reproductive capabilities and is known as a *poorly differentiated* or *undifferentiated* cell. Malignant cells grow faster, invade normal cells, and last longer than normal cells.

Frozen Section
When a biopsy specimen of a nodule has been removed, or a total specimen has been excised, the tissue is quickly frozen and sliced very thin. The pathologist then studies the specimen under a microscope. This examination can be performed while the client remains anesthetized. The pathologist reports the findings to the surgeon, who then decides on the appropriate surgery.

> **NCLEX Alert**
>
> Clients with various stages of cancer are commonly seen in clinical situations. The NCLEX would require that the nurse be able to educate the client regarding the aspects of diagnostic studies as well as inform the client regarding the signs and symptoms of treatment.

TREATMENT MODALITIES FOR CANCER
Cancer treatments are individual or combinations of four main modalities: surgery, chemotherapy, immunotherapy, and radiation therapy.

Surgery
Ideal surgical treatment would be the complete removal of all malignant tissue before it metastasizes. In many types of cancer, *surgery* can prevent the spread of the disease and offer cures. Surgery can involve not only removal of the tumor, but also may include small or large areas of surrounding tissue.

An *incisional tissue biopsy* will help establish diagnosis and staging criteria. The biopsy may be followed by more extensive surgery, radiation, and/or chemotherapy.

An *excisional biopsy* will remove the tumor as well as some of the margin of the tumor, to determine if the cancer has spread and to remove any malignant cells that may have spread to the surrounding area. In cases of small tumors, this procedure can be curative.

To prevent growth and spread, malignant tissues may be frozen (**cryosurgery**), burned (**electrocauterization**), or destroyed by high-frequency current (**fulguration**).

Some tumors may be removed by *en bloc resection,* which involves removal of the tumor and surrounding tissues and lymph nodes. Larger tumors may be treated by *exenteration* (removal of the tumor, the organ involved, and surrounding tissues).

> **Key Concept**
>
> Cancer cells can learn how to hide from the effects of chemotherapy and radiation therapy by changing their size and shape to mimic neighboring, normal tissues. Additionally, cancer cells can hide among healthy cells by coating their outer layer with a protein that resembles normal tissue.

Laser Surgery
Laser surgery can be used to excise precise areas of tumors, such as on the glottis. *Laser-induced interstitial thermotherapy* (**LITT**) shrinks or destroys a tumor with heat. Laser surgery can be curative or *palliative.*

In a laser technique known as *photodynamic therapy* (**PDT**), a chemical is introduced to the body. This photosensitizing agent will remain in or around a tumor cell longer than around normal cells. The photosensitized cancer cells are then exposed to the laser, and the laser light is absorbed by the photosensitizing (chemical) agent in or around the tumor. The advantages of this therapy are that cancer cells can be selectively destroyed, damage to normal cells is minimal, and side effects are fairly mild.

Photodynamic therapy is used mainly on tumors under the skin or on the lining of internal organs that can be reached by fiberoptic instruments such as a bronchoscope or endoscope. The skin and eyes of clients receiving PDT therapy are very sensitive to direct sunlight and bright indoor lighting for at least 6 weeks after treatment.

Prophylactic Surgery
Prophylactic (preventive) surgery may also be used when certain tumors are known or suspected to be precancerous.

Cystic tumors of the ovaries and polypoid tumors from the colon may be removed as preventive measures against progression to cancer.

In addition, some of the endocrine glands known to influence the development of specific cancers can be removed, such as in testicular cancer. In some types of familial breast cancer, when cancer is discovered in one breast, both breasts are removed as a prophylactic measure.

Palliative Surgery

Palliative surgery may be performed to relieve some of the complications of malignancies that cannot be totally excised. The goal of this type of surgery is not to cure but to promote comfort for the client. For example, with metastatic lung cancer, a tumor putting pressure on the trachea may be removed to facilitate breathing. Palliative surgery may also be done to promote quality of life and to improve longevity.

Hematopoietic Stem Cell Transplant

Hematopoietic stem cell transplantation (**HSCT**) is discussed in Chapters 82 and 72. In review, the client receives HSCT from their own (autologous) or from donated (allogenic) bone marrow after receiving chemotherapy and/or radiation. Preliminary results may be seen in 2–4 weeks. However, complete recovery with successful transplants may take 6 months to a year.

Chemotherapy

The term *chemotherapy* implies the use of chemical agents to destroy cancerous cells. Under normal circumstances, healthy cells have the self-destruction of DNA-related processes leading to cell death, called **apoptosis**. Apoptosis is a genetically determined process of cell self-destruction that limits cell life; it is also called *programmed cell death*. Cancerous cells lack apoptosis which causes uncontrolled cell growth and tumor formation. Cancerous cells cannot physiologically function as normal cells. The goal of chemotherapy is to damage the DNA within these abnormal cells and cause apoptosis, that is, cell destruction, or set about other changes in cellular DNA which enables them to be destroyed. There are several therapeutic indications for chemotherapy, including:

- To treat widespread or metastatic disease because chemotherapy is a systemic, rather than a local, treatment
- To provide a cure for clients with certain types of cancer, even in advanced stages; for example, acute leukemias, some types of lymphomas, and testicular cancer
- To control or *palliate* (relieve) temporarily tumor-related difficulties—palliative treatment does not cure
- To use as an **adjuvant** (*assistive*) **therapy** after surgery to treat metastases or to attempt to prevent metastases from occurring

Pharmaceutical companies search for these weaknesses of cancerous cells in order to achieve a method of destruction of the abnormal cells.

Chemotherapeutic agents are designed to be effective during one or more of the phases of cell division. Because of their abnormal replication process, malignant cells are very susceptible to chemotherapeutic agents.

Chemotherapy can also destroy normal cells. Bone marrow and the cells that line the GI tract also have rapid replication processes. Therefore, the normal cells of the bone marrow and GI tract can suffer considerable damage from the potent **antineoplastic** (anticancer) drugs. However, it is known that cancerous cells may be present and have been known to hide among normal cells.

Protocols (a written plan) for the administration of chemotherapy have been developed with extensive research and experience. Protocols dictate detailed directions as to specific routes of drug administration, the amount of time between doses, the total dosage of a particular drug, and the types of drugs that should be given in combination. The drugs are continued until the client is in remission. **Remission** is indicated by absence of all signs of the disease. Remission may be partial or complete. Some clients may have a permanent remission and the malignancy never returns (i.e., a cure). Unexplained, spontaneous remissions occasionally occur in clients without treatment.

Chemotherapeutic Agents

Chemotherapeutic agents are classified into five basic categories:

1. Alkylating agents
2. Antibiotics
3. Antimetabolites
4. Antimitotics
5. Hormonal agents

Most chemotherapeutic agents are associated with **myelosuppression** (bone marrow depression) (see In Practice: Important Medications 83-1). Several types of cancer are brought about by the body's own hormones. Therefore, *hormone therapy,* removing or inhibiting the action of causative hormones from the body, will interfere with the growth of these types of cancer. *Targeted drug therapy* focuses on the abnormalities of the cancerous cells. If the DNA abnormality can be targeted, the malignant cell may lose its ability to survive or to reproduce. *Clinical drug trials* are used to investigate the effectiveness of new forms of cancer treatments. If a client has not had success in treatment of cancer, the individual may qualify (be eligible) to be a part of an investigational study.

In addition to the five major classifications, other drugs such as corticosteroids (e.g., prednisone, dexamethasone) may be used. The goal of antiangiogenic drugs (e.g., endostatin, angiostatin) is to interfere with the formation and growth of blood vessels, which has been shown to be effective in some cases. In Practice: Nursing Care Guidelines 83-1 highlights important aspects of caring for a client receiving chemotherapy.

Immunotherapy

Immunotherapy, also known as **biotherapy**, uses the body's own defenses either directly or indirectly against tumor cells. The immune system may ignore cancerous cells because these cells may not be identified as intruders, which would happen when the body is invaded by a foreign virus or pathologic bacteria. Biologic response modifiers (**BRMs**) are produced by normal cells and help the immune system to recognize and attack the abnormal cells. BRMs repair,

IN PRACTICE
IMPORTANT MEDICATIONS 83-1 — For Chemotherapy[a]

Antimetabolites (Inhibit Metabolic Functions Needed for DNA Synthesis or Replication)
cytarabine (Ara-C)
    fludarabine (Fludara)
    fluorouracil, 5-fluorouracil, 5-FU (Efudex)
    gemcitabine (Gemzar)
    methotrexate, methotrexate sodium (Otrexup, Xatmep, Trexall)

Antimitotics: Vinca Alkaloids (Interfere With Cellular Mitosis)
vinblastine sulfate (Velban)
    vincristine sulfate (Oncovin)
    vinorelbine (Navelbine)

Alkylating Agents (Interfere With DNA Synthesis)
carboplatin (Paraplatin)
    cisplatin (Platinol)
    cyclophosphamide (Cytoxan)
    dacarbazine (DTIC)
    ifosfamide (Ifex)
    thiotepa (Tepadina)

Alkylating Agents: Nitrosoureas (Interfere With DNA Synthesis)
carmustine (BCNU)
    lomustine (Gleostine)
    streptozocin (Zanosar)

Antitumor Antibiotics (Prevent DNA Replication)
Bleomycin (Bleo 15K)
    doxorubicin HCl (Adriamycin)
    idarubicin (Idamycin PFS)
    mitomycin (Mitosol)
    plicamycin (Mithracin)

Taxanes
docetaxel (Taxotere)
    paclitaxel (Taxol)

Miscellaneous Agents
cladribine (Leustatin)
    topotecan HCl (Hycamtin)
    tretinoin (Retin-A Micro)

Hormonal Agents (Produce Temporary Regression of Metastatic Cancers)
finasteride (Proscar)
    flutamide (Eulexin)
    leuprolide (Lupron)
    tamoxifen (Soltamox)

Examples of Combination Chemotherapy Regimens
CAF: (cyclophosphamide) Cytoxan, (doxorubicin HCl) Adriamycin, fluorouracil (Efudex)
    CHOP: (cyclophosphamide) Cytoxan, (doxorubicin HCl) Adriamycin, vincristine sulfate Oncovin, prednisone (Deltasone)
    CMF: (cyclophosphamide) Cytoxan, methotrexate (Otrexup), fluorouracil (Efudex)
    CMV: cisplatin (Platinol), methotrexate (Otrexup), vinblastine (Velban)

[a]Most clients receive combinations of agents (regimens).

IN PRACTICE
NURSING CARE GUIDELINES 83-1 — Providing Care for the Person Receiving Chemotherapy

- Provide both emotional and physical support. The client may become discouraged or physically ill and may wish to discontinue treatment. Help by listening to the client and providing encouragement. A support group or a visit from a cancer survivor may be helpful.
- Assist the client with strategies for managing side effects, such as constipation, diarrhea, and fatigue.
- Manage nausea and vomiting, the main side effect of chemotherapy. Strategies include the use of antiemetics and distractors.
- Encourage good oral hygiene. Perform frequent mouth checks to check for mucositis.
- Encourage adequate fluid intake of at least eight glasses per day. Vary the fluids.
- Provide a dietary consultation that includes information on a high-calorie, high-protein diet. Frequent small meals, snacks, and nutritional supplements may provide a solution for a poor nutritional status.
- Provide emotional support when there are changes in body image or sexual dysfunction. For example, when hormonal therapies are used, men's breasts may become enlarged; women may develop a deeper voice and facial hair may appear. There may be a loss of sexual interest, impotence, or vaginal dryness, which may add to decreased self-esteem.
- Plan for a wig, turban, scarf, or hat if hair loss becomes problematic.
- Instruct the client in the implications of low blood counts, such as the potential for infection, fatigue, or abnormal bleeding.
- Stress the importance of open and honest communication between the client and family members. Emphasize the overall long-term results of the treatment.

stimulate, or enhance substances within the immune system to kill cancer cells. The BRMs, used in biotherapy, work either directly or indirectly to stimulate or enhance the client's immune system.

Biologic agents that can be produced in a laboratory are referred to as the BRMs. They can be listed in the following categories:

- *Monoclonal antibodies (MOAB)* (e.g., rituximab [Rituxan], trastuzumab [Herceptin])
- *Interferons (IFN)* (e.g., interferon-α 2a [Roferon, Intron])
- *Colony-stimulating factors (CSF)* (e.g., filgrastim [Neupogen], erythropoietin [Epogen])
- *Interleukins (ILs)* (e.g., aldesleukin [Proleukin])
- *Retinoids* (e.g., acitretin [Soriatane], tretinoin [Retin-A])

Monoclonal Antibodies

Monoclonal antibodies (**MOAB**, **MoAb**) are produced by genetically fusing cancer cells with normal cells. They are highly specific antibodies that seek out, and bind to, specific targets on cancer cells, causing apoptosis.

The MOABs can improve the client's immune response to cancer and interfere with the growth of cancer cells. They can be designed to deliver radioisotopes, other BRMs, or other substances that are toxic to cancerous cells. MOABs may be used as part of the treatment and therapy for HSCT, formerly called bone marrow transplantation (**BMT**) as discussed in Chapter 72.

Currently, MOABs are used to combat leukemia, lymphoma, and renal transplant rejection. Additionally, because they can carry radioisotopes to specific areas, they can be used as diagnostic aids for colorectal, prostate, and ovarian cancers.

When MOABs are used, the nurse needs to be aware of the possibility of acute anaphylactic reactions. Anaphylaxis would present initially as generalized flushing, followed by pallor. Respiratory distress may also occur. Other side effects include fever, chills, rigors, diaphoresis, malaise, urticaria, pruritus, nausea, vomiting, dyspnea, and hypotension.

Interferons

Interferons (**IFN**), made by lymphocytes, enhance the effects of the immune system. The three major types of interferon are alpha (α), beta (β), and gamma (γ). They protect normal cells from invasion by intracellular parasites, including viruses. Interferons are used to treat leukemia, acquired immunodeficiency syndrome-related Kaposi sarcoma, melanoma, non-Hodgkin lymphoma, multiple sclerosis, and chronic myelogenous disease. How interferons exert their effects is unknown and unclear; however, all three types appear capable of inducing antitumor activity.

Nursing considerations include client teaching about the usual side effects of flu-like symptoms. However, each client will usually adjust to these symptoms over the course of treatment. These symptoms include chills, fever spikes, fatigue, headaches, myalgia (muscle aches), arthralgia (joint pain), and malaise. Side effects become more severe as the dose becomes higher.

Hematopoietic Growth Factors

Hematopoietic growth factors (**HGFs**) consist of substances that have the ability to support tissues that are involved in the production of blood, bone marrow, and lymph nodes. The three main groups of HGFs are *colony-stimulating factors* (**CSFs**), *interleukin 3*, and *erythropoietin*. CSFs and interleukin 3 encourage growth and maturation of blood cell components. Erythropoietin stimulates production of erythrocytes (RBCs).

When growth factors are successful, myelosuppression (bone marrow suppression) is reduced. Accelerated growth of cells, following damage caused by cancer treatment, decreases the resulting *neutropenia* (decreased neutrophils), thereby leading to a decrease in the incidence of infection. HGFs are used in aplastic anemia and after chemotherapy because with less myelosuppression, the client can receive higher doses of other chemotherapy agents.

Nursing considerations for CSFs generally are influenced by the dose and route of administration. Be alert for low-grade fever, bone pain, fatigue, and anorexia.

Interleukins

Interleukins (**ILs**) promote the immune response of the T lymphocytes to stimulate the immune system to destroy neoplasms. High-dose therapy can create severe toxicity. ILs have shown some success in the treatment of metastatic renal cancers, lymphoma, and melanoma.

When ILs are administered, be alert for possible hypotension, edema (including pulmonary edema), tachycardia, dyspnea, and tachycardia. Other side effects include chills, fever, headache, malaise, myalgia, arthralgia, fatigue, nasal congestion, and GI upset.

Retinoids

Retinoids are a group of compounds derived from retinol or vitamin A. Although not always officially listed as a biotherapy agent, the effects of retinoids include antibody and immune responses. In cancer, retinoids induce cell differentiation and suppress proliferation. Types of cancer that appear to respond to retinoids include promyelocytic leukemia, melanoma, neuroblastoma, and various epithelial cancers. Topical retinoic acid may be used to treat skin lesions from Kaposi sarcoma, which can accompany AIDS.

Retinoic acid syndrome is a serious side effect of this therapy. It can include fevers, respiratory distress, interstitial pulmonary infiltrates, pleural effusions, and weight gain.

Radiation Therapy

Radiation therapy, or *radiotherapy,* is indicated in many types of cancer and may be used as a primary therapy, as a combined modality with chemotherapy, or as a palliative treatment for symptom relief (e.g., pain management). X-ray studies are also used to diagnose tumor sites. The purpose of radiotherapy is to direct ionizing radiation to target tissues for damage or destruction of the cells. Radiation damages both normal and abnormal cells. Thus, the therapies must be aimed as directly as possible at the cancerous tissues.

Proton Therapy

Proton therapy or *proton-beam therapy* is a type of radiation therapy (discussed below). A *particle accelerator* is needed for proton therapy. It is a large device that uses electromagnetic fields to propel charged particles to high speeds and to contain them in a well-defined beam of protons. The proton beam will deposit radiation into malignant tissue with minimal damage to neighboring normal tissues. The goal is to damage the DNA of the cancerous cells, which will destroy the cells or stop their ability to reproduce new malignant cells. Proton beam therapy avoids most normal tissue and reduces the severity or incidence of side effects. It is commonly used for head and neck cancers, lung cancer, melanoma, and prostate cancer.

Three types of rays are involved in radiation diagnosis and therapy: alpha, beta, and gamma rays. Alpha and beta rays penetrate only the upper layer of the skin. Gamma rays, on the other hand, penetrate deeply into body tissues.

Safety considerations are a priority for both the client and the healthcare workers when working around any radioactive substance. The critical components to safety when working around any radiation are time, distance, and shielding. Limit the time spent near the source of radiation. Increase the distance the individual stands from the source, and use available shielding to block radiation. To monitor exposure to radiation, healthcare workers in radiology units must wear badges (Fig. 83-2).

Nursing Alert If not correctly managed, radiation can be hazardous to the nurse and client. Radiation is particularly dangerous for pregnant women.

There are two main types of radiation therapy. *External-beam radiation* uses a treatment machine placed away from the body. *Internal brachytherapy, interstitial irradiation,* or *intracavity irradiation* are radioactive implants that deliver the ionizing radiation directly from within the tumor or a body cavity.

External Radiation

External radiation uses both deep and surface x-rays, as well as cobalt, radium, and radioactive isotopes of other elements.

Extreme precautions are taken to protect clients, staff, and healthy cells from the hazards involved in administering radiation therapy. Linear accelerators and betatrons have made delivery of high doses of irradiation to deep-seated malignancies possible, without damaging critical organs or causing severe surface skin reactions.

Direct nursing care toward ensuring the client's safety and carrying out measures that provide relief of side effects (see In Practice: Nursing Care Guidelines 83-2). Side effects depend on the area irradiated and may include decreased appetite, abdominal cramping, diarrhea, and local cutaneous irritation.

Internal Radiation

Brachytherapy is the placement of radioactive substances directly into a tumor site. The goal is to deliver large amounts of radiation to a specific site. Internal radiation is an attempt to destroy the cancer cells from within. Radioactive sources are encapsulated so that they do not contaminate body fluids.

Cancers that may be treated with brachytherapy include those of the brain, tongue, lips, esophagus, lung, breast, vagina, cervix, endometrium, rectum, prostate, and bladder.

NURSING CONSIDERATIONS FOR CLIENTS WITH CANCER

Procedures and Surgery

Diagnostic procedures and treatments for clients with cancer can be mildly uncomfortable to nearly intolerable. Before the procedure or treatment, it is important that the nurse administer medications that may be necessary to suppress nausea, vomiting, and diarrhea.

Supportive care after treatment is important because the client may feel that the side effects of the therapy are too great to endure. Depression may need to be treated with counseling and medications.

Nursing considerations in cancer surgery include all normal components of preoperative and postoperative teaching (see Chapter 56). In many cases, the client will be very anxious about the results of the surgery. Was the cancer removed, partially removed, or inoperable and not removed? Additionally, the client will be concerned about changes in

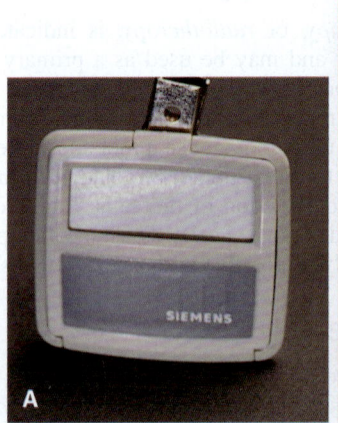
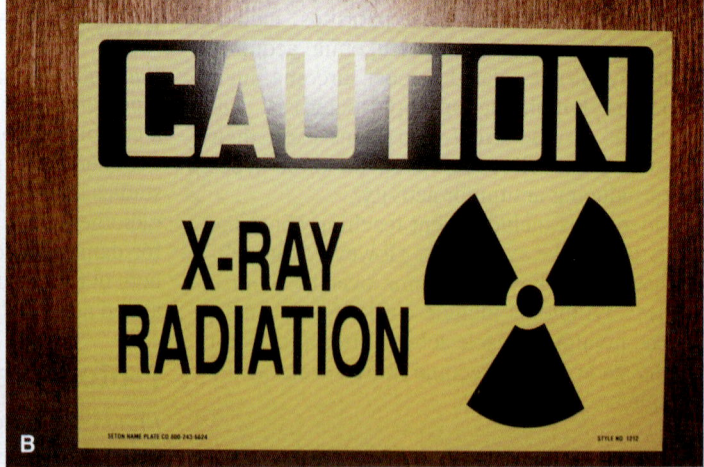

Figure 83-2 Radiation from x-ray machines is a health hazard. **A.** A dosimeter badge is worn by anyone working close to radiation sources. It helps to monitor the amount of exposure by healthcare workers. **B.** Radiation must be identified by warning signs. Note the universal symbol of radiation.

IN PRACTICE
NURSING CARE GUIDELINES 83-2: Providing Care for Clients Receiving External-Beam Radiation Therapy

- Provide frequent rest periods. *Rationale: The treatment and the disease often cause fatigue.*
- Individuals vary in their tolerance to food during radiation therapy. Encourage nutrient intake. *Rationale: A diet high in calories, protein, and vitamins is recommended to increase strength and help offset nausea and diarrhea. Proteins are needed to build new tissue.*
- Provide good oral hygiene. *Rationale: This helps to prevent breakdown of oral mucosa.*
- Provide special skin care (see In Practice: Educating the Client 83-1; also Chapter 50).
- Keep the radiation site dry and free from irritation. The client's clothing should fit loosely. *Rationale: Friction may cause irritation.*
- Avoid invasive procedures, such as injections and rectal temperatures, if possible. These measures must be particularly avoided within the radiation field. *Rationale: The client's skin is fragile due to radiation. Invasive procedures also introduce a possible route for infection.*
- Follow supportive routine nursing measures for side effects, such as gastrointestinal symptoms. If these symptoms are severe, radiation treatment may need to be discontinued or postponed. *Rationale: Typically, fear and anxiety accompany radiation therapy. The client will need psychological and physical support.*

NURSING PROCESS

DATA COLLECTION
Establish baselines for future comparison and determine the presence of suspected disorders. Report any changes in baseline levels.

With a neoplasm, a client may report a change in elimination habits or other normal functions. In addition, observe the client's emotional and physical response to the disorder or disease.

Data collection will generally include questions that provide information about the client's self-care abilities and support systems. For example, does the client need assistance to meet daily needs? Does the disorder affect social activities or self-esteem? Is the disorder life threatening? Is the client anxious or fearful of the outcome? Is ongoing counseling, rehabilitation, or home care needed? Is a support group available? What are the reactions of family members? Will the client be a candidate for hospice care?

PLANNING AND IMPLEMENTATION
The client with cancer requires assistance to meet many needs. Education and support are important so that the client and family better understand the disease, treatments, and side effects. The nursing care plan should consider all these needs.

Together with the client, family, and other members of the healthcare team, care is planned to meet the client's needs effectively. Planning for further nursing care should consider prognosis, treatments and their potential complications, as well as the client's functional status.

EVALUATION
The healthcare team, client, and family should evaluate outcomes of care. Have short-term goals been met? For example, is the client's pain controlled? Are long-term goals still realistic? For example, will the client be able to return to work? What types of therapy or rehabilitation will the client need?

> **Key Concept**
> Early detection promises the highest rate of survival for clients with cancer. Periodic physical examinations and self-examinations are important components of early detection.

body image, such as with mastectomy; possible loss of sexual function, such as with prostate surgery; or the presence of ostomies, as is possible with colorectal surgery or kidney surgery.

The importance of education and client teaching cannot be overemphasized. If postoperative exercises are recommended, such as those after mastectomy, teach the client the exercises before surgery, which will enable the client to perform them more effectively after surgery.

Allow clients to participate in their own treatment plan as much as possible. Individualized adaptations depend on each person's security and self-image. Kindness, understanding, and therapeutic communication techniques can provide an atmosphere in which clients are free to express themselves.

Chemotherapy

Providing care during chemotherapy requires knowledge about the drugs and their side effects. Only nurses who receive special instruction about chemotherapy should administer these potent agents. They must follow safe handling procedures during administration because chemotherapeutic agents are extremely toxic and can affect the normal cells of a healthcare worker in addition to the cancerous cells of a client. Some facilities have special precautions and limitations for the pregnant nurse who may be on a designated cancer unit or work with chemotherapeutic agents.

Some chemotherapeutic agents can be administered orally. Special handling precautions with oral drugs are generally not considered necessary. However, the nurse must understand the side effects of such agents.

For the nurse who is administering parenteral chemotherapy, the specific guidelines to follow are as follows:

- Wear gloves, gowns, and protective eyewear during preparation and administration. *Rationale: These items protect the nurse against personal injury.*
- Do not allow these agents to come in contact with the eyes or mucous membranes. If such events should occur, rinse the affected part thoroughly with clear water for at least 5 min. Obtain first aid immediately. *Rationale: These agents are extremely toxic and irritating.*
- Be knowledgeable about the medications being administered. *Rationale: Knowledge of the drugs is essential in providing quality client care.*
- Do not administer any chemotherapeutic agent without carefully reviewing administration guidelines and side effects. *Rationale: Administration of chemotherapeutic agents is often based on protocols that must be followed to ensure the maximum effectiveness of the therapy* (see also In Practice: Nursing Care Guidelines 83-1).

> **Key Concept**
>
> The person undergoing chemotherapy will experience both physical and emotional needs. Follow the treatment regimen, protocol, and procedures as established by the healthcare facility and be supportive. A referral to professional counseling or chaplaincy services may be beneficial to the client and family.

Chemotherapy Administration

Chemotherapeutic agents may be given via the following routes: oral, intramuscular, intracavitary, intraperitoneal, topical, intra-arterial, intrapleural, and intravenous (IV).

Vascular access devices are often used if chemotherapy is to be given routinely IV or intra-arterially. Because chemotherapeutic agents can damage tissue, and many cancer clients have poor veins, these devices are ideal. They are more convenient and more comfortable and eliminate the danger inherent in repeated venipunctures.

Selection of a vascular access device should take into consideration the frequency of use, length of treatment, integrity of veins, and the client's preference. Vascular access devices include:

- Peripheral access device, peripheral indwelling catheter (**PIC**) line, peripherally inserted central catheter (**PICC**)
- Central venous access device (subcutaneous port)
- External catheters (Hickman, Groshong)

In some cases, chemotherapeutic agents are administered on a constant basis by means of a chemotherapy infusion pump. A pump may be surgically implanted or worn externally.

Nursing Considerations

Chemotherapeutic medications typically have administration protocols. Many of these medications can cause irritation and inflammation to the linings of veins, leading to the inability to use standard IV sites for chemotherapy drugs. Specialized nurses or healthcare providers may be assigned to start longer term IVs using specific catheters (e.g., PIC lines). When administering chemotherapeutic drugs, never mix them with other medications. Over time and depending on the solutions being administered, most IVs tend to become occluded, which results in a loss of patency and potential for infiltration of IV solutions. All nurses (RNs and LVN/LPNs) are responsible for monitoring IV sites for signs of infiltration or inflammation. If your facility allows for the IV-trained LVN/LPNs to work with chemotherapy solutions, be sure that all protocols are observed. When testing for patency of the IV site, never insert a chemotherapeutic drug as the testing solution. If the site were infiltrated, the drug would be pushed into tissue, which could result in major tissue damage or tissue death.

Radiation Therapy

Providing care during radiation therapy requires special care for the client and specific precautions for the healthcare providers (see In Practice: Nursing Care Guidelines 83-2).

Adequate explanation of therapy to the client is necessary. The client should understand that the treatment will not hurt, will take only a few minutes, and that the area being treated will not feel hot. The client has a right to understand the goal of therapy and its possible side effects. In addition, the client needs teaching about properly caring for the skin in the area being irradiated (see In Practice: Educating the Client 83-1).

The client may be afraid to be alone during radiation therapy. Minimize anxiety by explaining that healthcare personnel must avoid radiation exposure for personal protection.

When caring for a client who has a radioactive implant (and in some cases after IV administration of a radioactive isotope), first become familiar with the institution's policies and procedures. Take proper precautions to protect staff, family members, and visitors from excessive radiation (see In Practice: Nursing Care Guidelines 83-3).

Management of Side Effects

Nausea and Vomiting

Nausea and vomiting can be extremely unpleasant side effects of chemotherapy and radiation. Some clients are so affected by nausea and vomiting that they decide to postpone or forego treatment.

Many new antiemetics can help to prevent nausea and vomiting. Determine the client's reaction to treatment during each visit or encounter. Become knowledgeable about various medications that are available, and administer antiemetics according to the healthcare provider's orders. In Practice: Important Medications 83-2 lists some commonly used antiemetics.

Stomatitis

The client receiving radiation or chemotherapy is susceptible to *stomatitis* (inflammation of the mouth). *Mucositis* (inflammation of the mucous membranes, such as in the mouth and throat) and esophagitis are also common.

Instruct the client to avoid alcohol or foods that may cause irritation. The client should avoid alcohol-containing commercial mouthwashes and flossing. They should use only a soft brush when cleaning the teeth and should rinse the mouth thoroughly after meals and at bedtime.

If the client develops inflammation, a healthcare provider may recommend that the client use a swish-and-swallow solution that often contains a mixture of diphenhydramine

IN PRACTICE
EDUCATING THE CLIENT 83-1 Skin Care During Radiation Therapy

- Use only plain, tepid water on the skin. *Rationale: The skin may be very sensitive to temperatures. Some individuals may not be able to feel heat or cold.*
- Use a soft washcloth. Do not scrub. *Rationale: Avoid damaging the skin, which may be very sensitive and tear or bruise easily.*
- Inspect the skin in the treatment area for erythema, pain, and dry or moist peeling. *Rationale: Due to the possibility of skin damage, it should be checked for signs and symptoms of damage, redness, blanching, pallor, or other problems.*
- If a moisturizing lotion is prescribed, be sure the healthcare provider determines the type of lotion to use. *Rationale: Some lotions may interfere with the action of the therapy.*
- Do not remove marks placed on the skin by the radiologist. *Rationale: These marks are used as the guide for locating the treatment site.*
- Do not apply deodorant, powder, soap, perfume, cosmetics, scented lotion, or other skin preparations on the treatment area. *Rationale: Some chemicals in these products may interfere with the action of the therapy.*
- Do not place tight clothing over the treatment area. *Rationale: The skin can be overly sensitive or not sensitive to pressure changes. Swelling can cause constriction of affected areas.*
- Wear cotton clothing next to the skin. *Rationale: Wool or synthetics may irritate the skin.*
- Do not use any heating or cooling devices on the treatment area. Take steps to prevent burning, such as hot water in the shower. *Rationale: The skin may not be able to differentiate between normal, cold, or hot temperatures, which can lead to damaged skin.*
- Do not shampoo every day. *Rationale: Shampooing can dry and damage the fragile hair follicles and the hair that has been affected by radiation and chemotherapy agents.*
- Do not use a "baby" shampoo. *Rationale: It may be advertised as a "baby" shampoo but it is not necessarily mild enough for cancer clients. A protein-based shampoo may be more beneficial.*
- Apply mineral oil, castor oil, or vitamin A and D ointment after shampooing. *Rationale: Hair can become dry and flaky. It may be necessary to protect the hair from breakage.*
- Protect the skin from sun: use at least an SPF 15 sunscreen. Protect from wind and cold. *Rationale: The skin in the treatment area may be permanently hypersensitive and is at risk for burns or frostbite.*

IN PRACTICE
NURSING CARE GUIDELINES 83-3 Providing Care for Clients With Implanted Radioactive Isotopes

If the nurse is pregnant, consider asking for a different assignment that does not involve radioactive isotopes. In some facilities, pregnant nurses are not encouraged to work with chemotherapeutic agents. *Rationale: The fetus is very sensitive to radiation and many types of drugs. Not all clients diagnosed with cancer have the potential of being hazardous to a pregnancy. The nurse should check with hospital protocol and their personal obstetrical healthcare provider.*

- When giving nursing care, do not stay with the client longer than necessary. *Rationale: Limit immediate and accumulated exposure to radiation.*
- Plan ahead to make as few trips as possible into the client's room.
- Keep a record of time spent with the client or wear a "radioactive sensor" badge. Usually, a chart is placed on the door of the room, and nurses and healthcare providers sign in and out.
- Do not stand close to the client longer than necessary. Use lead aprons or shields to minimize radiation exposure.
- In addition to Standard Precautions, handle drainage and dressings with extra care. *Rationale: There may be residual radioactivity.*
- Check whether the implant is in place after necessary nursing measures have been completed. Routinely check all equipment, such as bedpans, emesis basins, and linens, before removing them from the client's room. *Rationale: The implant might become dislodged, in which case it could be lost. If not handled properly, it is dangerous to others. In addition, the client would not be receiving the needed treatment.*
- If an implant does fall out, do not touch it unless absolutely necessary. Notify Radiology Department staff at once. If an implant must be moved, touch it only with a long forceps. A lead container is kept at the bedside for storage, in the event of an emergency. *Rationale: The implant is highly radioactive.*
- Provide diversionary activity for the client. Encourage friends and family to telephone, if the client's physical condition allows. Provide a television. Encourage friends to write. Offer reading materials or crafts. *Rationale: These actions help to decrease the client's sense of isolation.*
- Teach family members the procedures to follow. Visiting time is limited. *Rationale: Safety must be ensured.*
- Ensure that the Radiology Department has checked the room and declared it safe before another client is admitted. Sometimes, the room is not cleaned by housekeeping until declared safe by radiology personnel.

Sometimes, clients respond to nonpharmacologic therapies, such as guided imagery, massage, distraction, and relaxation techniques.

IN PRACTICE
IMPORTANT MEDICATIONS 83-2: For Chemotherapy-Induced Nausea and Vomiting

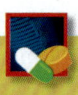

5-Hydroxytryptamine Receptor Antagonists
- granisetron (Sustol)
- ondansetron (Zofran)
- dolasetron (Anzemet)
- palonosetron (Aloxi)

Benzodiazepines
- lorazepam (Ativan)
- alprazolam (Xanax)

Dopamine Agonist: Prokinetic GI Agent
- metoclopramide (Reglan)

Dopamine Antagonists
- promethazine (Phenergan)
- prochlorperazine (Compro)

Glucosteroids
- dexamethasone (Decadron)

Neurokinin 1 Receptor Agonists
- aprepitant, fosaprepitant (Emend)
- rolapitant (Varubi)
- netupitant (Akynzeo)

Miscellaneous Agents
- olanzapine (Zyprexa)
- gabapentin (Neurontin)
- cannabinoids

(Benadryl), viscous lidocaine (Xylocaine), and antacid. Another alternative would be to apply vitamin E to affected areas in the mouth.

> **Nursing Alert** Caution the client to swallow only very small amounts of the swish-and-swallow solution at a time. *Rationale: The mixture will anesthetize the throat and may cause difficulty in swallowing, talking, or even breathing.*

Fatigue
Fatigue is known to affect almost all people with cancer at one time or another. It may result from the disease, treatment, or psychological distress. After pain, it is the second most distressing symptom reported.

Monitor and consider each client's unique condition. Make recommendations based on your findings, including:

- Optimal nutrition with supplements
- Planned rest and activity periods
- Assistance with prioritization of daily activities
- Support for psychological distress, such as depression and anxiety
- Regulation of pain, such as acute, chronic, and breakthrough episodes
- Increase fluids to avoid accumulation of cellular wastes
- Medical management if fatigue is related to anemia (e.g., blood transfusions)

Alopecia
Clients receiving radiation to the upper torso, or chemotherapy, often have *alopecia* (hair loss) because both therapies affect all frequently dividing cells (including cells of the hair follicles in addition to cancerous cells). Hair loss may include eyelashes, eyebrows, pubic hair, and body hair.

One intervention is to encourage clients to purchase attractive wigs before hair is lost so that wigs can be matched to natural hair in color and style. Instruct clients to use only mild shampoos and to avoid all harsh chemicals (e.g., dyes and permanents) during this time.

Hair loss may be the first visible sign that a client has cancer. It can also be an emotional side effect to devastatingly stressful situations.

Secondary Infections
Radiation or chemotherapy frequently renders the client more susceptible to infections because the WBC count is depressed (*neutropenia*). As dead tissue sloughs, it may leave raw open areas or ulcers. Such open surfaces provide excellent portals of entry for pathogens.

Instruct clients to avoid all activities that could injure cutaneous or mucous tissues. Teach clients precautions to prevent breakdown of skin or mucous membranes. Do not take rectal temperatures or give suppositories. Avoid multiple IV access attempts, and instruct clients to avoid anything that may lead to injury (e.g., shave with an electric razor, rather than a blade razor).

Inform clients that they should avoid persons and places that present increased risks for infection (e.g., outpatient treatment centers). Most importantly, be sure to use proper handwashing technique and to instruct clients and all visitors to do the same.

> **Nursing Alert** Bone marrow is typically affected in clients receiving radiation or chemotherapy. These therapies lower platelets and RBCs and WBCs (myelosuppression), and therefore, clients have an increased risk of bleeding, anemia, and infection. Families and caregivers need to know the importance of good handwashing technique.

Pain
Most clients diagnosed with cancer experience pain related to the disease, procedures, or treatments. Studies have proved that nearly all cancer pain is controllable.

Use subjective pain scales (e.g., 0–10) and medicate the client according to the provider's orders related for the administration of analgesics. Give medications around the clock to consistently control pain.

Try to prevent, rather than treat, pain. Educate the client and family about the myths related to narcotics and addiction; assure them that reporting pain and taking recommended medications are appropriate and safe measures.

SPECIAL CONSIDERATIONS Lifespan

Pain

Misconceptions related to pain may affect pain management in older adults. Healthcare providers may misperceive pain as deriving from the normal aging process. Believe and evaluate any report of pain a client makes.

Physiologic responses to pain medication with regard to absorption, metabolism, and excretion may be a major concern in the elderly population. Increasing age is associated with a decrease in the hepatic and renal clearance of many medications; therefore, this population may be at higher risk for toxicity.

Many clients in acute pain assist in managing their own pain using patient-controlled analgesia (**PCA**), which is helpful for break-through pain (pain that "breaks through" an existing analgesia regimen). The type and dose of pain medication prescribed by the healthcare provider are influenced by the pain's origin and severity.

Stress

A diagnosis of cancer, in combination with its various treatments and lifestyle changes, is stressful. Several techniques are known to be helpful in the reduction of stress.

Therapeutic visualization or guided imagery can provide forms of stress relief as well as pain relief. Clients use audio- or videotapes to guide themselves toward teaching their bodies to respond to cues and to become more proficient at lessening stress, relieving pain, or combating cancer cells.

Diversional activities are important. The client may enjoy massage therapy, music therapy, art therapy, or exercise as stress relievers.

Hormone-Related Effects

The most common side effects that women receiving tamoxifen therapy for breast cancer experience are those related to menopause. These side effects include amenorrhea, hot flashes, insomnia, and depression. For men receiving antiandrogen therapy for prostate cancer, the most frequently related side effect is hot flashes.

Drug therapy with clonidine HCl (Catapres) or a combination of belladonna, phenobarbital, and ergotamine may be effective in eliminating hot flashes for clients receiving hormone therapy. Vitamin E may also be useful.

Many herbal products claim to eliminate hot flashes and may be sold in combination: these include ginseng, cohosh, dong quai, wild yam root, and primrose oil.

Advise the client who is interested in trying an herbal remedy to speak with the provider first and to check for side effects related to these remedies.

Late Effects

Late effects are health problems that occur months or years after the treatment has been completed for a disorder such as cancer. Survival rates for cancer have increased significantly in the last few decades of healthcare, which has increased the longevity of cancer victims and the presentations of late effects. The treatments for cancer have known immediate and long-term side effects. The late effects can be the result of a new cancer or related to therapies for the initially treated cancer. The late effects will be related to the age of the individual during therapy, the type of cancer, and the therapies used to treat the cancer. Children who have had treatments for cancer are at significant risk for additional late effects.

Chemotherapy and radiation therapy are associated with late effects in the following areas: heart, lung, liver, and the reproductive organs. In addition, radiation therapy can lead to the development of cavities, tooth decay, skin changes, thyroid problems, lymphedema, and memory problems. Children have problems in the same anatomic systems as adult cancer survivors but may also have problems associated with early osteoporosis, short stature, memory problems, learning disabilities, or vision and hearing loss. Late effects that occur in both the adult and child include cataracts, osteoporosis, lung problems, and heart and vascular problems. All individuals who have survived cancer must be rechecked routinely, as designated by the healthcare provider, for the development of additional problems or other cancers.

Nutritional Needs

Cancer can deplete the body of proteins and affect overall nutritional status. **Cachexia**, a form of severe malnutrition and body wasting, may result. Cachexia occurs when proteins are depleted because of anorexia, chronic nausea, taste changes, and physiologic chemical changes. The client may experience oral complications, such as **stomatitis** (inflammation of the mucous membranes of the mouth and lips with or without ulceration) and **xerostomia** (dry mouth). Alternate forms of fluids, such as popsicles, or foods, such as liquid supplements, can be helpful. Taste and smell can be affected secondary to chemotherapy and radiation. Polypharmacy is a major factor in the development of problems of dry mouth. Thus, nutrition education and management of side effects are important components of the total nursing plan of care. In Practice: Nursing Care Plan 83-1 highlights the care of a client who is experiencing inadequate nutrition because of cancer therapy.

The diet must be high in proteins, carbohydrates, and vitamins. Stress the importance of good nutrition and maintenance of fluid and electrolyte balance to the client and family, particularly with clients who are receiving intensive radiation or chemotherapy. Several small meals a day are recommended for such clients. Note that many cultures have different food practices, beliefs, and rituals. Therefore, work within the food practices of a client's culture. By doing so, you will improve compliance, communication, and nutritional status.

> **NCLEX *Alert***
>
> Nursing care of oncology clients involves many approaches. An NCLEX scenario may require knowledge and prioritization of the aspects of care, such as pain management, the side effects of chemotherapy and radiation therapy, and the ability to listen to concerns.

IN PRACTICE
NURSING CARE PLAN 83-1   The Client With Cancer and Inadequate Nutrition

Medical History: H.B., a 36-year-old woman who was diagnosed with breast cancer and underwent a modified radical mastectomy, is now receiving chemotherapy. Radiation therapy is scheduled to begin in 2 weeks. Client has lost approximately 15 lb (6.8 kg) since their diagnosis 4 months ago. Weight currently 115 lb (52.2 kg). Client's partner reports that client is having trouble eating.

Medical Diagnosis: Breast cancer; chemotherapy-related weight loss due to poor nutrition.

DATA COLLECTION/NURSING OBSERVATION

Client is thin and appears frail. Skin pale pink, returns slowly when pinched. They state, "I'm so tired. It's so hard for me to do anything, especially eat. Nothing tastes good. I've lost so much weight." Client's receiving chemotherapy, currently in their third cycle. They report occasional nausea, but no vomiting. "The medicine that I get before the chemotherapy helps with the vomiting." Dietary history reveals intake of 1 piece of toast with jelly and tea for breakfast, sandwich with 4-oz milk for lunch, and only bites of food at dinner. Partner states, "I don't know how they can survive. They eats like a bird."

NURSING DIAGNOSIS

(Although other nursing diagnoses may be appropriate, a priority nursing diagnosis is addressed below.)

Deficient nutrition, less than recommended intake related to effects of chemotherapy as evidenced by client's limited intake on dietary history, weight loss, and client's statements about lack of taste.

PLANNING (Outcomes/Goals)	IMPLEMENTATION (Nursing Actions)	EVALUATION
Short-Term Goals **A.** Client will choose food that is high in calories, nutrients, and easy on gastrointestinal system. *See Evaluation: Revised Goal A—rescheduled teaching session.*	• Ask client to discuss the problems that they have with current food choices (e.g., nausea or vomiting, no taste to food, cannot swallow). • Ask client to state a selection of foods that they like and dislike, which can be put into a list. • Ask client for their preferred food preparation style (e.g., cooking at home, fast food, eating out, or mixture). • Review client's nutritional needs. • Determine the need for any specific food-related cultural considerations. • Discuss with client and client's partner the client's current energy needs vs. their current functioning capacity at this energy level, related to ADLs such as shopping, preparation of food, and eating. *Rationale:* Reviewing client's typical patterns provides a basis for teaching. The client and any family caregivers need to comprehend the fatigue that accompanies normal ADLs such as cooking and shopping. Making plans around personal physical abilities will help maintain energy needs. Cancer has a significant effect on the client's perception of taste, texture, and sense of smell. Stomatitis is a very annoying sensation and can cause multiple dental disorders. Therefore the mouth should be kept moist. >*Rationale:* Cultural considerations can prohibit foods that may be beneficial. If problems do occur, it may be possible to ask a religious leader for advice or permission for permission to take the food during the time of illness. • Suggest the use of commercial supplements such as Ensure or protein bars. • Suggest use of popsicles, over-the-counter aids for dry mouth, and frequent sips of fluid. *Rationale:* Supplements provide an additional source of necessary nutrients. They are readily available and convenient. They do not typically cause gastrointestinal distress. Dry mouth is a very annoying sensation and can be the source of significant dental disorders, which, in combination with chemotherapy and radiation therapy, could result in tooth loss, gingivitis, and expensive dental treatments. Suggest putting a popsicle into a cup with a handle which will be easier for the client to hold and not have to worry about fluids melting onto linens. Many over-the-counter products are available to help treat the symptoms of xerostomia.	In hospital—Week 1 Day 1—0900 hr • Client seems to tire easily when talking with nurse. • Partner seems very anxious. • Unable to obtain list of food likes/dislikes or to review nutritional needs. • Unable to complete client teaching session. **Goal A not met.** *Reschedule teaching session.*

PLANNING (Outcomes/Goals)	IMPLEMENTATION (Nursing Actions)	EVALUATION
B. Client and partner will verbalize ways to increase nutritional intake.	• Encourage client's partner, other friends, or family caregivers to attend during teaching sessions. • Encourage consultation with dietitian. • Encourage the use of foods high in protein, carbohydrates, vitamins, with focus on increased caloric needs. • Have snacks available that do not need food preparation. • Encourage rest periods several times per day. • Suggest small, frequent meals several times per day or whenever hungry. • Recommend fluids after meals. • Offer suggestions for ways to enhance nutritional value of foods, such as adding wheat germ to toast or ice cream to milk. • Encourage fluid intake to at least 2 L per day. *Rationale: Cancer and its therapies can deplete the body of proteins, affecting overall nutritional status and weight loss. Fluids are lost during therapies. Fatigue can interfere with appetite and desire to eat. It is important that the client and family know that rest periods are part of the overall therapy and not time limited to laziness. Smaller, more frequent meals prevent overtiring during eating and call for less use of energy than do big meals. Consuming fluids with meals may cause feelings of fullness, interfering with the client's ability to complete the nutrient-filled meal. Fluids between meals help prevent xerostomia.*	In hospital—Week 1 Day 2—1,030 hr • Client reports liking peanut butter, cheese, and fruit. • Partner will try adding ice cream to milk at lunch. • Client agrees to try to eat 2–3 peanut butter crackers as afternoon snack. • States that they are less fatigued today. • Client and partner able to discuss food needs as per A. • Unable to meet with dietician due to fatigue but states will make an appointment "in the next couple of weeks." ***Goal A in process of completion.*** ***Goal B partially met.***
Long-Term Goals **C.** On next office visit, client will report a weight gain of 2 lb.	• Encourage client and partner to keep a record of food intake for next visit. • Suggest that client weigh themselves once a week and record this weight, bringing the information with them at the next visit. • Recommend that the client have a family member or friend present during a teaching session. *Rationale: Keeping a diary helps in evaluating client's compliance with nutrition, and provides a means for offering additional suggestions and teaching. Caregiver support can benefit overall goals. Weekly weights provide evidence of the client's status. Adults under stress may have short-term memory loss, vision and hearing problems, and depression that could impede success when applying to new concepts (i.e., nutrition).*	Office Visit—Week 3 Day 3—1,300 hr • Family caregivers and client met with dietitian. Stated that they found the information very useful. • Client and partner report slight increase in intake supported by client's food diary. • Current weight = 116 lbs showing weight gain of 1 lb. • Family caregiver accompanies client to office visit and states, "They are trying to eat better since they know they won't get better without food." • Client states that they are eating several times a day, but "only a little each time." ***Goals A, B completed.*** ***Goal C partially met.***

PLANNING (Outcomes/Goals)	IMPLEMENTATION (Nursing Actions)	EVALUATION
D. Client will maintain at least current weight through remainder of chemotherapy regimen.	• Stabilize dietary intake to ensure no further weight loss. • Encourage weight gain of 5 lb in 2 months. • Recognize the long-term need of nutritional therapy in conjunction with cancer therapies. • Recognize need for alternate types of therapies such as medical marijuana to decrease nausea and increase appetite. *Rationale:* Food loses its social and desirable preferences. Food becomes part of the problem and may be thought of as an adversary to be overcome. The client and the family caregivers can provide much emotional support. Energy that formerly was available must be spared for eating. Additional energy consumption related to food such as shopping, preparation, and eating must be balanced with the client's personal abilities to eat. Nutrition is critical in the overall ability for the body to sustain and improve health. This concept is important for every day as well as during the day since each day offers different or new challenges.	Office Visit—Week 6 Day 4—1,530 hr • Client states that their energy level is "much better." • Family caregiver states that they are eating better, at least half the amount of food on their plate. • Client's weight per office scale shows a 3-lb weight gain. • Client and family caregivers state that they have a better understanding of the importance of nutrition during this time of cancer therapies. **Goal C ongoing, partially met.** **Goal D ongoing, partially met.**

Client and Family Teaching

Cancer screening guidelines are available to encourage the public to participate in decisions regarding screening tests based on age, sex, and risk factors (see Box 83-4). Healthcare protocols per the American Cancer Society or the CDC will advise the public and healthcare providers when to obtain vaccines and physical examinations, for example, mammogram, pelvic examination, and Pap smear. Teaching breast self-examination or testicular self-examination techniques can be beneficial. Pamphlets that reinforce client teaching techniques are readily available from the American Cancer Society. The nurse will benefit the client by providing information that can be taken home and read. Explanations of treatment options, various procedures, management of side effects, and other related issues cannot be learned or understood during a single teaching session. Supply written information along with verbal explanations that pertain to the specific client, for example, names, locations, and local resources. Repeat information during future meetings. Have the client and the family caregivers repeat information that they have just heard. Ensure that clients receive information in a manner they can understand, especially if English is their second language. Have the client and the client's family prepare questions to ask the healthcare team.

Key Concept

The mere diagnosis of cancer generates fear in most people. Remember to offer reassurance and support. Emphasize that most cancers are curable, especially if treatment begins early. When caring for persons with cancer, interpersonal skills are used in conjunction with nursing skills.

STUDENT SYNTHESIS

KEY POINTS

- Cancer is characterized by excessive growth and proliferation of cells that lack the capabilities of normal cellular function.
- Benign tumors do not metastasize, but they can interfere with structure and function of tissues. Metastatic tumors are composed of undifferentiated (poorly differentiated) cells that lack orderly growth.
- Carcinomas develop from epithelial tissues, and sarcomas develop from connective tissues.
- Carcinogenesis can be caused by chemicals, radiation, and viruses.
- To assist with the cancer regimens and protocol of various levels of treatment, cancers are graded and staged.
- Tumor markers are specific enzymes, antigens, proteins, hormones, or genes that can indicate malignancies.

- Surgical therapies can include biopsy, cryosurgery, electrocauterization, fulguration, exenteration, and laser, preventive, or palliative surgery.
- The main chemotherapeutic agents include alkylating agents, antibiotics, antimetabolites, antimitotics, and hormones.
- Immunotherapy uses biologic response modifiers to enhance the immune system and destroy cancerous cells.
- Radiation can be used externally as well as inserted as radioactive devices internally.
- The common side effects of cancer therapies include myelosuppression, nausea, vomiting, fatigue, alopecia, pain, and infections.

CRITICAL THINKING EXERCISES

1. Your client has been diagnosed with colon cancer. They tell you that their cousin had lung cancer and that the cousin's treatment was different from the treatment they have been undergoing. Your client is very worried about their own diagnosis and prognosis. What would you tell your client regarding the differences between the two cancer types, including treatment, prognosis, and expectations?

2. A colleague tells you that an older adult client that they are caring for has become confused and somnolent over the last 24 hr. The client is receiving chemotherapy for ovarian cancer and morphine for pain control. The family has become concerned that the disease is progressing. Your colleague asks your advice. Discuss your actions and the interventions you would present.

3. You have been caring for a client with breast cancer on an outpatient basis. They are currently receiving radiation therapy after lumpectomy. Your client tells you that normal daily activities are becoming difficult, they feel depressed most of the time, and all they want to do is sleep. Develop a therapeutic listening and communication project for this situation. As part of your discussion, include your plan of care, including education, and what interventions, if any, you would suggest.

NCLEX-STYLE REVIEW QUESTIONS

1. A sexually active 22-year-old woman client arrives in the clinic for a wellness visit. Which procedure will the nurse prepare this client for?
   a. A Pap smear
   b. A chest x-ray
   c. A CT scan of the abdomen
   d. A barium enema

2. The nurse is preparing a client with colon cancer for palliative surgery. Which outcome does the nurse expect for this client?
   a. Complete recovery
   b. Better quality of life
   c. Damage to cancer cells
   d. Remission

3. A client is undergoing photodynamic therapy. Which education would the nurse reinforce to prevent complications?
   a. Avoid direct sunlight and bright indoor lighting for 6 weeks.
   b. Maintain isolation for 6 weeks.
   c. Apply antibiotic cream to the area after treatment.
   d. Drink ten 8-oz glasses of fluids per day.

4. A client undergoing chemotherapy states to the nurse, "I am ready to give up. I can't take this anymore." Which is the most therapeutic response by the nurse?
   a. "I will let your primary care provider know you are canceling your chemotherapy."
   b. "You sound discouraged. Would you like to talk about it?"
   c. "What is the problem with the chemotherapy?"
   d. "You need to ask your family what you should do."

5. A client is receiving radiation therapy for the treatment of breast cancer. Which information would the nurse provide the client to prevent skin damage during treatments? Select all that apply.
   a. Use only tepid water on the skin.
   b. Use baby shampoo to wash the skin.
   c. Wear cotton clothing next to the skin.
   d. Do not use heating or cooling devices next to the skin.
   e. Use at least an 8 SPF sunscreen when going outdoors.

CHAPTER RESOURCES

Enhance your learning with additional resources on thePoint!

Student Resources related to this chapter can be found at thePoint.lww.com/Rosdahl12e.

84 Allergic, Immune, and Autoimmune Disorders

Learning Objectives

1. Differentiate the following: allergy, antigen, immunogens, antibody, and histamine.
2. Demonstrate the procedure for intradermal skin testing.
3. Discuss three components of the medical history and the physical examination that relate to the detection of allergies.
4. State three possible skin and three possible respiratory manifestations of the allergic response.
5. Discuss five possible gastrointestinal manifestations of the allergic response.
6. Discuss three possible manifestations of the allergic response that relate to drugs.
7. State three methods for treating multisystem allergy response.
8. Discuss five nursing considerations related to prevention and treatment of anaphylaxis.
9. Compare and contrast organ-specific and non–organ-specific autoimmune diseases.

Important Terminology

allergen, allergic rhinitis, allergy, anaphylaxis, antibody, antigen, atopy, autoimmune disorder, eczema, histamine, hives, immunogen, immuno-suppression, immunotherapy, induration, leukotrienes, monoclonal antibodies, urticaria, wheal

Acronyms

IgE, mAb, moAb, SLE

The complex human immune system protects individuals against "foreign invaders" (*antigens*). This protection is called the *immune response*. Sometimes, however, the immune system works against a person's best interests, and an allergy, immune, or **autoimmune** disorder results.

Allergy, a common problem, is defined as a hypersensitivity disorder of the immune system involving one or more substances such as is found in the environment, in medications, or in foods. The healthcare provider who treats allergies is called an *allergist,* although internal medicine and family practice specialists also treat clients with allergies. In addition, pediatricians see many children with allergies.

Normal immunity is based on the body's ability to recognize foreign proteins (**antigens**) and to marshal its defenses to destroy them. **Antibodies** (or *immunoglobulins*) are protein molecules produced by specialized white blood cells. As part of the immune response, their goal is to recognize and bind to identified antigens, for example, specific bacteria or viruses. Once identified, the antibody (immunoglobulin) helps destroy the antigens. Immune mechanisms are not always positive or beneficial to the body. The *antigen–antibody* reaction releases chemical mediators, the most common being histamine. These mediators initiate a series of physiologic events in the body's organs. Because antibodies form after initial contact with an antigen, an allergic reaction cannot occur at the first exposure to an antigen. Subsequent contact with the antigen may cause an allergic reaction with a wide variety of symptoms. One type of immune disorder is an *autoimmune disorder.* Normally, the body is able to distinguish "self" from "not-self" and takes steps to eliminate substances in the "not-self" category. The difficulty in an autoimmune disorder is that the body fails to recognize its own cells as "self" and begins to destroy normally healthy cells. Autoimmunity is discussed in more detail below.

> **Nursing Alert** Two terms are often misunderstood: *antibody* and *antigen*. An antibody, also known as immunoglobulin, is a specialized protein produced by the body's immune system to recognize and combat infectious agents or other foreign invaders, for example, bacteria or viruses. An antigen is the foreign substance that triggers the production of antibodies (or immunoglobulins).

DIAGNOSTIC TESTS

Determining the cause of an allergy, immune, or autoimmune disorder is often difficult. A person's antigen–antibody response may vary with fatigue, seasons, or hormones. A detailed medical history and physical examination are needed to help establish a diagnosis (Box 84-1). To further establish a diagnosis, laboratory and skin tests are performed.

Laboratory Tests

Laboratory tests that are initially reviewed include a complete blood count (CBC) with a white blood cell differential, an eosinophil count, an eosinophil smear of secretions, and an erythrocyte sedimentation rate (ESR, sed rate). The blood

CHAPTER 84 Allergic, Immune, and Autoimmune Disorders

Box 84-1 Important Medical History and Physical Examination Information for Diagnosing Allergies and Immune Problems

Medical history information
- Onset, duration, nature, and progression of symptoms
- Factors that aggravate and alleviate symptoms
- Possible environmental or occupational exposures, such as smoking, hobbies, household activities, and animals
- History of family allergies
- Medication usage

Physical signs and symptoms
- **Skin observations**
  - Color, for example, erythema, cyanosis, pallor
  - Temperature
  - Rashes
  - Pruritus (itching)
  - Urticaria (hives)
- **Respiratory observations**
  - Nasal edema and congestion
  - Sneezing
  - Rhinorrhea
  - Edema of the oropharynx
  - Hoarseness
  - Stridor
  - Cough
  - Dyspnea
  - Wheezing
- **Ear observations**
  - Tympanic membrane bulging or retraction
  - Fluid levels
- **Gastrointestinal tract observations**
  - Nausea, vomiting
  - Altered peristalsis
  - Cramping
  - Diarrhea
- **Cardiovascular observations**
  - Tachycardia
  - Hypotension
  - Syncope (fainting)
  - Signs of shock
- **Nervous system observations**
  - Anxiety
  - Confusion
  - Seizures
  - Temperature elevation
  - Behavioral changes

levels of immune response factors, such as immunoglobulin E (**IgE**), antinuclear antibody tests, and a C-reactive protein (CRP), provide additional data. Many disorders have one or more specific autoantibody tests, which can help differentiate the type of autoimmune disorder.

Skin Tests

Skin tests are done to confirm suspected disorders or to determine the causes of allergic reactions. Several antigens are tested at one time, with each antigen injected intradermally (Fig. 84-1) or applied to a small scratch on the skin (*epicutaneous method*). These areas are then labeled or otherwise identified. After 20 min, the provider reads the skin tests in much the same way as in a tuberculin test. *Erythema* (redness) and most commonly an **induration** (a lump, wheal, or edema) indicate a positive skin test. The degree of edema, measured in millimeters, indicates the severity of the reaction. In this way, the provider can identify which substances are causing the client's reaction and to what extent the client reacts. Skin testing is not 100% accurate. A substance may or may not initiate an allergic reaction. A healthcare provider may order prescription or over-the-counter antihistamines, immunotherapy (allergy shots or sublingual drops), or both for treatment of allergies.

Observe the client closely during a skin test because occasionally a test will cause a severe reaction. Such a reaction is unusual because the amount of the antigen used is very small; however, it may occur if the client is highly sensitive to it. Emergency airway management and epinephrine need to be available in case of severe or anaphylactic reactions.

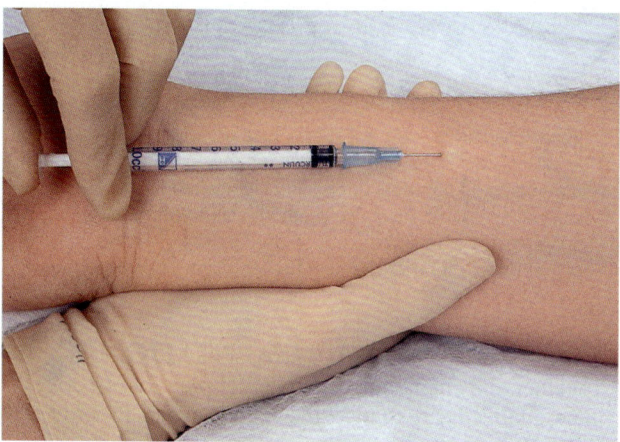

Figure 84-1 Skin testing by intradermal injection. With the needle held nearly flat against the skin and the bevel up, the needle is inserted approximately one-eighth of an inch under the epidermis. The test agent is injected slowly as a small blister appears. Signs of positive reaction to the agent will appear in 24–48 hr.

NURSING PROCESS

DATA COLLECTION

Carefully observe and assess the client with an allergic or immune disorder. Perform a head-to-toe assessment to establish a baseline for future comparison. Question the client for symptoms, such as pruritus, shortness of breath, numbness, and tingling. Examine the client for signs such as a rash, urticaria, excessive tearing, rhinorrhea, sneezing, wheezing, or other respiratory signs, and localized edema or erythema. Document and report any abnormal findings or changes in this baseline level.

Report any allergies a client describes or exhibits. For the client's protection, note any medication allergies in large letters on the front of the chart and on the medication record when the client is admitted. A client with allergies usually also wears a special identification band. Keep in mind that a person can have an allergic reaction to any medication. The reaction will occur faster and more dramatically if the medication is administered parenterally. Give no medication without first making sure that the client is not allergic to it. If there are any doubts, or if the client has a history of allergies or asthma, the healthcare provider may perform a skin (*intradermal*) test first. Even then, be prepared to deal with possible anaphylaxis.

The client with an immune disorder will generally present with vague symptoms such as fatigue or dyspnea, frequent or recurrent infections, slow wound healing, joint pain, skin rashes, or visual disturbances. Ask the client about any family history of cancer or immune disorders. The healthcare provider can further evaluate any reported abnormalities.

Observation of the immune system also includes the administration and evaluation of skin tests. The client's medical history is particularly important in determining allergic and immune disorders. In addition, observe the client's emotional response. Does the disorder interfere with the person's daily life? What assistance does the client need?

> **NCLEX Alert**
>
> When reading NCLEX questions, be alert for clues suggesting an allergic disorder. Clinical scenarios may provide information that indicates potential or ongoing allergic reactions, especially anaphylaxis. Also, you must be able to prioritize appropriate medication administration during anaphylaxis (e.g., epinephrine, diphenhydramine (Benadryl), or corticosteroids).

PLANNING AND IMPLEMENTATION

Together, the client, nurse, and family plan for effective individualized care to meet the client's needs. Provide supportive care and continuously monitor the client's status. The client may require assistance with activities of daily living and in dealing with the emotional aspects of having a chronic disorder. Teach the client and family about the disorder, its prognosis, and treatment.

EVALUATION

Evaluate outcomes of care with the client, family, and other members of the healthcare team. Have the short-term goals been met? For example, are the client's acute allergic symptoms controlled? Are long-term goals still realistic? Planning for further nursing care considers the client's prognosis, as well as any complications and the client's response to care given. For example, is the client complying with medications prescribed? The seriousness of the disorder influences the future planning for care and rehabilitation.

ALLERGIES

Antigens that cause an immune response in the body are known as **immunogens**. Sometimes, a tissue reaction may occur, in which case the antigens are called **allergens**. When a person has a tissue reaction to a specific substance, the person is called *sensitive or allergic* to the allergen. Allergens can enter the body in various ways, via:

- *Inhalation:* Pollen, dust, mold, grass, various plants, animal dander
- *Ingestion:* Medications (aspirin, penicillin), foods (chocolate, eggs, seafood, strawberries, nuts), preservatives
- *Injection:* Medications (e.g., antibiotics), insect stings or bites, immunization with animal serum, blood transfusions
- *Direct contact:* Poison ivy, cosmetics, dyes, metals, latex rubber, nylon, wool

Researchers believe the tendency toward allergic response is inherited, but this does not mean that specific allergies are inherited. The manifestation of allergy relates to many factors, including hormonal responses, type and concentration of allergen, body part involved, exposure to the allergen, and concurrent illness. Allergy symptoms can occur at any age and vary in response from mild to life-threatening (as in anaphylaxis).

Allergic reactions can affect the skin and mucous membranes, the respiratory passages, and the gastrointestinal tract. They can result in rash, edema, itching, dyspnea, contractions of the smooth muscles, and, in severe cases, total shock and death (as may occur in anaphylaxis).

Edema may occur in one part of the body, such as the lips and eyelids, or it may be generalized. If the swelling presses on a vital organ, such as the larynx, it can severely impair the person's ability to function.

Allergies With a Skin Response

Urticaria (Hives)

Reddened areas (*erythema*), itching (*pruritus*), and burning around swollen patches on the skin may appear. The swellings are called **hives**, **wheals**, or **urticaria**. Figure 75-1 shows diagrams of common skin lesions. They appear suddenly and may disappear after a few hours or may last for days or weeks. Hives may result from a variety of causes, including foods; additives; medications; viral, bacterial, or parasitic infections; or stress factors, for example, heat, sun, cold, emotional stress. Management includes identification of the causative factor and the administration of medications, such as antihistamines, epinephrine, or steroids.

Eczema

In **eczema** (atopic dermatitis), tiny blisters that itch and ooze cover the skin, usually in the folds of the neck, elbows, and knees. In *chronic eczema,* the skin becomes scaly and thickened (see Chapter 75).

Contact Dermatitis

Contact dermatitis can result from contact with plant oils (e.g., poison ivy, poison oak, poison sumac), soaps, detergents, perfumes, cosmetics, metals in jewelry, leathers, wool, and latex products. Contact with the skin results in itching, swelling, redness, and blisters. In Practice: Nursing Care Plan 84-1 describes the care for a client with contact dermatitis.

Asthma

Asthma is a chronic airway disorder that involves inflammation and narrowing of the airways. Wheezing, a high-pitched whistling sound of the narrowed upper airways, is commonly heard. The client is often short of breath and coughing. The attacks can be episodic, for example, happening after exposure to an irritating substance, occurring at night, or appearing early in the morning. The reversible airway obstruction results from bronchospasms, increased mucus secretions, and mucosal edema. Attacks can be mild or life-threatening. Multitudes of environmental substances trigger allergies (*allergens*) or cause flare-ups of symptoms. Triggers that induce asthma attacks include a variety of environmental, chemical, or physical substances such as:

- Environmental pollutants and irritants, for example, tobacco smoke
- Seasonal allergens and pollens from kapok trees, grasses, weeds, and flowers
- Sulfites and preservatives as food additives, for example, shrimp, dried fruit, processed potatoes, beer, and wine
- Household environments including dust, dust mites, mold, animal dander, feather pillows, or cockroaches
- Cold air
- Respiratory infections, for example, the common cold
- Physical activity that can promote exercise-induced asthma
- Some medications, such as beta-blockers, aspirin, ibuprofen (Motrin), and naproxen (Aleve)
- Strong emotions and stress
- Gastroesophageal reflux disease (GERD)

Research demonstrates that asthma is probably linked to both genetic and environmental factors. A familial tendency to develop allergies is called **atopy**. This genetic tendency includes atopic dermatitis, allergic rhinitis (hay fever), and asthma. Atopy involves the capacity to produce IgE in response to the proteins that produce allergies. Environmental exposure, often occurring early in life, affects the immune system during the system's growth and developmental stages, leaving the individual more prone to sensitivity to irritants. Infants and children who are exposed to secondhand smoke are more likely to develop asthma than other individuals who have not been exposed to smoke. Asthma is also found in children who have had certain respiratory infections or whose parents have had asthma. Asthma is also discussed in Chapters 72 and 86.

Signs and Symptoms
Allergens can cause spasms of the smooth muscles of the bronchi. Edema of the nasopharyngeal passages causes breathing difficulties, such as a cough, mucous accumulation, and wheezing. Signs and symptoms of asthma include periods of visible dyspnea, tightness in the chest, inspiratory and expiratory wheezing, cough, tenacious sputum, cyanosis, profuse diaphoresis (perspiration), diminished breath sounds, and increased pulse rate and respiration. Attacks can be frightening; the person can have a sensation of suffocation. In a severe attack, the client may become cyanotic. Respiratory failure and cardiac arrest can occur.

> **Nursing Alert** Notify the healthcare provider immediately if a client who was wheezing suddenly stops wheezing. This may indicate severely limited airflow.

Allergic Rhinitis

Allergic rhinitis (*hay fever*) is an inflammation of the nasal passages caused by an allergen. Additional responses include sneezing; watery rhinorrhea; edema; burning, itching, and watery eyes; fullness and itching of the ears; and itching of the throat and palate. Potential allergens include all inhalants, pollen, molds, dust, dust mites, perfumes, and animal dander. Symptoms may be seasonal or perennial.

Food Allergy

In food allergy, also called *food sensitivity*, the immune system reacts to an otherwise harmless substance. Common food allergens include dairy products, eggs, wheat, soybeans, fish, shellfish, chocolate, tree nuts (e.g., peanuts, pecans, pistachios, pine nuts, walnuts), seeds (e.g., sesame seeds, poppy seeds), corn, beer, citrus fruits, and many food additives and preservatives. Common manifestations include nausea and vomiting, diarrhea, abdominal pain and tenderness, swelling of the lips and throat, itching of the palate, rhinoconjunctivitis, sneezing, wheezing, urticaria, and migraine headaches.

> **Key Concept**
> Lactose intolerance, which is fairly common, is not a form of milk allergy. Some people do experience allergic reactions to dairy products, for example, cow's milk, and beef, which contain a similar protein. These allergic reactions often take the form of migraine headaches.

> **Nursing Alert** Latex allergies are noted in individuals who have hypersensitivities to bananas, avocados, kiwis, and chestnuts. Symptoms include local urticaria, for example, a rash inside latex gloves, and itching of the hands or face. More severe symptoms, including anaphylaxis, can also occur.

IN PRACTICE

NURSING CARE PLAN 84-1: The Client With Contact Dermatitis

Medical History: P.R., a college-aged student, comes to the student health center complaining of severe itching and a rash. Rash is located around the neck, both arms, back, and anterior abdomen. Wrists are red and scratched. Client stated, "It just started this morning after I put on my turtleneck sweater that I just washed yesterday." Client denies any history of other health problems.

Medical Diagnosis: Contact dermatitis

DATA COLLECTION/NURSING OBSERVATION

Several small, blister-like areas noted on the neck, both arms, back, and anterior abdomen. Lesions averaging in size from approximately 4 to 12 cm in diameter. Body is red with scratches on both wrists where client states he has been scratching. Denies any known allergies. Further investigation reveals client used a new laundry soap to wash their clothes. They state, "The itching is terrible, and I've been scratching a lot."

NURSING DIAGNOSIS

(Although other nursing diagnoses may be appropriate, a priority nursing diagnosis is addressed below.)

Compromised skin integrity related to contact dermatitis as evidenced by lesions, urticaria, and excoriated areas.

PLANNING (Outcomes/Goals)	IMPLEMENTATION (Nursing Actions)	EVALUATION
Short-Term Goals		
A. Client will have symptomatic relief of pruritus to avoid scratching of irritated areas, which could lead to infection.	• Monitor the client for signs of anaphylaxis. • Obtain vital signs. • Monitor respirations for signs of wheezing or dyspnea. • Remove shirt and any other clothing that seems to be irritating the skin. • Wash skin with cool water and mild soap. • Explain to client that the cause of the rash is most likely related to use of new laundry detergent. • Urge client to refrain from scratching the rash. • Administer medications for allergic rash, analgesics for pain, and prophylactic antibiotics for potential skin infection. *Rationale: Severe allergic reactions are possible if client has a lot of the body exposed to the irritant. Removal of clothing and washing of the skin is a priority to prevent development of respiratory response to allergen. Pruritus is very distressing. The client's skin needs to be washed gently in order to remove any allergen left on the skin from exposure from clothing against the skin. Explanations aid in helping the client understand suspected cause of the rash.* • Suggest that client take tepid shower when he gets home. • State the importance of putting on clothing that has not been washed with suspect detergent. • Offer suggestions to control itching, such as cool compresses or showers. • Encourage the client to keep the area clean and dry but to avoid vigorous rubbing. • Inform student that he will need to rewash all articles that have been washed in the problematic detergent. Extra rinsing cycles suggested. • Suggest consultation with allergist. *Rationale: Continued scratching promotes continued itching, which could lead to further irritation and skin breakdown. Keeping the area clean helps to reduce the risk of infection. Vigorous rubbing could exacerbate the itching. Severity of response for this episode may indicate possible hypersensitivity to other items.*	Student center Day 1—09:30 hr. • Vital signs stable; no respiratory difficulties. • Client states relief of itching and pain after medications (#8 on 1–10 scale). • Clothing removed and bagged and given to client for home rewashing. • Client states, "I won't ever use that cheap detergent again." • Cool compresses applied at clinic with stated relief. • Remind client to rewash clothing to remove allergenic detergent. • Notify client of signs and symptoms of anaphylaxis. • Tell client to seek help immediately if rash worsens or respiratory distress is noticed. • Follow-up visit with allergist scheduled for next week. *Goal A met.*

PLANNING (Outcomes/Goals)	IMPLEMENTATION (Nursing Actions)	EVALUATION
Long-Term Goals		
B. Provide teaching plan related to possible long-term consequences of exposure to allergens.	• Discuss possible acute vs chronic allergic responses. • Establish client's understanding of the possible outcomes of allergic responses. • Teach client about over-the-counter topical medications. • Discuss signs and symptoms of possible skin infection. • Teach client signs and symptoms of infection. *Rationale: The client had a significant allergic response to detergent that involved the trunk, arms, and neck. Unless treated quickly, this type of response could evolve into severe allergy or anaphylaxis. Follow-up care should include examination by the allergist to determine hypersensitivity. Teaching about signs and symptoms of infection allows for prompt identification and treatment should infection occur.*	Student center Day 3—14:30 hr. • States they understand the reasons to be aware of the onset of allergies. • Denies itching or scratching from problem seen in Goal A. • No signs of inflammation or infection of the skin. *Goal B partially met and continues in progress.*

Drug Allergy

Allergic Versus Adverse Reactions

A true drug allergy results from the antigen–antibody response. An *adverse drug reaction* is a noxious or unintended effect of a medication. For example, nausea and vomiting are common noxious side effects, whereas edema, dyspnea, or anaphylaxis occurs in allergic reactions. Symptoms vary depending on the drug. Pay close attention if a client claims to be allergic to a substance or drug. Obtain a careful history of the previous reaction and document it in the client's medical record. Encourage persons who are allergic to certain medications or who have had severe reactions to wear a medical alert identification bracelet or tag.

Serum Sickness or Serum Reaction

Administration of certain drugs may cause a serum reaction. For example, the antiserum used for rabies treatment may cause a severe serum reaction. The client's body mounts a reaction and immunologic attack on the serum or medication administered. Symptoms occur 7–14 days after receiving a drug against which the client has no antibodies. Symptoms include itching and inflammation at the point of injection, skin rash, enlarged lymph nodes, and sometimes swollen joints, as well as a feeling of general weakness and an elevated temperature. Treatment usually includes antihistamines. Corticosteroids are given in more severe cases.

Allergy With Multisystem Response

Some allergies produce symptoms in more than one body system. Initially, the client may experience localized itching and edema, but soon, systemic gastrointestinal or respiratory symptoms may appear. Latex sensitivity is an example of this type of allergic response. Early manifestations include symptoms of contact dermatitis, such as pruritus, erythema, and edema, but may progress to vesicles, papules, and skin crusting. Respiratory, cardiac, and gastrointestinal symptoms may follow and, in some instances, the life-threatening symptoms of anaphylaxis can occur. The client develops wheezing, dyspnea, laryngeal edema, bronchial spasm, tachycardia, and eventually cardiac arrest.

Treatments

Initial treatment for allergies is the identification and removal of the offending substance. Identification of the allergen can be done by eliminating suspected allergens, for example, dander, dust, or by slowly adding suspected allergens, for example, foods. Controlling other precipitating factors is also essential, such as food allergies. Dietary control may be necessary for persons sensitive to products containing peanuts, wheat, milk, beef, eggs, shellfish, soy, or fruits. Unseen chemical additives to food can initiate allergic responses and may be difficult to identify. Exercise is encouraged rather than discouraged. Instruct clients to use their inhalers before exercise (to avoid bronchospasm). Caution clients to wear a face mask in extremely cold weather.

Avoidance of the Substance

Avoiding allergens may be difficult. For instance, a person who is allergic to chocolate can simply stop eating it. But eliminating white flour from the diet or dust from the environment is more complicated. In many cases, when complete avoidance of the allergen is impossible, modifications are helpful. For example, foam rubber or polyester fiber can substitute for feather pillows, and antiallergenic or hypoallergenic cosmetics are available. People who are allergic to pet dander may have to give up their pets. When nurses or clients are allergic to latex, they must avoid rubber gloves, catheters, and other latex-based materials. Studies have shown that severe emotional reactions can precipitate or aggravate allergic reactions (see In Practice: Educating the Client 84-1).

> **Nursing Alert** Do not confuse antihistamines (H_1-receptor antagonists) with medications in the classification of H_2-receptor antagonists. H_2 antagonists (e.g., cimetidine, ranitidine) are used to treat gastric and duodenal ulcers.

IN PRACTICE
EDUCATING THE CLIENT 84-1: Understanding Allergic Conditions

Key Data Collection and Observation Areas
- History of allergic or anaphylactic responses
- Knowledge of allergens that trigger allergic or anaphylactic responses
- Understanding of treatment plan
- Name of allergen and how and where it occurs
- Relationship between symptoms and exposure to causative allergens
- Modifications to environment to reduce exposure to allergens
- Comprehension and careful reading of medication and food labels
- Proper administration of medications, including inhalers and self-injections
- Observations for delayed responses to immunotherapy (allergy shots)
- Compliance and self-responsibility
- Understanding that it may take weeks to months to obtain optimal results

Key Teaching Concepts for the Client and Family
- Decrease airborne particles if the allergens are dust or pollen.
- Remove dust-collecting draperies, venetian blinds, upholstered furniture, and carpeting.
- Vacuum and wet-mop floors and surfaces daily.
- Place hypoallergenic covers on mattresses and pillows.
- Remove houseplants and pets.
- Avoid contact with grasses, weeds, and dry leaves.
- Avoid stuffed animals, pillows, and tufted materials.
- Wear a mask when cleaning or when outdoors during seasons of high pollen counts.
- Remain in air-conditioned environment during high pollen counts.
- Heat home with steam or hot water rather than forced air, if possible.
- Replace filters frequently.
- Circulate room air through clean air filters.
- Avoid smoke-filled environments.
- Modify diet if the allergens are found in food substances.
- List all foods or food substances that cause allergic responses and remove from diet.
- Select alternative sources of nutrition.
- Identify the purpose and use of medications prescribed to treat the allergy.

Immunotherapy

Immunotherapy, also called *desensitization* or *hyposensitization*, consists of giving minute doses of allergens subcutaneously. The doses of "allergy shots" are gradually increased to enable the client to slowly develop an immunologic tolerance to the allergen. Sometimes, this treatment eliminates the allergy.

Clients may receive injections weekly or more often. If desensitization is done to treat a seasonal allergy, it must start at least 3 months before the specific allergy season. If the allergy is not seasonal, injections should continue throughout the year. Treatment is fairly expensive but can be helpful to those who have pollen or dust allergies. Treatment may last from 1 to 2 years or longer. Some treatments last for 5 years.

> **Nursing Alert** Clients should remain in the healthcare provider's clinic for 20 min following injections for desensitization because of the possibility of severe reactions.

Medication Therapy

In general, medical treatment includes the use of antihistamines, bronchodilators, corticosteroids, and anticholinergics. Symptomatic relief medications are types of medications that a client uses depending on the symptoms. Decongestants may be used to alleviate symptoms of nasal congestion. Many medications are available over the counter.

Inhalation therapy with adrenergic agonists, cromolyn sodium (Gastrocrom), and steroids is convenient and easy to perform.

Numerous medications may be given specifically to counteract an allergy or to treat symptoms (In Practice: Important Medications 84-1). H_1-receptor antagonists or H_1-blockers are also known as *antihistamines*. Antihistamines are effective because they inhibit the action of **histamine**, a major chemical mediator involved in the allergic response. These agents provide only temporary relief, however, and clients must use antihistamines frequently if they are to remain free of symptoms. Clients should not use antihistamines for perennial allergies because prolonged use is associated with undesirable effects. These medications may cause drowsiness. In clients who have asthma, antihistamines may dry up the secretions so much that clients cannot swallow or expectorate.

Leukotrienes are chemical mediators that are 100–1,000 times more potent than histamine in causing bronchospasm. Released by mast cells, they initiate the inflammatory response, causing smooth muscle contraction, bronchi constriction, and mucus secretion. *Leukotriene antagonists* or *modifiers* are the classification of medications that are effective in treating these inflammatory respiratory complications and commonly used for clients with asthma.

Clients may receive epinephrine in emergencies to neutralize the adverse effects of histamine. Epinephrine relieves or reduces bronchospasms and reduces congestion of bronchial mucosa by dilating the bronchi. It constricts small blood vessels in the skin and counteracts symptoms of shock. Epinephrine is also used in severe anaphylaxis to treat vasodilation and bronchial constriction. Bronchodilators and

CHAPTER 84   Allergic, Immune, and Autoimmune Disorders

IN PRACTICE
IMPORTANT MEDICATIONS 84-1 — For Treatment of Allergy Symptoms

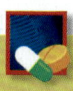

H₁-Receptor Antagonists (H₁-Blockers) (Antihistamines)

Sedating Drugs
- Diphenhydramine (Benadryl)
- Chlorpheniramine (Chlor-Trimeton)
- Hydroxyzine (Atarax)
- Promethazine (Phenergan)

Nonsedating Drugs
- Cetirizine (Zyrtec)
- Fexofenadine (Allegra)
- Loratadine (Claritin)

Leukotriene Antagonists or Modifiers
- Montelukast (Singulair)
- Zafirlukast (Accolate)
- Zileuton (Zyflo)

Adrenergic Decongestants
- Phenylephrine (Neo-Synephrine)
- Pseudoephedrine (Sudafed)

---

expectorants may relieve respiratory symptoms. Cortisone preparations and other anti-inflammatory agents may reduce itching and inflammation in skin lesions. External medications applied to the skin may have cooling and antiseptic effects and reduce itching and other symptoms.

Anaphylaxis

Anaphylaxis refers to a severe hypersensitivity reaction to an antigen (In Practice: Data Gathering in Nursing 84-1). Severe reactions can lead to vascular collapse, laryngoedema, shock, and death. Any allergen can cause anaphylaxis. Common causes of anaphylaxis include the use of antibiotics, aspirin, other medications, vaccines, foods, and insect venom, and exposure to x-ray contrast media containing iodine.

> **Nursing Alert**   Treatment for anaphylaxis must start immediately because the reaction can become severe very quickly. Death can result from laryngospasm and laryngeal edema, leading to blockage of the airways and suffocation.

Treatment
The immediate problems are airway obstruction caused by laryngeal edema and vasodilation, resulting in hypotension and hypoperfusion of organs. The cardiac output falls and the heart cannot pump sufficient blood and oxygen to the tissues. The result is anaerobic metabolism and lactic acidosis.

Treatment of anaphylactic shock involves removal of the causative agent and administration of antihistamines to block the effects of histamine on the blood vessels, bronchioles, and gastrointestinal tract. In severe cases, epinephrine may be used to counteract the vasodilation that occurs. Epinephrine also relaxes the smooth muscle of the airways and inhibits further mediator release. An ice pack to the site can slow absorption.

> **Nursing Alert**   During skin testing and allergy shots, clients are at risk for anaphylaxis. Keep epinephrine in 1:1,000 concentration, TB syringe, and emergency equipment available. Self-administration units are available for sensitive clients (Epi-pen).

Nursing Considerations
Follow the *ABC* emergency protocol when dealing with anaphylaxis:

- ***A**dminister medications*—Epinephrine, aminophylline (Theophylline), antihistamines, and corticosteroids are the drugs of choice.
- ***B**reathing (open the airway)*—This step may require an endotracheal tube, oxygen, or suction. A tracheostomy may be needed.
- ***C**irculation*—Maintain cardiovascular circulation. Intravenous fluids, placing the client in Trendelenburg position, or initiating cardiopulmonary resuscitation may be necessary to support circulation.

IN PRACTICE
DATA GATHERING IN NURSING 84-1 — Signs and Symptoms of Anaphylaxis

- Edema and itching at the site of injection or sting
- Rash (hives)
- Severe dyspnea; gasping respirations
- Continuous sneezing
- Apprehension
- Feeling of choking or suffocation
- Airway obstruction
- Hypotension
- Weak, rapid, thready pulse
- Diaphoresis (profuse sweating)
- Pallor or cyanosis
- Pupillary dilation (eyes)
- Seizures
- Loss of consciousness

IMMUNE DISORDERS

Immunity is the body's normal adaptive state designed to protect itself from disease. Usually, the immune system works on the body's behalf. The point at which a person becomes ill is when, for some reason, the immune system fails to operate as it should. Some immune disorders involve the following:

- *Infectious diseases:* The invading microorganisms are more *virulent* (stronger) or more numerous than the immune system antibodies.
- **Immunosuppression**: The immune system function is depressed, perhaps, because of disease, injury, shock, radiation, or drugs. Immunosuppression may also be congenital (*agammaglobulinemia*).
- *Overproduction of gamma globulins:* Malignant blood diseases or chronic infections may be indicated.
- *Severe immune response to an invading antigen (anaphylaxis).*
- *Rejection response:* A beneficial foreign substance placed in the body is rejected, such as graft-versus-host disease after organ or tissue transplant.

Rejection of a Transplanted Organ

A transplanted organ is a foreign substance, and the recipient's immune system will reject this foreign substance unless specific measures are taken to prevent it. Before the transplant, tissue typing is done to obtain the most genetically compatible match between donor and recipient. Tissue typing is conducted in much the same manner as blood typing. Another measure taken to suppress the rejection is the lifetime use of immunosuppressive drugs. Signs of rejection, which can be similar to other antigen–antibody responses, include fever, chills, diaphoresis, hypertension, hypotension, edema, and signs of organ involvement. If the immunosuppressive drugs are not effective, the organ will be rejected.

AUTOIMMUNE DISORDERS

An *autoimmune disorder* is a disease that results when the functions of the immune system mistakenly attack the body's own tissues, which leads to self-destruction. The immune system normally can differentiate between *self,* existing normal cells or tissues, and *nonself,* for example, foreign tissue such as a virus or bacteria. Usually, the immune system has various methods of attacking a foreign invader, the nonself tissues. With autoimmune disorders, the immune mechanisms produce *autoantibodies,* which attack normal cells by mistake. As a result, the body begins to produce antibodies against its own healthy cells or to inhibit normal cell function. This process is called *autoimmunity* or **autoimmune disorder**, and it results in damage to the body tissues by the immune system. The misguided attacks against the *self*-tissues result in damage to a variety of parts of the body. The most commonly affected parts of the body include joints, muscles, skin, red blood cells, blood vessels, connective tissue, and endocrine glands. Table 84-1 summarizes a variety of autoimmune diseases and disorders and their major symptoms.

SPECIAL CONSIDERATIONS — Culture and Ethnicity

Eighty percent of people affected by autoimmune diseases are women. The ratio of women to men with autoimmune disorders include Hashimoto disease, 10 women to 1 male (or 10-1); lupus (8-1 ratio); Graves disease (7-1 ratio); multiple sclerosis (3-1 ratio); and rheumatoid arthritis (2.5-1 ratio) (Mayo Clinic, 2016). Several autoimmune diseases are rare in less developed countries but are common in highly developed countries. Examples include Crohn, ulcerative colitis, multiple sclerosis, lupus, and rheumatoid arthritis.

Risk Factors

Risk factors for autoimmune disorders are genetic, environmental, or a combination of both. The individual may have a genetic tendency toward a disease and, under specific conditions, an invader, for example, a virus, may trigger the autoimmune process. Resulting damage from autoimmunity can affect anyone in almost any body cell or tissue, but women are more commonly affected than men. Although researchers do not yet completely understand the mechanisms behind autoimmunity, they have suggested the following risk factors:

- Women of childbearing age.
- Family genetics.
- Environmental exposures—Radiation, for example, sunlight; chemicals, for example, tobacco smoke; viral and bacterial infections.
- Racial and ethnic backgrounds—African American, Hispanic American, Native American, and European American.

Key Concept

Similarities of symptoms of autoimmune disorders:

Flares—Symptoms can appear suddenly and be severe.

Remission—Symptoms disappear for an unspecified period of time.

Intensity—Symptoms vary in intensity ranging from mild to severe.

Diagnosis

Initially, a diagnosis is formed on the observations and findings of the healthcare provider. Autoimmune diseases classically present with inflammation in one or more areas of the body. The disease can affect almost any part of the body, which creates a great diversity of problems. For example, if the joints are attacked, pain and swelling will occur in one or more joints. Loss of function may occur if these symptoms are severe. Often many parts of the body are affected. For example, lupus affects the major organs, including the skin, kidneys, heart, and blood vessels. Type 1 diabetes has vast effects on the heart and kidneys, the eyes, and the pancreas. The diagnosis of an autoimmune disorder can sometimes be made by diagnostic laboratory studies. Family history is sometimes helpful, with special emphasis on female relatives' history of autoimmune disorders.

Treatment

Generally, treatment of autoimmune diseases is, for the most part, *symptomatic,* which means that specific symptoms are

TABLE 84-1 Types of Autoimmune Disorders or Diseases and Their Symptoms

DISORDER OR DISEASE	SYMPTOMS
Addison disease (adrenal hormone insufficiency) Addison disease results if the adrenal cortex does not make enough hormones that would normally regulate water and salt balance.	• Weight loss • Muscle weakness • Fatigue that gets worse over time • Low blood pressure • Patchy or dark skin
Alopecia The immune system attacks hair follicles resulting in areas of hair loss.	• Patchy hair loss on the scalp, face, or other areas of the body • Affects body image
Antiphospholipid A disease that causes problems in the inner lining of blood vessels resulting in blood clots in arteries or veins.	• Blood clots in veins or arteries • Multiple miscarriages • Lacy, net-like red rash on the wrists and knees
Autoimmune hepatitis The immune system attacks and destroys the liver cells. This can lead to scarring and hardening of the liver and possibly liver failure.	• Fatigue • Enlarged liver • Yellowing of the skin or whites of eyes • Itchy skin • Joint pain • Stomach pain or upset
Celiac disease A disease in which individuals cannot tolerate gluten, a substance found in wheat, rye, and barley, and also some medicines. When this occurs, the lining of the small intestine is damaged.	• Abdominal bloating and pain • Diarrhea or constipation • Weight loss or weight gain • Fatigue • Missed menstrual periods • Itchy skin rash • Infertility or miscarriages
Diabetes type 1 A disease in which the immune system attacks the insulin-producing beta cells. Without insulin, too much sugar stays in the blood and is not available as energy.	• Polydipsia • Polyuria • Feeling very hungry or tired • Unexplained weight loss • Having sores that heal slowly • Dry, itchy skin • A tingling or loss of feeling in feet • Blurry eyesight, vision loss • Multiple cardiovascular problems • Multiple renal problems including kidney failure
Graves disease (hyperthyroid) A disease that causes the thyroid to make too much thyroid hormone. The most important thyroid hormones are thyroxine (T_4) and triiodothyronine (T_3).	• Insomnia • Irritability • Weight loss • Heat sensitivity • Sweating • Fine brittle hair • Muscle weakness • Light menstrual periods • Bulging eyes • Shaky hands • Sometimes there are no symptoms
Guillain–Barré syndrome The immune system attacks the peripheral nervous system (nerves that connect the brain and spinal cord with the rest of the body). Damage to the nerves inhibits transmission of nerve signals. As a result, the muscles have trouble responding to the brain.	• Weakness or tingling feeling in the legs that might spread to the upper body • Paralysis in severe cases • Symptoms often progress relatively quickly, over a period of days or weeks, and often occur on both sides of the body

(Continued)

TABLE 84-1 Types of Autoimmune Disorders or Diseases and Their Symptoms (Continued)

DISORDER OR DISEASE	SYMPTOMS
Hashimoto disease (hypothyroid) A type of thyroiditis seen as an inflammation, but not an infection, that inhibits thyroid hormone production. The most important thyroid hormones are thyroxine (T_4) and triiodothyronine (T_3).	• Fatigue • Weakness • Weight gain • Sensitivity to cold • Muscle aches and stiff joints • Facial swelling • Constipation • Enlarged thyroid gland, which decreases in size with thyroid hormone replacement • Thyroid antibodies present and often diagnostic for disorder • Thyroid antibodies remain even after adequate thyroid replacement
Hemolytic anemia The immune system destroys red blood cells faster than the body can make new RBCs. As a result of the loss of oxygen carrying ability, the body lacks perfusion of oxygen into the tissues which leads to an increased workload on the heart.	• Fatigue • Shortness of breath • Dizziness • Headache • Cold hands or feet • Paleness • Yellowish skin or whites of eyes • Heart problems, including heart failure
Idiopathic thrombocytopenic purpura (ITP) A disease in which the immune system destroys blood platelets, which are needed for blood to clot.	• Very heavy menstrual period • Tiny purple or red dots on the skin that might look like a rash • Easy bruising • Nosebleed or bleeding in the mouth
Inflammatory bowel disease (IBD) A disease that causes chronic inflammation of the digestive tract. Most common: *Crohn disease* and *ulcerative colitis.*	• Abdominal pain • Diarrhea, which may be bloody • Rectal bleeding • Fever • Weight loss • Fatigue • Mouth ulcers (in Crohn disease) • Painful or difficult bowel movements (in ulcerative colitis)
Inflammatory myopathies A group of diseases that involve muscle inflammation and muscle weakness, e.g., *polymyositis* and *dermatomyositis.*	• Slow but progressive muscle weakness beginning in the muscles closest to the trunk of the body • Polymyositis affects muscles involved with making movement on both sides of the body • With dermatomyositis, a skin rash comes before or at the same time as muscle weakness • Fatigue after walking or standing • Tripping or falling • Difficulty swallowing or breathing
Multiple sclerosis A disease in which the immune system attacks the protective coating around the nerves of the central nervous system. The damage affects the brain and spinal cord.	• Weakness and trouble with coordination, balance, speaking, and walking • Paralysis • Tremors • Numbness and tingling feeling in arms, legs, hands, and feet • Symptoms vary because the location and extent of each attack vary
Myasthenia gravis A disease in which the immune system attacks the nerves and muscles throughout the body.	• Double vision, trouble keeping a steady gaze, and drooping eyelids • Trouble swallowing, with frequent gagging or choking • Weakness or paralysis • Muscles that work better after rest • Drooping head • Trouble climbing stairs or lifting things • Trouble talking

TABLE 84-1 Types of Autoimmune Disorders or Diseases and Their Symptoms *(Continued)*

DISORDER OR DISEASE	SYMPTOMS
Pernicious anemia *(vitamin B_{12} deficiency anemia)* A decrease in red blood cells caused by inability to absorb vitamin B_{12} due to a lack of a substance called intrinsic factor.	• Fatigue • Shortness of breath • Dizziness • Numbness or tingling in your hands and feet • Muscle weakness • Personality changes • Unsteady movements • Mental confusion or forgetfulness
Primary biliary cirrhosis The immune system slowly destroys the liver's bile ducts. The damage causes the liver to harden and scar and eventually stop working.	• Fatigue • Itchy skin • Dry eyes and mouth • Yellowing of skin and whites of eyes
Psoriasis A disease that causes new skin cells that grow deep in your skin to rise too fast and pile up on the skin surface.	• Thick red patches, covered with scales, usually appearing on the head, elbows, and knees. • Itching and pain, which can make it hard to sleep, walk, and do ADLs. May have • A form of arthritis that often affects the joints and the ends of the fingers and toes. • Back pain, if the spine is involved.
Rheumatoid arthritis A disease in which the immune system attacks the lining of the joints throughout the body.	• Painful, stiff, swollen, and deformed joints • Reduced movement and function • Fatigue • Fever • Weight loss • Eye inflammation • Lung disease • Lumps of tissue under the skin, often the elbows • Anemia
Scleroderma A disease causing abnormal growth of connective tissue in the skin and blood vessels.	• Fingers and toes that turn white, red, or blue in response to heat and cold • Pain, stiffness, and swelling of fingers and joints • Thickening of the skin • Skin that looks shiny on the hands and forearm • Tight and mask-like facial skin • Sores on the fingers or toes • Trouble swallowing • Weight loss • Diarrhea or constipation • Shortness of breath
Sjögren syndrome A disease in which the immune system targets the exocrine glands that make moisture, such as tears and saliva.	• Dry eyes or eyes that itch • Dryness of the mouth, which can cause sores • Trouble swallowing • Loss of sense of taste • Severe dental cavities • Hoarse voice • Fatigue • Joint swelling or pain • Swollen glands • Cloudy eyes

(Continued)

TABLE 84-1	Types of Autoimmune Disorders or Diseases and Their Symptoms (Continued)
DISORDER OR DISEASE	**SYMPTOMS**
Lupus (systemic lupus erythematosus, **SLE**) A disease that can damage the joints, skin, kidneys, heart, lungs, and other parts of the body.	• Fever • Weight loss • Hair loss • Mouth sores • Fatigue • "Butterfly" rash across the nose and cheeks • Rashes on other parts of the body • Painful or swollen joints and muscle pain • Sensitivity to the sun • Chest pain • Headache, dizziness, seizure, memory problems, or change in behavior
Vitiligo The immune system destroys the cells that give your skin its color. It also can affect the tissue inside the mouth and nose.	• White patches on areas exposed to the sun, or on armpits, genitals, and rectum • Hair turns gray early • Loss of color inside your mouth

Adapted from U.S. Department of Health and Human Services, Office on Women's Health, ePublications. Autoimmune diseases fact sheet. https://www.womenshealth.gov/a-z-topics/autoimmune-diseases and https://www.endocrineweb.com/conditions/hashimotos-thyroiditis/hashimotos-thyroiditis-overview

treated as they occur, especially during flare-ups. It includes the use of mild analgesics to provide pain relief and to reduce inflammation, corticosteroids to treat more severe or chronic inflammation, and radiation to suppress the body's abnormal antigen–antibody responses. The goal of drug therapy for autoimmune disorders is to manage symptoms and help achieve remission.

Newer medications include the DMARDs (disease-modifying antirheumatic drugs), which have been shown to produce symptomatic relief and improve quality of life. Two main types of DMARDs are useful for autoimmune disorders: chemotherapy and biotherapy. These two types of therapy may be used in combination, which has the effect of attacking the disorder from different perspectives (Arthritis Foundation, n.d.).

Chemotherapy, typically known for its use as an anti-cancer treatment, has the capability to be an immunosuppressant, also referred to as having immunomodulating properties. A common side effect of chemotherapy is neutropenia, an abnormally low neutrophil count. In contrast to treatments for cancer, treatment for autoimmune disorders can often benefit from low neutrophil levels.

Biotherapy alters the process of inflammation that occurs between the body and the body's immune system, which is the main feature of autoimmune disorders. Most biotherapy drugs used for autoimmune diseases are **monoclonal antibodies (mAb, moAb)**. Monoclonal antibodies are laboratory-produced antibodies that are carefully engineered to mimic natural antibodies, which will identify and destroy abnormal cells. The following lists provide a summary of some of the chemotherapy and biotherapy agents used in the treatment of autoimmune diseases.

Examples of chemotherapy drugs include

- *Cyclophosphamide* (*Cytoxan*)—used in rheumatoid arthritis, multiple sclerosis, lupus, and sarcoidosis
- *Mercaptopurine* (*Purinethol, Purixan*)—used for inflammatory bowel diseases, including Crohn disease and ulcerative colitis
- *Methotrexate* (*Otrexup PF, Xatmep, Trexall*)—used in multiple sclerosis, lupus, sarcoidosis, rheumatoid arthritis, and psoriasis
- *Mitoxantrone* (*Novantrone*)—used in multiple sclerosis

Examples of biotherapy drugs include

- *Rituximab* (*Rituxan*)—used in rheumatoid arthritis
- *Infliximab* (*Remicade*)—used to treat rheumatoid arthritis and Crohn disease (in pediatric clients)
- *Natalizumab* (*Tysabri*)—used for multiple sclerosis and Crohn disease

Nursing Considerations

Autoimmune disorders are long-term disorders with acute and chronic episodes that have no cure. Chronic illnesses involve constant variations of flare-ups, remission, and intensity of symptoms. Nursing care will involve symptomatic relief of pain and fatigue plus emotional empathy. The malaise that accompanies long-term illness often instills depression. Thoughtfulness of the totality of symptoms is an important aspect of personal understanding and family caregiver support. It is not uncommon for healthcare professionals and family caregivers to judge the client on the basis of appearance. That is to say, if the individual appears to look well, the caregiver often assumes that the person is doing well. Appearances can be deceiving. Clients with long-term illnesses, such as autoimmune disorders, have constant physical and emotional symptoms. The clients learn to adapt. Part of this adaptation is adjusting to daily pain, physical disabilities, medication regimens, and trying to function at work or in a home environment. These clients may have a very different and limited perspective of doing well than do their caregivers. The nurse and family caregivers need to understand that long-term symptoms exist but may not be as obvious as acute symptoms.

Medication administration for chemotherapy and biotherapy agents typically has detailed instructions and regimens. The side effects of these drugs can interfere with the immune system, which can result in significant unanticipated problems. Monoclonal antibodies can result in serious intravenous-related reactions, which can be life-threatening. The client's history, medication list, and laboratory levels need to be known before giving these drugs. A CBC, serum creatinine level, and liver function tests are routinely ordered to help evaluate drug metabolism and excretion. Toxicity and undesirable immunosuppression may indicate that the medications should be withheld until instructions from the healthcare provider are received.

STUDENT SYNTHESIS

KEY POINTS

- The immune system leads the "battle" against invading microbes and malignant cells that contact or enter the body.
- Antigens are foreign protein substances that enter the body and stimulate the production of antibodies or immunoglobulins.
- Latex allergies are noted in individuals who have hypersensitivities to bananas, avocados, kiwis, and chestnuts.
- Common manifestations of allergic reactions vary; they may range from mild to life-threatening (anaphylaxis).
- Treatment of allergies is directed toward removal of the allergen and counteracting the antibody response.
- Autoimmune disorders occur when the body fails to recognize its own cells as "self" and begins to destroy those cells.
- Chemotherapy and biotherapy are often effective in the treatment of autoimmune disorders.

CRITICAL THINKING EXERCISES

1. Consider the various symptoms of allergic disorders. In addition to the physical impact of allergies, discuss the possible chronic effects on finances, emotions, relationships, and future plans.
2. C.G. has just been diagnosed with an autoimmune disorder. They come to you in the healthcare facility and tell you that they do not understand what is meant by an autoimmune disorder. How would you explain the condition? Which teaching measures would you use to outline the differences between immunity and autoimmunity?

NCLEX-STYLE REVIEW QUESTIONS

1. The nurse administers an "allergy shot" to a client in the clinic. Which is the nurse's priority action?
   a. Have the client eat a small meal.
   b. Administer epinephrine before discharging the client.
   c. Have the client wait 20 min in the clinic after the injection.
   d. Administer ibuprofen (Motrin) 400 mg after injection for pain.

2. A client arrives in the emergency department reporting severe hives and wheezing after eating shrimp. The nurse observes the client experiencing symptoms of laryngeal edema. Which is the priority action by the nurse?
   a. Administer epinephrine.
   b. Administer montelukast (Singulair).
   c. Administer loratadine (Claritin).
   d. Administer pseudoephedrine (Sudafed).

3. The nurse is reinforcing education prior to discharge for a client that has had a kidney transplant. Which statement made by the client indicates that education about rejection is understood?
   a. "I will take a laxative if I am unable to have a bowel movement."
   b. "I will report fever, chills, and profuse sweating to the primary care provider."
   c. "I will take my immunosuppressant drugs whenever I feel I am developing an infection."
   d. "I don't have to see my nephrologist any longer since I am cured of kidney disease."

4. A client is taking methotrexate (Otrexup) for the treatment of rheumatoid arthritis. What expected finding does the nurse observe when reviewing laboratory results?
   a. Low neutrophil count
   b. Low hemoglobin
   c. Elevated leukocyte count
   d. Elevated sedimentation rate

5. A client suspects an allergy to latex. When gathering data from the client, which questions would be appropriate for the nurse to ask? Select all that apply.
   a. "Are you allergic to dairy products?"
   b. "Are you allergic to bananas?"
   c. "Are you allergic to kiwi?"
   d. "Are you allergic to chestnuts?"
   e. "Are you allergic to avocados?"

CHAPTER RESOURCES

Enhance your learning with additional resources on thePoint!
Student Resources related to this chapter can be found at
thePoint.lww.com/Rosdahl12e.

85 HIV and AIDS

Learning Objectives

1. Define the following: retrovirus, HIV, and AIDS.
2. State the routes of transmission for HIV. Identify the body fluids that do carry HIV and those that do not.
3. Discuss the critical nature of T cells and B cells in the immune system.
4. Describe the effect of HIV on CD4 cells.
5. Differentiate the three stages of HIV: primary acute infection, chronic latent infection, and AIDS.
6. State eight common signs and symptoms of HIV and four signs and symptoms of HIV specific to women. Differentiate between the symptoms of HIV infection and the onset of AIDS.
7. Name the three classes of antiretroviral drugs used to treat HIV.
8. Discuss the development and consequences of the onset of opportunistic infections. Define wasting syndrome, AIDS dementia complex, Kaposi sarcoma, and HIV-associated nephropathy.
9. Differentiate between PrEP and PEP.
10. Discuss the circumstances in which HIV-positive tests are reported.

Important Terminology

AIDS dementia complex
antiretroviral therapy
B cells
HIV-associated neurocognitive disorders
HIV-associated nephropathy
Kaposi sarcoma
opportunistic infections
rapid test
retrovirus
T cells
viral load
wasting syndrome
Western blot test
window period

Acronyms

ADC
AIDS
ARV
CD4
CMV
ELISA or EIA
HAART, ART
HAND
HIV, HIV-1, HIV-2
HIVAN
HIV-RNA
HPV
MAC
OIs
PCP
PEP
PID
PrEP
PJP
RNA
STI

The immune system protects the body from the adverse effects of invasion by microorganisms and other foreign substances. It also regulates the removal of damaged cells and disposes of abnormal cells that arise within the body. One disorder that affects the functions of the immune system is the **h**uman **i**mmunodeficiency **v**irus or **HIV**. HIV invades the body due to the fact that the immune system is unable to function. The virus invades, multiplies, and proliferates throughout the body, becoming increasingly destructive because the protective mechanisms of immunity are ruined. HIV is treatable but not curable. Many medications that significantly slow the progression of the disease are available.

There are two types of HIV: *HIV-1* and *HIV-2*. **HIV-1** is the viral form of HIV that causes the majority of infections in the United States and worldwide. Unless specified differently, the acronyms *HIV-1* and *HIV* are used interchangeably in the United States. Endemic to West Africa, **HIV-2** is a less virulent form of HIV that infects fewer individuals. Both forms are transmitted through direct contact with HIV-infected body fluids or via the HIV-infected mother to child during pregnancy, delivery, or breastfeeding. HIV-2 infection generally takes longer to progress to symptomatic HIV/AIDS and has a lower mortality rate than HIV-1 infection. **A**cquired **i**mmuno**d**eficiency **s**yndrome (**AIDS**) is the most advanced and final stage of HIV. Not all persons with HIV will advance to this stage of the disease.

HISTORY OF HIV/AIDS

An international team of researchers has concluded that HIV was introduced to human populations when hunters became exposed to infected blood from a subspecies of chimpanzees native to west equatorial Africa. The chimpanzee virus is known as simian immunodeficiency virus (SIV). The animal virus was transmitted to humans and mutated into HIV. Additional studies suggest that HIV had been transmitted from apes to humans in the late 1800s. The virus spread across Africa into other parts of the world. In the United States, the virus is known to have existed in the mid-to-late 1970s. By 1982, public health officials developed the term *acquired immunodeficiency syndrome* or *AIDS*, which associated particular conditions occurring in individuals. In 1982, AIDS was added to the list of conditions that are formally tracked by the Centers for Disease Control and Prevention (CDC). In 1983, an international team of scientists discovered the virus that leads to AIDS. This virus was eventually given the name of human immunodeficiency virus or HIV.

Action of HIV

HIV is an infectious human **retrovirus** that invades a healthy, normal white blood cell. The virus uses its own ribonucleic acid (**RNA**) to change the healthy cell's existing deoxyribonucleic acid (DNA) into cells that replicate; that is, the virus overtakes the biosynthesis of existing cells to duplicate and

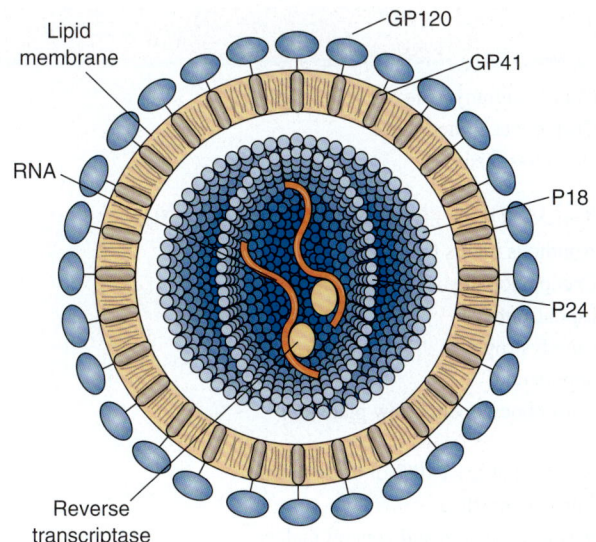

Figure 85-1 The human immunodeficiency virus (HIV).

spread HIV within the body. A reverse transcriptase enzyme is necessary to convert the virus's RNA into DNA. HIV invades a normal cell, inserts its RNA into the cell, and uses that cell's life-sustaining biomechanisms to convert RNA into DNA. Thus, HIV cells are created and are then able to reproduce new HIV cells. The original purpose or function of the normal WBC is destroyed. HIV has a highly sophisticated structure (Fig. 85-1). This retrovirus commonly invades two types of white blood cells: **T cells** (lymphocytes that mature in the thymus) and **B cells** (lymphocytes that originate in the bone marrow). Lymphocytes are one of the five types of white blood cells (Fig. 23-1). Lymphocytes become many types of specialized cells, for example, T cells, B cells, and CD4 cells. Normally, T cells and B cells function to fight infection and to produce antibodies for specific immune responses. The main cells affected by HIV are the helper T4 lymphocytes, better known as **CD4** cells. HIV destroys CD4 cells. The immune system is increasingly depleted as CD4 cells are destroyed. When the HIV-infected person's CD4 count falls below 200 and/or the client has developed unusual infections (see opportunistic infections below), the diagnosis of AIDS is confirmed. HIV differs from most viruses for a variety of reasons. It reproduces and mutates rapidly, which results in a multiplicity of HIV genetic variations in a single person. Several variations can occur within one client at any particular time. HIV has three main stages: primary infection (acute HIV), chronic latent infection (clinical latency or inactivity), and AIDS.

Primary acute infection occurs typically 2–4 weeks after initial exposure to the virus. The client may complain of flu-like symptoms such as sore throat, mild fever, aches, mouth ulcers, rashes, and night sweats. Some individuals have no symptoms. The immune system brings the virus to the lymph nodes where most viruses are destroyed. However, HIV has begun to invade the cells within the lymph nodes and starts making copies of itself, which are released to the general circulation, and travel to the bloodstream to release more invaders. At this time, the viral count or **viral load**, that is, the amount of the virus in the body, is significantly high.

HIV-positive individuals are very infectious. Since the person often ignores or is unaware of symptoms, the chances of transmitting the virus are quite high.

Chronic latent infection follows the acute phase. The virus becomes less active. The individual appears to be healthy, often for many years following the initial infection. The viral load may be "clinically undetectable," but HIV is active and infectious. If untreated, HIV depletes an individual's immune system over a number of years, allowing the development of both minor and major infections and cancers, eventually leading to death. In an *untreated* person, the average time from acquisition of HIV until a diagnosis of AIDS is made is about 10 years. However, this time frame varies from years to decades among individuals who are *treated* with the highly active sets of medications.

AIDS is the last stage of the disease. It is characterized by severe damage to the immune system. Life-threatening infections, which would not occur in the individual with a normal immune system, take advantage of an ailing immune system and develop into **opportunistic infections** (**OIs**). As a direct consequence of the HIV invasion, the individual is vulnerable to many OIs. OIs and cancers account for a large proportion of deaths related to HIV. The list of these infections is found in Box 85-1.

Since the mid-1990s, strong combinations of medications called **antiretroviral therapy** have become available. These medications are specifically designed to combat the retrovirus. They have exerted a profound effect on the progression of HIV disease to AIDS. HIV processes make pharmaceutical destruction of the virus difficult because most agents are designed to attack only one phase of a virus's life cycle. Individuals who take antiretroviral medications often see a drop in the amount of circulating virus and a restoration of immune function as measured by T-cell count (In Practice: Important Medications 85-1). Medication therapies have resulted in a significant decrease in the frequency of OIs and the numbers of deaths in persons infected with HIV. In Practice: Important Medications 85-2 lists the medications used for OIs.

TRANSMISSION

HIV is transmitted through contact with infected body fluids, which can be found inside the mouth, rectum, vagina, and the opening of the penis. These areas have mucous membrane linings that have the potential to be abraded, cut, or damaged, which will result in leakage of blood. Contaminated body fluids include blood, semen, preseminal fluid, rectal fluids, vaginal fluids, and breast milk. The majority of cases of HIV involve unprotected vaginal, oral, and anal sexual contact. If an uninfected individual has an open wound, for example, cuts, sores, abrasions, or inflamed or bleeding mouth or throat, this person can be infected by the blood of an HIV-positive person.

HIV is *not transmitted* in body fluids such as *saliva, sweat,* or *tears*. The virus cannot survive in insects; HIV cannot be transmitted through mosquito bites. Kissing does not transmit HIV unless there is deep, open-mouth kissing along with open sores or bleeding gums, which can enable an exchange of blood. As HIV and STIs are often coinfections, consider

Box 85-1 Opportunistic Infections and Conditions Related to HIV/AIDS

BACTERIAL INFECTIONS
- Bacterial diarrhea (Salmonellosis, Campylobacteriosis, Shigellosis)
- Bacterial pneumonia (especially recurrent)
- *Mycobacterium avium* complex (MAC)
- *Mycobacterium kansasii*
- Syphilis and neurosyphilis
- Tuberculosis (TB)

VIRAL INFECTIONS
- Cytomegalovirus (CMV)
- Hepatitis C
- Herpes simplex virus (oral and genital herpes)
- Herpes zoster virus (shingles)
- Human papillomavirus (HPV, genital warts, anal/cervical dysplasia/cancer)
- Molluscum contagiosum
- Oral hairy leukoplakia (OHL)
- Progressive multifocal leukoencephalopathy (PML)

PROTOZOAL INFECTIONS
- Cryptosporidiosis
- Isosporiasis
- Microsporidiosis
- Pneumocystis pneumonia (PJP)
- Toxoplasmosis

FUNGAL INFECTIONS
- Aspergillosis
- Candidiasis (thrush, yeast infection)
- Coccidioidomycosis
- Cryptococcal meningitis
- Histoplasmosis

OTHER CONDITIONS AND COMPLICATIONS
- Aphthous ulcers (canker sores)
- Encephalopathy (HIV related)
- Lipoatrophy
- Lipodystrophy
- Septicemia
- Thrombocytopenia (low platelets)

WASTING SYNDROME
- A loss of at least 10% of body weight
- Chronic diarrhea
- Severe weakness and general malaise
- Fever

MALIGNANCIES (CANCERS)
- Anal dysplasia/cancer
- Cervical dysplasia/cancer
- Kaposi sarcoma (KS)
- Lymphomas

NEUROLOGIC CONDITIONS
- AIDS dementia complex, HIV-associated neurocognitive disorders
- Peripheral neuropathy

U.S. Department of Health and Human Services. (2019). *Guidelines for Use of Antiretroviral Agents in HIV-1-Infected Adults and Adolescents. Aids Education and Training Center.* https://aidsetc.org/resource/guidelines-use-antiretroviral-agents-hiv-1-infected-adults-and-adolescents

IN PRACTICE
IMPORTANT MEDICATIONS 85-1 — HIV Medications

These Classifications Are Effective After Entering a CD4 Cell
- Nucleoside reverse transcriptase inhibitors (NRTIs)
- Nonnucleoside reverse transcriptase inhibitors (NNRTIs)
- Protease inhibitors (PIs)

These Classifications Prevent HIV From Entering CD4 Cells
- Entry inhibitors (including fusion inhibitors)
- Integrase inhibitors

---

also that STIs can be transmitted in some situations that are not infectious for HIV.

A contaminated needle or syringe can directly inject HIV-infected blood from infected individuals, who share intravenous drug use equipment with an uninfected person.

HIV transmission from an infected pregnant individual to the fetus and to the child during breastfeeding is possible. Protection for the infant is possible and is very effective in the prevention of HIV/AIDS development when the child is treated during pregnancy. Pregnant clients who are infected with HIV need to be treated for HIV because this greatly reduces the risk of infection in the newborn.

Standard Precautions are the healthcare worker's primary protective measures against infections carried by bodily fluids. These precautions are to be used for every client. Additional precautions, based on mode of transmission, that is, Transmission-Based Precautions, are to be used in addition to Standard Precautions when the client has a known infection (e.g., hepatitis or measles). Rarely, a healthcare worker has an accidental exposure to infected blood, most commonly via a contaminated needle. Effective prophylactic measures are available but must be started as soon as possible after exposure or in less than 3 days. To protect yourself against needle sticks, never recap a needle. Occupational preexposure and postexposure prophylaxis guidelines are maintained by the Centers for Disease Control. These situations are discussed below.

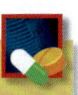

IN PRACTICE
IMPORTANT MEDICATIONS 85-2: Medications to Treat or Prevent Common Opportunistic Infections

Antiviral for Chronic Herpes Simplex Infections and for Shingles
acyclovir (Zovirax)

Antifungal for Severe Oral Thrush, Candida Esophagitis, Vaginal Candidiasis
fluconazole (Diflucan)

Antifungal for Mild Oral Thrush, Vaginal Candidiasis, Candida Skin Infections
clotrimazole (Mycelex) troche, cream, and vaginal suppositories

Antivirals to Treat CMV Retinitis
cidofovir (Vistide)
foscarnet Na (Foscavir)
ganciclovir Na (Cytovene)

To Treat or Prevent Tuberculosis
isoniazid (Niazid)
rifampin (Rifadin)
rifabutin (Mycobutin)
pyrazinamide
ethambutol (Myambutol)
streptomycin

To Treat Diarrhea
loperamide (Imodium)

To Treat or Prevent *Mycobacterium avium* (MAC) Infections
azithromycin (Zithromax)
clarithromycin (Biaxin)
rifabutin (Mycobutin)
ethambutol (Myambutol)

To Treat or Prevent *Pneumocystis jirovecii* (*Pneumocystis carinii*) Pneumonia
trimethoprim/sulfamethoxazole (Septra, Bactrim)
dapsone (Avlosulfon)
aerosolized pentamidine (NebuPent)

SPECIAL CONSIDERATIONS Lifespan

Prevention of HIV/AIDS in Infants

Early detection and treatment of HIV/AIDS as part of maternal prenatal care can prevent HIV infection in the newborn. Nurses must strongly advocate for HIV testing for all pregnant clients.

Before 1985, blood transfusion was associated with HIV transmission. This rarely occurs now because blood banks test donors for HIV. Transplant recipients are also potentially at risk, so transplant donors are tested for HIV infection before organ donation.

SIGNS AND SYMPTOMS OF HIV INFECTION

HIV can be entirely asymptomatic for many years. Many symptoms are associated with numerous disorders. These symptoms are listed below. HIV testing should be considered when there is a history of risk factors, for example, unprotected sex, sharing needles, or known sexual relationships with an HIV-positive individual. Generally, the more mild symptoms occur in the primary and chronic stages but, if untreated, AIDS will develop. As AIDS manifests, specific disorders are prevalent. **Kaposi sarcoma**, a malignant tumor of the walls of the blood vessels, is rarely seen in a nonpositive HIV individual, but it is very often associated with HIV-positive individuals. **Wasting syndrome**, a loss of at least 10% of body weight, accompanied by diarrhea, chronic weakness, and fever, can be reduced by aggressive treatment protocols. AIDS does not appear to infect neurons (nerve cells), but AIDS complications can severely affect the nervous system. Neurologic complications lead to the development of confusion, forgetfulness, depression, anxiety, and difficulty walking. **AIDS dementia complex** (**ADC**), also known as **HIV-associated neurocognitive disorders** (**HAND**), includes behavioral changes and diminished mental functioning. HIV-associated kidney disease, referred to as **HIV-associated nephropathy** (**HIVAN**), is an inflammation of the renal filters that affects the kidney's ability to remove fluids and waste products.

SPECIAL CONSIDERATIONS Culture and Ethnicity

A genetic predisposition puts those of African descent throughout the world at a higher risk of developing HIV-associated nephropathy (HIVAN) than other demographic populations.

In the presence of these disorders, antiretroviral therapy may be started even if the CD4 count is adequate. Generally, the characteristic signs and symptoms associated with infection include:

Symptoms suggesting primary HIV or AIDS:

- Fatigue
- Recurring fever
- Headache
- Lymphadenopathy—persistent enlargement of lymph nodes
- Diarrhea
- General malaise—profound or unexplained fatigue
- Anorexia
- Dry cough
- Rash
- Elevated viral load—seen in primary HIV and AIDS
- Oral thrush
- Herpes zoster infection or shingles
- Pneumonia
- Memory loss
- Soaking night sweats
- White spots or unusual lesions on tongue or in mouth
- Skin rash or bumps

Symptoms suggesting AIDS:

- Kaposi sarcoma—a cancerous tumor of the blood vessel walls. Appearing as red, brown, pink, or purple spots on or under the skin, inside the mouth, nose, or eyelids, and internal organs such as the gastrointestinal tract and lungs
- Tuberculosis
- AIDS dementia complex or HAND
- HIVAN
- Wasting syndrome—excessive weight loss with chronic diarrhea, weakness, and fever
- Lymphomas—a cancer of the WBCs originating in the lymph nodes seen as painless swelling of the lymph nodes of the neck, armpit, or groin
- Lipoatrophy—loss of fat in face, arms, legs, and buttocks
- Lipodystrophy—excessive fat buildup on back of neck and shoulders, breasts, or abdominal areas

> **Key Concept**
>
> The symptoms listed above can be linked to an assortment of infections or disorders and are not exclusively found with HIV or AIDS. The only way to identify actual infections is by accurate testing for HIV.

Diagnostic Tests

The accuracy of laboratory tests, especially if the tests are diagnostic, is critical for the healthcare of individuals. HIV testing offers additional scrutiny and has lifetime implications. The Centers for Disease Control provides recommendations for HIV testing by laboratories recognized as official testing sites in the United States (CDC, 2019). Testing for HIV is done in stages or per an algorithm. An algorithm is a sequence of tests used in combination to improve the accuracy of the laboratory diagnosis of HIV. The first phase is to confirm the presence of HIV, which may be done more than once. Initial testing may be a false positive or, rarely, a false negative. The second tier of testing determines the specific type of HIV, that is, HIV-1 or HIV-2. Healthcare and medication decisions are based on the results of these tests.

Diagnostic testing for HIV includes *antibody tests, antigen/antibody tests,* and *nucleic acid (RNA) tests.* Antibody tests detect antibodies that are made as an *indirect* response to HIV. Antigen and RNA tests detect HIV *directly.* The first tier of testing for HIV will be an antibody test or an antigen/antibody test. Blood or oral fluids are examined in a laboratory for a rapid test. Blood tests can detect HIV infection sooner after exposure than oral fluid tests because the level of antibody in blood is higher than it is in oral fluids. Antigen/antibody and RNA tests detect HIV infection in blood before antibody tests. A test for the HIV antigen, a protein produced after being infected, can quickly confirm a diagnosis. Some antigen/antibody laboratory tests can find HIV as soon as 3 weeks after exposure to the virus. No antigen/antibody or RNA tests are available for oral fluid.

> **Key Concept**
>
> Remember that antigens are proteins that stimulate the immune system to make a specific antibody. Antibodies act specifically against the antigen as part of the immune response.

Enzyme-Linked Immunoassay

The first test usually ordered to test for HIV is the enzyme-linked immunoassay (**ELISA or EIA**). A false positive may occur if the individual has syphilis, lupus, or Lyme disease. If the test is positive, another HIV test is usually done to confirm the diagnosis. A false-negative HIV result may mean that the testing has been done too early, that is, before the body has produced enough antibodies to the virus to be detected. This early stage is referred to as the *window period.* The **window period** can range from 2–8 weeks or about 25 days on average. In some cases, months may be needed before an accurate HIV-positive result is obtained. During this time, the healthcare providers may initiate therapy based on lifestyle and possible risk factors. If the test is a **rapid test**, a test done in a home or clinic, the next test will be done in a laboratory.

Typically the **Western blot test** confirms the HIV diagnosis. Both ELISA and Western blot tests detect HIV antibodies in the blood. If the initial test is negative, a future test may be scheduled after antibodies have had a chance to develop. Retesting is usually rescheduled for 4–6 weeks, 3 months, or 6 months after exposure to HIV, depending upon the clinical situation.

> **Key Concept**
>
> A *rapid test* is the term for a preliminary HIV test that is performed outside the typical laboratory, for example, in the home or in a clinic. It can give results in less than 30 min. Rapid test results can vary and may not be accurate. All positive results must be followed up by additional laboratory confirmation tests. An initial negative result may not be accurate and additional testing may be necessary.

If HIV is suspected, preliminary testing includes the following:

- ELISA (EIA) followed by Western blot
- CD4 count
- Viral load
- Complete blood count
- Blood chemistries (e.g., liver and kidney function tests)
- Urinalysis
- Testing for sexually transmitted infections (STIs)
- Testing for hepatitis, tuberculosis, and toxoplasmosis

Nursing Considerations and HIV Testing

Testing for HIV is associated with many legal implications. Although the laws vary from state to state, they generally hold the following:

- An informed consent must be obtained from the client before testing.
- Pre- and posttest counseling (usually by a state-approved HIV counselor) is required regardless of the test results.
- Results cannot be given over the telephone. Most laws identify specific standards for when and how the results can be given and to whom.
- Ensuring client confidentiality is essential. Most laboratories use a coding system rather than the client's name.
- The laboratory must be approved by the state for HIV testing.

> **Nursing Alert** Persons with HIV can be asymptomatic for many years, and individuals who have not been tested may not know they are infected.

Women's Concerns

Women should be aware that HIV infection may be overlooked and attributed to other disorders, such as genital ulcer disease, **STIs**, human papillomavirus (**HPV**) infections, and pelvic inflammatory disease (**PID**). Although women may experience the characteristic signs and symptoms, more commonly women experience gynecologic problems as the initial clinical manifestations. In women, other common HIV-related signs and symptoms include the following:

- Recurrent vaginal candidiasis
- Menstrual abnormalities, including *amenorrhea* (absence of periods) or bleeding between periods
- Abnormal Pap tests
- Cervical cancer

Treatment

The main treatment concepts of HIV therapy are to use medications specifically designed to combat a part of the retroviral replication cycle of HIV. The current antiretroviral drugs include five classifications. Therapy consists of a combination of these five classes. The drugs are collectively referred to as antiretrovirals (**ARVs**) or highly active antiretroviral therapy (**HAART** or **ART**), or just as "the cocktail." Because each classification is designed to attack a different developmental cycle of the virus, the use of different drugs simultaneously is more effective in controlling the amount of the virus in the individual. This often results in a lowering of the viral load. Refer to Table 85-1 and In Practice: Important Medications 85-1 for a listing of current classifications and some examples of each. The table also summarizes the main course of action of each classification.

With strong suppression of the virus via multiple drug therapies, the immune system may be able to repair. Clients often have an increase in their T cells. As a consequence, they are less susceptible to OIs. Some OIs can be treated and/or prevented with medications.

> **Key Concept**
> HIV is not curable; it is only treatable.

Antiretroviral therapy is often associated with significant problems. Many of the drugs produce side effects, such as severe gastrointestinal upset with nausea, vomiting, and diarrhea; lipoatrophy, lipodystrophy, and bone marrow suppression; and peripheral neuropathy. Treatment for HIV requires knowledgeable and experienced professionals. Medical regimens usually mean lifestyle changes, at least initially. Illnesses, such as diabetes, and increased cholesterol or triglyceride levels, can become life threatening. Some clients can tolerate medications for only a short period because of toxicity.

ACQUIRED IMMUNODEFICIENCY SYNDROME

HIV-positive individuals with a T-cell count below $200/mm^3$ belong in the group of individuals who may be considered to have the diagnosis of AIDS. As the virus progressively destroys the immune system, a variety of infections and cancers can develop. Persons with HIV and certain OIs or cancers also are considered to have AIDS. AIDS occurs during the later stages of HIV infection. Some individuals seem to maintain a healthy immune system for many years despite HIV infection, without the use of medications. The reasons for the delayed development of AIDS are not completely understood.

> **Key Concept**
> Early detection of HIV, OIs, and AIDS allows for more options in treatment of infections and preventative healthcare.

> **NCLEX Alert**
> NCLEX clinical scenarios may involve a variety of nursing issues related to the HIV client, for example, daily care, medication therapies, hospice care, caregiver concerns, or medication side effects. As part of these situations, you could be asked to identify in-home education of Standard Precautions, specific concerns of caregivers, or treatment of side effects. As with all scenarios, prioritization of needs for each individual's situation must be considered.

Opportunistic Infections

When an HIV-positive person's T-cell count falls between 200 and $400/mm^3$, the first OIs may appear. Initial infections of the skin and mucous membranes, such as oral thrush, shingles, and severe athlete's foot, may develop. As immunity diminishes further, more life-threatening infections are likely to occur (Box 85-1). A variety of fungal, viral, parasitic, and bacterial infections may occur, causing problems such as *wasting syndrome,* HIVAN, and neurologic disorders (e.g., AIDS dementia complex or HAND). Figures 85-2 and 85-3 show wasting syndrome and Kaposi sarcoma. The nurse and caregivers need to be aware of the more common OIs, which include the following:

- *Candidiasis:* Yeast-like fungus causing thick, white coating on the mucous membranes of the mouth (thrush), tongue, esophagus, or vagina.
- *Cryptococcal meningitis:* A fungus found in the soil causing inflammation of the membranes and fluid surrounding the central nervous system (i.e., the brain and spinal cord [meninges]).
- *Cryptosporidiosis:* An intestinal parasite commonly found in animals that is passed through contaminated food or water. It grows in the intestines and bile ducts leading to the severe, chronic diarrhea of AIDS.
- *Cytomegalovirus (CMV):* A herpes virus transmitted in body fluids such as saliva, blood, urine, semen, and breast milk. If it develops, it causes damage to the eyes, digestive tract, lungs and other organs.

TABLE 85-1 Classifications of HIV/AIDS Medications

CLASSIFICATION	HOW THEY WORK	EXAMPLES
Nucleoside/nucleotide reverse transcriptase inhibitors (NRTIs)	NRTIs replace part of HIV's genetic material with alternate enzymes, which means that the virus does not have access to normal developmental life cycle growth. Thus, the cell is prevented from producing new virus.	• abacavir sulfate (Ziagen) • didanosine (Videx) • emtricitabine (Emtriva) • lamivudine (3TC) (Epivir) • stavudine (Zerit) • tenofovir disoproxil fumarate (Viread) • zidovudine (Retrovir)
Nonnucleoside reverse transcriptase inhibitors (NNRTIs)	NNRTIs attach themselves to reverse transcriptase and prevent the enzyme from converting RNA to DNA. As a consequence, HIV's genetic material cannot be incorporated into the normal genetic material of the invaded cell. The cell is prevented from producing new virus.	• efavirenz (Sustiva) • etravirine (Intelence) • nevirapine (Viramune)
Protease inhibitors (PIs)	PIs disable a protein (protease) that the HIV needs for replication.	• atazanavir sulfate (Reyataz) • darunavir ethanolate (Prezista) • fosamprenavir calcium (Lexiva) • indinavir sulfate (Crixivan) • lopinavir/ritonavir (Kaletra) • nelfinavir mesylate (Viracept) • ritonavir (Norvir) • saquinavir mesylate (Invirase) • tipranavir (Aptivus)
Entry inhibitors (including fusion inhibitors)	Entry inhibitors work by preventing HIV from entering healthy CD4 cells by blocking specific proteins on CD4 cells. This classification may be especially beneficial to HIV-positive individuals who have become resistant to some other classifications.	• enfuvirtide (Fuzeon) • maraviroc (Selzentry, Celsentri)
Integrase inhibitors	Integrase inhibitors work by blocking a protein that the HIV uses to infect a CD4 cell.	• raltegravir (Isentress) • elvitegravir (Vitekta) • dolutegravir (Tivicay)
Immune-based therapies	Research is suggesting that an HIV-infected person can benefit from therapies that combat the virus by using one's own immune system. Important proteins called cytokines, such as interleukin-2 (IL-2), can affect immune cells. Immune-boosting drugs may be found in vaccines or hormones.	• aldesleukin, interleukin-2 (Proleukin) • Remune—a therapeutic vaccine. (HIV-1 immunogen, Salk vaccine) • Serostim—human growth hormone

- *Herpes simplex:* Viral infection causing a variety of problems including colitis, pneumonitis, and retinitis.
- *Histoplasmosis:* Fungal infection caused by inhaling spores of a fungus often found in bird and bat droppings.
- *Mycobacterium avium-intracellulare* (**MAC**): Bacterial disease with fever, malaise, night sweats, anorexia, diarrhea, weight loss, and lung and blood infections.
- *P. jirovecii (P. carinii) pneumonia* (**PJP**), formerly **PCP**: One-celled organism causing infection of the lungs, with cough, fever, chest pain, and sputum production.
- *Toxoplasmosis:* Parasitic infection spread by cat's stool, which can spread to other animals and humans. It involves the brain, lungs, and other organs, causing fever, chills, visual disturbances, confusion, hemiparesis, and seizures.
- *Tuberculosis (TB):* A bacterial infection causing the growth of nodules (tubercles) in the tissues especially the lungs. This is the most common OI and a leading cause of death of individuals with AIDS.

Treatment

The ideal approach to the management of AIDS involves the prevention of OIs when possible and the early treatment of such infections when they occur. The prevention of HIV in noninfected individuals is referred to as *preexposure prophylaxis (PrEP)* and *postexposure prophylaxis (PEP),* which are discussed below. The use of antiretroviral medications has resulted in the decline or delay in the number of individuals who progress from HIV to AIDS. When T-cell counts are low, prophylaxis is commonly given to prevent OIs, including PJP and MAC.

Mortality

HIV remains in the top ten leading causes of death for individuals aged 25–44 years (Kaiser Family Foundation, 2019). Mortality due to HIV rapidly increased in the 1980s and peaked in 1994–1995 (Kaiser Family Foundation, 2019).

CHAPTER 85 HIV and AIDS

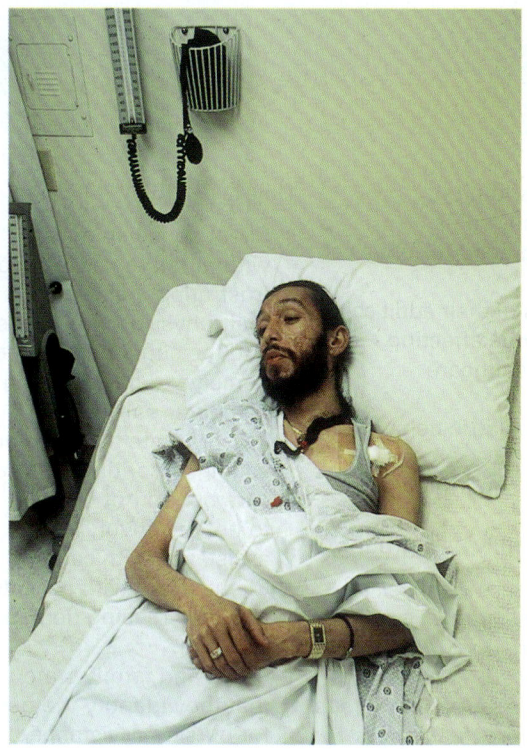

Figure 85-2 The wasting syndrome of acquired immunodeficiency syndrome (AIDS). In the later stages of AIDS, the client loses weight and is susceptible to many opportunistic infections.

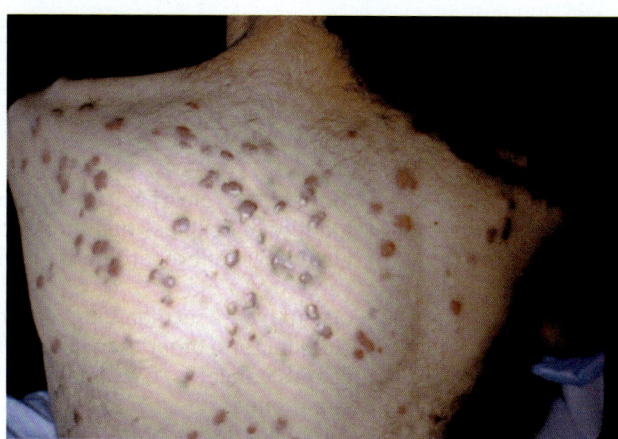

Figure 85-3 Lesions called *Kaposi sarcoma,* an acquired immunodeficiency syndrome (AIDS)–related malignancy common in later stages of the disease.

Due to a variety of available medications and aggressive treatment, the mortality rate decreased rapidly through 1997 and has continued a slow decline since then. Demographic groups of concern for HIV morbidity and mortality include women, African Americans, residents of the South, and individuals aged 45 years or older. HIV clients can delay the onset of AIDS for several years if properly treated with antiretroviral agents.

IN PRACTICE

NURSING CARE PLAN 85-1   The Person With AIDS-Associated Weight Loss and Wasting

Medical history: C.H., a 39-year-old client, was admitted to the hospital complaining of anorexia, weight loss, and diarrhea secondary to AIDS. History reveals the use of multiple antiretroviral therapies without success. "Either I had such terrible side effects that I couldn't tolerate them or I developed a resistance to them." Client's condition is considered terminal.

Medical diagnosis: AIDS, anorexia, wasting syndrome.

DATA COLLECTION/NURSING OBSERVATION

Client is 5′5″ tall, weighing 94 lb. Client reports episodes of persistent anorexia and diarrhea. Skin thin, pale, and transparent; turgor slow to return when pinched. Skin in perianal area and buttocks reddened and irritated. Client repeatedly talking about the fact that they seem to be getting progressively sicker, and that their weight loss, fatigue, and pain were also increasing in severity. Client states that they know that they are dying. They cried about the fact that their family is becoming exhausted with the increasing demands of physical care. For the last year, they lived at home with their retired parents who provide all of the client's care. "My mom is 70 years old and has really bad arthritis. My dad is 73 years old and has high blood pressure and a heart condition. Last month he was unable to speak for several minutes. I think he had a little stroke. I don't know how much more they can take." When questioned, parents report being tired, stating, "But we want to do everything that we can for our child." Client has no siblings or friends who can assume the duties of an in-home caregiver.

NURSING DIAGNOSIS

(Although other nursing diagnoses may be appropriate, a priority nursing diagnosis is addressed below.)

Stressed caregiver role (risk for) related to prolonged disease progression and increasing care responsibilities in conjunction with parental age and physical condition as evidenced by client's statements about current status and parents.

PLANNING (Outcomes/ Goals)	IMPLEMENTATION (Nursing Actions)	EVALUATION
Short-Term Goals		
A. Client will verbalize concerns to their parents.	• Identify the role of self in current family situation. • Identify how illness has changed the family roles. • Listen to client regarding their increasing need for physical care. • Listen to parents regarding terminal status of their adult child. • Note factors, other than illness, that may be affecting client's concerns, e.g., finances, lack of healthcare experience. • Ask client if they prefer professional psychiatric help, grief counselor, or neither at this time. • Consider counseling sessions with client separately and parents separately. • Consider counseling sessions with the family as a group. *Rationale:* Emotional needs are as important as physical needs. The client is aware of their terminal status. Acceptance that the family is having more difficultly caring for client both physically and psychologically is part of the grieving process. Past history of the family dynamics needs to be understood as some factors will affect the family's decisions including past family interrelationships, finances, available space, and the parent's personal health. • Encourage client to talk with parents about the increasing demands on them. • Help family differentiate between concerns of increasing physical care and the grief of impending death. *Rationale:* Having the client talk with their parents opens the channels of communication for future action. Feelings of guilt are not uncommon. The family's frustrations may diminish as they realize that they are not able to prevent their adult child from dying.	Day 1—14:15 hr. • Client spoke at length with nurse regarding their frustrations related to their physical care needs and the situation that they perceive to be occurring with their parents. • Parents state that they are willing to continue home care but do not object to options involving assistance with care. • Client spoke with parents about increasing demands on them. • Client and family state that they identify the need for outside assistance. **Goal A met.**
B. Client and family will understand the difference between in-home healthcare and hospice care.	• Provide information to the family regarding resources for additional healthcare. • Contact discharge planner for discussion with family and preparation of discharge. • Contact home health nursing for predischarge consultation regarding available services for in-home care. • Contact hospice nurse for discussion regarding available assistance from hospice and to differentiate this service from home health nursing. • Confirm client's understanding of in-home care. • Differentiate in-home healthcare with hospice services. *Rationale:* The discharge planner, home healthcare coordinator, and hospice coordinator can provide specific information related to the types of services that can be provided for this client in the various locations. Many individuals believe that a nurse will be available at all times, which is rarely an option for in-home nursing. The family needs the realistic information that will enable the family to comprehend what types of physical needs will be ongoing. The family needs to understand that feelings of guilt are normal. Discussions with clients and staff in a hospice facility will provide support for the situation and, hopefully, assist with the resolution of conflicting emotions.	Day 2—12:30 hr. • Family spoke with discharge planner. • Plan for home healthcare confirmed in family/nurse conference. • Home healthcare agency contacted. • Home healthcare visit scheduled prior to client's discharge from hospital. • Family stated that they would think about options and return the next day with their choice. **Goal B partially met.** Ongoing discussions continue.

PLANNING (Outcomes/Goals)	IMPLEMENTATION (Nursing Actions)	EVALUATION
Long-Term Goals		
C. Client and family will prepare for client's discharge to a hospice facility.	• Use active listening skills to gain understanding of client's individual desires for care. • Schedule time for group conference with family, primary nurse, and discharge coordinator. • Support client's and parent's decisions. *Rationale: After discussions with healthcare resource personnel, options are better understood. If the client elects to go to a local hospice facility, nursing care is available at all times and parents can visit at any time. The client's concerns about their parent's health will decrease. To minimize guilt, it is important that client and family understand that hospice referral is appropriate. There is a significant positive role available from hospice environments that assist clients and families in late-stage disease.*	Day 3—17:45 hr. Conference with client and parents: • Family expressing concerns about not being able to continue care at home. • Client states worry about their parent's health status, "My father had a ministroke last month" and "I don't want them to suffer any more because of me." • Client tells nurse that they prefer to go to hospice facility. **Goals B and C completed.**

IN PRACTICE

EDUCATING THE CLIENT 85-1 — Key Teaching Topics for Understanding HIV and AIDS

- Disease process, signs and symptoms
- Ways for transmitting and not transmitting HIV
- Infection control measures
- Proper disposal for sharps and contaminated objects
- Maintenance of hygiene in kitchen
- Possible side effects of medication
- Nutritional plans, including the use of dietary supplements
- Psychological support
- Available community resources and services to provide home management
- Sources for hospice care

NURSING PROCESS

DATA COLLECTION

Carefully observe and monitor the client who has been diagnosed with HIV. Refer to earlier section: Signs and Symptoms of HIV Infection. In addition to careful nursing observations, take note of medications. Determine if medication regimens and requirements for taking anti-HIV medications are being followed. Observe for evidence of depression, anxiety, or other symptoms, which may indicate psychological dysfunction or lack of coping mechanisms. When a person has AIDS, specific signs and symptoms may be difficult to identify because this disorder can affect many body systems. Establish a baseline for future comparison and determine the presence of suspected complications. Document and report any changes in this baseline level. Data collection generally includes specific legal concerns, such as consents to obtain HIV infection status.

Acquired immunodeficiency syndrome is a chronic condition and is ultimately fatal. Evaluate the client's physical and emotional response to the disease. What information or help does the client need to cope with the prognosis? Does the client need assistance to meet daily needs? How does the disorder affect social activities or self-esteem? Is the client taking medications as prescribed? What support services do the client and family need? Is professional counseling or a support group available? What rehabilitation or home care services are necessary?

PLANNING AND IMPLEMENTING

Plan together with the client, family, and other members of the healthcare team for effective individualized care to meet the client's needs. The client may require assistance in meeting all basic and healthcare needs, as well as in dealing with the chronic or terminal nature of the disorder. Teach the client and family about the disorder and prescribed medications and treatment. Counseling, social services, home care, and other community agencies are often involved. A nursing care plan is developed to meet identified needs (In Practice: Nursing Care Plan 85-1).

In addition to the physical effects of HIV infection, many persons with this diagnosis have experienced stigma, loss of job and insurance, depression, anxiety, and adjustment problems. All of these issues must be considered when working with HIV-infected individuals. Legal issues, especially related to confidentiality, are priority considerations.

> **Nursing Alert** Confidentiality is always a concern for healthcare professionals. For clients with HIV/AIDS, nurses must be diligently alert to the confidential nature of the disease.

Nursing Implications for Clients With HIV

Although many HIV-infected persons can function fully and do not require specialized care beyond that provided by their primary care providers, nursing care can be very helpful in many instances. For example, it is essential to take prescribed antiretroviral agents as directed, and persons with HIV often require assistance with medication adherence. The nurse can help in planning with the client how to take each dose; provide suggestions for pill boxes and calendars; assist in the management of side effects; aid in obtaining refills on time; and teach so that the client and family understand interactions that might occur with food and other drugs. The nurse plays a key role in client and family teaching about all aspects of the disease and care (In Practice: Educating the Client 85-1).

> **Key Concept**
> HIV cannot invade the body through intact skin; therefore, skin is an excellent barrier to HIV.

> **Key Concept**
> HIV/AIDS medication therapy demands strict adherence to a complicated regimen. The client and the nurse must be aware of the requirements of each medication.

The psychosocial aspects of being infected with HIV may be significant; persons are stigmatized, may lose the support of friends and family, and may find the restraints on sexual activity difficult. Support from healthcare professionals can assist HIV-positive clients to adjust to the diagnosis. The nurse can make referrals for psychosocial care to counselors and support groups. Some HIV-infected individuals choose to return to school and work and may benefit from referral to retraining programs or educational counselors. In addition, it is important that those who are infected know how to prevent transmission of HIV to family, friends, and sexual partners.

SPECIAL CONSIDERATIONS Lifespan

HIV and Aging
HIV and its treatment can complicate the aging process. Healthcare for the older population typically includes heart disease, hypertension, diabetes, cancer, and respiratory problems, which may need pharmaceutical or surgical therapies. Potentially hazardous drug interactions may occur.

> **Nursing Alert** Condoms do not guarantee safe sex. They provide safer sex.

Nursing Implications for Clients With AIDS

Individuals in later stages of the disease are more likely to require special nursing care. Because of their weakened condition, they many require total nursing care. Some may be able to stay home during their final days. Family members need education about what this entails. Box 85-2 has information on home care for a client with HIV/AIDS.

OIs require special medications, and clients may need assistance in taking these properly or in contacting the healthcare provider when problems develop. Intravenous medications may be used and with such medications comes the associated care of venous access lines. When a person is in the terminal stages of AIDS, the focus is on providing the client with comfort. Emotional support, combined with technical skills, will help clients and families cope with the illness. The nurse may need to schedule regular meetings to provide education and resources.

EVALUATION

The entire healthcare team, client, and family will evaluate outcomes of care. Have short-term goals been met? For example, is the client adhering to the prescribed medications? Are the client and family beginning to discuss the disease and its care? Are long-term goals still realistic? What community services are required? Is the client in need of home care services? Does the client need financial assistance? Is a referral for psychiatric care indicated? Planning for further nursing and healthcare considers the client's prognosis and responses to care.

Box 85-2 Home Care for the Person With HIV/AIDS

It is important that the client and family understand how the human immunodeficiency virus (HIV) is transmitted. Infection controls are essential, so always use standard precautions:

- Gloves should be worn during contact with blood or other body fluids or any time blood, or body fluids, including urine, feces, or vomit, may be present.
- Cuts, sores, or breaks on the caregiver's and client's exposed skin should be covered with bandages.
- Hands and other parts of the body should be washed immediately after contact with blood or other body fluids, and surfaces soiled with blood should be disinfected appropriately.
- Practices that increase the likelihood of blood contact, such as sharing of razors and toothbrushes, should be avoided.
- Needles and other sharp instruments should be used only when medically necessary and handled according to recommendations for healthcare settings.
- Do not put caps back on needles by hand or remove needles from syringes. Dispose of needles in puncture-proof containers out of the reach of children and visitors.

Adapted from Saint Luke's. (n.d.). *Discharge instructions for HIV infection and AIDS*. https://www.saintlukeskc.org/health-library/discharge-instructions-hiv-infection-and-aids

HIV EXPOSURE GUIDELINES

Prevention is the key to future HIV outcomes. Currently, there are no cures or vaccines available. Consider that about 37,968 new cases occurred in 2018 in the United States (CDC, 2020). The healthcare needed for an infection that devastates the immune system involves high levels of daily care, psychological adjustment, financial obligations, and approaches to personal relationships that include acknowledgment of HIV status.

PrEP and PEP

There are two basic types of information available regarding protection against HIV infection: *before exposure* or *PrEP* and *after exposure* or *PEP*. According to the CDC, the word "prophylaxis" means to prevent or control the spread of an infection or disease.

PrEP is used for prevention of infection with HIV. PrEP is intended for individuals who are at high risk of getting HIV, for example, a sexually active partner of an individual who is HIV positive. The PrEP method is designed to be used consistently, a pill every day, and to be used with other prevention options (e.g., condoms). PrEP may be an option for individuals who are exposed to HIV frequently. The individuals who may initiate PrEP need to understand that they must take the medication daily and use other prevention tools such as condoms. Side effects of the medication include headaches and GI distress, which seem to diminish in about a month.

PEP is used within 72 hr or 3 days after a single, high-risk event. PEP is used for healthcare workers who have had a single event of exposure to blood or body fluids that are infected or whose infection status is unknown. The goal is to stop HIV from making copies of itself and spreading throughout the body. It is imperative to take the antiretroviral medicines as soon as possible to prevent becoming HIV positive. Two to three types of medications are taken for a duration of 28 days. Nausea is the most common side effect. After the 28 days of treatment, the individual is rescheduled for HIV testing at 4–6 weeks, 3 months, and 6 months. PEP is not 100% effective; it does not guarantee that a person newly exposed to HIV will not become HIV positive if exposed to the virus. It will be necessary for the individual to continue to use condoms until HIV-negative status is confirmed by a laboratory at the sixth month. Refer to the CDC Website on HIV at www.cdc.gov/hiv/guidelines/preventing.html.

In addition to the CDC protocols, individual clinical facilities typically have regimens for situations involving possible or probable exposure to HIV. As a nurse, it will be your responsibility to be aware of these protocols. Counseling, laboratory tests, and follow-up testing will be included as part of PrEP and PEP.

Disclosure of HIV Status

Disclosure of HIV is a difficult personal responsibility and may also be a legal requirement. Notification begins with a positive HIV test. If the HIV test is positive, the clinic, laboratory, or other testing site will report the results to the state health department. State health officials, also known as public health officials, use this information to monitor the status of the epidemic of HIV, as well as many other infectious diseases, for example, syphilis, pertussis, or measles. Federal and state funding for HIV/AIDS services is often based on prioritization of needs, that is to say, where the need is greatest and the epidemic is strongest. The state health department will remove all personal information from the information, which is then sent to the Centers for Diseases Control and Prevention (CDC). The CDC is responsible for tracking epidemics and providing resources to healthcare personnel as well as to the American public. The CDC does not share this information with anyone, including insurance companies.

Partner-notification laws are available in many states, and some cities do require the HIV-positive individual to tell specific people of their HIV status. These laws required that a positive HIV test must be reported by the individual or the healthcare provider to any sexual partner(s) or any person(s) with whom the HIV-positive person has shared needles. Keep in mind the legal obligation to notify the appropriate agencies and individuals in order to prevent the spread of the disease. Failure to provide notification of positive HIV-positive status is a crime. If the contact information is known, some health departments require healthcare providers to report positive HIV results to the individuals who shared sex or needles with an HIV-positive person.

A *third-party notification* requires that healthcare personnel report the HIV status to an individual who has a significant risk for exposure to HIV by someone who is known to be HIV infected. While it may be the moral and legal responsibility of an HIV-infected person to notify any significant other, not all individuals will comply. The *duty to warn* is designed to show good faith efforts to notify a partner of an individual who has HIV/AIDS.

Notifying others may not be an easy task. Exposure to HIV may mean revealing personal information such as sexual relationships or drug use. Sexual partners need to know that they may have been exposed. The benefits of reporting can be lifesaving. By notifying the individual or the public health department, an HIV infection may be prevented. The sexual partner may be able to receive PrEP or PEP. Educating friends can help others to be more conscientious of the need for protected sex (e.g., the use of condoms). Since STIs often coexist with HIV, all individuals should seek healthcare advice and treatment, if needed.

The consequences of HIV exposure present a multitude of economic and social concerns. The HIV-positive individual can prevent others from getting this disease. Since HIV is a lifelong disease, all future contacts need to be notified. According to the CDC (2020), "as of 2020, 37 states have criminalized HIV exposure" (para 1).

STUDENT SYNTHESIS

KEY POINTS

- The terms *HIV* and *AIDS* are not synonymous. HIV is the virus responsible for causing the infection. AIDS is the third and terminal stage of HIV infection.
- HIV is a retrovirus, a virus that overtakes the biosynthesis of living cells to duplicate itself.
- HIV invades a normal cell and uses that cell's biomechanisms to reproduce new HIV cells.
- The Centers for Disease Control and Prevention include in the classification of AIDS diagnosis based on a T-cell count of fewer than 200 cells/mm^3, the presence of opportunistic infections, and the presence of some cancers.
- Follow Standard Precautions in caring for all clients, for self-protection, and to minimize the risk of contracting HIV and other infections, such as hepatitis B and C.
- ELISA (EIA) and Western blot testing are typically the first two laboratory tests done to detect and confirm HIV infection.
- Treatment for HIV includes a variety of antiretroviral medications that will be continued for life.
- Signs and symptoms of the primary stage of HIV may include headache, fever, fatigue.
- Symptoms of AIDS include malaise, diarrhea, Kaposi sarcoma, dementia, wasting syndrome, and several other opportunistic infections.
- PrEP and PEP are prophylaxis guidelines for individuals who may be exposed to HIV.

CRITICAL THINKING EXERCISES

1. You are working in a clinic. A coworker comes to you and is frantic. They have just accidentally stuck themselves with a used needle. Which measures would you take? How would you emotionally support the coworker? What should they do?

2. You are working in the home of a client with AIDS. You have provided care to this client for several months. The client is extremely depressed and mentions a few times that he is seriously contemplating suicide. You have worked with the client's family members as well, who are extremely supportive. Last week, the client's adult child mentioned to you that they are worried about their father's emotional state. How would you handle this situation? Give explanations for your response.

NCLEX-STYLE REVIEW QUESTIONS

1. The nurse is reinforcing education for a female client, who is HIV positive, about transmission of the virus. Which statement made by the client demonstrates that further education is required?
   a. "If I become pregnant, I must continue to take my antiretroviral medication."
   b. "I should not kiss anyone while I have an open sore in my mouth."
   c. "I will be able to breastfeed if my baby and I are taking antiretroviral drugs."
   d. "I may be able to transmit HIV if someone uses a glass after I drink from it."

2. The charge nurse is observing a new graduate providing care to a client who is HIV positive. Which action by the new graduate would require immediate intervention by the charge nurse?
   a. Recapping a needle after giving an injection
   b. Using gloves when changing a soiled dressing
   c. Wearing a face shield when irrigating a sacral wound
   d. Discarding gloves when exiting the client's room

3. A client arrives at the clinic requesting testing for HIV. Which response by the nurse is best?
   a. "Did you have sex with multiple partners?"
   b. "The test results won't be back for a while."
   c. "You will need to sign a consent form prior to testing."
   d. "We will call you with the results."

4. The nurse is teaching a client with human immunodeficiency virus (HIV) to understand the importance of medication adherence. Which information would the nurse include when reinforcing the education? Select all that apply.
   a. The use of pill containers and calendars
   b. Interaction with foods and other drugs
   c. Management of medication side effects
   d. Obtaining refills on time
   e. When to discontinue medications

5. A nurse is prescribed postexposure prophylaxis (PEP) antiretroviral medication after a needle stick from an HIV-positive client. Which side effect would the nurse likely experience when taking this medication?
   a. Fatigue
   b. Nausea
   c. Swollen lymph nodes
   d. Constipation

CHAPTER RESOURCES

Enhance your learning with additional resources on thePoint!
Student Resources related to this chapter can be found at **thePoint.lww.com/Rosdahl12e**

86 Respiratory Disorders

Learning Objectives

1. State the rationale for the use of each of the following: sputum, lavage, throat culture, ABG, CXR, lung scan, lung perfusion scan, pulmonary angiography, PFT, and skin testing.
2. Demonstrate the positions of postural drainage.
3. Differentiate the following: thoracentesis, paracentesis, and thoracotomy.
4. Identify four nursing considerations related to closed water-seal chest drainage.
5. Identify five alterations in normal respiratory status.
6. Identify 10 interventions that can assist the client who is in respiratory distress.
7. Differentiate the following infectious respiratory disorders: acute rhinitis, streptococcal throat infection, influenza, laryngitis, bronchitis, lung abscesses, pneumonia, pleurisy, histoplasmosis, tuberculosis, and empyema.
8. Compare and contrast the following pulmonary diseases: asthma, bronchiectasis, chronic bronchitis, and emphysema.
9. Identify three nursing considerations for a client with ARDS.
10. State three common sources of trauma to the lungs, along with three nursing considerations for each.
11. Differentiate between the two types of malignant lung tumors and state the names of three forms of NSCLC.
12. Identify three common inflammatory disorders and four structural disorders of the nose.

Important Terminology

anergic, asphyxiation, asthma, atelectasis, bronchiectasis, bronchitis, bronchoscopy, empyema, epistaxis, eupnea, group A streptococci, hemothorax, histoplasmosis, hyperventilation, incentive spirometer, laryngectomy, lobectomy, otitis media, paracentesis, pharyngitis, pleurisy, pneumonectomy, pneumonia, pneumothorax, postural drainage, pulmonary emphysema, rhinitis, rhinoplasty, sinusitis, strangulation, streptococcal pharyngitis (strep throat), suffocation, thoracentesis, thoracotomy, tracheostomy, tuberculosis

Acronyms

ABG, ARDS, ATT, BCG, COPD, CPAP, CPT, CT, CXR, GAS, IGRA, INH, IPPB, NSCLC, $PaCO_2$, PaO_2, PJP (formerly PCP), PFT, PJP, PPD, TST, SCLC, SOB, SOBOE, TB

The respiratory system is vital to sustaining life. Respiration requires a patent (open) airway for oxygen to reach the lungs and lungs that are physically capable of exchanging oxygen for carbon dioxide. Healthcare professionals may specialize in the field of respiratory care. A healthcare provider specializing in respiratory disorders is called a *pulmonologist*. A related field of respiratory care is *respiratory therapy,* which involves *respiratory therapists* and *respiratory technicians*.

The respiratory system consists of the upper respiratory tract (nose, sinuses, pharynx, and trachea) and the lower respiratory tract (bronchi and lungs) (Chapter 25). Because blood carries oxygen and carbon dioxide, both the cardiovascular system and the respiratory system must function for life to continue. A person can survive for only a few minutes without oxygen; it is the most vital, basic need of people and animals.

DIAGNOSTIC TESTS
Laboratory Tests

Sputum Specimen

Sputum specimens help determine the presence of organisms or blood in a person's sputum. Specimens are best early in the morning, when they are most likely to contain sputum, rather than just saliva (Chapter 52).

Nursing Alert Take precautions in the care and disposal of sputum. Wear gloves when collecting specimens. Wear a mask and eye shield if splashing is likely. Using gloves, discard all used facial tissues as contaminated material. Discard gloves in contaminated waste. Wash hands after removal of gloves.

Lavage Specimen

If the client is unable to cough up sputum, the healthcare provider may order that either the nurse or the respiratory therapist obtain a specimen by bronchoalveolar lavage. In this procedure, sterile saline is instilled into a bronchus. Then, cells and fluid from the bronchioles and alveoli are removed by endoscopy along with the saline. The cells are analyzed in the laboratory, most often to diagnose pulmonary tuberculosis.

1533

Throat Culture

A sore throat, or **pharyngitis**, is inflammation, but not necessarily infection, of the pharynx. It is most commonly due to a virus, which does not respond to antibiotics. However, a significant proportion of children with pharyngitis and many adults have bacterial infections of the throat that can have significant consequences if not treated. To test for the presence of infection, a sample of both mucus and secretions from the back of the client's throat is obtained. A specimen collection system consisting of a sterile cotton-tipped applicator inside a specimen tube is used. The back of the throat is swabbed with the cotton tip and inserted back into the closed system. The specimen needs to be sent to the laboratory quickly, usually in less than 30 min, or the bacteria can dehydrate and not be useful. In the laboratory, the cotton tip is swiped onto a slide or culture medium, which is then incubated to determine the presence of organisms. Drug sensitivity determinations may also be done by placing the specimen on solid media with different concentrations of medications or in various liquid dilutions of medications to determine which medication is most effective against the organism. This procedure is called a *culture and sensitivity* (C&S) test or *throat culture*.

A complete culture will determine all organisms present in the specimen. This test takes 48 hr because the organisms must have time to grow. However, a specific version of the throat culture may be done within a matter of hours to rule out the presence of streptococci. This test does not rule out any other organisms. The *rapid strep test* or *rapid antigen detection* test is done in cases of suspected **group A streptococci** (**GAS**) infection can have results in a few minutes so that appropriate antibiotic therapy can be initiated quickly.

Blood Gas Determinations

The best indicator of oxygen deficiency is the level of arterial blood gases (**ABGs**). The partial pressure of oxygen (**PaO$_2$**) value is generally considered normal when it is between 80 and 100 mm Hg (millimeters of mercury). The laboratory can analyze an arterial blood sample and determine the PaO$_2$, partial pressure of carbon dioxide (**PaCO$_2$**), and hydrogen ion concentration (pH) of the blood. The healthcare provider, nurse, and respiratory therapist then evaluate the blood gas results and plan the most effective treatment for the client. A noninvasive method for continually or intermittently monitoring oxygen saturation of hemoglobin, without the use of a blood sample, is *pulse oximetry*. (For additional information, see the Hypoxia section later in this chapter as well as in Nursing Procedure 46-6 and Chapter 87.)

> **Key Concept**
>
> Hypoxemia is considered a PaO$_2$ of less than 60–70 mm Hg on ABGs or a hemoglobin oxygen saturation of less than 90% on pulse oximetry. Always consider the client's actual clinical condition, which may not accurately reflect any relative mechanical value. The presence of iron deficiency anemia often yields misleading results.

X-Ray and Fluoroscopy Examinations

Chest X-Ray

The *chest x-ray* (**CXR**) examination is no longer done routinely for all clients who are admitted to acute care facilities. It is ordered to determine lung or heart abnormalities. Abnormalities that can be observed on x-ray study include lung tumors or other growths, lung abscesses, pulmonary tuberculosis, foreign objects in the lungs, pneumonia, or an enlarged heart.

Computed Tomography Scan

The *computed tomography* (**CT**) scan is a series of x-ray films taken to provide a cross-sectional view of the chest or other body part. CT scanning is valuable in the diagnosis of TB, lung abscesses, or tumors.

Lung Scan

After a radioactive medication is introduced into the system by injection or inhalation, a *lung scan* (*scintiscan*) is done. This test yields a two-dimensional map of various organs and tissues. Disorders are revealed as a difference in density from normal tissue. After the client inhales a special gas, this scan is called a *ventilation scan*.

Lung Perfusion Scan

Albumin tagged with a radioactive material is injected intravenously. These particles pass through the client's venous system and heart, but when they reach the lungs, they lodge in the capillaries. The *lung perfusion scan* illustrates different views through which lesions, pneumonia, and other disorders can be located.

Pulmonary Angiography

Pulmonary angiography involves injection of radiopaque dye into the pulmonary blood vessels to determine pathology (Box 47-2 for signs and symptoms of dye-related problems).

Other Diagnostic Tests

Magnetic Resonance Imaging

As with many other body systems, *magnetic resonance imaging* (MRI) can be used to diagnose disorders in the lungs and bronchi. This noninvasive nuclear procedure can produce images of tissues with high fat and water content, which often cannot be seen with conventional x-ray study. Thus, MRI is useful in the diagnosis of lung disorders. It allows the healthcare provider to distinguish among cancerous, trauma-induced, and normal tissues because it gives information about their chemical composition.

Pulmonary Function Test

The *pulmonary function test* (**PFT**) measures how much air a client inhales (*inspiration*) and exhales (*expiration*) in one breath and assesses the client's general respiratory status. Many large hospitals have pulmonary function laboratories for this purpose.

The PFT measures total lung capacity, *vital capacity* (amount of air that is forcibly exhaled after a maximum breath), and *residual volume* (amount of air remaining in the lung after forced exhalation). PFT also measures *tidal volume* (volume of air in an average breath), inspiratory volume, and expiratory volume. The ratios between specific measurements can be determined. The machine used for these tests is the *spirometer*.

> **Key Concept**
>
> Do not confuse the spirometer with the incentive spirometer. The spirometer measures pulmonary function. The incentive spirometer also measures pulmonary function, in a sense, but it is used by the client. The incentive spirometer helps the client, such as after surgery, to perform respiratory exercises to maintain lung function.

The PFT is used to diagnose disorders and to assess effectiveness of therapy. The test helps in determining pulmonary pathology at an early stage and indicates whether the person has a cardiac or a respiratory disease. The test can evaluate the effectiveness of respiratory therapies and bronchodilator medications and can indicate the surgical risk involved in many cases. When administering this test, encourage the client to breathe as deeply as possible or to follow other instructions.

Bronchoscopy

Bronchoscopy is an invasive procedure in which a *bronchoscope* (a lighted endoscope) is advanced through the pharynx into the trachea and bronchi. The purpose of this test may be to observe lung tissue, obtain a biopsy or bronchial washings, remove mucous plugs or foreign objects, or determine the location and extent of a mass (tumor). Photographs may be taken. Two types of bronchoscopes are used: the rigid and the fiberoptic. The fiberoptic scope is smaller and more flexible, making it more comfortable for the client and allowing the healthcare provider better visualization of the lung within the smaller airways (Fig. 86-1).

Before the test, the person's throat is anesthetized and medications (e.g., midazolam) are administered intravenously (IV) to promote relaxation. These medications may cause a client to experience amnesia about the test. Alert the client to this possibility before the test to prevent concern later.

Food and fluids are withheld for 6–8 hr before a bronchoscopy. Give mouth care immediately before the procedure. Explain the procedure to the client, who will most likely remain awake. Be sure that any dentures are removed.

Note any loose natural teeth because the bronchoscope may loosen or dislodge a tooth, which could lead to aspiration.

After bronchoscopy, the client takes nothing by mouth (NPO) until the gag reflex returns. The anesthetic numbs the throat, so reflexes are not functional and do not allow the person to cough out secretions. The client needs to be in a side-lying position. *Rationale: Doing so keeps the airway open and helps to prevent choking and aspiration.* The side-lying position also helps to facilitate drainage. Note any edema of the throat, bleeding, or dyspnea because if the airway becomes obstructed, an emergency **tracheostomy** (opening into the trachea) may be needed. A sterile endotracheal tube is kept at the bedside until the client is fully awake and reflexes return. In a respiratory emergency, the endotracheal tube can be inserted to assist in keeping the airway open temporarily.

After the client's gag reflex returns, offer clear liquids and monitor the client's ability to tolerate them. Gradually increase the client's diet to soft foods. Encourage the client to rest and to eat soft foods for 24 hr after this procedure.

Because most bronchoscopy procedures are done on an outpatient basis, be sure to teach the client and family to be alert for possible complications, especially the following:

- Swelling of the throat
- Difficulty swallowing
- Difficulty breathing
- Bleeding

Be sure to document all teaching completely.

> **NCLEX Alert**
>
> Testing of various respiratory functions is commonly done as inpatient or outpatient procedures. It is important that you are aware of nursing actions for these procedures, including pre- and postprocedure teaching and reactions to emergency situations.

Skin and Blood Tests

Skin tests are commonly used to determine if a person has been exposed to tuberculosis or other disorders, such as *histoplasmosis*. The procedure is the same as that for administering tests to determine allergies to medications or other allergens. Blood testing may be available for some diseases.

Skin Tests

The *purified protein derivative* (**PPD**) tuberculin test, also known as the *Mantoux tuberculin skin test* (**TST**), indicates whether a person has ever been exposed to the tubercle bacillus. The acronyms TST and PPD may be used interchangeably. Approximately 0.1-mL tuberculin serum (PPD) is injected intradermally, with a TB syringe and needle in the lower part of the arm. The injection site is examined for edema with induration (firmness) and redness (erythema) 2–3 days (48–72 hr) after the injection. The skin is usually circled with an indelible ink pen so the area will be remembered with accuracy. Erythema alone does not indicate a positive reaction; the degrees of positive readings are based on the area of induration, sometimes combined with erythema. If the client's test results are not read within the appropriate time frame, the test must be repeated. To ensure accuracy

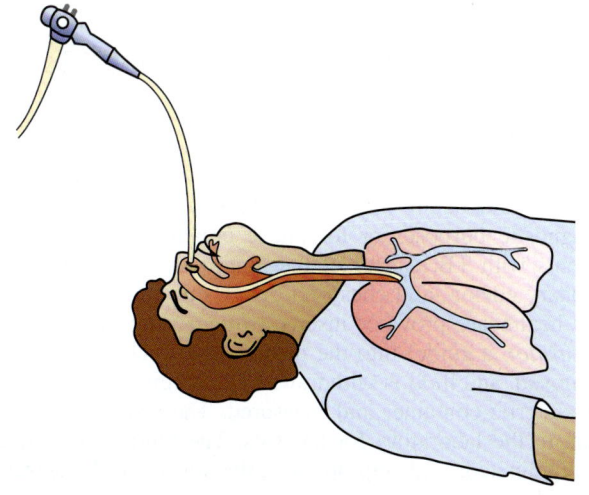

Figure 86-1 Fiberoptic bronchoscopy.

of administration and reliable results, the TST requires standardized TST administration procedures, training, and practice. Being diagnosed with TB, based on the TST, will have significant consequences for the individual; therefore, healthcare personnel need experience and the assistance of a knowledgeable person when initially reading any test results.

Another method of tuberculin skin testing is the *tine test*, which uses a prepackaged sterile stainless steel disk with four to six short needles (sharp prongs) that are coated with TB antigens, that is, the tuberculin, usually PPD tuberculin. The tines are pressed into the person's forearm. The disks are packaged individually and are disposable; thus, they offer a practical advantage when testing a large group of people. The injection method is simply to push the prongs into the skin and to read the results in 2–3 days, as would be done for the TST.

The tine method is somewhat controversial, as not all agencies consider it to be as reliable as the Mantoux TST, stating possible differences in the amount of tuberculin injected. The American Thoracic Society and the Centers for Disease Control and Prevention do not recommend the tine test. On occasion, an individual may not react to an antigen on a skin test. As a result, candida and mumps antigen sera may be injected at the same time as the TST (or PPD) to determine a person's ability to respond to any foreign agent (antigen). Persons with a healthy immune system should respond to candida or mumps or both. In the immunosuppressed individual, a response often does not occur. The term used is *anergy*, and the person is considered **anergic** (unable to respond to the foreign agent). In this case, the TST may have been mistakenly read as negative. The false-negative reaction occurs even though the individual carries the tuberculosis bacteria but is not able to have a positive reaction to the skin test. If the person is judged to be anergic, a two-step TST test may be necessary. The two-step TST test involves doing two TST tests, 1 or 2 weeks apart. This method attempts to boost the person's immune system to respond appropriately to the antigen. The two-step process may be used for individuals who are retested periodically such as residents in long-term care facilities or healthcare workers.

SPECIAL CONSIDERATIONS   Lifespan

False-Negative and Anergic Reactions to TST (or PPD) Tests

Anergy, the inability to create a reaction to skin tests, may cause *false-negative results*. This reaction can occur in persons who are immunocompromised, have HIV/AIDS, or a senior or elder adult with health issues. False-negative results are also a result of improper technique or incorrect reading of the results. Individuals who have recently been exposed to TB (within 8–10 weeks), have had a TB infection for many years, or have a current overwhelming TB are likely to have false-negative results. Additionally, an individual who is less than 6 months old or who has had a recent live-virus vaccination, for example, measles, will also have false-negative reactions.

A positive test means that the person has been exposed to the bacillus or that the individual has TB antibodies (e.g., BCG vaccinations). Individuals who have received the BCG vaccination as a protocol for TB prophylaxis may have either a positive or a negative TST reaction depending upon when the last BCG test was completed. A person who is a positive reactor usually remains so for life. Thus, once positive, the TST test is usually not repeated. If a person has a positive reaction to the testing, a CXR and a sputum culture should be done to determine if the lungs are affected. In addition, some individuals may develop a severe allergic reaction to the test.

Tuberculin Blood Tests

TB blood tests are called *interferon-gamma release assays* (**IGRAs**), which measure how the immune system reacts to the TB bacterium. Test available include QuantiFERON-TB Gold In-Tube test (QFT-GIT) and T-SPOT. Results from blood testing are generally available within 24–48 hr. A positive result to an IGRA indicates infection with the TB bacteria. Additional testing is needed to determine if the infection is latent or active.

COMMON MEDICAL TREATMENTS

Postural Drainage

Postural drainage uses position and gravity to drain secretions and mucus from the individual's lungs. This procedure is not often done by licensed vocational nurses or licensed practical nurses (LVN/LPNs) or registered nurses (RNs), but rather by respiratory therapists (Fig. 86-2). The procedures are commonly taught to family members for home care.

The person adopts a head downward position, which allows the secretions to run far enough into the trachea from the bronchi so that they can be coughed out. The client's exact position will depend on the portion of the lung to be drained. Treatments generally last about 15–20 min. The procedure is called chest physiotherapy (**CPT**). The nurse must receive specific instructions from a respiratory therapist, physical therapist, or pulmonary healthcare provider before performing this procedure (In Practice: Nursing Care Guidelines 86-1).

Often postural bronchial drainage is done in combination with other respiratory treatments, such as inhalations, to loosen and bring up secretions from the lungs and to prevent respiratory complications.

COMMON SURGICAL TREATMENTS

Thoracentesis

Thoracentesis involves puncturing the chest wall to remove excess fluid or air from the pleural cavity. It is done for diagnostic purposes or to relieve breathing difficulties in clients with TB, cancer of the lung, pleural effusion, pulmonary edema, and chest injuries. Using sterile technique, the healthcare provider inserts a *trocar* (large needle with *obturator*, a guide) into the pleural cavity. The obturator is removed, and fluid is withdrawn. The specimen is collected in a sterile container and measured. The specimen is then sent to the laboratory for analysis. The fluid is considered contaminated, and appropriate infection control measures should be taken.

CHAPTER 86 Respiratory Disorders 1537

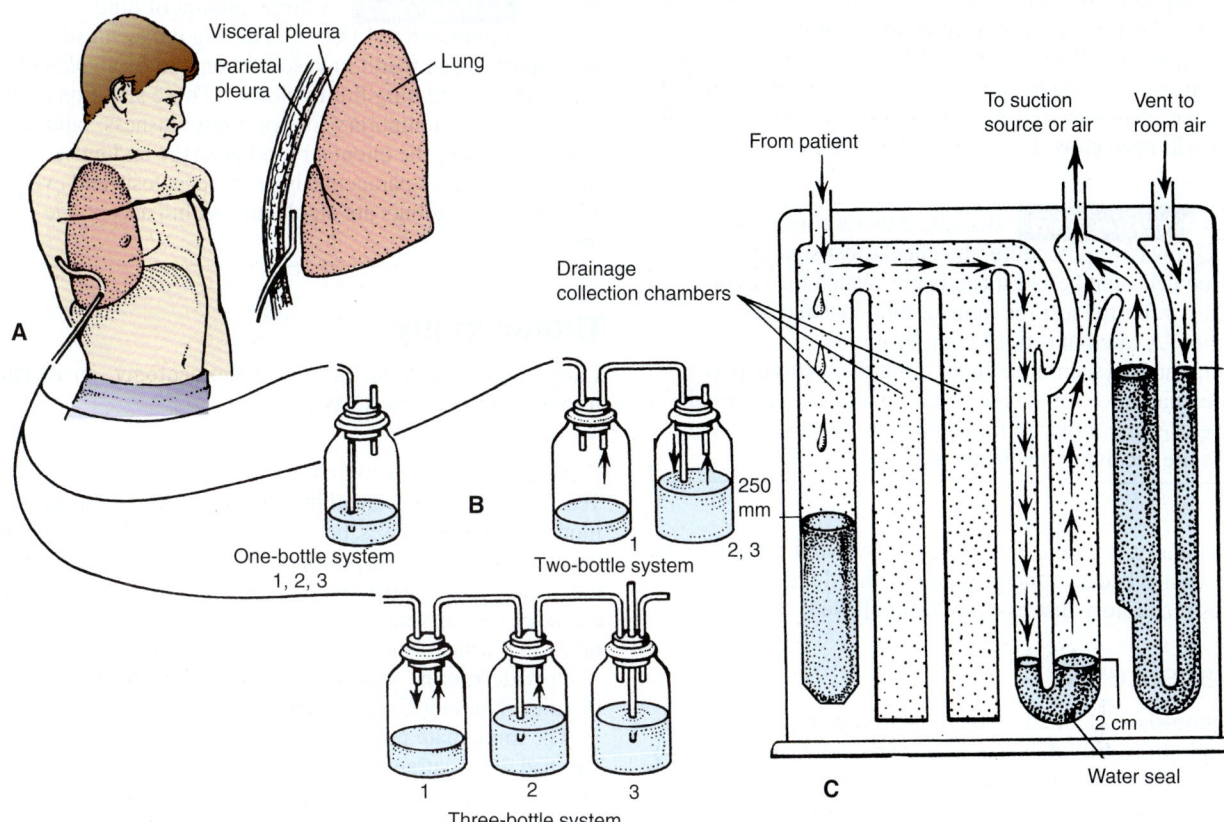

Figure 86-2 Chest drainage systems. **A.** Strategic placement of a chest catheter in the pleural space. **B.** Three types of mechanical drainage systems. **C.** A Pleur-Evac operating system: (1) the collection chamber, (2) the water-seal chamber, and (3) the suction control chamber. The Pleur-Evac is a single unit with all three bottles identified as chambers. (Nettina, 2006.)

IN PRACTICE
NURSING CARE GUIDELINES 86-1 | Assisting With Postural Drainage

- Always wash hands. **Rationale:** *Handwashing helps prevent the spread of infection.*
- Always wear gloves and handle all soiled tissues as contaminated material. **Rationale:** *This client may be infectious. Observe Standard Precautions.*
- Explain to the client why the head downward position is necessary for much of the treatment. **Rationale:** *This position may be uncomfortable, but if the client understands the reason, they will be more likely to cooperate.*
- Improve drainage by striking the client between the shoulder blades with cupped hands (*pummeling*) or by vibrating the client. **Rationale:** *These techniques help to loosen the secretions.* Be sure to receive instructions in these techniques.
- Have tissues available. **Rationale:** *The person will probably cough up secretions.*

- Have pillows and pads available. **Rationale:** *The various positions are easier to assume if a movable bed and pillows are available.*
- Perform this procedure before the person eats. **Rationale:** *The client may gag, choke, or vomit. Performing postural drainage before eating helps to prevent vomiting and aspiration.*
- Give the client oral hygiene following the procedure. **Rationale:** *The stagnant or infected mucus may have a foul taste and odor.*
- Dispose of all materials properly and wash hands. **Rationale:** *Proper disposal of materials and handwashing help reduce the risk of infection transmission.*
- Document the procedure and the client's reactions. **Rationale:** *Documentation provides for communication and continuity of care.*

Throughout the procedure, assist the client and offer support. The procedure is similar to abdominal paracentesis (Chapter 88). The person will be most comfortable in a sitting position while leaning on a padded overbed table. The healthcare provider will need very little assistance, but the client will need considerable emotional support.

> **Nursing Alert** Because a thoracentesis is an invasive procedure, the client must sign an informed consent before it can begin. Watch the client carefully after the test for signs of fluid leakage or infection. A rare but serious complication is pneumothorax (accumulation of air in the pleural space). Clients may have some pain, which analgesics can usually relieve. Be sure to watch for respiratory depression when clients are receiving medications.

Generally, after the procedure, the individual can breathe more easily because the pressure of the fluid, which often causes respiratory distress, has been relieved.

Paracentesis

Paracentesis is defined as the puncturing of a body cavity for aspiration of fluid; however, this process most commonly refers to puncture of the abdominal cavity. Abdominal distention caused by excess fluid immobilizes the diaphragm and interferes with breathing. Therefore, removing fluid from the abdomen can relieve breathing difficulties.

> **Nursing Alert** A large amount of fluid withdrawn (>1,000 mL) during paracentesis or thoracentesis can result in vasodilation and *hypovolemia* (decreased circulating fluid volume). These situations can cause *syncope* (temporary loss of consciousness, fainting) and shock. Take the client's blood pressure and pulse immediately after paracentesis or thoracentesis and every 15 min until readings are stable and within acceptable levels.

Thoracotomy

Lung surgery is done through a **thoracotomy**, an incision into the thorax or chest cavity.

Caring for the Client After Chest Surgery

Teach the client deep breathing techniques, as well as range of motion (ROM) exercises, before chest surgery. The extent of the client's participation in postoperative care will directly reflect the quality of preoperative instruction given. Postoperative exercises can be vital to recovery and help prevent complications (In Practice: Nursing Care Guidelines 86-2).

Provide routine preoperative and postoperative care (In Practice: Nursing Care Guidelines 86-2).

The immediate postoperative concern for the person who has had lung surgery is to maintain an adequate airway. Direct care at preventing respiratory complications.

Record vital signs frequently; turn the client often to prevent complications of immobility. Encourage the client to

---

IN PRACTICE
NURSING CARE GUIDELINES 86-2 — Caring for the Person Who Has Had Chest Surgery

- Always wash hands and wear gloves. **Rationale:** Handwashing and gloves help to prevent infection transmission.
- Turn the client often. **Rationale:** Turning helps to facilitate drainage and prevent hypostatic pneumonia and other complications. The wound will drain the most when the client is lying on the affected side; however, because this can be uncomfortable, coordinate turning to this side with the time when the pain medication effectiveness is optimum.
- Be sure the client turns and coughs and uses the incentive spirometer, as ordered. **Rationale:** These actions help to prevent stasis of secretions.
- Monitor for signs of dyspnea, changes in rate of respiration, cyanosis, increased heart rate, chest pain, restlessness, orthopnea, or hemoptysis. **Rationale:** These symptoms could indicate that the chest suction is malfunctioning.
- Help the client to sit comfortably in the chair while the chest suction is operating. **Rationale:** Getting the client out of bed helps to minimize the risk for developing complications, in particular, respiratory complications. Sitting in the chair helps to promote lung expansion.
- If the client is up walking with tubes and drainage bags or bottles, be sure that the hemostatic clamps go along. **Rationale:** The client must always be within reach of the clamps in case of accidental dislodgement of tubes.
- Make sure the client is passing flatus rather than having gas pains or distention difficulties. **Rationale:** Abdominal distention can cause difficulty in breathing and extreme discomfort.
- Encourage ambulation and exercise. **Rationale:** Ambulation and exercise help the client recover more quickly and decrease any risks of complications.
- Maintain a level of comfort acceptable to the client, so that deep breathing and coughing can and will be done. **Rationale:** Ease of breathing enhances the client's ability to comply with treatment.
- Remove and discard gloves and wash hands. **Rationale:** Washing hands is the most effective method of preventing cross contamination, even if gloves are worn during a procedure.

breathe deeply and to cough at least every 2–4 hr and to use the incentive spirometer. Coughing is easiest if the person is in an upright position and they splint the incision with a pillow.

The client must exercise soon after surgery because many muscles are incised during chest surgery, and function must be restored; exercise also prevents complications related to immobility. Carry out passive ROM exercises for the client; within a few days, they should be able to participate actively in ROM. Full ROM exercises, including *isometric* (muscle-setting) exercises, must be provided for the shoulder and arm on the operative side; these exercises may be initiated immediately following surgery. Discontinue any exercises that cause pain or great resistance. Do not overextend or overtire the client's muscles.

> **Nursing Alert** If a person with any disorder of the respiratory system is receiving a narcotic, be particularly watchful for respiratory depression. Depressed respirations can be an undesirable side effect in anyone, but the situation is most dangerous for the client whose respiratory function is already compromised.

Chest Suction
Following most types of lung surgery, the client will have large catheters called *chest tubes* inserted into the chest cavity and attached to suction. The breathing mechanism of the lungs works because the pressure of the chest cavity is lower than the pressure of the air outside the lungs. This negative pressure creates a vacuum, which causes air to rush into the lungs and keep them inflated. After the chest cavity has been opened, a vacuum must be created within the chest to reestablish negative pressure. The purpose of suction is to restore the negative pressure within the chest cavity and reinflate the lungs or to prevent loss of negative pressure and keep the lungs inflated. In addition, secretions and blood that may have accumulated in the chest cavity must be removed.

Closed Water-Seal Drainage
The most common method of reestablishing negative pressure is by *closed water-seal chest drainage*. In this procedure, one or more catheters are inserted into the chest cavity. If more than one catheter is inserted, each may be connected to a separate suction setup, or they may all be joined and attached to one suction setup.

> **Nursing Alert** Maintain the integrity of the suction apparatus and water seal at all times. Refill the water chamber if the fluid level gets low. Report at once any client who complains of severe pain or dyspnea. *If a bottle or connection breaks, the closed system will be disrupted, and this is an emergency.* Clamp the chest tubes immediately and summon help.

The water-seal drainage system must remain closed (airtight) so that no air is allowed to enter the chest cavity; otherwise, the lungs collapse. By putting the drainage tubes under water, air is prevented from backing up into the chest. One widely used apparatus of disposable chest drainage systems is called the Pleur-Evac (Fig. 86-2C).

This system comes assembled and sterile with instructions for use. It can be connected to suction and provides a water seal. When the chamber is full of blood, it is discarded and replaced with a new one; this is done *only by a trained professional.*

Nursing Implications
Monitor the client closely for signs of shock, dyspnea, pain in the chest, or a rapid increase in chest tube drainage, and report these symptoms immediately. *Rationale: The most serious postoperative complications are hemorrhage into the lung cavity (*hemothorax*) or collection of air in the pleural cavity, causing collapse of all or part of a lung (*pneumothorax*).* In hemothorax, the fluid (blood) collects in the lower part of the pleural cavity. In pneumothorax, the air rises to the top. In Practice: Data Gathering in Nursing 86-1 highlights danger signs for a person with a chest tube. In Practice: Nursing Care Guidelines 86-3 outlines care measures.

IN PRACTICE
DATA GATHERING IN NURSING 86-1 — Danger Signs for a Person With a Chest Tube

Be alert for the following:
- Leakage of air into the drainage system, whether in a simple water-seal type or a mechanical suction type, is indicated by constant bubbling in the water-seal system, after the client's lungs initially have been expanded. There will be bubbling in the control bottle—the one connected to suction. If bubbling stops, the suction pressure is too low.
- Air leaks can occur at the chest tube insertion site, in connections, in the bottles, or in the stoppers in three-bottle suction or in the closed drainage system itself.
- To check the location of an air leak, pinch the tubing for a few seconds at intervals between the chest tube and drainage connection. If the bubbling stops, the air leak is due to the system (check all connections). If the bubbling continues, pinch off tubing at intervals between the client and the system; when the pinching is between the source of the air leak and the water chamber, the bubbling will stop.
- Keep all tubes, bags, and other devices below the level of tube insertion. *Rationale:* This position prevents reflux.
- If the client shows signs of cyanosis or dyspnea, or complains of chest pain, investigate the situation immediately. This is an emergency!

IN PRACTICE

NURSING CARE GUIDELINES 86-3: Caring for the Person With Chest Suction

- Always wash your hands and wear gloves and wash hands after removing gloves. *Rationale: Handwashing and gloves help to reduce the risk for infection.*
- Never attempt to set up any chest suction without assistance. *Rationale: In most facilities, at least two people must check a suction setup before it can be connected to the client. This is a safety precaution.*
- Never disconnect or change chest suction without being absolutely certain about what to do. *Rationale: The person's life depends on the ability to maintain the integrity of the pleural space.*
- Never disconnect chest tubes! *Rationale: These tubes provide the suction that keeps the lungs inflated. If they are disconnected, the lungs will collapse.*
- Keep clamps or hemostats with the client, either clipped to the bedding or to the client's gown (when using the three-bottle system). With the disposable system, a clamp is attached with the tubing. Thus, additional clamps are not necessary. If the client gets out of bed, the clamps go along. *Rationale: The tubes are clamped as an emergency measure in case the tubes become accidentally disconnected.*
- If the tubes become disconnected, double-clamp all tubes close to the chest wall and summon assistance immediately. *Rationale: This is an emergency situation requiring prompt intervention. If air enters the chest cavity, the person's lungs will collapse!*
- Be aware that clamping chest tubes for more than a few minutes may cause a tension pneumothorax. *Rationale: If any untoward symptoms occur, call for help immediately.*
- Never empty drainage in a closed system. Note the amount as ordered. Discard the entire system when full. *Rationale: The integrity of the closed system must be maintained to prevent lung collapse.*
- Never use pins to fasten the tubes to the bed. *Rationale: A pin might puncture the tube.*
- Never change a chest dressing. *Rationale: The dressing may help maintain the integrity of the chest wall.*
- Never take the plugs out of the bottles without assistance and never pull on chest tubes. *Rationale: These actions may result in air entering the chest cavity.*
- Tape all connections to make sure they are airtight. *Rationale: Taping connections reduces the risk that the tubes may become disconnected.*
- If a chest tube becomes kinked, report it immediately. *Rationale: Kinking could disrupt the system and prevent drainage.*
- To set up the drainage after the tube is inserted, wrap a piece of cloth tape around the tube and then attach the tape to the edge of the bed, so the tube hangs straight down into the bottle. Keep the remainder of the tubing in the bed with the client. *Rationale: Straight drainage provides the best drainage flow. The excess tubing allows the client to turn in bed and move about.*
- Be sure the client does not lie or pull on the tubing. *Rationale: This might obstruct the flow of the drainage.*
- Keep drainage containers lower than the level of the client at all times. *Rationale: This position facilitates drainage and prevents backflow.*
- Observe and report accurately. Notify the healthcare provider if there is a marked change. *Rationale: The amount, color, and consistency of the drainage are vital information.*
- Observe for excessive bleeding or for abrupt absence of drainage. *Rationale: Hemorrhage is a dangerous complication, and abrupt absence of drainage often means that the system is not operating properly.*
- Document any changes in respiratory status, or respiratory distress, and any milking of the tubes. *Rationale: Documentation provides for communication and continuity of care.*
- Discard all drainage tubes and other equipment as required by Standard Precautions. *Rationale: Proper disposal of equipment helps prevent the spread of infection.*

> **Nursing Alert** Do not "strip" a chest drain (occlude the chest tube with one hand while quickly squeezing and moving the other hand down the tube to move fluid down the tube into the drainage chamber) because intraluminal pressures can rise dangerously high, which may convert a simple pneumothorax to a life-threatening pneumothorax and cause tissue trauma and unnecessary discomfort. Avoid other tubing manipulation, such as milking, fanfolding, and tapping, which do not improve fluid drainage from the chest.

NURSING PROCESS

DATA COLLECTION

Carefully observe the client with a respiratory disorder for changes in respiratory status. Document abnormal findings and notify the charge nurse and/or the healthcare provider of changes that indicate potential respiratory difficulties, such as dyspnea, tachycardia, tachypnea, or skin color changes. Because adequate oxygenation is vital to life, a disorder in the respiratory system can quickly become life threatening. An initial nursing observation with documentation establishes a baseline for future comparison and determines the presence of suspected complications. Report any changes in the baseline level.

When monitoring and charting a client's respiratory status, note the client's breathing and oxygenation level (In Practice: Data Gathering in Nursing 86-2).

In addition, observe the individual's emotional response to the disorder or disease. Does the client need assistance to meet daily needs? Does the disorder affect social activities or self-esteem? Is the person anxious or fearful about the outcome?

Noting Alterations in Respiratory Status

Various events, such as illness or injury, can alter a client's respiratory status. Table 86-1 lists possible alterations from **eupnea** (normal breathing).

Aspiration

Pathologic aspiration is the inhalation or movement of fluid, mucus, or another unwanted substance into the lungs. It can cause lung disorders or death.

Hyperventilation

In **hyperventilation**, the person breathes abnormally quickly or deeply, resulting in too little carbon dioxide in the blood. The usual cause is anxiety or overexcitement. The hyperventilating person may have muscle spasms, dizziness, or faintness because of excessive oxygen and the depletion of carbon dioxide in the body. The easiest treatment is asking the client to breathe into a bag. The air the client rebreathes will contain excess carbon dioxide, replacing that which was lost.

Hypoxia

The tissue cells must have a constant oxygen supply to remain alive. Because the body does not store oxygen, the person normally obtains oxygen from the air (air is approximately 21% oxygen). In some types of illness, the body is unable to take in sufficient oxygen or cannot use it effectively. When the oxygen level in body tissues is inadequate, the client is said to have *hypoxia* (Box 86-1).

One of the most obvious signs of hypoxia is shortness of breath (**SOB**). Earlier signs of hypoxia may be seen with shortness of breath on exertion (**SOBOE**). When the client expresses this feeling, SOB is called *dyspnea*. The nurse may also observe SOB in the client through clinical observation. Signs include restlessness, apprehension, an anxious facial expression, panic, fatigue, or impaired coordination. As the need for more oxygen continues, the client's rate and depth of respiration may increase.

Severe oxygen deficiency may be manifested by the person's use of accessory breathing muscles of the neck and upper chest. Gasping, wheezing, or retractions of the breastbone or intercostal spaces are also late signs of hypoxia.

Other manifestations include the following:
- Mental changes, confusion, stupor, and unconsciousness
- Cardiac symptoms, such as rapid pulse, dysrhythmias, fibrillation, and cardiac standstill (cardiac arrest), owing to the heart's inability to provide blood, and thus oxygen, to the tissues, causing the heart to overwork
- Changes in skin color, such as cyanosis of skin, nail beds, and mucous membranes (resulting from either a marked lack of oxygen or severe blood loss) or pallor

Hypoxemic Hypoxia

Hypoxemic hypoxia is a state of decreased blood oxygen level, leading to a decreased amount of oxygen in the tissues. Many situations can result in hypoxemic hypoxia: The client's airway may be blocked, in which case respiration ceases or is ineffective; the lungs may be congested, in which case respiration is difficult and gradually worsens; an injury to the chest or lungs may cause difficulty in breathing; or chronic or acute infections in the lungs may interfere with breathing.

In these instances, oxygen decrease may be sudden or gradual. For example, if a person chokes on a piece of meat, oxygen supply is suddenly cut off, and the person will die if the airway is not restored within a matter of minutes. In many infectious or chronic conditions of the lungs, breathing is impaired but not stopped completely. In these instances, most of which are not emergencies, the nurse can assist the person to breathe or to obtain oxygen.

Circulation Hypoxia

Circulation hypoxia is caused by inadequate blood circulation. If blood cannot get to tissues, the body's oxygen supply is cut off. The two chief circulatory disorders that account for a decrease in oxygen supply are failure of the heart to pump and blockage or rupture of a blood vessel.

Failure of the heart to pump may be caused by a lack of blood to the heart itself; weakening of the heart muscle; stoppage; or very irregular and rapid beating of the heart (*fibrillation*). If blood cannot get through a vessel because of a clot or stricture or developing atherosclerosis, the blood supply is reduced or stopped. This happens in a stroke and in a thrombosis. In a ruptured aneurysm, the vessel explodes, and the channel for blood is absent.

Anemic Hypoxia

Anemic hypoxia is caused by reduction in the blood's oxygen-carrying capacity. Hemoglobin, a constituent of red blood cells (RBCs), carries oxygen to the tissues. Anemia can result from decreased blood volume, decreased hemoglobin within the RBCs, or the inability of hemoglobin to take on oxygen. In sickle cell anemia, the malformed (sickle-shaped) RBCs cannot pass through the capillaries. Carbon monoxide poisoning is a form of anemic hypoxia because the carbon monoxide combines with hemoglobin, leaving no room for oxygen.

Histotoxic Hypoxia

Histotoxic hypoxia is caused by an inability of the tissues to use oxygen. Under the influence of certain chemicals, the cells are unable to use oxygen. The most common example is cyanide poisoning. Persons who have suffered smoke inhalation often have inhaled cyanide gas and may have histotoxic hypoxia.

PLANNING AND IMPLEMENTING

Together, the client, family, and healthcare team plan for effective individualized care to meet the client's needs. For the client undergoing lung or chest surgery, provide preoperative and postoperative teaching and care. The client with a respiratory disorder may be anxious. This person may also require assistance in the management of portable oxygen. They may need assistance in meeting some or all basic needs, in dealing with emotional problems, and understanding more about the disorder, its prognosis, and its treatment.

Relieving Respiratory Distress

Orthopneic Position

Orthopneic position is a position in which a person who has difficulty breathing (orthopnea) may utilize positioning to lessen the physical weight and gravity of the body during breathing. In orthopneic position, the intrathoracic spaces are opened and breathing is easier for the client with chronic lung diseases. In a hospital, the client may be in a high Fowler position leaning over pillows on top of a bedside table (Table 48-1). In the home, a lounge chair with high back is helpful. Pillows under the arm and shoulders can also be helpful.

Turning, Coughing, and Deep Breathing

Turning, coughing, and deep breathing (TCDB) are vital for anyone who is in bed for a long period. Lung complications can occur when a person is immobile and develop more quickly when a respiratory problem is present (In Practice: Nursing Care Guidelines 56-3 for specific instructions).

Administering Respiratory Treatments

Postural Drainage

Because *postural drainage* uses gravity, the person is placed in a head downward position (In Practice: Nursing Care Guidelines 86-1). Request training from the respiratory therapist specific to the individual. *Rationale: Positions vary according to the specific disorder and the lung area being drained.*

Breathing Exercises and Incentive Spirometer

The healthcare provider will probably order breathing exercises to help the client build up respiratory capacity. These are usually done with the aid of the **incentive spirometer** (In Practice: Nursing Care Guidelines 56-3). Instructions will depend on the particular type of device the client uses. A major reason for postoperative incentive spirometry is to prevent **atelectasis** (deflated or collapsed alveoli), which can potentially obstruct small or large sections of pulmonary tissues.

Breathing Treatments

Several types of breathing treatments may be used. Intermittent positive pressure breathing (**IPPB**) treatment is not often used today, unless aerosolized medications are to be given. The most common uses of IPPB are in cystic fibrosis and neuromuscular disorders. Aerosol nebulizer (mini-nebulizer) treatments provide aerosolized medication via a mask or mouthpiece apparatus attached to oxygen or compressed air (Chapters 63 and 87).

Oxygen

Many people with respiratory and other problems receive supplemental oxygen by cannula or mask, which assists them to breathe more easily and provides a higher concentration of oxygen than that of room air. Understand the precautions used when oxygen is administered (Chapter 87). Provide emotional support because it may be a frightening experience for clients and their families.

Administering Nasal Treatments

People with respiratory disorders often use nasal sprays and nose drops (In Practice: Nursing Care Guidelines 63-6). In addition, if the client has a purulent discharge that forms crusts in the nose, a nasal irrigation may be ordered. The irrigation solution flows into one nostril and out through the other. The important point to observe in giving a nasal irrigation is to use the correct amount of pressure. Too much pressure may force the fluid into the sinuses and the Eustachian tubes, thus spreading the infection. This procedure is uncommon.

Suctioning to Remove Oral–Nasal Secretions

Many people with respiratory problems require suctioning to remove excess secretions and mucus from the airway (In Practice: Nursing Procedure 86-1). Suctioning may also be indicated in the unconscious person or in clients with ineffective cough. Use a new, sterile suction kit each time to avoid introducing pathogens into the lungs. The client who cannot swallow may require only oral suctioning. In this case, use a tonsil suction device and follow clean technique. The procedure for suctioning a tracheostomy is similar and is presented in Nursing Procedure 87-6.

> **Nursing Alert** Suctioning can cause *arrhythmias* (irregular heartbeats) and *desaturation* (loss of oxygenation). Continuously monitor the person being suctioned for symptoms of respiratory distress, decreased oxygenation, or cardiac arrhythmias.

EVALUATION

Evaluate outcomes of care with the client, family, and other members of the healthcare team. Have short-term goals been met? Has the client shown evidence of improvement in their respiratory status? Are long-term goals still realistic? Planning for further nursing care considers the client's prognosis, as well as any complications and the client's response to care given.

IN PRACTICE

DATA GATHERING IN NURSING 86-2 — The Client With a Possible Respiratory Disorder

- Note respiratory rate, depth, and character.
- Determine respiratory status.
- Observe for signs of respiratory distress, dyspnea, or poor oxygenation.
- Be alert for signs or symptoms of *hypoxia* (lack of oxygen).
- Note any symptoms, such as cough, hemoptysis, and cyanosis.
- Listen to lung sounds and breath sounds.
- Check results of skin tests related to tuberculosis or other lung conditions.
- Observe mouth and throat by visualization and palpation.

TABLE 86-1 Possible Alterations in Respiratory Status

TERM	SIGN/SYMPTOM
Dyspnea: Labored or difficult breathing, painful breathing	Inadequate ventilation, lowered oxygen level in blood
Orthopnea: Difficulty breathing while lying down, relieved by sitting upright (*orthopneic* position)	Cardiac disorders, pulmonary emphysema, heart failure
Tachypnea: Very rapid breathing	High fever, pneumonia, alkalosis, salicylate overdose, brain stem lesions
Hyperpnea: Increase in depth of breaths; may be increase in rate (no feeling of increased respiratory effort)	Strenuous exercise
Bradypnea: Respiration slower than normal, regular in rhythm	Normal during sleep; sign of drug overdose, disturbance in respiratory center of brain, metabolic disorder
Hypoventilation: Respirations that have a reduced rate and depth (shallow), often irregular	Obesity; neuromuscular disorders affecting the thorax (e.g., multiple sclerosis, muscular dystrophy); damage to lung tissue (e.g., emphysema)
Hyperventilation: Increased rate and depth of respirations often leading to decreased carbon dioxide levels (hypocapnia)	Exercise, asthma, early emphysema, fever, multiple central nervous system disorders, anxiety, pain
Cheyne–Stokes breathing: Abnormal respiratory pattern that may start as slow and shallow that changes to deep and rapid respirations, followed by 10–20 s of apnea between cycles. Each cycle may last from 45 s to 3 min.	Brain stem lesion, heart failure, brain damage
Biot respirations: An abnormal respiratory pattern that may be sequences of 3–4 slow and deep or rapid and shallow breaths followed by periods of apnea, often accompanied by sighing.	Brain stem lesion, heart failure, brain damage, overdose of hypnotic or narcotic drug Meningitis or increased intracranial pressure
Apnea: Cessation of breathing for brief periods of time. Apneic periods may increase in length as with Cheyne–Stokes breathing.	Sleep apnea, Cheyne–Stokes respiration, sudden infant death syndrome
Central apnea: No brain drive to breathe *Obstructive apnea:* No airflow owing to upper airway obstruction *Mixed apnea:* Central apnea immediately followed by obstruction *Adult sleep apnea:* Prolonged and frequent episodes of apnea during sleep	Undeveloped respiratory center in preterm infants, adult brain stem lesion, high spinal cord injury Foreign object in airway, excessive secretions, absent cough reflex Obstructive (tongue or throat structures relax), obesity Central (brain damage, brain lesion)
Kussmaul respirations: Dyspnea with rapid (>20/min) gasping breaths, air hunger, panting, labored respirations	Associated with diabetic ketoacidosis (metabolic acidosis), renal failure

Box 86-1 Signs and Symptoms of Hypoxia

- Short of breath on exertion
- Tachycardia
- Mild increase in blood pressure
- Cool, moist skin
- Confusion
- Delirium
- Difficulty in problem solving
- Loss of judgment
- Euphoria
- Unruly or combative behavior
- Sensory impairment
- Mental fatigue
- Drowsiness
- Cyanosis
- Stupor and coma (late)
- Hypotension (late)
- Bradycardia (late)

INFECTIOUS RESPIRATORY DISORDERS

The Common Cold

The common cold or *acute rhinitis* is a viral illness of the upper respiratory tract, that is, the nose and throat. *Rhinitis* is a term that means inflammation of the nasal mucous membranes causing a *runny nose*. As many as 100 cold viruses have been identified. The common cold is generally harmless, having a great variety and severity of symptoms. The virus in the cold is infectious to others and is easily spread by talking, coughing, or sneezing. Individuals are contagious 48 hr before the appearance of the first symptoms. If fatigue, chilling, or substances that continually irritate the nasal membranes (e.g., exposure to secondhand smoke or to smog) lower the person's resistance, susceptibility to the virus is increased. The cold is most common in preschool aged children, but most adults have a few instances of the common cold each year. Recovery occurs in about 2 weeks; if not improved or conditions worsen, a healthcare provider should be consulted.

Signs and Symptoms

The most common symptoms include rhinitis, watery eyes, sore throat, and a mild cough or sneezing. In addition, the individual may have nasal or lung congestion, itchy or sore throat, general malaise, body aches, a mild headache, and a mild fever. Due to inflammation of the nasal mucous membranes, the senses of smell and taste can be blunted. **Otitis media**, infection behind the eardrum in the middle ear, is a frequent complication of a cold, especially in children. **Sinusitis**, the inflammation or infection of the mucous membrane lining the sinuses, is painful and a common side effect of a cold or flu. Medical treatment needs to be taken to prevent further complications such as permanent ear damage, deafness, and the development of scar tissue in the sinuses. Sinusitis is discussed in more detail later in this chapter.

The person should consult a healthcare provider if the fever continues for more than 2 days, if mild analgesics fail to relieve severe headache, or if severe coughing, earache, or chest pain occurs. The client should immediately consult a healthcare provider if they cough up dark or bloody sputum. If a fever becomes greater than 100.4 °F (38 °C) in children or 103 °F (39.4 °C) in adults, a healthcare provider should be consulted. Additional symptoms of worsening conditions include wheezing, diaphoresis, a cough with thick, yellow or green mucus, swollen lymph nodes, and severe pain, which may indicate development of additional problems, such as *sinusitis* or *otitis media*. Commonly, a child will react to either of these situations with cries of pain, which may not respond to OTC analgesics. Children often do not react to pain in the same manner as do adults; therefore, be alert for changes of behavior, such as restlessness and inability to sleep, plus elevations of temperature, and yellow or green discharge from the nose. Strep throat (streptococcal pharyngitis—see below), pneumonia, laryngotracheobronchitis (LTB or croup), and assorted bronchitis infections may also occur in children, rarely in adults.

Treatment

The most important treatment for a cold is rest. Rest also keeps the person from infecting others. Rest during a cold is especially important for infants, older adults, and debilitated clients because they are more susceptible to serious complications. Drinking plenty of fluids is essential to help reduce fever, replace lost fluids, and thin secretions. Aspirin, acetaminophen, or ibuprofen helps to relieve discomfort and reduce fever. Some authorities believe that vitamin C is helpful in preventing and treating colds. A more comprehensive list of symptomatic relief measures can be found in Box 72-1, Nursing Considerations: Symptom Relief.

Remind the client to give strict attention to handwashing and using disposable tissues to prevent spreading the infection to others. The client should blow the nose gently to prevent the infection from spreading into the sinuses, ears, or Eustachian tubes. Antibiotics are not effective against cold viruses; however, antiviral agents may be prescribed. Sometimes, a throat culture is done. Culture can indicate strep throat, but a negative culture for streptococci does not necessarily mean that a strep infection is not present. (See the section on Throat Culture.) The person with a chronic respiratory condition, such as asthma, should consult a healthcare provider at the first sign of a cold.

If the infection enters the lower respiratory tract, complications, such as laryngitis, bronchitis (inflammation of the bronchi), and pneumonia, can result.

> **Nursing Alert** Usually, nurses who have colds may continue working if they feel well. However, it is essential that they follow all principles of infection control, especially proper handwashing. Some facilities require such nurses to wear masks and not to be assigned to high-risk clients.

Streptococcal Sore Throat

In *streptococcal pharyngitis* or **strep throat**, physical symptoms are more widespread than with ordinary sore throat, with general physical weakness and malaise, high fever, pus on the tonsils, and a headache. Many adults who have recurrent streptococcal throat infections have permanently plugged Eustachian tubes; any change in atmospheric pressure is uncomfortable for them. Penicillin is the specific antibiotic prescribed for strep throat unless the person has an allergy or a penicillin-resistant streptococcal infection. The most dangerous complications of strep throat are rheumatic fever and glomerulonephritis (Chapters 72 and 89).

Influenza

Influenza, commonly called *the flu,* is an active contagious respiratory disease caused by one of several strains of filterable viruses: types A, B, C, D, and others. Flu strains may also be described using the name of the place of origin. Influenza occurs in periodic epidemics, usually due to virus types A and B. Most people recover, but some die from complications, such as heart disease, pneumonia, or encephalitis. Influenza viruses change, resulting in new strains of viruses regularly. The immune system has made antibodies for viral strains that an individual has had in the past; however, no antibodies are available for a new recent viral strain. Annually in the United States, a predicted flu strain is prepared for vaccination of the population. The flu shot is designed to promote the formation of antibodies that will enable the individual's immune system to quickly defend itself if exposed to the virus. The best method of prevention of the flu is by vaccination.

Transmission of flu viruses is by direct or indirect transmission. Direct transmission includes inhaling air from a cough, sneeze, or talking. Indirect transmission occurs when the virus travels by a droplet that has fallen onto objects and contaminated them. For example, touching a doorknob, ATM machine, or restaurant menu is common modes of indirect transmission. The individual touches the contaminated item and then touches an area of the mouth or nose, bringing along flu virus. Handwashing is the most effective way of preventing transmission. The individual who is infected with the virus is contagious starting about the day before the onset of symptoms and will remain contagious for about 5–10 more days, or longer. Children and immunocompromised individuals may be infectious for longer periods.

Risk factors for the flu include the following:

- Age—younger children and older adults at higher risk
- Health status—weakened immune systems and chronic illness, for example, HIV/AIDS, autoimmune diseases, cancer therapy, diabetes, or asthma
- Lifestyle—institutions such as a long-term care facility, military facilities, or dormitories
- Pregnancy—especially in second or third trimesters
- Obesity—a BMI of 40 kg/m^2 or more

SPECIAL CONSIDERATIONS *Lifespan*

Complications in Influenza

Infants, older adults, and immunocompromised people are at a much higher risk for developing complications from influenza.

Signs and Symptoms

A common concern is how to differentiate between the common cold and the flu. A cold tends to develop over a couple of days, the feeling of "coming down with something."
The flu tends to appear suddenly, feels worse than with a cold, and tends to have a higher temperature. Other signs and symptoms include suddenly feeling very ill, with muscle pains, fever, headache, sensitivity to light, burning eyes, and chills. The person may sneeze, cough, have a nasal discharge, complain of sore throat, feel nauseous, and vomit often. Fever is high (100 °F–103 °F [37.8 °C–39.4 °C]) and lasts for 2–3 days. Other symptoms, especially the cough, persist longer. A cough may persist for several weeks after a person has had the flu.

A dangerous complication of influenza is pneumonia. A person is particularly susceptible to any lung disorder after the flu because of general debility. Other complications are chronic disorders, such as bronchitis, sinusitis, and ear infections.

Treatment and Nursing Considerations

Rest, fluids, and symptomatic medications are the most common approach to treatment. Rest can be in bed, on the couch watching TV, or wherever the client does not have to exert energy. Clients should keep warm and avoid exposure to other diseases. To promote healing and avoid dehydration, encourage the client to drink adequate quantities of fluids, including fruit juices, soups, and plenty of water. Fluids help the body to flush out wastes created by the virus. Milk may not be helpful because it can form a film in the throat. Clients may follow a regular diet, although they may be *anorexic* (without appetite). Soups can provide calories and fluids. Symptomatic medications include over-the-counter (OTC) analgesics such as acetaminophen (Tylenol) or ibuprofen (Advil, Motrin IB), which help with muscle aches and general pain. Do not give aspirin to children or teens because of the risk of Reye syndrome, which is a rare but potentially fatal illness. Decongestants and antitussives (for coughs) are available OTC. Cough syrups are also available by prescription if they contain a narcotic such as codeine, which is helpful when the individual has severe dry coughing episodes.

Antiviral medications may be prescribed if they are started soon after the onset of symptoms. Examples of antivirals include an oral oseltamivir (Tamiflu) or the inhaled zanamivir (Relenza). However, zanamivir (Relenza) should not be used by individuals with chronic respiratory problems such as asthma or lung disease. Side effects to antiviral agents include nausea and vomiting, which may be decreased if taken with food. Antiviral medications, for example, oseltamivir, have been shown to have other, more disturbing side effects, such as mental changes and suicidal ideation in teenagers.

> **Nursing Alert** Antiviral agents, such as oseltamivir (Tamiflu), are given with *caution*. It has been associated with *delirium and self-harm behaviors in teenagers.*

Respiratory isolation may be ordered. Watch for signs of secondary infection, such as chest pains, purulent or rose-colored sputum, a rise in temperature, or an increase in pulse rate.

Prevention

Prevention is best achieved by an annual flu vaccination and avoidance of exposure. The CDC recommends annual vaccinations for anyone over 6 months of age. Vaccination should be encouraged for individuals who are at a high risk for exposure to the flu. Included in this list are older adults, persons with chronic disease, immunosuppressed persons, and healthcare workers. During a flu outbreak, urge people to stay away from crowds. Sometimes, public gatherings are suspended. If an individual is exposed and does not have symptoms, the individual should use caution when visiting an infant or an older adult.

Laryngitis

Laryngitis is an inflammation of the larynx (voice box). It may accompany a respiratory infection or result from overuse of the voice or excessive smoking. The person coughs, is hoarse, and may lose the voice. They should avoid talking and smoking and should receive high-humidity inhalations to soothe the throat's mucous membranes. If laryngitis is a complication of another infection, antibiotics may be prescribed. If laryngitis is viral in origin, it is highly contagious; the client should avoid exposing others.

Chronic laryngitis may be a complication of chronic sinusitis or chronic bronchitis or may follow repeated attacks of acute laryngitis. Continued irritation of the throat by public speaking, smoking, or irritating gases may contribute to the problem. People with chronic laryngitis must be carefully examined for signs of cancer, particularly if they smoke cigarettes.

Bronchitis

Bronchitis is an inflammation of the bronchial tubes (bronchi). *Acute bronchitis* often follows a respiratory infection, especially during the winter months. A dry cough is an early symptom; later, the cough produces mucus and pus. Other symptoms include fever and malaise.

Treatment includes bed rest, a nutritious diet, and plenty of fluids. Humidifiers help by moistening the air, whereas dry air aggravates the cough. Antibiotics are given to treat the infection, and precautions are taken to prevent the infection from spreading. Salicylates are sometimes given.

As in any respiratory disease, instruct the client to cover the mouth when coughing. Dispose of sputum and tissues using Standard Precautions. Acute bronchitis, if untreated, will often develop into *chronic bronchitis*.

Lung Abscess

A *lung abscess* is a localized area of infection in the lung that breaks down and forms pus. It can be caused by a foreign body or by aspiration of oral fluids or respiratory secretions and may follow pneumonia. Symptoms include chills and fever, with weight loss and a productive cough with foul, purulent sputum.

Surgery may be required to drain the lung abscess. If the cause of the abscess is an aspirated object, bronchoscopy can usually remove the object. Antibiotics usually are an effective treatment after the cause is eliminated.

Pneumonia

Pneumonia is an inflammation of the lung with consolidation or solidification (Fig. 86-3A). The lung becomes firm as the air sacs are filled with exudates. Pneumonia can be classified according to the source of infection, such as community acquired, hospital acquired, healthcare acquired, or aspiration. *Community-acquired pneumonia* is the most common type of the disease. Generally, pneumonia is listed according to the causative agent, which may be bacterial, viral, fungal, or chemical in origin. Hospital and healthcare-acquired pneumonia are associated with institutions, and both types are associated with antibiotic-resistant strains of bacteria. *Hospital-acquired pneumonia* relates to the individual who may develop pneumonia as a result of another problem while as a client in a hospital, such as postoperative pneumonia. *Healthcare-acquired pneumonia* occurs in facilities where immunocompromised individuals may live or cluster, such as long-term care facilities, dialysis centers, outpatient clinics, or rehabilitation centers. *Aspiration pneumonia* is a consequence of a foreign material getting into the lungs.

 SPECIAL CONSIDERATIONS Lifespan

Pneumonia

Pneumonia often occurs as a complication of another condition and is often a cause of death in older adults.

Types
Bacterial Pneumonia

Streptococcus pneumoniae is the most common causative agent and can occur as a consequence of a cold or the flu. It typically affects one lobe of the lung, referred to as lobar pneumonia. Persons who are in poor general health, or who are physically inactive, as well as older people and those with chronic lung disorders, are most susceptible to bacterial pneumonia. Substance abuse, which may be a risk factor, becomes part of the overall problem because the individual tends to ignore personal health in lieu of lifestyle choices.

Bacterial-Like Organisms

Some pathogens are not specifically labeled bacteria or viruses. *Mycoplasma pneumoniae*, which may be called walking pneumonia, results in milder symptoms.

Viral Pneumonia

A variant of the influenza virus causes *viral pneumonia*. The person is treated symptomatically. Viral pneumonia is rarely fatal, but it may leave the client in a weakened condition. However, viral pneumonia can occasionally be very serious. A virus is the most common cause of pneumonia in children younger than 5 years.

Fungal Pneumonia

Individuals with chronic health conditions or who are immunocompromised are most likely to be contaminated by an inhaled fungus. The organisms are found in soil or bird droppings.

Pneumocystis jiroveci pneumonia (**PJP**), formerly called *pneumocystis carinii pneumonia* (**PCP**), is caused by a fungus whose mechanisms are not totally understood. PJP is most commonly seen as one of the opportunistic diseases in the person with HIV/AIDS infection, or with other individuals receiving immunotherapy, such as cancer or organ

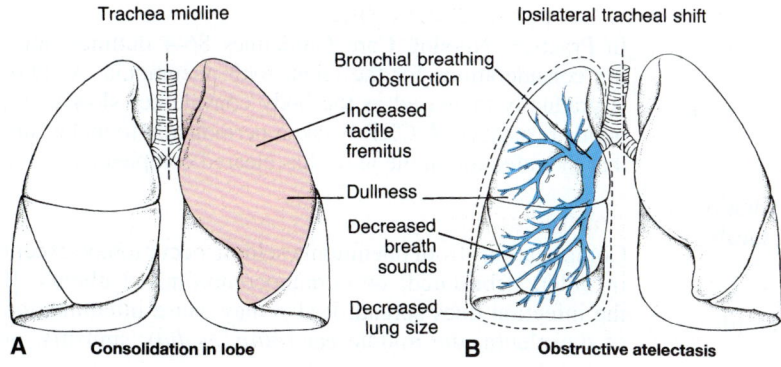
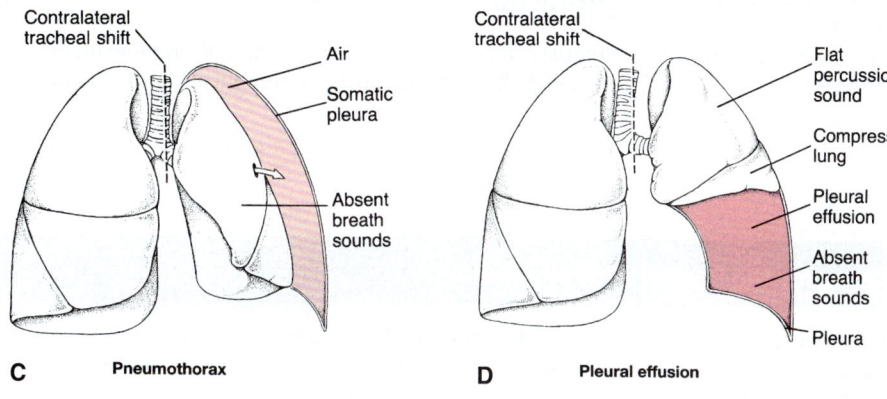
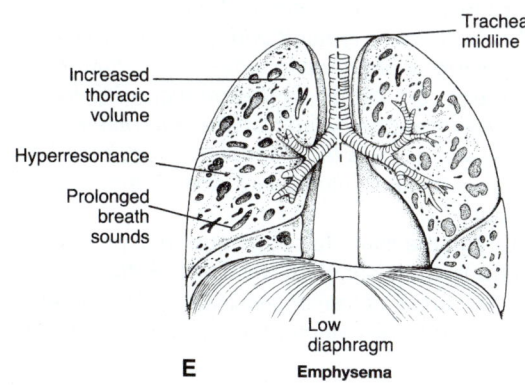

Figure 86-3 Respiratory system disorders and their comparative effects on the lungs. **A.** *Consolidation* within a lobe: trachea in center, dull sound in affected lobe. **B.** *Obstructive atelectasis:* trachea shifts to affected (ipsilateral) side; decreased lung size, decreased breath sounds. **C.** *Pneumothorax:* trachea shifts to other (contralateral) side; breath sounds absent on affected side. **D.** *Pleural effusion or hemothorax* (fluid or blood pooling in pleural cavity): trachea shifts to other side; absent breath sounds in affected lobe; lung compressed. **E.** *Emphysema:* enlarged (barrel) chest, prolonged breath sounds, *hyperresonance* (echo), trachea in center.

replacement. PJP does not respond to antifungal treatment. PJP is best treated with trimethoprim/sulfamethoxazole (TMP/SMX).

Chemical Pneumonia
Chemical pneumonia is largely associated with aspiration of a chemical substance. Be aware that a person may aspirate into the lungs without any obvious evidence of vomiting. Some people are at an extremely high risk, including older adult or postoperative clients, clients who abuse substances or are debilitated, and those with swallowing impairments.

Aspiration Pneumonia
If the person vomits or inhales a foreign object or substances, such as water or large amounts of mucus, the material may be drawn into the lungs. Complications also occur because gastric contents contain high acidity, which further irritates the lung tissues. Aspiration initiates the inflammatory process, which causes fluid accumulation and edema with a resulting pneumonia. Typical foreign materials may include emesis, saliva, food, drink, or, on occasion, a reaction to an irritant in gaseous form that is inhaled, such as gas fumes.

Signs and Symptoms
The onset of pneumonia is characterized by a severe, sharp pain in the chest and chills, followed by fever that may be as high as 105 °F or 106 °F (40.6 °C or 41.1 °C). A painful cough, tenacious sputum, and pain on breathing are present. The person's pulse is rapid. Respiration is rapid, and expiration is difficult. The individual feels very ill and may be cyanotic. The white blood cell count is high. Mental changes, such as delirium or anxiety, may be present.

Blood cultures and sputum cultures are sent for analysis to determine the causative organism. Sensitivity tests are done to determine which antibiotic is most effective. A CXR will show what part of the lung is affected and to what degree.

Treatment

Treatment focuses on the following:

- Administering appropriate antibiotic therapy
- Observing respiratory status and indicators of the effectiveness of therapy
- Administering oxygen
- Administering adequate fluid intake to ensure hydration
- Providing adequate nutrition via small, frequent meals
- Positioning to aid breathing
- Turning, coughing, and deep breathing
- Maintaining accurate intake and output (I&O) records
- Providing frequent mouth care for comfort

Antibiotics have revolutionized the treatment of pneumonia. They are usually administered IV for rapid action and to maintain a blood level that is effective in eradicating the causative organism. In 24–48 hr, the fever usually disappears and the other symptoms dramatically decrease.

Nursing Considerations

In Practice: Nursing Care Guidelines 86-4 outlines nursing considerations for the client with pneumonia. Activity is gradually increased as the body convalesces slowly and builds resistance. A CXR is taken periodically to make sure that the infection in the lungs has cleared completely.

Complications

Complications from pneumonia seldom occur today, except in older, debilitated, or immunocompromised clients. If the infection does spread, it also may cause inflammation of the pleura, the middle ear (*otitis media*), sinusitis, or bronchitis.

Pleurisy

Pleurisy, an inflammation of the pleura (the double membrane covering the lungs), can be a complication of pneumonia,

---

IN PRACTICE
NURSING CARE GUIDELINES 86-4 — Caring for the Person With Pneumonia

- Always wash your hands and wear gloves, if indicated. **Rationale:** *Proper handwashing and gloves help to prevent the spread of infection.*
- Be alert for increasingly labored respirations. **Rationale:** *If the person has difficulty breathing, they are given oxygen, usually by mask or cannula.*
- Adjust the client's position. An orthopneic position may be necessary. **Rationale:** *Proper positioning helps the person to be more comfortable and to breathe more easily.*
- Place a pillow lengthwise under the back. **Rationale:** *This action encourages fuller chest expansion.*
- Place a blanket around the shoulders if the person has chills. **Rationale:** *A blanket provides comfort and warmth, minimizing energy expenditure.*
- Keep the client's bed dry. **Rationale:** *Wet bed linens can chill the client.*
- Take the client's vital signs at least every 4 hr. **Rationale:** *Frequent monitoring is necessary to allow for prompt detection and early intervention if problems arise.*
- Attempt to control fever and discomfort with acetaminophen or ibuprofen, if ordered. Tepid sponges may also be ordered. **Rationale:** *Fever is often very high and can be dangerous.*
- Maintain the intravenous (IV) site or heparin lock. **Rationale:** *This client is probably receiving IV antibiotics.*
- Consider putting up the side rails if any sign of confusion exists. The clinical facility should have specific policies regarding limitation of movement and raised bedrails. Specific circumstances might need to exist, that is, a hazard or unsafe environment for the client. Safety is a priority nursing concern. **Rationale:** *Elevated side rails can be considered a type of restraint, that is, a legal consideration. However the safety of the client must also be considered. You need to follow facility policy and consult with your supervisor if any questions or concerns arise. Many medical conditions can lead to confusion including hypoxia, fever, medications, head trauma, and disease processes. Injury, a legal consideration, may be a consequence of inadequate attention to the situation.*
- Encourage the client to cough and to expectorate secretions while splinting the chest. **Rationale:** *Keep the lungs as free of secretions as possible. Splinting the chest helps to relieve the discomfort of coughing.*
- Encourage deep breathing. Aerosolized treatments or incentive spirometry may be prescribed. **Rationale:** *The lungs must be expanded as much as possible.*
- Measure intake and output (I&O) and daily weights, if ordered. **Rationale:** *Some clients may have edema. Others will need total parenteral nutrition (TPN) to maintain hydration and nutrition.*
- Give small amounts of fluids frequently. **Rationale:** *Fluids help to encourage hydration.*
- Provide frequent mouth care; put water-soluble lubricant (not oily) on the client's lips. **Rationale:** *A fever causes the mucous membranes to be very dry; probably, this person also has been breathing through the mouth. Oil might be aspirated and is not used with oxygen.*
- Keep the client's surroundings quiet. **Rationale:** *Rest promotes healing.*

caused by a spread of the infection from the lungs. The pleura becomes thickened, and the two membrane surfaces scrape together.

The client feels sharp pain with every breath. Later, as fluid forms, the pain diminishes, and a dry cough replaces it, accompanied by SOB and exhaustion after the slightest effort. Pleuritic pain may occur with other diseases, such as rheumatic fever, systemic lupus erythematosus, and polyarteritis.

Treatment of pleurisy is similar to that of pneumonia: bed rest and restriction of activity, along with anti-inflammatory agents. Encourage the person to cough, but because coughing may be painful, apply hot or cold packs over the area or have the person lie on the affected side for comfort.

When fluid collection in the pleural space increases, the person is said to have a *pleural effusion* (Fig. 86-3D). The client may exhibit the same symptoms as those seen with pleurisy, but they often become dyspneic and have a rapid pulse. Pleural effusion can result from heart failure, pulmonary infections (including TB), and malignancies. Treatment relates directly to the underlying cause and may be geared toward specific symptoms.

Histoplasmosis

Histoplasmosis, which mimics "summer flu" and is often misdiagnosed, is caused by inhaling *spores* of the fungus *Histoplasma capsulatum*. The spores are carried in dust from soil rich in the fungus, such as that in chicken houses, barns, or bat caves. The disease is not passed between individuals. Typically, only the lungs are infected; if other organs are infected, the disease is referred to as disseminated histoplasmosis and can be fatal if left untreated. The disseminated disease is more commonly seen in individuals who have cancer or AIDS or are otherwise immunocompromised. In the United States, histoplasmosis is most common in the eastern and central states. Positive skin tests may be common in up to 80% of the endemic population of these areas. Prevention is possible by wearing appropriate personal protective equipment.

SPECIAL CONSIDERATIONS Lifespan

Histoplasmosis
Very young children and older men are most likely to contract histoplasmosis, and they are especially susceptible to the form that spreads (disseminates) from the lungs to other body parts.

Signs and Symptoms
Many infected individuals have no obvious symptoms. Respiratory symptoms, such as chest pains, dry cough, or nonproductive cough, may develop. Many people are infected with the disease without knowing it because symptoms are so mild. Most people recover after a few weeks. Histoplasmosis can resemble tuberculosis. Chest x-rays typically show a distinct pattern. The lungs become inflamed because of invasion by foreign material, which damages the lymph glands and lungs. In more severe cases, weight loss and weakness occur, requiring a very long convalescence. In the chronic form, the disease spreads throughout the body, causing weight loss, bleeding, and other severe problems. Scar tissue and calcium deposits may form. Occasionally, histoplasmosis is fatal.

The fungus may be identified by isolation in culture, and, occasionally, both sputum and urine must be cultured. A skin test, administered intradermally, can indicate the presence of the fungus.

Treatment
In the disease's mild form, treatment is similar to that for the flu. Usually, symptoms clear by themselves. In more severe cases, amphotericin B or another antifungal medication is given IV for several weeks.

Tuberculosis

Tuberculosis (**TB**), an infectious disease, is caused by the acid-fast bacillus *Mycobacterium tuberculosis*. This organism encases itself in a waxy coating (*spore*) that makes its destruction difficult. When found in the lungs, the bacilli are encased in a lump called a *tubercle*. The tubercle (known as the *primary lesion* or *primary TB*) may remain inactive for life. Many people have tubercle bacilli in their bodies, but do not actually have active TB disease. There are two categories of TB: *latent* or *inactive* and *active*, which are discussed below.

Tuberculosis spreads by inhalation of infected droplets that a person with an active infection releases into the air. Physical contact with an infected person and contact with contaminated utensils or equipment can spread TB. The tubercle bacilli most frequently attack the lungs, but the blood can carry the organisms to other body parts, including the kidneys, spine, brain, and bones.

Persons with the following conditions or status and who have compromised (weak) immune systems have an increased risk for active TB disease:

- HIV (coinfection with TB)
- Substance abuse
- Chronic renal failure
- Infants, youth, or advanced age
- Immunosuppression from steroids or cancers
- Diabetes mellitus
- Unclean living conditions or crowded living conditions with one or more occupants having TB
- Homelessness
- Poor diet
- Living or visiting parts of the world with endemic tuberculosis

Key Concept
The number of cases of active TB disease has increased during the last several decades because of the increase in multidrug-resistant TB organisms, increasing numbers of persons with HIV infection, substance abuse, homelessness, and poor compliance with medication treatment plans. Healthcare workers must maintain diligence and use appropriate personal protective equipment (e.g., specialized masks) when working with known or suspected respiratory diseases such as TB.

Types
Latent (Inactive) Infection and Active TB Disease
For most individuals who inhale TB bacteria and become infected, the body's defense mechanisms surround the

bacteria to prevent them from growing and spreading. The bacteria remain in a dormant spore state (alive but inactive). This condition is called *latent (inactive) TB* infection. For many individuals, the TB bacillus remains inactive for a lifetime without causing disease. Active TB disease develops when disease, poor nutrition, stress, or a multitude of other factors lower the person's resistance. The person becomes immunocompromised and can no longer prevent the spore from developing into a TB infection. The organisms multiply and become active, spreading throughout the lungs. It is possible to stop the destructive progress of the disease to the point where it is not infectious and remains inactive.

Typically individuals with latent (inactive) TB infection:

- Have no symptoms.
- Do not feel sick.
- Are not infectious to other individuals.
- Usually have a positive skin test reaction.
- Can develop active TB disease if they do not receive treatment for latent (inactive) TB infection.

Active TB disease occurs if the individual's defense mechanisms become weakened, at which point the body may not be able to control and segregate the TB spore. When the capacity of the body's defense mechanisms is compromised (weakened), the TB bacillus will start to grow, invade, and destroy tissues, especially the lungs.

Pulmonary Tuberculosis

When the bacillus enters the lungs, it precipitates an infection called *pulmonary TB*. It may be so mild that it produces no symptoms, in which case the infection clears and the person is unaware that they were infected. However, the tuberculin test is positive, and a CXR will reveal a small scar, a sign that at some time the bacillus was active, but now is considered latent TB. The scar is the result of efforts of the white blood cells to surround and destroy the bacilli. Active TB will result if the person's resistance is lowered. The capsule enclosing the tubercle breaks down and the bacilli spread and cause active illness.

Pott Disease and Miliary Tuberculosis

Tuberculosis of bones and joints is another form. Should the bloodstream carry bacilli to the spine, the resulting disease is called *Pott disease*. The vertebrae collapse, and there is pronounced spinal curvature (*kyphosis* or *humpback*). This disease rarely occurs in the United States or Canada today. Seeding by the bloodstream may carry the bacilli to other bones and joints, especially the hips and the knees. If disease spreads throughout the body, it is called *miliary TB*.

Infection may spread to the oviducts, ovaries, and uterus; surgical removal of the diseased organ may be required. The gastrointestinal tract, the kidneys, and the meninges are other possible sites.

Atypical Tuberculosis

Atypical TB is often spread to individuals who are immunosuppressed. Coinfection with HIV has become more common because of the increased numbers of persons infected with HIV. It may also occur in the person undergoing chemotheraphy or radiation treatment for cancer. Atypical TB is highly resistant treatment.

Multidrug-Resistant Tuberculosis

Multidrug-resistant TB is on the rise. In a small percentage of cases, the treatment regimen does not successfully eliminate the TB. This may be owing to the client's noncompliance with the medication program, the medication may not be absorbed properly, or the individual may have contracted TB from a person with multidrug-resistant TB. This type is very difficult to treat. The individual will remain on different medications for a much longer period.

Signs and Symptoms and Diagnosis

Tuberculosis usually develops slowly. Signs and symptoms of pulmonary TB include the following:

- Cough
- Lack of pain (presence of pain may indicate extension to the pleura)
- Thick sputum (possibly blood streaked)
- Expectoration of blood (indicating pleural hemorrhage)
- Positive or negative sputum culture
- Fatigue
- Gradual weight loss (may lead to emaciation, if not treated)
- Low-grade fever, especially in the afternoon
- *Nocturnal diaphoresis* (profuse sweating at night)
- Severe chest pains, persistent cough, and dyspnea as disease progresses

The tuberculin skin test or the IGRA blood tests may indicate the presence of the tubercle bacillus in the body, but the positive test result is not necessarily an indicator that the person has active TB. In conjunction with preliminary tuberculin tests, CXR and positive sputum cultures for the tubercle bacillus are the most reliable means of detecting pulmonary TB.

Treatment

Medication therapy is the specific treatment for active TB, regardless of the organ involved. The goal of medication therapy is to arrest the growth of the bacillus so that natural body defenses (leukocytes and antibodies) can take over and eliminate the disease (In Practice: Important Medications 86-1).

Tuberculosis infection is usually treated with isoniazid (**INH**) alone because it is quite effective. INH has few toxic effects, although in rare instances it has been known to cause anemia, neutropenia, gastrointestinal distress, and hepatitis. In combination with other medications, INH is prescribed in almost all cases of TB disease. Rifampin is highly effective in the treatment of TB as well; however, it is more toxic than INH and much more expensive. Ethambutol is usually given with INH and has low toxicity. Vitamin B_6 is commonly given with INH in the treatment of TB to prevent peripheral neuropathy.

 SPECIAL CONSIDERATIONS **Lifespan**

Tuberculosis
The initial treatment of tuberculosis in children and pregnant women will be with INH alone for 6–9 months. Sputum cultures must be followed up closely.

The regimen for medication administration is important and must be followed faithfully. It may be necessary to treat the client with two to four medications for a period of

IN PRACTICE
IMPORTANT MEDICATIONS 86-1 Drugs of Choice for Tuberculosis

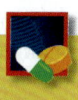

There are several approved drugs for treating TB, including the core drugs listed below.

The initial phase is at least 6 months with daily or weekly oral doses of:
- isoniazid (INH; Hyzyd), rifampin (Rifadin), and pyrazinamide
- plus ethambutol (Myambutol) or streptomycin in some cases
- after 2 months, pyrazinamide can be stopped if the client is responding

Second-line drugs include the following:
- capreomycin (Capastat Sulfate)
- ethionamide (Trecator)
- aminosalicylic acid (para-aminosalicylic acid [Parasol])
- pyrazinamide
- cycloserine (Seromycin)

Alternative agents for treatment of multidrug or highly drug-resistant TB include the following:
- levofloxacin (Levaquin)
- moxifloxacin hydrochloride (Avelox)
- linezolid (Zyvox)
- meropenem-clavulanate

6–12 months. Treatment time may be longer for immunosuppressed individuals, possibly taking as long as 2 years for those with drug-resistant TB.

Surgical procedures include *total* **pneumonectomy** (removal of an entire lung), *partial pneumonectomy* (removal of the affected part of a lung), **lobectomy** (removal of a lobe of a lung), and *wedge resection* or *segmental resection* (removal of one or more bronchopulmonary segments). Because effective medications are now available, surgery is rarely necessary.

Nursing Considerations
Tuberculosis is a long-term illness. Nursing care consists of several elements:

- Carefully administering medications; following a time schedule is important to maintain a constant blood level of the medications. Give medications at the same time each day, if a daily dose, or spread doses throughout the day. (If twice daily, instruct the person to take every 12 hr; if three times daily, take every 8 hr; if four times daily, take every 6 hr, rather than four times during waking hours.)
- Teaching the client about the importance of continuing medications, even if symptoms seem to have subsided; home care nursing intervention may be indicated
- Encouraging the client to follow a well-balanced diet that is high in protein and vitamins A and C
- Prevention of spread of the disease, with careful handwashing, and use of personal protective equipment
- Use of Transmission-Based Precautions (airborne precautions) if disease is active
- Encouraging the client to get plenty of rest
- Ensuring a smoke-free environment
- Providing the client with diversionary activities

Prevention
Nurses can take an active part in community health by seeking ways to prevent TB. The following are some suggestions:

- Educate the public in good, general health practices.
- In home care, burn all used tissues (the TB bacillus can survive for months in dried sputum). If unable to burn tissues, follow community guidelines for the disposal of biohazardous waste.
- Trace active cases and start early treatment of contacts to stop spread of the disease.
- Follow-up with all persons who have had active TB. Regular examination is necessary for life to determine if there is a recurrence and to treat it immediately.
- Screen members of high-risk groups, such as individuals with immunocompromised systems (e.g., HIV/AIDS), travelers, and immigrants from underserved medical areas and low-income populations.
- Give long-term residents of nursing homes, mental institutions, and correctional facilities the TST tuberculin test on admission and at intervals thereafter.
- Screen healthcare workers yearly.

Vaccine
A live TB vaccine, known as Bacille Calmette-Guérin (**BCG**), is available. It is a weakened strain of the bacterium. This should be used prophylactically on TB-negative persons who are repeatedly exposed to people with untreated or ineffectively treated TB. BCG is not generally used in the United States, but it is used in many countries that have a high incidence of TB. It does not prevent all cases of TB and may cause a false-positive TST skin test. Individuals who have had BCG vaccinations are generally guided to get CXRs, rather than skin testing, because false-positive results are common.

Empyema

Empyema, sometimes called *pyothorax*, is a collection of *purulent* (pus-containing) exudate in the pleural cavity. It can be acute or chronic.

Acute Empyema
Acute empyema is a secondary infection that may follow TB, lung abscess, or pneumonia. It may also result from an infection of the chest wall or other surrounding tissue or may be introduced directly by a chest wound or surgery. Because it is almost always a secondary infection, empyema is difficult to diagnose. The primary problem usually masks symptoms.

Symptoms of empyema include chest pain (usually on one side), cough, fever, dyspnea, and general malaise. If empyema is suspected, more decisive information can be obtained by CXR and thoracentesis. The offending organism can also be determined by a C&S test on fluid aspirated by thoracentesis.

Antibiotics to combat the infection and measures to drain the empyema cavity are started. The latter may be done by closed drainage or by thoracentesis, in which case an antibiotic may be injected directly into the pleural cavity. Bed rest and sedative cough preparations are also given. If this is not successful, open drainage is done.

Chronic Empyema

Chronic empyema may be a complication of acute empyema or may be caused by bronchopleural fistula, osteomyelitis of the rib cage, or an aspirated foreign body. It may also be a complication of TB or a fungal infection of the lungs.

Soft rubber drainage tubes are inserted in the wound, and large, absorbent dressings and pads are applied. Usually, the drainage is profuse at first, so the dressings must be changed frequently. In open drainage, usually a rib is removed, causing some pain.

CHRONIC RESPIRATORY DISORDERS

Snoring

Snoring (or *stertorous breathing*) is a respiratory disorder that is common in some people when they sleep. Not usually a serious problem, snoring is considered a pathologic condition if the person cannot stop snoring, no matter what sleeping position they use; if others can hear the snoring two or three rooms away; or if another person has to leave the room to be able to sleep. In extreme cases, surgery may be done. A procedure called *palatopharyngoplasty*, which removes extra material from the upper throat, has been successful in some cases. A relatively new, inexpensive external device (a tape strip) can be applied to the nasal bridge to help open the nasal passages. Other remedies include elevating the head of the bed; using a special pillow; sewing an object such as a ball on the back of the pajamas (so the person does not sleep on the back); avoiding heavy evening meals, smoking, sleeping pills, or alcohol; losing weight; and using decongestants.

Sleep Apnea Syndrome

Sleep apnea syndrome causes the person to wake up many times during the night, resulting in inadequate amounts of deep sleep. It is most common in middle-aged, overweight men but is also seen in women. The formal definition of sleep apnea is more than five cessations of airflow for at least 10 s each per hour of sleep. It is believed to occur because soft tissues at the back of the throat fall back and occlude the airway. This airway occlusion can last as long as 90 s. The person suddenly awakens owing to lack of oxygen. Hundreds of episodes can occur during a single night.

Diagnosis is based on symptoms and history, including the following:

- Extreme tiredness all day
- Difficulty in concentration
- Memory loss
- Inability to perform one's job
- Falling asleep during the day
- Episodes witnessed by sleeping partner

Almost all people with sleep apnea snore, although the reverse is not necessarily true. The person is at risk for auto or industrial accidents, high blood pressure with related disorders, or social and employment problems.

Treatment

Recommended treatment includes the following:

- Weight reduction
- Smoking cessation
- Avoidance of alcohol, especially before bedtime
- Elevation of the head of the bed
- Use of continuous positive airway pressure (**CPAP**) oxygenation (Box 86-2)

Possible surgery (*uvulopalatopharyngoplasty*) can now be done with lasers. Only about half the people who have this procedure done find significant improvement, however. Respiratory stimulant medications have not proved helpful. In severe cases, tracheostomy (which is plugged during the day) may be required to bypass upper airway obstruction.

Allergic Rhinitis

Rhinitis is an inflammation of the nasal mucous passages. Allergic rhinitis ("hay fever") is a condition that occurs when inflammation results from an allergic reaction to a protein substance. It may be caused by pollen from weeds, flowers, or grasses at certain seasons, or it may be a reaction to dust, feathers, or animal dander. People with a family history of allergy are more susceptible to hay fever, as are those who have asthma or eczema. In the United States, at least 10% of the population has a hereditary tendency. Persons of all ages are affected; hay fever may appear suddenly at any age and may just as suddenly disappear.

Signs and Symptoms

Allergic rhinitis is disagreeable and inconvenient. Symptoms include edema, an itchy nose, excessive sneezing, and profuse, watery discharge from the nose and eyes. The condition worsens on windy days and in the mornings and evenings. Determining the cause is difficult, and detailed questioning and many skin tests may be needed to identify the offending

---

Box 86-2 | Continuous Positive Airway Pressure (CPAP) Oxygenation

The continuous positive airway pressure (*CPAP*) apparatus is commonly used to assist persons with sleep apnea. This machine looks like an oxygen delivery system and is used at night, so the person can sleep. It delivers air, and sometimes oxygen, to the person at a continuous positive pressure that holds the alveoli open. (They usually close at the end of expiration.) This positive pressure prevents respiratory obstruction, increases oxygenation, and reduces breathing effort.

substance. Sometimes, several substances are the offenders (Chapter 84).

Treatment

The first step in treatment is to avoid the offending substance. It may mean eliminating a food from the diet, avoiding contact with animals, or avoiding dusty places. Air conditioning or filtering or purifying air can also help. Antihistamines relieve symptoms, and desensitization injections may eliminate them entirely. Corticosteroids may be given for severe attacks. An untreated allergy of this kind may lead to asthma, sinusitis, or nasal polyps.

Pneumoconioses

Pneumoconioses are "dust diseases" caused by habitual inhalation and retention in the lungs of certain heavy, harmful dusts. The most common disease is *silicosis,* common in miners, which is caused by breathing silica, or quartz dust. *Asbestosis* is another common form. As the person inhales dangerous dusts, the dusts eventually slow down or stop the ciliary action in the nose and lungs, and the dusts accumulate there. The dusts can cause irritation or allergic and chemical reactions.

Usually, the first symptom of dust diseases is dyspnea. Later, the person develops a chronic cough and expectorates the offending particles in thick mucus. Chest pains are often a later result. Serious complications include TB, pneumonia, chronic bronchitis, and emphysema. Vast evidence now indicates that the presence of asbestos directly relates to a specific lung cancer (*mesothelioma*).

Treatment focuses on prevention because these diseases are difficult to treat after extensive areas of the lungs are involved. The only treatment at present is to reduce exposure to the dust. Damage previously done cannot be reversed.

Chronic Obstructive Pulmonary Disease

Chronic obstructive pulmonary disease (**COPD**) is a general classification of progressive respiratory diseases, such as emphysema and chronic bronchitis, which are disorders that involve decreased airflow that worsens with age. COPD is treatable but not curable. Asthma is one of the risk factors for the development of COPD; about 40% of the individuals diagnosed with COPD also have asthma. Symptoms of both COPD and asthma include chronic coughing, wheezing, and dyspnea (SOB) that worsen with age. (Refer to asthma later in this chapter.)

Advanced stages of COPD have traditionally been placed into two categories based on physical manifestations of the disease. Two general clinical appearances are of note for clients with emphysema. Some clients have a chest that is usually hyperinflated or barrel like. Their face coloring can appear to be ruddy, pinkish, or flushed. These clients tend to be dyspneic, appearing to be gasping or puffing rather than breathing regularly. Other clients with COPD often have chronic bronchitis, which manifests as a cyanotic (blue) skin tone with edematous, bloated extremities. Available medical and oxygen therapies have lessened the differences between the two disorders so these features are not as distinctive now as in the 20th century. The general features of these two disorders are found in Table 86-2.

Care of the client with COPD involves physical, psychological, and environmental measures. The goals of treatment are to improve ventilation and to overcome hypoxic states through the following measures:

- Avoidance of irritants: smoking, allergens, industrial chemicals
- Use of medications: bronchodilators, expectorants, liquefying agents
- Postural drainage
- Increased fluid intake (1,000–2,000 mL/d)
- Cautious use of oxygen
- Breathing exercises
- Activity, as tolerated
- Avoidance of extremes of heat and cold
- Positioning to facilitate breathing (Fowler or orthopneic)
- Small, frequent meals

Fluid intake is important. Encourage the client to drink at least 2–3 quarts (2–3 L) of water daily to thin mucus and make it easier to expectorate (unless contraindicated).

Oxygen must be administered with caution. The amount should not exceed 3 L/min because many people with COPD retain carbon dioxide. Too high a level of oxygen could suppress the person's respiratory drive (i.e., the person loses the natural stimulus to breathe). Some clients may need to be reminded of the dangers of smoking in the presence of supplemental oxygen.

Breathing exercises, combined with other respiratory treatments, increase the volume of air the person is able to exhale. Inhaling and holding the breath also improves breathing. Practicing pursed lip breathing, especially during periods of dyspnea, is effective. *Rationale: This technique forces air into the lungs.* Avoid rapid or forceful exhalation because it may cause the terminal bronchioles to collapse. The person must be faithful in consistently carrying out breathing exercises.

Advise the person to keep active, but to pace activity with rest before and after activities. *Rationale: Give the client support and direction to enable them to accept that therapy is a lifelong commitment.* Teach the client to limit activities to whatever the heart and breathing capacities can tolerate. The individual has the potential to lead a fairly active life if they choose.

Persons with COPD have special needs because of the chronic nature of the disease. Help these individuals to live optimally through the following measures:

- Assist with developing energy-conserving measures in daily living.
- Teach relaxation techniques to use in situations of respiratory distress.
- Teach management of acute exacerbations of the disease and when to call for help.
- Help to identify situations or other factors that "trigger" symptoms and assist to find ways to modify or remove these triggers.

If the client is having difficulty with one or more aspects of managing COPD, a pulmonary rehabilitation program

TABLE 86-2 Chronic Obstructive Lung Disease: Characteristics of Emphysema and Chronic Bronchitis

CHARACTERISTICS	PULMONARY EMPHYSEMA	CHRONIC BRONCHITIS
Smoking history	Usually	Usually
Age of onset	40–50 years	30–40 years; disability in middle age, right heart failure common
Clinical features	Thin build, face may look flushed or pink	Stocky build, face may look cyanotic or bluish
• Barrel chest (hyperinflation of the lungs)	Often dramatic hyperinflated chest	May be present
• Weight loss	Advance disease—muscle wasting	Infrequent except for weight gain due to dependent edema
• Shortness of breath	May be absent early in disease Dyspnea progressive resting in disabling dyspnea	Predominant early symptoms, insidious in onset Exertional Productive cough
• Decreased breath sounds	Characteristic	Variable
• Wheezing	Usually absent	Variable, wheezes may be present
• Rhonchi	Usually absent or minimal	Often prominent
• Sputum	May be absent or may develop late in the disease course	Frequent early manifestation, frequent infections, abundant purulent sputum
• Cyanosis	Often absent, even late in the disease course when there is slow PaO_2	Often dramatic
• PaO_2	Slightly reduced	Markedly reduced Hypercapnia may be present Hypoxemia may be present
• Cor pulmonale (right heart failure)	Only in advanced cases	Frequent Peripheral edema
• Polycythemia	Only in advanced cases Hematocrit normal	Frequent Hematocrit increased
• Prognosis	Slowly debilitating disease	Numerous life-threatening episodes owing to acute exacerbations

Adapted from materials obtained from https://emedicine.medscape.com/article/297664-clinical#b3; National Emphysema Foundation (2020); and https://www.medicalnewstoday.com/articles/325616#symptoms

may be helpful. This is a program that includes medical management, breathing retraining, emotional support, exercise, nutritional information, and education about living with this disease. A multidisciplinary team of pulmonary experts works with the client to optimize quality of life.

Asthma

Asthma, also known as *bronchial asthma*, is a chronic airway condition characterized by inflammation of the lining of the bronchial airways. Asthma generally starts in childhood but can affect people of any age. Asthma is characterized by wheezing, difficulty in expiration, coughing, and bronchospasm, with a feeling of constriction in the chest. Coughing episodes are more common at night or early in the morning. Refer to the discussion of allergic asthma in Chapter 84. Triggers for asthma include sudden change in temperature, extreme physical exertion, contact with animal dander, overeating, emotional stress, and exposure to antigens.

When the airway is inflamed, swollen, and narrowed, it becomes more sensitive to things that may trigger an asthma attack. Obstruction of the airway is further complicated by tightening and narrowing of the surrounding muscles (*bronchospasms*). In some cases, mucous glands in the airways secrete thick mucus, which further obstructs the airways.

Research has not identified a single causative factor, but asthma seems to be related to genetic and environmental factors. Some families have a greater tendency to develop allergies. Individuals who are exposed to some viral infections in infancy or early childhood seem more likely to develop allergies. Some childhood respiratory infections may be linked with the development of asthma. The majority of asthma cases begin in the young. The rationale for this seems to be related to the health status and development of the immune system. Exposure to irritants, such as tobacco smoke, is known to cause the tissues in young airways to react, that is, to become inflamed and irritated.

Asthma Versus COPD

Asthma and COPD are conditions with airway obstruction. Asthma has fully reversible airway obstruction, whereas COPD does not. Asthma is typically diagnosed in childhood, whereas COPD is most prevalent in adults older than 40 years who are current or former smokers. The triggers of COPD and asthma are different. Asthma triggers include exposure to allergens, cold air, and exercise. COPD is made worse by respiratory tract infections, for example, a cold virus, the flu, or pneumonia. Environmental pollutants can affect both disorders, as can be seen in *airway hyperresponsiveness,* a condition in which the airways become very sensitive to things that are inhaled, such as pollens. Individuals with asthma or COPD often have additional conditions, known as comorbidities, for example, hypertension, insomnia, sinusitis, migraine, depression, cancer, or impaired mobility.

Signs and Symptoms

Onset of an asthma attack is sudden, also referred to as *paroxysmal.* The person experiences coughing, wheezing, SOB, and chest tightness and may be very pale and dyspneic, especially on expiration. As the attack subsides, the person may cough up thick, white mucus. Flare-ups and exacerbations are common. Asthma attacks may be occasional or frequent, but the individual is often symptom free between episodes. Those who have hay fever or chronic bronchitis are especially susceptible. Asthma can occur at any age and at any time. Chronic, severe respiratory conditions may lead to the clubbing of fingers (Fig. 86-4).

Acute severe asthma, formerly referred to as *status asthmaticus,* is a severe asthma attack that is unresponsive to the usual therapeutic medications such as subcutaneous epinephrine or inhaled albuterol, in addition to oral or parenteral corticosteroids. It is a medical emergency that can lead to death unless recognized and treated. Most acute severe asthma attacks are preceded by upper respiratory infections, nonadherence to medical treatment plans, exposure to allergens (especially pets), exercise, environmental pollutants such as smoke or paint, and insufficient use of inhaled or oral corticosteroids.

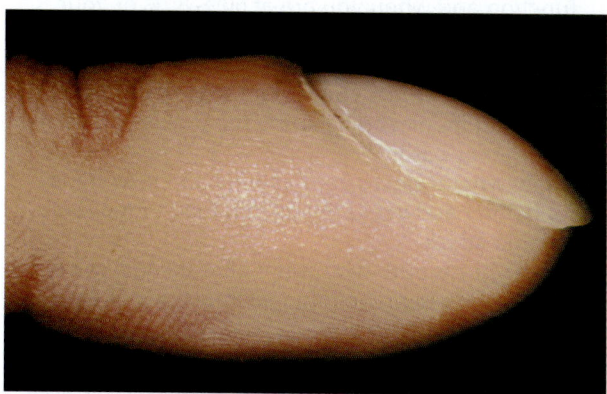

Figure 86-4 Clubbing of the finger. Normally, there is an obtuse angle of about 160° between the base of the nail and the adjacent dorsal surface of the finger; with clubbing, this angle exceeds 180°.

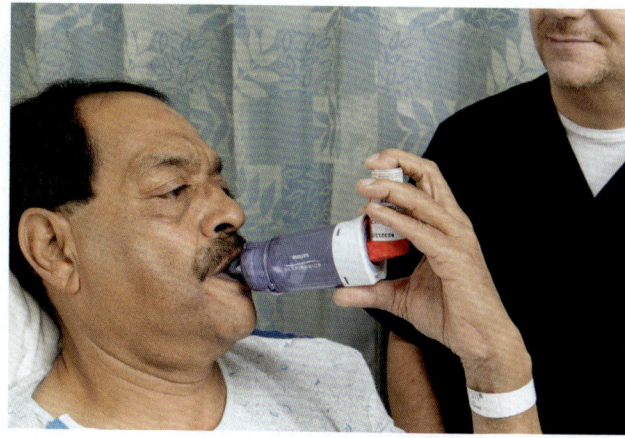

Figure 86-5 A metered-dose inhaler and spacer in use. (Smeltzer, Bare, Hinkle, & Cheever, 2010.)

Treatment

The main treatment objective in an acute attack is to relieve breathing difficulties. In the long term, it is important to assist the client in proper medical management of asthma to improve overall quality of life. This strategy will include the use of several classifications of medications. All people with moderate to severe asthma should be taking anti-inflammatory inhalers as frontline therapy. The inhaled steroids improve lung function, decrease inflammation, and decrease asthma symptoms and flare-ups (attacks) (Fig. 86-5 and In Practice: Important Medications 86-2).

> **SPECIAL CONSIDERATIONS** Lifespan
>
> **Asthma in Pregnancy**
>
> The pregnant client must take their medications faithfully and follow their asthma action plan. If their asthma is not under control, they are not getting enough oxygen to their lungs or to the baby's lungs.

Goals include decreasing symptoms and complications, improving physical conditioning and emotional well-being, and encouraging self-management (which will reduce hospitalizations). These goals can be accomplished by the introduction of an action plan (or crisis intervention plan) that assists the client in the determination of how best to manage their asthma. Education, with full understanding noted by the client and family, is essential. Many people with asthma have the condition well controlled. Teaching must include the following:

- Use of routine (maintenance) medications and emergency (rescue) medications
- Use of a peak flow meter, a small piece of equipment used to determine lung function by showing how fast a person can exhale after deep inhalation
- When to call the healthcare provider
- When to go to the hospital for emergency care

IN PRACTICE
IMPORTANT MEDICATIONS 86-2: Medications Used for Treating Asthma

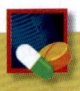

Anticholinergics
These bronchodilators work on the nervous system to control airway size:
- tiotropium bromide (Spiriva)
- ipratropium bromide (Atrovent)

Long-Acting Beta-Agonists
These medications dilate bronchial airways by working on the nervous system that controls the muscle tissue around the airway:
- salmeterol xinafoate (Serevent)
- formoterol fumarate (Foradil)
- fluticasone furoate (Veramyst)
- budesonide and formoterol fumarate (Symbicort)

Corticosteroids
These act as anti-inflammatory agents:
- beclomethasone (Qvar)
- budesonide (Rhinocort)
- mometasone (Asmanex)

Leukotriene Antagonists
These medications block the inflammatory biochemical pathway, making the airway less sensitive to asthma triggers:
- montelukast sodium (Singulair)

Monoclonal Antibodies
Monoclonal antibodies block cytokines and reduce airway inflammation in difficult cases of chronic asthma not relieved by other medications:
- omalizumab (Xolair)

Nursing Considerations

Asthma can be frustrating and frightening. Be calm and supportive and promptly administer the prescribed medications during an attack. Chapter 63 gives guidelines for the use of inhalers. Adherence to medical treatment plans is a beneficial preventative method of maintenance and prevention of acute attacks. Client and family teaching are highlighted within In Practice: Educating the Client 86-1.

Bronchiectasis

Bronchiectasis is a chronic dilation of the bronchi in which the walls become permanently widened, distended, flabby, and scarred. The main causes are infections or conditions that injure the bronchial airways or prevent the airways from clearing mucus. Mucus is an essential substance produced by the mucous membranes that helps remove inhaled dust, bacteria, or other environmental particles. If the airways cannot clear the slimy covering, mucus accumulates and creates environments that grow bacteria, which leads to serious lung infections. Airways lose their abilities to move air via inhalation and exhalation, which leads to hypoxia. Chronic hypoxia can preclude atelectasis, respiratory failure, and heart failure. Often, bronchiectasis begins in early adulthood and progresses slowly over a long period. Bronchial disorders in young adults are linked to exposure to secondhand smoke in childhood. In a child, it may be a complication of cystic fibrosis and immunodeficiency diseases. It is rarely fatal, but may have serious complications with life-threatening potential.

Signs and Symptoms

The characteristic symptom is a chronic cough, most often occurring when the client arises in the morning. The cough produces greenish-yellow sputum with a foul odor. As the disease progresses, the amount of sputum increases. Sometimes the person coughs up blood. In fact, bronchiectasis is the most common cause of *hemoptysis* (bloody sputum). The person loses weight because of poor appetite and may experience chronic fatigue.

IN PRACTICE
EDUCATING THE CLIENT 86-1: Asthma

- Have an action plan for asthma management.
- Know what medications you are using.
- Use the peak flow meter to determine how your lungs are functioning.
- Know your values for your personal best lung function and when you are at 50%–80% of your personal best.
- Check with your primary healthcare provider about situations in which you should start adding or changing medications, notify the provider, or seek emergency care.
- Know what triggers your asthma and take steps to identify and avoid things that may trigger an asthma attack.
- Rinse your mouth with water after using a steroid inhaler to help prevent fungal infections of the mouth.
- Rinse your inhaler mouthpiece daily.
- Use your inhaler properly as shown. Inhalers are not helpful if used incorrectly.
- Take your medications on time. Using medications regularly helps to prevent difficulties and complications.

> **IN PRACTICE**
> **EDUCATING THE CLIENT 86-2** Prevention of Bronchiectasis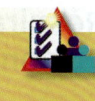
>
> - Have children vaccinated against pertussis (whooping cough) and measles.
> - Avoid exposure to passive smoke.
> - Have adults vaccinated against influenza.
> - Maintain general health at optimum level.
> - Seek prompt attention if a foreign object or fluid is aspirated into the lungs, or if a respiratory infection develops.

Treatment

Drainage of the purulent material is part of the treatment. Drainage is accomplished by postural drainage, in which the head is lower than the chest. Encourage the person to cough and breathe deeply. Humidification of air is recommended to help thin secretions and make expectoration easier. Expectorant cough medicines may be prescribed. Give ordered antibiotics to control the infection. Good nutrition, fresh air, and rest are also important. The person should not smoke. Give special mouth care to overcome the offensive taste and breath odor and to make food more palatable.

Prompt attention to such conditions as bronchial asthma and bronchitis helps to prevent bronchiectasis (In Practice: Educating the Client 86-2).

Surgical intervention may be necessary for individuals who continue to have bouts of pneumonia after treatment. Because bronchiectasis can be prevented, it is seen less frequently than in the past.

Chronic Bronchitis

Chronic bronchitis is more serious than acute bronchitis. It often develops so gradually that the person disregards its most significant symptom, a chronic cough. Consequently, the disease is firmly established before the person decides that treatment is needed. Chronic bronchitis is a form of COPD. It usually leads to pulmonary emphysema. Repeated attacks of acute bronchitis may lead to a chronic condition, or it may develop after an acute respiratory infection such as influenza or pneumonia.

Signs and Symptoms

Chronic bronchitis begins with a dry cough (also known as "smoker's cough") that is most severe when the person rises in the morning. As time goes on, the person coughs up mucus and pus, sometimes with streaks of blood. SOB becomes apparent with exertion. As the disease progresses, it persists even when the individual is quiet. The client's history of a cough, as well as their living habits, helps the healthcare provider in making a diagnosis. CXR, fluoroscopic examinations, and sputum tests also aid in diagnosis. Table 86-2 lists characteristics of chronic bronchitis and emphysema.

Treatment

Treatment is slow and continuous; no medication will work a miracle cure. However, treatment reduces symptoms and helps prevent complications. Untreated, the disease may progress until the bronchioles of the lungs are permanently damaged, or it may lead to asthma, emphysema, or heart failure.

Aerosolized treatments, postural drainage, and chest percussion are done. These treatments help to facilitate secretion removal. Build up the person's general health and remind the client to use precautions to avoid exposure to infections. The individual should have plenty of rest and be free from emotional stress. Assist the client with measures to help avoid situations of excessive dust or other factors that aggravate the bronchitis. The client must avoid cigarette smoking. Antibiotics will help to clear coexisting respiratory infections that complicate the condition.

Pulmonary Emphysema

Pulmonary emphysema is abnormal, permanent enlargement of the alveoli and alveolar ducts, with destruction of the alveolar walls, which results in lack of elasticity. It is a form of COPD. The number of cases of emphysema relates directly to cigarette smoking.

In emphysema, air that is normally exchanged becomes trapped in the alveoli. The client is unable to exhale, the lungs become distended, and the muscles suffer from lack of oxygen, becoming less elastic. The condition worsens as more and more air becomes trapped in the alveoli. As a result, the heart must work harder to pump blood through the body and get oxygen to the muscles and other body tissues. The end result of emphysema is often heart failure or right-sided heart failure.

Alpha-1 antitrypsin (α_1-antitrypsin) deficiency, also referred to as *ATT deficiency*, is a genetic deficiency of the plasma protein ATT that causes another type of emphysema. Symptoms begin to be obvious in young adulthood. The lack of ATT allows normal white blood cells to continuously damage lung and liver tissue. The damage to lungs worsens significantly if the individual smokes. Augmentation therapy is the main treatment for ATT deficiency in which the client receives replacement ATT from human donors.

Signs and Symptoms

The first symptom of emphysema is difficulty in breathing after exertion. As the condition progresses, the person has persistent difficulty in breathing. Other symptoms include wheezing and a chronic cough. The person is pale and drawn and is afraid of choking. Many individuals use abdominal muscles as well as other accessory muscles to aid in breathing. The person is afraid to lie down and instead sits up, leans forward, and contracts the neck muscles with every breath. The individual looks anxious. The person also raises the shoulder girdle and shows retraction above the clavicles when breathing. Over time, the chest becomes barrel shaped. In the advanced stages, as carbon dioxide accumulates in the blood, the person becomes listless and drowsy. The disease runs its course over a period of many years.

Prevention

Preventive treatment is most important to correct the conditions that cause emphysema because changes in lung tissue or the blood vessels of the lungs are irreversible. This means, for one thing, alerting the public to the danger signs, such as "morning cough" or "smoker's cough."

> **Key Concept**
> Cigarette smoking and secondhand smoke cause or predispose individuals to many diseases of the respiratory system and other systems.

Acute Respiratory Distress Syndrome

Acute respiratory distress syndrome (**ARDS**) is also called *noncardiogenic pulmonary edema*. ARDS is a state of progressive oxygen deprivation following a serious illness or injury. Causes include aspiration, medication overdose, cardiac surgery (especially bypass), pancreatitis, end-stage renal disease, embolism, major surgery, and trauma. The person is in acute respiratory failure and usually requires mechanical ventilation and blood pressure medications. If the cause can be determined, it can be treated. However, the mortality rate is greater than 50%.

TRAUMA

An accident may cause respiratory problems or death. If there is no air exchange in the lungs, the person will die within a matter of minutes.

Absence of Air Exchange

Asphyxiation is the condition in which the blood lacks oxygen and the blood and tissues contain excess carbon dioxide. Any form of **suffocation**, or stoppage of breathing, can cause asphyxiation. Suffocation may result from externally applied pressure to the throat (*strangulation*), drowning (*aspiration*), electric shock, or gases (e.g., carbon monoxide or gases in smoke from a house fire) that enter the lungs and prevent the exchange of oxygen and carbon dioxide. Choking on a foreign object that plugs the airway or covering the nose and mouth with an object (e.g., a pillow or plastic bag) can also cause suffocation.

Strangulation refers to respiratory arrest caused by an obstruction of the air passage. Most commonly, this term applies to trauma caused by another person, hanging, or an accident.

Chest Trauma

Asphyxiation can result from a sudden blow to the chest. It may cause pneumothorax or airway blockage. Accumulation of blood in the lungs can cause asphyxiation by drowning.

A puncture wound to the chest from a knife or a bullet is an emergency. If a foreign object is in place, do not remove it. Get emergency assistance immediately. *Rationale: The object may plug the hole and maintain the negative pressure within the lungs until help arrives.*

If an object, such as a bullet, has caused an open hole in the chest wall, plug the hole immediately. *Rationale: If the hole is left open, the lungs will collapse because the negative pressure will have been lost.* Keep the hole plugged until emergency assistance arrives.

> **Nursing Alert** Cardiopulmonary resuscitation (CPR) is ineffective if the person's airway is blocked or if there is an open chest wound. Clear the airway and/or apply pressure to occlude an open chest wound before initiating CPR.

Respiratory Complications in Drug Poisoning

In many cases of drug overdose, the person's respirations are depressed. In some cases, depression of the respiratory system to the point of apnea causes death. This development is called *respiratory arrest*. Drugs most likely to cause respiratory arrest include narcotics (e.g., codeine, morphine, and heroin) and depressants (e.g., barbiturates).

> **Nursing Alert** If a person is not breathing, CPR is necessary. It is done with an airway and a manual breathing bag, if available. *Rationale: This is less strenuous for the rescuer and prevents the spread of infection from the client to the healthcare worker.* If an airway and manual breathing bag are unavailable, mouth-to-mouth breathing is required.
>
> In the case of an overdose of stimulants (e.g., cocaine or amphetamines), respirations may increase. In this type of overdose, overstimulation may lead to seizures, hypertension, stroke, and death.

Drowning/Near Drowning

The medical term for fluid in the lungs is *aspiration*. Fluid or foreign bodies aspirated into the nose, throat, or the lungs during inspiration can prevent adequate air exchange in the lungs. This leads to *aspiration pneumonia*, a serious complication.

Near drowning occurs when an individual has been submerged under water without ventilation. The person will be hypoxic. Begin rescue ventilation and perfusion as quickly as possible. Do not attempt to clear the airway of water because the body can aspirate only a small amount into the lungs and quickly absorbs it into the bloodstream. A small percentage of victims will not aspirate at all, owing to breath holding or laryngospasm. In such cases, individuals die because of the lack of oxygen and inability to breathe, but no water is actually in the lungs.

> **Nursing Alert** Be careful in giving fluids to a person who has difficulty swallowing or who is confused. Never give fluids by mouth to an unconscious person. Aspiration can cause pneumonia or death. If aspiration occurs, notify the healthcare provider immediately and take measures to prevent complications.

Pneumothorax

Pneumothorax is the presence of air in the pleural cavity or between the pleura and the chest wall. It may result from trauma or be a complication of chest surgery or chest tube drainage. It usually causes the collapse of a lung, which is a serious complication because less air is exchanged. Pneumothorax is an emergency. Check for the following signs of pneumothorax:

- SOB or severe dyspnea
- Asymmetrical chest

- Mediastinal shift toward the affected side
- Sudden, sharp chest pain
- Drop in blood pressure
- Weak, rapid pulse
- Cessation of breathing (chest) movement on affected side
- Cyanosis
- Change in level of consciousness

Immediately report if any of these signs occur. If the client has chest tubes, clamp them and get help as soon as possible.

NEOPLASMS

Benign Neoplasms

A *benign lung tumor*, or *cyst*, is characterized on the x-ray film by smooth edges and sharply defined margins. Peripheral tumors usually have no symptoms. If the tumor is in the bronchi, there may be obstruction, causing infection or atelectasis distal to the obstruction (Fig. 86-3B). Bronchoscopy and biopsy are usually done to determine the reason for an abnormal shadow in the lung. Treatment is symptomatic.

Lung Cancer

Lung cancer, also known as carcinoma of the lung or pulmonary carcinoma, is a malignant lung tumor characterized by uncontrolled cell growth of lung tissues. It is the leading cause of cancer deaths in both men and women. Based upon their appearance under the microscope, there are two basic types of lung cancer: *small cell lung cancers* (**SCLC**) and *non–small cell lung cancers* (**NSCLC**). SCLC is the most aggressive and rapidly metastasizes to other sites quickly and extensively. Cigarette smoking has occurred in 99% of the individuals with this form of lung cancer. NSCLC is the most common form of lung cancer; three types are seen, designated by the type of cells found in the tumor. These include adenocarcinoma, squamous cell carcinoma, and large cell carcinoma.

Risk factors include cigarette smoking; exposure to secondhand smoke; exposure to carcinogenic and industrial air pollutants (asbestos, arsenic, chromium, coal dust, iron oxides, nickel, radioactive dust, and uranium); and a genetic predisposition. From available research, stopping or not smoking is the best preventive measure.

> **Key Concept**
> Individuals who smoke have the greatest risk of lung cancer. The risk increases with the length of time and number of cigarettes smoked. Quitting smoking will reduce the chances of developing lung cancer.

Signs and Symptoms

Many early lung cancers are asymptomatic. The first indication of trouble generally occurs when the person begins to cough up mucus and blood-streaked sputum. The client may experience dyspnea, chills, and fever. Typically, a person who smokes may think that the problems is excess smoking and may resolve to cut down. Later, fatigue, unexplained weight loss, and chest pains occur. By the time the client consults a healthcare provider, the disease is likely to be in an advanced stage. In summary, the common symptoms of lung cancer include the following:

- Shortness of breath
- Wheezing
- Hoarseness
- A persistent cough that gets worse over time
- Hemoptysis (coughing up blood)
- Constant chest pain
- Fatigue
- Weight loss and anorexia
- Episodes of respiratory infections
- Pleural effusion
- Swelling of the neck and face

Diagnosis

Detecting lung cancer in the early stage is difficult because symptoms may not appear until the disease is well advanced. A routine CXR will often reveal the cancer and can show a lesion up to 2 years before signs and symptoms appear. Lung cancer usually arises in the bronchi and produces no symptoms until it enlarges. Diagnosis is confirmed by a bronchoscopy, CT or MRI, sputum examination, and lung scan.

Treatment

Surgery, chemotherapy, and radiation are the general approaches to cancer. If the tumor is localized, immediate surgery, with removal of part (*lobectomy*) or all of the lung (*pneumonectomy*), may be curative. If the tumor is extensive and involves lymph nodes, radiation or chemotherapy (or both) may be used. These treatments will not usually cure the disease, but they often improve the individual's quality of life.

If the person has widespread lung cancer, with metastasis to other organs, a combination of chemotherapeutic medications may be instituted. Responses to this treatment vary. At this time, chemotherapeutic agents cannot cure lung cancer, but they are useful in controlling pain and in reducing the pleural effusions caused by the cancer.

DISORDERS OF THE NOSE

Inflammatory Disorders

Sinusitis

Sinusitis is inflammation of one or more of the sinuses located in the head. The maxillary sinus (*antrum*) is most frequently affected by infection spreading from the nasal passages. If the individual's resistance is low, the person is more susceptible to sinus infection. A sinus infection is uncomfortable. Allergy, frequent colds, and nasal obstruction of any kind increase susceptibility to repeated attacks. If neglected, sinusitis becomes chronic and damages the mucous membranes; treatment is then less effective. Of all possible complications of sinusitis, infections of the middle ear and the brain are most serious. Sinusitis may also lead to bronchiectasis or osteomyelitis in the adjacent bone. Early treatment is important to prevent these complications.

Acute Sinusitis

Acute sinusitis begins with pain and pressure. The person feels pain in the cheek or the upper teeth if the maxillary sinuses are affected. Frontal sinus pain occurs over the eyes. The person may have a low-grade fever, fatigue, and a poor appetite. A purulent nasal discharge accompanies postnasal drip, causing throat irritation. Sinus congestion shows on x-ray examination.

Treatment includes increased fluids, antibiotics to control infection, analgesics to relieve pain, and, in severe cases, bed rest. Nose drops containing phenylephrine (Neo-Synephrine) may be prescribed to shrink the swollen turbinates and to encourage drainage; antihistamines are also used. Steam inhalation or hot, moist packs to the forehead can be effective.

If drainage is obstructed in an acute sinus infection, the sinus may be irrigated with warm saline solution, a comparatively painless procedure. However, it may be necessary to puncture the bony wall between the nose and the sinus cavity or to enter the frontal sinus through the inner aspect of the eyebrow. These surgical procedures are painful for the client, who may become frightened and feel dizzy or faint.

Chronic Sinusitis

Many people mistakenly think that nothing can be done for sinusitis and unfortunately allow it to become chronic. *Chronic sinusitis* is characterized by repeated flare-ups of the infection, despite treatment. Symptoms include the following:

- Cough, caused by postnasal drip
- Chronic headaches in the affected area
- Facial pain
- Nasal stuffiness
- Fatigue

Sometimes, a relatively simple operation to create a new sinus opening may be ordered. Because many cases of chronic sinusitis are allergic in nature, allergy tests may be done and desensitization injections given.

Structural Disorders

Deviated Septum

The nasal septum is a partition made of bone and cartilage that divides the nose into right and left cavities. The septum is rarely absolutely straight, but unless the deviation is marked, it usually causes no trouble. An unusually crooked septum can interfere with drainage in one nostril or with insertion of a nasogastric tube. An injury that causes a deformity in the septum should have a healthcare provider's attention; if left uncorrected, the deformity can cause sinusitis. The operation to correct such a deformity is called a *submucous resection* or *septoplasty*.

Nasal Polyps

Polyps are tumors that look like small bunches of tiny grapes. Nasal polyps obstruct breathing and sinus drainage. They are easily removed through surgery under local anesthesia, but tend to return, in which case the operation must be repeated. A biopsy of the tissue should be done to determine if the growth is malignant.

Plastic Surgery

Plastic surgery of the nose (**rhinoplasty**) may be done for cosmetic reasons or to correct deformities resulting from injury.

Care of the Client Undergoing Nasal Surgery

Most surgery on the nose is performed on an outpatient basis. Therefore, client and family teaching is essential. Be sure to document all teaching carefully and completely.

The nose is highly vascular; hemorrhage is always a possibility. Therefore, teach the client and family important signs and symptoms for which to observe. The procedure can also be painful. In addition, nasal procedures can interfere with normal respiration and can cause anxiety. In Practice: Nursing Care Guidelines 86-5 discusses nursing care in nasal surgery.

Nasal Trauma

Fractures

A fractured nose is a relatively common occurrence. It should be set (moved back into place) promptly to avoid later deformity. Usually, no other treatment is needed.

Epistaxis

Irritation or injury to a small mass of capillaries on the nasal septum may cause nosebleed or **epistaxis**. The vast majority of nosebleeds are *anterior nosebleeds* meaning that they occur in the anterior portion of the nose as a result of a cracked, damaged, or irritated capillary or vein located near the front part of the nose. These nosebleeds tend to occur in the dry winter months and in cold, dry climates, especially between the ages of 2 and 10 years. Most of these can be contained by home measures. *Posterior nosebleeds* are more serious and less common, occurring mostly in the older adult. Posterior epistaxis occurs when an artery in the back of the nose ruptures. It may indicate a hypertensive emergency. Hypertension can give rise to bleeding, in which case the bleeding is more likely to be severe and not easily controlled. Certain blood disorders, cancer, and rheumatic fever are other possible causes. Other causes of epistaxis include therapy with blood thinners such as warfarin (Coumadin), acetylsalicylic acid (Aspirin), or NSAIDs. Some individuals have blood clotting disorders, including liver disorders or diseases. Nosebleeds are fairly common, but when severe, they can be serious.

Treatment for a posterior nosebleed is usually done in the emergency department by an otolaryngologist (ear, nose, and throat specialist). First aid for epistaxis consists of initially applying pressure or pinching the anterior section of the nose for 10 min without interruption.

If bleeding continues, additional therapy will be required. It is important to monitor the client for syncope, hypotension, tachycardia, hypoxia, and signs of shock. If the client has a history of easily bruising or frequent episodes of epistaxis, the cause of the problem may be include clotting disorders, chemotherapy, or blood-thinning medications.

Prolonged therapy will include packing the nasal cavity with gauze to create pressure on the bleeding area. This can usually be accomplished by passing a string through the nose and bringing it out through the mouth. The pack on the string is pulled back through the nose until the packing is in the back of the nasal cavity. The other end of the string extends out through the nostril.

Bleeding points may also be painted with silver nitrate or other solutions that tend to stop bleeding, or they may be cauterized to cause coagulation.

IN PRACTICE
NURSING CARE GUIDELINES 86-5: Caring for the Person Who Has Had Nasal Surgery

- Always wash your hands.
- Wear gloves.
- Teach precautions to the client or family and carefully document teaching. **Rationale:** *Most nasal surgery is done on an outpatient basis. The person will be going home immediately after surgery.*

Promoting Respiration
- Keep in mind that the client is often very uncomfortable. **Rationale:** *The initial postoperative period can be very painful. The person will probably have to breathe through the mouth.*
- Give frequent oral hygiene. **Rationale:** *Breathing through the mouth is very drying to the mucous membranes.*
- Elevate the head of the bed. **Rationale:** *Head elevation facilitates breathing.*
- Observe carefully for choking. Suctioning may be needed. **Rationale:** *Considerable mucous drainage is usual because the nasal mucosa has been irritated.*
- Observe for signs of respiratory distress. **Rationale:** *Swelling or bleeding may cause respiratory difficulties. Aspiration into the lungs is always a threat.*

Observing for Hemorrhage
- Observe for nausea, coffee-ground emesis, dark-colored emesis, frequent spitting of blood, blood on the dressing, and any signs of shock. **Rationale:** *The nose is very vascular and may bleed profusely.*
- At regular intervals, examine the back of the throat for draining of blood by using a flashlight and tongue depressor. **Rationale:** *In surgery of the nose or nosebleed (epistaxis), blood may run down the back of the throat and be swallowed.*
- Remember that the nostrils are usually packed with gauze, which is removed 24–48 hr following surgery. Observe carefully for hemorrhage after removal of a pack. **Rationale:** *The nose is very vascular and may bleed profusely.*
- Apply a mustache dressing (a gauze pad impregnated with petrolatum and held in place with strips of adhesive), beneath the nostrils, if necessary. **Rationale:** *This dressing is applied to absorb drainage.*

DISORDERS OF THE THROAT

The throat (*pharynx*) is the muscular tube communicating with the nasal cavity (*nasopharynx*), the oral cavity (*oropharynx*), and the laryngeal cavity (*laryngopharynx*). Two throat disorders, common in children but occurring occasionally in adults, are tonsillitis and streptococcal sore throat (Chapter 72).

Trauma

Aspiration of Foreign Bodies
A foreign body lodged in the trachea that obstructs breathing is an emergency. In most cases, a sharp blow between the shoulder blades while the person's head is lowered, or the abdominal thrust, will dislodge the object. If these measures fail and the person cannot breathe, an emergency tracheostomy or intubation with an airway must be done by trained personnel (Chapter 87). Artificial ventilation will probably be required after the airway is opened. A client may aspirate a small object into the lung without causing asphyxiation; it will result in infection and atelectasis of all or part of the lung (Fig. 86-3B) and must be removed. For this, bronchoscopy usually is effective. Open-lung surgery may be performed if the object has lodged deep in a bronchus.

Cancer of the Larynx

Cancer of the larynx most often afflicts men older than 45 years. Age increases the chances of developing cancer; women are less likely than men to develop this disease. Those who have chronic laryngitis, strain their voices, or are heavy drinkers or smokers are those most likely to develop laryngeal cancer. Theorists believe that heredity may also play a role. Symptoms are chronic hoarseness and, in some instances, inability to speak above a whisper.

Treatment
If the condition is detected early, radiation may be effective. Surgery is often successful in inducing a complete cure. The operation consists of removing either the tumorous part or the entire larynx. The surgery is called **laryngectomy**. A person who has a total laryngectomy is referred to as a *laryngectomee*. If the cancer has spread beyond the vocal cords, a simple or radical neck dissection is done.

After the larynx is removed, air enters and leaves through the trachea. Provision for this is made by inserting a tube into the trachea through an opening in the lower part of the neck. This procedure is called a *tracheostomy;* it is permanent, even after the airway tube is removed.

Nursing Considerations
Client teaching and support are important (In Practice: Educating the Client 86-3). The person not only faces the knowledge that they must permanently breathe through a hole in the neck but also must deal with the diagnosis of cancer. Reduce the client's fears about loss of speech by assuring the individual that, although they will lose the natural voice, voice training (esophageal or pharyngeal speech) or a mechanical device will make conversation possible. If only a partial laryngectomy was performed, reassure the client that speech usually returns quickly. A visit from another person who has made a good recovery after a laryngectomy may help.

Because esophageal reconstruction is likely, inform the client that, for a time, feeding may be done through a nasal

IN PRACTICE

EDUCATING THE CLIENT 86-3 After Laryngectomy

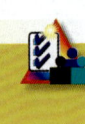

While the client recovers from laryngectomy, the client and family are able to:
- Describe care of the tube, such as cleaning and suctioning (if necessary), and how to handle emergencies.
- Explain or demonstrate various communication techniques.
- Identify support groups available for persons and families after laryngectomy or a diagnosis of cancer.
- Show how the permanent laryngectomy opening may be covered by a necktie, a crew or turtleneck shirt, a scarf, or jewelry.
- Demonstrate how to prevent aspiration of fluids or foreign objects into the laryngectomy tube.
- Explain why showering must be done with care and swimming is often prohibited.
- Identify the need to wear a scarf over the opening in extremely cold weather and to avoid thin, filmy scarves because they may be sucked into the tracheostomy and obstruct breathing.

---

or gastrostomy tube (until the esophagus heals) and that the tracheostomy opening will be permanent. The client needs good oral hygiene, which provides comfort and helps keep the surgical site as clean as possible.

When respiratory passages become irritated, mucus secretions increase; they must be removed frequently by suction through the tracheostomy tube. Keep a suction machine at the bedside, and never leave the client alone without a call light. A family member may stay with the client for the first few postoperative days. Because the client cannot cry out for help, they may fear choking and being unable to breathe. If oxygen is to be administered, apply it by mask or by T-piece (blow-by) over the tracheostomy tube. There is also the danger of hemorrhage, as evidenced by *hemoptysis* (coughing or spitting up of blood) or by symptoms of shock. Give the client a signal bell or call light.

Drainage from the wound following a neck dissection, or other procedure in this area, is usually handled with a portable wound suction device, such as Hem-O-Vac. This device stays with the individual at all times. Empty and measure the drainage. Follow the facility's protocol.

The client probably will be allowed out of bed the first postoperative day and soon will learn how to suction the tube and take care of it. Everyone involved in the client's care should know how to perform this procedure. When the airway becomes obstructed, the individual quickly becomes cyanotic and could die within a few minutes if the obstruction is not removed. In this emergency, call for help and suction the tracheostomy opening. Unless the healthcare provider has previously instructed the nurses as to what emergency procedures to use, nursing staff should consult the healthcare provider to see if the tracheostomy tube can be removed as an emergency measure.

The person usually loses the sense of smell temporarily after surgery. However, it will begin to return as they learn to breathe through the tracheostomy tube. The sense of smell will be best recovered in the individual who learns esophageal speech.

Key Concept
Sometimes, the person must write notes to communicate. In this case, make sure the person's dominant hand is not encumbered with an IV. A child's "Magic Slate" or a white board often works well temporarily. Alphabet and picture cards may also be useful. Be sure to answer this person's signal light immediately; they will be unable to tell the nurse what is wrong on the intercom. (A tap bell may be used for emergencies.)

Communication and Speech

Before the surgery, discuss the method of postoperative communication with the client. Clients who know that some type of communication will be available after surgery will be less anxious. Immediately after surgery, set up a workable communication system. Provide the client with writing materials. If the client tries to tell you something, make every attempt to find out what it is.

Speech therapy should begin as soon as possible. The technique of *esophageal speech* consists of swallowing air and using it to make speech sounds while regurgitating the air. It takes patience and constant practice to learn how to do this; some individuals learn the technique in 2–3 weeks. Esophageal speech is not smooth, although it is the easiest to learn.

Most people progress to *pharyngeal speech*. The air they use in this case is that which enters the nose and mouth; it is blocked by quick tongue action. The pharynx becomes the sounding board. Pharyngeal speech takes much more practice, but it is smoother and has a more natural sound than esophageal speech.

The third speech technique devised for the person who is unable to learn esophageal or pharyngeal speech is the *artificial larynx*. This is an electronic device that the person holds against the throat. Currently, many healthcare providers during surgery are implanting an electronic device that aids in making speech sound more normal.

Tracheoesophageal puncture is another speech alternative after a total laryngectomy. Movement of air from the lungs through a puncture in the posterior wall of the trachea, into the esophagus, and out of the mouth makes sounds. A prosthesis is placed over the puncture site after it has healed. In some individuals, speech is possible by placing a finger over the tracheostomy opening after taking a breath.

Identification as a Laryngectomee

Identification as a laryngectomee is important. The individual must wear an identifying tag, such as a MedicAlert tag, so others will know that they breathe through a neck opening. This consideration is especially important if the client has not yet begun speech training. Remember, if the opening is plugged, the laryngectomee will die of asphyxiation.

Supportive Resources

Supportive resources, such as clubs and organizations for laryngectomees, are available in some communities. Members give each other encouragement and emotional support. They are often willing to visit new laryngectomees in hospitals, encouraging them to begin rehabilitation.

Water Dangers

Anyone who has a tracheostomy or a permanent laryngectomy tube must always be careful to prevent water from getting into the opening. This person must use great caution when showering. A snorkel device is available to fit over the laryngectomee's stoma to allow for swimming. Strenuous water sports are contraindicated.

> **NCLEX Alert**
>
> All clinical NCLEX questions require accurate observations and initiation of priority actions relating to the "ABCs" or airway, breathing, and circulation. Therefore, the respiratory status of the client must be recognized in each question. The correct nursing interventions must be appropriate and quick.

STUDENT SYNTHESIS

KEY POINTS

- The respiratory and cardiovascular systems are vital to the entire body's functioning because they transport oxygen to cells and wastes away from cells.
- Nursing observations of a client with a respiratory disorder are critical in determining the severity of respiratory distress, the immediacy of the situation, and the priority of care.
- Disorders of the respiratory system may be caused by infections (bacteria, virus, fungi), irritants (smoking, allergens, environmental chemicals), masses (cancerous tumors), or trauma.
- Respiratory disorders may be characterized by multiple clinical manifestations, such as cough, changes in respiratory pattern, and abnormal breath sounds.
- When hypoxia (lack of oxygen) occurs, subsequent changes in the neurologic and cardiovascular systems may develop.
- Key elements in the treatment of respiratory disorders include medications specific to the disease; oxygen administration; postural drainage; positioning; turning, coughing, and deep breathing; and breathing exercises.
- The goals of nursing management for persons with respiratory disorders are a patent (open) airway, effective breathing pattern, and improved gas exchange.

CRITICAL THINKING EXERCISES

1. Your client and their partner are discussing general health concerns with you during the client's checkup. The client mentions that their snoring has worsened and is causing problems between the couple. Which factors may contribute to snoring? Which measures might help the client and their partner?

2. You are asked to design a prevention program for junior high school students about the dangers of cigarette smoking. Which strategies would you use? How would you encourage these students not to smoke? Which measures would you use to encourage their families to support these children?

NCLEX-STYLE REVIEW QUESTIONS

1. The nurse is preparing a client for a bronchoscopy. Which nursing actions are essential prior to the procedure? Select all that apply.
   a. Administer an enema.
   b. Detail the complications that can occur.
   c. Give mouth care.
   d. Observe for any loose teeth.
   e. Explain the procedure.

2. A client has a positive tuberculin skin test. Which action by the nurse is appropriate?
   a. Administer another tuberculin skin test.
   b. Administer a tine test.
   c. Prepare the client for a chest x-ray.
   d. Prepare the client for a bronchoscopy.

3. The nurse is assisting a client with chest tubes to the bedside commode when the tube becomes disconnected and falls on the floor. Which is the priority action by the nurse?
   a. Reconnect the tubing.
   b. Double-clamp tube close to the chest wall.
   c. Allow the client to ambulate to the bathroom.
   d. Place the client in the supine position.

4. The nurse is preparing a client for abdominal surgery. Which action by the nurse can prevent postoperative atelectasis?
   a. Suction the client every 2 hr.
   b. Administer supplemental oxygen.
   c. Administer an inhaled bronchodilator.
   d. Instruct the client about the use of incentive spirometry.

5. The nurse is caring for a client in the clinic who is diagnosed with the common cold. Which education would the nurse reinforce to help alleviate symptoms?
   a. Take antibiotics as prescribed.
   b. Drink plenty of fluids.
   c. Increase activity level.
   d. Avoid contact with others for 2 weeks.

CHAPTER RESOURCES

Enhance your learning with additional resources on thePoint!

Student Resources related to this chapter can be found at thePoint.lww.com/Rosdahl12e.

Welcome Steps

Look at healthcare provider's orders.

Protocol for procedure.

Necessary equipment/supplies.

Wash hands using proper hand hygiene; put on gloves.

Explain the procedure and reassure the client.

Locate two identifiers to confirm correct client.

Comfortable and efficient position for nurse and client.

Obtain privacy.

Make sure to follow correct steps and body mechanics with good technique.

Ensure safety and observe deviations from normal.

End Steps

Ensure comfort and safety.

Note questions or concerns from client or nurse; note significant data.

Dispose of materials properly.

Disinfect the area and your hands.

Document and report the procedure and your findings.

IN PRACTICE

NURSING PROCEDURE 86-1 — Suctioning to Remove Secretions

Supplies and Equipment
Sterile, disposable suction tube
Gloves
Sterile suction machine in the room

Steps
Follow LPN WELCOME Steps and Then

1. Place the conscious client in semi-Fowler position. *Rationale:* This position prevents aspiration.

2. Perform hand hygiene and set up equipment, opening the sterile suction package. *Rationale: Proper hand hygiene helps to prevent the spread of infection; proper technique is necessary to maintain the sterility of the equipment.*

3. Put on sterile or clean gloves, as ordered. *Rationale: Using gloves helps prevent introducing pathogens into the client's respiratory tract.*

4. Wear eye protection when performing deep suctioning procedures. *Rationale: This action adheres to Standard Precautions.*

5. Pick up the sterile catheter and connect it to the suction tubing being held by your nondominant hand, which now becomes unsterile (sterile to clean = contaminated). *Rationale: The suction tubing is considered contaminated. After this is touched, that hand then is considered contaminated.*

6. Moisten the catheter with sterile saline. *Rationale: Moistening the catheter lubricates the catheter and helps to minimize trauma to the mucous membranes and increase the client's comfort. Check the suction machine's functioning.*

7. Gently insert the catheter through the client's nostril with the suction off. *Rationale: Both the catheter and the suctioning can irritate mucous membranes.*

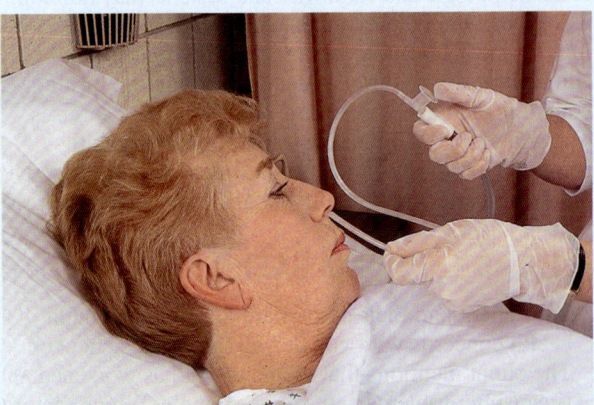

Insert catheter without applying suction. Here a "whistle-tip" catheter is left open to air as the catheter is inserted.

8. Insert the catheter down to the end of the trachea (stimulating the cough reflex); pull the catheter back a few millimeters to reduce irritation to the *carina* (the ridge at the lower end of the trachea that separates the openings of the two bronchi). Begin suctioning, for about 10–15 s. The entire process of entering, suctioning, and withdrawal should not exceed a total of 20 s. *Rationale: Suctioning stops oxygen inhalation and hypoxia may result. It is also very uncomfortable.*

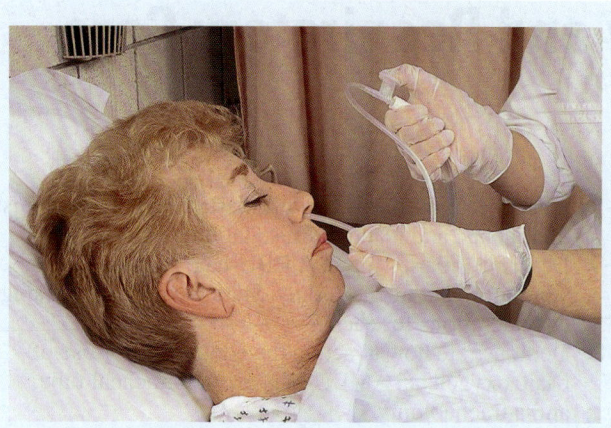

Suction the client by closing the system and creating a vacuum by putting a thumb over the opening as you pull out the catheter.

9. Withdraw the catheter fairly rapidly in a rotating motion while suctioning continues. *Rationale: Rotation helps clean all surfaces of the respiratory passageways.*

10. Repeat suctioning until no mucus returns. Give the client time to rest and breathe normally between suctionings. Give the client oxygen before and after passage of the catheter to relieve panic and reduce the risk of hypoxia. *Rationale: These actions help to prevent hypoxia.*

11. Flush the catheter with sterile normal saline between suctionings. Use suctioning pressures of 80–100 mm Hg for the adult client. *Rationale: Flushing cleans and clears the catheter and lubricates it for the next suctioning. A vacuum pressure in excess of 120 mm Hg causes trauma to the delicate respiratory mucosa; bleeding can result.*

Follow ENDDD Steps

87 Oxygen Therapy and Respiratory Care

Learning Objectives

1. State the three major goals of oxygen therapy.
2. Discuss four key safety factors and hazards in oxygen administration.
3. Describe the use of the pulse oximeter.
4. Identify five sources of oxygen and describe how they differ.
5. List eight key points of nursing observations of the client who is receiving oxygen.
6. Differentiate between low-flow and high-flow oxygen delivery systems. Describe the nursing interventions needed for the following types of oxygen delivery systems: simple mask, partial-rebreathing mask, nonrebreathing mask, Venturi mask, IPPB, aerosol mist treatments, and manual resuscitation bag.
7. Describe the uses for an AMBU-bag, mechanical ventilator, and tracheostomy. State the primary nursing considerations for each.
8. Demonstrate how to set up the equipment for use of basic oxygen, an AMBU-bag, an endotracheal tube, and a tracheotomy.
9. Discuss five nursing considerations for the client receiving oxygen on mechanical ventilation using an ET tube and using a tracheostomy.

Important Terminology

atelectasis
endotracheal (tube, ET tube)
hyperbaric (oxygenation)
hypoxemia
intubation
manual resuscitator, manual resuscitation bag
mechanical ventilator (respirator, breathing machine)
nasal cannula
pulse oximeter
simple mask
tracheostomy
Venturi mask
weaning

Acronyms

ABC
ABG
AMBU-bag
BVM
COPD
CPAP
ET, ET tube
HBO
IPPB
L/min
LPM
NRM
O_2 saturation, "O_2 sat"
PRM
psi
PSV
SIMV

Oxygen is a gaseous element that is essential to life. If a person is deprived of oxygen, death will occur in a matter of minutes. Normally, all people extract sufficient oxygen from the air they breathe. *Therapeutic* (supplemental) oxygen is necessary only when a client is unable to obtain sufficient oxygen for the body's needs because of a breathing or blood deficiency.

Excess oxygen is not helpful; in fact, it can be harmful. Therefore, oxygen is prescribed as a medication and is administered under controlled conditions. Oxygen is necessary for anything to burn, and increasing oxygen allows common flammable materials to burn faster and hotter. Thus, the more the oxygen in the air, the greater the danger for fire. Therefore, safety is of the utmost importance. This chapter discusses the client who is receiving supplemental oxygen, as well as the person whose breathing is supported by a *mechanical ventilator* (machine that forces air into the lungs) or who has a **tracheostomy** (artificial opening in the trachea through which a tube is inserted to aid a person in breathing).

OXYGEN PROVISION

Oxygen, an element abbreviated as O_2, makes up about 21% of the atmosphere, or as stated in healthcare, room air is 21% O_2. On occasion, a person's body needs to have more than the standard amount of O_2, and therefore the amount or concentration of oxygen the person inhales is increased. Usually higher concentrations of oxygen are needed temporarily, as during an illness. Oxygen may be administered to clients with pneumonia, carbon monoxide poisoning, severe asthma, heart failure, or myocardial infarction, or after chest or abdominal surgery. It provides comfort and allows the client to breathe more easily.

Goals of Oxygen Therapy

Increasing the concentration (or percentage) of oxygen the client inhales accomplishes three goals:

- Reverses **hypoxemia** (low oxygen concentration in the blood)
- Decreases the work of the respiratory system: If the client receives supplemental oxygen, the respiratory muscles do not work as hard to pump air in and out of the lungs and to maintain a sufficient blood oxygen supply.
- Decreases the heart's work in pumping blood: The heart tries to compensate for hypoxemia by increasing output; supplemental oxygen can ease the heart's load.

Hazards of Oxygen Therapy

As with all medications, oxygen must be administered safely. Oxygen given in high concentration over many days can result in oxygen toxicity, manifested as changes in lung tissue. In newborns, excess oxygen can cause vision difficulties and blindness. In some people, increased oxygen concentrations also affect their ventilatory drive control mechanism, which actually weakens the stimulus to breathe. Increasing the concentrations of O₂ for clients diagnosed with COPD can be fatal. Therefore, treat oxygen like a medication and administer it with the same care used in administering any medication.

A healthcare provider evaluates the client's need for oxygen and writes a specific order for oxygen therapy with the appropriate dosage. Administration of oxygen by mask or cannula is expressed in liters per minute (**LPM** or **L/min**); some devices control the specific oxygen concentration to be administered. When using mechanical ventilators, oxygen concentration can be controlled more easily.

Everyone, including the client, visitors, and others in the unit, must know and follow the necessary precautions when oxygen is administered. If oxygen comes in contact with any combustible material, even a small spark can ignite an explosive (flash) fire. Precautionary measures to be followed when providing oxygen are presented in In Practice: Nursing Care Guidelines 87-1.

Determination of Respiratory Status

When a client is receiving oxygen, the client's respiratory status must be continually monitored to ensure that treatment

---

IN PRACTICE
NURSING CARE GUIDELINES 87-1 | Providing Oxygen

- Explain about the dangers of lighting matches or smoking cigarettes, cigars, or pipes. Be sure the client has no matches, cigarettes, or smoking materials in the bedside table. *Rationale: Oxygen is highly combustible.*
- Make sure that warning signs are posted on the client's door and above the client's bed (even if the entire facility is nonsmoking). *Rationale: All persons coming in contact with the client need to be aware that oxygen is in use.*
- Use caution with all electrical devices, such as heating pads, electric blankets, or the ordinary call light. Many healthcare facilities provide call lights with grounding devices or give such clients tap bells instead. *Rationale: Oxygen is highly combustible.*
- Do not use oil on oxygen equipment. Be sure no traces of oil are on hands before adjusting an oxygen apparatus. *Rationale: Oil can ignite if exposed to oxygen.*
- Be aware of all potential sources of sparks, especially when administering oxygen by means of a containment device (e.g., a tent or isolette). *Note:* Items that appear innocuous (e.g., friction toys, electric razors) have caused explosive fires. *Rationale: Oxygen is highly combustible.*
- With all oxygen delivery systems, turn the oxygen on before applying the mask.
- Gain the client's cooperation. Inform the client of the therapeutic uses of oxygen before bringing equipment into the room. Reassure the client and family. *Rationale: They may be afraid that the use of oxygen is a sign of deteriorating condition. The client's need for oxygen will be reduced if they relax.*
- Instruct the client not to change the position of the mask, cannula, or any of the equipment after it is in place. *Rationale: Changing position could alter the amount of oxygen being delivered.*
- Maintain a constant oxygen concentration for the client to breathe; monitor equipment at regular intervals. *Rationale: Maintaining the appropriate flow rate enhances effectiveness of oxygen therapy.*
- Give pain medications, as needed; prevent chilling and try to ensure that the client gets needed rest. Be alert to cues about hunger and elimination. *Rationale: The client's physical comfort is important, and it decreases the demand for oxygen by the tissues.*
- Watch for respiratory depression or distress. *Rationale: Oxygen can depress the respiratory drive in some clients.*
- Encourage or assist the client to move about in bed. Many clients are reluctant to move because they are afraid of the oxygen apparatus. *Rationale: Movement helps to prevent hypostatic pneumonia or circulatory difficulties.*
- Make sure the tubing is patent at all times and that the equipment is working properly. *Rationale: To be effective, the client needs to receive the proper concentration of oxygen.*
- Monitor, document, and report the client's condition regularly. *Rationale: Regular observations and detection of potential or existing problems are necessary to determine the effectiveness of oxygen therapy.*
- Provide frequent mouth care. Make sure the oxygen contains proper humidification. *Rationale: Oxygen can be drying to mucous membranes.*
- Keep in mind that oxygen does not control every breathing difficulty, but where it is indicated, it can dramatically improve a client's condition. The person breathes more easily, the pulse rate drops, and an anxious attitude may change to a relaxed one.
- Discontinue oxygen use only after a healthcare provider has evaluated the client. Generally, you should not abruptly discontinue oxygen given in medium to high concentrations (>30%). Gradually decrease it in stages, and monitor the client's arterial blood gases or oxygen saturation level. *Rationale: These steps determine whether the client needs continued support.*
- Wear gloves any time there is a possibility of coming into contact with the client's respiratory secretions. *Rationale: Proper use of gloves helps prevent the spread of infection.*

IN PRACTICE
DATA GATHERING IN NURSING 87-1: Respiratory Status of a Client Who Is Receiving Oxygen

- Observe the client's respirations. Determine their rate, depth, and character.
- Document difficulty in breathing: abnormal movements, retractions, irregular breathing patterns, and abnormal breathing sounds.
- Auscultate lung sounds and document adventitious (abnormal) lung sounds.
- Determine the client's level of comfort. Pain may lead to hyper- or hypoventilation.
- Be aware of conditions such as anxiety or restlessness. Lack of oxygen may be the cause of these symptoms.
- Measure the client's pulse rate often. In respiratory distress, the pulse rate often rises.
- Monitor results of arterial blood gases (ABGs).
- Check pulse oximeter readings frequently.
- If indicated, monitor the client electronically (pulse, respiration, blood pressure, oxygen saturation).
- Observe for evidence of cyanosis.
- Monitor the oxygen delivery device for proper fit and usage. Check for signs of leakage.
- Document the settings of any equipment being used and your observations related to the client's condition.
- Closely observe the client whose oxygen has been discontinued. If the client becomes short of breath, shows signs of cyanosis, or has a markedly increased pulse rate, resume oxygen and call the healthcare provider at once.

has the desired effects (In Practice: Data Gathering in Nursing 87-1). If any signs of respiratory difficulty or distress occur, notify a healthcare provider immediately.

Use of the Pulse Oximeter

The **pulse oximeter** is a convenient monitor that measures the amount (percentage) of oxygen saturation in the blood. Commonly referred to as a "pulse ox," the probe (sensor) is attached to a fingertip, forehead, bridge of the nose, or an earlobe via specially designed clips or tape. The sensor detects changes in the amount of oxygen that is attached (or saturated) to hemoglobin by monitoring signals generated by the probe's beam of light. The result is an indication of oxygen saturation levels of hemoglobin by estimating blood pulsing (blood perfusion) through soft tissues at the probe site. This measurement is noninvasive (unlike drawing blood for arterial blood gas [ABG] analysis), and it can be used continuously or intermittently. The oximeter is read as percent oxygen saturation (O_2 sat), often notated as SpO_2 or SaO_2. Normal pulse oximetry levels range from 95%–100%. Values less than 90% need rapid intervention, usually supplemental oxygen. Values less than 85% generally need immediate intervention.

The pulse oximeter has limited accuracy. Readings are unreliable for a client who has moderate to severe anemia because the client's hemoglobin can be fully saturated with a resulting pulse oxygen percentage of more than 95%, but the readings do not take into account that the client may not be getting enough *total* oxygen to the tissues owing to an *overall* lack of hemoglobin. Clients with high carbon monoxide (CO) levels and those in cardiac arrest or in various types of shock do not have accurate readings. Inaccurate pulse oximetry readings are also possible with clients who have just received dyes, such as methylene blue for diagnostic testing purposes, or who are being treated for hypotension with vasoconstrictor medications. Readings must be interpreted with an awareness of these variables. Still, it is a useful adjunct to other evaluations of respiratory status for an acute care hospital, long-term care facility, and home settings.

> **NCLEX Alert**
>
> Multiple situations and options are possible on an NCLEX regarding the respiratory status of the client and/or the need for oxygen. Consider the client's overall clinical condition (e.g., dyspnea with anemia [Hgb and Hct]), versus pulse oximetry or ABGs. Remember all safety precautions that are needed with the use of oxygen, the teaching concepts of oxygen therapy, and home care use of oxygen.

Sources of Oxygen

Large healthcare facilities most frequently use the large bulk storage tank, with its convenient in-room piping system. They normally also have smaller oxygen tanks (cylinders) and oxygen strollers available to provide portable or emergency oxygen supplies. Some smaller facilities that use oxygen supplies less frequently have cylinders.

Wall Outlets

With bulk storage and in-room piping systems, a wall outlet is installed next to each bed. Wall outlets and adapters vary, not only by the type of gas they supply but also in terms of shape, color, and connection method. Be familiar with the wall outlet system used in the facility. Practice inserting the adapter into the outlet so that it can be done quickly and easily during an emergency. Use the following steps:

- Obtain a flowmeter and firmly and quickly push the adapter into the outlet.
- Give a gentle pull outward. *Rationale: This action ensures that the adapter is locked in place.*
- After the adapter is inserted, check to see that no oxygen leaks around the edges. If oxygen is escaping, remove and reinsert the adapter.
- To remove the adapter, push it in slightly, then firmly pull it out. Do not be startled by the loud popping sound—it is the release of pressure of the contained oxygen behind the wall source.

Oxygen Cylinders

Oxygen cylinders are available in many sizes, but are grouped into two main categories: large and small. A large cylinder is identifiable not only by its size but also by the presence of a metal cap screwed onto its top to protect the valve from damage. The valve itself also has an attached handle and threaded connection site. Large cylinders are generally used when high flow rates are essential or when a client requires oxygen for an extended period.

A small cylinder is identifiable by its rectangular valve with no handle and three holes on one side. Small cylinders are used when transporting clients or for short-term emergencies. Many clients also use small cylinders at home.

Careful handling and use of cylinders provide for safety. Because the gas contained within a cylinder is under extremely high pressure, the pressure must be reduced to a safe level before the cylinder is connected to a person. A regulator is a device that can reduce this pressure. A flowmeter and pressure gauge are attached to most regulators. The flowmeter is either round or similar to the flowmeter used with wall outlets. It indicates the oxygen flow to the client in LPM. The pressure gauge is round but usually smaller than the (round) flowmeter. It indicates the pressure in the cylinder in pounds per square inch (**psi**) of pressure.

Safety in using oxygen cylinders is vital. They are under high pressure. If a cylinder must be moved, secure it in a cylinder cart. If the top breaks off, the cylinder becomes "jet propelled." Turn off the valve when the cylinder is not in use. Keep all cylinders away from heat. If asked to administer oxygen or another gas using a cylinder, request instruction in oxygen administration, including the use and management of regulators.

Oxygen Strollers

Portable oxygen can also be provided by a liquid oxygen stroller, also nicknamed a "walker" or "companion" by manufacturers. The liquid oxygen portable unit consists of a thermos-type vessel in a shoulder bag or small carrying case. Liquid oxygen is denser than gaseous oxygen, so a portable stroller can carry more oxygen and yet be lighter and more compact than a steel gas cylinder. Liquid oxygen is allowed to evaporate within a warming coil into its gaseous state. It is then metered to the person through tubing connected to an oxygen delivery device. Liquid oxygen strollers are generally quite safe.

Remember the following guidelines when operating a portable liquid oxygen stroller:

- The tank must be kept upright at all times. **Rationale:** *If tipped, the tank will vent the oxygen contents quickly.*
- Strollers can be refilled from a larger stationary reservoir unit.
- A stroller is considered full or empty, depending on its relative weight.
- As liquid oxygen warms, it evaporates. Thus, strollers gradually empty by themselves.

For this reason, strollers cannot totally replace cylinders as sources of emergency portable oxygen.

Oxygen Concentrators

Oxygen concentrators are widely used in home and extended care settings. They compress room air and extract oxygen, providing concentrated oxygen flows in the range of 1–5 LPM. An oxygen concentrator is much safer and more convenient to use than an oxygen tank. It also does not need to be refilled with oxygen. However, it requires periodic maintenance by a technician and electricity to operate. There are several types of commercially available concentrators suitable for a variety of individual needs. Battery-powered concentrators are relatively lightweight and are often small enough to be carried like a handbag or tote bag. Others are on wheels and are portable in a home environment.

Hyperbaric Chamber

Some large facilities have a **hyperbaric** chamber, which simulates deep-sea diving by increasing atmospheric pressure. This method is called *hyperbaric oxygenation* (**HBO**) or *high-pressure oxygenation.* In the chamber, the person can take oxygen into the body in concentrations higher than is possible at normal atmospheric pressure. With the increased pressure, the client's hemoglobin and other blood components can carry more oxygen. HBO is used to treat air or gas embolism, carbon monoxide poisoning, and anaerobic infections (e.g., gas gangrene); administer some types of radiation therapy for cancer; and perform some surgeries (especially, heart surgery). It is also used to treat crush injuries or traumatic ischemias and enhance wound healing in necrotizing soft-tissue infections, compromised skin grafts and flaps, thermal burns, and chronic osteomyelitis.

THE CLIENT WHO IS HAVING DIFFICULTY BREATHING

When administering oxygen to an individual who is having difficulty breathing, the type of device that is used is critically important. The primary concern is delivery of the desired concentration (percentage) of oxygen. Monitoring the client's blood gases and detecting problems related to comfort, compliance, and safety are essential.

Oxygen delivery devices can be classified into two types: low-flow and high-flow devices. Low-flow devices do not provide exact oxygen concentrations; the client's breathing pattern influences the concentration of oxygen obtained. With high-flow oxygen devices, the oxygen percentage is constant (as long as the device is set up properly).

With most oxygen devices, humidification is provided. **Rationale:** *Oxygen from a tank or bulk system is absolutely dry and can be irritating to the respiratory mucosa.* A humidifier sends oxygen through small holes into water that creates bubbles and adds water molecules to the gas. The humidifier is connected to the threaded outlet at the bottom of the flowmeter or regulator. A small universal connector extends from the front or top of the humidifier for connection to the oxygen device. Oxygen delivery systems can be divided into *low-flow systems* that allow for oxygen percentages ranging from about 23% to nearly 100% and *high-flow systems* that reach an oxygen concentration of 100%.

Low-Flow Delivery Systems

Nasal Cannula

The **nasal cannula** (nasal prongs) is a device used to deliver small to moderate increases in oxygen concentration. The cannula has two short tubes that fit into the nostrils. This low-flow device can deliver 24%–40% oxygen at flow rates of 1–6 LPM. Humidification should be provided with flow rates greater than 4 LPM. Most people prefer cannulas because they are less confining and do not interfere with eating or talking (In Practice: Nursing Procedure 87-1).

> **Nursing Alert** Use cannulas with caution for clients who have irregular breathing patterns.
> *Rationale: The percentage of oxygen that reaches the lungs depends on the rate and depth of respirations.*

Simple Mask

The **simple mask** is a transparent mask with a simple nipple adapter. It fits over the client's nose, mouth, and chin. It is a low-flow device that provides an oxygen concentration of 35%–50%, with a flow of 6–10 LPM (In Practice: Nursing Procedure 87-2).

> **Key Concept**
>
> A healthcare facility may stock only one type of multipurpose mask, which is adapted according to specific needs of the client. A three-in-one mask setup can be established to become a simple mask, a partial-rebreathing mask, or a nonrebreathing mask. Therefore, it is important that the nurse be aware of exactly what type of oxygen delivery system is being utilized. Always check and document your client's type of oxygen delivery system and the flow (LPM), and check the flow against the healthcare provider's written orders.

> **Nursing Alert** The simple mask requires a minimum oxygen flow rate of 6 LPM to flush expired carbon dioxide from the mask so that the client does not rebreathe it.

Partial-Rebreathing Mask

The *partial-rebreathing mask* (**PRM**) is a low-flow device that can be identified by the presence of a bag and the absence of valves (Fig. 87-1A). This device can achieve oxygen concentrations between 60% and 90%, with a suggested flow rate of between 8 and 11 LPM. The bag must remain inflated during inspiration and expiration, with special attention given to ensure that the bag does not collapse during inhalation (In Practice: Nursing Procedure 87-3).

> **Key Concept**
>
> The PRM is never run at a specific oxygen flow rate; rather, it is run at whatever flow rate is necessary to keep the bag at least one-third inflated. *Rationale: The correct flow rate prevents the client from rebreathing their own carbon dioxide. However, a minimum flow rate of 6 LPM is required with this mask.*

Nonrebreathing Mask

The *nonrebreathing mask* (**NRM**) can be distinguished from the PRM by the presence of valves on the outside of the mask, as well as valves between the mask and bag (Fig. 87-1B). The NRM can provide oxygen in the 60%–80% range at a suggested flow rate of 12 LPM. As with the PRM, the NRM is never run at a specified flow rate. The bag of the NRM must also remain at least one-third inflated.

To use the NRM, follow the same procedures as for the PRM. Continuous observation of the client's respirations and proper bag deflation are essential. Cardiac monitoring with alarms is strongly recommended. Because the NRM produces extremely high oxygen concentrations, oxygen toxicity may occur in as little as 72 hr. Never leave the person who is wearing an NRM alone. Because of inherent dangers with this mask, some facilities may not permit use of NRMs.

> **Key Concept**
>
> Both the partial-rebreathing mask and the nonrebreathing mask can deliver high concentrations of oxygen; however, they are both classified as low-flow system oxygen administration devices because it is difficult to get the mask to fit tightly enough to ensure 100% oxygen delivery.

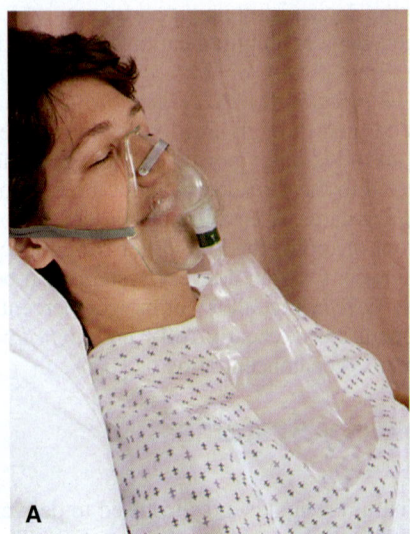
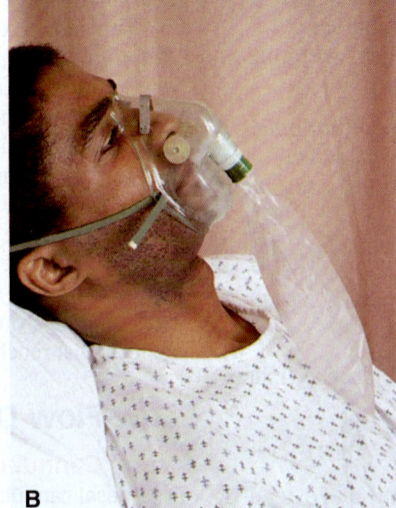
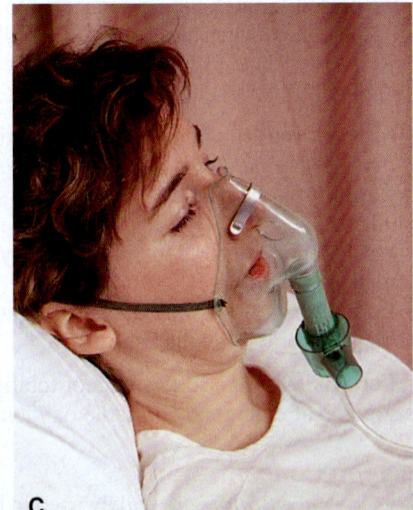

A B C

Figure 87-1 Types of oxygen masks. **A.** Partial-rebreathing mask. **B.** Nonrebreathing mask. **C.** Venturi mask. (Photos © Ken Kasper.)

> **Nursing Alert** The NRM is used only in an intensive care unit or in one-to-one client care situations. *Rationale: Insufficient or interrupted oxygen flow will seal the mask against the person's face, potentially suffocating them. The client needs constant monitoring.*

High-Flow Delivery Systems

Venturi Mask

Of all the facial devices, the high-flow **Venturi mask** provides the most reliable and consistent oxygen enrichment. This mask can be identified by the presence of a hard plastic adapter, with large windows on the adapter's sides (Fig. 87-1C). Because the Venturi mask has the ability to provide consistent, low levels of supplemental oxygen, it is often used for a client with chronic obstructive pulmonary disease (**COPD**).

> **Key Concept**
> High oxygen levels in clients with COPD can decrease the client's hypoxic drive. For some clients, too much oxygen can lead to respiratory arrest.

Venturi masks offer specific oxygen concentrations ranging from 24%–50% that match specific adapters for flow rates of 4, 6, or 8 LPM. Exact concentrations vary with manufacturers, and the flow rate adapters are often color coded. By drawing room air in through its windows, the Venturi mask mixes a low flow of gas (oxygen) with a high flow of room air. The resulting effect is a high flow of gas to the client with a specific oxygen concentration. Oxygen concentrations can be changed by changing adapters, window openings, or both. Always refer to the specific manufacturer's directions. The directions should specify the oxygen flowmeter setting to use for each desired oxygen percentage. Consult respiratory care personnel with any questions and concerns (In Practice: Nursing Procedure 87-4). Other high-flow systems include the aerosol mask, a tracheostomy collar, and a face tent.

> **Nursing Alert**
> - Do NOT use a humidifier with a Venturi mask. *Rationale: Significant back pressure may activate the safety pressure valve on the humidifier, causing it to burst. The large amount of room air that a Venturi mask uses will humidify the gas adequately.*
> - Ensure that the windows of the Venturi mask remain exposed to room air. Sheets or blankets must not cover the windows or the end of the adapter. *Rationale: Prevent occlusion of the oxygen flow, which would alter the desired oxygen concentration.*

Intermittent Positive Pressure Breathing

Intermittent positive pressure breathing (**IPPB**), also known as *intermittent positive pressure ventilation,* is a type of respiratory therapy for individuals who chronically hypoventilate and may need a ventilator. Hypoperfusion of the lungs can result in poor chest expansion and *atelectasis*. **Atelectasis** is a complete or partial collapse of a lung or a lobe of a lung due to the collapse of the alveoli (tiny air sacs). The amount of lung tissue involved in atelectasis is widely variable depending upon the cause of hypoperfusion. Atelectasis is common in individuals who do not cough and deep breathe after surgery. Cystic fibrosis, lung tumors, and chest injuries can be the primary cause of respiratory weakness and fluid buildup in the lungs, due to the inflammatory process, which lead to hypoperfusion, hypoxia, and alveoli collapse.

IPPB is used to expand the lungs and to deliver aerosol medications to individuals such as children or adults who have chronic lung conditions. IPPB uses pressure during the inspiratory phase of respiration, which helps the client breathe more deeply. The IPPB mechanical device forces room air or oxygen-rich air, combined with medications, deep into the client's airway. The client's lungs expand more completely. Secretions, such as thick mucus, become more liquid and are easier to expectorate or to remove by suctioning. IPPB can be set to deliver a specific volume or inhalation pressure as well time-limited ventilations. It may be used when less expensive or less invasive forms of respiratory therapy are not effective. This form of respiratory therapy is commonly used in individuals who have cystic fibrosis.

Aerosol Mist Treatment

Aerosol mist treatment refers to suspension of microscopic liquid particles in the air. It serves the following purposes:

- Adds humidity to certain oxygen delivery devices
- Hydrates thick sputum
- Administers bronchodilator medications to relax bronchioles narrowed by bronchospasm
- Administers anti-inflammatory or antiasthma medications
- Delivers antibiotics to the lungs to fight infection

The *mini-nebulizer* is a handheld apparatus commonly used for aerosol therapy. People with COPD and asthma commonly use mini-nebulizers to deliver inhaled medications. A mask or mouthpiece apparatus is attached to a chamber containing the prescribed solution. The chamber is attached via tubing to oxygen or a compressed air source. When used, a visible mist appears. The person inhales the medication in the form of mist.

THE CLIENT WHO IS UNABLE TO BREATHE

The process of breathing utilizes a considerable number of interrelated body functions, such as diaphragmatic muscular control, cardiopulmonary integrity, neurologic functioning, and useable caloric energy. A client may be unable to breathe for an extensive variety of reasons. Occasionally, a client is placed in an "induced coma," that is to say, placed on ventilator support to lessen the body's workload of breathing for itself. During times of artificial respiratory assistance, the individually is manually ventilated or "bagged." Manually ventilating a client uses assorted oxygen delivery systems and equipment. *Handheld resuscitation devices* with names such as an *AMBU-bag* or *VentiSure* are available. Manual *resuscitation devices* are available in sizes for an infant, child, and adults. These devices can deliver room air or be attached to supplemental oxygen via tubing.

As a student and a nurse, you are taught cardiopulmonary resuscitation (CPR) as a standard component of working in a clinical facility. Typically, healthcare providers are given training in the basic uses of handheld devices during their CPR training. Be prepared to initiate manual ventilation and be able to use manual airway resuscitation devices. Manual ventilation may also be required during airway tubing changes, before and after suctioning some clients, and during transport of a client who is in severe respiratory distress.

> **Nursing Alert** Every nurse must be able to initiate the **ABCs**—**A**irway, **B**reathing, and **C**irculation—as part of emergency CPR training. To achieve proficiency before an emergency occurs, airway and breathing techniques require knowledge of the use of the equipment and practice in a clinical laboratory. The cost to the client for poor technique is hypoxia, brain damage, and brain death.

AMBU-bag

The **AMBU-bag** is a proprietary name for a *bag valve mask* (**BVM**) device known generically as a **manual resuscitator** or **manual resuscitation bag** (Fig. 87-2). Other proprietary BVM brands are available, for example, the VentiSure. The bag has a nonrebreathing valve and holds about 1–1.5 L of air. It is a self-inflating, handheld device commonly used to provide positive pressure ventilation to individuals who need artificial ventilator support. The device can deliver high oxygen concentrations and provides more effective and sanitary resuscitation than the mouth-to-mouth method of air delivery during an emergency. The face mask of the AMBU-bag is first placed over the client's nose, followed by the mouth. Room air may be used. For more oxygenation, the bag can be connected to an oxygen source.

Resuscitation must be initiated at once or brain death will result within 4–6 min. The most important considerations are to ensure that the client's airway is *patent* (open) and to start treatment immediately. Children generally have a respiratory arrest before a cardiac arrest; therefore, if a child is the client, consider loss of airway (e.g., blockage due to a toy) or a sudden inflammation and blockage of the throat due to an upper respiratory disorder. When you first notice that a client is not breathing, immediately call for assistance and start CPR. Immediate assistance may be available by "calling a code" according to facility policy.

> **Nursing Alert** When you first notice that a client is not breathing, immediately call for assistance, then initiate chest compressions and respirations.

> **Nursing Alert** Stabilize, but do not hyperextend or turn, the neck of a person who has experienced possible neck or back injury. *Rationale: Doing so may cause further injury.*

Endotracheal Tubes

An **endotracheal** tube (**ET** or **ET tube**) is a flexible plastic tube used as a temporary device to maintain a patent airway during a process called **intubation** (Fig. 87-3). Specially trained personnel (e.g., emergency medical service providers, healthcare providers, respiratory technicians, nurses) use a metal *laryngoscope* to insert the ET into the trachea past the vocal cords. An ET is inserted for most surgeries

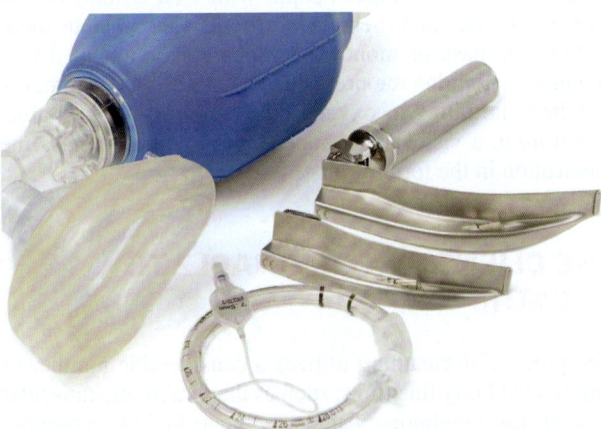

Figure 87-2 Bag, valve, mask device, laryngoscope, and endotracheal tube. A *bag valve mask device* (e.g., AMBU-bag) is used when the client cannot breathe without respiratory assistance. In the photo, note the adult-sized mask and the blue air reservoir of the AMBU-bag. The mask of the AMBU-bag can be used over the mouth and nose. If an endotracheal tube (ET) is in the client's trachea, the mask is removed and the AMBU-bag is connected directly to the ET. The silver-colored laryngoscope, which is inserted into the oropharynx, assists placement during the insertion of the ET.

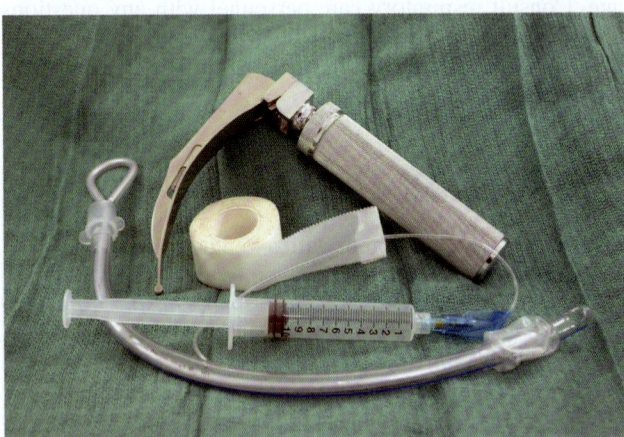

Figure 87-3 Laryngoscope and endotracheal tube. A laryngoscope is used during the insertion of an endotracheal tube (ET). Both endotracheal tubes and laryngoscope blades come in various sizes (e.g., child, small adult, adult). The ET tube in the photo has a guidewire already inserted. The ET is then ready for insertion alongside of the laryngoscope, which is in the client's oropharynx. When the ET has been verified for correct placement, its small cuff is inflated, which stabilizes the ET inserted inside the trachea. A special endotracheal guard (not shown) or tape holds the ET in place.

requiring general anesthesia, during emergency resuscitative procedures for cardiac or respiratory arrest, and for clients whose respiratory status is inadequate or is deteriorating, which occurs in respiratory situations such as acute severe asthma, also known as status asthmaticus.

There are strict protocols for intubation relative to choosing, sizing, and placing an ET. After placement, bilateral lung sounds are auscultated and, usually, a chest x-ray is obtained to verify proper placement. After correct placement is confirmed, the ET is secured in place. It is vital to check placement immediately on insertion because incorrect placement (e.g., in the esophagus) prohibits oxygenation and can promote gastric distention. Once the client is intubated, the ET can be connected to supplemental oxygen via a ventilator or the client can be manually ventilated using an AMBU-bag.

While the client is intubated, nursing care consists of providing oral care every 2 hr, monitoring respiratory status and placement of the ET (it can slip out of position), and repositioning the client to prevent hazards of immobility (e.g., pneumonia). More information about ETs is provided during CPR or advanced cardiovascular life support (ACLS) courses. Most acute care facilities require that employees take one or both of these courses.

Mechanical Ventilation

Mechanical ventilation, or artificial respirations via use of a machine, is used for individuals in a state of actual or pending respiratory failure. For some reason, the individual is unable to maintain adequate oxygenation or to breathe effectively alone. This individual needs support from a **mechanical ventilator**, also referred to as a **respirator** or *breathing machine*. A mechanical ventilator is a machine that forces supplemental oxygen, air, or both into the lungs. Mechanical ventilation is necessary when a client is unable to provide enough oxygen to the lungs or the client is unable to expire adequate amounts of carbon dioxide. A ventilator can be used when the client has severe dyspnea or cannot breathe because of an injury to the brain or spinal cord. An illness that interferes with or stops the effort to breathe is also an indication for respiratory assistance. A ventilator cannot fix a primary disease or injury, but it can allow for life support of the client until other therapies, such as medications, surgery, or healing of tissues, have had a chance to benefit the client. A ventilator is considered advanced life support, and for some individuals, the benefits of this type of therapy do not balance with the life-sustaining complications and consequences related to being placed on this type of machine. Some individuals may have refused or requested the use of advanced life-support mechanisms when they prepared and signed an advance directive.

The ventilator is connected to the client via an ET or a tracheostomy tube. The ventilator is used for the minimal amount of time possible. Some conditions make it difficult to *wean* the client off the mechanical support of ventilation. **Weaning** is a protocol, ordered by the healthcare providers, of slowly decreasing the individual's dependency on the machine so the ventilator may be removed. This process may take a few hours or several days to several weeks, or more. Some individuals may be permanently on a ventilator, as they have lost the physical mechanisms to breathe on their own, for example, in the case of high spinal cord injury. Complications of mechanical ventilation include infections (especially pneumonia), a pneumothorax (collapsed lung), and lung trauma.

The ventilator has different settings that are used for airway management and support. There are several types of machines, and some types of ventilators have multiple settings that can be used to meet a variety of clinical needs. The healthcare provider sets the parameters of the needed settings according to the client's respiratory needs. Often a respiratory therapist maintains or adjusts the settings per medical orders. In rehabilitation or some long-term care settings, the client can be maintained on a ventilator ("life support") for indefinite periods. The nurse, either a registered nurse (RN) or licensed practical nurse or licensed vocational nurse (LVN/LPN), has responsibility for overall management of the client, including, in many cases, the ventilator.

Nursing Considerations

Check for the existence of an advance directive to see if the client has made a choice about being placed on mechanical ventilation. Care for a client on a ventilator will include scrupulous infection control and continual monitoring of the tubing connecting the client to the machine. Any time the tube is disconnected, the client is at risk for hypoxia and brain damage. After about a week or two with an ET tube, a client may have a tracheostomy tube surgically inserted to replace the ET tube. The "trach" is used for clients who need longer periods of time connected to the machine. The client with a tracheostomy will need specific care, especially a newly inserted tube, because it has a fresh incision that is more prone to infection than a long-standing tracheostomy tube. See the tracheostomy discussion below and In Practice: Nursing Procedure 87-5 for a discussion of tracheostomy care. Remember that an ET or tracheostomy tube both disrupt functioning of the vocal cords. The client cannot speak or eat by mouth when an ET tube or tracheostomy tube is inserted, so nursing care must ensure other means of communication. The presence of the tube and its attachment to a ventilator is not overtly painful, but it can be quite uncomfortable. With some severe lung conditions, it is necessary to paralyze the breathing muscles by medications. Sedatives or analgesics are given to make the client more comfortable.

Negative Pressure Ventilator

The *negative pressure ventilator* (e.g., the iron lung) encloses all or part of the body. It may be used when normal muscle control has been lost or the client cannot breathe without artificial support. By lowering pressure around the chest, it causes the chest to expand and air to flow into the lungs. Because negative pressure ventilators are cumbersome and restrict access to the client, they are seldom used today. A small device of this type may be used in the home, however.

Positive Pressure Ventilator

The *positive pressure ventilator* pushes air into the lungs through a circuit that joins the machine and the client. Positive pressure ventilators may be operated in *volume* or *pressure* modes. Modes of operation are further classified as to whether they assist in or control breathing:

- *Volume ventilation:* Delivers a consistent, preset volume of air with each breath, ensuring adequate breathing.
- *Pressure ventilation:* Pushes air into the lungs until a preset pressure is achieved. (The pressure mode is not always as effective as the volume mode.)

- *Assisted-breath ventilation:* Helps support clients who are breathing on their own, but inadequately; this support may be necessary to avoid ventilatory failure or hypoxia.
- *Controlled-breath ventilation:* Breathes for the client, forcing a breath at set time intervals. (Controlled-breath ventilation prevents the person from controlling their own breathing.)

Care for the Client Receiving Mechanical Ventilation

A client is placed on a mechanical ventilator when they are unable to achieve adequate tissue oxygenation. Clients may require mechanical ventilation in acute situations, such as surgery, trauma, or drug overdose, and in certain disease processes. Some clients require chronic mechanical ventilation because of neuromuscular disease (e.g., spinal cord injury) or lung disease (e.g., emphysema). Most clients need ventilatory support for short periods and are withdrawn from it as their condition improves. Consult respiratory care staff for any questions about care or operation of a ventilator.

Assisting the Client on a Mechanical Ventilator

Assist the client who is on a ventilator to turn from side to side at least every 2 hr. *Rationale: Turning helps to improve lung function and to prevent immobility disorders, such as pressure wounds or thrombophlebitis.* Many of these clients are on special airflow beds. They may require suctioning of lung secretions that they are unable to mobilize. Carefully observe any secretions that the client expectorates or that are suctioned.

> **Nursing Alert** Immediately report any blood in a client's mucus.

Weaning the Client From the Ventilator

As the client's condition improves and they begin to breathe without assistance, the number of positive pressure breaths is gradually reduced. The person who has been on a ventilator for some time may need gradual removal (*weaning*) from it. Weaning can be done in several ways, depending on the situation. Some people have a difficult time breathing after having been on a ventilator. The problem may result from a true physical inability to breathe. However, it also may have an emotional basis (ventilator dependency and fear). These clients need emotional support and encouragement. If a client has required a high degree of ventilatory and oxygen support, they may show signs of acute respiratory distress syndrome (ARDS), which may make weaning more difficult (Chapter 86).

One strategy to facilitate weaning from the ventilator is *synchronized intermittent mandatory ventilation* (**SIMV**). SIMV gives the client a preset number of mechanical breaths at a certain volume. In addition, the client can take as many breaths at their own volume as desired. With progress, machine-controlled breaths are decreased in volume or rate. Thus, the client takes on more work of breathing gradually and progresses to breathing without mechanical assistance.

Another ventilatory mode is called *pressure support ventilation* (**PSV**). In PSV, constant pressure is applied as the person inspires, which lessens the inspiratory effort or work needed. *Continuous positive airway pressure* (**CPAP**) allows inspiratory and expiratory airway pressures to be maintained above atmospheric pressure. CPAP helps keep the client's lungs inflated and tends to improve lung function, although breathing is spontaneous.

> **Key Concept**
> Clients on ventilators are usually sedated, which will decrease their responsiveness and ability to communicate. Sedation may also depress respiratory effort. In addition, artificial airways prevent clients from speaking. Be sensitive to the needs of these clients. For clients on long-term ventilation, use various communication aids (e.g., chalk board, letter-pointing board, Magic Slate) and continue to talk to the clients, explaining everything that is being done.

Tracheostomy

Insertion of the Tracheostomy Tube

A *tracheostomy* tube, commonly called a "trach," may be inserted directly into a person's trachea as a lifesaving measure when there is sudden blockage of the mouth or throat (Fig. 87-4). A tracheostomy may also be a permanent breathing orifice (opening) for the person who has had the throat incision (a *tracheotomy*) or for anyone who requires

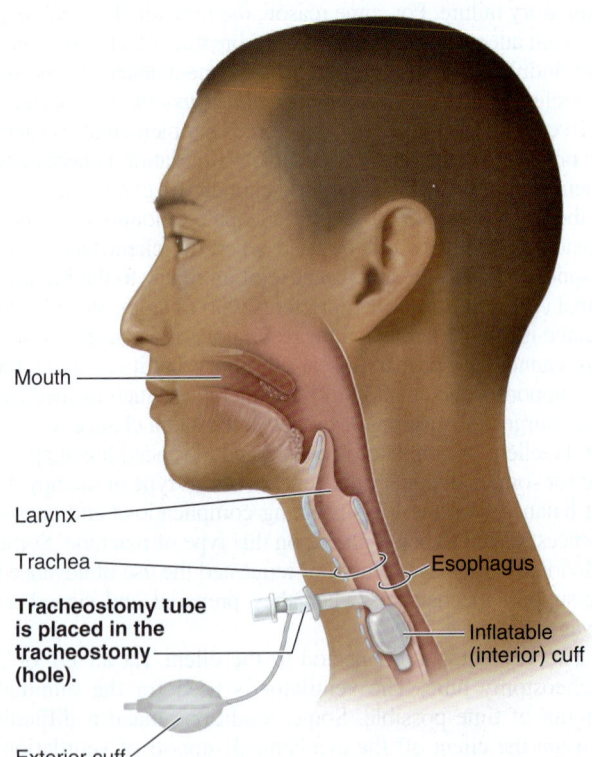

Figure 87-4 The diagram shows a tracheostomy tube in place. Note the *inflatable cuff* (a balloon) near the bottom of the tracheostomy tube, to stabilize and seal the trachea as well as to protect against air leakage and aspiration of gastric contents. It is directly connected to a smaller pilot balloon by a cuff inflation line, thus it is inflated as the interior cuff inflates. Also notice that the tracheostomy tube is in the trachea, which is anterior (in front of) the esophagus.

CHAPTER 87 Oxygen Therapy and Respiratory Care

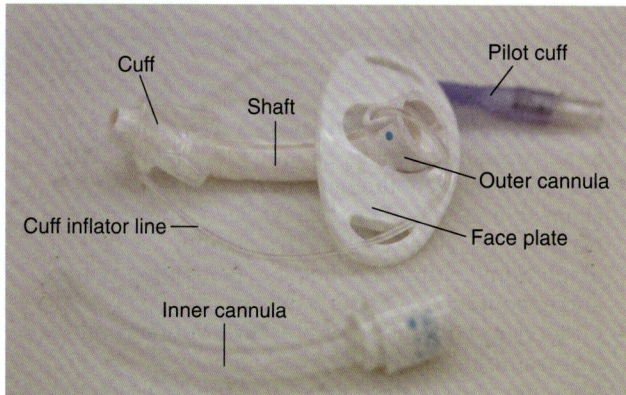

Figure 87-5 Parts of a tracheostomy tube. A typical tracheostomy tube has several parts. The tracheostomy tube has an *inner cannula*, which is inserted using an obturator (not shown). After being checked for placement, the *cuff* and its attached smaller *pilot cuff* (in the blue area) are inflated via the *cuff inflator line*. The inner cannula (bottom of photo) is removed once the outer cannula is inserted in the trachea. The oval white faceplate rests against the neck. Small cloth ties are threaded into the holes on either side of the faceplate and are tied together at the side (not the back) of the neck.

long-term mechanical ventilation. Nurses in an intensive care unit or emergency department may be asked to assist healthcare providers with the tracheostomy procedure (In Practice: Nursing Procedure 87-5). Most often, an endotracheal airway is inserted first and the person is transported to the operating room for the sterile tracheostomy procedure. There are occasions when the upper airway is blocked or swollen as with epiglottitis, and an ET tube insertion is not physically possible, thus a tracheostomy is a surgical emergency. When a tracheostomy is no longer needed, the tube is removed and the hole is allowed to close with or without surgical intervention.

The tracheostomy tube has three parts: an outer tube (*outer cannula*), sometimes with a cuff (an inflatable attachment designed to occlude the space between the trachea walls and the tube for mechanical ventilation), an inner tube (*inner cannula*), and a solid round-ended obturator (*guide*) (Fig. 87-5). The healthcare provider inserts the obturator into the outer cannula. Next, the outer cannula and obturator are inserted, as one unit, into the client's tracheal opening. When the outer cannula is in place, the healthcare provider withdraws the obturator and replaces it with the inner cannula (tube), which is locked into position. Cloth tape attached to each side of the outer tube and tied behind the neck holds the apparatus firmly in position. A cuff is inflated with air. Supplemental oxygen is connected to the tracheostomy tube in acute care cases; persons with long-term tracheostomies may not need supplemental oxygen.

Care of the Tracheostomy Tube

If a client accidentally coughs out the cannula, a healthcare provider or nurse trained in the procedure must replace the cannula immediately. An extra tracheostomy set should remain in the client's room at all times, in case of emergency.

Keep all equipment for cleaning and caring for the tube at the client's bedside. Each facility has a specific routine for tracheostomy care. For the person with a temporary tracheostomy tube, a humidifier must artificially warm and moisten the air to be breathed. Humidified air can be provided by a tracheostomy collar or tracheostomy mask. *Rationale: In normal breathing, the action of the nose and throat warms and cleans the air. Humidification helps to prevent secretions from becoming dry and tenacious.* If a person has a permanent tracheostomy, the body gradually adjusts to room air and, generally, supplemental oxygen and humidification are not needed.

Suctioning should be done using a new catheter each time with strict sterile technique. Typically, sterile gloves and a sterile container for the solution are found in the suctioning kit. The client needs continued reassurance. *Rationale: Until they are accustomed to breathing through the tube, the client may be very apprehensive, easily upset by coughing, and concerned about being unable to communicate verbally.* Keep a call light within the client's reach at all times. *Rationale: This person cannot talk or call out for help.* Provide the client with some means of communicating (e.g., Magic Slate, talking board, white board [dry erase], or pad and pencil). Sometimes, a client can whisper into a stethoscope for the nurse to hear and understand them.

Monitor closely for signs of respiratory difficulty, and take immediate action if respiratory distress occurs. Suctioning may be needed (In Practice: Nursing Procedure 87-6). Follow the facility's protocols.

Home Care of the Mechanically Ventilated Client

Clients today are able to receive mechanical ventilation at home. Mechanical ventilation and the care of the client on a ventilator must be ordered by a healthcare provider. However, continuous monitoring and daily care in the home may be provided by the person, family members, or other caregivers. This care is provided in conjunction with the healthcare provider, RN, LVN/LPN, respiratory therapist, and other home healthcare team members, as necessary. The client and caregivers must be able to recognize abnormalities or problems so that prompt attention and intervention can be initiated. All healthcare team members involved with the client's care must be able to do the same, within the level of the individual's training. Be sure to include all aspects of care that are pertinent to this client in the nursing care plan (In Practice: Nursing Care Guidelines 87-2).

IN PRACTICE
NURSING CARE GUIDELINES 87-2: Nursing Care Priorities for the Client Receiving Mechanical Ventilation

- Maintain ventilator settings as ordered.
- Observe for endotracheal tube misplacement. Tape tube securely in place.
- Observe respiratory rate and depth regularly because increased work of breathing adds to fatigue.
- Observe chest motion and auscultate lung sounds.
- Inspect chest wall for symmetry of movement. Asymmetry may indicate pneumothorax or hemothorax.
- Monitor arterial blood gases (ABGs) test results and pulse oximeter readings.
- Determine level of consciousness, listlessness, or irritability because these signs may indicate hypoxia.
- Observe and document skin color and capillary refill to determine that there is adequate flow of oxygen to tissues.
- Ascertain the client's level of comfort by direct questioning and/or noting the client's body language. Pain may prevent them from coughing and deep breathing. Medicate for pain, as needed.
- Observe for obstruction. Suction, as needed, because there may be a mucous plug and inadequate ventilation.
- Monitor amount, consistency, and color of secretions.
- Turn and reposition client every 1–2 hr, which helps to perfuse and ventilate all lung lobes adequately.
- If allowed, elevate the head of the bed or have the client sit in a chair. Some specialized critical care beds can become "chairs." This position facilitates diaphragm contraction, helps prevent pneumonia, and encourages good airway exchange.
- Observe skin integrity for pressure wounds and use a pressure-relief mattress.
- Maintain muscle strength with range of motion exercises—this client is at high risk for developing contractures.
- Be aware of possible psychosocial alterations. Symptoms may include anxiety, depression, confusion, inability to communicate, isolation, and change in family dynamics.
- Ensure that an emergency manual resuscitation bag, extra tracheostomy tubes, 10-ml syringe, tracheostomy tape, dressing supplies, and normal saline are at the bedside.
- For home care, ensure that there is a list of emergency phone numbers for the healthcare provider, local hospital emergency department, mechanical ventilation equipment dealers, and family/other caregivers for the client.

STUDENT SYNTHESIS

KEY POINTS

- Oxygen deficits to the brain occur within a few minutes. Without oxygen, hypoxia initiates brain damage; brain death will happen in a matter of minutes.
- Administration of oxygen reverses hypoxemia, assists the capacity of the respiratory system, and decreases cardiac workload getting oxygenated blood to the cells.
- Therapeutic oxygen is like a medication. It requires a healthcare provider's prescription and has associated safety considerations that must be understood and followed.
- Oxygen supports combustion; care must be used when using oxygen because a fire can start and be explosive.
- Oxygen is administered to support breathing using several devices or methods: nasal cannula, simple mask, partial-rebreathing mask, nonrebreathing mask, Venturi mask, intermittent positive pressure breathing, and aerosol mist.
- Endotracheal tubes, AMBU-bags, ventilators, and tracheostomy tubes are devices that support the airway and provide assistance to the person who is in severe respiratory distress or who has lost the capacity to breathe independently.
- A tracheostomy can be temporary or permanent. Nursing care includes maintaining a patent airway, prevention of infection, and emotional support to the client who cannot speak or eat when a tracheostomy is in place.

CRITICAL THINKING EXERCISES

1. Client L.A. is in respiratory distress with wheezes, coughing, dyspnea, and cyanosis. They are receiving oxygen by nasal cannula. Design a client teaching plan pertaining to oxygen therapy for them. Which safety and teaching measures would you address with family and visitors?

2. Client P.L. needs a tracheostomy due to an injury to their neck in an auto accident. P.L.'s family asks if this is considered advance life support and if they will have it permanently. The family insists the client does not want to be "attached to a machine" and states that P.L. has an advance directive. Discuss the moral, legal, and ethical implications of inserting a tracheostomy in this situation. How would you describe the tracheostomy procedure to the client's family? What are your nursing responsibilities during the procedure?

NCLEX-STYLE REVIEW QUESTIONS

1. The nurse is applying an oxygen cannula to a client with pneumonia. Which information would the nurse be sure to include when reinforcing education about oxygen administration? Select all that apply.
   a. Use an electric razor instead of a straight razor around oxygen.
   b. Do not use oils around the oxygen, especially on hands.
   c. Avoid smoking around oxygen.
   d. Do not adjust the cannula after it is applied.
   e. Discontinue the oxygen if there is nasal dryness.

2. A client with chronic obstructive pulmonary disease (COPD) is admitted with an exacerbation of the disease and requires a low-level consistent oxygen concentration. Which method of oxygen delivery will the nurse apply?
   a. Partial-rebreathing mask
   b. Nonrebreather mask
   c. Venturi mask
   d. Nasal cannula

3. The nurse is caring for a client who is intubated and mechanically ventilated. Which is a priority nursing intervention?
   a. Provide oral care every 2 hr.
   b. Suction the client every hour.
   c. Apply petroleum jelly to the lips to prevent dryness.
   d. Deflate the cuff and reposition the tube.

4. The nurse applies oxygen at 2 L/min via nasal cannula as prescribed for a client with dyspnea and an oxygen saturation of 90%. Which is a priority nursing action after oxygen administration for this client?
   a. Adjust the amount of oxygen flow every 4 hr.
   b. Continually monitor the client's respiratory status.
   c. Remove the oxygen cannula when ambulating in the room.
   d. Maintain the client in the supine position.

5. The nurse is gathering data for several clients. When obtaining pulse oximetry readings, the nurse determines that this method is ineffective for which client?
   a. A client on oxygen via nonrebreather mask
   b. A client with pneumonia
   c. A client with chronic obstructive pulmonary disease (COPD)
   d. A client with severe anemia

CHAPTER RESOURCES

Enhance your learning with additional resources on thePoint!

Student Resources related to this chapter can be found at thePoint.lww.com/Rosdahl12e.

Welcome Steps

Look at healthcare provider's orders.

Protocol for procedure.

Necessary equipment/supplies.

Wash hands using proper hand hygiene; put on gloves.

Explain the procedure and reassure the client.

Locate two identifiers to confirm correct client.

Comfortable and efficient position for nurse and client.

Obtain privacy.

Make sure to follow correct steps and body mechanics with good technique.

Ensure safety and observe deviations from normal.

End Steps

Ensure comfort and safety.

Note questions or concerns from client or nurse; note significant data.

Dispose of materials properly.

Disinfect the area and your hands.

Document and report the procedure and your findings.

IN PRACTICE

NURSING PROCEDURE 87-1: Supplying Oxygen With the Nasal Cannula

Supplies and Equipment
Flowmeter
Oxygen source
Nasal cannula and tubing
Humidifier and sterile water (optional)
"Oxygen in Use" sign
Gloves

Steps
Follow LPN WELCOME Steps and Then

1. Prepare the oxygen equipment:
   a. Plug the flowmeter into the wall outlet or oxygen tank.
   b. Attach the humidifier to the flowmeter.
   c. Fill the humidifier with sterile water.
   d. Attach the cannula with the connecting tubing to the adapter on the humidifier. *Rationale: Humidification prevents drying of the nasal mucosa. The agency's policy will dictate whether low flow of oxygen (≤3 L) requires humidification.*

2. Adjust the flowmeter's setting to the ordered flow rate. Check that oxygen is flowing out of the prongs. The flow rate via the cannula should not exceed 6 L/min (LPM). *Rationale: Higher rates may cause excess drying of nasal mucosa.*

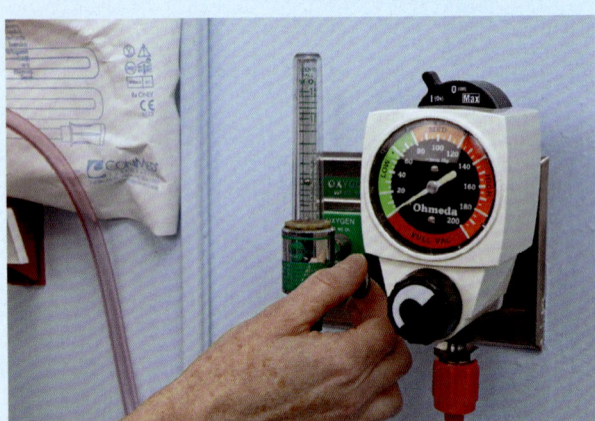

Regulating oxygen flow rate.

3. Insert the prongs into the client's nostrils. Adjust the tubing behind the client's ears, and slide the plastic adapter under the client's chin until they are comfortable. *Rationale: Proper positioning allows unobstructed oxygen flow and eases the client's respirations.*

CHAPTER 87 Oxygen Therapy and Respiratory Care

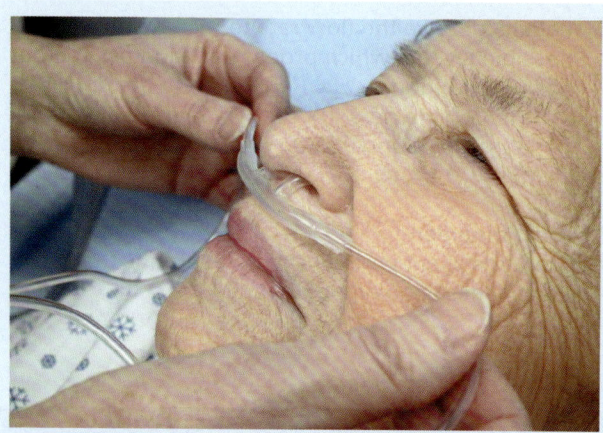

Applying the nasal cannula.

through the nose allows the client to inhale more oxygen that will move into the trachea and, thus, is less likely to be exhaled through the mouth.

5. Place "Oxygen in Use" sign at entry into the room. *Rationale: This sign reminds the client and visitors to use care.*

Follow ENDDD Step

Special Reminder
- Frequently check the oxygen setup, including the water level in the humidifier. Clean the cannula and examine the client's nares at least every 8 hr. (*Sterile water must be added when the level falls below the line on the humidification container. Nares may become dry and irritated and require the use of a water-soluble lubricant.*)

4. Encourage the client to breathe through the nose rather than the mouth. *Rationale: Breathing*

IN PRACTICE
NURSING PROCEDURE 87-2 — Using the Simple Mask

Supplies and Equipment
Oxygen mask
Source of oxygen
Gloves, if needed

Steps
Follow LPN WELCOME Steps and Then

1. Attach the humidifier to the threaded outlet of the flowmeter or regulator, and connect the tubing from the simple mask to the nipple outlet on the humidifier. *Rationale: Proper setup is necessary for proper functioning.*
2. Set the oxygen at the prescribed flow rate. *Rationale: The oxygen must be flowing before the mask is applied to the client.*
3. To apply the mask, guide the elastic strap over the top of the client's head. Bring the strap down to just below the client's ears. *Rationale: This position will hold the mask most firmly.*
4. Gently, but firmly, pull the strap extensions to center the mask on the client's face with a tight seal. *Rationale: The seal prevents leaks as much as possible.*

Follow ENDDD Steps

Special Reminder
- Check periodically for depressed respirations, increased pulse, and reddened areas under the straps. *Rationale: Be alert to signs that the oxygen may not be effective or that the client is experiencing further respiratory problems. The straps could place undue pressure on the underlying skin areas.*

IN PRACTICE
NURSING PROCEDURE 87-3 — Applying the Partial-Rebreathing Mask

Supplies and Equipment
Mask
Oxygen source
Gloves, if needed

Steps
Follow LPN WELCOME Steps and Then

1. Do not connect a humidifier unless specifically ordered to do so, which may be unnecessary and often is not recommended. *Rationale: The humidifier can restrict airflow so much that the device cannot keep up with the client's demand.*
2. Attach the mask to the oxygen source and the oxygen flow rate at 12–15 LPM. (*Attaching the mask and setting the flow rate must be done before applying the mask to the client to ensure that the equipment is functioning properly.*)
3. Place a finger inside the mask over the hole that leads out of the bag. *Rationale: Doing so will cause the bag to inflate with oxygen.*

4. Place the mask over the bridge of the client's nose. Bring the mask down over the client's chin. Guide the elastic strap over the client's head and secure it as for the simple mask. *Rationale: This position will hold the mask most firmly.*
5. Ask the client to take a few breaths, and observe to make sure that the bag deflates with each inspiration, but not to less than one-third full. *Rationale: If the bag does not inflate and deflate, it is either malfunctioning or incorrectly sealed.*
6. Reduce or raise the flow rate to the minimum possible level at which proper deflation occurs (but not <6 LPM). *Rationale: Regulation of the flow rate is based on the person's breathing, as related to the bag's deflation and inflation.*

Follow ENDDD Steps

Special Reminder
- Check the client periodically to determine the effectiveness of oxygen therapy.

IN PRACTICE
NURSING PROCEDURE 87-4 Applying the Venturi Mask

Supplies and Equipment
Mask
Oxygen source
Gloves, if indicated

Steps
Follow LPN WELCOME Steps and Then

1. Attach the wing nut and tailpiece to the flowmeter's threaded outlet. Then connect the tubing from the Venturi mask to the tailpiece. Attach the mask to the oxygen source. *Rationale: Properly setting up of the device ensures proper function.*
2. Attach the appropriate adapter or set the window openings, in accordance with the manufacturer's directions for the prescribed oxygen percentage. *Rationale: This ensures that the client will receive the prescribed amount of oxygen.*
3. Set the flowmeter to the manufacturer's recommended flow rate for the prescribed oxygen percentage. *Rationale: This ensures that the client receives the appropriate oxygen concentration.*
4. Place the mask over the bridge of the client's nose and then down onto the chin. Guide the elastic strap over the client's head and secure it as you would the simple mask. *Rationale: This action ensures a snug fit without leaks.*

Follow ENDDD Steps

Special Reminders
- Be sure the bed linens do not cover the Venturi adapter. *Rationale: The linens could plug the windows and disrupt the desired oxygen concentration.*
- Check periodically for depressed respirations, increased pulse, and reddened pressure areas under the straps. *Rationale: This ensures that the client does not experience further respiratory or skin integrity problems.*

IN PRACTICE
NURSING PROCEDURE 87-5 Assisting at a Tracheostomy

Supplies and Equipment
Sterile, disposable tracheostomy tray
Local anesthetic, such as procaine hydrochloride or lidocaine (Xylocaine)
Syringes and small-gauge needles
Sterile and clean gloves for healthcare provider and nurse
Strong light
Emergency breathing apparatus (e.g., manual resuscitation bag)
Source of oxygen
Source of suction

Steps
Follow LPN WELCOME Steps and Then

1. Hold the client's head during the procedure, if requested by the healthcare provider. If necessary, place a folded towel behind the client's neck to hyperextend it and to expose the surgical site. *Rationale: The site must be immobilized during the procedure.*
2. Provide strong emotional support. *Rationale: The client must lie very still throughout this frightening procedure. A lack of oxygen may cause extreme apprehension.*
3. Provide oxygen through an endotracheal tube while the tracheostomy is being done. This is most often done using a manual-breathing bag. *Rationale: The client needs to maintain an adequate supply of oxygen to their tissues.*

Follow ENDDD Steps

Special Reminder
- Monitor the site for swelling. Check to see if the client is able to breathe freely or has difficulty swallowing or is bleeding. *Rationale: These situations could impede respiration.*

CHAPTER 87 Oxygen Therapy and Respiratory Care

IN PRACTICE
NURSING PROCEDURE 87-6 Suctioning and Providing Tracheostomy Care

Supplies and Equipment
Tracheostomy suctioning kit containing the following sterile supplies:
Gloves
Suction catheter
Basins or containers
Sterile normal saline
Portable or wall suction apparatus
Sterile tracheostomy dressing
Twill tape or Velcro tracheostomy ties
Mild liquid soap and water
Sterile gauze pads
Disinfectant pad
Disposable inner cannula (optional)
Goggles and gown (optional)
Clean towel or plastic drape (optional)

Steps
Follow LPN WELCOME Steps and Then

1. Assist the conscious client to a semi- or high-Fowler position. Place the unconscious client on their side, facing the nurse. *Rationale: Upright positions promote drainage and prevent airway obstruction.*

2. Place a towel or drape across the client's chest. Put on a gown or goggles (optional). Turn on suction to the appropriate level. Put on gloves. *Rationale: Gown, goggles, and gloves act as barriers and protect the nurse from the client's secretions; the towel or drape protects the client.*

3. Prepare the suction equipment:
   a. Open the sterile tracheostomy suctioning kit and cleaning supplies on the bedside tray or table.
   b. Pick up the sterile container, open it, and pour sterile saline into it.
   c. Put on sterile gloves.
   d. Pick up the sterile suction catheter with your dominant hand.
   e. Use your nondominant hand to connect the wall or portable suction catheter tubing to the sterile suction catheter. *Rationale: Surgical asepsis decreases the potential for introducing organisms into the client's respiratory tract. The nondominant hand is unclean after it touches the nonsterile tubing.*

4. Dip the suction catheter into the basin with sterile saline. Use the thumb on your nondominant hand to occlude the suction port. *Rationale: Occluding the port applies suction and ensures that equipment is functioning.*

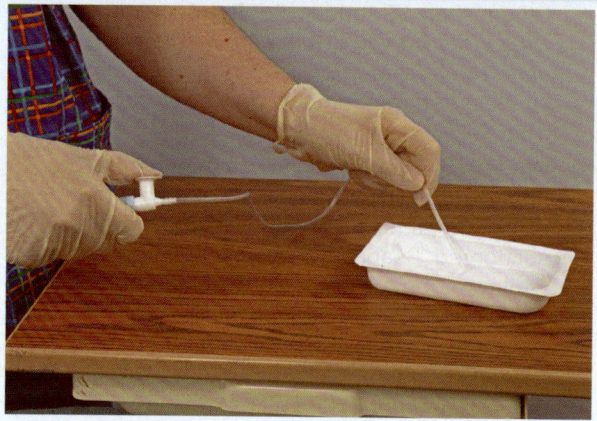
Dipping the suction catheter into the saline solution.

5. Preoxygenate the client with 100% oxygen for 30–60 s. Use a handheld resuscitation devise or, if able, ask client to take two to three deep breaths. *Rationale: Suctioning decreases oxygen supplies in the lungs. Preoxygenating increases the client's oxygen levels in the lungs, thus preventing hypoxia and unnecessary oxygen loss during the procedure.*

6. Remove the oxygen delivery system with the nondominant hand. *Rationale: Doing so facilitates tracheostomy tube suctioning while maintaining the sterility of the dominant hand.*

7. Use the dominant hand to insert the catheter into the tracheostomy; do not apply suction while inserting the catheter to prevent hypoxia. For deep suctioning, insert the suction catheter until you meet resistance and then withdraw the catheter 1 cm; for shallow suctioning, insert the catheter to a predetermined length, usually the length of the tracheostomy (plus the adapter if present). *Rationale: Applying suction while inserting the catheter may damage mucosa in the trachea and promote hypoxia.*

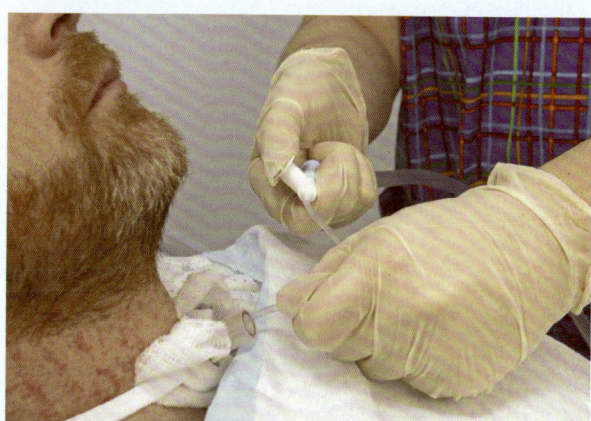
Inserting the suction catheter into the tracheostomy.

8. Occlude the suction port with the nondominant thumb while rotating and removing the catheter. Ensure that suctioning does not continue for longer than 15-s intervals. *Rationale: Rotating the catheter provides effective removal of secretions from the trachea. Limiting suctioning to 15-s intervals reduces the development of hypoxia.*

9. Dip the catheter into saline solution while applying the suction. Repeat the suctioning procedure, if necessary. Allow 1 min between suctioning. Reapply the oxygen delivery system while waiting to continue the procedure. *Rationale: Saline clears the catheter. Intervals between suctioning reduce development of hypoxia. Reapplying the oxygen system maintains the oxygen supply.*

10. Inspect the secretions:
    a. Normal sputum tends to be watery and white or translucent.
    b. Tenacious or thick secretions may indicate dehydration.
    c. Yellow, tan, or green-colored secretions may indicate infection.
    d. Brown-colored sputum may indicate prior bleeding.
    e. Red-colored sputum indicates active bleeding.

11. Before removing gloves, cleanse the cannula. If the inner cannula is disposable, remove it and replace it with a clean cannula. For the replaceable cannula:
    a. Unlock the cannula and carefully remove it.
    b. Hold it over the sterile basin.
    c. Rinse it with sterile saline.
    d. Gently replace the inner cannula and lock it in place. *Rationale: Rinsing with saline or replacing the cannula prevents accumulation of tracheal secretions.*

12. Cleanse around the tracheostomy stoma and under the tracheostomy tube faceplate with sterile cotton-tipped swabs dipped in normal saline. *Rationale: Normal saline aids in the removal of accumulated and encrusted secretions.*

13. Dry the area with a dry, sterile, gauze pad. *Rationale: Moisture provides a medium for growth of bacteria.*

14. Change the tracheostomy tube tape, if necessary:
    a. Have an assistant hold the tracheostomy tube in place with a sterile hand. If unassisted, leave the soiled tapes in place until new ones are inserted and secured. *Rationale: Keeping the tracheostomy tube secure while changing the tape prevents the client from accidentally coughing up the tube.*
    b. Pass the ends of the tape through the opening on the faceplate and bring them behind the client's neck to the other opening on the opposite side of the faceplate.
    c. Insert tape through the opening, pull securely, and tie or Velcro into place.
    d. If necessary, remove the soiled tape.

15. Place a sterile tracheostomy dressing under the faceplate. Tegaderm also may be applied under the gauze. *Rationale: Sterile dressing absorbs drainage.*

16. Reattach the oxygen delivery system over the tracheostomy tube. *Rationale: This provides for adequate oxygenation.*

Follow ENDDD Steps

Special Reminders
- When removing gloves, pull them over the suction catheter.
- Document the suctioning procedure, the nature and amount of secretions, the client's response, and observations of respiratory status following the procedure.

88 Digestive Disorders

Learning Objectives

1. Identify eight common liver function tests and two types of breath testing. State the rationale for using breath testing to determine gastrointestinal problems.
2. Describe the preparation that the client needs to complete for an upper and lower GI series using barium contrast medium.
3. Discuss nursing considerations for endoscopic procedures.
4. Describe nursing considerations for care of the client with a nasogastric and orogastric tube. State the names of four types of gastric tubes and differentiate the rationale for the use of each.
5. Define and differentiate between enteral tube feedings and TPN.
6. Differentiate between an ostomy bowel diversion and a continent bowel diversion.
7. In the nursing skills laboratory, demonstrate the care needed to change an ostomy. Discuss the nursing considerations for the types of bowel diversions.
8. Describe the nurse's role in caring for the client with stomatitis.
9. Discuss nursing considerations related to the care of both the client with GERD and the client with peptic ulcers.
10. Define and differentiate three nursing considerations related to the care of clients with IBS and IBD.
11. Describe risk factors for colorectal cancer.
12. Identify the types and causes of the major types of hepatitis.
13. Identify nursing concerns related to a client who is obese, anorexic, or bulimic.

Important Terminology

anastomosis
anoscope
ascites
bariatric surgery
cachexia
colostomy
dental caries
double-balloon enteroscopy
dumping syndrome
dyspepsia
endoscope
endoscopic ultrasonography
endoscopy
eructation
evisceration
fistula
gastrectomy
gastric bypass surgery
Helicobacter pylori (*H. pylori*)
hernia
ileostomy
insufflation
intussusception
melena
paralytic ileus
parenchymal cells
peritonitis
polypectomy
steatorrhea
stoma
tenesmus
video capsule endoscopy
volvulus

Acronyms

ALP
ALT (SGPT)
AST (SGOT)
EGD
ERCP
ET
EUS
GERD
GGT
HAV
HBV
HCV
HDV
HEV
IBD
IBS
LDH
LEP
LES
LFT
NG
PEG
PICC
PPI
TPN
UBT, C13-UBT, C14-UBT
VCE
WCON
WOCN

The major organs of digestion are those within the gastrointestinal (GI) tract, which begins with the mouth and ends with the anus. The accessory organs of digestion include the liver, gallbladder, and pancreas. The digestive system is responsible for digestion (mechanical and chemical) of food, absorption of nutrients and vitamins, and elimination of waste materials (Chapter 26).

Digestive disorders can be caused by structural malfunction, infection, inflammation, or disease. The healthcare provider who specializes in treating digestive disorders is called a *gastroenterologist*, although specialists in internal medicine also treat clients with GI conditions. GI tests and procedures may be done in an outpatient setting or a clinic called a GI laboratory. The *enterostomal therapist* (**ET**) also referred to as wound ostomy and continence nurse (**WOCN**) or wound care ostomy nurse (**WCON**) is a nurse who assists people with learning to care for surgically adapted openings, called ostomies, into the stomach (*gastrostomy*), intestine (*ileostomy*), or colon (*colostomy*).

DIAGNOSTIC TESTS

Laboratory Studies

Digestive disorders are diagnosed through laboratory studies, including blood tests, urine studies, and stool tests (In Practice: Data Gathering in Nursing 88-1 for additional considerations). Urine tests, such as urine bilirubin and urobilinogen, can estimate liver function. Urine amylase and lipase levels may also increase in pancreatitis.

Blood Tests

Blood studies are performed to assess, diagnose, and monitor the digestive system. The healthcare provider will start with generalized tests, such as a complete blood count (CBC), urinalysis (UA), and routine chemistries, to obtain basic data; more specialized tests, including carcinoembryonic antigen (CEA), serum cholesterol, and triglycerides, may then be ordered.

IN PRACTICE
DATA GATHERING IN NURSING 88-1 — Digestive Disorders

- Nutritional history
- Recent weight gain or loss
- Ability to purchase, prepare, and store food
- Ability to chew and swallow
- Any symptoms of digestive disorders
- Pattern of bowel elimination

Liver function tests (**LFT**) are valuable as indicators of liver function and for evaluating trends of abnormal liver processes. When the healthcare provider orders LFT, check your facility's laboratory manual to determine exactly which tests will be included. Some of the most commonly ordered LFT include the following:

- Albumin
- Total protein
- Alkaline phosphatase (**ALP**)
- Serum γ-glutamyl transpeptidase (**GGT**)
- Serum aminotransferase (**AST**), formerly serum glutamic oxaloacetic transaminase (**SGOT**)
- Serum alanine aminotransferase (**ALT**), formerly serum glutamate pyruvate transaminase (**SGPT**)
- Lactate dehydrogenase (**LDH**; isoenzyme differentiation may also be ordered)
- Cholesterol
- Triglyceride levels
- Prothrombin

Hepatitis profiles are done to identify the presence of antibodies or antigens for the hepatitis A, B, or C virus. Pancreatic enzyme tests, such as serum amylase and lipase, may be ordered to detect inflammation or disease of the pancreas or obstruction of surrounding ducts.

Breath Tests

Several types of diagnostic testing using breath analysis are available. The presence, absence, or concentration of certain substances, for example, hydrogen, can be a predictor of several types of GI disorders. Breath testing is noninvasive, accurate, and can confirm a diagnosis relatively quickly. A breath test may be considered for symptoms such as abdominal pain and bloating, cramping, gas, and diarrhea.

Common breath tests include *hydrogen and/or methane gas test, lactose intolerance testing, fructose intolerance testing,* and *bacterial overgrowth syndrome.* Anaerobic bacteria in the colon are capable of producing hydrogen and methane in the presence of unabsorbed foods. The basic mechanisms of breath testing depend on the process of fermentation of simple sugars and carbohydrates. If a problem exists with digestion or absorption of food in either the small intestine or the colon, large amounts of hydrogen can be produced. The hydrogen is absorbed into the blood that circulates in the blood vessels of the walls of the intestine or colon. This hydrogen-containing blood becomes part of the circulating blood, thus traveling to the lungs, where the hydrogen is released and exhaled in the client's breath where it can be collected and measured.

The *urea breath test* (**UBT**) is a test for the chemical composition resulting from the bacteria *Helicobacter pylori (H. Pylori)*. There are two types of UBT: **C13-UBT** does not use a radioactive isotope, but the **C14-UBT** does use a radioactive isotope. C14-UBT needs a clinical facility, usually a large hospital, which performs isotope testing. *H. pylori* are found in the mucosal lining of the stomach or duodenum. *H. pylori* can be a source of chronic inflammation, peptic ulcers, stomach atrophy, and gastric cancer. The *H. pylori* test can be done before treatment as a diagnostic aid and as a follow-up confirmation that the bacteria have been eliminated by therapeutic antibiotics. Eradication of the bacteria consists of 1 or 2 weeks of two antibiotics used simultaneously, combined with a proton pump inhibitor (PPI, which blocks acid production in the stomach).

Stool Tests

Stool tests are performed to detect the presence of pathogens, parasites, eggs (ova), blood, and fat. A culture and sensitivity study may be ordered for suspected pathogenic causes of severe diarrhea, such as *Salmonella, Shigella dysenteriae, Staphylococcus aureus,* or *Clostridium difficile.*

Fecal occult blood testing is used to test for *occult* (hidden or not visible) blood. The Hematest is the most inexpensive and simplest test used to detect occult blood in the stool; the client can perform the test at home, or the nurse or healthcare provider can perform the test in the office, clinic, or hospital. HemoQuant stool testing not only determines the presence of blood but also quantifies the amount (*fecal hemoglobin*). The HemoQuant can be done only in the laboratory. Thus, it requires more time and is less convenient than the Hematest. Each method of testing has its own manufacturer's instructions that must be followed to obtain accurate results (Chapter 52).

Radiographic Evaluations

Radiography (x-ray) is commonly ordered in addition to laboratory tests to diagnose and assess digestive disorders, including suspected abscesses, bowel obstructions and perforations, or intestinal paralysis (**paralytic ileus**). Angiography and arteriography may be done to evaluate vascular structures, and computed tomography (CT) scans are used to identify various abnormalities or tumors. Nuclear uptake scans using a radionuclide, such as technetium 99 (Tc-99m sulfide), will show size, structure, and abnormalities of the stomach, liver, and hepatobiliary system. Abdominal ultrasounds may be performed to visualize the liver, gallbladder and biliary system, pancreas, and abdomen. Ultrasound can identify gallstones or abdominal tumors. This test is becoming the preferred diagnostic tool, especially to rule out gallstones, pancreatic cysts, and cancerous tumors. No preparation, other than nothing by mouth (NPO) after midnight, is required for ultrasound.

Barium Studies

Two barium studies used to visualize the GI tract are the upper GI series and the lower GI series. Before the start of any procedure using barium, chest and/or abdominal ultrasounds and CT scans must be completed; barium may interfere with the visualization of the GI structures.

Upper GI Series

An *upper GI series*, often called a *barium swallow*, is conducted to examine the esophagus, stomach, and duodenum. A radiopaque or contrast material, such as barium or dye, is used to view the contours of the GI tract. Before the start of the procedure, the client will be given a drink containing barium, which is thick and chalky. Several flavored commercial preparations are available, such as diatrizoate meglumine and diatrizoate sodium solution (Gastrografin).

To examine structures under study, fluoroscopy, a type of x-ray examination, is used to visualize the contrast material. The outline of the esophagus, stomach, sphincters, and intestinal tract may be observed as the barium progresses. After 1–2 hr, x-ray films are taken of the small bowel. The rate at which the barium travels through the small intestine is significant in some diseases of the GI tract.

Lower GI Series

A *lower GI series*, or *barium enema*, is given to examine the contours of the lower bowel. The barium preparation is given rectally by enema. The client may worry about being able to retain the solution. Tell the client that they will have a chance to go to the bathroom immediately after the procedure. One more x-ray film will be taken after the client expels the solution.

Nursing Considerations

Client teaching is important before and after barium studies. The client must understand the appropriate dietary and bowel preparations and should know what the procedure entails.

> **Key Concept**
>
> The bowel preparation for a GI evaluation may be considered harsh for the client, but without a thorough evacuation of the intestines, the radiologist cannot visualize abnormal or malignant structures; the procedure may have to be canceled and repeated later starting with a new bowel preparation.

Generally, the entire GI tract is prepared, emptying it as thoroughly as possible, using liquid diets for several days before the procedure, and using enemas or cathartic drinks the day before and/or the morning of the procedure. After the procedure, check with the radiology department to make sure that the GI series has been completed before giving the client anything to eat or drink (In Practice: Nursing Care Guidelines 88-1).

A substance commonly used to cleanse the bowel for many procedures is often referred to as a product called GoLYTELY. It contains electrolytes that help maintain normal levels of these important chemicals, which can be washed out during a complete bowel evacuation. The client is required to drink several quarts of this mixture in divided doses the evening before the procedure. This is commonly called the "bowel prep." Tell the client to mix the solution beforehand, carefully following the package instructions. The solution is usually easiest to drink if it is chilled first. Caution the client to be close to a bathroom during the preparation process. With GoLYTELY or similar commercial products, the nurse should instruct the client to eat a light supper (some healthcare providers require clear liquids) in the evening and then to be NPO, except for the bowel prep, after supper. The client may brush the teeth but no water is allowed.

If the client is unable to drink the large amount of fluid required for GoLYTELY, an alternative is Fleet Phospho-soda or magnesium citrate (citrate of magnesia). This procedure involves drinking about two thirds of a glass of fluid in the evening and again in the morning. This preparation is considered a purgative because it forces evacuation of the bowel. It is contraindicated in clients with abdominal pain, heart disorders, impaired renal function, rectal or anal lesions, or in those who are pregnant. This preparation removes electrolytes and can cause dehydration.

Cholecystogram

A *cholecystogram* (gallbladder series) may be ordered to show the outline of the gallbladder and any existing gallstones. Before a cholecystogram, the client must prepare by:

- Eating a fat-free supper the night before the x-ray study.
- Taking a radiopaque dye by mouth. The liver excretes the dye into the bile, which then goes to the gallbladder. The healthcare provider will specify the time it is to be taken.
- Eating nothing for the next 12 hr (after taking the radiopaque dye), which allows time for the dye to concentrate in the gallbladder. The client may have water until bedtime, after which they are NPO.
- Stopping smoking and chewing gum, which cause premature emptying of the dye from the gallbladder.
- Administering an enema in the morning, if ordered.

If the client vomits before the test, postponement may be necessary because they may have lost some of the dye, rendering the test inaccurate. Provide a high-fat meal sometime after the initial x-ray study, if ordered. Another x-ray film may be obtained, as indicated, to show how well the gallbladder is emptying.

IN PRACTICE
NURSING CARE GUIDELINES 88-1: Providing Care Before and After Barium Studies

- Obtain a signed, informed consent. **Rationale:** An informed consent is required for any invasive procedure.
- Following the procedure, observe the client's stools. **Rationale:** Note if the client passes the barium, which will be white and chalky.
- Observe for constipation or signs of bowel obstruction, such as loss of bowel sounds and abdominal pain. Encourage the client to drink fluids. **Rationale:** Barium often causes uncomfortable constipation. Constipation can lead to other problems, such as impaction and infarction. Fluids will be lost owing to the bowel preparation and during the procedure. Fluids help the intestines pass the barium and stool.
- Give laxatives or stool softeners, as ordered. **Rationale:** Prevention and early treatment of constipation because of barium in the intestines will facilitate evacuation of the barium.

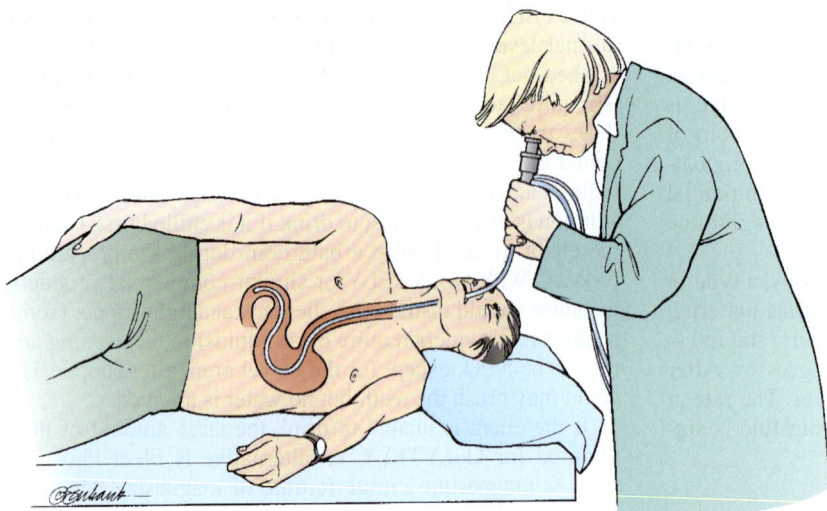

Figure 88-1 The flexible endoscope has been inserted through the mouth, down the esophagus, and into the stomach and duodenum to visualize these organs.

Endoscopic Procedures

Endoscopy is direct visualization of the body's interior through the intestinal tract using specialized instruments called **endoscopes** (Fig. 88-1). A capsule containing a camera for endoscopic visualization is also available (see video capsule endoscopy [VCE] below). Endoscopes are soft, flexible tubes containing specially designed fiberoptic strands connected to a light source. The endoscopic procedures can transmit light rays or sound waves to obtain an image of the GI tract. The healthcare provider manipulates the scope and can take pictures using the attached miniature video camera. The examination is usually performed in an endoscopy department by a trained endoscopist. This healthcare provider may be a gastroenterologist, surgeon, or internist. Routine endoscopic procedures do not involve making incisions, but tissue specimens may be obtained and polyps may be removed (*polypectomy*).

The introduction of video imaging allows viewing of internal tissue on a monitor or television-like screen. The healthcare provider, nurse, assistant, and even the client can see inside the intestinal tract. Excellent colored photography is possible. It can document a client's condition and healing process. Rapid advancement of endoscopic technology and its related equipment makes endoscopy a safe and effective diagnostic and treatment tool.

These procedures allow identification of growths, strictures, ulcers, or inflammatory disease. In addition to identification of abnormal conditions, endoscopy may be used to *biopsy* or *excise* (cut out) polyps or tumors; *dilate* (stretch) strictured areas; localize and stop active hemorrhaging or bleeding; and remove or crush biliary stones. In addition, palliative measures, such as stent and feeding tube placement, can ease the symptoms caused by a tumor obstructing the biliary tract and allow nutritional support to a debilitated client.

The endoscope will pass through the client's mouth or rectum. However, different types of fiberoptic scopes are used, depending on the part of the digestive tract to be examined. Because they are invasive, endoscopic procedures require informed consent. ERCP and colonoscopy are discussed below. Nursing interventions for other endoscopic procedures are similar.

The most common procedures for visualization of the GI tract include the following:

- *Esophagoscopy*—for direct visualization of the esophagus
- *Esophagogastroduodenoscopy* (**EGD**)—for direct visualization of the esophagus, stomach, and duodenum
- *Endoscopic retrograde cholangiopancreatography* (**ERCP**)—an extended version of the EGD plus direct visualization of the ducts of the pancreas and biliary tract structures
- *Gastroscopy*—for direct visualization of the stomach and duodenum
- *Colonoscopy*—for direct visualization of the large intestine (colon)
- *Sigmoidoscopy* or *flexible sigmoidoscopy*—for the direct visualization of the anus, rectum, and sigmoid colon
- **Endoscopic ultrasonography** (**EUS**) is similar to an endoscopy or colonoscopy because both procedures use long, thin, flexible tubes with a light and a camera at the distal end of the scope. However, the EUS uses sound waves to create visual images of the GI tract. The EUS can examine either the upper GI tract (the esophagus, stomach, and duodenum) or the lower GI tract (the colon, anus, and rectum). The pancreas and gallbladder can also be examined. During the procedure, the healthcare provider may obtain a small tissue specimen by using the procedure called a *fine needle aspiration*. A EUS is typically done using intravenous sedation and will need an escort to travel home after the procedure.
- **Video capsule endoscopy** (**VCE**) involves swallowing a capsule about the size of a large vitamin pill. The capsule has a miniature camera that takes multiple pictures of the small intestine, which are sent to a device (recorder) that the client wears. The VCE is disposable and remains inside the body for about 24–48 hr, after which it is passed out of the colon.
- **Double-balloon enteroscopy** is a procedure that examines the small intestine via an oral or an anal route. It is used to examine parts of the small intestine that cannot be seen clearly with other GI procedures. The device has double balloons that are inflated and deflated with air, which help the endoscope to advance far into the small intestine. Indicators for this procedure include individuals with altered GI anatomy, such as Roux-en-Y, a type of gastric

bypass surgery; individuals with GI bleeding, unexplained diarrhea, or Crohn disease; and if pancreatic or biliary disease is considered.

ERCP

Endoscopic retrograde cholangiopancreatography uses side-viewing flexible scopes to view the bile duct, pancreatic duct, and hepatic ducts to look for pancreatitis, tumors of the pancreas, stones of the common bile duct, and biliary tract disease. If the healthcare provider notices the presence of stones that block ducts, it is possible to enlarge the opening (*sphincterotomy*) to facilitate the passage of the stone. Stones in the area of the common bile duct can be removed mechanically with the endoscope or crushed using a lithotripter. Surgical intervention is indicated if passage of the stone is not accomplished by ERCP with sphincterotomy.

Before the test, the client may be instructed to avoid acetylsalicylic acid (Aspirin), ibuprofen (Motrin), or anticoagulants for 5–7 days because these medications prolong bleeding times and may cause excessive bleeding if tissue is removed during the procedure. A technique called *conscious sedation* is used for these procedures. The adult client is usually sedated with a short-acting intravenous (IV) analgesic, such as fentanyl (Sublimaze), or a sedative, such as midazolam. The medication allows introduction and manipulation of the endoscope, yet relaxes the client, who can respond and maintain vital functions.

A mouthpiece protects the client's mouth and the endoscope tube. Inform the client that the endoscope tube will not hinder normal breathing. The procedure takes 15 min–1 hr.

During the procedure, air is instilled into the stomach. The client will feel fullness and pressure, which is necessary to expand the stomach fully so that the entire interior surface can be visualized.

Nursing Considerations

As part of preparatory teaching, tell the client that another driver must be available to take them home after the procedure because of possible sustained effects of conscious sedation. Carry out any prescribed preparations for the client. Do not give any food or fluids until the client's gag reflex returns and they are fully aware.

> **Key Concept**
>
> Client teaching before any endoscopy is important. Clients need to know what to expect before, during, and after the procedure and what complications are possible. Be sure to document the content and client understanding of teaching sessions.

After oral endoscopy, observe the client closely for *dyspnea* (difficult breathing) because the passage of the tube may have irritated the throat or caused swelling. If the client has undergone a *dilatation* (stretching) procedure, observe for bleeding, pain, *dysphagia* (difficulty in swallowing), dyspnea, or a change in vital signs.

Because the dye is sequestered in the GI tract, diarrhea is a common side effect. Pancreatitis and hemorrhage are the most common complications. After an ERCP with sphincterotomy, closely monitor the client's pain intensity and effective response to analgesics. Routine vital signs, IV hydration, antibiotics, and follow-up laboratory work are important for the next 12–24 hr.

Colonoscopy

Colonoscopy can be used to follow-up on abnormal x-ray examinations. It can help identify growths and inflammatory disease of the lower GI tract. Small polyps and lesions may be *excised* (cut out) or *cauterized* (sealed off by heat or electric current). Growths may also be biopsied.

These excising and cauterizing techniques are possible because of the availability of various specialized tools for use with endoscopes. These tools are built so that they can be passed down the lumen of the fiberoptic scope.

Conscious sedation may be used in fiberoptic examinations of the lower GI tract. A colonoscopy is performed with the client lying on the back or left side (Fig. 88-2).

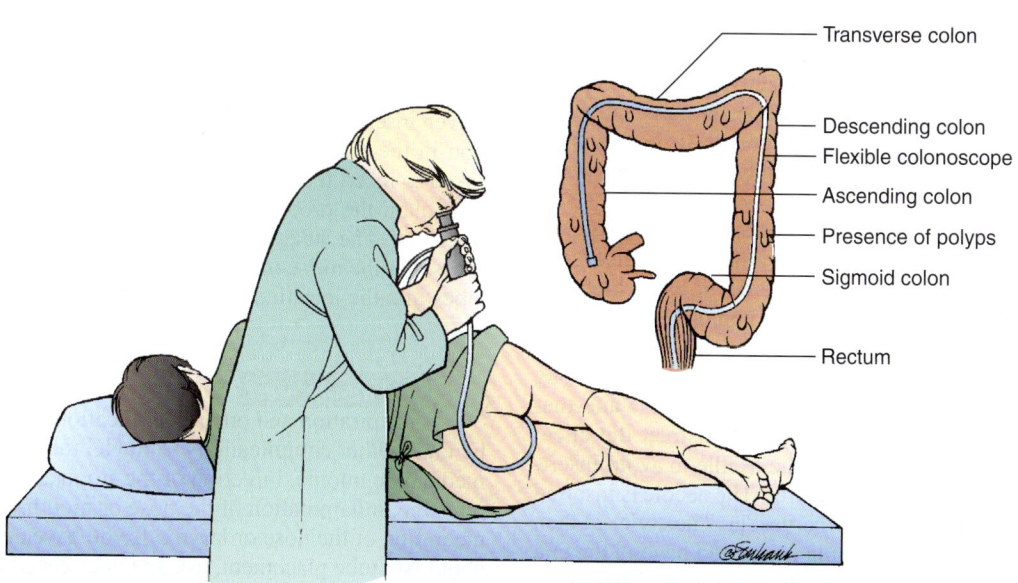

Figure 88-2 In colonoscopy, a flexible scope is passed through the rectum and sigmoid colon into the descending, transverse, and ascending colon.

The procedure takes 30 min–1 hr. The colonoscopy procedure is most uncomfortable when the scope "goes around the turns" in the colon. Most clients feel the air being instilled into the bowel (**insufflation**) and the endoscope tube being passed. Clients usually describe a mild cramping sensation or pressure. This sensation is mainly caused by the passage of the tube through the anal sphincter and the colon.

Nursing Considerations
Assist by encouraging the client to take a few deep breaths and to relax each time the scope passes through the colon, particularly around the curves in the large bowel. After the procedure, take and document vital signs.

Teach the client that lying on the right side after the test, with the knees bent and relaxed, will promote the passage of residual air in the colon. Measures to increase peristalsis and comfort include rolling from side to side to stimulate passage of air out of the colon, walking, and a warm bath. Be sensitive to the client's privacy at this time.

The first meal after the procedure should be light; the client should avoid highly concentrated fats. To avoid the feeling of being gaseous, the client should eliminate foods that cause gas production. Accumulated air in the lower GI tract may cause cramps. Instruct the client to observe stools for gross bleeding for 2–3 days after the procedure, particularly if polyps were removed or if biopsy was performed.

> **Nursing Alert** A rare complication of any endoscopy is perforation of the GI tract. Instruct the client and family to contact a healthcare provider if the client experiences fever, chills, bleeding, vomiting of blood, or severe abdominal pain.

COMMON MEDICAL AND SURGICAL TREATMENTS

Biopsy
Many endoscopic procedures of the lower bowel allow biopsy samples to be taken concurrently. The removed tissue is examined for the presence of cancer cells and other abnormalities. **Polypectomy** allows polyps to be removed and examined. In many cases, polyps are considered precancerous.

Liver biopsies are most often performed to verify suspected liver cancer or to detect other liver disorders. However, a biopsy is not done if the client has a bleeding tendency because of the possibility of hemorrhage; the liver is a highly vascular organ.

A small sample of liver tissue is obtained using a long needle with an inner, cutting cannula. The skin is anesthetized before the large needle is inserted. Instruct the client not to breathe during insertion of the needle to avoid inserting the needle into adjacent structures. The needle is inserted with the aid of a stylet inside the needle. The stylet is then withdrawn, and the inner cannula is inserted beyond the end of the needle and rotated to obtain a specimen. The specimen is then withdrawn. A sample may also be obtained by suction. The sample is examined microscopically. Locating a specific liver site or suspected tumor can require radiologic or ultrasound assistance to aid the healthcare provider in performing the liver biopsy.

Nursing Considerations
Explain the procedure and assist the client to maintain the proper position while the procedure is in progress. Wear gloves. This procedure is often uncomfortable. Stay with the client, and offer encouragement and support during the procedure.

Following a liver biopsy, position the client on the right side. Apply pressure to the biopsied site (usually the right side) for 4–6 hr, using a sandbag or folded bath blanket to help prevent bleeding.

Take vital signs every 15 min for 1 hr; every 30 min for 4 hr; and then hourly for 8 hr. Observe the client closely for signs of bleeding. Hemorrhage may be into the abdomen (watch for signs of shock) or from the puncture site.

Gastrointestinal Intubation
GI intubation involves the insertion of a tube through the nostrils, mouth, or abdominal wall (*gastrostomy* or *jejunostomy*) into the stomach, duodenum, or intestines. Gastrostomy and jejunostomy are used for long-term tube feedings. Tubes inserted through the nose into the stomach are called nasogastric (**NG**) tubes (Table 88-1). NG tubes are short and are used predominantly for suctioning stomach secretions; they may be used for short-term feedings and medication administration. The Levin tube, a single-lumen multipurpose plastic tube, is the most common NG tube (Fig. 88-3). A Salem sump tube is a double-lumen tube with a "pigtail"; this tube is often used for intermittent or continuous suction.

Tubes passed from the nostrils into the duodenum or jejunum are called *nasoenteric*. Their length can be either medium or long. Medium-length nasoenteric tubes (e.g., Dobbhoff) are generally used for feeding. Long, rubber nasoenteric tubes (e.g., Miller–Abbott and Cantor) are used for decompression, for aspiration, and to help unblock intestinal obstructions.

Nursing Considerations
Never insert an NG tube without previous careful instruction in the procedure. The nursing student generally is not asked to insert the tubes, but may be asked to assist. Be sure to explain the procedure to the client before beginning the insertion. The healthcare provider will insert nasoenteric tubes, but the nurse may need to assist with advancing these tubes into the intestines.

> **Nursing Alert** NG tube insertion can result in aspiration and other complications. Aspiration can be fatal. Other complications from NG tubes include otitis media, pneumonia, infection of the stomach or small intestine, inflammation of the nose or mouth, and ulceration of the nose or larynx. If you have any question about NG tube placement, ask an experienced nurse or healthcare provider for assistance. An x-ray examination may be required to determine tube placement.

CHAPTER 88 Digestive Disorders

TABLE 88-1 Common Gastrointestinal (GI) Suction Tubes[a]

TUBE TYPE	DESCRIPTION	PURPOSE	NURSING CONSIDERATIONS
Levin or Wangensteen	• Single lumen • Short tube (20–24 in.) • Multiple holes at distal tip (Fig. 88-3)	• Provides intermittent suction of gastric contents	• Irrigate frequently with small amounts of saline or air to keep patent.
Salem Sump	• Double lumen (two ports) • Short tube (20–24 in.) • Multiple holes at distal tip	• One port provides airflow. • Second port allows suction of gastric contents with continuous suction.	• Clear the air port with air to keep open and prevent distal tip from sucking against the wall of the stomach, which causes irritation.
Sengstaken-Blakemore	• Triple lumens, consisting of one channel and two balloons	• The channel provides irrigation and intermittent suction of gastric contents. • One balloon provides pressure on the cardiac sphincter area when inflated just inside the stomach. • Second balloon provides pressure along the wall of the esophagus to stop bleeding varices.	• Rarely utilized due to client discomfort, dangers of tube movement within the esophagus that may cause respiratory distress, and newer more effective treatments to eliminate esophageal hemorrhage • Nasotracheal suction is often needed because swallowing is impossible.

[a]Mercury-weighted tubes are no longer used for any internal body placement (because of the risk of mercury poisoning). Tungsten-weighted tubes may be used.

Providing Oral and Skin Care

Give soothing mouth rinses, and apply a lubricant to the client's lips and nostril. Apply a water-soluble jelly (e.g., K-Y Jelly) to the catheter where it touches the nostril because the client's nose and throat may become irritated and dry.

Do not use a humidifier because of bacteria in the air. If possible, the client should brush their own teeth; instruct the client to rinse the mouth well with mouthwash but not to swallow. Be sure to reposition the tape and give good skin care to prevent skin breakdown on the nose or cheek.

Verifying NG Tube Placement

At least two methods of testing for placement should be used. Evidence-based clinical practice has demonstrated that long-standing, traditional methods of verifying NG tube placement may not be currently acceptable or safe methods of verification. However, some of these practices may still be seen in use. The most common traditional practices are first to aspirate the tube, which should yield a small amount of watery-colored fluid (i.e., stomach contents), followed next by auscultation of air. About 15–20 mL of air is instilled at the same time as the nurse listens with a stethoscope placed approximately 3 in. (8 cm) below the sternum. If the tube is in the stomach, you should be able to hear the air enter, often with a "whooshing" sound. Checking by auscultation may be inaccurate because it is not always possible to differentiate between respiratory air sounds and stomach air sounds.

Evidence-based practice and research have shown other, often more accurate, methods of testing NG placement. Capnography can be used to detect carbon dioxide if the tube is in the respiratory tract. The pH of aspirates can *probably* detect the normally high acidity content of the stomach. There are exceptions to the pH testing method, which make pH testing misleading at times. *Providing that the radiograph is read correctly,* the most reliable method is x-ray visualization. In Practice Nursing Procedure 88-1 provides guidelines for checking the NG tube after insertion, and for irrigation.

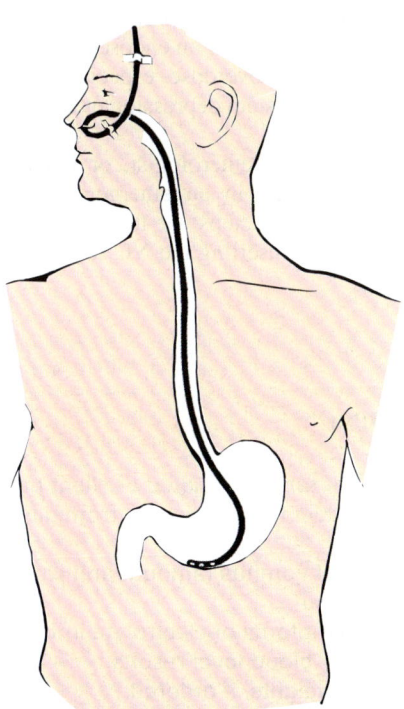

Figure 88-3 One type of nasogastric (NG) tube: Levin. It remains in place in the stomach. The tube is taped to the face and attached to suction. It is used to keep the stomach emptied or to obtain a specimen of stomach contents.

Removing the Tube

Temporarily clamp the tube before removal to make sure the client can tolerate its absence. Usually, the healthcare provider removes the long nasoenteric tubes. You may be instructed to remove shorter tubes. If a tube with any type of balloon is being used, be sure to remove any substance that keeps the balloons inflated.

Ask the client to hold their breath to close the epiglottis and remove the tube by simply pulling it out, slowly at first, then more rapidly when the client begins to cough. Crimp or pinch the tube as it exits to prevent leakage of the tube contents. Resistance is seldom encountered; however, do not remove the tube if you encounter any resistance. Generally, another attempt in an hour or so will be successful.

Place the tube in a towel after you have removed it and discard it in the appropriate receptacle. Be sure to remove any tape marks from the client's face. Provide mouth care and be alert for complaints of discomfort, distention, or nausea after tube removal. Do not give liquids or food without a healthcare provider's order.

Gastric Suction

Suction is used for periodic or continuous drainage in many GI conditions, such as the following:

- To obtain a specimen of stomach or intestinal contents for examination
- To treat intestinal obstruction
- To prevent and treat postoperative distention by removing gas and toxic fluid materials from the stomach or intestines
- To empty the stomach before emergency surgery or after poisoning
- To protect the suture line after GI surgery

The *proximal* (outer) end might have a clamp attached to keep it closed. To connect the NG tube to suction, a plastic connector might link it to a longer tube attached to an electric suction machine. Suction may be continuous or intermittent, depending on the type of tube or the needs of the client. NG suction is usually intermittent and low pressure unless the healthcare provider specifically orders otherwise.

Nursing Considerations

Note the amount of drainage of gastric fluid and consider it as part of output when calculating fluid intake and output (I&O). The plastic containers of gastric fluid are discarded generally every 24 hr or according to facility policy. Report vomiting at once; it often indicates a malfunction of the suction apparatus. If the apparatus appears to be functioning improperly, report it at once, and note the situation on the client's chart.

The NG tube will be connected to a mechanical intermittent suction machine, such as the Gomco suction. Be alert to the mechanical functioning of the machine. Document the amount of suction pressure used and what was suctioned (e.g., "NG tube attached to low intermittent suction at 30 mm Hg via Gomco; light green watery fluid noted in suction container"). The nurse must be aware of the continual output of fluid as well as its color, consistency, and amount (In Practice: Data Gathering in Nursing 88-2).

NG Tube Irrigation

A healthcare provider's order is needed for irrigating the NG tube. This order should include the type and amount of solution to use and the frequency of irrigation (sometimes it is "as needed" or PRN). The client's condition and different types of surgical procedures may require specific irrigating needs or techniques. In Practice: Nursing Procedure 88-1 details NG tube irrigation.

Gastric Lavage

Gastric lavage flushes the stomach and removes ingested substances through a tube. The procedures can help empty the stomach in preparation for an endoscopic examination or after poisoning or drug overdose, especially in clients who have central nervous system depression or an inadequate gag reflex.

A practitioner, gastroenterologist, or nurse most often performs gastric lavage in an emergency department or intensive care unit. The steps for this procedure are basically the same as for inserting the NG tube, except that the

---

IN PRACTICE
DATA GATHERING IN NURSING 88-2 — Checking Drainage in Gastric Suction

- Check the hookup of the bottle and its fluid level.
- Check the drainage for the following characteristics:
  - *Color:* Normal (greenish-yellow); more yellow after injury or surgery and becoming darker and brownish as bile secretion returns; maroon or red (with smell like blood) if blood is present.
  - *Odor:* Normal (acidic or sour); foul (indicates presence of infection); bloodlike (indicates gastric bleeding).
  - *Consistency:* Thin, thick, tenacious, presence of chunks or particles, strands of mucus.
  - Monitor fluid intake and output (I&O), including drainage:
- Amount (if tube is irrigated or client has oral fluids, deduct these amounts from gastric output).
- Presence of vomitus (amount and character) — add to output.
- Check for symptoms of electrolyte imbalance. Monitor daily blood level results.
- Check daily weights, if ordered.
- Monitor time, amount, and characteristics of stools, if any.
- Be observant for any other symptoms (including pain, cramping, nausea, edema, or jaundice).

lavage tube is larger and is often inserted through the mouth instead of the nose. Due to the size or type of the NG or orogastric device (e.g., an *Ewald tube*), special training may be needed to insert this tubing. The stomach is then irrigated or "washed" of its contents, which is known to the layperson as "pumping the stomach."

For some poisonings or drug overdoses, *activated charcoal* is added to the lavage solution to limit the amount of toxins in the stomach and bloodstream. Available as a prepared commercial powder, activated charcoal is diluted with water and instilled into the stomach. Charcoal absorbs poisons dissolved in the stomach and intestines, which limits the amount of toxins being transferred to the bloodstream. The normal amount of charcoal is 50–100 g for adults or about 5–10 times the amount of the suspected poison. The most beneficial effect occurs when charcoal is given as soon as possible after ingestion of the toxin. Substances that are not well absorbed by charcoal include toxic amounts of alcohol and most metals, for example, iron and lithium. Instead of charcoal, a specific antidote or isotonic polyethylene glycol solution may be instilled. After administering a specific solution, the tube can either be clamped for a few minutes and then allowed to drain via gravity, attached to intermittent suction, or removed.

Gastric lavage is controversial, even contraindicated, after ingestion of some poisons, hydrocarbons, and corrosive substances, for example, lye, petroleum distillates, ammonia, alkalis, and mineral acids. Lavage, in these circumstances, can cause the tube to perforate or cause trauma to the already-compromised esophagus. Aerosolized substances, in clients without a protected airway, can be inhaled into the trachea and lungs, causing aspiration pneumonia. The healthcare provider needs to consider benefits versus risks of gastric lavage in some circumstances. Contraindications for GI lavage include an unprotected airway, which increases the risk for aspiration, and GI hemorrhage or GI perforation due to disease or a recent surgery. Gastric lavage is controversial as a countermeasure for active bleeding from the upper GI tract. It may be contraindicated for the individual who refuses to cooperate during the insertion of the tube or during the lavage procedure because of the increased risk of complications such as aspiration or damage to the tissues.

Enteral Nutrition

Enteral nutrition, also known as *tube feedings*, assists the client to obtain nutritional intake when they are unable to obtain adequate calories, appropriate nutrients, solid foods, or liquids by mouth. For enteral tube feedings, it is essential that the client have a normally functioning GI tract. Good nutritional status greatly assists the client by providing shorter healing and recovery times. In some cases, enteral nutrition is life sustaining or lifesaving.

Long-term tube feeding is accomplished either via the nose by utilizing a small-bore, tungsten-weighted nasoenteric catheter (e.g., Dobbhoff) or by endoscope-guided tube placement through a "stab wound" in the stomach (*gastrostomy*). Direct insertion of tubes into the stomach can be done via gastric tubes, a percutaneous endoscopic gastrostomy (**PEG**). Figure 88-4 shows a typical dressing for a gastric tube. Give site care to maintain the skin surrounding a through-the-skin feeding tube.

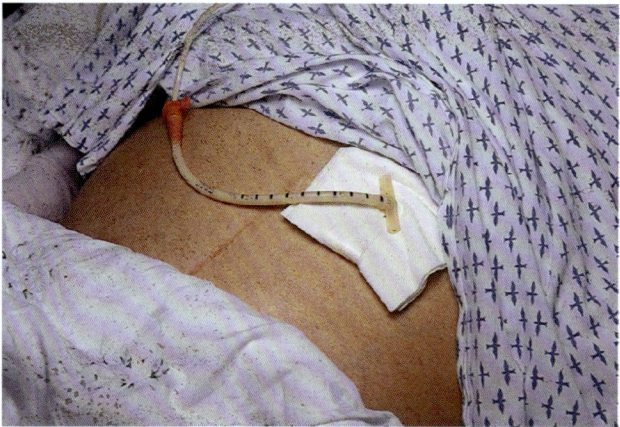

Figure 88-4 Protection at the gastrostomy site. A percutaneous endoscopic gastrostomy (PEG) tube may be protected by a dressing that allows access to the tube, but covers the exit site. Typically, the tube is stabilized with tape over the dressing.

Parenteral Nutrition

Parenteral nutrition involves direct IV administration of fluids and nutrients into the circulatory system. This method is referred to as parenteral nutrition because it does not access the digestive system (the enteral route). *Total parenteral nutrition* (**TPN**) is sometimes called *total parenteral alimentation*. *Hyperalimentation* is incorrect terminology because the amounts given are not excessive. If the stomach is functioning normally, it is safer and more appropriate to use enteral nutrition. However, parenteral nutrition may be necessary for many clients. TPN may provide total nutritional support, or it may be supplemental. TPN provides large quantities of fluids and nutrients, including proteins, fats, water, electrolytes, vitamins, and minerals. Each client will have a specifically prescribed TPN solution designed for their use.

> **Nursing Alert** TPN can provide all nutrients needed to sustain life, which is not true for traditional IV therapy. Never use the TPN line to administer medications or blood.

Various access devices are used as infusion devices for TPN. A *central line* involves surgical placement of a small catheter directly into a large blood vessel, often the superior vena cava; the catheter is then sutured in place. This central line allows long-term accessibility and unrestricted movement of the client when the line is not being used. Central lines may be temporary or semipermanent. The *Hickman catheter* is an example of a central line (Fig. 88-5A). It leaves a small-caliber tube exiting 10–14 in. from the upper chest. The *Port-A-Cath* system is accessible by a special needle and is placed just under the skin's surface, again on the upper chest. Both systems require periodic heparinization (injection of a dilute solution of IV heparin) to keep the blood from coagulating inside the lumen of the catheter.

Another central line is the *peripherally inserted central catheter* (**PICC**) line. A long catheter is inserted into a blood vessel, usually the subclavian vein (Fig. 88-5B). The catheter

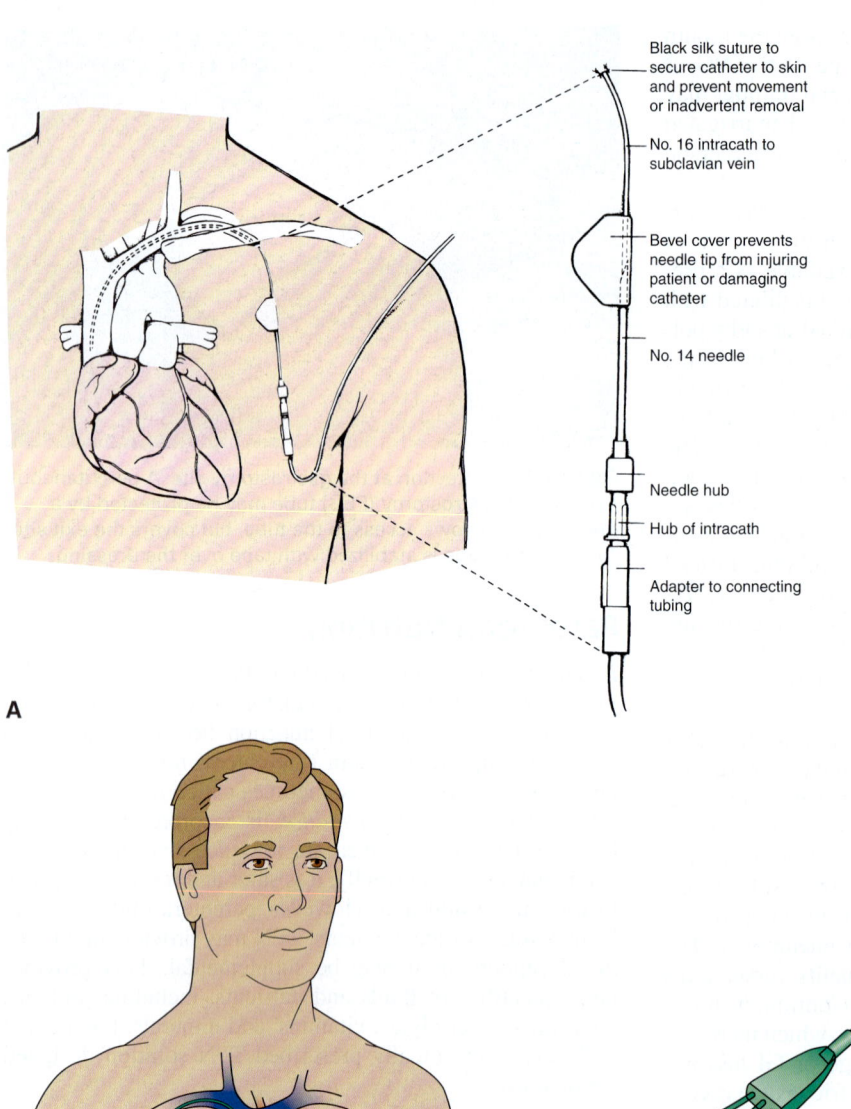

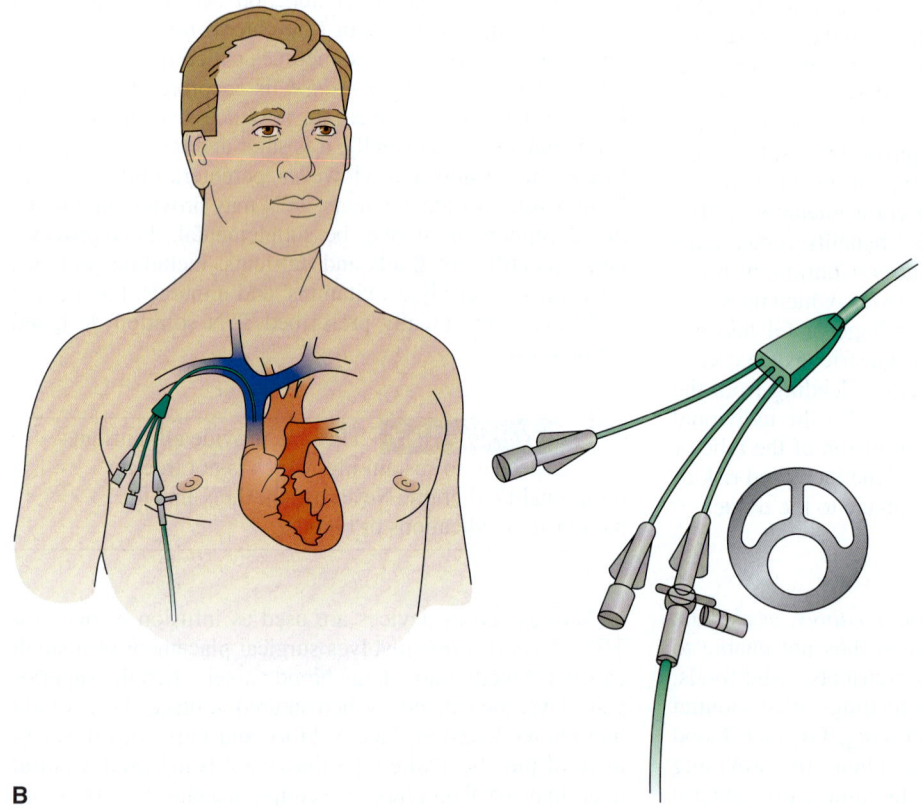

Figure 88-5 Total parenteral nutrition (TPN) catheters. **A.** Hickman catheter central line for TPN. The central line enters a large blood vessel, such as the subclavian vein, which has access to the superior vena cava. Monitor for bleeding at the site. Always use sterile dressing changes according to hospital policy. **B.** Subclavian triple-lumen catheter used for TPN and other adjunctive therapy. This catheter is threaded through the subclavian vein and placed in the vena cava (*left*). Each lumen is an avenue for solution administration; these are secured with Luer-Lok caps when not in use. Hemorrhage and contamination of the catheter or insertion site are major complications (*right*).

can be made of several substances, including plastic and Teflon. A trained healthcare provider inserts the catheter under strict sterile techniques and advances it into the superior vena cava.

Nursing Considerations

Several precautions are essential when caring for the client receiving TPN (In Practice: Data Gathering in Nursing 88-3). First, be sure to check your agency's procedure manual regarding TPN. Most healthcare facilities have specific protocols for administration of nutrients by TPN. In addition, facility policies often require specialized training to work with central lines and TPN solutions.

Follow strict sterile technique when changing bottles, tubing, filters, and dressings. Contamination can quickly

IN PRACTICE
DATA GATHERING IN NURSING 88-3 | The Client Receiving TPN

- Monitor vital signs frequently, especially temperature, for signs of infection.
- Auscultate lung sounds and monitor carefully for signs of pneumothorax, hemothorax, internal bleeding, or cardiovascular difficulties (especially during the first 24 hr).
- Monitor rate of infusion at least every hour. *Rationale: Ensure a constant rate of flow and prevent circulatory overload.*
- Monitor intake and output (I&O). *Rationale: Prevent edema or circulatory overload.*
- Check daily weights.
- Check for dislocation of the catheter.
- Change site dressing and inspect site according to agency protocols.
- Check for signs of bleeding.
- Check for patency of the centrally inserted intravenous catheter.
- Monitor electrolyte levels as well as blood and urine glucose levels.

---

disseminate throughout the client's body, leading to sepsis, because the catheter is placed directly into a large blood vessel. Dressings at the insertion site must be sterile. To prevent external hemorrhage from a disconnected central line, tape the catheter securely at the insertion site. To prevent dislodgment internally, use extreme care when working with the catheter or around the site. All connections must be secure. The client's hands may need to be restrained if pulling on the tube is a problem. Monitor and document the skin's integrity and the tube at least once each shift.

The infusion rate for TPN must be constant to prevent episodes of circulatory overload, hypoglycemia, or hyperglycemia. The flow rate is carefully controlled using a volumetric infusion pump. Discard any unused nutrient solution after 24 hr to reduce the chance of infection. Blood glucose monitoring may be ordered routinely because the solutions contain glucose as well as insulin. Clients may go home on TPN and manage lines there. Teach the client and family how to manage and become confident in the care of the lines. Document all teaching.

Gastric Surgery

Gastric surgery may be used as surgical intervention for gastric cancer, as treatment for ulcers with uncontrolled bleeding, or for *bariatric surgery* (types of weight-loss techniques). Box 88-1 reviews common gastric and bariatric surgeries.

Bariatric surgery, the collective name types of weight-loss surgery, is specifically performed to promote significant weight loss in clients who have previously tried and failed to lose weight without surgical methods. The goal of bariatric surgery is to restrict food intake by decreasing the size of the stomach and, in some cases, the length of the small intestine, thereby physically limiting the body's ability to absorb and use food intake. There are many types of weight-loss surgery; **gastric bypass surgery** is one of the most common types of bariatric surgery. Clients must be physically and psychologically prepared for the lifelong effects of these surgeries. The individual must be willing to commit to lifestyle changes, such as healthy eating, regular exercise, and the possibility of multiple minor and/or major side effects of the surgery. The obese person must be aware that they can lose weight only to regain it later if personal choices are not maintained.

These types of surgeries are not usually considered unless the candidate has several existing concerns, such as a body mass index (BMI) of 40 kg/m², sleep apnea, or is 80–100 lb overweight. The existing obesity may have created operative risks, such as cardiovascular disease, diabetes, dehiscence or evisceration, and increased risk for infections. The healthcare provider and the client must discuss the increased possibility of operative risks.

Postoperative Complications

Be aware of the possible development of anemia, such as pernicious anemia or iron-deficiency anemia (Chapter 82). Short-term or long-term electrolyte disturbances may also result from NG suction, malabsorption, anemia, diarrhea, and vitamin and mineral deficiencies. Pellagra, beri beri, and kwashiorkor may develop and lead to permanent nervous system damage.

Malnutrition is not uncommon after bariatric surgeries, especially if clients are not compliant with their new needs for vitamin and mineral supplements.

The suture line is delicate and may rupture and hemorrhage. Signs of shock will appear with massive hemorrhage. Examine the gastric drainage carefully for signs of bright-red or partially digested blood. The NG tube must operate properly to avoid distention.

Overeating or eating foods that are not recommended will usually cause immediate discomfort. This condition is called **dumping syndrome**. Foods most likely to cause the dumping syndrome are those high in carbohydrates and electrolytes, especially salt. Food containing monosodium glutamate is often particularly irritating. Symptoms include palpitations, sweating, faintness, excessive weakness, and diarrhea or vomiting. Signs of shock may also develop. Small, frequent, dry meals (without liquids) usually prevent this problem. Antispasmodic medications also help.

Dehiscence is separation of a surgical incision. **Evisceration** is protrusion of abdominal contents out of the body through the suture line. Both of these conditions are possible, although rare, complications, especially with abdominal surgery. Should either occur, contact a healthcare provider immediately. First aid consists of applying a large, sterile compress soaked in saline. Observe sterile technique. Never attempt to push the abdominal contents back into the abdomen.

> **Box 88-1** **Types of Gastric and Bariatric Surgeries**
>
> **GASTRIC SURGERIES**
>
> - *Total gastrectomy:* Removal of entire stomach. It may be used in advanced cancer of the stomach, when other treatments fail.
> - A *subtotal gastrectomy* is removal of two thirds to three fourths of the stomach, the pylorus, and the first part of the duodenum.
> - *Vagotomy:* Resection of vagus nerves; may be done to reduce the stimulus to create hydrochloric acid secretion in selected segments of the stomach. A vagotomy is usually done at the same time as gastric surgery because it limits the stomach's ability to produce secretions.
> - *Gastroduodenostomy (Billroth I):* A subtotal gastrectomy with removal of distal stomach; anastomosis to duodenum.
> - *Gastrojejunostomy (Billroth II):* A subtotal gastrectomy with removal of distal stomach and antrum; anastomosis to jejunum.
> - *Pyloroplasty:* Incision made into the pylorus to enlarge the outlet and relax the muscle; may be done with vagotomy to produce less gastric acid and promote gastric emptying.
>
> **BARIATRIC SURGERIES**
>
> - *Laparoscopic adjustable gastric banding (LAGB):* An inflatable, bracelet-like band is placed around the top of the stomach. When inflated, the band acts like a belt and separates the stomach into two parts. The top area or *pouch* is smaller and limits the amount of food that can be eaten. Weight loss is typically less than other, more intensive procedures. The band may need to be modified periodically. LAGB is considered a minimally invasive bariatric procedure and, unlike most bariatric surgeries, is generally adjustable and reversible.
> - *Roux-en-Y gastric bypass:* The most common method of gastric bypass surgery; it is not reversible. A smaller stomach or pouch is surgically cut from the existing stomach, forming a gastric pouch. The pouch is about the size of a walnut and can hold about an ounce of food. The pouch is connected directly to the jejunum (bypassing the rest of the stomach and the duodenum). Food goes directly from the pouch into the jejunum.
> - *Biliopancreatic diversion with duodenal switch:* This is similar to a Roux-en-Y gastric bypass. It is an effective, more complex procedure and is often limited to individuals with a BMI of >50 kg/m². A large portion of the stomach is removed (about 80%). The second part of the surgery is to bypass a large part of the intestine (duodenal switch and biliopancreatic diversion); the small intestine plus the bile and digestive juices are diverted. The amount the client can eat at one sitting is minimized and the absorption of nutrients from the intestine is reduced. Malnutrition and vitamin deficiencies are the major postoperative complications.
> - *Sleeve gastrectomy or vertical sleeve gastrectomy:* This surgery is the first part of the surgical procedure for the multipart process of the biliopancreatic diversion with duodenal switch. The stomach structure is changed to the shape of a banana or a tube, which restricts caloric intake. The second part of the biliopancreatic diversion is not needed for some individuals to achieve significant weight loss. (See biliopancreatic diversion above.)
> - *Vertical banded gastroplasty:* Also known as stomach stapling, the stomach is divided into two parts. The smaller stomach space limits the amount of food that can be eaten in one sitting. The upper pouch is small and empties into the lower pouch, that is, the rest of the stomach. Long-term weight loss is not as great as with other types of bariatric surgery.

Some clients, especially those who have had a vagotomy, are susceptible to diarrhea, which may become chronic. Treatment is symptomatic. Other complications specific to **gastrectomy** include a leaking **anastomosis** (the place where the two ends of the digestive system are joined together). Fever and abdominal distention may be the initial signs of problems. Also, obstruction may cause regurgitation. Long-term consequences of gastric surgeries include development of hernias, adhesions, and strictures.

Nursing Considerations

Preoperative nursing considerations for the client undergoing gastrectomy include the administration of antibiotics or sulfonamides, as ordered. They eliminate bacteria from the bowel and lessen the likelihood of postoperative infection.

Encourage the client to maintain adequate nutrition. The client may need additional vitamin and mineral supplements. TPN may be ordered to provide necessary nutrients. An NG tube may be ordered preoperatively for several days to suction drainage. The NG tube and TPN help to rest the stomach.

The stomach and colon must be empty when the client arrives in the operating room. Therefore, enemas may be ordered preoperatively. Explain to the client that after surgery they may need to follow a new dietary regimen that may require changes in meal schedules, nutrient consistency, and types of foods eaten. Allow time for therapeutic conversations to help the client to verbalize feelings and to relax as much as possible. A social worker or chaplain might help the client solve personal, financial, and family problems.

Postoperative nursing considerations include the following:

- Keep the client NPO, as ordered.
- Use NG suctioning for 2–3 days, as ordered. *Rationale: Keeps the operative area clean and eliminate pressure from accumulated fluids.*
- Keep the NG tube patent at all times. Irrigate the NG tube, as ordered (usually with approximately 20 mL normal saline). *Rationale: Irrigating the NG tube incorrectly could disrupt the suture line.*
- Observe NG drainage carefully. It may be tinged with bright-red blood at first. Report if the amount of red blood increases or remains bright red. *Rationale: Blood is a sign of hemorrhage.* The NG fluid should progress toward a normal greenish-yellow color.

- Keep the client in semi-Fowler position to facilitate drainage.
- Monitor chest tube drainage and chest tube suction. *Rationale: The chest may be opened during the surgery, necessitating the use of chest tubes and suction after surgery.*
- Provide routine postoperative care, including attention to mouth care and to early ambulation.
- Include deep breathing and incentive spirometer exercises. Encourage the client to cough gently. Support the incision with a small pillow.
- Monitor and control postsurgical pain. Give pain medications, as prescribed. The client may be reluctant to breathe deeply or cough because of incisional pain. Medications facilitate exercise, which decreases postoperative complications.
- Monitor dressings for excess drainage. Reinforce dressings, as needed. Usually, the surgeon observes the incision and does the first dressing change. Excess drainage indicates infection or a rupture of the suture line.
- When bowel sounds return to normal, an order will be given to clamp the NG tube for 6–8 hr. Monitor for potential complications, such as nausea, vomiting, abdominal pain, and decreased bowel sounds. If no complications occur, then the order may be given to remove the NG tube.
- Give clear liquids when bowel sounds are present. The diet progresses as tolerated.
- Decrease feedings if the client complains of nausea or abdominal distention. *Rationale: Such complaints are signs of complications. The NG tube may need to be reinserted.*
- Malnutrition may cause anemia or deficiency disorders. Vitamins and minerals are usually supplemented; the client must receive vitamin B_{12} for life. *Rationale: The stomach is no longer present to secrete the intrinsic factor necessary to metabolize vitamin B_{12} from foods.*
- Instruct the client to increase gradually the amount of food they eat at one time until they can tolerate three meals a day.
- Teach the client to plan regular rest periods. *Rationale: Prevent overexertion.*
- Regular medical follow-up is essential.

NCLEX Alert

Nursing considerations commonly consist of care for a client who has one of the many types of gastric surgeries, gastric tubes, TPN infusions, fecal diversions, or fecal appliances. For the NCLEX, the nurse must be very comfortable with their knowledge of insertion, maintenance, complications, and psychosocial aspects of care for all of these gastric concerns. Pre- and post-surgical nursing care and knowledge of normal electrolyte values are also of major importance.

Bowel Diversion

A bowel diversion (also known as fecal diversion) occurs when a portion or all of the ileum or bowel is removed, creating the need for an artificial opening for bowel elimination. An incision is made in the abdomen, and a loop of intestine is brought through the incision and opened to allow for drainage of feces. The opening is called a **stoma** or *ostomy*. The person with an ostomy of any type is referred to as an *ostomate*. Ostomy surgeries may be performed to remove all or part of the small or large intestine.

A **colostomy** is an opening into the colon, whereas an **ileostomy** is an opening into the ileum. A stoma may be an end (one stoma), double-barreled (two stomas—both cut ends of the intestine are brought to the outside), or loop (the bowel is not completely severed, so the one stoma has two openings).

The new stoma, which is mucous membrane, should be moist. It ranges from dark red to rich pink, looks like pursed lips, and immediately after surgery, is swollen and may bleed occasionally. External placement of the stoma depends on how much bowel is removed. In Practice: Data Gathering in Nursing 88-4 provides more detail about conditions and care of a new stoma.

A colostomy or an ileostomy may be temporary if treatment to eliminate or relieve the underlying condition is successful. A colostomy in the transverse colon is usually temporary and is located on the abdomen's right, left, or midline. A temporary stoma may be in place for several weeks to several months, depending on the underlying disease or disorder. Sometimes, an anastomosis is possible, which allows the diseased segment to be removed and the normal tissue

---

IN PRACTICE
DATA GATHERING IN NURSING 88-4 — Stoma Condition in the New Colostomy or Ileostomy

Abnormal and Danger Signs
- Abnormal sounds
- Excessive bleeding (more likely to occur in ileostomy)
- Darkening in color (indicating stenosis around the stoma, which cuts off the blood supply)
- Blanching or extreme lightening in color (indicating lack of circulation to the stoma)
- Drying of the stoma
- Edema of the stoma
- *Prolapse* (stoma pulls back into abdomen)
- Skin irritation around stoma
- Signs of infection
- Herniation around stoma (peristomal hernia)

Routine Observations and Documentation
- Size of the appliance (must be large enough so that it does not cut off circulation, but small enough so that it does not leak)
- Input and output (I&O) records
- Daily weights
- Electrolyte balance or imbalance; results of blood work
- Amount, character of stool
- Vital signs

ends to be reconnected. A *wedge resection* is the removal of only a small amount of bowel. A *bowel resection* is the removal of a larger portion of the bowel. A temporary stoma often consists of a double-barrel stoma. With the double-barrel stoma, the proximal end drains fecal material into the stoma appliance. The distal end does not receive nutrients, so it does not contain feces. When the underlying condition is healed, a takedown procedure is performed to reconnect (*anastomose*) the cut ends of the double-barrel intestine and close the abdominal wall. The goal is to have the individual resume excretion through the normal rectal outlet.

The colostomy or ileostomy will be permanent if surgery necessitates removal of the colon or the rectum. A permanent colostomy is usually made at the level of the descending or sigmoid colon and it is usually located on the abdomen's left side. An ileostomy indicates that the entire large intestine has been removed. The stoma is usually located on the abdomen's lower right side.

Colostomy Irrigation

Colostomy irrigation is a type of bowel management. Before the widespread use of disposable, odor-proof ostomy equipment, nearly all clients with colostomies used irrigation for control of bowel movements.

Colostomy irrigation is similar to an enema (Chapter 51). It is usually done with a cone tip and bag; the fluid drains into the toilet through an irrigating sleeve. The enterostomal (ET) nurse often teaches the client the procedure. You may be asked to perform this procedure if you are working in home care. Clients who wish to regulate their bowel by irrigating typically do not learn to do so until at least 6 weeks after surgery, to allow healing. Colostomy irrigation can be time consuming because it usually takes 1–1.5 hr to irrigate all stool from the bowel. Regular irrigation may enable the client to avoid the continual wearing of an ostomy appliance.

Ostomy Appliances

When the client returns from the operating room, a plastic disposable bag, called a *pouch*, covers the stoma. A faceplate on one end of the pouch has a hole that is the size of the stoma cut into it; the faceplate is then secured to the area around the stoma with a skin barrier that creates a seal (Fig. 88-6).

The opposite end of the pouch, which is not sealed, must be closed with either a special ostomy clamp or binder clip. Stool drains through the stoma and collects in the pouch. Ideally, a snug fit of the faceplate and effective application of a skin barrier prevent stool from coming in contact with the skin. Leaking of fecal material onto the skin causes *peristomal* (around the stoma) skin irritation and can result in skin breakdown.

When the pouch is one third to one half full with stool or flatus, it is emptied into a bedpan or other receptacle. *Rationale: This protects the client from skin irritation from leakage around the pouch and prevents it from falling off the abdomen. If ambulatory and able, the client sits on the toilet, removes the closure clamp, and empties the pouch contents between their legs into the toilet.*

As it heals, the stoma decreases in size. After approximately 6 weeks, the stoma can be measured for a permanent appliance, if one is indicated. A permanent appliance is a faceplate combined with pouch that is secured to the skin with a barrier for extended periods of time. A disposable appliance is a pouch that can be secured to a faceplate or wafer and removed as needed. This avoids repeated irritation of the peristomal skin, which can happen with frequent changing of the pouch–faceplate combination.

Ostomy appliances with a faceplate and pouch come in different styles and sizes. The ET nurse and the staff nurse will assist the client in choosing the appropriate appliance, depending on the person's abdominal contours and amount and type of drainage. The client will be fitted with a cut-to-fit pouch while in the healthcare facility (so the size of the stoma opening can be adjusted as stoma edema decreases).

Other permanent appliances have both faceplate and pouch; both must be removed regularly, emptied, rinsed, and replaced over the stoma. For most ostomies, the client can use disposable pouches if a secure seal can be achieved. After a prescribed number of days, the entire appliance is removed and discarded.

Skin barriers on appliance and pouching systems eventually deteriorate. Depending on the brand used, the person should change the appliance one to two times per week (In Practice: Nursing Procedure 88-2). Following the recommended time guidelines will prevent deterioration of the skin adhesive and prevent skin breakdown around the stoma.

After approximately 4–6 weeks, the nurse can fit the client into a precut appliance, which will eliminate the need for cutting out each pouch before changing it. Ostomy equipment is stocked at medical suppliers, although many pharmacies also carry it.

Nursing Considerations

Nursing considerations for ostomy care are summarized within In Practice: Nursing Care Guidelines 88-2. The most commonly discussed topics follow.

Clothing

If possible, it is highly beneficial for the ET nurse and the surgeon to discuss the placement of the stoma preoperatively so that long-term care can be anticipated. Immediately after surgery, many clients choose to wear loose-fitting clothing. However, clients will discover that even when wearing tight-fitting clothing or jeans, the presence of the pouch underneath is not noticeable. Most clients will return to wearing the same clothes as before surgery. The client should not wear a leather belt over the stoma, to prevent irritation. Clients who have their stoma site at the beltline may need to use suspenders. Clients can wear the ostomy pouch tucked into their underwear, or they can wear bikini underwear beneath the pouch.

Bathing

All pouching systems are waterproof, so clients can bathe, shower, or swim while wearing them. Clients may choose to remove soiled pouches and shower without them; this is not advisable for the person with an ileostomy. Bowel function with an ileostomy is fairly frequent and unpredictable.

Activity

Heavy lifting is prohibited for 6–8 weeks after any abdominal surgery. The person should not lift anything heavier than

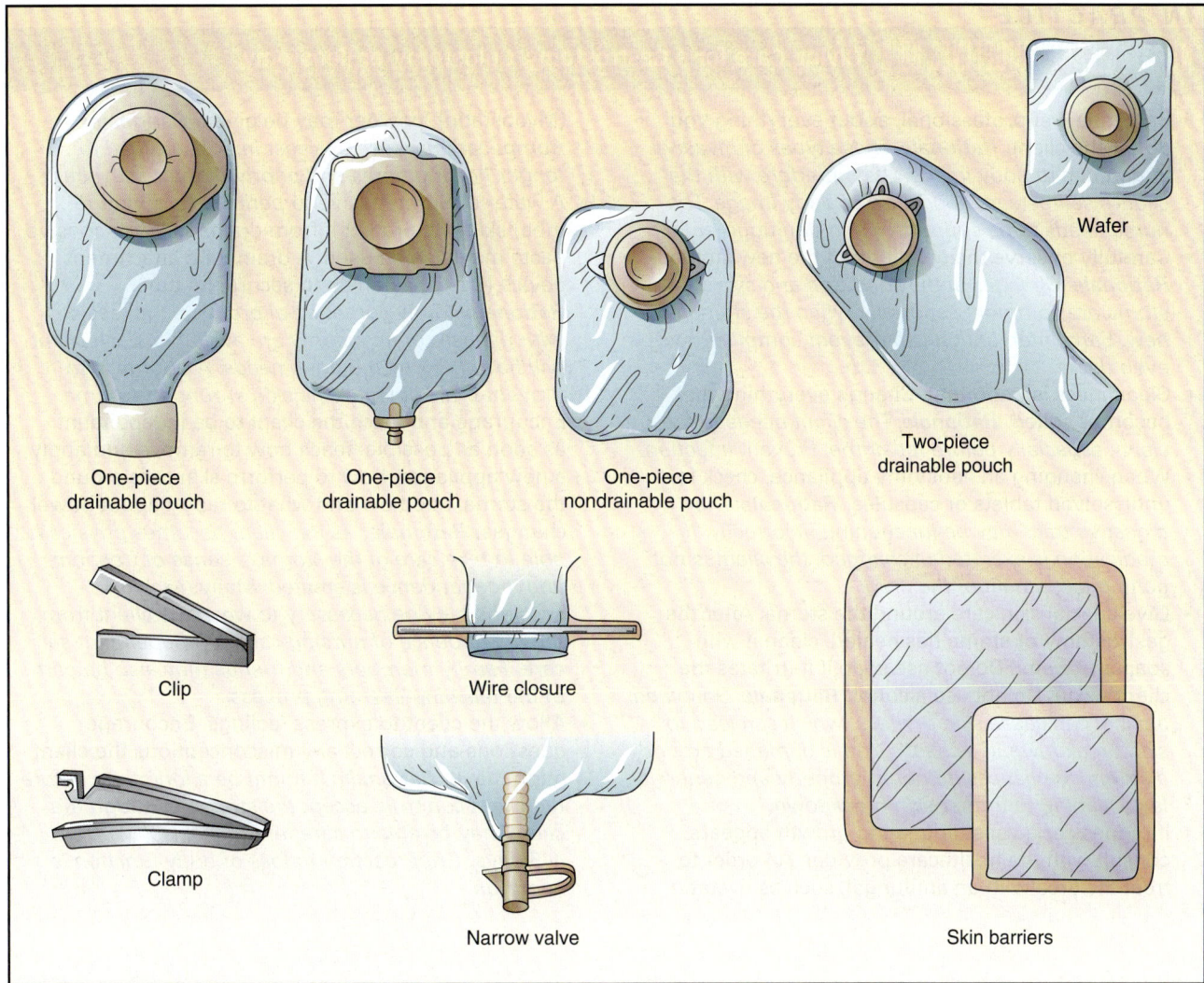

Figure 88-6 Selected ostomy pouches and accessories.

5 lb during this important period of tissue healing. Following this restriction is particularly important for the ostomate to avoid a **hernia** (an abnormal protrusion of intestine through the muscle), which can develop in the incision or around the stoma. After the initial postoperative period, the ostomate has no activity limitations.

Diet
After any bowel surgery, the client should follow a low-fiber diet for approximately 1 month. The bowel is generally edematous after surgery, and high-fiber foods may have difficulty passing through it. After 1 month, the person with a colostomy can follow a regular diet.

The person with an ileostomy needs to monitor the diet more closely. The most common complication following an ileostomy is food blockage. Foods that tend to cause blockage include dried fruits, popcorn; many vegetables and nuts; and meats in casings, such as frankfurters. Undigested food obstructs the bowel just prior to the stoma, preventing stool passage. A person with an ileostomy must chew food very well. This person may also have difficulty with odor from flatus; eliminating common gas-forming foods usually helps.

The person with an ileostomy needs plenty of fluids. This person has less formed stools and, therefore, loses more fluids during elimination. In addition to losing increased water, this person tends to lose sodium and potassium in the stool. Therefore, the person should drink not just plain water but also fluids that contain electrolytes, such as Gatorade and broth.

Skin Care
Ileal drainage is much more irritating than colostomy drainage, so give special attention to skin care and protection. Cleanse the skin carefully to prevent irritation and dry it thoroughly (In Practice: Nursing Care Guidelines 88-2). If the skin is not completely dry, the appliance will not stick. Remove the pouch gently and carefully to avoid pulling or tearing the skin.

Client and Family Teaching
The client who is to have a colostomy or ileostomy may need assistance with adjustment. Naturally, the client wonders how life will be disrupted and may be particularly concerned about the effect on sexual relationships, care of

IN PRACTICE
NURSING CARE GUIDELINES 88-2 — Giving Care for a Gastrostomy, Colostomy, or Ileostomy

- Be gentle, yet professional, about everything you do for the client. *Rationale:* These types of invasive alterations to body image often interfere with the client's self-esteem and sense of body image. The nurse needs to be supportive and nonjudgmental.
- Carefully observe the condition of the new stoma. *Rationale:* Changes in the condition and size of a stoma are common, especially when the stoma is new. Early intervention can prevent complications or even death.
- Cleanliness is important. Change everything that becomes soiled. *Rationale:* The client needs to feel clean, especially before mealtime. Prevent infection.
- When changing an ileostomy appliance, check for undissolved tablets or capsules. *Rationale:* The digestive tract may be functioning incorrectly. If medication is excreted unchanged, the client is not getting the benefit of the drug.
- Give special skin care around the stoma. After the gastrostomy or stoma has healed, clean it with soap and water. Do not use soap if it irritates the client's skin. Do not use alcohol. *Rationale:* Soap and alcohol can cause skin dryness, which can lead to skin breakdown. If a client's skin is damaged around a stoma, appliances do not fit properly and generally leak, leading to further skin breakdown.
- If redness or a yeast-appearing growth appears, consult with the healthcare provider. An order to treat the area with an antifungal, such as nystatin (Mycostatin), powder may be given. *Rationale:* Complications, such as yeast infections, lead to longer healing times and poorly fitting appliances.
- A wafer of Stomahesive to *peritube* (around the tube) skin will protect it from drainage. Stomahesive paste may also be used. A drain tube attachment device (DTAD) can help to secure the tube. *Rationale:* Many commercial products that assist with the care of an ostomy are available. Each client will have their own unique needs. A priority is to prevent breakdown of the skin around the stoma.
- Encourage and teach the client to be independent as soon as possible: Teach how to remove and apply a new appliance, how to perform skin care around the stoma, and how and what to report about bowel changes. *Rationale:* As the client becomes physically able to take care of the stoma, a sense of freedom and independence is created. Many teaching sessions may be necessary to wean the client from the dependence of nursing care to independent self-care. Family members and friends may also be part of the teaching–learning process.
- Allow the client to express feelings. Encourage questions and correct any misconceptions the client might have. *Rationale:* It might be a long time before the client can truly accept the stoma, although the client may be able to care for it physically within 4–5 days. Grief reaction to loss of body function is common.

the colostomy or ileostomy, and acceptance of family and friends.

Every nurse must be trained to care for an ostomy. Many healthcare facilities have certified ET nurses who are specially trained to teach clients with ostomies and to provide supportive counsel. The ET nurse is a resource and support person who is commonly called to assist with new, difficult, or unusual conditions that may need special training. However, the ET nurse will not be available at all times. Therefore, the staff nurse must be able to care for an ostomy.

The staff nurse should contact the ET nurse before the client's surgery. Teaching is started prior to surgery and continued for several months after surgery, depending upon the individual's needs and capacities. The healthcare provider, the staff nurse, and the ET nurse assist the client and family with the various aspects of ostomy care. As the stoma changes after surgery, the type of care will change. Teaching sessions, usually done in the home, will be necessary to enable the client and family to make adjustments for life with an ostomy (In Practice: Nursing Care Guidelines 88-2).

Continent Bowel Diversions

In some cases, the use of surgical techniques results in the removal and rerouting of intestinal tissues internally with the goal of avoiding external ostomies. In these instances, the client's own tissues may be formed into internal receptacles for stool. Many of these cases result in fecal control without the use of external stoma appliances. Complications of internal pouch procedures include stool seepage and *pouchitis* (inflammation of the internal pouch). Each of these surgeries is highly individualized to the client, the disease, condition of available tissues, and surgical capabilities.

Ileoanal Reservoir

The *ileoanal reservoir* is the surgical creation of a colon-like pouch fashioned from the small intestine (ileum) that collects ileal drainage. The reservoir is also known as a *pelvic pouch* or *J-pouch*. Procedures usually are done in two stages. In stage 1, the entire colon and lining of the rectum are removed, and the reservoir is fashioned. The anal sphincter is retained, and the reservoir (pouch) is sewn to it. A temporary ileostomy is done. The client then eliminates stool through the ileostomy stoma for 6 weeks–3 months, while resting the bowel. Stage 2 is surgical takedown of the ileostomy. The reservoir acts as the sigmoid colon, and the client usually achieves control of bowel movements.

The ileoanal reservoir procedure requires a longer recuperation time than the standard ileostomy, but it greatly improves the quality of life for clients in whom it can be used. The person will pass stool four to eight times in 24 hr and does not have a permanent stoma.

Kock Pouch

Another procedure called the *Kock pouch* or the *continent ileostomy* is often more surgically acceptable than the standard ileostomy. This procedure is usually impossible if the client is obese, is at high risk, or has Crohn disease, toxic megacolon, diabetes mellitus, or active colitis. The Kock procedure removes the colon, rectum, and anus. A permanent ileostomy is created from the end of the ileum, making an internal abdominal reservoir, which will collect stool. Additionally, a stoma is created and connected to the Kock pouch.

Nursing care after surgery includes catheterizing the pouch and irrigating it with 20–50 mL of normal saline every 2 hr. The return flows out by gravity. Check the skin around the stoma and the tube several times daily and change dressings as needed.

The client is usually able to achieve the same continence as with a colostomy by daily catheterization of the pouch by inserting a tube through the stoma. The stoma is covered by a patch (but not an ostomy appliance) when not being drained.

Abdominal Paracentesis

Abdominal paracentesis (*abdominal tap*) is a procedure that may be necessary for diagnostic purposes or to relieve **ascites** (fluid accumulation in the peritoneal cavity). It is considered diagnostic when fluid is withdrawn for microscopic study or for culturing when bleeding or infection is suspected. Therapeutic abdominal tap is done when the client is distended with ascitic fluid. The abdominal cavity is punctured to obtain a specimen for analysis or to drain excess fluid. Because the client may also have difficulty breathing, removal of this fluid will frequently relieve the condition. Ultrasound may be utilized to guide the aspiration of fluid from the abdomen with a large syringe and needle. Sometimes, a catheter is inserted into the abdominal cavity for continuous drainage.

Nursing Considerations

Nursing considerations for an abdominal paracentesis include the following measures:

- Ask the client to void immediately before the procedure. *Rationale: This helps to avoid rupture of the urinary bladder by the needle.*
- Assist the client into a comfortable position for the procedure.
- Perform sterile scrub of the abdomen in preparation for needle insertion.
- Monitor vital signs during and after the procedure. Watch for fainting or dizziness.
- Measure the amount of fluid obtained.
- Send the appropriate specimens to the laboratory.
- After the procedure, observe the client for bleeding or any signs of shock.
- Check the dressing to make sure it is tightly applied and dry. *Rationale: Prevent and check for bleeding.*
- Keep the client in Fowler position, unless ordered otherwise. *Rationale: Facilitate drainage and assist breathing.*
- Observe urine output. Check the male client's scrotum for edema. *Rationale: Evaluate the effectiveness of the procedure and determine if complications exist.*
- Tell the client to observe for any signs of infection.
- Carefully document the procedure and all teaching.

NURSING PROCESS

DATA COLLECTION

Using the skills of physical examination and nursing observations and data collection, observe and monitor carefully the client who has a digestive disorder. This establishes a baseline for future comparison and determines the presence of suspected digestive-related complications. Report any changes in baseline levels.

Compare the client's height in ratio to weight and ask about eating habits and recent weight gain or loss. Determine whether the person is able to chew and swallow and whether food preparation is a problem. In addition, observe the client's emotional response to the disorder or disease. Does the client need assistance to meet daily needs? Does the disorder affect social activities or self-esteem (e.g., does the client have a colostomy)? Is the disorder life threatening? Is the client anxious or fearful about the outcome? Are a support group, home care nursing, Meals on Wheels, and other community programs appropriate?

PLANNING AND IMPLEMENTING

Plan with the client, family, and other members of the healthcare team for effective care to meet the client's needs based on the nursing diagnoses. Provide pre- and postoperative care for the client undergoing endoscopy, liver biopsy, or surgery on the stomach or related organs.

The client with a digestive disorder may also require assistance in meeting nutritional or self-care needs. Many digestive disorders have strong emotional components that may aggravate the disorder or be related to the disease's course. Clients often need assistance to understand more about the disorder, including its prognosis and treatment. The client may need to perform special procedures at home; thus, client teaching is vital. Develop a nursing care plan to meet each client's needs.

EVALUATION

Evaluate outcomes of care by answering the following questions: Have short-term goals been met? Are additional teaching or rehabilitative measures needed? Is additional treatment or surgery necessary? Are long-term goals still realistic? Are community services required? Is a support group available? Planning for further nursing care considers the client's prognosis, complications, and responses to care given.

DISORDERS OF THE MOUTH

Mouth disorders are uncomfortable, often painful, and at times disfiguring or cosmetically unattractive. They can also disrupt nutritional intake or lead to other undesirable or more serious conditions and lifestyle changes.

Dental Problems

Dental **caries** (tooth decay) result from an erosive process that breaks down tooth enamel and later invades the dental pulp; this causes discomfort and sometimes necessitates tooth removal. The major cause of decay is bacteria nourished by food particles left on the teeth as a result of faulty brushing and lack of flossing. Acids in the mouth and their effectiveness in destroying bacteria; presence of plaque on the teeth and sugar in the mouth promoting bacterial growth; susceptibility of the teeth to decay; and the length of time between brushings play a part in the decay process.

Good brushing is essential to preserve a healthy mouth and prevent tooth decay. Many dentists recommend using fluoridated water or having the dentist apply fluoride. Flossing helps to clean between teeth and to prevent gum disease. Professional dental care also is important. Adults should have their teeth checked and cleaned professionally twice a year.

Dentures are better known as "false teeth." The term for "without teeth" is *edentulous*. Many people delay or ignore dental care. People often mistakenly believe that dentures are a normal part of aging. They may not have access to appropriate gum and dental care, which leads to infected teeth and tooth loss that could have been avoided. Additionally, the individual is being exposed to infection that can become systemic.

In some cases, dentures are the best solution for dental problems. At other times, reconstructive partial inserts can be used. Dentures may be slightly uncomfortable when they are first fitted, but the dentist can remove sources of irritation. The only way to become accustomed to dentures is to wear them all the time, especially when awake. Dentures also help preserve the face's normal shape.

Periodontal Disease

Periodontal disease affects the bones and tissues around the teeth. It can result from poor oral hygiene, inadequate dental care, or poor nutrition.

Gingivitis

Gingivitis, a form of periodontal disease, is inflammation of the gums. General symptoms include bleeding and erythematous, edematous, and tender gums. Gingivitis has many causes, but it is most frequently associated with accumulation of bacterial plaque on the teeth as a result of ineffective oral hygiene. Gingivitis may also be a sign of vitamin deficiencies, diabetes mellitus, anemia, and leukemia. It can lead to more serious disorders, such as inflammation of tissues that directly surround a tooth. Proper care of the teeth and gums, including daily flossing and an adequate diet, is the best preventive measure.

Pyorrhea Alveolaris

Pyorrhea alveolaris is an inflammation of the gums and teeth, sometimes with a purulent discharge. It usually begins with *periodontitis* (inflammation of the tissues around and supporting the teeth). Pyorrhea is caused by the collection of food, bacteria, and tartar deposits between the gum line and the tooth root. Untreated periodontitis spreads to the underlying bony structure. The teeth loosen because their support structure breaks down, making chewing impossible.

Treatment includes impeccable tooth, gum, and mouth care: regular flossing, surgical scraping and drainage of the infected area, antibiotics, or extraction of the affected teeth. Surgical scraping is painful, so other measures are tried first. Left untreated, pyorrhea can result in an abscess or a systemic infection.

Stomatitis

Causes of *stomatitis* (inflammation of the mouth) include primary lesions of the mouth; secondary lesions of the mouth (as a result of chemotherapy or radiation); mechanical trauma (mouth breathing, cheek biting); and chemical trauma (sensitivities/allergies of the oral mucosa to ingested substances).

Stomatitis may be a clinical manifestation of a systemic condition or the result of an infection in the oral cavity. Nutritional disorders and bone marrow disorders are some of the systemic causes of inflammation of the oral mucosa. Treatment of this problem depends on the cause and usually involves avoiding oral irritants and providing comfort with frequent oral hygiene. Topical antibiotic ointments may be prescribed to treat bacterial infections.

Canker sores (*aphthous stomatitis*) are recurrent, small, white, painful ulcers that appear on the inner cheeks, lips, gums, tongue, palate, and pharynx. No one knows their exact cause; however, many local and systemic factors, such as food and drug allergies (immune reaction) and physical and emotional stress, have been suggested. Canker sores have been linked to highly salted foods and some forms of nuts. Dental trauma is the most common factor in recurrent canker sores. Premenstrual flare-ups are common. Canker sores may be associated with chronic ulcerative colitis, Crohn disease, and malabsorption syndromes.

No effective treatment has been found. The sores usually heal without intervention in a few days. The use of topical anesthetics (e.g., benzocaine or lidocaine) may help to relieve pain. Silver nitrate stick application destroys nerve endings and may provide pain relief. Application of a solution of tetracycline may improve healing in some clients. Oral L-lysine also is believed to be helpful.

Candidiasis

Candidiasis, known as *thrush* or *moniliasis*, is a fungal infection caused by the organism *Candida albicans*, which is part of the normal flora of the oral cavity. It is common in newborns, immunosuppressed clients, and clients with chronic debilitating diseases such as HIV/AIDS, diabetes, STDs, or alcoholism. Antibiotic therapies also can lead to candidiasis. The infection appears as small, white patches on the mucous membranes of the mouth or tongue. It may extend into the entire GI tract. See Chapter 70 for additional information.

Oral pharyngeal cultures are recommended when this infection is suspected. Prophylactic treatment of high-risk clients is indicated. Treatment consists of nystatin, saline, and hydrogen peroxide mouth rinses, or vaginal suppositories.

Herpes Simplex Infections

Herpes simplex is a viral infection caused by either or both types of herpes: herpes simplex virus type 1 (HSV-1) and type 2 (HSV-2). The mouth, face, and genital areas are the most common sites of infection. Oral herpes may also be called *cold sores* or *fever blisters* and can be confused with canker sores (*aphthous stomatitis*). It is often difficult to differentiate between orofacial herpes (HSV-1) and genital herpes (HSV-2). Either type of herpes can be found in the common sites of infection where they go through active periods ranging from 2 days–weeks followed by periods of remission. Herpes simplex is most easily transmitted by direct contact with a blister, body fluid of an infected individual, or skin-to-skin contact during periods of asymptomatic shedding. The blisters that develop during the active phase of the disease contain infectious virus particles that are transported along sensory nerves (e.g., the trigeminal or cranial nerve V). Because of the virus's ability to be transported, it can cause very serious infections of the eye and brain or pass onto a newborn causing neonatal herpes. The virus can become active when the individual is immunocompromised either via medications or by severe illness. Typically, episodes of active disease reduce in frequency and severity over time. No cure exists and the virus will remain in the body for life (also review the discussion on STIs and herpes in Chapter 70).

Treatment
Antiviral drugs can reduce both the severity of active infections and shedding of the virus. Some individuals can become *perpetually asymptomatic* and will no longer experience outbreaks; however, they still may be contagious to others. Analgesics may be prescribed for comfort. Acyclovir (Zovirax; 5%) ointment may be applied to the lesions. The lesions are infectious, so wear gloves when treating them. Although the ointment may not speed healing, it may decrease virus shedding. The dietary supplement L-lysine may be palliative. Drying agents, such as benzoin or alum, may also be applied to the lesions to speed healing of the blisters.

Trauma
Various types of injuries, such as fracture of the jaw, laceration of the lips, and traumatic loss of teeth, can cause mouth injury. Chapter 43 describes first aid for traumatic tooth loss (*avulsion*).

With simple suturing, lacerations of the lips heal without complications because of a good blood supply. However, if the entire lip is severed, the person may experience problems with lip movement. For lip and other types of facial surgery, a plastic surgeon may perform the suturing.

For a jaw fracture, usually the upper and lower jaws are wired or fastened together so that they heal without displacement. This is called *intermaxillary fixation*. This client cannot open his or her mouth. Consequently, you must be ready to assist, as necessary. The client needs help with meals because they sip foods through a straw or from a spoon. NG tube feedings or TPN may be necessary.

If the client has their jaws wired or fastened together, keep a wire cutter with the client at all times for emergency use. If the client is choking or vomiting, the wires must be cut, or the client could die from lack of oxygen. The client's head is kept slightly elevated, and oral suctioning equipment is nearby. Antiemetic drugs are usually administered for the first few days after injury. A tracheostomy or a nasal or oral intubation procedure by a healthcare provider may be required to establish an airway as an emergency measure.

If an *extraoral* (outside the mouth) device is in place, give special attention to the position of the client's head for maximum comfort. The device often goes around the client's head. Teach the client not to roll onto the device, which might result in bending or dislodging the wires.

Precancerous Lesions
Leukoplakia buccalis (smoker's patch) is the most common precancerous lesion. It is a creamy white, nonsloughing patch on the mucous membranes of the mouth or tongue. This lesion is common in middle-aged people who smoke or who have extensive dental caries. It often disappears if the client stops smoking. A biopsy or oral cytology study is usually recommended.

Cancer of the Mouth
Many cancers of the mouth are asymptomatic until they have spread. Mouth cancer can be treated successfully if discovered early. Those who ingest large amounts of alcohol or engage in risky behaviors, such as smoking or using forms of smokeless tobacco (leaf, plug, or snuff), have an increased risk for developing oral cancer. Many people tend to ignore sores or irritations in the mouth because they think such symptoms are insignificant.

Treatment
Cancer of the mouth may be treated with surgery, radium implants, or deep x-ray therapy. Combination therapies with chemotherapy are also common. If possible, the malignancy is removed with as wide an excision as necessary to remove all affected structures and lymph nodes. NG or gastrostomy feedings might be indicated. The operation is often followed by reconstructive surgery to correct facial defects.

Nursing Considerations
Nursing considerations revolve around caring for the client pre- and postoperatively. Before surgery, design communication techniques because the client may be unable to speak as they did before surgery. After surgery, observe for hemorrhage and airway obstruction caused by facial edema or aspiration. Suction secretions and elevate the head of the bed to make breathing easier. As you support the client's head by placing your hands on either side, instruct the client to breathe deeply and to use the incentive spirometer. Do not encourage coughing unless congestion is present. These measures are needed to prevent hypostatic pneumonia. An emergency airway should be available at the client's bedside.

Give mouth care carefully to improve the client's comfort and prevent odor. Take great care to prevent disruption of the suture line. Give liquids through an NG tube until the client is able to swallow. Self-care is the goal.

DISORDERS OF THE ESOPHAGUS

Esophageal Varices
Esophageal varices are abnormal dilations of the blood vessels of the esophagus. They are most often associated with cirrhosis of the liver, which is a serious and chronic condition. Treatment is imperative; untreated varices can

hemorrhage profusely, and the client may die. An EGD may be used in the diagnosis and treatment of esophageal varices. *Sclerotherapy* is an endoscopic procedure whereby caustic agents are injected into the tissue near the varices. This procedure, done in a series of treatments, causes scar tissue to form and stops the hemorrhaging. Monitor the client closely for hemorrhage after each treatment and before and after surgery. *Band ligation* is another endoscopic procedure in which small rubber bands are placed on and around bleeding varices on the esophageal wall. These bands stop the bleeding; when the tissue is healed, they slough off, leaving scar tissue, which is less likely to bleed.

Esophageal Diverticulum

Esophageal diverticulum or *Zenker diverticulum* is an outpouching of the esophagus, usually where the esophagus passes through the neck area. The client first complains of bad breath, which is caused by bits of food that have accumulated in the diverticulum. X-ray studies determine the nature and location of the outpouchings.

In most cases, the diverticulum is small, causes no dysfunction, and requires no treatment. In more serious cases, the client's dietary status is evaluated. The client can be treated medically with a bland diet, antacids, and other measures to prevent *reflux* (return flow) of food and fluid. Surgery may be necessary if symptoms do not diminish with conscientious medical management or if the client is debilitated and aspiration of the food or fluid trapped in the diverticulum is considered a danger.

Nursing considerations include placing the client in a semi-Fowler position, serving small meals, and fitting the client with loose clothing. Encourage the client to maintain an appropriate weight to prevent an enlarged stomach or excess fatty tissue from pushing up on the esophagus.

Hiatal Hernia

Hiatal hernia is a condition in which part of the stomach protrudes through the diaphragm's esophageal hiatus (gap or cleft through which the esophagus passes). Weakening of the diaphragmatic muscles at the gastroesophageal junction, trauma, or congenital causes may contribute to development of a hernia.

Factors that increase intra-abdominal pressure, such as coughing, straining at stool, bending, or lifting heavy objects, may exacerbate the condition. Many people older than 50 years have asymptomatic hiatal hernias. A large hiatal hernia is likely to cause symptoms, such as a feeling of fullness, abnormal stomach sounds, ulceration, bleeding, and pain. Hiatal hernia does not cause heartburn, although a person with a hiatal hernia may have heartburn from another cause.

Treatment

Management is directed at keeping the stomach's acid contents from maintaining long contact with the esophageal lining. If a hernia is small and causes little distress, treatment is unnecessary. When surgical treatment is indicated, postoperative edema of the stomach and esophagus may make eating a problem for the first few days. Therefore, the client may receive IV fluids or TPN for several days.

Nursing Considerations

After surgery, observe the contents of the NG tube drainage carefully, looking particularly for blood. A small amount of blood may be evident immediately after the operation, but after this disappears, the drainage should have the yellowish-green color of normal gastric secretions. Frank bleeding signals a hemorrhage.

If the client has had chest surgery, give special attention to chest tube management and deep breathing. The client should use the incentive spirometer. Administer oxygen and give care to the chest's drainage site. Observe carefully for vomiting or aspiration, particularly when the client begins to take solid or semisolid foods. *Rationale: Regurgitated food may irritate the suture line, and aspiration can cause postoperative pneumonia.* Other postoperative care is routine.

Achalasia

Achalasia is a motility disorder of the lower portion of the esophagus in which food cannot pass into the stomach. Causes include absence of effective or coordinated esophageal peristalsis or failure of the cardiac sphincter to relax.

The most prominent symptom of achalasia is difficulty swallowing. Achalasia is chronic and progressive. Clients often use large volumes of fluids or bulk in an attempt to force open the cardiac sphincter and allow food to move into the stomach. Thus, they may develop malnutrition and vitamin deficiencies. These clients also are susceptible to respiratory problems caused by aspiration of regurgitated esophageal contents.

A special test called *esophageal manometry* is used to measure and record the motility patterns of the esophagus. A barium swallow with esophagoscopy may be done to assist in diagnosis. These procedures also can be used to monitor the disorder's progression.

Treatment

Surgical treatment often involves dilation of the cardiac sphincter to the point of weakening or disrupting its ability to close. Dilation is done by endoscopy with a variety of balloons and dilators. Medical treatment is directed toward educating the client.

Nursing Considerations

Teaching involves improving dietary and eating habits. Teach the client to eat slowly and in a peaceful setting. Chewing food thoroughly and drinking plenty of liquids during the meal help food move into the stomach.

Heartburn

Heartburn (also called *indigestion*, **dyspepsia**, and *pyrosis*) is a common clinical manifestation of esophageal disease. Heartburn is an uncomfortable burning sensation in the lower chest, which often radiates upward toward the neck. It is exacerbated by postural changes, ingestion of alcohol, and gulping of food or fluids. Clients often state that the pain is cramping and wavelike. Other symptoms include nausea, indigestion, belching, a bloated feeling, and a sore throat owing to acid reflux.

As a healthcare provider, determine exactly what "heartburn" means to the client who uses it to describe a symptom because "heartburn" may be used to describe many different sensations. Treatment of heartburn is directed at alleviating or minimizing the causes.

> **Nursing Alert** Differentiating between heartburn and heart attack pain is difficult. If a person has any question, they should seek medical attention immediately. Symptoms of heart attack that differ from heartburn include intense chest pain that radiates to the neck, jaw, back, or arms; difficulty breathing or breathlessness; fainting; limb numbness; sudden nausea and vomiting; and cold, clammy skin accompanied by sweating.

Gastroesophageal Reflux Disease

Esophageal reflux or gastroesophageal reflux disease (**GERD**) occurs when the lower esophageal sphincter (**LES**) leading into the stomach is weak or relaxes inappropriately. Typical symptoms of GERD include heartburn, regurgitation and dysphagia, pain when swallowing, nausea, and chest pain. With a sphincter that does not close firmly, acidic stomach contents can move back up into the esophagus and may be the cause of injury or *esophagitis*, which is acute or chronic inflammation and irritation of the lining of the esophagus.

Esophagitis can lead to reflux esophagitis, esophageal strictures, a precursor to cancer called Barrett esophagus, or esophageal adenocarcinoma. Esophageal injuries may lead to additional problems, including chronic cough, laryngitis, asthma, sinusitis, and damaged teeth. The presence of a hiatal hernia may aggravate the condition. Many medications and foods aggravate GERD or esophagitis, including acetylsalicylic acid (Aspirin), chocolate, peppermint, spicy foods, coffee, tomato products, citrus fruits, and fried foods. Cigarette smoking greatly decreases LES pressure and aggravates heartburn. Drinking alcohol and overeating exacerbate the condition. Hot or cold liquids may intensify the sensation. Bacterial or yeast infections may also be causes.

Treatment

Initially, treatment is designed to monitor and treat esophageal pH. An EGD is common. If the client's diet is aggravating the condition, nutritional counseling is in order. Medications that may help include H_2 blockers, PPIs, GI stimulants, cholinergics, and antacids, such as Mylanta, Rolaids, or Tums.

Surgical treatment is reserved for those clients who do not respond to medical management. Surgical procedures may be completed by either a laparoscopic or an open surgical approach.

Nursing Considerations

Nursing considerations center around client teaching and postoperative care. The client should stop smoking, elevate the head of the bed, avoid gastric irritants, eat small meals, and maintain proper weight. Explain that drinking adequate fluids and chewing food thoroughly assist in food passage. Instruct the client not to lie down for at least 2 hr after meals and not to wear tight belts or waistbands. Encourage those with GERD to move away from their desks and stretch intermittently to discourage reflux.

When an open surgical approach is used, postoperative nursing considerations are similar to those for hiatal hernia repair. Clients who undergo a surgical procedure for GERD are still encouraged to follow an antireflux regimen of lifestyle changes, medications, and diet changes because of a significant recurrence rate.

Barrett Esophagus

Barrett esophagus is a condition of extreme and chronic irritation of the lower esophagus. It changes the esophageal lining's cell formation from the normal squamous cell type to the columnar cell type, which is found in the stomach's wall. Barrett esophagus is thought to be a precancerous condition that requires careful medical management and annual endoscopic surveillance for the development of a malignancy.

Esophageal Cancer

Esophageal malignancies usually consist of squamous cell carcinoma or adenocarcinoma of the esophageal mucosa. The incidence of adenocarcinoma of the esophagus and upper stomach has increased significantly in the past few decades. Cancer of the esophagus is most common in men and in smokers. It is also associated with alcoholism. Esophageal cancer often is diagnosed late in its development, and the client's prognosis is usually poor.

Signs and Symptoms

One early clinical manifestation is dysphagia, which progresses from mild and intermittent in the first stages of the disease to constant and accompanied by an increase in salivation and mucus in the throat. As obstruction becomes more evident, the client may even be unable to swallow liquids. Any attempt at swallowing causes the person to regurgitate the food, creating discomfort and a disagreeable taste and odor in the client's mouth.

Diagnosis is made on the basis of an esophagogram, upper GI series, and laboratory cytology. Fiberoptic esophagoscopy may be done to visualize the tumor and to take a biopsy sample. CT scans can be used to define the size of the primary lesion and reveal nodal involvement.

Treatment

Surgery is the only effective treatment for esophageal cancer that allows the client to eat normally. Innovative developments in chest surgery have resulted in rapid advances in treatment. Surgery may be performed for cure or palliation, depending on the extent of the disease. Even if removing all the cancerous tissue is impossible because the disease has spread, surgery may help the client eat normally.

Often the malignancy is incurable because it is in an inoperable area or is discovered after the cancer has metastasized. Metastasis is fairly common because the esophagus is close to other vital structures. All malignant tissue that can be isolated is removed. Three common surgical treatments include esophagectomy with graft replacement, esophagogastrostomy, and esophagoenterostomy (colon interposition). Often the client requires parenteral fluids and TPN after surgery. Radiation therapy is a palliative treatment usually included before or after surgery or both. Chemotherapy and photodynamic therapy may be used to inhibit growth of the malignant lesion (Chapter 83).

Nursing Considerations

Nursing considerations relate to management of symptoms, providing sources of nutrition, and routine postoperative care.

DISORDERS OF THE STOMACH

Gastritis

Gastritis (stomach inflammation), commonly called *indigestion*, occurs in acute, chronic, and toxic forms. Gastritis may be a primary symptom of many disorders. Overeating, ingesting irritating medications (e.g., acetylsalicylic acid [Aspirin] or steroids) or poisonous food, abusing alcohol, or microbial infection (e.g., *H. pylori*) are causes of acute gastritis. *Acute gastritis* is characterized by abdominal pain, often with *anorexia* (refusal to eat), nausea, *enteritis* (intestinal inflammation), and *dyspepsia*. Dyspepsia includes symptoms such as heartburn, bloating, nausea, and abdominal pain. Temporary relief may be found by the use of a bland diet of liquids or soft foods, along with antacids. Treatment involves removing offending foods, medications, and *H. pylori*. *H. pylori* is linked to several disorders of the GI tract. It is found in some infections of the stomach, ulcers of the stomach and duodenum, and stomach cancer. *Chronic gastritis* continues over time. Pain may occur after eating, but often the person has no pain. Causes include excessive alcohol use, vitamin deficiencies, hiatal hernia, ulcers, and abnormalities in gastric secretions. Treatment is similar to that for peptic ulcer.

Toxic gastritis follows ingestion of poison. It is characterized by burning stomach pain, cramps, nausea, vomiting, and diarrhea. Emesis or diarrhea may be bloody. Toxic gastritis is an emergency. Poison control specialists in the emergency department treat the client by either flushing out the poison by lavage or neutralizing the poison, if possible, with a substance such as activated charcoal.

Peptic Ulcer Disease

An *ulcer* is an open sore in the skin or mucous membrane that is accompanied by sloughing of inflamed and necrotic tissue. The general term *peptic ulcer* refers to a break in the integrity of the mucosa of the esophagus, stomach, or duodenum. Peptic ulcers include gastric ulcers and the more common duodenal ulcers. Less common peptic ulcers include the esophageal ulcer and the Meckel diverticulum ulcer.

The presence of the gram-negative bacteria *H. pylori* is strongly associated with peptic ulcer disease. *H. pylori* can be detected by a UBT known as C13-UBT or C14-UBT. (See earlier section on breath testing.) *Gastric ulcers* (stomach ulcers) are thought to result from a break in the mucous barrier mechanisms that normally protect the stomach's lining. *Duodenal ulcers* are characterized by increased gastric secretion of hydrochloric acid. Ulcers can be caused or worsened by use of nonsteroidal anti-inflammatory drugs (NSAIDs), including acetylsalicylic acid (Aspirin), ibuprofen (Motrin), or clopidogrel (Plavix).

SPECIAL CONSIDERATIONS Lifespan

Bleeding Ulcers

The risk of bleeding is greater in older adults, especially if they are taking NSAIDs, such as ibuprofen (Motrin) or acetylsalicylic acid (Aspirin).

Signs and Symptoms

Table 88-2 compares the signs and symptoms of gastric and duodenal ulcers. The stool should be tested for occult blood. **Melena** (black, tarry stool containing blood) from bleeding in the stomach may occur and is a significant finding. Gastroscopy and x-ray examination help diagnose peptic ulcer and differentiate it from a cancerous lesion. Diagnosis of *H. pylori* infection can be accomplished by a gastric mucosal biopsy procedure, a serum blood test for antibodies to the *H. pylori* antigen, or a breath test.

Complications

In the event of complications, an NG tube attached to suction will be inserted. The client will be kept NPO for at least 24 hr, and IV fluids will be administered.

There are four major types of complication:

Abdominal infection: Abdominal infections will require massive doses of antibiotics. Continued distention without passage of flatus or feces is a sign of serious disruption of peristalsis, causing paralytic ileus.

Obstruction: Obstruction may occur when scar tissue builds to the point where it obstructs food passage through the pyloric sphincter. Symptoms include vomiting undigested food and stomach pain. Only vomiting relieves the pain. Peritonitis is a major threat.

Hemorrhage: Hemorrhage is another serious and frequent complication of ulcers, occurring when an ulcer penetrates a blood vessel. If the blood vessel is small, bleeding may be so slight that the client does not notice it. Vomiting blood or passing melena is evidence of more extensive hemorrhage. If bleeding is massive, signs of shock appear, which include pallor, weak and rapid pulse, low blood pressure, faintness, and collapse. A significant sign of hemorrhage is *coffee-ground emesis* (emesis of partially digested blood). If blood loss is great and sudden, the client is most likely to vomit; if it is small and gradual, the client will most likely pass blood in the stool.

Endoscopic procedures can be performed to seal off bleeding vessels with a small heat probe or bipolar cautery probe passed down an inner channel of an endoscope. Injection of epinephrine by sclerotherapy technique also will stop acute bleeding. Treatment of a bleeding ulcer includes rest, enforced by sedatives. Blood transfusion and IV fluids are often necessary. Surgery probably will be necessary if bleeding continues.

Perforation: Perforation occurs when an ulcer penetrates the wall of the stomach or intestine, allowing the contents to escape into the abdomen, causing *peritonitis* (inflammation of the serous membrane lining the walls of the pelvis and abdomen).

TABLE 88-2 Peptic Ulcer Disease: Comparing Gastric and Duodenal Ulcers

	GASTRIC ULCER	DUODENAL ULCER
Etiology	• Most common in people older than 65 years • Most common in older women • High mortality rate; higher incidence of malignancy than duodenal ulcer	• Most common in people younger than 65 years • Three times more common in men than women • Four times more common than gastric ulcer
Risk factors	• Stress • Alcohol abuse • Smoking • Nonsteroidal anti-inflammatory drugs and acetylsalicylic acid (Aspirin) use (commonly prescribed for arthritis), which contributes to gastric ulcer formation • Infection with *Helicobacter pylori*	• Stress • Alcohol abuse • Smoking • Pulmonary disease • Cirrhosis of the liver • Chronic pancreatitis • Chronic renal failure • Infection with *H. pylori*
Symptoms	• High epigastric pain 1–2 hr after meals; eating may not relieve pain • Weight loss	• Mid-epigastric pain 2–4 hr after meals and during night; often relieved by eating • Weight gain • More likely to perforate than gastric ulcer

Symptoms of perforation begin with sudden, viciously sharp abdominal pains. Physical signs include pallor and diaphoresis. The abdomen hardens and is tender and painful. The client breathes rapidly and draws up the knees in an attempt to relieve the pain. The client's face later becomes flushed and feverish. This condition can be fatal. It requires immediate surgery to close the perforation. A perforation can occur without warning and may not be preceded by marked signs of digestive disturbance.

Treatment

A variety of treatment modalities are available, depending on symptom severity. Diet and medications are effective treatment in most cases. Rest and stress management are also generally indicated. More invasive treatments are indicated in the event of complications.

Medications

Regimens using bismuth compounds (e.g., Pepto-Bismol) and a single or a combination of antibiotics (e.g., amoxicillin [Amoxil, Moxatag, Trimox], clarithromycin [Biaxin], tetracycline [Actisite, Panmycin], metronidazole [Flagyl]) to eradicate *H. pylori* are effective in healing and preventing recurrence of ulcers and gastritis. Other medications used include antacid preparations, histamine (H₂) receptor antagonists, PPIs, and cytoprotective agents, including misoprostol (Cytotec) and sucralfate (Carafate). See text further on for additional details regarding medications.

Antacid preparations act to *buffer* (neutralize) gastric hyperacidity. Antacids that contain aluminum hydroxide (e.g., Amphojel) may cause constipation, and those that contain magnesium hydroxide (e.g., Mylanta) may cause diarrhea. Aluminum hydroxide (Maalox), simethicone, magnesium hydroxide, and aluminum hydroxide (Gelusil) combine magnesium and aluminum salts and are less likely to cause electrolyte depletion.

Because antacids can disrupt a person's electrolyte balance, they are often rotated to maintain acid–base balance. Inform the client not to use bicarbonate of soda (baking soda) regularly because it upsets the body's acid–base balance more so than do commercial antacids. The client must chew antacid tablets slowly before swallowing them to obtain their maximum benefits. See Table 88-3 for more information about GI drugs.

Histamine (H₂) receptor antagonists inhibit acid secretion in response to all stimuli. Therefore, they reduce gastric acid secretions. The H₂ blockers are well absorbed from the GI tract and begin working within 30–60 min. IV administration is possible for faster effects. The H₂ blockers usually provide healing for acute gastric and duodenal ulcers in 6–8 weeks. They also have been proved safe and effective in long-term management of chronic gastric ulcers and related conditions, such as esophagitis and gastritis.

PPIs inhibit the secretion of gastric acid by binding to the proton pump of the stomach's parietal cells. PPIs are potent and widely used because of their effectiveness and the lack of side effects associated with their use. PPIs may be safely administered via NG tube by dissolving them in an alkaline solution.

Misoprostol (Cytotec), a synthetic prostaglandin (hormone-like medication), and the PPI lansoprazole (Prevacid) may be prescribed in conjunction with NSAID therapy to prevent and treat NSAID-related gastric ulcers for individuals who take these medications routinely. They enhance gastric mucosal defenses and inhibit gastric secretion to prevent gastric ulcers. Clients with arthritis are at the greatest risk for gastric ulcers, especially if they are female and older than 65 years. Diarrhea and loose stools are the most commonly reported side effects of misoprostol use. Sucralfate (Carafate) provides an additional protective mucous coating to the lining of the stomach and duodenum. It allows healing of ulcers or gastritis. Its most common side effect is constipation.

Diet

Recent research in diet therapies has shown that the frequency of meals is as important as their content. The client may follow a bland diet while pain is present. For the

TABLE 88-3 Classifications of Medications for the Gastrointestinal System

CLASSIFICATIONS AND NURSING CONSIDERATIONS	EXAMPLES OF DRUGS	COMMENTS	MAIN INDICATIONS FOR USE
Antacids Can decrease absorption of sucralfate, anticholinergics, H_2 blockers, fluoroquinolones, iron, INH, phenothiazines, and tetracycline. Can cause loss of effect for enteric-coated tablets.	aluminum hydroxide (Amphojel) magnesium hydroxide (milk of magnesia) aluminum hydroxide and magnesium hydroxide combinations: Gelusil, Maalox, Mylanta	Neutralize gastric acid, inhibit gastric acid secretions, or provide mucosal protection Can cause constipation or diarrhea, depending on drug and/or dosage	Used for indigestion, reflux esophagitis, and peptic ulcers and other gastric irritants[a]
Histamine$_2$-receptor antagonists (H_2 blockers) Remind the client to allow at least 1 hr between eating or taking doses of antacid and taking H_2 blockers. May cause dizziness and confusion. Use with caution in older adults.	cimetidine (Tagamet) famotidine (Pepcid) ranitidine (Zantac) nizatidine (Axid)	Cimetidine has many interactions leading to increased blood levels and toxicity of many drugs, such as theophylline, diazepam, and anticoagulants. Antacids and food delay absorption of the H_2 blocker, although the therapeutic effect will eventually be the same.	Used for heartburn, prevention or treatment of active duodenal ulcers, and gastric hypersecretion Used as prophylaxis for stress ulcers
Proton pump inhibitors (PPI) Capsules need to be swallowed whole. May interfere with metabolism and/or absorption of other drugs; check each drug for specific side effects.	esomeprazole (Nexium) lansoprazole (Prevacid) omeprazole (Prilosec) pantoprazole (Protonix) rabeprazole (Aciphex)	Interactions with other drugs may cause poor absorption of some drugs (e.g., iron) and increased serum levels of other drugs (e.g., diazepam, phenytoin, warfarin).	Depending on specific drug: used to treat esophagitis, GERD, gastric and duodenal ulcers, NSAID-related ulcers, and *Helicobacter pylori*
Cholinergic blockers Monitor for frank or occult GI bleeding and abdominal pain. Teach client to avoid GI irritants, such as smoking, alcohol, acetylsalicylic acid (Aspirin)–containing products, caffeine, NSAIDs, and some foods.	glycopyrrolate (Robinul) mepenzolate bromide (Cantil) methscopolamine bromide (Pamine) propantheline	Inhibits GI motility and gastric secretions. Causes tachycardia, dry mouth, constipation, urine retention, or hesitancy.	Used as adjunct therapy for peptic ulcer disease
Miscellaneous antiulceratives Sucralfate may decrease absorption of cimetidine, phenytoin, tetracyclines, and warfarin. Antacids may decrease the effectiveness of sucralfate. Do not use misoprostol during pregnancy; avoid pregnancy if taking this drug.	bismuth subsalicylate (Pepto-Bismol) misoprostol (Cytotec) sucralfate (Carafate)	Bismuth subsalicylate may darken tongue or stools. Misoprostol protects against drug-induced ulcer formation. Sucralfate helps the healing of stomach ulcers by adhering to an ulcer. Its soothing, topical protective coating on the stomach mucosa protects against stomach acids and digestive enzymes.	Used for short-term treatment and prevention of gastric, duodenal, and stress ulcers Used separately or in conjunction with other antacids/antiulceratives to destroy gastric acid by neutralizing all or part of the acid, absorbing the acid, or making the acid inactive
Peptic ulcer disease due to *H. pylori* Teach the client to complete all antibiotic therapies as well as use of H_2 blockers or PPIs.	Antibiotic therapy: combinations of amoxicillin, clarithromycin (Biaxin), tetracycline, and/or metronidazole (Flagyl) with H_2 blocker (e.g., lansoprazole [Prevacid]) or PPIs, or bismuth (Pepto-Bismol)	*H. pylori* is found in about 75% of duodenal ulcers. Most of the remainder of ulcers are caused by NSAIDs. Many individuals infected with *H. pylori* do not develop an ulcer.	Used to kill the microorganism *H. pylori*, which is the underlying cause of most ulcers in peptic ulcer disease and is also related to cancer of the stomach

CHAPTER 88 Digestive Disorders

TABLE 88-3 Classifications of Medications for the Gastrointestinal System (Continued)

CLASSIFICATIONS AND NURSING CONSIDERATIONS	EXAMPLES OF DRUGS	COMMENTS	MAIN INDICATIONS FOR USE
Antidiarrheals Monitor skin turgor and electrolytes because diarrhea may lead to fluid and electrolyte imbalance.	loperamide (Imodium) diphenoxylate (Lomotil) bismuth subsalicylate (Pepto-Bismol) kaolin and pectin mixture (Kapectolin) polycarbophil (FiberCon)	Loperamide (Imodium) and diphenoxylate (Lomotil) have the potential for drug dependence. They may cause sedation, dizziness, constipation, and drying of the mucous membranes.	Used to reduce motility of the GI system
Antiemetics Provide antiemetic therapy before the symptoms start to occur. Preventing the GI upsets from chemotherapy helps to promote compliance with the cancer medication therapies. Because of additive effects with other drugs, may cause CNS depression.	dimenhydrinate (Dramamine) metoclopramide meclizine (Antivert) ondansetron (Zofran) trimethobenzamide (Tigan) **Phenothiazines:** • chlorpromazine (Thorazine) • perphenazine (Trilafon) • prochlorperazine (Compazine) • promethazine (Phenergan)	Dimenhydrinate (Dramamine) and meclizine (Antivert): Used to prevent motion sickness. Metoclopramide: Promotes gastric emptying. The following are used for management of nausea and vomiting associated with chemotherapy: • aprepitant (Emend) • palonosetron (Aloxi) • ondansetron (Zofran) • granisetron • dronabinol (Marinol)	Used to prevent nausea and vomiting by acting on the inner ear (motion sickness) or the CNS (chemotherapy) Phenothiazines have significant side effects, including hypotension, constipation, blurred vision, dry mouth extrapyramidal reactions, and photosensitivity.
Laxatives and cathartics (Box 88-3) Because of reduction of time in small intestine and colon, may have reduced absorption of some orally administered drugs. Fluid and electrolyte imbalances possible.	**Bulk forming:** • methylcellulose (Citrucel) • polycarbophil (FiberCon) • psyllium (Metamucil) **Lubricant:** • mineral oil (Fleet Mineral Oil Enema) **Hyperosmotic:** • lactulose (Enulos, Generlac) **Saline cathartic:** • magnesium sulfate, polyethylene glycol-electrolyte solution (GoLYTELY) **Cathartic/purgative:** • senna (Senokot) • bisacodyl (Dulcolax) • sodium phosphate and sodium biphosphate (Fleet Phospho-soda) **IBS:** • tegaserod maleate (Zelnorm)	For short-term use only; long-term use may lead to electrolyte imbalances and laxative dependence because of the loss of normal gastric motility. Tegaserod maleate (Zelnorm) is used during constipation phase of IBS for women.	Used to treat or prevent constipation Used to prepare for bowel radiologic diagnostic studies Lactulose also used to help manage hepatic encephalopathy
Stool softeners (fecal softeners) May take 1–3 days to see effect; thus, do not use when rapid elimination needed. Can be used for most clients with cardiac conditions.	docusate calcium (Surfak) docusate sodium (Colace, Correctol) docusate sodium with casanthrol (Peri-Colace, Doxidan)	Sometimes a stool softener is combined with a more potent (irritant, bulk, cathartic) laxative for more rapid elimination.	Used to make stool softer for easier elimination Cause elimination without irritating the gastric mucosa or increasing bulk content of intestine

(Continued)

TABLE 88-3 Classifications of Medications for the Gastrointestinal System (Continued)

CLASSIFICATIONS AND NURSING CONSIDERATIONS	EXAMPLES OF DRUGS	COMMENTS	MAIN INDICATIONS FOR USE
Antilipidemic Teach the client that diet modification measures to reduce cholesterol should be considered first.	Cholestyramine (Questran)	Cholestyramine (Questran) may cause constipation, nausea, bloating, abdominal pain, and rash. Cholesterol levels are determined by both food and genetics, so diet restrictions alone may not be effective to reduce cholesterol levels.	Used to lower serum cholesterol by binding bile acids in the intestine

^aGastric irritants include smoking (nicotine), alcohol, acetylsalicylic acid (Aspirin)–containing products, NSAIDs, caffeine, and certain foods. These should be avoided in clients with, or susceptible to, gastrointestinal ulcers and GI bleeding. Cigarette smoking increases gastric acid secretion.
CNS, central nervous system; GERD, gastroesophageal reflux disease; GI, gastrointestinal; IBS, irritable bowel syndrome; NSAIDs, nonsteroidal anti-inflammatory drugs.
From Karch, A., & Tucker, R. (2021). *2020 Lippincott pocket drug guide for nurses*. Wolters Kluwer.

---

first few weeks, the client should eliminate gas-forming and highly seasoned foods and foods high in roughage (e.g., fresh fruits, popcorn, and nuts).

The client should also omit coffee, tea, cola beverages, chocolate, alcohol, and cigarette smoking because they stimulate secretion of hydrochloric acid. The client can include milk and cream, although not in large quantities. Daily eating habits and ulcer management consist of three normal meals and a bedtime snack.

> **Key Concept**
> Cigarette smokers are twice as likely to have ulcers as nonsmokers. Alcohol use also predisposes a client to ulcer formation.

Rest and Stress Management

Rest is important, but it does not necessarily have to be bed rest. Relaxation is even more important; many clients are hospitalized at the onset of treatment to force relaxation. Tranquilizers may also be prescribed. After the course of treatment is established, the client maintains the routine at home.

Nursing Considerations

The goals in ulcer treatment are to prevent irritating the lesion, lessen acidic secretions, reduce activity of the stomach and intestine, and manage emotional stress. Client teaching is an important component. Encourage the client to verbalize their concerns, rather than to internalize them. Physical activity may also help to alleviate frustrations. Stress management workshops and support groups often are beneficial (In Practice: Educating the Client 88-1).

> **NCLEX Alert**
> GI problems are commonly seen in healthcare facilities. NCLEX questions may require knowledge of the medications used for treatments, signs and symptoms of disorders, complications of GI problems, and interventions by the nurse.

Stomach Cancer

Stomach cancer is known as the "silent neoplasm" because it is usually not detected until after metastasis to adjacent structures. Thus, the client's prognosis is often poor. Signs and symptoms include sudden *dyspepsia* (indigestion) unrelieved by eating, which is the most important symptom. In addition, the person experiences unexplained weight loss and generalized weakness. Coffee-ground emesis and the absence of free hydrochloric acid in the stomach are other significant findings. Breath testing for UBT can indicate the presence of *H. pylori*, which is associated with gastric cancer. Diagnosis is generally made after microscopic examination of gastric contents shows cancer cells. Other routine laboratory and x-ray studies confirm the presence of a neoplasm

---

IN PRACTICE
EDUCATING THE CLIENT 88-1 — Ulcer Management

- Follow healthcare provider's treatment plan for elimination of *H. pylori*, if present.
- Three meals and a bedtime snack should be routine.
- Meal size and portions should be at a comfortable and tolerated level. Avoid overdistention.
- Determine and eliminate gastric irritants (foods that aggravate symptoms).
- Eat foods slowly and chew them well.
- Contact a healthcare provider if diarrhea or increased discomfort occurs, or if the condition is not improving.
- Avoid long-term use of over-the-counter medications unless recommended by healthcare provider.
- Use methods of relaxation.
- Verbalize concerns.
- Establish a personal balance between exercise and physical and emotional rest, especially during stressful periods.

Box 88-2 Symptoms of Ulcers and Stomach Cancer

ULCERS
- Frequent dyspepsia
- Burning sensation in stomach (may be seasonal)
- Pain that always begins in same place
- Pain relieved by eating or, possibly, vomiting
- Black, tarry stools (*melena*)
- Free hydrochloric acid in stomach
- Tenseness, irritability
- Difficulty sleeping
- Weight often maintained

STOMACH CANCER
- Sudden dyspepsia
- Absence of pain until cancer is advanced ("silent neoplasm")
- Pain unrelieved by eating or vomiting
- Coffee-ground emesis
- Absence of free hydrochloric acid in stomach
- Weakness, lethargy, tiredness much of the time
- Unexplained weight loss
- Cancer cells possibly visible in slides of gastric contents

and its exact location. Box 88-2 compares the symptoms of ulcers and stomach cancer.

Treatment generally involves surgery to remove the tumor completely. A total or subtotal gastrectomy may be performed, depending on the tumor's size and location. The spleen and many structures surrounding the stomach may be removed as well. Metastasis to the spleen, lymph nodes, liver, pancreas, and esophagus is common. Nursing considerations will include pre- and postoperative teaching as previously discussed for gastric surgeries. Client and family grief counseling may be necessary.

DISORDERS OF THE SMALL OR LARGE BOWEL

Diverticulosis and Diverticulitis

Diverticulosis refers to a condition in which outpouches (ruptures) occur along the intestinal wall. Diverticula can occur anywhere in the GI tract. Symptoms that accompany diverticular disease are vague or absent. Diverticula often are found during diagnostic procedures performed for other problems. A barium enema can confirm the presence of diverticula, but the barium may become trapped in the diverticula and form hard masses. Endoscopy can confirm the diagnosis by permitting direct visualization of the lesions.

Diverticulitis occurs when the diverticula become inflamed, usually because of diverticula obstruction and bacterial invasion. Signs and symptoms of diverticulitis include nagging, cramping pain and tenderness in the left lower abdomen, abdominal distention, flatulence, and elevated temperature. Increased pressure within the lumen of the bowel can cause rupture of the diverticulum and result in abscess formation and peritonitis.

Treatment
Treatment of diverticulosis and diverticulitis consists of dietary management of symptoms, medications, and possible surgery. Consumption of high-residue foods is recommended to prevent the formation of diverticula and to prevent acute onsets of diverticulitis. When diverticula are present and inflamed, stool softeners and bulk-forming agents, such as psyllium (Metamucil), help to produce soft, nonirritating, and unforced bowel movements.

When fever and abdominal pain are present, indicating infection along with inflammation, antibiotics are prescribed. A low-residue diet, including avoidance of milk products, is recommended. During an acute episode of diverticulitis, the client may be assigned NPO status and have an NG tube in place for suctioning to allow the bowel to rest. When acute diverticulitis resolves, the client should begin to add high-fiber foods to the diet and continue to use bulking agents.

Nursing Considerations
Client and family dietary teaching are important aspects of attack prevention, symptoms management, and treatment during attacks. Adequate water intake of six to eight glasses each day is important. Regular bowel habits, regular exercise, and plenty of fruit, vegetables, and fiber are key factors in preventing future problems. Teach the client when to use high-fiber and low-fiber foods.

Hernias

Hernias develop when abdominal muscle weakness causes a portion of the GI tract to protrude through muscle. Herniation often occurs when intra-abdominal pressure increases because of obesity, heavy lifting, coughing, blunt trauma to the abdomen, or pregnancy. A hernia may be reducible, irreducible, incarcerated, or strangulated. A *reducible hernia* is one that may be pushed back into the intestine by lying down and pressing on the abdomen. An *irreducible hernia* cannot be manipulated back into the body cavity. An *incarcerated hernia* occurs when the intestine's peristaltic flow is obstructed. A *strangulated hernia* requires immediate surgical intervention because it interrupts blood flow to the tissue, resulting in tissue necrosis (infarction).

Types of Hernias
Types of hernias include hiatal, inguinal, femoral, umbilical, abdominal, and incisional. Congenital defects are responsible for many hernias; these are often detected soon after birth. An acquired hernia may result from heavy lifting, pregnancy, coughing, or sneezing. Later in life, obesity and muscle weakness may cause hernias.

Hiatal hernias were discussed earlier in the section on the esophagus. *Inguinal hernias* are the most common type of hernia. They protrude through the inguinal area in the groin, especially in males. *Femoral hernias* are weaknesses of the femoral canal that carries blood vessels and nerves into the thigh. *Umbilical hernias* protrude through the umbilicus. An *abdominal hernia* is a protrusion of the intestine through the abdominal wall. The abdominal wall is weak in spots, and it is at these points that a hernia can develop. An *incisional hernia* may develop in an incisional area following surgery.

Signs and Symptoms
Signs and symptoms of hernia vary, depending on the location. Some hernias are asymptomatic, although if they are left untreated, they often enlarge and cause pain. If the condition is allowed to progress, the intestine may become constricted, and the blood supply is cut off (a *strangulated hernia*). This development is an emergency.

Treatment
The person may wear a truss or abdominal support over the herniated area to minimize or reduce the hernia. *Herniorrhaphy* is performed to repair a hernia surgically. It can be done using a laparoscopic extraperitoneal approach (**LEP**) after abdominal insufflation with carbon dioxide. The client will have only two or three small "stab wounds," instead of an incision, resulting in less pain and a shorter postoperative recovery period. This method also results in higher success rates than with traditional herniorrhaphy and in less recurrence.

If the hernia has gone untreated for many years, herniorrhaphy may not hold because the tissues are weakened and do not heal easily. In this case, a *hernioplasty* may be done. This reconstructive repair includes reinforcement with mesh to prevent future weakness and herniation.

Nursing Considerations
Nursing care after herniorrhaphy typically is not complicated; the client is allowed out of bed the day of the operation and can have food and fluids. In many cases, this procedure is done on an outpatient basis. Make sure that the client has voided after surgery; urinary retention is a common problem. Encourage the client to move around, but to avoid straining and lifting for several weeks or months. Returning to routine activities after laparoscopic surgery, especially if mesh reinforcement was used, occurs quickly. The male client's scrotum may become swollen and painful after inguinal hernia repair. An ice pack and a scrotal support may be ordered for relief.

The client's return to work depends on the hernia's nature and extent and the client's age, weight, and type of employment. If the work is heavy or strenuous, vocational counseling and retraining may be necessary. If a repair with mesh has been done, the person will most likely not have any long-term lifting restrictions. A referral to local vocational rehabilitation services and public health nursing services may be helpful.

Intestinal Obstruction

Ileus is obstruction of the intestine. It may be caused by a mechanical or functional difficulty, and it occurs when gas or fluid cannot move normally through the bowel. *Mechanical obstructions* occur when there is a blockage in the lumen or pressure exerted from outside the intestine. Examples include the following:

- Stenosis, strictures, and adhesion scars from previous surgery
- **Volvulus** (twisting of the bowel)
- Foreign bodies, such as a fruit pit
- **Intussusception** (telescoping of the bowel)
- Polyps and tumors (e.g., diverticulosis)
- Abscesses

Functional obstructions occur when the intestinal motility (*peristalsis*) is defective. Examples include the following:

- Paralytic ileus
- Muscle spasms (*spastic ileus*)
- Disorders (e.g., muscular dystrophy, diabetes mellitus, and Parkinson disease)

A vascular obstruction, such as atherosclerosis or thrombus formation, also can cause gradual cessation of peristalsis owing to decreased blood supply. Pneumonia, pancreatitis, and peritonitis can produce obstruction of infectious origin. A decrease or interruption of the nerve stimulus, which may result from postanesthesia paralysis, trauma to the autonomic nervous system, complications from peritonitis, inactivity, large doses of narcotics, or other nerve damage, causes paralytic obstruction (*paralytic ileus*) of the intestine.

Signs and Symptoms
Clinical manifestations of intestinal obstruction depend on the type of lesion causing the obstruction, the level and length of bowel involved, the extent to which the obstruction interferes with the blood supply to the intestine, and the completeness of the obstruction. Early paralytic ileus is marked by decreased or absent bowel sounds.

Abdominal distention, severe cramps, nausea, and vomiting are typical. When listening to abdominal bowel sounds with a stethoscope, the sounds may be high pitched at first and then become silent or absent in one or more quadrants of the abdomen. If the obstruction is high in the GI tract, the client will vomit to empty the stomach of accumulated digestive fluids. As these materials continue to accumulate, the vomitus becomes thick, dark, and foul smelling because the number of bacteria normally present in the digestive tract increases. If the obstruction is further down, vomiting may be absent. The client is listless, generally weak, thirsty, and has a feeling of fullness and constipation. Symptoms of small bowel obstruction develop and progress rapidly; symptoms of large bowel obstruction progress more slowly. If left untreated, the client will become very ill, with symptoms of dehydration and shock.

> **Key Concept**
>
> When auscultating (listening) the abdomen for bowel sounds, be sure to place the stethoscope carefully and listen carefully in all four quadrants. A healthy bowel can have the sounds of peristalsis ranging from 1–4 min apart. In an obstruction, you may hear sounds in some, but not all, quadrants, depending on the location of the blockage. Also, note that if gastric suction is in use, the suction must be turned off before listening for bowel sounds. *Rationale: The sound of the suction can be mistaken for bowel sounds.* Be sure to turn on the suction apparatus again once auscultation is completed.

> **Nursing Alert** An intestinal obstruction can be an emergency; it must be treated immediately. As a tumor in the intestine becomes larger, it may block the lumen of the intestine. An abdominal series will indicate large quantities of fluid or gas in the bowel. Laboratory studies may show infection, electrolyte disruptions, and dehydration.

Treatment

Treatment of the obstruction depends on its cause. Complete obstruction in the small intestine usually necessitates surgery; obstruction in the lower part of the large intestine may be treated medically.

Medical treatment of large bowel obstruction includes intestinal decompression, involving intubation with a nasoenteric tube. Constant suction via a rectal tube may be used to keep the intestine empty. The bowel is allowed to rest. A colonoscopy may be done to attempt to untwist or unblock the bowel.

Nursing Considerations

Assist with fluid and electrolyte replacement. It is important to note the quality of bowel sounds. If the client's condition deteriorates, emergency surgery becomes necessary. Postoperative nursing care follows the protocol for abdominal surgery.

Irritable Bowel Syndrome

Irritable bowel syndrome (**IBS**) is also known as *spastic colon, spastic colitis, mucous colitis,* and *irritable colon.* This condition is the most common functional disorder of the GI tract, which causes increased motility of the small or large intestine. It affects the intestine's structure, but its specific cause is unknown. IBS does not lead to, or cause, ulcerative colitis or cancer.

Signs and Symptoms

IBS causes alternately tense and flaccid bowel segments. Resulting symptoms can include nausea, abdominal pain, cramps, *flatulence* (gas), altered bowel function (constipation or diarrhea), and hypersecretion of colonic mucus. Symptoms vary in intensity and pattern and may be aggravated by foods, alcohol ingestion, stress, and fatigue.

Diagnosis is accomplished by tests, such as the upper GI series and barium enema. Colonoscopy is appropriate for adults because these tests also eliminate other pathologies with similar symptoms.

> **Nursing Alert** Rectal bleeding and fever are not associated symptoms of IBS. The person with these symptoms should report to a healthcare provider for evaluation.

Treatment

An integrated, individualized approach is recommended for the treatment of IBS. Clients must be willing to explore their lifestyle patterns and emotional stressors. They may require lifestyle changes to manage this chronic and frustrating condition. Counseling may be needed, along with biofeedback and relaxation training, which has proved helpful for people with IBS.

A high-fiber diet and agents that add bulk (e.g., psyllium [Metamucil]) help to promote an even and consistent stool to pass through the bowel. The diet also should include adequate oral fluids and regular meal patterns. If the client is subject to lactose intolerance, limitation of dairy products is helpful.

Medications may be prescribed to provide symptomatic relief. For example, sedatives or tranquilizers, such as alprazolam (Xanax), help to quiet the bowel's activity and provide relaxation. Dicyclomine hydrochloride (Bentyl) is an antispasmodic agent that can relieve pain and cramping symptoms if used routinely during periods of increased bowel irritability. Common side effects are dry mouth, blurred vision, and dizziness. Some clients require occasional antidiarrheal agents, such as loperamide (Imodium), to help them maintain normal activity (Box 88-3).

Nursing Considerations

Remind the client to be consistent and follow the prescribed treatment plan closely. Many times clients with IBS get discouraged by seemingly slow improvement or small setbacks, which may keep them from allowing the bowel to establish a more normal pattern. Keeping a log or diary can help the client track progress or identify needed changes.

Constipation

Constipation is a condition in which the client has infrequent, hard bowel movements accompanied by mucus. Constipation may be an acute or chronic condition. The client may have a fecal impaction with loose, watery stool and mucus traveling around the constipated stool. Dehydration, cancer, chemical dependency, or mechanical obstruction may cause this condition. It may also be a psychosomatic disorder. Because prolonged constipation can be a sign of serious difficulty, such as intestinal obstruction or paralytic ileus, immediate action is needed to determine the cause.

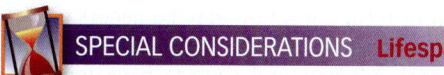

SPECIAL CONSIDERATIONS — Lifespan

Constipation

Older adults are especially susceptible to constipation and its complications. They commonly take multiple medications, which may decrease peristalsis, cause water loss, or interfere with intestinal absorption. In addition, they may have limited mobility or exercise, limited access to proper dietary fiber, and difficulty with chewing, swallowing, or digesting. Daily stool softeners are often suggested; however, regular laxative use should be avoided. An older client complaining of abdominal pain may be constipated, and such concerns should not be ignored. Constipation may lead to the serious complications of impaction and infarction.

Warn the client not to strain while having a stool. Encourage the client to avoid worrying about constipation because undue concern can compound the problem. Teach the client to drink a great deal of fluids, drink prune juice or eat bran, increase dietary bulk, exercise, and follow a regular schedule for defecation. Explain the importance of evacuating the bowel whenever the client feels the urge; postponing the act desensitizes the bowel to the presence of feces.

Removal of feces and flatus can be accomplished by enemas. The client with a disorder of the digestive system may need an enema to prepare for a diagnostic test or surgery, to alleviate symptoms of constipation or distention, or to administer specific medications and fluids.

Box 88-3 Summary of Palliative Medications for Symptomatic Relief of Some GI Disorders

- **Aminosalicylate**
  - sulfasalazine (Azulfidine)
  - mesalamine (Asacol)
  - balsalazide (Colazal)
  - olsalazine (Dipentum)
- **Analgesic**
  - acetaminophen (Tylenol)
- **Antianxiety**
  - diazepam (Valium)
- **Antibiotic**
  - rifaximin (Xifaxan)
  - metronidazole (Flagyl)
  - ciprofloxacin (Cipro)
- **Antidepressant**
  - Selective serotonin reuptake inhibitor (SSRI)
    - fluoxetine (Prozac)
    - paroxetine (Paxil)
  - Tricyclic antidepressant
    - desipramine (Norpramin)
    - imipramine (Tofranil)
    - nortriptyline (Pamelor)
- **Antidiarrhea**
  - diphenoxylate (Lomotil)
  - loperamide (Imodium)
- **Antispasmodic, anticholinergic**
  - atropine (Atropen)
  - dicyclomine (Bentyl)
  - hyoscyamine (Levsin)
- **Bile acid binding agent, bile acid binder**
  - cholestyramine (Prevalite)
  - colesevelam (Welchol)
- **Corticosteroid**
  - prednisone (Deltasone)
  - hydrocortisone (Cortef)
- **Osmotic laxative**
  - magnesium hydroxide (milk of magnesia)
  - lactulose (Enulose, Generlac)
  - polyethylene glycol (MiraLAX)
- **Stimulant laxative**
  - senna glycoside (Senokot)
  - linaclotide (Linzess)
- **Supplemental medication**
  - calcium
  - vitamin D
  - vitamin B_{12}
  - iron supplement
  - fiber supplement
    - psyllium (Metamucil)
    - methylcellulose (Citrucel)

Digital removal of fecal impaction may be necessary for severely constipated or paralyzed clients. The procedure is done only after stool softeners and enemas have failed to remove the mass.

Fecal impaction can develop after a barium enema or barium swallow and should be considered a possible complication of these procedures (Chapter 51).

Nursing Alert Loose, watery stools may not be diarrhea; they may signify severe constipation with leakage of water around the blockage, which can be an indicator of a fecal impaction. A fecal impaction can be the etiology (cause) of a fecal infarction, which can be fatal.

Diarrhea

Diarrhea consists of stools that are liquid or semiliquid and often very light colored. They may be foul smelling and contain mucus, pus, blood, or fats. Diarrhea often is accompanied by flatus and severe, painful abdominal cramps or spasms (**tenesmus**), which defecation relieves. Complications of severe or chronic diarrhea include dehydration, electrolyte disturbances, cardiac dysrhythmias, and hypovolemic shock.

SPECIAL CONSIDERATIONS Lifespan

Giardiasis

Giardiasis, caused by the protozoan *Giardia lamblia*, is commonly associated with contaminated water or food. Daycare centers have experienced outbreaks of diarrhea associated with poor hand-washing between diaper changes and children sharing toys that have been in their mouths. Symptoms may be mild or severe, with nonbloody diarrhea, abdominal pain, and distention. Metronidazole (Flagyl) for adults and furazolidone for children are the usual antibiotic treatments. The entire family or daycare may need stool testing to completely eradicate Giardia infection.

Diarrhea can be a symptom of some underlying condition, such as bacterial invasion by *S. dysenteriae* or *Salmonella*, which may be found in contaminated food. *C. difficile* is an anaerobic bacterium that can be normal in the intestine, but when exposed to antibiotics, it can produce extensive amounts of the bacterium and lead to the development of toxin A and toxin B. *C. difficile* (or "*C. diff*") is often the cause of severe, watery, and bloody diarrhea. This infection occurs frequently as a nosocomial infection in acutely ill hospitalized clients who have received numerous courses of antibiotics. *C. difficile* is also found outside of hospitals as well as being endemic to several cities worldwide. *Pseudomembranous colitis* is related to antibiotic-related diarrhea and is frequently caused by *C. difficile*. These types of severe diarrhea are characterized by offensive-smelling diarrhea, fever, abdominal pain, bleeding disorders, hemorrhage, septic or hypovolemic shock, and toxic megacolon.

IBS or *inflammatory bowel disease* (IBD) often is the cause of diarrhea. Medications, such as certain antibiotics, can cause diarrhea that stops when treatment stops.

Diagnosis

If chronic and not self-limiting, diarrhea symptoms must be evaluated for possible causes (particularly before the client self-medicates). Diarrhea that continually awakens a client from normal sleep often indicates intestinal pathology. A bacterial infection and IBS or IBD should be ruled out.

Stool tests, including cultures, occult blood tests, and ova and parasite (O&P) smears, are performed. Hematology studies indicate infection or inflammatory processes. Lower GI barium examinations are done to rule out pathologic causes.

Treatment

Treatment is geared toward eliminating the cause of the diarrhea. IV fluids and electrolytes may be needed, especially in the young and in older clients (Table 88-3).

Nursing Considerations

Obtain the client's fluid I&O and weight. Monitor for signs and symptoms of electrolyte disturbances and electrolyte levels because diarrhea can severely disrupt electrolyte balance. Record the exact time, amount, and character (TAC) of each stool. You may need to restrict the client's diet to clear liquids and then reintroduce fluids and foods slowly to observe for improvement or worsening. Client and family teaching include criteria to prevent food contamination with *S. aureus* and *Salmonella*, which are often sources of diarrhea.

Inflammatory Bowel Disease

IBD is a general term for ulcerative colitis and Crohn disease. Research suggests that environmental, immunologic, hereditary, age, and cultural factors influence this disease. However, the cause and cure of IBD are unknown. Review the information provided in Chapter 73 regarding IBD.

Ulcerative colitis involves inflammation and ulceration of mucosa and submucosa (the colon's lining). This disease can span the entire length of the colon, but most frequently begins in the rectum and distal colon. *Chronic ulcerative colitis* (CUC) implies long-standing disease. A client's risk of colon cancer increases if CUC lasts longer than 8–10 years.

Crohn disease can occur in any part of the intestinal tract, the most common location being the terminal ileum. Unlike colitis, it involves inflammatory processes of the entire thickness of the bowel wall. It is usually patchy and often skips segments of healthy bowel. The risk of cancer for the client with Crohn disease is the same as that for the general population. Table 88-4 compares ulcerative colitis with Crohn disease.

Signs and Symptoms

Typical symptoms of ulcerative colitis and Crohn disease are diarrhea, blood and mucus in the stool, abdominal pain, cramps, urgency, bowel incontinence, appetite loss, weight loss, fever, nausea, and vomiting. Electrolyte imbalance may result from loss of body fluids. Symptoms may develop gradually or suddenly. Most clients experience patterns of *exacerbation* (attacks) and remission.

Complications

In IBD, bowel obstruction and perforation are threats. They may result from scar tissue or a fistula (abnormal channeling between loops of bowel) and are the most serious complications of these diseases. Perforation is an emergency. Hemorrhage and peritonitis may develop; removal of the colon and permanent ileostomy are often necessary. Symptoms of perforation include rapid, thready pulse; extreme anxiety; severe abdominal pain; fever; abdominal rigidity (boardlike); and cold, clammy skin.

Treatment

Advances in medical treatment allow most clients to manage and cope with IBD. Antidiarrheal medications can allow the client to maintain normal work and daily activity patterns.

Steroids, such as cortisone, which reduce inflammation and generate healing, are given IV, orally, or rectally (foam, suppositories, or enema). Aminosalicylates (sulfasalazine [Azulfidine], mesalamine [Pentasa], and olsalazine [Dipentum]) are the most commonly used drugs to treat IBD, especially ulcerative colitis. Mercaptopurine (Purinethol), methotrexate (Otrexup), and azathioprine (Azasan) are potent immunosuppressants that are useful in treating IBD, especially Crohn disease. Infliximab (Remicade) blocks tumor necrosis factor, which acts to suppress intestinal inflammation. Close monitoring of blood counts and the client's clinical condition is necessary with these medications. IV antibiotics may be indicated during severe flare-ups. Table 88-3 reviews the variety of medications used for gastric problems, especially disorders of the small intestine and the colon.

> **Nursing Alert** Clients are weaned off steroid medications slowly and systematically. They must not stop these medications suddenly. Steroids suppress normal secretions of the adrenal gland, and abrupt discontinuation can trigger life-threatening adrenal insufficiency problems. Milder withdrawal symptoms include yawning, gooseflesh, and muscle aches and pains.

Ulcerative colitis is eliminated by removal of the entire colon, which is the treatment of choice when surgery is necessary. The standard ileostomy allows fecal waste to collect in an appliance attached to the abdomen. Approximately 66% of clients with Crohn disease require surgery, and 40% of these require a second surgery. These high percentages are owing to the typical recurrence of Crohn disease in another bowel segment. The continent bowel diversion procedure of ileoanal reservoir has been effective for those with Crohn disease.

Nursing Considerations

The client who presents with severe symptoms is weak, miserable, and often frightened. Nursing care and medical

TABLE 88-4 Comparison of Inflammatory Bowel Diseases

	ULCERATIVE COLITIS	CROHN DISEASE
Also known as	Ulcerative proctitis	Transmural colitis Regional enteritis Granulomatous colitis
Cause	Unknown, possibly *Escherichia coli*	Unknown, possibly altered immune system
Influences	Environment, heredity, allergies, age, culture, women more than men	Same as for ulcerative colitis
Location	Mucosa and submucosa of colon and rectum; may be localized, but ultimately spreads throughout colon, commonly in left colon and rectum	Entire thickness of wall of small or large intestine in segmented areas; commonly in right colon and ileum
Pathology	Recurrent inflammation and ulceration of colon, with formation of abscesses, purulent drainage, and sloughing of mucosa; capillaries become weak and bleed	Acute and chronic inflammation that erodes wall of intestine; fistulas, fissures, and abscesses form
Signs and symptoms	Nausea, vomiting, anorexia, weight loss, fever, abdominal pain and cramping, diarrhea with pus and blood, bowel incontinence; stenosis is common Stools: 10–20 liquid stools per day with blood and pus (no fat)	Nausea, vomiting, anorexia, weight loss, abdominal pain and cramping, diarrhea, mostly without blood, steatorrhea (fat in stool); stenosis is uncommon Stools: Three or more times per day; diarrhea not as severe as ulcerative colitis, occasional blood, steatorrhea
Complications	*Toxic megacolon* (severe dilation of colon), electrolyte disturbances, abscesses, fistulas, perforation of colon, increased risk of colorectal cancer	Malabsorption of nutrients, electrolyte disturbances, abscesses, fistulas, bowel obstruction, perforation of colon, increased risk of cancer with age
Medical interventions	Bowel rest, low-residue and increased protein diet, decreased lactose intake, vitamin supplements, IV therapy with electrolyte replacement, TPN, sedation, antidiarrheal medications, sulfonamides, antibiotics, corticosteroids	Same as for ulcerative colitis
Surgical interventions	Colostomy (curative if entire colon is removed)	Segmental or total colectomy, removal of diseased areas with anastomosis of bowel (not curative)
Nursing implications	Avoid laxatives and enemas; monitor I&O, nutrient status, laboratory values; encourage client to express feelings; offer support and encouragement	Same as for ulcerative colitis

I&O, intake and output; IV, intravenous; TPN, total parenteral nutrition.

treatment, including the use of anticholinergic, antidiarrheal, and antispasmodic agents, are used to promote optimal bowel rest.

The client is NPO or limited to clear liquids. TPN is often used when a client has not responded to medical intervention and is being prepared for, or has undergone, intestinal resection. The client may receive oral supplements only if tolerated.

Nutritional deficiencies are very common in IBD. The prescribed diet for the person with IBD will probably be high in protein and calories, low residue, and lactose restricted. Anemia and vitamin deficiencies can be treated nutritionally or with supplements.

Although recent studies have indicated that emotional stress does not contribute to the development of the disease, emotional stress can aggravate and stimulate physical symptoms. Be sensitive and supportive to help the client cope with disease-related stressors, which include symptoms, diagnostic tests, bowel preparation, dietary restrictions, activity limitations, and medication side effects.

Appendicitis

Appendicitis is an inflammation of the approximately 4 in. (10 cm) of slender blind tube that open off the tip of the cecum. The appendix may become obstructed by a hard mass of feces, with subsequent inflammation, infection, gangrene, and possible perforation. A ruptured appendix is serious because intestinal contents can escape into the abdomen and cause peritonitis or an abscess.

Signs and Symptoms

An acute attack of appendicitis usually begins with progressively severe generalized abdominal pain, which later localizes as pain and tenderness in the lower right quadrant midway between the umbilicus and the crest of the ilium (*McBurney point*). An attack of appendicitis may subside and then recur.

Ultrasound can often diagnose an enlarged appendix. Rebound tenderness usually is present: when the examiner quickly releases pressure during a palpation assessment, the pain becomes greater than when the pressure was directly on the site.

The quality of the tenderness relates to the exact location of the appendix. Usually nausea, vomiting, a mild to moderate fever, and an increase in leukocytes accompany the pain. A ruptured appendix will result in more severe symptoms associated with peritonitis.

Treatment

Prompt surgical treatment is necessary to remove an acute appendix before it ruptures. Trends toward minimally invasive surgery techniques, such as laparoscopic appendectomy, have lessened the chances of wound infection. Incisions are smaller, and recovery periods are shorter.

In most instances, the client recovers rapidly, is permitted fluids and food, and is allowed out of bed soon after the operation. The client may return to work in 10–15 days, with cautions to avoid heavy lifting.

If the appendix ruptures, treatment for peritonitis is necessary. Treatment includes an incisional drainage tube and large doses of IV antibiotics. Rupture is a serious and possibly fatal complication. However, modern treatment with suction devices, irrigation of the peritoneum, IV fluids, and antibiotics has greatly reduced this danger.

Nursing Considerations

Many people mistake abdominal pain, nausea, and vomiting as a temporary intestinal upset. Teach all clients what to do, and especially what not to do, for severe abdominal pain (In Practice: Educating the Client 88-2).

PERITONITIS

Peritonitis is inflammation of the peritoneum, the membrane that lines the abdominal cavity and covers the abdominal organs. Peritonitis usually results from perforation of the intestine or appendix, through which intestinal contents escape into the abdomen. Because the intestinal tract is normally filled with bacteria, the resulting perforation can cause inflammation and peritoneal infection. The most common causes of perforation are appendicitis, ulcer, IBD, abscessed diverticula, and cancer. An infected uterine tube, a ruptured tubal pregnancy, or a ruptured uterus may cause pelvic peritonitis. Peritonitis may be generalized, extending throughout the peritoneum, or it may be localized as an abscess.

Signs and Symptoms

Peritonitis often develops suddenly, with severe abdominal pain, nausea, and vomiting; a gradual temperature increase; a weak and rapid pulse; and low blood pressure. The client's respirations are shallow because breathing hurts the abdomen; the client tries to avoid moving the abdomen and draws up the knees to prevent pressure from the bedclothes and to relieve pain. The abdomen is tense and boardlike and becomes very distended.

Flatus and intestinal contents are stationary in the intestinal tract, and paralytic ileus may develop. If the infection does not respond to treatment, the client grows weaker. The pulse is thready, breathing becomes shallow, temperature falls, and death follows. Diagnosis of peritonitis is made by evaluation of symptoms, laboratory studies, abdominal x-ray examination, ultrasounds, or CT scans. White blood cell counts can be quite high, and the client presents as acutely ill.

Treatment

Surgery is sometimes necessary to close the perforation and promote drainage, although the perforation may close by itself. During surgery, the peritoneum is irrigated, usually with a saline and antibiotic solution. Peritonitis is less common today, and recovery is more likely, largely because of improvements in surgery and the use of antibiotics.

Nursing Considerations

Nursing considerations focus on postoperative care of the client. Administer antibiotics to fight infection and analgesics to relieve pain and provide rest. Elevate the head of the bed to the semi-Fowler position, and closely observe the abdominal wound, pulse, and temperature. Monitor incisional or drainage tube output (amount and type), vomiting, drainage through the GI tube, and fluid I&O; replace fluids and electrolytes.

Document bowel sounds and gas and feces passing through the rectum; these signs indicate return of normal GI function. Prevent abdominal distention by using a rectal or NG tube; excess distention is uncomfortable and can disrupt the suture line or cause other difficulties owing to pressure. Give special attention to mouth care because the client has no fluids by mouth; fever and the GI tube make the mouth dry and parched. Encourage early, progressive activity to promote peristaltic movement and normal GI function.

IN PRACTICE
EDUCATING THE CLIENT 88-2 — Actions to Take in Severe Abdominal Pain

- Do not take an enema or a cathartic. *Rationale:* They increase peristalsis, and the result may be a perforated appendix and peritonitis. If an enema is ordered as a preoperative measure, it must be given low and very slowly.
- Do not take anything by mouth, not even water.
- Call a healthcare provider for any attack of severe pain or for pain that persists.
- Do not apply heat to the abdomen. *Rationale:* Heat could spread infection.
- Do not take acetylsalicylic acid (Aspirin) or any other analgesic. *Rationale:* They tend to mask symptoms. Acetylsalicylic acid (Aspirin) and ibuprofen (Motrin) are anticoagulants.

Cancer of the Small Intestine

Cancer occurs rarely in the small intestine. However, an increased risk of cancer accompanies ulcerative colitis. If cancer does occur in the small intestine, the person's prognosis is usually poor because the disease is difficult to discover in its early stage. Usually it is asymptomatic. As the cancer advances, pain may be present. The client may have diarrhea (with or without blood), anorexia, nausea, and vomiting. Perforation or obstruction may occur.

The portion of the bowel containing the tumor may be removed and the ends of the bowel joined. Such anastomosis is impossible if malignancy is extensive. Suction relieves distention, IV fluids are given, and antibiotics may be prescribed. Postoperative nursing care is routine.

Colorectal Cancer

Colorectal cancer includes cancerous growths of the colon, rectum, and appendix. The etiology is typically mushroom-shaped polyps that are usually benign, but are known to become malignant over time. Early detection by colonoscopy is the preferred method of surveillance for polyps. Diagnosis is made by colonoscopy with biopsy of polyps. Rectal cancer is not as common as colon cancer. Risk factors include the following:

- Family history of cancer, especially of the rectum, bowel, or female reproductive organs
- Family history of ulcerative colitis or Crohn disease
- Presence of precancerous or bleeding polyps
- Change in bowel habits (constipation and diarrhea)
- Rectal bleeding or blood in the stool
- High-fat diet
- Low-residue diet

> **Key Concept**
>
> Screening tests, such as rectal examination, proctoscopy (sigmoidoscopy), and colonoscopy, can discover colorectal cancer early. Monitoring for occult blood may also be done as part of screening. These tests are often recommended for clients older than 40 years who are at risk.

Signs and Symptoms

Signs and symptoms include nausea, vomiting, weight loss, abdominal cramping or fullness, change in bowel habits (diarrhea, constipation, or both), tenesmus (ineffective, painful straining at stool), excessive flatus, anemia, rectal bleeding, rectal pain, anorexia, and **cachexia** (general ill health and malnutrition).

Treatment

Treatment generally consists of various regimens of chemotherapy, radiation, and surgery (Chapter 83). If a cancerous growth is in the upper part of the rectum, it can be removed without removal of the rectal sphincter; ultimately, the bowel will function normally. If the tumor involves the rectal opening, a dual operation is necessary through the abdomen from above (including a colostomy) and through the perineum from below. This second type of surgery is called an *abdominal–perineal resection*. With surgical staplers and other newer instruments, some surgeons have successfully retained the rectal sphincter, performing a low resection and anastomosis to eliminate the need for a permanent colostomy.

Nursing Considerations

Nursing considerations relate to the stage of the disease and the course of treatment. Nursing care for the client who has had surgery for rectal cancer is extensive. Carefully monitor the trends of vital signs to detect early signs of hemorrhage. Check dressings for bleeding at regular intervals. The danger of shock after this surgery is great. Nursing measures often include caring for a colostomy, administering parenteral fluids (including blood transfusion), NG suctioning, caring for bladder drainage (a Foley catheter is usually inserted in the bladder), and irrigating and caring for drainage from the perineal wound. Turn the client frequently to prevent respiratory complications and thrombophlebitis; finding a comfortable position may be difficult. If the client's condition permits, encourage them to ambulate as soon as possible after surgery, usually within 2 days. Recovery is much faster if the client ambulates soon; however, they will require your assistance.

DISORDERS OF THE SIGMOID COLON AND RECTUM

Hemorrhoids

Hemorrhoids are swollen (*varicose*) veins of the anus or rectum. *External hemorrhoids* protrude as lumps around the anus. They are painful, especially if the client is constipated and strains to have a bowel movement. They may alternately appear and disappear.

Signs and Symptoms

Usually, external hemorrhoids do not bleed, but they may become large, painful, and itchy. Uterine pressure on the rectum during pregnancy, intra-abdominal tumors, constipation, diarrhea, obesity, heart failure, and portal hypertension are major causes. *Internal hemorrhoids* develop inside the anal sphincter; they may bleed, but are unlikely to be painful if they do not protrude. Signs of bleeding may be no more than a drop of blood on the toilet paper, or bleeding may be so extensive and continuous that it causes anemia. Internal hemorrhoids almost always protrude on defecation, but at first the client can push them back with the finger. As hemorrhoids grow larger, pushing them back is no longer possible, and they discharge blood and mucus. The proctoscope allows the provider to inspect inside the rectum, to visualize hemorrhoids, and to take a biopsy sample.

Treatment

Prophylactic treatment of minor hemorrhoids involves the use of warm sitz baths, prescription and nonprescription anesthetic ointments or suppositories, or witch hazel compresses such as Tucks. Proper diet that involves roughage (i.e., high fiber) foods helps. Stool softeners can be used in addition to other measures. Eliminating chronic constipation can help prevent the development or exacerbation of painful hemorrhoidal episodes. If surgery is necessary, the options include the tying off and excision of the veins (*hemorrhoidectomy*), the banding of the most problematic hemorrhoids, or the cauterization of one or more hemorrhoids. A nonsurgical method of shrinking hemorrhoids is *infrared coagulation (IRC) therapy*. The client is positioned on the left side and the healthcare provider inserts an **anoscope**, a speculum specifically used for the anus and rectum. Through the anoscope, an infrared light wand is inserted. The infrared light is applied to the tissues for a few seconds; the client may feel a burning discomfort for a few seconds. Sometimes a solution is injected to shrink (*sclerose*) the tissues. Occasionally, hemorrhoidectomy must be done if the hemorrhoid is thrombosed, causing vascular obstruction. This situation is not life threatening; surgery is done to relieve moderate to severe chronic pain.

Nursing Considerations

Follow any other presurgical protocol such as cleansing enemas, cleansing the area with antimicrobial wash, and a shave of the local area. When the client returns from the operating room, position them on the side or abdomen to relieve pressure on the operative area. Give analgesics, as ordered. A liquid diet is permitted for the first meal after the operation; thereafter, a full diet is allowed.

Allow the client to sit up. Relieve pressure on the operative area using appropriate comfort aids. The client needs to move as soon as possible to prevent postoperative complications. On the operative day or the next day, the healthcare provider will want the client to ambulate. Sitting for long periods of time is not recommended because the rectal area becomes edematous and painful.

Several daily sitz baths may be ordered. If a porcelain sitz bath is used, be aware that the heat of the bath may cause vasodilation and make the person feel faint. Most facilities have eliminated the permanent, in-place sitz bath structures and replaced them with personal, portable sitz units that fit on top of the commode. The client should continue therapy for about 20 min, with the water's temperature at 110 °F (43.3 °C). It is best if the water circulates.

Because removal of hemorrhoids involves excision of portions of blood vessels, bleeding may occur. Monitor and document any signs of bleeding, either on the dressings or as indicated by symptoms of faintness, weakness, lowered blood pressure, or other signs of shock.

The client will need assistance with the first bowel movement following any rectal surgery. The client is naturally apprehensive. Explain that stool softeners are given to make the bowel movement easier. The client may feel some pain, but probably much less than they imagine beforehand.

Encourage the client to heed the urge to defecate; otherwise, constipation may develop. They should not use toilet paper because it may damage the suture line. Tucks are often used to cleanse and soothe the anal area and to relieve itching.

Petrolatum applied around the rectal area when moist compresses are being used helps maintain the skin's elasticity and integrity. If the client is unable to defecate by the second postoperative day, report this finding to the healthcare provider. If defecation has not occurred by the third day, an enema will probably be ordered.

Because the surgery was performed in close proximity to the urinary structures, anesthesia or manipulation may make voiding difficult. If the client does not void, distention could cause complications and discomfort, and catheterization will be needed.

Anal Fissure

An *anal fissure* is an ulcer in the skin of the anal wall. It causes severe pain on defecation and sometimes slight bleeding. The client may dread the pain so much that they delay defecation and become constipated. Sitz baths and local anesthetic ointments are commonly used to treat anal fissure; a stool softener also helps. The only cure for this condition is surgical removal of the ulcer.

Anal Abscess and Anal Fistula

An *anal abscess* is caused by infected tissue around the rectal area. This condition is painful and may be accompanied by fever and chills. The abscess is usually incised and drained, or it may rupture spontaneously. An *anal fistula* usually develops as a result of an anal abscess. A small tunnel forms in the tissues and discharges pus and feces through one or more openings onto the skin.

Treatment

Surgery is necessary to open the fistulous tract; medication-impregnated packing is inserted to keep the wound's edges apart. These measures allow the tissues to heal by granulation, thus eliminating the fistula. The fistula must heal from the inside out, or another abscess will form.

Nursing Considerations

Generally, nursing care is similar to that for any client after rectal surgery, with the following differences. Pack the fistula wound with petroleum gauze and change the dressing every day. Drainage from the abscess is profuse, purulent, and foul smelling. You need to change the dressing on the wound frequently. Dispose of dressings properly and wear gloves to prevent the spread of disease. Keep the fistula draining. If it stops draining before the entire area is filled in with granulation tissue, another abscess will form.

DISORDERS OF THE LIVER

Liver Failure

Liver failure (hepatic coma) occurs when the liver cells fail to clear toxins. The waste products build up in the body, resulting in diminished cerebral function. Liver failure can be an acute or chronic condition. The liver has the ability to repair some of its **parenchymal cells**, that is, those cells that perform the normal functions of the liver; therefore, damage can be chronic and ongoing. Causes include extensive damage to liver cells and hepatomegaly, such as may occur after massive GI hemorrhage, as a complication of anesthesia, secondary to sepsis or massive infections, and following an overdose of certain drugs. It also occurs in the client with alcoholic liver disease such as cirrhosis.

SPECIAL CONSIDERATIONS — Lifespan

Overdose on Acetaminophen

Clients who overdose on acetaminophen (Tylenol) are at risk for fulminant hepatic failure. Small children who accidentally ingest even a few tablets could have significant problems. Appropriate therapy should begin within 24 hr of ingestion.

Signs and Symptoms

Liver failure is characterized by tremors and mental changes, including seizures, stupor, and coma. Fulminant hepatic failure involves progressive multisystem failure resulting from massive liver cell death. Acute hepatitis B infections may be the initial causative agent. Clients are confused, *somnolent* (very sleepy), or comatose and usually have ascites, edema, *coagulopathy* (clotting disorder), and a shrinking liver. The mortality rate from this condition is high, and care is supportive. Diagnosis is made by LFT. Blood ammonia levels are high because the liver cells cannot convert ammonia to urea. Ammonia, a by-product of protein metabolism, is toxic to the brain.

Treatment

Treatment of liver failure is symptomatic, including control of bleeding, a low-protein diet, and careful management of fluid and electrolyte balance. Antibiotics may be given, and, in some cases, corticosteroids. The client's prognosis is guarded, and the possibility of successful treatment decreases with each episode. See In Practice: Nursing Care Guidelines 88-3 for nursing care of the client with a liver disorder.

Cirrhosis

Cirrhosis is a chronic, degenerative disease of the parenchymal cells of the liver. Due to the damaged parenchymal cells, the liver ultimately will lose its ability to function as a liver cell. The hepatocytes become infiltrated with fatty and fibrous tissue (nonparenchymal tissue) that cannot detoxify body waste. *Intrahepatic obstructive jaundice* results when hepatocytes are no longer able to function. All body functions eventually deteriorate.

Uncontrolled cirrhosis may result in *hepatorenal syndrome* and *hepatic coma*. Toxins absorbed by the GI tract are not metabolized properly and are allowed to circulate freely in the brain, producing *hepatic encephalopathy*.

In an effort to repair itself by creating new liver cells, the liver may become enlarged, which is known as *hepatomegaly*. Due to the backup and poor flow of fluids within the portal circulatory system, *portal hypertension develops*. Portal hypertension can accompany systemic hypertension, which exacerbates the overall situation. Disturbed liver metabolism also permits the accumulation of hormones that regulate sodium and water, which can lead to a further increase in portal hypertension and ascites.

Increased pressure in the hepatic portal system, combined with decreased production of albumin by hepatocytes and the development of ascites, leads to the formation of esophageal varices. Esophageal varices often rupture, causing massive *hematemesis* (bloody emesis) and hypovolemic shock. If the person survives the hemorrhage, the body's defenses are reduced, and they are more susceptible to infection.

Cirrhosis is more prevalent among men than women and occurs most often in people between the ages of 45 and 65 years. Chronic, long-term alcohol abuse is the most common cause of liver failure, cirrhosis, ascites, and esophageal varices. Drugs, toxins, and certain general anesthetics, as well as several types of viral hepatitis, also can lead to liver dysfunction, cirrhosis, and ascites.

Signs and Symptoms

Cirrhosis may develop so gradually that the client may not realize that anything is wrong and may experience only indigestion and anorexia. The client may be unaware of a low-grade fever or of weight loss because an increase in abdominal girth (caused by ascites) offsets the weight loss. As cirrhosis advances, the client has abdominal pain and a rapid pulse, and breathing becomes difficult because of the enlarged abdomen.

The client tends to bleed easily; blood appears in vomitus or as a nosebleed, and veins are dilated because of portal

---

IN PRACTICE

NURSING CARE GUIDELINES 88-3 — Caring for the Client With a Liver Disorder

- Use starch baths, calamine lotion, and tepid sponging for relief from itching. Place calamine lotion and cotton at the bedside, so the client can apply lotion to spots that itch. Make sure that nails are trimmed. *Rationale: Pruritus is a common symptom in liver disorders.*
- If ascites is present, place the client in a high- or semi-Fowler position. *Rationale: These positions facilitate respiration and gas exchange.*
- Look for signs of blood in the stool and urine or on the toothbrush when the client brushes the teeth. Look for black and blue marks. *Rationale: These are signs of a bleeding disorder, a common complication of liver disease.*
- Exert pressure on the puncture site for a longer time than usual after the needle is withdrawn during any procedure. *Rationale: This prevents a hematoma that would ooze blood and makes it impossible to use the vein again. This is important because people with liver conditions need frequent blood tests.* A central line or heparin lock is often in place. (Apply pressure to the site of an intramuscular injection as well.)
- Provide support and explain jaundice. *Rationale: The sense of self-worth can be impaired because of the client's yellow appearance.*

hypertension. The client is jaundiced, and the skin is dry. They feel weak and confused. Hemorrhaging and infection may develop. Diagnosis is made on the basis of symptoms, medical history, x-ray studies, and biopsy. Serial LFTs are usually done to monitor the extent of the condition.

Treatment

Treatment for liver cirrhosis aims at helping the liver repair itself to maximize liver function. It extends over a long period. In the client with liver failure, at least 2 months are needed before improvements can be noted. The treatment goal is to stop or delay the progression of symptoms.

Alcohol avoidance is a must. Client teaching and referrals to proper agencies that may assist the client to abstain from drinking alcoholic products are important initial steps. Dietary management may require the restriction of dietary protein. Maintaining electrolyte balance will also help lower the ammonia levels. The medication lactulose will promote ammonia retention and excretion through the GI tract. To relieve pressure from the fluid of ascites, an abdominal paracentesis may be performed.

Providing a safe and controlled environment will prolong life and stabilize the condition. Care must be taken to prevent complications associated with the client's activity intolerance, such as pneumonia and thrombophlebitis.

Nursing Considerations

Teach the client that compliance with dietary and fluid restrictions is necessary to promote health. The diet is high in vitamins, moderate in carbohydrates and fats, and low in sodium; the amount of protein depends on the liver's functional level. If these essential nutrients are not supplied, the body burns up its store of protein, thus increasing accumulation of ammonia (a waste product) in the blood. Teach the client to omit alcohol, tobacco, and fatty foods (pork, bacon, gravies, pastries). Give small liquid or semisolid meals frequently because they are usually more appealing to the person with a poor appetite. Frequent oral hygiene may promote an increase in appetite. The diet is often supplemented with multivitamins and vitamin B_{12}. Vitamin K is given (usually subcutaneously) to reduce the risk of hemorrhage. Watch for bruising on the skin (*petechiae*) and bleeding following an injection.

Diuretics and reduced sodium intake are ordered. Monitor daily weights and accurate I&O, which will indicate if the liver is functioning. Take abdominal girth measurements as often as ordered. Position the client in a semi-Fowler position to aid breathing. Good skin care is important. Emollient baths may be ordered to reduce *pruritus* (itching) and to soothe the skin (In Practice: Nursing Care Guidelines 88-3). Clients who show signs and symptoms of hepatic encephalopathy need much attention and monitoring because of their altered level of consciousness.

> **Nursing Alert** When caring for a client with cirrhosis of the liver, nutrients such as salt are often restricted. During client teaching sessions, encourage a diet rich in vitamins. A moderate amount of carbohydrates is needed. Protein intake may be monitored.

Hepatitis

Hepatitis is an acute or chronic condition of liver inflammation that may also be accompanied by liver tissue damage. Viruses are the most prevalent causes of hepatitis, affecting several hundred million people throughout the world. Alcohol, some drugs, and some autoimmune conditions also cause forms of hepatitis (Table 88-5).

Signs and Symptoms

Signs and symptoms of hepatitis are varied and often subtle, making diagnosis and prevention difficult (Box 88-4). Diagnosis is made by general LFTs and specific antibody testing for viruses. Blood tests can distinguish among many of the viruses that cause most cases of hepatitis.

TABLE 88-5 Comparing Types of Hepatitis

	HEPATITIS A	HEPATITIS B	HEPATITIS C	HEPATITIS D	HEPATITIS E	TOXIC HEPATITIS
Routes of transmission	Enteric (oral–fecal); close contact with contaminated person; ingestion of contaminated food or drinks	Blood, semen, and body fluids from contaminated person; contaminated needles; maternal–neonate transmission	Blood, semen, and body fluids from contaminated person; contaminated needles	Blood semen and body fluids from contaminated person; contaminated needles	Enteric (oral–fecal); contaminated water supply	Inhalation, ingestion, injection of anesthetic gases, chemicals
Notes	Self-limiting; may be asymptomatic; frequently found in daycare centers before use of vaccine	Linked to chronic hepatitis; increased risk of liver cancer	Linked to chronic hepatitis; increased risk of liver cancer and cirrhosis	Linked to chronic hepatitis; coinfection with hepatitis B	Self-limiting; rare in the United States	Chemicals damage liver tissue or cannot be excreted
Vaccination available	Yes	Yes	No	No	No	No

Adapted from https://www.cdc.gov/hepatitis/index.htm

> **Box 88-4 Common Presenting Signs and Symptoms of Hepatitis**
>
> - Fatigue and lethargy
> - Nausea (sometimes vomiting and diarrhea)
> - Loss of appetite
> - Abdominal pain
> - Joint and muscle aches
> - Mild fever (more common in hepatitis A)
> - Malaise (generalized feeling and complaint of illness)
> - Jaundice
> - Liver enlargement (*hepatomegaly*)
> - Dark urine

Types of Hepatitis

Hepatitis A

Hepatitis A virus (**HAV**) is the most common form of viral hepatitis. It is spread by the oral–fecal route and is transmitted through contaminated food, water, or infected food handlers. Oral–anal sexual practices also can transmit the virus. HAV primarily affects children and young adults. This disease is attributed to poor sanitation, crowded conditions, and difficulty in recognizing disease carriers. It is preventable by immunization against hepatitis A. In HAV, the greatest excretion of the virus occurs before jaundice appears. As the disease runs its course, the person becomes less infectious. Thus, the client may unknowingly spread the disease to others. A person who has been exposed may be given immune serum globulin as a prophylactic measure.

Generally, the client is noninfectious approximately 1 month after becoming ill. A person may harbor the virus without actually having the clinical disease. No adequate protection against carriers is known. Clients generally recover fully in 4–6 weeks with rest and supportive care. They acquire a lifelong immunity to HAV infection and do not develop chronic hepatitis.

Hepatitis B

Hepatitis B virus (**HBV**) is transmitted by three mechanisms:

1. Percutaneous transmission through infected blood, blood products, needles, or other invasive instruments. Blood transfusions are rarely a source of HBV contamination
2. Sexual transmission in semen or saliva
3. Perinatal transmission from an infected mother to their child at birth

Those at increased risk of exposure include IV drug users who share needles, sexually active homosexual individuals, clients receiving hemodialysis, individuals in mental institutions, and infants of women who are HBV carriers. Vaccination is recommended for infants, children, adolescents, and adults. Healthcare workers are at significant risk and should follow standard precautions rigorously to protect themselves. Pre-exposure HBV vaccination is highly recommended for people working in a healthcare field, such as medicine, nursing, physical therapy, dentistry, or medical laboratories.

The synthetic vaccinations Recombivax-B or Engerix-B are given in three intramuscular injections at 0, 1, and 6 months. A titer blood test confirms the presence of antibodies. If the vaccine recipient does not produce antibodies, they may receive a booster. If the person still does not form antibodies, they are classified as a "nonreactor." A significant percentage of healthy people are nonreactors; the reason is unknown. Many institutions are providing these vaccinations for their at-risk healthcare workers free of charge.

Tracing the exact source of the disease is often difficult because the incubation period of HBV is from 60 to 110 days. The acute symptoms of HBV are more clinically severe and longer lasting than are those of HAV, although they may include any of those listed in the previous section.

Recovery and resolution of HBV infection occurs in all but approximately 17% of infected people. Overwhelming acute HBV infection and liver tissue damage can progress to fulminant hepatic failure and death within weeks of clinical onset. Also, a small percentage (5%–10%) of people do not clear the virus from their blood within 6 months and become chronic carriers of HBV. Persistent HBV infection also increases one's risk of liver cancer.

Hepatitis C

*Hepatitis C is caused by the hepatitis C virus (**HCV**). Individuals with the greatest risk of contracting HCV are IV drug users and individuals who received blood products before changes in laboratory testing for HCV. At least four different subtypes of HCV are active within the United States. There is no vaccine for HCV.*

The incubation of the virus ranges from 35 to 70 days. The clinical manifestations of HCV are typical of the other viral hepatitis infections. Often, symptoms are mild enough for the affected individual to overlook and not seek medical intervention. However, 50% of these clients later present with chronic disease and, of those, 20% develop liver cirrhosis. Half of all people newly infected with HCV will become lifetime carriers of the virus. Liver cancer is also associated with HCV. Interferons, such as interferon alfa-2b (Intron A) and ribavirin (Copegus), an antiviral medication, are used to ease symptoms and slow the progression of chronic hepatitis. These clients are often good candidates for liver transplant.

Hepatitis D

The hepatitis D virus (HDV) causes serious liver disease and relies on HBV to replicate. Individuals infected with HBV contract **HDV** as a *coinfection* or a *suprainfection* (at the same time). The severity of HDV seems to be related to the severity and virulence of the HBV infection. Interferon is helping those who have developed the chronic form of HDV. Transmission, expected recovery outcomes, and prevention are the same as for HBV. There is no vaccine for HDV.

Hepatitis E

Although hepatitis E virus (**HEV**) is rare in the United States, it is sporadically epidemic in countries with contaminated water supplies and inadequate sanitation systems. The mode of transmission is oral–fecal. Typically, HEV is an acute infection and does not develop into a chronic infection. There is no vaccination for HEV available in the United States. Individuals who are traveling to foreign countries need a clear understanding of prevailing conditions and take necessary precautions for safe and healthy visits. Precautions for travelers are available on Websites for the World Health

Organization and the Centers for Disease Control and Prevention. On return from visiting vulnerable countries, the individual should be alert for signs and symptoms of illness and seek medical assistance as early as possible. Recovery is usually complete, and lifetime immunity to HEV occurs. However, a high mortality rate exists in infected pregnant women.

Drug-Induced or Toxic Hepatitis

Liver injury can result from ingestion or exposure to known or unknown drugs, chemicals, or fumes. These chemicals damage liver tissue or collect in the body and the liver cannot excrete them. These events may cause no symptoms other than elevated LFTs; however, a person may exhibit fully developing fulminant hepatic failure. The liver has great regenerating ability, and treatment focuses on clearing the offending agent.

Nursing Considerations

Supportive rest and care while monitoring liver function and electrolyte balance are necessary. Treatment and nursing care are similar for all forms of viral and nonviral hepatitis.

Reduce fatigue by emphasizing bed rest and avoidance of any strenuous physical activity during the acute phase of infection and when symptoms are present, especially jaundice, abdominal discomfort, and abnormal liver tests.

Too much activity too soon is likely to bring on a symptom recurrence. This period may be boring for the client, especially if they were active before the illness. Helping the client to gain knowledge of liver disease and understanding of the particular viral infection will help the person consider possible consequences and lifestyle changes. This time can be frightening or enlightening. Supportive listening is an effective tool to help clients recover.

Older adults or those who develop ascites or encephalopathy may require in-hospital treatment. This treatment includes maintenance of a nutritionally balanced diet, which includes IV hydration and electrolyte management. Injections of vitamin K and fresh frozen plasma may be beneficial. These individuals should use medications sparingly and avoid alcohol completely.

Closely observe Standard Precautions when caring for clients with hepatitis. Warn clients never to donate blood if they have ever had an HBV or HCV infection. *Rationale: The virus can be present in the blood and body fluids for an entire lifetime.*

Liver Abscess

Liver abscesses are caused by the spread of infection from some part of the intestinal tract, perhaps the appendix or gallbladder, or by obstruction of the bile tracts. Symptoms are chills, fluctuating temperature (intermittent fever), extreme weight loss, nausea and vomiting, abdominal distention, and right-sided pain in the abdomen and shoulder. Jaundice occurs frequently. Pain over the liver is a later symptom.

If the abscess bursts, it scatters infection through the abdominal or chest cavity. Antibiotics are given, and the outcome depends on how successful the person is at combating the infection. Sometimes, an attempt is made to establish drainage by surgery. Standard Precautions help prevent the spread of infection.

Trauma

Frequently, the liver is injured in an accident. Extensive damage is likely to be fatal, and the client may die of hemorrhage before reaching an emergency department. Signs and symptoms may include orthostatic hypotension, low blood pressure, tachycardia, and shock. Diagnosis may be made using these symptoms and a history of recent trauma. Many clients with a ruptured liver die.

Generally, surgery is necessary to control bleeding or to remove a portion of the damaged liver. One great danger accompanying liver surgery is hemovolemic shock because the liver is such a vascular organ. Nursing considerations include careful monitoring of vital signs, abdominal inspection, and assisting in treating shock. Use careful sterile technique to prevent infection. Observe the color of wound drainage for indications of bile or blood; either could indicate a rupture of the suture line.

Liver Transplantation

Life-threatening end-stage liver diseases have been treated with transplants. The success of the transplant relates closely to the body's acceptance of the foreign organ, technical difficulties, the hazards of immunosuppression, and the availability of a functioning liver for transplant. The transplanted liver may be a total replacement or a liver segment. During the surgical procedure, hemorrhage is likely, and many units of blood are needed.

Liver Cancer

The liver is rarely the site of a primary cancer; more often, cancer of the liver is metastatic. A cancer that does begin in the liver can be removed surgically by removing the affected part of the liver. If cancer is due to metastasis, surgery usually is not indicated; the client is treated palliatively with radiation or chemotherapy. Antineoplastic drugs may be infused directly into the liver (*intrahepatic*).

DISORDERS OF THE GALLBLADDER

Cholecystitis and Cholelithiasis

Cholecystitis and cholelithiasis are common forms of gallbladder disease. *Cholecystitis* is inflammation of the gallbladder, and *cholelithiasis* indicates gallstones. These often occur together, and each aggravates the other. The stones may block the duct that leads from the gallbladder. They may injure the wall, leading to infection. Bacterial contamination of bile often develops, causing serious complications.

The most likely victims of gallbladder disease are women older than 45 years who are obese. Changes in the form of diet (e.g., the use of processed cheese vs. natural cheese) are suspected causes of the significant increase in gallbladder diseases in first-generation Hispanic American individuals. Frequent pregnancies also seem to make women more susceptible. Asian American individuals seldom have cholecystitis or cholelithiasis.

The cause of gallstones (*calculi*) is unknown. Formation of most gallstones is believed to result from abnormally thick bile, which is high in cholesterol and low in bile acids.

The gallbladder absorbs water, causing the bile to change into crystals, then sludge, and then form gallstones. Some gallstones also have a calcium base; these are harder than cholesterol-based stones.

> **Nursing Alert** Strenuous dieting and rapid weight loss can precipitate a gallbladder attack or the formation of stones. Lack of fat in the diet causes bile to pool in the gallbladder because it is not needed for fat digestion.

Sometimes the infected gallbladder fills with pus (*empyema* of the gallbladder) and may rupture, causing peritonitis. Chronic gallbladder disease may also permanently damage the liver.

Signs and Symptoms
The symptoms of cholecystitis or cholelithiasis include the following:

- Sudden onset of acute pain, called *gallstone colic*, in the upper right abdominal quadrant that may radiate to the back or right shoulder; pain usually begins a few hours after eating, although some individuals have no pain
- Indigestion and complaints of feeling "full" after eating; fatty foods make this condition worse
- Light-colored stools, **steatorrhea** (fatty stools that float), excessive flatus, and foul-smelling stools
- Nausea, vomiting, **eructation** (belching), fever, jaundice, and malaise

Diagnosis is usually made by evaluation of symptoms and laboratory, ultrasound, or x-ray study. A cholecystogram will be done if time permits. EGD or ERCP of the duodenum or biliary ducts may be performed.

> **Key Concept** Some clients describe the pain of gallstone colic as the feeling of a "huge bubble" in the upper abdomen or chest area. It is important to differentiate between gallstone colic and the chest pain related to heart attack.

Treatment
The diet is restricted to nonfat foods. Such foods as cheese, cream, greasy fried foods, fatty meats, and gas-forming vegetables are not given. The client may have lean meat (never fried), plain mashed or baked potato, or rice. Alcoholic beverages are contraindicated. Immediately after an attack, the client receives liquids only. If the attack is severe, meperidine (Demerol) may be given. Morphine should not be used because it is believed to increase the spasms.

In some cases, drugs may be effective in dissolving cholesterol-based gallstones. Chenodeoxycholic acid (Chenodiol) has been used for several years. Another drug, ursodiol (Actigall), is a naturally occurring bile acid that is taken orally and dissolves noncalcium stones by diluting the thick bile that is present.

Surgical procedures include *cholecystostomy* (opening and draining the gallbladder), *cholecystectomy* (removal of the gallbladder), *choledochostomy* (incision into the common bile duct), and *choledocholithotomy* (incision into the duct and removal of calculi). Cholecystectomy is often done through a laparoscope as an outpatient procedure. The gallbladder is excised by laser and removed through the scope. Recovery is usually fast following this procedure.

Nursing Considerations
Assist with various diagnostic tests. Preoperative preparations are similar to those for other abdominal procedures. Tell the client about the tubes and drains that will be in place after abdominal surgery.

Postoperative nursing care for the client after a cholecystectomy depends on what surgical approach is used. If abdominal laparotomy is done, nursing care is essentially the same as for any major surgery, with the additional responsibilities of observing the quantity, color, and amount of bile drainage, protecting the skin around the tube, and providing client teaching regarding bile drainage and tube care. The client is expected to turn, deep breathe, and use the incentive spirometer to prevent pneumonia.

An NG tube is often in place to empty the stomach immediately after surgery. Many surgeons place a tube into the wound for drainage following surgery. Others allow the ducts to readjust and take over bile drainage spontaneously.

If the client has a drainage tube (most often a T-tube), the healthcare provider may order the drainage bag to remain at floor level for a short time to allow the release of excess bile. Later, the bag is raised. Note the level of the container on the nursing care plan, and gradually wean the client from the drainage tube. Measure and record the amount and character of the bile every 24 hr. If the amount does not diminish in a few days, it may indicate that the bile is not entering the intestine properly.

Protect the skin surrounding the tube with zinc oxide or petrolatum. Observe the client's stools and urine for the presence or absence of bile. The bile should disappear, and the stools and urine should become normal in color and consistency as function returns. Document accurate fluid I&O.

Teach the client to maintain low-Fowler position to facilitate drainage. Monitor the tube closely to prevent blockage or dislodgment of the T-tube. After the T-tube has drained for 24 hr, you may be asked to clamp it for 1–2 days before removal.

The client may go home with the T-tube in place. Teach the client clamping procedures and what to watch for before discharge. Document all teaching. The client must watch for signs of jaundice or discomfort when the tube is clamped or removed.

On discharge, most healthcare providers order a regular diet, as tolerated. Most clients have no trouble digesting a small amount of fat. Generally, the client who has had gallbladder surgery should avoid foods that caused preoperative discomfort, such as gas-forming foods and alcohol. The client may be referred to a dietitian for counseling.

Common Bile Duct Obstruction
A client may retain or develop biliary stones that block bile flow within the common bile duct. Flow blockage may even follow a cholecystectomy. The client with a common bile duct obstruction is very ill. They report severe abdominal

pain, nausea, and vomiting. On examination, other symptoms include fever, jaundice, elevated white blood cell count, or elevated liver and pancreatic enzymes.

Cancer of the Gallbladder

Early cancer of the gallbladder is not detected easily. Symptoms are similar to those of cholecystitis. Surgery might be attempted, but because the liver is often invaded as well, prognosis is usually poor. More women than men develop cancer of the gallbladder.

DISORDERS OF THE PANCREAS

Pancreatitis

Pancreatitis is inflammation of the pancreas. It may develop from infectious or traumatic damage, alcohol, or drugs. Cysts may occasionally occur. Pancreatitis can be acute or chronic. Normally, bile does not enter the pancreas; if it does, the pancreas may become acutely inflamed. This process destroys pancreatic tissue and leads to hemorrhage, edema, steatorrhea, and severe pain. Pancreatic enzymes being secreted directly into the pancreas, rather than into the duodenum, also cause pancreatitis. Another cause is a gallstone that traveled backward in the duct.

Signs and Symptoms

Signs and symptoms include intractable pain in the epigastric area that may radiate to the back or upper left side. Fever, anorexia, nausea, and vomiting are common. Jaundice may exist if the common bile duct is obstructed.

Diagnosis is made by ultrasound, CT scans, and/or endoscopic examinations in combination with physical examination and results of laboratory pancreatic enzyme tests. ERCP can diagnose the presence and specific location of a tumor in the head or tail of the pancreas, which is helpful preoperative information for the surgeon.

Treatment

Treatment includes analgesics to relieve pain and spasm. The prescribed diet is low in fat and high in protein and carbohydrates. If the islets of Langerhans are affected, treatment for diabetes mellitus is also necessary. If distress is severe, an NG tube may be inserted to remove gastric secretions, and the client may be given IV fluids or TPN. Rest and freedom from emotional strain and upsets are important. Because the pain is so intense, non–morphine-type narcotics are usually necessary. Surgery may be necessary to remove an inflamed gallbladder, neighboring ducts, or *cystadenomas* (nonmalignant tumors) that could be the cause of the pancreatitis.

Pancreatic Cancer

Tumors of the pancreas are usually malignant. Cancer of the body or tail of the pancreas is usually not detected until metastasis has occurred. The client's prognosis is poor. In addition to other symptoms of biliary obstruction and pancreatitis, jaundice is sometimes the first symptom of pancreatic cancer. Diagnosis and treatment are the same as for pancreatitis. Surgery (*pancreatectomy*) is necessary to remove any cancerous growth. Before the operation, attention is given to building the client's nutritional status.

Nursing considerations focus on postoperative care. Pain management is important because postoperative pain can be excruciating. The client may need to gain weight; however, their appetite is usually poor. TPN is often used to restore nutritional deficits. After surgery, the client must be maintained with insulin and digestive enzymes.

CONDITIONS OF OVERNUTRITION AND UNDERNUTRITION

Obesity

Definitions of obesity vary, but generally the terms *overweight* and *obesity* are labels for ranges of weight compared to height and total body fat. In essence, obesity is the condition of being overly fat, not necessarily overweight. Another method of quantifying obesity is to use the calculated BMI. Charts of "desirable weight" and BMI are available on the Internet. Details listing desirable weights are compared in relation to height, bone structure, sex, and age. Some people, such as athletes, may be technically overweight, but the weight may be from muscle tissue and not excess fat. BMI is discussed in more detail in Chapter 30.

Complications

Obesity is a contributing factor to many medical and surgical complications. For example, the person with cardiovascular disorders, such as arteriosclerosis, atherosclerosis, hypertension, heart attacks, and stroke is at greater risk for circulatory disorders. The individual with diabetes mellitus has a four times greater risk (than persons of normal weight) of developing complications. Respiratory problems are very common in the obese, for example dyspnea and pneumonia.

The obese person often suffers from musculoskeletal disorders and is more susceptible to contagious diseases. *Hyperlipidemia* (excess fat in the blood) develops, and fat is deposited in the liver, causing liver damage. Dermatitis in moist skinfolds, chafing, excessive perspiration, and heat intolerance are associated problems.

Treatment

If a physical cause for obesity is found, it is treated. A nutritionally sound diet and exercise program are planned. The client must see a provider at regular intervals to ensure that they are maintaining weight loss and adhering to new eating patterns and that no other physical problems develop. Any person wishing to lose a large amount of weight should do so under a healthcare provider's supervision.

> **Nursing Alert** Weight-loss programs requiring ingestion of large amounts of water may be dangerous to the person with glaucoma (it may increase intraocular pressure) or certain kidney or liver disorders. The nursing mother should not be on a drastic weight-loss program because toxins and pollutants, which are stored in fat tissue, enter the mother's blood and can pass to the baby.

Various diets and group counseling systems (e.g., WW, formerly Weight Watchers) are available. They may help a person reach and maintain a sensible body weight. If such a program is unsuccessful, the client may seek medical assistance. Many healthcare providers prescribe diets. Morbidly obese clients need much emotional support as well.

Surgery may be performed for extremely obese individuals in whom all other forms of treatment have failed. Common procedures include gastric partitioning, banding, or stapling, which can significantly reduce the stomach's capacity to hold food, and/or remove a large portion of the intestine. The goal is to eliminate the body's ability to absorb calories. Surgery for morbid obesity (>100 lb [>45 kg] overweight) is normally considered high risk. Discussed earlier in this chapter, it is necessary for the client to receive in-depth teaching and preoperative and postoperative counseling for bariatric surgeries. The person must understand the added surgical risk and must alter eating patterns or they will regain the weight. Complications of gastric stapling or intestinal bypass include fluid and electrolyte imbalance, malnutrition, and dumping syndrome. (See Box 88-1, which summarizes common gastric and bariatric surgeries.)

Nursing Considerations

In Practice: Nursing Care Guidelines 88-4 lists measures for obese clients receiving care in the hospital. Client and family teaching concepts include the knowledge that obesity occurs when the number of calories a person takes into the body exceeds the number of calories they expend. Exercise can be highly beneficial for the obese person. Explain that the types of exercise do not have to be high intensity, but should be routine, at least three to four times per week. In addition, teach the client that eating the wrong types of foods (especially fats) and emotional stress contribute to obesity.

IN PRACTICE
NURSING CARE GUIDELINES 88-4 — Caring for the Hospitalized Client Who is Obese

- Two gowns may be needed, one facing forward and one facing backward. Obtain a larger size gown, if possible. Help tie the gown. *Rationale: The standard sized hospital gown may not fit.*
- One hospital bed may not be large enough; securely tie two beds together and place the mattresses crosswise. Keep the beds in low position and the side rails up at the foot of the bed. *Rationale: Some hospitals have larger beds or beds that can be adjusted. Many hospital beds cannot accommodate an individual who is morbidly obese.*
- An overbed trapeze helps the client to move in bed. The person may need to sit up to breathe. You may place blocks under the head of the bed because the gatch mechanism is not appropriate. If the person is in one bed, they may be too heavy to lift if using a crank-style bed, or the electric gatch may not work. *Rationale: Accommodations must be made to facilitate nursing care and to promote self-care from the client.*
- When assisting the client to get up, get help if needed. *Rationale: You will not be able to support the client alone. Always use a transfer belt; you can join two together, if needed.*
- Put the bed in a position so the client's feet just touch the floor. *Rationale: If it is too high, the client may fall; if it is too low, the client may not be able to stand up.*
- Have the client wear rubber-soled shoes (not slippers); use loafers or assist the person to tie the shoes. *Rationale: For safety reasons, use only shoes that will limit the possibility of slipping. Slip-on shoes facilitate self-care and promote self-esteem when it is difficult for that person to get dressed independently.*
- Use a heavy-duty walker, wheelchair, or stretcher. A commode or wheelchair with removable arms may be needed if a large device is unavailable. *Rationale: This strategy will allow the client to fit.*
- Assist the person with personal care; dressing alone may be impossible. *Rationale: The client may not be able to assist with their own activities of daily living (ADLs).*
- Skin care is particularly important in skinfolds and the perineum. *Rationale: The client often cannot reach to do self-care, and chafing or dermatitis is common.*
- Daily skin care can be facilitated by assisting the client to take a shower. *Rationale: A shower is usually safer than a bath in the tub.*
- Use an appropriate sized blood pressure (BP) cuff, and keep the cuff at the bedside to ensure consistency. Most facilities have a large adult cuff, a thigh cuff, and/or an obese cuff. *Rationale: Determine the correct size of BP cuff by estimating 40% of the circumference of the arm. A cuff that is too narrow will yield a blood pressure reading that may be higher than is accurate. A cuff that is too wide tends to produce a BP that is lower than is accurate.*
- Use longer needles for intramuscular injections. *Rationale: If the needle is too short, you might be giving a subcutaneous injection, rather than an intramuscular injection.*
- Assist the client in collection of urine specimens. *Rationale: The person may not be able to position the bottle or bedpan properly.*
- If the apical pulse is difficult to hear, use the bell side of the stethoscope, and mark the chest at the optimum location. *Rationale: Hearing apical pulse may be easier if the bell is used. Marking the space where the heart rate is best heard will assist other care providers.*
- Consider the self-esteem needs of the person. Accentuate the person's achievements and skills. *Rationale: Research has shown that obesity has multiple causes, not all of which can be eliminated by telling the client to lose weight. The client needs physical and psychological support.*

Reinforce the concept that obesity usually occurs with time, and successful weight loss also takes time.

> **Key Concept**
>
> Most diet recommendations include reduction of fat in the diet. Controlling fat gram intake is important. Many obese people try "crash diets," but many of them fail because the person never learns how to change long-term eating habits. After the person stops the diet, they usually regain the weight. This "yo-yo" effect of fast weight loss and immediate weight regain can be as dangerous as the original obesity. Education is vital in the long-term maintenance of weight loss.

Anorexia Nervosa and Bulimia

Anorexia nervosa is characterized by self-imposed starvation. No physiologic cause has been found. Anorexia often begins during the adolescent years, and 95% of clients with anorexia are women. Persons who are anorexic believe that they are fat, when actually they are very thin, often to the point of emaciation. This eating disorder usually results in being severely underweight, with significant functional malnutrition along with electrolyte imbalances. Other conditions include dental caries, muscle wasting, slow pulse and hypotension, blotchy skin, loss of hair (*alopecia*) or abnormal hair growth (*hirsutism*), and susceptibility to infections. Anorectic women almost always experience amenorrhea (absence of menses). They may be hyperactive, even though they are undernourished. Mortality is usually caused by circulatory collapse or cardiac failure secondary to the electrolyte imbalances. Additional information regarding eating disorders (anorexia nervosa, bulimia, and binge-eating) is also discussed in Chapter 73.

Bulimia is known as the "binge" syndrome. As in anorexia nervosa, a high percentage of clients with bulimia are young women. The client with bulimia may either *binge* (gorge with food) or binge–purge. In the *binge–purge* form of the disorder, the client eats thousands of calories at one sitting and, in an effort to avoid weight gain, purges the body of food, either by self-induced vomiting or by excessive doses of laxatives. The nonpurging bulimic often is obese. The person who binges and purges is usually thin, sometimes to the point of starvation.

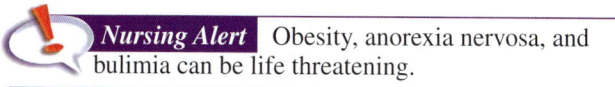 **Nursing Alert** Obesity, anorexia nervosa, and bulimia can be life threatening.

Signs and Symptoms

Symptoms and conditions common to anorexia nervosa and bulimia are as follows:

- Higher incidence of depression, obesity, and chemical dependency in the family than in the general population
- Overprotective parents with rigid rules and high expectations
- Usually very good students and school leaders
- Feeling of helplessness or being out of control, yet with manipulative behavior
- Intense fear of becoming "fat"
- Inaccurate self-image
- Low self-esteem, but unrealistically high goals
- Often great weight loss in a short time with no physical disorder
- Electrolyte imbalances
- Hiding or hoarding of food
- Preoccupation with food or gourmet cooking
- "Playing" with food; moving it around on the plate without eating it
- Shyness about eating with others
- Secretive behavior
- Going to the bathroom immediately after each meal
- Spending a great deal of time locked in the bathroom
- Going to various healthcare providers, requesting prescriptions for vague physical complaints
- Hiding medications

No specific laboratory test can diagnose anorexia nervosa or bulimia. Diagnosis is made by evaluation of the client, nutritional status, and risk factors.

Treatment

Treatment can be difficult: it consists of behavioral counseling, inpatient treatments, and diet therapy.

Nursing Considerations

During a crisis, treatment is symptomatic with enforced feeding, tube feeding, or TPN or oral replacement of missing electrolytes. The nurse may give oxygen to assist with respirations. Daily nursing observations and data collections include regular vital signs, weight, total calorie count, and I&O. Be sure to explain all procedures and the reasons for them to gain the client's cooperation. Explain the abnormal laboratory findings and their relationship to diet and to physical well-being.

The person needs to understand the functions of electrolytes in the body and the consequences of starvation. Offer small amounts of high-protein food or fluids often. High-protein, high-calorie liquids may be more tolerable than solids. Monitor fluid intake, so the person takes a variety of fluids, including fruit juices; make sure the person does not drink excessive amounts of plain water. *Rationale: Avoid electrolyte imbalance.* After the crisis, extensive psychotherapy and family counseling are needed. Group therapy often is helpful.

STUDENT SYNTHESIS

KEY POINTS

- Diagnostic tests for disorders of the GI tract include liver function tests, blood urea nitrogen, creatinine, and a CBC. Invasive testing of the GI tract includes endoscopies, EGD, and ERCP.
- Nursing care of the client with a digestive disorder includes management of NG tubes (e.g., lavage, suction, irrigation), stoma care (e.g., colostomies and ileostomies), and the ability to obtain data concerning nutritional history and disorders.
- Peptic ulcer disease includes ulcers that are found in both the stomach and the duodenum. Medical management is commonly successful. Surgical intervention may be necessary to prevent or treat hemorrhage.
- IBS is annoying and usually treated symptomatically. IBD (i.e., ulcerative colitis and Crohn disease) is long term, progressive, and often life threatening.
- The liver is subject to several forms of debilitating illness. Toxins, drugs, and many viruses can result in acute forms of hepatitis. Alcohol is related to cirrhosis and esophageal varices.
- Diseases of the accessory organs of the GI tract include cholecystitis, cholelithiasis, pancreatitis, and appendicitis.
- Cancer of many areas of the GI tract is often not found until metastasis has occurred. Common signs of GI cancer include alterations in eating habits and bowel elimination, weight loss, and rectal bleeding.
- Obesity, anorexia, and bulimia are risk factors for multiple physical and emotional disorders.

CRITICAL THINKING EXERCISES

1. State the role endoscopy has in diagnosing and treating GI disorders. Contrast its use with x-ray studies and incisional surgery.
2. List factors that are known to aggravate digestive conditions. Explain how you can use these factors in instructing a client how to prevent problems with hiatal hernia.
3. Alcohol is a known toxin of the liver. Develop a teaching project for high school students discussing the health hazards of alcohol.

NCLEX-STYLE REVIEW QUESTIONS

1. The nurse inserts a nasogastric tube (NGT) for a client. Which is the most reliable action that the nurse should take to ensure correct placement?
   a. Aspirate stomach contents.
   b. Obtain a chest x-ray.
   c. Instill 14–20 mL of air and auscultate.
   d. Test the pH of gastric contents.

2. The nurse is providing ileostomy care for a client and observes redness and a yeast-like growth around the site. After notifying the healthcare provider and receiving an order, which intervention will the nurse most likely provide?
   a. Application of Neosporin ointment
   b. Application of alcohol to the area
   c. Application of nystatin (Mycostatin) powder
   d. Washing the area with soap and water

3. A client has a new colostomy created during surgery to remove a mass in the sigmoid colon. The client is very upset and states, "I can't look at that!" Which is the best response by the nurse?
   a. "Would you like to talk about it? I can answer questions you may have."
   b. "You will have to look at it sometime. You are going to care for it."
   c. "You should be thankful this procedure removed your tumor and saved your life."
   d. "You don't have to look at it. Let's get a family member to learn the care."

4. A client is being discharged after the creation of an ileostomy. Which dietary information would the nurse reinforce? Select all that apply.
   a. Maintain a clear liquid diet for 1 month.
   b. Chew food very well.
   c. Avoid meat that is in a casing such as hot dogs.
   d. Eliminate gas-forming food.
   e. Blend all foods.

5. The nurse is preparing a client for an abdominal paracentesis. Which priority action by the nurse will help prevent complications?
   a. Have the client void before the procedure.
   b. Ensure the client has had a bowel movement within 24 hr.
   c. Have the client lie in the supine position.
   d. Insert an indwelling catheter.

CHAPTER RESOURCES

Enhance your learning with additional resources on **thePoint**!

Student Resources related to this chapter can be found at **thePoint.lww.com/Rosdahl12e**.

CHAPTER 88 Digestive Disorders

Welcome Steps

Look at healthcare provider's orders.

Protocol for procedure.

Necessary equipment/supplies.

Wash hands using proper hand hygiene; put on gloves.

Explain the procedure and reassure the client.

Locate two identifiers to confirm correct client.

Comfortable and efficient position for nurse and client.

Obtain privacy.

Make sure to follow correct steps and body mechanics with good technique.

Ensure safety and observe deviations from normal.

End Steps

Ensure comfort and safety.

Note questions or concerns from client or nurse; note significant data.

Dispose of materials properly.

Disinfect the area and your hands.

Document and report the procedure and your findings.

IN PRACTICE

NURSING PROCEDURE 88-1 Irrigating the NG Tube

Supplies and Equipment
Irrigation set
Room temperature tap water or saline
Stethoscope
Disposable pad or bath towel
Clamp
Disposable gloves

Steps

Follow LPN WELCOME Steps and Then

1. Wash your hands, following clean technique, and put on gloves. (When supplies are set up for the first time, they are sterile.) In many facilities, a new setup is used each time. Precautions are needed to prevent the spread of infection from person to person, but sterile technique is not necessary. *Rationale: The digestive tract is not sterile.*

2. Pour the ordered solution into the irrigation bottle. The most commonly used solutions are tap water or sterile normal saline at room temperature. Measure the amount of solution used. *Rationale: Subtract the amount of any solution not aspirated from the total amount of drainage for the day so that the intake and output (I&O) record will be accurate.*

3. Observe for signs of respiratory distress, for example, coughing and dyspnea. If distress is noted, seek assistance and be prepared to remove the NG tube. If no distress is noted, disconnect the nasogastric (NG) tube from the suction. Use at least two methods to make sure the NG is in the stomach.
   - Visually inspect the characteristics of the solution being aspirated from the NG tube. Secretions are aspirated from the NG tube using a catheter tip or bulb syringe. Gastric secretions can be a variety of colors.
   - Monitor pH of aspirate. If the pH is 5 or less, the NG is likely to be in the stomach because stomach contents are usually acidic. However, not all facilities allow or accommodate pH testing as it is not always accurate. *Notes regarding stomach pH:* Clients receiving gastric acid inhibitors may have a pH higher than 5 and gastric aspirate occasionally has a high pH. Therefore, a low pH is not always a sign of stomach intubation nor is a high pH indicative of malposition of the NG tube.
   - Use capnography, if available, to detect carbon dioxide, which indicates inadvertent tracheal insertion. *Rationale: If the tube is in the lungs, aspiration pneumonia or death can result. The methods for checking NG placement for a lavage are the same as the methods used after the initial insertion of the NG.*

4. Slowly introduce the solution, using the specified irrigating syringe. Do not use excessive force. *Rationale: Avoid damage to the stomach mucosa or a suture line.*

5. Reconnect the tube to low or intermediate continuous or intermittent suction, as ordered. The tube should remain *patent* (open) without putting undue stress, due to suction, on the gastric mucosa. The gastric contents should return freely when the tube is reconnected to suction. *Rationale: A tube*

that is not patent can lead to further abdominal distention, pain, and surgical complications.

6. Note the amount, color, and consistency of any drainage. Fluids that do not return freely may signify a plugged NG tube. Report such a finding immediately. **Rationale:** *Distention can cause discomfort and respiratory compromise and pull sutures apart.*

Special Reminder
- Note the amount of fluid instilled or aspirated on the I&O sheet.

IN PRACTICE
NURSING PROCEDURE 88-2 Changing the Ostomy Appliance

Supplies and Equipment
Pouch or pattern
Pouch adhesive wafer
Closure clip
Stomahesive paste (optional)
Cotton balls or gauze
Scissors
Pen or pencil
Tissues
Water
Soft towel
Liquid deodorant
Plastic waste bag
Gloves

Steps
Follow LPN WELCOME Steps and Then

1. Locate the stoma size pattern drawn by the enterostomal (ET) nurse. With a pen, trace this size hole on the paper backing of the pouch adhesive. Cut out the opening. **Rationale:** *The pouch opening should be only in or about 2 mm larger than the stoma size to prevent skin irritation from chronic exposure to stool.*
2. Remove the paper backing from the pouch adhesive (wafer). Apply a thin bead of Stomahesive paste to the edge of the adhesive you have just cut. **Rationale:** *The paste is a kind of caulking to help seal the pouch around the stoma and prevent leakage.*
3. Gently remove the old appliance and wipe around the stoma with tissue. **Rationale:** *You want to remove mucus or fecal drainage.*
4. Dispose of the old appliance in a plastic bag. Save the closure clip. **Rationale:** *Control odor and contamination.*
5. Inspect the skin. Wash the area with warm water, but do not use soap. **Rationale:** *Soap can leave a residue on the skin that interferes with pouch adhesion.*
6. Carefully dry the skin. Apply the new appliance. Hold your hand on the appliance for 2 min. **Rationale:** *The warmth of your hand helps warm the skin barrier and paste so the adhesives seal well to the client's abdominal wall.*
7. Add a few drops of the deodorant to the pouch and clamp it closed. **Rationale:** *The deodorant neutralizes odors.*

Follow ENDDD Steps

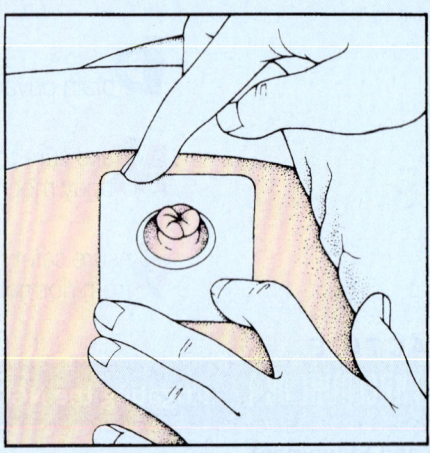

Stomahesive wafer with flange (1 ½, 1 ¾, 2 ¼, 2 ¾, -in openings) can be applied directly to the periostomal area after it has been thoroughly cleaned and dried.

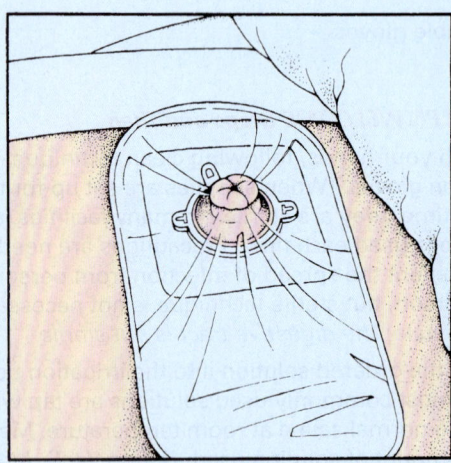

An opaque or transparent drainable pouch is positioned at the desired angle over stoma.

Special Reminder
- Observe the stoma every 6–12 hr or more frequently for a new stoma. **Rationale:** *The condition of the stoma may change, the pouch may become loose, or the pouch may become too full.*

89 Urinary Disorders

Learning Objectives

1. Identify the components of a normal urinalysis.
2. Discuss the rationale for using the following tests of renal function: BUN, serum creatinine, creatinine clearance, and uric acid.
3. Describe the role that the following imaging studies play in diagnosis of urinary disorders: KUB, IVP, radioactive renogram, cystogram, voiding cystogram, retrograde pyelogram, and renal arteriogram.
4. Identify the nursing considerations related to pre- and postprocedure cystoscopy care.
5. Describe the role of urodynamic tests in diagnosing urinary disorders.
6. Discuss medical and surgical approaches to treat incontinence.
7. Discuss the topics necessary for client teaching sessions for the individual with recurrent cystitis.
8. Define and discuss the nursing considerations for cystitis, pyelonephritis, interstitial cystitis, glomerulonephritis, hydronephrosis, ureterolithiasis, and nephromas.
9. Prepare a nursing care plan for a client who has been recently diagnosed with a metastatic kidney tumor.
10. Identify nursing considerations for the client with calculi and for the client with a urinary diversion.
11. Define and differentiate between acute renal failure and ESRD.
12. Identify nursing considerations for a client receiving dialysis.

Important Terminology

anuria
bacteriuria
bruit
calculi (calculus)
casts (cylinders)
crystalluria
cystectomy
cystoscope
dysuria
fistula
hematuria
hypotonic
incontinence
lithiasis
lithotripsy
micturition
nephritic syndrome
nephrolithiasis
nephroma
oliguria
pessary
precipitate
pyuria
reflux
shunt
stent
suprapubic
thrill

Acronyms

BUN
CAPD
CMG
C&S
EMG
ESRD
ESWL
ET
GFR
IC
IVP
K
P
TURBT
UA
UNOS
UPP
UTI
VCUG
WCON
WOCN

The urinary tract can be divided into the *upper tract* (kidneys and ureters) and the *lower tract* (bladder and urethra). The upper urinary tract filters the by-products of metabolism and adjusts the body's fluid and electrolyte balance. It also delivers urine to the lower tract. The lower urinary tract acts as a storage area until **micturition** (voiding, urination) occurs. Urine then flows through the structures of the lower urinary tract and out of the body (see Chapter 27).

Common problems affecting the lower urinary tract include infection and incontinence. Damage to the lower tract, although rarely life-threatening, can greatly affect a client's quality of life. Damage to the upper urinary tract usually stems from obstruction, which causes **reflux** (backflow) of urine into the kidneys. In addition, infection and inflammation can damage the sensitive tissues of the nephrons, resulting in decreased kidney function. Damage to the upper urinary tract is life-threatening. Any systemic condition that affects blood flow will affect kidney functioning. Examples of such conditions include hypertension, heart failure, trauma, and changes in small blood vessels related to diabetes mellitus or collagen/vascular diseases.

Key Concept
Many kidney disorders result from circulatory disorders that result in vascular insufficiency to the kidneys. For example, hypertension causes damage or destruction of the delicate parenchymal tissues of the kidney that make urine.

The *urologist* is a healthcare provider who treats diseases and disorders of the urinary tract system. A *nephrologist*, who specializes in medical aspects of kidney disease, may treat some disorders of the urinary tract. A *dialysis nurse* assists clients in a dialysis clinic or may bring dialysis equipment to the bedside of a hospitalized client. Because many terms in urology are similar, they can be confusing. Common combining forms that appear in this chapter are listed in Table 89-1.

NCLEX Alert
NCLEX questions very commonly require knowledge of the definitions of medical terminology. Combining forms, prefixes, and suffixes make up the key words in many clinical scenarios and their options. For example, what are the differences of nursing care for a cystoscopy versus a cystectomy or nursing actions for anuria, hematuria, or oliguria? Before taking your NCLEX, review and be able to apply medical terms. (Medical terminology is found in Appendix C which is available online.)

TABLE 89-1 Combining Forms in Urology

PREFIXES/SUFFIX	MEANING
• cyst(o)-	Pertaining to any bladder
• lith(o)-	Stone
• nephr(o)-	Pertaining to the kidney
• pyel(o)-	Pertaining to the renal pelvis
• ureter(o)-	Pertaining to the ureter (tubes from kidneys to bladder)
• urethr(o)-	Pertaining to the urethra (from bladder to outside of body)
• vesic(o)-	Pertaining to a bladder, usually the urinary bladder
• -tripsy	Crushing

Urinalysis

A *urinalysis* (**UA**) provides much information about the condition of the bladder and kidneys as well as other body systems. Abnormal readings on a UA can reflect disorders in many body systems; for instance, an elevated blood glucose can indicate diabetes mellitus, a disorder of the pancreas. The urinalysis shows whether pathogens are causing infections in the kidney or bladder, or whether dysfunctions of the liver permit breakdown products of protein (albumin) to escape into the urine instead of being eliminated by normal digestive routes.

SPECIAL CONSIDERATIONS Lifespan
Urinary Tract Infections in Older Adult Clients

- A change in mental status may be the only presenting symptom of urinary tract infections in older adults. Always monitor and report older clients who present with subtle or sudden, acute changes in mental status.
- Older adult clients metabolize medications more slowly than do younger clients. Consider this fact when choosing doses and times for as needed (PRN) medications.
- Older adult clients often have several chronic disorders. Always be aware of how these disorders and their treatments influence kidney function. Be alert to subtle changes in behavior, personality, or daily functioning. Report these changes to the healthcare provider. Document your observations carefully.

SPECIAL CONSIDERATIONS Lifespan
Taking a Complete History in Pediatric Clients

Obtain an accurate history when admitting pediatric clients. Voiding patterns and behaviors may be your only clue to detecting abnormalities. When possible, monitor the child during voiding and encourage vocalization of toileting habits that have been taught. *Rationale: Children do not always recognize a habit that is harmful. Frequently, children do not recognize that something is abnormal, so they do not know to tell family members about their symptoms. However, family members can also give valuable information.*

A *routine* or *random UA* includes tests for pH, specific gravity, glucose (sugar), ketones, albumin (protein), blood (**hematuria**), and bilirubin. This information is generally provided on a diagnostic test strip inserted briefly into the urine and then read.

Urine normally has a specific gravity of 1.010–1.025 and a pH of 4.6–8. No glucose, ketones, bacteria, albumin, or bilirubin should appear in normal urine. When examined microscopically, urine should contain no (or very few) red blood cells (RBCs) or white blood cells (WBCs). RBCs seen under the microscope could indicate hemorrhage. The bleeding could be seen as trace amounts with numerous RBC or as frank hemorrhage. Frank hemorrhage usually can be noted by gross inspection (visual inspection) of the urine. The presence of WBCs indicates infection.

A routine UA also will check for urine color, appearance, odor, and foam content. Table 89-2 lists conditions that are

DIAGNOSTIC TESTS

Laboratory Tests

Blood and urine tests are commonly ordered as screening tools for many urinary tract disorders. Chemistry levels may indicate normal ranges of electrolytes (e.g., potassium, calcium, and sodium). Serum and urine glucose and protein levels are also often obtained. These levels help indicate the body's overall fluid and electrolyte balance. Blood and urine levels can help evaluate the nature of renal diseases, such as renal failure.

TABLE 89-2 Conditions Indicated by Abnormalities in the Urine

ABNORMALITY OR ABNORMAL SUBSTANCE IN URINE	POSSIBLE CONDITIONS
Abnormal pH	Gout, calculi, infections
Abnormal specific gravity	Kidney disease, electrolyte imbalances, liver disorders, burns
Proteinuria or albuminuria (protein)	Nephritis, kidney stones, renal circulatory difficulties, infection, trauma, preeclampsia (of pregnancy)
Glycosuria (sugar)	Diabetes mellitus, shock, head injury
Ketonuria (ketones)	Diabetes, starvation, bulimia, other digestive disturbances (e.g., faulty fat metabolism)
Bilirubin	Liver dysfunction, biliary obstruction, hepatitis
Hemoglobinuria or hematuria	Infection, calculi, cancer, trauma, overdose of an anticoagulant, bleeding disorder

indicated by abnormalities found in urine. The laboratory also will test the urine for **casts** (*cylindruria*). Casts are epithelial, fatty, or waxy tissue abnormally forced out of the renal tubules. Additional abnormal findings include the presence of crystals (**crystalluria**) or pus (**pyuria**). Urine calcium may be measured to help detect bone disease; high amounts of calcium indicate degeneration of bone tissue. The urine also may be tested for the presence of other minerals, various drugs, and abnormal components.

> **Key Concept**
> Bacteria in a urinalysis sample will reproduce if the specimen is not refrigerated shortly after being obtained. To prevent false readings, be sure that biologic specimens (urine, stool, wounds) are processed according to facility protocols.

The laboratory performs a *urine culture* by placing small amounts of a urine sample on a culture medium and allowing it to *incubate* (grow). The culture will reveal organisms present in the urine. If a culture reveals the presence of an organism in the urine, the organism is tested with various medications (usually, an antibiotic) to see which one is most effective in eradicating it (*sensitivity test*). The client then receives that medication. Culture and sensitivity (**C&S**) tests for urine are usually ordered together.

Nursing Considerations

Collected urine may consist of a single random specimen or an accumulated fractional specimen, such as a 24-hour collection. Obtain a clean-catch midstream urine sample from the client for a C&S. Instruct the client to clean the perineal area. In a woman, teach them to separate and clean the area with the openings to the urethra and vagina. For a man, teach them to clean the tip of the penis. Teach the client to start voiding and then to insert the collection container under the urine stream to obtain the sample.

Wear gloves while packaging the urine, and be careful not to contaminate the specimen with any outside organisms so that a true culture of only the client's urine is performed. Contamination commonly occurs when replacing the cap on the specimen container. After the urine is collected for culture, send it to the laboratory immediately. If urine is allowed to stand, microorganisms can grow in it, thereby altering the test's accuracy. If a sterile specimen is required and a question exists to the client's ability to collect it, the specimen may be obtained by urinary catheter.

Renal Function Tests

The most common diagnostic studies for evaluation of kidney function are blood urea nitrogen (**BUN**), serum creatinine, urine creatinine, creatinine clearance, a serum BUN-to-creatinine ratio, and a glomerular filtration rate (**GFR**). Serum and urine uric acid levels also may be ordered. The GFR is a measurement of the rate of urine formation as blood is filtering through the glomeruli of the kidney.

The BUN test determines how efficiently the glomeruli remove the nitrogenous wastes (*urea*) that result from protein metabolism. The most common cause of an elevated BUN is kidney disease, although BUN also may be elevated in clients with high dietary protein intake, diabetes, some malignancies, or improper protein metabolism. Fluid loss, as seen in physical dehydration, can manifest as an elevated BUN on a urinalysis.

Serum creatinine, a product of protein metabolism, is related to muscle mass and excreted by the kidneys. *Creatinine* is the chief nitrogenous waste of protein (muscle) metabolism. The glomerular filtration rate must be reduced by at least 50% for significant elevation of serum creatinine to occur. Therefore, serum creatinine is a much more accurate indicator of renal function than serum BUN. An elevated serum creatinine level usually indicates a serious kidney disorder, such as impaired kidney function or obstruction. Additional information can be obtained by a BUN:creatinine ratio.

The *creatinine clearance test* uses a collected urine specimen to indicate glomerular filtration rate and renal insufficiency. Commonly, a creatinine clearance test is ordered in addition to a *morning serum creatinine*. *Serum creatinine* is found at a basically constant level. Serum and urine creatinine levels are compared, and a creatinine clearance ratio is calculated. Creatinine clearance is one of the most valuable tests to identify early kidney disease, and it is useful in monitoring the renal function of clients with known kidney disease. To obtain a creatinine clearance test, a 12- or 24-hour urine collection is made, noting the exact time the collection started and ended. *Rationale: Exactness is vital to obtain the full 24-hour specimen.*

Uric acid studies may be obtained from urine or serum. The main diagnostic purpose of obtaining a uric acid level is to evaluate the client for gouty arthritis or kidney disease. A urine uric acid study is generally performed with a 24-h collected specimen.

Imaging Studies

General imaging studies include x-ray and ultrasound examinations, computed tomography (CT) scans, and magnetic resonance imaging (MRI); more specialized imaging studies used to study the urinary tract include intravenous pyelogram, radioactive renogram, bone scan, nephrotomogram, renal arteriogram, cystogram and voiding cystourethrogram (**VCUG**), and retrograde pyelogram. In addition, a bone scan (*scintiscan*) is indicated when bony metastases are suspected in cases of renal, bladder, or prostatic cancer.

The kidney–ureter–bladder x-ray examination, commonly referred to as a "KUB flat plate of the abdomen," is a good screening test for kidney or bladder stones. Ultrasound may be used to view the kidneys and other urinary structures. CT scans will reveal any kidney abnormalities, such as cysts, tumors, or *calculi* (stones). Spiral CT is used to image the kidneys to evaluate tumors and stones. In addition, MRI may be used to distinguish normal from abnormal tissue.

Intravenous Pyelogram

Intravenous pyelogram (**IVP**) is composed of a series of x-ray films taken after a radiopaque dye has been injected intravenously. These films reveal the outline of the client's kidneys, ureters, and bladder. Before the IVP is done, the healthcare providers must determine whether the client is allergic to iodine or shellfish because the dye is iodine based. The client is given nothing by mouth (NPO) for 8–10 hr before the test. They usually receive a laxative the night before to rid the bowel of any feces or gas that could obstruct the view of urinary structures. The client may brush the teeth in the morning but should not swallow any water.

The radiology technician takes and develops one x-ray film, commonly a KUB. A radiopaque dye is then administered via the IV route into the client. The technician takes several more x-ray films at intervals to visualize the dye concentration in the kidneys.

A *nephrotomogram* may be performed along with IVP; it allows x-ray films to be taken of kidney layers and the structures within the layers, using a rotating x-ray tube after IV injection of a contrast medium. Preparation and care of the client are the same as for IVP.

Nursing Considerations
Notify the Radiology Department of known allergies and if the client is diabetic. Clients who have diabetes often have decreased renal function and cannot clear the dye quickly through the kidneys. Monitor and observe the client for untoward reactions to the dye. Instruct the client and family to provide at least 2–4 L of fluids for 24 hr after the test to help remove the dye and relieve any dehydration that may have resulted from the client's NPO status before the test. Contrast dye can damage the kidneys if not flushed out quickly.

Radioactive Renogram
A *radioactive renogram (renal scan)* tests the kidneys by means of radioactive substances. The scan will show blood vessels, obstructions, and each kidney. Tumors may be detected because they "pick up" more of the radioactive substance than normal tissue does.

Cystogram and Voiding Cystourethrogram
A *cystogram* is an x-ray study of the bladder and urethra made possible by instillation of dye directly into the bladder through a catheter. Using fluoroscopy, the x-ray cystogram will show the bladder's outline and the ureters (if reflux is present). It is used to evaluate the degree of *vesicoureteral reflux* (backflow of urine into the ureters) and the presence of bladder injury.

A *voiding cystourethrogram* (VCUG) is a fluoroscopic test done to diagnose vesicoureteral reflux. The first part of the test is very similar to the cystogram, in that a contrast agent is instilled into the bladder via a urethral catheter. When the client feels the urge to void, the catheter is removed and the client voids while x-ray films are taken (reflux often occurs when the client voids).

Retrograde Pyelogram
A *retrograde pyelogram* is used to show the kidneys and ureters. After the bladder is outlined on x-ray film by instillation of dye by catheter, smaller catheters are introduced into the ureters and then passed into the kidney pelvis, where dye is injected into them. X-ray films are then taken that show the kidneys and ureters.

This procedure is combined with cystoscopy. Preparation includes giving the client a low-residue diet the day before and a laxative or enema in the evening and immediately before the test. Observation following the test is the same as that required for any other test using dye.

Renal Arteriogram
Renal arteriogram is obtained by injecting a contrast dye through a catheter into the aorta at the level of the renal blood vessels. The kidneys are thereby visualized to determine

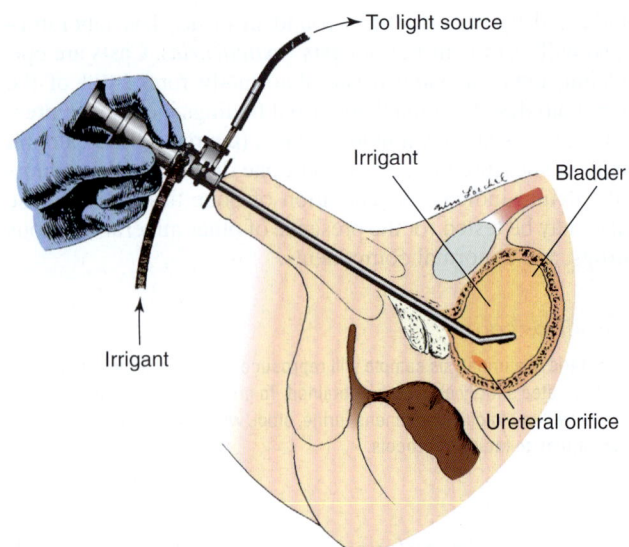

Figure 89-1 Examination of the inside of the bladder using a cystoscope.

the presence of a pathologic condition (e.g., a tumor). Care of the client after this examination is the same as for any arteriogram.

Endoscopic Procedure: Cystoscopy
A *cystoscopy* examination allows the healthcare provider to view the inside of the bladder through a tubular instrument, the **cystoscope**, which has a mirror and an electric lamp or a fiberoptic lens on its end (Fig. 89-1). The healthcare provider passes the cystoscope into the client's bladder through the urethra. This examination can detect inflammation or a tumor that may be causing blood to appear in the urine.

Cystoscopy also enables visualization of the openings of the ureters into the bladder; fine, opaque wax catheters can be threaded into these openings for collection of separate urine specimens from each kidney to determine which kidney is diseased. Dye also may be instilled through these catheters. Because the fluid medium is infused into the bladder at high pressures, infected urine can be forced up into the kidney, causing an infection of the kidney. Therefore, it is important to obtain a urinalysis and urine culture before this procedure to determine if a client has a kidney infection.

The healthcare provider may use a cystoscope to view the ureters while inserting ureteral catheters. Cystoscopy also may be used to remove a polyp or a tumor, perform a biopsy, or remove kidney stones. The surgeon may conduct electrosurgery (*fulguration*) through a cystoscope to remove small tumors or to coagulate (*cauterize*) small, bleeding blood vessels.

Because a cystoscopy is usually done in an operating room, the client requires routine preoperative preparation. A cystoscopy may be performed with general anesthesia. Local anesthesia involves administering a tranquilizer or sedative before the examination to relax the client and instilling lidocaine (Xylocaine) jelly into the urethra. Make sure the client is not allergic to lidocaine (Xylocaine), procaine (Novocain), or bupivacaine (Marcaine) before using these agents.

Urine specimens obtained are examined in the laboratory. A mild analgesic may be prescribed after the procedure because voiding may be uncomfortable for 1–2 days. The urine occasionally has a reddish tinge immediately after cystoscopy.

Nursing Considerations

Nursing considerations will include reporting blood-tinged urine for more than 24 hr or darkening urine. Encourage the client to drink fluids to prevent urinary stasis and flush any remaining dye from the body. Help the client with sitz baths to ease voiding and to soothe the affected area. Remind the client to report signs or symptoms of a urinary tract infection or increasing blood in the urine.

Biopsy

Following identification of a mass by imaging studies, a needle biopsy of the kidney may be done for a specific diagnosis. The kidney is located by x-ray or ultrasound, and the client's back is marked so that the needle can be inserted at the correct place.

Give the client a sedative as ordered. Place the client in a prone position, with a sandbag under the abdomen. *Rationale: The sandbag helps bring the kidney into a more accessible position.* A local anesthetic is injected into the skin, and the biopsy needle is inserted.

After the procedure, apply pressure to the site to minimize bleeding. Keep the client lying flat for 24 hr and watch them very carefully for any signs of hemorrhage. *Rationale: Hemorrhage is a complication of needle biopsy because the kidney is very vascular.* Take blood pressure, pulse, and respirations and document them at frequent intervals.

Urodynamic Tests

Urodynamic testing is a series of tests that best determines the actual function of the *detrusor muscle* of the bladder (which pushes the urine out), the external sphincter muscle, and the pelvic (pubococcygeal) muscles. Urodynamic tests also evaluate the ability of these muscles to work in sequence.

> **Key Concept**
> Because urodynamic tests are safer than x-ray procedures that require an IV dye, they are the tests of choice in many cases.

A urodynamic evaluation is usually done in two phases: phase one is the filling phase of the study; phase two is the emptying phase of the study. The *filling phase* tests sensation of the bladder, capacity, muscle activity, and stretch of the bladder wall (*accommodation or compliance*), as well as the ability of the bladder and pelvic muscles to hold the urine in without leaking. The *emptying phase* (*voiding or micturition studies*) tests how well the bladder empties and what strategies the client uses to empty it completely.

Uroflowmetry

Uroflowmetry is a noninvasive assessment of the status of micturition and generally the first test done in a urodynamic evaluation. The client voids into a funneled commode connected to an electronic measuring device. This device calculates the volume of the urine flow and the time it takes the client to void, in order to determine a flow rate. This information is recorded on a graph.

Before the test, instruct the client to void in the same fashion as usual. Leave the client alone (if possible) to prevent "bashful bladder syndrome" (the client is too tense to urinate). Further testing will be needed to differentiate between bladder outlet obstruction and **hypotonic** bladder (poor muscle tone).

Residual Urine Volume

A *residual urine volume* test is done to determine if the client emptied the bladder completely. Before obtaining a residual volume, the client voids as much as possible using whatever techniques they usually use to empty as well as possible. Some healthcare facilities require the client to void, followed by a second voiding 5 min later. This procedure is referred to as *double voiding technique*. The client is then immediately catheterized with a straight catheter (one that is inserted to obtain a specimen and then removed) to collect whatever urine remains in the bladder.

A noninvasive technique called *bladder scanning* may also be used to measure residual volume. The client voids as discussed above; then the nurse moves the ultrasound scanning device over the bladder area to determine the urine volume in the bladder.

If residual volume is greater than 150–200 mL, a disorder of the bladder or urethra is probably causing urinary retention. The healthcare provider may order a catheter to remain in place if the residual volume is over a certain amount, or the nurse may be ordered to teach the client how to intermittently catheterize themselves at home.

Cystometrogram

A *cystometrogram* (**CMG**) is a measurement of bladder pressure during filling. A urethral catheter is inserted, and the bladder is filled either with a liquid, such as normal saline, or with x-ray contrast media. Instruct the client to notify the healthcare provider when they begin to feel a sense of fullness, again when the bladder actually feels full, and again when the client can hold no more fluid because of discomfort or a feeling that they will leak. Normally, bladder pressure remains the same during bladder filling until the volume is approximately 500 mL.

If the urodynamic evaluation is being done to evaluate the continence status of the client, the filling phase may be interrupted several times during the test to have the client cough or bear down. If the client leaks urine during these maneuvers, a leak-point pressure is obtained. The leak-point pressure assists the surgeon in determining if the client is suitable for anti-incontinence surgery.

Urethral Pressure Profile

A *urethral pressure profile* (**UPP**) is another way to evaluate the smooth muscle activity along the urethra. This procedure is often done following a CMG. For the UPP, the bladder is filled either with a fluid, such as normal saline or water, or with contrast media using a catheter. A puller mechanism provides a slow, even rate of catheter withdrawal, while resistance exerted by the urethral wall is registered as a pressure rise on a graph. If the client is found to have a low-pressure urethra, a procedure that improves urethral closure is appropriate.

Perineal Electromyogram

The *perineal electromyogram* (**EMG**) is a test of pelvic muscle (pubococcygeal or levator muscle) function. Several methods are used to record perineal EMG. Patch electrodes are used more commonly today than needle electrodes, and they are more comfortable for the client.

The perineal EMG is usually combined with the CMG because the major function of the EMG is to evaluate the relationship of perineal muscle activity and detrusor muscle contraction. If the pelvic muscles are inappropriately relaxed during the filling phase of the urodynamic evaluation, then the client may leak urine. If the pelvic muscles cannot relax during the emptying phase of the study, the client may not be able to empty the bladder at all or may have a residual volume remaining after micturition. A *voiding study* also may be done. The CMG sensor is usually left in place along with the abdominal sensor and the EMG patches. The client is then asked to void. Measurements are taken during the procedure.

NURSING PROCESS

DATA COLLECTION

Carefully observe for abnormalities and document changes for the client with a urinary disorder. This initial observation establishes a baseline for future comparison and determines the presence of suspected complications. Report any changes in the baseline level, and try to recognize and treat kidney malfunctions early. In Practice: Data Gathering in Nursing 89-1 lists some components of the urologic nursing assessment.

IN PRACTICE

DATA GATHERING IN NURSING 89-1 — **Urinary System**

- Urinary history, including previous providers and treatments
- General health history
- Family health history
- Exposure to toxins
- Presence of related disorders (e.g., type 1 diabetes mellitus, heart or blood vessel disorders, infections, cancer)
- Character of urine, abnormal components
- Intake and output amounts
- Urinary residual
- Difficulty or pain in voiding
- Any incontinence and type
- Sudden weight gain or loss
- Diet and fluids
- Presence of symptoms, such as edema or poor skin turgor

In addition, observe the client's emotional response to the disorder or disease, asking the following questions. Would a support group be helpful? Does the client need assistance to meet daily needs? Do family caregivers understand needed medications and treatments? Is home care or public health nursing necessary? Does the disorder affect social activities or self-esteem? Is the condition chronic or life-threatening? Is it reversible or treatable? Does the client need periodic dialysis or other regular treatment? Is the client anxious or fearful of the outcome? Does the client need financial assistance?

PLANNING AND IMPLEMENTING

Plan with the client, family, and other members of the healthcare team for effective care based on the nursing diagnoses. Provide preoperative and postoperative care for the client undergoing **lithotripsy**, renal surgery, dialysis, or invasive diagnostic tests. The client with a urinary disorder also may require total assistance in meeting daily needs, dealing with emotional problems, and understanding more about the disorder, its prognosis, and treatment.

Renal disease may require regular dialysis or a kidney transplant, or it may be life-threatening, with minimal available treatment. A nursing care plan is developed to meet the individual's needs. Damage to the kidneys can be life-threatening if not recognized and treated promptly. The goal of nursing care is to prevent further damage or decline in function.

General Nursing Considerations

General nursing considerations when caring for clients with urinary tract disorders include monitoring vital signs and results from diagnostic tests, as well as the effects and side effects of medications. Assistance with activities of daily living (ADL) may be necessary in some clients. However, encourage clients to provide self-care whenever possible. Major nursing considerations include:

- Obtaining frequent vital signs, especially blood pressure
- Managing related symptoms, such as diarrhea, nausea, vomiting, headache, anemia, and pain
- Administering prescribed diuretics, mineral supplements, and antibiotics
- Providing skin and mouth care (because of dehydration, edema, and general tissue friability)
- Managing pruritus
- Observing and documenting skin condition, tissue turgor, and presence of edema or dehydration
- Measuring and recording intake and output (I&O), color and clarity, and urine-specific gravity; monitoring for urinary retention
- Taking daily weights, which provide an indication of overall fluid status related to edema
- Monitoring fluid intake with maintenance of fluid restrictions (to help control edema and electrolyte imbalances)
- Encouraging fluid intake, when indicated, to dilute urine and lessen **dysuria** (painful urination)
- Assisting with voiding and with continence training
- Providing medications and emotional support for dysuria and painful intercourse
- Inserting urinary catheters using appropriately ordered catheters; urologists may order specific types of indwelling catheters and may insert these catheters themselves
- Managing and caring for an indwelling catheter or **suprapubic** cystocath

- Managing incontinence, frequency, urgency, and other urinary symptoms
- Giving sitz baths and warm moist packs to offset pain
- Providing movement and activity to prevent disorders of immobility, such as deep vein thrombosis, pneumonia, and urinary tract infections

> **Key Concept**
> Infection of the urinary tract can result in life-threatening damage to the kidney if not treated promptly; therefore, prevention or early treatment is vital.

Postoperative Care

Provide postoperative care for the client after lithotripsy, renal surgery, dialysis, or invasive diagnostic tests. Whether surgery is done for stone removal, cancer, or kidney transplantation, deep breathing and turning can be painful postoperatively. *Rationale: A flank incision is usually made for a ureterolithotomy or a nephrotomy and is done through a number of major muscle groups.* Care of the client who has undergone urologic surgery follows usual postoperative nursing care.

> **Nursing Alert** Instruct the client and family members to report chills and fever. *Rationale: They are signs of infection.* Other symptoms of complications include sharp abdominal pain, hematuria, *anuria* (absence of urine formation), *dysuria* (painful urination), or urine retention.

Additional measures include
- Clients need prescribed pain medications before turning and deep breathing. Encourage the use of the incentive spirometer.
- The client may have multiple tubes for urinary drainage postoperatively. Be aware of the location, size, and kind of tubes and expected drainage from each. Check each tube for patency and monitor its drainage regularly.
- Careful observations of vital signs and the color of urinary output are needed to look for any indication of excessive bleeding. Hemorrhage can easily occur after surgery for renal calculi because the kidneys are so vascular.
- Large amounts of urinary drainage may be present on dressings after urologic surgery but drainage should not be bright red; bright-red drainage indicates frank bleeding. The color most often used to describe normal bloody discharge following nephrolithotomy is "rose."
- The client will often have a urinary catheter or suprapubic cystocath postoperatively.

> **Key Concept**
> Because many diagnostic and minor urologic surgical procedures are performed on an outpatient basis, aggressive client and family teaching is required. Clients and families must know how to perform preoperative preparation and untoward signs to look for after the procedure. Carefully document this teaching.

EVALUATION

Evaluate outcomes of care with the client, family, and other members of the healthcare team. Have you met short-term goals? Are long-term goals still realistic? Will the client receive care at home? Are additional home care services required? Is a support group indicated? Do the client and family understand the treatment plan? Does the client have a way to get to dialysis or will it be done at home? Planning for further nursing care considers the client's prognosis, any complications, and the client's and family's responses to care given.

URINARY INCONTINENCE

Urinary **incontinence** refers to involuntary voiding or urine loss. In men, two well-defined sphincter muscles control voiding. The *internal sphincter* controls the bladder's opening into the urethra, and the *external sphincter* (the pelvic muscles) controls the opening of the urethra below the prostate. In women, there is little definition between the internal and external sphincters. Normally, sufficient urine collects in the bladder and stimulates the involved nerve endings, causing the urge to urinate. When a person loses control of this function, incontinence results.

Types of Incontinence

Transient (Temporary) Incontinence

Transient (temporary) incontinence refers to incontinence that can be reversed with diagnosis and treatment. Factors causing transient incontinence include reversible contributing factors such as changes in mental status, infections, medications, fluid intake, mobility problems, or stool impaction. After the precipitating cause is discovered and treated, the incontinence usually resolves without further intervention. A type of transient incontinence, *iatrogenic incontinence*, is similar to transient incontinence in that the cause of the incontinence is usually the result of outside factors. However, iatrogenic incontinence is specifically caused by medical interventions or treatments. A new medication, restraints, or postsurgical mobility problems are the most common reasons for this type of incontinence. Sometimes, iatrogenic incontinence can be reversed, and other times it may be permanent (e.g., when medications cannot be changed).

True or Total Incontinence

True or *total incontinence* is defined as urinary leakage that is nearly continuous.

The most common cause of true incontinence in men is surgical removal of the prostate (*prostatectomy*) (see Chapter 90). Other causes of true incontinence include:

- Injury to the male's external (voluntary) urethral sphincter
- Injury to the female's perineal musculature (muscles)
- Congenital or acquired neurogenic disease (e.g., spina bifida or spinal cord injury)
- Congenital anomaly in which the urinary bladder is exposed on the lower abdomen (*exstrophy*)
- Abnormally placed ureteral orifices in the female (opening distal to the neck of the bladder or into the vagina)

- *Vesicovaginal fistula* secondary to situations such as injuries during delivery or surgery (may include defects caused by an infection after surgery)
- Invasive cancer of the cervix or prostate
- Radiation injury after treatment of cervical cancer
- Abdominal perineal resection for rectal cancer in men and women

Stress Incontinence

Stress incontinence is urinary leakage following a sudden increase in intra-abdominal pressure (e.g., coughing, sneezing, or other physical strain). Urine leakage may be a few drops or a stream of urine; however, clients can almost always tell the healthcare provider when it occurs and what they do to prevent the leakage. Stress incontinence primarily affects women with pelvic relaxation caused by childbirth, trauma, loss of tissue tone, or aging. Men frequently have stress incontinence after surgery to the prostate. Urodynamic tests are often used to confirm or rule out stress incontinence.

Reflex Incontinence and Urge Incontinence

Reflex incontinence and urge incontinence are similar in that in both types clients experience urgency before voiding caused by bladder spasm. *Reflex incontinence* is caused by bladder instability as a result of upper motor lesions or neuropathies. *Urge incontinence* is caused by irritation of the bladder wall, possibly because of urine components. In both conditions, involuntary loss of urine follows a sudden, strong desire to urinate. Clients usually cannot stop their urinary stream once it starts and often cannot get to a bathroom in time.

The client often reduces fluid intake to decrease incontinent episodes. However, this concentrates the urine further and increases spasms. Clients with urge incontinence also use the toilet frequently and void small amounts to prevent incontinent episodes. Again, however, this frequency ultimately decreases the bladder's functional capacity. If the client continues this practice for a long time, the detrusor muscle weakens. Distention of the bladder then causes it to spasm at lower volumes of urine.

Overflow Incontinence

Overflow incontinence happens when the bladder overfills with urine and is not able to release it because either the detrusor muscle no longer contracts (usually because of local nerve injury, as in diabetes or central spinal cord injury) or a blockage is preventing the urine from emptying. Examples of obstruction include benign prostatic hyperplasia (BPH), cancer of the prostate that presses on the urethra, and postoperative urinary retention (see Chapter 90).

The client typically has a large, distended bladder but dribbles urine either continuously or with stress maneuvers such as coughing or bearing down. If the incontinence is caused by a blockage, it is very important to either remove the blockage or bypass the blockage by using a catheter before reflux of the urine into the kidneys causes kidney damage. In addition, clients who have this type of incontinence are generally more susceptible to urinary tract infections because the stagnant urine provides an ideal place for bacteria to grow.

Treatment

Treatment will depend on the underlying cause of the urinary incontinence. Conservative (medical) treatment is effective in milder cases of incontinence, especially for young people, in clients who are poor surgical risks, or in clients who do not wish to undergo surgery. Conservative treatment includes use of a bladder-retraining program, Kegel exercises, electrical stimulation, pessaries, medication therapy (e.g., urinary antispasmodics), Credé maneuver, and a catheter to empty the bladder completely (in cases of incontinence caused by neurogenic bladder). Treatment for overflow incontinence caused by obstruction is to relieve the obstruction; surgical intervention may be necessary.

Credé Maneuver

Credé maneuver is used to manage overflow incontinence. In *Credé maneuver*, the healthcare provider applies firm, gentle pressure above the bladder. The technique involves placing hands on the abdomen to press down with flat hands, starting at the umbilicus and moving down to the symphysis pubis. The procedure is repeated several times, applying the final pressure directly over the client's bladder, thus causing the urine to flow out of the bladder.

Kegel Exercises

Kegel exercises often are used as a treatment for stress and urge incontinence. They are effective and practical methods to manage incontinence (see In Practice: Educating the Client 91-3). *Kegel exercises* are designed to increase sphincter tone and to help the client prevent leaking on the way to the bathroom. The client will need to wear a disposable pad during the training period to catch any urine. If after 3–6 months of working on an exercise program there is no noticeable improvement in the level of incontinence, the client may opt for surgery or medications for better management of incontinence. *Biofeedback* may be used if Kegel exercises are ineffective in controlling urine flow. Biofeedback uses a computer or other electronic device to help monitor how well the client can do Kegel exercises.

Electrical Stimulation

Electrical stimulation (pelvic muscle stimulation) is another method of helping the client to strengthen the pelvic muscles and decrease the bladder activity that causes urge incontinence. A small electrode connected to a generator is placed in the vagina or rectum. When an electrical impulse occurs, the pelvic muscles contract; when no impulse is sent, the muscles relax. This treatment is very comfortable and easy to do at home. It is very useful in clients with neurologic problems or in those who have difficulty figuring out which muscles to use in Kegel exercises.

Pessary

A **pessary** is a small, plastic device that is inserted into the vagina. The pressure of the pessary pushing against the vaginal walls will support the neck of the bladder and inhibit urinary leakage. Pessary placement is a nonsurgical option for females with stress urinary incontinence. These devices vary in size and shape and can be left in the vagina for long periods of time (4–8 weeks) without the need for removal for cleaning or maintenance.

If used to help support a prolapsed bladder, the client may improve their ability to empty the bladder completely. A pessary can also be used to help push the neck of the bladder closed, thereby lessening incontinence. Pessaries are useful devices for both the short- and long-term management of incontinence when clients either do not wish to have surgery or are not considered good surgical risks.

Medications

Medications often are used in conjunction with bladder retraining techniques, Kegel exercises, and biofeedback. Urinary antispasmodics are effective in many cases to decrease bladder muscle spasms and urinary incontinence; for example, tolterodine (Detrol) or oxybutynin.

Tricyclic antidepressants (e.g., imipramine) also are used to treat stress incontinence because this classification can increase bladder neck resistance. Other drugs used to treat stress incontinence include pseudoephedrine and phenylpropanolamine. Another medication treatment choice is estrogen therapy for women with vaginal atrophy.

Surgery

When a *fistula* (connection) between the bladder and another organ is the cause of incontinence, surgery is almost always needed to repair the opening. Electrocautery may be used to seal the hole. *Electrocautery* refers to both the procedure and the instrument that is used. In this procedure, the urologist *cauterizes* (destroys) defective tissue with an electrode that emits either alternating or direct electrical current. Larger holes may require a more major surgery to patch the hole or correct the defect.

If a fistula is large or is caused by radiation therapy or invasive cancer, the client may require a urinary diversion to correct the incontinence. *Surgical ureteral reimplantation* can correct abnormally placed ureteral orifices. In this procedure, the urologist attaches the ureters to the urinary bladder.

Many operative procedures are used to correct stress incontinence. The underlying principles of these procedures are the same—elevating the neck of the bladder and suturing it into place to restore the bladder's normal curvature. With the curvature of the bladder neck restored, the person usually regains continence. If the client has an open bladder neck because of nerve damage or scarring from previous surgeries, the goal is to close the bladder neck rather than to elevate it to a more functional position.

Another option for the client with a nonfunctioning urethra is the placement of an artificial sphincter. This artificial device consists of a cuff, which is placed around the bladder neck and is connected to a reservoir bulb. The bulb is implanted in the pelvis. The operating button is implanted in the scrotum or labia. The cuff is inflated with fluid from one of the reservoirs to maintain continence and then deflated when the client wants to empty the bladder.

If the above measures do not work, surgery for increasing the bladder size, *augmentation cystoplasty*, may be considered to increase the bladder's functional capacity. This is a measure of last resort in a population without neurologic problems and is rarely done unless the problem of urgency is extreme.

An implantable electrical stimulation (InterStim) device was approved for cases of severe urgency and frequency. The device uses a fine electrode attached to the sacral spinal cord to deliver an electrical current that is believed to both relax the bladder and block the sensation of urgency from the bladder.

Nursing Considerations

Nursing considerations for urge and reflex incontinence include encouraging fluids to dilute the urine and to flush irritating substances from the bladder. The nurse also can teach the client measures to empty the bladder completely (see In Practice: Educating the Client 89-1). Bladder retraining can increase the time between voiding episodes and increase the bladder's functional capacity. Biofeedback and Kegel exercises are recommended to assist with bladder retraining, so that the client learns to contract the pubococcygeal muscles until they reach toileting facilities.

Bladder incontinence is more difficult to control than bowel incontinence, but with perseverance, many clients can establish control. For the client's physical and emotional well-being, achieving continence is important. The client may choose to continue to wear incontinence briefs for urinary containment. See In Practice: Educating the Client 89-2 for management of chronic incontinence.

The nurse is responsible for assisting the person to manage a urethral or suprapubic catheter (see Chapter 51). The healthcare provider inserts suprapubic and other types of catheters. In some cases, the client learns to perform regular self-catheterization. In Practice: Nursing Procedures 57-3 and 57-4 discuss catheterization of a female and a male client.

URINARY TRACT INFECTIONS

Acute Cystitis

Cystitis means inflammation of the urinary bladder. It is probably more commonly called a *urinary tract infection*

IN PRACTICE
EDUCATING THE CLIENT 89-1 Emptying the Bladder Completely

- Teach clients to take ample time to toilet. If they try to rush through toileting, the pelvic muscle will tighten before their bladder is empty.
- Encourage the client who has "shy bladder syndrome" to find a private, quiet bathroom to toilet.
- The sound of running water will help the bladder that has difficulty starting to urinate.
- Tapping above the pubic bone, tapping the clitoris, or tickling the base of the bladder are all techniques that can be used to initiate a stream.
- It is better to avoid bearing down to empty, but rather push on the belly above the pubic bone during the stream (Credé maneuver) to empty the bladder completely.
- The client can use a double-void technique to empty the bladder completely.
- In female clients who have prolapsed bladder, the client can lift the base of the bladder using a finger in the vagina to tip it into a position that will help emptying.

IN PRACTICE
EDUCATING THE CLIENT 89-2: Management of Chronic Incontinence

- Incontinence is often correctable and usually can be reduced.
- Use an incontinent pad on the bed and wheelchair to prevent soiling.
- Teach principles of bladder retraining, including Credé maneuver, if necessary.
- Self-catheterization may be required for long-term management.
- The client may wear an appliance, condom catheter, or incontinent briefs or pads.
- Wash appliances regularly.
- Skin care is important to maintain good skin integrity.
- Female clients should wipe from front to back to help prevent urinary tract infections.
- Wash hands after toileting.

(UTI). A UTI is an infection along any part of the urinary tract. Women are more susceptible to cystitis than are men because their urethra is shorter.

Normally, the inside of the bladder is sterile, but microorganisms can enter from the urethra (the most common route), through the bloodstream, or directly through a fistula. The UTI may then ascend from the bladder into the ureters and into the kidney structures causing serious, often lifelong renal complications. The most common causative agent is *Escherichia coli*, followed by occasional cases caused by *Staphylococcus saprophyticus*, *Klebsiella* spp., *Proteus mirabilis*, or *Chlamydia trachomatis*.

Factors that may make a person more susceptible to UTI include catheterization, which can advance bacteria into the bladder (sterile technique during catheterization is a must), systemic disease (e.g., diabetes), and changes in the vaginal pH in women.

Signs and Symptoms
The cardinal signs of UTI are frequency, dysuria, hematuria, or other abnormal components of urine, such as WBCs or pus and a positive urine culture. Many times, the symptoms of UTI are missed, especially in an older adult client or during pregnancy.

The client with cystitis has an urge to urinate frequently even though the bladder does not need emptying. The client voids very small amounts each time. A painful, burning sensation accompanies urination; sometimes blood is in the urine, and the client complains of a "heavy feeling" in the abdomen or perineum. Diagnosis of UTI is made by urinalysis and C&S.

Treatment
Antibiotics or sulfonamides are ordered as a result of sensitivity testing. Mild analgesics may be necessary for a few days. Drugs given for UTI may cause urinary discoloration; for example, phenazopyridine hydrochloride (Pyridium), a urinary analgesic (but not antibiotic), causes the urine to appear orange-red.

Nursing Considerations
Teach preventative measures, such as the importance of fluids, avoiding tight-fitting nonabsorbent underwear, and avoiding irritants, such as soaps and bubble baths. Also explain that diets high in sugar promote bacterial growth and cystitis. Explain to women that sexual activity increases the risk of acquiring a UTI; voiding immediately after sexual intercourse reduces the risk. Teach women and girls to wipe the perineal area from front to back, which minimizes contamination of the urinary meatus with microorganisms from the rectum or vaginal areas.

Tell the client that warm packs can help alleviate the pain associated with infection. Explain the importance of taking antibiotics as ordered to eliminate the causative agents. During antibiotic treatment, fluid intake of 3–4 L daily is recommended, unless contraindicated. *Rationale: Additional fluid helps dilute the urine, thus lessening burning on urination.* Fluid intake also encourages elimination, thus preventing urinary stasis, in which bacteria can multiply. Flushing out the urinary system prevents the formation of crystals that may develop from sulfonamide therapy. Inform clients of the possibility of a change in color of urine to orange-red when taking phenazopyridine hydrochloride (Pyridium). This discoloration may stain fabric and toilet fixtures.

Chronic Cystitis

Clients will occasionally develop *recurrent UTI* or *chronic cystitis*. Signs and symptoms include urinary frequency, nocturia (nighttime voiding), and incontinence; dysuria will probably not be present. High bacterial counts often are obtained in a culture, yet the client may not be aware of the problem. Infections must be treated before damage is done to the kidneys. Clients with chronic cystitis often will be placed on long-term antibiotic therapy lasting 3–6 months.

Nursing Considerations
Nursing care of the client with chronic cystitis is the same as for clients with acute cystitis, but additional client teaching is necessary. The client who is susceptible to chronic cystitis should shower instead of bathe to avoid pushing bacteria up the urinary tract. In addition, remind female clients to empty their bladder before and after intercourse and to use a lubricant with intercourse if the vagina is dry. *Rationale: Friction irritates the urethra, increasing the risk of infection.*

Teach women to wipe from front to back to prevent sweeping bacteria into the urethra. Monitor the client on long-term antibiotics for *Candida* or yeast infection, also known as moniliasis. Signs and symptoms of yeast infection need to be explained. See Chapter 70's section on candidiasis or vulvovaginal candidiasis for a more in-depth discussion of signs and symptoms of yeast infections. Sometimes clients on long-term antibiotic therapy have breakthrough infections. Provide the client with a sterile container to bring in a specimen if the individual experiences increased urinary symptoms. For best urine culture results, obtain a clean-catch, midstream specimen, or obtain the specimen with intermittent straight catheterization.

Acute Pyelonephritis

Acute pyelonephritis, inflammation of the renal pelvis and medulla, is the most common form of kidney disease. Pyuria is noted in a urinalysis. It usually stems from infection with microorganisms that have migrated from another body part; *E. coli* contamination is common. Pyelonephritis may result from an ascending infection from the lower urinary tract or from an indwelling urinary catheter. Microorganisms also may reach the kidney through the bloodstream, causing inflammation, edema, and, sometimes, many small abscesses.

Signs and Symptoms

Signs and symptoms of acute pyelonephritis are rapid onset of fever and chills, with flank pain, pyuria, nausea, vomiting, and headache. The client with this condition is very ill. If the bladder also is infected, the client will have a desire to urinate frequently, and burning will accompany voiding. A urine test reveals bacteria in the urine (**bacteriuria**) as well as WBCs and casts.

> **Nursing Alert** Because many diagnostic and minor urologic surgical procedures are performed on an outpatient basis, aggressive client and family teaching is required. Clients and families must know how to perform preoperative preparation and untoward signs to look for after the procedure. Carefully document this teaching.

Treatment

Treatment is antimicrobial therapy for at least 10–14 days. Antibiotics, sulfonamides, or urinary antiseptics are ordered to combat the specific causative microorganisms. If the client has nausea or vomiting, an IV line to prevent dehydration may be ordered.

Nursing Considerations

The client with flank pain, fever, and nausea requires immediate medical attention. Bed rest, plenty of fluids, attention to mouth and skin care, proper nourishment, pain management, and change of position are needed to provide comfort and prevent deformities or further infection (see In Practice: Educating the Client 89-3).

IN PRACTICE
EDUCATING THE CLIENT 89-3 Signs of Infection

- Dysuria
- Frequency
- Nocturia
- Cloudy urine
- Hematuria
- Fever, chills, flank pain
- Mental status changes, for example, confusion in an older adult

---

Chronic Pyelonephritis

Chronic pyelonephritis may develop if an acute infection recurs or if an obstruction prevents the passage of urine. The kidney becomes permanently damaged and, because kidney tissue is not replaced, renal function is lost. Chronic pyelonephritis develops more slowly after the initial acute infection. Relapses of pyelonephritis are common. Causes may be related to obstructions. Treatment consists of long-term antimicrobial therapy and continued efforts to prevent more damage. Chronic pyelonephritis may advance to renal failure and death.

INFLAMMATORY DISORDERS

Interstitial Cystitis

Interstitial cystitis (**IC**) is a disease of the bladder that may be both autoimmune and inflammatory in nature. The lining of the bladder becomes "leaky" and allows irritants from the urine to contact the muscular wall of the bladder, causing irritability. This disease is more common in women, usually occurring between the ages of 20 and 50. Researchers have indicated that men who have a bacterial prostatitis may actually have IC.

Signs and Symptoms

The client experiences a strong urge to void extremely frequently (every 5–30 min), often for many days without relief. The client may also experience pelvic pain and have painful intercourse. Unlike cystitis, voiding is usually not painful; instead, it provides relief from the bladder pain and spasms. Men with this problem may have penile-tip pain and perineal pain. The major characteristic of IC is that the urine is free of bacteria, although the client experiences urgency, frequency, and pain. Clients usually can recall the exact time that their symptoms began, and the onset usually is associated with either a UTI or instrumentation of the bladder.

Diagnosis

In a small percentage of clients undergoing hydrodistention of the bladder, when the bladder is distended with fluid, lesions called *Hunner ulcers* appear. More typically, petechial hemorrhages occur. Either of these findings is diagnostic of IC. Bladder biopsy examination shows changes typical of IC.

Treatment

Treatment of this chronic disease is difficult and consists of symptom management; there is no cure. Hydrodistention may improve symptoms several weeks after it is initially done, although the client may experience increased symptoms the first few weeks after the procedure.

Pentosan polysulfate (Elmiron) can be helpful for interstitial cystitis. This medication prevents irritation of the bladder walls. Major side effects are known to occur with pentosan polysulfate (Elmiron), including bleeding, hair loss, and moodiness.

Bladder irritants should be removed from the diet and reintroduced gradually one at a time to see if symptoms lessen. Fluids should be encouraged to help dilute the urine and remove toxic wastes from the bladder; avoid fluids with an inherent chemical basis, such as some sodas, teas, or coffees. Physical therapy and stress reduction techniques are helpful in the long-term management of the disease.

Nursing Considerations

Clients with IC should see the same provider at each visit while a urology specialist coordinates the long-term care and management of their disease. Instrumentation frequently causes flare-ups of symptoms, so it is important to do as little manipulation of the pelvic area as possible.

Intercourse is usually painful (*dyspareunia*), and clients are often severely depressed, causing long-term relationships to suffer. The disease worsens when the client is under stress, so it is important to work with employers and family members to help them understand how stress affects the client's symptoms. Social support is very important for these clients.

In advanced cases, the pain caused by this disease can be extreme. These clients should be under the care of a urologist and may need counseling and support groups to help them cope with the disease.

Glomerulonephritis

Glomerulonephritis is a group of diseases in which the kidneys are damaged and partly destroyed by inflammation of the glomeruli. Glomerulonephritis may be a result of an acute bacterial, viral, or parasitic infection. Exposure to hydrocarbon solvents, diabetes, and blood or lymphatic disorders is a known risk factor for the disorder. It can be acute (temporary and reversible) or it can become chronic, leading to permanent kidney disease. Common symptoms include blood in the urine plus generalized edema with fatigue and malaise. Symptoms may not be noticed until renal failure has begun streptococcal infections of the skin or pharynx may result in inflammation of the glomeruli; this type of glomerulonephritic inflammation can result in an antigen and antibody reaction (i.e., an autoimmune response). *Nephritic syndrome* (*nephrosis*) may result from glomerulonephritis and is characterized by marked protein in the urine and edema.

Acute Glomerulonephritis

Acute glomerulonephritis is a disorder of the glomeruli that starts with inflammation of the glomeruli and can become a serious chronic condition. Glomeruli are the parenchymal cells that filter blood from urine. This makes the glomeruli extremely important for the process of urine formation because they filter blood and remove excess fluids, electrolytes, toxins, and many other substances. The returned clean blood goes back into the bloodstream while leaving the filtrates to become urine that exits the body. The causes and the process of inflammation can be sudden and acute or a long-term, gradual disorder. Primary glomerulonephritis is often due to infection, frequently caused by streptococcal infection of the throat (i.e., strep throat), which is more common in children. (Refer to Chapter 72 for more information on streptococcal infections and glomerulonephritis in children.) Bacterial endocarditis, often causing infection in the heart valves, can trigger glomerulonephritis. Viral infections such as HIV, hepatitis B, and hepatitis C are also associated with glomerulonephritis. Many disorders, such as lupus or diabetes, are the main causes of secondary kidney diseases. Diabetes and hypertension are common causes of scarring of the parenchymal glomeruli cells. Glomerulonephritis, by itself, can lead to hypertension, damaged glomeruli, and decreased kidney function. Sometimes, often for unknown reasons, an acute condition leads to a chronic condition. It is not uncommon for the first symptom of a renal problem to be kidney failure.

Signs and Symptoms

The client may not notice the initial symptoms of glomerulonephritis, which will differ depending upon whether the disease is acute or chronic. Family members may be the first to sense that something is wrong when they become aware of the client's pale, puffy face and swollen tissues (*edema*). The client gets up many times at night to void. Other signs and symptoms may include hypertension, headaches, edema, irritability, loss of appetite, general malaise, and body aches. Anemia, due to the loss of RBCs related to kidney failure, may be significant and be the cause of fatigue. Urine may present as pink or dark-colored as a result of RBCs leaking into the urine via damaged glomeruli. Proteinuria tends to result in foamy urine. In the absence of treatment, serious complications, and possibly death, may follow.

Complications of glomerulonephritis can be severe, life-threatening, long-term disorders such as acute kidney failure, which typically needs dialysis at least temporarily; chronic kidney disease; hypertension; and *nephrotic syndrome*, all of which usually result in sustained dialysis. **Nephritic syndrome** is a condition characterized by too much protein in the urine and too little protein in the blood, high cholesterol levels, and severe edema of the eyelids, feet, and abdomen. (Refer to nephritic syndrome in Chapter 72.)

Diagnosis

Diagnosis is made initially by urinalysis. The UA will show the urine to be more dilute, meaning that the urine consists of more water than normal. Dilute urine is due to the lack of filtration in the glomeruli, which results in more water loss during the brief time that blood passes through the damaged glomeruli. Hematuria or smoky urine may be present. Albumin, RBCs, WBCs, protein, and casts are present in the urine. Further testing will evaluate blood levels of creatinine, BUN, and CBC levels. Physical signs and symptoms will show edema. Imaging studies include an ultrasound, kidney x-ray, and CT of the pelvis. A kidney biopsy can confirm the diagnosis by showing a microscopic amount of the inflamed and damaged glomeruli.

Treatment

The treatment goal is to restore the kidney to its best possible function. The type of treatment will depend upon the cause of the kidney failure. Antibiotics are given to counteract any existing infection. Corticosteroids and immunosuppressant drugs may assist symptoms (e.g., inflammation). Control of hypertension is very important as well as the treatment for underlying diseases. Diuretics such as furosemide (Lasix) and antihypertensive drugs are given to treat causative problems. Antihypertensive agents include angiotensin-converting enzyme inhibitors (ACE inhibitors) and angiotensin II receptor blockers. Plasmapheresis may be used for immune-related glomerulonephritis. The client must maintain low-energy status, such as resting in bed or on the couch, sometimes for several weeks. The body needs a lot of rest and as little strain on the urinary system as possible. Fluid and dietary management is determined by laboratory test results. Restrictions may include the monitoring of dietary intake of protein and salt.

With treatment, almost all clients recover from acute glomerulonephritis. They are not considered well, however, until their urine has been continuously free of albumin and RBCs for several months. The treatment for long-term or end-stage renal failure is dialysis or kidney transplant.

Nursing Considerations
Document the client's daily I&O and weight. Give fluids to balance output. Provide skin care and oral hygiene to prevent skin breakdown and infection; remember that this client's skin is fragile. Passive or active exercises help prevent respiratory and circulatory complications. The healthcare provider and the nurse will observe for albumin in the urine, GFR, BUN, and creatinine levels, which can indicate intolerance to nutritional protein intake.

Chronic Glomerulonephritis
Chronic glomerulonephritis may develop immediately after an acute episode or after the client has been free of symptoms for an extended time. It also is possible for a person to contract chronic nephritis without having been aware that they had acute nephritis. Chronic glomerulonephritis is much more serious than acute glomerulonephritis because it permanently damages the kidney by destroying nephrons and thereby disrupting function.

> **Nursing Alert** Chronic glomerulonephritis can have serious complications, including pulmonary edema, increased blood pressure, anemia, cerebral hemorrhage, heart failure, and ultimately, renal failure.

Signs and Symptoms
Signs and symptoms are similar to those of the acute stage. In the beginning, few physical symptoms occur other than mild general malaise, albumin in the urine, pale and dilute urine, slight anemia, hypertension, and marked edema or anasarca (generalized body edema).

The disease flares up at intervals, but the client usually feels well between attacks. During the course of the disease, which maybe 10–30 years (with symptoms under control), signs of renal insufficiency develop. In advanced stages, complications include blurred vision followed by blindness. Nosebleed (*epistaxis*) and gastrointestinal bleeding are common in terminally ill clients.

Treatment
Treatment includes treating edema with diuretics, monitoring blood pressure with antihypertensive medications, and dietary restrictions of salt and water. Protein in the diet is typically minimized, which will reduce the amount of protein breakdown products such as ammonia.

Nursing Considerations
When signs of a flare-up of chronic glomerulonephritis appear, place the client on bed rest to reduce metabolic waste and preserve strength. Lower the client's salt and fluid intake. Instruction for the need of a low-protein diet may be necessary.

Avoid exposing the client to infection of any kind. Transfusions may be given for anemia. Place the client in the orthopneic position to facilitate breathing. With this treatment, symptoms usually subside in approximately 3 weeks, and the client gradually returns to normal. In the absence of dialysis or a kidney transplant, however, prognosis is poor.

> **Key Concept**
> The person with chronic glomerulonephritis is very ill and needs close observation and skilled nursing care to monitor for and treat related renal failure.

End-stage renal disease (**ESRD**) may develop in some cases of chronic glomerulonephritis. ESRD is preceded by chronic kidney disease or chronic renal failure (discussed below); terminology depends on the capability, if any, of kidney function.

OBSTRUCTIVE DISORDERS

Calculi, growths, spasms of the ureter; kinks in the ureter; or infectious scarring can obstruct the urinary system. An enlarged prostate gland (benign or malignant) can interfere with passage of urine. Other causes of obstruction may be meatal stenosis, blood clots, tumor, fibrosis, urethral stricture, neurogenic bladder, and adhesions, or scar tissue. In urine, the chemical process called *precipitation*, that is, the creation of a solid from a solution, occurs. A **precipitate** is the solid matter of the liquid urine that falls out of suspension. Typically few problems exist if a precipitate remains in suspension, but if the particles become larger solids, they can occlude the ureters or bladder.

> **Key Concept**
> Complete obstruction anywhere in the urinary tract system is a medical emergency and must be treated quickly before renal damage occurs.

Hydronephrosis

Hydronephrosis develops when urinary obstructions block the outflow of the kidneys. Hydronephrosis may be gradual, partial, or intermittent.

Signs and Symptoms
In this condition, urine forms, but the flow of urine from the kidney is obstructed. Depending on where the obstruction occurs, waste products accumulate in the kidney and back up into the blood, leading to ESRD. If the obstruction is in the ureter, only one kidney is involved; if it is in the urethra, the bladder abnormally retains urine and both kidneys usually are affected. A bladder infection also is likely because the urine is allowed to stagnate. In addition, stagnant urine is the ideal environment for stone formation.

Treatment
Generally, *acute hydronephrosis* is reversible. The cause of obstruction must be removed as soon as possible to prevent the development of *chronic hydronephrosis*.

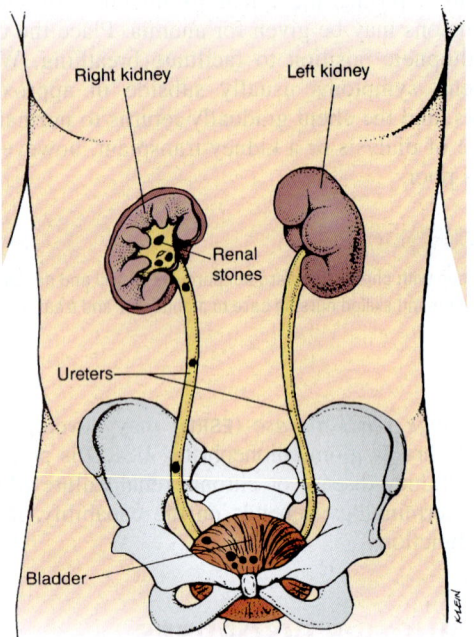

Figure 89-2 Locations of calculi formation in the urinary tract.

Ureterolithiasis

Ureterolithiasis, **renal lithiasis**, or **nephrolithiasis** include the conditions of stones or renal calculi in part of the urinary tract. **Calculi** (meaning pebble or stone) and **lithiasis** (meaning stone) form primarily in the kidneys and descend through the urinary passages (Fig. 89-2). Commonly grouped together under the name *kidney stones*, calculi are more common in men and occur most often in people between the ages of 20 and 40.

No single etiology for the development of stones has been identified, but theorists believe that risk factors such as infection, dehydration, low calcium intake, and urinary stasis contribute to the formation of stones. Calculi formation is related to the presence of concentrated urine, which allows minerals to crystallize and adhere (stick together), becoming larger precipitates. Clients with long-term indwelling catheters, multiple sclerosis, or diabetes are at risk for formation of bladder stones. Clients with urinary stasis owing to long-term immobilization are at high risk for ureterolithiasis, which is one of the hazards of immobility. Calculi are seen in individuals who have had gastric bypass surgery, inflammatory bowel disease, and chronic diarrhea due to changes to the body's ability to absorb calcium and water. Clients who are obese, have a high body mass index (BMI), large waist size, and weight gain are more likely to have kidney stones than others who do not have these conditions. Kidney stones may be the initial symptoms of some clients with metabolic conditions, such as hyperparathyroidism, or clients with Crohn disease.

Urine contains three basic types of crystal-forming substances (precipitates) such as *calcium oxalate*, *oxalate*, and *uric acid*. Stones in the urinary tract are generally made from substances such as calcium oxalate, calcium phosphate, struvite, uric acid, and cystine stones. The most common type of stones are calcium stones in the form of *calcium oxalate*, and less often, *calcium phosphate*. Oxalate is a natural substance found in food, such as nuts, chocolate, fruits, and vegetables. High doses of vitamin D, intestinal bypass surgery, and several metabolic disorders can increase the concentration of calcium or oxalate in urine, which promotes stone development. *Struvite* stones generally accompany a UTI. They can become large quickly, often with few symptoms. *Uric acid* stones often are seen in individuals with gouty arthritis, who are dehydrated, who eat a high-protein diet, or who have certain genetic factors. *Cystinuria* is an uncommon, genetic disorder that causes stones to form in the kidneys, ureter, and bladder due to excess precipitation of the amino acid *cystine*.

Diagnosis

Diagnosis of lithiasis occurs with imaging studies that include KUB x-ray examination, IVP, ultrasound, a CT scan of the abdomen and pelvis, or a CT urogram. A ureteroscopy can be done to view the urethra, bladder, and ureter; sometimes, a stent is inserted into the ureter to prevent recurrent episodes of pain. A cystoscopy is used to investigate the bladder for lesions, stones, and inflammation. Blood testing will test for calcium and uric acid in the blood. A 24-hour urine collection will look for stone-forming minerals or for too few stone-preventing substances. The stones may be analyzed for mineral content. If no stones are viewed, the client is typically treated symptomatically and monitored.

Signs and Symptoms

With kidney stones, pain in the region of the obstruction is the primary symptom. Often this pain is called *colic*, an excruciating pain that comes in waves as the ureter tries to force the obstructing stone onward. This pain is violent and unbearable. Gross hematuria may occur if the stone traumatizes the ureter. Signs of UTI may be present including nausea, vomiting, and chills. If the stone is very small, the spasm may move it along, allowing the client to pass it spontaneously.

> **Nursing Alert** Investigate hematuria because it is a sign of infections, stones, and cancers. The usual investigation starts with a clean-catch specimen or by a single catheterization in women for urinalysis and culture.

Bladder stones are generally less troublesome than are kidney or ureteral stones. Stones in the bladder may be asymptomatic or may cause mild hematuria or urgency and urge incontinence. If they do not obstruct the urethra, the client is generally unaware of them until they are found incidentally in diagnostic testing. Removal of bladder stones often relieves symptoms such as urgency, frequency, and recurrent UTIs.

Treatment

Treatment of stones begins with adequate hydration (3–4 L of fluid per day). Medications can help prevent the development of stones by helping to control the amounts of minerals and acid in the urine. The type of medication will depend on the content of the stone. Calcium stones may be helped by a thiazide diuretic or a phosphate-containing preparation. Uric acid stones may be minimized or dissolved by allopurinol (Zyloprim), which helps reduce uric acid levels in the blood and urine, plus an alkalizing agent, which helps keep urine more alkaline. Struvite stones, which are associated with UTIs, may require long-term use of antibiotics. Cystine stones are more difficult to treat and may require large amounts of diluting fluids plus medication to decrease the amount of cystine in the urine.

Only a strong analgesic will relieve the pain associated with kidney stones; antispasmodics also may be ordered. After a stone passes through the ureter into the bladder, the client usually has no difficulty passing it out of the body in the urine. If the stone does not pass through the ureteral channel spontaneously, it must be removed. Most of the time a stone passes on its own. However, depending on the location of the stone, there are surgical or lithotripsy options for treatment of urinary calculi, as follows:

Bladder Stones
One method is surgical removal of bladder stones and temporary use of a suprapubic tube to drain urine. Unless bladder stones are symptomatic or cause obstruction, they are not treated. However, bladder stones can grow quite large and may need to be removed surgically. If this is the case, the client will need a suprapubic tube to drain the bladder until the suture line is healed. Smaller stones can be removed using a cystoscope.

Ureter or Bladder Stones
Lithotripsy refers to the crushing of stones. It can be done in the bladder or the urethra by passing a crushing instrument into the urethra or urinary bladder through the urethroscope. The purpose of crushing the stone is to make the fragments small enough for the client to pass in the urine.

Ureter Stones
In some cases, a ureteroscopy is used for urethroscopic calculi removal. Stones are removed without crushing. The surgeon grabs the stone and pulls it out of the client's ureter, using a special tong-like instrument called a *stone basket*. Some bleeding is common after this procedure because of the trauma caused by the passing of the scope and/or stone. After urethroscopic calculi removal and lithotripsy, a **stent** (a hollow tube used to support structures) is placed so that it *bridges the* area where the stone was. The tube supports the structures and allows urine to drain easily. It is important that remaining fragments are washed out. The area will be swollen and traumatized after stone manipulation. It is important that the client returns for follow-up treatments for stent removal or changing of the stent.

Kidney or Ureter Stones
Extracorporeal (outside the body) *shock wave lithotripsy* (**ESWL**) is used in cases of calculi in the kidney or upper ureter (Fig. 89-3). In this treatment, the stones are "blasted" by shock waves that are so intense that they break the stones into small, gravel-like fragments. If a stone is in the lower ureter, it can be pushed up into the upper ureter or kidney and treated with ESWL. ESWL is not used in the lower ureter or bladder because it can be traumatic, and these tissues are more delicate. The client may find that ESWL is uncomfortable or painful; therefore, mild sedation and analgesia may be used during the procedure. ESWL is a specialized and potentially hazardous procedure that must be performed by carefully trained healthcare providers and technicians.

Kidney Stones
The procedure of percutaneous nephrolithotomy removes stones from the kidney. A small "stab wound" is made in the flank and a catheter is inserted. An ultrasonic probe is inserted through the catheter. Then, ultrasound waves are directed at the stone. These waves break the stone into pieces that are small enough to be withdrawn through the catheter. After the procedure, the catheter is left in place for 1 or 2 days until edema subsides. At this time, normal passage of urine into the ureter and bladder can resume.

Surgical Removal
A *ureterolithotomy*, surgical removal of calculi in the ureter, may be done in a few cases in which a stone blocking a ureter requires an incision for removal. Surgical *nephrolithotomy* is the method of kidney stone removal least likely to be used today. This major surgery includes an incision into the kidney and removal of the stone.

Nursing Considerations
Straining Urine for Calculi
If kidney or other urinary tract stones are suspected, the healthcare provider will order all urine to be strained. You can do this by pouring the urine through gauze, cheesecloth, or a strainer. Save any calculi. Calculi that are passed spontaneously may be as small as grains of sand or as large as pebbles. Measure and discard the urine, and save any material strained out of it for examination by the healthcare provider or laboratory personnel. See In Practice: Nursing Care Plan 89-1 for care of the client with renal calculi and hypertension.

Caring for the Client Undergoing Stone Removal
Pre- and postoperative care for surgical removal of stones is basically the same as for other abdominal procedures, with careful observation and straining of the urine; analysis of a stone can discover the causative agent. When the type of stone is known, appropriate preventative measures can be taken. Sterile technique is necessary when caring for drainage tubes postoperatively.

For the client undergoing ESWL, explain the procedure. Depending on the method of ESWL used, the client will either be placed on a treatment table that has a built-in water cushion or the client will be immersed in a tub of water. If using the submersion tank, place small water wings on the client's arms to keep the arms afloat and out of the way. A mild sedative is usually ordered before the procedure, and general anesthesia may be administered. The procedure is not totally without discomfort. Document all teaching.

Nursing care after ESWL includes observation of urine, which will be slightly bloody for 24–48 hr. The color is most often described as "rose." The bleeding results from ureteral trauma caused by the gravel-like stone fragments passing through in the urine. Strain the urine and encourage fluids. The client may be bruised in the area of the lateral pelvic bones.

The client must follow certain precautions after discharge from the healthcare facility. Urge the client to force fluids and strain all urine. Teach the client how to monitor for signs of infection and hematuria and to report these findings to the healthcare provider. Explain that medications must be taken as prescribed and that the client may find comfort by applying warm packs.

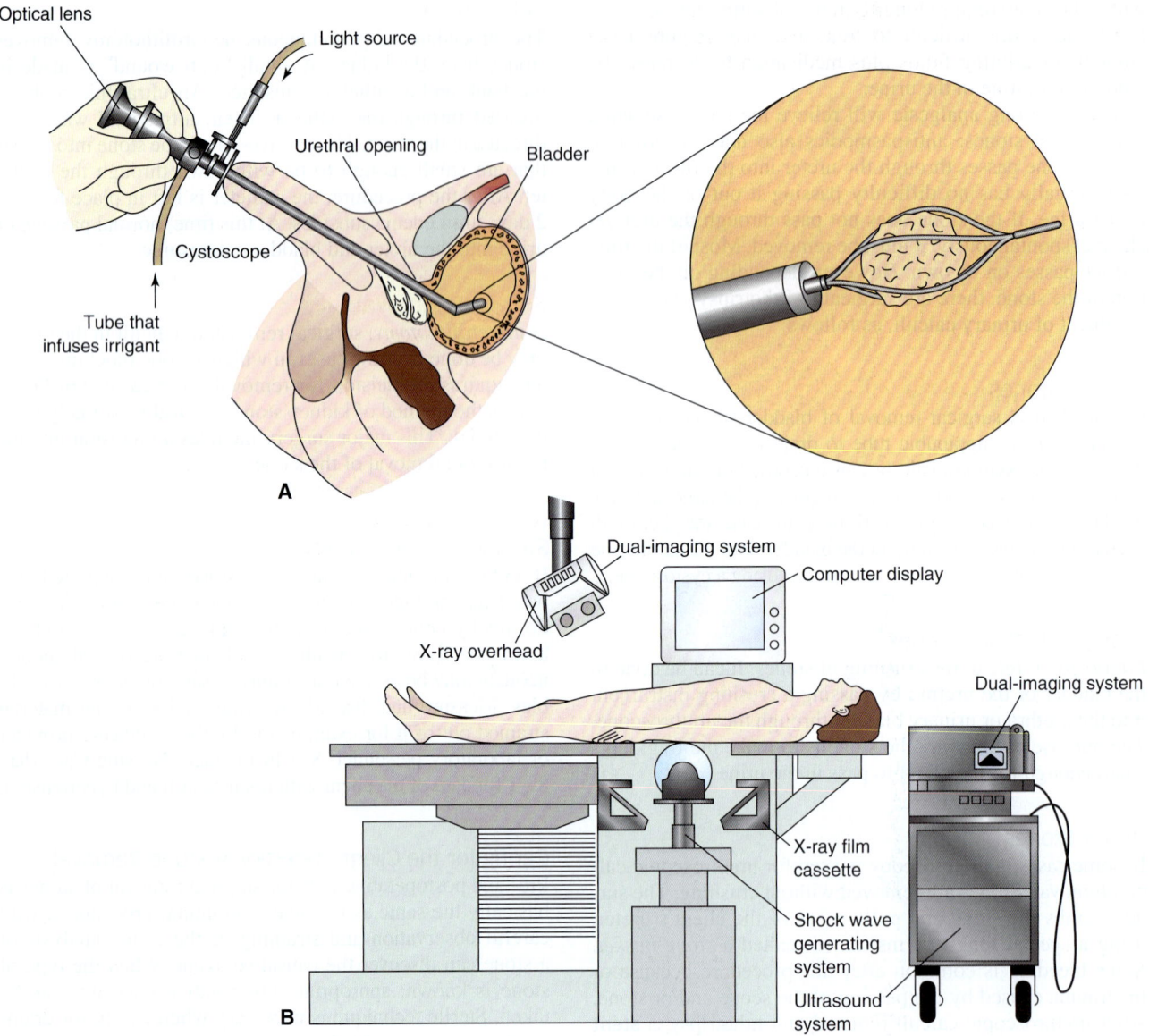

Figure 89-3 Removal of urinary and renal stones. **A.** Stone is removed using a ureteroscope, which captures the stone. **B.** Extracorporeal shock wave lithotripsy (ESWL).

Client Teaching
The client who has had one kidney stone has an increased chance of forming another one. A key factor in preventing kidney stone formation is intake of water. Encourage the client to drink at least eight 8-oz glasses of water every day to dilute the urine. Teach the client to increase fluid intake in hot weather to avoid dehydration. Also, depending on the analysis of the stone, have the client consult with a dietician to learn how to limit intake of certain foods (e.g., foods rich in oxalate).

Ureteral or Urethral Strictures
Fibrous bands can form anywhere along the ureters or the urethra, narrowing it and interfering with urine passage. This condition is more common in men than in women because the male urethra is longer. *Strictures* cause difficulty in voiding. The client feels the need to void frequently but an intense burning sensation accompanies voiding. A thorough medical history, urodynamic flow testing, and other diagnostic studies are used to diagnose strictures.

Treatment
A stricture can be stretched by inserting metal instruments (*sounds, bougies*) of graduated sizes into the urethra, beginning with the size that goes past the strictures and gradually increasing to larger ones. Because strictures have a tendency to reform, the client will need to return to the healthcare facility periodically to have this dilatation process repeated.

Sometimes, surgery is necessary to cut the constricting bands; this procedure is referred to as an *urethrotomy*. Recurrence of the stricture is rare after urethrotomy.

Nursing Considerations
Monitor clients for bleeding after treatment with bougies or urethrotomy. Other postoperative care is routine, including monitoring urinary output for symptoms of UTI.

CHAPTER 89 Urinary Disorders

IN PRACTICE
NURSING CARE PLAN 89-1 The Client With Renal Calculi and Hypertension

Medical History: R.M., a 61-year-old man, comes to the Emergency Department complaining of severe colic-like pain in the left flank area that radiates to the thigh. Client states, "I feel like I have to urinate, but then when I try, only a little urine comes out, and it hurts." Urinalysis shows hematuria and RBCs. Hypertension of 178/110 noted. KUB diagnostic tests reveal the presence of several stones in the kidney and ureter. Client's family history is negative for renal disease.

Medical Diagnosis: Renal calculi; hypertension.

DATA COLLECTION/NURSING OBSERVATIONS

Client is a well-nourished man, visibly in pain, holding side and lower back area, rubbing left flank area. He states, "The pain is terrible." He rates pain as 10 on a scale of 1–10. Urine appears cloudy and concentrated; client states he has "had a headache all day." Reports dysuria and frequency with small amounts of rose-colored or dark urine passed with each voiding. Voiding amounts ranging from 50 to 75 mL each time. Temperature 100.8 °F (38.2 °C), BP 178/110, pulse 128, respirations 28.

NURSING DIAGNOSIS

(Although other nursing diagnoses may be appropriate, a priority nursing diagnosis is addressed below.)

Impaired urinary elimination related to possible renal disease as evidenced by hypertension and client's complaints of dysuria, frequency, and voiding in small amounts.

Planning (Outcomes/Goals)	Implementation (Nursing Actions)	Evaluation
Short-Term Goals		
A. Client will verbalize that flank pain has decreased.	• Administer analgesic morphine sulfate prescribed for intravenous administration. • Monitor effect of analgesic. • Assist client to assume a position of comfort. • Apply warmth to flank area. *Rationale: The pain associated with renal calculi can be severe. Pain relief is essential for the client's comfort and cooperation and may lower BP. Since the BP is at hypertensive levels, the nurse must be alert for sudden changes of BP after administration of MS. BP may decrease quickly if hypertension when pain relief is achieved but the BP may diminish minimally if hypertension is due to renal disease.* • Obtain stat laboratory tests and x-ray per orders. • Be alert for appearance of additional problems due to kidney disease such as a stroke or renal failure. *Rationale: The healthcare provider typically looks for signs of infection, anemia, or signs of renal failure, which can be noted in preliminary studies. The client may have renal calculi as well as kidney diseases as evidenced by uncontrolled hypertension.*	Emergency Department Day 1–1930 hr. • Client rates pain as 7 on a scale of 1–10 after second dose of 3 mg MS: BP 175/110. • Client reports continued dysuria. • Repeat dose of 3 mg MS IVP. • After third dose of MS, pain stated to be at 2 on pain scale; BP 175/100. *Goal A partially completed. Ongoing observations.*
B. Hypertension will be decreased to less than 150/80 while continuing evaluation of etiology of hypertension.	• Monitor client's vital signs ½ hr. after administration of MS. • Notify healthcare provider of VS. • Repeat administration of MS for pain if client states pain has returned. *Rationale: It is important to determine if hypertension is due to pain or kidney disease or both. Pain relief is a priority for a client with lithiasis.* • Show client how to do strain urine. • Monitor urine output for any signs of calculi. • Maintain visual check of urine for hematuria or calculi. • Maintain I&O of urine *Rationale: Straining urine helps to gather and to identify the causative factor of stones, which then, perhaps, can be prevented in the future.*	Emergency Department Day 1–2345 hr. • VS: 160/95, 92, 24 s/p (status post) MS. • Client states, "I think I passed some stones." • Urine checked; small granules noted and sent to laboratory. • Urologist notified of pain, calculi, and VS. • Client to be admitted to medical/urology unit for evaluation of kidney function. *Goal B in process of completion.*

Planning (Outcomes/Goals)	Implementation (Nursing Actions)	Evaluation
Long-Term Goals		
C. Prevent further damage to renal structures and evaluate kidney function.	• Monitor VS. • Medications for anxiety, BP, and antibiotics initiated. • Order laboratory studies and CT of kidneys and pelvis. • Assist client with ADLs. • Explain importance of quiet environment, rest, and oral fluids to client and his partner. • Monitor oral and IV fluid intake. • Observe face, arms, and legs for signs of edema. • Notify healthcare provider of significant changes of status. • After laboratory analysis of renal calculi, consult dietitian regarding potential dietary changes. *Rationale: The client with kidney disease needs a restful environment and fluids. It is important to protect damaged glomeruli so that they may heal.* Reinforce urologist's explanation of rationale for hospitalization.	Medical Unit—Urology Day 2–02:30 hr. • Client expresses concern and denial regarding diagnosis of renal disease, "I've never had any problems before and don't think I have any now." • Teaching care plan regarding causes and care for renal disease initiated for client and his partner. • Client states he will remain in hospital for diagnostic testing. Goals A and B met. Goal C in process with continued observations and testing.

URINARY TRACT TUMORS

Benign Renal Cysts

Cysts of the kidney may be single (*monocystic*) or multiple (*polycystic*). *Monocystic kidney disease* or a single cyst is usually benign and asymptomatic. However, depending on the size of the cyst, it can cause pain or decrease kidney function.

Polycystic kidney disease consists of multiple clusters of benign tumors on the kidneys; it is a genetically inherited problem. The extent of the disease is much greater than with a single cyst. Generally, but not always, diagnosed shortly after birth, the cysts become so enlarged within the kidney that a mass is often palpable. With polycystic disease, the hormone erythropoietin increases, causing an overproduction of RBCs. (Usually, individuals with chronic kidney disease are anemic.) This disorder may start with abdominal pain, flank pain, hematuria, nocturia, and frequent UTIs. The disease will progress, developing high blood pressure, kidney stones and kidney infections, and ESRD. Treatment includes diuretics, low-salt diets, antihypertensive medications, drainage of cysts (if possible), and dialysis. The disorder can persist for years, even decades, but may eventually progress to ESRD. Emotional support for the client, siblings, and family is crucial.

Cancer of the Kidney

Nephroma is cancer of the kidney. Cancer of the kidneys has two principal origination sites: the renal tubule and the renal pelvis. The location and cellular type of cancer are important because prognosis and treatments differ. Kidney tumors are almost always malignant. They occur more frequently in men. Age differences occur. They are rare in people younger than 30 years and are increased in incidence in people over the age of 65. Some nephromas have a hereditary risk factor. Renal cancer is aggressive, often invading the aorta or vena cava. Clients often have distant metastases and local invasion of nearby organs. Kidney tumors in children are generally Wilms tumors (Chapter 72).

Signs and Symptoms

Cancer of the kidney is usually advanced before signs appear. The first sign may be blood in the urine (painless hematuria). Other symptoms are fever, loss of weight, and malaise; a palpable flank mass and pain may appear later. X-ray, CT scan, renal arteriography, or ultrasound study confirms the diagnosis.

Treatment

If the kidney is a primary site, the cancer is discovered early enough, and the other kidney is healthy, then removal of the kidney using nephrectomy may be curative. Before surgery, the kidney function is brought to as normal a level as possible. Radiation, chemotherapy, or both are used when the cancer has spread to the lymph nodes.

> **Key Concept**
> Neoplasms may present with problems to renal function by obstructing urinary flow. Chemotherapy may damage renal function.

Bladder Tumors

The bladder is the most common site of urinary system cancer. Bladder cancer occurs most often in men between the ages of 50 and 70. Tumors may be embedded in the bladder wall or may appear as small warts on the inside surface. Most bladder tumors are malignant.

Occupational exposure to chemicals increases the risk of this cancer. Cigarette smoking and lung cancer also are associated with increased incidence of bladder cancer.

Signs and Symptoms

Most often, the presenting sign of bladder cancer is painless hematuria. Bladder cancer is diagnosed with a combination of CT scan, x-ray, cystoscopy with biopsy, or urine cytology studies.

Treatment

Treatment for bladder cancer varies, depending on the tumor's extent. Carcinoma in situ may be treated using chemotherapy instilled into the bladder through a catheter and then allowed to remain in the bladder for an hour. Treatments take place weekly for 6 weeks and then are repeated at 3-month intervals for a year.

A transurethral resection of a bladder tumor (**TURBT**) is removal of a superficial tumor by endoscopic *resection* (cutting out) or *fulguration* (destruction by electricity). The surgeon uses a special cystoscope called a *resectoscope*, which is inserted into the bladder through the urethra. Laser therapy also may be used. Clients with this type of tumor return at 6-month intervals for cystoscopic examination to determine recurrence or further tumor development.

Cystotomy, an incision made into the bladder, can remove larger or more extensive tumors. If the bladder is not totally removed, a catheter may be placed in the bladder and brought out through the skin as a cutaneous cystostomy or suprapubic cystocath.

If the tumor is large and invasive, the entire bladder may be removed (**cystectomy**), necessitating urinary diversion (discussed below). Anytime the bladder is removed, a *stent* (tube- or spring-shaped support) is placed in the ureters, where they are connected to the ileum to keep them open and prevent edema or excess drainage from causing urinary obstruction during the postoperative period. The stents are usually removed about 2 weeks postoperatively.

Bladder tumors often metastasize to the lymph nodes, then to the bones of the pelvis, ribs, and vertebrae, and sometimes to the kidneys, liver, or lungs. Radiation therapy and chemotherapy are usually combined with tumor removal to prevent or minimize metastases. If the client receives radiation therapy, changes in the bladder wall (if the bladder was not totally

---

Box 89-1 | Types of Urinary Diversion

Urostomy—artificial pouch required to collect and drain urine
- **Ileal conduit urinary diversion:** Segment of ileum close to the ileocecal valve resected; ureters reanastomosed to it. Proximal end of ileal segment closed; distal end brought to abdominal wall as stoma.
- **Cutaneous ureterostomy:** Ureters brought to abdominal wall as stoma.

Continent Diversion—creation of internal pouch or internal bladder using part of digestive tract
- **Continent cutaneous diversion (Indiana pouch):** Segment of cecum and ileum resected from the bowel to build reservoir. Ureters tunneled into reservoir. Ileum brought to skin as small stoma. Urine flows downward to prevent urinary backup and kidney infections. Catheter is regularly inserted into external stoma to drain internal reservoir of urine.
- **Neobladder to urethra diversion:** Internal urinary reservoir that empties through urethra. Some incontinence normal for up to 1–1½ years after surgery. Persistent incontinence is possible.

---

removed) make it appear roughened and reddened. In addition, the bladder will lose its compliance and will not hold as much urine. These typically permanent changes are called *radiation cystitis* and can make the client miserable. Treatments used for urge incontinence can be used to help these clients.

Urinary Diversions

A urinary diversion is the general name for one of several types of surgical procedures that reroute urine flow from normal anatomic pathways. Diversions are done to divert urine flow from diseased or defective ureters, bladder, or urethra. The diversion can be temporary or permanent, depending on the etiology of the problem. Most commonly, some type of ureteroenteric anastomosis is done. That is, the ureters are anastomosed (joined) with an intestinal segment. There are basically two types of urinary diversion—a urostomy or cutaneous diversion and continent urinary diversion. Box 89-1 summarizes types of the most common urinary diversions. Many factors influence the type of urinary diversion that is used. See In Practice: Educating

---

IN PRACTICE
EDUCATING THE CLIENT 89-4 | Care of the Ileal Conduit Urinary Diversion

- Change appliance every 5–7 days.
- Use solvent to loosen appliance; do not "tear" off the appliance.
- Clean the skin with water and mild soap.
- To remove encrustations, use gauze soaked with a 1:3 part solution of vinegar and water.
- Examine the stoma; healthy stoma tissue is deep pink to dark red and shiny. If the stoma is macerated, dusky, or wet-looking, notify the healthcare provider.
- Dry the skin area gently, but thoroughly, before applying a new appliance.
- If the tissue is excoriated, apply medication, as ordered by the wound, ostomy, and continence nurse (enterostomal therapist).
- Use a synthetic barrier cream that contains little or no karaya (urine destroys karaya).
- Strands of mucus may appear in the urine (from the mucus-producing cells of the ileum).
- Increase fluid intake to 3 L/day (to flush out sediment and mucus and to prevent clogging of the stoma).

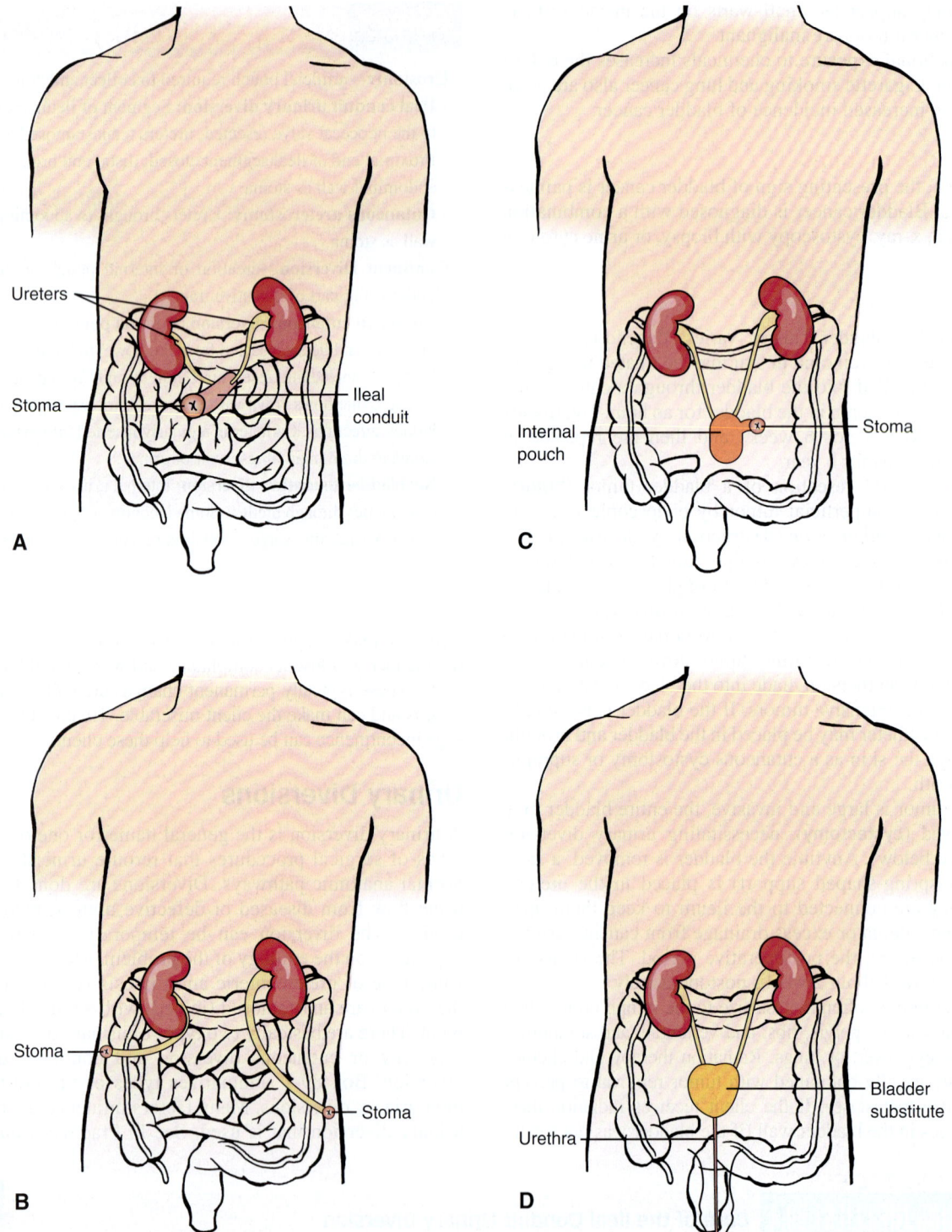

Figure 89-4 **A, B.** Examples of urostomies (cutaneous urinary diversion) procedures, after which the client must wear a urinary collecting device. **C, D.** Examples of continent diversions: Indiana pouch and a neobladder.

the Client 89-4, for more information on caring for an ileal conduit urinary diversion.

Many medications are available today to suppress rejection, and clients with transplanted organs have a much greater prospect for success. The rejection syndrome in kidney transplantation is usually easier to manage than that in other organ transplants.

Cutaneous Diversions

Cutaneous diversions involve the drainage of urine through a surgical opening (*stoma*) created in the abdominal wall. Several versions of cutaneous diversions are seen in Figure 89-4. The client must wear an appliance at all times over the surgically designed stoma, which continuously collects urine drainage. The client often has no voluntary control of urinary flow. Chapter 88 provides information on ostomy appliances and nursing care.

Continent Diversions

Continent diversions involve surgical creation of a new reservoir for urine from a portion of the intestine. This type of diversion is done depending on the client's preference and anatomy (see Box 89-1). Various methods of urinary diversions may provide the client with voluntary bladder control as shown in Figure 89-4.

Nursing Considerations

Pre- and postsurgical consultations with the wound, ostomy, and continence nurse or wound care ostomy nurse (**WOCN**, **WCON**), who may also be referred to as the enterostomal therapy (**ET**) nurse, is one of the primary steps in preparation for long-term physical and emotional adaption to diversions. Urinary diversion may strongly affect the person's body image. Bladder removal for men is often associated with permanent sexual dysfunction. Adapting to cancer, loss of the bladder, and loss of body image can be devastating. Be supportive. Listening to the client's concerns is an important aspect of nursing care.

> **Key Concept**
> Urinary diversions are provided to promote the elimination of urine from the body. Unobstructed, intact stomas or other urinary structures are crucial, along with good skin care, emotional support, and client teaching.

URINARY TRACT TRAUMA

Trauma to the kidney can be dangerous because the kidney receives a large amount of blood from the abdominal aorta. Because a small kidney laceration can cause massive hemorrhage, the client will need immediate surgery to repair the tear. Occasionally, a damaged kidney must be removed to prevent further hemorrhage. Bruising of the kidney can result in edema and blocked urine flow.

A fairly common injury sustained in motor vehicle and other accidents is *bladder rupture*, which results in shock, sepsis, and hemorrhage. The client must have emergency surgery, after which a urinary drainage system and other drains will be in place. Postoperative care is routine, with special attention to urinary drainage. Complications may include impotence or incontinence.

General health teaching includes attention to frequent voiding and the necessity of keeping the bladder empty when the client is traveling or participating in sports or other activities.

RENAL FAILURE

Changes in renal function often are graded on a continuum. *Renal impairment* is identified by specific urine concentration and dilution tests. *Renal insufficiency* becomes apparent when the kidneys cannot meet the demands of dietary or metabolic stress. *Renal failure* (or *kidney failure*) exists when the kidneys no longer meet everyday demands, and there is a significant decrease in the glomerular filtration rate. As renal function diminishes (see end-stage renal disease below), the kidneys lose their ability to adapt to varying intakes of foods and fluids.

Early in renal failure, the creatinine clearance test evaluates effectiveness of treatment. In chronic renal failure, the serum creatinine level reflects the level of renal function; as the disease progresses, the serum creatinine level increases. The phases of renal failure may be characterized by oliguria (lack of urine) or diuresis (increased urine), or they may fluctuate, depending on the cause.

In renal failure, the kidneys become unable to remove waste products from the blood and body cells and excrete them in the urine. This toxic condition is associated with renal insufficiency and retention of nitrogenous substances in the blood (azotemia). Abnormal levels of potassium, calcium, and phosphate are found in the blood. Anemia is typical. In the urine, abnormal amounts of protein (proteinuria) and blood (hematuria) are common. Renal failure may result from injury, kidney disease, urinary tract disturbances, or conditions that decrease blood supply to the kidneys. It may follow acute glomerulonephritis, drug overdose or poisoning, excessive inhalation of a highly toxic substance (e.g., sulfur or carbon tetrachloride), severe transfusion reactions, and other severe shocks to the system. The vascular changes of diabetes mellitus often lead to chronic renal failure. Renal failure also may occur more slowly as a result of nephrotoxic drugs given for unrelated disorders (Box 89-2).

> **Box 89-2 Common Drugs and Substances That Can Become Nephrotoxic**
>
> Common drugs and possible renal damage
> - Penicillins: Allergic reactions
> - Sulfonamides: Allergic reactions
> - Cephalosporins (e.g., cefaclor, cefazolin sodium, cefoxitin sodium, cephalothin sodium, cephradine): Damaged kidney cells
> - Allopurinol (Zyloprim, Lopurin): Allergies; also altered liver function
> - Aminoglycosides (e.g., gentamicin, neomycin, streptomycin): Damaged kidney cells
> - Amphotericin B (Fungizone): Used to treat fungal infections; can cause permanent renal damage
> - Lithium (psychiatric drug): Renal toxicity
> - Cimetidine (Tagamet): Used to treat peptic ulcer; can cause creatinine elevation
> - Phenytoin (Dilantin): Used to control seizures; can cause toxic hepatitis
> - Nonsteroidal anti-inflammatory drugs, analgesic drugs (e.g., ibuprofen, indomethacin [Indocin]): Used to control pain; can cause acute renal failure or nephrotic syndrome
> - Antineoplastics: Used to treat cancers; can damage renal cells
>
> Other substances toxic to the kidneys
> - Heavy metals
> - Aniline dyes
> - Iodine-based contrast media
> - Carbon tetrachloride
> - Ethylene glycol
> - Benzene

> **Key Concept**
>
> The nephrotoxicity of a drug must be determined before the agent is given to a client. Whenever administering medications, watch for signs of kidney dysfunction and report them to the healthcare provider at once.

Acute Kidney Injury

Acute kidney injury, also referred to as *acute renal failure*, is due to injury, hemorrhage, or severe reactions to some medications. The injury causes the sudden interruption of kidney functioning due to damage of the parenchymal cells of the kidneys. Without the ability to make urine, the result is a decline in the glomerular filtration rate, retention of urea and other nitrogenous waste products, and interrupted regulation of extracellular fluid volume and electrolytes. Some types of acute kidney injury may be reversible with medical treatment. If not treated, kidney failure typically progresses to permanent end-stage kidney disease, uremia, and death (see below). Acute kidney injury normally occurs in three distinct phases: oliguric-anuric, diuretic, and recovery.

Obstructions in urinary flow that damage the proximal structures or damage the kidney tissue itself are other possible causes. Tubular damage, referred to as *acute tubular necrosis*, is another form of renal dysfunction.

Signs and Symptoms

Oliguria is common in the early phases of renal failure (*prerenal failure*); it occurs when the urinary output is less than 400 mL in a 24-h period (in newborns, <1 mL/kg/hr). **Anuria**, output of less than 100 mL/day, may also occur. Laboratory values for serum sodium are decreased, and the serum creatinine and BUN levels are elevated. This phase may last from 8–14 days.

In obstructive failure, the client may experience an initial diuresis when production of urine increases. The client may be *polyuric* with urine output greater than 6 L/day.

Although urine volume eventually increases in most clients who are anuric or oliguric, the quality of this urine is inadequate, and the client's body is retaining waste products. This is evidenced in the remaining elevation of BUN and serum creatinine levels. The recovery phase begins when the client's BUN level stabilizes or is in the normal range. In this case, urine volume is normal, and the client returns to normal activity. This process may take several months. Some clients do not improve and develop ESRD.

> **Key Concept**
>
> Recognize signs of acute kidney injury and treat them promptly to prevent progression to permanent renal failure. Symptoms vary but close monitoring of intake and output as well as creatinine, BUN, GFR levels, and electrolytes can provide valuable data to try to arrest the disorder.

Treatment

During acute kidney injury, laboratory studies are performed frequently to monitor BUN, creatinine, and sodium and potassium levels. Treatment for kidney failure will include maintaining homeostasis of fluid and electrolytes. IV fluids will be given in cases of fluid volume deficiency, and diuretics are given when the client has fluid volume excess that results in edema, especially of the arms and legs. The healthcare provider will monitor electrolyte levels and glucose. Hyperkalemia (high potassium) causes arrhythmias and muscle weakness; it can lead to fatal heart arrhythmias. To regulate potassium levels in the blood, medications are given that help filter and prevent accumulation of this electrolyte. Calcium, glucose, and sodium polystyrene sulfonate (Kayexalate, Kionex) are examples of potassium-regulating medications. Blood tests will monitor calcium, which may need to be supplemented with calcium infusions. Phosphorous levels may also be monitored. Temporary dialysis may be initiated at an early stage of renal failure to help maintain homeostasis and to permit the parenchymal tissues of the kidney to heal, to eliminate excess potassium and fluids, and to remove toxins. Dialysis is discussed in more detail in a following section.

> **Key Concept**
>
> Do not confuse the mineral elements *potassium* and *phosphorus*. Potassium is chemically abbreviated with a "K" and phosphorus's initial is "P." Serious medication errors could result if potassium were given in place of phosphorus.

Nursing Considerations

Nursing considerations will involve client teaching regarding the importance of self-regulation of one's diet. A dietitian should review the client's individual's eating habits. Avoid foods with extra sodium chloride (table salt, KCl), which includes most convenience foods and processed foods. Suggest low-potassium foods such as apples, grapes, strawberries, cabbage, and green beans. High-potassium foods, which need to be avoided, include bananas, oranges, potatoes, spinach, and tomatoes. Phosphorus (P), a mineral, also needs to be limited because hyperphosphatemia can weaken bones and causes itching. Phosphorus is found in milk and milk products, canned vegetables, nuts (including peanut butter), and processed meats. Very accurate measurements of I&O are essential: use a measuring device that has specific demarcations in lieu of the more general type of I&O markings that require an estimation of fluids. To help the client conserve energy, assist with ADLs.

End-Stage Renal Disease

ESRD occurs when the kidney failure is permanent; dialysis or a kidney transplant is lifesaving. Most cases of ESRD are caused by diabetes, hypertension, inherited disorders, side effects of polypharmacia or of specific medications, and severe kidney trauma. Chronic kidney disease, such as glomerulonephritis, may lead to ESRD. Control of diabetes and hypertension can prevent some cases of chronic kidney disease and ESRD. If ESRD occurs, as evidenced by previous symptoms and elevated BUN and serum creatinine levels, the client receives the same treatment as for chronic renal failure. (See In Practice: Data Gathering in Nursing 89-2 for symptoms of ESRD.)

Nursing Considerations

Nursing and medical care plans are designed to treat the primary cause of ESRD and to treat symptoms as they occur. Keep the client in as normal a state as possible, and make

IN PRACTICE
DATA GATHERING IN NURSING 89-2: Symptoms of End-Stage Renal Disease (ESRD)

Symptoms of ESRD include any or all of the following:
- Anemia
- Itching (*pruritus*)
- Uremic frost (waste products crystallizing on the skin)
- Loss of appetite (*anorexia*)
- Hiccups (*singultus*)
- Nausea
- Vomiting
- Fatigue
- Fluid accumulation (*edema*)
- Generalized body edema (*anasarca*)
- Potassium retention
- Sodium retention
- Hypertension
- Gastrointestinal bleeding
- Bleeding disorders
- Bone disease
- Nerve-conduction defects
- Heart failure
- Inflammation of the pericardial sac
- Decreased immune response
- Decreased platelet function
- Retardation of growth (in children)
- Dementia
- Sexual dysfunction
- Malnutrition
- Decreased vitamin metabolism
- Metabolic acidosis

---

every attempt to prevent further kidney damage. The individual is typically a client at high risk because of existing diseases; therefore, medical examinations and regular testing of kidney function are necessary. Existing drug regimens should be evaluated by the healthcare providers or a pharmacist.

Nursing considerations in ESRD include the following:

- Give sedatives for restlessness, transfusions for anemia, and cardiac medications for tachycardia or dysrhythmias, as ordered.
- Restrict fluids because the kidneys are not excreting urine. Vary fluids. Urge the client to spread fluid allowance throughout the day.
- Monitor diet. A diet high in fat and carbohydrates and low in protein, sodium, and potassium is helpful, although restrictions may vary for each client.
- Maintain fluid and electrolyte balance as much as possible. Frequent blood chemistry studies will be done, and the healthcare provider needs reports as soon as possible. Make adjustments as needed for electrolytes given IV.
- Accurately document I&O: Determining exactly how much urine the kidneys are secreting helps to determine the extent of the disease.
- Take daily weights to detect fluid retention or edema.
- Provide good skin care and mouth care. To relieve the itching and crusting brought on by pruritus and uremic frost, the client should bathe with tepid water, use no soap, and place a small amount of vinegar or baking soda in the bathwater.
- Prevent chilling and exposure to infections because the client has few natural defenses to fight off infection. Also, many antibodies are excreted through the kidneys.
- Be alert for respiratory or cardiac complications.

Key Concept
A healthy kidney produces the hormone erythropoietin that is necessary for production of RBCs. A person with kidney disease may be short of breath, anemic, or chronically fatigued because they do not have enough hemoglobin molecules to carry oxygen. Be aware of using a pulse oximeter to establish a rationale for dyspnea because a pulse oximeter reflects the capabilities of existing hemoglobin levels, which can be misrepresented as normal oxygenation (above 90%).

NCLEX Alert
NCLEX clinical scenarios often include symptoms that the nurse observes, such as shortness of breath, cyanosis, pallor, diaphoresis, or anuria. The correct option will generally relate to the priority symptom(s) at the moment of observation. Read all options carefully because more than one answer can be correct; you are looking for the best correct answer.

Dialysis

Dialysis is a process that assumes the work of a damaged, nonfunctioning kidney. Two types of dialysis, *peritoneal dialysis* and *hemodialysis*, remove body wastes through a semipermeable membrane by osmosis, diffusion, and ultrafiltration. Dialysis may be performed in a hospital, dialysis center, or in-home, depending upon the individual's acute or chronic needs and current situation. It can be a long-term procedure for chronic disorders, such as kidney disease secondary to shock, diabetes mellitus, or chronic hypertension. Clients with severe drug overdose or poisoning may be treated with dialysis for relatively short periods during the acute phases of the illness. Some people are maintained for many years on intermittent dialysis. People who are awaiting kidney transplants are maintained on dialysis until a suitable kidney is available.

The purposes of dialysis are to:

- Remove waste products of protein metabolism from the blood.
- Remove poisons or toxins from the blood.
- Remove excess water.
- Establish or maintain proper levels of electrolytes.
- Maintain acid–base balance.
- Instill medications (e.g., antibiotics), electrolytes, or other substances.

Peritoneal Dialysis
In peritoneal dialysis, the connective tissue of the intestine (*peritoneum*), which lines the abdominal cavity, serves as the semipermeable membrane. Peritoneal dialysis is not used if

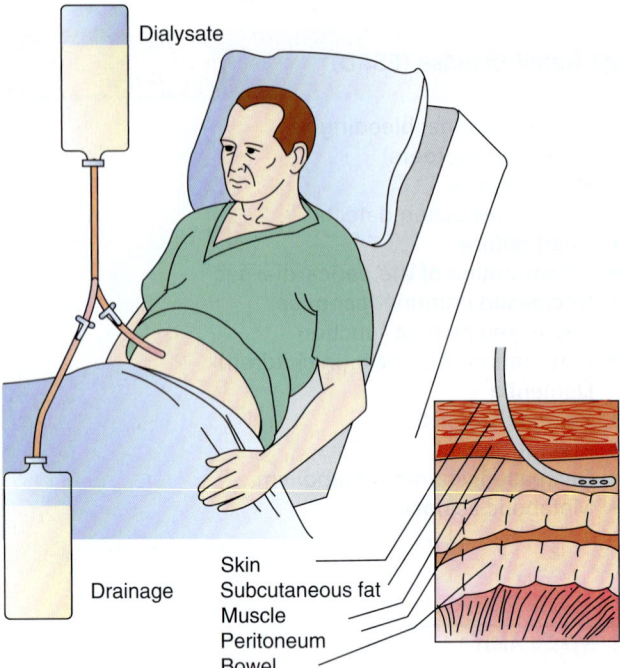

Figure 89-5 Peritoneal dialysis, in which the dialysate is infused into the peritoneal cavity by gravity. After remaining in the peritoneum for a period of time, the drainage tube is unclamped and the peritoneal cavity is drained by gravity.

including the client's I&O, through normal body orifices and a complete record of the dialysate (type and amounts taken in and released out). Continually record the total amounts of I&O, medications or electrolytes added, and times the solution was instilled and drained. The facility may have a specific documentation form for use during this procedure.

Continuous Ambulatory Peritoneal Dialysis (CAPD)
CAPD is used in the home when the client's condition, electrolytes, and hematologic status are stable. The peritoneum (lining of the abdomen) acts as the dialysis membrane. During an outpatient procedure, the healthcare provider will insert a catheter that will be used for fluid insertion and waste fluid drainage. The dialysate remains intraperitoneally for 3–5 hr, and the client exchanges the dialysate four to five times per day and once during the night. This procedure requires faithful commitment and the ability to do the process. A specially trained person will provide instruction and support. The benefits of this at home procedure include less time traveling and sitting for dialysis. Other advantages are that stable blood chemistry levels are more easily achieved, the process is shorter and less expensive, and training is less complicated than for home hemodialysis.

Hemodialysis
Hemodialysis is performed by circulating the client's blood through a machine outside the body using specialized cannulas or **shunts** that will be the connection between the client and machine. This procedure is also known as *extracorporeal hemodialysis*. An external shunt consists of an implanted U-shaped, large-bore cannula designed to facilitate repeated hemodialysis. The shunt allows blood to circulate in the machine, bypassing the body's central circulation, but it provides access to the arterial system. At the time of dialysis, two-needle punctures are made into the shunt. One needle into the shunt will act as arterial output to the external dialysis device, and the other acts as the venous input for the replacement of the filtered blood back into the body. Hemodialysis is conducted within the dialysis machine by means of blood flow from the client. This shunt remains in place because the client needs dialysis treatment two to three times per week for 3–8 hr per treatment to maintain life.

Home Hemodialysis
Occasionally, clients have a hemodialysis machine at home and do their dialysis during the day or at night. In this case, a family member must learn to assist and recognize complications. In some cases, specially trained dialysis nurses assist in the home.

Types of Shunts
The two main types of external shunts are an arteriovenous (AV) fistula or an AV graft. Joining a large vein into an artery creates a *fistula*. Generally, the client's nondominant arm at the radial artery and cephalic vein provides the location for a surgically created anastomosis (connection). A graft is similar to the AV fistula, but with a graft, a synthetic or biologic-based cannula (usually of animal origin) is surgically placed into the client. A *bruit* (whooshing sound) and a *thrill* (fine vibration) should be detected at the site of an AV shunt.

the client has known peritonitis or has had recent abdominal surgery. It is most often used on a short-term basis (e.g., in the case of poisoning) in an acute-care facility.

A trained healthcare provider inserts a specific catheter into the visceral cavity through which the dialysis solution (*dialysate*) is instilled into the abdominal cavity. The solution remains in the peritoneum for the time specified by the healthcare provider. Using continuous sterile technique, the dialysate is allowed to flow freely out of the catheter into an attached container, which is lowered to facilitate gravity drainage flow. This process may be continuous or repeated intermittently (Fig. 89-5).

Possible complications of peritoneal dialysis include

- Bacterial or chemical *peritonitis* (inflammation of the peritoneum)—cloudy, odoriferous outflow
- Septicemia
- Pain—abdomen, back, or shoulder (referred)
- Shortness of breath
- Protein loss
- Fluid overload or loss
- Electrolyte imbalance
- Constipation
- Infection
- Bleeding—the return looks bloody

Nursing interventions during peritoneal dialysis include observation for signs of drug reactions, abdominal distention or pain, bleeding or shock, respiratory problems, infection, and leakage around the catheter leading into the peritoneum. During the peritoneal dialysis procedure, keep the puncture site and dialysate sterile. The dialysate is warmed before the treatment, often using a warm-water bath. Do not use the microwave to warm dialysate. Document the process,

> **Key Concept**
> Whether the client has an AV graft or an AV fistula, they should be taught to check its patency daily by feeling the **thrill** (vibration) and hearing the **bruit** (whooshing sound of high-volume blood flow). Clients should also be taught to avoid venipuncture and having blood pressure measured in the affected arm.

An alternative dialysis device is a *subclavian or jugular IV catheter*, which is fairly large and is placed into blood vessels in the subclavicular region of the chest or the jugular region of the neck. This catheter has at least two ports, one for the arterial blood source and one for venous return. These sites are generally temporary, pending need of further dialysis and placement of a more permanent shunt.

> **Nursing Alert** Cannula separation is a life-threatening emergency. The client can exsanguinate (lose extreme amounts of blood) in a matter of minutes. Whenever a client has a cannula placement, they should be taught to have two clamps always attached to the dressing, to clamp the ends of the separated cannula quickly until they can be reattached.

Possible complications of hemodialysis are provided in Box 89-3 and below:

- *Exsanguination* (severe, immediately life-threatening hemorrhage)
- Septicemia
- Air emboli
- Hemolytic anemia
- Disequilibrium syndrome
- Hepatitis
- Hypotension

> **Box 89-3 Complications of Continued Dialysis**
>
> - The cannula can fall out and the client might bleed to death. More severe bleeding can also occur because the cannula is heparinized.
> - The membrane within the dialysis machine can rupture, causing hemorrhage.
> - If the chemical agents used are the wrong ones, or if the chemistry workup is incorrect, the client's electrolyte balance will be disrupted even further.
> - Because most clients on dialysis have high blood pressure (caused by renal damage), they may go into shock when connected to the machine.
> - The blood in the machine must be warm, or the client can suffer cardiac arrest from the shock of cold blood.
> - Infection or septicemia is always a possibility. Because this client has especially low resistance, infection can be dangerous.
> - Blood can clot in the cannula and cause phlebitis.
> - Male clients often become impotent, although this problem may correct itself as the condition is stabilized.
> - Excesses in alcohol or food intake will not be excreted between dialysis runs.

- Pain, cramps
- Nausea and vomiting

Nursing Considerations

The nurse may be asked to prepare a client for dialysis or to care for the client after a dialysis treatment. Before the dialysis "run" (treatment), be sure the client is wearing a name band. The client is often NPO after midnight for a morning dialysis run. Blood may be drawn just before dialysis.

Initially, specially trained personnel will monitor the hemodialysis run. If you are the client's primary nurse, you can provide vital information to the dialysis nurse regarding the client's baseline status, particularly if you suspect changes in neurologic status, an early sign of deteriorating hemodynamic status. Discuss the administration of any routine medications the client requires because dialysis can filter out the medication during the dialysis run. Many smaller healthcare facilities are served by regional dialysis centers that either send personnel to assist on a rotating basis or the client may go to the center several times per week. In this way, clients can be treated in their own hometown.

Specialty nursing considerations for all types of dialysis include the routine monitoring and documentation of the following:

- Intake and output
- Vital signs
- Daily weight
- Level of consciousness
- Patency of blood flow in an arm with a shunt. *Rationale: Constriction of blood flow can lead to clotting of the shunt.*
- Check for the presence of a bruit (use a stethoscope on a shunt)
- Check for the feel for the thrill (use the tips of your fingers on a shunt)
- Avoid taking blood pressure or withdrawing blood specimens on treated arm

Following the dialysis treatment, take vital signs frequently. The nursing care plan should include frequent turning, deep breathing, good skin care, and careful oral hygiene. The client generally feels better the day after dialysis than immediately following dialysis.

When a client is on dialysis, enforce strict dietary restrictions. For example, the client cannot excrete alcohol; therefore, they should not consume it. Intake of sodium and potassium varies depending on the client's status, type of renal failure, and type of dialysis.

Use meticulous sterile technique when caring for the hemodialysis shunt. *Rationale: Because the shunt is inserted within the circulatory system, any infection would quickly spread throughout the body.* Keep the shunt clean and dry and observe it frequently for clotting and signs of infection. (See In Practice: Nursing Care Guidelines 89-1 for more information.)

Kidney Transplant

More kidney transplants are done than any other type of transplant, and a high percentage of them are successful. The United Network of Organ Sharing (**UNOS**) is a private, nonprofit, contracted federal organization used by the Organ Procurement and Transplantation Network (OPTN). UNOS collects, stores, analyzes, and publishes information for clients on a waiting list for organ matching and transplants. The UNOS online network is https://www.unos.org/

With kidney transplantation, a major advantage is that a live donor can sacrifice one kidney and continue to live without difficulty. Also, cadaver donors can supply two kidneys for two potential clients. Moreover, the client can be carefully prepared for a long time because they can be maintained by renal dialysis.

Surgeons can take a kidney from a well human being or a recent cadaver and transplant it into the body of another person to replace a diseased kidney. The kidney is "typed" before transplant for as good a match between donor and recipient as possible. This process is similar to blood typing for a transfusion. Tissue typing of this sort allows the most suitable match for the client. Often, the client's living relatives have compatible tissue matches and are considered as kidney donors. The donor must have two well-functioning kidneys and no underlying disease.

Medical authorities, in conjunction with UNOS, have agreed that a kidney transplant should be attempted only when it has a reasonable chance to succeed and when all other options have been attempted and failed. Transplant surgeons have special training.

Key Concept

Kidney transplantation represents a potential cure for the client with renal failure. Proper matching of recipient and donor is crucial.

Rejection of Transplanted Organs

The chief difficulty with all transplants is the body's natural reaction—to reject the foreign substance. Certain factors cause rejection. For example, if the person has been exposed to foreign proteins in the process of previous transplant attempts or multiple blood transfusions, rejection is more likely.

Complications of Antirejection Medications

Side effects of medications that suppress tissue rejection are common because these drugs also suppress the client's immune response.

Observe for the following:

- Development of malignancies
- Susceptibility to viruses
- Susceptibility to infections of all types
- Gastric ulcers
- Gastrointestinal bleeding

IN PRACTICE
NURSING CARE GUIDELINES 89-1   Caring for the Client Receiving Dialysis

- Always wear gloves. *Rationale:* You will be exposed directly to the client's blood. Many people double-glove.
- Check the shunt every 2–4 hr for vibration (thrill), which you can feel. Listen with a stethoscope for the whooshing sound of blood moving through the shunt (bruit). *Rationale:* The feel of the thrill and the sound of the bruit indicate that the blood is flowing normally.
- Notify the healthcare provider immediately if you detect a change in the intensity of these sounds or sensations or if they are absent. *Rationale:* This could be life-threatening.
- Keep two clamps on the dressing over the external cannula at all times. *Rationale:* In case of cannula separation.
- Do not draw blood on the arm with a cannula or fistula. *Rationale:* To avoid disturbing the shunt.
- Do not measure blood pressure on the arm with a cannula or fistula. *Rationale:* To prevent cannula separation.
- You may need to take the client's blood pressure with an electronic device. *Rationale:* You may be unable to hear it with a stethoscope.
- If an arteriovenous fistula bleeds, apply pressure until the bleeding stops. *Rationale:* Bleeding can be a life-threatening emergency.
- Usually, you will not flush the port. *Rationale:* It is not likely to clot and you want to avoid further possibility of infection.
- Many clients on dialysis are diabetic and require insulin. *Rationale:* Hyper- or hypoglycemia can occur during dialysis. Blood sugar levels need to be monitored frequently.
- These clients usually will not void. *Rationale:* They do not produce urine because of lack of kidney functioning.
- Do not give these clients orange juice. Give apple or grape juice instead. *Rationale:* Orange juice is high in potassium. Elevated potassium, which is common in these clients, is dangerous. Hyperkalemia (elevated potassium) can cause fluid overload, shortness of breath, and irregular heartbeat, which can lead to cardiac arrest.
- Blood for potassium and other electrolyte-level tests is usually drawn daily. *Rationale:* To determine what should be included in the next run (treatment).
- Follow medication times exactly. *Rationale:* To maintain therapeutic blood levels and to avoid overload.
- Measure the client's daily weight. *Rationale:* To evaluate fluid retention.
- The client's blood pressure may be elevated. *Rationale:* Monitor blood pressure carefully.
- "Guaiac all stools" is often ordered. *Rationale:* To check for internal bleeding from the vascular kidney.
- Teach the client and family about care of the cannula or fistula and other aspects of dialysis. *Rationale:* They must understand that disconnection of these devices is an emergency, requiring immediate attention.
- Carefully and completely document all teaching. *Rationale:* For best compliance with a difficult life event, education is vital.

- Psychiatric disorders
- Bone disorders

If a client rejects the first kidney transplant, a second transplant may be performed. A concern in all transplants today is that of transmission of diseases, such as human immunodeficiency virus or acquired immunodeficiency syndrome (HIV/AIDS) or viral hepatitis, to the recipient. Specific diagnostic tests have become very accurate in detecting microscopic pathogens, thus preventing most transplanted infected organs.

STUDENT SYNTHESIS

KEY POINTS

- Blood tests to detect renal function include BUN, serum creatinine, urine creatinine, creatinine clearance, a serum BUN-to-creatinine ratio, and a glomerular filtration rate.
- Incontinence can be temporary, iatrogenic, total, stress, reflux, or paradoxical.
- Nursing care of the client with a urinary disorder focuses on maintaining and preserving renal function, decreasing discomfort, preventing infection, promoting skin integrity, maintaining fluid balance, and restoring and maintaining the client's self-esteem.
- Early symptoms of renal disease are subtle. The nurse's ability to detect small changes in the client is crucial to early treatment.
- A urinary tract infection is often referred to as cystitis and is often related to *E. coli*. Interstitial cystitis may be both an inflammatory and an autoimmune disorder.
- Nephrolithiasis can be treated by ESWL and percutaneous nephrolithotomy.
- Glomerulonephritis can be acute or chronic and have no symptoms or have significant problems, such as hypertension, hematuria, edema, anemia, malaise, and fatigue.
- Common urinary diversions include the ileal conduit and the Kock pouch.
- Kidney and bladder tumors are often metastatic before they are discovered.
- Cancer of the urinary tract is most often found in the renal tubules or the renal pelvis.
- The consequence of renal failure is end-stage renal disease, which typically involves long-term care and dialysis.

CRITICAL THINKING EXERCISES

1. Identify the critical elements you would include in a nursing assessment tool to determine urinary function. Explain why each is important.
2. A client has renal calculi. Explain how nutritional intake could contribute to the development of different renal calculi.
3. Discuss when dialysis might be used for clients who are not in chronic renal failure.

NCLEX-STYLE REVIEW QUESTIONS

1. The nurse at the long-term care facility observes that an older adult client has an acute change in behavior, exhibiting lethargy and confusion. Which action should the nurse take first?
   a. Obtain an order for a head CT scan.
   b. Monitor and report immediately to the healthcare provider.
   c. Document the behavior.
   d. Administer a prn dose of acetaminophen.

2. The nurse is preparing a client for discharge after having a cystoscopy. Which statement made by the client demonstrates an understanding of the discharge instructions?
   a. "I will report blood in my urine if it occurs over 24 hr."
   b. "I will limit my fluid intake for 24 hr."
   c. "I should expect a slight infection after the procedure."
   d. "I cannot use a tub bath for 1 week."

3. The nurse is preparing a client for a renal biopsy. Which position will the nurse assist the client to maintain during the procedure?
   a. High-Fowler
   b. Lithotomy
   c. Supine with the head flat
   d. Prone position with sandbags under the abdomen

4. A female client reports urinating incontinently when coughing, laughing, or sneezing. Which instructions should the nurse reinforce to initially manage the incontinence?
   a. Biofeedback
   b. Kegel exercises
   c. Care of the indwelling catheter
   d. Administration of tolterodine (Detrol LA)

5. Which measures should the nurse suggest to the female client to prevent repeated urinary tract infections (UTIs)? Select all that apply.
   a. Ensure adequate fluid intake.
   b. Avoid tight-fitting, nonabsorbent underwear.
   c. Avoid bubble baths.
   d. Void immediately after sexual intercourse.
   e. Wipe from the front to back after bowel movements.

CHAPTER RESOURCES

Enhance your learning with additional resources on **thePoint**!
Student Resources related to this chapter can be found at thePoint.lww.com/Rosdahl12e.

90 Male Reproductive Disorders

Learning Objectives

1. Identify the uses for the following laboratory tests: testosterone level, PSA level, and free PSA level.
2. Describe the circumstances that would be necessary for the healthcare provider to order an NPT test, a duplex Doppler ultrasonography, and a prostatic biopsy.
3. Differentiate between the medical and surgical treatments for erectile dysfunction. Identify the medications used for ED and state their major side effects.
4. Define and discuss the causes and treatment options for each of the following: priapism, phimosis, hypospadias epispadias, varicocele, and hydrocele.
5. Compare and contrast the signs and symptoms of the following: Peyronie disease, cryptorchidism, and testicular torsion. State the nursing considerations for each of these disorders.
6. Identify the similarities and differences between the following disorders: epididymitis, orchitis, and the following types of prostatitis: acute, chronic, chronic abacterial, and asymptomatic inflammatory.
7. Describe the differences and similarities between BPH and cancer of the prostate. State the classifications of drugs that are used to treat BPH.
8. In the skills laboratory, demonstrate how to care for a three-way bladder irrigation.
9. Discuss postoperative nursing considerations when caring for a client who has had TURP.
10. Differentiate and discuss the signs and symptoms of prostate cancer as compared with testicular cancer and penile cancer. Identify the types of treatment and nursing considerations for each.

Important Terminology

cryptorchidism
digital rectal examination
epididymitis
epispadias
erectile dysfunction
hydrocele
hypospadias
orchiopexy
orchitis
phimosis
plication
priapism
prostatectomy
prostatitis
varicocele

Acronyms

ABP
BPH
CBP
DRE
ED
NPT
PSA
TSE
TURP

The male reproductive system is closely linked to the urinary system (Chapters 27, 28, and 89). For this reason, *urologists* often treat male reproductive disorders.

DIAGNOSTIC TESTS

Testosterone Level

A *testosterone level* or levels of other hormones may be checked in cases of erectile dysfunction (sometimes called *impotence*) or sexual dysfunction. Testosterone is partly responsible for sperm production and *libido* (sexual desire).

Prostate-Specific Antigen

The *prostate-specific antigen* (**PSA**) is a blood test that detects a glycoprotein found only in the tissue of the prostate gland. PSA can be elevated in *prostatitis* (inflammation of the prostate gland), benign prostatic hyperplasia (**BPH**), and malignant prostatic tissue as well as metastatic prostate cancer. Factors that can affect the PSA levels include age, African ethnic origin, prostate infection, and an individual's relative normal level. PSA is best used in combination with a digital rectal examination (DRE) for early detection of prostate cancer. For more information regarding PSA testing, refer to the later section discussing prostate cancer.

> **Key Concept**
> To avoid falsely elevated PSA levels, collect the blood sample either before the digital prostate examination or at least 48 hr after the examination.

Nocturnal Penile Tumescence Tests

Nocturnal penile tumescence (**NPT**) tests help determine if a client is having nighttime erections. Some NPT systems can often show the degree and duration of the erection and provide definitive clues to the cause of the condition.

Duplex Doppler Ultrasonography

Duplex Doppler ultrasonography relies on imaging the cavernous arteries at the base of the penis before and after injection of a vasodilator into the corpora cavernosa of the penis. An ultrasound study of the penile arteries may detect an arterial problem of the penis. This test can also suggest a venous problem by ruling out the arterial problem.

Nursing Considerations

The client may experience some discomfort when the medication is injected. Tell the client that these injections usually induce an erection that may not go away. The client will need to be monitored until the erection has resolved or has been medically reversed by the healthcare provider.

Prostate Gland Biopsy

Prostate gland biopsy is a needle excision of a prostate tissue specimen for histologic examination. A biopsy is often performed to diagnose prostate cancer after a suspicious rectal examination. It may be performed via three possible approaches: perineal, transrectal, or transurethral. Another type of prostatic biopsy is performed through endoscopy. The endoscope is inserted through the urethra to the prostate, where a small tissue sample is removed.

Another method uses an ultrasound probe. The probe can be combined with a special biopsy needle that is activated by a rapidly firing spring. The biopsy needle obtains a tissue sample in a fraction of a second. The client feels pressure and mild discomfort during the ultrasound and biopsy procedures. The urologist inserts the probe through the rectum for a clear picture of the prostate on a television screen. The urologist can then guide the biopsy needle to the location of the suspected cancer.

COMMON MEDICAL TREATMENTS

Because the urethra passes through the prostate gland as it empties urine from the bladder, *bladder irrigation* is performed to maintain patency of the urethra after prostate surgery. *Radiation therapy* may be used following removal of a cancerous prostate to destroy any remaining malignant cells.

> **Nursing Alert** Urinary catheterization is done either prior to or as a part of prostate surgery. The indwelling catheter remains in place according to the healthcare provider's postoperative orders. Bladder irrigation may be done to keep the urinary catheter patent and to help reduce any postoperative bleeding.

NURSING PROCESS

DATA COLLECTION

Carefully observe the male client who has a reproductive system disorder. Establish a baseline for future comparison and determine the presence of suspected complications. Report any changes in the baseline level. In Practice: Data Gathering in Nursing 90-1 provides additional information about key areas. Because of the close relationship between the urinary and reproductive systems in the male, many of the questions are asked to evaluate needs in both areas. Remember that some clients are uncomfortable discussing their sexual or urinary systems, which they consider personal and private concerns.

Observe the client's emotional response to the disorder or disease. Does the client need assistance to meet daily needs? Is the disorder correctable? Does it affect social activities or self-esteem? Is it life threatening? Is the client anxious or fearful of the outcome? What additional services does he need?

IN PRACTICE

DATA GATHERING IN NURSING 90-1 — Male Reproductive System

- Urinary and reproductive history
- General health history
- History of sexually transmitted infections or exposure
- Erectile dysfunction
- Urinary dysfunction
- Inspection of external reproductive structures
- Prostate examination
- Testicular examination

PLANNING AND IMPLEMENTING

Together, the members of the healthcare team plan with the client and family for effective individualized care to meet the client's needs. Be sure to provide pre- and postoperative care and teaching for clients undergoing surgical procedures. The male client with a reproductive system disorder may also require assistance in meeting daily needs, dealing with emotional problems, and understanding more about the disorder, its prognosis, and treatment.

EVALUATION

Periodically evaluate outcomes of care with the client, family, and other members of the healthcare team. Have short-term goals been met? Are long-term goals still realistic? Planning for further nursing care takes into consideration the client's prognosis, as well as any complications and the client's response to care given. Be sure to deal with the emotional aspects that accompany reproductive disorders; refer the client or family member to an appropriate support group or counselor.

> **Key Concept**
> The client may be embarrassed and concerned about any disorder related to the reproductive system. The disorder may negatively influence the client's body image and self-esteem. Nurses should be especially conscious of such concerns and be sensitive to the client's feelings.

ERECTILE DISORDERS

Erectile Dysfunction

Erectile dysfunction (**ED**), often referred to as *impotence,* refers to the inability to achieve or maintain an erection sufficient to complete sexual intercourse. ED may be classified as *primary* or *secondary.* In *primary ED,* the client has never achieved sufficient erection. In *secondary ED,* the client has achieved erection and completed intercourse in the past. Causative factors for ED can be organic in origin, meaning

Box 90-1 Factors Contributing to Erectile Dysfunction

- **Drug use:** Tobacco, alcohol, hormones, immunosuppressive agents, diuretics, antiparkinsonian agents, antihypertensives, antidepressants, psychotropics, amphetamines, barbiturates, marijuana, cocaine
- **Chronic diseases:** Renal failure, heart failure, atherosclerosis, multiple sclerosis
- **Endocrine disorders:** Diabetes mellitus, thyroid disorders, adrenal disorders, pituitary disorders
- **Trauma:** Spinal cord injury
- **Cardiovascular disorders:** Stroke, heart disorders, inadequate vascularization
- **Surgery:** Prostatectomy, ileostomy, colostomy

IN PRACTICE
IMPORTANT MEDICATIONS 90-1 — To Treat Erectile Dysfunctions

Oral Medications
- tadalafil (Cialis)
- vardenafil (Levitra)
- sildenafil citrate (Viagra)

Intraurethral Suppositories
- alprostadil (MUSE)

Vasoactive Intracorporeal Pharmacotherapy
- alprostadil, prostaglandin E_1 (Caverject)
- phentolamine HCl (Regitine)

Transdermal Agents
- nitroglycerin paste

---

it is caused by disease, medication, or environmental factors (Box 90-1). It also can be psychogenic in origin, although most specialists believe that organic causes are more likely. All men with ED, except those who have a specific known cause for their ED (e.g., diabetes or prostate surgery), need an evaluation of hormone levels; nocturnal rigidity measurement; or duplex Doppler ultrasonography to determine causes and identify treatment options.

SPECIAL CONSIDERATIONS Lifespan

Sexual Problems
Many men remain sexually active throughout life. However, ED and loss of libido are common in older adults, particularly when illness is present (e.g., diabetes). The incidence of ED increases with age. The erection can take longer to achieve, and ejaculation can be less intense with aging—this mainly stems from medication side effects, neuropathy, or vascular problems. Although sperm viability decreases with age, sperm production continues at the same level throughout life. As the prostate enlarges, the amount of seminal fluid decreases.

Medical and Surgical Treatment
An *erection* is caused by spinal reflex arcs activated by tactile stimuli and *psychogenic* factors (auditory, visual, and psychological stimulation). If the client's ED is determined to be truly psychogenic in nature, counseling in conjunction with treatment options may help the client regain function. In cases of organic impotence, counseling also may be valuable along with treatment.

A variety of different treatment options are available. Give a nonjudgmental overview of the pros and cons of each option and let the client select what is best for the client and their partner.

Oral Medications
Oral medications include sildenafil citrate (Viagra), vardenafil (Levitra), and tadalafil (Cialis). These medications are vasodilators taken in pill form that help the penis to fill with blood. They must be taken with caution because of possible systemic side effects. Other medications also may be used (In Practice: Important Medications 90-1).

Nursing Alert Many medications used to treat ED, for example, tadalafil (Cialis) or sildenafil (Viagra), are contraindicated for clients who use nitroglycerin (Nitrostat) products. Life-threatening hypotension may result.

Intraurethral Suppositories
Medications such as alprostadil (MUSE) are urethral suppositories, smaller than a grain of rice, which the client self-injects into the urethra. The pellet melts, and the medication is absorbed into the corpora cavernosa. The medication causes the tissue to vasodilate, pulling blood into the area, which causes an erection. This drug has a more localized arteriole-dilating effect than does sildenafil citrate (Viagra) or tadalafil (Cialis).

Vasoactive Intracorporeal Pharmacotherapy
Medications, such as alprostadil (Caverject), can be used to induce an erection. The client self-injects a vasodilating medication into the penis.

Nursing Alert The client who receives vasodilating medications such as sildenafil citrate (Viagra), tadalafil (Cialis), and alprostadil (MUSE, Caverject) may have a side effect known as *priapism* (a prolonged, uncomfortable erection lasting for 2–3 hr or longer). The client should be educated to seek medical interventions for sustained erections lasting 3–4 hr.

Mechanical Devices
Mechanical devices, such as *vacuum erection devices* or *vacuum constriction devices,* are noninvasive. They create an erection by mechanically pulling blood into the penis.

Penile Implants
Several types of devices can be implanted in the penis to help the client achieve and maintain an erection. The device may be malleable or be a two- or three-piece inflatable prosthesis.

With the malleable device, the penis looks erect all the time. The inflatable prosthesis can be inflated and deflated, thus simulating a natural erection.

Each device has advantages and disadvantages. These, along with the risk of the implant procedure, need to be clearly explained to the client by their healthcare provider. Counsel the client who has a penile implant to avoid sexual activity until their healthcare provider gives medical clearance for intercourse. **Rationale:** *The site needs time to heal completely.*

Penile Revascularization

Only about 5% of all men with ED are candidates for *penile vascular surgery,* which involves reconstruction of the arterial blood supply or removal of veins that drain blood from the penis too rapidly. However, because this procedure rarely produces a successful outcome, it is rarely performed.

Priapism

Priapism refers to an abnormal and persistent penile erection without sexual stimulation. It is extremely painful and may last several hours or even days. The client must seek immediate medical attention.

Priapism can have many causes, including penile or spinal cord injury, tumor, and cerebrospinal syphilis. Pelvic vascular thrombosis is most often identified as the cause. However, priapism may also result from prolonged sexual activity, leukemia, sickle cell anemia, or other blood disorders. Priapism is common in infections such as prostatitis, urethritis, and cystitis, particularly if renal calculi are also present. It may be a side effect of medications, including trazodone (Desyrel), chlorpromazine (Thorazine), prazosin (Minipress), tolbutamide (Orinase), certain antihypertensives, anticoagulants, and corticosteroids. This condition may also be an undesirable result of therapy for ED, particularly with sildenafil (Viagra), alprostadil (MUSE, Caverject), and injection therapy.

Signs and Symptoms

The client has an erection that will not go away, along with penile pain and tenderness. The condition is emotionally upsetting. The corpora cavernosa contain thick, dark, venous blood; the corpus spongiosum and glans penis are not involved.

Medical and Surgical Treatment

Priapism can be difficult to treat, and sometimes treatment may be unsuccessful. The goal is to improve the venous drainage of the corpora cavernosa while preventing ischemia that may result in impotence. Injection of a solution of phenylephrine into the corpora cavernosa may reverse priapism. *Cavernostomy* with a butterfly needle (to allow drainage) and irrigation may be used, or surgery may be required. Caudal or spinal anesthesia may relieve priapism. Certain medications, such as anticoagulants, may be effective if used immediately. Surgical approaches include creation of a *fistula* (connection) between the glans penis and corpus spongiosum, and semipermanent diversion with a saphenous vein shunt.

Premature Ejaculation

Premature ejaculation is a consistent problem in which the client ejaculates before, during, or immediately after penetration. Evaluation and treatment are recommended if the client believes the problem affects their ability to have intercourse. Treatment may include wearing condoms, performing a special squeeze technique, application of lidocaine gel, and medications such as serotonin reuptake inhibitors.

Peyronie Disease

Peyronie disease is an accumulation of plaques or scar tissue along the corpora cavernosa, causing a painful curvature of the penis when erect. This plaque or scar tissue formation is idiopathic and benign. The erect penis curves in varying degrees and directions, resulting in painful or sometimes impossible penetration. Treatment includes oral medications: clostridium histolyticum (Xiaflex), vitamin E, and nonsteroidal anti-inflammatory drugs (NSAIDs). The plaque or scar tissue may be removed by surgery.

> **NCLEX Alert**
>
> NCLEX clinical situations for males may involve nursing observational skills or options relating to difficulties with urination, urinary procedures, side effects of medications, and discharge teaching. You also need to know normal laboratory levels, normal urinary output, and normal changes with aging.

STRUCTURAL DISORDERS

Undescended Testicle (Cryptorchidism)

Normally, the testes of the male fetus descend into the scrotal sac during the third trimester of pregnancy. A small percentage of male babies, however, are born with a testicle or testicles that have not descended to their normal position in the scrotum, a condition called *undescended testicle* or **cryptorchidism**. This may be a unilateral or bilateral condition, although it is unusual for both testes to be undescended. Sometimes the testicles descend without treatment. If this does not occur, they should be correctly positioned early in life to allow for successful sperm production because internal body temperature is too warm for the development of viable sperm. If one testis is normally descended, the man will most likely be able to reproduce.

If both testes remain in the client's abdomen past puberty, they may be malformed or progressively atrophy. The client may not develop secondary sex characteristics because the testes cannot secrete the appropriate hormones. The client may need to receive hormones throughout life. Testes that lodge in the inguinal canal may secrete adequate hormones, but most likely will not produce spermatozoa.

Hormonal therapy is an appropriate medical treatment for this condition. If hormonal therapy is ineffective, corrective surgery (*orchiopexy*) is usually done between the ages of 5 and 7 years. **Orchiopexy** involves suturing the testes to the scrotal sac to secure them.

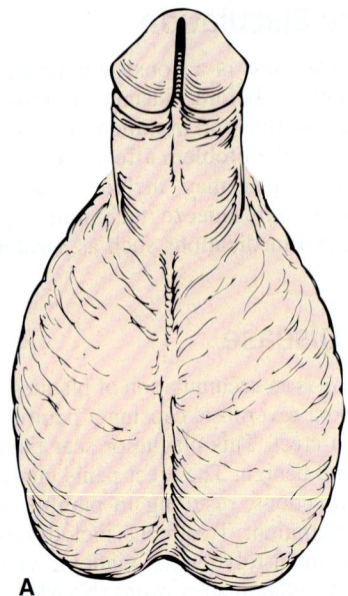

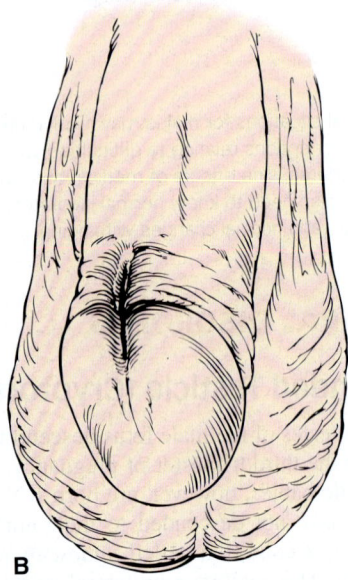

Figure 90-1 **A.** Hypospadias. **B.** Epispadias.

Abnormal Urethral Placement

A urethral meatus located on the underside of the penis is called **hypospadias**. A meatus located on the upper surface is called **epispadias** (Fig. 90-1). These congenital conditions are usually repaired surgically at a young age if they are severe.

Phimosis

Men who have not been circumcised at birth can develop a condition known as **phimosis**. The foreskin becomes so tight that it will not retract over the glans penis. Injury may also cause phimosis. Circumcision can relieve the condition.

Testicular Torsion

Torsion (twisting) of the testicle is caused by a twisting of the spermatic cord, resulting in an interruption in blood flow to the testicle. Torsion is uncommon and occurs most often in adolescents and young men. It may be caused by bilateral and congenital absence of the lateral attachments of the testes and epididymis to the scrotum. Torsion can follow an activity that puts a sudden pull on the cremasteric muscle, which elevates the testis. Extreme cold, such as with jumping into very cold water, may also cause torsion. Occasionally, torsion is spontaneous or occurs during sleep.

Signs and Symptoms

Symptoms of torsion include an acute onset of sudden severe scrotal pain, vomiting, abdominal pain, and nausea. This condition can cause testicular infarction and necrosis if left untreated for more than a few hours. Thus, it is considered a surgical emergency.

Surgical Treatment

Surgical *detorsion* (untwisting) and bilateral *orchiopexy* (surgical fixation of the testes) are treatments to fixate each testis and prevent recurrence. If torsion has caused testicle necrosis, the testicle must be removed (*orchiectomy*). An orchiopexy is then performed on the unaffected side to prevent torsion of that testis.

Varicocele

A **varicocele** is an abnormal dilatation of the testicular veins in the scrotum, causing a reflux of blood down to the scrotum when standing or straining. The scrotal temperature is higher than normal because of the blood pooling in the area. Heat impairs spermatogenesis and sperm storage, resulting in a low sperm count and infertility. Infertility clinics report an incidence of varicoceles in 30%–40% of men with male factor infertility.

Signs and Symptoms

Varicocele can cause pain in the testicle or pain radiating to the other side. Symptoms of varicocele include swelling and a nagging dull pain in the scrotum. A varicocele may not be clinically evident until puberty. The veins become dilated and tortuous and, on palpation, are often described as similar to a "bag of worms." Varicocele may be unilateral or bilateral. However, this condition is more commonly seen on the left side. This is probably because the left spermatic vein is longer than the right. Presence of a right-sided varicocele may suggest obstruction of the intra-abdominal venous drainage, which could be caused by a tumor.

Surgical Treatment

Correction is done surgically through a number of different types of incisions, laparoscopically, and radiographically. Surgical repair of varicocele may be necessary to eliminate or control pain. Repair can improve the semen count in 60% of men with infertility. However, if semen analysis is normal, infertile men with varicoceles do not require treatment.

Hydrocele

A **hydrocele** is an accumulation of fluid in the space between the membrane covering the testicle and the testicle itself (Fig. 90-2). It may be caused by infection (*orchitis*) or an injury. The scrotum enlarges; pain and swelling may be present. However, the client with a hydrocele is often asymptomatic.

Hydrocele may be treated by aspirating the fluid, although this treatment is rarely satisfactory in the adult. Sometimes the sac requires surgical removal. **Plication**, the stitching of

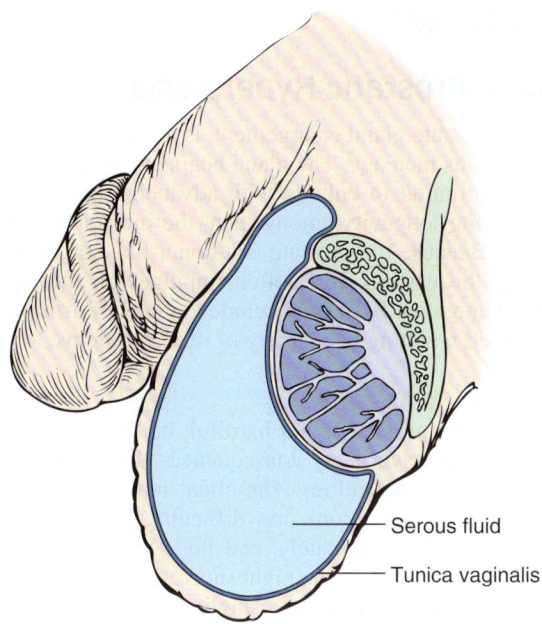

Figure 90-2 Hydrocele.

folds or tucks in the hydrocele wall to reduce its size, will usually prevent redevelopment of the hydrocele.

Symptomatic treatment includes applying cold packs, providing support for the scrotum, and providing emotional reassurance that the condition will resolve and will not affect future fertility. A drain is often used if a plication is not performed.

INFLAMMATORY DISORDERS

Epididymitis

Epididymitis is inflammation of the epididymis, which is the coiled tube at the posterior of the testicle that stores and carries sperm. When the testicle also becomes inflamed, the condition is called *epididymo-orchitis*. Epididymitis is usually an acute infection, but if it last 6 weeks or longer, it can become a chronic problem. Males of any age can develop this disorder, but it is most often caused by bacterial infections due to STIs such as gonorrhea, syphilis, or chlamydia. Other causes include organisms such as staphylococci, streptococci, and *Escherichia coli*. Epididymitis may follow an infection of the urinary tract or prostate gland. For clients who are not sexually active, the source of the problem is usually related to an infection spread from the urinary tract, including urine, urethra, prostate gland, or seminal vesicles. Other risk factors include urethral instrumentation, an indwelling urinary catheter, anal intercourse, brachytherapy for prostatic cancer, HIV/AIDS, and unprotected sexual intercourse with more than one sexual partner. Straining or strenuous exertion in conjunction with a full bladder can cause problems, for example, prolonged periods of sitting, bicycle riding, and motorcycle riding. Sports or trauma injury can be the source of the inflammation. A specific heart medication, amiodarone (Pacerone), can cause inflammation of the epididymis.

Symptoms include redness, pain, and unilateral scrotal swelling. Dysuria (painful urination), blood in the semen, enlarged lymph nodes in the groin, and pain in the lower abdomen and pelvic area are also seen. The bacterium chlamydia can be the cause of a burning sensation and penile discharge. In addition to chlamydia, signs and symptoms of other STIs will need to be identified and treated. The scrotum can enlarge greatly, and the condition can even interfere with the client's ambulation. Intercourse or ejaculation can be painful. It can affect a man's fertility. Chronic or untreated epididymitis can involve complications such as abscesses in the scrotum.

Diagnosis involves a physical examination including a check of the prostate gland, enlarged lymph nodes of the groin, and unilateral enlargement of a testicle. The healthcare provider will need to know the individual's sexual history and will obtain a culture and sensitivity (C&S) of any discharge. Laboratory analysis of blood and urine can rule out other disorders. Imaging tests include an ultrasound with color Doppler, which will indicate blood flow and possibly any testicular torsion.

Treatment involves a C&S of any penile discharge. Administer antibiotics and analgesics as ordered, provide scrotal support, and apply cold packs to the scrotum. Antibiotic therapy usually continues for 3 months, or longer if the infection is chronic. Surgery may be necessary to drain an abscess or remove part or all of the epididymis, known as an *epididymectomy*.

Nursing considerations will relate to both the physical and emotional aspects of this problem. The client needs to be aware that this is a relatively common problem and is typically treatable with medications. In many situations, the disorder can be avoided (e.g., by wearing condoms). The client may be embarrassed and reluctant to discuss the problem with a female nurse; consider asking a male nurse to participate with scrotal and testicular care as well as having male-only teaching sessions.

Orchitis

Orchitis, inflammation of the testes, may result from infection or injury. It is common in clients who have epididymitis. Mumps after puberty may cause orchitis, resulting in sterility. Risk factors, diagnosis, and treatment are similar to epididymitis (see above). Symptoms include pain and swelling in the scrotum and sometimes urethral irritation. A scrotal support is used. An ice bag applied to the scrotum is helpful. Heat is not used.

Prostatitis

Prostatitis is characterized by pain, swelling, and inflammation of the prostate gland. This gland is the size of a walnut and is located directly below a man's bladder. Its purpose is to produce the semen that nourishes and transports sperm. This disorder can occur in men of any age but typically is seen in men younger than 50 years. Prostatitis can be classified as *acute bacterial, chronic bacterial, chronic abacterial* (also known as *chronic pelvic pain syndrome*), and *asymptomatic inflammatory*. Urinalysis is often helpful in determining the cause of acute and chronic prostatitis. Bacteria and numerous white blood cells are present in the urine. A urine culture and sensitivity test is positive in acute bacterial prostatitis and negative in nonbacterial prostatitis.

Acute Bacterial Prostatitis

Acute bacterial prostatitis (**ABP**) usually results from an ascending urinary tract infection, such as with *E. coli*. Symptoms develop quickly, showing typical flu-like symptoms. The client may also complain of chills, fever, *myalgia* (muscle pain), general malaise, scrotal and low back pain, perineal pain, and pain after ejaculation. The client with acute prostatitis has a very tender, enlarged, and asymmetrical prostate on DRE. Urinary symptoms include *hematuria* (blood in the urine) and urgency on urination or obstructive symptoms such as *nocturia* (frequent voiding at night), hesitancy, or dribbling.

Treatment for ABP includes wide-spectrum antibiotics, analgesics, and sitz baths. A urine culture and/or ultrasound may be done to determine the cause. Clients should receive a long course of an appropriate antibiotic. If inadequately treated, chronic prostatitis may develop. The client may require hospitalization until afebrile.

Chronic Bacterial Prostatitis

Chronic bacterial prostatitis (**CBP**) develops after episodes of ABP are unsuccessfully treated with antibiotics. The hallmark of chronic bacterial prostatitis is a history of relapsing urinary tract infection. Recurring bouts and difficult-to-treat infections are common. The client with chronic prostatitis is usually asymptomatic, but may complain of back or perineal pain or other relatively minor symptoms. The prostate is usually normal on palpation. Diagnosis is established with isolation of bacteria from the expressed secretions obtained from prostatic massage. The client's serum white blood cell count also is elevated. The urine culture is usually negative. However, if bacteriuria is present, the initial treatment is a short course of antibiotics. If not successful, additional antibiotic therapy may last 3–6 months.

Chronic Abacterial Prostatitis

Chronic abacterial prostatitis, also called *chronic pelvic pain syndrome*, is the most common cause of prostatitis. As a type of nonbacterial prostatitis, it is not caused by bacteria and its etiology is often unknown. Symptoms range from mild to severe and vary over time. Empirical treatment includes long periods of antibiotics.

Asymptomatic Inflammatory Prostatitis

Asymptomatic inflammatory prostatitis does not have symptoms and may be found as a result of being tested for another problem. No treatment is required.

Nursing Considerations

Nursing measures for the client with prostatitis include pain control and warm compresses or sitz baths. Remind the client to increase fluid intake to flush bacteria out of the bladder. Stool softeners help prevent constipation.

NEOPLASMS

Benign Prostatic Hyperplasia

BPH, or prostate gland enlargement, is a common condition that occurs as men age. The gland begins to grow at adolescence, continuing to enlarge with advancing age. Because of increasing longevity among men, the incidence of BPH is rising. Because the prostate is a donut-like structure surrounding the urethra, BPH often impinges on the urinary stream. Untreated, BPH can occlude the flow of urine out of the bladder, resulting in a variety of renal problems.

Signs and Symptoms

Growth of the prostate is not harmful, but the symptoms it produces may have many consequences. Initial symptoms may be urinary difficulties. The client may not be able to urinate (urinary retention), has difficulty voiding or emptying the bladder completely, and finds that he must void frequently, often during the night (nocturia). The client may also find starting to void increasingly difficult (straining) or painful and may notice traces of blood in their urine. They may not be able to empty their bladder and may dribble at the end of urination. Although uncommon, complications include cystitis, urinary tract infections, hematuria, and bladder stones due to urinary stasis.

Diagnostic Tests

The healthcare provider, often an urologist, will start by reviewing the client's personal and familial history followed by a basic physical examination for a male. Part of the male's physical is a **digital rectal examination** (**DRE**). The digital examination provides basic knowledge about the size of the prostate. The examination is done by inserting a gloved hand into the rectum and feeling the tissues of the rectal wall, which are adjacent to the prostate (Fig. 90-3D). An enlarged prostate can be felt by the experienced healthcare provider. The general laboratory tests are ordered, for example, CBC, UA, and blood chemistries. BPH will show changes in the urinalysis, urine culture, serum creatinine, and blood urea nitrogen.

The test related to prostate issues is the test that measures PSA, a protein produced by the cells of the prostate. PSA levels increase when the prostate is enlarged, or the prostate area has had recent urologic procedures, an infection, surgery, or prostate cancer. Urinary testing may include a *post void residual volume test,* which measures the client's ability to completely empty their bladder. Normally, after voiding, any remaining (residual) urine indicates an enlarged prostate. A *urinary flow test* may be done; the client voids directly into a receptacle that measures the strength and amount of urine flow, which is typically abnormal with BPH. A specific urinary flow test can determine if the client's condition is changing, for example, after being on medications or after a surgical procedure. If the client has significant nocturia, a 24-hr voiding diary is done. The diary is done to document the amounts and times of voiding and how much it occurs at night (or when the client usually sleeps). Imaging studies may include a cystoscopy, transrectal ultrasound, or prostate biopsy. To determine bladder pressure and the strength of

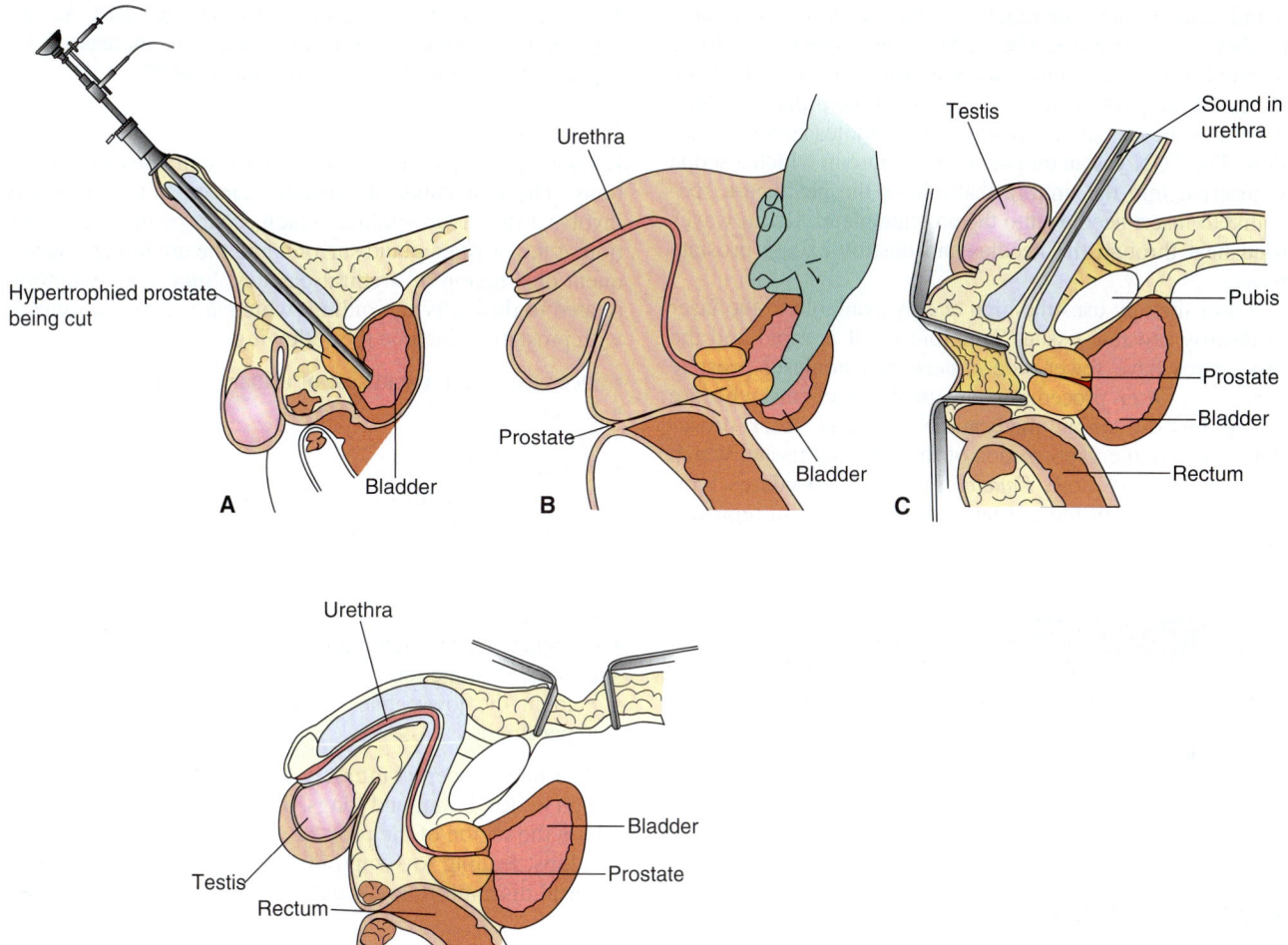

Figure 90-3 Types of prostatectomy. **A.** In a transurethral resection of the prostate (TURP), the surgeon connects a wire to a loop of current that is rotated in a cystoscope to remove shavings of the prostate. **B.** In suprapubic prostatectomy, the surgeon enters through the client's abdomen and uses their fingers to shell out the prostate. **C.** In perineal prostatectomy, the surgeon uses retractors to view the prostate. **D.** In retropubic prostatectomy, the surgeon makes a low abdominal incision and, working behind the pubic bone, removes the prostate.

bladder muscles, a *urodynamic and pressure flow study* may be indicated. This type of testing is done by inserting a catheter through the urethra into the bladder, followed by water or air, and the pressures are measured. Intravenous pyelogram and a CT urogram may also be indicated, depending upon initial findings.

Medical and Surgical Treatment

Medications that can be beneficial for these BPH symptoms include alpha blockers, such as doxazosin (Cardura), tamsulosin (Flomax), alfuzosin (Uroxatral), silodosin (Rapaflo), and finasteride (Proscar). Some medications can shrink the prostate by preventing hormonal changes that encourage prostate enlargement. These medications include the 5-alpha reductase inhibitors such as finasteride (Proscar) and dutasteride (Avodart), which may take up to 6 months to be effective. Combination therapy using an alpha blocker and a 5-alpha reductase inhibitor simultaneously may also be effective. The medication tadalafil (Cialis), which is designed for ED, can be effective in some men who have ED and BPH.

Prostate size can be reduced by a number of minimally invasive techniques or several different surgical methods. These options vary as to whether they are inpatient or outpatient procedures, in their ability to destroy specific amounts of prostate tissue, in the length of time needed for healing, and their degree of success in reestablishing urinary flow. The method selected depends on the status of the prostate and the severity of the client's symptoms. These methods include the *transurethral resection of the prostate* (TURP), *transurethral incision of the prostate* (TUIP), *transurethral microwave thermotherapy* (TUMT), *transurethral needle ablation* (TUNA), and laser therapy. The **TURP** remains the standard surgical treatment for obstructive BPH. Additional discussion of prostate surgeries is found below in the prostate cancer section. Figure 90-3 shows various ways to access the prostate for a prostatectomy. The TURP and the TUIP are done in the hospital using a lighted scope inserted into the urethra. With the TURP, the surgeon removes most of the prostate gland. It requires a temporary urinary catheter to drain the bladder. Symptomatic relief is generally good. With the TUIP, only small cuts are made of the prostate gland, which allow for relief of moderate problems related to obstruction of urine. The TUMT uses a special electrode inserted into the prostate via the urethra. Microwaves from the electrode pass to the inner portion of the prostate, which decreases the size of the prostate and promotes better urinary flow. The TUNA is an outpatient procedure in which a scope is inserted into the urethra that allows the healthcare specialist to insert needles into the prostate gland. Radio waves send heat through the needles and destroy excess prostate tissue.

Laser therapy uses the high energy available to the laser to destroy prostate tissue. Symptom relief is rapid and the procedures have fewer side effects than nonlaser prostate surgeries. Laser procedures are useful in clients who are taking blood-thinning medications. *Ablative laser* procedures involve the vaporization of the enlarged tissue, which increases urinary flow. *Enucleative laser* procedures typically remove all of the prostate tissue and prevent regrowth of tissue.

> **Nursing Alert** If a client experiences an episode of acute urinary retention at home, they can try a warm shower or bath to relax the sphincter muscles. Advise the client to allow the urine to flow in the shower or tub. If a shower or bath does not work, the client should go to the emergency department for immediate treatment.

Cancer of the Prostate

Prostate cancer is almost always an *adenocarcinoma*, a gland cell cancer that is fairly common in men, especially African American men. Most cancers grow slowly, initially being confined to the gland itself, and need little, if any, treatment. Some types of prostate cancer are aggressive and metastasize quickly. Cancer that is detected and treated early has an improved chance of being controlled. Prostate cancer is not often noted in men younger than the 40 years, but by the age of 60 years, the chances of developing this adenocarcinoma significantly increase.

Risk factors for prostate cancer include the following:

- Age—Incidences increase after the age of 40 years.
- Race—African American men are 60% more likely to develop prostate cancer than European or Hispanic men.
- Family history—Chances increase if an immediate blood relative has prostate cancer.
- Lifestyle—A diet high in animal fats, for example, saturated fats.
- Obesity—Obese men are more likely to have advanced prostate cancer.
- High testosterone levels—Men who use testosterone therapy for other disorders have an increase in development of prostate cancer because testosterone stimulates the growth of the gland.
- Prostatic intraepithelial neoplasia (PIN)—Prostate gland cells look abnormal under the microscope, but the man may not have any symptoms until around age 50 years, when cancer may be diagnosed.
- Genome changes—If genes BRCA1 and BRCA2 are present, the risk for prostate cancer is increased; the presence of other genes has also been noted.

Signs and Symptoms

Early cancer of the prostate does not usually produce symptoms. The first signs of prostatic cancer, if any, typically involve difficulty in voiding, which occurs owing to the position of the prostate gland surrounding the urethra and subsequent obstruction of urethral patency. Signs and symptoms related to difficulty in voiding, which are often the same as with prostatitis, include the following:

- Decrease in force and size of urinary stream
- Urgency
- Frequency
- Nocturia
- Hesitancy (difficulty in starting the stream)
- Dysuria (painful voiding)
- Dribbling
- Urine retention
- Hematuria
- Complete urinary retention—a medical emergency
- Erectile dysfunction
- Pain in the lower back (spine), chest (ribs), pelvis, or upper thighs

Prostate cancer commonly metastasizes to the bones, lymph nodes, brain, and lungs. The bones involved are usually in the region of the prostate and include the lower spine and hips, leading to symptoms such as backache, hip pain, perineal discomfort, and weakness.

Diagnostic Tests

Testing asymptomatic men for prostate cancer is controversial because it may or may not be beneficial to the individual. Some healthcare providers prefer to do prostate cancer screening for men in their 50s, or sooner if risk factors have been identified. Testing typically involves a DRE and a PSA test. Routine PSA screening for cancer is not recommended. On examination, a cancerous prostate feels irregular and may have hard nodules. A PSA blood test is performed to look for an elevation of PSA levels. However, there are several reasons for an elevated PSA, so a diagnosis of cancer cannot be confirmed by a DRE and/or PSA. A biopsy is the method most likely to distinguish cancer from prostatitis.

Treatment Options

Treatment depends on the disease's stage and the client's age and symptoms. Options for therapy include radical prostatectomy, radioactive seed implantation, cryosurgery, radiation therapy, or hormone ablation therapy. Treatment may lead to ED in the majority of clients; incontinence is less common.

Prostate Surgery

Preoperative Nursing Considerations

As part of the preoperative preparation for a radical prostatectomy, alert the client to the strong possibility of postoperative ED. Encourage the client who wishes to have children to consider sperm banking before the surgery. Review the types of available treatment options for ED and how they work.

Discuss the possibility that the client will have a suprapubic cystoscopy catheter and some sort of continuous bladder irrigation for approximately 2–3 days after surgery.

Before the prostatectomy, the client may have a catheter inserted for continuous urinary drainage to prevent accumulation of stagnant urine in the bladder. Give the client plenty of fluids, with proper diet and rest. Antibiotics are often given prophylactically.

Transurethral Resection of the Prostate

This is the most common procedure. Figure 90-3 illustrates common techniques. In TURP, the surgeon removes prostate tissue through the urethra by means of a *resectoscope*, which has a cutting edge or electric wire that slices the prostate away bit by bit (Fig. 90-3A). Because the surgeon does the operation through the urethra, no incision is necessary. Complications of TURP include hemorrhage, urinary retention, stress incontinence, and ED.

Prostatectomy

Another surgical treatment for prostatic cancer (and also BPH) is removal of the excess or abnormal prostate tissue (**prostatectomy**) through various approaches. The surgeon can dissect the prostate through an incision through the bladder (*suprapubic prostatectomy* or *suprapubic resection*), a perineal incision (*perineal prostatectomy* or *perineal resection*), or an incision below the bladder (*retropubic prostatectomy*). Dissection is also possible using a *cystoscope* (resectoscope) through the urethra.

Suprapubic prostatectomy: The surgeon usually performs the suprapubic procedure if the client's gland is greatly enlarged (>100 g). Surgery may be done in two stages. First, the surgeon performs a *cystostomy* (incision into the bladder) to relieve urinary retention; second, the prostate tissue is removed (Fig. 90-3B). After the two-stage suprapubic operation, the client returns with two indwelling catheters in place, one in the urethra and the other in the suprapubic wound (a *suprapubic cystocath*). These catheters are attached to separate drainage containers, allowing for more accurate output measurement. The urethral catheter is attached to a closed drainage system, and the wound catheter is attached to an irrigation apparatus. (The surgeon may prefer that any bladder irrigation be done through the urethral catheter.)

Perineal prostatectomy: If the surgeon removes gland tissue through an incision in the perineum, catheter drainage is through the perineal incision only (Fig. 90-3C). In this case, the client will find sitting up to be difficult. Fecal contamination of the incision may occur because of its location.

Nerve-sparing radical prostatectomy (retropubic prostatectomy): Nerve-sparing radical prostatectomy removes the prostate through an incision below the umbilicus and above the symphysis pubis (Fig. 90-3D). This procedure causes less ED, incontinence, and bleeding than do other methods.

Radical prostatectomy: A *radical prostatectomy* (removal of the prostate gland, seminal vesicles, and part of the urethra) sometimes cures prostatic cancer that has not metastasized. A radical prostatectomy is an open procedure because an abdominal incision is necessary. Complications of radical prostatectomy include stress incontinence, epididymitis, urethral stricture, fistula, and ED.

Cryosurgery

A less invasive procedure used to remove prostatic cancer is *cryosurgery*. An incision is made in the perineum, and a special tool is inserted to the area of the prostate cancer to freeze the tissue. This procedure is believed to kill the cancer. The risks involved in cryosurgery are similar to those for other prostate removal procedures. The success of the procedure is still under investigation.

Postoperative Nursing Considerations

The client will require routine postoperative care, such as antiembolism stockings, early ambulation, and incentive spirometry. Encourage fluid intake and monitor intake and output. Give stool softeners, as ordered. Help the client and their partner deal with any psychological and emotional problems. In Practice: Educating the Client 90-1 provides pertinent instructions for discharge and home care.

A urethral catheter is left in place for about 2 weeks after a radical prostatectomy. The catheter helps put pressure on the *vesicoureteral* (bladder and ureter) incision to control bleeding. Keep the catheter straight to avoid obstruction of urine flow. Accidental catheter removal may require the client to return to surgery for its reinsertion.

After TURP, the client will return from the operating room with a bladder irrigation in place. (This procedure may also

---

IN PRACTICE

EDUCATING THE CLIENT 90-1 **At Home After Prostatectomy**

Priorities for Home Care

- Review discharge instructions with the client.
- Have client demonstrate measures for catheter maintenance, including cleaning and changing of equipment per instructions.
- Explain bowel maintenance program, including use of stool softeners.
- Encourage ambulation.
- Encourage fluids.
- Demonstrate wound cleaning and dressing changes and have client return-demonstrate procedure using clean technique and sterile dressing as appropriate.
- Teach client about bladder retraining and Kegel exercises.
- Assist client with setting up necessary follow-up appointments, including postoperative appointments, appointments for evaluation and treatment of erectile dysfunction (ED), when necessary, and appointments for counseling, when necessary.
- Assist client and their significant others to understand that depression is common. Often the client will benefit from psychological counseling because the reality of cancer, loss of sterility, loss of sexual function, and/or incontinence are very real and lifetime changes.

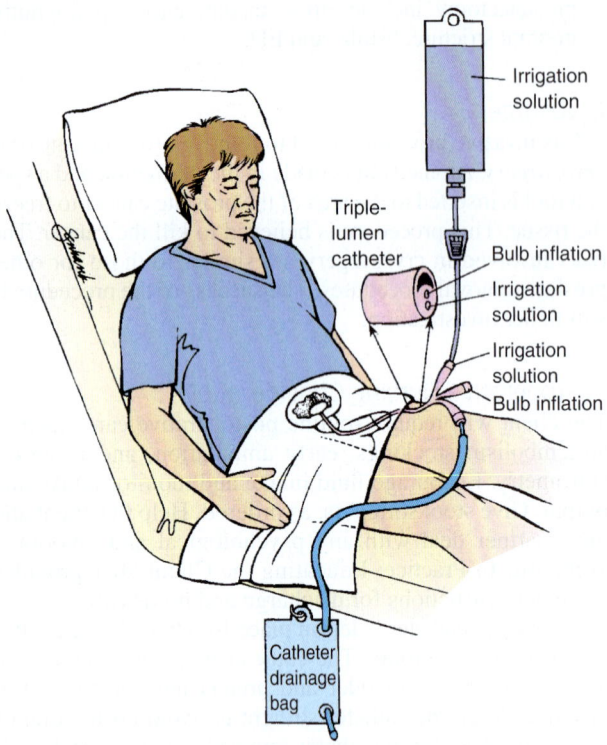

Figure 90-4 Three-way bladder irrigation used after prostate or bladder surgery.

be used after other genitourinary procedures.) The surgeon inserts a *triple-lumen catheter* (with three separate tubes or openings) immediately after the prostate is removed in the operating room. One lumen inflates the balloon that holds the catheter in place, whereas a second lumen drains the bladder into a drainage bag (similar to a Foley catheter). The third lumen is used to instill a bladder solution that irrigates the bladder.

Irrigation may be continuous to intermittent after surgery. Continuous irrigation washes out blood before it can form clots; intermittent irrigation washes out clots that plug the catheter. When the catheter becomes clogged, overdistention of the bladder may cause the client great discomfort. In many cases, a pump or controller regulates the flow of irrigant. Figure 90-4 illustrates TURP irrigation, which is used after the procedure. In Practice: Nursing Care Guidelines 90-1 provides information related to TURP irrigation.

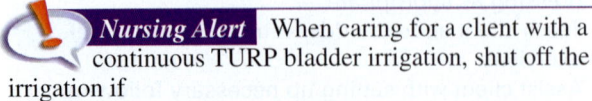 When caring for a client with a continuous TURP bladder irrigation, shut off the irrigation if
- The client complains of bladder fullness, urinary urgency, or bladder or flank pain.
- Drainage from the TURP tube stops.
- Check to see if an order exists for a manual irrigation; irrigate tubing to check for blood clots.

Carefully monitor intake and output in the immediate postoperative period. Pay particular attention to the color of the draining urine. The postoperative client will have bloody drainage, which should steadily decrease. Because hemorrhage is a major postoperative complication, report and document any sudden increase of blood in the drainage. If urinary flow slows or stops, the catheter may require irrigation to remove obstructing tissue or clots. If the drainage becomes bright red with gushes of fresh bleeding, report to the charge nurse immediately.

After catheter removal, clients usually are incontinent until they are able to train their external urethral sphincter to do the work of both the internal and external sphincters. Assist in sphincter retraining by instructing the client in Kegel exercises.

Sitz baths are usually ordered after a perineal prostatectomy. After a bowel movement, take care to avoid contaminating the wound. Use meticulous aseptic technique to cleanse the perineum.

A wound catheter may be in place following radical prostatectomy. Some urine will dribble onto dressings after removal of the wound catheter. Keep the skin clean and dry by frequent dressing changes. The wound may take a month or more to heal.

Painful bladder spasms are common after a client has had prostate surgery. Antispasmodics are administered to control this pain. Relief for incisional pain is also needed, but aspirin is avoided because of its anticoagulation effects. If the client has metastasis, pain management becomes a priority. If the client is able to swallow, narcotic analgesics are given orally on a routine schedule, not the "as needed" schedule, which will be ineffective in maintaining sustained pain relief. Intravenous narcotics, commonly morphine sulfate, will be given.

Medical Treatments
Radiation Therapy
Radiation may be used for cancer of the prostate to reduce tumor size or actually to cure some stages of cancer. It may also be considered a palliative measure for the client with bony metastases, thus alleviating some pain.

Radioactive seed implantation is a common method of treating prostate cancer. Small radioactive seeds (about the size of a grain of rice) are implanted directly into the prostate. This procedure puts radiation in the exact location of the cancer, thereby reducing side effects and risks associated with other types of radiation therapy.

Radiation cystitis is a common problem following radiation therapy after prostatectomy. Antispasmodics, analgesics, and increased fluid intake are forms of treatment. Monitor the client's skin condition during radiation therapy. Clients are susceptible to excoriation and yeast infections.

The client may experience *proctitis,* an inflammation of the rectum and anus, with preoperative chemotherapy. Use of a low-residue diet and antidiarrheal medications may help alleviate symptoms. The client may experience urethral stricture, due to scarring. Teach the client signs of urinary retention and monitor urine output closely.

Hormone Ablation Therapy
Prostate cancer needs testosterone to grow. Therefore, removing testosterone will destroy the prostate cancer's chance of survival and growth. An orchiectomy will simply solve this problem, and clients do, in some cases, choose this option. A *partial orchiectomy* can also be performed to remove the portion of the testicle that produces testosterone. There are also medications clients can take to decrease or stop testosterone production.

IN PRACTICE
NURSING CARE GUIDELINES 90-1 | Managing Continuous TURP or Bladder Irrigation

- Record the amount of irrigating solution instilled into the bladder and the total output. *Rationale: An accurate record of the client's actual urinary output is needed. Subtract the amount of irrigation solution from the total output to determine urine volume.*
- Carefully monitor the transurethral resection of the prostate (TURP) setup to make sure all the tubes are open and that they are not twisted or kinked. *Rationale: The tubing needs to remain patent and drain freely to prevent overdistention of the bladder.*
- Because many men who have TURPs are older and may become confused, make sure clients do not pull on the catheters or change rates of flow of the solutions. Catheters must remain taped in place. *Rationale: Damage may occur to the operative site.*
- Often, the surgeon orders that traction be placed on the penis, which is kept taped securely in place on the hip or abdomen and is not allowed to hang down. *Rationale: Traction facilitates drainage and prevents clotting, but may be uncomfortable.*
- It may be necessary to irrigate the catheter manually. Be sure the surgeon has written an order for manual irrigation. There is often a standing order to irrigate the catheter as needed. *Rationale: Manual irrigation helps to dislodge any clots that may be obstructing the catheter.*
- Take special note if the client complains of a feeling of fullness, urgency, or bladder or flank pain, or if the drainage stops flowing from the tube. In any of these situations, shut off the continuous irrigation and notify the team leader or surgeon immediately. *Rationale: The client is at risk for hemorrhage.*

Testicular Cancer

Testicular cancer occurs in the testicles (also known as testes), which are inside the scrotal sac. The testicles produce androgens (male sex hormones) such as testosterone. Testicular cancer is the most common form of cancer in younger European American males between 15 and 35 years of age. Testicular cancer grows rapidly and can often metastasize before diagnosis. The incidence of testicular cancer is higher in men with cryptorchidism. The cause of testicular cancer is unknown. It is not uncommon for the client to notice a lump or abnormal growth before being seen by a healthcare professional. Testicular self-examination may detect a new growth (In Practice: Educating the Client 90-2) and may be suggested as a cancer screening measure. However, major health agencies do not recommend a monthly routine screening for testicular or prostate cancer for the adolescent or adult male because the results are not consistent. Risk factors for testicular cancer include the following:

- Age 15–35 years most common but can occur at any age
- Cryptorchidism (undescended testicle at birth)
- Abnormal testicle development
- European American

Symptoms appear gradually. A painless mass or lump develops as the testis enlarges. A sudden collection of fluid is noted in the scrotum and a feeling of scrotal heaviness occurs. As the cancer grows, the man may feel a dull ache in the abdomen or groin, have pain in a testicle or the scrotum, or have enlargement or tenderness of the breasts. Advanced symptoms of metastatic disease include backache, pain in the abdomen, weakness, and weight loss.

There are two categories of testicular tumors, each of which is treated differently. The first type of testicular tumor is the *seminoma*. The seminoma is not as aggressive as the second type of tumor, the *nonseminoma*. Nonseminoma tumors develop at an earlier age and spread quickly. There are several subtypes of nonseminomal tumors.

If the cancer is found early, surgery may be the only treatment necessary. If treatment begins after onset of significant symptoms, chemotherapy and radiation are considered. Both chemotherapy and radiation may cause sterility; therefore, the client may want to be informed of options, such as preserving sperm, prior to beginning treatments. Two types of surgery may be used: radical inguinal orchiectomy (total removal of the testicle) and retroperitoneal lymph node dissection (removal of lymph nodes). During surgery, it is possible that nerves that affect ejaculation can be damaged.

Cancer of the Penis

Cancer of the penis is relatively rare, especially in circumcised men. Circumcision is the removal of the foreskin that covers the head of the penis. The vast majority of penile cancer is epidermoid or squamous cell carcinoma. It usually begins on or under the foreskin. When diagnosed at an early stage, this type of cancer can usually be cured. The human papillomavirus, which has been implicated in cancer of the cervix, also increases the risk of penile carcinoma.

Signs and symptoms of penile carcinoma may be a growth or lesion on the glans, foreskin, or shaft of the penis. The color of the penis may change, a reddish rash can be seen beneath the foreskin, and the penile skin can become thicker. Blood may be seen at the tip of the penis or under the foreskin. Unexplained pain of the penis, swollen lymph nodes in the groin, and irregular swelling at the end of the penis may also be noted.

Diagnosis is usually made after examination of biopsy tissue. Standard laboratory and imaging studies are typically done to confirm the diagnosis and to rule out any other problems such as infection from STIs.

Treatment generally involves surgical removal of the tumor and the marginal tissues (around the edges), called Mohs surgery. A circumcision may be done if the tumor is on the foreskin. Depending upon the stage of the cancer, *cryosurgery*, which uses liquid nitrogen to freeze and kill cells,

IN PRACTICE
EDUCATING THE CLIENT 90-2 — Notes on the Testicular Self-Examination

1. The procedure is simple and painless if the client uses gentle pressure.
2. The normal testicle is smooth, rubbery, and uniform in consistency.

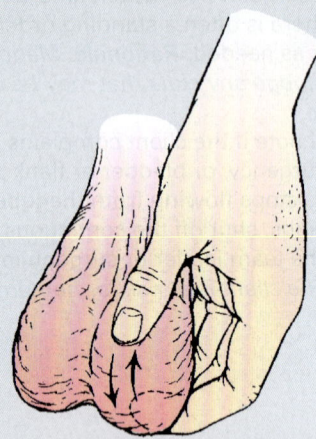

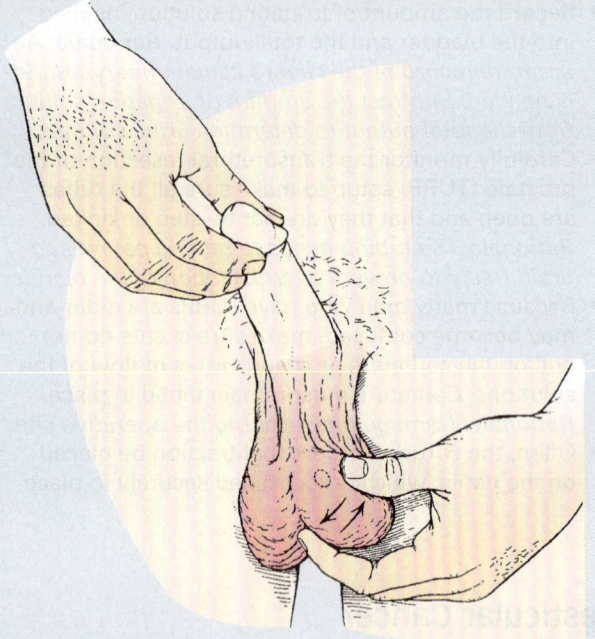

Testicular self-examination

3. The testicular self-examination (TSE) is best performed after a bath or shower because warm water relaxes the scrotal sac.
4. Use both hands to palpate the testis. The epididymis is on top of and behind the testicle.
5. Avoid touching the scrotum with cold hands; it may stimulate the cremasteric reflex, which causes the scrotum to contract close to the body.
6. If possible, stand in front of a mirror

The Testicular Examination

NOTE: It is normal to find that one testicle is somewhat larger than the other and for one testicle to hang lower than the other.

1. Check one side of the scrotal sac for swelling and then follow by checking the other side.
2. Locate the epididymis, a soft, rope- or cord-like structure on the top and back of the testicle, which feels like a small bump on the upper or middle outer side of the testicle. Normal testicles also have blood vessels, supporting tissues and vessels to carry sperm.
3. Once the structure or feel of the epididymis is known, the client will be less likely to think that it is a tumor or abnormal lump of the testicle.
4. Examine each testicle. Place the index and middle fingers under the testicle with the thumbs placed on top.

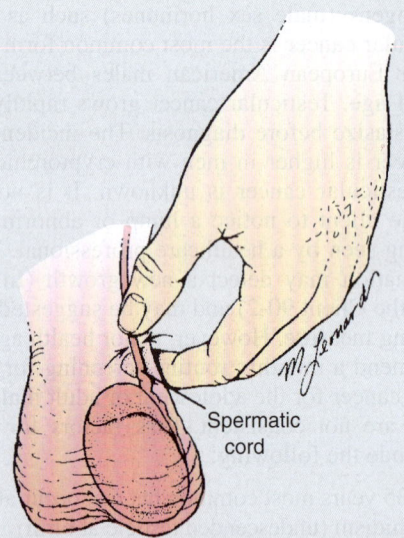

Spermatic cord

5. With the thumb on top and the testicle between the thumbs and first two fingers, palpate the structures, one side at a time. Use a firm touch and gently roll the testicle between the thumbs and fingers to feel for irregularities on the surface or texture of the testicle.
6. Feel for any evidence of a small lump or abnormality on both sides of the scrotum.

Adapted from http://www.cancer.org/cancer/testicularcancer/moreinformation/doihavetesticularcancer/, https://www.mayoclinic.org/tests-procedures/testicular-exam/about/pac-20385252.

or a *penectomy* (partial or complete removal of the penis) may be done.

Nursing considerations for the client with penile cancer include the client's concerns for sexual activity and the client's ability to have children. Coping strategies such as support from a partner and groups that have mutually beneficial discussions are helpful. Early treatment is essential; fear of their diagnosis may interfere with acceptance of this disorder.

STUDENT SYNTHESIS

KEY POINTS

- Conditions that affect male reproductive function potentially affect body image and self-esteem.
- Erectile dysfunction is generally organic in nature.
- Testicular torsion of the spermatic cord is an emergency; if unrelieved, it may cause necrosis of the affected testicle.
- Sexually transmitted diseases are often the cause of recurrent or chronic infection of the genitourinary tract, which may eventually affect fertility.
- Prostatitis is a common male problem that has a variety of medication and treatment strategies.
- Inform clients contemplating surgical treatment of benign prostatic hyperplasia that they may experience some incontinence and/or erectile dysfunction after surgery.
- Prostate cancer screening may not be desirable or effective for all men; the healthcare provider and the man need to discuss the risks and benefits of screening and review individual treatment options.

CRITICAL THINKING EXERCISES

1. Your 75-year-old client has a three-way bladder irrigation system in place following a TURP procedure. Identify the most common complication of TURP and this type of drainage. Describe when to stop continuous irrigation. Develop a teaching plan for the client and their family.

2. A client presents with a complaint of scrotal edema. Review the possible causes. Design a treatment plan for each suspected diagnosis.

NCLEX-STYLE REVIEW QUESTIONS

1. A client arrives in the emergency department reporting dizziness and lightheadedness after taking sildenafil citrate prior to sexual activity. The nurse obtains a BP of 86/48 mm Hg. Taken in combination with sildenafil citrate (Viagra), which medication is the most likely cause of these symptoms?
   a. Nitroglycerin (Nitrostat)
   b. Albuterol (Ventolin HFA)
   c. Lisinopril (Prinivil)
   d. Ibuprofen (Motrin)

2. A young male client with no history of health problems has difficulty achieving or maintaining an erection. The healthcare provider has ordered evaluations to diagnose the problem. Which activities would be appropriate actions for the nurse? Select all that apply.
   a. Prepare the client to have blood drawn for hormone levels.
   b. Prepare the client for surgery.
   c. Reinforce education for nocturnal rigidity measurements.
   d. Prepare for duplex Doppler ultrasonography.
   e. Inform the client to abstain from sexual contact prior to testing.

3. A client with erectile dysfunction (ED) is prescribed the drug sildenafil citrate (Viagra). Which information would the nurse be sure to include when reinforcing education of this medication?
   a. Seek medical intervention for erections lasting 3–4 hr.
   b. Take the medication with nitroglycerin (Nitrostat) to further dilate the arteries.
   c. If one pill does not work, double the prescribed dose.
   d. Prior to sexual activity, apply cool compresses to the penis.

4. A client is diagnosed with benign prostatic hyperplasia and prescribed the 5-alpha reductase inhibitor finasteride (Proscar). Which information would the nurse be sure to include when reinforcing education regarding this medication?
   a. The medication will eliminate bacteria in the prostate.
   b. The medication will take approximately 6 months to be effective.
   c. The medication will assist with achieving and maintaining an erection.
   d. The medication will prevent the formation of kidney stones.

5. A client is receiving continuous bladder irrigations after having a transurethral resection of the prostate (TURP). While the irrigation is in process, the client reports a feeling of fullness and right flank pain. Which is the first action by the nurse?
   a. Administer analgesics as prescribed.
   b. Turn the client on the left side to improve flow.
   c. Increase the amount of flow of the solution.
   d. Shut off the continuous irrigation and notify the team leader or surgeon.

CHAPTER RESOURCES

Enhance your learning with additional resources on thePoint*!*

Student Resources related to this chapter can be found at **thePoint.lww.com/Rosdahl12e**.

91 Female Reproductive Disorders

Learning Objectives

1. Describe the rationale, procedure, and nursing implications for the following diagnostic tests: pelvic examination, Pap test, clinical breast examination, mammography, breast ultrasound, and ultrasonography.
2. Define the following: laparoscopy, culdoscopy, colposcopy, cervical biopsy, and conization.
3. Describe the nursing implications for the client who needs a D&C.
4. List the factors involved in the nursing observations of a breast or reproductive disorder.
5. Relate the teaching components associated with each of the following: feminine hygiene and breast self-examination.
6. Demonstrate in the skills laboratory the following procedures: providing perineal care, providing sitz baths, inserting a vaginal suppository, and performing a vaginal irrigation.
7. Differentiate the following menstrual disorders: amenorrhea, menorrhagia, metrorrhagia, dysmenorrhea, and extreme irregularity.
8. Describe the causes, signs and symptoms, and the teaching components of nursing care for PMS, PMDD, and TSS.
9. Identify common client concerns related to menopause and hormone therapy.
10. Define the following structural disorders: vaginal fistula, cystocele, rectocele, prolapsed uterus, and abnormal flexion of the uterus.
11. Differentiate the following disorders: vulvitis, vaginitis, trichomoniasis, candidiasis, bacterial vaginosis, atrophic vaginitis, cervicitis, endometriosis, PID, vulvodynia, and STIs.
12. Compare and contrast ovarian cancer, uterine cancer, and cervical cancer.
13. Identify the preoperative and postoperative nursing care of a client undergoing a hysterectomy.
14. Explain the steps of breast self-examination.
15. Explain the preoperative and postoperative nursing care of a client undergoing breast biopsy, mastectomy, or reconstructive breast surgery.

Important Terminology

amenorrhea, cervicitis, colposcopy, conization, culdoscopy, cystocele, dysmenorrhea, dyspareunia, endometriosis, gynecology, hysterectomy, laparoscopy, leukorrhea, mammography, mammoplasty, mastalgia, mastectomy, menorrhagia, metrorrhagia, Pap (Papanicolaou) test (smear), pelvic exenteration, prolapse, rectocele, sentinel node biopsy, vaginitis, vulvitis

Acronyms

AP, BRCA1, BRCA2, BSE, CA125, CA 125, CBE, D&C, HCG, IUD, JP, LEEP, OB/GYN, PID, PMDD, PMS, TSS

The medical specialty that focuses on the female reproductive system is called **gynecology**. Healthcare providers who work in this area are called *gynecologists*. Gynecologists who also perform childbirth management are called *obstetrician–gynecologists* (**OB/GYN**; Unit 10).

General nursing interventions involving the female reproductive system include teaching about anatomy, self-care related to hygiene, and breast self-examination (**BSE**). Nurses who are specially trained in sexual counseling may provide more detailed care measures.

The female reproductive system comprises a complex and specialized set of organs (Chapter 29). (Refer to Chapter 70 for additional information on sexuality, fertility, and sexually transmitted infections.)

DIAGNOSTIC TESTS

Pelvic Examination

A pelvic examination is a procedure that is used to check the vulva, vagina, cervix, uterus, rectum, and pelvis for palpable abnormalities such as benign or malignant tumors. In preparation for the examination, ask the client to empty their bladder. The procedure takes only a few minutes and is done in an examination room. Encourage the client to breathe deeply, which helps the muscles to relax and minimizes the discomfort associated with the examination. The client is placed in lithotomy position (Fig. 91-1). A speculum is inserted by the healthcare provider, who examines external

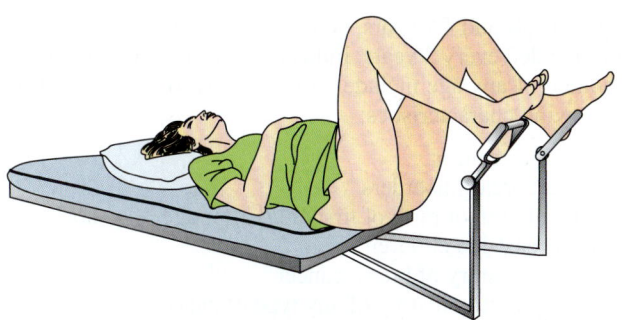

Figure 91-1 Lithotomy position. The nurse places drapes around the client to preserve privacy.

structures visually and palpates internal structures. A female attendant stays in the room and assists the healthcare provider by handing the examiner a water-soluble lubricant (K-Y jelly), vaginal speculum, and gloves, plus the materials needed for a Pap smear (see next section), which may be done at this time. The healthcare provider palpates the abdomen to feel the ovaries for masses, growths, or other abnormalities. Next, the uterus and ovaries are palpated after the healthcare provider inserts a gloved finger into the vagina and places the other hand on the abdomen. The procedure may also include rectovaginal examination, in which the healthcare provider places one finger in the client's vagina and another finger into the client's rectum. Palpating in this manner allows detection of abnormalities in the rectal area and problems of the posterior genital organs.

Generally speaking, every client past the age of puberty should have a complete pelvic examination, including a Pap test, every 1–3 years. When any pathology is present or the client has a family history of pathology, they should have the examination more as often as recommended. A cervical biopsy also can be done during a pelvic examination. Additionally, cauterization, removal, or coagulation of a portion of the cervix using electricity or laser can be performed during a pelvic examination.

Laboratory Tests

Pap Test

The most common test for cervical cancer, usually done during a pelvic examination, is known as the **Pap** (**Papanicolaou**) test or *Pap smear*. The Pap test is used as a preliminary method of detecting cancer of the endometrium or of the uterus. A malignant growth in the uterus or cervix sometimes sheds cancerous cells into uterine and vaginal secretions. A Pap test looks for cervical cells. A broader assessment of a client's reproductive organs includes a breast examination and a pelvic examination (with or without a Pap test), which are included in the standard procedure known as a "pelvic examination." Microscopic examination of a smear from these secretions may help detect cancer before symptoms appear. *Cervical cancer* is one of the most commonly occurring cancers in women. When cervical cancer is found and treated early, it is highly curable. Healthcare providers may recommend annual pelvic examinations (not always including the pelvic smear) for sexually active women. *Rationale: A Pap test looks only for cervical cells. A broader assessment of a client's reproductive organs includes a breast examination and a pelvic examination (with or without a Pap test), which are included in the standard procedure known as a "pelvic examination."*

> **Key Concept**
> All clients with a cervix are at risk for cervical cancer. Clients who have had a hysterectomy (uterus removed) may still have a cervix and need to have Pap tests.

The procedure for positioning the client is the same as for any routine pelvic examination. In addition to equipment needed for the pelvic examination, necessary Pap test equipment includes glass slides and the applicator or Y-shaped wooden stick that is inserted through the speculum to obtain a smear of cervical mucosa. This material is smeared onto the glass slide; a spray fixative is sprayed over the slide so that the specimen adheres to the glass. Pap smear cytology results may be reported in the range of low-grade lesions to high-grade lesions, which may be compared and differentiated from histologic biopsy results described as mild, moderate, or severe dysplasic precancerous cervical lesions.

> **Nursing Alert** Pap tests should be done between a client's menstrual periods. Tests are less accurate when a client is menstruating. Some clients have a higher than normal chance of contracting cervical cancer. These clients require regular screening, sometimes more often than once a year.

> **Key Concept**
> All clients must understand the importance of regular Pap tests. A client may not have physical symptoms with early cancer, but may have abnormal cells of the cervix, which could be early indicators of cancer. Early detection and treatment of cervical cancer is effective in a high percentage of cases. Teach clients that abnormal Pap tests do not necessarily indicate cancer, but further testing and evaluation are necessary.

> **Nursing Alert** Several types of cervical cancer are caused by the human papillomavirus (HPV). A vaccine is available that can prevent certain cervical cancers but does not treat cervical cancer if it has developed. Vaccination does not substitute for routine Pap testing and pelvic examinations.

Tests for Endometrial Cancer

A positive Pap test may indicate endometrial cancer. A Pap test can show a false-negative result for this type of cancer. Therefore, aspiration of the *endocervix* (the internal portion of the cervix) provides more accurate information. A biopsy of the endometrium itself is the best option for accuracy.

Blood Tests

Blood testing for cancer of the uterus, fallopian tubes, ovaries, and breast includes the widely used tumor marker known as *cancer antigen 125*, more often seen as **CA125** or

CA 125. Elevated levels of CA125 can also indicate cancer of the pancreas, lungs, or colon. While receiving therapy for cancer, a decrease in CA125 levels can indicate that treatment is effective. Rising levels of CA125 can indicate growth of a malignant tumor, recurrence of a previously treated tumor, or a tumor on the peritoneum. It is not used routinely as a screening tool because CA125 is also seen in many noncancerous conditions, such as menstruation and uterine fibroids. In a client who has very high-risk factors for the development of ovarian cancer, CA125 may be used to look for early signs of ovarian cancer. Human chorionic gonadotropin (HCG) is another tumor marker used as an aid in diagnosing testicular and ovarian cancers.

Clinical Breast Examination

A client between the ages of 20–39 years should have a *clinical breast examination* (CBE) performed by their healthcare provider at least every 3 years (National Breast Cancer Foundation, 2019). Clients who have a cystic disorder or who are aged 40 years and older should check with their healthcare providers to ascertain if the CBE needs to be done in conjunction with a mammogram. Recommendations vary and some authorities suggest monthly BSEs. At any age, if any unusual symptoms appear, a client should have their breasts examined immediately. Palpation by the healthcare provider is essentially the same as that done by the client during BSE. Signs and symptoms of breast cancer are discussed in the later section on breast neoplasms and In Practice: Educating the Client 91-5.

> **SPECIAL CONSIDERATIONS   Culture and Ethnicity**
>
> The CDC's National Breast and Cervical Cancer Early Detection Program (NBCCEDP) provides breast and cervical cancer screenings and diagnostic services to low-income, uninsured, and underinsured women across the United States (CDC, 2021). As part of the affordable Care Act, Medicare covers the full cost of a screening mammogram once a year for women with Medicare aged 40 years and older. Refer to www.cdc.gov and search for NBCCEDP or the National Breast and Cervical Cancer Early Detection Program. The American Cancer Society can provide more information regarding State and Federal regulations regarding costs for mammograms. More information can be found on the Website of the American Cancer Society (www.cancer.org).

Mammography

Mammography is an x-ray examination of the breasts that is capable of detecting some cancers 1–2 years before they reach palpable size. In previous decades, monthly BSEs and yearly clinical breast examinations were recommended; however, research has shown that these do not decrease the risk of dying from breast cancer. The best way to find breast cancer is with a mammogram. Professional guidelines change for initial and routine testing; refer your client to their healthcare provider or provide information available at www.cdc.gov and search for the latest guidelines on breast cancer. In 2020, recommendation for initial or routine mammogram screening for women between the ages of 40 and 49 years is based on the individual's background of cancer and the history of the client's female relatives. Discussion should occur between healthcare providers and client. Between the ages of 50 and 74 years, screening mammograms are recommended every 2 years. Indications for mammography for women of any age include individuals who have any of the following characteristics:

- Previous cancer
- Cystic breast disorders
- No children or birth of first child after age 30 years
- No breast-fed children
- Family history of breast cancer
- Strong family history of any type of cancer
- Hormone (estrogen) therapy
- Extreme fear of cancer (need mammography for reassurance)

Procedure

The procedure is simple and does not require the injection of dye. However, a specially trained radiologist must interpret the mammary x-rays.

Some laboratories request that the client refrain from using deodorant or powder before the test because they may contain zinc or other metals that will interfere with the x-rays. The client wears a gown that opens in front and is asked to remove neck jewelry and clothing above the waist. Help by explaining that they will be asked to assume several positions and that their breasts will be flat on the x-ray plate. A compressor is pressed from above or the side to flatten each breast as much as possible. The procedure may be uncomfortable, but should not be painful.

A more definitive diagnosis can be obtained by xerography (xeroradiography). However, this test exposes the client to higher radiation levels.

Interpretation

Tumors may appear on mammography as denser than normal breast tissue. However, not all breast abnormalities are identified on a mammogram. Mammography only identifies abnormal breast architecture or tumors with calcium deposits (approximately 70% of the breast tumors that can be diagnosed). The radiologist can speculate whether a tumor is malignant or benign based on its shape, location, and size. If a lesion is present, a biopsy is usually done.

Breast Ultrasound

The ultrasound examination can distinguish a breast cyst from a solid mass, which usually requires a biopsy examination to determine malignancy. Breast ultrasound is not used for routine screening. Ultrasound is being used more frequently with young women with dense breast tissue who present with breast lumps.

Breast Biopsy

Breast biopsy definitively determines the presence of cancer. The pathologist examines breast tissue or fluid to determine the presence and type of cancer cells. In the case of tissue, a *frozen section* is usually done and it is examined microscopically. Breast biopsy can be performed in several ways:

- *Aspiration (fine-needle aspiration):* Cells from a lump are drawn into a syringe. (In the case of some cysts, fluid is aspirated, collapsing the cyst. Often, this cyst requires no further treatment but, in chronic cystic disease, the procedure may be routinely repeated.)

- *Needle biopsy:* A needle with a cutting edge is inserted into a lump and rotated to remove a core sample.
- *Excisional biopsy:* An entire lump is removed and analyzed. If cancer is localized in this lump, no further treatment may be required.
- *Incisional biopsy:* Part of a lump is removed as a sample.

Other Diagnostic Tests

Abdominal or Pelvic Ultrasonography

Ultrasonography uses high-frequency sound waves directed back at a transducer placed over the client's abdominal or pelvic region. The sound waves are converted into electrical impulses, which can be viewed on a special monitor. By scanning the abdomen and viewing the results on the screen, the healthcare provider can evaluate reproductive conditions, such as tumors, cysts, and other pelvic diseases. A secondary approach using ultrasound is with a special probe through the vagina (*vaginal ultrasound*) to view pelvic organs that cannot be seen any other way.

X-ray Examinations

Several x-ray procedures determine patency of the oviducts or the presence of abnormalities in the uterus and oviducts. The most common is the *hysterosalpingogram*, in which the uterus and oviducts can be visualized following an injection of contrast dye. The ovaries may also be visualized. These procedures are most often necessary to locate the cause of infertility or to determine the presence of a tumor.

Laparoscopy

Laparoscopy is a diagnostic technique that provides direct visualization of the uterus and accessory organs, including the ovaries and oviducts (Fig. 91-2).

For this procedure, a small incision is made in the area of the umbilicus, and the abdomen is then distended (*insufflated*) with approximately 2 L of carbon dioxide or oxygen. Gas is used because it allows for a clear view of the organs, separate from the intestines. The laparoscope is inserted into the peritoneal cavity, and the internal organs are viewed.

Laparoscopy is usually performed using general or spinal anesthesia. Two or three small incisions may be made in more extensive procedures; an absorbable suture is placed in the incisions.

The client usually ambulates on the operative day. Document client and family teaching. Usually, the client will be discharged from the day-surgery center to home.

> **Nursing Alert** Following a laparoscopy, severe pain, such as "shoulder strap pain," may be felt as pain under a clavicle. Report pain to the healthcare provider. This type of referred pain may result from either gas instilled during the procedure, which is temporarily trapped under the diaphragm, or from blood accumulating under the diaphragm. Gas pain is temporary, but is quite uncomfortable. Pain from accumulated blood can be symptomatic of a life-threatening hemorrhage.

Culdoscopy

Culdoscopy furnishes direct visualization of the uterus, oviducts, broad ligaments, colon, and small intestine. An endoscope is passed through the vaginal wall behind the cervix after a small incision is made in the posterior vaginal cul-de-sac. The procedure is usually done in the operating room with the client in a knee-chest position. The client may have local, regional, or general anesthesia. Usually, no sutures are involved, and routine postoperative care is given.

During the culdoscopy, photographs may be taken of the cervix and the vaginal vault; cold *conization* (removal of a cone-shaped portion of the cervix) may also be done. This procedure is also used to diagnose pelvic pain, tubal pregnancy, and pelvic masses.

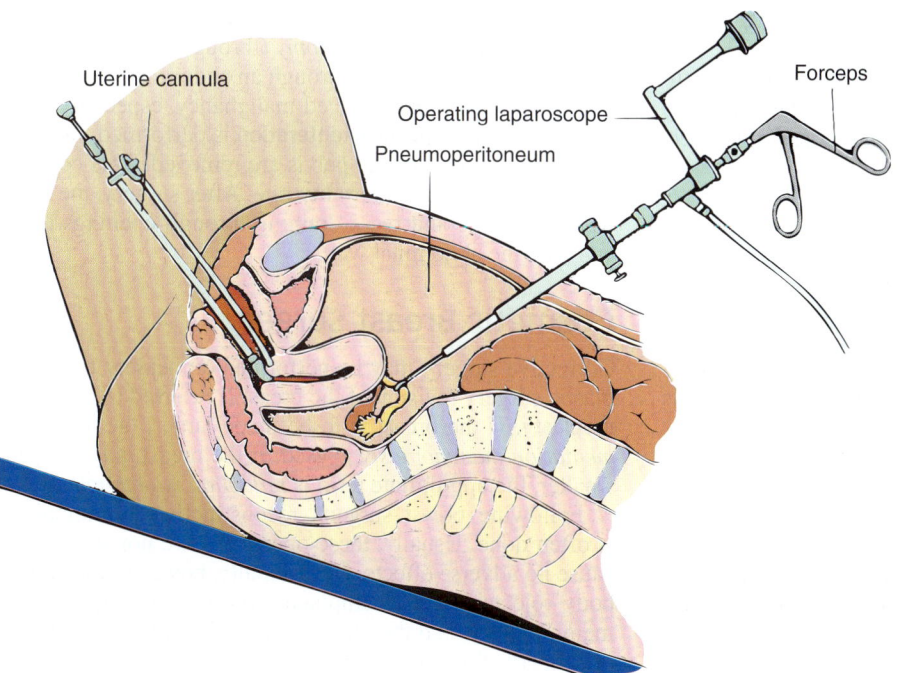

Figure 91-2 Laparoscopy. The laparoscope is inserted through a tiny incision near the umbilicus.

Colposcopy

High-risk clients often are screened routinely with **colposcopy**, which allows better visualization of the vagina and cervix than with the regular speculum. The colposcope is a lighted, magnifying speculum that is inserted into the vaginal vault. Many believe that the results are more reliable than those from the Pap test. Accurate diagnosis often requires biopsy, however.

Cervical Biopsy

A *cervical biopsy* involves the microscopic examination of a small piece of cervical tissue. It is performed when the healthcare provider observes cervical irregularities or when a Pap test is questionable. One means of obtaining this tissue is through a punch procedure (punching out a button of tissue for examination).

The loop electrosurgical excision procedure (**LEEP**) is a common office procedure in which tissue is removed for diagnosis and treatment of cervical abnormalities. A wire loop and a low level of electricity are used to remove a lesion. Minimal bleeding and cramping are the only side effects.

Conization (Cone Biopsy)

Conization is usually done in an operating room with the client under general or spinal anesthesia. The surgeon removes a cone-shaped piece of the cervix for examination. *Cold conization* is done with a specially cooled knife and it sometimes preserves the cells better. A small percentage of clients may have some bleeding after cervical conization. Watch for symptoms. The client should also check for delayed bleeding after the procedure.

> **Key Concept**
> Some clients who have had cervical conizations or other biopsies have difficulty in later pregnancies. They may need a special procedure, called cerclage, to prevent premature dilation of the cervix, leading to a spontaneous abortion (miscarriage; Chapter 68).

COMMON SURGICAL TREATMENTS

Some diagnostic surgical procedures mentioned previously may also be used for treatment. These procedures include laparoscopy, culdoscopy, colposcopy, and biopsy of the cervix, uterine lining, or breasts.

Dilation and Curettage

Dilation and curettage (**D&C**) is the most frequently performed gynecologic surgery. It can be used to diagnose disorders and to treat some disorders. In D&C, the cervix is *dilated* (widened) using calibrated rods. A spoon-shaped instrument (*curette*) is then passed into the uterus, and the endometrial lining is scraped out (*curettage*). D&C takes approximately 15 min; it is often done in a day-surgery department on an outpatient basis.

Purposes

A D&C is used as a diagnostic procedure in clients with abnormal vaginal bleeding or to obtain tissue for examination after a positive Pap test. The uterine scrapings are examined for evidence of malignant or nonmalignant growths or other abnormalities. Sometimes, a D&C is done just before the menstrual period in an effort to find the cause of infertility. D&C is frequently used to evaluate *endometrial hypoplasia* (incomplete development of the uterine lining), *menorrhagia* (excessive menstrual flow), and *metrorrhagia* (bleeding between menses). In some cases, the D&C is all that is needed to eliminate the problem.

A D&C is used as treatment in other instances. It may be used after an abortion, whether spontaneous or therapeutic, to remove the retained products of conception. A D&C is always performed after an incomplete abortion.

Nursing Considerations

Preoperative preparation is similar to that for any person about to receive anesthesia. In many cases, general anesthesia is used.

The client usually makes an uneventful postoperative recovery. The client will need to wear a perineal pad and receive perineal care. A mild analgesic, such as acetaminophen (Tylenol) or ibuprofen (Advil), usually relieves minor discomforts.

In rare instances, the vagina is packed with gauze at the time of the surgery, which may make voiding difficult. The pack is usually removed the next day. Carefully monitor the client to make sure that they can void and that they do not experience urinary retention.

Because the D&C is often done on an outpatient basis, teaching is vital. Vaginal discharge will be bloody at first, but should quickly become serosanguineous. This drainage typically does not last more than a few days. Teach the client signs of abdominal distention and how to perform perineal care. Instruct the client to call the healthcare provider if any problems occur. Carefully document all teaching.

Hysterectomy and Pelvic Exenteration

A **hysterectomy** is the surgical removal of the uterus. It may be performed for a variety of reasons: cancer of the cervix, ovaries, or uterus or to treat uterine fibroids, severe endometriosis, or a *prolapsed* ("fallen") uterus. In some cases, such as a ruptured uterus during labor, an emergency hysterectomy must be performed. The uterus may be removed by means of a *vaginal hysterectomy* (through the vagina) or an *abdominal hysterectomy* (through an abdominal incision).

In some cases of advanced malignancy, especially if the client is young, a **pelvic exenteration** is performed, in which the entire contents of the pelvis are removed. This complex procedure has a high mortality rate. After surgery, the client will have urine and feces draining through openings (*ostomies*) on the abdominal wall.

Cosmetic Breast Surgery

Corrective surgery may be performed on healthy breasts. A plastic surgery revision of the breast is referred to as a **mammoplasty**. If the breast is to be made larger, the term *augmentation mammoplasty* is used; if the breast is to be made smaller, the appropriate term is *reduction mammoplasty*.

Following breast surgery, reconstructive mammoplasty is often done. Usually, these operations are not serious and cause no adverse effects. Occasionally, however, the client's body rejects materials implanted during the augmentation mammoplasty, and the materials must be removed. Because of concerns for safety, implants must be used cautiously with follow-up monitoring.

Mastectomy

Mastectomy is surgical removal of a breast. It is discussed in the section on breast cancer later in this chapter.

> **NCLEX Alert**
>
> NCLEX clinical scenarios can present inpatient or outpatient situations in which knowledge of the reproductive system is prevalent. Options for these clinical scenarios can include observational skills regarding postprocedure recovery, pre- or postprocedure teaching, and communication skills for the client and their family.

NURSING PROCESS

DATA COLLECTION

Carefully observe the client with a reproductive disorder. The information obtained from the physical examination and data collection forms a baseline that is used for future comparison and determines the presence of suspected disorders and complications. Report any changes in the baseline level (In Practice: Data Gathering in Nursing 91-1).

Many clients are reluctant to discuss sexual or reproductive concerns. One nursing goal is to express concern and to put the client at ease when discussing sexuality or sexually related concerns. In addition, observe the client's emotional response to the disorder or disease. Does the client need assistance to meet daily needs? Is the disorder life-threatening? Does the disorder affect social activities, sexual identity, or self-esteem? Is the client anxious or fearful of the outcome?

PLANNING AND IMPLEMENTING

Together with the client, family, and other members of the healthcare team, plan for effective individualized care to meet the client's needs. Provide pre- and postoperative care for the client undergoing procedures, such as hysterectomy and mastectomy. The client with a reproductive disorder may also require teaching about preventive measures, such as BSE. The client may need assistance in meeting needs, dealing with emotional problems, and understanding more about the disorder, its prognosis, and treatment.

> **IN PRACTICE**
> **DATA GATHERING IN NURSING 91-1** — Female Reproductive System
>
> - Sexual history
> - Reproductive history (pregnancies, abortions)
> - Method of birth control used
> - Menstrual history; date of last menstrual period
> - History of sexually transmitted infections (STIs), pelvic inflammatory disease (**PID**), or other gynecologic infections
> - Visual observation of external genitalia
> - Breast examination; teaching of breast self-examination

Teaching Feminine Hygiene

Nurses are in an excellent position to teach clients about personal hygiene. Many women do not realize that after urinating or defecating they should wipe from front to back to prevent urinary tract and vaginal infections. Caution the client who is susceptible to infections against using bubble baths, bath oils, and nylon panties or pantyhose. Also stress the importance of thorough handwashing and perineal care, especially during menses. Menstrual discharge is an excellent culture medium for microorganisms. Techniques to prevent vaginal infections are presented in In Practice: Educating the Client 91-1.

> **IN PRACTICE**
> **EDUCATING THE CLIENT 91-1** — Prevention of Vaginal Infections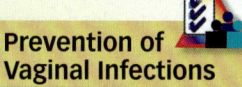
>
> - Wipe from front to back after going to the bathroom.
> - Wash hands thoroughly after using the bathroom or changing perineal pads.
> - Change tampons or sanitary pads frequently. Dispose of them safely. Place them in sealed plastic bags in the trash.
> - Pull panties, with perineal pad attached, straight down to avoid spreading infection during menses.
> - Remove a tampon immediately and call a healthcare provider if fever, nausea, vomiting, diarrhea, or weakness (signs of toxic shock syndrome) appear. Do not use deodorant tampons.
> - Do not use vaginal deodorant sprays or scented powders.
> - Douche only when absolutely necessary. Use the cleanest technique possible. Dispose of all equipment each time in a safe way.
> - Clean the bathtub carefully before use or take showers.
> - Do not use bubble bath or bath oil, especially if susceptible to infection.
> - Do not use colored or scented toilet tissue.
> - Wear only cotton panties, ventilated pantyhose, or hose with garters; avoid nylon panties.
> - Avoid tight pants or jeans, nonventilated clothes, or tight exercise clothing.
> - Change out of a wet bathing suit immediately after swimming. Stay out of swimming pools or hot tubs if you are susceptible to infection. (The chlorine in the pool may predispose to infection. An infected person also can spread the infection to others.)
> - Cut down on intake of sugar.
> - Wear a condom when having sexual intercourse. A water-soluble lubricant, such as K-Y jelly, may be needed to increase comfort and prevent irritation.
> - Check with a healthcare provider at the earliest sign of pain or infection. (Sexual partner should also be checked.)
> - Consult healthcare provider regarding use of oral contraceptives or other hormones.

Teach the client the procedure for BSE (In Practice: Educating the Client 91-2) and reaffirm the necessity of a yearly Pap test, breast examination, and serology tests for sexually transmitted infections (STIs). Stress the need for adequate nutrition, including vitamin D and calcium intake, as well as fruits and vegetables. Teach the client about the dangers of smoking.

Providing Perineal Care
Give perineal care to women after any perineal surgery. Many clients need instruction in this procedure.

Providing Sitz Baths
Sitz baths are frequently ordered for a client following a vaginal hysterectomy or delivery (Chapter 54). Remember to clean equipment after each use and to inform the client why the procedure is necessary (whether it is done to cleanse the area, to aid in the healing process, or to make the client more comfortable).

Performing a Douche or Vaginal Irrigation
The *douche* or *vaginal irrigation* is generally not recommended. Frequent douching disrupts the normal flora inside the vagina, irritates the vaginal mucosa, and generally increases the risk of a vaginal infection. Douching will not cure a vaginal infection. The normal secretions from the mucous membrane protect the area from infection. Therefore, it is not desirable to wash away these secretions unless the healthcare provider includes douching as part of a therapeutic treatment.

If a vaginal irrigation is ordered, explain the procedure and purpose to the client. Tell the client not to overfill the vagina with douche solution because it may push fluid into the uterus, which could cause inflammation or infection. Douching during pregnancy is not typically recommended, as it may harm the fetus. Vaginal irrigation cleanses the vaginal canal of excess discharge, supplies heat or medication, and relieves pain and inflammation.

In the clinical setting, the healthcare provider orders the solution to use. As the nurse, you are generally the individual who describes and sometimes assists the client with this procedure. Many clients douche for personal reasons. If there are questions about the procedure or which type of solution to use, check with the healthcare provider. Common solutions include saline solution, sterile water, or a solution of acetic acid (two tablespoons of cider vinegar in one quart of tepid water). Occasionally, the healthcare provider may suggest a solution of ½ tsp of povidone-iodine (Betadine) in one cup of water twice a day for a week to relieve symptoms and treat resistant or recurrent cases of bacterial infections such as bacterial vaginosis. In the home setting, equipment may be used more than once. To prevent cross contamination, it is very important that any douche tips or bags are cleaned and dry between uses. Over-the-counter disposable douches also are available (In Practice: Nursing Procedure 91-1).

Inserting a Vaginal Suppository
Medication is applied to the vaginal canal by means of vaginal suppositories. Most suppositories must be kept refrigerated until ready for use.

EVALUATION
Evaluate outcomes of care with the client, family, and other members of the healthcare team. Have short-term goals been met? For example, is the client ready for discharge following a hysterectomy? Are long-term goals still realistic? Does the client need follow-up care or education? Is long-term therapy required; for example, radiation therapy or chemotherapy for cancer? Planning for further nursing care takes into consideration the client's prognosis, any complications, and the client's response to care given.

DISORDERS RELATED TO THE MENSTRUAL CYCLE

Amenorrhea
Amenorrhea is the absence or abnormal stoppage of menses (*menstruation*). If an adolescent has not begun to menstruate by their 15th year, they should be examined. The difficulty may be hormonal, requiring a specialist's attention. Amenorrhea may also be caused by nutritional or emotional factors or by malformations of the organs. Temporarily after pregnancy and after completion of menopause, menses are normally absent. Treatment is prescribed based on the cause of the client's amenorrhea.

> **Nursing Alert** Clients who are starving often experience amenorrhea, a serious symptom, which is also a sign of anorexia or bulimia. Clients in intensive athletic training may experience amenorrhea. They should be under the supervision of an experienced sports medicine specialist.

Menorrhagia
Menorrhagia is excessive bleeding in amount or duration during menstruation. The excessive blood loss results in anemia. If this irregularity occurs in a young girl, it may adjust itself. However, monitoring is necessary. If it occurs during menopause, it may indicate pathology. Menorrhagia may also occur in the client using an intrauterine device (**IUD**) for birth control. In excessive bleeding unexplained by organic causes, hormone therapy may be helpful. A D&C may also be performed as therapeutic treatment.

Metrorrhagia
Metrorrhagia is bleeding between menstrual periods. It is abnormal and should be brought to a healthcare provider's attention because it may indicate cancer or retained placental tissue in the postpartum client or in the client who has had a spontaneous or induced abortion. Metrorrhagia may indicate fibroid tumors and is frequently associated with the use of oral contraceptives; in this instance, it is referred to as *breakthrough bleeding*.

CHAPTER 91 Female Reproductive Disorders 1677

IN PRACTICE
EDUCATING THE CLIENT 91-2 Breast Self-Examination

NOTE: The best way to find breast cancer is by having a mammogram.

Before a Mirror
1. Inspect the breasts with your arms at the sides.
2. Raise your hands above the head. Breast movement should be free and equal on both sides. Look for changes in the contour of each breast (discharge, puckering, dimpling, or scaling of the skin).

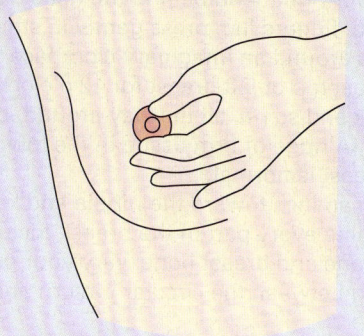

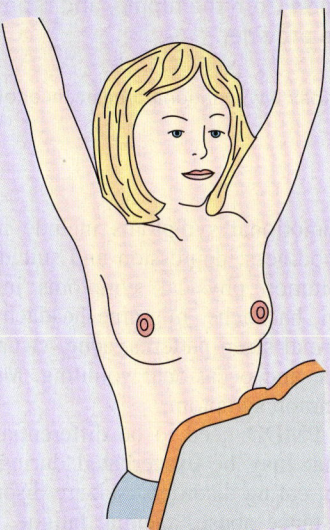

In the Shower
1. Keeping your fingers flat, move them gently over each part of the breast. Use the right hand to examine the left breast, and the left hand to examine the right breast. Check for any lump, hard knot, or thickening.

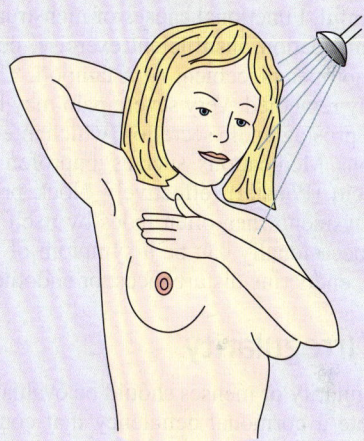

3. Press your hands firmly on the hips and bow slightly toward the mirror, pulling your shoulders and elbows forward. Note any changes in breast contours.

2. Check the axillae for any unusual signs (rash, lesions, lumps, absence of hair, unusual pigmentation).

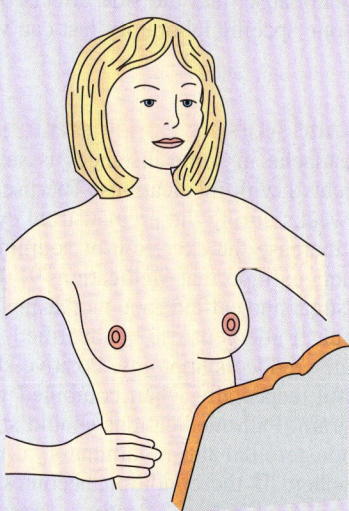

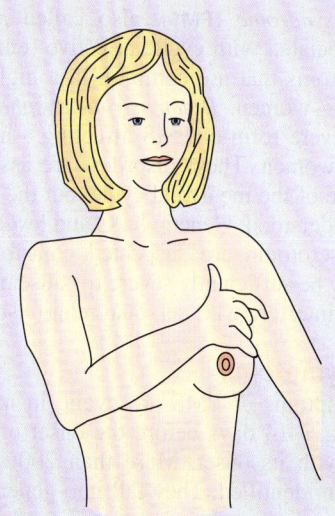

4. Squeeze the nipple of each breast gently between the thumb and index finger. Report any discharge (clear or bloody) to the healthcare provider immediately.

Lying Down
1. To examine the right breast, put a pillow or folded towel under the right shoulder.
2. Place your right hand behind the head. With your left hand, fingers flat, press gently in small circular motions around an imaginary clock face. Begin at outermost top of left breast for 12 o'clock. Move to 1 o'clock and so on, all the way around, back to 12 o'clock. (A ridge of firm tissue in the lower curve of each breast is normal.)
3. Move in an inch toward the nipple and keep circling to examine every part of the breast, including the collar bone and breast bone. Vary your pattern of checking between the circular pattern and a vertical pattern.

4. Repeat the above steps for the left breast.

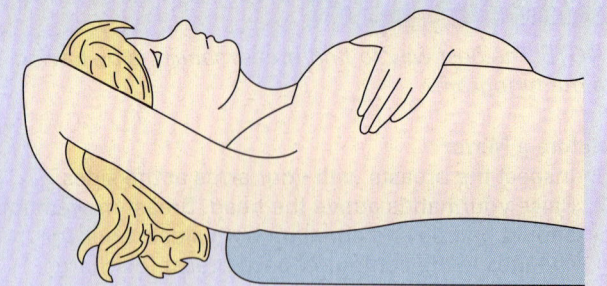

5. If you find any abnormalities, measure the distance and direction from the nipple, and report to the healthcare provider.

Adapted from https://www.breastcancer.org/symptoms/testing/types/self_exam; https://www.nationalbreastcancer.org/breast-self-exam

Dysmenorrhea

Dysmenorrhea is painful menstruation. Normal menstruation is not painful. Functional causes of menstrual pain may stem from constipation, insufficient exercise, poor posture, fatigue, or improper placement of a tampon. These conditions are easily remedied. Very severe pain may be owing to an increase in prostaglandin secretion, which intensifies uterine contractions. Medications, such as ibuprofen (Motrin) or mefenamic acid (Ponstel), effectively block prostaglandin production. Dysmenorrhea often fades by itself after childbearing, but occasionally can be a symptom of a displaced uterus, tumor, endocrine disturbances, or endometriosis.

Extreme Irregularity

Extreme irregularity of menses should be evaluated because it may indicate a hormonal deficiency that could result in later sterility.

Premenstrual Syndrome

Premenstrual syndrome (**PMS**), also called *premenstrual tension*, is associated with cyclic affective (emotional) and physical symptoms that are common in a high percentage of menstruating women. *Premenstrual dysphoric disorder* (**PMDD**) is a severe form of PMS affecting a much smaller percentage of women. These disorders are associated with the luteal phase of the menstrual cycle, but the exact causes are not well understood. Genetic links and levels of the neurotransmitter serotonin are suspected contributors. These conditions may be sufficiently severe to cause physical incapacitation and interfere with personal relationships.

Signs and Symptoms

Signs and symptoms of PMS are cyclic in nature, generally developing 7–14 days before the onset of menses and disappearing with its onset. More than 200 symptoms of PMS have been identified. They fall into general categories of mood alterations, symptoms related to fluid retention, and neurologic, vascular, gastrointestinal, and respiratory symptoms. Emotional symptoms include irritability, sadness, and moodiness; depression and suicidal ideation are possible. Common physical symptoms include abdominal distention, backache, migraine headaches, generalized edema, abnormal sleep patterns, acne, visual disturbances, food cravings, and occasional vomiting. **Mastalgia** (breast pain) is a common symptom.

PMS and PMDD need to be differentiated from other conditions that may be exacerbated during menses, such as depression, eating disorders, seizure disorders, hypothyroidism, substance abuse, anemia, fatigue, irritable bowel syndrome, asthma, and allergies. Problems that may have symptoms similar to PMS or PMDD need to be excluded before diagnosis is made. Several conditions that mimic PMS or PMDD can be diagnosed and successfully treated. These alternate conditions include dysmenorrhea, endometriosis, perimenopause, and the side effects of oral contraceptives. No one specific laboratory test can verify PMS or PMDD.

Treatment and Nursing Considerations

Menstrual headache in some instances is severe and may need to be treated with medications. The use of a low-salt diet for 1–2 weeks during the premenstrual cycle and medications that increase the excretion of sodium ions may be useful (In Practice: Important Medications 91-1). Decreasing the intake of sugar and caffeine and increasing protein intake may be helpful. If allergens can be identified, their elimination can greatly reduce symptoms. Positive stress management is helpful, especially when combined with an active exercise program. Pain medications should start with over-the-counter nonsteroidal anti-inflammatory drugs (NSAIDs) or acetaminophen. If the condition becomes severe, analgesics, antianxiety, and/or selective serotonin reuptake inhibitor (SSRI) agents may be prescribed. When painful symptoms are present, mild heat to the back or the abdomen often is beneficial. The nurse needs to be supportive of the client and their condition, especially because some individuals may ineffectively tell the client their symptoms are "all in your head."

IN PRACTICE
IMPORTANT MEDICATIONS 91-1: For Premenstrual Syndrome (PMS)

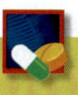

Diuretic Medications
- hydrochlorothiazide (Microzide)

Hormones
- oral contraceptives
- progesterone

Antianxiety Agents
- alprazolam (Xanax)
- diazepam (Valium)

Supplements
- vitamin B supplements, especially pyridoxine (B_6)
- magnesium supplements
- calcium and vitamin D supplements

Selective Serotonin Reuptake Inhibitors (SSRIs)
- citalopram hydrobromide (Celexa)
- fluoxetine hydrochloride (Prozac)
- paroxetine hydrochloride (Paxil)
- sertraline hydrochloride (Zoloft)

> **Key Concept**
> Provide the client with reassurance and informational counseling. If the client has not had a thorough medical evaluation, suggest that they seek the advice of a healthcare provider experienced in women's healthcare issues.

Toxic Shock Syndrome

Toxic shock syndrome (**TSS**) is caused by superantigen toxins that developed from bacterial skin infections from either *Staphylococcus aureus* or *Streptococcus pyogenes*. The infection manifests in typically healthy individuals who can quickly become very ill. Hospitalization is generally necessary because of the need for aggressive supportive treatments, such as intravenous (IV) fluids, medications to treat life-threatening hypotension (e.g., inotropic drugs, such as IV dopamine), endotracheal ventilation, and management of renal failure and/or multiple organ failure.

Symptoms initially seen include a characteristic rash in TSS caused by *S. aureus*. The rash resembles a sunburn that will blanch when touched. It can be seen in any region of the body, including palms and soles of the feet, lips, mouth, and eyes. Other symptoms include high fever, hypotension, general malaise, confusion, and altered level of consciousness, which can rapidly progress to stupor and coma, followed by multiple organ failure and death. When the client's condition improves, the rash will desquamate (peel off) in about 10–24 days.

Cases of TSS caused by the bacterium *S. pyogenes* differ from those caused by *S. aureus* in that the individual generally has a preexisting skin infection with the bacteria and may not develop a skin rash. The client complains of severe pain at the source of the skin infection that is accompanied by the TSS symptoms described above.

Treatment includes removal or drainage of the source of infection, if possible. If a client is wearing a menstrual tampon, it must be removed. If the source of the infection is not identified, the morbidity rate increases. Antibiotic therapy needs a culture and sensitivity test to ensure treatment of the appropriate organism. Multiple antibiotics are typically required. These include cephalosporins, penicillins, vancomycin (Vancocin), clindamycin (Cleocin), and gentamicin (Gentak). Recovery can occur in 2–3 weeks if therapy is successful. TSS can be fatal within hours if not diagnosed or treated.

Discomforts of Menopause

Menopause (*climacteric*), the cessation of menstruation, usually occurs between the ages of 45 and 50 years, although it may occur earlier or later. Menopause signifies that the client's production of estrogen and progesterone has stopped and that ovulation has ceased. Menopause is a normal body change that should not be viewed as an illness. However, some women experience difficulties as a result of changes in hormonal balance, particularly the decrease in estrogen and progesterone.

One of the first signs of approaching menopause is a change in the menses. The amount of flow lessens, and the cycle becomes irregular. Finally, the menses stop altogether. In a few clients, bleeding becomes heavier for a time. Because the ovaries produce less estrogen, levels may be inadequate, resulting in symptoms.

The most common symptom is the *hot flash*, with accompanying perspiration, palpitations, and fatigue. Although hot flashes are not serious, they are annoying and may embarrass the client. Another possible symptom of menopause is vaginal dryness and atrophy. The vagina loses its normal lubrication and elasticity. Some women also experience weight gain, skin dryness, sagging breasts, and signs of calcium deficiency (*osteoporosis*).

Sometimes clients experience symptoms during menopause that affect their sense of psychological well-being or quality of life. These include insomnia, anxiety, crying spells, fatigue, mood swings, and depression.

Treatment

Hormone therapy, formerly referred to as hormone replacement therapy (HRT), may be prescribed to treat severe symptoms and discomforts, under certain conditions. It is not used for disease prevention, such as heart disease or memory loss, as it was in the 20th century because research demonstrated that the hormones created more health risks than health benefits. If the client is a healthy client between the ages of 40 and 45 years, systemic estrogen therapy may be considered an effective treatment for specific menopausal symptoms. These circumstances include experiencing moderate to severe hot flashes, having a significant loss of bone mass, having premature menopause, or having premature ovarian insufficiency.

Systemic estrogen is available as a pill, skin patch, gel, cream, or spray. These modes of delivery provide adequate to good relief of menopausal hot flashes and night sweats. Vaginal dryness, itching, burning, and pain with intercourse are particularly distressing symptoms accompanying menopause. Estrogen is approved by the FDA for the treatment of osteoporosis but medications such as bisphosphonates (Actonel, Actonel+Ca, Aredia) should also be considered. Low-dose vaginal products with estrogen are available in cream, tablet, or ring form and are effective in treating some urinary symptoms but not hot flashes, night sweats, or as protection against osteoporosis.

Many over-the-counter products are available for treatment of symptoms. A client may use other products to make sexual intercourse easier, such as water-based lubricants (e.g., K-Y jelly). For women with vaginal atrophy, a vaginal dilator may be helpful before intercourse.

Nursing Considerations

A client often needs emotional support during menopause. Teach them to realize that menopause is a normal physiologic function. Instruct them about helpful health measures: a balanced diet, stress-relieving exercise, adequate rest, leisure activities, and relaxation techniques.

Induced Menopause

After hysterectomy and *bilateral oophorectomy* (removal of both ovaries) or radiation therapy for cancer, an artificial or surgical menopause occurs. If only the uterus is removed, the client will have no menstrual flow; however, normal hormonal cycles will continue. A young client who has had both ovaries and the uterus removed will often be maintained on estrogen therapy.

> **Key Concept**
> The premenopausal client who experiences surgical menopause may have more difficulties than the older client who undergoes a normal menopause. The younger the client is, the more likely they are to have difficulties with surgical menopause without estrogen replacement therapy.

STRUCTURAL DISORDERS

Vaginal Fistula

A *fistula* is an opening between two organs that normally do not open into each other. It results from an ulcerating process, such as cancer or irritation, or from a childbirth injury. A fistula may develop between the ureter and vagina (*ureterovaginal*), bladder and vagina (*vesicovaginal*), or vagina and rectum (*rectovaginal*).

Any fistula is troublesome. If it is ureterovaginal or vesicovaginal, urine will leak into the vagina. If it is rectovaginal, it will cause fecal incontinence. A long-standing fistula is difficult to repair successfully because the tissues are eroded. Infection can become an additional problem.

In many cases, particularly in young women, an attempt is made to repair the fistula surgically. A successful repair is difficult because of the associated problems. The incision must granulate from the inside out to prevent an abscess. The closeness of the urinary tract to the bowel makes infection a common postoperative complication. Repaired fistulas tend to recur because of continued irritation.

Make efforts to assist the healing process by building up the client's resistance and by keeping them as clean as possible, without perineal irritation. The client with a fistula that cannot be repaired is distressed by the odor and constant drainage. Sitz baths and deodorizing douches help maintain cleanliness.

Cystocele

Cystocele is the downward displacement of the bladder toward the vaginal orifice. It is most often seen in women who have experienced frequent deliveries or deliveries close together. Sometimes it results from injuries during childbirth.

Cystocele can cause nagging discomforts—pelvic pain, backache, fatigue, and a sagging pelvic weight. The client may experience stress incontinence or dribbling of urine on coughing, straining, sneezing, or laughing. They may also have urinary urgency and frequency and residual urine.

If the condition is not advanced, perineal exercises, for example, *Kegel exercises*, may be prescribed to strengthen the muscles (In Practice: Educating the Client 91-3). Surgery may be necessary, whereby the anterior vaginal wall is repaired (*anterior colporrhaphy* or *anterior repair*) and the bladder is returned to and secured in its normal position.

Rectocele

Rectocele is the upward displacement of the rectum toward the vaginal orifice. Rectocele is most often the result of injuries during childbirth. The client with rectocele will experience backache, fatigue, heaviness in the pelvic region, and bowel difficulties. They will have incontinence, flatus, and alternating constipation and diarrhea. Surgical repair of the posterior vaginal wall, with a return of the rectum to its normal position, is known as *posterior colporrhaphy* or *posterior repair*, and it is often very painful. The client who has had repair of a cystocele *and* a rectocele is said to have had an anteroposterior (**AP**) repair.

Another procedure sometimes performed is called the *Marshall-Marchetti*. In this surgery, the urethra is supported by sutures through the anterior wall of the vagina on either side of the urethra. The sutures are then passed through the outer covering layer (*periosteum*) of the pubic bone and secured.

Nursing Considerations

Before an AP repair or other gynecologic procedure, the client may receive an enema and have a catheter inserted,

> **IN PRACTICE**
> **EDUCATING THE CLIENT 91-3** **Kegel Exercises**
>
> - Locate the muscles surrounding the vagina by sitting on the toilet and starting and stopping the flow of urine.
> - Test the baseline strength of the muscles by inserting a finger in the opening of the vagina and contracting the muscles.
> - Exercise A: Squeeze the muscles together and hold the squeeze for 3 s. Relax the muscles. Repeat.
> - Exercise B: Contract and relax the muscles as rapidly as possible 10–25 times. Repeat.
> - Exercise C: Imagine sitting in a pan of water and sucking water into the vagina. Hold for 3 s.
> - Exercise D: Push out as during a bowel movement, only with the vagina. Hold for 3 s.
> - Repeat exercises A, C, and D 10 times each and exercise B once. Repeat the entire series three times a day.
>
> Regular practice of Kegel exercises can restore muscle tone. Benefits include control of stress incontinence, increased vaginal lubrication during sexual arousal, relief of constipation, increased flexibility of episiotomy scars, and stronger gripping of the base of the penis during intercourse.

unless a suprapubic cystocath will be used. For the anterior colporrhaphy, the catheter is left in place for several days, and a residual urine volume test or culture may be ordered when the catheter is removed. Showers and sitz baths promote comfort and healing. Instruct the client to avoid lifting, sexual intercourse, and prolonged sitting and standing until full healing has occurred (usually 6–8 weeks).

Prolapsed Uterus

A **prolapsed** uterus is one that sags or herniates into the vagina or, in severe cases, even falls outside the vagina. The most common cause is damage during childbirth. A prolapsed uterus is most frequently seen in menopausal women or women nearing menopause. The client is examined while standing or bearing down. The prolapse is classified as *first degree* (the cervix can be seen when labia are spread, without straining or traction); *second degree* (the cervix protrudes out to the level of the perineum); or *third degree* (also called *procidentia*; the entire uterus or most of it protrudes out the vagina onto the perineum).

The client with a prolapsed uterus complains of nagging backache, constipation, and stress incontinence. They may feel pain with intercourse (**dyspareunia**). Underwear rubbing may irritate the cervix. A hysterectomy may be performed to eliminate a severe prolapse. Some surgeons prefer to resuspend the uterus back into its normal position, particularly for younger women.

If surgery is contraindicated because the client is an older adult or in poor physical condition, one of the several types of pessaries (*pessary*—a ring-shaped device) may be needed. It is inserted snugly, similarly to a diaphragm, against the cervix and prevents the uterus from moving downward. The client may feel some discomfort when the pessary presses on the vaginal muscles because it is larger and firmer than a diaphragm. Teach the client how to insert and remove the pessary, and to clean it with warm, soapy water at least once a week. Most pessaries also must be removed for comfortable sexual intercourse and sometimes for bowel movements.

Abnormal Flexion of the Uterus

A displaced uterus is usually congenital, but it may result from childbearing. Forward displacement can be termed *anteversion* or *anteflexion*. Backward displacement can be termed *retroversion* or *retroflexion* (Fig. 91-3).

A displaced uterus may cause backache, dysmenorrhea, or sterility. Surgery can correct uterine displacement. With surgery, the uterus is sutured in its proper position.

INFLAMMATORY DISORDERS

Vulvitis

Vulvitis, inflammation of the vulva, may result from trauma caused by scratching, improper cleansing, birth control pills, or irritating vaginal discharge. Most often, its cause is some type of infection. Common signs and symptoms include severe itching and burning; pain during urination, defecation, or intercourse and swelling and redness. The goal of treatment is to determine and eliminate the cause.

Vaginitis

Vaginitis is inflammation of the vagina. Normally, vaginal secretions protect against infection. However, two organisms often cause vaginal infection: *Trichomonas vaginalis* or trichomoniasis and *Candida albicans* or candidiasis (formerly known as *monilia;* commonly known as *yeast infection*). Trichomoniasis, which is caused by protozoa, is likely to be transmitted sexually, whereas candidiasis, which is caused by fungus, is more easily spread in other ways. However, both are considered STIs. Many STIs cause inflammation (Chapter 70).

The most prominent symptom of vaginitis is a whitish vaginal discharge called **leukorrhea**. The discharge is odorous and profuse (more so in trichomoniasis), causing burning and itching in the perineum, vagina, and urethral area. In trichomoniasis the discharge is foul smelling and greenish-yellow or gray. With candidiasis, the discharge is white and like cottage cheese. The sexual partner must be treated at the same time so that the infection will not be spread back and forth (In Practice: Important Medications 91-2). Circumcision of the male may be necessary to help control a recurring infection.

Vaginitis can be difficult to cure. It can be extremely irritating and persist for a long time. Recurrence is fairly common. Early and persistent treatment is the only way to prevent this disorder from becoming chronic. The client may find that wearing sanitary napkins is necessary to absorb the profuse drainage. Frequent napkin replacement, perineal care, and sitz baths will help prevent odor and irritation. Sometimes, mild antianxiety agents or analgesics lessen the effects of *pruritus* (itching).

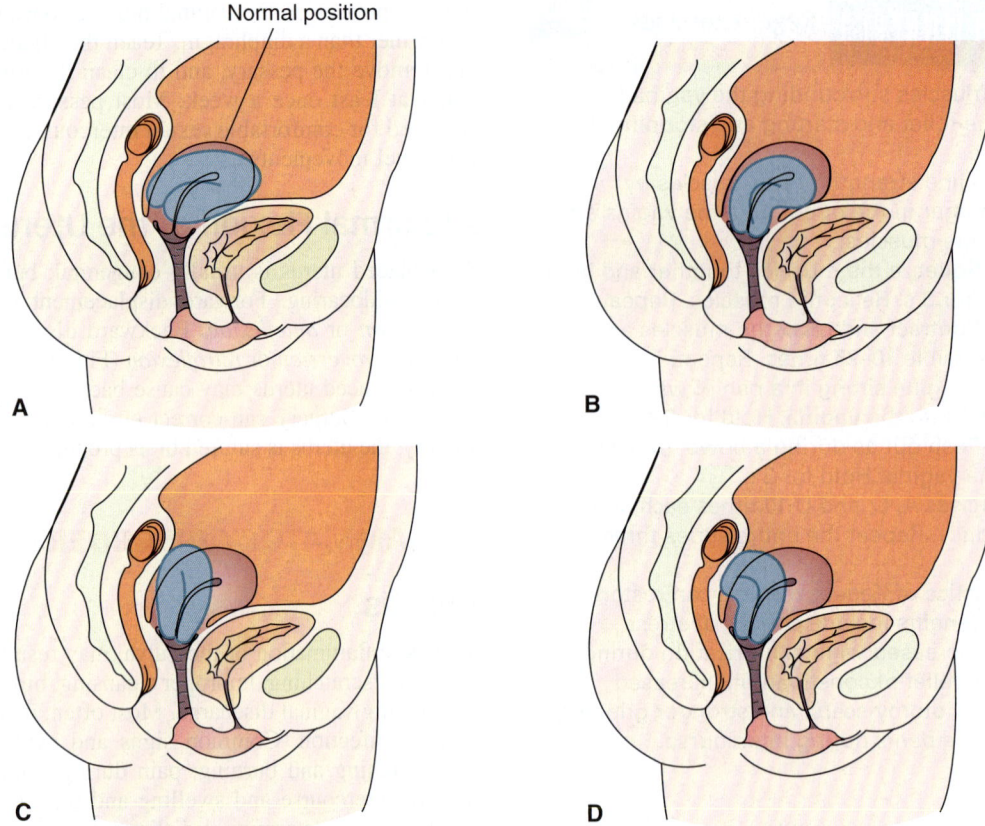

Figure 91-3 Variations in uterine position. **A.** Anteversion. **B.** Anteflexion. **C.** Retroversion. **D.** Retroflexion.

IN PRACTICE
IMPORTANT MEDICATIONS 91-2 — For Vaginal Infections

Trichomonas and Bacterial Vaginosis
- metronidazole (Flagyl)

Candidiasis
- nystatin (Mycostatin)
- miconazole nitrate (Micatin)

 Nursing Alert If a pregnant client contracts trichomoniasis, treatment is necessary, although it can be postponed until the second or third trimester because of the unknown effects of the drug on the developing fetus. Untreated trichomoniasis can lead to a fragile cervix that will be unable to maintain pregnancy or withstand delivery.

Nursing Considerations

Frequent bathing provides temporary relief from irritation and itching. Over-the-counter medications, such as nystatin and miconazole nitrate, are available. These medications are supplied in various systems of delivery, including creams with several different types of applicators, tablets that dissolve inside the body, and suppositories. A combination pack containing suppositories and cream is available to treat internal and external symptoms.

Teaching is particularly important because many women will treat their own infections at home and may not see a healthcare provider. Instructions are basically the same in all treatment systems (In Practice: Educating the Client 91-4).

IN PRACTICE
EDUCATING THE CLIENT 91-4 — Self-Care With a Yeast Infection

- Read and follow the instructions on the medication package carefully.
- Insert the full dosage of medication.
- Use cream during the day to control external itching.
- Use the treatment for specified consecutive days.
- Do not skip treatment during menses.
- Refrain from sexual intercourse during treatment and for at least 3 days after treatment is completed.
- Remember that a condom or diaphragm used during treatment will not be effective to prevent pregnancy because the medication weakens latex.
- Use only unscented sanitary napkins during treatment.
- Do not use tampons during treatment because they absorb some medication, reducing the dosage, and can be irritating.

Clients who are self-treating a vaginal infection should consult their primary care provider when there is

- No sign of improvement after 3 days of treatment
- Worsening of symptoms within 3 days
- No relief of symptoms after 7 days of treatment
- Return of symptoms within 2 months

The latter cases indicate the presence of an infection or condition other than candidiasis.

Atrophic Vaginitis

Atrophic vaginitis often occurs in postmenopausal clients. It is caused by atrophy of the vaginal mucous membranes and decreased mucus and other vaginal secretions, resulting from lowered estrogen production.

Atrophic vaginitis is treated by using a water-soluble lubricant, for example, K-Y jelly, during intercourse. An estrogen-based cream may also be helpful.

CERVICITIS

Several organisms cause **cervicitis** (inflammation of the cervix), notably *Staphylococcus*, *Streptococcus*, and *Gonococcus*. Cervicitis is often diagnosed after childbirth because of trauma to, and sometimes tearing of, the cervix. It also can be related to frequent douching, STIs, or a forgotten tampon. Cervicitis may also result from continued use of contraceptive foams or jellies. The main symptoms are leukorrhea and bleeding. Pain on sexual intercourse may also occur.

Unless cervicitis is treated promptly, it may be difficult to cure. Periodic vaginal examinations help in diagnosis. Antibiotics are the mainstay of treatment. Sometimes the cervix must be cauterized. After cauterization, a watery discharge appears, which may become foul smelling. It takes about 6–8 weeks for the area to heal after cauterization. Some precautions taken to prevent vaginal infection also help prevent cervical infection.

Endometriosis

Endometriosis is a painful disorder in which the tissues that line the uterus, known as the endometrium, travel to areas outside of the uterus. Normally, endometrial tissue is the layer that regularly detaches and flows from the uterus into the vagina as a routine part of the menstrual cycle. With endometriosis, the cells of endometrial tissue become transplanted in areas outside of the uterus, for example, the abdomen. Implanted endometrial tissue also acts as normal endometrial tissue within the uterus, that is, it thickens, breaks down, and bleeds with each menstrual cycle. Unlike the uterus, which has the cervix as an exit portal, displaced endometrial tissue cannot exit the body and it becomes trapped inside the abdomen. Areas that are most commonly affected include the ovaries and the bowel. Endometrial tissue can spread beyond the lower pelvic region into the *peritoneum*, a membrane that lines the walls of the abdominal and pelvic regions. The membrane surrounds the peritoneal cavity, which contains the internal organs of the abdomen such as the intestines and reproductive organs. The location of the organs affects the transit and transplant of the endometrial tissues, which causes varying levels of pain and general discomfort to a client. Cysts called *endometriomas* may form when endometriosis involves the ovaries. Over time, the cysts cause the surrounding tissue to become irritated. As part of the inflammatory process, scar tissue, also known as *adhesions*, develops. Adhesions and the endometriosis cause pain ranging from moderate to quite severe, especially during a menses. Fertility and reproduction are problematic; these subjects are discussed in Chapter 70. Endometriosis tends to develop several years after the onset of menarche (menstruation).

The cause of endometriosis is related to the mechanism of transit of endometrial cells from their original source, the interior of the uterus, to another source, back into the fallopian tubes and ovaries. *Retrograde menstruation* is the most likely cause, in which displaced cells stick to pelvic walls and tissues, where they act as typical endometrial cells. The mechanism of retrograde menstruation involves menstrual blood, which contains endometrial cells that flow backward into the fallopian tubes (retrograde) in lieu of flowing down into the vagina via the uterus. Other ways that endometrial cells develop into endometriosis are by embryonic cell growth, transport of endometrial cells by the lymphatic system, and hysterectomy or C-section surgeries. Risk factors include never giving birth, familial history of endometriosis, pelvic infections and inflammatory problems, and uterine abnormalities.

Signs and Symptoms

Signs and symptoms of endometriosis are pelvic pain that worsens with the menstrual period. Pain tends to increase over time, as the endometrial tissue spreads. The severity of pain may not be a reliable indicator of the amount of tissue that has been transplanted. Mild endometriosis may have severe pain, while moderate to severe pain may be associated with advanced disease. Relief of pain occurs with pregnancy, after menopause, and during estrogen therapy. General symptoms that are most noticeable during menses include fatigue, diarrhea, constipation, bloating, and nausea. *Dyspareunia*, pain during or after sex, differs from *dysmenorrhea*, cramping and pelvic pains of a typical period, but both may occur with endometriosis. Symptoms of menses commonly are associated with some degree of discomfort or pain; the pain of endometriosis typically is more severe. It begins earlier in a client's cycle and ends several days after the end of a period. Sometimes, endometriosis includes the abdomen and lower back areas. Additionally, endometriosis involves pain with defecation and urination, especially during a period. *Menorrhagia*, heavy periods, and *menometrorrhagia*, excessive or heavy bleeding between periods, are seen with endometriosis. Sometimes the first diagnosis is made because the client is seeking assistance for infertility. For more information on women's reproductive issues, refer to Chapter 70.

Treatment

Treatment is directed toward symptomatic relief starting with over-the-counter pain medications, heat to the abdomen, and rest. If the client desires children, healthcare providers may recommend pregnancy as a type of treatment for two reasons. First, endometriosis may eventually result in sterility, and second, because endometriosis is influenced by hormonal changes, symptoms often improve during and after pregnancy. Supplemental hormones may reduce or eliminate the pain of endometriosis because hormones may slow growth and prevent new tissue transplantation. Hormonal contraceptives, as supplemental hormones, can be given as birth control pills, patches, and vaginal rings. Another approach is to lower estrogen levels and prevent menstruation, which can be done by administration of drugs containing gonadotropin-releasing hormone (*Gn-RH*), such as leuprorelin (Lupron). Gn-RHs can force endometriosis into remission, which, in effect, creates an artificial menopause. Therefore, Gn-RH drugs may be given with low-dose estrogen or progestin, which decrease menopausal side effects. Menarche and the ability to get pregnant will return if the Gn-RN is stopped. Two other medical treatments are available: medroxyprogesterone (Depo-Provera) and danazol (Danocrine). Medroxyprogesterone (Depo-Provera) is injected and will stop menses, eliminate future growth of endometrial implants, and relieve signs and symptoms of endometriosis during the time that the client is taking the drug. (See birth control methods in Chapter 70.) Danazol (Danocrine) is a drug that suppresses the growth of the endometrium by blocking ovarian-stimulating hormones, which will also prevent menses and symptoms of endometriosis. However, it is important that the client know and understand that *danazol (Danocrine) can cause serious side effects and can be harmful to a fetus*, if the client becomes pregnant while taking this drug.

If pregnancy is undesirable, medications may shrink the endometrial tissue, thereby decreasing the symptoms (In Practice: Important Medications 91-3). Sometimes, endometriosis recurs when medication is stopped. Extensive and chronic endometriosis may require drastic surgical treatment, such as hysterectomy, *salpingectomy* (removal of oviducts), and oophorectomy. A client experiencing endometriosis will require a great deal of emotional support.

Pelvic Inflammatory Disease

Pelvic inflammatory disease is an infection of the ovaries (*oophoritis*), oviducts (*salpingitis*), uterus, or pelvic cavity. The most common causes of PID are two forms of STIs: *Chlamydia trachomatis* (chlamydia) and *Neisseria gonorrhoeae* (gonorrhea). Many other STIs and the bacterial strain of *Streptococcus* may also cause PID. The microorganisms most often pass up through the reproductive tract, entering the body through the vagina, peritoneum, lymphatic system, or bloodstream (Fig. 91-4). PID may develop following unprotected sex, a therapeutic or spontaneous abortion, the insertion of an IUD, childbirth, douching, or inadequate hygiene during menstruation, especially when tampons or pads are not applied hygienically or are used for time periods that are too lengthy. Regular douching upsets the balance of normal and abnormal bacteria within the vagina and can lead to infections that are hidden or masked.

The client who has multiple partners or is in a relationship with a partner who has more than one partner, does not use a condom, or has a past history of a PID or STI has a higher risk of developing STIs and PID. (Refer to Chapter 70 for additional information on STIs.)

Signs and Symptoms

Symptoms may be vague, mild, or severe, or the client can be completely asymptomatic. The client with mild symptoms or with no noticeable symptoms is most likely infected with chlamydia. Commonly, initially noticed symptoms include a foul-smelling vaginal discharge. The client also complains of backache, abdominal or pelvic pain, fever, chills, malaise, nausea, and vomiting. Painful urination, painful intercourse, and irregular menstrual bleeding may be noticed. The client may have a heavy vaginal discharge with an unpleasant odor. The healthcare provider should be seen if the client has signs of shock, such as vomiting, severe pain low in the abdomen, fainting, or a high fever (>101 °F or 38.3 °C). They may be developing sepsis, a life-threatening complication. Long-term consequences of PID are due to untreated

IN PRACTICE
IMPORTANT MEDICATIONS 91-3 For Endometriosis

- Combination (estrogen–progestin) oral contraceptives
- Progestins
- Synthetic estrogen, danazol (oral Danocrine)
- Gonadotropin-releasing hormone agonists (cause lowered estrogen levels):
  - leuprolide (Lupron)
  - nafarelin acetate (Synarel)

Note: Medications used to treat endometriosis can cause any or all of the following side effects: abdominal swelling, breast tenderness, breakthrough bleeding, atrophic vaginitis, weight gain, edema, hot flashes, and emotional lability.

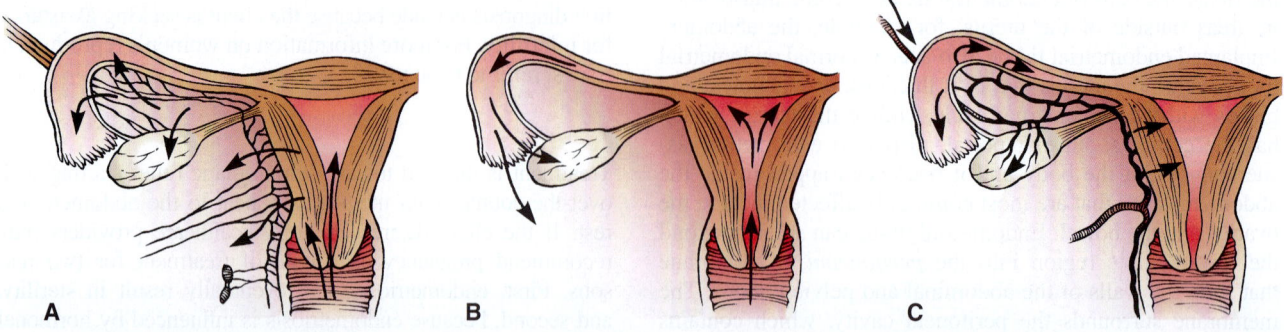

Figure 91-4 Pathways by which microorganisms enter the pelvis. **A.** Bacteria enter through the vagina into the uterus and through the lymph system. **B.** Gonorrhea spreads from the vagina into the uterus and into the tubes and ovaries. **C.** Bacterial infection may enter the reproductive organs through the bloodstream.

infection, the development of abscesses, and scar tissue in the fallopian tubes, plus damage to the reproductive organs. Complications include chronic pelvic pain, infertility, ectopic pregnancies, abscess formation, sepsis, and death. The reproductive tract, especially the fallopian tubes, can be permanently scarred, leading to chronic PID infections and permanent infertility.

Diagnosis

Diagnosis of PID is based on the results of a pelvic examination, and cultures and sensitivities of vaginal or cervical discharge and a urinalysis. Imaging studies may include an ultrasound or CT scan. A laparoscopy may be done to visualize the pelvic organs. The healthcare provider may remove a sample of the uterine lining, the endometrium, to obtain tissue for examination.

Treatment

Treatment includes combinations of clinical observations and antibiotics. PID can be caused by more than one organism; thus, combination antibiotic therapy is common. PID caused by the herpes virus is not affected by antibiotics. The sexual partner is also examined and treated, if necessary. Sexual intercourse is discouraged as long as the client has any trace of infection. The longer the time that PID is not treated, the greater the likelihood of chronic pain and sterility because of the increasing formation of scar tissue that blocks the oviducts. Pelvic ultrasound or a laparoscopy may be used to confirm diagnosis. No laboratory test can specifically identify PID, but a white blood count is typically elevated in acute infections. Serum pregnancy testing may be ordered (which will not differentiate between normal or ectopic pregnancies).

> **Nursing Alert** A client who has had PID is more likely to have an ectopic pregnancy (a fertilized egg that implants in the fallopian tubes rather than the uterus). An ectopic pregnancy is likely to cause rupture of the fallopian tubes, which results in life-threatening hemorrhage. Treatment of sudden, spontaneous abdominal pain in a reproductive-aged client is an emergency.

Nursing Considerations

Antibiotics and pain relief are important nursing concerns. The client hospitalized with PID is commonly placed in the Fowler position. *Rationale: This position helps encourage pelvic drainage and relief of abdominal pain.* Mild heat to the abdomen or sitz baths may be ordered. *Rationale: They help relieve pain and promote drainage.* Follow Standard Precautions with the disposal of soiled pads and dressings. The healthcare provider may order perineal care for the client after removing the pad and after the client uses the bedpan. Sometimes, an abdominal or perineal abscess forms, and the surgeon institutes drainage through an incision.

During the active disease process, the client should avoid douches and sexual intercourse. Prevention of PID is by sexual abstinence or having a long-term monogamous relationship with an uninfected partner. Correct and consistent use of male latex condoms reduces the transmission of chlamydia and gonorrhea. Teaching and the cooperation of the sexual partner are vital in the treatment of PID.

Vulvodynia

Vulvodynia is chronic vulvar pain. The vulva (or pudendum) consists of the external genitals, including the labia majora, labia minora, clitoris, the Bartholin glands, the vaginal opening, and the vestibule of the vagina. The pain is unexplainable by any known vulvar or vaginal disorder or infection (e.g., PID or STIs). Specific etiology is unknown, but the condition may occur in women who have had chronic moniliasis or who have been on long-term antibiotic therapy. Other factors may include nerve injury or irritation, muscle spasms, allergies, frequent sexual intercourse, oxalates in the urine, or hormonal changes. It can occur in women of any age and of any ethnic background.

Signs and Symptoms

Symptoms typically begin suddenly and they include burning (most universal), aching, itching, stinging, irritation, or sharp or severe pain when the vulva area is touched, or in the presence of pressure, such as attempted sexual intercourse, sitting, bike riding, or when tampons are inserted. Vulvodynia lasts at least 3 months and can last for years. The pain can be constant, intermittent, or happen only when the vulva is touched. On examination, the healthcare provider may find localized erythema and swelling of the vestibule. The emotional impact can be overwhelming because the disorder can severely impair sexual relationships, social interactions, exercise, and employment.

Treatment

Treatment should include a thorough physical examination and emotional history by a healthcare provider who is experienced in women's healthcare issues. Medications that are most helpful tend to have anti-inflammatory effects, such as NSAIDs. Local application of lidocaine creams may be helpful. Because of the intense impact the disorder has on everyday life, the client may need to be treated for depression. Additionally, biofeedback and relaxation techniques can reduce the client's feeling that things are "out of control." At home, the client needs to avoid using products that contain chemical irritants, such as scented toilet paper, body soaps, hot tubs, or detergents and fabric softeners. Underwear should be 100% cotton. The client should be taught to cleanse the vulva area with cool water after sex and after urinating, and to avoid activities that put direct pressure on the painful areas (e.g., use pressure-reducing pillows, lie on their side, or lie prone whenever possible). A cool or tepid water sitz bath can be helpful, as can either cool packs or warm packs applied to the affected area. Over-the-counter lubricants used daily or before sex may provide relief, but some types can contribute to yeast infections. Combinations of treatments tend to have the best results.

Nursing Considerations

The nurse needs to use active listening communication techniques. The client may have the feeling that there is nothing that can be done or that the pain is psychosomatic in origin. The nurse can help the client review home-based treatments suggested above because the use of many commercial products (e.g., scented tissues or bubble baths) has become so habitual that the consequences of their use are not at all considered. Numerous self-help aids are found in In Practice: Educating the Client 91-1 and 91-4.

NEOPLASMS

Tumors of the Ovary

Benign Ovarian Tumors

Also known as *cysts*, these benign growths may form from fluid retained in the ovary or from other causes. Although they usually do not cause any trouble, cysts may enlarge and press on other abdominal organs and cause pain if they rupture or twist.

Malignant Ovarian Tumors

Women who have a personal or family history of cancer have a higher than average chance of developing ovarian cancer. Cancers that seem the most predictive of ovarian cancer include those of the breast, uterus, colon, and ovary. If a client has had a tubal ligation, their chances of ovarian cancer seem to decrease to one third the risk of other women. Some researchers believe this is because carcinogens travel up the oviducts to the ovaries.

Vaginal ultrasound and the CA125 blood test can make the diagnosis. Cancer of the ovary often displays no early symptoms and usually is detected only after metastasis has occurred. Ovarian cancer is a fairly frequent cause of death in young women because it is often not discovered in time to provide a long-term cure.

Cancer of the ovary is treated surgically. The procedure involves a total abdominal hysterectomy and removal of both tubes and both ovaries. Hormones are not given because they seem to nourish this particular type of cancer cell. Radiation therapy and chemotherapy are usually prescribed after the surgery.

Table 91-1 provides an overview of the major cancers of the reproductive system.

Tumors of the Uterus

Benign Uterine Tumors

The *fibroid tumor* is the most common type of benign uterine tumor. Fibroid tumors range in size, usually growing slowly

TABLE 91-1 Cancers of the Reproductive System

	WARNING SIGNS	RISK FACTORS	EARLY DETECTION	TREATMENT (DEPENDENT ON INVOLVEMENT)
Breast cancer	Breast changes: Lump, pain, thickening, swelling, tenderness, distortion, retraction, dimpling, scaliness	Age older than 40 years (risk increases with age), history of breast cancer, early menarche, nulliparity, first birth at late age	Mammograms Monthly self-examination; clinical breast examinations	Lumpectomy, mastectomy, radiation therapy, chemotherapy, hormone manipulation therapy
Cervical cancer	Often asymptomatic; symptoms, if present, can include irregular bleeding or abnormal vaginal discharge	Intercourse at an early age, multiple sex partners, cigarette smoking, history of certain sexually transmitted infections, such as human papillomavirus	Annual Pap test for women older than 18 years or who are sexually active; after three consecutive normal tests, Pap tests may be done less often at the healthcare provider's discretion	Carcinoma in situ: Cryotherapy, electrocoagulation, local excision Metastatic cancer: Surgery or radiation therapy or both
Endometrial cancer	Irregular bleeding outside of menses, unusual vaginal discharge, excessive bleeding during menstruation, postmenopausal bleeding	Obesity, early menarche, multiple sex partners, late menopause, history of infertility, anovulation (not ovulating), unopposed estrogen or tamoxifen therapy, family history of endometrial cancer	Endometrial biopsy at menopause (for high-risk women)	Precancerous changes: Progesterone therapy Diagnosed cancer: Surgery or radiation therapy or both
Ovarian cancer	Often asymptomatic; symptoms, if present, can include abdominal enlargement, vague digestive disorders, discomfort, gas distention	Risk increases with age (especially after age 60 years), nulliparity, history of breast cancer	Periodic, complete pelvic examination; cancer-related checkup every year after age 40 years	Surgery, including oophorectomy (excision of an ovary), hysterosalpingo-oophorectomy, salpingo-oophorectomy, excision of all intra-abdominal disease; radiation therapy; chemotherapy

Adapted from www.cdc.gov

and arising from muscle cells. They are believed to result from hormonal influences. The first symptom is abnormal vaginal bleeding, associated with a feeling of heaviness and pressure in the pelvic region. A fibroid tumor, or *myoma*, may become so large that it presses on the urethra or bowel, causing urinary retention or constipation.

Treatment

Treatment for fibroids depends somewhat on the client's age. Often it is possible to remove a nonmalignant tumor from the uterus without removing the uterus itself, an especially important consideration for a client of childbearing years. Other treatments include medroxyprogesterone (Depo-Provera) injections or oral contraceptives to suppress the uterine lining, thus shrinking the tumors. Leuprolide (Lupron) injection therapy is showing promise in shrinking fibroids as well.

> **Key Concept**
> Most nonmalignant tumors shrink after menopause; thus, postmenopausal bleeding is seldom caused by a myoma.

Cancer of the Fundus or Endometrium

The *fundus*, which is the body of uterus, is not attacked as frequently by cancer as the cervix. However, malignant growths do occur in the endometrium and fundus. Cancers of the fundus and the endometrium are most likely to occur in postmenopausal women. Women who have previously taken estrogens also are at an increased risk. Therefore, hormone therapy is prescribed with caution.

Vaginal bleeding is the first sign of uterine cancer, possibly beginning as a watery, blood-tinged discharge. If it occurs before menopause, it may be mistaken for menstrual irregularity. A diagnostic curettage to obtain uterine scrapings is performed if the Pap test suggests cancer. If the results of the tests of the scrapings are positive, a hysterectomy is performed, followed by radium implantation, x-ray therapy, or both, to the pelvic cavity. This client may have postoperative chemotherapy, but usually not hormone therapy.

Cancer of the Cervix

Of the cancers affecting the reproductive system, cancer of the cervix is common, being surpassed only by breast cancer. Cervical cancer occurs most commonly in women between the ages of 40 and 55 years. Box 91-1 lists factors that place women at a higher risk of developing cervical cancer.

Signs and Symptoms

Bleeding is the first sign of cervical cancer, but it does not occur in the early stages, when a positive Pap test would indicate the presence of cancer cells. The bleeding usually appears first as spotting between periods or after intercourse. Gynecologists should follow up carefully with women at risk. These clients should have frequent Pap tests. The condition also can occur after menopause.

Staging of Cervical Cancer

Cervical cancer can be staged differently depending on the professional agency providing the information. (Staging is

> **Box 91-1 Risk Factors for Developing Cervical Cancer**
>
> - Infection with human papillomavirus (HPV)
> - Sexual activity at a young age
> - Frequent sexual activity
> - Multiple sex partners
> - Presence of genital warts (condyloma)
> - Presence of herpes virus II
> - Maternal history of cancer, especially cervical cancer
> - Maternal use of diethylstilbestrol (DES) during pregnancy with this daughter (especially if mother had toxicity to DES)

defined and discussed in Chapter 83.) Pap tests are identified differently, but are commonly used as preliminary guides to identify cervical cancer. This cancer is commonly staged similarly to many other types of cancer, which will help to standardize treatments that depend on location and extent of spread of the cancerous growth:

- Stage 0: Carcinoma in situ (cancer limited to the epithelial layer with no signs of invasion of deeper tissue or of surrounding area)
- Stage I: Cancer is confined to cervix
- Stage II: Cancer extends beyond the cervix, but not into the pelvic wall, or involves vagina but not the lower one third
- Stage III: Cancer extends to the pelvic wall and involves lower one third of the vagina
- Stage IV: Cancer is widely spread throughout the pelvic region or throughout the body.

Treatment

Early cervical cancer (in situ and some types of stage I) is susceptible to radiation therapy (usually radon implantation). In addition, early cervical cancer is more easily localized and, therefore, more easily excised. In these early states, conization with cryosurgery or laser surgery is frequently used. If conization is performed, Pap tests should be done every 3 months for the first year and every 6 months after that time. These procedures may be done on an outpatient basis in selected cases. Hysterectomy may also be done for early cervical cancer if the client does not wish to remain capable of childbearing.

In the early and middle stages, conization or hysterectomy may be done. In the middle stages, hysterectomy is the treatment of choice. Many of these surgical procedures are combined with radiation or chemotherapy, particularly in stages other than cancer in situ.

Cervical Cancer in the Pregnant Client

If a client is pregnant and cervical cancer in situ is discovered, treatment is delayed until after delivery, which may be allowed to occur vaginally. If invasive cancer is discovered early in the pregnancy, the pregnancy is terminated, and the cancer is treated as in the nonpregnant client. If invasive cancer is discovered late in pregnancy (third trimester), treatment is delayed until the fetus is viable, and cesarean delivery is done.

> **Nursing Alert** The importance of the Pap test for clients past puberty, particularly sexually active clients, cannot be overstated. Cervical cancer is almost 100% curable if it is discovered early and treated before it spreads.

Caring for the Client Undergoing a Hysterectomy

Hysterectomy is a term that describes the removal of portions or all of the reproductive system. The type of hysterectomy depends on which organs are affected and the goal of surgery. If the entire uterus, including the cervix, is removed, it is called a *total hysterectomy (panhysterectomy)*. Today, the cervix is rarely left in place. However, if it is, and the body and fundus of the uterus are removed, it is called a *subtotal hysterectomy*. Removal of the attached oviducts as well is called a *salpingectomy;* the total procedure is called a *panhysterosalpingectomy*. Removal of both ovaries combined with total removal of the uterus and both oviducts is known as a *panhysterosalpingo-oophorectomy*. If one ovary is removed, the operation is a *unilateral oophorectomy;* if both are removed, it is *bilateral*.

If cancer has metastasized to the entire abdomen, radiation therapy with or without chemotherapy may be used palliatively, and surgery may be unnecessary. In some cases, however, radical surgery is performed.

Preoperative Considerations

In addition to the usual preparation for abdominal or perineal surgery, the client may have a vaginal irrigation or douche. They will most likely have at least one enema to cleanse the colon of feces. The client must receive instruction in the administration of the enema and other procedures to be done the evening before surgery. They will be allowed nothing by mouth (NPO) after midnight. This client will probably come into the healthcare facility on the morning of the surgery.

A Foley catheter is often inserted in the client surgical preparation room to lessen the danger of bladder perforation during removal of the uterus. The Foley catheter is usually removed on the first postoperative day and is not replaced unless the client is unable to void. If the bladder is also repaired, the surgeon may insert a suprapubic cystocath during surgery to drain urine and rest the bladder. Antiembolism stockings are usually applied to the legs to prevent thrombophlebitis.

Be sure to answer all the client's questions fully. Include the client's husband or partner in teaching. A hospital chaplain or the client's spiritual leader can be a source of needed support and reassurance. Be sure to document all teaching.

Postoperative Nursing Considerations

Plan nursing care according to the type of hysterectomy performed. Provide the same postoperative care for the client who has had an abdominal hysterectomy as for any person who has had an abdominal incision. The client recovers more quickly from the vaginal procedure than from the abdominal procedure.

Give routine postoperative care to prevent complications. Antiembolism stockings may be ordered; they need to be removed and reapplied at least every 8 hr. Encourage early ambulation. The client often has a urethral catheter in place. After it is removed, report any difficulty in voiding. If the client cannot void within 6–8 hr, the surgeon needs to be notified.

Perineal pads are worn after surgery. Teach the client to pull the underwear and pad straight down to avoid fecal contamination of the operative area. Check the amount, color, and odor of vaginal drainage. Some bloody drainage is normal. However, notify the surgeon of unusual bleeding. Give perineal care, if ordered. The use of the peri bottle can help to keep the perineum clean and the client more comfortable. Teach the client how to perform perineal self-care.

Vaginal packing may be inserted during surgery. This is usually removed on the first or second postoperative day. The client may complain of severe back pain while the pack is in place. Reassure the client that removal of the packing will relieve much of the pain.

Before discharge from the healthcare facility, inform the client of complications that might occur and when to notify the healthcare provider. Carefully document all teaching.

Breast Neoplasms

Most breast lesions are benign. Benign lesions tend to be round or oval with a smooth border and usually show no secondary signs. Furthermore, benign lesions are likely to be movable. Malignant lesions are more likely to be irregularly shaped and hard and often show secondary signs, such as enlarged lymph nodes in the axillary area, asymmetry of the breast, retraction of the nipple, bloody discharge, dimpling, or elevation of one breast. Additionally, malignant lesions are often attached to the surrounding skin, underlying structures, or breast tissue. Diagnosis, however, requires a laboratory analysis of tissue or biopsy study.

Benign Neoplasms
Chronic Cystic Mastitis

Cystic disease is the most common breast disorder in women between the ages of 30 and 50 years. It is believed to result from a hormonal imbalance and is related to the activity of the ovaries. Cyst formation decreases after menopause.

Breast tissue cells collect together and form a mass. This cell mass shuts off the ducts and forms cysts. These masses may form fibrous tumors (*fibromas*) or breast lumps. A biopsy may be performed to rule out cancer. Most lumps removed from the breast are benign. A cyst may be excised or drained without removal of any of the surrounding tissue. On rare occasions, particularly if the client is extremely anxious, the surgeon may perform a simple mastectomy, in which only the breast is removed as a preventive measure. Caffeine aggravates cyst formation. Women with a cystic condition are therefore advised to avoid coffee, tea, chocolate, and cola drinks. Encourage the client to perform BSEs. Researchers suggest that these women have a yearly mammogram or ultrasound or both.

Breast Cancer

Breast cancer is the cancer that forms in the cells of breast tissue. The cause of breast cancer is probably related to interactions of genes, lifestyle, and environmental factors, but no specific cause has been identified. Some women with

Box 91-2 Risk Factors for Developing Breast Cancer

The following characteristics are associated with an increased risk for developing breast cancer (*NOTE: Most women diagnosed have no family history of breast cancer and may have no known risk factors*):

- Being female—Breast cancer rarely occurs in men.
- Age—Risk increases with age.
- Personal history of breast cancer—The risk increases with previous occurrence of cancer in one breast or previous treatment for breast cancer.
- Family history of breast cancer; age younger than 40 years (female relatives such as a mother, sister, maternal grandmother, or maternal aunt). If a client has a familial history of breast cancer, the chances are increased if cancer occurs at an age younger than 40 years.
- Inherited genes—BRAC1 and BRAC2 are the most common genetic mutations that can greatly increase the risk of breast cancer and other cancers. However, the presence of these genes does not make the presence of cancer inevitable.
- Sedentary lifestyle
- Alcohol consumption
- Oral contraceptive use
- Long menstrual cycles
- Nulliparous—Has never had children
- Pregnant for the first time after age 35 years
- Menarche started before age 12 years
- Late menopause—Beginning menopause later in life
- Postmenopausal obesity
- Postmenopausal hormone therapy
- Radiation exposure—Radiation treatment for cancer that occurred as a child or young adult increases the risk factor of cancer in the older adult. Accidental exposure to massive radiation contamination, as in nuclear power plant disasters.

risk factors never develop breast cancer and some women with no risk factors do develop cancer. Some breast cancers are linked to inherited mutated genes. For example, *breast cancer gene 1* (**BRCA1**) and *breast cancer gene 2* (**BRCA2**) are the most commonly known genes that significantly increase the risk of both breast and ovarian cancer. Factors predisposing to breast cancer are presented in Box 91-2.

Many healthcare professionals recommend that each client examine their breasts, preferably every month, approximately 1 week following menses, to check for any lumps, nodules, or thickening. If the client is postmenopausal, they should examine their breasts on the same date each month. The key is to note any change from the previous month. Self-examination of the breasts is done in several steps using the flat of the fingers, rather than the fingertips. Keep in mind that breast cancer can occur in women with no known risk factors.

SPECIAL CONSIDERATIONS   Culture and Ethnicity

Breast cancer incidence is highest in white women, lower in black and Hispanic women, and lowest in American Indian and Alaskan Native women. Breast cancer rarely occurs in men.

Screening mammography is able to detect some breast cancers as long as 2 years before they can be identified through palpation or other signs and symptoms. A radiologist often works up such abnormalities in a diagnostic breast center. The workup might include specialized mammography (compression views, magnification views, cone down views), ultrasound, and stereotactic core needle biopsies. The goal of such diagnostic breast centers is to decrease the period of anxiety for a client with an abnormality by carrying out the entire workup within 24–48 hr.

Signs and Symptoms

Signs of breast cancer usually become more evident as cancer advances. Prompt action may mean the difference between life and death. Women are urged to consult a healthcare provider if they notice a lump, thickening, or any other change in the breast. Possible noticeable changes include nipple discharge (particularly bloody discharge), history of pain or tingling without a palpable mass, breast enlargement or thickening, nipple retraction, redness with swelling and heat, or puckering in any area of the breast. In Practice: Educating the Client 91-5 summarizes the warning signs and symptoms of breast cancer.

Diagnostic Tests

The healthcare provider will do a clinical breast examination, checking the breast and lymph nodes of the armpit. The most accurate device for diagnosis is the screening mammogram, which will often, but not always, show a mass or other abnormality. If a mass is found, a diagnostic mammogram may be done to assist with the diagnosis. In addition, a breast ultrasound may be done to help distinguish between a solid mass and a fluid-filled cyst. Breast ultrasonography may also help differentiate between malignant and nonmalignant lesions. Breast biopsy is the only diagnostic test for breast cancer. At the time of biopsy, tests are done on the tissue to help determine the appropriate type of treatment. In an outpatient setting, the healthcare provider may next require a biopsy of the breast cells, which are examined by a pathologist. The biopsy tissue can show the type of cells involved, the aggressiveness of the tumor, and the presence of receptors, including hormone receptors, which will influence treatment choices. An "MRI with contrast" may be ordered. The contrast is a dye that can help visualize the vasculature of a tumor.

Treatment

The healthcare provider's first concern in treating breast cancer is to remove the cancer from the breast. Local treatment includes surgery and radiation therapy. Most women have a choice in selecting local treatment. The *lumpectomy*, also known as *breast-sparing surgery*, or *partial mastectomy*, is used to remove smaller tumors and some of the surrounding healthy tissue. Radiation to the remaining breast tissue is as effective as *total mastectomy* (removal of the entire breast) in treating many breast cancers. The mastectomy removes all of the breast tissue, including the lobules, ducts, fatty tissue, some skin, and the nipple and areola. A mastectomy may be necessary if more than one tumor is in a breast or if the tumor is extremely large or fast growing. Occasionally the decision is to remove the cancerous breast and the healthy breast in the procedure called a *contralateral prophylactic*

IN PRACTICE

EDUCATING THE CLIENT 91-5: Warning Signs and Symptoms of Breast Cancer

- New lump, mass, or thickening that feels different or from surrounding tissue or armpit
- A change in size, shape, or symmetry of the breasts
- Painful hard mass with irregular-shaped edges
- Painless lump or mass
- Round, soft, tender lump
- Any lump or thickening that does not shrink or lessen after a period
- Swelling or thickening of all or part of a breast (even if no distinct lump is felt)
- Skin over the breast that is irritated, dimpling, or puckering
- Breast or nipple pain, scaliness, or thickening
- Peeling, scaling, or flaking of the areola (pigmented area around the nipple) or breast skin
- Nipple retraction, that is, turning or drawing inward or pointing in a new direction
- Nipple or breast skin with redness or pitting (like the skin of an orange)
- A liquid discharge that drains from a nipple (not including breast milk) which may be bloody or clear and sticky
- Sometimes breast cancer can spread to lymph nodes under the arm or around the collar bone and cause a lump or swelling there, even before the original tumor in the breast tissue is large enough to be felt.

Note: The client is encouraged to do breast self-examinations at home and follow-up with a healthcare provider who is experienced in diagnosing breast disease if signs or symptoms are noticed.

Adapted from https://www.breastcancer.org/symptoms/testing/types/self_exam; https://www.nationalbreastcancer.org/breast-self-exam; and https://www.mayoclinic.org/tests-procedures/breast-exam/about/pac-20393237

---

mastectomy. In these instances, the client tends to have a high risk of cancer due to genetic findings and a strong family history of breast cancer. Most women who develop cancer in one breast do not develop cancer in the other breast. A *skin-sparing mastectomy* is done if the location and size of the tumor are not cancerous. This surgery allows the skin over the breast to be left intact, which is beneficial for later reconstruction and cosmetic appearance.

A procedure called **sentinel node biopsy** removes a limited number of priority lymph nodes that are most likely to become cancerous. The objective of the procedure is to determine if the lymph nodes are cancerous. If these nodes are cancer free, then it is assumed that no cancer cells are in the other nodes either; thus, they are not removed. If cancer is found in the sentinel nodes, an axillary lymph node dissection is done, in which removal of several lymph nodes may be necessary, including into the armpit.

Once the initial diagnostic procedures are completed, the healthcare professionals will "stage" the cancer. Staging is a method of stating the extent of the cancer. Knowing the stage of the cancer will determine the treatment options. Complete staging information may not be available until after breast surgery.

Before surgery for a malignant lesion, the surgeon discusses the safety of the surgery or surgery/radiation option with the client and their partner. The recommended treatment mode includes consideration of the client's preferences (e.g., accessibility to a radiation center), cultural and personal beliefs about radiation, and the client's feelings about keeping their breast. Oncology clinical nurse specialists often assist clients in making surgical decisions by discussing options and helping clients clarify their personal preferences and values.

Another consideration in the care of the person with breast cancer is the identification, prevention, and treatment of systemic or metastatic disease. If the cancer has spread from the breast to another part of the body, the client is said to have *metastatic disease*. Metastatic disease requires systemic treatment, such as chemotherapy or hormonal therapy. Determining which clients should receive systemic treatment requires diagnostic skill and a knowledge of prognostic factors. The tumor's size and the presence of cancer cells in the lymph nodes under the arm are the two best predictors of metastatic disease. For this reason, many surgeons remove some lymph nodes at the time of surgery.

Removal of the lymph nodes is a diagnostic procedure, but it does have long-term complications. Women who have had the lymph nodes removed can develop a condition called *lymphedema*, in which lymphatic fluid accumulates in the tissues, leading to arm discomfort and disability. For this reason, removal of the lymph nodes is becoming a controversial practice in the oncology field. Many healthcare providers believe that lymph node dissection should be done only when the information gained from testing the nodes will influence treatment.

Most premenopausal women with invasive breast cancer are treated with chemotherapy, regardless of evidence of positive lymph nodes or metastases.

Chemotherapy regimens for breast cancer include the use of *combination therapy* (the simultaneous use of multiple drugs). Preparing the client for chemotherapy is important and is often done by the oncologist, clinical nurse specialist, or chemotherapy nurse. Ensuring that the client has access to expert preparation falls within the role of the nurse who is responsible for the client.

Hormone therapy is used in addition to chemotherapy, radiation, and surgery to treat breast cancers that are sensitive to the hormones estrogen and progesterone. The term *hormone therapy* is more accurately termed *hormone-blocking therapy* because the medications block hormones from attaching to cancer cells. The hormone-sensitive cancers can also be referred to as estrogen receptor positive (ER positive) and progesterone receptor positive (PR positive) cancers. Examples include *selective estrogen receptor modulator* (*SERM*) medications such as tamoxifen, raloxifene (Evista), and toremifene (Fareston). The goal of hormone therapy is to decrease the chances of the cancer returning or, if the cancer has already spread, the goal would be to shrink and control the cancer (In Practice: Important Medications 91-4). Side effects include hot flashes, night sweats, and

CHAPTER 91 Female Reproductive Disorders

IN PRACTICE
IMPORTANT MEDICATIONS 91-4 — For Breast Cancer Chemotherapy

Anthracyclines
- doxorubicin (Adriamycin)
- epirubicin (Ellence)

Taxanes
- paclitaxel (Taxol)
- docetaxel (Taxotere)
- trastuzumab (Herceptin)

HER2 (human growth factor receptor 2)
- trastuzumab (Herceptin)
- ado-trastuzumab (Kadcyla)
- pertuzumab (Perjeta)
- lapatinib (Tykerb)

SERM (selective estrogen receptor modulator)
- tamoxifen (Nolvadex)
- raloxifene (Evista)
- toremifene (Fareston)

Aromatase inhibitors
- anastrozole (Arimidex)
- letrozole (Femara)
- exemestane (Aromasin)

Destroy estrogen receptors
- fulvestrant (Faslodex)

Other chemotherapy drugs
- paclitaxel (Abraxane)
- platinum agents (cisplatin, carboplatin)
- vinorelbine (Navelbine)
- capecitabine (Xeloda)
- liposomal doxorubicin (Doxil)
- gemcitabine (Gemzar)
- mitoxantrone (Novantrone)
- ixabepilone (Ixempra)
- albumin-bound paclitaxel (nab-paclitaxel or Abraxane)
- eribulin (Halaven)

vaginal dryness, that is, the same symptoms that occur with menopause. Significant risks include blood clots, stroke, uterine cancer, and cataracts.

Another classification of hormone medications is called *aromatase inhibitors*, which are used in postmenopausal women. They block the action of an enzyme that converts androgens into estrogens. Examples of aromatase inhibitors include anastrozole (Arimidex), letrozole (Femara), and exemestane (Aromasin). Side effects of aromatase inhibitors include postmenopausal symptoms plus an increased risk of osteoporosis. The drug fulvestrant (Faslodex), which destroys estrogen receptors, is used in postmenopausal women; it causes similar symptoms to the above drugs, plus joint pain. Some drugs can attack specific abnormalities within cancer cells; these are used in what are termed *targeted drug treatments*. A protein called human growth factor receptor 2 (HER2) helps breast cancer cells survive and grow. There are drugs that target HER2, including trastuzumab (Herceptin), pertuzumab (Perjeta), ado-trastuzumab (Kadcyla), and lapatinib (Tykerb). Surgery to remove the ovaries or medications to stop the ovaries from producing estrogen can be influential in hormone therapy.

Women taking these medications must have periodic biopsy or ultrasound of the uterine lining performed. Hormonal treatments have been shown to manage breast cancer effectively when used alone and in combination with chemotherapy. Hormone therapies are generally given for 5 years.

Radiation therapy is often given after breast reconstruction surgery to help reduce the chance that the cancer will recur in the breast or lymph nodes. It may also be recommended after mastectomy in clients with a cancer larger than 5 cm or when cancer is found in the lymph nodes. External ration therapy is the most common type of radiation therapy for women with breast cancer. The extent of the radiation depends on whether lymph node involvement is present and whether a mastectomy or breast reconstructive surgery was performed.

The client must discuss all therapy choices thoroughly with the oncologist. Decisions about therapy are made on the basis of the type and extent of the tumor and the client's wishes.

Reconstructive Surgery

Women who have had a mastectomy have the option of breast reconstruction. National laws require insurance companies to cover the costs of reconstruction in women who lose a breast to cancer. There are two major types of reconstructive breast surgery. The plastic surgeon may implant a saline-, silicone-, or soy-filled envelope under one of the chest muscles to form a breast. Or, the surgeon may move skin, muscle, and fat from another part of the body to the breast area and shape it to form a realistic-looking breast. Later the surgeon can form a nipple by bunching up tissue and create an areola by tattooing the tissue to create color.

Breast reconstruction can be done at the time of surgery, or it can be delayed to a later time. The client will make this decision in discussion with the healthcare providers involved in their care. It is often viewed as better to wait, if the client will be receiving chemotherapy or radiation therapy. Because a reconstructed breast never looks completely like the original breast, many women decide to have a bilateral mastectomy and reconstruction for symmetry.

Prosthesis

A *prosthesis* is an artificial breast form that is inserted in a bra. It must be fitted to match the remaining breast. A prosthesis creates a natural appearance in clothing. For large-breasted women, prostheses are problematic because they may be made of silicone, which can be heavy. Many women purchase a prosthesis, but later decide not to wear it because of resulting shoulder pain. For these women, lighter-weight prostheses are available, but many elect to use cotton forms.

The client generally does not purchase a prosthesis until all swelling is gone from the surgical area and healing is complete. A cancer survivor volunteer often recommends a particular store or medical supply house where the prosthesis can be fitted. The cost of the prosthesis and the special bras that hold it may be covered by insurance if the healthcare provider writes a prescription.

Nursing Considerations

Preparation begins as soon as the client learns that they will need a breast biopsy or surgery. They must understand the procedure for the biopsy and that most breast lesions are benign. If they are to have a frozen section performed at the time of biopsy, she will want to know when they will receive the test's results. Most surgeons will see the client as soon as they get the result (usually, 15–20 min after surgery) and tell them the result and what the next steps are, if any.

In a presurgical suite, physical preoperative preparations are done, such as shaving and preparing the client for the type of anesthesia to be used. The client should understand that if the frozen section is positive, the surgeon may need to do more extensive surgery later. Discuss the safety of the alternatives presented to them by the surgeon and the implications of the various surgical alternatives (lumpectomy with radiation, mastectomy, and mastectomy with reconstruction). If the client will need future surgery, they will need assistance with decision-making before scheduling it.

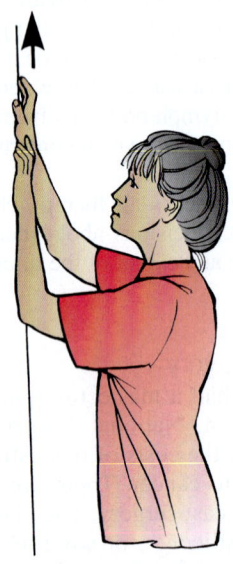

1. *Wall handclimbing*: Stand facing the wall with feet apart and toes as close to the wall as possible. With elbows slightly bent, place the palms of the hand on the wall at shoulder level. By flexing the fingers, work the hands up the wall until arms are fully extended. Then reverse the process, working the hands down to the starting point.

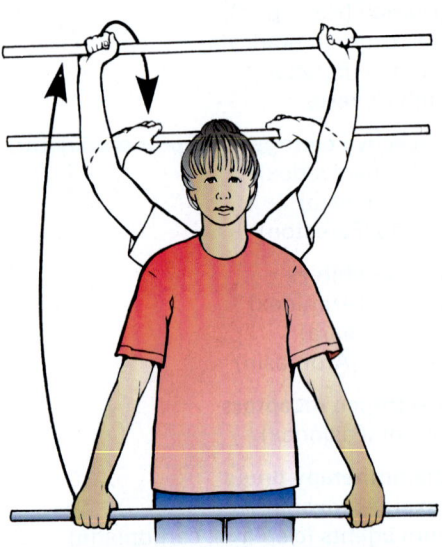

3. *Rod or broomstick lifting*: Grasp a rod with both hands, held about 2 feet apart. Keeping the arms straight, raise the rod over the head. Bend elbows to lower the rod behind the head. Reverse maneuver, raising the rod above the head, then return to the starting position.

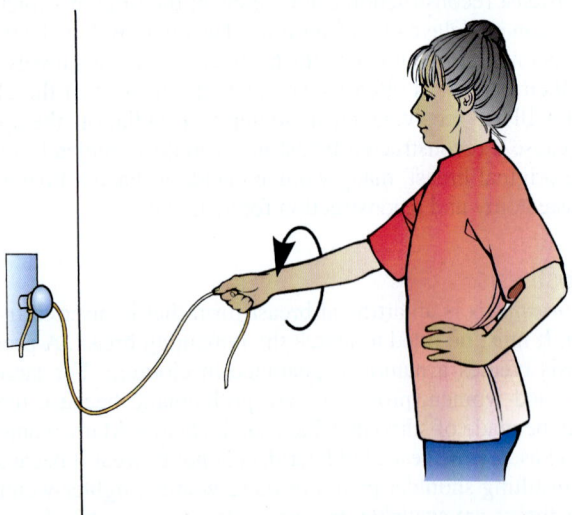

2. *Rope turning*: Tie a light rope to a doorknob. Stand facing the door. Take the free end of the rope in the hand on the side of surgery. Place the other hand on the hip. With the rope-holding arm extended and held away from the body (nearly parallel with the floor), turn the rope, making as wide swings as possible. Begin slowly at first; speed up later.

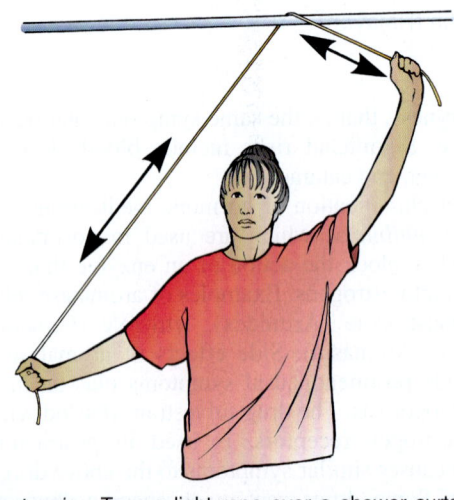

4. *Pulley tugging*: Toss a light rope over a shower curtain rod or doorway curtain rod. Stand as nearly under the rope as possible. Grasp an end in each hand. Extend the arms straight and away from the body. Pull the left arm up by tugging down with the right arm, then the right arm up and the left down in a see-sawing motion.

Figure 91-5 Postoperative exercises for the mastectomy client.

Preoperative teaching includes information about the care of any drains, such as a Jackson-Pratt (JP) drain, if they are to be inserted during surgery. In many facilities, lumpectomy is a same-day procedure, so teaching must be done before surgery. If lymph node surgery is to be done, teach postoperative exercises of the arm and allow the client to practice. Include the client's partner and other family members in discussions, if possible.

The client who is going to have a breast biopsy is understandably apprehensive about the possibility of breast cancer. Listen with understanding and support the client and family. Extreme emotional reactions are possible. Breast cancer affects the entire family, and each family member may need assistance with coping. Almost all women who are diagnosed with breast cancer, no matter how good the prognosis, respond with thoughts and fears of dying. Women who are to have a mastectomy are fearful about how they will adjust. They may be concerned about their sexual appeal to their partners. Those who are about to have the lymph nodes removed are anxious about possible metastases.

If the biopsy sample reveals the presence of breast cancer, assist the client to verbalize their fears and allow them to express emotion. The client is often in such shock that they hear nothing other than the word cancer. Assist by providing anticipatory guidance and focusing on the next steps. Taking action is one of the best ways of coping, and many actions will be taken and decisions to be made in the next few days. After the biopsy procedure, apply an ice bag to the area to reduce bleeding and swelling. At home, the client may want to continue the cold application.

Following definitive surgery, give routine postoperative care. Encourage the client to walk and move around. Monitor drains that are placed in the surgical wound to drain excess fluid and prevent edema. Note the amount of drainage and determine its character. One complication of mastectomy may be excessive bleeding. If this occurs, the client may need to return to surgery to stop the bleeding. Check dressings frequently for drainage around the drain insertion site.

Elevate the affected arm for several days to minimize development of edema. Expect some edema if surgery involves the lymphatic system. Surgeons differ in their beliefs about the value of postoperative arm exercises for the client who has had lymph node surgery. Some encourage exercise to prevent the loss of arm function. Others prohibit exercise because it can lead to formation of a *seroma* (serum-filled mass) in the axillary area. Mild shoulder shrugging and movement of the elbow and hand are usually permitted. Occasionally, a snug elastic sleeve will be used to decrease or prevent swelling. A low-sodium diet and diuretics may also be ordered.

> **Nursing Alert** The most common cause of lymphedema in the client who has had their lymph nodes removed is infection. Many precautions are necessary to prevent damage to the skin and tissues. Avoid taking blood pressure, giving injections, or drawing blood on the operative side. Protect the arm against future infection. Report signs of infection in the arm or the hand immediately. In many facilities, a pink arm band is applied to the affected arm to alert staff to these precautions.

The client will need emotional support after mastectomy. They are likely to experience grief over the loss of their breast. They may direct anger at the surgeon, nursing staff, or family members. Many clients are relieved that the surgery is over and do not exhibit negative emotions in the immediate postoperative period. Because of preoperative tension and anxiety, many clients are exhausted after surgery.

The client can combine some exercises with ordinary daily activities, such as sliding a towel back and forth to wipe the back, brushing the hair, and reaching with the arms when making a bed. The client should know how to exercise the muscles before they go home (Fig. 91-5). Some facilities offer postmastectomy classes so that clients can exercise together.

Key Concept

A visit from a support group representative may help while the client is still in the hospital or shortly after they go home. This person can assist clients with postoperative exercises and answer common questions about the breast cancer experience. Volunteers can recommend places that sell prostheses for women who have had a mastectomy. They also can offer much-needed emotional support and answer questions.

STUDENT SYNTHESIS

KEY POINTS

- Diagnostic studies help to determine the diagnosis. The nurse is an important intermediary in the preparation for diagnostic studies and helping the client prepare for any examinations.
- Nursing skills performed to assist the client include perineal care, vaginal irrigation, and insertion of vaginal suppositories.
- Explanation and follow-up with a client who must undergo surgical treatment is important. The client may not have heard or understood all that was explained to them.
- Endometriosis may be frustrating and painful. It is not uncommon for the diagnosis to be missed because the symptoms are similar to other disorders.
- Menopause and hormone therapy have benefits and risks.
- High cure rates exist in certain cancers if discovered early (especially, breast and cervical cancer).

CRITICAL THINKING EXERCISES

1. Suggest how you would approach and reassure an adolescent who is having their first pelvic and clinical breast examination. What would you say to the girl before the procedure begins? Do you need to know if the girl is sexually active? Would you show them the equipment and tell them the steps of the examinations? What would you tell the healthcare provider, who is going to do the examinations, before seeing the adolescent? As part of discharge teaching after the examinations, what topics need to be discussed with the girl?

2. A 28-year-old client has found a lump, doing a breast self-examination while at home. The healthcare provider confirms that there is a lump and has scheduled them for a mammogram. Which steps are taken next if the examination confirms a mass in the breast? Which steps are to be taken if a mammogram does not reveal a mass? To contrast the previous scenario, which differences would occur if the client were aged 60 years?

3. A 22-year-old client has frequent vaginal irritation and infections. What are the important topics that you would use to inform them of ways to prevent frequent vaginal infections?

4. A 38-year-old client states they have frequent severe abdominal pain that worsens during their period. Their description of symptoms suggests endometriosis. The client states that they have seen healthcare providers on several previous occasions, but they "cannot fix their problems." The client's sister has had the same problem, which went away after a hysterectomy. Discuss your approach to this situation.

NCLEX-STYLE REVIEW QUESTIONS

1. A client is scheduled for a pelvic examination. In preparation for the procedure, which intervention by the nurse is appropriate?
   a. Ask the client to empty their bladder.
   b. Instruct the client to hold their breath when the speculum is inserted.
   c. Place the client in the prone position.
   d. Have a Vaseline-based gel available to lubricate the speculum.

2. A client requests an office visit for a Pap test. When is the best time for the nurse to schedule the client?
   a. The timing of the test is not significant and the appointment can be scheduled at any time.
   b. The appointment should be scheduled while the client is on their menstrual period.
   c. The appointment should be scheduled the day after the client's menstrual period.
   d. The appointment should be scheduled between the client's menstrual periods.

3. A client is having a breast biopsy with the entire lump to be removed and analyzed. Which type of breast biopsy would the nurse prepare the client for?
   a. Needle biopsy
   b. Excisional biopsy
   c. Incisional biopsy
   d. Aspiration biopsy

4. A client is postoperative after a laparoscopy. After the procedure, the client reports severe pain under the right clavicle. Which is the priority action by the nurse?
   a. Prepare the client to return to surgery.
   b. Turn the client on the right side.
   c. Notify the healthcare provider.
   d. Administer an analgesic.

5. A client reports frequent vaginal infections. Which suggestions can the nurse make to decrease the risk of infection in this client? Select all that apply.
   a. Douche daily.
   b. Wipe from front to back after voiding.
   c. Avoid the use of bubble bath.
   d. Thoroughly wash hands, especially during menses after voiding.
   e. Wear nylon panties.

CHAPTER RESOURCES

Enhance your learning with additional resources on thePoint!

Student Resources related to this chapter can be found at **thePoint.lww.com/Rosdahl12e**.

CHAPTER 91 Female Reproductive Disorders

Welcome Steps

Look at healthcare provider's orders.

Protocol for procedure.

Necessary equipment/supplies.

Wash hands using proper hand hygiene; put on gloves.

Explain the procedure and reassure the client.

Locate two identifiers to confirm correct client.

Comfortable and efficient position for nurse and client.

Obtain privacy.

Make sure to follow correct steps and body mechanics with good technique.

Ensure safety and observe deviations from normal.

End Steps

Ensure comfort and safety.

Note questions or concerns from client or nurse; note significant data.

Dispose of materials properly.

Disinfect the area and your hands.

Document and report the procedure and your findings.

IN PRACTICE

NURSING PROCEDURE 91-1 Performing a Vaginal Irrigation (Douche)

Supplies and Equipment
Gloves
Irrigating bag, tubing, and clamp, or disposable douche
Disposable douche tip
Bedpan
Solution, as prescribed
Standard (short intravenous stand)
Bath thermometer
Protective waterproof pad for the bed
Perineal pad (sanitary napkin), if needed
Tissues
Bath blanket
Mineral oil, if needed

Steps
Follow LPN WELCOME Steps and Then

1. Ask the client to void. *Rationale: A full bladder will interfere with the insertion of the douche nozzle and may cause discomfort. The douche may stimulate voiding if the bladder is full.*

2. Protect the bed with a waterproof pad. Have the bedpan ready before preparing the solution. *Rationale: Some fluid might spill; using a waterproof pad protects the bed from becoming wet and avoids having to change the linens.*

3. Prepare approximately 1,500 mL of the prescribed solution at the required temperature, 100 °F–110 °F (37.8 °C–43.3 °C), according to the treatment's purpose. *Rationale: The fluid will cool; be sure to administer it at the correct temperature. Heat relieves inflammation, but a solution that is too warm will burn the mucous membranes and the skin around the meatus when flowing back.*

4. If the solution is ordered at a temperature above 105 °F (40.6 °C), apply mineral oil or petrolatum to the vulva and perineum. Maximum temperature is 115 °F (46.8 °C). *Rationale: The vulva and perineum are more sensitive than the vagina.*

5. Carefully inspect the douche tip to make sure it is not cracked or rough. *Rationale: This action prevents injury to delicate vaginal tissue.*

6. Have the client lie back with a rolled bath blanket under their head, and place them on the bedpan or if the client is on the toilet, ask them to lean back. *Rationale: In this position, gravity will help direct the solution over the entire vagina.*

7. Place the irrigating bag slightly above the level of the client's hips, never more than 18 in. (48 cm). *Rationale: This placement ensures a continuous, but gentle, flow of solution. If the bag is higher, it can drive infection into the uterus.*

8. Release the clamp to let air out to the tubing before inserting the nozzle. *Rationale: Air might distend the uterus or vagina.*

9. Separate the labia, and gently insert the nozzle, directing it downward and backward. If necessary, lubricate the tip of the nozzle with water-soluble lubricant. *Rationale: This direction is the same as the slant of the vaginal canal; a small amount of water-soluble lubricant, such as K-Y jelly, aids insertion.*

10. Gently release the clamp, and allow the fluid to flow slowly. Rotate the nozzle gently during treatment. *Rationale: A natural pocket forms between the cervix and the vagina's rear wall. Rotating the douche tip rinses material out of this pocket and directs fluid over all parts of the vagina.*
11. Clamp the tubing, and gently withdraw the tip from the vagina. *Rationale: Clamping the tubing prevents the solution from spilling as the tip is removed.*
12. Discard the entire douche system in the prescribed manner. *Rationale: Proper disposal helps prevent the spread of infection.*
13. If the client is able, have them sit up on the bedpan or toilet for a few minutes. *Rationale: This position will help the fluid drain from the vagina.*
14. Place a sanitary pad over the vulva. *Rationale: The sanitary pad helps protect the bed and client from additional drainage.*

Follow ENDDD Steps

Gerontologic Nursing | UNIT 13

92 Gerontology: The Aging Adult

Learning Objectives

1. Discuss how the wording and terms of aging may contribute to stereotypes of individuals of specific ages. Note how the terms may influence gerontology and geriatrics.
2. Identify the nursing measures that assist the older adult to meet nutritional, elimination, and personal hygiene needs.
3. Differentiate between the needs of the adult who has normal concerns related to aging and one who has significant health issues. Discuss the different aspects of their IADLs and their ADLs.
4. List common mental health problems in adults that may become apparent as they age.
5. Explain why depression and chemical dependency are important concerns in the older adult.
6. Discuss the nursing considerations for adults who need psychological therapies.
7. Compare and contrast adults who have few health concerns and adults who have multiple health concerns. Describe how this phenomenon affects society's needs, individual family's concerns, and the overall concepts of aging.
8. Define presbyopia and presbycusis. List nursing measures to assist an adult to meet communication needs.
9. State the nursing measures needed to assist an older person to compensate for impaired proprioception. Discuss the relationship between proprioception and injuries due to falls.
10. State five warning signs of elder abuse. Identify three nursing interventions that are necessary for suspected elder abuse.
11. Name five areas of loss that impact lifestyle as individuals age.
12. Discuss the concept of cumulative loss in adults.

Important Terminology

aphasia
aspiration
caregiver stress
chemical restraint
elder abuse
friable
geriatrics
gerontology
halitosis
hirsutism
instrumental activities of daily living (IADLs)
kyphosis
older adult
paradoxical effect
polypharmacy
presbycusis
presbyopia
proprioception
respite care
Sjögren syndrome
synergistic interaction
vulnerable adult

Acronyms

ADLs
IADLs
LTC

Gerontology is the study of the effects of normal aging and age-related processes, including diseases and disorders. As discussed in Chapter 13, gerontology looks at the physical, psychological, economic, sociologic, and spiritual dimensions of the aging process. **Geriatrics** is the branch of medicine concerned with the problems and illnesses of aging and their treatment. Both terms (*gerontology* and *geriatrics*) refer to the study and healthcare of the adult as the individual progresses through the dynamic changes known as the aging process. The branch of nursing that assists people to age in a healthy manner, to promote and maintain wellness in later life, and to care for people in times of sickness and death is called *gerontological nursing*. Chapter 13 discusses many issues related to aging, one of which pertains to the terminology that defines the specific delineation of "who is the older adult," and whether that definition is different from the "aging adult." In the United States, the average lifespan of both men and women has nearly reached the age of 80 years. A major issue of gerontology involves the general philosophical question, "At what point in life is a person considered older?" Review Chapter 5 for Maslow concepts of *hierarchy of needs*. Chapter 13 discusses Erikson's concepts of *generativity versus self-absorption* and *ego integrity versus despair*.

Words pertaining to a specific number of years, or chronological aging, are often used to define whether a person is considered an older adult. A major CDC report on aging defines the "older population" as individuals who are aged 65 years and older. Many adults have more than one chronic illness early in their adult life. When individuals reach the age of 50 years, their chances of having one or more chronic illnesses increase. The effects of chronic illness can also confer an aspect of aging. In general, the wording and the terms relating

1697

to age are not standardized. The dilemma is how to define a changing population. When people are categorized simply by chronological age, there is often a stereotyped assumption of age-related issues and limitations, which arises from an association of advancing age and declining health. In nursing, we are concerned with the holistic components of healthy aging that are involved with gerontology.

The current world population has a great mixture of adults who are older than 65 years and who are actively working and functioning members of society. Many countries have defined the age of 65 years as the age of retirement and have based their social retirement system upon this age. As healthcare advances, the actual number of years that an individual lives becomes a factor in retirement age. Thus, an arbitrary age that has been a guideline associated with retirement and becoming an older adult is becoming more individualistic and related to the person's ability to function independently in society. Additionally, an individual's functional age may be very different from that individual's chronological age, biological age, or psychosocial age.

For clarification of some of these issues, in this chapter, the generalized term *older adult* is defined as the person whose age ranges approximately between 70 years and above. Some older adults have one or more chronic illnesses that can increase the effects of normal aging. These clients may be less independent and might be in need of assistance with some or all of the instrumental activities of daily living (IADLs) as well as with the standard activities of daily living (ADLs).

Nursing in the 21st century will be affected by three coinciding and interrelated events:

1. A proportionally higher number of the baby boom generation will reach age 65 years. (Baby boomers are individuals born between 1946 and 1964.)
2. The number of citizens reaching the age of 85–100 years or even older is significant.
3. The social, financial, and healthcare needs of these age groups will affect existing family units, healthcare services, and governmental allocation of finances.

This chapter discusses health-related needs that result from the normal aging process. Normal aging does not cause specific illnesses; however, aging does cause changes of normal physiology. Most of the older adults are active and healthy and able to perform basic *activities of daily living* **(ADLs)**. However, as they age, it is not uncommon for them to have increasing difficulty in performing more complex tasks, such as household maintenance, managing money, or using modern technologies, such as cell phones or computers. These types of more complex activities are referred to as **instrumental activities of daily living (IADLs)**.

Chronic illnesses are more common in older adults compared with the general population. When caring for adults, the nurse will need to understand the process of normal aging versus pathologies associated with disease. Normally, older adults retain the ability to learn, adapt, and change, even when the aging process requires modifications. Table 92-1 summarizes the common effects of aging on the systems of the body.

Our society emphasizes age-related changes and common health problems as diseases experienced by older people, when actually they are normal consequences of aging. These include the following:

- Decreased functioning of organs
- Changes in visual and auditory acuity
- Decreased reaction time
- Unsteady gait; decreased sense of balance
- Decreased tactile sensations
- Stiff joints
- Decreased capacity for recovery from wounds, injury, or illness

> **NCLEX Alert**
>
> Common changes in aging are typically seen in NCLEX scenarios. Questions or options may relate to what is normal versus what is not a normal part of aging. Therefore, it is important that you become very familiar with normal and nonnormal physiological changes.

GERIATRIC CARE SETTINGS

The development of a plan of care for geriatric individuals requires observation and an understanding of the person's current lifestyle. Remember that a very high percentage of adults live in their own homes; however, some need assistance or special care. Sometimes the care may be permanent, whereas at other times the individual might be recovering from an acute illness. Care settings for older adults vary depending upon the acute or chronic nature of a problem, the availability of local facilities, and the expected outcome of the diagnosis. Options have advantages and disadvantages. Cultural considerations, personal and governmental financial resources, and personal preferences often dictate available choices. The person's ability for ADLs or IADLs and potential for rehabilitation are also issues that require information from the healthcare providers, nursing interventions, and the availability of assistance either at home or in a residential facility. Care settings include home care, adult daycare centers, retirement communities, assisted-living facilities, acute care hospitals, long-term facilities, and hospice care.

Factors determining the choice of residence for the adult with geriatric medical or psychological issues and who needs healthcare and/or personal assistance include the following:

- The expected time frame of recovery, that is, from recovery of a chronic or acute illness or the combination of chronic illnesses and acute illnesses.
- The person's ability to provide for physical, financial, and emotional self-care needs.
- Physical, financial, and emotional support that might be available from family and friends.
- Access to healthcare and rehabilitation services, including availability and transportation.
- Need for protection and supervision.

Home Care

Most adults live in their own homes and are able to care for their own needs independently. For those with manageable conditions, the current trend in healthcare is to provide needed care in the client's home. To some degree, measures such as financial aid, Medicaid, Medicare, rental and fuel assistance, and the Food Stamp Program help adults to remain in their homes.

When complicated physical needs require ongoing assistance, home care agencies have a substantial variety of services available 24 hr a day. Other services, such as home

TABLE 92-1 Effects of Aging on Body Systems

	SYSTEMIC CHANGES	MANIFESTATIONS	CLIENT TEACHING
Integumentary system	Thinning of epidermis, Loss of subcutaneous fat Decrease in melatonin production Loss of elasticity Decreased dermis vascularity	Increased incidence of bruising or skin tears Wrinkling, sagging, decreased ability to maintain hydration, less protection against temperature changes Paler skin, loss of hair color—graying hair, less protection against sun damage	Encourage the client to drink plenty of fluids and dress appropriately for climate changes. Encourage the use of sunscreens with appropriate ultraviolet (UV) protection. Suggest using good lubricating lotions and bathing less often. Caution the client to guard against injuries because they take longer to heal.
	Slower reproduction of new hair and skin cells Diminished oil and sweat production	Sallow skin, thicker nails Balding; thin, fine hair; slower healing Dry, fragile skin; intolerance to heat	Suggest ways to guard against injuries. Encourage the client to use good lubricating lotions and bathe less often. Suggest ways to avoid becoming overheated.
	Erratic pigment and cell production	Senile lentigines (liver or age spots) and keratoses (scaly, slightly raised, pale or brown harmless growths on skin)	Show the client how to conduct skin checks and consult a dermatologist with any concerns.
Musculoskeletal system	Loss of muscle strength and size	Loss of strength, flexibility, and endurance	Suggest frequent exercise appropriate to the client's age and ability.
	Loss of bone density	Vertebral compression with diminished height and a dowager hump (abnormal spinal curvature); osteoporosis (abnormal bone porosity) with frequent fractures	Educate the client regarding weight-bearing exercises. Encourage the client to conduct a home safety check to avoid falls. The healthcare provider may recommend calcium supplements, dietary consultations, or estrogen replacement.
	Cartilage thins	Joints may be painful, inflamed or stiff.	
Nervous system	Slower nerve conduction	Slower reaction time, slower learning; diminished sensation, or slower perception of pain, with resulting increase in injuries	Allow extra time, as needed, and educate the client about possible hazards of delayed reaction times. Aim teaching at comprehension level. Encourage the client to conduct home safety checks.
	Reduced neurons and neurotransmitter activity	Balance may be impaired and reaction time decreases. Less time spent in deep sleep	Have the client install bath rails; conduct a home safety check. Encourage the client to use ambulatory aids. Allow client rest periods, as needed.
Eyes	Diminished adjustment of lens to accommodation	Presbyopia (farsightedness)	Allow the client rest periods, as needed. Obtain a referral to an ophthalmologist. Provide adequate lighting and use large-print books.
	Increased density and yellowing of lens	Lens cloud and cataracts gradually form (lens opacity) that dim vision as less light reaches the retina	Provide adequate lighting. Use yellow, orange, or red on signs; violet, blue, and green colors are more difficult to see.

(Continued)

TABLE 92-1 Effects of Aging on Body Systems (Continued)

	SYSTEMIC CHANGES	MANIFESTATIONS	CLIENT TEACHING
	Pupils decrease in size	Dark and light adaptation takes longer; intolerance to light or glare, poor night vision	Provide adequate lighting and have the client avoid night driving.
Ears	Loss of auditory hair cells (organ of Corti)	Ability to hear tones in upper frequencies diminishes	Speak clearly, facing the client, in an area with few distractions.
	Cerumen increases	Increased risk of cerumen impaction	Teach importance of keeping regular doctor appointments.
Other senses	Diminished sense of smell Diminished sense of taste	Loss of appetite, Diminished ability to taste bitter, salt, and sour, may increase use of salt or spices	Encourage frequent emptying of trash. Encourage the use of spices rather than salt.
Cardiovascular system	Arteries become less elastic, capillary walls thicken, thus slowing exchange between blood and tissues narrowing of vessels	Loss of peripheral circulation, cold extremities, slower healing time, hypertension	Encourage the client to exercise as able and to eat a balanced, low-fat, low-salt diet. Have the client dress appropriately for temperature changes.
	Slower response time to demands for increased output	Complaints of fatigue on exertion	Help the client pace exercise and exertion.
	Diminished cardiac muscle strength, heart valves thickened and more rigid	Presents as weaker heart contractions, blood volume decreases and cardiac output declines	Educate the client regarding low-salt diets and maintaining an *orthopneic* or semivertical position.
Respiratory system	Stiffening costal cartilage	Decreased expansion and contraction, decreased lung capacity	Educate the client about smoking hazards and emphysema. Encourage moderate exercise.
	Functioning alveoli decreases	Fatigue and breathlessness on exertion, shallow breathing patterns affect gas exchange	Encourage the client to exercise, as appropriate, with short rest periods during activity. Caution the client to guard against upper respiratory infections.
	General loss of muscle mass and strength and postural changes	Difficulty coughing deeply (may lead to pneumonia)	Encourage the client to drink adequate fluids to liquefy respiratory secretions.
Gastrointestinal system	Drying of secretions, including saliva	Dry mouth, dysphagia (difficulty swallowing)	Educate the client regarding oral hygiene and adequate fluid intake.
	Decreased enzyme activity	Incomplete digestion, poor conversion of nutrients with malnourishment	Encourage the client to eat small, frequent, well-balanced meals.
	Slower peristalsis	Constipation, flatulence, indigestion	Suggest the client increase fluid and fiber intake. Have the client avoid laxative dependency.
	Reabsorption of bone in the jaw may loosen teeth or cause a loss of teeth	Poor chewing function, loss of appetite, poor nutrition	Refer the client to a dentist and provide instruction regarding good oral hygiene. Suggest dietary counseling.
Urinary system	Decreased bladder capacity	Urinary frequency	Encourage the client to respond to the initial urge to void.
	Decreased bladder muscle tone	Urinary retention with resulting urinary tract infections or incontinence	Suggest exercises for strengthening the pelvic floor. Urge the client to empty the bladder completely with each voiding.

TABLE 92-1 Effects of Aging on Body Systems (Continued)

	SYSTEMIC CHANGES	MANIFESTATIONS	CLIENT TEACHING
	Fewer functioning nephrons	Less blood flowing through the kidneys to be cleaned of wastes, creating possible lethal levels of medications or normal body wastes	Have the client increase fluid intake to maintain hydration. Healthcare provider may lower dosage of some medications.
Endocrine system	Decreased enzyme activity	Menopause, slower metabolism	The healthcare provider will supplement hormones as needed.
Immune system	Diminished production and function of T cells and B cells	Less resistance to illness	Encourage the client to obtain immunizations as age appropriate.
	Diminished ability to distinguish self from other	Increase in autoimmune diseases	Educate the client regarding symptoms of autoimmunity.
	Diminished defenses elsewhere (e.g., gastrointestinal enzymes)	Overload on compromised immune system and more frequent serious illnesses	Encourage the client to obtain immunizations as age appropriate and to guard against communicable diseases.
Female reproductive system	Decreased egg production	Menopause or climacteric	The healthcare provider may prescribe supplemental estrogen.
	Decreased estrogen production	"Hot flashes"; thinner, drier vaginal walls with vaginal itching and painful intercourse.	The healthcare provider may prescribe supplemental estrogen.
	Poor perineal muscle tone	Stress incontinence	Suggest exercises for strengthening the pelvic floor.
Male reproductive system	Decreased testicle size	Reduced sperm count	This should not affect physical ability to achieve erection or ejaculation.
	Benign prostatic hyperplasia (BPH)	Urgency, frequency, nocturia, retention	Encourage the client to have yearly checks for BPH, and provide instruction regarding testicular self-examination.

health aides, homemakers, or occupational, physical, speech, or respiratory therapists, also are available. These services, plus delivered meals and transportation, also help individuals remain in their homes.

Circumstances may require older adults to move into the home of one of their children. In this situation, roles can reverse, as the child becomes the caregiver and the parent is the care receiver.

Senior Centers

Senior centers provide social interaction and opportunities for peer group relationships. Many centers provide travel, educational discussions, recreational games, meals, and other services. Some centers also provide adult daycare. Caregivers of older adults can obtain **respite care** (temporary relief and rest) from the responsibilities of caring for relatives who are now frail adults.

Resident Housing and Apartment Complexes

An increasing number of independent-living complexes are being designed and built exclusively for adults. Living spaces for residents include homes or apartment complexes that are designed with special features such as wide doorways that can accommodate wheelchairs or walkers. The bathroom may be designed to accommodate individuals who have arthritis or coordination problems. Special safety features are typically installed, such as handrails and safety lighting. These facilities may be governed by a home owner association (HOA), with a fee per each house (or unit) paid to a general fund. The fees from the HOA usually pay for general maintenance of the public areas. Therefore, the residents are not responsible for the majority of lawn or pool maintenance, which can be physically demanding. Adults who live in residential homes or retirement complexes have the advantage of living in close proximity to others of their age group, which promotes physical activity and socialization. These communities may offer services desired by aging adults, such as the freedom and privacy of their own space, while providing conveniences, security, and assistance with their ADLs or IADLs, if needed.

Age qualifications and limitations of the numbers of residents may be part of the admission requirements. For example, some HOAs may apply age-specific requirements. Families with dependents might not qualify for admission. Such complexes are not nursing homes, although many have assorted assisted-living options reserved for clients with dementia and nursing care units available for the resident whose health declines, requiring various levels of skilled nursing care. Some assisted-living facilities have small apartments for the geriatric consumer; these units are often in one building with a nursing staff available at all times. Ambulatory and semi-dependent residents may be able to eat meals in a common dining room, although a kitchen may be available in the living quarters as well. Laundry services are often available. Some of these complexes require a deposit or "buy-in" fee in addition to a monthly charge. Individuals may face confusing choices when searching for a place to live that is different from their family home. Nurses may be called on to help families and clients understand the specific differences between living facilities.

Long-Term Care Options

Some of the traditional long-term healthcare facilities have developed specialized areas for care of adults with significant medical problems, such as Alzheimer's disease. Chronically ill younger people, such as individuals with amyotrophic lateral sclerosis, may also live in long-term care facilities because they need access to a professional healthcare staff and facilities. Some rehabilitation facilities are intended for clients of many ages who, for example, are in a permanent coma (permanent vegetative state), have paraplegia or quadriplegia, or have other problems that affect the individual's lifestyle. Choosing a facility depends on the availability of services, finances, and client needs. Some facilities have separate units in one building that serve the different requirements of the clients. All facilities should provide the best possible nursing care in as homelike an atmosphere as possible (Box 92-1).

Long-term facilities offer four general options or levels of care:

1. An assisted-living facility provides room and some meals, laundry, and some personal assistant services and the privacy of living in their own apartment; standards and regulations vary. The facility may or may not have employees who are licensed nurses or nurses' aides.
2. A rehabilitative care facility is often a unit within another facility; a client may transfer from an acute care facility or hospital and receive physical, occupational, or speech therapy. The facility provides 24-hr care for a few weeks or months. Typically the client returns home after recovery from a disabling experience, such as a stroke, traumatic injury, or hip fracture. There are facilities where the neurologic client remains as a long-term resident.
3. A long-term care (**LTC**) facility is often referred to as a nursing home. Clients are generally referred to as residents because the facility is their home or residence. The facility offers care from nurses, nurses' aides, and other healthcare workers who function as an interdisciplinary team. Each facility has a medical director and a director of nurses and functions similarly to an acute care facility. However, LTC facilities generally do not have some of the onsite services that can be found in an acute care facility (e.g., radiology). Services, such as occupational therapy, physical therapy, rehabilitation, and hospice, may be available and used according to each resident's individual needs. Other services are brought into the facility, as needed (e.g., portable x-ray equipment), or the resident may be transported to the location of the service (e.g., a CT scan).

> **Box 92-1** **Characteristics of a High-Quality Skilled Long-Term Care Facility**
>
> - Is licensed and regularly inspected by state or local government and is free of serious deficiencies
> - Meets Medicare and/or Medicaid requirements
> - Has a medical director (healthcare provider) who makes regular visits and is actively involved
> - Has a staff of licensed nurses available 24 hr a day, 7 days a week
> - Provides other healthcare and therapeutic care
> - Provides special services for residents, such as a beautician or barber
> - Provides rehabilitation services by trained personnel and encourages all residents to work toward rehabilitation
> - Has an in-service program for all staff members
> - Conducts routine staff member evaluations
> - Maintains high standards of safety for residents and staff
> - Provides nutritionally adequate food and special diets, as needed
> - Provides for social needs of the residents in a homelike atmosphere
> - Has a well-planned and purposeful activities program
> - Provides a recreational program
> - Develops and maintains a medical record and nursing assessment and care plan for each resident
> - Makes provisions for obtaining necessary diagnostic laboratory and radiology services for the residents
> - Encourages family and friends to visit often
> - Encourages visits by young children and pets; focuses on pet therapy
> - Recognizes and provides for spiritual needs of individual residents

Residents of LTC facilities have an attending healthcare provider who provides monitored care. In recent years, extensive governmental regulations have been instituted for LTC facilities, and the care given in such facilities has improved because of nursing interventions and regulatory agencies. Nurses who work in LTC facilities have a significant amount of responsibility. These nurses, often LVN/LPNs, require special knowledge of the normal and abnormal progressions of aging, the nursing process, physical and mental dysfunctions, nutrition, and pharmacology.

The LTC facilities encourage family members to visit and provide care whenever appropriate. Healthcare professionals must be aware of the importance of family and friends.

4. A subacute care facility is available in most LTC facilities. Typically, residents require more complex care and higher staffing levels than the usual LTC resident, but not the intensity of care provided by an acute hospital. Usually a registered nurse (RN) must be present or available by phone 24/7 in this type of facility. A subacute care unit can be a separate section within a hospital or LTC facility or a separate facility that exists solely for this purpose.

HELPING THE OLDER ADULT MEET BASIC NEEDS

Because of cumulative losses caused by aging, individuals may need assistance from nurses or other healthcare workers to meet their basic needs. Clients have a tremendous diversity of needs. For example, some need assistance with daily physical requirements; priorities for others may include financial, emotional, or social needs. The nurse must be aware of specific variations in a client's needs. Each environment in which an older adult lives has advantages and resources, as well as disadvantages and limitations. Living at home helps the client retain independence. However, the home environment may limit social interaction, or it may not provide adequate physical resources to maintain basic hygiene, nutritional, and healthcare needs. The client who is terminally ill and is dying at home will need a different approach to physical care and basic needs, called hospice care. Table 14-1 in Chapter 14 summarizes the care of the dying client.

Nutritional Needs

Individuals must maintain lifelong satisfactory nutritional status to prevent the premature deterioration of body systems. Estimates are that one-third to one-half of all health problems of older adults relate directly or indirectly to inadequate nutrition and fluid intake. Balanced nutrition results in increased energy and a healthy mental outlook. In addition, medical or surgical conditions heal more rapidly with fewer complications when clients meet their nutrient needs (Unit 5). Proper nutrients must be available to build the thousands of compounds needed to maintain the body. The body must absorb, store, reorganize, or otherwise convert consumed nutrients into useful substances. To do so, the gastrointestinal system, pancreas, and liver must be healthy.

As a consequence of aging, older adults absorb nutrients more slowly, and their caloric needs are reduced owing to the slowing of metabolism. In general, they need to consume fewer calories while meeting their specific nutrient requirements, which vary only slightly from those of younger people. Protein requirements do not change: a minimum of 1 g of protein per kilogram of body weight is necessary for maintenance. A person whose body needs to build and repair tissues after injury (e.g., pressure wound) or during illness (e.g., cancer) has greatly increased daily protein requirements. Fat intake should not exceed approximately 35% of total caloric intake. Fats with essential fatty acids are more nutrient dense than empty calorie fats, such as those in fried foods or chocolate. Vitamins and minerals are important; most can and should be obtained through a healthy diet, rather than supplements.

Factors, such as the inconvenience and effort of food shopping, storage, and preparation, also affect a person's nutritional status. The aging process may influence an adult's appetite; a reduced appetite occurs because taste perception declines. The individual may be less physically active or unable to shop or cook food as often. Poorly fitting dentures often limit a client's ability to eat. In care settings other than the home, a client may feel rushed during meals or may not like to eat at the times meals are served.

Weight control is harder as a person ages. The body's overall metabolic rate declines, making fat more difficult to eliminate than in younger years. Excess weight can seriously affect self-esteem and health. Disorders, such as diabetes mellitus, hypertension, myocardial infarction, stroke, back and joint pains, and falling, are related to obesity. To help control weight, a low-fat, low-calorie, nutrient-dense diet may be recommended. The quality versus the quantity of food intake becomes important. Increasing caloric expenditure through regular exercise can greatly assist in weight control.

Understanding the Nutritional Status of the Older Adult

Understanding the nutritional status of an older adult includes not only observing the person's food and fluid intake but also understanding other factors that affect specific nutrients needed and consumed. Such factors include the following:

- Availability of food
- The client's ability to purchase, shop for, and prepare food
- Health conditions that change nutritional needs
- Oral health
- Elimination patterns
- Independence in eating
- Mood and mental status
- Energy level
- Activity
- Cultural preferences
- Food likes and dislikes
- Effects of medications
- Presence of symptoms, for example, pain, fatigue, and shortness of breath

You should compare the client's current weight with the past history of weight gain or loss. Weight loss within the past month that is greater than 5% of the total body weight, or a loss of 10% or more of body weight within the past 6 months, is significant. Report and discuss such findings with the client's healthcare provider. Encourage the client to eat. For clients with eating problems, try to determine why they do not want to eat, rather than forcing nutrition.

Special Considerations
Teeth and Chewing

Although tooth loss is not a normal event of aging, many older adults wear dentures or have few teeth. These individuals must adapt food so that they can chew it and eat it. Oral care and denture care can facilitate the eating success of clients. Food that is adapted (e.g., chopped, pureed, liquid) must be nutritionally balanced and attractively served.

Swallowing Difficulties

Older adults may have conditions that impair their swallowing mechanisms. Make certain that provided food is of a consistency that clients can swallow. Clients may better tolerate semisolid foods and thickened liquids; they may prefer small, frequent meals to large, less-frequent meals.

For meals, elevate the head of the bed or, if possible, have the client sit in a chair. Cutting food into edible bites will enable the client to chew it easily and helps prevent choking. Suggesting that the client bend the chin toward the chest while swallowing can help in preventing *aspiration* (inhaling food into the airway). Having a suction apparatus available at meals may be helpful. The client who has great difficulty swallowing or who refuses to eat can use special adaptive techniques; a speech therapist can provide suggestions for the client's specific condition.

Medications and Supplements

Table 92-2 describes implications of medication administration as related to the changes of aging. The nurse must be aware of the unique risks associated with medications for older adults. Because older adults have a high risk of complications associated with medications, be certain to educate clients and caregivers about their purpose, proper administration, expected side effects, adverse effects, and special precautions.

Do *not* crush enteric-coated tablets because they are not meant to be digested in the stomach. Be aware of medication–food interactions, including contraindications and side effects. "Tricking" a person into taking a medication by hiding it in food is illegal. Every person has the right to refuse medications unless a specific court order exists stating otherwise.

In a home setting, establishing a routine for medication administration is important. Additionally, the client is more likely to be compliant with a complicated medication regimen if a system is established. Inexpensive organizers can be set up for the client for a day, a week, or longer (Fig. 92-1). A list of current medications, times, and doses should be placed on the refrigerator where emergency personnel can see it and put into the client's wallet or purse near any insurance cards. Encourage the client or caregiver to make and update any list of medications. The list should include the generic and trade name, dose, how many times given, and the prescribing healthcare provider's name. The list should be kept with emergency papers.

Nursing Alert Observe for unexpected or unusual side effects when giving medications to older adults. The usual adult dose of an antidepressant may be toxic to an older adult. In addition, a **paradoxical effect** may occur. A *paradoxical effect* means that a drug causes an effect that is opposite to or different from what would normally be expected.

Supplementation with vitamins and minerals is an area of continuing research. Vitamin deficiencies can greatly affect nutritional status in older adults. Excessive quantities of vitamins and minerals, however, are potentially harmful. Calcium supplementation with vitamin D is often combined with exercise and estrogen as part of postmenopausal therapy for women. Self-administration of supplements is common. Teaching is an important nursing consideration in the use of medications and supplements.

Water

Adults need encouragement to drink adequate amounts of water. Generally, older adults have lower fluid reserves to protect them during periods of excess fluid loss or reduced fluid intake. Many older adults do not experience thirst as strongly as younger people. Immobile adults often do not drink adequate fluids. Sometimes, the individual avoids

TABLE 92-2 Changes in Aging as Related to Medication Administration

FACTOR	NURSING IMPLICATIONS
Decreased sense of thirst, dry oral mucosa	Difficulty swallowing medications; decreased absorption; offer water prior to giving first medication
Decreased total body fluid volume or percentage	Higher concentration of water-soluble drugs in blood, increasing risk for toxicity
Decreased muscle tissue	Slower or decreased absorption of intramuscular (IM) medications, shorter needle may be needed
Increased percentage of fatty tissue	Accumulation of fat-soluble drugs; more difficulty locating site for IM injection, may need longer needle
Decreased general circulation	Slowed absorption; slowed transport of drugs to cells; slowed removal of drugs or wastes from cells
Decreased circulation to colon, vagina	Slower melting of suppositories
Decreased blood flow to liver and kidneys; decreased liver enzymes	Slowed metabolism and absorption; slowed excretion
Fewer functioning (kidney) nephrons; decreased tubular reabsorption	Slowed or faulty excretion; retention of drugs in body for longer time leading to toxicity
Decreased stomach acids and other digestive fluids; lower stomach pH	Slowed absorption
Confusion, forgetfulness	Noncompliance with medication program leads to over or under medicating

CHAPTER 92 Gerontology: The Aging Adult

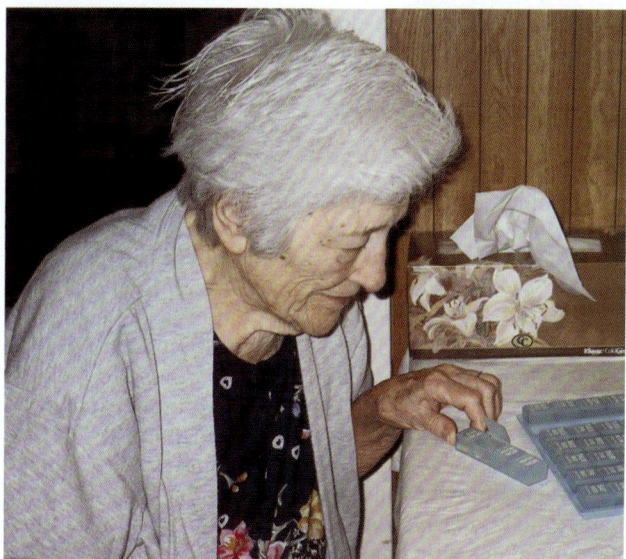

Figure 92-1 This client uses a multiple-dose, multiple-day medication dispenser to ensure that she takes her prescribed medications on time and in safe doses.

drinking fluids because of problems with urinary incontinence, urinary retention, or frequency. Dehydration is a serious and frequently overlooked problem. The nurse should offer a variety of fluids and provide assistance to clients who are unable to consume fluids independently.

> **Key Concept**
> Older adults are at risk for dehydration because of inadequate fluid intake, not feeling thirsty, medications, perspiration, and/or chronic diseases. Dehydration is dangerous and can happen within a few hours.

Supplementing Oral Intake
In many cases, an individual, particularly one who is ill, cannot eat and drink sufficiently to maintain adequate nutritional status. In this event, an alternate means of supplying nutrients is needed to supplement or replace oral intake. The first choice involves oral supplements that are commercial or blended formulas. Many different brand names, such as Ensure, are available. If this is not possible, other means must be used. Three major types of mechanical nutrient supplementation are intravenous (IV) therapy, usually short-term; total parenteral nutrition (TPN), an RN is responsible for maintenance and monitoring; and *enteral*, tube feedings when a physician places a tube directly into the GI tract through the abdomen.

> **Key Concept**
> Tube feedings can be controversial in some situations. An individual's advance directive, which hopefully has been completed by the client, may state refusal of nutrition while the family prefers the initiation of enteral or parenteral feedings.

Personal Hygiene Needs

Skin Care
Changes in the skin and circulatory system may cause older adults to be more susceptible to the development of pressure areas and skin breakdown. Because aging skin has few oils and is fragile, daily bathing is not always necessary and, in fact, can be harmful. Bed baths or sponge baths at the sink can be alternative hygiene measures. Waterless bath sponges and shampoo cloths are commercially available. Daily hygiene measures remain important throughout the lifespan and promote feelings of normalcy and independence. To promote circulation and a sense of independence, encourage clients to do as much of their own hygiene as possible. Care can progress through the stages of dependent bed bath, sitting in a chair at the sink, assisted shower or bath, and finally self-care. This progression is a therapeutic measure to increase activity and promote self-esteem.

If a client is incontinent, keep the skin clean and dry to prevent irritation and breakdown. An older person's skin can become very dry, thin, and *friable* (easily bruised/broken). The nurse may apply lotion to keep the client's skin soft and to promote peripheral circulation. Special bath oils are available to keep the skin supple; the client should avoid harsh soaps.

> **Key Concept**
> When bath oil is used, the tub may become slippery. Be careful to prevent falls.

Oral Hygiene
Encourage the client to care for the mouth to prevent dental difficulties and *halitosis* (bad breath). Clients with natural teeth need to brush and floss regularly; the use of mouthwash or swabs alone is not sufficient. Clients who have arthritis, strokes, altered mental status, or other difficulties often require assistance with oral care. They may be embarrassed or unable to ask for assistance; therefore, you must actively provide the opportunity for oral hygiene. Make sure that the confused person does not lose any dentures.

> **Nursing Alert** Encourage clients with dentures to check the condition of their gums regularly. Irritation can result from poorly fitting dentures. Cancer of the mouth sometimes occurs and may go undetected.

Hair Care
Clients should shampoo their hair, as needed, to promote comfort and cleanliness. Because the hair may become dry and brittle, especially in the older years, it is generally not necessary to shampoo as often as in earlier years. A fresh hairdo or haircut may give the client a more positive self-image and improve self-esteem. Massaging the scalp during a shampoo can be relaxing. Most LTC facilities and retirement communities have a hair salon with hairdressers available for the residents.

Key Concept
Self-care of the hair is an excellent opportunity for active range of motion exercise.

Nail and Foot Care
As we age, our fingernails grow more slowly and are more brittle. Toenails often become hard and thick, requiring a podiatrist to trim and care for them, and, in many institutions, toenail cutting must be done by a podiatrist. Nails should be cut straight across. Corns and calluses can be soaked in warm water, but are never cut; they also require a podiatrist's care and treatment. Encourage clients to wear proper-fitting flat or low-heeled shoes and comfortable hosiery. Clients should wash, thoroughly dry, and inspect their feet daily. When caring for a client's feet, document any injuries or discolored areas and report them to the client's healthcare provider. Even in healthy older adults, infection is possible, and wound healing is often slow in the extremities.

> **Nursing Alert** Most healthcare facilities do not allow nurses to cut the toenails or fingernails of diabetic clients. Check your facility's protocols.

Shaving
The self-esteem of clients may benefit from regular shaving. Allow clients to do as much for themselves as possible. Be sure they are safe and responsible. Assist, when needed, remembering that the skin may be more sensitive than that of a younger adult. Be careful to prevent cuts. Postmenopausal clients may occasionally develop **hirsutism** (increased facial hair), which the client may want removed for cosmetic purposes.

Clothing
When choosing clothing, consider physical limitations, environmental needs, functionality, and ease of dressing. Buttons and zippers may not be appropriate choices because of the loss of finger dexterity owing to arthritis or other problems. Clothing should be easy to remove and reapply when the client has to use the bathroom. Keeping warm due to loss of subcutaneous fats is often noted in older adults. Layering of clothing is very beneficial and helps the client maintain internal warmth. Allow residents of nursing homes to wear their own clothes, and encourage clients to dress in street clothes each day. Compliment their efforts to appear clean and well groomed. Sometimes, a new shirt or dress can greatly enhance morale. Encourage and assist clients to apply cosmetics, if this has been part of their daily routine.

Elimination Needs
Difficulties with elimination stem from many causes. Peristalsis slows with age. Many people exercise less and lack a good diet that promotes normal elimination. Foods, such as whole grains, fruits, and vegetables, provide needed fiber, complex carbohydrates, vitamins, and minerals. Generally, older clients do not consume sufficient fluids. They may deliberately reduce fluid intake as problems with voiding and defecation develop. Foods that they once tolerated now may be irritating.

Constipation
Many older adults are misinformed about or preoccupied with bowel function. A daily bowel movement is not necessary for all individuals; if the client is eliminating regularly without discomfort and straining, they are not constipated. Discourage excessive use of laxatives or enemas because they can disturb or even eliminate the normal urge to defecate. Encourage clients to respond to the urge to defecate as soon as possible. If they are dependent on assistance, nurses and nursing assistants must be quick to respond to their needs. Changes in fluid and food intake can often eliminate constipation. Individuals with chronic pain, who regularly take narcotic pain medications, often have problems with constipation. Prune juice, bran flakes, oatmeal, or fresh fruit are good alternatives to laxatives. Sometimes a laxative or mild stool softener, for example, docusate sodium (Colace), is required. Three or more days without a stool may indicate constipation, impaction, or infarction of the bowel. Nursing care in acute and long-term care facilities requires daily monitoring of gastrointestinal function.

> **Nursing Alert** Impaction in older adults with chronic health problems can become very serious. Impaction can cause infarction of the bowels, which leads to death of intestinal tissue, and soon the client becomes critically ill. Death is not uncommon due to an unrecognized sequence of events: constipation → impaction → infarction = death. Constipation can occur gradually. However, impaction, infarction, and death may result within a few hours, unless treated.

Bladder or Bowel Incontinence
Adults of many ages may have difficulty controlling bladder and bowel functions. To overcome this problem, retraining is possible by following a regular schedule. Most clients eagerly accept a bladder or bowel retraining program because it can help alleviate embarrassment. Medications, such as tolterodine (Detrol, Detrol LA), are designed to minimize urinary frequency and incontinence.

Incontinence may embarrass clients and can be a source of social isolation because of a fear of leaving the security of a ready bathroom. Be sensitive to treating this situation with dignity and discretion. Do not chide or scold anyone for episodes. Provide assistance in cleaning the skin and changing clothes, as needed. Evaluate incontinence to identify its cause; some forms can be eliminated with correction of the underlying problem. Many incontinence protection products are available over the counter. Clients may be able to purchase and wear protective garments. Catheters are not the treatment of choice for urinary incontinence because they can introduce infection-causing microorganisms into the urinary tract.

Difficulty in Voiding

Anatomic changes in aging adults may cause difficulties with normal voiding. Weaker bladder muscles can contribute to the bladder retaining some urine after voiding. Fecal impaction is a common cause of urinary retention. Accurate intake and output records may be required to monitor excretory status.

Many men, at some time in their life, have difficulty voiding because the prostate gland enlarges and obstructs urinary flow. This problem can be painful and embarrassing. Men with prostate problems must be examined on a regular basis, to rule out prostate cancer. Surgery may be necessary in some cases. Refer to Chapter 90 for more information regarding problems with the male urinary tract.

> **Key Concept**
> Even if the urine has dried, the skin of the incontinent client needs thorough cleansing to prevent skin breakdown from the irritating substances contained in urine.

HELPING THE OLDER ADULT MEET EMOTIONAL NEEDS

Psychological health is just as important as physical health. Because in later life adults often face cumulative losses (physical, financial, social), mental health problems are common. Healthcare providers may overlook or misdiagnose symptoms. Symptoms, such as depression, anxiety, and chemical dependency, may be undertreated. Suicide or suicidal gestures are possible. Box 92-2 identifies possible nursing interventions when working with a client at risk for depression.

Encourage clients to remain self-sufficient and mentally active. Keeping mentally active helps prevent feelings of boredom and depression. Older adults should maintain as much independence as possible. During times of illness, be sure to include the individual in the care and planning of activities. Provide maximum opportunities for them to participate in decision making. Offer options rather than telling or announcing that a decision has been made.

> **Box 92-2 Signs and Symptoms of Depression in Older Adults**
>
> - Feelings of pessimism, worthlessness, or helplessness
> - Lack of interest or ability to concentrate
> - Tearfulness or irritability
> - Withdrawal, anxiety, or paranoia
> - Insomnia (cannot sleep) or hypersomnia (can/does fall asleep at any time)
> - Fearfulness about finances or ability to care for oneself
> - Statements about suicide
> - Suicidal gestures

Mental Health Concerns

Anxiety

Anxiety is a feeling of uneasiness or apprehension in response to some threat. The threat can be real, such as disease pathology, or perceived, such as fear of the unknown. Some anxiety is normal and can stimulate an individual to take purposeful actions. Excessive or chronic anxiety can interfere with rational thinking and independent functioning. For those who are feeling the effects of the aging process, threats to self-image and self-esteem are common. Anxiety increases. These individuals may face loss of health, independence, the familial home, family contacts, and life itself. Anxiety can result in withdrawal, isolation, confusion, or combative or maladaptive behaviors. Anxiety is especially evident in adults who are physically ill and who have not developed adequate coping skills in earlier years.

Treatment

The nurse should first determine the level of the client's anxiety (mild, moderate, or panic-like). Available physical and emotional defense mechanisms should then be identified. Many times, increased knowledge reduces stress; the fear disappears because the stressor is identified and understood. Remain calm, provide outlets for excess energy, answer questions honestly, and give reassurance to the client. In some instances, referral of the client to a psychiatrist or other mental healthcare professional is necessary for evaluation and treatment. Reassure the client that anxiety and depression are very common during periods of change. A truth of aging is that change will occur.

Depression

Depression is not a normal part of aging. However, depression is a very common occurrence because of the risk factors of aging related to loss. Cumulative losses and numerous changes, most of which are beyond a person's control, can lead to depression. Many older adults are reluctant to admit they are depressed. The negative stigma attached to psychiatric diagnoses is more pronounced for individuals born in the 20th century than for those born in this century. Individuals may believe that depression, fear, and loneliness are normal aspects of aging, they may assume that they should be able to solve their own problems, or they may not even realize that they are depressed.

Educate the client and the family about the many aspects of depression. Clinical depression is often underdiagnosed or misdiagnosed in older adults. Disease processes, side effects of medications, or adjustment to life cycle changes are possible causes of depression. Do not confuse clinical depression with dementias, which often contain an element of depression (Chapter 93). Symptoms of depression include lack of interest in surroundings and in self-care; lack of energy and appetite changes; and altered sleep patterns. Loneliness, helplessness, guilt, worthlessness, and loss of interest are significant contributors to feelings of depression. Depression in the older adult is also commonly associated with physical complaints, such as chronic pain, chronic fatigue, anorexia, or insomnia (In Practice: Educating the Client 92-1). Suicidal ideation is a possibility. The nurse should always take threats or gestures of suicide seriously.

IN PRACTICE

EDUCATING THE CLIENT 92-1   Activities That Promote Feelings of Self-Worth

- *Pursue* an active social life with people of all ages. A place of worship usually has social gatherings. Senior citizen centers offer appropriate activities and encourage people to meet other people.
- *Return* to school. Educational programs stimulate the mind and offer opportunities for socializing.
- *Join* a support group. Share concerns, and gain insight from others in the group.
- *Volunteer* at the local hospital or civic organization. Some communities have babysitting services or daycare centers.
- *Acquire* a pet. This builds a sense of being needed and provides companionship.
- *Work* part time. Many companies are encouraging retired people to come back to work. The older adult worker is reliable and dependable. It is also therapeutic to have a place to go and to have responsibility and pride in having a job.
- *Maintain* good health practices (balanced diet, exercise, adequate rest).

Depression may be precipitated by a specific event, but usually results from a combination of risk factors, including the following:

- Chemical imbalance
- Dehydration
- Poor nutrition
- Financial difficulties
- Poverty-level subsistence
- Loss of spouse, friends, pets, or roles
- Serious, chronic illness
- Debilitating disease
- Lack of mental or physical exercise
- Medication side effects; over sedation
- Drug or alcohol abuse

Treatment

Reluctance to seek assistance, or failure of caregivers/healthcare providers to recognize symptoms, can hinder treatment for geriatric depression. The lack of medical professionals who specialize in geriatric psychiatry also limits therapy. The goal of therapy aims at increasing the client's self-esteem and/or relieving the underlying cause (e.g., pain). Involvement in social, recreational, and cultural events can be motivating. Participating in volunteer services and caring for pets may be helpful. Many general suggestions for stress relief also relate to the treatment of depression. Encourage the individual to get adequate exercise and to eat a balanced diet. Be sure that any general physical problems are being treated. Sometimes referral to a psychiatrist or other mental health provider is necessary. Various antidepressant medications also may be helpful.

> **Nursing Alert**   Remind clients and their caregivers that clients will need to use most antidepressants for 1 month (or more) before therapeutic levels are reached. Equally important is to teach clients not to discontinue the medication abruptly.

Substance Abuse

Substance abuse or chemical dependency can be a result of loneliness, depression, or many, often interrelated, factors. It is important to remember that **polypharmacy** is common for older adults. The use of many medications for one or more conditions (*polypharmacy*) will commonly result in a variety of side effects; *medications commonly react differently in older persons*. Many individuals have little knowledge of medication interactions. Some see no harm in sharing medications with friends or a spouse or in using medications after the expiration date. They may mix several different medications in the same container or misuse over-the-counter medications. They may forget how much medication they took or even if they took medications. They may be using chemicals as self-medication and taking doses larger than those prescribed; some may deliberately visit several healthcare providers to obtain added prescriptions. Even conscientious older adults can experience difficulties related to polypharmacy. Duplication of prescriptions occurs because some are labeled in generic names, whereas others use brand names. Many adults have several healthcare providers who prescribe separate, and often conflicting, medications.

> **Key Concept**
>
> The use of a single pharmacy that can maintain a drug profile for the client can prove useful and spare the adult unnecessary expense and complications. Pharmacists are often able to counsel the client on the use of over-the-counter medications as well as prescribed medications.

Risk factors for substance abuse among older adults include being widowed or being retired and alone. This individual may feel there is "nothing to do," promoting a lack of purpose, self-esteem, or self-actualization. The theorists Maslow and Erikson provide discussions related to the concepts of aging. Some older adults try to deal with these feelings by overusing chemicals, most often alcohol or prescription drugs. They may also abuse substances to cope with anxiety. Like much of the general public, they may believe that substance abuse is a problem of the young, denying the possibility that they or others of their age group could have a chemical dependency problem.

Alcoholism in older adults may be difficult to detect. Family and friends may not be aware of their loved one's situation. For those who do not have frequent visitors, covering up chemical dependency during occasional visits is not difficult to accomplish. Relatives may think the person is "just confused" when, in fact, the person is under the influence of alcohol. If the person is widowed, the former spouse may have covered up and enabled the alcoholism for a long time. The lack of a known alcohol problem can cause family members to disbelieve that their older adult relative has alcoholism. The situation often does not get out of control until the person is alone or retired.

Treatment of substance abuse in older adults can be difficult. They may be more resistant to the recognition of a problem than might a younger person who is chemically dependent, or they may resent the younger population, especially their own children, telling them what to do. Denial of the problem is common. Before treatment can be effective, the individual must accept the idea of help and be prepared to change lifestyle patterns.

Measures for Emotional and Psychological Support

> **Key Concept**
> Evaluate confusion in older adults for organic pathologies and substance abuse.

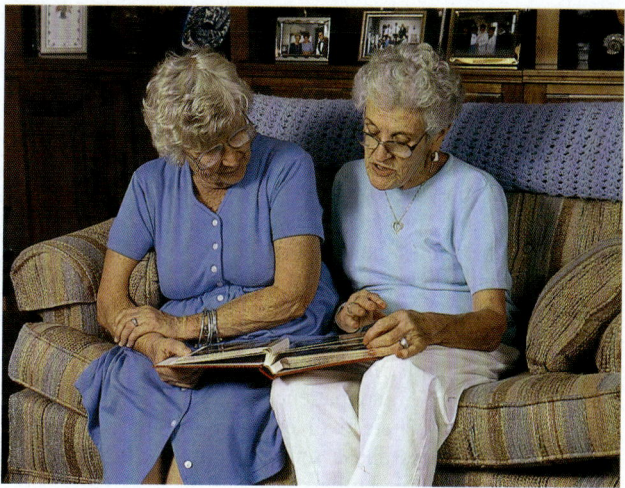

Figure 92-2 These women are using reminiscence to fulfill needs for friendship and stimulation.

Remotivation/Reminiscence Techniques

Remotivation is an important adjunct to therapy. This reality orientation attempts to focus attention on the present by calling on memories from the client's past (reminiscence). Sharing memories encourages participation. Reminiscence and reality orientation are useful strategies to promote mental stimulation and validation of life's past events (Fig. 92-2).

Recreation

Recreation is important at any age. In LTC facilities, an activity or recreation director plans and directs events designed to promote creativity. The goal is to motivate individuals to use their physical and mental capabilities.

Cognitive Function

Age alone does not result in a loss of cognitive function; older adults normally comprehend and appropriately use and understand language, perform basic calculations, and retain and recall information. Intelligence does not decline with age, but rather it reflects lifelong intellectual capacity. Although short-term memory loss is common, exercise of memory function helps to maintain and improve it. Adults maintain the ability to learn as they age, although they require adjustments for slower responses, sensory deficits, and physical limitations. Motivation and readiness to learn are important. Lack of direction and decreased stimulation contribute to decreased mental alertness and comprehension. Changes in cognitive function can accompany a wide range of physical and mental health problems. When cognitive changes are noted, evaluation is warranted.

Social Life and Activities

Encourage the client to carry on a normal social life and to engage in as many activities as possible. Include family members in the plan of care. Encourage them to visit and to take their relative with them on trips and outings.

Older adults typically love to see their grandchildren, as well as other children. They usually are interested in young people and will enjoy sharing their own youthful recollections with them. Often, nursing students are favorites among residents of LTC centers.

Pet Therapy

Many older adults welcome pets. Pets can provide companionship, stimulate the sense of touch, facilitate interactions, and encourage a sense of responsibility. Many confused clients respond to animals, even when they fail to respond to other people. Pet therapy has proved beneficial in geriatrics and is an accepted activity in many nursing homes.

Religious Support

Religious practices can be extremely therapeutic. Studies have shown that those who engage in religious practices have higher levels of health and function than those who do not. Support clients in their religious practices. Provide privacy for any desired religious practice. Many hospitals and facilities have visiting clergy who conduct religious services; encourage residents to attend if they so desire. If attending services is impossible because of limitations, you may be able to arrange tape recordings of services or arrange for visitors to interact with residents in ways that support their religious beliefs.

Use of Volunteers

Most community organizations for adults have volunteers who assist in the agency's activity programs. These volunteers are essential; always encourage their participation when you work with them. Volunteers provide many important services to clients, such as visiting those who have no other visitors, taking residents of LTC facilities on outings, helping with craft activities, providing parties and entertainment, and assisting with reading or writing letters.

Church groups or service clubs often work with nursing home residents as a special service. Because nursing home residents especially enjoy the company of younger people, teens and young adults should be encouraged to assist in the activities of local nursing homes. Not only is this practice meaningful to the residents but it is also rewarding for young people.

A staff member should coordinate the duties of volunteers to make certain they are helping residents. Encourage all volunteers to keep confidences and to treat clients with respect. If a volunteer makes a commitment to be at the facility on a certain day, they need to meet this obligation. Residents rely on, and look forward to, visits and may become upset when volunteers miss their appointments. Volunteers should develop empathy. They need patience to help residents perform independently because it is not helpful just to do things for them.

Many older adults make good volunteers as well. They often have the time and patience required to make valuable contributions. Their involvement as volunteers can add meaningful activities and a sense of purpose to their own lives, while also helping others.

SPECIAL CONCERNS OF THE ADULT RELATED TO INCREASING AGE

Communication

The senses of older adults are less acute than those of younger people owing to the physiologic changes of aging. Hearing and visual deficits can cause many adult to have difficulties in communication. Conditions, such as stroke and dementia, can alter language comprehension and use.

Age barriers may add to the difficulties of engaging in social interaction. Older adults can avoid feelings of isolation and rejection if they regularly talk with others. In a hospital or nursing home setting, placing people in double rooms is usually best, to help prevent isolation and provide more environmental stimulation. Encourage adults with whom you work to participate in social events.

Communication is a two-way process. Therapeutic and social communications have different approaches. Be aware of the meanings of touch and body language. Make appropriate eye contact and show genuine interest when visiting. Listen attentively and sit down when speaking to demonstrate interest and respect. Encourage visits from family, friends, and family pets.

Visual Impairment

Although many older adults have difficulty seeing because of cataracts or other eye disorders, encourage their participation in activities as much as they are able. Provide aids for the visually impaired, such as large numbers on the telephone and calendar, or magnifying glasses for reading. Remove obstacles that could cause falls, for example, throw rugs, footstools, extension cords. Be particularly careful around animals that may be the unwanted cause of a fall. Make sure there is adequate lighting in the home. Arrange for a safety check of the adult's home as the individual may be unaware of safety risks in their environment. Teach them what hazards exist and how to avoid them.

Presbyopia

Presbyopia is the specific name for impaired vision that results from normal aging. Presbyopia is caused by a loss of elasticity in the lens of the eye. As the person ages, the lens becomes more inflexible and, therefore, does not become sufficiently convex to focus on nearby objects. The first symptom often is an inability to read small print, such as the telephone book. Eyeglasses can usually correct this condition. The client will probably need bifocals to allow for far and near vision.

The older person will find that they need more light for reading because the pupils cannot adapt as well. Night blindness also increases with age. A night-light in the client's room helps prevent injury. Lamps, not necessarily a small wattage night-light, should be kept on at critical locations throughout the house, such as in a bathroom or hallway. Automatic timers for off and on settings of lamps are beneficial.

> **Key Concept**
> Clients should clean eyeglasses daily with soap and water or a cleaning solution and a soft, dry cloth. Teach them to avoid using paper products to clean because they may scratch the lenses.

Dry eyes can be uncomfortable and irritating, thereby affecting vision. Although dry eyes are a common outcome of normal aging, for some individuals they result from an autoimmune disease called **Sjögren syndrome**. This disease causes a drying of the mucous membranes, including the eyes. Persons with Sjögren syndrome often feel that something is in their eyes and may rub them, causing irritation. To alleviate symptoms, the use of over-the-counter or prescription eye drops are often helpful.

Hearing Loss

A specific hearing disorder of aging is called **presbycusis**. It begins at approximately age 40 and progresses with age. Presbycusis is a sensorineural hearing problem that first affects the client's ability to hear high-frequency sounds (e.g., ch, s, sh, and z sounds). As presbycusis progresses, other sounds are affected as well.

Evaluate the client who has a hearing loss to determine if a hearing aid can assist. If so, encourage the client to wear the hearing aid, even if the client is reluctant to do so. Special devices are available for telephones and televisions to enable hearing-impaired persons to hear them better.

Encourage the client to let people know if speech is not heard. Sometimes, using different words to communicate the same message can be helpful. Eliminate distracting background noises. If a client totally loses hearing, communication can be written or signed with the hands. The Internet, TV, newspapers, and magazines can help keep the hearing-impaired client aware of current events.

Speech Impairment

Aphasia is the inability to use or understand speech. It is often a mixture of deficits, such as slow speech, incorrect speech, or the use of incorrect words and sounds. Aphasia is always due to a brain injury. The client may be unaware of the communication problem. They may not be able to understand speech or writing or may have trouble naming objects. Remember to converse with the client, even if the client is unable to speak. Encourage the client to communicate in other ways (gestures, picture boards, diagrams, writing). Speech therapy is often helpful. Patience is necessary when communicating with clients who have aphasia; they are probably frustrated, and hurrying makes the situation worse.

> **Key Concept**
> Talk *to* the person, not about the person. Often, the person with aphasia has clear thinking processes.

Safety

Accidents, particularly falls, increase significantly with age and are a leading cause of disability and death after age 65 years. In addition to falls, the greatest dangers are fire, suffocation, and poisoning. The most common locations for accidents are the bedroom, bathroom, and kitchen. Most accidents are preventable.

As individuals age, they may be unsteady on their feet or may misjudge their physical capabilities. Medications or age-related changes can contribute to *orthostatic* (postural) hypotension. The client may become light-headed and fall when getting out of a bed or a chair. Changes in visual acuity and depth perception disturb the person's ability to judge distance. A safety check of the home environment to look for the presence of risk factors for falls can be useful in identifying risks and planning measures to reduce them.

Educate the client and family about home hazards. Safety teaching is important (In Practice: Educating the Client 92-2). Be sure all people on the staff of the healthcare facility know about these safety measures.

IN PRACTICE
EDUCATING THE CLIENT 92-2 — Safety Precautions for the Aging Adult

In the Home
- Move with caution, especially on stairs and at curbs.
- Stand up slowly to avoid postural hypotension or dizziness.
- Safe-proof the house. Remove or rearrange cords that might cause falls. Place furniture where it will not be tripped over. Grab bars should be placed on tubs, showers, toilets, and stairways.
- Ensure adequate lighting in all living areas. Night-lights must be used at night in bedroom, bathroom, and stairs.
- Use ambulatory devices (canes, walkers, wheelchairs), as needed.
- Follow good housekeeping practices. Clean clutter and spills.
- Establish an emergency calling system with family and friends, neighbors, and local emergency medical services.
- Place a telephone near the bed for night emergencies.
- Place a fire extinguisher in the kitchen, and know how to use it. Know how to use smoke detectors, and check batteries regularly. Do not smoke in bed.
- Carry a list of medications. Understand the use of medications and their side effects. Review use of medications periodically. Do not drive while taking medications that cause drowsiness or dizziness.
- Wear suitable and safe clothing: Avoid flowing robes and nightgowns, flowing sleeves, floppy slippers, long shoelaces.
- Understand that the lack of proprioception can be the cause of falls. *Proprioception* is the body's ability to sense its position and maintain equilibrium when in motion. For example, tilting the head backward, when looking up into a cupboard, can cause the individual to get dizzy and result in a fall.
- Obtain help with banking, especially with Social Security checks, or get direct deposit. Ensure safety on the street when coming from the bank, going to the mailbox, and so forth.
- Avoid scams. Caution the client about financial "deals," especially from strangers. Banks can establish an "alert" if a great amount of money is withdrawn or if more than a certain amount is withdrawn.

In the Hospital
- Use call light and ask for assistance, especially if getting out of bed at night to go to the bathroom.
- Keep bed in low position.

Loss of Proprioception

Proprioception is the awareness of posture, movement, and changes in equilibrium in relation to other objects. As people age, they may lose or experience alterations in their sense of proprioception. Often, they are unsure of where they are stepping, especially if they are walking on dark floors, bare ground, or dark paved areas. They have more difficulty staying erect without looking. Older adults who have a loss of proprioception may lose their balance when hyperextending the neck to look up at a clock or a high shelf. Lost balance is hard to regain. Teach clients to be aware of obstacles and uneven ground. When walking with older persons, allow them to take your arm and do not push or pull. Also, avoid quick turns to prevent loss of balance.

> **Nursing Alert** Many people are afraid of falling and may grab you or furniture when they are lifted or moved. Never rush or frighten an individual when assisting them.

Safety Devices

Numerous safety devices for the home and healthcare facility are available. Bathtubs and showers can be equipped with anti-slip surfaces, hand bars, and rails. Night-lights are essential for bathrooms and bedrooms. Adaptive devices that make getting on and off the toilet more safely are available. A cane, walker, or other assistive device may assist with balance.

> **Nursing Alert** Whenever you use a mechanical lift to assist a client into or out of a tub or bed, you must have thorough familiarity with the equipment's operation and safety factors.

Restraints (Client Safety Devices)

A restraint is anything that limits the client's free movement, such as a bed side rail, wrist restraint, or waist restraint. For example, a tray attached to a wheelchair that prevents the client from freely moving is a restraint. Another type of restraint is a **chemical restraint**, in which medications are given to control behavior. All healthcare providers and families need to learn about the laws related to the use and potential abuse of restraints.

If restraints are necessary, use them only after alternatives have failed to help and have been documented. Usually, a healthcare provider's order is required to apply restraints. Consult with the healthcare provider when you and other healthcare providers have exhausted other options. Explain to both the client and family or visitors that the purpose of the restraint is to keep the client safe. **Never** use restraints for your own convenience. A call light must always be within the client's reach if restraints are used. Proper application and frequent monitoring are required to prevent injury and ensure safety. Most clinical facilities have special forms for documentation of restraint use, the times that the restraint is checked, the steps required for their removal, and the behaviors that necessitate a restraint.

Although intended to reduce accidents, restraints can result in serious injury or death, such as strangulation, which may be a risk if a client attempts to escape from the physical restraint. Clients who feel powerless and frustrated will often exert much energy fighting against the restraint in an attempt to get out, causing self-injury. A chemically restrained adult often becomes confused and suffers impaired mental function; this client can fall and become injured. *Chemical restraints (medications used to control behavior)* should only be used as a last resort in a violent situation that could result in harm to the client or others. Medicare stated in 2000 in relation to LTC facilities that "*Chemical Restraints* is defined as any drug that is used for discipline or convenience and not required to treat medical symptoms" and prohibited their use at that time (Centers for Medicare and Medicaid Services, 2000). Because of these potential hazards, federal and state agencies that monitor and regulate healthcare facilities have placed significant restrictions that discourage the use of restraints of any nature. Nurses need to be aware of the policies of their facilities as well as any governmental regulations.

Frequently remind the client to ask for assistance and provide reassurance that someone is available and willing to assist, if needed. This information may help the individual feel more empowered. If the client is awake, aware, and cooperative but is at risk of falling because of physical weakness or impairment, a protective device or client reminder device may be used (Chapter 48). Side rails are another form of restraint. Both side rails should not be up on beds unless legal documentation exists. However, keep in mind that having one side rail up may assist the client when moving in or out of bed. To prevent falls, beds should remain in the lowest possible position. Instruct the client to ask for assistance when getting out of bed. Hospital beds are available for home use.

> **Nursing Alert** In some situations, the client is in more danger with the bed side rails up. A bed left in low position is safer than the client climbing over the side rails and falling.

Physical Activity and Exercise

Physical activity is an important part of a total health program for all people (Table 92-3). Exercise is vital to maintain circulation, muscle tone, and general health and to prevent disuse deformities. The older adult should participate in exercise that complements a former lifestyle. The ambulatory person can walk, stretch, swim, do tai chi or yoga, or participate in competitive activities. Exercises may be modified to suit individual needs such as after a stroke, loss of a limb, or a respiratory problem. Encourage clients of all ages to participate in active range of motion exercises; if this is not possible, provide passive range of motion exercises.

> **Key Concept**
> Walking is the single most highly recommended exercise for older adults.

> **NCLEX Alert**
> A situation on the NCLEX exam may include observation and education of safety issues. Discharge instructions or topics taught to the client prior to leaving the hospital are common clinical situations. NCLEX situations also focus on preventive measures, such as teaching the importance of exercise, avoidance of tobacco, and vaccinations for adults.

Immobility is a significant threat to older adults. The dangers of bed rest, even of short duration, and lengthy sitting include contractures, pressure wounds, constipation, renal and pulmonary complications (especially, pneumonia), cardiovascular disorders, depression, and social isolation.

Osteoporosis (a medical condition in which bones become brittle, often related to hormonal changes) is very common. Radiologic examination may detect loss of bone density, fractures, or loss of vertebral height (Fig. 92-3). Bone tissue loses density and strength without exercise; thus, fractures may occur very easily. Exercise can assist in reducing mineral loss from the bones. **Kyphosis** (curvature of the spine) can be associated with osteoporosis; this typically causes a humpbacked appearance ("dowager hump" or "widow hump"). Appropriate diet, increased calcium intake, supplementary vitamin D, and fluoride may be helpful. Postmenopausal women may be treated with calcium and cyclic estrogen administration. Physical activities promote physical and mental stimulation and help prevent such problems from developing.

CHAPTER 92 Gerontology: The Aging Adult

TABLE 92-3 Benefits of Exercise

SYSTEM TARGETED	BENEFITS
Cardiovascular	Increases endurance
	Lowers cholesterol to avoid atherosclerosis
	Maintains vascular elasticity to delay arteriosclerosis
Musculoskeletal	Increases bone mass to reduce osteoporosis
	Decreases fat-to-muscle ratio to maintain metabolism
	Retains strength and flexibility to ensure mobility and improve posture
Nervous	Improves mental health by reducing stress, fatigue, tension, and boredom
	Maintains or restores balance to reduce falls

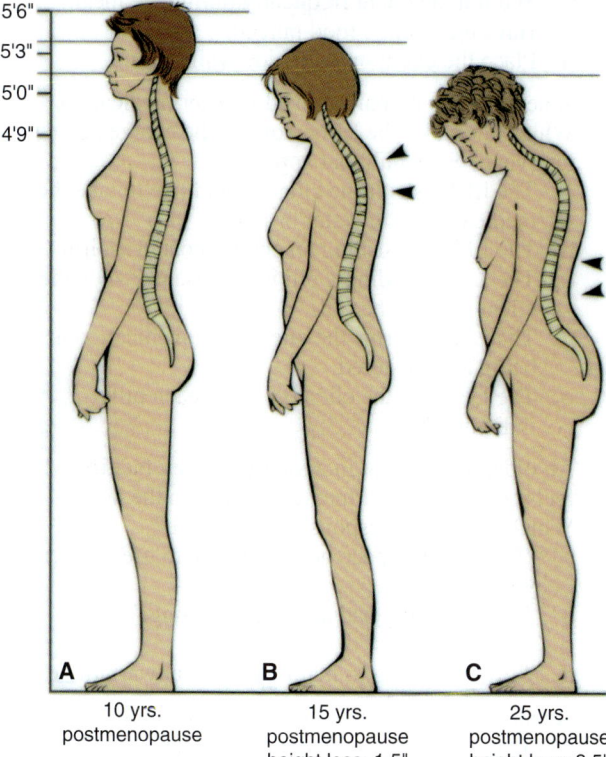

Figure 92-3 Typical loss of height associated with osteoporosis and aging. **A,** Height at 10 years after menopause. **B,** Loss at 15 years after menopause: 1.5 in. **C,** Loss at 25 years after menopause: 3.5 in.

Sexuality

Individuals generally maintain the ability and desire to engage in sexual activity as they get older. Physical changes caused by aging may require some modifications. Menopause does not affect sexual desire. Physical acts of affection, with or without intercourse, are important for an individual's physical and emotional well-being. The closeness of hugging and holding hands can alleviate feelings of loneliness. Touch can be therapeutic and beneficial at any age. Recognize the value of physical contact for older adults and assure them that the desire to be sexually attractive and active is normal. Encourage clients to discuss with their healthcare provider the impact of health conditions on sexual activity.

ELDER ABUSE

Elder abuse includes emotional, physical, and sexual abuse, financial exploitation, or neglect of older persons. Abuse or neglect may relate to health status and care, personal freedom, property, or income. Abuse takes many forms—any action that places a person in jeopardy may be considered abusive or neglectful. For example, sales gimmicks, medical quackery, fear tactics, and "con games" are considered exploitation of the older person. Organizations, such as insurance companies, mail-order sales companies, or religious groups, may defraud older adults intentionally or accidentally. Many oldest adult individuals (individuals who range in age from 80 to 100+ years) are considered **vulnerable adults**. Abuse of vulnerable adults is a crime, and all people, including family members and healthcare workers, are subject to laws protecting vulnerable adults.

The most common abusers of older adults are caregivers, which include adult children, other relatives, spouses, service providers, friends or neighbors, grandchildren, and siblings. The exhaustion and frustration of daily obligations related to caregiving can be overwhelming and is called **caregiver stress**. Be alert to signs of caregiver stress in a family because it may lead to mistreatment. Older adults, who are the victims, often fail to report abuse. Witnesses are difficult to obtain and many victims fear retaliation. Box 92-3 lists signs and symptoms of elder abuse.

Prevention of elder abuse begins with the recognition of high-risk families, including those families with a recent disruption in lifestyle or living arrangements, financial problems, substance abuse, a history of violence, or mental illness. The greater the number of risk factors, the greater the tendency

Box 92-3 Signs and Symptoms of Elder Abuse

- Frequent or no visits to healthcare personnel
- History of unexplained injuries
- Unacknowledged or untreated conditions or wounds
- Malnutrition or weight loss
- Inability to or lack of interest in self-care
- Inappropriate medication administration
- Depression, withdrawal, fearfulness to talk with healthcare professional
- Talks less about self
- Substance abuse of older adult or caregiver
- Nontypical spending or donating money

toward abuse. When working in such situations, remember to address the needs of caregivers as well as those of the client. Caregivers need to know what resources are available; a respite from daily care can offer them relief. Accessible community resources include social service agencies, home healthcare and homemaker services, and Meals on Wheels.

Key Concept

Be observant and aware of the possibility of elder abuse. In most states, it is illegal for a healthcare professional not to report abuse.

STUDENT SYNTHESIS

KEY POINTS

- The normal aging process does not cause specific illnesses. Lifestyle adjustments are necessary, however, to compensate for physical changes.
- Most older adults live at home. Some live in specially adapted living situations.
- Many health problems in older adults relate directly or indirectly to nutrition.
- As adults age, illnesses become more common and more debilitating for the individual. Adjustments are needed to maintain the instrumental events of the individual's daily life, and, sometimes, basic care measures, such as personal hygiene measures, are needed.
- Appropriate preventive care for constipation includes adequate fiber and fluids. Clients should avoid dependence on laxatives.
- Medications are a primary cause of problems for older clients. Responses to medications include confusion, dizziness, increased *potentiation or synergistic interaction* (one or both drugs' effects are greatly increased by the use of the other drug), increased sensitivity to drug dosages, and an increased number of side effects.
- Anatomic changes can lead to problems with continence.
- Presbyopia, presbycusis, and aphasia are three conditions that may hinder an older person's ability to communicate.
- Safety is an important consideration. Changes due to aging are often the cause of falls, for example, presbyopia, presbycusis, changes in proprioception, and decreased reflex reaction times.
- All adults must remain as physically and mentally active as possible to prevent anxiety, depression, and disorders related to immobility.
- By law, the nurse must report cases of suspected elder abuse.

CRITICAL THINKING EXERCISES

1. A diabetic male, H.Y., 72 years of age, is being treated at home for a foot ulcer. He lives with his daughter, her husband, and their two children. H.Y. has been living in his daughter's house for 8 months. What are the advantages for the client, for married couple, and for the children to have H.Y. reside in this home? What are possible disadvantages? What additional information would be needed?

2. Your neighbor, G.K., age 79 years, states that she is so stiff she can hardly move in the morning. During your conversation, she says that she still drives but states she does not bother to get groceries unless it is absolutely necessary. She asks you if you can help her move the TV. Would you have any concerns about this individual? Discuss the concerns that might need further investigation? State the reasons for your responses.

3. At the local department store, you meet a friend you have not seen for a long time. She is a retired adult female, aged 66 years. You notice that she has bruises on both her arms and seems to have lost a lot of weight. As a nurse, what might be the approach of your conversation? Are you obligated to report your observations to adult protective services? Debate and discuss this situation with your classmates. What additional information is necessary?

NCLEX-STYLE REVIEW QUESTIONS

1. A client has developed a large pressure wound on the right trochanter. How can the nurse best ensure this client's nutritional needs are met to assist with healing?
   a. Encourage the client to drink 2 L of fluid per day.
   b. Increase fat intake to 50% of total caloric intake.
   c. Give vitamin and mineral supplements.
   d. Increase daily protein requirements.

2. The nurse is caring for a client at risk for aspiration. What action would be best for the nurse to take when assisting the client with the meal to prevent aspiration?
   a. Have the client bend the chin toward the chest when swallowing.
   b. Suction the client frequently during the meal.
   c. Have the client's food pureed.
   d. Place the client on their side while eating.

3. A new LPN is preparing to administer medication. Which action by the LPN requires the charge nurse to intervene? Select all that apply.
   a. The LPN asks if the client would like to take the medication with water or juice.
   b. The LPN is crushing an enteric-coated aspirin.
   c. The LPN is hiding a pill in applesauce when the client refuses the pill.
   d. The LPN informs the client what medication is being administered.
   e. The LPN has the client swallow each pill individually.

4. An older adult client in a long-term care facility, who feels cold all of the time, reports this to the nurse. Which is the best response by the nurse?
   a. "I will find a space heater for you to use to warm you up."
   b. "Use a heating pad at a higher setting."
   c. "Take hot baths."
   d. "Layer clothing to maintain internal warmth."

5. An alert, oriented client voided incontinently, soiling clothing. What action by the nurse is a priority?
   a. Inform the client to use the bathroom next time.
   b. Provide assistance with washing and changing clothing.
   c. Tell the client that an adult diaper must be worn.
   d. Insert an indwelling catheter.

CHAPTER RESOURCES

Enhance your learning with additional resources on thePoint!
Student Resources related to this chapter can be found at thePoint.lww.com/Rosdahl12e.

93 Cognitive Impairment in the Aging Adult

Learning Objectives

1. Define and discuss the following terms: cognitive impairment, cognitive deficit, and intellectual disabilities.
2. State the risk factors for cognitive impairment. Compare the risk factors with those actions that can reduce the risk of cognitive impairment.
3. Discuss the signs and symptoms of confusion.
4. State how sundown syndrome can be identified. What actions can be taken to prevent sundown syndrome?
5. Differentiate confusion, delirium, and dementia.
6. Identify several causes of reversible dementia.
7. Describe the sign and symptoms of dementia and compare those symptoms with Alzheimer's disease.
8. Describe nursing interventions needed for the family and caregivers of clients with dementia.
9. Name common medications used to treat Alzheimer's disease and common adverse reactions to the medications.
10. Provide three reasons why medication use in older adults may differ from medication use in the younger population.
11. Identify how vascular dementia differs from Alzheimer's disease.
12. Differentiate between the three stages and the seven stages of dementia. Provide reasons why the seven stages of identification are most descriptive of the client's status.
13. Differentiate the following types of dementia: vascular dementia, frontotemporal disorders, Lewy body dementia, Parkinson dementia, Wernicke–Korsakoff syndrome, Creutzfeldt–Jakob disease, and HIV-associated neurocognitive disorder.
14. Discuss the nursing considerations for a client with dementia concerning ADLs, communication, behavior management, and family caregivers.

Important Terminology

agnosia, akinesia, aphagia, aphasia, apraxia, balking, catastrophic reaction, cognitive deficits, cognitive impairment, confabulate, confusion, delirium, dementia, dysphagia, idiosyncratic effects, infarction, intellectual disability, late-day confusion, mini-cognitive examination, mini-mental status examination, plaques, pseudodementia, respite care, sundowning, sundown syndrome, tangles, tau

Acronyms

AD, ADC, CJD, FTD, HAND, MCI, MMSE, MRI, NPH, PDD, PET, SPECT

This chapter examines various forms of *cognitive impairment*, also known as *cognitive deficits*, in the older adult. The normal aging process is responsible for some visual, hearing, and sensorimotor changes, for example, presbyopia, presbycusis, and arthritis. These changes will affect the ways in which adults behave and process information. Most individuals who have reached the young-old adult and oldest adult levels have productive, independent lives. A mild decline in some areas of the ability to think is considered normal, especially in the oldest adults. Normal decline tends to include some areas of visual and verbal memory, the ability to judge space (visuospatial abilities), short-term (immediate) memory, and the ability to name objects. Review the basic concepts of growing older in Chapters 13, 14, and 92.

Cognitive impairment may take the form of poor thinking skills, which are seen as basic aspects of confusion, delirium, or dementia. *Intellectual disabilities*, which typically are noted in early childhood, are also aspects of cognitive deficits. Children are usually diagnosed with intellectual disabilities by about the age of 5. These individuals had trouble learning as children and will continue having problems as they become adults. Therefore, individuals with permanent intellectual disabilities will be affected by new forms of cognitive impairment that are due to dementias as well as to the normal changes of aging. Every age group has both cognitive impairments and intellectual disabilities. Normal changes associated with aging can occur in addition to any pathologies of cognitive functioning. Sometimes the changes can be stopped and reversed. In other instances, the cognitive impairment may be a gradual neurologic decline, which is usually permanent.

COGNITIVE IMPAIRMENT

Cognitive impairment, sometimes called **cognitive deficit**, is an inclusive term used to describe a vast range of abnormalities in an individual's mental processes that lead to difficulty in the acquisition of knowledge and information. No single condition is responsible for cognitive impairment nor is it limited to any specific age group. Cognitive functioning provides the understanding and knowledge that enables the adult to learn, communicate, and interact with others. The term *cognitive deficit* tends to infer the person's ability to use intellect, that is, cognition is declining. When referring to someone who has difficulty with intellectual functioning, the term **intellectual disability** is more often used than cognitive impairment.

Individuals are unique in their ability to use their intellect. Intellectual disabilities are found in several areas of learning, that is to say, the ability to utilize cognitive functioning. Such disabilities will be affected by education, training, environment, genetics, past medical history, injuries, and age, plus a myriad of assorted detailed factors, such as the presence of stress or the availability of healthcare resources. Most of the time, the individual with intellectual disabilities has difficulty gaining knowledge, maintaining focus, and paying attention. Making appropriate decisions may be difficult for the person with intellectual disabilities because this cognitive function uses a high level of intellect, involving analysis and understanding of specific circumstances. Judgment, language, memory, perception, and reasoning are affected in ways unique to each person. However, new intellectual disabilities can be an adult problem related to genetic disorders, brain trauma or infection, and neurologic degeneration as found in Alzheimer's disease. It is also important to be mindful that the child with intellectual disabilities will grow into an adult who will have to cope with the changes of aging.

Cognitive impairment involves many risk factors. It is not caused by any one disease or condition nor is it limited to a specific age group.

Risk factors for cognitive impairment include the following:

- Increasing age—the primary risk factor
- Sex—female > male for Alzheimer's disease; male > female for mild cognitive impairment
- Genetics—family history and having a specific form of a gene known as APOE e4
- Down syndrome
- Low educational level
- Lifestyle: stressful, isolation from mentally or socially stimulating activities
- Brain disorders (e.g., tumor, trauma, infection, seizures, cerebral ischemia, normal-pressure hydrocephalus [age-related hydrocephalus])
- Exposure to toxins, air pollution, and pesticides
- Smoking or secondhand smoke
- Disorders (e.g., hypertension, sleep apnea, depression, diabetes)
- Lack of exercise—mental and physical
- Sleep deprivation or disturbances
- Medications—sudden stopping or starting of new drugs, idiosyncratic effects, paradoxical effects
- Changes in environment (e.g., being moved from home to church or from home to a hospital)
- Alcohol or substance abuse; withdrawal; Wernicke–Korsakoff syndrome
- Fluid and electrolyte imbalance
- Malnutrition or nutritional deficiencies (especially niacin, vitamin D, thiamine [B_1], or vitamin B_{12})
- Obesity
- Poorly controlled diabetes
- Hypercholesterolemia
- Neurodegenerative conditions, for example, Parkinson disease, Huntington disease, Pick disease,

> **Box 93-1** **Factors That Reduce the Risk of Cognitive Impairment**
>
> - Maintain good relationships with friends and family
> - Physical activity
> - Mental activity—memory games and exercises
> - Adequate time for sleep and rest
> - Healthy diet
> - Healthy weight
> - Manage health problems, including diabetes, high blood pressure, and high cholesterol
> - Use of protective clothing and safety devices (e.g., wearing helmets, using seat belts)
> - Protective adult vaccinations and booster vaccinations
> - Quiet, safe environment, especially around bedtime

Creutzfeldt–Jakob dementia (CJD), dementia with Lewy bodies (DLB), vascular dementias caused by hypertension, heart failure, stroke, diabetes

Factors that reduce the risk of cognitive impairment are listed in Box 93-1. There are various signs and symptoms of cognitive impairment.

Common signs and symptoms of cognitive impairment include the following:

- Confusion
- Changes in mode or behavior
- Memory loss
- Inability to stay focused on a topic
- Easily distracted; cannot focus; inattentive
- Continuously changing subjects during a conversation
- Being withdrawn or hyperactive
- Unable to make decisions or judgments
- Difficulty starting or completing a task—preparing a meal, writing a letter
- New behaviors related to changes in medications (addition or deletion)
- Idiosyncratic effects of medications
- Change in bowel or bladder habits
- Edema; respiratory distress; pain; fever
- Frequently asking the same question; repetition of the same story
- Failure to recognize familiar individuals
- Getting lost in a familiar environment

Confusion

Confusion is a loss of orientation to time, place, situation, and person, which is often combined with poor judgment and loss of memory. The confused individual may lack orderly thought processes or be unable to make decisions. Depending upon the causative factors, confusion may develop quickly or gradually. Confusion may be a symptom of an acute temporary problem, such as dehydration or severe emotional stress, and, with appropriate therapy, disappear without long-term consequences. Sometimes confusion is permanent and not curable, as may be seen with cases of early dementia. These disorders may gradually worsen and have permanent consequences, as occurs with chronic, organic progressive disorders such as Alzheimer's disease (**AD**). Confusion is always an abnormality because loss of cognitive function is not an expected component of the aging process.

Sundowner's syndrome, **sundowning**, or *late-day confusion* are terms that refer to a state of confusion developing at the end of the day and into the night. A nurse may see this type of phenomenon during the evenings and at nighttime in a hospital in adults with dementia. The person's behavior changes from its normal pattern to a state of confusion, anxiety, aggression, or combativeness. It is most often seen in clients who have mid-stage or advanced dementia. Typically, in the morning, the individual no longer demonstrates this level of confusion. The fading light that occurs at sunset seems to be a trigger for the problem. Risk factors that may aggravate late-day confusion include fatigue, low lighting, increased shadows, disruption of the body's internal clock, and difficulty maintaining a sense of reality versus a dreamlike state. Nursing considerations for individuals with this form of dementia include the following:

- Maintain a routine for daily hygiene, meals, activities, and bedtime.
- Limit daytime sleeping so that the adult is sleepy at nighttime.
- Limit sugar and caffeine in the afternoons and evenings.
- Use night lights.
- Provide a quiet environment that is free of stimulating activities.
- Use the same person, whenever possible, to provide care.

Delirium

Delirium is a serious disturbance of cognitive ability that begins with confusion, a reduced awareness of the environment, sleep disturbances, and restlessness. It progresses to anxiety, delusions, hallucinations, or fear. Delirium has a sudden onset (often hours or days) and may be reversible. Three main types of delirium are identified: hyperactive, hypoactive, and mixed delirium. *Hyperactive delirium* includes symptoms such as pacing, restlessness, agitation, and rapid mood swings. *Hypoactive delirium* may include reduced physical activity, sluggishness, and abnormal drowsiness. *Mixed delirium* includes symptoms of the other types, and the individual may rapidly switch from one mode to the other.

Causes of delirium include severe or chronic physical illness, hypoglycemia, metabolic and electrolyte disturbances, such as hyponatremia (low sodium), an infection (outside the brain), with high fevers, surgery complications due to anesthesia, drug or alcohol toxicity, long-term alcoholism (*Wernicke–Korsakoff syndrome*), dehydration, malnutrition, head trauma, sensory deprivation or overload, systemic infection, stress, severe sleep deprivation, and reaction to being in an unfamiliar environment (e.g., hospitalization, especially being in ICU, or admission to a nursing home). A key concept of delirium is inattention with a confusion that fluctuates, often dramatically, during the day.

Although delirium can occur at any age, older adults are more vulnerable to occasional episodes. Delirium does not result from the normal aging process. Older clients simply have decreased physiological reserve, that is to say, more physical and metabolic difficulties because of anatomical system deteriorations and can easily experience conditions that disrupt the body's balance and cause altered mental status. In addition, older persons are more likely to take multiple medications, which can produce delirium as an adverse effect. Delirium and dementia can be confused because the individual living with dementia commonly also has delirium; symptoms between the two are often indistinguishable. Occasionally, the agitation that accompanies delirium and confusion can pose a threat to health or safety to the client or a caretaker, including nurses. At this time, a low dose of a specific antipsychotic, haloperidol (Haldol), may be prescribed. *Idiosyncratic effects* (unexpected or unusual) and *paradoxical effects* (opposite to the expected reaction) are not uncommon side effects of medications in the adult, especially in older adults. Early recognition of the signs of delirium will ensure timely treatment and usually reverse the problem.

> **NCLEX Alert**
>
> A clinical scenario on the NCLEX can relate to the ability to differentiate between temporary conditions and permanent, progressive disorders. Also, be observant of the need for nursing interventions related to hydration, electrolyte disturbances, nutritional deficiencies, head trauma, and safety.

Mild Cognitive Impairment

Mild cognitive impairment (**MCI**) may be considered a transitional or intermediate stage between expected cognitive decline due to normal aging and the more serious mental impairment of dementia. Symptoms of MCI include ongoing problems in reasoning, judgment, perception, attention, language, reading, and writing. Some individuals have difficulties in some areas but not others. Some individuals have no difficulty with activities of daily living (ADLs). Friends and family may notice a change in mental processing, but typically the adult maintains the abilities to perform ADLs. As impairment progresses, the ability to perform the more detail-oriented instrumental activities of daily living (IADLs) will accompany confusion, frustration, forgetfulness, and depression. Diagnosis is made after a thorough review of mental performance. Normal aging often is accompanied by forgetfulness. However, MCI should be considered when the changes are consistent and increasing. Forgetfulness occurs more and often includes forgetting appointments, getting lost in a conversation, or after starting a task. Being overwhelmed by decisions or being unable to make decisions, depression, impulsivity, and increasingly poor judgment are more severe symptoms. If the individual gets lost in a familiar environment, such as the home, this is a significant symptom of MCI as well as of a more serious dementia.

The causes of MCI are not well understood, but evidence from autopsy or brain biopsy results suggests that mild cognitive impairment is a type of brain disruption as seen in AD and other dementias. Plaques, tangles, and Lewy bodies (which are discussed later on) may be found in the brain, which are abnormal clumps of protein similar to those associated with many dementias, including AD. A reduced blood flow will cause ischemia and may lead to strokes or a myocardial infarction (heart attack).

Treatment of MCI remains elusive, as no drugs or other therapies are specifically approved by the Food and Drug Administration (FDA) for this disorder. Sometimes the healthcare provider will prescribe cholinesterase inhibitors, which are designed for AD if the client's main symptom is memory loss. Cognitive impairment can be affected by other conditions such as hypertension, depression, and sleep apnea. Hypertension can damage blood vessels in the brain resulting in damaged brain tissue, leaving memory deficits. The results of hypertension can be mild (e.g., transient ischemia) to severe (e.g., a stroke). Depression is often accompanied by forgetfulness and loss of mental acuity. Sleep apnea results in excess fatigue, forgetfulness, and a lack of the ability to concentrate.

As stated earlier in this chapter, healthy lifestyles benefit the brain. A diet that is low in fat; has adequate fruits, vegetables, vitamins, and minerals; and heart-friendly omega-3 fatty acids promotes a healthy heart and brain. As a part of educating the client, remind the client that the diet has proteins, fats, vitamins, and minerals that are essential for nerve transmission and a healthy brain. These days, as the baby boomer population reaches the age of 65 years, many types of memory exercises or enhancements, also known as "brain games," are available. Suggest that a client take a memory training game along when they go for an appointment; the waiting room can be a place to play the game. Computer games, reading, and being involved in the community help preserve functioning and prevent cognitive decline. Encourage your clients to write out a list of things that they would like to accomplish.

> **Nursing Alert** Normal aging has a minor degree of memory loss, such as forgetting where you put your car keys or the name of someone you have not seen for a while. Concerns should be noted when a pattern of forgetfulness develops; when the quality and quantity of memory deficits increase with time.

Dementia

Dementia describes a group of symptoms that reflect progressive damage to the neurons (brain cells) until they die. This condition affects cognitive function, which is the ability to think, understand, and react appropriately to daily events. Typically, to determine the diagnosis of dementia, at least two of the following core mental functions must be affected, including memory, communication and language, ability to focus and pay attention, reasoning and judgment, and/or visual perception. Changes tend to begin with memory loss and continue to progress until cognitive impairment in multiple areas is noted. Dementia is not a specific disease and many disorders can cause dementia.

Dementia is not an expected part of aging. Normally, adults have some age-associated memory impairments as an expected part of aging. Dementias have a progression of physical abnormalities that affect memory and cognition; the neurons are damaged and eventually will die. For example, a normal aging adult may occasionally have difficulty finding the right words or expressions. Individuals with dementia have frequent pauses in conversation and substitute stories (*confabulate*) when they cannot find the right words. In a normally aging adult, the individual may be worried about memory loss, but close friends of family members do not seem to be concerned about any mental deterioration.

In contrast, the adult who has no concerns about memory problems is more likely to have dementia if the family and friends are concerned but the individual is not. Eventually dementia interferes with a person's ability to have normal social relationships or to perform self-care. Dementias are characterized by deterioration of emotional control, intellect, memory, judgment, basic arithmetic abilities, language, and independence. Dementia does not affect level of consciousness.

ASPECTS OF DEMENTIA

Dementia occurs in two main areas of the brain: the cortex and the subcortex. The neurons in the affected areas will typically show some pathology, such as tangles, plaque, infection, or Lewy bodies.

The first area of the brain to be affected is the *cerebral cortex*, the outer layer of the brain, where *cortical dementias* develop. Affected individuals with cortical dementias have memory loss and cannot remember words or understand language; therefore, the healthcare provider is more likely to see aphasia, amnesia, agnosia, and apraxia. Box 93-2 lists some common terminology associated with dementias. Alzheimer's dementia, frontotemporal dementia, and Creutzfeldt–Jakob disease are examples of cortical dementias.

Box 93-2 Dementia's Common Terminology

Agnosia—inability to recognize objects or persons via auditory, visual, sensory, or tactile sensations, such as not able to recognize the feeling of a full bladder or be able to identify familiar smells

Akinesia—difficulty moving; may be complete or partial loss of muscle movement

Amnesia—an inability to make new memories as seen in Alzheimer's disease

Aphagia—inability to or refusal to swallow

Aphasia—impaired communication via speech or writing due to a cognitive loss as with a stroke or a dementia

Apraxia—affects the body's physical ability to function: such as loss of familiar bodily movements; or to use familiar objects properly, such as in forgetting how to hold a comb

Compulsions—repetitive behaviors

Confabulation—fabricating details of events to cover up lack of memory

Delusional—having beliefs that are contradicted by reality, such as "I own the Empire State Building."

Dysphagia—medical term for swallowing difficulties

Emotional lability—rapid, unexplained, or inappropriate mood shifts

Hallucination—an experience involving the apparent perception of something (see, hear, feel, smell, taste) that is not, in reality, present; visual hallucinations are the most common for the client with delirium or dementia

Paranoid—irrational, obsessive distrust of others

The second area of the brain to be affected is below the cortex. *Subcortical dementia* is considered a clinical syndrome that is characterized by slowness of mental processing, clumsiness, forgetfulness, cognitive impairment, irritability, apathy, and depression. Examples include Parkinson disease, Huntington disease, and HIV-associated neurocognitive disorders.

The terms *cortical* and *subcortical* can be misleading because both classes of dementia can cause damage to both cortical and subcortical areas. Differentiation of these two classes depends upon the recognition that impairments in high-level behavior—that is, memory, language, problem-solving, and reasoning—are present as the earliest symptoms of the cortical dementias. Subcortical dementia is more likely to affect attention, motivation, and emotions. Early symptoms of subcortical dementia include depression, clumsiness, irritability, and apathy. As subcortical dementia progresses, symptoms that reflect cortical dementia will appear, such as problems with memory and judgment. The end stages result in the total breakdown of brain function of both the cortical and subcortical areas.

The types of dementias are more often associated with their underlying pathology or the causative problems than the area of the brain in which they occur. The most commonly known form of dementia is *AD*, with its *pathological plaques, tangles*, or *tau*, which may also be linked to other dementias. *Vascular dementia*, due to ischemic attacks in the brain, causes brain damage, which may result in signs of dementia. *Lewy body dementia* results from the formation of abnormal clumps of a protein called *alpha-synuclein*, which are called Lewy bodies, in the cortex of the brain. *Frontotemporal dementia, Creutzfeldt–Jakob disease, Parkinson disease,* and *Huntington disease* have similar and overlapping dementia symptoms. *Young onset dementia* (YOD) occurs before the age of 65 years in about 1 out of 1,000 people who have dementia. It typically starts in the fourth or fifth decade. People with Down syndrome have a much higher rate of developing dementia at a young age. *Infections of the central nervous system* include disorders such as meningitis, Creutzfeldt–Jakob disease, and HIV. HIV infections that occur in the later stages of AIDS are known as *HIV-associated neurocognitive disorders* (**HAND**). *Long-term alcohol abuse* can lead to Wernicke–Korsakoff syndrome. *Long-term substance abuse* due to street drugs or prescription medications produces a variety of problems. Normal-pressure hydrocephalus (**NPH**) is a type of hydrocephalus that occurs in adults older than 60 years caused by a slow accumulation of cerebrospinal fluid of the ventricles of the brain. The term *normal pressure* can be misleading; age-related hydrocephalus is more often related to blockages that develop slowly with aging. NPH can be confused with Alzheimer's disease or Parkinson disease. However, NPH can be successfully treated, unlike the other two diseases, if it is correctly diagnosed.

The causes or types of dementia may be reversible or permanent. Early diagnosis is an important aspect of treatment for all types of dementias. In some cases, if the underlying etiology is fixed, the dementia will disappear, for example, in thyroid disorders or hypoglycemia. Sometimes, the brain damage of dementia can be permanent but does not progress (e.g., head trauma). *Traumatic brain injury* (TBI) results from accidents, explosions, falls, or direct hits to the brain. Most of these injuries are preventable. Sometimes the brain injury will improve with time but, often, the damage is extensive and permanent. Repeated blows to the head, such as boxing traumas, with injury to the brain can cause *chronic traumatic encephalopathy* (CTE), which may occur decades or years after the brain injuries. An autopsy is needed to determine CTE.

> **Key Concept**
>
> When first meeting an individual who has a cognitive dysfunction, the nurse may find it difficult to determine if the disruption is owing to confusion, delirium, or dementia. Learning about the history of onset and observing the client's level of consciousness and cognitive abilities can help differentiate the condition.

Signs and Symptoms

Signs and symptoms of most dementias are listed earlier in this chapter in the section on cognitive impairment. In the early stages, individuals and their families may ignore or not notice the signs or symptoms. Often, observations of the client's behaviors and a discussion with the family caregivers will reveal early symptoms. Early signs of dementia include apathy, depression, poor judgment, confusion, disorientation, difficulty speaking, swallowing, and walking. Changes are usually *insidious* (gradual and cumulative). As the condition progresses, the person has increasing difficulty with social interactions and functional skills. Personality changes occur; exaggerated emotions are common.

More noticeable early symptoms include changes of behavior, such as getting verbally abusive, moody, or irritated in situations that were not previously bothersome. Difficulty in using mental processes, such as making a phone call or engaging in a conversation, will become more pronounced, with the individual showing increased frustration, anger, or apathy. These changes of behavior tend to gradually become more frequent. The individual may **confabulate**, which means to fabricate or make up imaginary experiences to make up for loss of memory. Sometimes the fabrications may be subtle; other times, they may be quite bizarre. The individual is generally confident about the truth of the story despite evidence to the contrary.

It is not uncommon to have symptoms that mimic dementia. Medical intervention and diagnosis can help differentiate between true dementias and dementia-like symptoms. These are conditions that are typically temporary and may be reversed. Examples of temporary conditions include adverse or unexpected responses to medications, metabolic or endocrine problems, nutritional deficiencies, infections, brain tumors, and hypoxia. **Pseudodementia** is used to describe the condition in which depression causes cognitive deficits that masquerade as dementia. Usually, the confusion clears when the depression is treated.

Diagnosis

Testing for Organic Causes

Before a diagnosis of any form of dementia is made, including AD, organic causes need to be considered and treated.

Diagnosis for several types of dementia depends upon ruling out other possible problems. Organic causes include electrolyte imbalance, hypothyroidism, hypoglycemia, and vitamin B_{12} deficiency. Individuals who take street drugs or many types of prescribed medications are also at risk for confusion and the early signs of dementia. If these deficiencies are repaired, there is a good chance that the problem will be reversed. Some organic problems, such as a brain tumor, HIV-associated neurocognitive disorder (HAND; which has several alternative names), subdural hematomas, normal-pressure hydrocephalus (NPH), and substance abuse can often be managed or even reversed with early diagnosis and treatment. If these disorders become chronic, the brain damage can become permanent. The prevalence of dementia and specific causative pathophysiology increases with age. Laboratory tests (Table 93-1) are performed to rule out and treat reversible causes of cognitive impairment. They are helpful in identifying risk factors associated with some forms of dementia.

Computed tomography (CT) scanning and magnetic resonance imaging (**MRI**) provide visualization of the brain's anatomy. Imaging studies such as CT and MRI scans will look for growths, abnormalities, general brain shrinkage. Progressive atrophy may be seen, which indicates changes beyond that of normal aging. These tests are helpful in identifying conditions such as strokes, closed-head trauma, hydrocephalus, vascular disease, tumors, and hematomas. They are not reliable, however, in confirming any diagnosis of dementia. Atrophy of the brain's hippocampus is one of the first signs seen in AD. (The *hippocampus* is the area of the brain associated with short-term memory and consolidation of short- and long-term memory.) Positron emission tomography (**PET**) may show decreased metabolism in some areas. A scan called single-photon emission computed tomography (**SPECT**) is helpful in evaluating blood *perfusion* (flow) to the brain and the brain's metabolic activity. PET scans, plus a special form of MRI, can increase the accuracy of diagnosis of various types of dementias. The electroencephalograph (EEG) records the brain's electrical activity. This test is not always performed, but it may rule out seizure disorders or other brain pathology. In AD, the EEG shows a generalized slowing of brain-wave activity. Distinctive EEG changes are also seen in CJD.

TABLE 93-1 Laboratory Studies and Causes of Dementia

TEST	POSSIBLE CAUSE OF PROBLEM	RATIONALE
Complete blood count	Anemia	Lack of oxygen (ischemia) in brain causes confusion.
Chemistry screening	Toxicity	Metabolic disturbances, kidney disease, and liver disease cause toxic, confused states.
Fasting blood sugar and other tests for insulin-dependent diabetes mellitus	Diabetes mellitus	Excessively high or low blood sugar levels can cause mental disturbances; nutritional disorders also can contribute to delirium and dementia.
VDRL, RPR, MHA-TP, or FTA-ABS	Syphilis	Tertiary syphilis causes dementia.
Erythrocyte sedimentation rate	Infection, immune disorders	Infectious agents can lead to toxicity; chronic inflammation can lead to ischemia.
Urinalysis	Urinary tract disorders	Uremia, infections, and toxicity can lead to dementia.
Thyroid panel	Hyperthyroidism, hypothyroidism	Confusion and depression can occur with abnormal thyroid levels.
Vitamin B_{12} and folate	Anemias	Inability to make or use red blood cells can cause ischemia to brain; also folate and vitamin B_{12} are low in chronic alcoholism.
Plasma homocysteine level	A high level usually caused by low vitamin B_{12} or folate	High level of homocysteine can cause arterial damage and blood clots.
Cerebrospinal fluid analysis	Meningitis, meningeal cancer, encephalitis	In rapidly progressive dementias.
Autoimmune testing	Vasculitis	Elevated in some cases of multi-infarct dementias.
Tests for HIV	AIDS	Later stages of AIDS can cause dementia.
Alcohol (ETOH); other chemical screening	Drug- or alcohol-related dementia	Rule out Wernicke–Korsakoff syndrome, crack-related dementias, and other chemical toxicities.
Electrolyte levels	Electrolyte imbalance	Excess or deficiency of some electrolytes can cause dementia.

AIDS, acquired immunodeficiency syndrome; FTA-ABS, fluorescent treponemal antibody absorption; HIV, human immunodeficiency virus; MHA-TP, microhemagglutination assay for *Treponema pallidum*; RPR, rapid plasma reagin; VDRL, Venereal Disease Research Laboratory.

> **Key Concept**
> The healthcare provider must perform a comprehensive physical and mental status evaluation to determine the cause of dementia. Definite diagnosis of dementia can only be made by brain biopsy or autopsy, but a thorough examination can rule out other, more treatable, disorders.

Psychometric Testing

Usually, the healthcare provider will perform a brief mental status examination as a screening tool to test the client's orientation to time and place; ability to register and recall information; attention, concentration, and calculation ability; and language skills. If a client fails the *mental status examination* (MSE), a psychologist can then perform more comprehensive *psychometric* (neuropsychological) testing. Tests could include standardized intelligence scales, memory scales, testing for judgment and planning abilities, and more comprehensive language testing. (Results of these tests are compared against those of unimpaired people in the same age group.) Neurological tests that evaluate a client's balance, reflexes, eye movements, and senses are also performed by the healthcare provider. Psychiatric testing may also be conducted to rule out psychoses.

An initial screening tool that is used in mental health and drug rehabilitation facilities, and periodically in long-term care facilities, is known as the **Mini-Cog**. The client is asked to identify three objects, draw the face of a clock from memory, and then recall from memory the three items identified earlier. The **mini-mental status examination** (**MMSE**) is a brief evaluation tool that is used in identifying problems with short-term memory and other areas of weakness. During the MMSE, the client is asked to state the time, date, street, city, and state of the location of the testing. Additionally, the client is asked to count backward, identify familiar objects, repeat common phrases, and perform basic skills in math, use of language, and comprehension. Finally, the client is asked to perform some basic motor skills. This tool is also used frequently in the above facilities.

Functional Assessment

A *functional assessment* is part of the diagnostic workup for dementias. The client is evaluated for the ability to perform basic skills (ADLs) required for daily functioning. Included in this assessment is the ability to perform the more complex skills or IADLs, such as meal preparation, shopping, telephone use, and transportation. Nursing considerations related to ADLs and IADLs are discussed in the Nursing Process section later in this chapter.

> **Key Concept**
> The person with dementia who resides in a long-term care facility may state, "I want to go home." Do not try to convince the resident that this is the home that has been part of the person's past life. It is not the "home" that the individual remembers. The nurse can make statements, such as "You are staying here. You are safe here." Distracting the person by initiating an activity may also help.

Progression of Dementia

The disease progression of dementia, particularly AD, is typically separated into stages, which should only be used as a general guide for the needs of care. AD is the most common form of dementia. More than one system is available to describe the gradual progression of loss of abilities. The categories may be listed as stages of dementia or of AD, since these terms are often used interchangeably. Be aware that it may be difficult to place a person with dementia, such as Alzheimer's disease, in a specific stage, as stages may overlap.

A common system of staging AD or dementia involves three stages:

1. *Mild AD* (early-stage): In the earliest stage, the individual remains independent, may work, and continues to participate in social activities. Early problems involve becoming forgetful of names, words, or objects. Concentration is difficult and the individual tends to forget what was just read or loses a valuable object. Difficulties start becoming obvious and the person cannot work with money, make travel plans, or organize a party.

2. *Moderate AD* (middle-stage): Memory problems worsen and the individual has greater difficulty performing tasks and remembering details and becomes increasingly forgetful. Emotional lability is noted; the person may be happy then angry or socially engaged then depressed and withdrawn. All these will have little to do with what is happening with the person. Personal details and life history are gradually forgotten. This stage is the longest, often lasting several years but with a steady rate of decline noted. The individual will need increasingly more advanced assistance with ADLs and is unable to do IADLs. The person generally has periods of hostility and frustration with periods of acting out, such as throwing things. He or she may be suspicious, have delusions, or exhibit repetitive behaviors such as tissue shredding or hand-wringing. Symptoms are noticeable to family and friends. Bowel and bladder control is gradually lost. The individual wanders and gets lost easily in a familiar environment such as a home or grocery store.

3. *Severe AD* (late-stage): In the final stage, the person has lost the ability to respond to the environment, cannot control muscle movement, and rarely speaks in sensible ways. The nurse needs to discern that the client is in pain using observation skills, vital signs, and individual behaviors. The individual needs extensive help with ADLs. Full-time assistance is needed. The person becomes vulnerable to the hazards of immobility, such as skin problems, contractures, and pneumonia. Family caregivers typically need emotional support from other caregivers or groups.

Another system that describes the gradual loss of abilities in more detail involves seven levels. These levels provide a more detailed overview of how abilities will change as individuals progress through each segment than does the three-stage classification of symptoms.

The seven stages of AD or dementia are as follows:

1. *No impairment:* The individual may have no obvious symptoms but testing may reveal a problem.
2. *Very mild decline:* Slight but noticeable changes in behavior but individual remains independent.
3. *Mild decline:* Trouble making plans with noticeable changes in thinking and reasoning. *Amnesia* or short-term memory loss. May repeat things a lot and have difficulty remembering recent events.

4. *Moderate decline:* Increasing problems making plans and remembering recent events. Traveling and handling money become difficult. Impaired communication (*aphasia*) may be noticed, which makes talking, listening, and writing much more difficult.
5. *Moderately severe decline: Agnosia,* or loss of the ability to correctly understand information, such as cannot utilize reminders such as important numbers and names of family or friends, a daily calendar/clock on the nightstand, or even recognize loved ones and may not be able to recognize words. Assistance needed with most ADLs.
6. *Severe decline:* Cannot remember the name of spouse. ADLs become more difficult; *apraxia,* the body's decreased physical ability to function, which includes difficulty with buttons and zippers, forget how to do basic grooming, and difficulty walking and eating. Changes noted in personality and emotions.
7. *Very severe decline:* Spends most of the time in bed unable to speak and cannot walk.

> **Key Concept**
> The pattern and progression of symptoms can vary greatly among clients with AD. There are four words beginning with *A* that you will find used frequently to describe the presenting symptoms of Alzheimer's disease: *amnesia, aphasia, agnosia,* and *apraxia.* See Box 93-2 for further descriptions.

Alzheimer's Disease

AD is a progressive, irreversible, fatal neurologic disorder and one of the most common types of dementia. Behavioral, intellectual, and emotional changes develop in fairly regular patterns, which are discussed in the previous section. AD has been called the "dementia from which the client dies twice": first in mind and then in body. AD has a progression of common patterns or stages. During a period known as *preclinical AD,* changes in the brain are discernible, typically several years before any onset of symptoms; this period can last for several years. On average, the person with AD lives between 3 and 11 years *after* diagnosis, depending upon the presence of other risk factors and chronic, coexisting disorders that were present at the time of diagnosis. The earlier section on cognitive impairment and Box 93-3 show the typical risk factors related to AD.

Signs and Symptoms

In addition to the discussion of symptoms and stages of dementia that have previously been discussed, the appearance of these symptoms is an important healthcare consideration to the family. Symptoms are minimally observable in the early stages, but they continue to progress until the individual is grossly impaired and unable to handle any component of self-care. The first mental functions clients lose are memory of recent events, abstract reasoning, mathematic calculations, and the ability to concentrate and complete complex tasks. Box 93-4 lists some factors to consider in the identification of AD.

> **Key Concept**
> Although the incidence of AD increases with each decade of life, this condition is not a normal outcome of aging.

> **Box 93-3 Risk Factors for Alzheimer's Disease**
>
> Researchers suggest that there is not one, but a combination of risk factors for Alzheimer's disease:
> - Age
> - Genetics—family history
> - Smoking and alcohol use
> - Changes in the brain, for example, trauma, infection
> - Atherosclerosis, for example, buildup of plaque (fatty deposits) in arteries
> - High cholesterol levels
> - Diabetes mellitus
> - Low levels of the vitamin folate
> - High plasma homocysteine level, for example, a type of amino acid
> - Decreased training/education or use of intellectual abilities
> - Diseases that affect cerebral blood flow, such as stroke, heart disease, and hypertension
> - Decreased physical, mental, and social activities which are seen as protective factors against Alzheimer's disease
>
> Adapted from the CDC Healthy Brain Initiative: Alzheimer's Disease – Aging Website: http://www.cdc.gov/aging/aginginfo/alzheimers.htm

Causes of Alzheimer's Disease

The vast majority of cases of AD are suspected to be caused by a combination of risk factors, including genetics, lifestyle, and environment. In a small proportion of the population, currently estimated at less than 5%, AD is caused by specific genetic changes. Individuals with genetic changes are highly likely to develop AD. It is important to know the family medical history so that early detection and treatment of genetic-based AD can be initiated. When compared with a healthy brain, the unhealthy brain has fewer *neurons* (brain cells) and a significant percentage of lost brain connections among surviving cells. In general, the brain of the AD victim actually shrinks due to the loss of neurons.

The specific pathology that initiates the start of the brain damage that results in dementias is not well understood. Microscopic examination will reveal damage to the neurons. Two types of abnormalities, known as *plaques* and *tangles,* are the key features of this type of dementia.

Plaques are "sticky" clumps and abnormal clusters of a beta-amyloid protein that accumulate between nerve cells. Small clumps of plaques damage and destroy cells by blocking the cell-to-cell transmission of signals at synapses. The clumps of plaques may also activate the immune system, trigger the inflammatory process, and destroy the disabled cells.

Tangles are twisted fibers made of **tau**, a protein that normally helps to maintain the transport system in the brain. When AD occurs, threads of tau proteins twist into abnormal tangles inside brain cells, and the messaging ability of the neurotransmitters is decreased. AD is characterized by a significant reduction in the brain's ability to make *acetylcholine,* which is a major neurotransmitter. Eventually, the transport system fails, and the decline leads to the death of the neurons. Most adults develop some plaques and tangles as part of the process of aging. Individuals with AD develop many more plaques and tangles that occur in a predictable pattern (Fig. 93-1). The

CHAPTER 93 Cognitive Impairment in the Aging Adult

Box 93-4 Signs and Symptoms of Alzheimer's Disease

Every person has difficulty remembering or doing things occasionally, but when these episodes become frequent or dangerous, medical intervention should be sought. The following represent some typical behaviors, but these examples do not represent behaviors for every individual:

- Gradual, but progressive loss of memory, starting with recent events (e.g., forgetting appointments)
- Loss of balance and proprioception (where things are in relationship to the individual)
- Difficulty paying attention (e.g., cannot follow directions)
- Gets lost, wanders, or forgets how to get somewhere in a familiar environment
- Becomes disoriented to time, place, and situation
- Asks the same question repeatedly
- Inability to work with money accurately (e.g., balance checkbook, make change)
- Unable to perform complex tasks (e.g., driving a car, shopping for food)
- Forgets to do important things (e.g., turn off stove, lock doors, close windows)
- Personality changes (e.g., moody, irritable, less trusting)
- Unable to think through a problem to a solution
- Loss of motivation and initiative
- Isolates self from others
- Unable to stand or sit unsupported
- Unable to dress or feed self
- Unable to recognize friends, family, and common items
- Loss of language skills:
  - Difficulty finding words or expressions
  - Inability to remember everyday words
  - Use of nonsense words
  - Repeating the last sound or word said by someone else

Adapted from various sources from the Administration of Aging (www.aoa.gov) and the Centers for Disease Control and Prevention (www.cdc.gov/aging).

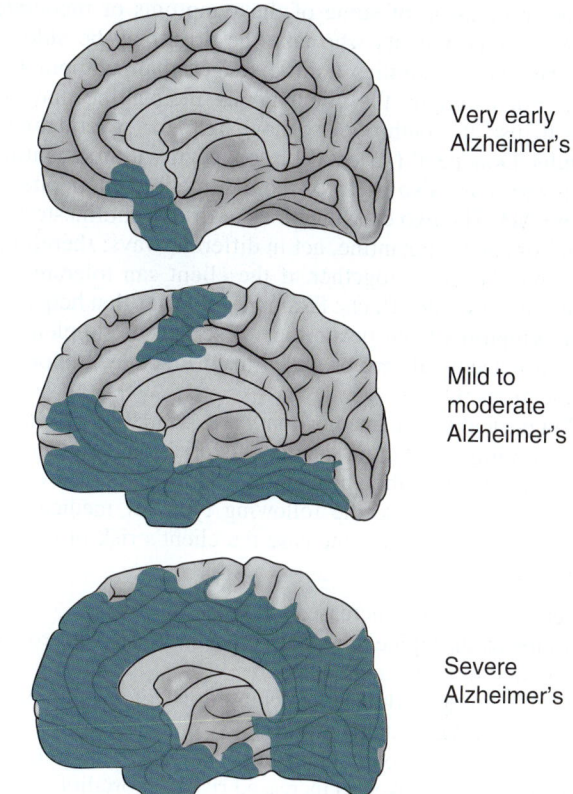

Figure 93-1 Progressive damage of Alzheimer's disease (Redrawn with permission from https://www.drrahulchakor.com.)

damage begins in the areas that are necessary for learning and memory and then spread to other areas of the brain.

> **Nursing Alert** It is important that the nurse remember to maintain gentle touch and eye contact with the client who has AD (Fig. 93-2).

Key Concept
The following are the most common symptoms of AD:
- Memory loss
- Inability to learn and retain new information
- Loss of judgment and planning skills
- Personality and mood changes
- Decreased reasoning and abstract thinking skills
- Loss of language skills
- Inability to care for self

Pharmacologic Treatment

No current medical treatment will stop the progression of AD. Medication therapy is generally palliative rather than curative. Current medications can relieve or delay the onset of some symptoms, which might slow the progressive mental deterioration. The goal with medication therapy is to delay the appearance of cognitive impairment and to improve the quality of life for both individuals and their caretakers. Delaying the deterioration of cognitive problems means that clients and their caregivers can have a more productive life for a longer period. The client will have comfort, dignity, and independence that, without the medicinal therapies, would be lost.

There are two classifications of drugs available to treat the symptoms of AD: cholinesterase inhibitors and memantine. Cholinesterase inhibitors are used for individuals with mild to moderate AD. The inhibition of cholinesterase helps prevent the breakdown of acetylcholine, which is considered important for normal memory and thinking. They only work for a limited time because the AD brain has less and less acetylcholine and, eventually, the drugs lose their effect. Examples are galantamine (Razadyne), rivastigmine (Exelon), and donepezil (Aricept). These medications are beneficial in delaying or preventing symptoms from becoming worse for a limited period time frame. They may be given to help control some behavioral symptoms.

A drug used to treat moderate to severe AD would be memantine (Namenda), an N-methyl-D-aspartate (NMDA) antagonist. Memantine is available as a pill or in a syrup form. As with cholinesterase inhibitors, memantine can delay progression of some of the symptoms of moderate to severe AD. Clients who take the drug may be able to perform daily activities a little longer than without the drug. For example, the client taking memantine may be able to use the bathroom without help for several more months. Donepezil (Aricept) or donepezil with memantine (Namzaric) are also used for the treatment of moderate to severe AD. The two classifications of drugs, cholinesterase inhibitors and memantine, act in different ways; therefore, they may be given together, if the client can tolerate the drugs and any side effects. Examples of drugs that help prevent symptoms from becoming worse and of supplemental pharmaceuticals are provided in In Practice: Important Medications 93-1.

Many additional medications are available to assist in controlling agitation, anxiety, depression, wandering, sleeplessness, or other behavioral disturbances. However, it is important to use the following types of medications minimally, as they may increase the client's risk of certain outcomes:

- Benzodiazepines (increased fall risk)
- Nonbenzodiazepine prescription sedatives (linked to impaired thinking and balance)
- Anticholinergics (linked to increased risk of developing or worsening Alzheimer's disease)
- Antipsychotics/mood stabilizers (dampen brain function and have been linked to increased risk of mortality)

Female hormones have seemed to help in some clients. With the proper use of medications, clients with AD and their caregivers may find it easier to cope with everyday activities. All medications must be used with caution in older people, who metabolize medications less rapidly than do younger people. For the older adult client, medications may have **idiosyncratic effects** (unusual or unexpected) or *paradoxical effects* (opposite effects to what is expected). It is not unusual for medications to increase confusion.

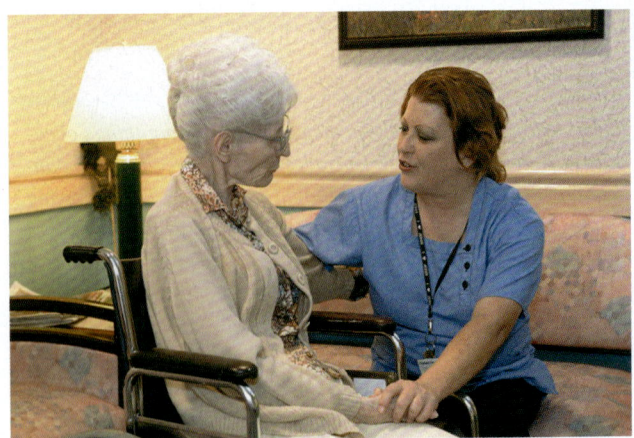

Figure 93-2 The nurse speaks calmly and distinctly to the client with Alzheimer's disease.

> **Nursing Alert** Be aware that medications should be a *last resort* in managing behavior problems in AD because of their numerous side effects. Attempt nursing management approaches to these problems *before* the use of chemicals.

Vascular Dementia

Vascular dementia, formerly called multi-infarct dementia, is caused by having ischemia and brain **infarcts**, which are localized areas of ischemic necrotic (dead) tissue due to anoxia, usually the result of an occlusion or an inadequate blood supply. This type of dementia is commonly part of overall, systemic vascular problems. Cerebrovascular disease and hypertension are the most common causes of vascular dementia. Adults who have had a series of small strokes can lose mental abilities as nerve cells die from lack of oxygen and nutrients. It is possible to have both AD and vascular dementia. Vascular dementia has a faster onset than AD and progresses differently. Additionally, vascular dementia usually coexists with other systemic conditions such as diabetes, hypertension and a history of strokes, heart failure, and vascular disease. An MRI can usually detect a stroke but may not be able to differentiate AD. If identified and treated early, this type of dementia can have a more positive outcome than AD.

Parkinson Disease Dementia

Parkinson disease dementia (**PDD**), or *Parkinson disease,* is a chronic, progressive neurological condition. In its later stages, cognitive impairment can become significant. Not all people with Parkinson disease will develop dementia. PDD may be difficult to distinguish from AD. Lewy bodies are seen with PDD. The client with Parkinson disease has a history of tremors before the onset of dementia. Resembling AD, the symptoms include problems with speech, reasoning, memory, and judgment, but individuals with AD do not typically have the tremors and muscle stiffness associated with Parkinson disease.

IN PRACTICE
IMPORTANT MEDICATIONS 93-1 — For Alzheimer's Disease (AD)

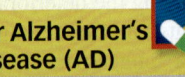

- *Slows memory impairment:* donepezil (Aricept); rivastigmine (Exelon); and galantamine (Razadyne)
- *Treats moderate to severe AD:* memantine (Namenda); memantine; and donepezil (Namzaric)

Additional Symptomatic Medications
- *Antipsychotics:* haloperidol (Haldol); thiothixene (Navane); thioridazine HCl (Mellaril); and chlorpromazine hydrochloride (Thorazine)
- *Antidepressants:* trazodone hydrochloride (Desyrel) and fluoxetine HCl (Prozac)
- *Hypnotics/sedatives:* estazolam (ProSom); quazepam (Doral); temazepam (Restoril); flurazepam hydrochloride (Dalmane); and chloral hydrate
- *Antihypertensives:* useful in prevention of vascular dementias, which can accompany AD

Wernicke–Korsakoff Syndrome

Wernicke–Korsakoff syndrome is the most common type of alcohol-related dementia. It is thought to result from direct damage to the brain by alcohol. It may be caused by nutritional factors, or it may result indirectly from liver damage. Short-term memory is most impaired, although people with this syndrome also may demonstrate poor judgment, lack of insight, diminished attention, and slowed thinking. They may not have the language or perceptual problems common in AD. The characteristic belligerent behavior patterns of some clients with Wernicke–Korsakoff syndrome can be problematic and require patience.

Frontotemporal Dementia

Frontotemporal dementia (**FTD**), also known as *Pick disease*, is rare and may be mistaken for AD. Symptoms are similar to those of AD; however, FTD involves primarily the brain's frontal and temporal lobes. Thus, symptoms may present in some clients as socially inappropriate behavior, impulsivity, and emotional indifference. In others, it may present as difficulty using language properly. FTD disease has an earlier onset than AD, most commonly between ages 40 and 50 years. It has a strong genetic component. The disease progresses steadily and generally more rapidly than AD, ranging from 2–10 years.

Creutzfeldt–Jakob Disease

Creutzfeldt–Jakob disease (**CJD**) is a rare dementia caused by a slow virus, meaning that the incubation period for harboring the organism and developing the disease is measured in years, rather than days, weeks, or months. CJD is an infectious dementia that is considered transmissible. Despite its long incubation period, its course is rapid; death almost always occurs within 2 years of onset. The type called *variant CJD* is known as "mad cow disease," which occurs in cattle but is known to be transmitted to people in specific circumstances. Both types are rare.

HIV-Associated Neurocognitive Disorder

HIV-associated neurocognitive disorder (**HAND**) has several alternative names including *HIV-associated dementia, AIDS dementia complex* (**ADC**), or *HIV/AIDS encephalopathy*. HAND occurs in late-stage HIV/AIDS. Dementia does not occur in all clients with AIDS; in some people with AIDS dementia, periods of lucidity remain until late in the disease. Cognitive impairment for individuals with HAND includes forgetfulness, reasoning skills, judgment, concentration, and problem-solving. HIV/AIDS dementia also shows personality and behavioral problems, difficulty with speech, and problems with movement such as poor balance with general clumsiness.

Other Causes of Dementia

Numerous physical disorders can cause brain injury that results in dementia. *Toxic dementias* are related to drug overdoses. *Metabolic dementias* can occur after untreated end-stage renal disease (*uremia*), hypoglycemia, hyperglycemia, hypothyroidism, hyperthyroidism, or hepatic failure. Structural problems caused by closed-head trauma, brain tumors, Huntington disease, and irradiation to the frontal lobes may also cause dementia. *Neurosyphilis dementia* may result from late-stage syphilis. This dementia can show deterioration in cognition and behavioral disturbances. This cognitive impairment can be treated with penicillin and sometimes reversed. See the Nursing Process display at the end of this section.

> *Key Concept*
>
> There is no way to predict which skills a client with dementia will lose. One part of the brain may be affected, but not another. Some clients retain specific skills until late in the disease. A thorough evaluation is necessary to determine the disease's extent and progression.

NURSING PROCESS

DATA COLLECTION

The healthcare team initially establishes baseline data for the client with AD or any other dementia for later comparison with deterioration trends. A discussion with the client's support systems (family, friends) is essential when determining short- and long-term treatment options.

Physical Assessment

History and Physical

After the healthcare provider performs a thorough history and physical, the nurse will complete the assessment. Include basic information, such as the client's immunizations, particularly flu shots, and protection against pneumococcal pneumonia, on the client's chart. Knowledge of a variety of other areas, particularly sensory deficits, is also important. Be sure to obtain substantial information about the client. The following information from the client or family will aid in determining the overall picture.

Visual Acuity Examination

Determine the date of the client's last vision examination. Determine if the client has been checked recently for glaucoma or cataracts and whether the person wears glasses. People with dementias often neglect personal healthcare measures. Perceptual problems are common. (They often believe something is wrong with their glasses and refuse to wear them.) They may lose or break their glasses. They may find it difficult to position themselves in relation to objects and may misperceive the edges of chairs or stairs, resulting in frequent falls.

Audiometric Testing

Find out if the client's hearing has been evaluated. Determine whether the client has had a hearing aid prescribed and whether the individual wears it. Also ask if it works; be sure that batteries are functional. (Limited or misinterpreted stimuli may contribute to confusion.)

Nutritional Status

Discuss the history of weight gain or loss and the time frame in which it occurred. Clients may forget to eat or forget that they just ate. Ask about ability to chew and swallow. Ask if the client wears dentures.

Sleep Pattern Disturbances
Ask about the total number of hours of rest the client gets at night and during the day. Ask if the person gets up during the night and, if so, how many times and for what reasons. Determine if a client's sleep problems are disruptive for family members.

Skin Care
Evaluate the client's skin condition. Check for dryness, bruises, sores, pressure areas, and cracked heels. Check fingernails and toenails.

Oral Care
Determine whether the client is able to brush the teeth or care for dentures. Ask if dentures fit properly, if the client wears them regularly, and if the gums have been checked recently for sores or irritated areas.

Psychological Assessment
Psychological assessment includes identification of past and present behaviors. Identifying behavior problems allows the healthcare team to develop a realistic nursing care plan, which includes family education. Behaviors are often responses to environmental cues; clients with dementia may be confused by these cues or may easily misinterpret them. Also, the nurse should try to avoid over- or understimulating all clients with dementia. Some common behaviors seen in AD and some other dementias are listed below.

Aggression or Agitation
Some clients undergo personality changes. A previously mild-mannered person may become loud, begin to curse and swear, and lash out at people. *Verbal abuse* (using hostile language, cursing, or making verbal threats) is the most common aggressive behavior found in clients living in community-based care settings. Clients also can be *physically aggressive,* especially with strangers (e.g., healthcare workers) who invade their personal space. Many hostile behaviors are responses to situations that confused clients perceive as threatening. Using a calm approach and keeping the environment and activities as stable and consistent as possible can assist in relieving anxiety.

Key Concept

Be sure to monitor the bowel elimination patterns of clients who have altered cognition. They often are unable to identify and communicate the absence of regular bowel movements. Fecal impactions may result.

Anxiety or Paranoia
As clients lose short-term memory and time orientation, they cannot understand what has recently happened or what will happen next. They may show *anxiety* by rummaging through drawers, wringing their hands, pacing, or displaying worried looks. As they misplace things or cannot recall their location, clients may believe that items have been stolen. *Paranoia* may lead to accusations. Some clients may cover windows and move furniture in front of doors because they are afraid. In nursing facilities, simple tasks, such as bathing or showering, may frighten clients because they do not understand what is happening. Breaking activities into simple steps and providing short comments may help (e.g., "I'm going to wash your face now.").

Hallucinations and Delusions
Hallucinations are false sensory perceptions that may be auditory (e.g., hearing voices) or visual (e.g., seeing a person). Hallucinations may also involve the senses of taste, touch, and smell. Sometimes, clients believe that people on television are in the room with them or that their own reflection is another person. *Delusions* may cause confused ideas, such as believing that a bank has confiscated all of the client's money or that a spouse is going to kill the client. These symptoms are usually related to organic changes in the brain; trying to reason with the client will not work.

Withdrawal and Depression
Clients who retain insight into their cognitive and physical losses may become depressed. Report a client's feelings of worthlessness to a healthcare provider. *Suicide* (accidental or intentional) is a risk during the early stages of AD. Some clients respond to antidepressants. In many clients, symptoms of depression seem to decrease as the dementia progresses.

Determination of Abilities to Perform Functional or Basic ADLs
An important part of nursing care is determining a client's ability to carry out basic daily tasks.

Dressing, Bathing, and Grooming
Determine if the client is able to dress appropriately. Danger signs include soiled clothes worn repeatedly, and clothes put on in an incorrect sequence (e.g., clients may wear two dresses or underwear on the outside). Determine whether the client bathes. Danger signs include an inability to set water temperature or a lack of grooming. The nurse makes observations and documents the client's ability to do ADLs, such as shaving, combing hair, brushing teeth, or using makeup. Determine if these abilities have changed recently.

Nursing Alert The most common cause of burns in older people is hot water. Take steps to control the water temperature available to clients with dementia. These clients also may be afraid of water and may be particularly confused in the shower.

Toileting: Bowel and Bladder Control
Evaluate whether the client is able to remain continent, locate and use the bathroom independently, perform the tasks in the right order, and accomplish basic hygiene practices. If incontinence exists, determine if it can be managed by scheduled toileting.

Drugs, such as the antipsychotic haloperidol (Haldol), can cause urinary retention. Reducing the Haldol dose may help prevent overflow incontinence. Regular toileting helps to maintain usual urinary function.

Ambulation and Transfer
Determine if the client can walk without assistance. If the client uses a cane or walker, evaluate the ability to use it safely. Danger signs include a history of falls or unsteady gait, wandering off and getting lost, unexplained cuts and bruises, or several falls within the past year.

The family (or the long-term care facility, if the client resides there) also should have a recent photo of the person, in case this person becomes lost and police need to assist in the search. (A photo will help with identification.)

> **Nursing Alert** Clients with dementia must wear some sort of identification in case they wander and become lost. They can wear ID bracelets or sewn-on name tags. Hospital identification bands may work well because they cannot be removed easily. Placing bands around ankles rather than wrists might be better because the bands are then out of a client's sight. At least two telephone numbers should be on the identification. Identify the client as memory impaired.

Eating
Determine whether the client can use utensils and cut food. If the client needs to be fed, determine whether the individual is cooperative, is able to chew, and remembers to swallow. Danger signs include a history of choking, confusion with utensils, and refusal to eat. Be sure to monitor food and fluid intake and weight.

Communication Skills
Although variable for each client, language skills gradually deteriorate as dementia progresses. To determine the ability of the client to communicate, notice if the client repeats questions or stories, has difficulty finding words or naming objects, or makes up nonsense words or phrases. Skills deteriorate in different ways and at different times. For example, some people lose the ability to speak, but still understand written language; others lose the ability to understand all forms of language. Music and social skills tend to remain intact until late in the process.

Determination of Abilities to Perform Complex or Instrumental ADLs

Management of Finances
Determine if the person is able to handle a checkbook, pay bills, and make change. Clients with dementia may pay bills more than once or forget to pay them at all. They may make large contributions to charity because requests look like bills. They also may become victims of con artists. Clients may hide or lose checks. Danger signs include many unpaid bills, disconnected utilities, or misplacing or donating large amounts of money. Solutions include having Social Security checks deposited directly, bills sent to a family member or guardian, and a cosigner required for all checks.

Driving
Determine if the client is able to drive safely. Is the person having accidents, getting lost, or trying to get out of moving cars? Danger signs include near misses, accidents, or signs of poor judgment. It may be necessary to request that the state remove the person's driver's license or retest him or her. The family may need to remove any car keys from the client so that driving is not possible. In some cases, the person's car must be sold or taken from the home.

Public Transportation
Evaluate whether the person can take a bus or train without getting lost, can make correct change, and can get transfers.

Food Preparation
Determine whether the client is able to follow recipes and instructions. Check if items are left on burners, pots or pans are burned, or food stored unsafely. Danger signs include spoiled foods, evidence of fires or burned pans, or hoarding large amounts of food. A solution may be to contact Meals on Wheels for assistance and disconnect the stove.

Shopping, Housekeeping, and Laundry
Determine the client's ability to shop. Note if there has been a change from previous patterns of cleaning. Can the individual remember how to use common household machines? For example, is the individual able to use the settings on the washing machine, measure detergent, and load clothes? Danger signs include large amounts of the same items in the house, items stored in the wrong places (e.g., frozen foods in the cupboard), messy home environment (in a previously neat home), presence of insects and rodents, washing everything by hand, and soiled clothing in closets or drawers. The solution is for family members to perform or to supervise these tasks or to arrange for help through homemaker services.

Telephone Use
Determine the client's ability to dial and recall phone numbers for emergencies. Danger signs include inability to dial telephones, repeated calls, or calls in the middle of the night to others. The solution is to keep a list of numbers near the telephone. Install a computer dialing device and have family members or friends call often to check on the client and caregiver.

Safety in the Community
Determine if the client can take measures to remain safe in home and out in the community. Danger signs include opening doors to strangers, giving money to strangers or neighbors, and becoming victims of scams. Persons with AD also may have problems in neighborhoods, such as walking into other people's houses, hitchhiking, or requesting money from neighbors.

Determination of Support Systems

The Family
AD and other dementias are overwhelming for family members. In many ways, the disease strikes not only the client but the family as well. An important part of assisting the person with dementia includes understanding the

needs of family members and other primary caregivers. Sometimes, complex networks of friends and neighbors provide necessary supervision or care for clients affected with dementia. The entire family or caregiver needs a great deal of support and education about caring for the client as the disease progresses.

Caring for a person with AD in the early stages interferes with the family's recreational time. In later stages, caregivers spend most of their time supervising confused and emotional clients, and this can be exhausting. They need to balance their caregiving with personal activities that bring pleasure. Without respite and balance in their own lives, the incidence of elder abuse by caregivers is significant.

Aging Caregivers
Conflicts can arise among the demanding roles of caregiver, spouse/partner, parent, and employee. Spouses of people with dementias are often older adults themselves. Caregivers may be unable to handle the physical and psychological demands necessary to manage the constantly increasing level of care. Support groups and respite care can prove beneficial to the health and well-being of caregivers.

PLANNING AND IMPLEMENTING
Management of the person with dementia includes caring for basic personal needs, but it also requires a basic understanding of communication and behavior management techniques. Teach caregivers and serve as a role model. Daily routines may help clients. Monitor the client's ability to perform IADLs because when these higher level abilities are lost, the client will have increasing difficulty performing ADLs. Many nursing interventions are provided in the next section. Listen to their concerns and be aware of problems that are arising. In Practice: Nursing Care Plan 93-1 highlights a priority nursing diagnosis for the client with AD who is hospitalized. See also In Practice: Educating the Client 93-1.

IN PRACTICE
NURSING CARE PLAN 93-1 — The Client With Alzheimer's Disease Who Is Hospitalized

Medical history: J.S. is a 73-year-old married man with a history of AD who is admitted to the hospital with a fever of 102.5 °C (39.1 °C), confusion, and periods of agitated behavior. Does not respond appropriately to time, place, or situation. Can state his name and his wife's name. Laboratory studies show a WBC of 13,500, Hgb 11.3, and Hct 37%. UA is concentrated and has bacteria TNTC (too numerous to count) noted. Culture results pending. Chemistry results pending. CT scan of brain scheduled for after admission to hospital. Referral to neurologist Dr. Y.H. made for information r/t diagnosis and stage of AD. Referral to urologist for UTI, possible sepsis.

Medical diagnosis: Urinary tract infection, rule out sepsis; Alzheimer's disease.

DATA COLLECTION/NURSING OBSERVATION

Nursing Admission Note 0945: Client and his wife of 32 years were oriented to hospital room and electronic bed. Husband does not seem to understand how to work the controls. Client responds appropriately to simple questions but cannot state why he was brought to the urgent care center or admitted to the hospital. Wife remains with husband in hospital room and asks if she can stay the night. Client is alert at present and able to state his name, but unable to state day of week, month, or year and unable to state the reason for his current situation. Sitting up in bed, he seems anxious and asks inappropriate questions. Wife states that this behavior is not typical. Currently, client lives at home with wife. She states, "His doctor has said that he is progressively getting worse." She reports increasing problems with memory, reasoning, judgment, and social interaction. "A few weeks ago he got lost inside the house. He frequently roams and paces around the room." She reports that her husband wakens frequently at night and has difficulty voiding. Wife reports that she used to be able to coach him to wash and dress, but his behaviors have changed in the last few weeks. "Sometimes he gets so irritable. When I talk to him and try to get him to get dressed or to eat, he refuses. I don't know what to do to make him better." At 10:00, Tylenol given for fever of 102.5 °C (39.1 °C). At 10:30, temperature of 101.2 °C (38.4 °C). Client sitting in bed looking out window; wife at bedside.

NURSING DIAGNOSIS

(Although other nursing diagnoses may be appropriate, a priority nursing diagnosis is addressed below.) ADL deficit (bathing/hygiene, dressing/grooming) related to altered thought processes secondary to febrile state and stated advancing history of Alzheimer's disease as evidenced by wife's statements about difficulty with washing and dressing.

Planning (Outcomes/Goals)	Implementation (Nursing Actions)	Evaluation
Short-Term Goals		
A. Prevent urinary tract infection from becoming septic.	• Treat urinary tract infection with ordered antibiotics and antipyretics. • Monitor culture results from UA. • Monitor change in fever during the next 24 hr. • Obtain blood cultures. • Explain each intervention, test, or treatment clearly and calmly to the client. *Rationale: The priority of nursing actions is to treat the most life-threatening problem which, at this juncture, is the UTI because it could develop into sepsis. Blood cultures results may take 2–3 days before sepsis can be ruled out as a diagnosis. Sepsis has a high mortality rate, especially in the elder adult. When the fever is less than 100 °F (37.7 °C), the client may become less confused. If not, the confusion may be due to pathology in the brain r/t Alzheimer's disease. Nursing care would be to ensure infusions of IV antibiotics and PO antipyretics are given as ordered. Maintaining a safe environment may be difficult due to client's combined risk factors of confusion, fever, and AD. Having his wife stay in room and assigning a room close to the nurses' station may be helpful.* • Provide for client's safety. • Promote wife's support. • Share plan of care with wife. • Provide in-room stay for wife as requested. *Rationale: The 32-year relationship between wife and husband may help prevent further deterioration from reality r/t new hospital environment, fever, illness, and AD. The relationship between couple promotes trust that may include nursing staff.*	Admitted to hospital room Day 1—10:00 hr • Client's temperature dropped to 101.2 °F (38.4 °C) after Tylenol, which shows improvement from initial admission temperature. • Client confused r/t environment. For the first 6 hr after admittance, he thinks that he is at home. • At 8 hr after admission, client is less confused and able to talk to wife about being in the hospital. • UTI seems to be responding to antibiotics. *Goal A complete. Observations ongoing.*
B. Client will participate in self-care activities within the limits of his disease.	• Discuss with client's wife the client's usual routine of care. • Provide slow, step-by-step instructions for the client when providing hygiene. • Provide positive comments. • Encourage wife to bring in personal care items from home. • Label client's articles that have been brought from home, ie, toothbrush, comb, brush, socks, and pajamas. *Rationale: Familiarity helps to allay anxiety. Reduction of the number of new situations is important as this will greatly aggravate client's sense of trust and decrease incidences that might make the client feel threatened. Slow, step-by-step instructions help the client to focus on the task and complete it with minimal frustration.* • Assign nursing staff to maintain consistent care for client. • Minimize the number of people going into and out of room. • Attempt to maintain an atmosphere and routine of care similar to that experienced by the client at home. *Rationale: It is unlikely that only one nurse can be assigned to client, but utilizing the same people will support the concepts of routine and consistence, which is needed for clients with AD. Routine and consistency help promote trust and security for the client with dementia.*	In hospital Day 2—1,900 hr • Blood cultures preliminary report does not indicate sepsis. • Hygiene activities scheduled in evening as per client's usual routine at home. • Client's articles brought in from home and labeled. • Client participated in washing face and hands with verbal guidance. • Per wife's statement, he seems to be "adapting to hospital routine." • Client seems to have an improved sense of well-being and comfort. • No signs of anxiety noted in day 2. Cannot state reason for being in hospital; remains confused to place and situation. *Progress to meeting Goal B.*

Planning (Outcomes/Goals)	Implementation (Nursing Actions)	Evaluation
Long-Term Goals C. Prepare client and wife for postdischarge actions r/t disease progression.	• Describe stages of AD to wife; explain current stage of AD progression • Teach wife the signs and symptoms of UTI. • Ask wife to state her ability to aid in care of husband. • Discuss expected future behaviors of a client with AD. • Discuss with wife the possibility of having the client transferred to a long-term care facility after discharge from the acute care hospital. • Discuss the care that the husband will need if he is transferred to home. • Arrange for wife to receive respite care. *Rationale: Having the client's wife present can help to allay the client's anxiety and fears.* Encourage the client to verbalize feelings of fear, frustration, and anger when they occur. Verbalization helps to reduce these feelings. Acceptance of client's progression of AD in order that plans can be made is often difficult for the client and family members.	In hospital—Predischarge Day 3—1,630 hr • Client's physical and psychological assessment monitored for 2 days. With wife's help, he is able to assist with some parts of ADL. • Team meeting including wife for discussion of future. Wife states that she "can still take care of him at home for now." • Morning UA specimen reveals no infection. • Client's dementia has not improved or worsened in the last 2 days. • Most of the time, the client remains confused to time, place, and situation but does follow simple directions and responds to name. • Discharge planning preparing wife for home care at this time because she does not want to admit husband to LTC. • Wife states she will continue to monitor temperature at home for potential reoccurrence of UTI. *Progress to meeting Goal C. Ongoing observations. To continue contact with family with home healthcare visitations.*

IN PRACTICE
EDUCATING THE CLIENT 93-1 — Provision of a Safe Environment for People With Cognitive Dysfunction

- Do not allow the client to drive (remove keys, disable car, revoke license).
- Remove guns and ammunition from the house.
- Supervise smoking; lock up supplies; use only ashtrays that will not tip or melt. Encourage smoking cessation.
- Disable stove or supervise cooking.
- Supervise use of knives and forks; lock up utensils.
- Turn down temperature of water heater.
- Remove dangerous power tools; supervise use of small power tools.

- Supervise use of razors (allow only an electric razor) and supervise use of electrical appliances; do not allow appliance use around water; do not allow use of dangerous appliances (food processor, garbage disposal).
- Supervise use of electric fans or air conditioners.
- Lock up all medications, over-the-counter remedies, poisons, paints, and cleaning solutions. Make sure the primary caregiver knows how and when to administer medications; do not leave with client to take unsupervised.
- Supervise use of china and glass dishes to prevent injury from breakage.
- Put a control on thermostat or disable it to prevent the person from constantly adjusting temperature.
- Reduce potential for falls by keeping floors clear of debris (but not highly polished), wiping up spills, and not using throw rugs. Have good railings on stairways. See that the person's shoes fit well. Have halls and stairs well-lighted.
- Install safety locks and buzzers on doors (in case person wanders). Make sure person has identification at all times. Many persons can get through locks and dismantle doors. Fence yard; control access to dangerous areas (swimming pool, beach, highway).
- Keep emergency numbers next to each phone; a preprogrammed phone is a good idea.
- Find a good home for pets, if this person is no longer able to care for a pet safely.

Assisting With Daily Care

Bathing
Bathing is frightening for clients with dementia. The client might tolerate a bed bath much better. When assisting with baths, schedule a preferred time for clients and be calm. Rested clients are more cooperative than those who are overtired or overstimulated. Use low water levels and have everything prepared before the client enters the bathtub. Avoid the noise and confusion of a whirlpool or shower. Pad the walls to reduce echoing (overstimulation). Use positive reinforcement ("You look so handsome!"). Use gestures; do not shout to be heard. A smile is understood by the confused individual.

Dressing
For clients with dementia, dressing becomes complicated. Lay out clean clothes, and remove dirty clothes (to prevent confusion). Offer clothing in sequence, one piece at a time. Do not give several verbal commands at once because they can overwhelm clients. Use simple clothing (Velcro, elastic waistbands). Suggest that clients wear cardigan or button-down shirts or blouses instead of those put on over the head (covering the head is frightening). Clients may be unable to manage buttons without help.

Pain Control
Pain control may be difficult to quantify in the person with dementia but pain control is very important. Individuals in pain may have aberrant behaviors such as anger, withdrawal, apathy, depression, or aggression because they cannot verbally state their sensations. Keep the concept in mind that clients with dementia may experience pain, but be unable to express it. Older clients often have arthritis, chronic back pain, chronic neck pain, or many other physical disorders. Give pain medications before performing care measures, such as bathing or dressing. The effectiveness of pain control may be seen as a change of behavior, for example, improvement from aggressiveness to being cooperative.

Nursing Alert Monitor the client's weight. If weight loss is evident, the client is probably forgetting to eat. Agitation and pacing also take a great deal of energy. Remind the client to chew and swallow. Observe for choking.

Nutrition and Hydration
Maintaining nutrition and hydration is important. As people age, their sense of thirst becomes less acute. Many older people tend to forget to drink or eat. Offer small amounts of fluid each time you interact with clients. Vary choices by providing gelatins, ices, juices, herbal teas, and soups; do not give plain water all the time. Avoid very hot liquids (people with poor judgment are likely to spill liquids and be burned). Limit the variety of foods to prevent confusion. Cut meats to appropriate sizes to prevent choking. Place clients near people they should mimic. If a client is able to self-feed, place the spoon (forks may be dangerous) in the client's dominant hand. Give finger foods if the person cannot manage the utensil.

The person living at home is in danger due to the stove. Gas is particularly dangerous. Remove the knobs or install a master shut-off for either electric or gas stoves.

See In Practice: Nursing Care Guidelines 93-1 for monitoring hydration.

Bladder and Bowel Management
Bladder and bowel management often becomes necessary for clients with dementia because incontinence is common in later stages. Clients can avoid daytime episodes by regular toileting. Label the bathroom; give one-step instructions, and make each step simple, identifying one activity with each step. ("Come with me. Pull down your pants. Sit down.") Families need education in the use of continence products at home. Document bowel movements; be alert for constipation or impaction. If a client develops diarrhea, check for lactose intolerance, constipation, or drug reactions. Blood electrolyte levels may be ordered if diarrhea continues.

UNIT 13 Gerontologic Nursing

IN PRACTICE
NURSING CARE GUIDELINES 93-1 — Monitoring a Client's Hydration Status

- Monitor intake and output.
- Remind/assist the client to take a drink every time caregivers come into the room.
- Increase fluids for clients who have dementia to prevent urinary tract infections and to allow the bladder (which is a muscle) to contract properly.
- Some medications promote urinary retention; therefore, closely monitor clients who are taking such medications.
- Check for edema and test skin turgor for signs of "tenting."
- Documenting "skin turgor +1" indicates that the skin stays pinched for about a second and indicates that the client is somewhat dehydrated.
- Documenting "skin turgor +4" on the client's chart means that the skin stays elevated ("tenting") for about 4 s and that the client is very dehydrated.

Assisting With Communication
Use all the communication skills you have learned. Your verbal and nonverbal communication skills greatly influence how others respond. If you remain calm, you will have a calming effect on clients. If you are quiet and gentle, clients are more likely to cooperate with you. If you are agitated and in a hurry, clients may respond to your behavior and become upset and belligerent. See In Practice: Nursing Care Guidelines 93-2 for communication guidelines.

Assisting With Behavior Management

Anxiety
Anxiety is common in persons who have dementias. Often, these clients display frustrating behaviors, such as pacing or rummaging through closets or drawers, which help them to feel more in control. Reassure anxious clients. Keep commands simple, and reward successes. Work in small groups, and encourage family members to visit one or two at a time. Keep the client's environment and daily routines consistent; assign the same caregivers daily if possible. Allow clients to move around. Eliminate caffeine and limit sugar in the diet. Avoid overstimulation.

FAMILY VISITS WITH THE CLIENT WHO HAS DEMENTIA

Balking
Balking, which means refusing to do things, often occurs when clients do not understand what is expected. If a client balks, go away briefly, and come back later with a pleasant tone of voice. Model expected behavior or have clients mimic others (e.g., eating at a table with others).

Persons with dementias commonly display **catastrophic reactions** in which they become overly agitated when confronted with situations that are too overwhelming or too difficult for them. The best approach when this occurs is to cease the activity and allow quiet time or time out.

Paranoia
Paranoia or fearfulness is common. Keep the environment calm and predictable; remove excess stimulation or items that can contribute to misperceptions (e.g., mirrors, intercoms, lamps that cast shadows). Do not try to reason with paranoid clients, but reassure them that they are safe.

Aggressiveness
Aggressiveness can be physical (striking out), verbal (name calling, cursing), or sexual. Use a calm approach. Do not confront or try to reason with clients; scolding aggravates aggressive responses. If necessary, remove clients from the group (to avoid upsetting others). Validate their feelings ("You seem angry or frightened."). Give reassurance ("You are safe."). If a client strikes out when you try to perform nursing care, leave temporarily. Allow the client time to calm down, and then return. Remember that your tone of voice can either soothe or upset clients. Try to identify factors (triggers) that cause these outbursts so that you can plan to avoid or minimize them. Consider the possibility that the client is in pain or needs to void or defecate.

Assisting Caregivers
Someone should be enlisted to check on the primary caregiver of the demented person, particularly if the caregiver also is an older person. A neighbor or relative should call at least twice a day to make sure everything is under control. If something should happen to the primary caregiver, help may be delayed because the demented person may not know what to do.

Support Groups
Clients and family members can obtain support from many areas. The Internet provides access to many professional organizations as well as the ability to communicate with other individuals who have similar circumstances. Help them to identify their needs and be open to adaptations. Some needs are educational; for example, learning what the family needs to know to care for the client. Practical solutions, such as transportation assistance, legal assistance, answers for insurance and Medicare questions, medical equipment, and meal services at home are available in most locations. The family as a unit may need counseling because the situation is overwhelming.

Respite Care
Respite care allows caregivers some time to themselves by having others care for clients on a short-term basis. *Respite is crucial for caregivers*—they need relief from the constant responsibility of caring for their loved one, to maintain their own physical and mental health. Many long-term care facilities arrange short-term stays to provide respite. Community alternatives exist, including senior volunteers, home health services, and adult daycare. Adult daycare programs afford caregivers a break from their caregiving responsibilities for a portion of the day so that they can work or fulfill other responsibilities. Sometimes caregivers feel guilty about not providing care or assistance or cannot afford to provide it. A referral to social service may be needed. Caregivers may be willing to try a supplemental service on a temporary basis. When they find how helpful it is, they may be less reluctant to seek help in the future.

Education
The healthcare team helps with a plan for the family. Document all teaching. Many professional associations provide free literature regarding the assorted dementias. These resources provide group support and education. Caregivers can learn that many other people are having similar problems and can share experiences. It is important that the caregiver does not feel isolated and alone with an overwhelming situation.

Advance Directives
Normally, individuals make their own decisions and grant consent for healthcare, diagnostic, and treatment options.

CHAPTER 93 Cognitive Impairment in the Aging Adult

IN PRACTICE
NURSING CARE GUIDELINES 93-2   Communicating With the Person Who Has Dementia

- Identify yourself—do not make the client guess. *Rationale: The client may not remember you or be able to read your name tag.*
- Tell the client what you are going to do in simple language. *Rationale: Clients with dementia are often afraid of people (paranoia). Communication should be at a level that does not require complex thinking skills from the client.*
- Do not rush the client. *Rationale: The client may become resistant, more confused, and distressed.*
- Approach the client from the front and maintain direct eye contact (unless cultural considerations suggest other methods). *Rationale: It is important that the client can see you approach. If surprised, the client can become defensive and strike out.*
- Stay at the client's eye level. If the client is in a wheelchair, kneel or sit. *Rationale: Clients are less intimidated by someone who physically remains at their level.*
- Use a low-pitched voice; speak slowly. *Rationale: The client will mirror an angry or tense tone of voice.*
- Gently touch the person (unless this is frightening to them). *Rationale: Appropriate physical contact can be very soothing. However, if the client is agitated, any physical contact can be perceived as a threat.*
- Eliminate background noise. *Rationale: Extraneous noise adds to the individual's feeling of paranoia and fear. Avoid overstimulating the confused client.*
- Use short, simple sentences; give one-step commands. Speak clearly and make sure the client can hear you. *Rationale: The client's brain cannot process multiple steps. Too many commands add to confusion, frustration, and fear.*
- Avoid using questions, such as "Why did you... ?" or "What do you want?" *Rationale: The client cannot process or think through questions because those abilities are lost with increasing brain damage.*
- Label the environment if the client can read ("John's closet," "Caroline's bathroom"). *Rationale: The client feels more secure having and using things that are familiar.*
- Give the person "reassurance cards" (e.g., "Your wife is coming at 3 PM."). *Rationale: The client typically has short-term memory loss and will not remember facts or verbal conversations. These cards help decrease anxiety.*
- Post a simple daily schedule to structure the day. Post the day and date. Have a clock visible. *Rationale: These actions help the client to be oriented to time, place, and situation.*
- Be aware of nonverbal language; smile, nod your head. Use gestures, such as waving goodbye. *Rationale: The person can often respond to nonverbal cues, even after speech is lost. Your body language might be the only thing the person can perceive.*
- Avoid restraining the person. *Rationale: Restraints should be used only as a last resort. Restraining a client with dementia often causes more aggression. If the client becomes combative or hostile, have a safe place or room the client can stay and be monitored but not physically restrained.*

Persons with dementias are unable to give informed consent for procedures, and responsibility for decision making often falls on the family. The family may feel uneasy making decisions or may be unsure of the client's preferences. A means to ease their burden is to recommend that the client complete an advance directive while still mentally competent to understand and make health decisions. An *advance directive* states the client's preferences for caregiving procedures, treatments, and life-sustaining measures. At a later time, if the client is unable to make decisions competently, the family can make decisions on behalf of the client, using the client's expressed preferences. All individuals should be encouraged to complete advance directives.

Decision Making
The family may need assistance to come to the understanding that the person they knew is really gone and a childlike person has replaced their loved one. This procedure parallels the nursing process:

Identify problems: Realize the ambiguity of the situation. The adult is now like a child; the former decision maker is no longer able to make decisions.

Validate their perceptions: Verify their feelings and perceptions to make sure they correctly understand the situation.

Clarify: Restate and clarify their perceptions and feelings to make sure you understand how they are feeling.

Devise solutions: Assist the family to create solutions for the problems presented.

Test: Test the solutions.

Evaluate: Evaluate by determining if goals have been met or not and revise the care plan.

EVALUATION
The healthcare team, along with the client and family, evaluate outcomes of care. Have short-term goals been met? Are long-term goals still realistic?

When planning for further nursing care, consider the client's prognosis, as well as any complications and the client's response to care given. Is the person able to maintain self-care in a familiar environment? Evaluate the client to see how well the person is coping with changes. Working with the caregivers and asking for their input is often helpful.

Key Concept

It is important that both the older adult client and their family members know and consider the advantages of having an advance directive and, depending on the state, a power of attorney for healthcare *before* health issues become a concern.

NCLEX Alert

Nursing interventions must be prioritized in any clinical situation. An NCLEX clinical scenario might provide nursing interventions that are all accurate, but the correct answer relates to which action should be taken *first* for the situation given.

STUDENT SYNTHESIS

KEY POINTS

- Cognitive impairment may take the form of a client having trouble remembering, learning new things, concentrating, or making decisions that affect their everyday life. It can range from mild to severe.
- Intellectual impairment or disabilities are aspects of cognitive deficits but are more commonly associated with intellect and the ability to learn and are usually diagnosed long before a person is 18 years.
- Many reversible causes of confusion and delirium exist, including physical illness, metabolic disturbances, drug or alcohol toxicity, malnutrition, increased stress, and sensory deprivation.
- Although confusion can occur at any age, the older adult is more vulnerable because of decreased physiological reserves and the number of medications taken.
- Dementias affect the neurons of the brain but may have different etiologies, such as formation of plaques, tangles and taus, or the presence of Lewy bodies.
- The most common dementia is Alzheimer's disease. Other dementias that have similar symptoms but different etiologies include vascular dementia, Parkinson disease, Wernicke–Korsakoff syndrome, FTD, CJD, HAND, NPH, and Huntington disease.
- Diagnosis of a neurodegenerative disease (e.g., Alzheimer's disease) is often difficult. A brain or tissue biopsy can confirm the diagnosis but most clients are tested by ruling out treatable factors that result in confusion and dementia caused by factors such as hypoglycemia, malnutrition, or head trauma.
- Alzheimer's disease develops in stages, beginning with memory difficulty and progressing to increasing difficulties with memory, language, and movement. In the final stage, the client is no longer conscious of anything around them and is usually bedfast.
- Treatment for Alzheimer's disease is palliative; there is no known cure.
- The two types of drugs used to treat Alzheimer's disease include the cholinesterase inhibitors, which are used for early to moderate stages, and the drug memantine, or a combination of the two types may be used for moderate to severe stages.
- Nursing observations and interventions related to physical and mental abilities, needs, and resources are integral in the treatment of dementia.
- One nursing goal is to determine the client's abilities to perform ADLs and IADLs.
- When caring for the client with moderate to severe stage dementia, nursing actions include assisting with ADLs, providing a safe environment, and providing dignity to the client.
- The family or caregivers of the client with dementia require understanding of their own needs, of the progression of dementia, and of the importance of respite care with referrals to support groups.

CRITICAL THINKING EXERCISES

1. Some long-term care facilities have special units for residents with dementias, whereas others mix these residents with residents who have normal cognitive function. Discuss the pros and cons of these approaches.
2. The wife of a client with AD confides in you that she feels guilty because she promised her spouse that she would never put them in a nursing home, but she is now considering it. She says that she is feeling exhausted and gets so overwhelmed with the situation that she has slapped her spouse several times when they have resisted care. Discuss your response to her and the options you could recommend.
3. Review the causes of some dementias and describe lifestyle changes people can make early in life to decrease their risk for developing these dementias.

NCLEX-STYLE REVIEW QUESTIONS

1. A client with Parkinson disease is experiencing subcortical dementia. Which early findings does the nurse expect to observe? Select all that apply.
   a. Language impairment
   b. Depression
   c. Clumsiness
   d. Irritability
   e. Apathy

2. The nurse is talking with a family member of an older adult client with dementia. The family member reports that the client becomes more confused, aggressive, and combative in the evening. Which suggestions can the nurse provide to the family member to decrease this behavior? Select all that apply.
   a. Sedate the client every evening before mealtime.
   b. Have the client restrained to avoid injury.
   c. Maintain a routine for the client.
   d. Limit daytime sleeping.
   e. Limit sugar and caffeine intake.

3. A client with dementia at the long-term care facility states to the nurse, "I want to go home." What is the best response by the nurse?
   a. "You have repeatedly asked me the same question."
   b. "You can't live at your house anymore. It isn't safe."
   c. "You are safe here. Let's go eat lunch."
   d. "No one can take care of you at home anymore."

4. The nurse observes that a client with dementia does not recognize a grandchild and now requires assistance with most ADLs. Which phase of dementia does the nurse determine the client is experiencing?
   a. Mild decline
   b. Moderate decline
   c. Moderately severe decline
   d. Severe decline

5. A client with moderate Alzheimer's disease (AD) is prescribed memantine (Namenda). When explaining to the caregiver how the drug will be beneficial for the client, what information should the nurse provide?
   a. The drug will prevent aggressive and combative behavior.
   b. The drug can delay progression of some of the symptoms of AD.
   c. The drug will arrest any further cognitive impairment.
   d. The drug will cure AD.

CHAPTER RESOURCES

Enhance your learning with additional resources on thePoint!

Student Resources related to this chapter can be found at **thePoint.lww.com/Rosdahl12e**.

Mental Health Nursing | UNIT 14

94 Psychiatric Nursing

Learning Objectives

1. Explain normal defense mechanisms and results if they are overused.
2. Differentiate between functional and organic mental illness. List organic causes of mental illness.
3. Describe the role of neuropsychological and neurodiagnostic testing.
4. List general symptoms of a mental disorder. Describe the diagnostic criteria for a mood disorder.
5. Explain the differences between a major depressive episode and dysthymia.
6. Describe typical behavioral characteristics of the person with bipolar disorder.
7. List and describe personality disorders. Describe in detail common behaviors of people with borderline personality disorder.
8. Define psychosis and list common symptoms.
9. Describe relationships between substance abuse and mental illness.
10. Identify key members of the mental healthcare team and describe their roles.
11. Describe outpatient services commonly available for people with mental illnesses.
12. Identify types of structured living available to clients with mental disorders.
13. Discuss legal categories of admission to the acute mental healthcare setting.
14. Discuss therapies available to clients with mental illness, including electroconvulsive therapy, indications for its use, and associated nursing implications.
15. Identify and give examples of the most commonly used classifications of medications in psychiatry. Describe the undesirable side effects of neuroleptic or antipsychotic therapy, including neuroleptic malignant syndrome and tardive dyskinesia.
16. Describe approaches for dealing with aggressive or assaultive persons.
17. State the people most likely to attempt suicide and describe suicide precautions in the acute mental healthcare setting.
18. Discuss nursing responsibilities when working with each of the following clients: overactive, withdrawn, depressed, hypomanic, regressive, or self-injuring.

Important Terminology

affect
akathisia
anhedonia
antipsychotic
anxiety
assault
athetoid
benzodiazepine
bipolar disorder
catatonia
cogwheeling movement
commitment
compulsion
cyclothymic
delusion
dual diagnosis
dyskinesia
dysthymia
dystonia
entitlement
euthymia
factitious
forensic
functional disorder
grandiosity
hallucination
hypersomnia
hypervigilance
hypomania
intrusive thoughts
labile affect
malingering
mania
milieu/milieu therapy
neologism
neuroleptic/antipsychotic drugs
neuroleptic malignant syndrome
neuropsychiatrist
obsession
oculogyric crisis
opisthotonos
organic disorder
paranoid
perseveration
phobia
polydipsia
psychiatrist
psychometric
psychosis
psychotropic or psychoactive drugs
rapport
regression
schizophrenia
tardive dyskinesia
vulnerable adult

Acronyms

AH
AIMS
AMSIT
ANAD
APE
ASD
AWOL
BDI
BPD
BPRS
CHI
CHT
CMHC
DISCUS
DSM-5
ECT
EP
EPSE
ETOH, EtOH
FOI
GP
HID
Li+
MAOI
MI/CD
MMPI
MMSE
NEC
NMS
NOS
OCD
OD
ODT
PADS
Ψ
PMDD
PTSD
SCAD
SIB/SIW
SP
U-Tox
VH
W/D

1735

Most clients with alterations in mental health are treated in the community; community-based mental healthcare is expected to expand (Fig. 94-1). Some clients, however, with severe problems or sudden exacerbations of mental illness, receive inpatient care in acute or long-term facilities. Basic principles of mental health apply to all nursing care, no matter what the setting. People with physical illnesses may develop emotional/psychiatric problems that interfere with recovery. If individuals display unpredictable, dangerous behavior, their mental health and safety (and sometimes, the safety of others) is threatened. There are many signs of mental health disturbances. Remember that everyone experiences stress and worries, but when things spin out of control, intervention is needed. Talking about concerns early can help prevent further stress and abnormal use of defense mechanisms, as introduced in Chapter 6. Encourage clients to seek counseling for stress, before it becomes a greater concern. (Remember: We all may need counseling at times.)

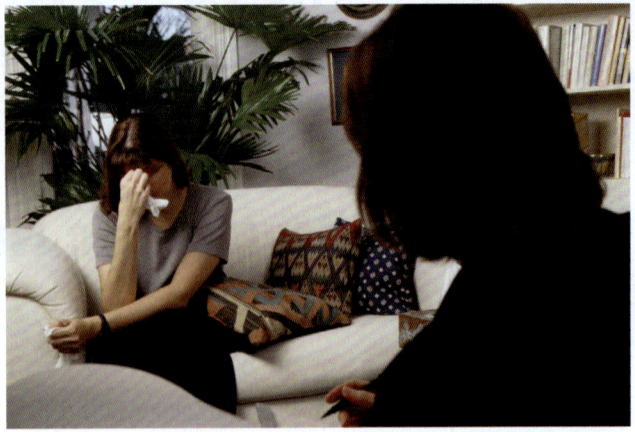

Figure 94-1 As a nurse, you will find that most people with mental health issues are not hospitalized. You will see many of the "worried well" in outpatient settings. (Carter, 2012.)

Key Concept

As a nurse, you will use concepts learned in psychiatry/mental health in all interactions with clients and others throughout your career.

MENTAL HEALTH

Understanding the term *mental health* is basic to the study of psychiatry. The World Health Organization (WHO) defines health as "a state of physical and mental well-being." Following are possible definitions of a mentally healthy person:

- Responsible for personal behavior
- Able to manage activities of daily living (ADLs): eating, grooming, managing money, and finding a safe place to live
- Able to adjust to new situations and handle stress without severe discomfort, yet still maintain sufficient energy to be a constructive member of society
- Possessing insight into personal strengths and weaknesses; able to accept weaknesses and use strengths positively
- Able to accept frustration and change without resorting to harmful, self-defeating, or dangerous behavior (against themselves or others)

In the early 1900s, Sigmund Freud, a pioneer in psychiatry, called certain reactions to stress *defense mechanisms*. Defense mechanisms help individuals resolve mental conflicts, reduce anxiety (fear of impending danger), protect *self-esteem* (self-value), and maintain a sense of security and balance (Fig. 94-2). All people use defense mechanisms at times. When they are used to excess *or are used exclusively*, however, they threaten that individual's mental health. Definitions and examples of common defense mechanisms are described in Table 94-1. It is important to recognize the use of defense mechanisms in yourself and your clients, in order to plan effective nursing care.

MENTAL ILLNESS

Everyone has feelings and behaviors they must control. *Mental illness* often means a difference in *degree of behavior*, rather than completely different behavior. Many people with mental disorders cannot control their socially unacceptable behavior. It is believed that nearly half of all Americans will experience a deviation from mental health at some point

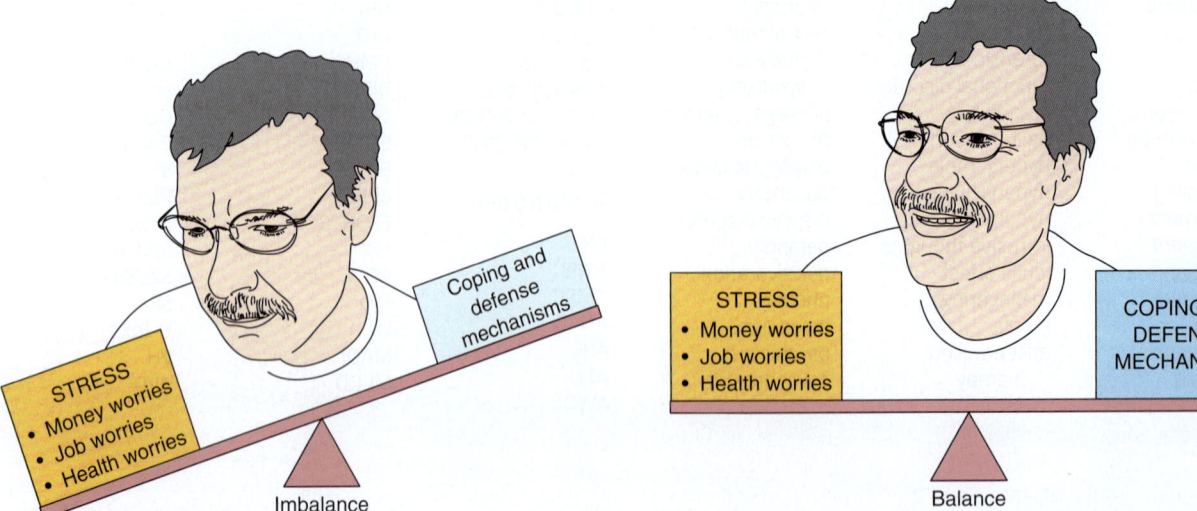

Figure 94-2 The mentally healthy person can maintain a state of *emotional balance* most of the time (**right**). If stress or change occurs (**left**), the mentally healthy person might tip out of balance for a short time, but is able to adjust and to return to homeostasis. (Carter, 2012.)

TABLE 94-1 Defense Mechanisms

DEFENSE MECHANISM	DEFINITION	EXAMPLE
Suppression	*Consciously* inhibiting an impulse or emotion that is unacceptable to the person	Joe does not want to discuss his mother's recent death and continually tells his spouse, "We'll talk about it later."
Repression	*Unconsciously* inhibiting an impulse or emotion that is unacceptable to the person	Lauren, who was in an automobile accident in which she did not lose consciousness or suffer any brain damage, cannot recall anything that happened directly before, during, or after the event.
Reaction formation	Displaying a behavior, attitude, or feeling opposite to that which one would normally exhibit in the same situation	Peter does not like his stepfather, but is excessively polite to him.
Rationalization	Trying logically to justify irrational, socially, or personally unacceptable behaviors or feelings	Twelve-year-old Jill fails to get elected to student council. She says that "The elections were probably fixed, and student council is for nerds, anyway."
Displacement	Unconsciously transferring feelings onto another person or object	Michelle is upset with her spouse, but yells at her preschool-age child, who in turn kicks the family dog.
Denial	Disavowing the existence of unpleasant realities	Gordon, recently diagnosed with terminal cancer, tells his family that he feels fine and the doctors do not know what they are talking about.
Projection	Attributing to another person one's unacceptable thoughts and feelings	Chuck accidentally erases files from his computer. He yells at his child, "See what you made me do with all that noise," and calls the computer names.
Sublimation	Diverting unacceptable urges into personally and socially acceptable channels	Madeline has an urge to be unfaithful to her partner, but rechannels her feelings into gardening.
Intellectualization	Unconsciously transferring emotions into the realm of intellect; using reasoning as a means of avoiding confrontation with objectionable impulses	Lincoln, going through a messy divorce, refuses to become emotional. He continually philosophizes about the meaning of relationships and love, saying things like "Nothing lasts forever."

in time. Psychiatric disorders can arise from external conditions, life stressors, metabolic changes, or brain disorders. Some mental disorders arise from unknown causes. The Greek letter *psi* (Ψ) is used sometimes to denote psychiatry. Mental illness affects all spheres of a person's life, including physical health, employment, housing, finances, and relationships. It may be influenced by, or may be a contributing cause to, substance abuse and other addictions.

 SPECIAL CONSIDERATIONS   Culture and Ethnicity

Reactions to and Treatment of Mental Illness
A client's cultural practices and ethnicity can influence beliefs and behaviors. "Normal" and "abnormal" behaviors often depend on one's cultural perspective. Conditions such as schizophrenia, bipolar disorder, and major depression are believed to occur worldwide. However, cultural reactions to them differ. For example, in some cultures, guilt and suicidal ideation do not accompany depression. North America has examples of culture-bound illnesses (e.g., "nervous breakdown" or anorexia nervosa) that are not common in other cultures. *Misdiagnosis* (no diagnosis or an incorrect one) is common in clients who differ from the typical behaviors of North American culture.

Different cultures also have varying customs and beliefs related to such concepts as eye contact, personal space, or causation of illness. In some cultures, the person experiencing hallucinations is believed to be directly communicating with God, and this is considered to be a special "gift." Many of the world's people believe in the effect of the "evil eye," in "possession by demons," or in the "hot and cold" effects of various disorders. These factors influence beliefs regarding causation and treatment of illness, including mental illness. It is important to consider cultural beliefs in caring for clients, both in the mental health unit and elsewhere. The client who holds the beliefs of the people in their cultural group should not be considered mentally ill just because their beliefs differ from traditional Western beliefs.

Diagnosis

The psychiatrist, psychologist, advance practice nurse, physician assistant, and other team members work together to determine if a client has a deviation in mental health and its cause and type. *Neuropsychiatrists*, a growing area of additional training that brings integrative thinking about brain and behavior, may also be included in the care team. Emphasis is often on behavior and any known neurological or brain injury, rather than specific diagnoses. Nursing observations are very important input for these evaluations. A complete physical examination is done to rule out any possible physical cause of the illness. Specific diagnoses are described in the American Psychiatric Association's (APA) reference book, the *Diagnostic and Statistical Manual of Mental Disorders* (**DSM-5**). It is important to note that psychiatric diagnoses are based on observation of behavior and client reporting. A client may have more than one diagnosis, and these diagnoses may change, as more is learned about the client. In some cases, a firm diagnosis cannot be made and the diagnosis is classified as *not elsewhere classified* (**NEC**); this category was formerly "not otherwise specified" (**NOS**).

Organic Versus Functional

In some cases, the healthcare team identifies a physical (organic) cause for the client's mental disorder (**organic disorder**). In an organic disorder, evidence from the person's history, physical examination, and laboratory findings indicates that the mental disturbance is a direct consequence of a medical condition. An endocrine disorder (especially of the thyroid), infection, high fever, hypoglycemia (low blood sugar), abuse of drugs/alcohol and/or overdose (**OD**), cerebrovascular disease, brain lesion or stroke, and conditions, such as tertiary syphilis, Huntington disease, or AIDS dementia, may cause organic disorders. Closed-head trauma (**CHT**), also known as a closed-head injury (**CHI**), may also cause temporary or permanent *psychosis* (when thoughts and emotions are so impaired that contact is lost with external reality). (CHT is often the result of a motor vehicle accident [MVA] or assault.) If an organic cause is identified, its treatment *may* alleviate the mental illness. If no specific causative agent is identified, this mental illness is known as a **functional disorder**.

Psychometric Tests

The *psychologist* (an expert in the field of psychology) and *psychometrist* (a professional who administers and scores psychological tests) aid the psychiatrist in making a differential diagnosis of mental illness. *Neuropsychiatric* (brain function/behavior) testing includes an in-depth interview and various tests. Commonly used tests include the Beck Depression Index (BDI), Brief Psychiatric Rating Scale (**BPRS**), and Mini Mental Status Examination (**MMSE**). Sometimes, the results of a mental status examination are stated/documented as **a**ppearance, **m**ood, **s**ensorium, **i**ntelligence, and **t**hought process (**AMSIT**) in the client record. Psychometric tests evaluate the client's orientation to time and place and require the person to perform specific tasks. A common abbreviation to describe orientation is *A&O × 3* (alert and oriented to person, place, and time). If the client is oriented to only one or two of these, the specific orientation must be identified. ("Client is oriented only to person.") Other projective and memory tests include the Rorschach inkblot, "Draw-a-Person," sentence completion, Bender–Gestalt, word association, and thematic apperception tests (TAT). Personality inventories, such as the Minnesota Multiphasic Personality Inventory (**MMPI**), are used extensively. Intelligence tests may also be given.

The client's living situation is evaluated; for example, it is determined whether a client needs assistance with ADLs. One such test is the Kohlman Evaluation of Living Skills (KELS). The Millon Clinical Multiaxial Inventory (MCMI-4) helps identify a level of personality functioning. Many other tests are used to analyze more deeply areas that were revealed by the neuropsychiatric tests mentioned above. (Some of these tests are available in languages other than English.)

Neurologic Tests

Neurodiagnostic tests can rule out organic causes of psychiatric disorders. These tests include the computed tomography (CT) scan, magnetic resonance imaging (MRI), positron emission tomography (PET, PETT), single-photon emission computed tomography (SPECT), and the transcranial Doppler (TCD). In addition, a cerebral angiogram (brain x-ray study, using contrast media), digital subtraction angiogram, or *electroencephalography* (EEG) may be used. Measurement of *evoked potentials* of the cerebral cortex (auditory brain response [ABR] or auditory-evoked response [AER]) is also made in the EEG department, as are *sleep studies*. These tests can often rule out conditions such as brain tumor, abscess, cerebral vascular disease, cerebral atrophy, some forms of dementia, sleep disorders, some metabolic disorders, and sometimes, organic changes associated with schizophrenia. Tests can diagnose some cases of Parkinson syndrome or seizure disorders and locate the origination site of some seizures. Changes resulting from TBIs can be identified. A lumbar puncture (LP) may be done. In this invasive procedure, a needle is introduced into the subarachnoid space around the spinal cord (Chapter 78). LP can determine intracranial pressure (ICP) or the presence of microorganisms, blood, or abnormal proteins in the cerebrospinal fluid (CSF). Elevated ICP or abnormal substances in CSF can help diagnose underlying disorders contributing to mental disorders.

> **Key Concept**
>
> The person who is sleep deprived can exhibit severe psychiatric symptoms, commonly known as delirium. In some cases, symptoms disappear or are markedly reduced when the person is able to sleep. (This is true of all people, including nurses.)

Symptoms

Often, certain behavioral patterns signify a mental disorder. These symptoms affect a person's identity and public image and may contribute to low self-esteem. Examples of significant behaviors include the following:

- Noticeable behavioral changes—exaggerated feelings, inappropriate responses, unexplained depression, inappropriate elation
- Overuse of defense mechanisms
- Sudden lack of concern about physical appearance; inability to perform basic ADLs
- Not eating, binge eating, purging, or excess fluid intake (polydipsia)
- Not sleeping or sleeping all the time
- Physical symptoms, without apparent medical cause
- Loss of contact with reality—altered perceptions and sensory changes, such as increased watchfulness (**hypervigilance**), **hallucinations** (hearing, seeing, feeling, tasting things that are not there), misperceptions, distorted thinking, difficulty in filtering out irrelevant stimuli, **paranoia** (unreasonable fears), *delusional* thinking (false beliefs)
- Cognitive confusion—disorientation, thought blocking, loose associations, poor abstract thinking, illogic thinking, inability to solve problems, inability to cope with stress,

preoccupation, poor concentration, poor memory, speech latency (the time between a thought and its verbal expression), speech aberrations (e.g., word salad, flight of ideas, alliteration, echolalia), talking/laughing to oneself
- Morbid fascination with death—talk of wanting to die or of committing suicide; thoughts of hurting oneself or others; incapacitating depression
- Religious preoccupation—constant praying, unreasonable fear of dying, constant preaching
- Total immobility (including catatonia); suddenly becoming mute

> Key Concept
> It is important to remember that these and other symptoms may be caused by organic disorders and may be reversible or treatable. In addition, medications are often helpful in managing overwhelming symptoms.

Types

Mental illness varies considerably in degree and type. Clinical diagnosis is often stated as one of the following:

- Acute or chronic
- In remission
- Prior history

The following text describes general psychiatric categories.

Mood Disorders

Mood disorders are a group of clinical conditions characterized by disturbance of mood (internal, subjective emotional state), along with a loss of control and a subjective feeling of distress. (**Euthymia** is the term for normal mood.)

Major Depressive Episode and Major Depressive Disorder

Depression is the most common mood disorder in the United States. The majority of suicides can be attributed to a depressive disorder. Diagnosis of a major depressive episode (MDE) includes signs and symptoms, which must be present frequently and must represent a change from previous functional levels. (Many of these signs and symptoms are observable by other people.) At least one symptom must be *depressed mood most of the day* or markedly diminished/loss of interest or pleasure (**anhedonia**) in all, or most, activities. A major depressive disorder (MDD) is recurrent and consists of more than one MDE. (There must be a period of at least 2 months between episodes for a diagnosis of MDD.)

Additional signs and symptoms of depressive disorders include the following:

- Weight/appetite changes—significant weight loss when not dieting; significant weight gain; marked appetite decrease or increase; inability to eat/drink (all without physical cause)
- Sleep disturbances—*insomnia* (difficulty falling or staying asleep) or **hypersomnia** (sleeping too much); severe nightmares; sleeping only in the daytime
- *Psychomotor retardation* (very slow or abnormal movements/responses), *catatonia* (lack or movement, rigidity), or psychomotor agitation
- Fatigue; loss of energy
- Feelings of worthlessness (*low self-esteem*) or excessive, inappropriate guilt—may be **delusional** (fixed, false belief not shared by others)
- Diminished ability to think/concentrate; indecisiveness; thought blocking (difficulty finishing sentences or thoughts); preoccupation
- Recurrent thoughts of death or suicidal ideation, with or without a specific plan
- The nurse may observe other signs of depression in clients, including crying, poor grooming, anxiety, self-blame, isolation, loneliness, irritability, and vague physical complaints. Symptoms of depression cause significant distress or impairment in social, occupational, and other areas of functioning.

Physical (organic) causes of depression may be found. For example, some medications cause depression (e.g., corticosteroids). Disorders, such as hypothyroidism, stroke, head trauma, and multiple sclerosis, often lead to depression, as does the use of drugs (e.g., cocaine, alcohol).

Situational depression is caused by a specific event or factors in one's life. Examples include depression following the death of a loved one or loss of a job or home. Sometimes, several stressors occur simultaneously, and the person feels overwhelmed. Resolution of stressors or therapy to help deal with them can often relieve situational depression. The person who recovers from situational depression often never has another episode.

Depression in older adults is increasing. Older adults often have situational stressors, such as loss of a spouse, loneliness, financial problems, physical disorders, chronic illness, pain, and fear of death.

Dysthymia

Dysthymia is defined as a persistent, mild, depressive disorder over time. The client subjectively describes this state, signs of which may be observed by others. Additional symptoms include sleep disturbances, appetite changes, decreased energy, low self-esteem, poor concentration, and feelings of hopelessness. Dysthymia tends to be less severe, but longer lasting, than MDD.

Bipolar Disorder

Unusual shifts in mood, energy, and activity levels from elation to major depression are symptoms of a disorder known as **bipolar disorder** (**BPD**), formerly called *bipolar affective disorder* (*BPAD*) or manic depression. Mood swings are drastically different from normal behavior and may vary from person to person. In **mania**, the person shows accelerated thinking and speaking, **grandiosity** (feelings of invincibility and exaggerated self-importance), intrusiveness, distractibility (inability to concentrate), aggressiveness, and excessive involvement in pleasurable activities that have a high potential for painful or undesirable consequences. Excessive use of methamphetamine, cocaine, or other drugs (substance-induced mania) is common. Mania and depression *alternate* in BPD.

Some people have short periods of mania alternating with short periods of depression, which is sometimes referred to as *rapid cycling*. Others have much longer cycles or stay mostly in the manic or the depressed end of the scale. Some people have periods of normal behavior between cycles, particularly if medications are effective. This disorder is often evidenced in the late teen years or early adulthood, but may also develop in children (and these children are at high risk for suicide). Often, several members of a family will display BPD.

Personality Disorders

All people have specific personality traits, but when these characteristics become dysfunctional, this is described as a *personality disorder*. Personality disorders follow a pattern of thinking and outward behavior that deviates markedly from cultural expectations. This deviation may manifest in several ways:

- Cognition (how a person thinks)
- Affectivity (**affect** [pronounced af'-ekt]: the outward manifestation of subjective emotions)
- Interpersonal functioning (relationships with others)
- Poor impulse control; **intrusive** (interfering) behavior; bizarre behavior
- Unstable moods, behavior, and relationships—*labile* behavior (out of control emotions)
- Paranoia (extreme hypervigilance or watchfulness), fear
- Detachment from *schizoid* behavior or detachment from personal relationships

Although personality disorders may be of several types, an individual may exhibit characteristics of more than one type. Personality disorders may range from slight deviations from normal to highly unacceptable and dangerous behaviors. In some cases, the person demonstrates *grandiosity* and excessive attention to clothing and makeup, and a sense of **entitlement** ("the world owes me everything"). People with personality disorders are often difficult and frustrating to work with. One reason is that many of them are blind to their behaviors and tend to create more distress for others than for themselves. All these behaviors may become stable over time. In some situations, behaviors can be triggered again by a life event in the person with a personality disorder. Many clients on the mental health unit have a condition known as *borderline personality disorder*. This client demonstrates personality deviations in several extremes. These clients are often female, and a history of sexual abuse is common. They may have frequent hospitalizations and have many physical complaints. Cognitive behavioral therapy (CBT) can be a more effective treatment than medications, but often the client chooses not to remain in therapy. A client with borderline personality disorder may pack a suitcase with clothing and a teddy bear, then cut their wrists, and call 911. The person with borderline personality disorder may be very hostile toward others, demonstrating pathological personality traits and poor impulse control with marked impulsivity. Other characteristics include the following:

- Displays of self-destructive or self-injurious behavior (**SIB**), self-inflicted wounds (**SIW**), and suicidal gestures (not lethal attempts)
- Unstable mood or very poor self-image; self-criticism
- Lack of goals or plans; lack of values
- Difficulty with intimacy; mistrust, needy behaviors, preoccupation with abandonment, and extreme separation anxiety. There is a pervasive pattern of instability in interpersonal relationships.

Anxiety Disorders

Some clients exhibit *anxiety disorders*. Components of anxiety disorders can be present in other disorders as well.

Panic Attacks

The *panic attack* is characterized by intense fear and anxiety, with no known cause. Symptoms include shaking, diaphoresis (excessive sweating), a smothering or choking feeling, nausea, chest pain, tachycardia, and dizziness. This person may believe that he or she is having a heart attack or dying.

Phobias

A specific **phobia** is a persistent, excessive, unreasonable, and severe fear of a particular thing or event. The object of fear (*phobic stimulus*) may be anything; exposure to this stimulus causes severe, disabling panic. The person realizes intellectually that the fear is illogical, but is powerless to control it, without therapy. Examples of specific phobias are as follows:

- *Agoraphobia* (irrational fear of crowds, public places, or places from which escape would be difficult). This client may be unable to leave home.
- Social anxiety disorder (fear of embarrassment), including fear of public speaking or performing.
- Specific phobias—related to a well-defined situation or object, such as flying (aerophobia), snakes (ophidiophobia), heights (acrophobia), animals (zoophobia), spiders (arachnophobia), or enclosed places (claustrophobia).

Obsessive-Compulsive Disorder

Obsessive-compulsive disorder (**OCD**) is marked by **obsessions**—recurrent, persistent, intrusive thoughts, or beliefs that the person cannot ignore, and **compulsions**—repetitive behaviors (e.g., handwashing, cleaning), or mental acts (e.g., counting, praying) that the person feels driven to perform, sometimes constantly. Newly defined types include *excoriation disorder* (constant skin picking) and *hoarding disorder*. The person with OCD usually imposes rigid rules onto the acts. OCD can cause great distress; the ritualistic behaviors can interfere partially or totally with the person's life. In some cases, the person spends the entire day performing these rituals and cannot do anything else. The person realizes that these obsessions and compulsions are products of their own mind, but cannot achieve change without therapy.

Eating Disorders

Several severe disturbances in eating and weight regulation exist, either independently or as a symptom of another mental disorder. Eating disorders include *anorexia nervosa*, *bulimia nervosa*, and *binge-eating disorder*. In anorexia nervosa, clients see themselves as overweight, although they are extremely thin. They may refuse to eat or follow extreme diets. Bulimia nervosa involves binge eating and purging. Both anorexia and bulimia may involve self-induced vomiting, overuse of laxatives or enemas, or extreme exercise. Binge-eating disorder involves huge caloric intake, not followed by purging. These disorders are treated with counseling, behavior modification therapy, art therapy can be very helpful, medication therapy (often antidepressants), and close medical supervision. All of these disorders can be life-threatening (Chapter 88).

Trauma and Stress-Related Disorder: Posttraumatic Stress Disorder

Trauma and stress-related disorder, commonly called **PTSD**, is an anxiety disorder that is increasing in prevalence, particularly among veterans returning from war zones. The person with PTSD has been exposed to a traumatic event or series of events (e.g., sexual abuse, severe injury, wartime events, disasters, torture, or sudden death of a loved one) in which the response was intense fear or helplessness. (This can also occur if a family member experienced these events.) Symptoms of PTSD include recurrent and intrusive flashbacks to, or dreams of, the event, insomnia, inability to concentrate, persistent avoidance of stimuli associated with the event, and/or inability to recall all or part of it. The person often exhibits symptoms, such as hypervigilance, paranoia, exaggerated startle response (or constant hyperarousal), guilt, and irritability that were not present before the trauma. Many clients with PTSD isolate themselves and avoid activities that they previously enjoyed; they feel lonely and as though they have no future. They may be unable to concentrate or care for themselves and are often suicidal or self-injurious. (A milder form of this disorder is *acute stress disorder* [**ASD**], which resolves after a few weeks.) Children may react differently to traumatic events (e.g., bedwetting, mutism, acting out the event during play, running away, rebellion, or being very clingy and insecure). PTSD is treated with psychotherapy and medications, such as sertraline (Zoloft) and paroxetine (Paxil).

Factitious Disorders

A **factitious** disorder is one with no basis in fact. The client deliberately shows repeated feigning (pretending) or exaggeration of physical or psychiatric symptoms (which may be done unconsciously). The motivation for this behavior is often to assume the "sick role" and obtain attention. (A factitious disorder differs from **malingering** because there is no apparent external motive for feigning the illness.) Types of factitious disorders include those in which symptoms described are physical, those with psychological symptoms, and those with a combination.

In *Ganser syndrome*, the client's symptoms are psychological and may take the form of factitious hallucinations or amnesia, or may involve *conversion reactions* (e.g., blindness or paralysis), with no organic basis. This syndrome is very rare and has been removed from the DSM-5 as it has long been argued as to whether it was a true mental illness with many referring to it as a specific type of malingering. A specific type of factitious disorder is *Munchausen syndrome*. In this case, the client seeks frequent treatment for claimed acute physical illness or disease. The client gives a dramatic history and expresses severe physical symptoms, all of which are false, or which have been produced by the client (such as altering a urine specimen or injecting fecal material to produce an abscess). The client may agree to undergo life-threatening surgeries or tests. *Munchausen by proxy* involves another person, usually the client's child. The parent, usually the mother, fabricates or induces severe physical or psychological symptoms in the child, in order to obtain sympathy and attention. This child may be subjected to needless procedures (which may be life-threatening).

Psychosis Disorder

Marked deviation from normal behavior and seriously inappropriate conduct may indicate **psychosis**, a thought disorder that interferes with one's ability to recognize and deal with reality and to communicate effectively. Psychosis can be *organic* (caused by a physical disorder) or *functional* (unknown cause). The DSM-5 offers the following classifications of symptoms: *hallucinations* (false sensory perceptions), *delusions* (fixed, false beliefs), *disorganized speech, abnormal psychomotor behavior, negative symptoms* (restricted emotional expression), *impaired cognition* (thinking), and *mania*.

Some additional descriptive terms are helpful is describing behavior:

Paranoia: Fears and suspicions, for example, about being injured or followed
Mutism: Refusal to speak
Posturing: Voluntary assumption of inappropriate or bizarre positions
Echolalia: Repetition of another person's words or phrases
Echopraxia: Repetition of another person's movements

Psychotic behavior is unusual and noticeable in severe cases. The person who is severely disturbed is said to be having an acute psychotic episode (**APE**). Severity of the disorder is ranked by the practitioner on a scale of 0 to 4, with 0 being "not present" and 4 being "present and severe."

Hallucinations are common and include the following:

- Auditory (**AH**)—hearing voices, music, or other sounds (the most frequent hallucination)
- Visual (**VH**)—seeing things that others do not see; images, shadows, visions (the second most common)
- Tactile (haptic)—feeling of being touched or something crawling on/in the body
- Gustatory—hallucination of tastes
- Olfactory—hallucination of smell, odors

"Command auditory hallucinations" are those that instruct clients to do something, often to hurt themselves or others.

Schizophrenia Spectrum Disorder

Schizophrenia is a spectrum of psychotic disorders, characterized by abnormal interpretation of reality. The person with schizophrenia has a profound disruption in the way he or she acts, including distortion of cognition and emotions, affecting language, thought, perceptions, affect (basic sense of being), and sense of self, as well as occupational and social dysfunction. The following *positive* (or greater than normal) symptoms are often present: delusions, hallucinations, disorganized speech (derailment, incoherence), abnormal psychomotor behavior and/or movement, and/or **catatonia** (stupor, muscle rigidity). *Negative* (or less than normal) symptoms of schizophrenia indicate restricted emotional expression and include social and emotional withdrawal, isolation, apathy, lack of spontaneity, poor hygiene, lack of insight, a flat/blunted affect, poor judgment, poverty of speech, and *anhedonia* (inability to feel pleasure).

The second criterion for the diagnosis of schizophrenia is that the person's level of functioning is significantly below their prior level. (The first symptom of schizophrenia is often *withdrawal* from friends and activities.) Symptoms interfere with social, occupational, and self-care abilities and must be present for at least 6 months for a diagnosis of schizophrenia. If symptoms are present for 1–6 months, this is known as a *schizophreniform* disorder; if less than 1 month, the condition is referred to as a *brief psychotic disorder*. (A brief psychotic disorder may occur with a marked stressor—a brief *reactive psychosis*, without a specific stressor, or with postpartum onset.)

Schizophrenia must be differentiated from schizoaffective disorder (described below), as well as autism spectrum disorders or communication disorders. In addition, it must be determined that the disorder is not caused by drug abuse or a medical condition.

> **Key Concept**
>
> Acute lethal catatonia (*ALC*) exists when the person does not move and is unable to eat or care for themselves. In this case, prompt medical intervention is required. A *medical emergency* may be declared and medications forced. Tube feeding or IVs may be required to save the client's life.

Other Psychoses

Substance-induced psychosis may be characterized by prominent hallucinations, delusions, or other symptoms of schizophrenia, described above, that develop during or within a month of substance intoxication or withdrawal (Chapter 95). *Schizoaffective disorder* (**SCAD**) is a psychotic disorder with symptoms of both a mood disorder (e.g., major depression, mania, or both) and schizophrenia. There are two types of SCAD: bipolar type and depressive type. A *delusional disorder* is characterized by persistent, nonbizarre delusions involving situations that may occur in real life. The person may believe that they are being followed, poisoned, infected, diseased (*somatic delusion*), loved by a distant admirer (*erotomania*), or deceived by a lover (*jealous-type delusion*). Delusions may also be *grandiose* (e.g., believing that one has a special relationship with God or is royalty, "delusions of grandeur"). The person may also feel that he or she is being treated in an evil way (*delusions of persecution*). Apart from the impact of delusions, everyday functioning is not markedly impaired, and behavior is not obviously odd. Delusions are often fixed and of long standing; they may be very difficult to treat. A person may have a fixed delusion for life and may expand and elaborate on it as time goes on.

> **Key Concept**
>
> A person can have symptoms of several mental disorders simultaneously. For example, a person with depression may also have hallucinations. An individual's diagnosis may change over time. Therefore, the nurse must learn to *deal with various behaviors* and not to classify people in terms of their diagnosis.

Dual Diagnosis

The term *dual diagnosis* literally means that the person has two separate chronic conditions. This can be a combination of any two factors, such as mental illness and sexual addiction or anorexia nervosa and substance abuse disorders. Some people with mental illness also exhibit some level of intellectual disability (ID). However, the term *dual diagnosis* is most commonly used to describe mental illness, combined with a substance abuse disorder, formerly called chemical dependency (**MI/CD**). People with serious mental illness are at high risk for substance abuse or dependency (Chapter 95).

Identifying whether substance abuse or mental illness occurred first is difficult. Some clients drink or use drugs to mask voices or other psychotic symptoms. Others become psychotic after using chemicals. People with no previous psychosis may experience psychiatric symptoms during withdrawal from alcohol or drugs. Long-standing abuse of alcohol can also cause *organic psychosis* (such as Korsakoff syndrome), secondary to brain damage. Other psychoses can result from abuse of other drugs. Substance abuse often aggravates existing mental illness. For example, alcohol is a depressant; when combined with underlying depression, symptoms worsen. People with normal moods may become depressed when drinking. When working with clients with a dual diagnosis, consider the following factors:

- Many psychiatric clients are *polysubstance abusers* (abuse more than one substance).
- In many cases, chemical abuse *exacerbates* (worsens) mental illness.
- Alcohol (**ETOH**, **EtOH**) and other mood-altering chemicals have adverse reactions with *neuroleptic* (antipsychotic) and other prescribed medications. These chemicals may negate the desired effects of these medications or may dangerously increase their effects. These combinations seriously interfere with treatment and can be life-threatening.
- Many psychiatric clients are particularly susceptible to the effects of drugs because of their underlying mental instability.
- The presence of mental illness may make it difficult for the client to understand or to follow a substance abuse treatment program.
- Clients are often vulnerable and easy prey for those who distribute drugs.
- Clients may be inappropriately told by lay people not to take their prescribed psychiatric medications instead of encouraging them to avoid alcohol and other chemical substances.

> **Key Concept**
>
> Whenever a client is admitted to a mental health unit (or any other unit of the hospital), consider the possibility of alcohol or drug withdrawal. Substance abuse is very common, and withdrawal can be life-threatening, particularly from alcohol (Chapter 95).

THE MENTAL HEALTHCARE TEAM

Mental illness affects the client's entire life and that of the family. The team approach is vital to provide the best assistance.

Psychiatrist

A **psychiatrist** or neuropsychiatrist is a healthcare provider (MD or DO) who has completed advanced education in the treatment of mental disorders. Psychiatrists direct the mental healthcare team and often treat both mental and physical disorders. Physical disorders are classified as causative, coexisting, or secondary. Some areas employ physician assistants (PA-C), to work with psychiatrists. They usually may prescribe medications and treatments.

Nurse

The *nurse* is an important member of a mental health team. By creating a therapeutic environment (**milieu**), nurses help to assist people to return to as near-normal functioning as possible. Many mental health facilities hire LPNs/LVNs to work on the units. Master's-prepared registered nurses (RNs) can receive national clinical certification in Psychiatric and Mental Health Nursing (RNBC—RN Board Certified). The clinical nurse specialist, advanced practice registered nurse (APRN), or psychiatric nurse practitioner is a master's or doctorate degree–prepared nurse with a specialty in psychiatry. This person is often licensed to provide psychiatric therapy and prescribe medications.

Other Team Members

Psychiatric technicians, *mental health workers*, or *human service workers* also deal directly with clients on a mental health unit. These workers, certified, licensed, or unlicensed, may provide a large proportion of the daily care required by clients. In some states, these workers are authorized to give medications.

Psychologists usually have a doctorate degree in psychology and provide testing, counseling, and therapy. (They are not MDs and do not prescribe medications.) *Psychometrists* administer psychological tests.

Recreational therapists and *music therapists* provide diversional and personal growth activities and often take clients on outings. *Art therapy*, when facilitated by a professional art therapist, can be beneficial for clients with very diverse needs. *Occupational therapists* evaluate and instruct clients in ADLs, homemaking, crafts, and sometimes, job-retraining or employment skills. *Vocational rehabilitation* and *veteran's services* sometimes make further education or employment possible. Physical therapists assist with movement disorders and specialized exercises. *Chaplains* offer spiritual counseling and support. *Social workers* prepare clients for, and assist with, discharge. They often act as the liaison among clients, family members and friends, and the community. Social workers are usually the main therapists who may also help clients find a safe place to live, obtain financial assistance, or access other community resources.

Other specialists may assist with individual cases. These specialists include those in *substance abuse disorders, medical/surgical specialties, interpreters, wound care, diabetic or stoma care, hearing or vision professionals, dentists, dietitians, pharmacists,* and *respiratory therapists. EEG, ECG, laboratory,* and *radiologic (X-ray) technicians* perform specialized examinations. *Volunteers* may provide pet therapy, gifts for holidays, puzzles, games, magazines, escorts, and other services.

Treatment Centers and Resources

Many resources are available today to assist people with mental health concerns, including a variety of community agencies, as well as acute and semiacute inpatient units. The range of care varies from independent living to total care.

Community-Based Programs

The trend is toward the *least restrictive treatment possible.* Therefore, most people with mental illnesses are currently treated and managed in the community.

Outpatient Mental Health Clinics or Centers

An *outpatient mental health clinic* or *community mental health center* provides ongoing therapy and counseling for people who do not require hospitalization. Clients visit regularly; staff home visits may be included. Medications are prescribed, and compliance and effectiveness are evaluated. In some cases, blood work is done (for example, clozapine [Clozaril] maintenance, lithium to maintain therapeutic levels and avoid toxicity).

Psychiatric Home Care/Community Outreach

The trend toward community living for people with chronic, persistent mental illness has necessitated the initiation of home care services. One of the major goals is to prevent rehospitalization. Usually, a nurse, a community health team, and other workers visit regularly, to help with management. Box 94-1 lists factors involved in successful

---

Box 94-1 Mental Health Management in the Community

Most clients with mental illnesses are managed in the community. Certain factors contribute to successful community living. These include the following:

- Involvement in school, work, or volunteering
- Association with community resources, such as a drop-in center, AA, or church
- Knowledge of how to obtain reasonably priced items, such as food and clothing
- Ability to manage money (or having a payee, if needed)
- Medication compliance; attention to adverse side effects
- Supportive people, such as family and friends
- Keeping appointments with the counselor, nurse, and/or psychiatrist
- Maintaining good health (e.g., managing physical disorders; seeking help when ill; having blood tests as needed; eating a well-balanced diet; exercising; smoking cessation)
- Involvement in safe (and inexpensive) recreational activities and hobbies
- Having a safe place to live
- Access to safe transportation
- Having a case manager, social worker, or payee, as needed
- Abstinence from alcohol and street drugs
- Having a personal care attendant, homemaking services, or other caregiver, as needed
- Having a pet (if able to care for the pet safely)

community living. If a client experiences symptoms or problems, a short stay in a nursing home or group home may be helpful. In some cases, an outreach worker refers clients for acute inpatient care. If necessary, police may force transfer to a hospital for clients who are combative or suicidal or who refuse voluntary admission and are considered dangerous to themselves or others. An *involuntary transportation hold* usually involves getting a person to a hospital or mental health facility where precautions are in place to maintain safety, and where assessment/evaluation can occur. The client is usually kept for 72 hr or less, and often the person must appear before a judge prior to being discharged or to remain as inpatient. Different states have different laws or practices related to this situation. Be sure you know your state's laws.

Challenges are involved in delivering home care to clients with mental illnesses. Care must focus on rehabilitation and teaching. Because care is provided in the client's home, staff can get a clearer picture of daily challenges for the client and family. Nurses address issues such as medication setup and compliance, symptom recurrence, sleep disorders, homemaking and home safety, and eating habits. They help clients keep appointments, structure time, and attend treatment or support groups. Nurses assist with interpersonal skills and teach family members. It is also important for home care nurses to be alert to their own safety. They may visit in pairs, and they always carry a cell phone. If a situation feels unsafe, they should leave and consult the supervisor. *Never* enter a potentially unsafe situation without backup. (See Chapter 98 and Box 98-3.)

> **NCLEX Alert**
> Follow-through and aftercare may be among nursing actions to be selected on an NCLEX examination.

Some clients need physical care or assistance with homemaking. The personal care attendant/aide (PCA), also known as a healthcare attendant/aide (HCA) or home health aide (HHA), makes home visits to assist clients. PCAs remind clients to take medications and make sure they eat properly. Some homemaking assistance may also be available (e.g., homemaker services; Chapter 98).

Telephone Services

Telephone services are often available; people can call and consult knowledgeable persons about concerns. Such services have proved particularly effective in crisis intervention, such as suicide, drug, and rape counseling. Advantages include anonymity and immediate accessibility. If the situation is considered dangerous, the caller may be referred immediately for help.

Other Community Services

Federally mandated *community mental health centers* (**CMHC**) exist throughout the country. These drop-in centers provide clients with structured recreation and opportunities to meet others with similar disorders. They often assist clients with employment, volunteer opportunities, money management, and housing. Community programs assist clients with training in independent living, so that they can live safely, either alone or in a minimally supervised situation. CMHCs often sponsor dances, parties, and outings for clients. Usually, there are games and other recreational materials in the center, as well as computers for client use. Individual communities have organizations that offer speakers and support groups to clients and families. National organizations, such as the National Alliance on Mental Illness (www.NAMI.org) and the National Mental Health Association (www.NMHA.org), also have local affiliates that offer various services.

Community-Based Living Facilities

Clients who do not need care in a hospital or extended-care facility are discharged into the community. Some live alone in apartments or subsidized housing. Others live in shelters, boarding houses, or foster homes. Additional supervision is sometimes necessary for those with chronic and persistent mental illnesses. Some of the facilities providing extra care are discussed below.

Adult Residential Care, Board-and-Care, Licensed Group Homes, and Nursing Homes

Some clients need structure and supervision to remain safe in the community. Adult residential care has many names and some differences in what is provided. They may live in a *board-and-care* home that provides meals and other services, with minimal supervision. *Licensed group homes* provide more structure by supervising medications and offering group activities. Most group homes require the client to attend a day program, have a volunteer position, or be employed for a minimum number of hours per week. If a client needs more supervision and physical care, a *nursing home* may be necessary. In some cases, the client requires a locked nursing home unit, particularly in the case of dementia.

Halfway Houses

Many communities offer "halfway houses" for mentally ill and/or chemically dependent clients. This facility provides a buffer between the inpatient facility and the community. The client lives there for a short time after discharge, making readjustment into the community less traumatic.

Adult Foster Care

Some states have adult foster care programs for clients with mental illness. These homes provide housing, often for an extended time. The client becomes part of the family and learns to live in a family and a community, with the guidance of foster parents.

Sheltered Workshops and Vocational Rehabilitation

A client may need assistance with employment. *Sheltered workshops* provide an entry into the working world. In many cases, they provide skill training, often paying clients a small wage during training. Some clients continue to work in sheltered workshops; others are able to seek competitive employment.

Vocational Rehabilitation Services

These services may be available to train clients for competitive employment. Vocational rehabilitation counselors also consult with employers to assist them to understand mental illness.

Respite Care

Supervision of a chronically mentally ill person is stressful. Clients may be placed in an inpatient area for a short time, so family caregivers can obtain rest and a chance to regroup. This *respite care* gives caregivers a *respite*, or break. Sometimes, respite care is covered by third-party payors.

> **Key Concept**
>
> A number of clients with chronic and persistent mental illness are unable to find or maintain an adequate living situation and become homeless. Outreach workers often attempt to locate homeless mentally ill people and assist them to find safer places to live. In some cities, single room occupancy apartments are available at a subsidized rate. In addition, free medical and dental care, examinations, immunizations, and medication therapy are often provided by community health centers. Organizations, such as the Salvation Army, sometimes deliver meals to shelters and homeless camps and provide basic health screening.

Partial Hospitalization Programs

Some psychiatric treatment centers have a service whereby clients spend nights at the facility and hold employment or volunteer positions during the day (*night hospital*). This provides some client supervision, while removing them from potentially dangerous living situations. In other cases, clients live at home and attend *intensive outpatient programs* (IOP) or *partial hospitalization programs* (PHP). Activities include groups, occupational, and recreational therapies. Clients learn about their medications and illnesses. For chemically dependent individuals, group therapy after discharge from the acute treatment center is vital and often continues indefinitely.

Emergency Services

Many healthcare facilities offer emergency evaluation and assistance to people with disruptions in mental health. Crisis intervention centers, acute psychiatric services (APS) centers, or emergency mental health clinics are different names for what is often part of a hospital's emergency department (ED). Crisis centers offer many services, including prescription of medications and referral of clients to mental health centers for therapy and case management. These centers also facilitate admission to inpatient psychiatric units for people who are seriously disturbed and present a danger to themselves or others.

The Inpatient Psychiatry Unit

If mental illness is severe, making the person dangerous to self or others, he or she is admitted to a hospital's *acute care* or *inpatient psychiatry unit*. Hospitalization helps prevent the illness from escalating by reducing emotional stress and offering medication and other therapies. The hospital provides a safer environment (*therapeutic milieu*) for a client in danger. The goal is to help the person learn to function effectively and safely in the community upon discharge.

Admission Status

The terms of admission to a mental health facility vary among states and provinces and even within an area. Several general types of admission exist:

Voluntary admission ("vol"): Person comes to the hospital voluntarily.

Involuntary transportation hold: Placed by a professional, which may be the police, to bring the person to the hospital in an emergency.

Emergency hold: Placed by a primary provider, the emergency hold (usually 3 days/72 hr), is for evaluation of clients who are judged to be dangerous to themselves or others. This gives the psychiatric team time to evaluate the client and place a court hold, if needed. This client is not allowed to leave the facility. Usually, this hold does not count weekends and holidays (because courts are closed).

District court hold (DCH): Placed by a court to hold the person before a preliminary commitment hearing.

Assessment hold: Placed by the court while determining a client's competency to stand trial for a crime.

Medical emergency: Placed by a primary provider to force medical treatment in the case of a critical medical condition, to prevent the client's further deterioration (discussed elsewhere).

Court commitment: Forced admission to a state, veteran's administration (VA), or county hospital, CD treatment center, or other care facility for treatment. If the court determines the client is currently able to manage, a *stay of commitment* may be issued. The client is able to remain in the community, as long as he or she is safe. Conditions are set up and if the client violates the conditions of the stay, the stay is *vacated* (revoked) and the client is placed in custody.

Mentally ill/chemically dependent (MI/CD): Dual diagnosis, both of which need treatment.

Mentally ill and dangerous (MI&D): Court commitment to a more restrictive "security hospital." (The MI&D commitment is difficult to obtain, but if obtained, usually remains with the person for life.)

Admission Procedures

Some clients refuse to talk when being admitted to a mental health unit. However, it is *vital* to obtain the following data, if at all possible. Try to get the client to answer at least the five questions below. If the client will not answer, try looking at old records or talking with relatives.

1. Do you have allergies?
2. Are you feeling like hurting yourself (*suicidal ideation*) or anyone else (*homicidal ideation*)?
3. Are you hearing voices (*auditory hallucinations*) or seeing things that others do not see (*visual hallucinations*)?
4. Why did you come to the hospital? Did you come voluntarily?
5. What medications are you taking (or are supposed to be taking)? When did you last take them?
6. Do you drink alcohol? If so, when did you last drink?

Commitment

Long-term hospitalization may be conducted at a state facility (state hospital or local treatment center), although the trend is toward closing state hospitals. Some of these facilities may admit people voluntarily, sometimes for special treatment (e.g., substance abuse disorders), but more people are admitted involuntarily (**commitment**). Commitment is imposed by the court and often follows a stay in another facility, such as an acute care hospital. Most committed clients are supported by public funds, availability of which varies between states and provinces.

Special Circumstances

A client may be admitted to a mental health unit under "no information status." This client does not want anyone to know they are there, and no information can be given out regarding the person, including that the person is there. No flowers or mail will be delivered, and visitors or callers will be told that no such person is registered. In other cases, a high-profile client, such as a movie star or celebrity, may be admitted under an *alias* (not the client's true name). This person is "also known as" (AKA), and all records are filed under the alias. If a client has legally changed their name or has been previously admitted under other names, this also is an AKA situation and all names are noted in the client record. In other cases, an unknown person is admitted and registered as "John Doe" or "Jane Doe" until the person's identity is established.

Discharge Planning

Planning for discharge begins on admission to a facility, with the goal of discharge as soon as possible. However, the hospital has a responsibility to both the client and the community. Clients cannot be discharged unless the treatment team feels that they are not dangerous to themselves or others. Everything possible is done to facilitate readjustment into the community and prevent readmission after discharge. Management of symptoms and client safety are of primary concern; efforts are made to place people in safe and comfortable living situations.

Provisional Discharge

A person may be discharged on a provisional basis. This may include those committed because the court found them incompetent to stand trial. The *provisional discharge* (PD) may discharge the person to jail. The terms of the PD are spelled out. If the client does not meet these terms, they are returned to the hospital (*revoked PD*). Common terms of a PD include medication compliance, keeping follow-up appointments, maintaining sobriety, attending a day-treatment program or support group, and avoiding legal trouble.

Payment for Mental Healthcare

Third-party payors may cover part or all of the cost of mental healthcare, including treatment for substance abuse disorders. However, requirements for inpatient care have become more stringent. Inpatient hospital stays are usually short, covering the crisis period only. Persons with chronic persistent mental illness often receive governmental financial assistance. It may be from Social Security Disability Income (SSDI), Medicaid, general assistance, another funding program, or the Affordable Care Act.

METHODS OF PSYCHIATRIC THERAPY

The goal of therapy is to alleviate symptoms and modify clients' behavior so they can meet life's demands and return to optimum wellness. (Safe return to the community is usually the goal of psychiatric care.) Therapy is based on specific behaviors and individual needs. Because therapists and nurses work together, nurses need to be aware of therapeutic goals and incorporate them into nursing care.

> **Key Concept**
>
> The major goal of all psychiatric care is *safety* of the client, their family, and others in the community.

Psychotherapy

Many different methods and theories of *psychotherapy* have been developed. Examples are presented here.

Individual Psychotherapy

Individual psychotherapy is based on a personal relationship between client and therapist, in a therapeutic, nonthreatening environment. The goal is to relieve symptoms and resolve the underlying factors that caused them. Treatment encourages people to tell their stories, express concerns and feelings, discuss problems, and work with the therapist to devise socially acceptable and healthy ways of dealing with issues. Many people are more willing to reveal thoughts and feelings to one person than in a group. It is most helpful for a client to have the same staff person for several sessions, in order to build trust. Guidelines for therapeutic communication are listed in Chapter 44. Hypnosis, psychoanalysis, counseling, and medication therapy are among methods that may be used in individual therapy.

Group Psychotherapy

Group psychotherapy involves several clients and provides an opportunity for all to participate by discussing individual concerns. Each client is drawn out of their private world and assisted to focus on others and the concerns of others. Clients often have keen insight and often, peers can relate to each other's concerns and offer constructive ideas. Group members usually have a special empathy and learn that they are not alone in their feelings and behaviors. They are often very accepting of suggestions and constructive criticism from peers, perhaps more so than from staff. Group therapy is especially effective for the treatment of addictive behaviors and for grief and loss counseling. Support groups are often available for families as well. This helps them to understand and learn how best to support their loved one who is dealing with mental health issues.

Verbal and Other Therapies

Many therapy methods are used in mental health settings. Below are selected examples. It is important to note that *combinations* of these therapies may be used.

Behavior Modification

Also known as *behavior shaping*, behavior modification is used primarily to deal with attention deficit hyperactivity disorder (ADHD), obsessive-compulsive disorder (OCD), phobias, generalized anxiety disorder (GAD), and autism spectrum disorder (ASD). *Behavior modification* is based on the theory that people respond well when rewarded for *positive behavior*. This *positive reinforcement* encourages the person to perform the same activity again to win another reward. To be effective, the expected task or behavior must be geared to the client's abilities; success must be possible. Show the person what you want, help the person accomplish it, then reward the person for a job well done. Rewards are most effective if given *immediately*. An effective form of positive reinforcement is a special reward. This may be a special hand lotion, stickers, deck of cards, special coffee, hair decoration, scented shampoo, special pass, puzzles, coloring book, or another special magazine or book. Almost any other reward, including attention from staff, can be reinforcing when used correctly. What is rewarding for one client may not necessarily be rewarding for another. *Negative reinforcement (punishment) is usually not effective* because it does not promote and teach positive behavior; *rewarding appropriate behavior and ignoring inappropriate behavior is most effective.* (Giving attention for negative behaviors reinforces the undesirable behavior.) Gradually let the person assume more independence. Consistency is important. Another technique used in behavior modification is guided relaxation.

> **Nursing Alert** Food is often not an appropriate reward. *Rationale: The client may have diabetes or be on another type of special diet. In addition, many clients are overweight, often as a side effect of psychiatric medications.*

Remotivation

Many units use *remotivation technique* or *reality orientation*, especially for clients with dementia or intellectual impairment. Groups are structured so clients discuss topics meaningful to them. To stimulate conversation, scrapbooks with pictures of familiar items can be helpful. Photo albums, newspapers, or videos of recent events can also spur discussion. Everyone is included in the discussion and encouraged to participate. The level of the discussion depends on the group's abilities. For example, in a group of clients with severe regression or dementia, the discussion would be simple, and the leader would ask many questions, to maintain the discussion.

> **Key Concept**
> All individuals need to know who they are, where they are, who other people are, and what day it is, in order to be comfortable.

Reality Therapy

People need to love and be loved, and to feel worthwhile to themselves (*self-esteem*) and others (*acceptance*). If a person is unable to meet these needs in a socially acceptable way, they may act inappropriately. The goals of *reality therapy* are to help people face reality, reject irresponsible/inappropriate behavior, and learn new and more socially acceptable behaviors. Reality therapy differs from conventional psychotherapy by concentrating on the present, rather than the past. In reality therapy, understanding the reasons behind client behaviors are less important than solving immediate problems and dealing with behaviors. The reality therapist approaches behaviors as they occur, rather than examining feelings or underlying causes. It is important for the client to learn that what happened in the past cannot be changed. Clients are encouraged to look toward the future and live accordingly. Behaviors can be taught, which will be helpful in meeting future goals and in learning to live comfortably outside the treatment center. A slogan commonly used is, "Today is the first day of the rest of your life."

Rational Emotive Behavior Therapy

Rational emotive behavior therapy (REBT), *rational recovery*, or *cognitive behavior therapy* is used in psychiatry, treatment for substance abuse disorders, and rehabilitation. Group members can usually relate to each other because they share similar concerns. REBT disputes irrational beliefs and accentuates rational/positive behaviors.

The principles of REBT are as follows:

- People are accepted unconditionally.
- Nothing is awful or terrible, even though it may be frustrating and difficult.
- Support is helpful in learning and practicing new ways to react to stress.

This approach is less effective if the client is out of contact with reality, highly manic, brain injured, or intellectually challenged. Chapter 95 discusses the REBT approach in CD treatment, as well as dialectical behavior therapy (DBT; sometimes also used in treatment of certain psychiatric disorders, such as BPD, chronic suicidality, and eating disorders).

Transactional Analysis

All interactions between people have meaning and are based on the way people feel at the moment. The goal of *transactional analysis* (TA) is to teach people to react in ways that produce positive responses from others, rather than hostility. TA is based on the concept that all people react, at different times, as the child, the parent, or the adult. At any particular time, one of these roles predominates. Two roles, those of parent and child, are actually from a person's past. When persons assume the parent role, they often react as their own parents did. When persons assume the child role, they often react as they did when they were a child. The goal is to react as a *reasonable adult* in as many situations as possible.

Psychodrama

The use of *role-playing* (acting out feelings) offers many people, especially children, the opportunity to release emotions. Many people are able to act out life situations that they are unable to verbalize, such as relationships with a spouse or parents. Close observation of *psychodrama* by staff is an aid in determining the client's underlying problems and planning the most effective measures for treatment and nursing care.

Occupational Therapy

Not only is *occupational therapy* (OT) highly therapeutic, it also acts as a source of enjoyment for many people. Clients are able to participate in creative projects, such as arts and crafts, while socializing with staff and peers. Through the creative process, people gain a sense of success and increased self-esteem. The overactive person is able to release some energy working on a project; the underactive person is encouraged to participate. Projects can be designed to be appropriate for any skill level. Fine motor skills and coordination can be developed and evaluated. The OT staff also evaluates the client's concentration, ability to plan, follow instructions, and relate to others. The non–English-speaking person can also comfortably participate in OT. Professional OTs also evaluate an individual's ability to function independently, using the KELS, as described previously. Another tool is the Functional Assessment Inventory (FAI). These tests help determine the safest living situation for each client after discharge. In many facilities, OT staff members assist in career planning, occupational skill training, or training in daily living skills, such as cooking, laundry, managing money, or grocery shopping. Occupational therapists may also work in a sheltered workshop, group home, or halfway house, assisting clients who have been discharged from acute psychiatric settings.

Drawing and Art

Children and adults can be encouraged to draw pictures of their families, their life situation, or thoughts and feelings. Often, these drawings can provide insight into the client's mental status. In addition, many people enjoy special art projects, just for fun. Often, very intricate designs are made and colored. Special media is available for clients to use. Art group serves as an adjunct to OT, but is different, because clients are encouraged to express their creative talents in any way they choose. The goal of the free art group is entertainment and free expression, more than specific therapy.

Recreational Therapy/Therapeutic Recreation

Recreational therapy, also known as *therapeutic recreation*, is an important component of the treatment program. Through planned recreational activities, on and off the mental health unit, the person is helped to safely reenter the community. A group may go bowling, to a sports event or movie, or out to eat. They may also engage in games, activities, and music on the inpatient unit, or they may assist in cooking a meal or dessert. Going to the gym or swimming pool or participating in an active game, such as bowling or shuffleboard, can help work off excess energy and assist in weight loss. Games such as "Life Stories" help clients share feelings. Games requiring scorekeeping help the person to regain math skills. Reading the newspaper together or celebrating holidays and birthdays helps clients keep up with current events. A grooming group encourages clients to look their best; being well-groomed and dressed appropriately adds to client self-esteem. Often, a relaxation group is held in the evening, to prepare clients for sleep. By using activities, RT staff assist clients to adapt and gradually become reaccustomed to interacting with others. The person who does not speak English can comfortably participate in many RT activities.

Music Therapy and Video Games

Music is a universal language. Many nonverbal or non–English-speaking people enjoy music and enthusiastically join in by singing or playing rhythm instruments. All clients are able to communicate and develop social skills, without being forced to speak. Sometimes, clients use music to help drown out "voices." Encourage the use of headphones; this is less disruptive to others. Video games and computer use are popular with many clients. It is important for staff to monitor the use of these modalities, to prevent viewing violence or inappropriate websites. *Computers must be blocked so clients cannot access medical records.*

Pet Therapy

Many facilities encourage helper animals. Many clients, regardless of condition, respond positively to an animal. Many people with mental illness relate better to animals than to other people; they may see animals as less threatening than other people. *Pet therapy* can help prepare individuals for future human interactions and responsibilities. Many mental health units have a resident pet, and clients can assist in its care. (It is important to closely supervise interactions with pets, to prevent injury to clients or the animals. Helper or service animals must be specially trained and certified, as discussed in Chapter 97.)

Play Therapy

There are two types of *play therapy*. The first is used to assist children (and occasionally adults) with disruptions in mental health. The play therapist guides their behavior, slowly helping them to socialize with others and adjust to the outside world. The therapist can also learn about the children and origins of their mental disorders by observing their play. The second type of play therapy is used with adults. One example is the "New Games" approach. These games are designed for various activity and attention levels and numbers of participants. Many are incorporated into activities for clients in mental health, rehabilitation, geriatric, and substance abuse disorder units. The games utilize rules that can apply to the real world. People are taught to take safe psychological and physical risks, to develop trust and a sense of community, to realize that winning is not as important as effort, and to emphasize challenge, rather than competition. Imagery and ritual promote a sense of freedom and decrease inhibition. Staff must be flexible and able to change to another game if the one chosen is not therapeutic. Games can also be adapted to suit the group. "Play hard, play fair, nobody hurt" is the slogan of the New Games Foundation.

Hydrotherapy

Many large mental health units have *hydrotherapy* facilities or swimming pools. Often, swimming or relaxing in a whirlpool can help clients work off frustrations or relax. Always *closely supervise* anyone who is swimming, in a whirlpool tub, or in a bathtub.

Electroconvulsive Therapy

Electroconvulsive therapy (**ECT**) is not used unless other methods have been used to decrease depression and have failed. In a carefully monitored procedure with a physician, anesthesiologist, and nurse present, the client is sedated and prepared for a short seizure (usually less than a minute), which is induced by sending a small amount of electricity through a precise location of the brain. It is believed that the seizure affects the brain's neurotransmitters, radically improving the person's mood. ECT has also more recently been used for bipolar disorder and schizophrenia. The person may experience anxiety before treatment and short-term memory loss afterward (In Practice: Nursing Care Guidelines 94-1). In rare cases, ECT may be administered against the client's will. This procedure may only be done involuntarily in severe situations and requires a specific court order by a judge.

Repetitive transcranial magnetic stimulation (rTMS) was approved in 2008 by the FDA as a treatment for major depression in clients who do not experience relief with the trial of at least one antidepressant. Some countries are using rTMS for intractable depression (does not respond to treatment) instead of ECTs. In this procedure, the client is not anesthetized. The procedure lasts about 30 min and the client may feel a slight knocking on the head. There is no preparation needed and the client may wear headphones to listen to music during the procedure. Its side effects appear to be minor.

> **Nursing Alert** Benzodiazepines and antiseizure medications are usually not given before ECT. These medications are held, beginning at approximately 6 PM the prior evening. Blood pressure medications are usually given in the morning, as ordered. The client is also not allowed to chew gum, including Nicorette gum, the morning of ECT. These procedures are in addition to NPO (nothing by mouth) after midnight, shower/shampoo the night before, and any other local protocols. If these procedures are not followed, the ECT may need to be canceled, for client safety.

IN PRACTICE
NURSING CARE GUIDELINES 94-1: Caring for the Client Who Is to Have ECT

- Make sure a signed surgical permit is on file (see Chapter 56 for preoperative preparations). *Rationale: This is required before any invasive procedure.*
- Be sure the client's weight (in kilograms) is recorded. *Rationale: Medication dosages are often calculated based on weight.*
- The client wears hospital garb (usually including pajama bottoms) and removes items such as dentures, contacts, jewelry, piercings, hearing aids, and artificial nails. *Rationale: This allows access to the client in case of emergency and helps prevent injury.*
- The morning's vital signs should be documented before the client goes to the treatment. *Rationale: This establishes a baseline for anesthesia personnel during the procedure.*
- The client *must* be wearing a name band and an allergy band. This is mandatory, not optional. *Rationale: The client will not be permitted to have ECT if these are not present.*
- ECT is usually carried out in the recovery room or a special treatment room. *Rationale: Emergency equipment and personnel are available, if needed, for client safety.*
- The person must void before the treatment. *Rationale: Incontinence may occur.*
- A mental status (cognitive skills) examination is performed before and several hours after ECT. *Rationale: This helps determine changes in cognitive skills resulting from ECT. Short-term memory loss is fairly common.*
- Explain the procedure to the client/family. A CD may be available to aid in teaching. *Rationale: This informs the client and helps reduce anxiety.*
- The client is transported to and from the treatment in a wheelchair or on a gurney. *Rationale: This helps avoid falls, if the client feels faint or excessively sleepy.*
- An IV is started. *Rationale: Routine medications are administered. The IV is also available in case of emergency.*
- A tourniquet is applied to one limb. *Rationale: This prevents a total body seizure, helps prevent injury, and provides visualization and confirmation of a seizure. (The tourniquet obstructs entry of anesthetic into the limb, restricting the seizure to only this limb.)*
- Paralysis is achieved by using short-acting anesthetics. *Rationale: This promotes safety and rapid recovery.*
- Clients commonly fear suffocation. Make sure the person understands that respiration will be supported during the procedure. *Rationale: Extreme panic can interfere with ECT. The client must understand that he or she will not stop breathing.*
- The person may complain of a sore throat after ECT. *Rationale: This may result from endotracheal tube placement.*
- Prevent injury during and after ECT. Monitor vital signs during ECT and report deviations. *Rationale: ECT is an invasive procedure.*
- After ECT, continue to monitor vital signs frequently until the client is stable. *Rationale: Although complications are rare, it is important to prevent injury.*
- Allow the person to sleep after ECT. *Rationale: Most clients are tired; sleeping can help prevent after-ECT complaints, such as headache.*
- Some clients require ibuprofen or muscle relaxants, such as cyclobenzaprine (Flexeril), or a specific antimigraine drug, such as sumatriptan (Imitrex) for side effects of ECT. If the client has severe problems, Imitrex may be administered IM one-half to 1 hr before ECT, as a preventive measure. *Rationale: Headache and myalgia (muscle pain) are side effects of ECT that may be effectively treated.*
- The client often complains of a dry mouth after ECT. *Rationale: Atropine is given to reduce secretions during the treatment.*

Medication Therapy

Introduced in the 1950s, *antipsychotic medications* revolutionized the treatment of mental disorders. Certain medications decrease or greatly alleviate the adverse symptoms of many psychiatric disorders, enabling clients to function better (Table 94-2). As a result of these medications, the number of long-term clients in inpatient facilities at all levels has greatly decreased. However, *medication noncompliance is a major concern* in psychiatry. To address this issue, several forms of medication are used to increase compliance (Box 94-2). In Practice: Nursing Care Guidelines 94-2 includes information on administering medication therapy in psychiatry.

The client who tries to avoid taking medications may be placed on "cheeking precautions." The client is observed carefully after taking medications. In some cases, the client must remain visible for a specified length of time after taking medications and show an open mouth, to make sure medications are swallowed or dissolved. The client's bathroom may also be locked for a specified length of time, to prevent the client from spitting out or vomiting medications. These actions by the client may occur when the medication has not yet reached therapeutic levels and the client is not yet feeling the benefits of the medication. Remember, legal and ethical issues accompany healthcare providers' actions, especially in the care of clients with mental illness.

> **Nursing Alert** Medications taken must be determined on admission to a facility. A "medication reconciliation" form is usually used. Information is obtained from the client, the family, and/or the client's previous home or pharmacy. Whether or not the client was compliant with medications and when the last doses were taken is vital, to avoid drug interactions and determine initial dosages.

In addition, it is vital to determine the client's allergies. An allergy band is worn by all clients, whether they have allergies or not. If the client refuses to wear an allergy band and/or a name band, this must be documented in the client's record. Medication compatibilities must be determined before medications are ordered or given.

Psychotropic Drugs

Psychotropic drugs (mood modifiers) include antipsychotics, antianxiety, sedative-hypnotics, mood stabilizers, stimulants (ADHD drugs), and antidepressants. These drugs are used primarily by psychiatric clients. However, clients may also use them in other healthcare settings—epilepsy or pain disorders. Pregnant clients should not take these medications without medical supervision. *Rationale: Many of these drugs are damaging to a fetus.*

Antipsychotic (Neuroleptic) Drugs

Antipsychotics, also known as **neuroleptics**, are pharmacological agents used to control the symptoms of schizophrenia and other disorders characterized by impaired reality testing, as evidenced by severely disorganized thought, speech, and behavior. They work on the nervous system to reduce confusion and agitation. They fall into two classes: first-generation (typical) antipsychotic medications and second-generation (atypical) antipsychotics. First-generation drugs were developed in the 1950s. These drugs (e.g., haloperidol [Haldol], chlorpromazine [Thorazine], fluphenazine [Prolixin], perphenazine [Trilafon]) are used to treat *positive symptoms* of psychosis (hallucinations, delusions, and thought disorders—paranoia, severe agitation, hyperactivity, combativeness, and feelings of unreality). These medications act on the brain's postsynaptic dopamine receptors. Older antipsychotics are generally less effective in treating *negative symptoms*, as listed in the discussion of schizophrenia. Second-generation antipsychotics were developed in the 1980s. However, second-generation or atypical medications, such as aripiprazole (Abilify), clozapine (Clozaril), olanzapine (Zyprexa), paliperidone (Invega), ziprasidone (Geodon), and risperidone (Risperdal), can be effective against both positive and negative symptoms (Table 94-2). Many of the newer medications also work selectively on the brain's dopamine receptors. Generally, they have fewer *extrapyramidal symptoms* (**EPS**), or drug-induced movement disorders, than the older medications and are less likely to cause *tardive dyskinesia*, cognitive impairment, and other unwanted symptoms (see later discussion). In addition to new medications, new forms of medications have been introduced in recent years. Most of these are aimed at *improving medication compliance*. They are designed to be difficult to "cheek" or are given as injections. Some injectable medications are available in long-acting form (*decanoate*), so the client needs to receive an injection only 1–2 times per month. Extended release, delayed release, and sustained release tablets and capsules reduce the number of times per day the client is required to take medications. Recent innovations also include the orally disintegrating tablet (ODT), the transdermal patch, and medication sprinkles (Table 94-2).

Side Effects

Multiple side effects are associated with the use of neuroleptics/antipsychotics (Box 94-3). For example, clozapine (Clozaril) has the potential to cause bone marrow suppression and blood dyscrasias; these clients must have weekly blood work performed, which significantly increases treatment costs. Because of this, clients must have at least two failures with other classes of antipsychotics/neuroleptics before beginning clozapine. Clozapine must not be given with any other medications that have similar adverse effects. In addition, it can cause postural hypotension; this client should be on fall precautions. Adverse neurologic and other unwanted side effects may also occur as a result of administration of other antipsychotic medications (Box 94-3).

Anticholinergic Medications

These medications are used to prevent or treat many side effects of antipsychotics although there are concerns about their being used for prevention. The most commonly used anticholinergic medications are amantadine (Symmetrel), benztropine mesylate (Cogentin), and trihexyphenidyl (Artane). The antihistamine diphenhydramine (Benadryl) and biperiden (Akineton), an antiparkinsonian drug, are also used to prevent side effects.

Tardive Dyskinesia

Tardive dyskinesia (**TD or TDK**) is a neurologic disorder, characterized by involuntary movements, especially of the

TABLE 94-2 Examples of Medications Used in Psychiatry

NAME OF DRUG[a]	FORMS AND DOSAGES AVAILABLE	NOTES AND INDICATIONS FOR USE
Benzodiazepines/anxiolytics (some are also antiepileptics)		Used in seizure disorders, anxiety, delirium. Phenothiazines used in agitated psychotic states, hallucinations, anxiety (also in tetanus, hiccups, itching).
alprazolam (Xanax, Apo-Alpraz [Can], Novo-Alprazol [Can])	Tablets: 0.25–2 mg; ER tablets: 0.5–3 mg; ODT tablets: 0.25–2 mg; oral solution: 1 mg/mL.	Panic attacks, anxiety.
chlordiazepoxide HCl (Librium)	Capsules: 5–25 mg.	Anxiety disorders, acute agitation, preoperative anxiety, acute alcohol withdrawal (DTs, hallucinosis, severe tremors).
clonazepam (Klonopin)	Tablets: 0.5–2 mg; ODT wafers: 0.125–2 mg.	Anxiety disorders, panic attacks, specific seizures, tic disorders, BPD.
diazepam (Valium, Diastat, Diazemuls [Can])	Tablets: 2–10 mg; oral solution: 5 mg/mL; rectal gel: 2.5–20 mg; injectable (IM, IV): 5 mg/mL.	Anxiety disorders, acute alcohol withdrawal, muscle relaxant, adjunct in status epilepticus (IV), preoperative—to promote relaxation. May be used in night terrors, tetanus.
lorazepam (Ativan, Novo-Lorazem [Can]) midazolam HCL (Versed)	Tablets: 0.5–2 mg; oral solution (Intensol): 2 mg/mL; injectable (IM, IV): 2–4 mg/mL. Syrup: 2 mg/mL; injectable: 1–5 mg/mL.	Anxiety, insomnia, preoperative sedation, status epilepticus (IV). Intermediate acting; may be given IM to control dangerous behavior (not psychiatric related). Injectable solution may be given orally. Conscious sedation and amnesia for minor surgery.
oxazepam (Novoxapam [Can]—not used in the United States) temazepam (Restoril)	Capsules: 10–30 mg. Capsules: 7.5–30 mg.	Alcohol withdrawal; anxiety. Hypnotic—short-term treatment of insomnia
Miscellaneous		
hydroxyzine (Vistaril, Atarax)—anxiolytic	Hydroxyzine HCl—tablets: 10–50 mg; capsules: 25–50 mg; oral syrup: 2–10 mg/5 mL; injectable (given deep IM only): 25–50 mg/mL. Hydroxyzine pamoate: capsules: 25–100 mg; oral suspension: 25 mg/5 mL.	Anxiety, tension, management of acutely disturbed client (IM). Also antiemetic, antihistamine—used to manage pruritus (itching), alcohol withdrawal, and as premedication and after general anesthesia.
pregabalin (Lyrica)—anticonvulsant	Capsules: 25–300 mg; oral solution: 20 mg/mL.	Generalized anxiety disorder; management of acute pain, fibromyalgia, diabetic neuropathy, specific seizures.
Antipsychotic drugs		Used in schizophrenia, psychosis, depression or mania in BPD, autism.
aripiprazole (Abilify) (second generation—atypical antipsychotic)	Tablets: 2–30 mg; oral solution: 1 mg/mL ODT (Discmelt): 10–15 mg; injectable; long-acting injection (Abilify, Maintena): 160–400 mg, give monthly.	Schizophrenia, bipolar mania, agitation, irritability (especially in autism), MDD (used in addition to antidepressants). Maintena: Give in *gluteus medius only.*
chlorpromazine HCl (first generation—phenothiazine)	Tablets: 10–200 mg; injectable: 25 mg/mL.	Psychosis, mania, nausea, vomiting, intractable hiccups, tetanus. Full effects may take up to 6 months. Infrequent use in the United States.
clozapine (Clozaril) (second generation)	Tablets: 12.5–200 mg; oral suspension; ODT (Fazaclo): 12.5–200 mg.	Schizophrenia and schizoaffective disorders (not responsive to other drugs).
fluphenazine HCl (Modecate, Moditen) (first generation—phenothiazine, formerly Prolixin in the United States)	Tablets: 1–10 mg; oral concentrate: 5 mg/ml; oral elixir: 2.5 mg/5 mL; injectable—IM: 2.5 mg/ml; (+ long-acting [decanoate]— every 1-3 weeks): 25 mg/mL; 100 mg/mL	Psychosis. Can cause blood dyscrasias, EPS (rarely used).

(Continued)

TABLE 94-2 Examples of Medications Used in Psychiatry (Continued)

NAME OF DRUG[a]	FORMS AND DOSAGES AVAILABLE	NOTES AND INDICATIONS FOR USE
haloperidol (Haldol, Novo-Peridol [Can]) (first generation)	Tablets: 0.5–20 mg; oral concentrate (Haldol lactate): 2 mg/mL; injectable: 5 mg/mL; +long-acting (Haldol decanoate—every 3–4 weeks): 50–100 mg/mL.	Psychosis, muscle spasms, control of tics in Tourette syndrome. High risk of EPSE. Low sedative properties. Risk of EPS. Decanoate: do not exceed 3 ml/site.
loxapine succinate (first generation)	Capsules: 5–50 mg.	Psychosis; observe carefully in respiratory D/O, glaucoma, epilepsy, or ulcers.
olanzapine (Zyprexa) (second generation)	Tablets: 2.5–20 mg; ODT (Zyprexa Zydis): 5–20 mg; powder (must be reconstituted) for injection: 10 mg; extended-release injection: 210–405 mg/vial.	Schizophrenia, bipolar mania (often combined with lithium or valproate), management of violent clients (IM). Sedative effects (give at HS). Significant side effect: weight gain, diabetes. Not recommended for psychotic dementia in older adults.
paliperidone (Invega)—atypical antipsychotic	ER tablets: 1.5–9 mg. Long-acting injection—INVEGA SUSTENNA: 39–234 mg.	Schizophrenia. Long-acting: give; then give 1 week later; then once monthly.
pimozide (Orap) (first generation)	Tablets: 1–2 mg.	Suppression of disabling motor or phonic tics in Tourette. Not used in schizophrenia.
prochlorperazine (Compro) (first generation—phenothiazine) edisylate and maleate	Tablets (maleate): 5–25 mg; rectal suppositories; (edisylate): 25 mg; (prochlorperazine) 10 mg [Can]; injectable: 5 mg/ml.	Psychosis, nonpsychotic anxiety, severe nausea, and vomiting.
quetiapine (Seroquel) (second generation)	Tablets: 25–400 mg; ER/XR tablets: 50–400 mg.	Schizophrenia (older than 18 years); BPD, short-term treatment of acute mania (combined with lithium or divalproex), depression.
risperidone (Risperdal) (second generation) thioridazine HCl (first generation)	Tablets: 0.25–4 mg; oral solution: 1 mg/ml; ODT (M-Tabs): 0.25–4 mg; powder (to be reconstituted) for injection (must use designated syringe)—long-term injection (Risperdal Consta), given approximately every 2 weeks. Tablets: 10–100 mg.	Schizophrenia, acute bipolar mania (alone or in combination with lithium or valproate—oral only), OCD, irritability in autism, Tourette syndrome. Low risk of EPSE. Schizophrenia—used only if client fails two other drugs.
thiothixene (Navane) (first generation—phenothiazine)	Capsules: 1–10 mg.	Psychosis. Risk of EPSE and other serious side effects. Older than 12 years only.
Ziprasidone HCl (Geodon) (second generation)	Capsules: 20–80 mg; IM injection: 20 mg/ml, give with food.	Atypical antipsychotic. Schizophrenia, acute mania, rapid control of severe agitation (IM). Lower risk of EPS; less likely to cause weight gain; monitor for diabetes. Not for dementia-related psychosis in elderly.
Antidepressants[b]		SSRIs used in major depression, OCD, bulimia nervosa, panic disorder, PTSD. Tricyclics especially used in depression, OCD.
bupropion (Wellbutrin, Aplenzin) (for smoking cessation—Zyban)	Bupropion HCl (Wellbutrin, Zyban): ER tablets: 150–450 mg; IR: 75–100 mg; SR: 50–200 mg. Bupropion hydrobromide—(Aplenzin): ER tablets 174–522 mg.	Depression, including MDD—(Aplenzin only); seasonal affective disorder. Unrelated to other antidepressants.
buspirone (Buspar)	Tablets: 5–30 mg.	Anxiety disorders, traumatic brain injury.
citalopram hydrobromide (Celexa)—SSRI clomipramine HCl (Anafranil)—TCA	Tablets: 10–40 mg; oral solution: 10 mg/5 mL. Capsules: 25–75 mg.	Depression, especially MDD. May be used in OCD, social phobia. OCD, panic disorder, enuresis (bedwetting) in children older than 6 years.
desvenlafaxine succinate (PRISTIQ)	ER tablets: 50–100 mg.	Depression, including MDD.
doxepin HCl (Sinequan, Silenor)—TCA	Capsules: 10–150 mg; oral concentrate: 10 mg/mL. Tablets: 3–6 mg.	Depression, especially bipolar depression, anxiety, insomnia.

TABLE 94-2 Examples of Medications Used in Psychiatry (Continued)

NAME OF DRUG[a]	FORMS AND DOSAGES AVAILABLE	NOTES AND INDICATIONS FOR USE
duloxetine HCl (Cymbalta)—SSNRI	DR capsules: 20–60 mg.	MDD, anxiety, fibromyalgia, diabetic neuropathic pain, stress incontinence.
escitalopram (Lexapro)—SSRI	Tablets: 5 mg; oral solution (5 mg/ml).	Depression, including MDD, generalized anxiety, panic disorder, PTSD. Contraindicated with MAOIs. Caution in elderly.
fluoxetine HCl (Prozac, Sarafem)—SSRI	Tablets: 10–60 mg; capsules: 10–40 mg; oral liquid: 20 mg/5 mL, DR capsules: 90 mg. For premenstrual dysphoric disorder (PMDD)—Sarafem.	Bulimia nervosa, BPD, bipolar depression, PTSD, panic disorder, OCD, menopausal hot flashes.
fluvoxamine (Luvox)—SSRI	Tablets: 25–100 mg; ER capsules: 100–150 mg.	OCD, social anxiety disorder, bulimia nervosa, panic disorder.
imipramine (Tofranil), (Novo-pramine [Can])—TCA	Tablets: 10–50 mg. Imipramine pamoate: capsules: 75–150 mg.	Depression, intractable pain, especially neuropathic, childhood enuresis—older than 6 years, ADHD.
mirtazapine (Remeron) nortriptyline HCl (Aventyl, Pamelor)	Tablets: 7.5–45 mg; ODT (Soltab) 15–45 mg. Capsules: 10–75; oral solution: 10 mg/5 mL.	MDD, may assist in sleep. Depression, postherpetic neuralgia, IBS.
paroxetine HCl (Paxil; paroxetine mesylate [Pexeva])—SSRI	Tablets: 10–40 mg; CR tablets: 12.5–37.5 mg; oral suspension: 10 mg/5 mL.	Depression, OCD, panic disorder, social phobias, PTSD, premenstrual dysphoric disorder (PMDD).
selegiline (Emsam)—MAOI	Capsules or tablets: 5 mg; ODT tablets: 1.25 mg; transdermal patch: 6–12 mg/patch—applied daily. (The first *transdermal* antidepressant.)	Depression. At *lowest dose*, dietary restrictions are not necessary.
sertraline (Zoloft)—SSRI	Tablets: 25–100 mg; oral concentrate: 20 mg/mL.	Depression, OCD, panic disorder, PTSD, PMDD, social phobias.
trazodone HCl (Desyrel, Oleptro)	Tablets: 50–300 mg; ER tablets: 150–300 mg.	Depression, sleep aid in depression (especially in elderly). Priapism is side effect.
venlafaxine HCl (Effexor)—SSNRI	Tablets: 25–100 mg; ER tablets: 37.5–225 mg; ER capsules: 37.5–150 mg.	Depression (including MDD), generalized anxiety, panic disorder, PMDD, and diabetic neuropathy. Social anxiety disorder (ER form only).
Mood stabilizers and antiepileptics		
carbamazepine (Tegretol; Carbatrol)	Tablets: 200 mg, chewable tablets: 100 mg; ER tablets: 100–400 mg; ER capsules: 100–300 mg; oral suspension: 100 mg/5 mL.	Antiepileptic. Also used in BPD (acute mania), trigeminal neuralgia, alcohol withdrawal.
gabapentin (Neurontin)	Tablets: 100–800 mg; capsules: 100–400 mg; ER tablets: 300–600 mg; oral solution: 250 mg/5 mL.	Partial seizures, RLS, neuralgia, diabetic neuropathy.
lamotrigine (Lamictal)	Tablets: 25–200 mg; chewable tablets: 2–25 mg; ER tablets: 25–300 mg; ODT: 25–200 mg.	Antiepileptic. Long-term management of bipolar disorder.
lithium citrate, lithium carbonate (Lithobid, Eskalith, Carbolith [Can])	Capsules: 150–600 mg; tablets: 300 mg; ER tablets: 300–450 mg; oral syrup (lithium citrate, sugarless): 8 mg/5 ml.	Bipolar mania, BPD.
oxcarbazepine (Trileptal) topiramate (Topamax)	Tablets: 25–200 mg; capsules/sprinkles: 15–25 mg; ER capsules: 25–200 mg. Tablets: 25–200 mg; capsules/sprinkles: 15–25 mg; ER capsules: 25–200 mg.	Antiepileptic. May be used in bipolar disorder. Antiepileptic. Anxiety, bulimia nervosa, migraine headache.

(Continued)

TABLE 94-2 Examples of Medications Used in Psychiatry (Continued)

NAME OF DRUG[a]	FORMS AND DOSAGES AVAILABLE	NOTES AND INDICATIONS FOR USE
valproate Na+, valproic acid, divalproex Na+ (Depacon, Depakene, Depakote, Epival ECT [Can])	Valproate Na+: injection: 100 mg/mL; syrup: 250 mg/5 ml. Valproic acid: capsules: 250 mg, DR capsules: 125–500 mg; EC tablets: 200–500 mg; syrup: 200 mg/5 ml. Divalproex Na+: DR tablets: 125–500 mg; ER tablets: 250–500 mg; capsules/sprinkle: 125 mg.	Antiepileptic. Bipolar disorder, simple and generalized seizures, mania, prophylaxis for migraine headache, symptom management in schizophrenia, ADHD. Dangerous if given to young females.
Other drugs		
cyclobenzaprine HCl (Flexeril, Amrix)	Tablets: 5–10 mg; ER capsules: 15–30 mg.	Skeletal muscle relaxant (may be used in ECT), antidepressant effects (structurally related to tricyclics).
methylphenidate HCl (Ritalin, Concerta, Methylin, Daytrana [transdermal]).	Various forms including tablets, chewable tablets, capsules, oral solution, and transdermal patch.	CNS stimulant. Adults: Narcolepsy, ADHD, geriatric depression.
phenytoin Na+ (Dilantin, Phenytek)	ER capsules: 30–300 mg; chewable tablets: 50 mg; oral suspension: 125 mg/5 mL; injectable: 50 mg/mL.	Anticonvulsant—for generalized tonic–clonic and psychomotor seizures, status epilepticus.
sumatriptan (Imitrex)	Tablets: 25–100 mg; nasal spray: 5–20 mg/0.1 mL; injectable: 4–6 mg/0.5 mL.	Severe migraine headaches; headaches associated with ECT (may be given as prophylactic before ECT).

[a]A trade name appears in parentheses following the generic name of the drug. Examples of Canadian trade names [Can] are included.

[b]Tricyclics (antidepressants) such as amitriptyline, imipramine, and doxepin can cause severe side effects (i.e., ECG changes, tachycardia, hypertension).

Special note: All medications, particularly in psychiatry, must be used with extreme caution if combined with over-the-counter drugs or herbal supplements. Specifically, the following herbals can cause serious interactions with psychiatric drugs: *chamomile, evening primrose, ginkgo, ginseng, kava, ma huang, passionflower vine, St. John wort, thyme, valerian root, and yohimbe.*

Caution clients not to use alcohol or street drugs with any psychiatric drugs. Alcohol and some street drugs increase the risk of drug toxicity and often reduce the effectiveness of the prescribed medications.

Many psychiatric medications can contribute to kidney and/or liver disorders. Other possible serious side effects include diabetes mellitus, extreme weight gain, hypertension, and sexual side effects, including impotence. Clients must be carefully monitored.

Certain psychiatric medications *interact* negatively *with grapefruit juice.* (Grapefruit juice causes delayed and/or decreased metabolism of the drug, which can lead to drug toxicity or reduce the effectiveness of the drug.) These drugs include alprazolam (Xanax), buspirone (Buspar), carbamazepine (Tegretol), fluoxetine (Prozac), fluvoxamine (Luvox), and sertraline (Zoloft).

The dosage of most psychiatric medications must be titrated up and tapered down gradually to avoid severe problems. Some drugs are very dangerous if stopped abruptly or if the dose is titrated up too fast.

A number of drug forms and specific drugs cannot safely be cut, crushed, or chewed. These include CR, DR, XR, ER, and SR forms; capsules; enteric-coated tablets; gel caps; and certain specific drugs (e.g., bupropion, divalproex, fluphenazine, paroxetine CR, and valproic acid derivatives).

Orally disintegrating tablet (ODT) forms usually should not be cut. The client should be taught to dissolve the tablet first and then to swallow the medication.

Tyramine-rich foods to avoid when taking MAOIs include aged cheese, avocados, bananas, beer, bologna, caffeine, chocolate, herring, liver, meat tenderizer, pepperoni, pickled foods, raisins, red wine, ripe fruit, salami, smoked foods, yeast, and yogurt.

Many of these drugs can have adverse effects on a fetus. Because some of these drugs are hormone-based or interact with hormones, women of child-bearing age are strongly advised to use barrier methods of fertility control, rather than "birth control pills."

The atypical antipsychotics are not recommended for elderly clients with dementia-related psychoses because of increased risk of death.

face and jaw. It is a serious side effect resulting from long-term use of neuroleptics. It affects more women than men and is more common in older clients. Many clients treated with first-generation neuroleptics developed TD; this is less common with newer medications. TD rarely results within the first year of neuroleptic use and may occur after the medication is discontinued. Almost any antipsychotic/neuroleptic can cause TD. TD may also occur as a result of taking amoxapine (Asendin), an antidepressant; the gastric drug metoclopramide (Reglan); or the antinausea drug prochlorperazine (Compazine). Early identification of TD is essential, to prevent worsening of involuntary movements. TD usually cannot be reversed and may continue even after the causative drug is discontinued. To be diagnosed with TD is devastating and, in some cases, the involuntary muscle movements are disfiguring and disabling.

The person with TD most often has oral–lingual–buccal dyskinesias—obvious abnormal mouth and tongue movements. The first sign is a small, wriggling movement under the surface of the tongue. Other signs of TD are listed below. TD movements usually stop during sleep; they may be aggravated when the person tries to perform a purposeful movement or speak. (If no other effective psychotropic drug can be found, the client with TD may opt to continue with a lower dose, to control psychotic symptoms.) Because clozapine (Clozaril) has not been found to cause TD, this drug may be used. No effective treatment exists for TD, but its progression can usually be arrested by decreasing or discontinuing the offending medication. One medication used to treat symptoms of TD, particularly tremors, is propranolol HCl (Inderal). Fear of TD (or existing symptoms of TD) is a common reason for clients to refuse or stop taking medications.

Box 94-2 Forms of Medications Used in Psychiatry

ORAL MEDICATIONS
- Tablet, capsule: available in IR (immediate release), ER and XR (extended release), DR (delayed release), CR (controlled release) forms
- Chewable tablets: if difficulty swallowing tablets or capsules
- Crushed tablets: administered in food. (All the food must be taken, to ensure administration of full dose.)
- Liquid forms: aid in compliance and act faster than tablets. May be put in juice (not grapefruit) or applesauce, to disguise taste. (Available as syrup, suspension, concentrate, elixir.)
- Sprinkle: usually contained in a special capsule; may need to be measured. Sprinkled over food.
- **ODT** (orally disintegrating tablet) form: dissolves on contact with tongue (Chapter 63)
- Nasogastric (NG) tube administration

TRANSDERMAL PATCH
- Some antidepressants (and pain control medications) available in this form. Requires once-a-day application (or off for 12 hr, new patch on for 12 hr).

INJECTIONS
- Intramuscular (IM) injections
- Powder for injection—must be reconstituted (follow manufacturer's instructions)
- Long-lasting injections (last several weeks)
- Intravenous (IV) injections (in emergency, to control extremely dangerous behavior or reverse life-threatening side effects)

Key Concept

A person may have early tardive dyskinesia, but mild symptoms may be masked by neuroleptic medications that he or she is taking. Only when symptoms become worse do they "break through" and become obvious. At that point, it is usually not possible to reverse existing symptoms.

Several evaluation scales, such as the **DISCUS** (Dyskinesia Identification System Condensed User Scale) and **AIMS** (Abnormal Involuntary Movement Scale), are used to assess the presence or absence and severity of TD. Special training in administration of these tests is required. Most long-term facilities require each client on a neuroleptic medication be assessed at regular intervals. Tests for TD determine if *specific abnormal movements* are present most of the time, including the following:

- Facial tics, grimaces, or rhythmic movements of lips, eyes, or face, including facial tics
- Chewing or sucking; lip smacking
- Excessive blinking or bursts of blinking
- Abnormal tongue movements (including tongue tremors), intermittent darting in and out of the mouth, tonic "tongue in cheek," stationary protruding tongue
- Abnormal twisting or jerking of fingers or arms (not including tremor), slow writhing (**athetoid** movements), or pill rolling
- Abnormal toe or foot movements, writhing toes, or overlapped toes caused by cramping
- Abnormal head or neck movements or jerking (usually to the same side), constant shrugging of the shoulders
- Abnormal, rigid body posturing
- In rare cases, breathing or walking may be affected

Certain common EPS are not considered specifically indicative of TD. These include, but are not limited to the following:

- Arm or hand tremors
- **Cogwheeling** (ratcheting, when arms are passively moved)
- **Akathisia** (extreme motor restlessness), pacing, leg jerks
- Rocking
- **Opisthotonos** *(spasm, with head and heels bent toward each other, trunk bowed forward)*
- **Oculogyric crisis** (abnormal circular movement of eyeballs)
- Stiff neck
- Difficulty swallowing
- Difficulty breathing
- Abnormal verbalizations

The person with milder manifestations of these symptoms, such as tremor, usually does not need to have the medication discontinued or changed. More severe symptoms indicate a need to stop the antipsychotic medication. The most frightening of these symptoms, particularly opisthotonos, oculogyric crisis, or difficulty breathing, can usually be quickly reversed by administration of benztropine (Cogentin) or diphenhydramine (Benadryl), either orally (in liquid form) or by intramuscular (IM) injection.

Neuroleptic Malignant Syndrome

Neuroleptic malignant syndrome (NMS) is a rare, life-threatening complication of certain neuroleptic medications. It is believed to be caused by a dopamine blockage in the hypothalamus. NMS is a medical emergency, with a mortality rate as high as 20% (most frequently caused by respiratory failure, then renal failure or pulmonary embolism). NMS can occur soon after first administration of an antipsychotic/neuroleptic medication or can occur later. If you suspect NMS, stop the medication and provide emergency care. If NMS is detected and treated early, symptoms usually resolve in several days, with no permanent damage. Symptoms of NMS include the following:

- Sudden altered level of consciousness (LOC); mental status changes
- Rapid onset of muscle rigidity (client often describes as "feeling like a lead pipe")
- Cogwheeling
- General **dyskinesia** (impaired voluntary movement)
- Opisthotonos
- Oculogyric crisis
- Autonomic nervous system disturbances. Examples:
  - Sudden unexplained hyperthermia (fever)
  - Diaphoresis (excessive perspiration)
  - Tachypnea (rapid breathing—approximately 25 breaths per minute)

IN PRACTICE
NURSING CARE GUIDELINES 94-2: Administering Medication Therapy in the Mental Health Unit

- Follow all general steps for administering medications (see Chapter 63, In Practice: Nursing Care Guidelines 63-1 and 63-2; for injections, see Chapter 64, In Practice: Nursing Procedures 64-3, 64-4, and 64-5).
- Leave medications in their packages until you reach the client. *Rationale: Allow the person with paranoia to see the package being opened or to open it themselves. Medication need not be wasted if it is refused, and the nurse can more easily identify and teach about medications. If a client loses control and hits the medication tray or cup, the medications will not be lost.*
- Use clear, plastic medication cups, not paper soufflé cups. *Rationale: The nurse will be able to see if there are any pills remaining, and plastic cups are harder to crush in an effort to hide pills.*
- If liquid medication is ordered, pour it shortly before administration. If it is supplied in a brown bottle, it must be covered while on the medication tray. (*Rationale: These medications are not stable when exposed to air or light.*)
- Some liquid medications cannot safely be combined. If there is any doubt, use a separate medicine cup for each.
- Identify the person carefully before giving any medication. "Check two for safety." Always check or scan the person's name band and check the MAR or computer. You may ask the person's name, but this may not be reliable. Another staff member may be asked to identify the client. *Rationale: The client may be confused or may deliberately try to mislead you. (This may be more common in psychiatry than other areas.)* Follow the previously outlined guidelines if the person refuses to wear a name band. In some cases, the client will wear the name band on an ankle.
- Ask the client to drink an entire cup of water. It may be necessary to look in the client's mouth, under the tongue, and in the cheeks. Watch to make sure the client does not spit out or vomit medications. *Rationale: Many psychiatric clients attempt to "cheek" (hide) medications and not take them.*
- Document the effectiveness of medications. Desired effects include the following:
  - Lessening hallucinations.
  - Decreasing delusional thinking.
  - Diminishing distortions in the thought process.
  - Lessening of destructive behavior to self or others.
  - Improvement in self-care, sleep, or eating habits.
  - Ability to carry on a logical conversation.
  - Improvement in socialization with peers and staff.
- Observe and document the client's willingness to take medications. Some clients argue about taking medications but do take them. If the person refuses, document this and the reasons the person gives for refusing. Most clients have the right to refuse medications. *Rationale: The client's reasons for refusal or reluctance to take medications are important because they are often related to side effects. If there is a court order to force medications, they may be given by injection. (This may be called a "Jarvis" order in Minnesota.)*
- The client with a history of medication noncompliance may be given the liquid or instantly dissolving form of a medication (orally disintegrating tablet—ODT), may have medications crushed in foods, or may receive long-acting injections, which are given every 2–3 weeks.
- If the ODT form of a medication is to be given, it should not be touched or exposed to the air. *Rationale: It will disintegrate, especially if it becomes damp.*
- Observe and document any side effects. Carefully describe the side effect, how it progressed, and how it was treated. *Rationale: Major reasons for medication refusal are fear of undesirable side effects, especially tardive dyskinesia (impairment of muscle movement, a potentially disabling side effect), unwanted weight gain, and sexual side effects (e.g., impotence).*
- Teach the client/family about medications, the importance of following administration times and dosages, possible side effects, and what to do if these occur. *Rationale: Side effects can occur suddenly, even after the client has been taking a medication for some time.*
- Warn clients about discontinuing medications abruptly or about increasing or decreasing their dosage without consulting the provider. *Rationale: These situations can be life-threatening.*
- Clients also need to know that some factors such as smoking and taking antacids adversely affect medication absorption. Most antipsychotic medications should be avoided during the first trimester of pregnancy (to avoid birth defects) and within 10 days of delivery (to avoid EPSE in the infant).

Note: In some cases, medications are administered against the client's will. This is the case if the client is out of control and a danger to self or to others. A "medical emergency" can also be declared or the court may order the client to take medications. In these cases, medications will be forced. Usually, forced medications must be given by injection until the client agrees to take them orally. The injection is usually intramuscular (IM), but may be given intravenously (IV) if the situation is critical. A nasogastric tube (NG) may also be used, but this is uncomfortable for the client and difficult to monitor. When the client agrees to take oral medications, usually liquid or ODT medications are administered, to make sure the client is not trying to cheek them. Long-acting injections may also be used. *Rationale: In an emergency, the client does not have the right to refuse treatment. In some cases, forcing medications is lifesaving.*

> **Box 94-3** Potential Side Effects of Antipsychotic/Neuroleptic Drugs (Including Extrapyramidal Side Effects—EPSE)
>
> - *General dyskinesia:* Involuntary, continual rhythmic movements; jerking; tremors; twisting; abnormal tongue movements; tonic tongue; toe movements; tics (severe form: tardive dyskinesia)
> - **Dystonia**: Involuntary and irregular movements of muscles of the trunk and extremities; impaired muscle tone
> - *Akathisia:* Extreme inability to sit still, motor restlessness (tapping, rocking, pacing), or muscle-quivering tremors
> - *Parkinsonian syndrome:* Symptoms similar to Parkinson disease (resting tremor, rigidity, slowness in motor activity, and postural abnormalities)
> - *Other muscular side effects:* Jaw spasms, impaired breathing or swallowing, involuntary grimaces
> - *Nonmovement side effects:* Dry mouth, blurred vision, constipation, incontinence, thick tongue, constant hunger and rapid weight gain, sleepiness, tachycardia, impotence, decreased libido, insomnia, or hypersomnia
> - *Orthostatic hypotension:* Decrease in blood pressure and rise in heart rate on standing, dizziness
> - *Cogwheeling movements:* When the client relaxes the arm and the examiner moves it, the movement is jerky and seems to catch (ratcheting)
> - *Opisthotonos:* Uncontrollable and severe head and neck extension, with trunk bowed forward
> - *Oculogyric crisis:* Involuntary upward rolling of eyes or prolonged fixation of eyeballs
> - Tardive dyskinesia and neuroleptic malignant syndrome are serious side effects that are discussed within the chapter.
> - Other conditions may result from these medications (e.g., diabetes mellitus, hypertension, obesity, kidney and liver disorders, extreme sedation, and sexual side effects, including impotence).

- Tachycardia (rapid pulse—approximately 30 beats greater than usual)
- Fluctuating blood pressure—generally elevated—about 20 mm rise in diastolic pressure
- *Dystonia* (sustained contractions of axial or appendicular muscles, cramps) and flexor–extensor posturing
- Choreiform movements (constant rapid and jerky involuntary movements)
- Incontinence
- Difficulty swallowing
- Excessive salivation and drooling
- Akathisia
- Poor response to anticholinergic medications
- Sleep disturbances
- Abnormal laboratory values: elevated white blood cell (WBC) count and creatine phosphokinase (CPK) level, indicating muscle damage caused by rigidity (can affect heart muscle), and myoglobin in the urine, also indicating muscle damage
- Frequent respiratory distress; may be life-threatening
- Other disorders must be ruled out. These include parkinsonism, encephalitis, meningitis, lethal catatonia, and drug allergy. It is believed that NMS is more common in clients who are receiving long-acting injections and in those who are dehydrated. Others at higher risk for developing NMS include younger clients, males, those who are physically ill, and those with prior neurologic instability.

> **Nursing Alert** Some symptoms of NMS are the same as those of TD. However, a combination of symptoms and greater severity of these symptoms indicate NMS. *Changing blood pressure and sudden elevation of temperature* are some of the first significant signs of NMS. If you have any question, immediately consult the primary provider.

Treatment of NMS

Treatment involves immediately discontinuing antipsychotic/neuroleptic medications, maintaining the person's airway, and monitoring vital signs (particularly temperature, BP, and LOC). Ongoing treatment includes monitoring the client's intake and output (I&O), nutritional status, daily weight, and lowering of body temperature. Specific medication therapy may include bromocriptine mesylate (Parlodel), although this drug may interact with specific antipsychotics, and/or dantrolene sodium (Dantrium). The client's hypertension may be symptomatically treated with a medication such as captopril (Capoten), clonidine HCl (Catapres), or nitroprusside sodium (Nitropress). This client will need to be maintained on an unrelated neuroleptic medication in the future.

Sedative-Hypnotic Agents

Inability to sleep (insomnia) is a significant problem, particularly for clients with disturbances in mental health. Even persons without psychiatric disorders can become psychotic if they are severely sleep deprived. A number of medications are prescribed to assist clients to sleep. In the past, barbiturates were used, but their many adverse side effects, including habituation (less effect at same dose/or addiction) and danger of overdose when used with alcohol or other drugs. These adverse effects have caused other medications to be preferred. Commonly used medications include zolpidem (Ambien), eszopiclone (Lunesta), and trazodone, as well as medications with sedative side effects, such as mirtazapine (Remeron) and over-the-counter diphenhydramine (Benadryl). Short-acting benzodiazepines, such as triazolam (Halcion) and Temazepam (Restoril), are used for sleep issues also. A newer drug called ramelteon (Rozerem) is also being used for insomnia, especially for those who find getting to sleep difficult. It works similarly to melatonin.

Antianxiety Agents

Antianxiety agents (*anxiolytics*) are central nervous system (CNS) depressants. Table 95-2 lists commonly used anxiolytics. **Benzodiazepines** are uniquely effective for anxiety, especially when taken orally. They are also effective for preventing panic attacks. Long-lasting benzodiazepines, such as chlordiazepoxide (Librium), clonazepam (Klonopin), diazepam (Valium), and alprazolam (Xanax), are especially effective. *Barbiturates*, such as phenobarbital and secobarbital, were formerly used to attain behavioral control. However, they have disadvantages, compared with benzodiazepines, including rapid development of tolerance and physical dependence. Therefore, barbiturates are rarely prescribed today.

Other medications are used to treat anxiety. *Buspirone (Buspar)* is an antianxiety medication that is not a CNS depressant and does not cause euphoria or sedation. It has a lag of several weeks before effects begin, so is not useful as an emergency (PRN) medication. Another commonly used anxiolytic is *venlafaxine (Effexor)*, which takes effect within about 12 hr. Side effects of these medications are usually mild, but can be troublesome. They include hypotension, headache, nausea, dry mouth, refusal to eat, flatulence, constipation, decreased libido, and impotence. A commonly used PRN anxiolytic is *hydroxyzine (Vistaril, Atarax)*, which takes effect in 15–30 min and has many fewer side effects. (Hydroxyzine is also used to treat pruritus [itching], nausea, and alcohol withdrawal, and for preoperative sedation.)

Disadvantages of Antianxiety Medications

Alcohol potentiates the effects of antianxiety agents, often causing severe depression. In addition, individuals become dependent, both emotionally and physically, on benzodiazepines and barbiturates. Severe withdrawal symptoms follow abrupt discontinuation. (Withdrawal must be done carefully with a physician's assistance.)

Mood Stabilizers

Mood stabilizers are used to treat both elevated mood (*mania*) and depressed mood (*major depression*). These medications also help prevent instability when the client is in a *euthymic* (normal) mood. They work by chemically stabilizing the brain's membranes. Other medications used in this manner include anticonvulsants, such as divalproex, carbamazepine, and lamotrigine, and antipsychotics such as aripiprazole, olanzapine, quetiapine, risperidone, and ziprasidone.

Lithium

Lithium (Li^+) is a naturally occurring element. It is very commonly used in the treatment of bipolar mania and borderline personality disorder. It is also used to reduce impulsivity and **lability** (sudden changes) when treating personality disorders. It is available in several forms (Table 94-2). The client taking lithium must maintain adequate daily fluid intake (about eight glasses), salt should not be restricted without medical supervision, and these clients should not use nonsteroidal anti-inflammatory drugs (NSAIDs) because they can lead to lithium toxicity. Clients should be monitored for changes in renal and thyroid function at least annually. There are a number of side effects attributed to lithium including renal insufficiency and other urinary problems, GI upsets, edema of the extremities and face, hypothyroidism, excessive weight gain, sexual dysfunction, and mild hypoglycemia. In some cases, adult enuresis (bedwetting) occurs and is treated with sublingual atropine or desmopressin acetate (DDAVP), given at bedtime.

Anticonvulsants as Mood Stabilizers

Another group of medications, the *anticonvulsants*, have proved effective in treating mood disorders. Medications, such as carbamazepine (Tegretol) and valproate (Depakote), are used, alone or in conjunction with lithium. These medications also have side effects, which may lead to medication noncompliance.

> **Key Concept**
>
> Several classifications of medications used in psychiatry have sexual side effects, such as impotence and decreased libido, in all clients. These and other side effects are a major reason clients refuse medications or stop taking them after discharge from the hospital.

Antidepressants

Antidepressants are commonly used to treat major depression and in conditions such as panic disorders, eating disorders, PTSD, and OCD. These drugs increase activity of norepinephrine or serotonin (or both) at the brain's postsynaptic membrane receptors. The major classifications of antidepressants are tricyclics (imipramine), selective serotonin reuptake inhibitors (SSRIs, such as citalopram and escitalopram), monoamine oxidase inhibitors (**MAOIs**), and other non-MAOI antidepressants. The SSRI and non-MAOI antidepressants are most frequently used. Tricyclic antidepressants (TCAs) are quite successful, but have more side effects and can be lethal in overdose. MAOI antidepressants are very effective, but require the client to adhere strictly to dietary restrictions.

> **Key Concept**
>
> Antidepressants generally take 1–6 weeks from initiation of administration for symptom relief or full therapeutic effect to occur. This client is at risk of being overwhelmed by depressive symptoms while waiting for relief.

> **Nursing Alert** Warn clients taking MAOIs against eating foods with high tyramine content (e.g., aged cheese, avocados, bananas, beer, bologna, caffeine, chocolate, liver, pepperoni, pickled foods, red wine, ripe fruit, salami, smoked foods, yeast, meats prepared with tenderizer, raisins, herring, and yogurt). Clients taking MAOIs should also avoid over-the-counter (OTC) medications, such as many cold and hay fever products, which can lead to hypertensive crises. In addition, some herbal preparations can cause serious side effects if combined with MAOIs. (The exception to this restriction is the lowest dose of transdermal selegiline [Emsam], an MAOI used in MDD.)

Side effects of all antidepressants include dry mouth, which can be very bothersome. (This is sometimes relieved by eating sugarless hard candy or chewing gum. Drinking excess water is discouraged.) Many of these medications also cause sexual dysfunction. Other side effects of tricyclics include urinary hesitancy or retention, constipation, tachycardia, sedation, and orthostatic hypotension. Side effects of SSRIs include nausea, vomiting, headache, sedation, nervousness, and insomnia. Side effects of MAOIs are orthostatic hypotension, edema, and insomnia. Other non-MAOI antidepressants can cause sweating, seizures, and nausea (Table 94-2).

> **Key Concept**
>
> Excessive weight gain is a significant side effect of many psychiatric medications, particularly lithium, tricyclic antidepressants, and MAOIs. This weight gain is a major reason given by clients for not taking their medications. This can also be life-threatening. **Rationale:** *The client may gain weight so fast that the cardiopulmonary systems cannot compensate; the client may die of fluid overload and cardiac arrest.*

THE CLIENT IN AN INPATIENT SETTING

Although this chapter is geared primarily to the care of the person diagnosed with a serious disruption in mental health, many of these skills apply to clients in other areas as well. The nurse will encounter people experiencing threats to mental health in all areas of the healthcare facility, as well as in daily life. Remember: People who are ill or injured often regress or respond in ways that differ from their usual behavior. You may find symptoms of a mental health disorder in many general medical-surgical clients. Often, their undesirable behavior disappears after their medical problem is under control. It may be more difficult to manage a client's serious deviation from mental health in the general areas of the hospital or other healthcare facility than it would be in a more controlled psychiatric unit.

The Therapeutic Environment

The therapeutic environment (**milieu therapy**) is one in which physical and social aspects of the surroundings are designed to promote health and safety and to prepare clients to cope with life's demands. The eventual goal is *safety and comfort in the community after discharge* from a facility. The *therapeutic environment* is a community within the facility that encourages people to interact with one another and to improve interpersonal relationships. They are assisted to gain insight into their actions and to change undesirable behaviors. Clients form a "government" and, with supervision, express concerns and set up guidelines. In this way, they are able to test methods of coping. The therapeutic environment can fulfill its function only if people learn to live in such a way as to prepare them for eventual discharge.

Rights of the Client

Chapter 4 described the Bill of Rights that applies for all healthcare clients. Some differences exist in mental health units. Because safety must be maintained, limitations to a client's freedom (by seclusion or giving medications or treatments against the client's will) are sometimes necessary. Clients may also be held in a facility against their will, if they pose a danger to themselves or others.

Civil Rights Legislation

Civil rights laws provide for equal treatment of all clients, regardless of ethnic or religious background. Clients can refuse treatment, unless a medical emergency has been declared, there is a court order, or a client is out of control or dangerous to others. A healthcare facility cannot violate a client's civil rights, even though the person is committed by law to the facility. For example, clients must be allowed to receive mail and telephone calls without being censored. They have the right to see visitors. These rights change only if preserving them would compromise the safety of the client or others (e.g., clients are not allowed to use cell phones, as described below).

Vulnerable Adult Legislation

Legislation is in place to protect people who cannot protect themselves. Clients with mental illness or intellectual impairment are considered **vulnerable adults** and are protected by these laws. Physical, sexual, or verbal abuse or neglect of any client is illegal. Clients must also be protected from abuse or harassment by other clients (peers). It is also illegal for staff to have social contact with clients outside the facility.

Confidentiality

As in any other area of a healthcare facility, it is vital to protect the client's privacy and healthcare information. This may be even more important in psychiatry because many people do not want anyone to know they have a mental health disorder. Be sure to determine if the client will allow people to know that he or she is in the facility before taking calls or admitting visitors. Clients and visitors are never allowed to have cameras, *including cell phones with photo capability*, in order to maintain each client's privacy.

Advocacy

Most healthcare institutions employ counselors or advocates (*ombudspersons*) who advise people about their civil rights. These advocates act as effective "watchdogs" and pursue complaints. Any suspected abuse must be reported, or the person who observed the abuse, in addition to the abusive person, may be prosecuted.

Prevention of Dehumanization

A mental health unit is a controlled environment. To maintain safety for everyone in the group, all members must follow protocols. As in all healthcare facilities, measures must be taken to prevent a dehumanizing atmosphere. All clients must be treated with dignity. In Practice: Nursing Care Guidelines 94-3 discusses ways to prevent dehumanization.

> **Key Concept**
>
> Clients and staff are usually encouraged to wear street clothes on the inpatient psychiatric unit to reinforce the feeling of normalcy. In some cases, forensic clients or those at high risk for escape must wear specific identifying clothing.

IN PRACTICE
NURSING CARE GUIDELINES 94-3: Maintaining the Client's Dignity in Mental Health Units

- Allow clients as much choice as possible (clothes, hairstyle, food, and hours—bathing, etc.).
- Encourage clients to participate in and help plan activities.
- Make sure clients have privacy in the bathroom, when bathing, and performing other personal care (within safety limits).
- Allow clients to keep as many personal possessions as is possible and safe. Make sure clients have hearing aids, false teeth, or glasses, if needed. (Space limitations may influence this.)
- Allow freedom in sending/receiving mail and gifts and receiving visitors (within safety limits).
- Ask the client what they want to be called. Do not use nicknames, unless requested, and use only appropriate nicknames.
- Help people to look as good as possible. Assist with personal cleanliness, makeup, and hairstyling, if necessary.
- Encourage clients to keep their personal bed areas neat.
- Encourage clients to strive for recovery or management of the illness.
- Give positive reinforcement; encourage a positive self-image. Do not be punitive.
- Explain treatments before they are given; make clients active participants in their care.
- Be consistent. Enforce rules equally for everyone.
- Be respectful and truthful—keep promises; be on time.
- Do not set inappropriate limits, but do maintain safety (for the client and staff).

Visitors

Nurses work with clients' visitors. The client's family and other visitors can provide valuable background information and observations of the client's current behavior, compared with their baseline. Visitors may be upset by the client's condition and need support and reassurance. They may have been dealing with the person's unpredictable or difficult behavior for many years; families can be very frustrated. To avoid surprises, tell clients about upcoming visits. Help them bathe and dress, if needed. Refer all requests from visitors about a client's condition to the client, the client's nurse, or the charge nurse. See In Practice: Nursing Care Guidelines 94-4 for specific ways to monitor client visits.

> **Nursing Alert** Be sure the client (or guardian) has signed a release of information (ROI) before talking with the client's loved ones. It is illegal to give any information without a signed consent, except to other legal medical personnel. (Everyone must have a valid reason to access information.)

IN PRACTICE
NURSING CARE GUIDELINES 94-4: Supervised Visits

The following procedures help protect the rights of vulnerable clients and maintain safety:

- Check to see if the client wants to see the visitor.
- Ask visitors to sign in and state their relationship to the client.
- Usually purses, bags, and coats must be left in a locker or at the desk. Make sure to obtain cell phones from visitors.
- Visits are usually conducted in the lounge, not the client's room (particularly if the client has a roommate).
- Conjugal visits are usually not allowed.
- Have clients open packages or suitcases in the nurse's presence; keep all dangerous items in a safe place away from clients. Record all items on the client's property sheet. Take cash, checks, credit cards, and other valuables to the vault. Try to send excess property back with visitors.
- Prevent other clients from interfering with the visit.
- Flowers and plants must not be in ceramic or glass pots. Balloons are usually not allowed because of latex allergies and because of the strings.
- Watch for suicide attempts or efforts of clients to escape.
- If the client is on a special diet, monitor food brought by visitors. Be particularly aware of clients' special diets (e.g., candy brought to clients with diabetes). Caffeine may not be allowed.
- Terminate the visit if the client becomes unduly disturbed. Make sure the client does not attempt to attack visitors.
- Observe to make sure visitors are not taking advantage of vulnerable clients (e.g., pressuring the client to give them money, let them use a car or apartment, or buy drugs).
- Observe to make sure visitors are not bringing drugs, other contraband, or weapons onto the unit. Usually bottled beverages are not allowed because they may have been tampered with.
- If a visitor has been drinking, is under the influence of drugs, is abusive, or is otherwise inappropriate, request that the visitor leave. They may need to be escorted out by security. (Most clients are too vulnerable or fearful to ask visitors to leave; staff will need to do this.)
- If a visitor brings small children onto the unit, make sure there is a safe place for them to visit. Pets are not allowed unless they are certified service animals.
- Thank visitors for coming and encourage them to come again, if the visit seemed to go well.
- Document the visit, noting the client's reaction and comments before, during, and after the visit.

Outings

A provider's order is required before clients can leave a mental health unit at any time; make sure orders are entered and signed. Clients must also sign a "pass waiver," in which they promise to return and release the facility from liability while they are gone. The staff is responsible if any client is allowed to leave without an order, without signing a pass waiver, or without signing out *against medical advice* (AMA). Make sure clients understand the expectations applying to outings. Usually, clients must sign out and indicate where they are going and with whom. Clients may be allowed to leave only with staff, may be given independent passes, passes with family, or with case managers. Inform clients of the curfew and consequences if they are late.

When clients return from outings, note whether or not they return on time and who accompanied them. Ask what they did and how the outing went. Ask clients if they brought anything back, and if they did, check it in. Document comments, nonverbal behaviors, physical appearance, and any unusual reactions. Be sure to note, for example, if the person seems unusually agitated or depressed, if you can detect alcohol on their breath (AOB), or if they seem to be under the influence of other drugs. In some cases, the provider orders a routine urine toxicology screen (**U-Tox**) for drugs or a breathalyzer test for alcohol on return from passes. If a client does not return, absent without leave (AWOL) procedures usually take effect (see later discussion).

Security

Persons with mental illness need a secure environment and protection against harm to themselves, other clients, personnel, and visitors. The healthcare facility is responsible for providing this protection. Personnel must always maintain safety. Be alert to what is going on and be ready to assist if there is a threat to a client or anyone else. People with mental disorders are usually not dangerous to others; nevertheless, all facilities treat some clients who could be physically **assaultive** (threatening to hurt others or striking someone). Try to anticipate acting-out behavior before it occurs. Most hospitals have security personnel available to assist in an emergency. Remember, however, that it may take a few minutes for them to get to the unit; you must maintain safety until help arrives. Some hospitals have an emergency response team (sometimes called the "BERT" team; behavioral emergency response team) that can be called to assist in a dangerous situation. They respond, much as would the code team, and assist in restoring control.

In addition, some clients attempt actions of *self-mutilation* (self-injurious behavior [SIB]). This includes scratching, cutting, biting, burning, beating themselves, or attempting suicide. In a unit where people may become violent or self-injurious, it is helpful to carry an electronic signal (if available) that can be used to summon assistance. Letting clients know this device is being used will help prevent violence. Most units also have a "panic button" for use in emergency only. The staff needs to intervene and set firm limits on inappropriate behavior as quickly as possible. Some facilities have closed circuit cameras in place, so security personnel can monitor the units. If a client is becoming more agitated (e.g., yelling and hitting the wall) but is not injuring anyone, it is best to wait until help arrives to restore control.

> **Nursing Alert** Often a gentle touch can be soothing. However, it is important to ask permission before touching a client. If this person is surprised, it could be perceived as invasive or threatening, and the client may strike out.

Seclusion

Sometimes, a client can bring undesirable behavior under control if he or she is placed in a room alone. Try a voluntary time-out first. If the person does not cooperate, it may be necessary to place him or her in a locked seclusion room (LSR), also called the locked quiet room (LQR), with or without restraints. This process is called *seclusion;* it should be used with care. A written order is required for locked seclusion. *Safety within the milieu is the primary goal of all treatment.* Observe the person in seclusion carefully; one-to-one observation is usually required, but video observation may be substituted, if the client is not restrained and it is permissible, per protocol. (See In Practice: Nursing Care Guidelines 94-5 for procedures and safeguards.) As soon as possible, release the client. The room temperature should be comfortable, with plenty of fresh air. Give water or juice. Serve meals on nonfragile dishes. The person should have exercise and frequent opportunities for toileting; however, the bathroom is usually kept locked when not in use, for safety.

Restraints and Client Safety Devices

Today, there is a concerted effort to avoid restraining clients, if possible. The least restrictive method should always be used. However, in addition to enforced seclusion, *restraints* (*client safety devices* and *reminder devices*) may be necessary, to keep clients from hurting themselves or others, to prevent clients from destroying property, interfering with necessary treatments, or removing dressings or IV lines. Civil rights laws are intended to prevent the use of inappropriate client safety devices. (Hospital funding agencies are now moving toward abolishing the use of all physical restraints.) Mental Health America (MHA) believes that involuntary treatment and forced medication administration should be only be used in rare situations. So always be sure to follow the policies and procedures of your facility. Categories of restraints or safety procedures used in psychiatry:

- *Emergency chemical restraints* (ECR) or *pharmacologic restraints:* Drugs can be given to help control dangerous behavior. A combination frequently used is Benadryl 50 mg, Haldol 5 mg, and Ativan 2 mg (colloquially known as a "B_{52}"). This combination may be given orally as pills or liquid or may be injected IM and with a physician's order may be given without the client's consent.
- *Emergency physical restraint* (EPR) or *client safety device:* This is used only if absolutely necessary. If a client must be physically restrained, a device, such as the waist belt, may be used. Sometimes leg and arm cuffs are required as well. If any restraint becomes necessary, take specific precautions (In Practice: Nursing Care Guidelines 94-5). Substitutes for physical restraint are therapeutic treatments (e.g., verbal intervention and de-escalation), routine drug therapy, diversion, and seclusion. *Use EPR as a last resort only.*

IN PRACTICE
NURSING CARE GUIDELINES 94-5: Using Safety Devices for the Client With Mental Illness

Stringent efforts are made in mental health units to avoid the use of physical or chemical restraints. However, in extreme cases, restraint may be necessary, to maintain client, visitor, and staff safety. Be aware that any time a client is held down (as for an injection or blood draw), *locked* in seclusion, placed in a safety device, or given a medication to control behavior, this is a *restraint*.

- Leather restraints are rarely used today. Less painful safety devices may be required to control extremely assaultive or dangerous behaviors. *Note:* Restraint is a last resort *after all other measures have been attempted.*
- The client's family must be notified after any restraint is used.
- Wear gloves while doing any restraint. Wear eye goggles if the client is likely to spit. Be careful not to be bitten or kicked.
- Restrained clients are vulnerable because they cannot defend themselves. They must have one-to-one nursing observation and are usually also under constant camera surveillance.
- A specific written order to use any type of restraints must be in place. (In an emergency, this may be obtained *immediately after an incident.*) This order must be written for a specified number of hours, according to facility protocol. Carefully document all de-escalation techniques that were tried first, any restraint used, the reason for the action, and all observations of the person. (An order is also required for hands-on, such as forcing medication by IM injection.)
- A provider must see the client *face-to-face* within 1 hr after any physical restraints are applied.

If Physical Restraint is Necessary
- When restraining the arms and legs (*four-point restraints*), be careful not to make the device too tight. Apply restraints to the client's arms and legs before attaching them to the bed (or wheelchair). *Rationale: This allows safety and convenience in positioning of arms and legs.*
- Fasten the arms and legs in as comfortable a position as possible. If a person must be quickly placed in an uncomfortable position to prevent injury to others, change the position as soon as possible. Remove safety devices every hour, one limb at a time, and allow the person to exercise limbs. Keep the other limbs secure. *Rationale: These procedures help prevent injury to staff or client.*
- Clients usually are first placed on the stomach, without a pillow. *Rationale: This helps prevent the client from smothering, choking, spitting, or biting. It also offers better control of the client and facilitates intramuscular (IM) injections.*
- The client may be carried into the room in a face-down position. *Rationale: This helps to prevent injury to staff and to maintain better control of the client.*
- Use a stockinette, clothing sleeve or leg, or soft bandage under any safety device. *Rationale: This helps prevent injury.*
- Do not apply a safety device over the chest. *Rationale: This can cause the person to panic and restrict breathing.*
- Never restrain only one side of the body. Even if it seems unnecessary to restrain both hands or both feet, restrain the hand and foot on the opposite side, too. In some facilities, limbs on "opposite corners" can be restrained (e.g., left foot and right arm). (Some facilities never allow only two limbs to be restrained.) *Rationale: These procedures help prevent the client from turning and falling out of bed.*
- When releasing the person from restraints, release one extremity at a time, and alternate "corners." Do not release both extremities on the same side at the same time. *Releasing the client carefully can help prevent assault of staff and provide safety to the client.*
- Some facilities require a waist restraint if limbs are restrained. (The person is then in *three- or five-point restraints.*)
- Client safety devices are usually locked on psychiatry. Every nurse must have a key available. *Rationale: This ensures that the client can be immediately released in an emergency (such as a fire).*
- Be sure all staff members know how to manipulate restraints used in the facility and to practice using them before they are needed. *Rationale: Staff must know what to do in an emergency.*
- When applying restraints, check the buckle to make sure it is locked. *Rationale: If the client gets out of the restraint, the client could be injured or could be dangerous to others.*
- If a client is out of control, medications may be forced (by IM injection), unless the person then agrees to take them orally (liquid medications are usually used in this case).
- Offer the client an opportunity to use the urinal or bedpan or go to the bathroom at least every 1–2 hr. *Rationale: Restraint cannot be used as punishment or retaliation. Basic needs of the client must be met.*
- Offer fluids and food frequently. Use Styrofoam trays and dishes, to prevent injury to staff or to the client. Some clients cannot ever be given plastic flatware. *Rationale: These could be used as weapons.*
- Be sure to document the type of restraint used and attempts to discontinue or reduce the extent of restraints. *Rationale: It is important to keep the client in full restraints for as short a time as possible. Continuous attempts should be made to release the restraints, if possible. Documentation is necessary*

NURSING CARE GUIDELINES 94-5 Using Safety Devices for the Client With Mental Illness (Continued)

to indicate what restraint device was used and what attempts were made to reduce them.
- Frequently feel the pulse of the person in restraints, particularly if they are struggling, and watch the client's general condition carefully. *Rationale: Death can result from exhaustion. The person also can work down in the bed and strangle on a restraint.*
- Be aware that the person may try to do destructive things while restrained, such as tearing the bed linens or biting holes in the mattress. It is also possible for a severely agitated client to chew through a restraint. The person also may try to harm themselves, or the staff. For example, if the person in full restraints bites their shoulder, a cervical collar ("whiplash" collar) can be used, to maintain client safety.
- Whenever a client is placed in locked seclusion or restraints, they must be *thoroughly searched* for dangerous objects. This includes matches/lighters, tableware, plastic bags, pens, pencils, paper clips, staples, any sharps, liquids such as shampoo or hand lotion, headphones, belts, shoelaces, gowns with ties, and any other potentially dangerous items. Usually, glasses, jewelry, and shoes are removed as well. *Rationale: This helps keep the client safe.*
- If a client is out of control, do not attempt to carry out a restraint without assistance. Sometimes, a "show of force" is sufficient. *Rationale: The team must be prepared for violence on the part of the client. The team must be ready to apply involuntary restraints, if needed, for safety and to maintain the safety of others.*
- If a staff member or client is injured during a restraint, report it immediately and file an incident report. Tests for infectious diseases or a checkup in the emergency department may be required. *Rationale: This helps protect the staff and client.*
- If a client is extremely dangerous, but has been in restraints for some time, they may be allowed to be on the unit wearing a device called **PADS** (preventive aggression device system). PADS are a form of self-contained personal assault prevention device. The arms are restrained by wrist straps locked onto a waist belt. The amount of movement of the arms to be allowed can be adjusted by staff. If the client is likely to kick, locked ankle restraints (shackles) are also worn. When used in combination with a behavior modification program, clients may be weaned off ambulatory restraints. *Rationale: A client cannot be safely or humanely kept in bed in restraints for an extended period. Allowance must be made for exercise and readjustment to the unit, while protecting others from injury.*
- All clients must be interviewed after any seclusion or restraint. *Rationale: This is done to determine if the client understands the reasons for this, to obtain the client's feelings and suggestions, and to determine if there was any alternative.* Staff members often hold a "posting" meeting following a seclusion or restraint, to discuss what happened and determine if there might have been an alternative way of handling the situation.
- Careful documentation, according to facility protocol, is a must.
- Remember that the person in any type of locked restraint must have one-to-one supervision.

In some facilities, a room with exercise equipment and a punching bag is provided, as an alternative to seclusion. This allows the client to work out aggressions in a socially acceptable manner. The client must always be supervised in this area, to provide safety.

Nursing Care of the Severely Disturbed Client

Nursing care for the severely disturbed client involves three areas: physical care, teaching safe life skills and recreation, and building occupational or employment skills, if possible.

Physical Care

Encourage clients to bathe regularly and provide them with suitable clothing. Even the most deteriorated people often respond positively to having their hair fixed, getting new clothes, or having their clothes laundered. Disregard for personal appearance hastens disorganization; therefore, pay attention to helping people keep themselves presentable. Assist, as needed, in caring for a client's nails, hair, and teeth. Encourage clients to perform as much self-care as possible. The nurse is responsible for seeing that clients carry out self-care; these activities should be performed only for clients who cannot do so themselves. In rare cases, a bed bath or forced shower may be necessary. Sometimes, a forced haircut is also necessary (e.g., if hair is extremely matted and/or treatment for pediculosis [lice] must be instituted).

Because some people are unable to care for themselves, incontinence can be a problem. At regular intervals, take disorganized clients to the bathroom. Prevent dehumanization as much as possible. Persons who refuse or who cannot get out of bed may need special skin care, to prevent breakdown (Chapter 58). Incontinence briefs and heavy bed pads can help manage incontinence. Assist women to maintain feminine hygiene during menses.

Teaching Life Skills and Recreation

The goal of hospitalization is to prepare clients to return to the community. In some cases, clients need to learn acceptable social behaviors and how to care for personal needs. Eating may present problems. Many people eat too much and too rapidly; others eat insufficient amounts of food. Some clients drink too much or too little water. Clients often must learn how to buy and prepare food for themselves before going home. Flatware in the hospital is usually plastic, unless even this is a safety consideration. (Plastic knives are often not allowed.) If necessary, monitor a client's intake. Table manners can be taught, if possible.

Behavior modification techniques are often used with severely disturbed clients; usually retraining in ADLs is successful. Long-term clients often benefit from remotivation therapy and from contact with others. Recreation and activity at an appropriate level are important for all clients, who often enjoy simple activities, such as walks, games, and crafts. Such activities also tend to lessen combative and destructive behavior, as clients work off tensions in a healthy manner. Recreational activities also help teach social skills. Remember: Everyone needs some social contacts, no matter how ill they are. Many people with mental illnesses are very lonely, increasing their vulnerability.

Building Employment or Occupational Skills

People benefit from exposure to the world of work, particularly those in long-term care facilities. A duty in the unit, such as maintaining one's own living quarters, may be the first attempt. The client may progress to helping in the laundry, kitchen, coffee shop, garden, or gift shop. Many clients in long-term facilities receive a small stipend for such work. As a person's abilities improve, a sheltered workshop may be an option. Employment and earning money can improve a person's self-esteem. Before discharge from the system, most people need vocational rehabilitation training, if they can be employed. Many people also benefit from volunteering. Some clients are too ill to be employed, even as volunteers. However, they can learn to spend leisure time in safe, low-cost, and beneficial ways (e.g., going to a nearby drop-in center).

MENTAL HEALTH NURSING SKILLS

Mental health knowledge and skills in dealing with deviations in behavior are needed in all nursing fields. Care of clients with serious deviations in mental health, however, provides a particularly challenging opportunity. By working closely with these clients, the nurse becomes a source of stability and consistency. The nurse must be emotionally available, able to listen, nonpunitive, supportive, understanding, and encouraging. Nurses must also carry out many technical psychiatry nursing skills, as well as medical-surgical skills. Some skills are common to all areas of nursing. Other skills are specific to mental health nursing (which can apply to clients in all settings).

Key Concept

Common orders for *precautions* on the mental health unit include the following:

- **GP/SP:** General and suicidal precautions
- **AP:** Assault
- **EP:** Escape (elopement)
- **SIB:** Self-injurious behavior
- **Fall:** Risk of falls
- **SX:** Sexually inappropriate
- **SZ:** Seizure
- **Cheeking:** Not swallowing medications
- **Dismantling:** Taking things apart
- **Hoarding:** Collecting large amounts of food or other items
- **W/D** *(EtOH, ETOH W/D):* Withdrawal or alcohol withdrawal
- Other precautions may include phone restrictions, fluid restrictions, and dietary restrictions.

Physical Care

The nurse may need to assist clients with severe mental disorders to perform routine physical care. Aspects of this care include the following:

- Assisting with ADLs that the person cannot perform without encouragement or assistance; teaching, supervising, and evaluating ADLs. Urge the client to do as much as possible for himself or herself. Make sure the client's nutritional and hydration status are adequate. Some clients drink excessive amounts of fluids (*polydipsia*); fluids will be restricted. Some are on calorie-controlled diets. Others must be encouraged to take food and fluids; some need nutritional supplements or tube feedings. I&O or calorie counts may be ordered. Clients may be on special diets, as in the case of the diabetic client. Certain medications, such as MAOIs, also require dietary restrictions.
- Handling inappropriate or dangerous behaviors. Staff must protect themselves from injury, while also preventing injury to the inappropriate client, as well as to other clients and visitors. A behavioral control and/or self-defense class is usually provided for all psychiatry staff.
- Administering prescribed medications, observing for side effects, and teaching clients about medications. Offering PRN medications for side effects or behavior control.
- Assisting the sleep deprived client to sleep. Administering PRN medications, as ordered, and offering measures to assist in sleep: relaxation tapes, a snack or milk before bedtime, or a place to sleep where the client feels safe (Fig. 94-3).
- Administering physical treatments, as ordered. (Many clients have a physical disorder, as well as a mental disorder.)

Emotional Support

The client and family need emotional support. The nurse can be supportive in many ways:

- Establish **rapport** (harmonious relationship). Box 94-4 lists aspects of positive nurse–client relationships.
- Create a therapeutic and safe environment within the mental health setting.
- Provide emotional support to the client and family.

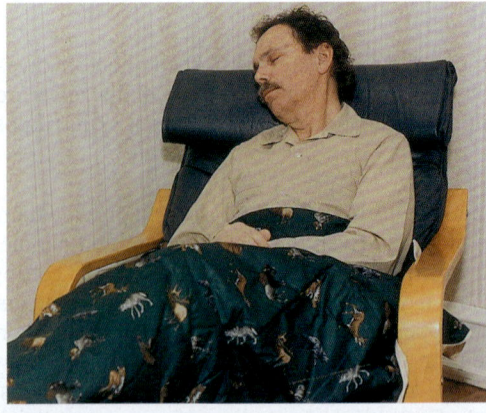

Figure 94-3 This paranoid client is afraid to sleep in his own room because of hallucinations and paranoid delusions. He can sleep in the lounge or commons area near the desk, where he feels more secure, until he becomes less fearful.

Box 94-4 The Nurse–Client Relationship

To establish a good relationship with any person, the nurse should do the following:
- Introduce yourself and offer to shake hands (but do not force physical contact).
- Be truthful but not brutally so. Be consistent and not evasive.
- Be even-tempered and uncritical; remember, the person is ill.
- Demonstrate poise to instill confidence in both nurse and client.
- Be an *interested* listener. Sit down to visit with clients. Do not stand over them. (Sometimes it is necessary to pace with a client.)
- Display empathy. It is not enough to imagine how *you* would feel in the person's situation; try to understand how *the client* feels.
- Concentrate on the person's strengths and not on weaknesses.
- Appreciate individual differences. Not everyone has the same goals and values.
- Treat adults as adults. Do not argue or get into power struggles.
- Set appropriate limits.
- Reward positive behaviors and steps toward wellness.
- Remember "The Patient's Bill of Rights."
- Do not force a client to have a long interview if it is uncomfortable. Initiate several short interactions.
- Respect the client's living quarters as private. Allow appropriate personal space; avoid being intrusive; knock before entering.
- Never have any outside social contact with current or discharged clients.
- Maintain confidentiality (e.g., if you meet a former client, allow the person to acknowledge you first).
- Be cordial to visitors.
- Always maintain safety.
- Do not talk loudly or yell in response to a client who yells. Maintain your voice calm, the volume low, and the tone modulated. Sometimes, talking even softer is effective.

- Provide leadership in socialization activities with a person or group.
- Aid in group therapy sessions.
- Conduct remotivation therapy in small groups.
- Assist the client and family to access other resources, such as Alcoholics Anonymous, a community drop-in center, or community social worker.

Other Skills

In psychiatry, nurses function not only as nurses but also as leaders, teachers, and support persons (Chapter 2).

- As a *socializing agent*, the nurse helps clients to participate in group activities and interact appropriately with others.
- As a *leader*, the nurse listens and encourages clients to work through problems.
- As a *teacher*, the nurse helps guide people into socially acceptable activities and teaches about medications, healthy eating habits, and treatments.
- As a *support person*, the nurse provides physical and emotional care, while encouraging people to face reality independently and to perform self-care.

Key Concept

Under no circumstances can the nurse have social contact with a client outside the healthcare setting or as an assigned home care nurse. This client is considered a vulnerable adult, and the nurse would be subject to legal charges.

NCLEX Alert

Integrated into the NCLEX are many aspects relating to care of clients with mental illnesses. Be alert to the importance of meaningful observation of these clients in any setting and the importance of excellent documentation skills.

If a Client Escapes

Even if the nursing unit is locked and a client is on escape/elopement precautions, it is still possible to escape (*elope*). A client may walk away from a recreation group, may leave when another person leaves the unit, or may take staff keys. This client is said to be AWOL, and certain measures are taken. The provider, other specific staff, and the client's family must be notified. If the client was on a court hold or legally committed, the police are notified. The nurse must describe the client (including birth date, height, weight, general appearance, and clothing) and identify where they might have gone. Some facilities have a photo of each client for identification purposes. Often, clients escape and then return in a short time or are brought back by a family member or the police.

In a *forensic unit*, additional security is needed. **Forensic** clients are those from a jail or prison, or with legal charges against them. In many cases, forensic clients have been charged with a serious crime, such as murder. They may be in the hospital to determine if they are *competent to stand trial*. Forensic units often have *sally port doors*, similar to those in a jail. In order to get in and out, people must pass through a sally port, an area with a locked door on each end. One door must be closed and locked before the other can be opened. This way, if a client escapes through the first door, they can be held in the sally port, to help prevent escape. Some clients also have around-the-clock guards.

Nursing Actions in Specific Behaviors

Although broad psychiatric diagnoses were presented earlier in this chapter, not all people can be easily categorized. Therefore, nursing care involves *dealing with behaviors*. The following behaviors and approaches are specific to mental health nursing but can be adapted to other areas. *These are only guidelines: the nurse must adapt to each person and situation.*

Observation

Observations that are documented carefully, objectively, and accurately can greatly assist the therapist, provider, or social worker. Observations provide information regarding the client's ongoing behavior (Fig. 94-4). Documentation consists

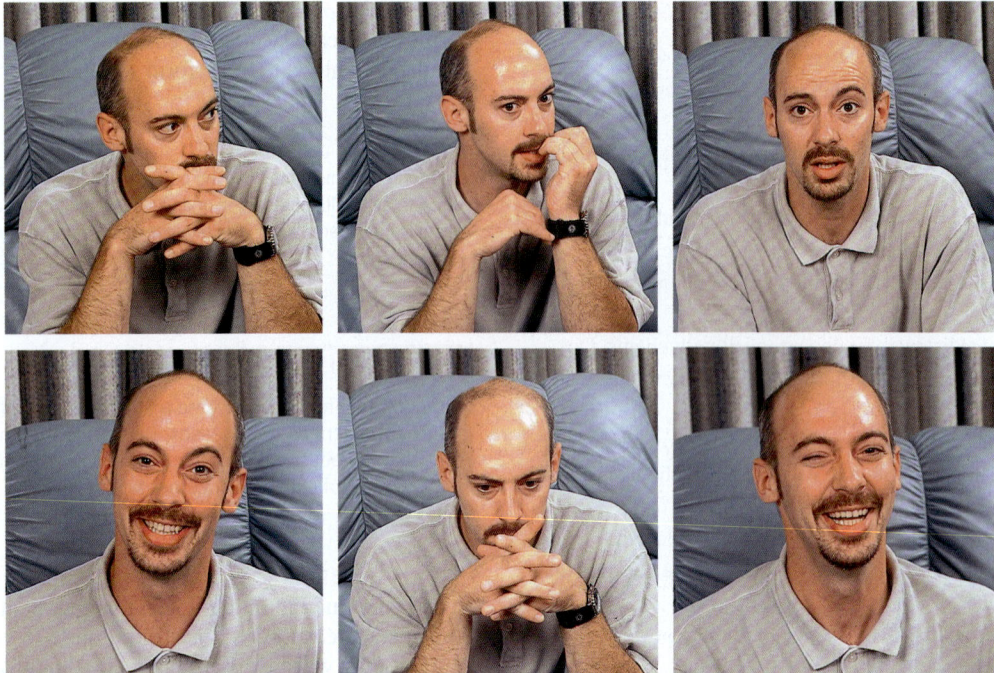

Figure 94-4 Nonverbal cues, such as body language and eye contact, are observed and documented. They can give clues to how the client is feeling. The client's affect may be described using terms such as "anxious," "fearful," "bright," "blunted," "flat," "irritable," or "labile." Document if the client has a wide range of affect or constricted affect, and if the affect is appropriate to the situation. Document if the client laughs inappropriately, talks to himself, or is tearful.

mostly of behavioral descriptions; this may be done without the client's knowledge. Clients usually have the right to review their medical records. (Often, a provider's order is required because to read the record may be detrimental to the client's care.) A staff member should be present whenever a client is reading their record, to interpret data, answer questions, and prevent the client from defacing or destroying any part of the record. In some settings, clients document their own feelings, thoughts, and activities, for the benefit of the healthcare team. Individuals often have more insight into their behaviors than does the staff. Many clients find it easier to write thoughts than to express them verbally. Place all such documents in the client's chart or scan them into the computer after dating and initialing them. In Practice: Data Gathering in Nursing 94-1 lists factors to consider when observing, planning care, and documenting behavior.

Some behaviors and speech patterns strongly indicate that individuals are responding to internal stimuli (auditory ["voices"] or visual hallucinations ["visions"]). Examples include talking to themselves, thought blocking, speech latency, and preoccupation. Some clients use a radio, headphones, earmuffs, or cotton in the ears to try to block out voices. Some clients experiencing hallucinations feel distracted, irritable, and hopeless. Psychotropic medications may help.

The nurse should observe the *client* in the following ways:

- Carefully and accurately document behaviors while in the mental health unit and on outside outings.
- Observe personal appearance and grooming, and other ADLs.
- Observe what the client eats or if the client refuses to eat.
- Note weight gain or loss.
- Note excessive food or fluid intake.
- Ask about pain whenever vital signs are taken, and document.
- Evaluate and document fall risk each shift.
- Record any physical symptoms.
- Carefully observe and document the client's interactions with others. Note if differences exist in interactions with certain other clients, staff, or family members. Observe the client's interactions on the phone. Document direct statements in quotes.
- Measure vital signs, including pain, at least twice daily and weight at least weekly. Orthostatic blood pressure and pulse is usually measured daily. Oxygen saturation may also be ordered. Note and report abnormal vital signs immediately.
- Document attempts to escape, or clients who return late from passes.
- In most cases, the client who is absent without leave (**AWOL**) is discharged at midnight. If this client returns later, they must be readmitted. (Third-party payors may not pay for subsequent hospitalization after a client goes AWOL. See discussion later.)

The Suicidal Person

Suicidal ideation (**SI**), suicide attempts (**SA**), and suicidal gestures (along with depression) are very frequently the reasons for admission to inpatient mental health units. These clients present a nursing challenge. They are placed on suicide precautions (**SP**) or general precautions (**GP**) until the provider determines they are no longer a danger to themselves. (See also section on childhood suicide in Chapter 74 and www.cdc.gov.). The National Suicide Prevention hotline number is 1-800-273-TALK (8255).

IN PRACTICE
DATA GATHERING IN NURSING 94-1 The Person in the Mental Health Unit

Appearance
- Is the client neat and clean, or dirty and untidy? Are the client's clothes appropriate for the weather, situation, and current activity? Check makeup and hair for appropriateness and cleanliness.
- Record lack of adequate grooming. Describe bizarre or inappropriate clothing or makeup. Does the client remain in hospital clothing all day?
- Describe the client's room order: messy and dirty, or neat and tidy? Is the client's bathroom clean? Does the client void or defecate on the floor? Does the client leave the sheets and mattress on the bed, use a pillowcase, and use towels appropriately? Is the client able to do their own laundry? Change their own bed? Does the client sleep on the floor? Are large amounts of food and other items collected in the room?
- Does the client display any rituals? *Rationale: These factors help determine if the client is safe to live independently after discharge and if the client needs assistance while in the facility.*

Sociability
- Does the client associate freely with others or isolate? Is interaction only with staff, with peers, or with visitors? Is the demeanor different on the phone than in person?
- Does the client stay in bed all day? Is he or she asleep or awake in bed? *Rationale: Sociability within the healthcare setting helps determine how the client will respond to others after discharge.*

Behavior
- Is the client orderly or disorderly, still or restless, quiet or noisy, friendly or indifferent, interested or uninterested, cooperative, assaultive, or destructive? Document irritability, intrusiveness, and threatening behavior. *Rationale: These behaviors help determine if the client is a danger to self or others. For example, intrusiveness and threatening others are dangerous behaviors because this client would be vulnerable to being assaulted in the community or potentially could assault someone else.*
- Does the client take things apart (dismantling) and/or destroy property?
- How does the client spend time: is the conduct always the same; does he or she comply with treatments and medications? Is the client able to occupy themselves appropriately (e.g., reading, watching TV)? *Rationale: It is important to assist clients to develop recreational activities they can continue after discharge.*
- Document group attendance or refusal and group participation. *Rationale: This could indicate willingness to continue treatment after discharge.*

Emotional Reactions
- How does the client express emotions (e.g., crying, anxiety, depression, fear, suspicion, happiness, sadness, loneliness, anger)? Is the client irritable, hostile, or excited? Does the client act impulsively or have unprovoked bursts of excitement, temper tantrums, or assaultive tendencies?
- Observe the client's overall emotional state. Are their emotions relatively consistent? *Rationale: Some of these observations indicate the client's response to stress and change and how well the client might do in the community.*

Speech
Determine answers to the following questions—Does the client:
- Follow normal speech patterns? Is speech rapid, loose, disorganized and disconnected, or slow?
- Speak English? Does the client speak with a "faked" accent or in several accents? Does speech indicate understanding of what is said or requested?
- Repeat or rhyme words or phrases; repeat someone else's words (echolalia)? Does the client coin new words that are not really words (**neologisms**)?
- Pause before speaking when asked a question (*speech latency*)? Document the length of any latent periods. (Time this with a second hand.) Does the client stop talking halfway through a sentence and seem unable to continue (*thought blocking*)?
- Talk or laugh to themselves? How loudly? Is the client argumentative? Does the client seem frightened? Does the client seem preoccupied?
- Demonstrate a specific speech defect (e.g., stuttering, lisping, stammering)?
- Demonstrate adequate hearing and vision?
- Talk constantly or very little? Does the client initiate conversation, or respond only when questioned? Is speech pressured and/or loud? Are answers only in monosyllables?
- Make sounds constantly (words, singing, or just sounds)? Does the client not speak (mutism)? If the client is mute with staff, does this continue with peers, with visitors, and on the phone?
- Make sense when talking? Does the client dwell on one subject (perseverate) or shift subjects constantly? Is the client able to concentrate? Is speech tangential and loose?
- Do meaningless *word salad* sentences occur? Does the person use unusual profanity without being able to be redirected? Are responses relevant and coherent? Does the client's conversation jump from one subject to another without order or apparent connection—*flight of ideas*? Is the client religiously preoccupied?
- Demonstrate adequate memory? Is there memory loss for recent events or events in the past? Is he or she oriented to person, time, date, and place?
- Acknowledge hearing voices? Having visual hallucinations? Describe what the client tells you about this. For example, are the voices telling the client to hurt himself or herself or to hurt someone else? Can the client identify whose voice he or she is hearing?

Document pertinent statements as direct quotes (in quotation marks), as much as possible. *Rationale: Speech patterns and mannerisms often indicate the client's thought process. Speech can help identify confusion, lack of contact with reality, hallucinations, and other factors relating to the client's mental illness.*

DATA GATHERING IN NURSING 94-1 The Person in the Mental Health Unit (Continued)

Nonverbal Behavior
- Does the client react differently when staff is not there, as opposed to when they know staff is watching? Does the client act out when being observed or when they think no one is looking?
- Document a client's inappropriate behavior, such as smearing of feces or food, eating garbage, masturbating in public, undressing in public, or writing on walls.
- Document any characteristic, ritualistic, and repeated gestures, posturing, or mannerisms.
- Determine if the client looks at a person when talking and makes *eye contact*. (Consider culture.) (Fig. 94-4).
- Describe the client's *affect* (external expression of emotions). Is it flat, blunted, bright, anxious, or fearful? (See Fig. 94-4.) Does the client cry often?
- How does the client respond to children? To animals? To people of the same and different genders? To older people? To younger people? To people of another race? To visitors, as opposed to staff? *Rationale: How clients behave is often more important than what they say. Posture, facial expression, and personal hygiene can indicate a great deal about self-image and is often a clear indicator of the client's thinking patterns and inner thoughts.*

Physical Complaints
- Carefully document any complaints of pain or discomfort, including voiding difficulties, drooling, gastrointestinal (GI) complaints, dizziness, or blurred vision. Never ignore a complaint of chest pain.
- Document specific signs of extrapyramidal medication side effects (Box 94-3).
- Document vital signs and report abnormalities at once. Orthostatic vital signs may be required. *Rationale: Physical symptoms may be an indicator of drug side effects or toxicity. In addition, many clients have physical disorders, as well as mental disorders. It is important to consider the whole person. A formal evaluation of pain must be made at least daily for each client.*

Physical Condition
- Note the client's general physical condition. Many clients have not been able to care for themselves or have not had access to adequate medical care.
- Many clients may experience homelessness and suffer from problems such as malnutrition, frostbite, or parasitic infestation. They may have several other unrelated physical disorders. Physically ill clients will have orders for medications and treatments, in addition to psychiatric orders.
- The nurse helps manage physical disorders such as diabetes: for example, nurses perform blood sugar testing, encourage ADA diet, and administer medications, including insulin. Diabetic teaching is particularly important. *Rationale: The nurse helps clients manage physical illnesses, under the direction of the provider. Many psychiatric clients have coexisting physical conditions.*

Movements
- Is the client coordinated? Does the person move quickly or slowly? Does the client pace continuously or march in place? Is the gait even and controlled?
- Document and describe tremors.
- Does the client remain in one position for long periods? Does the person seem to get "stuck" in one position (*catatonia*)?
- If the person's arm is moved, will he or she maintain that position (*waxy flexibility*)?
- Is there unusual posturing (e.g., ritualistic movement, karate stances, boxing)? *Rationale: Movements and posturing can indicate medication side effects, tardive dyskinesia, or more serious problems, such as neuroleptic malignant syndrome. In addition, some movement disorders are indicative of specific mental illnesses.*

Sleep
- Determine the client's sleep pattern, including length and frequency. Is it normal? Disturbed?
- Does the client talk or cry out at night? Are nightmares reported? Does the person sleepwalk/talk?
- Is it difficult to awaken the client in the morning? Is the client unusually sedated? Does he or she want to stay in bed all day? Stay up all night?
- Is he or she afraid at night? Sleep-deprived?
- Does the client snore? Has the client been tested for sleep apnea?
- Document the number of hours the client sleeps during the day, as well as at night. *Rationale: It is important for clients to obtain adequate sleep. Everyone who becomes sleep deprived is in danger of developing deviations from desirable mental health. Extreme sedation can be a side effect of some medications. In addition, the client who sleeps or lies in bed all day is often using this to isolate or escape from others. Some clients are afraid at night, so sleep all day and stay up at night.*

Appetite
- Does the client eat willingly, or must the staff encourage the client to eat? Does the client think food is poisoned?
- Is the person losing or gaining weight? Was weight gained or lost immediately prior to admission?
- Does evidence exist of an eating disorder, such as anorexia nervosa and associated disorders (**ANAD**)? Does the client eat constantly? Is the client obese or extremely thin?
- Note any peculiar behaviors or rituals in relation to food or eating.
- Document the client's table manners (or lack thereof).
- Does the client drink constantly? Drink only plain water? Is the client on a fluid restriction or intake and output (I&O)? Does he or she follow special dietary orders? Does he or she refuse to eat? If so, will the person eat food brought in by family members or in sealed food packages? *Rationale: Many clients have eating disorders, such as anorexia nervosa or bulimia nervosa; others eat*

DATA GATHERING IN NURSING 94-1 The Person in the Mental Health Unit (Continued)

huge amounts of food as a side effect of psychiatric medications. Some medications cause dry mouth and thirst—medications can be rendered ineffective by excessive fluid intake. It is also possible to upset the fluid and electrolyte balance of the body by drinking too much, particularly plain water. Some clients refuse to eat because they believe food is poisoned. It is helpful if these disorders are recognized and treated as soon as possible.

Elimination and Menstruation
- Observe elimination habits. Does the person maintain cleanliness? Continence?
- Document menstruation and menstrual hygiene. *Rationale:* The nurse can assist with maintaining hygiene if the person is unable to do so independently.

Other Observations
- Document any unusual occurrences, such as injuries or altercations between clients, along with names of witnesses.
- Document attempts to escape.
- Document any short or overnight visits and passes outside the facility. What was the client's response to the pass?

- Does the client acknowledge that he or she is feeling suicidal? Is there a plan? Is the plan lethal? Is this person able to contract for safety?
- Does the person lose things? Give things away? *Rationale:* The nurse in psychiatry is an important person in helping protect the client and keep him or her safe. Vulnerable adults may make inappropriate decisions or may fall prey to other clients (e.g., inappropriately giving away their property or spending excessive amounts of money on gifts). Reactions to time away from the healthcare facility will help determine how well or poorly the client will be able to manage on discharge. Evaluation of suicidality is an ongoing nursing responsibility.

Safety
- In addition to regular rounds of all clients, in many acute facilities, a "safety check" of all client rooms is performed regularly. The room is searched for contraband or for any dangerous items. Staff fully enter the room, look in waste baskets, under the mattress and pillow, and in drawers or shelves. Any inappropriate items are removed, and any faulty equipment can be reported.

> **Key Concept**
>
> Women attempt suicide more often than men; however, men are more likely to complete an attempt. The National Alliance on Mental Illness (NAMI) suggests steps to preventing suicide: *Question, Persuade, and Refer.* To connect the suicidal person to resources: Apply the "talk" method: *Tell, Ask, Listen, Keep Safe.* Teach families to restrict access to lethal means of suicide.

Risk Factors
Certain factors place clients at higher risk for suicidal attempts than normal (In Practice: Nursing Care Guidelines 94-6).

Reporting and Documentation
Consider any attempt at suicide to be serious: *report any suicide threat or attempt*, however minor it seems. Document and report any conversation in which a client expresses hopelessness or a desire to die. Suicide prevention involves constant and effective supervision and continuous, undemanding emotional support. Carefully document a client's SI (suicidal ideation). Document, in quotes, any statement the client makes about feeling suicidal, wanting to die, or "not wanting to be around anymore." Ask if the client has a suicide plan and document the response. Document any related statements made by friends and family about the client. They may detect subtle changes in the client's behavior. If the client expresses any form of SI, take immediate precautions to maintain safety and notify the provider. Document safety measures taken and who was notified.

> **Nursing Alert** If a client who is suicidal has a plan, this is more serious than the client who is feeling vaguely suicidal. Can this plan be put into action here and now? And would this plan be lethal? This is information that must be known by the healthcare team.

If the client has set a time to act, this is particularly dangerous. Nurses in *all areas of a healthcare facility* should be aware of the possibility of depression and suicidal ideation in their clients. Clients at greatest risk include those who have been diagnosed with a chronic illness or who are terminally ill and women who have had a spontaneous abortion or an ill or dying child. Many hospice clients and chemically dependent people consider suicide. If symptoms of depression are observed in any client, report it immediately and carefully observe the person.

Suicide Attempts
People who injure themselves or others may have been given increased privileges too soon. Sometimes, self-injurious behavior is aimed at getting attention, or it may be in response to *command hallucinations.* People may attempt suicide in the healthcare facility using readily available articles or materials, as listed above. Early morning hours are crucial for people with depression because they often dread facing another day. Deeply depressed people are often too exhausted to attempt suicide. However, as they take the medications, *begin to recover and regain energy*, they become more likely to attempt. Depressed clients who are recovering appear more optimistic than previously; nurses may fail to watch them as closely. Such persons may seem optimistic because they have devised a suicide plan. Routinely observe clients for signs of suicidal plans or attempts particularly during the early stages of illness and during convalescence. Be especially alert at changes of nursing shifts and at night, when fewer staff may be on duty. Actively suicidal clients should be "one-to-one" (observed by one staff person during each shift). A client on one-to-one observation in a mental health unit is always within arm's length and never left alone (In Practice: Nursing Care Guidelines 94-6).

NURSING CARE GUIDELINES 94-6: Suicide Prevention

Certain symptoms are considered significant in predicting suicidality. For example, the cluster of headache, insomnia, and depression (**HID**) may point to suicidal ideation. Tests are available to help identify and quantify depression. These include the Beck Depression Inventory (**BDI**) and the Hamilton Depression Rating Scale (HDRS).

Risk Factors and Warning Signs
- Newly admitted to the facility
- Low self-esteem (e.g., guilt, self-hatred), low motivation, poor support system, lack of religious beliefs, worry
- Homelessness; unemployment
- Recent loss (e.g., divorce; death of parent, spouse, child, or pet; bankruptcy)
- Anniversary of serious loss, such as a death
- Feeling hopeless, like there is no way out; personality change, apathy
- Long-standing depression; thinking about hurting/killing self; talking about death/dying
- Looking for ways to kill self
- Self-destructive behavior (e.g., collecting weapons, high-risk behaviors)
- Insomnia or sleep deprivation
- Change in eating patterns (e.g., overeating, refusing to eat/drink)
- Loss of interest in activities, friends, sex; loss of religious faith
- Constant negative hallucinations; nightmares
- Alcohol abuse, especially during withdrawal; withdrawal from other drugs
- Drug abuse, especially depressants (including alcohol; oxycontin and related drugs; and cocaine and related drugs)
- Paranoia and certain types of delusions (e.g., persecution); bipolar disorder
- Anxiety, agitation, mood swings, withdrawing from friends; giving possessions away
- Terminal or serious illnesses (e.g., AIDS, cancer) or chronic pain (e.g., low back pain, arthritis)
- Age (teenagers and senior citizens)
- Confusion; extreme mood swings
- Previous suicide attempt (25% more likely to try again)
- Self-injurious behaviors (may accidentally commit suicide)
- Borderline personality disorder (may accidentally commit suicide)

Suicide Methods Attempted in the Hospital
Almost anything can be used by a client to injure themselves. Some methods include the following:
- Cutting with plastic, glass, or sharp instruments (including scissors)
- Hanging by sheets, blankets, belts, electrical cords, ties, shoelaces, etc.
- Standing in high places and falling; banging the head or tipping over backward in a chair while sitting
- Drinking toxic substances, including hand sanitizer; saving up medications and taking them all at once
- Biting and swallowing foreign objects or putting objects in body orifices
- Bribing privileged clients or visitors to obtain destructive articles
- Drowning in the toilet, bathtub, or swimming pool
- Setting fires
- Suffocation (*be extremely careful with plastic bags*)

Preventive Measures
- Always know the whereabouts and condition of each client; 15-min checks are a minimum. (The extremely suicidal client may require 1:1 observation.)
- Make sure each client is breathing. If a client is in the bathroom or shower, make sure they answer you, or go in.
- All clients should have regularly scheduled one-to-one time with their staff at least each shift and whenever requested.
- If a client is in bed with covers pulled up over the head, make sure the client is breathing.
- Many psychiatric clients smoke. Although healthcare facilities are smoke free, sometimes clients are allowed to smoke outdoors. Staff may be expected to dispense cigarettes. Make sure clients follow smoking rules. (Often, privileges are lost if rules are not followed.) Make sure all smoking takes place in a designated smoking area and during limited smoking times.
- Keep all medications, not just narcotics, under lock and key.
- Because people who are suicidal are integrated into the general psychiatric population, sharp and dangerous objects are removed from *all* people on the mental health unit. Cans and glass items are not allowed. Often, shoelaces, belts, and clothing with ties are not allowed. If the client has hard boots, they also may not be allowed.
- Keep doors locked.
- Question clients about suicidal or self-injurious ideation and have clients contract for safety. (This includes promising not to hurt themselves and promising to let staff know if they feel like hurting themselves later.) If a client cannot contract for safety, he or she should remain in view of staff or will probably require one-to-one observation.

Care of Clients in One-to-One Observation
- Carefully watch every movement of the client. The nurse must always stay within arm's length.
- Do not allow the client to use sharp objects, electrical appliances, and other dangerous items.
- Encourage the client to be independent and get out of bed and dress each day.
- Encourage group attendance.
- Wait until relief arrives before reporting off duty or going on break.

NURSING CARE GUIDELINES 94-6 — Suicide Prevention—(Continued)

- Supervise bathroom use. Leave the door ajar. Listen carefully. Usually, tub baths are not allowed, but showers are required. If there is any question, a staff person must go into the bathroom with the client.
- Occupy the client when possible. Encourage reading, but do not read to the client. Inspire the client to accomplish things.
- Anticipate behavior by being aware of mood changes. Occasionally, clients will pretend improvement, to gain an opportunity for suicide.
- Be sure the client is given prescribed medications.
- Encourage adequate intake, including fluids.
- Find out if remotivation therapy or reorientation techniques are available.
- This client usually is not allowed to leave the unit, except for electroconvulsive therapy (ECT) or a special test. They must always be accompanied, on or off the unit.

Suicide Prevention Centers

Some cities have established suicide prevention centers and telephone hotlines to help people who are contemplating suicide. The caller can speak with a knowledgeable person who will listen and discuss the situation; the counselor tries to persuade the person to delay acting. Some centers will rush help—often the police—to the person to prevent him or her from carrying out the suicide threat. Statistics of how many suicides are prevented through crisis prevention centers are unavailable; many callers remain anonymous. However, theorists believe that just talking with another person when the crisis is most severe stops many people from taking their own life. (The suicide crisis counselor also attempts to refer the caller for continuing assistance after the crisis call.) In many cases, clients who attempt suicide or express suicidality state that they are grateful to be alive after the crisis passes.

The Overactive Person

Activity is a normal characteristic of life. Some people are more animated and forceful than others by nature. Other factors, such as illness or medications, can influence a person's activity level. Just as the degree of activity varies among people, so does the overactive behavior of people with certain types of mental illness. Activity levels range from overactive (*hyperactive*) to agitated and excitable (*hypomanic*) to extreme states of frenzy (*mania*). Marked changes may occur in the same person at different times; nursing care is adjusted accordingly. A quiet atmosphere is important. Use a calm, soft voice; do not talk loudly (even though the client may be shouting); and avoid long discussions. Do not force issues or get into power struggles. Set limits, be consistent, and prevent harm and injury. The person may need a "time-out," to prevent injury to self or others. The person may benefit from large-muscle activities (e.g., basketball, dancing, a workout in the gym, a punching bag, or swimming). Medications may need to be forced to control unsafe behavior, or PRN medications may be accepted or requested by the client.

The Hypomanic or Manic Person

The two degrees of mania are *hypomania* and *mania*, disorders characterized by elation, agitation, hyperactivity, hyperexcitability, and accelerated thinking and speaking (e.g., *flight of ideas* [FOI]). Clients may experience grandiosity, believing, for example, that they are God, royalty, or millionaires. They may have spent thousands of dollars more than they could afford or may have "maxed out" a number of credit cards. They are sometimes "airport admissions," having flown thousands of miles, with no specific destination. When confronted by airport security officers, they may become hostile and aggressive and are brought to the hospital. **Hypomania** (below mania) has less-intense characteristics than mania and usually does not require hospitalization when it occurs alone. However, hypomania can cause the person to lose a job or to be evicted and can be difficult for loved ones.

Manic people can be challenging. Often, they are witty, breezy, and enterprising; because of their keen memory and quick conversation, others may not recognize them as disturbed. As the disorder escalates, they become intrusive, domineering, and irritable. They may have rapid mood swings and *labile affect* (rapid changes in expressions). They rarely accept hospitalization voluntarily and may feel very entitled, believing everyone should wait on them, even though their demands are unreasonable. The nursing challenge is channeling their behavior because of their overactivity. They are usually oriented to time and place, but may have delusions, often *delusions of grandeur*. They often are unable or unwilling to sleep. As they become more sleep deprived, they become more irritable and intrusive and may become assaultive (In Practice: Nursing Care Guidelines 94-7).

The Highly Disturbed Person

Management and nursing care of the highly disturbed person includes protection for the client and others. These clients require a variety of activities, to channel surplus energy. They often need direct physical care or supervision of ADLs, which will need to be encouraged. These clients often need encouragement to bathe and remain clothed. Offer adequate food and fluids and observe and record the client's intake. Encourage good mouth and skin care and pay attention to cuts or bruises. Nursing care is directed toward *limiting overstimulation*. Do not force group attendance. (This person is usually very disruptive to the group.)

The Hostile or Combative Person

Hostile persons may threaten to injure others and may become physically violent. These individuals usually require assault precautions. Document if a client has homicidal ideation, threatening to injure or kill others. This person may be threatening to everyone or may have a specific person who is the target of their hostility. If the client is targeting or has threatened a specific person, the person must be notified by the provider (In Practice: Nursing Care Guidelines 94-8). When working with a highly disturbed client, be sure you have adequate assistance. Staff must work together to maintain safety. (Sometimes a "show of force" is needed.) Set firm limits on undesirable and dangerous behavior. Use time-outs in the client's room (5–30 min) to assist the person to calm; this provides stability for the entire unit. In an emergency, medications may be administered without consent by a physician's order to

IN PRACTICE

NURSING CARE GUIDELINES 94-7 — Care of the Client Who Is Manic/Hypomanic

- A small unit is recommended for this client. *Rationale: This limits stimulation and allows activity to be controlled.*
- Be firm, but kind; avoid familiarity.
- Do not argue or confront.
- Control behavior. Try to keep the client from irritating others; provide safe means to keep the person safely occupied.
- If the client cannot safely participate in groups or outings, try using crafts, writing, reading material, cards, or board games for activity.
- Some clients may enjoy using a punching bag or stationary bike or may benefit from competitive games, such as badminton, ping pong, or foosball. Remember to provide careful supervision. Avoid contact sports. *Rationale: These clients are likely to play too rough and hurt others.*
- Remember: Their attention span may be quite short. *Rationale: These clients are easily distractible.*
- Supply extra nourishment and fluids. *Rationale: These clients expend much energy and require additional calories.*
- Treatment usually involves mood stabilizer medications. The client may be resistant to taking medications and may need a great deal of encouragement to take medications early in treatment. *Rationale: Such clients usually feel they are not ill and do not want to be sedated. Many people enjoy being hypomanic; they may become uncontrollable and uncomfortable when they progress to mania. Watch for cheeking of medications.*
- Medications may need to be forced. *Rationale: This is required to maintain safety.*

Medications commonly used include the following:

- Lithium carbonate in oral tablets/capsules and extended release; lithium citrate syrup (to ensure compliance). Note: Syrup is more concentrated than the tablets.
- Valproate valproic acid, divalproex (Depakote and other brand names) available in tablets, including extended release tablets, injection, capsules (sprinkle), and in syrup form.
- Benzodiazepines and neuroleptic medications may be used during the acute phase to control behavior and maintain safety (Table 94-2).

IN PRACTICE

NURSING CARE GUIDELINES 94-8 — Care of the Combative or Assaultive Client

If a Client Is Argumentative

- Carry an electronic signaling device and tell the client you have it.
- In a verbal confrontation, avoid becoming excited, self-defensive, or making statements or using body language that can be interpreted as a challenge (e.g., eye contact may be misinterpreted). *Rationale: A defensive or challenging response will further escalate the combative person's behavior.*
- Recognize the client's feelings without judgment. Do not belittle or punish the client. Allow the client to talk and express feelings. Do not argue. *Rationale: A firm but understanding approach may prevent a hostile client from acting aggressively.*
- Do not allow the client to move behind a staff person or between staff and the door. Protect yourself physically, but do not injure or insult the client. Try to look beyond a client's anger and determine the cause. Try to get the client to help solve problems. Emphasize the positive and reward appropriate behavior. *Rationale: Punishing negative behavior is much less effective.*
- Choose appropriate and safe outlets for physical energy. *Rationale: Large muscle activities are often helpful. Supervise carefully.*
- Set limits; try not to get into power struggles. Explain reasons for limits (even though the client may not listen). You may need to be very assertive if there is a specific danger. *Rationale: Clients who are confused, out of touch with reality, hearing unwelcome voices, or experiencing delusions are often reacting to their situations in the only way they know. They may be terribly upset by being locked in and may feel "trapped" and afraid.*
- Seclusion and/or client safety devices may be needed; to maintain safety, medications may need to be forced.

Note: If a client is out of control but is not hurting themselves or anyone else, get help before trying to intervene. Rationale: It is dangerous to try to de-escalate this person without adequate staff present. The client and/or staff could be injured.

If a Client Strikes Out

- If a person becomes assaultive, threatening to hurt others or striking someone, use seclusion (to protect the client and others). Seclusion requires written provider's orders and one-to-one nursing supervision, as described previously.
- Neuroleptic or antipsychotic medications can usually control the client, although he or she may refuse to take them orally. Medications may be forced (by injection) in an emergency.
- In an extreme case, a powerful antipsychotic, benzodiazepine, or sedative may be used. *Rationale: These medications help clear thinking and diminish hallucinations. They also promote sleep, which the client often needs; many of these clients are sleep deprived.*

IN PRACTICE

NURSING CARE GUIDELINES 94-9 Assisting the Client Who Has Delusions or Hallucinations

- Try not to reinforce false perceptions. Ask the client to describe the delusion or hallucination, but state calmly that you do not see or hear what the client perceives. It may be helpful to say, "That seems to be part of your illness."
- Remember that hallucinations and delusions are very real to the client, but it is therapeutic for the client to realize that others do not hear, see, or believe the same things they do.
- Do not argue about delusions or hallucinations.
- Build the client's trust by being consistent.
- Use a soothing voice.
- Document exactly what the client says, in quotes.

---

control dangerous behavior. Immediate de-escalation of dangerous behavior is vital. Try to anticipate behavior, to prevent the client from losing control. (Most people do not want to lose control.)

Always use the least restrictive methods of behavior control first. For example:

- Talk to the client.
- Encourage a voluntary time-out.
- Force a time-out.
- Place the client in locked seclusion.
- Use physical or chemical restraints.

Release the client from any seclusion or restraint as soon as possible.

The Person With Delusions or Hallucinations

People may have false beliefs (*delusions*) or perceive false sensory stimuli (*hallucinations*).

Delusions

A *delusional* belief may be anything, from the client's situation to that of the entire world. If a person has a fixed delusion about another person, that individual may need to be warned. Delusional clients may harass or stalk love objects or believe that the person is in love with them. They may also seek to hurt the person in their delusion.

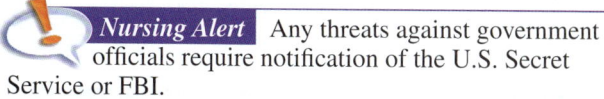 **Nursing Alert** Any threats against government officials require notification of the U.S. Secret Service or FBI.

Hallucinations

Many clients experience *hallucinations*, sensory perceptions, not based in reality, and delusions, as described previously. Delusions and hallucinations often occur simultaneously (In Practice: Nursing Care Guidelines 94-9).

The Confused or Demented Person

Many people with mental illnesses are confused as a result of their illness. In addition, some medications or ECT can contribute to disorientation. A person can also show dementia as a result of a condition such as Alzheimer's or Huntington syndrome or brain damage caused by an accident, drug abuse, or an infection, such as encephalitis or AIDS (In Practice: Nursing Care Guidelines 94-10 and Chapter 93).

The Withdrawn Person

People who are withdrawn choose to be left alone. Matters of concern to other people, such as food, grooming, and elimination, are often unimportant to withdrawn people. Conversations are difficult; therefore, withdrawn individuals do not interact with peers. They may choose to spend the entire day in bed, often with covers over their heads. Documentation often describes such persons as *isolating themselves*. The withdrawn person may be depressed and suicidal and should be monitored carefully, to maintain safety (In Practice: Nursing Care Guidelines 94-11).

The Depressed Person

In MDD, the person is usually inactive and shares many characteristics with the withdrawn person. A major treatment objective is suicide prevention; therefore, this person requires particularly close observation. Other nursing care is the same as for other withdrawn people (In Practice: Nursing Care Guidelines 94-6 and 94-11). A new treatment, *Light Therapy*, is showing promise in MDD. It is used as an adjunct to medications and may speed their effectiveness. (Chapter 55 discusses depression as it relates to chronic pain.)

> **Key Concept**
>
> Remind the client that it takes several weeks for antidepressant medications to take effect. This will be a difficult time for the client, and he or she will need a great deal of encouragement.

IN PRACTICE

NURSING CARE GUIDELINES 94-10 Assisting the Client Who Is Confused or Demented

- Provide a calm, quiet environment, regulated by routine and free from danger and anxiety.
- The major treatment goal is to reorient the client to reality, as much as possible (Chapter 93). Try to involve the person in activities; encourage remotivation therapy and occupational therapy (OT) groups. Mark off each day on a calendar. Provide a clock. Remind the client about birthdays and holidays. Although it is appropriate to encourage these clients to participate and converse with others, do not force socialization. The client may be able to talk to one other person but may be uncomfortable in a group.

- Nursing care includes helping maintain grooming, bowel and bladder continence, and menstrual hygiene. It may be necessary to document intake and offer nutritional supplements, such as Resource, Boost, or Ensure. Weigh the client regularly. Encourage the client to eat by sitting with them or by allowing the client to eat in their room. Notify the provider if the client has insufficient intake. An intravenous (IV) line or feeding tube may be needed in extreme cases.
- Check for constipation, a frequent side effect of medications. *Rationale: This client might not volunteer this information.*
- Observe clients for symptoms of physical disease; monitor vital signs. *Rationale: The client may not complain of pain or other symptoms.*
- The client may relate to a pet or children who visit. Be sure to monitor visits very carefully. *Rationale: It is important to prevent injury to the child, the pet, or the client.*
- Display a large sign on the client's door ("Judy's room"). *Rationale: This can remind the client not to enter other rooms.*
- Speak in short, clear, simple sentences; have the person repeat them, if necessary. Question the client's statements for clarity and try to understand what the client is saying. *Rationale: Try to avoid further confusion.*
- Give instructions one at a time; assist the client to perform tasks, as needed. *Rationale: This client will not be able to carry out complex tasks.*
- The nursing staff may need to manage assaultive behavior in this person. Medications may or may not be helpful in managing behavior, particularly in the older person. *Rationale: Some older people have a paradoxical (opposite) reaction to medications. In other cases, medications disinhibit the person, causing even more antisocial behavior.*

IN PRACTICE
NURSING CARE GUIDELINES 94-11 Assisting the Client Who Is Withdrawn or Depressed

- Speak softly and calmly.
- Encourage the client to eat. It may be necessary to monitor intake and output (I&O).
- Provide a cheerful, well-lighted living area.
- Encourage the client to spend time out of bed or out of their room.
- Try not to place these clients in groups of exuberant people in efforts to cheer them. *Rationale: This attempt usually has the opposite effect and tends to make them more conscious of their own unhappiness.*
- Encourage participation in activities, but do not force. As convalescence progresses, reading, games, puzzles, and small parties are helpful. Although occupational therapy (OT) is of great value, it should be simple and brief. *Rationale: These clients often tire quickly and have short attention spans.*
- Introduce the client to *one other person* at a time, not to large groups. *Rationale: A large group is usually threatening to these clients.*
- Give the person only one or two choices. *Rationale: Indecision is typical in these clients.*
- If the person is suicidal, follow the guidelines presented in In Practice: Nursing Care Guidelines 94-6.
- It may appear that the client is not listening to what you say. *Rationale: Clients may be preoccupied, often as a result of auditory hallucinations.*

IN PRACTICE
NURSING CARE GUIDELINES 94-12 Assisting the Client Who Is Regressed

- Remotivation therapy and behavior modification therapy are useful. Assist clients to focus on reality. Present current events to reorient the person. Design interesting and simple activities. Reward appropriate behavior; do not reprimand. *Rationale: This assists the client to learn to live comfortably in the world. Some clients are extremely sensitive and become embarrassed, despite seeming oblivious to everything.*
- Allow the person to do as much for themselves as possible. *Rationale: Help encourage self-respect.*
- Be truthful; keep promises. *Rationale: It is important to gain the client's trust.*
- Set up a bathroom schedule, reward and praise success. Adult diapers may be helpful at first, but try to eliminate them as soon as possible. *Rationale: Encourage the client to have pride in achieving self-care.*
- Encourage contact with peers, one or two at a time. Initiate games and participate in them with clients.
- Be alert for violent outbursts or suicide attempts. *Rationale: Clients often require assistance to remain safe.*
- Encourage verbalization of feelings; accept any verbalization, no matter how minimal. If the client uses profanity, gently guide them to more acceptable language. Discourage inappropriate behaviors by distracting the client, rather than criticism.
- All clients *should* be up and out of bed and dressed for the day, unless physically ill. *Rationale: Being dressed in street clothes, rather than hospital garb, helps reinforce appropriate adult behaviors.*

NURSING PROCESS

DATA GATHERING

Nursing History
- Expressions of feeling sad, unhappy, blue, "down in the dumps"; loss of interest or pleasure in usual activities (*anhedonia*); thoughts of suicide
- Anxiety
- Feelings of inadequacy, helplessness, inability to make decisions
- Feelings of fatigue, lassitude, wanting to stay in bed or sleep all day or inability to sleep
- Pessimism, hopelessness, feelings of worthlessness, self-reproach, or excessive or inappropriate guilt
- Complaints of sleep disturbances, gastrointestinal disturbances, decreased *libido* (sexual drive), extreme weight changes (±10%), unusual aches and pains

Data Collection
- Psychomotor agitation or retardation
- Posture
- Personal hygiene
- Excessive tearfulness
- Verbalizing suicidal ideation, with or without plan or intent
- Sudden change in activity level—becomes hyperactive or, if highly agitated, suddenly becomes calm

POSSIBLE NURSING DIAGNOSES
Impaired adjustment
Anxiety
Ineffective individual coping
Dysfunctional grieving
Altered health maintenance
Hopelessness
Altered nutrition: more or less than body requirements
Powerlessness
Self-care deficit
Self-esteem disturbance
Sexual dysfunction
Sleep pattern disturbance
Social isolation
High risk for self-directed violence

PLANNING
Following are goals of care:
- Meeting physical needs, including nutrition
- Meeting safety needs
- Verbalization of appropriate emotions
- Evidence of interest in life, including ADLs and independent self-care
- Coping skills
- Goals for the future
- Increased self-esteem

IMPLEMENTATION
Implementation is aimed toward
- Maintenance of safety; contracting for safety
- Meeting physiologic needs, assisting with ADLs and cleanliness
- Encouraging the client to express feelings
- Encouraging interest in the world, outside activities, and socialization
- Increased self-esteem and healthy interpersonal relationships
- Assisting to determine healthier ways of coping
- Encouraging involvement of community and family support systems and resources
- Administration of medications and teaching about them
- Assisting with treatments such as ECT; supporting and teaching the family

EVALUATION
If the client is unable to meet key goals, the plan must be modified. Key evaluative criteria include the following:
- Healthy resolution of depression with return to independent, meaningful living
- Absence of self-inflicted harm
- Verbalization of goals and plans for the future

The Person With Both Overactive and Underactive Behavior
In some disorders, the client's behavior alternates between overactivity (hypomania or mania) and underactivity (withdrawal or depression). A **cyclothymic** disorder is a mild form of this condition; the more severe form is *bipolar disorder.* Behavior extremes require symptomatic treatment. Medications are often helpful in controlling behavior, although the person often stops taking them after leaving the facility, causing a relapse.

The Regressed Person
Regression is a return to infantile or childish behavior. Examples include eating with the hands, urinating on the floor, soiling instead of using the toilet, openly masturbating, and being naked in public. Reteaching basic social skills to regressive adults takes patience and usually involves a number of people (In Practice: Nursing Care Guidelines 94-12).

STUDENT SYNTHESIS

KEY POINTS

- Today, most people with disruptions of mental health are managed in the community.
- Everyone uses defense mechanisms. When they are used to an extreme, a deviation from mental health exists.
- Several organic causes of mental illness exist. If an organic cause can be identified, treatment is often successful. The organic disorder is usually treated before treating mental deviations.
- Neurologic and neuropsychological tests help establish the diagnosis of mental illness and help determine the treatment plan.
- A common mood disorder is major depressive disorder, which often leads to suicide.
- The person with bipolar disorder experiences mood swings, from mania to depression.
- Clients with personality disorders may be very difficult to work with.
- Psychosis is a thought disorder, with major deviations from normal behavior and lack of contact with reality. Hallucinations, delusions, and paranoia are common symptoms.
- Many mentally ill people are also chemically dependent. The two conditions (MI/CD) complicate and contribute to one another.
- Outpatient and emergency services are available to serve clients with mental illness. They include a variety of structured and less-structured living situations.
- Clients may come into the healthcare facility voluntarily or may be brought in under one of the several legal categories.
- Electroconvulsive therapy (ECT) is used in some cases of intractable depression and other conditions, or when medication is contraindicated. Nurses are responsible for monitoring the client before and after the treatment and for evaluating any loss of short-term memory or cognitive changes.
- People receiving treatment for mental illness have the same rights as all other clients. Sometimes, a court order to force treatment is required, in order to protect the client and others.
- Many medications used in psychiatry have unpleasant side effects, some of which are life-threatening.
- Many appropriately medicated psychiatric clients live productively in the community.
- Client safety devices are never used unless absolutely necessary; careful safety measures must be used, to avoid injury. Accurate documentation is vital.
- Clients on a mental health unit are legally considered vulnerable adults.
- It is illegal and unethical for the nurse to have social contact with vulnerable clients.

CRITICAL THINKING EXERCISES

1. Mohamed, 43 years old, brings himself to your community mental health center for the first time. He says he "feels like killing himself" and recently bought a gun. He states, "My mother talked me into coming here." Mohamed's wife recently left him, taking their two children with her. Since then, he has been depressed and has been using drugs. He says he also "used a little khat (which is similar to amphetamines) yesterday." He denies long-term substance abuse. He says, "I don't know what to do. I feel hopeless. I can't even work. I'm afraid my boss is going to fire me. Nothing like this has ever happened to me before."
   a. Describe your initial nursing actions on meeting Mohamed. Make a list of pertinent factors to consider when his nursing care plan is developed.
   b. How does Mohamed's case differ from a case of chronic, severe depression, lasting about 10 years or more?
   c. How would you rate the severity and lethality of his suicidal ideation? What precautions are likely for him in the mental health unit?

2. The police bring an unidentified older woman into the crisis center. She is wearing handcuffs and leg shackles. She has reportedly lived in the city park for several years. She has two shopping bags of dirty clothes and other belongings, including cash. Reportedly, she has been extremely agitated, talking to herself and threatening passersby. Today, she entered a church and threw several statues. "Jane Doe" is wearing two dirty dresses, a sweater, jacket, knitted cap, unmatched socks, and dirty tennis shoes. (The temperature today is 92 °F.) Her gray hair is snarled, and she scratches her head often. She is malodorous; her breath is stale. She is thin and missing her front teeth. She appears to have a partially healed wound on her left lower leg. When asked her name, she replies, "God." She is uncommunicative, except to demand cigarettes. When placed in a holding room, she seems fearful and moves into a far corner, striking out when anyone approaches. She refuses to sit on the bed. Ms. Doe refused most of her vital signs, but her weight is 97 lb, her pulse is 120 beats per minute, and respiration rate is 22 breaths per minute. She has a productive cough.
   a. Describe ways to approach Ms. Doe. What immediate nursing actions are likely? List important factors to consider when her nursing care plan is developed. (Consider short- and long-term goals.) What medical and psychiatric diagnoses are likely?
   b. Describe safety measures that might be used in this client's care.
   c. What medications might be prescribed to control the client's behavior and help make her more comfortable?
   d. Identify possible community resources for Ms. Doe on discharge.
   e. Identify physical disorders that must be evaluated and/or ruled out in planning her care.

NCLEX-STYLE REVIEW QUESTIONS

1. The nurse is caring for a client who is on the behavioral health unit. What cluster of symptoms reported by the client should the nurse recognize indicates suicidal ideations?
   a. Headache, insomnia, depression
   b. Nausea, vomiting, diarrhea
   c. Vomiting, mania, coughing
   d. Flat affect, catatonia, hallucinations

2. A parent brings her 2-year-old child to the emergency department frequently, reporting seizure activity that has not been witnessed by anyone other than the parent. Diagnostic tests reveal no organic cause. What should the nurse monitor the parent for?
   a. Obsessive-compulsive disorder
   b. Posttraumatic stress disorder
   c. Borderline personality disorder
   d. Munchausen syndrome by proxy

3. The nurse is caring for a client with schizophrenia who is experiencing positive symptoms. Which symptoms observed by the nurse will be documented as positive? Select all that apply.
   a. Anhedonia
   b. Delusions
   c. Hallucinations
   d. Disorganized speech
   e. Apathy

4. The nurse says to a client, "How are you today?" The client repeats, "Today, today, today, today." How will the nurse document this behavior?
   a. Echopraxia
   b. Echolalia
   c. Mutism
   d. Posturing

5. A client treated for a substance abuse disorder is being discharged from an inpatient facility to a facility that will help make the transition into the community less traumatic. Where should the nurse ensure the client has a room?
   a. A homeless shelter
   b. A long-term care facility (LTC)
   c. A halfway house
   d. A hospice

CHAPTER RESOURCES

Enhance your learning with additional resources on thePoint*!*

Student Resources related to this chapter can be found at **thePoint.lww.com/Rosdahl12e**.

95 Substance Use Disorders

Learning Objectives

1. List the categories of substance use disorders.
2. Discuss theories related to development of substance use disorders. Identify common characteristics of the person with this disorder.
3. List specific steps in managing substance use disorders, including withdrawal.
4. Describe signs indicating substance use disorders, including characteristic behavioral changes and physical signs. Describe common steps in progression to the disorder.
5. Identify pertinent questions related to substance use in nursing data gathering.
6. Describe nursing measures in detoxification of different chemicals, including alcohol. Identify the most life-threatening withdrawal.
7. Define refeeding syndrome; describe related precautions.
8. Describe programs/theories for long-term treatment of substance use disorders.
9. Describe the stages of unmanaged alcohol withdrawal, including delirium tremens and alcohol hallucinosis. Describe specific related nursing care.
10. Describe the role of the codependent in alcohol misuse. Identify how the cycle of dependence can be interrupted.
11. List signs of misuse and withdrawal symptoms for sedatives, cannabis, narcotics, cocaine, hallucinogens, anabolic steroids, nicotine, and caffeine.
12. Describe adverse effects of methamphetamine misuse; identify related nursing actions and precautions.
13. Explain how opiate agonists function in maintenance programs for narcotic substance use disorders.
14. Discuss dangers of hallucinogen and volatile substance use disorder.
15. Describe problems related to misuse of OTC and prescribed drugs.
16. Discuss special problems associated with drug misuse in pregnant women, adolescents, and older adults.
17. Discuss legal obligations of nurses who believe coworkers are abusing drugs or alcohol.

Important Terminology

aftercare
agonist therapy
alcohol hallucinosis
aversion therapy
blackout
cirrhosis
codependency
detoxification
enabler
huffing
macropsia
micropsia
mydriasis
refeeding syndrome
remission
substance use disorder
tolerance
tweaker
Wernicke–Korsakoff syndrome
Withdrawal symptoms

Acronyms

AA
ARLD
BAL
CBD
CIWA-Ar
DBT
DOM
DTs
DUI/DWI
FAS
GBA
HPPD
HR
LSD
MDA/MDMA
MgSO$_4$
MJ
NA
OBS
PCP
THC
W/D

Individuals respond to stress in numerous ways, sometimes by using harmful, mood-altering chemicals. Another factor often related to use of these substances is *low self-esteem*. (Although these disorders are most often related to chemicals, such as alcohol and other drugs, they may also include obsessions with activities such as work, sex, food, or gambling.) Many people use these behaviors to avoid relationships and painful problems. Substance use disorders know no racial, religious, gender, age, or socioeconomic barriers. Recognizing and caring for these clients requires high-level data gathering, nursing skills, patience, and compassion. This chapter is primarily devoted to misuse of chemicals, but many concepts apply to other situations as well.

SUBSTANCE USE DISORDERS

Diagnosis of Substance Use Disorders

The American Psychiatric Association (2013), in the new edition of the DSM-5, replaced the terms *abuse* and *dependence* with the term *substance use disorder*. They then classify and describe each specific type of substance (alcohol, opioids, stimulants, hallucinogens, and tobacco) and identify three levels of severity. These levels are *Mild, Moderate,* and *Severe.* The "recurrent use of alcohol or drugs causes clinically and functionally significant impairment," as evidenced by:

- Health problems
- Disability

- Failure to meet major responsibilities and obligations in work, school, social, or family life
- Impaired control, resulting in social impairment, risky behaviors (e.g., driving or using heavy machinery), and specific pharmacologic criteria
- Other factors, such as legal problems and arrests; or continued use, despite related problems.

Any drug can be misused, including alcohol, marijuana, street drugs, nicotine, or drugs prescribed by a healthcare provider. Substance use disorder is now considered a long-term, chronic illness. The person with this disorder:

- Needs more of the drug to cause intoxication or experiences decreased effects from previously sufficient amounts—**tolerance**
- Experiences characteristic **withdrawal** symptoms if he or she stops using the drug or must take the same or related substances to avoid withdrawal symptoms
- Uses the drug in larger amounts or for a longer time than planned (e.g., goes on a "binge" and cannot stop)
- Wishes to stop using or cut down but is unable to do so
- Spends much time and energy planning to obtain and use the drug (e.g., obtaining prescriptions from multiple healthcare providers, traveling out of town to get medications/drugs, burglary to get money or drugs, hiding bottles)
- Gives up important activities (e.g., organizations, entertainment, family), secondary to drug use
- Continues to use, even though he or she knows the drug is causing significant physical, psychological, legal, or interpersonal problems
- Spends increasing amounts of money on the drug, even though this jeopardizes personal and family finances
- Combines overuse of substances with other compulsive behaviors, such as gambling

> **Key Concept**
> Note that use can be daily or episodic and still be considered a substance use disorder.

Substance use disorders have been considered disorders since the 1950s. Untreated, these disorders can be fatal and usually will worsen without intervention. Classifications related to recovery include the following:

- Active
- In **remission** (not currently active)
- On agonist/blocking therapy
- In a controlled environment

The healthcare industry is continually learning better ways to describe and treat these disorders. It is important to note that they can lead to various disruptions in mental health, including delirium, dementia, psychosis, and sleep disorders. In addition, various physical disorders can result, including cirrhosis of the liver, nutritional deficiencies and eating disorders, sleep disorders, organic brain damage, pancreatitis, and sexual dysfunction.

Causes

Despite all that has been written about the causes of substance use disorders, a sole causative factor has not been identified. The following are current theories.

Physical Factors Theory

This theory states that excessive consumption of substances is the most obvious cause of these disorders. For example, some investigators believe that a nutritional deficiency or an endocrine factor (similar to diabetes) can lead to excessive alcohol use. (It is known that nutritional deficiencies *result from excessive use*.) Another theory is that ingestion of alcohol and certain other drugs cause an *allergic response,* or an altered reaction of body tissues, to a specific substance (e.g., alcohol) that would not produce the same effect in nonallergic people.

Genetic Theory

Considerable research has been conducted to target genetic causes. It has yet to be determined whether overuse of alcohol and other drugs is based on direct biologic transmission or is a learned behavior in children who constantly interact with family members with substance use issues.

Emotional and Psychological Theories

Psychological explanations of substance use disorders vary in detail, but experts generally agree that stress is a contributing factor. In addition, *low self-esteem* is often considered to be the most potent precipitating factor. The person needs the drug to feel good about life and self. The stress theory is compatible with this theory because stress can be caused by low self-worth, as the person continuously tries to be good enough to satisfy personal ideals. Many people use substances "just to feel better," to "stop being depressed or hearing voices," or to "escape from life and its problems."

Some generalizations about personality traits related to substance use disorders include the following:

- Low self-esteem
- Difficulties in interpersonal relations
- General uneasiness and dissatisfaction with life
- Low tolerance for frustration
- Tendency toward excessive and self-destructive, risky behaviors
- Coexisting mental illness (in many cases)

> **Key Concept**
> As with most psychological theories, it is unclear whether these characteristics are typical of the person with a *potential* for substance use disorder or if they are the *result* of the disorder.

Dual Disorders

As discussed in Chapter 94, many people with substance use disorders also have a coexisting mental illness that complicates both conditions. This dual disorder or *dual diagnosis* has been called "mental illness combined with chemical dependency" (*MI/CD*). Many people with mental disorders are depressed and use chemicals in an attempt to ease depression or to commit suicide. Many of these people also suffer from "voices" (auditory hallucinations) and use chemicals in an effort to "make the voices go away." In addition, it is often difficult to locate therapists or support groups that understand the need for continuing to take psychiatric medications while abstaining from other drugs and

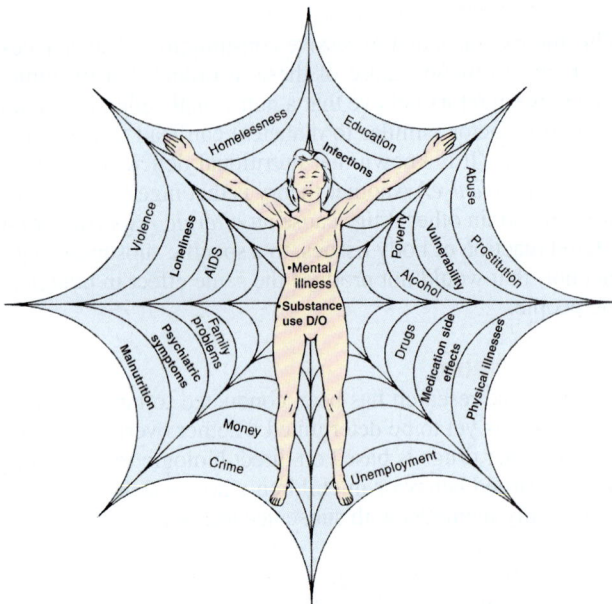

Figure 95-1 Clients with a dual diagnosis of mental illness and a substance use disorder are often confronted with a myriad of social, financial, physical, and relationship problems (SAMHSA, n.d.).

alcohol, although this is not as difficult as it was in the past. Preexisting depression often deepens after substance use and may also be accompanied by guilt. Figure 95-1 illustrates the complexity of interrelated social factors that contribute to and result from MI/CD.

> **Key Concept**
> Most people are not aware that many commonly misused drugs, including alcohol, sedatives, and narcotics, are depressants and *compound* the person's original depression.

Nature of Substance Use Disorders

Progressive Nature
The *progressive nature* of these disorders corresponds to their psychological causes. The typical progression is as follows:

1. "I use it to feel better." In the early stages of substance use, the chemical temporarily alleviates the person's feelings of low self-worth and stress; the person uses it to escape and feel better.
2. "I use it to keep from feeling bad." As the disorder progresses, the person must use *increased amounts* of the substance to stop feeling sick or depressed. The person begins to need the substance to keep from feeling bad, but he or she never really feels good.
3. "I'm losing control." The person now finds that even a small amount of the chemical causes illness or severe intoxication. In other cases, even a small amount of the chemical renders the person unable to stop using until he or she passes out or runs out of the drug and is unable to get more. **Blackouts** (periods of total amnesia) often occur with excessive use. At this point, immediate intervention is vital, often to save the person's life.

Defense Mechanisms
Of the many defense mechanisms people use (see Chapter 94), denial, rationalization, and projection are commonly used and are the most pertinent to substance use disorders.

Denial
The person who misuses substances denies using drugs, denies any difficulty in controlling intake, or denies that drug use is causing problems long after others realize that the person is out of control.

Rationalization
Many people who misuse substances argue that they could not possibly have a problem, and they offer rationalizations, such as "I cannot have an alcohol problem, because…": "I do not use during the day," "I have a good job," "I only use on weekends," "I don't hide bottles or drink at home," "I never drink before 5 o'clock," "I only drink beer," "I can quit whenever I want," or "I can go for months without drinking."

Projection
Whether or not the person admits to having a problem, they often blame others. A typical complaint is projected onto the family: "If you were a better parent or spouse, I would not have to drink," "If my kids were better behaved, I would not need drugs," or "It's not my fault, it's ____'s fault."

Management
The following concepts are basic to management of all substance use disorders:

1. *Recognition:* Someone must recognize the condition. The first person to do so is very often someone other than the person with the disorder.
2. *Intervention:* Active intervention must occur. If no one intervenes in the process, it usually escalates.
3. *Treatment:* These disorders often respond to structured therapy. The person may need a specific milieu to gain control. In rare cases, the person sees the impact of the destructive behavior and stops using. *Usually, however, the client needs assistance to stop using.* (Often, if the person stops using without treatment, the positive emotional changes resulting from successful treatment do not occur. This person may present to a physician as being severely anxious and get prescriptions for benzodiazepines. People who have been on antianxiety medications for a long time may be referred to as a "dry drunk," as there has been no therapy or work done to deal with the low self-esteem and many undesirable personality traits and concerns that still exist.) In addition to positive self-enhancement and abstinence, treatment should address such issues as malnutrition, heart and liver dysfunction, brain damage, general health, social changes, and interpersonal relationships.
4. *Recovery:* Many therapies assist people with substance use disorders to lead a successful and productive life. Many such programs use the 12-step approach of Alcoholics Anonymous **(AA)** or apply principles of behavior modification.

NURSING CARE MEASURES

Caring for clients dealing with substance use disorders occurs in various settings, including outpatient treatment, extended-care facilities, specific treatment centers and clinics, and hospitals.

> **Key Concept**
>
> It is important to note that up to 45% of clients receiving care for general medical-surgical conditions have underlying substance use disorders; the great majority of these clients overuse alcohol. Research shows that more than one-third of Emergency Department admissions and about one-fifth of acute hospital admissions can be traced to complications related to substance use.

Because many insurance plans no longer cover inpatient treatment for substance use disorders, many people are admitted under another diagnosis, either associated with or directly resulting from substance use. These diagnoses include depression and suicide attempts; pancreatitis, diabetes, cirrhosis, and other liver problems; gastrointestinal (GI) disorders; headaches; and cardiovascular disorders, such as suspected heart attack and hypertension. In addition, motor vehicle accidents (MVAs) are often directly attributable to substance use. (See the Nursing Process at the end of this section for more information on working with these clients.)

Identification of the Person With a Substance Use Disorder

Many people routinely use defense mechanisms. They often convince healthcare professionals that their medical disorder is not related to any form of substance use; therefore, the underlying disorder goes undetected. Be aware of stereotypes; it is not possible to identify a person with a substance use disorder by appearance. Be alert for signs and symptoms of substance overuse or withdrawal *in all clients*. Many people are admitted for non–chemical-related problems. Clients in the healthcare facility who are deprived of their substance of choice may suddenly begin having serious or life-threatening withdrawal symptoms. **Remember:** Clients in the Emergency Department, Day Surgery, Labor and Delivery, or any other area may experience withdrawal symptoms. Also, be alert to cross-dependence: clients who misuse one substance often have built up tolerance to related drugs. (This includes prescription drugs, such as pain killers, tranquilizers, and sleeping pills.)

> **NCLEX Alert**
>
> After reading the NCLEX scenario, be alert to suggested options that offer questions that could be asked when obtaining the nursing history or interview data. Substance use disorders can affect any population, from birth to old age.

Nursing Data Gathering

Several formal evaluation tools are used to identify a substance use disorder. In addition, the nurse gathers relevant information to assist the provider in making a diagnosis. It is important to know what items to include. The LPN/LVN often assists with the admission and talks with the client and family. Report pertinent observations to the person who is doing the written admission assessment and writing the nursing care plan. Initial data gathering regarding the client's use of mood-altering chemicals can be incorporated naturally into every nursing interaction. Ask the person, "How much alcohol do you use? What other drugs do you use? How often? How much?" If the person responds negatively to these questions, ask him or her, "When was the last time you used alcohol or drugs?" (When you ask nonjudgmental questions, clients are less likely to deny use.) If a client acknowledges any use, ever, obtain additional information. Ask open-ended questions such as, "Tell me about your drinking or drug use." (It is usually not as effective to ask a question such as, "Do you drink alcohol?" It is too easy for the client to just say, "No.")

If this approach does not yield enough information, probe further by asking specific questions:

What do you take to relieve stress? Pain? When you get nervous?
Do you drink or use chemicals alone or with others? Are you usually at home or in a bar?
What type of beverages do you drink?
Do you combine alcohol and other drugs?
Do you drink at work?
Do you drink and drive? Have you ever had a **DUI/DWI** (driving under the influence, driving while intoxicated)?
Have you had any legal problems because of drug/alcohol use? Have you been in jail/prison? What for?
How often do you miss work? On what day of the week do you usually call in sick? (Routinely calling in sick on Mondays [or Fridays] is a danger signal for substance use disorders.) Are you unemployed? Experiencing homelessness?
At what age did you start using? What did you use first? What was the progression?
How much of each chemical (alcohol, marijuana, cocaine, amphetamines, or other chemicals) do you use in a day? How much in a week? How much does it cost? Where do you get the money?
In what form do you use the drug (e.g., cocaine, crack, crank, speed, rock)? Do you inhale, smoke, snort, or inject the drug?
Have you ever been through treatment for substance use? How many times? Where? What is your longest period of sobriety (in your life)?
Have you ever been told you had a physical disorder related to alcohol/drug use? Have you had relationship problems related to your use?
When was your last drink? Drug use?
Have you ever had problems with withdrawal? Seizures? DTs?

The last two questions are particularly important in terms of predicting withdrawal. (For example, the person who has been drinking alcohol in the past few days must be closely observed for *life-threatening withdrawal symptoms* for at least 96 hr.) These questions are significant for clients who are being prepared for surgery or to deliver babies. They can suddenly go into unexpected withdrawal. **Remember:** How often and how much a person drinks or uses drugs are not always the best criteria for determining whether someone has a substance use disorder. Rather, explore the role of the substances in the individual's life. Loss of control or inability to stop drinking/using is a cardinal sign of the disorder. If a person's use affects his or her job, interpersonal relationships, or

IN PRACTICE
DATA GATHERING IN NURSING 95-1 | Signals of Childhood or Adolescent Substance Use Disorder

Signs that a child or adolescent may have a substance use disorder include the following:
- Extreme changes in dress
- Sudden loss of interest in personal appearance
- Sudden change in friends
- Extreme changes in eating or sleeping patterns
- Radical changes in normal behavior patterns or interests
- Extreme changes in relationships with family members
- Tardiness or absenteeism
- Unexpected or unusual failure in school
- Seclusion and withdrawal in room for extended periods
- Slurred speech, glazed look, other physical symptoms
- Defense of the right to use alcohol or drugs
- Prominent mood changes
- Sudden refusal to work; not showing up for work or school
- Feelings of being sad or "bummed out"
- Dishonesty, stealing, hiding things
- Wearing dark glasses during the day to hide the eyes
- Wearing long sleeves to hide needle marks
- Sudden need for large amounts of money
- Sudden, unexplained disappearance of items in the home, such as money or jewelry
- Trouble with the law, speeding tickets, driving while intoxicated (DWI) tickets
- Leaving home for several days at a time, unexplained absences

family, that person has a substance use disorder. Young people are particularly vulnerable to societal influences. In Practice: Data Gathering in Nursing 95-1 identifies some signals of substance use disorder, particularly in young adults.

Dealing With an Intoxicated Person in the Healthcare Facility

Admission of an intoxicated person, either in the emergency department, mental health unit, general hospital, nursing home, or outpatient clinic, is a nursing challenge. In Practice: Nursing Care Guidelines 95-1 identifies nursing skills used in an emergency department. Many of these skills apply to other settings as well. Remember the following general points:

Key Concept
Visitors may enter a healthcare facility in an intoxicated state. Allowing them to enter the client unit or a client's room is unwise. Call the nursing supervisor, charge nurse, or security personnel if such a situation arises. The intoxicated person may be excitable and dangerous. Do not attempt to force an intoxicated person to leave without assistance.

- The healthcare staff have no way of truly knowing what drugs a client has used without specific laboratory tests. (Some drugs are difficult to identify. In addition, many

IN PRACTICE
NURSING CARE GUIDELINES 95-1 | Caring for the Alcohol- or Drug-Using Person in the Emergency Department

- Remain with the person at all times. Provide a quiet, calm environment. Speak softly and calmly. Remove as much stimulation as possible. Tell the client frequently where they are, what the date is, and who you are. *Rationale: The person may be very frightened, disoriented, or combative. People are more comfortable if they know where they are. Also, clients are often hyperirritable and overly sensitive to environmental stimuli. If you are afraid, the client will probably sense your fear. Request security assistance, if needed.*
- Monitor level of consciousness (LOC) and orientation. Check neurologic eye signs and other responses. *Rationale: Lowering of LOC is a dangerous sign.*
- Watch for tremors, involuntary movements, or seizures. *Rationale: Withdrawal symptoms may occur without warning and may be life-threatening.*
- Monitor the client's cardiac and respiratory status. Monitor vital signs, oxygen saturation, and pain levels. *Rationale: Arrhythmias are common. Artificial respiratory support or ventilation may be necessary. The person may have depressed reflexes or secretions that block his or her airway. Emesis and aspiration may occur. Respirations may be dangerously depressed in cases of an overdose. Elevated or fluctuating vital signs are often the first indicator of withdrawal, especially from alcohol. Pain often occurs with withdrawal from certain drugs.*
- Try not to use any type of restraint unless absolutely necessary. Remove harmful objects from the immediate environment. *Rationale: The person may become more frightened and may be injured while fighting restraints. In a confused or agitated state, the client might not recognize familiar objects or may attempt to harm themself or others. Maintain safety.*
- Do not touch the client unless necessary. Make sure the client understands what you are going to do. *Rationale: The person may misperceive your action to be a threat and react violently.*
- If a client begins to lose control, get assistance. Bring the situation under immediate control. *Rationale: A person on certain drugs can quickly become violent. Prevent injury to clients and others.*
- Report any unusual signs or symptoms immediately. *Rationale: Many people misuse several drugs. Therefore, almost any unusual reaction can be a sign of withdrawal. Some drug withdrawals can be life-threatening.*
- **Remember:** An injury, accident, surgery, or delivery can precipitate withdrawal symptoms.

drugs are not included in a routine toxicology screen.) *Anticipate all possible behaviors.*
- A thorough history is required for safety during detoxification and in the event of complications related to detoxification or withdrawal. (Not all clients will be willing or able to give an accurate drug/alcohol use history.)
- It is particularly important to determine when the last alcohol or drug use was and if the person has ever had serious withdrawal symptoms.
- Carefully document all information. The provider usually orders blood alcohol and drug testing (*toxicology [tox] screen*) and/or urine toxicology (*U-Tox*). These laboratory tests include many drugs, both illegal and legal, over-the-counter (OTC), and prescribed. Orders for these tests are written, based on the physical examination, client history, history given by the family, and admission of nursing history and diagnosis. Careful data gathering is a vital component of this process.
- It may be necessary to obtain a *witnessed urine specimen* for drug testing. In this case, a staff member must watch the specimen being obtained. Be aware of the use of devices, such as the "Whizzinator," designed to thwart the accuracy of the specimen.
- It is vital to closely observe all clients in the event of unexpected withdrawal symptoms.

NURSING PROCESS

DATA COLLECTION

Behavior Changes
- Erratic or inappropriate behavior: sudden changes in mood, anhedonia
- Poor school or job attendance or performance
- Illegal acts, such as stealing, embezzling, prostitution, or selling drugs
- Declining social status or an incongruent economic situation
- Avoidance of previously enjoyed activities
- Frequent visits to an emergency department for depression or suicide threats

Physical Signs
- Withdrawal symptoms (see Table 95-1)
- Needle tracks, often covered by long sleeves
- Chronic nasal congestion and cold symptoms with drug snorting; after heavy use, the septum may perforate
- Dilated pupils (**mydriasis**), often masked by sunglasses
- Unkempt appearance (unusual for this client)
- Unexplained weight loss
- Abnormal electrolyte levels, anemia, extreme weight loss

Complications With Overdose
- Cerebrovascular spasm, as shown by hemorrhage, seizures, hypertensive or hypotensive crisis; angina; myocardial infarction; dysrhythmias; abnormal respirations (e.g., Cheyne–Stokes, hyperpnea); hyperthermia; tachycardia or bradycardia
- Use urine or blood toxicology studies to identify drugs of misuse

POSSIBLE NURSING DIAGNOSES
Anxiety
Ineffective individual coping
Altered growth and development (fetal)
Altered health maintenance
High risk for infection
High risk for injury
Knowledge deficit (specify)
Altered nutrition: Less than body requirements
Altered parenting
Powerlessness
Self-care deficit
Self-esteem disturbance
Sensory/perceptual alterations
Impaired social interaction
Altered thought processes
High risk for violence: Self-directed or directed at others

PLANNING
A plan of care is designed with the client to achieve general goals including those in the following list. The person will
- Safely detoxify
- Admit that use of substances has been a problem and that he or she needs help to stop using
- Agree to participate in a treatment program
- Show behavior and physical signs demonstrating decreased or discontinued substance use
- Test drug free (urine tests, toxicology screening)
- Agree to continue with aftercare

IMPLEMENTATION
- Refer the client to a psychiatric liaison nurse or drug treatment counselor.
- Support the client's family; encourage them to seek help by contacting a support group, such as AA.
- In some cases, intervention and forced treatment may be required.
- Strongly recommend client follow-up in a support group, such as AA or Narcotics Anonymous (NA).

EVALUATION
The adequacy of the plan is determined by evaluating the client's achievement of stated goals.

DETOXIFICATION AND RECOVERY

Detoxification is the process of removing a drug and its physiologic effects from the body. Total detoxification may take many days, depending on the drug(s) used, amounts, dependence level, liver and kidney function, and the client's size and general health. The most important goals in detoxification management are *comfort and safety.* Use sedation and emotional support to allow the client to rest and recover and prevent injury or exhaustion. Treatment depends in part on the specific substance(s) used. *Remember that detoxification must occur before long-term treatment can begin.*

TABLE 95-1 Withdrawal Pointers for Selected Substance Use Disorders

SIGNS AND SYMPTOMS DURING UNMANAGED WITHDRAWAL	NURSING CONSIDERATIONS
Alcohol Acute detoxification usually completed in 5-7 days; milder symptoms may continue: ≥10 days. (Acute detox usually begins within 48-72 hr of last ingestion.) Alcohol when combined with mood-altering drugs—withdrawal may include unexpected symptoms Suicide risk increases during detox Tremors (internal first, then hands, then entire body); agitation, irritability, depression; anxiety; diaphoresis Delusions, hallucinations (auditory/visual—delirium tremens); tonic–clonic seizures possible Hypertension, tachycardia, hyperthermia; mydriasis Nausea, vomiting, anorexia Sleep disorders, especially insomnia; sexual dysfunction Vitamin deficiency (especially thiamine and folate); hypoglycemia; electrolyte imbalance Confusion, disorientation, coma, delirium, amnesia, blackouts, memory loss; dementia may be exacerbated Exhaustion and cardiac arrest	Carefully observe vital signs, level of consciousness, oxygen saturation, and pain. Follow detoxification protocol of facility. Client evaluated for other health problems (malnutrition, liver damage, cardiac malfunction, infection, tuberculosis, vitamin deficiencies, brain damage). Follow seizure precautions. Monitor blood sugar levels. Encourage food and fluid intake; monitor intake and output. Administer vitamins, as ordered. (Avoid refeeding syndrome.) Follow suicide precautions; monitor client carefully. Manage nausea and vomiting. Reorient client, as needed. Give as needed (PRN) prescribed medications, to manage symptoms and control blood pressure. (Alcohol often causes fetal alcohol syndrome when used during pregnancy.) Document frequently.
Sedatives, Hypnotics, Anxiolytics—including depressants, such as barbiturates, benzodiazepines; and illegal drugs, such as GHB and flunitrazepam (Rohypnol) Anxiety, diaphoresis, hypervigilance, tachycardia, hypertension, paranoia, and severe insomnia. These symptoms may quickly progress to severe withdrawal, with extreme agitation and combativeness, paranoia, and delirium (or loss of consciousness). These symptoms may alternate with somnolence and coma.	
Other symptoms vary and may include tonic–clonic seizures; extreme psychological and physical effects, including slurred speech, unsteady gait, nystagmus; decreased memory and attention span; mydriasis; urinary/fecal incontinence Sleep disorders, particularly insomnia Confusion, delirium, amnesia, hallucinations; psychotic disorders, mood disorders; severe anxiety; tremors; sexual dysfunction Electroencephalogram (EEG) changes; slowed/absent reflexes; respiratory slowing, apnea; weak, rapid pulse; abnormal lung sounds Coma and death may result; dementia *may persist after withdrawal*. (Arousal from coma may be dangerous, resulting in *emergence delirium*.) Withdrawal symptoms may last 7-12 days and may be fatal if untreated. GHB symptoms also include: facial tics, fist-clenching, self-injurious behavior (e.g., head-banging), "chain-saw" snoring, hypothermia, bradycardia	Follow specific protocol of facility, including seizure precautions. Determine vital signs, oxygen saturation, pain, and level of consciousness often. Reorient client, as needed. Keep client from hurting self or others. Monitor respiratory status; maintain patent (open) airway; support respirations, if needed. Give PRN medications to manage symptoms.
Heroin (and Other Narcotics)—morphine, codeine, opium, heroin, oxycodone, Percocet, Vicodin Symptoms resemble those of a cold or an allergic response, with sore throat, rhinorrhea, *lacrimation* (tearing of eyes), diaphoresis, and insomnia. Yawning and mydriasis are specific signs.	
Nausea, vomiting, severe abdominal cramping; diarrhea (sometimes explosive); anorexia Tremors, weakness; muscle/joint pain Flushing, sometimes followed by chills; gooseflesh Depression or irritability and hyperactivity Confusion, disorientation, delusions, hallucinations Insomnia, sleep disturbances; sexual dysfunction Fast, weak, irregular pulse; mild hypertension; usually lowered temperature (may also be increased) *Overdose:* pinpoint pupils; cold, clammy skin; seizures; depressed respirations and heart rate; extreme drowsiness; coma and possible death.	Follow specific protocol of facility. Frequently determine vital signs, pain, oxygen saturation, and level of consciousness. Withdrawal more life-threatening if a concurrent medical diagnosis is present (e.g., heart or lung disease, diabetes). Client often malnourished. May have infections, abscesses, and other complications of injections. Blood tests for human immunodeficiency virus (HIV), hepatitis, hemoglobin, etc. Follow seizure precautions. Reorient client, as needed. Give PRN medications to manage symptoms. A specific antidote for narcotic overdose is naloxone (Narcan).

TABLE 95-1 Withdrawal Pointers for Selected Substance Use Disorders (Continued)	
SIGNS AND SYMPTOMS DURING UNMANAGED WITHDRAWAL	**NURSING CONSIDERATIONS**
Amphetamines/Stimulants and Related Drugs—methamphetamine, cocaine, crack, uppers, "speed, crank," khat, bath salts Highly unpredictable behavior, including irritability, agitation, anxiety, erratic behavior, hyperactivity, unpredictability, assaultiveness, intrusiveness, rapid and pressured speech, crying jags, obsessive and repetitive behaviors. Depression may occur. Confusion, poor memory, and poor judgment Headache, bone pain, muscle cramps, tremors Low urine output (oliguria) increased appetite Fatigue and increased need for sleep, vivid and frightening nightmares Sexual dysfunction Psychiatric symptoms: extreme mood swings, blunted affect or euphoria, hallucinations (tactile = "cocaine bugs"), hypervigilance, paranoia, grandiosity, delirium, irritability, anxiety, as well as depression and other mood disorders Lack of enjoyment (anhedonia) Possible permanent organic brain syndrome *Life-threatening symptoms* include respiratory depression, cardiac arrhythmias, extreme hypertension, sudden hyperthermia, seizures, and coma. (All of these symptoms are usually more severe in meth use disorder.)	Follow facility protocol. Provide safety for client and others. Keep client in private room. Maintain calm, quiet atmosphere. Anticipate the client's acting out; *this client may be very dangerous.* PRN medications given to prevent injury to client and others. (Do not physically restrain, unless absolutely necessary.) Give consistent, calm, and nonthreatening care In cases of meth overdose, assess level of consciousness and orientation, oxygen saturation, pain, and vital signs frequently. Reorient, as needed. Monitor respiratory status (respiratory depression can be dangerous). Respiratory stimulants may be needed. Specific withdrawal symptoms treated with PRN medications. Seizure precautions observed. Hypertension and hyperthermia controlled with medications. Encourage adequate nutrition and fluid intake. Monitor intake and output; report oliguria (a serious sign). Manage nausea and vomiting. Assess sleeping habits; give sedatives as needed.

Motivation for Treatment

Several reasons exist for the person with a substance use disorder to seek treatment. The person may really want to stop and may realize that employment, loved ones, and health are in jeopardy if the practice continues. The person who misuses substances may want to "cut down" but must realize that *avoiding relapse is almost impossible while using any amount of the drug.* A person might be ordered by a court to enter treatment. In many states, people involved in an MVA while intoxicated or arrested for DUI/DWI are ordered into treatment. (Usually, jail is the only other option.) When the person enters treatment, they are often truly angry and lack the motivation and desire to succeed. An underlying rationale for the court order is the hope that exposure to a good treatment program will encourage the person to participate in recovery. Peer pressure can be strong; in many cases, the person gradually begins to take the program seriously. **Remember**: Abstinence is the only sure method for detoxification and recovery.

> **Nursing Alert** When a person stops taking drugs, such as barbiturates or cocaine, the danger of future overdose exists. After the person stops the drug for a period of time, tolerance is reduced. If the person then takes the usual dose, this often constitutes an overdose and can cause death.

The Detoxification Center

A person with a substance use disorder may initially be admitted to a *detoxification center.* Often, the person is transported to "detox" by police. Here, detoxification is supervised. Hopefully, the emphasis is on supportive care and referral to continuing therapy after detoxification, so the person can deal with the underlying motivations that led to the condition.

The Therapeutic Community

In a *therapeutic community,* clients are isolated from the substance-oriented environment. Their lifestyle is encouraged to change, as they learn drug-free coping skills. Recovering clients organize and administer many such programs. Clients are assigned to work or study groups and given assigned readings to help them learn more about the disorder and assume personal responsibility. Group therapy is a common component of treatment programs. Sometimes, the groups are gender-specific and focus on particular concerns to each gender. The goals of treatment are to assist clients to address physical and emotional problems associated with the disorder and understand the cycle of dependence. When clients have accomplished these goals, they are ready to begin recovery. Clients in early stages of withdrawal often show common signs and symptoms, including anxiety, uncontrollable fear, tremors (internal and external), irritability, agitation, hyperactive reflexes, GI disturbances (especially nausea and vomiting), diaphoresis, and insomnia. In alcohol or benzodiazepine withdrawal, *all vital signs are usually elevated*; in withdrawal from some other drugs such as stimulants, vital signs may be depressed or fluctuate.

> **Nursing Alert** Detoxification requires careful and correct management, especially for those who misuse alcohol. *Rationale: If managed improperly, the client may progress to a dangerous withdrawal that includes terrifying hallucinations and/or seizures. Aspiration, coma, and death may follow.*

Immediate Treatment in Detoxification

A complete medical workup is important. Blood work determines liver, kidney, and thyroid function. Blood chemistry levels indicate vitamin deficiencies, lipid (fat) levels, uric acid levels, and enzyme levels that might indicate physical (especially muscle) damage. Urine toxicology reveals which common drugs the client has used. In some cases, blood tests are also done to determine more exact drug levels.

Before administering medications (e.g., benzodiazepines), the client is evaluated for severity of withdrawal symptoms. The decision to administer or withhold medications is based on the presence or absence of specific factors. Several formal rating scales are available to assist in determining the severity of withdrawal symptoms. One such scale is the Clinical Institute Withdrawal Assessment-Alcohol Revised (**CIWA-Ar**). This scale systematically itemizes and quantifies the most common alcohol withdrawal symptoms and allows healthcare staff to determine if medications are needed. These symptoms include nausea and vomiting, tremors, *paroxysmal sweating, anxiety, agitation* tactile disturbances, auditory disturbances, visual disturbances, headache/fullness in head, and orientation to reality (rated 0-4). These factors, except orientation, are rated from 0 to 7, denoting severity (maximum score = 67). Any score greater than 18 indicates severe withdrawal. Generally, a client with a total score of 10 or more is eligible to receive benzodiazepines, such as Librium (for younger clients) or Valium (for older clients and those with liver or pulmonary dysfunction). Clients with other physical disorders, such as liver failure, esophageal varices (enlarged blood vessels in esophagus; varicosities), brain damage, or heart failure, may need different evaluation measures or medications. Repeat the CIWA-Ar every hour until score is less than 10 during the intensive detoxification period. See In Practice: Important Medications 95-1 for a list of medications used in detoxification.

> **Nursing Alert** Medications are given as ordered. Many chemically dependent people experiencing withdrawal are medication-seeking and ask for medications. Report their requests and document carefully.

Withdrawal Symptoms

To begin detoxification, the client's body is denied access to the drug of choice. When this drug is removed, most people with substance use disorders experience withdrawal (**W/D**) symptoms of varying severity. Some clients withdraw with minimal discomfort; others experience very difficult and/or dangerous withdrawals. Intensity depends on several factors, including the drug used, amount, and general health and nutritional status. Liver function and the client's history of previous withdrawal episodes are especially important. Predicting the progression of any individual's withdrawal episode at any given time, however, is impossible.

Those experiencing withdrawal are in psychological and medical jeopardy. They immediately present many potential nursing problems. Detoxification from alcohol and certain other drugs, such as central nervous system depressants, is a serious medical problem; the process can be fatal. (*Alcohol withdrawal is one of the most dangerous.*) Table 95-1 lists common withdrawal signs/symptoms and selected drugs used. In Practice: Nursing Care Guidelines 95-2 describes general nursing measures used to assist clients during withdrawal. Remember: Withdrawal can occur in any healthcare area. Always be alert for withdrawal symptoms.

Nutrition and General Health

In addition to treatment for the disorder, health care must address the client's nutritional status and general health. Many clients are seriously malnourished as a direct result of substance use. Usually, liver function tests (to rule out cirrhosis and other disorders) and evaluation of GI function (to rule out conditions such as ulcers, diverticulitis, esophageal varices, or colon cancer) are necessary. If the client is severely malnourished, weight gain is carefully supervised (see later discussion of refeeding syndrome). Supplemental vitamins are often given. Any coexisting conditions, such as injuries, skin rashes, hypertension, and diabetes mellitus, are treated. Many times, physical disorders require immediate medical attention. Some clients require long-term treatment for generalized infections, including tuberculosis and AIDS, which often relate directly to misuse of drugs.

Refeeding Syndrome

If a person is deliberately limiting their food intake, overusing drugs or alcohol, is severely malnourished or starving, careful dietary management is vital. These clients should be rehydrated very slowly, with small and carefully planned fluids and feedings. Carbohydrates, such as dextrose intravenous (IV) solutions, tube-feeding mixtures, and liquid dietary supplements, must be given very carefully. A sudden influx of carbohydrates stimulates insulin production and other events that may seriously upset electrolyte balance. Failure to follow the above guidelines can cause **refeeding syndrome**, which if not appropriately identified and treated, may also cause cardiac failure, hypertension, peripheral edema, neurologic complications (including seizures or coma), respiratory failure, and death.

Long-Term Follow-Up and Treatment

The period after detoxification is vitally important. Usually, the client remembers vividly the extreme discomfort experienced and may now be willing to enter treatment. The role of the nurse includes discussing the possibility of a comprehensive drug evaluation. A person may be diagnosed as having mild, moderate, or severe substance use disorder. The person may also have a **polysubstance use disorder** (having overused several drugs). Many are also **codependents**, living with or caring for another person who overuses alcohol or other drugs. A substance use disorder specialist is available in many healthcare facilities to evaluate the client's drug use and recommend treatment options.

Inpatient or Outpatient Treatment

Treatment for substance use disorders may be as an inpatient in a treatment center or as an outpatient. The client's

IN PRACTICE
IMPORTANT MEDICATIONS 95-1 Selected Medications Used in Detoxification and Substance Use Disorders

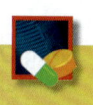

To Control/Prevent Seizures; to Provide Sedation (Benzodiazepines)

Clients are evaluated for severity of withdrawal symptoms before benzodiazepines are given because of their *misuse potential.* Most people who overuse drugs have cross-tolerance to many drugs used in detoxification. (*Explanation in text.*)

Long-Acting

chlordiazepoxide HCl (Librium) Capsules, IM or IV injectable	Helpful in acute agitation, delirium tremens (DTs), hallucinosis. Oral/IV preferred.
diazepam (Valium) Tablets, oral solution, rectal gel, injectable	Commonly used in acute alcohol withdrawal. IV may be given.

Short-Acting

lorazepam (Ativan) Tablets, injectable, oral solution	Preferred in older adults or if the liver is damaged; oral or IM preferred—may be given IV. Avoid sudden discontinuation.
oxazepam (Serax) Capsules	Acute tremulousness, especially in alcohol withdrawal.

Nursing Considerations

The goal is safe, comfortable withdrawal.
- Monitor vital signs; *do not overmedicate*—the medications used depress the CNS. Death may occur due to respiratory depression or cardiovascular collapse. Physical symptoms, such as tachycardia or hypertension, are also treated.
- Give lorazepam (Ativan) or diazepam (Valium) until the client is mildly sedated. When the client is stable, the dose is usually divided into four doses daily and then tapered down.
- When medications are discontinued, they must be slowly tapered down. Benzodiazepines should be tapered down as soon as possible, usually within 2 to 4 days, to avoid misuse, and are often contraindicated in heart failure, asthma, and diabetes mellitus.
- Give nutritional supplements to reduce nutritional deficiencies and electrolyte imbalances and to arrest brain damage (vitamin C, thiamine, folate, multivitamins, and iron).
- For long-term seizure prevention, phenytoin (Dilantin) or divalproex sodium (Depakote) may be used.
- In an emergency, magnesium sulfate ($MgSO_4$) may be given IV, to prevent or treat seizures. Antiseizure medications also help promote sleep.

Adjunct Medications

β Blockers	Help reduce autonomic nervous system hyperactivity (e.g., tachycardia, diaphoresis, hypertension)
atenolol (Tenormin) and other drugs	Control blood pressure

Adjunct Medications

clonidine (Catapres)	Control blood pressure in chronic methadone use and in alcohol or benzodiazepine withdrawal
guanfacine HCl (Tenex)	Reduce hypertension and withdrawal symptoms in heroin withdrawal

Medications Used in Alcohol Use Disorders
Relapse Prevention

acamprosate (Campral): DR	Antialcoholic drug; GABA analog
disulfiram (Antabuse):	Antialcoholic drug; enzyme inhibitor
naltrexone (Revia, Vivitrol—inj. only):	Opioid antagonist

Vitamins

Multivitamins	To treat malnutrition
supplemental iron	To treat anemia
vitamin B_9 (folate)	Not well absorbed in alcoholism; folate given to prevent neurological disorders
vitamin B_1 (thiamine)	To treat thiamine deficiency. Folate helps prevent or treat Wernicke–Korsakoff syndrome
vitamin C (ascorbic acid)	To treat nutritional deficiency

Nursing Considerations

- Many people with substance use disorders are malnourished. The vitamins listed above are given to other persons with substance use disorders, particularly those who misuse alcohol.
- In chronic alcohol use disorder, IV glucose can worsen thiamine depletion. The IV fluid of choice is usually $D_5$1/2NS. Thiamine is often added, and $MgSO_4$ may be added, to prevent seizures.

Specific Drugs Used to Counteract Overdose

Drug Overdose	Antidote
Depressants/sedatives/hypnotics	Doxapram HCl (Dopram)—injectable respiratory stimulant
Benzodiazepines (e.g., diazepam [Valium], lorazepam [Ativan])	Flumazenil (Romazicon)—IV benzodiazepine receptor antagonist. (May be contraindicated in mixed substance overdose or chronic benzodiazepine use.)
Narcotics/opiates: (e.g., opium heroin, codeine, morphine, oxycontin)	Naloxone HCl (Narcan)—IV opioid antagonist. (Action is shorter than that of opioids, so continued IV maintenance is often required.)

Drug Overdose	Antidote	Drug Overdose	Antidote
Opiates	Methadone or Buprenorphine (Buprenex, Subutex) may be used in withdrawal and for relapse prevention Buprenorphine and Naloxone (Suboxone), combination drug, may be used for both detoxification and maintenance.	**Smoking Cessation** Smoking deterrent—a semisynthetic narcotic analgesic	Bupropion HCL (Zyban): tablets. Given for 7-12 weeks; adverse side effects include increased agitation and irritability, insomnia, headache, dizziness, tremors, dry mouth, and constipation. A helpful side effect is anorexia and weight loss, which may help offset hunger.
Stimulants: (e.g., methamphetamine, amphetamines, cocaine)	Lorazepam (Ativan); in severe cases, haloperidol (Haldol). Antidepressants may assist in relapse prevention.	Smoking deterrent–nicotine receptor antagonist Nicotine replacement	Varenicline (Chantix): capsules. The client can smoke for the first few days, thus easing the cessation process. This drug may be dangerous in pregnancy or lactation and may cause suicidality. Nicotine (NicoDerm CQ; Nicotrol); transdermal patch, nasal spray, inhaler. Nicotine polacrilex (Commit, Nicorette); chewing gum, lozenges.
Hallucinogens: (e.g., acid, LSD, mescaline, MDMA, "Ecstasy," psilocybin/ mushrooms, PCP, spice)	"Talking down" and quiet environment used first; then benzodiazepines, such as diazepam or lorazepam; use haloperidol, if not effective, try not to restrain the client.		
Heroin	Methadone (Dolophine): tablets, ODT tablets, oral concentrate, injectable. Opioid agonist analgesic. Used for detoxification and temporary maintenance of opioid sobriety.		

Nursing 2021 Drug Handbook (2021). Wolters Kluwer; Lieberman, J. A. & Tasman, A. (2006). Handbook of Psychiatric Drugs. Wiley. Rosemary Rosdahl, RPh, Watertown Pharmacy, Minnesota.

attitude, family support, insurance coverage, and work and personal situation often determine what type of treatment is recommended or possible. (The client may also be legally committed to a treatment program depending on the situation.)

Treatment centers usually base their treatment on one or more of the following programs:

- The 12-step program, based on AA
- Rational recovery therapy
- Dialectical behavioral therapy
- Health realization theory

In addition, most treatment programs also include the following:

- Personal and group counseling
- Client and family education
- Family counseling
- Improving nutritional and general health

Programs often include general group therapy, gender-related issues, goal setting, grief management, anger management, esteem building, and referrals to sexual assault or violence anonymous groups. Groups may teach relaxation skills, financial management, stress management, safer sex practices, or other special topics. For example, a writing group teaches therapeutic benefits of creative expression and keeping a journal. Special programs are available for young children, adolescents, seniors, and persons with mental illness, combined with substance use disorders. Family groups are common. Programs are offered at various times during the day. An adjunctive treatment may be the administration of an agonist or adverse conditioning medication (see In Practice: Important Medications 95-1).

12-Step Programs

Twelve-step groups, such as AA and Narcotics Anonymous (**NA**), teach that an untreated substance use disorder is a progressive, incurable disease. The disease is considered to be *arrested* or *in remission* when the person is not using. *The dependent person is never cured.* Twelve-step programs do not sponsor or endorse any particular treatment program; rather, they are based on helping the individual admit their powerlessness over the chemical and that their life has become unmanageable because of it. The person then accepts the existence of a "higher power," determines whom they have harmed and makes amends, turns their life over to their individual higher power, and assists others to do the same. The premise of 12-step programs is, "I have a disease. It's not my fault. I need assistance to stop using." Other examples of therapies used in treatment for substance use disorders follow.

IN PRACTICE
NURSING CARE GUIDELINES 95-2 Nursing Care in Alcohol Withdrawal

Following are general nursing measures for the client withdrawing from alcohol. *Most of these procedures apply to withdrawal from other drugs as well:*

- Develop an individual nursing care plan, based on close observation. Set clear client goals. *Rationale: If withdrawal symptoms occur, they usually begin within 12 to 36 hr.*
- Follow a detoxification protocol/checklist that includes careful observation. *Rationale: Each client withdraws differently. A specific protocol is followed, to avoid missing symptoms.*
- Make observations, including frequent vital signs, with apical pulses and orthostatic blood pressures (and occasional oxygen saturation), as ordered. As the client stabilizes, observations may be less frequent. Monitoring continues until at least 96 hr (4 days) after the person's last drink or use. Report pain and any changes in LOC, neurologic eye signs, or vital signs immediately. Give ordered medications. *Rationale: The client's condition can deteriorate rapidly. A change in vital signs is one of the first signs of inadequate detoxification. Medications (e.g., diazepam) can help control blood pressure and other symptoms; administration is based, in part, on vital signs and CIWA-Ar scores. Dilated pupils (mydriasis) are common in withdrawal from most substances.*
- It is important not to lower blood pressure too quickly. *Rationale: Hypertension is caused by hyperactivity of the autonomic nervous system. Peripheral circulatory collapse may occur if blood pressure drops too rapidly.*
- Provide a quiet atmosphere and subdued lighting. *Rationale: Reduce stress and stimuli.*
- Stay with the client as much as possible; family or friends may assist. *Rationale: The client's condition can change rapidly. This client is also at risk for suicide.*
- Document intake and output (I&O), calorie count, and daily weights. Encourage a variety of fluids. Evaluate skin turgor and look for other signs of dehydration. *Rationale: Restoring fluid and electrolyte balance improves nutritional status. Drinking only plain water can contribute to electrolyte imbalance.*
- Frequent, small feedings are usually given. Manage malnourished clients carefully. *Rationale: Small meals place less stress on the body; the client usually has a decreased appetite and may be nauseated. Refeeding syndrome is life-threatening and must be prevented.*
- The client's blood sugar levels are monitored; carefully planned supplements may be given. Many clients who use alcohol crave sugar. *Rationale: Hypoglycemia may occur during withdrawal because alcohol depletes glycogen stored in the liver. Overuse of alcohol also impairs glycogenesis, due to liver damage, as in cirrhosis. However, excess sugar can cause refeeding syndrome and worsen thiamine depletion, so sugar intake must be carefully balanced.*
- Intravenous (IV) fluids are often given. Electrolytes are closely monitored and may be given IV (often with $D_5 1/2NS$). *Rationale: Dehydration and electrolyte imbalances often result from intestinal malabsorption, starvation, diaphoresis, vomiting, and client hyperactivity. Diluted saline solution helps restore electrolyte balance.*
- Body temperature is carefully monitored. *Rationale: Life-threatening hyperthermia may occur.*
- Routinely prescribed vitamins, particularly in alcohol use disorder, include thiamine (vitamin B_1), folic acid (vitamin B_9, folate), a multivitamin with iron, and sometimes vitamin C. A high-protein diet is often ordered. *Rationale: Many clients are malnourished. Specific vitamin deficiencies are caused by the inability of the proximal small intestine to absorb certain vitamins and sugars. Chronic thiamine deficiency can lead to life-threatening Wernicke–Korsakoff syndrome.*
- Report respiratory or cardiovascular distress and any deviations in blood tests immediately. Electrocardiograms (ECG) and liver function tests are often done. *Rationale: Complications include respiratory distress, pneumonia, liver damage and disease, cardiac failure, and infections.*
- The client usually is not restrained but should have bedside rails up and be observed on fall precautions. *Rationale: Restraints could agitate the person further and can cause death. The absence of restraints requires close observation to prevent falls.*
- The client is turned and repositioned at least every 2 hr, if confused or unconscious. *Rationale: Prevent disorders related to immobility.*
- Position the person on either side if he or she is nauseated or vomiting. *Rationale: Prevent aspiration.*
- Seizure precautions are usually ordered; anticonvulsant drugs are often given. *Rationale: Seizures are a life-threatening complication of unsuccessful detoxification.*
- Other common symptoms (e.g., diaphoresis and dry mouth) are treated symptomatically. *Rationale: They are not life-threatening.*
- If the client becomes agitated or threatening, or if you have any questions, request assistance. *Rationale: It may be dangerous to attempt to control this person, who may injure himself or herself or staff.*
- If the client experiences hallucinations, a medication such as haloperidol (Haldol) may be given. *Rationale: Hallucinations can be life-threatening and are frightening. Haldol must be used very carefully.*

Rational Recovery

Rational emotive therapy (RET) or rational emotive behavior therapy (REBT) was introduced in Chapter 94. REBT is built on the premise that an individual's values and beliefs influence behavior. Therefore, a person's *illogical beliefs influence irrational behaviors*. For example, a person who overuses substances may believe he or she is weak, worthless, or unworthy of happiness. Therefore, the person continues harmful behavior, even though he or she knows it is dangerous, because of their derogatory self-perceptions and low self-esteem. The treatment premise in REBT is helping the person recognize that "I am the only one who can control my behavior and I need to remove irrational behaviors by rejecting my irrational beliefs."

Dialectical Behavioral Therapy

Dialectical behavioral therapy (**DBT**) was developed by Marsha Linehan to treat individuals with borderline personality disorder. It has since been adapted to provide therapy to other clients, including those with substance use disorders. DBT emphasizes the "here and now" and assists individuals to take charge of their own lives. Linehan identifies the goal as the "wise mind," a midway point between being totally rational and totally emotional. The essential elements of DBT are as follows:

- *Individual therapy*, which discusses self-damaging behaviors, behaviors that interfere with therapy, and quality-of-life issues. The goal is to work toward improving one's total life.
- *Group therapy*, in which clients learn to use specific skills, including *core mindfulness* ("Who am I?"—self-awareness), *interpersonal effectiveness* (asking for what one needs, learning to say no, and coping with conflict), *distress tolerance* (nonjudgmentally accepting oneself and the current situation, dealing with stress), and *emotion regulation* (becoming aware of emotions and taking steps toward positive emotions, using stress tolerance techniques).

Health Realization

Health realization (**HR**) is a psychological/spiritual therapy model. HR is based on the theory that each person possesses inborn or *innate (inner) health* and has the *capacity* or ability to lead a healthy life. HR helps the person learn to do this. This therapy draws on the natural resiliency (recuperative powers) of all people and teaches them to gain awareness and insight to bring about positive change. As the person gains insight, they begin to view life from a healthier perspective and can make better life choices and thus have a more positive impact on others. The person who changes from the "inside out" learns to stop living life "reactively" and learns to be more self-directed. The goal of HR therapy is to assist the client gain *self-esteem*.

Family Counseling

Treating only the client is not sufficient; significant others also need intensive counseling. Treatment centers offer family programs conducted simultaneously with the client's treatment. The person and family must realize that they all need follow-up care, which is vital if the client is to maintain sobriety. The client and family need encouragement and support to deal with normal familial stressors, plus added challenges of recovery. The person's recovery is less likely to be successful if significant others are not also in the recovery mode. Referrals to social service agencies may assist in locating support groups, education/retraining, employment, financial assistance, or housing.

Aftercare

Following detoxification and/or intensive treatment, **aftercare** is often the most important factor in maintaining sobriety. The client needs to work with AA or another specific program, for at least 2 years, and often for life, after completing intensive treatment.

ALCOHOL USE DISORDER

Overuse of alcohol (ETOH, EtOH) is a major public health problem, causing or contributing to over 88,000 deaths (5% of all deaths) yearly in the United States, many of which are alcohol-related MVAs (1/3 of all traffic fatalities). Groups such as *MADD* (Mothers Against Drunk Driving) have initiated programs strongly encouraging people not to drive while drinking or using drugs. They have lobbied for stricter laws, and now severe penalties for DUI are in place in most states. Groups also sponsor designated driver programs and offer free taxi rides on holidays such as St. Patrick's Day and New Year's Eve. A program sponsored by law enforcement, *DARE* (Drug Abuse Resistance Education), encourages school-age people to avoid alcohol and drugs. However, The U.S. Public Health Service (PHS) and National Safety Council estimate that at least 15 million Americans, including many young people, have problems with alcohol.

> **Nursing Alert** It is important for the person with any substance use disorder to realize that beverages called "alcohol-free" or "near beer" still contain a small amount of alcohol and should be avoided. This is also true of certain mouthwashes and other substances, such as elixir-type medications.

Palcohol

Palcohol, powdered alcohol, has been introduced, although over 30 states have opposed it. One ounce of Palcohol contains 80 calories and the same amount of alcohol as one drink. Sale of this product follows the same regulations as sale of any other alcohol product (www.palcohol.com).

Signs and Symptoms

Alcohol is a CNS depressant. Signs and symptoms that a person is under its influence include slurred speech, unsteady gait, confusion, and behavioral changes, including aggression. The person who chronically misuses alcohol may have a swollen nose, prominent or spidery veins (*spider angiomas*) on the nose and/or cheeks, and thickened and reddened palms (*palmar erythema*). Chronic alcohol use disorder can also lead to impaired attention, confusion, dementia, amnesia, sleep disorders, and psychotic symptoms, including delusions and hallucinations. Suicide is a major risk.

Alcohol absorption varies and is influenced by many factors. For example, carbonation increases absorption; therefore, faster intoxication occurs from drinking champagne. Medications such as aspirin, cimetidine (Tagamet), and ranitidine (Zantac) enhance absorption of alcohol. Women become intoxicated faster than men because their GI absorption rate is faster, their body fluid composition is different, the ratio of muscle to fat is different, and they are usually smaller.

Diagnosis

It is important to note that drug use (including alcohol) within 4 to 12 hr can be determined with blood and breath testing. Urinalysis can identify substance use, other than alcohol, within the past 24 to 72 hr. Saliva testing is becoming more commonly used because it is convenient. Other tests, such as microscopic hair examination, for chronic, long-term use are available.

It is important to know blood alcohol levels (**BAL**) for detoxification. The maximum legal blood alcohol level for driving varies among states but generally is 0.08 to 0.10 grams per deciliter (g/dL). This represents approximately 4 drinks in 2 hr for a woman or 5 for a man. A person with a level of 0.3 g/dL will usually be vomiting and incoherent, aggressive, or in a stupor. Coma usually occurs at about 0.4 g/dL, and severe respiratory depression and death can occur at 0.5 g/dL and above. The nurse may be asked to perform a Breathalyzer to determine a person's blood-alcohol level. (Follow instructions on the machine.) Thresholds for these symptoms depend on the person's tolerance level.

> **Nursing Alert** Suspect alcohol use disorder if the Breathalyzer level is 0.08 to 0.15 g/dL and the person does not appear to be impaired. It is important for nurses to realize that *sleep deprivation* can imitate the signs and symptoms of alcohol use. Sixteen hours without sleep = 0.05 BAL; 24 hours = 0.10 BAL (Center for Disease Control and Prevention, 2017). The horizontal nystagmus test may be used as a field test when an officer asks a driver to use his eyes to follow his penlight. Nystagmus (involuntary jerking of the eyes) may occur if the person has a high blood-alcohol level. Other things beside alcohol can cause nystagmus too.

Routine blood work to determine the physical status of a person who uses alcohol usually includes evaluation of liver function and enzyme levels (aspartate transaminase [AST], alanine transaminase [ALT], lactic dehydrogenase [LDH], alkaline phosphatase [ALP], and γ-glutamyl-transpeptidase/serum γ-glutamyl-transferase [Gamma = G; GGTP/SGGT]). Elevated enzyme levels indicate liver damage. GGTP/SGGT is elevated in about 75% of people with alcohol use disorder. Specific dietary deficiencies usually exist, including malnutrition, as described below. RBC and blood sugar levels are typically low (anemia and *hypoglycemia*). Lipid and uric acid levels are often increased (*hyperlipidemia* and *hyperuricemia*).

Specific Disorders Caused by Alcohol Misuse

Dietary Deficiencies

Alcohol disrupts nutrient absorption in the proximal small intestine, causing dietary deficiencies. Most common are deficiencies in vitamin B_1 (thiamine) and vitamin B_9 (folic acid, folate). Routine administration of these, in addition to iron and a multivitamin, is usually part of the detoxification treatment protocol.

Sequelae of Thiamine Deficiency

Thiamine (vitamin B_1, thiovitamin, "sulfur-containing" vitamin) is vital in the breakdown of sugars. Untreated thiamine deficiency causes a severe neurological disorder called **Wernicke–Korsakoff syndrome** (*WKS*). Many untreated persons with chronic alcohol overuse exhibit symptoms of WKS, including dementia, *diplopia* (double vision), ataxia, *somnolence* (extreme sleepiness), stupor, and *horizontal nystagmus* (rapid eyeball movement from side to side). Ocular symptoms are treatable, but ataxia and dementia are often irreversible. The mortality rate in the acute phase of WKS is as high as 15%. Prophylactic administration of oral thiamine can prevent WKS if started early enough.

Cirrhosis of the Liver and Hepatitis

Chronic liver **cirrhosis** (hepatic cirrhosis), leading to liver failure, is commonly associated with chronic alcohol use disorder (*Laennec cirrhosis*). The person may also have *acute alcoholic hepatitis,* with fever and dehydration. These disorders are sometimes referred to as *alcohol-related liver disease* (**ARLD**). Because the liver has many vital functions, prompt treatment is particularly important (see Chapter 88).

Other Disorders

Other disorders directly related to alcohol misuse are esophageal varices and bleeding; cancer of the mouth and esophagus; gastritis, gastric ulcers, and other GI disturbances; also kidney disorders, and heart disorders, including coronary artery disease. Sexual impotence is common. Newborns of clients who misuse alcohol are often burdened with fetal alcohol syndrome (**FAS**) (see Chapter 69).

> **Key Concept**
>
> A person who has built up alcohol tolerance is likely to be cross-tolerant to other CNS depressants, such as benzodiazepines, commonly used to treat mental illnesses. Analgesics, such as morphine, given for pain, will also have less potent or desired effects.

Treatment

Treatment of alcohol use disorders is complex. After the person completes detoxification and general medical conditions are treated, ongoing follow-up begins. The client and family are referred to an ongoing support program. In addition to vitamin replacement and other nutritional and electrolyte replacement therapies, specific medications are available to assist clients with severe dependence to maintain sobriety. (See In Practice: Important Medications 95-1 and later discussion of *aversion therapy*).

> **NCLEX Alert**
>
> Healthcare professionals must be alert for signs of withdrawal, such as from alcohol or other substances. NCLEX options may relate to providing safe, emergency care in various life-threatening situations or basic nursing care in an acute care, rehabilitation, or a home-based setting.

Stages of Withdrawal

Many factors determine the severity of alcohol withdrawal (ETOH W/D), including the individual's physical makeup, how much the individual drinks and how often, what other drugs the person combines with alcohol, history of previous severe withdrawal symptoms, and other underlying disorders, such as liver damage or diabetes mellitus. *Uncomplicated withdrawal* is usually completed within 3 to 7 days.

Unlike withdrawal from most other drugs, alcohol withdrawal progresses through three distinct stages *if medical management is ineffective*. The goal of alcohol detoxification is to keep the client as comfortable and safe as possible and prevent progression into the second and third stages of withdrawal, which are *life-threatening*. Following are the stages of *unmanaged alcohol withdrawal:*

1. *Autonomic hyperactivity:* Symptoms include elevated vital signs (temperature over 37.7 °C [100 °F], pulse over 100 BPM, respirations over 20-22/min, and BP over about 160/95 mm Hg). Other symptoms include nervousness, restlessness, and psychomotor agitation. This stage includes anxiety, sleep disturbances (including insomnia and vivid nightmares), irritability, diaphoresis, flushed face, anorexia, and nausea (with copious vomiting and later "dry heaves"). A significant sign is the presence of tremors ("shakes"). *Subjective,* internal tremors occur first. The client can describe these tremors, but they are not observable to others. Hand tremors are the first objective sign observed. (*Stage 1 usually occurs within 8-12 after the person's last drink.*)
2. *Neuronal excitation:* Symptoms include severe tremors (internal and external), panic, insomnia, and increased agitation. The person may experience transient hallucinations of frightening events (e.g., drowning while drunk) or frightening auditory hallucinations. The person may become paranoid, depressed, and is at extremely high risk for suicide. (*Stage 2 usually occurs within 24-36 hr after the last drink, without treatment.*)
3. *Sensory-perceptual disturbances:* Symptoms include vivid visual hallucinations (e.g., "pink elephants," flashing lights), generalized tonic–clonic seizures, and severe agitation and panic, leading to profound confusion and coma. Death may occur during a seizure or as a result of aspiration or exhaustion. This stage is a *life-threatening and medical emergency.* Untreated, the mortality rate is 25% in this stage. (*Stage 3 usually occurs within 3-4 days after the person's last drink, without successful treatment.*) An indicator of a severe toxic state in stage 3 is the presence of *delirium tremens* (**DTs**). Symptoms include delusions and vivid and terrifying auditory and tactile hallucinations called **alcohol hallucinosis** (e.g., "bugs crawling on the skin"), which may last a few days to several weeks. The person often retains consciousness during DTs, so the experience is extremely frightening.

Vomiting may be present; severe diarrhea is common. Vital signs are unusually high; fever may be as high as 37.7 °C to 39.4 °C (100 °F-103 °F) or even higher. Tachycardia is present, with pulse in the range of 130 to 150 bpm. Seizures may be present. Alcohol withdrawal seizures or "rum fits" exist when the person has two to eight tonic–clonic seizures close together; this may progress to *status epilepticus.* Death may occur in this stage because of exhaustion, circulatory collapse (resulting from blood volume depletion), aspiration, or *hyperthermia* (very high fever).

> **Nursing Alert** The nurse working in a healthcare facility's medical-surgical unit or ED must be aware of the possibility of serious withdrawal symptoms in a client who is admitted for an acute infection or severe injury. Whenever a client has a seizure in the ED, they should be questioned as to alcohol use. Evaluate especially all people who have been involved in serious MVAs, fights, or street crime for possible alcohol or drug use. Surgery or newborn delivery may also precipitate DTs in an alcohol-dependent person. *Any other client* could also experience withdrawal. *Avoid stereotypes.* Remember: The client withdrawing from alcohol often may have also misused other drugs. *Be alert for mixed withdrawal signs and symptoms.* Detoxification from alcohol is dangerous and can be life-threatening, *particularly if combined with withdrawal from another substance.*

Family Considerations

Alcohol use disorder involves the entire family. In addition to the client, the people most affected are the spouse or significant other and children or the client's parents, particularly if the client lives with them. The following are characteristics of the family of the client who misused alcohol (many of these characteristics are also present in families of persons with other substance use disorders as well):

- Control—The person who misuses alcohol often attempts to control the rest of the family.
- Rigidity or perfectionism (or both)—Everyone tries too hard to avoid angering the person who misuses substances. Everyone is afraid of the person's sudden rages and mood swings.
- Mistrust of others on the part of the client and family.
- Tension, or overly cheerful and social behavior by the family, that seems forced—Constant coverup, hiding of real feelings, and denial of the inappropriate behavior displayed by the person who misuses alcohol.
- Abuse of family members by the person who misuses alcohol (particularly psychological abuse).
- Overuse of certain defense mechanisms, particularly *projection, rationalization, and denial,* by the family and the client.

Young people raised in the family of a person with a substance use disorder have unique issues including low self-esteem, feelings of failure, and a sense of responsibility to take care of everyone else. Many falsely believe that they somehow caused their loved one's disorder. Adult Children of Alcoholics (*ACOA*) is an organization to assist children now grown who are often clinically depressed or suicidal. Without intervention, they frequently suffer from a substance use disorder themselves later in life.

The Codependent or Enabler

Most persons with alcohol use disorder have one or more *codependents*. Hazelden, a well-known treatment center, defines a codependent, also called an **enabler**, as "one who has let someone else's behavior affect him or her. The codependent is obsessed with controlling or being responsible for (the person who misuses) behavior." The codependent (often the spouse, partner, child, or friend of the person who misuses substances) tries to keep the family together, fends off creditors, maintains a full-time job, drives the intoxicated person home after a party, and helps while the intoxicated person vomits the next morning. The codependent calls in sick for the person and may make excuse, telling others that the person "can't cook tonight because they have headache" or encourage others to not bother the person because they "don't feel well." The codependent, however, is often whom the person who misuses substances blames for the entire problem; in turn, the codependent accepts that blame, thinking, "Maybe if I took better care of myself and looked better, the person wouldn't have this problem."

> **Key Concept**
> Codependents usually do not play as strong a role in the misuse of most other mood-altering chemicals as they do in alcohol use disorder.

Recovery for the Codependent

To break the cycle of dependence, codependents must realize that monitoring another person's behavior and being honest about their own feelings are impossible to reconcile. Preventing crises and shielding the person with an alcohol use disorder will *not solve the problem*. Many persons with alcohol use disorder, as well as those who misuse other substances, become motivated to seek help only when their well-being or "status quo" is threatened. Sometimes, when the children begin to suffer, the codependent will act. To begin recovery, codependents must stop covering up and protecting the person who misuses substances. Codependents must come to understand that this individual (mother, father, brother, or daughter) has a severe disorder but is not a bad person. Codependents must also realize that some people who misuse alcohol will not stop; they then must decide to "let go" in whatever way is comfortable. Often, when codependents get help for themselves and stop enabling, individuals with a substance use disorder no longer continue the cycle of abuse, because no one is available to blame for their problems but themselves. *Enabling allows a life-threatening condition to continue and progress.*

Family Programs

Al-Anon, Al-A-Tot, and Al-A-Teen, sponsored by AA, offer support and encouragement to families of persons with alcohol use disorders. Al-Anon is usually for the client's spouse or significant other. Al-A-Tot and Al-A-Teen are designed for children of these clients (see Chapter 73). Some programs are available for young children, as young as 3 to 4 years. There are also special programs for adult children of alcoholics (ACOA). In making referrals to treatment programs, consideration is given to programs targeting specific ethnic groups, gender-specific groups, as well as those for gay clients, religious and military personnel, and for couples and families. Offering options helps clients better assimilate into and accept the treatment process.

> **SPECIAL CONSIDERATIONS** **Culture and Ethnicity**
>
> **Culture and Treatment of Substance Use Disorders**
> A major goal in caring for all clients is to be knowledgeable and respectful of all cultures and beliefs. In many cultures, substance use disorder is hidden or denied. In other cultures, alcohol and illegal drug consumption is culturally acceptable and expected. Often, the best resource is the client or family. Awareness of cultural practices assists in providing appropriate care. (However, it is important to avoid stereotypes about an entire cultural or ethnic group.)

Medication Management of Alcohol Abstinence

Clients *must be detoxified before beginning any of these medications.*

Disulfiram (Antabuse)

As listed in "Important Medications 95-1," a medication, *disulfiram* (Antabuse), is an alcohol *antagonist*. It is sometimes used as **aversion therapy** or *adverse conditioning* in the person with a chronic alcohol use disorder who is unable to maintain sobriety. It is used only if the client is preoccupied with or craving alcohol and has had multiple failed treatments. The relapse history often includes impulsive, unpremeditated use. Antabuse may also be court ordered. Disulfiram (Antabuse) should never be administered until the client has abstained completely from alcohol for more than 12 hr. The oral loading dose is 500 mg/day PO for 1 to 2 weeks, followed by a daily, uninterrupted maintenance dose of about 125 to 250 mg until a basis for self-control is established. Maintenance therapy may be necessary for months to years. If a person taking disulfiram drinks alcohol, even a very small amount, they become violently ill. (Disulfiram blocks oxidation of ethanol [alcohol], causing buildup of acetaldehyde.) Resulting symptoms include flushing, throbbing headache, dyspnea, hypotension or fluctuating blood pressure, nausea with violent and copious vomiting, tremors, diaphoresis, thirst, anxiety, weakness, dizziness, and confusion. In a severe reaction, respiratory depression, cardiovascular collapse, heart attack, seizures, coma, and death can result. Obviously, *this drug is used only when everything else has failed.* It is implemented only under close medical supervision. The person with ARLD (liver disease) is usually not eligible to use Antabuse, and it is also contraindicated in heart disease, after a stroke, and in diabetes. The client must be motivated to stop drinking and agree to cooperate fully with the program. For more information see In Practice: Nursing Care Guidelines 95-3.

Acamprosate Calcium (Campral)

Acamprosate calcium (Campral) is a drug developed in 2004, used to reduce craving for alcohol after withdrawal. The method of action is not known, but when used with a person who has expressed a desire to quit and has recently completed alcohol withdrawal, acamprosate calcium has sometimes been successful. It is strongly suggested that it be part of a counseling and support program. The usual dose is

666 mg three times daily, often with meals. (It does not cause alcohol aversion, as does Antabuse.) Campral must be used with caution in clients with impaired renal function. Clients with a history of depression should be monitored. All older adults lose some renal function; they should also be monitored. Its adverse side effects include GI symptoms (constipation, nausea), headache, insomnia, weakness, decreased libido, weight loss or gain, depressed mood. This drug is not known to adversely interact with other medications. If the client resumes drinking alcohol, he or she should *continue the medication*, continue therapy and contact the provider.

Naltrexone (Revia, Vivitrol)

Naltrexone (Revia, Vivitrol, Depade) is a blocking agent, originally used to treat opioid misuse but now also used as an adjunct treatment for alcohol misuse after detoxification. It reduces subjective effects of alcohol and other mood-altering substances, reducing the enjoyable effects. Naltrexone is not used in those with hepatitis or liver failure.

Kudzu

Kudzu, a plant-based remedy native to Eastern Asia, has proved effective in reducing the craving for alcohol in some cases.

IN PRACTICE

NURSING CARE GUIDELINES 95-3 — Nursing Considerations in Antabuse Therapy

(Some of these are also considerations with other aversion therapies.)

Client/family teaching is vital in disulfiram (Antabuse) therapy:

- Do not give disulfiram (Antabuse) within 12 hr of alcohol ingestion. A reaction may even occur up to 2 weeks after disulfiram is discontinued.
- Adverse interactions occur with several other drugs, in addition to alcohol.
- The drug is contraindicated during pregnancy and lactation.
- Liver function, complete blood count (CBC), and SMA-12 must be monitored.
- Complete physical and psychological workups are required before beginning the disulfiram program; acceptable physical condition is required.
- All sources of alcohol must be avoided, including cooking sauces, vinegars, cough syrup, some mouthwashes, elixir medications, and possible transdermal sources, such as after-shave lotion, liniments, and rubbing alcohol.
- Adverse side effects may occur, including impotence, decreased libido, fatigue, and an unpleasant taste in the mouth. These usually disappear within a few weeks.
- Any alcohol-disulfiram reaction necessitates immediate medical care. Important are unusual bleeding/bruising, jaundice, chest pain, difficulty breathing, or any alcohol ingestion.
- The client should wear a medical alert tag identifying disulfiram use.

OTHER SUBSTANCE USE DISORDERS

Overuse of substances other than alcohol ranges from common drugs found in the home medicine cabinet to illegal "street" drugs, including methamphetamine, crack, or heroin. Many people also overuse substances such as nicotine and caffeine. It is also common that more than one substance is overused (substance use disorder). Alcohol, in particular, is often combined with other mood-altering chemicals, such as cocaine and/or marijuana. There are many commonalities between persons with alcohol use disorders and those with substance use disorders.

Ethnicity and peer pressure can affect chemical use, sometimes influencing a person's drug of choice. Drugs are widely available but finances and geography may influence what a person is able to obtain. Advertising may also influence a person's drug use, and some substances seem to be more commonly used in the general population than others. For example, heroin use was declining but now seems to be increasing, especially in young adults. This is thought to be because heroin is cheaper and more easily available than prescription opioids. Sometimes, people try drugs like cocaine or methamphetamine for excitement, but, unfortunately, dependence can occur very quickly, and the person may be unable to stop using.

Counseling and psychological treatment for the person with any substance use disorder is the same, as is physical care during detoxification. Check your facility's protocols.

Remember: With use disorders of alcohol or any other substance, detoxification *must precede* counseling and long-term recovery/remission.

Sedatives, Hypnotics, and Anxiolytic Drugs

This large group of drugs includes barbiturates and antianxiety agents. The illegal street use of these drugs is increasing. Most of these drugs are prescription drugs with legitimate medical uses. However, the concern here is their misuse. It is important to destroy any prescribed medications no longer being used to prevent their diversion to the illegal drug market. Frequently misused sedatives, hypnotics, and anxiolytic drugs include the following:

Barbiturates: Secobarbital Na (Seconal, "reds"), and "yellow jackets"

Benzodiazepines: Alprazolam (Xanax), chlordiazepoxide HCl (Librium), diazepam (Valium), and lorazepam (Ativan)

Others: Oxycodone (OxyContin, "oxy," many other names), zolpidem (Ambien), hydroxyzine (Vistaril), and gamma-hydroxybutyrate (GHB, many nicknames). Many combination drugs are also misused. Some of these are hydrocodone with acetaminophen (Vicodin), oxycodone with acetaminophen (Percocet), hydrocodone and ibuprofen (Vicoprofen), and oxycodone with aspirin (Percodan)

Symptoms of Substance Use Disorders

Drugs in these groups are processed by the liver, as is alcohol. They cause symptoms of generalized body depression, coma, or extreme lability. *A particular danger of overdose with these sedatives, hypnotics, and opioids is life-threatening respiratory depression and cardiopulmonary arrest.* (In Chapter 94, Table 94-2 lists many mood-altering drugs used in psychiatry. Many of these drugs also have serious side effects.) All such drugs have a potential for physical and psychological dependence. Effects of many of these drugs are potentiated when combined with alcohol, which can speed the progress of liver damage.

> **Nursing Alert** Many persons with substance use disorders have severely damaged livers that cannot properly process drugs, causing toxic wastes to accumulate. Therefore, combining any drug with alcohol is particularly dangerous. In some cases, combining drugs and alcohol *potentiates* the effects of both. (The combined effect is greater than the sum of the individual drugs.) Potentiation can cause overdose and death.

Withdrawal

In acute ("cold turkey") withdrawal from sedative, hypnotic, or anxiolytic drugs, seizures are possible. Withdrawal must be gradual (although this withdrawal is not as life-threatening as is that from alcohol). Overdose and acute withdrawal are medical emergencies, often requiring hospitalization. A specific antidote for overdose of benzodiazepines is flumazenil (Romazicon—see In Practice: Important Medications 95-1).

GHB (Gamma-Hydroxybutyrate)

A dangerous street drug showing increasing misuse is GHB, also known as "the date-rape drug," "G," and "liquid ecstasy" (it is *not the same* as "ecstasy"). GHB is colorless, odorless, and tasteless. It is available alone and is also contained in several dietary supplements, many of which are marketed on the Internet. (The active ingredient may be listed as *furanone* or *lactone*.) GHB causes a decrease in inhibitions and often *amnesia*. However, death may occur, even with first-time use. Precursors of GHB are marketed on the Internet as "cleaning products" but are used as drugs of misuse. The sale, manufacture, or possession of GHB is illegal (DEA, 2017).

Symptoms of GHB Overuse

Acute toxicity symptoms are highly variable and unpredictable. The person may be extremely labile, alternating abruptly between combativeness and somnolence (the characteristic presentation.) Other signs and symptoms exist, demonstrating lack of control. Symptoms of *overdoses* are considered dangerous because they affect the respiratory system. The person who has overdosed may breathe at such a slow shallow rate that the brain does not get enough oxygen. Other symptoms of overdose include incoherency, profuse sweating, vomiting, and involuntary muscle contractions. Many people who use GHB come to the ED following an MVA or rape. Other trauma, such as a fracture, can occur as a result of sudden loss of muscle control ("head-snap") or collapse ("carpeting-out"). A number of fatalities have been documented, particularly when GHB is combined with alcohol or other depressants.

Withdrawal

Withdrawal symptoms may be similar to the DTs of alcohol withdrawal, but vital signs are often normal or only slightly elevated. Because continued dependence on GHB requires around-the-clock dosing, withdrawal may begin within 2 to 5 hr. Withdrawal symptoms are listed in Table 95-1. Nursing and medical care are supportive. High doses of sedatives, including benzodiazepines and/or anesthetics, may be needed and intubation may be required to support respiration. Recent studies have shown that baclofen (Lioresal) may be used to prevent relapse in clients with GHB dependence after detoxification.

> **Nursing Alert** MVAs, DUIs, and sexual assault are common with GHB use. If GHB use is suspected, collect 100 mL of the first voiding, as well as a blood sample. *Refrigerate both and report immediately.* (GHB is not detected in most routine U-tox screening tests and requires a special test.)

Cannabis Use Disorder

The major active ingredient in cannabis-related drugs is tetrahydrocannabinol (**THC**), sometimes referred to as *cannabis,* although there are more than 100 other cannabinoids in marijuana. Cannabis drugs are classified as mood-altering (*psychoactive*) drugs or hallucinogens. Preparations include bhang, marijuana ("ganja, Mary Jane, **MJ**, bud, pot, weed"), hashish ("hash, hash oil"), and Wax (a specific way of processing marijuana that makes it more potent). Marijuana is usually dried and smoked ("joint, pipe, bong, or blunt") or brewed as tea. Hashish, much more potent than marijuana, is usually smoked or chewed. Marijuana cigarettes dipped in formaldehyde ("wets") often cause permanent brain damage. A very concentrated form of THC, which has been created by using butane, is called Wax and can be up to 99% pure THC. To be used, Wax is vaporized, and it is believed that "one hit of Wax, which is the size of a pinhead, can equal 2 high-grade marijuana joints" (Street Drugs, 2020).

> **Nursing Alert** If a person obtains hashish, believing it is marijuana, a fatal overdose is likely.

Symptoms of Misuse

The most common effect of THC is a dreamy state, characterized by euphoria; the person's perception of space and time may be distorted, although signs and symptoms vary among people. The person with a cannabis use disorder often shows impaired motor coordination, impaired attention, judgment, and other neurocognitive functions, tachycardia, anxiety, hunger, sleep problems, chronic cough, and dry mouth while intoxicated Cannabis can induce psychological and physical dependence. There is no empirical evidence that smoking marijuana directly leads to the use of opiates or other drugs. However, most people who use "harder" drugs smoked marijuana first. In addition, the person who regularly smokes MJ often has the same disorders as those who smoke tobacco. Some studies indicate that use of marijuana has been linked to an increased risk of developing certain disorders, such as depression, schizophrenia, anxiety, and substance use disorder; however, the "…extent it actually causes these conditions is not always easy to determine," (Street Drugs, 2020).

Medical Marijuana (THC)

Several cannabinoids are used medically. These have been tested for purity and freedom from mold, pesticides, and other harmful chemicals, and efforts have been made to reduce the "high" of street THC. In addition to medical THC, other preparations currently used in the United States include cannabidiol (**CBD**), dronabinol (Marinol), and nabilone (Cesamet), a synthetic cannabinoid. (Sativex is a combination of THC and CBD and is approved in several European countries to treat disorders such as MS.) New forms are in development, and it is believed that medical THC will be used widely in the future. Many states have approved the use of medical THC for disorders such as nausea and vomiting associated with cancer chemotherapy and to treat anorexia in AIDS. In some cases, it is used to treat intractable seizures in children and to reduce pain, spasticity, and inflammation. (THC may exacerbate bipolar illness, schizophrenia, hypertension, and heart disease.)

Withdrawal

Withdrawal symptoms related to THC misuse usually do not appear until about 1 week after use (but may begin within 12 hr). Therefore, these symptoms often are not recognized as being related to the use of THC. Symptoms include cravings, flu-like symptoms, headache, depression, restlessness, irritability, insomnia, changes in appetite—weight loss or gain. Withdrawal is not usually life-threatening.

Opiate Use Disorders

This group includes major derivatives of opium: morphine and codeine, derived from the opium poppy. Semisynthetic/synthetics include heroin—"horse" (including "black tar"), oxycodone (Oxycontin), hydrocodone, and hydromorphone (Dilaudid). Others in this general group are methadone (Dolophine), butorphanol tartrate (Stadol), and pentazocine (Talwin). A number of combination drugs are also considered to be narcotics: Vicodin, Percocet, and Percodan. Except for codeine, all these drugs are highly addictive and rapidly induce tolerance and physical and psychological dependence. In some cases, these drugs are prescribed to treat pain and are later misused. They are also sold as street drugs and sometimes are snorted or injected with a high risk of overdose.

Symptoms of Opiate Use Disorder

The person who misuses opiates has a strong, uncontrollable desire for the drug and builds up a tolerance, requiring increasing doses. Symptoms of opiate intoxication include drowsiness or coma, euphoria or dysphoria, confusion, nausea, constipation, slurred speech, decreased memory and attention span, *bradypnea* (respiratory depression), and depression. Suicide is a great risk. In our country's current opioid epidemic, most states have responded by creating laws that make naloxone (Narcan, Evzio) widely available to emergency medical teams, firefighters, police, and now friends and family of those known to be at-risk for opioid overdose. There are three types available for administration: injection, auto-injector, and prepackaged nasal spray. The last two types are available for the general public. Because of newer state laws, these can often be obtained from a pharmacist without a prescription. Before or right after administering Narcan, 911 must be activated. Narcan works almost immediately by blocking all opioid activity on the receptors; however, Narcan's effects only last about 30 to 90 min. This is why it is imperative that the emergency rescue system be notified, as the person to whom Narcan was administered will now need careful monitoring and support for at least 2 hours to ensure breathing does not slow or stop.

Withdrawal

Opiate withdrawal, although extremely uncomfortable, is less dangerous than barbiturate or alcohol withdrawal. Symptoms and nursing care are listed in Table 95-1. A nonopioid medication called lofexidine (Lucemyra) was approved by the FDA in 2018 to reduce withdrawal symptoms (stomach cramps, muscle spasms, runny eyes, trouble sleeping, heart pounding). It is now the only non-narcotic approved for use during detox. Lofexidine is not a treatment for opioid use disorder; it is considered part of the first-line intervention in abrupt withdrawal from opioid use.

> **Nursing Alert** A narcotic or benzodiazepine overdose may occur accidently or intentionally (as a *suicide attempt*). This life-threatening emergency requires immediate medical attention.

Agonist and Drug Replacement Therapy

Opiates, such as heroin, are very addictive; withdrawal is difficult. Outpatient therapy alone is often ineffective. Inpatient therapy accomplishes detoxification, but clients often relapse when released from the controlled environment. Several drugs, some without pharmacologic effects of their own, are used as adjunct therapy in selected cases. They act in differing ways. Some are longer lasting and do not present the desired high (**agonist therapy**); some displace previously administered opioids (*opioid blockers or antagonists*) such as the following.

Naltrexone (Revia)

Although now also used to treat alcohol use disorders, naltrexone was originally developed as a treatment for narcotic use disorders (see In Practice: Important Medications 95-1). The client usually takes this long-acting opioid blocker three times weekly. This medication blocks the brain's specific opiate receptors, so clients do not experience the addicting subjective effects (euphoria, psychological dependence) of opiate use. These clients must be completely detoxified to prevent severe withdrawal symptoms. Persons using short-acting opioids (e.g., heroin) must wait at least 7 days before administration; those using longer-acting drugs, such as methadone, must wait 10 days. This client must continue treatment on a long-term basis. This drug may cause liver damage and other adverse effects. If the client taking naltrexone has pain, opioid analgesics should not be used, except in an emergency. It is preferable to use nonopioid analgesics, such as NSAIDs. If this client has surgery, naltrexone should be discontinued 3 days prior. Postoperatively, opioids must be carefully titrated, and the client closely monitored. Postoperatively, decreased LOC and impaired respiratory function are danger signs. Readdiction is also a strong possibility. Its use has been limited due to poor adherence and tolerability by clients. In 2010, Vivitrol, an injectable, long-acting form of the medication was approved for treating opioid use disorder. Vivitrol is a good option for those who have difficulty taking their medications regularly.

Methadone Therapy

Methadone (Dolophine, Methadose), an opiate-agonist analgesic, is used in heroin use disorder (see In Practice: Important Medications 95-1). It binds with opiate receptors in the CNS. It substitutes for heroin (or IV morphine) because it does not produce heroin's "high" or sedation. It suppresses opiate withdrawal symptoms for 24 to 48 hr. Side effects include sedation, nausea, diaphoresis, hypotension, constipation, and urine retention. Life-threatening side effects include seizures (with large doses) and respiratory depression. Some healthcare providers are reluctant to use methadone because it is addictive; withdrawal can be dangerous (although it is usually milder than withdrawal from other narcotics). After a client reaches a maintenance dose of methadone, they can be discharged from a treatment facility and receive the drug daily as an outpatient. Doses are highly individualized; a dose greater than 120 mg requires state/federal approval. Clients usually are not told their dose. Oral administration (usually liquid) is required by law, and orange juice or another liquid is used to mask the taste and dosage. Tablets and ODT tablets are available but usually must be dispensed daily at a methadone clinic or specialized opioid treatment program. Regular, supervised urine specimens are required and are analyzed for opiates, barbiturates, or other drugs. Evidence of other drug misuse usually results in dismissal from a methadone program. Many methadone programs also require group participation, to assist the client to live comfortably in a drug-free environment. Health and occupational issues may also be included.

Buprenorphine Therapy

Buprenorphine (Belbuca, Subutex) is a partial opioid agonist. This means that it binds to the same receptors as opioids but activates them less strongly without producing a high. Like methadone, it can reduce cravings and withdrawal symptoms. Clients tend to tolerate it well. Research has found it is similarly effective to methadone. The difference is that the FDA approved it to be prescribed by certified physicians, so it does not have to be obtained through a specialized treatment center. It is available as a tablet, as a sublingual film, a once-monthly injection, and as a 6-month subdermal implant. The last two formulations can be administered after the client has stabilized on buprenorphine. There is also a combination drug, buprenorphine/naloxone (Suboxone, Bunavail) that works in the brain to treat dependence on opioids. This medication can only be absorbed and activated in the body if it is administered as a sublingual tablet or film. Some serious adverse effects can occur, so it is vital that clear teaching is done with this medication.

> **Key Concept**
>
> Clients are carefully selected for opiate-blocker programs. Generally, the person must have been opiate dependent for at least a year and must have failed other treatment programs. Many have misused multiple drugs and have coexisting mental health disorders and medical problems.

Stimulant Use Disorders

The CNS (cerebral) stimulants include amphetamines and cocaine-related drugs. These drugs are taken orally, snorted, or injected and induce tolerance and psychological dependence. Caffeine is considered a milder cerebral stimulant.

Amphetamines

Amphetamines are mood elevators and appetite depressants, and they combat fatigue. Caffeine potentiates the action of amphetamines. A number of drugs in this class (or related drugs) are used medically. These include methylphenidate (Ritalin), amphetamine/dextroamphetamine (Adderall), and dextroamphetamine (Dexedrine, Dextrostat), which may be prescribed for narcolepsy or for children with ADHD. Any of these drugs may be misused. Many of the drugs in this class are now illegal but are sold as street drugs; these include benzphetamine ("Benzedrine," "bennies") and gamma butyric acid (GBA).

Methamphetamine HCl

Although it can be legally prescribed, this amphetamine is commonly misused and is becoming a serious public health problem. Known by street names such as "meth, crank, speed, tweak, and STP," it is usually a white, crystalline powder taken orally, snorted, smoked, or injected. *Crystal meth* ("glass, crystal, ice") is produced from the powder and is typically smoked. (When combined with caffeine, crystal is called "Yerba".) Since crystal is very pure, its effects can last up to 12 hr. Methamphetamine is a powerful, highly addictive CNS stimulant, causing a cascading release of norepinephrine, dopamine, and some serotonin. It often results in rapid dependence, requiring ever-higher doses to obtain a high. This causes intense behavioral, psychiatric, and physical symptoms:

Behavioral symptoms: Euphoria ("rush"), blunted affect, confusion, anger, irritability, and poor judgment.
Psychiatric symptoms: Hypervigilance, paranoia, depression, and delirium; *GI symptoms* are nausea, vomiting, and weight loss. Physically, meth may cause permanent brain damage and heart disorders.
Physical symptoms: Dilated pupils, pulse and blood pressure disturbances, muscle weakness, sexual dysfunction, sleep disorders, tooth destruction ("meth mouth"), and skin lesions (caused by impurities). The client may have the sensation of insects or snakes crawling on the skin (*formication,* "meth mites").

People who use meth may stay awake for many days; the combination of the drug and sleep-deprivation exacerbates the drug's negative effects. Prolonged sleeplessness and meth use may result in "**tweaking**." A "tweaker" is a person who uses meth who has not slept for days and is in acute withdrawal. They may appear normal, except for rapid eye movements or quick, jerky body movements. (Post-withdrawal syndrome may last for months.)

> **Nursing Alert** A "tweaker" is *extremely dangerous*. This person may be very paranoid and is susceptible to unprovoked, violent outbursts (see Table 95-1). NEVER use the term "tweaker" when speaking to a client, and always take measures to protect yourself and others when working with this person.

Another danger of meth is that it may be used by people who would not otherwise be abusing drugs. For example, adolescents may use the drug to promote weight loss. Others may use the drug to stay awake. They may be unaware of the drug's potency and may quickly become addicted. Meth labs are also dangerous, in that they emit dangerous fumes and other wastes that can cause CNS and liver damage, cancer, permanent brain damage, immune and respiratory problems, and can cause dangerous explosions.

Withdrawal

Withdrawal from amphetamines usually causes many psychological symptoms, as described in Table 95-1. People in withdrawal from amphetamines are highly unpredictable and can be very dangerous. Those who misuse amphetamine alternate amphetamines with sedatives, such as barbiturates or alcohol. They take sedatives to "even out" the high and avoid the "crash" of stimulant withdrawal or to help them sleep. Then they must take amphetamines to wake up. This necessitates simultaneous withdrawal from several drugs. These alternating "highs" and "lows" are quite complicated and may be life-threatening, if continued. It is important to prevent these clients from injuring themselves or others.

Cocaine and Related Drugs

Cocaine HCl ("coke, snow, flake, blow") is an alkaloid derived from the coca plant or manufactured synthetically; it can be absorbed by all mucous surfaces and stimulates the release of dopamine. (Cocaine combined with heroin is called a "speedball.") Two types of cocaine are available: water-soluble HCl salt, injected or snorted, and the water-insoluble form ("freebase, crack"), which can be smoked and is even more dangerous and addictive. Cocaine is one of the most widely used drugs across all socioeconomic groups in the United States. Since it directly affects the brain, it is very addictive; dependence occurs quickly and *may occur with first use*. Derivatives such as "crank" and "rock" continue to emerge (Street Drugs, 2020.)

> **Nursing Alert** Because cocaine is often snorted, the person may have chronic inflammation of nasal mucous membranes, perforation of the nasal septum, loss of the sense of smell, and nosebleeds. Severe bowel gangrene also may result from reduced blood flow caused by the drug.

The use of cocaine and related drugs is particularly dangerous in pregnancy; it often leads to premature birth, low birth weight, and often, later cognitive impairment of the child (see Chapter 69). Child Protection often is involved if a pregnant client is identified as a person who uses cocaine. After giving birth, the clients usually are not allowed access to their babies until they have detoxified and entered a long-term treatment program. A cocaine habit is expensive because its effects rapidly disappear, requiring constant dosing. A person often must resort to illegal means, such as burglary or prostitution, to support the habit. Many violent crimes are related to cocaine, crack, and crank activity.

Symptoms of Cocaine Use Disorder

Many symptoms of cocaine intoxication or overuse are comparable to those of amphetamines. Cocaine frequently causes delirium and mood and anxiety disorders. Even small amounts of cocaine can cause *permanent brain damage,* causing psychosis. The organic brain syndrome (**OBS**) that results cannot be reversed. Many clients experience vivid hallucinations and grandiose delusions, with paranoia. Seizures, coma, and death may follow. Acute detoxification from many of the stimulants takes 4 to 5 weeks; approximately the fourth week, intense craving occurs that comes with high risk for relapse.

> **Nursing Alert** Cardiac arrest, severe hypertension, and very high fever can result from cocaine overdose, which can be rapidly fatal (and is becoming more common).

Withdrawal

The client in severe cocaine withdrawal usually needs intensive care or 1:1 staffing (see Table 95-1). Exhaustion and depression render this client in great danger of suicide. These clients often relapse after detoxification, even a long time later, because cocaine is so addicting. If the person with a cocaine use disorder also uses heroin, naloxone (Narcan) may be given as prophylaxis.

Catha Edulis (Khat)

Catha edulis (*khat,* pronounced "cot") has been used as a stimulant for centuries in some countries such as parts of Africa, Yemen, Somalia, the Arabian Peninsula, and much of the Middle East; it is prohibited in Saudi Arabia. Because of increased immigration from source countries, its use is increasing in the United States and Canada. Khat is usually chewed, although it also can be brewed as tea, to release cathinone, a stimulant. Street names include qat (Yemen), chat (Ethiopia), jaad (Somalia), and miraa (Kenya), as well as "kat, gat, kus-es-salahin, tohai, tschat, catha, quat, Abyssinian tea, and African tea." Khat is a sympathomimetic; its pharmacological effects are believed generally to parallel those of amphetamines, although khat is not as potent.

Symptoms of Khat Use Disorder

Khat is used for euphoric and stimulant effects. Most of its effects parallel those of other stimulants, although its effects may be less severe. In some documented cases, it has induced psychosis, including hallucinations and/or a feeling of being liberated from space and time. In some cultures, khat is used to stay awake or to aid in fasting. It can also produce depression, sedation, and semi-coma. If used chronically, khat can lead to a form of DTs. Other undesirable effects are intense thirst, constipation, tachycardia, increased respiratory rate (tachypnea), and epigastric pain, as well as decreased cardiovascular function and hypertension.

Withdrawal
Withdrawal from khat produces drowsy (hypnagogic) hallucinations, lethargy, mild depression (similar to withdrawal from cocaine), nightmares, and tremor. Withdrawal is managed in much the same way as that for amphetamines but is not as dangerous.

Hallucinogen Use Disorders

Hallucinogenic drugs are found in plants or produced synthetically. They are not believed to cause actual physical dependence but do produce psychological dependence and mild tolerance. There are several types of hallucinogens, including traditional psychedelics (e.g., lysergic acid diethylamide [**LSD**, "acid"]; phencyclidine hydrochloride [**PCP**]; and mescaline/peyote). Other amphetamine-like drugs (including **DOM**, **MDA/MDMA**, GBA ["ecstasy," XTC] and sometimes Khat), and anticholinergics (e.g., belladonna, methantheline bromide [Banthine], and scopolamine [Hyoscine]) produce similar effects and symptoms.

LSD, Mescaline, and "Mushrooms"
Between LSD, mescaline/peyote ("buttons, cactus"), and psilocybin ("mushrooms"), LSD is the most potent. Tolerance to such drugs is highly variable. Their most characteristic effects are altered perceptions of time and space, auditory hallucinations, and intense visual hallucinations (e.g., vivid colors, light flashes, or geometric shapes). The person may see "trails of light" or "halos" around objects. Objects may appear larger (**macropsia**) or smaller (**micropsia**) than normal. Medications are not usually used in detoxification. Major problems associated with hallucinogens are "flashbacks" (*hallucinogen persisting perception disorder* [**HPPD**]), sometimes years later, causing severe panic attacks. The uses LSD also may injure themself by thinking that they can fly, walk on water, or stop traffic on a busy freeway. Providing a safe, controlled environment is essential. If a person has a "bad trip," speak calmly and quietly; give reassurance. This person can also have permanent brain damage, especially if several drugs are combined.

Phencyclidine Hydrochloride
Phencyclidine hydrochloride (**PCP**, "angel dust") is a hallucinogen that was originally developed as an animal anesthetic. It has been misused for about 40 years because of its low cost and availability. Because it has a simple chemical structure, it is believed that most PCP on the streets is illegally manufactured. Its effects resemble those of hallucinogens and CNS stimulants; the person becomes overwhelmed by environmental stimuli. The drug's most characteristic effect is an alteration in body image, frequently accompanied by uncomfortable feelings of unreality. Some individuals experience intense feelings of loneliness and isolation. It can result in permanent brain damage. The most effective way to assist a person on a "bad trip" caused by PCP or another hallucinogen is to provide a quiet environment with reduced stimuli. Verbal reassurance will not benefit the person on PCP; do not talk at all (an approach that differs from the treatment of withdrawal from other hallucinogens).

> **Nursing Alert** Do not touch any detoxifying person without warning the person first. It is easy for them to misperceive the actions and strike back, resulting in serious injury to staff. Physical restraints are particularly dangerous in these detoxifications.

Inhalant Use Disorder
Volatile substances, CNS depressants, are inhaled ("**huffing**") and are found in thousands of household items, such as air freshener, spray paint, and other vaporized products (known as "boppers, whippets, moon gas, poppers"). The substance can be inhaled from the mouth, sniffed, or snorted. When inhaled from a balloon or plastic bag, the practice is known as "bagging." Inhalants are often the first drug used by younger adolescents and children (formerly called "glue sniffing"). When inhaled, they quickly produce altered states of consciousness and varied degrees of intoxication and euphoria, as well as hearing and vision difficulties (including nystagmus and diplopia [double vision]). They can also cause slurred speech, loss of coordination and other nervous system disorders, lessening of inhibitions, irritability, lethargy, muscle weakness, and dizziness. More serious effects include hallucinations, marked behavioral and personality changes, impaired perception and judgment, memory loss, permanent brain damage, and depression, as well as lung, liver, and kidney damage. If the person is pregnant, fetal development can be seriously impaired. Many of these effects are *irreversible*. Because the inhaled chemicals spread to the brain within minutes, the intoxication lasts a very short time, often resulting in repeated huffing, thus greatly increasing the dangers. Death can occur quickly ("*sudden sniffing death*"), even with first use, due to burns, irregular heart rhythms and heart failure, sudden cardiac arrest, asphyxiation, or aspiration of vomitus. Clues to inhalant use include the odor of chemicals on the breath (the most important clue), as well as spots on the clothing and spots and sores around the mouth.

> **Key Concept**
> New drugs of misuse are constantly becoming available. These include materials with names such as NBome, Kratom, Flakko, and 25D. Those who misuse these substances are also inventing new uses for common materials. For example, blotter paper on the tongue mimics LSD and is marketed as being "safer," although several deaths have occurred.

Steroid Use Disorder

Anabolic-androgenic steroids (AAS) ("Arnolds, juice, stockers") derive synthetically from the male hormone, *testosterone*, and are available (usually illegally) in many forms, including tablets, liquid, and transdermal or injectable forms.

The most frequently misused are testosterone, nandrolone, stanozolol, methandienone, and boldenone. They promote growth of skeletal muscles and increase lean muscle mass in the body. They may be misused by athletes to increase strength and athletic performance and to improve physical appearance. Those who misuse steroids usually take steroids intermittently (*cycling*), often combining several types. Undesired side effects include liver damage and cancer, endocrine and sexual dysfunction, impaired judgment, electrolyte imbalance, acne, edema, headache, fatigue, and insomnia. Withdrawal can be difficult and uncomfortable. Relapse is common.

> **Nursing Alert** The person who misuses steroids can become very irritable, aggressive, and violent and can be very dangerous, especially during withdrawal. The person may also develop psychiatric symptoms, such as mood *lability* (rapid changes) and *paranoia* (fear or panic not based in reality). Death can occur due to endocrine imbalances, MI, endocarditis, or stroke; depression and suicide can result.

Tobacco Use Disorder

Nicotine is contained in cigarettes, cigars, pipe tobaccos; and in snuff, chewing tobaccos, smokeless tobacco, and most e-cigarettes contain nicotine. According to the United States Public Health Services (USPHS), approximately one-fourth of Americans smoke cigarettes; this percentage is higher in persons with mental illness. According to the FDA, more than 800 youth under the age of 18, start using smokeless tobacco, although in 2019 the legal age to buy tobacco was raised to 21 years. Nicotine and other additives in tobacco are considered to be the most addicting drugs available. Nicotine contributes to or causes cancer, particularly of the lungs, lips, mouth, throat, esophagus, or larynx, and clients who smoke also have a higher than normal risk of cancer of the stomach, kidney, pancreas, bladder, or skin. Nicotine also contributes to heart and blood vessel disorders (hypertension, narrowing of blood vessels, tachycardia, increased blood clotting, arteriosclerosis, increased incidence of stroke, and heart attack) and congenital disorders. Coughing, dizziness, and burning of the eyes and respiratory tract are early signs that smoking is causing physical damage. (It is important to note that the use of smokeless tobacco can cause many of the same physical reactions and disorders as smoked tobacco. This includes cancers of the mouth, throat, esophagus, or stomach, as well as other system disorders.) Smoking particularly increases health risks in persons with diabetes, hypertension, or high cholesterol. (More than 480,000 people in the United States die yearly from illnesses caused by smoking [CDC, 2020].) In response to the Surgeon General's Report in 1964, each cigarette pack must carry a warning such as "SURGEON GENERAL'S WARNING: Smoking causes lung cancer, heart disease, emphysema, and may complicate pregnancy."

Nicotine withdrawal causes dysphoria and depression, as well as insomnia, irritability, restlessness, and anxiety. Heart rate decreases (*bradycardia*), and the person often feels hungry and gains weight. The relapse rate is high and "cutting down" usually is not effective. Many smoking cessation materials are available, such as nicotine patches, lozenges (troches), nasal sprays, inhalers, or nicotine gum (see In Practice: Important Medications 95-1). The client may need assistance with calorie control. Hypnosis/acupuncture may be helpful.

> **Key Concept**
> In addition to nicotine, other harmful substances are contained in cigarettes. For example, cigarette smoke contains approximately 1% carbon monoxide, which binds with hemoglobin which reduces the blood's oxygen-carrying capacity, thus reducing tissue oxygenation. A quick test, the "Cotinine" COT rapid test device tests urine and can determine if a person has been smoking. Some states have laws prohibiting smoking in a car containing a child.

E-cigarettes

Recently, electronic cigarettes (e-cigs, personal vaporizers [*PV*], electronic nicotine delivery systems [*ENDS*], or vapor cigarettes) have been developed and are very popular. (Their use is known as "*vaping*.") E-cigarettes are battery-powered vaporizers that simulate the feeling of smoking without burning tobacco. Instead of inhaling smoke, the person inhales an aerosol or vapor. E-cigs are believed to contain about the same amount of nicotine as smokeless tobacco. In addition, those who use e-cigs can vape other substances, such as marijuana. Many people who vape also smoke cigarettes. A single pod contains as much nicotine as a whole pack (20) of regular cigarettes. There is currently less governmental oversight over e-cigarettes, even though recent findings show the health risks of e-cigarettes are very concerning. Some brands of e-cigarettes are shaped like a USB flash drive, making them easy to disguise (CDC, 2020).

Caffeine

Caffeine is found not only in coffee but also in tea, chocolate, some alcoholic beverages, and soft drinks (e.g., colas and "energy" drinks—see Table 95-2). Caffeine is also a component of many OTC and prescription analgesic preparations such as Anacin, Excedrin Extra-Strength, and Fiorinal. Ergotamine and caffeine are combined in Cafergot, and caffeine is combined with other drugs, for the treatment of migraines and sold OTC as NoDoz and other trade names ("stay awake pills"). Caffeine is available as tablets capsules, lozenges, oral solution, or injection. Caffeine may be used medically as a respiratory stimulant, particularly in an overdose of a CNS depressant, and to treat newborn apnea. Caffeine acts directly on blood vessels, causing them to constrict, thus triggering the *fight or flight response*. It is effective as a mild stimulant and diuretic. Evidence shows that 200 to 300 mg will partially offset fatigue, may enhance a person's capacity to function, and increase attention span. Symptoms of overuse include restlessness, nervousness, agitation, insomnia, flushed face, and GI discomfort. Caffeine does not reverse alcohol's intoxicating or depressant effects and may actually add to depression. (A person may temporarily become more alert, but the overall effect is that of general physical and mental depression.)

Caffeine is not without dangerous side effects. At levels of 500 mg or higher, heart rate increases and may become

TABLE 95-2 Caffeine Levels of Common Substances[a]

SUBSTANCE	CAFFEINE LEVELS
Beverages (per 12 oz, unless otherwise stated)	
Pepsi Cola	37.5 mg
Coca-Cola Classic	34 mg
Red Bull (8.2 oz)	80 mg
Mountain Dew	55 mg
5-hour Energy (1.9 oz.)	208 mg
Brewed coffee and drip (8 oz)	80-175 mg
Starbucks Instant coffee (8 oz)	135 mg
Decaffeinated coffee (8 oz)	2-10 mg
Regular tea (8 oz)	40-60 mg
Pepsi One	55.5 mg
Diet Pepsi	36 mg
Caffeine-free Pepsi and Coke	0 mg
Diet Rite, 7-Up, Minute Maid Orange, A&W Root Beer, Fresca, etc.	0 mg
Medications	
NoDozand Vivarin, Ultra Pep Back (maximum strength) (Injectable caffeine also available for medical use)	200-mg tablets
Regular Anacin	32 mg
Excedrin (Extra Strength, Migraine)	65 mg
Excedrin PM	0 mg

12 oz = 355 mL.
[a]Some soda manufacturers refused to divulge the amounts of caffeine in their products.
U.S. Food & Drug Administration. (2018b). Center for Science in the Public Interest (https://cspinet.org/eating-healthy/ingredients-of-concern/caffeine-chart).

irregular. In a person with limited tolerance, even a small amount of caffeine makes falling asleep difficult and interferes with normal sleep patterns. Aggravation of cystic breast disease is also related to caffeine use.

> **Key Concept**
>
> Physical dependence on caffeine is possible. Withdrawal symptoms include tiredness, sleep disorders, severe headache, anxiety, and irritability. Cardiac arrhythmias are possible. These symptoms are not usually life-threatening.

Over-the-Counter Drugs and Herbals

Over-the-counter (OTC) drugs are those available without a prescription. Many medications, dietary supplements, and herbal preparations can be purchased OTC at local stores or on the Internet. In some cases, self-medication is dangerous, especially if used to excess. Some supplements adversely interact with prescribed medications (see Chapters 56 and 62) and can also cause or aggravate medical conditions. Herbal supplements can inhibit blood clotting, increase hypertension, adversely affect diabetes, or cause kidney/liver damage. Many of these products also have adverse effects when combined with certain prescribed drugs (see Chapter 62). Nurses have many opportunities to teach clients about dangers related to self-medication.

> **Key Concept**
>
> Any substance has the potential for misuse, including mouthwash (especially those containing alcohol) and caustic substances (e.g., rubbing alcohol and cleaning solutions). Various nontobacco items can be smoked. Anything in excess can be harmful. Some practices may cause serious health problems and death. The misuse of anything, chemicals and drugs, can also include sex, gambling, overeating, and constant overuse of exercise.

SPECIAL POPULATIONS

Pregnant Clients

Drug, alcohol, or nicotine use greatly complicates pregnancy, labor, and delivery, with profound effects on both the client and fetus. Babies born to clients who overuse drugs or alcohol are often of low birth weight with many related problems. Preterm labor is common. Heroin withdrawal symptoms in a newborn may occur within hours after delivery; most affected babies demonstrate symptoms within 24 hr. The number of cocaine- and crack-dependent babies continues to increase. Many babies born to clients with chemical use disorders have permanent physical and/or mental disorders, including birth defects. Long-term adverse effects on the child as in fetal alcohol syndrome (FAS) are particularly evident when the pregnant client misuses alcohol during pregnancy. In addition, many of the clients lack parenting skills because of their drug or alcohol use. Chapters 68 and 69 describe some disorders in newborns related to maternal drug use. Sometimes, children born to clients with substance use disorders are cared for in foster homes until the client can properly care for them.

Adolescents

Substance use disorders present a serious problem among adolescents and school-age children. Peer pressure and low self-esteem contribute to chemical use. Cigarette smoking and alcohol use are also on the increase among adolescents (see Chapter 73).

Older Adults

Many older adults take large amounts of prescribed and OTC medications. The senior client may be confused and accidently take a double dose of medications or may intentionally take extra sleeping pills or tranquilizers to counteract loneliness, depression, worries about health problems or financial status,

Box 95-1 Signs of Substance Use Disorder in a Nurse

THIS NURSE
- Consistently signs out more controlled drugs than other staff.
- Consistently wants to be the medication nurse.
- Opens medication cabinet only when alone.
- Frequently breaks, drops, or spills drugs and must dispose of ("waste") them; "forgets" to have a witness observe wasting of medications.
- Makes medication errors.
- Spends a great deal of time in the bathroom.
- Always wears long sleeves.
- Spends much time on the unit when not on duty; "hangs around."
- Volunteers for extra night shifts.
- Has clients who report less relief gained by medications than do these clients when they have other nurses.
- Consistently has medication count discrepancies; often has difficulty with medication dispensing machine; has frequent "overrides" to obtain medications.
- Does not "scan" medications, as per protocol.
- Requests to be assigned to clients who are receiving narcotics.
- "Forgets" to dispose of single-dose medication packages properly.
- Puts unopened medication packages and vials into their pocket.
- Exhibits behavior that might indicate substance use, illogic or unreadable charting, consiste arriving late to work, extreme mood swings, defensiveness, frequent absences (especially Monday or Friday), overuse of sick leave.
- Sometimes appears to be under the influence of alcohol/drugs at work.

or feelings of loss and hopelessness. Alcohol use disorder is fairly common among older adults and is a rapidly growing national health problem. Alcohol is particularly dangerous when combined with sleeping pills or tranquilizers. Because many older adults live alone, problem use may not be recognized until it has become very serious. Suicide attempts with medications and/or alcohol may occur. Many older adults overuse medications such as cathartics and antacids. In addition, it is not unusual for older people to change their own medication dosages without consulting a healthcare practitioner. Remember that older people often have a *paradoxical reaction* or opposite reaction to drugs or alcohol. For example, they may become very agitated, confused, or assaultive when given a benzodiazepine instead of becoming sedated. Always remember that an accurate drug history is an important part of data collection in nursing (see Chapter 92).

Nurses

Drugs are readily available in healthcare facilities; nurses are at high risk for substance use disorders (Box 95-1). This is a serious problem. Research indicates that nurses are often more likely to overuse drugs than the general population, partially because of stress and overwork. Nurses are bound by law, the nursing code of ethics, and the pledge taken on entering nursing, to report any staff person suspected of abusing drugs or alcohol. Reporting is necessary to assist others to get help and to protect clients with whom the nurses might come in contact. The safe care of all clients rests in each nurse's hands. *Not reporting can be prosecuted as a crime.*

Nursing Alert The nurse who is using controlled substances not prescribed for them usually prefers to open the medication cabinet alone so that others do not see what medications and amounts are being retrieved.

Key Concept
Remember: Substance use disorders can occur despite knowledge. Some states have special programs to assist nurses who are using drugs or alcohol. One such program is the Tennessee Peer Assistance Program (TAP), funded by a portion of nurse licensure fees. This program offers a resource for nurses who request help without action being taken by the licensing agency and without jeopardizing the nurse's license. If you have a concern about yourself or a peer, check with your local licensing agency.

STUDENT SYNTHESIS

KEY POINTS

- Substance use disorders are serious public health problems, costing millions of dollars and taking many lives yearly.
- Major precipitating factors related to overuse of chemicals include stress and low self-esteem.
- The person with a dual disorder, such as mental illness and a substance use disorder, may experience more difficulty in achieving a successful recovery.
- Management of substance use disorders involves recognition, intervention, treatment, and ongoing recovery.
- Clients admitted to any healthcare facility may be overusing substances. Watch for withdrawal symptoms in all clients. Do not assume that any client is exempt from the possibility of a substance use disorder.
- Care of a client during detoxification requires excellent observation and nursing skills.
- Detoxification differs, depending on the misused drug and other physical and emotional factors.
- Certain blocker or agonist medications may be used as adjunct treatment for long-term management of chronic, intractable substance use disorders, including smoking.
- Most clients require long-term follow-up and aftercare following detoxification and intensive treatment.

- The codependent or enabler can be a key figure in alcohol use disorder.
- Substance use disorders are particularly serious in selected groups, including pregnant women, adolescents, and older adults.
- Nurses are more likely than the general population to overuse drugs and other substances.

CRITICAL THINKING EXERCISES

1. M., 15 years of age, is 6 months pregnant. She states that she does not know "for sure" who the father is. She comes to your clinic for her first prenatal visit. She says that she never uses condoms and has had two previous abortions. She acknowledges that she drinks alcohol ("only a few beers a day") and "smokes weed once in a while." Her weight is well below that expected for her height. She has a constant, hacking, and productive cough. She smokes two packs of cigarettes and drinks four to five cups of coffee each day. She has recently been living at the Salvation Army shelter in their "special needs" area. She has no contact with her family and does not know what immunizations she had as a child. She wants to have "a healthy baby" and plans to keep her child. She refuses to discuss treatment for substance use. What implications do alcohol, marijuana, caffeine, and tobacco use have for M.'s general health and for that of her fetus? What are the social implications of her age and lifestyle?

   Describe your approach to this client. What nursing measures should you perform? What medical, laboratory, and other examinations or tests would you expect to be ordered? What disorders would you expect to be ruled out? What are the nurse's legal obligations? What services could you offer to assist M. to learn parenting skills? What community resources might be available to assist with housing, medical care, education, financial support, and other needs for M. and her baby in your community? What is your personal reaction to this situation?

2. Mr. O., was admitted to your facility's surgical unit following a major gastric resection. He performed his preoperative preparation at home and reportedly was in good spirits while on the way to the OR. His vital signs on admission were BP 122/82 mm Hg, temperature 37 °C (98.6 °F), heart rate 70, respirations 12, and oxygen saturation 98%. Mr. O. received IV morphine in the Operating Room to prevent immediate pain. Since then, he has received other pain-relieving injections; he consistently asks for them more frequently than they are ordered. He is becoming restless and irritable and says he feels "shaky." He has slept about 3 hr in the past 24 hr, once waking up after a nightmare. You are assigned to care for Mr. O. When you enter his room, he is irritable and demanding. His face is flushed, and he complains of severe pain, although it has been only 2 hr since his last pain medication. He begins crying when talking about the pain. Mr. O.'s vital signs are now BP 152/92, temperature 38 °C (100.4 °F), HR 104, respirations 20, and oxygen saturation 90%. When you took his blood pressure, you noticed his hand was shaking. He complained that the "cuff was too tight." He also says his "insides feel shaky all over" and his "chest hurts." He says he feels nauseated and has a "terrible headache."

   Describe your interpersonal approach to Mr. O. What questions might you ask to gather helpful data? What specific nursing actions do you think should be taken and why? Would you call the primary healthcare provider, notify the team leader, or simply document your observations at the end of the shift? If you call the team leader or provider, what would you report (consider the SBAR format presented in Chapter 96)? What new orders might be written? Describe potential implications of Mr. O.'s condition since surgery. What important points would you expect to be included in the nursing care plan? What is your personal reaction to this situation?

3. Contact your local licensing agency. What programs do they have to assist nurses who are overusing alcohol or drugs? What steps are taken if the nurse does not receive treatment? If a license is suspended or revoked, what is the process for reinstatement?

NCLEX-STYLE REVIEW QUESTIONS

1. A client with alcoholism states to the nurse, "I can't be an alcoholic. I can quit whenever I want." What defense mechanism does the nurse recognize the client is displaying?
   a. Rationalization
   b. Denial
   c. Projection
   d. Recognition

2. When attempting to obtain information regarding a client's alcohol use, what statement will be most effective?
   a. "Do you overuse alcohol?"
   b. "Where do you drink?"
   c. "How much do you drink?"
   d. "Tell me about your alcohol use."

3. The nurse is caring for a group of clients in a behavioral health unit. Which client would be documented as having a dual disorder?
   a. A client with diabetes and hypertension
   b. A client with depression and substance use disorder
   c. A client with schizophrenia and visual impairment
   d. A client with borderline personality disorder and chronic kidney disease

4. The nurse is caring for a client admitted for alcohol detoxification. When assisting with the development of a care plan, what priority goals should be addressed?
   a. Nutrition and hydration
   b. Maintenance of acid–base balance
   c. Comfort and safety
   d. Maintenance of skin integrity

5. A client arrives in the emergency department with reports of an overdose of oxycodone. The healthcare provider has issued an order for an antidote. What antidote would the nurse likely need to prepare for administration?
   a. Buprenorphine (Suboxone)
   b. Lorazepam (Ativan)
   c. Haloperidol (Haldol)
   d. Naloxone (Narcan)

CHAPTER RESOURCES

Enhance your learning with additional resources on thePoint!

Student Resources related to this chapter can be found at **thePoint.lww.com/Rosdahl12e**.

UNIT 15
Nursing in a Variety of Settings

96 Extended Care

Learning Objectives

1. Describe the continuum of healthcare from acute care to independent living.
2. Differentiate among major types of long-term facilities.
3. Describe and discuss the concept and purpose of transitional facilities.
4. List some community resources available to persons living in their own homes.
5. Identify optional services or amenities that may be available at an extended-care facility.
6. State at least three publicly reported quality measures used to evaluate nursing homes and other continuing care facilities.
7. Describe procedures and tools used to improve care transitions (handover) from one level of care to another, from one healthcare facility to another, or to home care.
8. Discuss the concept of hospital readmission and steps taken to avoid this.

Important Terminology

assisted living
congregate housing
handover/handoff
medically complex nursing unit
ombudsperson
payee
subacute care
transitional care

Acronyms

AARP
CCRC
CM
CMS
CNA
COE
CON
ECF
ICF
LOS
LTC
LTCCC
NAHC
P4P
PHR
PPACA
PRQM
QIN
SNF
TOC
UAP
UTF

This chapter describes selected lifestyle and housing options available to clients outside acute care settings. These range from skilled nursing facilities to independent living. Individuals may require different options on this continuum at different times, depending on their particular needs.

A continuum of lifestyle options (the continuing care retirement community—CCRC) is available for clients of all ages, very often seniors. Options include independent living, with or without community-based services, assisted living or home care in one's own home, subacute placement, skilled nursing care, and short- or long-term rehabilitation in a healthcare facility. Sometimes, a single corporation owns/manages several levels of these facilities; residents can move among them easily. It is important to remember that, regardless of the setting, staff must understand disease prevention (e.g., the prevention of respiratory, cardiovascular and infectious/communicable diseases, including the importance of vaccines [including immunization for people of all ages and for healthcare workers, as well as clients]).

SPECIAL CONSIDERATIONS — Lifespan

People are living longer today than in previous generations, presenting unique healthcare challenges. For example, an older person or one with disabilities may have lost their caregiver to death or illness. Consider the 75-year-old adult child who can no longer care for their 98-year-old parent or the 80-year-old parent with a 58-year-old adult child who has profound intellectual impairment. Often, these situations must be addressed by community healthcare and social services systems.

Extended-care facilities and **assisted living** services provide many nursing opportunities for nurses; these opportunities are increasing daily. National groups are addressing nurse staffing, particularly in facilities requiring high-level nursing skills. From the nurse's standpoint, extended-care nursing provides the opportunity to integrate many nursing skills and practice total nursing care. This often allows the nurse to work with clients over a longer period of time, to work more closely with the client's family, and to observe client–family interaction.

1805

> **Nursing Alert** Remember: Basic principles of asepsis, rationales for nursing procedures, Standard Precautions, interpersonal communication, confidentiality, and safety apply in every setting.

This chapter is intended only as an introduction to extended-care options. Nurses working in these areas must determine the specific procedures, rules and regulations, and documentation practices there. Certification in long-term care is available for the LVN/LPN (see Chapter 103).

EXTENDED-CARE OPTIONS

The hospital is rapidly becoming the site dealing almost exclusively with acute injury or illness. Clients with chronic conditions or requiring crisis aftercare are seen elsewhere. A broad continuum of care and assistance is available *after the acute phase* of illness or injury. The term *continuing care retirement community* (**CCRC**) denotes a continuum of living and care situations (Fig. 96-1). Other facilities, *extended-care facilities* (**ECFs**), "extend" or continue care started in the acute care facility. Facilities that are considered ECFs include the following:

- Subacute care or transitional facilities
- Medically complex care facilities
- Short-term rehabilitation units
- Long-term care (**LTC**) facilities or *skilled nursing facilities* (**SNFs**) (e.g., "nursing homes")

The acute care hospital may be the first step in the continuum of care for persons who are ill, injured, or disabled. The hospital stabilizes the person during acute illness, performs surgery, or cares for the client immediately after an injury. The client then enters another facility or accesses community resources while living at home, to continue toward achieving the maximum possible level of functioning. It is important to realize that, as hospital lengths of stay decrease, the in-hospital client is treated primarily for the admitting diagnosis. The other transitional facilities consider *comorbidities* (other factors) as well. Length of stay (**LOS**) often differs between types of facilities and may vary among states, commonwealths, or provinces, depending on local legislation and available services. Even within a particular type of facility, there may be different levels of care. Facilities may also include a locked area specifically designated for clients with dementia or mental illness.

Subacute Care or Transitional Facilities

Subacute care, *transitional care*, or *continual care* facilities provide an "in-between" level of care. (This term may also refer to level of reimbursement.) Although they often provide highly sophisticated care, these facilities are less costly to operate than hospitals. Many free-standing skilled nursing facilities have departments providing subacute care. A person designated as a *subacute client* may require only one procedure classified as *skilled nursing care*, with the remainder of their care being less complex. (A client may be classified as "subacute" for only a specific number of days under Medicare; then, the person's status is reevaluated. Regulations are constantly changing.)

Generally, clients/residents remain in subacute care facilities for 1-4 weeks. It is very beneficial if nurses in these settings have previous experience in an intensive care unit, emergency department, or acute medical–surgical unit. Functions in subacute care include intravenous (IV) therapy, cardiac monitoring, ventilator and/or tracheostomy care, tube feedings, dialysis, colostomy/ileostomy care, and management of severe wounds. These facilities have access to medical laboratories, x-ray facilities, and the capability of filling medication prescriptions quickly. Examples of clients in subacute care facilities include people recovering from extensive surgery, stroke, joint replacement, or hip fracture. When their condition improves, these clients may then be released to an assisted living facility, or to independent living, with or without home care assistance. Others may enter LTC facilities or rehabilitation units from the subacute care facility.

Medically Complex Care Units

A specialized step in the continuum of care is the **medically complex nursing unit**. Here, we see clients requiring more specialized, high-tech care than that provided in traditional skilled nursing facilities, while still not requiring hospitalization or care in subacute units. The medically complex unit is often a section in the SNF; nursing procedures here include IV therapy, specialized wound care, and some daily nursing care.

Short-Term Rehabilitation Units

Facilities may have *short-term rehabilitation units* specially designed to serve residents recovering from accidents, joint surgery, heart attacks, or other acute illnesses. These units usually provide physical, occupational, and speech therapy, as well as other services (see Chapter 97).

Long-Term Care Facilities

There are two major types of LTC facilities in the center of the CCRC continuum. Sometimes called *nursing homes* or *nursing care centers*, these are the *SNF* and the *intermediate care facility* (**ICF**). Both are licensed by the state, commonwealth, or province, and must follow prescribed regulations. Nursing assistants must be trained according to

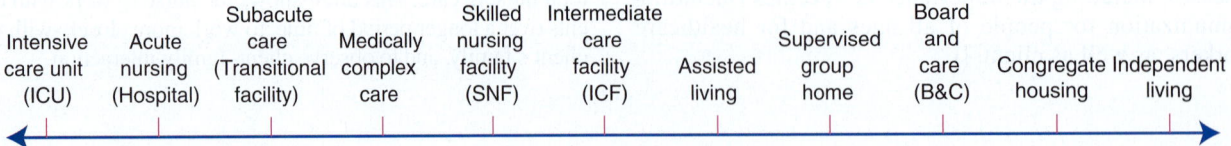

Figure 96-1 Many lifestyle options are available for older adults and those with physical or mental challenges. Options range from total care to total independence.

a prescribed curriculum and, in most states, certified (as a **CNA**—Certified Nursing Assistant). Facilities are expected to provide a clean, safe, and homelike environment. Room, board, and a range of nursing care are provided. Emergency medical care must also be available, often as an on-call service (see Chapter 92).

The Skilled Nursing Facility

The SNF provides 24-hr care and must have a licensed nurse (often an RN) on duty 24 hours a day. The SNF provides rehabilitation services, special diets, and access to pharmacy, x-ray, and laboratory services. Occupational, physical, recreational, and speech therapists are usually on staff or serve as consultants. Other services that may be provided include podiatry, dentistry, optical, social services, music therapy, and the services of counselors and psychologists. In addition, services such as reminiscence therapy or pet therapy may be available. Nursing care in the SNF includes such procedures as IV therapy, enteral feeding, ostomy care, wound care, pain management, diabetes management, bowel and bladder retraining, and physical rehabilitation. Primary care or "medical oversight" is often provided by an advance practice nurse (nurse practitioner) or physician assistant. Healthcare providers or osteopaths are on call and are required to make regular visits to residents, as well as to provide supervision for the medical oversight staff. Facilities often provide for consultations with specialists in internal medicine, endocrinology, urology, dermatology, ophthalmology, and orthopedics.

Various situations may have brought residents to the SNF. Some plan to live there indefinitely; others come to recuperate following injury, surgery, or severe debilitating illness, but plan to return to independent living. (A stay in an ICF may occur between the SNF and the client's home.)

The Intermediate Care Facility

The ICF provides fewer services and less extensive care than the SNF. ICFs provide room, board, and some nursing care. Generally, a licensed nurse is not required to be on duty 24 hr a day, although a nurse is usually required to be on call. LVN/LPNs often work with the more stable residents in the ICF or SNF.

Components of LTC Facilities

Meal Programs

Meal programs in LTC facilities vary. Often, residents can select a meal program. Choices may include three full meals a day, with snacks; a certain number of meals per week; or one full meal each day. Another type of program issues a "meal ticket" with a specific dollar amount; the ticket is used as a debit card.

> **Nursing Alert** Elective meal programs can cause problems in that the resident may feel that they cannot afford the full meal program or may skip meals with the "punch card" system. The case manager must oversee the person's dietary intake, to make sure the resident is receiving sufficient nutrition.

Activities and Services

The best facilities have many activities and services available, including physical, occupational, and recreational therapy (Fig. 96-2A). Support groups, libraries, van transportation for shopping or recreation, and resident councils are common. Many facilities also have lounges, fireplaces, and TV/video rooms for residents and their families. Gardening in raised garden beds is popular, as are aviaries and aquariums. Some facilities have a resident dog or cat, to provide comfort and a sense of responsibility to the residents. Special services, such as a snack bar, gift shop, small convenience store, bank, ATM, beauty/barber shop, therapeutic massage, or exercise room, as well as a supervised swimming pool, may be provided. Most facilities provide access to high-speed Internet service and/or a staffed computer room.

A planned recreation program is a *requirement* in LTC facilities. The program's complexity is often based on the functional level of the residents. Common recreational activities include crafts, scrapbooking, quilting, book clubs, cards and other games, and supervised outings. Sports activities such as golf, fishing, or boating may be available. Some facilities have carnivals, with games and food for residents, their families, and the community. Residents may enjoy displays of antique cars or model trains, fashion shows, musical programs, or plays. The residents may form a dance band, orchestra, or choir to perform for fellow residents and guests. Guest rooms are often available for a small fee, so the residents' families can visit overnight. Often, family can also share a meal in the dining room at a reasonable price. Some LTC facilities have a day care center for employees' and community children; residents often enjoy interacting with children and may assist in the center. In some facilities, particularly those sponsored by a religious organization, a chaplain and formal chapel may be available for regular services, counseling, and individual prayer (Fig. 96-2B). Time and space for religious observances should be provided for each resident in any facility.

Often, a swimming pool, whirlpool, and/or sauna is available. Therapeutic swimming programs play a part in rehabilitation, by providing exercises that are less painful to perform. Sometimes, a person who is otherwise unable to walk is able to "walk" in the pool, providing exercise and entertainment, as well as therapy. Aquatic exercise helps prevent disabilities associated with inactivity and builds self-esteem. Many facilities have a client lift that can lower the resident safely into the water (as do some hotels). A qualified lifeguard must be in attendance at all times.

A wellness clinic in an LTC facility is a plus. In some cases, specialists are available on certain days. Some facilities have a full healthcare center on site, with a complete medical office and pharmacy, staffed with healthcare providers, advance practice nurses, podiatrists, dentists, mental health professionals, pharmacists, and other healthcare professionals. Residents can receive their primary healthcare here. In some cases, these clinics are designated as *community health centers* and serve the wider community as well (see Chapter 99).

Skin and Wound Care

All healthcare facilities are charged with providing careful and appropriate skin care to clients/residents. The Centers for Medicare/Medicaid Services (**CMS**) continues to stress the importance of pressure wound prevention, as well as meticulous skin and wound care. In most cases, a facility will not be reimbursed for the treatment of pressure wounds originating in the facility. Remember to assess for pressure

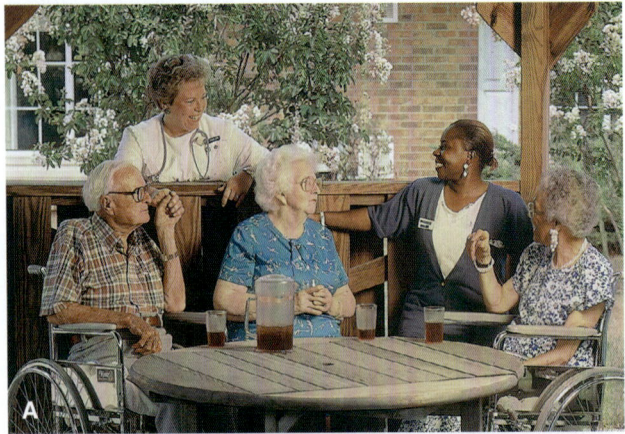

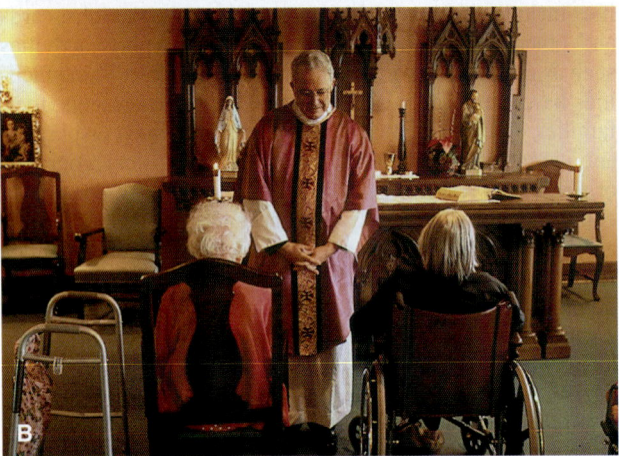

Figure 96-2 A good long-term care facility offers many programs for its residents. Opportunities are provided for (A) walks out of doors and other outings and (B) expression of one's religious faith.

wounds, irritated skin areas, or any disruption in skin integrity when a client/resident is admitted to any facility, and regularly thereafter. Skin care is so important that a separate chapter (Chapter 58) addresses that topic.

The Ombudsperson

Federal law requires each state to have an LTC **ombudsperson** (*client advocate*) to provide assistance and information to residents and families. Most clients in healthcare facilities are designated as *vulnerable adults* and are protected by law from abuse or neglect. The ombudsperson is responsible for protecting their rights. Complaints are first referred to the facility's administration. If these complaints cannot be resolved at the local level, the state ombudsperson is consulted.

Payment for Long-Term Care

Private insurance and other third-party payors, such as Medicare, may cover all or part of the cost of LTC facilities. However, Medicare was designed to pay for acute illnesses or injuries, rather than chronic conditions (see Chapter 98). Medicaid was designed for financially needy people, but coverage is not consistent among the states. New laws attempt to ensure that all people have insurance coverage, but this is not always adequate. Therefore, some people are unable to obtain or pay for LTC. In many cases, clients must exhaust their private insurance and nearly all financial resources before government funds can be applied. Many people are purchasing individual LTC insurance for this reason. The American Association of Retired Persons (**AARP**), Alzheimer's Association, and National Association for Home Care (**NAHC**) have established the Long Term Care Community Coalition (**LTCCC**), which is reviewing LTC financing and the devastating financial burdens placed on individuals and their families. Medicare and Medicaid are often unable to cover all the costs. The LTCCC, as well as other agencies and the federal government, work to help ensure that Americans will have access to the healthcare they need. The goal of the LTCCC is to "help maximize personal independence, self-determination, dignity, and fulfillment."

A Medicare program, "Pay for Performance" (**P4P**), bases a facility's reimbursement on quality of care provided. The facility's performance is evaluated on preestablished quality measures. Four of these *publicly reported quality measures* (**PRQM**) include the *percentage of residents* with

- Moderate to severe pain. (Goal: through appropriate care measures and/or medication administration, the person will not experience "break-through pain"; their pain will be managed.)
- Pressure wounds. (Goal: care provided should aid in healing of wounds existing on admission and should prevent new pressure areas from developing.)
- Physical restraints in place. (Goal: facilities are encouraged to work toward a restraint-free environment.)
- Increasing depression or anxiety. (Goal: counseling and medications should be provided, to help alleviate mental health concerns.)

Preventing Readmission

Great emphasis is currently being placed on *prevention of facility readmission* (within 30 days of discharge). The CMS is placing increased emphasis on reported quality measures, along with the importance of collaborative goals for improvement for hospital, nursing home, and home care settings. The "handoff" or "handover" procedure when a client is transferred within the system is very important and is discussed later in this chapter. Box 96-1 includes information about Medicare Part D and the Patient Protection and Affordable Care Act, designed to help Americans handle the rising costs of medications and healthcare.

> **Key Concept**
>
> Information about Medicare services is available at www.Medicare.gov. This Website provides a "compare" link for evaluation of nursing homes and other LTC facilities, basic Medicare benefits, including Part D, and supplemental insurance plans for clients on Medicare. Citizens can search for the services that would best meet their needs.

The Quality Innovation Network

Each state, U.S. territory, and the District of Columbia must have a quality improvement network (**QIN**) (formerly called quality improvement organization [QIO]), contracted with CMS, to provide support and oversight to LTC facilities. The goal is to improve care, particularly that provided to Medicare recipients. Although the names of these networks differ, the goals are the same. Examples of QINs are as follows: Superior Health Quality Alliance (IL, MN, WI, MI) and Quality Insights (WV, DE, PA, and NJ). Facilities are

> **Box 96-1 Medicare**
>
> Medicare Part D is designed to lower prescription costs for participants. The initial goal was to improve clients' adherence to medication regimens, thus improving their health and reducing healthcare costs. Although this program is part of a federal program, it is implemented and managed by private third-party payors, and the specifics vary between states and insurance companies. Options offered are different, and costs to the client vary, depending on the insurer's drug formulary, monthly charge, and co-pay required. Although the program is considered to be voluntary, a person must register for a plan when becoming eligible for Medicare, or he or she may be penalized later. Some seniors have been able to save money with this program, although others have been required to pay during the federally mandated time period known as the "gap" or "doughnut hole." All insurance programs are currently undergoing evaluation and revision.
>
> The current Healthcare Act, the **PPACA** (*Patient Protection and Affordable Care Act*), also called the Affordable Care Act, was established to protect consumers and is still in a state of flux. (Resources include Websites for Medicare, Centers for Medicare and Medicaid Services [www.CMS.gov], state and local health departments, local Offices on Aging [OOA], healthcare facility outreach programs, insurance companies, and organizations such as American Association of Retired Persons [AARP] and Families USA.)

rated based on quality of care and client reporting. STAR ratings are given, so the public can understand. Functions of QINs include the following:

- Providing educational materials and resources to facilities for staff development
- Guidance for quality improvement for facility managers and staff (to improve care)
- Monitoring techniques and intervention strategies, to improve care
- Recommendations for training and/or certification of nonlicensed personnel

The Case Manager or Care Manager

Each client in the LTC system should have a *case manager* or *care manager* **(CM)** who oversees the client's case, regardless of the length of care or whether the client is cared for in a facility or the community. (In a short-term stay, the head nurse or nursing director often serves as case manager.) The CM is the local advocate for the client and must ensure that the client is receiving appropriate care. The CM often evaluates the client's money management skills, and the CM or another person may be designated as the client's **payee**, receiving the client's monthly check and disbursing funds appropriately. (Family or friends serving as payees require oversight, to avoid dishonesty.)

Specialized Communities/Population Health

Some corporations are developing communities for specific groups of clients (e.g., young clients, or persons with specific disorders, such as multiple sclerosis, head injury, Huntington disease, Parkinson disease, clients on permanent ventilators, or particular cultural ethnic, religious, or fraternal groups).

The Centers of Excellence **(COE)** programs have developed centers to accommodate groups with special needs, which include assessment, treatment, and rehabilitation therapy. One such COE program is the Shepherd Program in Atlanta for clients with multiple sclerosis. In addition, *population health* includes persons covered by a particular insurer, such as persons living within the service area of a health system or those with a specific disease or condition, such as diabetes.

Restraint-free policies have caused changes in treatment of clients with memory loss and mental illness. Clients with dementia disorders often live in a special memory care unit that is locked and alarmed, as are the elevators. In many cases, these units are specially designed to provide a safe and secure space for the person to wander and pace without feeling "hemmed in." The client who may accidently leave the unit may wear a special WanderGuard or Ambularm device (Fig. 96-3), which warns staff if the person tries to leave the unit without permission. Another device may be a sensor located under the chair pad or mattress; a buzzer warns staff if a client at risk for falling attempts to get out of bed or a wheelchair (see Fig. 48-22B and C). *The ultimate goal is to provide safety for clients.*

Respite Care and Daycare Programs

Medical daycare programs may be private or government-sponsored nonprofit organizations providing respite care for families. The client spends part of the time in a daycare facility, giving family caregivers time to themselves (a *respite or break*). Respite programs often provide family support groups as well. However, caregivers must be available to care for the client before and after the respite.

Services Provided to the Community by Long-Term Care Facilities

LTC facilities may provide home care or assisted living services to the wider community. Meals, respite care, parish nursing, or hospital visitations are often provided. Some facilities belong to a consortium of healthcare providers, allowing community residents to receive dental, hearing, and vision care; podiatry; pharmacy services; and acute hospital care without being residents of an LTC facility.

Volunteers

Most healthcare facilities, including long-term facilities, have a cadre of volunteers who provide many services. They may run the gift shop, help with craft activities, provide beauty and barber shop services, take residents on outings, or visit with residents who do not have family. They may read to residents or help them write letters. The volunteers often organize fund-raising programs for special activities and may provide special items, such as craft materials, quilts, sweaters, toiletries, or stationery and stamps. Volunteers often give parties on holidays and birthdays and provide entertainment. Some facilities have volunteers who help with daily care of residents, serving as bed-makers or helping to feed residents, allowing more time for nursing staff to provide skilled nursing care.

> **Key Concept**
>
> The goal of all care is to provide the least restrictive living arrangement possible, while providing maximum safety and quality of life. Emphasis is on client-centered care, including the client's family—*family engagement*.

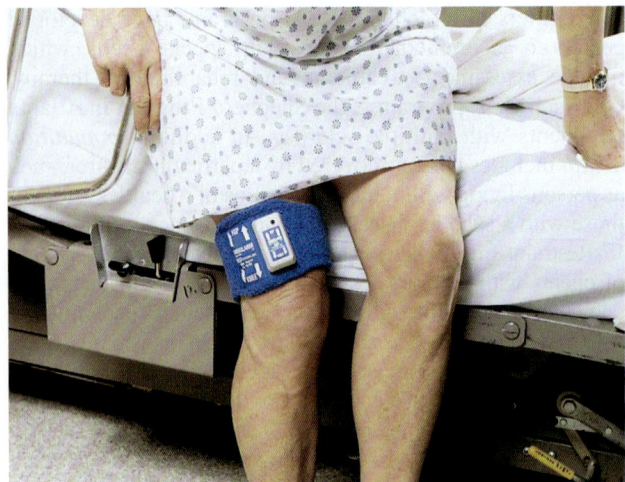

Figure 96-3 To provide safety, this client is wearing an Ambularm device, which will alert the staff if the client tries to leave the immediate safe area. (Photo courtesy of AlertCare, Inc.)

Independent Living Options

Many older adults and people with physical or mental disabilities do not need to be in an ECF but still need help to live independently. (See Fig. 96-1 for the continuum of CCRC living options.)

The Continuing Care Retirement Community

Community programs can help clients remain independent. Many services are available, including subsidized and **congregate housing**, assisted living, home nursing care, and homemaker services. (Chapters 98 and 99 discuss home care and ambulatory nursing; and Chapter 100, hospice care.)

Senior and Other Special Housing Programs

A variety of housing options are available for older adults and individuals with disabilities. A special building (**congregate housing**) may be designated for a specific group. These buildings may contain free-standing apartments and may have only minimal or no supervision. Meals and activities may be provided. In many cases, each unit has a call button for emergency assistance, and in some facilities, each client is checked daily. A person must qualify to live there, and in most cases, the resident pays a sliding scale, *government-subsidized rent,* based on income (sometimes known as "Section 8" housing). A person may live in a *board-and-care home,* which provides room, board, and minimal supervision. *Adult foster care* is also available for selected clients. Many people with mental illnesses and/or physical disabilities live in board-and-care or adult foster care homes.

The next level of housing is the *supervised group home.* In this facility, clients are supervised regarding medications and are often required to participate in a treatment program or to work or volunteer a specific amount of time weekly. Meals and activities are provided (see Chapter 94).

Other types of congregate living facilities, such as senior apartment complexes, provide more services for older clients or for those with disabilities. Facility personnel usually check on each resident at least daily. Each apartment or room has a signal bell, so the resident can call for help in an emergency. *Hospice care, end-of-life care,* or *advanced illness care* may be provided to individuals in congregate living facilities. However, most hospice care is provided in the client's home (see Chapter 100).

Assisted Living

Assisted living is a major area of growth in LTC and is one way to facilitate independent living for seniors and for younger people with mental and physical disabilities. These programs give clients an opportunity to *age in place,* usually in their own homes or apartments. Clients, together with their case managers, can choose necessary services. Available services often include Meals on Wheels, laundry, transportation to appointments or shopping, visiting pet programs, grocery and medication delivery, or assistance with finances or housekeeping. Home care nurses may visit to evaluate clients or perform treatments, such as drawing blood for tests or changing dressings (see Chapter 98). Nurses may set up a daily medication reminder box for clients, to promote medication compliance and help prevent duplicate dosing. Each day's medications are placed into compartments marked for that day and for administration times during the day (see Fig. 92-1). Home care assistants help clients with activities of daily living (ADLs), such as bathing, laundry, and food preparation. They may check the client's food/fluid intake, run errands, or provide companionship. (Some clients require reeducation in basic homemaking skills before they can live independently.)

Some states have formal statewide assisted living facilities. These facilities require a *certificate of need* (**CON**), and each site manager must be certified. Manager certification requires classroom instruction, community clinical experience, and satisfactory performance on a state-administered examination. (This may be controversial because unlicensed staff administer certain medications at many sites.) Visiting nurse associations may monitor *unlicensed assistive personnel* (**UAP**), as well as certified site managers. People who regularly receive services from UAP usually live alone or have inadequate outside support. In other cases, family members may learn to administer medications and provide certain treatments for their loved ones.

> **Key Concept**
>
> Older adults and people with disabilities spend less time in nursing care facilities today. The average stay is expected to continue to drop in the future. A great majority of these people now live independently (with or without outside services).

THE CONCEPT OF TRANSITIONAL CARE

A safe and appropriate transition of care (**TOC**) between agencies and facilities and between departments in a single facility is vital, whether in acute or long-term care. One goal is to prevent unnecessary hospital readmission of clients after discharge from a facility. Often, the hospital readmission of a client results from the lack of appropriate assessment and transmission of information about the client when they are transferred from one facility or service to another (Box 96-2). Communication skills are vital between settings. Causes of hospital readmission include respiratory issues, falls, and inappropriate wound care. Ways to prevent hospital readmission include the following:

- Ongoing education of clients and families about the disease process and care needed
- Increasing the ability of clients/families to self-manage chronic conditions
- Better discharge planning during the stay
- Medication reconciliation
- Better communication between settings and persons providing care
- Increased use of telehealth
- Utilization of electronic medical records between facilities, agencies, and providers' offices
- Better utilization of palliative care and hospice services
- Encouraging primary providers to be truthful with clients/families who have progressive diseases and to offer options other than hospital care.

The concept of **transitional care** refers to the transfer of clients between healthcare practitioners and settings, as their conditions and care need change. Remember that, as a nurse, *you are responsible for the client until the next setting has the needed information to safely assume care* of the client. The goals of TOC include medication and medical condition management and client and family confidence in care being given. Accurate TOC helps meet these goals. Home care is often involved in providing continuing care, particularly to older adults with complex healthcare needs (see Chapter 98).

The term **handover or handoff** implies transfer of information, as well as the professional responsibility to *make sure information is understood by the receiver.* The SBAR process, shown in Box 96-2, presents a method of organizing information in preparation for a handover. Transitional care is so important that a national coalition exists to provide education and coordination among agencies. A Universal Transfer Form **(UTF)** is used in several states to improve the handover/transition process. Each client is also encouraged to maintain a personal health record **(PHR)** to share with providers. This record should contain a list of medications and dosages, including all over-the-counter (OTC) medications, herbal remedies, and dietary supplements, as well as pertinent information about allergies, surgical procedures, past illnesses, and specific treatments.

Box 96-2 Communication Using the SBAR Process

It is important for healthcare personnel to communicate clearly with each other. The SBAR process offers a tool for organizing one's thoughts for concise and accurate communication. SBAR is used when "handing over" a client from one level of care to another or when calling the primary provider for assistance or instructions.

- Have all relevant information available and organized. This includes team discussions and a review of all client documentation. You need the client's full name, medical record number, birth date, date of admission, and primary provider's name and number.
- Other information required includes the client's diagnosis and mental status, current medications and allergies, most recent vital signs (including pulse oximeter readings and blood glucose determinations), pertinent laboratory results, any signs or symptoms, and DNR or DNI status. Communicate such factors as an intravenous (IV) or tube feeding, tracheostomy, catheter, or supplemental oxygen.

THE SBAR PROCESS
- **S**ituation: Who are you and why is contact being made?
- **B**ackground: Pertinent information, as listed above
- **A**ssessment: What is the situation, as reported by nursing staff?
- **R**ecommendations: What should be done for the client? Why is the transfer being made or what instructions are you seeking from the healthcare provider? These recommendations must be clearly communicated to all staff involved.

STUDENT SYNTHESIS

KEY POINTS

- Many lifestyle options are available for people who do not need care in the acute facility.
- Clients may move from one type of lifestyle option to another, as their needs change.
- The least restrictive type of care should be given, to promote the client's independence.
- Most older adults and people with physical and mental challenges live independently.
- Today's LTC facilities offer safe and comfortable living, with a wide variety of amenities.
- Quality improvement organizations exist in each state, territory, and the District of Columbia, to provide support and oversee the care given, particularly to Medicare beneficiaries.
- Specific information must be given when a client is handed over from one type of care to another. SBAR provides a framework for organizing this information. This information transfer helps prevent avoidable hospital readmissions.

CRITICAL THINKING EXERCISES

1. Imagine that your aunt is 79 years old and her memory is failing. Her physical health is generally good, except she is overweight and has type 2 diabetes mellitus. She smokes one to two packs of cigarettes a day and has a chronic cough. Your uncle (her husband) is living with her and is in good health. He stopped smoking more than 20 years ago. Knowing that you are a nurse, your uncle calls you in despair and says, "I can't take care of her anymore!" The couple's only child (your cousin) is widowed and lives 75 miles away. Your cousin has one teenage child at home and one in college.
   a. Which additional information do you need from your uncle in order to help him? Which agencies or people would you suggest he call for advice and information?
   b. Identify community resources that are most likely to be available in your uncle's hometown (or the nearest large city).
   c. Which questions should he ask his family healthcare provider?
   d. If nursing home placement is needed, how can the best one be selected?
   e. Which level of long-term care or community assistance do you think would be recommended for your aunt?
   f. Which role could your cousin play in planning care for their mother?
   g. What are your personal feelings about this situation?

2. Interview a person in an assisted living program and one in a nursing home. Which services do they receive? Compare and contrast the two in terms of the following:
   a. Client self-esteem
   b. Relationships with family
   c. Cost
   d. Services provided and desired
   e. Social interactions with peers
   f. Independence
   g. Role of the nurse

3. Interview a nursing home client and family about their experience of transfer or handover from the hospital to the nursing home. Was the transition smooth? Were there concerns? Which forms or paperwork accompanied the client to the nursing home? How much input did the client/family have? How could the communication between the two facilities have been improved?

NCLEX-STYLE REVIEW QUESTIONS

1. The new LVN/LPN is searching for employment options in the extended-care facility (ECF). Which type of facility would the nurse research? Select all that apply.
   a. Subacute care
   b. Medically complex care facility
   c. Hospital emergency department
   d. Short-term rehabilitation unit
   e. Skilled nursing facility

2. A client is injured in a boating accident sustaining a femur fracture. Which facility would be the first step in the continuum of care?
   a. Transitional facility
   b. Short-term rehabilitation unit
   c. Skilled nursing facility
   d. Acute care facility

3. An older adult client in a healthcare facility develops a large sacral pressure wound. Which outcome does the nurse anticipate will occur from this incident?
   a. The facility will be mandated to close.
   b. Nursing personnel caring for this client will be terminated.
   c. The facility will not be reimbursed for care.
   d. The client will have to pay out-of-pocket expenses.

4. An adult child of a client has a complaint regarding the care their parent has received at an extended-care facility. To whom should the family member first state the complaint?
   a. State ombudsperson
   b. Facility administration
   c. The state's attorney
   d. The client's insurance company

5. An older adult client in assisted living after recovering from an illness is having difficulty remembering what medication to take. Which option would be appropriate for this client to avoid complications?
   a. The client will have to live with a family member.
   b. The client will need to live in a long-term care facility to obtain medications.
   c. Request that the pharmacy put all of the medication in a daily pill reminder.
   d. Have a home health nurse come and set up a daily medication reminder box.

CHAPTER RESOURCES

Enhance your learning with additional resources on thePoint*!*

Student Resources related to this chapter can be found at thePoint.lww.com/Rosdahl12e.

97 Rehabilitation Nursing

Learning Objectives

1. Define rehabilitation and explain its goals.
2. Describe stages of adjustment to a disabling illness or injury; compare to Kubler–Ross stages of dying.
3. Identify key members of the rehabilitation team and their roles.
4. Relate rehabilitation to Maslow hierarchy of needs.
5. Differentiate between functional and instrumental activities of daily living (ADLs).
6. Describe examples of adaptive equipment and home modifications that assist clients to independently perform ADLs.
7. Describe rehabilitation, as it relates to mobility.
8. Discuss the major elements of a continence program.
9. Briefly describe general rehabilitation for people with disabling musculoskeletal, cardiovascular, or neurologic disorders.
10. Give examples of community resources for people with physical and mental disabilities.
11. Define the term *architectural barrier* and identify several in your community.
12. Identify factors interfering with rehabilitation for individuals and communities.

Important Terminology

architectural barriers
comorbidity
exoskeleton
hemiplegia
mainstreaming
neurogenic
orthotics
paraplegia
physiatrist
prosthetics
quadriplegia
rehabilitation

Acronyms

ADA
ALS
FADL
FES
IADL
PM&R
TBI
TENS

In many cases, long-term rehabilitation is needed when a person is physically or mentally disabled, often as a result of injury or debilitating illness. Other clients undergo a short period of rehabilitation, for example, following joint replacement surgery, minor stroke (cerebrovascular accident–CVA), or heart attack (myocardial infarction–MI). Many people, in addition to the client, are involved in rehabilitation, including nurses, therapists, and family members. Many nurses are employed in rehabilitation nursing. Rehabilitation can occur in a healthcare facility, community health center, "rehab" center, or in the client's home.

DEFINITIONS OF REHABILITATION

Many definitions of *rehabilitation* exist. In general, **rehabilitation** is defined as assisting a person to regain former abilities, as much as possible, or to adjust to a disability and live as independently as possible. Rehabilitation emphasizes coping with physical or mental disabilities and learning to adapt one's environment, to facilitate independence and safety.

Another definition states that the goal of rehabilitation is to restore the person to a satisfactory quality of life. Rehabilitation should offer clients optimal happiness and the ability to *use all available assets*. Clients should be assisted to achieve the most independence possible, not just survival or pain relief. Outcomes of rehabilitation are measured in terms of improvement in function resulting from the intervention. Each individual is assisted to become independent and a participating member of society, *as much as is possible*.

It is important to differentiate between treatment for acute illness or injury and long-term rehabilitation. An *acute illness or injury* is treated, and the person often recovers and returns to normal activities, having encountered only a brief interruption or having received a short term of rehabilitation. In *long-term illness or disabling injury,* the person must be assisted over time (long-term rehabilitation) and may never recover fully to the level that was enjoyed before the event. The person requiring long-term rehabilitation often has a number of physical and emotional problems (**comorbidities**). For example, the person who has had a *major stroke* often must overcome paralysis. Rehabilitation of this person often includes challenges such as spasticity and muscle atrophy, maintenance of skin integrity (prevention of skin breakdown), *aphasia* (difficulty in speaking), *dyspraxia* (difficulty in performing coordinated movements), *dysphagia* (difficulty swallowing), vocational concerns, sexuality, incontinence, emotional lability, and prevention of complications, such as pneumonia or contractures.

Key Concept
Most long-term rehabilitation occurs in the community. Only the initial phase of the process occurs in rehabilitation facilities.

REHABILITATION AND MASLOW HIERARCHY OF NEEDS

Rehabilitation is based on early recognition and individualized planning for each client. When Maslow hierarchy of needs is applied to rehabilitation, the person in the acute

Box 97-1 Goals Set Forth by a United Nations Proclamation for the Disabled[a]

1. Help people with disabilities in their physical and psychological adjustment to society.
2. Promote all national and international efforts to provide them with proper assistance, training, care, and guidance to make available opportunities for suitable work and to ensure full integration into society.
3. Encourage study and research projects designed to facilitate practical participation in daily life, such as improving access to public buildings and transportation.
4. Educate and inform the public of the rights of all people to participate in and contribute to various aspects of economic, social, and political life.
5. Promote effective measures for the prevention of disabilities and the rehabilitation of people who are disabled.

World Health Organization (2019).
[a]These are appropriate goals for any rehabilitation program.

stage of illness or injury first requires assistance with basic survival needs, such as maintaining an open airway and an adequate oxygenation level, obtaining food and water, and eliminating wastes. Next, activities of daily living (ADLs) are addressed, such as being able to feed, dress, and bathe oneself; the ability to move independently; and being able to communicate effectively. Later, the person learns to work toward self-actualization and to be independent, and a creative and contributing member of society. (See Chapter 5 for discussion of Maslow hierarchy of needs.)

Rehabilitation presents many challenges and opportunities for members of the healthcare team. An extensive discussion of rehabilitation nursing is beyond the scope of this book, but this introduction emphasizes that the principles and purposes of rehabilitation remain the same, *regardless of the person's specific situation*. Many nursing skills and procedures utilized in rehabilitation have been presented elsewhere in this book and throughout your nursing program. The goal of all rehabilitation nursing is to assist clients to approach normal functioning as much as possible, that is, to minimize the person's limitations and maximize their capabilities. Emphasis should be placed on *quality of life* (Box 97-1).

STAGES OF ADJUSTMENT TO A DISABILITY

During adjustment to a long-term physical or mental disability, a person usually experiences grief reactions similar to those experienced when dealing with any loss, including end-of-life issues (Chapter 14).

- Early reactions may be defense, shock, and denial. ("This can't be happening to me!") The person often is confident of recovery and may also experience fear and anxiety.
- Next, the client often experiences anger and wants to retaliate, asking, "Why me? I'll get even with someone for this!"
- Many people try to bargain with God or make deals. "I will be a better person if I can just recover."
- Eventually, the client with any permanent disability must face reality (and may experience severe depression).
- It is hoped the client will come to accept limitations and actively participate in developing *realistic* long-range goals. Some people have great difficulty in attaining acceptance. Sometimes, psychiatric assistance or counseling is an essential part of rehabilitation.

 SPECIAL CONSIDERATIONS Lifespan

Children and adolescents who have been injured or who have degenerative diseases face additional challenges because they are dealing with disability or disease along with the usual challenges of maturation. Their parents often go through the same stages of grief as the child.

THE REHABILITATION TEAM

Healthcare providers who specialize in rehabilitation are sometimes called **physiatrists** or physical medicine and rehabilitation (**PM&R**) specialists. The rehabilitation team includes the healthcare provider, physiatrist, nurse, advance practice nurse or certified rehabilitation nurse, UAPs, and therapists (physical, occupational, speech, music, recreation, sexual), as well as the vocational counselor, social worker, and psychologist. The client's *case manager* or care manager is becoming an increasingly important member of the team. Team conferences are held regularly during the rehabilitation process so all members can establish common goals. The family and the client should be involved in these team conferences.

Preparation for Rehabilitation

Home Assessment

Clients *and their families* are vital members of the healthcare team. A home assessment helps determine the appropriateness and possibility of home-based rehabilitation. Questions, such as the following, must be answered: Is it possible for the client to live at home safely? Is it necessary to negotiate stairs if the person has movement limitations? Are most areas of the home accessible to the client? Is it possible for the person to shower/bathe/go to the bathroom? Are floors too slippery to be safe? Do adaptations need to be made in the home? Can the client access the outside, get into the car, and move through doors? Are family/caregivers able and willing to provide needed care? Can the client be safely left alone for short periods of time, so the family can shop, work, and run errands? Is the family capable and willing to provide adequate nutrition, medication administration, skin care, and other necessary daily needs?

In many cases, physical adaptations must be made, to prepare the home for client care. Ramps may be needed; railings in hallways, stairs, and bathrooms may need to be installed; and doors may require expansion, to accommodate a wheelchair or walker. An open shower, without a curb, may need to be constructed so the client can use a walker or wheelchair

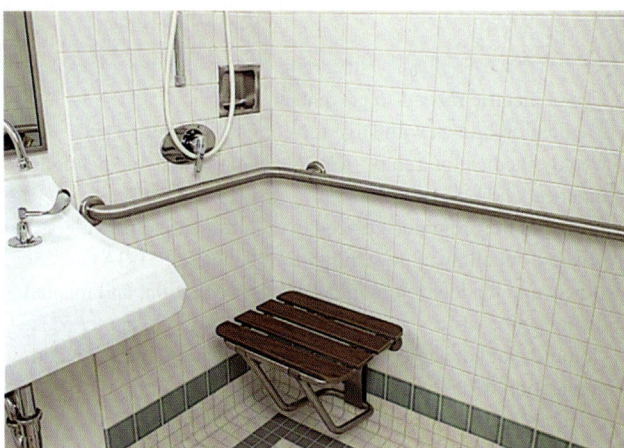

Figure 97-1 Simple adaptations allow a client to return home after an illness or injury or to care for themselves on a long-term basis. This remodeled bathroom includes an open shower, shown with a built-in seat, sturdy handrails, and a handheld shower spray. Lever-type faucets on the sink are easier to operate, and a high faucet allows free movement underneath.

to enter (Fig. 97-1). A handheld shower is easier to use than a wall-mounted shower head. A shower chair or built-in seat or side-opening bathtub may be necessary (Nursing Procedure 50-11). Sinks and countertops may need lowering or open space below them, to accommodate a wheelchair. If the client is required to go upstairs, an elevator or lift may be required. Toilet seats may be raised, to allow the person to sit down and stand up again more easily (Fig. 51-3A) or a bedside commode may be needed. Bed rails provide security and a handhold to assist in turning and getting out of bed (Fig. 51-3B). Box 97-2 identifies many adaptations and available equipment to assist the person with a disability.

Availability of Primary Caregivers

In addition to the physical layout of the home, home assessment includes an evaluation of available caregivers. Taken into consideration are caregivers' availability, skill level, and willingness and commitment to assist in the rehabilitation process. The family or significant other usually becomes the primary caregiver (Chapters 98–100). They must understand the responsibilities and dedication involved and must be willing to make a commitment to providing it. The client's motivation is also an important determining factor in the decision for the client to live at home.

> **Key Concept**
>
> The lack of an appropriate caregiver usually prevents the client with a disability from living independently, particularly during the initial rehabilitation process.

Evaluation of the Disability

Before rehabilitation can begin, the client is evaluated to determine their abilities and needs. This evaluation *should begin during the acute phase* of illness or injury. Common tests performed include *electromyography* (EMG) (to determine electrical activity and potential of muscles) and a *motor nerve conduction* study (at rest, or stimulated [*elicited*]). *Gait analysis* evaluates how well, or if, the person can walk. Vision, hearing, speech, and language production are assessed. Studies such as voiding and continence evaluation, electroencephalogram (EEG) studies, and other tests are done. Psychological and neurologic testing determines the person's motivation, attitudes, and neurologic deficits. A functional evaluation determines the client's ability to perform ADLs. Vocational assessment identifies skills, potential for homemaking or employment, and retraining needs. The team gathers all information and makes a plan for care.

> **Key Concept**
>
> It is important for the nurse to ask the client about the use of complementary therapies, such as acupuncture, herbal therapy, or chiropractic care. These therapies can significantly influence the rehabilitation process.

> **NCLEX Alert**
>
> As in other chapters, it is helpful to consider the normal functioning of a body system, such as the musculoskeletal or sensory system, when considering appropriate nursing actions for clients beginning a rehabilitation program. Assisting clients to adapt to health alterations, whether related to mobility/immobility, personal hygiene, managing other ADLs, or communication, may be involved in choosing appropriate responses to test questions.

NURSING CONSIDERATIONS IN REHABILITATION

Rehabilitation begins with treatment to halt destructive processes and repair functional damage. It continues with preventing further injury and then with restoring normal functions whenever possible. Increasing strength is often a goal of rehabilitation—this is important to regain or maintain independence, allow mobility (walking, crutch walking, wheelchair, scooter), and to reduce the possibility of falls. Because insurance may not cover the cost of a physical therapist, the nurse may be called on to perform or supervise muscle-strengthening exercises. In addition to physical support, rehabilitation nursing provides clients with *emotional support*. The rehabilitation nurse's most important quality is *empathy;* it is important to be sensitive and to offer encouragement and assistance. When working in rehabilitation, nurses assist clients to meet unique, complex, and multi-dimensional needs, to build interventions based on client strengths and resources, and to envision rehabilitation as a logical and essential component in the health process across the lifespan. The scope of rehabilitation nursing extends from primary prevention, through acute and subacute levels, including specific treatments, and beyond tertiary intervention into community and lifelong care.

ACTIVITIES OF DAILY LIVING

It is important to encourage clients to become as independent as possible. Assist clients by providing physical care and positive reinforcement and by strongly encouraging

Box 97-2 Adaptive or Assistive Devices Used in Rehabilitation

Many items have been developed or modified for use by people with disabilities. Some general types of equipment are listed here.

PERSONAL CARE AND ADL ADAPTATIONS

- Long-handled comb or brush—allows person with limited or painful arm mobility to comb the hair
- Long-handled or regular shoe horn—allows person to put on shoes without assistance
- Velcro closures—on shoes, pants, blouses, and other clothing simplifies dressing for person with limited manual dexterity
- Clothing that opens down to the waist or bottom hem—to facilitate dressing and removal
- Elastic waistbands—make dressing easier
- Elastic shoelaces—convert tie shoes to slip-ons, for easier access
- Large rings or zipper pulls on zippers—for easier grasping
- Garter clips on long ribbon and loose-fitting stockings—to aid in pulling on stockings
- Front-hooking bra or bra without hooks—to make dressing easier
- Gowns or slips with front zippers—for ease in putting them on
- Gowns or dresses that fasten at the shoulder, instead of in the back
- Electric toothbrush—allows person to brush teeth with minimal physical effort
- Padded or enlarged handles on silverware or toothbrush, rubber handles, and handles with a loop for the entire hand—allow person with difficulty grasping to feed themselves or brush teeth (Fig. 97-2)
- Rocking knife—allows cutting by rocking the knife, instead of using a sawing motion. The food does not need to be secured with the other hand (Fig. 97-3)
- Plate holder—to keep plate in place so a person can eat with one hand; or a person with spasticity will not move the plate
- Plate guard—acts as edge on the plate so food will not be pushed off (Fig. 97-2)
- Child's "sippy" cup or cup with handles on both sides—to prevent spills and make it easier to grasp (Fig. 97-2)
- Smaller spoon, fork—for person with arm or hand weakness
- Angled spoon, fork—for easier picking up of food and easier access to mouth (Fig. 97-2)
- Divided plate—for person with spasticity
- Shower stool or chair—to provide safety and independence for person with weakness or instability. Some chairs have suction-cup feet, to further prevent falls.
- Stool or bench in the shower—for comfort and safety (Fig. 97-1)
- Bedside commode—for use at night, to prevent falls (Fig. 51-3B)
- Flame-resistant, flame-retardant materials in clothing and bedding—for added safety
- Various slings and braces—to facilitate movement
- Long-handled back scratcher—to allow person to reach the back or feet, to provide comfort
- Long-handled bath brush—to facilitate washing the back
- Availability of "bag bath"—for use between tub or shower baths
- Use of tooth flosser device or toothpick with attached floss—to facilitate flossing teeth
- Use of electric razor—to prevent cuts
- Medication bottles with large tops or easy-open tops and weekly medication setup—to allow client to take medications independently (Fig. 92-1)
- Free-standing commode placed over toilet seat, to provide privacy, but allow more stability for client (Fig. 51-3A)
- Bowel and bladder retraining, self-catheterization, and manual disimpaction of feces—to facilitate elimination (Chapter 51)
- Commercial hot and cold packs—to facilitate preparation and application (Chapter 54)
- Adequate pain management—to facilitate movement and comfort (Chapter 55)
- Use of electronic, temporal, or chemical thermometer—to facilitate temperature measurement (Chapter 46)

HOME ADAPTATIONS

- Ramp, instead of stairs—facilitates entry into home by wheelchair, walker, scooter, or crutches
- Lever-style doorknobs—allows person who cannot grasp a conventional doorknob to open doors
- Electronic door locks—to make it easier to lock and unlock doors
- Emergency alarm button worn around the neck—to facilitate calling for assistance
- Lever-style faucet handles—allows person to easily turn on and off water (Fig. 97-1)
- Raised electrical plug-ins—allow person to reach from wheelchair, without bending over
- Closets and cupboards with automatic lights—light goes on when door is opened, to avoid searching and reaching for light switch
- Wider doors—to facilitate wheelchairs, walkers, or scooters
- Low pile on carpet—allows easier movement of wheelchairs, walkers, or scooters
- Removal of scatter rugs and low coffee tables—for easier wheelchair access and to prevent falls or stumbling
- Electric lift or home elevator—allows people who cannot climb stairs to go up and down or send items up and down
- Raised toilet seat—allows people to sit down and stand up easier (Fig. 51-3A)
- Location of toilet paper holder—may need to be moved to client's stronger side
- L-shaped toilet paper holders—facilitate changing rolls
- Curtain or "barn door"-type door, instead of bathroom door—gives easier access and more room for wheelchair or walker
- Flush mechanism on toilet—must be easy to maneuver and reach. Foot pedal may be used for those with limited hand mobility. Electronic automatic flush mechanism may also be used. Automatic seat raising and lowering device is helpful.
- Large shower—to facilitate bathing on shower stool, chair, or wheelchair. Many people cannot safely get in and out of conventional bathtub (see Fig. 97-1).
- Bathtub with side door—for safer access to tub (Nursing Procedure 50-11)
- Special-color and fluorescent tape on the edge of each stair and at the edge of top stair—to warn person of stairs and prevent falls

Box 97-2 Adaptive or Assistive Devices Used in Rehabilitation (Continued)

- Small lights in darker areas—to prevent falls. Tap lights and motion sensor lights may be used for small corners and areas without lights.
- Tile instead of carpet, especially in bathroom and kitchen—to facilitate cleaning (and make movement easier)
- Elimination of scatter rugs and use of motion lights—to prevent falls
- Flotation pads, egg crate mattresses, adjustable "Sleep Number" beds, incontinence pads, elbow and heel pads, etc.—to help prevent skin breakdown
- Seizure pads and/or side rails on beds—to prevent falls and assist person to turn over (Fig. 51-3B)
- Large toggle light switches—to allow person to turn on and off lights
- Phone headset, Bluetooth, or speakerphone—so person does not have to hold handset
- Gas fireplace, especially with remote control—so person does not need to handle wood and lighters
- Long-handled propane lighter—to facilitate lighting candles or barbecue
- Snap-in or L-shaped toilet paper holder—to facilitate changing rolls
- Remote control draperies, window blinds, and shades—to allow adjustment of light and privacy
- Motion lights outside—to provide safety and security
- Photo sensor light (photocell)—to turn lights on at night and off during daylight
- Remote control with large numbers for all systems, such as TV, DVD/Blu-ray, DVR, and so on—to allow easier operation
- Handheld shower spray—to allow person to shower while sitting (Fig. 97-1)

HOMEMAKING ADAPTATIONS

- Food preparation board—protruding spikes or nails hold foods for peeling and slicing (Fig. 97-3)
- Stationary scrub brush—brush mounted inside sink, to facilitate scrubbing hands, dishes, or vegetables
- One-handed equipment—various items are adapted for use with one hand. These include rolling pins, can openers, and egg beaters (Fig. 97-3)
- Use of larger electric mixer on stand—to eliminate need to hold hand mixer
- Bowl holder—a stationary board containing a hole, used to hold a bowl while mixing foods
- Adjusted height—stoves, countertops, and sinks lowered to accommodate homemaker in a wheelchair
- Use of walker with seat—to allow homemaker to sit while preparing food or if becoming tired
- Removal of cupboard doors or swing-away doors—for easier visibility and access
- Burner knobs and dishwasher controls placed in front—for easier wheelchair access
- External ice maker on refrigerator—to provide easy access
- Lift-type or electronic faucet controls—for those who cannot grasp knob
- Foot controls to operate faucets or soap dispensers—for person with limited hand movement or weakness
- Combination clothes washer and dryer—so clothes do not need to be transferred from washer to dryer
- Front-loading washer/dryer (raised on platform, with controls in front)—for the person in a wheelchair
- Dishwasher that contains garbage disposal—so dishes do not need to be scraped or prerinsed
- Toaster that operates based on weight and thickness of bread—to eliminate need to push down lever
- Electric can opener or one-handed can opener—to allow one-handed use (Fig. 97-3)
- Prepackaged meals—to facilitate preparation
- "Lazy Susan" devices or pull-out shelves in cupboards—to prevent reaching and allow ease in locating items
- Toaster or microwave that beeps when food is ready—for person with limited vision
- Toaster oven—for smaller baking jobs, eliminating need to reach into large oven
- Wheels on garbage cans—to facilitate moving
- Step-on opening garbage cans—to avoid having to lift cover
- Microwave or convection oven—to make cooking easier and faster
- Blender or food processor—to prevent having to chop or use mixer
- Grill built into range—so person does not have to go outside

MOBILITY ADAPTATIONS

- Canes, crutches, and walkers—to give support and provide safety (Fig. 48-11)
- Braces, splints, foot/leg prostheses—to allow greater mobility and/or support and facilitate movement (Fig. 97-6)
- Use of hand rolls, trochanter rolls, and footboards—to prevent further deformity (Chapter 48)
- Use of bed trapeze and side rails—to allow person to exercise and move about in bed (Nursing Procedure 48-11)
- Handihook or mechanical arm—for person who has had an amputation or who has paralysis or weakness of arm and/or hand
- Wheelchairs and walkers; basket on wheelchair or walker—to facilitate carrying items; seat on the walker—to allow person to sit when tired
- Motorized scooters and wheelchairs
- Use of knee scooter—to avoid use of wheelchair or walker, for person with one strong leg
- Wheelchair and walker tables—attached tables allow person to work while seated
- Backpack and fanny pack purse—allows person to carry items and have both hands free
- Purse hook for the table—so purse is not placed on the floor
- Railings and grab bars—should be installed in bathrooms, hallways, stairs, and wherever needed. The person must be able to maneuver and feel safe in the home. It is important to prevent falls.
- Telescoping cane—may be used when needed and collapsed, for easy storage; also allows adjustment for client's height

(Continued)

Box 97-2 Adaptive or Assistive Devices Used in Rehabilitation (Continued)

- Must have secure rubber tip (A cane with 4 ft is more secure than a straight cane with single end. See Fig. 48-11A)
- Cane spikes—to place on tip of cane, for snowy or icy conditions
- Chair lift or elevator chairs—lift the person, so they can stand up easier
- Spikes for shoes or boots—for safety in slippery outdoor conditions
- Automobile lift for wheelchair—to allow access to car
- Hand controls to operate automobile—for person with limited leg movement
- Foot controls for automobile—for person with limited arm movement
- Key fob that locks and unlocks car doors and/or opens trunk and side doors
- Remote starting for vehicles
- Foot operated tailgate on van—to prevent leaning
- "Handicapped/wheelchair" permits for automobile—to allow safer and more convenient parking
- "Geri chair"—to provide safe movement and work or eating surface; helps prevent falls that might occur if wheelchair is used
- Bluetooth telephone technology—making it easier to hear and answer the phone
- Voice-activated dialing on phones—for those unable to dial because of limited vision or dexterity
- iPod downloads—allowing person to listen to books or have a large music library readily available

ADAPTED EQUIPMENT FOR PEOPLE WITH LIMITED VISION OR HEARING
- Hearing aid—to assist in hearing
- Bluetooth device integrated into hearing aid—to facilitate using phone
- Magnifying glasses—to allow person with limited vision to read
- TV remote control with large numbers—allows person with limited vision to see numbers
- Large numbers on phone and alarm clock (or talking clock)—for person with limited vision
- Playing cards with large numbers or Braille numbers—allow people with limited vision to play cards
- Card holder—so person does not need to hold cards while playing
- Appliance knobs in large print or Braille—for vision impaired
- Appliance instructions and recipes on tape or computer—for vision impaired (type can be enlarged on computer)
- Volume control on telephone—allows people to hear better
- High-wattage light bulbs in lamps, with dimmer switches—allow clients with vision impairments to obtain more light; others can turn down the lights
- Talking thermometer—allows the nonsighted person to take temperature
- Talking/chiming watch—for person with limited vision or who is nonsighted
- Service animals—to assist and provide safety (for many conditions)
- TTY telephone service—allowing person with limited hearing to communicate

RECREATIONAL ITEMS
- TV remote control—facilitates changing channels and volume, or operating DVD or video player
- Magnetic game boards, boards with pegs, or boards with holes to hold game pieces—allow people with spasticity or severe tremors to play games without losing pieces
- Games and puzzles with larger pieces—for easier handling and visibility
- Prism eyeglasses—allow people to read while lying down, without having to hold book up
- Checkers or chess pieces with loops—for easier grasping
- Handheld computer games—easy to hold and manipulate
- Books on CD or iPod—for entertainment
- Voice-activated television—to provide entertainment, without client effort
- Cell phone with voice-activated dialing—to facilitate use of phone
- Phone or computer with voice-activated dictation ability or access to Google—to facilitate research
- Closed captioning of TV or movies—for persons with limited hearing

MISCELLANEOUS ITEMS
- Long-handled tongs or specially designed grasping device ("grabbers")—allow people to reach and pick up items easier
- Computer—multiple uses. Helps people with aphasia to communicate. Enables visually impaired people to read because print can be enlarged. Allows homebound people to communicate or work via email, Facebook, etc.
- Electronic voice synthesizer—to facilitate speech for people with mechanical speech disorders or following laryngectomy
- Pill splitter—allows accurate dividing of pills
- Pill crusher—to facilitate swallowing of large pills
- Daily medication box—allows client's medications to be identified by day and time, to help client remember to take medications and prevent duplication of doses
- Electronic medication carousel and dispenser—sounds alarm when medications are due, to remind client; dispenses correct dosage
- Panic alarms and automatic telephone dialers—allow client to call for help in emergency
- Home alarm system, with remote control—to provide security and alert person to intruders, fire, or other security factors and to call for assistance in an emergency
- Smoke and carbon monoxide alarms in the home; possibly a sprinkler system—to provide safety
- Hip, knee, or elbow pads—to prevent injury if client falls; helps prevent skin breakdown
- Helmets—to prevent head injury

| Box 97-2 | Adaptive or Assistive Devices Used in Rehabilitation (Continued) |

- "Handicap-accessible" buses, trains, and taxis—to increase mobility
- Self-adjusting, digital, wrist blood pressure cuff—to facilitate blood pressure measurement
- Easy-to-use blood glucose testing equipment
- Ambularm—for persons who are confused, to provide safety and alert caregivers if the person leaves a particular area; provides more freedom for client
- Large ashtray—for easier access and more safety (*teach clients never to smoke in bed;* encourage clients to quit smoking, provide smoking cessation materials—gum, patch, etc.)
- Automatic pet feeder and waterer—allow person to care for pet or service animal more conveniently
- Fenced yard—to allow client to let dog out without having to use leash
- Self-cleaning litter box—to make it easier to care for pet cat

and reinforcing self-care. It is vital for all clients to perform as much self-care as possible. Help clients to move as quickly as possible through the stages of adjustment, in order to maximize their self-care abilities. Patience and perseverance are necessary. Clients and families must understand the extent of the disability and how it is possible to regain some—perhaps all—normal functions. Even in progressive or degenerative disorders, clients should be encouraged in self-care for as long as possible. Basic nursing care is often required for the person with a disability and is contained in Unit 8. Many disorders and specific condition-related procedures and protocols are described in Unit 12. The paramount goal of rehabilitation is to assist the client to regain the ability to perform as many ADLs as possible. This enhances the client's self-esteem, which is of primary importance. When the rehabilitation team has thoroughly evaluated the client and determined what functional capacity is realistic, a program of retraining in ADLs is initiated.

Functional ADLs

The basic functional ADLs (**FADLs**) include aspects of self-care, such as dressing, bathing, toileting and continence, transfer, mobility, and eating. Because of disability, adaptations may be necessary so clients can perform these self-care activities (Fig. 97-2). Not all clients will be able to care for themselves or to live independently. Box 97-3 contains examples of FADLs.

Instrumental ADLs

Instrumental ADLs (**IADLs**) are more complex living skills, such as food preparation, laundry, taking medications, money management, and moving about the community. These IADLs may or may not be achievable by individual clients. One important IADL is being able to purchase groceries and prepare meals.

Healthcare staff members maintain an ADL record that informs all members of the healthcare team of the activities the client is able to do and those that they are attempting. Nursing care plans are continually updated, with improvements or regressions in progress. (Box 97-3 gives examples of IADLs.)

Modified Equipment and Adaptive Devices

A great deal of adaptive equipment is available to people with disabilities. Much of this equipment has been invented and developed by people with disabilities to help themselves and others. It is important to emphasize that many of the items listed in Box 97-2 used to make life easier for persons with disabilities are also used by able-bodied people. We use many of these things in our everyday life.

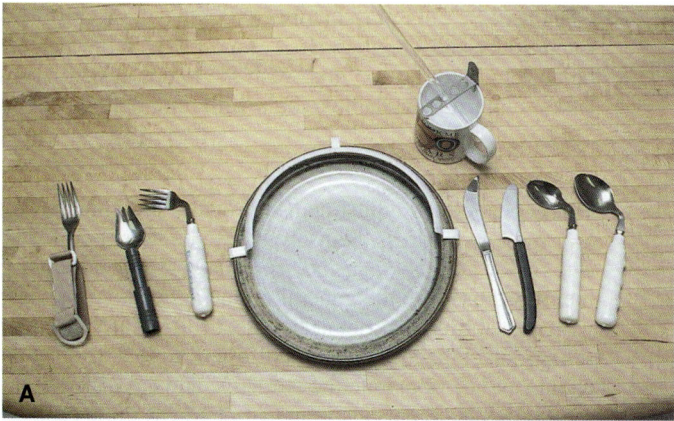
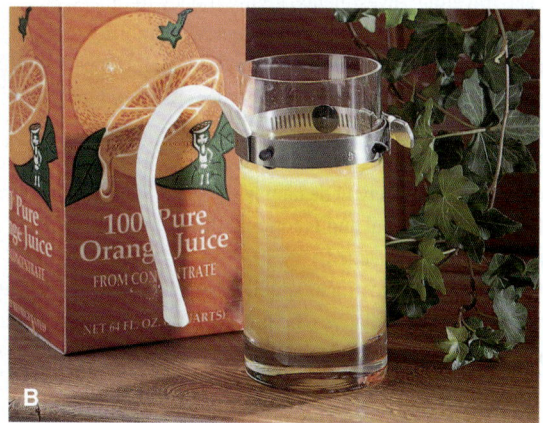

Cup holder

Figure 97-2 Many devices are available to allow clients with disabilities to feed themselves. **A.** Shown here (*left to right*) are a fork with a hand strap, a combination fork/spoon ("spork"), an angled fork, a plate guard to prevent food from being pushed off the plate, a partially covered cup with easy-to-grip handle and drinking straw, a small easy-to-handle knife, a partially rocking knife, and angled spoons with enlarged handles. **B.** A cup holder with a large, easy-to-grip handle can be attached to almost any cup or glass. (Carter & Lewsen, 2005.)

Box 97-3 Examples of ADLs

FUNCTIONAL ADLS (FADLS)
- Dressing skills (amount of assistance needed)
- Cleanliness and self-care (bathing, grooming, care of teeth, nails, and hair; amount of assistance needed)
- Elimination (toileting skills, continence level, management of incontinence)
- Taking of food and fluids (self-feeding, ability to chew and swallow, assessment of dysphagia)
- Communication (ability to talk or communicate in other ways)
- Activity and mobility levels (walking and transfers; use of walker, wheelchair, or scooter; maintaining intact skin and reporting change in skin condition; prevention of falls)
- Ability to obtain rest and sleep

INSTRUMENTAL ADLS (IADLS)
ADL skills needed at home or work (homemaking, laundry, vocational rehabilitation/retraining). The person must be able to
- Use telephone and/or computer.
- Shop for groceries and essentials or order home delivery.
- Prepare appropriate meals.
- Manage money (pay bills, write checks, use an ATM).
- Drive or use public transportation safely.
- Read and write.
- Make appropriate choices of clothing for weather conditions, safety, and activities.
- Monitor medications (take medications daily and on time), order medication refills when needed, report adverse side effects.
- Manage special sleep problems (as needed [PRN] sleep medications, equipment to manage sleep apnea).
- Manage special medical problems (e.g., diabetes, emphysema, need for supplemental oxygen).
- Manage special elimination devices (e.g., incontinence pads, catheters, ostomy bags).
- Make and keep appointments with healthcare providers and therapists.
- Make wise decisions about savings, major purchases (e.g., car), traveling, investments, giving money to others, etc.
- Maintain personal safety and reduce vulnerability (e.g., prevention of falls and/or skin breakdown, intruder avoidance, safety in one's own home—use good judgment; use a security system).
- Maintain appropriate behavior (e.g., public behavior, avoidance of legal issues, safety in dealing with others, safer sex practices).
- Recognize physical and emotional difficulties and seek assistance when needed.
- Participate in recreational and diversional activities, visiting with friends and relatives, being comfortable and safe when going out in public.

The Homemaker With a Disability

Devices have been designed to assist homemakers in caring for themselves, their homes, and their families. Box 97-2 describes some of these adaptations. It is important to protect the homemaker with a disability from injuries. The

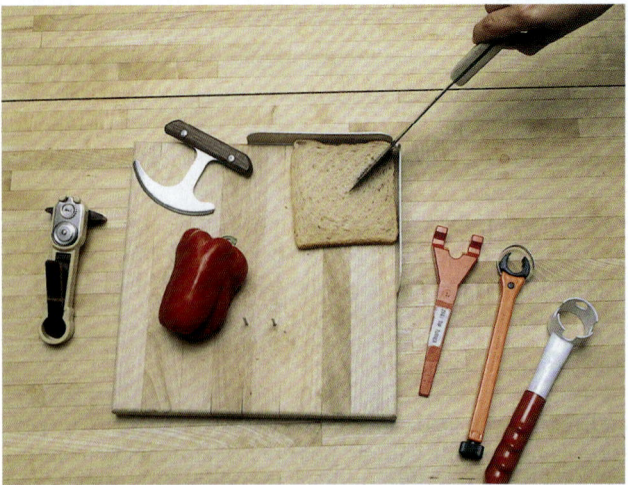

Figure 97-3 Adapted equipment can assist the homemaker with a disability to be independent in meal preparation. Shown here (*left to right*) are a one-handed can opener, a rocking knife, and a food preparation board. This board has rubber feet on the bottom (to prevent movement) and spikes on top to hold food for peeling or chopping. A food guard is in the corner, to allow bread or other items to be buttered or cut. Items shown to the *right* assist in opening bottles and other containers.

person is taught to use a walker for support and to keep a fire extinguisher handy. The stovetop may be lowered, with controls in the front, to accommodate the homemaker in a wheelchair.

Adaptive Equipment

Clients with disabilities often need equipment modifications (Fig. 97-3). Occupational therapists can assist in suggesting, locating, or improvising equipment. It is important to provide as much independence as possible, to increase the client's independence and self-esteem.

Home Modifications

Adaptations to the home may be necessary to make it more comfortable and convenient for the client. For example, bathrooms and kitchens may be modified, to allow wheelchair access. This may involve enlarging the room or lowering sinks and counters. It is important for the person to be able to bathe, cook, and wash the hands easily. In some cases, funds are available to help with remodeling expenses.

Adaptive Clothing

A few changes or adjustments to regular clothing can often allow clients to dress themselves or to be more comfortable. The major goal is *client independence*. Many modified garments are used by the general public as well, so the person with a disability does not need to feel "different." Companies selling specialized clothing will often meet with groups of clients and demonstrate the attractive and easy-to-use clothing available. Clients also can learn to dress more easily. For instance, clients with **hemiplegia** (paralyzed on one side of the body) are taught to place clothing on the affected arm or leg first and to undress the unaffected arm or leg first. The strong side is thereby free to help the weak side. Much of this teaching is logical. For example, clients can learn to put

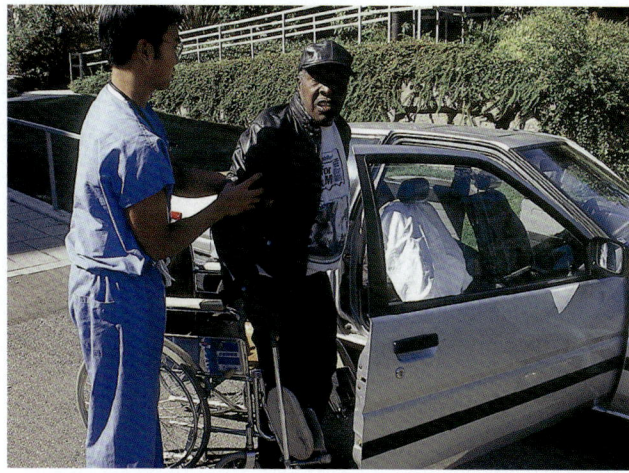

Figure 97-4 To regain mobility in the community, a ramp is usually needed, and the client must be taught to transfer safely from wheelchair to car.

on socks before pants, so toenails will not catch on the pants. (Toenails should be kept short, to avoid catching on socks.)

Mobility

Clients can be taught basic position changes in bed and transfers from bed to chair, onto the toilet, and into the bathtub or shower. Independence is further enhanced when the client can leave home. Teaching transfer from the wheelchair to the car is an important component of this independence (Fig. 97-4).

> **Key Concept**
> Not only does mobility enhance independence and self-esteem, it also helps prevent complications, such as hypostatic pneumonia, pressure areas and skin breakdown, thrombophlebitis, and constipation.

Wheelchairs and Scooters

Some clients are confined to wheelchairs or motorized scooters. Motorized wheelchairs are also available for those with limited hand or arm strength. Some can be driven using only the client's breath. (Be aware that the weight limit of bariatric wheelchairs is usually 550 lb.) Some clients can move about their homes using a walker, but need a wheelchair or scooter when outside the home.

Special wheelchairs are available for racing and sports (Fig. 97-7). You will find that many persons in wheelchairs take part in marathons, sports, and other activities, along with able-bodied people. Some wheelchairs are equipped with various adaptive devices. A "rescue" wheelchair is available to assist in evacuation of wheelchair-bound individuals in an emergency (Chapter 39). A standing wheelchair, although expensive, allows the client to meet people at eye level, providing additional mobility and self-esteem. Wheelchair lifts and hand controls are available for cars, enabling many clients to maintain independence in transportation. Various types of slings and pulleys exist, which allow the person with upper extremity weakness to write, eat, or perform other ADLs.

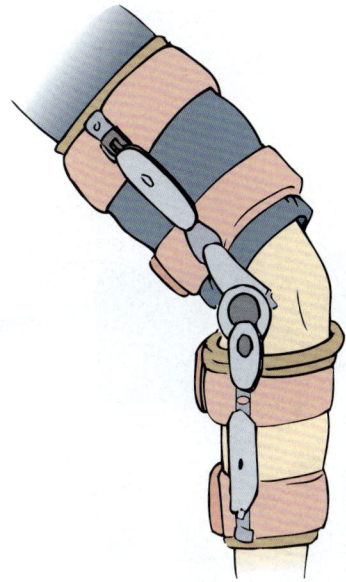

Figure 97-5 A supportive brace can be used temporarily after a knee injury or knee surgery, or it may be used permanently to support the knee. (Timby, 2005.)

> **Key Concept**
> When talking with clients confined to wheelchairs or scooters, sit or kneel, so you are at the client's eye level.

Canes and Walkers

Many clients can achieve mobility just by using a cane or walker for support. Chapter 48 describes and illustrates many of the more commonly used mobility devices for clients with disabilities. Several types of canes are available (Fig. 48-11A). Many people paint or otherwise decorate their canes or use fancy canes to express their individuality. Several varieties of walkers are also available (Fig. 48-11B). Each client is evaluated to determine which type of walker will be the most comfortable and safe to use. The reverse walker is encouraged for long-term use, when possible, to enable the client to stand more upright (Fig. 48-11C). It is important to encourage the client to move independently as much as possible.

Braces and Splints

Clients may need special braces or splints to support affected limbs or maintain correct and safe positioning. The medical specialty involved in the fabrication of braces and splints is called **orthotics**. *Splints* are available in two forms: *resting splints,* which hold the body part stationary and prevent the hand or limb from becoming contracted, and *dynamic* (moving) *hand splints,* which enable clients to function more easily than would be possible without them. Some splints are attached to sling-type devices, one on each finger. These allow the client with arm and hand weakness or paralysis to use the hands. Another type of splint is combined with a hook device for grasping objects.

Braces are often applied to the legs for support, especially for clients with **paraplegia** (lower limb paralysis) or hemiplegia. In some cases, a special brace is used to support a joint after an injury or reconstructive surgery (Fig. 97-5).

UNIT 15 Nursing in a Variety of Settings

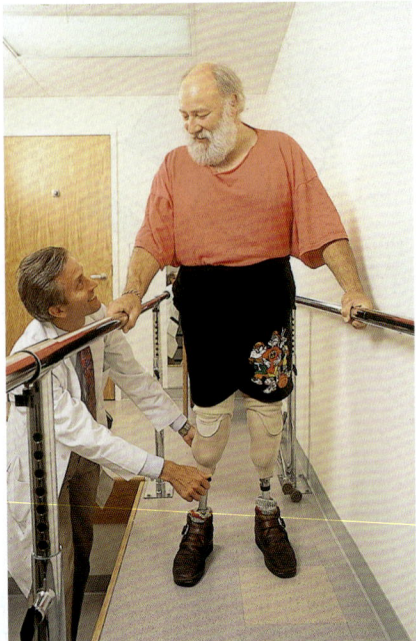

Figure 97-6 Persons with amputated lower limbs often receive prostheses soon after surgery. Therapists and specially trained nurses assist the person in learning to walk with the new prostheses.

The brace may be adjusted to allow limited movement; this helps protect the joint while it heals. This type of brace may also be used on a permanent basis, to support a weak joint. Many people who would otherwise be immobilized are able to walk with the aid of braces.

Physical therapists teach clients to apply and remove braces, and nursing personnel reinforce this teaching. If a client has **quadriplegia** (all four extremities and, possibly, the trunk paralyzed), they may need a neck or back brace. In rare cases, this client may use a type of inflatable trousers (**exoskeleton**) to maintain an upright position and prevent vascular collapse. Many clients also require special shoes or shoe inserts. Some clients will require breathing assistance on a permanent basis.

Artificial Limbs

People who have had all or part of a leg or arm amputated are often fitted with artificial limbs. This specialty is called **prosthetics**, the fabrication and adjustment of *prostheses* (artificial body parts). You may be familiar with the arm prosthesis that resembles a hook. This prosthesis provides movement and control similar to normal thumb–finger opposition. A leg prosthesis fitted over the amputation stump allows the person to walk and participate in sports (Fig. 97-6). Today's technology has advanced the science of prosthetics. Artificial hands are available that look much like a natural hand, but still have thumb–finger opposition. Some prostheses are electronic and/or computer driven. Clients with leg prostheses often participate in running or other sports.

 SPECIAL CONSIDERATIONS Lifespan

Children may be fitted with prostheses or braces. These are enlarged as needed, to accommodate the child's growth.

Range of Motion and Flexibility

Clients must perform range of motion (ROM) exercises, to build muscle strength and maintain joint mobility (Chapter 48). *Rationale: These exercises prevent joint stiffness, muscle shortening, and atrophy.* ROM exercises are either *passive* or *active,* depending on the client's level of ability. Clients also may use the continuous passive motion (CPM) machine in their rehabilitation program (Fig. 48-8). Clients who spend long periods lying in bed or sitting in wheelchairs may become *hypotensive* (low blood pressure—postural hypotension) when they stand. They may be assisted to adjust gradually to being upright by using a *tilt table*.

Fall Assessment

A formal fall assessment should be done on each client on a regular basis, whether they are in a rehabilitation program or not. It is very important to prevent all clients from falling. This is particularly true of the client with physical limitations; it is vital to prevent further injury. The process of formal fall assessment of all clients is described in Chapter 48. One such formal assessment uses the Hendrich Fall Risk Tool.

Skin Care

Clients with impaired sensation or mobility are particularly vulnerable to skin breakdown, due to impaired circulation, pressure areas due to immobility, difficulty in obtaining adequate nutrition and fluids, problems with elimination, impaired mental functioning, and other related factors. A number of nursing measures related to skin care do not require a provider's order.

These include keeping the skin and linens dry and clean, application of barrier creams for the client with incontinence, repositioning the client, and giving a backrub. Some measures, such as special pads and beds, require a provider's order. These and other measures are described in Chapters 49–51, and 58. The "Braden Scale for prediction of pressure sore risk" is illustrated in Figure 58-5. Chapter 58 also discusses skin and wound care and prevention of skin breakdown in detail. *Prevention of skin breakdown is a primary nursing function.*

> **Key Concept**
>
> Clients may see an *enterostomal therapist,* to assist in skin and wound care, as well as the care of a colostomy or ileostomy. Clients are often referred to *wound care or burn centers* for evaluation, treatment, and teaching, to restore and maintain skin integrity. Excellent skin care is vital in clients who lack sensation in a portion of the body, who are unable to move independently, who are incontinent, or whose skin is particularly *friable* (fragile).

Elimination

A rapidly growing area of rehabilitation services involves caring for and treating clients with bowel and/or bladder incontinence. Management of incontinence is a major factor in a person's quality of life. Fortunately, treatment is available for most types of incontinence, and nursing is actively involved (Chapter 89). By increasing the care and treatment provided, many clients are able to increase their social contacts. As they gain continence, they are often able to move out of the nursing home; some of these clients become eligible for government-funded housing facilities.

> **Key Concept**
>
> A person's independence and ability to live at home, rather than being required to live in a healthcare facility, is often directly related to that person's ability to maintain continence.

A client who is paralyzed may have a **neurogenic** (lacking nerve stimulation) bladder or bowel. This may be caused by a spinal cord injury. The lower the level of injury, the less likely the client is to have difficulty with elimination. If the injury is high in the spinal cord, the client will often need bowel or bladder retraining, to reestablish independent elimination patterns (Chapters 51 and 89). In some cases, bladder continence is not possible. This client may wear a leg bag or special underwear for urine collection (Figs. 51-7 and 51-8) or may perform self-catheterization.

Bowel Elimination

If a person is paralyzed or lacks sensation below the waist, *fecal impaction* (blockage) can cause difficulties. Some people manually disimpact themselves daily, as part of their bowel program (Nursing Procedure 51-5). A well-balanced diet high in fiber, adequate fluids, exercise, and regular times for bowel elimination are helpful preventive measures.

Bladder Elimination

Care of the client with a neurogenic bladder is complex. Voiding studies are often performed to determine the cause of incontinence. During a bladder retraining program, the provider may order nursing actions, including measures such as encouraging fluid intake, establishing regular voiding schedules, and administration of specific medications, as well as teaching self-catheterization. A treatment recently approved for insurance reimbursement involves Botox injections into the bladder. In some cases, a special diet that eliminates bladder irritants is prescribed. (These bladder irritants include caffeine, aspartame artificial sweetener, dairy products, tomato products, citrus fruits, spicy foods, alcoholic beverages, and sugar.) Chapter 51 describes bladder and bowel retraining in more detail.

> **Key Concept**
>
> Some nurses specialize in continence care and set up programs for continence rehabilitation. They assist clients with bowel or bladder incontinence to achieve control and to manage their own elimination programs.

Vocational Rehabilitation

Clients often benefit from vocational testing and retraining. Testing helps determine what the client would enjoy and what options are possible. Counselors help clients search out appropriate employment possibilities. The client can then be educated in particular job skills. For example, if a formerly mobile client has become paralyzed, they may choose to be retrained for a desk job. If a client has lost vision, a job as a transcriptionist or answering phones may be an option. Clients with severe intellectual impairments may enjoy working in a sheltered situation of some type. Often, special funding is available to assist with costs of retraining.

Diversional Activities

All people, whether or not they have disabilities, must find activities to occupy free time and increase self-esteem. Occupational and physical therapists assist clients to find activities of interest and initiate exercises for specific muscles, build strength, and help prevent deformities. Computers can assist many clients who have aphasia and other speech problems and those with impaired vision or hearing to communicate more easily.

Recreation and Sports

Many games have been adapted for people with various disabilities. Occupational or recreational therapists will have suggestions for diversional activities. Some activities have specific goals in mind. Examples include improving fine motor skills and eye–hand coordination by tying fishing flies or crocheting or improving large-muscle strength by weaving on a large loom with weights attached.

A young woman, Jessica Cox, has demonstrated that physical differences need not prevent activities enjoyed by nondisabled people. She was born without arms and is an accomplished pianist, a black belt in Taekwondo, and a licensed pilot (https://www.jessicacox.com/). National and local athletic events for people with physical and intellectual disabilities are increasing (Fig. 97-7). Marathons and other races have wheeled divisions for persons confined to wheelchairs. Many wheelchair-bound individuals also enjoy bowling, playing golf or tennis, or going fishing or sailing. Skiing, swimming, horseback riding, bowling, and many other activities are available to persons with disabilities. A growing number of wheelchair sports teams in basketball, table tennis, softball, and other sports are available. Adaptations of golf carts are available to allow golfers who cannot walk to enjoy the game. Some people also play golf or softball one-handed. The National and International Special Olympics offer fun and competition and allow large numbers of people with physical or intellectual disabilities to participate. Most of these people would otherwise be unable to compete in athletic events. The emphasis here is not on winning but on "doing your best" and "fair competition."

Various programs and camps provide outdoor experiences for people with disabilities. With the availability of cell phones and satellite phones, camping and wilderness experience has become much safer. Wilderness Inquiry is one such program that provides an opportunity to camp and canoe in the wilderness. Camp Courage is a camp in Minnesota designed specifically for clients with disabilities. Medical specialists are on hand during each session to provide therapy and handle emergencies. Programs and camps such as these exist in all parts of the country, and many have volunteer opportunities for nurses and nursing students. For information, contact your local YMCA, Red Cross, Easter Seals Society, Huntington's Disease Society, or County Social Services department.

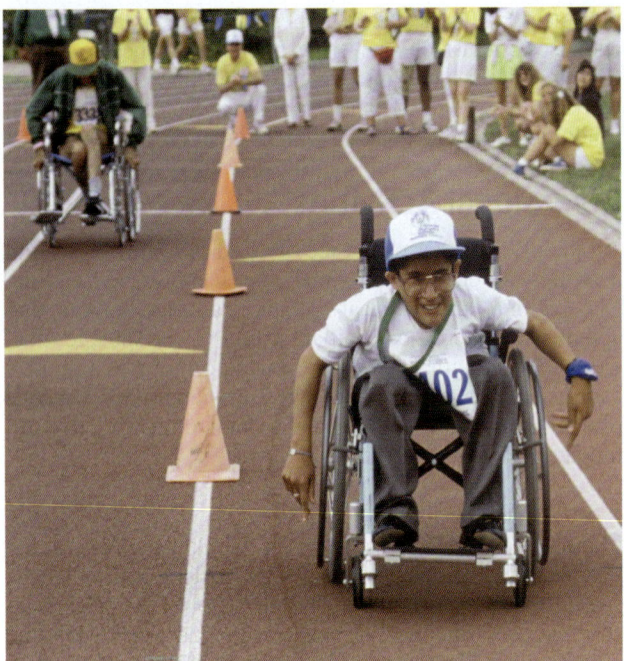

Figure 97-7 People of all ages who have physical disabilities enjoy participating in sports and other physical activities. Many activities and sports are available for persons with disabilities. (Photo by Joseph Sohm/Shutterstock.)

Pet Therapy

Many clients benefit from having pets to provide diversion and companionship and encourage responsibility. In addition, some residence facilities have pets who live there or who visit regularly. It is important to verify that these pets have received required immunizations.

The pet must be gentle and not afraid of strangers. Resident and visiting cats are usually declawed and not allowed outside. Most of the pets are neutered or spayed. Training is required on the part of the pet and the owner, before they are allowed to make therapeutic visits to healthcare facilities. The residents in many long-term care facilities help care for pets. Often, a person who does not respond to other people will respond favorably to an animal. An example of the helpfulness of therapy dogs occurred during the World Trade Center crisis in 2001. These dogs provided needed diversion for overworked firefighters, police officers, and other rescue workers. (Other dogs provided search and rescue services.)

Service Animals

Service animals are useful as aids to persons with special challenges. These animals are very valuable; the cost of training can exceed $30,000. Leader or guide dogs assist nonsighted persons to move safely about the community. (Recently, a service dog saved their master's life when they fell in front of a train.) Hearing dogs assist deaf persons by alerting them to the telephone, doorbell, or intruders. Dogs can be trained to warn their master about situations such as an impending seizure or a dangerous blood sugar (glucose) level. Dogs and simian monkeys assist clients with limited mobility by performing tasks such as delivering items, turning on lights, and opening doors. Often, animals provide comfort and security to clients with serious disabilities. For example, at "Nature's Edge Therapy Center" in Rice Lake,

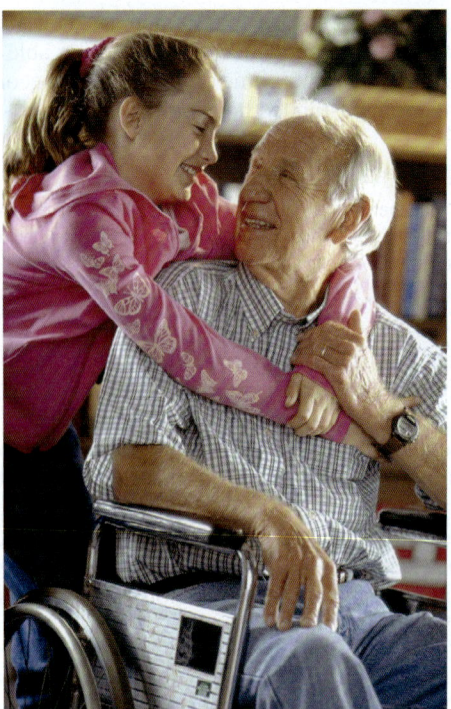

Figure 97-8 The importance of family and friends to the rehabilitation process cannot be overestimated. Both the grandparent and the grandchild benefit from a cozy time together. (Eliopoulos, 2001.)

Wisconsin, animals help severely disturbed children with autism and head injuries to relate to the world. Service animals are exempt from restrictions against pets in situations such as entering public buildings and restaurants, flying in the cabin on commercial airlines, living in college dormitories, or sailing on cruise ships, by mandate of the *Americans with Disabilities Act* (ADA), 1990. It is illegal to ban service animals from these places. Service animals are often identified by a special vest when they are "on duty" (specific certification is not available). Remember: Service animals are "working" and *should not be petted by strangers* without permission. (It is also possible to obtain a healthcare provider's letter allowing an "emotional support" animal in all places.)

The Importance of Family and Friends

All people need to feel worthwhile and part of a social group. Encourage the client's family and friends to visit and take the client on outings. Often, clients are lonelier living at home than in a facility with other people; visits at home are even more important. Special relationships often develop between generations; both "grandpa" and the family can benefit from special time spent together (Fig. 97-8).

THE SCOPE OF REHABILITATIVE SERVICES

Many clients receive care from inpatient rehabilitation services at one time or another. Clients in rehabilitation facilities may have chronic conditions, such as cystic fibrosis (CF), progressive multiple sclerosis (MS), Huntington disease (HD), muscular dystrophy (MD), acquired immunodeficiency syndrome (AIDS), or dementia. These clients may remain in extended care for an extended period. Other clients may be recovering from acute situations, such as a gunshot wound, traumatic brain injury (**TBI**), severe burn, stroke, or hip joint replacement, and may leave the facility fairly quickly. Therefore, nurses in rehabilitation have an opportunity to perform a myriad of skills.

Burn Rehabilitation

The person who has been severely burned faces many challenges. After the initial crisis, maintaining mobility, preventing deformities and infection, maintaining hydration, and managing pain and itching are primary concerns. Restoring skin integrity is particularly important. Nurses assist clients first with passive and later with active ROM and strengthening exercises. *Rationale: It is vital to prevent contractures and muscle hypertrophy.* Clients may use braces and other orthotic appliances. Various means help prevent scarring and contractures, including special tight gloves, face masks, or body wraps. Skin and other grafting may be done. Special medicinal substances are often used, and whirlpool treatment (hydrotherapy) is common. Surgery and therapeutic exercise may be required to release contractures. Clients must deal with many emotional concerns; they often benefit from counseling and group therapy. They may also need teaching to learn to perform ADLs or to gain employment, considering their disability. (Chapter 75 discusses burns and their treatment in more detail.) Return to work or school following a severe burn, especially to the face, can be emotionally challenging. This person needs much support; professional counseling is often beneficial to both the client and their employment supervisor.

Rehabilitation for Musculoskeletal Disorders

A broad range of therapies are used to assist in movement and relieve pain. Chronic conditions, such as arthritis and low back pain, often require ongoing nonpharmacologic pain management, as well as strengthening and stretching exercises. Clients who have fractured a hip or had a stroke will often need gait training and may need assistive devices to walk. Clients with spinal column disorders (e.g., scoliosis, spinal cord injuries, or spina bifida) require varying levels of therapy, depending on the severity of the disorder. (Chapter 77 discusses musculoskeletal disorders in more detail.)

Therapeutic heat and cold are used extensively (Chapter 54). Heat is provided by special heating pads and blankets, diathermy, and ultraviolet light (e.g., sun lamps, black light), as well as ultrasound and lasers.

Transdermal electrical nerve stimulation (**TENS**) assists with pain management (Chapter 55), as do acupuncture and self-hypnosis, with guided imagery. Functional electrical stimulation (**FES**) sends a stimulus to the nerves to move muscles; this therapy assists clients to move or walk, improve their gait, reduce spasticity, or better use hands and fingers. In many cases, corrective or reconstructive surgery is performed. Joints, such as the hip, knee, and shoulder, are routinely replaced. Clients with amputations are fitted with prostheses and learn how to use and care for them (Chapter 77). Therapeutic exercise and physical therapy are essential treatments to help clients maintain mobility of joints and muscles, develop coordination, and build strength and endurance.

Rehabilitation for Neurologic Disorders

Clients with spinal cord injuries or severe head trauma usually require extensive rehabilitation. Many cities have special centers or specific home care programs for rehabilitation of persons with traumatic brain injuries. When a client faces permanent *paralysis* (inability to move a part of the body), serious physical and emotional complications can occur. Major complications include contractures, pressure areas, impotence, and bladder and bowel disturbances, as well as depression and threat of suicide. Many people with progressive neurologic disorders, such as Alzheimer's disease (AD), HD, or amyotrophic lateral sclerosis (**ALS**) also can benefit from rehabilitation (Chapter 78).

Sexuality

Sexuality may be a concern for persons who are paralyzed or otherwise disabled. Many people with varying degrees of paralysis are able to participate in sexual activity. Paralyzed men may need a penile implant or other device (Chapter 90). S*exual health clinicians* or *sex therapists* are counselors specially trained in dealing with sexuality. They conduct workshops and seminars to discuss specific sexual problems of paralyzed individuals. Family members should also be encouraged to attend counseling sessions, and to speak freely, express their feelings, and ask questions (Chapter 70). Proper positioning may facilitate intercourse. Women who are paralyzed can have sexual intercourse, become pregnant, and deliver healthy children. Delivery may be vaginal or via cesarean delivery. Women with limited mobility and sensation may more easily contract vaginal or bladder infections and require frequent examinations to detect the presence of infection, before it becomes a serious problem. Teach clients to maintain an adequate fluid intake. Dietary prevention of bladder infections often includes drinking cranberry juice and taking acidophilus.

> **Key Concept**
>
> Clients require individual counseling regarding sexuality because each case is different. The client and their partner should be carefully interviewed by a qualified sexual health clinician. The client and partner may require instruction regarding safe and comfortable positions for intercourse or alternate means of sexual expression. Love and understanding are necessary on the part of both partners.

Rehabilitation for Sensory Disorders

Clients with limited vision or who are nonsighted can learn to perform ADLs. They may receive instruction in the use of Braille for reading or use "talking books" (books on CD or other electronic device). They may learn to use guide or leader dogs. In selected cases, surgery and/or the implantation of a special electronic device enables nonsighted people to have some very limited vision. Clients with hearing disorders may use hearing aids. Changing technology in the development of hearing aids has provided hearing to many people who were not able to hear in the past. In the case of deafness, surgical procedures, such as the cochlear implant, may be effective. Specialized rehabilitation teams help clients adjust to the world of sound and teach them how to care for and use the equipment involved (Chapter 80). Computers are helpful to people with limited sight or hearing, as well as to those who have difficulty speaking.

Cardiovascular Rehabilitation

Following MI (heart attack) or heart surgery to insert stents, replace valves, or bypass vessels, clients often need rehabilitation to return to normal activities. Prevention is important; the client is counseled about specific high-risk behaviors (e.g., obesity, poor diet, smoking, lack of exercise). A change in behavior can help prevent another heart attack or further cardiac damage. However, it is important not to make clients so fearful they are unable to perform normal daily activities. It is important to build endurance, without overtaxing the damaged heart. These clients need much encouragement and reassurance to overcome fear of another MI. Sexual issues may also be a major concern; counseling by a sexual health clinician is often helpful. Following a stroke, clients often need extensive rehabilitation. Hemiplegia and aphasia are frequent challenges. These clients often need assistance with transfers, walking, speaking, and eating and may have visual impairment. They may be confused or emotionally labile. Vocational rehabilitation often helps them to function independently in the home or at work (Chapter 81).

Cancer Rehabilitation

Cancer is quickly becoming a chronic, rather than acute, illness. Many people each year are diagnosed with cancer; these clients often require rehabilitative services. For example, men may require a penile implant after prostatectomy. After radical mastectomy, women may require special exercises and compression appliances to reduce *lymphedema* (swelling of lymph nodes). Breast reconstruction or breast prostheses are often used following mastectomy. The person with either a malignant or a benign brain tumor may have symptoms and require rehabilitation similar to that of a client who has had a stroke. The person with lung cancer may need pulmonary rehabilitation or chest physiotherapy. The person with cancer of an extremity may need assistance in learning to use a prosthesis. The possibilities for rehabilitation are extensive, because cancer can be located in any part of the body (Chapter 83).

Rehabilitation in Respiratory Disorders

The rehabilitation team has intense involvement with clients who have chronic respiratory disorders, such as CF, or a chronic obstructive pulmonary disease (COPD), such as emphysema. These clients need chest physiotherapy, postural drainage, breathing exercises, inhalation treatments, spirometry exercises, and special medications (Chapter 86).

Psychiatric Rehabilitation

Most people with disorders in mental health are now living as members of the greater community, rather than in institutions. Some require a payee (Chapters 95 and 96) to manage money. Others only require instruction and supervision in IADLs, such as grocery shopping, meal preparation, laundry, money management, medication administration, and managing public transportation. They are then able to live on their own, or with minimal guidance, without further formal services. Other clients require ongoing community services and support and may require a more structured living situation. Programs, such as assisted living, homemaking, meal delivery, and ombudsperson/social service contacts, may be all that are needed for the client to stay out of the hospital. A case manager, the first line of contact, helps to determine the services needed. A major nursing role in management and rehabilitation of the client with mental health issues often involves assistance with medication setup, supervision of medication compliance, or biweekly injections of long-acting antipsychotic medications. The nurse often sets up the client's medications weekly and can determine if the client has been taking their medications as ordered. Clients taking the medication clozapine (Clozaril) require a weekly blood draw, in order to continue receiving the medication. The nurse also observes clients for adverse medication side effects. The home nurse or case manager evaluates all clients to determine if they are managing adequately in the community or if hospitalization is needed. Some mental health clients also need assistance in managing physical problems such as diabetes, asthma, high blood pressure, urinary incontinence, or electrolyte imbalance. If a client with a psychiatric disability cannot live independently, they may live in an extended-care facility, such as a nursing home, group home, or board-and-care home. These facilities are briefly described in Chapters 94 and 95.

> **Key Concept**
>
> Be respectful to any person who is physically or mentally disabled. Allow all people to maintain personal dignity. Offer to assist clients, if needed, but do not force your help. Do not touch the person's equipment or service animal. *Rationale: Many clients consider equipment as an extension of themselves. It is important not to distract the service animal.* (In addition, the service animal is often trained to protect the client and may misunderstand your intentions.) It is recommended to refer to such clients as "a person with a disability," rather than as a "disabled person." (Each person has many abilities and only a few disabilities.)

COMMUNITY RESOURCES

Members of the rehabilitation team help explore community resources with the client and family, to plan for care and discharge. Public health nurses can be involved in preparing clients for home care, giving clients and their families complete instructions and required teaching. It is important to give them opportunities to return demonstrations (Chapter 98). Family members are encouraged to be active participants in care while clients are in a rehabilitation center. By doing so, family members will have a clear understanding of the client's limitations and capabilities and of how to perform needed treatments after discharge. Public health nursing and home care services can assist these clients and caregivers. Available home care services include home nursing; home health aide or homemaker services; social work; and physical, occupational, and speech therapy.

The Case Manager

Nearly all clients require a *case manager* or *care manager* (CM), at least early in the rehabilitation process. This is a specific requirement for reimbursement by Medicare and Medicaid. However, agencies appoint case managers for other clients as well. The case manager oversees the care and treatment of the client and acts as the client's advocate.

> **Key Concept**
>
> Facilities to assist people with disabilities are available at no cost or for a minimal fee. For example, Shriners Hospitals throughout the country provide free hospitalization, surgery, and rehabilitation for children with physical disabilities. Rehabilitation facilities, such as the Courage (Sister) Kenny Institute in Minneapolis, often operate on a sliding-fee scale, based on the client's ability to pay.

Various health agencies, service organizations, and private companies have equipment, such as hospital beds or wheelchairs, available for loan, rent, or purchase. Almost every person can regain a certain amount of function by using special devices and aids. An occupational therapy assessment of the home is particularly helpful in recommending adaptations for the homemaker (Chapter 96). The government provides vocational rehabilitation testing and counseling services and financial aid for retraining.

Most young people who are physically or mentally disabled attend regular classes in schools. This is called **mainstreaming**. These young people participate in school activities and mingle with others their own age. In some cases, they have a full-time aide to assist them.

Legislation

The Americans with Disabilities Act of 1990 sets many standards to assist persons with disabilities. Many laws exist to reduce discrimination against people with disabilities and assist them to live more independently. Not only does this reduce tax burdens but it also enhances client self-esteem.

Architectural Barriers

Legislation is in place to make public buildings accessible and safe for all people. All new construction of public buildings in the United States must include wheelchair ramps, elevators, and pneumatic doors. Streets must have graduated areas, rather than curbs, to accommodate wheelchairs and walkers. This reduction of **architectural barriers** has enabled many people with disabilities to become employed and to lead more satisfying and productive lives. Removal of architectural barriers also allows people to do everyday things such as shopping, going to school and places of worship, or attending athletic events and concerts. Legislation to prevent architectural barriers varies somewhat between the states and provinces. It is important to evaluate the laws in your area; you can then contact local lawmakers if there are inappropriate situations.

Parking for People With Disabilities

Clients with mobility limitations are eligible for special parking permits. Areas near all public buildings must have designated parking for people with "handicap" parking stickers or license plates. These areas must have ramps over curbs and extra space for car doors to open and for wheelchairs and scooters to maneuver. It is illegal for anyone else to park in designated "wheelchair" spots, even for a few minutes. Most states impose substantial fines for violations.

Report anyone who illegally uses these designated parking spaces.

Preferential Seating

Airlines and other public transportation vehicles are required to reserve easily accessible seats for people with disabilities. For example, bulkhead seats on an airplane may be more comfortable for persons with leg braces or artificial limbs. Many buses have lifts, allowing the loading of persons in wheelchairs; they also designate special seating. Sports arenas, restaurants, and theaters have spaces for people using wheelchairs, with adjacent seats for persons accompanying them.

Rest Rooms

Public buildings are required to have rest rooms that are accessible to persons with disabilities. In some cases, these are used by all people; in other cases, separate rest rooms are set aside for persons in wheelchairs and with other disabilities. Able-bodied people should not use separate specially designated rest rooms, so they remain available for those who particularly need them. Most hotels have at least one room designated for use by persons with disabilities. However, these rooms vary in appropriateness and are not always totally accessible.

BARRIERS TO REHABILITATION

Some clients encounter obstacles that interfere with their access to rehabilitation services.

Legislative Barriers

The laws relating to delivery of, and reimbursement for, rehabilitation and long-term care services are continually changing. Changes in the *prospective payment system* (PPS) are continually being proposed and written into law and into the rules and regulations of agencies such as Medicare. For example, since October 2000, home care services have been paid on a PPS basis by Medicare (Chapter 98). This system also exists in most extended-care facilities. As eligibility requirements change, the pool of clients served also will change. Clients may find this confusing and cumbersome, as well as frightening.

> **Key Concept**
>
> With the aging of the population in the United States and Canada, the need for rehabilitation services is increasing and will continue to increase in the future. Nurses will find many opportunities for employment in these areas. It is important to keep informed about changing legislation and regulations.

Agencies delivering rehabilitation services often find the amount of required paperwork overwhelming. Nurses may be frustrated by the amount of time spent filing reimbursement requests and filling out forms, instead of delivering client care.

Financial Barriers

The cost of long-term care and rehabilitation services is staggering. Many families do not have adequate insurance coverage and cannot afford needed care. In many cases, a person's entire life savings is used to pay for one illness or rehabilitation after an injury. Many people now have long-term care insurance to assist with this possibility. (See also Chapter 99.) Some financial reimbursement/assistance programs exist to help with payment for rehabilitation services:

- Private insurance
- Medicare or Medicaid reimbursement
- Organizational support, such as homes sponsored by an organization, church, or an employer. If the resident's funds are depleted, the client will continue to be cared for by the organization.
- Subsidized coverage; payment based on a "sliding scale"
- Long-term care insurance
- Care paid for totally by personal finances

Attitudinal Barriers

Some clients and families are embarrassed about requiring rehabilitation services. They may feel they should be able to take care of a family member without assistance and may feel guilty when this is not possible. Many people feel they should be able to keep aging family members at home, even though they require full-time nursing care.

A client may also feel guilty about the amount of family time and money being spent on their care; this affects the entire family dynamics. Some clients become very depressed and may "give up," making rehabilitation difficult, increasing their risk of suicide. These clients may be so devastated by the illness or injury that they do not have the energy to begin or continue the slow process of rehabilitation. Body image is often greatly affected by a disability, especially if a young person has been seriously injured or paralyzed. This constitutes a barrier to rehabilitation, if the person is not able to accept the situation and the limitations it imposes. Rehabilitation is hard work and requires the client's cooperation and effort. In some cases, family members are not supportive or are unable to assist with care. In the case of many older people, a suitable primary caregiver is not available. The spouse and any children the couple have may also be older and unable to care for their family member. The person's younger relatives are often living in another area, may have small children, and may be working full time, making them unable to provide care.

> **Nursing Alert** Be aware that suicide is a genuine concern for the client who must undergo a long rehabilitation or who has a progressively worsening condition. Assess the client and refer them to a counselor, if necessary.

Educational Barriers

Some people may not realize the benefits of rehabilitation services. It is also difficult for some people to understand that the sooner the rehabilitation begins, the more likely it is to be effective. An important component of nursing care is to educate clients and their families about the goals and benefits of rehabilitation.

It is the job of the rehabilitation team to work with clients and families in an effort to eliminate the barriers to rehabilitation and to encourage the client to live a happy and productive life.

> **Key Concept**
> Remember to consider the client's ethnic and religious background when planning, carrying out, or evaluating rehabilitation or long-term care. Reactions to illness or injury or to the rehabilitation process may be cultural, rather than personal.

STUDENT SYNTHESIS

KEY POINTS

- Rehabilitation aims to restore a person to full functioning or to maximize the client's remaining abilities.
- It is important to focus on *abilities,* rather than disabilities. Everyone has skills and positive attributes, no matter what they can and cannot do. Reinforce the positives with all clients.
- Professionals from many different disciplines function as part of the rehabilitation team.
- The client and primary caregivers are vital members of the rehabilitation team.
- Clients and families often work through predictable stages of grief in dealing with serious illness or disabling injury.
- Rehabilitation team members assist clients in performing strengthening exercises, to prevent falls or other injuries and to provide mobility.
- A multitude of adaptive materials are available to assist the person with a disability to perform ADLs and engage in diversional activities.
- Many pieces of equipment, including wheelchairs, scooters, walkers, splints, braces, lifts, and adapted automobile controls, help provide mobility to people with disabilities. Many of these items may be used by able-bodied people as well.
- It is important to work toward an environment free of architectural barriers.
- Continence management is a major component of rehabilitation and may determine whether or not the client can live at home.
- Many community resources and agencies are available to assist people who have disabilities or chronic conditions and their families.

CRITICAL THINKING EXERCISES

1. A young married client with paraplegia is concerned about their sexuality and sexual activity. Anticipate what questions they might ask. Formulate possible answers.

2. A.Y., a 34-year-old from Ethiopia, has been in the United States for 7 months. A.Y.'s family is still in Ethiopia. A.Y. was planning to return home next week, when their visa expires. Three weeks ago, A.Y. sustained a severe spinal cord injury and a fractured right femur in a motor vehicle crash. They were transferred to your rehabilitation unit after the acute period of stabilization. They have been classified as paraplegic, although they have some sensation in his legs. The healthcare providers believe they will eventually be able to achieve bowel and bladder control, but will require extensive rehabilitation (at least 3–4 months). They will also require special equipment, such as a motorized wheelchair. A.Y. has no difficulty breathing or eating. Their skin is intact, except for one small reddened area on their coccyx. They speak almost no English. They are unemployed and experiencing homelessness.
   a. Describe major aspects of A.Y.'s care that the team needs to address in the care plan.
   b. How would you expect A.Y.'s care plan to evolve in your rehabilitation unit?
   c. Discuss the following aspects of A.Y.'s care: mobility, bowel and bladder continence, sexuality, skin integrity, nutrition, communication, diversion, emotional and financial support, and spirituality.
   d. Which type of living arrangements might be available for A.Y. after discharge from the rehabilitation unit?
   e. Research immigration laws to determine which steps need to be taken on A.Y.'s behalf. Which options are available to A.Y. regarding remaining in the United States for rehabilitation?
   f. Explore options for assisting A.Y. to return to Ethiopia for rehabilitation.
   g. Which continuing care and services might be required for A.Y. after discharge from the rehabilitation center?

3. Imagine you are caring for a client who uses a wheelchair. Go to several public buildings in your area that the client may need to access on a regular basis. Which architectural barriers do you notice? What resources might be needed for this client? Discuss your findings and your personal feelings with your classmates.

NCLEX-STYLE REVIEW QUESTIONS

1. The nurse is caring for a client who is admitted to the rehabilitation facility after a stroke. Which outcome does the nurse anticipate will be achieved for this client? Select all that apply.
   a. The client will not require assistance with activities of daily living (ADLs).
   b. The client will not have another stroke.
   c. The client will regain former abilities.
   d. The client will regain a level of independence.
   e. The client will adjust to the disability.

2. The nurse in a rehabilitation facility is caring for a client who sustained a cervical spine injury resulting in quadriplegia. Which action is the highest priority of care?
   a. Ensuring adequate bowel/bladder function
   b. Providing diversional activities
   c. Maintenance of a patent airway
   d. Providing skin care

3. A client with hemiplegia is being taught how to dress more easily and independently. How would the nurse demonstrate this skill to the client?
   a. Use a tool, such as tongs, to place the clothing on the body.
   b. Place the clothing on the unaffected arm or leg first.
   c. Have someone else dress the client.
   d. Place clothing on the affected arm or leg first.

4. According to Maslow hierarchy of needs, which need would be a priority in the acute phase of rehabilitation?
   a. Maintenance of a patent airway
   b. Bathing the client
   c. Dressing in appropriate clothing
   d. Adequate communication

5. The nurse is performing passive range of motion exercises for a client who is immobile. Which response by the nurse is best when the client states, "Why are you doing this?"
   a. "It will prevent you from developing pneumonia."
   b. "It will improve appetite and increase metabolism."
   c. "It will prevent skin breakdown."
   d. "It will prevent joint stiffness and muscle atrophy."

CHAPTER RESOURCES

Enhance your learning with additional resources on thePoint!

Student Resources related to this chapter can be found at **thePoint.lww.com/Rosdahl12e**.

98 Home Care Nursing

Learning Objectives

1. Identify the reasons for, and benefits of, home care.
2. Describe situations in which home care might be most appropriate.
3. Identify healthcare workers who might be involved in home care.
4. Identify common nursing functions in home care.
5. Discuss important safety practices for home care nurses.
6. Describe and discuss the influences of regulatory and funding agencies on delivery of home healthcare.
7. Describe recent changes in reimbursement for home care; discuss the impact of these changes on clients and on the healthcare system.
8. Discuss the concept of self-management of chronic conditions.
9. Describe the importance of family caregivers in home care.

Acronyms

ACH
CHHA
CNO
DME
FFS
HCA
HCSF
HHA
HHRG
ICD
NAHC
OASIS-D
PPS
PRM
UTF
VBP

Home care is very important in the trend to offer most healthcare within an individual's own community. Some people are able to receive all healthcare while living at home and are never admitted to the acute care hospital. Thus, fewer clients are being admitted to acute care hospitals, and those who are admitted are being discharged sooner, with more technical healthcare needs. These clients are then transferred to a skilled nursing facility (*SNF*) or directly to home care, as a *complex client*. Home care agencies report that they are receiving an increasing number of referrals from SNFs. Home healthcare consists of part-time, medically necessary skilled care (including nursing, physical, occupational, and speech-language therapy), and specialties, such as wound care, ordered by a primary provider. Home care has also expanded to include more complex procedures, such as tapping a client's lungs to remove fluid, caring for drainage tubes, saline locks, intravenous (IV) lines with pumps, patient-controlled analgesia (PCA) pumps, catheters, supplementary oxygen, and other complicated equipment. Many ventilator-dependent children live at home. Home care nurses teach clients and families how to operate all types of equipment and reinforce teaching given in hospitals, as well as supervising and documenting care given at home. The instrument/data collection tool used to collect and report performance data by home health agencies is called OASIS-D, discussed later.

Home care continues to be one of the fastest-growing fields in nursing today. According to U.S. Government data (www.cms.gov), in 2017, there were 11,593 Medicare-certified home health agencies in the United States, and nearly 4.5 million clients were served, with nearly 122.6 million visits made (Centers for Disease Control, 2016). The employment growth rate for home care is greater than that for the overall healthcare industry. (Hospital employment is expanding the least.) In addition to community-based home care agencies, extended-care facilities (ECFs) may also offer home care as one of their services. The National Association for Home Care (**NAHC**) is concerned with the delivery of home care. In some states, for example, in New Jersey, "Hospice" has been added to agency names (e.g., Home Care and Hospice Agency). Able Care Connect Home Health in Minnesota states they offer "...a large scope of services ranging from minimal assistance to skilled clinical professionals." Services includes skilled nursing, occupational therapy, home health aides, fall prevention, case management, and medication set up. (Able Care Home Health, n.d.). Another agency, *Visiting Angels*, states, "We're all About Relationships," and offers many services (www.visitingangels.com).

REASONS FOR HOME CARE

The scope of work (SOW) of the *CMS* (Centers for Medicare and Medicaid Services) gives home care agencies the directive and responsibility to *reduce unnecessary and avoidable hospital readmissions*. (Approximately one fifth of clients return to the hospital within 30 days; many have not seen their primary provider since discharge.) Because acute care hospitalization (**ACH**) is one of the publicly reported measures (**PRM**) or *quality indicators* of home care, the avoidance of unnecessary hospital readmissions is vital for home health agencies (**HHAs**) and SNFs. Funding of these agencies depends partially on the percentage of ACH readmissions. HHAs are being asked to consider their role along the healthcare continuum—particularly their role in preventive care (Fig. 96-1). HHAs are charged with preparing the client/caregivers to be better able to *self-manage chronic conditions* upon discharge from the HHA. There is also increased interest in providing all primary care in clients' homes, particularly for those clients who would find it physically difficult or too expensive to get to the provider's office (e.g., those requiring special "handicap" transportation). However, there are also related liability concerns. For example, it is difficult to monitor care being given by family members.

In rare cases, home care nurses and assistants provide 24-hr nursing care in the client's home. Most often, services are intermittent. Clients may receive assisted living services, which allow them to live independently (Chapter 96). Home care may be given on a long-term basis, as intermittent services, or on a short-term basis for just a few visits. Box 98-1 lists selected characteristics and advantages of home care.

TYPES OF AGENCIES AND SERVICES

Several types of agencies provide home care services. If an agency is called a "home health agency" or "visiting nurse service," it is usually certified as a Community Nursing Organization (**CNO**). (If Medicare reimbursement is used for funding, the pay for performance [P4P] program must be in place [Chapter 96].) In some cases, the term *value-based purchasing* (**VBP**) is used. Some agencies also are certified by The Joint Commission (formerly: Joint Commission on Accreditation of Healthcare Organizations [JCAHO]). Other agencies are licensed by their state, province, or territory health department. The services provided by agencies vary and range from total physical care to homemaking or shopping assistance only. Other services include mental health counseling; social work; hospice care; occupational, physical, and speech therapy; companions; and the administration of IV medications or drawing blood. Some agencies also provide respite care for caregivers. Many home care agencies also have access to rental equipment, such as hospital beds or wheelchairs. (This equipment, called durable medical equipment [**DME**], is now being highly regulated because of fraud and previous abuse of the system.)

Long-Term Home Care

Older clients or people with chronic, disabling conditions (often cardiac disorders) may require long-term care in their homes. Long-term services include periodic nursing assessment and case management, with homemaking and personal care services provided. Nurses may assist with "restorative nursing," such as assisting with exercises to maintain muscle integrity (Chapter 97). In some cases, clients with multiple chronic conditions can receive palliative care, while still receiving curative care. Some clients requiring long-term services receive care 24 hr a day or for 8- or 12-hr shifts, but usually this total care is not provided by the home care agency. In some cases, families participate by providing care during the day, with nurses on duty at night so the family can rest. Hospice care, to assist terminally ill clients and their families, is usually delivered in the client's home, although it may also occur in a nursing home, shelter, or other facility, such as a jail. Third-party payors often pay for all or part of hospice care (Chapter 100).

Box 98-1 Characteristics of Home Care

- Third-party payors require early discharge from hospitals, so clients are discharged while they are still ill or recovering. Clients often need assistance with postoperative care and/or self-care activities.
- New mothers may require assistance during the first few days at home because obstetrical stays are usually 24 hr or less.
- Some people are never admitted to the hospital but receive their entire care at home or as outpatients. This includes same-day/ambulatory surgical clients.
- The aging population is increasing. Older people often have physical disorders and require high-level management and assistance for chronic illness and *comorbidity* (coexisting disorders).
- Clients may not have available family caregivers, requiring more healthcare attention from nurses, aides, and volunteers.
- Sophisticated electronic equipment allows clients to receive complex care at home. Most of this equipment can be managed by nonprofessionals after receiving adequate instruction. The nurse is available to supervise and answer questions.
- Telehealth (telemedicine) allows nurses and clients to transmit information (e.g., electrocardiograms [ECGs], blood pressure readings) by telephone, computer, or video to hospitals or providers' for interpretation. Many client conditions can be monitored electronically. Telehealth is not used only in rural areas but is an excellent way to supplement (not replace) home care in all areas. It is vital in management of chronic conditions and helps prevent unnecessary hospital readmissions. Regularly scheduled phone visits between the nurse and client can help the client to self-manage care between actual home visits.
- Digital cameras record information, such as the condition of a wound, and the image is transmitted electronically for evaluation. It can also be saved and used to compare with past and future photos, to evaluate wound healing (or lack of healing).

ADVANTAGES OF HOME CARE
- Home care is less expensive than hospital or nursing home care.
- Nurses, support personnel, and caregivers can provide continuous care from hospital to home and until the client's recovery or death.
- Many people are more comfortable receiving care in their own home, surrounded by loved ones, friends, and pets. The surroundings and foods are familiar and comfortable.
- Many clients prefer to die at home. Home care agencies often provide hospice care (Chapter 100).
- Clients and families experience less emotional strain at home because they avoid separation.

There is a limited role for LVN/LPNs in Certified Home Health Agencies. However, there is a role in Health Care Service Firms (**HCSF**). This includes working with special needs children and adults and LTC clients without "high-level skilled" needs. This depends somewhat on the licensing agency, either the Division of Consumer Affairs or the Department of Health.

TELEHEALTH

The concept of *telehealth* (health monitoring and counseling via telephone or video) is described briefly in Chapter 99. Telehealth is particularly useful in home care for the management of chronic illnesses, providing contact with healthcare staff and monitoring of data, such as vital signs, between home visits. This frequent contact can help greatly in preventing unnecessary hospital readmissions. Clients can also make appointments with the home care nurse for planned telehealth counseling between home visits. In addition, the nurse is available on call, if the client has concerns or questions.

Children With Special Healthcare Needs

As stated above, some children with special needs require nursing care, around the clock or for part of the day. This provides an increasing employment opportunity for LVN/LPNs, as the acuity level for clients in home care increases. (A home health aide is often not qualified to care for these children.) The child with severe disabilities usually will need an attendant in school as well. In rare situations, home care staff is in the client's home 24 hr a day. This may continue for a long time. Unique adjustments are required for this family, who is never alone.

SELF-MANAGEMENT OF CHRONIC CONDITIONS

Self-management of chronic conditions has become a *major priority* in healthcare. The client and caregivers learn how to manage special equipment and to perform special procedures needed by the client. They are also taught to recognize deviations from the client's baseline condition and request assistance when needed. Medication reconciliation and management are essential components of self-management. The home care nurse is vital in client self-care—teaching the client and caregivers, monitoring the delivery of care, and responding when questions or concerns arise. In this way, many clients are managed at home, thus avoiding costly, uncomfortable, and unnecessary rehospitalization.

> **NCLEX Alert**
> It is important to be alert to the need for clients/families/caregivers to learn to manage chronic conditions at home—their ability to deliver care and monitor signs and symptoms of the client's status. Your role in teaching self-management skills may be integrated into the NCLEX examination.

Intermittent or Short-Term Home Care

When a client receives short-term services or intermittent care, the nurse provides care in the home for a short time or provides care at specific intervals. Examples include the following:

- Home visits two to three times a week for assessment, administration of special medications or treatments, or to draw blood
- Weekly home visits to assist in setting up medications for the next week
- A very limited number of home visits to assist a new parent
- Dressing changes and wound inspection once or twice daily, for 1–2 weeks after surgery
- Administering IV medications
- Administering and reading skin tests, such as PPD for tuberculosis or allergy tests, or administering immunizations (e.g., flu shots to seniors)
- Administering a periodic electrocardiogram (ECG), usually transmitted electronically for interpretation
- A periodic home visit, to evaluate care given by family caregivers

> **Key Concept**
> Many clients can self-manage care with only weekly medication setup. Each day's medications are placed in a marked box, with divisions for time of day (Fig. 92-1). This helps clients to remember to take medications and avoid double-dosing. The nurse checks the box, to see if medications have been taken.

Centers of Excellence

The center of excellence (COE) concept has been previously described, in connection with rehabilitation. (These COEs are sometimes called *institutes*.) The COE concept also functions in home care. A team of nurses with specific expertise assists local nurses with procedures. COE nurses may make home visits or may serve as consultants to local home care nurses.

The expertise of a COE team may include the following:

- Wound care
- Continence care and bowel/bladder retraining
- IV and other high-technology care
- Psychiatric management and crisis intervention
- Maternal–child healthcare or maternity consultation
- Pediatric high technology, including care of ventilator-dependent children

PAYMENT FOR HOME CARE

A prospective payment system **(PPS)** for home care was instituted by Medicare in October 2000 and represented a major change in home care reimbursement (called **FFS**—fee for service). FFS is now by *episode*, rather than for each visit, as it was previously. Clients with managed Medicare or another insurer may be charged a co-pay, either per visit or per day. Payment for several services in 1 day saves money but requires collaboration among disciplines, so they all visit on the same day (avoiding multiple co-pay fees). It is important to note that when too many professionals visit on the same day, this can be very exhausting for the client and family. Clients may also deny needed home care because of cost and because they do not understand the importance of home care. (Clients tend to see home care as optional, whereas they consider hospital care necessary.)

Another development in the reimbursement system is called P4P (Chapter 96). In P4P (pay for performance), payment is based not only on diagnosis but also on the quality of care provided to Medicare beneficiaries. This care is evaluated by a number of *publicly reported measures* (PRM), aimed at improving clients' quality of life, while reducing costs.

Payment is based on selected **OASIS-D** (**O**utcome and **AS**sessment **I**nformation **S**et) measures, new versions of which become effective periodically. These measures are based on *outcome, process, and utilization of resources* (based on effectiveness, efficiency, equity, safety, timeliness, and client-centeredness).

OASIS considers the total client by looking at the client's functional ability and available support systems (service needs). OASIS requires minimum baseline data to be obtained on all Medicare clients at Start of Care, Resumption of Care, Follow-up Assessments, Transfer to an Inpatient Facility, and Discharge from a Home Health Agency (not to an inpatient facility). OASIS outlines specifics, to encourage providers to be more consistent in their assessments and to use the same terminology, particularly for pressure wound assessment. (Usually, the initial assessment is performed by an RN or physical therapist, with interim data gathered by other healthcare workers, including LVN/LPNs.) All PRMs (Publicly Reported Measures) are aimed at improvement in the percentage of clients who are able to self-manage all or part of their own care. The global health information standard for mortality and morbidity statistics is called the **ICD** (International Classification of Diseases). The ICD is used to define diseases, study disease patterns, and to manage healthcare and monitor results. In 2015, the ICD-10 became the version universally used. Key PRMs include the following (in all cases, the goal is *improvement in self-care*):

- Improvement in ambulation
- Improvement in bathing
- Improvement in transferring (e.g., bed to chair, chair to toilet)
- Improvement in management of oral medication (independent, safe, and correct administration)
- Reduction in pain interfering with daily activities
- Reduction in acute care hospital readmissions
- Reduction in use of emergent care (e.g., urgent care or emergency department)
- Discharge to the community (total self-management of care)
- Improvement in dyspnea (shortness of breath)
- Improvement in urinary incontinence (increase in percentage of previously incontinent clients who are now continent)
- Improvement in wound status (percentage of clients with improvement and/or healing of wounds). A *negative PRM* is the percentage of clients who need unplanned medical care related to wounds that are new, are worse, or have become infected.
- Reduction in use of care for wound deterioration (worsening wounds)

Prospective payment systems (PPS and P4P) begin by evaluating the case mix, according to clinical, functional, and service needs. After OASIS data are collected, the client is assigned to a home health resource group (**HHRG**) for a given episode of care, which is usually a 60-day period. Predetermined and standardized reimbursement rates are established for each client, based on data from the OASIS and the ICD. Another factor in development of the PPS was the realization that the nurse cannot do everything for the client. It is the role of the nurse to educate and prepare the family to learn about, understand, and manage their loved one's care. The family is included in the system, rather than the nursing staff trying "to do it all."

National programs aimed at improvement of home healthcare quality are as follows:

- INTERACT II, developed by the Georgia QIO: to decrease avoidable hospital readmissions from home care and SNFs
- Home Health Quality Improvement National Campaign and Advancing Excellence in America's Nursing Homes: to improve clients' self-management of oral medications and improve care and transfers from one healthcare setting to another

The CMS is working to ensure that beneficiaries receive the *right care at the right time in the right setting*, while reducing avoidable or unnecessary hospital readmissions. It is vital that providers understand the environment and processes of each type of care, in order to recommend appropriate and safe care. Communication between sites is essential.

MEMBERS OF THE HOME CARE TEAM

In addition to healthcare providers and other primary providers, family caregivers, RNs, LVN/LPNs, and many other members compose the home care team. They include physical, occupational, and speech therapists; wound care and cardiovascular specialists, social workers; dietitians; chaplains; healthcare assistants (**HCAs**) or personal care attendants (PCAs); home health aides or certified home health aides (**CHHAs**); companions; and volunteers. All these individuals work with clients. Some agencies employ a gerontology specialist because many home care clients are seniors (Chapters 92 and 93). Team members hold regular meetings to discuss each client's case. (Not all members serve on all cases.) Team members report the client's progress and plan future care. The client/family, case manager, and team jointly determine when and if the client should be discharged from the service. In some cases, a third-party payor determines the number of visits allowed for a specific type of case.

> **NCLEX Alert**
>
> It is important to know who the members of the home care team are and the importance of communication among them, to develop, implement, and evaluate the client's plan of care. This may impact the identification of your nursing role as you review NCLEX examination scenarios, relating to principles of safe and effective care and coordination/continuity of care.

Case Management

As presented in Chapter 96, each home care client has a case manager or care manager (CM). In many states and provinces, this must be an RN. In some cases, the CM is a social worker or physical therapist. The CM makes an initial home assessment visit and evaluates the safety of the home and competency of available caregivers. Often, the CM determines the client's eligibility for services, sometimes in conjunction with the team, and the necessary and available nursing/therapy care needs are determined. The team assists caregivers to obtain needed equipment and makes suggestions about the home setup to provide optimal client care. The CM is required to visit the client at specific intervals, to determine if the client's healthcare goals are being met and documented appropriately and if funding requirements are being satisfied. (The CM may be the primary home care nurse, or some responsibilities may be delegated.) It is important to note that when care is delegated to aides or other members of the team, this care must be within the scope of practice of the delegated person.

> **Key Concept**
>
> Remember that the client and family caregivers are vital members of the team and are considered "co-care managers." It is important to reinforce self-management of chronic conditions. This includes teaching regarding medications and interpretation of test results, demonstrating procedures, observing return demonstrations, providing pertinent and constructive feedback, and rechecking periodically to make sure appropriate care is still being given.

Role of the LVN/LPN

Federal Medicare regulations identify the following standard duties of the LVN/LPN in home care:

- Furnish services, in accordance with agency policies.
- Prepare clinical and progress notes.
- Assist providers and RNs to perform specialized procedures.
- Prepare equipment and materials for treatments, observing aseptic technique as required.
- Assist clients in learning appropriate self-care techniques.

LVN/LPNs are required to practice within the guidelines of the state, commonwealth, territory, or province's nursing practice legislation and according to specified agency policies. LPNs and CHHAs serve as team members, under the supervision of the CM. All staff working in home care encounter special challenges and should possess specific qualifications. These include the ability to get along with people, high motivation, self-direction, the ability to make sound decisions, and maturity. Home care staff need to know when to ask questions or request assistance and must be familiar with community and medical resources. It is important to remember that *excellent communication* is vital in home care. This includes the entire spectrum—communication with the client and family, with the primary provider, and with therapists and other healthcare workers. In addition, communication must exist between home care nurses and all workers in the client's previous or subsequent settings. (Remember: Care takes place in many places other than the client's home, including ECFs, jails, homeless shelters, and schools.)

> **Nursing Alert** It is highly recommended that the new graduate, whether LPN or RN, gain added clinical experience before being employed in home care. The level of autonomy requires a very sound clinical background, which often must be enhanced after graduation.

NURSING DUTIES IN HOME CARE

The nurse working in home care will be required to perform many skills learned in the basic nursing program. However, the home care nurse functions *independently* and must possess a high level of independence, as well as sound judgment. Working in the home setting, the nurse is more isolated than in the hospital or ECF. Therefore, it is important that home care nurses have a thorough knowledge of state and agency policies and protocols. It is also important to maintain personal safety.

Functions of the Home Care Nurse

The LVN/LPN performing home care must work closely with the CM. Nursing activities and skills commonly used in home care include the following:

- Coordinating care with hospital and medical staff and agency resource people.
- Providing client and family teaching about procedures and recognition of symptoms. It is important to call the CM first with any questions, so the CM can add or adjust a visit and prevent a trip to the ED or hospital readmission. The CM can instruct caregivers when to report to the primary provider. Document all teaching.
- Completing and submitting required forms and records to the healthcare agency.
- Counseling the client. The nurse is the liaison between the client and the healthcare system.
- Accurately gathering information about the client. Report untoward symptoms to the appropriate person.
- Evaluating the client's total home situation. Observe and evaluate care being given; safety, cleanliness, and appropriateness of the home; adequacy of the client's food and fluid intake; administration of medications; and diversionary activities. It is important to evaluate ongoing relationships between the client and caregivers.
- Performing nursing treatments, drawing blood for routine tests, supervising medication setup, documenting care, and evaluating client progress.
- Working in psychiatric outreach, visiting clients in the community, and recommending hospitalization when necessary. Screen for depression, medication side effects, or other untoward symptoms (Chapter 94).
- Performing a formal fall risk assessment on admission to the home care service and periodically thereafter (Chapter 48). Falls in the home are common and are often preventable.
- Evaluating the client's risk for skin breakdown; evaluating the healing process of existing wounds (Chapter 58).
- Suggesting necessary equipment or changes that might improve client care and the safety of the home. In some cases, the nurse will help improvise equipment (e.g., use a plastic lawn chair for a shower chair).
- Assisting caregivers to prepare the home for the client's arrival from the hospital or other facility.
- Observing for possible client abuse.
- Reassuring the client on the telephone. On days when visits are not scheduled, call and give support or answer questions, as necessary.

Box 98-2 Community Services Available to Home Care Clients

- Meals on Wheels, homemaking services, food shelf, free meals
- Transportation (specially equipped vans/buses) and escort services
- Grocery shopping and delivery; medication delivery
- Visiting pet therapy; helper animals
- Telephone safety, electronic alert equipment (e.g., "lifeline")
- Adult daycare and respite care for caregivers, senior centers
- Outpatient rehabilitation services
- Community centers, such as YMCA, for exercise and swimming; exercise groups; walking programs
- Outings and field trips for seniors and people with disabilities
- Internet resources, including support groups
- Free educational programs
- Support groups and therapy for clients and caregivers, chaplain and parish nurse services
- Low-cost medical, diabetic, and continence care supplies, rental/loaned equipment
- Adaptive equipment (Chapter 97)
- Equipment, such as computers or telephone aids, for persons with hearing or vision loss
- Screening for vision, hearing, diabetes, blood pressure, scoliosis, osteoporosis
- Free clinics and community health centers
- Volunteer services (including home repair and maintenance)
- Ombudsperson services and payee services (to help manage money)
- Programs to assist with housing (e.g., Habitat for Humanity, Domestic Peace Corps)
- Telehealth visits between home visits
- Telephone transmission of medical data for interpretation

- Determining how primary caregivers are doing. Are they having difficulty with the stress of caring for a loved one? Do they need respite care?
- Demonstrating knowledge of community resources (Box 98-2). Social workers often can make referrals. In some cases, a provider's order is required.

Nursing Alert When a client is admitted to home care, a risk assessment for hospital readmission is done. As discussed previously, this is becoming increasingly important, particularly in terms of reimbursement. In most cases, home care staff members have electronic access to previous hospital records, at least for a short time after hospital discharge. Some states have a Universal Transfer Form (*UTF*), to be completed when the client transfers from one facility to another or to home care.

In some cases, the client pays for home nursing. However, in most cases, a third-party payor is involved. In this case, the number and length of visits will be limited and strictly

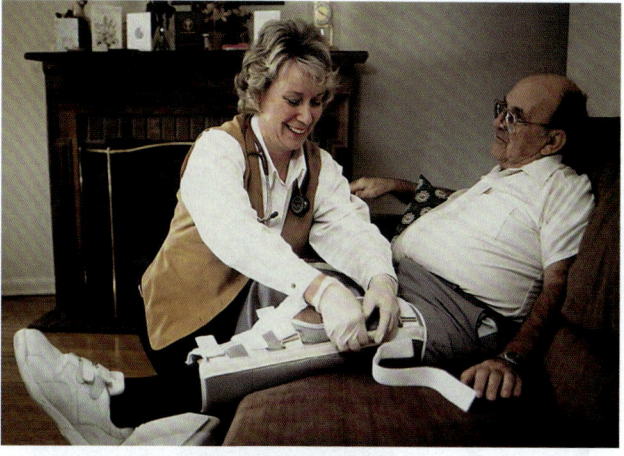

Figure 98-1 The home care nurse must exhibit effective communication skills, personal self-direction, and sound clinical judgment. A certified wound specialist or field nurse may take a photo of a wound while care is being given and transmit this information electronically to a specialist for evaluation.

regulated by the funding agency. The nurse will be expected to document the exact length of each visit and what procedures were performed.

Choosing Home Care as a Career

There are many reasons for a nurse to choose to work in home care. Hospital employment is less available. In addition, most clients are discharged from the hospital earlier, with many healthcare needs. These situations contribute to the many opportunities for the LVN/LPN to work in home care.

Advantages of working in home care include the following:

- The unique opportunity to care for a small number of clients. In the home, the nurse can get to know the client and family better.
- Greater flexibility in planning the workday.
- Being able to assist the client to remain at home, where they are most comfortable.

Disadvantages of working in home care include the following:

- Working alone much of the time
- Being required to be on call
- Providing personal transportation. (In some cities, public transportation is available; some agencies provide cars.)
- Personal safety issues
- The large amount of documentation required for the agency and third-party payors

Requirements for Home Nursing

The home care nurse must always use good judgment. This nurse must make independent decisions, but it is vital to base these decisions on sound nursing practice (Fig. 98-1). It is important to consult the CM if there are any questions or concerns. One of the most important responsibilities for the home care nurse is *dependability*. Clients

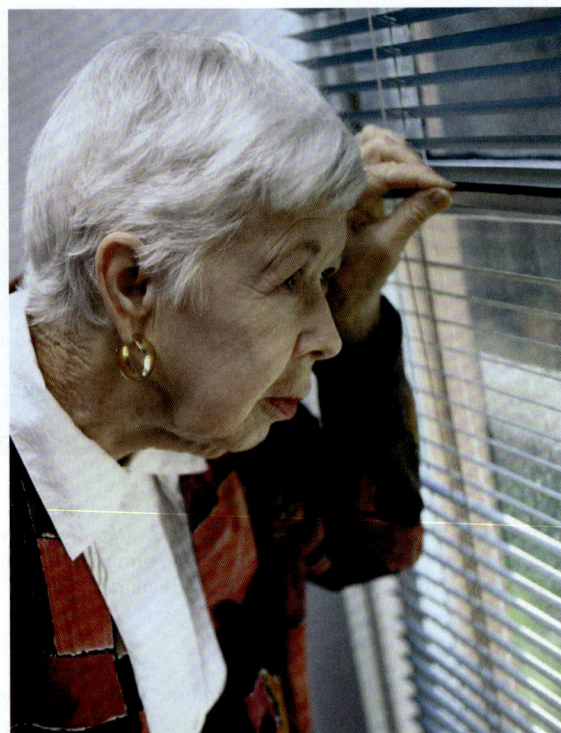

Figure 98-2 The home care client is often lonely and depends on the nurse's visit. If you leave a client alone and without adequate assistance, you are guilty of *abandonment*. (Carter, 2005.)

and families look forward to the arrival of the home care nurse. It is important to let them know when you are coming and to always come at the appointed time (Fig. 98-2).

Protocols and Procedures

Nurses in home care perform many of the same procedures used in other healthcare settings. Home care agencies have guidelines or nursing protocols for specific procedures. A number of reference books that can assist the nurse to adapt nursing care to the home setting are also available. Home care agencies have equipment available to be used when making home visits. It is important to know what equipment and supplies you need and to ensure they are available. Always use Standard Precautions and guard against spreading contamination among clients.

In many agencies, electronic health records (EHR) are used. Computer linkage among providers, pharmacists, therapists, home care staff, and other agencies provides greater communication between agencies and greater safety for clients. For example, a "red flag" may come up signaling a potentially inappropriate medication, a drug interaction, or client allergy.

> **Key Concept**
>
> It may be necessary to adjust procedures when caring for a client at home. However, it is important to remember the *underlying rationales* behind procedures. Although the nurse may need to adjust the way a procedure is performed in the home, it is vital not to jeopardize the client's safety. Always consult the CM or supervisor if you have a question.

Transition Between Care Sites

When a client is transitioned from one care site to another, communication between sites is vital, to ensure safe and appropriate care and follow-up. The CMS encourages the increased use of technology, as a means of improving management of chronic illnesses, with the ultimate goal of reduction of avoidable hospital readmissions. The CMS also promotes activities such as increased immunization of seniors for diseases such as influenza and pneumonia, as well as improved communication at time of transition or "handover" (handoff) from hospital to ECF to home care or from provider to nurse. The UTF is helpful in standardizing information and preventing or identifying a deterioration of the client's condition. The QIOs in each state are also contracted by CMS to work with home care agencies (Chapter 96). An excellent resource for clients, caregivers, and home health staff is the Website, *Next Step in Care*. This site provides questions to ask when transitioning from one site to another. Review the SBAR communication technique in Box 96-2. The term *handover* implies involvement by both sender and receiver when a client is transferred from one care site to another. It is vital that the receiving caregiver hears and understands what the client needs and is able to provide that care. It is also important to allow the receiving caregiver to ask questions and clarify concerns. The client's information and health status *remains the responsibility of the sender* until the receiver understands and is able to provide needed care for the client or the client is able to perform self-care. It is also important for the nurse to understand client/caregivers' rights in the provision of primary care under the auspices of managed care.

SAFETY FOR THE HOME CARE TEAM

Preventing injury to healthcare workers is very important. When going into a home, the nurse is responsible for maintaining personal safety. Nurses often work alone. The agency usually conducts a risk assessment before sending a nurse into a home. In some cases, two healthcare workers visit together. Box 98-3 lists safety tips for nurses making home visits.

> **Key Concept**
>
> Be sure to "trust your instincts." If you are to visit a home and it does not look safe or feel right, check before entering. You always have the right to maintain your own safety.

SUGGESTIONS FOR PRIMARY CAREGIVERS

Many people care for their loved ones at home (Fig. 98-3). Often, the client has a long-standing disorder. Although rewarding, caring for someone is exhausting and challenging for caregivers, responsible for the client 24 hr a day. Caregivers need support and reassurance and often need a *respite* (break) to maintain their own physical and emotional health.

Box 98-3 Examples of Safety Guidelines for Home Care Nurses

- Wear a name badge that clearly identifies your name and employer. It is suggested to use only a first name and last initial, for safety reasons. Your professional status should be on the name tag (LPN, LVN, RN).
- Dress professionally. Dress slacks may be worn, to enable you to move more easily. (Jeans, shorts, sandals, halter tops, and bare midriffs are not appropriate.)
- Notify clients in advance, alerting them to the approximate time of your home visit and come on time. Obtain directions and ask about parking, if necessary.
- If a client owns a pet, ask the client to secure the animal properly before you come. If you are confronted with an aggressive dog or other animal, back away, but do not turn around and do not run. Do not make direct eye contact with a threatening dog. *Rationale: The dog may misinterpret this as a threat, precipitating an attack.*
- Some home care nurses carry mace or pepper spray. Be very careful with these items; make sure you are not downwind or that it is not stolen.
- Some agencies request that firearms be removed from the home before care can begin.
- Be alert to your surroundings, including other people in the home and when driving.
- Carry a cell phone and ensure that it is always charged. Have a car charger.
- Keep your vehicle in good working order, with plenty of gas. Always wear your seat belt.
- Lock your car at all times, with windows rolled up, both when driving and when parking.
- Park your car in a well-lighted place, in full view of the client's residence. Avoid parking in alleys or deserted streets, if at all possible.
- When exiting the car, have all equipment you need ready.
- Walk in a brisk, professional, businesslike manner directly to the client's residence. (Escort services may be available.)
- When passing a group of strangers, cross to the other side of the street, as appropriate, and keep eye contact with those in the group.
- Look before entering an elevator; in buildings, use common walkways, avoiding isolated stairs.
- Always knock or ring the doorbell and be acknowledged before entering a client's home.
- Have your car keys and cell phone in your hand when approaching your car. Look into your car before getting in, to make sure it is empty. Lock the car immediately on entering, before putting things away or starting the car. If someone threatens you, use the panic button on your car key fob.
- Check your agency's guidelines before giving a ride to a client or family member. *Rationale: Your insurance might not cover this situation.*
- Take a self-defense class. Learn to protect yourself. (Remember: An attacker cannot defend against a hard blow to the *side of the knee*, only to be used as a last resort.)

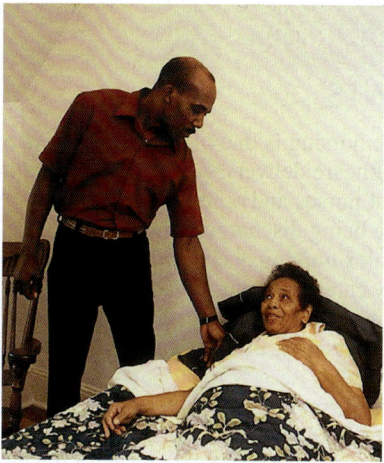

Figure 98-3 The role of family caregiver is vital in managing chronic illness at home. Many clients would not be able to live at home if a caregiver were not available.

Following are suggestions for caregivers, to fulfill their own needs:

- Manage stress. Plan daily recreational activities. If the client cannot be alone, the caregiver can do something such as read, knit, work puzzles, or call a friend while at the client's bedside.
- Maintain a sense of humor. It is often helpful to read cartoons or joke books or to watch comedies.
- Get plenty of exercise and as much fresh air as possible.
- Stretch and relax at intervals.
- Listen to soothing music while at the bedside. The client will also enjoy this.
- Eat a well-balanced diet (Chapter 30).
- Take vitamins or minerals, as prescribed.
- Maintain energy by eating several small meals daily.
- Use a minimum of salt, sugar, and caffeine.
- Avoid large weight gain or loss.
- Drink a variety of liquids, not just plain water.
- Avoid smoking and alcohol.
- Protect the back by using lift equipment and good body mechanics.
- Get plenty of rest and take naps.
- Get a checkup for physical complaints. Maintain immunizations, including flu, shingles, pneumonia, and other immunizations.
- Encourage the client's friends and family to visit. This provides a break for the caregiver and is enjoyable for the client.
- Take an occasional respite or time away. Hire someone to come in and help, if necessary. In some cases, volunteers are available.
- Keep a journal; this can be a tension reliever.
- Attend a support group or see a counselor. It is often very helpful to share one's feelings with others and learn that you are not alone.
- Respite care may be available at a local nursing home or other facility.

Always remember that primary caregivers are vital members of the healthcare team. To continue caring safely and comfortably for their family member, they must be able to maintain their own physical and emotional health.

STUDENT SYNTHESIS

KEY POINTS

- Home care nursing is one of the fastest-growing segments of the healthcare delivery system, employing increasing numbers of nurses and other workers.
- Clients are being discharged from acute care facilities with complex nursing needs, which home care workers and family caregivers must meet.
- Home care nurses sometimes have the opportunity to schedule hours and, in some cases, to structure their time.
- Home care nurses must be alert to untoward signs and symptoms and report them to the appropriate person.
- Many clients opt for home care because it is cost-effective and often more comfortable than hospital care.
- Various regulations often determine services available to Medicare clients.
- Quality of care given is evaluated by a definitive process, using specific outcome measures.
- Home care nurses are ultimately responsible for their own personal safety.
- Caregivers need to maintain their own health.

CRITICAL THINKING EXERCISES

1. L.J., an 82-year-old client, lives alone in a senior apartment complex. You are assigned to visit them once a week for a medication setup. Their prescribed medications include metformin (Glucophage), lisinopril (Prinivil), furosemide (Lasix), KCl (potassium chloride), and a multivitamin. When you stop at their home on Tuesday, you find that medications for 2 days last week are still in their daily containers. Their main supplies of lisinopril (Prinivil) and furosemide (Lasix) are gone. They state that they went with their family "for a few days to visit," but cannot remember when they returned. The client is "worried about money." They have very little food in the refrigerator. They are not wearing their TED socks. Their vision is quite poor, and they do not like to wear their hearing aids. They say their dentures "hurt their mouth." Their blood pressure is 210/148 mm Hg and her blood glucose is 184 mg/dL.
   a. Which actions would you take? In which order? Which client teaching is needed? What immediate actions are required?
   b. List nursing procedures that need to be performed.
   c. Which items might be on the agenda for a team meeting about L.J.? Who is likely to be invited to the meeting? What suggestions would you have? What possible outcomes can you envision for the meeting?
   d. Which medical conditions do you think L.J. is likely to have, based on the medications they are receiving? Which signs and symptoms would you particularly look for?
2. Describe ways to adapt a client's home to maximize the safety and independence of clients.

NCLEX-STYLE REVIEW QUESTIONS

1. The nurse is preparing to transition a client from the acute care facility to home with assistance from home health services. Which action is important for the nurse to do to take to ensure safe and appropriate follow-up care?
   a. Have a representative from the hospital go home with the client.
   b. Call the client the day after discharge to be sure the client is well.
   c. Communicate with the home health nurse prior to discharge.
   d. Call social service to make a home visit the next day.

2. The home health agency is preparing to dispatch the nurse to perform a new admission for home care. Which intervention would the nurse be sure is done before making this home visit?
   a. A risk assessment for the home has been performed.
   b. Make sure the client is able to pay for the visit.
   c. Have a police officer arranged to meet the nurse at the house.
   d. Have social service visit the client before the nurse is dispatched.

3. A family member caring for a client at home informs the nurse that caring for the client is exhausting because the client is unable to be left alone. Which suggestion can the nurse offer to alleviate the risk of caregiver burnout?
   a. Make a referral for respite care.
   b. Inform the caregiver that the client will not be around much longer.
   c. Tell the family member to leave the client home alone for brief periods.
   d. Tell the family member to find someone else to care for the client.

4. The LVN/LPN would like to work for a home health agency. Which opportunity is best for this nurse?
   a. Working with a child with special needs
   b. Working as a home health supervisor
   c. Working as a contract nurse to perform admissions
   d. Working to administer IV medications via vascular access

5. The home health nurse requires the assistance of center of excellence (COE) nurses for a client. Which client would benefit the most from this specialized nurse?
   a. A pediatric client who is ventilator dependent
   b. A client with a small sacral pressure wound
   c. A client requiring teaching of insulin administration
   d. A client who requires indwelling catheter changes monthly

CHAPTER RESOURCES

Enhance your learning with additional resources on thePoint!

Student Resources related to this chapter can be found at thePoint.lww.com/Rosdahl12e.

99 Ambulatory Nursing

Learning Objectives

1. Explain what is meant by the "trend toward community-based healthcare delivery."
2. Describe some functions of the nurse working in a medical provider's office, an emergency department or urgent-care center, and a same-day or ambulatory surgery center.
3. Briefly outline the benefits of same-day or ambulatory surgery.
4. Differentiate the "minute clinic" from the traditional clinic; list some services provided in the minute clinic.
5. State examples of scientific developments that have made ambulatory surgery possible.
6. List and describe the classifications of potential clients for ambulatory surgery.
7. Describe the particular importance of client and family teaching in ambulatory healthcare.

Important Terminology

cardioversion
endoscopy
managed care
protocol
minute clinic
stabilization
(stable) room
telemonitoring
teletriage
urgent-care center
vertical clients

Acronyms

ACO
ACS
CHC
EHR
EHS
FHC
HMO
LHI
NACHC

The early chapters of this text introduced you to the concept of community-based healthcare. Chapters 96 and 97 discussed nursing in extended-care and rehabilitation settings and Chapter 98 described home care. In the current chapter, nursing in other selected community-based settings is discussed. Community-based (*ambulatory*) healthcare is, by far, the fastest-growing segment of the healthcare industry. In community-based settings, the nurse encounters many exciting challenges and learning opportunities. Graduates of all types of nursing programs are finding employment in ambulatory healthcare. The LVN/LPN in these settings usually works under the supervision of an RN or primary provider.

Chapter 7 introduced the community health center as a major provider of primary healthcare. It also briefly referred to public health departments and visiting nurse organizations. This chapter continues that discussion by focusing on ambulatory healthcare. The term *ambulatory healthcare* refers to the care of clients who do not need to be in an acute care hospital or long-term care setting. Many clients receive their entire basic healthcare in community-based facilities and are never in a residential or acute healthcare facility. It is understood that primary client care may be delivered by either a healthcare provider, an osteopath, or by another primary care provider (PCP). Persons, such as the clinical nurse specialist, the advance practice nurse, or the physician assistant, may deliver primary healthcare. This person is considered to be the client's PCP. PCPs usually work under the auspices of a healthcare provider or osteopathic healthcare provider.

THE ROLE OF THE NURSE

In ambulatory clinics or community healthcare centers, nurses have the opportunity to use many skills learned in basic nursing programs. In addition to routine client care skills, nurses in ambulatory settings perform other duties not usually performed by nurses in acute care settings.

Nursing Alert Remember: The underlying principles of nursing care, such as Standard Precautions, safety, asepsis, interpersonal communication, and confidentiality, apply in all healthcare settings.

Some functions of the nurse in ambulatory care are unique. This nurse often will

- Make appointments and set up schedules for providers.
- Call to remind clients of their appointments (Fig. 99-1).
- Check the client's insurance card and make a copy.
- Qualify clients for third-party payor reimbursement and process insurance claims.
- Initially triage all clients to determine clinical acuity and the need to be seen immediately. (In some states, initial triage must be performed by a registered nurse [RN].) Triage by telephone is known as **teletriage**.
- (If paper charts are used), make sure the client's charts are all pulled and complete before the client sees the PCP.
- Gather baseline data, including height, weight, and vital signs, and possibly other tests, such as pulse oximetry or blood glucose determination, when a client enters the clinic.
- Ask the client about any wounds or open or irritated areas in the skin. The PCP may examine the client to determine skin integrity.
- Make sure a fall risk assessment has been done on each client. (If the client is at risk for falling, appropriate precautions should be taken.)
- Ask the client about pain. If pain is present, document this, ask the level of pain, and document what was done

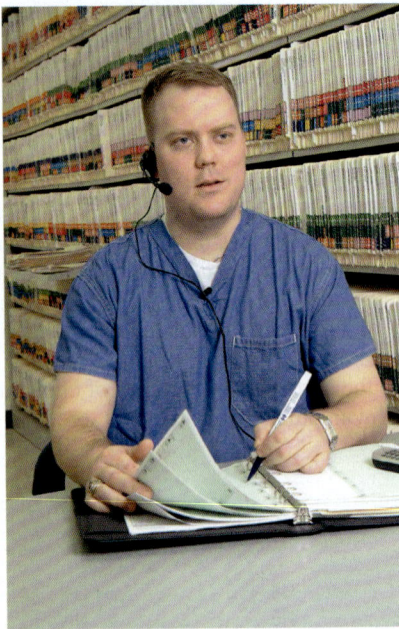

Figure 99-1 The nurse in a healthcare provider's clinic may perform duties such as making appointments for clients or pulling client records or x-rays before the client is seen by the primary provider.

to alleviate the pain, as well as the client's reaction to the intervention. In some cases, this client should be seen immediately.
- Make sure the client is carefully identified. (The client must be wearing a name band for any invasive procedure.)
- Make sure any allergies are documented; double-check at each visit, especially for new allergies. (The client must be wearing an allergy band for any invasive procedure, whether or not they have allergies.)
- Perform *medication reconciliation* to determine the client's current medications and medication compliance.
- Interview the client to determine the client's "chief complaint," the reason for today's visit to the clinic or care center. Document any special concerns or symptoms.
- Ask the client if any procedures or immunizations have been done since last seen, including dental or eye examinations and chiropractic care.
- Ensure that clients are seen quickly, efficiently, and with a minimum of paperwork or waiting.
- Assign clients to examining rooms and keep the schedule moving. Notify waiting clients if the wait will be long and let them know why (e.g., an emergency case).
- Instruct clients as to what will be required. For example, "Take off all your clothes above the waist and put on this gown, with the opening in the front."
- Assist with examinations, including gynecologic, general physical, and neurologic.
- Assist with sterile procedures, including placement of sutures and some ambulatory surgery. Assist with cast application.
- Perform special procedures, as ordered by the PCP. These procedures might include suture removal, cast removal, catheterization, or flushing the client's ears. The nurse may draw blood for special tests or may do a finger stick for laboratory examination.
- Perform routine hearing and vision screening and report to the PCP.
- Prepare and collect specimens and slides.
- Administer special treatments, such as ultrasound, bladder scanning, heat treatments, or application of medicinal creams and ointments.
- Take basic x-rays in some settings.
- Perform special, nontraditional nursing procedures, such as laboratory tests, electrocardiograms (ECGs), postural drainage, and inhalation/nebulizer treatments.
- Assist with teaching clients and families. Answer their questions.
- Call in prescriptions to pharmacies, following specific orders from a healthcare provider, osteopathic healthcare provider, dentist, physician assistant, or advanced practice nurse. (In some states, only RNs can make such telephone calls.)
- Schedule clients for additional tests or surgery.
- Assist with referrals to other healthcare providers and specialists.
- Teach clients how to use special equipment, such as blood pressure apparatus or a continuous positive airway pressure (CPAP) machine.
- Arrange for hospital admission when necessary.
- Wrap and sterilize supplies by autoclave or other methods.
- Keep records, including billing, appointments, and laboratory reports.
- Track preventive and health-promotion procedures, such as immunizations and periodic health screenings. Notify clients when these are due.
- Administer injections, such as antibiotics, tetanus toxoid, and various immunizations.
- Administer skin-scratch tests and intradermal screening tests, such as the purified protein derivative (PPD) (for tuberculosis [TB]) and appropriate controls, as well as allergy skin tests.
- Clean and restock rooms and order supplies.
- Follow-up with clients by telephone to see how they are doing, following surgery or other procedures.
- Enter all data on the client's electronic health record (EHR).
- Receive data from telemonitoring sources and forward the information to the appropriate person for interpretation and/or follow-up.
- Collect data for research projects.

TYPES OF AMBULATORY FACILITIES

There are several general types of ambulatory healthcare facilities. These include private clinics, specialized clinics, minute clinics, community health centers, emergency care centers, and ambulatory/same-day surgery centers.

Private Clinics

Private healthcare providers or groups of healthcare providers often practice in a clinic, which may be associated with hospitals or may be free-standing. Other professionals who work in these clinics include advance practice nurses, nurse practitioners, physician assistants, general staff nurses (RNs and licensed practical/vocational nurses [LVN/LPNs]), and various specialists and office personnel. Some of these clinics have walk-in services, but most require appointments. Services are usually provided on a fee-for-service basis, and clients may be required to have insurance coverage for nonemergency care. Some clinics handle one specialty, such as urology, gynecology, mental health, or neurology; others see a variety of health concerns. Because community health centers are rapidly becoming the healthcare provider for many special populations, private clinics tend to see only clients with insurance. Special populations, such as the homeless and older adults, are more likely to receive primary care at the community health center, as are many neighborhood residents.

The Accountable Care Organization

In some areas, groups of providers, including physicians and other healthcare providers, are formed to deliver coordinated, high-quality care to Medicare clients. These are called **ACOs** or Accountable Care Organizations. The ACO "investment model" uses prepayment as an approach to reducing costs of healthcare.

Public Reporting

Under the PPACA, the "Affordable Care Act," all providers must report specific results as well as clients' evaluations, and these are published on the CMS (Centers for Medicare and Medicaid Services) Website (http://www.cms.gov). This information can be used by potential clients to make informed decisions about their healthcare.

The Minute Clinic or Walk-In Clinic

Some pharmacies, such as CVS, have small clinics on-site ("**minute clinics**"), usually staffed by an advance practice nurse, that handle nonacute health concerns. These may include (http://www.cvs.com) the following:

- Minor illnesses, such as allergies, bronchitis, cough, earache and infections, flu symptoms, pinkeye and styes, sinus infections, coughs, sore and strep throats, upper respiratory infections, and urinary tract infections.
- Minor injuries, such as bug or tick bites and stings, minor burns, sunburn, minor cuts, blisters, splinters, sprains and strains, and suture or staple removal.
- Screenings and monitoring, including A1c check, diabetes monitoring and screening, cholesterol screening and monitoring, hypertension evaluation, and basic and comprehensive health screening.
- Skin conditions and testing, including acne, eczema, athlete's foot, chicken pox, cold and canker sores, impetigo, lice, poison ivy and oak, ringworm, scabies, shingles, swimmer's itch, and warts.
- Immunizations and injections, including birth control injections, and immunizations such as DTaP, hepatitis A and C, HPV, polio, meningitis, MMR, pneumonia, Td, Tdap, and flu shots, as well as specialized injections, such as vitamin B_{12}.
- Wellness, athletic, and other physical examinations, such as college, camp, sports, and DOT (Department of Transportation) examinations, ear wax removal, EpiPen and Auvi-Q refills, motion sickness prevention, one-time medication renewal, pregnancy evaluation, smoking cessation, TB tests, and weight-loss programs. If a person comes to the minute clinic with a condition that would not be appropriate for the Minute Clinic, they are referred to an Urgent-Care Center or Emergency Department.

Specialized Clinics and Services

Target Populations and Mobile Clinics

Specialized clinics serve target populations. For example, they may be open a few days a week in a shelter or downtown area, specifically to serve homeless or older adults. In other situations, a mobile outreach clinic is housed in a van and comes into the community to provide healthcare. The van may visit retirement centers, soup kitchens, homeless shelters, group homes, and single-room occupancy (SRO) hotels (Fig. 99-2). They may also set up in a shopping mall, pharmacy, or busy downtown district on certain days of the week and may also serve health needs of prison inmates. An immunization clinic may be set up in a large grocery store or mall. When the demand has passed (e.g., for common flu or H1N1 immunizations), the clinic no longer exists. Another specialized service is a health screening clinic or "health fair." This may occur at a shopping center, state fair, car show, church, or other community building. This screening tests for common disorders, such as diabetes and high blood pressure. Other tests, such as vision, hearing, testing for TB, hepatitis, or human immunodeficiency virus (HIV), and scoliosis screening may be included. Sometimes, a mobile clinic is set up for more advanced screening. This may include ultrasound screening of the carotid arteries or aorta, electrocardiograms (ECGs), bone density tests, and other specific tests. The results of this screening may be sent to the client's primary provider or to the client, in which case it is the client's responsibility to follow-up, if needed.

Clients can receive basic healthcare and screening at these sites, often without appointments. The mobile clinic or community clinic is the only source of healthcare for many clients. Here, staff members perform basic tests, keep records, and perform a great deal of health promotion and teaching.

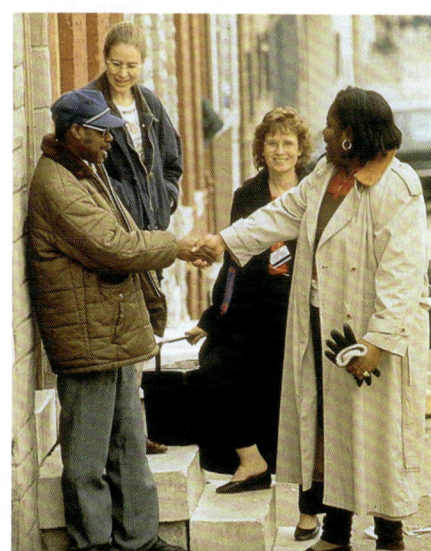

Figure 99-2 Community healthcare can be delivered wherever people are located. This may include a shopping center, pharmacy, retirement center, homeless shelter, prison, or single-room occupancy hotel.

In some rural counties, vans visit different towns each day to provide needed services not available in the local small hospital or clinic. Examples include computed tomography (CT) scan, magnetic resonance imaging (MRI), colonoscopy, dialysis, or mammography. Another type of specialized mobile clinic is provided for a particular ethnic group, such as Native Americans or Alaska Natives. In Alaska, for example, a healthcare team flies to a different village each day to provide primary healthcare (including vision and dental care) to the residents. Telemonitoring (discussed later) is often used to determine needed treatment for these clients.

Clinics for Particular Conditions

Some clinics or resource centers specialize in particular disorders or diseases. Examples include HIV and AIDS, including confidential testing for the virus. Other clinics specialize in conditions such as closed head trauma, cystic fibrosis, scoliosis, or Huntington disease.

The School-Based Health Service

The school-based health service is becoming increasingly important in the delivery of healthcare. This may be located at the preschool center, the elementary school, middle school, high school, or college. In addition to school nurses, many of these programs employ an advance practice nurse or physician assistant who can provide primary healthcare. In some cases, LVN/LPNs are employed as *assistants,* with a limited scope of functions, under the supervision of a certified school nurse or other licensed provider. School sites may also be designated as *community health centers.* This service helps reduce school absenteeism.

Services provided by school-based health services often include the following:

- Administration of basic first aid
- Diagnosis and treatment of common minor illnesses
- Basic hearing and vision screening and referral
- Administration of routine immunizations and skin tests for TB
- Administration of medications, following a primary provider's orders
- Treatments such as dressing changes, care of a colostomy or ileostomy, management of a urinary catheter, aerosolized nebulizer treatments, pulmonary physiotherapy, or assistance with special orthopedic exercises
- Screening for conditions such as scoliosis, diabetes, high blood pressure, or asthma
- Assistance with splints, casts, crutches, and management of skin breakdown or related problems
- Analysis and correction of architectural barriers within the facility
- Accident reduction
- Diagnosis of complex medical conditions and referral to specialists
- Services to adolescent parents and their babies
- Services for children with severe disabilities. (In some cases, an attendant is provided for a child with a disability to assist during the entire day)
- Follow-up of students with excessive absences
- Reporting of suspected child abuse
- Health counseling for students regarding concerns such as eating disorders, weight-loss, prevention of pregnancy and sexually transmitted infections (STIs), smoking cessation, anger management, or rape prevention
- Support groups and counseling for students dealing with specific issues such as drug abuse; groups include programs for students recovering from abuse of alcohol and/or other drugs, as well as other addictions
- Support groups for students related to death or serious illness of friends or family, crime in the community or the school, depression and suicidal ideation, and other concerns
- Teaching in all areas of health and wellness, including sex education and teaching of safer sex practices
- Transmitting data to appropriate locations for telemonitoring of students' health concerns
- Counseling and support groups may be held for teachers and staff as well

The school nurse may also make home visits, assist with contests regarding health or science, teach health classes or CPR classes, and organize a "medical interest club" for students.

The Employee Health Service

Many employers have an employee health service (**EHS**) that provides some primary healthcare to the employees. Immunizations, health screening, health counseling, and referrals to specialists are usually available. In some companies, the EHS must assess the employee who has been ill and issue "return to work" permission. The EHS often works with Workers' Compensation and the Occupational Safety and Health Administration (OSHA) and usually is in charge of obtaining or generating safety data sheets (SDS; see Chapter 39).

Teletriage and Telemonitoring

Many hospitals, health maintenance organizations (**HMOs**), insurance companies, and visiting nurse services offer call-in services, which may be called crisis lines or "nurse lines" (*teletriage*). These services provide general health information, counseling, and referrals, as well as evaluation and referral in cases of suicidal ideation. Using a computerized database, each call is triaged to determine its disposition. The caller may be referred immediately to emergency services, instructed to see their PCP the next day, or given suggestions for managing current healthcare concerns. Callers may be given names of healthcare providers and medical facilities in their local area. Insurance questions, sometimes, maybe answered if the telehealth program is under the auspices of an insurance company. (In some cases, the triage nurse must be an RN.)

Telemonitoring refers to the management of medical situations remotely, using electronic technology. Transmission of data, including blood pressure, oxygenation levels, ECG readings, and electroencephalogram (EEG) readings, are transmitted from a client's home to a provider in another location for evaluation. Data may also be transmitted by a PCP in a remote location to a specialist for interpretation.

Support Groups

Some community agencies facilitate support groups. Common group designations include coping with cancer, grief and loss (*bereavement groups*), and mutual support groups for primary caregivers and families of mentally ill people or people with long-term disorders, such as dementia or Huntington disease, as well as chemical abuse and dependency. Many hospitals and clinics conduct groups aimed at weight-loss, exercise, smoking cessation, or cardiac rehabilitation and may provide space for group meetings such as Alcoholics Anonymous (AA) or Narcotics Anonymous (NA).

The Community/Family Health Center

The government publication, *Healthy People 2030* (https://health.gov/healthypeople), prepared and sponsored in part by the Centers for Disease Control and Prevention (CDC) in Atlanta, describes the community/family health center (**CHC** or **FHC**) as a provider of primary care for a large segment of the population, particularly underserved populations (Fig. 99-3). Many people consider the CHC to be their family healthcare provider. The centers provide access to high-quality primary and preventive care in a cost-effective manner, assist clients to manage chronic illnesses, improve birth outcomes, and provide employment for members of the local community.

Some of the goals of *Healthy People 2030* include the following:

- Cancer—"to reduce the number of new cases, as well as illness, disability, and death caused by cancer"
- Disabilities—"improve health and well-being in people with disabilities"
- Food Safety—"to reduce foodborne illnesses"

The initial goals have been expanded, as discussed below. The CHCs play a major role in helping citizens to meet healthcare goals. CHCs differ from other healthcare providers because:

- Clients are involved in service delivery, with local residents serving on governing boards.
- CHCs are located in "high-need" communities (e.g., elevated poverty, higher-than-average infant mortality, or where few healthcare providers practice).
- CHCs target medically underserved areas or populations and offer services such as transportation, translation (nearly one-third of clients speak a language other than English), case management, health education, and home visitation. About half the clients are in rural areas.
- CHCs must provide comprehensive primary care services and related support services, tailored to the special needs and priorities of the community.
- Care must be available to all residents, regardless of insurance status. Even with the Affordable Care Act, a large portion of the U.S. population remains uninsured.
- Fees must be adjusted, in relation to ability to pay.

The National Association of Community Health Centers (**NACHC**) estimates that CHCs are the only available source of primary healthcare for millions of people in the United States. This number continues to increase; therefore, CHCs must be available as major providers of ambulatory and primary care. According to data compiled by the Henry J. Kaiser Family Foundation, in January 2018, there were 1,362 separate federally funded CHC/FHCs in the United States and its territories. California, the state with the most CHCs (177), serves over 4 million clients yearly (National Association of Community Health Centers, 2020). These centers were and still are *nonprofit* and are federally designated and funded. Many people are not aware of the availability of healthcare at these centers or choose not to take advantage of this care. Public health officials are working to address this issue by strengthening existing CHCs; managing the growth of new CHCs; and managing quality improvement in all CHCs.

A number of government regulations apply to the CHCs, and these regulations must be followed carefully for the facility's funding to continue. Reimbursement for healthcare in the CHC varies, with some clients having insurance (most often, Medicaid) or by a managed care contract with the local community. In some cases, the state reimburses the center for some of the cost of care for the uninsured. Local communities, sometimes, pay for some care for clients who receive general assistance. Many centers offer a sliding fee scale. Many rural clients are low-income, and many have no insurance or have only Medicaid and/or Medicare. These people frequently are homeless as well. Many clients are members of racial and ethnic minority groups and, in many cases, are very old or very young. However, many of the centers appeal to other members of the local community, and most of the residents in that neighborhood may receive their primary care at the center, whether or not they are low income.

The CHC/FHCs are staffed by healthcare providers, physician assistants, advance practice nurses, other nurses, dentists, therapists, pharmacists, and other health professionals. The centers employ more than 110,000 people nationwide, many of whom live in the neighborhoods they serve. Many centers employ LVN/LPNs. Sometimes, staff members are volunteers.

The CHC/FHCs offer a wide range of services similar to other health centers, including primary and preventive healthcare and education. Preventive services include testing for HIV, cholesterol, pap tests, and mammograms, as well as prenatal care. Other services include social services and various therapies (e.g., physical therapy, occupational therapy and job retraining, dietetic and weight-loss counseling, diabetic teaching, smoking cessation, speech therapy, and mental health counseling). Support services, such as translation services and transportation, are also provided. These centers are also involved with community outreach and educational

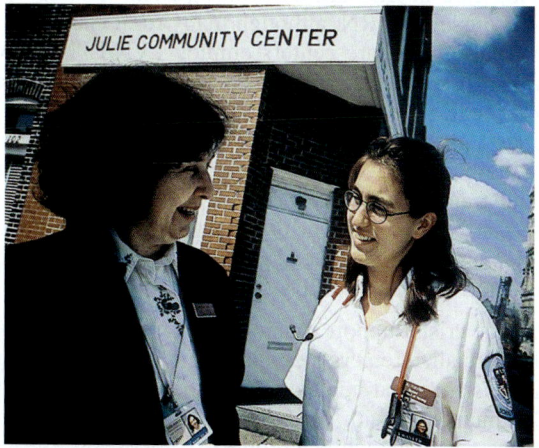

Figure 99-3 Community health centers provide primary healthcare. Here, an advance practice nurse orients a student to the center.

programs, including literacy programs. They cooperate with other community agencies, such as schools, homeless shelters, and Head Start programs. The centers serve millions of children per year, and nearly one-fifth of all births in the United States are under the auspices of a CHC/FHC. Since the inception of the CHC/FHCs, the services have expanded to include dental services, as well as programs to assist clients who have a history of substance abuse.

Specialized Populations

Some CHCs have a specialized population focus. For example, they may target teenagers, such as the West Suburban Teen Center in Wayzata, Minnesota. Other clinics may specialize in family planning or in testing and treating persons who are positive for HIV. These centers may be part of the federal CHC program or maybe "look-alikes" (funded by other sources). Migrant healthcare centers serve migrant worker populations. Other specialized centers include centers in public housing units, homeless shelters, shelters for women who have been abused, and prisons.

The Role of the Advance Practice Nurse

Advance practice nurses, nurse practitioners, or physician assistants provide most of the primary care to clients of all ages in the CHC/FHC. In other words, they act as general family healthcare providers. Some conditions are considered ambulatory care sensitive (**ACS**), and clients with these conditions are often seen in these settings. Examples include asthma, diabetes mellitus, seizure disorders, and hypertension. For many chronic disorders, providers are required to follow specific **managed care protocols**. These formally established guidelines are based on national criteria and detail the required management of specific disorders. The publication, *Healthy People 2030*, sets forth two major goals: "to increase quality and years of healthy life…and to eliminate health disparities." This publication identifies *Leading Health Indicators* (**LHI**), which separates indicators by age. LHIs in the category for all ages include oral health, hunger and food insecurity, overweight and obesity, drug overdose deaths knowledge of HIV status, homicides, suicides, environmental quality, immunization, and access to healthcare. LHIs for infants include infant deaths. Children and adolescent LHIs include obesity, tobacco use among adolescents, subpar reading skills for fourth grade and above, and adolescents with major depressive episodes who receive treatment. LHIs for adults and older adults focus on alcoholism, physical activity, colorectal cancer screening, hypertension, cigarette smoking, employment, maternal deaths, and new cases of diagnosed diabetes. These LHIs are the basis for a comprehensive list of objectives for healthcare in the future. Information regarding *Healthy People 2030* can be obtained at www.healthypeople.gov and the CDC Website.

The Emergency Department and Urgent-Care Center

Most hospitals have an emergency department (ED) or emergency room (ER) where they care for clients with traumatic or life-threatening conditions. Some hospitals also have urgent-care departments as part of the ED or in a separate area, which care for less critically ill clients. Free-standing **urgent-care centers** (*emergi-centers, urgi-centers*) are also available but not attached to hospitals. Hospitals may also designate an area of the ED for pediatric clients or may have a specific area that handles the triage and treatment of all clients. Most large hospitals have a separate area designated to handle psychiatric emergencies, called *mental health crisis centers, acute psychiatric services (APS)*, or *crisis intervention centers* (CIC). These areas may also maintain a nurse line, crisis line, or teletriage center.

Many urgent-care centers are open longer hours than are healthcare providers' offices; sometimes, they are open 24 hr a day. The fees and insurance copayments are usually lower in the urgent-care center than in the ED. All types of urgent-care or minute clinics usually treat only **vertical clients** (clients with noncritical conditions); they refer more critically ill or injured clients to hospital EDs. Follow-up information for the PCP is becoming increasingly important. In many cases, community health centers, specialized clinics, and PCP offices transfer information to one another by computer or fax or maybe in the same computer network. If a PCP has questions, they can access additional information.

> **Key Concept**
>
> A client's PCP usually must give permission for the client to receive care from an emergency department or other clinic if the client belongs to a Health Maintenance Organization (HMO). (This permission may be given retroactively, in an emergency.) HMOs evaluate PCPs based on how many of their clients are seen in emergency rooms or how many times an individual client goes to the ED/ER.

> **Nursing Alert** It is important when working in the ED to look for the client's emergency medical information. This might be a MedicAlert tag or information in the client's wallet. This information can help identify a client or inform the facility that the client has health insurance, special health concerns, a living will, or wishes to be an organ/tissue donor. Next-of-kin information is usually contained there also.

Nursing Care

Nursing care in EDs differs from inpatient nursing. Often, the ED nurse is an RN, although many rural and small hospitals and urgent-care centers employ LVN/LPNs as well. Advance practice nurses, physician assistants, and emergency medical technicians (EMTs) treat clients with less emergent problems. Life-threatening illnesses and injuries are usually treated by healthcare providers or osteopaths. Special training and experience are necessary before any nurse can be employed in the ER. In addition to performing many routine and special procedures as in the outpatient clinic, staff members in EDs also

- Provide crisis support and counseling to families
- Use specialized emergency equipment, such as endotracheal airways and hand-held ventilating bags (AMBU bags)
- Communicate with ambulance, helicopter, and other rescue personnel while en route
- Open and use supplies and equipment contained in the crash cart or storage areas. (Nurses must know where all supplies and equipment are kept for immediate access)

- Set up examination and treatment areas appropriately to receive clients when ambulances or helicopters arrive, and assemble necessary equipment and supplies
- Notify appropriate personnel to prepare for arrival of incoming clients
- Work with law enforcement personnel to preserve evidence, notify next of kin, and related procedures
- Assist in the **stabilization (stable) room** while clients are being triaged and stabilized for transfer to an operating room (OR) or other area
- Assist with **cardioversion** (defibrillation) or other emergency procedures
- Take primary responsibility for monitoring intravenous (IV) lines (after specialized training)
- Call all family members and appropriate clergy members
- Continuously monitor critically ill clients while they are being examined
- Notify appropriate individuals if difficulties arise
- Obtain necessary permits for treatments or surgery from the client or next of kin
- Perform triage in the event of multiple admissions at one time to determine which clients require immediate attention
- Keep accurate records of emergency procedures performed and medications given, by whom, and at what time (*documentation is so essential that one nurse may be assigned only to document, without any other duties*). In most facilities, documentation is done on the electronic record
- Arrange for special tests, such as MRI, CT scan, ultrasound, x-ray examination, or emergency transfer to the OR
- Take clients to x-ray or other diagnostic areas: many nurses assist with x-ray, ultrasound, or other examinations in emergencies
- Assist withdrawing blood or obtaining other specimens for laboratory analysis: In some situations, nurses draw blood and perform some laboratory tests
- Perform ECGs for evaluation by healthcare providers
- Coordinate transcription of healthcare provider's orders (see Chapter 101), fill out requests, or enter information into computers for laboratory tests, x-ray examinations, and other procedures
- Make arrangements for hospital admission
- Assist with nonsterile procedures, such as cast, splint, or traction application
- Assist with emergency sterile procedures, such as suturing, removal of foreign objects, or catheterization
- Apply cold or warm packs and perform other noninvasive procedures
- Administer medications, as ordered: This may include emergency medications during triage, as well as more routine injections, such as tetanus toxoid, immunizations, or antibiotics
- Assist with adjusting crutches or canes and with teaching the client to use these devices (see Chapter 48)
- Obtain necessary permissions from HMOs or other third-party payors for emergency care to be given, if possible
- Approach family members regarding organ/tissue donation (following specialized training)
- Assist with care of the client's body after death (see Chapter 59)

Nursing Alert Remember that, even though a person has designated themselves as a "donor" on their driver's license or on a donor card, the next of kin must give permission for donation after a person's death.

The steadily increasing volume of cases coming into ERs and urgent-care centers has increased the load on each staff person. The length of time a noncritical client spends in the ER has increased as well. A client may be required to spend several hours in the ER during triage and stabilization before being treated and discharged. The triage process enables the staff to see those clients with life-threatening problems first. Therefore, the person with a severe asthma attack or diabetic reaction or who is hemorrhaging will be seen before the person requiring a tetanus injection and several sutures in a nonhemorrhaging wound.

The Same-Day Surgery or Ambulatory Surgery Center

Some centers are called same-day surgery, day-surgery, or ambulatory surgery centers. Clients visit here for many procedures that once required inpatient hospitalization. In addition to pressure from third-party payors, the development of specialized equipment and innovative procedures has contributed to this trend. Some specialized equipment and procedures in ambulatory surgery centers are as follows:

Endoscopy: (visualization of an internal structure through a scope); for example, *laparoscope* (to visualize internal abdominal structures), *cystoscope* (to visualize within the bladder), or *arthroscope* (to visualize within joints). This allows visualization and manipulation of internal structures and removal of organs/tissues and biopsy samples through a small "stab wound" or "port"

Laser: Provides cutting and vessel cauterization, controlled from a distance; many eye surgeries are performed via laser

Fiberoptics: Provide light and magnification at a distance

Ultrasound, MRI, CT, and positron-emission tomography (PET/PETT) scans: Allow accurate visualization and location of internal structures and their functioning and of tumors and other lesions

Procedures, such as extracorporeal lithotripsy: To pulverize kidney or bladder stones without open surgery

Stent placement: To eliminate the need for blood vessel bypass (e.g., following a heart attack [MI]) or vessel blockage (e.g., coronary arteries, femoral artery)

Increased sophistication of local, spinal, and block anesthesia: Eliminates the need for general anesthesia

Client-managed pain-control pump systems (patient-controlled analgesia [PCA]): Allows the client to self-manage pain

Operating microscope: Allows accurate visualization and manipulation of tiny structures

Specialized implant materials, joints, bone stabilization, and so on: Require shorter recovery time

Robotic procedures: Assist surgeons to perform procedures using robots; these procedures were previously impossible

External fixators, halo devices, etc.: Often eliminate the need for bed rest, traction, or a cast for a fracture or neck injury; the device provides immobilization

Computerization: Enables performance of many specialized procedures and functions

Use of today's equipment and procedures eliminates, in many cases, the need for a large incision or any incision. Local anesthesia greatly reduces the risk of postoperative complications. The PCA pump allows the client to manage pain effectively. All these factors speed the recovery process, add to client comfort, and eliminate the need for inpatient hospitalization. In addition, clients often find visiting an ambulatory surgery center for the surgery and then recovering at home to be more comfortable and conducive to relaxation than recuperating in a hospital.

> **Key Concept**
> The use of ambulatory surgery allows clients to be up and moving sooner. This helps prevent disorders of immobility (e.g., pneumonia, contracture, constipation, blood clots, etc.).

Ambulatory or same-day surgery clinics are often located in the operative area of a hospital or are managed by an operating room staff. Free-standing ambulatory surgery centers have also been established by groups of surgeons. All such centers must be licensed and are inspected and regulated in much the same manner as are hospitals.

Endoscopy

Endoscopy has been one of the most important factors in changing the way in which surgery is performed. Complex surgery with endoscopes can be done, using several entry points (ports) via small *"stab wounds."* Surgeons can use various angles and several instruments simultaneously. For example, one port accommodates suction, another, the scalpel, and another, the cautery. Other ports accommodate fiberoptics, lasers, crushing instruments, various equipment for obtaining biopsies, clamps, pickup forceps, and retractors. Surgeons can insert materials, such as reinforcement meshes for hernia repair, through the ports. They can also remove tissue, such as the gallbladder or uterus, and biopsy samples through the ports.

> **NCLEX Alert**
> Understanding the determination of clients' appropriateness for outpatient surgery (Classes I–III) and benefit of ambulatory surgery may help you understand the role of the nurse in these settings, as well as to assist in educating and preparing clients/families for procedures performed in these settings and for their postoperative self-care. NCLEX questions may incorporate the above considerations.

Procedures Performed

Criteria have been established to assist in determining appropriate clients for outpatient surgery (Box 99-1). It is important to remember that the appropriateness of a client for ambulatory surgery is determined not only by the *complexity of the surgery* but also by the *underlying physical and mental condition* of the client and the *availability of appropriate after-care* (see Chapter 56). The number of procedures performed in day-surgery is expanding continuously. Many procedures performed in ambulatory surgery today were inpatient procedures just a few years ago. It is vital for the client to have a caregiver at home to assist in follow-up postoperative care. Ambulatory surgery centers may refer clients to home care services for a few visits to ensure safe follow-up. However, finances may preclude the availability of home care services.

> **Key Concept**
> The determination of candidates for ambulatory surgery is based on factors such as:
> - Client condition
> - Client age
> - Complexity of the procedure (usually shorter than 90 min)
> - Availability of a driver to take the client home
> - Availability of aftercare
> - Existence or absence of underlying physical or mental disorders

Nursing Care

Because most third-party payors do not give clients choices about whether or not to have ambulatory surgery, the nurse plays a vital role in assisting clients and family members to feel comfortable. Assure clients that ambulatory surgery reduces the overall risk for postoperative complications, including infection, and reduces adverse reactions to anesthesia. Teaching the client and family is one of the most important functions of the nurse in the day-surgery center. The nurse is responsible for the following:

- Teaching clients and caregivers about preoperative preparation, which will almost always be done at home before coming to the surgery center. Clients or family members must perform many preoperative measures at home, including following special diets, maintaining nothing by mouth (NPO) status for a specified number of hours before surgery, giving an antiseptic scrub or shower, using a product such as CHG/Hibiclens, and administering enemas or other types of bowel preparation. (Home care nurses may help clients perform some of these procedures and may help provide preoperative teaching.)
- Obtaining a medication list from the client, including supplements and vitamins.
- Obtaining information about client allergies, including latex.
- Determining which of the client's scheduled medications should be taken the morning of surgery.
- Making sure the client has a preoperative physical several days before the procedure and that this is filed with the client's legal papers.
- Explaining the surgery clearly and making sure the client has signed the operative permit, and it is in the record. (Usually, this is the responsibility of the surgeon.) All operative permits must be signed *before the client receives any medications.*
- Telling the client to bring insurance cards, photo identification, living will, guardianship papers, and money for copay, if applicable.

> **Box 99-1**   **Client Criteria for Outpatient (Same-Day) Surgery**
>
> **CLASS I**
> - No major underlying organic, physiologic, psychological, or biochemical condition (e.g., absence of brittle insulin-dependent diabetes, emphysema, multiple sclerosis, bleeding disorders, immune disorders, such as acquired immunodeficiency syndrome [AIDS], seizure disorders, serious eating disorders, mental illness, or previous adverse reactions to anesthesia)
> - No underlying adverse factor such as morbid obesity, chronic chemical abuse and dependency, or extreme age (very old or very young)
> - No serious psychiatric disturbance or uncontrollable fear
> - Absence of severe dementia or intellectual impairment
> - Conditions requiring surgery are localized (nonsystemic)
> - Client has primary caregivers available
>
>   *Examples of appropriate class I procedures include* wound debridement, tonsillectomy, tubal ligation, vasectomy, biopsy, cervical conization, corneal transplant, cataract removal and lens implant, ptosis correction, cryosurgery removal of nonmalignant lesions, arthroscopy and joint repair, kidney stone removal, polyp removal, hemorrhoid removal, breast lumpectomy, cranial burr holes, dilation and curettage (D&C), open reduction and internal or external fixation of simple fracture, and other orthopedic procedures (e.g., carpal tunnel release, toe amputation, or bunion repair).
>
> **CLASS II**
> - Increasing levels of systemic disturbance with class I-type procedures (client may have mild diabetes, essential hypertension, controlled asthma, etc.)
> - More complex surgery without complicating physiologic or psychological factors.
>
>   *Examples of appropriate class II procedures include* removal of tubal pregnancy, hysterectomy, stent placement (in blood vessel), cholecystectomy, coronary artery arthroplasty (balloon or "Roto-Rooter" procedures), lobectomy (lung), hernia repair, partial bowel resection, simple nephrectomy (kidney), biopsy of brain tumor, patent ductus repair, and partial foot amputation.
>
> **CLASS III**
> - Serious underlying organic disorder that is life-threatening
> - Severe psychosis or intellectual impairment, rendering the client unable to cooperate or to care for themselves following surgery
> - Systemic condition requiring extensive surgery
> - Absence of a caregiver for postoperative care
>
>   *Examples of class III procedures include* total colon resection, radical mastectomy, coronary artery bypass, hysterectomy with anterior and posterior repair, total gastric (stomach) resection, total pneumonectomy (lung removal), craniotomy and removal of brain tumor, limb amputation, bone marrow transplant, repair of coronary septal defects, replacement of heart valves, and heart, liver, or lung transplant.
>
>   *Note:* Nearly all clients in class I and some clients in class II are candidates for outpatient (same-day) surgery. Clients in class III are too ill or the surgery is too complex or life-threatening for them to be candidates. In some cases, the lack of an available caregiver may move the client to a higher classification and rule out same-day surgery.

- Telling the client to wear comfortable, loose-fitting clothing.
- Referring the client and family to appropriate sources for equipment and supplies that will be needed after surgery.
- Documenting all teaching. (If teaching is not accurately documented, it is considered, in a court of law, not to have been done.)
- Instructing clients to call if any change occurs in their physical status. For example, canceling surgery or conducting it in an acute care facility may be necessary if a client has an infection, a cold, or influenza or is extremely fearful of the procedure.
- Making sure the client knows if they will be awake during the procedure. Explain that many clients are given conscious sedation, such as midazolam (Versed), to help them relax and provide some amnesia about the procedure.
- Letting the client know that, in many cases, they will be allowed to play tapes or radio with headphones during the procedure. This helps many clients to relax.
- Telling the client not to wear jewelry, nail polish or artificial nails, or to bring valuables to the procedure. (A wedding ring may be taped in place.) The client will usually be asked to remove any body piercings.
- Teaching clients what to expect after surgery and helping them practice postoperative exercises before surgery.
- Taking the client and caregiver on a tour of the operating suite before surgery, if permitted.
- Making sure the client brings along a driver. (Clients are not allowed to drive after any procedures involving sedation.)
- Letting the client know that they may stay overnight for stabilization.
- Making sure the client has someone to stay with them at home for at least 24–48 hr after surgery.
- Providing postoperative client and family teaching the day of the procedure. Explain postoperative care; describe untoward symptoms and medication side effects to watch for.
- In the case of a child, the child may bring a favorite toy or blanket and a sippy cup or bottle.

> **Nursing Alert**   The presence of an infection such as a common cold could result in cancellation of minor surgery, such as a tonsillectomy. A condition such as high blood pressure, unless it could not be controlled with medication, would not cause cancellation of this type of surgery.

> **Key Concept**
>
> It is very important to provide instructions in the client's first language. Provide an interpreter, if necessary. Written instructions should be provided in the person's first language or in Braille if the client is blind or is visually impaired. If the client cannot read or does not know Braille, recorded instructions should be provided. Verbal instructions must be given by signing for clients who are deaf or hard of hearing. Be sure to have the client and/or family *repeat instructions back to you* to make sure they understand. Just asking if they understand is not sufficient because many people will say "yes" to avoid embarrassment or to be polite, even if they do not understand. (This is particularly true if the client does not speak English.)

> **Nursing Alert** The client is instructed that no acetylsalicylic acid (Aspirin), ibuprofen (Motrin), or other NSAID be taken for 7 days before any surgical procedure. Other medications, including blood thinners, such as clopidogrel (Plavix), are contraindicated. In addition, the client should avoid certain herbal or dietary supplements. In particular, St. John wort reduces the effectiveness of some commonly used medications, such as midazolam (Versed). Other herbal supplements can contribute to bleeding after surgery; these are listed in Chapter 56.

On the day of surgery, the nurse will:

- Check in the client's clothing and personal property.
- Double-check to make sure the client has a signed operative permit (before any medications are given) and physical examination on file.
- Perform specific preparations, such as the preoperative scrub and shave or drawing of blood, as ordered.
- Follow the preoperative checklist. Make sure laboratory and ECG results are on the client's chart. Remove devices such as the client's dentures, contact lenses, and prostheses, and remove all jewelry (and/or tape a wedding ring in place).
- Measure the client's height, weight, vital signs, and pulse oxygenation. Be sure to ask about pain.
- Allow the client to wear glasses and a hearing aid until all permits are signed and all explanations given. Then, these are placed with the client's other property. (In some cases, these are worn in the OR to facilitate communication during the procedure.)
- Make sure the client is wearing one or two name bands and an allergy band (even if the client has no allergies), per protocol.
- Have the client state their name and birth date and what procedure is being done. Double-check this with the client's name bands and medical record.
- Check with the client to make sure the correct site has been marked by the surgeon.
- Check to make sure the client's skin is intact and there are no pressure areas.
- Assist the client into appropriate attire (e.g., hospital garb), if needed.
- Apply pressure stockings, pulse oximeter, IV, and other needed items, as ordered.
- Double-check about possible allergies; compare with the allergy band and client record to detect any differences.
- Make sure the client voids immediately before surgery.
- Make sure all required information is entered into the client's electronic or paper chart.
- Assist the family by answering questions and show them where they may wait. Often, they will be given a pager, so they can be called when surgery is over. Tell them where they can get coffee or tea and/or lunch, and where they can access the Internet.
- Tell the family that someone will talk to them after the procedure; provide a private place for this conference.
- Introduce the client to anesthesia and operating room personnel, and make sure the client is comfortable in the preinduction room.
- Assist surgeons as needed. The nurse may be asked to "scrub in" and assist with the procedure.
- Support and remain with clients during induction of general anesthesia or remain for the entire procedure if done under local anesthetic.

The nurse in ambulatory surgery will also function as the recovery room nurse after surgery if the client is not to be admitted to the hospital:

- Stay with clients after surgery until they are fully awake. Observe for any complications.
- Monitor vital signs and perform other routine postoperative procedures.
- Assist the client who is vomiting.
- Supply warm blankets. (After anesthesia, nearly all clients feel chilled.)
- Give the client ice chips or oral fluids, as ordered.
- Administer pain medications, as ordered.
- Make sure the client/family have prescriptions for pain medications and other medications needed after surgery.
- Check dressings to make sure there is no excessive bleeding.
- Check to make sure drains, IVs, and other equipment is working properly.
- Verify again that the family understands the postoperative care and when to call for assistance. Tell them undesired signs to watch for.
- Give the client/family printed instructions to make sure they understand procedures.
- Tell the client and family that you will call tomorrow to see how the client is doing. Make sure you have their preferred telephone number.
- Assist the client to dress and help them into a wheelchair for transport to the car. (Clients are not allowed to walk.) Assist the client into the car. Be sure to furnish an emesis basin or box of tissues, as needed.
- Tell the client they are not allowed to drive for at least 24 hr.
- The client must be reachable for at least 48 hr after surgery.
- Telephone clients on the first postoperative day. Determine if they are having any complications. Know what questions to ask. The nurse must be knowledgeable about possible complications and when to instruct the client to see the healthcare provider. (In many cases, some of these procedures are contained in a standard postoperative computer program.)
- Make recommendations for necessary referrals to public health or home care services.

- Make sure the client has an appointment with the surgeon or primary provider for postoperative follow-up.
- Assist with admission to the hospital if the client will be admitted following ambulatory surgery.

Benefits of Same-Day Surgery

A relaxed, friendly atmosphere in the ambulatory day-surgery center is conducive to confidence and recovery. Clients may not need preoperative medications because of the more relaxed atmosphere; they can walk into the OR feeling more in control. Many clients recover faster and have fewer complications after same-day surgery because they have local anesthesia; they have only small incisions or no incision; they do not receive heavy sedation; and they are more comfortable at home. Clients are also able to ambulate sooner after surgery, helping to prevent the complications of immobilization. Most people are strongly motivated to recover and cooperate. Ambulatory surgery will continue to be more and more common in the future.

USE OF THE ELECTRONIC HEALTH RECORD

The use of the electronic health record (**EHR**) is becoming increasingly widespread. In some locations, hospitals, clinics, laboratories, and pharmacies are all using compatible systems and can access each others' records. This greatly enhances communication between agencies and facilities, improves client care, and increases safety. Clients can also access their own information and ask informed questions. Providers can access client information from remote areas. For example, the healthcare provider in a clinic or community health center can access all the clients' records from a recent hospital stay or visits to other clinics. The provider can also access client records from their home or from another city. The use of the EHR also allows clients to receive ordered medications when they are in a different part of the country, using a nationwide system, such as Walgreen or CVS.

> **Nursing Alert** With today's computerized records, it is vital to have a safeguard to protect client confidentiality. Special passwords are used, changed often, and only appropriate personnel are allowed to access client records. It is important for the nurse to know that it is illegal and unethical to access a client's information unnecessarily. This can be cause for *termination of employment*.

STUDENT SYNTHESIS

KEY POINTS

- Ambulatory nursing care may be delivered in a healthcare provider's office or clinic, urgent-care center, community health center, day-surgery center, or in the client's home. In addition, temporary clinics may be set up in shopping centers, prisons, homeless shelters, and other community sites.
- Nurses function as direct assistants to healthcare providers in many ambulatory care settings.
- Nurses who work in ambulatory settings need multiple skills. They may require additional training to perform some skills.
- The family/community health center provides primary care and secondary services for many people. These centers employ large numbers of nurses.
- Clients coming in for ambulatory same-day surgery or in the morning for inpatient surgery need a great deal of instruction because most preoperative preparation is done at home.
- Ambulatory surgery clients and many clients discharged soon after surgery (as well as their caregivers) need follow-up care after discharge to ensure proper recovery.
- Documentation is vital in all phases of ambulatory care, as it is in inpatient settings.

CRITICAL THINKING EXERCISES

1. Visit a healthcare provider's clinic. Talk to a nurse about their duties and responsibilities. What are the types and ages of clients who visit? Which disorders are most commonly seen? Which in-service education or special training did the nurse need before working there? What are the differences between this type of nursing and nursing in a hospital or nursing home?

2. Observe in an ambulatory surgery center and interview several clients. What were their feelings about same-day surgery? Have any of them previously had inpatient surgery? How did it compare? What are the feelings of the nurses who work there? How well prepared do you feel you would be to function as a nurse in these settings?

3. Visit a community health center. Describe the specific programs available there. Identify the staff qualifications and education. How many are paid and how many are volunteers? Which types of care are available in the center? Obtain a list of fees and charges to share with your classmates. Discuss the concept of a sliding scale for payment.

NCLEX-STYLE REVIEW QUESTIONS

1. A client arrives in the ambulatory care unit to have a procedure performed and informs the nurse, "I have pain." Which is the priority action by the nurse?
   a. Ask the client to rate their pain using a numeric scale.
   b. Obtain the rest of the client data.
   c. Obtain vital signs.
   d. Administer an analgesic for the pain.

2. The nurse is preparing a client for an ambulatory surgical procedure. Which statements are true regarding the benefits to the client having a procedure done in this way? Select all that apply.
   a. There is a faster recovery time.
   b. There are fewer complications.
   c. More medications will be required during the procedure.
   d. Ambulation is quicker.
   e. There is no requirement to stop home medications.

3. The nurse is caring for a group of clients in an urgent-care center. Which client would be immediately transferred to a hospital Emergency Department?
   a. A client with a migraine headache
   b. A client with a productive cough
   c. A client with a rash on the genital area
   d. A client with chest pain radiating to the jaw

4. The LVN/LPN has been assigned to assist the RN with obtaining vital signs in the triage area in a busy Emergency Department (ED). Which client presenting to the ED would the nurse triage first?
   a. A client having an asthma attack
   b. A client with a nosebleed that is controlled
   c. A client with a 2-cm laceration on the leg
   d. A client who thinks they are pregnant

5. A client is being prepared for a surgical procedure in 1 week. Which medication would the nurse instruct the client to abstain from 7 days prior to the procedure?
   a. Diuretics
   b. Antihypertensives
   c. Anticoagulants
   d. Thyroid hormone replacement

CHAPTER RESOURCES

Enhance your learning with additional resources on **thePoint!**

Student Resources related to this chapter can be found at **thePoint.lww.com/Rosdahl12e**.

100 Hospice Nursing

Learning Objectives

1. Describe the evolution of the hospice movement.
2. Name four areas of human needs on which the hospice concept is based.
3. List the criteria a program must meet to be classified officially as a hospice, and explain criteria for a client's admission to a hospice program.
4. Define respite care; explain its purpose.
5. Describe the concept and objectives of palliative care.
6. Define interdisciplinary care in hospice; identify major disciplines usually involved.
7. Describe the functions of the case manager, hospice nurse, and other healthcare team members. Discuss the role of primary caregivers in hospice.
8. Describe emotional and spiritual support for the client and family. Discuss depression and anxiety, as related to hospice clients and caregivers.
9. Discuss measures used to treat respiratory distress, anorexia, nausea and vomiting, constipation, diarrhea, and skin breakdown, and describe measures for odor management.
10. Identify medications commonly used for pain management and other symptoms in hospice.
11. List and briefly describe three psychosocial modalities and two physical modalities used in pain management.
12. Discuss considerations when caring for children in a hospice program.
13. Explain the nurse's role after the client dies.

Important Terminology

ablative surgery
adjuvant
bereavement
compassion
fatigue
debulking
hospice
integrative care
palliative care
primary caregivers
respite (care)
somnolent
tapering down
titration up

Acronyms

BSC
COP
CRNH
DME
DNH
DNI
DNR
IAHPC
IDT, IDG
NAHC
NHPCO
PAD
PCA
POC

The term *hospice* does not signify a specific care setting, but rather a *philosophy of care*. (It is also known as *advanced illness care* or *end-of-life care*.) Hospice is based on the concept that many people prefer to die at home or in a homelike setting, free of pain, and among their loved ones. Hospice care can occur at home, in a hospice center, a hospital, or a skilled nursing facility. Physical and emotional comfort and quality of life are primary concerns of hospice, *not cure*. Hospice programs care for terminally ill persons, allowing them to die with dignity. Clients do not only have cancer but may also select hospice care for chronic situations such as end-stage renal disease (ESRD), end-stage cardiac disease, chronic obstructive pulmonary disease (COPD), and Alzheimer's disease. The goal of hospice care is to provide as much pain relief as possible, while helping the client to remain alert and to meet basic needs. In addition, the client often needs assistance with control of other physical symptoms and with emotional concerns. Hospice care promotes the idea that if the client's symptoms are controlled, he or she becomes emotionally and spiritually at peace. In this way, clients can move toward self-actualization on Maslow hierarchy of human needs (Chapter 5). The family is also provided with support and, sometimes, respite. Nurses working with hospice clients and their families use many skills learned during the entire nursing program. As a nurse working in a hospice program, it is important to examine personal values and feelings about death. Chapter 59 describes end-of-life physical care in more detail.

Key Concept

It is important to note that many people are discharged alive from hospice programs, more than 16.7% in 2017 (Medicare Payment Advisory Commission, 2019).

EVOLUTION OF THE HOSPICE MOVEMENT

The term *hospice* derives from a medieval word meaning "to provide shelter for travelers on difficult journeys." The hospice concept acknowledges that not all illnesses are curable and emphasizes management of uncomfortable symptoms. The primary force behind the modern hospice movement was Dame Cicely Saunders, who founded St. Christopher's Hospice in London in 1967. She stated that healthcare providers should do everything possible not only to help people die peacefully but also to help them "to live until they die." Another way to put it is, "to live as long and as well as possible." In 1974, Florence Wald initiated the first U.S. hospice as a home care program in New Haven, Connecticut, later called the Connecticut Hospice. Other early hospice projects were located in Boonton, New Jersey, and Tucson, Arizona.

> **Key Concept**
>
> In some European countries, hospice programs advocate euthanasia by healthcare providers ("mercy killing"), which is illegal in the United States. The concept of physician aid in dying (**PAD**), "assisted suicide" allows the client to self-administer medication causing death; PAD is allowed in a small number of U.S. states.

Legislation has greatly influenced the U.S. hospice movement and laws continue to change. For example, government funding, managed care plans, and private insurance now often pay for hospice care. The Patient Self-Determination Act (PSDA) of 1991 (Chapter 4) allowed people more say regarding their end-of-life care. "Of the 2.6 million people who died in 2014 in the United States 2.1 million are ages 65 and older, making Medicare the largest insurer of healthcare provided during the last year of life" (Cubanski et al, 2016, para 1). Medicare states *conditions of participation* (**COP**), which set out specific requirements for a program or client to receive funding. Included is the requirement for quality improvement (QI) standards, which have increased, because of changes in COP. Many hospice programs were doing active and appropriate QI, but in some cases, improvements were required. The Affordable Care Act is also concerned with hospice care, with recommendations and requirements in a state of flux.

A number of organizations are specifically concerned with hospice care. The World Health Organization (WHO) is involved in advising hospices and setting standards for pain control. The National Hospice and Palliative Care Organization (**NHPCO**) establishes criteria for hospices and offers information and education to healthcare professionals and the public. The National Association for Home Care & Hospice (**NAHC**) assists hospices and other healthcare agencies with regulations governing hospices. For example, federal regulations state that hospices must make every effort to control clients' pain. Numbers of hospice clients continue to grow (Box 100-1).

Box 100-1 Hospice Care in the United States (and Puerto Rico)

Number of U.S. Hospice Programs, by Year

Year	Number
1974	1
2015	4,199
2016	4,382
2017	4,488
2018	4,639

Number of Medicare Clients Served, by Year

Year	Number
2015	1.38 million
2016	1.43 million
2017	1.49 million
2018	1.55 million

Services Provided (2018)

Routine home care	98.2%
General inpatient care	1.2%
Continuous home care	0.2%
Inpatient respite care	0.3%

Principal Diagnosis of Decedents (2018)

Cancer	29.6%
Circulatory/heart	17.4%
Dementia	15.6%
Other	14.7%
Respiratory	11.0%
Stroke	9.5%
Chronic kidney disease	2.2%

Trends:

- Clients are slightly older
- Percentage of Asian/Pacific islander and Hispanic clients have increased since 2014
- Increasing numbers of noncancer clients
- Increasing length of service at home since 2014 (3.4% increase)
- Increasing percentage of for-profit hospice providers

Reprinted with permission from National Hospice and Palliative Care Organization. (2020). *Facts and figures.* https://www.nhpco.org/wp-content/uploads/NHPCO-Facts-Figures-2020-edition.pdf

THE HOSPICE CONCEPT

Most U.S. hospice programs are independent and community based or are divisions of hospitals, home health agencies, or nursing homes. Most hospices admit people with cancer, as well as other diagnoses, although the overall percentage of cancer clients is declining (Box 100-1). Many admit persons with acquired immunodeficiency syndrome (AIDS), and about 90% of hospices in the United States admit terminally ill children. Hospices encourage the presence of primary caregivers at home, but individual cases are considered. Many U.S. hospices admit people who need high-tech therapies, such as intravenous (IV) medications, tube feedings, or supplemental oxygen. The average age of hospice clients is increasing.

Goals of Hospice

Hospice care focuses on four areas of human needs:

- Physical
- Psychological/emotional
- Social/cultural
- Spiritual

Hospice programs eliminate the emphasis on "saving lives" that permeates acute care settings and emphasize *quality of life.* Much of the high-tech equipment commonly found in acute care units is not commonly used in hospice. Physical and emotional comfort is emphasized instead.

The goals of hospice are as follows:

- Relief of distressing symptoms (physical and emotional)
- Provision of expert care and a protective environment
- Assurance that the client and family will not be abandoned

A hospice program may be located in a place other than the client's or a family member's home. For example, the National Prison Hospice Association (NPHA) has been instrumental in developing a number of programs in prisons. Locations include Texas, Connecticut, and Angola Prison in California. Hospice care also exists in nursing homes and in free-standing inpatient hospice residences. Wherever the client lives is considered to be the *client's home at that time.*

> **NCLEX Alert**
>
> Be alert to the goals of hospice, as listed above. Consideration of these goals as you read the test scenarios during your examination may help you select appropriate nursing actions and considerations. The goals provide the nurse with the conceptual understanding to adapt nursing principles during this state of a client's illness.

> **Box 100-2 Sample Criteria for Admission to a Hospice[a]**
>
> - A diagnosis of progressive, terminal illness. Primary care provider, client, and family agree that control of symptoms is the primary goal, after determining no curative treatment is available or desirable.
> - Life expectancy is usually no more than 6 months.
> - Primary caregiver(s) agree to be responsible for care 24 hr a day.
> - In most cases, client and caregivers have agreed on DNR/DNI status. DNH status is also very common.
> - Hospice care can be discontinued with the agreement of the client, family, and primary care provider.
> - Admission can be directed primarily toward meeting the needs of the family.
>
> DNH, do not hospitalize; DNI, do not intubate; DNR, do not resuscitate.
> [a]Courtesy of Good Samaritan Hospice Care, Kellogg Community College, Battle Creek, Michigan, and Abbott-Northwestern Home Care, Hospice Unit, St. Louis Park, Minnesota.

Characteristics of a Hospice

To be classified as a legitimate hospice, an agency must meet the following criteria:

- The hospice must be a centrally administered, autonomous program. Staff members and family caregivers primarily provide care, with backup inpatient services.
- The goal is *symptom control* (intensive **palliative care**), not curative measures. The term *advanced illness care* applies here. Clients should remain as alert and comfortable as possible.
- The major unit of care should be the client and his or her family. The term *family* refers to a client's significant others, whether related by blood or not. These significant others are designated as *primary caregivers.*
- Team members should practice interdisciplinary (integrative) care, under a qualified healthcare provider's direction (discussed later). Consultation must be available at all times, day or night, and specially trained volunteers must be available to provide assistive services.
- Support should be available for hospice staff and the client's caregivers.
- Hospice services must be extended to the family during the time of bereavement (following the client's death) for at least 1 year.
- Hospice services must be based on a client's needs, not on financial resources.

> **Key Concept**
>
> The term *palliative care* encompasses nursing care and medical treatments that relieve or reduce *physical and psychological symptoms,* to make the client more comfortable. It does not aim to "cure" a disease. Principles of palliative care aid the terminally ill person toward the end of his or her life (advanced illness care).

Clinical practice guidelines for palliative care include "assessment and treatment of pain and other symptoms, help with patient-centered communication and decision making, and coordination of care" (National Coalition for Hospice and Palliative Care, 2018). Palliative care and hospice begin with the diagnosis of a life-limiting condition and follow the client and family through curative modalities, chronicity, and end-of-life care. Pain management is a vital component (Sholjakova et al, 2018). (Some components of this care are not reimbursable under Medicare; skilled care usually can be provided, however. The Affordable Care Act also aims to alleviate discrepancies.)

Box 100-2 lists criteria for a person's admission to a hospice. If a client experiences a remission, the client may be discharged from the hospice program, to resume aggressive medical treatment. If another exacerbation occurs, the client can reenter the hospice program. (Many living people are discharged from hospice programs each year—see Box 100-1.)

> **Key Concept**
>
> The hospice concept attempts to make the dying process an experience of coming together for clients and families.
>
> Common terms used by hospice programs to reference services or levels of care are as follows:
>
> - Routine
> - Respite
> - Continuous care
> - General inpatient (GIP)

Service Coordination

Usually, hospice staff members attempt to coordinate a client's care at home as long as possible. Many clients choose to die at home; staff members assist with this decision. Primary caregivers must be willing and able to assume responsibility for home care. Hospice staff members meet with clients/caregivers to determine feasibility and provide information about available supplementary services.

> **Key Concept**
>
> The goal of hospice care is *not to speed death, nor to unduly prolong life*. Team members assist clients and caregivers to manage pain and other symptoms. Hospice's goal for the client is a safe and comfortable passage through terminal illness, while maintaining self-esteem and attaining self-actualization.

Funding

Various means are used to fund hospice care. Some clients have private insurance. In addition, the federal Social Security Act (Title XXII) provides Medicare and Medicaid assistance to clients meeting COP requirements, as introduced earlier. Services are usually covered on a per diem (by the day) basis, paying for various levels of services, including home care, skilled nursing facility (SNF), and hospital care, as well as family respite care. The Affordable Care Act also addresses payment for hospice care.

Equipment

Durable medical equipment (**DME**) may be covered by third-party payors. DME includes the hospital bed, bedside commode (**BSC**), overbed table, trapeze, or wheelchair, as well as high-tech equipment, such as an IV pump or oxygen concentrator. Community agencies, such as the American Cancer Society or County Social Services, often have DME to loan or rent to hospice clients.

Symptom Management

The person at the end of life often has many physical symptoms requiring nursing management, some of which are discussed in Chapter 59. Remember, however, that symptoms related to hospice care often span a longer period or require management different from that in other settings. The client, caregivers, and the hospice team plan together, to manage pain and other symptoms. Usually, clients discontinue radiation therapy or chemotherapy before admission to a hospice program. As per the PSDA of 1991, hospice clients are often encouraged to designate *Do Not Resuscitate* (**DNR**) and *Do Not Intubate* (**DNI**) status. Clients also often choose to be on *Do Not Hospitalize* (**DNH**) status. The philosophy of hospice is that suffering is not prolonged; client comfort is the goal. Symptoms are managed as noninvasively as possible.

Client and Family as Care Unit

The client and family, along with the hospice team, decide on the most appropriate care. A specially trained nurse (usually a registered nurse [RN]) makes an initial home visit, to assess the home's physical setup and family dynamics. This assessment includes an evaluation of the willingness, ability, and motivation of caregivers and client to participate. The client is particularly encouraged to use medications and other modalities for control of pain and other symptoms. After the initial visit, other hospice team members make most of the home visits and assist caregivers to prepare for their loved one's death. They help with matters such as funeral planning, as well as referrals for services, such as writing a will and financial planning. Clients and caregivers are encouraged to join support groups. Usually, if a client has a peaceful terminal phase of life, family members feel less guilt and grief. (Staff members also observe and report on family members who experience unhealthy grieving, so they can receive assistance.) The client remains in control of his or her care for as long as possible. This is "autonomous decision making at the end-of-life" (Houska & Loucka, 2019).

Compassion Fatigue

Compassion fatigue is a natural reaction to stress but may result in a caregiver's inability to continue caring for a loved one. In this situation, caregivers suffer emotional and sometimes, physical breakdown, resulting from the stress of constant care of a loved one. (This can also occur in nurses, due to the extreme stress of constantly caring for terminally ill clients.) The signs and symptoms of compassion fatigue include reduced ability to understand client needs, personal nightmares and/or flashbacks, exhaustion, irritability, depression and hopelessness, difficulty making decisions, and problems concentrating. Some caregivers increase their use of drugs, alcohol, and tobacco. Some may even consider suicide. Caregivers may reach the point where they can no longer separate caregiving functions from their personal life. The nurse can be helpful to caregivers and fellow nurses by encouraging them in self-care and encouraging them to participate in diversional activities, crafts, scrapbooking, journaling, meditation, or yoga, as well as to obtain adequate rest and proper nutrition. Respite care for caregivers is included in most hospice programs. Caregivers must maintain their own physical and mental health at optimum level, in order to be beneficial to their loved one.

Respite Care

Caring for a dying person may cause financial hardship as well as be exhausting and frustrating. Caregivers may be required to take excessive time away from work, or the client may have been the primary breadwinner. **Respite** means that caregivers "take a break," usually for 2 to 4 weeks, but it may be just for 1 day. Respite care is accomplished by admitting clients to inpatient hospice settings or by arranging for supplemental home care. Some hospice programs have contracts with inpatient facilities to provide family respite; this cost may be covered by third-party payors. Family caregivers should be encouraged to utilize respite services. In this way, they will be physically and emotionally better able to continue with the difficult task of caring for their loved one.

> **Key Concept**
>
> In some cases, client rehospitalization is necessary because caregivers can no longer physically or emotionally care for their loved one. They may also lack the necessary technical skills to manage equipment, such as oxygen, feeding tubes, IVs, etc.

Integrative Care

Integrative care addresses healing the whole person, mind, body, and spirit. Integrative care combines conventional

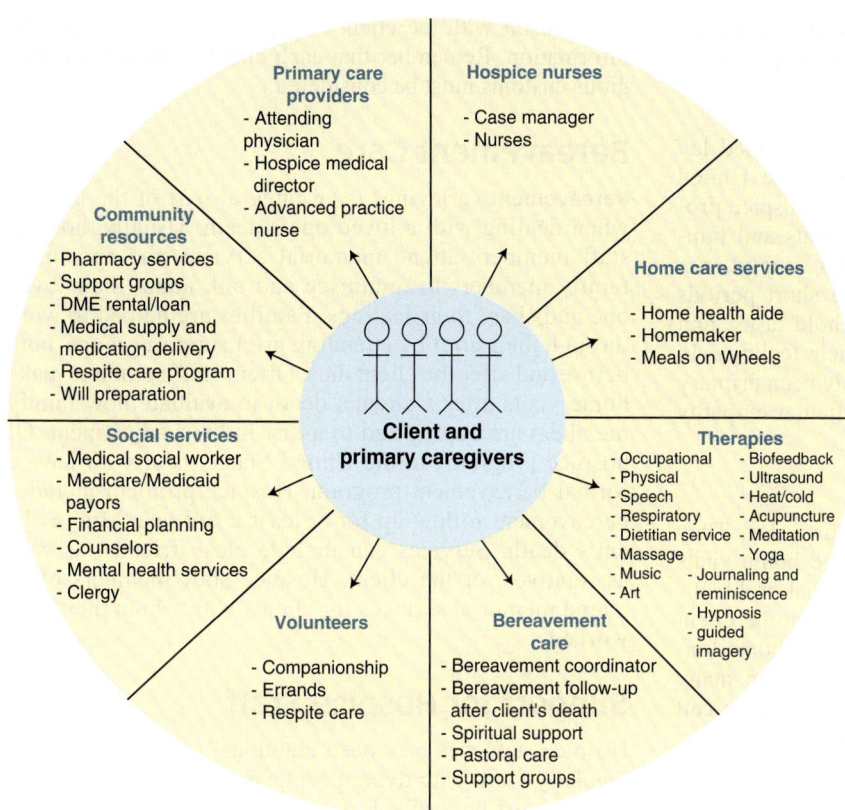

Figure 100-1 Integrative care in hospice. Note that the client, along with the caregivers, is the center of all hospice care. The care under the direction of a healthcare provider, physician assistant, and/or advance practice nurse is carried out by staff nurses, volunteers, and other members of the hospice team. DME, durable medical equipment.

medicine with an array of other therapies. An interdisciplinary team or group (**IDT** or **IDG**) consisting of healthcare providers, nurses, social workers, therapists (occupational, physical, speech, respiratory, massage), clergy, bereavement coordinators, dietitians, pharmacologists, home health aides, homemakers, and volunteers integrates the care of the client, *with the client always at the center.* IDTs today also include acupuncturists, and specialists in therapies such as hypnosis, biofeedback, ultrasound, guided imagery, music, and art. Figure 100-1 depicts **integrative care** in hospice.

Although approved provider-directed services are required, the client is the center of care; the interdisciplinary team responds to each client's needs. A plan of care (**POC**) is established for each client; input is obtained from the client, primary caregivers, and members of the IDT. The primary provider establishes the diagnosis and signs the initial certification of terminal illness. The healthcare provider, physician assistant, or advance practice nurse performs the admission history and physical examination, orders required tests and medications, and follows the client throughout the illness. (Often, the primary caregiver or the client is first to suggest that hospice care might be appropriate.)

Role of the Nurse

An RN does the initial admission and assessment of the client and the home and is the case manager. A nationally certified RN is entitled to use the initials **CRNH** (Certified RN, Hospice). LVN/LPNs, the client, and other caregivers are vital members of the team; communication between team members is vital.

Nurses set up medications, as ordered, evaluate the client's compliance, and determine their effects and/or side effects. Questions involving medications include the following:

Is the client taking medications as ordered?
Are medications effectively controlling pain and other symptoms?
Are there any unwanted side effects?

Hospice nurses answer caregivers' and clients' questions and assist other team members. Nurses perform functions, such as drawing blood or teaching caregivers to use specialized equipment. Nurses also serve as client advocates, ensuring that each client's care is maximized.

Role of Home Health Aides and Homemakers

Home health aides and homemakers work under the overall guidance of the case manager but may be directly supervised by LVN/LPNs. Home health aides and homemakers assist with daily client needs, such as cleanliness and nutrition. For example, the client may receive a bed bath three times a week, given by a home health aide, or a homemaker may assist with cleaning the home or preparing meals.

Role of Primary Caregivers

Primary (family) caregivers are vital to the client's care, providing constant liaison between the client and the hospice team and suggesting appropriate approaches to care. Caregivers often can identify subtle changes in the client's condition that need to be addressed. Some functions of daily care are performed by primary caregivers. For example, after medications are set up by the nurse for the week, their daily administration is supervised by the client and caregivers.

Role of Volunteers

Integral to any hospice program are specially trained lay volunteers. More than 400,000 volunteers in the United States donate over 19 million hours yearly to hospice programs (NHPCO, n.d.). Volunteers assist clients and families in many ways; they provide emotional support, run errands, assist with physical care, provide short periods of respite, help with child care and household tasks, and allow caregivers and clients to express their feelings. In many cases, these volunteers have previously been primary caregivers; therefore, they can provide particular empathy and understanding.

Role of On-Call Services

Services of hospice staff are available 24 hr a day. They answer questions or concerns and may make home visits to help families deal with physical or emotional problems. Hospice staff members come to the home when the client dies. Many caregivers are able to keep clients at home longer, knowing that on-call services are available. In many cases, hospice clients are able to die at home, with on-call assistance from hospice staff.

Emotional Support

The greatest fear of many clients is that they will die alone. It is important for caregivers to realize this and to provide more support as illness progresses. Volunteers can assist by staying with clients, to relieve the family. The second greatest fear of most clients is that of having uncontrolled pain. It is important for them to know that physical pain can usually be managed successfully. It is important to address emotional and spiritual pain, as well as physical pain.

Empathic communication with hospice clients is essential. Remember to be aware of nonverbal cues. It is important for the family to let the client know that they care and that they are sad about the situation. It is OK to cry with the client. If no one shows emotions, the client may believe that no one cares that he or she is dying. Caregivers may be more distressed than clients when the client's status deteriorates (often an unnecessary cause of hospital readmission). Therefore, caregivers also need emotional support and need to discuss their concerns and feelings. Referrals to spiritual support or social services may be helpful. Hospice programs assist clients and families individually to explore the meaning, purpose, and value of their own lives. One goal is that clients can reconcile with estranged loved ones, heal relationships, and complete other important personal tasks before they die.

Spiritual Support

Most hospice teams have chaplains or spiritual advisors available for consultation if clients are interested. Various religious groups have different rituals and procedures related to illness, death, and care of the body after death (Chapter 14). It is important for the hospice team to determine the client and family wishes early in the process. The hospice team can also consult with the client's religious advisor for specific information. Remember that each client's cultural and religious customs must be considered.

Bereavement Care

Bereavement (grieving) is an integral part of the process when dealing with a loved one's death. Usually, hospice staff members attend memorial services and encourage family members to reminisce and talk about their loved one and share their feelings. Families are helped to work through their grief by attending grief support groups, both before and after the client dies. Often, staff members make home visits after a client's death to evaluate how family members are coping and to assist in their adjustment. Of hospice programs in the United States, nearly all have a formal bereavement program. Hospice protocol includes bereavement follow-up for at least a full year after a client's death. Services can include close friends, as well as relatives, of the client. Hospice staff members often attend memorial services for clients with whom they have worked.

Support for Hospice Staff

Hospice staff members need emotional support when they regularly work with dying people. Support groups or other outlets must be available for team members, to help deal with the loss of people for whom they have cared (compassion fatigue). Grieving when clients die is normal and appropriate. Family members often appreciate staff members who are able to express their grief.

ASSISTING THE HOSPICE CLIENT TO MEET BASIC NEEDS

The hospice client has basic needs, as do all people. The hospice nurse assists in helping clients to meet basic needs that have been compromised by illness. Hospice nurses usually do not provide most of the direct physical care. Their focus is on identifying family and client needs and helping to find ways to meet these needs. The case manager coordinates the client's care with hospice team members and caregivers (Fig. 100-1). A major component of all hospice care is that of symptom control—to make the client as comfortable as possible. A hospice nurse plays a major role in symptom control (Box 59-3). In Practice: Important Medications 100-1 lists medications often used to help clients meet basic needs and achieve greater comfort. Most hospice clients have several symptoms simultaneously. It is important to address all symptoms, while determining those that are most problematic. The goal is to alleviate those symptoms that interfere with the client's quality of life, without causing unnecessary, unpleasant side effects. Unneeded, invasive, and painful treatments or examinations are eliminated, as much as possible. Staff members must continuously monitor the client and adjust treatment, as necessary. To help the client meet basic needs, the hospice nurse teaches caregivers how to provide the best care. In Practice: Nursing Care Guidelines 100-1 provides additional information.

> **Key Concept**
>
> Review Chapter 59 for an overview of general end-of-life care. Most of the procedures identified in that chapter apply in hospice care as well. One major function of the hospice nurse is to teach caregivers to assist the client to meet basic needs and to be as comfortable as possible. Box 59-3 describes some signs of approaching death, with their causes.

Oxygen and Airway

Maintaining a patent (open) airway is probably the most important factor in promoting client comfort. Many clients have lung involvement, causing dyspnea. Stress reduction, position changes, such as raising the head of the bed, and circulating air with a fan or air conditioner to cool the room may help. Frequently evaluate the client's vital signs, including pain, oxygen saturation, and level of consciousness. Supplemental oxygen may be helpful; oxygen concentrators, rather than tanks, are commonly used in the home (Chapter 87). Thoracentesis, to remove fluid, may relieve pressure, and medications (including aerosolized inhalers and nebulizer treatments, cough medicines, and decongestants) may decrease secretions and improve respiration. A low dose of morphine may help reduce the tissue oxygen demand, as well as reduce pain. Postural drainage helps eliminate lung secretions; surgery may help relieve obstructions. The client may be able to breathe only when sitting upright (*orthopnea;* Table 48-1). Hospice programs rarely use heroic measures, such as mechanical ventilators.

IN PRACTICE
NURSING CARE GUIDELINES 100-1 — Providing Care in Hospice Nursing

- The client is encouraged to "live as long and as well as possible" (http://hospiceofrockland.org/).
- Emphasize the positive; consider difficulties as *challenges and opportunities,* not problems. Focus on what *can* be done.
- Provide practical solutions for care.
- Control the client's symptoms, as much as possible.
- Do not try to predict the exact time of death.
- Do not get involved in family disputes.
- Allow the client and family to express spirituality in the way they desire.
- Respect the client's cultural customs and beliefs.
- Maintain your sense of humor.
- Allow the client to be alone or stay with the client, depending on what he or she desires.
- Recognize that acting out behaviors by the family and the client are normal factors in grieving.
- Be honest. Explain what is happening.
- When in doubt, be quiet.
- Allow the client and family to maintain hope, at whatever level.
- Encourage the client to reminisce, tell family stories, or assist with a scrapbook or photo album.
- Remember: *Comfort* is the goal of all therapy (physical and emotional).
- Refer the family and client to counseling, if appropriate.

Seizures

Clients may be at risk for seizures, secondary to primary or metastatic lesions. Seizures may cause falling or threaten the client's airway or mobility. Medications are available to help control seizures (In Practice: Important Medications 100-1).

Nutrition and Hydration

The client is assisted to maintain nutrition and hydration, as much as is desired and comfortable for the client. It is important to note that dehydration may be the cause of unnecessary rehospitalization if caregivers do not understand the active dying process (Box 59-3).

Anorexia

Many terminally ill people are unable to eat because of fatigue, pain, anxiety, depression, odors, dehydration, nausea, or general discomfort. Clients may be encouraged to eat or take fluids, to preserve strength and improve quality of life. However, studies indicate that most clients benefit from low oral intake in late stages of illness. Reassure the family about this. Vitamins, tranquilizers, antidepressants, *antiemetics* (antinausea medications), appetite stimulants, or small amounts of alcohol may help and are most effective if given about a half hour before meals. Be sure the client receives good mouth care before and after meals (Chapters 31 and 32).

Mealtimes are usually enjoyed more if free of unpleasant odors and if music, television, mail, or socializing is available. Bright lights, loud noises, or a stuffy room may be annoying. Dietitians and staff can teach caregivers ways to encourage clients to eat. In rare cases, nasogastric tube feedings are given. Late in the process, clients may not eat or drink; they only receive mouth care. These clients may enjoy sucking on prepared mouth swabs, a wet washcloth, ice chips, or hard candy, providing liquid and numbing the mouth.

Try to give the client frequent, small meals and snacks, presented attractively. Consider food preferences; soft foods are often preferred. Fluids are often better tolerated than solids. High-protein, high-calorie liquid supplements such as Ensure, Boost, or Resource are often preferred to solids, as are clear liquids. (Milk, creamed milk products, or very sweet drinks may cause problems.) Offer ice pops, sherbet, and ice chips. (Remember: most clients prefer cold liquids, but this depends heavily on cultural preferences.)

Nausea and Vomiting

Hospice clients often experience nausea and vomiting caused by anorexia, tumor invasion, pain, inner ear involvement, reaction to narcotics, increased intracranial pressure, or previous radiation or chemotherapy. Many procedures suggested to treat anorexia also apply to nausea. Evaluate nausea for patterns and remove causes whenever possible. Lying on the right side and guided relaxation (including meditation and hypnosis) are effective, as are companionship, music, backrubs, mouth breathing, and cool cloths on the forehead. Antiemetics and other medications are often helpful and should be given approximately one half hour before meals (In Practice: Important Medications 100-1). Clients may want carbonated beverages or tea; dry foods, such as popcorn or soda crackers, are often helpful. Ice chips may be soothing. (Teach caregivers to wear gloves when caring for this client.)

IN PRACTICE
IMPORTANT MEDICATIONS 100-1: The Hospice Comfort Pack

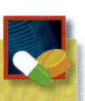

One hospice uses a combination of medications to promote client comfort. These medications are given regularly, rather than waiting for discomfort to occur, to help prevent "breakthrough pain." Other hospices have similar medication configurations. The "comfort pack" includes the following:

- Morphine—to manage pain and dyspnea (helps to reduce tissue oxygen demand, especially related to acute sedation)
- Haldol—to treat delirium and nausea (used as dopamine antagonist)
- Lorazepam (Ativan)—to treat anxiety and dyspnea
- Metoclopramide (Reglan)—antiemetic (to prevent nausea and emesis)
- Acetaminophen (Tylenol)—to reduce fever
- A fiber or laxative may be added, to reduce constipation caused by morphine
  https://www.vnsny.org/article/comfort-pack-convenient-medication-relief/

Symptom Control (Other Than Pain) in Hospice Care

Nausea—Antiemetics (Some Are Used During and After Chemotherapy as Well)
- ABHR (combination of lorazepam [Ativan], diphenhydramine [Benadryl], haloperidol [Haldol], metoclopramide [Reglan]), aprepitant (Emend)
- chlorpromazine HCl—also anxiolytic[a]
- dolasetron mesylate (Anzemet)
- dronabinol (tetrahydrocannabinol)—also appetite stimulant (Marinol)
- hydroxyzine HCl—also anxiolytic, antipruritic[b] (Vistaril)
- meclizine HCl—also antihistamine (Antivert, Bonine)
- metoclopramide HCl—also gastrointestinal (GI) stimulant (Reglan, Apo-Metoclop [Can])
- ondansetron HCl (Zofran)
- prochlorperazine—also anxiolytic (Compro)
- promethazine HCl—also antihistamine, sleep aid (Promethegan)
- trimethobenzamide HCl (Tigan, Ticon)
- antispasmodics also used

Stomach Distress and Flatulence
- aluminum hydroxide (Amphogel)
- calcium carbonate (Alka-Seltzer, Rolaids, Tums)
- magnesium oxide (MagOx 400)
- ranitidine HCl (Zantac)
- Simethicone—antiflatulent (Flatulex, Gas-X, Maalox, Mylicon)

Diarrhea
- bismuth subsalicylate (Kaopectate, Pepto-Bismol)
- loperamide HCl (Imodium)
- octreotide acetate (Sandostatin)

Constipation (Laxatives)

Bulk-Formers
- calcium polycarbophil (FiberCon, Konsyl Fiber)

Osmotic Agents
- glycerin (Fleet)
- lactulose (Constilac)
- polyethylene glycol (PEG; MiraLAX)

Saline Laxative
- magnesium hydroxide—milk of magnesia (MOM)
- magnesium sulfate—Epsom salts

Stimulant Laxatives
- bisacodyl (Dulcolax, Ex-Lax Ultra, Feen-a-Mint)
- senna

Stool Softener
- docusate sodium (Colace)

Combination Agents
- docusate sodium and senna concentrate (Senokot-S, Peri-colace)
- docusate sodium and casanthranol (DSS 100 Plus)

Bladder Spasm
- belladonna suppositories

Diuretics (to Treat Edema)
- acetazolamide (Diamox)
- furosemide (Lasix)
- indapamide (Lozo, Lozide [Can])—also treats hypertension

Seizures (Many Are Available in Tablet, Liquid, or Injectable Forms)—See Also Table 94-2

Many of These Medications Also Used to Manage Neuropathic Pain
- carbamazepine—also used to manage neuropathic pain (Tegretol)
- diazepam—also anxiolytic and skeletal muscle relaxant (Valium)
- gabapentin—also treats postherpetic neuralgia, neuropathic pain (Neurontin)
- phenytoin (Dilantin)
- pregabalin—also analgesic (Lyrica)
- primidone (Mysoline)
- topiramate—also antimigraine (Topamax)
- valproic acid/divalproex sodium—also causes sedation and manages pain (Depakote, Depakene syrup, Deproic [Can], Depacon [injection])

Depression—See Also Table 94-2 and In Practice: Important Medications 100-2
- bupropion HCl (Wellbutrin, Aplenzin)
- citalopram hydrobromide (Celexa)
- doxepin HCl (Silenor)
- fluoxetine HCl (Prozac)
- imipramine HCl and pamoate—also treats pain (Tofranil)
- mirtazapine—also sedative effects (Remeron)
- nortriptyline HCl (Pamelor, Aventyl)—also treats pain
- paroxetine HCl and mesylate (Paxil, Pexeva)
- sertraline HCl (Zoloft)
- trazodone HCl—also treats insomnia (Desyrel, Oleptro)
- venlafaxine HCl—also anxiolytic; treats pain (Effexor)

IN PRACTICE
IMPORTANT MEDICATIONS 100-1: The Hospice Comfort Pack (Continued)

Anxiety (Many Also Used to Prevent Seizures)—See Also Table 94-2
- buspirone HCl (BuSpar)
- chlorpromazine HCl—also antiemetic (Thorazine)
- diazepam—also skeletal muscle relaxant (Valium, Diastat, Diazemuls [Can])
- doxepin HCl—also antipruritic, sleep aid (Silenor, Sinequan)
- hydroxyzine HCl and pamoate—also antiemetic, antipruritic (Vistaril, Atarax)
- lorazepam—also sedative (Ativan)

Insomnia
- diphenhydramine—also antihistamine (Benadryl)
- eszopiclone (Lunesta)
- temazepam (Restoril)
- zolpidem tartrate (Ambien, Zolpimist—oral spray)

Edema (Most Also Used to Treat Hypertension)
- furosemide (Lasix)
- hydrochlorothiazide (HCTZ, Apo-Hydro [Can], Microzide, Urozide [Can])
- torsemide (Demadex)
- triamterene/hydrochlorothiazide (Dyazide, Maxzide)

[a]Anxiolytic: treats anxiety.
[b]Antipruritic: treats itching.
Antiemetic: treats nausea and vomiting.
Resource: Karch, A. & Tucker, R. (2019). *2020 Lippincott pocket drug guide for nurses*. Wolters Kluwer.
Rosemary Rosdahl, RPh, Watertown Pharmacy, Minnesota.

Dehydration

Many clients become dehydrated shortly before death, which is often unavoidable. Studies indicate that these clients usually do not feel hunger or thirst and have also shown that some dehydration can be beneficial. *Rationale: Dehydration dries secretions and reduces choking, nausea, ascites, pulmonary edema, and breathing difficulties.* However, when clients retain fluid, feces may become hard and impacted, causing constipation and bowel obstruction. Observe and report dehydration and complications. The hospice team determines if treatment is appropriate for dehydration or electrolyte imbalance. The major area of discomfort for the dehydrated client is a dry mouth. This can be alleviated by ice pops, ice chips, drops of water, or sucking on a wet washcloth or hard candy.

In rare cases, a client may receive supplemental IV fluids containing dextrose (sugar), electrolytes (e.g., potassium), vitamins, or medications (e.g., morphine). An IV pump or controller is the safest, and caregivers regulate the rate of flow. IV bags are usually delivered to the client's home and nurses, or pharmacists add medications and electrolytes to the solution. Caregivers are taught to hang the bags, adjust the pump or controller, troubleshoot the machine, and know whom to call for questions.

Elimination

The client is assisted with elimination. Bladder and/or bowel incontinence often occurs near the end of life. It is important to keep the client clean and dry, to promote comfort and prevent skin breakdown. Sometimes, medications are helpful; some substances, such as caffeine, acidic and spicy foods, and the artificial sweetener, Aspartame, can aggravate incontinence (Chapters 51 and 89).

Diarrhea

Clients may develop diarrhea from lesion involvement, inadequate intake, bowel obstruction, fecal impaction, or infection or as a side effect of previous chemotherapy, radiation, or medications. A low-residue diet lessens stimulation. Eliminate foods causing gas or cramps. (Clients often know what foods bother them.) Encourage clients to drink a variety of fluids. Good skin care is necessary. (Remind caregivers to wear gloves when giving care to this client.)

Constipation

Many clients are constipated because of inactivity, low food/fluid intake, dehydration, a low-residue diet, or tumor invasion. Constipation is a frequent side effect of narcotics, especially morphine and codeine. Before constipation is treated, it is necessary to determine if a bowel obstruction exists. *Rationale: A bowel obstruction can be life threatening; laxatives can cause a bowel perforation. Diarrhea may be a sign of bowel obstruction, with liquid stool flowing around the obstruction.*

Treatment for constipation includes a high-residue diet, as long as tolerated. Many hospice clients routinely receive laxatives or a stool softener (In Practice: Important Medications 100-1). Suppositories also encourage peristalsis. If constipation is severe, cathartics and hyperosmotic agents may be necessary. In severe cases, the client may require an enema or manual disimpaction of stool (Chapter 51). Most hospices routinely use a bowel regimen, sometimes called a "colon cocktail." An example is 1 cup applesauce, 1 cup prune juice, and 1 cup miller's bran; the client is given 1 tablespoon twice daily. This "cocktail" is usually effective, providing relief without harsh laxatives and cathartics.

> **Key Concept**
> Sometimes, clients think they are constipated because they are not having daily bowel movements. They need to know that a bowel movement every 2 to 3 days is common because of physical inactivity and low oral intake.

Sleep and Rest

It is important to promote sleep and rest, which helps the client to be more alert and comfortable during the day.

Insomnia and Hypersomnia

Sleep disturbances are common, including *insomnia* (difficulty falling asleep or staying asleep long enough). Insomnia may result from anxiety or pain. *Sleep deprivation* can be serious and may lead to further agitation and discomfort, as well as acceleration of the disease process. Extreme sleep deprivation can also lead to paranoia, hallucinations, and other mental disorders. Assist the client to sleep by providing comfort measures, such as fresh bedding, a backrub, soft music and relaxation tapes, or self-hypnosis and guided imagery. Medications are given only if other measures do not help. Depressed clients may sleep too much (*hypersomnia*). The goal of hospice, especially early in the process, is for clients to sleep adequately at night, while maintaining normal activity and as much mobility as possible during the day.

Personal Care and Comfort

As the client's disease progresses, he or she will likely require more assistance with performing activities of daily living (ADLs). The nurse and caregivers are vital in helping to provide this assistance.

Skin Breakdown

A major challenge in the physical care of hospice clients is preventing skin breakdown and pressure areas. Nonintact skin can be a source of infection and pain. Clients with terminal illnesses are often too uncomfortable or weak to move and may choose to remain in one position. They should be encouraged and assisted to change position as much as possible. In addition, the client's nutritional status and hydration may be inadequate to maintain skin integrity; the disease process may have made the skin *friable* (fragile). Stress the importance of frequent position changes and protecting pressure points when teaching caregivers and remind them to wear gloves when dealing with nonintact skin. It is vital to keep the client's skin clean and dry. If possible, clients should be assisted to be out of bed occasionally, to relieve pressure. Special mattresses may help prevent skin breakdown; some special beds allow clients to remain in bed continually without sacrificing skin integrity (Fig. 49-6). Regular pain medications provide maximum comfort and help the client to move more comfortably. (Chapter 58 describes special skin care and wound care in detail.)

Management of Odor

In some cases, the disease process causes a disagreeable odor (Chapter 59). Aerosolized sprays, a few drops of wintergreen oil on a cotton ball, or a mechanical air filter may be used to help cover or eliminate odor. Another device used is the charcoal filter dressing; odors pass through the filter before entering the atmosphere. These dressings are expensive and are usually only used when odors are very disturbing.

Emotional Concerns

Depression

Clients and/or caregivers may experience depression. Hospice staff can assist by listening with empathy and validating feelings. Clinical depression, with or without suicidal ideation (SI), may require antidepressant medication. It is normal to be sad, but continuing clinical depression is usually treated and should be prevented as much as possible

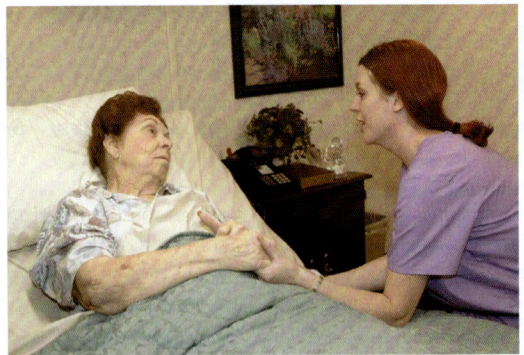

Figure 100-2 The person with a terminal illness may be depressed and may feel that no one cares. It is important for hospice staff and caregivers to be available, to allow this person to express feelings, and to refer the client to professional counseling if necessary. (Timby, 2005.)

(Fig. 100-2). The hospice social worker or chaplain is a possible resource. A referral to a psychologist or psychiatrist may also be necessary. Chapter 94 describes care of depressed or suicidal persons in more detail.

Anxiety

Major causes of anxiety include fear of severe pain, fear of being alone, and fear of dying. Many clients are concerned about the future for their loved ones. Anxious clients may become overly agitated or paranoid. Listen and offer reassurance. Some clients need antianxiety medications (anxiolytics), many of which help control other symptoms as well. (See In Practice: Important Medications 100-1.)

Self-Actualization and Acceptance

The long-term goal of hospice is *death with dignity* that is as comfortable as possible. At the top level of Maslow hierarchy of needs is that of *self-actualization*. The person doing end-of-life work is encouraged to reminisce with the client. The goal is that the person will feel that they have accomplished important things and has lived a worthwhile life (Fig. 100-3). Remember that having raised a family and maintained a household constitutes an important contribution to society. The fully functioning person will be more comfortable and able to achieve the *acceptance* stage in the dying process. The hospice nurse and caregivers play an important role in encouraging and supporting the client and listening to the client (Fig. 100-2).

PAIN MANAGEMENT

Many clients experience chronic, severe, and unremitting pain that differs from occasional, temporary pain caused by other conditions (Chapter 55). Aggressive pain management is a primary goal of hospice nursing. The hospice concept encourages clients to take advantage of available pain control measures, but this is not required. Morphine is very commonly used and works well, although a number of other modalities are also available to assist in pain control (In Practice: Important Medications 100-2 and Table 100-1). Addiction is not a concern; the client may be physically dependent, but does not display addictive behavior.

Evaluation of Pain

Remember to assess pain frequently as the *fifth vital sign*. Listen to the client's self-report; this is considered the most reliable indicator of pain. Only the client knows how the pain feels, what makes it worse, and what gives relief. Pain and its level of interference with activities, rest, and general comfort are evaluated. Pain is very common in the client with cancer, the most common source being the invasion of the lesion. Classify and document pain—its *character, onset, location, duration, severity, pattern,* and *associated factors* (COLDSPA) (Chapter 55).

> **Key Concept**
> Sometimes clients want to experience pain because pain reminds them they are still alive. These clients may refuse adequate pain control measures; this is their right.

> **SPECIAL CONSIDERATIONS** **Culture and Ethnicity**
> It is important to remember the expression of pain is influenced by culture. Some people are stoic in the face of severe pain and others react extremely to mild pain.

Pharmacologic Therapy

Medications are often used to control pain. A three-step analgesic ladder developed by the World Health Organization suggests nonopioids, weak opioids, and strong opioids for mild, intermediate, and severe pain, respectively (Table 100-1). **Adjuvant** (assisting) medications may be added to *potentiate* (enhance) the opioid's effects or to treat other symptoms. The goal is to manage pain with the *least amount and potency of medication and the highest possible level of client consciousness.* Medications are increased as pain intensity increases (In Practice: Important Medications 100-2). Lesser amounts of medication are often needed if clients self-administer their medications (patient-controlled analgesia [**PCA**]).

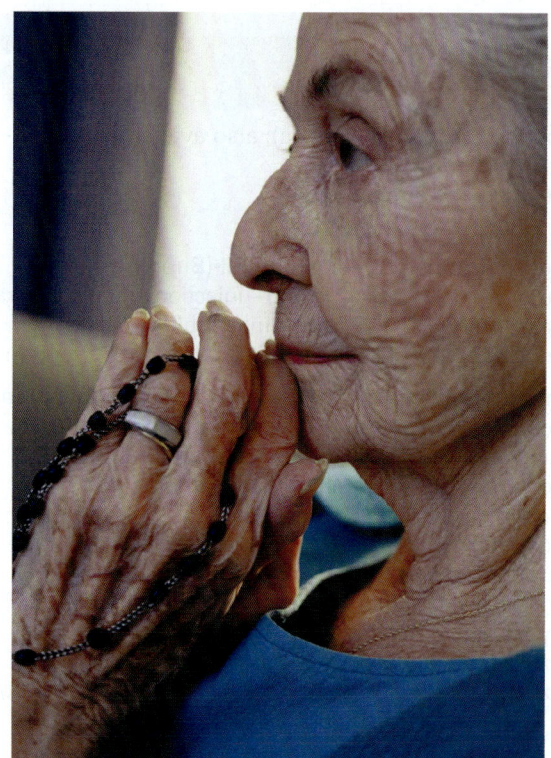

Figure 100-3 The goal of hospice is death with dignity, as a self-actualized person. The client is assisted to explore feelings and beliefs derived from his or her religious/spiritual background, ethnicity/culture, and heritage and reconcile these with his or her personal values (Carter & Lewsen, 2005).

> **NCLEX Alert**
> In this chapter, you will notice references to cultural and religious considerations, as well as pediatric considerations. Be aware of these, as they may be reflected in the NCLEX examination and influence your response to test scenarios/questions.

TABLE 100-1 An Analgesic Ladder[a]

	MEDICATION	PAIN CONTINUES	COMMENTS
Severe pain[b] (7-10) ↑	Strong opioid	Add stronger opioid (e.g., morphine SR; oxycodone IR; OxyContin—SR; hydromorphone; methadone; levorphanol; fentanyl).	Client may now be NPO; use sublingual, rectal, or transdermal fentanyl (patch), SQ morphine, etc.
Moderate pain[b] (4-6) ↑	Weak opioid	Add strong opioid (e.g., acetaminophen combinations with codeine, oxycodone, hydrocodone, morphine IR). Also increase dose, shorten interval between doses.	
Mild to moderate pain[b] (1-3)	Nonopioid	Administer aspirin, acetaminophen, or nonsteroidal anti-inflammatory drug	Opioid-sparing effect—less opioid needed

Nursing considerations
- Addiction is not a concern in hospice—the client may be physically dependent, but does not display addictive behavior.
- Other medications and therapies are often combined with the above.
- Use the least-invasive management and the mildest medications first.
- Rectal suppositories or parenteral medications are usually given if the client is nauseated.

IR, immediate release; NPO, nothing by mouth; SQ, subcutaneous; SR, sustained release. Note: Start at bottom of ladder and add medications as needed.
[a]Initially developed by WHO (the World Health Organization).
[b]Client report of pain on a scale of 1 to 10, with 10 being most severe.

IN PRACTICE
IMPORTANT MEDICATIONS 100-2 Medications Used in Pain Management[a]

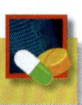

Remember: Pain, as the fifth vital sign, should be assessed whenever other vital signs are assessed and, more often, as needed. The client's self-report is the most reliable indicator of pain. Document the intensity of pain (Chapter 55) and the client's ability to function. Federal guidelines state that "every reasonable effort should be made to control pain."

Nonopioid
- acetaminophen (APAP, Mapap, Aspirin Free Anacin, Atasol [Can], Genapap, Tylenol)—because it is not an anti-inflammatory, it is not as effective as others

Nonsteroidal Anti-Inflammatory Drugs
- aspirin (ASA)
- celecoxib (Celebrex)—fewer GI complications
- etodolac (Lodine)
- ibuprofen (Advil, Motrin)
- indomethacin (Indocin, Novo-Methacin [Can])
- ketoprofen
- naproxen (Naprosyn) and naproxen sodium (Anaprox)

Opioids

Mild Opioids
- hydrocodone bitartrate and acetaminophen (Norco)
  Often added to NSAIDs as combination agent. (Codeine is not used often because of undesirable side effects, see note below.)

Midrange Opioid
- oxycodone (OxyContin)

Strong Opioids
- morphine sulfate, the most commonly used—use IR first, SR later (Astramorph PF, Avinza and Kadian [timed release], Duramorph PF, M-Eslon [Can], MS Contin [controlled-release], Statex [Can])—available in many forms and many combinations).

  Note: Opioid side effects include respiratory depression, sedation, nausea and vomiting, constipation, confusion, urinary problems, dry mouth, and pruritus (itching).

Morphine-Like Agonists (and Opioid Analgesics)
- codeine—may be combined with acetaminophen (Tylenol #3)
- codeine—combined with acetaminophen, butalbital, and caffeine (Fiorinal)
- Various forms of fentanyl citrate (Sublimaze), including injection; nasal spray (Lazanda), sublingual spray (SUBSYS), transdermal (Duragesic patch); transmucosal and lozenge (Actiq)
- hydromorphone HCl (Dilaudid)
- meperidine HCl (Demerol, Pethidine [Can])
- methadone HCl (Dolophine)
- oxycodone HCl (Roxicodone, OxyContin)
- oxycodone (two types) and ASA (Percodan)
- oxymorphone HCl (Opana); also available in crush-resistant form
- pentazocine and naloxone

Mixed Agonist/Antagonists
- buprenorphine HCl—parenteral (Buprenex)
- butorphanol tartrate (Stadol)—injection and nasal spray
- nalbuphine HCl (Nubain)—injectable
- pentazocine HCl (Talwin); with naloxone

Combination Opioid/NSAIDs and Other Combinations
- acetaminophen and hydrocodone (Vicodin, Norco, Anexsia, Co-Gesic, Norco)
- acetaminophen, butalbital, and caffeine (Fioricet, Repan)
- acetaminophen and tramadol (Ultracet)
- codeine and Fiorinal (Fiorinal with codeine)
- codeine and acetaminophen (Tylenol with codeine)
- hydrocodone and ibuprofen (Vicoprofen)
- oxycodone and ASA (Percodan, Roxipirin)
- oxycodone and acetaminophen (Percocet, Endocet)

Adjuvant Drugs Used for Pain Management
- baclofen, combined with anticonvulsants

Anticonvulsants (Manage Neuropathic Pain)
- carbamazepine (Tegretol)
- clonazepam (Klonopin)
- gabapentin (Neurontin)
- pregabalin (Lyrica)
- valproate (Depakote)

Antidepressants (Manage Neuropathic and Musculoskeletal Pain, May Potentiate Effects of Opioids)
- amitriptyline HCl (Levate [Can])
- desipramine HCl (Norpramin)
- doxepin HCl
- duloxetine (Cymbalta)
- imipramine HCl (Tofranil)
- nortriptyline HCl (Aventyl, Pamelor)
- paroxetine HCl (Paxil)

Corticosteroids (Produce Mood Elevation; Other Actions Include Anti-Inflammatory, Antiemetic, Appetite Stimulation, Reduction of Spinal Cord Edema, and Management of Bone Pain and Arthralgia)
- prednisolone (Orapred)
- prednisone (Winpred [Can])

Muscle Relaxants (Help With Muscle Pain)
- baclofen (Gabiofen, Lioresal—intrathecal)
- carisoprodol (Soma)
- chlorzoxazone (Lorzone, Parafen Forte DSL)
- cyclobenzaprine HCl (Amrix, Flexeril)

Neuroleptics and Others (Help With Psychiatric Symptoms)
- hydroxyzine (Vistaril) (also for anxiety, insomnia, nausea, itching)
- many others—Chapter 94

IN PRACTICE
IMPORTANT MEDICATIONS 100-2 Medications Used in Pain Management (Continued)

Anesthetics, Analgesics, and Benzodiazepines (Used as Secondary Treatment for Neuropathic Pain and Anxiety)
- clonazepam (Klonopin)
- clonidine (Catapres, Duraclon)—antihypertensive, also used in severe cancer pain, refractory to other therapies
- lidocaine HCl—antiarrhythmic, also used for pain refractory to other medications; available also as transdermal patch

Adjuvant Medications (Used for Deep Bone Pain)
- bisphosphonate (e.g., pamidronate disodium [Aredia], given IV)
- octreotide acetate—used for deep visceral pain, flushing, and diarrhea

[a]Based in part on CME Course #9713, "Assessment and Management of Pain at the End of Life." Accreditation Council for Continuing Medical Education; 2012.
Intrathecal, administered within the spinal column; IR, immediate release; IV, intravenous; SR, sustained release.
Resource: Karch, A. & Tucker, R. (2019). *2020 Lippincott pocket drug guide for nurses*. Wolters Kluwer.
Rosemary Rosdahl, RPh, Watertown Pharmacy, Minnesota.

Consider several points when administering medications to hospice clients:

- The appropriate dose, route, and interval of administration are carefully chosen.
- The lowest dose of medication is tried first.
- Pain medications are chosen to correspond with the client's report of pain intensity.
- The dose of a narcotic (opiate) may be aggressively increased, if necessary ("**titration up**" of the dose).
- Dosages of opiates should decrease slowly ("**tapering down**") if the medication is to be discontinued. (Withdrawal symptoms are usually reduced in this case.)
- It is important to prevent pain and to relieve breakthrough pain. Pain medications should be administered around the clock to maintain a blood level, not waiting for the client to have breakthrough symptoms. These clients are usually more comfortable and survive longer and less medication is needed, in most cases. Appropriate co-analgesics (and nonpharmacologic modalities) are used, to minimize use of opiates as much as possible.
- It is important to prevent unwanted side effects of medications, as much as possible.
- When routes change (e.g., from oral to rectal or intramuscular [IM]), dosages usually change as well.
- The client's tolerance to other medications is taken into account, as well as previous use of alcohol and street drugs, smoking, exercise, and other physical conditions. Opiate-naïve clients usually respond to even small doses of medication. People who smoke, abuse drugs and other substances, or have been very athletic often require more medication than others to achieve comfort. *Rationale: Substance abuse causes the client to build up tolerance to medications; thus, this client requires higher doses to obtain relief. Exercise increases production of endorphins, natural pain relievers. Endorphin production decreases as clients become less active.*
- People with severe liver or kidney damage may require higher dosages of pain-relieving medication. *Rationale: These clients usually metabolize medications more slowly and not as completely as those with normal liver and/or kidney function.*
- A hospice client taking narcotics is not considered an "addict," although withdrawal symptoms will occur if the drug is discontinued.

> **Nursing Alert** Many nonopioid drugs (especially NSAIDs and aspirin) are mild anticoagulants and must be used with caution.

Administration Routes

Oral medications are the first choice for pain management. Clients usually administer their own oral medications, based on pain severity. Some oral medications are very effective for mild pain; NSAIDs and combination medications are commonly used. Clients often find that liquid medications are easier to swallow than tablets. In some cases, medications are administered by the *sublingual* (under the tongue), *buccal* (inside the cheek), or rectal (suppository) route. Some drugs, such as fentanyl may also be administered *transdermally*, by use of a skin patch, as well as orally in a liquid, a lozenge, or a lozenge on a stick.

When oral, rectal, or transdermal medications no longer control pain, parenteral medications may be administered subcutaneously, intramuscularly, intravenously, or intrathecally. In some cases, clients administer their own subcutaneous injections. (The IM route is used only when medications given by another route are not effective because IM absorption is variable, due to muscle tissue deterioration and decreased circulation. It is also painful and inconvenient.) In the case of IV administration, a saline or heparin lock is routinely placed, to preclude repeated venipuncture. Caregivers and clients are taught to administer medications via the lock and to flush it (Chapter 64). PCA pumps allow clients to control their own parenteral medication administration. Some clients have implanted, pre-programmed pumps that automatically dispense medications and provide constant blood levels. Routes of administration (oral, injectable, rectal, transdermal) may also be combined. Clients who regulate their own medication usually use less; use of a morphine pump is very common. Allowing the person to have this control also increases self-esteem.

> **Key Concept**
> Morphine is very commonly used in hospice and is available in several forms, including oral solution and tablets, rectal suppositories, and injectable forms (IV, IM, SQ, epidural [lumbar], and intrathecal [spinal cord area]). It is available in immediate-release and timed-release forms. Oral administration is one third to one sixth as effective as parenteral administration. There is no upper limit to the dose of morphine in hospice, if it is needed.

Management of Side Effects

A side effect of opiates (opioids) may be sedation, although most clients quickly build up tolerance. When the client is more comfortable, sedation usually is not bothersome. Blood pressure and respirations may be reduced; when administering morphine or other opiates, regularly evaluate the client's respiratory status and level of consciousness. In oversedation, the dose may be reduced. Evaluate the client's sedation as follows (nursing actions are in parentheses):

- Awake, alert
- Drowsy, easily aroused
- Asleep, easily aroused
- Drowsy most of the time, may go to sleep during conversation (give less "as needed" [PRN] medication; consult the provider)
- **Somnolent**: very difficult or impossible to arouse; shallow respirations (fewer than 10-12 per minute); pinpoint pupils (hold medication and consult the provider—an antidote, such as naloxone [Narcan], may be prescribed if client does not respond)

Another common side effect of opiates is constipation, which can result in fecal impaction or bowel obstruction. Usually, clients receive scheduled laxatives and/or stool softeners along with opiates.

> **Key Concept**
> Remember that hospice clients usually do not have daily bowel movements. Reassure the client and caregivers that this is normal.

Long-term treatment with opiates can cause other undesirable side effects, such as nausea and vomiting, dry mouth, itching, difficulty voiding, and sleep disturbances. These conditions are treated symptomatically.

Psychosocial and Other Nonpharmacologic Modalities for Pain Management

Although medications are used very commonly in pain management, other nonpharmacologic modalities can also be helpful, alone or in combination with medications. Some of these also help the client to sleep. Nonpharmacologic modalities include relaxation, massage, guided imagery, self-hypnosis, visualization, distraction, ultrasound, skin stimulation, biofeedback, and acupuncture/acupressure. Relaxation helps reduce muscle tension, promotes sleep, reduces anxiety, and enhances the effectiveness of medications. It is helpful to lie or sit comfortably in a quiet place and systematically relax all the muscles in the body. Gentle massage in the painful area may be combined with relaxation. Controlled breathing is vital. Guided imagery is often combined with relaxation techniques; this involves visualizing the pain or disease as small and weak and the body as strong and powerful. Self-hypnosis can assist the client gradually to "move pain out of the body." Audio relaxation and visualization exercises are available on CD or for podcasts. Skin stimulation involves the use of massage, vibration, pressure, friction, temperature changes (heat/cold), and menthol-type creams (e.g., Bengay, Icy Hot, Mineral Ice, Salonpas) to stimulate the skin's nerve endings. Sometimes, applying ice on the *contralateral* side (opposite the pain) helps. A TENS unit may be activated by the client, to apply electrical stimulation directly to nerves, interrupting pain transmission. This *biofeedback* allows the client to anticipate pain and deliver the impulse at the first hint of discomfort, for maximum effectiveness. This strategy can also assist the client to assess pain intensity to determine how much medication, if any, to use. Acupuncture and acupressure provide *counterstimulation* (against the pain) and can also help block pain transmission.

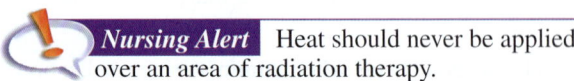

> **Nursing Alert** Heat should never be applied over an area of radiation therapy.

Many clients also benefit from psychotherapy, support groups, or pastoral counseling. Education is important. Clients should visit with family and friends, play with pets, read, sew, watch television, listen to or play music, or pursue other hobbies and activities. These activities help to distract the client; this distraction can be increased by keeping time to music or turning up the volume. Encourage clients to maintain physical activity and exercise as long as possible. Movement prevents stiffness and other problems related to immobility, as well as increasing endorphin levels. Immobilizing or supporting an affected part or repositioning the body is often helpful. Cutaneous (skin) stimulation modalities help promote exercise.

Palliative Radiation, Medications, and Surgery

Palliative radiation may arrest tumor growth or reduce its size, usually in a specific area. IV injection of radioactive materials can help relieve severe pain of widespread bony metastases. In specific cases, usually related to the reproductive system, medications, such as hormones, are given to reduce the size of a tumor and thereby relieve pain.

Surgical interventions to control intractable pain include nerve block and neurosurgery. A temporary nerve block is applied with a local anesthetic (e.g., lidocaine). Permanent nerve block is achieved with a neurolytic agent (e.g., ethanol, phenol), which "kills" the nerve. Both types of medications are injected directly into nerves transmitting pain sensations. In rare cases, neurosurgery is performed to *sever* (cut) the pain pathway—this procedure is called **ablative surgery** or *surgical ablation*. Palliative surgery may also be performed in any body part, to relieve pressure or obstruction by removing part of a tumor (**debulking**). *Hypophysectomy* (pituitary gland removal) may relieve deep bone pain.

CHILDREN IN HOSPICE PROGRAMS

Staff members must consider dying children in terms of their developmental levels and levels of understanding (Unit 3). Very young children may be unable to differentiate death from other types of separation (e.g., sleep). As children get older, their understanding of death's permanence evolves. Children often respond to nonverbal cues such as play, drama, art, music, other children, pets, or stuffed toys more easily than they respond to adults. Children and their families must communicate, and children should be involved as much as possible in decisions regarding their care. When working with dying children, be specific in explaining death. For example, talking about "going to sleep" can be confusing and frightening. *Rationale: This may cause the child to be afraid to go to sleep at night.* Help children to understand that they have contributed to the world and to their family, even though they have lived a short time. Let them know that they will be greatly missed. The family should be encouraged to explain death to the child in terms of their religious beliefs.

Key Concept

Approach dying children at their appropriate developmental level. Children usually understand what is happening but need their questions answered truthfully. They need to discuss their feelings, perhaps more so than do adults. Allow children to see your feelings about them and the situation. Let them know you care. Remember that medication doses are adjusted according to a child's size and reactions.

Family members are naturally devastated by a child's illness. They need a great deal of support and reassurance. Encourage them to cry and express their grief. Refer the family to a support group. An appropriate support group is "The Compassionate Friends," which has chapters in many cities (www.compassionatefriends.org). This group is particularly targeted toward families who have lost a child. The organization, Children's Hospice and Palliative Care Coalition (www.chpcc.org), "places priority on the needs of the entire family." Their mission is to "ensure that children with life-threatening conditions can *live well and die gently.*" Their belief is that "when a child has a serious illness, medicine is not enough… [they] need strong families to support them…throughout the long and difficult treatment, and families…need ongoing and compassionate grief support." A "Caring Bridge" (www.caringbridge.org) blog can be established, to allow friends to express their concern for the child (or adult) and the family.

WHEN THE CLIENT DIES

Many hospice clients choose to die at home. Assisting loved ones with end-of-life work is a special privilege and a great challenge for nurses and caregivers. Nursing's responsibility is to assist in this process and ensure that caregivers know what to expect and what to do when death occurs. Encourage caregivers to participate in the process as much as possible.

When a client dies, caregivers have been instructed to call the hospice nurse (In Practice: Educating the Client 100-1). If you are working with the family, go to the home to assist with postmortem care (Chapter 59). Caregivers may wish to wash the client's hands and face, comb the hair, or more. Support the family's wishes and assist with technical details.

Following are nursing functions performed for a client who dies at home:

- Remove all equipment.
- Allow the family time alone with their deceased family member.
- Encourage the family to do as much postmortem care as they wish.
- Prepare the body for transportation to the funeral home. Assist in notifying the funeral home, if needed.
- Count narcotics, IVs, and other medications and dispose of them, per agency policy.
- Listen to and validate the family's need to talk about the loved one's final moments.

Key Concept

Remember that grief is natural when a loved one dies, even if the death was anticipated. Allow the family to express their grief. It is appropriate for you to show your grief as well. It is also important to remember that the hospice staff needs time to "debrief" and grieve together following the death of a client.

Most hospice programs conduct memorial services during the year to remember their clients and families.

IN PRACTICE
EDUCATING THE CLIENT 100-1 When the Client Dies at Home

Family teaching in preparation for the client's death at home includes the following:
- Call the hospice nurse—keep the telephone number handy.
- Tell the family to provide the following information:
  - Time of death
  - Last medications administered, dosage, time given
  - Client's condition during last 8 hr
  - Name, address, and phone number of funeral home
  - Name, address, and phone number of next of kin
  - When client was last seen by a registered nurse and/or case manager
- Document all information.
- Make sure the provider and coroner have been notified. (The coroner is usually not required to come to the home of a registered hospice client.) In many states, the RN case manager or advance practice nurse can sign the death certificate.
- Assist the family, as needed, to make arrangements for the body's transfer.
- Assist the family to make arrangements for the return of rented or borrowed medical equipment.
- Refer the family to a bereavement support group.
- Make sure the family knows that you wish to be notified of the time and date of any memorial service and that hospice staff will attend.
- Let the family know they will continue to be involved in the hospice program for at least the next year. They will be invited to hospice memorial services during the year.

STUDENT SYNTHESIS

KEY POINTS

- Hospice care is designed for advanced illness care. Its focus is providing aggressive, intensive palliative care and assisting with physical, psychological, social, and spiritual needs.
- Clients can be discharged from a hospice program, if their health improves. They may also be readmitted if their health deteriorates.
- The client is assisted toward self-actualization, as much as is possible.
- Respite care may be necessary for family members.
- Several disciplines work together with clients and families to deliver compassionate end-of-life care.
- Most hospice programs hold annual or semiannual memorial services, to remember their clients.
- Hospice programs follow up with families for a full year after a loved one's death, to assist with bereavement. Support group membership is encouraged.
- Education and support of family caregivers is a major hospice nursing goal.
- Consider the client's ethnicity and culture when planning and administering hospice care.
- The goal of pain and symptom management is relief, without unwanted side effects.
- Hospice care is very difficult. Clients and caregivers can experience deviations from mental health, such as depression and anxiety (compassion fatigue).
- The nurse and family caregivers work together to perform final care and make final preparations after the client dies.
- Hospice staff members need assistance and support to help them deal with the emotional stress of continuously working with dying people and their families.

CRITICAL THINKING EXERCISES

1. Mr. B., a 43-year-old man, has been admitted to the home care hospice where you work. His primary diagnosis is colon cancer, with metastases to the skeletal system. He is a Christian Scientist, and his primary caregivers are his wife and 20-year-old son. Describe a possible pain management plan for Mr. B. that includes alternatives to medication and surgery. Consider the physical, psychosocial, emotional, ethnic/cultural, and spiritual aspects of care.

2. R.G. is a 68-year-old man from Puerto Rico who is just being admitted to your hospice program. He speaks some English. He has lung cancer, with widespread metastases. He has had extensive surgery, radiation, and chemotherapy. He continues to smoke three packs of cigarettes per day. He has two sons and one daughter in the area, all of whom are married with children. They speak varying amounts of English. R.G. lives in a small two-story home with his wife, who does not speak English. R.G. has worked as a carpenter all his life. Develop an agenda for the first family meeting to discuss his care. In your agenda, list major topics and indicate subcategories and challenges to consider. Who else needs to be involved in the meeting?

3. Using the above situations as examples and considering ethnic/cultural aspects, describe major considerations in planning and carrying out hospice care for the following clients:
   a. A 53-year-old Jewish woman with breast cancer and lung metastases who follows kosher dietary practices.
   b. A 33-year-old gay man with end-stage AIDS, including AIDS dementia. His family is Christian, but he states he is an atheist. He has a strained relationship with his father and his mother has died. He has an older brother who is married.
   c. A 4-year-old African American girl with an inoperable, fast-growing brain tumor. Her family is Muslim.
   d. A 98-year-old Asian man who lives alone. All his children and close relatives have died. He is Buddhist.

NCLEX-STYLE REVIEW QUESTIONS

1. Which statements are true regarding hospice care in the home? Select all that apply.
   a. The client will have relief of distressing symptoms.
   b. The client will have no financial responsibilities.
   c. The client will receive expert care and a protective environment.
   d. The client will receive nursing care 24 hr a day 7 days a week.
   e. The client and family will not be abandoned.

2. After the death of a hospice client, the spouse states to the nurse, "I don't know what I will do without you here." Which response by the nurse is best?
   a. "We will continue our service with you for at least 1 year."
   b. "Now that your spouse has passed, there is no need for our service."
   c. "You should seek the service of a support group."
   d. "Do you have any family members that can see you through this period?"

3. The nurse is concerned that the primary caregiver is experiencing "compassion fatigue." Which behaviors exhibited by the caregiver lead the nurse to suspect this occurrence? Select all that apply.
   a. The caregiver reports having a problem with frequent nightmares.
   b. The caregiver is depressed.
   c. The caregiver wants to continue to care for the client.
   d. The caregiver displays hopelessness.
   e. The caregiver has a difficult time concentrating.

4. Which nonpharmacologic methods can the nurse use to help manage pain in the client receiving hospice services?
   a. Provide relaxation therapy.
   b. Administer morphine sulfate.
   c. Take the client out for a drive.
   d. Administer acupuncture.

5. A family member caring for a client who is receiving home hospice expresses concern to the nurse regarding the client's decrease in appetite. Which response by the nurse is best?
   a. "The client will benefit from low oral intake during this stage."
   b. "You should try to encourage the client to eat three meals per day."
   c. "We can discuss inserting a nasogastric feeding tube with the healthcare provider."
   d. "The client is probably trying to commit suicide by not eating."

CHAPTER RESOURCES

Enhance your learning with additional resources on thePoint!

Student Resources related to this chapter can be found at **thePoint.lww.com/Rosdahl12e**.

UNIT 16 — The Transition to Practicing Nurse

101 From Student to Graduate Nurse

Learning Objectives

1. Describe why the nursing license is vital to the practicing nurse.
2. Explain how the NCLEX examination relates to the nursing process.
3. List and describe categories of client needs measured by the NCLEX.
4. Name just causes for which a nurse's license may be revoked or suspended.
5. Identify the entry-level competencies expected of an LVN/LPN.
6. Describe the use of computers and the Internet in nursing.
7. Discuss the differences in activities or client behavior that may occur during evening or night shifts, as opposed to daytime hours.
8. Describe ways in which a nurse can protect their health while working the night shift.
9. Identify the components and importance of a personal nursing file.

Important Terminology
career mobility
Internet

Acronyms
AJN
CAT
CEU
EHR
NCLEX
NCSBN

On completing a basic nursing program, the graduate nurse is eligible to sit for (take) the licensing examination to obtain a nursing license. This chapter introduces you to the licensure examination, the general procedure for obtaining the initial nursing license, and the responsibilities involved in maintaining this license. In addition, this chapter describes changes in the role and functions from nursing student to graduate nurse, as an entry-level nurse within the healthcare team. Professional activities, continuing education, and ways to balance work and personal responsibilities are also included.

NURSING LICENSURE

Chapters 2 and 4 introduced nursing licensure, differences in licensing laws, and legal aspects of licensure. When a nursing student completes an approved nursing program, they are eligible to apply to take the licensure examination. On passing this examination, the individual is licensed as a licensed vocational nurse, licensed practical nurse (LVN/LPN), or a registered nurse (RN) in that state, territory, or province. The nursing license is one's passport to employment. It is vital for each nurse to obtain a license and to maintain it if they plan to work as a nurse.

> **Key Concept**
> In nearly all states, territories, and provinces, it is *illegal to perform nursing functions* without a license, even if the person does not refer to themselves as a "nurse." (The *specific functions are protected by law*.)

Permit to Practice

In some states, new nursing graduates are issued a "permit" to practice and are called "graduate nurses" or "graduate practical nurses" until they receive a license. Other states do not issue permits; new graduates are required to practice as nursing assistants until licensed. Usually, these nurses are paid less until they prove they have passed the licensure examination. If a nurse working under a permit does not pass the examination on the first writing, the permit is often revoked and the person is required to work as a nursing assistant until fully licensed. (Procedures vary among states.) In some cases, this person is allowed to continue to practice as a "graduate nurse." Most states allow only a limited number of attempts to pass the examination (usually two); then if the graduate has not passed, they must take a refresher course and pay an additional fee to be allowed to take the examination again.

Probationary Status

In most healthcare facilities, new graduates are required to practice for a certain period, often 6 months, as a "nurse intern," "orientee," or "nurse resident." This employment is considered *probationary*, and full employment status begins after the person satisfactorily completes probationary requirements. Usually, this nurse does not receive paid vacation or full benefits until the probationary requirement is met. Each healthcare facility specifies criteria for removing probationary status. Many facilities require the new graduate to pass a written and skills test in medication administration and/or mathematics. Some facilities require the nurse to pass an examination in a specialty area, such as pediatrics or obstetrics, before being allowed to work in that area. In addition, facilities sometimes require a mentor or orientation instructor to work with and evaluate the probationary nurse on commonly performed nursing skills (Fig. 101-1). The probationary period gives both the employer and employee an opportunity to determine if this job placement is appropriate. Such factors as punctuality, dependability, minimal use of sick leave, and ability to get along with coworkers and clients are considered, in addition to basic nursing skills. In most cases, an employee in the probationary period can be terminated without due process. After the new nurse has successfully passed probation, they are usually eligible to use vacation time and cannot be terminated without cause and without due process.

> **Key Concept**
> If a new graduate has not become licensed during the probationary period, a facility may automatically terminate the person's employment.

Licensure Examination (NCLEX)

To become licensed as an RN, LPN, or LVN, a nursing graduate is required to pass the National Council Licensure Examination (**NCLEX**). This test is a computer adaptive test (**CAT**), rather than paper-and-pencil. It is based on a job analysis of tasks that most nurses perform in the course of their employment. In most states, a specific score is not given; the graduate is simply notified that they have "passed" or "not passed."

Application to Sit for NCLEX

To be eligible to apply to take the licensure examination the first time, the student must reasonably be expected to graduate from an approved nursing program. (In some states, the candidate must have actually graduated.) A completed application, transcript of the student's records, and the required fee is sent from the school to the State Board of Nursing, or the authority responsible for issuing licenses. The school must certify the applicant's expected graduation date. If the student does not graduate, they will not be allowed to take the examination. If a nursing graduate must repeat the examination, they are usually responsible for submitting the necessary information. The application to retake the examination is less complicated because the licensing authority already has the pertinent information, but an additional fee is usually required. Because the NCLEX is taken via computer, it is available frequently and at various sites. The applicant specifies preferences for time and location of the examination, choosing from a list prepared by the licensing agency.

Components of the NCLEX

The NCLEX measures entry-level competencies in nursing. The NCLEX-PN must be passed in order to be licensed as an LVN/LPN; the NCLEX-RN leads to RN licensure. Having passed the test verifies that a nurse possesses *minimum competencies for practice*. The examination includes questions measuring knowledge, comprehension, and application. Each examination question represents a phase of the nursing process as it relates to client need. The NCLEX-RN is similar to the NCLEX-PN examination, with more emphasis on assessment and planning.

The *four phases of the nursing process* (Unit 6) associated with the NCLEX-PN examination include the following:

- Data collection (establishing a database)
- Planning (assisting in setting goals for meeting client needs and designing strategies to meet these goals)
- Implementation (actions necessary to achieve goals)
- Evaluation (determining the extent to which goals have been achieved)

> **Key Concept**
> The LVN/LPN does not perform nursing assessment per se and does not independently develop the nursing care plan.

Following are the *categories of client need* addressed by the NCLEX-PN examination (according to NCLEX, clients are defined as individuals, families, and significant others):

1. Safe, effective care environment—collaboration with healthcare team, to facilitate effective client care
   - Coordinated care (including advance directives, client assignments and rights, management, confidentiality, continuity of care, priorities, ethics, informed consent, legalities, quality assurance, and referrals)

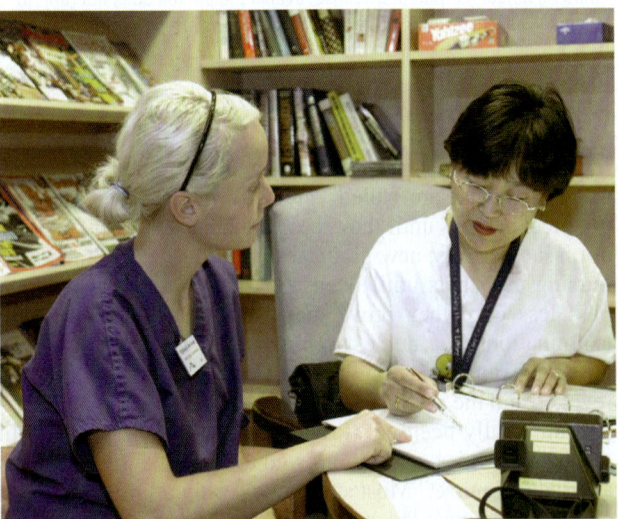

Figure 101-1 After graduation, the new nurse will benefit by having a more experienced nurse as a mentor. The mentor can assist the new graduate in accessing important information, such as the facility's nursing protocols, and operation of the facility's computer system. In addition, the mentor can serve as a "sounding board" for the new graduate's questions and concerns. (Carter, 2005.)

- Safety and infection control—protection from health/environmental hazards (including accident/error prevention, hazardous materials, safety, disaster plans, asepsis, incident reporting, variances, precautions, and safety devices)
2. Health promotion and maintenance—growth and development; prevention/early detection of health problems (including aging, ante/intra/postpartum/newborn care, developmental stages, disease prevention, body image changes, family interaction, family planning, risk behaviors, sexuality, immunizations, and self-care)
3. Psychosocial integrity—promotion/support of emotional, mental, and social well-being (including abuse/neglect, behavioral/crisis intervention, coping, cultural awareness, end-of-life, grief/loss, religious/spiritual influences, sensory/perceptual alterations, stress management, substance-related disorders, disruptions in mental health, suicide, therapeutic communication, and body image changes)
4. Physiologic integrity—reducing clients' risk potential; assisting with management of health alterations, considering all body systems
   - Basic care and comfort—assistance with activities of daily living (ADLs) (including assistive devices, elimination, mobility, nonpharmacologic interventions, nutrition/hydration, palliative/comfort care, hygiene, and rest/sleep)
   - Pharmacologic therapies—administration of medications; monitoring of clients receiving parenteral therapies (including pharmacologic agents/administration/actions, therapeutic effects, and unwanted side effects)
   - Reduction of risk potential—reduces potential for clients to develop complications/health problems related to treatments, procedures, or existing condition (including diagnostic tests/treatments/procedures/surgery, laboratory values, therapeutic procedures, and vital signs)
   - Physiologic adaptation—providing care for clients with acute, chronic, or life-threatening physical conditions (including alterations in body systems, pathophysiology, fluid/electrolyte imbalances, emergencies, and unexpected response to therapies)

The NCLEX licensing examination requires knowledge of all courses studied in the nursing program. It also requires *application of knowledge* by using critical thinking skills to make nursing judgments, within the parameters of the licensure involved. When taking the licensure examination, the computer selects individual test items from a large test pool. Each examination measures knowledge and skills pertaining to phases of the nursing process and categories of client needs. A candidate completes items until the computer determines that the person has either passed the examination or statistically cannot pass. The computer then terminates the examination. Therefore, each candidate receives different questions and a different number of questions and spends a different length of time taking the examination. The results will be sent by email or U.S. mail to the candidate.

> **Key Concept**
>
> When you are taking the examination, do not be alarmed when the computer terminates the examination. This is normal. It is not possible to predict if this means passing or not passing the examination. Maintain a positive attitude.

Preparation for the NCLEX

The best way to ensure success on the examination is to study throughout the entire basic nursing program. If material is mastered during the program, the student should have little difficulty passing the examination. Try not to "cram" for the examination just before taking it.

If desired, review and practice materials are available, including outline review books, practice questions (and answer explanations, describing why an answer is correct or not correct), and CDs with questions and answers. Computerized test banks with questions (and accompanying answers) actually simulate the test-taking experience. There are a number of ancillary materials accompanying this textbook, as well as related Websites, to assist students in preparing for the examination.

On the night before the test, relax and get plenty of sleep. On the morning of the test, eat a good breakfast and dress comfortably. Make sure to have the agency-issued identification information and your government-issued photo ID (e.g., driver's license or passport) for admittance to the examination. Know beforehand how to get to the examination site and where to park; allow ample travel time.

> **NCLEX Alert**
>
> It is a good idea to make a "practice run" to the examination site, unless you are positive you know how to get there and where to park. If you are late, you may not be admitted. In addition, you will not be admitted without proper credentials and photo identification.

If you do not pass the examination the first time, several options are available. Maintain a positive attitude and remember you can repeat the examination. Consider taking a review course before repeating the examination—helping recall skills in areas of concern and building your self-confidence. Most review courses include practice tests that can help you overcome "test anxiety" and make you more comfortable when retaking the examination. (Often, a review or preparation course is required before a candidate is allowed to retake the examination. This varies among states, but is usually required if the candidate needs a third attempt.)

The Nursing License

On passing the NCLEX examination, the individual will receive notification from the state, commonwealth, territorial, or provincial Board of Nursing or other agency responsible for nursing licensure and will receive the first license. (This may be a paper license or may be online notification.) The individual can then use the appropriate title: LPN, LVN, or RN.

> **Key Concept**
>
> If the nurse is employed, the licensure information is often sent to the employer online. It is each nurse's responsibility to make sure this occurs. (In some states, a small fee is charged if a nurse wants a paper copy of the license.) The employer keeps a record of each nurse's current license. This procedure must be followed each time the license is renewed, or the nurse will be practicing illegally and both the nurse and employer may be fined.

Nursing licensure may sometimes be obtained by waiver for graduates of approved Canadian nursing programs. Nurses will be required to verify their education, and, if it is determined to be comparable, they may be licensed in the United States. The waivered license may or may not be transferable to another state. (In the case of nurses from other countries, specific courses usually must be taken and the nurse required to sit for the U.S. licensure examination. Upon passing the examination, a regular license is issued.) Procedures may vary between states and provinces.

Maintenance of the Nursing License
Each person is responsible for keeping their nursing license current, in order to legally practice nursing.

License Renewal
Most states and provinces require renewal of a nursing license about every 2–3 years. *Always* inform the licensing agency of changes in name, address, or employment status, because license renewal applications usually cannot be forwarded, per Board of Nursing regulations. If a nursing license lapses, the nurse is *not allowed to practice*, under penalty of law. In addition, requirements for relicensure are usually more stringent than are renewal requirements. This often includes a refresher course, supervised clinical experience, and an additional fee.

> **Nursing Alert** It is *always* the nurse's personal responsibility to maintain current licensure. Particularly if you move or change your name without notifying the licensing agency, it is your professional responsibility to renew your license independently.

Continuing Education Requirements
Most states require a specified number of hours or continuing education units (**CEUs**) for licensure renewal. In some states, specific courses, such as infection control, are required as part of the CEU courses. Usually, a record of the presenter's name and professional credentials, the objectives and length of the course, and the certificate of completion must be kept on file. Other information may also be required by your licensing agency. This information may be sent in with the license renewal or may only be needed for an audit. The CEU requirement is an opportunity to stay updated; the goal is to improve the quality of nursing care. Take advantage of these courses to improve skills. Many healthcare facilities offer educational opportunities free or at a low cost. The **Internet** offers a wide variety of continuing education courses for nurses. In addition, articles providing CEUs are found in nursing journals, such as the *American Journal of Nursing* (**AJN**). Many private companies offer continuing education courses free or for a small fee. Satisfactory completion of a test may be necessary to obtain CEUs, if the course was taken by correspondence or on the Internet. In many cases, CEUs can be awarded immediately on completion of the course, and the person can print out a certificate online; in other cases, a certificate of completion will be mailed. If results are needed immediately, most educational organizations will fax the certificate for an additional fee. Each nurse is required to keep CEU information on file, in case it is required by the licensing agency.

License Revocation
Every licensed nurse is responsible for practicing within the rules and regulations of the Nurse Practice Act and within the laws of the state, province, or territory in which the nurse works. In most U.S. states and territories and in Canada, the Board of Nursing or other licensing authority has the right to revoke or suspend a nurse's license for just cause. Following are examples of just causes:

- Conviction of a felony
- Conviction of other crimes, such as child or elder abuse
- Substance use disorder, compulsive gambling, or other addictive behavior (until it is controlled), including several arrests for driving while intoxicated or driving under the influence of alcohol or other drugs (DWI/DUI) or arriving at work under the influence
- Stealing medications, particularly "schedule" drugs
- Stealing from a client
- Sexual harassment of a coworker or client
- Mental incompetence/uncontrolled mental illness
- Fraudulent acquisition of, or renewal of, a nursing license
- Violation of the state Nurse Practice Act (e.g., practicing medicine or prescribing medications without a license)
- Suspended or revoked license in another state
- Willful neglect or abuse of a client
- Sexual activity with, or sexual harassment of, a vulnerable client (nearly all clients are considered to be vulnerable)
- Inappropriate contact with a client after discharge from the hospital, particularly those deemed to be vulnerable (e.g., children and psychiatric clients)
- Proven negligence in nursing practice
- Conviction as a sexual predator

The state board must notify the nurse before it takes action to suspend or revoke a license. Usually this is published and the nurse and involved others have an opportunity to present their case at a formal hearing. Actions that may be taken include: denial of license renewal, denial of first license, letter of reprimand, suspension or revocation of license, or placement of the nurse on formal probation. In some cases, specific conditions for full reinstatement are set out. If the nurse is convicted of serious misconduct, willful negligence, or a felony related to nursing care, the license may be permanently revoked, with no opportunity to reinstate. However, this is rare.

> **Key Concept**
> If a nurse's license is suspended or revoked, the nurse cannot legally practice nursing until the license is reissued. A valid license is known as an *unencumbered license*.

License Transfer Between States

After becoming licensed, a nurse may wish to move and transfer their licensure to another state, territory, or province. This procedure is known by several terms, including *interstate endorsement, reciprocity,* or *licensure without examination.* To become licensed in another state, a request must be made to the new state's licensing/regulating agency. The nurse is required to complete an application and pay a fee. Because the NCLEX examination is used in all states and territories, license transfer is usually very easy. Most states do not require an examination, if the nursing program from which the nurse has graduated meets the new state's educational requirements and the NCLEX has been passed.

> **Key Concept**
>
> If you plan to transfer your license to another state, allow plenty of time. It may take 4–6 weeks to receive the new license.

To locate the proper agency to contact for initial licensure or transferring a license, look on the Internet for the agency, usually in the state or territory's capital city. In Canada, contact the Canadian Nurses' Association in Ottawa. The National Council of State Boards of Nursing (**NCSBN**) Website lists names, addresses, phone numbers, and Websites of all licensing agencies in the United States and its territories (www.NCSBN.org). (This Website also describes the NCLEX examination.) In addition, some textbooks list all state licensing agencies. Usually, the application to transfer a license can be obtained via the Internet and printed out on one's computer. In many states and territories, the licensing agency for nurses is called the *State Board of Nursing* or simply the *Board of Nursing.* Examples of other names of licensing agencies, at the time of this writing, are listed in Box 101-1.

> **NCLEX Alert**
>
> It is important to review NCLEX scenarios and test question options, using a variety of NCLEX review sources, starting early in your nursing program. When combined with your textbook, the review sources can help define key areas of knowledge content and provide practice in critical thinking.

ROLE TRANSITION

Functions

The LVN/LPN is prepared to function as a member of the healthcare team by exercising sound nursing judgment, based on preparation, knowledge, skills, understanding, and past experiences in nursing situations. The LVN/LPN participates in the planning, implementation, and evaluation of nursing care in all settings where nursing takes place. Generally, this means "providing for the emotional and physical comfort and safety of clients; (and) observing, recording, and reporting to appropriate persons, changes in clients' symptoms and conditions; (and) performing more specialized nursing functions, such as administering medications and therapeutic treatments, and assisting with rehabilitation." The Website goes on to give examples of LVN/LPN nursing functions.

According to the U.S. Bureau of Labor Statistics, the role of the LVN/LPN is to

- "Monitor patients' health—for example, by checking their blood pressure
- Administer basic patient care, including changing bandages and inserting catheters
- Provide for the basic comfort of patients, such as helping them bathe or dress
- Discuss the care they are providing with patients and listen to their concerns
- Report patients' status and concerns to registered nurses and doctors
- Keep records on patients' health" (2020, para 2).

Entry-Level Competencies

The LVN/LPN needs to demonstrate the following entry-level skills (*competencies*):

Data collection: Collects data about clients' basic physical, emotional, spiritual, and sociocultural needs; uses knowledge of normal values to identify deviations; documents data collection; communicates findings.

Box 101-1 Names of Licensing Agencies for Nurses

- Board of Nursing or State Board of Nursing (most states)
- Department of Safety and Professional Services (Wisconsin)
- Board of Nurse Examiners (Guam, Maritime Provinces, Puerto Rico, Mariana Islands)
- Board of Examiners for Nursing (Connecticut)
- Board of Nurse Registration and Nursing Education (Rhode Island)
- Board of Registration in Nursing (Massachusetts)
- Board of Nurse Licensure (Virgin Islands)
- Nursing Care Quality Assurance Commission (Washington)
- Health Services Regulatory Board (American Samoa)
- California, Louisiana, Texas, West Virginia, and Georgia have separate boards for licensed vocational/practical nurses (LVN/LPNs) (e.g., California Board of Vocational Nurse and Psychiatric Technician Examiners) and RNs (California Board of Registered Nursing).
- Nevada has separate boards for licensure and for "administration, discipline, and investigation."
- In most Canadian provinces, the agency is known as the Association of Nurses or College of Nurses

This information, as well as addresses, phone numbers, and Websites, is available on the Website of the National Council of State Boards of Nursing Inc. (www.ncsbn.org) or by writing to them at: 111 East Wacker Drive, Suite 2900 Chicago, IL 60601-4277.

Planning: Contributes to development of nursing care plans; prioritizes nursing care needs; assists in review and revision of nursing care plans.

Implementation: Provides nursing care; communicates effectively; collaborates with team members; instructs clients and families.

Evaluation: Seeks guidance, as needed; modifies nursing approaches, based on evaluation of nursing care.

Member of the healthcare team: The LVN/LPN complies with standards of practice outlined in the Nurse Practice Act of the state, territory, or province in which licensed; describes the role of the LVN/LPN to others; maximizes educational opportunities; identifies personal potential and considers **career mobility** (additional education, responsibility, and status); identifies personal strengths and weaknesses; adheres to a nursing code of ethics; functions as a client advocate.

Managing/supervising: The LVN/LPN appropriately manages own actions when providing nursing care; assumes responsibility for nursing care delegated to unlicensed assistive personnel (UAP), particularly in the nursing home.

Political activism: Is aware that as a nurse they affect nursing and healthcare through political, economic, and societal activities.

The graduate nurse is expected to perform these skills. These skills are not isolated to one client or one situation. Rather, they are intertwined, requiring the graduate nurse to be focused, adaptable, flexible, and organized.

Role as a Member of the Healthcare Team

No matter what the setting, several levels of nurses and many other workers make up the total healthcare team. All members work together, under the direction of the healthcare provider, advance practice nurse, physician assistant, or other primary provider, to help clients return to optimum functioning as soon as possible.

The RN has more formal education than the LVN/LPN. Therefore, they will almost always be the nurse manager, team leader, or charge nurse in an acute care setting. In home care, the case manager is nearly always required to be an RN. In addition, many RNs give direct client care, as do LVN/LPNs. In complex nursing situations, the LVN/LPN is expected to assist the RN. In the nursing home setting, the LVN/LPN may function as a charge nurse and may supervise other workers, such as unlicensed assistive personnel (UAP). Remember: The UAP are very valuable members of the nursing team, particularly in long-term care and community settings.

Organizing Workload

Typically, a new graduate nurse will provide care for more clients for more hours at a time than they did as a student. Whatever the situation, organization is key to providing efficient and safe care for all clients. Organizational skills come with experience and practice, and supervisors and experienced coworkers can provide helpful hints and guidelines. Box 101-2 highlights some key aspects for organizing the workload and practicing safely.

Box 101-2   Organizing the Workload

Organization requires preparation and effective use of time. The following guidelines may assist in organizing your workload:

- Establish goals, plans, and priorities for your shift; evaluate the "what," "how," and "when" for each. Consider the nursing care plan for each client.
- Set up or print out a "to-do" list, in order of importance or need; check off tasks as completed. Include times when medications and treatments are due.
- Stay focused; avoid procrastinating.
- Assist in general activities of the unit (e.g., making rounds, taking vital signs, disposing of laundry, conducting client activities, serving meals, etc.). Be aware of the general climate of the unit.
- When in doubt about a technique or procedure, *ask questions*. Know where nursing protocols are located; review protocols in advance; refer to them as needed.
- Know when and to whom to report significant symptoms/medication side effects, or other concerns.
- Know where to find information about medications and treatments.
- Be thoroughly knowledgeable about the institution's emergency, fire, and disaster procedures. Locate fire extinguishers and exits wherever you are assigned. Know the various "codes" of your facility and how to call them.
- Follow agency protocol for disposing of hazardous wastes, cleaning up spills, or reporting defective equipment.
- Follow nursing procedures, as taught in the nursing program, while adapting them safely to your facility. Always consider the underlying rationales and facility protocols. Use the facility procedure manual or computer program.
- Plan your break times so they do not conflict with specific procedures scheduled for your clients. Report off to another nurse when going on break or leaving the unit for any reason.

Maintaining Confidentiality

Maintaining client confidentiality is vital in any nursing setting. The licensed nurse not only is personally responsible for maintaining confidentiality but also must be aware of the actions of the unlicensed personnel and others with whom they work. It may be necessary to teach others the importance of safeguarding the client's privacy. Some ways to protect client confidentiality are as follows:

- When documenting client information, keep the screen turned away, so passersby cannot see it; "exit" or clear the screen when moving away.
- Keep your password confidential; prevent unauthorized people from accessing information.
- Be aware that communication via Internet, Facebook, and other social media is not secure.
- Keep information boards (e.g., vital signs or rounds boards) facedown when not in use.
- Use only client first names on door, bed, or other labels.
- Do not discuss clients anyplace where inappropriate people may overhear (e.g., the elevator or cafeteria).

- Never access information about a client unnecessarily or for personal reasons. (Remember: This could be grounds for termination of employment.) There may be a "break the glass" provision in a high-profile client's chart. In this case, employees must prove that they legally need to access the chart.

> **Nursing Alert** Cell phones often are not allowed in client care areas because they contain cameras. Photos of clients would violate their privacy.

Working With Providers' Orders

The licensed nurse needs to know how to check providers' orders and needs to check for new orders regularly throughout the shift. In most facilities, orders are entered directly into the computer (the electronic health record [**EHR**]). In this way, medication orders are transmitted directly to the pharmacy; orders for tests, special procedures, or special equipment are submitted directly to the appropriate department. The computer identifies client allergies and can alert staff to inappropriate medication dosages or incompatible medications. Medications, with dosages and times of administration, are automatically printed on the client's medication administration record (MAR). These important safeguards help protect clients from errors and help the nurse to organize the work day.

In rare cases, including the nursing home, healthcare provider's orders may be handwritten. If this is the case, the nurse or secretary may be expected to *transcribe orders* (write orders on the chart). No matter who transcribes orders, the nurse is responsible for their accuracy and for ensuring that they are carried out appropriately. Because the EHR is universally used, if your agency or facility utilizes handwritten orders, in-service education will be required. Remember: In nonacute settings, *standing orders* are often in place, and the provider augments these orders to meet specific needs of individual clients. Make sure you know the protocol for caring for clients within standing orders. Box 101-3 provides an example of guidelines for acknowledging or responding to orders for medications and treatments.

> **Key Concept**
> Remember, the charge nurse or client's nurse must double-check and acknowledge all orders for accuracy. The computer automatically records who acknowledges orders. Orders for discontinued medications and treatments are also acknowledged. If there is any question about an order, the nurse must clarify it with the provider.

Telephone or Verbal Orders

Ideally, all orders are "signed" by a provider on the computer or paper. In emergencies, verbal or telephone orders may be necessary (Chapter 61). Healthcare facilities vary regarding who may legally take telephone or verbal orders. The LVN/LPN in acute care may take telephone or verbal orders only if the practice is clearly permitted by institutional policies. (LVN/LPNs usually may receive verbal/telephone orders in long-term care, the clinic, or ambulatory care.) *Rationale: Verbal/telephone orders are more subject to errors and disagreement than written or computerized orders. The nurse taking them and carrying them out must take responsibility for their accuracy. The nurse taking a verbal order must be sure the order is clearly understood and should question anything that is unclear. If an order is questioned, it cannot be carried out until it is clarified. It is important to* "read back" all telephone or verbal orders. The order is then written or entered into the computer. TORB indicates "telephone order, read back," and VORB indicates "verbal order, read back." The nurse adds the ordering person's name and title and cosigns the order. The provider giving a verbal or telephone order must sign or acknowledge it (no later than 24 hr after given, in acute care). Orders, such as those for certain client safety devices/restraints, must be cosigned by the provider within 1 hr.

> **Nursing Alert** The nursing student or other unlicensed personnel *never* takes verbal or telephone orders.

Using Technology

Today's nurse must interact comfortably with computers and other electronic equipment (Fig. 101-2). Much of this equipment is familiar to you, including computer documentation

---

Box 101-3 Responding to Medication/Treatment Orders Via Computer

To ensure client safety, follow these guidelines when acknowledging medication or treatment orders:
- Check the computer at least every hour, to make sure no new orders have been written.
- Acknowledge new orders as soon as possible.
- Check for one-time dated orders (e.g., reading of a PPD test).
- Check time due for any new medication or treatment orders.
- Read all orders and verify them. Usually, each nurse will check and acknowledge all orders for their clients.
- Always do "stat" orders first. Document these immediately after they are carried out.
- Make sure a medication order is verified by the pharmacy.
- Double-check the name of the medication, dose, route, and frequency of administration.
- Note the date of a medication's discontinuation. Many medications must be reordered every 48 hr or every 7 days. Some are ordered for a specific period (e.g., 3 days).
- Notify the person giving medications, if it is someone other than yourself.
- When medications arrive, check them against the medication administration record (MAR).
- If there are any questions, always ask.

When a medication is discontinued:
- Acknowledge this on the computer.
- Notify the nurse involved.
- Return leftover medications to the pharmacy.

Orders for tests, procedures, and treatments are acknowledged in the same manner and documented when carried out.

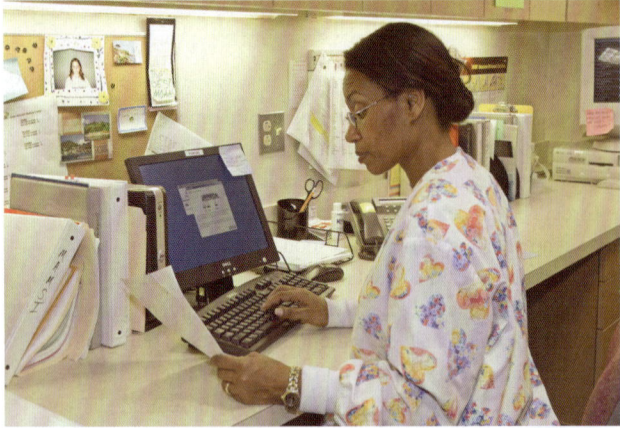

Figure 101-2 In nearly all inpatient facilities and many clinics, you will find that all documentation is done on the computer. It is important to learn how to access and enter data. Classes are usually offered to help new graduates. (Carter, 2005.)

and research and other equipment, such as the electronic thermometer, blood pressure and glucose testing equipment, medication scanner, electronic medication dispenser, pulse oximeter, computerized scale, computerized infusion or tube feeding pump, and apnea or automatic vital signs monitor. As technology advances, other electronic equipment will become available. Be sure to look up information or ask questions about the safe operation of a particular piece of equipment. Usually, healthcare equipment has accompanying instruction books, often attached to the equipment. Scientific advances improve client care, by ensuring greater accuracy of diagnoses and treatment and greater efficiency and safety in care delivery.

Computers

Computers (including medication scanners) serve many purposes in healthcare facilities. They are used to

- Monitor the client's condition and assist in diagnosis.
- Store medical records, bookkeeping records, and order supplies and equipment.
- Quickly locate pertinent client information; often, clinic records and records of previous hospitalizations are available.
- Generate charts/tables of pertinent client information, such as blood pressure, weight, laboratory results, oximeter readings, or blood glucose determinations.
- Interact with the laboratory and the client's record to document blood glucose readings.
- Generate a list of medications to be given during the shift, including times of administration, dosages, route of administration, etc.
- Interact with medication administration machines, to make sure correct medications are pulled for each client (Fig. 61-1).
- Record medications, as given, in the client's record.
- Regulate specialized machines and equipment, such as continuous electrocardiogram (ECG) or blood pressure monitoring, rotating pressure cuffs, or an intravenous (IV) or tube feeding pump; an alarm is sounded if readings deviate from previously determined parameters (or if an IV or tube feeding bag is empty).
- Generate healthcare provider's orders and forward them to nursing staff and to the pharmacy, laboratory, operating room, ECG, and elsewhere.
- Renew clients' prescriptions; check for medication interactions.
- Conduct quality assurance research.
- Teach students; conduct literature searches.
- Offer continuing education courses and seminars.
- Supply medication and healthcare information to students an d clients.
- Assist in nursing tasks, such as developing nursing care plans, documenting care.
- Generate advance directives and other forms, such as living wills; store living wills and other advance directives for quick retrieval.
- Make appointments for x-ray examinations and diagnostic tests.
- Generate instructions for clients for special tests.
- Generate medication information for clients.
- Order laboratory tests and retrieve results; display normal parameters.
- Schedule the operating room and other specialized areas.
- Send messages via email, fax, or alpha page; transmit client records.
- Assist in telephone triage of clients; provide guided questionnaires and protocols for triage nurses to use in assisting clients.
- Assist in client triage in the clinic or emergency department.
- Generate lists of hospitalized clients or clients assigned to a particular nurse; generate a daily schedule of care.
- Transmit pertinent client information (e.g., blood pressure [BP], blood sugar readings, or ECG) from client to healthcare provider or the laboratory.
- Obtain audio/video consultations with specialists in other locations; facilitate conference calls.
- Apply for nursing positions or a nursing license.
- Assist with general administrative functions, such as scheduling staff, generating paychecks, and authorizing insurance payments.

Most communities and facilities offer courses for staff unfamiliar with computers. In addition, numerous self-help books and aids are available. Specific instructions about how to use a facility's computer system are usually provided during the nurse's orientation to the facility. Also, remember that operation manuals for computers and computerized equipment are usually available.

The Internet

The Internet (World Wide Web [WWW]) is an enormous source of information about medications, diseases, or new nursing procedures. Chat rooms, forums, and discussion boards allow communication with experts who will answer questions and give additional information. (These experts may be in countries other than the United States, providing an international perspective.) Interactive forums and webinars relating to nursing and medical topics are offered. Most nursing organizations, state boards of nursing, voluntary health agencies, health promotion agencies, and health maintenance organizations (HMOs) have Websites. Some Websites provide abstracts of journal articles, entire articles, bibliography lists, clinical updates, and speeches from medical conferences. Many journals, book reviews, and books are available online. Signing up for a specialty mailing list via an electronic mailing list (Listserv) allows one to send and receive information related to that specialty. The participant can communicate with individuals in the group via email. Nursing Listserv topics include home care, IV therapy, maternal–child, surgery, psychiatry, neurology, nursing education, research, and many other subjects. The Internet is particularly valuable to students, people in rural areas, and those who do not have access to a large library. Remember too that Websites are usually updated regularly.

Continuing education programs are offered via Internet, and applications for specialized credentials are available. A certificate of completion can usually be printed at the end of online classes. Various Websites online may also contain job boards that list employment opportunities. In most cases, the résumé and application is submitted via the Internet.

A great deal of client-teaching information can be downloaded from the Internet. The nurse must screen this material before giving it to the client, to ensure it is not too overwhelming or too technical. Be sure to be available to answer questions.

> **Nursing Alert** It is important to exercise appropriate media literacy. Double-check Internet information for accuracy and access information from reputable Websites to ensure accuracy.

Maintaining a Current Knowledge Base

Although a new graduate has completed the general nursing program, their education in healthcare is *just beginning*. Continuing to learn throughout one's entire nursing career is essential in order to deliver safe and up-to-date care. In addition to the Internet, sources of current information are readily available. Books and magazine articles provide information about new scientific discoveries. Nursing journals, textbooks, radio programs, podcasts, and television programs provide information on health problems and new procedures and equipment. Workshops, conferences, and conventions are available in many general and specialty areas, to provide updated information. Healthcare facilities usually maintain ongoing in-service programs and libraries for employees. Take advantage of these sources to stay current.

Adjusting to the Workplace

The clinical arena may present the new graduate with unexpected challenges. Nursing continues around the clock, providing clients with continuity of care. While a student, clinical experience during evening or night hours or a full 8- or 12-hour experience is usually not included. A new graduate is often expected to work during times other than the day shift. The requirement may be to work only evenings, nights, or *rotating shifts*—that is, days, evenings ("relief," "swing shift"), and nights ("graveyard shift", "overnights") or two of these, on a rotating (alternating) basis. Many acute care and extended-care facilities require nurses to work weekends, often every other weekend. A new graduate's first job may be totally on weekends or during "off hours" and may also include holidays, giving more senior nurses time off.

Work Schedules

Many nursing employment opportunities exist; employers may offer incentives to attract nurses. However, you may not be able to begin with your first choice of location or shift. However, nursing offers unique scheduling opportunities; rotating shifts or nonday shifts may be an advantage to an individual nurse.

Flexible Schedules

Many nurses find working flexible hours fits well into a family schedule. A number of scheduling options are available. Examples include the following:

Part time or full time
Scheduled or casual (or on call)
Straight evenings or straight nights
Weekends only: Variations of a scheduling plan, the Baylor Plan, exist at many facilities. The nurse usually works 3 days every weekend (Friday, Saturday, and Sunday). In most cases, either a bonus is paid to weekend-only nurses or the nurse working part time is paid a full-time wage. This allows time off during the week.
Twelve-hour shifts: Working three 12-hour shifts per week is nearly full time. Adding one 8-hour shift every 2 weeks makes the contract equal to full time. The nurse working 12-hour shifts is usually required to work only every third, instead of every other, weekend. This plan gives the nurse more days off. Twelve-hour shifts are usually from 7 AM to 7 PM, and two nurses are partners, one working days and one working nights. These two nurses may alternate shifts, so one does not work all nights or all days.
Ten-hour shifts: These are much less common in inpatient facilities; however, clinics, home care, and industries often offer 10-hour shifts.
Shared contracts: Two nurses can share a single full-time position, allowing each to have more free time.
Flex time: In some situations, the nurse is allowed to set their own hours, fitting the work schedule around family responsibilities, perhaps beginning at 9 AM, rather than 7 AM.

Scheduling Challenges

A growing concern in nursing is *mandatory overtime*. Because clients need 24-hour care, nurses from a shift may be forced to stay and cover the next shift, if no nurses are available. This has become such a concern that hospitals have been forced to turn away clients if they do not have adequate staffing. Nurses have negotiated and, in some cases, gone on strike, to ensure competent and safe nursing care for clients, including the abolishment of mandatory overtime. Union contracts often allow the filing of a grievance if contract stipulations are violated. Voluntary double-shifts may be available, with time-and-a-half or double-time salary paid. Working conditions and salaries continue to improve, as nurses express their concerns and negotiate to improve client care.

The 24-Hour Day

Because nursing occurs around the clock, working the evening or night hours may be different than working during the daytime. When working in the evening or at night, keep in mind the following:

- Clients may exhibit different behavior, compared with that during the day. For example, the person with dementia or paranoia is often more confused or afraid after dark (the "sundowner" phenomenon).
- Many clients are more anxious or worried at night, when it is quiet and they are alone.
- Psychotic clients may be more likely to act out at night.
- Many clients experience an elevation of fever and/or exacerbation of illness in the evening.
- Pain may be accentuated by fear or by being alone and free of distractions in the evening or night.
- Visitors often come in the evenings, providing an excellent opportunity for nursing staff to meet clients' loved ones.
- Fewer staff members are usually on duty during nonday shifts. Each nurse may be responsible for a greater number of clients. Accessing security assistance, special laboratory, x-ray, or other tests, or a specialized healthcare provider may be more difficult.
- It is quieter on nonday shifts. Usually, there is less confusion and fewer nonnursing staff (healthcare providers, social workers, students, etc.) on the unit. Fewer orders are written, and fewer special tests and procedures performed. (Clients are usually discharged during the day. In addition, admissions often take place during the day shift, unless they are emergency admissions.)
- In rare cases, clients come into the hospital to be prepared for surgery or another procedure the next morning. (Usually, however, clients come to the facility the morning of surgery.)
- Clients coming in the morning for surgery or procedures may have questions and may call for information.
- Hospitalized clients may be nothing by mouth (NPO) after midnight for procedures, such as electroconvulsive therapy (ECT), surgery, or various diagnostic tests.
- Clients who have had surgery during the day may require special attention during the evening or night.
- Clients are more likely to fall when it is darker and/or they are more confused.
- Clients who are continent in the daytime may be incontinent at night. It is important to check them frequently.
- Assisting clients to sleep at night is important. Sometimes, a warm shower or soothing backrub helps; medications to relieve pain or enhance sleep may be necessary. Some clients drink warm milk to promote rest. (Remember that noises, including nurses' conversations or slamming doors, seem louder at night and may keep clients awake.) Some people fall asleep more easily if soft music is playing in the background. The lights in the hallways and other areas may be dimmed. (Be sure a night light is on in each client room.)
- A client's roommate may snore, keeping the client awake. Provide earplugs to assist clients.
- Some medications, such as sedating psychotropic medications, laxatives, and vaginal suppositories, are routinely given in the evening.
- In most facilities, the night nurse performs routine once-a-day record-keeping at midnight. Intake and output, IV fluids, and caloric intakes are checked on the computer. Laboratory procedures may be ordered or vital signs documented.
- It is important to double-check all scheduled surgical, ECT, or special laboratory procedures, to ensure that clients are properly prepared (and NPO) for the next morning. Indicate wake-up times for clients.
- The night nurse and other staff often order missing medications, tube feedings, and IV fluids; replenish supplies for the unit; check the crash cart and refrigerator temperatures; and perform quality control tests on the blood glucose testing or blood pressure equipment. These machines are plugged in to charge at night.
- The night staff is required to perform frequent rounds on the unit, to make sure all clients are comfortable and safe and to turn clients. Be sure to check for breathing.
- In long-term facilities, nonnarcotic medications may be set up for the next morning.
- Early morning medications, such as thyroid preparations, are given at the end of night shift.
- AM blood glucose checks may be done by the night staff.
- Staffing for the next day is checked; arrangements are made to fill vacant spots.
- Client assignments may be prepared for the next day.
- The night nurse may be required to prepare a comprehensive report to be given to the day nurses or the medical team.

> **Key Concept**
>
> Remember: Nurses are only in the healthcare facility for a work shift. The client is there 24 hr a day, and the environment is different in the evening or night. It is important to make the client feel safe and comfortable, whatever the time of day.

Working the Night Shift

In some instances, new graduate nurses may be required to work the night shift. Some individuals may choose to work nights because this fits their lifestyle. Regardless of the reason, Box 101-4 highlights general suggestions to aid the nurse in working the night shift. Working nights can be advantageous. Usually, there is a pay differential, traffic to and from work is less, and parking is easier and often less expensive. Days and evenings are free for other activities, for example, attending school or family activities, shopping when stores are less crowded, or walking and exercising during safer daytime hours. It is possible to make daytime appointments for services, such as dental care and car repair. Access to child care services may not be necessary because one's partner is home at night. The work may be less physically demanding. Although, typically, fewer medications and treatments are given at night, more time may be available to talk with clients, if they are awake. If a nurse is taking classes, there may be time to study or do research on the Internet.

There are also disadvantages to working nights, some of which have been mentioned. The work may be less interesting, and it is possible that the nurse may not be able to interact with clients because they are sleeping. The nurse's family members may have difficulty adjusting to the routine. Managing one's sleep schedule may be challenging and may contribute to obtaining less total sleep. Nurses with specific health challenges (e.g., diabetes, seizure disorders, gastrointestinal disorders, bipolar disorder, chronic obstructive pulmonary disease, and heart disorders) may be at risk when working nights. However, many nurses work permanently at night by choice.

Box 101-4 Working the Night Shift

To help in adjusting to working the night shift, keep in mind the following:

- Eat healthy meals. Get plenty of exercise. Plan recreational time. Drink plenty of fluids, varying the types of fluids.
- Eat a snack or meal during the shift. Limit caffeine intake after about 3 am.
- Eat a light, nonfat meal before going to bed during the day.
- Be sure to allow adequate time for uninterrupted sleep during the day.
- Take medications at prescribed times. Adjust personal medications, such as insulin, psychotropics, and antiseizure medications, as appropriate for the individual schedule.
- Plan a suitable sleep schedule; for example, it may be easiest to sleep immediately after work, to stay up for a few hours and go to bed about midday, or to sleep a few hours in the morning and take a nap before returning to work. Try to get your usual amount of total sleep daily.
- If possible for you, arrange to work straight nights. This is easier for the body to adjust to than rotating shifts. If you are working full-time nights, sleep days when possible, even when off duty, to help maintain a steady biorhythm.
- Involve family members when planning the schedule. Make sure they understand that you need to sleep during the day.
- Make your bedroom as dark as possible; wear an eye mask.
- Keep the bedroom quiet. Turn off the telephone and doorbell or put a sign on the door. Use a fan or soft music to provide "sound masking."
- Make sure friends and relatives know about the night shifts and do not call or visit during sleep time. Allow calls to go to the answering machine.
- Bring a sweater to work; most people get chilly in the middle of the night because of normal body cycles.
- While at work, keep the nursing desk area well lighted. (The body's biorhythms are based in large part on light and darkness.)
- If there is a choice between 8-hour and 12-hour shifts, choose the 8-hour shift. It is less exhausting and usually begins about 11 pm, allowing for participation in evening activities and being with one's children.
- Bring something interesting to do, if any free time becomes available. It will help in maintaining alertness.
- Try not to snack on junk food, sugary or salty foods, or caffeine; this promotes weight gain and prevents sleep during the day. It is better to snack on fruits or vegetables. Some nurses eat one of their daily meals during the night.
- If there is a break during the night, take a nap. A short nap can help greatly in staying awake. Use an alarm on the cell phone or clock; sleep will be more relaxed without worrying about waking up on time.
- Make sure to be safe during the trip home. If you drive, listen to the radio or books on CDs, sing, or eat popcorn, sunflower seeds, or peanuts to remain alert. Stop and rest for a few minutes if becoming too tired. Call for assistance or take a bus/train, if you are unable to stay awake while driving.

Professional Activities

A graduate nurse is responsible for keeping up with current trends in nursing, particularly within one's nursing specialty. By being an active member of a nursing organization, a graduate nurse will be aware of current trends and new advancements, as well as changing employment trends.

State and National Nursing Organizations

Chapter 2 provided an introduction to state and national nursing associations. It is important to support and participate in their activities. Nursing organizations publish journals offering updated healthcare information and continuing education by correspondence or in one's local community. The local nursing association may be the bargaining unit for nurses. By working collectively, a group can accomplish things that one person could not accomplish alone. A representative of the local association may speak at your school or place of employment about the association's function and activities and how graduates can join. (Often, students join nursing organizations as student affiliates.) Instructors also have information about nursing associations. In some states, recognition is given for exceptional scholarship in PN/VN programs. Request information from your local program if you are interested.

Alumni Associations

Many schools have alumni associations. Among their activities are student recruitment programs, speaking to potential students at career days, and fund-raising events to provide student scholarships. Attending reunions provides graduates with a chance to have fun and renew friendships. Classmates and instructors are also valuable networking resources, possibly providing information about employment or advancement opportunities.

Personal Nursing File

Keeping nursing records organized is important when transitioning from nursing student to licensed nurse. Start a personal nursing file immediately on graduation and keep it updated. This information will be needed when applying for the initial license, renewing the license, and seeking employment. This file will also be needed if the nurse's CEUs are audited by the licensing agency. Have the following materials readily available in your personal nursing file:

- A copy of the original nursing license and of each renewed license, as well as the NCLEX notification of initial licensure. (These documents are particularly important when seeking licensure in more than one state or in another country. Each state may require a copy of the license or license number.) Keep track of the license's expiration date and make sure to renew in a timely manner.
- A record of all continuing education courses; in some states, a copy of completion certificates must be submitted with license renewal applications. Requirements for continuing education vary among the states and provinces. Make sure you keep a file of all required information, in case you are audited.
- A copy of any advanced or specialized certification received.
- Copies of immunization records and most recent tuberculin testing (or negative chest x-ray) and rubella titer information. (Some employers require or strongly

recommend hepatitis and other specialized immunizations, in addition to routine immunizations.)
- A copy of a current cardiopulmonary resuscitation (CPR) certification. Most facilities require current CPR certification for continued employment.
- Copies of all high school, college, and nursing school transcripts, as well as any additional education received.
- A complete record of previous work experience, with dates of employment, copies of written evaluations, and name, address, and telephone number of immediate supervisor(s), and other references. (Make sure your references have agreed to be listed if you apply for employment.)
- A copy of your personal resume (keep it updated).
- A copy of your professional liability insurance policy.
- Birth certificate and/or passport or resident alien card/work permit ("green card"). (These documents are required for employment in the United States and in most other countries.)
- Social Security card (required for employment in the United States).
- Any other pertinent information, such as volunteer work, organizational offices held, and pertinent community activities.
- Records of income and job-related professional expenses for tax purposes. (Professional expenses include malpractice insurance premium, fees and expenses for continuing education, licensure renewal fee, and costs of required uniforms and professional journals and books required for continued employment or licensure. These may be tax deductible.)
- If your license application is audited, you will greatly benefit from having an organized professional file.

Networking: Personal and Professional Contacts

The term *networking* refers to a person's personal and professional connectedness. The electronic address book, BlackBerry, Facebook, email, chat rooms, and other Internet sources are invaluable tools in finding employment, learning about new opportunities and classes, and learning about new developments in medicine and nursing. This is a person's *professional network*, which usually contains a number of contacts, many of which may be superficial and related only to work. Keep this network up to date for future reference. The *personal network*, which includes family and close friends, is more close-knit and involves interdependence with a smaller number of people. This is marked by closer interaction. Both types of networking involve contact with other people, either in person, by mail, or electronically. The difference lies in the depth and intimacy of the contacts. The new nurse will find that keeping track of contacts throughout a career can prove very beneficial—both for the nurse and for the other people. It is impossible to predict when a question or concern will surface that can be addressed by one of the people in one's network of contacts.

PERSONAL LIFE

One's work life is interrelated with one's personal life. Be sure to have regular health, dental, and eye examinations. Maintain current immunizations and tests such as purified protein derivative (PPD), mammograms, or prostate-specific antigen (PSA) determination. (Most employers have health, dental, disability, and life insurance plans available at low cost to the employee and sometimes to their family.) All these factors help to ensure a safer and happier life (Fig. 101-3).

Balancing of Work and Personal Responsibilities and Activities

Although an individual will spend a great deal of time at work or thinking about work, it is important to have outside interests and hobbies. It is important to be able to relax and have fun after the busy day at work. There are many low-cost ways to do this. The new graduate will find that the flexibility of scheduling in nursing can fit very well into family and personal life. Often, the new income as a nurse helps enhance the quality of family life as well. Be sure to include physical activities in the recreational plan.

Financial Planning and Retirement

Financial security is important, so plan a personal budget. Be realistic—money never goes as far as one thinks it will.

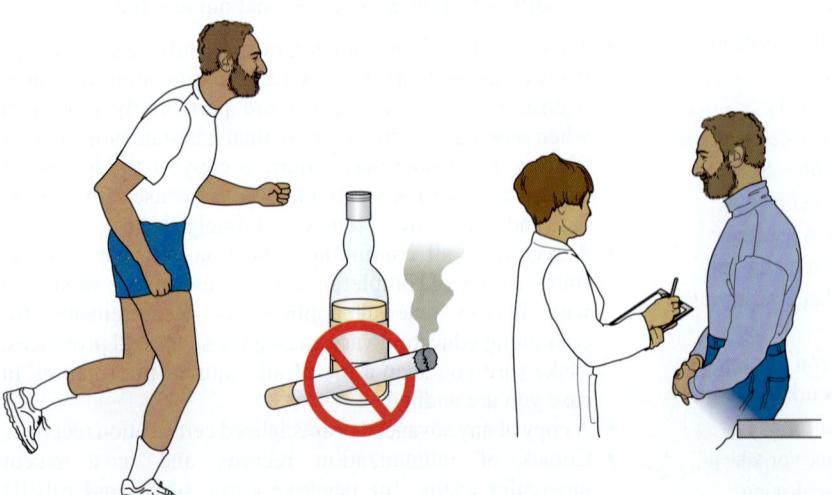

Figure 101-3 It is each nurse's responsibility to maintain healthy lifestyle practices. It is important to get enough sleep; eat well-balanced meals and maintain a healthy weight; exercise regularly and participate in recreational activities; avoid smoking and excess alcohol consumption, the use of recreational drugs, or overuse of prescription drugs; and to have regular physical, eye, and dental examinations. (Carter, 2005.)

Although it is difficult for a new graduate to think of retirement, early planning is essential. Be aware that to receive Social Security payments and Medicare at retirement, a certain number of eligible quarters must be worked and entered into the system. Even if the employer has a private or employer-sponsored retirement or investment plan, it is a good idea for the employee to pay into Social Security as well, if this option is available, even if this is not required by local law. Social Security benefits continue to change. Younger workers need to be in the system longer before becoming eligible for benefits. In addition, Social Security benefits are usually not sufficient to support oneself without a supplemental source of income after retirement.

It is important to build up as much retirement security as possible. Some healthcare facilities, particularly those administered by governmental units, have a built-in retirement plan. If this is not the case, it is important to invest in some sort of retirement and/or annuity plan. (These plans are available to those who have other retirement plans as well.) These funds can grow quickly when an amount from each paycheck is set aside and put into the fund. Many employers provide access to funds such as 401(k), Roth IRA, or tax-sheltered annuities. These provide a convenient and secure way to build a growing fund. In addition, many nurses have access to a credit union through their employer. Credit unions provide a number of benefits to their members, including automatic payroll savings deductions, free checking accounts, and low-interest loans.

There are often employment incentives for nurses. Some employers offer a sign-on bonus, if the nurse stays for a specified length of time. These bonuses may be based on the area in which the nurse chooses to work. In addition, nurses may receive a referral bonus if they recruit another nurse to the facility or agency and that person is hired. In some areas of the country, a nursing shortage exists. Sometimes, nurses are paid a moving allowance or a monthly housing allowance if they come to work there. Some employers are willing to help new graduates pay student loans, as well as paying for additional education for employees. Some facilities pay educational costs for nursing assistants to become LVN/LPNs and then go on to become RNs. (Many LVN/LPNs are able to go back to school and become RNs in this way.) The Armed Forces often also financially assist persons to become nurses, if they enlist for the service after graduation.

Self-Fulfillment

Several factors contribute to the nurse's feelings of satisfaction and fulfillment, both professionally and personally. These factors include the following:

- Knowing one's self and one's values and goals
- Living in the present, but having a plan for the future and working toward future goals
- Being self-reliant; taking responsibility for one's own actions
- Desiring to help others
- Considering situations to be challenges and opportunities, not problems
- Demonstrating self-direction and self-improvement
- Learning how to manage money
- Developing leisure time activities and friendships
- Maintaining flexibility and a positive attitude

STUDENT SYNTHESIS

KEY POINTS

- Nurses must pass the NCLEX examination, to obtain nursing licensure and to practice nursing.
- The NCLEX examination, a CAT, rather than a paper-and-pencil test, is based on a job analysis of tasks that actual nurses perform in the course of employment.
- A person must be licensed to perform certain nursing tasks or to be known as a "nurse."
- Most states require renewal of a nursing license every 2–3 years, along with evidence of continuing education. Each nurse is responsible for maintaining a current license.
- After becoming licensed, a nurse may wish to move and transfer their licensure to another state or country.
- Entry-level skills of the LVN/LPN include data collection, and assisting in planning, implementation, and evaluation of client care. Nurses are integral members of the healthcare team.
- After experience is gained, management and supervision opportunities are available to LVN/LPNs in some settings.
- Maintaining client confidentiality, organizing workload, appropriately acknowledging and interpreting orders, using technology, and maintaining a current knowledge base are important for every nurse.
- Nurses are responsible for continuity of client care 24 hr a day; the atmosphere and some activities in the healthcare facility during the evening and night hours may differ from those during day hours.
- All nurses are responsible for keeping up with current trends in nursing and being professionally responsible.
- Nurses must learn to balance the demands of work with their personal responsibilities and activities.

CRITICAL THINKING EXERCISES

1. Talk to three recently licensed nurses about the licensing examination. What were their reactions to the examination? Which suggestions do they have for students? What are your feelings about taking the examination? How do you plan to prepare?

2. As a new nursing graduate, you have not yet received your license. On your fourth day of employment in a local skilled nursing facility, the evening charge nurse, who is the only licensed person on duty, calls in sick. The administrator asks you to be in charge in their place. Describe what you would say and do and why. State who you might use as a resource in your facility.

NCLEX-STYLE REVIEW QUESTIONS

1. The new graduate taking the NCLEX-PN examination receives a question asking about a client's advance directives. Which category of client needs is the question addressing?
   a. Safe and effective care environment
   b. Coordinated care
   c. Safety and infection control
   d. Health promotion and maintenance

2. A new graduate was unsuccessful when taking the NCLEX-PN examination the first time. What can the graduate do to improve the chance of success when repeating the test?
   a. Audit all of the nursing courses.
   b. Wait 1 year to take the test again.
   c. Read all of the nursing books again.
   d. Take a review course.

3. The charge nurse should intervene immediately when which observation is made?
   a. A nurse is documenting and the computer screen is visible to others.
   b. A nurse refuses to allow a coworker access to the nurse's password.
   c. The vital sign clipboard is facedown and not visible to others.
   d. A nurse is obtaining data from a client and has the curtain drawn and the door closed.

4. The nurse delegates the transcription of healthcare providers' orders to the unit secretary. Who will maintain responsibility for accuracy and implementation?
   a. The healthcare provider
   b. The certified nursing assistant
   c. The unit secretary
   d. The nurse

5. The nurse is taking a telephone order from the healthcare provider, but the order is unclear to the nurse. Which is the priority action by the nurse?
   a. Carry out the order without question.
   b. Discuss the order with the charge nurse.
   c. Read back the order to clarify.
   d. Inform the healthcare provider that a written order is required.

CHAPTER RESOURCES

Enhance your learning with additional resources on thePoint!

Student Resources related to this chapter can be found at thePoint.lww.com/Rosdahl12e.

102 Career Opportunities and Job-Seeking Skills

Learning Objectives

1. List types of healthcare facilities or related agencies, other than hospitals, in which LVN/LPNs might seek employment.
2. Describe employment opportunities for LVN/LPNs in the long-term care facility; describe differences from hospital nursing.
3. List some specialized areas of nursing available to the LVN/LPNs.
4. Name sources of employment information for nurses. Describe the function of a placement service, nursing pool, or registry.
5. Explain how a nurse might conduct a job search or apply for a position, using the Internet.
6. Identify your important personal and professional considerations in choosing a place of employment.
7. List items to include in a résumé. Demonstrate the ability to prepare a personal résumé.
8. Describe the letter of application (cover letter) and procedures for filling out the application form; demonstrate the ability to complete an application for a position.
9. Describe preparation for and protocols during a job interview.
10. Identify the proper protocol for resigning from a position.

Important Terminology
nurse registry

Acronyms
EHS
HBO
PTO

As graduation approaches, decisions about future career plans enter the picture. This chapter describes selected employment opportunities available to a licensed vocational or licensed practical nurse (LVN/LPN) and suggestions for securing employment.

EMPLOYMENT OPPORTUNITIES

Most graduates of nursing programs seek employment soon after graduation. This may be the first step in a career or a means to earn money for additional education. After graduating from an approved nursing program, arrangements are made to take the NCLEX licensing examination to practice as a registered nurse (RN) or LVN/LPN (Chapter 101). (In some states, the student may apply for the test near the end of the program, if they reasonably expected to graduate.)

According to the U.S. Bureau of Labor Statistics (2020) in 2019, "Employment of LPNs is projected to grow *much faster than average for all occupations*" (approximately 9%) between 2019 and 2029. Overall job prospects are expected to be *very good,* but job outlook varies by location. Current data show that the largest employers of LVN/LPNs occur in long-term nursing facilities (38%), in hospitals (15%), in medical providers' offices (13%), and home healthcare services (13%). Demand for nurses, particularly LPNs, "will be driven by the increase in the share of the older population." This source goes on to state that "*median* annual wages of (LPN/LVNs) were $47,480 in May, 2019." The highest 10% earned more than $63,360. These statistics vary in different parts of the country and in different types of facilities. The individual nurse will need to explore employment opportunities in the area of the country where they prefer to work.

Entry Level Role

The LVN/LPN's role differs slightly in each state and in every facility. Currently, most are traditionally employed as members of the healthcare team, working with RNs, physicians, and other primary healthcare providers. A number of LVN/LPNs are also receiving special educational preparation to assume advanced positions or to become RNs.

Numbers of Nurses

The demand for LVN/LPNs continues. Job prospects are especially favorable for LVN/LPNs in medically underserved areas (U.S. Bureau of Labor Statistics, 2020). In 2019, there were approximately 721,700 LPNs employed in the United States. The total number of employed LVN/LPNs is expected to increase by 9% over the next 10 years. The National Council of State Boards of Nursing (2020b) states that 41,299 new LVN/LPNs were licensed in 2019. In 2020, there were roughly 3 million registered nurses (RNs) employed in the United States and an additional 721,700 LVN/LPNs.

Men in Nursing

Until the mid-1800s, nursing was a male-dominated profession. Then, during the U.S. Civil War, men were needed in the Army and women took over nursing roles. More men are again entering nursing, with about 6%–12% of all nurses being male.

General Employment Opportunities

Extended-care facilities (ECFs) of various types are a major source of new jobs for LVN/LPNs, as well as for RNs. Continued and rapid growth is expected in nursing homes, board-and-care homes, and community group homes. These areas include extended care for seniors and people with disabilities. Projections are that a greater percentage of jobs in these areas will continue to be filled by LVN/LPNs, rather than RNs. Other nonhospital settings will also provide expanded employment for LVN/LPNs. These include areas such as home care, community health centers, same-day surgery, physicians' offices, and schools. Some hospitals are hiring LVN/LPNs, although hospitals reflect the slowest growth for employment of all nurses, including LVN/LPNs.

Elder Care and Rehabilitation

Because of the continued growth of senior citizens, various segments of long-term and elder care are rapidly expanding (Fig. 102-1—see also Chapter 96). These include ECFs (including nursing homes) and assisted living facilities, as well as retirement communities. Many older citizens, as well as younger people, also receive rehabilitation and nursing services, either in their own home or in a rehabilitation center. Many staff positions for all levels of nurses are available in these ambulatory and home care services and ECFs. As the level of client acuity in these facilities increases, nurses will have many opportunities to use their medical-surgical and advanced nursing skills.

A number of specialized opportunities are available to the LVN/LPN in an ECF. This nurse may be employed as a:

- Medication nurse
- Treatment nurse
- IV nurse
- Charge nurse/nurse manager
- Client advocate/case manager
- Staff development person
- Assistant director of nursing

Some of these positions do not require further education beyond the basic LVN/LPN program or may require only in-service education. (National certification is available for LVN/LPNs in gerontology, pharmacology, and IV therapy. However, many states include certification of pharmacology and IV therapy within their curriculum now.)

Hospitals

Nurses also find positions in hospitals as staff nurses, giving bedside care and performing various nursing procedures. In many cases, the new graduate will not have priority and may not be able to work immediately in the preferred area or at the preferred time of day. As stated previously, hospital nursing in general is not expanding as fast as other types of healthcare. The LVN/LPN may be employed in a specialized area of the hospital or may function in a specialized role. This often requires additional education or training. Examples include the following:

- Special procedures
- Behavioral emergency response team
- Intravenous (IV) team
- Phlebotomy nurse
- Gerontology services
- Hospice unit
- Treatment nurse
- Medication nurse
- Emergency department or urgent care nurse
- Psychiatry nurse
- Clinic nurse

Home Care

A growing number of nurses, both RNs and LVN/LPNs, are finding employment in home care. The certified public health nurse (PHN) is an RN with a baccalaureate degree. PHNs supervise other nurses and unlicensed assistive personnel (UAP), such as home health aides and homemakers. Each client must have a designated case manager, usually required to be an RN. The case manager makes the initial evaluation visit, admits clients to the service, and writes a nursing care plan. The case manager then assists other nurses and UAP, makes regular assessment visits to evaluate client progress, supervises other caregivers, and updates nursing care plans. The LVN/LPN may be employed in home care to deliver routine daily care. In some cases, this nurse supervises UAP and volunteer caregivers. Home health nursing requires high-level skills, independent motivation, and a sense of professionalism; these nurses often work alone (Chapter 98). Home care is a career opportunity for experienced nurses and is not recommended for new graduates.

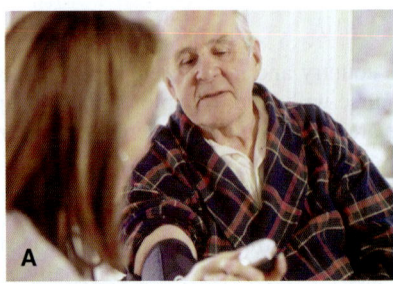

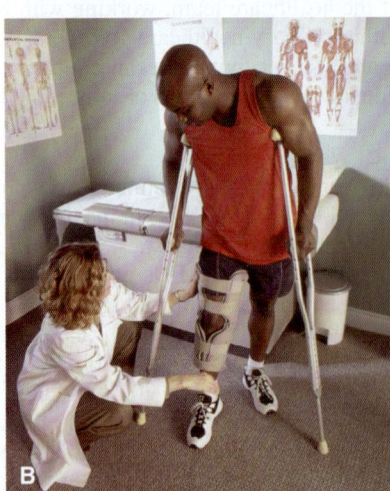

Figure 102-1 **A.** A large percentage of new LVN/LPNs and RNs will be employed in elder care—assisted living, skilled nursing facilities, and nursing homes. **B.** Many other LVN/LPNs will find employment in areas such as rehabilitation centers, schools, group homes, and other community-based facilities. (Carter, 2008.)

Community Health Centers

More and more U.S. healthcare is being provided in community health centers. In many cases, these centers provide all primary healthcare for a family or for most residents of a neighborhood. Although this has not been a primary source of employment for LVN/LPNs in the past, opportunities are expanding as the centers are growing in number and importance (Chapter 99).

Private Duty and Travel Nursing

A *private duty nurse* cares for one client in the client's home, an institution, or during travel, but rarely in a hospital. This nurse is often paid directly by the client or family; insurance usually does not cover this service. Private duty nursing offers the opportunity to practice basic bedside and teaching skills and to meet one client's total needs. Because this practice area often includes care for clients with long-term illnesses or those who are physically or emotionally challenged, private duty often offers nurses long-term employment.

A number of agencies recruit nurses for private duty or as travel companions for elderly or disabled clients. The nurse working as a travel companion may be "on duty" all the time. In addition, "travel nurse" agencies recruit nurses to work in understaffed parts of the country. In this case, a bonus, moving expenses, and a monthly housing allowance may be paid. In some cases, nurses are recruited to follow "snow birds" going south for the winter. This nurse has an opportunity to travel and earn money at the same time; employment may be contracted for 2–5 months, sometimes longer. The travel nurse may work with an individual client or in a healthcare facility.

Hospice Care

Hospice nursing involves providing end-of-life, or advanced illness, care and is located in hospitals, long-term care facilities, other sites (e.g., hotels, shelters, or prisons), or the client's own home. In rare cases, a client is in a hospital or hospice facility. Hospice nurses help clients and their families work through the final stages of life. The goal of hospice is to help clients die with dignity and to assist family members in the loss of their loved one (Chapter 100). Nurses working in a home care agency may encounter hospice clients as part of a regular caseload. In many agencies, the hospice program is separate and employs its own staff.

Substance Use Disorder Programs

Substance use disorders (chemical dependency [CD]) programs allow the nurse to assist with treatment and rehabilitation of clients who misuse drugs, alcohol, and other substances (Chapter 95). These nurses may work in hospitals, private treatment centers, or detoxification (detox) centers. (Remember that detoxification, particularly from alcohol, can be life threatening and requires a high degree of nursing competence.) These areas employ nurses at all levels, to function as nurses, group leaders, and substance use disorder counselors. In many cases, the employees are themselves recovering from a substance use issue.

Mental Health Nursing

Mental health and psychiatric settings provide opportunities for employment of both RNs and LVN/LPNs. These settings include state-run institutions, psychiatric units housed in acute care facilities, free-standing psychiatric hospitals, clinics, day treatment or partial treatment programs, specialized group homes, and community mental health centers (Chapter 94). Some long-term care facilities also have specialized units for adults with mental health concerns, including dementia. In some facilities, such as long-term or state treatment centers, the length of stay may be several months or longer. This allows the nurse to work with clients on a long-term basis. Community mental health is a growing field. Some community mental health centers are designed to treat clients with the *dual diagnosis* of mental illness and substance use disorders (MI/CD) (Chapter 94). In some cities, crisis nurses make home visits to clients with mental health and psychiatric problems.

Assisting Children With Disabilities

Nurses also have many opportunities for employment with developmentally delayed and intellectually challenged children and adults in institutions, group homes, and schools. The employment of nurses to work with children in schools is a growing field. In many cases, a child with severe disabilities requires medications, as well as treatments such as oxygen, ventilator care, or chest physiotherapy. In some cases, funds cover one-to-one nursing care while children are at school. In other cases, nursing care is funded 24 hr a day.

Residential Treatment Centers

Nurses may find employment in specialized residential treatment centers or group homes that serve specific client populations. In addition to substance use disorder programs, the nurse might be employed in a group home for persons who are developmentally delayed or intellectually challenged or those who have a chronic and persistent mental illness (CPMI). Employment is also available at halfway houses for clients discharged from psychiatric hospitals or other treatment centers, but who are still unable to live independently. Many of these facilities have a licensed nurse on duty for at least part of the day. Nursing functions include supervision of the setup and administration of medications and provision of first-aid care.

Correctional Facilities

Prisons and many large jails employ nurses (RNs and LVN/LPNs) who monitor inmates with special needs, such as those who may be contemplating suicide or who receive medications on a regular basis. These nurses also assist with diabetic management and teaching, perform routine health screenings, and provide health-related counseling. If an inmate appears too physically or mentally ill to be managed in jail, the nurse consults a healthcare provider for referral to a hospital. Nurses also may teach classes on topics such as sex education, safer sex, nutrition, and healthy lifestyles. In some cases, support groups are also included.

Physicians' Offices

Nurses are often employed in a physician's office or clinic, to assist with physical examinations, dressings, and minor surgical procedures and to perform routine screening (e.g., hearing, vision, TPR, blood pressure [including orthostatic evaluation], oxygen saturation, blood glucose, bladder scanning, height, weight, and levels of pain). Nurses are involved in medication teaching and lifestyle counseling. In addition to nursing skills, clinical duties may include answering telephones, making appointments, assisting clients into examination rooms, performing some laboratory tests or simple x-rays, processing items for billing, keyboarding letters, and serving as a receptionist. Computer skills are usually required. Office nurses must be skilled in triage, so clients receive necessary care in a timely manner. Many clinic nurses in physicians' offices are LVN/LPNs. Work is usually during daytime hours and may include part of the weekend, but usually does not involve evenings, nights, Sundays, or holidays (Chapter 99).

Ambulatory/Day-Surgery Clinics

Many clients go to ambulatory/day-surgery clinics for surgical procedures. Some of these procedures are fairly extensive and require the nurse to be skilled in pre- and postoperative care and in client and family teaching. In addition, the nurse in ambulatory/day surgery often assists the surgeon during the surgical procedure. The nurse calls the client before the procedure to make sure the client is properly prepared and does not have additional questions. In addition, this nurse performs telephone follow-up after clients return home. Nurses in day surgery may be LVN/LPNs. Hours are usually Monday through Friday. Although the nurse may begin work very early in the morning, in many cases, the surgical schedule is completed by midday or early afternoon (Chapter 99).

Health Maintenance Organizations/Third-Party Payors

Employment for LVN/LPNs exists in the area of preapproval or reimbursement for healthcare. Health maintenance organizations, insurance companies, and other third-party payors train these nurses to research each client's healthcare needs, to determine if the cost of a particular surgical or diagnostic test can be paid by their company. This *claims analyst* works with physicians and other healthcare professionals to ensure that quality care is given in the most cost-effective manner. This is primarily a sedentary position, involving extensive use of the computer, telephone, fax, and e-mail. In some cases, the analyst will visit the healthcare facility to interview healthcare personnel or clients or to review client records. Hours are most often during the day, Monday through Friday, not including holidays.

Telehealth

"Telephone nursing" or *telehealth* is a growing area of nursing employment. (In some states, this field is limited to RNs.) Third-party payors and health maintenance organizations often provide this service in the form of "Nurse Lines" or "Dial-a-Nurse," using computerized triage systems. Clients call about symptoms and with questions and nurses answer questions and make appropriate referrals, following carefully prescribed computerized protocols. Many telehealth systems include a medical information library, with educational materials available for members. Referrals to primary providers or community health centers may also be made. (Often, members can access services via the telehealth's own Website, as well.) If the telehealth program is run by a third-party payor, these nurses may preapprove care for insurance purposes. Crisis lines and suicide prevention lines are other examples of telehealth. Many such services are available 24 hr a day. Goals of telehealth programs include cost effectiveness, increased medication compliance, decreased physician and emergency room visits, and fewer rehospitalizations. Telehealth is particularly valuable in remote areas where residents have limited access to primary healthcare services. As previously stated, many day-surgery centers use a form of telehealth nursing where nurses call clients the day before surgery to answer questions and conduct preoperative teaching and again the day after surgery to ensure that recovery is progressing without complications.

Occupational Health

Positive health maintenance is a goal of many companies, hospitals, and industries. These sites are interested in their employees' health and welfare, as well as promoting minimal absenteeism. Nurses may act as wellness coordinators for such industries, teaching preventive care and health maintenance to employees. In many situations, nurses are responsible for enforcing safety measures and Occupational Safety and Health Administration (OSHA) regulations, as well as managing worker's compensation claims and providing safety data sheets (SDS) for employees. The occupational health nurse must be knowledgeable in first aid. These nurses often chair safety committees and may manage employee-assistance programs, including CDC education and prevention. In rare cases, the industrial nurse may perform home visits to employees.

Both RNs and LVN/LPNs are employed in occupational health, although the team leader is usually an RN. As a nursing student, you may come in contact with the employee health service (EHS) of your school or the facilities where clinical experience is gained. Employees of healthcare facilities usually are seen by the EHS for various reasons, including the initial physical examination, yearly tuberculin (PPD) testing, routine immunizations and other routine screenings, and return-to-work permits after illness or injury. EHS personnel in the healthcare facility are responsible for investigating any reports of unusual or unexpected exposure of employees to communicable disease, including needlestick incidents or cases of the assault of a nurse by a client. The EHS may also be responsible for teaching cardiopulmonary resuscitation (CPR) and other classes. Nurses who develop latex sensitivity would also be assisted by the EHS to locate safe materials and equipment and an acceptable work environment. The EHS is usually open only during daytime and early evening hours and may be closed on weekends.

Armed Forces

The active armed forces and reserves offer employment opportunities for all levels of nurses. After basic training, licensed nurses may enter the armed forces at a level higher than that of other enlisted persons. Usually, they are assigned to hospitals or clinics and may be assigned to duty in another country. The nurse in the military is trained in CPR and may also be trained as an emergency medical technician (EMT). Specially trained combat medics may be RNs or LVN/LPNs. In many cases, qualified individuals receive salary and expenses while attending nursing programs, in exchange for enlistment. Nurses, while in service, can often earn "credits" to help pay for additional education after leaving the service and can also take college courses free of charge while on active duty.

Schools

In addition to nurses employed to assist specific students with disabilities, school systems and colleges may employ nurses and other healthcare personnel to work with the general student body. LVN/LPNs may be employed as *assistants* or *school health aides* in the Student Health Service. In most states, schools are required to have a public health nurse (PHN) or licensed/certified school nurse in charge of the program. Duties are varied and interesting. Assistant nurses help with vision and hearing screening, immunization clinics, and athletic physical examinations. The nurse or assistant nurse also performs routine first aid, with additional education/training, and assists with record keeping. The nurse may help teach nursing assistants on work-release programs and may assist with student support groups regarding weight loss, eating disorders, conduct disorder, smoking cessation, and related topics. This nurse may also oversee a student "medical interest" club or may accompany the band or a sports team on an out-of-town trip, as a first-aid resource. The nurse may help students deal with such issues as violence in school or the death of a classmate and may be called on to help teach topics such as sex education, safer sex, and pregnancy prevention. The nurse works with teen parents and their children and may make supervised home visits.

Parish Nursing

Many religious congregations have *parish nurses,* who may be paid employees or volunteers. Parish nurses facilitate a congregation's holistic health, combining physical, emotional, and spiritual dimensions. A local hospital or public health agency may provide a case manager or nurse coordinator to help develop the concept, support the parish, and provide in-service education to the nurse. Specific parish nursing courses are available; this nurse is usually an RN; the LVN/LPN may function as an assistant. The functions of the parish nursing service often include health screenings (particularly blood pressure), educating individuals or groups on health and wellness topics, writing newsletter articles, and visiting parishioners in hospitals and nursing homes (and sometimes performing home visits). Parish nurses provide counseling, make referrals, and serve as client advocates, but usually do not provide hands-on nursing care. They may assist in training family caregivers. They sometimes accompany congregation members to healthcare providers' offices or hospitals for test results or surgery. Parish nurses provide support to terminally ill clients and their families and often participate in funerals for deceased parishioners. They often facilitate bereavement support groups. Occasionally, churches sponsor healthcare clinics or "health fairs" for parishioners and the local community. Services may be limited, or the clinic may be an ongoing community health center. The parish may also sponsor an outside agency brought in to provide screenings, including bone density, carotid artery ultrasound, and ECGs. Parish nurses may oversee such programs and coordinate volunteers. The parish nurse may also oversee a program in the community, such as Meals on Wheels or the local blood drive.

Nursing in Unique Locales

Employment is available for a limited number of nurses, both RNs and LVN/LPNs, in such unique locations as cruise ships or large resorts, particularly those catering to older people. In these positions, nurses function under "standing orders" from a healthcare provider, who may not be on site. In an emergency, the nurse must be able to contact the provider, but must be able to perform first aid or life-support measures, to stabilize the person for transport or until emergency services arrive.

In many countries, nurses educated in the United States or Canada are in great demand. Sometimes, the host country's government will pay moving and living expenses, as well as a high salary. The American nursing license is often sufficient, although a local license may be required as well. Nurses who anticipate seeking employment in other countries would benefit from learning languages other than English. Understanding the customs for appropriate personal and professional behavior and apparel in the host country is also essential in preparation for these positions (e.g., there are strict taboos and protocols for behavior of women in many Middle Eastern countries). Additional immunizations may be required.

Volunteer Service

The nurse is a member of the larger community. Opportunities exist for volunteer service to give back to that community. Service opportunities include teaching others about healthcare or assisting in times of disaster. The events of September 11, 2001, Hurricane Katrina in 2005, and earthquakes in Haiti in 2010, and Nepal in 2015, as well as tsunamis and earthquakes in Japan, serve to emphasize the need for first-aid volunteers in every community and around the world.

Nurses may also be involved in the local community by teaching first aid, babysitting, or expectant parents' classes at local hospitals, or in teaching adult or community education classes. Some positions utilize volunteers; some positions are paid.

The American Red Cross, a large national organization, uses nurse volunteers to assist with well-baby and immunization clinics, as well as to provide first-aid services for community events and during disasters. Red Cross nurse volunteers also teach CPR, first aid, childcare, babysitting, and other classes. Volunteer nurses assist with blood drives and health fairs. All major stadiums, sports arenas, and other venues have a cadre of first-aid volunteers and paid rescue personnel who work during games, concerts, and other events. Nurses can receive special training to serve in either a paid or volunteer capacity at these events.

AmeriCorps/Volunteers in Service to America (AmeriCorps VISTA) celebrated its 50th anniversary in 2015. This organization provides care and education to people in need in the United States, especially those whose incomes are below the federal poverty threshold or those in medically underserved areas (americorps.gov). Usually, volunteers serve for 1 year as part of a specific project at a partner organization (nonprofit organization or public agency). One goal is to "improve health services." A summer associate program of 8–10 weeks is also available. The Peace Corps (Global Leadership Adventures) offers a volunteer opportunity for needed human services in many parts of the world (www.experiencegla.com). This organization also has a teen program. Other volunteer opportunities in the United States and around the world include Habitat for Humanity and teams providing surgery or eye care in underserved areas in the United States and other countries. Churches often sponsor mission trips to assist with delivering healthcare and other services in underserved areas. Most of these programs welcome all nurses as volunteers.

Other Opportunities
Other potential employment opportunities may include the following:

- *Head Start programs:* Head Start employs nurses in schools as assistant instructors in programs for very young children.
- *Weight-loss clinics:* Weight loss clinics employ nurses as support persons or counselors. These nurses are often LVN/LPNs. They weigh clients, measure skinfold thickness, calculate body mass index (BMI), take blood pressure, teach classes, and perform other functions.
- *Camp programs:* Most camps are required to employ nurses. The lead nurse is often an RN, but LVN/LPNs may also be on staff. Camp nurses share many functions with school nurses, although many illnesses and disorders they encounter are different. Campers may have poison ivy or oak; insect or snake bites; fractures; lacerations; and various infections. They may be sunburned, windburned, or burned by campfires. A near drowning may occur, or a child may be thrown from a horse. Camp nurses also assist homesick children. They often teach wilderness safety, survival, and first aid. A camp may also focus on a particular condition, such as asthma or diabetes. This is typically a summer position, allowing the nurse ample time to further their education during the school year or pursue other employment.

Specialized Employment Opportunities

Some positions are available for nurses with special qualifications and the ability to meet the demands of a particular job. Most of these positions require further education or training beyond the basic nursing program.

Specialized Training Programs
Specific education (and sometimes, certification) is available to LVN/LPNs in areas such as pharmacology, intravenous (IV) therapy, and gerontology. Practical nursing programs in many states now include medication administration and IV therapy training in their certification degree. Nurses may also receive additional education in areas such as emergency medicine technician (EMT) or phlebotomy (drawing blood). Specially trained nurses are practicing in acute care settings, including intensive care units, coronary care units, emergency departments, and operating rooms. (Advanced education in nursing is addressed in Chapter 103.)

Practical Nursing Programs
To become an instructor in a practical nursing program, the nurse must have a Bachelor of Science in Nursing (BSN) degree. Qualifications also include a sound educational background, recent and pertinent clinical nursing experience, proficiency in nursing skills, patience, and the ability to work with people. A previous degree in education and teaching experience is always an advantage. Hours are usually days, Monday through Friday.

Operating Rooms
Hospitals may employ LVN/LPNs or newly graduated RNs in operating rooms. These nurses, following postgraduate training as a surgical technician, function as *scrub nurses*. (In most states, the lead *circulating nurse* must be an RN.) The hours are usually Monday through Friday during the day, often starting at 4 or 5 AM. However, operating room staff members are often on call for emergencies.

Dialysis Centers
Nurses may be specifically trained to work in hospital dialysis units, ambulatory dialysis centers, or on mobile teams that administer dialysis to clients in their homes. Some clients have their own in-home dialysis units. Nurses teach clients and family members how to operate machines; in some cases, nurses operate the machines. Dialysis nurses must have a thorough understanding of the complications and emergency measures associated with this treatment.

Hyperbaric Medicine
Additional hospitals are developing *hyperbaric chambers*. Here, oxygen is administered, under pressure to clients, including those with anaerobic diseases, such as gas gangrene or tetanus. In addition, hyperbaric oxygenation (**HBO**) is often helpful in cases of carbon monoxide poisoning; in conjunction with some types of cancer chemotherapy; in cases of near drowning; and in cases of rapid reentry into the earth's atmosphere, such as the fighter pilot or hot air balloonist who crashes from a high altitude or a deep-sea diver who ascends too fast. Some types of surgery are also performed under HBO. The nurse, either RN or LVN/LPNs, requires special instruction to work in the hyperbaric chamber or with the supporting team outside the chamber. Because very high concentration oxygen is delivered, *special safety measures must be carefully observed*. People working in the chamber also must have patent (open) auditory tubes, in order to adequately equalize the pressure in the middle ear with the surrounding atmosphere in the chamber and thereby to avoid severe discomfort. (Former Navy divers also have found hyperbaric medicine to be a good career opportunity.)

Pharmaceutical Sales
Pharmaceutical companies sometimes employ nurses in sales and marketing positions. Nurses working there have an advantage over other salespeople because they understand the actions and side effects of medications and may be better able to communicate information to physicians. The salesperson is often required to travel and must provide a professional wardrobe and a car. Hours can be long, but the salesperson often works on commission, with the potential for high earnings.

Veterinary Clinics
Veterinarians may hire nurses as assistants. Many nursing techniques for humans are useful in veterinary medicine and surgery as well.

Chiropractic Clinics and Acupuncture Centers

Chiropractic clinics and acupuncture centers often employ nurses as assistants. In some cases, nurses receive instruction to perform some treatments, such as diathermy and ultrasound. Nurses may also return to school to receive advanced training to perform therapies, such as homeopathy, flower essence therapy, acupressure/acupuncture, and other complementary therapies.

Dental, Ophthalmology, and Other Specialty Clinics

Nurses may be employed by dentists or eye specialists, particularly those who perform surgery. These nurses assist with procedures such as biopsies, LASIK eye surgery, or various dental procedures. Other *specialty clinics* may employ nurses to assist with procedures, such as colonoscopy or vasectomy; this often involves on-the-job training. Functions include preprocedure teaching, starting IVs, administration of medications before and during the procedure, handing instruments and supplies to the practitioner during the procedure, receiving and preserving biopsied material, monitoring client vital signs, and emotional support of the client. The nurse also monitors the client after the procedure until they are stable, makes sure the client is safe to return home, and carries out postoperative instruction, including signs of complications. This position involves daytime hours during the week, but the staff may be on call for emergencies.

Emergency Rescue

Some nurses work with clients who are injured or suddenly become ill. An additional paramedic or EMT course is often required to be employed in ground rescue services for nonemergent cases. Most states require an RN license and 3–5 years in ICU/ED to be eligible for flight nurses. Employment in this area requires calmness under pressure, quick thinking, and accurate decision making. Emergency rescue personnel use medical-surgical equipment and must be familiar with a variety of high-tech equipment. Other opportunities for nurses with paramedic or EMT training include military service, park ranger rescue services, and ski patrol programs. EMTs and paramedics may be employed or may be volunteers at parades, races, sports events such as golf tournaments and football games, concerts, and other large gatherings and may provide rescue services in the event of a disaster.

Self-Employment

Some nurses are self-employed entrepreneurs. Examples include running a shop that sells or rents medical equipment or uniforms, assisting clients to manage equipment, such as home oxygen or CPAP machines, contracting nurses to provide home care, developing and marketing a specialty health-related product, operating a health food or herbal medicine store, or acting as a personal trainer in a gym. The person may specialize in prostheses, including breast prostheses and specialized clothing for people with disabilities. Nurses might work from home doing medical transcription or medical literature searches and research on the Internet for others. Specialized educational programs are available to train nurses to do legal consulting. A nurse might contract with a city or county to provide testing services for contaminants, such as radon or lead; many large cities have such programs. Practical/vocational nurses often sit as members of their State or Province Board of Nursing.

Key Concept

The possibilities for entrepreneurship and related volunteer activities are unlimited. The individual nurse's imagination, available time, financial resources, and personal energy are pertinent factors.

OBTAINING EMPLOYMENT INFORMATION

Nursing provides a unique opportunity for employees to choose work schedules and locations that best suit their lifestyle. Examine personal and family needs to choose the most suitable work situation (Chapter 101). There are many Websites with advice on how to apply for and select your first job. However, try to "…go with the company that feels like the best fit, where you feel you'll learn the most, and find good mentors. Odds are, this first job won't be your last" (Schrager, 2019).

A very large percentage of jobs are never advertised in print media or are filled by the time an advertisement publishes. Be sure to build networks to learn about positions as they become available. If an internship, student learning experience, or volunteer opportunity is available, take it. Future employees are often chosen from those who have had some exposure to the facility and are known to the staff. Take advantage of any on-campus career days or recruiter visits. Many schools also have a placement officer who will help with job applications.

Key Concept

Remember that approximately 90% of all positions are filled based on personal contacts. Many positions are not advertised or are advertised after the employer already has a prospective employee in mind. Doing homework and expanding one's professional network increases the chances of obtaining the desired position.

Medical Float Pool or Registry Service

A medical pool/**nurse registry** recruits nurses to work in facilities that need extra help for vacation coverage or during busy periods, maternity leaves, or illness. A nurse registers with the agency, which calls when a job is available. The nurse has the option of declining, which is an advantage for those who do not wish to work full time. (Nurses who decline too often, however, risk losing future opportunities with the agency.) Agencies may offer insurance, vacation pay, and free in-service education to nurses who accept a required number of shifts. Some agencies have regular posts to fill in healthcare facilities, home care, and schools and can provide nurses with full-time employment. There are advantages and disadvantages in working for a pool. The nurse is often paid a higher hourly wage but may be without benefits. The nurse has more choice as to when and where to work. Disadvantages include not knowing if one will be working or not; unpaid time off; and difficulty in establishing strong bonds with coworkers unless the nurse is regularly assigned to the same location. Often the pool nurse is assigned to an extremely busy area, which may be a positive challenge or may be very difficult. In addition, nurses in the facility may resent the pool nurse, knowing that the salary is higher.

Most hospitals and some long-term facilities have their own *internal nursing pool* (*float pool*). This has the advantage of continuity and stability and the nurse's familiarity with the physical setup, nursing protocols, computerized recording system, and staff at the facility. This nurse may also be able to build seniority with the facility and is often eligible for benefits.

State Employment Services

Each state's jobs or employment service is affiliated with state or local government (www.statelocalgov.net). This agency provides free job information, both in private industry and government positions. In addition to helping workers find employment, they also "promote the well-being of the state's workers,…deal with issues confronting special populations, such as veterans, migrants, youth, seniors, or disabled workers,…and provide retraining and rehabilitation." Positions in other areas are also accessible, via this same Website.

Many large organizations, healthcare facilities, counties, or states maintain an Internet job hotline. A person can call or access the service 24 hr a day. Many of these entities are required by law to post all positions, so the person accessing the service can peruse all available positions. An application for employment is obtained and usually submitted online.

Nursing Journals

Nursing journals also advertise positions. Some positions are in specialty areas; others are for general staff nurses, including new graduates. Specific positions advertised in a journal are often filled by the time they are published. However, these ads can provide some insight into which healthcare facilities are currently hiring and the geographical areas that seem to have the most available positions. Nursing journals list facility addresses, e-mail addresses, and Websites for obtaining further information.

Newspapers, Bulletin Boards, and Other Sources

Newspapers publish available positions, both in print and online. Although print ads are becoming less common, they do provide some resources. Even if a particular position is filled by the time an application is filed, related positions may be available. Newspapers may have articles regarding job searches, and application or interviewing techniques. Do not forget to look on facility bulletin boards, either paper postings or Internet bulletin boards.

Internet

Nearly all job postings today are found on the Internet. Several national employment Websites are available, some of which are specific to healthcare careers. The Internet also provides information about online job fairs and about many employers. Many hospitals and other facilities have Websites with employment information. Usually, applications for employment are obtained and sent via the Internet, a particularly useful service if you plan to work in a part of the country, or another country, different from your current residence. Websites also exist where you can post your résumé for potential employers to review. (Often, the only way to apply for a position is online.)

In addition to individual Websites, online versions of several journals' career directories are available. These directories typically include a large number of positions, as well as articles related to job seeking. (They may also be available in printed form.) The *American Journal of Nursing* publishes a career issue yearly. Although most positions advertised are for RNs, pertinent articles give hints on job seeking. The LVN/LPN can also get a good feeling for where jobs are located by reading this issue. Websites devoted to writing résumés and cover letters, job interviewing, and other pertinent topics for employment seekers also are available. In addition, many Websites link to other helpful sites. In the search for employment, the Internet offers several advantages. For example, an individual can search for opportunities in a particular part of the country. A wide range of potential employers can be searched. One of the most important advantages of using the Internet is that all searching can be completed from home. In addition, communicating with potential employers via the Internet demonstrates one's experience and proficiency with computer technology. To help focus and narrow the search, books are also available, which list specific Websites and helpful suggestions, to guide the electronic job search.

> **Key Concept**
> Although many nursing opportunities exist for the new graduate, be aware of the importance of choosing a first job in a setting that gives you experience in applying your basic nursing skills and knowledge.

> **Nursing Alert** Be sure that your social media profile does not include anything you would not want a prospective employer to see you doing or writing. Be sure that you maintain strict privacy settings and exercise caution on whichever platforms you are using. It is better to be very careful than to miss a great opportunity due to embarrassing or unprofessional social media posts.

JOB-SEEKING SKILLS

Before deciding on the type of employment to seek, individual personal requirements must be evaluated. Consider such factors as geographic location, shift rotation, childcare, transportation, and housing in the decision-making process (Fig. 102-2). Unwillingness to compromise about where to work or desired hours of work may lead to difficulty in obtaining a job. Develop a job search plan that includes the following:

- Decide on the types of jobs desired, in relation to what is available.
- Complete a self-evaluation: What are your greatest skills and assets? Where is the best fit? Consider factors such

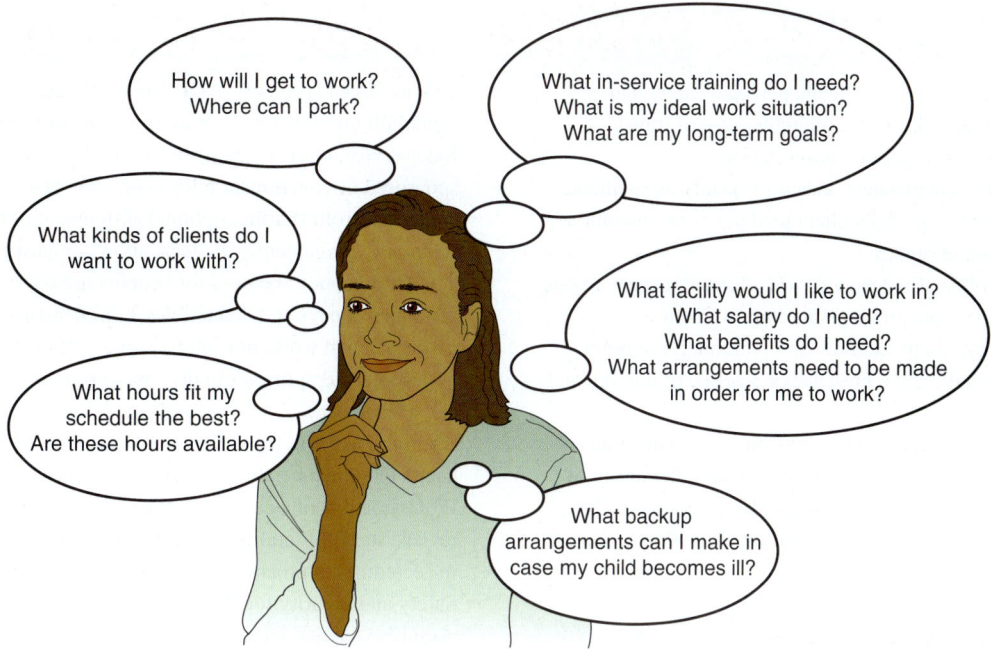

Figure 102-2 It is important to think about what type of nursing position will best fit your personality, lifestyle, and interests.

as desire to work alone or with others; freedom and flexibility versus structure; and desire to be a leader or a team member.
- Spend at least 5 hr a day in the job search. Finding a job is your "job" now.
- Set a goal for the number of contacts per day.
- Be sure the résumé and cover letter are neatly printed and error free. Use your spell check and make sure you are using the correct word. (Spell check only determines if it is a word, but not the meaning.) Usually, these will be submitted online.
- Prepare for interviews with appropriate dress and a plan for answering difficult questions.
- Emphasize the positive—what you can contribute to the organization, your education, and all former positions, paid or volunteered.
- Use networking skills to find unadvertised positions.
- Arrange issues, such as transportation and daycare ahead of time.

The first job is important. It forms the basis for future opportunities. Performing well the first time provides a sound basis and good references that will help in acquiring future positions.

Choosing a Place of Employment

Many factors must be considered when choosing possible places of employment. The first job may not be the perfect job. Consider what is most important and choose the best job available. Box 102-1 lists specific items to consider when choosing where to work. Try to match skills, needs, and personal goals with available positions, as much as possible.

Applying for a Position

After targeting positions of interest, the next step is to apply. Because competition may be fierce for the most desirable jobs, how the application process is completed can greatly affect an employer's decision about whom to hire.

Letter of Application

The value of the letter of application, sometimes referred to as the "cover letter" (if it accompanies a résumé), cannot be overestimated. The letter is the first thing employers see. The application may not be considered if the letter fails to have a positive effect. Remember that the focus is on convincing employers that you are the best candidate. The opening paragraph should call attention to the résumé, *but not repeat the information in the résumé*. If you were referred by someone, state that in the first sentence. The letter should be informative and concise. Limit it to two or three paragraphs.

The letter of application should

- State the position for which you are applying and how you found out about it.
- Explain briefly why you feel you are qualified and what special skills and attributes you bring to the position.
- Describe applicable job experience, skills, and education. Remember to include volunteer positions.
- Conclude by informing the employer of availability for a personal interview and for employment and the easiest method for contact.

If being submitted by mail, print out the letter neatly on conservative stationery and enclose it along with a concise, up-to-date personal résumé. If via Internet or fax, include the cover letter with the résumé.

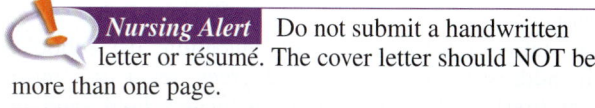 **Nursing Alert** Do not submit a handwritten letter or résumé. The cover letter should NOT be more than one page.

If access to a high-quality printer is not available or knowledge about composing an appropriate résumé is lacking, use

Box 102-1 Factors to Consider When Looking for a Place of Employment

- Personal factors: childcare, hours, personal career and educational goals, distance from home, ease of travel, including parking or public transportation
- Quality of care: client safety, means of quality assessment, legal support, average daily client load per nurse, nonnursing duties expected of nurses
- Teamwork: collegiality, general work climate, respect among coworkers, participation in quality improvement
- Type of facility: client care, research, teaching; nonprofit, proprietary; small, large; presence or absence of nursing and other students
- Available shifts: day, evening, night; full time, part time; permanent shift assignment or rotating shifts; flexibility of honoring special hours requests; mandatory double shifts
- Length of shifts: choices of 8-, 10-, and 12-hr shifts; special incentives, such as Baylor plan or weekend contract, bonuses, option for a shared position
- Chances for advancement and leadership opportunities; available teaching and committee opportunities; use of computers in daily care—documentation, ordering treatments and medications, calling up information, e-mail, Internet access
- Educational opportunities and professional growth: internships, in-service education, continuing education courses, library facilities, computer availability, pay or reimbursement for advanced education and continuing education courses, training in use of new equipment, incentive pay for special certification
- Salary: opportunities and requirements for moving up the salary scale; shift/weekend differential; charge nurse pay, overtime pay, job stability, financial security
- Benefits: insurance (health, dental, vision, disability, life, individual, and family), sick leave, vacation time, holidays (holiday bonuses, number of paid holidays, "holiday back policies"), paid time off (**PTO**), onsite childcare (including the availability of care for ill children), adult daycare, parking, food service, worker's compensation, 401(k), employer-sponsored or government retirement plan, tax-sheltered annuities, profit sharing, optional assignment of benefits. (*Optional assignment of benefits* allows employees to set aside a dollar amount to be used for benefits not covered, such as insurance copays and deductibles, complementary healthcare, glasses, dental work, or elective surgery. If the total amount is not used, the employee usually loses the unused portion at the end of the year.)
- Ability to use sick leave time to pay for health promotion (e.g., health club membership, exercise equipment)
- Professional feedback and evaluation: periodic review, peer review, status of facility accreditation, participation of nurses in accreditation process, praise, and recognition
- Safety and security for staff: parking lot escort, assistance with assaultive clients, security in home care, providing nurse with beeper or phone for home care, "panic button" on dangerous units, camera surveillance in dangerous areas (with connection to security)
- Extra "perks": payment of professional dues, subscription to nursing journal, choir, theater group, discount tickets, group travel, Weight Watchers, gift shop, staff tournaments, holiday teas, retirement parties, recognition for years of service, use of gym, health club or swimming pool, pharmacy, credit union, payment for preventive healthcare, immunization programs, free or reduced-rate parking or bus passes, housing allowance, Internet access, payment for unused sick leave or option to convert to vacation time
- Professional association membership: required or voluntary; bargaining agent, contract for nurses
- Presence or absence of a nurses union; requirement to belong or pay "fair share"

a professional résumé service. Such services can help compose and print a professional-looking résumé at a relatively low cost. It is recommended that you use "bullet points" to accent your skills and how they would be beneficial to the position for which you are applying. Your communication skills will usually be judged by the quality of your cover letter.

Résumé

The two types of résumés are (a) emphasizing strengths and abilities or (b) listing experience chronologically. When seeking a first nursing position, usually the second type is used. List education, previous employment, and relevant experience.

In stating information about education, list schools, their addresses, diplomas or degrees received (most recent first), and licenses and certificates held (and in what states). *Dates can be omitted.* List work experience, with the most recent position first (name of facility; dates employed; title of position; and supervisor's name, address, e-mail, and/or telephone number). Identify special skills, training, honors, or volunteer positions, and be sure to provide references. (If you attended your nursing program immediately after high school, describe honors and leadership positions held in high school. Include part-time jobs and volunteer activities.) Many nursing programs offer guidelines on what to include in a good résumé. They also may have keyboarding and printing services available to students and graduates. Box 102-2 gives further tips for composing a résumé.

Interview

Routine procedure usually includes a personal interview with a prospective employer. It is important to prepare for the interview by finding out as much about the position and the facility as possible. For the interview, wear tailored, conservative clothes (a suit or dress shirt and tie is usually best) and simple jewelry (Fig. 102-3). Be sure shoes are neat and clean, and polished, if necessary. Avoid extremes in makeup and nail polish. Clean and neatly styled hair and clean, short

CHAPTER 102 Career Opportunities and Job-Seeking Skills

> **Box 102-2 Guidelines for Writing a Résumé**
>
> - Clearly list name, mailing address, telephone number (home phone, cell phone); include e-mail address.
> - State your career objective.
> - Be positive. (Do not mention shortcomings.)
> - Be specific and accurate. Make sure no errors exist in dates of employment or school; make sure there are no "typos" or spelling errors. Use a spell check. Also check grammar.
> - Be creative.
> - Be brief. Keep to one page, if possible.
> - *Print out* neatly on good quality paper. A handwritten résumé is usually not accepted. Space the résumé so it looks attractive. Use a high-quality printer. Print an original and a copy for your files. Do not send a carbon copy or photocopy. (If you apply for a second position, make another copy, stating that job objective.)
>
> **SPECIAL TIPS**
> - Briefly state special circumstances while in school (worked 20 hr a week, commuted 50 miles, perfect attendance, high-grade point average, special awards, participation in governing board, activities).
> - Emphasize the past 5 years.
> - Include nonnursing and related volunteer positions.
> - If a veteran, list length of service, branch of service, and rank; be sure to indicate health-related experience (e.g., medic or tech). State honorable discharge.
> - List memberships in organizations and offices held; include nursing and community organizations (a limited number).
> - List selected special interests and skills.
> - If you are fluent in a language other than English, state this fact.
> - List references on a separate sheet. References are not always sent with the résumé. (Be sure to contact references and get permission to list them.)
> - *Do not* list personal data, such as married or single, number of children, age, sex, religion. (A professional-looking photograph may be included but is usually not recommended. It is illegal for prospective employers to require a photo or to ask personal questions.)
> - Have another person read and react to the résumé before sending it.
> - If necessary, rearrange the résumé or emphasize specific factors to fit the needs of different employers.

fingernails are essential. Men should be clean shaven or should make sure that moustaches or beards are clean and neatly trimmed. A short haircut and a minimum of jewelry are recommended. Facial or tongue piercings and more than two ear piercings are not recommended. Practice giving a firm handshake. Remember: The first impression is made in just a few seconds. Arrive at least 5 minutes early for the interview. Make a practice run the day before or be sure to have good directions and know where to park. Arriving late to an interview leaves the prospective employer with a

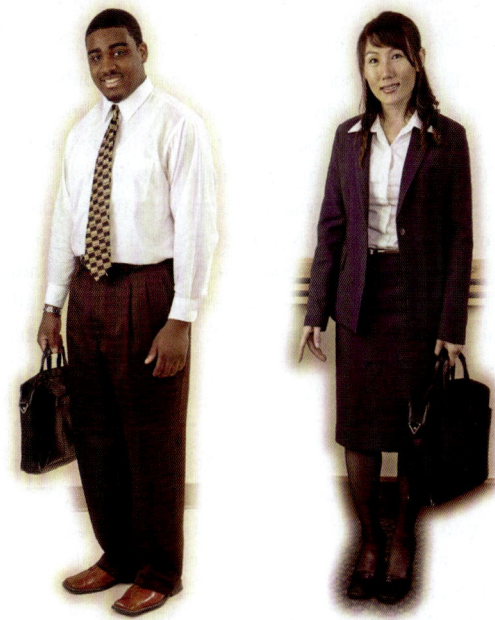

Figure 102-3 How you dress for a personal interview makes an instant first impression. Here, one applicant wears a dress shirt, tie, and pants with a belt. Another applicant wears a business suit with dress shirt and minimal jewelry. Both carry only a briefcase. (Carter, 2008.)

negative impression and will probably result in not being considered for the job.

The nursing transcript can be brought to the interview. If it is in narrative form, you may need to interpret it, if asked. Commonly, you will be asked to sign a release that permits the potential employer to contact your references. (It is illegal for schools or individuals to release information about a prospective employee without that person's written consent.) Proof of citizenship, legal residence, or a work permit ("green card") is necessary to work in the United States. You should also bring a form of photo identification, your Social Security card, CPR card, evidence of a negative PPD or chest x-ray examination, and nursing license, if received. You may be asked to sign a release for a background check. (Many times this information has already been submitted as part of the online application form.)

A prospective employer is interested in past employment, school record, punctuality, attendance records, ability to work with others (teamwork), willingness to accept assignments, and reactions in emergencies. Box 102-3 lists guidelines for the job interview. Be prepared to answer the following questions:

- What shift will you work?
- Will you work part time?
- What are your rotation choices (e.g., day–night, day–afternoon)?
- What salary do you expect?

Remember that most beginning nursing positions require rotating or night shifts and often working every other weekend. Many facilities require medical-surgical nursing experience before being assigned to a specialty area, such as obstetrics or psychiatry.

Box 102-3 Guidelines for the Job Interview

- Prepare for the interview: practice to gain self-confidence. Find out who will be doing the interviewing and memorize the interviewer's name(s). Get plenty of sleep the night before and have tissues or cough drops available, if needed.
- Dress neatly and conservatively to project a professional image. If a smoker, be sure your clothes and breath do not smell of smoke—ask someone else to check. Wear a minimum of jewelry. Make sure fingernails are clean (artificial nails and bright polish are not recommended) and shoes are clean and, if necessary, polished.
- It is recommended to remove visible piercings, other than one pair of earrings.
- Write down questions and review them ahead of time. Take notes during the interview.
- Be sure to arrive a few minutes *early*.
- Do homework on the agency before going. Be able to ask intelligent questions.
- Know in advance how to handle difficult questions, such as "Why do you want to work here?" "What can you offer us?" "What are your strengths?" "What is unique about you?" "What are your weaknesses?" "What was your biggest mistake?" "What are your long-term career goals?" "What was the last book you read (or your favorite book)?" "How do you handle conflicts?" "How would you describe your proficiency in spoken or written English (or the prevailing language of the facility)?"
- If you have held several positions, let the employer know in a positive way why you changed jobs. For example, "to accept a promotion, higher pay, or to return to school." (Employers are often wary about a person who seems to be a "job-hopper.")
- If there are any gaps in your job experience or education, be prepared to explain them in a positive way. For example, "to care for young children, to obtain further education."
- Be prepared to answer questions about technical competence. The employer may ask about experience with specific nursing procedures or with particular types of clients. Be honest about your skills. State that you would appreciate in-service education in procedures if you are not comfortable.
- Be aware that many interviewers will still offer to shake hands. Make sure your handshake is *firm,* but not crushing. Use your whole hand, *not* just the fingertips.
- Let the interviewer indicate where to sit. Wait to sit until the interviewer has been seated.
- Put purse or briefcase on the floor—not on the interviewer's desk. (Do *not* bring both purse and briefcase; this is too burdensome.)
- Sit up straight. Keep hands folded on the lap or in front on the table.
- If possible, leave your coat outside the interview room to avoid having to take it off and then having to find a place to put it.
- Do not smoke or chew gum. Make sure not to have bad breath.
- Do not accept coffee or food.
- Look at the person when speaking, but do not stare.
- Listen carefully to questions and *think* before talking.
- Do not act as though getting this job is critical.
- Inform the interviewer of any special skills and preferences, but do not exaggerate. Let the employer know about any computer expertise or experience.
- Do not talk too much; give concise answers, and, when finished with an answer, stop, and let the interviewer résumé with further questioning.
- Be prepared to ask pertinent questions, for example, about the specific job description as well as about opportunities for advancement, evaluation policies, and available in-service education or tuition reimbursement. Ask if there is a formal employment contract.
- If the salary and benefits are not known, ask these questions *last*.
- Do not complain about previous employers. Speak of any previous positions in the most positive way possible.
- Avoid the use of negative terms in responses. Speak of "challenges" and "opportunities," instead of "problems" and "issues".
- Thank the interviewer for their time. Use the person's name that they introduced themselves with, including titles such as doctor, as appropriate ("Dr. Smith," "Ms. Jones").
- Bring your nursing license, school transcript, record of tuberculin test, driver's license, birth certificate (or passport or resident alien card), CPR card, and Social Security card, in case any are needed.
- If written evaluations from previous employment (even if not nursing related) are available, bring *copies* of them to leave with the interviewer. It is good to show a good previous work history, whether in nursing-related jobs or not.
- If possible, have letters of reference already written to leave with interviewers. This will save them the time of contacting the references.
- If letters of reference are not available, have a neat list of names, addresses, professional positions, and telephone numbers of references readily available to leave with interviewers. *Contact these references in advance.*
- If currently employed, be prepared to tell the interviewer if it is acceptable to call the current employer. (Be sure to ask the current employer ahead of time.)
- Ask the interviewer when notification about the position will be made and the starting date.

Crosby, O. (2016). Employment interviewing: Seizing the opportunity and the job. *Career Outlook*, U.S. Bureau of Labor Statistics. https://www.bls.gov/careeroutlook/2016/article/employment-interviewing.htm?view_full

> **Nursing Alert** Be prepared to be interviewed by a committee or to have the interview recorded. Make eye contact with each member of the interview team and use their names.

Informational Interview

Even if a facility has no positions available, a member of the human resources department may be willing to conduct an *informational interview*. In this case, the interviewee is not applying for a position, but simply gaining practice and information. Informational interviews allow an individual to practice the interview process, get an idea what job interviews are like, and meet the interviewers for future reference. Interviewers may provide feedback on how they felt the individual handled the interview and may be willing to give suggestions for improvement. If a position becomes available in that facility later, an interviewer may consider the interviewee over other candidates because they met that person and because the person has shown initiative. In addition, the interviewee will be better prepared when participating in other interviews.

Application Forms

As part of the job-seeking process, a prospective employee is almost always required to fill out an application form. When filling out a standard application form, have your Social Security number, résumé, and nursing license (if received) available. Properly worded responses, with careful, neat handwriting or printing in ink, make a favorable impression. Emphasize computer skills. Employers often use the way in which an individual completes an application as one of the criteria for evaluation of the person as a prospective employee. Think before writing. *Be neat.*

Be prepared to give references to potential employers. Have the addresses and telephone numbers of the individuals acting as references neatly printed. *Always contact these references in advance* to ask permission before listing them. ("May I list your name on my résumé for a positive reference?")

Testing

In some instances, the prospective applicant may be asked to take aptitude tests or baseline tests in subjects such as medication administration. You may also be asked to demonstrate some basic nursing skills, such as measuring blood pressure. Relax and try not to be anxious. Generally, it is best not to change a test answer after it is written. If taking a timed test, go through the entire test as quickly as possible, answering the questions known. Then, go back and work on the other questions. Do not spend too much time on any one item.

Follow-Up After the Interview

After the interview is completed, follow up with a letter thanking the interviewer(s) for their time and stating your interest in the position. Briefly restate your qualifications. Be sure this letter is as neat as the letter of application. Write the thank-you letter within 24 hr.

Drug Testing and Physical Examination

Nearly all employers require negative drug testing as a condition of employment and may require routine spot checks throughout the employee's tenure. Expect to sign a release for this information. A urine sample will be collected in a carefully controlled environment. Future employees will often be required to pass a physical examination. This will usually include TB (PPD) testing, an ECG, hearing and vision screening, and laboratory and other tests. Many employers draw a blood sample, to keep frozen, for conditions such as the human immunodeficiency virus (HIV). (This will not be used unless the employee later files a claim stating that they contracted HIV while working at the facility.) Specific immunizations may be required of all employees. Many employers require a background check before employment. This will include such things as a criminal record, including convictions for DUI or as a sex offender.

Accepting the Position

When an individual accepts a position, they are entering into an agreement. Be familiar with pertinent personnel policies. Every institution establishes local personnel policies, although there are many commonalities. Salaries may vary, according to a facility's size, type, and location. Salaries are usually higher in large cities and in certain areas of the country. Government hospitals (e.g., Veterans Administration, county, state, and university hospitals) may offer higher salaries than do private hospitals or ECFs. Clinics and home care tend to have lower salaries than hospitals, but often have the advantage of daytime hours and minimal weekend assignments. Larger facilities may offer extra compensation to nurses who have additional education. Additional responsibility and higher pay may be available, based on a nurse's education level and length of service. Most facilities have a graduated salary schedule and credit may be given for previous experience. (Sometimes, a bonus is paid to new employees hired in difficult-to-fill positions.) When offered a position, the nurse is usually given a day or two to decide. If offered more than one position, it is important to notify each employer of the final decision, including positions declined.

Contracts and Agreements

When accepting a position, the nurse should notify the employer as soon as possible. Make sure you both agree on factors such as hours, salary, starting date, and benefits. In some facilities, time off is combined as paid time off (**PTO**). This includes vacation, sick leave, and holidays. This can be an advantage or a disadvantage. Sometimes, salary and benefit information is presented as a contract or letter of agreement to be signed. It is a good idea to write a letter of acceptance to verify the start date, shifts to be worked, salary, benefits, and other pertinent information.

Salary and Contract Negotiation

Some hospital systems or cities have a standard nurses' contract, renegotiated on a regular basis. The terms and conditions are written, but in most cases, cannot be negotiated individually. Recently, nurses' groups are negotiating working conditions and client safety, as well as salaries. Some nurses' contracts allow nurses to determine when a unit or hospital can no longer accept new clients because of staff shortage. Most nursing contracts forbid mandatory overtime. Some facilities are considered "union"; the local unit of the American Nurses Association (ANA) often serves as the negotiating agent for RNs and, sometimes, for LVN/LPNs. In some situations, nurses have gone on strike, but nurses in "safety net" hospitals, those providing emergency care for the area, are usually not allowed to strike.

Employer Responsibilities

The employer is responsible for providing a safe working environment, which

- Is free from unusual dangers and observes conditions such as OSHA guidelines and provides SDS information sheets, indicating hazards in the area.
- Is safe, regarding protection from assaults by clients.
- Is not discriminatory.
- Negotiates in good faith.
- Does not allow sexual or other forms of harassment.
- Does not interfere with legal rights of employees.
- Provides regular employee evaluations.
- Follows federal, state, and local guidelines on pay, hours worked, break time, and time off.
- Provides a grievance, mediation, and arbitration process for disputes.
- Follows due process in all dealings with employees.
- Offers assistance and guidance in the case of unfounded legal action against the nurse.
- Provides a health service or some means for employees to obtain minimum healthcare, immunizations, and screenings.

Employee Responsibilities

It is important to know what is expected of employees before accepting a position. All employers have the right to expect that employees will

- Work on assigned days and report on time.
- Call in sick only when truly ill.
- Maintain client confidentiality; will not access client charts without a specific need to do so.
- Practice within the parameters of their license and within the limits of individual training and experience.
- Seek assistance, if needed; utilize nursing protocols.
- Practice with integrity (e.g., honest documentation, observation of appropriate client–nurse boundaries, proper care and administration of medications, and immediate reporting of medication errors, injuries, or incidents).
- Observe the regulations of the facility, regarding matters such as continuing education or participation in committees.
- Maintain the nursing license and other required certificates, such as PPD testing and CPR certification.
- Practice as a collaborative member of the healthcare team.
- Follow rules and guidelines of the facility.

After Obtaining the Position

How an individual functions after being hired will affect their professional status and references for the future. Having good references increases opportunities for obtaining future positions. Chances are also greater that this individual will be recommended for leadership positions, salary advancement, and further education.

Orientation

Facilities usually provide orientation programs for new employees. Discuss with instructors any procedures about which you are unsure. Your instructor or supervisor can provide knowledge, experience, and sources of information. Orientation programs include information about disaster, fire, and emergency code procedures. Other topics include instruction in computer documentation and access to medication dispensing machines and scanners, personnel policies, evaluation procedures, nursing protocols, facility organizational charts, and safety and security procedures.

Internship

The recent graduate is usually required to serve a period of internship or "nurse residency" before being considered a regular employee and a benefit-earning member of the staff. Ask about these probationary policies when discussing salary and benefits (Chapter 101).

Continuing Education

Many facilities provide continuing education for nurses. Take advantage of this opportunity, both for personal enhancement and to gain CEUs for license renewal (if your state requires CEUs). In addition, advanced education and certification are available to LVN/LPNs in several specialty areas (Chapter 103). Many LVN/LPNs go on to become RNs and employers often help fund this education.

Resigning From a Position

When leaving a position, the employer should be given *written advance notice*—at least 2 weeks and preferably a month. Notice gives the agency adequate time to find a replacement. Advance notice requirements are sometimes stated in personnel policies. A letter of resignation should be as neat and professional as was the letter of application. Customarily, if an individual leaves before the designated time or without notice, that person will be paid up to the time of departure only. Although it is generally illegal to give a poor reference, the employer may refuse to give a reference or may give an obviously neutral reference, for the nurse who leaves a job without proper notice (or whose performance has not been satisfactory). Try not to "burn bridges." Always continue your professionalism and leave in a positive manner. One never knows when a reference might be needed or when one might wish to return.

STUDENT SYNTHESIS

KEY POINTS

- Multiple employment opportunities exist in nursing and other healthcare fields.
- Nurses can choose employment to fit personal needs—different practice areas, structured or less-structured settings, self-employment, and different parts of the country or world.
- The Internet provides a means of conducting a job search, applying for a position, and taking continuing education courses.
- Completing and updating the professional résumé is an integral component of the job search.
- First impressions are established in a few seconds; a positive first impression is vital in obtaining employment.
- The personal interview allows the applicant and potential employer to learn about each other. Always follow up an interview with a thank-you letter.
- Employers provide orientation for new employees. A part of any orientation program includes learning about disaster, fire, and emergency code procedures. Other topics include personnel policies, evaluation procedures, nursing protocols, facility organizational charts, and safety and security procedures.
- A written advance notice of at least 2–4 weeks should be given when resigning from a position.

CRITICAL THINKING EXERCISES

1. Conduct informational interviews in two different healthcare facilities or other occupational areas near the geographic area in which you plan to work after graduation. Make a list of factors important to you. How many of these relate to compensation? How many to other benefits? How many relate to personal and professional growth? Compare and contrast the conditions of employment in the two places. Discuss your findings with classmates.

2. Survey your local area and identify as many "nontraditional" positions for nurses as possible. What are your feelings about nursing in these areas?

NCLEX-STYLE REVIEW QUESTIONS

1. A new graduate LVN/LPN is searching for a job. What should the nurse understand will be the best opportunity available at this time?
   a. Long-term care nursing
   b. Emergency department nursing
   c. Intensive care nursing
   d. Case management

2. An LVN/LPN applies for a position as an assistant to a school nurse. What should the anticipated job responsibilities encompass? Select all that apply.
   a. Substitute teach when the teacher is out of the class.
   b. Assist with vision and hearing screenings.
   c. Perform routine first aid.
   d. Assist with record keeping.
   e. Prescribe medications for students.

3. The new graduate LVN/LPN is beginning the search for a job. Prior to obtaining employment, what is important for the graduate to do?
   a. Purchase new uniforms.
   b. Inquire at a temporary agency.
   c. Pick the job where the nurse will work for the duration of a career.
   d. Examine personal and family needs.

4. The nurse determines that working on a PRN basis in a community medical pool or personnel service pool is the best choice of employment at this time. What are some possible disadvantages that may come with this type of position? Select all that apply.
   a. Less salary than full time
   b. Working in only one unit
   c. No paid time off
   d. Lack of insurance benefits
   e. Inconsistent work schedule

5. The new graduate nurse is preparing to attend an interview with a facility. What should the nurse do to prepare?
   a. Determine what salary to ask for.
   b. Bring a neatly handwritten résumé.
   c. Find out as much about the facility and the position as possible.
   d. Determine what hours the nurse will ask for.

CHAPTER RESOURCES

Enhance your learning with additional resources on thePoint!

Student Resources related to this chapter can be found at thePoint.lww.com/Rosdahl12e.

103 Advancement and Leadership in Nursing

Learning Objectives

1. Describe how an LVN/LPN can become nationally certified in gerontology, IV therapy, and other specialty areas.
2. Compare and contrast the terms *leader* and *manager*.
3. Discuss characteristics of a good manager.
4. Describe leadership roles that may be available to the LVN/LPN.
5. Describe four leadership styles.
6. Describe further educational opportunities available to LVN/LPNs.
7. Describe duties and responsibilities of the team leader/charge nurse/manager in a nursing home/ECF.

Important Terminology

autocratic leadership
bureaucratic leadership
democratic leadership
due process
laissez–faire leadership
leader
manager
oral reprimand
performance review
plan of assistance
written reprimand

Acronyms

CLTC
IVT
NCP
OBRA

Graduation and employment are just the beginning steps in a nursing career. Opportunities are available for advancement if the individual nurse wishes to further their career. Opportunities include national certification and further education; nearly all states require nurses to take continuing education courses to maintain the nursing license. As the nurse advances in their career, opportunities arise for assuming positions of leadership. This chapter briefly addresses some of the areas of advancement and leadership in nursing.

ADVANCEMENT IN NURSING

Some nurses choose to advance their careers. Others wish to continue delivering competent, caring, and safe bedside care, without added responsibilities. Some career paths lead to higher salaries, additional certification, and/or college degrees, whereas other activities enhance the nurse's professional recognition or personal satisfaction.

National Certification

As of 2013, the National Association of LPNs (NALPN) offered several certifications for licensed practical nurses (LVN/LPNs) (www.nalpn). There are also national certification courses available through National Association for Practical Nurse Education and Service, Inc. (NAPNES).

1. Long-term care (*gerontology*): The nurse who qualifies for and passes this examination is then eligible to use the initials, **CLTC** (Certified in Long-Term Care), after their name, in addition to LPN or LVN. This certification was developed specifically for LVN/LPNs. To qualify for this examination, the nurse must hold an active LVN/LPN license in the United States or its territories and must have practiced in long-term care for 6 months. The examination, which consists of multiple-choice questions, similar to the NCLEX, is most often taken online. A period of 150 min is allowed for the examination. On successful completion of the examination, the nurse receives a certificate and lapel pin. The certification period lasts for several years and can be renewed by meeting established requirements, including 20 or more units of specific continuing education. Nurses who are members of NALPN pay a discounted fee for the examination. The content of the test includes the following goals:

    - Physiologic integrity (promotion of quality of life)
    - Psychosocial integrity (quality of life, as related to mental health)
    - Specialty practice issues (improvement of quality of life, related to serving as a resource to others)
    - Leadership and management (utilizing the nursing process, communication, and organizational skills, as a resource person. Team leading is included.)

2. Pharmacology: The pharmacology application and examination processes are similar to the long-term care certification. The successful candidate is authorized to use the initials, **NCP** (NAPNES Certified in Pharmacology), after their name, along with LVN/LPN.

    Components of this examination are as follows:

    - General principles of pharmacology
    - Pharmacology and the role of the LVN/LPN
    - Drug therapy affecting specific body systems
    - Drug therapy in infection
    - Drug therapy in cancer

3. Intravenous (IV) therapy: Attainment of this certification allows the LVN/LPN to add **IVT** after their name.

Current information regarding these certification programs can be obtained via the NALPN Website or NAPNES Website.

Other certifications have been proposed, but were not available as of this writing. Some of the proposed certifications are rehabilitation, fetal heart monitoring (FHM), Alzheimer's disease, cardiology, phlebotomy (blood drawing), dialysis, human immunodeficiency virus (HIV) care, and wound care. A few LVN/LPNs are certified in such related fields such as massage therapy, Lamaze delivery, and Reiki therapy.

NAPNES offers courses in pharmacology, long-term care, and IV therapy. The LVN/LPN pays a fee to take self-study modules. Once the nurse has completed the course, an examination is taken. If passed, certification is awarded. The certification is good for 3 years. Any individual can take the course, but only an LVN/LPN can receive certification. Forty-five hours of continuing education are awarded for licensed nurses.

Nurse Mobility Programs

A number of programs throughout the country offer an accelerated route to nursing. In some cases, the programs give credits for previous nursing education and experience. In some cases, they give credit for life experiences. A number of LVN/LPNs continue their education to become registered nurses (RNs). LVN/LPNs are often encouraged to go on to become RNs, and this number is continually increasing.

One-Plus-One Programs

You may be enrolled in a one-plus-one program. In this program, usually lasting 2 years, students are eligible to take the NCLEX-PN examination after the first year. These nurses are then licensed as LVN/LPNs. The second year of the program builds on the first year, and graduates of the 2-year program are eligible to take the NCLEX-RN examination and become licensed as RNs. A one-plus-one program has the advantage of allowing the nurse to work as an LVN/LPN after approximately 1 year of education. The nurse can work during the second year of the program or may choose to work for a period before returning for the second year of the program.

Other Types of Advanced Standing Programs

One-plus-one programs may also recruit students from other postsecondary programs or with applicable life experiences. In this case, entering students may test out of specific skills or classes. The "test out" usually includes both written and clinical demonstration components and is designed to establish that the student is able to meet the objectives of the original basic-level course. The nurse enrolling from another nursing program may not be able to test out of all classes and may be required to retake classes to meet the requirements of the new school.

Advanced Education and Specialized Training

Numerous opportunities exist for LVN/LPNs to obtain further education in nursing or in specialized programs, such as emergency rescue or surgical technician. Employers may provide tuition reimbursement to help cover the cost of additional education. Often, in return for this reimbursement, the employee agrees to continue to work for the employer for a specified period after completion of the education. This period is often dependent on the amount of the reimbursement. Information about special courses may be obtained from local and national nursing organizations and schools, healthcare facilities, or the Internet. In addition, many nursing journals provide information.

Associate Degree to Baccalaureate Degree RN Programs

The associate degree RN or LVN/LPN with an associate or baccalaureate degree in another field can often obtain a bachelor's degree in nursing in less time than the usual required 4 years. Local 4-year colleges vary in their admission requirements and offer differing credits for previous education.

Bachelor's Degree to RN or Master's Programs

Some nursing programs enroll students who have a bachelor's degree in a major other than nursing. In these programs, graduates are eligible to take the RN licensure examination after a shorter period because they have already taken their general liberal arts courses. Therefore, the student is not required to repeat many of the courses typically offered in the first 2 years of study and can focus primarily on clinical courses. These accelerated RN courses usually last about 2 years. In some specialized courses, the graduate receives a master's degree, in addition to the RN.

> *Key Concept*
>
> As a student or practicing nurse, you are strongly encouraged to consider further education. Additional education offers a wider variety of employment opportunities. One such opportunity is teaching in nursing (which often requires a master's degree). Many nursing faculty will be retiring within the next few years, leaving many positions available nationwide. This trend is expected to continue for some time.

Refresher Courses

There are several reasons for taking "nurse refresher" courses:

- A nurse may have stopped working for some time to pursue further education, travel, or raise a family. Refresher courses are a good idea when nurses have not been actively employed in nursing for several years. An employer may also require this if the nurse has not been working recently.
- A nurse whose license lapses or is revoked or who is on inactive licensure status for some time may be required to take a refresher course as a requirement to be relicensed.
- A new graduate who does not pass the licensure examination in two or three attempts is usually required to take a refresher course, to qualify to retake the examination.

Practicing nurses teach refresher courses, which include overviews of several nursing areas, such as medical-surgical, pediatrics, and obstetrics. These courses may review basic sciences, such as body structure and function, nutrition, microbiology, and child development. Other topics may include pharmacology and mathematics, new equipment, and general nursing procedures. A refresher course often includes several hours of clinical experience, in addition to theory classes.

Continuing Education

As stated previously, most states require continuing education units (CEUs) or credits, in order to renew the nursing license. There are many sources of these credits, including formal classes, online classes, and courses provided in nursing journals. The nurse who is nationally certified may be required to obtain additional CEUs for renewal of that certificate.

LEADERSHIP

Today, the LVN/LPN is expected to assume a leadership role in some healthcare settings. The NALPN and other organizations have reported that this increased responsibility is most evident in long-term or extended-care facilities (ECFs). According to the NALPN Career Center Website (www.nalpn.org), opportunities for LVN/LPN advancement include employment in critical care settings on the "IV team, as treatment nurses, and as special procedure nurses…In some instances, at other facilities, such as nursing homes, LVN/LPNs practice in the charge nurse supervisory role."

> **Key Concept**
>
> It is important to remember that client acuity in extended care is steadily increasing. Therefore, nurses in this area must continuously upgrade skills and competencies to meet the growing responsibilities.

Effective Leadership and Management

As the need for various levels of nurses to function as leaders increases, effective leadership skills become more critical. A competent leader must be able to direct effectively and influence the actions of others. Leadership styles and basic management skills are presented here. It is advisable to obtain postgraduate training in leadership skills, but leaders need other knowledge and attributes as well. The nurse expected to function as a charge nurse or to assume another leadership position must decide if they are prepared for this responsibility. The person may need assistance in planning and implementing client care and in coordinating and directing activities of other staff members. The leader must be able to evaluate nursing care given, as well as their personal leadership abilities. Any new nurse assuming a leadership position would be wise to consult other people with more experience. The LVN/LPN in a leadership position will usually report to a higher authority, for example, a department supervisor or the director of nursing.

In an ECF, the nurse/leader requires information about legislation, such as Medicare, Medicaid, the Affordable Care Act, and the Omnibus Budget Reconciliation Act *(OBRA)*. Information about third-party reimbursement policies, such as regulations of the Centers for Medicare and Medicaid Services (*CMS*), will also be necessary. This nurse/leader is also responsible for maintaining client confidentiality throughout the facility and will be involved in reaccreditation of the facility. It is important to know how to access information, if there are questions.

> **Key Concept**
>
> The nurse working in a charge capacity or other leadership position must have *strong clinical expertise*, in addition to *excellent judgment* and *sound leadership skills*. It is highly discouraged for the new nursing graduate to assume a leadership role, without additional clinical experience as a licensed nurse, under the guidance of a more experienced nurse. Some nurses may choose never to assume leadership positions.

Leader Versus Manager

The terms *leader* and *manager* refer to two distinct roles. These terms may be inappropriately used interchangeably. A leader is not necessarily a manager, but can be. A manager is not necessarily a leader, but can be a leader.

A **leader** is a person who uses specific skills, such as role modeling, to influence others to accomplish a task or do the work. A **manager** coordinates and controls the work of others. A manager is involved with organizing, planning, directing, and controlling.

> **Key Concept**
>
> The leader influences others.
> - The manager controls others.

Although the roles of leader and a manager are typically separate, they often overlap. These roles may include the following:

- Role model
- Educator
- Advocate
- Decision maker
- Planner
- Counselor
- Change agent

Characteristics of an Effective Manager

Being a good manager requires sound communication, decision making, and problem-solving skills (Fig. 103-1). The following characteristics are necessary in an effective manager:

- A desire to manage—Comfort with the position is important
- Trust in one's own judgment—Ability to work without constant guidance from others
- Ability to perform research to determine pertinent information and skills needed for the position

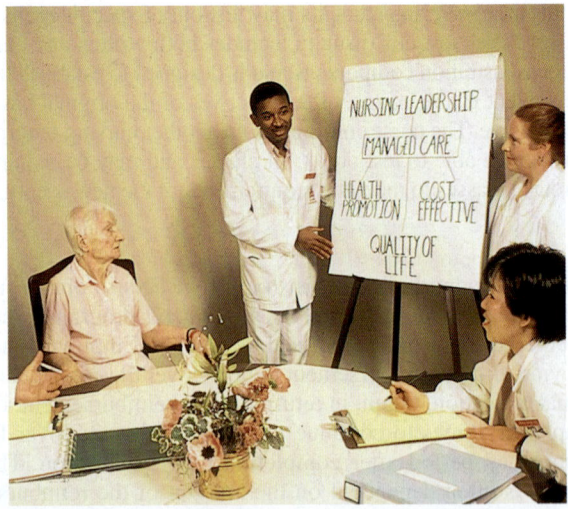

Figure 103-1 An effective manager communicates on a regular, consistent basis with other members of the staff. Planning is a joint effort.

- Ability to choose competent coworkers and allow them to perform their tasks independently, rather than "micromanage"
- Skills in stress management—To assist self and others
- Ability to understand and consider feelings and opinions of others
- Independence and self-direction
- Motivation to guide and work with people, not just to attain power
- Ability to handle different situations
- Ability to make competent decisions, especially in emergencies
- Ability to channel others' feelings and hostility into constructive problem solving
- Ability to competently and fairly evaluate the work of others, to identify deficiencies, and to determine appropriate solutions

Effective Leadership

One needs to develop leadership skills, to supervise others effectively. Nurses develop organizational skills in daily client care; as a new graduate, additional leadership skills are needed. The following qualities or attributes are required of an effective leader:

- Self-confidence
- Self-awareness
- Strong personal values
- Skills of *values clarification* (choosing freely from alternatives, prizing the choice, and acting consistently on that choice)
- *Advocacy* (providing information and support to those being led)
- *Accountability* (taking responsibility for values and actions)
- Ability to *inspire* others, so they want to follow
- Ability to discipline others, recommending termination of their employment, if necessary

> **Nursing Alert** Nursing leaders and managers must possess comprehensive nursing knowledge, as well as the nursing skills required in the particular facility. A sound knowledge of the rationales underlying nursing procedures is vital.

Leadership Styles

Leadership style refers to behavior used by a leader in a specific situation. Various situations in healthcare dictate the most appropriate leadership style, but a strong knowledge base is essential to all styles. The most effective leader often blends leadership styles and can move from one style to another, as the situation dictates.

Autocratic Leadership

Autocratic leadership/management is self-directed; this style calls for little or no input from staff. In its extreme form, autocratic leadership may be compared with a dictatorship, in which the leader makes decisions and the group is expected to carry out orders. In certain situations, such as a "code blue" or other life-threatening emergency, this style is appropriate for the nurse leader. New graduates may feel more comfortable with an autocratic leader until they gain additional self-confidence.

Bureaucratic Leadership

Bureaucratic leadership is policy minded. Bureaucratic leaders rely on established protocols for decision making. The policy and procedure manual of the facility offers step-by-step instructions; a bureaucratic leader will consider them as iron-clad rules. This style may be helpful for new graduates who need detailed instructions. In addition, some procedures, such as sterile technique, require strict guidelines, and make no allowance for deviations in basic principles/underlying rationales.

Democratic Leadership

Democratic leadership is people-oriented and tries to *guide staff* in the right direction. Some nursing approaches, such as team nursing, benefit from democratic leadership, by fostering team spirit in an atmosphere of mutual respect and shared responsibility. Democratic leaders consider group input, but are able to make final decisions themselves, when no consensus is achieved. This style allows for a free flow of ideas, plans, and information between leader and followers.

Laissez–Faire Leadership

The leadership style with the least structure is **laissez–faire leadership**. This leader has loosely structured goals, with no firm guidelines. They encourage followers to choose their own goals and plans for implementation. Although leaders who continuously use this style may be well liked, their team may have difficulty in accomplishing specific goals. However, laissez–faire leadership encourages creativity and independence and allows people to try new things, without fear of mistakes.

> **NCLEX Alert**
>
> Opportunities may exist in the future for you, as an LVN/LPN, to become certified in LTC or another specialty, or to become a manager/team leader. As you complete this stage of your education and prepare for the NCLEX examination, be alert to the responsibilities of a team leader. This may be helpful as you review examination questions and select nursing actions or item answers. Being a member of the healthcare team or a team leader relates directly to the *coordination of care*, as provided to clients.

Team Leader/Charge Nurse Role

In ECFs, such as nursing homes, many LVN/LPNs assume charge nurse positions and oversee the work of nursing assistants and other ancillary staff. These nurses also function in leadership positions in other areas, such as clinics, insurance companies, and the military.

The role of the *team leader/charge nurse* has many facets, those of both a leader and a manager. The responsibilities of this person include the following:

- Obtaining shift reports and determining client acuity
- Assigning clients to staff members

- Handling emergencies
- Coordinating all the unit's activities
- Assigning staff breaks, coverage for breaks, attendance at team conferences, family meetings, and other special meetings
- Monitoring client tests and procedures
- Ensuring availability of needed supplies and equipment
- The team leader or charge nurse also performs other activities, such as counting narcotics or checking the medication dispensing machine, counting scissors or mirrors, checking the crash cart, reporting to the nursing supervisor and primary providers, checking staffing for the next shift, sending client acuity reports to administration, checking the temperature of the medication refrigerator, and performing quality control checks on blood sugar testing equipment.
- Some of these activities may be assigned to other staff by the team leader.

The team leader/charge nurse must have leadership and administrative abilities, a thorough knowledge of nursing, and an intuitive understanding of behavior. The new LVN/LPN or RN should not attempt to assume this role without further in-service education and experience after graduation.

The Vocational/Practical Nurse as Manager

LVN/LPNs often function as managers in specific areas, most commonly clinics, long-term care facilities, and the military (Chapter 102).

Functions include the following:

- Supervision of other nursing and health-related personnel, including UAPs
- Functioning as a charge nurse or team leader
- Functioning as a medication or treatment nurse
- Serving as client advocate/ombudsperson
- Assisting in staff development instruction

In addition, LVN/LPNs may be trained in specialty areas (Chapter 102). NFLPN recommends that LVN/LPNs meet the following requirements, in order to serve as leaders in specialty areas:

- Have at least 1 year experience as a staff nurse in that area
- Present personal qualifications that indicate leadership abilities, particularly in the specialty area
- Demonstrate evidence of completion of appropriate in-service education or a formal course approved by an appropriate agency (to provide knowledge and skills necessary to function safely in the specialized field)
- Meet all standards of nursing practice, as set forth by NALPN and the State Board of Nursing

Clinics

In addition to the many previously listed functions (Chapters 99 and 102), the nurse working in a *leadership position* in a primary provider's clinic or community health center is expected to:

- Follow-up on quality assurance
- Train other staff
- Attend team leader meetings
- Write policies
- Assist in conflict resolution between staff members
- Assist in hiring new staff, ongoing evaluation, and dismissal from positions
- Establish and update procedures and protocols
- Establish training programs
- Function as the safety officer or OSHA representative

The nurse in the clinic often receives telephone calls and must determine what action to take first. *Telephone triage* involves sorting calls, to determine if a life-threatening situation must be immediately referred to emergency services. The triage nurse must differentiate between clients who require immediate care and those who can make future appointments. Less urgent calls are referred to the appropriate provider. Clinics may have a computerized protocol to guide the triage nurse. (In some situations, the triage nurse must be an RN.)

Long-Term Care

By far, most LVN/LPNs management or leadership positions are in extended-care/nursing homes. The U.S. government has established a standard for a charge nurse in the skilled nursing facility (SNF). This standard states that at least one RN or LPN must be present in the facility and in charge at all times. In some subacute care facilities, a licensed nurse is not required to be on duty 24 hr a day, but is required to be on call for emergencies at all times. It is desirable that each charge nurse be trained or experienced in areas such as nursing administration and supervision, rehabilitation, and psychiatric or geriatric nursing. The charge nurse must be able to recognize significant changes in the condition of clients and take necessary action, regardless of the time of day or night.

> **Nursing Alert** The charge nurse is ultimately responsible for the *total nursing care* of all clients while they are on duty.

Duties of the team leader/charge nurse in ECFs parallel those listed previously and also include making rounds and assessing clients, directing administration of medications and treatments, supervising nursing care given by UAP, conferring with team members regularly throughout the shift, and communicating with the primary provider when necessary. (Box 96-2 identifies guidelines to use when communicating information to the primary provider, using the SBAR method—Situation, Background, Assessment, Recommendations.) Box 103-1 briefly identifies the role and some of the functions of the charge nurse in the long-term care facility. A number of helpful books and instructional CDs are available for the new nurse assuming a leadership position.

> **Key Concept**
> The role of the team leader or charge nurse parallels the steps in the nursing process.

Staff Assignments

The charge nurse is often expected to assign duties to other members of the team. They should know the clients and the staff members (and their strengths). Each person has special abilities that can be matched to specific client needs. This

Box 103-1 Functions of the Charge Nurse in Long-Term Care

PLANS CLIENT CARE
- Demonstrates ability to identify total needs of each client
- Identifies therapeutic goals for each client
- Receives and interprets verbal, written, and computerized reports about clients
- Observes clients and identifies changing and stable daily needs
- Assists the primary provider with examinations and treatments
- Serves as a member of the care team with the provider, nursing administrators, and other staff
- Develops or assists in developing nursing care plans for individual clients
- Determines placement of new clients
- Participates in in-service education and activities, to improve nursing practice
- Serves on facility committees

COORDINATES STAFF ACTIVITIES
- Demonstrates the ability to understand behavior
- Demonstrates basic leadership techniques
- Follows good management practices
- Communicates effectively
- Demonstrates the ability to motivate staff
- Allows staff to independently formulate and carry out solutions in nursing care

IMPLEMENTS CLIENT CARE
- Follows previously developed care plans; ensures that other staff do so as well
- Teaches staff appropriate actions in an emergency
- Assists in teaching in-service classes
- Matches staff members with appropriate clients for daily care
- Assists staff to care for clients with special needs, including the client who is dying
- Coordinates nursing services with other departments
- Recognizes the limits of one's own nursing practice and seeks advice when needed
- Prepares and gives verbal, written, and computerized reports about clients, as well as special reports

EVALUATES CLIENT CARE
- Determines effectiveness of client care, using sound evaluation practices
- Recommends changes in nursing care procedures
- Modifies client care plans, as needed
- Performs self-assessment on a regular basis and sets long-term personal goals for nursing practice
- Observes and documents the performance of those being supervised
- Discusses performance reviews with staff members
- Ensures that quality assurance goals are being met
- Evaluates safety of care given and reports safety concerns

---

helps ensure that the best possible care is given to clients. (Usually, it is advantageous to the client and staff to have a consistent client assignment from day to day, if possible.)

Making rounds is usually the first activity, either immediately before or after the change-of-shift report. The clients may be involved in this rounding activity. At this time, staff can introduce themselves and determine immediate client needs. The team leader/charge nurse is responsible for explaining and demonstrating procedures to staff members and assisting in planning their workload, so all clients receive optimum care. The charge nurse also checks periodically with staff to make sure they are not having difficulty completing their assignments.

> **Key Concept**
> Not every nurse has the ability or desire to be a charge nurse or team leader. Do not feel inadequate if you are unable or unwilling to assume this role.

Performance Reviews of Staff

The charge nurse is often responsible for writing summary evaluations or **performance reviews** of staff members and for going over this information with them. This is a challenging function for those in leadership. Steps in the evaluation process include the following:

- Letting the staff person know that observations will be done; sometimes, the staff is notified of the specific time the observation will occur.
- Observing the staff person in a number of different situations and in delivering care to a variety of clients.
- Dating each observation (include the client's initials and a brief description of care).
- Writing a few notes *immediately after each observation*. (Describe what was observed. Identify both positive and negative observations and suggestions.)
- Holding a very short, informal "debriefing" session with the staff person after each observation. (If concerns were noted, let the person know, so they can work to improve performance.)
- Writing a summary evaluation/performance review of the employee after the interval designated by the facility. (Many facilities use a specific format for these reviews.)
- Scheduling a time to meet alone with the staff person and go over the evaluation, asking for their input. (The employee may write comments, agreeing or disagreeing.) Notes about this meeting and the evaluation document itself must be dated and signed by the evaluator and staff person. A copy is given to the staff person for their files. The original is kept on file by the facility.

If an employee is showing deficiencies, the first step in *due process* is an **oral reprimand**. If the deficiency continues, a **written reprimand** is given to the employee. **Due process** procedures ensure fair labor practices and prevent frivolous or punitive actions against employees by employers.

> **Key Concept**
> The due process procedures described here apply to employees in most facilities. This includes RNs, LVN/LPNs, nursing assistants, and others. After the probationary period, due process must be followed to terminate employment, except in very special circumstances. In general, employees cannot be terminated without just cause (which might be a cutback in staffing).

The Plan of Assistance

If, after an oral and written reprimand, serious deficiencies are still noted, the evaluator/supervisor writes a **plan of assistance** for the employee. The plan of assistance is dated and signed by the evaluator/supervisor.

A plan of assistance includes the following:

- Statement of deficiency, noting potential consequences to clients
- Employee actions needed to correct the deficiency
- Timeline for improvement to be apparent
- Consequences to the employee, if the plan of assistance is not followed and improvement not shown

The evaluator presents the plan of assistance to the employee and discusses it with them. The employee is given a copy and asked to sign the original, to signify that they have read it and received a copy. (The employee's signature does not imply agreement, but simply acknowledges receipt of the information.) In many cases, employees have the right to add their interpretation of the situation to the written plan of assistance.

For an evaluator, it is important to continue to observe the employee, to determine if the conditions set out were met by the timeline. If so, the plan of assistance is ended. (If the staff member repeats the deficiency at a later time, the plan of assistance is reactivated.) If the staff member does not meet the stipulations of the plan of assistance, further actions, as set out in the plan and within the policies of the facility, are taken. The nurse evaluating the work of others has a very serious responsibility. The evaluator needs to be mature, observant, fair, and tactful.

> **Nursing Alert** If the charge nurse observes life-threatening or illegal deficiencies on the part of an employee, the director of nursing should be notified at once. The employee should be suspended, pending investigation. During suspension, retraining or treatment may occur. However, if the employee's act was very serious, termination of employment is often the only legal option open to the facility. Many of the just causes for suspension or immediate termination of employment are similar to those for suspending or revoking a nursing license (Chapter 101).

Decision Making

The nurse in a leadership position is required to make many decisions, ranging from assigning staff, to managing an assaultive client, to calling a code on a lifeless client. Whatever leadership style is used, the leader should be able to make and communicate competent decisions. In life-and-death situations, decisions must be made quickly. The client and other team members depend on the team leader/charge nurse to determine what to do. In non–life-threatening situations, team members can give input and take part in the decision-making process. However, remember that the leader takes ultimate responsibility for any decision.

Follow basic problem-solving steps to work toward decisions (Chapter 33). Determine the problem, set goals, gather relevant information, and determine what action to take. In an emergency, act quickly and communicate the situation's urgency. Seek advice or assistance from others, when necessary and when possible; remember to follow the "chain of command" in the facility. Follow personal intuition; if the situation seems critical, act accordingly. After a decision is made, follow through, and make sure the situation is safely resolved. Evaluate the situation as it evolves, keeping in mind that revisions may need to be made continuously. After a crisis, such as a code, debrief the entire team, to allow venting of feelings and to determine the best action to take in the event of another similar emergency.

STUDENT SYNTHESIS

KEY POINTS

- The role of all nurses, including LVN/LPNs, is expanding.
- LVN/LPNs can be nationally certified in long-term care, IV therapy, and pharmacology. Other specialty certifications are being proposed.
- Many LVN/LPNs work as charge nurses or team leaders, especially in ECFs.
- As a new graduate of a nursing program, additional education and experience are needed before assuming a leadership role.
- Several leadership styles exist. There is no right or wrong style; any of them can be effective—a particular style may be needed in a certain situation.
- All employees are entitled to regular evaluations. Specific evaluation and plan of assistance procedures must be followed, to ensure due process for deficient employees.

CRITICAL THINKING EXERCISES

1. Do a survey in your local area. What leadership or management opportunities exist for LVN/LPNs in sites other than hospitals and nursing homes? (Examples include home care, third-party payors, various types of clinics, armed forces, industry, and schools.)
2. Investigate nursing journals and the Internet for courses related to nursing leadership and develop a list of potential opportunities.
3. Do an Internet search to determine areas of specialization or certification available to LVN/LPNs. Identify steps needed to attain these.
4. Research your local area and determine advanced educational/training opportunities that are available.

Identify requirements for entry into these programs. Include online classes.

5. Research opportunities in your area for the LVN/LPN to become an RN. Identify related funding that may be available.

6. Identify procedures for performance evaluation and the nurse's related responsibilities.

NCLEX-STYLE REVIEW QUESTIONS

1. The LVN/LPN is interested in obtaining certification in gerontology through NALPN. Which qualifications is the nurse required to meet? Select all that apply.
   a. Have an active LVN/LPN license
   b. Have 6-year, full-time practice in long-term care
   c. Work as a charge nurse in long-term care
   d. Have 40 hr of continuing education credits related to long-term care
   e. Have 5 years of medical-surgical nursing experience

2. A nurse supervisor carefully follows the acute care facility's policy and procedure manual and expects the same from the new graduate nurse. Which type of leadership style is this supervisor most likely using?
   a. Autocratic
   b. Democratic
   c. Laissez–faire
   d. Bureaucratic

3. The nurse is working on a unit that will begin implementing team nursing. Which type of leadership style would this unit best benefit from?
   a. Autocratic
   b. Democratic
   c. Laissez–faire
   d. Bureaucratic

4. The nurse is assigning duties to members of the team. Prior to making the assignments, which information would the nurse consider?
   a. How busy the unit is
   b. The request of the staff for their pick of clients
   c. Knowledge of the client population and the staff abilities
   d. The break times of the nurses

5. The new graduate is asked to be a team leader on a unit at the long-term care facility. Which response by the new graduate is best?
   a. "I am not ready for that so I will have to resign."
   b. "I would require at least 1 year of experience prior to serving as a leader."
   c. "I was a good student so should be able to fulfill the role as leader."
   d. "I will do it if I can work the day shift."

CHAPTER RESOURCES

Enhance your learning with additional resources on thePoint*!*

Student Resources related to this chapter can be found at **thePoint.lww.com/Rosdahl12e**.

BIBLIOGRAPHY

Able Care Home Health. (n.d.). *Minnestoa*. https://ablecareconnect.com/mn-twin-cities/

Abrams, A., Pennington, S., & Lammon, C. (2007). *Clinical drug therapy: Rationales for nursing practice* (8th ed.). Lippincott Williams & Wilkins.

Academy of Nutrition & Dietetics. (2013). *Food and nutrition topics: "Common food-drug interactions"*. www.eatright.org

Academy of Nutrition & Dietetics. (2018). *Vegetarianism: The basic facts*. https://www.eatright.org/food/nutrition/vegetarian-and-special-diets/vegetarianism-the-basic-facts

Accreditation Council for Continuing Medical Education. (2012). *#9713: Assessment and management of pain at the end of life*. http://www.accme.org/moclist/97141-assessment-and-management-pain-end-life-139

Acute Pain Management Guide Panel, Agency for Healthcare Research and Quality. (n.d.). *Pain distress scales*. www.ahrq.gov

Administration for Community Living. (2018). *Profile of older Americans 2018*. https://acl.gov/sites/default/files/Aging%20and%20Disability%20in%20America/2018OlderAmericansProfile.pdf

Administration on Aging, U.S. Department of Health and Human Services. (2009). *A profile of older Americans 2009*. http://www.aoa.gov/aoaroot/aging_statistics/profile/2009/docs/2009profile_508.pdf

Administration on Aging. (2001). *Profile of older Americans 2000*. http://www.aoa.gov/aoa/stats/profile

Agency for Healthcare Research and Quality. (2018). *Race, ethnicity, and language data: Standardization for health care quality improvement*. https://www.ahrq.gov/research/findings/final-reports/iomracereport/reldata5.html

Agency for Healthcare Research and Quality. (2019). *Electronic health records*. https://psnet.ahrq.gov/primer/electronic-health-records

Alagiakrishnan, K., & Chopra, A. (2010). Health and health care of Asian Indian American elders. In *Curriculum in ethnogeriatrics: Core curriculum and ethnic specific modules*. http://www.stanford.edu/group/ethnoger/asianindian.html

Alcohol.org. (2020a). *Alcohol induced psychosis, hallucinations, and delusions*. https://www.alcohol.org/comorbid/psychotic-disorder/

Alcohol.org. (2020b). *Alcohol withdrawal symptom severity*. https://www.alcohol.org/treatment-types/withdrawal-signs/

Alejandro, R. G. (1999). *Food of the Philippines*. Periplus Editions.

Alfleesy, O. (2020). *Café coronary death is a misleading medical term that had been put and applied wrongly by Haugen in 1963, instead of choking death*. https://irispublishers.com/ctcms/pdf/CTCMS.MS.ID.000518.pdf

Almohanna, H. M., Ahmed, A. A., Tsatalis, J. P., & Tosti, A. (2019). The role of vitamins and minerals in hair loss: A review. *Dermatology and Therapy, 9*(1), 51–70. https://doi.org/10.1007/s13555-018-0278-6

Alzheimer's Europe. (2019). *How is it diagnosed?* https://www.alzheimer-europe.org/Dementia/Alzheimer-s-disease-and-Alzheimer-s-dementia/How-is-Alzheimer-s-disease-diagnosed

American Academy of Dermatology Association. (2020). *How to care for your skin during and after radiation therapy*. https://www.aad.org/public/diseases/skin-cancer/types/common/melanoma/radiation-care

American Academy of Family Physicians. (2007). *Tobacco statistics*. http://www.aafp.org

American Academy of Orthopaedic Surgeons. (2020). *Diseases and conditions: Perthes disease*. https://orthoinfo.aaos.org/en/diseases--conditions/perthes-disease

American Academy of Pediatrics. (2016). SIDS and other sleep-related infant deaths: Updated 2016 recommendations for a safe infant sleeping environment. *Pediatrics, 138*(5), e20162938. https://doi.org/10.1542/peds.2016-2938

American Academy of Pediatrics. (2020). *Types of families*. https://www.healthychildren.org/English/family-life/family-dynamics/types-of-families/Pages/default.aspx

American Addiction Centers. (2020). *Signs of drug use in the eyes*. https://americanaddictioncenters.org/health-complications-addiction/signs-drug-use-eyes

American Association for Clinical Chemistry. (2016). Syphilis tests. *Lab Tests Online*. https://labtestsonline.org/tests/syphilis-tests

American Association of Neurological Surgeons. (n.d.). *How neurosurgeons perform a stereotactic brain biopsy*. https://www.aans.org/en/Patients/Neurosurgical-Conditions-and-Treatments/Stereotactic-Brain-Biopsy

American Association of Retired Persons (AARP). (n.d.). *Planning for your retirement*. https://www.aarp.org/retirement/planning-for-retirement/

American Cancer Society. (2019). *Signs and symptoms of melanoma skin cancer*. https://www.cancer.org/cancer/melanoma-skin-cancer/detection-diagnosis-staging/signs-and-symptoms.html

American Cancer Society. (2020a). *Advanced directives*. https://www.cancer.org/treatment/finding-and-paying-for-treatment/understanding-financial-and-legal-matters/advance-directives/types-of-advance-health-care-directives.html

American Cancer Society. (2020b). American Cancer Society recommendations for the early detection of breast cancer. *Cancer A-Z*. https://www.cancer.org/cancer/breast-cancer/screening-tests-and-early-detection/american-cancer-society-recommendations-for-the-early-detection-of-breast-cancer.html

American Cancer Society. (2020c). *Leukemia*. https://www.cancer.org/cancer/leukemia.html

American Cancer Society. (2020d). Lung cancer risks for non-smokers. *News*. https://www.cancer.org/latest-news.html

American Cancer Society. (2020e). Lung cancer. *Cancer A-Z*. https://www.cancer.org/cancer/lung-cancer.html

American Cancer Society. (2020f). American Cancer Society lung cancer screening guideline. *Screening Criteria*. https://www.cancer.org/health-care-professionals/american-cancer-society-prevention-early-detection-guidelines/lung-cancer-screening-guidelines.html

American Cancer Society. (2020g). *Skin cancer*. https://www.cancer.org/cancer/skin-cancer.html

American Cancer Society. (2020h). *Spend time outside and stay sun-safe*. https://www.cancer.org/latest-news/stay-sun-safe-this-summer.html

American College of Allergy, Asthma, and Immunology. (n.d.). *Urticaria*. https://acaai.org/

American College of Obstetricians and Gynecologists. (2019). *Endometrial cancer*. https://www.acog.org/womens-health/faqs/endometrial-cancer

American Diabetes Association (ADA). (1997a). Committee report: Report of the expert committee on the diagnosis and classification of diabetes mellitus. *Diabetes Care, 20*(7), 1183–1197.

American Diabetes Association (ADA). (1997b). Position statement: Diabetes mellitus and exercise. *Diabetes Care, 20*(12), 1908–1912.

American Diabetes Association. (2020). *Overview*. https://www.diabetes.org/diabetes

American Diabetes Association. (n.d.). *Get to know carbs*. https://www.diabetes.org/nutrition/understanding-carbs/get-to-know-carbs

American Heart Association. (2012). *Why rush? TIA is an emergency*. http://www.strokeassociation.org/STROKEORG/AboutStroke/TypesofStroke/TIA/Why-Rush-TIA-is-an-Emergency_UCM_310729_Article.jsp

American Heart Association. (2013). *Medication interactions: Food, supplements and other drugs*. www.heart.org/conditions

American Heart Association. (2014). *Medication interactions: Food, supplements, and other drugs*. https://www.heart.org/en/health-topics/consumer-healthcare/medication-information/medication-interactions-food-supplements-and-other-drugs

American Heart Association. (2016). *What is cardiac rehabilitation*. https://www.heart.org/en/health-topics/cardiac-rehab/what-is-cardiac-rehabilitation

American Heart Association. (n.d.). *What is a TIA*. https://www.stroke.org/en/about-stroke/types-of-stroke/tia-transient-ischemic-attack/what-is-a-tia

American Hospital Association. (1992). *A patient's bill of rights*. American Hospital Association.

American Hospital Directory. (2020). *Departments*. https://www.ahd.com/departments.php?hcfa_id=0e6ed911d02223fd12ca9d-585a2c3af1&ek=51e36f85366ee68aed4903b62848db2b

American Liver Foundation. (2017). *Diseases of the liver*. https://liverfoundation.org/

American Lung Association. (2018). *Your aging lungs*. https://www.lung.org/blog/your-aging-lungs

American Lung Association. (2020). Acute respiratory distress syndrome (ARDS). *Lung Health and Diseases*. https://www.lung.org/lung-health-diseases/lung-disease-lookup/ards

American Nurses Association. (2020). *The nursing process*. https://www.nursingworld.org/practice-policy/workforce/what-is-nursing/the-nursing-process/

American Optometric Association. (n.d.). *Adult vision: Over 60 years of age*. https://www.aoa.org/healthy-eyes/eye-health-for-life/senior-vision?sso=y#:~:text=Regular%20eye%20exams%20are%20even,any%20changes%20in%20your%20vision

American Physical Therapy Association. (2017). Face, legs, activity, cry, consolability (FLACC) behavioral pain scale. *Tests and Measures*. https://www.apta.org/patient-care/evidence-based-practice-resources/test-measures/face-legs-activity-cry-consolability-flacc-behavioral-pain-scale#:~:text=FLACC%20is%20a%20behavioral%20pain,activity%2C%20cry%2C%20and%20consolability

American Pregnancy Association. (2019a). *Medication and pregnancy*. https://americanpregnancy.org/medication/medication-and-pregnancy/

American Pregnancy Association. (2019b). *What is a doula?* https://americanpregnancy.org/healthy-pregnancy/labor-and-birth/having-a-doula-616/

American Pregnancy Association. (2020a). *Braxton hicks contractions*. https://americanpregnancy.org/healthy-pregnancy/labor-and-birth/braxton-hicks-762/

American Pregnancy Association. (2020b). Fetal development. *Healthy Pregnancy*. https://americanpregnancy.org/healthy-pregnancy/fetal-development

American Pregnancy Association. (2020c). Signs and symptoms. *Am I Pregnant?* https://americanpregnancy.org/getting-pregnant/am-i-pregnant/pregnancy-symptoms

American Psychiatric Association (APA). (2000). *Diagnostic and statistical manual of mental disorders* (4th ed., revised). American Psychiatric Association.

American Psychiatric Association. (2013). *Diagnostic and statistical manual of mental disorders (DSM-5)* (5th ed.). American Psychiatric Association.

American Psychiatric Association. (2018). *Diagnostic and statistical manual of mental disorders (DSM-5)*. https://www.psychiatry.org/psychiatrists/practice/dsm

American Psychological Association. (2017). *Parenting styles*. https://www.apa.org/act/resources/fact-sheets/parenting-styles

American Psychological Association. (2020a). *Publication manual of the American Psychiatric Association* (7th ed.). American Psychological Association.

American Psychological Association. (2020b). *Work, stress, and health & socioeconomic status*. https://www.apa.org/pi/ses/resources/publications/work-stress-health

American Psychological Association. (2020c). *APA dictionary of psychology*. https://dictionary.apa.org/

American Society of Hematology. (2020a). *Blood basics*. https://www.hematology.org/education/patients/blood-basics

American Society of Hematology. (2020b). *Anemia*. https://www.hematology.org/education/patients/anemia

American Stroke Association. (2019). *F.A.S.T. materials*. https://www.stroke.org/en/help-and-support/resource-library/fast-materials

American Therapeutic Recreation Association (ATRA). (n.d.). *What is recreational therapy?* https://www.atra-online.com/page/AboutRecTherapy#:~:text=Recreational%20therapy%2C%20also%20known%20as%2C%20recovery%20and%20well%2Dbeing

American Thoracic Society. (2020). Interpretation of ABGs. *Clinical Education*. https://www.thoracic.org/professionals/clinical-resources/critical-care/clinical-education/abgs.php

American Thoracic Society. (n.d.). *Patient information series: Mechanical ventilation*. http://www.thoracic.org/patients/patient-resources/resources/mechanical-ventilation.pdf

American Thyroid Association. (2020). *Thyroid function tests*. https://www.thyroid.org/thyroid-function-tests/

Andrews, M., Boyle, J., & Collins, J. (2020). *Transcultural concepts in nursing care* (8th ed.). Wolters Kluwer/Lippincott Williams & Wilkins.

Ansong-Assoku, B., & Ankola, P. A. (2020). *Neonatal jaundice*. In *StatPearls* [Internet]. StatPearls Publishing. https://www.ncbi.nlm.nih.gov/books/NBK532930/

Apothecary, household, and metric systems of measurement. (n.d.). George Brown College. https://my.georgebrown.ca/uploadedFiles/TLC/_documents/Apothecary,%20Household%20 and%20Metric%20Systems%20of%20Measurement.pdf

Arthritis Foundation. (n.d.). *DMARDs.* https://www.arthritis.org/drug-guide/dmards/dmards

Association for Professionals in Infection Control and Epidemiology (APIC). (2020a). Break the chain of infection. *Infection Prevention and You.* https://professionals.site.apic.org/protect-your-patients/break-the-chain-of-infection/

Association for Professionals in Infection Control and Epidemiology (APIC). (2020b). What are transmission-based precautions? *Infection Prevention and You.* http://professionals.site.apic.org/what-are-transmission-precautions

Baker, J., & Baker, R. (2000). *Healthcare finance.* Aspen.

Ballstaedt, L., & Woodbury, B. (2020). *Bladder post void residual volume.* StatPearls Publishing. https://www.ncbi.nlm.nih.gov/books/NBK539839/

Baranoski, S., & Ayello, E. A. (2012). *Wound care essentials: Practice principles* (3rd ed.). Lippincott Williams & Williams.

Barnett, J. (2020). 11 types of senior living options: How to choose the best senior living option. *Consumer Affairs.* https://www.consumeraffairs.com/health/senior-living-options.html

Basu, G., Costa, V., & Jain, P. (2017). Clinicians' obligations to use qualified medical interpreters when caring for patients with limited English proficiency. *AMA Journal of Ethics, 19*(3), 245–252. https://doi.org/10.1001/journalofethics.2017.19.3.ecas2-1703

Bauldoff, G., Gubrud, P., & Carno, M. (2020). *Medical-surgical nursing: Clinical reasoning in patient care* (7th ed.). Pearson.

Bayer Pharmaceuticals. (2019). The four types of MS. *Multiple Sclerosis: Better Questions Lead to Better Answers.* https://www.multiplesclerosis.com/global/treatment.php

Berman, A., Snyder, S., & McKinney, D. S. (2011). *Nursing basics for clinical practice.* Pearson.

Bernard, J., & Schneider, M. (1996). *The true work of dying: A practical and compassionate guide to easing the dying process.* Avon Books.

Berríos-Torres, S. I., Umscheid, C. A., Bratzler, D. W., Leas, B., Stone, E. C., Kelz, R. R., Reinke, C. E., Morgan, S., Solomkin, J. S., Mazuski, J. E., Dellinger, E. P., Itani, K. M. F., Berbari, E. F., Segreti, J., Parvizi, J., Blanchard, J., Allen, G., Kluytmans, J. A. J. W., Donlan, R., Schecter, W. P., & Healthcare Infection Control Practices Advisory Committee, . (2017). Centers for Disease Control and Prevention Guidelines for the prevention of surgical site infection. *JAMA Surgery, 152*(8), 784–791. https://doi.org/10.1001/jamasurg.2017.0904

Beurmanjer, H., Kamal, R. M., de Jong, C., Dijkstra, B., & Schellekens, A. (2018). Baclofen to prevent relapse in gamma-hydroxybutyrate (GHB)-dependent patients: A multicentre, open-label, non-randomized, controlled trial. *CNS Drugs, 32*(5), 437–442. https://doi.org/10.1007/s40263-018-0516-6

Bigatello, L. M., & George, E. (2002). *Hemodynamic monitoring.* http://ncbi.nlm.nih.gov/pubmed/12024086

BJA-National Training and Technical Assistance Center. (2017). *Does naloxone reverse any overdose?* https://bjatta.bja.ojp.gov/naloxone/does-naloxone-reverse-any-overdose

Blackmer, A. (2018). *Fluids and electrolytes.* In PedSAP 2018 Book 2. American College of Clinical Pharmacy. https://www.accp.com/docs/bookstore/pedsap/ped2018b2_sample.pdf

Blood Types. (n.d.). American Red Cross. https://www.redcrossblood.org/donate-blood/blood-types.html

Bowden, V. R., & Greenberg, C. S. (2014). *Children and their families: The continuum of nursing care* (3rd ed.). Wolters Kluwer Health/Lippincott Williams & Wilkins.

Bowden, V. R., & Smith Greenberg, C. (2010). *Children and their families: The continuum of care* (2nd ed.). Wolters Kluwer Health/Lippincott Williams & Wilkins.

Brainline. (2019). What is the Glasgow Coma Scale? https://www.brainline.org/article/what-glasgow-coma-scale

Branum, A. M., & Lukacs, S. L. (2008). *Food allergy among U.S. children: Trends in prevalence and hospitalizations. NCHS data brief, no. 10.* National Center for Health Statistics.

Brooks, A. (2019). *What is a nursing intervention? A beginner's guide.* Rasmussen College. https://www.rasmussen.edu/degrees/nursing/blog/nursing-intervention-beginners-guide/

Bureau of Labor Statistics. (2020). *Occupational outlook handbook: Licensed practical and licensed vocational nurses.* https://www.bls.gov/ooh/healthcare/licensed-practical-and-licensed-vocational-nurses.htm

Burgess, A. W., & Lanning, K. V. (1995). *An analysis of infant abductions.* National Center for Missing and Exploited Children.

Burrell, L. O., Gerlach, M. J., & Pless, B. S. (1997). *Adult nursing: Acute and community care* (2nd ed.). Appleton & Lange.

By the numbers: Braden score interventions. (2004). *Advances in Skin & Wound Care, 17*(3), 150. http://journals.lww.com/aswcjournal/pages/toc.aspx?year = 2004&issue = 04000

Canwest News Service. (2007). *Canada tops U.S. in health care comparison study.* http://www.canada.com/topics/bodyandhealth/story.html?id = 7af65822–8a73–46cc-afb6–808e49be3eff

Carter, P. J. (2008). *Lippincott's textbook for nursing assistants: A humanistic approach to caregiving* (2nd ed.). Lippincott Williams & Wilkins.

Carter, P. J. (2012). *Lippincott's textbook for nursing assistants: A humanistic approach to caregiving* (3rd ed.). Lippincott Williams & Wilkins.

Carter, P. J. (2016). *Lippincott's textbook for nursing assistants: A humanistic approach to caregiving* (4th ed.). Lippincott Williams & Wilkins.

Carter, P., & Lewsen, S. (2005). *Textbook for nursing assistants: A humanistic approach to caregiving.* Lippincott Williams & Wilkins.

Case-Lo, C. (2019a). Medication administration: Why it's important to take drugs the right way. *Healthline.* https://www.healthline.com/health/administration-of-medication#routes

Case-Lo, C. (2019b). What causes heart murmurs? *Healthline.* https://www.healthline.com/health/heart-murmurs

Cay, D. (2019). Contemporary issues in law and ethics: Exploring the family veto for organ donation. *Journal of Perioperative Practice, 29*(11), 361–367. https://doi.org/10.1177/1750458918818998

Center for Disease Control and Prevention. (2019). *CDC's environmental public health tracking: Children's environmental health.* https://www.cdc.gov/nceh/multimedia/infographics/childrens_environmental_health.html

Center for Disease Control and Prevention. (2020a). *Vaccine information statements (VISs).* https://www.cdc.gov/vaccines/hcp/vis/index.html

Center for Disease Control and Prevention. (2020b). *Vaccines: Healthcare providers/professional resources.* https://www.cdc.gov/vaccines/hcp/

Center for Disease Control and Prevention. (2020c). *Overweight and obesity: Defining childhood obesity.* https://www.cdc.gov/obesity/childhood/defining.html

Center for Disease Control and Prevention. (n.d.). *Preventing abusive head trauma*. https://www.cdc.gov/violenceprevention/childabuseandneglect/Abusive-Head-Trauma.html#:~:text=What%20is%20Abusive%20Head%20Trauma,because%20of%20a%20child's%20crying

Center for Disease Control. (2019, October 11). *CDC's environmental public health tracking: Children's environmental health*. https://www.cdc.gov/nceh/multimedia/infographics/childrens_environmental_health.html#:~:text=The%20environment%20affects%20children%20differently,of%20body%20weight%20than%20adults

Center for Disease Control. (2020). *Diphtheria, tetanus, and pertussis vaccine recommendations*. https://www.cdc.gov/vaccines/vpd/dtap-tdap-td/hcp/recommendations.html

Center for Science in the Public Interest (CSPI). (n.d.). *Caffeine chart*. https://cspinet.org/eating-healthy/ingredients-of-concern/caffeine-chart

Centers for Disease Control and Prevention and Association of Public Health Laboratories. (2014). *Laboratory testing for the diagnosis of HIV infection: Updated recommendations*. http://stacks.cdc.gov/view/cdc/23447

Centers for Disease Control and Prevention. (2001). HICPAC guidelines for isolation procedures in hospitals. *American Journal of Infection Control, 24*, 24.

Centers for Disease Control and Prevention. (2003). *Prostate cancer screening: A decision guide for African Americans*. http://www.cdc.gov/cancer/prostate/pdf/aaprosguide.pdf

Centers for Disease Control and Prevention. (2005). *Standard precautions*. http://www.cdc.gov/about/cio.htm

Centers for Disease Control and Prevention. (2006). *CDC organization*. http://www.cdc.gov/about/cio.htm

Centers for Disease Control and Prevention. (2007). *Autism spectrum disorders overview*. http://www.cdc.gov/ncbddd/autism/overview.htm

Centers for Disease Control and Prevention. (2008). *CDC childhood injury report: Patterns of unintentional injuries among 0–19-year olds in the United States, 2000–2006*. Centers for Disease Control and Prevention, National Center for Injury Prevention and Control.

Centers for Disease Control and Prevention. (2010a). *A closer look at African American men and high blood pressure control: A review of psychosocial factors and system-level interventions*. U.S. Department of Health and Human Services.

Centers for Disease Control and Prevention. (2010b). U.S. medical eligibility criteria for contraceptive use. *Morbidity and Mortality Weekly Report, 59*(2–4), 7–82.

Centers for Disease Control and Prevention. (2013a). *The state of aging and health in America 2013*. U.S. Department of Health and Human Services. http://www.cdc.gov/aging/index.html

Centers for Disease Control and Prevention. (2013b). *Asthma facts—CDC's national asthma control program grantees*. U.S. Department of Health and Human Services.

Centers for Disease Control and Prevention. (2013c). Deaths: Final data for 2010. *National Vital Statistics Report, 61*(4), 1–117.

Centers for Disease Control and Prevention. (2015a). *Guide to infection prevention for outpatient settings: Minimum expectations for self-care*. www.cdc.gov/HAI/settings/outpatient/outpatient-care-gl-standarded-precautions.html

Centers for Disease Control and Prevention. (2015b). *HIV/AIDS: Basic statistics*. http://www.cdc.gov/hiv/basics/statistics.html

Centers for Disease Control and Prevention. (2015c). *Finding a screening provider near you*. http://www.cdc.gov/cancer/nbccedp/screenings.htm

Centers for Disease Control and Prevention. (2015d). *Growth chart training, division of nutrition, physical activity, and obesity*. https://www.cdc.gov/nccdphp/dnpao/growthcharts/index.htm

Centers for Disease Control and Prevention. (2016a). Standard precautions for all patient care. *Infection Control*. https://www.cdc.gov/infectioncontrol/basics/standard-precautions.html

Centers for Disease Control and Prevention. (2016b). *Home health care*. National Center for Health Statistics. https://www.cdc.gov/nchs/fastats/home-health-care.htm

Centers for Disease Control and Prevention. (2017a). *Pregnancy and rubella*. Rubella (German Measles, 3 Day Measles). https://www.cdc.gov/rubella/pregnancy.html

Centers for Disease Control and Prevention. (2017b). *Scabies*. https://www.cdc.gov/parasites/scabies/fact_sheet.html

Centers for Disease Control and Prevention. (2017c). *Syphilis fact sheet. Sexually transmitted diseases (STDs)*. https://www.cdc.gov/std/syphilis/stdfact-syphilis.htm

Centers for Disease Control and Prevention. (2017d). *Drowsy driving*. https://www.cdc.gov/sleep/about_sleep/drowsy_driving.html

Centers for Disease Control and Prevention. (2018a). *The state of STDs - infographic*. https://www.cdc.gov/std/stats18/infographic.htm

Centers for Disease Control and Prevention. (2018b). *Violence prevention*. https://www.cdc.gov/violenceprevention/index.html

Centers for Disease Control and Prevention. (2018c). *Immunity types*. https://www.cdc.gov/vaccines/vac-gen/immunity-types.htm

Centers for Disease Control and Prevention. (2018d). *Adolescent and school health*. https://www.cdc.gov/healthyyouth/disparities/index.htm

Centers for Disease Control and Prevention. (2018e). *Productive aging and work*. The National Institute for Occupational Safety and Health. https://www.cdc.gov/niosh/topics/productiveaging/

Centers for Disease Control and Prevention. (2018f). The role of potassium and sodium in your diet. *Salt*. https://www.cdc.gov/salt/potassium.htm

Centers for Disease Control and Prevention. (2019a). *2007 Guidelines for isolation precautions: Preventing transmission of infectious agents in healthcare settings*. https://www.cdc.gov/infectioncontrol/pdf/guidelines/isolation-guidelines-H.pdf

Centers for Disease Control and Prevention. (2019b). Basic information about gynecologic cancers. *Gynecologic Cancers*. https://www.cdc.gov/cancer/gynecologic/basic_info/index.htm#:~:text=The%20five%20main%20types%20of,treatment%20can%20be%20most%20effective

Centers for Disease Control and Prevention. (2019c). Benefits of routine screening. *Screening for HIV*. https://www.cdc.gov/hiv/clinicians/screening/benefits.html

Centers for Disease Control and Prevention. (2019d). *Ebola (Ebola virus disease)*. https://www.cdc.gov/vhf/ebola/index.html

Centers for Disease Control and Prevention. (2019e). *Infertility FAQs*. https://www.cdc.gov/reproductivehealth/Infertility/

Centers for Disease Control and Prevention. (2019f). *Lice*. https://www.cdc.gov/parasites/lice/

Centers for Disease Control and Prevention. (2019g). Infant mortality. *Reproductive Health*. https://www.cdc.gov/reproductivehealth/maternalinfanthealth/infantmortality.htm

Centers for Disease Control and Prevention. (2019h). Preventing new HIV infections. *HIV Guidelines*. https://www.cdc.gov/hiv/guidelines/preventing.html

Centers for Disease Control and Prevention. (2019i). *Isolation precautions.* https://www.cdc.gov/infectioncontrol/guidelines/isolation/index.html

Centers for Disease Control and Prevention. (2020a). *Things to know about the COVID-19 pandemic.* https://www.cdc.gov/coronavirus/2019-ncov/your-health/need-to-know.html

Centers for Disease Control and Prevention. (2020b). *National diabetes statistics report.* https://www.cdc.gov/diabetes/data/statistics-report/index.html?CDC_AA_refVal=https%3A%2F%2Fwww.cdc.gov%2Fdiabetes%2Fdata%2Fstatistics%2Fstatistics-report.html

Centers for Disease Control and Prevention. (2020c). *HIV surveillance report, 2018 (Updated): Vol. 31.* http://www.cdc.gov/hiv/library/reports/hiv-surveillance.html

Centers for Disease Control and Prevention. (2020d). *Cancer.* https://www.cdc.gov/cancer/breast/basic_info/screening.htm

Centers for Disease Control and Prevention. (2020e). *Common eye disorders and diseases. Vision Health Initiative.* https://www.cdc.gov/visionhealth/basics/ced/index.html

Centers for Disease Control and Prevention. (2020f). *Hazardous drug exposures in healthcare.* https://www.cdc.gov/niosh/topics/hazdrug/default.html

Centers for Disease Control and Prevention. (2020g). *HPV vaccine recommendations. Vaccines and Preventable Diseases.* https://www.cdc.gov/vaccines/vpd/hpv/hcp/recommendations.html

Centers for Disease Control and Prevention. (2020h). *About us. Global Health Protection and Security.* https://www.cdc.gov/globalhealth/healthprotection/about.html

Centers for Disease Control and Prevention. (2020i). *Viral hepatitis.* https://www.cdc.gov/hepatitis/index.htm

Centers for Disease Control and Prevention. (2020j). HIV and STD criminal laws. *HIV Legal Landscape.* https://www.cdc.gov/hiv/policies/law/states/exposure.html

Centers for Disease Control and Prevention. (2020k). HIV basics. *HIV.* https://www.cdc.gov/hiv/basics/index.html

Centers for Disease Control and Prevention. (2020l). *Immunization schedules.* https://www.cdc.gov/vaccines/schedules/index.html

Centers for Disease Control and Prevention. (2020m). *Malaria* [Brochure]. https://www.cdc.gov/malaria/resources/pdf/fsp/cdc_malaria_program_2020.pdf

Centers for Disease Control and Prevention. (2020n). *Minority health.* https://www.cdc.gov/minorityhealth/index.html

Centers for Disease Control and Prevention. (2020o). National breast and cervical cancer early detection program (NBCCEDP). *Cancer.* https://www.cdc.gov/cancer/nbccedp/

Centers for Disease Control and Prevention. (2020p). *Overweight and obesity.* https://www.cdc.gov/obesity/index.html

Centers for Disease Control and Prevention. (2020q). *Smoking and tobacco use.* https://www.cdc.gov/tobacco/basic_information/e-cigarettes/Quick-Facts-on-the-Risks-of-E-cigarettes-for-Kids-Teens-and-Young-Adults.html

Centers for Disease Control and Prevention. (2020r). *Sun safety.* https://www.cdc.gov/cancer/skin/basic_info/sun-safety.htm#

Centers for Disease Control and Prevention. (2020s). What is PRAMS? *PRAMS.* https://www.cdc.gov/prams/index.htm

Centers for Disease Control and Prevention. (2020t). *When and how to wash your hands.* https://www.cdc.gov/handwashing/when-how-handwashing.html

Centers for Disease Control and Prevention. (2020u). Who is at risk for prostate cancer? *Prostate Cancer.* https://www.cdc.gov/cancer/prostate/basic_info/risk_factors.htm

Centers for Disease Control and Prevention. (2021). *What is breast cancer screening?* https://www.cdc.gov/cancer/breast/basic_info/screening.htm

Centers for Disease Control and Prevention. (n.d.). *Smoking and tobacco use.* U.S. Department of Health and Human Services, National Institutes of Health. https://www.cdc.gov/tobacco/index.htm

Centers for Disease Control and Prevention. (n.d.). *Healthy aging: Data and statistics.* http://www.cdc.gov/aging/index.htm

Centers for Disease Control and Prevention. (n.d.). *Children's mental health.* https://www.cdc.gov/childrensmentalhealth/basics.html

Centers for Disease Control and Prevention. (n.d.). *Tuberculosis.* https://www.cdc.gov/tb/default.htm

Centers for Disease Control and Prevention. (n.d.). *Economic trends in tobacco.* https://www.cdc.gov/tobacco/data_statistics/fact_sheets/economics/econ_facts/index.htm#spending

Centers for Disease Control and Prevention. (n.d.). *National action plan for child injury prevention.* https://www.cdc.gov/safechild/nap/index.html

Centers for Disease Control. (2006). *Mass casualties: Burns.* http://www.bt.cdc.gov/masscasualties/burns.asp

Centers for Medicare and Medicaid Services. (2000). *Medical state operations manual provider certification.* U.S. Department of Health and Human Services, Health Care Financing Administration (HCFA).

Centers for Medicare & Medicaid Services. (2014). *ICD-10-CM/PCS. The next generation of coding.* http://www.cms.gov/Medicare/Coding/ICD10/Downloads/ICD-10Overview.pdf

Centers for Medicare & Medicaid Services. (2015). *Community mental health centers.* https://www.cms.gov/Medicare/Provider-Enrollment-and-Certification/CertificationandComplianc/CommunityHealthCenters

Centers for Medicare and Medicaid Services. (2019a). *Medicare program-general information.* https://www.cms.gov/Medicare/Medicare-General-Information/MedicareGenInfo/index

Centers for Medicare and Medicaid Services. (2019b). *Home health PPS.* https://www.cms.gov/Medicare/Medicare-Fee-for-Service-Payment/HomeHealthPPS

Centers for Medicare and Medicaid Services. (2020a). *ICD-10-CM official guidelines for coding and reporting FY 2020.* https://www.cms.gov/Medicare/Coding/ICD10/Downloads/2020-Coding-Guidelines.pdf

Centers for Medicare and Medicaid Services. (2020b). *Hospital readmission reduction program (HRRP).* https://www.cms.gov/Medicare/Medicare-Fee-for-Service-Payment/AcuteInpatientPPS/Readmissions-Reduction-Program

Centers for Medicare and Medicaid Services. (2020c). *Quality improvement organizations (QIOs).* https://www.cms.gov/Medicare/Quality-Initiatives-Patient-Assessment-Instruments/QualityImprovementOrgs

Centre for Addiction and Mental Health. (2016). *Opioid agonist therapy.* https://www.camh.ca/-/media/files/oat-info-for-clients.pdf

Chabner, D. E. (2014). *The language of medicine* (10th ed.). Elsevier Saunders.

Chemocare. (n.d.). *Types of chemotherapy.* http://chemocare.com/chemotherapy/what-is-chemotherapy/types-of-chemotherapy.aspx

Chichirez, C. M., & Purcărea, V. L. (2018). Interpersonal communication in healthcare. *Journal of Medicine and Life, 11*(2), 119–122.

Children's Hospital of Philadelphia. (2019). *Parts of the immune system.* https://www.chop.edu/centers-programs/vaccine-education-center/human-immune-system/parts-immune-system

Children's Hospital of Pittsburg. (2020). *Building your child's self-esteem.* https://www.chp.edu/for-parents/health-tools/parent-resources/parenting-tips/building-your-childs-self-esteem

Children's Medical Center of Dallas. (2006). *Understanding the basics.* http://www.childrens.com/basics.htm

Chopik, W., Bremner, R., Johnson, D., & Giasson, H. (2018). Age differences in age perceptions and developmental transitions. *Frontiers in Psychology, 9,* 67. https://doi.org/10.3389/fpsyg.2018.00067

Cleveland Clinic. (2017a). *Musculoskeletal system: Normal structure and function.* https://my.clevelandclinic.org/health/articles/12254-musculoskeletal-system-normal-structure--function

Cleveland Clinic. (2017b). *Osteomyelitis.* https://my.clevelandclinic.org/health/diseases/9495-osteomyelitis

Cleveland Clinic. (2018a). *The structure and function of the digestive system.* https://my.clevelandclinic.org/health/articles/7041-the-structure-and-function-of-the-digestive-system

Cleveland Clinic. (2018b). *True versus false labor.* https://my.clevelandclinic.org/health/articles/9686-true-vs-false-labor

Cleveland Clinic. (2019a). *Blood clotting disordes (hyercoagulabule states).* https://my.clevelandclinic.org/health/diseases/16788-blood-clotting-disorders-hypercoagulable-states

Cleveland Clinic. (2019b). *Female reproductive system.* https://my.clevelandclinic.org/health/articles/9118-female-reproductive-system

Cleveland Clinic. (2019c). *Mechanical ventilation.* https://my.clevelandclinic.org/health/articles/15368-mechanical-ventilation

Cleveland Clinic. (2019d). *Skeletal system.* https://my.clevelandclinic.org/health/articles/21048-skeletal-system

Cleveland Clinic. (2020a). *Respiratory system.* https://my.clevelandclinic.org/health/articles/21205-respiratory-system

Cleveland Clinic. (2020b). *Urinary tract infections: Prevention.* https://my.clevelandclinic.org/health/diseases/9135-urinary-tract-infections/prevention

Cleveland Clinic. (n.d.). *Fetal positions for birth.* https://my.clevelandclinic.org/health/articles/9677-fetal-positions-for-birth

Clinical review update: Concomitant anticholinergic and antipsychotic use, 2019 *Clinical review update: Concomitant anticholinergic and antipsychotic use.* (2019). https://files.medi-cal.ca.gov/pubsdoco/dur/Articles/dured_28115.01.pdf

Cohen, B., & Wood, D. (2000). *Memmler's structure and function of the human body* (7th ed.). Lippincott Williams & Wilkins.

Cohen, B., & Wood, D. (2005). *Memmler's structure and function of the human body* (8th ed.). Lippincott Williams & Wilkins.

Colorado Department of Human Services. (2018). *Involuntary transportation for immediate screening rules.* https://www.colorado.gov/pacific/cdhs/involuntary-transportation-immediate-screening-rules

Covered California. (2014). *Covered California participant guide. Introduction to covered California. (Version 2.0).* www.steveshorr.com

Cox, J. (n.d.). *Possible thinking: Achieve the impossible.* https://www.jessicacox.com/

Craven, R. F., & Hirnle, C. J. (2003). *Fundamentals of nursing: Human health and function* (4th ed.). Lippincott Williams & Wilkins.

Craven, R. F., & Hirnle, C. J. (2007). *Fundamentals of nursing: Human health and function* (5th ed.). Lippincott Williams & Wilkins.

Crossroads Hospice and Palliative Care. (n.d.). *A guide to understanding end-of-life signs and symptoms.* https://www.crossroadshospice.com/hospice-resources/end-of-life-signs/

Cubanski, J., Neuman, T., Griffin, S., & Damico, A. (2016). *Medicare spending at the end of life: A snapshot of beneficiaries who died in 2014 and the cost of their care.* https://www.kff.org/medicare/issue-brief/medicare-spending-at-the-end-of-life/

Currie, G. (2018). Pharmacology part 2: Introduction to pharmacokinetics. *Journal of Nuclear Medicine Technology, 46*(3), 221–230. https://doi.org/10.2967/jnmt.117.199638

CVS Pharmacy. (n.d.). *Minute clinic.* https://www.cvs.com/minuteclinic/?icid=CVS-HOME-PWRZN-MINUTECLINIC

Dahlkemper, T. R. (2016). *Caring for older adults holistically* (6th ed.). F. A. Davis.

Danesh, A., Carlos, T., Mark, P., Thomas, C. (2020). Efficacy of lofexidine for mitigating opioid withdrawal symptoms: Results from two randomized, placebo-controlled trials. *Journal of Drug Assessment, 9*(1), 13–19. https://doi.org/10.1080/21556660.2019.1704416

Department of Health and Human Services. (2014). *Healthy people 2020 leading health indicators: Progress update March 2014.* U.S. Department of Health and Human Services.

Department of Health and Human Services. (2019). *Guidelines for use of antiretroviral agents in HIV-1 infected adults and adolescents.* AIDS Education and Training Center. https://aidsetc.org/resource/guidelines-use-antiretroviral-agents-hiv-1-infected-adults-and-adolescents

Department of Health and Human Services. (2020). Healthcare associated infections. *Healthy People 2020.* https://www.healthypeople.gov/2020/topics-objectives/topic/healthcare-associated-infections

DiBaise, M., & Tarleton, S. (2019). Hair, nails, and skin: Differentiating cutaneous manifestations of micronutrient deficiency. *Nutrition in Clinical Practice, 34*(4), 490–503. https://doi.org/10.1002/ncp.10321

Dictionary.com Unabridged. (n.d.). *Ethnic.* http://dictionary.reference.com/browse/ethnic

Doka, K. (2018). Should children attend funerals? *Psychology Today.* https://www.psychologytoday.com/us/blog/good-mourning/201805/should-children-attend-funerals

Dorvil, B. (2018). The secrets to successful nurse bedside shift report implementation and sustainability. *Nursing Management, 49*(6), 20–25. https://doi.org/10.1097/01.NUMA.0000533770.12758.44

Dosage Help. (n.d.). *Dosage calculations tutorials.* http://www.dosagehelp.com/

Dudek, S. (2017). *Nutritional essentials for nursing practice* (8th ed.). Wolters Kluwer/Lippincott Williams & Wilkins.

Durbin, D. R., & Hoffman, B. D. (2018). Child passenger safety. *Pediatrics, 142*(5), e20182460. https://doi.org/10.1542/peds.2018-2460

Ead, H. (2019). Application of the nursing process in a complex health care environment. *Canadian Nurse.* https://canadian-nurse.com/en/articles/issues/2019/september-2019/application-of-the-nursing-process-in-a-complex-health-care-environment

Eliopoulos, C. (2001). *Gerontological nursing* (5th ed.). Lippincott Williams & Wilkins.

Ellis, J. R., & Bentz, P. M. (2007). *Modules for basic nursing skills* (7th ed.). Lippincott Williams & Wilkins.

Ellis, J. R., & Hartley, C. L. (2012). *Nursing in today's world: Trends, issues, and management* (10th ed.). Wolters Kluwer/Lippincott Williams & Wilkins.

Ely, D. M. & Driscoll, A. K. (2020). Infant mortality in the United States, 2018: Data from the period linked birth/infant death file. *National Vital Statistics Reports, National Center for Health Statistics.* https://www.cdc.gov/nchs/data/nvsr/nvsr69/NVSR-69-7-508.pdf

Emery, R., & Dillon, P. (1994). Conceptualizing the divorce process. *Family Relations, 43*(4), 374–380.

Engelkirk, P. G., & Burton, G. R. W. (2006). *Burton's microbiology for the health sciences* (8th ed.). Lippincott Williams & Wilkins.

Epilepsy Society. (n.d.). *About epilepsy*. https://www.epilepsysociety.org.uk/about-epilepsy/epileptic-seizures

Erikson, E. (1963). *Childhood and society* (2nd ed.). Norton.

Erikson, E. (1980). *Identity and the life cycle*. Norton.

Ervin, R. B. (2009). Prevalence of metabolic syndrome among adults 20 years of age and over, by sex, age, race and ethnicity, and body mass index: United States, 2003–2006. *National Health Statistics Reports, 13*, 1–7.

Etafy, M. H., Saleh, F. H., Ortiz-Vanderdys, C., Hamada, A., Refaat, A. M., Aal, M. A., Deif, H., Gawish, M., Abdellatif, A. H., & Gadalla, K. (2017). Rapid versus gradual bladder decompression in acute urinary retention. *Urology Annals, 9*(4), 339–342. https://doi.org/10.4103/0974-7796.216320

Evans-Smith, P. (2005). *Taylor's clinical nursing skills: A nursing process approach*. Lippincott Williams & Wilkins.

Fader, R., Engelkirk, P., & Duben-Engelkirk, J. (2019). *Burton's microbiology for the health sciences* (11th ed.). Wolters Kluwer.

Ferner, R. E., Huson, S. M., & Kirby, A. (2007). Guidelines for the diagnosis and management of neurofibromatosis 1. *Journal of Medical Genetics, 44*(2), 81–88.

Ferrell, K. (2015). *Nursing 2015 drug handbook*. Wolters Kluwer Health.

Finkel, M., & Stanmeyer, J. (2007). Raging malaria: The rapidly spreading disease affects more people than ever before. But until recently, the outcry has been muted. *National Geographic, 212*, 32.

Fitzsimmons, S. (2014). *Healthy aging. Western schools CE express home study, #1434*. Nurses Continuing Education.

Fleck, C., & Chakravarthy, D. (2010). Newer debridement methods for wound bed preparation. *Advances in Skin and Wound Care, 23*, 313–315.

Flynn, J. T., Kaelber, D. C., Baker-Smith, C. M., Blowey, D., Carroll, A. E., Daniels, S. R., de Ferranti, S. D., Dionne, J. M., Falkner, B., Flinn, S. K., Gidding, S. S., Goodwin, C., Leu, M. G., Powers, M. E., Rea, C., Samuels, J., Simasek, M., Thaker, V. V., Urbina, E. M., & Subcommittee on Screening and Management of High Blood Pressure in Children, . (2017). Clinical practice guideline for screening and management of high blood pressure in children and adolescents. *Pediatrics, 140*, e20171904.

Follin, S. A., & Springhouse Corporation. (2004). *Nurse's legal handbook*. Lippincott Williams & Wilkins.

Food and Drug Administration. (2018a). *Bed rail safety*. https://www.fda.gov/medical-devices/consumer-products/bed-rail-safety

Food and Drug Administration. (2018b). *Spilling the beans: How much caffeine is too much?* https://www.fda.gov/consumers/consumer-updates/spilling-beans-how-much-caffeine-too-much

Food and Drug Administration. (2019). *Statistics about smokeless tobacco product use*. https://www.fda.gov/tobacco-products/products-ingredients-components/smokeless-tobacco-products-including-dip-snuff-snus-and-chewing-tobacco

Food and Drug Administration. (2020). *How to understand and use the nutrition facts label*. https://www.fda.gov/food/new-nutrition-facts-label/how-understand-and-use-nutrition-facts-label

Ford, S. M., & Roach, S. S. (2014). *Roach's introductory clinical pharmacology* (10th ed.). Wolters Kluwer, Lippincott Williams & Wilkins.

Foundations Recovery Network. (n.d.). *Dual diagnosis treatment*. https://dualdiagnosis.org/

Fountain, J., & Lappin, S. (2020). *Physiology, renin angiotensin system*. StatPearls Publishing. https://www.ncbi.nlm.nih.gov/books/NBK470410/

Fudin, J. (2018). Opioid antagonists, partial agonists, antagonists: Oh my! *Pharmacy Times*. https://www.pharmacytimes.com/contributor/jeffrey-fudin/2018/01/opioid-agonists-partial-agonists-antagonists-oh-my

Garcia, L. (2019). Charting by exception: What to be aware of when taking shortcuts. *Berxi*. https://www.berxi.com/resources/articles/charting-by-exception/

Garmo, C., Bajwa, T., & Burns, B. (2020). *Physiology, clotting mechanism*. StatPearls Publishing. https://www.ncbi.nlm.nih.gov/books/NBK507795/

Garner, J. S., & Hospital Infection Control Practices Advisory Committee (HICPAC), . (2001). *Guideline for isolation precautions in hospitals*. Public Health Service.

Gavin, M. (2018). My food plate guide. *Kids Health*. https://kidshealth.org/en/parents/myplate.html

Gavin, M. (2019). Leadership vs. management: What's the difference? *Harvard Business School Online*. https://online.hbs.edu/blog/post/leadership-vs-management

Gay and Lesbian Alliance Against Defamation (GLADD). (2016). *GLADD media reference guide* (10th ed.). https://www.glaad.org/sites/default/files/GLAAD-Media-Reference-Guide-Tenth-Edition.pdf

Gee, E. (2019). How to apply antiembolism stockings to prevent venous thromboembolism. *Nursing Times, 115*(4), 24–26.

Genetics Home Reference. (2014). *Lactose intolerance*. ghr.nlm.nih.gov

Gerontological nursing definition. https://encyclopedia.thefreedictionary.com/gerontological+nursing

Giger, J. N., & Davidhizar, R. E. (2004). *Transcultural nursing: Assessment and intervention* (4th ed.). Elsevier/Mosby.

Giger, J. (2016). *Transcultural nursing: Assessment and intervention* (7th ed.). Elsevier/Mosby.

Godfrey, A. (2017). *Leaving against medical advise. A clinician's dilemma. In Practice: Reflections from NPs and PAs*. https://blogs.jwatch.org/frontlines-clinical-medicine/2017/05/11/leaving-medical-advice-ama-clinicians-dilemma/

Goodheart, H. P. (2003). *Goodheart's photoguide of common skin disorders: Diagnosis and management* (2nd ed.). Lippincott Williams & Wilkins.

GoodTherapy. (2019). *Codependency*. https://www.goodtherapy.org/learn-about-therapy/issues/codependency

Gordon, S., Bernadett, M., Evans, D., Shapiro, N. B., & Patel, U. (2011). *Asian Indian culture: Influences and implications for health care*. The Molina Institute for Cultural Competency. http://www.molinahealthcare.com/

Gore, D. R., Passhel, R., Sepic, S., & Dalton, A. (1981). Scoliosis screening: Results of a community project. *Pediatrics, 67*(2), 196–200.

Grap, M. J., & Munro, C. (2017). Oral care for acutely and critically ill patients. *Critical Care Nurse, 37*(3), e19–e21. https://doi.org/10.4037/ccn2017179

Gregory, C. (2019). *The five stages of grief*. https://www.psycom.net/depression.central.grief.html

Griffith, C., Akers, W., Dispenza, F., Luke, M., Farmer, L. B., Watson, J. C., Davis, R. J., & Goodrich, K. M. (2017). Standards of care for research with participants who identify as LGBTQ+. *Journal of LGBT Issues in Counseling, 11*(4), 212–229. https://doi.org/10.1080/15538605.2017.1380549

Gudgel, D. (n.d.). *Recognizing and treating eye injuries*. American Academy of Ophthalmology. https://www.aao.org/eye-health/tips-prevention/injuries

Haddad, L. M., & Geiger, R. A. (2019). *Nursing ethical considerations*. StatPearls Publishing. https://www.ncbi.nlm.nih.gov/books/NBK526054/

Harding, M. (2020). *Lewis's medical-surgical nursing: Assessment and management of clinical problems* (11th ed.). Mosby.

Hartford Institute for Geriatric Nursing. (n.d.). *Fall risk assessment for older adults: The hendrich II fall risk model*. https://hign.org/consultgeri/try-this-series/fall-risk-assessment-older-adults-hendrich-ii-fall-risk-model

Hartney, E. (2020). *DSM-5 criteria for substance use disorders*. https://www.verywellmind.com/dsm-5-criteria-for-substance-use-disorders-21926

Harvard Health Publishing. (2019). *Benzodiazepines (and the alternatives)*. https://www.health.harvard.edu/mind-and-mood/benzodiazepines_and_the_alternatives

Harvard Health Publishing. (2020). *Diagnostic tests and medical procedures*. https://www.health.harvard.edu/diagnostic-tests-and-medical-procedures

Haskins, D. R., & Wick, J. Y. (2017). Medication refusal: Resident rights, administration dilemma. *The Consultant Pharmacists, 32*(12), 728–736. https://doi.org/10.4140/TCP.n.2017.728

Hatfield, N. T. (2014). *Introductory maternity & pediatric nursing* (3rd ed.). Wolters Kluwer Health/Lippincott Williams & Wilkins.

Hatfield, N. T., & Kincheloe, C. A. (2018). *Introductory maternity & pediatric nursing* (4th ed.). Wolters Kluwer Health/Lippincott Williams & Wilkins.

Havighurst, R. J. (1972). *Developmental tasks and education* (3rd ed.). David McKay.

HCPro. (2019). Steps for maintaining patient privacy. *Nurse Leader Insider*. https://www.hcpro.com/NRS-204070-868/Steps-for-maintaining-patient-privacy.html

Health Disparities. (n.d.). *Health Disparities Among Youth*. www.cdc/gov/healthyyouth/disparities

Health Resources and Services Administration. (n.d.). *How organ donation works*. https://www.organdonor.gov/about/process.html

Health Resources and Services Administration. (n.d.). *What is a Health Center?* https://bphc.hrsa.gov/about/what-is-a-health-center/index.html

Healthline. (2019). *What's aversion therapy and does it work?* https://www.healthline.com/health/mental-health/aversion-therapy

Healthwise. (2019). *Thumb-sucking*. https://www.uofmhealth.org/health-library/hw170183

Heerema, E. (2019). *The 4 A's of Alzheimer's disease*. https://www.verywellhealth.com/the-4-as-of-alzheimers-disease-98591#:~:text=5%EF%BB%BF-Agnosia,feeling%20of%20a%20full%20bladder

Hein, E. C. (2001). *Nursing issues in the 21st century: Perspectives from the literature*. Lippincott Williams & Wilkins.

Heitz, E. (2017). Nasal cannulas and face masks. *Healthline*. https://www.healthline.com/health/nasal-cannulas-and-face-masks#1

Heller, B. R., Oros, M. T., & Durney-Crowley, J. (2001). The future of nursing education: Ten trends to watch. *Nursing and Health Care Perspectives, 21*(1), 9–13. http://www.nln.org/nlnjournal/infotrends.htm

HER Foundation. (2020). About hyperemesis gravidarum. *About HG*. https://www.hyperemesis.org/about-hyperemesis-gravidarum/

Herdman, H. T., & Kamitsuru, S., (Eds.). (2014). *NANDA International Nursing diagnoses: Definitions and classification 2015–2017* (10th ed.). Wiley Blackwell.

Hinkle, J., & Cheever, K. (2013). *Brunner & Suddarth's textbook of medical-surgical nursing* (13th ed.). Lippincott Williams & Wilkins.

Hinkle, J., & Cheever, K. (2018). *Brunner & Suddarth's textbook of medical-surgical nursing* (14th ed.). Lippincott Williams & Wilkins.

Hirsch, L. (2019a). Immune system. *Kids Health*. https://kidshealth.org/en/parents/immune.html

Hirsch, L. (2019b). Male reproductive system. *Teens Health*. https://kidshealth.org/en/teens/male-repro.html

Hockleberry, M. J. (2005). *Wong's essentials of pediatric nursing* (7th ed.). Mosby.

Holden, W. (2014). *Haatchi and Little B: The inspiring true story of one boy and his dog*. Macmillan.

Holland, T. (2018). What is holistic health care, anyway? *Dignity Health*. https://www.dignityhealth.org/articles/what-is-holistic-health-care-anyway

Holland, K. (2019). All about electrolyte disorders. *Healthline*. https://www.healthline.com/health/electrolyte-disorders#causes

Hormone Health Network. (2020a). *Glands and hormones A-Z*. https://www.hormone.org/your-health-and-hormones/glands-and-hormones-a-to-z

Hormone Health Network. (2020b). *Rare endocrine genetic diseases*. https://www.hormone.org/diseases-and-conditions/rare-endocrine-genetic-diseases

Hosley, J., Jones, S., & Molle-Matthews, E. (1997). *Lippincott's textbook for medical assistants*. Lippincott-Raven.

Hospice Foundation of America. (2020). *Signs of approaching death*. https://hospicefoundation.org/Hospice-Care/Signs-of-Approaching-Death

Houska, A., & Loucka, M. (2019). Patients' autonomy at the end of life: A critical review. *Journal of Pain and Symptom Management, 57*(4), 835–845. https://doi.org/10.1016/j.jpainsymman.2018.12.339

Hoyert, D. L., & Xu, J. (2012). Deaths: Preliminary Data for 2011. Abstract from *National Vital Statistics Reports, 61*(6).

Huether, S., McCance, K., & Brashers, V. (2020). *Understanding pathophysiology* (7th ed.). Elsevier.

Institute for Safe Medication Practices. (2017a). *Despite technology, verbal orders persist, read back is not widespread, and errors continue*. https://www.ismp.org/resources/despite-technology-verbal-orders-persist-read-back-not-widespread-and-errors-continue

Institute for Safe Medication Practices. (2017b). *List of error-prone abbreviations*. https://www.ismp.org/recommendations/error-prone-abbreviations-list

International Association for the Study of Pain. (2020). IASP announces revised definition of pain. *Publication and News*. https://www.iasp-pain.org/PublicationsNews/NewsDetail.aspx?ItemNumber=10475

Jarvis, C. (1996). *Physical examination and health assessment* (2nd ed.). W. B. Saunders.

Jauch, E. C., Saver, J. L., Adams, H. P., Jr., Bruno, A., Connors, J. J., Demaerschalk, B. M., Khatri, P., McMullan, P. W., Jr., Qureshi, A. I., Rosenfield, K., Scott, P. A., Summers, D. R., Wang, D. Z., Wintermark, M., Yonas, H., American Heart Association Stroke Council, , Council on Cardiovascular Nursing, , Council on Peripheral Vascular Disease, , & Council on Clinical Cardiology, . (2013). Guidelines for the early management of patients with acute ischemic stroke. *Stroke, 44*, 870–947. http://stroke.ahajournals.org/content/44/3/870.full

Jensen, D., Wallace, S., & Kelsey, P. (1994). Latch: A breastfeeding charting system and documentation tool. *Journal of Obstetric, Gynecologic, and Neonatal Nursing, 23*, 27–32.

Job-Hunt.org. How employers view your online presence. https://www.job-hunt.org/job-search-mindset/how-employers-view-your-online-presence.shtml

Johns Hopkins Medicine. (2020a). Disorders of the immune system. *Health*. https://www.hopkinsmedicine.org/health/conditions-and-diseases/disorders-of-the-immune-system

Johns Hopkins Medicine. (2020b). Fetal heart monitoring. *Health*. https://www.hopkinsmedicine.org/health/treatment-tests-and-therapies/fetal-heart-monitoring

Johns Hopkins Medicine. (2020c). Fractures. *Health*. https://www.hopkinsmedicine.org/health/conditions-and-diseases/fractures

Johns Hopkins Medicine. (2020d). 24-hour urine collection. *Health*. https://www.hopkinsmedicine.org/health/treatment-tests-and-therapies/24hour-urine-collection

Johns Hopkins Medicine. (2020e). Calculating a due date. *Health*. https://www.hopkinsmedicine.org/health/wellness-and-prevention/calculating-a-due-date

Johns Hopkins Medicine. (2020f). Cytology. *Health*. https://www.hopkinsmedicine.org/health/treatment-tests-and-therapies/cytology

Johns Hopkins Medicine. (2020g). *Anatomy and function of the heart's electrical system*. https://www.hopkinsmedicine.org/health/conditions-and-diseases/anatomy-and-function-of-the-hearts-electrical-system

Johns Hopkins Medicine. (2020h). Anatomy of the urinary system. *Health*. https://www.hopkinsmedicine.org/health/wellness-and-prevention/anatomy-of-the-urinary-system#:~:text=The%20urinary%20system's%20function%20is,and%20converts%20them%20to%20energy

Johns Hopkins Medicine. (2020i). Constipation. *Health*. https://www.hopkinsmedicine.org/health/conditions-and-diseases/constipation

Johns Hopkins Medicine. (2020j). Gestational trophoblastic disease. *Health*. https://www.hopkinsmedicine.org/health/conditions-and-diseases/gestational-trophoblastic-disease#:~:text=A%20hydatidiform%20mole%20is%20also,but%20can%20sometimes%20turn%20cancerous

Johns Hopkins Medicine. (2020k). The growing child: Adolescent 13 to 18 years. *Health*. https://www.hopkinsmedicine.org/health/wellness-and-prevention/the-growing-child-adolescent-13-to-18-years

Johns Hopkins Medicine. (2020l). Heart attack. *Health*. https://www.hopkinsmedicine.org/health/conditions-and-diseases/heart-attack

Johns Hopkins Medicine. (2020m). Hospital discharge. *Health*. https://www.hopkinsmedicine.org/health/treatment-tests-and-therapies/hospital-discharge#:~:text=When%20you%20leave%20a%20hospital,hospitals%20have%20a%20discharge%20planner

Johns Hopkins Medicine. (2020n). Ice packs vs. warm compresses for pain. *Health*. https://www.hopkinsmedicine.org/health/treatment-tests-and-therapies/ice-packs-vs-warm-compresses-for-pain

Johns Hopkins Medicine. (2020o). Liver: Anatomy and functions. *Health*. https://www.hopkinsmedicine.org/health/conditions-and-diseases/liver-anatomy-and-functions

Johns Hopkins Medicine. (2020p). Transurethral resection of the prostate (TURP). *Health*. https://www.hopkinsmedicine.org/health/treatment-tests-and-therapies/transurethral-resection-of-the-prostate-turp

Johns Hopkins Medicine. (n.d.). Fall risk assessment. *Institute for Johns Hopkins Nursing*. https://www.hopkinsmedicine.org/institute_nursing/models_tools/fall_risk.html

Johnson, S. (2020). "A changing nation: Population projections under alternative migration scenarios." *Current population reports* (pp. 25–1146). U.S. Census Bureau. https://www.census.gov/content/dam/Census/library/publications/2020/demo/p25-1146.pdf

Johnson, J. (2017). Hemothorax: What you need to know. *Medical News Today*. https://www.medicalnewstoday.com/articles/318184

Johnson, S. (2019). Syphilis. *Healthline*. https://www.healthline.com/health/std/syphilis#symptoms-by-stage

Joint Commission on Accreditation of Healthcare Organizations. (2000). *Accreditation standards for management of pain*. www.jcaho.org

Joint Commission on Accreditation of Healthcare Organizations. (2006). *National patient safety goals for hospitals*. www.jcaho.org

Joint Committee on Administrative Rules. (2019). *Standards for pharmacology/administration of medication course for practical nurses*. https://www.ilga.gov/commission/jcar/admincode/068/068013000B02400R.html

Journal of Emergency Dispatch. (2020). *New protocol T helps stop the bleed*. https://iaedjournal.org/new-protocol-t-helps-stop-the-bleed/

Kaiser Family Foundation. (2018). Community health center delivery sites and patient visits. *State Health Facts*. https://www.kff.org/other/state-indicator/community-health-center-sites-and-visits/?currentTimeframe=0&sortModel=%7B%22colId%22:%22Location%22,%22sort%22:%22asc%22%7D

Kaiser Family Foundation. (2019). *The HIV/AIDS epidemic in the United States: The basics*. https://www.kff.org/hivaids/fact-sheet/the-hivaids-epidemic-in-the-united-states-the-basics/#:~:text=Still%2C%20more%206%2C000%20people%20died%20of%20HIV%2FAIDS%20in%202016.&text=While%20HIV%20is%20not%20a,for%20those%20ages%2035%2D44

Kaiser Permanente. (2019). Learning about how to shave an adult. *Health Encyclopedia*. https://healthy.kaiserpermanente.org/health-wellness/health-encyclopedia/he.learning-about-how-to-shave-an-adult.abs2285?kpSearch=circle

Kalil, A., & Bailey, K. (2020). Septic shock treatment and management. *Medscape*. https://emedicine.medscape.com/article/168402-treatment#d10

Karch, A., & Tucker, R. (2021). *2020 Lippincott pocket drug guide for nurses*. Wolters Kluwer.

Karch, A. M. (2003). *2003 Lippincott's nursing drug guide*. Lippincott Williams & Wilkins.

Karch, A. (2011). *2012 Lippincott's nursing drug guide*. Lippincott Williams & Wilkins.

Katulka, L. (2019). How to set SMART goals for your nursing career. *Berxi*. https://www.berxi.com/resources/articles/setting-smart-nursing-goals/

Kellahear, A. (1990). *Dying of cancer: The final year of life*. Harwood Academic Publishers.

Kernisan, L. (n.d.). *Cognitive impairment in aging*. https://betterhealthwhileaging.net/cognitive-impairment-causes-and-how-to-evaluate/

KidsHealth. (2014). *Abusive head trauma (shaken baby syndrome)*. http://kidshealth.org/parent/medical/brain/shaken.html

Kittler, P. G., Sucher, K. P., & Nelms, M. (2011). *Food and culture* (6th ed.). Cengage Learning.

Klossner, N. J., & Hatfield, N. (2006). *Introductory maternity and pediatric nursing*. Lippincott Williams & Wilkins.

Koznjak, B. (2017). Kuhn meets Maslow: The psychology behind scientific revolutions. *Journal for General Philosophy of Science, 48*(2), 257–287. https://doi.org/10.1007/s10838-016-9352-x

Kübler-Ross, E. (1969). *On death and dying*. Macmillan.

Kübler-Ross, E. (1986). *The final stage of growth*. Touchstone.

Kulkarni, K. (2004). Food, culture, and diabetes in the United States. *Clinical Diabetes, 22*(4), 190–192.

Laino, D., Mencaroni, E., & Esposito, S. (2018). Management of pediatric febrile seizures. *International Journal of Environmental Research and Public Health, 15*(10), 2232. https://doi.org/10.3390/ijerph15102232

Larson, E. (1996). *APIC infection control and applied epidemiology: Principles and practice*. Mosby-Year Book.

Latha, K. S. (2010). *The noncompliant patient in psychiatry: The case for and against covert/surreptitious medication*. https://www.ncbi.nlm.nih.gov/pmc/articles/PMC3031933/

Lawton, S., & Shepherd, E. (2019a). Procedure for washing patients' hair in bed. *Nursing Times, 115*(6), 60–62.

Lawton, S., & Shepherd, E. (2019b). The underlying principles and procedure for bed bathing patients. *Nursing Times, 115*(5), 45–47.

Levinson, D. J. (1986). *The seasons of a man's life*. Ballantine.

Levy, B. L., Schiffrin, E. L., Mourad, J. J., Agostini, D., Vicaut, E., Safar, M. E., & Struijker-Boudier, H. A. (2008). Basic science for clinicians: Impaired tissue perfusion. A pathology common to hypertension, obesity, and diabetes mellitus. *Circulation, 118*, 968–976. http://circ.ahajournals.org/content/118/9/968.full

Lewis, S. M., Collier, I. C., & Heitkemper, M. M. (1996). *Medical-surgical nursing: Assessment and management of clinical problems* (4th ed.). Mosby-Year Book.

Lilley, L., Collins, S., & Snyder, J. (2020). *Pharmacology and the nursing process* (9th ed.). Elsevier.

Lippincott Nursing Center. (2019). *Neurovascular assessment*. https://www.nursingcenter.com/getattachment/Clinical-Resources/nursing-pocket-cards/Neurovascular-Assessment/Neurovascular-Assessment.pdf.aspx

Lippincott Solutions. (2018). *Interdisciplinary care plans: Teamwork makes the dream work*. Wolters Kluwer. http://lippincottsolutions.lww.com/blog.entry.html/2018/09/06/interdisciplinary-ca-z601.html

Litholink. (2013). *Instructions for 24-hour urine collection*. Litholink.

Louise, B. (2015). *When Fraser met Billy: How the love of a cat transformed my little boy's life*. Simon & Schuster (Atria Books).

Lowey, S. (2020). Management of severe pain in terminally ill patients at home: An evidence-based strategy. *Home Healthcare Now, 38*(1), 8–15. https://doi.org/10.1097/NHH.0000000000000826

Lucile Packard Children's Hospital at Sanford. (2007). *Facts about sunburn*. http://www.lpch.org/diseasehealthinfo/healthlibrary/burns/sunburn.html

Lynch, J. (2017). Home care nurses at unique risk for workplace violence. *Nurse.com*. https://www.nurse.com/blog/2017/08/22/home-care-nurses-at-unique-risk-for-workplace-violence/

Lynch, J. (2018). AONE leader describes characteristics of a good nurse manager. *Nurse.com*. https://www.nurse.com/blog/2018/03/21/aone-leader-describes-characteristics-of-a-good-nurse-manager/

Lynn, P. (2008). *Taylor's clinical nursing skills: A nursing process approach* (2nd ed.). Lippincott Williams & Wilkins.

Lynn, P. (2011). *Taylor's clinical nursing skills: A nursing process approach* (3rd ed.). Lippincott Williams & Wilkins.

Lynn, P. (2018). *Taylor's clinical nursing skills: A nursing process approach* (5th ed.). Wolters Kluwer (Lippincott Williams & Wilkins).

Lyon, S. (2020). Stay independent with these assistive technologies. *Verywell Health*. https://www.verywellhealth.com/assistive-technologies-for-independence-4065357

MacAllister, L., Zimring, C., & Ryherd, E. (2019). Exploring the relationships between patient room layout and patient satisfaction. *Health Environments Research & Design Journal, 12*(1), 91–107. https://doi.org/10.1177/1937586718782163

MacGill, M. (2017). What are the benefits of a sitz bath? *Medical News Today*. https://www.medicalnewstoday.com/articles/312033

Mai, C. T., Kucik, J. E., Isenburg, J., Feldkamp, M. L., Marengo, L. K., Bugenske, E. M., Thorpe, P. G., Jackson, J. M., Correa, A., Rickard, R., Alverson, C. J., Kirby, R. S., & National Birth Defects Prevention Network, . (2013). Selected birth defects data from population-based birth defects surveillance programs in the United States, 2006 to 2010: Featuring trisomy conditions. *Birth Defects Research Part A: Clinical and Molecular Teratology, 97*(11), 709–725. http://www.ncbi.nlm.nih.gov/pubmed/24265125

Male nursing statistics. (2019). https://www.statisticsstats.com/health/male-nursing-statistics/

Marks, M. G. (1998). *Broadribb's introductory pediatric nursing* (5th ed.). Lippincott Williams & Wilkins.

Marroquin, B., Vine, V., & Morgan, R. (2020). Mental health during the COVID-19 pandemic: Effects of stay-at-home policies, social distancing behavior, and social resources. *Psychiatry Research, 293*, 113419. https://doi.org/10.1016/j.psychres.2020.113419

Maslow, A. (1970). *Motivation and personality* (2nd ed.). Harper.

Mayo Clinic Laboratories. (2019). *Specimen collection and preparation guide*. https://www.mayocliniclabs.com/it-mmfiles/specimen-prep-guide.pdf

Mayo Clinic. (2014). *Drug-eluting stents: Do they increase heart attack risk?* http://www.mayoclinic.org/diseases-conditions/coronary-artery-disease/in-depth/drug-eluting-stents/art-20044911

Mayo Clinic. (2015). *Thermometers: Understand the options*. http://www.mayoclinic.org/diseases-conditions/fever/in-depth/thermometers/art-20046737

Mayo Clinic. (2016). *Autoimmune diseases*. http://www.mayo.edu/research/centers-programs/womens-health-research-center/focus-areas/autoimmune-diseases

Mayo Clinic. (2017a). *Bacterial vs. viral infections: How do they differ?* https://www.mayoclinic.org/diseases-conditions/infectious-diseases/expert-answers/infectious-disease/faq-20058098

Mayo Clinic. (2017b). *Herbal supplements and heart medicines may not mix*. https://www.mayoclinic.org/healthy-lifestyle/consumer-health/in-depth/herbal-supplements/art-20046488

Mayo Clinic. (2017c). *Molar pregnancy*. https://www.mayoclinic.org/diseases-conditions/molar-pregnancy/symptoms-causes/syc-20375175#:~:text=A%20molar%20pregnancy%20%E2%80%94%20also%20known,pregnancy%20and%20partial%20molar%20pregnancy

Mayo Clinic. (2017d). *Foot drop*. https://www.mayoclinic.org/diseases-conditions/foot-drop/diagnosis-treatment/drc-20372633#:~:text=Physical%20therapy.Nerve%20stimulation

Mayo Clinic. (2018a). *Albinism*. https://www.mayoclinic.org/diseases-conditions/albinism/symptoms-causes/syc-20369184

Mayo Clinic. (2018b). *Hyperbaric oxygen therapy*. https://www.mayoclinic.org/tests-procedures/hyperbaric-oxygen-therapy/about/pac-20394380

Mayo Clinic. (2018c). *Living wills and advance directives for medical decisions*. https://www.mayoclinic.org/healthy-lifestyle/consumer-health/in-depth/living-wills/art-20046303

Mayo Clinic. (2018d). *Rh factor blood test*. https://www.mayoclinic.org/tests-procedures/rh-factor/about/pac-20394960

Mayo Clinic. (2018e). *Testicular exam*. https://www.mayoclinic.org/tests-procedures/testicular-exam/about/pac-20385252

Mayo Clinic. (2019a). *Gallstones*. https://www.mayoclinic.org/diseases-conditions/gallstones/symptoms-causes/syc-20354214

Mayo Clinic. (2019b). *Alzheimer's stages: How the disease progresses*. https://www.mayoclinic.org/diseases-conditions/alzheimers-disease/in-depth/alzheimers-stages/art-20048448#:~:text=On%20average%2C%20people%20with%20Alzheimer's,diagnosis%20can%20affect%20life%20expectancy

Mayo Clinic. (2019c). *Bladder stones*. https://www.mayoclinic.org/diseases-conditions/bladder-stones/symptoms-causes/syc-20354339

Mayo Clinic. (2019d). *Blood pressure chart: What your reading means*. https://www.mayoclinic.org/diseases-conditions/high-blood-pressure/in-depth/blood-pressure/art-20050982

Mayo Clinic. (2019e). *Blood transfusions*. https://www.mayoclinic.org/tests-procedures/blood-transfusion/about/pac-20385168

Mayo Clinic. (2019f). *Cushing syndrome*. https://www.mayoclinic.org/diseases-conditions/cushing-syndrome/symptoms-causes/syc-20351310

Mayo Clinic. (2019g). *Drug eluting stents: Do they increase heart attack risk?* https://www.mayoclinic.org/diseases-conditions/coronary-artery-disease/in-depth/drug-eluting-stents/art-20044911#:~:text=Drug%2Deluting%20stents%20have%20a,compared%20to%20bare%20metal%20stents

Mayo Clinic. (2019h). *LASIK surgery: Is it right for you?* https://www.mayoclinic.org/tests-procedures/lasik-eye-surgery/in-depth/lasik-surgery/art-20045751

Mayo Clinic. (2019i). Symptoms and causes. *Syphilis*. https://www.mayoclinic.org/diseases-conditions/syphilis/symptoms-causes/syc-20351756

Mayo Clinic. (2019j). Symptoms and causes. *HPV Infection*. https://www.mayoclinic.org/diseases-conditions/hpv-infection/symptoms-causes/syc-20351596

Mayo Clinic. (2019k). *Fingernails: Do's and don'ts for healthy nails*. https://www.mayoclinic.org/healthy-lifestyle/adult-health/in-depth/nails/art-20044954

Mayo Clinic. (2019l). *Latex allergy*. https://www.mayoclinic.org/diseases-conditions/latex-allergy/symptoms-causes/syc-20374287

Mayo Clinic. (2019m). Menstrual cycle: What's normal, what's not. *Women's Health*. https://www.mayoclinic.org/healthy-lifestyle/womens-health/in-depth/menstrual-cycle/art-20047186

Mayo Clinic. (2019n). *Tracheostomy*. https://www.mayoclinic.org/tests-procedures/tracheostomy/about/pac-20384673

Mayo Clinic. (2019o). *Puncture wounds*. https://www.mayoclinic.org/first-aid/first-aid-puncture-wounds/basics/art-20056665

Mayo Clinic. (2019p). *Urinary incontinence*. https://www.mayoclinic.org/diseases-conditions/urinary-incontinence/symptoms-causes/syc-20352808

Mayo Clinic. (2020a). *Biopsy: Types of biopsy procedures used to diagnose cancer*. https://www.mayoclinic.org/diseases-conditions/cancer/in-depth/biopsy/art-20043922

Mayo Clinic. (2020b). *Eating disorders*. https://www.mayoclinic.org/diseases-conditions/eating-disorders/symptoms-causes/syc-20353603

Mayo Clinic. (2020c). *Allergy skin tests*. https://www.mayoclinic.org/tests-procedures/allergy-tests/about/pac-20392895

Mayo Clinic. (2020d). Cast care: Dos and don'ts. *Healthy Lifestyle Children's Health*. https://www.mayoclinic.org/healthy-lifestyle/childrens-health/in-depth/cast-care/art-20047159

Mayo Clinic. (2020e). *Hypothermia*. https://www.mayoclinic.org/diseases-conditions/hypothermia/symptoms-causes/syc-20352682#:~:text=Hypothermia%20is%20a%20medical%20emergency,95%20F%20(35%20C)

Mayo Clinic. (2020f). *Asthma*. https://www.mayoclinic.org/diseases-conditions/asthma/symptoms-causes/syc-20369653

Mayo Clinic. (2020g). *Bedsores (pressure ulcers)*. https://www.mayoclinic.org/diseases-conditions/bed-sores/symptoms-causes/syc-20355893

Mayo Clinic. (2020h). *Breast self-exam for breast awareness*. https://www.mayoclinic.org/tests-procedures/breast-exam/about/pac-20393237

Mayo Clinic. (2020i). *Caregiver stress*. https://www.mayoclinic.org/healthy-lifestyle/stress-management/in-depth/caregiver-stress/art-20317392

Mayo Clinic. (2020j). *Cystitis*. https://www.mayoclinic.org/diseases-conditions/cystitis/symptoms-causes/syc-20371306

Mayo Clinic. (2020k). *Diarrhea*. https://www.mayoclinic.org/diseases-conditions/diarrhea/symptoms-causes/syc-20352241

Mayo Clinic. (2020l). *Dehydration*. https://www.mayoclinic.org/diseases-conditions/dehydration/symptoms-causes/syc-20354086

Mayo Clinic. (2020m). *Gastroesophageal reflux disease (GERD)*. https://www.mayoclinic.org/diseases-conditions/gerd/symptoms-causes/syc-20361940

Mayo Clinic. (2020n). *Hearing loss*. https://www.mayoclinic.org/diseases-conditions/hearing-loss/symptoms-causes/syc-20373072

Mayo Clinic. (2020o). *Malignant hyperthermia*. https://www.mayoclinic.org/diseases-conditions/malignant-hyperthermia/symptoms-causes/syc-20353750

Mayo Clinic. (2020p). *Nutrition and healthy eating*. https://www.mayoclinic.org/healthy-lifestyle/nutrition-and-healthy-eating/in-depth/vegetarian-diet/art-20046446

Mayo Clinic. (2020q). *Osteomalacia*. https://www.mayoclinic.org/diseases-conditions/osteomalacia/symptoms-causes/syc-20355514#:~:text=Osteomalacia%20refers%20to%20a%20marked,adults%20can%20lead%20to%20fractures

Mayo Clinic. (2020r). *Overactive bladder*. https://www.mayoclinic.org/diseases-conditions/overactive-bladder/symptoms-causes/syc-20355715

Mayo Clinic. (2020s). Placenta: How it works, what's normal? *Pregnancy Week by Week*. https://www.mayoclinic.org/healthy-lifestyle/pregnancy-week-by-week/in-depth/placenta/art-20044425#:~:text=The%20placenta%20is%20an%20organ,umbilical%20cord%20arises%20from%20it

Mayo Clinic. (2020t). *Preeclampsia*. https://www.mayoclinic.org/diseases-conditions/preeclampsia/symptoms-causes/syc-20355745#:~:text=Preeclampsia%20is%20a%20pregnancy%20complication,blood%20pressure%20had%20been%20normal

Mayo Clinic. (2020u). *Prostatectomy*. https://www.mayoclinic.org/tests-procedures/prostatectomy/about/pac-20385198

Mayo Clinic. (2020v). *Psoriasis*. https://www.mayoclinic.org/diseases-conditions/psoriasis/symptoms-causes/syc-20355840

Mayo Clinic. (2020w). *Seizures*. https://www.mayoclinic.org/diseases-conditions/seizure/symptoms-causes/syc-20365711

Mayo Clinic. (2020x). Stages of labor and birth: Baby, it's time! *Labor and Delivery, Postpartum Care*. https://www.mayoclinic.org/healthy-lifestyle/labor-and-delivery/in-depth/stages-of-labor/art-20046545

Mayo Clinic. (n.d.). *Hypothyroidism (underactive thyroid)*. https://www.mayoclinic.org/diseases-conditions/hypothyroidism/symptoms-causes/syc-20350284

Mayo Clinic. (n.d.). *Stroke*. https://www.mayoclinic.org/diseases-conditions/stroke/diagnosis-treatment/drc-20350119

McCaffery, M. (1968). *Cognition, bodily pain and man–environment interactions*. University of California.

McCall, R. E., & Tankersley, C. M. (2007). *Phlebotomy essentials* (4th ed.). Lippincott Williams & Wilkins.

McCall, R. E. (2003). *Phlebotomy essentials* (3rd ed.). Williams & Wilkins.

McLeod, S. (2018). Erik Erikson's stages of psychosocial development. *Simply Psychology*. https://www.simplypsychology.org/Erik-Erikson.html

McLeod, S. (2020). Maslow's hierarchy of needs. *Simply Psychology*. https://www.simplypsychology.org/maslow.html

Medicaid.gov. (2020). *Eligibility*. https://www.medicaid.gov/medicaid/eligibility/index.html

Medical News Today. (2018). *What is refeeding?* https://www.medicalnewstoday.com/articles/322120

Medicare Payment Advisory Committee (MEDPAC). (2019). *Report to the congress: Medicare payment policy*. http://www.medpac.gov/docs/default-source/reports/mar19_medpac_ch12_sec.pdf

Medicare state operations manual. (2000). https://www.cms.gov/Regulations-and-Guidance/Guidance/Transmittals/downloads/R20SOM.pdf

Medi-Smart. (n.d.). *Palliative care, pain*. www.medi-smart.com

Medline Industries, Inc. (2013). *Proper application and care of Medline transfer/gait belts*. Medline Industries, Inc.

Medline Plus. (2014). *Birth weight*. https://www.nlm.nih.gov/medlineplus/birthweight.html

Medline Plus. (2020). *Aspiration*. https://medlineplus.gov/ency/article/002216.htm

Medline Plus. (n.d.). *Seizures*. http://www.nlm.nih.gov/medlineplus/seizures.html

MedLink—Neurology. (2020). *Alcohol withdrawal seizures*. https://www.medlink.com/article/alcohol_withdrawal_seizures

Medscape. (2015). *Macrosomia*. http://emedicine.medscape.com/article/262679-overview

Medscape. (2017). *Aggression*. https://emedicine.medscape.com/article/288689-overview#a1

Medscape. (2018a). *Anaphylaxis clinical presentation*. https://emedicine.medscape.com/article/135065-clinical#:~:text=Anaphylaxis%20is%20an%20acute%20multiorgan,is%20grouped%20by%20organ%20system

Medscape. (2018b). *Animal bites in emergency medicine medication*. https://emedicine.medscape.com/article/768875-medication

Medscape. (2019). *What is the clinical institute withdrawal assessment for alcohol revised (CIWA-Ar) and how is it used?* https://www.medscape.com/answers/166032-46107/what-is-the-clinical-institute-withdrawal-assessment-for-alcohol-revised-ciwa-ar-and-how-is-it-used-in-the-evaluation-of-delirium-tremens-dts

Medscape. (2020). *Extremely low birth weight infant*. http://emedicine.medscape.com/article/979717-overview

Meehan, T. C. (1998). Therapeutic touch as a nursing intervention. *Journal of Advanced Nursing, 28*, 117–125. https://doi.org/10.1046/j.1365-2648.1998.00771.x

Meinke, H. (2019). *Nurses share the pros and cons of working 12-hr shifts*. Rasmussen College. https://www.rasmussen.edu/degrees/nursing/blog/working-12-hour-shifts/

Mental Health America. (2015). *Involuntary mental health treatment*. https://www.mhanational.org/issues/position-statement-22-involuntary-mental-health-treatment

Merck Manual Consumer Version. (n.d.). Complications of labor and delivery. *Women's Health Issues*. https://www.merckmanuals.com/home/women-s-health-issues/complications-of-labor-and-delivery/introduction-to-complications-of-labor-and-delivery

Merriam-Webster. (n.d.). Ethnic. In *Merriam-Webster.com dictionary*. https://www.merriam-webster.com/dictionary/ethnic

Merriam-Webster. (n.d.). Race. In *Merriam-Webster.com dictionary*. https://www.merriam-webster.com/dictionary/race

Michigan Medicine. (2019a). *Ear problems and injuries, age 12 and older*. https://www.uofmhealth.org/health-library/earp4

Michigan Medicine. (2019b). Sponge bath for a child's fever. *Topic Overview*. https://www.uofmhealth.org/health-library/not59770

Michigan Medicine. (2019c). *Sprained ankle: Using a compression wrap*. https://www.uofmhealth.org/health-library/te7620

Microbiology Society. (2020a). *Fungi*. https://microbiologysociety.org/why-microbiology-matters/what-is-microbiology/fungi.html

Microbiology Society. (2020b). *Protozoa*. https://microbiology-society.org/why-microbiology-matters/what-is-microbiology/protozoa.html

Milas, K. (2020). *Hashimoto's thyroiditis overview: The most common cause of hypothyroidism*. https://www.endocrineweb.com/conditions/hashimotos-thyroiditis/hashimotos-thyroiditis-overview

Miller, B. F., & Keane, C. B. (1997). *Miller-Keane encyclopedia and dictionary of medicine, nursing and allied health* (6th ed.). W. B. Saunders.

Miller-Keane, B. F., & O'Toole, M. T. (2005). *Encyclopedia and dictionary of medicine, nursing and allied health* (7th ed.). W. B. Saunders.

Minnesota Department of Human Services. (2020). *Provisional discharge of direct care and treatment patients*. https://www.dhs.state.mn.us/main/groups/publications/documents/pub/dhs-308039.pdf

Mleziva, P., Mleziva, L. J., & Johnson, E. G. (2018). Sensory processing disorder and vestibular rehabilitation: A pediatric case report. *Physical Therapy Rehabilitation, 5*, 6. https://doi.org/10.7243/2055-2386-5-6

Molle, E. A., & Kronenberger, J. (2005). *Comprehensive medical assisting* (2nd ed.). Lippincott Williams & Wilkins.

Mona, M. (2017). Types of bedmaking in nursing, purpose of bedmaking, principles of bedmaking. *Nursing Exercise*. http://nursingexercise.com/bed-making-nursing-purpose-principles/

Mongrain, C. (2019). Hospital beds components and safety: Expert overview. *Robson Forensic*. https://www.robsonforensic.com/articles/hospital-bed-safety-expert/

Moon, R. Y., & Task Force on Sudden Infant Death Syndrome, . (2016). SIDS and other sleep-related infant deaths: Evidence base for 2016 updated recommendations for a safe infant sleeping environment. *Pediatrics, 138*(5), e20162940. https://doi-org.ezp.slu.edu/10.1542/peds.2016-2940

Moore, K. L., Agur, A. M., & Dalley, A. F. (2014). *Essential clinical anatomy* (5th ed.). Wolters Kluwer Health.

Morgan, M., Degenstein, V., Moser, K., Radzwill, K., & Weisenberger, P. (2018). The intervention of bed alarms with fall risk patients. *The North Dakota Nurse, 87*(2), 13.

Mosenifar, Z. (2020). Chronic obstructive pulmonary disease clinical presentation. *Medscape*. https://emedicine.medscape.com/article/297664-clinical#b3

Moule, P., Armoogum, J., Douglass, E., & Taylor, J. (2017). Evaluation and its importance for nursing practice. *Nursing Standard, 31*(35), 55–63. https://doi.org/10.7748/ns.2017.e10782

Mount Sinai. (n.d.). *What is urgent care and when should you use it*. https://www.mountsinai.org/locations/urgent-care/what-is-urgent-care

Mueller, C., Bruggraf, V., & Crogan, N. L. (2020). Growth and specialization of gerontological nursing. *Geriatric Nursing, 41*(1), 14–15. https://doi.org/10.1016/j.gerinurse.2020.01.013

NANDA-I approved diagnoses list. (2020). *Health conditions*. https://ar.israa.edu.ps/uploads/documents/2020/02/4gcM0.pdf

NANDA-International. (2020). *Problem-focused diagnosis*. https://kb.nanda.org/article/AA-00492/0/How-do-I-write-a-diagnostic-statement-for-risk-problem-focused-and-health-promotion-diagnoses.html

National Aphasia Association. (2020). https://www.aphasia.org/aphasia-definitions/

National Association for Continence. (n.d.). *Kegel exercises*. https://www.nafc.org/kegel

National Association for Licensed Practical Nurses. (n.d.). *Certification programs*. https://nalpn.org/certifications/

National Association for Practical Nurse Education and Service (NAPNES). (2000). *Licensed practical nursing: The work of the caregiver*. NAPNES.

National Association for Practical Nurse Education and Service (NAPNES). (2005). *Standards of practice and code of ethics for licensed practical/vocational nurses*. NAPNES.

National Association for Practical Nurse Education and Service, Inc. (n.d.). *NAPNES cert prep*. https://napnescertsprep.com/home

National Association of Community Health Centers. (2015). *Key health center data by state: Federally-funded health centers only*. http://nachc.com/state-healthcare-data-list.cfm

National Association of Community Health Centers. (2020). *California health center fact sheet*. https://www.nachc.org/wp-content/uploads/2020/02/California-2282020.pdf

National Association of Licensed Practical Nurses. (n.d.). https://www.govserv.org/US/Manitowoc/97999949911/National-Association-of-Licensed-Practical-Nurses%2C-Inc

National Breast Cancer Foundation, Inc. (2015). *Symptoms and signs*. http://www.nationalbreastcancer.org/breast-cancer-symptoms-and-signs

National Breast Cancer Foundation. (2019). *Clinical breast exam*. https://www.nationalbreastcancer.org/clinical-breast-exam

National Breast Cancer Foundation. (2020). *Self-breast exam*. https://www.nationalbreastcancer.org/breast-self-exam

National Cancer Institute. (2020). *Pain threshold. NCI dictionary of cancer terms*. https://www.cancer.gov/publications/dictionaries/cancer-terms/def/pain-threshold

National Cancer Institute. (n.d.). *Bronchi, bronchial tree, and lungs*. https://training.seer.cancer.gov/anatomy/respiratory/passages/bronchi.html

National Cancer Institute. (n.d.). *Larynx and trachea. Seer training modules*. https://training.seer.cancer.gov/anatomy/respiratory/passages/larynx.html

National Coalition for Hospice and Palliative Care. (2018). *Clinical practice guidelines for quality palliative care*. https://www.nationalcoalitionhpc.org/wp-content/uploads/2018/10/NCHPC-NCPGuidelines_4thED_web_FINAL.pdf

National Commission on Correctional Healthcare. (n.d.). *Therapeutic communication and behavioral management*. https://www.ncchc.org/cnp-therapeutic-communication#:~:text=Therapeutic%20communication%20is%20defined%20as,support%20and%20information%20to%20patients

National Consumer League. (2017). *Avoid food-drug interactions*. https://curehht.org/wp-content/uploads/2017/11/Food_and_Drug_Interactions_FDA.pdf

National Council of State Boards of Nursing. (2020a). *2020 NCLEX-PN test plan*. https://www.ncsbn.org/2020_NCLEX-PN_TESTPLAN.htm

National Council of State Boards of Nursing. (2020b). *The 2019 interactive year in review*. https://yearinreview.ncsbn.org/nclex.htm

National Council of State Boards of Nursing. (2020c). *2019 NCLEX examination statistics*. https://www.ncsbn.org/2019_NCLEXExamStats.pdf

National Council of State Boards of Nursing. (2020d). Find your nurse practice act. *Policy and Government*. https://www.ncsbn.org/npa.htm

National Council on Aging. (2014). *Healthy aging: Fact sheet*. www.ncoa.org/press-room/fact-sheets/healthy-aging-fact-sheet.html?

National Council on Aging. (2020a). *Fall prevention facts*. https://www.ncoa.org/news/resources-for-reporters/get-the-facts/falls-prevention-facts/#:~:text=Falls%20are%20the%20leading%20cause%20of%20fatal%20injury%20and%20the,and%20more%20than%2027%2C000%20deaths

National Council on Aging. (2020b). Chronic disease. *Healthy Aging Facts*. https://www.ncoa.org/news/resources-for-reporters/get-the-facts/healthy-aging-facts/

National Eczema Association. (2020). *Patient fact sheets*. https://nationaleczema.org/eczema/patient-fact-sheets/

National Emphysema Foundation. (2020). *Emphysema vs chronic bronchitis: Understanding the differences*. http://www.emphysemafoundation.org/index.php/about-uss/privacy/83-copd-emphysema-articles/428-emphysema-vs-chronic-bronchitis-understanding-the-differences

National Eye Institute. (2019). *Color blindness*. https://www.nei.nih.gov/learn-about-eye-health/eye-conditions-and-diseases/color-blindness

National Foundation for Infectious Diseases. (2020). *Immunization*. https://www.nfid.org/immunization/

National Hospice and Palliative Care Organization. (2019). *NHPCO facts and figures*. https://www.nhpco.org/wp-content/uploads/2019/07/2018_NHPCO_Facts_Figures.pdf

National Hospice and Palliative Care Organization. (2020). *Facts and figures*. https://www.nhpco.org/wp-content/uploads/NHPCO-Facts-Figures-2020-edition.pdf

National Hospice and Palliative Care Organization. (n.d.). *Hospice volunteers*. https://www.nhpco.org/patients-and-caregivers/about-hospice-care/volunteering-for-hospice/

National Institute of Deafness and other Communication Disorders. (2017). *Meniere's disease*. https://www.nidcd.nih.gov/health/menieres-disease

National Institute of Deafness and Other Communication Disorders. (2018). *Age related hearing loss*. https://www.nidcd.nih.gov/health/age-related-hearing-loss

National Institute of Diabetes and Digestive and Kidney Diseases. (2020). *Endocrine diseases*. https://www.niddk.nih.gov/health-information/endocrine-diseases

National Institute of Health, National Institute of Diabetes and Digestive and Kidney Disease. (2020). *Irritable bowel syndrome in children*. https://www.niddk.nih.gov/health-information/digestive-diseases/irritable-bowel-syndrome-children

National Institute of Mental Health. (2016). *Brain stimulation therapies.* https://www.nimh.nih.gov/health/topics/brain-stimulation-therapies/brain-stimulation-therapies.shtml

National Institute of Mental Health. (2020). *Eating disorders.* https://www.nimh.nih.gov/health/topics/eating-disorders/index.shtml

National Institute of Mental Health. (n.d.). *What is post-traumatic stress disorder (PTSD)?* http://www.nimh.nih.gov/health/topics/post-traumatic-stress-disorder-ptsd/index.shtml

National Institute on Aging. (2017a). *What is menopause?* https://www.nia.nih.gov/health/what-menopause

National Institute on Aging. (2017b). What is respite care? *Caregiving.* https://www.nia.nih.gov/health/what-respite-care

National Institute on Aging. (2018a). Getting your affairs in order. *Advance Care Planning.* https://www.nia.nih.gov/health/getting-your-affairs-order

National Institute on Aging. (2018b). *Heart health and aging.* https://www.nia.nih.gov/health/heart-health-and-aging

National Institute on Aging. (2019). Vitamins and minerals. *Healthy Eating.* https://www.nia.nih.gov/health/vitamins-and-minerals

National Institute on Deafness and Other Communication Disorders. (2014). *American sign language.* http://www.nidcd.nih.gov/health/hearing/pages/asl.aspx

National Institute on Deafness and Other Communication Disorders. (2015). *Hearing, ear infections, and deafness.* http://www.nidcd.nih.gov/health/hearing/Pages/Default.aspx

National Institute on Drug Abuse. (2015). *Can marijuana use during and after pregnancy harm the baby?* http://www.drugabuse.gov/publications/research-reports/marijuana/can-marijuana-use-during-pregnancy-harm-baby

National Institutes of Health (NIH). (2014). *Tourette syndrome fact sheet.* http://www.ninds.nih.gov/disorders/tourette/detail_tourette.htm

National Institutes of Health (NIH). (2017). *Cultural respect.* https://www.nih.gov/institutes-nih/nih-office-director/office-communications-public-liaison/clear-communication/cultural-respect

National Kidney Foundation. (2020a). *How your kidneys work.* https://www.kidney.org/kidneydisease/howkidneyswrk

National Kidney Foundation. (2020b). *Religion and organ donation.* https://www.kidney.org/atoz/content/religion-organ-donation

National Multiple Sclerosis Society. (n.d.). *Symptoms and diagnosis.* http://www.nationalmssociety.org/Symptoms-Diagnosis

National Multiple Sclerosis Society. (n.d.). *What is MS?* https://www.nationalmssociety.org/What-is-MS/Types-of-MS

National Pressure Injury Advisory Panel. (2017). *NPIAP pressure injury stages.* https://cdn.ymaws.com/npuap.site-ym.com/resource/resmgr/npuap_pressure_injury_stages.pdf

National Pressure Ulcer Advisory Panel. (1998). *Stage I assessment in darkly pigmented skin.* www.npuap.org

National Public Radio. (2015). *At VA hospitals, training and technology reduce nurses' injuries.* http://www.npr.org/2015/02/25/387298633/at-va-hospitals-training-and-technology-reduce-nurses-injuries

National Stroke Association. (2016). *Act FAST.* http://www.stroke.org/understand-stroke/recognizing-stroke/act-fast

NCLEX—before the exam. https://nalpn.org/aboutnalpn/

Nelson, L. (2020). How to become a flight nurse. *Nurse.org.* https://nurse.org/articles/flight-nurse-salary/

Nettina, S. M. (2006). *Lippincott's manual of nursing practice* (8th ed.). Lippincott Williams & Wilkins.

Nightingale, F. (1992). *Notes on nursing: What it is and what it is not* (commemorative edition 1859). J. B. Lippincott.

NIH: National Institute on Drug Abuse. (2018a). *Prescription opioids and heroin research report.* https://www.drugabuse.gov/publications/research-reports/prescription-opioids-heroin/heroin-use-driven-by-its-low-cost-high-availability

NIH: National Institute on Drug Abuse. (2018b). *How do medications to treat opioid use disorder work?* https://www.drugabuse.gov/publications/research-reports/medications-to-treat-opioid-addiction/how-do-medications-to-treat-opioid-addiction-work

NIH: National Institute on Drug Abuse. (2019). *Is marijuana safe to use while pregnant or breastfeeding?* https://www.drugabuse.gov/publications/marijuana-safe-to-use-while-pregnant-or-breastfeeding

NIH: National Institute on Drug Abuse. (2020). *Opioid overdose reversal with naloxone (Narcan, Evzio).* https://www.drugabuse.gov/drug-topics/opioids/opioid-overdose-reversal-naloxone-narcan-evzio

Nowak, T. (2019). *Training day: 4 hemorrhage control solutions that stop the bleed.* https://www.ems1.com/ems-products/ambulance-disposable-supplies/articles/training-day-4-hemorrhage-control-solutions-that-stop-the-bleed-pslpp6ko8kpAwsyq/

Nurse Licensure Compact. https://www.ncsbn.org/nurse-licensure-compact.htm

Nursing Central. (n.d.). Bandage. *Taber's Medical Dictionary.* https://nursing.unboundmedicine.com/nursingcentral/view/Tabers-Dictionary/731000/all/bandage

Nursing Process. (2020). *Five steps of the nursing process.* https://www.nursingprocess.org/Nursing-Process-Steps.html

Occupational Safety and Health Administration (OSHA). (2014). *Data & statistics.* https://www.osha.gov/oshstats/index.html

Occupational Safety and Health Administration (OSHA). (2020). *Data and statistics.* https://www.osha.gov/data

Office of Women's Health. (2019). *Menopause.* https://www.womenshealth.gov/menopause

Ogoina, D. (2011). Fever, fever patterns and diseases called 'fever' – A review. *Journal of Infection and Public Health, 4*(3), 108–124. https://doi.org/10.1016/j.jiph.2011.05.002

O'Neill, J. E., & O'Neill, D. M. (2007). *Health status, health care and inequality: Canada vs. the U.S.* NBER Working Paper No. 13429. http://www.nber.org/papers/w13429

Oral Cancer Foundation. (2020). *Commercial formulas for the feeding tube.* https://oralcancerfoundation.org/nutrition/commercial-formulas-feeding-tube/

Oren-Sosebee, M. (2007). *Prevent pressure ulcers.* The Kids' Campaign 2007 Pediatric Webcast Series. http://www.docstoc.com/docs/15077857/Microsoft-PowerPoint—Prevent-Pressure-Ulcers—The-Kids

Ortman, J. M., Velkoff, V. A., & Hogan, H. (2014). *An aging nation: The older population in the United States, current population reports* (pp. 25–1140). U.S. Census Bureau.

Pancreatic Cancer Action Network. (2020). *What is the pancreas?* https://www.pancan.org/facing-pancreatic-cancer/about-pancreatic-cancer/what-is-the-pancreas/

Parkinson's Foundation. (n.d.). 10 early signs of Parkinson's disease. *Understanding Parkinson's.* https://www.parkinson.org/understanding-parkinsons/10-early-warning-signs

Patel, S. J., & Teach, S. J. (2019). Asthma. *Pediatrics in Review, 40*(11), 549–567. https://doi.org/10.1542/pir.2018-0282

Patton, K., & Thibodeau, G. (2019). *Structure & function of the body* (16th ed.). Elsevier/Mosby.

Pennsylvania Patient Safety Authority. (2006). Confirming feeding tube placement: Old habits die hard. *PA-PSRS Patient Safety Advisory, 4*(3), 23–30. http://patientsafetyauthority.org/ADVISORIES/AdvisoryLibrary/2006/Dec3(4)/documents/23.pdf

Pew Research. (2015). *Division of labor in households with two full-time working parents.* https://www.pewsocialtrends.org/2015/11/04/raising-kids-and-running-a-household-how-working-parents-share-the-load/st_2015-11-04_working-parents-02/

Pfizer. (2019). *Rheumatoid arthritis versus osteoarthritis.* https://www.arthritis.com/about-arthritis/rheumatoid-arthritis-vs-osteoarthritis

Physicians' Disability Services and PDS Disability Facts. (2005). *Fifteen key questions about disability benefits.* http://www.disabilityfacts.com/faqs.html

Pillitteri, A. (2007). *Maternal and child health nursing: Care of the childbearing & childrearing family* (5th ed.). Lippincott Williams & Wilkins.

Pimentel, J. (2009). What the doctor ordered: Filipinos need better diet. *Asian Journal.*

Planned Parenthood. (2020). *Sex and gender identity.* https://www.plannedparenthood.org/learn/gender-identity/sex-gender-identity

Porth, C. (2013). *Pathophysiology: Concepts of altered health states* (9th ed.). Lippincott Williams & Wilkins.

Postpartum Support International. (n.d.). *Pregnancy & postpartum mental health overview.* https://www.postpartum.net/learn-more/pregnancy-postpartum-mental-health/

Potter, P., Perry, A., Stocker, P., & Hall, A. (2017). *Fundamentals of nursing* (9th ed.). Mosby Elsevier.

Practical Recovery. (2020). *Health realization compared to 12-step programs in drug rehab.* https://www.practicalrecovery.com/health-realization-compared-to-12-step-programs-in-drug-rehab/

Practicalnursing.org. (2020). *LPN instructor careers with BSN.* https://www.practicalnursing.org/lpn-instructor-careers-bsn#

Preminger, G. (2019). *Obstructive uropathy.* https://www.merckmanuals.com/professional/genitourinary-disorders/obstructive-uropathy/obstructive-uropathy

Prescriber's Digital Reference. (2020). *Drug information.* https://www.pdr.net/

Pressure injury risk factors in special populations. (2019). *Wound Source.* https://www.woundsource.com/blog/pressure-injury-interventions-in-special-populations

Prochnow, J., Meiers, S., & Scheckel, M. (2018). Improving patient and caregiver new medication education using an innovative teach-back toolkit. *Journal of Nursing Quality, 34*(2), 101–106. https://nursing.ceconnection.com/ovidfiles/00001786-201904000-00003.pdf

Psychiatry Database. (2020). *Extrapyramidal symptoms (EPS).* https://www.psychdb.com/meds/antipsychotics/eps

Pullen, R. L., Jr. (2014). Communicating with patients from different cultures. In *Nursing made incredibly easy.* Wolters Kluwer/Lippincott Williams & Wilkins.

Queensland Brain Institute. (2017). *The spinal cord.* https://qbi.uq.edu.au/brain/brain-anatomy/spinal-cord

Queensland Brain Institute. (2018a). *Central nervous system: Brain and spinal cord.* https://qbi.uq.edu.au/brain/brain-anatomy/central-nervous-system-brain-and-spinal-cord

Queensland Brain Institute. (2018b). *Types of neurons.* https://qbi.uq.edu.au/brain/brain-anatomy/types-neurons

Reeve, C. (1998). *Still me.* Random House (Cambria Publications).

Reynolds, F. W., Mohr, C. F., & Moore, J. E. (1946). Penicillin in the treatment of neurosyphilis: II. Dementia paralytica. *Journal of the American Medical Association, 131*(16), 1255–1260. https://doi.org/10.1001/jama.1946.02870330001001

Rezaie, S. (2017). Urinary retention: Rapid drainage or gradual drainage to avoid complications? *REBEL EM Blog.* https://rebelem.com/urinary-retention-rapid-drainage-gradual-drainage-avoid-complications/

Rhoads, J. (2006). *Advanced health assessment and diagnostic reasoning.* Lippincott Williams & Wilkins.

Ria Health. (2019). *Kudzu for alcohol addiction: Can a natural remedy help you drink less?* https://riahealth.com/2019/06/11/kudzu-for-alcohol/

Ricci, S. S. (2007). *Essentials of maternity, newborn, and women's health nursing.* Lippincott Williams & Wilkins.

Richards, W. A. (2017). Abraham Maslow's interest in psychedelic research: A tribute. *Journal of Humanistic Psychology, 57*(4), 319–322. https://doi.org/10.1177/0022167816670997

Ridgeview Medical Center. (2013). *Client information.* Ridgeview Medical Center.

Robert Wood Johnson Foundation. (1996). *Chronic care in America: A 21st century challenge.* Robert Wood Johnson Foundation.

Rogel Cancer Center. (n.d.). *Alternative medicine.* https://www.rogelcancercenter.org/support/symptoms-and-side-effects/alternative-medicine

Rondinelli, J., Zuniga, S., Kipnis, P., Kawar, L. N., Liu, V., & Escobar, G. J. (2018). Hospital-acquired pressure injury: Risk-adjusted comparisons in an integrated healthcare delivery system. *Nursing Research, 67*(1), 16–25. https://doi.org/10.1097/NNR.0000000000000258

Rubin, E., Gorstein, F., Rubin, R., Schwarting, R., & Strayer, D. (2005). *Rubin's pathology: Clinicopathologic foundations of medicine* (4th ed.). Lippincott Williams & Wilkins.

Russell, G., & Jarrett, C. (2020). Pelvic fractures treatment and management. *Medscape.* https://emedicine.medscape.com/article/1247913-treatment#d10

RxList. (2019a). *Antabuse.* https://www.rxlist.com/antabuse-drug.htm#description

RxList. (2019b). *Campral.* https://www.rxlist.com/campral-drug.htm

Saint Luke's. (n.d). *Discharge instructions for HIV infection and AIDS.* https://www.saintlukeskc.org/health-library/discharge-instructions-hiv-infection-and-aids

Salimbene, S. (2005). *What language does your patient hurt in? A practical guide to culturally competent patient care* (2nd ed.). EMC Paradigm.

Salimbene, S. (2015). *What language does your patient hurt in? A practical guide to culturally competent patient care* (3rd ed.). EMC Paradigm.

Sanmartin, C., Ng, E., Blackwell, D., Gentleman, J., Martinez, M., & Simile, C. (2003). *Joint Canada/United States survey of health, 2002–03 statistics Canada (Catalogue 82M0022-XIE).* http://www.cdc.gov/nchs/about/major/nhis/jcush_mainpage.htm

Scher, C., Meador, L., Van Cleave, J. H., & Reid, M. C. (2018). Moving beyond pain as the fifth vital sign and patient satisfaction scores to improve pain care in the 21st century. *Pain Management Nursing: Official Journal of the American Society of Pain Management Nurses, 19*(2), 125–129. https://doi.org/10.1016/j.pmn.2017.10.010

Schildkrout, B., & Frankel, M. (2016). *Neuropsychiatry: Toward solving the mysteries that animate psychiatry.* https://www.psychiatrictimes.com/view/neuropsychiatry-toward-solving-mysteries-animate-psychiatry

Schnelder, D. (2019). *Ganser syndrome*. https://emedicine.medscape.com/article/287390-overview

Schrager, A. (2019). *How to weigh the risks when choosing your first job*. https://hbr.org/2019/10/how-to-weigh-the-risks-when-choosing-your-first-job

Science Direct: Avulsion injury. (2017). https://www.sciencedirect.com/topics/medicine-and-dentistry/avulsion-injury

Science Direct: Pseudodementia. (2016). https://www.sciencedirect.com/topics/medicine-and-dentistry/pseudodementia#:~:text=Pseudodementia%20may%20be%20defined%20as,associated%20with%20apparent%20cognitive%20decline

ScyMed: eH&P. (2019). *Fever patterns*. http://www.scymed.com/en/smnxkd/kdcdbdc9.htm

Senior Care. (n.d.). *Benefits of home care: Reasons to select home care as a senior option*. https://www.seniorcare.com/home-care/resources/benefits-of-home-care/

Shaheen, N. A., Alqahtani, A. A., Assiri, H., Alkhodair, R., & Hussein, M. A. (2018). Public knowledge of dehydration and fluid intake practices: Variation by participants' characteristics. *BMC Public Health, 18*(1), 1346. https://doi.org/10.1186/s12889-018-6252-5

Sheehy, G. (1984). *Passages: Predictable crises of adult life*. Bantam.

Sholjakova, M., Durnev, V., Kartalov, A., & Kuzmanovska, B. (2018). Pain relief as an integral part of the palliative care. *Open Access Macedonian Journal of Medical Sciences, 6*(4), 739–741. https://doi.org/10.3889/oamjms.2018.163

Shouse California Law Group. (2020). *The horizontal gaze nystagmus test*. https://www.shouselaw.com/ca/dui/fst/horizontal-gaze-nystagmus/

Siegel, J. D., Rhinehart, E., Jackson, M., Chiarello, L., & Healthcare Infection Control Practices Advisory Committee, . (2007). *Guideline for isolation precautions: Preventing transmission of infectious agents in healthcare settings*. http://www.cdc.gov/hicpac/2007IP/2007isolationPrecautions.html

Silverman, W. A., & Andersen, D. H. (1956). A controlled clinical trial of effects of water mist on obstructive respiratory signs, death rate and necropsy findings among premature infants. *Pediatrics, 17*(4), 1–9. (Copyright by the American Academy of Pediatrics.)

Sissons, B. (2019). Emphysema vs chronic bronchitis. *Medical News Today*. https://www.medicalnewstoday.com/articles/325616#symptoms

Skin Cancer Foundation. (2020). *Advanced squamous cell carcinoma treatment*. https://www.skincancer.org/skin-cancer-information/squamous-cell-carcinoma/advanced-scc/

Skolnik, R. (2021). *Global health 101: Essential public health* (4th ed.). Jones and Bartlett.

Slater, D. (2020). *Middle cerebral artery stroke*. https://emedicine.medscape.com/article/323120-overview

Smeltzer, S., & Bare, B. (2004). *Brunner & Suddarth's textbook of medical–surgical nursing* (10th ed.). Lippincott Williams & Wilkins.

Smeltzer, S., Bare, B., Hinkle, J., & Cheever, K. (2008). *Brunner & Suddarth's textbook of medical–surgical nursing* (11th ed.). Lippincott Williams & Wilkins.

Smeltzer, S., Bare, B., Hinkle, J., & Cheever, K. (2010). *Brunner & Suddarth's textbook of medical–surgical nursing* (12th ed.). Lippincott Williams & Wilkins.

Smith, M., & Segal, J. (2020). Family caregiving. *HelpGuide*. https://www.helpguide.org/articles/parenting-family/family-caregiving.htm

Society for Human Resource Management. (2020). *Managing disability benefits*. https://www.shrm.org/resourcesandtools/tools-and-samples/toolkits/pages/managing-disability-benefits.aspx

Solberg, H., & Naden, D. (2019). *It is just that people treat you like a human being: The meaning of dignity for patients with substance abuse use disorders*. https://onlinelibrary.wiley.com/doi/full/10.1111/jocn.15108?af=R

Sood, M. (2020). Chronic functional constipation and fecal incontinence in infants, children and adolescents: Treatment. *UpToDate*. https://www.uptodate.com/contents/chronic-functional-constipation-and-fecal-incontinence-in-infants-children-and-adolescents-treatment#H25

Spector, R. E. (2004). *Cultural diversity in health and illness* (6th ed.). Pearson/Prentice Hall.

Spector, R. E. (2016). *Cultural diversity in health and illness* (9th ed.). Pearson/Prentice Hall.

Srinath, S., Jacob, P., Sharma, E., & Gautam, A. (2019). Clinical practice guidelines for assessment of children and adolescents. *Indian Journal of Psychiatry, 61*(suppl 2), 158–175. https://doi.org/10.4103/psychiatry.IndianJPsychiatry_580_18

Standardized Usage of Military Time. (2020). *Military time chart*. http://militarytimechart.com/common-use-of-military-time/

Standl, T., Annecke, T., Cascorbi, I., Heller, A. R., Sabashnikov, A., & Teske, W. (2018). The nomenclature, definition and distinction of types of shock. *Dtsch Arztebl Int, 115*(45), 757–768. https://doi.org/10.3238/arztebl.2018.0757

Stanford Childrens Health. (2020). *Fetal monitoring*. https://www.stanfordchildrens.org/en/topic/default?id=fetal-monitoring-90-P02448

Stanford Health Care. (n.d.). *Types of arthroplasty*. https://stanfordhealthcare.org/medical-treatments/a/arthroplasty/types.html

Stanford Health Care. (n.d.). *Dementia*. https://stanfordhealthcare.org/medical-conditions/brain-and-nerves/dementia.html

Stanford School of Medicine. (n.d.). *Signs of impending death*. https://palliative.stanford.edu/transition-to-death/signs-of-impending-death/

Stanton, M. W., & Rutherford, M. K. (2005). *The high concentration of U.S. health care expenditures*. Research in Action, Issue 19. AHRQ Pub. No. 06–0060. Agency for Healthcare Research and Quality.

Staton, G. W. (2009). *Chronic obstructive pulmonary disease*. www.medscape.com/viewarticle/707973

Stewart, P. (2019). *Implicit biases in evaluating information gathered during social network screenings*. University of Houston/Libraries. https://uh-ir.tdl.org/handle/10657/4633

Stibich, M. (2020). *Cognitive impairment risk factors*. https://www.verywellmind.com/preventing-cognitive-impairment-2224108

STOP THE BLEED Legislative Updates. Federal and State Legislation. https://www.stopthebleed.org/learn-more/advocate-promote-support

Straight A's in nursing pharmacology: A review series. (2007). Lippincott Williams & Wilkins.

Street Drugs. (2020). *An online drug identification guide*. Publishers Group West, LLC.

Substance Abuse and Mental Health Services Administration (Ed). (n.d.). *Treatment for alcohol and other drug abuse: Opportunities for coordination*. DHHS Publications No. (SMA) 94–2075.

Suneja, M. (2019). *What is the trousseau sign in patients with hypocalcemia?* https://www.medscape.com/answers/241893-20151/what-is-the-trousseau-sign-in-patients-with-hypocalcemia

Taylor, C., Lillis, C., LeMone, P., & Lynn, P. (2005). *Fundamentals of nursing: The art and science of nursing care* (5th ed.). Lippincott Williams & Wilkins.

Taylor, C., Lillis, C., LeMone, P., & Lynn, P. (2008). *Fundamentals of nursing: The art and science of nursing care* (6th ed.). Lippincott Williams & Wilkins.

Taylor, C., Lillis, C., LeMone, P., & Lynn, P. (2011). *Fundamentals of nursing: The art and science of nursing care* (7th ed.). Lippincott Williams & Wilkins.

Taylor, C., Lillis, C., LeMone, P., & Lynn, P. (2015). *Fundamentals of nursing: The art and science of nursing care* (8th ed.). Lippincott Williams & Wilkins.

Taylor, C., Lynn, P., & Bartlett, J. (2018). *Fundamentals of nursing: The art and science of person-centered care* (9th ed.). Lippincott Williams & Wilkins.

Tellado, M. (2019). Head lice. *Kids Health*. https://kidshealth.org/en/parents/head-lice.html

Temple Health. (n.d.). *Crohn's disease vs. ulcerative colitis*. https://www.templehealth.org/services/conditions/crohns-disease-versus-ulcerative-colitis

Texas Medical Association. (2020). *Positive pressure: Physicians promote hemorrhage control training*. https://www.texmed.org/Template.aspx?id=53954

The Anatomical Chart Company. (2002). *Atlas of pathophysiology*. Springhouse.

The Joint Commission. (2017). Joint commission enhances pain assessment and management requirements for accredited hospitals. *The Joint Commission Perspectives, 37*(7), 2–3. https://www.jointcommission.org/-/media/tjc/documents/standards/jc-requirements/2018-requirements/joint_commission_enhances_pain_assessment_and_management_requirements_for_accredited_hospitals1.pdf?db=web&hash=1DFAA78F3C6ED-D8AA2A1A152D18D4409

The Joint Commission. (2018). *New joint commission advisory on pressure injuries related to medical devices*. https://www.jointcommission.org/en/resources/news-and-multimedia/news/2018/07/new-joint-commission-advisory-on-pressure-injuries-related-to-medical-devices/

The Joint Commission. (2019). *Official do not use list*. https://www.jointcommission.org/-/media/tjc/documents/fact-sheets/do-not-use-list-fact-sheet-06-28-19.pdf?db=web&hash=043C-80759207C3EC9616DDD3D5557113

The Joint Commission. (2020a). Two patient identifiers: Understanding the requirements. *Standards*. https://www.jointcommission.org/en/standards/standard-faqs/home-care/national-patient-safety-goals-npsg/000001545/

The Joint Commission. (2020b). *Ambulatory health care: 2020 national patient safety goals*. https://www.jointcommission.org/-/media/tjc/documents/standards/national-patient-safety-goals/2020/simplified_2020-ahc-npsg-eff-july-final.pdf

The Merck Manual of Medical Information—Second Home Edition. (2003). *Seizure disorders*. http://www.merck.com/mmhe/print/sec06/ch085/ch085a.html

Thibodeau, G. A., & Patton, K. T. (2012). *Structure and function of the body* (14th ed.). Elsevier/Mosby.

Thompson, N. E. (2013). Chemotherapy and biotherapy drugs for autoimmune disease. *American Nurse Today, 8*(9), 22–27. https://www.myamericannurse.com/chemotherapy-and-biotherapy-drugs-for-autoimmune-disease/

Timby, B. K. (2009). *Fundamental nursing skills and concepts* (9th ed.). Lippincott Williams & Wilkins.

Timby, B. K., & Smith, N. E. (2014). *Introductory medical-surgical nursing* (11th ed.). Wolters Kluwer/Lippincott Williams & Wilkins.

Timby, B. K., & Smith, N. E. (2018). *Introductory medical-surgical nursing* (12th ed.). Wolters Kluwer/Lippincott Williams & Wilkins.

Timby, B., Carmack, A., & Rupert, D. L. (2011). *Lippincott's review for NCLEX-PN*. Lippincott Williams & Wilkins.

Timby, B. K. (2005). *Fundamental nursing skills and concepts* (8th ed.). Lippincott Williams & Wilkins.

Timby, B. K. (2013). *Fundamental nursing skills and concepts* (10th ed.). Lippincott Williams & Wilkins.

Toney-Butler, T. J., & Thayer, J. M. (2019). *Nursing process*. StatPearls Publishing. https://www.ncbi.nlm.nih.gov/books/NBK499937/

Toney-Butler, T. J., & Unison-Pace, W. (2020). *Nursing admission assessment and examination*. StatPearls Publishing. https://www.ncbi.nlm.nih.gov/books/NBK493211/

Toney-Butler, T. J. (2019). *Nursing admission assessment and examination*. StatPearls Publishing. https://www.ncbi.nlm.nih.gov/books/NBK493211/

Tortora, G. J., & Grabowski, S. R. (1996). *Principles of anatomy and physiology* (8th ed.). HarperCollins.

Trauma System News. (2017). *Stop the bleed: 8 pitfalls to avoid in hemorrhage control*. https://www.trauma-news.com/2017/09/stop-bleed-8-pitfalls-avoid-hemorrhage-control/

U.S. Bureau of Labor Statistics. (2019). *Occupational outlook handbook: Healthcare*. https://www.bls.gov/ooh/healthcare/licensed-practical-and-licensed-vocational-nurses.htm

U.S. Bureau of Labor Statistics. (2021). *Labor force statistics from the current population survey: Employed persons by detailed occupation, sex, race, and Hispanic or Latino ethnicity*. https://www.bls.gov/cps/cpsaat11.htm

U.S. Census Bureau. (2000). *Poverty in the United States*. http://www.census.gov

U.S. Census Bureau. (2014). Estimates of the components of resident population change by race and Hispanic origin for the United States*: April 1, 2010 to July 1, 2013*. https://www.census.gov/data/tables/time-series/demo/popest/2010s-national-detail.html

U.S. Census Bureau. (2019). *What we do*. https://www.census.gov/about/what.html

U.S. Department of Agriculture. (2005). *Dietary guidelines for Americans*. http://www.health.gov/dietaryguidelines/dga2005/recommendations.htm

U.S. Department of Agriculture. (2006). *MyPyramid food guidance system education framework*. http://www.mypyramid.gov/downloads/MyPyramid_education_framework.pdf

U.S. Department of Agriculture. (2015). *2015–2020 Dietary guidelines for Americans* (8th ed.). U.S. Department of Agriculture. https://health.gov/our-work/food-nutrition/2015-2020-dietary-guidelines/guidelines/

U.S. Department of Agriculture. (2020). *My plate messages*. https://www.choosemyplate.gov/WhatIsMyPlate

U.S. Department of Agriculture. (n.d.). Start simple with my plate. *My Plate*. https://www.choosemyplate.gov/eathealthy/start-simple-myplate

U.S. Department of Health and Human Services, Office of Women's Health. (2012a). *Infertility fact sheet*. https://www.womenshealth.gov/publications/our-publications/fact-sheet/infertility.html

U.S. Department of Health and Human Services, Office of Women's Health. (2012b). *Autoimmune diseases fact sheet*. http://womenshealth.gov/publications/our-publications/fact-sheet/autoimmune-diseases.html?from = AtoZ

U.S. Department of Health and Human Services. (2019a). Infertility fact sheet. *Office of Women's Health*. https://www.womenshealth.gov/publications/our-publications/fact-sheet/infertility.html

U.S. Department of Health and Human Services. (2019b). Autoimmune diseases. *Office of Women's Health*. https://www.womenshealth.gov/a-z-topics/autoimmune-diseases

U.S. Department of Health and Human Services. (2020a). *Health information privacy*. https://www.hhs.gov/hipaa/index.html

U.S. Department of Health and Human Services. (2020b). Objectives and data. *Healthy People 2030*. https://health.gov/healthypeople/objectives-and-data

U.S. Department of Health and Human Services/National Institutes of Health. (2014). *Eating disorders: About more than food*. http://www.nimh.nih.gov/health/publications/eating-disorders-new-trifold/index.shtml

U.S. Department of Health and Human Services/National Institutes of Health. (n.d.). *Attention deficit hyperactivity disorder (ADHD)*. http://www.nimh.nih.gov/health/topics/attention-deficit-hyperactivity-disorder-adhd/index.shtml

U.S. Food and Drug Administration. (2020). *How to understand and use the nutrition facts label*. https://www.fda.gov/food/new-nutrition-facts-label/how-understand-and-use-nutrition-facts-label

U.S. Food and Drug Administration. (n.d.). *Drug safety and availability*. https://www.fda.gov/drugs/drug-safety-and-availability

U.S. Legal. (n.d.). *Good samaritans*. https://definitions.uslegal.com/g/good-samaritans/

U.S. National Library of Medicine. (n.d.). Medication search. *Daily Med*. https://dailymed.nlm.nih.gov/dailymed/index.cfm

U.S. Pharmacist. (2017). Polypharmacy and drug adherence in elderly patients. *U.S. Pharmacist, 42*(6), 13–14. https://www.uspharmacist.com/article/polypharmacy

UCLA Pain Management Clinical Resource Guide. (2004). *Pain rating scales for patient assessment*. www.anes.ucla.edu/pain

UNICEF. (2017). *A familiar face: Violence in the lives of children*. https://www.unicef.org/publications/files/Violence_in_the_lives_of_children_and_adolescents.pdf

United Nations. (n.d.). *About the sustainable development goals*. https://www.un.org/sustainabledevelopment/sustainable-development-goals/

United Network for Organ Sharing (UNOS). Deceased donation. https://unos.org/transplant/deceased-donation/

United States Bureau of Labor Statistics. (2020). What licensed and practical and licensed vocational nurses do. *Licensed Practical and Licensed Vocational Nurses*. https://www.bls.gov/ooh/healthcare/licensed-practical-and-licensed-vocational-nurses.htm#tab-2

United States Department of Labor. (n.d.). Electrical safety. *Occupational Safety and Health Administration*. https://www.osha.gov/Publications/electrical_safety.html#:~:text=Electrical%20Safety,or%20appears%20to%20be%20insulated

United States Department of Labor. (n.d.). Hazard communication safety data sheets. *Occupational Safety and Health Administration*. https://www.osha.gov/Publications/HazComm_QuickCard_SafetyData.html

United States Drug Enforcement Agency (DEA). (2017). *Drugs of abuse, a DEA resource guide*. https://www.dea.gov/sites/default/files/drug_of_abuse.pdf

United States Drug Enforcement Agency (DEA). (n.d.). *Drug schedules*. https://www.dea.gov/drug-scheduling

United States Food and Drug Administration. (2019). *Schedules of controlled substances*. https://www.accessdata.fda.gov/scripts/cdrh/cfdocs/cfcfr/CFRSearch.cfm?CFRPart=1308

University Hospitals. (2018). *How microtears help you to build muscle mass*. https://www.uhhospitals.org/Healthy-at-UH/articles/2018/02/microtears-and-mass

University of Minnesota School of Nursing. (2008). The changing face of nursing. *Minnesota Nursing (Fall/Winter)*.

University of Rochester Medical Center. (2020). External and internal heart rate monitoring of the fetus. *Health Encyclopedia*. https://www.urmc.rochester.edu/encyclopedia/content.aspx?contenttypeid=92&contentid=P07776

University of Wisconsin Health. (2019). Comparing rheumatoid arthritis and osteoarthritis. *Health Information*. https://www.uwhealth.org/health/topic/special/comparing-rheumatoid-arthritis-and-osteoarthritis/aa19377.html

Urology Care Foundation. (2018). Erectile dysfunction. *Urological Conditions*. https://www.urologyhealth.org/urologic-conditions/erectile-dysfunction(ed)

Urology Care Foundation. (2019). *What is an intravenous pyelogram (IVP)?* https://www.urologyhealth.org/urologic-conditions/intravenous-pyelogram-(ivp)

Urology Care Foundation. (2020a). *What are undescended testicles (cryptorchidism)?* https://www.urologyhealth.org/urologic-conditions/cryptorchidism

Urology Care Foundation. (2020b). *Urinary incontinence*. https://www.urologyhealth.org/urologic-conditions/urinary-incontinence

Venes, D., & Thomas, C. L., (Eds.). (2001). *Taber's cyclopedic medical dictionary* (19th ed.). F. A. Davis.

Verywell Mind. (2020). *How long does withdrawal from marijuana last?* https://www.verywellmind.com/what-to-expect-from-cannabis-withdrawal-22304

Vikas Mehta. (2020). The new proxemics: COVID-19, social distancing, and sociable space. *Journal of Urban Design, 25*(6), 669–674. https://doi.org/10.1080/13574809.2020.1785283

Viljoen, A., Foster, S., Fantner, G., Hobbs, J., & Dufrene, Y. (2020). Scratching the surface: Bacterial cell envelopes at the nanoscale. *American Society for Microbiology, 11*(1), 19. https://doi.org/10.1128/mBio.03020-19

Walker, M. (2016). Fluid and electrolyte imbalances. *Journal of Infusion Nursing, 39*(6), 382–386. https://doi.org/10.1097/NAN.0000000000000193

Watson, S. (2018). Is postpartum bleeding normal? *Healthline*. https://www.healthline.com/health/pregnancy/is-postpartum-bleeding-normal

Weber, J., & Kelley, J. (2014). *Health assessment in nursing* (5th ed.). Lippincott Williams & Wilkins.

Weber, J., & Kelley, J. (2018). *Health assessment in nursing* (6th ed.). Lippincott Williams & Wilkins.

WebMD. (2015). *Pain management: Palliative care*. http://www.webmd.com/pain-management/guide/palliative-care

WebMD. (2016). *The vape debate: What you need to know*. http://www.webmd.com/smoking-cessation/features/electronic-cigarettes

WebMD. (2019a). *Psychosis and psychotic episodes*. https://www.webmd.com/schizophrenia/guide/what-is-psychosis#1

WebMD. (2019b). *Vaginal bleeding after birth*. https://www.webmd.com/women/vaginal-bleeding-after-birth-when-to-call-doctor#main-container

WebMD. (2020). *Tests and exams for dementia diagnosis*. https://www.webmd.com/alzheimers/diagnose-dementia#2

White, J. (2015). No. 1 threat to your nurses: Injuries from lifting patients. *Healthcare Business and Technology*. http://www.healthcarebusinesstech.com/nurses-safe-lifting-patients/

Wilkins, N., Tsao, B., Hertz, M., Davis, R., & Klevens, J. (2014). *Connecting the dots: An overview of the links among multiple forms of violence*. National Center for Injury Prevention and Control, Centers for Disease Control and Prevention, Prevention Institute.

Williamson, E. (2017). What's your leadership style? *Nurse.com.* https://www.nurse.com/blog/2017/07/07/whats-your-leadership-style/

Willis, L. M., (Ed.). (2018). *Anatomy and physiology made incredibly easy!* (5th ed.). Lippincott Williams & Wilkins.

Willis, L. (2019). *Fluid and electrolytes made incredibly easy!* (7th ed.). Lippincott Williams & Wilkins.

Wintersgill, W. (2019). Gait belts 101: A tool for patient and nurse safety. *American Nurse.* https://www.myamericannurse.com/gait-belts-101-a-tool-for-patient-and-nurse-safety/

World Health Organization. (2006). *Defining sexual health.* www.who.int/reproductivehealth/topics/sexual_health/sh_definitions/en/

World Health Organization. (2009). *Eleventh general programme of work 2009.* http://www.who.int/research/en/

World Health Organization. (2015). *Definition of an older or elderly person.* www.who.int/healthinfo/survey/ageingdefnolder/en/

World Health Organization. (2019). *Rehabilitation in health systems: A guide for action.* https://www.who.int/publications/i/item/rehabilitation-in-health-systems-guide-for-action

World Health Organization. (2020). *Immunization, vaccines and biologicals: Rubella and congenital rubella syndrome (CRS).* https://www.who.int/immunization/monitoring_surveillance/burden/vpd/surveillance_type/passive/rubella/en/

World Health Organization. (2021). *Violence against women.* http://www.who.int/mediacentre/factsheets/fs239/en/

World Health Organization. (n.d.). Gender and human rights. *Sexual and Reproductive Health.* https://www.who.int/reproductivehealth/topics/gender_rights/sexual_health/en/

World Health Organization. *Gender.* https://www.who.int/genomics/gender/en/index1.html#Gender%20Assignment%20of%20Intersex%20Infants%20and%20Children

Wound, Ostomy and Continence Nurses Society. (2011). *Guideline for management of wounds in patients with lower-extremity venous disease.* WOCN. (Level VII).

Wound Reference. (2017). Medfix montgomery straps. *Technology and Product Assessment.* https://woundreference.com/app/topic?id=medfix-montgomery-straps

Xu, J. Q., Murphy, S. L., Kochanek, K. D., & Arias, E. (2020). *Mortality in the United States, 2018.* (NCHS Data Brief, no 355). National Center for Health Statistics. https://www.cdc.gov/nchs/data/databriefs/db355-h.pdf

Xu, J., Murphy, S., Kochanek, K., & Arias, E. (2020). Mortality in the United States in 2018. *NCHS, 385,* 6.

Yoder-Wise, P. S. (2019). Chapter 16: The impact of technology. In *Leading and managing in nursing* (7th ed., pp. 274–297). Mosby Elsevier.

Yogman, M., Garner, A., Hutchinson, J., Hirsh-Pasek, K., & Golinkoff, R. M. (2018). The power of play: A pediatric role in enhancing development in young children. *Pediatrics, 142*(3), e20182058. https://doi.org/10.1542/peds.2018-2058

Younas, A. (2017). The nursing process and patient teaching. *Nursing Made Incredibly Easy, 15*(6), 13–16. https://doi.org/10.1097/01.NME.0000525549.21786.b5

Young Dementia UK. (2020). https://www.youngdementiauk.org/young-onset-dementia-facts-figures

Zimmermann, K. A. (2018). *Nervous system: Facts, function & diseases.* https://www.livescience.com/22665-nervous-system.html

GLOSSARY

A

abdominal thrust the force a rescuer exerts when treating obstructed airway (Heimlich maneuver).

abduct (abduction) to move away from the centerline, as to *abduct* the arm.

ablation surgical removal or deadening of body tissues, particularly abnormal tissues or nerves conducting pain impulses.

ablative surgery neurosurgery performed to sever or cut pain pathways.

ABO incompatibility a type of hemolytic disease of the newborn; can arise if the client's blood type is A and the fetus's is B or AB; if the mother is B and the fetus is A or AB; and if the mother is O and the fetus is A, B, or AB.

abort to prematurely halt a developmental process, as to *abort* a pregnancy.

abrasion scraping or rubbing off of the skin.

abruptio separation, as *abruptio placentae*.

abruptio placentae condition in which the placenta tears abruptly and prematurely from the uterus.

abscess collection of pus in a localized area.

absorption transfer of food into the cardiovascular circulation for transport.

A1c a test that measures average blood sugar.

acceptance the final stage of the Kübler-Ross' stages of grief demonstrated when the client wishes to plan for life after death or for their family after they die. The feeling could be summarized as saying *I am at peace with the diagnosis*.

accommodation ability to focus, as the *accommodation* of the lens of the eye.

accountability responsibility for all actions that one performs.

accountability measures developed by The Joint Commission and Centers for Medicare and Medicaid Services, they are evidence-based quality indicators that focus on client care and the improvement of the outcomes of care. See also *core measures*.

accreditation status given to a program that meets approved standards (voluntary).

acculturation the process of adopting cultural beliefs, values, and practices.

acetabulum the depression into which the rounded head of the femur fits; also known as the hip socket.

achalasia failure of the smooth muscles of the gastrointestinal tract to relax, especially in the lower esophagus.

acid a chemical compound with a pH below 7.

acidosis pathology resulting from acid accumulation or alkali depletion.

acme time during which the contraction is at full intensity. This phase becomes longer as labor progresses.

acne skin disorder characterized by papules or pustules; also called acne vulgaris.

acquired immunity immunity that one obtains through natural or artificial sources.

acrocyanosis newborn condition in which the extremities appear cyanotic.

acromegaly condition resulting from the overproduction of a pituitary hormone.

acronym a word formed by combining the letters of a word or phrase.

acrosclerosis scleroderma of the distal extremities and face.

action potential state that results when a stimulus causes an organized, rapid exchange of sodium and potassium ions across a cell membrane, which spreads like an electric current along the membrane.

active range of motion exercises in which the client is able to move without assistance.

active transport moving substances against the normal gradient through cell walls into cells using a power source, such as ATP.

activities of daily living (ADLs) normal activities, such as eating, dressing, walking, bathing.

acuity clearness or a disorder's level of severity; minimum level or need for healthcare services that must be met for a client to be admitted to an acute-care facility.

acute of short duration but with severe symptoms; sharp.

acute coronary syndrome (ACS) a group of coronary disorders or conditions such as an acute myocardial infarction (AMI), diagnostic ST changes on an ECG, and unstable angina.

acute illness/disease disease or illness that develops suddenly and runs its course in days or weeks; disorders that interfere with the health–illness continuum for a relatively short period of time.

acute pain See *nociceptive pain*.

Addison disease a condition caused by the destruction or degeneration of the adrenal cortex. Symptoms include a darkening of the skin and oral mucous membranes, dehydration, anemia, weight loss, low blood pressure, and thinning hair.

Adduct to draw toward the center, as to *adduct* the arm.

adenohypophysis the anterior lobe of the pituitary gland.

adenosine triphosphate (ATP) a power source for active transport.

adhesions areas of scar tissue that have formed on mucous membrane linings of body tissues causing tissues to adhere together.

adjuvant therapy assisting or enhancing therapy given, especially in cancer, to prevent further growth or pain; therapy used which was originally intended for another purpose.

adolescence time between puberty's onset and cessation of physical growth, ages 11–19.

adrenal near or above the kidney.
adrenal glands two glands, each consisting of an adrenal medulla and a cortex, of which one sits atop each kidney. The adrenal medulla secretes catecholamines, including epinephrine and norepinephrine, which mimic the action of the sympathetic nervous system and help stimulate the "fight or flight" reaction. The adrenal cortex secretes corticosteroids.
advance directive written instructions clients give in advance about the types of healthcare they desire should they become unable to decide for themselves.
advanced cardiac life support techniques that include starting IV lines, administering fluids and medications, using defibrillation and cardiac monitoring, administering oxygen, and opening and maintaining the airway.
advanced practice registered nurse (APRN) a nurse with postgraduate education and training in nursing who specializes in some areas of healthcare, such as pediatrics, obstetrics, or family practice.
adverse effect a response to a medication that is not intended or desired; a side effect.
advocate a person who works to gain or preserve the rights of others; a defender (as in client *advocate*) (verb: to work for the rights of others, to assist).
aerobe microorganism that requires oxygen for growth; also called obligate aerobe.
aesthetic needs essentials of life that are more advanced or complex than the simple physical needs necessary for survival; needs met to give quality to life.
affect the expression of emotion or feelings shown to others through facial expressions, hand gestures, voice tone, laughter, or tears.
afferent sensory neurons that receive messages from all parts of the body and transmit them by way of sensory nerves to the central nervous system; conducting toward the center, as *afferent* nerves; also applies to blood vessels.
Affordable Care Act a comprehensive healthcare reform law enacted in March 2010.
after-care continued follow-up and therapy after discharge, especially from chemical dependency treatment or psychiatric hospitalization.
afterload the amount of pressure or resistance the ventricles of the heart must overcome to empty their contents.
afterpains abdominal discomfort or cramping after delivery caused by uterine contractions.
ageism prejudice against people based on age.
age-related macular degeneration (AMD or ARMD) a painless disorder associated with aging, which results in gradual or rapid destruction of the macula, which is the part of the eye, which is responsible for sharp, central vision.
agglutination clumping of blood cells.
agnosia inability to recognize objects, faces, voices, or places via auditory, visual, sensory, or tactile sensations. Usually affects only a single information pathway in the brain.
agonist a muscle that contracts to move a body part and is opposed by another muscle (the antagonist); a medication that produces a desired response.
agonist therapy drug therapy that uses specific long-acting opioid drugs to replace the shorter-acting opioids the person is addicted to. Long-acting means the drug acts more slowly, which prevents withdrawal for 24–36 hr without causing a person to get high. They also help to reduce or eliminate cravings for opioid drugs.
agoraphobia fear of being in a place from which escape may be difficult or embarrassing.
agranulocytosis an acute disorder, often caused by drug toxicity, in which granulocyte production greatly decreases, causing neutropenia and rendering the body defenseless against bacterial infections. (Also called malignant neutropenia.)
AIDS acronym for acquired immunodeficiency syndrome.
AIDS dementia complex neurologic complications of HIV that cause confusion, forgetfulness, depression, anxiety, and difficulty walking, behavioral changes, and diminished mental capability.
airborne precautions precautions taken when a person has an illness that can be carried in the air or on dust particles. Common measures include special air handling and ventilation.
akathisia a state of agitation, distress, and restlessness; that is, an occasional side effect of antipsychotic and antidepressant medications.
akinesia loss of ability to move the muscles voluntarily as in Parkinson disease.
albumin a protein substance found in animal and vegetable tissues.
alcohol hallucinosis vivid and terrifying, typically auditory hallucinations, but may manifest as visual and tactile hallucinations a person may experience with acute intoxication or during alcohol withdrawal. Symptoms usually appear quickly and resolve quickly especially if the person stays off alcohol
alias an assigned name under which certain clients are admitted to (and records kept in) a healthcare facility in order to maintain anonymity.
alimentary canal tube-like structure responsible for digestion and absorption of food, also known as the digestive tract.
alkalosis a serious condition caused by accumulation of bases or loss of acids; a decrease in hydrogen ion concentration (pH) (opposite of acidosis).
allergen a substance capable of producing hypersensitivity (allergy).
allergic rhinitis also known as hay fever, an allergic response resulting in a runny nose, itching eyes, and sneezing.
allergy a state in which the body is hypersensitive to a substance, usually a protein.
allogeneic persons who are not genetically related. See also *allograft*.
allograft a graft between individuals of the same species (as in two unrelated persons).
alopecia abnormal hair loss or baldness.
alveolar duct place in the bronchi where the bronchioles first branch.
alveolar sac grape-like clusters in the bronchi where the bronchioles end.

alveoli the lung sacs where gas exchange takes place.

Alzheimer's disease a common form of dementia, most often occurring in older adults.

ambiguous loss the debilitating confusion a family may experience when a living loved one is still physically present but psychologically absent, as in dementia or psychological disorders.

amblyopia subnormal vision in one eye, which may fail to develop due to lack of stimulation as a child continues to use the stronger eye for vision; also called lazy eye.

AMBU-bag Artificial manual breathing unit (AMBU); a proprietary name for a bag valve mask (BVM) device, which when accurately pressed over the nose and mouth and squeezed, air is forced into the lungs. The bag then refills itself with air when released.

ambulatory walking or able to walk (noun: ambulation).

amenorrhea absence or abnormal stoppage of menses (menstruation).

amino acids building blocks of proteins, comprised mainly of carbon, hydrogen, oxygen, and nitrogen.

amnihook special sterile hook used to artificially rupture membranes to stimulate the beginning of true labor or to speed up the active labor process.

amniocentesis insertion of a needle through the maternal abdominal wall into the amniotic sac to withdraw amniotic fluid.

amnion the inner membrane and fluid surrounding the fetus (bag of waters).

amniotic fluid fluid that suspends the fetus within the amnion, cushioning the fetus from injury, regulating temperature, and allowing the fetus to move freely.

amniotomy surgical rupture of fetal membranes; artificial rupture of membranes (AROM).

ampule small, glass-sealed flask, often containing medication.

amputation removal of a limb or other body part.

anabolism the constructive phase of metabolism, which involves synthesis of substances to form new, larger substances.

anaerobe microorganism that cannot survive in the presence of oxygen; also called obligate anaerobe.

analgesic medications that relieve pain; usually most effective when given on a regular basis or at the very onset of pain.

anaphylaxis serious, potentially life-threatening allergic reaction that can occur within seconds of exposure; also called anaphylactic effect.

anaplastic cell cell which lacks orderly growth, arrangement, and does not function normally; these cells are found in malignant tumors.

anasarca generalized, total body edema.

anastomose communication between two blood vessels (see also anastomosis).

anastomosis the joining together of two normally distinct spaces or organs.

anatomic position a standard reference point used by medical texts to present the body, in which the model stands erect with the arms at the sides and the palms turned forward.

anatomy science dealing with body structure.

androgen a hormone that stimulates male characteristics (steroid).

anemia a blood deficiency in quality or quantity; reduction in hemoglobin.

anencephaly congenital disorder in which the skull and brain are absent.

anergic unable to respond to antigens by producing antibodies; weak, lacking energy.

anesthesia complete or partial loss of sensation.

anesthetic a substance that produces loss of feeling or sensation.

aneurysm a dilation of the wall of a vessel that causes the formation of a sac; a life-threatening situation, as an aortic *aneurysm*.

anger second stage of Kübler Ross' stages of grief; the individual is angry and may have periods of acting-out or rage. Individual may ask: *Why did this happen to me?*

angina a spasmodic, severe attack or pain, as *angina pectoris*.

angina pectoris literally "pain in the chest;" occurs when extra exertion calls for the arteries to increase blood supply to the heart, and narrow or obstructed arteries are unable to provide the necessary supply and the heart muscle suffers.

angiocardiogram an x-ray of the heart and major vessels.

angioedema localized edema deep within or under the skin, producing giant wheals (lumps).

angiogram a radiograph of any blood vessel.

angioma birthmark.

angioplasty surgical repair of a blood or lymph vessel; often refers to repair of coronary vessels.

anhedonia markedly diminished or lost interest or pleasure in all or most activities. (One of the negative symptoms of schizophrenia.)

anion a negatively charged ion.

ankylosis abnormal consolidation of a joint causing immobility.

anorexia lack or loss of appetite for food, refusal to eat.

anorexia nervosa a condition in which a person refuses to eat because he or she wants to be thin, although he or she is already very thin.

anoscope a speculum specifically used for the anus and rectum.

antagonist a muscle that exerts an action opposite that of another muscle; a medication that blocks or reverses the action of another medication.

antepartal occurring before childbirth (in reference to the pregnant woman); antepartum.

anterior toward the front or belly of the body.

antiarrhythmic a medication that helps regulate the heart's rhythm.

antibiotic substance produced by a living organism that can destroy or weaken other organisms.

antibody a specific protein that neutralizes foreign antigens (essential to the immune response).

antibody-mediated immunity immunity that results when an antibody changes an antigen, making it harmless to the body.

anticipatory guidance education about expected changes prior to them happening.
anticonvulsant a medication that reduces, controls, or stops seizure activity.
antidote an agent that counteracts the effects of a specific poison.
antiembolism stockings also called TED socks; elastic stockings that cover the foot (not the toes) and the leg, up to the knee or mid-thigh.
antiemetic antivomiting medication or substance.
antigen a substance that stimulates the production of antibodies.
antihypertensives medications that reduce blood pressure.
antimicrobial agent a chemical that decreases the number of pathogens in an area by suppressing and destroying their growth.
antineoplastic an agent that inhibits the growth of malignant cells.
antipsychotic any pharmacological agent used to control the symptoms of schizophrenia and other disorders characterized by impaired reality testing, as evidenced by severely disorganized thought, speech, and behavior.
antiretroviral (ARV) agents that act against retroviruses such as HIV.
antiretroviral therapy medications to specifically combat the retrovirus.
antitussive an agent that reduces coughing.
anuria complete suppression of urine secretion in the kidney.
anus opening of the rectum on the body surface.
anxiety apprehension, uneasiness, worry, or dread (may be marked by physiologic signs, such as sweating, tension, or increased pulse).
aorta the largest artery of the body.
aortic valve valve which separates the left ventricle from the aorta.
apex inferior tip of the heart's left ventricle—the point of maximal impulse (the heart sounds loudest here).
Apgar score a method of determining a newborn's condition at birth by rating the baby's respiration and responses.
aphagia an abnormal neurologic or psychogenic condition that results in the inability to swallow.
aphasia an impairment of language, either of speech or comprehension of speech and/or the ability to read or write. It is usually caused by an injury to the brain. It can present very differently, as severe or very mild.
apical pulse pulse normally heard at the heart's apex, the left side of the heart, which usually gives the most accurate assessment of pulse rate.
apical–radial pulse reading done by measuring both the apical and radial pulses simultaneously, used when it is suspected that the heart is not effectively pumping blood. The apical pulse should always be the higher number; if not, do it again.
apnea cessation of breathing for at least 10 s.
apnea monitor machine used to monitor respiratory activity and patterns, especially of infants.

apoptosis cell self-destruction.
apothecary one of the oldest measurement systems based on volume and weight.
appendicitis inflammation of the appendix.
appendix small finger-like projection of the cecum, which has no known function; also called vermiform appendix.
approval status given to a program that allows its graduates to obtain a license (required).
apraxia a defect in the brain pathways that contain memory of learned patterns of movement (no longer knows how to hold a comb correctly).
aquathermia pad the pad which produces dry heat by the use of temperature-controlled water flowing through a waterproof shell.
aqueous humor liquid that flows through the anterior and posterior eye chambers in the space between the cornea and the lens.
architectural barriers building structures that make certain areas inaccessible to individuals with physical disabilities.
arrhythmia irregularity in the heartbeat's rhythm.
arterial blood gases the levels of oxygen and carbon dioxide in the blood.
arteriogram an x-ray of any artery.
arteriosclerosis a condition of the arteries that produces abnormal loss of elasticity and hardening of the walls, especially in the middle layer; also called hardening of the arteries.
artery any vessel through which blood passes from the heart to all body parts.
arthritis joint inflammation.
arthrocentesis aspiration of synovial fluid, blood, or pus from a joint cavity.
arthrogram x-ray of a joint.
arthroplasty joint repair.
arthrosclerosis stiffening of the joints.
arthroscope an endoscope used to examine or do surgery within a joint (arthroscopy).
arthrostomy creation of an opening drain.
articular pertaining to a joint.
articulation point at which bones attach; also known as a joint.
artificial insemination process in which male sperm is artificially implanted into a woman's cervix or into an egg.
artificial sphincter a cuff placed around the bladder neck and connected to a reservoir bulb implanted in individuals with a nonfunctioning urethra.
artificially acquired immunity immunity that occurs when a person is deliberately exposed to a causative agent, such as during vaccination.
ascites edema in the peritoneal cavity generally associated with liver damage.
asepsis practices that minimize or eliminate organisms that cause infections or disease.
aseptic free from germs that cause infection or disease.
asexual without sex; a person who has no interest in sex.
asphyxia suffocation; deficiency of oxygen (asphyxiation).

aspiration breathing in a foreign object as in sucking food into the airway; a medical procedure that removes something from an area of the body (can be body fluids or air).

assault an act that threatens harm, either physical or verbal, whether or not actual harm is done.

assaultive violent physical action which can cause immediate physical harm to self or others.

assertiveness confidence without aggression or passivity, an important skill for a nurse to possess in interpersonal communication; the ability to express positive and negative ideas and feelings in an open, honest, and direct way.

assessment phase of the nursing process in which the nurse systematically and continuously collects and analyzes data about a client.

assisted living programs that allow older adults to age in place, maintain independence, and choose services they want and need.

assisted reproductive technology (ART) *Also known as in vitro fertilization.* ART procedures involve removal of a woman's eggs, which are surgically taken from her ovaries and combined with sperm in a laboratory for fertilization.

assisted suicide helping an individual who wants to end his or her life to do so.

asthma a disease marked by breathing difficulty, caused by spasmodic contractions of the bronchial tubes; bronchial *asthma.*

astigmatism condition in which the eye cannot bring horizontal and vertical lines into focus at the same time, causing blurry vision, as a result of irregularities in the curvature of the cornea and lens.

ataxia loss of voluntary coordination of muscle movements.

ataxic cerebral palsy type of cerebral palsy that results in tremors, unsteady gait, lack of coordination and balance, rapid repeated movements of the eyeball, muscle weakness, and lack of leg movement during infancy.

atelectasis a complete or partial collapse of a lung or a lobe of a lung due to the collapse of the alveoli (tiny air sacs).

atherectomy type of angioplasty in which a sharp device is used to shave away plaque from the coronary or other artery.

atherosclerosis arteriosclerosis characterized by deposits of cholesterol, fatty acids, or plaques on the inner wall of the artery.

athetoid movements slow, involuntary convoluted, writhing movements of fingers, toes, or extremities (see *athetosis*).

athetoid cerebral palsy (dyskinetic cerebral palsy) a type of CP characterized by slow, writhing involuntary movements such as twisting, grimacing, and sharp jerks that disappear during sleep and increase with stress.

athetosis abnormal, involuntary writhing movements, particularly of the arms and hands; abnormal muscle contractions.

atom the smallest particle of an element that retains the original properties of that element.

atony lack of firmness, as in the uterus.

atopy the genetic tendency to develop atopic dermatitis, allergic rhinitis, and asthma. Atopy produces IgE in response to allergens.

atrial ablation procedure which uses a catheter to determine the location of the abnormality within the heart and using radiofrequency energy, destroys the diseased tissue.

atrioventricular valves valves that lie between the atria and the ventricles.

atrium entrance (usually refers to upper chambers of the heart) (plural: atria).

atrophy to waste away.

audiology the science concerned with the sense of hearing.

auditory tube See *eustachian tube.*

aura a subjective sensation prior to a seizure, such as before an epileptic attack or a migraine headache; a warning.

aural pertaining to the ear (otic).

auricle flap of the cartilage and skin that comprises the outer ear, external ear, pinna. A portion of the atrium of the heart. (Sometimes used to refer to the entire atrium.)

auscultation externally listening to sounds from within the body to determine abnormal conditions, as *auscultation* of blood pressure, or breath sounds, or bowel sounds with a stethoscope.

autism a condition marked by preoccupation with inner thoughts and withdrawal from the outside world.

autistic savant an individual who has severe mental disabilities but has exceptional abilities in areas such as mathematics, art, memory, or music.

autoclave a pressure steam sterilizer.

autocratic leadership leadership style that is self-directed and calls for little input from others.

autograft a graft that is transplanted from one place to another on the same person's body.

autoimmune allergic response of one's own body to cells or organs within the body; inability of the body to differentiate between "self" and "nonself."

autoimmune disorder disorder in which the body fails to recognize its own cells as "self" and begins to destroy them.

autologous related to self, pertaining to the same person or organism, as an *autologous* skin graft from another place on one's own body.

automated external defibrillator (AED) a portable defibrillation device designed to recognize specific cardiac dysrhythmias and initiate defibrillation (electroshock) therapy; user-friendly and available in medical facilities or public places (such as airports) for emergency treatment of major cardiac events such as asystole or severe cardiac dysrhythmias.

autonomic not subject to voluntary control, as the *autonomic* nervous system, "automatic."

autonomic dysreflexia (AD) hyperreflexia or exaggerated autonomic nervous system reflexes occurring, for example, in clients with a spinal cord injury, especially injury above T6.

autopsy examination of the body after death; postmortem.

aversion therapy a type of therapy or conditioning used to help a person give up a behavior or habit by having them associate it with something unpleasant. Has been criticized.

avulsion injury the tearing away of a structure or part of the body is pulled away from the bone. Can happen at numerous sites—forceful rotation of the head/neck away from a part of the shoulder and a knocked-out tooth are most common.

axillary relating to the armpit.

axon outgrowth of the body of a nerve cell that conducts impulses away from the cell body.

B

B cells lymphocytes that originate in the bone marrow; B lymphocytes.

Babinski reflex a reflex caused by scraping the sole of the foot (normal in a newborn; a sign of neurologic damage in an adult).

bacillus a rod-shaped bacterium (plural: bacilli).

bacteremia presence of bacteria in the blood.

bacteria microorganisms, some of which are disease-causing; common forms are staphylococci, streptococci, bacilli, and spirochetes.

bacterial vaginosis infection of the vagina caused by a gram-negative bacteria, *Gardnerella vaginalis;* also called nonspecific vaginitis; formerly known as *Haemophilus vaginalis.*

bactericidal a substance that kills bacteria.

bacteriology the study of bacteria, commonly used to denote the study of all organisms.

bacteriophage virus that destroys bacteria by lysis.

bacteriostatic a substance that arrests bacterial growth.

bacteriuria bacteria in urine.

balking refusing to do something: to stop and refuse to proceed.

Ballard score (Ballard maturational assessment) a tool used shortly after birth to assess neuromuscular maturity and physical maturity. The scores are assigned and compared with a variety of capabilities from gestational ages 26–44 weeks. The new Ballard score can assess premature maturation starting at the age of 20 weeks.

ballottement a specific palpation to test for a floating object, such as a fetus.

bandage a strip of material (gauze, tape, cloth, etc.) used to cover a wound or to hold a dressing in place, in order to give support or to apply pressure (verb: to apply a bandage, to bandage).

bargaining third stage of Kübler-Ross' stage of grief; involves developing awareness of the situation. An individual makes deals or bargains with God or with themselves. (e.g., "If I live just 2 more weeks, I can see my son get married.")

bariatric surgery the type of surgery used for weight loss.

baroreceptors sensory receptors in blood vessel walls stimulated by blood pressure changes.

Bartholin glands glands in the vagina that provide it with lubrication.

basal metabolism minimum amount of energy the body uses at rest.

base also called an alkali, a compound that contains the hydroxyl ion (OH−).

base of support balance or stability provided by the feet and their positioning.

basic cardiac life support life-saving measures such as rapid entry into emergency medical services, performance of CPR, and use of techniques to clear obstructed airway.

basic metabolic panel (BMP) various combinations of fundamental laboratory tests as defined by a specific laboratory that commonly include electrolytes (sodium, potassium, chloride), glucose, bicarbonate, carbon dioxide, plus assorted liver enzymes or kidney studies. See *comprehensive metabolic panel (CMP).*

battery physical striking or beating, as assault and *battery.*

Becker muscular dystrophy a form of muscular dystrophy that is similar to Duchenne muscular dystrophy but with less severe symptoms.

bed cradle a frame used to prevent bedclothes from touching all or part of a person's body.

beliefs concepts that a person or group thinks are true.

benign results from the growth of cells similar to the tissue in which it appears and is often surrounded by a capsule. Once removed, the tumor usually does not recur. It may be disfiguring, but it is not dangerous

benign prostatic hyperplasia (BPH) narrowing of the urethra, which results as the prostate continues to grow throughout a man's life.

benzodiazepine class of common antianxiety or minor tranquilizers medication. (Most generic names end in –pam or –lam.)

bereavement normal period of mourning or grieving following the death of a loved one.

beriberi disease of the nervous system that can lead to paralysis and death from heart failure, caused by a severe thiamine deficiency.

beta (a) endorphins hormones that have the same effect as opiate drugs, whose release is stimulated by stress and exercise.

bicuspid (mitral) valve valve between the left atrium and left ventricle formed of two tissue flaps.

bile fluid produced by the liver and stored in the gallbladder that aids in fat digestion.

biliary atresia defect in the bile ducts that prevents bile from escaping the liver.

binge drinking defined as a pattern of drinking that brings a person's blood alcohol concentration (**BAC**) to 0.08 g percent or above. See also *blood alcohol concentration.*

binuclear family a family in which a separation or divorce of the adult partners occurs, but both adults continue to assume a high level of childrearing responsibilities.

biofeedback using an electronic device to measure the effectiveness of internal exercises, such as Kegel, or to expand one's ability to control the autonomic nervous system.

biohazardous harmful to humans or animals; infectious.

biological death permanent and irreversible cessation of the body's physical and chemical processes: death at the cellular level. Organ donation is permissible and accepted within stipulated time.

biologic response modifiers (BRMs) used in immunotherapy (biotherapy). BRMs are produced by normal cells and are designed to treat assorted cancers and to repair, stimulate, or enhance substances within the immune system to kill cancer cells. See *immunotherapy*.

bionomics study of the environment and its relationship to living things.

biopsy removal of a sample of body tissue or fluid for diagnostic examination, usually microscopic; most often used to detect the presence of cancer.

biotherapy the use of biologic response modifiers (BRM) in cancer treatment.

bipolar disorder serious mental illness in which behavior alternates between extremes of happiness, energy and clarity to sadness, fatigue, and confusion.

birth assistant (sometimes also known as *doula*.) A respected individual in a community who provides emotional support, basic advice, and healthcare during pregnancy

birth attendant an individual who "attends" the expectant woman by providing basic and emergency healthcare during the prenatal months, childbirth, and the postpartum period. A variety of educational requirements, clinical training, and possible licensure examination requirements may be necessary to be called a birth attendant who, in many cases, may be called a midwife, certified midwife, or an RN specialized in obstetrics and delivery of a healthy newborn and pre- and postnatal care of the mother. See also *doula* or *birth assistant*.

birth center a free-standing option where an individual can choose to give birth.

birth plan written document in which the expectant mother expresses her desires for labor and birth.

birthing room room in a hospital in which both labor and delivery take place; also called labor/delivery/recovery/postpartum (LDRP) rooms.

bisexual sexual attraction to persons of both sexes; exhibiting both heterosexuality and homosexuality.

blackout temporary loss of vision and consciousness due to lack of blood supply to the brain and retina; sometimes refers to fainting. In relation to excessive alcohol intake, blackout refers to a total loss of memory that cannot be recalled under any circumstances.

bladder a membranous muscular sac, as the gall- or urinary-*bladder*.

bland diet diet that is limited in gastric acid stimulants.

blastocyst thin-walled hollow structure of early embryonic growth and development.

blastoma malignant tumors of immature or embryonic tissue.

blended family family that results when two people who already have children marry, blending two families into one.

blepharitis inflammation of the eyelid.

blood alcohol concentration the concentration of alcohol in blood, used as a measure of the degree of intoxication. In many states, **BAC** at 0.08% is considered intoxication for legal purposes. This level can be reached when a man consumes five or more alcoholic drinks in about 2 hr or a woman consumes four drinks in this time.

blood glucose monitoring a laboratory or home-base blood test used to determine the level of blood glucose. Often done several times per day to monitor serum glucose in a diabetic client.

blood pressure pressure of the blood on the walls of the blood vessels, expressed as systolic (contraction phase) over diastolic (relaxation phase).

body cavity a space within the body that contains internal organs.

body cue feelings experienced in response to body rhythms, self-monitoring.

body language the use of physical behavior, expressions, and mannerisms to communicate nonverbally, often done instinctively rather than consciously.

body mass index weight in kilograms divided by height in meters squared.

body mechanics use of safe and efficient methods of moving and lifting.

body temperature measure of heat inside a person's body; balance between heat produced and heat lost.

bolus a rounded mass, as an amount of food in the intestine, a pill, or a rounded pad. A dose of IV medication given quickly, as a *bolus* dose.

bonding the development of a close emotional tie, as between the parent and child.

bore a needle's inner diameter.

bottle mouth a condition of tooth erosion in infants that occurs when an infant is allowed to sleep with a bottle of milk or juice. Sugars in milk or juice cause erosion of the enamel of the teeth leading to the development of dental caries (also known as nursing bottle caries).

bowel obstruction a partly or completely blocked portion of the intestine, which may result in tissue necrosis and infarction.

Bowman capsule funnel-shaped structure that encloses the glomerulus of the kidney.

bradycardia abnormally slow heart action; slow pulse—usually defined as less than 60 bpm.

bradykinesia slowness of movement.

bradypnea condition in which breaths are abnormally slow and fall below 10 per minute.

braille an alphabet system for the nonsighted, with raised dots that one can feel with the fingers.

brain death the irreversible loss of all measurable functions or activity of the brain including the brain stem. Three main criteria apply coma, absence of brainstem reflexes, and apnea. This definition excludes comatose clients and clients in a persistent vegetative state.

brainstem part of the brain that connects the cerebral hemispheres and the spinal cord.

brain-type natriuretic peptide (BNP) laboratory test helps to confirm or exclude the diagnosis of heart failure. See also *N-terminal (NT) pro-BNP*.

brand name copyrighted name assigned by a company that makes a medication; also called trade name.

Braxton–Hicks contractions during pregnancy, naturally occurring tightening and relaxing of uterine muscles in preparation for labor and delivery; usually irregular and painless.

BRCA1, BRCA2 inherited mutated genes that can increase the likelihood of breast cancer and ovarian cancer.

breakthrough pain pain that occurs even when the client is taking around-the-clock medication for severe pain.

breech positioning of the fetus in which the buttocks or either or both feet present rather than the head.

broad-spectrum antibiotic classification of an antibiotic that is effective against many different organisms.

bronchi tubular-shaped air passages that connect the trachea and lungs (sing.: bronchus).

bronchiectasis chronic dilation of the bronchi, with large amounts of sputum production.

bronchioles smaller bronchi.

bronchiolitis inflammation of the bronchioles.

bronchitis inflammation of the bronchi.

bronchodilator a medication that causes the bronchioles to expand (dilate), thus improving respiration.

bronchoscope a lighted instrument used to examine the interior of the bronchi (bronchoscopy).

bronchoscopy invasive procedure in which a *bronchoscope* (a lighted endoscope) is advanced through the pharynx into the trachea and bronchi.

brown fat stored fat occurring only in infants born at term, used to produce heat; once it is used, the baby cannot create more.

bruit whooshing sound of high-volume blood flow

bruxism grinding of the teeth during sleep.

buccal pertaining to the cheek or mouth.

buffer a chemical system set up to resist changes, particularly in the level of hydrogen ions.

bulbourethral glands glands that secrete an alkaline mucus that lubricates the penis and neutralizes the pH of urine residue, also known as Cowper gland.

bulimia a condition in which a person eats huge amounts of food and then self-induces vomiting or uses large amounts of laxatives (binge–purge syndrome); also called bulimia nervosa.

bureaucratic leadership leadership style that is policy-minded and relies on established protocols for decision-making.

bursae a small, fluid-filled sac that prevents friction, as in *bursae* of the shoulder (plural bursae).

bursitis inflammation of a bursa.

butterfly needle a device used to draw blood from a vein or deliver IV therapy to a vein; it consists of two flexible wings, which gives the device the name "butterfly" needle attached to a connector and needle.

C

cachexia severe ill health and malnutrition; debilitated state.

Caduceus modern symbols of medicine, two sets of wings atop two serpents entwined around a staff, based on mythical figures (also known as the staff of Aesculapius).

cafe coronary misleading term for a person who dies by choking while eating.

calcaneus the largest tarsal bone located in the heel (os calcis).

calcium most abundant mineral element in the body; found especially in bones and teeth.

calculi formed from substances normally excreted by the body, such as calcium, or when certain conditions (e.g., infection, urinary retention, or prolonged immobility) are present (i.e., urinary calculi (stones), renal calculi, cystic calculi).

calices See *calyces*.

calyces cup-like extensions of the renal pelvis into which urine flows from the collecting tubules (sing.: calyx).

cancer a malignant growth, neoplasm, carcinoma.

cancer pain specific type of pain identified by IASP, caused by a malignancy; often intractable and severe; usually chronic.

candidiasis the most common cause of vaginitis, resulting primarily by an overgrowth of the normal population of the fungus *Candida albicans;* also known as moniliasis, thrush, fungal infection, and yeast infection.

canthus (inner and outer) angle at either side of the corners of the eye.

capitation fee a monthly or yearly payment made by a participant in an HMO.

Caplet a tablet in the shape of a capsule, making it easier to swallow.

capsule a small gelatinous case for holding a dose of medicine; a membranous structure enclosing another body structure, as the articular *capsule* in a joint.

caput pertaining to the head, as *caput succedaneum*.

caput succedaneum accumulation of fluid within the newborn's scalp caused by pressure to the head during delivery.

carbohydrate most widely used energy source in the world; found mostly in sugars and starches. (Made of carbon, hydrogen, and oxygen [CHO].)

carbohydrate-controlled diet approach to eating which focuses on consistency in the amount of carbohydrates consumed, especially useful in maintaining healthy blood sugar and fat levels for diabetics.

carbuncle a cluster of boils (furuncles).

carcinogen/carcinogenic an agent that causes cancer.

carcinogenesis transformation of a normal cell into a malignant cell.

carcinoma cancer, a malignant neoplasm (new growth).

cardiac pertaining to the heart.

cardiac catheterization procedure in which a catheter is passed into the heart through a large blood vessel to assess its structures or output.

cardiac sphincter muscle that guards the stomach opening.

cardinal movements mechanisms of a spontaneous delivery involving a specific spontaneous or overlapping sequence of events. The events include engagement, descent, flexion, internal rotation, extension, restitution and external rotation, and expulsion.

cardinal symptoms functions necessary to life; vital signs (temperature, pulse, respiration, and blood pressure).

cardiogenic shock a life-threatening complication sometimes occurring with an MI. The heart cannot pump effectively, and the body's unmet oxygen needs result in life-threatening hypotension and organ failure.

cardiology field of medicine that examines the cardiovascular system and its disorders.

cardiopulmonary resuscitation (CPR) a combination of external cardiac massage and artificial ventilation.

cardioversion delivery of an electric shock to the heart to restore normal rhythm; countershock; precordial shock; sometimes called defibrillation.

caregiver-controlled analgesia analgesia activated by a trained caregiver (often a family member) when the client is unable to activate their PCA pump independently.

care map plan that outlines protocols for the management of a specific disorder.

career ladder (program) community college programs that lead LPNs to an RN.

career mobility ability of a person to advance or diversify within his or her profession; career ladder.

caregiver stress a condition characterized by physical, mental, and emotional exhaustion. Usually results from a person neglecting their own physical and emotional health while they focus on caring for an ill, injured, or disabled loved one.

dental caries tooth decay.

carotene yellowish pigment contained in many foods such as squash, carrots, and green, leafy vegetables; converted to vitamin A in the body.

carotid pulse pulse felt on either side of the neck, over the carotid artery.

carpal pertaining to the wrist (carpus).

cartilage fibrous connective tissue in joints.

case management providing high-quality care while effectively using healthcare resources and controlling costs.

case manager a person who plans and directs all necessary activities to coordinate a client's care.

cast an appliance used to immobilize displaced or injured parts; a fatty, waxy, or epithelial substance formed in the urinary system and found (abnormally) in urine; a mold or impression, as of the jaw, used to make braces or dentures.

catabolism the destructive phase of metabolism; breaking down.

catalepsy state in which a person maintains the body position in which he or she is placed.

cataplexy abrupt attacks of muscular weakness and decreased strength.

cataract an opacity of the lens of the eye or its capsule.

catastrophic reaction display of excessive agitation that a person with dementia may experience when confronted with a difficult, overwhelming situation, or just feeling rushed and confused.

catatonia stupor (a state of insensibility or responsiveness) and muscle rigidity associated with mental illness. May involve repetitive or purposeless overactivity.

catecholamines neurotransmitters that increase cardiac output, constrict peripheral blood vessels, increase blood pressure, and cause bronchodilation in response to stress.

cathartic a medicine that causes bowel evacuation, laxative, purgative.

catheter a flexible tube that is passed into the body, usually through body channels, for the withdrawal or instillation of fluids; most often refers to urinary catheter.

catheterization procedure to insert a catheter into the client's body.

cation an ion that carries a positive electrical charge.

caustic something that is able to burn or corrode organic tissue by chemical action.

cavity a hollow space within the body or one of its organs.

cecum a pouch 2–3 in. long that forms the first portion of the large intestine.

celiac disease chronic intestinal disorder which involves small bowel inflammation and is the most common nutrient malabsorption syndrome in children of European descent.

cell the minute protoplasmic building unit of living matter; the body's basic structural unit.

cell membrane surface layer that surrounds the cells' outer boundary and regulates what enters and leaves the cell, also known as the plasma membrane.

cell-mediated immunity type of immunity in which T cells have proliferated and become capable of combining with specific foreign antigens.

cellular respiration exchange of oxygen for carbon dioxide within the cells.

Celsius temperature scale in which water boils at 100 degrees and freezes at zero (formerly centigrade). "Normal" oral body temperature is 37 °C. Celsius scale is most often used in healthcare facilities.

center of gravity the center of one's weight; half of one's body weight is below and half above, and half to the left, and half to the right of the center of gravity. This concept is important in body mechanics.

central line Devices that can be used long-term to deliver fluid into a large central vein or directly into the heart.

central nervous system brain and spinal cord.

central venous pressure a type of hemodynamic monitoring that provides a general estimation of the amount of blood returning to the heart and the ability of the heart to pump blood into the arterial system; it provides treatment guidelines for disorders such as heart failure and acute pulmonary edema.

cephalalgia head pain.

cephalhematoma newborn condition in which blood accumulates between the bones of the skull and the periosteum.

cephalocaudal literally, "head to toe" (used to denote developmental progression in infants).

cerclage nonabsorbable suture placed around an incompetent cervix to hold it closed for the duration of pregnancy.

cerebellum part of the brain located on the back of the brain stem. It has three lobes, one median (*vermis*) and two laterals (hemispheres).

cerebral cortex outside of the brain made of soft gray matter containing mostly nerve cell bodies.

cerebral lobes four lobes of the brain that enable humans to associate impressions and information, which becomes knowledge.

cerebrospinal fluid a lymph-like fluid that forms a protective cushion around and within the central nervous system.

cerebrum the major portion of the brain, comprising 80% of its volume.

certified nurse midwife (CNM) a nursing specialty and designation in obstetrics indicating that a registered nurse has received specialized, advanced training in the management of pregnancy, labor, and birth. To use this designation, the RN must successfully complete advanced theory and clinical nursing education and have passed the comprehensive nursing certification requirements.

cerumen waxy substance that collects in the outer ear canal; ear wax.

ceruminal glands specialized glands found only in the passage that leads into the ear that function to protect the eardrum by producing cerumen.

cervical os mouth or opening of the cervix.

cervicitis inflammation of the uterine cervix.

cervix the narrow lower end of the uterus, which opens into the vagina.

cesarean delivery surgical procedure to deliver a baby through an incision in the abdomen and uterus.

Chadwick sign a cervix that looks blue or purple which may occur as early as the sixth week of pregnancy.

chain-of-command hierarchy of an organizational structure.

chalazion a small mass on the eyelid caused by inflammation of a meibomian gland.

chancre hard, primary lesion which is the first sign of syphilis.

chancroid soft sore caused by *Haemophilus ducreyi* and generally spread by sexual contact.

change-of-shift reporting a means of exchanging information between outgoing and incoming staff on each shift.

chart audit an evaluation of outcomes of care from the client's point of view.

charting by exception type of narrative charting that usually uses a flow sheet listing the body systems and their typical findings, such as lung sounds: clear, crackles, or rhonchi. The nurse checks the correct finding in the preprinted box.

chelation a process for treating poisoning with a metal such as lead (plumbism), in which the chelating agent and the metal combine, become soluble, and can be eliminated. (Also used to remove excess iron in sickle cell anemia.)

chemical change a change that alters a substance's chemical composition.

chemical dependency substance abuse, with tolerance, withdrawal, and other indicative symptoms.

chemical name medication name that describes its chemical composition (often same as generic name).

chemical restraint medications that are given to control behavior when a client poses a threat to himself or others. Should only be used as a last resort in a violent situation.

chemotherapy use of chemical agents to destroy cancerous cells.

chest the thorax; the part of the body that lies between the neck and the abdominal cavity.

Cheyne–Stokes respiration breathing characterized by deep breathing alternating with very slow breathing or apnea; indicative of brain damage; often precedes death.

chlamydia sexually transmitted infection caused by the bacteria *Chlamydia trachomatis,* that is, the leading cause of preventable infertility in women and the most common STI in the United States. "Silent STI"

chloasma hyperpigmentation (darker coloration) in particular skin areas, such as the "mask of pregnancy" or the linea nigra in pregnancy (*chloasma gravidarum*). (Also called melasma.)

chloride elemental ion needed for the production of stomach acid and the body's complex buffering system.

choanal atresia condition in which the newborn's nostrils are closed at the entrance to the throat so that air cannot pass through to the lungs.

cholecystic pertaining to the gallbladder.

cholelithiasis gallstones.

cholesterol a steroid alcohol found only in animal tissues, needed to produce hormones, vitamin D, and bile acids; has been connected with atherosclerotic disease.

chorea nervous condition characterized by twitching in the limbs or face, as in Huntington chorea (also known as Huntington disease).

choriocarcinoma type of cancer of the uterus or at the site of an ectopic pregnancy that may develop as the result of hydatidiform mole.

chorion the outermost cell layer that surrounds the embryo and fluid cavity.

chorionic villus sampling a prenatal test in which a sample of chorionic villi from the placenta is obtained.

chromosome body in the nucleus of the cell that carries genetic factors.

chronic a condition that remains for a length of time, maybe progressive.

chronic disease/illness a disease of long duration that generally manifests itself in an individual as recurring problems that tend to worsen in severity over time.

chronic pain pain that lasts more than 6 months; neuropathic pain.

chronic ulcerative colitis relatively common disorder in adolescents and young adults characterized by inflammation of the colon and rectum.

Chvostek sign abnormal spasms of the facial muscles in response to light taps on the facial nerve; indicative of tetany following thyroidectomy.

chyme partially digested food as it enters the duodenum.

cilia hair-like threads that sweep materials across a cell.

circumcise/circumcision usually refers to surgical removal of the foreskin (prepuce) of the penis.

circumduction circular movement of a limb or the eye.

circumoral cyanosis darkening of skin color, particularly around the eyes, nose, and mouth due to poor oxygenation.

cirrhosis a late stage of scarring (fibrosis) of the liver caused by many forms of liver diseases and conditions, one of which is excessive alcohol consumption.

claudication cramps that occur because of an insufficient supply of oxygen, as in intermittent *claudication*.

clavicle the collar bone.

clean in medical asepsis, devoid of all gross contamination and free of many microorganisms.

cleft lip vertical opening in the upper lip.

cleft palate congenital split in the roof of the mouth.

client a person who is a participant in his or her healthcare.

client-oriented focused on meeting individualized needs.

client reminder/safety device See *protective device*.

client unit area where most client care is provided.

climacteric cessation of reproductive function in the female (menopause), and decreased testicular activity in the male.

clinical breast examination a breast examination conducted by a healthcare provider.

clinical care path planning method that identifies the optimal sequencing and timing of healthcare interventions; designates interventions for all members of a healthcare team, not just nurses.

clinical death absence of heartbeat and cessation of breathing: may be reversible if achieved within 4–6 min. Organ donation is permissible and accepted within stipulated time

clitoris small structure of erectile tissue in the female at the anterior junction of the labia that is stimulated by sexual excitement.

clonic phase rhythmic jerking movements which alternate with a tonic phase of rigid contraction of body muscles during a seizure; known as tonic-clonic or grand-mal seizure (most life-threatening seizure).

closed bed bed used when preparing a unit for a new client—an unoccupied bed.

closed-ended questions questions that can usually be answered by one word, such as "yes" or "no," or a rating scale (such as from strongly agree to strongly disagree); they usually give limited insight.

cluster care nursing care planned so that several nursing functions can be done during each episode of contact with a high-risk infant.

coagulation the changing of a liquid to thickened, curd-like form.

coccus a round or spherical bacterium (plural: cocci).

coccyx tailbone.

cochlea snail-shaped organ of the inner ear; the essential organ of hearing.

code a predetermined phrase or term used by healthcare professionals in an emergency situation that is activated to alert specific personnel to act in the identified situation.

codependency a behavioral condition where the person takes on a "caretaker" role, often to the loss of ones-self; this can happen when the loved one is involved in addiction or abuse.

cognitive involving knowledge, understanding, and perception; in the mind.

cognitive function ability to think and reason.

cognitive deficits describes any characteristic that acts as a barrier to the cognition process.

cognitive impairment trouble remembering, learning new things, concentrating, or making decisions that affect everyday life. May range from mild to severe.

cogwheeling movements abnormal muscular rigidity that manifests as jerky movements when the muscle is passively moved; can be a side effect of psychotropic medications.

cohabitation unmarried individuals in a committed partnership living together, with or without children.

coitus interruptus withdrawal of the penis from the vagina before ejaculation.

colic paroxysmal abdominal pain, most commonly occurring in the first 3 months of an infant's life; or severe, penetrating lower back pain, caused by a stone becoming lodged in the ureter (renal colic).

collaborative problem problem in which nurses work with physicians or other healthcare providers.

collagen white, tough, fibrous structural protein found in tendons, bone cartilage, skin, and other connective tissues, as well as in the vitreous humor of the eye.

collagen diseases diseases of the connective tissue.

collateral circulation circulation that occurs when one blood vessel is plugged and another evolves to take over its function, usually in the heart.

colloid solutions solutions used to replace circulating blood volume; also called plasma expanders.

colon a continuous tube divided into three parts that forms the longest portion of the large intestine.

colonization microorganisms present in a person who shows no signs or symptoms of illness.

colonoscopy procedure in which a scope is passed into the rectum to allow visualization of the colon.

colostomy an artificial opening from the colon to outside the body by way of a stoma.

colostrum the first fluid secreted by the mammary (breast) glands just before or after childbirth.

colposcopy Insertion of a lighted, magnified speculum (colposcope) into the vaginal vault, which allows better visualization of the vagina and cervix than with the regular speculum.

command center place that provides overall direction of a facility's activities in a disaster.

commitment/civil commitment involuntary admittance to a mental healthcare facility following certification by appropriate mental health authorities. The process may be voluntary but is generally involuntary.

commode toilet; bedside toilet.

communal family family where many people live together, strive to be self-sufficient, and minimize contact with the outside society.

communicable disease a disease that can be transmitted from one person to another.

communication giving, receiving, and interpreting information (may be verbal or nonverbal).

community a collection of people who interact with one another and whose common interests or characteristics form the basis for a sense of unity or belonging.

community health aggregate health of a population.

commuter family a family in which both adults are usually professionals, one of whom lives in another city because of employment, and the partners must travel a long distance, usually on weekends, to be together.

comorbidity coexisting disorders.

compartment syndrome disorder that results from inadequate or obstructed blood flow to muscles, nerves, and tissue; may also stem from compression of the muscle compartment or from an increase in contents related to edema, hemorrhage, fracture, or soft tissue injury.

compassion fatigue caregivers suffer emotional and sometimes, physical breakdown, resulting from the stress of constant care of a loved one; this is also common in nurses who deal with death and dying on a frequent basis.

complement a group of proteins normally present but inactive in the blood.

complement fixation mechanism for antigen destruction by which activated complements destroy invaders.

complementary healthcare methods and beliefs other than traditional Western medicine.

compliance muscle activity and stretch of the bladder wall; also known as accommodation.

complication an unexpected event in a disease's course that delays a person's recovery.

compound substance composed of two or more elements united according to chemical weights; they undergo chemical change (elements lose their original characteristics).

comprehensive metabolic panel (CMP) various combinations of fundamental and specific laboratory tests that commonly include electrolytes (sodium, potassium, chloride), glucose, bicarbonate, carbon dioxide, plus assorted liver enzymes or kidney studies. See *basic metabolic panel (BMP)*.

compulsion a repetitive behavior or mental act that a person feels driven to perform, sometimes constantly.

conception union of two sex cells: the ovum (female) and the sperm (male).

concussion violent jar or shock, or the injury that results.

conduction carrying or conveying energy, such as heat, electricity, or sound.

conduction anesthesia a form of regional anesthesia, also known as conduction block.

condylomata acuminata venereal warts that grow in warm, moist body areas and are often spread by sexual contact.

cones specialized neurons concentrated in the retina's center that receive color, add visual acuity, and require a significant amount of light to function.

confabulate to fabricate or make up imaginary experiences to make up for loss of memory.

confidentiality information a client shares with a professional, expecting the information to remain with that person alone.

confusion a symptom that causes difficulty focusing, making decisions, thinking clearly, or feeling safe.

congenital disorders existing at birth (may be genetic/inherited or acquired), as in *congenital disorders*.

congenital syphilis pertains to infants who are born with syphilis. They may not have symptoms at birth but develop them within a few weeks. Infected infants may be stillborn. Infants who survive infancy tend to have skeletal deformities, neurologic problems, speech and motor delays, or seizures.

congregate housing a special high rise or other building designated for a specific group.

congruence agreement, consistency, or compatibility with other information.

congruent communication when the words, tone, and body language are completely aligned to make one message.

conization removal of a cone-shaped portion of the cervix.

conjunctiva transparent mucous membrane covering the anterior eye (front).

conjunctivitis commonly called pink eye; inflammation and redness of the conjunctiva.

conscious sedation condition in which internal sedative medications are used alone or in conjunction with local anesthetics and the client has a depressed level of consciousness but is still able to breathe and respond to verbal stimuli.

consortium public and private organizations who share data and workers to provide more cost-efficient healthcare.

constipation difficult or infrequent and hardened bowel movements.

consumer fraud misleading the public.

contact precautions precautions taken against diseases that can be transmitted through direct contact between a susceptible host's body surface and an infected or colonized person. Common measures include the use of personal protective equipment.

contagious able to be transmitted from one person to another, infectious.

contaminate to make unsterile or unclean.

contaminated anything that is not sterile.

continuous passive motion (CPM) machine that provides exercise for a limb without active participation by client or nurse.

contraceptive artificial prevention of pregnancy.

contractility ability to shorten and become thicker.

contractions tightening of the muscle fibers of the uterus to bring about the birth of the fetus.

contracture a condition of shortened, hardened muscles, tendons, or other tissue that leads to deformity and rigidity of joints.

contralateral the opposite side.

contusion injury without breaking the skin; a bruise.

convection spread/transmission of heat in a liquid or gas by circulation of heated particles.

convoluted tubule long, twisted tube extending from Bowman capsule, through which water travels in the kidneys.

copay predetermined fee that is charged to HMO clients at the time of an office visit.

coprolalia continuous uttering of obscenities.

copulation sexual intercourse between male and female.

core measures reclassified as accountability measures, they are sets of actions based on evidenced-based quality of care and best possible outcomes. See also *accountability measures.*

corium the dermis, "true skin," the fibrous inner layer of skin just under the epidermis; thickest skin layer

cornea the transparent front covering of the eye, as in corneal transplant.

coronary artery disease (CAD) cardiovascular disease involving narrowing of the arteries.

coronary sinus opening in the heart which returns blood to the right atrium.

corpus callosum a band of approximately 200 million neurons connecting the brain's right and left hemispheres.

cortex outer layer. See also *renal cortex.*

corticosteroids compounds secreted by the outer part of the adrenal glands.

crackle on auscultation, an abnormal discontinuous nonmusical respiratory sound heard on inspiration; formerly called rale.

cranial pertaining to the skull, as *cranial* nerves.

cranial nerves one of two sets of nerve groups that comprise the peripheral nervous system; these nerves originate in the brain.

craniotomy any operation into the cranium (skull), "brain surgery."

crash cart a cart or rolling chest containing emergency medications and equipment.

crime an illegal act; a felony or misdemeanor; an offense which is against the law.

crisis the turning point of a disease; sudden drop of fever and improvement of client's symptoms.

critical thinking mix of inquiry, knowledge, intuition, logic, experience, and common sense.

cross-match testing of donor blood against a recipient's blood to determine compatibility.

cross-sensitivity the characteristic of a medication that reacts similarly to a related drug; common adverse effects.

crowning in childbirth, the appearance of the top of the baby's head at the vaginal opening.

cryosurgery removal of tissue by destroying it through freezing.

cryptorchidism undescended testicles.

crystalluria crystals in the urine.

cue feeling that one experiences by listening to one's body rhythms.

culdoscopy examination of the (internal) female viscera by means of an endoscope inserted through the posterior vaginal fornix.

cultural competence sensitivity to cultural factors involved in a person's health or illness.

cultural diversity state in which a group has members from many different cultural, ethnic, and religious backgrounds.

cultural sensitivity understanding and tolerating all cultures and lifestyles.

culture growing of microorganisms in specific media; the product of culture growth; the concepts, habits, skills, and institutions of a given group of people (civilization).

cultured epithelial autograft grafts made from a biopsy of unburned skin and grown on new skin; useful in covering extensive burns.

curandero a layperson, in Latino cultures, who assists a client with herbs and counseling during an illness.

Cushing syndrome condition that results from overproduction of hormones secreted by the adrenal gland. Signs and symptoms include a rounded face, heavy abdomen, thin arms and legs, weakness, soft bones, edema, hypokalemia, and urinary retention.

cutaneous pertaining to the skin.

cyanosis blueness or duskiness of the skin usually caused by oxygen deficiency and excess carbon dioxide in the blood.

cyclothymic disorder mild form of bipolar disorder (i.e., characterized by less extreme periods of overactivity and depression).

cylindruria cylinders (casts) in the urine.

cystectomy removal of the entire bladder.

cystic fibrosis congenital multisystem chronic and incurable condition characterized by the dysfunction of the exocrine glands. Mucus producing glands secrete abnormal quantities of thick mucus which collect in the lungs, pancreas, and liver, disrupting their normal functioning.

cystitis inflammation of any bladder (most often refers to urinary bladder).

cystocele herniation of the urinary bladder into the vagina.

cystogram a radiograph of the bladder and urethra.

cystometrogram measurement of bladder pressure during filling.

cystoscope device which has a mirror and an electric lamp or fiberoptic lens on its end used to examine the bladder.

cystoscopy examination of the inside of the bladder.

cytokine a specific protein involved in cell-to-cell communication that coordinates antibody and T cell immune interactions and/or amplifies immune reactions (e.g., colony-stimulating factors, interferons, interleukins, and lymphokines [secreted by lymphocytes]).

cytology the study of cells.

cytomegalovirus, CMV a group of host-specific herpes viruses, causing many different symptoms.

cytoplasm area of the cell not located in the nucleus.

D

dangling positioning of a client so that he or she is sitting on the edge of the bed with legs down and feet supported by a footstool or the floor. This is an exercise in preparation for sitting in a chair and/or walking.

data analysis analyzing each piece of information to determine its relevance to a client's health problems and its relationship to other pieces of information.

debridement removal of foreign, dead, and contaminated material from a wound, so as to expose healthy underlying tissue and aid in healing.

debulking removing part of a tumor.

decanoate injectable long-lasting psychotropic medications.

decidua the endometrium during pregnancy.

decimal fraction fraction in which ten is always the denominator.

decrement A phase of labor during which the uterine contraction eases until the resting state is achieved.

decubitus ulcer See *pressure wound*.

decussation crossing.

defecation excretion of feces.

deficiency needs An individual's basic (physical) needs and are a priority.

defense mechanisms reactions to stress that help individuals resolve mental conflicts, reduce anxiety, protect self-esteem, and maintain a sense of security.

deglutition swallowing.

dehiscence opening or separation of the surgical incision.

dehumanization to make a person/client feel like an object, to remove one's dignity.

dehydration lack of fluid/water in the body.

delirium a sudden change in mental status, usually temporary, marked by forgetfulness, wandering speech, delusions, excitement, and at times, hallucinations.

delirium tremens symptoms that appear in the third stage of alcohol withdrawal that include delusions, vivid hallucinations, along with severe physical effects.

delivery forceps double-bladed curved instruments that fit around the fetal head and are used to increase traction and assist in rotating the fetus during delivery.

delusion a false belief that cannot be corrected by reason. Delusion maybe transient, as in delirium, or highly elaborate as in delusional disorders. They are not primarily logical errors but are usually derived from emotional material.

dementia gradual organic loss of intellectual function; A collective term used to describe various symptoms of cognitive decline. It is not a single disease in itself.

democratic leadership leadership style that is people-oriented and tries to guide others in the right direction.

demography study of population trends, including births, deaths, and diseases.

demographics study of characteristics and changes in a population.

dendrite nerve branch that conducts impulses toward the cell body.

denial preliminary stage of Kübler-Ross' stage of grief occurs when the person does not believe that the diagnosis is correct: *This can't be happening to me*.

denominator bottom number in a fraction.

dentin bone-like substance, which is the bulk of tooth material.

deoxyribonucleic acid (DNA) a complex acid occurring in the nucleus of all cells, which is the basic structure of genes and carries the genetic code.

dependent actions actions that nurses must follow explicitly according to healthcare provider's orders.

dependent edema a type of swelling promoted by body positioning. If the client is sitting up or walking, the feet, ankles, or legs swell. If the client is supine, the edema is in the posterior muscles, for example, buttocks.

depressant medication that slows down certain mental and physical processes.

depression fourth stage of Kübler-Ross' stage of grief in which the person realizes that they are going to die and that nothing can be done to stop it. The sentiment of this phase would be *I am so sad, I have no hope of recovery*.

dermabrasion surgical means of smoothing the skin, used to minimize scarring.

dermatitis inflammation of the skin; rash.

dermatology study of the skin and its diseases.

dermis the "true skin," or thickest skin layer; corium.

desquamation the shedding or scaling of the skin or cuticle; peeling.

detachment the final stage of dying when an individual gradually separates from the world, so that a two-way communication no longer exists with those around them; becoming disconnected.

detoxification a therapeutic procedure that reduces or eliminates toxic substances (often alcohol, opioids) in the body; procedures vary relating to which toxic substance was imbibed; also called *detox*.

detrusor muscle of the bladder that pushes urine out.

development change in body function.

developmental delay a significant delay in the achievement of childhood developmental milestones (tasks) that may affect language or speech, motor coordination, social and emotional development, and cognitive skills. It does not refer to slight or temporary lapses of development. See *developmental milestone (tasks)*.

developmental disability assorted physical, cognitive, psychological, sensory, and speech impairments that affect about 17% of children under 18 years of age.

developmental milestone a specific ability that marks a particular stage of development, in such areas as cognitive skills, language, speech, fine and gross motor coordination, and social and emotional skills. Developmental milestones are reached in predictable patterns and within general age-related timeframes. See *developmental task, developmental delay*.

developmental task See *developmental milestone*.

diabetes a disease characterized by great increase in urinary discharge and increased blood glucose; usually refers to *diabetes* mellitus; may also refer to *diabetes insipidus*.

diabetes insipidus disease that results from an underproduction of antidiuretic hormone.

diabetes mellitus metabolic condition involving elevated levels of glucose in the blood.

diabetic ulcer ulceration occurring in persons with diabetes mellitus, partly as a result of impaired circulation, usually difficult to heal (diabetic neuropathic ulcer).

diagnosis recognition of a disease by its signs and symptoms, made by a healthcare provider.

diagnosis-related group (DRG) grouping of medical diagnoses to determine level of payment by an agency such as Medicare.

dialysis diffusion of dissolved molecules through a semipermeable membrane (most often refers to treatment given to remove waste products from the blood of a client who suffers from renal failure).

diaparesis weakness affecting the symmetrical parts of the body.

diaphoresis perspiration or sweating, particularly profuse perspiration.

diaphragm the muscular partition between the thoracic and abdominal cavities, important in breathing; a type of female contraceptive device; a part of a stethoscope.

diaphysis shaft of a long bone.

diplegia symmetrical paralysis of corresponding parts on both sides of the body (e.g., both legs or both arms).

diarrhea expulsion of loose, watery, unformed stools.

diastole a rhythmically recurrent expansion especially the atrial and ventricular relaxation, which allows the chambers of the heart to fill with blood.

diastolic pressure of the blood against the arterial walls when the heart is at rest between beats (the lower number recorded in a blood pressure reading).

differentiation the process of growth and development that occurs in immature or stem cells that have recently left their origination site, for example, bone marrow. The stem cell becomes more complex, altered, or changed to suit the specific needs of tissues. A normal cell is well-differentiated.

diffusion state of being widely spaced; the process whereby molecules move in an effort to equalize the concentration of a liquid or gas.

digestion process of converting food into chemical substances for assimilation and absorption by body tissues.

digital rectal examination (DRE) part of the male's physical examination to gain basic knowledge about the size of the prostate; performed by inserting a gloved hand into the rectum and feeling the tissues of the rectal wall, which are adjacent to the prostate

dilation action of expanding, as in *dilation* and curettage or *dilation* of blood vessels, vasodilation. (Dilation and dilatation are often used interchangeably.)

dilation and curettage expansion of the cervix and scraping of the walls of the uterus to remove material such as polyps or as in an abortion.

diluent liquid solution used to reconstitute injectable medications that have been prepared as powders.

diphtheria contagious infection characterized by sore throat, fever, and malaise. Manifestations also include throat inflammation followed by formation of a whitish-gray membrane that cannot be removed without causing bleeding and a possible weakening of cardiac muscles.

diplopia double vision.

dirty any object or person that has not been cleaned or sterilized for removal of microorganisms.

disaccharide a double sugar molecule.

disaster medical assistance team (DMAT) team that provides assistance and support in emergencies both inside and outside healthcare facilities.

discharge planning process by which a client is prepared for continued care after discharge from a healthcare facility.

discipline area (multidisciplinary) documentation documentation style that includes a separate note for healthcare providers, nurses, and other healthcare team members, such as dietary, respiratory therapy, physical therapy, occupational therapy, or home health providers.

disease a deviation or departure from normal body structure or function that is characterized by certain signs and symptoms; cause and prognosis may be known or unknown; illness.

disease management program plan that outlines protocols for the management of a specific disorder.

disinfection cleaning process that destroys most pathogens but not necessarily their spores.

dislocation separation of two bones where they meet at a joint; a dislocated joint is a joint where the bones are no longer in their normal positions.

distal furthest from the origin of a part.

distention swelling or fullness, as in urinary distention.

diuresis increased urinary output.

diuretic medication that increases the amount of urine excreted by the kidneys.

diverticulitis inflammation of a diverticulum (outpouching or sac in a mucous membrane), often referring to the colon (plural: diverticula).

diverticulosis the condition of having diverticula, without inflammation.

domestic violence abuse or violence that occurs within the home. See *intimate partner violence.*

Doppler electronic stethoscope, which converts ultrasonic frequencies into either audible frequencies or projects them onto a video monitor, used to detect fetal heart tones as early as the 10th week of pregnancy.

dorsal posterior or backside.

dorsal recumbent lying on the back with knees flexed.

dorsiflexion bending a body part toward the dorsum (backward), as in moving the foot, so the toes are pulled toward the knee and thus facing backward.

dosage an amount in a prescription that contains the dose and the scheduled time.

dose a single amount of a medication administered to achieve a therapeutic effect.

double-balloon enteroscopy procedure that examines the small intestine via an oral or an anal route.

doula also known as a birth assistant, birth worker, labor support person, or childbirth educator, who is traditionally a respected woman in the community who provides emotional support, basic advice, and healthcare during pregnancy. This woman assists the birth attendant or the midwife.

Down syndrome congenital abnormality characterized by specific physical defects and by varying degrees of intellectual impairment; also called trisomy 21.

drain tube or strip of material inserted into a wound to aid in elimination of exudate.

drainage discharge from a wound.

droplet precautions precautions taken to prevent the spread of diseases transmitted by microorganisms propelled through the air from an infected person and deposited on the host's eyes, nose, or mouth.

drowning suffocation from submersion in liquid.

drug substance other than food used to prevent disease, to aid in the diagnosis and treatment of disease, and to restore or maintain functions in body tissues. Also called medication.

drusen yellow, lipid deposits that develop between the retinal epithelium and the choroid layer; often the first signs of age-related macular degeneration.

dual-career/dual-earner family nuclear family in which both parents work.

dual diagnosis two separate distinct disorders that are present at the same time; has commonly come to mean mental illness, such as depression, coexisting with substance dependence disorder.

Duchenne muscular dystrophy the most common degenerative muscle disorder in children; symptoms include developmental delay, using upper extremities to compensate for weak hip muscles, walking on the toes, or falling frequently.

ductus arteriosus connection between the pulmonary artery and aorta that allows for shunting of blood around the fetal lungs.

ductus deferens tubes that transport sperm from the epididymis to the ejaculatory ducts.

ductus venosus short duct is found only in the fetus and atrophies after birth.

due process procedures that ensure fair labor practices and prevent frivolous or punitive actions against employees by employers.

dumping syndrome immediate discomfort caused by overeating or eating foods that are not recommended after surgery.

duodenum proximal (first) portion of the small intestine.

duration spanning a length of time, as in *duration* of a contraction during labor.

dysarthria speech and language disorder.

dysfluency interruption in the natural flow of speaking.

dysfunctional abnormal or impaired action or interaction.

dysfunctional family family whose coping systems disintegrate as stressors build.

dyskinesia involuntary (unintended) movements or rapid and jerky movements of the muscles such as a tic or spasm.

dyskinetic cerebral palsy type of cerebral palsy characterized by abnormal involuntary movements and difficulty with speech caused by involuntary facial movements; also called athetoid cerebral palsy.

dyslexia disorder in which one has difficulty reading, spelling, or writing words and often reverses letters or numbers.

dysmenorrhea difficult or painful menstruation.

dyspareunia pain upon sexual intercourse.

dyspepsia indigestion.

dysphagia difficulty in swallowing.

dysphasia difficulty in understanding or expressing language.

dysphonia difficulty speaking due to a physical disorder of the mouth, tongue, throat, or vocal cords.

dysplasia abnormal development; alteration in shape.

dyspnea difficulty in breathing—a tightening of the chest, air hunger, breathlessness, or a feeling of suffocation; may be caused by very strenuous exercise, extreme temperatures, obesity, and higher altitude in a healthy person.

dysrhythmia lacking rhythm, without rhythm, as in an irregular heartbeat.

dysthymia any depressed mood that is mild or moderate in severity. Also called minor depression.

dystocia ineffective contractions.

dystonia impairment of normal muscle tone, causing prolonged muscle contraction that results in abnormal posture, twisting, or repetitive movements.

dysuria difficult or painful urination or voiding.

E

ecchymosis bleeding into the tissues under the skin, leaving small bruises.

echocardiography recording of activity and location of the heart by means of ultrasound.

echolalia automatic repeating of what has been said.

echopraxia involuntary imitation of the movements of other people.

eclampsia seizure disorder with high blood pressure, usually related to a complication of pregnancy, pregnancy-induced hypertension (PIH).

ecology study of the interrelationship of organisms and their environment.

ectopic pregnancy pregnancy which implants outside the uterus.

ectropion turning outward (eversion) of an edge.

eczema an inflammatory skin rash, characterized by itching, redness, weeping, oozing, and crusting, and later by scaling.

edema abnormal fluid accumulation in the intercellular tissue spaces of the body; fluid excess.

effacement thinning of the cervix in preparation for delivery.

effectors neurons that carry out activity in response to messages relayed by sensory neurons.

efferent conducting away from the center, as an *efferent* nerve.

egestion process by which wastes are eliminated (also known as defecation).

egg-crate mattress a foam pad, shaped like an egg carton, which is used on the top of a regular bed mattress to provide comfort.

ejaculation forceful expulsion of semen from the ejaculatory ducts to the urethra during sexual excitement.

elasticity ability to return to normal length after stretching.

elder abuse emotional, physical, sexual abuse, financial exploitation, or neglect of older adults.

elective (surgery) case in which the client's condition is not life-threatening and may choose whether or not to have surgery; also called optional surgery.

electrical stimulation use of an electrical impulse to strengthen pelvic muscles and decrease bladder activity that causes urge incontinence.

electrocardiogram (ECG) the graphic record of minute electrical currents generated within the heart's conduction system, indicating *depolarization* and *repolarization* as the heart beats.

electrocauterization destruction of malignant tissues by burning.

electroconvulsive therapy (ECT) administration of an electric shock to induce convulsions (seizures) as a treatment, usually for clinical depression.

electrodesiccation removal of tissue using intermittent electric sparks.

electroencephalogram (EEG) recording of the brain's electrical activity.

electrolyte a chemical substance that dissociates into electrically charged ions (positive ions are called *cations*; negative ions are called *anions*) when melted or in solution (becomes capable of conducting electricity).

electromyogram (EMG) recording of electrical activity of muscles.

electron subatomic particle carrying a negative electrical charge.

electronic medical records rapid form of documentation in healthcare facilities using various, individualized, computerized formats

element a chemical substance made of atoms that cannot be further divided without losing the characteristics of the substance; the physical and chemical properties of a particular element are always the same.

elimination the act of expelling wastes from the body, voiding and defecation.

emaciation a wasting away of the flesh, causing extreme leanness, starvation (adjective: emaciated).

embolus a blood clot that is carried through the circulation to some vital organ; it can lodge in a blood vessel and cause death. (embolism; plural: emboli).

embryo a new organism in the first stage of development.

emergency medical service service to contact in life-threatening situations.

emergi-center free-standing facility that provides urgent care for clients with noncritical conditions. May also be called an urgent care center.

emerging adulthood the period between the age of about 20 years to middle age, when an individual transitions from adolescent behaviors and choices to those of a mature adult. Choices during this period include adult lifestyle (e.g., single vs. married), occupation/career, and values.

emesis the act of vomiting; the product of vomiting, vomitus.

emetic an agent that causes vomiting.

emission accumulation of sperm cells and secretions in the male urethra.

emphysema inflation or swelling of tissues due to the presence of air; usually refers to chronic pulmonary *emphysema,* a severe lung disorder.

employee right-to-know laws laws that state that employees have the right to be aware of dangers associated with hazardous substances or harmful physical or infectious agents they might encounter in the workplace.

empty calories foods that supply calories with few or no nutrients.

empyema accumulation of pus in a body cavity, often the pleural (lung) cavity.

en face **position** two individuals with heads aligning as they look at one another, as in a mother and baby in the beginning stages of bonding.

enabler a person who passively permits or unknowingly encourages maladaptive or pathological behavior (child abuse, substance abuse) in another person; person may be aware of the destructiveness of the other person's behavior but feels powerless to prevent it.

encephalalgia pain in the head; headache, cephalalgia.

encephalitis inflammation of the brain.

encephalocele condition in which the bones of the fetal skull do not close correctly.

encopresis incontinence of feces not caused by age, disease, or physical disorder.

endemic microorganisms that do not produce disease under normal conditions or are not present most or all of the time in the environment or the body.

endocarditis inflammation of the endocardium.

endocardium the inner lining of the heart and connective tissue bed around it.

endocrine pertaining to internal secretions (not into ducts or tubes); applies to organs.

endocrine glands located throughout the body, and each contains a group of specialized cells that secrete hormones, chemicals that regulate body processes, in response to body signals; these glands secrete hormones directly into the bloodstream, where they are transported throughout the body.

endocrinologist healthcare provider who specializes in the treatment of disorders of the endocrine system.

endocrinology specialty that studies endocrine glands, their secretions, and related disorders.

endocytosis engulfing of particles or dissolved substances to move them through cell walls by active transport.

endogenous normally occurring or existing within the body or in the community.

endometriosis presence of endometrial tissue in places where it is not normally found.

endometrium mucous layer of the uterus, which forms the maternal portion of the placenta during pregnancy.
endorphin a naturally occurring analgesic that the body produces in response to exercise and other stimuli.
endorsement process by which a licensed nurse in one state may receive a license to practice in another state without retaking the licensing examination.
endoscopes long, thin, flexible tubes with a light and camera at the distal end of the scope, used to view the small and large intestines.
endoscopic ultrasonography a diagnostic endoscopic procedure using sound waves to visualize the intestinal tract.
endoscopy direct visualization and photographic images of the body's interior through the intestinal tract using specialized instruments (*endoscopes*).
endotoxin a heat-stable toxin (poison) that is released when a bacterial cell is disrupted (less potent than exotoxins).
endotracheal tube (ET, ET tube) a flexible plastic tube that is used to access the upper portion of the trachea just below the vocal cords, which permits manual or mechanical ventilation of the lungs. See *intubation*.
enema an injection of solution into the rectum, usually to induce evacuation of the bowel.
engagement state in which the presenting part of the fetus has moved downward so that it cannot be pushed up and out of the pelvis.
engorgement local congestion or distention with fluids, as in *engorgement* of the breasts during pregnancy and lactation.
enteral within the intestine.
enteric pertaining to the small intestine. *Enteric-coated* tablets are covered with a substance that prevents their digestion in the stomach.
entitlement unreasonable claims to special consideration, especially as a disturbance of self-concept in *narcissistic personality disorder*.
entropion inversion, turning inward, as the turning under of the eyelid.
entry-level skills basic competencies.
enucleate to remove whole and clean; often refers to removal of an eye.
enuresis involuntary urine discharge, usually occurring during sleep; bedwetting.
environment one's surroundings, the situation in which a person lives (as opposed to heredity).
enzyme a protein produced in a cell that activates or speeds up a chemical reaction.
epicardium the inner layer of the pericardium, which is in contact with the heart.
epidemic widespread disease in a certain geographical region.
epidermis the outermost layer of the skin; protective layer.
epididymis tightly coiled tube approximately 20 ft (6 m) long; stores sperm cells.
epididymitis inflammation of the epididymis (coiled, cord-like structures in the testes through which spermatozoa are carried).
epidural common method of anesthesia during labor and delivery in which a small catheter is inserted into the epidural space within the spinal column and anesthesia is administered via this route.
epiglottis cartilage that covers the entrance to the larynx.
epilepsy a chronic disease marked by attacks of convulsions; a convulsive or seizure disorder.
epiphysis the end of a long bone.
episiotomy surgical incision into the perineum and vagina, usually during childbirth.
epispadias absence of the upper wall of the urethra resulting in an abnormal location of the urethral opening, usually occurring in the male.
epistaxis a nosebleed.
eponym a word or term based on the name of a person, such as Parkinson disease.
Epstein pearls white or grayish bumps found on the mouth's hard and soft palate in newborns.
eradicated eliminated.
erectile dysfunction inability to achieve or maintain erection sufficient to complete sexual intercourse.
erection process of the penis becoming engorged with blood and firm.
eructation belching
erythema skin redness produced by capillary congestion, as may follow a tuberculin test; bright red color associated with capillary dilation can indicate fever or infection.
erythema toxicum red raised rash that appears on the skin of some sensitive newborns.
erythroblastosis fetalis condition in which Rh-positive red blood cells from a fetus cross the placental barrier into an Rh-negative woman, causing the woman to form antibodies which return to the fetus, destroying fetal erythrocytes. *Erythroblastosis fetalis* is this condition as it manifests itself in the newborn.
erythrocyte red blood cell.
erythropoietin glycoprotein hormone produced in the adult's kidney and in the child's liver which stimulates red blood cell production; also known as renal erythropoietic factor.
eschar dead skin and tissue that slough off after a chemical or thermal burn.
esophageal atresia newborn abnormality in which the upper end of the esophagus ends in a blind pouch, making it impossible for the baby to obtain food.
esophagoscopy visualization of the esophagus through the intestinal tract using a specialized instrument.
esophagus passageway for digestion that extends from the pharynx to stomach.
essential nutrients nutrients a person must obtain through food because the body cannot make them in sufficient quantities to meet its needs.
estimated average glucose (eAG) a laboratory test that reports HA1c levels using the same units as standard handheld glucose monitors.
estrogen female hormones.
ethics code or rules of behavior.

ethnicity sense of identification of a collective cultural group based on common heritage.
ethnocentrism belief that one's own culture is the best and only acceptable way.
ethnonursing an approach to nursing that considers a client's religious and sociocultural backgrounds during treatment, also known as ethnic sensitive nursing.
etiology specific cause of a disease.
eukaryote multicellular organism, including plants and animals.
eupnea normal, good, unlabored respiration.
eustachian tube the passage from the throat to the middle ear; auditory tube.
euthanasia an easy or painless death (may be induced), often referred to as mercy death or mercy killing; deliberate ending of the life of a person who has an incurable or painful disease.
euthymia a mood of well-being and tranquility; often used to refer to a state in clients with bipolar disorder that is neither manic nor depressive, but in between.
evaluation in nursing process, measuring the effectiveness of the other steps.
evaporation process of changing a liquid or solid into a vapor (gas); to give off moisture.
eversion turning inside out; turning outward, as *eversion* of the foot.
evidence-based practice the collection and correlation of scientific research studies, clinical expertise, and client perspectives. Nursing research integrates scientific evidence with clinical and client data to achieve high-quality outcomes that formulate nursing interactions or nursing protocols.
evisceration the protrusion of the intestines through an abdominal wound; removal of the internal body contents.
exocrine secreting externally through a duct (as opposed to endocrine).
exocrine gland secrete special substances (hormones and/ or other materials) into ducts that open onto the body's external or internal surfaces and include sweat, mammary, and salivary glands, as well as mucous membranes and lacrimal (tear) glands
exogenous referring to organisms that enter from outside the body and cause infection.
exophthalmos abnormal protrusion of the eyes, most often caused by hyperthyroidism.
exoskeleton type of inflatable trousers used to help an individual maintain an upright position and prevent vascular collapse.
exotoxin a potent toxin (poison) formed by a bacteria, which can cause severe illness.
expected outcome measurable behavior that indicates whether a person has achieved the expected benefit of nursing care.
expectorant medication that liquefies secretions in the bronchi, making it easier to cough up and expel mucus.
expectoration (expectorate) spitting out and coughing up mucus or other fluid from the lungs and the throat.

expiration exhalation of air from the lungs; sometimes used to refer to death.
exstrophy congenital defect in which an organ is turned "inside out," a result of abnormal development causing exposure of the urinary bladder to the abdominal wall.
extended care facilities that extend or continue care that begins in a hospital.
extended family one's family beyond that of parents and siblings.
extensibility ability to stretch.
extension increasing the angle between two bones; the straightening of a flexed limb (opposite of flexion).
external chest compressions measures to resume the heart's action.
external condom latex, plastic, or animal sheath applied to the erect penis before sexual intercourse and used as a barrier method.
external disaster a disaster occurring outside a healthcare facility that impairs normal operation.
external respiration lung breathing.
extracellular outside the cell wall, as *extracellular* fluid.
extracorporeal outside the body.
extracorporeal membrane oxygenation (ECMO) the use of heart–lung mechanical assistance to promote and sustain cardiac and respiratory functioning for seriously ill infants.
extrapyramidal causing adverse neurologic side effects.
extremely low-birth-weight (ELBW) infants born with a birth weight of less than 1,000 g (about 2 lb 3 oz).
extrication emergency removal of a victim, performed only when the danger of injury by remaining in the same place is greater than the risk of aggravating existing injuries by moving. Also, the process of removing a person from an entrapment, usually from a motor vehicle, often requiring the use of special tools.
exudate material that escapes from blood vessels and is deposited in tissues or on tissue surfaces; usually contains protein substances.
eye contact looking another person in the eye as in keeping eye contact with the person you are talking with shows you are actively listening and paying attention. We use our eyes as a form of communication at all times.

F

facet small, flat area where bones articulate, as between vertebrae.
factitious disorder physical or mental symptoms that a client intentionally produces or feigns solely to assume the sick role.
Fahrenheit temperature scale in which water boils at 212 degrees and freezes at 32 degrees. Conversion is: Fahrenheit # subtract 32 = ___ divided by 1.8 = Celsius #
failure to thrive (FTT) a condition in which an infant or young child demonstrates inadequate physical growth and other symptoms; can result from neglect or physical disorders; marasmus.
fallopian tube See *oviducts*.

false labor also called prodromal labor; the term for Braxton Hicks contractions occurring toward the end of the pregnancy.

family two or more persons who are joined together by bonds of sharing and emotional closeness and who identify themselves as being part of that family.

fasciotomy excision of the fibrous membranes that cover and support muscles (fascia).

fat a component of foods that is composed of fatty or greasy material and that yields the highest caloric value per gram; lipid material; adipose tissue.

fat-controlled diet approach to eating which focuses on altering both the total amount and type of fat consumed in order to lower elevated levels of blood lipids.

fatigue weariness resulting from overexertion; extreme tiredness.

febrile pertaining to a fever; pyrexia.

fecal impaction stool that is so hard and dry or putty-like that it cannot be expelled by the client, even after administration of laxatives and/or enemas. See also *impaction*.

feces the residue, consisting of bacteria, secretions (chiefly of the liver), and a small amount of food residue which is discharged from the intestines; stool, bowel movement.

feedback the receipt of external stimuli as a result of output (can be verbal, nonverbal, and emotional). Physical feedback is involved in the self-regulation of hormones and electrolytes within the body.

felony a crime more serious than a misdemeanor, usually punishable by imprisonment for more than a year. Felonies include murder, euthanasia, kidnapping, and blackmail.

femoral pulse pulse felt in the groin over the femoral artery.

femur thigh bone.

fetal alcohol spectrum disorder (FASD); fetal alcohol syndrome (FAS) a group of conditions causing physical deformities, learning difficulties, and behavioral disorders relating to alcohol consumption by a mother during pregnancy.

fetal monitor electronic device that monitors the rate and quality of the fetal heartbeat during labor.

fetoscope special manual stethoscope used to detect fetal heart tones around the 18th–20th week of pregnancy.

fetus the unborn offspring in the postembryonic period from the ninth week after fertilization through birth, which is usually at about the end of the 40th week of pregnancy.

fever abnormally high body temperature. For clinical purposes when temperature is above 100.4 °F (38 °C).

fiber group name for the portion of plants resistant to digestion by human enzymes.

fibrillation a quivering of muscle fibers.

fibrin insoluble threads created by the thrombin conversion of fibrin, which form a net to entrap RBCs and platelets to form a blood clot.

fibrinogen a protein in blood plasma that is converted into fibrin by the action of thrombin. (Also called clotting factor I.)

fibrostenosis a narrowing of the intestinal lumen due to scaring and inflammation of the tissue.

fibula bone in the lower leg which is not weight-bearing.

filtration transport of water and dissolved materials through a membrane from an area of higher pressure to an area of lower pressure; this operates like a sieve.

fimbriae fringe-like ends of the oviducts that catch the ovum as it bursts from the ovary into the pelvic cavity.

fissure type of skin lesion resembling a slit or furrow.

fistula an abnormal tube-like passage that connects two internal organs, or connects an internal organ to the surface of the body; A fistula is often difficult to heal, the most common being an anal fistula in the rectal area

flaccidity brief loss of muscle tone, as in a seizure.

flagellum cellular organelle resembling a long whip which can propel bacteria in different directions in response to chemical changes in the environment (plural: flagella).

flatulence condition of having intestinal gas.

flatus gas in the intestines or stomach; gas expelled through the anus.

flexion decreasing the angle between two bones or bending a part on itself, as in bending the leg at the hip.

flotation mattress mattress or pad filled with a gel-type material which supports the body in a way to provide comfort and avoid creating pressure points, thereby helping to prevent skin breakdown.

flow sheet a form used to document client care (often contains check-off spaces for assessments/review of systems and nursing care items, as well as spaces to record items such as IV fluids, vital signs and weight, fluid intake, and client teaching).

fluid volume deficit a deficiency of fluid and electrolytes in the ECF.

fluid volume excess excessive retention of water and sodium in the ECF.

focal point specific location, as in the certain place in the brain where a seizure originates.

focus point of origin.

focus charting charting that focuses on specific problems, for example, a client reports a headache charting will focus on documentation of pain.

folliculitis staphylococcal infection starting around the hair follicle.

fontanel a soft spot in a baby's skull.

footboard vertical support at the foot of a bed helps to prevent foot drop.

foot drop contracture deformity that prevents the client from putting the heel on the floor; results from improper positioning or anterior leg muscle paralysis; abnormal plantar flexion of the foot.

foramen a natural opening or passage, as the *foramen ovale* in the fetal heart.

foramen ovale opening between the right and left atria in the fetal heart which permits most blood to bypass the right ventricle since the fetus' lungs are not yet functioning.

forceps a two-pronged surgical instrument for grasping or clamping tissues.

foremilk milk produced at the beginning of a nursing session which is relatively low in fat.

forensic pertaining to legal matters.
foreskin a loose fold of skin covering the glans penis (removed in circumcision), also called prepuce.
foster family family in which children temporarily live with paid caregivers.
Fowler examination position in which the client is lying on his or her back with the head elevated.
fraction a portion or a piece of a whole that indicates the division of that whole into equal parts; fractions can be either common fractions or decimal fractions.
fracture a break, usually in a bone.
fragile X syndrome genetic sex-linked abnormality of the X chromosome resulting in cognitive impairment and distinct physical features; the most common form of inherited mental retardation.
fraud dishonesty, cheating, deceit, misrepresentation.
freckle brown or tan macule-type spot, often accentuated by exposure to the sun, formed by patches of melanin clustered together.
frequency number of occurrences within a defined time period, as in *frequency* of contractions during labor.
friable fragile or easily bruised, torn, or broken, skin.
friction superficial abrasion, resulting from the skin rubbing another surface (results in scrape, abrasion, or blister)
frontal pertaining to the forehead or the front, anterior, or ventral portion of the body when divided longitudinally from side to side.
frontal lobe cerebral lobe that is larger in humans than in all other animals and allows for higher levels of mental functioning, including conceptualization, judgment, communication, and body movements.
frontotemporal dementia (FTD) also known as Pick disease, a type of dementia thought to be genetic, primarily affecting behaviors and language.
frostbite freezing of skin and underlying tissue caused by exposure to cold; most common on fingers, toes, nose, ears, cheeks, and chin.
fulguration destruction of malignant tissues using a high-frequency current.
functional affecting body function but not structure; also called idiopathic.
functional disease disorder in which a structural cause cannot be identified.
functional disorder a disorder for which there is no known physiological basis.
functional family a family that uses its resources to cope and become stronger under stress.
fundal height measurement of the size of the uterus.
fundus upper curve of the uterus.
furuncle a painful, localized, pus-filled skin infection originating in a gland or hair follicle (boil).

G
gait manner or style of walking.
gait belt See *transfer belt*.
galactosemia genetic absence of the enzyme necessary for metabolizing galactose.
gallbladder muscular sac on the liver's undersurface, which stores and releases bile.
gamete germ cell; reproductive cell (sperm or ova) that can unite with a gamete of the opposite sex to form a zygote (fertilized egg).
gamma globulin a type of immunization given after disease exposure that results in only short-term immunity, not specific for a certain disease; also known as immunoglobulin IgG.
ganglion a collection of knot-like nerve cell bodies located on the dorsal root of each spinal nerve (plural: ganglia).
gangrene necrosis of tissue due to insufficient blood supply.
Ganser syndrome disorder in which the client displays factitious psychological symptoms.
gastrectomy surgical procedure to remove the entire stomach (total gastrectomy) or a portion of it (partial gastrectomy; subtotal gastrectomy).
gastric bypass surgery one of the most common types of bariatric surgery, creating a small gastric pouch.
gastric lavage pumping out the stomach.
gastroscopy endoscopy of the stomach.
gastrostomy creation of an artificial opening into the stomach for the instillation of food and fluids.
gavage passing food into the stomach through a tube; forced feeding.
gay homosexual; sexually attracted to the same sex.
gay or lesbian family partners of the same sex who live or own property together, with or without children.
gene a unit of heredity within a chromosome.
general anesthesia the blockage of all body sensations, causing unconsciousness and loss of reflexes.
generalized existing throughout a system (as opposed to localized).
generativity passing on and sharing skills with younger generations.
generic name name assigned by a drug's first manufacturer; may be called the brand or proprietary name.
genetics the study of heredity in biology; the study of genes, heredity, and variation of living organisms.
genital herpes viral infection caused by herpes simplex virus type 2 (HSV-2) is characterized by recurrent episodes of painful genital sores and systemic flu-like symptoms.
geriatrics branch of medicine that focuses on healthcare of elderly people while aiming to promote health.
gerontology the study of the social, cultural, psychological, cognitive, and biological aspects of aging.
gestation period of development from fertilization to birth.
gestational age (GA) the weeks between conception and birth; the first day of the woman's last menstrual cycle to the current date determines the GA, normally from 38–42 weeks.
gestational carrier a woman who is pregnant with the embryo of a couple who are not able to give birth to an infant but who are able to donate a fertilized egg (surrogate).
gestational diabetes diabetes that a woman develops for the first time during pregnancy.

giantism (gigantism) excessive bone growth, resulting from overproduction of somatotropin (growth hormone).

giardiasis illness caused by ingesting water contaminated by human excrement.

gingival pertaining to the gum.

gland an organ that secretes or excretes hormones and other substances.

glans penis smooth cap of the penis.

glaucoma eye disease characterized by increased intraocular pressure.

glial cells See *neuroglia*.

globulin proteins that are insoluble in water or highly concentrated saline solution but which dissolve in isotonic (normal) saline.

glomerular filtration rate (GFR) a measurement of the rate of urine formation as blood is filtering through the glomeruli of the kidney.

glomerulonephritis a group of diseases in which the kidneys are damaged and partly destroyed by inflammation of the glomeruli.

glomerulus small, twisted mass of capillaries, as the *glomerulus* of the kidney (plural: glomeruli).

glucagon hormone secreted by the alpha cells, which raises blood sugar.

glucocorticoid corticosteroid that has an important influence on the synthesis of glucose, amino acids, and fats during metabolism and depresses immune response and decreases inflammatory response.

glucose simple sugar, dextrose; it is the end product of carbohydrate metabolism and the primary energy source for living organisms, found in the normal blood of all animals.

glycemic index a measurement of how foods containing carbohydrates (starchy foods such as potatoes, bread, or cereals) raise blood glucose levels. Carbohydrates are compared to a standard known carbohydrate such as glucose or white bread.

glycogen a multiple sugar (polysaccharide) that is stored in the body; animal starch.

goal-oriented establishment of objectives or specific desired outcomes early in the nursing process.

goiter an enlargement of the thyroid gland, causing a swelling in the front part of the neck.

gonad a sex gland or organ.

gonadotropic hormones hormones secreted by the gonads, which provide males and females with secondary sex characteristics and enable reproduction; also known as gonadotropins.

gonorrhea sexually transmitted disease that generally affects the genital area and urinary function of either sex and, if left untreated, can spread to bones, joints, or the bloodstream.

Good Samaritan Act law in effect in most states that protects healthcare providers from liability when performing emergency care within the limits of first aid if they act in a "reasonable and prudent manner."

Goodell sign softening of the cervix at about the eighth week of gestation.

gout arthritic condition caused when the body is unable to metabolize purines, and uric acid accumulates in the bloodstream and forms crystal deposits in the joints.

Gowers sign positive sign of muscular dystrophy exhibited by a child's need to use upper extremity muscles to compensate for weak hip muscles.

graft transplant of skin placed on clean viable tissue.

gram metric system measurement of weight.

Gram stain series of dyes used to stain a microorganism so that its features become more clearly visible and is able to be classified as either "gram negative" or "gram positive."

grandiosity an exaggerated sense of one's greatness, importance, or ability. In extreme form, it may be regarded as a *delusion of grandeur*.

grand multipara pregnant woman who has given birth at least five times.

granulation tissue new tissue that forms when old destroyed tissue is sloughed off.

Graves disease a condition that includes goiter, thyrotoxicosis, exophthalmos, and sometimes skin changes.

graphic flow sheet graph, form, or picture that records large amounts of information collected at intervals over a specified period in brief, concise entries.

gravida the number of pregnancies a woman has had.

gravital plane See *line of gravity*.

grief deep sorrow.

group A streptococci (GAS) a group of illnesses caused by group A streptococci, such as strep throat, impetigo, necrotizing fasciitis, or streptococcal toxic shock syndrome.

growth change in body structure or size; formation of abnormal tissue, such as a tumor.

growth needs secondary needs which must be met to maintain quality of life.

guaiac stool examination for blood; also known as Hemoccult.

guided imagery a type of complementary or alternative intervention; a process through which the client receives a suggestion that helps control his or her pain or disease. The person learns to visualize himself or herself as powerful and able to conquer pain or disease.

gurney See *litter*.

gustation sense of taste.

gynecology the branch of medicine that treats diseases of the genital tract in women.

H

Hagar sign softening of the lower uterine segment that occurs at about the sixth week of pregnancy.

hair follicle shaft or opening on the surface of the skin through which hair grows.

halal any object or action that is permissible to use or engage in, according to Islamic law; denotes foods that are religiously acceptable to Islam. See also *kosher*.

halitosis Technical term for bad breath.

hallucination a false sensory perception that has a compelling sense of reality despite the absence of an external stimulus;

may affect any of the senses, but auditory hallucinations and visual hallucinations are most common.

halo device form of skeletal traction applied to the skull that allows the client to ambulate and perform self-care activities.

halo sign a positive test for cerebrospinal fluid.

handover/handoff transfer of information, as well as the professional responsibility to *make sure information is understood by the receiver.*

hand sanitization cleansing the hands using a chemical agent or thorough handwashing.

Harris flush return-flow enema.

Hashimoto thyroiditis hypothyroidism believed to be autoimmune in origin.

Hawaii Early Learning Profile (HELP) charts designed to help determine a child's developmental assessment. These charts contain curriculum-based assessments, including cognitive, language, gross motor, fine motor, social–emotional, and self-help.

health optimum functioning of body, mind, and spirit; absence of disease.

healthcare providers also referred to as health professionals, are individuals who provide a wide variety of allied health services including treatment and cure of diseases and disorders, surgical interventions, preventative care and teaching, and rehabilitation. Examples of healthcare providers include but are not limited to physicians, nurses, pharmacists, dentists, dietitians, chiropractors, phlebotomists, emergency medical technicians, and physical, respiratory, or occupational therapists. Health professionals have various levels of clinical skills and academic training which enable them to function in specific areas of the allied health professions, for example, internal medicine, mental health, optometry, obstetrics, or midwifery.

health interview way of soliciting information from the client; may also be called a nursing history.

health maintenance approach to healthcare in which disease prevention is emphasized; also called health supervision.

health maintenance organization (HMO) an agency that provides prepaid healthcare, as needed, to members (as opposed to fee paid as service is given). The emphasis is on prevention.

health record manual or electronic (computer) account of a client's relationship with a healthcare facility.

health supervision See *health maintenance.*

heart block condition associated with diseases of the coronary arteries and rheumatic heart disease in which heart contractions are weak and lack sufficient force to effectively pump blood.

heat cramps painful, involuntary muscle spasms that usually occur during heavy exercise in hot environments. Fluid and electrolyte loss often contribute to these cramps

heat exhaustion occurs when a combination of high temperatures, high humidity, and strenuous physical activity limits the body's ability to sweat enough to cool the blood and body. Heavy sweating and a rapid pulse can be seen. Untreated, this can lead to heatstroke.

heat index is a measure of how hot it really feels when relative humidity is factored in with the actual air temperature.

heat stroke *classic heat stroke* occurs when the body's heat-regulating mechanisms fail and core temperature soars; *exertional heat stroke* develops from an increased internal heat load due to muscular exertion, along with high external temperatures and humidity. A core body temperature that rises above 104 °F (40 °C) accompanied by hot, dry skin and CNS abnormalities such as delirium, convulsion, or coma is an emergency. Call 911 immediately

Hegar sign at about 6 weeks, the lower uterine segment (the portion between the body of the uterus and the cervix) softens.

***Helicobacter pylori* (*H. pylori*)** the bacteria known to cause chronic inflammation, peptic ulcers, stomach atrophy, and gastric cancer.

hemangiomas overgrowths of blood vessels.

hematemesis vomiting of blood.

Hematest a test for occult (hidden) blood in stool or body secretions.

hematocrit the volume percentage of packed red blood cells in whole blood.

hematologist a healthcare provider educated in the hematologic and lymphatic systems.

hematology study of blood and blood-forming tissues.

hematoma a mass of coagulated blood (internal or under the skin) due to a break in the wall of a blood vessel; a mild form is a black eye or a bruise.

hematopoiesis process of manufacturing blood cells, mostly occurring in the bone marrow.

hematuria blood in the urine.

hemianopsia blindness in half the visual field of one or both eyes.

hemiparesis weakness of the entire left or right side of the body.

hemiplegia paralysis on one vertical half of the body.

Hemoccult a test for occult (hidden) blood in stool or body secretions.

hemodialysis dialysis by way of an arterial shunt and using an artificial kidney; used to remove toxic wastes from the blood in kidney disorders.

hemodynamic monitoring specialized device used to evaluate the pressure in the heart chambers.

hemofiltration slow continuous renal replacement therapy that is effective in removing solutes and fluids in unstable newborns; also called hemodiafiltration.

hemoglobin the oxygen-carrying pigment in blood that gives blood its red color

hemophilia a congenital condition in males characterized by spontaneous or traumatic bleeding and very slow clotting.

hemorrhage the medical term for bleeding, usually excessive bleeding (internal or external); escape of blood from nonintact blood vessels.

hemorrhoid a dilation of the veins (varicose veins) of the anal region (may be internal or external).

hemostasis stoppage of bleeding (naturally or artificially).

hemothorax fluid or blood pooling in the pleural cavity; also called pleural effusion.

heparin (hep) lock IV catheter that is inserted into a vein and left in place for intermittent administration of medicine or as an open line in case of emergencies. Similar to a saline lock, which is flushed with saline versus heparin.

hepatitis inflammation of the liver. Types include A, B, C, D, and E, some of which are transmitted via blood or body secretions.

hereditary genetically determined, transmitted from parent to child, inherited (not acquired).

heredity the genetic transmission of physical or mental characteristics from parent to offspring.

hernia abnormal protrusion of an organ or tissue through the structure usually containing it, as an inguinal *hernia* or hiatal *hernia;* rupture; condition is called herniation.

herpes an inflammatory skin disease characterized by the formation of small vesicles in clusters (caused by a virus). (*Herpes simplex virus type I* causes fever blisters and canker sores in the mouth; *herpesvirus II* [herpesvirus genitalis] causes genital lesions; *herpes zoster* is also known as shingles.)

herpes zoster condition in adults caused by the same varicella virus that causes chickenpox in children; commonly known as shingles.

hesitancy inability to start the stream of urine.

heterograft a graft obtained from an animal and received by a person; also called xenograft.

heterosexual pertaining to different sexes; sexually attracted to the opposite sex.

hiatal pertaining to an opening or gap, as a *hiatal* hernia.

hierarchy of needs established by Maslow, the hierarchy categorizes human needs from the most basic vital needs, survival needs (necessary to life), up through higher-level needs such as beauty, love, and learning.

highly active antiretroviral therapy (HAART, ART) therapies for HIV/AIDS consisting of a combination of the five classes of drugs collectively referred to as antiretrovirals (ARVs).

high-risk newborn newborn with special problems related to maturity, hemolytic conditions, birth injuries, alterations in structure and function, infections, or chemical dependency.

high-risk pregnancy this term is used when physiologic or psychological factors could significantly increase the chances of mortality or morbidity of the client or fetus.

hindmilk milk produced near the end of a nursing session that is higher in fat and calories than the milk produced in the beginning.

Hippocratic oath pledge based on the principles of Hippocrates repeated by healthcare providers when they enter the field of medicine.

Hirschsprung disease condition in which a child's colon lacks parasympathetic nerve supply and the abdomen becomes enlarged with stool and flatus due to lack of peristalsis; also called megacolon or *aganglionic megacolon.*

hirsutism having excessive facial and/or bodily hair; may be a side effect of medications or point to an underlying hormonal imbalance.

histamine an amine found in all body tissues that stimulates dilation of small blood vessels and production of gastric juice. It is involved in inflammation and allergic reactions.

histology study of tissues.

histoplasmosis specific fungal infection.

hives swollen patches on the skin as a result of an allergic reaction.

HIV-associated nephropathy (HIVAN) an inflammation of the renal filters, which results in loss of removal of excess fluid and wastes from the bloodstream.

HIV-associated neurocognitive disorders (HAND) behavioral changes and diminished mental functioning.

HIV-related encephalopathy dysfunction of the brain as a result of HIV infection; also known as AIDS dementia complex.

Hodgkin lymphoma also known as Hodgkin disease (HD), is a malignancy of the lymphatic system; has a high cure rate when treated.

holistic healthcare healthcare that emphasizes care of the whole person.

Homan sign a test for thrombophlebitis in which pain occurs behind the knee when the foot is hyperflexed upward (dorsiflexion).

home healthcare a nurse monitoring a client in his or her home, often after being discharged while completing recovery from surgery or an illness.

homeostasis stability, balance, or equilibrium in normal body states.

homograft a graft from one person to another; also called allograft.

homosexual a person who is sexually attracted to members of the same sex, gay.

hookworm type of roundworm that usually enters the host through bare feet, migrating through the body to the mouth and throat, destroying red blood cells and causing anemia.

hormone chemical substance secreted, usually from a ductless gland, that regulates body processes.

hospice a facility or program of care that is specifically designed to provide emotional and physical support to end-of-life clients and their families.

hospitalist a term introduced in 1996, is a doctor, typically a general internist, who works mainly or exclusively for a hospital whose responsibility includes the care of hospitalized individuals. See also *healthcare provider, physician.*

huffing is a common term for inhalant abuse (such as solvents, aerosols, gases, or nitrites). Inhalants produce a very short-lived high; continued use to maintain a high can slow down brain activity.

human immunodeficiency virus (HIV) virus that lowers normal immune response, rendering the person susceptible to otherwise harmless (opportunistic) organisms.

humerus single long bone found in each upper arm.

humoral immunity immunity created by the B lymphocytes and is the body's resistance to circulating disease-producing antigens and bacteria.

hydatidiform mole rare condition of pregnancy characterized by abnormal growth of trophoblasts; the cells that normally develop into the placenta. There is typically not a formation of a fetus, but in the case there is a formation of a fetus, the fetus is not able to survive but is miscarried early in the pregnancy.

hydramnios excessive amniotic fluid surrounding a fetus; polyhydramnios.

hydrocele painless swelling of the scrotum caused by fluid collection.

hydrocephalus fluid accumulation in the skull; it is typically characterized by enlargement of the head if a shunt is not successful; also called water on the brain.

hydrodistension bladder that is stretched out with fluid.

hydrogenated a liquid oil to which hydrogen has been added to make it more stable and decrease the chance of rancidity.

hydrometer urinometer (used to measure the specific gravity of a liquid, such as urine).

hydronephrosis distention of the pelvis and calices of the kidney with urine as a result of obstruction of the ureter or other urinary structure.

hydrospadias condition in which the urinary meatus is located on the bottom of the penis.

hymen a fold of membrane sometimes found at the vagina's external opening.

hyperbaric high-pressure; as in hyperbaric oxygenation (HBO).

hyperbilirubinemia condition that results from elevated bilirubin levels in a newborn.

hyperemesis excessive vomiting.

hyperemesis gravidarum pernicious vomiting in pregnancy.

hyperextension increasing the angle of an extremity beyond normal, as in bending the head back to look at the ceiling or bending the fingers back.

hyperglycemia abnormally high blood sugar.

hyperlipidemia excess fat in the blood.

hyperopia condition in which light rays focus behind the retina; farsightedness.

hyperparathyroidism condition that stems from an excess of parathormone causing elevated blood calcium levels, resulting in calcium depletion in the bones.

hyperplasia enlargement, as in benign prostatic *hyperplasia*.

hyperpnea abnormal increase in rate and depth of respirations.

hypersomnia excessive sleepiness during daytime hours.

hypertension elevated blood pressure; also called high blood pressure. Persistently above normal: systolic more than 139 and diastolic above 89.

hyperthyroidism excessive functioning of the thyroid gland, causing excessive thyroid hormone in the body.

hypertonic a solution that is stronger than what is found on the opposite side of a membrane.

hypertrophy enlargement.

hyperventilation abnormally fast and deep breathing, usually caused by anxiety, resulting in reduction of carbon dioxide and an increase in oxygen.

hypervigilance state of abnormally heightened alertness.

hyphema hemorrhage into the anterior chamber of the eye.

hypnotic a drug or agent that induces sleep.

hypodermis also called subcutaneous tissue, a single layer of fat below the dermis that cushions, supports, nourishes, and insulates the skin.

hypoglycemia abnormally low blood sugar.

hypomania generally, a state of enhanced mood and increased energy and activity that has not reached the level of mania; usually does not require hospitalization.

hypoparathyroidism condition that stems from parathormone deficiency, with a consequent reduction in the amount of calcium available in the body and an accumulation of phosphorus in the blood.

hypophysectomy surgical removal of the pituitary gland.

hypospadias abnormal male condition in which the urethra opens on the underside of the penis or onto the perineum.

hypotension chronic depression in blood pressure; abnormally low blood pressure that may or may not be accompanied by s/s such as dizziness and lightheadedness.

hypothalamus a tiny but complex portion of the brain believed to be the "master controller" of the hormones.

hypothermia low body temperature; when the body loses heat faster than it can produce heat and body temperature falls below 95 °F (35 °C), which may be fatal. Hypothermia may also be induced for therapeutic purposes, such as surgery, or pathological as a result of faulty thermoregulation (temperature control).

hypothermic blanket cooling blanket; also called hypothermia blanket.

hypothyroidism condition that occurs as a result of a deficiency in thyroid secretion, which lowers metabolism.

hypotonic a solution that is less concentrated than that found on the opposite side of a membrane.

hypovolemic shock shock caused by excessive blood loss.

hypoxemia low oxygen concentration in the blood.

hypoxia abnormal reduction of oxygen in the tissues.

hysterectomy surgical removal of the uterus.

I

iatrogenic iatrogenic refers to an inadvertently acquired problem due to medical or surgical treatments, such as newborn blindness due to oxygen therapy or the acquisition of some types of infections.

iatrogenic incontinence urinary leakage caused by medical interventions or treatments.

ice cap a flat, oval, bag with a leakproof, screw-in top.

idiosyncratic effects drug reactions are adverse reactions that do not occur in most people at any dose and do not involve known pharmacological properties of the drug.

ileal diversion urinary diversion.

ileostomy surgical opening of the ileum onto the abdomen by means of a stoma.
ileum distal portion of the small intestine (adjective: ileal).
ileus intestinal obstruction, usually as a result of inadequate peristalsis.
ilium upper flaring portion of the bones that form the pelvis, usually identified as the hip bone.
illness pronounced deviation from normal health.
imam Muslim clergy person.
immunity condition of being nonsusceptible to a certain disease.
immunization the process of providing protection against infection from a particular disease; vaccination, inoculation.
immunogen a substance capable of initiating or stimulating an immune response.
immunoglobulins antibodies.
immunosuppressive referring to deliberate suppression of the natural immune system, as in chemotherapy for cancer (adjective: immunosuppression).
immunotherapy also known as biotherapy. It uses the immune system directly or indirectly against cancerous tumor cells via biologic response modifiers (BRMs). See *biologic response modifiers* (*BRM*).
impaction a condition in which a tooth or stool (feces) is lodged in a body cavity or passage, usually requiring dental or medical attention to prevent pain, tissue damage, or death. See also *fecal impaction*.
imperforate anus congenital defect in which the newborn's rectum ends in a blind pouch, obstructing the normal passage of feces.
impetigo bacterial infection of the skin; also called impetigo contagiosa.
implant burrowing of the future embryo into the endometrium.
implementation in nursing process, the carrying out of nursing care plans; also called interventions.
impotence a male's inability to achieve or sustain an adequate erection for sexual intercourse.
inborn immunity immunity that is inherited or genetic.
incentive programs rewards given to employees by their employers for practicing healthy habits such as smoking cessation, weight loss, and having regular physical examinations.
incentive spirometer a device used to force the client to concentrate on inspiration and promote full inflation of the lungs while providing immediate feedback; used particularly after surgery and in lung disorders.
incise to cut; to make a surgical incision (noun: incision).
incontinence inability to hold urine or stool.
increment phase of labor during which the contraction builds from the resting phase to full strength is longer than the other two combined.
incubation disease period between exposure to a pathogen and manifestation of clinical symptoms.
incus the "anvil," one of three tiny bones within the middle ear which are set in motion by sound waves.

independent actions nursing actions that do not require a healthcare provider's order.
induction stimulating the beginning of labor by using a medication such as oxytocin (Pitocin); beginning stage of anesthesia.
induration swollen area; a hardened place, a lump, as in the skin in a positive reaction to a tuberculin test.
infancy a child from 1–12 months of age.
infant mortality an estimate of the number of infants who die before their first birthday estimated to be six deaths for every 1,000 live births.
infarction the formation of an area of tissue death, an infarct, due to lack of oxygen. Infarcts are caused by obstruction of blood flow to the tissue as a result of a thrombus or an embolus.
infection the invasion and multiplication of infective agents in body tissues with a resultant reaction (illness or injury) to their presence and/or their toxins.
Infectious disease occurs if the chain of infection remains intact; it is not interrupted.
inferior below or in a lower position.
infertility inability to produce offspring; lack of fertility or productivity; barren.
infiltration the diffusion or accumulation in the tissues or cells of substances not normally present or found in those amounts.
inflammation a condition resulting from irritation in any body part, marked by pain, heat, redness, and swelling.
inflammatory bowel disease general term for ulcerative colitis and Crohn disease.
inflammatory process the initial healing response to damage to the body, for example, cut, bruise, infection, and surgery. Classical signs of this process are redness, localized heat, swelling, and pain. An overabundance of the inflammatory process can lead to autoimmune disorders.
informed consent giving full information and making sure the client understands before the client consents to surgery or other medical procedures.
infrared rays rays that relax muscles, stimulate circulation, and relieve pain.
infusion slow induction of fluids (not blood) into a vein, as an intravenous (IV) *infusion*.
ingestion to take a material into the digestive tract.
inhalant medications that are inhaled or breathed in.
injectable medications that are administered via a needle into the subcutaneous tissues, muscles, or blood vessels.
insensible not perceptible to the senses.
insignia a distinguishing badge of authority or honor.
insomnia sleeplessness; chronic inability to fall asleep or to stay asleep, with no apparent external cause.
inspection careful, close, and detailed visual examination of a body part.
inspiration inhalation; drawing air into the lungs.
instrumental activities of daily living (IADL) the indicators of an individual's ability to function using more complex skills than standard activities of daily living (ADLs) such as the ability to manage an income, the ability to sustain and maintain a household, or the ability to shop for food, prepare food, and serve meals.

insufflation feeling of air being instilled into the bowel
insulin a hormone which is vital in carbohydrate metabolism and is secreted by the islets of Langerhans of the pancreas.
insulin resistance a decreased tissue sensitivity to insulin that occurs in people who have type 2 diabetes mellitus.
integrative care addresses healing the whole person, mind, body, and spirit while working with multiple disciplines.
integument the skin, the integumentary system.
integumentary covering.
intellectual disability demonstrating below average intellectual abilities accompanied by difficulty functioning independently; originates before the age of 18.
intellectual skills knowing and understanding essential information.
intensity strength.
interaction when a drug reacts with either another drug or food; can cause an increased or decreased absorption of the medication or various reactions.
intercom system that allows clients in their rooms to communicate directly with healthcare providers at the nursing station; also known as an intercommunication system.
intercostal muscles muscles located between the ribs.
interdependent depending on one another; one action occurs because of another. Activities of various organ systems (e.g., the nerves, muscles, and bones) are *interdependent.*
interdependent actions nursing actions that occur in cooperation with healthcare providers and other team members.
interdisciplinary care team of individuals from different disciplines acting together to care for a client under a healthcare provider's direction.
intermediate care facilities facilities that provide room, board, and nursing care.
intermittent positive pressure breathing treatment method that assists a person to breathe more easily by liquefying mucus.
internal condom previously referred to as *female condom;* a pouch made of thin latex attached to two flexible rings that is inserted into the vagina prior to intercourse; is a mechanical and chemical barrier method.
internal disaster a disaster in which a healthcare facility itself is in danger or damaged and its function is impaired.
internal respiration cellular breathing.
Internet a global system of electronic, wireless, or optically interconnected computers and other technologic devices that access and transmit information.
interneuron a neuron between the first afferent neuron and the last motor neuron; neurons whose processes are all in a specific area, such as the olfactory lobe.
interpersonal skills the abilities that an individual possesses that provide for communication and interaction between individuals. These include language, behaviors, listening, delegation, and leadership. Sometimes referred to as "people skills."
interstate endorsement procedure in which a nurse transfers licensure from one state to another.

interstitial situated in the interspaces of tissue, as in interstitial or extracellular fluid (not blood or lymph).
interstitial cells small clusters of specialized endocrine cells which secrete testosterone and other androgens.
interstitial cystitis disease in which the bladder's lining allows for irritants from the urine to contact the bladder wall, causing extreme irritation.
interval in labor, the time from the start of one contraction to the start of the next.
interview a goal-directed or structured conversation in which one person seeks specific information from the other.
intimacy establishing relationships with others.
intimate partner violence (IPV) describes threats or acts of physical violence, sexual violence, coercive tactics, stalking, or physical aggression by a current or former partner or spouse. Also known as *domestic violence.*
intracellular within the cells, as in *intracellular* fluid.
intracranial pressure (ICP) the pressure of subarachnoidal fluid in the space between the skull and the brain and around the spinal cord. Elevated, increased intracranial pressure (↑ICP) is a significant sign in determining neurologic disorders.
intractable (intractable pain) that which cannot be relieved; continuous, relentless, as in *intractable* pain.
intradermal within the substance of the skin (dermis); intracutaneous, as an *intradermal* tuberculin or allergy test.
intramuscular within the muscle substance, as an *intramuscular* injection.
intraoperative occurring during a surgical operation.
intrapartum occurring during childbirth.
intravascular within the blood vessels.
intravascular fluid (IVF) fluid within the cardiovascular system of arteries and veins and the fluid within the lymphatic vessels.
intravenous within a vein, as *intravenous* infusion.
intravenous therapy injecting into a vein any number of sterile solutions that the body needs, including medications and electrolytes.
intrusion injury an injury in which a structure or part is pushed out of place into the body; often refers to a sports-related tooth injury when the tooth is driven back up or away from the jawline.
intrusive thoughts in psychiatry, mental events interrupt the flow of task-related thoughts in spite of efforts to avoid them, common in *obsessive-compulsive disorder* (*OCD*).
intubation a procedure by which an endotracheal tube (ET) is inserted through the mouth down into the trachea past the vocal cords and into the airway so that the person receives breathing assistance, often during anesthesia, sedation, or when receiving CPR.
intussusception the telescoping or prolapsing of one part of the intestine into an adjacent part.
in utero within the uterus.
invasive term used to describe surgery and some diagnostic tests that involve an incision or puncture through the skin, insertion of an instrument (such as an endoscope), or

injection of a foreign substance (such as dye) into the body; quickly spread widely throughout the body, such as *invasive* cancer.

inversion turning a body part so that it faces medially or inside, such as turning the ankle so that the sole of the foot faces the opposite foot.

involution turning inward; a retrograde change of the entire body or in a particular organ, as *involution* of the uterus after childbirth.

ion an atom with an electrical charge; positive (cation), negative (anion). Substances forming ions are called electrolytes.

iris pigmented section over the front of the eyeball that gives the eye its color.

iron an essential part of every body cell and a constituent of hemoglobin, which carries oxygen.

irritability ability to respond to a stimulus.

ischemia decrease or lack of blood supply to a body part as a result of the obstruction or constriction of blood vessels.

islets of Langerhans 500,000–1,000,000 small islands of cells scattered throughout the endocrine portion of the pancreas that secrete the pancreatic hormones.

isograft A graft in which the donor and recipient are genetically identical.

isolation separation from others; separation of people with infectious diseases from others.

isometric having the same length or dimensions, as isometric exercises (pushing against stable resistance); also called muscle setting.

isotonic of equal tension; normal, as *isotonic* saline that is the same tonicity as body fluids; exercise that shortens the muscle but does not change the force of contraction.

isotope an element with an altered number of neutrons; important in diagnosis and treatment of some disorders, such as cancer.

J

jaundice yellowish skin discoloration due to excess bile.

jejunum portion of the small intestine.

joint point at which bones attach to one another.

The Joint Commission establishes quality and appropriate care standards for hospitals, community health centers, and home care agencies.

jugular venous distention an indicator of heart failure manifested by distention or bulging of the jugular veins in the neck.

K

kangaroo care a technique to promote bonding between mother or father and child, the placement of a newborn's naked body directly against the mother's/father's skin.

Kaposi sarcoma opportunistic malignancy associated with AIDS that primarily affects the skin.

Kardex a flip-file with card slots or a notebook for each client on a unit or nursing care team; a system for recording background information and care related to a client's treatment.

karma Buddhist/Hindu belief that an individual's life can be a result of past life actions that present when the individual is reborn through reincarnation; a belief that actions and reactions (i.e., "karma") are significant to an individual's health or are the cause of disease.

Kawasaki disease febrile, multisystem disorder in which platelets in the blood tend to be caught in the vessels and can develop into serious cardiac problems; also called mucocutaneous lymph node syndrome.

Kegel exercises exercises designed to increase sphincter tone by tightening, holding, and releasing the muscles of the pelvic floor and sphincter, used to improve incontinence.

keloid scar or scar tissue.

keratin protein that is a major component of hair, nails, and the epidermis and is the organic matrix of tooth enamel. (Keratin is sometimes used as the coating for enteric-coated tablets.)

keratoplasty plastic surgery of the cornea of the eye, corneal grafting, corneal transplantation.

Kerlix proprietary name of a type of stretchy gauze used to hold dressings in place.

ketoacidosis also called *diabetic ketoacidosis* (DKA); results from a lack of effective insulin, causing hyperglycemia. Glucose no longer enters the muscle cells. To make up for the loss of sugar as a source of energy, the body uses more fats and proteins, which it breaks down into ketones and sends to the muscles. If too many ketones accumulate (*ketosis*), body fluids become imbalanced, and a condition called ketoacidosis follows.

ketogenic diet approach to eating that is extremely low in carbohydrates and very high in fat, aimed at controlling seizures, especially in children.

ketosis an increase in ketone bodies in the body tissues and fluids; also called ketoacidosis, a complication of diabetes mellitus.

kidneys two bean-shaped organs located at the small of the back at the lower edge of the ribs on either side of the vertebral column. Urine is formed in the kidneys and levels of many electrolytes are regulated by the kidneys. Blood pressure is greatly influenced by the kidneys.

kilocalorie unit of measurement that specifies the heat energy in a particular amount of food (1 kcal = 1,000 cal).

Koplik spots bluish-white pinpoint spots with a red rim that appear around the mouth about day 2 or 3 after being infected with rubella.

Korotkoff sounds blood flow sounds heard when measuring blood pressure with a stethoscope (auscultation).

kosher food that has been ritually prepared and served according to Jewish law.

Kussmaul respiration deep, rapid, and labored breathing. This distinct abnormal breathing pattern can result from certain medical conditions, as in diabetic acidosis and coma.

kwashiorkor condition caused by a severe protein deficiency.

kyphosis an increased front to back curve in the upper spine, resulting in a bulge in the upper back.

L

labia literally means lip, as the *labia* minora and *labia* majora of the external female genitalia.

labia majora two rounded folds of skin of the female genitals, posterior to the mons pubis.

labia minora thin pair of skin folds of the female genitals, medial to the labia majora.

labile affect highly variable, suddenly shifting emotional expression.

labor the process by which the uterus contracts and expels the fetus.

labor contractions rhythmic contracting and relaxing of the uterus during the four stages of labor; also called uterine contractions.

labyrinth the inner ear, including the vestibule, cochlea, and semicircular canals.

labyrinthitis inflammation of the inner ear.

laceration a wound produced by tearing or ripping (as opposed to an incision made in surgery).

lacrimal gland pertaining to tears, as the *lacrimal* glands of the eyes.

lacrimation tearing of the eyes.

lactation milk secretion by the mammary glands (breasts).

lacteal dead-end lymph capillaries within each villus that absorbs fat-soluble nutrients.

lacto-ovo vegetarian a person who eats plant foods, dairy products, and eggs.

lactose sugar found in milk; commonly called milk sugar.

lactose intolerance genetic absence of the enzyme necessary for metabolizing lactose in milk and dairy products (lactase).

laissez-faire leadership style that has loosely structured goals and no firm guidelines.

laminectomy type of lumbar decompression that exposes the spinal canal and allows for relief of compression of the spinal cord and spinal nerve roots.

lanugo fine, downy hair covering the body of a fetus.

laparoscope endoscope used to examine the peritoneal cavity (laparoscopy).

laparoscopy diagnostic technique that provides direct visualization of the uterus and accessory organs, including the ovaries and oviducts.

laryngectomy surgical removal of the larynx; the person is then called a laryngectomee.

laryngopharynx the lowest portion of the pharynx, extending from the epiglottis to the opening of the larynx and esophagus. It is divided to provide separate passages for food and air.

larynx box-like structure of cartilage in the midline of the neck; also called voice box.

lateral further from the midline, toward the side.

lateral (position) side-lying.

lavage washing out of an organ, such as the stomach or bowel; irrigation.

law formal, written rules of behavior that govern conduct and are enforced by an authority.

leader individual who is able to effectively direct and influence the actions of others.

leak point pressure pressure at which one can no longer hold one's urine, used to assess continence status.

learning disability disorder in one or more of the processes involved in understanding or using language.

legal death death, usually declared by a healthcare provider, as total absence of activity of any of the body's systems.

legend drug a drug that requires a provider's prescription.

lens a transparent, crystalline eye structure that converges or scatters light rays before they focus as images on the retina.

lesbian a female homosexual.

let-down sensation in the breasts of a lactating woman when she hears or thinks about her baby. *Let-down* reflex: flowing of milk into the breasts when the mother begins to nurse (milk-ejection reflex).

leukemia malignant disease of blood-forming organs; may be classified as acute or chronic and also in relationship to the specific blood cell affected, as acute lymphoid (lymphocytic), myelocytic, or granulocytic *leukemia*.

leukocyte white blood cell (WBC).

leukocytosis condition in which white blood cells increase in number.

leukopenia condition in which white blood cells decrease in number.

leukoplakia disorder characterized by white patches on the mucous membrane of the cheeks, gums, or tongue that cannot be rubbed off, as *leukoplakia buccalis*.

leukorrhea whitish vaginal discharge, which is a symptom of vaginitis.

leukotrienes chemical mediators, which are 100–1,000 times more potent than histamine in causing bronchospasm. Released by mast cells, they initiate the inflammatory response causing contraction of smooth muscle, constriction of the bronchi, and secretion of mucus.

levator pelvic muscle.

liability something one is required to do, an obligation, often financial; being found guilty of inappropriate or illegal acts.

libel a false or damaging written statement or photograph.

licensure status that says a nurse has the minimum requirements for competence and practice—can be lost or revoked.

lie term used to compare the position of the fetal spinal cord to that of the woman.

lifestyle factor one of many patterns of living one follows, including levels of exercise, nutrition, smoking, substance abuse, stress, and violence.

ligament fibrous band connecting bones or cartilages.

lightening feeling of decreased abdominal distention caused by the descent of the pregnant uterus deeper into the pelvis, usually 2–3 weeks before delivery.

limbic system part of the brain largely responsible for maintaining a person's level of awareness.

line of gravity direction of gravitation pull; an imaginary vertical line through the top of the head, center of gravity, and base of support.

linea narrow ridge or line. *Linea alba:* a white line, the vertical line in the center of the abdomen. *Linea nigra:* black line, the linea alba when it is darkly pigmented during pregnancy.

linoleic acid one of the omega-6 fatty acids is required but cannot be synthesized by humans and thus is considered essential in the diet. Primary sources are liquid vegetable oils including soybean oil, corn oil, and safflower oil.

linolenic acid linolenic acid is an omega-3 fatty acid that is required because it is not synthesized by humans and thus is considered essential in the diet. It is obtained from plant sources including soybean oil, canola oil, walnuts, and flaxseed.

lipid fat.

lipoma benign tumor composed of fatty tissues.

liquid diet approach to eating that consists entirely of liquids, used mostly during acute illnesses or certain body disturbances such as gastrointestinal irritation.

liter metric system measurement of liquid volume.

lithiasis condition of having stones (calculi), as in *cholelithiasis* (stones in the gallbladder).

lithotomy examination position in which the client is lying on his or her back with the feet in stirrups.

lithotripsy crushing or breaking up of stones (calculi) in the urinary tract or gallbladder. Extracorporeal shock wave *lithotripsy* (ESWL): noninvasive breaking up of stones by means of shock waves directed onto the outside of the body.

litter four-wheeled cart; also called gurney, wheeled stretcher. A *litter* scale is used to weigh clients who cannot stand.

liver largest glandular organ in the body; plays an important part in many bodily functions.

living will legal form a person signs requesting no extraordinary measures to be taken to save his or her life in terminal illness; a form of advance directive.

lobectomy removal of a lobe of the lung.

local limited to one part or place; not general, as *local* infection or *localized* pain.

local anesthesia disruption of sensation to a specific body area without causing unconsciousness; caused by infiltration or topical application of anesthetic, usually to a small area; not general.

local effect an effect restricted to the area in which it was administered.

lochia vaginal discharge that occurs for 1–2 weeks following childbirth.

lochia alba white or yellow discharge that begins about the 10th day after delivery.

lochia rubra red, bloody discharge seen for the first two days after client gives birth. It should smell like blood (slightly metallic); a foul odor indicates infection.

lochia serosa pink or brown-tinged discharge that begins after bleeding diminishes, around the second through the ninth day after delivery.

logroll turn method of turning a client that keeps the body in straight alignment, used for clients with injuries to the back and/or spinal cord.

long-term goal an outcome or goal that a client hopes to achieve but may require an extended amount of time to do so.

loop of Henle middle portion of the convoluted tubule, with ascending and descending loops.

lordosis an abnormal increase in the lumbar curvature of the spine; sometimes called swayback.

loss the fact or process of no longer having someone or something in your life.

lower tract division of the urinary tract that includes the bladder and urethra.

low-residue diet approach to eating composed of foods that the body can absorb completely so that little residue is left over for the formation of feces and is prescribed for severe diarrhea, colitis, diverticulitis, other gastrointestinal disorders, intestinal obstruction, and before and after intestinal surgery; also known as a fiber-controlled diet or low-fiber diet.

lumpectomy removal of a node or lump from the breast, without removing the breast.

lung one of two cone-shaped organs that fills the chest cavity; the organ of respiration.

Lyme disease bacterial illness carried by the deer tick and transferred to humans through its bite.

lymph transparent fluid that circulates throughout the body tissues to filter wastes; can be a means by which a malignancy spreads.

lymph nodes small bundles of special lymphoid tissue that remove bacteria and toxins from the blood and may assist in the formation of antibodies.

lymphangiomas overgrowths of lymph vessels.

lymphocyte particular type of leukocyte that is formed in lymphoid tissue and participates in cell-mediated immunity, as in T cells or T *lymphocytes*.

lymphoma a group of blood cell tumors that derive from lymphatic cells.

lysis destruction due to a specific agent, as *lysis* of red blood cells; also, a gradual recovery from disease (as opposed to crisis); or an elevated temperature that gradually returns to normal.

M

maceration softening of a solid due to soaking until connective tissue fibers are dissolved, such as *maceration* of the skin under a cast or bandage.

macronutrients carbohydrates, fats, and proteins.

macrophage large cell derived from a monocyte.

macropsia a visual illusion in which an object appears to be larger than it is in reality (may occur with illicit drug use.

macrosomia condition in which a newborn is born large-for-gestational-age; may also refer to an oversized fetus.

macule (macula) a flat discolored spot on the skin (also, macule); an area surrounding the fovea near the center of the retina; the region of greatest visual acuity.

magnesium mineral found in the bones of the body.

mainstreaming bringing physically and intellectually challenged people into school or activities involving nonchallenged people of their own age.

malaise feeling of illness; general bodily discomfort.

malignant wild and disorderly growth of cells that is unlike the tissue from which it arises. Malignant cells tend to spread to other parts of the body

malingering faking illness or disability to achieve a particular desired outcome: to stay in the hospital, to win compensation, as defense in a trial, or otherwise receive desired attention.

malleolus protrusions where the lower ends of the tibia and fibula meet the ankle bones.

malleus the "hammer," one of three tiny bones within the middle ear which are set in motion by sound waves.

malnutrition poor intake or inadequate use of food by the body; faulty nourishment.

malocclusion incorrect tooth positioning, often corrected by orthodontia.

malpractice injurious or faulty treatment; professional misconduct.

mammary pertaining to the mammary gland (breast).

mammary glands glands within the female breast that are stimulated by hormones after childbirth to release milk.

mammography special x-ray examination of the breasts, capable of detecting some breast cancers.

mammoplasty plastic surgery of the breast. Augmentation mammoplasty: enlarging or lifting of the breast. Reconstruction mammoplasty: repair following mastectomy or injury. Reduction mammoplasty: decreasing the size of the breast.

managed care a plan for continual monitoring and maintenance of an individual's health.

managed care payment financial reimbursement for healthcare services by a third-party, that is to say, all or part of the healthcare costs are billed to a designated agency or service, not the beneficiary (individual/client).

managed care protocols formally established guidelines are based on national criteria and detail the required management of specific disorders.

manager individual who coordinates and controls the work of others.

mandatory licensure regulation that makes it illegal for any nurse to practice nursing for pay without a license.

mandatory reporter an individual legally required to report child maltreatment, including nurses and other healthcare workers, teachers, and day care workers. *Voluntary reporters* of abuse are referred to as "permissive reporters."

mandible lower jaw bone.

mania disordered mental state of excitement; exaggerated hyperactivity as a phase of bipolar disorder; often accompanied by overoptimism, impaired judgment, or grandiosity. Can be preoccupation with a particular activity or ideas, especially when used as a suffix (e.g. *kleptomania, pyromania*).

manual resuscitator, manual resuscitation bag the generic name for the bag, valve, mask device known as the Ambu-bag (proprietary name).

marasmus particular form of malnutrition usually seen in infants; also called failure to thrive, often due to a protein deficiency.

marrow sponge-like material in the hollow cavities in bones. (The red bone marrow produces many blood cells.)

mastalgia breast pain.

mastectomy surgical removal of all or part of the breast. (Removal of a lump only is called lumpectomy.)

masticate to chew.

mastitis inflammation of the breast.

masturbation handling one's own genitals for erotic stimulation.

maxilla two bones that fuse to create the upper jaw bone.

mayo stand stand that holds equipment used in examination or surgery.

mean arterial pressure approximately the value of the diastolic blood pressure plus one-third of the pulse pressure.

meatus opening, as in the urinary meatus.

mechanical ventilation device that moves air in and out of the lungs.

Meckel diverticulum congenital disorder in which a small portion of the ileum ends in a blind pouch just before its junction with the colon.

meconium dark green or black fecal substance in the intestines of the fully grown fetus or newborn passed as the first one or two stools after birth.

medial nearer the midline, toward the middle.

mediastinal shift shift of the heart, great vessels, and trachea toward the side opposite the injury. Can occur during a traumatic injury (tension pneumothorax), pleural fluid pressure, or with the growth of mediastinal mass or tumor.

mediastinum the cavity containing the heart; between the lungs and second and sixth ribs.

Medicaid public, tax-supported health insurance program for which people must qualify, a joint effort of federal and state governments.

medical asepsis practice of reducing the number of microorganisms or preventing and reducing transmission of microorganisms from one person (source) to another; also referred to as "clean technique."

medical diagnosis statement formulated by a primary healthcare provider that identifies the disease a person is believed to have, which provides a basis for prognosis and treatment decisions.

medical terminology vocabulary used in the healthcare field.

medically complex nursing unit unit that cares for clients who require specialized care but who do not require hospitalization or care in subacute units.

Medicare federal health insurance program available to nearly everyone over the age of 65, regardless of financial status, and to younger people who qualify.

medication substance other than food used to prevent disease, to aid in diagnosis and treatment of disease, and to restore or maintain functions in body tissues; also called drug.

medication administration record (MAR) document that lists all medications that a healthcare provider orders for a client with spaces for marking when medications are given.

medulla inner portion of an organ, as the *medulla* oblongata (a center portion of the hindbrain) or the renal *medulla*.

megacolon See *Hirschsprung disease.*

meiosis cell division that produces eggs or sperm containing half the number of needed chromosomes.

melanin dark pigment that may be present in a tumor (melanoma) or may be excreted in the urine (melanuria).

melanoma the most dangerous type of skin cancer, which originates in the pigment-producing melanocytes.

melasma a "sun-tanned" or bronze-like masking across the face that may occur during pregnancy; also called *chloasma gravidarum* or the "mask of pregnancy."

melena passage of dark-colored stools containing partially or fully digested blood; also used to mean abnormal blood in the stool or vomitus.

membrane a thin layer of tissue covering a surface (as cell or plasma *membrane*), covering a body part or lining a body cavity (as mucous *membrane*). Drum membrane: tympanic membrane (eardrum). Fetal membranes: membranes that protect the embryo, "bag of waters."

membranous labyrinth set of tunnels and chambers in the inner ear.

menarche establishment of menstruation; the first menses.

Ménière disease a disorder of the labyrinth of the inner ear causing vertigo, headache, tinnitus, and hearing loss.

meninges membranes that cover the brain and spinal cord (dura mater, arachnoid, pia mater).

meningitis inflammation of the meninges.

meningocele condition in which one or more layers of the meninges (spinal cord covering) protrude through an opening in the vertebral column.

meningomyelocele herniation of a portion of the spinal cord, meninges, spinal fluid, and nerves through a defect in the spinal column.

menopause cessation of menstruation; also called climacteric, change of life.

menorrhagia abnormally profuse menstrual flow.

menstrual cycle two interrelated cycles (ovarian and uterine) that cause the flow of blood and other materials approximately every 28 days in the nonpregnant woman.

menstruation periodic vaginal discharge of blood and tissues from the nonpregnant uterus; also called period, menses.

mesophile prokaryote that survives at room temperature or body temperature.

metabolic acidosis a condition that results from a deficit in bicarbonate ions or an excess of hydrogen ions.

metabolic alkalosis a condition that results from an excess of bicarbonate, often due to excess administration or a loss of acids.

metabolic syndrome a combination of at least three conditions that are commonly found in a prediabetic or diagnosed diabetic state, to include abdominal obesity, hypertension, low HDL, elevated cholesterol, elevated triglyceride levels, high blood glucose, and/or insulin resistance.

metabolism ability to process, obtain energy from, and create new products using the chemicals found in foods.

metastasis transfer of disease organisms or cells from one organ or body part to another not directly connected with it; often refers to cancer cells or tuberculosis.

meter metric system measurement of length.

metric measurement system based on the number 10.

metrorrhagia uterine bleeding at irregular intervals and sometimes for a prolonged time.

micelles glue-like (colloid) particles that transport digested fats to the intestinal villi for absorption.

microbe an individual living animal or plant that is so small, it can be seen only with the aid of a microscope. Also known as a microorganism.

microbiology scientific study of microorganisms.

microcirculation blood flow through the capillaries.

microencephaly congenital condition characterized by a small skull and small amount of brain tissue.

micronutrients water, minerals, and vitamins.

microorganisms minute living cells not visible to the human eye but found almost everywhere in the environment.

micropsia a visual illusion in which an object appears to be smaller than it is in reality. Usually caused by disorders in the eye, central nervous system, migraines, epilepsy, or by drug effects.

micturition passage of urine from the urinary bladder; also called voiding, urinating.

midbrain brain area that functions as an important reflex center.

midlife transition sense that arises in middle adulthood that others of the same age have achieved more and that one must contribute to society before it is too late.

midline an imaginary line dividing the body into right and left halves, as a *midline* incision.

milia pinhead-sized white spots that may appear on the nose and cheeks of a newborn, caused by unopened sweat and oil glands.

milieu environment, atmosphere, surroundings that affect the personality and adjustment of the individual.

milieu therapy psychotherapeutic treatment based on modification or manipulation of the client's immediate environment in order to promote healthier, more adaptive cognitions, emotions, and behavior.

mineral a nonorganic chemical element or compound vital for building bones and teeth, maintaining muscle tone, regulating body processes, and maintaining acid–base balance. Common minerals in the body include calcium and iron.

mineralocorticoid corticosteroid that regulates the amount of electrolytes in the body.

Mini-Cog 3-min screening for cognitive impairment in older adults.

minim apothecary system unit of measurement of liquid, approximately equal to one drop.

Mini-Mental Status Examination (MMSE) a widely used test of cognitive function in older adult clients; it includes tests of orientation, attention, memory, and language.

minimum data set a form that measures a client's ability to perform activities of daily living and identifies functional losses that affect this ability.

minister Christian clergy person (Protestant); pastor (Catholic or Protestant). Also to provide care to a person, to minister to a person's needs.

minute clinic types of urgent-care clinics used to treat vertical clients (clients with noncritical conditions); critical clients are referred to the ED.

misdemeanor a crime less serious than a felony, usually punishable by a fine or imprisonment for less than a year.

mitered the type of beveled or diagonal corners used when making a hospital bed.

mitosis cell division.

mitral valve valve between the left atrium and left ventricle formed of two tissue flaps.

mittelschmerz "middle pain" a client may experience during ovulation or midway between menstrual periods.

mixture a blend of two or more substances that have been brought together without forming a new compound.

moderate sedation formerly known as conscious sedation.

modified diet approach to eating that has been specifically altered (whether in vitamins, nutrients, serving size, etc.) to meet the individual needs of a client.

molding temporary elongation of the head of a newborn, caused by the overlap of skull bones due to the pressure of traveling through the birth canal.

molecule the smallest division of a substance that still possesses the characteristics of that substance; if divided further, it breaks down into its individual chemical elements (atoms).

Mongolian spots dark blue areas of discoloration that may appear on the buttocks, lower back, and upper legs of nonwhite babies, which usually disappear by early childhood.

monoclonal antibodies laboratory-produced antibodies engineered to mimic natural antibodies, which will identify and destroy abnormal cells.

monocyte a particular type of white blood cell that has one nucleus.

mononucleosis contagious infection characterized by flu-like symptoms and often an enlarged liver or spleen.

monosaccharide a single sugar molecule.

mons a raised area, prominence, as the *mons* pubis.

mons pubis fatty pad overlying the pubic area.

Montgomery straps easily removable straps that stay in place to facilitate dressing removal.

mood internal, subjective emotional state.

morbid inducing disease or having a disease; thoughts of death or severe disease, as *morbid* thoughts.

morbidity number of people with an illness or disorder relative to a specific population.

morgue a place for keeping dead bodies temporarily until they are identified or claimed by relatives or until an autopsy is done.

mortal terminating in death as a *mortal* wound.

mortality death, or rate of death per certain number of population; a personal realization that one will eventually die.

morula the fertilized zygote when it has divided rapidly and formed a ball of about 16 identical cells.

motility the ability to move, one of the characteristics of specific cells; motion.

mottling a skin coloring appearing as a purplish or blotchy red-blue. Typically beginning as a red-blue coloring on the knees and/or the feet. In the dying client, mottling is often a sign of imminent death.

mullah healer in some Muslim faiths.

multifetal pregnancy of twins or more.

multigravida pregnant woman who has given birth at least once.

mumps viral disease that affects the salivary glands, especially the parotids; also called *epidemic parotitis*.

Munchausen syndrome disorder in which the client seeks treatment for acute factitious mental or physical illness. (*Munchausen syndrome by proxy:* seeking treatment for a factitious disorder in another person, usually the client's child.)

muscle tone state of slight contraction with the ability to spring into action.

mutism refusal or inability to speak.

mycosis disease caused by a fungus.

mycology study of fungi.

mydriasis a dilation of the pupil that continues even in bright environments, usually having a nonphysiological cause, such as disease, trauma, or the use of stimulant drugs such as cocaine, hallucinogenics, and crystal meth.

myelin fatty covering of some nerve fibers, as the *myelin* sheath; electrically insulate one nerve call from another.

myelogram a radiograph showing the differential count of various cells in the bone marrow.

myelomas (from *myelo,* for bone marrow) are cancers of the plasma cells (mature forms of B cells). Multiple myeloma is an example.

myelosuppression reduction in bone marrow function.

myocardial pertaining to the myocardium, as in *myocardial* infarction ("heart attack").

myocarditis inflammation of the heart's muscular walls.

myocardium the middle and thickest layer of the heart wall, the muscular layer.

myopia nearsightedness; light rays focus in front of the retina.

myotonic muscular dystrophy (MMD) the most common type of muscular dystrophy in adults.

myringotomy surgical incision into the eardrum.

myxedema a condition that results from hypothyroidism (lack of the hormone thyroxine). (The adult form is cretinism.)

N

Nägele rule method of determining a client's due date; adds seven days to the date of the first day of the woman's LNMP, then subtract 3 months. The resulting date is the EDD.

narcolepsy a condition characterized by uncontrollable sleep.

nares nostrils.

narrative charting type of nurses' notes that essentially documents what is occurring throughout the day in a chronological manner.

narrow-spectrum antibiotic classification of antibiotics that are specific or effective in fighting only a few microorganisms.

nasal cannula a device used to administer small to moderate increases in oxygen concentration.
nasopharynx section of the pharynx that extends from the nares to the uvula that is used for air passage only.
naturally acquired immunity immunity that occurs when a person is accidentally exposed to a causative agent.
near-drowning recovery that occurs after submersion in liquid and apparent cessation of body processes.
necrosis tissue death.
needleless system an injection system that prevents needle sticks by allowing medication to be drawn up into a syringe and injections made into IV tubing without an exposed needle
negative feedback system a system by which once a gland stimulates another gland to produce a hormone and the hormone level rises highly enough, the first gland stops stimulating the target gland and stops the hormone release.
negative pressure wound therapy (NPWT) a system that consists of a vacuum unit, foam wound coverage, and negative pressure which combine to seal the edges of the wound. It promotes healing by minimizing excessive blood and fluids, promotes the development of new blood vessels, and increases the chances that the wound graft will be successful.
negligence harm done to a person because of failure to do something that a responsible person would do; doing something a responsible person would not do; irresponsible care.
neologism new word or expression whose origins and meanings are usually nonsensical and unrecognizable: typically associated with *aphasia* or *schizophrenia*.
neonate a newborn during the first 28 days of life.
neoplasm tumor, new growth (may be benign or malignant); often refers to cancer (adjective: neoplastic).
nephrectomy kidney removal.
nephritic syndrome (nephrosis) results from glomerulonephritis and is characterized by marked protein in the urine and edema.
nephrolithiasis kidney stones (calculi).
nephrologist a healthcare provider who specializes in medical aspects of kidney disease.
nephroma cancer of the kidney.
nephron the functional unit of the kidney.
nephropathy kidney disease.
nephrotic syndrome a condition of too much protein in the urine and too little protein in the blood.
nephrotoxicity kidney damage, which can be caused by aminoglycosides and manifested by blood and protein in the urine.
nerve a macroscopic cord-like structure that contains individual nerve fibers that carry impulses within the body. Sensory (afferent) nerves carry information to the brain; motor (efferent) nerves carry impulses from the brain to muscles. Some nerves are mixed sensory and motor.
neuralgia pain that extends along one or more nerves, as trigeminal *neuralgia* (tic douloureux).

neurodiagnostic hospital department that performs and records "brain wave" tests, administers evoked potential examinations, does specialized sleep studies, and monitors clients who have seizures; also called the electroencephalography (EEG) department.
neurogenic originating in the nervous system.
neuroglia supporting structure of nerve tissue; also called glial cells.
neurohypophysis the posterior lobe of the pituitary gland.
neuroleptic See *antipsychotic*. An agent that modifies psychotic behavior.
neuroleptic malignant syndrome (NMS) rare, life-threatening complication with conventional (typical or first-generation) antipsychotic or neuroleptic medications; a medical emergency.
neurology medical specialty related to the nervous system.
neurons cells that make up nervous tissue.
neuropathic pain chronic pain or discomfort that continues for 6 months or longer and interferes with normal functioning.
neuropathy nerve damage.
neuropsychiatrist specialist who is trained in the study of both psychiatric and neurologic disorders and they approach treatment from.
neurosyphilis invasion of the nervous system by the bacterium that causes syphilis (*Treponema pallidum*).
neurotransmitter a chemical that an axon releases to allow nerve impulses to cross the synapse and reach the dendrites.
neurovascular checks a systematic method of monitoring the function and status of nerves and blood vessels, as well as the movement of muscles that could be damaged. Also known as CMS checks because they include observations and documentation of the client's circulation, motion, and sensation; generally performed on sites distal to an injury or fracture.
neutron subatomic particle carrying a positive electrical charge.
neutropenia decreased neutrophils in the blood. Malignant neutropenia is called agranulocytosis.
neutropenic isolation See *protective isolation*.
nevus mole.
newborn a human being in the first 4 weeks of life.
Nightingale lamp a standard in nursing insignia (also known as the *Lamp of Nursing*).
nirvana Buddhist/Hindu state of enlightenment in which the soul no longer lives in the body and is free from desire and pain.
nits lice eggs.
nociception pain transmission with four components; transduction, transmission, perception, and modulation.
nociceptive pain acute pain; a pain sensation that results abruptly.
nocturia excessive voiding (urination) during the night.
nocturnal emission involuntary discharge of semen while sleeping.

nodule type of skin lesion appearing as a small knot or protuberance.

non–organ-specific a disease that affects one or more organs.

nonpitting edema swelling that does not result in a persistent indentation if pressure is applied. Occurs usually in lymphatic disorders such as lymphedema after a mastectomy.

nonproductive term used to describe a dry cough in which the person does not cough up any sputum or other material.

nonrebreathing mask device that can deliver high doses of oxygen.

nonseminoma a type of testicular tumor.

nonspecific immunity immunity that helps fight against a variety of foreign invaders; also known as nonspecific defense systems which include the skin, tears, neutrophils, and monocytes, etc.

nonverbal communication conveying information or messages without speaking or writing. Components include items such as therapeutic touch, gestures, body language, facial expressions, and eye contact (or lack thereof).

normothermia normal body temperature.

norms "rules" for behavior in a group.

nosocomial originating in a healthcare facility; that is, a *nosocomial* infection.

N-terminal (NT) proBNP laboratory test that helps to confirm or exclude the diagnosis of heart failure.

nuchal cord loops of umbilical cord that may have become wrapped around a baby's neck during delivery.

nuchal rigidity stiff neck.

nuclear dyad a married couple who live together without children.

nuclear family a two-generation unit consisting of a husband, wife, and their immediate children—biologic, adopted, or both—living within one household.

nuclear medicine diagnosis and treatment of body disorders using radioactivity (includes x-ray, scintillation scan, and radiation therapy).

nucleus body within the cell that contains chromosomes (sometimes referred to as the regulator).

numerator top number of a fraction.

Nurse Practice Act the law to govern and guide nursing practice in a state or territory.

nurses' notes type of nurses' notes that essentially documents what is occurring throughout the day in a chronological manner.

nurse registry Sometimes refers to an agency, either local or state, that assists with job placement for full-time, part-time, or as needed (PRN) positions. Other times, the words refer to the national registry of nursing, NRSYS, a list of nurses who are legally licensed to practice nursing. It can be found at www.nrsys.com.

nursing action nursing interventions; these may be performed dependently, interdependently, or independently.

nursing assessment systematic and continuous collection and analysis of information about the client.

nursing bottle mouth a serious dental condition resulting from regularly placing an infant in bed with a bottle of breast milk, formula, or juice propped on a blanket or towel.

nursing care plans guidelines used by healthcare facilities to plan the care for clients.

nursing diagnosis a statement about the client's actual or potential health concerns that can be managed through independent nursing intervention.

nursing history way of soliciting information from the client; may also be called a health interview.

nursing implementation a part of the nursing process in which the nurse performs actions or initiates interventions on behalf of the client; may be referred to as nursing intervention or nursing action.

nursing intervention nursing actions; dependently, interdependently, or independently.

nursing peer review an evaluation of nursing activities and client outcomes as demonstrated in the nursing documentation.

nursing process systematic method in which the nurse and client work together to plan and carry out effective nursing care. (The steps include assessment, nursing diagnosis, planning, implementation, and evaluation.)

nursing progress notes documentation by nurses of care given and observations made; charting data input.

nursing unit hospital area that contains several client units.

nutrient substances needed for growth, maintenance, and repair of the body.

nutrient density significant amounts of key nutrients per volume consumed.

nutrition the selection, preparation, ingestion, and assimilation of foods by the body.

nystagmus rapid, repetitive involuntary movement of the eyeball; may be horizontal, rotating, vertical, or a combination of these.

O

obese overweight; morbid obesity or gross obesity is usually considered to be more than 100 lb overweight or twice normal weight.

object permanence the knowledge that an object seen in a particular spot but temporarily hidden from view continues to exist and will return to view.

objective able to be perceived by another person by means of the senses (a rash is an *objective* sign, as opposed to subjective); a goal or criterion (as *objectives* for each book chapter); a test item that has a definite answer (open to only one interpretation).

objective data all measurable and observable pieces of information about a client and his or her overall state of health.

observation looking at the client or watching for *general characteristics,* such as overall appearance, skin color, grooming, body posture, gait, mood, interactions with others, and other factors that do not require closer scrutiny or the use of measurement aids (e.g., a stethoscope)

obsession a persistent, intrusive thought idea, image, or impulse that the person experiences as intrusive or inappropriate and results in marked anxiety, distress, or discomfort.

obstetrics branch of medicine that deals with pregnancy, labor, delivery, and the puerperium.

obstetrician is a healthcare provider who specializes in obstetrics.

occipital lobe cerebral lobe that directs visual experiences.

occult hidden.

occupational therapy (OT) department that rehabilitates clients so they can perform activities of daily living (ADLs) and return to work and leisure following an injury or illness.

occupied bed bed holding a client that is unable to get up as a result of his or her condition or generalized weakness.

oculogyric crisis prolonged fixation of the eyeballs in a single position for minutes to hours. Also called *oculogyric spasm.*

official name a medication's name as identified in the United States Pharmacopeia and the National Formulary.

older adult describes those who have reached an age which nears the life expectancy of human beings.

oldest adult individuals ranging from age 80–100+ years of age.

olfaction sense of smell.

oliguria deficient urinary secretion or infrequent urination of less than 500 ml daily.

ombudsperson state required representative who provides assistance and information to residents of long-care facilities and their families.

oncogene a cancer-causing gene.

oncologist cancer specialist.

oncology study of tumors; the study of cancer, as *oncologic* nursing.

oocyte ova at a female baby's birth.

open bed bed that allows linens to be turned down, making it easier for a person to get into or out of.

open-ended questions questions used in therapeutic communication and interviews that don't invite one-word responses but rather encourages clients to talk about themselves and their concerns in a way that makes them feel safer.

ophthalmia neonatorum blindness in the neonate.

ophthalmic medications that are instilled or administered directly into the eye.

ophthalmology medical specialty related to the study of the eye and vision.

ophthalmoscope a lighted instrument used to inspect the eye.

opiate analgesic derived from the seeds of a certain species of poppy plant or a synthetic derivative with similar pain-blocking effects.

opisthotonos a type of spasm in which the back is rigid and arches and the head is thrown backward. If in a supine position, only the back of the head and the heels would touch the surface they are on.

opportunistic causing disease under certain circumstances.

opportunistic infection (OI) infections or cancers that do not generally cause disease in a person with a normal immune system. Commonly found in later stages of HIV or part of diagnosed AIDS.

opsonize the action of an antibody on a complement split product that attaches to and coats foreign material, antigens, or other microorganisms, enhancing phagocytosis of the foreign material by macrophages, such as leukocytes.

optic disk eye region that is not light sensitive.

oral of or pertaining to the mouth, as in the *oral cavity.* An oral solution is a solution to be administered by mouth.

oral/written reprimand respectively, the first and second steps in due process informing an employee of deficiencies.

orbit ball-shaped cavity in the skull that contains the eye.

orchiectomy removal of one or both testes.

orchiopexy corrective surgery in which undescended testes are sutured, so they remain in the scrotum.

orchitis inflammation of the testicles.

organ a group of body tissues having a particular function.

organ of Corti small but intricate organ in the inner ear where the transmission of nerve stimuli begins.

organic pertaining to an organ.

organic brain syndrome irreversible condition that affects cognitive function; now called dementia, formerly called senility.

organic disease a disorder in which a detectable structural change has occurred in one or more organs, also alters usual function (as opposed to a psychogenic disorder).

organic disorder mental illness that is caused by an actual physical disorder.

organ-specific having an effect only on a particular organ.

orgasm climax of sexual excitement.

oropharynx part of the pharynx extending from the uvula to the epiglottis that carries food to the esophagus and air to the trachea; commonly called the throat.

orthodontia branch of dentistry that deals with malocclusion (misplaced teeth) and other jaw and facial deformities.

orthopedic pertaining to the correction of deformities of the musculoskeletal system.

orthopnea feeling short of breath while recumbent or lying flat; usually relieved by sitting up or standing.

orthopneic position position that facilitates breathing; is achieved by placing the overbed table across the bed or in front of a chair with one or two pillows on top of the table. The client leans forward across the table with the arms on (or beside) the pillows and rests his or her head on the pillows. Pillows can also be placed behind the client's back, for additional support. In the alternative orthopneic position, the client sits up straight, with arms supported by pillows.

orthostatic hypotension drop in blood pressure upon standing, often causing dizziness.

orthotics the practice that deals with the application of braces or appliances to the body; closely related to prosthetics (the science that deals with the fabrication of braces and other orthopedic devices).

os opening; any body orifice. Specifically refers to the mouth and the cervical opening (cervical *os*).

osmosis passage of a solvent from one side of a selectively permeable membrane to the other due to the relative pressures on both sides.

ossicle collectively, the three tiny bones in the middle ear (the malleus, incus, and the stapes) which are set in motion by sound waves.

ossification the process of bone formation.

osteoblast a cell that is associated with bone production; a "bone cell."

osteoclast large multinuclear bone cells that assist in the resorption or breakdown of bone.

osteocyte hardened, mature muscle cell.

osteomalacia adult form of vitamin D deficiency which results in a softening of the bones.

osteomyelitis bone inflammation caused by a pyogenic (pus-forming) infection.

osteoporosis a chronic bone disorder caused by mineral loss, especially of calcium, in the bone (often occurs with aging).

ostomate one who has a stoma outside the abdomen to drain feces or urine.

ostomy an opening.

otic pertaining to the ear.

otitis externa inflammation of the external ear; also called swimmer's ear.

otitis media inflammation or infection of the middle ear.

otology study of the anatomy and physiology of the ear and related disorders.

otorrhea leakage of CSF from the ear may occur.

otosclerosis abnormal spongy bone formation in the labyrinth of the ear (often causes hearing loss because the ossicles become fixed and unable to transmit sound waves).

otoscope a lighted instrument used to inspect the ear.

ototoxic drugs used to treat conditions unrelated to the ear that may harm the inner ear.

ototoxicity damage to the eighth cranial nerve which can be caused by aminoglycosides and manifested by dizziness, tinnitus, and gradual hearing loss.

outcome-based care quality management in which delivery of care is judged by results achieved.

outercourse refers either to the abstinence from sexual activity or to the activities of an intimate relationship without vaginal intercourse. May also be used to mean sexual activity without any vaginal, oral, or anal penetration.

ova female gametes (eggs).

ovaries female gonads.

over-the-counter medications that may be purchased without a prescription.

overflow incontinence that occurs when the bladder overfills with urine but is not able to release it; also called paradoxical incontinence.

overhydration excess water in the extracellular spaces.

overweight ten percent over the desirable weight for the body's frame.

oviducts passageways for ova between the ovaries and the uterus. Also called ovarian tubes, uterine tubes (formerly called fallopian tubes).

ovulation process by which an ovum (egg cell) ruptures the ovary's surface and is expelled into the pelvic cavity.

oximeter instrument used to measure the oxygen saturation or concentration in the client's arterial blood usually attached to a finger or toe, or ear (expressed in a percentage). Also called *pulse oximeter.*

P

packing material placed (packed) into a wound to assist healing from the inside-out and to prevent pockets of infection (abscesses) from forming.

pain feeling of suffering, distress, or agony, caused by stimulation of specialized nerve endings, a protective device of the body; a *subjective* sensation (reported by the client).

pain modulation inhibitory response of the body to effects of pain.

pain perception recognition of pain impulses and response of the body.

pain threshold lowest intensity of a stimulus that causes a subject to recognize pain.

pain tolerance point at which a person can no longer tolerate pain.

pain transduction painful stimulus in nerve endings changed to neural impulses.

pain transmission neural pain impulses carried to the brain for interpretation.

palliative care measures that give relief but are not curative (as chemotherapy is palliative for some types of advanced cancer). The goal is comfort and pain control.

pallor absence of skin pigment; paleness.

palpation the act of feeling with the hand, placing the fingers on the skin with light pressure to determine the condition of underlying parts.

pancarditis widespread, general inflammation of the heart.

pancytopenia having a decreased number of platelets.

pandemic widespread epidemic of disease.

PAOP or PAWP pressure within the pulmonary arterial system when a specialized catheter tip is "wedged" in the tapering branch of one of the pulmonary arteries.

Pap smear (aka **Pap test**) a method of examining body secretions from the cervical area for malignant cells; also called Pap test or Papanicolaou test.

papule a small, solid, circumscribed skin elevation, less than 0.5–1.0 cm in diameter.

para refers to the parting of mother and baby or the birth itself.

paracentesis surgical puncture of a body cavity for the aspiration of fluid (often refers to abdominal paracentesis). (Removal of fluid from the thoracic cavity is called thoracentesis.)

paradoxical opposite reaction.

paradoxical effect opposite reaction to that expected, usually in relationship to the effects of a medication.

parallel play two children playing side-by-side with the same or similar toys, without interacting with each other (common in toddlers).

paralysis motion loss or impairment of sensation in a body part.
paralytic ileus intestinal paralysis.
paranoid exhibiting extreme distrust or suspiciousness (*paranoid personality disorder*), or relating to delusions (*paranoid schizophrenia*).
paraplegia paralysis from the waist down; a person with this condition is called a paraplegic.
parasites plants or animals that live on or within another organism, taking something from that other organism.
parasympathetic division of the autonomic nervous system that produces body responses that are normal while at rest or under normal conditions.
parathyroid small glands lying on either side of the undersurface of the thyroid gland.
parenchymal cells the cells and tissues of an organ that perform the normal functions for that organ, as distinguished from cells that make up the architecture or framework of the organ (connective tissue).
parenteral administered into the body in a way other than through the alimentary canal (subcutaneous, intravenous, intramuscular), as *parenteral* medications.
paresis slight or incomplete paralysis or loss of sensation.
parietal lobe cerebral lobe responsible for sensations of touch, spatial ability, speech, and communication.
parietal pleura outer layer of pleura that lines the chest cavity.
parkinsonism chronic progressive neurologic disease affecting the dopamine producing cells in the brain; also called Parkinson disease; symptoms similar to Parkinson disease caused by some medications.
partial rebreathing mask a low-flow oxygen device.
passive submissive or not produced by active efforts, as *passive* range-of-motion exercises.
passive immunity immunity that occurs during pregnancy and lactation when a woman passes protection to the baby through the placenta or breast milk.
passive range of motion range-of-motion exercises with which the client may need physical assistance.
patella kneecap.
patent unobstructed, open, as a *patent* drainage tube or *patent* airway.
pathogen a disease-producing agent or organism (adjective: pathogenic).
pathology study of changes in body tissues or organs as a result of disease; also used to mean a disease process. (The healthcare provider who specializes in this field is a pathologist.)
pathophysiology study of disorders in functioning.
patient individual being treated by a healthcare provider, also referred to as a "client" when the usage relates to a consumer of healthcare.
payee person designated to receive a client's monthly check and disburse funds appropriately if the client is unable to do so for him- or herself.
pedal pulse pulse in the foot felt over the dorsalis pedis artery or the posterial tibial artery, used to determine status of circulation in the lower extremities.

pediatrics branch of medicine concerned with disorders of children. (Pediatrician: healthcare provider who treats children.)
pediculi lice.
pediculosis infested with lice.
pediculosis pubis pubic lice or parasites that attach themselves to pubic hair follicles and cause intense itching.
peer group contemporaries and friends; the group of people with whom one is associated.
pellagra disease in which the mucous membranes of the mouth and digestive tract become red and inflamed, and lesions appear on the skin (in severe cases can lead to dermatitis, diarrhea, dementia, and even death) due to a marked niacin deficiency.
pelvic exenteration surgical procedure in which the entire contents of the pelvis are removed.
pelvis supports the spinal column and protects parts of the digestive, urinary, and reproductive systems.
penis the male sex organ.
percentage figure denoting the number per 100; the ratio of a given amount to 100.
percussion tapping a body part with short sharp blows to elicit sounds or vibrations that aid in diagnosis; often refers to the use of a percussion hammer to elicit a reflex.
percutaneous endoscopic gastrostomy insertion of a small tube (PEG) through the abdominal wall directly to the stomach, acting as a feeding tube.
performance review written evaluation of an employee's work performance which is discussed in an interview between the individual and his or her supervisor.
perfusion the process of delivering blood to a capillary bed.
pericardial fluid small amount of fluid contained in the space between the visceral and parietal layers in the pericardium that acts as a lubricant and reduces friction between the layers as the heart contracts and relaxes.
pericarditis inflammation of the pericardium.
pericardium the sac enclosing the heart and the roots of some of the great vessels.
perinatal relating to the time around childbirth, may be considered to start around the 20- to 28-gestational week and ending around 1–4 weeks after birth.
perinatologist an obstetrician with special training in high-risk pregnancy care; a maternal-fetal medicine specialist.
perineal care bathing the genitalia and surrounding area.
perineum the pelvic floor and associated structures (from the symphysis pubis to the coccyx).
periodontitis inflammation of tooth sockets.
perioperative the period surrounding surgery; includes the preoperative, intraoperative, and postoperative periods.
periosteum the specialized connective tissue that covers all bones. Periosteum is able to form bone in some cases.
peripheral pertaining to the outward part of surface; further from the center, as *peripheral* nervous system.
peripheral neurovascular assessment method for evaluating the status of an extremity in a bandage or case.
peristalsis wave-like contractions of the intestines by which they propel their contents through the GI tract.

peritoneum serous membrane that lines walls of body cavities and encloses viscera.

peritonitis inflammation of the peritoneum.

permeability allowing passage of a substance, as a *permeable* membrane.

permissive licensure practicing nursing without a license; rarely occurs today.

pernicious tending to be fatal unless treated, as *pernicious* anemia.

perseveration to dwell on one subject or task; also used to describe the inappropriate repetition of behavior that is often associated with damage to the frontal lobe of the brain.

personal protective equipment pieces of equipment that serve as barriers against organisms from entering or leaving the respiratory tract: gloves, eye protection, gowns, and masks.

personal space an invisible, mutually understood area or zone around a person that is considered inappropriate for strangers to violate (varies between cultures). If a person invades another's personal space (comes too close), it may cause discomfort. Much nursing care must occur within the client's personal space. It is vitally important that nurses maintain awareness and respect for the client's personal space.

pertussis highly contagious respiratory disease; also known as whooping cough.

pessary device inserted into the vagina to support the organs of the pelvis.

pH symbol for hydrogen ion concentration (use of the symbol with a number denotes whether a substance is acidic [below 7.0] or basic [above 7.0]).

phagocyte a cell that ingests or engulfs other cells, microorganisms, or foreign particles. This process is called phagocytosis.

phagocytosis engulfing of particulate matter.

phalanges bones of the fingers and toes (singular: phalanx).

pharmacokinetics actions of drugs.

pharmacology the study of chemicals (drugs, medications) and their effects.

pharyngitis inflammation, but not necessarily infection, of the pharynx.

pharynx tube-shaped passage for food and air.

phenylketonuria (PKU) a congenital disease caused by a defect in metabolism of phenylalanine (an essential amino acid) that, if not treated, leads to intellectual impairment.

pheochromocytoma a catecholamine-secreting tumor.

phimosis constriction in the foreskin or prepuce so that it cannot be drawn back over the glans penis.

phlebitis inflammation of a vein. (Thrombophlebitis is inflammation *and* blood clots.)

phlebotomy removal of blood through a vein.

phobia a persistent, irrational fear of a specific situation, object, or activity. (Claustro*phobia* is fear of small, enclosed places.)

phoropter instrument that simulates different corrective lenses during an eye examination in order to better test vision and select glasses.

phosphorus an important mineral found in every body cell.

photophobia intolerance to light.

photosensitivity sensitivity to light.

phototherapy treatment with light, as in physiologic, nonhemolytic jaundice of the newborn.

physiatrics branch of medicine involved with physical medicine, physical therapy, and rehabilitation.

physical change a change in a substance's outward properties (e.g., ice into water).

physical therapy (PT) department that rehabilitates clients with limited physical mobility, using physical modalities, exercises, and assistive devices. Chest physiotherapy is a form of respiratory therapy that uses percussion and postural drainage to loosen and drain secretions from the lungs.

physician also known as a medical doctor (MD), is a health professional or healthcare provider who has received advanced and specialized clinical and academic training to practice medicine. A physician promotes, maintains, and/or restores health by the use of diagnosing a problem, recommending treatment, and providing medical or surgical interventions.

physiologic pertaining to physiology, the function of the body; normal.

physiologic jaundice newborn condition in which the baby's immature liver cannot handle bilirubin, and thus bilirubin levels increase in the body.

physiologic needs needs required to sustain life such as oxygen, food, water, and elimination; survival needs.

physiology science that deals with body functions.

phytochemical previously unidentified naturally occurring components in plant foods that may help protect against disease.

pica a craving to eat inedible items or unnatural food items, such as *pica* in pregnancy.

piggyback infusion a supplemental IV added to a primary IV.

pilonidal having a group of hairs, as in *pilonidal* cyst or sinus tract.

pilonidal cyst cyst above the anus, often believed to result from an infolding of the skin in which hair continues to grow.

pincer grasp the ability of an infant to use the forefinger and thumb to hold small objects.

pineal shaped like a pine cone, as the *pineal* body within the brain or the *pineal* gland.

pineal gland small cone-shaped structure located at the top portion of the brain's third ventricle that produces melatonin.

pinna external ear; auricle.

pinocytosis engulfing of extracellular fluids.

pinworms a common parasitic infestation in children causing anal and perineal itching.

pitting edema swelling in an extremity that persists after pressure (e.g., socks) is applied. Often indicates cardiovascular and tissue perfusion problems, such as heart failure.

pituitary gland a tiny gland located at the base of the brain that secretes or releases several hormones, including growth hormone; called the master gland.

placenta an organ joining woman and fetus during pregnancy in human beings and other mammals. The placental blood furnishes nutrients, oxygen, hormones, and other substances to the fetus and carries away wastes. (Also called afterbirth.)

placenta accreta condition in which a placenta fails to separate and be expelled within 20–30 min after delivery or leaves remnants in the uterus; also called retained placenta.

placenta previa low implantation of the placenta so that it partially or completely covers the cervical os.

plan of assistance third step in due process in which a supervisor writes a statement describing a deficiency, employee actions needed to correct it, timeline for improvements, and consequences to employee if the plan is not followed and improvement is not shown.

plane an imaginary flat surface that divides the body into sections.

planning in nursing process, developing goals to prevent, reduce, or eliminate problems and identifying nursing interventions that will assist in meeting these goals.

plantar flexion bending the foot so that the toes are pointed downward.

plaque the buildup of cholesterol and other fats on the inner surface of blood vessels.

plaques, tangles, and tau (in relation to Alzheimer's) abnormal clusters of protein fragments that build up between nerve cells decreasing communication; tangles form inside neurons and interfere with ability to create normal proteins, called tau, and the cell dies.

plasma the fluid portion of the blood.

plasma membrane See *cell membrane*.

platelet type of blood cell composed of cell fragments that provide a major step in the blood clotting process.

pleura membrane covering the lungs and lining the walls of the chest cavity, as the parietal *pleura*.

pleural cavity space between the two layers of the pleura; also called pleural space.

pleurisy inflammation of the pleura.

plexus a network or tangle, as of veins or nerves.

plication surgical pleating or taking of tucks to shorten a structure, as in treatment of retinal detachment.

plumbism chronic lead poisoning.

***Pneumocystis jiroveci* pneumonia** an interstitial plasma cell pneumonia, one of the most common opportunistic diseases of AIDS.

pneumonectomy removal of an entire lung.

pneumonia lung inflammation, with consolidation and drainage.

pneumothorax collapse of a lung due to air or gas into the space between your lung and chest wall. This air pushes on the outside of the lung causing it to collapse.

poison any substance that through its chemical action kills, injures, or impairs an organism.

poliomyelitis contagious viral disease that attacks the CNS and can cause temporary or permanent paralysis or weakness; commonly known as "polio."

pollution act of contamination or making impure by noxious substances; may refer to air, food, water, or noise contamination.

polycythemia vera disorder in which the total number of RBCs, WBCs, and platelets are increased; also called primary polycythemia.

polydactylism condition in which an individual is born with an extra finger or toe.

polydipsia excessive thirst as in *diabetes* or as related to psychological factors as in *psychogenic nocturnal polydipsia*

polyhydramnios excessive amniotic fluid.

polymerase chain reaction test (PCR) a specific laboratory test for HIV that can identify HIV within 2–3 weeks as well as identify the genetic material of the HIV.

polyneuritis inflammation of many nerves.

polypectomy removal of polyps from the lower bowel.

polyphagia an abnormal craving for all kinds of food.

polypharmacy the use of several medications concurrently by one individual; often consistent with adverse drug reactions and commonly seen in the chronically ill and the elderly.

polysaccharide long chain of many sugar molecules; a complex carbohydrate.

polysubstance abuse abuse of two or more substances.

polyuria voiding an excessive amount of urine.

pons brain area that contains nerve tracts that carry messages between the cerebrum and medulla.

popliteal pulse pulse located posteriorly to the knee, sometimes used as an alternative means of assessing blood pressure with a large leg cuff.

pores tiny openings in the skin that release oil and sweat.

ports entry or exit points.

port-wine stain a permanent birthmark consisting of a flat, purple-red area with sharp borders.

positive Homans sign pain that occurs on the knee upon dorsiflexion, which may be indicative of thrombophlebitis.

posterior toward the back.

postmortem examination after death, as *postmortem* examination (autopsy); "post."

postnatal the period for a newborn occurring after birth.

postoperative after surgery.

postoperative bed bed prepared for a client who is returning from surgery or another procedure that requires transfer into the bed from a stretcher or wheelchair.

postpartum a timeframe of about 4–6 weeks for the newly delivered mother, starting after giving birth.

postpartum hematoma bleeding into the subcutaneous tissue in the perineal area after delivery.

postpartum hemorrhage any blood loss from the uterus after delivery in the amount of 500–1,000 mL within 24 hr.

post-term fetus remaining in the uterus beyond 42 weeks.

postural drainage method of drainage that uses position and gravity to drain secretions and mucus from a person's lungs.

potassium chemical element that plays a major role in the acid–base and water balance in the body; a major ion in the intracellular fluid, symbol is K^+.

potential needs in the nursing process, needs which may occur; identified as *at risk for…*

potentiation enhancement (multiplication) of one agent by another, so that the combined action is greater than the sum of the two (e.g., alcohol and Valium *potentiate* each other); synergism.

practical nurse a licensed practical nurse (LPN) who cares for the acute and chronically ill individual under the direction and supervision of healthcare providers and registered nurses; referred to as a licensed vocational nurse (LVN) in Texas and California.

preadolescence early adolescence (approximately ages 11–14).

prebiotic nondigestible food ingredients that selectively feed probiotic bacteria. These are found in whole foods, supplements, and specialized food products. Prebiotics and probiotics work to maintain a healthy digestive system and may boost immune function.

precipitate the solid matter of liquid urine (or another liquid) that falls out of suspension. The process is called *precipitation,* that is, the extraction of a solid from a solution.

preconception period in time before the woman is pregnant, as in *preconceptional* care.

prediabetes the condition of *impaired glucose homeostasis* (IGH) that occurs when blood glucose levels are higher than normal but not high enough for the definitive diagnosis of diabetes mellitus; may also be referred to as impaired fasting glucose (IFG) or impaired glucose tolerance (IGT).

preeclampsia condition in which a woman whose pregnancy was previously progressing normally develops hypertension with either edema, proteinuria, or both, usually after the 20th week of gestation.

prefilled syringe a single medication dose prepared by a manufacturer or pharmacy.

pregnancy the state of having a developing embryo or fetus within the uterus; being with child; gravid.

pregnancy-induced hypertension (PIH) an abnormal complication of pregnancy, and for a short time following delivery, characterized by hypertension (high blood pressure), edema, and proteinuria. Seizures may occur if not successfully treated. Also called gestosis, toxemia of pregnancy, and preeclampsia–eclampsia syndrome. May be fatal to woman and/or fetus.

prejudice an opinion formed without knowing the facts.

preload the amount of pressure or "stretching force" against the ventricular wall at end diastole.

premature cervical dilation a condition in which the cervix is unable to support a pregnancy and the weight of the fetus is enough to force it to dilate, causing a spontaneous abortion.

premenstrual dysphoric disorder (PMDD) a severe form of premenstrual disorder (PMS). Compared to PMS, PMDD has more significant physical symptoms, more severe affective (emotional) symptoms, and noted dysfunction in personal relationships.

prenatal care before birth.

preoperative before surgery.

preparatory depression depression that occurs when a person realizes the impact of a loss before it happens.

prepuce foreskin of the penis.

presbycusis gradual hearing loss associated with aging, often starting in middle age and becoming noticeable by the mid-60s.

presbyopia a visual disorder associated with aging due to the loss of flexibility of the lens, making it difficult to see close objects.

prescription written formula for preparing and administering medication.

presentation part of the fetus that lies closest to the pelvis and will first enter the birth canal, usually the head.

pressure external force sufficient to occlude blood in capillaries, resulting in tissue anoxia (lack of oxygen) and tissue death (necrosis).

pressure injury, also known as pressure ulcer, pressure wound, pressure sore ulcerated sore often caused by prolonged pressure on a bony prominence or other area, especially if the client is allowed to lie in one position for an extended period. (Formerly referred to as decubitus ulcer, pressure ulcer, or bedsore.)

preterm birth born early, prior to the end of the 37th week of gestation.

priapism continued erection accompanied by pain.

priest Catholic or Episcopal clergy person.

primary caregivers a client's significant others whether blood related or not.

primary disease a disease that occurs independently, not related to another disease.

primary healthcare family-focused healthcare that emphasizes health education and wellness to promote healthy lifestyles and decrease the potential for illness.

primary needs needs that must be satisfied before attempting to meet other needs (such as oxygen, food, water, and elimination); *physiologic needs, survival needs.*

primigravida a woman pregnant for the first time.

primipara a woman who has had one live birth (often used interchangeably with primigravida).

priority needs needs which must be met to sustain life (physiological, survival, or primary needs).

prioritization in the nursing process, following specific steps to determine the client's most important needs.

probationary an internship period a recent graduate nurse is required to serve before becoming a full-fledged RN or LVN/LPN.

probiotic healthy live bacteria found in whole foods, supplements, and specialized food products.

problem-oriented medical records a type of charting focused on specific problems; is sometimes called focus charting. Used to support collaborative healthcare teams in identifying and solving priority problems.

prodromal the period before actual symptoms occur; may involve a premonition that a disease is about to occur. Some disorders, such as genital herpes virus, are more contagious during the prodromal period.

products of conception the placenta and fetus.
progesterone female hormone that functions primarily during pregnancy.
prognosis projected client outcome.
progress note form nurses fill out at regular intervals to summarize a client's condition or response to treatment.
projectile vomiting emesis expelled with great force.
prokaryote unicellular organism without separate nucleus. Prokaryotes are divided into archaea and bacteria. Each cell of a type is identical and can function independently.
prolapse condition in which an organ or internal part drops or sags.
prolapsed cord umbilical cord that precedes the baby in delivery.
pronation turning the hand so that the palm faces downward or backward.
prone positioning a client so that he or she is lying on the stomach.
prophylaxis medications given to prevent infections.
proportion two ratios separated by an equal sign or a double colon.
proprioception the unconscious awareness of how one's body is positioned when standing, sitting, or moving in a space (i.e., *spatial orientation*).
prospective predetermined, before the fact.
prospective payment reimbursement for healthcare made by third-party payors according to a formula or average reimbursement of actual costs per case.
prostaglandins fatty acids that are widespread in body tissues and that generally stimulate contraction or relaxation of smooth muscles.
prostate a doughnut-shaped gland lying just below the bladder in the male.
prostate specific antigen (PSA) a glycoprotein found only in the tissue of the prostate gland; elevated PSA level is indicative of a prostate disorder.
prostatectomy removal of the prostate.
prostatitis inflammation of the prostate gland.
prosthesis the replacement of a missing part by an artificial substitute (e.g., an artificial eye, arm, or leg is a prosthesis).
prosthetics the manufacture of prostheses, splints, and braces for limbs and the back.
protection ability of cells to prevent injury to themselves (includes spore formation, mutation).
protective device piece of equipment, most often a vest or a belt, used to ensure the safety of the client (i.e., helping client to remain in a chair without falling); also called a client reminder device.
protective isolation attempts to prevent harmful microorganisms from coming into contact with the client; also called reverse or neutropenic isolation.
protein groups of amino acids in complex compounds that are vital to life. Protein-rich foods are essential to building and repairing all body tissues and include meat, eggs, fish, legumes, and dairy products.
prothrombin a plasma protein that is converted to thrombin during blood clotting. (Also called clotting factor II.)

protocol specific policies outlining a healthcare facility's standards for care.
proton subatomic particle carrying a positive electrical charge.
protoplasm the essential component of the living cell.
protraction moving forward or anteriorly, as in jutting out the jaw.
proxemics the study of human use of space and the effects that population density has in relationship to communication.
proximal nearest the origin of a part.
proximodistal from the center or core outward. (Refers to the pattern of development and achievement of motor control of the infant.)
pruritus itching.
pseudodementia a condition in which a person appears to have dementia but is actually suffering from depression.
pseudomenstruation small amount of vaginal bleeding in newborns caused by maternal hormones.
psoriasis a chronic skin disorder that involves red macules and patches covered with flakes or silvery scales. It is believed to have a hereditary or autoimmune origin in some cases.
psyche the mind.
psychiatrist a healthcare provider who specializes in the treatment of mental disorders and typically will write prescriptions for psychiatric medications.
psychological pertaining to the mind, behavior, or thoughts rather than to the physical body.
psychological needs those human needs related to safety and security.
psychometric type of testing for mental disorders that includes an in-depth interview and various other tests; also may be called neuropsychiatric testing.
psychosis a mental disturbance when thought and emotions are so impaired that contact is lost with external reality. Maybe temporary or permanent.
psychoactive or psychotropic drug any drug that has significant effects on psychological processes, such as thinking, perception, and emotion. These include drugs used deliberately to produce an altered state of consciousness and therapeutic agents designed to help a mental condition. *Psychotropic* is the term usually used in clinical settings.
psychrophile prokaryote that can live in very cold temperatures.
ptosis drooping or sagging of an organ or part from its normal position (usually refers to eyelid).
ptyalism increase in salivation during pregnancy.
puberty period in life when a person becomes sexually able to reproduce.
pubic arch opening of the pelvis.
pubococcygeal pelvic muscles.
puerperal complication occurring following the birth of a baby.
puerperium period immediately after childbirth, continuing through involution (return of the uterus to its nonpregnant state).

pulmonary artery occlusion (wedge) pressure reflects the degree of severity of many cardiovascular problems such as heart failure, pulmonary hypertension, pulmonary vascular resistance, and cardiovascular–pulmonary circulation; uses a pulmonary artery catheter (PAC), also known as a Swan-Ganz catheter, to measure internal pulmonary pressures which provide estimates of tissue perfusion.

pulmonary edema excess fluid in the lungs.

pulmonary emphysema abnormal, permanent enlargement of the alveoli and alveolar ducts with destruction of the alveolar walls.

pulmonic valve valve that separates the right ventricle from the pulmonary aorta, also called the pulmonary semilunar valve.

pulse the heartbeat as felt through the walls of the arteries and the skin or as heard at the apex of the heart with a stethoscope. The rhythmic dilation of an artery that results from beating of the heart.

pulse deficit a difference that exists between the apical and the radial pulse.

pulse oximeter a convenient monitor that measures the amount (percentage) of oxygen saturation in the blood.

pulse pressure difference between systolic blood pressure minus diastolic blood pressure. The normal range of pulse pressure is between 40–60 mm Hg.

pulse rate measure of how often a person's heart beats.

pulse rhythm spacing between heartbeats.

puncture a hole made by a pointed object; penetration.

pupil black center of the eye that regulates the amount of light that enters it.

purified protein derivative the solution used for intradermal testing for tuberculosis. See *tuberculin skin test*.

purulent consisting of or secreting pus.

pus the liquid product of inflammation made up of leukocytes, liquid, and cellular debris.

pustule a small elevation of the skin filled with pus or lymph.

pyelonephritis potentially dangerous infection of the kidney and renal pelvis.

pyloric sphincter circular muscle that controls the opening between the stomach and the duodenal portion of the small intestine.

pyloric stenosis a congenital anomaly in which an increase in the size of the musculature at the junction of the stomach and small intestine occurs, causing the pyloric opening to constrict and block food passage.

pylorus lower narrow portion of the stomach, which attaches to the small intestine.

pyorrhea copious discharge of pus. *Pyorrhea alveolaris*, a purulent mouth infection.

pyrexia fever; abnormally high body temperature.

pyuria pus in the urine.

Q

quadrant one of four corresponding quarters, as of the abdomen or buttock. For example, the appendix is in the lower right abdominal *quadrant*.

quadriplegia paralysis of both arms and both legs; also called tetraplegia.

quality assurance standards of care that represent acceptable, expected levels of performance by nursing staff and other staff members.

quickening first fetal movements a woman feels in pregnancy; signs of life.

R

rabbi Jewish clergy person.

rabies an acute viral disease of the central nervous system that can be transmitted by a rabid animal's bite. Prophylaxis treatment is available, so any bite by a wild animal should be reported immediately.

race term used to differentiate large groups of humankind that share common genetic characteristics associated with having ancestors from a specific part of the world.

radial pulse pulse rate measured above the radial artery or thumb side of the wrist.

radiation giving off infrared heat rays; radioactive energy.

radius the small bone of the forearm.

radon a by-product of the disintegration of radium that contributes to diseases.

range of motion ability to move various joints and structures of the body.

rape violent crime in which an individual is sexually assaulted without his or her consent.

rapid test a rapid, preliminary laboratory test that is performed outside the typical laboratory, for example, in the home or in a clinic, and can give results in 30 min or less.

rapport a warm relaxed relationship of mutual understanding, acceptance, and sympathetic compatibility between or among individuals. A desirable element in the therapist/client relationship.

ratio relationship of one quantity to another; may be written as a fraction or separated by a colon.

rationale reason or underlying principle behind a nursing procedure.

reabsorption the process of absorbing again; it allows bones to grow and change shape.

reactive depression depression that results when an individual concentrates on past losses.

receptor a sensory nerve ending that responds to stimuli.

reciprocity states known as compact states, who by mutual agreements set in place by the nurse licensure compact (NLC), grant a license to practice nursing to any person licensed to practice in another compact state.

recommended dietary allowance recommendations for average daily amounts of nutrients considered adequate in meeting the nutritional needs of all healthy people.

recovery position used in emergency rescue, in which the person is rolled to the side, so the head, shoulders, and torso move simultaneously, without twisting.

rectocele herniation of part of the rectum into the vagina.

rectum distal portion of the large intestine between the sigmoid colon and the anal canal (adjective: **rectal**. accurate temperature may be assessed at this site, and some medications are administered rectally).

refeeding syndrome set of symptoms that results when a starving person, or one who has been receiving insufficient nutrition related to alcohol or drug abuse, receives carbohydrates too quickly, overstimulating insulin production and seriously upsetting electrolyte balance; can be fatal.

referred (referring to pain) pain that is felt at a location other than its origination; when one healthcare provider sends (refers) a client to another healthcare provider or specialist.

reflex an automatic movement in response to a particular stimulus, as the knee jerk in response to a tap below the kneecap.

reflex arc circle in the spinal cord that receives and sends messages through nerve fibers.

reflex incontinence urinary leakage due to bladder instability as a result of upper motor lesions or neuropathies.

reflux backing up of urine into the kidneys as a result of a bladder obstruction.

refraction determination of refractive errors of the eye and their correction.

regional anesthesia interruption of sensory nerve conductivity to specific area of the body (includes conduction block, field block, nerve block).

registered nurse a person who is licensed to practice nursing after completion of a registered nursing program and has passed the national council licensure examination (NCLEX-RN).

registered pharmacist a healthcare professional who is licensed to prepare and to dispense medications upon the order of a licensed practitioner of medicine.

registry a service that recruits nurses to work in facilities that need extra help for special duty clients, during busy periods, or for vacation coverage.

regression return to a former state as a child *regresses* when ill. Regression of a disease process refers to its relief or subsiding. In psychiatry, when an individual reverts to immature behavior or developmental stage when threatened with overwhelming external problems or internal conflicts

rehabilitation restoration of a person to as normal as possible body structure and/or function after an injury or illness.

reminder device See *protective device*.

reminiscence remembering past joys and successes.

remission in relation to drug or alcohol use: early remission means the person has not used for more than 3 months and sustained remission means the person has not used for greater than 12 months.

renal pertaining to the kidney, as *renal* failure.

renal colic severe, penetrating lower back pain caused by a stone becoming lodged in the ureter.

renal cortex outer portion of the kidney.

renal erythropoietic factor See *erythropoietin*.

renal failure disorder in which the kidneys can no longer meet everyday demands.

renal medulla kidney portion that contains the renal tubules, loops of Henle, and collecting tubules.

renal pelvis end of the ureter that receives urine from the calyces.

renal threshold maximum amount of a substance that the renal tubules can reabsorb back into the body before the excess is excreted into the urine.

renin hormone that is important in blood pressure regulation.

replantation reattachment of a completely severed body part back to the body.

replication reproduction of cancer cells.

reproduction ability of cells to form colonies or of individual cells to increase in size and/or replicate themselves.

rescue breathing one component of CPR that of blowing breaths into the victim who has stopped breathing.

research laboratory laboratory where studies and experiments on animals are conducted to understand, cure, or prevent human disease.

resection excision of a portion of an organ or structure, as a gastric (stomach) *resection*.

reservoir any place where a microorganism can multiply or survive before moving to a place where it can multiply.

resident term used to refer to the client, particularly in a nursing home or other long-term facility; term used to refer to a healthcare provider who is studying in a medical specialty.

resident assessment protocol form that aids the nursing care team to create an individualized plan of care for every client; often used in long-term care.

residual amount remaining or left behind, as *residual* urine after voiding.

residual urine volume amount of urine that remains in the bladder after voiding at least once.

respiration the total process of the exchange of oxygen and carbon dioxide between the air and body cells. (External respiration denotes the exchange of gases in the lungs; internal respiration denotes exchange of gases between the blood and body cells.)

respirator a machine that forces air into the lungs; also called a ventilator.

respiratory acidosis condition that stems from an increase in carbon dioxide in the blood.

respiratory alkalosis condition that stems from a deficit of plasma CO_2 or carbonic acid.

respiratory distress syndrome (RDS) leading cause of death in premature newborns in whom the lungs have not fully developed and do not expand for adequate breathing. Also called hyaline membrane disease.

respiratory therapy (RT) (respiratory care) department concerned with treatment, management, and care of clients with respiratory disorders through use of oxygen and other gases and assistive devices for breathing and maintenance of ventilation.

respite care temporary institutional care of a sick, elderly, or disabled person, providing relief for their usual caregiver.

resting energy expenditure total calories a person needs to maintain his or her body processes.

resume document that emphasizes a person's strengths and abilities and/or that lists a person's employment and educational experiences and achievements.

retention inability to void.

retina the innermost tunic of the eyeball that contains rods and cones and is the origin of the optic nerve. Light rays focus at the retina in normal vision.

retinitis inflammation of the retina, as *retinitis* pigmentosa.

retinopathy any noninflammatory disorder of the retina of the eye, as diabetic *retinopathy* (which may lead to blindness).

retinopathy of prematurity (ROP) condition commonly seen in a preterm infant in which the retinal blood vessels are abnormal and immature. A second causative factor is the use of high concentrations of oxygen.

retraction moving backward or back into anatomic position.

retrovirus one of a large group of RNA-based viruses that tend to infect immunocompromised persons.

reverse isolation See *protective isolation.*

Reye syndrome acute and potentially fatal childhood disease, which often follows a viral illness and may be related to aspirin use during that time.

Rh factor the presence or absence of the D antigen on RBC, used to determine ABO compatibility.

Rh sensitization a condition in which a pregnant Rh-negative woman has had Rh-positive RBCs from the fetus cross the placental barrier, stimulating the formation of antibodies within her circulatory system, which then return to the fetus and destroy fetal erythrocytes. This condition is prompted by, but does not occur, during the first pregnancy but does so with increasing sensitivity in subsequent pregnancies.

rheumatic carditis complication of rheumatic fever in which valvular lesions impair valve efficiency and increase the heart's workload.

rheumatic fever autoimmune reaction to group A beta-hemolytic *Streptococcus,* believed to develop as a result of continued streptococcal infections.

rhinitis inflammation of the mucous membrane lining the nasal cavity.

rhinoplasty plastic surgery/repair of the nose.

rhinorrhea a runny rose; leakage of cerebrospinal fluid from the nose

rhonchi low-pitched rattling sounds in the throat that resemble snoring (singular: rhoncus).

ribonucleic acid genetic material responsible for taking messages from DNA and transporting them to the ribosomes in the cytoplasm.

rickets a condition in children caused by lack of vitamin D.

risk factors factors that increase a person's likelihood of developing a certain disease.

rituals practices that provide a group with comfort, acceptance, and inclusion.

rods specialized neurons dispersed throughout the retina, suited to dim light and especially useful in night vision.

roseola rose-colored rash. *Roseola infantum,* an acute viral disease that usually occurs in children under age 2 and disappears suddenly; *exanthem subitum.*

rotation process of turning about an axis, as *rotation* of the hand or of the fetus in preparation for delivery.

roundworm intestinal parasite common to warm climates and unsanitary conditions, which mature in the intestines and can cause diarrhea, intestinal obstruction, and sometimes intestinal rupture.

rubella mild disease with fever and a mild rash; German measles (in English); 3-day measles.

rubeola measles (in English); German measles (in French and Spanish). Preventable by immunization.

rugae (singular: ruga) folds of the stomach when it is empty (they allow the stomach to distend when food is eaten).

S

sacrum solid bone in the spinal column of adults that anchors the pelvis.

sagittal an imaginary vertical plane that divides the body into right and left sides, from top to bottom. The midsagittal plane divides the body into equal, symmetrical halves. (Also means shaped like an arrow, as the coccyx or xiphoid process of the sternum.)

saline lock provides continuous peripheral IV access without continuous infusion. A seal or cap is attached to the hub (end) of the IV catheter, "locking" it. To reduce the possibility of clotting, the lock may be flushed with 2–3 ml of saline every 8 hr or as ordered. (Also referred to as a heparin lock or hep lock.)

saliva thin, watery fluid secreted into the mouth which moistens food particles and begins the digestive process by breaking down starch into smaller sugar molecules.

salivation secretion of saliva.

sally port a system of two doors, only one of which can be opened at a time, used to prevent escape of disturbed or incarcerated clients.

salt any compound of a base or an acid; table salt (sodium chloride); a purgative, as Epsom salt.

sanguineous drainage made up mostly of blood.

saprophyte live off the organic remains of dead plants and animals.

sarcoma connective tissue tumor, often malignant, as Kaposi *sarcoma.*

saturated fat a fat, such as an animal fat, which already contains its full complement of hydrogen.

scabies contagious skin disorder caused by the itch mite. Often sexually transmitted.

scabies scraping a diagnostic tool obtained by shaving the top of a suspected lesion, placing the specimen on a microscope slide that has been covered with immersion oil, and examining the slide under a microscope.

scapula shoulder blade.

schizophrenia a psychotic disorder characterized by disturbances in thinking (*cognition*), emotional responsive, and behavior.

scientific problem-solving precise method of investigating problems and arriving at solutions.

sclera outer coating of the eyeball.

sclerodactyly scleroderma of the fingers and toes.

scleroderma chronic hardening and shrinking of the connective tissues of any body organ; often refers to thickened, hard, and darkened skin.

scoliosis lateral curvature of the normally straight, vertical line of the spine, sometimes is S-shaped ("curvature of the spine").

scrotum sac-like structure that encloses the testes.

scurvy disease caused by a vitamin C deficiency. Lesser deficiencies cause listlessness, irritability, and lowered resistance to disease; greater deficiencies cause bleeding gums, loose teeth, sore and stiff joints, tiny hemorrhages, and great weight loss.

sebaceous pertaining to sebum (the oily, fatty secretion of the sebaceous gland).

sebaceous glands oil-secreting glands located close to the hair follicles into which they usually drain.

sebum oily secretion of the sebaceous (oil) glands composed of fat and dead skin and released into the hair follicles.

secondary disease a disease that directly results from or depends on another disease.

secondary needs needs, according to Maslow, that do not sustain life, but enhance quality of life (such as beauty, learning, and love). A person must meet primary needs before attempting to meet secondary needs.

secondhand smoke smoke from someone else's cigarette; the chemicals found in smoke that a nonsmoker breathes are more dangerous than the smoke inhaled by the smoker.

sedation allaying irritability or excitement, usually by administration of a sedative medication; *conscious sedation* is used for some surgical procedures in which the client remains awake.

sedative a remedy that has a quieting effect, sometimes enabling sleep.

seizure a sudden attack or recurrence of a disease, as in epilepsy (cerebral seizure), formerly called convulsion.

seizure disorder repeated episodes of seizures.

self-actualized according to Maslow, state of being fulfilled, complete, and reaching full potential.

self-esteem how one feels about oneself; self-respect, self-worth, self-image.

semen fluid that carries spermatozoa which are manufactured in the male's testes.

semicircular canals section of the inner ear that contains hair-like nerve endings that respond to movement and control the sense of balance.

semilunar valves heart valves with three crescent (half-moon) shaped cusps.

seminal vesicles convoluted, sac-shaped glands that store semen.

seminiferous tubules the functional units of the testes, where sperm cells are produced and mature.

seminoma malignancy of the testis.

senescence the symptoms or changes associated with normal aging; growing old, aging.

senility See *dementia*.

senior, senior citizen a common, generalized expression for an old or older person; may refer to citizens who have retired or are over the age of 65.

sensitivity test performed on a culture to discern which medication is most effective in treating an organism; also called a culture and sensitivity (C & S) test.

sentinel lymph node node that drains the area of a breast involved by tumor.

sentinel lymph node biopsy removes a limited number of priority lymph nodes that are most likely to become cancerous.

separation anxiety a behavior associated with distress in children less than 24 months of age due to a caregiver leaving the sight of the child. Behaviors include fussiness, crying, clinging, screaming, and tantrums. See *stranger anxiety*.

septicemia generalized infection (sepsis) throughout the body.

septum dividing wall between two cavities, as the nasal *septum* or the *septa* (plural) between the chambers of the heart.

sequela an illness or injury that follows as a direct result of a previous condition or event.

sequestration abnormal separation of a part from the whole, as a part of a bone.

serosanguinous fluid drainage composed of serum and blood.

serous containing clear fluid; drainage made up of serum.

severe maternal morbidity (SMM) the most severe complications of maternal morbidity, which includes physical and psychological conditions that result from or are aggravated by pregnancy and have an adverse effect on a woman's health.

sex can be defined as the rhythmic movements of *coitus*, also known as *sexual intercourse* or *sexual activity*. Also refers to biologic characteristics that divide humans into different categories.

sexual dysfunction the inability to enjoy or to engage in sexual activity.

sexual health a state of physical, emotional, mental, and social well-being in relation to sexuality.

sexual orientation term referring to which gender a person finds sexually desirable.

sexual rights embrace certain human rights that are already recognized in international and regional human rights documents and other consensus documents and in national laws.

sexual violence sexual activity that is not obtained by freely given consent.

sexuality the way in which individuals physically, mentally, emotionally, and socially experience and express themselves as sexual beings.

sexually transmitted infection (STI) a disease that can be (and most often is) transmitted by sexual intercourse or other intimate contact.

shaman a Native American medicine man or woman.

shearing (force) friction, as applied to the skin, usually caused by moving the client's body across bedding without proper protection.

shingles See *herpes zoster*.

shock a life-threatening condition that occurs when cells and organs do not get enough oxygen and nutrients due to decreased circulation or loss of blood. Can be caused by many things but signs and symptoms of shock are similar despite the cause.

shock wave treatment used to blast stones in the kidney into small gravel-like fragments that are more easily passed from the body.

short-term goal an expected outcome or goal that a client can reasonably meet in a matter of hours or days.

show discharge of blood, usually as a beginning sign of labor (bloody show).

shunt a bypass; u-shaped tube inserted into blood vessels to facilitate repeated hemodialysis; also called a fistula.

siblings two or more people having at least one parent in common.

sickle cell an abnormal crescent-shaped erythrocyte. (*Sickle-cell* anemia is a genetic blood defect that is most commonly found in African Americans, also known as sicklemia.)

sickle cell crisis severe, painful episodes of sickle cell anemia due to clumping and occlusion of blood vessels.

sickle cell disease genetic disorder characterized by the formation of abnormally curved RBCs which are ineffective as oxygen-carriers (thereby causing anemia) and because of their shape are able to clump together (causing further anemia and circulatory occlusion).

side effect a result from a therapeutic agent other than originally intended (often refers to the result of a prescribed medication).

sign objective evidence of disease that another person can note (as opposed to symptom, which only the client can describe).

significant figure term used to refer to numbers that have practical meaning; in determining doses, rounding up or down to a certain decimal place.

signs indications of disease or illness that can be seen by someone other than the client, for example, excessive bleeding, cough, or weight loss; objective evidence. See also *symptoms*.

simian line abnormal crease appearing straight across the palms in the hands of children with Down syndrome.

simple mask a transparent green mask with a simple nipple adapter that fits over a client's nose, mouth, and chin, which provides low-flow oxygen.

simple triage and rapid treatment (START) system that identifies people who will die quickly if they don't receive immediate medical care.

Sims position examination position in which the client is lying on his or her left side with right knee flexed.

single-adult household adults who live alone in their own apartments or houses with no children.

single-parent family a family in which one adult is head of household with dependent children. The adult who is single may be single by choice or as a result of separation, divorce, or death.

sinus a cavity or channel, often refers to the paranasal *sinuses;* may also refer to fistula (a sinus tract).

sinusitis inflammation of the sinuses.

sitz bath a bath used to apply heat to the pelvic area.

Sjögren syndrome an immune system disorder characterized by dry eyes and a dry mouth.

skeletal traction form of directly applying traction to a client's bones by surgically inserting metal pins or wires into the bones.

skilled nursing facility facility that provides 24-hr care to clients who live there or stay there temporarily to recover from injury or severe illness.

skin traction traction applied to the skin, which transmits the pull to the musculoskeletal system.

skin turgor tension or fullness of the skin.

slander malicious and false verbal statements.

sleep apnea a sleep disorder characterized by transient absence of spontaneous respirations that occur during a sleeping cycle.

slough to shed; to cast off (noun: slough—a mass of dead tissue).

smegma sebaceous gland secretion that may collect under the foreskin of the penis in an uncircumcised male.

social needs needs for love and belonging.

sodium a chemical element that is a major ion in extracellular fluids (common table salt is composed of sodium [Na^+] and chloride).

soft diet a nutritionally adequate diet that is low in fiber, connective tissue, and fat.

solitary play children playing alone with their own toys in the same general area but not next to each other and with no interaction (common in infants).

solute a substance dissolved in a solvent.

solvent a liquid that dissolves a solute.

somnambulism sleepwalking.

somniloquism sleeptalking.

somnolent state in which a person is very difficult or impossible to rouse.

Somogyi phenomenon condition in diabetes mellitus in which overtreatment with insulin causes hypoglycemia. This is followed by a compensatory period of rebound hyperglycemia as the body tries to correct the initial problem by increasing glucose production.

sordes foul, brownish deposits that collects around the teeth and lips in low-grade fevers.

soul food cooking style and particular foods commonly eaten by people in the southeastern United States.

spastic cerebral palsy most common type of cerebral palsy, characterized by increased muscle tone or spasticity, partial or full paralysis, and sensory abnormalities.

special respiratory precautions/special respiratory isolation protection for healthcare staff and visitors against TB and other diseases if the client is still considered communicable. *Personal respiratory protection* (PRP) in this case consists of a special *high-filtration particulate respirator* (N95 or HEPA-filtered) or a *powered* (*positive*) *air-purified respirator* (PAPR) as per CDC recommendations.

specific gravity a substance's weight, as compared with another. Fluids, such as urine, are compared to pure water, which has a specific gravity of 1.000.

specific immunity immunity in which specific defense mechanisms are able to recognize and act against particular harmful substances.

spermatozoa sperm cells; male reproductive cells.
spermicide chemicals that immobilize or kill sperm and block the cervix to inhibit sperm from traveling to an egg.
sphincter circular muscle that guards an opening.
sphygmomanometer device used in conjunction with a stethoscope to measure blood pressure, consisting of an inflatable bladder attached to a bulb or pump, enclosed in a cuff, with a deflating mechanism.
spina bifida congenital anomaly in which the vertebral spaces fail to close.
spinal anesthesia anesthetic injected into the subarachnoid space of the spinal cord providing an extensive conduction block. Many types of surgery can be performed in this manner.
spinal bifida occulta an opening in a child's vertebral column with no apparent symptoms.
spinal cord a long mass of nerve cells and fibers extending though a central canal from the brain's medulla to the approximate level of the first or second lumbar vertebra.
spinal nerves nerves that originate in the spinal cord.
spinal stenosis narrowing of the intervertebral space.
spirillum spiral shaped bacteria (plural: spirilla).
spirometry spirometry and pulmonary function tests help determine a client's respiratory status.
spleen an organ containing lymphoid tissue that is designed to filter blood. Its functions in an adult including destroying old RBCs, forming bilirubin, producing lymphocytes and monocytes, and acting as a reservoir for blood.
splint an appliance, either rigid or flexible, that immobilizes body parts in place, as an arm fracture *splint* (verb: splint—to provide firm support as postoperative splinting or a splint to immobilize a fracture).
splinting (incision) use of a pillow or large towel to provide support along a suture line.
spore protective capsule formed by some microorganisms to safeguard themselves.
sprain twisting a joint with stretched or torn ligaments (not a fracture) and possibly other damage to blood vessels, tendons, or nerves.
squamous scaly, plate-like, as *squamous* epithelium.
stabilization (stable) room room in an emergency facility in which clients are triaged and stabilized for transfer to an operating room or other area.
stages of labor process of delivery that spans from the onset of true labor to the stabilization of the mother afterward; the four stages are, specifically, dilation, expulsion, placental, and recovery.
stagnation according to Erikson theory, stagnation involves adults who focus on personal pursuits and interests.
Standard Precautions safety precautions designed for the care of all clients regardless of diagnosis or infection status.
stapes the "stirrup," one of three tiny bones within the middle ear which are set in motion by sound waves.
stasis standstill, stationary, or not moving.
station level of descent of the fetal presenting part into the birth canal.
status asthmaticus dangerous condition that exists when medications do not relieve an acute episode of asthma.
status epilepticus a medical emergency; convulsions with intense muscle contractions and dyspnea lasting 15 min or more.
steatorrhea excess fecal fat; occurs in malabsorption syndromes or deficiencies of pancreatic enzymes, often causes floating stools.
stenosis narrowing or constriction of an opening or tube, as aortic *stenosis* or pyloric *stenosis*.
stent a wire coil similar to the coil in a ballpoint pen used to keep open an artery.
stepfamily the reconstruction of more than one family into a single family unit; for example, when a divorced person with children remarries, the new family is called the stepfamily. Also referred to as a *blended* family or *reconstituted* family.
stereotype classifying or categorizing people; believing that all those who belong to a certain group are alike.
sterile free of microorganisms, aseptic; unable to bear children, infertile, barren.
sterility absolute inability to procreate.
sterile technique surgical asepsis.
sterilization process that destroys all microorganisms and spores.
sternal pertaining to the sternum, as a *sternal* puncture.
sternum breast bone.
steroid adrenocortical hormone produced by the adrenal glands or a synthetic derivative that mimics its action.
stertorous breathing breathing that occurs when air travels through secretions in the air passage; sometimes used to describe snoring. May be heard after a seizure.
stethoscope instrument used to amplify internal body sounds, especially heartbeat, lung, and bowel sounds.
stimulant any agent that increases activity in the body or one of its parts—mental or physical (stimulus).
stoma an opening on a free surface, such as a pore; an artificially created opening between a body cavity and the body's surface, such as the stoma of a colostomy, ileostomy, or tracheostomy.
stomatitis the inflammation of the mucous membranes of the mouth and lips with or without ulcerations.
stool feces, discharge from the bowels.
stork bite birthmark that appears on the newborn's eyelid or forehead that usually fades during infancy.
strabismus a deviation of the eye; squint. (Convergent strabismus is called cross-eye; divergent strabismus is called exotropia or walleye. Other types include cyclotropia, esotropia, hypertropia, and hypotropia.)
strain a stretched or torn muscle or tendon. Back and hamstring strains are common.
stranger anxiety condition seen in infants and children, in which unfamiliar people, places, and events upset them.
strangulated closed because of constriction, as a *strangulated* hernia.
strangulation suffocation resulting from externally applied pressure to the throat.

***Streptococcal pharyngitis* (strep) throat** infection caused by the *Streptococcus* bacterium that is common in children and responds well to antibiotic therapy if treated promptly; otherwise, it may develop more serious complications such as rheumatic fever, rheumatic heart disease, and nephritis.

stress pressure; reaction to adverse stimulus, as emotional stress or as physical stress placed upon the body by injury, pregnancy, chemicals, or disease, as a *stress* fracture.

stress incontinence urinary leakage following a sudden increase in intra-abdominal pressure such as coughing or sneezing.

stress test (1) method of evaluating the response of the fetal heart to contractions and providing information as to how well the placenta is supplying oxygen to the fetus; also known as the oxytocin challenge test (OCT). (2) method of evaluating the severity of heart disease by measuring the heart's response to physical activity and/or medication.

stressor an agent that produces stress and disrupts homeostasis.

striae stretch marks.

stricture fibrous band that can form along the ureters or urethra, narrowing it and interfering with urine passage.

stridor an abnormal, high-pitched musical breathing sound (usually refers to the inspiratory sound that occurs when the larynx or voice box is obstructed).

stroke also known as cerebrovascular accident (CVA). sudden or gradual interruption of blood supply to a vital center in the brain. A stroke can cause complete or partial paralysis or death.

subacute between an acute or chronic state, with some acute features.

subacute care facilities that provide an "in-between" level of care for a client for approximately two to four weeks between hospitalization and return to independent living or a long-term care facility; also called transitional or continual care.

subculture groups within a dominant culture who share a characteristic such as profession, religion, geographical origin, age, etc.

subcutaneous beneath the skin.

subcutaneous tissue tissue that lies below the dermis and binds the skin to the underlying muscle tissue.

subdural hematoma slow-forming clot in the skull, below the dura, caused by an accumulation of blood, usually from a torn vein on the brain's surface.

subjective perceived only by the affected individual (pain is a subjective sign); also refers to a test item that requires judgment and interpretation as to the correct answer, open to more than one interpretation.

subjective data information that consists of the client's opinions and feeling about what is happening, conveyed to the nurse either directly or through body language.

sublingual under the tongue; nitroglycerin is administered sublingually; oral thermometer placement is sublingual.

substance use disorder patterns of symptoms resulting from the use of a substance that a person continues to take despite experiencing problems as a result.

sudden death a situation in which breathing and heartbeat stop; also called cardiopulmonary arrest.

sudden infant death syndrome (SIDS) crib death, cot death, infantile apnea syndrome. Thought to be a result of untreated prolonged infantile apnea (PIA) or "near miss."

sudoriferous glands glands conveying or transmitting sweat.

suffocation stoppage of breathing; asphyxia.

suicidal ideation thoughts or ideas of killing oneself, which usually precede an actual suicide attempt.

sundowner syndrome, sundowning, or late-day confusion a term that refers to a state of confusion at the end of the day and into the night, when the behavior of a person with dementia may grow increasingly confused, anxious, aggressive, or combative.

superior above or in a higher position.

supination act of turning to the supine position; turning the hand so the palm is upward.

supine lying on the back.

suppository a conical mass to be introduced into the vagina, rectum, or urethra, usually containing medication (easily melted).

suppuration formation or discharge of pus (adjective: suppurative).

suprapubic above the pubic arch.

surfactant surface-active agent, such as soap; a mixture of phospholipids (mostly lecithin and sphingomyelin) in the respiratory passages, used as a test for fetal maturity.

surgical asepsis destruction of all pathogens, "sterile technique."

surgical incision an intentional wound with clean edges (caused from an operation).

surrogate a woman (substitute) who carries a pregnancy for another, usually by artificial insemination or surgical implantation of a fertilized egg.

survival needs according to Maslow, those needs that are vital to sustain life; primary needs, physiologic needs.

suture thread used to hold an incision together while it heals; also called stitches.

sympathetic division of the autonomic nervous system that responds to emergencies, pressure, danger, or extreme stress.

symphysis pubis juncture where the pubic bones meet in front and are joined by a pad of cartilage.

symptom functional evidence of a disease or condition that a client perceives subjectively (as opposed to signs, which the examiner or others perceive).

symptomatic treating symptoms as they occur rather than treating an underlying condition.

symptoms indications of disease or illness that are noticed by the client, for example, fatigue, nausea, or malaise; subjective observations. See also *signs*.

synapse the functional junction between two neurons (nerve cells) at which point the impulse is transmitted.

syncope medical term for fainting, caused by an insufficient supply of blood and oxygen to the brain, may be caused by a drop in blood pressure due to changing body position.

syndactylism condition in which an infant is born with two or more digits fused together.
synergism joint action of agents in which the combined effect is greater than the sum of the individual parts (synergistic medications enhance the action of each other); potentiation.
synovectomy excision of the synovial membrane.
syringectomy surgical removal of a fistula.
system group of organs.
systemic pertaining to the entire body, general, total (as opposed to local).
systemic effect Medication absorbed into the general circulation, affecting the entire body.
systole contraction of the heart; systolic blood pressure is the pressure of the blood against the walls of the arteries when the heart beats (the top number in the blood pressure reading).

T

T cells lymphocytes that mature in the thymus (T lymphocytes).
tablet a compressed, spherical form of a medication.
taboos practices or beliefs that a group's members cannot violate without discomfort and risk of exclusion.
tachycardia abnormally fast heart rate with no explanation, usually greater than 100 bpm.
tachypnea condition in which breaths are abnormally rapid, more than 20 per minute.
tactile sense sense of touch.
talipes condition in which one or both feet turn out of the normal position; commonly known as "club foot."
tangles twisted fibers made of **tau**, a protein that normally helps to maintain the transport system in the brain.
tapering down gradually decreasing the dose of a medication (as opposed to titrating up).
tardive dyskinesia a movement disorder that may occur with long-term use of conventional or first-generation antipsychotics/neuroleptics. A common symptom is obvious facial, mouth, and tongue movements.
target population subgroups in the community with unique or special healthcare needs.
T-binder a binder made of two strips of material, 3–4 in. wide, fastened together, forming a T and used to hold rectal or perineal dressings in place.
technical skills skills used to perform interventions, such as changing a sterile dressing or administering injections.
TED socks See *antiembolism stockings*.
telecommunications system that enables healthcare providers to communicate with clients in different locations using a telephone and a computer.
telehealth the ability to access a nurse or physician via telephone or computer audio/video link.
telemonitoring management of medical situations remotely using electronic technology.
telephone triage system of sorting calls to determine which needs immediate attention.

teletriage a nurse line or provider line clients can call to receive general health information, counseling, and referrals, as well as evaluation and referral in cases of suicidal ideation.
temperament the combination of an individual's characteristics, the way the person thinks, behaves, and reacts to the environment.
temporal temperature a temperature taken with a forehead or temporal scanner; is usually 0.5 °F–1 °F degree lower than an oral temperature.
temporal lobe cerebral lobe that controls hearing, auditory interpretation, and smell; pertaining to the temple, the side of the head.
tendon tough cords that attach muscle to bone.
tenesmus the unyielding feeling or need to pass stool accompanied by straining, pain, and cramping, even if the bowels are already empty.
tenosynovitis inflammation of a tendon sheath.
tension pneumothorax occurs when air leaks out of the lung into the chest cavity and cannot escape, causing pressure to build in the chest and the lung on the side of the leak to collapse.
tepid sponge bath sponge (bath) performed using moderately warm water (below body temperature), between 80 °F and 95 °F (26.6 °C and 35 °C) used to reduce fever.
teratogen an agent or factor that causes defects in a developing embryo, such as a medication a woman takes during pregnancy.
terminal illness a state in which an individual faces a medical condition that will end in death within a limited period.
testes the male gonad (singular: testis).
testosterone major male hormone.
tetanic contractions irregular, uncoordinated uterine contractions; also called tonic contractions.
tetanus a highly fatal disease characterized by muscle spasms and seizures ("lock-jaw"). Can be prevented by immunization.
tetraplegic a synonym for quadriplegic.
thalamus relay station between the cutaneous receptors and the cerebral cortex for all sensory impulses except smell.
theoretical framework . a structure of concepts or models on which to base understanding of the reason and purpose for nursing actions.
therapeutic communication the face-to-face process of interacting that focuses on advancing the physical and emotional well-being of a client.
therapeutic diet approach to eating that is prescribed as part of the treatment of more than one disease or condition.
therapeutic effect a medication's desired effect; produces the result for which it was given.
therapeutic soak moist heat may be applied by immersing the client's affected body part in warm water or medicated solution, a therapeutic soak or *warm soak*.
therapy treatment of disease (therapeutic).
thermophile prokaryote that can live at very high temperatures.

thermoregulation the regulation of temperature to support homeostasis, for example, thermoregulation of the newborn.

third-party payment system developed to help individuals pay for the cost of medical bills, usually a health insurance plan.

third-space (fluid) fluid found in the interstitial tissue spaces.

thoracentesis surgical puncture and drainage of the thoracic (chest) cavity.

thoracotomy incision into the thorax or chest cavity.

thorax the chest.

thrill a vibration felt upon palpation.

thrombin clotting agent created by the reaction of prothrombin activator and calcium ions, which converts fibrinogen into threads of fibrin.

thrombocytes blood platelets, which are essential for clotting.

thrombocytopenia platelet disorder characterized by too few thrombocytes.

thrombocytosis condition marked by an increased number of platelets.

thrombolytic therapy type of medication designed to dissolve a clot or thrombus. clear a blocked blood vessel, and prevent a stroke or pulmonary embolism; is usually administered by IV as quickly as possible after diagnosis of a life-threatening clot.

thrombophlebitis formation of a blood clot in a vein, with inflammation.

thrombus a stationary blood clot.

thrush fungal infection of the oral mucous membrane.

thymus small gland in the upper chest that functions as an endocrine gland.

thyroid resembling a shield. The thyroid gland, located in the neck, is the largest endocrine gland. It secretes hormones vital to growth and metabolism.

thyroidectomy surgical removal of the thyroid gland.

tibia shin bone, which is the long, weight-bearing bone of the lower leg.

tidal volume amount of gas passing into and out of the lungs during each respiratory cycle.

time out procedure procedure taken when the client arrives in the operating room. Includes pausing to ensure healthcare team have the correct client, procedure, and surgical site.

tinnitus ringing in the ears.

tissue a group of similar, specialized cells united to perform a specific function, as epithelial *tissue*.

titration up gradually increasing a medication's dose.

tocodynamometer pressure-sensitive device used to monitor the frequency of uterine contractions.

toddler a child from 1–3 years in age.

tofu soybean curd.

toileting various nursing interventions to assist the client with either bowel or bladder elimination.

tolerance a pharmacological concept describing a person's reduced reaction to a drug following its repeated use. Increasing the dosage may increase the drug's effects; however, this may accelerate further tolerance.

tongue tough skeletal muscle covered with mucous membrane whose function include sensing temperature and texture of food, mixing food with saliva, and moving food into position to be chewed and swallowed.

tonic phase periods of rigid contraction of body muscles during a seizure alternated with phases of rhythmic jerking movements (clonic phase); known as tonic-clonic or grand-mal seizure (most life-threatening seizure).

tonometer instrument which can indirectly measure intraocular pressure.

tonsil a ring of lymphatic tissue around the pharynx forming a protective barrier for infectious substances entering the oral and respiratory passages.

tonsillitis inflammation of the tonsils caused by a virus or bacteria.

topical medications that are applied directly to the skin or mucous membranes.

tort a wrong or injury committed against a person or property for which the injured person has the right to sue.

torticollis torsion (twisting) of the neck; "wry neck."

tortillas round, flat bread made from unleavened flour or cornmeal.

total incontinence nearly continuous urinary leakage.

total parenteral nutrition (TPN) method of nutrition in which a catheter is inserted into a large blood vessel and nutrient solution is administered by continuous drip.

tourniquet a device (a bandage twisted tight with a stick) used to check bleeding or blood flow in a specific area. If applied by rescue personnel, the tourniquet should not be released except by receiving hospital.

toxic pertaining to a poison or toxin.

toxic shock syndrome bacterial infection characterized by fever, vomiting, and/or diarrhea, believed to be facilitated by the use of tampons, especially those with plastic inserters.

toxicity undesired, harmful effect of medication that results from an increased blood level of the agent beyond its therapeutic level.

toxin poison or venom of plant or animal origin that causes disease when present in the body and is capable of inducing antibody formation. In the context of detox diets, toxin usually refers to pollutants, synthetic chemicals, and processed foods.

toxoplasmosis a congenital or acquired disease that can cause lesions in most body systems. It is particularly dangerous to pregnant women and can be prevented by careful cooking of meat and by avoiding the handling of cat litter.

trachea the windpipe, through which food and air pass.

tracheotomy incision into the trachea.

tracheostomy artificial opening in the trachea through which a tube is inserted to aid a person in breathing.

traction exertion of a pulling force; an apparatus attached to the client to maintain stability of a joint or aligned fracture or to exert a pulling force elsewhere, as in the lower back, to relieve pressure.

trade name the copyrighted brand name of a medication assigned by its manufacturer. (A medication with the same generic/chemical name can have several trade or proprietary names.)

transcribing orders reading a healthcare provider's order sheet and carrying out necessary actions.

transcultural nursing unbiased care of persons from all races, religions, and ethnic groups.

transdermal through the skin, a substance absorbed into the body after being placed on the skin, as *transdermal* administration of medication by ointment or patch; transcutaneous.

transection cut, divide, sever; can be incomplete (partial) or complete.

trans-fat process in which a polyunsaturated fatty acid is hydrogenated to make it solid at room temperature. These have fewer essential fatty acids than the original oil because unsaturated fat content is lowered.

transfer belt sturdy webbed belt used by the nurse to help provide support to the weak or unsteady person.

transfer board board made of hard plastic used to move clients who are unable to stand from the side of the bed to a chair.

transfusion injection of blood or blood components or substitutes into a person's circulation.

transient ischemic attack a sudden, short-lived attack of cerebral occlusion, which may be a warning of an impending stroke.

transient tachypnea of the newborn (TTN) a form of mild to moderate respiratory distress starting to occur at about 36 hr after birth; commonly seen in infants delivered by cesarean delivery.

transitional care facilities that provide an "in-between" level of care for a client for approximately two to four weeks between hospitalization and return to independent living or a long-term care facility; also known as subacute care.

transitioning process that some transgender individuals pursue in order to possess the physical characteristics of their gender.

translingual on the tongue, medication administered to be absorbed via the tongue.

transmission-based precautions precautions designed for clients with specific infections or diagnoses.

transmucosal tablet or gel is placed between the cheek and gum and absorbed through the oral mucosa.

transverse from side to side; crosswise.

transverse lie positioning in which the fetus lies across the woman's abdomen in the uterus.

trapeze horizontal bar suspended above and attached to the bed, which is used to pull up to a sitting position or to lift the shoulders and hips off the bed.

trauma a wound or injury to living tissue from an external source. Also, a disordered behavioral state resulting from severe mental or emotional stress or physical injury.

Trendelenburg position position with the head-down—with the head lower than the feet.

triage a process of sorting disaster victims to determine the urgency of their need for care.

trial and error problem-solving experimental problem-solving that tests ideas to decide which methods work and which do not.

trichomoniasis one of the three most common types of vaginitis; symptoms include itching and burning of the vulva and a foul-smelling greenish-yellow or gray bubbly discharge; usually sexually transmitted.

tricuspid with three cusps or points, as the *tricuspid* valve of the heart, between the right atrium and ventricle.

triglyceride a compound consisting of three molecules of fatty acids and one molecule of glycerol, which is the usual form of fat storage in the body.

trimester 3 months, as a *trimester* in pregnancy.

trisomy 21 See *Down syndrome*.

trochanter roll padding placed on sides of legs and feet of a client in bed, to prevent abnormal outward rotation and related sequelae.

troche a medicated tablet that dissolves in the mouth.

Trousseau sign an abnormal carpal spasm induced by inflating a sphygmomanometer cuff on the upper arm to a pressure exceeding systolic blood pressure for 3 min; indicative of tetany following accidental removal of the parathyroid glands during thyroidectomy, hypocalcemia, or hypomagnesemia.

true labor In true labor, the involuntary uterine contractions are rhythmic, grow stronger over time, and begin the true work of labor

tubal ligation most common and effective procedure for permanent sterilization in women; ligation of the oviducts.

tube feeding providing liquid nourishment through a tube into the intestinal tract.

tuberculin skin test (TST) also referred to as the Mantoux tuberculin skin test; test using 0.1 ml of tuberculin purified protein derivative (PPD) injected intradermally into the inner surface of the forearm. The site of induration (firmness) is read 48–72 hr after injection to test for tuberculosis.

tuberculosis (TB) a communicable disease caused by the tubercle bacillus (any organ may be affected, but it primarily affects the lung in human beings).

tumor an abnormal new tissue growth that has no physiologic use and grows independent of its surrounding structures. May be benign or malignant.

tunneling one or more channels within or underlying an open wound.

turgor skin resiliency and plumpness; also called skin turgor.

tweaker slang term describing a methamphetamine user who after using large doses or long periods of dosing, now displays the physical motions methamphetamine users engage in or, to their unpredictable mood swings or violent outbursts. This person can be *very dangerous*.

tympanic membrane eardrum. Tympanic temperature is obtained by placing an electronic probe in the ear canal with similar results to the body's core temperature.

tympanoplasty plastic reconstruction of the ossicles of the middle ear.

Tzanck smear examination of cells and fluids from vesicles, which are applied to a glass slide, stained, and examined under a microscope.

U

ulcer open sore on an external or internal body surface that causes gradual disintegration of tissues, often an ulcer of the stomach (peptic *ulcer*) or a pressure sore (decubitus *ulcer*).

ulna large bone of the forearm.

ultrasound a method of applying deep, penetrating heat to muscles and tissues; Ultrasound is the most common method used to evaluate fetal size, development, and due date.

ultraviolet rays rays used to treat skin infections and wounds.

umbilicus the navel, or site where the umbilical cord is joined to the fetus.

undermining process in which tissue recedes beneath the skin, creating a shelf of skin or free edge with a space underneath.

undifferentiated, poorly differentiated refers to a cell that has not developed into a specific, mature, normal cell. Most commonly occurring in cancerous cells.

United Network of Organ Sharing (UNOS) a private, nonprofit, contracted federal organization used by the Organ Procurement and Transplantation Network (OPTN) that collects, stores, analyzes, and publishes information for clients who are on a waiting list for organ matching and transplants. The UNOS online network is called UNet.å

units specific measurements used for certain nutrients and drugs.

universal healthcare the concept that every person has healthcare coverage/insurance.

unoccupied bed bed that is empty at the time it is made up.

upper tract division of the urinary tract that includes the kidneys and ureters.

ureter narrow tube that carries urine from the kidney to the urinary bladder.

urethra tube through which urine passes from the urinary bladder to outside the body.

urethral pressure profile technique used to evaluate smooth muscle activity along the urethra.

uretolithotomy surgical removal of a stone blocking a ureter.

urge incontinence urinary leakage due to irritation of the bladder wall or from urine components.

urgency desire or sensation of needing to void immediately.

urgent-care center free-standing facility that provides urgent care for clients with noncritical conditions. May also be called an emergi-center.

urinalysis examination of urine.

urinary catheter tube inserted into the bladder through the urethra to remove urine.

urinary frequency voiding more often than usual without an increase in total urine volume.

urinary incontinence involuntary voiding or urine loss.

urinary retention inability to empty the bladder of urine.

urinary suppression stopping or inhibition of urination. Suppression of *secretion*—urine is not formed. Suppression of *excretion*—urine is not expelled.

urination passing urine from the urinary bladder to outside; voiding; micturition.

urine fluid output of waste projects from the kidneys.

urinometer an instrument that determines urine's specific gravity; also called urometer, hydrometer.

urodynamics series of urination tests that best determines the actual level of functioning of the detrusor muscle, external sphincter muscle, and pubococcygeal muscles; also called urodynamic testing.

uroflowmetry noninvasive assessment of the status of voiding.

urology the study of urinary disorders in the female and genitourinary disorders in the male. A urologist is a healthcare provider who specializes in this area.

urticaria an allergic skin reaction characterized by superficial wheals and often accompanied by severe itching; also called hives.

uterine inertia insufficient, uncoordinated contractions that do not produce effective dilation for delivery.

uterine tubes See *oviducts*.

uterus hollow, pear-shaped organ in the female pelvis where the fetus develops and grows; also called womb.

V

vaccine an injection of a disease-causing agent into a person to induce immunity to the agent.

vaccine information statements informational fact sheets provided by the CDC that must be given to individuals or caregivers of individuals receiving immunizations.

vacuum extraction method of delivery in which a round soft plastic cup is gently suctioned to the fetal head and traction exerted to ease the fetus out of the birth canal.

vacutainer disposable plastic sleeve into which a double-ended needle setup or butterfly needle is inserted; device has a needleless connector on one end and a venipuncture needle or butterfly needle on the other end. The needleless end is screwed into the plastic sleeve, with the needle or butterfly outward and the needleless access device inside the sleeve. The needle often contains an articulated shield, which is pushed over the needle after the venipuncture. After the vein is accessed, the needleless connector is pushed into a vacutainer (vacuum) tube, which draws the blood into the tube.

vagina the female sex organ.

vaginismus involuntary contraction of the vaginal outlet muscles, preventing penetration during sexual intercourse.

vaginitis vaginal inflammation.

vagus nerve cranial nerve X (ten)—affects many body functions beyond conscious control.

values a person's or group's "rights" and "wrongs" or what is considered desirable or important.

values clarification examining values, beliefs, and feelings about life and healthcare issues.

variance an actual outcome that differs from an expected outcome.

varicella viral infection in children, which is characterized by an outbreak of rash that progresses into papules, vesicles, then pustules; also called chickenpox.

varices outpouching blood vessels.
varicocele scrotal swelling caused by varicosities in the spermatic blood vessels (described as feeling like a "bag of worms").
vasectomy surgical excision of the vas deferens that renders a male sterile.
vasoconstriction lessening a blood vessel's circumference.
vasoconstrictor medication that raises blood pressure by constricting or narrowing the blood vessels.
vasodilator medication that lowers blood pressure by causing dilation (enlargement of lumina) of blood vessels, used to treat hypertension (high blood pressure).
vector carrier, especially of a disease organism.
vegan a vegetarian who eats no animal-originated foods. (A lacto-vegetarian eats milk and dairy products; an ovo-vegetarian eats eggs.)
vegetarian diet based mainly on plant foods. Some vegetarians exclude all animal products from their diet (vegans); others vary on what animal products they consume.
vein blood vessel that returns blood from the body to the heart (in most cases, deoxygenated blood).
venipuncture puncture of a vein, usually with a needle. May be used to obtain a blood specimen or to start an intravenous infusion (IV).
venous access lock catheter used to maintain an open route to a client's venous system to give fluids and/or medications.
venous stasis ulcer wound or ulceration caused by venous insufficiency or pooling of blood in dependent veins (usually in the legs).
ventilation supplying oxygen to the body through the lungs; breathing.
ventilator a machine that supplies oxygen and forces breathing; also called a respirator.
ventilatory failure state of being unable to breathe adequately alone.
ventral anterior or front.
ventricles a small cavity or chamber; two lower chambers of the heart (pump blood to the body and lungs); small cavities within the brain, most containing cerebrospinal fluid.
Venturi mask mask with a hard plastic adapter, with large "windows" on the sides; this device provides the most reliable and consistent oxygen enrichment.
verbal communication giving and receiving information, news, or messages by speaking or writing.
vermiform appendix See *appendix*.
vernix (Latin) varnish.
vernix caseosa substance covering the fetus before and at birth.
version turning, as of the fetus during normal delivery.
vertebral column the spine.
vertex normal, head-first presentation.
vertical client a client who has a noncritical condition; ambulatory care client.
vertigo sensation of rotation or movement of self (subjective *vertigo*) or surroundings (objective *vertigo*). (Not all dizziness is true vertigo.)
vesicle small sac containing liquid; small blister.
viable state in which a fetus is mature enough to survive outside the woman's uterus (usually 24 weeks' gestation).
vial glass container equipped with a self-sealing rubber stopper that contains either a single or multiple dose of a medication.
video capsule endoscopy an endoscopic test to diagnose Crohn disease. The client swallows a capsule containing a camera; data obtained is transmitted and analyzed.
villi finger-like projections in the small intestine that provide greater absorption area for nutrients to enter into the bloodstream (singular: villus).
viral load amount and strength of the HIV virus in an individual; also called HIV-RNA.
virology the study of viruses and related diseases.
virulence ability of a microorganism to cause disease; strength, potency.
virus protein-covered sac containing genetic or other organic materials, which enters a living organism and uses the host cell for viral reproduction to cause an illness or disease.
viscera internal organs contained within a body cavity.
visceral pleura layer of the pleura that covers the lungs.
visualization guided imagery technique in which client visualizes or forms positive images, often used to manage pain.
vital signs measurements of temperature, pulse, respiration, and blood pressure.
vitamin various organic substances essential to life (includes fat-soluble vitamins [A, D, E, and K] and water-soluble vitamins [B-complex, C, and others]).
vitiligo skin condition in which the melanocytes stop producing melanin; characterized by distinct, localized areas of white patches on the skin.
vitreous humor a transparent, gelatin-like material that fills the space behind the lens of the eye.
vocal cords two triangular-shaped membranous folds that extend from the front to back of the larynx that vibrate and produce sound as air passes over them.
vocational nurse term used in place of licensed practical nurse (LPN) applied to the person practicing in California and Texas; more commonly called an LVN.
voiding (void) to cast out wastes, as to urinate, micturate.
voiding study use of sensors to measure detrusor pressure when voiding.
voluntary controlled by the will, as a *voluntary* muscle.
volvulus twisting of a loop of intestine; may or may not strangulate.
vomitus stomach contents expelled by vomitus.
von Willebrand disease most common hereditary bleeding abnormality; result of a lack of sufficient or poor quality von Willebrand factor, which is required for platelet adhesion.
vulnerable adult a person over the age of 18 who is at risk of harm or lacks some life skills.
vulva the external parts of the female genital organs.
vulvitis inflammation of the vulva.

W

walking rounds caregivers move from client to client, discussing pertinent information.

wart a skin tumor caused by a virus; verruca.

wasting syndrome a complication of AIDS defined as a loss of at least 10% of body weight accompanied by diarrhea, chronic weakness, and fever.

weaning a protocol consisting of slowly decreasing the individual's dependency on the machine so the ventilator may be removed. The gradual cessation of breastfeeding.

wellness state of physical and emotional well-being; optimum health.

Wernicke–Korsakoff syndrome a neurologic disorder leading to brain damage caused by a chronic deficiency of vitamin B_1 or thiamine, often related to chronic alcoholism, malabsorption, or chronic malnutrition.

Western blot test a second tier test done to confirm the diagnosis of HIV after receiving a positive ELISA (EIA).

wet-to-dry dressing saturated dressing that is wrapped around a wound and left to dry. Upon removal, the dressing pulls away tissue debris and drainage, making it a useful tool in debridement.

Wharton jelly soft jelly-like substance that protects the umbilical cord.

wheal a smooth, slightly elevated skin area, usually pale in the center with a reddened periphery, often accompanied by severe itching when caused by an allergic reaction; small elevation caused by injection of an intradermal medication, such as the PPD test for tuberculosis or other skin test.

wheeze a whistling respiratory sound, typical of asthma.

wide-spectrum (antibiotic) an antibiotic that is effective against a large number of pathogens.

Wilms tumor malignant adenosarcoma and common neoplasm of childhood, which usually affects only one kidney; also called nephroblastoma.

windchill factor mathematical calculation of temperature and wind speed to determine the intensity of cooling expected from the environment or the rate of heat loss on the body.

window period an early phase of HIV infection in which HIV testing results can be inaccurate due to insufficient antibodies. The period averages about 25 days but can range up to several months before an accurate HIV-positive result is obtained.

withdrawal symptoms abnormal physical or psychological features that follow the abrupt discontinuation of a drug that has the capability of producing physical dependence.

Wood light special high-pressure mercury lamp that produces long-wave UV rays used to diagnose abnormalities and infections of the skin.

worker's compensation program that provides financial compensation to a person who has been injured at work or who has contracted a disease that can be directly related to his or her job.

wound injury to any body structure caused by physical means.

wound sinus canal or passage leading to an abscess.

X

xenograft graft of tissue between animals of different species, as in the grafting of pigskin onto a human in burn treatment; also called heterograft.

xerostomia dry mouth in which saliva is reduced. May be caused by polypharmacy or chemotherapy and often causes tooth decay and/or gum disease.

Y

yin-yang belief system that emphasizes balance and its influence on illness and health.

young-old adult adults ranging from age 50–79 years of age.

Z

Z-track "zig-zag" method of injecting caustic medications deep into muscle tissue.

zygote cell that results from the fusion of two mature germ cells.

INDEX

Note: Page numbers followed by "f" indicate figures, "t" indicate tables and "b" indicate boxes.

A

AARP. *See* American Association of Retired Persons (AARP)
Abandonment of care, 34
Abbreviations
  in documentation, 450t–451t
  in obstetrics, 1024t
Abdomen
  auscultation, 637f
  enlargement of, in pregnancy, 1032
  muscles of, 210t
  quadrants of, 161f
  regions of, 161f
  ultrasound, 1672
Abdominal aorta, 264, 264t
  aneurysm of, 1461–1462, 1461f
Abdominal binder, 782
Abdominal data collection, 637t
Abdominal distention
  by excess fluid, 1536
  postoperative, 830–832
Abdominal (ABD) pads, 869, 869f
Abdominal paracentesis, 1599
Abdominal–perineal resection, 1616
Abducens nerve (CN VI), 249
ABG. *See* Arterial blood gas (ABG)
Ablation surgery, for chronic pain, 808
Abnormal breathing patterns, 590t
Abnormal heart sounds, 588–589
Abnormal plantar flexion, 689f
ABO incompatibility, 1115
Abortifacient, 1154
Abortion (AB), 1154, 1106
  complete, 1106–1107
  complications of, 1107
  illegal, 1107
  incomplete, 1107
  induced, 1107
  inevitable, 1107
  medically induced, 1106
  missed, 1107
  recurrent spontaneous, 1107
  septic, 1107
  spontaneous, 1106–1107
  therapeutic, 1107
  threatened, 1106
Above-the-elbow amputation (AEA), 1325
Above-the-knee amputation (AKA), 1325
Abrasion, 857
Abrupt awakening, postoperative, 830
Abruptio placentae, 1116
Abscesses, 867
  brain, 1370
Absence seizures, 1357b
Absorbable gelatin sponge (Gelfoam), 938
Abuse
  child, 1213–1219
  domestic, 64
  elder, 65
  emotional, 1217
  within families, 103
  physical, 1214
  reporting of, 1213
  sexual, 1217–1218

Acamprosate calcium (Campral), 1793–1794
Acarbose (Precose), 1401
Acceleration–deceleration injuries, 1374
Accessory glands, 334
Accessory structures, 172–174
  ceruminal glands, 174
  hair, 172–173, 173b
  nails, 173, 173f
  sebaceous glands, 173
  sudoriferous glands (sweat glands), 174
Accidental hypothermia, 583
Accidental stick, with contaminated needle, 501
Accidents, 67
Accommodation, 249, 252, 252f
Accountability, 436, 442–443
Accreditation, 12–13
Accredited record technician (ART), 464
Acculturation, 381
ACE. *See* Angiotensin-converting enzyme (ACE) inhibitors
ACE bandage. *See* All cotton elastic (ACE) bandage
Acetaminophen, 807, 921, 923t, 927, 962, 1248
Acetones, testing for, 1386
Acetylcysteine (Mucomyst), 1239
Acetylsalicylic acid (ASA), 921, 924t, 927
ACF. *See* Administration for Children and Families (ACF)
Achalasia, 1602
Acid–base balance, 190–192
  maintenance of, 1318–1319
  regulation of, 302
Acidosis, 1317
Acids, 190
ACL. *See* Administration for Community Living (ACL)
ACLS. *See* Advanced cardiovascular life support (ACLS)
Acne vulgaris, 1250–1251, 1251f
Acoustic/auditory nerve (CN VIII), 251
Acquired/adaptive immunity, 290–292, 291f
Acquired disorders, 1269–1270
Acquired immunodeficiency syndrome (AIDS), 59, 1520, 1525, 1531
Acrocyanosis, 1083
Acromegaly, 1387
Acrosclerosis, 1333
ACTH. *See* Adrenocorticotropic hormone (ACTH)
Action potential, 227–228
Activase, 835
Activated partial thromboplastin time (APTT), 1469
Active dying, 146
Active range of motion (AROM), 655
  in musculoskeletal disorders, 1323
Activities of daily living (ADLs), 423, 1267, 1269, 1698
  in nervous system disorders, 1354
Acuity, 20, 609
Acupressure, 29
Acupuncture, 29
Acupuncture centers, 1889
Acute bacterial prostatitis (ABP), 1662

Acute care facilities, 21, 61
Acute care hospitalization (ACH), 1830
Acute coronary syndrome (ACS), 1454
Acute hemorrhagic anemia, 1475, 1477
Acute infectious mononucleosis, 1249–1250, 1249f
Acute inflammatory demyelinating polyradiculoneuropathy (AIDP), 1372
Acute kidney injury, 1650
Acute lymphoid leukemia (ALL), 1235–1236, 1479
Acute myeloid leukemia (AML), 1235–1236, 1479
Acute myocardial infarction (AMI), 1454, 1456–1457
  mortality rate for, 66
Acute normovolemic hemodilution, 1470
Acute Psychiatric Services (APS), 462, 1844
Acute psychotic episode (APE), 1741
Acute respiratory distress syndrome (ARDS), 1558
Acute transverse myelitis, 1373
Acyclovir ointment, 1601
Adalimumab (Humira), 1332
Adam's apple, 297
Added sugars, 352b
Addiction, family stresses and, 103–104
Addison disease, 1385, 1392
Addisonian crisis, 1392
Adenohypophysis, 234, 235t
Adenosine triphosphate (ATP), 317, 323, 1318
Adequate intake (AI), 348
ADH. *See* Antidiuretic hormone (ADH)
Adhesions, 610, 1162
Adipose tissue, 166
Adjuvant medications, for pain relief, 807
Administration (facility), 463
Administration for Children and Families (ACF), 74
Administration for Community Living (ACL), 74
Admissions, 565b
  admitting department, 564–565, 565f
  advance directives, 565–566
  client's arrival on nursing unit, 566–569, 566f
    client into bed, assistance to, 566–567
    client's clothes, removal of, 566, 566f
    client to facility, orientation, 567–568
    dehumanization, prevention of, 568–569
    personal belongings, care of, 568
    skin integrity, inspection of, 566
  documentation, 570–573, 573b
  donor status, 565–566
  interview for, 422, 570
  reporting, 573
Admissions department, 464, 564–565, 565f
Adolescence, 122, 1801
  age-related concerns, 1179
  body image, 126
  developmental stages, 123–124
  early, 123–124
  Erikson's theory of psychosocial development, 122–123, 123t, 123f

1983

Adolescence (continued)
    food and eating habits in, 126
    growth and development, 122–123
    health concerns in, 67–68
    late, 124
    middle, 124
    motor vehicle accidents and, 67
    nutrition during, 373–374
    peer pressure in, 126
    physical growth, 124
    Piaget's theory of cognitive development, 123
    pregnancy in, 1118
    psychosocial developmental, 125, 126f
    risk behaviors common in, 67
    risk taking behavior of, 126
    sexual development, 124–125
Adrenal angiogram, 1385
Adrenal cortex gland, 1383t
Adrenal crisis, 931
Adrenal function tests, 1384–1385
Adrenal glands, 239–240, 1391–1392
    adrenal cortex, 239–240
    adrenal medulla, 240, 1383t
    neoplasms, 1392–1393
Adrenergics, 930–931
Adrenocorticotropic hormone (ACTH), 234, 1384
Adult foster care, 1744
Adulthood
    early
        adult identification, 130–131
        adult relationships during, 131
        career choices, 130
        career decisions, 131–132
        emerging, 130
        Erikson's theory of psychosocial development, 129, 130t
        leaving home, 130
        reappraising commitments during, 131
        settling in during, 131
        starting families during, 131, 131f
        women's issues during, 132
    middle
        equilibrium reestablished during, 133–134
        Erikson's theory of psychosocial development, 129–130, 130t
        perceptions of mortality during, 133
        physical aspects of aging, 133, 133f
        retirement planning during, 134
        role changes during, 132–133
        transitions during, 132–134
    nutrition during, 374–375
    older, 138–143. See also Older adults
        areas of concern, 138–141
        development in, 138–143
        physical changes, 139, 139b
Adult-onset diabetes, 1393
Adult residential care, 1744
Adult respiration patterns, 590t
Advanced cardiovascular life support (ACLS), 526, 1573
Advance directive (AD), 40–41, 40b, 881
Advanced practice nurse (APRN), 11, 1175, 1840
Adverse drug reaction, 1511, 1742
Adversive seizures, 1356b
Advocacy, 1759
AEA. See Above-the-elbow amputation (AEA)
Aerobes, obligate, 480
Aerobic exercise, 213
Aerosol mist treatment, 1571
Aesculapius, 2, 2f
Afebrile state, 583

Affordable Care Act, 20–21, 25–26
Afrezza, 1399
Afterload, 268
Aganglionic megacolon. See Megacolon
Ageism, 137
Agency for Healthcare Research and Quality (AHRQ), 74, 801
Agency for Toxic Substances and Disease Registry (ATSDR), 74
Age-related health concerns, 65–69
    adolescents and young adults, 67–68
    children, 66–67
    disease risk and, 609t
    infants, 66
    mature adults, 68–69
    older adults, 69
Agglutination, 278
Aggressiveness, 556–557, 556b, 1732
Aging, 102–103. See also Older adults
    cardiovascular system and, 269t–270t
    digestive system and, 317t–318t
    disease risk and, 609t
    endocrine system and, 244t
    hematologic and lymphatic systems and, 284t
    immune system and, 293t
    integumentary system and, 177t
    nervous system and, 229t–230t
    physical aspects of, 133, 133f
    reproductive system, 332t, 343t
    respiratory system and, 303t
    sensory system and, 256t–257t
    terms related to, 136–137
    urinary system and, 328t–329t
Agonist (medication), 907
Agonist therapy, 1796
Agoraphobia, 1740
Agranular leukocytes, 277
Agranulocytosis, 1479
AHA. See American Hospital Association (AHA)
AHRQ. See Agency for Healthcare Research and Quality (AHRQ)
AI. See Adequate Intake (AI)
AIDP. See Acute inflammatory demyelinating polyradiculoneuropathy (AIDP)
AIDS. See Acquired immunodeficiency syndrome (AIDS)
AIDS dementia complex (ADC), 1523
AIMS scale, 1755
Airborne precautions, 509–511, 510t
Airborne transmission, 509
Air pollution, 79–80
Airway maintenance, end-of-life care and, 883–884
AKA. See Above-the-knee amputation (AKA)
Akathisia, 1755
Alanine aminotransferase (ALT), 1584
Albino, 172
Albumins, 355
Albuminuria, 1448
Alcohol
    client education on, 380
    effects of, on fetus, 1272–1273, 1273f
    guidelines for intake of, 372b
Alcohol abuse, 63
    dietary deficiencies, 1791
    disease risk and, 609t
    thiamine deficiency sequelae, 1791
Alcohol-based hand sanitizers, 502t
Alcohol-related birth defects (ARBD), 1272
Alcohol-related liver disease (ARLD), 1791
Alcohol-related neurodevelopmental disorder (ARND), 1272
Alcohol use disorder, 1790–1794

Alcohol wipes, 502t
Alcott, Louisa May, 4
Aldosterone, 239, 324
Aldosteronism, 1392
Alendronate (Fosamax), 1334
Algae, 481
Alginates, 868t, 870
Alias, admission using, 36
Alimentary canal, 305
Alkaline phosphatase (ALP), 1584
Alkalosis, 1317, 1318t, 1319
All cotton elastic (ACE) bandage, 778f, 779
Allergens, 1508
Allergic reactions, 1508
Allergic rhinitis, 1509, 1552–1553
Allergies, 1506
    allergic conditions, 1512
    diagnostic tests, 1506–1508, 1507b
    laboratory tests, 1506–1507
    medications for, 939–940
    multisystem response, 1511
    signs and symptoms, 1513
    skin response, 1508–1509
    skin tests, 1507, 1507f
Allis sign, 1219
Allogeneic transfusion, 1470
Allograft, 1305, 1442
Allopurinol (Zyloprim), 1333, 1642
All-or-none law, 228
Alopecia, 172, 630f, 1235, 1500, 1625
ALP. See Alkaline phosphatase (ALP)
Alpha-1 antitrypsin deficiency (ATT deficiency), 1557
Alpha cells, 240
Alpha-tocopherol. See Vitamin E
Alprazolam (Xanax), 924t, 929, 1611
ALS. See Amyotrophic lateral sclerosis (ALS)
ALT. See Alanine aminotransferase (ALT)
Alteplase (t-PA), 835
Alternative and complementary techniques in pain management, 809
Alternative families, 100
Alveolar ducts, 299
Alveolar sacs, 299
Alveoli, 301, 1077
Alzheimer's disease, 1702, 1722–1724, 1723t, 1723f
    mortality rate for, 58
AMA (against medical advice), 37
Amblyopia, 1225
AMBU-bag, 524, 524f, 1571–1572
Ambularm system, 1810f
Ambulatory care centers, 21
Ambulatory care sensitive (ACS), 1844
Ambulatory facilities, types, 1840–1849
Ambulatory nursing, 1839–1849
Ambulatory Surgery Center, 1845–1849
Amenorrhea, 1031, 1261, 1387, 1676
American Association of Birth Centers (AABC), 1054
American Association of Retired Persons (AARP), 1808
American Board of Obstetrics and Gynecology, 1024
American Cancer Society, 78
American Diabetes Association, 78
American Heart Association, 78
American Hospital Association (AHA), 44
American Journal of Nursing (AJN), 16
American Nurses Association (ANA), 4, 11
American Nurses Credentialing Center (ANCC), 11
American Psychiatric Association (APA), 1737
American Red Cross, 5, 77
Amines, 232

Amino acids, 355–356
Aminoglycosides, 917t, 920
Amniocentesis, 1105, 1275
Amniohook, 1058
Amnion, 1030
Amniotic fluid, 1030
Amniotomy, 1058, 1121
Amphetamines, 1797–1798
Ampicillin, 1158
Ampule, 981, 981f
Amputation, 1323, 1325–1326
Amylase, 306, 1385
Amyl nitrate, 933t, 936
Amyotrophic lateral sclerosis (ALS), 1370, 1825
ANA. See American Nurses Association (ANA)
Anabolic-androgenic steroids (AAS), 1799
Anaerobes, obligate, 480
Anaerobic exercise, 213
Anal abscess, 1617
Anal fistula, 1617
Analgesic ladder, 1861t
Analgesics, 921
    narcotic agonist, 926–927, 926b
    nonnarcotic, 927–928
    for pain relief, 807
Anaphylactic (allergic) shock, 520b
Anaphylactoid reaction, 520b
Anaphylaxis, 540, 960, 1352, 1513
Anasarca, 182, 1313, 1449b
Anastomosis, 1594
Anatomic position, 158
ANCC. See American Nurses Credentialing Center (ANCC)
Androgen, 240, 331, 334, 948–950
Anemia, 1233–1234
    acute hemorrhagic, 1475, 1477
    aplastic, 1477–1478
    chronic hemorrhagic, 1477
    hemolytic, 1475
    iron deficiency, 1475
    pernicious, 1477
    sickle cell, 1478
    signs and symptoms, 1475b
Anemic hypoxia, 1542
Anencephaly, 1142
Aneroid manometer, 593, 593f
Anesthesia, 816–818
    administration, 817–818
    client care, 816–817
    during labor and delivery, 1063
    shock, 520b
    types of, 817, 818b
Anesthesiologist, 817
Anesthesiology, 816–817
Anesthetics, 816–817. See also Anesthesia
Aneurysm, 1461–1462, 1461f
Angina pectoris, 1452–1454
Angiocardiogram, 1436
Angioedema, 1295
Angiogram, 1352, 1436
Angiography, 614t
Angiomas, 1306
Angioplasty, 1438, 1441
Angiotensin-converting enzyme (ACE) inhibitors, 242, 1449
    for hypertension, 937, 1406
Angiotensin II receptor blockers (ARBs), for hypertension, 937
Anhedonia, 1739
Animal bites, 540, 1210
Anion, 185
Ankylosing spondylitis, 1331–1332
Ankylosis, 1330
Annuloplasty, 1442
Anorexia, 126, 400, 610t, 1604

Anorexia nervosa, 1262, 1625
    signs and symptoms, 1262b
Anorgasmia, 335
Anoscope, 1617
Anoxia, 1455
ANS. See Autonomic nervous system (ANS)
Antabuse therapy, 1793
Antacid, 943, 944t
Antagonist (medication), 907
Antepartum period, 1024. See also Pregnancy
Anterior pituitary gland, 1383t
Antianxiety agents, 1758
Antiarrhythmics, 933
Antiasthmatic medications, 940, 942t
Antibiosis, 492
Antibiotic-resistant organisms, 919
Antibiotics, 914–915, 919–921
    broad-spectrum, 915
    commonly anti-infective medications, 916t–918t
    effectiveness of, 919
    narrow-spectrum, 916
    preoperative, 824–825
    selection of, 919–921
Antibody (Ab), 287–288, 1506
Antibody-mediated immunity, 292
Anticholinergics, 1367, 1750
Anticipatory guidance, 107
Anticoagulants, 938–939
Anticonvulsants, 925t, 929–930, 1353, 1356
Antidiabetic agents, 1402b
Antidiarrheals, 945t, 947
Antidiuretic hormone (ADH), 181, 238, 323, 324, 1313, 1387
Antiembolism stockings, 780–781
    application of, 785–786
Antiemetics, 944t, 946
    end-of-life care and, 884
    postoperative, 830–831
Antiflatulents, 943
Anti-friction glide sheet, 665
Antifungals, 917t, 922t
Antigen–antibody reactions, 292, 1506
Antigen-presenting cells (APC), 280
Antigens, 287, 1506
Antihemophilic factor, 939
Antihistamines, 939, 941t–942t, 942, 1512
Antihypertensives, 934t, 936–937
Antimalarials, 1332
Antimicrobial agents, 501, 502t
Antimicrobial products, wound healing, 868t
Antimicrobial-resistant microorganisms, 487–488
Antineoplastic medications, 939, 1235
Antinuclear antibody tests, 1507
Antipsychotic agents, 1751t–1752t
Antipyretic analgesics, 927
Antirejection medications, complications of, 1654
Antiretroviral therapy, 1521
Antispasmodics, 944t, 946
Antistreptolysin-O (ASO) titer, 1208
Antitussives, 940, 941t
Antivirals, 918t
Anuria, 1650
Anus, 312
Anxiety, 110, 569, 1707, 1740–1741
Anxiety disorders, 1283
Anxiolytic drugs, 1784–1785
Aorta, 264, 264t
Aortic stenosis, 1233
Aortic valve, 262
Aortocaval compression, 1038
Apgar score, 1078
Aphasia, 552, 1463, 1710

Apheresis, 1472
Aphthous stomatitis, 1600–1601
Apical pulse (AP), 259, 587f, 588, 601–602
Apical–radial pulse (A-R), 587, 589, 589f
APIE charting, 446, 447t
Aplastic anemia, 1477–1478
Apnea, 590, 1542t
Apnea monitor, 1212
Apocrine sweat glands, 174
Apoptosis, 1493
Apothecary system, of measurement, 895, 896t
Appearance, mood, sensorium, intelligence and thought process (AMSIT) test, 1738
Appendectomy, 312
Appendicitis, 1614–1615
Appendicular skeleton, 205–207
    lower extremities, 206, 206f
    pelvic girdle/pelvis, 206–207
    upper extremities, 205–206, 206f
Appendix, 312
Aprepitant (Emend), 830
APS. See Acute Psychiatric Services (APS)
Aquathermia pad (Aqua-K pad), 788–790, 796–797
Aqueous humor, 248
Architectural barriers, defined, 1827
ARDS. See Acute respiratory distress syndrome (ARDS)
Area charting, 446
Areolar glands, 340
Areolar tissue, 166
Arm and anterior chest, muscles of, 210t
Armed forces emergency services, 77
Armed forces, employment with, 1886–1887
AROM. See Active range of motion (AROM)
Arrector pili, 172
Arrhythmia, 1436
ART. See Assisted reproductive technology (ART)
Arterial blood gas (ABG), 611, 615t, 1310, 1534, 1568
Arteriography, 612, 617, 1352, 1584
Arterioles, 264, 268
Arteriosclerosis, 591, 1405, 1444
Arteriovenous (AV) fistula, 1652
Arthritis, 1329–1332, 1330b
Arthrocentesis, 1322
Arthrogram, 1322
Arthroplasty, 1343
Arthroscope, 612, 1322
Arthroscopy, 1322
Artificial insemination (AI), 1150
Artificial larynx, 1562
Artificial limbs, 1822
Artificially acquired immunity, 290–292
Artificial rupture of the membranes (AROM), 1058
Asbestosis, 1553
Ascites, 182, 1599
Ascorbic acid. See Vitamin C
Asepsis, 494–495
Aseptic meningitis, 1371
Asian American, 84t, 382–383
Asian populations, India, 384
Asperger syndrome, 1278
Asphyxiation, 1558
Aspiration, 1541, 1558
    pneumonia, 832, 1546–1547
Aspirin, 927–928
Assertiveness, 556, 556b
Assisted reproductive technology (ART), 1152–1153
Asthma, 591, 1237, 1509, 1554–1556
Astigmatic keratotomy (AK), 248
Astigmatism, 252, 1257, 1423

Astrocytes, 219, 283
Ataxia, 1279–1280, 1366
Atelectasis, 832–833, 1348, 1543, 1571
Atherectomy, 1441
Atherosclerosis, 68, 591, 1444
Athetoid, 1281
Athetosis, 1280
Athlete's foot, 628f. *See also* Tinea pedis
Atomic mass, 156
Atomic number, 156
Atonic seizures, 1356b
Atony, 1116
Atopic dermatitis. *See* Eczema
Atopy, 1509
ATP. *See* Adenosine triphosphate (ATP)
Atrial ablation, 1447
Atrial fibrillation, 1447
Atrial natriuretic factor (ANF), 242
Atrial natriuretic peptide (ANP), 182, 242, 324
Atrial septal defect (ASD), 1142, 1230, 1231f
Atrioventricular heart block, 1446–1447
Atrioventricular (AV) valves, 260–261, 261f
Atrophic vaginitis, 1683
Atropine eye drops, 932
Atropine sulfate, 824
ATSDR. *See* Agency for Toxic Substances and Disease Registry (ATSDR)
ATT deficiency. *See* Alpha-1 antitrypsin deficiency (ATT deficiency)
Attention deficit disorder (ADD), 1276
Attention deficit hyperactivity disorder (ADHD), 1276, 1277
Attitudinal barriers, 1828
Atypical tuberculosis, 1550. *See also* Tuberculosis (TB)
Audiobooks, 1419
Audiology, 249
Audiometer, 253
Audiometry, 1414
Audition, 253
Auditory observation, 422
Auranofin (Ridaura), 1332
Auras, 1355
Auricle, 249
Auscultation
  abdomen, 637f
  diagnosis and, 619, 619f
  pulses, 588
Autism, 1276
Autism spectrum disorder (ASD), 1278–1279
Autoantibodies, 1514
Autoclave, 842
Autocratic leadership, 1901
Autograft, 1304, 1442
Autoimmune disorders, 1514, 1515t–1518t, 1518
Autolysis, 1293
Autolytic debridement, 870
Automated external defibrillator (AED), 526, 526f
Automatic thermometers, 584
Autonomic disturbances, 1463–1464
Autonomic dysreflexia, 1363
Autonomic hyperactivity, 1792
Autonomic nervous system (ANS), 226–227, 226f, 227t
Autonomic neuropathy, 1406
Autonomy, 43
Autopsy, 461, 890
Aversion therapy, 1793
Avulsed teeth, first-aid for, 535
Axial skeleton, 202–204, 203b, 203f
Axillary (Ax) temperature, 585
Azathioprine (Imuran), 1332

B
Babinski reflex, 1085
Baby boomers, 58
Baby bottle syndrome, 1229
BAC. *See* Blood alcohol concentration (BAC)
Bacille Calmette-Guérin (BCG), 1551
Bacillus anthracis, 483
Bacitracin ointment, 1304
Back and posterior chest, muscles of, 210t
Back pain, chronic, 1326–1328
Backrub, 710–711, 710f
Bacterial endocarditis, 1451–1452
Bacterial pneumonia, 1546
Bacterial skin infections, 1297
Bacterial vaginosis (BV), 1172–1173
Bacteria/prokaryotes, 482–484
  bacillus, 483
  cell envelope of, 482
  classification by shape, 483, 484f
  coccus, 483
  cytoplasm, 483
  flagella on, 482–483, 483f
  gram-negative, 482
  gram-positive, 482
  mesophiles, 482
  pathogenic, 483–484
  plasma membrane of, 482
  psychrophiles, 482
  reproduction and survival, 483
  Rickettsiae, 484
  spirillum, 483
  structure and function of, 482
  thermophiles, 482
Bactericidal agents, 915
Bacteriology, 482
Bacteriostatic agents, 915
Bacteriuria, 1639
Bag of waters (BOW), 1121
Bag valve mask (BVM), 1572
Balanced suspension traction, 1338, 1340f
Balanced traction, 1339
Balance scale, for weight, 624f
Baldness, 172
Ball-and-socket (spheroidal) joints, 200
Ballard score, 1130
Ballottement, 1032
Bandages, 777, 778f
  extremity status, evaluation of, 777, 779
  Kerlix, 779
  purposes and therapeutic benefits of, 779
  roller, 779
  stretch-net, 779
  wrapping of, 778t
Band ligation, 1602
Barbiturates, 924t, 929, 1158, 1758, 1794
Bare-metal stent (BMS), 1441
Bariatric surgery, 1593
Barium enema, 616t, 1585
Barium studies, 1584–1585
Barium swallow, 1585
Baroreceptors, 268
Barrett esophagus, 1603
Barrier methods, 1160
Bartholin gland, 337, 339
Barton, Clara, 4
Bartonella henselae, 1210
Basal body temperature (BBT), in pregnancy, 1032
Basal cell carcinoma, 1308
Basal metabolism, 317
Base, 190
Basic cardiac life support (BCLS), 526, 526f
Basic metabolic panel (BMP), 1310
Basilar artery, 283
Basilar skull fracture, 1375, 1375f

Basophils, 276–277
Bath
  bed, 713, 729–731
  end-of-life care and, 885
  infant, 1188
  partial, 713, 713f
  shower, 712, 713f
  sitz, 714
  sponge, 713
  therapeutic, 713
  towel, 714
  tub, 712, 713f, 727–729
Battle sign, 1375, 1375f
BBP. *See* Blood-borne pathogens (BBP)
B cells, 1521
BCG. *See* Bacille Calmette-Guérin (BCG)
BCLS. *See* Basic cardiac life support (BCLS)
BCPs. *See* Birth control pills (BCPs)
BEA. *See* Below-the-elbow amputation (BEA)
Beats per minute (BPM), 587
Becker muscular dystrophy (BMD), 1282
Bed baths, 713, 729–731
Bedbugs, 715, 1298
Bed cradle, 689
Bedsore. *See* Pressure wound
Bedtime insulin and daytime sulfonylureas (BIDS), 1401
Bed wetting. *See* Enuresis
Behavior modification, 1269
Behaviors, documentation of, 1765
Beliefs, cultural considerations, 86
Bell palsy, 1138, 1359
Belly bag, 846
Below-the-elbow amputation (BEA), 1325
Below-the-knee amputation (BKA), 1325
Bender–Gestalt test, 1738
Beneficence, 43
Benign neoplasms, 1559
Benign prostatic hyperplasia (BPH), 1656, 1662
Benign renal cysts, 1646
Benign tumors, 1487
Benzodiazepines, 924t, 929, 1500, 1751t, 1794
Beriberi, 366
Beta blockers, for hypertension, 937
Bethanechol chloride (Urecholine), 948
BGM. *See* Blood glucose monitoring (BGM)
Bicarbonate, 192
Bicarbonate buffer system, 192
Bicuspid valve, 260–261
BIDS. *See* Bedtime insulin and daytime sulfonylureas (BIDS)
Bifocals, 1423
Bile, 310, 311t
Bile duct, 310
Biliary apparatus, 314
Biliary atresia, 1224
Bilirubin, 1137
Binders, 777, 781–782
Binge drinking, 67
Binge-eating disorder, 1262
Binge syndrome, 1625
Binocular vision, 252
Binuclear families, 99–100
Biographical data, 482
Biohazardous medical wastes, disposal of, 81, 501
Biologic agents, 1254
Biological death, 526, 889
Biologic response modifiers (BRMs), 1254, 1493
Biologic valves, 1442
Biomedical electronics department, 464
Biomedical services, 77
Bionomics, 79

Biopsy, 612, 1290, 1586, 1588
  bone marrow, 613t, 1469
  lymph node, 1469
  in musculoskeletal disorders, 1323
Biosurgical debridement, 1293
Biotherapy, 1493
Biotin, 364t
Biot respiration, 590t, 1542t
Bipolar affective disorders (BPADs), 1739
Bipolar disorders (BPDs), 1739–1740
Birth, 1052–1061. *See also* Labor
Birth assistant (doula), 1053
Birth attendant, 1053
Birth centers, 1054
Birth control implant, 1153
Birth control pills (BCPs), 1157
Birthing room, 1053
Birthmarks. *See* Angiomas
Birth plan, 1054
Birth setting, 1053–1054
Bisexual, 1147
Bisphosphonate, 1334
BKA. *See* Below-the-knee amputation (BKA)
Black/African American, 84
Bladder, 325
  exstrophy, 1143
  rupture, 1649
  scanning, 1633
  stones, 1642
  tumors, 1646–1647
Bland diet, 396
Blanket warmers, 790
Blastic tumors, 1488
Blastocyst, 1025–1026
Bleeding
  assessment of, 528
  first-aid in, 538–540
    hemorrhage, 539
    minor wound, 539
    nosebleed, 538
  internal, 539–540
Blepharitis, 1424
Blind spot, 248
Blood, 165, 272–278, 274t
  formed elements, 274–277, 274f
  medications affecting, 937–939
    anticoagulants, 938–939
    coagulants, 938
    iron replacement preparations, 937–938
    products, 939
    vitamins, 938
  plasma, 273
  platelets, 277
  red blood cells, 274–275, 275b
  white blood cells, 275–277, 276b, 276f
Blood alcohol concentration (BAC), 67
Blood-borne pathogens (BBP), 508–509
Blood–brain barrier (BBB), 283
Blood circulation, 282
  cerebral circulation, 283, 283f
  hepatic–portal circulation, 282, 282f
  pulmonary circulation, 282
  systemic circulation, 282, 282f
Blood clotting, 277, 278f
Blood components, 939
Blood donation, 1470
Blood gas determinations, 1534
Blood glucose level, testing for, 1407
Blood glucose monitoring (BGM), 1393
Blood groups, 278, 279t
Blood lead level (BLL), 1280
Blood pressure (BP), 268, 581
  assessment of, 591–595
  children, 1182
  diastolic, 268, 592, 592f

  direct measurement of, 593
  indirect measurement of, 593
  measurement, 593f, 594–595
  normal, 592, 593t
  regulation, 268
  regulation of, 591–592
  systolic, 268, 592
Blood pressure regulation and kidney mechanism, 326
Blood products, 1470–1472
Blood sugar, 351
Blood tests, digestive system and, 1583–1584
Blood transfusions, 1470
Blood urea nitrogen (BUN), 1631
Blood vessels
  arteries and arterioles, 264, 264t, 264f
  capillaries, 265
  of heart, 262–263, 263f
  medications affecting, 935–937
  tissue layers within, 266
  veins and venules, 265–266, 265t, 266f
Bloody show, 1057
Blue spells, 1230
B-lymphocytes (B-cells), 277, 287–288
BMD. *See* Bone mineral density (BMD)
BMI. *See* Body mass index (BMI)
Board-and-care, 1744, 1810
Body alignment, 644–645
  Body cavities, 158–161, 160f–161f, 160t
Body cues, 809
Body directions, 158, 159f, 159t–160t
Body fluids, 180–186
  dehydration, 183
  edema and, 182, 182b
  electrolyte, 184–185, 186t
  extracellular fluid, 180–182
  intracellular fluid, 181
  ions and, 185–186
  location of, 181–182, 180f–181f
  normal intake and output, 182
  overhydration, 182
  transport of, 186–189
  water, 183–184, 183t, 183b, 184f
Body language, 552–553
Body mass index (BMI), 370, 1042, 1244, 1263
Body mechanics, 213–214, 643–645, 644b
Body movements, 652t–654t
  and posture, 554
Body planes, 158, 158f
Body position, 158, 159f, 159t–160t
Body regions, 158
Body temperature
  assessment of, 582–586
  elevated, 583, 483f
  equipment for measurement of, 584, 584f
  lowered, 583
  measurement of, 584–586, 585f–586f
  of newborn, 1077
  normal, 582–583, 583t
  regulation of, 582–583
Body weight, 370–371
Boil, 1297
Bolus, 306
Bonding, 111, 1061, 1061f
Bone conduction audiometry tests, 1414
Bone densitometry (DEXA/DXA), 613t
Bone marrow
  biopsy, 613t
  suppression, 1236
  transplantation, 1472
Bone mineral density (BMD), 613t
Bones, 195–198, 196f, 197t, 197f–198f
Bone scans, 613t–614t, 1322
Bone tissue, formation of, 211–212
Bone tumors, 1349

Borderline personality disorder, 1740
Bordetella pertussis, 1202
Boston brace, 1254
Bottle feeding, 1071
Bottle mouth, 112
Botulism, 543
Bowel diversion, 1595–1598
Bowel incontinence, 1706
Bowel obstruction, 1259
Bowel resection, 1596
Bowman capsule, 322–323, 322t, 323f
BPM. *See* Beats per minute (BPM)
Braces, 1821–1822
Brachial plexus injury, 1138
Brachial pulse, 587f
Brachytherapy, 1496
Braden scale, 862, 863f
Bradycardia, 587
Bradykinesia, 1366
Bradypnea, 590, 590t, 1542t, 1796
Braille alphabet, 1419
Brain, 220t
  abscess, 1370
  brainstem, 220t, 221
  cerebellum, 219
  cerebral cortex, 219, 221
  cerebral hemispheres, 221, 221f
  cerebrum, 222
  herniation, 1374
  hypothalamus, 222
  limbic system, 222
  thalamus, 221–222
  trauma, 1373
  white matter, 221
Brain death, 41–42, 889
Brain mapping, 1357
Brain natriuretic peptide (BNP), 242, 1436
Brain scan, 1352
Brain tumors, 1377
Brand name (medication), 906
Braxton Hicks contractions, 1057
Breast cancer, 1686t, 1688–1689
Breastfeeding, 1092–1095
  recommendations, 372
Breasts, 339–340
  changes in, 1068–1069
  data collection, 635t, 637t
Breath-holding spells, 1224
Breathing
  difficulty, 1569–1571
  exercises, 1543
  machine, 1573
  patterns, in dying person, 883
  treatments, 1543
Breath tests, 1584
Breckinridge, Mary, 5
Breech presentation, 1120
Bromocriptine mesylate (Parlodel), 1387
Bronchi, 298–299
Bronchial asthma. *See* Asthma
Bronchiectasis, 1556–1557
Bronchioles, 298–299
Bronchiolitis, 1238
Bronchitis, 1544
  acute, 1546
  chronic, 1557
Bronchoalveolar lavage, 1533
Bronchodilators, 940, 941t, 1512–1513
  for asthma, 1238
Bronchoscope, 612
Bronchoscopy, 615t, 1535
Broselow tape, 1191
Brown fat, 1077
Brudzinski sign, 1371, 1371f
Bruit, 1652

Brunner glands, 310
Bubbling (burping), 1096
Buck extension traction, 1338
Buck traction, 1339, 1339f
Buerger disease, 1447
Buffered regular, insulin, 1400
Buffers, 191–192
Building maintenance (facility), 464
Bulbourethral (Cowper) gland, 334
Bulimia, 126, 1625
Bulimia nervosa, 1262–1263
Bulk-producing agents, 947
Bulletin boards, 1890
Bumetanide (Bumex), 948
Buprenorphine therapy, 1797
Bureaucratic leadership, 1901
Bureau of Labor Statistics, 77
Burn care unit, 1301
Burn center, 462
Burns, 1299–1306
    characteristics of, 1301t
    classification, 1300
    depth and size, 1300
    first aid in, 532–533, 1300b
    injury management, 1301–1306
    nursing care plan, 1303
Burn shock, 520b
Bursae, 199
Bursitis, 1329
Business office, 464
Buspirone (BuSpar), 1752
Butterfly needles, 996
Button feeding device, 401
BVM. *See* Bag valve mask (BVM)

C

Cachexia, 1501, 1616
CAD. *See* Coronary artery disease (CAD)
CADD-Solis Intravenous Pump, 989
Caduceus, 2, 2f
Café coronary, 537
Caffeine, 1800
    in pregnancy, 1095
Calciferol. *See* Vitamin D
Calcitonin (CT), 239
Calcitrol (calciferol), 175
Calcium (Ca^{++}), 1317
    characteristics, 360
    deficiency, 357t, 1316t
    excess, 1316t
    functions, 357t, 360, 1316t
    imbalances, 1316t
    osteoporosis and, 375
    sources, 357t
    toxicity, 357t
Calcium channel blockers, for hypertension, 937
Calcium-modified diet, 400
Calculi, 1641
Call lights, 472
Calories
    client education on, 379
    empty, 350
    guidelines for intake of, 372b
    intake during pregnancy, 371
Calyx, 321
Cambodian populations, 383
Cambridge Color Test, 1270
Camp programs, 1888
Canadian Nurses' Association, 17, 1873
Cancer
    carcinogenesis, 1488, 1488b
    colorectal, 1616
    data collection, 1496
    development, 1486–1489, 1487b
    diagnostic tests, 1489–1492, 1491t
    esophageal, 1603–1604
    of gallbladder, 1623
    grading, 1488–1489
    incidence and risk factors, 1489
    kidney, 1646
    larynx, 1561–1563
    late effects, 1501
    liver, 1621
    lung, 1559
    mortality rate for, 58
    mouth, 1601
    nursing considerations, 1494, 1497–1504
    nutritional needs, 1501
    pain, 802
    pancreatic, 1623
    prevention and early detection, 1489
    of retina, 1258
    screening guidelines, 1490b
    small intestine, 1616
    smoking and, 62
    staging, 1488–1489, 1489b
    stomach, 1608–1609
    tobacco use and, 62
    treatment modalities, 1492–1497
    types, 1487–1488, 1487f
Candida albicans, 481, 481f, 1141, 1681
Candidiasis, 1171, 1172, 1525, 1600
Canes, 658, 659f, 1821
Canker sores, 1600
Cannabidiol (CBD), 1796
Cannabis drugs, 1795
Cannabis use disorder, 1795
Capacitance vessels, 265
Capillaries, 265
Capillary hemangioma, 1219
Capillary refill, 625, 626f
Capitation fee, 26
Caplet, 908
Capsule, 908
Caput succedaneum, 1082
Carbachol (Carbostat), 932
Carbamazepine (Tegretol), 925
Carbapenem-resistant *Klebsiella pneumonia* (CRKP), 488
Carbidopa-levodopa (Sinemet), 1367
Carbohydrate-controlled diets, 397
Carbohydrates (CHO)
    complex, 352–353
    counting, 1397
    digestion of, 351
    function of, 350–351, 351t
    guidelines for intake of, 372b
    simple, 351–352
Carbon dioxide (CO_2), 192
Carbuncle, 1297
Carcinogenesis, 1488, 1488b
Carcinogenic, 62
Carcinomas (CA), 1487
Cardiac arrhythmias, 1445–1446
Cardiac catheterization, 614t–615t, 1438
Cardiac conduction, 266–267, 267f
Cardiac cycle, 267–268
Cardiac flow studies, 615t
Cardiac glycoside, 1449
Cardiac output (CO), 268, 591
Cardiac sphincter, 308
Cardiogenic shock, 520b, 1454
Cardiopulmonary resuscitation (CPR), 38, 517, 525, 1447, 1572
    compression-only, 526
    team, 472
Cardiotonic drug digoxin (Lanoxin), 1451
Cardiotonics, 933, 935
Cardiovascular disorders. *See also* Cardiovascular system
    abnormal conditions, 1444–1445
    data collection, 1443
    diagnostic tests, 1436–1438
    medical treatments, 1438
    medications, 932–937, 933t–934t, 1439t–1440t
    prevention of, 1444
    signs and symptoms, 1443
    surgical treatments, 1438, 1441–1442
Cardiovascular emergencies
    assistance with, 527
    first-aid in, 537–538
        fainting, 537
        suspected cerebrovascular accident, 538
        suspected heart attack, 537–538
Cardiovascular medications, 932–937, 933t–934t
    antiarrhythmics, 935
    antihypertensives, 936–937
    cardiotonics, 933, 935
    vasoconstrictors, 935
    vasodilators, 935–936
Cardiovascular system, 259–270
    disorders of, 1229–1233
        acyanotic defects, 1229, 1229t
        coarctation of aorta, 1233
        cyanotic defects, 1229, 1229t
        and open-heart surgery, 1233
        patent ductus arteriosus, 1230, 1231f
        septal defects, 1230, 1231f
        stenosis, 1233
        tetralogy of Fallot, 1230, 1232f
        transposition of great arteries, 1230, 1231f
        tricuspid atresia, 1233
    effects of aging on, 269t–270t
    factors influencing, 269b
    function of, 259 260b
    physiology of, 266–269
    structure, 259
        blood vessels, 262–266
        heart, 259–262
Cardiovascular tests, 614t–615t
Career ladder program, 11
Caregiver-controlled analgesia (CCA), 807
Caregivers
    assistance, 1831b
    home assessment, 1810–1815
    hospice care, 1855–1856
    instruction, for children, 1176
    nursing duties, 1834–1836
    payment, 1832–1833
    protocols and procedures, 1836
    reasons for, 1830–1831
    transitions, 1836
Caribbean populations, 381
Caries, 1600
Carotene, 172
Carotid artery, 589
Carotid pulse, 589
Carpal tunnel syndrome, 1329
Cartilage, 202
Cartilaginous joints, 199
Case management, 20, 446, 464
Casts, 1335–1337, 1631
CAT. *See* Computerized adaptive testing (CAT)
Cataracts, 256t, 1225
Catecholamines, 239, 930
Catha edulis, 1798
Cathartics (Laxatives), 944t–945t, 946–947
Catheter-associated urinary tract infections (CAUTI), 515
Catheterization
    caring for client after, 846
    children, 1188
    female client, 845, 846f, 851–854

male client, 845–846, 854–855
urinary, 846
Catheters
removal, 846, 856
self-catheterization, 845
urinary, 845
Cation, 185
Cat scratch disease, 1210
CAUTI. *See* Catheter-associated urinary tract infections (CAUTI)
Cavernostomy, 1659
Cavernous hemangioma, 1219
CBC. *See* Complete blood count (CBC)
CBE. *See* Charting by exception (CBE)
CCU. *See* Coronary care unit (CCU)
CD4 cells, 1521
CDU. *See* Clinical decision unit (CDU)
Cecum, 312
Celecoxib (Celebrex), 924t, 928
Celiac disease, 1224
Cell-mediated immunity, 288, 290
Cell membrane, 163
Cell(s), 161–164
animal, 162f
enzymes, 164
of epidermis, 171t
Langerhans', 171
melanocytes, 171
Merkel, 171
properties, 161–162
reproduction, 163–164, 164f
structure and function of, 162–163, 163t, 163f
Cellular respiration, 301, 316
Cellulose, dietary fiber and, 353
Celsius (C) scale, 582, 582f
Center of gravity, 644
Centers for Diseases Control and Prevention (CDC), 57–58, 73–74, 509, 1531
Centers for Medicare & Medicaid Services (CMS), 74, 429, 1841, 1900
Centers of Excellence (COE), 1809, 1832
Central fovea (fovea centralis), 252
Central line associated blood stream infection (CLABSI), 515
Central nervous system (CNS), 219, 221–224, 1357
accessory structures, 223–224, 223b
brain, 219, 220t, 221f, 220–222
medications affecting, 921, 923t–926t, 926–931
adrenergics, 930–931
analgesics, 921, 926–928, 926b
anticonvulsants, 929–930
depressants, 921
hypnotics and sedatives, 928–929
selective depressants, 921
stimulants, 921
spinal cord, 222, 223f
Central parenteral nutrition (CPN). *See* Total parenteral nutrition (TPN)
Central service supply (CSS), 464
Central supply room (CSR), 464
Central venous pressure (CVP), 1448
Centrosomes, 162
Cephalgia (headache), 1354
Cephalic presentations, 1054
Cephalohematoma, 1082
Cephalopelvic disproportion (CPD), 1119
Cephalosporins, 916t, 920
Cerclage, 1107
Cerebral angiography, 1352
Cerebral circulation, 283, 283f
Cerebral embolism, 1459, 1462
Cerebral hemorrhage, 1462

Cerebral (brain) infarct. *See* Stroke
Cerebral palsy (CP), 1280–1282
Cerebral perfusion, 283
Cerebral thrombosis, 1462
Cerebrospinal fluid (CSF), 223–224, 223b, 614t, 1142, 1352, 1375f
Cerebrovascular accident (CVA), 538
Cerebrovascular disease, mortality rate for, 58
Certified home health aides (CHHAs), 1833
Certified in Long Term Care (CLTC), 1898
Certified nurse midwife (CNM), 1024, 1035
Certified nursing assistant (CNA), 11t
Certified registered nurse anesthetist (CRNA), 1061
Certified RN, Hospice (CRNH), 1855
Cerumen, 174
Cerumenolytics, 932
Cervical biopsy, 1674
Cervical cancer, 1170, 1686t, 1687
Cervical cap, 1160
Cervical halter traction, 1339, 1339f
Cervical os, 1053
Cervicitis, 1683
Cervix, 339
changes in, pregnancy and, 1057
Cesarean delivery, 1122–1123
Chadwick sign, 1032
Chancroid, 1166
Change-of-shift reporting, 453
Chaplaincy staff, 464
Chaplains, 1743
Charge nurses, 1901–1904, 1903b
Charting by exception (CBE), 446, 447t
Cheiloplasty, 1228
Cheilosis, 366
Chelation, 1270–1271
Chemical dependency unit, 462
Chemical methods, of tubal sterilization, 1161
Chemical name (medication), 906
Chemical pneumonia, 1547
Chemical thermometers, 584f
Chemistry and life, 155–157
Chemoreceptors, 254
Chemotaxis, 276
Chemotherapy, 1493–1494
in leukemia, 1235–1236
in malignant bone tumors, 1256
Chemotherapy-induced nausea and vomiting (CINV), 1500
Chenodiol, 1622
Chest
assessment, 633t, 635t
circumference, children, 1183
data collection, 631t, 633t
drainage systems, 1537f
pain, 1438
percussion, 1239
Chest injuries, 523
Chest physical therapy (CPT), 1238–1239
Chest physiotherapy (CPT), 1536
Chest radiograph (x-ray), 615t
Chest suction, 1539. *See also* Thoracotomy
Chest trauma, 1558
Chewing gum, 908
Cheyne–Stokes breathing, 1542t
Cheyne–Stokes respiration, 590t, 591, 883
Chief cells, stomach, 315
Child abuse, 1213–1219
emotional abuse, 1217
neglect, 1213–1214
nursing care plan, 1215–1217
physical abuse, 1214
reporting of, 1213
sexual abuse, 1217–1218

Childbearing stage, 101
Childbirth education, 1047
Childbirth, natural, 1047
Childbirth preparation, 1047
Childhood immunizations, 59
Childhood, nutrition during, 373
Child launching stage, 102
Childrearing stage, 101–102
Chinese populations, 382–383
Chiropractic therapy, 28
Chiropractor, 10b
Chlamydia, 1163–1164, 1164b, 1164f
Chloral hydrate, 929
Chlorhexidine, 502t
Chloride (Cl^-), 1318
deficiency, 356t, 1316t
excess, 1316t
functions, 356t, 357, 1316t
imbalances, 1316t
sources, 356t
toxicity, 356t
Chlorine, 502t
Chloroquine (Aralen), 1332
Chlorpheniramine (Chlor-Trimeton), 939
CHO. *See* Carbohydrates
Choanal atresia, 1143
Choking prevention, 1209
Cholecystectomy, 313–314, 1622
Cholecystitis, 610, 1621–1622
Cholecystogram, 1585
Cholecystokinin (CCK), 242, 310, 314–315
Cholecystostomy, 1622
Choledocholithotomy, 1622
Choledochostomy, 1622
Cholelithiasis, 1622
Cholesterol, 355, 369–370
Cholinesterase inhibitors, 1368
ChooseMyPlate.gov, 346, 346f, 347t–348t
Chordae tendineae (tendinous cords), 261
Chorea, 1369
Choriocarcinoma, 1108
Chorion, 1027
Chorionic villus sampling (CVS), 1106, 1272
Chorizo, 381
Chromium (Cr), 359t, 360
Chromosomes, 162
Chronic back pain, 1326–1328
Chronic diseases, 609
Chronic illnesses, 1698
Chronic lymphoid leukemia (CLL), 1235–1236, 1479
Chronic myeloid leukemia (CML), 1235–1236, 1479
Chronic obstructive lung disease, 1554
Chronic obstructive pulmonary disease (COPD), 1553–1558
asthma, 1554–1556
bronchiectasis, 1556–1557
chronic bronchitis, 1557
mortality rate for, 58
pulmonary emphysema, 1557–1558
risk factors, 1553
smoking and, 62
symptoms, 1553
treatment, 1553
Chronic pain, 802
Chronic shock, 520b
Chronic ulcerative colitis (CUC), 1613
Chvostek sign, 1390, 1390f
Chyme, 309
Cigarette smoking
and acne, 1250
and lung cancer, 1559
Cilia, cell, 163
Cilia, nose, 297

Circle of Willis, 283
Circulating nurse, 824
Circulation hypoxia, 1541
Circulatory disorders, postoperative, 835
Circumcision, 333, 1091
Circumoral cyanosis, 1189
Cirrhosis, 1618–1619, 1791
Cisgender, 1147
Civil rights legislation, 1759
CLABSI. *See* Central line associated blood stream infection (CLABSI)
Clean technique. *See* Medical asepsis
Clear liquid diet, 394t
Cleft lip and cleft palate, 1143, 1227–1229, 1228f
Client education department, 463
Client identification, before giving medications, 955
Client lift, 662–664
Client planning conference, 437
Client representatives, 24
Client unit, 455–458, 456f
    cleaning after use of, 458
    components of, 456–458
    examination room, 458
    furniture, 457–458
    linens in, 458
    neatness of, 458
    noise, 457–458
    odors, 457
    privacy in, 458
    restocking of, 458
    safety and nursing care equipment in, 457
    ventilation and air quality in, 457
Climacteric, 335t
Clindamycin (Cleocin), 921
Clinical care path, 444
Clinical death, 526, 889
Clinical decision unit (CDU), 463
Clinical hypothermia, 583
Clinical Nurse Specialist certifications, 11
Clitoris, 339, 342–343
Clonazepam (Klonopin), 925t, 930
Clonic seizures, 1356, 1356b
Clonidine, 829
Closed head trauma (CHT), 223, 1738
Closed-heart surgery, 1441
Closed procedure, arthroscopy, 1322
Closed reduction, 1335
Closed water-seal drainage, 1539. *See also* Thoracotomy
Clostridium botulinum, 543
Clostridium tetani, 483, 1202
Clozapine (Clozaril), 943, 1750
Clubfoot. *See* Talipes
Cluster headaches, 1355
CMG. *See* Cystometrogram (CMG)
CMP. *See* Comprehensive metabolic panel (CMP)
CMS. *See* Centers for Medicare & Medicaid Services (CMS)
CMV. *See* Cytomegalovirus (CMS)
CNS. *See* Central nervous system (CNS)
Coagulants, 938
Coarctation of aorta (COA), 1142, 1232f, 1233
Coarse crackles, breath sounds, 635t
Cobalamin. *See* Vitamin B$_{12}$
Cocaine HCl, 1798
Cocaine use disorder, 1798
Coccidioidomycosis, 481
Cochlea, 251
Cochlear implant, 1417
Cochlear nerve, 251
Codeine, 923t, 927
Codes, 881

Cognitive behavioral techniques, in pain management, 809
Cognitive deficit, 1715
Cognitive function, 627t, 629t
Cognitive impairment, 1715–1718, 1716b
Cogwheeling, 1755
Cohabitation, 100
Coitus, 335
Coitus interruptus, 1156–1157
Colchicine (Colcrys), 1333
Cold exposure, 1408
Cold humidity, 794
Cold receptors, 255
Cold-related injuries, first-aid in, 529–530
    frostbite, 529, 529b
    hypothermia, 530
    immersion foot, 530
Cold sores, 1601
COLDSPA mnemonic, 608b
Cold therapy, 792–794
    cold humidity, 794
    cold, moist compresses, 792–793, 794f
    hypothermia blanket, 794
    icecap or ice collar, 792, 800
    in pain management, 808
    rationale for, 792, 792f
    single-use and refreezable ice packs, 792
    tepid sponge, 793–794
Colectomy, 1260
Colic, 1240–1241
Collaborative problem, 431
Collagen, 171
Collagenase-based debridement, 1293
Collagen diseases, 1207
Collateral circulation, 263, 1454
Collodion, 1353
Colloid solutions, 1470
Colon, 312–313
Colonoscopy, 616t, 1587–1588, 1587f
Colony-stimulating factors (CSFs), 1479, 1495
Color blindness, 249, 1270
Colorectal cancer, 1616
Color vision deficiency. *See* Color blindness
Colostomy, 1595
    irrigation, 1596
    nursing care guidelines, 1598
    stoma condition in, 1595
Colostrum, 1031–1032, 1068
Colposcopy, 1674
Coma, irreversible, 42. *See also* Brain death
Combative person, 1771, 1773
Comfort measures, in pain management, 808
Commissurotomy, 1233
Commitment, mental illness and, 1745
Common bile duct obstruction, 1622–1623
Common cold, 1248, 1544–1545
Communal family, 100
Communicable diseases, 488, 1201, 1246–1250
    admission screening for, 611b
Communication, 88–90, 550f, 1710–1711
    barriers to effective, 552t
    with client speaking different language, 560
    components of, 550–551
    culture and subculture, 556–557, 556b
    documentation of, 441–442
    facilitate, 442b, 562
    factors influencing, 555–556
    with infants, 109–110
    interviewing, 557–559
        clarification, 558
        closed-ended question, 557, 558t
        nonverbal therapeutic techniques in, 557–558
        open-ended question, 557, 558t
        paraphrasing, 558
        reflection, 558
        summarizing, 558–559
        unfinished statement, use of, 559
        use of silence, 558
    nonverbal, 552–555
        body language, 552–553
        body movements and posture, 554
        COVID-19, 555
        eye contact, 554
        facial expressions, 554
        gestures and rituals, 554
        personal appearance and grooming, 554
        proxemics and personal space, 553
        therapeutic use of touch, 554, 554f
    and nursing process, 549–550
    person with aphasia, 559, 561b
    in special situations, 559, 559f
    with specific client behaviors, 560, 560f, 561b
    types of, 551–555
    verbal, 551–552, 551b, 551f
    with visually impaired/hearing-impaired person, 551
    with young child, 109–110
Community-based care, 1743–1744, 1743b
Community health, 23, 72–81
Community health centers (CHC), 79, 1843–1844
Community health services, 23
Community mental health centers (CMHCs), 1743
Community needs, 53
Community Nursing Organization (CNO), 1831
Community resources, 1826–1827
Community services, 77
Community violence, 64–65
Commuter family, 99
Compartment syndrome, 830, 1348–1349
Compassion fatigue, 1854
Complementary healthcare, 28–29, 608
Complement fixation, 292
Complements, 292
Complete blood count (CBC), 611, 1467–1468
Complete fractures, 1334
Complete proteins, 356
Complex partial (psychomotor) seizures, 1356b
Compound fractures, 1334
Compounds, 156–157
Comprehensive metabolic panel (CMP), 1310
Compression fractures, 1334
Compulsions, 1740
Computed axial tomography (CAT) scans, 611, 615t
Computed tomography (CT) scan, 611, 615t, 1534
    of lung abscesses, 1534
    in musculoskeletal disorders, 1322
    in nervous system disorders, 1351
Computerized adaptive testing (CAT), 38
Computerized medication dispensing unit, 904, 904f
Conception, 1106–1107
Concussion, 1374
Conditions of participation (COP), 1852
Condom catheter, 845
Condoms, 1160
Conduction block, 817, 818b
Condyloid joints, 200
Cones, 248–249
Confidentiality, 34
    client's right to, 43b
    violation of, 35
Confusion, 1716–1717
Congenital anomalies, 1027
Congenital defects, of spinal cord, 1362

Congenital disorders, 69–70, 1269–1270
Congenital glaucoma, 1225, 1258
Congenital hypertrophic pyloric stenosis. *See* Pyloric stenosis
Congenital hypothyroidism, 1389, 1389f
Congenital rubella syndrome (CRS), 1140, 1206
Congestive heart failure (CHF), 1448
Congregate housing, 1810
Conization, 1673
Conjunctiva, 247
Conjunctivitis, 629, 1141, 1164, 1248–1249
Connective tissue membranes, 167
Connective tissues, 165–166
Consistent carbohydrate diet, 397
Constant fever, 583
Constipation, 946, 1611–1612, 1706
    end-of-life care and, 884–885
    in older adults, 374–375
    postoperative, 831–832
Consulting nurse service (telehealth), 464–465
Consumer fraud, 30
Contact dermatitis, 1508–1509
Contact precautions, 511–512
Contact transmission, 511
Contagious (microorganisms), 69
Contagious diseases, 1206–1208
Contiguous (or continuous) quality improvement (CQI), 23
Continent bowel diversions, 1598–1599
Continent diversions, 1647
Continent ileostomy, 1599
Continual care facilities, 1806
Continuing care retirement communities (CCRCs), 1806, 1806f, 1810
Continuing education hours (CEHs), 38
Continuing education units (CEUs), 38, 1872, 1899
Continuity of care, plans for, 448
Continuous ambulatory peritoneal dialysis (CAPD), 1652
Continuous-chest-compression, 526
Continuous passive motion (CPM), 655, 1325
Continuous positive airway pressure (CPAP), 1137, 1552b, 1574
Continuous quality improvement (CQI), 464
Contraception, 1153–1162
    and abortion, 1154
    barrier methods, 1160
    birth control implant, 1156b, 1158
    breastfeeding, 1157
    continual abstinence, 1156
    Depo-Provera, 1158
    fertility awareness methods, 1157
    hormonal methods, 1157–1159
    intrauterine device, 1159
    oral contraceptives, 1157–1158
    sterilization, 1161
    transdermal patches, 1158
    vaginal ring, 1159
    withdrawal, 1156–1157
Contractions of uterine muscles, 1058–1059, 1058f
Contraction stress test. *See* Oxytocin challenge test (OCT)
Contracts, 1895–1896
Contracture, 1280, 1305–1306
Controlled release (CR) drugs, 915b
Controlled substances, 904–905
Controlled Substances Act, 904
Contusion, 1374
Convoluted tubule, 323
Convulsion. *See* Seizures
Cooley anemia, 1479
COPD. *See* Chronic obstructive pulmonary disease (COPD)

Copper (Cu), 359t, 360
Coprolalia, 1278
Copulation, 335
Cordocentesis. *See* Percutaneous umbilical blood sampling (PUBS)
Corium, 171
Cornea, 247–248
Corneal transplantation, 248
Coronary arteries, 262–263, 263f
Coronary artery bypass grafting (CABG), 1441
Coronary artery disease (CAD), 58, 68, 1452–1455
    physiologic differences and, 263
Coronary care unit (CCU), 463, 1435
Coronary embolus, 1459
Coronary heart disease (CHD), exercise and, 62
Coronary intensive care unit (CICU), 1435
Coronary rehabilitation unit (CRU), 463
Coronary sinus, 263
Coronary veins, 263
Corpus callosum, 221
Corpus cavernosum, 333
Corpus spongiosum, 333
Correctional facilities, 1885
Cortex, adrenal glands, 1391
Cortical dementias, 1718
Corticosteroid nasal spray, 939
Corticosteroids, 234, 239, 1332
Corticotropin. *See* Adrenocorticotropic hormone (ACTH)
Corticotropin-releasing hormone (CRH), 234
Cortisone, 931, 1332
Cosmetic breast surgery, 1674
Cotton-tipped applicator, 1415
Coudé-tip catheter, 845
Cough, 610t
Coughing, 302, 940
Counseling, 1834
Countertraction forces, 1338
Court commitment, 1745
CPAP. *See* Continuous positive airway pressure (CPAP)
CPR. *See* Cardiopulmonary resuscitation (CPR)
CPT. *See* Chest physiotherapy (CPT)
CQI. *See* Continuous quality improvement (CQI)
Cradle cap, 1219
Cranial nerves, 224–225, 224b–225b, 225t, 619
Craniocerebral disorders, 1353–1359
Craniotomy, 1366
Crash carts, 527, 527f, 1191
C-reactive protein (CRP), 1208, 1260, 1507
Creatinine, 1631
Credé maneuver, 1636
Cremasteric reflex, 333
Crepitus, breath sounds, 635t
Creutzfeldt–Jakob disease (CJD), 1719, 1725
Crisis intervention centers, 1148, 1844
Critical Access Standards, 518–519
Critical thinking, 412, 412f
CRKP. *See* Carbapenem-resistant *Klebsiella pneumonia* (CRKP)
Crohn disease, 1260, 1613
Cross-sensitivity, 913
Croup, 1237
Croupette, 794
Crowning, 1060
CRU. *See* Coronary rehabilitation unit (CRU)
Crutches, 658–662, 660f
Crutch-walking gaits, 660, 661f, 662
Cryoprecipitates, 1471
Cryosurgery, 1297, 1308, 1492, 1665–1666
Cryotherapy, 1171
    of retinoblastoma, 1258
Cryococcal meningitis, 1525
Cryptorchidism, 1244, 1659

Cryptosporidiosis, 1208, 1525
Crystalluria, 1631
CSF. *See* Cerebrospinal fluid (CSF)
C&S test. *See* Culture and sensitivity (C&S) test
Cuban populations, 382
Culdoscopy, 1673
Cultural assessment, 87b
Cultural competence, 85
Cultural considerations, death/dying and, 882, 883b
Cultural diversity, 85
Culturally competent care, 85–86
Cultural sensitivity, 86
Cultural shock, 520b
Culture, 78
    beliefs and values, 86
    characteristics of, 84b
    and communication, 556–557
    death and dying, beliefs about, 91
    diet and nutrition, 90–91
    elimination of wastes and, 91
    health and illness, 87–88
    language and communication, 88–90
    minorities, 73
    religious/spiritual customs and traditions, 91–92
    sensitivity to, 86
    subcultures, 83–84
    taboos and rituals, 86
Culture and sensitivity (C&S) test, 611, 919, 1631
Cultured epithelial autografts (CEA), 1305
Curettage, 1152
Cushing syndrome (hyperadrenalism), 1388
Cutaneous diversions, 1648–1679
Cutaneous stimulation, for pain management, 808
Cuts and punctures wounds, in children, 1210
Cyanosis, 591, 610t, 1212
Cyclophosphamide (Cytoxan), 1332, 1518
Cyclosporine (Gengraf), 1332
Cyclothymic disorder, 1775
Cyst. *See* Benign neoplasms
Cystadenomas, 1623
Cystectomy, 1647
Cystic fibrosis, 1238
Cystic Fibrosis Foundation, 78, 1239
Cystinuria, 1642
Cystitis, 1124
    acute, 1637–1638
    chronic, 1638
Cystocele, 1680
Cystogram, 1632
Cystometrogram (CMG), 616t, 1633
Cystoscope, 1632
Cystoscopy, 616t, 1632–1633
Cystotomy, 1647
Cystourethrogram, 616t
Cysts, 1271
Cytokines, 289
Cytology, 1489
Cytomegalovirus (CMV), 1140, 1169, 1525
Cytoplasm, 162, 483

D

Daily Food Intake Patterns, 349
Daily values (DV), 368
Dairy products, 379
Dandruff, 1299
Dangling, 656–657
DAPE charting, 446, 447t
Dapiprazole (Rev-Eyes), 932
DARE charting, 446, 447t
DARP charting, 446, 447t
DAT (diet as tolerated), 836

Data, 420
  biographical, 423
  objective, 420–421
  subjective, 421–422
Data analysis, 423
  data recognition, 423
  patterns/clusters recognition, 423
  reaching conclusions, 426–427
  strengths and problems, identification of, 426
  validate observations, 423
Data collection, 422–423
  in children, 638–641
  in client care, 607–641
  in endocrine disorders, 1386–1387
  factors influencing, 608–617
  of fluid and electrolytes, 1311
  health interview, 422–423, 424t–426t
  in musculoskeletal disorders, 1323
  in nervous system disorders, 1354
  in nursing, 622t–623t, 625t, 627t, 629t, 631t, 633t, 635t, 637t
  nursing care plans and, 608
  observation, 422
  in pediatrics, 1181–1183
  techniques in, 619f
Davol drain, 871, 872f
Daycare programs, 1809
Day-surgery centers, 21
DBP. *See* Diastolic blood pressure (DBP)
Death
  biological, 526, 889
  brain, 41–42, 889
  care following, 888–890
  caring for body after, 889–893
  caring for family after, 889
  clinical, 41, 889
  exceptions to determination of, 42
  family coping after, 889, 890f
  legal, 41
  pronouncement of, 889
  religious beliefs and practices related to, 150b
  signs of approaching, 888, 888b
Débridement, 1291
  in burn injuries, 1304
  injuries, 865, 870
Decidua, 1026
Decision making, 1904
Decongestants, 942t, 943
Decubitus ulcer. *See* Pressure wound
Decussation, 221
Deep relaxation techniques, in pain management, 809
Deep vein thrombosis (DVT), 1348, 1455
  postoperative, 832
Defecation, 317
Defense mechanisms, 64
Deficiency diseases, 69
Degenerative disorders, 1364–1370
Degenerative joint disease (DJD), 1329, 1331
Deglutition, 307
Dehiscence (surgical incision), 835–836, 836f, 1593
Dehumanization, 1759
  prevention of, 568–569
Dehydration, 183, 320
Dehydroepiandrosterone (DHEA), 239
Delayed awakening, postoperative, 830
Delayed release (DR) medications, 915b
Delayed union, 1349
Delirium, 1717
Delivery
  anesthesia during, 1060–1061
  cesarean, 1122–1123
  emergency, 1121–1122

  estimated date of, 1036
  forceps, 1122
  necessary documentation for, 1066b
Delta cells, 241
Delusional behavior, 1739
Delusions, 1286, 1741
Demeclocycline, 1387
Dementia, 1718
  causes of, 1720t
  data collection, 1725
  diagnosis, 1719–1721
  Parkinson disease dementia, 1724
  progression, 1721–1722
  signs and symptoms, 1719
  vascular, 1724
Democratic leadership, 1901
Demography, 72
Densford, Katherine J., 6
Dental caries, 701
Dental clinics, 1889
Dental hygienist, 10b
Dental injuries/missing teeth, first-aid in, 535
Dental malocclusion, 1255–1256
Dental problems, 1600
Denver-II Developmental Screening Test (DDST), 1176
Deoxyribonucleic acid (DNA), 162
Department of Agriculture, U.S. (USDA), 346
Department of Health and Human Services (HHS), 59, 74–75, 74f, 74b
Dependent edema, 1313, 1449b
Depressed skull fracture, 1374
Depression, 802, 1283–1284, 1707–1708, 1739, 1773
  chronic pain and, 802
  malnutrition and, 371
Dermatitis, 1291, 1296
Dermatology (DERM), 462, 1289
Dermis, 169, 171
Desensitization, 1512
Desmopressin acetate (DDAVP), 948
Desquamation, 170, 1205
Detergent, 502t
Detoxification process, 1783
Detrusor muscle, 1633
Developmental delays, 107
Developmental disability, 1267
Developmental dysplasia, 1142, 1219–1220
Developmental milestones, 107
Deviated septum, 1560
Dextrins, 351
Dextromethorphan (DM), 940
Dextrose, 351
5% dextrose in normal saline (D5NS), 987
5% dextrose in 0.45% normal saline (D5½NS), 987
5% dextrose in sterile water (D5W), 987
DHA. *See* Docosahexaenoic acid (DHA)
D.H.E. (dihydroergotamine mesylate), 928
Diabetes insipidus, 1387
Diabetes mellitus (DM), 68, 1393
  complications of, 1401–1406
  drugs classifications for, 1402t
  long-term management, 1406–1409
  mortality rate for, 58
  oral medications, 1400
  prediabetes, 68
  type 1, 1394–1401
  type 2, 1257
  ulcers, 1405f
Diabetic ketoacidosis (DKA), 1404
Diabetic ulcers, 862
Diagnosis-related groups (DRGs), 28
Diagnostic Adaptive Behavior Scale (DABS), 1267

Diagnostic and Statistical Manual for Mental Disorders (DSM), 1737
Diagnostic procedures, nurses and, 617
Diagnostic statement, 430–431
Diagnostic tests, 613t–617t, 1290
  client and family teaching, 612
  ears, 1414–1415
  eye, 1413–1414
  hearing, 1414–1415
  vision, 1414–1415
Dialectical behavioral therapy (DBT), 1790
Dialysis, 1212, 1651–1653
Dialysis centers, 1888
Dialysis unit, 462
Diapedesis, 276
Diaphoresis, 174, 190
Diaphragm, 158, 204, 299, 1153
Diaphragmatic hernia, 1239
Diarrhea, 1240, 1612–1613
  in children, 1188
  end-of-life care and, 885
  and ulcerative colitis, 1259
Diastole, 267
Diastolic blood pressure (DBP), 592, 592f
Diazepam (Valium), 924t, 929–930
Dicyclomine hydrochloride (Bentyl), 1611
Diet. *See also* Diet therapy; Nutrition
  added sugars in, 352b
  bland, 396
  carbohydrate-controlled, 397
  with controlled minerals and electrolytes, 399–400
  cultural considerations, 90–91
  digestive soft, 395
  disease risk and, 609t
  gluten-restricted, 399
  healthy, 368
  high- and low-fat, 397, 399
  high- and low-fiber, 395–396
  high-calorie, 396
  house, 393
  liquid, 393–395
  modified, 393–400
  planning of, 370–371
  protein-controlled, 397, 399
  reduced-calorie, 396
  soft, 395, 395T
  vegetarian, 384–386
Dietary department, 463
Dietary fiber, 352–353, 354b
Dietary guidelines, 372b
Dietary Reference Intakes (DRIs), 348
Diethylstilbestrol (DES), 1045
Dietitian, 10b
Diet therapy, 389–410
  between-meal and bedtime supplements, 391
  fluid intake, 392, 392b
  house diet, 393
  modified diet, 393–400
Difficult breathing (dyspnea), 591
Diffusion, 187
Digestion, 305
  chemical, 315
  and enzymes, 350
  mechanical, 315
  processes of, 315, 315t
Digestive disorders
  diagnostic tests, 1583–1588
  esophagus, 1601–1604
  gallbladder, 1621–1623
  large/small bowel, 1609–1615
  liver, 1617–1621
  medical treatments, 1588–1599
  mouth, 1599–1601
  overnutrition, 1623–1625

pancreas, 1623
peritonitis, 1615–1616
rectum, 1616–1617
sigmoid colon, 1616–1617
stomach, 1604–1609
surgical treatments, 1588–1599
undernutrition, 1623–1625
Digestive soft diet, 395
Digestive system, 305, 311t–312t
    accessory organs of, 313, 313f, 314t
        gallbladder, 313–314
        liver and spleen, 313
        pancreas, 314
        peritoneum, 314–315
    effects of aging on, 317t–318t
    function of, 305, 306f, 306b
    organs of
        cecum and appendix, 312
        colon, 312–313
        duodenum, 310
        esophagus, 308, 308f
        jejunum and ileum, 310
        large intestine, 310, 312
        mouth, 306–308
        palate, 306
        pharynx, 308
        rectum and anus, 313
        salivary glands, 306
        small intestine, 309–310, 310f
        stomach, 309, 309f
        teeth, 307, 307f
        tongue, 307–308
    physiology of, 315–316
        digestive process, 315–316
        elimination, 317
        energy synthesis and release, 317
        metabolism, 316–317
Digital mammography, 617t
Digoxin, 933, 933t, 935
Dilation and curettage (D&C), 1107, 1674
Diltiazem, 937
Diluent, 981
Dimenhydrinate (Dramamine), 946
Diparesis, 1281
Dipeptides, 355
Diphenhydramine (Benadryl), 929, 939
Diphtheria, 1202
Diphtheria, tetanus, acellular pertussis (DTaP), 1202, 1204
Diplegia, 1281
Diplopia, 1368
Direct Coombs test, 1467
Direct measurement of blood pressure, 593
Disabilities, 1266–1267
Disaccharides, 351–352
Disaster medical assistance team (DMAT), 474
Disaster plan, 473–476
    bomb threat, 474b, 475
    evacuation, 474–475, 475f
    implementation, 474
    infant/child abduction, 475–476
    internal vs. external disasters, 473–474
    triage in, 474
    work stoppages, 476
Discharge, 438–439, 439b, 574–575
    after delivery, 1072
    of children, 1181
    day of discharge, 574
    documentation of, 574–575
    in various facilities, 565b
Discipline area documentation, 446
Discoid lupus erythematosus, 1333
Discretionary calorie allowance, 349
DISCUS scale, 1755
Disease, 56, 60b–61b, 69–70

body's response to, 609–611
course of, 609
risk factors for, 608, 609t
signs and symptoms of, 610t
Disease-modifying antirheumatic drugs (DMARDs), 1254, 1518
Disinfection, 841–842
Diskectomy, 1327
Dislocations, 1334
Disposable electronic thermometers, 584, 584f
Disposal of medication packages, 959
Disseminated intravascular coagulation (DIC), 1117, 1471
Distal convoluted tubule (DCT), 323
Distraction, pain management, 809
Distributive shock, 520b
District court hold (DCH), 1745
Diuretics, 936–937, 947–948, 948t
Divalproex sodium (Depakote ER or DR), 930
Diversion
    death/dying and, 886
    in pain management, 809
Diversional activities, in healthcare facility, 1191
Diverticulitis, 1609–1610
Diverticulosis, 1609–1610
Divorce, 103
Dix, Dorothea Lynde, 4
DJD. See Degenerative joint disease (DJD)
DKA. See Diabetic ketoacidosis (DKA)
DM. See Diabetes mellitus (DM)
DMAT. See Disaster medical assistance team (DMAT)
DMC Pain Assessment Behavioral Scale, 806
DOA (Department of Agriculture), 74
Dock, Lavinia Lloyd, 4
Docosahexaenoic acid (DHA), 354b
Doctor of medicine (MD), 2
Documentation
    abbreviations used, 450t–451t
    accountability for, 442–443
    acronyms used in, 450t–451t, 452b
    of assessments, 444
    of client admissions, 570–573, 573b
    of communication, 441–442
    confidentiality of, 451
    contents of, 443–448, 445t, 447t
    criteria, 442
    diet/nutrition, 391
    discharge planning and, 439b
    discipline area, 446
    electronic medical records, 443
    of errors, 451–452
    formats, 444, 446, 448
    guidelines for, 448–453
    24-hour check, 449t
    24-hour clock and, 461
    medical information systems, 443
    narrative–chronological, 444, 446
    plans for care, 444
    purposes of, 441
    relevant information in, 449, 451
    symbols used in, 452b
    systems of, 443
    types of charting, 446
Documented evidence, 442
Docusate sodium (colace), 831, 1070
Dolasetron mesylate (Anzemet), 831
Domestic violence, 63
Do not hospitalize (DNH), 881
Do not intubate (DNI), 526, 881
Do not resuscitate (DNR), 518, 526, 881
Dopamine agonists, 1367
Dopamine, 240, 931, 1367
Doppler ultrasound, 594
Dorsalis pulse, 587f

Dosage calculation, 897–899
    formula method, 900
    fractions, 899
    percentages, 901
    ratio and proportion method for, use of, 897
    rules for, 897
    significant figure, 900–901
Dose, medication, 909
Double balloon enteroscopy, 1586–1587
Double voiding technique, 1633
Douching, 1038
Doula, 1053
Down syndrome (DS), 1140, 1274–1276, 1275f
Doxapram HCl (Dopram), 940
D-penicillamine, 1332
Drainage systems, 870–872
    closed, 871–872, 872f
    nursing considerations in handling, 872
    Penrose drain, 871, 871f
Drain tube attachment device (DTAD), 1598
Drawing, therapy using, 1748
Dressing reinforcement, 836–837
Dressings, 869–870
    after amputation surgery, 1325
    in burn injuries, 1323
    change, 836–837
    commercially prepared, 870, 871f
    dry, sterile, 869, 869f
        changing of, 875–879
    packing, 870, 870f
    wet-to-dry, 870
    wet-to-wet, 870
DRIs. See Dietary Reference Intakes (DRIs)
Dronabinol (Marinol), 1796
Droplet precautions, 511
Droplet transmission, 511
Drospirenone, 1157
Drowning, 1212, 1558
Drug allergy, 1511
Drug–drug interactions, 914
Drug-eluting stents (DES), 1441
Drug Enforcement Agency (DEA), 904
Drug overdose, 543
Drug poisoning, respiratory complications in, 1558
Drug references, 905–906
Drug replacement therapy, 1796–1797
Drug testing, 1895
Drying agents, preoperative, 824
Dual diagnoses, 1742
Dual disorders, 1779–1780
Dual-earner family, 99
Duchenne muscular dystrophy (DMD), 1282
Ductal system, 332–333
Ductless glands. See Endocrine glands
Ductus arteriosus, 1029
Ductus deferens, 332–333
Ductus venosus, 1029
Due process procedures, 1903
Dumping syndrome, 1593
Dunlop (side-arm) traction, 1339
Duodenal ulcers, 1604
Duodenum, 310
DuoDerm, 870
Duplex Doppler ultrasonography, 1656–1657
Durable power of attorney, 40, 881
Dust cells, 290
Dust diseases, 1553
DV. See Daily values (DV)
DVT. See Deep vein thrombosis (DVT)
Dyazide, 948
Dye procedures, older adults and, 1352
Dyes, 618b
Dying, 146–149
    end of life care, 146

Dying (*continued*)
  impact of, 148–149
  nursing considerations, 147t–148t
  stages of, 880
Dysarthria, 629, 1281
Dysfluency, 1268
Dysfunctional family, 103
Dyskinesia, 1280, 1281, 1755
Dyslexia, 1267
Dyslipidemia, 1393
Dysmenorrhea, 1260, 1678
Dyspareunia, 1149
Dyspepsia, 1602, 1604
Dysphagia, 308, 392, 1280, 1368, 1587
Dysphasia, 629t, 1368, 1463
Dyspnea, 299, 591, 610t, 1229, 1348, 1541
  signs and symptoms, 1542t
Dyspraxia, rehabilitation, 1813
Dysrhythmia, 587, 1436
Dystocia, 1117–1120
Dysuria, 1163, 1242, 1634

E

eAG. *See* Estimated average glucose (eAG)
EAR. *See* Estimated Average Requirement (EAR)
Eardrum, 250
Ear irrigation, 1415
Ears, 251f
  external, 249–250
  inner, 251
  medications affecting, 932
  middle, 250, 251f
  nerves, 251
Eating disorders, 67, 1262–1263
Ebola hemorrhagic fever, 487
Ebolavirus disease (EVD), 487
Eccrine sweat glands, 174
ECFs. *See* Extracellular fluids (ECFs)
Echocardiogram, 614t
Echolalia, 1278, 1741
Echopraxia, 1741
E-cigarettes, 1800
Eclampsia, 1109
Ecology, 79
Economic conditions, diet and, 387
Ectopic pregnancy, 1108, 1108f
Eczema, 1296, 1296f, 1508
Eczema herpeticum, 1219
Edema, 182, 182b, 320, 399, 610t, 1313, 1449b, 1508
  in pregnancy, 1036
Edentulous, 395, 1600
Edrophonium chloride (Tensilon), 1368
Educational barriers, 1828
Education and health promotion, 65
Eesophageal reflux, 1603
Effacement, 1057
EGD. *See* Esophagogastroduodenoscopy (EGD)
Egg cells, 340–341
Egg crate mattress, 691
E-HealthKEY, 881
Eicosapentaenoic acid (EPA), 354b
Ejaculation, 335
Ejaculatory ducts, 332
Ejaculatory fluid, 335
Elder abuse, 65, 1713, 1713t
Elective single-embryo transfer (eSET), 1153
Electrical defibrillation, 1447
Electrical stimulation, 1636
Electric heating pad, 790
Electric shock, 520b
Electrocardiogram (ECG), 267, 461, 1435
  in musculoskeletal disorders, 1323
  test, 614t

Electrocardiograph, 1436, 1437f
Electrocardiograph technician, 10b
Electrocautery, 1171, 1637
Electrocerebral silence, 1353
Electroconvulsive therapy (ECT), 1748–1749
Electrodesiccation, 1308
Electroencephalogram (EEG), 228, 1223
  in musculoskeletal disorders, 1323
  purpose, 614t
Electroencephalograph technician, 10b
Electroencephalography (EEG) department, 461
Electrolyte balance, 190
  aging effects on, 193t
  burn injuries and, 1302
  imbalances, 1316t
Electrolytes, 185
  characteristics, 356t–357t
  extracellular, 185
  food sources of, 186t
  functions of, 186t
  intracellular, 185
  serum values of, 187t
  transport of, 186–189
Electromyogram (EMG), 461, 613t, 1323
Electroneurography (ENG), 614t
Electronic blood pressure apparatus, 594
Electronic bracelets, 1080
Electronic cigarettes, 63
Electronic infusion controllers, 989
Electronic medical records (EMRs), 443
Electronic pacemaker, 1446
Electronic thermometers, 584, 584f
Electrons, 156
Electronystagmography (ENG), 1415
Electrophoresis, 1484
Electrophysiology study (EPS), 1438
Electroretinogram (ERG), 1414
Elements, 156–157
Elevated body temperature, 583
Elimination, 884–885, 910, 1037–1038, 1088
Elimination diet, 1219
Emaciation, 623t
Embolism, 835, 1348, 1458–1459
Embolus, 277, 283
Embryo, 340–341, 1025–1026
Emergence excitement, postoperative, 830
Emergency care
  assessment, 522–527
    of airway and cervical spine, 523
    of breathing, 523
    of circulation and bleeding, 523–524, 523f–524f
    disability, 523–524
    expose and examine site of injury, 525
  emergency medical service, 518
  emergency responders in, 519f
  first-aid measures, 527–547
    anaphylaxis, 540
    animal bites and scratches, 540–541
    back and neck injuries, 528–529, 528f
    in bleeding, 538–540
    in cardiovascular emergencies, 537–538
    chest injuries, 528
    cold-related injuries, 529–530
    dental injuries and missing teeth, 535
    exposure to hazardous materials, 541–542
    foreign objects, 535–537
    head injuries, 528–529
    heat-related injuries, 530–533
    musculoskeletal injuries, 534–535
    near drowning, 533–534
    poisoning, 542–543
    in psychiatric emergencies, 543–544

  principles of, 517–522, 518b
    identify problems, 518–519
    perform triage, 519
    safety assessment, 518
    during shock, 519–522, 520b–521b
    summon assistance, 518
  sudden death and life support, 525–527
    advanced cardiac life support, 526
    basic cardiac life support, 526, 526f
    client at home, 526–527
    code in healthcare facility, 527, 527f
    compression-only CPR, 526
Emergency chemical restraints (ECRs), 1761
Emergency contraception (EC), 1158
Emergency delivery, 1121–1122
Emergency department (ED), 463, 1844–1845
Emergency hold, 1745
Emergency medical service (EMS), 77, 518
Emergency medical technician, 10b
Emergency physical restraint (EPR), 1761
Emergency preparedness, 472–473
Emergency rescues, 1889
Emergency resuscitation, 472
Emergency services, 1745
Emergency signal, 472
Emergi-centers, 1844
Emerging adulthood, 130
Emesis, 309, 610t
Emetics, 946
Emission-computed axial tomography (E-CAT scans), 611, 615t
Emotional abuse, 1217
Emotional aspects, in burn injuries, 1229
Emotional balance, 1736f
Emotional factors, influence of, 387
Emotional health, 56
Emotionally neglected child, 1213
Emotional reactions, documentation, 1767
Emotional support, 886, 1764–1765
Employee health service (EHS), 1842, 1886
Employee right-to-know laws (ERTK), 469
Employees, responsibilities of, 1896
Employers, responsibilities of, 1896
Employment opportunities, 1883–1889
Empty calories, 350
Empyema, 1551–1552
EMS. *See* Emergency medical service (EMS)
Encephalitis, 1205, 1372
Encephalocele, 1221
Encephalopathy and plumbism, 1279
Encopresis, 118, 1240
Endocarditis, 1450
Endocrine disorders, 1257
  common medical and surgical treatments, 1386–1387
  diagnostic tests, 1382–1386
Endocrine glands, 232, 234f, 239, 1382, 1383t. *See also* specific glands
Endocrine system, 232–244, 1387
  effect of aging on, 244t
  feedback, 243
  functions of, 233–243, 233b
  medications affecting, 931–932
  physiology, 243
  secretions of, 235t–238t
  signaling effects, 243
  structure of, 233–243
Endocrinology, 232
Endocytosis, 276
End-of-life care, 146, 881f
  basic needs, dying person and, 883–886, 883b
    activity, 885
    elimination, 884–885
    environment, 886

hydration and nutrition, 884
hygiene, 885
oxygen and airway maintenance, 883–884
pain control, 885
client's wishes and, 880–882
advance directives, 881
choice to die at home, 882
cultural considerations, 882, 883b
ethics committee, 881
healthcare codes, 881
hospice, 882
organ and tissue donation, 881–882
failing circulation and, 888, 888f
failing senses and, 888
higher-level needs of dying person and, 886–887
nursing care, 887–888
stages of dying and, 880
End-of-life discussions, 149
Endogenous microorganisms, 495t
Endometrial cancer, 1671, 1686t
Endometrial cycle. *See* Uterine cycle
Endometriosis, 1260, 1683–1684
Endometrium, 339, 1025
Endoplasmic reticulum (ER), 162
Endorphins, 803
Endorsement, 13, 38
Endoscope, 612, 1586, 1586f
Endoscopic retrograde cholangiopancreatography (ERCP), 616t, 1586
Endoscopic tube, 401
Endoscopic ultrasonography (EUS), 1586
Endoscopy, 612, 1586, 1586f
Endotoxins, 491
Endotracheal tube (ET tube), 1137, 1572–1573
End-stage renal disease (ESRD), 1641, 1650–1654
Enema, 747–748
in children, 1188
preoperative, 823–824
Energy
kilocalories and, 349–350
modified diet for, 396–397
synthesis and release, 317
ENG. *See* Electroneurography (ENG)
Engerix-B, 1620
Engorgement, 1069
Enkephalins, 240
Ensure, 352
Entamoeba histolytica, 481
Enteral administration, 962–964
Enteral nutrition, 1591
Enteric-coated tablet, 908
Enteritis, 1604
Enterostomal therapist (ET), 1583
Entitlement, 1740
Enucleation, 1258, 1416
Enuresis, 118, 1241
Enzymatic debridement, 870, 1293
Enzyme-linked immunoassay (ELISA), 1524
Enzymes, 164, 352
for digestion, 311t–312t
EnzySurge, 873
Eosinophils, 276
Ependymal cells, 219
Epicutaneous method, 1507
Epidemic parotitis. *See* Mumps
Epidemiology, 488
Epidermis, 169–171, 170f, 171t
Epididymis, 332
Epididymitis, 1661
Epidural hematoma, 1376, 1376f
Epigastric shock, 520b

Epiglottis, 297, 308, 1237
Epilepsy, 929–930, 1356
Epinephrine, 240, 930
Episiotomy, 1065, 1065f
Epispadias, 1083, 1143, 1243
Epistaxis, 538, 1226, 1560
Epithelial membranes, 166
Epithelial tissues, 165, 165t
Epoetin alfa (erythropoietin), 937
Epstein–Barr virus (EBV), 1249, 1364
Epstein pearls, 1083
Erb–Duchenne paralysis, 1138
ERCP. *See* Endoscopic retrograde cholangiopancreatography (ERCP)
Erectile dysfunction (ED), 1149, 1657–1659
medications for, 949
Erection, 333, 335, 333
Erikson's theory, of psychosocial development, 108, 108t, 122–123, 123t, 129–130, 130t, 137, 137t
ERTK. *See* Employee right-to-know laws (ERTK)
Eructation, 1622
Erythema, 1507
Erythema migrans, 1250
Erythema toxicum, 1084, 1084f
Erythroblastosis fetalis, 1115, 1139–1140
Erythrocytes. *See* Red blood cells (RBCs)
Erythrocyte sedimentation rate (ESR), 1260, 1321, 1469
Erythromycin ointment, 1080
Erythropoiesis, 273, 324
Erythropoietin (EPO), 237t, 242, 273, 324, 1495
ESBLs. *See* Extended-spectrum β-lactamases (ESBLs)
Eschar, 865, 1291
Escherichia coli, 481, 520b, 1247
Esophageal adenocarcinoma, 1603
Esophageal atresia, 1143
Esophageal cancer, 1603–1604
Esophageal diverticulum, 1602
Esophageal reflux, 1603
Esophageal speech, 1562
Esophageal varices, 1618
Esophagitis, 1603
Esophagogastroduodenoscopy (EGD), 1586
Esophagoscopy, 1586
Esophagus, 308, 1601–1604
ESR. *See* Erythrocyte sedimentation rate (ESR)
Essential nutrients, 346
Establishment stage (family), 101
Estimated average glucose (eAG), 1386
Estimated Average Requirement (EAR), 348
Estimated date of confinement (EDC), 1036
Estimated date of delivery (EDD), 1036
Estimated Energy Requirements (EERs), 349
Estrogen, 240, 334, 337, 340, 949
Eszopiclone (Lunesta), 929
ET. *See* Enterostomal therapist (ET)
Etanercept (Enbrel), 1332
Ethambutol, in tuberculosis treatment, 1550
Ethical standards, healthcare, 42–44
Ethics committee, 43–44, 44f, 881
Ethnic heritage, 377–381, 380b
Ethnocentrism, 86
Etiology, 430, 488
Eukaryotes, 481
Eupnea, 299, 590, 1541
EUS. *See* Endoscopic ultrasonography (EUS)
Eustachian tube, 250, 297
Euthanasia, 33, 43
Evaluation of nursing care, 437–439, 438f
client response, analyzing, 437–438
discharge planning, 438–439, 439b
factors contributing to success/failure,

identification of, 438
Evidence-based practice, 442–443
Evisceration, 835–836, 836f, 1593
Evoked responses, brain, 1353
Ewing sarcoma family of tumors (ESFT), 1256
Exacerbation, 1259
Excisional biopsy, 1492, 1673
Excretory system. *See* Urinary system
Exenatide (Byetta), 1400
Exercise, 62, 212
arthritis and, 1332
disease risk and, 609t
in pain management, 808–809
postoperative, 833–834
in pregnancy, 1038
Exocrine gland, 232, 233t
Exophthalmos, 1388, 1388f
Exoskeletons, 1822
Expected outcome, 432, 433b
Expectorants, 940, 941t
Expiration, 299
Expressive aphasia, 552
Exstrophy, bladder, 1143
Extended care facilities (ECFs), 20, 22–23, 393, 455, 1806–1809
Extended families, 99
Extended release (ER) medications, 915b
Extended-spectrum β-lactamases (ESBLs), 488
External auditory canal, 1415, 1415f
External disaster, 473–474
External fixation, 1340
External genitalia, 339, 339f
Exteroceptors, 228
Extracellular fluids (ECFs), 180–182, 1311
Extracorporeal hemodialysis, 1652
Extracorporeal membrane oxygenation (ECMO), 1137
Extracorporeal shock wave lithotripsy (ESWL), 1643
Extrapyramidal side effects (EPSE), 1757b
Extrication, 528
Exubera, 1399
Exudate, 610, 859–860
Eyeball, 247–249, 248f
Eye care, death/dying and, 885
Eye contact, 554
cultural consideration, 90
Eyeglasses, 1422
Eye injuries, first-aid for, 536
Eyelids (palpebrae), 247
Eye patching, 1415
Eye protection, 499f, 500
Eye(s)
choroid layer, 248
disorders of, 1225
enucleation, 1258
light transmission, 253b
medications affecting, 932
muscles of, 252, 257t
nerves of, 252, 257t
protection, 248, 843
right, 247f
structure of, 247
tears, 247f
E-Z stand, 663

F
Face-brow presentation, 1120
Face tent, 794
Facial expressions, 554
Facial nerve (CN VII), 254
Facial paralysis, 1138
Factitious disorders, 1741
Fahrenheit (F) scale, 582, 582f
Failure to thrive (FTT), 1218–1219, 1218t

Index

Fainting (syncope), 537
Fallopian tubes, 338
Fall-risk assessment, 467–469, 468b
False labor, 1057, 1057t
False teeth, 1600
Families
    abuse within, 103
    alternative, 100
    binuclear, 99–100
    characteristics of, 97–99
    coping with stress, 103–104
    culture/ethnicity/religion, influence of, 100, 100b
    divorce and remarriage, 103
    extended, 99
    functions of, 98–99
    nuclear, 99
    parenting and, 97–98
    siblings within, 98, 102f
    single-parent, 99
    as social systems, 97
    socioeconomic stressors, 103
    stages of, 100–103, 101t
        contracting family stage, 102–103
        expanding family stage, 101–102
        transitional stage, 100
    stepfamily, 100
    structure of, 99–100
    tasks of, 98–99
    violence within, 103
Family-centered care, 1179
Family dynamics, 1047–1048
Family health centers (FHC), 1843–1844
Family of dying client, nursing care of, 887–888
Family planning, medications for, 949
Family respite, 887
Fascial membranes, 167
Fasciotomy, 1348
Fasting plasma glucose (FPG), 1385, 1393
Fat absorption, 316
Fat-controlled diet, 397
Fat embolism, 1348
Fatigue, 496, 610t
    in pregnancy, 1031
Fats (lipids)
    characteristics, 351t, 353
    client education on, 379–380
    digestion, 353–354
    guidelines for intake of, 372b
Fat-soluble vitamins, 361t–362t, 364–365
Fatty acids
    digestion, 353–354
    saturated, 354, 354b
    unsaturated, 354–355
F cells, 241
FDA. See Food and Drug Administration (FDA)
Febrile seizures, 1223–1224
Febrile state, 583
Febuxostat (Uloric), 1333
Fecal diversion. See Bowel diversion
Fecal occult blood testing, 1584
Fecal softening agents, 947
Feces, 316
Federally Qualified Healthcare (FQHC), 79
Feeding of newborns
    assisting nursing mother, 1092–1093
    bottle feeding, 1095–1096
    breastfeeding, 1092–1095
    and burping, 1096
    supplements to feedings, 1096
Fee for service plans, 26
Female condom, 1160
Female infertility, 1151–1152, 1152b
Female sexual dysfunction, 1149–1150
FemCap, 1160

Feminine hygiene, 1675
Femoral artery, 587
Femoral pulse, 587, 587f
Femur, 206
Fentanyl (Sublimaze), 923t, 927
Fentanyl patch, 968
Ferrous fumarate, 937
Ferrous sulfate (Feosol), 937
Fertility awareness methods (FAM), 1157
Fertilization, 1024, 1026f
Fetal alcohol spectrum disorder (FASD), 1140, 1272–1273
Fetal alcohol syndrome (FAS), 1140, 1272–1273
Fetal biophysical profile (FBP), 1106
Fetal heart rate (FHR), 1106
Fetal heart tones (FHTs), 1032, 1051
Fetal lung development, 299
Fetal monitor, 1063
Fetal positions and presentations, 1120
Fetal status, tests for assessment of, 1105–1106
Fetoscope, 1032
Fetus, 1027f
    blood circulation, 1029, 1030f
    disorders affecting, 1115
    growth and development, 1025–1026
        cephalocaudal, 1027–1028
    heartbeat, 1032, 1033f
    visualization of, 1032
Fever (pyrexia), 583, 610t
    management of, in children, 1191–1193
Fever blisters. See Cold sores
FHR. See Fetal heart rate (FHR)
FHTs. See Fetal heart tones (FHTs)
Fiber
    dietary, 352–353
    insoluble, 395
    soluble, 395
    sources of, 395b
Fibrillation, 1447
Fibrin, 277
Fibrinogen, 273, 939
Fibrostenosis, 1348
Fibrous connective tissue, 166
Fibula, 206
Filipino populations, 383
Film mammography, 617t
Filtration, 188, 189f
Fimbriae, 338
Fimbriae pili, 483
Financial barriers, 1828
Financial planning, 1880–1881
Fingernails, 626f
Firearms, use of, 67
Fire extinguishers, 477t
Fire plan, 476–477
Fires, protection from, 1299
First-aid measures, 527–547
    anaphylaxis, 540
    animal bites and scratches, 540–541
    back and neck injuries, 528–529, 528f
    in bleeding, 538–540
    in cardiovascular emergencies, 537–538
    chest injuries, 528
    cold-related injuries, 529–530
    dental injuries and missing teeth, 535
    exposure to hazardous materials, 541–542
    foreign objects, 535–537
    head injuries, 528–529
    heat-related injuries, 530–533
    musculoskeletal injuries, 534–535
    near drowning, 533–534
    poisoning, 542–543
    in psychiatric emergencies, 543–544
Fissures, 627t
Fistula, 611, 1259, 1617, 1637

Fixed joints, 198
Flaccidity, 1356
FLACC nonverbal pain scale, 806, 806f
Flagella, 482–483
Flat affect, 1218
Flatus, postoperative, 830
Fleet, 824
Flibanserin, 1150
Fliedner, Pastor Theodor, 3, 4
Flight of ideas (FOI), 1771
Flotation mattress, 691
Flowers, safety considerations, 472
Flu. See Influenza
Fluid balance, 190
    aging effects on, 193t
    in burn injuries, 1299
    maintenance of, 1312–1314
    monitoring of, 1312
Fluid intake, 391, 392b
    pediatric clients, 1180
Fluid loss, 1314–1315
Fluid volume deficit (FVD), 182, 1316t
Fluid volume excess (FVE), 1312–1313
Fluoride (Fl), 359t
Fluorocortisone acetate (Florinef), 1392
Fluoroquinolones, 916t
Flurazepam (Dalmane), 924t, 929
Foam, wound healing, 868t
Focal point, seizures, 1357
Focus charting, 446
Folate, 363t
Foley catheter, 845
Folic acid, 938
Follicle-stimulating hormone (FSH), 238, 334, 340, 1383
Follicular phase, 341
Folliculitis, 1297
Fomite, 1246
Fontanels, 1082–1083
Food
    added sugars in, 352b
    allergy, 1509
    ChooseMyPlate.gov, 346, 346f, 347t–348t
    fads, 387
    safety guidelines, 372b
Food and Drug Administration (FDA), 74, 75, 1267
Food-drug interactions, 403t, 404
Food poisoning, first-aid in, 543
Food safety, client education on, 380
Food sensitivity, 1509
Footboard, 689
Footdrop, 689, 1364
Footprinting, 1080
Foot soak, 706, 791
Foramen ovale, 1029
Forced-air warming blanket, 789f, 790
Forceps delivery, 1122
Foreign objects, 535–537, 1210
    airway obstruction by, 536–537, 537f
    in eyes, 535–536
    in nose/ears, 536
Forensic clients, 1765
Foreskin (prepuce), 333, 333f
Formula feeding, 371–372
Fornices, 339
Foster family, 100
Fovea centralis (central fovea), 252
FPG. See Fasting plasma glucose (FPG)
FQHC. See Federally Qualified Healthcare (FQHC)
Fractured clavicle, 1141
Fractures (Fx), 1210, 1334–1335
Fragile X syndrome (FXS), 1276–1277, 1276t
Freckles, 172

Frenulum, 307
Frequent vital signs sheet, 582
Fresh frozen plasma (FFP), 1471
Frontal lobe, cerebral cortex, 219
Frontotemporal dementia (FTD), 1718, 1725
Frostbite, 529, 529b
Fructans, 352, 368
Fructose, 351
Fruits, client education on, 379
Fruit sugar, 351
FSH. See Follicle-stimulating hormone (FSH)
Fulguration, 1492
Full liquid diet, 394t
Functional activities of daily living (FADLs), 1819, 1820b
Functional disease, 69, 1259, 1738
Functional electrical stimulation (FES), 1825
Functional families, 103
Fundal height, 1036
Fundal massage, 1069
Fundus, 1069
Fungal pneumonia, 1546–1547
Fungi, 481
Funic souffle, 1032
Furosemide (Lasix), 947, 1391
Furuncle, 1429
Furunculosis, 1297
Fusion process, casts, 1336
FVD. See Fluid volume deficit (FVD)
FVE. See Fluid volume excess (FVE)

G
Gait analysis, 1815
Gait belt, 656
Galactose, 351
Galactosemia, 1143
Gallbladder, 313–314, 1621–1623
Gallops, heart sounds, 588
Gamete (germ cell), 164, 334
Gamete intrafallopian transfer (GIFT), 1153
γ-Glutamyl transpeptidase (GGT), 1584
Gamma globulins (GG), 273
Gamma hydroxybutyrate (GHB), 1795
Gangrene, 1326
Ganser syndrome, 1741
Gardnerella vaginalis, 1172
GAS. See Group A streptococci (GAS)
Gas exchange, 295
Gastrectomy, 1594
Gastric analysis/tube gastric analysis, 615t
Gastric bypass surgery, 1593
Gastric inhibitory polypeptide (GIP), 241
Gastric lavage, 1590–1591
Gastric suction, 1590
Gastric surgery, 1593–1595, 1594b
Gastric ulcers, 1604
Gastrin, 242, 315
Gastritis, 1604
Gastroesophageal reflux disease (GERD), 308, 396, 1603
Gastrointestinal disorders, 1239–1241
Gastrointestinal intubation (GI), 1588–1590
Gastrointestinal obstructions, in newborn, 1143
Gastrointestinal suction tubes, 1589t
Gastrointestinal (GI) system
  disorders of, 1239–1241
    colic, 1240–1241
    congenital, 1143
    diarrhea, 1240
    encopresis, 1240
    hernia, 1239–1240
    intussusception, 1240
    lactose intolerance, 1240
    Meckel diverticulum, 1239
    megacolon, 1241
    pyloric stenosis, 1239
  medications affecting, 943, 944t–946t, 946–947
  medications for, 1606t–1608t
Gastrointestinal tests, 615t–616t
Gastrointestinal tract, 306
  hormones secreted by, 242
Gastroscopy, 1586
Gastrostomy
  nursing care guidelines, 1588
  tube, 401
Gatch bed, 687
Gauze, 868t
Gavage feeding, 1186–1187, 1187f
Gavage tube, 1138
Gay/lesbian family, 100
GCS. See Glasgow coma scale (GCS)
GDM. See Gestational diabetes mellitus (GDM)
Gender transition, 1147
General anesthesia, 817–818
Generalized scleroderma, 1333
Generativity, in middle adults, 129–130
Generic name, medication, 906
Genes, 162
Genetic counseling, 1370
  Tay–Sachs disease and, 1271–1272
Genetic disorders, 1272
Genital herpes, 1168–1169. See also Herpes simplex virus (HSV) infection
Genital warts, 1170
Genitourinary disorder, congenital, 1143
Genitourinary system (GUS), 320
Gentamicin, 962
Gentamicin-resistant Staphylococcus aureus, 1251
GERD. See Gastroesophageal reflux disease (GERD)
Geriatric care settings, 1698, 1701–1702
Geriatrics, 136, 1697
Geriatric (GERI) unit, 462
German measles. See Rubella
Gerontologic nursing, 136
Gerontology, 136, 1697–1713
Gestation, 1024
Gestational age (GA), 1129
Gestational carrier, 1153
Gestational diabetes mellitus (GDM), 371, 1115, 1393
Gestational surrogacy, 1153
Gestational trophoblastic disease, 1108
Gestures and rituals, 554
GGT. See γ-Glutamyl transpeptidase (GGT)
GH. See Growth hormone (GH)
GI. See Glycemic index (GI)
Giant papillary conjunctivitis (GPC), 1424
Giardiasis, 1208
Gigantism, 1387
GI. See Gastrointestinal intubation (GI)
Gingivitis, 1600
Gland, 232. See also Endocrine glands
Glans penis, 333
Glasgow coma scale (GCS), 1376, 1376t
Glass thermometer, 586, 586f
Glaucoma, 932, 1424–1425
Glial cells. See Neuroglia
Gliding (arthrodial, plane) joints, 200
Gliomas, 218
Global Disease Detection Centers, 75
Globulin, 273, 355
Glomerular capsule, 322
Glomerular filtration, 326
Glomerular filtration rate (GFR), 326, 1631
Glomerulonephritis, 1242–1243, 1640–1641
Glomerulus, 322–323, 322t, 323f, 324t
Glossitis, 362t–363t, 366

Glossopharyngeal nerve (CN IX), 254
Glottis, 297
Gloves, 499–500
  clean (nonsterile), 506–507
  closed gloving, 844
  latex allergies and, 499–500
  latex-free, 500
  putting on (open gloving), 850–851
  removal of, 844–845, 845f
  sterile, 844–845
GLP-1 receptor agonists, 1401
Glucagon, 236t, 240, 314, 1404
Glucagon-like peptide-I (GLP-I), 242
Glucocorticoid, 239
Gluconeogenesis, 240
Glucose, 351
Glucose monitoring, 1407
Glucose-6-phosphodehydrogenase deficiency, 1088
Glutaraldehyde, 502t
Gluteal muscles, 210t
Gluten-free diet, 1224
Gluten-restricted diet, 399
Glycated hemoglobin, 1386
Glycemic index (GI), 1386
Glycogen, 351, 352
Glycogenolysis, 240
Glycohemoglobin, 1386
Glycoproteins, 234
Glycosylated hemoglobin (HA1c, HbA1c, A1c), 1386, 1394
Goiter, 239, 1388
Gold salts, 1332
Golgi apparatus, 162
Golimumab (Simponi), 1332
GoLYTELY, 824, 1585
Gonad, 240, 334
Gonadotropic hormone, 238, 340
Gonadotropin, 238
Gonadotropin-releasing hormone (GnRH), 238
Gonococcus (GC), 1164
Gonorrhea, 1080, 1141, 1141f, 1684f
Goodell sign, 1032
Goodrich, Annie W., 6
Good Samaritan Act, 40
Gout, 1332
Gouty arthritis, 1332
Gowers sign, 1282, 1282f
Gowns/aprons, 501
Graafian follicle, 340–341
Graft, 1293
Graft-versus-host disease (GVHD), 1473
Grains, client education on, 379–380
Gram (g), 896
Grand multipara, 1024
Granisetron HCl (Kytril, Sancuso), 831
Granular leukocytes, 275–277
Granulation tissue, 611, 868
Granulocytopenia, 1479
Graphic flow sheet, 440–442
Graphic record, 581–582
Graves disease, 1388, 1388f
Gravida, 1024
Gravital plane, 644
Gray matter, nerve cell bodies, 1362
Great cardiac vein, 263
Greenstick fractures, 1335
Grief, 150
  Kübler-Ross stages of, 149–152
  and loss, 151t
Griseofulvin, 1158
Gross hematuria, 1242
Group A beta-hemolytic streptococcal infections (GABHS), 1207

Group A streptococci (GAS), 1534
Group therapy sessions, pain management, 809
Growth and development, 107–110
　adolescence, 123–127
　anticipatory guidance, 107
　Erikson's theory of, 108, 108t
　influences on, 107–108
　Piaget's theory of, 108–109
　role of play in, 109
　theories of, 108–109
Growth hormone (GH), 234, 1383
Growth hormone-inhibiting
　　hormone (GHIH), 234
Growth hormone-releasing
　　hormone (GHRH), 234, 238
Guaiac test, 611, 768
Guanethidine monosulfate (Ismelin), 937
Guided imagery, 809
Guide dogs, 1419
Guillain–Barré syndrome, 1372–1373
Gustation, 254
Gynecologic tests, 616t–617t
Gynecology (GYN), 462, 1670

H

Haemophilus influenzae meningitis type b, 1371
Haemophilus influenzae serotype b (Hib), 1204
Hair, 172–173, 173b
　inspection of, 630f
　loss, excessive, 630f
　protection, 843
Hair care, 707–709, 885
Halal diets, 384
Half-cast splints, 1335
Halflytely, 824
Halitosis, 701, 943, 1705
Hallucinations, 1286, 1738, 1773
Hallucinogen persisting perception disorder
　　(HPPD), 1799
Hallucinogen use disorders, 1799
Hallucinosis, 1792
Halo device, 1340–1341
Halo sign, 1375
HA-MRSA. *See* Healthcare-acquired MRSA
　　(HA-MRSA)
Hand antisepsis, 498b
Handbook of Drugs for Nursing Practice, 905
Handheld inhalers, 965
Hand massage, 705
Handovers, 1811
Hand sanitization, 499
Handwashing, 498–499, 499b, 505–506, 842
Haploid cell, 340
Hard connective tissues, 166
Harrington rods, 1254
Hashimoto thyroiditis, 1390
Hawaii Early Learning Profile (HELP) charts, 1176
Hay fever, 1509
Hazardous materials, exposure to, 541–542
HBO. *See* Hyperbaric oxygenation (HBO)
HCl. *See* Hydrochloric acid (HCl)
HDL. *See* High-density lipoproteins (HDL)
Head
　muscles of, 210t
　and neck examination, 621t, 627t, 629t
　trauma, 1373–1377
Headaches, 1353–1355
Head circumference, 1183
Head injuries, first-aid in, 528–529
Head start programs, 1888
Health and safety services, 78
Health Canada, 906
Healthcare
　Affordable Care Act and, 20–21
　community health center, 79
　complementary, 28–29
　consumer fraud and, 30
　delivery system, 19–30
　finances and, 58–59
　inconsistencies in, 56
　insurance and, 25–27
　legal and ethical standards of, 32–44
　at local level, 79
　multidisciplinary approach to, 9, 10b, 10f
　national level, 73–78
　preventive, 20
　and quality assurance, 23–24
　in school and industry, 23
　settings and services, 21–23
　at state level, 78–79
　transcultural, 83–93
Healthcare-acquired MRSA (HA-MRSA), 488
Healthcare assistants (HCAs), 1833
Healthcare-associated infections (HAI), 488
　clients and, 495–496
　Infection Control Committee, role of, 498
　nurses and, 495
Healthcare facilities, 21–23
Healthcare personnel
　immunizations for, 498b
　infection risks for, 496
　prevention of infection for, 497
　and services, 461–465
　　diagnostic and treatment
　　　departments, 461
　　direct client care departments, 461–465
　　nursing care units, 462–463
　　specialized client care departments, 463
　　support services, 463–465
　　surgery, 462
Healthcare team, culturally diverse, 92
Health information management (HIM)
　　department, 464
Health Insurance Portability and Accountability
　　Act (HIPAA), 34–35, 560
Health interview, 422–423
　samples of questions for, 424t–426t
Health maintenance, 1176–1178
Health maintenance organizations (HMOs), 20,
　　26–27, 1842, 1886
Health realization (HR), 1790
Health record, 39, 441. *See also* Documentation
　computerized, 443
　contents of, 443–448, 445t
　corrections in, 451
　as documented evidence, 442
　manual, 443
　purposes of, 441
Health Resources and Services Administration
　　(HRSA), 74
Health supervision, 1176
Healthy diets, 368–371
Hearing, 253
Hearing aids, 704, 704f, 1417
Hearing impairment, 1267
Hearing loss, noise-induced, 133
Heart
　apex, 259
　atria, 260
　base, 259
　blood vessels of, 262–263, 263f
　chambers, 260
　conduction system of, 266–267, 267f
　endocardium, 259
　epicardium, 259
　hormones secreted by, 242
　myocardium, 259
　pericardial fluid, 259
　pericardium, 259
　route of blood flow through, 262, 262f
　septum, 260
　structure of, 259
　valves, 260–261
　ventricles, 260
Heartburn, 1602–1603
Heart disease, 68, 1444
Heart failure, 1448
Heart rate (HR), 268, 587, 591
Heart sounds, 267
　abnormal, 588–589
　normal, 267
Heart transplantation, 1442
Heart valve surgery, 1441–1442, 1441b
Heat cradle, 790
Heat cramps, 531
Heat exhaustion, 531
Heat index, 530
Heat lamp, 790
Heat loss, mechanisms of, 174–175
Heat production/conservation,
　　mechanisms of, 175
Heat receptors, 255
Heat-related injuries, first-aid in, 530–533
　burns, 532–533
　heat cramps, 531
　heat exhaustion, 531
　heat stroke, 531–532, 532t
Heat stroke, 531–532, 532t
Heat therapy, 788
　dry, 789–790
　moist, 790–792, 791f
　rationale for, 788–789, 789b
Heat transfer, mechanisms of, 175t
Heel stick blood samples, infants, 1192
Hegar sign, 1032
Heimlich maneuver, 537
Helicobacter pylori (*H. pylori*), 1584
Helper T cell, 289
Hemangiomas, 1219
Hematemesis, 1618
Hematocrit, 275
Hematologic studies, 1469
Hematologic system
　blood, 272–278
　blood clotting, 277, 278f
　blood groups, 287, 279t
　functions of, 273b
　hemorrhage, 278
　Rh factors, 278
Hematoma, 1375–1376
Hematopoiesis (hemopoiesis), 273
Hematopoietic growth factors (HGFs), 1495
Hematopoietic stem cell, 275
Hematopoietic stem cell transplantation (HSCT),
　　1236, 1472–1473, 1478
Hematuria, 1630
Hematuria catheter, 845
Hemianopsia, 1463
Hemiarthroplasty, 1343
Hemicelluloses, 353
Hemiparesis, 1281
Hemiplegia, 664, 1281, 1360, 1462–1463, 1820
Hemoccult brand method, 768
Hemoccult test, 611
Hemochromatosis, 1270–1271
Hemodialysis, 1651
Hemodynamic monitoring, 1448–1449
Hemoglobin, 172, 275, 937
Hemoglobin A1c, 1386
Hemoglobin electrophoresis, 1234
Hemolysis, 1137
Hemolytic anemia, 1475, 1516t
Hemolytic disease of the newborn (HDN),
　　1139–1140
Hemolytic uremic syndrome (HUS), 1241–1242

Hemophilia, 1481–1482
Hemoptysis, 1348, 1556, 1562
HemoQuant stool testing, 1584
Hemorrhage, 278, 539, 610t
    assessment of, 524
    control, 524
    fractures and, 1348
    intraventricular, 1138
    maternal, 1118
    postoperative, 828–829
Hemorrhagic strokes, 1462
Hemorrhoidectomy, 1617
Hemorrhoids, 1617
Hemostasis, 277
Hemothorax, 1539
Hemovac drain, 871, 872f
Henry Street Settlement Visiting Nurse Society, 4
Heparin, 938
Hepatic coma, 1617. *See also* Liver failure
Hepatic duct, 314
Hepatic encephalopathy, 1618
Hepatic portal circulation, 282–283, 282f
Hepatic vein, 283
Hepatitis, 1619–1621, 1620b
Hepatitis A, 1206, 1620
Hepatitis B virus (HBV), 1202, 1620
Hepatitis C virus (HCV), 1620
Hepatitis D virus (HDV), 1620
Hepatitis E virus (HEV), 1620–1621
Hepatomegaly, 1618
Hepatorenal syndrome, 1618
Hereditary disorders, 69
Heredity, 107
Hernia, 1239–1240, 1597, 1602, 1609–1610
Herniated intervertebral disc disease, 1327
Herniated nucleus pulposus (HNP), 1327
Herniation, 637t
    brain, 1374
Herpes simplex virus (HSV) infection, 1141, 1162, 1168–1169, 1600–1601
    considerations related to, 1169b
    genital herpes, 1601
    orofacial herpes, 1601
    treatment, 1601
    vesicles, 628f
Herpes zoster, 1206, 1359, 1362
Heterograft, 1305
HFCS. *See* High-fructose corn syrup (HFCS)
HHS. *See* Department of Health and Human Services
Hiatal hernia, 1602
Hickman catheter, 1591, 1592f
HICPAC. *See* Hospital Infection Control Practices Advisory Committee (HICPAC)
Hierarchy of needs, 47, 48f. *See also* Human needs
High-calorie diet, 396
High-density lipoproteins (HDL), 355
High-fat diet, 397
High-fiber diet, 395
High-fructose corn syrup (HFCS), 351
High-pressure oxygenation. *See* Hyperbaric oxygenation (HBO)
High-protein diet, 397, 399
High-risk newborn, 1128–1144
Hilum, 321
Hinge (ginglymus) joints, 200, 201f
HIPAA. *See* Health Insurance Portability and Accountability Act (HIPAA)
Hip fractures, 1338, 1343–1344
Hip joint, 206f
Hip pinning, 1344
Hippocratic oath, 2

Hip replacements, 1344
Hirschsprung disease. *See* Megacolon
Hirsutism, 1387, 1625
Hispanic, 66
Histamine, 242, 1512
Histamine antagonists, 943
Histiocytes, 277
Histologist, 10b
Histoplasma capsulatum, 1549
Histoplasmosis, 481, 1549
History of Nursing, 4
Histotoxic hypoxia, 1542, 1543b
HIV. *See* Human immunodeficiency virus (HIV)
HIV and tuberculosis, 1549
HIV-associated nephropathy (HIVAN), 1523
HIV-associated neurocognitive disorders (HAND), 1523, 1719
Hives, 1295
HIV testing, in pregnancy, 1036
HMOs. *See* Health maintenance organizations (HMOs)
HNP. *See* Herniated nucleus pulposus (HNP)
Hodgkin lymphoma, 1236, 1482
Holistic healthcare, 2, 28–29
Homans sign, 631t, 1124
Home health aides, 1833, 1855
Home healthcare, 20, 22
Home health nurse, 20
Home health resource group (HHRG), 1833
Home hemodialysis, 1652
Homelessness, healthcare for, 51
Home nursing, 1835–1836
Homeostasis, 156, 179, 272, 302, 1310
    feedback in, 179–180
    impaired fluid, 183
Home owner association (HOA), 1701
Home pregnancy testing, 1032
Homograft, 1305, 1442
Hookworm infection, 1208
Hormonal axis, 232
Hormonal imbalances, and female sexual dysfunction, 1150
Hormonal methods, of birth control, 1157–1159
Hormone, 212, 232
    role of, 323–325
Hormone ablation therapy, 1666
Hormone levels, in pregnancy, 1034
Hormone-related effects, 1501
Hormone replacement therapy (HRT), 931, 1679–1680
Hormones, 1382, 1383t
Hormone therapy, 1690–1691
HOSA, 16
Hospice care, 22, 882
Hospice care unit, 463
Hospice nursing, 1851–1865
Hospice staff, 1856
Hospital-acquired infections (HAI), 1246
Hospital gown, 567
Hospital Infection Control Practices Advisory Committee (HICPAC), 508
Hospital room furnishings, 456f
Hostile persons, 1771, 1773
Host resistance, 491–492
Hot flashes, 1679
Hour of sleep (HS, bedtime) doses, 958
House diet, 393
Household Nursing School, 5
Housekeeping department, 463
Hoyer lift, 662–663
HR. *See* Heart rate (HR)
HRSA. *See* Health Resources and Services Administration (HRSA)
HSV infection. *See* Herpes simplex virus (HSV) infection

HTN. *See* Hypertension (HTN)
Huffing, 833–834
Human chorionic gonadotropin (hCG), 242, 1032, 1275
Human chorionic gonadotropin titer, 1108
Human development, stages of, 1025–1031
    conception and sex determination, 1025, 1026f
    embryo, 1026–1027, 1027f
    fetal circulation, 1029, 1030f
    fetus, 1027–1028, 1027f–1028f
    membranes and amniotic fluid, 1030–1031
    placenta and umbilical cord, 1028–1029, 1029f
    zygote and implantation, 1025–1026, 1026f
Human growth hormone (HGH), 234
Human immunodeficiency virus (HIV), 1163, 1520, 1521f. *See also* Acquired immunodeficiency syndrome (AIDS)
    action of, 1520–1521
    classifications, 1526t
    data collection, 1529
    history, 1520
    mortality, 1526–1527
    nursing implications for, 1527–1529
    opportunistic infections and conditions, 1522b
    signs and symptoms, 1523–1524
    transmission, 1521–1523
Human needs
    family and community needs, 53
    love, affection, and belonging, 51–52
    Maslow's hierarchy of, 51–52
    and nursing interventions, 48f
    physiologic needs, 48f, 49–50
    security and safety needs, 48, 48f
    self-actualization needs, 52–53
    self-esteem needs, 52
Human papillomavirus (HPV) infections, 1170–1171, 1297, 1306, 1525
Human placental lactogen (HPL), 1034
Humidity tent, 794
Humoral immunity, 287, 290, 292
Hunner ulcers, 1639
Huntington disease (HD), 1369, 1719
Hydatidiform mole, 1108
Hydralazine (Apresoline), 936
Hydration, end-of-life care and, 884
Hydrocele, 1244, 1660–1661, 1661f
Hydrocephalus, 1142, 1223
Hydrochloric acid (HCl), 309, 315
Hydrochlorothiazide (HCTZ), 947
Hydrocolloid dressing, 868t, 870, 871f
Hydrocortisone, 239, 931, 1332
Hydrogel, 868t
Hydrogenated fats, 354
Hydrogen ions (H^+), 1319
Hydromorphone hydrochloride (Dilaudid), 923t, 927
Hydronephrosis, 1641
Hydrotherapy, 1748
Hydroxychloroquine sulfate (Plaquenil), 1332
Hydroxyzine, 831, 1758
Hygiene, end-of-life care and, 885
Hymen, 339
Hyperactive delirium, 1717
Hyperalimentation, 403
Hyperbaric chamber, 463, 1569
Hyperbaric medicine, 1888–1889
Hyperbaric oxygenation (HBO), 275, 1569, 1888
Hyperbilirubinemia, 1137–1138
Hypercalcemia, 1317t
Hyperchloremia, 1317t
Hyperemesis gravidarum, 1031, 1109
Hyperextension, 1330

Hyperglycemia, 351, 1392, 1394, 1403t, 1404–1405
Hyperkalemia, 1316t
Hyperlipidemia, 1436, 1623
Hypermagnesemia, 1316t
Hypernatremia, 1316t
Hyperopia, 252, 1423t
Hyperoxygenation, 1441
Hyperparathyroidism, 1391
Hyperphagia, 1272
Hyperphosphatemia, 1316t
Hyperplasia, 1384
Hyperpnea, 1542t
Hypersomnia, 1739, 1860
Hypertension (HTN), 65, 591–592, 1444–1445
    nursing care plan, 1645–1646
    postoperative, 829
Hypertensive heart disease, 1444
Hyperthermia, postoperative, 830
Hyperthyroidism, 1388–1389
Hypertonic solution, 188
Hypertrophy, 1445
Hypertropic cardiomyopathy, 1450
Hyperuricemia, 1332
Hyperventilation, 590t, 1541, 1542t
Hypervigilance, 1738
Hypervitaminosis, 365b
Hypnosis, 1047
Hypnotics, 925t, 928–629
Hypoactive delirium, 1717
Hypoallergenic tape, 782
Hypocalcemia, 1316t
Hypochloremia, 1316t
Hypodermis, 169
Hypoglycemia, 351, 1385, 1401–1402
    versus hyperglycemia, 1403t–1404t
    insulin shock, 1402
Hypoglycemic shock, 520b
Hypoglycemics, oral, 932
Hypoinsulinism, 1393
Hypokalemia, 1316t, 1317
Hypomagnesemia, 1316t, 1318
Hypomania, 1771
Hyponatremia, 1316t, 1317
Hypoparathyroidism, 1391
Hypophosphatemia, 1316t
Hypophysectomy, 1388
Hypophysis. See Pituitary gland
Hyposensitization, 1512
Hypospadias, 1083, 1143, 1243
Hypostatic pneumonia, 832, 1348
Hypotension, 591–592, 1445
    postoperative, 829
Hypothalamus, 220t, 221–222
    temperature regulation and, 582–583
Hypothermia, 530, 583
    accidental, 530
    blanket, 793–794
    local, 530
    postoperative, 829–830
    surgical, 530
    treatment of, 530
Hypothyroidism, 1088, 1389–1390
Hypotonic bladder, 1633
Hypotonic dystocia, 1118
Hypotonic solution, 187–188
Hypoventilation, 590t, 1542t
Hypovolemic shock, 519, 520b, 521
    postoperative, 829
Hypoxemia, 829, 1566
Hypoxemic hypoxia, 1541
Hypoxia, 1144, 1541
    anemic, 1542
    circulation, 1541, 1542
    histotoxic, 1542
    hypoxemic, 1541
    postoperative, 829
    signs, 1543
Hysterectomy, 1161, 1674, 1688
Hysterosalpingogram, 1151, 1673
Hysteroscopic tube insertion, 1161

I

Iatrogenic incontinence, 1635. See also Transient (temporary) incontinence
Iatrogenic issues, 1140
IBD. See Inflammatory bowel disease (IBD)
IBS. See Irritable bowel syndrome (IBS)
Ibuprofen (Motrin, Advil, Nuprin), 807, 924t, 928, 1332
Ice collar, 792, 800
Ice packs, single-use, 792–793
ICRC. See International Committee of the Red Cross (ICRC)
Ictal phase, seizures, 1356
Ideal body weight (IBW), 370
Identification (ID) bands, 955, 1079
    checking of, 824
Idiopathic thrombocytopenic purpura (ITP), 1234, 1516t
Idiosyncratic effects, 1717
Ileoanal reservoir, 1598
Ileocecal valve, 310
Ileostomy, 1895
Imiquimod (Aldara, Zyclara), 1170
Immediate release (IR) medications, 915b
Immersion foot, 530
Immobilization devices, 1323–1324
Immune disorders, 1514
Immune response, 293b, 1506
    lymphocytes involved in, 289t
Immune system, 286, 293b
    antigen–antibody reaction, 292
    B lymphocytes, 287–288
    bone marrow and lymphocyte production, 286–289, 288f, 289t
    effects of aging on, 293t
    functions of, 286, 287b
    lymphoid organs, 290
    medications affecting, 939–940
    mononuclear phagocyte system, 290
    nonspecific defense mechanisms, 290
    specific defense mechanisms, 290–292
    structure of, 286, 287f
    T lymphocytes, 288–289
Immunity, 286, 1514
Immunization, 292, 1177, 1177b
Immunogens, 1508
Immunoglobulin E (IgE), 1507
Immunoglobulins, 287–288, 1471, 1506
Immunoglobulin therapy, 1372
Immunologic memory, 287
Immunosuppression, 1514
Immunosuppressives, 1332
Immunotherapy, 1493, 1495, 1512
Impaired fasting glucose (IFG), 1393
Impaired glucose homeostasis (IGH), 1393
Impaired glucose tolerance (IGT), 1393
Impaired reality testing, 1750
Imperforate anus, 1143
Impetigo, 1251–1252
Impetigo contagiosa, 1251, 1252f
Implanon, 1158
Implantable cardioverter-defibrillator (ICD), 1447
Implantation, 1025–1026
Implementation of nursing care, 435–437, 436f
Impotence, 335, 1149
Inactivated poliovirus vaccine (IPV), 1205
Inborn immunity, 290

Incentive programs, by employers, 27
Incentive spirometers, 834, 1543
Incisional biopsy, 1492, 1673
Incompetent cervix, 1107
Incomplete fractures, 1334
Incomplete proteins, 356
Incontinence, 328
    end-of-life care and, 884
    types, 1635–1636
    urinary, 1635
Incontinence-associated dermatitis (IAD), 862, 862t
Incretin mimetics, 1400
Incubation period, 1201
Incus, 250
Indapamide, 947
Independent living options, 1810
Independent nursing actions, 431
Indian Health Service (IHS), 74
Indigestion. See Gastritis
Indirect Coombs Test, 1467
Indirect measurement of blood pressure, 593
Indomethacin (Indocin), 924t, 928, 1332
Induction, labor, 1114
Induration, 627t
Indwelling catheter, 845
Infancy/infants (1-12 months), 110–113
    age-related concerns, 1178
    areas of concern, 112–113
    bathing, 1188
    blood–brain barrier, 219
    bottle mouth in, 112
    caregiver instructions, 1176
    childcare, 113
    cognitive and motor development, 111–112
    feeding to, 112
    nutrition for, 371–373
    oral hygiene for, 1188–1189
    oxygen hood for, 1191f
    physical growth, 110–111, 111f
    prenatal care and, 66
    psychosocial development, 111
    reducing anxiety in, 1180
    vital signs for, 1181–1183, 1181t
    weaning, 112–113
Infant care, client education for, 1048
Infantile glaucoma. See Congenital glaucoma
Infant mortality, 1128–1129
Infarction, 1234
Infection
    actions of pathogens in body, 491
    in burn injuries, 1302
    chain of, 488–491, 489
    communicable diseases, 488
    control, 1186. See also Infection control
    development of, factors influencing, 491–492
    in diabetes, 1405
    epidemic diseases, 488
    healthcare-associated, 488. See also Healthcare-associated infections (HAI)
    incubation period, 491
    normal course of, 491
    postoperative, 835
    prevention of
        barrier techniques for, 499–501
        clean and controlled environment, 501–503
        client and family education, 503
        handwashing, 498–499
        for nursing staff and clients, 497
    process of, 489f
    response to, 491–492
    transmission of, 490t
Infection control, 508–515

Infection Control Committee, 508
and isolation, 512–514
nursing procedures in pediatric, 512–514
standard precautions, 508–509
transmission-based precautions, 509–512
additional, 512
airborne precautions, 509–511, 510t
contact precautions, 511–512, 511f
droplet precautions, 511
Infection Control Committee, 498, 508
Infection control officer, 10b
Infectious diseases, 1247b
Inferior vena cava (IVC), 265, 283
Infertility, 1150
female, 1151–1152, 1152b
male, 1150, 1151b
Infiltration, 985, 987
Inflammation, 610
Inflammatory bowel disease (IBD), 1259–1260, 1613–1614, 1614t
Inflammatory disorders, 1329–1332, 1455, 1458–1459, 1639–1641. *See also* Nose
Inflammatory process, 1162
Inflatable splints, 1335
Infliximab (Remicade), 1332, 1518
Influenza, 1205, 1545–1546
morbidity and mortality rates for, 56
Informed consent, 34, 617
before surgery, 821
Infrared coagulation therapy (IRC), 1617
Infuse-a-Port, 992
Infusion ports, 992
Infusion pumps, 994
Infusions, 985, 987, 990, 1018–1021
Ingestion, 305
Inguinal canal, 333
Inguinal hernia, 333, 1239
INH. *See* Isoniazid (INH)
Inhalants, 965
Inhalant use disorder, 1799
Inhalation therapy, for cystic fibrosis, 1239
Inhaled insulin, 1399
Inhalers, 909
Inhibiting hormones (IH), 234
Injectable medications, administration of, 909, 978, 992–997
intradermal injections, 982
intramuscular injections, 982–983, 983f
intravenous administration, 985–992
preparations for, 981–982
subcutaneous injections, 982–985, 982f
syringes and needles, 979–981, 979f–981f
Inpatient psychiatry unit, 1745
Insignia, nursing, 3f, 6–7, 7f
Insoluble fiber, 395
Insomnia, 1261, 1860
Inspection, diagnosis and, 618
Inspiration, 299
Instant Glucose, 1404
Instillations, 908
Instrumental activities of daily living (IADLs), 138, 1269, 1698, 1820b
Insufflation, 1588
Insulin, 237t, 240, 241b, 314, 931–932, 1393, 1398–1399
Insulin-dependent diabetes mellitus (IDDM), 1257
Insulin-like growth factor (IGF), 242
Insulin pumps, 1400, 1400f
Insulin resistance, 1394
Insurance, healthcare and, 25–27
Integumentary system, 169, 1289
aging effects on, 177t
functions of, 169, 173b
medications affecting, 921

physiology, 174
protection, 174
structure of, 169
thermoregulation, 174–175, 175t
Intellectual disability, 1266–1267, 1716
Intellectual skills, in implementing nursing care, 437
Intelligence quotient (IQ), 1266–1267
Intensive care unit (ICU), 21, 463
Interbody fusion, 1327
Intercom, 472, 567
Intercostal muscles, 211, 299
Intercourse, 333
Interdisciplinary teams (IDTs), 1855
Interferon alfa-2b (Intron A), 1620
Interferon-gamma release assays (IGRAs), 1536
Interleukin-3, 1495
Interleukins (ILs), 289, 1495
Intermaxillary fixation, 1601
Intermediate care facility (ICF), 23
Intermediate care unit, 463
Intermittent catheter, 845
Intermittent fever, 583
Intermittent home care, 1832
Intermittent infusion device, 837
Intermittent/irregular pulse, 587
Intermittent positive pressure breathing (IPPB), 1191, 1543, 1571
Intermittent self-catheterization, 845
Intermittent sequential compression device (ISCD), 781
Internal carotid artery, 283
Internal disaster, 473–474
Internal fixation, types of, 1343f
International Association for the Study of Pain (IASP), 801
International Classification of Diseases, 10th Revision (ICD-10), 429
International Committee of the Red Cross (ICRC), 77
International Council of Nursing (ICN), 17
International Federation Red Cross and Red Crescent Societies (IFRC), 77
International normalized ratio (INR), 938
International Statistical Classification of Diseases and Related Health Problems, 429
Internet, 1876–1877
Internships, 1896
Interoceptors, 228
Interpersonal skills, in implementing nursing care, 437
Interstitial cells, 331
Interstitial cell-stimulating hormone (ICSH), 238, 334
Interstitial cystitis (IC), 1639–1640
Interstitial (tissue) fluid, 180
Intervertebral disc (IVD), 1327
Intervertebral disc disease (IVDD), 1327
Intestinal obstruction, 1610-1611
Intestinal preparation, preoperative, 823–824
Intestine, medications affecting, 946–947
Intimate partner violence (IPV), 64, 1148
Intimate space, 90
Intracavernous injection, for erectile dysfunction, 1149
Intracellular fluid (ICF), 180, 180f, 1312
Intracranial hematoma, 1376, 1376f
Intracranial pressure (ICP), 224, 528–529
increased, 1354, 1373–1374
monitoring, 1374f
Intractable angina, 1452
Intracytoplasmic sperm injection (ICSI), 1153
Intradermal injections, administration of, 982, 1001–1002

Intradermal test, 613t
Intramedullary nail, 1342
Intramuscular (IM) injections, 982–985, 983f
Intraocular pressure (IOP), 1414
medicines for reducing of, 932
Intraoperative care, 824, 827f
Intrapartum hemorrhage, 1118
Intrapartum period, 1118
Intrauterine device (IUD), 1159, 1676
Intrauterine growth restriction (IUGR), 1105, 1131
Intravascular fluid (IVF), 180
Intravenous (IV) moderate sedation, 816
Intravenous pyelogram (IVP), 1393, 1631–1632
nursing consideration, 1631
x-ray, 613t
Intravenous (IV) therapy, 985
caring for client receiving, 986–987
infiltration of IV fluid, 987
infusion ports, 990–992
infusions, 985
IV solutions, 987
medication administration, 992–997
converting continuous IV infusion to saline lock, 992–994
by IV bolus or push, 996
saline lock, 994–995
via piggy back, 995
via volume-controlled infusion, 996
midline catheter, 992
nursing considerations, 990
and phlebitis, 988
PICC line, 991–992
protective devices, 1187, 1187f
pumps and controllers, 989–990
Intraventricular hemorrhage (IVH), 1138
Intubation, 526, 1572
Intussusception, 1240, 1610
Invasive diagnostic techniques, 1492
Invasive therapy, 496
Invisible fats, 353
In vitro fertilization (IVF), 1152
Iodine (I), 360
Ionization, 185
Ions, 185–186
Iris, 248
Iron (Fe), 358t, 372
Iron deficiency anemia, 373, 1233–1234, 1475
Iron dextran (DexFerrum), 938
Iron replacement preparations, 937–938
Irreversible shock, 520b
Irrigation, wound, 873, 878–879
Irritable bowel syndrome (IBS), 1259, 1611
Irritant cathartics, 947
Ischemia, 1438
Ischemic heart disease, 1452
Ischemic strokes, 1462
Ishihara color blind test charts, 1270
Islets of Langerhans, 240
Isograft, 1305
Isometric contractions, 213
Isoniazid (INH), 1550
Isotopes, 156
Isthmus, 239
IVD. *See* Intervertebral disc (IVD)
IV piggyback (IVPB), 995, 995f, 1011–1012

J

Jacksonian seizures, 1356b
Jackson–Pratt drain, 871, 872f
Japanese populations, 383
Jaundice, 610t, 1137
intrahepatic obstructive, 1618
Jejunum and ileum, 310
Job safety analysis (JSA), 469

Job seeking, 1883–1896 John Doe admissions, 36
Joint Commission, 23, 804
Joint replacement surgery, 1323
Joints, 198–202
    classification, 198–199, 199t
    synovial, 200
Jugular venous distention (JVD), 1448
Juvenile chronic arthritis (JCA), 1254
Juvenile diabetes, 1393
Juvenile glaucoma, 1258
Juvenile Huntington disease, 1369
Juvenile idiopathic arthritis (JIA), 1254
Juvenile rheumatoid arthritis (JRA), 1254–1255
Juxtaglomerular apparatus (JGA), 242

K

Kaiserswerth School for Nursing, 3
Kangaroo care, 1133
Kaposi sarcoma, 1523
Kawasaki disease, 1233
KCl. See Potassium chloride (KCl)
Kegel exercises, 1636, 1666, 1680
Kelly clamp, 1079
Keloid, 611, 1304, 1306
Keratin, 171
Keratinocytes, 171
Kerlix, 779
Kernicterus, 1137
Kernig sign, 1371, 1371f
Ketoacidosis, 1404
Keto-Diastix test, 1386
Ketogenic diet, 397
Ketones, 1405
Ketoprofen, 1332
Ketorolac tromethamine, 1332
Ketosis, 1404
Kidney, 321
    cancer of, 1646
    failure. See Renal failure
    hormones secreted by, 240
    stones, 1642
    transplant, 1653–1655
Kidney/ureter stones, 1643
Killer T cells (cytotoxic T cells), 289
Kilocalories (kcal), 349–350
Kinesics, 553
Knee joint, 201f
Knowledge base, 1877
Kock pouch, 1599
Koplik spots, 1205
Korean populations, 383
Korotkoff sounds, 593f
Kosher diets, 384
Kübler-Ross stages, of grief and loss, 149–152
Kudzu, 1794
Kupffer cells, 290
Kussmaul respirations, 590, 883, 1542t
Kwashiorkor, 371, 1224
Kyphosis, 633, 1253, 1326, 1712

L

Labia majora, 339
Labia minora, 339
Lability, of mood, 1758
Labor, 1053
    anesthesia during, 1063
    average time frames of, 1059t
    cardinal movements, 1056
    danger signs in, 1062b
    and delivery, complications of, 1118–1120
    emotional and physical support during, 1062
    epidural anesthesia during, 1063
    false, 1057
    fetal well-being, assessment of, 1063–1064
    induction of, 1121
    maternal and newborn feeding, 1067
    neonatal care, 1065
    nursing care during, 1061–1072
        stage I, 1061–1064
        stage II, 1064–1065
        stage III, 1065
        stage IV, 1065–1067
    observations and data gathering, 1066–1067
    preterm, 1119
    procedures after admission of women in labor, 1061–1062
    process of, 1052–1061
    4 P's of, 1056
    rupture of membranes, 1058–1059
    signs of approaching labor, 1056–1057
    stages of, 1059
        stage I (dilation), 1059
        stage II (birth or expulsion), 1059–1060
        stage III (placental), 1060–1061
        stage IV (recovery), 1061
    transitioning after birth, 1067
    true, 1057
    uterine contractions, 1058–1059
Laboratory technician, 10b
Labor-delivery-recovery-postpartum (LDRP), 1085
Labor-delivery-recovery room (LDR), 1085
Labor pains, 1058
Labyrinth, 251
Laceration, 857, 1210, 1374
    during emergency delivery, 1122
Lacrimal ducts, 703
Lacrimal glands, 703
Lactate dehydrogenase (LDH), 1584
Lactation, 1033, 1048, 1068
Lacteals, 316
Lacto-ovo vegetarians, 384
Lactose, 352
    intolerance, 352, 1240
Lactose-restricted diet, 397
Lacto-vegetarians, 384
Laissez-faire leadership, 1901
La Leche League, 78
Lamaze method, of childbirth, 1047
Laminectomy, 1327
Lamp of Learning, 3, 3f
Land pollution, 80
Langerhans cells, 240
Lansoprazole (Prevacid), 1605
Lanugo, 1084, 1131
Laotian populations, 383
Laparoscope, 612
Laparoscopy, 1151, 1673, 1673f
Laparotomy, 1243
Large bowel, disorders of, 1609–1615
Large intestine, 310–312
    absorption in, 312
Laryngectomee, 1561
    identification as, 1562
Laryngectomy, 1561
    after, 1562
Laryngitis, 1546
Laryngopharynx, 1561
Laryngotracheobronchitis (LTB), 1237, 1544
Larynx, 297
    cancer of, 1561–1563
Laser angioplasty, 1441
Laser photocoagulation, 1258
Laser procedures, 1845
Laser soldering, 873
Last menstrual period (LMP), 1036
Lateral epicondylitis, 1329
Latex allergies, 499–500
Latino Americans populations, 381
Laundry, 513
Lavage specimen, 1533
Law enforcement, 1845
Laws. See also Legal issues, of nursing practice
    common sources of, 33t
    for practice of nursing, 37. See also Nurse Practice Acts
    for vulnerable persons, 41
Laxatives, 831
Lazy eye, 1225
LDH. See Lactate dehydrogenase (LDH)
LDL. See Low-density lipoproteins (LDL)
Leadership, 1898–1904
Leaders, roles of, 1900
Lead poisoning, 81
Leflunomide (Arava), 1332
Left anterior descending (LAD) artery, 262
Left circumflex (LCX) artery, 262
Left main coronary artery (LMCA), 262
Legal issues, of nursing practice, 32
    abandonment of care, 34
    abortion and sterilization, 37
    assault, 33
    battery, 33
    client information, release of, 36
    crime, 33
    crimes of omission, 33
    death in hospice, 37
    duty to provide treatment, 36
    emergencies and, 40
    experimentation, 37
    felonies, 33
    informed consent, 34
    liability, 33
    libel, 34
    malpractice, 33
    misdemeanor, 33
    negligence, 33
    related terminology, 33–34
    release from liability, 37
    right to privacy, 34
    slander, 34
    special healthcare concerns, 36–37
    tort, 33
Legend drug, 910
Leg exercises, postoperative, 834
Legg–Calvé–Perthes disease (LCPD), 1255
Legionella, 484
Legislative barriers, 1827–1828
Leg strength, 634f
Length of stay (LOS), 1806
Lens, 248
LES. See Lower esophageal sphincter (LES)
Lesbians, 1147
Let-down reflex, 1069, 1093
Lethal dose, medication, 909
Leukemia, 1235–1236, 1479–1480, 1488
Leukocytes. See White blood cells (WBCs)
Leukocytosis, 1468
Leukopenia, 1468
Leukoplakia buccalis, 1601
Leukorrhea, 1681
Leukotriene antagonists, 1512
Leukotrienes (LT), 1512
Level of consciousness (LOC), 521, 629t, 1354
Levetiracetam (Keppra), 930
Levodopa (L-dopa), 1367
Levothyroxine sodium (T4, L-thyroxine sodium), 1389
Levulose, 351
Lewy body dementia, 1719
Leydig cells, 240
LFT. See Liver function tests (LFT)
LH. See Luteinizing hormone (LH)
Lice, 1298
Licensed Practical Nurse (LPN), 12

Licensed vocational nurse (LVN), 9
Licensing laws, for nursing, 13. *See also* Nurse Practice Acts
Licensure of nurses, 13
Lidocaine hydrochloride (Xylocaine), 935
Lie, fetal, 1054–1056
Lifespan in 21st century, increase in, 73
Lifespan, nutrition across, 371–375
Lifestyle factors, 62–65
    in diabetes, 1407
Lifting techniques, 646f
Lifts, types of, 662–664
Ligaments, 201–202
Lightening, 1057
Light intensity lifestyle, 350
Lignin, 353
Linea nigra, 1032
Linear measurement, wound, 860
Line of gravity, 644
Lingual arteries, 585
Linoleic acid, 354b
Linolenic acid, 354b
Liothyronine sodium (Cytomel), 1389
Lipases, 1385
Lipids, 353–355
Lipodystrophy, 979
Lipoproteins, 354
Lipotropin, 238
Lippincott's Nursing Drug Guide, 905
Lip reading, 1422
Liquid diets, 393–395, 388t
Liquid medications, 908
Listening, 552
Liter (L), 896
Liters per minute (LPM), 1567
Lithiasis, 1642
Lithium (Li⁺), 1758
Lithium carbonate, 1387
Lithotomy, 649t
Lithotomy position, 1670, 1671f
Lithotripsy, 1634, 1643
Liver, 237t
    disorders of, 1617–1621
    hormones secreted by, 311t
Liver abscess, 1621
Liver cancer, 1621
Liver failure, 1617–1618
Liver function tests (LFTs), 1310, 1584
Liver transplantation, 1621
Living will, 40–41, 881
Loading dose, medication, 909
Lobar pneumonia, 1546
Lobectomy, 1551, 1559
LOC. *See* Level of consciousness (LOC)
Local anesthesia, 818, 818b
Local effects, medication, 960
Localized scleroderma, 1333
Lochia, 1067, 1123
Lochia alba, 1068
Lochia rubra, 1068
Lochia serosa, 1068
Locked quiet rooms (LQRs), 1761
Lockjaw. *See* Tetanus
Lofstrand crutch, 659
Logroll turn, 651
Lomotil, 947
Long Term Care Community Coalition (LTCCC), 1808
Long-term care facility (LTC), 61, 1702b, 1806–1809
Long-term home care, 1831
Loop diuretics, 948
Loop of Henle, 323
Loperamide (Imodium), 947
Lorazepam (Ativan), 924t, 929

Lordosis, 633t, 1033, 1219, 1253, 1326
Lotion bath, 714
Lou Gehrig disease, 1370
Low-density lipoproteins (LDL), 355
Lower esophageal sphincter (LES), 1603
Low-fat diet, 397
Low-fiber diet, 395–396
Low-molecular-weight heparins (LMWHs), 938
LP. *See* Lumbar puncture (LP)
LPM. *See* Liters per minute (LPM)
LPN. *See* Licensed practical nurse (LPN)
LS ratio, 1105, 1121
LTB. *See* Laryngotracheobronchitis (LTB)
Lubricant cathartics, 947
Lumbar decompression, 1327
Lumbar puncture (LP), 612, 1352–1353
    in children, 1352
    infants, 1192
    in myelography, 1352
    in nervous system disorders, 1353f
    test, 614t
Lumbar vertebrae, 201
Lung abscess, 1546
Lung cancer, 1559
Lung perfusion scan, 1534
Lungs, 190t
    sounds (abnormal), 533
Lung scan, 1534
Lung shock, 520b
Lung volumes and capacities, 301t
Lupus erythematosus, 1333
Luteal phase, 341–342
Luteinizing hormone (LH), 1152, 1387
LVN. *See* Licensed vocational nurse (LVN)
Lyme disease, 1250
    prevention of, 1251
Lymph, 191. *See also* Lymphatic system
Lymphangiomas, 1219
Lymphangion, 280
Lymphatic circulation, 283
Lymphatic organs, 281–282
Lymphatic system, 273b
    functions of, 272
Lymphatic vessels, 280
Lymph fluids, 1312
Lymph nodes, 279
Lymph nodules, 281
Lymphocytes, 274t, 1521
Lymphocytosis, 1468
Lymphomas, 1488
Lysis, 583

M

Maceration, skin, 782
Macrolide antibiotics, 920
Macronutrients, 346
Macrophages, 277
Macropsia, 1799
Macrosomia, 1114, 1130–1131
Macula, 249
Macular rash, 1207
Macules, 627t, 628f
Mafenide acetate, 1304
Magical thinking, 117
Magic Mouthwash, 943
Magnesium (Mg⁺⁺), 1317–1318
    characteristics, 357
    deficiency, 357t, 1316t
    excess, 1316t
    functions, 357t, 1316t
    imbalances, 1316t
    sources, 357t
    toxicity, 357t
Magnesium sulfate, 925t, 930
    in preeclampsia, 1109

Magnetic resonance imaging (MRI), 1415, 1492, 1534, 1720
    for lung disorder, 1534
    in musculoskeletal disorders, 1322
    in nervous system disorders, 1351
    test, 615t
Mainstreaming, 1827
Major depressive disorders (MDDs), 1739
Major depressive episode (MDEs), 1739
Malaise, 610, 610t, 1257
Malecot catheter, 845
Male genitalia, 637f
    data collection, 635t
Male infertility, 1150, 1151b
Male pattern baldness, 172
Malignant bone tumors, 1256
Malignant hyperthermia, 830
Malignant lymphomas, 1482
Malignant melanoma, 1308
Malignant tumors, 1487
Malingering, 1741
Malleus, 250
Malnutrition, 371
Malocclusion, 1255, 1328
Malpighian corpuscle. *See* Renal corpuscle
Malpractice insurance, 39
Maltose, 352
Malunion, 1349
Mammary glands, 174, 340
Mammograms, 1491
Mammography, 1672
Managed care, 20
Managed care payment, 20
Management information services (MIS), 464
Managers, roles of, 1900–1901
Mandatory licensure, 13
Mandatory reporter, 1213
Mandibular artery, 587
Mandibular pulse, 587
Manganese (Mn), 357t
Mania, 1739
Mannitol (Osmitrol), 1374
Manometry, 616t
Mantoux tuberculin skin test (TST), 1036
Manual resuscitation bag. *See* Manual resuscitator
Manual resuscitator, 1572, 1572f
MAO B inhibitors, 1367
MAP. *See* Mean arterial pressure (MAP)
MAR. *See* Medication administration record (MAR)
Marasmus, 371, 1224
Marijuana, 1144
Marshall-Marchetti procedure, 1680
Masks, 500
Maslow's hierarchy of human needs, 47, 1813–1814, 1851. *See also* Human needs
Mastalgia, 1678
Mastectomy, 1675–1676
Mastication, 301
Mastitis, 1042, 1094, 1124–1125
Materia Medica for Nurses, 4
Maternal dystocia, 1119–1120
Maternal hemorrhage, 1118
Maternal–infant bonding, 1046
Maternal serum α-fetoprotein (MSAFP), 1037, 1106
Mathematics, review, 895–902
Matter, 156
Maximal dose, medication, 909
McGill–Melzack Pain Questionnaire, 804, 805f
MDGs. *See* Millennium Development Goals (MDGs)
Meals. *See also* Diet; Nutrition
    planning for diabetics, 1399

Mean arterial pressure (MAP), 592, 592f
Measles. See Rubella
Measles, mumps, and rubella (MMR), 1205, 1278
Measurement, systems of, 895–896
Meatal stenosis, 1241
Mechanical débridement, 1293
Mechanical soft diet, 395
Mechanical valves, 1442
Mechanical ventilation, 1573–1574
Mechanical ventilator, 1566, 1573
Meckel diverticulum, 1239
Meconium, 1088
Meconium aspiration syndrome (MAS), 1139
Meconium ileus, 1238
Mediastinal shift, 528
Mediastinum, 299
Medicaid, 27
Medical asepsis, 494–502, 842
   vs. standard precautions, 495
Medical assistant, 10b, 37
Medical diagnosis, 429–430
   vs. nursing diagnosis, 429–430
MedicAlert, 518
Medical history, 519
Medical ICU (MICU), 463
Medical information system (MIS), 463
Medically complex care nursing units, 1806
Medically underserved areas (MUA), 79
Medical marijuana, 1796
Medical pools, 1889–1890
Medical record number, 564
Medical records (MR) department, 464
Medical secretary, 10b
Medical/surgical care units, 462
Medical terminology, 157
Medical transcriptionist, 10b
Medicare, 27, 1808, 1852
Medication administration, 951–977, 1312
   buccal administration, 962–964
   to children, 960, 1193
   client refusal, 959
   client teaching, 960
   crushing/splitting tablets, procedure for, 963
   disposal of medication packages, 959
   documentation of, 952–953
   ear (otic) administration, 965
   enteral methods of, 961t
   eye administration, 964
   "Five Rights, Plus Two" of, 954–959
   general principles of, 960–962
   by injection, 978–1021
   intravenous, 992–996
   medication compliance, 959
   medication errors, 959
   nasal/respiratory administration, 965–967
   nicotine replacement in chewing gum form, 964b
   oral administration, 962
   orally disintegrating tablets, 962
   parenteral methods of, 964–968
   preparation for, 951–953
   rectal administration, 964
      routes of, 961t
   rate of absorption and onset of action, 961
   safe, 953
      right client, 955–957
      right documentation, 958
      right dose, 957–958
      right medication, 957
      right programming, 959
      right route, 958
      right time, 958
      tips for, 954
   sublingual (SL) medications, 962
   through gastric tube, 964
   transdermal administration, 967–968
   translingual (TL) administration, 962–964
   vaginal administration, 964
Medication administration record (MAR), 445t, 952, 1875
Medication errors, 959
Medication poisoning, first-aid in, 543
Medications, 903. See also Medication administration
   action, 905
   adrenergics, 930–931
   analgesics, 921–928
   antibiotics/anti-infective agents, 914–921
   anticonvulsants, 929–930
   antihypertensives, 936–937
   antineoplastic, 939
   blood, medications affecting, 937–939
   cardiovascular, 932–937
   central nervous system, 921, 924t–926t
   clarification of orders, 911
   classification of, 914
   and client rights, 905
   controlled substances, 904–905
      management of, 926b
   dermatologic, 922t–924t
   discontinued/changed, 959–960
   dispensing and supply systems, 952
   dosage, 909
   drug–drug interactions, 914
   drug references, 905–906
   endocrine system and, 931–932
   factors affecting prescription, 909–910
   Federal Drug Standards, 903–905
   food and, interactions between, 907, 913
   gastrointestinal system and, 943–947
   with grapefruit juice, 915b
   Hazardous to Handle, 959
   herbal/dietary supplements and, 914b
   high-alert, 931b
   hypnotics and sedatives, 928–929
   immune system and, 939–940
   injectable, 978–1021
   interactions with herbal supplements and homeopathic remedies, 907
   noninjectable, 951–977
   nonnarcotic analgesics, 927–929
   nonsteroidal anti-inflammatory drugs (NSAIDS), 927–929
   nursing considerations, 906
   photo guides, 915f
   postoperative, 830–831
   preoperative, 824
   reproductive systems and, 948–949
   respiratory system and, 940–943
   self-administered, 952
   sensory system and, 932
   setting up, 953
   side effects/adverse reactions, 907
   speed of action of, 915b
   storage of, 951–952
   systems of measurement, 895–896
   urinary system and, 947–948
   verbal order, 911
   wound healing and, 868–869, 869t
Medication toxicity, 960
Mediport, 992
Meditation, 29
Medroxyprogesterone acetate (Depo-Provera), 949, 1158
Medulla, 1391
Megacolon, 1241
Megaloblasts, 367
Meiosis, 164
Meissner plexus, 310
Melanin, 172
Melanocyte-inhibiting factor (MIF), 234t
Melanocytes, 171
Melanocyte-stimulating hormone (MSH), 236t
Melanomas, 1487
   malignant, 630f
Melasma, 1032
Melatonin, 237t
Melena, 1604
Memantine, 1723
Membranes, 166–167
Membranous labyrinth, 251
Memory cells, 291
Men
   health issues in, 68–69
   reproductive system, 331–335
   urinary system, 322f
Menadione. See Vitamin K
Menarche, 341
Meninges, 223
Meningitis, 1206, 1221, 1370–1372
Meningocele, 1142, 1222, 1222f
Meningococcal infection, 1206
Meningococcal meningitis, 1371
Meningomyelocele, 1222
Menopause, 1679
Menorrhagia, 1389, 1676
Menses, irregularity in, 1687
Menstrual cycle, 341–342
   hormonal changes, 341f
Menstrual difficulties, 1260–1261
Menstruation, 1260–1261, 1769
Mental health, 1283
Mental health advance declaration, 41
Mental health crisis centers, 1844
Mental health nursing, 1885
Mental health unit (MHU), 462
Mental illness, 1283
   signs/symptoms of, 1283–1284
Meperidine hydrochloride (Demerol), 927, 1622
mEq/L. See Milliequivalents per liter (mEq/L)
Mercaptopurine, 1518
Mercury, 502t
Merkel cells, 171
Mesothelioma, 1553
Messenger RNA, 162
Metabolic acidosis, 193t, 1318t
Metabolic alkalosis, 193t, 1318t
Metabolic and nutritional disorders, 1224–1225
Metabolic dementias, 1725
Metabolic syndrome, 1393
Metabolism, 161
Metaraminol bitartrate (Aramine), 935
Metastasis, 70
Metastatic bone tumors, 1349
Meter (M), 896
Metered-dose inhalers (MDI), 965, 1238
Metformin (Glucophage), 1401
Methadone hydrochloride (Dolophine), 927
Methadone therapy, 1797
Methamphetamine HCl, 1797–1798
Methicillin-resistant *Staphylococcus aureus* (MRSA), 488, 919, 1251
Methotrexate (Abitrexate), 1332, 1518
Methyldopa, 937
Methylergonovine maleate (methergine), 1066
Metoclopramide HCl (Reglan), 831, 946
Metric system of measurement, 895
Mexican populations, 381
MG. See Myasthenia gravis (MG)
mg/dL. See Milligrams per deciliter (mg/dL)
Micelles, 316
Microcephaly, 1142
Microcirculation, 265

Microdiskectomy, 1327
Microdrip setup, 989, 989f
Microglia, 219
Micronutrients, 346
Micturition, 1629
Midazolam (Versed), 924t, 929
Middle adulthood, 374
Middle Eastern American populations, 384
Mifepristone (Mifeprex), 1154
Miglitol (Glyset), 1401
Migraine headache, 1355
Mild cognitive impairment (MCI), 1717–1718
Milia, 1083, 1084f
Miliary tuberculosis, 1550
Milieu therapy, 1759
Milk of magnesia (MOM), 947
Millennium Development Goals (MDGs), 56b
Milliequivalents (mEq), of potassium chloride, 1311
Milliequivalents per liter (mEq/L), 1314
Milligrams per deciliter (mg/dL), 1315
Milwaukee braces, 1254, 1326
Mineralocorticoid, 236t
Minerals, 356–360
Minimal dose, medication, 909
Minimally invasive valvular surgery, 1442
Mini-mental status examination (MMSE), 1721, 1738
Minimum data set (MDS), 444
Mini-pill, 1157
Minnesota Multiphasic Personality Inventory (MMPI), 1738
Minority populations, 82
Minoxidil (Rogaine), 412
Miotics, 932
MiraLax, 824
Mirena, 1159
Miscarriage. See Spontaneous abortion
Misoprostol (Cytotec), 1154, 1605
Mist tent, 1189–1191
Mitochondria, 163t
Mitosis, 163–164
Mitoxantrone, 1518
Mitral stenosis, 1450
Mittelschmerz, 1260
Mixed delirium, 1717
Mixtures, 156–157
Mobile clinics, 1841–1842
Mobility, 213–214
Moderate physical activity, 350
Modified diet, 393–400
    for allergens, 400
    consistency and texture of, 393–396
    for energy, 396–397
    modification of nutrients, 396–400
    by serving size, 400
Moist dressings, 1291
    nursing care guidelines, 1292
Molding, in newborn's head, 1082, 1082f
Molds, 481
Moles (nevus), 1306
Molybdenum (Mo), 359t
Mongolian spots, 1084, 1084f, 1219
Monilial infection, 1141, 1681
Moniliasis. See Thrush
Monoamine oxidase inhibitors (MAOIs), 1284, 1758
Monoclonal antibodies, 1495, 1518
Monocyclic arthritis, 1330
Monocystic kidney disease, 1646
Monocytes, 277
Mononuclear phagocyte system, 290
Mononucleosis, 1249
Monosaccharides, 351
Monounsaturated fatty acids (MUFAs), 354b

Mons pubis, 339
Montgomery straps, 780
    application of, 778t
Mood disorders, 1739–1740
Mood stabilizers, 1753t, 1758
Morbidity, 56
Morgue, 461
Morning serum creatinine, 1631
Morning sickness, 1031
Moro reflex, 1085, 1141
Morphine, 807, 923t, 926, 1622
Mortality, 57
Morula, 1025
Motor vehicle accidents (MVAs), 67
    mortality rate for, 58
Mouth, 306–307
Mouth cancer, 1601
Mouth care, death/dying and, 884
Mouth disorder, 1599–1601
Mouthwashes, 943
Movements, documentation of, 1768
MRI. See Magnetic resonance imaging (MRI)
MRSA. See Methicillin-resistant *Staphylococcus aureus* (MRSA)
Mucociliary escalator, 297
Mucocutaneous lymph node syndrome. See Kawasaki disease
Mucosa-associated lymphoid tissue (MALT), 279
Mucositis, 1498
Mucous blanket, 297
Mucous membranes (mucosa), 232
MUFAs. See Monounsaturated fatty acids (MUFAs)
Multidrug-resistant tuberculosis, 1550. See also Tuberculosis (TB)
Multifetal pregnancy, 1036
Multigravida, 1024, 1056b
Multipara, 1056b
Multiple myeloma, 1483–1484
Multiple sclerosis (MS), 1364–1366, 1366t
Multisystem response, 1511
Mumps, 1205–1206
Munchausen syndrome, 1741
Murmurs, heart sounds, 588
Muscle tone, 213
Muscular dystrophy (MD), 1282–1283, 1328
Musculoskeletal disorders, 1253–1256, 1321–1349
    congenital, 1141–1142
    tests, 642
    treatments, 1323
Musculoskeletal injuries, first-aid in, 534–535
Musculoskeletal system, 195–214
    aging effects of, 214t
    data collection, 622
    muscles, 207–211
    physiology, 211–214
    skeleton, 195–204
Mushroom catheter, 845
Music therapy, 1748
Mutism, 1741
MVAs. See Motor vehicle accidents (MVAs)
Myasthenia gravis (MG), 1368–1369
Mycobacterium avium-intracellulare (MAC), 1526
Mycobacterium tuberculosis, 484, 1549
Mycology, 481
Mycoplasma, 481
Mycosis, 481
Mydriatics, 932
Myelograms, 1322, 1352
Myelomas, 1488
Myelomeningocele, 1142
Myocardial infarction (MI), 1454–1455
    mortality rate for, 58

Myocardial ischemia, pain patterns, 1453f
Myocardial perfusion, 615t
Myocarditis, 1450
Myoclonic seizures, 1356b
Myopia, 1257
Myotonic muscular dystrophy (MMD), 1282
Myringoplasty, 1226
Myringotomy, 1226, 1226f
Myxedema, 1389

N
Nabilone (Cesamet), 1796
Nabumetone, 1332
Nägele rule, 1037
Nails, 173
Naloxone (Narcan), 923t, 940
Naltrexone, 1794, 1796–1797
NANDA-I. See North American Nursing Diagnosis Association International (NANDA-I)
NAPNES. See National Association for Practical Nurse Education and Service (NAPNES)
Naproxen (Naprosyn, Aleve), 807, 1332
Narcolepsy, 1262
Narcotic agonist analgesics, 926–927
Narcotic analgesics, for pain relief, 807
Narcotic antitussives, 940
Narcotics
    preoperative, 824
    safety considerations, 471–472
Nares, 295
Narrative charting, 444–446
Narrative-chronological documentation, 444–446
Nasal cannula, 1569–1570
    nursing procedure, 1578–1579
Nasal polyps, 1560
Nasal speculum, 621
Nasal sprays/drops, 967
Nasal surgery, 1560
Nasal swab, 770
Nasal trauma, 1560
Nasal treatments, 1543
Nasogastric (NG) tubes, 405–406, 1588, 1589f
    insertion of, 405–406
    irrigation, 1590
    nursing procedure, 1627–1628
Nasolacrimal ducts, 297
Nasopharyngeal swab, 770
Nasopharynx, 1561
Natalizumab, 1518
National Academy of Sciences, 346
National Association for Home Care and Hospice (NAHC), 1830, 1852
National Association for Practical Nurse Education and Service (NAPNES), 12
National Association of Community Health Centers (NACHC), 1843
National Center for Health Statistics (NCHS), 57, 429
National Council Licensure Examination (NCLEX), 13, 1870–1871
National Council of State Boards of Nursing (NCSBN), 37, 1873
National Easter Seal Society, 78
National Federation of Licensed Practical Nurses (NFLPN), 12, 1902
National Hospice and Palliative Care Organization (NHPCO), 1852
National Institute for Nursing Research (NINR), 76, 442
National Institutes of Health (NIH), 75–76
National League for Nursing (NLN), 12
National Safety Council (NSC), 77

National Society for the Prevention of Blindness, 78
Native American, 85t, 384
Natural killer (NK) cell, 289
Naturally acquired immunity, 291
Nausea, 1498
  end-of-life care and, 884
  postoperative, 832
  in pregnancy, 1031
NCHS. *See* National Center for Health Statistics (NCHS)
NCLEX. *See* National Council Licensure Examination (NCLEX)
NCSBN. *See* National Council of State Boards of Nursing (NCSBN)
Near drowning, 1558
  first-aid in, 533–534
Nebulizer, 909, 965, 1571
Neck, muscles of, 210t
Necrosis, 611
Necrotizing enterocolitis (NEC), 1139
Needle biopsies, 1673
Needleless systems (injection system), 980
Needles, 979
Negative feedback system, 1387
Negative pressure ventilator, 1573. *See also* Mechanical ventilation
Negative pressure wound therapy (NPWT), 872, 872f, 1305
Neglect, 1213
Neisseria gonorrhoeae, 1164, 1684
Neisseria meningitides, 485, 1206, 1371
Neonatal abstinence syndrome (NAS), 1144, 1273–1274, 1274b
Neonatal/infant pain scale (NIPS), 806
Neonatal intensive care unit (NICU), 1131
Neonatal/newborn ICU (NICU), 463
Neonatal resuscitation, 1079
Neonate care. *See* Newborn care
Neoplasms, 1306–1308, 1349, 1377–1378, 1559
  of pituitary gland, 1388
Neoplastic diseases, 70
Neostigmine methylsulfate (Prostigmin), 948
Nephritic syndrome (nephrosis), 1640
Nephroblastoma. *See* Wilms tumor
Nephrolithiasis, 1642
Nephroma, 1646
Nephron loop. *See* Loop of Henle
Nephropathy, 1406
Nephrotic syndrome, 1243
Nephrotomogram, 1632
Nephrotoxicity, aminoglycosides and, 920
Nerve, 166
Nerve impulses, transmission of, 227–229
Nerve tissues, 166
Nervous system, 216
  autonomic nervous system, 226–227
  cells of, 216
    neuroglia, 216–219
    neurons, 218–219
  central nervous system, 219–224
  disorders of, 1351–1381
  divisions of, 219–227
  effects of aging on, 229t–230t
  functions of, 217b
  peripheral nervous system, 224–226
  physiology of, 227–229
  structure of, 216
Networking, professional, 1880
Neuralgia, 1359
Neural tube defects (NTDs), 1142, 1142b
Neuro chairs, 1354
Neurodiagnostic department, 461
Neurofibromatosis (NF), 1271
Neurogenic bladder, 1823

Neurogenic shock, 520b
Neuroglia, 218–219
Neurohypophysis, 238
Neuroleptanalgesic, 818
Neuroleptic drugs, 1750–1757, 1757b
Neuroleptic malignant syndrome (NMS), 1755–1757
Neurologic assessment, 1354
Neurologic complications, postoperative, 830
Neurologic disorders, 1221–1224, 1825
Neurologic tests, 1738
Neurologists, 1351
Neurology, 1351
Neuronal excitation, 1792
Neurons, 166, 216–218
Neuropathic pain, 802
Neuropathy, 1406
Neuropeptide Y (NPY), 237t
Neuropsychiatric EEG-Based Assessment Aid (NEBA), 1277
Neuropsychiatric testing, 614t
Neuroscience nurses, 1351
Neurosurgeons, 1351
Neurosyphilis, 1166
Neurotransmitters, 228
Neurovascular checks, 1324
Neurovascular pressure, 1344
Neutral protamine hagedorn (NPH), 1398
Neutrons, 156
Neutropenia, 1479, 1495, 1500
Neutropenic isolation, 514
Neutrophils, 276
Nevus, 1219
Nevus vasculosus, 1219
Newborn. *See also* Newborn care
  appropriate for gestational age (AGA), 1129
  assisting with breathing, 1099
  bathing, 1101–1102, 1176
  extremely low–birth-weight (ELBW), 1129–1130
  head and body, 1082, 1082f
  heel stick procedure on, 1102–1103
  high-risk. *See* Newborn, high-risk
  large-for-gestational-age (LGA), 1130
  low–birth-weight (LBW), 1129
  movement and activities, 1085
  postterm, 1131
  preterm, 1131
  skin, 1083–1084
  small for gestational age (SGA), 1130
  substance abuse and, 1136
  very low–birth-weight (VLBW), 1129
  weight and length, 1081, 1082f
Newborn care, 1076–1103
  after delivery, 1085–1089
  Apgar score, 1078, 1078t
  body temperature, 1077
    maintaining, 1088
  bubbling (burping), 1096
  circulation, 1077
  clamping and cutting cord, 1079
  cleansing, 1088
  cord care, 1091
  crying, 1087
  daily, 1089–1091
  data gathering, 1089–1091
  discharge, 1096
  dressing and wrapping, 1091
  examination by healthcare provider, 1088
  eye prophylaxis, 1080
  genitals care, 1091
  handling newborn, 1091
  identification, 1079–1080
  immediate care, 1077–1081
  infection control, 1080

  initial observations, 1085–1087
  laboratory screening, 1088–1089
  measurements, 1085
  neonatal resuscitation, 1079
  nutrition, 1091–1096
  parental–infant bonding, promoting of, 1080–1081
  protection of newborn, 1089
  respiration, 1077
  respiratory status, 1087
  sleep, 1091
  sleeping position, 1089
  standard precautions, 1080
  umbilical cord, 1085
  vaccinations, 1080
  vital signs, 1085–1087
  vitamin K administration, 1080
Newborn, high-risk, 1128–1129
  birth weight and, 1129–1130
  cardiovascular defects, 1142
  categories of, 1129–1131
  causative factors for, 1136b
  complications in, 1136–1139
  conditions contributing to, 1130b
  gastrointestinal disorders, 1143
  genitourinary disorder, 1143
  gestational age and, 1130–1131
  hemolytic disease, 1139–1140
  hyperbilirubinemia, 1137–1138
  intrauterine disorders, 1140–1141
  meconium aspiration syndrome, 1139
  musculoskeletal disorders, 1141–1142
  necrotizing enterocolitis, 1139
  neural tube defects, 1142
  neurologic complications, 1138
  newborn of mother with diabetes, 1133
  nursing care, 1132–1133
  nursing observations, 1132–1133
  respiratory disorders, 1136–1137
  retinopathy of prematurity (ROP), 1138
  sudden infant death syndrome (SIDS), 1139
Newborn nursery, 1089
Newborn respiratory distress, signs of, 1088b
New Delhi metallo-beta-lactamase (NDM), 488
Newspapers, 1890
Nexplanon, 1158
NFLPN. *See* National Federation of Licensed Practical Nurses (NFLPN)
Niacin, 362t, 366–367
Nicotinamide, 366
Nicotine, 1800
Nicotine patches, 967
Nicotinic acid, 366
NIDDM. *See* Non-insulin-dependent diabetes mellitus (NIDDM)
Nifedipine (Procardia), 937
Nightingale lamp, 3, 3f
Nightingale School for Nurses, 3–4
Night shifts, 1878, 1879b
Night terrors, 1262
NIH. *See* National Institutes of Health (NIH)
NINR. *See* National Institute for Nursing Research (NINR)
Nipples, sore and cracked, 1094
Nissl bodies, 217
Nitrates, 935–936
Nitrazine test, 1058
Nitro-Bid, 936
Nitro-Dur, 936
Nitroglycerin (NTG), 936, 967
Nitro-Time, 936
Nits, 1298
NLN. *See* National League for Nursing (NLN)
N-methyl-D aspartic acid inhibitors, 1367
Nociception, 801. *See also* Pain

Nociceptive pain, 802
Nocturia, 329t
Nocturnal diaphoresis, 1550
Nocturnal emission, 331
Node of Ranvier, 217
Nodule, 627t
"No information" status, 36
Noise-induced hearing loss, 133
Noise pollution, 80
Noise trauma, 253
Noncatecholamines, 931
Non-Hodgkin lymphomas (NHLs), 1483
Non-insulin-dependent diabetes mellitus (NIDDM), 1257, 1393
Nonketotic hyperosmolar state, 1405
Nonnarcotic analgesics, 927–928
Nonnarcotic antitussives, 940
Nonnutritive sucking, toddlers, 115
Nonopioid–nonsteroidal anti-inflammatory drugs (NSAIDs), for pain relief, 807
Nonoxynol-9 (N-9), 1160
Nonpitting edema, 1313, 1449b
Nonrebreathing mask (NRM), 1570, 1570f
Nonsalicylate analgesics, 928
Non-small cell lung cancers (NSCLC), 1559
Nonspecific immunity, 290
Nonsteroidal anti-inflammatory drugs (NSAIDs), 927–928, 1254, 1329, 1331, 1604
Nonstress test (NST), 1106
Nonunion, 1349
Nonverbal communication (NVC), 551b, 552–555
Norepinephrine, 930
Norepinephrine bitartrate (Levophed, Levarterenol), 935
Normal blood pressure, 592
Normal body temperature, 582–583
Normal saline, 987
Normothermia, 788
North American Nursing Diagnosis Association International (NANDA-I), 428
Nose, 295–297
  disorders of, 1559–1560
Nosebleed, 538, 1560. See also Epistaxis
  nursing procedure, 538
Notes On Nursing: What It Is, and What It Is Not, 3
NPH. See Neutral protamine hagedorn (NPH)
NRM. See Nonrebreathing mask (NRM)
NSAIDs. See Nonsteroidal anti-inflammatory drugs (NSAIDs)
NSC. See National Safety Council (NSC)
NSCLC. See Non-small cell lung cancers (NSCLC)
Nuchal cord, 1065, 1121
Nuchal rigidity, 1221, 1371
Nuclear dyad, 99
Nuclear families, 99
Nuclear medical technician, 10b
Nuclear medicine department, 461
Nuclear scan, 1437
Nulligravida, 1056b
Nullipara, 1056b
Nurse-client relationships, 1764, 1765b
Nurse-controlled analgesia (NCA), 807
Nurse Practice Acts, 11, 13
Nurse practitioner (NP), 1053
Nurses (Registered) Act, Canada, 37
Nurse's aide, 11
Nurses' notes, 422
Nurse's Pledge, 13, 14b
Nursing, 1, 9
  adult learners, 15
  careers in, 9–17
  current trends in, 6
  dark ages of, 3
  early influences, 2, 2f
  Hippocrates, influence of, 2
  history of, 1–4
  insignia, 6–7
  legal issues, 32–37
  legal responsibilities in, 38–39
  military orders, 2–3
  monastic orders, 2
  Nightingale's, 3
  origins of, 1–7
  the Reformation movement and, 3
  Roman matrons and, 2
  school pins, 7
  theories of, 13–14, 14t
  uniforms, 6, 7f
  in United States, 4–6
  during wartime, 6
Nursing assessment, 420
  data collection, 420–427
Nursing assistant, 11
Nursing care
  barium studies, 1584–1585
  burns, 1300
  chest suction, 1539
  colostomy, 1596
  dialysis patient, 1629
  gastrostomy, 1588
  guidelines for, 453
  hospitalized obese patient, 1623
  hypertension, 1640
  ileostomy, 1595
  intellectually impaired child, 1268
  liver disorder, 1618
  mechanical ventilation, 1573
  moist dressings, 1302
  nasal surgery, 1561
  obesity, 1623–1625
  oxygen therapy, 1567
  pneumonia, 1548
  providing oxygen, 1567
  provision of, 458–461
  renal calculi, 1645–1646
  special needs, 1266
  suctioning to remove secretions, 1543
  therapeutic baths, 1300
Nursing care plan, 413
  in action, 417
  burns, 1303
  child abuse, 1215–1217
  data collection and, 420–422
  hypertension, 1645–1646
  renal calculi and hypertension, 1645–1646
  writing, 431
Nursing care units, 462–463
Nursing diagnosis, 428
  diagnostic statement, 430–431
  history of, 428–429
  medical diagnosis vs., 429–430
  purposes of, 430
  renal calculi and hypertension, 1645–1646
Nursing Drug Reference, 905
Nursing history, 423
  components of, 423
  nursing diagnoses and, 608
Nursing homes, 22–23
Nursing interventions
  in pain management, 808–809
  selection of, 569
Nursing organizations, 15–17
Nursing process, 411–419
  assessment, 418t
  characteristics of, 417–419
  data collection, 413
  in endocrine disorders, 1386–1387
  evaluation, 418
  implementation, 417
  in musculoskeletal disorders, 1323
  potential needs/potential problems and, 416
  steps in, 416–417
  vs. scientific problem-solving, 412
Nursing programs
  accredited, 12–13
  approved, 12
  types of, 9–12, 11t
Nursing unit, client's arrival on, 566–569
Nutrient broths, 480
Nutrient-Dense Foods, 349
Nutrient density, 370
Nutrient intake, pediatric clients, 1186–1187
Nutrition. See also Diet
  across the lifespan, 371–375
  added sugars in, 352b
  assistance with eating, 392–393
  basic, 345–375
  between-meal and bedtime supplements, 391
  bland, 396
  for breastfeeding mother, 1091–1096
  client and family, education of, 384
  client education, 463
  in diabetes, 1397
  documentation and reporting, 437
  end-of-life care and, 884
  ethnic heritage, 377
  feeding clients/patient, 391
  growth and development, influences on, 106–107
  and health, 59
  healthy diet, components of, 62
  high-fiber diet, 395
  for infants, 1094–1095. See also Feeding of newborns
  liquid diets, 393–395
  low-fiber diet, 395–396
  peripheral parenteral, 403–404
  postoperative, 825
  during pregnancy, 1041–1042
  problems relating to, 373
  serving food in hospital, 389–392
  soft diet, 394t, 395
  total parenteral, 403
  in young children, 1224–1225
Nutritional support, 400–404
  parenteral therapy, 403
  tube feeding, 400–101
Nutrition Facts Labels, 346
Nutrition Labeling and Education Act of 1993, 345
Nutting, Mary Adelaide, 5
NuvaRing, 1159
Nystagmus, 1270, 1281, 1414

O

OA. See Osteoarthritis (OA)
OASIS (Outcome and Assessment Information Set), 1833
Obamacare. See Affordable Care Act
Obesity, 1263, 1393, 1623–1625
  in children, 66
  disease risk and, 609t
  nursing care guidelines, 1624
Objective data, 420–421
Object permanence, 109
Oblique fractures, 1343f
Observation, 422
  diagnosis and, 429
Obsessive compulsive behaviors (OCD), 1277
Obstetric client, nursing process for, 1048–1049
Obstetric (OB) healthcare care, 1053
Obstetrician-gynecologist (OB/GYN), 1670

Obstetrics, 1024, 1024t
Obstetrics (OB) department, 462
Obstructive disorders, 1641–1644
Occipital–frontal circumference (OFC), 1176
Occipital lobe, cerebral cortex, 221
Occupational disorders, 70
Occupational hazards, 469t
Occupational Outlook Handbook, 12
Occupational Safety and Health Administration (OSHA), 23
    standards for client care, 509
Occupational skills, 1764
Occupational therapists, 10b, 1743, 1748
Occupational therapy (OT), 28, 462
Occupied bed, 689
Ocular hypertension, 932
Ocular ultrasound, 1414
Oculogyric crisis, 1755
Oculomotor nerve (CN III), 249
Odor control, end-of-life care and, 885
Odors, 1860
Official name, medication, 906
OGTT. *See* Oral glucose tolerance test (OGTT)
Oils, 349t, 354t
Oldest adults, 141
    areas of concern, 141–143, 142f–143f, 143b
    physical health of, 141
Olfaction, 254
Olfactory nerve (CN I), 254
Olfactory observation, 422
Oligodendrocytes, 219
Oligospermia, 335
Oliguria, 1235, 1650
Ombudsperson, 24
Omega-3 PUFAs, 354b
Omega-6 PUFAs, 354b
Omnibus Budget Reconciliation Act (OBRA), 1900
On-call services, 1856
Oncogene, 1488
Ondansetron (Zofran), 831, 946
Onset, insulin, 1398
Onycholysis, 1297
Oocyte, 340
Oogenesis, 340
O&P. *See* Ova and parasites (O&P)
Open-heart surgery, 1233, 1441
Open reduction, 1341–1343
Open reduction and internal fixation (ORIF), 1341–1343
Open skull fractures, 1374
Operating room (OR), 812, 1888
Operative obstetrics, 1122–1123
Ophthalmia neonatorum, 1080, 1141, 1249
Ophthalmic antibiotics, 932
Ophthalmic medications, 932
    administration of, 964
Ophthalmic nerve, 249
Ophthalmic zoster, 1359
Ophthalmologists, 1422
Ophthalmology, 247
Ophthalmology clinics, 1889
Ophthalmoscopes, 1414
Opiates, 926
Opiate use disorders, 1796–1797
Opioids, 1144
    for pain relief, 807
Opisthotonos, 1371
Opportunistic infections (OIs), 1525–1526
Optic chiasm, 249
Optic disk, 249
Optic nerve (CN II), 249
Optic tract, 249
Optometrists, 1422
Oral contraceptives, 949, 1157–1158

Oral endoscopy, 615t
Oral glucose tolerance test (OGTT), 1385–1386, 1394
Orally disintegrating tablets (ODT), 908, 962
Oral–nasal secretions, 1543
Oral poliovirus vaccine (OPV), 1205
Oral rehydration solution (ORS), 1240
Oral reprimands, 1903
Orbit, 247
Orchiopexy, 1244, 1659
Orchitis, 1661
Organ and tissue donation, 881–882
Organ, 156
Organelles, 162f
Organic disorders, 69, 1738
Organ of Corti, 251
Organ Procurement and Transplantation Network (OPTN), 1653
Orgasm, 335, 1149
ORIF. *See* Open reduction and internal fixation (ORIF)
Oropharynx, 1561
Orthodontia, 1255
Orthognathic surgery, 1256
Orthopedic beds, 691
Orthopedics (ORTHO), 456, 1321
Orthopnea, 299, 1542t
Orthopneic position, 1543
Orthostasis, in diabetes, 1406
Orthostatic blood pressure, 595
Orthostatic hypotension, 595
Orthotics, 1821
Ortolani sign, 1142
OSHA. *See* Occupational Safety and Health Administration (OSHA)
Osmosis, 187–188
Osmotic agents, 947
Osmotic pressure, 184
Osmotic shock, 520b
Ossicle, 250
Ossification, 212
Osteoarthritis (OA), 1331, 1332f
    versus rheumatoid arthritis, 1331t
Osteoblasts, 212
Osteoclasts, 212
Osteocyte, 212
Osteogenic sarcoma, 1256
Osteomalacia, 1333–1334, 1391
Osteomyelitis, 1344–1348
Osteoporosis, 69, 360, 1253, 1344
    calcium intake and, 360
    in women, 69
Osteosarcoma, 1256
Ostomate, 1595
Ostomy, 1595
    appliances, 1596–1597
    pouches and accessories, 1597f
OTC. *See* Over-the-counter (OTC)
Otitis media, 1205–1226, 1544
Otolaryngologist, 1226
Otology, 249
Otorrhea, 1375
Otoscopes, 458, 1414
Otoscopic examination, 1414
Ototoxicity, aminoglycosides and, 920
Ounce-Equivalent, 349
Outcome-based care, 23
Outercourse, 1156
Outings, mental health units and, 1761
Outpatient care centers, 21
Outpatient department (OPD), 463
Outreach staff, 465
Ova (female gamete), 337
Ova and parasites (O&P), 611
Ovarian cancer, 1686, 1686t

Ovarian cycle, 341–342
Ovarian tubes, 338
Ovary, 338, 341
    hormones secreted by, 1383t
Overactivity, 1771
Overflow incontinence, 1636
Overflow valves, heart, 261
Overhydration, 1312
Overnutrition, 370
Overriding aorta, 1230
Over-the-counter (OTC) drugs, 910, 1248, 1545, 1801
Overweight, 370, 1393
Oviduct, 338
Ovo-vegetarians, 384
Ovulation, 341
Oxidized cellulose (Oxycel), 938
Oximetry, 595
Oxybutynin (Ditropan), 948
Oxycodone, 923t, 927
OxyContin, 923t, 927
Oxygen, 1566–1569
    need for, 49
Oxygen administration, 1190t, 1190
Oxygen hood, 1191f
Oxygen therapy, 1566–1582
    in burn injuries, 1302
    delivery systems, 1569–1570
    hazards of, 1566–1567
    nursing care guidelines, 1567
Oxyhemoglobin, 275
Oxytocin (pitocin), 238, 1066, 1105
Oxytocin challenge test (OCT), 1105

P
Pacemaker cells, of heart, 267
Packing, wound, 870, 870f
$PaCO_2$. *See* Partial pressure of carbon dioxide $(PaCO_2)$
PACU. *See* Post-anesthesia care unit (PACU)
Pain, 801
    acute, 802
    cancer, 802
    causes of, 801
    chronic, 802
    cycle of, 802f
    data collection, 804–805
    documentation of, 808
    expression of, 804
    as fifth vital sign, 804
    intractable, 802
    management in burn injuries, 1302–1303
    neuropathic, 802
    perception, factors affecting, 802
    postoperative, 824
    rating scales, 804–806
    referred, 256, 802
    superficial, 255
    threshold, 803
    tolerance, 803
    transmission, 801–802
    types of, 802
    visceral, 255
Pain distress scales, 804f
Pain management, 801–810
    end-of-life care and, 885
Palate, 306
Palatopharyngoplasty, 1552
Palatoplasty, 1228
Palliative care, 146, 882
Pallor, 635t
Palmar grasp, 1093
Palmar grasp reflex, 1085
Palonosetron HCl (Aloxi), 831

Palpation
  blood pressure, 619
  diagnosis and, 594
  pulses, 587–588
  of skin, 626f
Palpebrae (eyelids), 247
Palpebral fissure, 247
Pancarditis, 1450
Pancreas, 311t
  disorders of, 1623
  transplantation, 1401
Pancreatectomy, 1623
Pancreatic cancer, 1623
Pancreatic enzymes, 1238
Pancreatic function tests, 1385
Pancreatic islets gland, 1383t
Pancreatitis, 1623
Pandemics, 1247
Panic attacks, 1740
Pantothenic acid, 363t, 367
PaO$_2$. *See* Partial pressure of oxygen (PaO$_2$)
Papain-based débridement, 1293
Papanicolaou (Pap) tests, 1671
PAPR. *See* Powered (positive) air-purified respirator (PAPR)
Papules, 627t
Paracentesis, 1538
Paradoxical effects, 960, 1704, 1717
Paradoxical reaction, 1802
ParaGard, 1159
Paralysis, in female clients, 1363
Paralytic ileus, 832, 1610
Paramedic, 10b
Paranoia, 1286, 1732, 1741
Paraplegia, 1362, 1821
Parasites, 480
Parasitic infestations, 1208–1209, 1298
  nursing considerations and, 1209b
Parasomnias. *See* Sleep disorders
Parathormone. *See* Parathyroid hormone (PTH)
Parathyroid function tests, 1384
Parathyroid gland, 1383t
  disorders, 1391
Parathyroid hormone (PH, PTH), 1384
Parenchymal cells, 1617
Parental–infant bonding, 1080–1081
Parenteral fluid administration, in children, 1187
Parenteral nutrition, 1591–1593
Parenting, 97–98
Paresthesia, 1319, 1327, 1372
Parietal cells, stomach, 311t
Parietal lobe, cerebral cortex, 224
Parish nursing, 1887
Parking, disabled, 1827
Parkinsonism, 1366
Parkinson disease, 1366–1368, 1367f, 1719
  mortality rate for, 58
Paroxysmal, 1555
Partial hospitalization programs, 1745
Partial pressure of carbon dioxide (PaCO$_2$), 1534
Partial pressure of oxygen (PaO$_2$), 1534
Partial-rebreathing mask (PRM), 1570, 1572f
  nursing procedure, 1579–1580
Partial simple seizures, 1356b
Partial thromboplastin time (PTT), 938, 1469
Partner-notification laws, 1531
Passavant Hospital, 4
Passive range-of-motion (PROM), 1323, 1458
Patch tests, 613t
Patent ductus arteriosus (PDA), 1142, 1230, 1231f, 1233
Pathologic fractures, 1347
Pathologic jaundice, 1138
Pathologists, 461
Pathophysiology, 158

Patient-controlled analgesia (PCA), 807, 885, 952, 989, 1845
Patient Safety Act, 35
Patient's Bill of Rights, 24
Patient Self-Determination Act (PSDA), 40, 881, 1852
Pavlik harness, infant in, 1220f
Pay for performance (P4P), 1808, 1832
PCM. *See* Protein-calorie malnutrition (PCM)
PCP. *See Pneumocystis carinii pneumonia* (PCP)
PCPs. *See* Primary care providers (PCPs)
Peak, insulin, 1398
Pedal pulse, 587f
Pedialyte, 1240
Pediatrician, 1175
Pediatric ICU (PICU), 463
Pediatric nursing, 1175–1199
  admission to healthcare facility, 1181
  catheterization, 1188
  daily cleanliness, 1188–1189
  data collection on admission, 1181–1183
  diagnostic procedures, 1192
  diarrhea treatment, 1188
  discharging children, 1183
  diversion and recreation, 1191
  documentation of information, 1183
  elimination, 1187
  enema administration, 1188
  family caregiver instruction for children, 1176
  fever management, 1191–1193
  health maintenance, 1176–1178
  hospitalization and, 1179
  immunization, 1177, 1177b
  infection control, 1186
  medication administration, 1193
  nutrient intake, 1186–1187, 1187f
  oxygen administration, 1190
  physical examination, 1177
    assisting with, 1181
  resuscitation, 1191
  safety of children, 1184
  specific care for age groups, 1177–1178
  suppositories, use of, 1188
  surgery and, 1194
    postoperative care, 1194
    preoperative care, 1194
  therapeutic procedures, 1191–1193
  transcultural considerations, 1180
  urine specimen collection, 1187
Pediatrics, 1175
Pediatrics (PEDS) unit, 462
Pediculosis, 511, 1209
Peer group, 122
PEG. *See* Percutaneous endoscopic gastrostomy (PEG)
Pellagra, 367
Pelvic/abdominal cramping, in pregnancy, 1034
Pelvic examination, 608t, 1670–1671
Pelvic exenteration, 1674
Pelvic inflammatory disease (PID), 1525, 1684–1685
  female infertility and, 1151
Pelvic pouch, 1598
Pelvic sling traction, 1339
Pelvic traction, 1339
Penetrating head injuries, 1376
Penicillin-resistant *Streptococcus pneumoniae* (PRSP), 488
Penicillins (PNS), 916t, 919–920
Penile implants, 1149, 1658–1659
Penile pump, 1149
Penile revascularization, 1149, 1659
Penis, 1667–1668
Penrose drain, 871, 871f
Pentosan polysulfate (Elmiron), 1639

Peptic ulcer disease, 1604–1608, 1605t
Percentages, 901
Percussion, 619
Percutaneous endoscopic gastrostomy (PEG), 1591, 1591f
Percutaneous transluminal coronary angioplasty (PTCA), 1438–1441, 1440f
Percutaneous tube, 401
Percutaneous umbilical blood sampling (PUBS), 1106, 1275
Performance reviews, 1903–1904
Perfusion, 1229
Periauricular ecchymosis, 1375
Pericardial space, 260
Pericarditis, 1452
Perinatologist, 1108
Perineal care, 1676
Perineal electromyogram (EMG), 1634
Perineum, 339
Periodic abstinence, 1157
Periodontal disease, 1600
Periodontitis, 1600
Perioperative period, 815
Periorbital ecchymosis, 1375
Peripheral access device, 1498
Peripheral blood smear, 1468
Peripheral blood stem cells (PBSC), 1472
Peripheral embolism, 1459
Peripheral indwelling catheter (PIC) line, 1498
Peripherally inserted central catheter (PICC), 990–992, 1187, 1498, 1591
Peripheral nervous system (PNS), 224–226
  cranial nerves, 224–225
  spinal nerves, 225–226
Peripheral neuropathy, 1406
Peripheral parenteral nutrition (PPN), 403–404
Peripheral pulses, sites of, 589
Peripheral vascular disease, 1459
Peripheral vision, 253
Peristalsis, 318t
Peritoneal dialysis, 1651–1652, 1652f
Peritonitis, 1604, 1615–1616
Periwound area, 860
Permeability, 187
  of membranes, 187–189
Permissive licensure, 5
Permit to practice, 1869
Pernicious anemia, 1477
Pernicious vomiting. *See* Hyperemesis gravidarum
PERRLA+C procedure, 525
Personal appearance and grooming, 554
Personal care, 1860
Personal health records (PHRs), 1811
Personal identification number (PIN), 904
Personality changes, 1463
Personality disorders, 1740
Personality inventories, 1738
Personal preparedness, in emergency, 473
Personal protective equipment (PPE), 496
Personal respiratory protection (PRP), 509
Personal space, 95, 553
  cultural consideration, 95
Pertussis, 1202–1204
Pessary, 1636–1637
PET. *See* Positron emission tomography (PET)
Petaling, 1336
Petechiae, 1084, 1234, 1480
Petri dishes, 480
Pet therapy, 1748, 1824
Peyer patches, 280
Peyronie disease, 1149, 1659
Pezzer catheter, 845
PFT. *See* Pulmonary function test (PFT)
Phagocytic cells, 277

Phagocytosis, 276f
Phantom pain, 1363
Pharmaceutical sales, 1888
Pharmacist, 10b
Pharmacokinetics, 905
Pharmacologic therapy, 1861–1864
Pharmacology, 903
    and mathematics, 895–901
Pharmacy, client care and, 463
Pharyngeal speech, 1562
Pharyngeal tonsils, 297
Pharyngitis, 1534
Pharynx, 297, 1535
Phenazopyridine, 948
Phencyclidine hydrochloride, 1799
Phenylephrine hydrochloride
    (Neo-Synephrine), 935
Phenylketonuria (PKU), 1088, 1143, 1224–1225
Phenytoin, 925t, 930, 1158
Pheochromocytoma, 1392
Phimosis, 1083, 1091, 1660
Phlebitis, 988, 1455
Phlebotomist, 10b
Phlebotomy, 1474. *See also* Venipuncture
Phobias, 1740
pH (potential of hydrogen in concentration), of
    blood, 1310
Phoropter, 1414
Phosphate (PO$_4^-$), 1318
    deficiency, 1316t
    excess, 1316t
    functions, 1316t
    imbalances, 1316t
Phosphorus (P), 357t 1316t, 1318
    characteristics, 361
Phosphorus-modified diet, 400
Photophobia, 1205, 1258, 1371
Photosensitivity, tetracyclines and, 920
Phototherapy, 1138
Physiatrists, 1814
Physical abuse, 1214
Physical activity
    client education on, 380
    importance of, 62
Physical evidence recovery kit, 1148
Physical health, 56
Physically neglected child, 1213
Physical measures, in pain management, 808
Physical medicine and rehabilitation
    (PM&R), 463
Physical therapist, 10b
Physical therapy (PT), 21b, 461, 1323
Physician assistant (PA), 10b, 1053
Physician's Desk Reference (PDR), 905
Physicians' offices, 1885–1886
Physics, 156
Physiologic anorexia, 1244
Physiologic jaundice, 1137–1138
Physiology, 157–158
Phytochemicals, 345
Phytonadione (Mephyton), 938
Phytonadione injection (AquaMEPHYTON),
    938
Piaget's theory, of cognitive development,
    108–109, 123
Pica, 1042
PICC. *See* Peripherally inserted central catheter
    (PICC)
PIE charting, 447t
Pigmentation loss, 623t
Pigment changes, in pregnancy, 1032
Pigmented nevi, 1219. *See also* Moles
Pilocarpine, 932
Pilomotor reflex, 172
Pincer grasp, of infant, 112

Pineal gland, 240
Ping-pong effect, 1164
Pink eye, 1164
Pinna, 249
Pinocytosis, 189f
Pinworms, 1208
Piroxicam (Feldene), 1332
Pitting edema, 1313, 1313f, 1449b
Pituitary function tests, 1383
Pituitary gland, 233–238
    anterior lobe, 234
    anterior lobe disorders, 1387
    hypothalamus, 234
    middle lobe, 238
    neoplasms, 1388
    posterior lobe, 238
    posterior lobe disorders, 1387–1388
Pivot joints, 200
PJP. *See Pneumocystis jiroveci pneumonia* (PJP)
PKU. *See* Phenylketonuria (PKU)
Placenta, 1028–1029, 1029f
    afterbirth, 1029
    delivery of, 1053
    hormones secreted by, 242
Placenta accreta, 1117–1118
Placental insufficiency, 1118
Placenta previa, 1116, 1116f
Placentography, 1116
Planimetry, wound, 861
Planned Parenthood of America, 78
Plans of assistance, 1904
Plaque, 1722
Plasma, 273
Plasma fluids, 1312
Plasmapheresis, 1369, 1372, 1471
Plasma protein fraction (PPF), 939
Plasma proteins, 273
Plasmids, 483
Plasmodium malariae, 481
Plaster cast, 1336
Plastic surgery, 1293, 1560
Platelet apheresis, 1236
Platelet count, 1468
Platelet disorders, 1480–1482
Platelets, 939
Play, in hospital setting, 1191
Play therapy, 1748
Pleura, 299
Pleural shock, 520b
Pleural space, 299
Pleur-Evac, 1539
Pleurisy, 299, 1548–1549
Plugged ducts, 1094
Plumbism, 81, 1211, 1279–1280
PMI. *See* Point of maximal impulse (PMI)
PM&R. *See* Physical medicine and rehabilitation
    (PM&R)
Pneumatic compression device (PCD), 781, 781f
Pneumococcal infection, 1204–1205
Pneumococcal vaccine (PCV), 1205
Pneumoconioses, 1553
Pneumocystis carinii pneumonia (PCP),
    1523, 1546
Pneumocystis jiroveci pneumonia (PJP), 1546
Pneumonectomy, 1551, 1559
Pneumonia, 1205, 1546–1548
    elderly female hospitalized with, 590
    postoperative, 832
Pneumothorax, 1558–1559
Podocytes, 322
Podofilox (Condylox), 1171
Point-Loc device, 980
Point of maximal impulse (PMI), 588
Point of service (POS) plan, 27
Poison, 542

Poison control center, 465
Poliomyelitis (polio), 1205
Polyarthritis, rheumatic fever and, 1207
Polycyclic arthritis, 1330
Polycystic kidney disease (PKD), 1271, 1646
Polycystic ovarian syndrome (PCOS), female
    infertility and, 1151
Polycythemia, 1473–1474
Polycythemia rubra, 1473
Polydactylism, 1142
Polydipsia, 1257, 1393, 1738
Polyethylene glycol electrolyte solution, 947
Polyethylene (PE) ventilating tube, 1226
Polyhydramnios, 1117
Polymorphonuclear leukocytes (PMNs). *See*
    Granular leukocytes
Polypectomy, 1588
Polypeptides, 233
Polyphagia, 1257, 1393
Polypharmacy, 1708
Polyps, 1560
Polysaccharides, 352
Polysomnogram, 1262
Polysubstance use disorder, 1786
Polyunsaturated fatty acids (PUFAs), 354b
Polyuria, 1257, 1393
PO (per os) medication, 962
POMR. *See* Problem-oriented medical records
    (POMR)
Popliteal pulse, 589
Pores, 174
Port-a-Cath, 992, 1591
Portal hypertension, 1618
Portal of entry, 490
Portal of exit, 489–490
Portal vein, 283
Ports, 1846
Port-wine stains, 1084, 1084f, 1219
Position, fetus, 1056–1057
Positioning, end-of-life care and, 883–884
Positive pressure ventilator, 1573–1574. *See also*
    Mechanical ventilation
Positron emission tomography (PET), 1352,
    1720, 1845
Post-anesthesia care unit (PACU),
    812, 827–828
Postanesthesia recovery (PAR), 812
Posterior descending artery (PDA), 263
Posterior pituitary gland, 1383t
Post-exposure prophylaxis (PEP), 1522
Postherpetic neuralgia, 1359
Postictal phase, seizures, 1356
Postlumbar decompression, 1328
Postmortem care of body, 889–890
Postmortem examination, 890
Postoperative shock, 520b
Postparenting stage, 102
Postpartum blues, 1125
Postpartum complications, 1123
Postpartum depression, 1125
Postpartum hematoma, 1123
Postpartum hemorrhage, 1123–1124
Postpartum period, 1070
Postpartum psychosis, 1125
Post-polio syndrome, 1205
Postterm newborn, 1131
Posttraumatic stress disorder (PTSD),
    1148, 1741
Post-treatment lyme disease syndrome
    (PTLDS), 1250
Postural defects, 1253–1254. *See also*
    Musculoskeletal disorders
Postural drainage, 1536, 1553
    assisting with, 1537
Postural hypotension, 595

Potassium (K⁺), 349t, 1317
    deficiency, 356t, 1316t
    excess, 1316t
    functions, 356t, 1316t
    guidelines for intake of, 356t
    imbalances, 1316t
    sources, 356t
    toxicity, 356t
Potassium chloride (KCl), 1319
Potassium hydroxide (KOH) test, 1171, 1173
Potassium-modified diet, 400
Potential of hydrogen (pH), 191
Potentiation, medication, 960
Pott disease, 1348, 1550
Pouchitis, 1598
Powered (positive) air-purified respirator (PAPR), 509
PP cells. *See* F cells
PPD. *See* Purified protein derivative (PPD)
PPE. *See* Personal protective equipment (PPE)
PPI. *See* Proton pump inhibitor (PPI)
PPN. *See* Peripheral parenteral nutrition (PPN)
Practical nurses, 11–12
Practical nursing programs, 1888
Prader–Willi syndrome (PWS), 1272
Pramlintide (Symlin), 1399
Prazosin HCl, 936
Preadolescence/pubescence, 123
Prebiotics, 367–368
Precancerous lesions, 1601
Precipitate, 1641
Precipitate labor and delivery, 1119
Precipitation, 1641
Precipitous labor, 1117
Preconceptional care, 1025
Preconceptional visits, 1025
Prediabetes, 68, 1393
Prednisolone (Hydrocortone), 931
Prednisone, 931, 1332
Preeclampsia, 1110
Pre-exposure prophylaxis (PrEP), 1526
Preferential seating, 1827
Preferred provider organizations (PPOs), 27
Prefilled syringes, 979f, 1009
Pregnancy, 68, 1023, 1033
    adapting to, 1046
    adolescent, 1118
    cardiac disorders in, 1115
    categories of drug safety in, 1046b
    chemical dependency in, 1115
    common concerns in, 1033
    common discomforts of, 1042–1045, 1043t–1045t
    danger signs, 1034b
    diabetes in, 1114
    driving during, 1040–1041, 1041f
    ectopic, 1108
    endometrium in, 1025
    existing conditions complicating, 1114–1115
    external changes in, 1033
    healthcare during, 1035–1045
    high risk, 1104–1126
    hormone levels in, 1034
    internal changes in, 1033–1034
    interrupted, 1106–1108
    maternal complications during, 1108–1114
    multiple, 1118
    as normal process, 1024–1035
    nutrition during, 1041–1042
    placental/amniotic disorders in, 1116–1118
    precautions, 1025
    preconceptional care, 1025
    preparing for labor and birth, 1046–1048
    prolonged, 1118
    sexual safety during, 1040
    siblings reaction to, 1047
    signs of, 1031–1033
    signs of possible problems during, 1034–1035
    teratogens, 1041
    terminology relating to, 1056b
    tobacco use and, 62–63
    weight gain during, 1042
    in woman older than 35 years, 1118
    woman's body during, changes in, 1031
Pregnancy-associated plasma protein-A (PAPP-A), 1275
Pregnancy-induced hypertension (PIH), 1034, 1109
    eclampsia, 1114
    preeclampsia, 1110
Pregnancy Risk Assessment Monitoring System (PRAM), 1108
Prejudice, 42
Preload, 268
Premature cervical dilation, 1107
Premature ejaculation, 1659
Premature rupture of membranes (PROM), 1118–1119
Premature ventricular contraction (PVC), 1446
Premenstrual dysphoric disorder (PMDD), 1261, 1678
Premenstrual syndrome (PMS), 1261, 1678
Prenatal care, 1024, 1035
    activity, 1038
    appetite, 1042
    breast care, 1038
    clothing, 1040
    components of, 1035–1045
    dietary counseling, 1042
    discomfort of pregnancy and, 1042, 1043t–1045t
    elimination and hygiene, 1037–1038
    exercise and posture, 1039
    healthcare provider, choice of, 1035
    health promotion, 1037–1042
    initial prenatal visit in, 1035–1036
    medical interventions, 1042, 1045
    oral hygiene, 1038
    rest, 1038, 1039f
    return prenatal visits in, 1036
    risk assessment in, 1035–1037
    sexual relations, 1040
    sleep, 1038–1039
    travel and employment, 1040–1041, 1041f
    vaginal infections, 1038
Prepuce, 1083
Presbycusis, 1710
Presbyopia, 1423, 1710
Preschoolers, 116–118
    age-related concerns, 1178–1179
    areas of concern, 117–118
    caregiver instructions, 1176
    care of, 1175
    cognitive and motor development, 117
    encopresis, 118
    enuresis in, 118
    masturbation, 117–118
    phobias and nightmares, 117
    physical growth, 116
    psychosocial development, 116–117
    reducing anxiety in, 1180
    sibling rivalry in, 117
    vital signs for, 1181t
Prescriptions, 910–911
Presentations, fetal, 1054
Pressure receptors, 256
Pressure support ventilation (PSV), 1574
Pressure wound, 867, 1289
    causes of, preventive measures for, 864t–865t
    classification of, 865, 866b
    common sites for, 859f
    and incontinence-associated dermatitis, 862t
    prediction of, 862–864
    prevention of, 865–866
    stages of, 861f
Preterm births, maternal smoking and, 68
Preterm infant, 1131
Preterm labor (PTL), 1034
Preterm premature rupture of the membranes (PPROM), 1034
Prevention, and healthcare, 59
Preventive care, benefits of, 20
Priapism, 1149, 1659
Primary aldosteronism, 1392
Primary bone tumors, 1349
Primary care providers (PCPs), 59
Primary diseases, 609
Primary healthcare, 79
Primary malignant bone tumors, 1349
Primary nephrogenic insipidus, 1387
Primary ovarian insufficiency (POI), female infertility and, 1151
Primigravida, 1024, 1056b
Primipara, 1056b
Private clinics, 1840–1841
Private duty nursing, 1885
PRM. *See* Partial-rebreathing mask (PRM)
PRN medication, 958
Probationary status, 1870
Probenecid (Probalan), 1333
Probiotics, 367–368
Problem-oriented medical records (POMR), 446
Problem-solving, 411
Procainamide hydrochloride (Pronestyl), 935
Prochlorperazine (Compazine), 946, 962
Prochlorperazine (Compro), 831
Proctitis, 1666
Proctocolectomy, 1260
Proctoscopy, 616t
Professional boundaries, 40
Progesterone, 236t, 949
Progestins, 240
Prognosis, 608
Programmed cell death, 1493
Progressive arthritis, 1330
Progress notes, 422
Projectile (forceful) vomiting, 1377
Projection, 1737t
Prolactin (PRL), 234t, 1387
Prolactin-inhibiting hormone or dopamine (PIH/DA), 234t
Prolactin-releasing hormone (PRH), 234t
Prolapsed cord, 1120–1121
Prolonged infantile apnea (PIA), 1212
PROM. *See* Passive range of motion (PROM)
Promethazine HCl (Promethegan), 825
Propranolol hydrochloride (Inderal), 935
Proprioception, 142, 1415, 1711
Proprioceptors, 228
Propylthiouracil (PTU), 1388
Prospective payment system (PPS), 28, 1832–1833
Prostaglandin, 232, 353
Prostaglandins A (PGA), 242
Prostate biopsy, 1657
Prostate cancer, 1664–1666
Prostatectomy, 1663f, 1665
Prostate gland, 334
Prostate-specific antigen (PSA) test, 1656
Prostatitis, 1661–1662
Prostheses, 1325
Prosthetic devices, for erection, 1149
Prosthetic grafts, 1305
Prosthetics, 1822
Protected Health Information (PHI/EPHI), 35

Protective device, 709–710
Protective isolation, 514
Protein-calorie malnutrition (PCM), 371
Protein-controlled diets, 397, 399
Protein-restricted diet, 399
Protein shock, 520b
Prothrombin, 314t
Prothrombin time (PT), 938
Proton-beam therapy, 1495
Proton pump inhibitor (PPI), 943, 1584
Protons, 156
Proton therapy, 1495–1497
Protozoa, 481–482
Provisional discharge (PD), 1746
Proxemics, 553
Proximal convoluted tubule (PCT), 324t
PRSP. See Penicillin-resistant *Streptococcus pneumonia* (PRSP)
Pruritus, 1290
Pseudodementia, 1719
Pseudoephedrine HCl (Sudafed), 943
Pseudomenstruation, 1083
Pseudomonas, 483
Pseudostrabismus, 1225
Psoriasis, 1296–1297, 1296f
PSV. See Pressure support ventilation (PSV)
Psychiatric disorders, 1826
Psychiatric emergencies, first-aid in, 543–544
Psychiatric nursing, 1735–1775
Psychiatric outreach, 1834
Psychiatric technicians, 1743
Psychiatric therapy, 1746–1759
Psychiatrists, 1743
Psychiatry unit (PSYCH), 462
Psychic (mental) shock, 520b
Psychodrama, 1747
Psychological health, 56
Psychological needs, 50. See also Human needs
Psychologist, 10b
Psychometric tests, 1721, 1738
Psychomotor retardation, 1739
Psychosis disorder, 1741
Psychotherapy, methods of, 1746
Psychotropic drugs, 1750
PTH. See Parathyroid hormone (PTH)
Ptosis, 257t, 1225, 1368
PTU. See Propylthiouracil (PTU)
Ptyalin, 351
Ptyalism, 1038, 1109
Puberty, 122
Public health centers, 79
Publicly reported measures (PRM), 1833
Puerperal infection, 1124
Puerto Rican populations, 382
PUFAs. See Polyunsaturated fatty acids (PUFAs)
Pulmonary angiography, 1534
Pulmonary artery, 282
Pulmonary artery occlusion pressure (PAOP), 1448
Pulmonary circulation, 282
Pulmonary edema, 1313, 1449b
Pulmonary embolism, 835, 1348, 1458
Pulmonary emphysema, 1557–1558
Pulmonary function test (PFT), 1534–1535
Pulmonary stenosis, 1233
Pulmonary tuberculosis, 1550
Pulmonary veins, 302
Pulmonic valve, 262
Pulmonologist, 1533
Pulse oximeter, 829, 1568
Pulse pressure, 592
Pulse rate, 587
    abnormal, postoperative, 829
Pump oxygenator, 1441
Puncture wound, 857

Pupil, 248
    assessment of, 629t
Pure tone audiometry tests, 1414
Purified protein derivative (PPD), 1535
Purines, 1332
Purkinje network, 1445
Purulent, 611
Purulent drainage, 860
Pustules, 625t, 628f
Pyelitis. See Pyelonephritis
Pyelonephritis, 1242, 1639
Pyloric sphincter, 309
Pyloric stenosis, 1143, 1239
Pyloromyotomy, 1239
Pyorrhea alveolaris, 1600
Pyothorax. See Empyema
Pyrexia (fever), 610t
Pyridoxine. See Vitamin B_6
Pyrimidines, 162
Pyuria, 1631

Q

Quadriparesis, 1281
Quadriplegia, 1281. See also Tetraplegia
Quality assurance (QA), 23–24
Quality improvement (QI) department, 464
Quality improvement organizations (QIOs), 1808
Quality indicators, 1830
Quality of life, 1814
Quickening, 1031
Quinidine sulfate (Quinidine), 935

R

RA. See Radiographic absorptiometry (RA)
Raccoon's eyes, 1375, 1375f
Race, 81
    American Indian and Alaska native, 82
    Asian, 82
    Black/African American, 82
    disease risk and, 609t
    Hispanic/Latino, 82
    native Hawaiian and other Pacific Islander, 82
    racial groups, 81
    White, 82
Radial artery, 587
Radial keratotomy (RK), 248
Radial pulse, 587
Radiation hazard, 81
Radiation therapy, 1495, 1498
    for leukemia, 1236
Radioactive iodine uptake (RAIU), 1384
Radioactive renogram, 1632
Radiographer, 10b
Radiographic absorptiometry (RA), 613t
Radiography, 1321–1322
Radioisotope, 1352
Radiology Department, 572
Radiotherapy, 1495
Radon, 80
Radon pollution, 80
RAIU. See Radioactive iodine uptake (RAIU)
Rales, breath sounds, 635t
Random blood glucose, 1385
Range-of-motion (ROM), 1291, 1538
    in musculoskeletal disorders, 1323
RAP. See Resident assessment protocol (RAP)
Rape, 1148
Rape kit, 1148
Rapid antigen detection test. See Rapid strep test
Rapid eye movement (REM), 1262
Rapid strep test, 1534
Rapid test, 1524
Rash, 1206
Rational emotive behavior therapy (REBT), 1747
Rational emotive therapy (RET), 1790

Rationalization, 1737t
Raynaud disease, 1460
Raynaud phenomenon, 1333
RBCs. See Red blood cells (RBCs)
RDAs. See Recommended Dietary Allowances (RDAs)
Reaction-formation, 1737t
Reality therapy, 1747
Receptive aphasia, 552
Receptors, 228
Reciprocity, 13
Recombinant human erythropoietin (RHE), 273
Recombivax-B, 1620
Recommended Dietary Allowances (RDAs), 346
Reconstructive surgery. See Plastic surgery
Recreational therapy, 1748
Rectal EMG, 613t
Rectal examination, 648t
Rectal (R) temperature, 583
Rectocele, 1680–1681
Rectum, 313
    disorder of, 1616–1617
Red blood cell count, 1468
Red blood cells (RBCs), 274–275, 360
Red Cross, 77
Reduced-calorie diet, 396
REE. See Resting energy expenditure (REE)
Refeeding syndrome, 1786
Referred pain, 802
Reflex arcs, 1362
Reflex center, 222
Reflexes, 229
    measuring of, 619
    newborn, 1085
Reflex hammer, 619
Reflex incontinence, 1636
Reflux, 1629
Refractive errors, 1257, 1422, 1423t
Refractive examination, 1414
Regional anesthesia, 818b
Regional preferences, 377
Registered nurse (RN), 9–10
    advanced certification, 11
    education, 10–11
    functions and role of, 10
Registered nurse anesthetist (RNA), 817
Registered nurse first assistant (RNFA), 817
Registered Pharmacist (RPh), 903
Registered record administrator (RRA), 464
Registered respiratory therapist (RRT), 462
Regression, 64, 1775
Regular diet as tolerated (DAT), 393
Rehabilitation, 213
Rehabilitation (REHAB) unit, 463
Reimbursement systems, 1806
Relapsing fever, 583
Relaxation and imagery, 29
Release of Information (ROI), 36
Releasing hormones (RH), 234t
Remarriage, 103
Remission, 1259
Remittent fever, 583
Remotivation techniques, 1709
Remotivation therapy, 1775
Renal arteriogram, 1632
Renal blood flow, 325
Renal calculi, nursing care plan, 1645–1646
Renal corpuscle, 322
Renal cortex, 322t
Renal failure, 1649–1655, 1649b
Renal function
    in burn injuries, 1302
    tests, 1631
Renal lithiasis, 1642
Renal medulla, 322t

Renal papillae, 321
Renal pelvis, 321
Renal pyramids, 321
Renal scan. *See* Radioactive renogram
Renal threshold, 327
Renin, 237t
Renin–angiotensin–aldosterone (RAA) system, 323
Repetitive strain injuries, 1329
Replantation, of limbs, 1326
Reporting, 453. *See also* Documentation
    change-of-shift, 453
    of client admissions, 500
    diet/nutrition, 346
    of incidents, 543
Repression, as defense, 1737t
Reprimands, 1903
Reproductive system
    disorders of, 1243–1244, 1260–1261
    medications affecting, 948–949
Reproductive system, female, 337–343
    breasts, 339–340
    effects of aging on, 343t
    external genitalia, 339
    hormonal influences, 340
    organs of, 337–339
    physiology, 340–343
    structure and function, 337–340
Reproductive system, male, 331–343
Resectoscope, 1647
Resident assessment protocol (RAP), 444
Residential treatment centers, 1885
Residual limb pain, 1325
Residual urine volume, 1633
Residual volume, 1534. *See also* Pulmonary function test (PFT)
Resignations, 1896
Resistance transfer factor (RTF), 483
Resource utilization groups (RUGs), 28
Respiration, 301–302
    assessment of, 589–591
    counting, 591
    external, 301
    internal, 301
    muscles of, 199t
    newborn and, 1077
    patterns in adult, 558t
    regulation of, 302, 589–591
    sounds, 591
Respiration rates, 590
Respirator, 1573
Respirator mask, 500f
Respiratory acidosis, 192, 1318t
Respiratory alkalosis, 193t, 1318t
Respiratory arrest, 1558
Respiratory complications, 832–833
Respiratory control, 589–590
Respiratory depression, narcotic overdose and, 927
Respiratory disorders, 1533–1565
    chronic, 1552–1558
    diagnostic tests, 1533–1536
    infectious, 1544–1552
    medical treatments, 1536
    neoplasms, 1559
    nursing process, 1540–1541
    surgical treatments, 1536–1544
Respiratory distress, sites of, 1189
Respiratory distress syndrome (RDS), 1137
Respiratory reflexes, 302
Respiratory status
    in burn injuries, 1302
    determination of, 1567–1568
Respiratory stimulants, 940
Respiratory syncytial virus (RSV), 1207

Respiratory system, 295
    effects of aging on, 139
    functions of, 295
    lower respiratory tract, 298–299
    medications affecting, 940–943
    physiology of, 157–158
    structure of, 162
    upper respiratory tract, 295–298
Respiratory tests, 615t
Respiratory therapist, 10b
Respiratory therapy (RT), 462
Respiratory tract, disorders of, 1237–1239
Respite care, 22, 887, 1809
Resting energy expenditure (REE), 350
Resting potential, 227–228
Rest, need for, 49–50
Rest position, during pregnancy, 1038, 1039f
Restraints, pediatric, 1185
Restrictive cardiomyopathy, 1450
Rest rooms, disabled persons and, 1827
Résumé, 1892, 1893b
Resuscitation of children, 1191
Retained placenta, 1117
Retention (urinary), 329t
Rete pegs, 171
Reticular activating system (RAS), 222
Reticuloendothelial system. *See* Mononuclear phagocyte system
Retina, 248–249
Retinal angiogram, 1414
Retinitis pigmentosa (RP), 1258
Retinoblastoma, 1258–1259
Retinoic acid syndrome, 1495
Retinoids, 1495
Retinol. *See* Vitamin A
Retinopathy, diabetic, 1406
Retinopathy of prematurity (ROP), 1138
Retrograde pyelogram, 1632
Retroplacental hemorrhage, 1117
Retrospective payment, 28
Retrovirus, 1520
Reversible ischemic neurologic deficit (RIND), 1462
Reye syndrome, 928, 1221
RF. *See* Rheumatoid factor (RF)
Rh antibody test, 1037
Rheumatic carditis, 1208
Rheumatic fever, 1207–1208
Rheumatic heart disease, 1207, 1450–1451
Rheumatoid arthritis (RA), 1329, 1330, 1518
    vs. osteoarthritis, 1331t
Rheumatoid factor (RF), 1321
Rh factors, 278
RH immune globulin (RhoGAM), 1036–1037
Rhinitis, 1544
    acute, 1544
    allergic, 1552–1553
Rhinoplasty, 1228, 1560
Rhinorrhea, 1248, 1375
RhoGAM (anti-D gamma globulin), 1115, 1139
Rh sensitization, 1106, 1139
Ribavirin (Copegus), 1207, 1620
Riboflavin, 349t, 366
Ribonucleic acid (RNA), 162
Ribosomal RNA, 162
Ribosomes, 483
Rickets, 1224, 1333–1334
Rickettsiae, 484
Rifampin, 1158
    in tuberculosis treatment, 1550
Right lymphatic duct, 283
Right to privacy, 34
Right ventricular hypertrophy, 1230
Rigidity, 1280
Ring splints, 1336

Ringworm of the foot. *See* Tinea pedis
Risk manager, 10b
Risperidone (Risperdal), 962
Rituals, 86
Rituximab (Rituxan), 1332, 1518
RN. *See* Registered nurse (RN)
Robotic procedures, 1845
Rods, 249t
ROI. *See* Release of Information (ROI)
Roller bandages, 539
Romberg test, 1378
Rooting reflex, 1085
Rorschach inkblot, 1738
Roseola, 1208
Rotator cuff injury, 1329
Rotavirus (RV), 1202
Roughage, 352
RRA. *See* Registered record administrator (RRA)
RRT. *See* Registered respiratory therapist (RRT)
RTF. *See* Resistance transfer factor (RTF)
Rubella, 1140, 1206
Rubeola, 1205
Rubin test, 1151
Rubs, heart sounds, 588
Rugae, 309
RUGs. *See* Resource utilization groups (RUGs)
Rule of Threes, 883, 883b
Ruptured uterus, 1119
Russell traction, 1339

S
Saccule, 251
Sacral edema, 1313
Saddle joints, 201
Safer sex, 1162
Safety Committee, 466
Safety Data Sheet (SDS), 470
Safety devices, 667
    of children, 1184
Safety syringe, 980, 980f
Salem sump tube, 1588
Salicylates, 927–928
Saline cathartics, 947
Saliva, 306
Salivary glands, 306, 350
Salivation, 306
Salmonella typhi, 485
Salpingitis, 1684
Salts, 375
Same-day surgery center, 812
Same-day surgery units (SDSUs), 1845–1849
Sanguineous drainage, 860
Saprophytes, 480
Sarcomas, 1256, 1488
SARS. *See* Severe acute respiratory syndrome (SARS)
Saturated fatty acids, 354b
SBAR process, 1811b
SBP. *See* Systolic blood pressure (SBP)
Scabies, 715, 1209, 1298
    scraping, 1290
Scarlet fever, 1207
Schiøtz tonometer, 1414
Schizoid personality disorder, 1740
Schizophrenia, 1285–1286, 1741–1742
    childhood, 1285
School-age child, 118–120
    age-related concerns, 1178
    areas of concern, 119–120
    care of, 1178, 1246–1263
    cognitive and motor development, 118–119
    nutritional aspect, 1263
    physical growth, 118
    psychosocial development, 118

School-age child (*continued*)
 responsibilities to, 119
 sex education to, 120
 sibling rivalry in, 119
 sleep deprivation, 1261–1262
 vital signs for, 1181t
School-based health services, 1842
Schools, violence in, 64
Schultze presentation, 1061
Schwann cells, 217
Scientific problem-solving, 412
 vs. nursing process, 418t
SCLC. *See* Small cell lung cancers (SCLC)
Sclera, 247–248
Sclerodactyly, 1333
Scleroderma, 1333, 1517t
Sclerose, 1617
Sclerotherapy, 1602
Scoliometer, 1254
Scoliosis, 633, 1253, 1253f, 1326
Scratch tests, 613t
Scrotum, 333
Scrub nurses, 1888
Scurvy, 366, 1224
SDS. *See* Safety Data Sheet (SDS)
Sebaceous cysts, 1298
Sebaceous glands, 173
 disorders of, 1298–1299
Seborrhea, 1299
Seborrheic dermatitis, 1299
Sebum, 173
Seclusion, mental health units and, 1761
Secobarbital (Seconal), 929
Secondary central diabetes insipidus, 1387
Secondary diseases, 609
Secondhand smoke, 62, 80
Secretagogues, 1401
Secretin, 237t
Security, 1761–1763, 1771
Sedatives, 928–929
Sedentary lifestyle, 373
Segmental resection. *See* Wedge resection
Segmented neutrophils (segs). *See* Granular leukocytes
Seizure disorders, 1355–1359
Seizures, 929
 classification of, 1356b
 client safety during, 1358
 precautions, 1357f
Selective serotonin reuptake inhibitors (SSRIs), 1758
Selenium (Se), 349t, 360
Self-actualization, 52–53
Self-actualization needs, 1860
Self-care unit, 463
Self-employment, 1889
Self-esteem, 52
 children's, promotion of, 102b
 death/dying and, 886
Self-inflicted wounds (SIW), 1740
Self-injurious behavior (SIB), 1740
Self-management, 1832
Self-monitoring of blood glucose (SMBG), 1395
Sella turcica, 233
Semen, 124
Semicircular canals, 251
Semilunar valve, 261
Seminal vesicle, 334
Seminiferous tubule, 334
Semisolid medications, 909
Senescence, 136
Senior housing, 1810
Sensory-perceptual disturbances, 1792
Sensory seizures, 1356b

Sensory system, 246–257
 balance and equilibrium, 253–254
 data collection, 1417
 disorders, 1413–1434
 documenting, 1418–1419
 effects of aging on, 256t–257t
 functions, 247b
 physiology of, 252–256
 structure, 246–247
Sensory system disorders
 data collection, 1417
 definition, 1413
 diagnostic tests, 1413–1414
 evaluation, 1420–1422
 medical treatments, 1415
 planning and implementation, 1418
 surgical treatments, 1415–1422
Sentence completion test, 1738
Separation anxiety, 1179–1180
Septicemias, 920
Septic shock, 520b
Septoplasty. *See* Submucous resection
Sequelae, 609
Sequential compression device (SCD), 781
Sequestration, 1347
Serosanguineous, 611
Serosanguineous drainage, 860
Serotonin and norepinephrine reuptake inhibitors (SNRI), 1284
Serous, 627t
Serous drainage, 860
Serous membranes, 167
Serum, 191
Serum albumin, 1471
Serum creatinine, 1631
Serum glutamic oxaloacetic transaminase (SGOT), 1584
Serum reaction, 1511
Serum shock, 520b
Serum sickness, 1511
Service animals, 1824
Severe acute respiratory syndrome (SARS), 488
Sex, 1147
 need for, 50
Sex education, to adolescence, 125
Sex hormones, 948–949
Sexual abuse, 1217–1218
Sexual assault evidence collection kit, 1148
Sexual assault forensic evidence kit, 1148
Sexual Assault Nurse Examiner (SANE), 1148
Sexual development, adolescence, 124–125
Sexual dysfunction, 1149–1150
Sexual health, 1147
Sexual intercourse, 1147
Sexuality, 1147–1150, 1713
 in diabetes, 1408
Sexually transmitted infections (STIs), 68, 1025, 1162–1173, 1256
 bacterial vaginosis, 1172–1173
 chlamydia, 1163–1164
 concerns related to, 1155
 cytomegalovirus, 1169
 genital herpes, 1169
 gonorrhea, 1164–1165
 prevention of, 1171
 syphilis, 1166
 treatment of, 1149
 trichomoniasis, 1171–1172
 vulvovaginal candidiasis, 1171
Sexual orientation, 1147–1148
Sexual response, female, 242–243
Sexual rights, 1148
Sexual violence (SV), 1148
SGOT. *See* Serum glutamic oxaloacetic transaminase (SGOT)

Shaken baby syndrome, 1214, 1267
Shaman (medicine man), 86
Shampoo, 707–709
Sharp debridement, wound, 870
Shell shock (battle fatigue), 521b
Sheltered workshops, 1744
Shingles, 1359–1362. *See also* Herpes zoster
Shock, 519–522
 assessment of, 519–522
 capillary refill test for, 524
 hemorrhagic, 519
 hypovolemic, 519–522
 nursing care guidelines, 522
 postoperative, 829
 primary, 519
 progressing, assessment for, 524
 secondary, 522
 treatment of, 519–522
 types of, 520b–521b
Shortness of breath (SOB), 1541
Shortness of breath on exertion (SOBOE), 1541
Short-stay surgical center, 812
Short-term home care, 1832
Short-term rehabilitation units, 1806
Shoulder presentation, 1054, 1120
Shoulders, muscles of, 199t
Shuffling, 1366
Shunt, 1652
 types of, 1652–1653
SIADH. *See* Syndrome of inappropriate antidiuretic hormone (SIADH)
Siblings, 98
Sickle cell crises, 1234
Sickle cell disease (SCD), 1234, 1478
Sickle cell trait, 1234
Sigh breath, 302
Sigmoid colon, disorder of, 1616–1617
Sigmoidoscopy, 1586
Significant figure, 900–901
Sign language, 1422
Sildenafil (Viagra), 1658
Silent neoplasm. *See* Stomach cancer
Silicosis, 1553
Silver nitrate, 1304
Silver sulfadiazine, 1304
Simethicone (Mylicon, Gas-X), 947
Simian line, 1275
Simple fractures, 1334, 1339b
Simple mask, 1570
Simple triage and rapid treatment (START) system, 474
Simpulse VariCare system, 873
SIMV. *See* Synchronized intermittent mandatory ventilation (SIMV)
Single-adult household, 99
Single energy x-ray absorptiometry (SXA), 613t
Single-parent families, 99
Single-photon emission computed tomography (SPECT), 1720
Single-voided urine specimen, 764
Sinoatrial node (SA node), 266
Sinus bradycardia, 1446
Sinuses, 297
Sinusitis, 1544
 acute, 1559–1560
 chronic, 1560
Sinusoids, 283
Sinus tachycardia, 1446
Sinus tract, packing, 868
Sitz bath, 791–792
Sjögren syndrome, 1517t, 1710
Skeletal traction, 1338–1341
Skeleton, 195–205
 appendicular, 205–207
 axial, 202–204

bones, 195–198
　divisions of, 202–204
　joints, 198–202
Skilled nursing facility (SNF), 23, 1807
Skin, 169–172
　biopsies, 613t
　care in musculoskeletal disorders, 1324
　color of, 172
　color variations, 613t
　communication, 170b
　data collection, 613t
　dermis, 171
　epidermis, 173
　hypodermis, 169
　inspection of, 624f
　lesions, 627t
　lifestyle to protect, 176
　maintenance of, 176
　palpation of, 613t, 624f
　sensory awareness, 176
　structures of, 172–174
　subcutaneous tissue, 171–172
　sunscreens for, 176
　tests, 613t
　turgor, 624f
　vitamin D production, role in, 175
Skin breakdown, 857. See also Wound
　causes of, 861
　prevention of, 867b
　types of, 862–867
Skin Bundle, 857
Skin cancer, 1306–1308, 1307f
Skin care, 709
Skin changes, in pregnancy, 1032
Skin disorders, 1250–1253, 1289–1308, 1290b
　eczema, 1219
　nevi, 1219
　nursing process, 1293–1295
　rash, 1219
Skin grafts, 1293
　in burn injuries, 1305
Skin preparation, preoperative, 823
Skin tests, 1507, 1507f, 1535–1536
Skin traction, 1338
Skull, 202–203
　bones of, 202b
　fractures, 1374–1375
Skull tongs traction, 1338–1341
Skyla, 1159
SLE. See Systemic lupus erythematosus (SLE)
Sleep apnea, 1261–1262, 1275
Sleep apnea syndrome, 1552
Sleep deprivation, 1261
Sleep disorders, 1261–1262
Sleep hygiene, 1261
Sleep, need for, 49–50
Sleep-onset anxiety, 1261
Sleep studies, 614t
Sling, applying, 535
Slit lamps, 1414
Slough, 865
Sloughed, 611
Small cell lung cancers (SCLC), 1559
Small-for-gestational-age (SGA) infants, 1212
Small intestine, 309–310
　absorption in, 239
　cancer, 1616
　digestion in, 239
SMBG. See Self-monitoring of blood glucose (SMBG)
Smegma, 1091
Smell, 225t
Smoker's cough, 1557
Smoker's patch. See Leukoplakia buccalis
Smoke, secondhand, 62–63

Smoking, 62
　cessation, 63
　and contagious illness, 1248b
　in diabetes, 1407–1408
　disease risk and, 609t
　hazards of, 63, 176
　medical conditions from, 63
Smooth-pursuit movement (SPM), 252
Sneezing, 224
Snellen chart, 1413
Snoring, 1552
SOAP charting, 446, 447t
SOAPE charting, 447t
SOAPIE charting, 447t
SOAPIER charting, 446, 447t
SOB. See Shortness of breath (SOB)
SOBOE. See Shortness of breath on exertion (SOBOE)
Social health, 56
Social Security Act, 1854
Social Security Administration (SSA), 77
Social Security Disability Income (SSDI), 27, 1746
Social services department, 464
Social workers, 10b, 1743
Sociocultural factors, 386–388
Sodium (Na$^+$), 360b, 1315–1317
　client education on, 463
　deficiency, 356t, 1316t
　excess, 1316t
　function of, 356t, 1316t
　guidelines for intake of, 372b
　imbalances, 1316t
　sources, 356t
　toxicity, 356t
Sodium-controlled diet, 399–400
Sodium-glucose transporter-2 inhibitors, 1401
Sodium–potassium pump, 189
Soft connective tissues, 166
Soft diet, 394t
Solid fats, 379b
Solid food, in young children, 1244
Solid medications, 908
Soluble fiber, 395b
Solvent, 184
Somatostatin, 237t
Somatotropin (STH), 1387. See also Human growth hormone (HGH)
Somnambulism, 1262
Somniloquy, 1262
Somnolence, 1385
Somnolent, 1862–1864
Somogyi phenomenon, 1404
Sonography, 617
Sore throat, 1248, 1544–1545
Soul food, 377
Sound amplification, 253
Southeast Asian populations, 382–383
Spastic diplegia, 1281
Spastic hemiplegia, 1281
Spasticity, 1280
Spastic quadriplegia, 1281
Special learning disabilities (SLD), 1267–1269
Special needs, 1265–1286
Special Olympics, 1823
Special respiratory precautions (SRP), 509–511
Specific immunity, 290
Speech, characteristics of, 448
Speech development, 1268
Speech impairment, 1268
Speech reading, 1422
Speech therapist, 10b
Speech therapy, 1562
Spermatic cord, 333
Spermatids, 334

Spermatogenesis, 334–335
Spermatozoa, 335
Sperm cells, 334–335
Sperm concentration/count, 1150
Spermicides, 1160
Sphygmomanometer, 421
Spica (body) cast, 1337
Spina bifida, 1142, 1222
Spinal anesthesia, 818b
Spinal cord, 1352
　disorders, 1362–1364
　injury to, 226
　tumor, 1362
Spinal fusion, 1327
Spinal nerves, 1362f
Spinal shock, 521b
Spinal stenosis, 1326, 1330
Spine range of motion, 450t
Spiral fractures, 1335
Spiritual health, 56
Spiritual support, 1856
Spirometer, 1534
Spirometry test, 612
Spironolactone (Aldactone), 948
Spleen, 265t
Splenectomy, 1234
Splinting, of incisions, 833
Splints, 1328, 1821–1822
Spontaneous abortion, 1034, 1106–1107, 1166
Spontaneous rupture of membranes (SROM), 1058
Spores, 481
Sports, disabled clients and, 1823
Sprains, 1334
Sputum specimen, 769, 1533
Squamous cell carcinoma, 1308
SRP. See Special Respiratory Precautions (SRP)
SSA. See Social Security Administration (SSA)
Stab wounds, 1846
Stagnation, in middle adults, 129–130
Standards of care, 442
Stannous fluoride, 943
Stapes, 250
Staphylococcus aureus, 485t
Staples, 873
　removal of, 873f
Starches, 397
State Board of Nursing, 37–38
State employment services, 1890
Static balance, 253
Stations of fetal head, 1054–1056
STAT medications, 958
Status asthmaticus, 940, 1555
Status epilepticus, 1356, 1357
Status epilepticus seizures, 1356
Steatorrhea, 1622
Stent, 1643, 1845
Step-down unit, hospital, 21
Stepfamily, 100
Stepping reflex, 1085
Stereophotogrammetry, wound, 861
Stereotype, 86
Stereotyping, 86
Sterile assistant, 824
Sterile gloves, 844–845, 844f
Sterile gown, 843–844
Sterile, meaning of, 843
Sterile packages, opening of, 848–849
Sterile technique, 842–845. See also Surgical asepsis
Sterile vaginal examination (SVE), 1062, 1116
Sterility, 1150
Sterilization, 841–842, 1161–1162
Steri-Strips, 873
Sternum, 202t

Steroids, 931
    long-term use of, side effects of, 931
Steroid use disorders, 1799–1800
Sterols, 355
Stertorous breathing, 591. See also Snoring
Stethoscope, 421
STH. See Somatotropin (STH)
Stillbirth, 1117, 1141
Stimulants, 1144
Stimulant use disorders, 1797–1799
St. John wort, 1158
Stoma, 1595
Stomach, 237t
    digestion in, 237t
    disorders of, 1604–1609
    medications affecting, 926
    wall of, layers of, 297
Stomach cancer, 1608–1609
    symptoms of, 1609b
Stomatitis, 1498–1500, 1600
Stool softeners, 945t
Stool specimen, 768
    for ova and parasites (O&P), 1208
Stool tests, 1584
Stork bite, 1084, 1084f
Strabismus, 1225
Strains, 1334
Stranger anxiety, infant, 110
Strangulation, 1558
Stratum corneum, 173
Strawberry tongue, 1233
Strep throat, 1544
Streptococcal infections, 1207–1208
Streptococcal sore throat, 1207, 1544–1545
Streptococcus pneumoniae, 1204, 1371, 1546
Stress, 1501
    cumulative, 63
    divorce and, 99
    in eldest adults, 130
    family coping and, 103–104
    family response to, 104b
    and health, 63
    and maladaptive behaviors, 63
    physical responses to, 63
    psychological responses to, 63
    remarriage and, 103
    socioeconomic, 103
Stress/emotional shock, 496
Stress incontinence, 1636
Stress management, pain and, 809
Stress test, 1437
Stretch-net bandages, 779, 781
Striae, 637t
Striae gravidarum, 1117
Stridor, 633t
Stroke, 1359, 1360, 1462
Stroke in evolution (SIE), 1462
Stroke volume (SV), 268
Structural disorders, 1560. See also Nose
Struvite stones, 1642
Subacute bacterial endocarditis (SBE), 1451
Subacute inflammation, 611
Subcortical dementia, 1719
Subcultures, 81
Subcutaneous injections, 982–985
Subcutaneous tissue, 171–172
Subdural hematoma, 1376, 1376f
Sublimation, as defense, 1737t
Sublingual (SL) medications, 962
Subluxation, 1330, 1331f
Submandibular gland prolapse, 306
Submucous resection, 1560
Substance abuse, 63, 1136, 1708–1709
Substance Abuse and Mental Health Services
    Administration (SAMHSA), 74

Substance abuse programs, 1885
Substance use disorders
    causes, 1779–1780
    diagnosis, 1778–1779
    evaluation, 1783
    management, 1780
    medications, 1787–1788
    nature, 1780
    nursing care measurement, 1781–1783
    treatment motivation, 1785
Sucking reflex, 113, 1085
Sucralfate (Carafate), 1605
Sucrase, 351
Sucrose, 351
Suctioning, end-of-life care and, 884
Sudden death, emergency care and, 525–527
    advanced cardiac life support, 526
    basic cardiac life support, 526
    client at home, 526–527
    code in healthcare facility, 527
    compression-only CPR, 526
Sudden infant death syndrome (SIDS),
    1089, 1139, 1212–1213
    maternal smoking and, 62
Sudden unexpected infant death (SUID),
    1212–1213
Suffocation, 1558
    in children, 1212
Sugar, 351
Suicidal ideation (SI), 1284b, 1285, 1766
Suicide, 67, 1284–1285
    attempts, 1766
    gesture, 1285
    risk factors for, 1284b
Sulfamethoxazole/trimethoprim, 921
Sulfasalazine (Azulfidine), 1332
Sulfonamides and urinary antiseptics, 920
Sulfonylureas (Diabinese, Glucotrol, DiaBeta,
    Micronase), 1401
Sulfur (S), 357t
Sulindac (Clinoril), 1332
Sundown syndrome, 1717
Sun protection factor (SPF), 1307
Superficial pain, 255
Superimposed infusion, 995
Superior vena cava (SVC), 265t
Supine hypotension syndrome, 1038, 1039f
Supine lift, 663
Supplemental oxygen, end-of-life care and, 884
Support groups, pain management, 809
Suppositories, 964, 1676
    children and, 1188
Suppression, as defense, 1737t
Suppuration, 611
Suprapubic, 1634
Suprarenal glands. See Adrenal gland
Surfactant, 299, 1077
Surgical asepsis, 842, 1107
Surgical débridement, 1293
Surgical hand scrub, 498b
Surgical hypothermia, 1441
Surgical ICU (SICU), 463
Surgical incision, 857, 858f
Surgical mask, 843
Surgical risk, in diabetes, 1405
Surgical shock, 521b
Surgical site infections (SSI), normothermia
    and, 788
Surgical technician/technologist, 10b
Surgical ureteral reimplantation, 1637
Surgi-Pads, 869, 875
Surrogacy, 1153
Survival needs, 49. See also Human needs
Susceptible host, 490–491
Sustained release (SR) medications, 915b

Swaddling, 1091
SXA. See Single energy x-ray absorptiometry
    (SXA)
Sydenham chorea, 1208
Symbiosis, 492
Synapse, 218f
Synchronized intermittent mandatory ventilation
    (SIMV), 1574
Syncytium, 266
Syndactylism, 1142
Syndrome of inappropriate antidiuretic hormone
    (SIADH), 1387
Synergistic medications, 907
Synovectomy, 1331
Synovial fluid, 180
Synovial joints, 200
Synthetic casts, 1336–1337
Syphilis, 1166
Syringes, 979–981
Systemic circulation, 282–283
Systemic lupus erythematosus (SLE),
    1329, 1518t
Systemic vascular resistance (SVR), 268
Systems (body), 167
Systole, 262, 592
Systolic blood pressure (SBP), 592

T
Tabes dorsalis, 1166
Tablet, 908
Taboo, 86
Tachycardia, 587
Tachypnea, 1348, 1542t
Tactile observation, 422
Tadalafil (Cialis), 1658
Talipes, 1141–1142, 1220–1221, 1220f
Tangles, 1722
Tape, 779
Tardive dyskinesia (TD, TDK), 1750–1755
Targeted drug therapy, 1493
Target populations, 79
Taste, 225t
Tay–Sachs disease (TSD), 1271–1272
TB. See Tuberculosis (TB)
T-binders, 782
TCDB. See Turning, coughing, and deep
    breathing (TCDB)
T cells, 1521
Team leaders, 1901–1904
Teamwork, in healthcare, 24
Technical nurse, 10
Technical skills, in implementing nursing care, 437
TED sox, 780
Teeth, 307
Tegaderm/OpSite, 870
Telangiectasia, 1461
Telecommunication department, 464
Telehealth, 22, 1832, 1886
Telemonitoring, 1842
Telephone order, read back (TORB), 1875
Temazepam (Restoril), 929
Temperament, 110
Temperature
    children, 1182
    physiology of, 157
Temperature, pulse, respiration (TPR), 350
Temperature regulation, need for, 50
Temporal artery (TA) temperature, 585
Temporal lobe, cerebral cortex, 251
Temporal pulse, 587
Temporomandibular joint (TMJ) disorders, 1328
Tendonitis, 610
Tendons, 167
Tenesmus, 1259, 1612, 1616
Tenosynovitis, 1329

Tenotomy, 1220
Tension pneumothorax, 528
Tenting, 1314
Tepid sponge, 793
Teratogens, 1140, 1267
Terminal disinfection, 502
Terminal illness, 150
Testes, 236t
    hormones secreted by, 1383t
Testicular examination, 426t
Testicular self-examination, 1667–1668
Testicular shock, 521b
Testosterone, 1799
Tetanus, 1202
Tetracyclines, 920, 1158
Tetrahydrocannabinol (THC), 1795
Tetralogy of Fallot (TOF), 1142, 1230
Tetraplegia, 1362
Tet spells, 1230
TFTs. See Thyroid function tests (TFTs)
THA. See Total hip arthroplasty (THA)
Thalassemia, 1478–1479
Thalassemia major, 1479
Thematic apperception tests (TAT), 1738
Theoretical framework, nursing actions, 14
Therapeutic baths, 1291
    nursing care guidelines, 1291
Therapeutic communication. See also Communication
    nursing care guidelines, 550
    techniques, 557–561
        communication in special situations, 559
        communication to client speaks different language, 550
        dealing with specific client behaviors, 560
        interviewing, 557–559
Therapeutic community, 1785
Therapeutic diet, 393. See also Modified diet
Therapeutic dose, medication, 909
Therapeutic environment, 1759–1761
Therapeutic recreation, 1748
Therapeutic soaks, 791
Therapeutic touch, 29
Thermometers
    automatic, 584
    chemical, 584f
    disposable electronic, 584
    electronic, 584
    glass, 586
Thermoregulation, 174–175
Thermotherapy, of retinoblastoma, 1258
Thiamin, 366
Thiazide diuretics, 947
Thigh and lower leg, muscles of, 210t
Third-party payment, 1886
Thirst, 1312
    postoperative, 830
Thirst center, 181
Thomas splints, 1338
Thompson Practical Nursing School, 5
Thoracentesis, 1536–1538
Thoracic (rib) cage, 204–206
Thoracic duct, 280
Thoracic-lumbar-sacral orthosis (TLSO), 1328
Thoracotomy, 1538–1539
Threatened abortion, signs of, 1034
Thrill, 1652–1653
Throat
    culture, 1534
    disorders of, 1561–1563
Thrombin, 277
Thromboangiitis, 1459
Thrombocytes. See Platelets
Thrombocythemia, 1480

Thrombocytopenia, 1480
Thrombocytosis, 1468
Thrombolytic agents, 835
Thrombolytic therapy, 1438
Thrombophlebitis, 938, 1124, 1455–1458
    postoperative, 835
Thromboplastin, 277
Thrombopoietin, 237t
Thrombosis, 1234, 1452
Thrombus, 277
Thrush, 1141, 1600
Thymectomy, 1369
Thymomas, 1368
Thymopoietin, 241
Thymosin, 241
Thymus, 237t
Thymus gland, 279
Thyrocalcitonin, 239
Thyroid crisis, 1391
Thyroidectomy, 1388
Thyroid function tests (TFTs), 1383–1384, 1384t
Thyroid gland, 239
    disorders of, 1388–1391
    hormones secreted by, 1383t
    neoplasms, 1388
Thyroid replacement hormones, 931
Thyroid-stimulating hormone (TSH), 1388
Thyroid storm, 1391
Thyroid ultrasound test, 1384
Thyrotoxicosis, 1391
Thyrotropin. See Thyroid-stimulating hormone (TSH)
Thyrotropin-releasing hormone (TRH), 234
Tibia, 197
Tics, 1278
Tidal volume, 1534. See also Pulmonary function test (PFT)
Tincture of benzoin, 873
Tinea pedis, 1252–1253
Tine test, 1536
Tinnitus, 254
Tissue fluids, 1312
Tissue grafts, 1293
Tissue plasminogen activator (t-PA), 1438
Tissues, 165–167
    subcutaneous, 171–172
TLSO. See Thoracic-lumbar-sacral orthosis (TLSO)
T-lymphocytes (T-cells), 241
TMJ. See Temporomandibular joint (TMJ)
Tobacco use, 62–63. See also Smoking
    pregnancy and, 63
Tobacco use disorder, 1800
Tocodynamometer, 1064
Tocolytic agents, 1119
Toddlerhood/toddlers (1–3 years), 113–116
    areas of concern, 114–116, 1178–1179
    care, 1177
    caregiver instructions, 1176
    cognitive and motor development, 114
    negativism in, 114
    physical growth of, 113
    psychosocial development, 114
    reducing anxiety in, 1180
    ritualism and, 114
    vital signs for, 1181t
Toenails, 705–706
Toilet articles, 567
Toilet training, toddlers, 114–115
Tolerable upper intake level (UL), 348
Tongue, 203
Tonic–clonic (grand mal) seizures, 1356b
Tonic neck reflex, 1085
Tonic phase, seizures, 1356
Tonic seizures, 1356b

Tonometers, 1414
Tonsillectomy, 1227
Tonsillitis, 1227
Tonsils, 290
Topical agents, in burn injuries, 1304
Topical dermatologic agents, 921
TORCH syndrome, 1131, 1140
Torticollis, 1221
Total hip arthroplasty (THA), 1343
Total hip replacement, 1343
Total parenteral alimentation. See Total parenteral nutrition (TPN)
Total parenteral nutrition (TPN), 992, 1187, 1305, 1591
    administration of, 992
    dying person and, 884
    patient receiving, 1591
Touch, 171
    cultural considerations, 95
    therapeutic use of, 443
Tourette syndrome (TS), 1277–1278
Tourniquet, 539
Toxic dementias, 1725
Toxic dose, medication, 909
Toxic megacolon, 1260
Toxic shock syndrome (TSS), 1160
Toxins, 491
Toxoplasmosis, 1140, 1208, 1526
TPN. See Total parenteral nutrition (TPN)
TPR. See Temperature, pulse, respiration (TPR)
Trace minerals, 358t
Trachea (windpipe), 239
Tracheobronchial tree, 298–299
Tracheoesophageal fistula, 1143
Tracheoesophageal puncture, 1562
Tracheostomy, 1535, 1562, 1566, 1574–1575, 1574f–1575f
    nursing procedure, 1580
Traction, 1337–1341
    caring for clients in, 1341
    forces, 1338
Trade name (medication), 906
Tramadol (Ultram), 928
Transactional analysis (TA), 1747
Transcellular fluids, 180
Transcultural healthcare, 81–98
    cultural assessment, 88b
Transcutaneous electrical nerve stimulation (TENS), 808, 1825
Transdermal medications, 909, 921
Transdermal (TD) patches, 921, 967, 977, 1158
Transdermal testing, 613t
Transducer, 616t
Transection, 1362
Trans fats, 398t
Trans-fatty acids, 354b
Transfer belt, 656
Transfer board, 665
Transfer, client, to another unit, 573–574
Transfer RNA, 162
Transfusion, 985
Transgender, 1147
Transient (temporary) incontinence, 1635
Transient ischemic attack (TIA), 1462
Transient tachypnea of the newborn (TTN), 1136–1137
Transitional care facilities, 1806, 1811
Transitioning, 1147, 1836
Transition of care (TOC), 1810
Translation services, 464
Translingual (TL) medications, 962
Transmission-based precautions, 1201
Transparent dressing, 870, 871f
Transplanted organs, rejection of, 1654
Transport maximum (TM), 327

Transposition of great arteries (TGA), 1230
Transradial catheterization, 1438
Transurethral resection of a bladder tumor (TURBT), 1647
Transverse fractures, 1342, 1343f
Trapeze, 690
Trauma, 1253, 1558–1559, 1601
　absence of air exchange, 1558
　care, 1335–1344
　chest, 1558
　drowning/near drowning, 1558
　drug poisoning, respiratory complications in, 1558
　head, 1373–1377
　pneumothorax, 1558–1559
　spinal cord, 1362
Trauma ICU (TICU), 463
Traumatic brain injury (TBI), 1719, 1825
Traumatic injuries, 70, 1334–1335
Traumatic shock, 520b
Travel, in diabetes, 1408
Travel nursing, 1885
Tremors, 1280
T₄ replacement, 1389
Treponema pallidum, 1166
Trial and error problem-solving, 411–412
Triamterene (Dyrenium), 948
Trichloroacetic acid, 1171
Trichomonas vaginalis, 1681
Trichomoniasis, 1171–1172
Tricuspid atresia, 1232f, 1233
Tricuspid valve, 262
Tricyclic antidepressants (TCAs), 1758
Trigeminal nerve (CN V), 249
Trigeminal neuralgia, 1359
Triglycerides, 397
Trimesters, 1024
Trimethoprim-sulfamethoxazole (TMP-SMX), 1547
Tripeptides, 355
Triple marker screen, 1037
Trisomy 21, 1140, 1275
Trocar, 1536
Trochanter rolls, 651f
Troche, 908
Trochlear nerve (CN IV), 249
Tropic hormones, 234
Trousseau sign, 1390, 1390f
True/total incontinence, 1635–1636
TSH. *See* Thyroid-stimulating hormone (TSH)
TST. *See* Tuberculin skin test (TST)
Tubal embryo transfer (TET), 1153
Tubal ligation, 1161
Tubal pregnancy, 1108. *See also* Ectopic pregnancy
Tub bath, 711–712
Tube feeding, 400–401
　administration, 403b
　liquid formulas for, 401
　nursing considerations, 402t
　placement sites for, 401
Tube feedings. *See* Enteral nutrition
Tubercle, 1549
Tubercle bacilli, 1549
Tuberculin blood tests, 1536
Tuberculin skin test (TST), 1550. *See also* Purified protein derivative
Tuberculin syringe, 982
Tuberculosis (TB), 1526, 1549
　active, 1549–1550
　admission screening for, 498b
　atypical, 1550
　causes, 1549
　diagnosis, 1550
　drugs for, 1551

　latent, 1549–1550
　latent infection and active, 1549–1550
　miliary, 1550
　multidrug-resistant, 1550
　nursing consideration, 1551
　prevention, 1551
　primary, 1549
　pulmonary, 1550
　risk for, 1549
　signs and symptoms, 1550
　treatment, 1550–1551
　vaccine for, 1551
Tuberculosis osteomyelitis, 1348
Tuberculosis testing, in pregnancy, 1036
Tubular damage, 1650
Tubular reabsorption, 326–327
Tubular secretion, 327
Tumor, 1306, 1487
　benign, 70
　malignant, 70
　markers, 1490–1491, 1491t
　nonmalignant, 1306
Tunics, 247
Tuning fork, 619
Tunneling, 860, 860f
Tunnel vision, 1258
Turgor, 623t, 1311
Turning, coughing, and deep breathing (TCDB), 833, 1543
Tweaking, 1798
T&X. *See* Typed and crossmatched (T&X)
Tympanic (TM) temperature, 586f
Tympanoplasty, 1226
Typed and crossmatched (T&X), blood, 611
Tzanck smear, 1290

U

UA. *See* Urinalysis (UA)
UAP. *See* Unlicensed assistive personnel (UAP)
UBT. *See* Urea breath test (UBT)
Ulcer, 857, 1604
　diabetic, 1405f
　management, 1608
　symptoms of, 1608b
Ulcerative colitis (UC), 1260, 1613
Ultrasonography (US), 1491–1492
　abdomen, 1673
　breast tissue, 1672
　for fetus visualization, 1032
　in musculoskeletal disorders, 1322
　in pregnancy, 1120
　test, 617
Ultrasound (US) treatment (heat application), 790
Umbilical arteries, 1029
Umbilical cord, 1029
　complications, 1120–1121
Umbilical hernia, 1239
Umbilical vein, 1029
Umbilicus, 1029
UN. *See* United Nations (UN)
Unclassified seizures, 1356b
Undermining, 860
Undescended testicle, 1659–1660
UNICEF. *See* United Nations Children's Fund; UN program, the United Nations Children's Fund (UNICEF)
Uniform Anatomical Gift Act, 882
Uniform Determination of Death Act, 1980, 41
Unit clerk, 10b
Unit-dose packages, 952
　opening of, 952, 952b
United Nations (UN), 72–73
United Nations Children's Fund (UNICEF), 73
United Nations Proclamation for the Disabled, 1814b

United Network of Organ Sharing (UNOS), 43, 1653
United States
　acquired immunodeficiency syndrome in, 59
　healthcare plans available in, 26t
　history of nursing in, 4–6
United States Department of Agriculture (USDA), 346
United States Pharmacopeia/National Formulary (USP-NF), 905
United States Pharmacopoeia (USP), 364
United States Public Health Service (USPHS), 73–74
Universal Transfer Forms (UTFs), 1811
Unlicensed assistive personnel (UAP), 11, 37, 462
Unoccupied bed, 687
UN program, the United Nations Children's Fund (UNICEF), 73
UPP. *See* Urethral pressure profile (UPP)
Upper respiratory infection (URI), 1212, 1237
UPT. *See* Urine pregnancy test (UPT)
Urea breath test (UBT), 1584
Ureter, 325
Ureteral/urethral strictures, 1644
Ureter/bladder stones, 1643
Ureterolithiasis, 1642–1644
Ureterolithotomy, 1643
Ureter stones, 1643
Urethra, 326, 1660
Urethral pressure profile (UPP), 1633
Urge incontinence, 1636
Urgent care department, 463
Urgi-centers, 1844
Urinalysis (UA), 1630–1631
　nursing consideration, 1631
Urinary and renal stones, removal of, 1644f
Urinary antiseptics, 920–921
Urinary bladder, 327
Urinary catheterization, 845–846
Urinary disorders, 1629–1655
　diagnostic tests, 1630–1635
　imaging studies, 1631–1633
　laboratory tests for, 1630–1631
　nursing process, 1634–1635
Urinary diversion, 1647–1649
　ileal conduit, 1647
　types of, 1647b
Urinary incontinence, 1635–1637
Urinary obstruction, 1242
Urinary retention, 329t
　end-of-life care and, 884
　postoperative, 832
Urinary system, 320–330, 1634–1635
　disorders of, 1241–1243
　effect of aging on, 328t–329t
　female, 320
　functions, 321b
　male, 328
　medications affecting, 947–948
　physiology of, 322f
　structure, 323f
Urinary tract infection (UTI), 1242, 1637–1639
Urinary tract trauma, 1649
Urinary tract tumors, 1646–1649
Urination, 326
　frequent, in pregnancy, 1031
Urine
　abnormalities in, 1630t
　characteristics and composition, 147t
　formation, 326–327
　glucose in, 1384
Urine pregnancy test (UPT), 611, 1032
Urine-specific gravity (SG), 764
Urine specimen, 762
　collection of, pediatric, 1187

Index

Urine testing, in pregnancy, 1036
Urine toxicology (UTox), 611
Urinometer, 764
Urodynamic tests, 1633–1634
Uroflowmetry, 1633
Urologic tests, 616t
Urology, 462, 1630t
Ursodiol (Actigall), 1622
Urticaria, 1295, 1508
US. *See* Ultrasonography (US)
U.S. Census Bureau, 82, 86b
U.S. Department of Labor (DOL), 76
U.S. Environmental Protection Agency's (EPA), 74
U.S. Food and Drug Administration (FDA), 903
Usher syndrome, 1258
USP. *See* United States Pharmacopoeia (USP)
USPHS. *See* United States Public Health Service (USPHS)
Uterine atony, 1124
Uterine changes, in pregnancy, 1032
Uterine contractions, 1058–1059
Uterine cycle, 342
Uterine fibroids, female infertility and, 1151
Uterine inertia, 1119–1120
Uterine rupture, 1119
Uterine souffle, 1032
Uterine tubes, 338
Uterus, 339
    hormones secreted by, 222
    medications affecting, 949
UTox. *See* Urine toxicology (UTox)
Utricle, 251
Uvulopalatopharyngoplasty, 1552

V

Vaccination for hepatitis B, 1080
Vaccine, 292
Vaccine Information Statements (VIS), 1177
Vacuum-assisted closure (VAC) device, 872, 872f
Vacuum constriction device, 1149
Vacuum extraction, 1122
VAE. *See* Ventilator-associated enterococcus (VAE)
Vagina, 334
Vaginal bleeding, in pregnancy, 1034
Vaginal ring, 1159
Vaginal speculum, 621
Vaginal sponge, 1160
Vaginal suppositories, 1676
Vaginismus, and female sexual dysfunction, 1150
Vaginitis, 1681–1683
Vagus nerve, 224
Valproic acid (Depakote), 930
Valsalva maneuver, 1373
Values, cultural considerations, 86
Vancomycin-resistant enterococci (VRE), 488
Vanillylmandelic acid (VMA), 1384
Variable decelerations, in fetal heart rate, 1064
Varicella zoster virus, 486t
Varicocele, 1660
Varicose veins, 1460–1461
Vascular dementia, 1719, 1724
Vascular headaches. *See* Migraine headache
Vascular nevus, 1219
Vasculitis, 1233
Vasectomy, 1161–1162
Vasoactive intestinal peptide (VIP), 241
Vasoconstrictors (vasopressors), 935
Vasodilators, 935–936
Vasogenic shock, 521b
Vasopressin, 1387
VCE. *See* Video capsule endoscopy (VCE)

Vector, 1246
Vegan diets, 384
Vegetables, dietary, 347t
Vegetarian diets, 384–385
Venereal warts, 1170
Venipuncture, 996–997
    butterfly needles, use of, 996, 997f
    in infants, 1192
    Vacutainer system, 996, 997f
Venlafaxine (Effexor), 1758
Venogram, 1385
Venostasis, 1348
Venous access devices (VAD), 997f
Venous access lock, 837
Venous insufficiency wound. *See* Venous stasis ulcer
Venous stasis, 835
Venous stasis ulcer, 862
Venous thrombosis, 1348
Ventilation (breathing), 299–301
Ventilation scan, 1534
Ventilator-associated enterococcus (VAE), 515
Ventricles, brain, 224
Ventricular dysrhythmias, 829
Ventricular fibrillation, 1447
Ventricular septal defect (VSD), 1142, 1230, 1231f
Ventriculostomy, 1374
Venturi mask, 1570f, 1571
    nursing procedure, 1580
Venules, 265
Verapamil hydrochloride, 935
Verbal communication, 437
Verbal medication order, 911
Verbal order, read back (VORB), 1875
Vergence movement, 252
Vernix caseosa, 1084
Vertebral column, 1362
Vertical clients, 1844
Vertigo, 1374
Vesicles, 627t
Vestibule, 251
Vestibulocochlear nerve, 253
Veteran's services, 1743
Veterinary clinics, 1888
Vial, 981
Vibrational remedies, 29
Video capsule endoscopy (VCE), 1260, 1586
Video games, 1748
Video telemetry monitoring, 1353
Vietnamese Americans, 383
Vigorous physical activity, 350
Villi, small intestine, 310f
Violence, 1148
    within families, 107
Viral meningitis, 1371
Viral pneumonia, 1546
Virology, 486
Virulence, 491
Viruses, 484–487
Visceral pain, 255
Visible fat, 353
Vision, 225t
    disorders, 1257–1259
    factors, 225t
Visiting Nurse Association of America (VNA), 78
Visitors, for children, 1183
Visual acuity, 1413–1414
Visual analog scale (VAS), 804f
Visual impairment, 1267–1268
    in diabetes, 1408
Visual observation, 422
Vital capacity, 1534. *See also* Pulmonary function test (PFT)

Vital signs (VS), 581–606
    in burn injuries, 1302
    of children, 1181–1183, 1181t
    frequent, 582
    graphic record, 581–582
    recording, 582
Vitamin A, 349t, 360
Vitamin B_1. *See* Thiamin
Vitamin B_2. *See* Riboflavin
Vitamin B_3. *See* Niacin
Vitamin B_6, 363t
    in tuberculosis treatment, 1550
Vitamin B_9. *See* Folate
Vitamin B_{12} (cyanocobalamin), 938, 367
Vitamin B complex, 366–367
Vitamin C, 364t
Vitamin D, 1391, 349t
    deficiency,
    functions of, 360
    urinary system and, 325
Vitamin E, 349t
Vitamin K, 362t
    administration of, after birth, 1080
    deficiency, 938
    functions of, 365
Vitamins, 346
    fat-soluble, 362t–363t
    intake during pregnancy, 364
    nutrients and, 346–368
    principles related to, 365b
    water-soluble, 362t–364t
Vitelline membrane, 338
Vitiligo, 1295–1296, 1518
Vitreous humor, 248
VMA. *See* Vanillylmandelic acid (VMA)
VNA. *See* Visiting Nurse Association of America (VNA)
Vocal cords, 297–298
Vocalization, 302
Vocational nurses, 11–12, 1902
Vocational rehabilitation, 1823
Voice box. *See* Larynx
Void, 325
Voiding cystourethrogram (VCUG), 1631–1632
Volkmann contracture, 1348
Volkmann paralysis, 1348
Voluntary admissions, 1745
Voluntary health agencies, 78
Volunteer services, 464
Volvulus, 1610
Vomiting, 1364, 1498
    medications for, 946
    pyloric stenosis and, 1239
von Willebrand disease (vWD), 1482
VRE. *See* Vancomycin-resistant enterococci (VRE)
VS. *See* Vital signs (VS)
Vulnerable adult legislation, 1759
Vulnerable persons, 41
Vulva, 337
    and vagina, changes in, pregnancy and, 1032
Vulvitis, 1681
Vulvodynia, 1685–1686
Vulvovaginal candidiasis (VVC), 1171, 1172f

W

Walkers, 1821
Walking pneumonia, 1546. *See also* Pneumonia
Walking rounds, 453
Warfarin sodium (Coumadin), 938
Warmed blankets, 790
Warm, moist compresses and packs, 790
Warm soak, 791
Warts, 1297
Waste products, need for elimination of, 49

Wasting syndrome, 1523
Water pollution, 80
Water reabsorption and ADH influence, 312
Water-soluble vitamins, 362t–364t
WCON. *See* Wound care ostomy nurse (WCON)
Weaning, 112–113, 1573
Weapons, safety considerations, 471–472
Wedge resection, 1551, 1596
Weight-bearing restrictions, 660
Weight, children, 1182–1183
Weight gain, during pregnancy, 1042
Weight-loss clinics, 1888
Well-child visit, 1176
Wellness, concept of, 56
Wellness–illness continuum, 59–61
Wernicke–Korsakoff syndrome, 1725
Western blot test, 1524
Wharton jelly, 1029
Wheals, 1295
Wheat, kernel, 353f
Wheelchairs, 1821
Wheeze, breath sounds, 635t
Wheezing, 1237
White blood cells (WBCs), 275–275
    agranular, 277
    characteristics, 276b
    count, 1468
    disorders, 1479–1480
    granular, 275–276
White canes, 1419
White matter, spinal cord, 1362
WHO. *See* World Health Organization (WHO)
Whole blood, 939, 1470
Whooping cough. *See* Pertussis
Wilms tumor, 1243
Wind chill factor, 529
Window period, 1524
Witch hazel (Tucks) pads, 1071
Withdrawal method, of contraception, 1160

Withdrawal symptoms, 1779
Withdrawn persons, 1773
WOCN. *See* Wound ostomy and continence nurse (WOCN)
Wolffian duct, 334
Women
    health issues in, 69
    reproductive system, 343t
    urinary system, 320
Women's shelters, 1148
Wong–Baker Faces Pain Scale, 805
Wood light examination, 1290
Word-association test, 1738
Word salad, 1286
Worker's compensation, 77
Workplace violence, 472
Workplace, violence in, 64
World Health Organization (WHO), 56, 72–73
    global issues and potential resolutions, 56b
    health-related functions of, 72–73
    on sexuality, 1147
Wound, 857
    accidental/unintentional, 857
    care, objectives of, 869t
    care products, 870
    characteristics of, 860–861
    debridement, 865, 1291–1293
    drainage, 859–860
    dressings, 869–870
    equipment in care of, 871–873
    healing, 867–873
    infections, 1344
    inspection of, 857–858
    intentional, 857
    irrigation, 836, 873
    measurement of, 860–861
    packing, 870, 870f
    photography, 861
    preventive measures, 864t–865t

    skin inspection, 857
    sutures/staples, 873
    tracing, 861
    types of, 857
Wound care ostomy nurse (WCON), 1583, 1649
Wound ostomy and continence nurse (WOCN), 1583
Wound, Ostomy and Continence Nurses (WOCN) Society, 865
Wound sinus, 611
Written reprimands, 1903
Wryneck. *See* Torticollis

X

Xenografts, 1305, 1442
Xerostomia, 1501
X-ray examination, 496, 1673
Xylocaine jelly, 1632

Y

Yawning, 302
Yeasts, 481
    infections, 1681
Yin-yang, 93b
Young onset dementia (YOD), 1719

Z

Zenker diverticulum. *See* Esophageal diverticulum
Zig-zag method. *See* Z-track method
Zinc (Zn), 352t, 386
Zinc lozenges, 943
Z-line, 308
Zolpidem tartrate (Ambien), 929
Zona pellucida, 338
Zoonotic diseases, 1247
Z-track method, 984–985, 985f
Zygote, 340, 1025
Zygote intrafallopian transfer (ZIFT), 1153